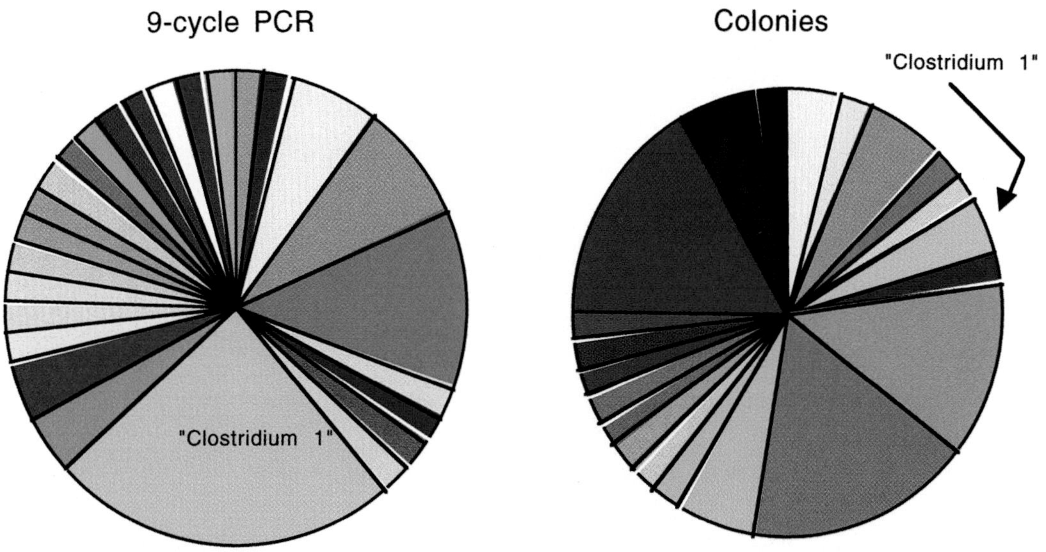

FIGURE 4.1. Relative diversity of bacterial ribosomal DNAs (rDNAs) in organisms cultured from a human fecal specimen and obtained by direct polymerase chain reaction amplification of rDNAs extracted from the same specimen. A more diverse set of rDNAs was recovered by direct amplification. However, some rDNAs commonly obtained from cultured bacteria did not appear in the directly amplified sample. Also, additional cycles of polymerase chain reaction expanded the proportion of sequences attributable to "*Clostridium* 1."

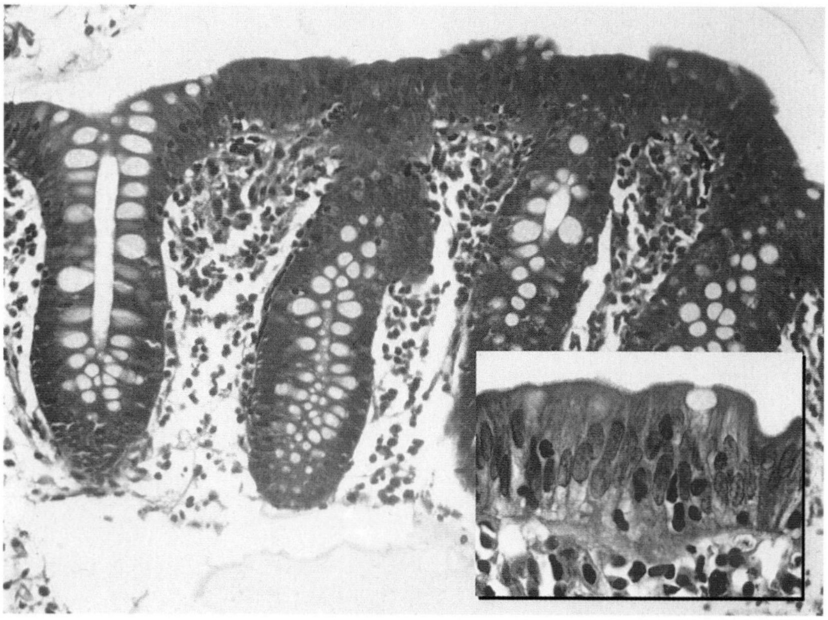

FIGURE 20.1. A case of colonic epithelial lymphocytosis in an outbreak of Brainerd diarrhea among passengers on a cruise ship to the Galapagos Islands. The architecture of the colonic crypts and surface epithelium is well preserved, without evidence of structural damage. Marginally increased lymphocytosis is seen in the lamina propria, but not in the crypt epithelium. The insert shows marked lymphocytosis of the surface epithelium, which retains its normal morphology. (Courtesy of Robert E. Petras, M.D., Department of Anatomic Pathology, Cleveland Clinic Foundation, Cleveland, Ohio.)

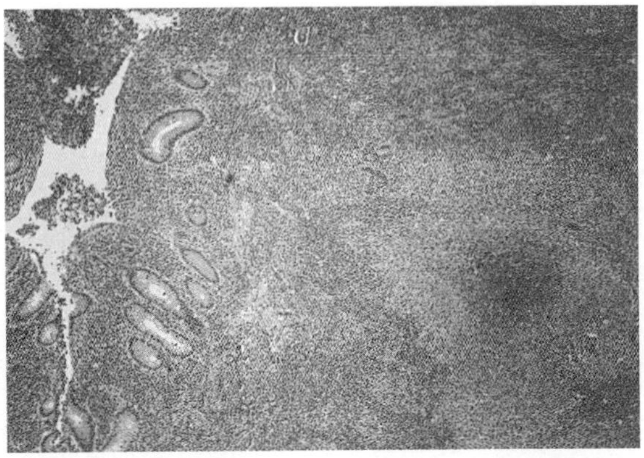

FIGURE 23.1. Appendicitis due to *Yersinia enterocolitica*. Diffuse inflammation and a submucosal granuloma with central necrosis are present in the vermiform appendix (H & E). (Courtesy of Dr. Rodger Haggitt.)

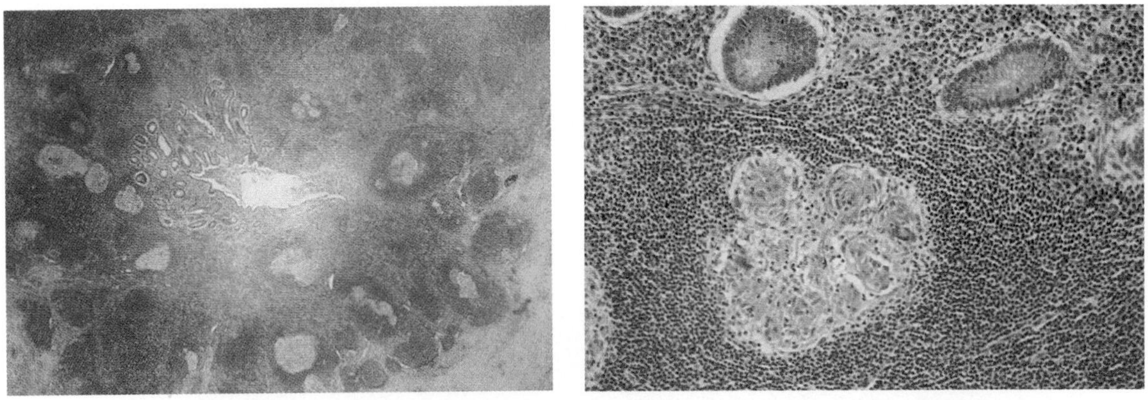

A

B

FIGURE 23.2. Granulomatous appendicitis. **A:** The presence of multiple granulomas in the mucosa and submucosa of the appendix characterizes granulomatous appendicitis (H & E). **B:** The granuloma is discrete, noncaseating, and composed of epithelioid histiocytes with occasional multinucleated giant cells (H & E). (Courtesy of Dr. Rodger Haggitt.)

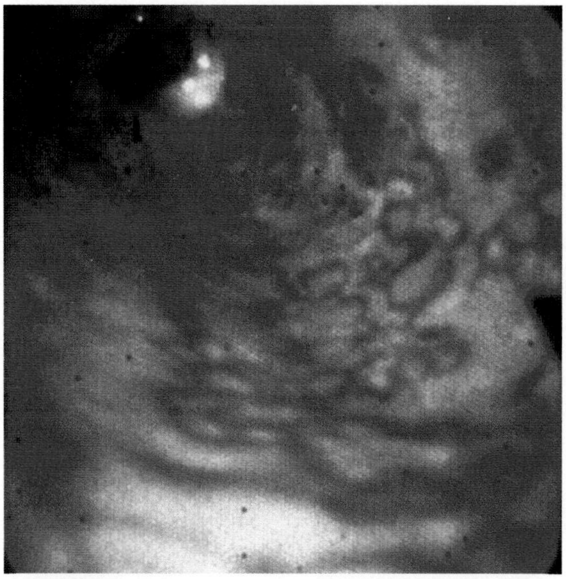

FIGURE 29.4. Endoscopic appearance of multiple vesicular erosions, some of which have coalesced into small superficial ulcers, due to herpes simplex virus esophagitis.

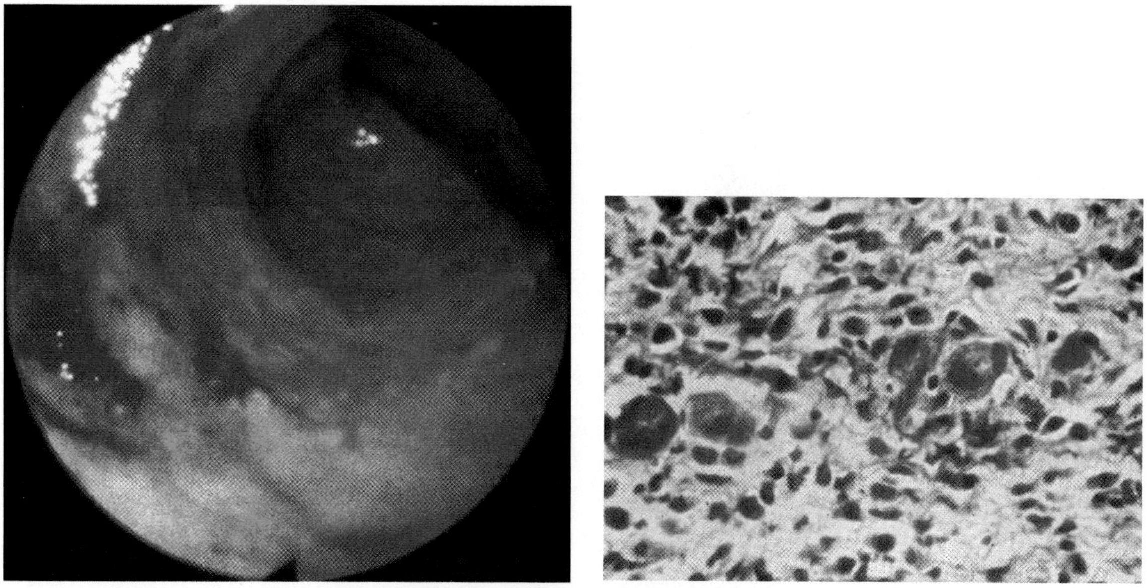

FIGURE 29.5. Endoscopic and light microscopic appearance of cytomegalovirus colitis in an HIV-1-infected man. Direct visualization **(left)** shows a diffusely ulcerated and bleeding mucosa with inflammation and exudates. Histology of the **(right)** lesion in left panel show numerous cytomegalic inclusion cells and inflammatory cells, ×125. (From Smith PD, Saini SS, Raffeld M, et al. Cytomegalovirus induction of tumor necrosis factor-α by human monocytes and mucosal macrophages. *J Clin Invest* 1992;90:1642–1648, with permission.)

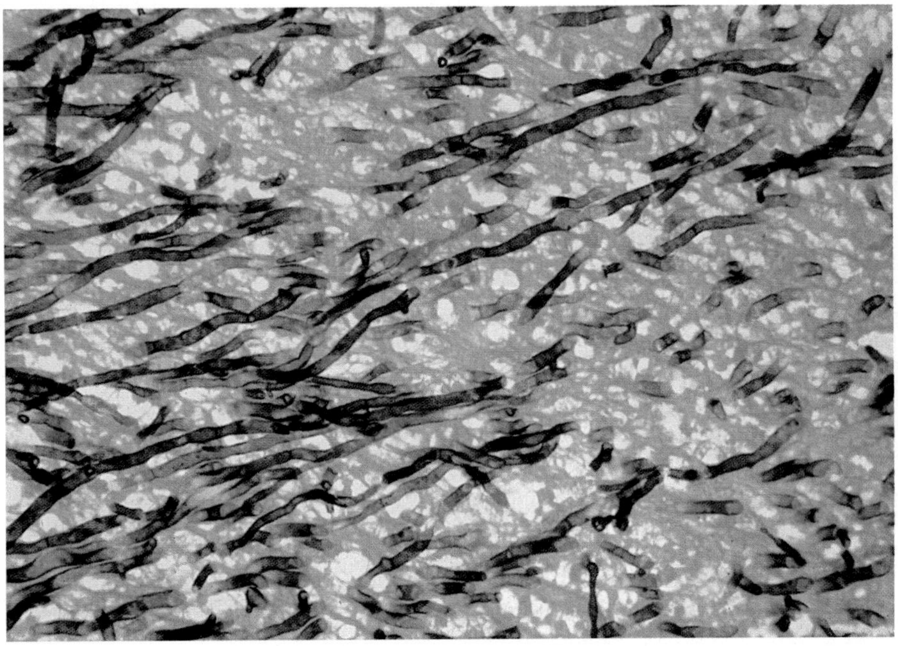

FIGURE 32.3. Bacterial esophagitis.

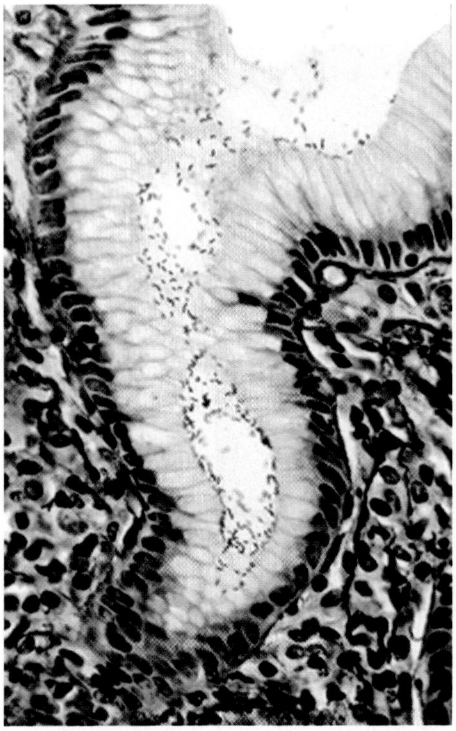

FIGURE 34.1. Colonization of the gastric mucosa with *Helicobacter pylori.* Modified Steiner silver stain.

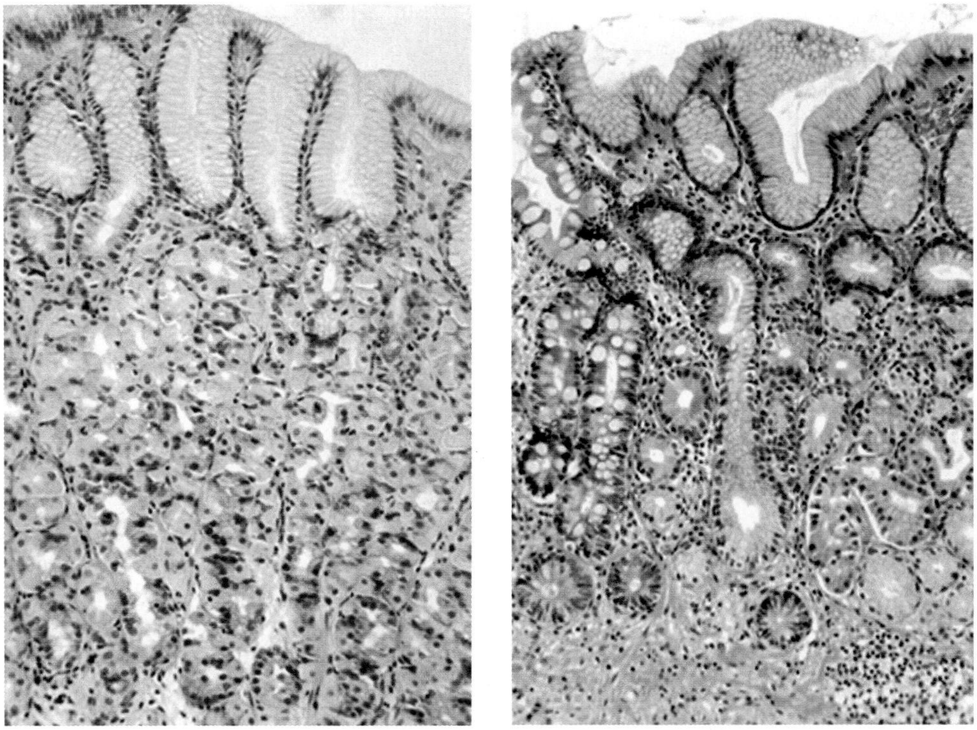

FIGURE 34.3. Two samples of gastric histology from the same *Helicobacter pylori*-positive person before and after 12 years of follow-up show the development of atrophic gastritis with intestinal metaplasia during follow-up. (From Kuipers EJ, Uyterlinde AM, Peña AS, et al. Long-term sequelae of *Helicobacter pylori* gastritis. *Lancet* 1995;345:1525–1528, with permission.)

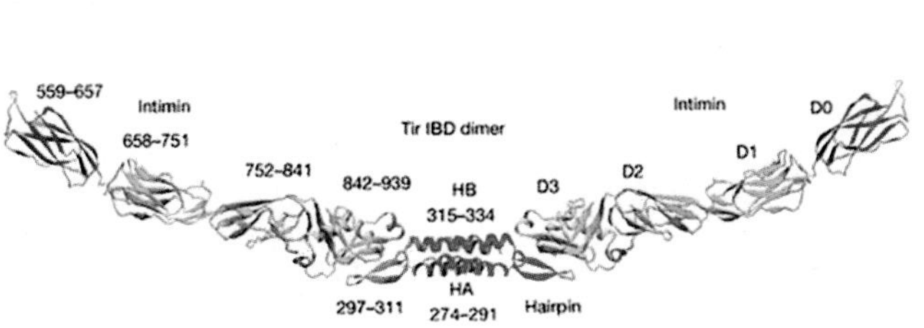

FIGURE 40.3. A RIBBONS representation of the intimin and Tir intimin-binding domain (IBD) dimer complex. The immunoglobulin-like (D0, D1, and D2) and lectin-like (D3) domains of the two intimin monomers are color coded by secondary structures (α helices in cyan, β strands in green, coils in brown). The predicted (but unresolved) immunoglobulin-like domain D0 is in red. The Tir IBD dimer in the center is color coded by chains (pink and dark blue, respectively). The amino acid residues corresponding to each domain are indicated. (From Luo Y, et al. Crystal structure of enteropathogenic *Escherichia coli* intimin-receptor complex. *Nature* 2000; 405:1073–1077, with permission.)

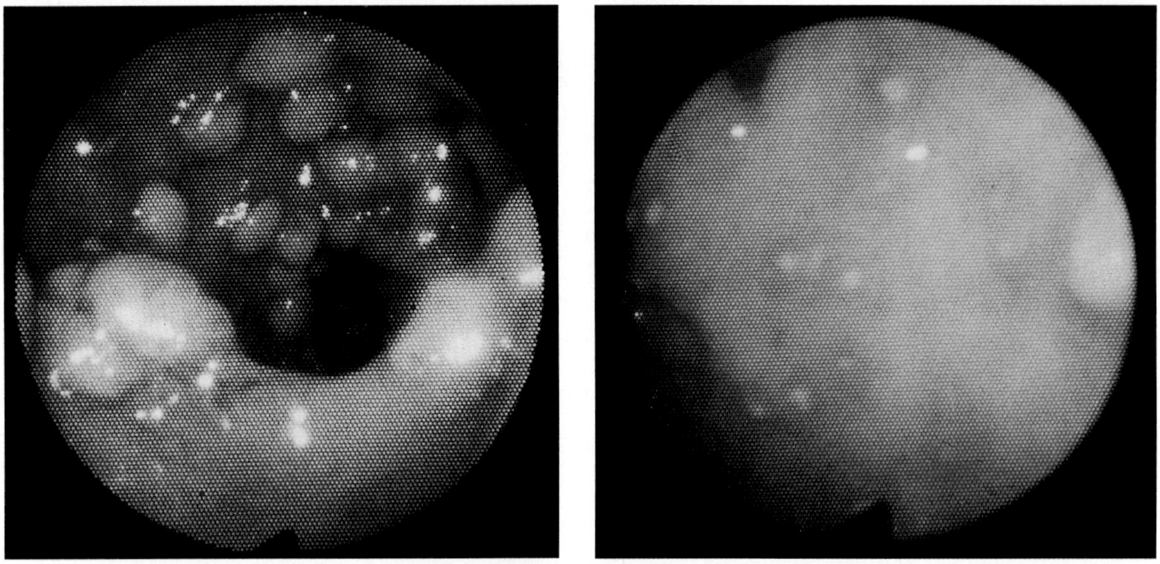

A B

FIGURE 48.4. Endoscopic appearance of pseudomembranous colitis (PMC). **A:** Multiple yellow-white, round, adherent, raised plaques 0.5 to 2 cm in diameter are apparent. **B:** Small raised aphthous-like lesions seen early in the course of disease after only 36 hours of diarrhea. These subtle changes are easily missed. Note the relatively normal-appearing mucosa between lesions. (From Gerding DN, Gebhard RL, Sumner HW, et al. Pathology and diagnosis of *Clostridium difficile* disease. In: Rolfe RD, Finegold SM, eds. Clostridium difficile: *its role in intestinal disease*. New York: Academic Press, 1988, with permission.)

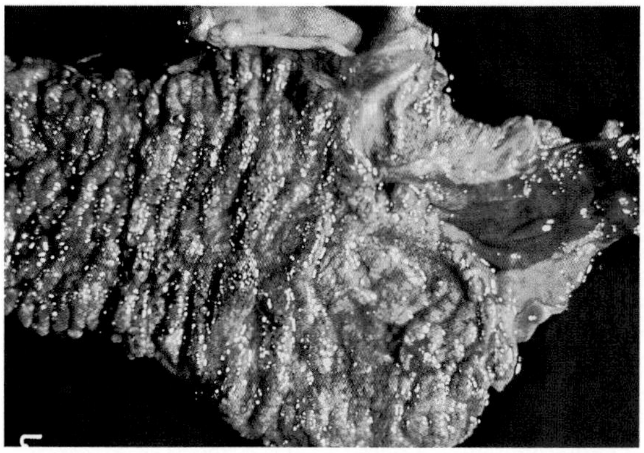

FIGURE 48.5. Pathologic specimen of the cecum and ileum demonstrating confluent pseudomembrane formation that involves the entire cecum, but stops abruptly at the ileocecal valve and spares the ileum. (From Gerding DN, Gebhard RL, Sumner HW, et al. Pathology and diagnosis of *Clostridium difficile* disease. In: Rolfe RD, Finegold SM, eds. Clostridium difficile: *its role in intestinal disease*. New York: Academic Press, 1988, with permission.)

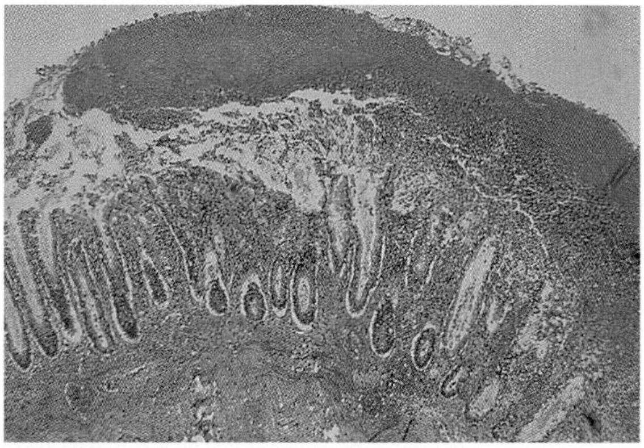

FIGURE 48.6. Large pseudomembrane comprised of cellular debris overlying inflamed colonic mucosa. There is marked polymorphonuclear leukocyte infiltration of the mucosa and submucosa. Attachment point of the pseudomembrane is at the lower left margin of the micrograph.

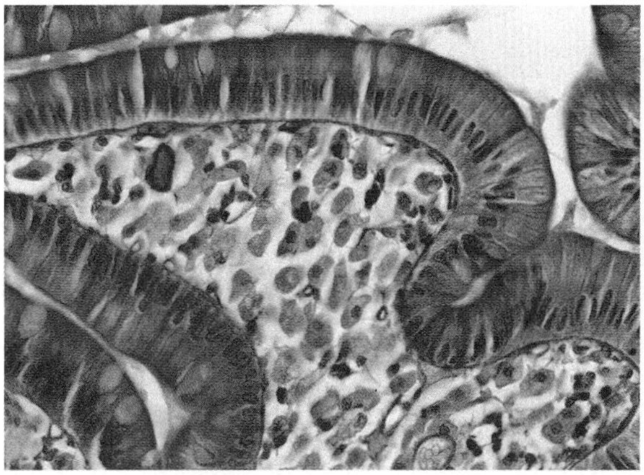

FIGURE 51.3. Typical histology of the duodenal mucosa in a patient with Whipple disease. Numerous vacuolated macrophages crowd the lamina propria. Hematoxylin and eosin stain, ×300. (From Relman DA, Schmidt TM, MacDermott RP, et al. Identification of the uncultured bacillus of Whipple's disease. *N Engl J Med* 1992;327:293–301, with permission. Courtesy of Dr. Donald Regula.)

A

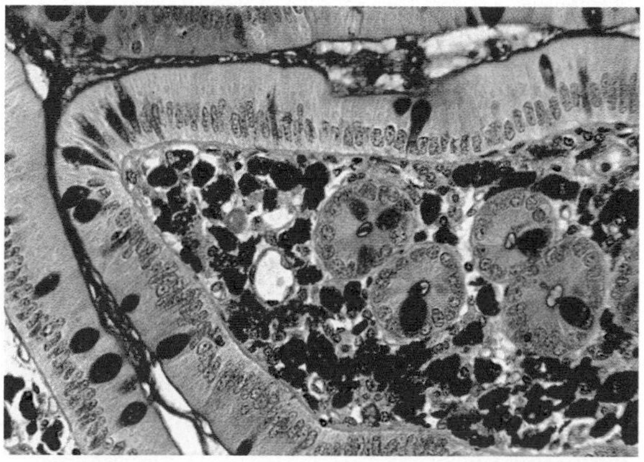

B

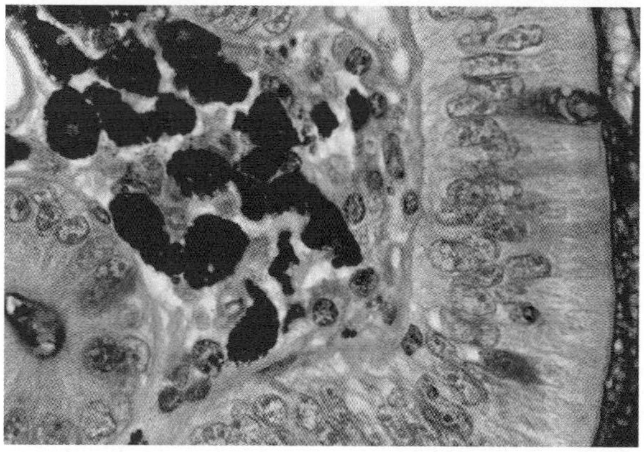

FIGURE 51.4. A: Duodenal mucosa of same patient as in Fig. 51.2 stained with periodic acid–Schiff (PAS) reagent. Vacuoles of the macrophages within the lamina propria react intensely and appear purple, indicating the presence of glycoprotein (in this case, bacterial cell wall). Epithelial goblet cells also stain with PAS, ×300. **B:** Same tissue at higher magnification, ×750. (From Relman DA, Schmidt TM, MacDermott RP, et al. Identification of the uncultured bacillus of Whipple's disease. *N Engl J Med* 1992;327:293–301, with permission. Courtesy of Dr. Donald Regula.)

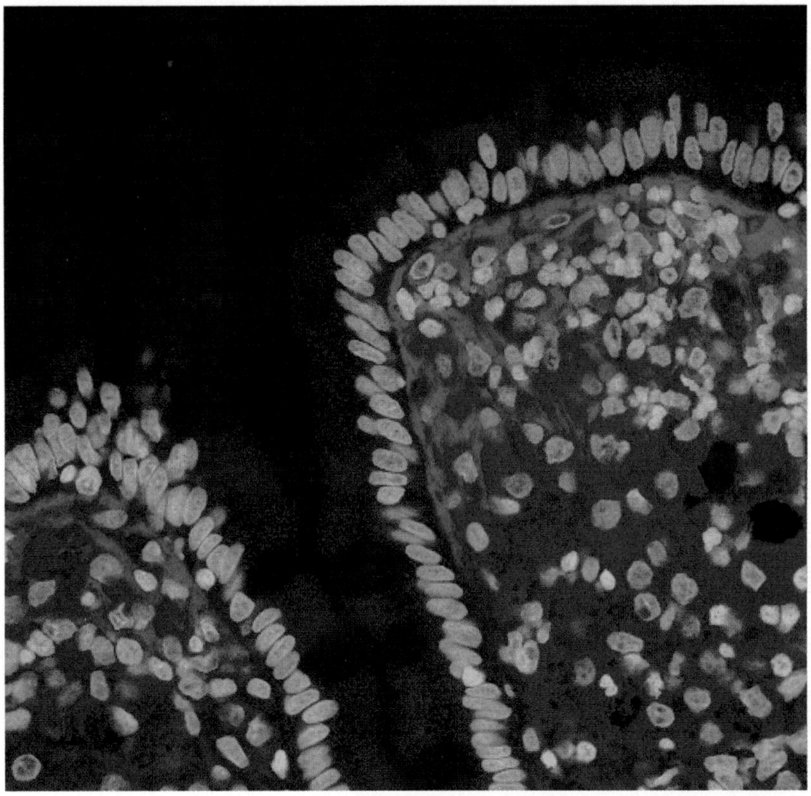

FIGURE 51.5. Fluorescence **in situ** hybridization of *Tropheryma whippelii* ribosomal RNA (rRNA) performed on a section of intestine from a patient with Whipple's disease and visualized by confocal microscopy. Cell nuclei appear green with YO-PRO 1 stain, the human intracellular cytoskeletal protein vimentin appears red with a Texas red-labeled antibody, and *T. whippelii* rRNA appears blue with a Cy 5-labeled DNA probe. Bacteria localize to the extracellular spaces of the lamina propria. Original magnification ×600.

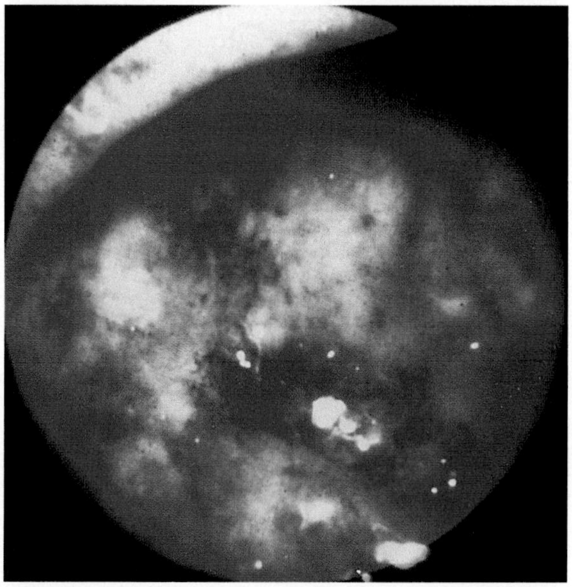

FIGURE 60.3. Patient with amebic colitis at colonoscopy. Note punctate hemorrhagic ulcers with normal-appearing mucosa. (Courtesy of H. Jinich, UCSD Medical Center.)

A

B

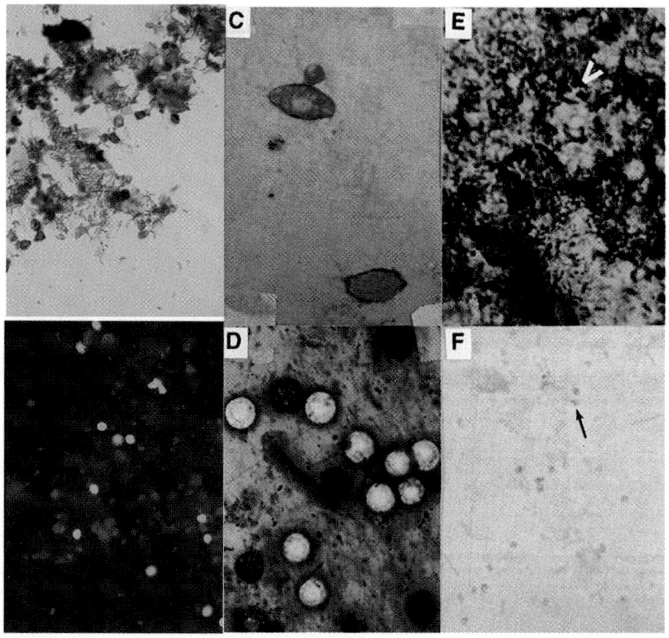

FIGURE 62.3. Causes of diarrhea in patients with AIDS. **A:** *Cryptosporidium*—acid-fast stain. **B:** *Cryptosporidium*—direct immunofluorescent stain. **C:** *I. belli* and *Cryptosporidium* together in the stool of a patient with AIDS. **D:** *Cyclospora* (formerly called "cyanobacterium-like organism") in the stool of a patient with AIDS and diarrhea. **E:** *Mycobacterium avium* complex organisms (*arrow*) in the stool of a patient with AIDS and protracted fever and diarrhea. **F:** *Microsporidia* C–E, acid-fast stain; F, chromotrope stain. (Courtesy of Rosemary Soave, Cynthia Sears, Earl Long, Madeline Boucy, and Ralph Bryan, with permission.)

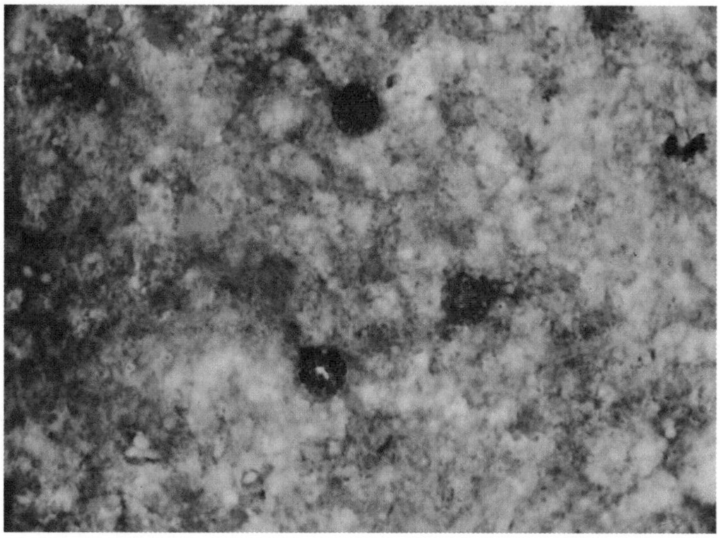

FIGURE 63.1. Oil immersion photomicrograph of a smear of concentrated stool specimen from a patient with chronic diarrhea shows three *Cyclospora* organisms with central morula containing nonrefractile globules and outer membrane. Organisms measure 9 to 10 μm in width. (Acid-fast stain; original magnification ×4,000.)

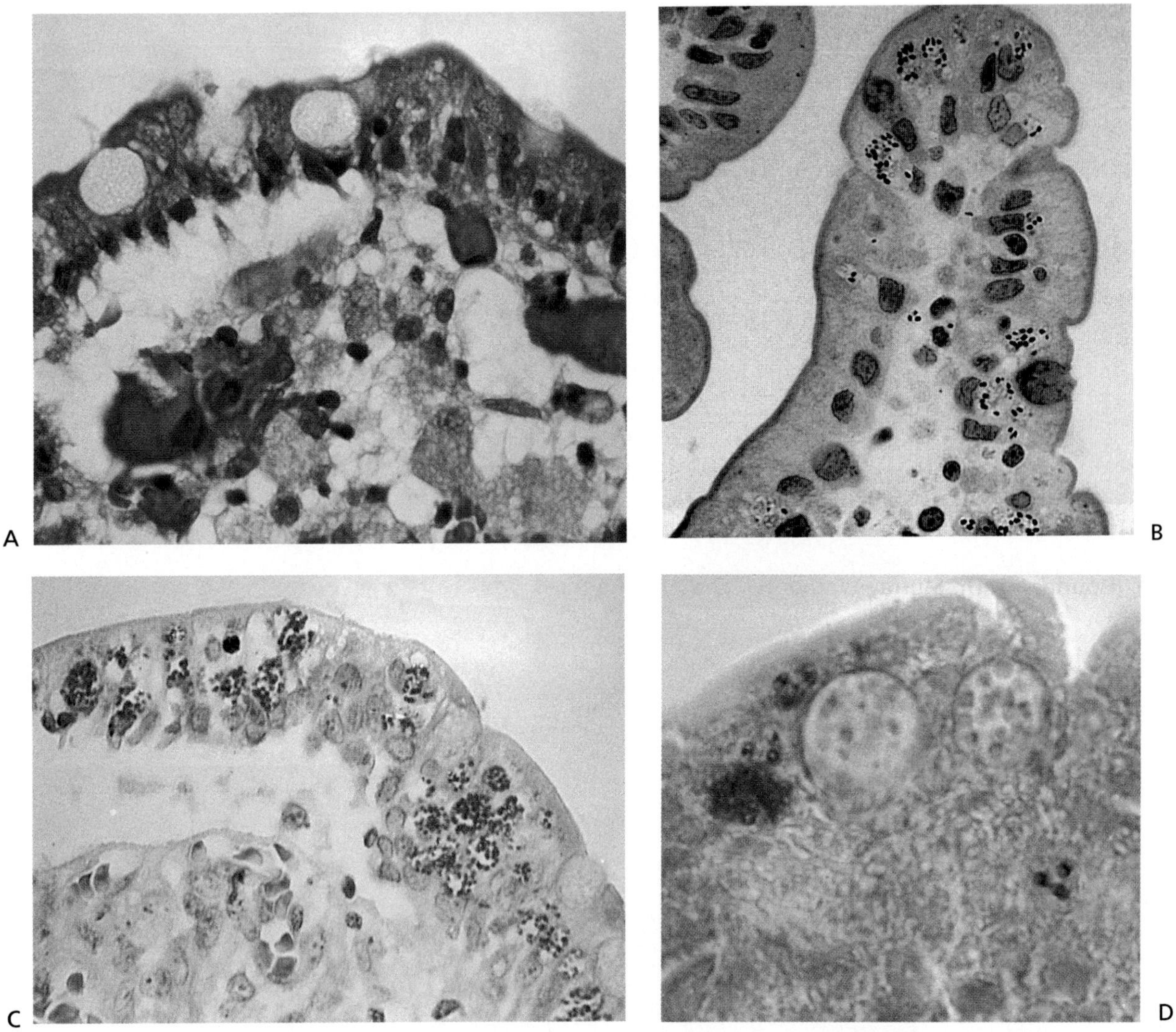

FIGURE 64.4. Light microscopy of *Encephalitozoon intestinalis.* **A:** Spores appear as supranuclear collections of refractile bluish bodies. Strips of enterocytes are frequently seen being shed from the mucosa. Some of the prominent lamina propria macrophages contain spores. Hematoxylin and eosin stain, ×640. **B:** In plastic sections, the spores stain dark blue. Stain, ×640. **C:** A partially polarized Brown–Brenn, Gram-stained section of an intestinal biopsy shows pink birefringence of some of the dark red-staining spores. Stain, ×640. **D:** A characteristic dark-staining central band is visible in some of the spores. Brown–Brenn-stained paraffin section, ×1,200.

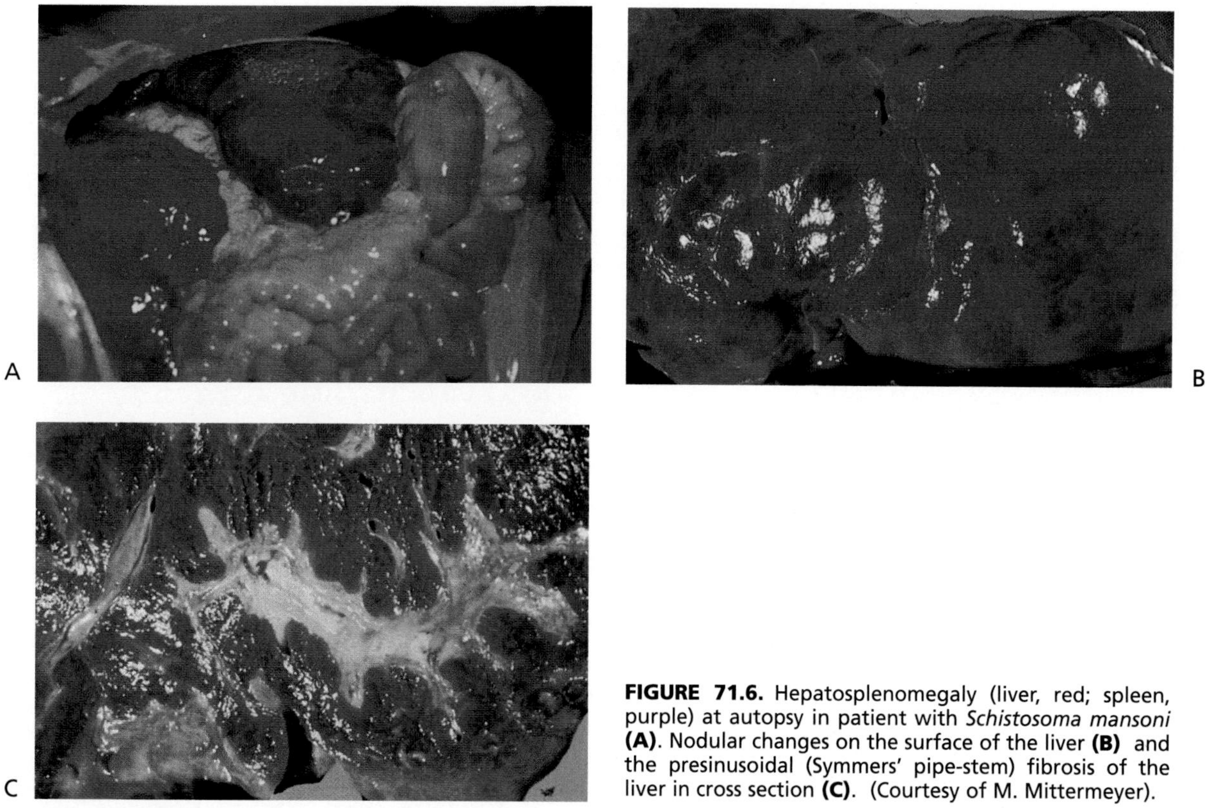

FIGURE 71.6. Hepatosplenomegaly (liver, red; spleen, purple) at autopsy in patient with *Schistosoma mansoni* **(A)**. Nodular changes on the surface of the liver **(B)** and the presinusoidal (Symmers' pipe-stem) fibrosis of the liver in cross section **(C)**. (Courtesy of M. Mittermeyer).

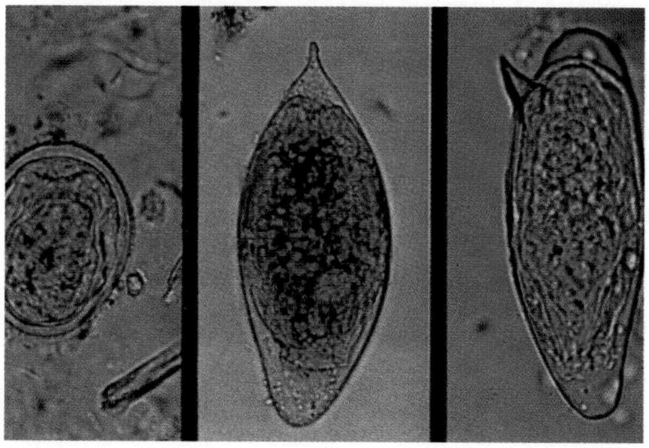

FIGURE 71.8. *Schistosoma japonicum* **(left)**, *S. haematobium* **(center)**, and *S. mansoni* **(right)** ova in the stool or urine.

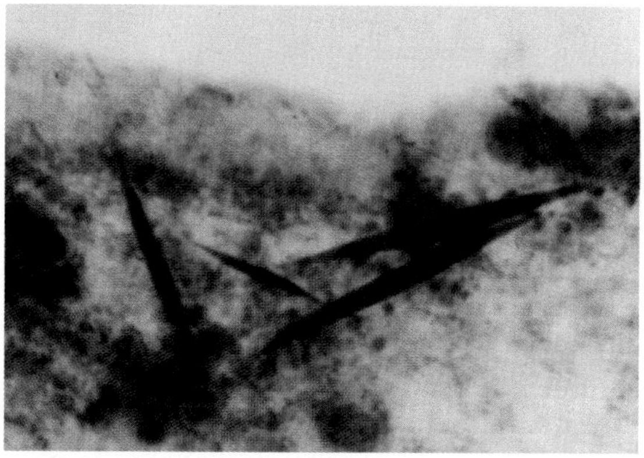

FIGURE 72.2. Charcot–Leyden crystals (trichrome stain, oil immersion). Note the characteristic shape; various sizes will be present in a single specimen. The presence of these crystals indicates the presence of eosinophils in the contents of the intestinal lumen. (Courtesy of L. Garcia and D. Bruckner.)

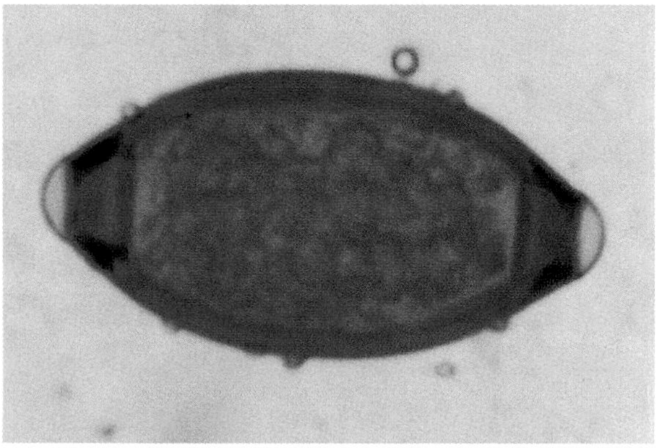

FIGURE 72.3. *Trichuris trichiura* egg; iodine stain, wet mount. (Courtesy of L. Garcia and D. Bruckner.)

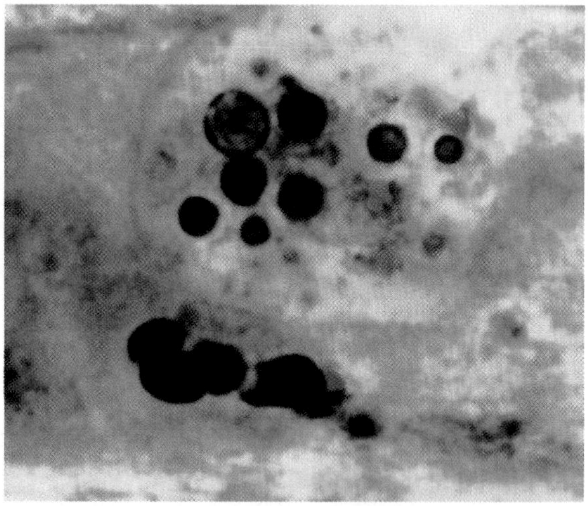

FIGURE 72.4. *Entamoeba histolytica* trophozoite; trichrome stain. Note the presence of ingested red blood cells in the cytoplasm, which stain red with trichrome stain. (Courtesy of L. Garcia and D. Bruckner.)

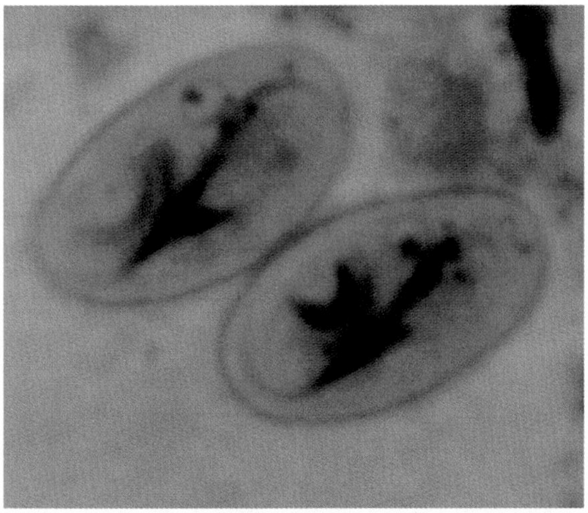

FIGURE 72.6. *Giardia lamblia* cysts; iron and hematoxylin stain. (Courtesy of L. Garcia and D. Bruckner.)

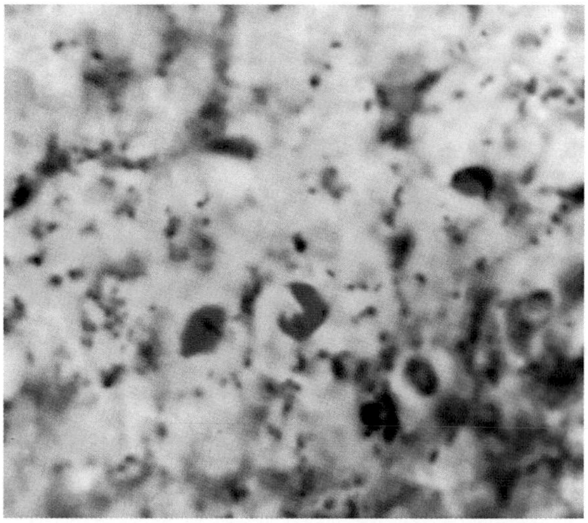

FIGURE 72.8. *Cryptosporidium parvum* oocysts; modified acid-fast stain. (Courtesy of L. Garcia and D. Bruckner.)

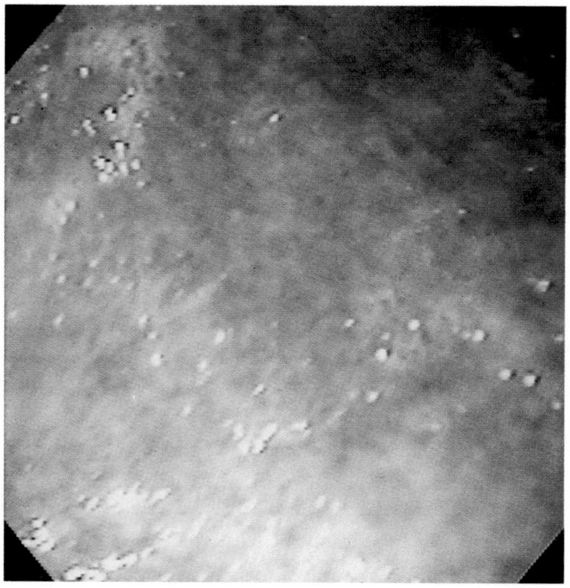

FIGURE 73.1. *Helicobacter pylori* gastritis.

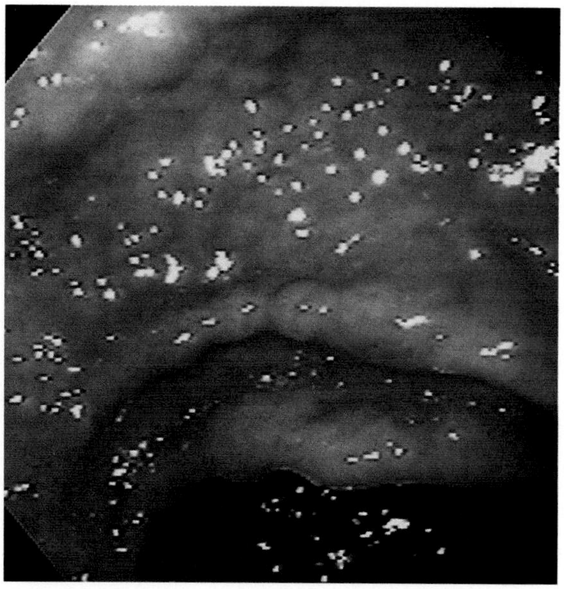

FIGURE 73.2. *Helicobacter pylori* nodular gastritis.

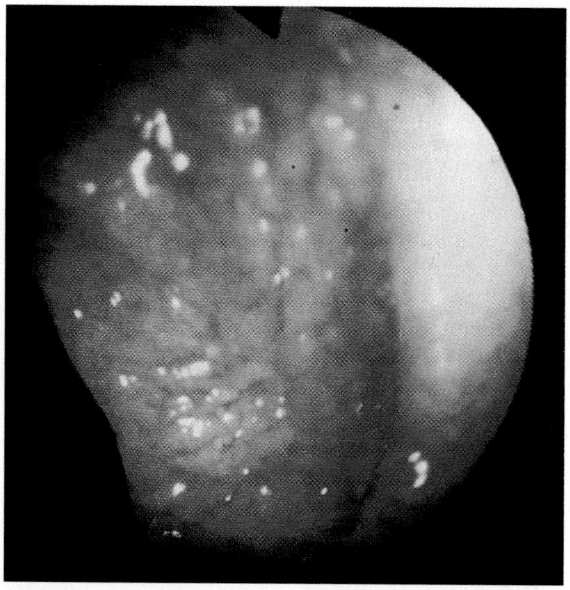

FIGURE 73.3. Whipple's disease. Note characteristic coarsening of the villous pattern and pale, yellow, shaggy mucosa. (From Silverstein FE, Tytgat, GNJ. *Atlas of gastrointestinal endoscopy.* Philadelphia: W.B. Saunders; 1987, with permission.)

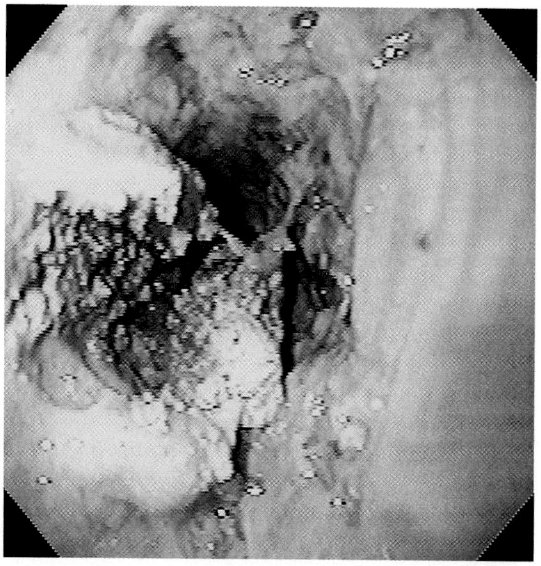

FIGURE 73.4 Pseudomembranous esophagitis.

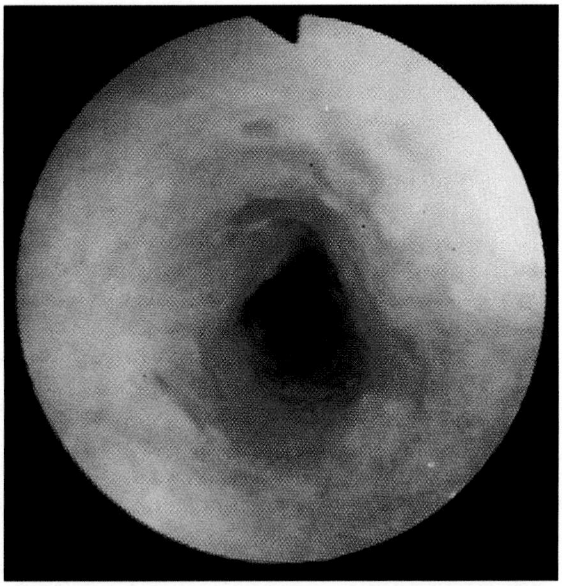

FIGURE 73.5. Herples simplex virus esophageal ulcer, early. Discrete punched-out ulcerations with normal intervening mucosa. (From Silverstein FE, Tytgat, GNJ. *Atlas of gastrointestinal endoscopy*. Philadelphia: W.B. Saunders; 1987, with permission.)

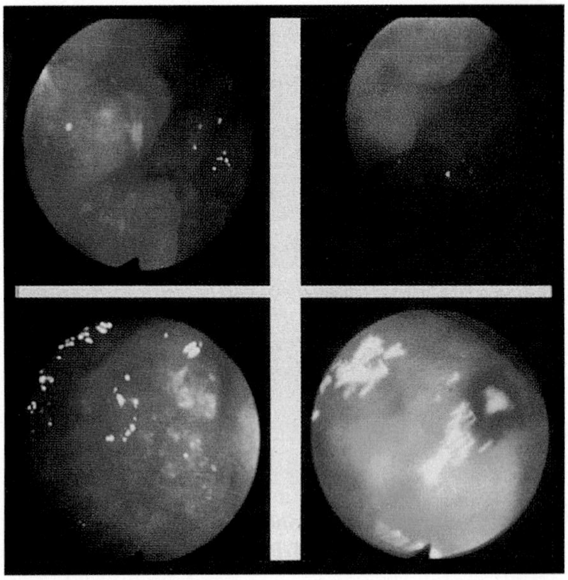

FIGURE 73.6. Varied endoscopic appearance of cytomegalovirus gastric lesions. **Top left:** Nodular gastritis with erosions. **Top right:** Nodular gastritis with minimal inflammation. **Bottom left:** Erosive gastritis. **Bottom right:** Gastric ulcerations. (From Kaplan CS, Petersen EA, Icenogle TB, et al. Gastrointestinal cytomegalovirus infection in heart and heart-lung transplant recipients. Arch Intern Med 1989;149:2095–2100, with permission.)

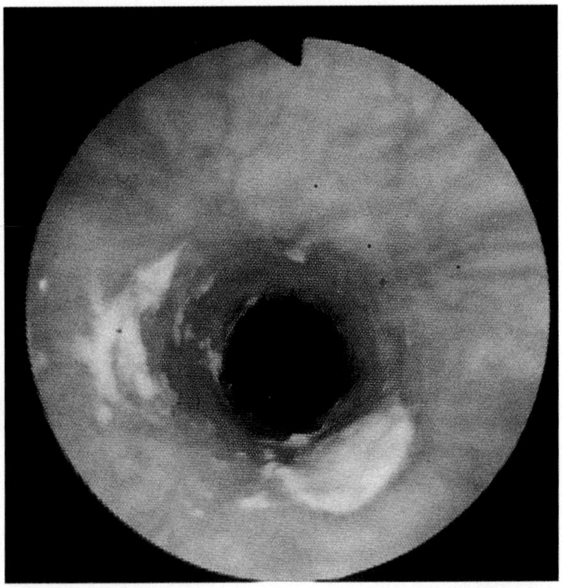

FIGURE 73.7. *Candida* esophagitis. Severe, with extensive exudate and erythema. (From Silverstein FE, Tytgat, GNJ. *Atlas of gastrointestinal endoscopy*. Philadelphia: W.B. Saunders; 1987, with permission.)

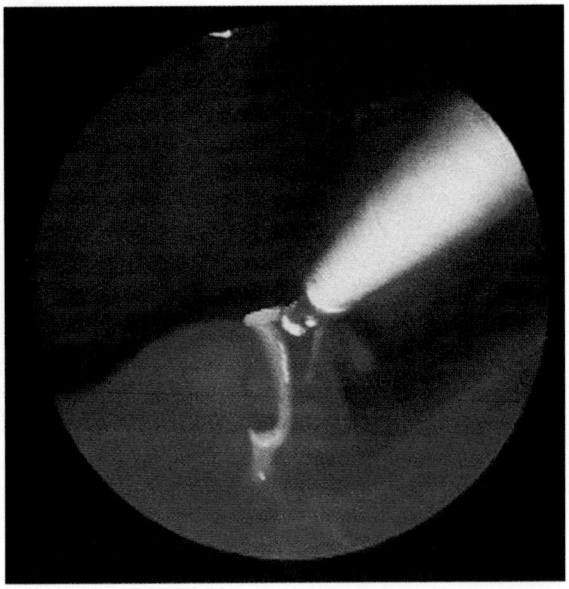

FIGURE 73.8. Gastric anisakiasis. Anisakis larva being removed from the top of the inflammatory nodule. (From Ikeda K, Kumashiro R, Kifune T. Nine cases of acute gastric anisakiasis. *Gastrointest Endosc* 1989;35:304–308, with permission.)

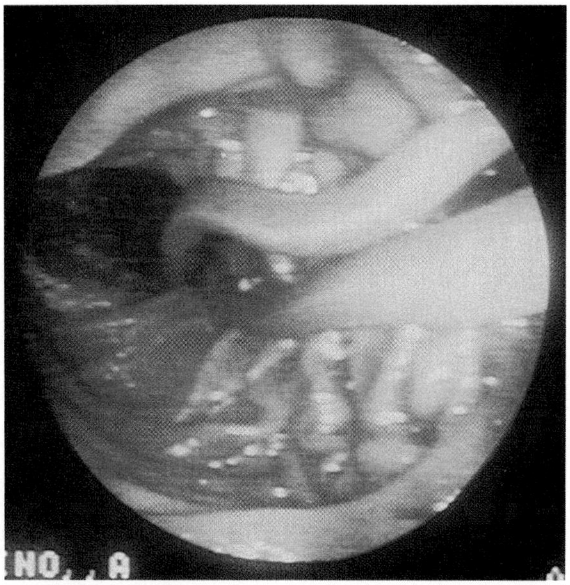

FIGURE 73.9. Ascaris in duodenum. (Courtesy of Dr. C. Michael Knauer.)

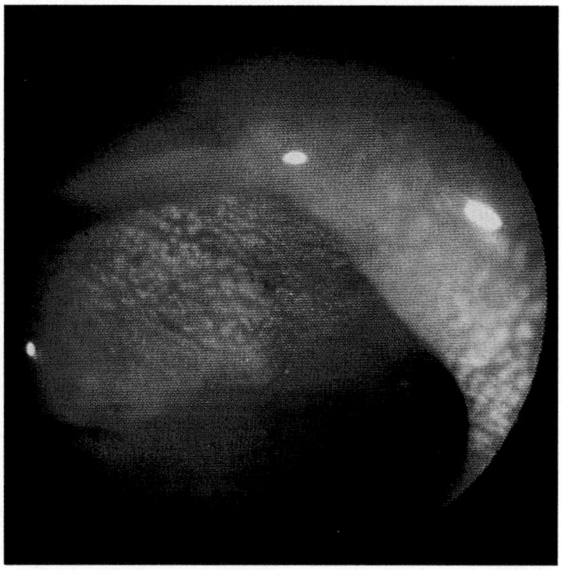

FIGURE 73.10. *Mycobacterium avium* complex of the duodenum. Coarse, pale whitish-yellow, granular mucosa resembling Whipple's disease. (From Cotton PB, Tytgat GNJ, Williams CB. *Slide atlas of gastrointestinal endoscopy*. London: Current Science; 1992, with permission.)

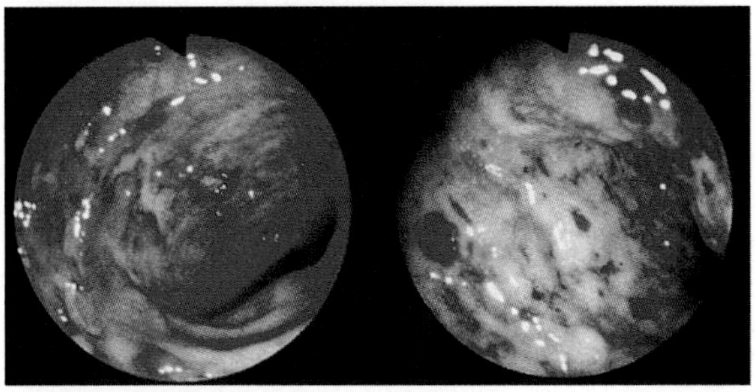

FIGURE 73.11. Left: Severe *Shigella flexneri* colitis with extensive coalescent superficial ulceration involving nearly the entire bowel circumference. **Right:** Improved appearance after 2 weeks of antibiotic therapy. (From Silverstein FE, Tytgat, GNJ. *Atlas of gastrointestinal endoscopy*. Philadelphia: W.B. Saunders; 1987, with permission.)

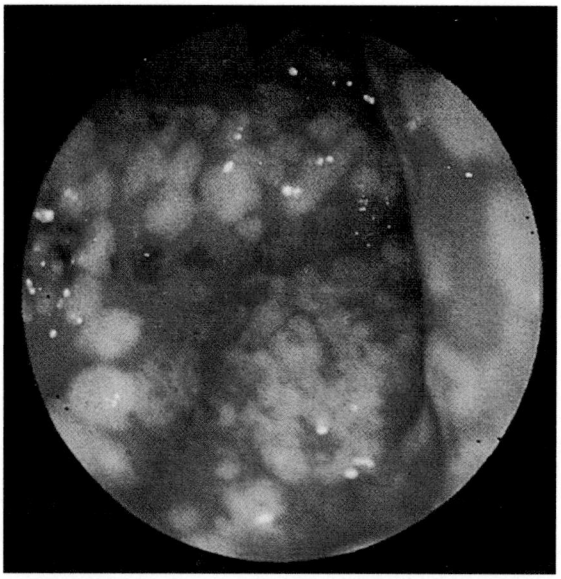

FIGURE 73.12. Pseudomembranous colitis. Confluent colonic inflammation with pseudomembrane formation. This colonoscopic view illustrates the greenish pseudomembrane overlying the inflamed mucosal surface. (From Pounder RE, Allison MC, Dhillon AP. *Colour atlas of the digestive system*. London: Wolfe Publishing; 1989, with permission.)

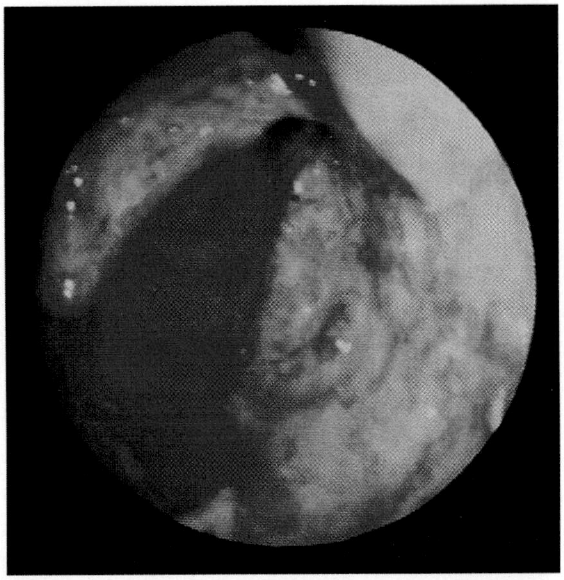

FIGURE 73.13. Herpes simplex virus proctitis. Confluent, nearly circumferential ulceration of the anal canal and distal rectum. (From Silverstein FE, Tytgat, GNJ. *Atlas of gastrointestinal endoscopy*. Philadelphia: W.B. Saunders; 1987, with permission.)

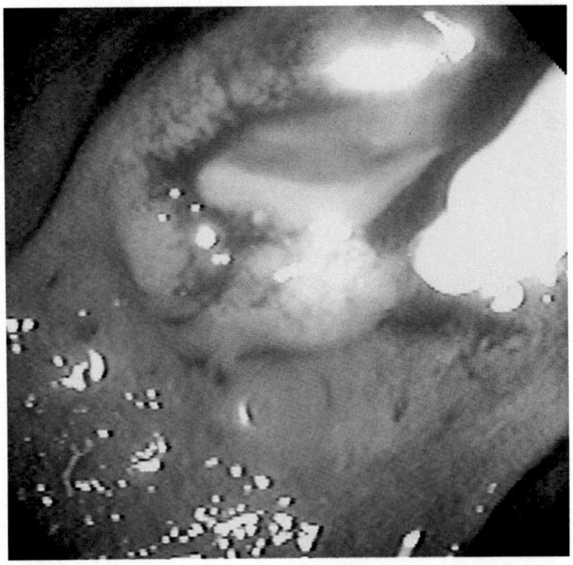

FIGURE 73.14. Pus extruded with balloon in cholangitis.

INFECTIONS OF THE GASTROINTESTINAL TRACT

SECOND EDITION

INFECTIONS OF THE GASTROINTESTINAL TRACT

SECOND EDITION

Editors

MARTIN J. BLASER, M.D.

Frederick H. King Professor of Internal Medicine
Chairman, Department of Medicine
Professor of Microbiology
New York University School of Medicine
Staff Physician
New York Harbor Veterans Affairs Medical Center
New York, New York

PHILLIP D. SMITH, M.D.

Mary J. Bradford Professor in Gastroenterology
Department of Medicine
University of Alabama at Birmingham
Medical Staff
University of Alabama Hospital
Birmingham, Alabama

JONATHAN I. RAVDIN, M.D.

Nesbitt Professor and Chairman
Department of Medicine
University of Minnesota
Minneapolis, Minnesota

HARRY B. GREENBERG, M.D.

Grant Professor of Medicine,
Microbiology, and Immunology
Stanford University Medical School
Professor
Veterans Affairs Palo Alto Healthcare System
Palo Alto, California

RICHARD L. GUERRANT, M.D.

Thomas H. Hunter Professor of International Medicine
University of Virginia School of Medicine
Chief, Division of Geographic Medicine
University of Virginia Hospital
Charlottesville, Virginia

LIPPINCOTT WILLIAMS & WILKINS
A **Wolters Kluwer** Company
Philadelphia • Baltimore • New York • London
Buenos Aires • Hong Kong • Sydney • Tokyo

Acquisitions Editor: Hal Pollard
Developmental Editor: Ellen DiFrancesco
Production Editor: Tony DeGeorge
Manufacturing Manager: Ben Rivera
Cover Designer: Mark Lerner
Compositor: Lippincott Williams & Wilkins Desktop Division
Printer: Courier Westford

530 Walnut Street
Philadelphia, PA 19106 USA
LWW.com

Printed in the USA
First edition published 1995

Library of Congress Cataloging-in-Publication Data

Infections of the gastrointestinal tract / editors, Martin J. Blaser ... [et al.].—2nd ed.
p. ; cm.
Includes bibliographical references and index.
ISBN 0-7817-2847-9
1. Gastrointestinal system—Infections. I. Blaser, Martin J.
[DNLM: 1. Gastrointestinal Diseases. 2. Communicable Diseases. 3. Infection.
WI 140 I43 2002]
RC840.I53 I54 2002
616.3'3—dc21

2002016166

Care has been taken to confirm the accuracy of the information presented and to describe generally accepted practices. However, the authors, editors, and publisher are not responsible for errors or omissions or for any consequences from application of the information in this book and make no warranty, expressed or implied, with respect to the currency, completeness, or accuracy of the contents of the publication. Application of this information in a particular situation remains the professional responsibility of the practitioner.

The authors, editors, and publisher have exerted every effort to ensure that drug selection and dosage set forth in this text are in accordance with current recommendations and practice at the time of publication. However, in view of ongoing research, changes in government regulations, and the constant flow of information relating to drug therapy and drug reactions, the reader is urged to check the package insert for each drug for any change in indications and dosage and for added warnings and precautions. This is particularly important when the recommended agent is a new or infrequently employed drug.

Some drugs and medical devices presented in this publication have Food and Drug Administration (FDA) clearance for limited use in restricted research settings. It is the responsibility of the health care provider to ascertain the FDA status of each drug or device planned for use in their clinical practice.

10 9 8 7 6 5 4 3 2 1

To our families for their patience and tolerance, and to our colleagues, students, and co-authors who continue to educate us.

CONTENTS

CONTRIBUTORS

Aws Abdul-Wahid, B.Sc., Ph.D. Institute of Parasitology, McGill University, Ste. Anne de Bellevue, Quebec, Canada

Sharon L. Abbott, B.A. Enteric Bacteriology Supervisor, Microbial Diseases Laboratory, Berkeley, California

David W.K. Acheson M.D. Director, The Food Safety Initiative at New England Medical Center, Boston, Massachusetts

Ban Mihsu Allos, M.D Assistant Professor, Department of Medicine and Preventive Medicine,Vanderbilt University School of Medicine, Nashville, Tennessee

Anne M.Anglim, M.D., M.S. Orlando, Florida

John C. Atherton, M.D., F.R.C.P. Professor in Gastroenterology, Division of Gastroenterology and Institute of Infections and Immunity, University of Nottingham; Honorary Consultant, Division of Gastroenterology, University Hospital, Nottingham, England

John N. Aucott, M.D. Department of Internal Medicine, Johns Hopkins at Green Spring Station, Towson, Maryland

Michele Barry, M.D., F.A.C.P. Professor, Department of Medicine and Public Health, Yale University School of Medicine; Director, International Health, Yale-New Haven Hospital, New Haven, Connecticut

Dorsey M. Bass, M.D. Associate Professor, Department of Pediatrics, Stanford University School of Medicine Stanford, California; Attending Physician, Pediatric Gastroenterology, Packard Children's Hospital, Palo Alto, California

John E. Bennett, M.D. Head, Clinical Mycology Section, Laboratory of Clinical Investigation, National Institute of Allergy and Infectious Diseases, National Institutes of Health, Bethesda, Maryland

Steven L. Berk, M.D. Regional Dean, Professor, Department of Medicine, Texas Tech School of Medicine, Amarillo, Texas

Robert E. Black, M.D., M.P.H. Edgar Berman Professor and Chair, Department of International Health, Bloomberg School of Public Health, Johns Hopkins University, Baltimore, Maryland

Neil R. Blacklow, M.D. Professor of Medicine, Molecular Genetics, and Microbiology, Department of Medicine, Division of Infectious Diseases, University of Massachusetts Medical School; Attending Physician, Department of Medicine, Division of Infectious Diseases, University of Massachusetts Memorial Medical Center, Worcester, Massachusetts

Martin J. Blaser, M.D. Frederick H. King Professor of Internal Medicine and Chairman, Department of Medicine; Professor of Microbiology, New York University School of Medicine; Director of Medical Services, Bellevue Hospital Center and Tisch University Hospital; Staff Physician, New York Harbor Veterans Affairs Medical Center, New York, New York

Joan R. Butterton, M.D. Assistant Professor, Department of Medicine, Harvard Medical School; Assistant Physician, Division of Infectious Disease, Massachusetts General Hospital, Boston, Massachusetts

Stephen B. Calderwood, M.D. Professor of Medicine, Harvard Medical School; Chief, Division of Infectious Diseases, Massachusetts General Hospital, Boston, Massachusetts

Michael Cappello, M.D. Associate Professor, Departments of Pediatrics and Epidemiology & Public Health, Yale University School of Medicine, New Haven, Connecticut

Kris Chadee, Ph.D Associate Professor, Institute of Parasitology, McGill University, Ste. Anne de Bellevue, Quebec, Canada

Eugene B. Chang, M.D. Martin Boyer Professor, Associate Director of Academic Programs and Training in Gastroenterology, Department of Medicine, Gastroenterology Section, University of Chicago, Chicago, Illinois

Tien-lan Chang, M.D. Division of Pediatric Gastroenterology and Nutrition, Department of Pediatrics, Massachusetts General Hospital for Children, Boston, Massachusetts

John Cello, M.D. Professor, Departments of Medicine and Surgery, University of California, San Francisco School of Medicine, San Francisco, California

Thomas G. Cleary, M.D. Director, Department of Pediatrics, Division of Infectious Diseases, University of Texas Medical School, Houston, Texas

Mitchell B. Cohen, M.D. Professor, Department of Pediatrics, University of Cincinnati College of Medicine; Professor, Department of Pediatric Gastroenterology, Children's Hospital Medical Center, Cincinnati, Ohio

Bradley A. Connor, M.D. Clinical Associate Professor, Weill Medical College of Cornell University; Associate Attending Physician, Department of Medicine, New York Presbyterian Hospital, New York, New York

Timothy L. Cover, M.D. Associate Professor, Department of Medicine, Division of Infectious Diseases, Departments of Medicine and Microbiology and Immunology, Vanderbilt University School of Medicine, Nashville, Tennessee

John K. Crane, M.D., Ph.D. Assistant Professor, Department of Medicine, University at Buffalo; Attending Physician, Division of Infectious Diseases, Erie County Medical Center, Buffalo, New York

Dickson D. Despommier, Ph.D. Professor, Environmental Health Sciences and Microbiology, Columbia University, New York, New York

Michael S. Donnenberg, M.D. Professor and Head, Division of Infectious Diseases, Department of Medicine, University of Maryland-Baltimore, Baltimore, Maryland

John S. Dummer, M.D. Professor, Departments of Medicine and Surgery, Vanderbilt University School of Medicine; Director, Transplant Infectious Diseases, Departments of Medicine and Surgery, Vanderbilt University Hospital, Nashville, Tennessee

Herbert L. DuPont, M.D. Clinical Professor, Department of Medicine, Baylor College of Medicine and University of Texas-Houston Medical School; Chief, Department of Internal Medicine, St. Luke's Episcopal Hospital, Houston, Texas

Charles O. Elson III, M.D. Basil Il Hirschowitz Chair in Gastroenterology and Professor, Department of Medicine, University of Alabama at Birmingham; Attending Physician, Department of Medicine, University Hospital, Birmingham, Alabama

Mark E. Engel, M.D. Medical Natural Scientist, Department of Pathology, Molecular Lab, Red Cross Children's Hospital & UCH-UCT, Cape Town, South Africa

Mary K. Estes, Ph.D. Professor, Department of Molecular Virology & Microbiology, Baylor College of Medicine, Houston, Texas

Barry M. Farr, M.D., M. Sc. William S. Jordan Jr. Professor of Medicine and Epidemiology, Department of Internal Medicine, University of Virginia School of Medicine; Hospital Epidemiologist, University of Virginia Hospital, Charlottesville, Virginia

Gaétan M. Faubert, Ph.D. Professor, Department of Parasitology, McGill University, Ste. Anne-de-Bellevue, Quebec, Canada

Sydney M. Finegold, M.D. Professor, Department of Medicine, VA West Los Angeles Medical Center, Los Angeles, California

David N. Fredricks, M.D. Assistant Professor, Department of Medicine, University of Washington; Assistant Member, Program in Infectious Diseases, Fred Hutchinson Cancer Research Center, Seattle, Washington

Glenn T. Furuta, M.D. Assistant Professor, Department of Pediatrics, Harvard Medical School; Attending Physician, Department of Pediatric Gastroenterology, Combined Program in Pediatric Gastroenterology and Nutrition, Boston, Massachusetts

Eugene J. Gangarosa, M.D. Professor Emeritus, Department of International Health, Rollins School of Public Health, Emory University, Atlanta, Georgia

Gabriel Garcia, M.D. Associate Professor, Department of Medicine, Stanford University Medical Center, Palo Alto, California

Bruce G. Gellin, M.D. Staff Director, IDSA/Vaccine Initiative, Vanderbilt University School of Medicine, Nashville, Tennessee

Robert M. Genta, M.D. Professor, Department of Pathology, Veterans Affairs Medical Center, Houston, Texas

Dale N. Gerding, M.D. Professor, Department of Medicine, Northwestern University; Chief, Medical Service, VA Medical Center-Lakeside Division, Chicago, Illinois

Ralph A. Giannella, M.D. Mark Brown Professor of Medicine and Director, Division of Digestive Diseases, Department of Internal Medicine, University of Cincinnati College of Medicine, Cincinnati, Ohio

Roger I. Glass, M.D., Ph.D. Chief, Viral Gastroenteritis Section, National Center for Infectious Diseases, CDC, Atlanta, Georgia

Gary M. Gray, M.D. Professor, Department of Medicine, Stanford University School of Medicine; Attending Physician, Department of Medicine, Stanford Hospital and Clinics, Stanford, California

Harry B. Greenberg, M.D. Grant Professor of Medicine, Departments of Medicine, Microbiology, and Immunology, Stanford University School of Medicine, Stanford, California

Patricia M. Griffin, M.D. Chief, Foodborne Diseases Epidemiology Section, Foodborne and Diarrheal Diseases Branch, Division of Bacterial and Mycotic Diseases, National Center for Infectious Diseases, Centers for Disease Control and Prevention, Atlanta, Georgia

Richard L. Guerrant, M.D. Thomas H. Hunter Professor of International Medicine, University of Virginia School of Medicine; Chief, Division of Geographic Medicine, University of Virginia Hospital, Charlottesville, Virginia

Michele E. Hardy, Ph.D. Veterinary Molecular Biology Laboratory, Montana State University, Bozeman, Montana

David W. Hecht, M.D. Professor and Division Chief, Department of Infectious Diseases, Loyola University Medical Center, Maywood, Illinois

Barbara A. Hendrickson, M.D. Sections of Infectious Diseases, Department of Pediatrics and Department of Medicine, University of Chicago, Chicago, Illinois

John E. Herrmann, M.D. Professor of Medicine, Molecular Genetics, and Microbiology, Division of Infectious Diseases and Immunology, University of Massachusetts Medical School, Worcester, Massachusetts

Barbara L. Herwaldt, M.D., M.P.H. Medical Epidemiologist, Division of Parasitic Diseases, Centers for Disease Control and Prevention, Atlanta, Georgia

C. Robert Horsburgh, Jr., M.D., M.U.S. Professor, Department of Epidemiology and Biostatistics, Boston University School of Public Health; Professor, Department of Medicine, Boston University School of Medicine, Boston, Massachusetts

Duane R. Hospenthal, M.D., Ph.D. Assistant Professor, Department of Medicine, Hebert School of Medicine, Uniformed Services University of the Health Sciences, Bethesda, Maryland; Clinical Associate Professor, Department of Medicine, University of Texas Health Science Center at San Antonio, San Antonio, Texas; Assistant Chief, Infectious Disease Service, Brooke Army Medical Center, Fort Sam Houston, Texas

Peter J. Hotez, M.D., Ph.D. Director of the Medical Helminthology Laboratory and Associate Professor, Division of Epidemiology of Microbial Diseases, Yale University School of Medicine, New Haven, Connecticut

Stephen P. James, M.D. Deputy Director, Division of Digestive Diseases and Nutrition, National Institute of Diabetes and Digestive and Kidney Diseases, National Institutes of Health, Bethesda, Maryland

J. Michael Janda, Ph.D. (ABMM) Chief, Microbial Diseases Laboratory, California Department of Health Services, Berkeley, California

Edward N. Janoff, M.D. Infectious Diseases Division, Minneapolis, Minnesota

Stuart Johnson Infectious Diseases Sections, VA Chicago-Lakeside Division, Northwestern University Medical School, Chicago, Illinois

Kevin C. Kain, M.D. Professor, Department of Medicine, University of Toronto; Director, Tropical Disease Unit, Department of Medicine, Toronto General Hospital, Toronto, Ontario, Canada

Allen B. Kaiser, M.D. Professor, Department of Medicine, Vanderbilt University Medical Center, Nashville, Tennessee

John E. Kellow, M.D., F.R.A.C.P. Associate Professor, Department of Medicine, University of Sydney; Director, Gastrointestinal Investigation Unit, Department of Gastroenterology, Royal North Shore Hospital, New South Wales, Australia

Gerald T. Keusch, M.D. Director, Fogarty International Center, National Institutes of Health; Bethesda, Maryland

Douglas S. Kernodle, M.D. Associate Professor, Department of Medicine, Vanderbilt University School of Medicine; Chief, Division of Infectious Diseases, VA Medical Center, Nashville, Tennessee

Jay S. Keystone, M.D. Professor, Department of Medicine, University of Toronto; Staff Physician, Centre for Travel and Tropical Medicine, Toronto General Hospital, Toronto, Ontario, Canada

David Kiang, Ph.D. Postdoctoral Fellow, Department of Medicine, Stanford University, Stanford, California; Research Scientist, Department of Gastroenterology, VA Palo Alto Health Care System, Palo Alto, California

Christopher L. King, M.D. Associate Professor, Department of Medicine and International Health, Division of Geographic Medicine, Case Western Reserve University and University Hospitals School of Medicine, Cleveland, Ohio

Donald P. Kotler, M.D. Professor, Department of Medicine, Columbia University College of Physicians and Surgeons; Chief, Gastrointestinal Division, Department of Medicine, St. Lukes Roosevelt Hospital Center, New York, New York

Jean-Pierre Kraehenbuhl, M.D. Professor, Department of Vaccinology and Mucosal Immunology, Swiss Institute for Experimental Cancer Research, Epalinges, Switzerland

Ernst J. Kuipers, M.D., Ph.D. Professor, Department of Medicine, Division of Gastroenterology and Hepatology, Erasmus Medical Center, Rotterdam, The Netherlands

Johannes G. Kusters Departments of Gastroenterology and Hepatology, Erasmus Medical Center, Rotterdam, the Netherlands

Michael E. Lamm, M.D. Joseph R. Kahn Professor, Department of Pathology, Case Western Reserve University, Cleveland, Ohio

Claudio F. Lanata, M.D., M.P.H. Senior Researcher, Instituto de Investigacion Nutricional, Lima, Peru

Albert J. Lastovica, M.D. Department of Medical Microbiology, University of Cape Town, Cape Town, South Africa

Adrian Lee, B.Sc., Ph.D., Melb., F.A.S.M. Pro Vice Chancellor, University of New South Wales, Sydney, New South Wales, Australia

Peter Lee, Ph.D. Student, Department of Parasitology, Institute of Parasitology, McGill University, Ste. Anne de Bellevue, Quebec, Canada

Myron M. Levine, M.D., D.T.P.H. Professor and Head, Department of Medicine, Division of Geographic Medicine; Professor and Head, Department of Pediatrics, Division of Infectious Diseases and Tropical Pediatrics; Director, Center for Vaccine Development, University of Maryland School of Medicine, Baltimore, Maryland

Erich R. Mackow, Ph.D. Associate Professor, Departments of Medicine, Molecular Genetics, and Microbiology, Stony Brook University, Stony Brook, New York; Research Scientist, Department of Research, Northport VA Medical Center, Northport, New York

Adel A.F. Mahmoud, M.D., Ph.D. President, Merck Vaccines, Merck & Co., Inc., Whitehouse Station, New Jersey

Barbara J. Mann, Ph.D. Associate Professor, Departments of Internal Medicine and Microbiology, University of Virginia, Charlottesville, Virginia

Suzanne M. Matsui, M.D. Clinical Associate Professor, Department of Medicine, Stanford University School of Medicine, Stanford, California; Staff Physician, VA Palo Alto Health Care System, Palo Alto, California

Paul S. Mead, M.D., M.P.H. Chief, Outbreak Response and Surveillance Unit, Foodborne and Diarrheal Diseases Branch, Centers for Disease Control and Prevention, Atlanta, Georgia

Jiri F. Mestecky, M.D., Ph.D. Professor, Departments of Microbiology and Medicine, University of Alabama at Birmingham, Birmingham, Alabama

Samuel I. Miller, M.D. Professor, Departments of Medicine and Microbiology, University of Washington, Seattle, Washington

Eric D. Mintz, M.D. Chief, Diarrheal Diseases Epidemiology Section, Foodborne and Diarrheal Diseases Branch, Division of Bacterial and Mycotic Diseases, National Center for Infectious Diseases, Centers for Disease Control and Prevention, Atlanta, Georgia

Darcy Moncada, Ph.D. Institute of Parasitology, McGill University, Ste. Anne-de-Bellevue, Quebec, Canada

Desiree E. Morgan, M.D. Associate Professor, Department of Diagnostic Radiology, University of Alabama at Birmingham, Birmingham, Alabama

J. Glenn Morris, Jr., M.D., M.P.H. & T.M. Professor and Chairman, Department of Epidemiology and Preventive Medicine, University of Maryland School of Medicine, Baltimore, Maryland

James P. Nataro, M.D., Ph.D. Professor, Center for Vaccine Development, University of Maryland School of Medicine; Associate Chairman, Department of Pediatrics, University of Maryland Hospital, Baltimore, Maryland

Ann Marie Nelson, M.D., Chief, AIDS Pathology Branch, Infectious and Parasitic Diseases Pathology, Armed Forces Institute of Pathology, Washington D.C.

Marian R. Neutra, Ph.D. Professor, Department of Pediatrics, Harvard Medical School; Director, Gastrointestinal Cell Biology Laboratory, Children's Hospital, Boston, Massachusetts

Richard A. Oberhelman, M.D. Associate Professor of Tropical Medicine and Pediatrics, Tulane School of Public Health and Tropical Medicine, New Orleans, Louisiana

Michael E. Ohl, M.D. Senior Fellow, Department of Medicine, Division of Allergy and Infectious Diseases, University of Washington, Seattle, Washington

Sonja J. Olsen, Ph.D. Epidemiologist, Foodborne and Diarrheal Diseases Branch, National Center for Infectious Diseases, Centers for Disease Control and Prevention, Atlanta, Georgia

Jan M. Orenstein, M.D., Ph.D. Professor, Department of Pathology, George Washington University, Washington, D.C.

Jani L. O'Rourke, Ph.D. Senior Research Officer, Department of Microbiology and Immunology, University of New South Wales, Sydney, New South Wales, Australia

Julie Parsonnet, M.D. Associate Professor of Medicine and Health Research and Policy, Division of Infectious Diseases and Geographic Medicine, Stanford University School of Medicine, Stanford, California

David A. Pegues, M.D. Associate Clinical Professor, Department of Medicine, UCLA School of Medicine; Hospital Epidemiologist, UCLA Medical Center, Los Angeles, California

David H. Persing, M.D. Medical Director, Infectious Disease Research Institute; Vice President, Department of Molecular Biology, Corixa Corporation, Seattle, Washington

Willam A. Petri, Jr., M.D., Ph.D. Chief, Division of Infectious Diseases, Professor of Internal Medicine and Pathology, Associate Director of Microbiology, Department of Pathology, University of Virginia, Charlottesville, Virginia

Larry K. Pickering, M.D., F.A.A.P. Senior Advisor to the Director, National Immunization Program, Centers for Disease Control and Prevention; Professor, Department of Pediatrics, Emory University School of Medicine, Atlanta, Georgia

Thomas C. Quinn, M.D., M.Sc. Professor, Department of Medicine, Johns Hopkins University School of Medicine, Baltimore, Maryland

Jonathan I. Ravdin, M.D. Nesbitt Professor and Chairman, Department of Medicine, University of Minnesota, Minneapolis, Minnesota

Sharon L. Reed, M.D. Professor, Departments of Pathology and Medicine, University of California San Diego School of Medicine; Chief, Division of Laboratory Medicine, University of California San Diego Medical Center, San Diego, California

David A. Relman, M.D. Associate Professor, Department of Medicine, Department of Microbiology and Immunology, Stanford University, Stanford, California; Acting Chief, Infectious Diseases, Department of Medicine, VA Palo Alto Health Care System, Palo Alto, California

Lee W. Riley, M.D. Professor, School of Public Health, University of California Berkeley, Berkeley, California

Roy M. Robins-Browne, M.B., B.Ch., Ph.D. Professor, Department of Microbiology and Immunology, University of Melbourne; Director, Department of Microbiological Research, Department of Microbiology and Infectious Diseases, Royal Children's Hospital, Parkville, Victoria, Australia

James K. Roche, M.D., Ph.D. Associate Professor, Department of Internal Medicine, University of Virginia Health System, Charlottesville, Virginia

Philippe Sansonetti, M.D. Professor, Department of Bacteriology and Mycology, Institut Pasteur, Paris, France

R. Balfour Sartor, M.D. Professor, Departments of Medicine, Microbiolog,y and Immunology, Division of Digestive Diseases, University of North Carolina, Chapel Hill, North Carolina

William Schaffner, M.D. Professor and Chairman, Department of Preventive Medicine, Professor of Medicine (Infectious Diseases), Vanderbilt University School of Medicine; Hospital Epidemiologist, Vanderbilt University Medical Center, Nashville, Tennessee

Cynthia L. Sears, M.D. Associate Professor, Department of Medicine, Divisions of Infectious Diseases and Gastroenterolgy, Johns Hopkins University School of Medicine, Baltimore, Maryland

Kent A. Sepkowitz, M.D. Associate Professor, Department of Medicine, Weill Medical College of Cornell University; Head, Clinical Infectious Disease, Department of Medicine, Memorial Sloan-Kettering Cancer Center, New York, New York

Afzal A. Siddiqui, M.Phil., Ph.D. Associate Professor, Department of Internal Medicine, Texas Tech University Health Sciences Center; Research Scientist, Department of Research and Development, Amarillo VA Health Care System, Amarillo, Texas

Sumath Sivapalasingam Foodborne and Diarrheal Diseases Branch, Division of Bacterial and Mycotic Diseases, National Center for Infectious Disease, Centers for Disease Control and Prevention, Atlanta, Georgia

Martin B. Skirrow, M.B., Ph.D., F.R.C.P., D.T.M&H, Honorary Emeritus Consultant Microbiologist, Public Health Laboratory Service, Gloucestershire Royal Hospital, Gloucester, United Kingdom

Laurence Slutsker, M.D., M.P.H. Division of Parasitic Research, Center for Disease Control and Prevention/ Kenya Medical Research Institute Research Station, Kisumu, Kenya

Phillip D. Smith, M.D. Mary J. Bradford Professor in Gastroenterology, Professor of Medicine and Microbiology, Professor, Department of Medicine, University of Alabama at Birmingham; Medical Staff, University at Alabama Hospital; Staff Physician Birmingham Veterans Affairs Medical Center, Birmingham, Alabama

John D. Snyder, M.D. Professor, Department of Pediatrics, University of California at San Francisco, San Francisco, California

Jeremy Sobel, M.D., M.P.H. Foodborne and Diarrheal Diseases Branch, Centers for Disease Control and Prevention, Atlanta, Georgia

Roy Soetikno, M.D. Assistant Professor of Medicine, Stanford University School of Medicine; Chief of Endoscopy and Associate Chief of Gastroenterology Section, VA Palo Alto Health Care System, Palo Alto, California

Ronald D. Soltis, M.D. Associate Professor, Department of Medicine, Division of Gastroenterology, University of Minnesota Medical School, Minneapolis, Minnesota

Theodore S. Steiner, M.D. Assistant Professor, Department of Medicine, University of British Columbia; Assistant Professor, Department of Medicine, Division of Infectious Diseases, Vancouver Hospital and Health Sciences Centre, Vancouver, British Columbia, Canada

Charles R. Sterling, Ph.D. Professor, Department of Veterinary Science and Microbiology, University of Arizona, Tucson, Arizona

Kathryn N. Suh, M.D. Department of Medicine, Division of Infectious Diseases, Queen's University, Kingston, Ontario, Canada

Christina M. Surawicz, M.D. Professor, Department of Medicine, Division of Gastroenterology, University of Washington; Section Chief, Department of Medicine, Division of Gastroenterology, Harborview Medical Center, Seattle, Washington

David Swerdlow, M.D. Chief, Clinical Outcomes Section, Surveillance Branch, Division of HIV/AIDS Prevention, Centers for Disease Control and Prevention, Atlanta, Georgia

Yi-Wei Tang, M.D., Ph.D. Assistant Professor, Departments of Medicine, Division of Infectious Diseases and Pathology, Vanderbilt University School of Medicine; Medical Director, Molecular Infectious Diseases Laboratory, Vanderbilt University Hospital, Nashville, Tennessee

Robert V. Tauxe, M.D., M.P.H. Foodborne & Diarrheal Diseases Branch, Centers for Disease Control and Prevention, Atlanta, Georgia

Nathan M. Thielman, M.D., M.P.H. Assistant Professor, Department of Medicine, Division of Infectious Diseases and International Health, Duke University Medical Center, Durham, North Carolina

Phillip P. Toskes, M.D. Professor and Chairman, Department of Medicine, Shands Hospital, University of Florida, Gainesville, Florida

Edmund C. Tramont, M.D., F.A.C.P. Director, Division of Acquired Immunodeficiency Syndrome, National Institute of Allergy and Infectious Diseases, Bethesda Maryland; Staff Physician, Department of Medicine, Clinical Center, National Institutes of Health, Bethesda, Maryland

George Triadafilopoulos, M.D. Professor, Department of Medicine, Division of Gastroenterology and Hepatology, Stanford University, Stanford, California; Chief, Section of Gastroenterology, Palo Alto VA Health Care System, Palo Alto, California

Janice R. Verley, M.D. Department of Medicine, Johns Hopkins University School of Medicine, Baltimore, Maryland

Duc J. Vugia, M.D. Chief, Disease Investigations and Surveillance Branch, Division of Communicable Disease Control, California Department of Health Services, Berkeley, California

W. Allan Walker, M.D. Conrad Taff Professor of Nutrition and Professor, Department of Pediatrics, Harvard Medical School; Chief, Combined Program in Pediatric Gastroenterology and Nutrition; Director, Mucosal Immunology Laboratory, Massachusetts General Hospital East; Department of Medicine, Children's Hospital, Boston, Massachusetts

Christine A. Wanke, M.D. Associate Professor, Departments of Medicine, Tufts University School of Medicine; Staff Physician, Department of Infectious Disease, New England Medical Center, Boston, Massachusetts

Kenneth H. Wilson, M.D. Professor, Department of Medicine, Duke University; Chief, Infectious Diseases Section, VA Medical Center, Durham, North Carolina

Harland S. Winter, M.D. Associate Professor, Department of Pediatrics, Division of Pediatric Gastroenterology and Nutrition, Pediatric GI Unit, Massachusetts General Hospital, Boston, Massachusetts

Harvey S. Young, M.D. Department of Medicine, Stanford University School of Medicine, Stanford, California

PREFACE TO THE SECOND EDITION

In the seven years between the first and second editions of this textbook, medicine has continued its relentless advance. The world is changing, and medical researchers and practitioners have been responding.

As has been a constant theme since the beginning of microbiology, pathogenic microbes continue to be discovered, and new consequences of already-known agents have become apparent. Although much progress has been made in the fight against the Human Immunodeficiency Virus (HIV) in the developed countries of North America and Europe, the range and extent of the misery caused by HIV continues to expand. As patients live longer, gastrointestinal pathogens play an increasingly important role in HIV-infected patients. With the worldwide trade in food, and the ever-increasing industrialization of food production, foodborne disease outbreaks grow larger. Outbreaks now often involve multiple states in the United States, and multiple countries in several continents. Now more than 60 years into the era of antibiotics, resistance continues to climb, and our microecology is changing in ways unbeknownst to us. These are some of the current and future challenges.

What about solutions, or are we hopelessly spiraling into an era of greater morbidity and mortality? Fortunately, there have been many advances. Two revolutions stand out. First has been the electronic revolution with computerization and the internet as the main tools. Physicians of tomorrow will be as comfortable in front of their personal computers as their ancestors were in their libraries and clinics. Clearly these processes affect all of medicine.

The second revolution, which is emerging with similar force, has been the breakthroughs in genetics, including the sequencing of the human genome. Equally important, but receiving less attention, has been the deciphering of the genomes of human pathogens, many of them the subject of this book. From this greater storehouse of information about humans and our pests will come new advances in the prevention, diagnosis, and treatment of disease.

These advances already are happening, and the following pages will bring the readers the latest information about state-of-the-art treatment in gastrointestinal infections. We, the authors and editors, have been privileged to participate in this undertaking. A text is a repository of human knowledge and we are pleased to share what we know with our readers. We hope that you will again find this a very useful book.

This book could not have come to fruition without the dedication and patience of Jonathan Pine. He and the members of the Lippincott team, including Ellen DeFrancesco, Tony DeGeorge, Denise Martin, and Penny Bice, prodded and poked at authors and editors alike to move us ahead on schedule. Without them, we might still be caught up in the very busy nature of the academic practice of medicine, and this edition would be a dream rather than a reality.

Martin J. Blaser
Phillip D. Smith
Jonathan I. Ravdin
Harry B. Greenberg
Richard L. Guerrant

March 2002

PREFACE TO THE FIRST EDITION

Gastrointestinal infections are a major cause of disease and death, particularly in the developing world. New etiologic agents, including bacteria, viruses, and protozoans, have been identified; new diseases, such as AIDS, have appeared; and the pathophysiologic mechanisms of old diseases have been newly characterized. Widespread travel to developing countries has brought diseases associated with contaminated food and water to the immunologically naive populations of Main Street. The increased number of immunocompromised persons and the pandemic of HIV-infection have turned once-rare infections into everyday occurrences for the busy practitioner. New techniques permit quicker and more complete diagnosis of many infections.

These developments have increased the importance of understanding gastrointestinal infections not only by gastroenterologists and infectious diseases specialists, but by internists, pediatricians, pathologists, and surgeons as well. The goal of this book is to provide a comprehensive source that combines the scientific basis and the art of medicine, relevant to enteric infections. It is intended for the health-care practitioner, the clinical investigator, and all who seek not only the latest clinical details but also an understanding of the breadth and limitations of our knowledge of enteric infections.

We recognize and reaffirm that medicine is both an art and a science; in this text we hope to emphasize both faces of this same coin. The clinician who understands the new technologies, be they preventive, diagnostic, or therapeutic, becomes their master, not their slave. Nevertheless, especially in this field, there are many opportunities for simple, low-technology, low-cost approaches for treating ill patients that must be considered as well.

This book is organized to permit readers to access information according to clinical presentation and by etiologic agent, as well as segregating information on infection in normal and immunocompromised hosts. This is a large text; to avoid dilution of interest and focus, we have not included the many infections that primarily involve the liver, which should be treated as a separate subject.

Part I provides an accounting of the importance of gastrointestinal infections in human history and reviews the major epidemiologic patterns of enteric infections today. Parts II and III cover the basic principles of gastrointestinal structure, physiology, and immunology, as they pertain to enteric infections. Parts IV, V, and VI consider the major clinical syndromes involving the gastrointestinal tract in normal and immunocompromised hosts. The pertinent features of each are described, emphasizing differential diagnosis and approach to therapy. Part VII describes the most important pathogens of the gastrointestinal tract. In this section, the emphasis is on microbiology of the agent, its epidemiology and pathophysiology, and the specific approaches to diagnosis and therapy. The final sections, Parts VIII, IX, and X provide information on special diagnostic and therapeutic considerations and prevention of gastrointestinal infections including new strategies in vaccine development.

Above all, we have tried to provide a volume that is both comprehensive and practical.

Martin J. Blaser
Phillip D. Smith
Jonathan I. Ravdin
Harry B. Greenberg
Richard L. Guerrant

INFECTIONS OF THE GASTROINTESTINAL TRACT

SECOND EDITION

1

CHOLERA, DYSENTERY, AND DIARRHEA: LESSONS OF HISTORY

EDMUND C. TRAMONT
EUGENE J. GANGAROSA

Probably because infectious diseases are not glamorous and remind us of our vulnerabilities, their impact on the history of humankind is underappreciated (1). It is not our purpose here to catalogue, examine, or discuss the numerous and well-documented effects of gastrointestinal illnesses on the course of history, or their role in determining military outcomes. Instead, we have focused on two examples—namely, cholera and dysentery. Cholera was chosen because it can be argued that this disease, more than any other, mobilized and focused the public health efforts that led to the "sanitary revolution." Through investments in safe water and sanitation, rich dividends were reaped; control of a host of gastrointestinal diseases, including cholera, contributed enormously to an improved quality of life. In addition, research on the pathophysiology of cholera led to the development of oral rehydration therapy, now the cornerstone of treatment of virtually all diarrheal illnesses. Dysentery was chosen because of its historic role in the epic battles at Gallipoli and El Alamein, the outcomes of which significantly affected world events in the twentieth century, which in turn influenced European and North American relationships and, hence, our daily lives.

CHOLERA: OLD SCOURGE AND NEW CHALLENGES

> "When Vasco da Gama rounded the southernmost point of Africa, which he called the Cape of Good Hope, with all the flags of his gallant little ships flying, his officers and men clad in their gayest clothes and brightest armor, and his trumpets sounding, he little thought he was soon to meet with a new and dreadful pestilence at the courts of the great King of Calicut, low down on the southwestern or Malabar coast of India. He landed in 1498, and in 1503 Gaspar Correa, an officer of Vasco da Gama, says 20,000 men of Calicut died of a disease which struck them suddenlike in the belly, so that some of them died in eight hours."
>
> J. C. Peters, 1885 (2)

Historically, cholera was a feared epidemic diarrheal disease.

> "Our citizens had heard and read much of the Asiatic scourge and all we knew of it had impressed us with a sense of its mysterious character, its rapid and erratic course, its unmanageable and incurable nature, and its certain and dreadful fatality. Its fearful devastation in India and elsewhere had filled the mind with horror at the bare recital of its ravages, and the rumor of its appearance on the shores of the St. Lawrence threw our population into consternation,... which in some instances became so intense as to dethrone reason itself, and impel to suicide."
>
> A physician's account, New York, 1833 (3)

Cholera or a similar disease was known during ancient times. The first recognizable mention of a cholera-like illness is in the writings of Hindu physicians about 400 B.C. (4). The word *cholera* is derived from the Greek words meaning "flow of bile." Thomas Sydenham is credited with distinguishing cholera from other forms of diarrhea in 1817, when the disease came acutely to European attention following an explosive outbreak in Calcutta (5). John Snow determined the mode of transmission in 1849, and 5 years later, Filippo Pacini described curved bacilli in the stools of cholera victims and coined the term *Vibrio cholerae.* Robert Koch verified his discovery in 1883. Today, new epidemics continue in different parts of the world, almost exclusively in underdeveloped regions, although sporadic cases occasionally occur in developed regions (6).

Cholera is an acute and potentially deadly diarrheal disease (see Chapter 36). Cholera diarrhea, often described as *purging* to underscore its severity, may result in the loss of 10% or more of the body's vital fluids and electrolytes. The

E. C. Tramont: Institute of Human Virology, University of Maryland Biotechnology Institute, University of Maryland, Baltimore, Maryland

E. J. Gangarosa: Department of International Health, Rollins School of Public Health, Emory University, Atlanta, Georgia responsible pathogen, *Vibrio cholerae,* causes diarrhea by elaborating an enterotoxin, known as *cholera toxin,* that poisons the upper small intestine through a cascade of chemical events resulting in a molecular derangement of the control of water and electrolytes. Hypersecretion of chloride and a partial block of sodium absorption ensue. The net result is an enormous outflow of fluid from the intestinal circulation into the lumen of the bowel (Fig. 1.1). Fluid mixed with mucus and containing large quantities of sodium, potassium, bicarbonate, and chloride gives the cholera stool its characteristic appearance of "rice water." Hypokalemia, hyponatremia, and metabolic acidosis develop. In severe cases, the victim progresses to shock. The process may be so fulminating as to cause death in a matter of hours, although for every severe case, many asymptomatic infections occur, or cases with milder diarrhea that are indistinguishable from other forms of secretory diarrhea. *V. cholerae* does not invade the intestinal wall; hence, few polymorphonuclear cells are found in the stool (see Chapter 36).

As with other pestilences, moralism, interwoven with theology and piety, pervaded medical thinking in the early pandemics (outbreaks extended in time and crossing many national boundaries), and cholera was explained in terms of divine displeasure. Rosenberg (7) noted the prevailing theme of the nineteenth century: "Sin, in the scientific guise of predisposition, could still induce a case of cholera." Others explained epidemic diseases like cholera in terms of the miasmic theory, attributing environmental influences as the cause. Built on the lessons of the Civil War and John Snow's critical observations in London, a change occurred during the pandemic that reached the United States after that war. Despite clinging to religious and miasmic theories into the late nineteenth century, some prominent medical leaders, especially in the military, began to recognize the importance of sanitation in transmission. For example, the health officer William Clendenin wrote in the *Cincinnati Daily Gazette* of July 23, 1866, that "before erecting statues, building opera houses and art galleries, and buying expensive pictures, towns should be relieved of bad odors and fermenting pestilence. Good privies are far higher signs of civilization than grand palaces and fine art galleries" (7).

Furthermore, the terror of cholera led to town meetings, which mobilized public support for change. Some actions taken, such as the implementation of fasting, played no role in control, but its important legacy is that communities recognized the need for standing committees to implement control measures. Many of these standing committees took on a life of their own and lasted well beyond the cholera crises when they evolved into boards of health and subsequently into municipal health departments. Thus, the 1866 pandemic in the United States spawned the beginnings of a scientific rationale for public health action and gave substance to early departments of health (1). Religious rhetoric was gradually replaced by rational actions; fast days were replaced by clean-up days, and eventually public health departments gained credibility as communities witnessed the success of their actions. Clearly, cholera provided considerable leverage in bringing about these changes and proved to be a powerful stimulus for the *sanitary revolution* (see below).

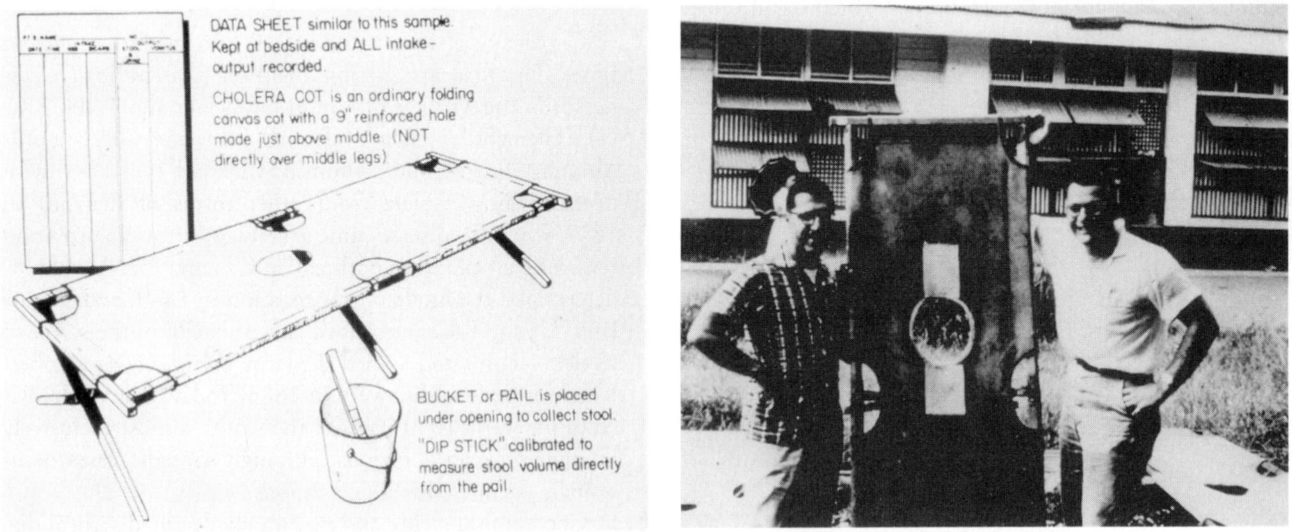

FIGURE. 1.1. The cholera cot was constructed for easy measurement of the volume of fluid loss to guide fluid replacement. One of the authors is shown holding such a cot. Since the advent of oral rehydration therapy, it has been relegated to the status of historical importance.

CHOLERA PANDEMICS

A pandemic is an epidemic outbreak that is extended in time and crosses many national boundaries. Beginning in 1817, medical historians described seven pandemics, the first six originating on the Indian subcontinent with subsequent extension to Europe and the Americas. It is uncertain whether the disease was confined to Asia before 1817, but during the following five decades, the disease spread in six pandemic waves out of India and across much of the world, including Europe and the Americas. This suggests that like smallpox, measles, and tuberculosis, which spread from Europe to the Americas, cholera spread from the Asian subcontinent to the Western World. Cholera receded after 1869, disappearing by the turn of the century from the Americas and most of Africa and Europe, so that by 1950, it remained only on the Asian subcontinent.

There is reason to believe that the first six pandemics may in fact have been a single pandemic caused by the classic strain, *V. cholerae* serotype O1 (8,9). The seventh pandemic was caused by the El Tor biotype of *V. cholerae* O1, which was described early in the twentieth century after being isolated at the El Tor quarantine station in Egypt from a pilgrim returning from Mecca. By 1960–1961, this strain had spread out of Indonesia, where an endemic focus had been described a quarter of a century earlier. In subsequent decades, the pandemic spread to Southeast Asia, the Western Pacific, South Asia, the Middle East, Africa, South America, and Latin America.

The pandemic extended into January 1991, when a new epidemic of cholera appeared explosively in villages, towns, and cities along the Peruvian coast (10). In the ensuing months, it spread swiftly throughout Latin America, challenging the health care infrastructure of all the countries of that continent. In its intensity, the epidemic resembled the great urban epidemics of the past century in Europe and the United States, but what was conspicuous was the velocity of its spread into neighboring areas, with transmission most likely facilitated by modern air, sea, and land travel. Subsequently, this cholera outbreak assumed the characteristics of the pestilence of the past in terms of its persistence in foci that lacked safe water and good sanitation. *V. cholerae* non-O1 has been isolated from the Gulf of Mexico (11). Cholera cases associated with travel, ingestion of foods from affected regions, and ingestion of raw shellfish have been reported in developed countries (12). Despite the extraordinary numbers of persons requiring emergency treatment and straining medical resources, the mortality rates were remarkably low. This can be attributed to the widespread use of fluid replacement therapy, especially *oral rehydration therapy* (ORT).

In October 1992, another outbreak occurred in Madras India, which quickly spread to the rest of India. Although it has thus far been contained in India and Bangladesh, it has sometimes been referred to as the eighth pandemic (6). The unique aspect of this outbreak is that it was caused by a newly recognized serogroup, O139, the first non-O1 *V. cholerae* to cause an extended outbreak (13).

UNIQUE CHARACTERISTICS OF THE CHOLERA ORGANISM AND ITS RESERVOIR

For years, traditional wisdom held that the only reservoir of the cholera organism was in humans. Fecal–oral transmission was thought to be the exclusive means of spread. However, nonhuman reservoirs exist. *V. cholerae* has a unique repertoire of mechanisms for survival and persistence in aquatic environments. It is a halophilic organism endowed with an ecologic niche in estuarine waters, an environment from which shellfish, which obtain their sustenance through filtration, are commonly harvested. In these waters, the organism has special relationships with a wide range of aquatic plants, such as water hyacinths and duckweeds, and a variety of phytoplankton and zooplankton (11,14–17). The organism persists and spreads from its niche periodically, especially during aquatic plumes, in a cycle involving seafood, especially shellfish, and humans.

The nature of the endemic foci of cholera around the world is such that the incidence of the disease can explode during facilitating environmental changes. Although humans play a central role as amplifiers and sources of fecal–oral transmission, the organism can persist in endemic foci and may cause disease when humans eat raw or undercooked seafood. In parts of the world where water treatment and the sanitation infrastructure are substandard, the two transmission mechanisms imperceptibly merge, causing food-borne and waterborne outbreaks. A combination of environmental conditions (e.g., sunlight, pH, temperature, salinity, availability of nutrients) affects marine microflora and the physiologic state and survival of *V. cholerae.* It has been postulated that manipulation of the environment by humans may have contributed to the emergence of cholera in Peru in the 1980s. Or, as in the well-recorded phenomenon of overgrowth or overpopulation when fauna or flora are transplanted on land, the organism may have arrived in the bilge of a ship, subsequently thriving in a permissive environment rich in coastal plankton fertilized by atmospheric and coastal nitrate deposits increased by global warming, the excessive use of agricultural fertilizers, the discharge of industrial wastes and domestic sewage, and soil erosion (18). Emergence may also be a normal or natural periodic phenomenon. Hence, it can be postulated that changing environments, not changing pathogens, are the main cause of so-called emerging infectious diseases (19,20). For example, the Ebola, Marburg, yellow fever, and Lassa fever viruses, hantaviruses, and HIV are normally nonhuman primate-, mosquito-, and rodent-specified pathogens that have escaped their normal ecologic niche through ecologic imbalances (e.g., created when forests are cleared).

CHOLERA: A DIARRHEAL DISEASE PROTOTYPE AND THE TREATMENT BREAKTHROUGH

At the beginning of the seventh pandemic in the 1960s, little was known about the pathogenesis of cholera. Without this understanding to guide therapy, mortality rates were high, often approaching 20% to 30% in hospitalized patients, and higher in victims treated at home. In the early 1960s, studies conducted in Southeast Asia radically changed this situation.

During an urban epidemic of cholera in Bangkok, Thailand, in 1959–1960, several landmark studies were conducted, the results of which led to an understanding of the basic pathophysiology of the disease. One of these showed, contrary to the views held at the time, that the intestinal epithelium remains intact throughout the disease process and that intestinal epithelial cells continue their normal function (21). Hence, a poisoned cellular function caused by a toxin rather than an infection-induced cytopathic effect was sought. Another study defined the physiologic deficits that occur when cholera patients purge (22). These studies subsequently provided the rationale for intravenous fluid and electrolyte replacement.

As the cholera pandemic moved quickly throughout Southeast Asia and across South Asia in the 1960s, the administration of intravenous fluids to replace electrolyte (physiologic) losses resulted in a dramatic reduction of mortality in these patients to nearly zero. However, this hospital-based therapy was expensive and out of the reach of the vast majority of cholera victims. Thus, the development of a simpler, less costly regimen became a high priority for research.

The success of the intravenous strategy naturally stimulated research focused on oral rehydration. The subsequent discovery that glucose is necessary for the absorption of orally administered electrolytes was a landmark in the history of the treatment of cholera (23).

Soon thereafter, it was recognized that these discoveries could be applied to the treatment of all diarrheal diseases because the physiologic electrolyte losses differ only in degree. Cholera is now recognized as the prototype of the so-called secretory diarrheas, which account for most of the diarrheal diseases associated with a high mortality rate.

Furthermore, it was found that infants with diarrheal illness of any etiology treated with ORT had a significant weight gain in comparison with those treated by conventional regimens that did not include oral fluids. It became evident that the vicious cycle of diarrhea/malnutrition and malnutrition/diarrhea could be successfully broken, at least in cases of acute, watery diarrhea (24).

The impact of ORT on diarrheal disease mortality and morbidity has been dramatic. The number of lives saved each year by this inexpensive, easily administered therapy can be measured in the millions. Perhaps the most prophetic comments relative to this breakthrough were made in an editorial in the *Lancet* in 1978, which heralded ORT as perhaps the most significant medical breakthrough in this century (25). For both clinician and victim, the development of fluid replacement therapy means that cholera is no longer perceived as the dreaded disease it once was. The transformation from a highly malignant to an easily managed disease permits the clinician to shift the focus from treating cholera as a single clinical entity to treating it as one of a generic group of acute secretory diarrheas that are all managed in essentially the same way. Today, anyone with cholera seen alive by a health care provider should survive!

However, the implications of this inexpensive, easy-to-administer treatment strategy extend well beyond cholera, other diarrheal diseases, or clinical medicine. ORT has provided the leverage and has proved to be the centerpiece in the development of multifaceted, multidisciplinary World Health Organization diarrheal diseases control programs now in place in most developing countries, which have contributed substantially to overall infant and child survival rates in these areas.

The "Sanitary Revolution"

Documentation of the waterborne transmission of cholera in the large urban outbreaks occurring in London, England, in the 1850s and Hamburg, Germany, in the 1890s, coincident with the urban outbreaks in the United States, set in motion the "sanitary revolution." The essence of this revolution was the commitment of communities to long-term investments in the delivery of safe water by establishing water treatment plants and sewage systems for the sanitary disposal of human wastes. Simultaneously, food-handling practices were improved as the food-producing and food-serving industries went through a slow process of improved food safety under the scrutiny of newly formed public health departments.

The sanitary revolution has had a profound impact on industrialized nations. Cholera and other epidemic gastrointestinal diseases have been virtually eliminated as a significant public health threat. As always, a few exceptions have occurred, such as the shellfish-related cholera outbreak in Naples, Italy, in 1973 (26) and the outbreak in Portugal in 1974 caused by noncarbonated water (27). Cases have also been imported into European and North American countries (28), but without subsequent transmission. These few exceptions serve to emphasize the rule that the development of community infrastructures ensuring safe water, safe food, and effective sanitation markedly reduces the threat of cholera. In addition to this benefit, investments in such infrastructures profoundly improve all other aspects of health, quality of life, and economic development. The solution for those countries that still bear the burden of cholera and other diarrheal diseases is to initiate their own sanitary revolution.

The argument that the resources necessary to address such issues are simply not available ignores the economic consequences of the disease. Decreases in foreign investment and tourism and quarantines and restrictions on imports are the result. In short, the economic disasters created by cholera underscore how tenuous economic investments can be when an insufficient and weak public health infrastructure is in place.

New Challenges

Whereas human actions upset the ecologic balance and lead to the emergence or reemergence of disease, the success of ORT and antibiotics in the treatment of diarrheal diseases has resulted in complacency and blurred the responsibilities of clinicians, microbiologists, and public health practitioners in regard to epidemic diarrheal diseases.

For example, the clinician needs to know that specialized media are required to isolate *V. cholerae* and that specific, nonroutine methods must be used to isolate other microbiologic causes of diarrhea. Unless the clinician alerts the laboratory of these possibilities, the likelihood of identifying the offending agent is significantly compromised. The clinician's awareness that contaminated water and foodstuffs spread diarrheogenic agents is also important in the enforcement of hand washing and other precautions to be taken regarding stool.

The challenge to the public health practitioner is to institute and maintain an effective water and sanitation infrastructure. Few diseases provide as much leverage to bring about a change in infrastructure as cholera.

IMPACT OF GASTROINTESTINAL ILLNESSES ON MILITARY CAMPAIGNS

> "Soldiers have rarely won wars. They more often mop up after the barrage of epidemics. And typhus with its sisters, plague, cholera, typhoid and dysentery, have decided more campaigns than Caesar, Hannibal, Napoleon and all the inspector generals of history. The epidemics get the blame for defeat, the generals, the credit for victory. It ought to be the other way around."
>
> Hans Zinsser, 1935 (29)

Although the ravages of smallpox on Amerindians in the sixteenth and seventeenth centuries and the devastating effects of plague and tuberculosis in Europe have been duly recorded (1,3,4), the most conspicuous impact of infectious diseases has been on military campaigns. Simply stated, food-borne, waterborne, and vector-borne diseases have accounted for the outcome of more battles than the instruments of war (30) (Fig. 1.2). As noted above, whenever the normal lifestyle and sanitation of a community are disrupted, intestinal infections become important and critical

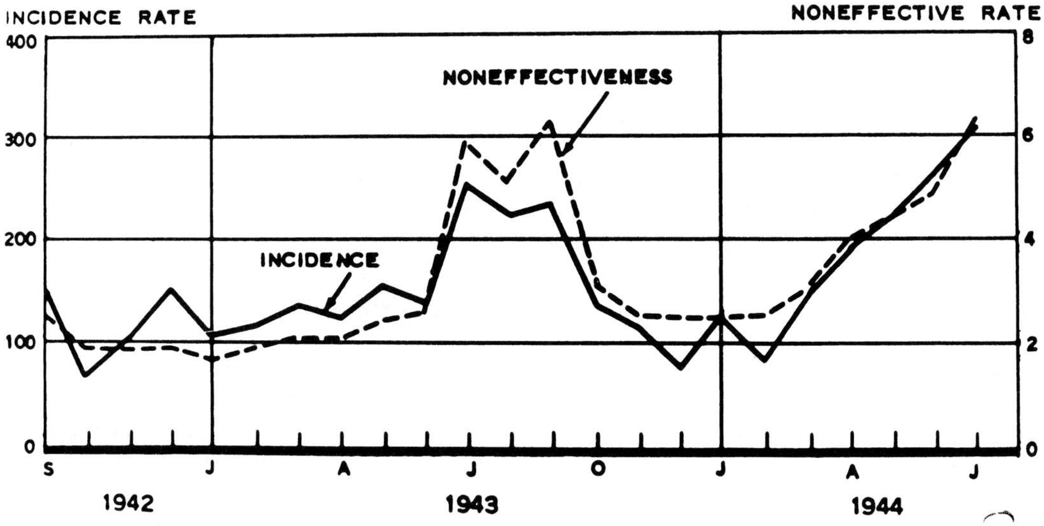

FIGURE 1.2. Impact of illnesses on troop effectiveness, Pacific Theater, World War II. In simple terms, troops cannot fight when they are sitting on their bottoms or weak from loss of fluid and electrolytes. The impact goes beyond individual patients; others are needed to care for the ill, and those who have to fill in become fatigued. Source: Monthly Progress Report, Army Service Forces, War Department, 31 Aug. 1944, Section 7: Health.

determinants of human functionality, and the legacy of war is just that!

Even if one argues that future conflicts will be conspicuous for the use of immensely destructive modern weaponry that may result in quick, decisive outcomes (as witnessed in military conflicts involving Western countries following the Vietnam War), the aftermath of destruction and occupation will set the stage for an overwhelmingly increased incidence of gastrointestinal infections, and the least immunologically experienced (i.e., Americans, Canadians, and Western Europeans) and the most immunologically dysfunctional (i.e., the malnourished) will be the most vulnerable. Furthermore, many "local" civil and regional wars continue to erupt. These occur primarily in underdeveloped countries. Hence, immediate destruction by missiles hurled through the air is not the norm; old-fashioned long and drawn-out conflicts remain the rule. The legacy of these conflicts is massive shifts in population, refugee camps, and poorly functioning water and sanitation infrastructures; hence, the prerequisites for massive food and waterborne outbreaks and associated malnutrition are in place (31,32).

Gallipoli

> "From June onwards dysenteric diarrhea spread through the Army and soon every man was infected by it. Many of the soldiers were able to endure it without reporting sick, but some soon became too weak even to drag themselves to the latrines, and by July, when over a thousand men were being evacuated every week, the disease had become far more destructive than the battle itself. Quite apart from the discomfort and the self-disgust, it created an overmastering lassitude. 'It fills me,' Hamilton wrote, 'with a desperate longing to lie down and do nothing but rest...and this, I think, must be the reason the Greeks were ten long years in taking Troy.' "
>
> Alan Moorehead, 1956 (33)

It is always dangerous to declare a single episode in any protracted military conflict to be the decisive event of that conflict, but some major battles have marked a turn of the tide in favor of the eventual "victor" (if there is such a thing in war). For example, the battles of Waterloo, Gettysburg, and Midway and the Tet offensive are considered, from a historical perspective, the turning points of the Napoleonic Wars, the United States Civil War, the Pacific Theater in World War II, and the Vietnam War (34,35).

In World War I, many historians consider the battle of Gallipoli in a similar light. The Allied failure doomed any potential victory for Czarist Russia, thereby helping to set the stage for the Bolshevik Revolution and the eventual creation of the Communist Soviet Union and the subsequent Cold War. Furthermore, Winston Churchill was cast into the backwaters of political influence, which arguably made it easier for Hitler to promulgate Nazism (36).

Gallipoli is a peninsula (Fig. 1.3) that guards the Dardanelles, the entrance into the Black Sea, and hence a key supply route to Russia. During World War I, the Allied Forces, under a plan drawn up by Sir Winston Churchill, then First Lord of the Admiralty of the British Navy, attempted to occupy Gallipoli and so secure a logistic pipeline to Russia and maintain a second front against Germany. The Turks, then allied with Germany, defended Gallipoli. The Allied Forces, made up primarily of Australians, were defeated despite having larger numbers of troops, superior battle equipment, and better training. The reason for the defeat was an epidemic of dysentery that disproportionately affected the relatively nonimmune Allied Forces in comparison with the local defenders (33).

El Alamein

> "General Montgomery says the Eighth Army won, but Rommel claimed the victory for dysentery."
>
> Sir Sheldon F. Dudley (37)

Soon after the United States entered into World War II, the brilliant German General Rommel was poised to gain control of the Suez Canal, thereby further blocking the transport of oil and other supplies to Great Britain and potentially crippling the British. But Rommel never accomplished his objective.

Perhaps because of the lessons learned at Gallipoli, or because of Great Britain's long-term occupation of the Middle East, the Allied forces took measures to practice superior preventive medicine; namely, they buried their excrement and so controlled spread by flies carrying *Shigella* and other diarrheogenic microorganisms. The Axis Forces, on the other hand, relied on the sun to "bake" their excrement in the sand, allowing flies ample time to become contaminated with diarrheogenic microorganisms and ultimately to contaminate the human food chain.

Indeed, during the fateful and decisive battle at El Alamein, which preserved British control of the Suez Canal, Rommel was convalescing from dysentery in Germany. "But, as the Germans learned at El Alamein, dysentery can still win battles when hygienic discipline on one side is slack" (37).

Other Conflicts

> "He who fails to learn from history is destined to repeat it."
>
> Anonymous

A review of the major conflicts in which the U.S. military has participated (Table 1.1)—the U.S. Civil War (38) (Table 1.2), the Spanish–American War (39), World War I (40), World War II (41,42) (Fig. 1.2, Table 1.3), Korea (43,44), Lebanon (45,46), Vietnam (47,48) (Fig. 1.4), and the Gulf War (Desert Storm) (49,50)—reveals that diarrhea/dysen-

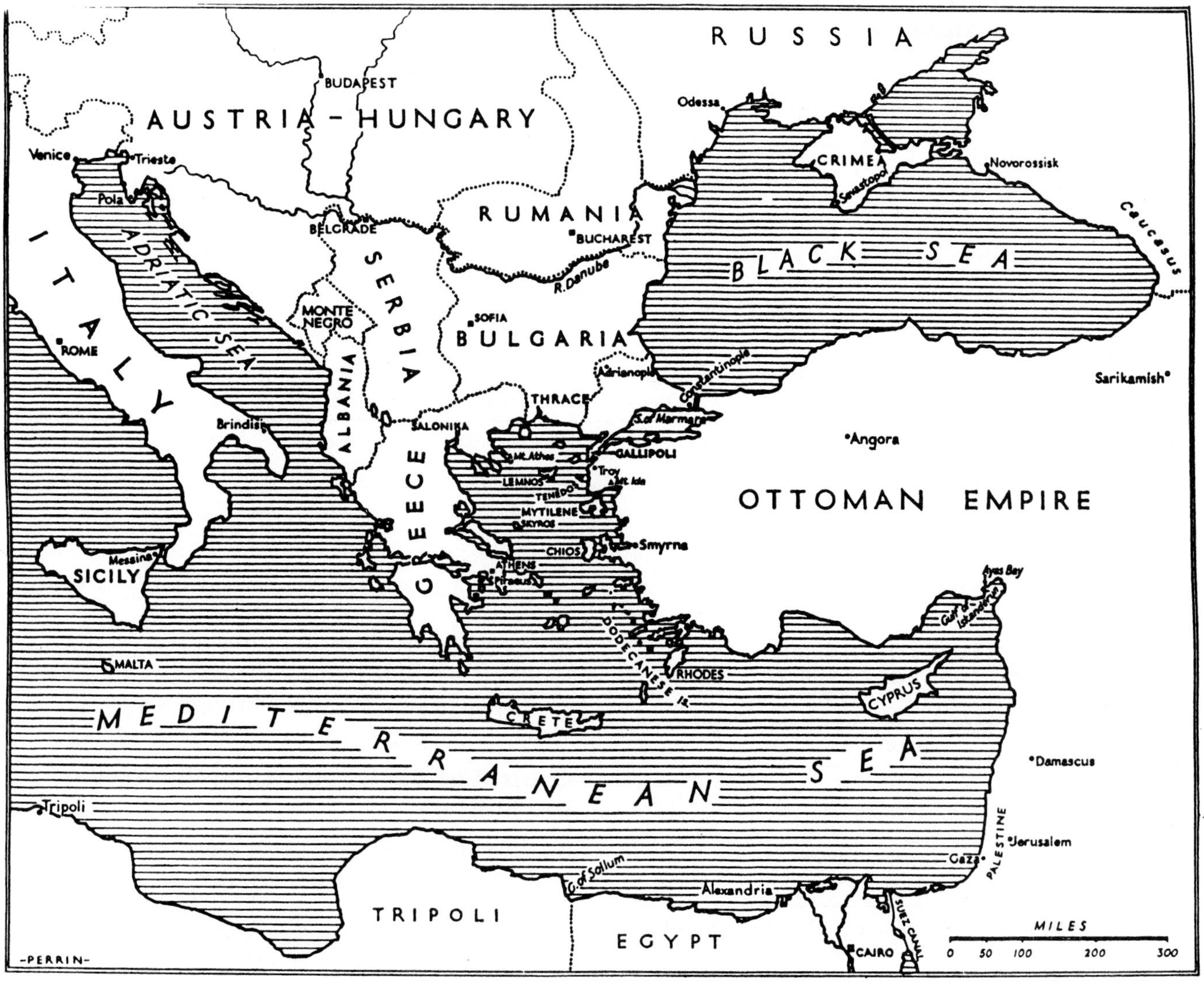

FIGURE 1.3. Eastern Europe and the Middle East, 1912.

TABLE 1.1. HOSPITAL ADMISSIONS FOR DIARRHEA/DYSENTERY[a] (PER 1,000 TROOPS PER YEAR)

Conflict	Incidence	Death Rate
Civil War	741	18
Spanish-American War	426	3.3
World War I	29	0.13
World War II	14	0.005
Korea	14	NA
Lebanon[b]	247	NA
Vietnam[c]	60	NA

[a]Includes all causes of diarrheal and dysenteric illnesses (infectious origin, gastroenteritis, ulcerative colitis, ileitis). Before the Spanish-American War, etiologic differences were not considered. Beginning with the Spanish-American War, typhoid fever was distinguished separately; amebiasis was considered separately during the Vietnam War.
[b]August 13 to September 24, 1958.
[c]January 1965 to March 1966.
NA, not available.

TABLE 1.2. INCIDENCE OF DIARRHEA AND DYSENTERY IN THE U.S. ARMY BY AREA AND YEAR PARALLELS THE AVAILABILITY OF SAFE LOCAL WATER AND SANITARY DISPOSAL OF FECAL EXCREMENT

	Number of Cases per 1,000 Troops per Year					
	1940	1941	1942	1943	1944	1945
Continental United States	7	15	8	12	9	9
U.K. and Continental Europe			17	12	13	14
Mediterranean			34	132	54	22
Middle East			229	179	114	89
Persian Gulf					115	56
China					68[a]	122
India and Burma					107[a]	86
Australia					23	5[b]
Philippine Islands	27	28			114	104
Latin America	8	13	21	21	17	16
Central America			104	86		

[a]November and December only.
[b]January through August only.
From Medical Department, U.S. Army. *Medical statistics in World War II.* Washington, DC: U.S. Government Printing Office, 1975.

TABLE 1.3. DEATH RATE FOR DIARRHEA/DYSENTERY PER 1,000 TROOPS PER YEAR IN THE CIVIL WAR

Year	Rate
1861–1862	4.2
1862–1863	16.0
1863–1864	26.7
1864–1865	28.8
1865–1866	21.5

Adapted from *Medical and surgical history of the War of Rebellion (1861–1865).* Washington, DC: U.S. Government Printing Office, 1879 (*Medical history,* parts 2 and 3).

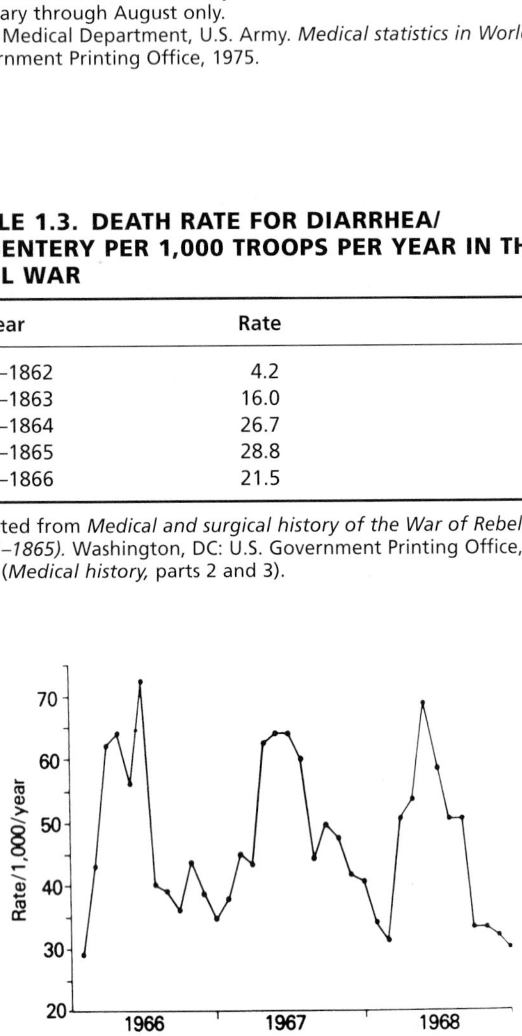

FIGURE 1.4. Monthly diarrheal disease as documented by the U.S. Army during the Vietnam War (cases per 1,000 troops per year). The highest incidence occurred during the warmest months. Diarrhea caused by *Escherichia coli* infection was demonstrated for the first time in a military setting (47). Source: USARV surgeons Monthly Command Health Reports to USARV commander: 1966–1968.

tery has been monotonously recorded as a major problem of morbidity and troop dysfunction. In the U.S. Civil War, it was a major cause of mortality (38) (Table 1.2).

Control of Gastrointestinal Illnesses by the Military

Every conflict leaves a legacy of improved medical care (30,51,52). The U.S. Civil War left us, among other advances, the nascent principles and practice of public health that are still valid today (53). For example, by quarantining U.S. troops in fortified camps and having them forego local foodstuffs in favor of previously prepared food rations (MREs), the U.S. military reduced the rates of gastrointestinal illnesses (and sexually transmitted diseases) in U.S. troops stationed in Somalia (1993) and maintained them at baseline levels. Mosquitoes, which obviously are not bound by such human-instituted policies, continued to spread malaria.

THE FUTURE

The importance of controlling intestinal infections has often been forgotten. Unless we heed history's lessons and intercede before the human gut is exposed to the omnipresent and ever-changing horde of intestinal pathogens, a weak link in the fortunes of all peoples and all military operations is the ever-present threat of gastrointestinal infection. Medical professionals practicing in every country must know and understand cholera as the prototype of diarrheal disease in every aspect—clinical and laboratory diagnosis, treatment, investigation and reporting of cases, outbreaks, and especially prevention.

Medical professionals must recognize their special leadership role when deficiencies involving the water–food–sewage infrastructure occur, and they must further recognize that careful investigation of an outbreak provides leverage to persuade decision makers who control resources to address deficiencies, reorder priorities, and ensure the commitment needed to correct the root problems. Experiences in all countries ravaged by cholera underscore the importance of a multisectorial, multidisciplinary approach to prevention. The actors on this stage must include political leaders and the ministries and departments responsible for health, agricultural development, transportation, and fisheries.

Countries that have already made the investments in the water–food–sewage infrastructure spawned during the sanitary revolutions of the past are generally protected. However, this infrastructure cannot be taken for granted; it must be nurtured, upgraded, and maintained. Obviously, countries where cholera and other diarrheal illnesses are actively transmitted must address the need for their own sanitary revolution if the long-term benefits of improved quality of life and enhanced economic development are to be realized.

REFERENCES

1. McNeill WH. *Plagues and peoples.* Garden City, NY: Doubleday Publishing, 1976.
2. Peters JC. Early history of Asiatic cholera in India as known to Europeans (A.D. 1503–1800). In: Wendt EC, ed. *Asiatic cholera.* New York: William Wood & Co., 1885.
3. Smith G. *Plague on Us.* New York: Commonwealth Fund, 1941.
4. Cartwright FF. *Disease and history.* New York: Thomas Y Crowell, 1972.
5. Baura D. History of cholera. In: Baura D, Greenough WB, eds. *Cholera.* New York: Plenum Publishing, 1992.
6. Swerdlow DL, Ries AA. *Vibrio cholerae* non-O1, the eighth pandemic. *Lancet* 1993;342:382–383.
7. Rosenberg CE. *The cholera years: the United States in 1832, 1849, and 1866.* Chicago: University of Chicago Press, 1987.
8. Blake PA. Epidemiology of cholera in the Americas. *Gastroenterol Clin North Am* 1993;3:639–660.
9. Politzer R. *Cholera.* Geneva: World Health Organization, 1959.
10. Reis AA, Vugia DJ, Beingolea L, et al. Cholera in Piura, Peru: a modern urban epidemic. *J Infect Dis* 1992;166:1429–1433.
11. Levine WC, Griffin PM. *Vibrio* infections on the Gulf Coast: results of first year of regional surveillance. *J Infect Dis* 1993;167: 479–483.
12. Finelli L, Swerdlow D, Mertz K, et. al.. Outbreak of cholera associated with crab brought from an area with epidemic disease. *J Infect Dis* 1992;166:1433–1435.
13. Sack RB, Albert MJ, Siddique AK. Emergence of *Vibrio cholerae* O139. *Curr Clin Trop Infect Dis* 1996;16:172–193.
14. Colwell RR, Kaper J, Joseph SW. *Vibrio cholerae, Vibrio parahaemolyticus* and other vibrios: occurrence and distribution in Chesapeake Bay. *Science* 1977;198:394–396.
15. Spira WM, Huq A, Ahmed QS, et al. Uptake of *Vibrio cholerae* biotype El Tor from contaminated water by water hyacinth (*Eichhoronia crassipes*). *Appl Environ Microbiol* 1981;42:550–553.
16. Khan MU, Shahidullah M, Haque MS, et al. Presence of vibrios in the surface water and their relation with cholera in the community. *Trop Geogr Med* 1984;36:335–340.
17. Islam MS, Drasar BS, Bradley DJ. Long-term persistence of toxigenic *Vibrio cholerae* O1 in the mucilaginous sheath of a blue-green algae, *Anabaena variabilis. J Trop Med Hyg* 1990;93: 133–139.
18. Epstein PR. Cholera and the environment: an introduction to climate change. *PSR Q* 1992;2:146–160.
19. Levine MM, Levine OS. Changes in human ecology and behavior in relation to the emergence of diarrheal disease, including cholera. *Proc Natl Acad Sci U S A* 1994;91:2390–2394.
20. Gibbons A. Where are "new" diseases born? *Science* 1993;261: 680–681.
21. Gangarosa EJ, Beisel WR, Benyajati C, et al. The nature of the gastrointestinal lesion in Asiatic cholera and its relation to pathogenesis. *Am J Trop Med Hyg* 1960;9:125–135.
22. Watten RH, Morgan FM, Phillips RA, et al. Water and electrolyte studies in cholera. *J Clin Invest* 1959;38:1879–1891.
23. Nalin DR, Cash RA, Islam R, et al. Oral maintenance therapy for cholera in adults. *Lancet* 1978;2:370–374.
24. Duggan C, Santosham M, Glass RI. The management of acute diarrhea in children: oral rehydration, maintenance, and nutritional therapy. *MMWR Morb Mortal Wkly Rep* 1992;41(RR-16).
25. Water with sugar and salt. *Lancet* 1978;2:300–301.
26. Baine WB, Zampiere A, Mazzotti M, et al. The epidemiology of cholera in Italy in 1973. *Lancet* 1974;2:1370–1374.
27. Blake PA, Rosenberg ML, Costa JB, et al. Cholera in Portugal, 1974. Modes of transmission. *Am J Epidemiol* 1997;105: 337–343.
28. Taylor JL, Tuttle J, Pramukul, T, et al. An outbreak of cholera in Maryland associated with imported commercial coconut milk. *J Infect Dis* 1993;167:1330–1335.
29. Zinsser H. *Rats, lice and history.* Boston: Little, Brown and Company, 1935.
30. Lacey SW. The arts of war and medicine: a study in symbiosis. *Am J Med Sci* 1993;305:407–420.
31. Swerdlow DL, Malenga G. Begkoyian G, et al. Epidemic cholera among refugees in Malawi, Africa: treatment and transmission. *Epidemiol Infect* 1997;118:207–214.
32. Shapiro RL, Otieno MR, Adcock PM, et al. Transmission of epidemic *Vibrio cholerae* O1 in rural western Kenya associated with drinking water from Lake Victoria: an environmental reservoir of cholera? *Am J Trop Med Hyg* 1999;60:271–276.
33. Moorehead A. *Gallipoli.* New York: Harper Brothers, 1956.
34. Summers HG. *On strategy: a critical analysis of the Viet Nam War.* Novato, CA: Presidio Press, 1982.
35. Karnow S. *Vietnam: a history.* New York: Viking Press, 1983.
36. Manchester W. *The last lion, Winston Spencer Churchill: visions of glory, 1874–1932.* Boston: Little, Brown and Company, 1983.
37. Philbrook FR, Gordon JE. Diarrhea and dysentery. In: Hoff EB, ed. *Preventive medicine in World War II,* vol 4. Washington, DC: Office of the Surgeon General, Department of the Army, 1958: 319–413.
38. *Medical and surgical history of the War of the Rebellion (1861–1865).* Washington, DC: U.S. Government Printing Office, 1879 (*Medical history,* parts 2 and 3).
39. Reed W, Vaughn C, Shakespeare EO. *Report on the origin and spread of typhoid fever in U.S. military camps during the Spanish War of 1898.* Washington, DC: U.S. Government Printing Office, 1900.
40. *Communicable and other diseases.* Washington, DC: U.S. Government Printing Office, 1928 (*The medical department of the United States Army in the World War,* vol 9).
41. U.S. War Department, Military Intelligence Division. *Merrill's marauders (February–May 1944).* Washington, DC: U.S. Army

Center of Military History, 1945 (*American forces in action series*).
42. Medical Department, U.S. Army. *Medical statistics in World War II.* Washington, DC: U.S. Government Printing Office, 1975.
43. Health of the Army, Office of the Surgeon General, U.S. Army. *Korea: a summary of medical experience, July 1950–December 1952.* Washington, DC: Office of the Surgeon General, 1953.
44. Crowdrey AE, ed. *The medic's war: United States Army in the Korean War.* Washington, DC: Center of Military History, U.S. Army, 1987.
45. Hurewitz S. Military medical problems of the Lebanon crisis. *Mil Med* 1960;125:26–35.
46. Long P. Office of the Surgeon General. *Preventive medicine: lessons learned in Lebanon.* Disposition form to Director, Historical Unit, January 26, 1960.
47. Gentry LO, Hedlund KW, Wells RF, et. al. Bacterial diarrheal diseases. In: Ognibene AG, Barrett O, eds. *Internal medicine in Viet Nam,* vol 2. Washington, DC: Office of the Surgeon General and Center of Military History, 1982.
48. Sheehy TW. Digestive disease as a national problem. VI. Enteric disease among United States troops in Vietnam. *Gastroenterology* 1968;55:105–112.
49. Hyams KC, Bourgeois AL, Merrell BR, et al. Diarrheal disease during operation Desert Shield. *N Engl J Med* 1991;325:1423–1428.
50. McCarthy M, Estes MK, Hyams KC. Norwalk-like virus infection in military forces: epidemic potential, sporadic disease, and the future direction of prevention and control efforts. *J Infect Dis* 2000;2:S387–S391.
51. Bayne-Jones S. *The evolution of preventive medicine in the United States Army: 1607–1939.* Washington, DC: Office of the Surgeon General, Department of the Army, 1968.
52. Key JD. U.S. Army Medical Department and Civil War medicine. *Mil Med* 1968;133:181–192.
53. Sartin JS. Infectious diseases during the Civil War: the triumph of the "Third Army." *Clin Infect Dis* 1993;16:580–584.

2

EPIDEMIOLOGY OF DIARRHEAL DISEASES IN DEVELOPING COUNTRIES

ROBERT E. BLACK
CLAUDIO F. LANATA

Diarrheal diseases are a serious public health problem in developing countries, especially in children, whose rates of diarrheal morbidity and related mortality are high (1,2). Under the conditions of poverty, poor environmental sanitation and hygiene, inadequate water supplies, and limited education prevalent in developing country settings, diarrheal diseases occur frequently and can have the lethal consequences.

Substantial global efforts were first directed at reducing diarrheal disease mortality in the 1980s (1). These efforts were based on the recognition that acute dehydrating diarrheas play a substantial part in fatal illnesses. Furthermore, it had been demonstrated that such dehydration can be treated with oral replacement of fluids and electrolytes, along with continued feeding, rather than by expensive and difficult-to-administer intravenous fluids (3). After this discovery, it became possible to make effective therapy much more widely available, and national diarrheal control programs were initiated in nearly all developing countries (1). These programs have led to greatly improved therapy for diarrhea in many settings and a subsequent reduction in diarrhea-related mortality (4). With the reduction in diarrheal deaths related to dehydration, additional attention is now being turned to the problems of dysentery and persistent diarrhea (often associated with malnutrition), which are also major causes of diarrhea-related morbidity and mortality (5,6). These illnesses require additional therapeutic interventions (7,8). Furthermore, control programs are increasingly turning their efforts toward preventive interventions. It is important to understand the etiologic and epidemiologic features of the diarrheal diseases because they may provide a basis for specific therapeutic and preventive measures.

R. E. Black: Department of International Health, Johns Hopkins University, Bloomberg School of Public Health, Baltimore, Maryland

C. F. Lanata: Nutrition and Infection Working Group, Instituto de Investigacion Nutricional, Lima, Peru

GENERAL EPIDEMIOLOGY

Definitions

Diarrhea is a symptom complex characterized by stools of decreased consistency and increased number. Although on a clinical basis diarrhea can be defined in relation to an individual patient's prior bowel habits, epidemiologic studies have commonly used a more precise definition for standardization (9). Most studies now consider diarrhea to be present when three or more liquid stools are passed during any 24-hour period. In the first 2 months of life, especially for breast-fed infants, the definition is more commonly based on what a mother considers to be a decrease in stool consistency or an increase in stool frequency for her child. At least 2 days free of diarrhea are usually required for an episode to be defined as terminated. Dysentery is a diarrheal disease defined by the presence of blood in loose or liquid stools.

Although most diarrheal episodes resolve during the first week, a small proportion continue for 2 weeks or more. Studies in children living in developing countries indicate that the distribution of episode durations is continuous, but skewed toward longer durations (7, 10–12). Thus, establishing a specific definition of persistent diarrhea as an illness of more than a given number of days is arbitrary. Nevertheless, doing so is useful for comparability in research studies and for implementing case management strategies. The World Health Organization (WHO) recommends that persistent diarrhea be operationally defined as an episode that lasts for at least 14 days. Furthermore, this definition of persistent diarrhea operationally identifies children who tend to have heavy diarrheal burdens (13,14). The term *persistent diarrhea* is intended to encompass episodes that begin acutely and continue for longer than the expected duration, but not to include infrequent chronic diarrheal disorders, such as hereditary syndromes, gluten-sensitive enteropathy, granulomatous diseases, or tumors producing gastrointestinal hormones (7).

Incidence and Duration of Diarrhea

Diarrheal incidence has varied in the different settings in which it has been studied. These variations may be a consequence of methodologic differences, such as the definition of diarrhea and surveillance techniques used (9,15), or of actual differences in the study populations. In a summary of prospective, community-based studies in developing countries, the median incidence of all diarrheal illness in children under 5 years of age was 2.6 episodes per child per year (2). Among these studies, the incidence was highest in those with a small number of children under surveillance and with frequent home visiting (e.g., two or three times per week), which suggests that larger studies with infrequent surveillance may have found lower rates because diarrhea was underreported. Although it is likely that incidences differ in different populations, methodologic variations may account for a substantial part of the apparent differences. A number of individual studies with intensive surveillance have found rates as high as 8 to 11 episodes per year per child (Table 2.1).

The incidence of diarrhea varies with the age of the child within the first 5 years of life (12–14,16–19). Generally, children in the first 2 years of life have the highest incidence, which then falls progressively with age. The peak incidence is often at 6 to 11 months of age. The incidence in boys and girls as determined by community-based studies is similar; however, in some countries, boys may be more commonly taken to health facilities, so that their rates of diarrhea appear higher.

Although rates of diarrhea may be high throughout the year in children in developing countries, in most settings, a peak occurs during hot or rainy months (18,20). The seasonality of all diarrheal illness is, in fact, a composite of the seasonality of individual agents causing diarrhea. Most of the bacterial causes of diarrhea appear to peak during the hot or wet months. Rotaviral illness may exhibit little seasonality in tropical areas but often peaks in the cool or dry season in more temperate climates (21). The seasonality must be largely a consequence of environmental influences on the transmission of infectious agents, although seasonal shifts in the health of children, such as seasonal deterioration in nutritional status, may also play a part.

In most settings, the majority of diarrheal episodes are self-limited and resolve within 1 week (Table 2.1). A small fraction take 2 weeks or more to resolve. The decline in incidence with age appears to be similar for persistent and all other diarrheas.

Impact of Diarrhea

It has long been appreciated that diarrheal diseases are an important cause of death in childhood. Case fatality rates in children under 5 years of age have been reported to be 0.1% in Bangui, Central African Republic (22), 0.3% in rural Egypt (23), 0.4% in rural North India (24), and 0.5% in rural Indonesia (25). The U.S. Institute of Medicine estimated a diarrheal case fatality rate in children under 5 years of age in developing countries of 0.2% (26). The case fatality rate varies substantially with age, being highest in the youngest children. In a study from rural India, the case fatality rate was reported to be 0.7% for acute diarrhea but 14% for persistent diarrhea (27).

The World Bank reviewed the health problems of developing countries and concluded that diarrheal diseases are the second most important cause, after respiratory infections, of disability-adjusted years of life lost (28). This is largely a consequence of high rates of childhood mortality from diarrheal diseases. It has been estimated that currently 3.2 to 3.5 million deaths from diarrhea occur in children in developing countries each year (2). The diarrheal mortality rate is highest in the first year of life, at about 20 deaths per 1,000 children. Although the rate of about 5 deaths per 1,000 children in the 1- to 4-year-old age group is lower, this age group still accounts for approximately half of the diarrheal deaths of childhood. Mortality rates appear to fall

TABLE 2.1. INCIDENCE AND DURATION OF DIARRHEAL EPISODES IN CHILDREN FROM COMMUNITY-BASED STUDIES

Study (reference)	Age Group (months)	Total Episodes	Diarrheal Incidence (per 100 child-years)	Diarrheal Duration (days)		
				1–7	8–14	≥15
Indonesia (16)	0–11	618	311	83%	14%	4%
Guatemala (17)	0–11	262	334	53	27	19
Bangladesh (11)	0–59	941	557	66	21	14
Brazil (18)	0–71	519	600	82	15	3
Peru (10)	0–11	1,299	984	79	14	7
India (44)	0–71	471	61	35	55	10
Brazil (13)	0–60	2,896	1,140	76	13	11
Peru (12)	0–35	5,302	807	88	9	3
Bangladesh (14)	0–59	2,609	455	71	22	7
Bangladesh (19)	0–71	1,074	195	50	27	23

to very low levels after the first 5 years of life, although a slight increase may occur in older adults.

The infectious diseases of childhood have been found to have adverse effects on growth (29). Of all the infectious diseases, diarrhea seems to have the greatest adverse effect, possibly because of reduced appetite, altered feeding practices, and decreased nutrient absorption, along with the very high prevalence of diarrhea in young children (30). In various studies of the magnitude of the effect of diarrheal diseases on growth, from 10% to 80% of the growth retardation has occurred in the first few years of life, in comparison with an international reference population (29). The true estimate in most settings is probably closer to the lower end of this range. Furthermore, certain factors may moderate the effect of diarrheal illnesses on growth. Appropriate treatment of the illness may reduce the adverse effects of diarrhea; fluid replacement, continued breast-feeding, and a good diet during diarrhea can prevent weight faltering (29). In addition, children with an adequate regular diet not only better withstand the illness but also have the potential to grow more rapidly after an illness, so-called catch-up growth, especially if they do not have subsequent episodes of diarrhea or other serious illness (31,32).

Diarrheal diseases are also an economic burden in developing countries because of the costs of medical care, medications, and lost work. Although the illnesses can largely be managed by fluid and nutritional therapy, with the selective use of antibiotics, pharmaceuticals are frequently inappropriately used for managing diarrhea (33). The administration of antibiotics and so-called antidiarrheal drugs represents an unnecessary expenditure of hundreds of millions of dollars in developing countries each year, and in addition to reducing the likelihood of appropriate therapy, it also contributes to antibiotic resistance among enteropathogens and other infectious agents (33).

MICROBIAL ETIOLOGIES

Relative Importance of Enteropathogens

A wide array of bacterial, viral, and parasitic agents have been associated with diarrhea in developing countries. Because the highest incidences of diarrhea and the most severe consequences are generally in young children, most studies have focused on this age group. Older children and adults may become ill from the same enteropathogens; however, the relative frequencies of these organisms may vary in different age groups because of immunity acquired from prior exposure.

Community-based studies are those in which household visits are made, usually at least once per week, to identify cases of diarrhea and collect fecal specimens for culture. Results from these studies best represent the overall occurrence of diarrheal illnesses, regardless of severity or care seeking. Based on 24 studies with comprehensive microbiology from 13 countries, enterotoxigenic *Escherichia coli* (ETEC) has been found to be associated with the largest proportion of episodes, with a median of 14% (Table 2.2). The next most commonly found has been *Giardia lamblia,* but the proportion infected with this protozoan has been highly variable. *Campylobacter* species and rotavirus are both found in a median of 6% of episodes. *Shigella* species and *Cryptosporidium parvum* have been found in 4% of episodes.

Studies in health facilities, either outpatient clinics or hospitals, evaluate a more selected group of patients for whom care has been sought, often for an illness of greater severity than those identified in community-based studies. Based on 73 studies with comprehensive microbiology from 33 countries, rotavirus has been the most frequent enteropathogen, with a median of 20% (Table 2.3). However, in these studies, bacterial enteropathogens predominated overall. ETEC (median, 11%), *Campylobacter* species (7%), and *Shigella* species (5%) were most commonly identified. *Aeromonas, Salmonella* species, and vibrios, especially *Vibrio cholerae,* may be frequent in some settings. *G. lamblia* has been infrequently and *Entamoeba histolytica* rarely found in childhood diarrheas in health facilities. *C. parvum* has been sought only more recently in studies of etiology, but it has been found in each of 10 studies seeking this agent, with a median identification rate of 4%.

Generally, the community-based studies have identified an enteropathogen in about half of the episodes, and the facility-based studies in 60% to 70%. The sensitivity of the tests employed to detect enteropathogens is not optimal, and many more enteropathogens are known than are evalu-

TABLE 2.2. PERCENTAGES OF SELECTED ENTEROPATHOGENS IDENTIFIED IN CHILDREN WITH DIARRHEA IN COMMUNITY-BASED STUDIES IN DEVELOPING COUNTRIES

Characteristic	*Aeromonas*	*Campylobacter*	*Cryptosporidium parvum*	*Entamoeba histolytica*	ETEC	*Giardia lamblia*	Rotavirus	*Salmonella*	*Shigella*	Vibriones
Number of studies	9	18	7	17	22	18	22	23	24	14
Median range	2 <1–13	6 1–24	4 2–7	<1 0–9	14 2–41	10 <1–24	6 2–29	1 0–6	4 1–27	<1 0–3

ETEC, enterotoxigenic *Escherichia coli.*

TABLE 2.3. PERCENTAGES OF SELECTED ENTEROPATHOGENS IDENTIFIED IN CHILDREN WITH DIARRHEA IN HEALTH FACILITIES IN DEVELOPING COUNTRIES

Characteristic	*Aeromonas*	*Campylobacter*	*Cryptosporidium parvum*	*Entamoeba histolytica*	ETEC	*Giardia lamblia*	Rotavirus	*Salmonella*	*Shigella*	Vibriones
Number of studies	22	56	10	42	51	43	58	71	72	40
Median range	2 <1–42	7 0–32	4 1–12	1 0–7	11 2–54	2 0–28	20 5–49	4 0–38	5 0–33	1 0–33

ETEC, enterotoxigenic *Escherichia coli.*

ated in most studies. These other agents may each account for a small proportion of the episodes in which one of the more common enteropathogens is not identified.

The identification of an enteropathogen in feces during diarrhea does not necessarily mean that that agent is causing the illness. In fact, studies in which comprehensive microbiology has been performed frequently find two or more enteropathogens simultaneously, and it is rarely possible to ascertain which is causing the illness or whether both are playing a role. These mixed infections may occur because a person is exposed simultaneously to more than one agent through a common vehicle of transmission or to more than one vehicle of transmission. A person may also have an asymptomatic infection with one enteropathogen when exposed to another.

Asymptomatic enteric infections are common in populations in developing countries. In community-based studies (10,11,13,19), the same children were examined for enteropathogens on a routine basis (e.g., once per month) and when they had diarrhea. *Campylobacter* species were found as frequently when study children did not have diarrhea as when they did (34). In most, but not all, studies, ETEC, *Shigella* species, and rotavirus were found more frequently during diarrhea, and the median values for percentage identification of these enteropathogens differed between diarrheal cases and controls.

In studies based in health facilities, the controls were usually children who came to the facility for a reason other than diarrhea. Generally, the differences between patients with diarrhea and controls were greater than in community-based studies. Most of the studies found *Campylobacter* species more frequently in children with diarrhea than in controls, and nearly all found ETEC and *Shigella* species more frequently in children with diarrhea than in controls (34). The different rates of identification for rotavirus in cases of diarrhea and in controls were quite striking; the median rate in controls was 4% versus 21% in patients with diarrhea, based on data from 31 studies (34).

Some of the asymptomatic infections might represent convalescent carriage after an illness but could also reflect exposures to enteropathogens that were insufficient to cause illness, perhaps because of a low number of ingested organisms or immunity (35). The immunity could have been either passively transferred through breast milk or acquired from previous exposure to the organism (35–37). The high prevalence of these asymptomatic infections appears to be more indicative of frequent exposure to the agents than of a long-term carrier state, which appears to be rare (10,11, 37,38).

Few studies have focused specifically on enteropathogens associated with dysentery and used recently developed microbiologic methods (11,39,40). However, older studies and more comprehensive recent studies have documented that *Shigella* species can be isolated in about half of dysenteric episodes. Given the evidence that these organisms can be isolated from a single stool culture in only 60% to 70% of cases of shigellosis (41), the proportion of dysentery cases caused by *Shigella* species is probably even higher. *Campylobacter* species may be the second most frequent cause of dysentery, but the importance of these organisms seems to vary by setting (39,42). Although enteroinvasive *E. coli* (EIEC) can cause dysentery, it has been isolated with very low frequency in the studies available. *E. histolytica,* a cause of amebic colitis (42a), appears to be an infrequent cause of dysentery, especially in children (11,39,40). Other organisms, such as *Salmonella* species, *Vibrio parahaemolyticus,* and *Plesiomonas shigelloides,* can be associated with dysentery with a low frequency (39,40). Enterohemorrhagic (O157:H7) *E. coli* produces a hemorrhagic colitis (43). The organism has not yet been adequately studied in developing countries, but the distinctive clinical syndrome seen with this infection is uncommon. Although a number of other enteropathogens, such as ETEC, rotavirus, and *V. cholerae,* have been isolated from the feces of patients with dysentery, it is likely that these were part of a mixed infection and did not cause the invasive diarrhea.

Because persistent diarrheal episodes have particularly severe consequences for nutritional status and survival, a special effort has been focused on identifying the enteropathogens associated with these episodes. To ascertain such an association, it is necessary to identify the enteropathogens present during the first week of diarrhea in episodes that resolve in less than 2 weeks and compare them with the enteropathogens in episodes that last longer; thus, a prospective study is required. Assessment of enteropathogens present during the third week of illness may also provide useful information if the organisms present in the initial stage of the same episode are known. Five studies using comprehensive microbiology provide data (19,44–47a). Rotavirus was not found to be more frequent in persistent diarrhea; in fact, it was more commonly found in acute diarrhea in two of four studies (19,45,46). *Aeromonas* species, *Campylobacter* species, and *G. lamblia* were identified at similar rates in acute and persistent diarrhea, and *E. histolytica* was rare in both. ETEC was frequently found in both acute and persistent episodes. *Shigella* species have been associated with longer episodes (11), and their lack of association with persistent diarrhea in these prospective studies may have been a consequence of early antibiotic therapy.

Attention has been given recently to types of *E. coli* demonstrating adherence properties in tissue culture assay that have been proposed as potentially important agents of acute or persistent diarrhea (47,48). These organisms have now been subclassified as enteropathogenic *E. coli* (EPEC), enteroaggregative *E. coli* (EAEC), and diffuse-adherent *E. coli* (DAEC) (49.50). EPEC has been shown to cause acute diarrhea, whereas EAEC has been associated with persistent diarrhea in some, but not all, studies (16,44–47,49,50). DAEC may be a heterogeneous group, and only some may cause diarrhea, but some studies have found associations between DAEC and either acute or persistent diarrhea (44,47,50).

Cultures of specimens obtained from patients with diarrheal episodes that have continued for more than 2 weeks have yielded enteropathogens in the same proportions as cultures of specimens obtained during the acute phase. However, examination of sequential cultures in the first and third weeks of same episodes in Bangladesh and Peru indicates that persistent infection with the same organism during an episode is uncommon (45,46). A new enteropathogen is often found in the third week, which suggests that a prolonged episode in some cases is caused by sequential infection with different pathogens.

In general, the infections of adults with diarrhea in developing countries seem to be predominantly bacterial (50,51). ETEC infections are probably the most frequent (52). *Salmonella* species, *Shigella* species, and *Vibrio* species are commonly found (53–55). In areas where *V. cholerae* O1 is endemic or where cholera epidemics are occurring, this organism may be frequent (52,56,57).

In developing countries, diarrhea is a common complication of other infectious diseases, such as measles and AIDS. Measles-associated diarrhea has generally been linked to the same enteropathogens that cause childhood diarrhea in that setting (58,59). In adults with AIDS in developing countries, a variety of pathogens, some uncommon causes of illness in normal hosts, have been associated with diarrhea. *C. parvum, Enterocytozoon bieneusi* (microsporidia), and *Isospora belli* may be especially important (60–62). However, in both adults and children, common bacterial enteropathogens also play an important part in AIDS-associated diarrhea.

It appears that nosocomial diarrhea is common in health facilities in developing countries. Rotavirus may be especially common in nosocomial infections in pediatric wards (63), but many bacterial organisms, even *V. cholerae*, can be transmitted in treatment centers (64).

Bacterial Agents

Bacterial enteropathogens account for most of the diarrheal illnesses in both children and adults in developing countries. Most of the responsible agents could not be detected until appropriate conditions for their isolation and assays to identify their virulence properties were developed in the last two decades.

Of the bacterial enteropathogens, diarrheogenic *E. coli* is clearly the predominant group causing illnesses in developing countries. Although *E. coli* organisms are an important part of the normal flora of the intestine, they can cause diarrhea by a variety of mechanisms if they possess the necessary virulence properties (65). Diarrheogenic *E. coli* organisms are designated based on the demonstration of virulence properties or laboratory characteristics felt to be associated with virulence properties (65). Some of the strains have been found to produce attaching and effacing lesions in the intestine and localized adherence in the HEp-2 cell assay and are now called EPEC (66,67). The pathogenic role of EAEC in acute and persistent diarrhea has been documented; however, the importance of *E. coli* with diffuse adherence (DAEC) to HEp-2 cells in acute or persistent diarrhea is not yet clear (68–73).

Strains of ETEC produce a heat-labile toxin (LT) or a heat-stable toxin (ST) or both, and a number of assays are now available to test for toxin production or the genetic capability of such production in *E. coli* (65). Although these assays are not optimally sensitive, the ETEC organisms are still the most commonly found enteropathogens. In addition, not all studies have sought both types of toxins, so that the frequency of ETEC has been underestimated in such studies. The relative frequencies of the production of each toxin by ETEC organisms have varied from study to study, but usually either ST-only or LT-only strains predominate, and strains producing both toxins are the least frequent. It has been demonstrated further that many ETEC organisms produce colonization factors that are important in pathogenesis, leaving open the possibility that not all toxin-producing strains are capable of causing diarrhea (65). This may be a partial explanation for the high frequency of asymptomatic infections in developing country populations; however, it is also clear that acquired immunity may protect from illness, but not colonization (74). Enteroinvasive and enterohemorrhagic *E. coli* organisms do not appear to be common in developing countries, although epidemics of hemorrhagic colitis caused by O157:H7 *E. coli* have occurred in South Africa and Swaziland.

Campylobacter jejuni or *C. coli* organisms (often encompassed in epidemiologic studies by the term *C. jejuni*) cause watery diarrhea and dysentery, especially in young children, in developing countries. Immunity acquired from *C. jejuni* diarrhea is the likely explanation for the low rate of illness in adults and the high prevalence of asymptomatic infection (75). Other species of *Campylobacter,* such as *C. hyointestinalis, C. lari,* and *C. upsaliensis,* may cause diarrhea, but their importance is unknown.

Of the *Shigella* species found in cases of diarrhea and dysentery in developing countries, *S. flexneri* is usually the most common, followed by *S. sonnei, S. boydii,* and *S. dysenteriae* (76,77). However, outbreaks caused by *S. dysenteriae* type 1, or Shiga bacillus, have occurred in many countries (77–79). The resulting illnesses are often severe, with high fatality rates, and the organisms may be resistant to most commonly used antibiotics, so that specific treatment is ineffective (80).

Cholera occurs seasonally in areas of endemicity, such as the Ganges River delta of India and Bangladesh, and in global pandemics (81,82). In areas of endemicity, cholera primarily affects children 2 to 15 years of age, but it may cause a large proportion of the cases of severe watery diarrhea in adults during the season of transmission (82). Immunity develops after an initial illness caused by *V. cholerae,* although asymptomatic infections may still occur. In areas without previous exposure to *V. cholerae,* the entire population is susceptible. Introduction of the organism into such a setting, if sanitation is poor and food and water are inadequately protected, can result in an explosive epidemic affecting the entire population (83). When the seventh pandemic of cholera, caused by the El Tor biotype of *V. cholerae* O1, spread to Peru, hundreds of thousands of known cases and several thousand deaths were reported in that country (57). Within 1 year, 18 countries in the Western Hemisphere reported cholera, including most of South and Central America (84).

While the El Tor biotype of *V. cholerae* O1 continues to spread, a new strain of *Vibrio* has recently caused a large epidemic of cholera-like watery diarrhea in Bangladesh and India (85). The involved non-O1 strain of *V. cholerae,* assigned to serogroup O139, produces an enterotoxin that is apparently identical to cholera toxin. Because this epidemic has affected all age groups, as when *V. cholerae* O1 is newly introduced to an area, it is thought that previous experience with *V. cholerae* O1 does not provide immunologic protection from the new *Vibrio* strain.

Aeromonas hydrophila is frequently and *P. shigelloides* is less frequently found during diarrhea in developing countries (86). At least in the case of *A. hydrophila,* the higher rate of isolation of the organism during diarrhea versus controls in some studies suggests a causative role (87). However, the role of the organisms as enteropathogens and the mechanisms by which they may cause diarrhea are still not resolved (88,89). *Yersinia enterocolitica* has been sought in a number of developing countries and appears to be found rarely in cases of diarrhea (90).

Clostridium difficile causes antibiotic-associated colitis and has been examined in this syndrome and also in acute childhood diarrhea in a few developing countries (91). Limited evidence suggests that the organism may be found in acute diarrhea, but the causative relationship is not clear.

Viral Agents

Rotaviruses are the most important cause of severe watery diarrhea in young children. The greater frequency of isolation of this agent in cases of diarrhea in health facilities than in the community undoubtedly reflects the greater severity of disease caused by rotaviruses (92). This has also been documented in community-based studies, in which rotaviruses have been associated with about 40% of cases of diarrhea with dehydration, a potentially life-threatening complication (11).

Enteric adenoviruses of serotypes 40 and 41 are also an important cause of diarrhea (93,94). In 14 studies in developing countries (all but one of childhood diarrhea in health facilities), enteric adenoviruses were found in a median of 3% (range, none to 6%) of episodes.

The Norwalk agent and related 27-nm caliciviruses (e.g., Hawaii and Snow Mountain agents) cause watery diarrhea and vomiting (95). Seroepidemiologic studies indicate that these agents occur worldwide (96,97). Several etiologic studies suggest that the Norwalk agent alone may account for 2% to 5% of cases of childhood diarrhea in developing countries (98–100). The importance of the other caliciviruses is unknown, but it is likely that they cause an additional small fraction of episodes (101).

Other viruses or virus-like particles have been proposed as causes of diarrhea. Astroviruses (102), in addition to 25- to 30-mm round virus-like particles, have been found during diarrhea (38). Pestivirus has also been suggested as a pathogen (103). However, the causative role of these agents and their importance in developing countries are still uncertain.

Parasitic Agents

G. lamblia is a ubiquitous protozoan with a very high carriage rate in many developing country populations, especially in children (103,104). Although it could be a cause of diarrhea in specific cases, it is unlikely to be an important diarrheal pathogen in most settings (104–106). Likewise, amebiasis caused by *E. histolytica* can be a serious disease with extraintestinal complications, such as liver abscess, but *E. histolytica* appears to be a very infrequent cause of childhood diarrhea or dysentery in developing countries (42, 107–109).

C. parvum, a small coccidian parasite, is a cause of acute diarrhea and may have a particular association with persistent diarrhea or diarrhea in malnourished or immunocompromised hosts (47a,110–112). It has a global distribution and may be the most important parasite causing childhood diarrhea in developing countries (110). Related organisms of the true coccidia, such as *I. belli,* may cause diarrhea but seem to be uncommon, except perhaps in association with AIDS (60–62). Diarrhea associated with microsporidia (*E. bieneusi*) also occurs with AIDS (113), but the role of this organism in immunocompetent persons is unknown.

Cyclospora cayetanensis organisms, also referred to as *Cyanobacteria-like bodies* and other names in the early literature, are recently described protozoan enteropathogens found in a number of developing countries (114,115). Infection is identified by the presence of spherical cystlike organisms measuring 8 to 10 μm in diameter (larger than *C. parvum* oocysts, which are 3 to 5 μm in diameter) (115). Because the staining characteristics are similar to those of *C. parvum* and size discriminations have not been made in most previous studies, some of the cases attributed to *C. parvum* may have been caused by *Cyclospora* species.

Other protozoan infections can be associated with diarrhea (116). *Balantidium coli* infection can cause diarrhea or dysentery, *Chilomastix mesnili* infection may result in mild diarrhea, and *Blastocystis hominis* is of uncertain pathogenicity.

Most intestinal helminthic infections are not associated with diarrhea, but dysentery and even rectal prolapse have been seen in severe *Trichuris trichiura* infections and diarrhea in infections with other intestinal parasites, such as *Capillaria philippinensis, Trichostrongylus* species, *Strongyloides stercoralis, Necator americanus,* and *Ancylostoma duodenale* (117). Although diarrhea has been considered to occur as one of the clinical manifestations of other parasitic infections, such as malaria and schistosomiasis, a causative relationship is not clear; many of these diarrheal illnesses may be caused by bacterial and viral enteropathogens.

RISK FACTORS AND TRANSMISSION ROUTES

Diarrheal diseases are a consequence of two factors: exposure to a pathogenic organism and the susceptibility of the host to development of the disease. Nearly all diarrheal diseases are transmitted by direct contact with feces or indirectly through contact between feces and water, food, utensils, fingers, flies, or the ground. These routes of transmission usually coexist in a given community, although the intensity of each may vary and one or two of them may dominate (118).

Socioeconomic Factors

Several studies have documented an association between indicators of socioeconomic status (SES) and diarrheal diseases (18,119,120). Economic status and educational level may determine exposure to a particular transmission route. Even more basically, poverty and limited education place families in poor environmental conditions, where they are exposed to multiple routes of transmission. A lower level of family income (119–121), lower SES (121,122), ownership of valuable objects (121–123), occupation of the household head (124), poorer quality of household construction (123,125,126), crowding (119,124,127), larger family size (128), lower level of maternal education (123,124,129), younger maternal age (130), less access to improved water and sanitation (127,129,131), and absence of the mother from the home (132) have been found to identify children at higher risk of diarrhea.

Socioeconomic status affects diarrheal incidence through different behaviors. In Lima, Peru (122), a low rating on an SES scale was significantly associated with behavioral factors such as children eating soil, adults not using latrines, and children defecating outside the home. A multivariate analysis suggested that the low SES rating was associated with diarrhea through the behavioral factors, not independently. A similar result was found in a study performed in rural Bangladesh (124).

Hygienic Practices

Hygienic practices are closely linked with person-to-person transmission of diarrhea, which usually occurs indirectly through contaminated fingers. Of the hygiene practices, hand washing is probably the most widely studied. The risk for transmission of diarrhea with a lack of hand washing, in particular by mothers after they have defecated or cleaned a child, has been documented (123,133,134). These findings have been confirmed by several studies documenting the efficacy of hand-washing interventions in reducing the incidence of diarrhea (124,133,135,136).

The level of hand contamination with fecal coliforms is associated with diarrheal incidence. The association is stronger in communities with unimproved water and sanitation facilities, which suggests that the impact of hand washing may depend on the level of sanitary facilities and hygiene available in the community. Not only bacteria but also viruses can adhere to the hands. Rotavirus was more frequently isolated from the hands of attendants of children with rotavirus diarrhea than from those attending children with non-rotavirus diarrhea in Bangladesh (137).

Hand washing with soap is effective in eliminating fecal contamination (133,138,139), even with viruses (140), and the absence of soap in the household has been found to be a risk factor for diarrhea (125). However, hand washing with ash, mud, or other agents that facilitate the removal of contaminants from the hands has also been found to be effective; rinsing with water alone is less so (123,141).

Another important hygienic behavior is the elimination of fecal material from the household environment. All major enteropathogens are shed by infected persons via the feces, and therefore hygienic disposal of human excreta plays an important role in the control of diarrheal diseases (142,143). Defecation by a child in the household area (134,144,145) or in the yard or open areas (122,146) and unhygienic methods of feces elimination (146,147) have been described as risk factors for diarrhea. Direct contact of a child with human feces (123) or eating human feces, reported in a child (122), has been documented as a risk factor for diarrhea. Crawling infants, especially those who crawl relatively far away or are more active, are at greater risk for fecal contamination, as demonstrated in a study in Bangladesh (123). After careful structured observations in Lima, Peru (148), it was determined that the presence of feces from other infants and toddlers in the household soil after defecation in open areas poses a major threat of direct fecal exposure for a susceptible child (149). Exposure of children to their own feces is not likely to cause diarrhea. Feces from older children and adults appear to be deposited very rarely in areas where susceptible children may be exposed to them. Fecal exposure to stools of chickens is also important.

Other aspects related to the handling of feces may be significant. The use of paper after defecation (138), scraping a baby's feces off the ground for disposal (123), and having a child defecate into a diaper or bucket (122) have been found protective. In a structured observation study in Lima, it was found that rates of diarrhea were lower in households in which an infant's feces deposited in potties were discarded in a pit latrine, whereas they were higher in households that did not discard the feces in a latrine (150). The use of pit latrines by adults may not be sufficient to reduce household rates of diarrhea (122), although households without pit latrines have been found to have higher diarrheal rates (18), and rates have been reduced in populations that moved to households with water and sanitation. Hygiene education is an important component. Interventions promoting hygienic disposal of feces may be more effective in the dry season, when water is scarce and sources more polluted, as suggested by a study in Nigeria (125).

Feeding Patterns

The increased incidence of diarrheal diseases at the age when weaning foods are introduced was recognized many years ago (151). An extensive review of the literature reported a median relative risk for diarrheal morbidity in infants not receiving breast milk, in comparison with those receiving exclusive or partial breast-feeding, ranging from 3.0 in infants ages 0 to 2 months to 1.5 for those ages 9 to 11 months (152). No protection was seen during the second year of life or after cessation of breast-feeding. Breast-feeding was protective irrespective of the hygiene level of the study areas (152).

Several studies have clarified the risk created by adding liquids and foods to breast milk. The simple addition of water or infusions to breast milk is associated with a 122% to 317% increase in diarrheal rates (153,154). The addition of other types of milk (128% to 235% increase) or solids (137% to 1,330% increase) and the cessation of breast-feeding (280% to 1,345% increase) were associated with higher rates of diarrhea in comparison with rates in exclusively breast-fed infants (18,125,153,154). Children who are not breast-fed are also at increased risk for diarrhea in comparison with partially breast-fed children and older infants. Interestingly, the protection of breast-feeding was greater in poor urban slums than in improved urban or rural areas (154,155), where diarrheal incidence is lower, which suggests that breast-feeding may be more protective in areas where the risk for diarrhea is higher.

Breast-feeding may affect the duration of diarrhea (125, 153). Children who are not breast-fed, in comparison with children who are at least partially breast-fed, have a diarrheal duration that is increased 25% to 200% (7,14,156, 157), or an incidence of persistent diarrhea that is increased 407% to 643% (156,158). Breast-feeding also reduces the severity of diarrhea. Several studies have documented an increased risk for hospitalization in children who are not breast-fed in comparison with those who are breast-fed (158–160). This impact on severity may explain the documented reduced risk for death in breast-fed children (152,161,162). Bottle-fed children appear to have higher case fatality rates for diarrhea, and in comparison with exclusively breast-fed children, they have a 25-fold increase in the relative risk for mortality in infants under 6 months of age (152). Non–breast-fed infants are 14.2 times more likely to die of diarrhea than exclusive breast-fed infants (161). Partially breast-fed infants have an intermediate risk for death. Breast-feeding also protects from deaths caused by persistent diarrhea, but not dysenteric illness (163).

Food and Liquids

Bacterial contamination of weaning foods in developing countries has been documented extensively (10,132, 164–169). However, the relationship between contaminated weaning food and diarrhea has not been shown as clearly. In developed countries, food-related outbreaks of diarrheal diseases are frequent (170), but they are not reliably reported in developing countries. The clear association between traveler's diarrhea and exposure to food from street vendors and restaurants and even food prepared at home shows that food transmits diarrheal diseases in developing countries (171,172). Adults in developing countries, however, do not commonly become ill when they eat the same foods, most likely because of the protection provided by acquired immunity. Nonimmune infants and young children are, however, at risk.

Children receiving much of their dietary intake from breast milk are at least partially protected from diarrhea (153,154,173), but the specific relationship to contaminated weaning foods has been somewhat more difficult to document. Some studies have shown an association between ETEC infection in children and ETEC- or *E. coli*-contaminated food and drinking water (74,165), but others have not (168,174). Community-based longitudinal studies also have obtained conflicting results when the contamination of weaning foods with fecal coliforms and the incidence of diarrhea were correlated (175,169). Part of the variability in results may be a consequence of a lack of sensitivity of the methods used in food microbiologic studies and sampling error (176).

Despite the lack of conclusive evidence, a wealth of data available indicates a very strong likelihood that weaning foods are an important route for the transmission of enteropathogens. Practically all major bacterial enteropathogens have been isolated from weaning food samples, in concentrations from 10^3 to 10^8 bacteria per gram or milliliter (10,164–169,177,178), a level that exceeds the known dose required to induce illness in a susceptible host (179,180). Moreover, food in itself reduces the need for a high inoculum to induce illness because it neutralizes gastric acid. For example, with cholera, instead of the 10^8 *V. cholerae* organisms required to induce illness in normal volunteers, only 10^3 organisms are needed when introduced with food (179).

The level and frequency of bacterial contamination vary by type of food. Foods that are cooked at high temperatures and eaten hot (e.g., soups and stews) are less frequently contaminated than those that are not (10,164,165). Food seems to be more frequently contaminated and have higher bacterial counts than drinking water (165). Among foods commonly given to young children, milk is more frequently contaminated and also has higher bacterial counts (10-fold higher) than other foods (10,165,166,181). One way of contaminating food is by practicing poor hygiene during handling. Dirty containers (181–183), contaminated water (10,165,181,184), and contaminated hands (10,168,181, 184) are the most likely routes for entry of fecal organisms into food. Some cooking practices, such as mashing weaning foods or premastication, also contaminate food (185).

The level of bacterial contamination is strongly influenced by storage time between preparation and eating (10, 164,165,174,175,182). Cooked foods cultured less than 1 hour after being prepared are often not contaminated or have low bacterial counts (10,165). The level of bacterial contamination rapidly increases after 4 to 6 hours, reaching a plateau at about 8 hours after preparation (10,164,174, 175,182). Bacterial proliferation is affected by ambient temperature, as demonstrated by a higher frequency of food contamination and higher counts in samples studied during warm than during cold seasons (164,165,168). The optimal temperature for the multiplication of most enteropathogens or toxin-producing organisms is between 6°C and 60°C. Temperatures below or above these values can be considered safe, whereas temperatures between 20°C and 40°C are more risky (186). An increase in ambient temperature, as observed during the El Niño phenomenon in Peru, has been associated with an increased number of hospital admissions for severe diarrhea (187), probably because of increases in the bacterial contamination of food, among other factors. Bacterial replication can be inhibited by keeping food at low temperatures, and the use of refrigerators for food storage has been found to be protective against diarrheal diseases (132). Inadequate cooking (164) or rewarming at temperatures up to 60°C (188) allows bacteria to survive, even in counts of up to 10^3/g (184). Cooking or rewarming food at high temperatures may destroy bacterial contaminants or reduce the content to a safe level (10,189). However, mothers in developing countries often do not warm foods to this level (i.e., >60°C), and this may not be a feasible intervention because of the need for extra time and fuel (190), as shown in a study in Nigeria, in which reheated leftover foods had significantly higher bacterial counts than freshly cooked food (191). Other alternatives might be the use of fermented foods (189,192) or yogurt (193) because these inhibit the growth of bacterial contaminants. Acid sauces (pH <4) have been shown to reduce the risk for contamination in salads (194,195), but these may not be acceptable for weaning foods.

Food may also be contaminated before it reaches the home; 30% to 80% of uncooked fruits and vegetables have been reported to be contaminated with fecal coliforms and other enteropathogens, in addition to a variety of other bacteria, viruses, and parasites (176,195–198). Vegetables that grow close to the soil are more frequently contaminated than fruits and vegetables that grow in trees or above the ground (198,199). Many farmers in developing countries use sewage-contaminated water to irrigate their fields because of the added fertilization value of its organic content (200). Fields irrigated with overhead sprinklers or contaminated water are more frequently contaminated (176,198,199,201), whereas vegetables grown in greenhouses irrigated with potable water are free of harmful bacteria (176,202). Polluted water has been found to contain a variety of bacteria, viruses, and parasites, which survive from 1 to 60 days (176). In the soil, fecal coliforms are more frequently isolated just after irrigation and in wet mud, whereas dry soil is sterile (176). Enteropathogens enter vegetables through the roots (176) or the stem, as documented in experiments with healthy tomatoes exposed to test bacteria (201,202).

Irrigation is not the only source of contaminants. It is a common practice to wash vegetables at the time of harvesting to remove soil particles. Also, vegetables are kept moist with sprayed water during transport and in markets. The water used for those practices is frequently of poor bacteriologic quality (176). The bacterial content of vegetables has been shown to increase sixfold in the market over the level in the field before harvest (176).

Washing does reduce to some degree the level of contamination of fruits and vegetables, but not always to a safe level (198). In a laboratory experiment, the microbiologic content of lettuce, tomatoes, celery sticks, green peppers, and cucumbers did not change after a 1-minute wash with plain or distilled water, a 0.01% bleach (chlorine) solution, and a 0.025% solution of potassium permanganate (C. Lanata, *unpublished data*). Meats and dairy products may also carry enteropathogens (170,203). Meat may be inoculated in the abattoir when it comes into contact with animal feces or internal organs or with unhygienic surfaces or washing containers (204).

Finally, specific constituents of foods may contribute to diarrheal diseases. It has been hypothesized that lectins, present in some foods, such as beans and lentils, facilitate the binding of bacteria with the intestinal mucosa, promoting the development of diarrhea or prolonging it (205,206). In contrast, other food components may prevent the development of diarrhea by modifying the colonization resistance of the gut to enteropathogenic organisms. The ingestion of specific bacteria (called *probiotics*) capable of colonizing the gut (e.g., *Lactobacillus casei* GG) has been found to reduce the duration and severity of diarrhea (207,208), and when ingested frequently, these bacteria prevent diarrhea (209). Some nondigestible sugar precursors (called *prebiotics*), such as fructo-oligosaccharides, may selectively stimulate the growth of certain gut bacteria, increasing the colonization resistance to human pathogens (210,211).

Feeding Utensils

Baby bottles (10,158,212,213), nipples (10,212–214), cups and spoons (10,212), and food containers (181–183) have frequently been found to be contaminated with fecal bacteria and specific diarrheogenic enteropathogens, including *E. coli, Salmonella* species, *Shigella* species, *Staphylococcus aureus,* and others (10,213,214), even after being cleaned by the mother. Baby bottles have been found to be more frequently contaminated and to have higher bacterial counts than other food utensils. This is probably related to the difficulty of eliminating all food residuals from bottles and to frequency of use, so that bottles do not dry completely. A small amount of liquid may permit bacteria to survive, and these bacteria replicate rapidly when milk or other liquids are added and kept at ambient temperature. This situation is complicated by the fact that poor mothers usually have very few bottles, which are used constantly and never allowed to dry (214).

Water

Waterborne transmission has been documented for most enteropathogens (142), especially *V. cholerae* (82,215,216), *Salmonella typhi* (142), *G. lamblia* (142), and 27-nm Norwalk agent (217). The use of contaminated sources of water has been associated with an increased risk for diarrhea or poor growth in numerous studies (142,146,160,218). The use of contaminated unboiled drinking water has been associated with diarrhea (74,125,219). In areas without tap water, poor handling of water stored in the house, with contaminated hands (220) and in contaminated buckets or jars (122), and in uncovered reservoirs (122,125) has been linked with an increased risk for diarrheal diseases. Contamination in water reservoirs at the home level is also indicated by the higher levels of fecal coliforms found in the home container than at the water source (132,221). Contaminated water may also introduce enteropathogens into food (181,184). As expected, boiling drinking water is associated with a reduction in the level of bacterial contamination (10,182,186), but because of the cost, this practice may be difficult to implement in poor areas (222). Carbonated water is safe, but uncarbonated bottled water, even in developed countries, may not be (223).

Several studies have now documented that water quantity is more important than water quality in diarrheal diseases (130,142,143,224), which suggests that the effect of water on diarrheal diseases is more through its use in hygiene behaviors than through ingestion. Nevertheless, water quality interventions have been effective in reducing diarrheal diseases (221,142,225), especially if combined with hygiene promotion (124).

Flies

Many health professionals and lay persons believe that flies transmit diarrhea. A variety of enteropathogens have been isolated from flies; these can survive up to 30 days (226–229). Survival appears longer for organisms ingested by the flies rather than carried on the surface (228). In one experiment, *Salmonella typhimurium* was picked up by flies from infected dog feces and inoculated into a beverage, which later infected human volunteers (228). Because flies feed once every 4 to 5 hours and deposit vomit and feces several times per hour, it is feasible that they transmit diarrheal pathogens.

The evidence that flies are a route of transmission of enteropathogens is becoming stronger. Initial studies that tried to correlate fly density with diarrheal rates provided conflicting results (228). In a case–control study, members of households in which food was left without fly covers were twice as likely to have diarrhea, although the association was not significant (229). Initial fly control interventions provided unconvincing results, mostly because of the limitations in study design. In a military camp, after an intervention to reduce the number of flies by 60%, the outpatient attendance for diarrhea was reduced by 42% (85% for shigellosis) (226). Moreover, the fly intervention reduced seroconversion for ETEC by 56% and for *Shigella* by 76%. A recent controlled intervention trial has clearly documented the efficacy of fly control in reducing diarrheal incidence in Pakistan (230), confirming the findings from Israel.

Animals

Animal feces have been reported to harbor a variety of enteropathogens, in particular *C. jejuni, Salmonella* species,

C. parvum, and ETEC (10,74,231). The relationship varies by enteropathogen because only a few cause diarrhea in both animals and humans. Most chickens living in or around households in developing countries harbor *C. jejuni* organisms (10,231–233). The presence of chickens in a household has been found to be a risk factor for *C. jejuni* diarrhea (234). Structured observation techniques were used in a periurban community in Lima, Peru, to document that within a 12-hour period, an infant crawling on a household floor had a mean of 2.9 contacts with chicken feces, and that hands or objects contaminated with chicken feces were introduced into the child's mouth a mean of 3.9 times (233). *C. jejuni* was shown to survive up to 48 hours in chicken feces deposited on the household floor (223). Corraling the animals was 100% effective in preventing such contamination. However, an intervention study evaluating the effect of corraling free-living chickens in the household, performed in Lima, failed to demonstrate any significant reduction of diarrheal rates or *C. jejuni* infections in children (C. Lanata, *unpublished data*). Therefore, other routes of transmission may be at least as important as the direct exposure to chicken feces.

Other Routes Of Transmission

Other routes of transmission for diarrheal diseases may also exist. Air-borne transmission has been suggested for rotavirus but has not been clearly shown (235).

HOST RISK FACTORS

Malnutrition

An association between malnutrition and diarrheal diseases has been identified, in part because both occur with a high frequency in children living in poor socioeconomic and environmental conditions (236). However, malnutrition may be a more direct risk factor for diarrheal diseases through compromise of host immune and nonimmune defenses and regenerative capabilities. The incidence of diarrhea in malnourished children, generally classified by a low anthropometric status on a variety of indicators, has been found in some, but not all, studies to be increased by 20% to 70% (237–242).

Prospective community-based studies in a number of countries have clearly documented that malnutrition is a risk factor for an increased duration of diarrheal episodes, whether all episodes or those caused by ETEC or *Shigella* species (242). The duration may increase by 200% or more in malnourished children. As might then be expected, malnutrition is also a risk factor for persistent diarrhea, increasing the incidence of persistent diarrhea in community-based studies by 200% to 300% (238,242–244).

Malnutrition may also be related to other measures of severity in diarrheal episodes. Relatively more malnourished children with rotavirus diarrhea have more severe dehydration (245) and a higher rate of diarrheal stool output (246). Furthermore, malnourished children have a higher case fatality rate for diarrhea, especially persistent diarrhea (27), and an increased diarrheal mortality rate (6,247).

Micronutrient Deficiencies

Specific micronutrient deficiencies may result in either a higher incidence or greater severity of diarrhea. Vitamin A deficiency is associated with a higher rate of severe diarrhea (248), and in a deficient population, vitamin A supplementation reduces diarrheal mortality (249–251). Zinc deficiency is also related to diarrhea (252,253). Supplemental zinc given during diarrhea shortens the duration of the episode and reduces stool output (252,254). Furthermore, zinc supplementation in children in developing countries reduces diarrheal incidence by 18% (255).

Previous Morbidity

In a subset of the population of children in developing countries, the prevalence of diarrhea is high (13,14,256). A strong predictor of an episode of diarrhea is a recent similar episode (239,241,243). This may reflect a high level of exposure to enteropathogens or reduced host resistance, or perhaps a prior episode actually contributes to reduced resistance through mucosal damage, micronutrient losses, or immunosuppression. These possible mechanisms also apply to measles, which is known to increase the risk for diarrhea for a month or longer following an episode (257).

Gastric Acid

The acidic contents of the stomach form an important barrier to ingested enteropathogens, especially many of the bacterial agents. Hypochlorhydria may increase the likelihood that an illness-inducing number of organisms will reach the small intestine. Indeed, hypochlorhydria has been shown to be a risk factor for cholera and has been hypothesized to be a risk factor for other diarrheal infections (258,259). It follows that medical conditions that reduce gastric acid or medications that neutralize acid may lead to a greater frequency or severity of diarrheal infections (260).

Blood Group

Persons of blood group O are at greater risk for cholera, at least for infection with the El Tor biotype of *V. cholerae,* and for more severe illness (261,262). The mechanism has not been determined. Few studies have been performed to examine such a relationship with other enteropathogens, but limited data suggest that a strong relationship does not exist for ETEC or for vibrios other than *V. cholerae* O1 (263,264).

Immunity

The immune defenses clearly play an important role in susceptibility to enteropathogens. Maternal antibody passively acquired by an infant through breast milk protects against a variety of enteric infections, and a child acquires active immunity as a result of symptomatic and asymptomatic infections with enteropathogens.

Evidence is accumulating that the competence of the immune system can be compromised, possibly reducing resistance to enteric infection and delaying recovery. Studies in Bangladesh and Peru have demonstrated depressed cell-mediated immunity in children, assessed by delayed-type hypersensitivity to common antigens (240,241,243). Even when anthropometric status or other variables were controlled for, anergy was associated with a 100% increase in all diarrhea and in persistent diarrhea.

The immunocompetence of a child can be compromised by previous viral infections, such as measles (or measles vaccine) and influenza, or by other infections, such as tuberculosis and typhoid fever (265,266). The immune system can also be affected by a deficiency of various micronutrients, notably vitamin A and zinc (267,268). Such deficiencies may place children at greater risk for diarrhea or severe illness through alterations in immune functions and a variety of other mechanisms.

STRATEGIES FOR CONTROL OF DIARRHEAL DISEASES

Reduction of mortality by prompt and appropriate treatment of diarrhea is the mainstay of diarrheal disease control programs (1). Prevention and correction of dehydration by oral rehydration therapy and maintenance of nutrition by continued feeding during illness are reducing the mortality rates associated with dehydrating diarrheas (2). Antibiotic therapy of dysentery as presumed shigellosis shortens the duration of illness and the dysentery case fatality rate (269). Finally, for persistent diarrhea, the most important diarrheal syndrome associated with mortality, dietary management can be effective, both to treat the episode and to correct the underlying nutritional deficits (7).

Breast-feeding and improved weaning practices are important means to prevent diarrhea. It has been estimated that successful programs to promote breast-feeding could reduce the prevalence of diarrhea by 40% in infants ages 0 to 2 months, 30% in those ages 3 to 5 months, and 10% in those ages 6 to 11 months (152). Diarrheal mortality rates in children under 5 years of age might be reduced by 8% to 9%. Improved weaning practices could have the dual advantages of improving nutrient content and decreasing microbial contamination (270). It has been estimated that weaning education could improve nutritional status and so reduce diarrheal severity and case fatality. A reduction of between 2% and 12% in childhood mortality could be expected by this indirect route (271). Improving the vitamin A status or zinc status of children living in areas with diets deficient in these micronutrients also prevents diarrheal mortality and morbidity (248–251,254,255). Reducing the transmission of food-borne enteropathogens should be successful in reducing diarrheal incidence, based on the results of epidemiologic studies of diarrheal transmission to young children (272). Because no intervention trials have been completed, it is not possible to estimate the magnitude of the reduction in incidence that would be achieved by improvements in food safety.

Improved water supply, sanitation, and hygiene behaviors could also be expected to reduce diarrheal incidence. If both water supply and sanitation were improved, it has been estimated that diarrheal incidence and mortality could be reduced by about 25% (142). Improvements in water availability or sanitation have been found to have a greater impact on diarrheal diseases than do improvements in water quality. Hygiene education might further enhance the impact. In fact, hand-washing education programs have been found to reduce diarrheal incidence by 14% to 48% (133). It is expected, then, that well-designed interventions combining water supply, sanitation, and hygiene education might reduce diarrheal morbidity by 35% to 50% (273).

Measles immunization, which is currently being widely implemented in developing country health programs, is likely to have a substantial effect. It has been estimated that measles vaccination with 60% coverage might reduce diarrheal incidence by 2% and diarrheal mortality by 13% (274).

Improved cholera vaccines are in development and undergoing field testing. If successful, these vaccines may benefit the public health in appropriate areas (275). A killed whole-cell vaccine with or without the B subunit of cholera toxin, given orally in three doses, has been shown to have 50% efficacy for at least 3 years (276). The vaccine may be useful for public health purposes in an area where cholera is endemic if given to young children or in an area where cholera has been recently introduced if provided to the entire population. The long-term protection afforded by this vaccine enhances its value. However, because of the lower level of protection shown in children (23% to 26% efficacy), the vaccine may be less useful in children in an area of endemicity or in an area not previously exposed, where its efficacy in the entire population may be similar to that in children in an area of endemicity. The cholera vaccines currently being developed must provide protection from the *V. cholerae* O139 that recently caused epidemics in South Asia (85). Modified vaccines containing antigens of this new strain are being developed.

Because of the importance of rotavirus as a cause of diarrhea mortality (possibly 20% of diarrheal deaths), the predominance of only four rotavirus serotypes in human disease, and the ability to use animal rotavirus strains to construct animal–human rotavirus reassortment vaccines, the development of a rotavirus vaccine has been given high priority. One such rhesus–human reassortment vaccine provided high-level protection against severe rotavirus diarrhea, but because intussusception occurred in some U.S. infants after vaccination, the vaccine was withdrawn (277,278). Other candidate rotavirus vaccines are still under evaluation (279,280).

It is critical to ensure that all children in developing countries receive effective case management for diarrhea. This will rightly remain the focus of diarrheal disease control programs in the next decade. However, a pressing need also exists to implement efficacious preventive interventions while the search for even more effective and feasible technologies, such as vaccines against the major enteropathogens, continues.

REFERENCES

1. Claeson M, Merson MH. Global progress in the control of diarrheal diseases. *Pediatr Infect Dis J* 1990;9:345–355.
2. Bern C, Martines J, de Zoysa I, et al. The magnitude of the global problem of diarrhoeal disease: a ten-year update. *Bull World Health Organ* 1992;70:705–714.
3. Santosham M, Brown KH, Sack RB. Oral rehydration therapy and dietary therapy for acute childhood diarrhea. *Pediatr Rev* 1987;8:273–278.
4. El-Rafie M, Hassouna WA, Hirschhorn N, et al. Effect of diarrhoeal disease control on infant and childhood mortality in Egypt. *Lancet* 1990;335:334–338.
5. Victora CH, Huttly SRA, Fuchs SC, et al. International differences in clinical patterns of diarrhoeal deaths: a comparison of children from Brazil, Senegal, Bangladesh, and India. *J Diarrhoeal Dis Res* 1993;11:25–29.
6. Fauveau V, Henry FJ, Briend A, et al. Persistent diarrhea as a cause of childhood mortality in rural Bangladesh. *Acta Paediatr* 1992;381[Suppl]:15–21.
7. Black RE. Persistent diarrhea in children of developing countries. *Pediatr Infect Dis J* 1993;12:751–761.
8. Richards L, Claeson M, Pierce N. Management of acute diarrhea in children: lessons learned. *Pediatr Infect Dis J* 1993; 12:5–9.
9. Baqui AH, Black RE, Yunus MD, et al. Methodological issues in diarrhoeal diseases epidemiology: definition of diarrhoeal episodes. *Int J Epidemiol* 1991;20:1057–1063.
10. Black RE, Lopez de Romana G, Brown KH, et al. Incidence and etiology of infantile diarrhea and major routes of transmission in Huascar, Peru. *Am J Epidemiol* 1989;129:785–799.
11. Black RE, Brown KH, Becker S, et al. Longitudinal studies of infectious diseases and physical growth of children in rural Bangladesh. II. Incidence of diarrhea and association with known pathogens. *Am J Epidemiol* 1982;115:315–324.
12. Lanata CF, Black RE, Gilman RH, et al. Epidemiologic, clinical, and laboratory characteristics of acute vs. persistent diarrhea in periurban Lima, Peru. *J Pediatr Gastroenterol Nutr* 1991;12: 82–88.
13. Schorling JB, Wanke CA, Schorling SK, et al. A prospective study of persistent diarrhea among children in an urban Brazilian slum: patterns of occurrence and etiologic agents. *Am J Epidemiol* 1990;132:144–156.
14. Baqui AH, Black RE, Sack RB, et al. Epidemiological and clinical characteristics of acute and persistent diarrhea in rural Bangladeshi children. *Acta Paediatr* 1992;381[Suppl]:15–21.
15. Martorell R, Habicht J-P, Yarbrough C, et al. Underreporting in fortnightly recall morbidity surveys. *Environ Child Health* 1976; June:129–134.
16. Joe LK, Rukmono B, Oemijati S, et al. Diarrhoea among infants in a crowded area of Djakarta, Indonesia. A longitudinal study from birth to two years. *Bull World Health Organ* 1966; 34:197–210.
17. Mata LJ, Urrutia JJ, Gordon JE. Diarrhoeal diseases in a cohort of Guatemalan village children observed from birth to age two years. *Trop Geogr Med* 1967;19:247–257.
18. Guerrant RL, Kirchhoff LV, Shields DS, et al. Prospective study of diarrheal illnesses in northeastern Brazil: patterns of disease, nutritional impact, etiologies, and risk factors. *J Infect Dis* 1983; 148:986–997.
19. Henry FJ, Udoy AS, Wanke CA, et al. Epidemiology of persistent diarrhea and etiologic agents in Mirzapur, Bangladesh. *Acta Paediatr* 1992;381[Suppl]:27–31.
20. Black RE, Merson MH, Rahman ASMM, et al. A two year study of bacterial, viral, and parasitic agents associated with diarrhea in rural Bangladesh. *J Infect Dis* 1980;142:660–664.
21. Cook SM, Glass RI, LeBaron CW, et al. Global seasonality of rotavirus infections. *Bull World Health Organ* 1990;68:171–177.
22. Georges MC, Roure C, Tauxe RV, et al. Diarrheal morbidity and mortality in children in the Central African Republic. *Am J Trop Med Hyg* 1989;36:598–602.
23. El Alamy MA, Thacker SB, Arafat RR, et al. The incidence of diarrheal disease in a defined population in rural Egypt. *Am J Trop Med Hyg* 1986;35:1006–1012.
24. Kumar V, Kumar R, Dutta N. Oral rehydration therapy in reducing diarrhoea-related mortality in rural India. *J Diarrhoeal Dis Res* 1987;5:159–164.
25. Nazir M, Pardede N, Ismail R. The incidence of diarrhoeal diseases and diarrhoeal diseases related mortality in rural swampy low-land area of south Sumatra. *J Trop Pediatr* 1985;31:268–272.
26. Institute of Medicine. Committee on Issues and Priorities for New Vaccine Development. *New vaccine development: establishing priorities,* vol 2. Washington, DC: National Academy Press, 1986 (*Diseases of importance in developing countries*).
27. Bhan MK, Arora NH, Ghai KR, et al. Major factors in diarrhoea-related mortality among rural children. *Indian J Med Res* 1986;83:9–12.
28. The World Bank. Health and developing countries: successes and challenges. In: *World development report 1993: investing in health.* Oxford: Oxford University Press, 1993;17–36.
29. Black RE. Would control of childhood infectious diseases reduce malnutrition? *Acta Paediatr Suppl* 1991;374:133–140.
30. Black RE, Brown KH, Becker S. Effects of diarrhea associated with specific enteropathogens on the growth of children in rural Bangladesh. *Pediatrics* 1984;73:799–805.
31. Black RE, Brown KH, Becker S. Influence of acute diarrhea on the growth parameters of children. In: Bellanti JA, ed. *Acute diarrhea: its nutritional consequences in children.* New York: Raven Press, 1983;75–84 (*Nestle nutrition workshop series,* vol 2).
32. Guerrant RL, Schorling JB, McAuliffe JF, et al. Diarrhea as a cause and effect of malnutrition: diarrhea prevents catch-up growth and malnutrition increases diarrhea frequency and duration. *Am J Trop Med Hyg* 1992;47(1 Pt 2):28–35.
33. Harris S, Black RE. How useful are pharmaceuticals in managing diarrhoeal diseases in developing countries? *Health Policy Management* 1991;6:141–147.
34. Black RE. Diarrheal disease. In: Nelson K, Williams CM, Graham N, eds. *Infectious disease epidemiology theory and practice.* Aspen Press, 2000:497–517.
35. Levine MM, Kaper JB, Black RE, et al. New knowledge on pathogenesis of bacterial enteric infections as applied to vaccine development. *Microbiol Rev* 1983;47:510–550.

36. Glass RI, Svennerholm A-M, Stoll BJ, et al. Protection against cholera in breast-fed children by antibodies in breast milk. *N Engl J Med* 1983;308:1389–1392.
37. Ferreccio C, Prado V, Ojeda A, et al. Epidemiologic patterns of acute diarrhea and endemic *Shigella* infections in children in a poor periurban setting in Santiago, Chile. *Am J Epidemiol* 1991; 134:614–627.
38. Cravioto A, Reyes RE, Trujillo F, et al. Risk of diarrhea during the first year of life associated with initial and subsequent colonization by specific enteropathogens. *Am J Epidemiol* 1990;131: 886–904.
39. Taylor DN, Echeverria P, Pal Tibor T, et al. The role of *Shigella* spp., enteroinvasive *Escherichia coli* and other enteropathogens as causes of childhood dysentery in Thailand. *J Infect Dis* 1986;153:1132–1138.
40. Echeverria P, Sethabutr O, Serichantalergs O, et al. *Shigella* and enteroinvasive *Escherichia coli* infections in households of children with dysentery in Bangkok. *J Infect Dis* 1992;165: 144–147.
41. Harris JC, DuPont HL, Hornick RB. Fecal leukocytes in diarrheal illness. *Ann Intern Med* 1972;76:697–703.
42. Salazar-Lindo E, Sack RB, Chea-Woo E, et al. Early treatment with erythromycin of *Campylobacter jejuni*-associated dysentery in children. *J Pediatr* 1986;109:355–360.
42a. Walsh JA. Problems of recognition and diagnosis of amebiasis: estimation of the global magnitude of morbidity and mortality. *Rev Infect Dis* 1986;8:228–272.
43. Riley LW, Remis RS, Helgerson SD, et al. Hemorrhagic colitis associated with a rare *Escherichia coli* serotype. *N Engl J Med* 1983;308:681–685.
44. Bhan MK, Bhandari N, Sazawal S, et al. Descriptive epidemiology of persistent diarrhoea among young children in rural northern India. *Bull World Health Organ* 1989;67:281–288.
45. Baqui AH, Sack RB, Black RE, et al. Enteropathogens associated with acute and persistent diarrhea in Bangladeshi children less than 5 years of age. *J Infect Dis* 1992;166:792–796.
46. Lanata CF, Black RE, Máurtua D, et al. Etiologic agents in acute vs. persistent diarrhea in children under three years of age in peri-urban Lima, Peru. *Acta Paediatr* 1992;381[Suppl]: 32–38.
47. Cravioto A, Tello A, Navarro A, et al. Association of *Escherichia coli* HEp-2 adherence patterns with type and duration of diarrhoea. *Lancet* 1991;337:262–264.
47a. Lima AA, Moore SR, Barboza MS Jr, et al. Persistent diarrhea signals a critical period of increased diarrhea burdens and nutritional shortfalls. *J Infect Dis* 2000;181:1643–1651.
48. Mathewson JJ, Cravioto A. HEp-2 cell adherence as an assay for virulence among diarrheogenic *Escherichia coli. J Infect Dis* 1989;159:1057–1060.
49. Nataro JP, Steiner T, Guerrant RL. Enteroaggregative *Escherichia coli. Emerging Infect Dis* 1998;4:251–261.
50. Levine MM, Ferreccio C, Prado V, et al. Epidemiologic studies of *Escherichia coli* diarrheal infections in a low socioeconomic level peri-urban community in Santiago, Chile. *Am J Epidemiol* 1993;138:849–869.
51. Korzeniowski OM, Dantas W, Trabulsi LR, et al. A controlled study of endemic sporadic diarrhoea among adult residents of southern Brazil. *Trans R Soc Trop Med Hyg* 1984;84:363–369.
52. Stoll BJ, Glass RI, Huq MI, et al. Surveillance of patients attending a diarrhoeal disease hospital in Bangladesh. *Br Med J* 1982;285:1185–1188.
53. Echeverria P, Pitarangsi C, Eampokalap B, et al. A longitudinal study of the prevalence of bacterial enteric pathogens among adults with diarrhea in Bangkok, Thailand. *Diagn Microbiol Infect Dis* 1983;1:193–204.
54. Choudari CP, Mathan M, Rajan DP, et al. A correlative study of etiology, clinical features and rectal mucosal pathology in adults with acute infectious diarrhoea in southern India. *Pathology* 1985;17:443–450.
55. Adkins HJ, Escamilla J, Santiago LT, et al. Two-year survey of etiologic agents of diarrheal disease at San Lazaro Hospital, Manila, Republic of the Philippines. *J Clin Microbiol* 1987;25: 1143–1147.
56. Sen D, Saha MR, Niyogi SK, et al. Aetiological studies on hospital in-patients with acute diarrhoea in Calcutta. *Trans R Soc Trop Med Hyg* 1983;77:212–214.
57. Ries AA, Vugia DJ, Beingolea L, et al. Cholera in Piura, Peru: a modern urban epidemic. *J Infect Dis* 1992;166:1429–1433.
58. Varavithya W, Aswasuwana S, Phuapradit P, et al. Etiology of diarrhea in measles. *J Med Assoc Thai* 1989;72:151–154.
59. Greenberg BL, Sack RB, Salazar-Lindo E, et al. Measles-associated diarrhea in hospitalized children in Lima, Peru: pathogenic agents and impact on growth. *J Infect Dis* 1991;163:495–502.
60. Colebunders R, Francis H, Mann JM, et al. Persistent diarrhea, strongly associated with HIV infection in Kinshasa, Zaire. *Am J Gastroenterol* 1987;82:859–864.
61. Guerrant RL, Bobak DA. Bacterial and protozoal gastroenteritis. *N Engl J Med* 1991;325:327–340.
62. Keusch GT, Thea DM, Kamenga M, et al. Persistent diarrhea associated with AIDS. *Acta Paediatr* 1992;381[Suppl]:45–48.
63. Lam BCC, Tam J, Ng MH, et al. Nosocomial gastroenteritis in paediatric patients. *J Hosp Infect* 1989;14:351–355.
64. Ryder RW, Rahman ASMM, Alim ARMA, et al. An outbreak of nosocomial cholera in a rural Bangladesh hospital. *J Hosp Infect* 1986;8:275–282.
65. Levine MM. *Escherichia coli* that cause diarrhea: enterotoxigenic, enteropathogenic, enteroinvasive, enterohemorrhagic, and enteroadherent. *J Infect Dis* 1987;155:377–388.
66. Robins-Browne RM. Traditional enteropathogenic *Escherichia coli* of infantile diarrhea. *Rev Infect Dis* 1987;9:28–53.
67. Nataro JP, Baldini MM, Kaper JB, et al. Detection of an adherence factor of enteropathogenic *Escherichia coli* with a DNA probe. *J Infect Dis* 1985;152:560–565.
68. Scaletsky IC, Silva MLM, Trabulsi LR. Distinctive patterns of adherence of enteropathogenic *Escherichia coli* to HeLa cells. *Infect Immun* 1984;45:534–535.
69. Scaletsky ICA, Silva MLM, Toledo MRF, et al. Correlation between adherence to HeLa cells and serogroups, serotypes, and bioserotypes of *Escherichia coli. Infect Immun* 1985;49: 528–532.
70. Mathewson JJ, Johnson PC, DuPont HL, et al. Pathogenicity of enteroadherent *Escherichia coli* in adult volunteers. *J Infect Dis* 1986;154:524–527.
71. Tacket CO, Moseley SL, Kay B, et al. Challenge studies in volunteers using *Escherichia coli* strains with diffuse adherence in HEp-2 cells. *J Infect Dis* 1990;162:550–552.
72. Wanke C. To know *Escherichia coli* is to know bacterial diarrheal disease. *Clin Int Dis* 2001;32:1710–1711.
73. Yamamoto T, Koyama Y, Matsumoto M, et al. Localized, aggregative, and diffuse adherence to HeLa cells, plastic, and human small intestines by *Escherichia coli* isolated from patients with diarrhea. *J Infect Dis* 1992;166:1295–1310.
74. Black RE, Merson MH, Rowe B, et al. Enterotoxigenic *Escherichia coli* diarrhoea: acquired immunity and transmission in an endemic area. *Bull World Health Organ* 1981;59:263–268.
75. Black RE, Levine MM, Clements ML, et al. Experimental *Campylobacter jejuni* infection in humans. *J Infect Dis* 1988; 157:472–479.
76. Thisyakorn USA, Rienprayoon S. Shigellosis in Thai children: epidemiologic, clinical and laboratory features. *Pediatr Infect Dis J* 1992;11:213–215.
77. Khan MU, Roy NC, Islam R, et al. Fourteen years of shigellosis

in Dhaka: an epidemiological analysis. *Int J Epidemiol* 1985; 14:607–613.

78. Ebright JR, Moore EC, Sanborn WR, et al. Epidemic Shiga bacillus dysentery in Central Africa. *Am J Trop Med Hyg* 1984; 33:1192–1197.
79. Rahaman MM, Khan MM, Aziz KMS, et al. An outbreak of dysentery caused by *Shigella dysenteriae* type 1 on a coral island in the Bay of Bengal. *J Infect Dis* 1975;132:15–19.
80. Munshi MH, Sack DA, Haider K, et al. Plasmid-mediated resistance to nalidixic acid in *Shigella dysenteriae* type 1. *Lancet* 1987;2:419–421.
81. Glass RI, Becker S, Huq MI, et al. Endemic cholera in rural Bangladesh, 1966–1980. *Am J Epidemiol* 1982;116:959–970.
82. Glass RI, Black RE. The epidemiology of cholera. In: Barua D, Greenough WB III, eds. *Cholera.* New York: Plenum Publishing, 1992:129–154.
83. Glass RI, Claeson M, Blake PA, et al. Cholera in Africa: lessons on transmission and control for Latin America. *Lancet* 1991; 338:791–795.
84. Gangarosa EJ, Tauxe RV. Epilogue: the Latin American cholera epidemic. In: Barua D, Greenough WB III, eds. *Cholera.* New York: Plenum Publishing, 1992:351–358.
85. Cholera Working Group, International Centre for Diarrhoeal Diseases Research, Bangladesh. Large epidemic of cholera-like disease in Bangladesh caused by *Vibrio cholerae* O139 synonym Bengal. *Lancet* 1993;342:387–390.
86. Rennels MB, Levine MM. Classical bacterial diarrhea: perspectives and update—*Salmonella, Shigella, Escherichia coli, Aeromonas,* and *Plesiomonas. Pediatr Infect Dis J* 1986;5:S91–S100.
87. Gracey M, Burke V, Robinson J. *Aeromonas*-associated gastroenteritis. *Lancet* 1982;2:1304–1306.
88. Pitarangsi C, Echeverria P, Whitmire R, et al. Enteropathogenicity of *Aeromonas hydrophila* and *Plesiomonas shigelloides*: prevalence among individuals with and without diarrhea in Thailand. *Infect Immun* 1982;35:666–673.
89. Holmberg SD, Farmer JJ III. *Aeromonas hydrophila* and *Plesiomonas shigelloides* as causes of intestinal infections. *Rev Infect Dis* 1984;6:633–639.
90. Samadi AR, Wachsmuth K, Huq MI, et al. An attempt to detect *Yersinia enterocolitica. Trop Geogr Med* 1982;34:151–154.
91. Torres JF, Cedillo R, Sánchez J, Dillman C, Giono S, Muñoz O. Prevalence of *Clostridium difficile* and its cytotoxin in infants in Mexico. *J Clin Microbiol* 1984;20:274–275.
92. Black RE, Merson MH, Huq I, et al. Incidence and severity of rotavirus and *Escherichia coli* diarrhoea in rural Bangladesh. *Lancet* 1981;1:141–143.
93. Gary GW Jr, Hierholzer JC, Black RE. Characteristics of noncultivable adenoviruses associated with diarrhea in infants: a new subgroup of human adenoviruses. *J Clin Microbiol* 1979; 10:96–103.
94. Kotloff KL, Losonsky GA, Morris JG, et al. Enteric adenovirus infection and childhood diarrhea: an epidemiologic study in three clinical settings. *Pediatrics* 1989;84:210–225.
95. Dolin R, Treanor JJ, Madore HP. Novel agents of viral enteritis in humans. *J Infect Dis* 1987;155:365–376.
96. Greenberg HB, Valdesuso J, Kapikian AZ, et al. Prevalence of antibody to the Norwalk virus in various countries. *Infect Immun* 1979;26:270–273.
97. Ryder WR, Greenberg H, Singh N, et al. Seroepidemiology of heat-labile enterotoxigenic *Escherichia coli* and Norwalk virus infections in Panamanians, Canal Zone residents, Apache Indians, and United States Peace Corps Volunteers. *Infect Immun* 1982;37:903–906.
98. Huilan S, Zhen LG, Mathan MM, et al. Etiology of acute diarrhoea among children in developing countries: a multicentre study in five countries. *Bull World Health Organ* 1991;69:549–555.
99. Black RE, Greenberg HB, Kapikian AZ, et al. Acquisition of serum antibody to Norwalk virus and rotavirus and relation to diarrhea in a longitudinal study of young children in rural Bangladesh. *J Infect Dis* 1982;145:483–489.
100. Tiemessen CT, Wegerhoff FO, Erasmus MJ, et al. Infection by enteric adenoviruses, rotaviruses, and other agents in a rural African environment. *J Med Virol* 1989;28:176–182.
101. O'Ryan ML, Mamani N, Gaggero A, et al. Human caliciviruses are a significant pathogen of acute sporadic diarrhea in children of Santiago, Chile. *J Infect Dis* 2000;182:1519–1522.
102. Walter JE, Mitchell DK, Guerrero ML, et al. Molecular epidemiology of human astrovirus diarrhea among children from a periurban community of Mexico City. *J Infect Dis* 2000;183: 681–686.
103. Yolken R, Dubovi E, Leister F, et al. Infantile gastroenteritis associated with excretion of pestivirus antigens. *Lancet* 1989;1: 517–520.
104. Gilman RH, Marquis GS, Miranda E, et al. Rapid reinfection of *Giardia lamblia* after treatment in a hyperendemic third world community. *Lancet* 1988;1:343–345.
105. Mason PR, Patterson BA. Epidemiology of *Giardia lamblia* infection in children: cross-sectional and longitudinal studies in urban and rural communities of Zimbabwe. *Am J Trop Med Hyg* 1987;37:277–282.
106. Sullivan PS, DuPont HL, Arafat RR, et al. Illness and reservoirs associated with *Giardia lamblia* infection in rural Egypt: the case against treatment in developing world environments of high endemicity. *Am J Epidemiol* 1988;127:1272–1281.
107. Reed SL. Amebiasis: an update. *Clin Infect Dis* 1992;14: 385–393.
108. Wanke C, Butler T, Islam M. Epidemiologic and clinical features of invasive amebiasis in Bangladesh: a case–control comparison with other diarrheal diseases and postmortem findings. *Am J Trop Med Hyg* 1988;38:335–341.
109. Nanda R, Bavaja U, Anand BS. *Entamoeba histolytica* cyst passers: clinical features and outcome in untreated subjects. *Lancet* 1984;2:301–303.
110. Current WL, Garcia LS. Cryptosporidiosis. *Clin Microbiol Rev* 1991;4:325–358.
111. Sarabia-Arce S, Salazar-Lindo E, Gilman RH, et al. Case–control study of *Cryptosporidium parvum* infection in Peruvian children hospitalized for diarrhea: possible association with malnutrition and nosocomial infection. *Pediatr Infect Dis J* 1990;9:627–631.
112. Petersen C. Cryptosporidiosis in patients infected with the human immunodeficiency virus. *Clin Infect Dis* 1992;15: 903–909.
113. Shadduck JA. Human microsporidiosis and AIDS. *Rev Infect Dis* 1989;11:203–207.
114. Hoge CW, Shlim DR, Rajah R, et al. Epidemiology of diarrhoeal illness associated with coccidian-like organism among travellers and foreign residents in Nepal. *Lancet* 1993;341: 1175–1180.
115. Ortega YR, Sterling CR, Gilman RH, et al. *Cyclospora* species—a new protozoan pathogen of humans. *N Engl J Med* 1993;328: 1308–1312.
116. Casemore DP. Food-borne protozoal infection. *Lancet* 1990; 336:1427–1430.
117. Genta RM. Diarrhea in helminthic infections. *Clin Infect Dis* 1993;16[Suppl 2]:S122–S129.
118. Briscoe J. Intervention studies and the definition of dominant transmission routes. *Am J Epidemiol* 1984;120:449–455.
119. Becker S, Black RE, Brown KH, et al. Relations between socioeconomic status and morbidity, food intake and growth in young children in two villages in Bangladesh. *Ecol Food Nutr* 1986;18:251–264.
120. Stanton BF, Clemens JD. Socioeconomic variables and rates of

diarrhoeal disease in urban Bangladesh. *Trans R Soc Trop Med Hyg* 1987;81:278–282.

121. Winikoff B, Laukaran VH. The influence of infant feeding practices on morbidity and child growth. In: Winnikoff B, Castle M, Lankaran V, eds. *Feeding infants in four societies. Causes and consequences of mother's choices.* Westport, CT: Greenwood Press, 1988:215–226.
122. Yeager BAC, Lanata CF, Lazo F, et al. Transmission factors and socioeconomic status as determinants of diarrhoeal incidence in Lima, Peru. *J Diarrhoeal Dis Res* 1991;9:186–193.
123. Zeitlin MF, Guldan G, Klein RE, et al. *Sanitary conditions of crawling infants in rural Bangladesh.* Report to the USAID Asia Bureau and the HHS Office of International Health, Bangladesh.
124. Alam N, Wojtyniak B, Henry FJ, et al. Mother's personal and domestic hygiene and diarrhoea incidence in young children in rural Bangladesh. *Int J Epidemiol* 1989;18:242–247.
125. Huttly SRA, Blum D, Kirkwood BR, et al. The epidemiology of acute diarrhoea in a rural community in Imo State, Nigeria. *Trans R Soc Trop Med Hyg* 1987;81:865–870.
126. Kournary M, Vasquez MA. Housing and certain socioenvironmental factors and prevalence of enteropathogenic bacteria among infants with diarrheal disease in Panama. *Am J Trop Med Hyg* 1969;18:936–941.
127. Rahaman M, Rahaman MM, Wojtyniak B, et al. Impact of environmental sanitation and crowding on infant mortality in rural Bangladesh. *Lancet* 1985;2:28–31.
128. Khan AZ. Impact of family size on the morbidity pattern in school children. *Indian Pediatr* 1981;18:107–111.
129. Betrand WE, Walmus BF. Maternal knowledge, attitudes and practice as predictors of diarrhoeal disease in young children. *Int J Epidemiol* 1983;12:205–210.
130. Esrey SA, Collett J, Miliotis MD, et al. The risk of infection from *Giardia lamblia* due to drinking water supply, use of water, and latrines among preschool children in rural Lesotho. *Int J Epidemiol* 1989;18:248–253.
131. Tomkins AM, Drasar BS, Bradley AK, et al. Water supply and nutritional status in rural northern Nigeria. *Trans R Soc Trop Med Hyg* 1978;72:239–243.
132. Molbak K, Hojlyng N, Jepsen S, et al. Bacterial contamination of stored water and stored food: a potential source of diarrhoeal disease in West Africa. *Epidemiol Infect* 1989;102:309–316.
133. Feachem RG. Interventions for the control of diarrhoeal diseases among young children: promotion of personal and domestic hygiene. *Bull World Health Organ* 1984;62:467–476.
134. Bartlett AV, Hurtado E, Schroeder DG, et al. Association of indicators of hygiene behaviour with persistent diarrhea of young children. *Acta Paediatr* 1992;381[Suppl]:66–71.
135. Black RE, Dykes AC, Anderson KE, et al. Handwashing to prevent diarrhea in day-care centers. *Am J Epidemiol* 1981;113: 445–451.
136. Khan MU. Interruption of shigellosis by hand washing. *Trans R Soc Trop Med Hyg* 1982;76:164–168.
137. Samadi AR, Huq MI, Ahmed QS. Detection of rotavirus in hand-washings of attendants of children with diarrhoea. *Br Med J* 1983;286:188.
138. Han AM, Nwe OO K, Aye T, et al. Personal toilet after defaecation and the degree of hand contamination according to different methods used. *J Trop Med Hyg* 1986;89:237–241.
139. Sprunt K, Redman W, Leidy G. Antibacterial effectiveness of routine hand washing. *Pediatrics* 1973;52:264–271.
140. Eggers HJ. Handwashing and horizontal spread of viruses. *Lancet* 1989;1:1452.
141. Hoque BA, Briend A. A comparison of local handwashing agents in Bangladesh. *J Trop Med Hyg* 1991;94:61–64.
142. Esrey SA, Feachem RG, Hughes JM. Interventions for the control of diarrhoeal diseases among young children: improving water supplies and excreta disposal facilities. *Bull World Health Organ* 1985;63:757–772.
143. Esrey SA, Habicht JP. Epidemiologic evidence for health benefits from improved water and sanitation in developing countries. *Epidemiol Rev* 1986;8:117–128.
144. Han AM, Moe K. Household faecal contamination and diarrhoea risk. *J Trop Med Hyg* 1990;93:333–336.
145. Clemens JD, Stanton BF. An educational intervention for altering water-sanitation behaviors to reduce childhood diarrhea in urban Bangladesh. 1. Application of the case–control method for development of an intervention. *Am J Epidemiol* 1987;125: 284–291.
146. Alam N, Wai L. Importance of age in evaluating effects of maternal and domestic hygiene practices on diarrhoea in rural Bangladeshi children. *J Diarrhoeal Dis Res* 1991;9:104–110.
147. Baltazar JC, Solon FS. Disposal of faeces of children under two years old and diarrhoea incidence: a case–control study. *Int J Epidemiol* 1989;18[Suppl 2]:S16–S19.
148. Huttly SRA, Lanata CF, Yeager BAC, et al. Feces, flies, and fetor: findings from a Peruvian shantytown. *Pan Am J Public Health* 1998;4:75–79.
149. Lanata CF, Huttly SRA, Yeager BAC. Diarrhea: whose feces matter? Reflections from studies in a Peruvian shanty town. *Pediatr Infect Dis J* 1998;17:7–9.
150. Huttly SRA, Lanata CF, Gonzales H, et al. Observations of handwashing and defecation practices in a shanty town of Lima, Peru. *J Diarrhoeal Dis Res* 1994;12:12–14.
151. Gordon JE, Chitkara ID, Wyon JB. Weanling diarrhea. *Am J Med Sci* 1963;130:345–377.
152. Feachem RG, Koblinsky MA. Interventions for the control of diarrhoeal disease among young children: promotion of breastfeeding. *Bull World Health Organ* 1984;62:271–291.
153. Brown KH, Black RE, Lopez de Romaña G, et al. Infant-feeding practices and their relationship with diarrheal and other diseases in Huascar (Lima), Peru. *Pediatrics* 1989;83:31–40.
154. Popkin BM, Adair L, Akin JS, et al. Breast-feeding and diarrheal morbidity. *Pediatrics* 1990;86:874–882.
155. Chakraborty AK, Das JC. Comparative study of incidence of diarrhea among children in two different environmental situations in Calcutta. *Indian Pediatr* 1983;20:907–913.
156. Munir M. Infantile diarrhoea: breast- and bottle-feeding compared with special reference to their clinical role. *Paediatr Indonesia* 1985;25:100–106.
157. Khin-Maung U, Nyunt-Nyunt W, Myo K, et al. Effects on clinical outcome of breast-feeding during acute diarrhoea. *Br Med J* 1985;290:587–589.
158. de Zoysa I, Rea M, Martines J. Why promote breast-feeding in diarrhoeal disease control programmes? *Health Policy Planning* 1991;6:371–379.
159. Clemens JD, Stanton B, Stoll B, et al. Breast-feeding as a determinant of severity in shigellosis. Evidence for protection throughout the first three years of life in Bangladeshi children. *Am J Epidemiol* 1986;123:710–720.
160. Clemens JD, Sack DA, Harris JR, et al. Breast-feeding and the risk of severe cholera in rural Bangladeshi children. *Am J Epidemiol* 1990;131:400–411.
161. Victora CG, Smith PG, Vaughan JP, et al. Evidence for protection by breast-feeding against infant deaths from infectious diseases in Brazil. *Lancet* 1987;2:319–322.
162. Victora CG, Smith PG, Vaughan JP, et al. Infant feeding and deaths due to diarrhea. A case–control study. *Am J Epidemiol* 1989;129:1032–1041.
163. Victora CG, Huttly SR, Fuchs SC, et al. Deaths due to dysentery, acute and persistent diarrhea among Brazilian infants. *Acta Paediatr* 1992;381[Suppl]:7–11.
164. Barrell RAE, Rowland MGM. Infant foods as a potential source

of diarrhoeal illness in rural West Africa. *Trans R Soc Trop Med Hyg* 1979;73:85–90.
165. Black RE, Brown KH, Becker S, et al. Contamination of weaning foods and transmission of enterotoxigenic *Escherichia coli* diarrhoea in children in rural Bangladesh. *Trans R Soc Trop Med Hyg* 1982;76:259–264.
166. Agarwal DK, Chandra S, Bhatia BD, et al. Bacteriology of weaning foods in some areas of Varanasi. *Indian Pediatr* 1982; 19:131–134.
167. Echevarria P, Verhaert L, Basaca-Sevilla V, et al. Search for heat-labile enterotoxigenic *Escherichia coli* in humans, livestock, food, and water in a community in the Philippines. *J Infect Dis* 1978;138:87–90.
168. Echevarria P, Taylor DN, Seriwatana J, et al. Potential sources of enterotoxigenic *Escherichia coli* in homes of children with diarrhoea in Thailand. *Bull World Health Organ* 1987;65:207–215.
169. Han AM, Oo KN, Aye T, et al. Bacteriological studies of food and water consumed by children in Myanmar: 2. Lack of association between diarrhoea and contamination of food and water. *J Diarrhoeal Dis Res* 1991;9:91–93.
170. Roberts D. Sources of infection: food. *Lancet* 1990;336: 859–861.
171. Merson MH, Morris GK, Sack DA, et al. Traveler's diarrhea in Mexico: a prospective study. *N Engl J Med* 1976;294:1299–1305.
172. Tjoa WS, DuPont HL, Sullivan P, et al. Location of food consumption and traveler's diarrhea. *Am J Epidemiol* 1977;106: 61–66.
173. Watkinson M. Delayed onset of weanling diarrhoea associated with high breast milk intake. *Trans R Soc Trop Med Hyg* 1981;75:432–435.
174. Lloyd-Evans N, Pickering HA, Goh SGJ, et al. Food and water hygiene and diarrhoea in young Gambian children: a limited case–control study. *Trans R Soc Trop Med Hyg* 1984;78: 209–211.
175. Bukenya GB, Nwokolo N. Transient risk factors for acute childhood diarrhoea in an urban community of Papua New Guinea. *Trans R Soc Trop Med Hyg* 1990;84:857–860.
176. Geldreich EE, Bordner RH. Fecal contamination of fruits and vegetables during cultivation and processing for market. A review. *J Milk Food Technol* 1971;34:184–195.
177. Kaul M, Kaur S, Washwa S, et al. Microbial contamination of weaning foods. *Indian J Pediatr* 1996;63:79–85.
178. Afifi ZE, Nasser SS, Shalaby S, et al. Contamination of weaning foods: organisms, channels, and sequelae. *J Trop Pediatr* 1998;44:335–337.
179. Levine MM, Black RR, Clements ML, et al. Volunteer studies in development of vaccines against cholera and enterotoxigenic *Escherichia coli*: a review. In: Holme T, Holmgren J, Merson MH, et al., eds. *Acute enteric infections in children: new prospects for treatment and prevention.* Amsterdam: Elsevier/North-Holland Biomedical Press, 1981:443–459.
180. Teunis PF, Nagelkerke NJ, Haas CN. Dose–response models for infectious gastroenteritis. *Risk Anal* 1999;19:1251–1260.
181. Barrell RAE, Rowland MGM. Commercial milk products and indigenous weaning foods in a rural West African environment: a bacteriological perspective. *J Hyg (Camb)* 1980;84:191–202.
182. Rowland MGM, Barrell RAE, Whitehead RG. The weanling's dilemma: bacterial contamination in traditional Gambian weaning foods. *Lancet* 1978;1:136–138.
183. Barrell RA, Kolley SSMI. Cow's milk as a potential vehicle of diarrhoeal disease pathogens in a West African village. *J Trop Pediatr* 1982;28:48–52.
184. Capparelli E, Mata L. Microflora of maize prepared as tortillas. *Appl Microbiol* 1975;29:802–806.
185. Imong SM, Jackson DA, Rungruengthanakit K, et al. Maternal behaviour and socio-economic influences on the bacterial content of infant weaning foods in rural northern Thailand. *J Trop Pediatr* 1995;41:234–240.
186. Motarjemi Y, van Schothorst M. *HACCP hazard analysis and critical control point principles and practice. Teacher's handbook.* WHO/SDE/PHE/FOS/99.3. Geneva: World Health Organization, 1999.
187. Checkley W, Epstein LD, Gilman RH, et al. Effects of El Niño and ambient temperature on hospital admissions for diarrhoeal diseases in Peruvian children. *Lancet* 2000;355:442–450.
188. Makukutu CA, Guthrie RK. Behavior of *Vibrio cholerae* in hot foods. *Appl Environ Microbiol* 1986;52:824–831.
189. Mensah PPA, Tomkins AM, Drasar BS, et al. Fermentation of cereals for reduction of bacterial contamination of weaning foods in Ghana. *Lancet* 1990;336:140–143.
190. Gilman RH, Skillicorn P. Boiling of drinking water: can a fuel-scarce community afford it? *Bull World Health Organ* 1985; 63:157–163.
191. Iroegbu CU, Ene-Obong HN, Uwaegbute AC, et al. Bacteriological quality of weaning food and drinking water given to children of market women in Nigeria: implications for control of diarrhoea. *J Health Popul Nutr* 2000;18:157–162.
192. Mensah PPA, Tomkins AM, Drasar BS, et al. Effect of fermentation of Ghanaian maize dough on the survival and proliferation of four strains of *Shigella flexneri. Trans R Soc Trop Med Hyg* 1989;82:635–636.
193. Ashworth A, Draper A. *The potential of traditional technologies for increasing the energy density of weaning foods.* WHO/ CDD/EDP/92.4. Geneva: World Health Organization, 1992.
194. St Louis ME, Porter JD, Helal A, et al. Epidemic cholera in West Africa: the role of food handling and high-risk foods. *Am J Epidemiol* 1990;13:719–728.
195. Rodríguez-Rebollo M. Coliformes y *Escherichia coli* en frutas y verduras de mercado. *Microbiol Españ* 1974;27:225–234.
196. Jiwa SFH, Krovacek K, Wadstrom T. Enterotoxigenic bacteria in food and water from an Ethiopian community. *Appl Environ Microbiol* 1981;41:1010–1019.
197. Kolvin JL, Roberts D. Studies on the growth of *Vibrio cholerae* biotype El Tor and biotype classical in foods. *J Hyg (Camb)* 1982;89:243–252.
198. Abdelnoor AM, Batshoun R, Roumani BM, et al. The bacterial flora of fruits and vegetables in Lebanon and the effect of washing on the bacterial content. *Zentralbl Bakteriol Mikrobiol Hyg* 1983;177:342–349.
199. Samish Z, Etinger-Tulkzynska R, Bick M. The microflora within the tissue of fruits and vegetables. *J Food Sci* 1963;28: 259–266.
200. Downs TJ, Cifuentes-Garcia E, Suffet IM. Risk screening for exposure to ground water pollution in a waste water irrigation district of the Mexico City region. *Environ Health Perspect* 1999;107:553–561.
201. Samish Z, Etinger-Tulczynska R. Distribution of bacteria within the tissue of healthy tomatoes. *Appl Microbiol* 1963;11:7–10.
202. Meneley JC, Stanghellini ME. Detection of enteric bacteria within locular tissue of healthy cucumbers. *J Food Sci* 1974; 39:1267–1268.
203. Rasrinaul L, Suthienkul O, Echeverria P, et al. Foods as a source of enteropathogens causing childhood diarrhea in Thailand. *Am J Trop Med Hyg* 1988;39:97–102.
204. Pether JVS, Gilbert RJ. The survival of salmonellas on fingertips and transfer of the organisms to foods. *J Hyg (Camb)* 1971; 69:673–681.
205. Banwell JG, Abramowsky CR, Weber F, et al. Phytohemagglutinin-induced diarrheal disease. *Dig Dis Sci* 1984;29:921–929.
206. Pistole TG. Interaction of bacteria and fungi with lectins and lectin-like substances. *Annu Rev Microbiol* 1981;35:85–112.

207. Isolauri E, Juntunen M, Rautanen T, et al. A human *Lactobacillus* strain (*Lactobacillus casei* sp strain GG) promotes recovery from acute diarrhea in children. *Pediatrics* 1991;88:90–97.
208. Raza S, Graham SM, Allen SJ, et al. *Lactobacillus* GG promotes recovery from acute nonbloody diarrhea in Pakistan. *Pediatr Infect Dis J* 1995;14:107–111.
209. Oberhelman RA, Gilman RH, Sheen P, et al. A placebo-controlled trial of *Lactobacillus* GG to prevent diarrhea in undernourished Peruvian children. *J Pediatr* 1999;134:15–20.
210. Gibson GR, Roberfroid MB. Dietary modulation of the human colonic microflora: introducing the concept of prebiotics. *J Nutr* 1995;125:1401–1412.
211. Gibson GR. Dietary modulation of the human gut microflora using prebiotics. *Br J Nutr* 1998;80:S209–S212.
212. Phillips I, Lwanga SK, Lore W, et al. Methods and hygiene of infant feeding in an urban area of Uganda. *J Trop Pediatr* 1969; 15:167–171.
213. Cherian A, Lawande RV. Recovery of potential pathogens from feeding bottle contents and teats in Zaria, Nigeria. *Trans R Soc Trop Med Hyg* 1985;79:840–842.
214. Elegbe IA, Ojofeitimi EO, Elegbe I, et al. Pathogenic bacteria isolated from infant feeding teats: contamination of teats used by illiterate and educated nursing mothers in Ile-Ife, Nigeria. *Am J Dis Child* 1982;136:672–674.
215. Tamplin ML, Parodi CC. Environmental spread of *Vibrio cholerae* in Peru. *Lancet* 1991;338:1216–1217.
216. Hughes JM, Boyce JM, Levine RJ, et al. Epidemiology of El Tor cholera in rural Bangladesh: importance of surface water in transmission. *Bull World Health Organ* 1982;60:395–404.
217. Taylor JW, Gary GW Jr, Greenberg HB. Norwalk-related viral gastroenteritis due to contaminated drinking water. *Am J Epidemiol* 1981;114:584–592.
218. Esrey SA, Habicht JP, Latham MC, et al. Drinking water source, diarrheal morbidity and child growth in villages with both traditional and improved water supplies in rural Lesotho, Southern Africa. *Am J Public Health* 1988;78:1451–1455.
219. Mertens TE, Fernando MA, Cousens SN, et al. Childhood diarrhoea in Sri Lanka: a case–control study of the impact of improved water sources. *Trop Med Parasitol* 1990;41:98–104.
220. Swerdlow DL, Mintz ED, Rodriguez M, et al. Waterborne transmission of epidemic cholera in Trujillo, Peru: lessons for a continent at risk. *Lancet* 1992;340:28–33.
221. Pinfold JV. Faecal contamination of water and fingertip-rinses as a method for evaluating the effect of low-cost water supply and sanitation activities on faeco-oral disease transmission. II. A hygiene intervention study in rural north-east Thailand. *Epidemiol Infect* 1990;105:377–389.
222. Gilman RH, Marquis GS, Ventura G, et al. Water cost and availability: key determinants of family hygiene in a Peruvian shantytown. *Am J Public Health* 1993;83:1554–1558.
223. Lalumandier JA, Ayers LW. Fluoride and bacterial content of bottled water vs. tap water. *Arch Fam Med* 2000;9:246–250.
224. Victora CG, Smith PG, Vaughan JP, et al. Water supply, sanitation and housing in relation to the risk of infant mortality from diarrhoea. *Int J Epidemiol* 1988;17:651–654.
225. Deb BC, Sirca BK, Senegupta PG, et al. Studies on interventions to prevent El Tor cholera transmission in urban slums. *Bull World Health Organ* 1986;64:127–131.
226. Cohen D, Green M, Block C, et al. Reduction of transmission of shigellosis by control of houseflies (*Musca domestica*). *Lancet* 1991;337:993–997.
227. Echeverria P, Harrison BA, Tirapat C, et al. Flies as a source of enteric pathogens in a rural village in Thailand. *Appl Environ Microbiol* 1983;46:32–36.
228. Levine OS, Levine MM. Houseflies (*Musca domestica*) as mechanical vectors of shigellosis. *Rev Infect Dis* 1991;13:688–696.
229. Knight SM, Toodayan W, Caique WJC, et al. Risk factors for the transmission of diarrhoea in children: a case–control study in rural Malaysia. *Int J Epidemiol* 1992;21:812–818.
230. Chavasse CD, Shier RP, Murphy OA, et al. Impact of fly control on childhood diarrhoea in Pakistan: community-randomised trial. *Lancet* 1999;353:22–25.
231. Blaser MJ, LaForce FM, Wilson NA, et al. Reservoirs for human campylobacteriosis. *J Infect Dis* 1980;141:665–669.
232. Georges-Courbot MC, Cassel-Beraud AM, Gouandjika I, et al. A cohort study of enteric *Campylobacter* infection in children from birth to two years in Bangui (Central African Republic). *Trans R Soc Trop Med Hyg* 1990;84:122–125.
233. Marquis GS, Ventura G, Gilman RH, et al. Fecal contamination of shanty town toddlers in households with non-corraled poultry, Lima, Peru. *Am J Public Health* 1990;80:146–149.
234. Grados O, Bravo N, Black RE, et al. Case–control study to identify risk factors for pediatric *Campylobacter* diarrhoea in Lima, Peru. *Bull World Health Organ* 1988;66:369–374.
235. Santosham M, Yolken RH, Quiroz E, et al. Detection of rotavirus in respiratory secretions of children with pneumonia. *J Pediatr* 1983;103:583–585.
236. Gordon JE, Guzman MA, Ascoli W, et al. Acute diarrhoeal disease in less developed countries. I. An epidemiological basis for control. *Bull World Health Organ* 1964;31:1–7.
237. Sepúlveda J, Willett W, Muñoz A. Malnutrition and diarrhea. A longitudinal study among urban Mexican children. *Am J Epidemiol* 1988;127:365–376.
238. Schorling JB, McAuliffe JF, de Souza MA, et al. Malnutrition is associated with increased diarrhoea incidence and duration among children in an urban Brazilian slum. *Int J Epidemiol* 1990;19:728–735.
239. El Samani EFZ, Willett WC, Ware JH. Association of malnutrition and diarrhea in children aged under five years. A prospective follow-up study in a rural Sudanese community. *Am J Epidemiol* 1988;128:93–105.
240. Black RE, Lanata CF, Lazo F. Delayed cutaneous hypersensitivity: epidemiologic factors affecting and usefulness in predicting diarrheal incidence in young Peruvian children. *Pediatr Infect Dis J* 1989;8:210–215.
241. Baqui AH, Black RE, Sack RB, et al. Malnutrition, cell-mediated immune deficiency and diarrhea: a community-based longitudinal study in rural Bangladeshi children. *Am J Epidemiol* 1993;137:355–365.
242. Black RE, Brown KH, Becker S. Malnutrition is a determining factor in diarrheal duration, but not incidence, among young children in a longitudinal study in rural Bangladesh. *Am J Clin Nutr* 1984;37:87–94.
243. Baqui AH, Sack RB, Black RE, et al. Cell-mediated immune deficiency and malnutrition are independent risk factors for persistent diarrhea in Bangladeshi children. *Am J Clin Nutr* 1993;58:543–548.
244. Bhandari N, Bhan MK, Sazawal S, et al. Association of antecedent malnutrition with persistent diarrhoea: a case–control study. *Br Med J* 1989;298:1284–1287.
245. Black RE, Merson MH, Taylor PR, et al. Glucose vs. sucrose in oral rehydration solutions for infants and young children with rotavirus-associated diarrhea. *Pediatrics* 1981;67:79.
246. Black RE, Merson MH, Eusof A, et al. Nutritional status, body size and severity of diarrhoea associated with rotavirus or enterotoxigenic *Escherichia coli*. *J Trop Med Hyg* 1984;87:83–89.
247. Bhandari N, Bhan MK, Sazawal S. Mortality associated with acute watery diarrhea, dysentery and persistent diarrhea in rural North India. *Acta Paediatr* 1992;381[Suppl]:3–6.
248. Sommer A, Katz J, Tarwotjo I. Increased risk of respiratory disease and diarrhea in children with preexisting mild vitamin A deficiency. *Am J Clin Nutr* 1984;40:1090–1095.

249. Sommer A, Dijunaedi E, Tarwatjo I, et al. Impact of vitamin A supplementation on childhood mortality. *Lancet* 1986;327: 1169–1173.
250. Daulaire NMP, Starbuck ES, Houstoni RM, et al. Childhood mortality after a high dose of vitamin A in a high risk population. *Br Med J* 1992;304:207–210.
251. Ghana VAST Study Team. Vitamin A supplementation in northern Ghana: effects on clinic attendances, hospital admissions, and child mortality. *Lancet* 1993;342:7–12.
252. Sazawal S, Black RE, Bhan MK, et al. Zinc supplementation in young children with acute diarrhea in India. *N Engl J Med* 1995;333:839–844.
253. Sazawal S, Black RE, Bhan MK, et al. Efficacy of zinc supplementation in reducing the incidence and prevalence of acute diarrhea—a community-based, double-blinded, controlled trial. *Am J Clin Nutr* 1997;66:413–418.
254. Zinc Investigators' Collaborative Group (S. Sazawal and R. E. Black, coordinators). Therapeutic effects of oral zinc in acute and persistent diarrhea in children in developing countries: pooled analysis of randomized controlled trials. *Am J Clin Nutr* 2000;72:1516–1522.
255. Zinc Investigators' Collaborative Group (S. Sazawal and R. E. Black, coordinators). Prevention of diarrhea and pneumonia by zinc supplementation in children in developing countries: pooled analysis of randomized controlled trials. *J Pediatr* 1999; 135:689–697.
256. Lima AAM, Fang G, Schorling JB, et al. Persistent diarrhea in northeast Brazil: etiologies and interactions with malnutrition. *Acta Paediatr* 1992;381[Suppl]:39–44.
257. Feachem RG, Koblinsky MA. Interventions for the control of diarrhoeal diseases among young children: measles immunization. *Bull World Health Organ* 1983;61:641–652.
258. Gitelson S. Gastrectomy, achlorhydria and cholera. *Isr J Med Sci* 1971;7:663–667.
259. Nalin DR, Levine RJ, Levine MM, et al. Cholera, non-*Vibrio* cholera, and stomach acid. *Lancet* 1978;2:856–859.
260. Sullivan PB, Thomas JE, Wight DGD, et al. *Helicobacter pylori* in Gambian children with chronic diarrhoea and malnutrition. *Arch Dis Child* 1990;65:189–191.
261. Glass RI, Holmgren J, Haley CE, et al. Predisposition for cholera of individuals with O blood group. Possible evolutionary significance. *Am J Epidemiol* 1985;121:791–796.
262. Levine MM, Nalin DR, Rennels MB, et al. Genetic susceptibility to cholera. *Ann Hum Biol* 1979;6:369–374.
263. Black RE, Levine MM, Clements ML, et al. Association between O blood group and occurrence and severity of diarrhoea due to *Escherichia coli. Trans R Soc Trop Med Hyg* 1987;81: 120–123.
264. van Loon FPL, Clemens JD, Sack DA, et al. ABO blood groups and the risk of diarrhea due to enterotoxigenic *Escherichia coli. J Infect Dis* 1991;163:1243–1246.
265. Mellman WJ, Wetton R. Depression of the tuberculin reaction by attenuated measles virus vaccine. *J Lab Clin Med* 1963;61: 453–458.
266. Starr S, Berkovich S. The depression of tuberculin reactivity during chickenpox. *Pediatrics* 1964;33:769–772.
267. Beisel WR. Single nutrients and immunity. *Am J Clin Nutr* 1982;35:417–468.
268. Shankar AH, Prasad AS. Zinc and immune function: the biological basis of altered resistance to infection. *Am J Clin Nutr* 1998;68[Suppl]:447S–463S.
269. Ronsmans C, Bennish ML, Weirzba T. Diagnosis and management of dysentery by community health workers. *Lancet* 1988; 2:552–555.
270. World Health Organization. Research on improving infant feeding practices to prevent diarrhoea or reduce its severity: memorandum from a JHU/WHO meeting. *Bull World Health Organ* 1989;67:27–33.
271. Ashworth A, Feachem RG. Interventions for the control of diarrhoeal diseases among young children: weaning education. *Bull World Health Organ* 1985;63;1115–1117.
272. Esrey SA, Feachem RG. *Interventions for the control of diarrhoeal diseases among young children: promotion of food hygiene.* WHO/ CDD/89.30. Geneva: World Health Organization, 1989.
273. Feachem RG. Preventing diarrhoea: what are the policy options? *Health Policy Planning* 1986;1:109–117.
274. Feachem RG, Koblinsky MA. Interventions for the control of diarrhoeal diseases among young children: measles immunisation. *Bull World Health Organ* 1983;61:641–652.
275. de Zoysa I, Feachem RG. Interventions for the control of diarrhoeal diseases among young children: rotavirus and cholera immunization. *Bull World Health Organ* 1985;63:569–583.
276. Clemens JD, Sack DA, Harris JR, et al. Field trial of oral cholera vaccines in Bangladesh: results from three-year follow-up. *Lancet* 1990;335:270–273.
277. Flores J, Perea-Schael I, Marino G, et al. Protection against severe rotavirus diarrhoea by rhesus rotavirus vaccine in Venezuelan infants. *Lancet* 1987;1:882–884.
278. Murphy TV, Gargiullo PM, Massoudi MS, et al. Intussusception among infants given an oral rotavirus vaccine. *N Engl J Med* 2001;344:564–572.
279. Bernstein DI, Sack DA, Rothstein E, et al. Efficacy of live, attenuated, human rotavirus vaccine 89-12 in infants: a randomized placebo-controlled trial. *Lancet* 1999;354:287–290.
280. Bresee JS, Glass RI, Ivanoff B, et al. Current status and future priorities for rotavirus vaccine development, evaluation and implementation in developing countries. *Vaccine* 1999;17: 2207–2222.

3

EPIDEMIOLOGY OF DIARRHEAL DISEASE IN DEVELOPED COUNTRIES

JEREMY SOBEL
ROBERT V. TAUXE

The nineteenth and twentieth centuries were marked by giant strides in the control of enteric diseases in the developed world. Typhoid fever, bacillary dysentery, and cholera, once leading causes of mortality, were essentially eliminated by the treatment and disposal of municipal water and sewage, pasteurization of milk, regulation of food safety, and general improvements in hygiene (1). Although mortality has been vastly decreased, diarrheal illnesses still affect everyone in the developed world. It is now appreciated that enteric illnesses are extensively propagated through the complex chain of industrial scale food production, processing, and distribution, and that their spread is abetted by an increasingly mobile population that is also more vulnerable by reason of age and medical comorbidities (2). The worldwide emergence of *Escherichia coli* O157:H7, *Salmonella* serotype *enteritidis, Listeria monocytogenes,* and multidrug-resistant *Salmonella typhimurium* DT-104 has demonstrated that an interplay of host, pathogen, and environment results in the adaptation of food-borne and bacterial pathogens to changing ecosystems. Entirely new pathogens continue to be recognized, such as the parasite *Cyclospora* and the increasing array of Norwalk-like viruses. Many food-borne illnesses are caused by pathogens whose association with food has been recognized only within the last 25 years. The movements of travelers and commodities across international boundaries are obscuring the demarcation between the developed and developing world, not least with regard to diarrheal diseases.

An understanding of the epidemiology of enteric infections is important for the practicing clinician. The dynamic panorama of diarrheal diseases means that clinicians will be treating patients with a broad variety of pathogens (3). These include pathogens imported from abroad by travelers or in foods, bacteria that are increasingly resistant to antimicrobial agents, and organisms that cause pandemic disease. Furthermore, public health surveillance for diarrheal diseases depends on the laboratory identification of pathogens from patient stool samples. Surveillance therefore fundamentally depends on the willingness and ability of clinicians to order these tests. By ordering such tests, clinicians do more than obtain a specific diagnosis in the case of one patient; they also contribute to the national surveillance and control of diarrheal diseases.

ROUTES OF TRANSMISSION

For an agent to cause diarrheal disease, a sufficient number of organisms must be transmitted from their reservoir to a susceptible host, and they must reach the site in the gastrointestinal tract where they can cause illness. The routes of transmission are often determined by the characteristics of an organism and its natural host. Descriptive and analytic epidemiology is useful in identifying the reservoirs and the routes and specific mechanisms of transmission of diarrheal disease. For an organism to persist, it must have an ecologic niche or reservoir where it can replicate. Such reservoirs may exist either in the environment or in animal or human populations. Reservoirs for diarrheal pathogens can be in animal populations (e.g., *Salmonella, Campylobacter*) (4,5), human populations (*Shigella,* Norwalk-like virus) (6), or elsewhere in the environment (*Vibrio cholerae* O1, *L. monocytogenes*) (7,8).

Investigations of outbreaks of diarrheal illnesses have been critical in identifying pathogens, their natural reservoirs, their routes of transmission, and ultimately approaches to their control. Clinicians play a key role in detecting outbreaks by reporting clusters of illness to public health authorities and ordering cultures of stool specimens.

Food-borne Route

Most diarrheal illnesses are caused by pathogens that originate in the digestive tracts of animals or humans, and therefore they fundamentally result from the ingestion of water or food contaminated with animal or human fecal microbes.

J. Sobel and **R. V. Tauxe:** Foodborne and Diarrheal Diseases Branch, Centers for Disease Control and Prevention, Atlanta, Georgia.

Some pathogens are closely associated with particular food vehicles that are derived from their natural reservoir. For example, the natural reservoir of *Yersinia enterocolitica* is the porcine digestive tract and oropharynx (9), and illness is typically caused by the ingestion of pork food products (10) or foods contaminated by contact with pigs (11). The identified reservoir of *E. coli* O157:H7 is the digestive tract of cattle, wild deer, and other ruminants (12), and transmission of this organism is often associated with the ingestion of ground beef or other beef products. Contamination of beef typically occurs at slaughter, and the mixing together of large volumes of meat from many animals in grinding facilities can produce widespread contamination and multistate outbreaks (13–15). The original site of infections in the animal can also be extraintestinal. For example, the ovary of the egg-laying hen is a natural niche of *Salmonella* serotype *enteritidis* (4), and human infection with this organism is largely the result of the ingestion of incompletely cooked eggs that were contaminated while still within the ovary (16–20).

In other cases, the infecting food may not be directly related to the animal that is the natural host of the infecting pathogen. For example, an increasing number of outbreaks of *E. coli* O157:H7 infection have been caused by the consumption of fresh produce and fruit juices (21,22–25); most dramatically, in Japan in 1996, thousands of cases were attributed to the consumption of contaminated radish sprouts (26). The organism is hardy and can survive for months outdoors (27). *E. coli* O157 in ruminant manures may contaminate non-animal foods, possibly when water contaminated with feces is used in produce growing and processing, or when deer invade apple orchards or fields.

Some pathogens are widespread in the environment and can be transmitted by many food sources. *S. typhimurium* appears to have bovine, porcine, and avian hosts, and consequently it can be transmitted by a broad range of foods (28). With other pathogens, the natural host or the relationship between several natural hosts and food vehicles is complex or poorly understood. For example, *Campylobacter* species are known to infect chickens, and most sporadic cases of campylobacteriosis are associated with the consumption of undercooked poultry. However, outbreaks of campylobacteriosis, which are rare, are associated with the consumption of raw milk or untreated water (5). This suggests different ecologic niches as sources of *Campylobacter* infection in sporadic and outbreak-related cases.

Still other pathogens are naturally encountered throughout the environment, but the modern food industry has created conditions that facilitate their introduction into the food supply through specific processes that favor their survival and multiplication. In particular, *L. monocytogenes,* a bacterium that causes severe systemic infection in immunocompromised persons and induces miscarriages in pregnant women (8), poses an increased risk because of two properties that allow it to thrive in a particular class of highly processed foods. Although refrigeration inhibits the growth of most food-borne bacterial pathogens, *L. monocytogenes* survives and reproduces in conditions of refrigeration (29). Additionally, *L. monocytogenes* is a tenacious environmental colonizer of food-processing factories, especially of drains and air-conditioning systems (30). The development of refrigerated foods with long shelf life, such as hot dogs, certain cheeses, and patés, has created a class of food vehicles in which *L. monocytogenes* organisms can grow and cause infection following storage at supposedly safe refrigeration temperatures during the long shelf life of the product (31,32).

Food-borne illnesses that result from the contamination of foods by infected food handlers, with consequent infection of food consumers, comprise a specific category. This type of transmission commonly involves pathogens whose principal natural reservoir is in humans and that are spread by person-to-person transmission; these include Norwalk virus, hepatitis A virus, and *Shigella sonnei,* although it occasionally also occurs with other pathogens. Earlier in the twentieth century, this phenomenon resulted in local "church supper" outbreaks (33); in the contemporary world, one sick food handler can affect consumers spread out over thousands of miles. For example, in February of 2000, car dealerships throughout the United States received catered banquet lunches from one supplier in Ohio. Salads in the banquet lunches were apparently contaminated with calicivirus from a sick food handler, and 334 illnesses among employees of 21 car dealerships in 13 states were the result (34).

Person-to-Person Route

Person-to-person transmission entails the ingestion of human fecal material through close personal contact. Transmission is facilitated by conditions of crowding and poor hygiene, which are common in some urban communities (35), day care centers (36), prisons, camps (37), long-term care facilities (38), military bases (39), ships (40), and religious communities (6,41). The organisms can also be transmitted sexually, particularly among male homosexuals. The organisms transmitted in this fashion typically are highly infectious, and small numbers of them can produce clinical infection. For example, the minimum infectious dose for *Shigella* is 10 to 100 organisms, and for hepatitis A virus and Norwalk virus a single virion (42); all three are commonly transmitted from person to person. A low infectious dose, however, is not the sole determinant of mode of transmission. *E. coli* O157:H7 and *Campylobacter* species, despite their very low infectious doses of about 100 bacteria, rarely spread by person-to-person transmission (5,12). Bacteria that are principally transmitted from person to person seem to be especially adapted to primate hosts, as in the case of *Shigella* and *S. typhi.*

Waterborne Route

Urban populations rely on centralized water sources; these can be effectively protected by chlorination or ozone treatment, processes that inactivate bacteria and some viruses, and by filtration, which removes parasites. Breakdowns in treatment systems in the developed world are rare, but they cause large outbreaks when they do occur because of the large number of persons exposed. Detection of community waterborne outbreaks may be delayed because illness is manifested diffusely throughout the population (43,44). Community-wide waterborne outbreaks of *E. coli* O157:H7 infection have produced high rates of morbidity; a spectacular outbreak of *Cryptosporidium parvum* infection in Milwaukee affected more than 400,000 persons, apparently because the filtration equipment was overwhelmed by a transient increase in turbidity (45). This outbreak was detected when pharmacies noted that stocks of antidiarrheal medication were depleted. These incidents serve as reminders of the vigilance required to prevent large outbreaks of diarrheal disease, in addition to the role pharmacists, clinicians, and others must play in detecting them.

Small-scale, rural, and temporary supplies of drinking water are the source of many outbreaks of diarrheal infection (46). Unlike large municipal supplies, they may be poorly maintained. In recent years, large outbreaks of *E. coli* O157:H7 infection in the United States have been associated with rural wells, county fairs, and other water sources not covered by the federal regulation of drinking water (47–49).

Swimming constitutes another potential exposure to waterborne diarrheal pathogens (46). Outbreaks are often caused by inadequate maintenance of swimming pools (50). Defecation by children of diaper age is a common cause of contamination. Like swimming pools, crowded public bathing areas of beaches, lakes, and streams have been the source of outbreaks. Monitoring microbial contamination will reduce the risk of swimming in sewage or manure runoff, but the most likely source of contamination is the bathers themselves. The provision of adequate toilet and diaper-changing facilities may be more important than periodic coliform monitoring. An outbreak of diarrheal illness in which different pathogens are isolated from the stools of multiple patients with the same exposure to water is suggestive of sewage contamination .

Animal-to-Person Route

Because many diarrheal pathogens have natural reservoirs in animals, they may be transmitted as contact zoonoses in occupational or recreational settings. Reptiles, which have become popular household pets, are asymptomatic carriers of many serotypes of *Salmonella* (51). Pet chicks and African pygmy hedgehogs have also been associated with salmonellosis (52,53). These infections are of particular concern when a child or an immunocompromised person lives in a household with such a pet (54). Contact with animals at established zoos, county fairs, and petting zoos has caused outbreaks of diarrheal diseases. It is not necessary to touch an animal. An outbreak of *S. enteritidis* infection occurred among visitors to a zoo exhibit of Komodo dragons, an exotic reptile species, who touched a contaminated wooden barrier (55). In 2000, an outbreak of *E. coli* O157:H7 infection was caused by contact between children and animals on a petting farm in Pennsylvania; 15 confirmed infections and cases of hemolytic–uremic syndrome were documented, among an estimated 7,000 cases of illness (49). In Scotland, contact with farm animals was the dominant risk factor identified in a recent case–control study of *E. coli* O157:H7 infections (56). These settings are of particular concern because of the frequently large number of exposed visitors, many of whom are in school groups. Occupational exposure is also a risk factor. In a recent study, sporadic infection with highly resistant *S. typhimurium* was associated with contact with farm animals (57).

International Travel

Huge numbers of adventurous tourists, business travelers, laborers, and immigrants revisiting their countries of origin cross national borders every year and are exposed to a variety of contaminated foods and water. A substantial proportion of enteric infections are travel-associated, particularly in countries with successful efforts at domestic disease control. For example, 81% of cases of salmonellosis in Sweden are associated with foreign travel, as are 69% of cases of shigellosis in Japan (58,59). In addition, large numbers of people travel involuntarily, fleeing to surrounding nations to escape war, famine, or poverty. These events intimately connect the developing and industrialized worlds. The array of pathogens from the developing world that cause traveler's diarrhea is only one manifestation of this trend; others include diseases brought by immigrants from refugee camps, nosocomial infections brought by orphanage children coming to the developed world for adoption, diseases of volunteer workers living in the developing world, and diseases of people in developed nations whose vegetables are harvested, pigs slaughtered, and oysters shucked by recent immigrants from the developing world. Contemporary immigrants differ from their predecessors in that relatively cheap and rapid air travel allows frequent visits to their homelands. Some carry back souvenir foods in their luggage, causing "suitcase outbreaks" (60).

INCIDENCE AND SURVEILLANCE IN THE DEVELOPED WORLD

Information about enteric infections in the developed world can be obtained in several ways. The incidence of diarrheal illness can be measured by direct survey of the population. The incidence of clinically significant illness can also be measured by such surveys or, in countries with a well-organized health care system, by a review of clinical visits for such conditions. Typically, the number of visits is a small fraction of the total number of diarrheal episodes, although how small depends on the availability and cost of medical consultation. Similarly, hospitalizations for diarrheal illness and deaths from such illness can be estimated from statistics collected from hospital discharge summaries and death certificates. The number of cases of a specific infection that occur in a population can be measured if sentinel physicians obtain appropriate cultures of all potential cases that come their way. It can also be extrapolated from the number of cases that are actually diagnosed in routine practice by making assumptions about the proportion of cases that go undiagnosed because no diagnostic study was undertaken. However, these extrapolations are acutely sensitive to differences in health care systems. In a nation where health care is free to the consumer and laboratory testing is liberally supported, more cases may be diagnosed than in another country where many lack insurance and laboratory testing is paid for out of pocket. Without comparable survey data, it is difficult to separate the effect of differences in health care systems from variations in underlying incidences from country to country.

Most information on the incidence of infections comes from routine public health surveillance. Disease surveillance for public health purposes requires clinicians to report clinically diagnosed infection, or microbiologists to report the laboratory isolation of certain pathogens. Local public health authorities track these reports, and if they suddenly increase, they may begin an epidemiologic investigation. Surveillance is monitoring linked to action, so the point of conducting surveillance is to guide public health decision making. As a result, the number and nature of infections under surveillance vary from one jurisdiction to another, depending on local interest, resources, and mandates. Population-based networks of sentinel sites can provide reliable and comparable information across jurisdictions about infections for which surveillance requirements may not be uniform. The food-borne disease surveillance network, or FoodNet, is one example of such a system (61). FoodNet gathers information directly about all diagnosed cases of nine intestinal infections from clinical laboratories that represented 11% of the U.S. population in 2000.

The value of reporting diagnosed infection can be greatly increased by further characterization of the infecting organism in a public health laboratory. For example, routine serotyping of *Salmonella* is now conducted for public health purposes in at least 61 countries worldwide to identify trends and outbreaks of one or another serotype (Centers for Disease Control, *unpublished data*). Comparison of the results from many states and provinces in the United States and Canada, and from many countries in Europe, is facilitated by electronic data collection and processing. *Shigella* strains are also routinely serotyped in many countries. To discriminate strains within a serotype, many public health laboratories use phage typing or other subtyping systems. New molecular tools are expanding the precision and power of subtyping to a broad range of pathogens. A multilaboratory assessment of subtyping methods for *L. monocytogenes* concluded that pulsed-field gel electrophoresis (PFGE) offers the best combination of reproducibility and practicality for the United States (62). The banding patterns that result from PFGE can be normalized and compared electronically with patterns generated by the same method in a variety of laboratories. This method can be used to subtype a variety of different bacterial pathogens and is the basis for the molecular subtyping network in the United States, PulseNet, that is now used routinely for *Listeria, E. coli* O157:H7, and *Salmonella* (63). This network is particularly useful for identifying widespread outbreaks that affect several jurisdictions at once and might be missed altogether by surveillance restricted to the local level; it is also useful for investigating outbreaks once they are recognized. A similar subtyping network is being developed for Norwalk-like viruses in the United States and Europe. However, routine subtyping is not necessarily of value for all infections. For example, *Vibrio* and *Campylobacter jejuni* are hugely diverse groups and rarely cause outbreaks; the usefulness of subtyping as part of routine surveillance remains to be demonstrated for infections with these organisms. The determination of antimicrobial resistance patterns can guide clinical practice, provide another epidemiologic marker to detect outbreaks, and be useful in judging the impact of antibiotic use in agriculture and human medicine. Monitoring antimicrobial resistance among enteric bacteria can also be a routine part of public health surveillance. For example, the Danish program DANMAP integrates data on resistance in zoonotic pathogens and antimicrobial use for agricultural purposes (64). In the United States, resistance in *Salmonella* and *Campylobacter* organisms is monitored by the National Antimicrobial Monitoring System for Enteric Bacteria (65). Again, the methods of public health surveillance are closely tied to the uses to which the data will be put.

With many enteric pathogens, prevention depends on understanding the precise route of transmission. It is often difficult to determine the source of an individual case. However, systematic investigation of unusual clusters of illness can often identify a common source and confirm a cluster as an outbreak. Rapid epidemiologic investigation can determine the etiology of an undiagnosed illness, identify the groups affected, and implicate a specific source. These investigations provide a scientific basis for emergency control measures to prevent further illness, such as closing restaurants, beaches, or food-processing plants. Careful tracing of the chain of events that have produced an outbreak often leads to a better understanding of how to prevent similar outbreaks in the future. Systematic tracing of the potential sources of contamination can identify the ultimate reservoir of infections among humans or animals.

Many countries systematically collect information about investigated food-borne or waterborne outbreaks. Such reporting of outbreaks is a surveillance activity in itself that can identify trends in specific pathogens and foods and be a powerful tool for the development of new regulatory strategies. As with any surveillance system, the degree of underreporting depends greatly on the available resources and interest of many jurisdictions.

The prospective investigation of sporadic cases can also identify sources of infection and risk factors for infection, even in the absence of a recognized outbreak. Such investigations can be conducted over months to years; patients are enrolled into the study as they appear, and their pre-illness exposures are compared with those of healthy persons. Such studies can help define the relative importance of various sources. In general, prospective case–control studies are more expensive and require more time to conduct than outbreak investigations; they are less driven by the pressure to respond to an emergency and less frequently performed. Where laboratory subtyping is performed systematically on isolates of pathogens, from both humans and potential food sources, the distribution of subtypes may offer important information about the relative contribution of various sources to human infections. *Salmonella* serotyping and phage typing have been used for this purpose in Denmark (66).

Public health surveillance data are limited in several important ways. Only those diseases that are routinely diagnosed can be included, and the diseases that are legally reportable vary from jurisdiction to jurisdiction. Variations in underreporting may occur because of differences in the availability of laboratory tests. For example, in the United States, some public health laboratories are able to identify the Norwalk-like viruses in an outbreak setting, whereas others are not, and very few clinical laboratories are able to make this diagnosis. As a result, the recognized contribution of these viruses to series of outbreaks and sporadic cases is particularly undercounted. The use of rapid diagnostic methods that do not require isolation of the organism may considerably affect the quantity and quality of public health data on diarrheal disease in the future. For example, the use of a rapid diagnostic test for Shiga toxin production may increase the detection of non-O157 Shiga toxin-producing *E. coli* but will be of value in protecting the public health only if the organism itself is also isolated from the specimen.

ESTIMATES OF DISEASE BURDEN FROM ENTERIC PATHOGENS IN THE DEVELOPED WORLD

Recently, studies employing prospective, population-based approaches have yielded estimates of the burden of diarrheal diseases in several developed nations. Although these data are superior to previous estimates, methodologic differences between the studies limit the degree to which figures from different countries can be compared.

United States

The burden of diarrheal illness in the United States has been estimated recently by Mead et al. (67), who incorporated data from various sources, including national laboratory-based surveillance, active population-based surveillance, hospital discharge and outpatient diagnoses, surveillance for food-borne disease outbreaks, and population surveys. Their analysis concluded that about 211 million cases of acute gastroenteritis occur annually in this country, of which 38 million (18%) are caused by known pathogens. Of these, 80% are viral, 8% bacterial, and 7% parasitic. The estimated incidence of gastroenteritis manifesting as diarrhea, vomiting, or both is 1.05 episodes per person per year. Of the affected individuals, an estimated 1 in 13 sought medical attention (Centers for Disease Control, *unpublished data*). The estimated frequencies of specific pathogens are given in Table 3.1. Viral testing of stools from patients with gastroenteritis is not routinely performed in the United States. Acute gastroenteritis results in an estimated 937,000 hospitalizations (3.5 hospitalizations per 1,000 person-years) and 6,400 deaths annually (67).

Using estimates of the proportion of enteric illnesses caused by viral, bacterial, parasitic, and unknown pathogens that are transmitted by food, Mead et al. (67) calculated that 76 million cases of food-borne illness occur per year in the United states, of which all but 300,000 manifest as acute gastroenteritis. Food-borne illness resulted in 323,000 hospitalizations and 5,200 deaths, of which 18,000 hospitalizations and 1,300 deaths were caused by non-gastroenteritis syndromes. The analysis suggested that 81% of food-borne illnesses and hospitalizations and 64% of deaths are caused by unknown agents. Of the 19% of illnesses caused by a known pathogen, 67% were caused by Norwalk-like viruses, which also accounted for 33% of hospitalizations and 7% of deaths. *Salmonella* and *Campylobacter* infections accounted for 26% and 17%, respectively, of hospitalizations of patients with food-borne illness of known etiology. Leading causes of death from food-borne illnesses were *Salmonella, Listeria,* and *Toxoplasma* organisms, which accounted for more than 75% of deaths caused by a known pathogen. Figures for deaths from *Toxoplasma* infection may be lower today as a consequence of improved therapies for HIV infection.

Data on outbreaks of food-borne disease in the United States are limited. The Centers for Disease Control Food-borne Disease Outbreak Surveillance System reported a yearly average of 550 outbreaks affecting about 17,000 persons between 1993 and 1997 (68). This represents a fraction of the true numbers. Most outbreaks of food-borne disease are not recognized, and of those that come to the attention of clinicians and public health officials, not all are

TABLE 3.1. ESTIMATED ILLNESSES, HOSPITALIZATIONS, AND DEATHS CAUSED BY KNOWN AND UNKNOWN FOOD-BORNE PATHOGENS, UNITED STATES, 1997

Pathogen	Incidence per 1,000 Person-Years	Illnesses	Hospitalizations	Deaths
Bacteria				
Bacillus cereus	0.1	27,360	8	0
Botulism, food-borne	0.0002	58	46	4
Brucella	0.006	1,554	122	11
Campylobacter	8.9	2,453,926	13,174	124
Clostridium perfringens	0.9	248,520	41	7
Escherichia coli O157:H7	0.3	73,480	2168	61
E. coli, non-O157 STEC	0.13	36,740	1,084	30
E. coli, enterotoxigenic	0.29	79,420	21	0
E. coli, other diarrheogenic	0.27	73,420	21	0
Listeria monocytogenes	0.009	2,518	2,322	504
Salmonella typhi	0.003	824	618	3
Salmonella, nontyphoidal	5.1	1,412,498	16,430	582
Shigella	1.6	448,240	6,231	70
Staphylococcus food poisoning	0.67	185,060	1,753	2
Streptococcus, food-borne	0.19	50,920	358	0
Vibrio cholerae, toxigenic	0.0002	54	18	0
Vibrio vulnificus	0.0003	94	86	37
Vibrio, other	0.029	7,880	99	20
Yersinia enterocolitica	0.35	96,368	1,228	3
Subtototal		5,204,934	45,826	1,458
Parasites				
Cryptosporidium parvum	1.1	300,000	1,989	66
Cyclospora cayetanensis	0.059	16,264	17	0
Giardia lamblia	7.2	2,000,000	5,000	10
Toxoplasma gondii	0.82	225,000	5,000	750
Trichinella spiralis	0.0002	52	4	0
Subtotal		2,541,316	12,010	827
Viruses				
Norwalk-like viruses	83.3	23,000,000	50,000	310
Rotavirus	14.1	3,900,000	50,000	30
Astrovirus	14.1	3,900,000	12,500	10
Hepatitis A virus	0.30	83,391	10,841	83
Subtotal		30,833,391	123,341	433
Known pathogens	140	38,629,641	181,177	2,718
Unknown etiology	625	172,370,359		
Grand total	765	211,000,000	—	—

Adapted from Mead P, et al. Food-related illness and death in the United States. *Emerging Infect Dis* 1999;5:607–625, with permission.

reported. More systematic surveillance of outbreaks of food-borne disease is carried out at FoodNet. In 2000, the incidence of food-borne outbreaks affecting 10 or more persons was 3.2 per million population, or approximately 900 per year for the United States (Centers for Disease Control, *unpublished data*). Of the outbreaks reported through this system, 32% had a known etiology, and of these, 75% were bacterial, 17% chemical, 6% viral, and 2% parasitic (68). Of the 68% of outbreaks with no reported etiology, the incubation period was reported for 75%, and this period was consistent with a viral etiology in most outbreaks. Between 1993 and 1997, multistate outbreaks caused by contaminated produce and outbreaks caused by *E. coli* O157:H7 were prominent; as in preceding years, *S. enteritidis* remained a leading cause of outbreaks, illnesses, and deaths, the latter particularly among residents of nursing homes. Because of the substantial underreporting inherent in these results, extrapolation of the data to gauge the panorama of outbreaks in the United States should be undertaken with caution.

United Kingdom

The burden of enteric illness in the United Kingdom was estimated recently by Wheeler et al. (69) in a study of two nationally representative cohorts: a community cohort and a cohort of gastroenteritis patients from a representative sample of general medical practices. In a prospective surveillance of the community cohort, 781 of 9,776 persons experienced gastroenteritis in 6 months. These figures yielded an estimate of 9.4 million cases of gastroenteritis per year, corresponding to a national incidence of 0.19 episodes per person per year. In this cohort, a pathogen was identified in 315 cases (40%), and of these, 64% were bacteria, 34% were viruses, and 2% were parasites. The frequencies of specific pathogens are given in Table 3.2. By comparing the community cohort with the cohort of persons presenting for care at medical practices, the authors demonstrated that about one in six persons with gastroenteritis sought medical care for their illness, corresponding to a national rate of 1.5 million consultations per year. By performing stool cultures on ill persons in the community and comparing isolation rates with rates of reporting to the national surveillance system, the authors demonstrated that the surveillance detected fewer than 1% of gastroenteritis, 32% of *Salmonella,* 8% of *Campylobacter,* 3% of Rotavirus, and 0.1% of small round structure virus cases.

TABLE 3.2. ESTIMATED INCIDENCE OF GASTROENTERITIS BY PATHOGEN, UNITED KINGDOM, 1999

Pathogen	Incidence per 1,000 Person-Years
Bacteria	
Aeromonas	12.4
Campylobacter	8.7
Clostridium difficile toxin	1.6
Clostridium perfringens endotoxin	2.4
Escherichia coli O157	0
E. coli (by DNA probe)	
Attaching and effacing	5.4
Diffusely adherent	6.2
Enteroaggregative	4.9
Enteroinvasive	0
Enteropathogenic	0.3
Enterotoxigenic	2.7
Verocytotoxigenic	0.8
Salmonella	2.2
Shigella	0.3
Staphylococcus aureus	0.3
Vibrio species	0
Yersinia species	6.8
Parasites	
Cryptosporidium parvum	0.8
Giardia intestinalis	0.5
Viruses	
Rotavirus	7.1
Small round structured viruses (Norwalk-like)	12.5
Adenovirus group F	3
Astrovirus	3.8
Calicivirus	2.2
Total known pathogens	30.5
Unknown etiology	163.5
Grand total	194

Adapted from Wheeler J, Sethi D, Cowden JM, et al. Study of infectious intestinal disease in England: rates in the community, presenting to general practice, and reported to national surveillance. *Br Med J* 1999;318:1046–1050, with permission.

The Netherlands

The incidence and burden of enteric illness in the Netherlands have been estimated in several studies. In 1991, de Wit and colleagues (70) enrolled 2,206 subjects in a 4-month population-based study. The calculated incidence of gastroenteritis was 45 per 100 person-years, or a total of 7.1 million episodes per year in Holland. This study also calculated that 12,000 work-years may be lost annually in Holland because of acute gastroenteritis, a figure that highlights the significant economic burden associated with this low-mortality syndrome. The burden of enteric illness among patients presenting for medical care in Holland was also explored in a more recent study by de Wit et al. (71). The authors prospectively examined patients presenting with diarrhea to a representative sample of general medical practitioners between 1996 and 1999. During 4 years, 2,264 persons presented with gastroenteritis, and of these, 857 provided stool samples. A pathogen was identified in 39% of stool samples, and of these, 40% were bacteria, 38% viruses, and 22% parasites. The frequencies of specific pathogens are given in Table 3.3. These figures yielded an estimate of 128,000 patients presenting for physician evaluation of gastroenteritis per year, or 0.008 physician visits per person per year. This study did not estimate the overall incidence of gastroenteritis in Holland—that is, the proportion of cases in which patients did not present for medical care, or the proportion of gastroenteritis cases evaluated by physicians in which a diagnosis was not attempted. A comparison of studies from the United Kingdom and Holland underscores the potential biases that can result from different health care practices. In the United Kingdom,

TABLE 3.3. FREQUENCY OF DIARRHEAL PATHOGEN ISOLATION IN A COHORT OF 857 PATIENTS WITH GASTROENTERITIS IN HOLLAND

Pathogen	No.	Percentage
Salmonella	33	3.9
Campylobacter	89	10.5
Yersinia	6	0.7
Shigella	1	0.1
VTEC	4	0.5
Rotavirus	45	5.3
Adenovirus	19	2.2
Norwalk-like viruses	43	5
Sapporo-like viruses	5	2.1
Giardia lamblia	46	5.4
Entamoeba histolytica/other	9	1.1
Cryptosporidium	18	2.1
Cyclospora	1	0.1
All known pathogens	332	39
Unknown etiology	525	61

VTEC, verotoxin-producing *Escherichia coli.*
From de Wit M, Koopmans MP, Kortbeek LM, et al. Gastroenteritis in sentinel general practices, the Netherlands. *Emerging Infect Dis* 2001;7:82–91, with permission.

about 1 in 6 patients with gastroenteritis consults a physician (69), whereas in Holland only between 1 in 10 and 1 in 50 does so (72,70). This may be a consequence of the standard practice of Dutch physicians of actively discouraging office visits for gastroenteritis in favor of managing the case over the phone (71).

Comparing Data from the United States, United Kingdom, and the Netherlands

Comparisons of rates of food-borne and diarrheal diseases from recent population-based studies in developed countries are intriguing but must be undertaken with caution. Rates differ considerably between the United States, the United Kingdom, and Holland, but methodologic differences quite likely account for some of the variations. The U.S. study incorporated data from many sources and relied on a series of assumptions and extrapolations that allowed the authors to present a very comprehensive picture of the burden of illnesses, although possibly at the cost of reduced precision (67). The British results are based on active gastroenteritis case finding in the community, so that very accurate population-based data are derived, but the nondiarrheal burden of infections has not been reported (69). The latest Dutch study is physician practice-based and therefore represents incidence data for the select group of physician-treated patients (70). True variations in incidence of diarrheal diseases between these three developed countries may be a consequence of differences in patterns of travel, population hygiene, and the food chain.

The sheer magnitude of the incidence of diarrheal diseases, which affect up to 1% of the population of the three representative countries in the developed world, is remarkable. Although mortality is low, the burden of illness in economic terms, including days lost from work and use of medical resources, amounts to tens of billions of dollars annually (73). Another striking observation is the proportion of illnesses with an unknown etiology: 82% in the United States, 60% in the United Kingdom, and 61% in Holland. Because this vast unexplained burden remains after common pathogens such as calciviruses, which are not routinely sought in clinical laboratories, have been accounted for, the gap likely represents yet-to-be discovered pathogens or unrecognized noninfectious causes. Understanding the etiologies of these hundreds of millions of cases is a central challenge of diarrheal disease research. A third observation is that in cases of known etiology, the bacterial-to-viral ratio is very low in the United States. The difference is largely explained by the nearly sevenfold higher calculated incidence of Norwalk-like viral infections in the United States than in the United Kingdom, but why Norwalk-like viruses appear to be so much more prevalent in the United States, contributing so massively to the incidence of gastroenteritis, is yet another research challenge.

PANDEMIC PATHOGENS

Global pandemics of cholera and other diarrheal pathogens have been well documented in the developing world. However, global pandemics also occur in the industrialized world. The vigorous international trade in food, animal feed, and live animals plays a major role in this dissemination. One well-studied example occurred early in the 1970s, when contaminated anchovy fish meal from a Latin American source caused a global outbreak of *Salmonella agona* infections (74). The meal was sold on the international commodity market as an ingredient for chicken feed. First, the chickens became ill, then the persons eating the chickens. Absent from the United States and many other countries before then, *S. agona* quickly established itself in the poultry reservoir, recycling through the rendered animal feed products and spreading to turkeys and other animals in the 1980s (75). Global dissemination of several major food-borne pathogens has occurred, although the mechanism of spread has been less clear. For instance, in the 1970s, serotypes O:3 and O:9 of *Y. enterocolitica* increased rapidly in Europe, Canada, and Japan at the same time (76). In the 1980s, *S. enteritidis* emerged as a major new public health threat, associated with eggs and poultry, almost simultaneously in North America, Europe, and Japan (77). The emergence was caused by the spread of several different strains of *S. enteritidis* among the egg-laying flocks; in Europe, the broiler chicken flocks were also affected. In the 1990s, a multiply resistant strain of the *Salmonella* serotype *typhimurium* phage type 104 appeared in North America and Europe (78). How and why this global dissemination occurred remains unclear. One clue is that to date, Australia and New Zealand have not been affected, which suggests that the pandemic is not transmitted through international travel of humans or migratory wild birds. Perhaps the vehicle has been live animals or animal feed, both of which are heavily regulated or quarantined down under.

The vehicle for widespread dissemination is not always animals or feeds. In the mid-1990s, a new serotype of *Vibrio parahaemolyticus,* O6:K3, spread from Southeast Asia to Japan, where it caused a large number of seafood-associated outbreaks. In 1997, this strain appeared in the oyster beds of Puget Sound, on the west coast of North America, and in 1998 in Texas (79,80). This organism was most likely brought to the New World in the ballast water of oil tankers, as the first cases were related to oysters harvested near the shipping lanes. Travelers can also disseminate diarrheal pathogens. In 1986, a wave of shigellosis followed the travel connections of a community of nomadic part-time hippies with links to India (81). In 1996, another wave followed the travel of communities of traditionally observant Jews connecting North America, Europe, and Israel (82). Even the sudden appearance of epidemic cholera in the New World in January 1991 was probably associated with a ship from the orient, although whether the epidemic was introduced by discharging ballast or via a clandestine cargo of immigrants is unclear (83).

MULTINATIONAL OUTBREAKS

More transient international dissemination of illness in the form of multinational outbreaks probably occurs frequently, although few are recognized. The apparent rarity is likely the consequence of a limited exchange of information rather than a lack of occurrence. Such outbreaks provide insight into how easily organisms can travel across boundaries. Investigating them can control a hazardous commercial product and may help spotlight an unsuspected problem in the source country.

For example, an outbreak of *Salmonella stanley* infections affected persons in the United States and Finland simultaneously in 1995 (84). Combining data from the two outbreaks made it possible to trace the source of contamination to a common lot of alfalfa seeds from a Dutch shipper, in which seeds from several other countries had been combined. In 1996, a multicontinental outbreak of *S. agona* infections was traced to a peanut candy produced in Israel, where a large and unexplained increase in *S. agona* infections among children that had been going on for many months disappeared as soon as the production was stopped (85,85a). In 1998, investigation of an outbreak of shigellosis in Denmark identified imported baby maize, eaten raw, as the source; after imports were halted and the producing country was notified, the incidence of sporadic domestic shigellosis in Denmark dropped substantially (86). In 1998, outbreaks of shigellosis in Canada and the United States were traced to shipments of parsley from one farm in Mexico that used local municipal water to wash and chill the parsley (87). In 1988, outbreaks of Norwalk-like virus infections in Finland and elsewhere were traced to frozen raspberries imported from central Europe (88). In an extraordinary example of how a new trade item can uncover a previously unknown problem, in 1995 and again in 1996, a large number of outbreaks of *Cyclospora cayetanensis* infection occurred in the United States and Canada associated with raspberries harvested in Guatemala (89). This was a new fruit crop for Central America that seems to have provided an efficient means of transmitting *Cyclospora* organisms to the suburbs of North America. *Cyclospora* was subsequently identified as a common cause of diarrheal illness in Guatemala. Efforts to modify production practices may have reduced the risk subsequently and have focused new attention on the health of the field workers themselves.

These outbreaks illustrate how efficiently global commerce can transport pathogens around the world. The problem may originate in either the developed or the developing world. The observations and investigations in one country may illuminate and even help control health problems in another country. Detecting, investigating, and controlling such problems require international collaboration and cooperation (90). The ability to recognize such outbreaks depends heavily on systematic and comparable subtyping of strains in different countries, such as *Salmonella* serotyping. Presumably, many pathogens can cause multinational outbreaks, but they are not likely to be detected without more routine diagnosis and standard subtyping.

APPROACHES TO CONTROL AND PREVENTION

The successful prevention of most enteric infections depends on understanding the routes of transmission well enough to intervene at the weakest link.

In the case of enteric infections that pass from one person directly to another, hand washing is a fundamental preventive strategy. Promoting hand washing aggressively in child care centers can prevent diarrheal illness and teach good hand washing habits. Hand washing in restaurant and institutional kitchens can prevent the direct transmission of pathogens from one person to the next through food, and the transfer of zoonotic pathogens from raw meat and poultry to other foods. Providing food workers with paid sick leave and educating them routinely in the basics of food safety would also prevent direct food contamination in commercial and institutional kitchens.

Contact with pets or farm animals is an important control point for some enteric pathogens. For example, in the 1970s, small pet turtles were thought to be the most common source of salmonellosis in the United States, until their sale and distribution were banned (91). The same turtles, still contaminated with *Salmonella,* continue to be exported to many other countries (92). Other reptiles can be sources of both rare and common serotypes of *Salmonella* (51,93). Educating new reptile owners may reduce the risk (94). *Campylobacter* infection has been repeatedly associated with drinking a glass of raw milk during a visit to a farm, an easily avoidable exposure (95). To prevent *E. coli* O157 infections after visits to farms and contact with farm animals, short of banning contact altogether, encouraging careful hand washing and separating animal contact from eating are cornerstones of prevention (49). When *Vibrio vulnificus* biotype 3 infections emerged in Israel in 1998, an epidemiologic investigation showed that they were wound infections that resulted from pricks with the spines of live, farm-raised tilapia fish. Simply freezing the fish before they were sold eliminated the problem (96).

However, many agents of diarrheal illness reach the patient at the end of a longer chain of food-borne or water-borne transmission. With these agents, infections can be prevented by control measures implemented all along the chain of production. For example, beginning in the 1970s, Sweden developed an extensive integrated control program that eliminated *Salmonella* from their food animal reservoirs; testing, decontamination, and prevention of reintroduction were carried out at every step of the food chain, including the farm environment, transportation vehicles, slaughter facilities, and venues of sales (97). The search for better and more effective control measures goes on.

Control at the Reservoir

Major programs can keep some pathogens from entering food or water in the first place. Large natural watersheds are protected to keep sewage and manure out of drinking water. Oyster beds are monitored and regulated to prevent contamination with sewage. Some pathogens that cause diseases in food animals, such as brucellosis and bovine tuberculosis, are controlled by monitoring the health of herds and eliminating those that are infected. Because other pathogens, such as *Campylobacter, Salmonella, E. coli* O157:H7, *Vibrio,* and *Y. enterocolitica,* can spread silently through food animal populations without causing apparent illness, herd- and flock-based measures to prevent spread can prevent illness in the final consumer. This means convincing farmers and fishermen that they are part of the food safety program. One approach is to screen, isolate, and separately process herds or flocks with an infection. For example, *S. enteritidis* infection in persons eating eggs or chickens is now being prevented by flock-based control programs in a number of countries. Long-standing and successful programs to control *Trichinella* have largely eliminated that parasite from pigs (98). A second approach is to increase the resistance of animals to colonization by zoonotic food-borne pathogens by enhancing their gut flora with mixtures of beneficial gut microbes, or probiotics. Giving pigs fermented, microbially rich feeds has been shown to protect them against salmonellosis, sufficiently that feeding practices are now changing in the Netherlands (99). Probiotic competitive exclusion products are now commercially available and are used routinely to reduce the spread of salmonellosis in poultry in Europe (100). In the future, it may be possible to vaccinate food animals to reduce infections and the spread of zoonotic food-borne pathogens (101). The general problem of the safety of animal feeds themselves has been largely neglected, a gap that is likely to change rapidly in the future because of concern about the transmission of bovine spongiform encephalopathy.

On fruit and vegetable farms, improved sanitation can prevent contamination. This involves controlling the quality of the water used in irrigating and washing produce, and providing toilets and hand-washing facilities and incentives to use them to agricultural workers engaged in harvesting and packing produce. Like restaurant workers, agricultural workers should be provided with paid sick leave when they suffer diarrheal illness. Although oyster beds are now generally well protected from point source sewage contamination, they are not yet protected from the sewage of the oyster workers themselves, nor from contamination by vibrios that live naturally in the warm water.

Prevention at the Processing Level

Contamination may occur or be increased after food has initially been harvested or drinking water collected. Methods for disinfecting municipal water supplies have received enormous attention from public health engineers and officials during the last century. In countries that do not routinely disinfect water supplies, waterborne outbreaks of *Campylobacter* infection fuel growing concern that protecting the reservoir or well is not enough (102). In countries that do routinely disinfect water, outbreaks of infections with cryptosporidia and other relatively chlorine-resistant organisms indicate that further improvements are needed (103). The detection of cryptosporidia in drinking water is leading to a general reevaluation of the effectiveness of standard drinking water protection and treatment in the United States (104). Unprotected rural water supplies remain a worrisome problem everywhere.

Some food technologies are bulwarks in the prevention of enteric illness. Two critical advances, milk pasteurization and pressure retort canning, date from the early part of the twentieth century and are now nearly universal in industrialized nations. More recently, pasteurization has been extended to juice and eggs, as a result of the otherwise unavoidable risk of outbreaks attendant on pooling many fruits or eggs together.

The safe production of meat remains a continuing challenge. Animals brought to slaughter can infect each other *en route.* The slaughter process may offer many opportunities for the spread of organisms from gastrointestinal tract to final product. The safety of the meat supply depends both on exclusion of ill animals and on efforts to reduce microbial contamination of the carcass during the slaughter process. Early in the twentieth century, the United States and many other countries developed systematic inspection processes to exclude visibly ill animals from the food supply. However, these visual inspections do little to prevent microbial contamination. Some countries, such as Denmark, screen animals serologically for evidence of infection with *Salmonella,* and animals from infected herds are slaughtered in separate facilities (105). In the United States, beginning in 1996, the meat safety program was enhanced to reduce the presence of pathogens in meat via the concept of "hazard analysis critical control point" (HACCP) (106). This safety process was initially developed by the National Aeronautical and Space Administration to reduce the possibility of food-borne illness during spaceflight, and it has proved to be generally applicable throughout the food industry. Inspectors now monitor critical safety elements of the slaughter process rather than inspecting meat with their own eyes, hands, and noses. A microbial standard for the finished product is an essential part of the program; it verifies that the overall process is working. Further systematic assessment of slaughter process may identify more specific control measures (107).

The food technologies used for prevention are evolving rapidly. In U.S. slaughter plants, steam scalding, acid rinses, and highly disinfected water baths can greatly reduce or prevent contamination with pathogens. Eggs that are pasteurized in the shell are now available in stores. Irradiation with either gamma rays or electron beams is a logical and available technology for meats and many other foods (108). Irradiated ground beef is already for sale commercially in the United States. In the produce arena, control strategies are also being tested. Careful monitoring of chlorine levels in wash water may prevent produce from becoming contaminated during processing (109). Soaking seeds in chlorine before sprouting them may reduce, although not altogether prevent, salmonellosis or other infections related to sprouts (21).

Consumer Self-defense

For some pathogens, control at the ultimate reservoir or during processing remains incomplete, and the last line of defense lies in the behavior of consumers themselves. Thus, although the presence of cryptosporidia in municipal water supplies has stimulated the search for better filtration and treatment methods, it has also led in the United States to recent recommendations that high-risk populations boil their water or drink water that has been sterilized (110). The basic principles of safe food handling and the risks associated with specific foods are again becoming part of the practical reality of living in industrial societies, as they still are in the developing world. In the United States, recent efforts have included a general education campaign, "Fight Bac!," that stresses the simple message of cooking foods properly, chilling leftovers promptly, separating raw from cooked foods, and washing up afterward (*www.fightbac.org*). Physicians and other health care providers can play an important role in advising patients at highest risk (111). Pregnant women can be counseled about the risks of *Listeria* infections associated with soft cheese, paté, and delicatessen meats, and about how to avoid other infections (112). Counseling AIDS patients and other immunocompromised persons may reduce their risk for diarrheal illness (113). Advising patients with severe liver disease about the risks of severe *Vibrio* infections associated with raw oysters may help protect them (114). The traveler to the developing world can be counseled regarding careful selection of food and drink; the traveler to other parts of the industrialized world can be advised of the specific risks of raw eggs and meats (115).

Vaccines and Colonization Resistance

Great strides being made in the development of vaccines against some infectious diseases continue to spark hope that effective vaccines will be developed against a variety of diarrheal illnesses. New and more effective vaccines against cholera and typhoid fever developed during the last decade are expanding the options for possible prevention of these infections in the developing world. Hepatitis A vaccine may have value in selected populations. The recent experience with a Rotavirus vaccine in the United States, where it was associated with intussusception in young children, halted the production of one commercial vaccine and has spurred efforts to develop vaccine alternatives (116). *Shigella* vaccines, such as one currently being tested in Israel, may be useful tools in the future (117).

As in food animals, nonimmune resistance of a human host to colonization, associated with the native gut flora, can be increased. In clinical settings, it has been observed that antibiotic treatment increases the risk for subsequent *Salmonella* infections (78,118), whereas with treatments that do not affect the gut flora, this important barrier to colonization is preserved. The beneficial effects of specific *Lactobacillus* preparations given to young children suggest that providing beneficial bacteria or probiotics early on may be effective in humans, as it is in chickens (119). Other nonantimicrobial prophylactic strategies may be useful, including milk-derived specific immune globulins (120). In general, dietary or other manipulations that increase or restore resistance to colonization or infection remain a relatively unexplored but potentially fruitful arena for future research.

Eradication: A Distant Hope

The complexity of transmission, extensive environmental reservoirs, frequency of silent infections, and lack of effective vaccines make the eradication of most diarrheal pathogens extremely unlikely in the developed world. However, eradication is at least theoretically possible for *Salmonella typhi,* the cause of typhoid fever, and *Shigella* because infections with these organisms are restricted to human or primates, without another animal reservoir. The difficulty of recognizing disease and carrier states and of breaking all chains of transmission in the world make this a remote possibility in the next decade. In contrast, the control of many food-borne infections through the irradiation of meat, poultry, and perhaps other foods offers the prospect of a definitive step toward pathogen reduction that may be as far-reaching as were the treatment of water supplies and the pasteurization of milk early in the last century.

CONCLUSION

Hundreds of millions of cases of food-borne and diarrheal disease occur in the United States each year, and comparable numbers in other developed countries. In recent years, a growing number of bacterial, viral, and parasitic agents have been identified as important causes of enteric infections, yet the majority of cases appear to be of unknown etiology (67). Traditional food and water safety measures, including milk pasteurization and water treatment, and food safety regulations have dramatically reduced the morbidity and mortality of this class of infections since the nineteenth century (1). However, where the public health infrastructure not adequately maintained, a rapid decline to presanitary revolution conditions may occur (83,44). Many infections of known etiology are caused by agents whose existence or routes of transmission have only recently been established. Even with well-established pathogens, increases in antimicrobial resistance and in the immunocompromised population are creating new clinical challenges in diagnosis and appropriate therapy (42). A better understanding of the complex reservoirs and mechanisms of transmission has led to a reduction in the incidence of specific pathogens where scientific data and political will have resulted in the implementation of improved prevention strategies from farm to table. Prevention depends in the first place on the willingness and ability of clinicians to order stool samples from patients because surveillance is based on laboratory-confirmed cases. The border between the developed and the developing world is blurring as we accelerate transfer through travel and trade. Industrialized nations export their pathogens to developing nations, and vice versa. Changing human ecology continues to open up new evolutionary niches for known and unsuspected pathogens, which will appear as new epidemics, new pathogens, and new vehicles of infection. It seems unlikely that we will ever know all the causes of diarrheal illness or how to prevent them. We should expect the unexpected.

REFERENCES

1. Centers for Disease Control. Achievements in public health, 1900–1999: safer and healthier foods. *MMWR Morb Mortal Wkly Rep* 1999;48:905–913.
2. Swerdlow DL, Altekruse S. Foodborne diseases in the global village: what's on the plate for the 21st century. In: Scheld WM, Craig WA, Hughes JM, eds. *Emerging infections.* Washington, DC: American Society for Microbiology Press, 1998:273–294.
3. Guerrant R, et al. Practice guidelines for the management of infectious diarrhea. *Clin Infect Dis* 2001;32:331–351.
4. Tauxe R. Salmonella enteritidis and Salmonella typhimurium DT104: successful subtypes in the modern world. In: Scheld W, et al., ed. *Emerging infections.* Washington, DC: American Society for Microbiology Press, 1999:37–52.
5. Friedman CR, et al. Epidemiology of *Campylobacter jejuni* infections in the United States and other industrialized nations. In: Nacharnkin I, et al., eds. *Campylobacter,* second edition. Washington, DC: American Society for Microbiology Press, 2000:121–138.
6. Sobel J, Mintz E. Shigellosis. In: Wallace RB, ed. *Diseases spread by food and water.* Stamford, CT: Appleton & Lange, 1998:239–240.
7. Mintz ED, Popovic T, Blake PA. Transmission of *Vibrio cholerae* O1. In: Wachsmuth K, Blake PA, Olsvik O, eds. Vibrio cholerae *and cholera: molecular to global aspects.* Washington, DC: American Society for Microbiology Press, 1994:345–356.
8. Slutsker L, Evans M, Schuchat A. Listeriosis. In: Scheld W, ed. *Emerging infections.* Washington, DC: American Society for Microbiology Press, 2000:83–106.
9. Tauxe RV, et al. *Yersinia enterocolitica* infections and pork: the missing link. *Lancet* 1987;1:1129–1132.
10. Lee LA, et al. *Yersinia enterocolitica* O:3 infections in infants and children associated with the household preparation of chitterlings. *N Engl J Med* 1990;322:984–987.
11. Ackers M, et al. An outbreak of *Yersinia enterocolitica* O:8 infections associated with pasteurized milk. *J Infect Dis* 2000;181: 1834–1837.
12. Griffin PM, Tauxe RV. *Escherichia coli* O157:H7 human illness in North America, food vehicles and animal reservoirs. *International Food Safety News* 1993;2:15–17.
13. Riley LW, et al. Hemorrhagic colitis associated with a rare *Escherichia coli* serotype. *N Engl J Med* 1983;308:681–685.
14. Centers for Disease Control. *Escherichia coli* O157:H7 infections associated with eating a nationally distributed commercial brand of frozen ground beef patties and burgers—Colorado, 1997. *MMWR Morb Mortal Wkly Rep* 1997;46:777–778.
15. Griffin PM, et al. Large outbreak of *Escherichia coli* O157:H7 infections in the western United States: the big picture. In: Karmali MA, Goglio AG, eds. *Recent advances in verocytotoxin-producing* Escherichia coli (E. coli) *infections.* New York: Elsevier Science, 1994:7–12.
16. St. Louis ME, et al. The emergence of grade A eggs as a major source of *Salmonella enteritidis* infections: implications for the control of salmonellosis. *JAMA* 1988;259:2103–2107.
17. Centers for Disease Control. Outbreaks of *Salmonella* serotype *enteritidis* infection associated with eating raw or undercooked shell eggs—United States, 1996–1998. *MMWR Morb Mortal Wkly Rep* 2000;49:73–79.
18. Centers for Disease Control. Outbreaks of *Salmonella* serotype *enteritidis* infection associated with consumption of raw shell eggs—United States, 1994–1995. *MMWR Morb Mortal Wkly Rep* 1996;45:737–742.
19. Mishu B, et al. *Salmonella enteritidis* gastroenteritis transmitted by intact chicken eggs. *Ann Intern Med* 1991;115:190–194.
20. Mishu B, et al. Outbreaks of *Salmonella enteritidis* infections in the United States, 1985–1991. *J Infect Dis* 1994;169:547–552.
21. Toarmina P, Beuchat L, Slutsker L. Infections associated with eating seed sprouts: an international concern. *J Emerging Infect Dis* 1999;5:626–634.
22. Centers for Disease Control. Outbreaks of *Escherichia coli* O157:H7 infections associated with eating alfalfa sprouts—Michigan and Virginia, June–July 1997. *MMWR Morb Mortal Wkly Rep* 1997;46:741–744.
23. Centers for Disease Control. Outbreaks of *Escherichia coli* O157:H7 and cryptosporidiosis associated with drinking unpasteurized apple cider—Connecticut and New York, October, 1996. *MMWR Morb Mortal Wkly Rep* 1997;46:4–8.
24. Cody S, et al. An outbreak of *Escherichia coli* O157:H7 infection from unpasteurized commercial apple juice. *Ann Intern Med* 1999;130:202–209.
25. Besser RE, Lett SM, Weber T, et al. An outbreak of diarrhea and hemolytic uremic syndrome from *Escherichia coli* 0157:H7 in fresh-pressed cider. *JAMA* 1993;269:2217–2220.
26. Mermin J, Griffin P. Invited commentary: public health in crisis: outbreaks of *Escherichia coli* 0157:H7 infections in Japan. *Am J Epidemiol* 1999;150:797–803.
27. Sargent J, et al. Prevalence of *Escherichia coli* O157:H7 in white-tailed deer sharing rangeland with cattle. *J Am Vet Med Assoc* 1999;215:792–794.
28. Centers for Disease Control. Multidrug-resistant *Salmonella* serotype *typhimurium*—United States, 1996. *MMWR Morb Mortal Wkly Rep* 1997;46:308–310.
29. Lou Y, Yousef AIL. Characteristics of *Listeria monocytogenes* important to food processors. In: Ryser T, Marth E, eds. *Listeria, listeriosis and food safety.* New York: Marcel Dekker Inc, 1999.
30. Gravani R. Incidence and control of *Listeria* in food-processing facilities. In: Ryser T, Marth E, eds. *Listeria, listeriosis and food safety.* New York: Marcel Dekker Inc, 1999.

31. Centers for Disease Control. Update: multistate outbreak of listeriosis—United States, 1998–1999. *MMWR Morb Mortal Wkly Rep* 1998;47:1117–1132.
32. Schuchat A, Swaminathan B, Broome C. Epidemiology of human listeriosis. *Clin Microbiol Rev* 1991;4:169–183.
33. Gross M. Oswego county revisited. *Public Health Rep* 1976;91: 168–170.
34. Garrett V, et al. Appreciation luncheons gone awry: a large, multistate outbreak of gastroenteritis associated with catered, shipped food. In: *Programs and abstracts of the 38th annual meeting of the Infectious Diseases Society of America,* Alexandria, Virginia, 2000(abst No. 513).
35. Farrar W, Eidson M, Wells J. Extensive urban outbreak caused by antibiotic-sensitive *Shigella sonnei. JAMA* 1976;235:1026–1029.
36. Mohle-Boetani JC, et al. Community-wide shigellosis: control of an outbreak and risk factors in child day-care centers. *Am J Public Health* 1995;85:812–816.
37. Lee LA, et al. An outbreak of shigellosis at an outdoor music festival. *Am J Epidemiol* 1991;133: 608–615.
38. Hunter P, Hutchings P. Outbreak of *Shigella sonnei* dysentery on a long-stay psychogeriatric ward. *J Hosp Infect* 1987;10:73–76.
39. Centers for Disease Control. Norwalk-like viral gastroenteritis in U.S. Army trainees—Texas, 1998. *MMWR Morb Mortal Wkly Rep* 1999;48:225–227.
40. Bohnker B, et al. Explosive outbreak of gastroenteritis on an aircraft carrier: an infectious disease mass casualty situation. *Aviation Space Environmen Med* 1993;64:648–650.
41. Porter B, et al. An outbreak of shigellosis in an ultra-orthodox Jewish community. *Soc Sci Med* 1984;18:1061–1062.
42. Sobel J, Swerdlow D, Parsonnet J. Is there anything safe to eat? *Curr Clin Top Infect Dis* 2001;21:114–134.
43. Angulo F, et al., A community waterborne outbreak of salmonellosis and the effectiveness of a boil water order. *Am J Public Health* 1997;87:580–584.
44. Mermin J, et al. A massive epidemic of multidrug-resistant typhoid fever in Tajikistan associated with consumption of municipal water. *J Infect Dis* 1999;179:416–422.
45. MacKenzie RW, et al. Massive outbreak of waterborne *Cryptosporidium* infection in Milwaukee, Wisconsin: recurrence of illness and risk of secondary transmission. *Clin Infect Dis* 1995; 21:57–62.
46. Barwick R, et al. Surveillance for waterborne disease outbreaks—United States, 1997–1998. *MMWR Morb Mortal Wkly Rep* 2000;49:1–44.
47. Olsen S, et al. A waterborne outbreak of *E. coli* O157:H7 infections and hemolytic uremic syndrome: implications for rural water systems. *Emerging Infect Dis* 2001 (*in press*).
48. Centers for Disease Control. Public health dispatch: outbreak of *Escherichia coli* O157:H7 and *Campylobacter* among attendees of the Washington County fair—New York, 1999. *MMWR Morb Mortal Wkly Rep* 1999;48:803–804.
49. Centers for Disease Control. Outbreaks of *Escherichia coli* O157:H7 infections among children associated with farm visits—Pennsylvania and Washington, 2000. *MMWR Morb Mortal Wkly Rep* 2001;50.
50. Centers for Disease Control. Epidemiologic notes and reports: swimming-associated cryptosporidiosis—Los Angeles County. *MMWR Morb Mortal Wkly Rep* 1990;39:343–345.
51. Mermin J, Hoar B, Angulo F, Iguanas and *Salmonella marina* infection in children: a reflection of the increasing incidence of reptile-associated salmonellosis in the United States. *Pediatrics* 1997;99:399–402.
52. Centers for Disease Control. *Salmonella* serotype *montevideo* infections associated with chicks—Idaho, Washington, and Oregon, spring 1995 and 1996. *MMWR Morb Mortal Wkly Rep* 1997;46:237–239.
53. Centers for Disease Control. Salmonellosis associated with chicks and ducklings—Michigan and Missouri, spring 1999. *MMWR Morb Mortal Wkly Rep* 2000;49:297–303.
54. Angulo FJ, et al. Caring for pets of immunocompromised persons. *J Vet Med Assoc* 1994;205:1711–1718.
55. Friedman C, et al. An outbreak of salmonellosis among children attending a reptile exhibit at a zoo. *J Pediatrics* 1998;132:802–807.
56. Locking M, et al. *Escherichia coli* O157: a case–control study of sporadic infection in Scotland. In: *Verotoxigenic* E. coli *in Europe: 5. Epidemiology of verocytotoxigenic* E. coli, *2001.* Dublin, Ireland: The National Food Centre.
57. Fey P, et al. Ceftriaxone-resistant *Salmonella* infection acquired by a child from cattle. *N Engl J Med* 2000;342:1242–1249.
58. Linders A. *Smittsamma sjukdomar 1999: epidemiologist enhetens oarsrapport.* Solna, Sweden: Swedish Institute for Infectious Disease Control, 2000:32.
59. Anonymous. Shigellosis, Japan, 1999–2000. *Infect Agents Surveillance Rep* 2001;22:81–82.
60. Finelli L, et al. Outbreak of cholera associated with crab brought from an area with epidemic disease. *J Infect Dis* 1992; 166:1433–1435.
61. Centers for Disease Control. Preliminary FoodNet data on the incidence of foodborne illnesses—selected sites, United States, 2000. *MMWR Morb Mortal Wkly Rep* 2001;50:241–246.
62. Graves L, Swaminathan B, Hunter S. Subtyping *Listeria monocytogenes.* In: Ryser T, Marth E, eds. *Listeria, listeriosis, and food safety.* New York: Marcel Dekker Inc, 1999:279–298.
63. Swaminathan B, et al. PulseNet: the molecular subtyping network for foodborne bacterial disease surveillance, United States. *Emerging Infect Dis* 2001;7:1–8.
64. Bager F. *DANMAP 1999.* Copenhagen: Danish Zoonosis Centre, 2000:52.
65. Marano N, et al. The National Antimicrobial Resistance Monitoring System (NARMS) for enteric bacteria, 1996–1999: surveillance for action. *J Am Vet Assoc* 2000;217:1829–1830.
66. Hald T, Wegener H. Quantitative assessment of the sources of human salmonellosis attributable to pork. In: *Proceedings of the third international symposium on the epidemiology and control of* Salmonella *in pork,* Washington, DC, 1999.
67. Mead P, et al. Food-related illness and death in the United States. *Emerging Infect Dis* 1999;5:607–625.
68. Centers for Disease Control. Surveillance for foodborne disease outbreaks—United States, 1993–1997. *MMWR Morb Mortal Wkly Rep* 2000;49:1–51.
69. Wheeler J, et al. Study of infectious intestinal disease in England: rates in the community, presenting to general medical practice and reported to national surveillance. *Br Med J* 1999; 318:1046–1050.
70. de Wit M, et al. A population-based longitudinal study on the incidence and disease burden of gastroenteritis and *Campylobacter* and *Salmonella* infections in four regions of the Netherlands. *Eur J Epidemiol* 2000;16:713–718.
71. de Wit M, et al. Gastroenteritis in sentinel general practices, the Netherlands. *Emerg Infect Dis* 2001;7:82–91.
72. Hoogenboom-Verdegaal A, et al. Community-based study of the incidence of gastrointestinal disease in the Netherlands. *Epidemiol Infect* 1994;112:481–487.
73. Archer D, Kvenberg JJFP. Incidence and cost of foodborne diarrheal disease in the United States. *J Food Protection* 1985;48: 887–894.
74. Clark G, et al. Epidemiology of an international outbreak of *Salmonella agona. Lancet* 1973;2:1–10.
75. Helfrick D, et al. An atlas of *Salmonella* in the United States: serotype-specific surveillance, 1968–1998. Atlanta: Centers for Disease Control, 2001:621.
76. World Health Organization. Worldwide spread of infections with *Yersinia enterocolitica. World Health Organ Chronicle* 1976; 30:494–496.

77. Rodrigue D, Tauxe R, Rowe B. International increase in *Salmonella enteritidis*: a new pandemic? *Epidemiol Infect* 1990;105:21–27.
78. Glynn M, et al. Emergence of multidrug-resistant *Salmonella enterica* serotype *typhimurium* DT104 infections in the United States. *N Engl J Med* 1998;328:1333–1338.
79. Centers for Disease Control. Outbreak of *Vibrio parahaemolyticus* infections associated with eating raw oysters—Pacific Northwest, 1997. *MMWR Morb Mortal Wkly Rep* 1998;47:457–462.
80. Daniels N, et al. Emergence of new *Vibrio parahaemolyticus* serotype in raw oysters: a prevention quandary. *JAMA* 2000; 284:1541–1545.
81. Wharton M, et al. A large outbreak of antibiotic-resistant shigellosis at a mass gathering. *J Infect Dis* 1990;162:1324–1328.
82. Sobel J, et al. A prolonged outbreak of *Shigella sonnei* infections in traditionally observant Jewish communities in North America caused by a molecularly distinct bacterial subtype. *J Infect Dis* 1998;177:1405–1409.
83. Tauxe RV, et al. The Latin American epidemic. In: Wachsmuth K, Blake PA, Olsvik O, eds. Vibrio cholerae *and cholera: molecular to global perspectives.* Washington, DC: American Society for Microbiology Press, 1994:321.
84. Mahon B, et al. An international outbreak of *Salmonella* infections caused by alfalfa sprouts grown from contaminated seeds. *J Infect Dis* 1997;175:876–882.
85. Killalea D, et al. International epidemiological and microbiological study of outbreak of *Salmonella agona* infection from a ready-to-eat savoury snack—I: England and Wales and the United States. *Br Med J* (clinical research edition) 1996;313:1105–1107.
86. Molbak K, Neimann J. Outbreak of *Shigella sonnei* infections related to uncooked "baby maize" imported from Thailand. *Eurosurveillance Weekly* 1998;2.
87. Centers for Disease Control. Outbreaks of *Shigella sonnei* infections associated with eating fresh parsley—United States and Canada, July–August, 1998. *MMWR Morb Mortal Wkly Rep* 1999;48:285–289.
88. Ponka A, et al. Outbreak of calicivirus gastroenteritis associated with eating frozen raspberries. *Eurosurveillance* 1999;4:66–69.
89. Herwaldt B. *Cyclospora cayetanensis*: a review focusing on the outbreaks of cyclosporiasis in the 1990s. *Clin Infect Dis* 2000; 31:1040–1057.
90. Tauxe RV, Hughes JM. International investigation of outbreaks of foodborne disease. *Br Med J* (clinical research edition) 1996; 313:1093–1094.
91. Cohen EA. Turtle-associated salmonellosis in the U.S: effect of public health action, 1970–1976. *JAMA* 1980;243:1247–1249.
92. Tauxe RV, et al. Turtle-associated salmonellosis in Puerto Rico: hazards of the global turtle trade. *J Assoc Med* 1985;254.
93. Olsen S, et al. The changing epidemiology of *Salmonella*: trends in serotypes isolated from humans in the United States, 1987–1997. *J Infect Dis* 2001;183:753–761.
94. Centers for Disease Control. Reptile-associated salmonellosis—selected states, 1996–1998. *MMWR Morb Mortal Wkly Rep* 1999;48:1009–1013, 1051.
95. Wood R, MacDonald K, Osterholm M. *Campylobacter* enteritis outbreaks associated with drinking raw milk during youth activities. A 10-year review of outbreaks in the United States. *JAMA* 1992;268:3228–3230.
96. Bisharat N, et al. Clinical, epidemiological, and microbiological features of *Vibrio vulnificus* biogroup 3 causing outbreaks of wound infection and bacteraemia in Israel. *Lancet* 1999;354: 1421–1424.
97. Wierup M, et al. Control of *Salmonella* enteritis in Sweden. *Int J Food Microbiol* 1995;25:219–226.
98. Schantz P. Trichinosis in the United States, 1947–1981. *Food Technol* 1983; :83–86.
99. van der Wolf P, et al. Herd level husbandry factors associated with the serological *Salmonella* prevalence in finishing pig herds in the Netherlands. *Vet Microbiol* 2001;78:205–219.
100. Deruyttere L, et al. Field study to demonstrate the efficacy of Aviguard against intestinal *Salmonella* colonization in broilers. In: *Salmonella and salmonellosis.* Ploufragan, France: Zoopole, Institut Supérieur des Productions Animales et des Industries Agro-alimentaires, 1997.
101. Gyles C. Vaccines and Shiga toxin-producing *Escherichia coli* in animals. In: Kaper J, O'Brien A, eds. Escherichia coli *O157:H7 and other Shiga toxin-producing* E. coli *strains.* Washington, DC: American Society for Microbiology Press, 1998:434–444.
102. Engberg J, et al. Waterborne *Campylobacer jejuni* infection in a Danish town—a 6-week continuous source outbreak. *Clin Microbiol Infect* 1998;4:648–656.
103. MacKenzie W, Hoxie M, Procter M. A massive outbreak in Milwaukee of *Cryptosporidium* infections transmitted though the public water supply. *N Engl J Med* 1994;331:161–167.
104. Cryptosporidium *and water: a public health handbook.* Atlanta: Centers for Disease Control and Prevention, 1997.
105. Mousing J, et al. Nationwide *Salmonella enterica* surveillance and control in Danish slaughter swine herds. *Prev Vet Med* 1997;29:247–261.
106. Anonymous. Pathogen reduction: hazard analysis and critical control point (HACCP) systems: the final rule. *Federal Register* 1996;61(144):38805–38989.
107. Hald T, et al. The occurrence and epidemiology of *Salmonella* in European pig slaughterhouses. 2001 (*in press*).
108. Tauxe R. Food safety and irradiation: protecting the public health from foodborne infections. *J Emerging Infect Dis* 2001;3:516–521.
109. Rushing JW, Angulo FJ, Beuchat LR. Implementation of an HACCP program in a commercial fresh-market tomato packinghouse: a model for the industry. *Dairy Food Environmen Sanitation* 1996;16:549–553.
110. Anonymous. *Preventing cryptosporidiosis: a guide for persons with HIV and AIDS.* 1999. www.cdc.gov/ncidod/dpd/parasites/cryptosporidiosis/factsht_crypto_prevent_hiv.htm.
111. Anonymous. Diagnosis and management of foodborne illnesses: a primer for physicians. *MMWR Morb Mortal Wkly Rep* 2001;50:1–69.
112. Anonymous. *What you can do to keep germs from harming you and your baby.* Atlanta, Centers for Disease Control, 1999.
113. Centers for Disease Control. *Safe food and water: a guide for people with HIV infection.* Atlanta: Centers for Disease Control, 1999.
114. Tuttle J, Kellerman S, Tauxe RV. The risks of raw shellfish: what every transplant patient should know. *J Transplant Coord* 1994; :60–63.
115. Centers for Disease Control. *Health information for international travel, 1999–2000.* Atlanta: Department of Health and Human Services, 2000.
116. Centers for Disease Control. Withdrawal of rotavirus recommendation. *MMWR Morb Mortal Wkly Rep* 1999;48:1007.
117. Ashkenazi S, et al. Safety and immunogenicity of *Shigella sonnei* and *Shigella flexneri* 2a O-specific polysaccharide conjugates in children. *J Infect Dis* 1999;179:1565–1568.
118. Pavia A, et al. Epidemiologic evidence that prior antimicrobial exposure decreases resistance to infection by antimicrobial-sensitive *Salmonella. J Infect Dis* 1990;161:255–260.
119. Gorbach S. Probiotics and gastrointestinal health. *Am J Gastroenterol* 2000;95[1 Suppl]:S2–S4.
120. Freedman D, et al. Milk immunoglobulin with specific activity against purified colonization factor antigens can protect against oral challenge with enterotoxigenic *Escherichia coli. J Infect Dis* 1998;177: 662–667.

4

NATURAL BIOTA OF THE HUMAN GASTROINTESTINAL TRACT

KENNETH H. WILSON

The human alimentary tract, like the alimentary tracts of all vertebrates studied thus far, is populated with complex, host-specific, natural communities of bacteria. After a decade of intense research on the biodiversity of our planet, it is surprising that these symbiotic ecosystems have not been more fully characterized by modern molecular analysis. Although it is clear that the organisms found in the human gastrointestinal tract do not belong to the plant kingdom (so that the term *flora* is outdated), we do not yet know the full diversity of community structure, nor do these bacteria have a nomenclature that withstands scrutiny. Fortunately, in the past, a great effort was made to use classic bacteriologic methods to characterize the gastrointestinal biota, so a strong foundation is available on which to build with current approaches.

DISTRIBUTION AND COMPOSITION OF THE BIOTA

The gastrointestinal tract consists of three distinctive ecosystems—the stomach, the small intestine, and the colon. The bacterial communities found in these environments differ in composition and total numbers of organisms.

Stomach

The presence of *Helicobacter* species is characteristic of the mammalian stomach, and each mammalian species exhibits a strong tendency to harbor a particular species of *Helicobacter* (1–4). In humans, the species of *Helicobacter* most commonly found in the stomach is *H. pylori* (5), although *H. heilmannii* is occasionally also present (6,7). The fact that helicobacters are found in large numbers almost exclusively in the gastric mucosa of many animal species and in most preindustrial humans (8) indicates that they are part of our normal biota. In Western industrialized countries, the rate of colonization is much lower, in the range of 25% during childhood and rising to around 50% after the age of 60 (9). Whether this decreased rate of colonization by a symbiont has been advantageous or disadvantageous for human populations is not known. Colonization with helicobacters is associated with an inflammatory response in the lamina propria, a finding sometimes cited as evidence of the organism's undesirability. However, this response in itself is not known to have any pathologic significance clinically, and studies of germ-free animals colonized with a wide variety of organisms indicate that an inflammatory response in the gastrointestinal tract is a normal reaction to bacterial colonization. The known involvement of *H. pylori* in the pathogenesis of peptic ulcers and gastric malignancies, and its protective effect against adenocarcinoma of the esophagus, are discussed in detail in Chapter 33.

Given the low pH of the stomach, one might expect it to contain members of the kingdom Archaea, microbes that are morphologically similar to bacteria and often populate environments at extremes of temperature or pH (10,11). However, when DNA samples extracted from gastric biopsy specimens were subjected to polymerase chain reaction (PCR) with primers directed at the 16S ribosomal DNA (rDNA) of the kingdom Archaea, no PCR products were detected. Ribosomal DNA sequences from *H. pylori* and α-hemolytic streptococci were found when eubacterial kingdom primers were used on the same specimens (K. H. Wilson and R. S. Brown, *unpublished data*).

Small Intestine

The small intestine has been thought to contain few bacteria. However, except for the pathogenic Whipple bacillus, identified by PCR of its rDNA (12,13), the bacterial community of the small bowel has been studied only with culture methods. Most organisms entering the stomach die in the acid environment, and the remaining organisms fail to

K. H. Wilson: Department of Medicine Duke University; Infectious Diseases Section, Veterans Affairs Medical Center, Durham, North Carolina multiply significantly in the small intestine before they are washed out. By standard culture methods, this community is sparse ($\leq 10^5$ organisms per milliliter) and consists of facultative (oxygen-tolerant) organisms such as yeasts, streptococci, lactobacilli, and enterobacteria, in addition to a variety of anaerobes (14–17). Unless stasis leads to bacterial overgrowth, the proximal small bowel is considered to be a paradoxical nutrient-rich ecologic vacuum. A gradual transition occurs between the sparsely populated proximal small bowel to the terminal ileum, where the populations increase in size to around 10^8/mL, become more diverse, and are dominated by anaerobes.

In contrast to the human proximal small intestine, the small intestines of other vertebrates are not a paradoxical nutrient-rich ecologic vacuum. They are populated with variable numbers of segmented filamentous bacteria (SFB) that adhere closely to the mucosa (18–21). These organisms have been observed in vertebrates as dissimilar as mammals, birds, toads, and fish. SFB from mice, rats, and chickens form a phylogenetic cluster, which suggests co-evolution with their respective hosts (22). Although not commonly reported, these organisms have been detected in the human small intestine (21). Given the fate of *H. pylori* in societies with fastidious hygienic practices and the fact that SFB cannot be cultured, it seems very likely that the natural biota of humans includes such organisms but that many individuals in our society no longer harbor them. The importance of SFB may be considerable. Gnotobiotic mice colonized with these organisms quickly exhibit an "explosion" of immunoglobulin A (IgA) plasma cells populating the lamina propria (23,24), a marked increase of secretory IgA production (23,25), and maturation of the T helper 1 (Th1) response (26). Most of the IgA appears to be directed at antigens not found in SFB. Thus, SFB nonspecifically up-regulate the mucosal immune system. Although the mechanism is not known, SFB may also serve as a defense against enterpathogenic organisms (27).

Colon

The vast majority of the bacterial biomass associated with the human body is located in the colon. Here, the bacterial population (approximately 100 billion bacteria per milliliter) is some 1,000 times denser than that in the terminal ileum. Investigators have estimated that about 200 species of bacteria typically coexist in the human colon, and that humans in the aggregate harbor more than 500 species (28,29). In the late 1960s and early 1970s, three factors stimulated research on this ecosystem. First, an explosion of information on the importance of anaerobic infections became available. Second, differences in composition of the colonic biota appeared to be a reasonable hypothesis to explain differences in rates of colon cancer in various populations. Third, a need was perceived to know what we were sending to the moon with the Apollo mission, so that we would know if new microbes came back. Methods were developed to recover in culture more than 90% of the bacterial cells counted microscopically (28–31), although most investigators fell short of this mark and continue to do so. Cultivation of community members from almost any natural ecosystem is extremely difficult, and the colonic biota is no exception. Many of the metabolic activities of the recovered organisms were characterized, and a taxonomic scheme was developed. However, the taxonomic methods are very cumbersome for these organisms, requiring around 100 analytic observations per isolate (32). The important details in the original investigations are often ignored. Because of the demanding nature of the methods, many investigators have omitted documenting the microscopic count or recovery rate, and identification is sometimes inaccurate. Consequently, studies of the composition of colonic biota that do not report that the majority of bacterial cells counted microscopically were actually recovered as colonies should be interpreted with skepticism. Unfortunately, this admonition applies to most reported studies of the topic.

The picture that has emerged from studies of the colonic biota (14,28,29,33) is one of a highly complex ecosystem in which anaerobes outnumber facultative bacteria by around 1,000:1. Species of nine genera (*Bacteroides, Bifidobacterium, Clostridium, Coprococcus, Eubacterium, Fusobacterium, Lactobacillus, Peptostreptococcus,* and *Ruminococcus*) dominate the ecosystem. Although a great deal of variability in composition occurs from person to person, the colonic biota of a single individual is sufficiently stable that it is often possible to identify the donor of a given sample (W. E. C. Moore, *personal communication*). Despite great differences in diet, no difference has been found between bacterial populations in persons at high and low risk for colon cancer (29,33,34). Interestingly, extreme dietary variation appears to have only minor effects on the composition of this ecosystem (35).

The advent of molecular taxonomy has greatly facilitated the evaluation of phylogenetic relationships among intestinal bacteria and made it possible to study the composition of a biota without performing cultures (36,37). Because of many of its properties (11,38) and because of the size of the database available, 16S rDNA is the most useful molecule for phylogenetic analysis. Direct sampling of rDNAs present in the human colon indicates that the biota is more complex than it appears when culture methods are used (39–41). Color Figure 4.1 (see color section) shows the diversity of 16S rDNA sequences found in bacterial colonies from a cultured fecal sample in comparison with sequences found when DNA extracted from the same sample was amplified directly by PCR (39). These data show that more sequences were present in the directly amplified specimen. Furthermore, 22% of sequences from direct PCR versus 38% of sequences from colonies matched sequences in public databases. Although the difference was not statistically significant, these findings suggest that at least some of the PCR-derived sequences were from unculturable species. In a similar study of 284 clones from a single specimen, 22% of the sequences matched known sequences (41). Among the remaining 78% of the sequences, the proportion derived from organisms not culturable by current methods is not known. Although most of the described species from human biota have now undergone 16S rDNA sequencing, we do not know the full range of rDNA sequences within these species. In addition, many isolates studied by the group at Virginia Polytechnic Institute were never formally described as new species (W. E. C. Moore and L. V. H. Moore, *personal communication*) and are therefore not separable from organisms that cannot yet be cultured. Color Figure 4.1 also shows that PCR does not increase the amounts of rDNA from all bacterial species equally. Thus, neither culturing nor sampling by PCR can be called unbiased.

The analysis of rDNA sequences has also revealed that the current taxonomic system does not correlate well with the phylogeny of many intestinal anaerobes. As in all natural communities of bacteria examined to date, most of the predominant colonic biota clusters into only a few phylogenetic groups. The genera *Bacteroides* and *Bifidobacterium* comprise two of these groups and hold together reasonably well in light of rDNA sequence analysis. A third group falls within a cluster related to *Clostridium coccoides.* The taxonomy of organisms within this cluster is misleading because it overstates the diversity of the organisms. Common, very closely related isolates in this group fall into the genera *Clostridium, Ruminococcus, Coprococcus,* and *Eubacterium,* with smaller numbers in *Roseburia, Butyrovibrio,* and *Lachnospira.* To illustrate the point, *C. coccoides* and *Ruminococcus productus* have exactly the same rDNA sequence, ferment the same sugars, make the same products of fermentation, and produce the same cellular fatty acids. The only difference is that one makes spores and the other does not. The fourth group, consisting of *Clostridium leptum* and relatives along with the closely related genus *Fusobacterium,* also comprises organisms named *Clostridium, Eubacterium, Fusobacterium,* and *Ruminococcus.* Clearly, extensive changes in nomenclature are needed. The distribution of bacterial isolates from the colonic biota of four individuals is shown in Fig. 4.2.

Smaller populations of bacteria coexist with the dominant groups. Some of these less numerous components are anaerobes, such as large, fast-growing clostridia not in a dominant group (e.g., *C. perfringens*). Other small populations include facultative bacteria such as *Enterococcus* and *Streptococcus* species and Enterobacteriaceae (e.g., *Escherichia coli*). These components are less numerous because they are suppressed by the dominant organisms. *E. coli,* for example, establishes a population of more than 10^{10} organisms per milliliter in the ceca of germ-free mice, whereas in the presence of the entire biota, the number is reduced by many logs (42,43). The phylogenetic distribution of the dominant populations and subpopulations is shown in Fig. 4.3. Table 4.1 presents some of the most numerous members of the dominant groups shown in this figure. "Invading" or "transient" strains of bacteria are also likely to be present in the gastrointestinal tract. These organisms maintain a population as long as they are being ingested but fail to maintain a steady population otherwise. Probiotic strains of *Lactobacillus* and *Bifidobacterium* are well-studied examples of such organisms (44,45). Many other strains of bacteria are ingested naturally on a daily basis but fail to colonize.

As in other ecosystems, the biota first goes through an ecologic succession before the mature, stable, "climax stage" populations are established. In the germ-free adult animal, this process takes about 2 weeks. In human infants, it takes much longer because diet and weaning seem to play a role. Newborns are colonized within days by facultative organisms, such as *E. coli* and streptococci (46). The first stages of ecologic succession are completed within a few weeks as infants ingest the requisite organisms. The process is significantly faster in vaginally delivered infants than in infants delivered by cesarian section (47). Infants show more variability in the composition of their intestinal biota than adults when individuals are compared and when the same

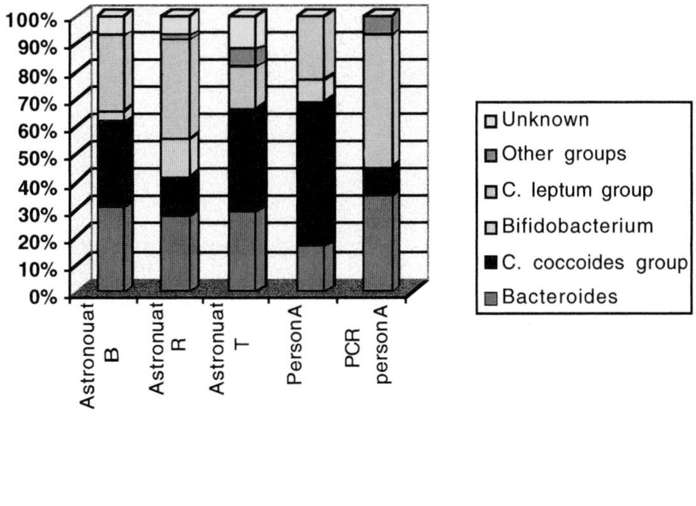

FIGURE 4.2. Phylogenetic distribution of organisms isolated from four individuals. Astronauts B, R, and T were studied by Holdeman et al. during the Apollo program. Person A was studied in the author's laboratory. This figure illustrates the variability of the colonic biota from person to person and the comparability of data from two eras of study despite differences in phylogenetic classifications. The distribution of directly amplified ribosomal DNAs from person A is shown for comparison. (From Holdeman LV, Cato EP, Moore WEC. Human fecal flora: variation in bacterial composition within individuals and a possible effect of emotional stress. *Appl Environ Microbiol* 1976;32:359–375, and Wilson KH, Blitchington RB. Human colonic biota studied by ribosomal DNA sequence analysis. *Appl Environ Microbiol* 1996;62:2273–2278, with permission.)

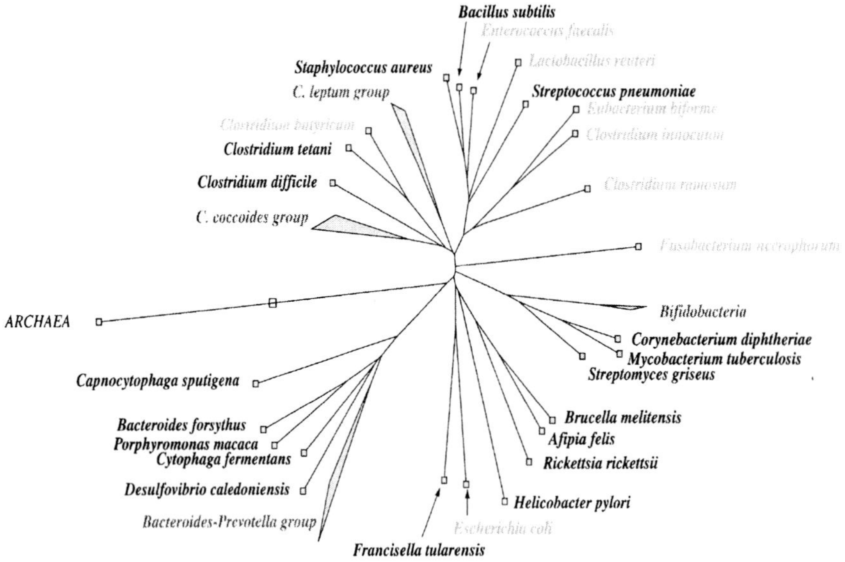

FIGURE 4.3. Phylogenetic distribution of organisms found in human colonic biota. Ribosomal DNA (rDNA) sequences from the Ribosomal Database Project were selected and placed in a tree with use of a neighbor-joining algorithm. Clusters shown in red represent more than 95% of organisms detected by culture methods or polymerase chain reaction (PCR) of rDNA. Bifidobacteria are not typically found by PCR of rDNA because of their high content of guanosine and cytosine (G+C), and they are difficult to amplify. Culture methods show such bacteria to be numerous. Table 4.1 presents some of the most numerous members of the dominant groups. Species shown in yellow are representative of organisms that comprise significant subpopulations. These organisms represent clusters of related species. Thus, *Escherichia coli* occurs in a cluster with other enteric gram-negative bacteria. *Fusobacterium necrophorum* represents the genus *Fusobacterium. Clostridium ramosum, Clostridium innocuum,* and *Eubacterium biforme* represent a cluster of anaerobes associated with *Anaeroplasma. Lactobacillus reuteri* represents the genus *Lactobacillus. Enterococcus faecalis* is clustered with other enterococci and members of the genus *Streptococcus. Clostridium butyricum* represents other fast-growing members of the genus *Clostridium,* including *C. perfringens* and *C. sporogenes.*

TABLE 4.1. COMMON BACTERIAL SPECIES OF THE PREDOMINANT COLONIC BIOTA[a]

Clostridium coccoides Group	*Clostridium leptum* Group	*Bacteroides* Group	*Bifidobacterium* Group
Ruminococcus productus	*Fusobacterium prausnitzii*	*B. vulgatus*	*B. adolescentis*
Coprococcus eutactus	*Ruminococcus bromii*	*B. thetaiotaomicron*	*B. longum*
Ruminococcus torques	*Eubacterium siraeum*	*B. distasonis*	*B. infantis*
Eubacterium rectale	*Clostridium leptum*	*B. eggerthii*	*B. breve*
Eubacterium formicigenerans	*Ruminococcus albus*	*B. fragilis*	*B. bifidum*
Eubacterium hallii	*Ruminococcus obeum*	*B. uniformis*	
Eubacterium ventriosum	*Ruminococcus callidus*	*Prevotella ruminicola*	
Clostridium clostridiiforme			
Lachnospira pectinoschiza			
Eubacterium eligens			
Ruminococcus hansenii			
Eubacterium ruminantium			
Clostridium nexile			

[a]These organisms have been detected by culture methods and by polymerase chain reaction. In addition to the described species, other organisms exist for which ribosomal DNA sequences are not available.

individual is resampled at different points in time. The first relatively stable bacterial community to become established tends to differ between breast-fed and formula-fed babies (47,48), although the composition of the biota among infants in both groups varies greatly. In breast-fed infants, the bifidobacteria tend to predominate over *E. coli* organisms and other Enterobacteriaceae by a factor of 100:1 to 1,000:1, although in some individuals, bifidobacteria do not predominate. Other anaerobic genera, such as *Bacteroides,* are also represented. In contrast, the Enterobacteriaceae tend to dominate the biota of formula-fed infants. In both groups, clostridia are present, although the numbers of clostridia tend to be much lower in communities dominated by bifidobacteria. This tendency may account for the less putrid smell of fecal material from breast-fed infants. *C. difficile* and *C. botulinum* are probably the best-studied of the clostridia. For unknown reasons, the former is a harmless commensal in normal infants (49–53), whereas the latter often causes infant botulism (54,55). As infants begin to ingest a solid diet, the infant biota gradually shifts to an adult biota, and the populations of these clostridia dwindle away. Interestingly, in one study of breast-fed infants in a preindustrial society, much less variation was noted in the numbers of bifidobacteria among individuals; all had populations in the range of 10^{10} to 10^{11}/g (56). This finding suggests that the biota in some infants in our very hygienic society may be incomplete.

INTERACTION WITH THE IMMUNE SYSTEM

A large proportion of antibody produced in the human body traverses the gastrointestinal mucosa and is passed in the feces (57). One-fourth of the mass of the gastrointestinal tract consists of lymphoid tissue that is highly organized, consisting of several components (58). Specialized epithelial M cells assist in sampling luminal contents for presentation to underlying dendritic cells and lymphoid follicles (59,60). Lymphocytes and plasma cells are present throughout the submucosa; the vast majority of plasma cells in the gastrointestinal tract produce IgA (57). Juxtaposed to this large collection of immune sensor and effector cells is the largest mass of bacteria that the host encounters. Despite the seeming importance of this encounter, the interactions between our biota and the immune system remain relatively unstudied.

Gnotobiotic Animal Studies

The study of germ-free animals has facilitated our understanding of how lymphoid tissue develops in the absence of bacteria. Mice and rats raised germ-free have very little of the inflammatory infiltrate normally present in the submucosa of the bowel (42,61). Lymphoid follicles are few, and the mesenteric lymph nodes of these animals do not have well-developed germinal centers (62). Serum immune globulin levels are extremely low and are even lower if the animals are fed an elemental diet (63). The B-cell repertoire lacks diversity (64), although the T-cell repertoire appears to be normal (65). The latter observation fails to explain the germ-free animal's defect in delayed-type hypersensitivity (66). In addition to stimulating the classic immune system in lymphoid follicles and Peyer's patches, the biota appears separately to induce a possibly more primitive response (67). This response is independent of lymphoid follicles and T-cell help and is manifested by IgA antibodies directed at components of the biota.

One of the characteristics of the host response to some orally ingested antigens is the development of a mucosal immune response in the setting of systemic immune tolerance to the same antigens. The study of mucosally induced tolerance in germ-free animals has been particularly interesting. Not only can the host manifest systemic tolerance to bacterial antigens in the gastrointestinal tract, but colonization itself appears to play an important role in oral tolerance in general. This phenomenon was first suggested by Mattingly et al. (68), who showed that suppressor cell activity in the spleens of conventional rats is absent in germ-free rats (68). It was subsequently observed that germ-free mice could not be rendered tolerant by the oral route to sheep erythrocytes given parenterally. However, tolerance could be established after the oral administration of lipopolysaccharide to the mice (69). Moreover, studies have repeatedly shown that germ-free rodents develop less mucosal tolerance involving the systemic T helper 2 (Th2) lymphocyte response in comparison with their conventional counterparts (70,71), although not all groups have been able to reproduce this finding (72). In general, mucosal tolerance has a greater effect on the Th1 than on the Th2 response, but the former has not been evaluated with respect to antigens of bacteria that colonize the gut. Thus, the emerging picture is complex. Although the host often responds to colonizing bacteria with a mucosal Th2 response, tolerance to bacterial antigens is manifested in the systemic compartment of the immune system, and the very existence of oral tolerance depends on bacterial colonization.

The tendency of the mucosal immune system to generate immunologic tolerance may seem paradoxical in light of the importance of the biota in generating a B-cell repertoire. However, it is believed that the well-known "translocation" of bacteria to regional lymph nodes may play a critical role in up-regulating the Th2 response, and it is possible that components of the organisms act as immunologic adjuvants. When germ-free mice were given only *Morganella morganii,* the germinal center response in the mucosa and translocation of bacteria peaked at about 2 weeks, and both decreased as IgA secretion increased (62). Thus, although an initial immune response to a mucosal antigen may be systemic, it may be more typical for the host to sustain an IgA response to indigenous bacteria than to maintain a systemic response. The work of Garg et al. (73), showing the development of systemic tolerance to ingested novel bacterial antigens, supports this contention and lends further evidence that the mucosal response to indigenous microbes is linked to systemic tolerance. The IgA coating of a large portion of bacterial cells in the human intestine is consistent with these data. Similar results were found when germ-free rats were colonized with a strain of *E. coli* that produced ovalbumin in the cytoplasm (74). In these animals, intestinal IgA formed that was measured in biliary secretions, but no systemic antibody response. This sustained IgA response to commensals contrasts sharply with the brief IgA response that is usually associated with intestinal infections.

Role of Enteric Biota in Inflammatory Bowel Disease

As noted above, the predominant host response to the antigens of bacteria that colonize the gut is one in which the secretion of antigen-specific IgA decreases the translocation of bacteria from the gut lumen to regional lymph nodes (62). This response is typically accompanied by antigen-specific down-regulation of the systemic immune response (tolerance), particularly the Th1 response to the same antigen (75), which tends to cause more tissue destruction than the Th2 response. Patients with inflammatory bowel disease differ from normal subjects in that they appear to have lost tolerance as they switch to a pathologic T-cell response to bacterial antigens (76,77). This switch is associated with a Th1-type inflammatory response in the bowel wall in Crohn disease with resultant tissue destruction and a mixed T-cell response in ulcerative colitis (78).

Whether bacterial antigens actually induce an inflammatory response is not known with certainty. However, circumstantial evidence supports causation. One line of evidence lies in work on the human leukocyte antigen (HLA)-B27 transgenic rat. Colitis develops in transgenic rats that express high levels of this major histocompatibility complex (MHC) class I antigen, but only if they are colonized with bacteria (79); germ-free animals remain disease-free. Importantly, the type of colonizing bacterium is a critical factor in this model. A strain of *Bacteroides vulgatus,* originally isolated from a guinea pig with carrageenan-induced colitis, is a particularly strong inducer of disease in gnotobiotic HLA-B27 transgenic rats, whereas *E. coli* does not induce such disease (80). Similarly, colitis or immune activation does not develop in mice deficient in interleukin 10 (IL-10) that are raised in a germ-free environment, but histologic evidence of colitis appears in the animals within 1 week after colonization with specific pathogen-free (SPF) mouse biota (without intestinal *Helicobacter* species) (81). The inflammation in these animals progressively increases, and a 50% mortality occurs by 5 weeks of colonization. The lack of intestinal inflammation in the absence of luminal bacteria appears to be a universal observation, substantiated in at least 10 different genetically engineered and induced rodent models. The population size of *B. vulgatus* and other species in the ceca of SPF mice, natural mice, and guinea pigs is not known. One appealing hypothesis is that the organisms normally predominant in the gastrointestinal tract are particularly unlikely to trigger a Th1 response, but that inflammation leads to overgrowth of "proinflammatory" bacteria. This switch in the biota could continue to induce the Th1 inflammatory response. Thus, inflammation would tend to perpetuate itself, and quiescence also would tend to remain stable. If substantiated, this hypothesis could help explain the exacerbations and remissions of Crohn's disease.

COLONIZATION RESISTANCE

High-level pathogens, such as *Yersinia pestis, Pseudomonas aeruginosa, Clostridium tetani, C. botulinum,* and *C. difficile,* are notably absent from the normal host. The fact that most pathogenic bacteria tested can colonize germ-free animals but not conventional animals (42,82–85) indicates that the biota suppresses them. Even the lower-level pathogens that are themselves members of the ecosystem, such as *Enterococcus* species, enteric gram-negative organisms, and *Candida albicans,* are able to maintain only small populations. Although some specialized pathogens are able to cause disease by adhering to or invading enterocytes, such organisms do not compete effectively within the lumen against an intact biota. Most antibiotics simplify the biota (86). The role of host defense was originally observed experimentally in rodents that had been treated with the antibiotic streptomycin, then challenged with *Salmonella* (87), *Shigella,* or *Vibrio cholerae* organisms (88). Similarly, nosocomial infections with *Enterococcus* species, pathogenic *E. coli, C. albicans, Staphylococcus epidermidis,* and other organisms able to establish large enteric populations develop in humans treated with antibiotics.

Animal models of *C. difficile* disease illustrate the defense function of the biota. The normal hamster is unaffected by even large challenges of either vegetative cells or spores (89), but *C. difficile* colonizes antibiotic-treated animals, reaching a population size of around 100 million colony-forming units (CFU) per milliliter within a matter of hours after inoculation. The host defense role of the biota has also been demonstrated in gnotobiotic mice. Germ-free mice can be stably colonized by *C. difficile* because they are much less susceptible than hamsters to the toxin (82). In mono-associated mice, *C. difficile* organisms maintain a population of about 400 million CFU/mL. However, by 2 weeks after the introduction of mouse biota into these mono-associated mice (about the length of time required for ecologic succession), *C. difficile* is suppressed to undetectable levels (43).

Mechanisms by Which the Biota Controls Pathogens

Our understanding of how the colonic ecosystem operates far exceeds our technical expertise in applying this knowledge clinically. The best theoretic framework for conceptualizing the ecology of the colon is Freter's theory (90,91), which is based on the chemostat [theoretically perfect continuous-flow (CF) culture], independently described by Monod (92) and Novick and Szilard (93). This theory holds that one metabolic substrate in a medium turns out to be growth-limiting, and if two organisms grown together in a chemostat are limited by the same substrate, the less fit organism will be forced to divide at a growth rate slower than the dilution rate and its population will diminish to zero. The theory is able to predict accurately the outcome of single-nutrient competition in chemostats (94). Freter observed that the ability of organisms to compete with *Shigella flexneri* in the gastrointestinal tract of gnotobiotic mice was predicted by their ability to compete in CF culture (95). Static broth cultures and cultures on solid media were not able to reproduce *in vivo* interactions with this fidelity. Thus, the fact that CF cultures succeeded as *in vitro* models of bacterial competition in the gastrointestinal tract suggested that bacteria compete for nutrients. Further study indeed showed this to be the case for both *S. flexneri* (96) and *E. coli* (97). These results have been confirmed repeatedly (98). Subsequent study showed that an environment-simulating medium is better than a standard laboratory broth medium (43). This result is not surprising because in the cases studied so far, a carbon source has been growth-limiting. The major carbon sources in the colon are unabsorbed plant carbohydrates and gastrointestinal mucin, neither of which is present in standard laboratory media. In the case of *C. difficile,* it was possible to determine which monosaccharides in colonic contents the pathogen could metabolize and to show that growth of the organism was indeed limited by these substrates (99).

Clearly, competition for nutrients is not the only mechanism of microbial competition in the colon, and the mathematical modeling of various other factors can become quite complex (90). Despite (or because of) these complexities in both theory and practice, the CF culture can be a highly useful model. Studies have been performed with the biota of mice (100), rats (101), humans (102), and chickens (103), and the results of all support the concept that the entire ecosystem can be modeled in this manner.

Ecologic Manipulations to Control Pathogens

In 1908, Metchnikoff noted the often disastrous results of ingesting putrefied food. On the other hand, foods prepared by fermentation with lactic acid bacilli seldom became putrefied and were safe to ingest. He reasoned that because putrefaction occurs in the human gastrointestinal tract, ingesting lactic acid bacilli could prolong life (104). Consequently, some investigators have believed that lactic acid-producing bacteria, such as *Lactobacillus acidophilus* (105), *Lactobacillus casei* (105,106), *Lactobacillus reuteri* (107), *Enterococcus faecium* (108), and various bifidobacteria (109), are beneficial to humans. Claims have included prevention of traveler's diarrhea (110) and colon cancer (111); treatment of antibiotic-associated diarrhea (112), lethal irradiation (113), and *C. difficile* colitis (114); and lowering of serum cholesterol (108). Most often, these claims either were not supported by clinical studies, the studies were not controlled, or the conclusions were supported by trends that did not reach statistical significance. Importantly, control organisms that do not produce lactic acid have virtually never been directly compared with lactate producers, and the studies involved do not provide a scientific rationale that reflects what we have learned of colonic micro-ecology since 1908.

An approach with a more firm rationale, interstrain competition, has been shown to be therapeutically effective at suppressing pathogens in both experimental animals and patients. Work in this area was pioneered by Shinefield and co-workers in the late 1950s (115) with *Staphylococcus aureus.* At that time, penicillin-resistant staphylococci of the 80/86 phage type were widely distributed in the United States and caused outbreaks of deep-seated infections in newborn nurseries. In eight outbreaks, further infections with 80/86 were prevented by intentionally colonizing newborns with a relatively nonpathogenic strain of penicillin-sensitive *S. aureus* (strain 502A), which was inoculated directly into the umbilical stumps and nares of the infants. The same group went on to show that replacement of the indigenous strain in patients with recurrent furunculosis is an effective treatment for that disorder (116). Other groups have demonstrated that interstrain competition is a generalized phenomenon that applies to strains of *E. coli* in the intestinal tract of gnotobiotic animals (117) and to *C. difficile* organisms in hamsters (118). Seal et al. (119) confirmed these results in humans, showing that recurrent *C. difficile* disease can be prevented by inoculation with a nontoxigenic strain.

The major disadvantage of using interstrain competition therapeutically is that the protective strain must be introduced before exposure to the pathogenic strain occurs. This requirement results from the fact that if both strains are equally fit, competition for space (adhesion sites) is the only control mechanism. Another approach to the ecologic manipulation of bacterial populations has been the use of "replacement biotas"—relatively large, random collections of organisms indigenous to the colon that can take over many functions of the entire ecosystem. This approach is more likely to succeed in suppressing a pathogen that has already become established in the colon because of the redundancy of control mechanisms involved and the relative power of substrate competition. In gnotobiotic animals, a collection of 95 anaerobes was required to suppress populations of *E. coli* and *S. flexneri* to nearly normal levels (42,120). Although a collection of 150 isolates suppressed *C. difficile* by only about three orders of magnitude, in comparison with eight orders of magnitude when the entire mouse biota was used, the collection protected gnotobiotic mice from disease when they were challenged with a hypertoxigenic strain of *C. difficile* (43). As an approach, biota replacement is difficult because of the unwieldy number of strains involved. Although the approach has not been tried in humans, some investigators have administered whole fecal biota and reported success (121–123). Although the rationale was not clear, Tvede and Rask-Madsen (124) treated five patients who had *C. difficile* diarrhea with a combination of 10 bacterial strains and noted resolution of symptoms in all subjects. These provocative human studies lacked adequate numbers of appropriate control subjects.

Using a reductionist approach to obtaining a competitor of *C. difficile,* investigators eliminated most organisms in mouse biota with erythromycin, cultured the surviving bacteria (125), and obtained one species with the ability to suppress *C. difficile* in the gnotobiotic animal. This organism belongs to the group *C. coccoides* and relatives.

We have tested the hypothesis that organisms from the *C. coccoides* group in human biota are able to suppress *C. difficile* (K. H. Wilson, *unpublished data*). A CF culture with a mucin-rich medium was inoculated with *C. difficile* organisms and a local strain of vancomycin-resistant *E. faecium* (VRE). Both organisms reached a population size of 10^8 to 10^9 CFU/mL. Six strains from the *C. coccoides* group, including *Ruminococcus obeum, Eubacterium rectale, Ruminococcus lactaris,* and three unnamed organisms, were then inoculated into the CF culture. The population size of the VRE did not change significantly, and as predicted, the population of *C. difficile* decreased by four logs. Entire fecal biota inoculated into a second CF culture run in parallel suppressed *C. difficile* by five logs. In CF cultures harboring entire biotas, the small remnant populations of *C. difficile* in the lumen appear to be daughter cells from relatively large wall-adherent populations. Thus, partial suppression in CF culture often translates into total suppression *in vivo,* where the wall population is less significant.

CROSS-TALK BETWEEN BIOTA AND HOST

In recent years, new research has focused on molecular signaling between the biota and its host (126–134), particularly the host response to colonization by symbionts. The effects of the biota on the immune system and the ability of SFB to up-regulate the Th2 immune responses in the murine gastrointestinal tract have been described above. At the molecular level, intercellular adhesion molecule 1 (ICAM-1) is decreased in the liver, intestine, and skin of germ-free animals, and these decreases can be corrected by associating the mice with their natural biota (132). Other adhesion molecules studied to date do not reflect the same pattern. Indigenous organisms may also affect the immune system by stimulating intestinal epithelial cells to elaborate immunoregulatory cytokines (135). *E. coli* or *Lactobacillus sakei* induce CACO-2 cells to elaborate IL-8, MCP-1, IL-1β, and tumor necrosis factor (TNF)-α messenger RNAs (mRNAs), but enteropathogenic *E. coli* induces the same cytokine messages much faster. In contrast, an intestinal isolate of *Lactobacillus johnsonii* reduces the production of message for the above proinflammatory cytokines and induces the antiinflammatory cytokine transforming growth factor (TGF)-β, which switches the B-cell isotype to IgA. Whether these results can be generalized to other commensals and to other proinflammatory and antiinflammatory cytokines is not known.

Studies in gnotobiotic NMRI mice have shown that colonization with the predominant anaerobe *Bacteroides thetaiotaomicron* induces expression of an $\alpha_{1,2}$-fucosyltransferase mRNA, which fucosylates glycans on the surface of mucosal epithelial cells in the ileum (136). Teleologically, induction is understandable because fucose is among the carbon sources that *B. thetaiotaomicron* can utilize. Further analysis of this phenomenon has revealed a complex interaction between the epithelial cells of the mouse ileum and *B. thetaiotaomicron* (129). An operon coding for enzymes in the metabolic pathway for fucose is repressed by the gene product of *fucR,* a gene in the same operon. De-repression of the operon by fucose leads to expression of *fucR* and the fucose-metabolizing enzymes. Data are also consistent with *fucR* repressing another genetic element, designated *csp.* In this case, it appears that rather than inducing *csp,* fucose is actually a co-repressor. The site designated *csp* actually leads to induction in mouse epithelial cells of $\alpha_{1,2}$-fucosyltransferase through a pathway yet to be determined. Thus, it appears that by coordinated regulation of the operons *fucRIAKP* and *csp, B. thetaiotaomicron* regulates the production of a fucose-containing metabolic substrate in its host as the bacterium regulates its own intracellular concentration of fucose.

The exquisite cross-talk between biota and host manifested in the regulation of fucose pathways is not unique. *B. thetaiotaomicron* is also able to induce expression of the metalloprotease matrilysin by epithelial cells that underproduce this enzyme in germ-free mice (133). With the use of microarrays of oligonucleotides, it has been possible to screen broadly for changes in mRNA expression under various conditions (137,138). This approach has been applied to measure changes in mRNA levels induced in germ-free mice colonized with several organisms, including *B. thetaiotaomicron, E. coli, Bifidobacterium infantis,* and conventional mouse biota (131). Mouse genes from several classes are up- or down-regulated, including those for the glucose/sodium transporter and several components of the lipid transport system. Another constellation of genes should make bacterial colonization less damaging by down-regulating complement activation and decreasing the permeability of the mucosa. Changes in mRNA have also indicated changes in drug-metabolizing enzymes, components of the myoenteric plexus, lactase production, levels of the IgA transporter protein, and levels of angiogenin 3. These changes occurred in specific cell types and varied as a function of which organisms were colonizing the mice. None of these differences was related to the fucose metabolic system described above.

Thus, the interactions between the various components of the enteric biota and physiologic mechanisms in the host promise to be exceedingly complex. Our biota appears more complex when studied by rDNA analysis rather than by culture techniques alone, and the collective human colonic biota probably greatly exceeds 500 species. These organisms interact with one another, with epithelial cells, and with the cells of the immune system. Given the new research tools available, including high-throughput sequencing, the photolithography chip, and fluorescent *in situ* hybridization, the study of human microbial ecology in the near future should be exceedingly productive.

REFERENCES

1. Marshall BJ, Warren JR. Unidentified curved bacilli in the stomach of patients with gastritis and peptic ulceration. *Lancet* 1984;1:1311–1314.
2. Fox JG, Cabot EB, Taylor NS, et al. Gastric colonization by *Campylobacter pylori* subsp. *mustelae* in ferrets. *Infect Immun* 1988;56:2994–2996.
3. Lee A, Hazell SL, O'Rourke J, et al. Isolation of a spiral-shaped bacterium from the cat stomach. *Infect Immun* 1988;56: 2843–2850.
4. Whary MT, Cline JH, King AE, et al. Monitoring sentinel mice for *Helicobacter hepaticus, H. rodentium,* and *H. bilis* infection by use of polymerase chain reaction analysis and serologic testing. *Comp Med* 2000;50:436–443.
5. Solnick JV, O'Rourke J, Lee A, et al. An uncultured gastric spiral organism is a newly identified *Helicobacter* in humans. *J Infect Dis* 1993;168:379–385.
6. Stolte M, Kroher G, Meining A, et al. A comparison of *Helicobacter pylori* and *H. heilmannii* gastritis. A matched control study involving 404 patients. *Scand J Gastroenterol* 1997;32: 28–33.
7. Andersen LP, Boye K, Blom J, et al. Characterization of a culturable "Gastrospirillum hominis" (*Helicobacter heilmannii*) strain isolated from human gastric mucosa. *J Clin Microbiol* 1999;37:1069–1076.
8. Anonymous. Ecology of *Helicobacter pylori* in Peru: infection rates in coastal, high altitude, and jungle communities. The Gastrointestinal Physiology Working Group of the Cayetano Heredia and the Johns Hopkins University. *Gut* 1992;33:604–605.
9. Dooley CP, Cohen H, Fitzgibbons PL, et al. Prevalence of *Helicobacter pylori* infection and histologic gastritis in asymptomatic persons. *N Engl J Med* 1989;321:1562–1566.
10. Barns SM, Fundyga RE, Jeffries MW, et al. Remarkable archaeal diversity detected in a Yellowstone National Park hot spring environment [see Comments]. *Proc Natl Acad Sci U S A* 1994;91:1609–1613.
11. Woese CR, Olsen GJ. Ribosomal RNA: a key to phylogeny. *FASEB J* 1993;7:113–123.
12. Wilson KH, Blitchington R, Frothingham R, et al. Phylogeny of the Whipple's-disease-associated bacterium. *Lancet* 1991; 338:474–475.
13. Mandell GL, Douglas RG, Bennett JE. *Principles and practice of infectious diseases.* New York: Churchill Livingstone, 1990.
14. Finegold SM, Sutter VL, Mathison GE. Normal indigenous intestinal flora. In: Hentges DJ, ed. *Human intestinal microflora in health and disease.* New York: Academic Press, 1983:3–31.
15. Justesen T, Haagen Nielsen O, Jacobsen IE, et al. The normal cultivable microflora in upper jejunal fluid in healthy adults. *Scand J Gastroenterol* 1984;19:279–282.
16. Plaut AG, Gorbach SL, Nahas L, et al. Studies of intestinal microflora. III. The microbial flora of human small intestinal mucosa and fluids. *Gastroenterology* 1967;53:868–873.
17. Gorbach SL, Plaut AG, Nahas L, et al. Studies of intestinal microflora. II. Microorganisms of the small intestine and their relations to oral and fecal flora. *Gastroenterology* 1967;53: 856–867.
18. Dewhirst FE, Chien CC, Paster BJ, et al. Phylogeny of the defined murine microbiota: altered Schaedler flora. *Appl Environmen Microbiol* 1999;65:3287–3292.
19. Smith TM. Segmented filamentous bacteria in the bovine small intestine. *J Comp Pathol* 1997;117:185–190.
20. Lowden S, Heath T. Segmented filamentous bacteria associated with lymphoid tissues in the ileum of horses. *Res Vet Sci* 1995;59:272–274.
21. Klaasen HL, Koopman JP, Van den Brink ME, et al. Intestinal, segmented, filamentous bacteria in a wide range of vertebrate species. *Lab Anim* 1993;27:141–150.
22. Snel J, Heinen PP, Blok HJ, et al. Comparison of 16S rRNA sequences of segmented filamentous bacteria isolated from mice, rats, and chickens and proposal of "Candidatus arthromitus." *Int J Syst Bacteriol* 1995;45:780–782.
23. Talham GL, Jiang HQ, Bos NA, et al. Segmented filamentous bacteria are potent stimuli of a physiologically normal state of the murine gut mucosal immune system. *Infect Immun* 1999;67:1992–2000.
24. Cebra JJ, Periwal SB, Lee G, et al. Development and maintenance of the gut-associated lymphoid tissue (GALT): the roles of enteric bacteria and viruses. *Dev Immunol* 1998;6:13–18.
25. Umesaki Y, Setoyama H, Matsumoto S, et al. Differential roles of segmented filamentous bacteria and clostridia in development of the intestinal immune system. *Infect Immun* 1999; 67:3504–3511.
26. Umesaki Y, Okada Y, Matsumoto S, et al. Segmented filamentous bacteria are indigenous intestinal bacteria that activate intraepithelial lymphocytes and induce MHC class II molecules and fucosyl asialo GM1 glycolipids on the small intestinal epithelial cells in the ex-germ-free mouse. *Microbiol Immunol* 1995;39:555–562.
27. Heczko U, Abe A, Finlay BB. Segmented filamentous bacteria prevent colonization of enteropathogenic *Escherichia coli* O103 in rabbits. *J Infect Dis* 2000;181:1027–1033.
28. Holdeman LV, Cato EP, Moore WEC. Human fecal flora: variation in bacterial composition within individuals and a possible effect of emotional stress. *Appl Environ Microbiol* 1976;32: 359–375.
29. Moore WEC, Holdeman LV. Human fecal flora: the normal flora of 20 Japanese-Hawaiians. *Appl.Microbiol* 1974;27:961–979.
30. Bryant MP, Robinson IM. An improved nonselective culture medium for ruminal bacteria and its use in determining diurnal variation in numbers of bacteria in the rumen. *J Dairy Sci* 1961;44:1446–1456.
31. Bryant MP. Nutritional features and ecology of predominant

anaerobic bacteria of the gastrointestinal tract. *Am J Clin Nutr* 1974;27:1313–1319.
32. Holdeman LV, Cato EP, Moore WEC. *Anaerobe laboratory manual.* Blacksburg, VA: Virginia Polytechnic Institute and State University, 1977.
33. Finegold SM, Attebery HR, Sutter VL. Effect of diet on human fecal flora: comparison of Japanese and American diets. *Am J Clin Nutr* 1974;27:1456–1469.
34. Finegold SM, Sutter VL, Sugihara PT, et al. Fecal microbial flora in Seventh Day Adventist populations and control subjects. *Am J Clin Nutr* 1977;30:1781–1792.
35. Moore WEC, Cato EP, Good IJ, et al. The effect of diet on the human fecal flora. In: Bruce WR, Correa P, Lipkin M, et al., eds. *Branbury report 7, gastrointestinal cancer: endogenous factors.* New York: Cold Spring Harbor Laboratory, 1981:11–24.
36. Pace NR, Stahl DA, Lane DJ, et al. The analysis of natural microbial populations by ribosomal RNA sequences. In: Marshall KC, Atlas R, Jorgesen BB, et al., eds. *Advances in microbial ecology,* vol 9. New York: Plenum Publishing, 1986:1–55.
37. Schmidt TM, DeLong EF, Pace NR. Analysis of a marine picoplankton community by 16S rRNA gene cloning and sequencing. *J Bacteriol* 1991;173:4371–4378.
38. Gutell RR, Weiser B, Woese CR, et al. Comparative anatomy of 16S-like ribosomal RNA. *Prog Nucl Acid Res Mol Biol* 1985; 32:155–216.
39. Wilson KH, Blitchington RB. Human colonic biota studied by ribosomal DNA sequence analysis. *Appl Environ Microbiol* 1996;62:2273–2278.
40. Cellini L, Allocati N, Angelucci D, et al. Coccoid *Helicobacter pylori* not culturable *in vitro* reverts in mice. *Microbiol Immunol* 1994;38:843–850.
41. Suau A, Bonnet R, Sutren M, et al. Direct analysis of genes encoding 16S rRNA from complex communities reveals many novel molecular species within the human gut. *Appl Environ Microbiol* 1999;65:4799–4807.
42. Freter R, Abrams GD. Function of various intestinal bacteria in converting germfree mice to the normal state. *Infect Immun* 1972;6:119–126.
43. Wilson KH, Freter R. Interactions of *Clostridium difficile* and *E. coli* with microfloras in continuous-flow cultures and gnotobiotic mice. *Infect Immun* 1986;54:354–358.
44. Alander M, Satokari R, Korpela R, et al. Persistence of colonization of human colonic mucosa by a probiotic strain, *Lactobacillus rhamnosus* GG, after oral consumption. *Appl Environ Microbiol* 1999;65:351–354.
45. Tannock GW, Munro K, Harmsen HJ, et al. Analysis of the fecal microflora of human subjects consuming a probiotic product containing *Lactobacillus rhamnosus* DR20. *Appl Environ Microbiol* 2000;66:2578–2588.
46. Tannock GW, Fuller R, Smith SL, et al. Plasmid profiling of members of the family Enterobacteriaceae, lactobacilli, and bifidobacteria to study the transmission of bacteria from mother to infant. *J Clin Microbiol* 1990;28:1225–1228.
47. Rotimi VO, Duerden BI. The development of the bacterial flora in normal neonates. *J Med Microbiol* 1981;14:51–62.
48. Lundequist B, Nord CE, Winberg J. The composition of the faecal microflora in breast-fed and bottle-fed infants from birth to eight weeks. *Acta Paediatr Scand* 1985;74:45–51.
49. Kotloff KL, Wade JC, Morris JG Jr. Lack of association between *Clostridium difficile* toxin and diarrhea in infants. *Pediatr Infect Dis J* 1988;7:662–663.
50. Thompson CMJ, Gilligan PH, Fisher MC, et al. *Clostridium difficile* cytotoxin in a pediatric population. *Am J Dis Child* 1983;137:271–274.
51. Zedd AJ, Sell TL, Schaberg DR, et al. Nosocomial *Clostridium difficile* reservoir in a neonatal intensive care unit. *Pediatr Infect Dis* 1984;3:429–432.
52. Torres JF, Cedillo R, Sanchez J, et al. Prevalence of *Clostridium difficile* and its cytotoxin in infants in Mexico. *J Clin Microbiol* 1984;20:274–275.
53. Rolfe RD, Iaconis JP. Intestinal colonization of infant hamsters with *Clostridium difficile. Infect Immun* 1983;42:480–486.
54. Midura TF, Arnon SS. Infant botulism: identification of *Clostridium botulinum* and its toxins in faeces. *Lancet* 1976;2:934–936.
55. Wilcke BW, Midura TF, Arnon SS. Quantitative evidence of intestinal colonization by *Clostridium botulinum* in four cases of infant botulism. *J Infect Dis* 1980;141:419–423.
56. Mata LJ, Urrutia JJ. Intestinal colonization of breast-fed children in a rural area of low socioeconomic level. *Am J Ophthalmol* 1971;176:93–110.
57. Conley ME, Delacroix DL. Intravascular and mucosal immunoglobulin A: two separate but related systems of immune defense? *Ann Intern Med* 1987;106:892–899.
58. Kagnoff MF. Immunology of the digestive system. In: Christensen J, Jackson MJ, Jacobson ED, et al., eds. *Physiology of the gastrointestinal tract.* New York: Raven Press, 1987:1699–1728.
59. Kelsall BL, Strober W. Peyer's patch dendritic cells and the induction of mucosal immune responses [Review; 65 refs]. *Res Immunol* 1997;148:490–498.
60. Kraehenbuhl JP, Hopkins SA, Kerneis S, et al. [Review; 57 refs]. *Behring Institute Mitteilungen* 1997:24–32.
61. Luckey TD. *Germfree life.* New York: Academic Press, 1963.
62. Shroff KE, Meslin K, Cebra JJ. Commensal enteric bacteria engender a self-limited humoral mucosal immune response while permanently colonizing the gut. *Infect Immun* 1997; 63:3904–3913.
63. Unni KK, Holley KE, McDuffie FC, et al. Comparative study of NZB mice under germfree and conventional conditions. *J Rheumatol* 1975;2:36–44.
64. Helgeland L, Vaage JT, Rolstad B, et al. Microbial colonization influences composition and T-cell receptor V beta repertoire of intraepithelial lymphocytes in rat intestine. *Immunology* 1996;89:494–501.
65. Vos Q, Jones LA, Kruisbeek AM. Mice deprived of exogenous antigenic stimulation develop a normal repertoire of functional T cells. *J Immunol* 1992;149:1204–1210.
66. MacDonald TT, Carter PB. Requirement for a bacterial flora before mice generate cells capable of mediating the delayed hypersensitivity reaction to sheep red blood cells. *J Immunol* 1979;122:2624–2629.
67. Macpherson AJ, Gatto D, Sainsbury E, et al. A primitive T cell-independent mechanism of intestinal mucosal IgA responses to commensal bacteria. *Science* 2000;288:2222–2226.
68. Mattingly JA, Eardley DD, Kemp JD, et al. Induction of suppressor cells in rat spleen: influence of microbial stimulation. *J Immunol* 1979;122:787–790.
69. Wannemuehler MJ, Kiyono H, Babb JL, et al. Lipopolysaccharide (LPS) regulation of the immune response: LPS converts germfree mice to sensitivity to oral tolerance induction. *J Immunol* 1982;129:959–965.
70. Sudo N, Sawamura S, Tanaka K, et al. The requirement of intestinal bacterial flora for the development of an IgE production system fully susceptible to oral tolerance induction. *J Immunol* 1997;159:1739–1745.
71. Moreau MC, Gaboriau-Routhiau V. The absence of gut flora, the doses of antigen ingested and aging affect the long-term peripheral tolerance induced by ovalbumin feeding in mice. *Res Immunol* 1996;147:49–59.
72. Furrie E, Turner M, Strobel S. The absence of gut flora has no effect on the induction of oral tolerance to ovalbumin. *Adv Exp Med Biol* 1995;371B:1239–1241.
73. Garg S, Bal V, Rath S, et al. The effect of multiple antigenic exposures in the gut on oral tolerance and induction of antibacterial systemic immunity. *Infect Immun* 1999;67:5917–5924.

74. Dahlgren UI, Wold AE, Hanson LA, et al. Expression of a dietary protein in *E. coli* renders it strongly antigenic to gut lymphoid tissue. *Immunology* 1991;73:394–397.
75. von Herrath MG. Bystander suppression induced by oral tolerance [Review; 95 refs]. *Res Immunol* 1997;148:541–554.
76. Duchmann R, Kaiser I, Hermann E, et al. Tolerance exists towards resident intestinal flora but is broken in active inflammatory bowel disease (IBD) [see Comments]. *Clin Exp Immunol* 1995;102:448–455.
77. Duchmann R, Schmitt E, Knolle P, et al. Tolerance towards resident intestinal flora in mice is abrogated in experimental colitis and restored by treatment with interleukin-10 or antibodies to interleukin-12. *Eur J Immunol* 1996;26:934–938.
78. Fuss IJ, Neurath M, Boirivant M, et al. Disparate CD4+ lamina propria (LP) lymphokine secretion profiles in inflammatory bowel disease. Crohn's disease LP cells manifest increased secretion of IFN-gamma, whereas ulcerative colitis LP cells manifest increased secretion of IL-5. *J Immunol* 1996;157:1261–1270.
79. Rath HC, Herfarth HH, Ikeda JS, et al. Normal luminal bacteria, especially *Bacteroides* species, mediate chronic colitis, gastritis, and arthritis in HLA-B27/human beta2 microglobulin transgenic rats. *J Clin Invest* 1996;98:945–953.
80. Rath HC, Wilson KH, Sartor RB. Differential induction of colitis and gastritis in HLA-B27 transgenic rats selectively colonized with *Bacteroides vulgatus* or *Escherichia coli*. *Infect Immun* 1999;67:2969–2974.
81. Sellon RK, Tonkonogy S, Schultz M, et al. Resident enteric bacteria are necessary for development of spontaneous colitis and immune system activation in interleukin-10-deficient mice. *Infect Immun* 1998;66:5224–5231.
82. Onderdonk AB, Cisneros RL, Bartlett JG. *Clostridium difficile* in gnotobiotic mice. *Infect Immun* 1980;28:277–282.
83. Raibaud P, Ducluzeau R, Dubos F, et al. Implantation of bacteria from the digestive tract of man and various animals into gnotobiotic mice. *Am J Clin Nutr* 1980;33:2440–2447.
84. Hazenberg MP, Bakker M, Burggraaf AV. Effects of the human intestinal flora on germ-free mice. *J Appl Bacteriol* 1981;50:95–106.
85. Wells CL, Balish E. *Clostridium tetani* growth and toxin production in the intestines of germfree rats. *Infect Immun* 1983;41:826–828.
86. Finegold SM, Mathison GE, George WL. Changes in human intestinal flora related to the administration of antimicrobial agents. In: Hentges DJ, ed. *Human intestinal flora in health and disease.* New York: Academic Press, 1983:356–438.
87. Bohnhoff M, Drake BL, Miller CP. Effect of streptomycin on susceptibility of the intestinal tract to experimental *Salmonella* infection. *Proc Soc Exp Biol Med* 1954;86:132–137.
88. Freter R. Fatal enteric cholera infection in the guinea pig achieved by inhibition of normal enteric flora. *J Infect Dis* 1955;97:57–64.
89. Wilson KH, Sheagren JN, Freter R. Population dynamics of ingested *Clostridium difficile* in the gastrointestinal tract of the Syrian hamster. *J Infect Dis* 1985;151:355–361.
90. Freter R, Brickner H, Fekete J, et al. Survival and implantation of *Escherichia coli* in the intestinal tract. *Infect Immun* 1983;39:686–703.
91. Freter R, Brickner H, Botney M, et al. Mechanisms that control bacterial populations in continuous-flow culture models of mouse large intestinal flora. *Infect Immun* 1983;39:676–685.
92. Monod J. La technique de culture continué: théorie et applications. *Ann Inst Pasteur* 1950;79:390–410.
93. Novik A, Szilard L. Experiments with the chemostat on spontaneous mutations of bacteria. *Proc Natl Acad Sci U S A* 1950;36:708–719.
94. Fredrickson AG. Behavior of mixed cultures of microorganisms. *Annu Rev Microbiol* 1977;31:63–87.
95. Hentges DJ, Freter R. *In vivo* and *in vitro* antagonism of intestinal bacteria against *Shigella flexneri*. I. Correlation between various tests. *J Infect Dis* 1962;110:30–37.
96. Freter R. *In vivo* and *in vitro* antagonism of intestinal bacteria against *Shigella flexneri*. II. The inhibitory mechanism. *J Infect Dis* 1962;110:38–46.
97. Ozawa A, Freter R. Ecologic mechanism controlling growth of *Escherichia coli* in continuous-flow culture and in the mouse intestine. *J Infect Dis* 1964;114:235–242.
98. Guiot HF. Role of competition for substrate in bacterial antagonism in the gut. *Infect Immun* 1982;38:887–892.
99. Wilson KH, Perini F. Role of competition for nutrients in suppression of *Clostridium difficile* by the colonic microflora. *Infect Immun* 1988;56:2610–2614.
100. Freter R, Stauffer E, Cleven D, et al. Continuous-flow cultures as *in vitro* models of the ecology of large intestinal flora. *Infect Immun* 1983;39:666–675.
101. Veilleux BG, Rowland I. Simulation of the rat intestinal ecosystem using a two-stage continuous culture system. *J Gen Microbiol* 1981;123:103–115.
102. Miller TL, Wolin MJ. Fermentation by the human large intestine microbial community in a semicontinuous culture system. *Appl Environ Microbiol* 1981;42:400–407.
103. Nisbet DJ, Ricke SC, Scanlan CM, et al. Inoculation of broiler chicks with a continuous-flow derived bacterial culture facilitates early cecal bacterial colonization and increases resistance to *Salmonella typhimurium*. *J Food Protection* 1994;57:12–15.
104. Metchnikoff E. *The prolongation of life. Optimistic studies.* New York: G.P. Putnam's Sons, The Knickerbocker Press, 1908.
105. Clements ML, Levine MM, Black RE, et al. *Lactobacillus* prophylaxis for diarrhea due to enterotoxigenic *Escherichia coli*. *Antimicrob Agents Chemother* 1981;20:104–108.
106. Silva M, Jacobus NV, Deneke C, et al. Antimicrobial substance from a human *Lactobacillus* strain. *Antimicrob Agents Chemother* 1987;31:1231–1233.
107. Talarico TL, Dobrogosz WJ. Chemical characterization of an antimicrobial substance produced by *Lactobacillus reuteri*. *Antimicrob Agents Chemother* 1989;33:674–679.
108. Zacconi C, Bottazzi V, Rebecchi A, et al. Serum cholesterol levels in axenic mice colonized with *Enterococcus faecium* and *Lactobacillus acidophilus*. *Microbiologica* 1992;15:413–417.
109. Hekmat S, McMahon DJ. Survival of *Lactobacillus acidophilus* and *Bifidobacterium bifidum* in ice cream for use as a probiotic food. *J Dairy Sci* 1992;75:1415–1422.
110. Oksanen PJ, Salminen S, Saxelin M, et al. Prevention of travellers' diarrhea by *Lactobacillus* GG. *Ann Med* 1990;22:53–56.
111. Gorbach SL. Lactic acid bacteria and human health. *Ann Med* 1990;22:37–41.
112. Siitonen S, Vapaatalo H, Salminen S, et al. Effect of *Lactobacillus* GG yoghurt in prevention of antibiotic-associated diarrhoea. *Ann Med* 1990;22:57–59.
113. Dong M-Y, Chang T-W, Gorbach SL. Effects of feeding *Lactobacillus* GG on lethal irradiation in mice. *Diagn Microbiol Infect Dis* 1987;7:1–7.
114. Gorbach SL, Chang T-W, Goldin B. Successful treatment of relapsing *Clostridium difficile* colitis with Lactobacillus GG. *Lancet* 1987;2:1519.
115. Shinefield HR, Ribble JC, Boris M, et al. Bacterial interference: its effect on nursery-acquired infection with *Staphylococcus aureus*. I. Preliminary observations on artificial colonization of newborns. *Am J Dis Child* 1963;105:146–154.
116. Boris M, Shinefield HR, Romano P, et al. Bacterial interference. Protection against recurrent intrafamilial staphylococcal disease. *Am J Dis Child* 1968;115:521–529.
117. Duvall-Iflah Y, Raibaud P, Rousseau M. Antagonisms among isogenic strains of *Escherichia coli* in the digestive tracts of gnotobiotic mice. *Infect Immun* 1981;34:957–969.

118. Wilson KH, Sheagren JN. Antagonism of toxigenic *Clostridium difficile* by nontoxigenic *C. difficile. J Infect Dis* 1983;147: 733–736.
119. Seal D, Borriello SP, Barclay FE, et al. Treatment of relapsing *Clostridium difficile* diarrhea by administration of a nontoxigenic strain. *Eur J Clin Microbiol* 1987;6:51–53.
120. Syed SA, Abrams GD, Freter R. Efficiency of various intestinal bacteria in assuming normal functions of enteric flora after association with germfree mice. *Infect Immun* 1970;2:376–387.
121. Delmee M, Bulliard G, Simon G. Application of a technique for serogrouping *Clostridium difficile* in an outbreak of antibiotic-associated diarrhoea. *J Infect* 1986;13:5–9.
122. Schwan A, Sjolin S, Trottestam U, et al. Relapsing *Clostridium difficile* enterocolitis cured by rectal infusion of normal faeces. *Scand J Infect Dis* 1984;16:211–215.
123. Guiot HFL, van der Meer JWM, Van Furth R. Selective antimicrobial modulation of human microbial flora: infection prevention in patients with decreased host defense mechanisms by selective elimination of potentially pathogenic bacteria. *J Infect Dis* 1981;143:644–654.
124. Tvede M, Rask-Madsen J. Bacteriotherapy for chronic relapsing *Clostridium difficile* diarrhoea in six patients. *Lancet* 1989;1: 1156–1160.
125. Su WJ, Bourlioux P, Bournaud M, et al. Mise au point d'un modèle expérimental animal permettant de la microflore coecale du hamster, antagoniste de *Clostridium difficile. Ann Inst Pasteur* 1986;137A:89–96.
126. Gordon JI, Hooper LV, McNevin MS, et al. Epithelial cell growth and differentiation. III. Promoting diversity in the intestine: conversations between the microflora, epithelium, and diffuse GALT [Review; 29 refs]. *Am J Physiol* 1997;273:G565–G570.
127. Haller D, Bode C, Hammes WP, et al. Non-pathogenic bacteria elicit a differential cytokine response by intestinal epithelial cell/leucocyte co-cultures. *Gut* 2000;47:79–87.
128. Hamzaoui N, Pringault E. Interaction of microorganisms, epithelium, and lymphoid cells of the mucosa-associated lymphoid tissue [Review. 53 refs]. *Ann N Y Acad Sci* 1998;859: 65–74.
129. Hooper LV, Xu J, Falk PG, et al. A molecular sensor that allows a gut commensal to control its nutrient foundation in a competitive ecosystem. *Proc Natl Acad Sci U S A* 1999;96: 9833–9838.
130. Hooper LV, Falk PG, Gordon JI. Analyzing the molecular foundations of commensalism in the mouse intestine [Review; 45 refs]. *Curr Opin Microbiol* 2000;3:79–85.
131. Hooper LV, Wong MH, Thelin A, et al. Molecular analysis of commensal host–microbial relationships in the intestine. *Science* 2001;291:881–884.
132. Komatsu S, Berg RD, Russell JM, et al. Enteric microflora contribute to constitutive ICAM-1 expression on vascular endothelial cells. *Am J Physiol Gastrointest Liver Physiol* 2000; 279:G186–G191.
133. Lopez-Boado YS, Wilson CL, Hooper LV, et al. Bacterial exposure induces and activates matrilysin in mucosal epithelial cells. *J Cell Biol* 2000;148:1305–1315.
134. Raupach B, Mecsas J, Heczko U, et al. Bacterial epithelial cell cross-talk [Review; 82 refs]. *Curr Top Microbiol Immunol* 1999; 236:137–161.
135. Kagnoff MF, Eckmann L, Yang S, et al. Intestinal epithelial cells: an integral component of the mucosal immune system. In: Kagnoff MF, Hiroshi K, eds. *Essentials of mucosal immunology.* New York: Academic Press, 1996:63–72.
136. Bry L, Falk PG, Midtvedt T, et al. A model of host–microbial interactions in an open mammalian ecosystem [see Comments]. *Science* 1996;273:1380–1383.
137. Notterman DA, Alon U, Sierk AJ, et al. Transcriptional gene expression profiles of colorectal adenoma, adenocarcinoma, and normal tissue examined by oligonucleotide arrays. *Cancer Res* 2001;61:3124–3130.
138. Li C, Wong WH. Model-based analysis of oligonucleotide arrays: expression index computation and outlier detection. *Proc Natl Acad Sci U S A* 2001;98:31–36.

5

PRODUCTION, STRUCTURE, AND FUNCTION OF GASTROINTESTINAL MUCINS

DARCY MONCADA
KRIS CHADEE

GENERAL PROPERTIES OF MUCINS

The gastrointestinal (GI) epithelium is covered by a thick viscous mucus blanket composed of water, salts, immunoglobulins, secreted proteins, and most importantly, mucins. Mucins are high-molecular-weight glycoproteins, which act as the main structural component, giving rise to the polymeric, visoelastic, and protective properties of the adherent mucus gel. The mucus gel layer is the most important protective component of the GI tract and all mucosal surfaces because of its ability to maintain epithelial barrier function. Not all mucins are alike; they are grouped into two major classes: membrane-bound mucins and secreted mucins. Secreted mucins contribute to the formation of the mucus gel and are produced from specialized epithelial cells found throughout the GI tract, including the salivary glands, stomach, pancreatic and bile ducts, small and large intestines, and colon. On the other hand, the role of membrane-bound mucins is still not entirely understood. As a class, mucins are extremely large glycoproteins with molecular masses ranging from 0.5 to 25×10^6 KDa. The protein core of a typical mucin molecule contains mucin domains, consisting of tandem repeats rich in the amino acids threonine, proline, and/or serine, and the hydroxyl residues are heavily substituted with *O*-linked oligosaccharides (1). The carbohydrate content of mucin may be responsible for more than 80% of its dry weight. The abundant glycosylation of the mucin domains give mucin its characteristic bottle-brush–like appearance. Additionally, the densely packed carbohydrates are responsible for protecting the protein core from damage. Many mucins also contain sialic acid and sulfate attached to sugars, giving it a negative charge under physiological conditions. The general properties of mucins, such as protease resistance, high charge density from sialic acid and sulfate residues, and a large water-holding capacity, are attributes of extensive glycosylation. In general, the amino and carboxyl terminal regions of mucin are less glycosylated than the mucin domains and contain a wide range of amino acids, most notably cysteine residues. The cysteine residues form intramolecular disulfide bonds within the carboxyl and amino terminal regions, as well as intermolecular disulfide bonds between mucin molecules, participating in the polymerization of mucin and enabling formation of the visoelastic mucus gel. Figure 5.1 depicts the major intestinal gel-forming secretory mucin, MUC2.

The surface of the GI epithelium is continually exposed to numerous macromolecules and microorganisms, including chemical irritants, digested foods, toxins, resident bacteria, and intestinal pathogens and their products. The meshlike structure of the mucin gel impedes the diffusion of offending macromolecules through it. The delicate single-cell thick epithelium lining the intestinal tract would be susceptible to injury from acids and luminal contents if it were not for the nonspecific protection provided by the mucus blanket (2). In addition, the gel also serves to protect the GI epithelium from mechanical damage by reducing shear stresses, serving to lubricate as well as aid in repair of the mucosal epithelium. Not only does the mucus gel protect against chemical insults, but it also provides a physical barrier against pathogens by containing binding sites for pathogens and resident flora while maintaining high concentrations of secretory immunoglobulin A (IgA; 3). Additionally, mucins act as nucleation sites for bile stones (4). Membrane-associated mucins may play a dual function in signaling cell-to-cell contact and possibly differentiation, as well as influencing cellular morphology, growth, tumor metastases, and recognition by the immune system.

Mucin plays a major role in infections of the GI tract by providing initial attachment sites for mucosal pathogens, allowing colonization and establishment of the organisms in the mucus layer. Many invading pathogens secrete

D. Moncada and K. Chadee: Institute of Parasitology of McGill University, Quebec, Canada

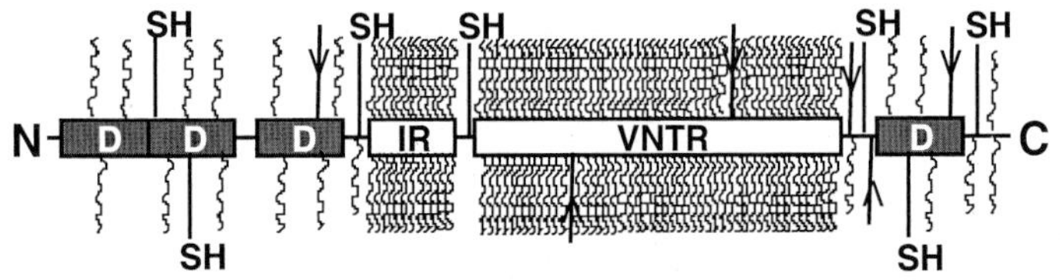

FIGURE 5.1. Hypothetical model of a MUC2 monomer. The heavily glycosylated mucin domains termed the irregular repeat (IR) region and the variable number tandem repeat (VNTR) region give mucin its bottle-brush–like appearance and protect the protein core from damage. The less glycosylated D-domains are rich in cysteine residues, forming intramolecular disulfide bonds and giving the carboxy and amino terminus a globular protein appearance. These unglycosylated regions are susceptible to damage. IR, irregular repeat; VNTR, variable number tandem repeat; D, von Willebrand factor–like domains; lines indicate areas of glycosylation. (Adapted from Gum JR Jr. Human mucin glycoproteins: varied structures predict diverse properties and specific functions. *Biochem Soc Trans* 1995;23:795–799.)

enzymes and putative mucin secretagogues that weaken the mucin barrier, facilitating access to the epithelial surface. Alternatively, mucins may prevent invading pathogens from gaining access to the mucosa by physically trapping and aiding in expulsion of the organisms. Goblet cells work in concert with other protective defenses of the GI tract by "flushing" out the offending organism. The ability of goblet cells to hypersecrete mucin, along with release of fluid from enterocytes, may aid in the rapid expulsion of pathogens. The fate of mucin-bound organisms depends on their ability to successfully colonize the intestinal tract. Most microorganisms are not able to colonize the mucin barrier and are sloughed away with peristaltic movements and expelled during defecation. In addition, nonpathogenic intestinal flora residing in the GI tract play an important role in preventing colonization of pathogens by occupying available microbial attachment sites. Alterations in the mucin barrier are most likely a contributing factor in the pathogenesis of many infections and disease states. An increase in mucin viscosity has been reported in such diseases as cystic fibrosis, inflammatory bowel disease, peptic ulcer, and chronic bronchitis, as well as trivial infections. The mechanisms leading to these altered mucin states and mucin-pathogen interactions are still poorly understood.

MORPHOLOGY AND PHYSIOLOGY OF GOBLET CELLS

Goblet Cell Morphology

The mucus layer is continually replenished by specialized cells, which produce large quantities of mucin and other components of the mucus blanket. These unique epithelial cells are termed *mucus* cells in the stomach and gallbladder, and *goblet* cells in the small and large intestine (5) (Fig. 5.2). Goblet cells function as exocrine cells and are specialized for the production and unidirectional transport of mucin to the lumen of the intestinal tract. These highly polarized columnar cells are the major mucus-producing cells in the small and large intestine. Goblet cells increase in number from the duodenum toward the ileum and are most numerous in the colon. These cells are able to store membrane-bound mucin granules in an intracellular compartment known as the *theca* (6). The apical cytoplasm is densely packed with numerous mucin granules, which constitute a major portion of the cell and fill the so-called cuplike region of the goblet cell. The mature mucin granules are tightly packed and separated from the plasma membrane and organelles by a thin layer of cytoplasm containing a complicated arrangement of cytoskeletal components making up the theca. By comparison, the mucin granules of mucus cells are not clearly separated from the rest of the cell, although they are apically located in the cell (7). Like other intestinal epithelial cells, goblet cells have microvilli on their apical surface but they are less predominant in comparison to absorptive cells. The basal area of the goblet cell displays the characteristic stem shape of a mature goblet cell (Fig. 5.3) and contains the mucin-producing machinery,

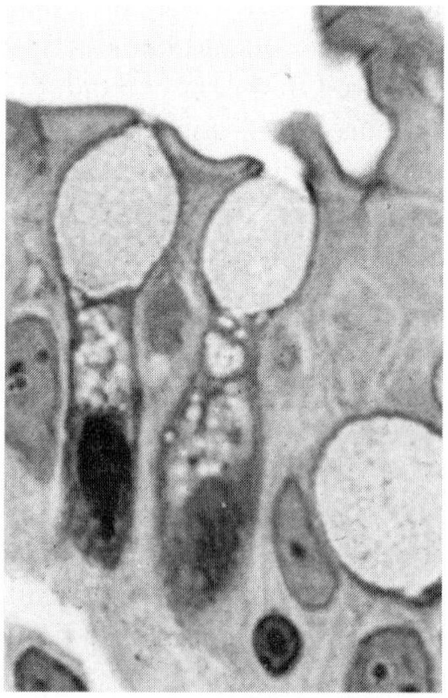

FIGURE 5.2. Light micrography of a colonic goblet cell. The nucleus resides in the basal aspect of the cell and is surrounded by basophilic cytoplasm. The supranuclear region appears lighter stained due to the presence of numerous condensing vacuoles and nascent granules. The upper region of the cell contains a tightly packed mass of mucin granules.

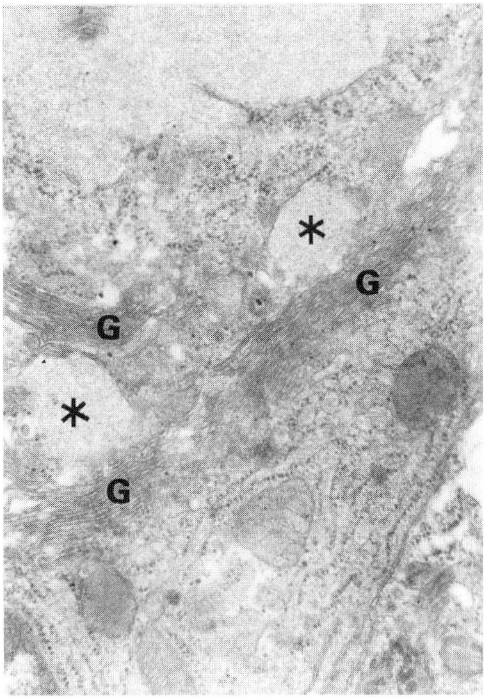

FIGURE 5.3. Transmission electron micrograph of a colonic goblet cell. Abundant RER is present surrounding the cell nucleus and along the periphery. The supranuclear region contains numerous Golgi stacks (G) and condensing vacuoles (*).

including the nucleus surrounded apically by the rough endoplasmic reticulum (ER) and Golgi complex. The cytoplasm surrounding the nucleus is highly basophilic as a result of the presence of free ribosomes (8). Newly formed mucin granules, which bud off of the trans region of the Golgi, are termed *condensing vacuoles* and mature granules are located in the theca (Fig. 5.3).

Goblet Cell Maturation and Changes in Cytoskeleton

Goblet cells undergo dramatic morphologic changes during their short lifespan of 3 to 5 days (Fig. 5.4*A*). Goblet cells arise by mitosis from pluripotent stem cells at the base of the crypt or poorly differentiated oligomucus cells in the lower third of the crypt having characteristics of both absorptive and goblet cells. Shortly after the cells arise, goblet cells start to synthesize and secrete mucin granules (Fig. 5.4*B*). Immature cells at the base of the crypt are large compared with mature goblet cells and they are pyramidal in shape and contain loosely organized organelles. The ER is located from the cell base to the apex. Elements of the Golgi apparatus are located primarily in the supranuclear region and mucin granules are scattered throughout the supranuclear and apical portions of the cell. During this early stage of their life, goblet cells have extensive contact with the basal lamina and make little contact with the lumen. The average volume of a typical goblet cell at this point is 1229 mm^3 (9). As the cells migrate upward from the crypt (Fig. 5.4*C*), the volume of the cells dramatically decreases as mucin granules are secreted and as cellular organelles and cytoplasm that are trapped between the densely packed mucin granules are shed. As the cells mature, they gain more access to the lumen and gradually lose contact with the basal lamina. The cellular organelles become more distinctly separated, although the cells are still pyramidal in shape compared with the mature goblet cell. Once the goblet cells have reached the top one-third of the villus, the apical portion of the cells become packed with mucin granules and the ER becomes more restricted to the basal and lateral portions of the cells. The Golgi can be easily distinguished in the supranuclear region. At the mouth of the crypt or the epithelial surface (Fig. 5.4*D*), the average cell volume decreases by 50% of its original volume, to 542 mm^3, with a corresponding decrease in the volume of organelles. The polarized goblet cell takes on the characteristic "goblet" shape, becoming elongated and having a narrow stemlike basal portion and a cuplike apical region packed with mature mucin granules. When the mature goblet cell reaches the tip of the villus or the surface of the colon, the cell loses all contact with the basal lamina and is sloughed off into the intestinal lumen, releasing all contents of the cell. Goblet cells continually produce mucin throughout their migration until they are sloughed away into the lumen (10).

Cytoarchitectural Organization

Dramatic morphologic changes occur in goblet cells because of their abundant cytoarchitectural reorganization that occurs during their migration upward toward the villus tip. These changes are most likely due, in part, to the baseline secretion of mucin, which results in a significant loss of goblet cell cytoplasm and cellular organelles (9). Once the mature goblet cell reaches the tip of the villus, it displays the typical goblet-shaped morphology. These cells are highly polarized and the cellular machinery is clearly organized and separated from the apical store of tightly packed mucin granules. The mucin granules are separated from the lateral plasma membrane and the Golgi apparatus by a dense network of filaments constituting the theca. The theca lies below the apical plasma membrane and is composed of intermediate filament (IF) bundles and microtubules intermeshed together in a basket-like structure. This network of keratin filaments is found from the cell base to the apex and confers the goblet shape of the cell. Neither loss of secretory granules nor elimination of other cellular components alters the mature goblet cell shape (11,12) (Fig. 5.5).A network of F-actin filaments forms the physical barrier between the granule mass and the apical plasma membrane, preventing contact of the mucin granules with the membrane inhibiting their release.

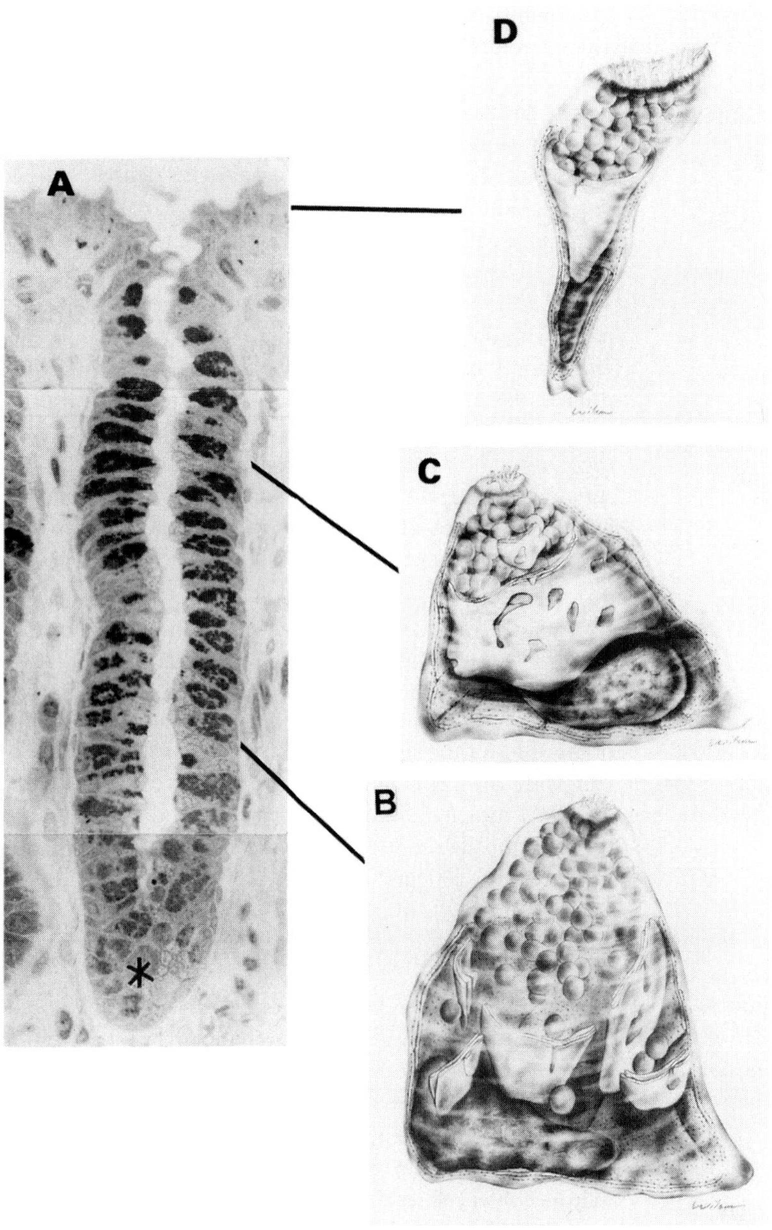

FIGURE 5.4. Maturation of colonic goblet cells during migration to the epithelial surface. **A:** Light micrograph of rabbit colonic crypt. The colonic crypt contains two predominant cell types: dark-staining goblet cells and light-staining vacuolated cells. Progenitor cells reside in the crypt base (*), and the crypt lumen communicates with the intestinal lumen that contacts the surface cells. **B:** Schematic representation of colonic goblet cell in the lower one-third of the crypt. The cell demonstrates a pyramidal shape with little luminal contact. The RER is spread throughout the cell and numerous Golgi stacks are present. These elements intermingle with the mucin secretory granules filling the cytoplasm. **C:** Schematic representation of colonic goblet cell in the upper one-third of the crypt. The cell remains pyramidal but has reduced its cell volume. RER is concentrating along the basolateral aspects of the cell. The Golgi stacks are coalescing centrally in the cell, and the mucin granules are becoming more tightly packed. **D:** Schematic representation of colonic goblet cell on the epithelial surface. The basal region of the cell has narrowed, and luminal contact is greater than basal luminal contact. The organelles have become well ordered; the Golgi apparatus has coalesced in the supranuclear region, and the RER surrounds the nucleus and Golgi along the periphery of the cell. The apical granule mass is tightly packed. (From Schmidt GH, Wilkinson MM, Ponder BAJ. Cell migration pathway in the intestinal epithelium: an *in situ* marker system using mouse aggregation chimeras. *Cell* 1985;40:425–429, with permission.)

Goblet cells from the human colon produce a heterogeneous population of mucins that can be separated into different species using ion-exchange chromatography (13). In addition, histochemical analysis has revealed that changes in the chemical composition of goblet cell mucin also occur as the cell migrates toward the villus tip (14). The sialic acid content of mucin increases in cells as they migrate from the crypt to the villus. The sialic acid residues are potential sites for further *N*- and *O*-acetylation. Differences in mucin content have been observed in goblet cells throughout the length of the colon.

Unregulated/Baseline Secretion

Under normal physiological conditions, goblet cells continually synthesize and secrete mucins that are not stored in the apical granule mass to replenish the mucus blanket covering the epithelium. This continual secretion is necessary to maintain the thickness of the mucus gel, which is constantly exposed to acids and irritants in addition to being sloughed away via peristaltic movements (15). The release of newly formed mucin granules during unregulated (baseline) secretion in not a receptor-mediated event. Mucosal

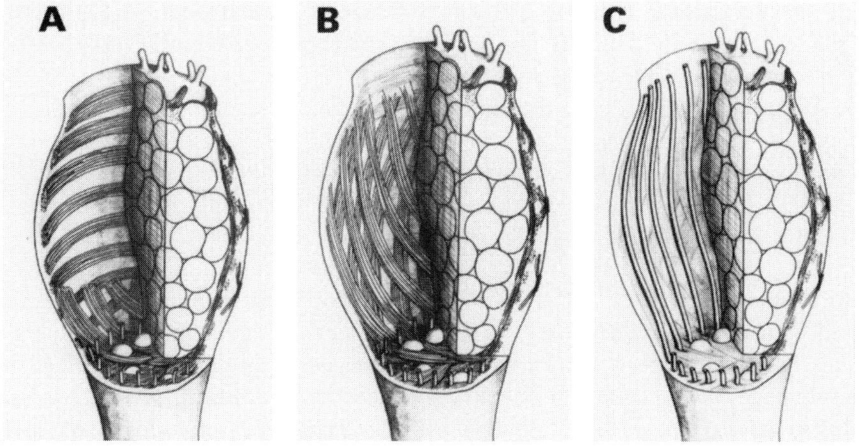

FIGURE 5.5. Schematic representation of the theca of a colonic goblet cell. **A:** The outermost layer of the theca consists of intermediate filament bundles that girdle the granule mass. **B:** The middle layer is comprised of IFs that spiral around the apical granule mass like a basket and delimit the face of the theca. **C:** The inner layer consists of vertically oriented MTs immediately adjacent to the peripherial mucin granules. The MTs arise below the theca and cross the intermediate filament network at the base of the theca. (From Phillips TE, Phillips TL, Neutra MR. Regulation of intestinal goblet cell secretion. III. Isolated intestinal epithelium. *Am J Physiol* 1984;247:G674–G681, with permission.)

explants of human and rat colon have been shown to continually incorporate radiolabeled mucin precursors into mucus glycoproteins (16). Following synthesis, labeled mucins are then packaged into granules, transported to the cell surface, and secreted into the lumen. Stored mucin granules are thought to play a role in unregulated secretion in that there is evidence for incorporation of newly formed mucins into storage granules (17). Little is known about the mechanism of unregulated secretion; however, it is dependent upon continuous transport of mucin granules from the Golgi vesicles to the cell surface, and movement of granules within the cell is a microtubule-dependent event (18). Baseline granule turnover is a result of the movement of newly synthesized mucin granules along the periphery of the theca to the apical plasma membrane for exocytosis. Microtubules play a major role in baseline secretion by maintaining the orderly movement of mucin granules from the Golgi to the apex of the cell. Monensin, which disrupts Golgi function, was found to almost completely inhibit baseline secretion in the colonic adenocarcinoma cell line LS180 (19). Nocodazole, a potent inhibitor of microtubule assembly, was also found to significantly inhibit baseline mucin secretion (20,21). These studies suggest that baseline secretion is entirely a result of newly synthesized mucin being transported from the Golgi to the cell surface with the assistance of microtubules.

Mucin granules are prevented from making contact with the apical plasma membrane by an actin cytoskeleton. Treatment of goblet cells with cytochalasin D, which disrupts the layer of F-actin filaments overlying the apical granule mass, was shown to cause a significant increase in baseline secretion of newly formed mucin granules, but had no effect on the release of stored mucin, implicating the involvement of actin filaments in baseline exocytosis (12). Therefore, baseline secretion of mucin granules from goblet cells is dependent upon their access to the plasma membrane. On the other hand, stored granules are thought to participate in accelerated exocytosis through a mechanism independent to baseline secretion (22).

Accelerated/Regulated Secretion

When goblet cells are exposed to a potential mucus secretagogue, mucin is released in an accelerated fashion (23,24) by either (a) the release of centrally stored mucin granules followed by compound exocytosis of granules and release of peripheral granules resulting in the cavitation of the deep apical membrane or (b) the release of a single mucin granule one at a time (11,25).

Mucus secretagogues induce a rapid increase in the number of mucin granules released from the goblet cell; a maximum rate of exocytosis is established after 1 to 3 minutes of stimulation, followed by a much slower release of mucin granules (26). Depletion of mucin stores take between 5 and 15 minutes. Crypt goblet cells respond more strongly to acetylcholine or cholinomimetic agents than do cells on the villi or colonic surface (11,27–30). A number of compounds elicit GI mucin secretion. Neurotransmitters, lipid and inflammatory mediators, and chemical agents all release mucin from stored pools. Cholinergic agents such as carbachol, acetylcholine, and pilocarpine have been shown to increase GI mucin secretion *in vivo* (27) and in mucosal explants (31). The purinergic agonist adenosine triphosphate increases the rate of mucin exocytosis from the same granule pool as cholinergic secretagogues (32). Several studies using mucus-secreting colonic cell lines have reported that vasoactive peptide (VIP; 25), nitric oxide (33), interleukin-1 (IL-1; 28, 34), prostaglandin E_2 (PGE_2; 35), and macrophage/monocyte and neutrophil derived secretagogues all stimulate mucin exocytosis (36).

Regulated/accelerated mucin secretion is linked to a receptor-mediated event. The arachidonic acid metabolite PGE_2 was shown to bind to the EP4 receptor to stimulate cyclic adenosine monophosphate ([cAMP]i)-dependent mucin exocytosis in LS174T cells (35,37). Similarly, PGD_2 evokes mucin secretion in LS174T cells via the DP receptor (38). Mucin secretagogues are known to signal through various secondary messengers such as intracellular Ca^{2+} ([Ca^{2+}]i), cAMP, and diacylglycerol for activation of protein kinase C (6,39) to stimulate mucin secretion (40). Many other biological macromolecules are linked to mucin secretion, such as the proteases, elastin, and chymotrypsin. Even some food constituents and their fermentation products have been shown to cause an increase in mucin secretion in the rat colon, including glucuronic acid, galacturonic acid (fibers), and the short chain fatty acids acetate and butyrate (41). A summary of the major mucin secretagogues and their modes of action are listed in Table 5.1. More extensive reviews on mucin secretion, secretagogues, and their mechanisms are provided in references 6, 17, 31, and 42 to 51.

Mucin Secretion in Response to Gastrointestinal Pathogens

The mucus blanket is the first line of host defense against invading GI pathogens. Goblet cells are responsible for maintaining the mucus blanket and are known to respond to various luminal pathogens and their products through an increase in mucus secretion. (43–51). This rapid secretion is thought to bestow an important mechanism of protection by trapping and flushing out intestinal pathogens. Bacteria and their toxins and end products are known to have a potent secretagogue effect on goblet cells; for example, in addition to causing severe diarrhea in humans, *Vibrio cholerae* enterotoxin was shown to markedly increase mucin secretion in the rat small intestine, colon, and HT-29 cells (52,53). The bacillus *Yersinia enterocolitica* is linked to an increase in mucin secretion in rabbit distal small intestine and the proximal colon (54). Perhaps the best example illustrating mucin-pathogen interactions may be observed during infection with the enteric protozoan parasite *Entamoeba histolytica*. The parasite colonizes the colon by binding galactose (Gal) and *N*-acetylgalactosamine (GalNAc) residues of colonic mucins and is known to evoke the release of LS174T cell mucins through protein kinase C activation (55) (Table 5.1). Not only do goblet cells respond to *E. histolytica* by secreting mucins, but the parasite also stimulates the release of both preformed and newly synthesized mucins (59), as well as both neutral and acidic mucin species (60). This rapid secretion does not result in expulsion of the parasite but may result in depletion of the mucus blanket at a rate that exceeds regeneration, allowing

TABLE 5.1. GASTROINTESTINAL MUCIN SECRETAGOGUES

Secretagogue	Second Messenger/Kinase	Receptor-mediated	Tissue/Cell Line	References
Dibutyryl cAMP	$[cAMP]_i$[a]	No	HT29	53
Forskolin	$[cAMP]_i$	No	HT29, T84, LS174T	39, 53
Cholera toxin	$[cAMP]_i$	No	HT29, rat small intestine and colon	45, 46, 52, 53
Vasoactive intestinal peptide	$[cAMP]_i$[b]	Yes	HT29, T84	39, 49
Serotonin	$[cAMP]_i$[b]	Yes	Rat small intestine	50
PGD_2	$[cAMP]_i$[b]	Yes	LS174T, colon	38, 39
PGE_2	$[cAMP]_i$[b]	Yes	Rabbit and rat gastric cells, rat colon, HT29, T84, LS174T	40, 48, 49, 35
Carbachol	$[Ca^{2+}]_i$	Yes	HT29, T84	39, 51
Neurotensin	$[Ca^{2+}]_i$	Yes	HT29	51
Ionophores	$[Ca^{2+}]_i$	No	HT29, T84, LS174T, LS180	18, 39, 55–58
Phorbol ester	PKC[c]	No	HT29, T84, LS174T, LS180	18, 38, 55

[a]Membrane permeable $[cAMP]_i$ mimetic.
[b]Based on the second messenger that the receptor activates.
[c]Phorbol esters mimic the second messenger diacylglycerol and directly activate protein kinase C.
Adapted from Belley A, Keller K, Goettke, et al. Intestinal mucins in colonization and host defense against pathogens. *Am J Trop Med Hyg Suppl* 1999;60:10–15.

the parasite to gain access to the colonic epithelium. Infection with *Helicobacter pylori* is associated with depletion of the gastric mucus barrier, but instead of causing mucin hypersecretion, the organism inhibits mucin biosynthesis (61). The thiol-activated exotoxin produced by the gram-positive facultative intracellular pathogen *Listeria monocytogenes* (62) has been shown to be an agonist of mucus secretion on HT29-MTX cells. Ironically, pathogens can cause a depletion of the mucus blanket, either inducing hypersecretion of stored mucin pools or decreasing mucin biosynthesis. This may be a novel strategy by which intestinal pathogens gain access to the underlying epithelial cells.

OTHER PRODUCTS PRODUCED BY GOBLET CELLS

Interactions between the Trefoil Factor Family of Proteins and Mucin

In addition to producing mucin, goblet cells also produce other important proteins. Trefoil factors are a family of small peptides expressed and secreted along the length of the GI tract and are implicated in the process of epithelial restitution following mucosal injury. The trefoil family is made up of the intestinal peptide TFF3 and the gastric peptides TFF1 and TFF2. These protease-resistant peptides share several structural features, including a distinctive motif of six cysteine residues termed *trefoil domains* (P domain), which contribute to the formation of intrachain loops. In addition, free cysteine residues in some trefoil peptides contribute to homodimerization or heterodimerization of the peptides (63). Mammalian family trefoil factor proteins contain one or two of these P domains (64). Evidence for coexpression of mucin and trefoil peptides has been suggested. TFF1 is expressed throughout the foveolar epithelial surface cells and stomach (65). TFF2 is expressed mainly in the distal stomach, the duodenum, and acini of Brunner glands (66). In addition, TFF3 (ITF) is expressed specifically by goblet cells along the length of the small and large intestines and colon (67,68). As trefoil factors colocalize with mucin, they may work in concert in repairing and protecting the GI mucosa. ITF was found to contain goblet cell–specific promoter elements and is specifically expressed by rat goblet cells (64). TFF1 was shown to interact with the cysteine-rich von Willebrand factor (VWF) C D-domains of MUC2 and MUC5AC in the murine model (69). These findings confirm the interaction between trefoil peptides and mucins and it was hypothesized that this interaction may help stabilize the mucus gel, in addition to playing a role in mucosal repair. Indeed, trefoil factors have been shown to promote epithelial restitution after injury, helping to maintain epithelial barrier function. Interestingly, trefoil factors and mucus glycoproteins together were shown to be far more effective at protecting epithelial cells *in vitro* when compared with either one individually (70). Mice deficient in ITF exhibited an increased sensitivity to intestinal damage. However, mice that overexpressed TFF1 in the jejunum were more resistant to mucosal injury in that area of the GI tract (71). Trefoil peptides were also suggested to play a role in tumor suppression, in that antropyloric adenoma and intramucosal or intraepithelial carcinomas develop in TFF1-deficient mice (67,72,73). However, there is still no general agreement on the mode of action of trefoil peptides on epithelial cells, although there is evidence that ITF activates the epidermal growth factor (EGF) receptor by an indirect mechanism (74).

Other bioregulatory peptides in addition to trefoil peptides are produced by goblet cells. Two serine proteases have been localized to goblet cells, the first, ingobsin, is produced by goblet cells in human and rat duodenum; release is stimulated by acetylcholine and vasoactive peptide (75). In contrast, the serine protease kallikrein is localized to and secreted by goblet cells of the human colon and cells of the pancreas and kidney. Colon kallikrein is identical to tissue kallikrein and is most likely transcribed from the tissue kallikrein gene (76). The biological function for these proteases in the GI tract is not yet understood, but there is speculation that they may play bactericidal roles in addition to regulating the thickness of the mucus layer via degradation of mucin.

STRUCTURE OF GASTROINTESTINAL MUCINS

Peptide Core

The peptide core of mucin ranges in size from approximately 1,500 to more than 5,000 amino acids in composition. The polypeptide backbone provides numerous sites for the addition of *O*-linked oligosaccharides through an abundance of serine, threonine, and proline residues. The amino acid composition of mucin contributes to only approximately 20% of the dry weight of a typical secretory mucin molecule and the remainder of the protein is composed of *O*-linked and *N*-linked oligosaccharides and a small percentage of sulfate residues. There are 11 recognized epithelial mucins in humans: MUC1, MUC2, MUC3, MUC4, MUC5AC, MUC5B, MUC6, MUC7, MUC8, MUC11, and MUC12. Evidence suggests that MUC3 mucin is transcribed from two different genes termed *MUC3A* and *MUC3B* although the gene products are not yet characterized (77). There is speculation that MUC3 may be present in the GI tract as a predominant membrane-bound form in addition to a minor soluble secreted form, making the classification of MUC3 as a secreted or membrane-bound mucin difficult. Reported mucin complementary DNA (cDNA) sequences are often incomplete because of their repetitive nature and the large size of the mRNAs. The complete cDNAs are available for secreted human GI mucins MUC2 (78,79) and MUC5AC (80, 81).

The complete cDNA sequence is available for the salivary mucin MUC7 (82), and partial cDNA sequences for GI mucins MUC5B (83), MUC3 (84), and MUC6 (85) are also available. Interestingly, MUC3 was found to contain one EGF-like domain and the putative function of this domain is not currently known (86). The complete cDNA sequences have also been cloned for membrane-bound mucins MUC1 (87) and MUC4 (88). The *C*-terminus of MUC4 contains two EGF-like domains and a transmembrane domain, although these mucins may not significantly contribute to the mucus gel, their biological functions are still under investigation and they may play a role in cytoprotection.

Advancements in the discovery and cloning of mucins have revealed several characteristics common among these molecules. Intestinal apomucins contain common structural domains, including a series of tandem repeats rich in threonine and proline and often serine residues. These mucin domains often contain numerous amino acid repeats and provide a scaffold for abundant *O*-glycosylation. These highly glycosylated domains take on a rodlike, extended conformation due to the presence of numerous oligosaccharides and proline residues. In addition, the amino and carboxyl terminal ends of secreted GI mucins are rich in cysteine residues, which play a role in polymerization and formation of the mucus gel. Salivary mucin MUC7 is devoid of cysteine-rich regions. The cysteine-rich flanking regions in secretory GI mucins contain D-domains sharing similarity to the D-domains in von Willebrand factor (VWF).

One of the most well studied and characterized GI mucins is MUC2. MUC2 is the major secretory mucin produced by goblet cells of the small and large intestines and is the predominant gel forming mucin. The structure of MUC2 is illustrated in Figure 5.1, at least 90% of *MUC2* alleles encode for a protein consisting of more than 5000 amino acid residues. The MUC2 apoprotein contains two mucin domains termed the variable number tandem repeat (VNTR) composed mainly of threonine and proline and an irregular repeat region (IR) rich in serine, threonine and proline residues. The VNTR is composed of a series of 23 amino acid repeats and provides several potential sites for *O*-linked glycosylation. The IR is composed of a 347-amino acid domain, providing several *O*-linked glycosylation sites that contribute to the domain's resistance to chemical and proteolytic damage (1). The amino terminus of MUC2 flanking the IR region contains three cysteine rich D-domains and the carboxyl terminal end of MUC2 flanking the VNTR possesses one cysteine rich D-domain. These regions are involved in the polymerization of MUC2 monomers into the characteristic large secretory mucin polymers. Potential *N*-linked glycosylation sites are also dispersed throughout the molecule, although much less prominent than *O*-linked oligosaccharides.

Amino Terminal End

There are several cysteine rich domains found in human secreted mucins, excluding MUC7. These domains are often at the terminal regions of mucin molecules and share a high sequence similarity in the position of the cysteines with VWF. These regions are also named similarly to the D-domains of VWF, termed *D1, D2*, and *D3*. In addition, a partial D′ domain is located between the D2 and D3 in all VWF-like secreted mucins as well as in VWF (89). Secretory mucins often contain three *N*-terminal flanking VWF-like domains as depicted in Figure 5.1 for MUC2. In addition, these regions may have as many as 30 cysteine residues involved in the assembly of mucins into multimers by the formation of disulfide bonds. All cysteine residues in VWF are thought to participate in intermolecular or intramolecular disulfide bond formation (89). The *N*-terminal of MUC2 and other mucins contains sites for potential *N*-linked glycosylation, which is essential in the proper processing and transport of mucins (90,91).

Carboxyl Terminal End

The C-terminal regions of most secreted mucins contain a single D domain that is rich in cysteine residues aligning similarly with those of the VWF domains. Most secreted mucins contain one C-terminal D-domain, termed *D4,* in keeping with the naming in order from N- to C-terminus. The carboxyl terminal D-domain of mucin most likely takes on the structure of a globular protein and is highly homologous to the cysteine knot motif family of proteins (91,92). It is believed that all available thiols participate in either intermolecular or intramolecular disulfide bond formation in a similar fashion to those in VWF (89). Sites for *N*-glycosylation may also be present in this region. On the other hand, there are little or no potential sites for *O*-linked glycosylation. Dimerization and subsequent polymerization of mucin is thought to occur in a similar fashion as VWF, through the C-terminal by a "tail-to-tail" assembly. Reducing agents disrupt the polymeric structure by breaking the intermolecular disulfide bonds between mucin molecules, although reduction insensitive bonds have been identified (1). MUC2 has a unique C-terminal region. Exposure of MUC2 mucin to reducing agents results in the release of a 118-kDa peptide from the C-terminus. Even though this reduction product of MUC2 was previously thought to be a link peptide, further analysis revealed the sequence to be part of the C-terminal peptide core. Proteolytic degradation of MUC2 mucin may release this peptide under normal conditions and this fragment may remain attached via disulfide bonds (92). The liberation of a 118-kDa peptide and other mucin glycopeptide fragments has been observed to occur during mucin purification. To explain these observations, there has been recent speculation that MUC2 possesses autoproteolytic activity or, alternatively, intestinal proteases may remain strongly associated with mucins during purification.

Membrane-bound mucins contain a unique C-terminal tail, which differs from secreted mucins. In addition to a cysteine-rich domain, membrane-bound mucins may possess putative transmembrane domains as well as one or more EGF-like domains, whose functions are still unknown (88,93,94).

Tandem Repeats

Epithelial mucins are characterized by their tandem repeat (TR) domains (Fig. 5.1), which can comprise more than 50% of the apomucin. The TRs provide sites for *O*-glycosylation; however, the content and order of threonine, proline, and serine residues influences the actual extent of oligosaccharide density. MUC1 contains less serine and threonine residues when compared with MUC5AC and, as a consequence, has less glycosylation sites available. In contrast, MUC2 TRs contain a greater concentration of threonine residues and therefore are more densely glycosylated. The 23 amino acid TRs of MUC2 contain 14 threonine residues, which have been reported to be glycosylated up to 78% in LS174T cells (95). The extent of glycosylation can have a dramatic effect on the physical properties of mucin and the TR can influence the rigidity and gel-forming properties of mucin, depending on the availability of glycosylation sites. The sequence of the repeat may vary between different mucins depending on the function of the molecule, but repeats from all mucins are known to contain threonine, proline, and serine residues. The size of the repeats have been reported to range from eight amino acids in MUC5AC to as many as 164 amino acids in MUC6 (96,97). The TR of various secretory mucins are depicted in Table 5.2. The presence of proline residues within these repeats appears to be important in determining the specificity of the polypeptide *N*-acetyl-galactosaminyltransferases (GalNAc transferases) catalyzing *O*-linked oligosaccharide addition. The six or seven flanking amino acids around the target hydroxy amino acid influence its acceptor function (98,99), especially proline at the position +3, favoring glycosylation of threonine.

Many tumor mucins show glycosylation patterns different from those of noncancerous cells. Several cancer-associated mucins, including breast, ovary, and colon tumor mucins (100) show marked changes in membrane-bound epithelial mucin MUC1 antigen. Antibodies specific to apomucin tandem repeat peptides usually do not react strongly with the mature mucin molecule because of the masking of the epitopes by oligosaccharides. However, mucins produced by tumors often undergo incomplete or truncated glycosylation of the tandem repeats (101,102), and, therefore, new epitopes become unmasked. These tumor-associated mucins are potential markers for cancer and there is good evidence that portions of these mucins will allow a directed approach to the development of a vaccine for the induction of immunity against tumors positive for cancer-associated mucins (103–105). Identification of newly exposed epitopes of the mucin tandem repeats in tumors may have diagnostic and immunotherapeutic significance.

Polymorphisms

Theoretically, mucins are the most polymorphic of all the biological macromolecules produced by eukaryotic organisms. They are even more polymorphic than immunoglobulin and T-cell receptors, resulting from the abundant potential sites for *O*-linked glycosylation and the numerous possibilities for unique and extended oligosaccharide chain combinations. Mucin genes exhibit genetic polymorphism and there are allelic variations between individuals. As a consequence, there are different protein isoforms. Polymorphism in the VNTR regions are a common feature of most mucins and there is a high level of genetically determined polymorphism due to variations in the number of copies of these tandem repeated sequences (VNTR). The TR sequences may undergo deletions or insertions through unequal sister chromatid exchange or unequal crossover, which can lead to highly polymorphic VNTRs containing more or less repeats for a given allele compared with the ancestral sequence (106). Interestingly, the secretory

TABLE 5.2. TANDEM REPEATS OF SECRETORY GASTROINTESTINAL MUCINS

Mucin	Repeat Sequence	Number of Residues
MUC2	PTTTPITTTTTVTPTPTPTGTQT	23
MUC3	HSTPSFTSSITTTETTS	17
MUC5AC	TTSTTSAP	23
MUC5B	SSTPGTAHTLTVLTTTATTPTATGSTATP	29
MUC6	SPFSSTGPMTATSFQTTTTYPTPSHPQTTLP THVPPFSTSLVTPSTGTVITPTHAQMATSAS IHSTPTGTIPPPTTLKATGSTHTAPPMTPTTS GYSQAHSSTSTAAKTSTSLHSHTSSTHHPEV TPTSTTTITPNPTSTGTSTPVAHTT	164
MUC7	TTAAPPTPSATTPAPPSSSAPPE	23

mucins MUC2 and MUC6 show an incredible degree of polymorphism in the VNTR region, with up to a twofold difference in length of the coding sequence and subsequently an increase in protein size (107). In contrast, MUC5B does not show any common allele length variation. Variations in the length of secreted mucin molecules could have a significant impact on the properties of the mucus gel.

Polymorphism in VNTR regions of genes encoding for biological molecules, excluding mucins, are linked with many abnormalities (108). Currently, there is little evidence linking mucin VNTR polymorphism with disease, although one study has found a significant increase in frequency of the longer MUC2 allele in nonasthmatic subjects when compared with asthmatics (109). There is also a report suggesting a possible link between a so-called rare VNTR allele of MUC3 with genetic predisposition to ulcerative colitis (106).

EXPRESSION AND REGULATION OF MUCIN GENES

The genes of several human-secreted mucins have been located to chromosome 11p15.5 (107). Both *MUC2* and *MUC5AC* have been mapped to this chromosome as well as *MUC5B* and *MUC6*, and there is reason to believe that these mucins may have a common ancestral gene (110). The secretory mucin MUC7 significantly differs structurally from other secretory mucins and the gene encoding it is located on chromosome 4q13-21. The gene encoding membrane-bound mucin MUC1 is located on chromosome 1q21-24, MUC3 on 7q22, and MUC4 on 3q29. Expression of specific mucin genes is relatively organ and cell specific. The tissue/cell distribution of secretory mucin expression is summarized in Table 5.3 In the normal stomach, *MUC6* is expressed in the mucus neck cells as well as the antral glands and *MUC5AC* is expressed at the surface/foveolar epithelium (111). In addition, *MUC5B* is primarily expressed in the gallbladder and pancreas and, to a lesser extent, in the colon (112). *MUC2* and *MUC3* are the most prominent mucin genes expressed in the human intestines. *MUC2* is constitutively expressed throughout the length of the intestines by goblet cells and is the major gel-forming mucin in the intestines (113). Goblet cells as well as columnar cells express *MUC3*, although it is more localized to the surface epithelium of the colon and the villus compartments of the small intestine (114). Expression of *MUC2* is almost completely specific to goblet cells and expression begins deep in the crypts, as would be expected since mucin production starts early in the development of a goblet cell. The 5′-flanking region of the *MUC2* gene has been identified and has been shown to have promoter activity in cultured cells as well as *in vivo* through the construction of transgenic mice containing a portion of the 5′-flanking region fused to a reporter gene (115,116). These studies suggest that differential expression of *MUC2* in the colon and small intestines is dependent on different regulatory elements within the 5′-promoter sequence of *MUC2*. It was speculated that *MUC3* expression might be related to the maturation of intestinal epithelial cells.

Transcriptional and Posttranscriptional Regulation of MUC2

In contrast to secretagogue-induced release of stored mucin granules, the constitutive release of mucins involves the translocation of newly synthesized mucins budding from the *trans*-Golgi face to the apical membrane to be secreted. This process is dependent upon the rate of synthesis and therefore gene expression (i.e., an increase in the transcriptional rate increases constitutive secretion). It seems plausible that increased *MUC2* gene expression may translate to increased secretion of MUC2, but, in contrast, it may be a mechanism whereby the cell replenishes its stored mucin pool quickly following exocytosis. Few studies have

TABLE 5.3. TISSUE DISTRIBUTION OF HUMAN SECRETED MUCINS

Mucin	Tissue/Cell Distribution
MUC2	Small and large intestine (goblet cells), salivary gland ducts, inferior turbinates
MUC3[a,b]	Jejunum, ileum, colon, gallbladder, goblet cells, and absorptive cells of intestine
MUC5AC	Colon (goblet cells), superficial stomach epithelium, bronchus (mucus glands and ciliated epithelium), inferior turbinates, endocervical epithelium
MUC5B	Submandibular glands, salivary glands, gallbladder (billiary epithelial cells), bronchus (mucus and serous glands), colon (goblet cells), endocervical epithelium, inferior turbinates (submucosal glands)
MUC6	Small and large intestine (goblet cells), gallbladder epithelium, stomach (mucus neck cells, antral mucus cells), seminal vesicle, pancreas (centroacinar cells and ducts), endocervical epithelium, endometrial epithelium, biliary epithelial cells
MUC7	Salivary glands (mucus cells), bronchial airways (submucosal glands), inferior turbinates (submucosal glands)

[a]Reports of both membrane and secreted forms produced by alternative splicing (84).
[b]Evidence for two genes encoding for MUC3 termed *MUC3A* and *MUC3B* (77).
Adapted from Perez-Vilar J, Hill RL. The structure and assembly of secreted mucins. *J Biol Chem* 1999;274:31751–31754.

addressed how *MUC2* is regulated transcriptionally and posttranscriptionally. Alterations in mucin gene expression have been noted in various disease states, including cystic fibrosis. Upregulation of the *MUC2* gene occurs in the airways of cystic fibrosis patients in response to the pathogen *Pseudomonas aeruginosa*. Lipopolysaccharide from *P. aeruginosa* has been shown to increase the expression of *MUC2* in transient transfection experiments employing the *MUC2* promoter (117). Subsequent studies revealed that *P. aeruginosa* promotes NF-κB binding to the NF-κB site at -1452 to -1441 of the *MUC2* promoter (118). Exoproducts from the bacterium were shown to increase expression of the airway mucin gene, *MUC5AC* (81). In addition, tumor necrosis factor-α (TNF-α) was shown to stimulate hypersecretion of MUC2 from human airway organ cultures and the human pulmonary mucoepidermoid carcinoma cell line NCI-H292 with accumulation of *MUC2* mRNA (119). The $[cAMP]_i$–elevating agent forskolin and the protein kinase C–activating agent 12-O-tetradecanoylphorbol-13-acetate, also caused the accumulation of *MUC2* mRNA but did not initiate transcription in human colonic HT29 cells differentiated *in vitro* to the goblet cell lineage (120). In contrast, other studies have revealed that activation of protein kinase C induces *MUC2* mRNA gene transcription (121). Cholera toxin, a $[cAMP]_i$–elevating agent, not only increased mucin secretion but caused the accumulation of *MUC2* mRNAs in HT-29 Cl.16E cells (53).

CARBOHYDRATE STRUCTURE

N-linked Oligosaccharides

N-linked oligosaccharides are present in most mucins, although they comprise only a small percent of the total carbohydrates present on mucin. These carbohydrates are mostly confined to the *N*- and *C*-terminal regions of the mucin molecule. Experiments using LS174T cells treated with tunicamycin, a potent inhibitor of *N*-linked glycosylation, revealed the importance of *N*-glycosylation in the synthesis of the MUC2 apomucin (37). Despite the lack of *N*-glycans, MUC2 monomers are able to form dimers in the ER but the rate of dimerization is delayed. There is a high probability that *N*-glycosylation may be important in mediating proper folding and disulfide bond formation in the MUC2 apomucin. In addition, the successful transfer of mucin dimers to the Golgi for further processing was also found to be dependent on *N*-linked glycosylation of mucin in the ER (91). In MUC2, there are several consensus sequences for potential *N*-glycosylation sites (asnX-ser/thr) and some of these sites are known to be occupied, although it is unknown whether all available sites are glycosylated. Few compositional or structural details concerning the *N*-linked branches in mucin are known, although at least some of them in rat and human intestinal mucins must have exposed oligomannosyl residues, based on their recognition of *Escherichia coli* type 1 (mannose sensitive) pili. (122).

O-Linked Oligosaccharides

The incorporation of *O*-linked oligosaccharides into mucins occurs following *N*-glycosylation and disulfide linked dimer formation (92). The functions of *O*-glycans are diverse and include maintaining protein conformation, controlling active epitopes and antigenicity, and acting as binding sites for microbes. The most prominent mucin oligosaccharides are of the *O*-glycan type. *O*-glycans are attached to the apomucin peptide TRs via an *O*-glycosidic linkage between the first carbon of GalNAc and the hydroxyl oxygen of threonine or serine. It is possible that these linkages are further stabilized, and the chains oriented with respect to the peptide, by a hydrogen bond between the amide group of GalNAc and the carbonyl oxygen of the threonine or serine (123). The addition of GalNAc serves to "stiffen" the TR domain of the peptide core in an extended conformation (124,125). GalNAc residues are important in maintaining a highly extended random coil configuration of mucin, and removal of the mucin oligosaccharide branches results in the denaturation and collapse of the molecule (124,126). These mucin-bound carbohydrates also have a large water-holding capacity, which allows for hydration of the mucin molecule. Although *O*-glycans are tightly packed side by side in the central TRs (Fig. 5.1), not all serine and threonine residues are necessarily glycosylated, and the carbohydrate chains may exist as clusters, possibly exposing regions of the TR to damage (126,127). A consensus sequence for the addition of GalNAc has not yet been found, although predicted algorithms do exist. Proline residues are responsible for breaking helix formation and instead may promote the formation of β sheets, and *O*-glycosylation is thought to occur at these predicted β turns. Alanine, serine, and threonine are often found adjacent to *O*-glycosylated residues and apparently charge distribution is the more major factor compared with actual charge (128). Studies conducted to predict glycosylation patterns in MUC2 mucin have been performed using synthetic peptides representing various sequences of the VNTR of MUC2. These peptides were incubated with LS174T cell microsome fractions to determine the maximum incorporation of GalNAc into threonine residues and it was revealed that maximum incorporation occurred in peptides containing consecutive threonine residues (129).

O-glycans contain GalNAc, *N*-acetylglucosamine (GlcNAc), fucose, galactose, and sialic acid. MUC2 contains 21 separate oligosaccharide groups including 10 acidic and 11 neutral structures ranging in chain length size from two to 12 sugars. Many of these may represent minor variations of a basic biantennary structure (130). Several hundreds of different *O*-glycan structures have been described in mucins, made possible by variations in linkage (α or β) and degree of branching, which amplify their potential to generate numerous recognition sites for lectins, viral, bacterial, or parasite adhesins. The carbohydrate composition of mucins are heterogeneous and vary in different regions of the intestine, even among different mucus cells of the same organ, such as the deep superficial mucus cells of the stomach (131) or the crypt and surface goblet cells of the colon (132). A detailed review of mucin oligosaccharide structure is provided in reference 133.

The initiating event of *O*-glycosylation is the addition of the monosaccharide GalNAc (from UDP-GalNAc) to serine or threonine residues. *O*-glycan synthesis is simpler than *N*-glycan synthesis because it does not use a lipid-linked oligosaccharide precursor for transfer of the oligosaccharide to the apomucin. When GalNAc is transferred to serine or threonine of the nascent peptide, the Tn antigen structure is formed (Fig. 5.6). This addition is catalyzed by a polypeptide GalNAc transferase (GalNAcT). There are several GalNAcTs expressed in various tissues. GalNAcT-1 expression seems to be widespread and abundant in human and other vertebrate cells and there are at least eight polypeptide GalNAcT genes, which are generally expressed in specific tissues and cell types. Specificity for glycosylation by GalNAcTs is regulated both by the enzyme source (organs) and by the apomucin sequence (134,135).

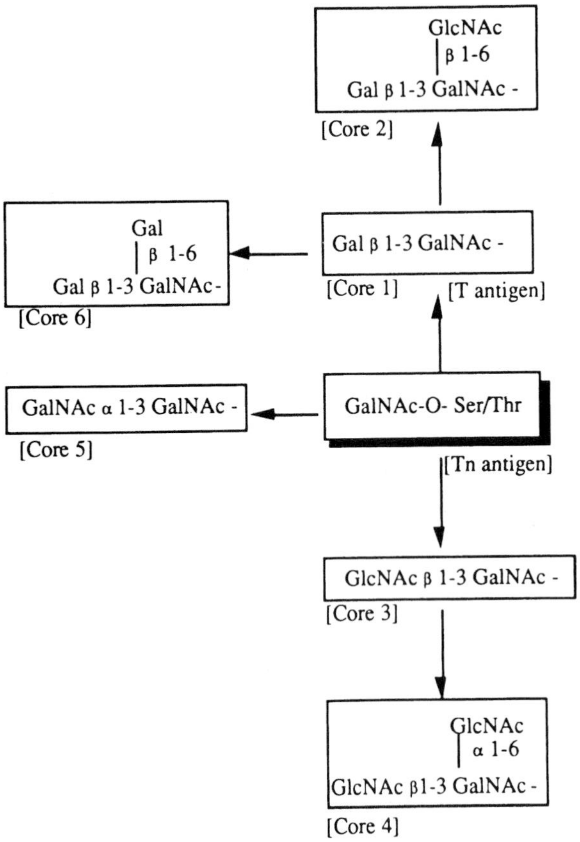

FIGURE 5.6. *O*-glycan core structures. The cores are synthesized from the precursor Tn antigen by addition of galactose (Gal), N-acetylglucosamine (GlcNAc), or both. Cores 1 to 4 are most common in normal mucins.

Typical core structures of mucin *O*-glycans consist of six different arrangements of Gal and GlcNAc bound to GalNAc (Fig. 5.6). Most *O*-glycans contain the core 1 subtype structure formed by the addition of galactose in a β1-3 linkage to the GalNAc. The first four cores are common, particularly cores 2 and 3 in intestinal mucins. Many mucins also express the sialosyl-Tn antigen (sialyl GalNAc), which is increased in tumor mucins and mucins produced in some cases of ulcerative colitis (136,137). The glycosyltransferase responsible for the core 1 subtype structure is known as core 1 β1-3 galactosyltransferase (core 1 GalT), core 2 GlcNAcT for the formation of the core 2 subtype, core 3 GlcNAcT for the core 3 subtype, and core 4 GlcNAcT for the core 4 subtype (138,139). The core structures are substrates for transferases, which add sugars and elongate the oligosaccharide chains. The production of core 2 *O*-glycans requires the core 1 as substrate, and production of core 3 *O*-glycans actually inhibits the ability of core 2 GlcNAcT to act. In addition, the core 2 structure can become elongated into either a mono- or biantennary form with the presence of multiple lactosamine (Galβ1-4GlcNAc) units, which become terminated by the addition of sialic acid or fucose. The core 3 *O*-glycans can be the building block for the formation of biantennary *O*-glycans by acting as a substrate for core 4 GlcNAc activity. Very few tissues besides those of the GI tract show high core 3 and 4 GlcNAc activities. As oligosaccharide elongation proceeds, the more proximal core structures become "masked," making them inaccessible to lectins, adhesins, or antibodies specific for them. A detailed review regarding *O*-glycosylation is provided in reference 140.

The final step in oligosaccharide synthesis is the transfer of sugars (fucose, galactose, GalNAc, and sialic acid) from their nucleotide sugar donors to terminal galactose residues of the backbones, completing oligosaccharide synthesis. The peripheral sugars bond via α-glycosidic linkages, which stop further elongation and give rise to the well-known ABH and Lewis blood group–specific mucins. The A-, B-, or H-specific sugars serve as nutrients for some colonic commensals (141,142). To some extent, the blood groups determine which species or strains inhabit the human colon. Alterations in peripheral sugars occur in mucins of malignant tumors (143,144), in colonic mucins during immune responses to parasitic infections (145), and in the macrophage, sialomucins produced in response to inflammatory stimuli (146). In addition, incomplete oligosaccharide chain synthesis occurs in many cancer cells and contributes to the prevalent expression of the Tn antigen (GalNAc-Thr/Ser) (147). Peripheral sialylation is a relatively late Golgi-mediated event, and, together with sulfate, sialic acid gives rise to a negative charge to the mucin chains. Sialic acid content of intestinal glycoproteins tends to be higher in the fetal and newborn period and decreases with aging (148). In addition, enhanced sialylation is one of the common abnormalities of tumor mucins (148).

Sulfation

Some of the peripheral or backbone residues (chiefly Gal or GlcNAc) of mucin oligosaccharides acquire sulfate at the level of the Golgi membranes during biosynthesis (149). The longest or most branched chains are likely to carry the most sulfate (150). In respiratory mucins, it was shown that sulfate and sialic acid could be expressed on the same oligosaccharide, although usually on different branches (151). Most goblet cells contain some sulfated mucin molecules and sulfation increases from the proximal to distal segments of the intestine and is highest in colonic areas that harbor high populations of fecal bacteria (152). Staining reactions with HID/Alcian blue pH 2.5 change from blue to brown-purple as the ratio of sulfate exceeds that of sialic acid in goblet cell granules (153). Sulfation of mucin is decreased in ulcerative colitis (154,155) and increased in cystic fibrosis (156,157). To date, there is no strong evidence suggesting that parasites, bacteria, or viruses use sulfate residues as receptors for attachment. The role of sulfation in mucin is thought to be one of protection against bacterial exoproducts (158). Gastric corpus and duodenal mucins are highly sulfated (159,160). It has been suggested that this confers resistance against gastric pepsin and pancreatic proteases; sulfation also rate-limits bacterial degradation of mucins (161,162). There is evidence that sulfation of *O*-glycans may play a role in cell adhesion and in the regulation of biosynthetic pathways. Other reports suggest that rotavirus uses sialic acid residues as sites for attachment (163).

MUCIN POLYMERS

The interactions of mucins at the intermolecular and intramolecular levels give rise to the polymeric and eventually the visoelastic properties of the mucus gel. To achieve this, mucin monomers must link together to form polymers. The formation of disulfide bonds between MUC2 mucin monomers is a crucial step in the assembly of mucins into multimers. The assembly of gel-forming mucin polymers is believed to occur in a similar fashion to that of VWF as a result of the high degree of sequence similarities in the positions of the cysteines in the carboxyl and amino termini. The initial dimerization of MUC2 has been shown to occur in the ER (91) through the formation of disulfide bonds between the carboxyl terminal regions of the mucin peptide. Transfer of the mucin monomers and dimers to the Golgi apparatus is an *N*-glycosylation–dependent event. Subsequent *O*-glycosylation of the mucin dimers and even monomers occurs in the Golgi, although the presence of mucin monomers in the Golgi is not entirely understood. Multimerization of the mucin dimers occurs through interchain disulfide bonds formed between the amino terminal D-domains of disulfide-linked dimers, forming very high-molecular-weight multimers (164,165) (Fig. 5.7). There may well be more than one biosynthetic pathway for the production and assembly of gel-forming mucins. For example, there is a difference between the interactions of the chaperones calreticulin and calnexin with MUC2 and MUC5AC in the ER. Even though calreticulin and calnexin are involved in proper folding and oligomerization of MUC2 (166), they appear not to interact with the gel-forming mucin MUC5AC. Although the two mucins are structurally similar, they may require the assistance of different chaperones for proper folding.

Once mucin polymers are assembled and fully glycosylated, they normally assume semiflexible "kinky" configurations, which, when extended by shearing stress and examined by electron microscopy, are seen to be extremely heterogeneous in length (167). Respiratory mucins are well studied and range from 0.2 to more than 10 μm in length. After reduction, they decrease in size to 200 to 600 nm (168).

GEL FORMATION

Within goblet cell granules, mucin polymers are physically constrained in a highly condensed form, which excludes water. Packing is enhanced by calcium ion neutralization of the fixed negative charges of sulfate and sialic acid. Upon secretion of the mature mucin granules, polymers uncoil, Ca^+ diffuses outward, and the mucin becomes rapidly

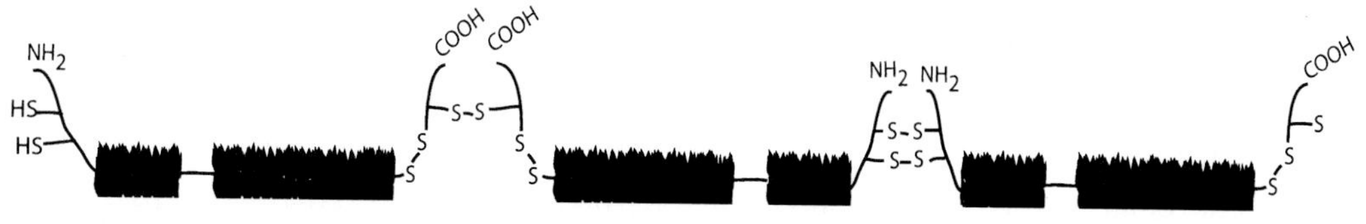

FIGURE 5.7. Hypothetical model of a MUC2 polymer. The sulfhydryl bonds at the carboxy- and amino-terminal ends link two MUC2 monomers to form a polymeric structure. The heavily glycosylated regions (IR and VNTR) are depicted as bottle-brush areas. (Adapted from Gum JR Jr. Human mucin glycoproteins: varied structures predict diverse properties and specific functions. *Biochem Soc Trans* 1995;23:795–799.)

hydrated and its volume greatly increases (169,170), becoming 80% to 90% hydrated. Mucin molecules in solution aggregate via H-bonding, electrostatic and hydrophobic interactions, and Van der Waals forces (171). Gel formation occurs as the number of cross-links between mucin molecules increases and the long polymer chains intertangle. The sol-gel-phase transformation from the solution of linear or branched molecules to a highly viscous and elastic gel occurs when mucin reaches a concentration of 30 to 50 mg/mL. Cross-linkage of the gel structure provides considerable resistance to flow and may explain why mucins are not completely cleared from the mucosal surface after a single fluid "flush."

Mucin forms a two-layer gel that is adherent to the intestinal epithelium: one layer is a loosely adherent layer, which is removable, and the other layer is firmly attached to the mucosa. The mucus gel flows slowly over the mucosal surface to form a blanket, which follows the surface of the mucosa. The visoelastic properties of mucus can withstand the large shear forces found in the digestive tract as well as the movement of particles and macromolecules over the epithelial surface (171). If subjected to a strong shear stress, a mucin gel may rupture, but if left undisturbed, it will reanneal because of its intrinsic elasticity. Thus, viscosity and elasticity are important properties for the continuity and stability of the mucus blanket covering the GI mucosal surface. The unstirred mucus layer provides a stable microenvironment at the mucosal surface, and, in the colon, the mucus layer provides an essential environment for microflora (172). The thickness of the mucus gel ranges from 50 to 450 μm (average 180 μm) in the human stomach and is thinner and possibly discontinuous in the small intestine. Studies measuring the thickness of intestinal mucus in the rat have shown that the mucus layer is thickest in the colon (830 μm) and thinnest in the jejunum (approximately 123 μm) (3,173). The mucus layer is decreased during starvation (174) and increased in bacterial overgrowth (175). Upon injury of the mucosa, a thick mucoid coat develops over the site of injury, which acts as a "cap" composed of mucin, fibrin, and necrotic cells and enables the rapid reepithelialization of the mucosa (127). The mucus gel does not cover Peyer patches, apparently not preventing the translocation of bacterial or other potentially antigenic luminal components across the bowel wall. Interestingly, there are reports that rabbit M cells contain various MUC2 carbohydrate epitopes, which are not expressed on dome enterocytes, and it has been suggested that these epitopes play a role in attachment of pathogens to the M-cell luminal surface (176). Indeed, this is significant because many pathogens and parasites attach via MUC2.

The lubricant properties of mucin gels are important, but the physiochemical basis is not well understood; it is assumed to reduce the frictional coefficients at mucosal surfaces. Mucin has the ability to adhere to the GI mucosa and particulate matter as well as spread over the mucosa (177). Hydrophobic interactions involving carbohydrates (178) may play a role in the adherence to the mucosa, although the level of hydration of the mucin layer may also be important to its functional adhesivity, in addition to determining viscosity. The ability of mucin to spread over the mucosa probably depends on anionic charge repulsion (sulfate and sialic acid) as well as repulsive hydration forces in the gel (177).

The mucus gel is composed of mucin, water, proteoglycans, electrolytes, DNA, and serum proteins such as IgA, albumen, and lysozyme (178,179). Some of these compounds are believed to enhance the adhesivity of mucus secretions, but they also tend to produce weaker gels than those formed of mucin molecules alone (180). The mucus gels that form under inflammatory conditions or in regions of high sloughing may be "mixed" gels, which are more vulnerable to disruption by acid, detergents (bile), and denaturing agents (180).

SUSCEPTIBILITY OF MUCINS TO DAMAGE

Both the peptide core and the oligosaccharides of GI mucins are fragmented and eventually completely degraded by enzymes liberated into the lumen from normal host tissue and colonic bacteria (Fig. 5.8). Degradation of mucin is a natural physiological process that plays a role in regulating the thickness of the GI mucus blanket. However, many pathogens and host cells elaborate enzymes that are mucolytic. An excess of these enzymes can alter the dynamic equilibrium between mucin production and degradation of mucin that can cause a structural weakening of the protective mucus gel layer. Some of the sites on mucin molecules, which are recognized to be particularly susceptible to damage, are discussed herein and are highlighted schematically in Figure 5.8.

Proteolysis

Solubilization of the intestinal mucus gel occurs throughout the gut by degradation of the mucin polymer into soluble degraded mucin units. The nonglycosylated regions of mucins are known to be susceptible to proteolytic cleavage by a wide range of proteinases. A large portion of the proteolysis of GI mucin takes place in the colon where there is a high content of intestinal microflora. In addition, mucin in the upper GI tract is continually degraded by host proteinases. Analysis of the amino acid sequence of MUC2 has revealed that the *N*- and *C*-terminal regions contain many arginine, lysine, and valine residues as well as a small number of aromatic residues such as phenylalanine, tyrosine, and tryptophan. Therefore, these domains may be highly susceptible to serine proteinases produced by the host as well as serine and cysteine proteinases produced by GI pathogens (181). Experimental studies support this conclusion in that mucins are readily fragmented by serine and cysteine pro-

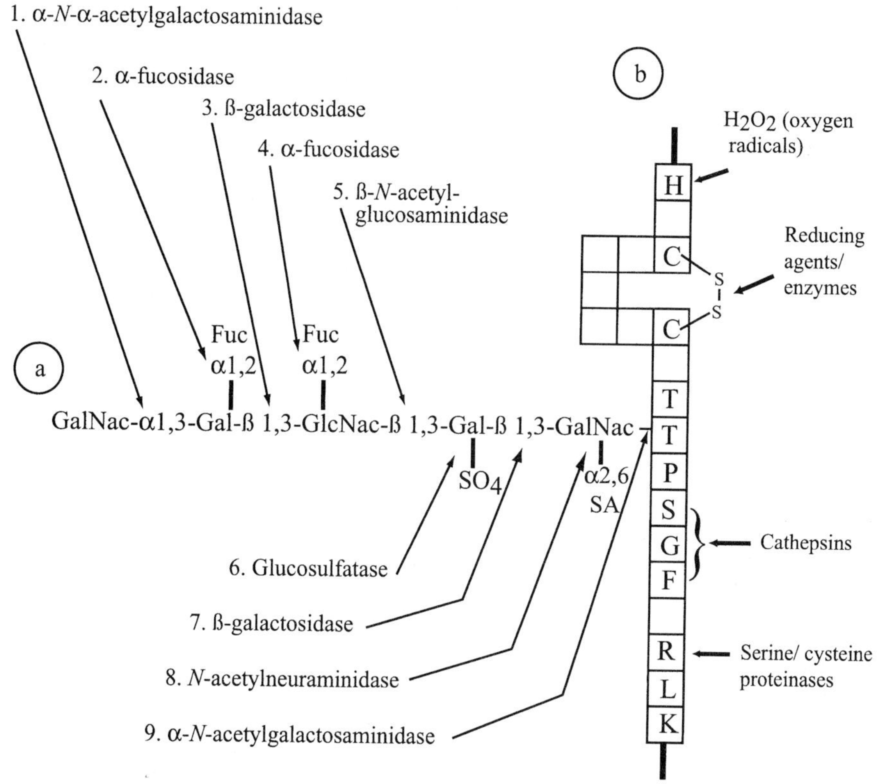

FIGURE 5.8. Degradation of intestinal mucin. **A:** A hypothetical mucin oligosaccharide to show the sequential action of bacterial exoglycosidases and glucosulfatate. **B:** A portion of the polypeptide core to show amino acids (*squares*) vulnerable to chemical and enzymatic rupture. H, histidine; T, threonine; S, serine; P, proline; R, arginine; F, phenylalanine; K, lysine; G, glycine; C, cysteine. Many serine and cysteine proteinases of bacterial and host epithelial cells are mucolytic.

teinases without any loss of carbohydrate (1,181–183). The enzymes cleave poorly glycosylated ("naked") peptide segments and disrupt the continuity of the linear polymers. Consequently, there is a dramatic reduction in the molecular mass of mucin, as well as a decrease in viscoelasticity and polymer length. Proteases capable of degrading mucin are produced in salivary, gastric, intestinal, and pancreatic tissues, including goblet cells (184) and colonic enterocytes (185). Fecal bacteria elaborate a mixture of proteinases (183), although serine proteinases are responsible for the majority of damage to mucin structure.

In vivo, some protection of mucins against luminal proteases may be afforded by weak interactions of mucins with nonmucin components such as proteins, constituents of bile, anionic proteoglycans, lipids, and products of sloughed cells (74,186). It is also likely that the normally folded state of the mucin peptide near the cysteine-rich terminals "buries" some protease-sensitive regions, which only become vulnerable after disulfide bonds are ruptured (187).

Proteolytic degradation of mucin has been observed during conventional purification steps. This degradation occurs even when mucins are purified in the presence of numerous protease inhibitors (188). For example, once the sequence of porcine submaxillary mucin was available from isolated cDNAs, it was realized that traditional purification procedures resulted in the loss of a long *C*-terminal domain of the mucin (189). In the case of rat MUC2, purification routinely allows for the "nicking" of a particular aspartyl-proline bond located in the *C*-terminal domain, releasing the 118-kDa peptide known as the link peptide. This cleaved fragment is thought to stay attached to the mucin molecule via disulfide bonds and is liberated in the presence of reducing agents. Generally, aspartyl-proline bonds in proteins are sensitive to heating in the presence of acids (190), but because acidic conditions are not used during mucin purification, this is unlikely to be the cause of cleavage at these sites. Purification of mucin in the presence of guanidinium chloride, to denature all proteases, is known to be an effective way to significantly prevent degradation during the purification and storage of mucin.

Various GI pathogens secrete proteases, some of which affect mucins. For example, the enteric protozoan parasite *E. histolytica*, which colonizes the mucus layer of the colon, is known to secrete an abundant amount of cysteine proteinases. These proteinases are thought to degrade the poorly glycosylated *N*- and *C*-terminal flanking regions of MUC2, destroying its polymeric structure (Fig. 5.8). It is hypothesized that once the polymeric structure has been lost, the mucus blanket is less effective at preventing amebic invasion of the colon (181). *V. cholerae* secretes a potent zinc-dependent metalloproteinase that lowers mucin viscosity and facilitates penetration of the enterotoxin to its GM1 ganglioside receptor on cell membranes (191). There is evidence that *H. pylori* secretes a protease that increases the movement of the organism through the mucus gel to the gastric cells (192). The mucus barrier may also be damaged in inflammatory bowel disease by fecal proteinases, which are increased by alteration in the normal resident bacterial populations (193,194). Additionally, it is likely that GI inflammation contributes to mucin damage by the action of neutrophil proteases (195), mast cell proteases (196), and proteases from other inflammatory cells.

Cysteine residues form disulfide bonds that stabilize the tertiary structure of mucins, and reducing agents are widely recognized to be capable of destroying mucin polymers and collapsing mucin gels. Although specific bacterial reductases for these bonds have not been identified, colonic flora and host cells produce reductases and glutathione, both of which are believed to participate in mucin depolymerization. Thiols in secretions can also activate cathepsins, which can damage the mucin peptide.

Mucins of the stomach and bile have also been shown to act as scavengers of oxygen radicals, thereby protecting the mucosa from damage by these agents (197). Mucin structure is compromised in the process, because a marked reduction in mucin viscosity occurs upon exposure to oxygen radicals (198). The antioxidant function of mucin is probably associated with the rupture of histidine residues in the core peptide; earlier studies revealed that hydrogen peroxide damages this amino acid (199). The effect was dependent upon the presence of Cu^{2+} (or Fe^{2+}), suggesting that an oxidation-reduction reaction is involved. Because mucin does contain numerous histidine residues, it is likely that they play a role in this event.

Glycosidases

Mucin oligosaccharides are degraded in a stepwise manner by the sequential removal of carbohydrates in a direction from the periphery to the internal core nearest the peptide linkage as shown schematically in Figure 5.8. Specific subpopulations of normal colonic flora elaborate the required exoglycosidases (194,200). Host mucins can also induce or regulate the expression of at least some of the enzymes required for mucin deglycosylation (200,201). Mucolytic exoglycosidases, including neuraminidases (194) and blood group–specific exoglycosidases (202,203), are increased in intestinal inflammation and infection. The importance of these enzymes as virulence factors, however, is largely speculative. Antibiotics decrease mucin degradation and alter mucin composition to resemble that of mucins found in the germ-free state (204). A glycosidase has been described in a strain of *Streptomyces* (205) and is expressed when the bacteria are grown in media containing mucin.

Proteinases, as well as glycosidases, have been shown to play a role in host-parasite interactions, in particular, mucus penetration. There is some evidence that the protozoan parasites *E. histolytica* and *Giardia lamblia* produce a β-*N*-acetylglucosaminidase that may aid in the penetration of the protective mucus layer. For organisms such as *G. lamblia* and *Trichomonas vaginalis*, motility alone is not sufficient for these pathogens to migrate through the mucus layer (206). Therefore, the concerted action of proteinases and glycosidases may be necessary for some pathogens to invade the mucosa, although glycosidases may not be a significant virulence factor in some infections, such as infection with *E. histolytica* (207). As mucin peptides become progressively deglycosylated, they are rendered more sensitive to rupture by proteolytic enzymes. Thus, alternating activities of bacterial (and host) glycosidases may gradually degrade mucin macromolecules. Bacterial glycosulfatases (201) participate by removing sulfate from its attachment to galactose, GlcNAc, or GalNAc of the oligosaccharides. Because sulfate is thought to decrease the rate of mucin damage by glycosidases and proteases, those pathogens that elaborate sulfatases may accelerate mucin fragmentation (208). A number of mucin-specific glycosulfatases have been reported in bacteria.

Mechanical Rupture

A heightened sensitivity to shear forces marks mucin gels as being different from highly structured gels of alginate, agarose, gelatin, or other conventional gels. During purification and handling, mucin polymers are easily broken (shortened) by shear forces, but in a physiological context, mucin fragility is an asset, in that *in vivo* mucin gels must be deformed and made to flow by shearing forces of peristalsis and the waving motion of the intestinal villi. Mechanical fragility may be a factor in the phenomenon termed *viscous fingering*. In this process, HCL injected through solutions of pig gastric mucin produced viscous fingering patterns dependent on pH, mucin concentration, and acid flow rate. HCL secreted by the gastric glands penetrates the mucus gel layer through narrow fingers (pH 5 to 7), which are formed as a result of the differences in viscosity between the mucus gel and acid secretion and HCL in the lumen (pH 2). The acid is prevented from diffusing back to the epithelium by the viscosity of the gastric mucus gel on the luminal side (209).

MUCINS IN HOST DEFENSE AGAINST INTESTINAL PATHOGENS

A number of microorganisms have been found to adhere to mucin carbohydrate moieties. Protection of the intestinal epithelium against pathogenic microorganisms including, bacteria, parasites, and viruses lies in the binding capacity of mucin carbohydrates to microbial adhesins. Binding sites on mucins are thought to compete with those on underlying epithelial cells, preventing attachment to the mucosal surface. In many instances, microorganisms are sloughed and swept out during peristaltic movements and defecation. Nonpathogenic organisms including the indigenous flora that reside in the adherent mucus blanket occupy an important niche within the intestine as a result of their ability to prevent attachment of pathogenic organisms by occupying available binding sites. The initial step in the pathogenesis of many intestinal pathogens is the binding of the microorganism to mucin. The fate of many mucin-bound organisms lies in their ability to colonize the intestinal tract. There are four possible outcomes in the interactions between pathogens and intestinal mucins (a) initial mucin binding followed by elimination of the pathogen through sloughing and peristalsis, (b) successful colonization with the pathogen retained in the mucus blanket and access denied to the underlying epithelium, (c) colonization of the mucus layer with elaboration of virulence factors, and (d) epithelial invasion where the mucus barrier is breached and the invading pathogen gains access to the intestinal epithelium (6). Perhaps the best example of this process is illustrated during infection with *E. histolytica*. The successful colonization of *E. histolytica* is mediated through its ability to adhere to Gal and GalNAc residues of colonic mucin via its Gal/GalNAc lectin. Interestingly, highly purified mucins from LS174T cells have been shown to inhibit amebic adherence to Chinese hamster ovary cells (CHO), demonstrating the ability of mucin to compete with binding sites found on target cells (210). In addition, the protective role of the intestinal mucus blanket has been demonstrated *in vitro* by comparing the ability of ameba to destroy monolayers of target cells with and without a mucus barrier. As expected, disruption of CHO cell monolayers occurred more rapidly when compared with monolayers composed of LS174T cells that produce an adherent mucus blanket (37). These findings reinforce the premise that the mucus blanket serves an important protective function. Several other pathogens including *Salmonella typhimurium* (211), *V. cholerae* (212), *Y. enterocolitica* (213), and *Candidia albicans* (214) are all known to adhere to intestinal mucin. Although the mechanisms enabling the penetration of the mucus layer by these organisms is still under investigation, release of proteinases and mucus secretagogues by pathogens may play a role in destroying the protective polymeric nature of the mucus gel. In most cases, mucus physically traps the organisms and entangles them. If mucus "flushing" rates exceed bacterial colonization rates and mucin proteolytic degradation, then the offending organisms are rapidly eliminated.

CONCLUSIONS AND FUTURE CONSIDERATIONS

This chapter deals mainly with the protective role of secretory mucins, including lubrication, hydration, epithelial repair, and protection against mechanical stresses, chemical irritants, and pathogens. Tremendous advancements have been made in the area of mucin gene discovery and cloning as well as in elucidating the primary structure and assembly of GI mucins. However, modern understanding of basic mucin biology and regulatory pathways involved in mucin biosynthesis and secretion is rudimentary.

An important area for future research is the mechanisms by which GI pathogens overcome the protective mucus barrier and the role of mucin heterogeneity in disease states. One can speculate that differences in mucins between individuals or even disease states could play a major role in the outcome of GI infections. There is little information regarding whether host mucins may become biosynthetically altered in response to infection, although this phenomenon is known to occur in experimental infections with helminths. Recently, there has been great interest in the regulation and expression of the *MUC2* gene in response to intestinal pathogens and GI inflammation. Even though *MUC2* is constitutively expressed by goblet cells, its expression is altered in response to various GI pathogens, possibly affecting the outcome of infection. Discovery of the regulatory elements in the promoter region of *MUC2* involved in regulating gene expression and protein production may be beneficial in treatment of disease. Moreover, some pathogens affect the host by causing hypersecretion and, thus, depletion of the mucus blanket. Research is needed to identify the putative mucin secretagogues released by pathogens to identify the receptors and intracellular signaling events involved in mucin exocytosis and to determine the intracellular mechanisms involved in accelerated secretion and the protein machinery involved in the release of stored as well as newly synthesized mucin. Knowledge is still rudimentary regarding the possible alterations of tissue-specific regulation of mucin gene expression but progress is being made rapidly. A pressing topic for future research includes the possible alterations of mucin glycosylation in response to infectious agents and inflammatory states. In addition, understanding the expression and glycosylation patterns with regard to mucus-producing adenocarcinomas is and will continue to be a key element in detecting and even treating cancer.

ACKNOWLEDGMENTS

The authors acknowledge financial support for this research from the Canadian Institutes of Health Research and the Crohn's and Colitis Foundation of Canada. Darcy Moncada is the recipient of a Canadian Institutes of Health Research Studentship.

REFERENCES

1. Hermann A, Davies JR, Lindell JR, et al. Studies on the "insoluble" glycoprotein complex from human colon: identification of reduction-insensitive MUC2 oligomers and *C*-terminal cleavage. *J Biol Chem* 1999;274:15828–15836.
2. Laboisse C, Jarry A, Branka D, et al. Recent aspects of the regulation of intestinal mucus secretion. *Proc Nutr Soc* 1996;55:259–264.

3. Cross CE, Halliwell B, Allen A. Anti-oxidant protection: a function of tracheobronchial and gastrointestinal mucus. *Lancet* 1984;16:1328–1330.
4. LaMont JT, Smith BF, Moore JR. Role of gallbladder mucin in pathophysiology of gallstones. *Hepatology* 1984;4[*Suppl* 5]: 51S–56S.
5. Forstner JF, Forstner GG. Gastrointestinal mucus. Physiology of the gastrointestinal tract, third edition. New York: Raven Press, 1994:1255–1283.
6. Belley A, Keller K, Goettke, et al. Intestinal mucins in colonization and host defense against pathogens. *Am J Trop Med Hyg Suppl* 1999;60:10–15.
7. Forstner JF, Oliver MG, Sylvester FA. Production, structure, and biologic relevance of gastrointestinal mucins. In: Blaser MJ, Smith PD, Ravdin JI, et al: Infections of the gastrointestinal tract. New York: Raven Press, 1995:71–88.
8. Ross MH, Romell LJ, Kaye GI. Histology—a text and atlas, third edition. Baltimore: Williams & Wilkins, 1995.
9. Radwan KA, Oliver MG, Specian RD. Cytoarchitectural reorganization of rabbit colonic goblet cells during baseline secretion. *Am J Anat* 1990;189:365–376.
10. Schmidt GH, Wilkinson MM, Ponder BAJ. Cell migration pathway in the intestinal epithelium: an *in situ* marker system using mouse aggregation chimeras. *Cell* 1985;40:425–429.
11. Specian RD, Neutra MR. Mechanism of rapid mucus secretion in goblet cells stimulated by acetylcholine. *J Cell Biol* 1980;85:626–640.
12. Oliver MG, Specian RD. Cytoskeleton of intestinal goblet cells: role of actin filaments in baseline secretion. *Am J Physiol* 1991;260:G850–G857.
13. Podolsky DK, Isselbacher KJ. Composition of human colonic mucin. Selective alteration in inflammatory bowel disease. *J Clin Invest* 1983;72:142–153.
14. Specian RD, Oliver MG. Functional biology of intestinal goblet cells. *Am J Physiol* 1991;260:C183–C193.
15. Akiba Y, Guth PH, Engel E, et al. Dynamic regulation of mucus gel thickness in rat duodenum. *Am J Physiol* 2000;279: G437–G447.
16. Neutra MR, Leblond CP. Synthesis of the carbohydrate of mucus in the Golgi complex as shown by electron microscope radioautography of goblet cells from rats injected with glucose-^{3}H. *J Cell Biol* 1966;30:119–136.
17. Forstner G. Signal transduction, packaging and secretion of mucins. *Annu Rev Physiol* 1995;57:585–605.
18. McCool DJ, Forstner JF, Forstner GG. Regulated and unregulated pathways for MUC2 mucin secretion in human colonic LS180 adenocarcinoma cells are distinct. *Biochem J* 1995; 312:125–133.
19. McCool DJ, Forstner JF, Forstner GG. Synthesis and secretion of mucin by the human colonic tumour cell line LS180. 1994;302:111–118.
20. Romisch K. Microtubules: fast tracks to secretion. *Trends Biochem Sci* 2001;26:281.
21. Specian RD, Oliver MG. Cytoskeleton of intestinal goblet cells: role of microtubules in baseline secretion. *Am J Physiol* 1991;260:G850–G857.
22. Ferro-Novick S, Jahn R. Vesicle fusion from yeast to man. *Nature* 1994;370:191–193.
23. Phillips TE, Phillips TL, Neutra MR. Regulation of intestinal goblet cell secretion. III. Isolated intestinal epithelium. *Am J Physiol* 1984;247:G674–G681.
24. Jackson AD. Airway goblet-cell mucus secretion. *Trends Pharmacol Sci* 2001;22:39–45.
25. Plaisancie P, Barcelo A, Moro F. Effect of neurotransmitters, gut hormones, and inflammatory mediators on mucus discharge in rat colon. *Am J Physiol* 1998;275:G1073–G1084.
26. Halm DR, Halm ST. Secretagogue response of goblet cells and columnar cells in human colonic crypts. *Am J Physiol* 2000;278:C212–233.
27. Specian RD, Neutra MR. Regulation of intestinal goblet cell secretion. 1. Role of parasympathetic stimulation. *Am J Physiol* 1992;262:G327–G331.
28. Phillips TE. Both crypt and villus intestinal goblet cells secrete mucin in response to cholinergic stimulation. *Am J Physiol* 1992;262:G327–G331.
29. Stanley CM, Phillips TE. Selective secretion and replenishment of discrete mucin glycoforms from intestinal goblet cells. *Am J Physiol* 1999;l;277:G191–200.
30. Kemper AC, Specian RD. Rat small intestinal mucins: a quantitative study. *Anat Rec* 1991;229:219–226.
31. Neutra MR, O'Malley LJ, Specian RD, et al. Regulation of intestinal goblet cell secretion. II. A survey of potential secretagogues. *Am J Physiol* 1982;242:G380–G387.
32. Bertrand CA, Laboisse CL, Hopfer U. Purinergic and cholinergic agonists induce exocytosis from the same granule pool in HT29-C1.16E monolayers. *Am J Physiol* 1999;276: C907–C914.
33. Branka JE, Vallette G, Jarry A, et al. Stimulation of mucin exocytosis from human epithelial cells by nitric oxide: evidence for a cGMP-dependent and cGMP-independent pathway. *Biochem J* 1997;323:521–524.
34. Jarry A, Vallette G, Branka JE, et al. Direct secretory effect of interleukin-1 via type1 receptors in human colonic mucous epithelial cells (HT29-CL.16E). *Am J Physiol* 1989;256: G223–G450.
35. Belley A, Chadee K. Prostaglandin E_2 stimulates rat and human colonic mucin exocytosis via the EP_4 receptor. *Gastroenterology* 1999;117:1352–1362.
36. Sperber K, Shim J, Mehra M, et al. Mucin secretion in inflammatory bowel disease: comparison of a macrophage-derived mucin secretagogue (MMS-68) to conventional secretagogues. *Inflamm Bowel Dis* 1998;4:12-17.
37. Belley A, Keller K, Grove J, et al. Interaction of LS174T human colon cancer mucins with *Entamoeba histolytica*: an *in vitro* model for colonic disease. *Gastroenterology* 1996;111:1484–1492.
38. Wright HD, Ford-Hutchinson AW, Chadee K, et al. The human prostanoid DP receptor stimulates mucin secretion in LS174T cells. *Br J Pharmacol* 2000;131:1537–1545.
39. McCool DJ, Marcon MA, Forstner JF, et al. The T84 human colonic adenocarcinoma cell line produces mucin in culture and releases it in response to various secretagogues. *Biochem J* 1990;267:491–500.
40. Roomi N, Laburthe M, Fleming N, et al. Cholera induced mucin secretion from rat intestine: lack of effective cAMP, cycloheximide, VIP, and colchicines. *Am J Physiol* 1984;247: G140–G148.
41. Barcelo A, Claustre J, Moro F, et al. Mucin secretion is modulated by luminal factors in the isolated vascularly perfused rat colon. Gut 2000;46:218–224.
42. Lundgren JD. Mucus production in the lower airways. *Dan Med Bull* 1992;39:289–303.
43. Tse SK, Chadee K. The interaction between intestinal mucus glycoproteins and enteric infections. *Parasitol Today* 1991;7: 163–172.
44. Hecht G. Innate mechanisms of epithelial host defense: spotlight on intestine. *Am J Physiol* 1999;277:C351–C358.
45. Forstner JF, Roomi NW, Fahim REF. Cholera toxin stimulates secretion of immunoreactive intestinal mucin. *Am J Physiol* 1981;240:10–16.
46. Chadee K, Keller K, Forstner J, et al. Mucin and nonmucin secretagogue activity of *Entamoeba histolytica* and cholera toxin in rat colon. *Gastroenterology* 1991;100:986–997.

47. Laburthe M, Augeron C, Rouyer-Fessard C, et al. Functional VIP receptors in the human mucus-secreting colonic epithelial cell line C1.16E. *Am J Physiol* 1989;256:G443–G450.
48. Seider U, Knafla K, Kownatski R, et al. Effect of endogenous and exogenous prostaglandins on glycoprotein synthesis and secretion in isolated rabbit gastric mucosa. *Gastroenterology* 1988; 95:945–951.
49. Phillips TE, Stanley CM, Wilson J. The effect of 16,16-dimethyl prostaglandin E_2 on proliferation of an intestinal goblet cell line and its synthesis and secretion of mucin glycoproteins. *Prostaglandins Leukot Essent Fatty Acids* 1993;48: 423–428.
50. Moore BA, Sherkey KA, Mantle M. Role of 5-HT in cholera toxin-induced mucin secretion in the rat small intestine. *Am J Physiol* 1996;270:G1001–G1009.
51. Bou-Hanna C, Berthon B, Combettes L, et al. Role of calcium in carbachol- and neurotensin-induced mucin exocytosis in a human colonic goblet cell line and cross-talk with the cyclic AMP pathway. *Biochem J* 1994;299:579–585.
52. Jarry A, Merlin D, Velcich A, et al. Interferon-γ modulated cAMP-induced mucin exocytosis without affecting mucin gene expression in a human colonic goblet cell line. *Eur J Pharmacol* 1994;267:95–103.
53. Lencer WI, Reinhart FD, Neutra MR. Interaction of cholera toxin with cloned human goblet cells in monolayer culture. *Am J Physiol* 1990;258:G96–G102.
54. Mantle M, Thakore E, Hardin J. Effect of *Yersinia enterocolitica* on intestinal mucin secretion. *Am J Physiol* 1989;256: G319–G327.
55. Keller K, Oliver M, Chadee K. The fast release of mucus secretion from human colonic cells induced by *Entamoeba histolytica* is dependent on contact and protein kinase C activation. *Arch Med Res* 1992;23:217–221.
56. Seider U, Pfeiffer A. Ca^{+2} dependent and –independent secretagogue action on gastric mucus secretion in rabbit mucosal explants. *Am J Physiol* 1989;256:G739–G746.
57. Yedgar S, Eidelman O, Malden E, et al. Cyclic AMP-independent secretion of mucin by SW1116 human colon carcinoma cells. *Biochem J* 1992;283:421–426.
58. Phillips TE, Wilson J. Signal transduction pathways mediating mucin secretion from intestinal goblet cells. *Dig Dis Sci* 1993;38:1046–1054.
59. Chadee K, Meerovitch E. The pathology of experimentally-induced cecal amebiasis in gerbils (*Meriones unguiculates*) *Am J Pathol* 1985;119:485–494.
60. Tse SK, Chadee K. Biochemical characterization of rat colonic mucins secreted in response to *Entamoeba histolytica*. *Infect Immun* 1992;60:1603–1612.
61. Byrd JC, Yunker CK, Xu QS, et al. Inhibition of gastric mucin synthesis by *Helicobacter pylori*. *Gastroenterology* 2000;118: 1072–1079.
62. Coconnier MH, Dlissi E, Robard M, et al. *Listeria monocytogenes* stimulates mucus exocytosis in cultured human polarized mucus secreting intestinal cells through action of listeriolysin O. *Infect Immun* 1998;66:3673-3681.
63. Chadwick MP, Westley BR, May FE. Homodimerization and hetero-oligomerization of the single-domain trefoil protein pNR-2/pS2 through cysteine 58. *Biochem J* 1997;327: 117–123.
64. Ogata H, Inoue N, Podolsky DK. Identification of a goblet cell-specific enhancer element in the rat intestinal trefoil factor gene promoter bound by a goblet cell nuclear protein. *J Biol Chem* 1998;273:3060–3067.
65. Rio M, Bellecq JP, Daniel JY, et al. Breast cancer-associated pS2 protein: synthesis and secretion by normal stomach mucosa. *Science* 1988;241:705–708.
66. Hanby AM, Poulsom R, Singh S, et al. Spasmolytic polypeptide is a major antral peptide: distribution of the trefoil peptides human spasmolytic polypeptide and pS2 in the stomach. *Gastroenterology* 1993;105:110–116.
67. Longman RJ, Douthwaite J, Sylvester PA, et al. Coordinate localization of mucins and trefoil peptides in the ulcer associated cell lineage and the gastrointestinal mucosa. *Gut* 2000; 47:792–800.
68. Podolsky DK, Lynch-Devany K, Stow JL, et al. Identification of human intestinal trefoil factor: goblet cell-specific expression of a peptide for targeted apical secretion. *J Biol Chem* 1993; 268:6694–6702.
69. Tomasetto C, Masson R, Linares JL, et al. pS2 /TFF1 Interacts directly with the VWFC cysteine-rich domains of mucins. *Gastroenterology* 2000;118:70–80.
70. Kindon H, Pothoulakis C, Thin L, et al. Trefoil peptide protection of intestinal epithelial barrier function: cooperative interaction with mucin glycoprotein. *Gastroenterology* 1995;109: 516–523.
71. Playford RJ, Marchbank T, Goodlad RA, et al. Transgenic mice that overexpress trefoil peptide pS2 have an increased resistance to intestinal damage. *Proc Natl Acad Sci U S A* 1996;93: 2137–2142.
72. Lefebvre O, Chenard MP, Masson R, et al. Gastric mucosa abnormalities and tumorigenesis in mice lacking the pS2 trefoil protein. *Science* 1996;274:259–262.
73. Giraud AS. Trefoil peptide and EGF receptor/ligand transgenic mice. *Am J Physiol* 2000;278:G501–G506.
74. Taupin D, Wu D-C, Jeon W-K, et al. The trefoil peptide family are coordinately expressed immediate-early genes: EGF receptor and MAP kinase-dependent interregulation. *J Clin Invest* 1999;103:R31–R38.
75. Nex E, Poulsen SS, Hansen SN, et al. Characterisation of a novel proteolytic enzyme localised to goblet cells in rat and man. *Gut* 1984;25:656–664.
76. Chen LM, Richards GP, Chao L, et al. Molecular cloning, purification and *in situ* localization of human colon kallikrein. *Biochem J* 1995;307:481–486.
77. Pratt WS, Crawley S, Hicks J, et al. Multiple transcripts of *MUC3*: Evidence for two genes, MUC3A and MUC3B. *Biochem Biophys Res Commun* 2000;275:916–923.
78. Gum JR Jr, Hicks JW, Toribara NW, et al. Molecular cloning of human intestinal mucin (MUC2) cDNA: identification of the amino terminus and overall sequence similarity to pre pro-von Willebrand factor. *J Biol Chem* 1994;269:2440–2446.
79. Gum JR Jr, Hicks JW, Toribara NW, et al. The human MUC2 intestinal mucin has cysteine-rich subdomains located both upstream and downstream of its central repetitive region. *J Biol Chem* 1992;267:21357–21383.
80. Van de Bovenkamp JHB, Hau CM, Strous GJAM. Molecular cloning of human gastric mucin MUC5AC reveals conserved cysteine-rich D-domains and a putative leucine zipper motif. *Biochem Biophys Res Commun* 1998;245:853–859.
81. Li JD, Gallup M, Fan N, et al. Cloning of the amino-terminal and 5′ flanking region of the human MUC5AC mucin gene and transcriptional up-regulation by bacterial exoproducts. *J Biol Chem* 1998;273:6812–6820.
82. Bobek LA, Tsai H, Biesbrock AR, et al. Molecular cloning, sequence, and specificity of expression of the gene encoding the low molecular weight human salivary mucin (MUC7). *J Biol Chem* 1993;268:20563–20569.
83. Keates AC, Nunes DP, Afdhal NH, et al. Molecular cloning of a major human gall bladder mucin: complete *C*-terminal sequence and genomic organization of MUC5B. *Biochem J* 1997;324:295–303.
84. Crawley SC, Gum JR Jr, Hicks JW. Genomic organization and

structure of the 3′ region of human MUC3: alternative splicing predicts membrane-bound and soluble forms of the mucin. *Biochem Biophys Res Commun* 1999;263:728–736.
85. Toribara NW, Ho SB, Gum E, et al. The carboxy-terminal sequence of the human secretory mucin, MUC6. *J Biol Chem* 1997;272:16398–16403.
86. Gum JR Jr, Ho JJL, Pratt WS, et al. MUC3 human intestinal mucin. Analysis of gene structure, the carboxyl terminus, and a novel upstream repetitive region. *J Biol Chem* 1997;272: 26678–26686.
87. Gendler SJ, Lancaster CA, Taylor-Papadimitriou J, et al. Molecular cloning and expression of human tumor-associated polymorphic epithelial mucin. *J Biol Chem* 1990;265: 15286–15293.
88. Moniaux N, Nollet S, Porchet N, et al. Complete sequence of the human mucin MUC4: a putative cell membrane-associated mucin. *Biochem J* 1999;338:325–333.
89. Perez-Vilar J, Hill RL. The structure and assembly of secreted mucins. *J Biol Chem* 1999;274:31751–31754.
90. Sadler JE. Biochemistry and genetics of von Willebrand factor. *Annu Rev Biochem* 1998;67:395–424.
91. Asker N, Axelsson AB, Olofsson SO, et al. Dimerization of the human MUC2 mucin in the endoplasmic reticulum is followed by *N*-glycosylation-dependent transfer of the mono- and dimers to the Golgi apparatus. *J Biol Chem* 1998;273:18857–18863.
92. Turner BS, Bhaskar KR, Hadzopoulou-Cladaras M, et al. Cysteine-rich regions of pig gastric mucin contain von Willebrand factor and cystine knot domains at the carboxyl terminal (1). *Biochim Biophys Acta* 1999;1447:77–92.
93. Khatri IA, Forstner GG, Forstner JF. The carboxyl-terminal sequence of rat intestinal mucin RMUC3 contains a putative transmembrane region and two EGF-like motifs. *Biochim Biophys Acta* 1997;1326:7–11.
94. Monaiux N, Escande F, Batra SK, et al. Alternative splicing generates a family of putative secreted and membrane-associated MUC4 mucins. *Eur J Biochem* 2000;267:4536–4544.
95. Byrd JC, Nardelli J, Siddiqui B, et al. Isolation and characterization of colon cancer mucin from xenografts of LS174T cells. *Cancer Res* 1988;48:6678–6685.
96. Sheehan JK, Brazeau C, Kutay S, et al. Physical characterization of the MUC5AC mucin: a highly oligomeric glycoprotein whether isolated from cell culture or *in vivo* from respiratory mucous secretions. *Biochem J* 2000;347:37–44.
97. Guyonnet D, Audie V, Debailleul V, et al. Characterization of the human mucin gene MUC5AC: a consensus cysteine-rich domain for 11p15 mucin genes? *Biochem J* 1995;305:211–219.
98. Tanpipat N, Mattice WL. Range of the influence of the carbohydrate moiety on the conformation of the poly (amino acid) backbone in glycosylated mucins. *Biopolymers* 1990;29:377–383.
99. Briand JP, Andrews SP, Cahill E, et al. Investigation of the requirements for *O*-glycosylation by bovine submaxillary gland UDP-N-acetylgalactosamine:polypeptide *N*- acetylgalactosamine transferase using synthetic peptide substrates *J Biol Chem* 1981;256:12205–12207.
100. Kim SY. Altered glycosylation of mucin glycoproteins in colonic neoplasia. *J Cell Biochem* 1992;16G:91–96.
101. Irimura T, Denda K, Iida SI, et al. Diverse glycosylation of MUC1 and MUC2: potential significance in tumor immunity. *J Biochem* 1999;126:975–985.
102. Mizue I, Takahashi S, Yamashina I, et al. High density *O*-glycosylation of the MUC2 tandem repeat unit by *N*-acetylgalactosaminyltransferase-3 in colonic adenocarcinoma extracts. *Cancer Res* 2001;61:950–956.
103. Shigeo K, Kashiwaba M, Chen D, et al. Induction of antitumor immunity by vaccination of dendritic cells transfected with MUC1 RNA. *J Immunol* 2000;165:5713–5719.
104. Finn OJ, Jerome KR, Bendt KM, et al. Cytotoxic T-lymphocytes derived from patients with breast adenocarcinoma recognize an epitope present on the protein core of a mucin molecule preferentially expressed by malignant cells. *Cancer Res* 1991;51:2908–2916.
105. Apostolopoulos V, Pietersz GA, McKenzie IF. MUC1 and breast cancer. *Curr Opin Mol Ther* 1999;1:98–103.
106. Kyo K, Parkes M, Takei Y, et al. Association of ulcerative colitis with rare VNTR alleles of the human intestinal mucin gene, *MUC3. Hum Mol Genet* 1999;307–311.
107. Vinall LE, Hill AS, Pigny P, et al. Variable number tandem repeat polymorphism of the genes located in the complex on 11p15.5. *Hum Genet* 1998;102:357–366.
108. Merry DE, Kobayashi Y, Bailey CK, et al. Cleavage, aggregation and cytotoxicity of the expanded androgen receptor in spinal and bulbar muscular atrophy. *Hum Mol Genet* 1998;7: 693–701.
109. Vinall LE, Fowler JC, Jones AL, et al. Polymorphism of human mucin genes in chest disease: possible significance of *MUC2. Am J Respir Cell Mol Biol* 2000;23:678–686.
110. Desseyn JL, Aubert JP, Porchet N, et al. Evolution of the large secreted gel-forming mucins. *Mol Biol Evol* 2000;17: 1175–1184.
111. Ho SB, Robertson AM, Shekels LL, et al. Expression and cloning of gastric mucin complementary DNA and localization of mucin gene expression. *Gastroenterology* 1995;109:735–747.
112. Van Klinken JWB, Dekker J, van Gool SA, et al. MUC5B is the prominent mucin in the human gallbladder and is also expressed in a subset of colonic goblet cells. *Am J Physiol* 1998;274:G871–G878.
113. Velcich A, Palombo L, Selleri L, et al. Organization and regulatory aspects of the human intestinal mucin gene (*MUC2*) locus. *J Biol Chem* 1997;272:7968–7976.
114. Weiss AA, Babyatsky MW, Ogata S, et al. Expression of MUC2 and MUC3 mRNA in the normal, malignant, and inflammatory tissues. *J Histochem Cytochem* 1996;44:1161–1166.
115. Gum JR, Hicks JW, Kim YS. Identification and characterization of the MUC2 (human intestinal mucin) gene 5′-flanking region: promoter activity in cultured cells. *Biochem J* 1997;325 (Pt 1):259–267.
116. Gum JR Jr, Hicks JW, Gillespie AM, et al. Goblet cell-specific expression mediated by the *MUC2* mucin gene promoter in the intestine of transgenic mice. *Am J Physiol* 1999;276: G666–G676.
117. Li JD, Dohram AF, Gallup M, et al. Transcriptional activation of mucin by *Pseudomonas aeruginosa* lipopolysaccharide in the pathogenesis of cystic fibrosis lung disease. *Proc Natl Acad Sci U S A* 1997;94:967–972.
118. Li JD, Feng W, Gallup M, et al. Activation of NF-κB via a Src-dependent Ras-MAPK-pp90rsk pathway is required for *Pseudomonas aeruginosa*-induced mucin overproduction in epithelial cells. *Proc Natl Acad Sci U S A* 1998;95:5718–5723.
119. Levine SJ, Larivee P, Logun C, et al. Tumor necrosis factor-alpha induces mucin hypersecretion and MUC2 gene expression by human airway epithelial cells. *Am J Respir Cell Mol Biol* 1995;12:196–204.
120. Velcich A, Augenlicht LH. Regulated expression of an intestinal mucin gene in HT29 colonic carcinoma cells. *J Biol Chem* 1993;268:13956–13961.
121. Hong DH, Petrovics G, Anderson WB, et al. Induction of mucin gene expression in human colonic cell lines by PMA is dependent on PKC-ε. *Am J Physiol* 1999;277:G1041–G1047.
122. Sajjan SU, Forstner JF. Role of the putative "link" glycopeptide of intestinal mucin in binding of piliated *Escherichia coli* serotype O157H7 strain CL-49. *Infect Immun* 1990;58: 868–873.

123. Mimura Y, Yamamato Y, Inoue Y, et al. NMR study of interaction between sugar and peptide moieties in mucin-type model glycopeptides. *Int J Biol Macromol* 1992;14:242–248.
124. Gerken TA, Butenhof KJ, Shogren R, et al. Effects of glycosylation on the conformation and dynamics of O-linked glycoproteins, carbon-13 NMR studies of ovine submaxillary mucin. *Biochemistry* 1989;28:5536–5543.
125. Sterk H, Fabian W, Hayn E, et al. Dynamic behavior of mucus glycoproteins—a ^{13}Cnmr relaxation study. *Int J Biol Macromol* 1987;9:58–62.
126. Shogren R, Gerken TA, Jentoft N. Role of glycosylation on the conformation and chain dimensions of *O*-linked glycoproteins: light scattering studies of ovine submaxillary mucin. *Biochemistry* 1989;28:5525–5535.
127. Allen A, Pearson JP. Mucus glycoproteins of the normal gastrointestinal tract. *Eur J Gastroenterol Hepatol* 1993;5:193–199.
128. Hansel JE, Lund O, Nielsen JO, et al. O-GLYCBASE: A revised database of O-glycosylated proteins. *Nucleic Acids Res* 1996;24:248–252.
129. Iida S, Takeuchi H, Kato K, et al. Order and maximum incorporation of *N*-acetyl-D-galactosamine into threonine residues of MUC2 core peptide with microsome fraction of human-colon-carcinoma LS174T cells. *Biochem J* 2000;347:535–542.
130. Podolsky DK. Oligosaccharide structures of human colonic mucin. *J Biol Chem* 1985;260:8262–8271.
131. Ishihara K, Hotta K. Comparison of the mucus glycoproteins present in the different layers of rat gastric mucosa. *Comp Biochem Physiol* 1993;104B:315–319.
132. Oliver MG, Specian RD. Intracellular variation of rat intestinal mucin granules localized by monoclonal antibodies. *Anat Rec* 1991;230:513–518.
133. Brockhausen I. Clinical aspects of glycoprotein synthesis. *Crit Rev Clin Sci* 1993;30:65–151.
134. Hennebicq S, Tetaert D, Soudan B, et al. Influence of the amino acid sequence on the MUC5AC motif peptide *O*-glycosylation by human gastric UDP-GalNAc:polypeptide *N*-acetylgalactosaminyltransferase(s). *Glycoconjugate J* 1998;15:275–282.
135. Wandall HH, Hassan H, Mirgorodskaya E, et al. Substrate specificities for three members of the human UDP-*N*-acetyl-α-D-galactosamine: polypeptide *N*-acetyl-galactosaminyltransferase family, GalNAc-T1, -T2, and T3. *J Biol Chem* 1997;272:23503–23514.
136. Morita H, Kettlewell MG, Jewell DP, et al. Glycosylation and sulfation of colonic mucus glycoproteins in patients with ulcerative colitis and in healthy subjects. *Gut* 1993;34:926–932.
137. Itzkowitz SH. Blood group-related carbohydrate antigen expression in malignant and premalignant colonic neoplasms. *J Cell Biochem Suppl* 1992;16:G97–G101.
138. Hennet T, Dinter A, Kunhert P, et al. Genomic cloning and expression of three murine UDP-galactose: β-*N*-acetylglucosamine β1-3 galactosyl transferase genes. *J Biol Chem* 1998;273:58–65.
139. Granovsky M, Bielfeldt T, Peters S, et al. UDP-galactose:glycoprotein-*N*-acetyl-D-galactosamine3-β-D-galactosaminyltransferase activity synthesizing *O*-glycan core 1 is controlled by the amino acid sequence and glycosylation of glycopeptide substrates. *Eur J Biochem* 1994;221:1039–1046.
140. Varki A, Cummings R, Esko J, et al., eds. Essentials of glycobiology. Cold Spring Harbor, NY: Cold Spring Harbor Laboratory Press, 1999.
141. Neutra MR, Forstner JF. Gastrointestinal mucus synthesis, secretion and function. In: LR Johnson, ed. Physiology of the gastrointestinal tract, second edition. New York: Raven Press, 1987:975–1009.
142. Hoskins LC, Augustines M, McKee WB, et al. Mucin degradation in human colonic ecosystems. Isolation and properties of fecal strains that degrade ABH blood group antigens and oligosaccharides from mucin glycoproteins. *J Clin Invest* 1985;75:944–953.
143. Schoentag R, Primus FJ, Kuhns W. ABH and Lewis blood group expression in colorectal carcinoma. *Cancer Res* 1987;47:1695–1700.
144. Hirohashi S, Ino Y, Kodama T, et al. Distribution of blood group antigens A, B, H, and 1 (Ma) in mucus-producing adenocarcinoma of human lung. *J Natl Cancer Inst* 1981;72:1299–1305.
145. Ishikawa N, Horii Y, Nawa Y. Immune-mediated alteration of the terminal sugars of goblet cell mucins in the small intestine of *Nippostrongylus brasiliensis*-infected rats. *Immunology* 1993;78:303–307.
146. Rabinowitz SS, Gordon S. Macrosialin, a macrophage-restricted membrane sialoprotein differentially glycosylated in response to inflammatory stimuli. *J Exp Med* 1991;174:827–836.
147. Brockhausen I. Pathways of O-glycan biosynthesis in cancer cells. *Biochim Biophys Acta* 1999;1473:67–95.
148. Shu-Heh WC, Walker WA. Bacterial interaction with the developing intestine. *Gastroenterology* 1993;104:916–925.
149. Strous GJ, Dekker J. Mucin-type glycoproteins. *Crit Rev Biochem Mol Biol* 1992;27:57–92.
150. Wesley AW, Forstner J, Forstner G. Structure of intestinal mucus glycoprotein from human post-mortem or surgical tissue: inferences from correlation analyses of sugar and sulfate composition of individual mucins. *Carbohydr Res* 1983;115:151–163.
151. Mawhinney TP, Landrum DG, Gayer DA, et al. Sulfated sialyl-oligosaccharides derived from tracheobronchial mucous glycoproteins of a patient suffering from cystic fibrosis. *Carbohydr Res* 1992;235:179–197.
152. Filipe MI. Mucins in the human gastrointestinal epithelium: a review. *Invest Cell Pathol* 1979;2:195–216.
153. Forstner J, Roomi N, Kharasani R, et al. Effect of reserpine on the histochemical and biochemical properties of rat intestinal mucin. *Exp Mol Pathol* 179;2:195–216.
154. Raouf AH, Tsai HH, Parker N, et al. Sulfation of colonic and rectal mucin in inflammatory bowel disease: reduced sulfation of rectal mucus in ulcerative colitis. *Clin Sci* 1992;83:623–626.
155. Van Klinken BJW, Van der Wal JWG, Einerhand AWC, et al. Sulfation and secretion of the predominant secretory human colonic mucin MUC2 in ulcerative colitis. *Gut* 1999;44:387–393.
156. Morrisey SM, Tymvios MC. Acid mucins in human intestinal goblet cells. *J Pathol* 1978;126:197–208.
157. Cheng PW, Boat TF, Cranfill K, et al. Increased sulfation of glycoconjugates by cultured nasal epithelial cells from patients with cystic fibrosis. *J Clin Invest* 1989;84:68–72.
158. Mian N, Anderson CE, Kent PW. Effect of *O*-sulfated groups in lactose and *N*-acetylneuraminyl-lactose on their enzyme hydrolysis. *Biochem J* 1979;181:387–389.
159. Goso Y, Hotta K. Types of oligosaccharide sulfation, depending on mucus glycoprotein source, corpus or antral, in rat stomach. *Biochem J* 1989;264:805–812.
160. Goso Y, Hotta K. Regional differences in sulfated oligosaccharides of rat gastrointestinal mucin as detected by two-dimensional chromatography. *Arch Biochem Biophys* 1993;302:212–217.
161. Brockhausen I, Kuhns W. Role and metabolism of glycoconjugate sulfation. *Trends Glycosci Glycotechnol* 1994;11:381–394.
162. Nieuw Amerongen AV, Bolscher JG, Bloemena E, et al. Sulfomucins in the human body. *Biol Chem* 1998;379:1–18.
163. Yolken RH, Willoughby R, Wee SB, et al. Sialic acid glycoproteins inhibit *in vitro* and *in vivo* replication of rotaviruses. *J Clin Invest* 1987;79:148–154.

164. Perez-Vilar J, Eckhardt AE, Hill RL. Porcine submaxillary mucin forms disulfide-bonded dimers between its carboxyl-terminal domains. *J Biol Chem* 1996;271:9845–9850.
165. Gum JR Jr. Human mucin glycoproteins: varied structures predict diverse properties and specific functions. *Biochem Soc Trans* 1995;23:795–799.
166. McCool DJ, Okada Y, Forstner JF, et al. Roles of calreticulin and calnexin during mucin synthesis in LS180 and HT29/A1 human colonic adenocarcinoma cells. *Biochem J* 1999;341: 593–600.
167. Sheehan JK, Oates K, Carlstedt I. Electron microscopy of cervical, gastric and bronchial mucus. *Biochem J* 1986;239: 147–153.
168. Sheehan JK, Thorton J, Somerville M, et al. The structure and heterogeneity of respiratory mucus glycoproteins. *Am J Respir Dis* 1991;144:S4–S9.
169. Verdugo P. Goblet cell secretion and mucogenesis. *Annu Rev Physiol* 1990;52:157–176.
170. Verdugo P. Mucin exocytosis. *Am J Respir Dis* 1991;144: S33–S37.
171. Bansil R, Stanley E, LaMont T. Mucin biophysics. *Annu Rev Physiol* 1995;57:635–657.
172. MacFarlane G, Allison C, Gibson SAW. Contribution of the microflora to proteolysis in the human large intestine. *J Appl Bacteriol* 1988;64:37–26.
173. Atuma C, Strugala V, Allen A, et al. The adherent gastrointestinal mucus layer: thickness and physical state *in vivo*. *Am J Physiol* 2001;280:G922–G929.
174. Sherman P, Forstner J, Roomi N, et al. Mucin depletion in the intestine of malnourished rats. *Am J Physiol* 1984;248: G418–G423.
175. Sherman P, Fleming N, Forstner J, et al. Bacteria and the mucus blanket in experimental small bowel bacterial overgrowth. *Am J Pathol* 1897;126:527–534.
176. Lelouard H, Reggio H, Roy C, et al. Glycocalyx on rabbit intestinal M cells displays carbohydrate epitopes from Muc2. *Infect Immun* 2001;69:1061–1071.
177. Jay GD. Characterization of a bovine synovial fluid lubricating factor I. Chemical, surface activity and lubricating properties. *Connect Tissue Res* 1992;28:71–88.
178. Sundari CS, Raman B, Balasubramanian D. Hydrophobic surfaces in oligosaccharides: linear dextrins are amphiphilic chains. *Biochim Biophys Acta* 1991;1065:35–41.
179. Girod J, Zahm JM, Plotkowski C, et al. Role of the physiochemical properties of mucus in the protection of the respiratory epithelium. *Eur Resp J* 1992;5:477–487.
180. Sellers LA, Allen A, Morris ER, et al. The rheology of pig small intestinal and colonic mucus: weakening of gel structure by non-mucin components. *Biochim Biophys Acta* 1991;1115: 174–179.
181. Moncada D, Yu Y, Keller K, et al. *Entamoeba histolytica* cysteine proteinases degrade human colonic mucin and alter its function. *Arch Med Res* 2000;31:S224–S225.
182. Carlstedt I, Sheehan JK. Mucus glycoproteins—a short course. In: Glantz PO, Leach SA, Ericson T, eds. Oral interfacial reactions of bone, soft tissue and saliva. Oxford: ILR, 1985:97–105.
183. Hutton DA, Pearson JP, Allen A, et al. Mucolysis of the colonic mucus barrier by faecal proteinases: inhibition by interacting polyacrylate. *Clin Sci* 1990;78:265–271.
184. Poulsen SS, Nex E, Olsen PS, et al. Localization of a new serine protease, ingobsin, in goblet cells in rat, pig and man. *Histochem J* 1985;17:487–492.
185. Schachter M, Peret MW, Billing AG, et al. Immunolocalization of the protease kallikrein in the colon. *J Histochem Cytochem* 1983;31:1255–1260.
186. Kvist N, Olsen PS, Poulsen SS, et al. Secretion of goblet cell serine proteinase, ingobsin, is stimulated by vasoactive intestinal polypeptide and acetylcholine. *Digestion* 1987;37:223–227.
187. Sheehan JK, Carlstedt I. Electron microscopy of cervical-mucus glycoproteins and fragments therefrom: the use of colloidal gold to make visible "naked" protein regions. *Biochem J* 1990; 265:169–178.
188. Khatri IA, Forstner GG, Forstner JF. Susceptibility of the cysteine-rich *N*-terminal and *C*-terminal ends of rat intestinal mucin MUC2 to proteolytic cleavage. *Biochem J* 1998;331: 323–330.
189. Gum JR Jr, Hicks JW, Lagace RE, et al. Molecular cloning of rat intestinal mucin. *J Biol Chem* 1991;266:22733–22738.
190. Marcus F. Preferential cleavage at aspartyl-proline peptide bonds in dilute acid. *Int J Peptide Protein Res* 1985;25:542–546.
191. Crowther RS, Roomi NW, Fahim REF, et al. *Vibrio cholerae* metalloproteinase degrades intestinal mucin and facilitates enterotoxin-induced secretion from rat intestine. *Biochem Biophys Acta* 187;924:393–402.
192. Slomiany BL, Murty VLN, Piotrowsky J, et al. Glycosulfatase activity in *Helicobacter pylori* toward gastric mucin. *Biochem Biophys Res Commun* 1992;183:506–513.
193. Schultz C, Van Den Berg FM, Ten Kate FW, et al. The intestinal mucus layer from patients with inflammatory bowel disease harbors high numbers of bacteria compared with controls. *Gastroenterology* 1999;117:1089–1097.
194. Corfield AP, Wagner SA, Clamp JR, et al. Mucin degradation in the human colon: production of sialidase, sialate *O*-acetylesterase, *N*-acetylneuraminate lyase, arylesterase, and glycosulfatase activities by strains of fecal bacteria. *Infect Immun* 1992;60:3971–3978.
195. Takahashi H, Nikiwa T, Yoshimura K, et al. Structure of the human neutrophil elastase gene. *J Biol Chem* 1988;263: 14739–14747.
196. Cole KR, Kumar S, Trong HL, et al. Rat mast cell carboxy peptidase: amino acid sequence and evidence of enzyme activity within mast cell granules. *Biochemistry* 1991;30:648–655.
197. Grisham MB, Von Ritter C, Smith BF, et al. Interactions between oxygen radicals and gastric mucin. *Am J Physiol* 1987;253:G93–G96.
198. Gong D, Turner B, Bhaskar KR, et al. Lipid binding to gastric mucin: protective effect against oxygen radicals. *Am J Physiol* 1990;259:G681–G686.
199. Mantle M. Effects of hydrogen peroxide, mild trypsin digestion, and partial reduction on rat intestinal mucin and its disulphide-bound 118kDa glycoprotein. *Biochem J* 1991;274:679–685.
200. Stanley RA, Ram SP, Wilkinson RK, et al. Degradation of pig gastric mucin and colonic mucins by bacteria isolated from pig colon. *Appl Environ Microbiol* 1986;51:1104–1109.
201. Rhodes JM, Black RR, Gallimore R, et al. Histochemical demonstration of desialylation and desulfation of normal and inflammatory bowel disease rectal mucus by faecal extracts. *Gut* 1985;26:1312–1318.
202. Prizont R. Degradation of intestinal glycoproteins by pathogenic *Shigella flexneri*. *Infect Immun* 1982;32:615–620.
203. Henderson IR, Czeczulin J, Eslava E, et al. Characterization of Pic, a secreted protease of *Shigella flexneri* and enteroaggregative *Escherichia coli*. *Infect Immun* 1999;67:5587–5596.
204. Carlstedt-Duke B, Hoverstad T, Lingaas E, et al. Influence of antibiotics on intestinal mucin in healthy subjects. *Eur J Clin Microbiol* 1986;5:634–638.
205. Ishii-Karakasa I, Iwase H, Hotta K, et al. Partial purification and characterization of an endo-α-*N*-acetylgalactosaminidase from the culture medium of *Streptomyces* sp. OH-11242. *Biochem J* 1992;288:475–482.
206. Paget TA, James SL. The mucolytic activity of polyamines and mucosal invasion. *Biochem Soc Trans* 1994;22:394S.

207. Spice WM, Ackers JP. The effects of *Entamoeba histolytica* lysates on human colonic mucins. *J Eukaryot Microbiol* 1998;45:24S–27S.
208. Robertson AM, Wright DP. Bacterial glycosulphatases and sulphomucin degradation. *Can J Gastroenterol* 1997;11:361–366.
209. Bhaskar KR, Garik P, Turner BS, et al. Viscous fingering of HCl through gastric mucin. *Nature* 1992;360:458–462.
210. Chadee K, Petri Jr WA, Innes DJ, et al. Rat and human colonic mucins bind to and inhibit adherence lectin of *Entamoeba histolytica. J Clin Invest* 1987;80:1245–1254.
211. Vimal DB, Khullar M, Gupta S, et al. Intestinal mucins: the binding sites for *Salmonella typhimurium. Mol Cell Biochem* 2000;204:107–117.
212. Yamamoto T, Yokota T. Electron microscopic study of *Vibrio cholerae* O1 adherence to the mucus coat and villus surface in the human small intestine. *Infect Immun* 1988;56: 2753–2759.
213. Mantle M, Husar SD. Binding of *Yersinia enterocolitica* to purified, native small intestinal mucins from rabbits and humans involves interactions with the mucin carbohydrate moiety. *Infect Immun* 1994;62:1219–1227.
214. Repentigny LD, Aumont F, Bernard K, et al. Characterization of binding of *Candidia albicans* to small intestinal mucin and its role in adherence to mucosal epithelial cells. *Infect Immun* 2000;68:3172–3179.

6

THE ROLE OF MICROBIAL ADHERENCE FACTORS IN GASTROINTESTINAL DISEASE

BARBARA J. MANN
WILLIAM A. PETRI, JR.

The first step in the pathogenesis of many infectious diseases is adherence of the microorganism to the host. Adherence to the host is often paramount in establishing colonization and facilitating events such as invasion, dissemination, toxin delivery, or host cell lysis. The harsh and dynamic environment found in the mammalian gastrointestinal (GI) tract presents a challenge to both pathogenic and commensal organisms that adhere to and colonize this site. Microbial adherence molecules (adhesins) must be protected against destruction by digestive enzymes and avoid recognition by the intestinal immune responses. Secretory immunoglobulin A (IgA) directed against adherence molecules may block colonization and therefore infection. Nonimmunologic protective barriers, including a mucous lining, periodic sloughing of the lining, peristaltic movements, and cleansing actions, also may block the establishment of infection by enteric pathogens. All of these factors necessitate that enteric microorganisms have specific means of attachment to the cells lining the GI tract in order to colonize and exert their pathogenic effects.

SPECIFICITY OF ADHESIN RECEPTOR INTERACTIONS

An adhesin is a microbial surface molecule that interacts with a specific host receptor to mediate attachment of the organism to host surfaces. Some adhesins may be capable of interacting with more than one receptor. This promiscuity allows organisms to adhere to different cell types and locations. The ability to recognize multiple receptors may facilitate the colonization and invasion of organisms that are able to penetrate the intestinal epithelium and establish infection at extraintestinal sites. Type 1 fimbrial adhesins of *Escherichia coli*, for example, recognize and bind to laminin, immobilized fibronectin, and the CD11/CD18 leukocyte adhesion molecules (1–3).

Microbial adhesins and host receptor molecules represent a diverse set of molecules. Host receptors can consist of protein, lipid, or carbohydrate moieties. Tables 6.1 and 6.2 list some examples of the various types of receptor and adhesin molecules. The diversity of receptor types reflects the role that the adherence event can play in the pathogenesis of disease.

The adhesin receptor interaction plays a part in both tissue tropism and species specificity. Restricted expression of a receptor in a specific cell, tissue, or species can determine whether colonization or pathogenesis, or both, will occur. Experiments in animal models suggest that many enteric pathogens use M cells to establish local or systemic infections (4). M cells are specialized epithelial cells of the intestine that transport macromolecules, particles, and microorganisms and act as a conduit to the mucosal immune system. Even though the data on human M cells is limited, M cells from other species show pronounced species and regional variation in glycoconjugate expression (5,6). Because glycoconjugates have been identified as receptors for a variety of adhesins, M cells may also help determine which portion of the intestine is colonized or invaded (5–8) (Table 6.1). A number of enteric organisms that are thought to target M cells also primarily colonize or invade specific regions of the intestine (5). Enteropathogenic and enterotoxogenic *E. coli* (EPEC and ETEC, respectively) and *Vibrio* colonize the proximal small intestine, while rabbit enteropathogenic *E. coli* (REPEC) are found in the distal small intestine. Other bacteria, such as enteroaggregative *E. coli* (EAEC) and *Shigella flexneri* prefer the large colon (5). A number of strains of *E. coli* are known to cause disease only in specific animal species. In several cases, the presence of a specific fimbrial type has been demonstrated to be required for infection. Strains of *E. coli* expressing K88 fimbria cause diarrheal illness only in certain strains of neonatal pigs. Once

B.J. Mann and **W.A. Petri, Jr.:** Departments of Internal Medicine and Microbiology, University of Virginia, Charlottesville, Virginia

TABLE 6.1. EXAMPLES OF HOST RECEPTORS AND MICROBIAL ADHESINS

Host Cell Ligand	Microbial Adhesin
Sugars	
Mannose	*Escherichia coli* type 1 fimbriae
Sialic acid	Influenza virus hemagglutinin
	Trypanosoma cruzi trans-sialidase
Galactose	*Entamoeba histolytica* lectin
Immunoglobulin superfamily	
ICAM-1	Rhinovirus capsid (major group)
CD4	HIV gp120/41
Carcinoembryonic antigen	Mouse hepatitis virus
Integrins	
VLA-2	Echovirus 1
Poliovirus receptor	Poliovirus
β_1 integrins	*Yersinia* sp. Inv protein
CD11/CD18	*E. coli* type 1 fimbriae
Growth factors/growth factor receptors	
EGF receptor	Vaccinia virus
IL-6	Hepatitis B virus envelope protein
Chemokine receptors	
CCR5, CXCR4	HIV gp120/40
Extracellular matrix components	
Laminin	*Toxoplasma gondii*
	E. coli type 1 fimbriae
Fibronectin	Streptococci
Transport proteins	
Basic amino acids	Ecotropic murine retrovirus
Phosphate transporter	Gibbon ape leukemia virus
Proteases	
Aminopeptidase N	Transmissible gastroenteritis virus
Complement receptors	
CR2	Epstein-Barr virus gp350/220
CR3	Leishmania
Glycosphingolipids	
GM_1	*E. coli* K88 fimbriae
Globoseries glycolipids	*E. coli* P fimbriae

TABLE 6.2. EXAMPLES OF DIFFERENT TYPES OF MICROBIAL ADHESINS

Adhesin Type	Organism
Fimbriae	
Type 1	*Escherichia coli*
P	*E. coli*
YadA	*Yersinia* sp.
BFP	*E. coli*
Nonfimbrial bacteria	
AIDA-1	*E. coli*
Invasin	*Yersinia* sp.
Glycoproteins	
Gal/GalNAc lectin	*Entamoeba histolytica*
gp120/41	HIV
gp350/220	Epstein-Barr virus
Glycolipids	
Lipoteichoic acid	*Streptomyces pyogenes*
Lipophosphoglycan	*Leishmania* sp.
Enzymes	
Trans-sialidase	*Trypanosoma cruzi*
Toxins	
Pertussis toxin	*Bordatella pertussis*

these pigs mature, they are no longer susceptible. Studies comparing the epithelial brush border cells from mature pigs and genetically resistant pigs correlate resistance with the lack of specific receptors for K88 fimbriae in the intestinal epithelial cells of resistant animals (9–11).

Another example of species restriction is demonstrated with poliovirus, which only infects primates. Poliovirus exhibits a limited tissue tropism, replicating primarily in the lymphoid tissues of the pharynx and gut as well as motor neurons. The receptor for poliovirus is a member of the immunoglobulin superfamily (12). Somewhat paradoxically, poliovirus receptor is detected in a wide variety of tissue types, including kidney, but poliovirus replication does not occur in these cell types. Transgenic mice expressing the human poliovirus receptor are susceptible to poliovirus infection by intracerebral inoculation, indicating that the receptor is primarily responsible for species restriction (13). However, transgenic mice are not susceptible to infection by an oral route. This result suggests that expression of the receptor is necessary but not sufficient for poliovirus infection and that there are other factors involved in species restriction in the gut (14).

A novel adhesin receptor interaction is exemplified by EPEC. Remarkably, EPEC transfer their own receptor to host cells using a type III secretion mechanism (15). The bacterial encoded receptor, Tir, inserts into the host membrane and binds to the bacterial adhesin intimin. In clinical trials, EPEC strains lacking intimin show reduced virulence, indicating a role for tir–intimin interaction in human disease (16).

IDENTIFICATION OF ADHESINS

The identification of a molecule as an adhesin is not always straightforward. The development of a relevant adherence assay is key. An important consideration for an assay is the selection of an appropriate target cell that best represents the physiologic situation. This would be especially true of organisms that exhibit cell, tissue, or species specificity for pathogenicity. One caveat in analyzing adherence properties of enteric organisms *in vitro* is that it is not possible to recreate the microenvironment of the GI tract *in vitro* including the influences of the mucous lining, commensal microbial flora, and peristaltic movements on adherence. Another important aspect of a meaningful assay is that conditions should be designed to measure only adherence and limit other activities such as motility, invasion, and cell lysis. The identification of an adhesin is often complicated by the fact that many organisms possess multiple adhesins that may be expressed simultaneously. Multiple adhesins may act independently or synergistically. The expression of some adhesins may be subject to specific regulatory controls that differ in microorganisms grown in cell culture versus microorganisms infecting animals.

In many bacterial species, the study of individual putative adhesins can be accomplished by genetic manipulation, including the ability to introduce and express a putative adhesin in a nonadherent strain of *E. coli*. For other organisms, such as protozoan parasites and viruses, the initial identification of an adhesin is usually accomplished by adherence inhibitory antibodies or by the carbohydrate recognition properties of the adhesin. Rigorous identification of a purified protein as an adhesin should include a demonstration that specific antibody inhibits adherence and that purified protein will competitively inhibit adherence. If carbohydrate specificity is known, a demonstration that the carbohydrate is capable of blocking the adhesive activity of the protein should also be presented.

CLASSIFICATION OF ADHESINS

In bacteria, the adhesin molecule is often part of an adherence organelle called fimbriae or pili (Fig. 6.1). The most common type of fimbriae is the type 1, or mannose-sensitive fimbriae, which has been found on at least 70% of wild-type strains of *E. coli* (17). Fimbriae can be generally classified into four groups based on the type of assembly pathway: the chaperone-usher pathway (type 1, P, K88), the generalized secretion pathway (type IV pili of EPEC and *Vibrio*), extracellular nucleation-precipitation pathway (curli found on *E. coli* and *Salmonella*), and alternate chaperone pathway (CS1 and CFA pili of ETEC) (18). *E. coli* fimbriae range from about 2 to 7 nm in diameter and can only be seen by electron microscopy. They are easily distinguishable from flagella, which are about 20 nm in diameter (19). The adhesive subunit can be the major subunit as in K88 fimbriae (20) or a minor component located at the tip of the organelle (21). In type 1 and P fimbriae, the adhesive subunit is located at the end of morphologically distinct tip structure, called fibrillae (22). A heterogeneous group of nonfimbrial types of bacterial adhesins such as AIDA-I (adhesin involved in diffuse adherence) and AFA I/III have also been identified but their contributions to bacterial adherence are not as well characterized (23,24).

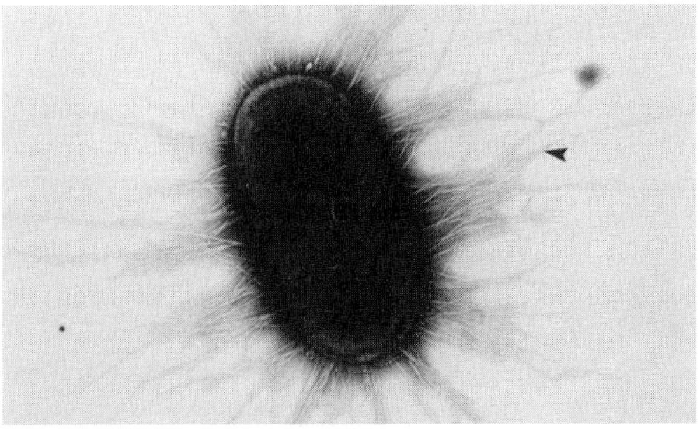

FIGURE 6.1. Electron micrograph of *Escherichia coli* expressing P fimbriae. Bar, 0.25 μ. (From Klemm P. Fimbrial adhesins of *Escherichia coli*. *Rev Infect Dis* 1985;7:321–340, with permission.)

Many microbial adhesins, including the fimbriae, can be classified as lectins because they bind specific carbohydrate moieties. The complexity of carbohydrate structures and linkages has resulted in the creation of a large diversity of structures that could potentially be specifically recognized by microbial adhesins. The subtlety and specificity of adhesin receptor interaction is illustrated by a study of the binding specificity of three allelic variants of P fimbrial-associated adhesins of *E. coli* that share antigenic cross-reactivity and sequence similarities (25). These three adhesin variants all recognize the same immobilized Gal (1-4) Gal β-containing globoseries glycosphingolipids (GSLs). However, when tested in solutions in hemagglutination assays, the adhesins differ in their ability to agglutinate erythrocytes with different GSLs in their membranes. Molecular modeling of the GSLs suggests that these GSLs have different saccharide orientations with respect to the membrane. Differential binding of the three P adhesins may result from differences in epitope presentation at the membrane by these GSLs (25).

EFFECTS OF ADHERENCE

The outcome of an adherence event may be colonization, invasion/internalization, toxicity, host cell lysis, rearrangement of host cytoskeleton, or stimulation of specific cytokine production. EPEC initially adhere to intestinal surfaces via a bundle-forming pilus (BFP) (26). This pilus appears to play a role in pathogenesis because strains lacking BFP were attenuated in human trials (27). This initial pilus-mediated interaction helps to facilitate an intimate interaction called an attaching and effacing (AE) lesion. During this intimate attachment, bacterial proteins are secreted directly into the host cell cytoplasm via a type III secretion mechanism (28). These secreted proteins, which are encoded on a pathogenicity island called LEE (locus of enterocyte effacement) activate signal transduction pathways in the host epithelial cell (29). One of these proteins is Tir, which acts as the receptor for intimin, the bacterial adhesin. The binding of Tir and intimin activates several host pathways, which result in gross rearrangements of the microvilli to form pedestal-like structures beneath adherent bacteria (30–32).

The invasin protein of *Yersinia* has been shown to mediate both adherence and invasion. Transfection of *E. coli* K12 with the invasin gene confers an adherence and invasion phenotype to the normally noninvasive strain (33,34). Receptors for invasin have been identified as members of the β1 integrin family (35). Members of the integrin family are transmembrane proteins associated with cytoskeleton proteins and focal adhesions. *Yersinia* invasion can be inhibited by cytochalsin D, suggesting that the invasion process involves cytoskeletal rearrangements facilitated by the interaction of the invasin protein with the β1 integrin (36). A "zipper" model of invasion has been proposed in which high-affinity binding of invasin to β1 integrins competes with the relatively low-affinity binding of the extracellular matrix to the integrins (37). As the number of invasin-integrin interactions grows, the bacteria become surrounded and internalized into an endosomal compartment. Although the invasin plays a key role in invasion of cultured cells, its role *in vivo* is more subtle (38). In a mouse model, bacteria lacking invasin have the same LD_{50} as wild-type cells. However these strains appear to invade Peyer patches less efficiently and infections have a delayed course (38). These studies suggest that invasin promotes entry during the initial stages of infection.

Toxin activity and cytolysis can occur after adherence by virtue of the host and microbial membranes being in close contact and enabling a separate toxin or cytotoxic molecule to be efficiently delivered to its target. However, some toxins can also function as an adhesin. Pertussis toxin of *Bordetella pertussis* mediates adherence to ciliated respiratory epithelium (39). Site-directed mutagenesis of the toxin subunits localized the adherence-mediating domains to the S2 and S3 subunits (40). A comparison of these regions revealed a significant amino sequence similarity with the carbohydrate recognition domains of calcium-dependent eukaryotic lectins.

The galactose/N-acetyl D-galactosamine-inhibitable (Gal/GalNAc) lectin of the protozoan parasite *Entamoeba histolytica* mediates adherence to host cells and has a role in contact-dependent killing (Fig. 6.2). This remarkable ability to kill host cells can be inhibited Gal, GalNAc, colonic mucins or lectin-specific antibody (41–43). Inhibition of cell killing is not merely due to a blocking adherence since apposition of the plasma membranes of amebas and target cells, as can be achieved by centrifugation, does not result in target cell lysis in the presence of galactose (42,44). The specific mechanisms by which *E. histolytica* kills cells is not understood, but, after contact, host cells show signs of apoptotic cell death such as nuclear chromatin condensation, DNA fragmentation, and caspase 3 activation (45).

Bacterial adherence can elicit inflammatory responses that include cytokine production. Uropathogenic *E. coli* stimulate the release of a number of cytokines from uroepithelial cells such as interleukin (IL)-1, IL-1β, Il-6, and IL-8 (46,47). The release of these cytokines causes a variety of responses, including activation of lymphocytes and recruitment of neutrophils, as well as other inflammatory processes.

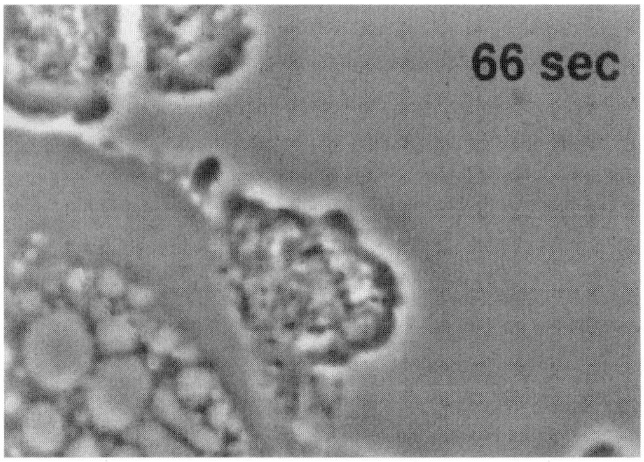

FIGURE 6.2. Still shot from a video of an *Entamoeba histolytica* trophozoite, shown in bottom left corner, in contact with and killing a human neutrophil. (Adapted from Petri WA Jr. Recent advances in amebiasis. *Crit Rev Clin Lab Sci* 1996;33:1–37, with permission.)

For instance, adherence of P and type 1—fimbriated bacteria to epithelial cell layers increases neutrophil migration by inducing IL-8 release and increasing the density of IL-8 receptors on the epithelial cells (47). Inflammatory responses contribute to many aspect of the disease process but it is unclear what advantages they provide for the bacteria.

Adhesins have additional biologic activities. Several adhesins, such as the invasin protein of *Yersinia*, mediate invasion as part of the adherence event (36,37). The galactose-specific adhesin of *E. histolytica* has a role in resistance to serum lysis by blocking assembly of the membrane attack complex of complement (48). The adhesin YadA, encoded by the virulence plasmid of *Yersinia* sp., also appears to have a role in resistance to complement-mediated lysis (49). YadA binds to complement factor H, which prevents C3b opsonization and results in reduced amounts of C5b-9 complexes deposited on the surface of the bacteria (49).

REGULATION AND EXPRESSION OF ADHESINS

Many organisms have developed mechanisms for regulating the expression or function of their adhesins. Because adhesins are prime targets for the immune system, it may be advantageous to turn off the expression of adhesin-encoding genes or to perhaps switch to a different adhesin. Many fimbrial adhesins are able to undergo phase variation, that is, to turn the expression of fimbrial genes off or on (50). This would help with immune avoidance; however, it may also allow the organism to adapt to a new environment or detach and disseminate to a different site. The expression of type 1 fimbriae is controlled by a 314–base-pair invertible element containing the promoter element of the *fim* operon that encodes the type 1 fimbrial subunits (50). In one orientation of the element, transcription of the *fim* genes occurs; in the opposite orientation, the transcription of the *fim* genes is turned off. The inversion of this element is controlled by two gene products: *fimB* and *fimE*. The products of these two genes presumably encode site-specific recombinases. The mechanism for phase variation of type 1 fimbriae is similar to the mechanism described for the switch of flagellar antigens in *S. enteriditis typhimurium*. Other genes, unlinked to the *fim* gene cluster, have also been implicated in regulating phase variation, acting presumably as auxiliary factors or regulating the expression of *fimB* and *fimE* (51). Phase variation in P fimbriae is controlled by a distinctly different mechanism involving site-specific differential DNA methylation in the promoter region of the gene cluster encoding the P fimbrial subunits (50). The methylation state of this DNA site influences the binding of different regulatory proteins, which then either promote or prevent transcription.

Some adhesins require posttranslational processing, especially proteolytic fragmentation, to manifest full biologic activity. The membrane fusion activity of the influenza virus hemagglutinin (HA), which is required for viral infectivity, requires processing of the intact hemagglutinin (HA_0) by a host protease, cleaving HA_0 into HA_1 and HA_2. This proteolytic fragmentation exposes a highly conserved hydrophobic sequence at the amino terminus of HA_2, which, at acidic pH, is involved in viral entry into the cell by fusion of the viral membrane to the endocytic vacuole cell membrane (52). Similar processing events are required for the gp160 adhesin of HIV to have functional cell fusion activity (53). The need for host proteases to activate the fusion activity of adhesins may partly account for the tropisms of microbial pathogens, because proteases required to activate the adhesins may only be present in certain tissues. This mechanism may help ensure that the virus will only infect the appropriate tissue type. Adhesin coreceptors may also account for cell tropism, as in the case of HIV. After initial adherence to CD4, interaction of gp120 with the HIV coreceptors CXCR4 and CCR5 is required for entry of the virus into T lymphocytes and macrophages, respectively (54).

Microbial adhesins may also exist in active and inactive conformational states. The Gal/GalNAc lectin *E. histolytica* has been shown to be regulated by inside-out signaling (55). Overexpression of the lectin cytoplasmic domain produces a dominant negative effect on lectin-mediated adherence to target cells. The regulation of mammalian integrin-mediated adherence involves the interaction with titratable cytoplasmic factors that regulate the affinity of the integrin for its ligand (56). The cytoplasmic domain of the Gal/GalNAc lectin shares sequence identity with critical residues in the cytoplasmic domains of β2 and β7 integrins (55,56). It is tempting to speculate that the Gal/GalNAc lectin may be regulated in an analogous manner.

ADHESINS AS VACCINES

Adhesins are potential candidates for protective vaccines. Because many adhesins are critical for the establishment of colonization or the pathogenic process, antibodies or antimicrobial agents that block this interaction would have the potential to block infection. Antibodies specific for fimbrial antigens have been shown to be protective. One of the first effective fimbrial vaccines was the use of K88 antigen to prevent diarrheal disease in newborn pigs (57). One potential problem is the variation of fimbrial antigens. An effective fimbrial subunit vaccine would have to include a number of different antigens (58). The galactose-specific adhesin of *E. histolytica* has been shown to function as a protective antigen in a gerbil model of amebiasis (59–62). Unlike the fimbrial proteins, the Gal/GalNAc lectin is quite conserved among different isolates. The potential to use DNA recombinant technology to alter, combine, or specifically express protective epitopes should help improve the effectiveness of these types of vaccines.

CONCLUSION

Adhesin molecules that mediate adherence and corresponding receptors have not been identified or well characterized for many pathogenic organisms. This should be an area of intensive research because it can provide practical information in identifying targets for preventing or containing disease. The study of adhesin receptor interactions can also contribute to modern understanding of intermolecular interactions, cell-cell communication, and signaling, which are important for many biologic activities.

REFERENCES

1. Gbarah A, Gahmberg CG, Ofek I, et al. Identification of the leukocyte adhesion molecules CD11 and CD18 as receptors for type 1-fimbriated (mannose-specific) *Escherichia coli*. *Infect Immun* 1991;59:4524–4530.
2. Korhonen TK, Vaisanen-Rhen V, Rhen M, et al. *Escherichia coli* fimbriae recognizing sialyl galactosides. *J Bacteriol* 1984;159: 762–766.
3. Sokurenko EV, Courtney HS, Abraham SN, et al. Functional heterogeneity of type 1 fimbriae of *Escherichia coli*. *Infect Immun* 1992;60:4709-4719.
4. Siebers A, Finlay BB. M cells and the pathogenesis of mucosal and systemic infections. *Trends Microbiol* 1996;4:22–29.
5. Edwards RA, Puente JL. Fimbrial expression in enteric bacteria: a critical step in intestinal pathogenesis. *Trends Microbiol* 1998; 6:282–287.
6. Jepson MA, Clark MA, Foster N, et al. Targeting to intestinal M cells. *J Anat* 1996;189:507–516.
7. Warner L, Kim YS. Intestinal receptors for microbial attachment. In: Farthing MJG, Keusch GT, eds. *Enteric infections*. New York: Raven Press, 1988:31–40.
8. Karlsson K. Animal glycosphingolipids as membrane attachment sites for bacteria. *Annu Rev Biochem* 1989;58:309–350.

9. Francis DH, Erickson AK, Grange PA. K88 adhesins of enterotoxigenic *Escherichia coli* and their porcine enterocyte receptors. *Adv Exp Med Biol.*1999;473:147–154.
10. Grange PA, Erickson AK, Anderson TJ, et al. Characterization of the carbohydrate moiety of intestinal mucin-type sialoglycoprotein receptors for the K88ac fimbrial adhesin of *Escherichia coli. Infect Immun* 1998;66:1613–1621.
11. R, Gibbons RA, Jones GW, Rutter JM. Adhesion of enteropathogenic *Escherichia coli* to pig intestinal brush border: the existence of two pig phenotypes. *J Med Microbiol* 1975;4:467–485.
12. Mendelsohn CL, Wimmer E, Racaniello VR. Cellular receptor for poliovirus: molecular cloning, nucleotide sequence and expression of a new member of the immunoglobulin superfamily. *Cell* 1989;56:855–865.
13. Ren R, Costantini F, Gorgacz EJ, et al. Transgenic mice expressing a human poliovirus receptor: a new model for poliomyelitis. *Cell* 1990;63:353–362.
14. Zhang S, Racaniello VR. Expression of the poliovirus receptor in intestinal epithelial cells is not sufficient to permit poliovirus replication in the mouse gut. *J Virol* 1997;71:4915–4920.
15. Kenny B, DeVinney R, Stein S, et al. Enteropathogenic *E. coli* (EPEC) transfers its receptor for intimate adherence into mammalian cells. *Cell* 1997;91:511–520.
16. Donnenberg MS, Tacket CO, James SP, et al. Role of the eaeA gene in experimental enteropathogenic *Escherichia coli* infection. *J Clin Invest* 1993;92:1412–1417.
17. Klemm P. Fimbrial adhesins of *Escherichia coli. Rev Infect Dis* 1985;7:321–340.
18. Soto GE, Hultgren SJ. Bacterial adhesins: common themes and variations in architecture and assembly. *J Bacteriol* 1999;181: 1059–1071.
19. Silverman M, Simon MI. Bacterial flagella. *Annu Rev Microbiol* 1977;31:397–419.
20. Jacobs AAC, Veneme J, Leeven R, et al. Inhibition of adhesive activity of K88 fibrillae by peptides derived from K88 adhesin. *J Bacteriol* 1987;169:735–741.
21. Lindberg F, Lund B, Johansson L, Normark S. Localization of the receptor-binding protein adhesin at the tip of the bacterial pilus. *Nature* 1987;328:84–87.
22. Kuehn MJ, Heuser J, Normark S, et al. P pili in uropathogenic *E. coli* are composite fibres with distinct fibrillar adhesive tips. *Nature* 1992;356:252–255.
23. Suhr M, Benz I, Schmidt MA.Processing of the AIDS-1 precursor: removal of AIDA[c] and evidence for the outer membrane anchoring as a β-barrel structure. *Mol Microbiol* 1996;22:31–42.
24. Goldhar J. Nonfimbrial adhesins of *Escherichia coli. Adv Exp Med Biol* 1996;408:63–72.
25. Stromberg N, Nyholm P, Pascher I, et al. Saccharide orientation at the cell surface affects glycolipid receptor function. *Proc Natl Acad Sci U S A* 1991;88:9340–9344.
26. Donnenberg MS, Giron JA, Nataro JP, et al. A plasmid-encoded type IV fimbrial gene of enteropathogenic *Escherichia coli* associated with localized adherence. *Mol Microbiol* 1992;6:3427–3437.
27. Bieber D, Ramer SW, Wu C-Y, et al. Type IV pili, transient bacterial aggregates, and virulence of enteropathogenic *Escherichia coli. Science* 1998;280:2114–2118.
28. Hueck CJ. Type III protein secretion systems in bacterial pathogens of animals and plants. *Microbiol Mol Biol Rev* 1998; 62:379–433.
29. Lai LC, Wainwright LA, Stone KD, et al. A third secreted protein that is encoded by the enteropathogenic *Escherichia coli* pathogenicity island is required for transduction of signals and for attaching and effacing activities in host cells. *Infect Immun* 1997;65:2211–2217.
30. Jarvis KG, Giron JA, Jerse AE, et al. Enteropathogenic *Escherichia coli* contains a putative type III secretion system necessary for the export of proteins involved in attaching and effacing lesion formation.*Proc Natl Acad Sci U S A* 1995;92(17):7996–8000.
31. Goosney DL, DeVinney R, Pfuetzner RA, et al. Enteropathogenic *E. coli* translocated intimin receptor, Tir, interacts directly with alpha-actinin. *Curr Biol* 2000;10:735–738.
32. Phillips AD, Giron J, Hicks S, et al. Intimin from enteropathogenic *Escherichia coli* mediates remodeling of the eukaryotic cell surface. *Microbiology* 2000;146:1333–1344.
33. Young VB, Miller VH, Falkow S, et al. Sequence, localization and function of the invasin protein of *Yersinia enterocolitica. Mol Microbiol* 1990;4:1119–1128.
34. Isberg RR, Voorhis DL, Falkow S. Identification of invasin: a protein that allows enteric bacteria to penetrate cultured mammalian cells. *Cell* 1987;50:769–778.
35. Isberg RR, Leong JM. Multiple $1 chain integrins are receptors for invasin, a protein that promotes bacterial penetration into mammalian cells. *Cell* 1990;60:861–871.
36. Young VB, Falkow S, Schoolnik GK. The invasin protein of *Yersinia enterocolitica*: internalization of invasin-bearing bacteria by eukaryotic cells is associated with reorganization of the cytoskeleton. *J Cell Biol* 1992;116:197–207.
37. Tran Van Nhieu G, Isberg RR. Bacterial internalization mediated by β1 chain integrins is deterined by ligand affinity and receptor density. *EMBO J* 1993;12:1887–1895.
38. Marra A, Isberg RR. Invasin-dependent and invasin-independent pathways for translocation of *Yersinia pseudotuberculosis* across the Peyer's patch intestinal epithelium. *Infect Immun* 1997;65: 3412–3421.
39. Tuomanen E, Weiss A. Characterization of two adhesins of *Bordetella* pertussis for ciliated respiratory epithelial cells. *J Infect Dis* 1985;152:118–125.
40. Saukkonen K, Burnette WN, Mar V, et al. Pertussis toxin has eukaryotic-like carbohydrate recognition domains. *Proc Natl Acad Sci U S A* 1992;89:118–122.
41. Ravdin JI, Guerrant RL. Role of adherence in cytopathic mechanisms of *Entamoeba histolytica.* Study with mammalian tissue culture cells and human erythrocytes. *J Clin Invest* 1981;68:1305–1313.
42. Guerrant RL, Brush JR JI, Sullivan JA, et al. Interaction between *Entamoeba histolytica* and human polymorphonuclear neutrophils. *J Infect Dis* 1981;143:83–93.
43. Chadee K, Petri WA Jr, Innes DJ, et al. Rat and human colonic mucins bind to and inhibit the adherence lectin of *Entamoeba histolytica. J Clin Invest* 1987;80:1245–1254.
44. Ravdin JI, Croft BY, Guerrant RL. Cytopathogenic mechanisms of *Entamoeba histolytica. J Exp Med* 1980;152:377–390.
45. Huston CD, Houpt ER, Mann BJ, et al. Caspase 3—dependent killing of host cells by the parasite Entamoeba histolytica. Cellular Microbiol 2000;2:617–625.
46. Abraham SN, Jonsson A-B, Normark S. Fimbriae-mediated host-pathogen cross-talk. *Curr Opin Microbiol* 1998;1:75–81.
47. Godaly G, Frendeus B, Proudfoot A, et al. Role of fimbriae-mediated adherence for neutrophil migration across *Escherichia coli*—infected epithelial cell layers. *Mol Microbiol* 1998;30:725–735.
48. Braga LL, Ninomiya H, McCoy JJ, et al. Inhibition of the complement membrane attack complex by the galactose-specific adhesin of *Entamoeba histolytica. J Clin Invest* 1992;90:1131–1137.
49. China B, Sory MP, N'Guyen BT, et al. Role of the YadA protein in prevention of opsonization of *Yersinia enterocolitica* by C3b molecules. *Infect Immun* 1993;61:3129–3136.
50. Henderson IR, Owen P, Nataro JP. Molecular switches—the ON and OFF of bacterial phase variation. *Mol Microbiol* 1999;33: 919–932.
51. Gally DL, Rucker TJ, Blomfiled IC. The leucine-responsive regulatory protein binds to the *fim* switch to control phase variation of type 1 fimbrial expression in *Escherichia coli. J Bacteriol* 1994; 176:5665–5672.

52. Wiley DC, Skehel JJ. The structure and function of the hemagglutinin membrane glycoprotein of influenza virus. *Annu Rev Biochem* 1987;56:365–394.
53. Hallenberger S, Bosch V, Angliker H, et al. Inhibition of furin-mediated cleavage activation of HIV-1 glycoprotein gp160. *Nature* 1992;360:358–361.
54. Choe H, Martin KA, Farzan M, et al. Structural interactions between chemokine receptors, gp120 Env and CD4. *Semin Immunol* 1998;10:249–257.
55. Vines RR, Ramakrishnan G, Rogers JB, et al. Regulation of adherence and virulence by the *Entamoeba histolytica* lectin cytoplasmic domain, which contains a beta2 integrin motif. *Mol Biol Cell* 1998;9:2069–2079.
56. Lub M, van Vliet SJ, Oomen SP, et al. Cytoplasmic tails of beta 1, beta 2, and beta 7 integrins differentially regulate LFA-1 function in K562 cells. *Mol Biol Cell* 1997;8:719–728.
57. Rutter JM, Jones GW. Protection against enteric disease caused by *Escherichia coli*—a model for vaccination with a virulence determinant? *Nature* 1973;242:531–532.
58. Lindberg AA. Vaccinations against enteric pathogens: from science to vaccine trials. *Curr Opin Microbiol* 1998;1:116–124.
59. Petri WAJ, Ravdin JI. Protection of gerbils from amebic liver abscess by immunization with the galactose-specific adherence lectin of *Entamoeba histolytica. Infect Immun* 1991;59:97–101.
60. Zhang T, Stanley SL Jr. Protection of gerbils from amebic liver abscess by immunization with a recombinant protein derived from the 170-kilodalton surface adhesin of *Entamoeba histolytica. Infect Immun* 1994;62:2605–2608.
61. Soong CJ, Kain KC, Abd-Alla M, et al. A recombinant cysteine-rich section of the *Entamoeba histolytica* galactose-inhibitable lectin is efficacious as a subunit vaccine in the gerbil model of amebic liver abscess. *J Infect Dis* 1995;71:645–651.
62. Mann BJ, Burkholder BV, Lockhart LA. Protection in a gerbil model of amebiasis by oral immunization with *Salmonella* expressing the galactose/N-acetyl D-galactosamine inhibitable lectin of *Entamoeba histolytica. Vaccine* 1997;15:659–663.
63. Petri WA Jr. Recent advances in amebiasis. *Crit Rev Clin Lab Sci* 1996;33:1–37.

7

ENTERIC BACTERIAL TOXINS

CYNTHIA L. SEARS
DAVID W. K. ACHESON

Bacteria that colonize the intestine and produce one or more toxins are important etiologic agents of diarrheal disease in both industrialized and developing countries. This chapter is intended to provide an overview of the toxins of enteric pathogens that are, in most instances, linked to and putatively important in the pathogenesis of human disease. The various criteria utilized to demonstrate pathogenicity of an enteric bacterial toxin are reviewed, after which the criteria used to classify a given bacterial enteric toxin are discussed. By means of these definitions, Table 7.1 classifies the enteric bacterial toxins according to their identified general mode of action(s) and also by genus and species. In a classification of the toxins, data derived from studies of toxins in potentially relevant models of disease have been emphasized—namely, intestinal mucosa *in vivo* and intestinal epithelial cells *in vitro.* More detailed information on each of these toxins is available in other chapters in this volume. The potential mechanisms by which enteric bacterial toxins contribute to intestinal secretion are displayed in Table 7.2. The most striking conclusion to be drawn from these latter data is that despite the elegance of the mechanistic data available for a few enteric bacterial toxins, knowledge of the secretory mechanisms of most toxins are incompletely understood.

CRITERIA FOR ESTABLISHING THE PATHOGENICITY OF AN ENTERIC BACTERIAL TOXIN

The most convincing criterion by which to determine whether an enteric toxin contributes to the pathogenicity of an organism is to demonstrate that the purified toxin causes diarrhea when ingested by human volunteers. Only one enteric bacterial toxin fulfills this stringent criterion: cholera toxin (CT). Ingestion of as little as 5 μg of CT resulted in diarrhea in four of five subjects with a mean stool volume of 2.5 L, and ingestion of 25 μg resulted in diarrhea in two of two subjects with a mean stool output of 21.9 L (1). These data unequivocally establish the potent secretory activity of CT in the human intestine but do not identify the mechanism(s) resulting in the secretory response.

An alternative strategy for establishing the significance of a toxin in volunteer trials is to feed subjects isogenic bacterial strains specifically engineered so that the only difference between the strains is expression of an active toxin. In studies with strains of *Vibrio cholerae* specifically mutated in genes encoding CT (*ctx*), volunteers who ingested the wild-type strain expressing CT experienced the severe diarrhea characteristic of cholera, whereas subjects who ingested the same strain mutated in the *ctx* genes did not experience clinical cholera (2). However, approximately 50% of the volunteers in the latter group did experience mild to moderate diarrhea with low volumes, which indicates that although CT is responsible for the severe diarrhea that is cholera, additional factors are produced by *V. cholerae* organisms that can stimulate secretion and cause mild diarrhea.

Volunteer trials are not always possible or ethical, and other criteria can be used to associate an enteric toxin with human disease. Supporting evidence for such an association can include (a) detection of a toxin directly in a clinical specimen, (b) measurement of an intestinal or serum antibody response to the toxin, and (c) an epidemiologic association of bacteria producing the toxin with clinical disease. Fulfillment of the first two criteria indicates *in vivo* production of the toxin. However, because enteric bacteria most often produce numerous virulence proteins in addition to an enteric toxin, such as attachment or invasion factors, the detection of toxin in a clinical specimen, the demonstration of an antitoxin response, or an epidemiologic association is only supportive and not definitive in determining that a toxin contributes to the intestinal secretion observed in an infection.

Examples of toxins that have been detected directly in stools from infected patients include the following: *Clostrid-*

C. L. Sears: Department of Medicine, Divisions of Infectious Diseases and Gastroenterology, Johns Hopkins University School of Medicine, Baltimore, Maryland

D.W. K. Acheson: Department of Epidemiology and Preventive Medicine, University of Maryland School of Medicine, Baltimore, Maryland

TABLE 7.1. ENTERIC BACTERIAL TOXINS: FUNCTIONAL CLASSIFICATION BY GENUS AND SPECIES[a]

Genus and Species	Enterotoxin	Cytoskeleton-altering	Cytotoxin	Neural Activity	Reference
Aeromonas hydrophila[b]					
Alt	+	+			94
Ast	+	+			94
Act[c]			+(s)[d]		94,95
Other toxins[e]	+	+			94
Bacillus cereus					
"Emetic toxin"				+(?)	81,121
"Diarrheal toxin"			+(s)		81,82,122
Bacteroides fragilis (ETBF)					
BFT		+(i,s)[f,g]			13,84,85,123,124,125
Campylobacter jejuni[b]					
Cytotoxin			+		126,127
CDT		+[h]	+(s)		128,129
Clostridium botulinum					
C2 toxin		+[h]	+(s)		36,98,130,131
Clostridium difficile					
Toxin A		+(i,s)	+(i,s)[i]	+	71,72,73,76
Toxin B		+(i,s)	+(i,s)		71,72,74,75,102
Clostridium perfringens type A					
CPE			+(i,s)		87–89
Clostridium perfringens type C					
β Toxin			+(i)		132,133
α Toxin[j]	+(?)		+(i)		134,135
"Enterotoxin" (CPE)			+(i,s)		136,137
Enteroaggregative *Escherichia coli* (EAEC)					
EAST	+				23,24
Plasmid-encoded toxin (Pet)	+	+	+(i,s)		138–142
Enterohemorrhagic *E. coli* (EHEC)					
Shiga toxin			+(i,s)		5,25,33
Enteroinvasive *E. coli* (EIEC)[b]					
Shigella enterotoxin (ShET-2)[k]	+				143,144
Cytotoxin			+		143
Enterotoxigenic *E. coli* (ETEC)[b]					
STa	+	+		+	17,20,21,55,68
STb	+[l]				22,114,117,146–148
LTI	+	+			30
LTII	+[m]	+[n]			149–152
Other *E. coli* toxins					
CDT	?	+[h]	+(i,s)		153
CNF-1 and -2[o]		+(s?)	+(i,s)		100,101,154–157
Plesiomonas shigelloides[b]					
Heat-labile enterotoxin	+[p]	+			110,158
Heat-stable enterotoxin	+[p]				158,159
Salmonella species (non-*typhi*)[b]					
Enterotoxin (Stn)	+	+[n]		+	28,29,160–163
Shigella dysenteriae[b]					
Shiga toxin			+(i,s)		5,25,33
CDT[q]	+(?)	+	+(i,s)		164
Other *Shigella* species[b]					
ShET-1[k]	+				165–167
ShET-2[k]	+				144
Sig A		+(i,s)			168
Staphylococcus aureus					
Enterotoxins A–E	+			+	35,169–172
δ Toxin	+		+(i,s)[r]		173–176
Vibrio cholerae O1/O139[b,s]					
CT	+	+(i,s)[n]		+	19,30,55
Zot		+(i,s)			43,97
Ace	+				26,44
Hemagglutinin/protease		+(i,s)			46,177,178
RTX toxin		+(i,s)			45,179
Hemolysin/phospholipase C			+		180,181

TABLE 7.1. (*continued*)

Genus and Species	Enterotoxin	Cytoskeleton-altering	Cytotoxin	Neural Activity	Reference
Vibrio cholerae non-O1, non-O139[b]					
ST-like	+	+[n]			56
Vibrio parahaemolyticus[b,t]					
TDH hemolysin[u]	+[v]		+(i,s)		16,90,91,183
Yersinia enterocolitica					
Heat-stable enterotoxins[w]	+	+[n]			15,56

[a]Ace, accessory cholera enterotoxin; Act, *A. hydrophila* cytolytic enterotoxin; Alt, *A. hydrophila* heat-labile toxin; Ast, *a. hydrophila* heat-stable toxin; BFT, *B. fragilis* toxin, also known as fragilysin; CDT, cytolethal distending toxin; CNF, cytotoxic necrotizing factor; CPE, *C. perfringens* enterotoxin; CT, cholera toxin; EAST, enteroaggregative *E. coli* heat-stable enterotoxin; EIEC, enteroinvasive *E. coli*; ETBF, enterotoxigenic *B. fragilis*; LT, enterotoxigenic *E. coli* heat-labile enterotoxin; Pet, plasmid-encoded toxin; RTX, "repeats-in-toxin"; Sen, *Shigella* enterotoxin; ShET-1 or -2, *Shigella* enterotoxin 1 or 2; ST, enterotoxigenic *E. coli* heat-stable enterotoxin; Stn, *Salmonella* enterotoxin; TDH, thermostable direct hemolysin; Y-ST, *Yersinia* heat stable toxin; Zot, zonula occludens toxin.

[b]Indicates that organism has been tested in volunteers (Table 7.2).

[c]Closely related to proteins designated as aerolysin, β-hemolysin, cholera toxin cross-reactive cytolytic enterotoxin (CTC cytolysin).

[d](s), Cytotoxin is secretory in animal intestine and/or Ussing chambers *in vitro.*

[e]Limited data suggest that *Aeromonas* species secrete additional proteins with enterotoxic and/or cytoskeleton-altering activity.

[f]BFT stimulates secretion in ligated intestinal segments in lamb, rabbit, rat, and calf. Histopathology of lamb intestine after 18 hours of exposure to ETBF or BFT reveals intestinal epithelial cell rounding and detachment from the lamina propria (13,84). Intestinal epithelial cell morphologic changes appear to precede the onset of secretion (84).

[g](i), Alteration of the cytoskeleton or change in cell morphology has been shown in intestinal cells *in vivo* or *in vitro.* (i,s), Alteration of the cytoskeleton as above, plus evidence for secretion or alteration of intestinal barrier function in an intestinal model, such as ligated intestinal segments or native intestinal tissue or monolayers of intestinal epithelial cells in Ussing chambers *in vitro.*

[h]Cells display altered morphology for up to 3 days with lethality (cytotoxicity) occurring later.

[i]In vivo studies with *C. difficile* toxin A demonstrate that secretion is consistently associated with inflammation and damage to the intestinal epithelium. However, *in vitro* studies with intestinal epithelial cells and nonintestinal cell lines have not revealed cytotoxic activity with *C. difficile* toxin A. Thus, it seems likely that this toxin stimulates a striking inflammatory response by as yet incompletely delineated mechanisms that are cytotoxic to the intestinal epithelium (71).

[j]The α toxin of *C. perfringens* type C has been reported to increase I_{sc} in Ussing chambers only when added to the serosal side of rat colonic mucosa. Histologic results are not available.

[k]The enterotoxin produced by EIEC is variably designated as ShET-2 (144), Sen or SenA (144,145), or OSPD3 (145). This enterotoxin is also produced by all *Shigella* species. In contrast, the ShET-1 protein is secreted only by *S. flexneri* 2a (165–167).

[l]In detailed studies, alterations in villous cell morphology have been identified in rat intestine after treatment with *E. coli* STb.

[m]*E. coli* heat-labile enterotoxin (LT) II, unlike *E. coli* LTI, does not stimulate secretion in rabbit ileal segments. However, *E. coli* LTII does stimulate secretion in the sealed adult mouse (SAM) model. Histologic studies of intestinal tissue are not available.

[n]Intestinal epithelial cell chloride secretion stimulated by increases in intracellular cyclic AMP and cyclic GMP has been shown to be dependent in part on rearrangement of F-actin (50,51,68). Thus, by analogy, it is postulated that enteric bacterial toxins that increase cyclic AMP or cyclic GMP may also be cytoskeleton-altering toxins in intestinal epithelial cells.

[o]Only CNF-2 has been shown to stimulate intestinal secretion and cytotoxicity to date (154).

[p]Culture filtrates of *P. shigelloides* may contain heat-labile or heat-stable secretory factors detectable in rabbit ileal loops that do not alter the histology of the intestine (158,159).

[q]Profuse secretion in suckling mouse noted with normal small-intestinal histology and damage in colonic tissue by histology.

[r]Delayed histologic damage is seen *in vivo* after treatment of the intestine with δ toxin. However, δ toxin rapidly (within minutes) alters intestinal transport by increasing potential difference and decreasing resistance in guinea pig ileum studied in Ussing chambers.

[s]O1/O139 refers to the O1 and O139 serogroups of *V. cholerae.* These serogroups comprise the epidemic strains of *V. cholerae* that produce cholera toxin and clinical cholera. Although some strains of *V. cholerae* belonging to serogroups other than O1 or O139 may express cholera toxin, the majority of strains in these serogroups are either nonpathogenic or express virulence factors other than cholera toxin.

[t]V. parahaemolyticus produces other potential toxins, such as the TDH-related hemolysin (TRH), but data are limited (182).

[u]Other species of *Vibrio* implicated in diarrheal disease—namely, *V. mimicus* and *V. hollisae*—have also been reported to produce TDH and possess the *tdh* gene.

[v]Low concentrations of TDH increase chloride current, whereas high cncentrations are cytotoxic.

[w]*Y. enterocolitica* organisms have been reported to produce three molecular species of ST. Data on the cGMP responses for each of these toxins are not yet available.

TABLE 7.2. ENTERIC BACTERIAL TOXINS: MECHANISTIC CLASSIFICATION

- I. Toxins with established mechanisms of action[a]
  - A. ADP-ribosylation
    - Adenylate cyclase
      - Cholera toxin (27,30,47)
      - *Escherichia coli* LTI and LTII[b] (30)
    - Actin
      - *Clostridium botulinum* C2 toxin (99)
  - B. Direct activation of guanylate cyclase
    - *E. coli* STa (17,20,56,62,198)
    - Enteroaggregative *E. coli* heat-stable enterotoxin (23,24,62)
    - *Yersinia enterocolitica* heat-stable enterotoxins[c] (56)
  - C. Inhibition of protein synthesis
    - Shiga toxins (5,33)
  - D. Calcium/calmodulin/protein kinase C signaling
    - *Vibrio parahaemolyticus* thermostable direct hemolysin (TDH) (90,91)
    - *Vibrio cholerae* zonula occludens toxin (Zot) (97)
  - E. Modification of Rho GTPases[d]
    - Glucosylation
      - *Clostridium difficile* toxins A and B (75,76,102)
    - Deamidation
      - *E. coli* cytotoxic necrotizing factors 1 and 2 (103)
  - F. Protease activity[e]
    - *Bacteroides fragilis* enterotoxin (BFT) (E-cadherin) (104)
    - *Clostridium perfringens* enterotoxin (CPE) (claudins 3 and 4) (89)
  - G. Pore formation
    - *Staphylococcus aureus* δ toxin (111)
    - *C. perfringens* enterotoxin (CPE) (87)
- II. Toxins with possible or postulated mechanisms of action
  - A. Cyclic AMP
    - *Aeromonas hydrophila* heat-labile toxin (Alt) (94)
    - *A. hydrophila* heat-stable toxin (Ast) (94)
    - *Plesiomonas shigelloides* heat-labile toxin (158)
    - *Salmonella typhimurium* heat-labile enterotoxin (Stn) (28,29,118)
  - B. Arachidonic acid cascade
    - Cholera toxin (52–54)
    - *C. difficile* toxin A (71,115,116)
    - *E. coli* STb (117)
    - *S. aureus* δ toxin (112)
    - *S. typhimurium* enterotoxin (Stn) (28,199)
    - *A. hydrophila* heat-labile toxin (Alt) (94)
  - C. Calcium/calmodulin/protein kinase C signaling
    - *E. coli* STb (114)
    - *V. cholerae* accessory cholera enterotoxin (Ace) (26)
    - *E. coli* STa (55,56,113)
    - *V. cholerae* non-O1 ST (56,119)
  - D. Pore formation
    - *V. cholerae* O1 accessory cholera enterotoxin (Ace) (26,44)
    - *A. hydrophila* cytolytic enterotoxin (Act) (94)
    - *C. perfringens* β toxin (132,133)
    - *Bacillus cereus* "diarrheal toxin" (122,200)
  - E. Protease activity[e]
    - Enteroaggregative *E. coli* plasmid-encoded toxin (Pet) (fodrin) (141)
    - *V. cholerae* hemagglutinin/protease (HA/protease) (occludin) (89)
  - F. Immune modulation[f]
    - Shiga toxins (5,33)
    - *Bacteroides fragilis* enterotoxin (BFT) (201,202)
    - *C. difficile* toxin A (71)
    - *S. typhimurium* Sip (203)
    - *Campylobacter jejuni* cytolethal distending toxin (CDT)[f] (204)
  - G. Other
    - *C. jejuni* cytolethal distending toxin (CDT)[g,h]
    - Cell cycle arrest in Caco-2 cells (205)
    - Deoxyribonuclease activity (129)

TABLE 7.2. *(continued)*

III. Toxins with unknown mechanisms of action
- A. Enterotoxins
  - *C. perfringens* α toxin (phospholipase C) (134,135)
  - Enteroinvasive *E. coli* enterotoxin (ShET-2)[i] (143,144)
  - *Plesiomonas shigelloides* heat-stable toxin (ShET-2)[i] (159)
  - *S. aureus* enterotoxins A–E (169–171)
  - *Shigella flexneri* 2a enterotoxin (ShET-1)[i] (165–167)
  - *Shigella* species enterotoxin (ShET-2)[i] (143–145)
- B. Cytotoxins
  - *C. difficile* toxin A[j] (71,72)
  - *C. difficile* toxin B[j] (71,72)
  - Enteroinvasive *E. coli* cytotoxin (143)
  - *C. jejuni* cytotoxin (126,127)
  - *Vibrio parahaemolyticus* TDH (91)
  - Enteroaggregative *E. coli* plasmid-encoded toxin (Pet) (141)
  - *V. cholerae* hemolysin/phospholipase C (180,181)
- C. Cytoskeleton-altering toxins[k]
  - Cholera toxin (50,51)
  - *E. coli* STa (68)[l]
  - *E. coli* LTI and LTII (50,51)
  - *S. typhimurium* enterotoxin (Stn) (50,51)
  - *A. hydrophila* heat-labile enterotoxin (Alt) (94,50,51)
  - *A. hydrophila* heat-stable enterotoxin (Ast) (94,50,51)
  - *S. flexneri* 2a Sig A (168)
  - *V. cholerae* O1 "repeats-in-toxin" (RTX)
- D. Neural activity
  - *B. cereus* "emetic toxin" (81,121)
  - Cholera toxin (reviewed in reference 55)
  - *C. difficile* toxin A (71,107)
  - *E. coli* STa (reviewed in reference 55)
  - *S. aureus* enterotoxins A–E (35,206)

[a]A toxin is considered to have an "established" mechanism of action if the molecular mechanism of action has been identified and the toxin stimulates intestinal secretion or alters the physiology of intestinal epithelial cells.
[b]LT, heat-labile enterotoxin; ST, heat-stable enterotoxin.
[c]*Y. enterocolitica* organisms have been shown to produce three molecular species of ST toxins. It is not yet demonstrated that all three toxins activate guanylate cyclase type C, similar to *E. coli* STa.
[d]One or more of the Rho family GTP-binding proteins (i.e., Rho ABC, Rac, and CDC-42) may be modified by the listed toxins. The Rho family proteins are key regulators of cellular actin. The toxin's enzymatic modification of a Rho family protein is listed in parentheses.
[e]The cellular protein cleaved by each toxin appears in parentheses. In the case of CPE, only a carboxyl terminal fragment of CPE has been shown to exhibit protease activity.
[f]Each of the listed toxins either has been reported to stimulate the release of the proinflammatory cytokine interleukin 8 and possibly other cytokines or has been shown to stimulate the migration of polymorphonuclear leukocytes across polarized monolayers of intestinal epithelial cells.
[g]Secretion of cytolethal distending toxin has also been reported for *Shigella dysenteriae* and some strains of *E. coli* (153,164).
[h]It is unclear whether the activities reported as cell cycle arrest and deoxyribonuclease activity for *C. jejuni* CDT represent the same mechanism of action.
[i]The enterotoxin produced by EIEC and all *Shigella* species is variably designated as ShET-2 (143), Sen or Sen A (144,145), or OSPD3 (145). Only *S. flexneri* 2a secretes the enterotoxin ShET-1 (166).
[j]The *C. difficile* toxins A and B appear to act as cytotoxins by stimulating an intestinal proinflammatory response (reviewed in reference 71).
[k]Chloride secretion in intestinal epithelial monolayers, stimulated by agonists such as vasoactive intestinal peptide, which increase cyclic AMP, is regulated by F-actin, most likely through the Na/K/2Cl co-transporter, which plays a key role in transepithelial Cl^- secretion (50,51). By analogy, a similar response to cholera toxin, *E. coli* LTI and LTII, the *S. typhimurium* enterotoxin, and *Aeromonas* toxins is hypothesized.
[l]*E. coli* STa has been shown to alter the appearance of F-actin in the basal portion of T84 cells, a human intestinal epithelial cell line, but the mechanism of this effect is unknown (68).

ium difficile toxin A (reviewed in reference 3), Shiga toxin (4,5), CT (reviewed in reference 6), and heat-labile toxin (LT) and heat-stable toxin (ST) from enterotoxigenic *Escherichia coli* (ETEC) (7). However, failure to detect toxins in stools may be a consequence of insensitivity of the detection assay, toxin-binding effects of free gangliosides present in mucin found in stools, proteolytic degradation of the toxin in the intestinal tract, or other reasons.

The production of an immune response against a toxin can be taken as evidence of *in vivo* toxin production, but failure to detect an immune response does not rule out *in vivo* toxin production. Although serum and intestinal antibody responses against CT and LT are seen, an antibody response against ST has not been demonstrated (reviewed in reference 1). Because of its small size, ST is not immunogenic unless it is experimentally conjugated to a larger carrier protein. Frequently, the immune response against Shiga toxins in patients infected with either *Shigella dysenteriae* 1 or Shiga toxin-producing *E. coli* is poor. The precise reasons for this are unclear, but it may be linked to the fact that Shiga toxin has been shown to kill immunoglobulin G (IgG)- and IgA-committed lymphocytes selectively, whereas most IgM-producing cells are resistant to Shiga toxin (8). Nevertheless, some studies have clearly demonstrated an immune response to Shiga toxin (9,10).

Many examples of an epidemiologic association of toxin production with human disease can be cited; such studies have been particularly useful for establishing the significance of LTI and STa-producing ETEC, enterotoxigenic *Bacteroides fragilis* (ETBF), and Shiga toxin-producing *E. coli. E. coli* and *B. fragilis* are both members of the normal intestinal flora, but the strains isolated from healthy persons usually do not produce enterotoxins. Epidemiologic studies have demonstrated that *E. coli* organisms producing LTI or STa (11,12) and ETBF organisms (13) are found significantly more often in patients with diarrheal disease than in healthy persons.

Additional methods of studying the pathogenicity of enteric bacterial toxins utilize one or more nonhuman experimental approaches, including animal models, Ussing chambers, and *in vitro* assays. Most data on the pathogenicity of bacterial enteric toxins are based on these approaches; by analogy, the toxin is then proposed to be important in human diarrheal disease. Although only gross intestinal secretion is typically measured, in a classic approach to determining whether an enteric toxin stimulates secretion, ligated intestinal segments or loops are used, as originally described by De (14). In this experimental approach, small intestinal (jejunal or ileal) or colonic ligated segments are inoculated with toxin preparations or bacterial cultures, and the subsequent presence or absence of secretion is assessed at time points up to 18 hours. For the reasons discussed above, inoculation of whole bacterial cultures is less definitive in establishing the importance of the toxin to pathogenesis unless the experiments are conducted with isogenic (toxin minus and toxin plus) mutant strains of bacteria. Such isogenic strains of enteric bacteria are a potent tool for establishing the pathogenicity of a toxin in animal models. For example, isogenic strains of *Yersinia enterocolitica* have been used to establish that the heat-stable enterotoxin produced by most pathogenic strains contributes to the severity of disease in a rabbit animal model (15). Similarly, isogenic strains of *Vibrio parahaemolyticus,* differing only in the production of thermostable direct hemolysin (TDH), were tested in ligated rabbit ileal loops to demonstrate the contribution of TDH in causing the secretion (16). An alternative approach to establishing the relevance to secretion of an enteric bacterial toxin is oral inoculation of an animal with the toxin and the demonstration of either diarrhea or the accumulation of intestinal fluid. Animal models in which this approach has proved valuable include suckling mice, in which oral inoculation of *E. coli* heat-stable enterotoxin (STa) stimulates intestinal secretion (17), and the sealed adult mouse model, which has been used, for example, to study the role of host genetics in modulating the secretory response to CT (18).

A valuable *in vitro* experimental approach used to identify secretory responses to enteric bacterial toxins is the Ussing chamber. For this technique, either native intestinal epithelium or monolayers of cultured intestinal epithelial cells are mounted between Lucite chambers under conditions of ionic, osmotic, and electric (voltage-clamped) equilibrium. The ability of an enteric toxin to stimulate anion (usually chloride or bicarbonate) secretion or inhibit sodium chloride absorption, both potentially contributing to net intestinal secretion, can be measured under these conditions. Three measurements related by Ohm's Law ($V = IR$) are made in Ussing chambers: (a) short circuit current (I_{sc} or I), (b) potential difference (PD or V), and (c) resistance (R). Increases in I_{sc} and PD in monolayers of intestinal epithelial cells indicate the secretion of chloride or bicarbonate. In native intestinal tissue, increases in I_{sc} and PD in combination with secretion in a ligated intestinal segment are consistent with net intestinal anionic secretion. This technique has been used extensively to identify and characterize the secretory potential of numerous enteric bacterial toxins, including CT (19), the *E. coli* heat-stable enterotoxins (STa, STb) (20–22), the enteroaggregative *E. coli* (EAEC) heat-stable enterotoxin (EAST-1) (23,24), Shiga toxin (25), and the accessory cholera enterotoxin (Ace) (26), to name a few.

In a third experimental approach to identifying the activities of enteric bacterial toxins, a wide variety of nonintestinal cell lines are used. Most often, the activity of a particular toxin is identified by a change in the shape of cells (sometimes referred to as a *cytotonic effect*) or by cytotoxicity (in which cells are killed) in response to treatment with an enteric toxin. For example, Chinese hamster ovary (CHO) and Y-1 adrenal cells have proved useful for identifying toxins that increase intracellular cyclic adenosine monophosphate (cAMP), such as CT (reviewed in reference 27), the *Salmonella* toxin (28,29), and the heat-labile enterotoxins of *E. coli* (reviewed in reference 30). In response to an increase in intracellular cAMP, CHO cells stretch (31) and Y-1 adrenal cells become round (32). Another example is the use of HeLa or Vero cells to identify cytotoxicity resulting from the inhibition of protein synthesis by Shiga toxins (5,33). Although the use of these cell lines has been very valuable in identifying one or more activities of enteric toxins, the experimental data do not help in determining the secretory activity of enteric toxins and thus must be interpreted with caution in discussions of the importance of the results to intestinal pathogenesis.

CLASSIFICATION OF ENTERIC BACTERIAL TOXINS

The term *toxin* is derived from the Greek term *toxikon* ("bow poison"). Thus, the classic definition of a bacterial toxin is a protein secreted into the culture supernatant by a bacterium and predicted to act at a distance from the site where it is produced *in vivo.* Recent data defining the action of bacterial proteins delivered to cells suggest a broader view of the concept of a bacterial toxin. Data on the pathogenesis of enteropathogenic *E. coli* (EPEC) exemplify this concept and are discussed later in this chapter.

The classification of enteric bacterial toxins is most often based on an identified general mode of action. However, a strict classification of enteric bacterial toxins is often problematic. In some instances, this is because the available data are incomplete; in other cases, it is because the mode of action is complex. For the purposes of this chapter, four classes of toxins are defined: (a) enterotoxins, (b) cytoskeleton-altering toxins, (c) cytotoxins, and (d) toxins that stimulate the nervous and immune systems. To be included within a particular class of toxin, only one of the listed criteria (see below) must be fulfilled. Several of the toxins can be placed in more than one category.

A toxin is classified as an *enterotoxin* if (a) the toxin stimulates net secretion in ligated intestinal segments without either histological evidence of intestinal damage by light microscopy (if data are available) or evidence in *in vitro* assays of injury to nonerythrocytic cells; or (b) the toxin stimulates secretion as measured in Ussing chambers.

The second class of enteric toxins are the *cytoskeleton-altering* (also known as cytotonic) toxins. This group of toxins, including *C. difficile* toxin A and the toxin produced by ETBF (*B. fragilis* toxin, or BFT), produce an alteration in cell shape without inducing significant cell injury. When studies are available, toxin-induced changes in cell shape have most often been shown to be the result of a rearrangement of filamentous actin (F-actin) in the affected cells.

The third class of enteric toxins are the *cytotoxins.* These toxins produce cellular damage, documented by either gross findings (e.g., intestinal hemorrhage), evidence of light microscopic intestinal damage, or studies identifying toxicity to cells (e.g., inhibition of protein synthesis, release of lactic dehydrogenase from cells). As delineated in Table 7.1, the activity of enteric cytotoxins may or may not be associated with secretion in *in vivo* or *in vitro* intestinal models of disease.

Lastly, enteric bacterial toxins may have *nerve-stimulating* or *immune-stimulating activity.* A toxin is classified in this group if available data suggest that at least part of the secretory activity of the toxin is attributable to (a) release of one or more neurotransmitters from the enteric nervous system, (b) alteration of smooth-muscle activity in the intestine, or (c) production of one or more immune modulators (e.g., cytokines) by either enterocytes or submucosal cells. At present, no enteric toxin has clearly been identified as stimulating secretion solely through these potential mechanisms. However, such mechanisms appear to augment the biologic activity of several enteric toxins (e.g., Shiga toxin, *C. difficile* toxin A, BFT).

ENTERIC BACTERIAL TOXINS CATEGORIZED BY GENUS AND SPECIES

Table 7.1 is a compendium of the enteric bacteria and the toxins they produce. These bacteria have been linked to human illnesses predominantly through epidemiologic studies and, in many cases, volunteer trials (Table 7.3). The clinical expression of disease associated with infection with the vast majority of these bacteria is diarrhea that is watery or, uncommonly, dysenteric. Exceptions are the following: (a) infection with *Bacillus cereus,* which produces two clinical syndromes, one dominated by emesis and the second by diarrhea (34), and (b) ingestion of food containing toxin(s) produced by *Staphylococcus aureus,* which results in a prominent emetic response that is sometimes accompanied by diarrhea (35). This latter food poisoning syndrome is an intoxication caused by the ingestion of preformed toxin, not an infection. Each bacterium listed in Table 7.1 has been identified to produce one or more toxins with biologic activity in either native intestinal mucosa, intestinal epithelial cell lines, or nonintestinal cell lines. These enteric bacterial toxins are categorized by the definitions previously described in the text, and data on the mode of action of the toxin derived from intestinal models of disease have been emphasized. Question marks indicate toxins for which the data are too limited for the general activity of the toxin to be classified with confidence. In limited instances, toxin-producing bacteria are listed in Table 7.1 that are not known to play a significant role in human disease or have only a weak association with disease. A pertinent example is the C2 toxin produced by *Clostridium botulinum,* which is secretory in mouse intestinal loops and not a neurotoxin like other *C. botulinum* toxins (36,37). The role of the C2 toxin in human disease is unknown. Similarly, strains of *E. coli* producing the cytolethal distending toxins and the cytotoxic necrotizing factor 1 (CNF-1) are associated with human disease only by limited anecdotal reports at present (38,39). As shown in Table 7.3, human volunteer data have established the pathogenicity of many of the important enteric bacterial pathogens; notable exceptions are Shiga toxin-producing *E. coli,* which cannot be studied for ethical reasons. In some instances (e.g., toxin-producing *Aeromonas hydrophila* and *Plesiomonas shigelloides*), pathogenicity could not be demonstrated in adults despite inocula as large as 10^9 to 10^{10} organisms administered with 2 g of sodium bicarbonate to neutralize gastric acid and enhance the likelihood of survival of the inoculum through the stomach. However, these trials were conducted in the 1980s, when considerably less was known about the potential virulence factors of *Aeromonas* species in particular. To provide a complete listing of enteric pathogens studied in human volunteers, Table 7.3 includes EPEC, diffusely adherent *E. coli,* and *Salmonella typhi.* For the most part, these bacteria have not been shown to produce cell-free toxins (i.e., present in culture supernatants) that stimulate an intestinal secretory response. EPEC, a pathogen primarily in children less than 1 year of age, caused diarrhea in adult volunteers (40,41). In contrast, diffusely adherent *E. coli,* which has been variably associated with diarrheal illnesses in children in epidemiologic investigations (38,42), did not cause diarrhea in adult volunteers. Infection with *S. typhi,* the etiologic agent of typhoid fever, predominantly causes a systemic illness.

Three general observations are apparent based on the data in Table 7.1, each of which is discussed separately below. First, although most enteric toxins have been reported to have one identified activity to date, recent data available for some of the best-studied toxins, in particular CT, *E. coli* STa, and *C. difficile* toxin A, highlight the potential complexity of toxin action in stimulating intestinal secretion. For example, *E. coli* STa and most likely CT can be classified as enterotoxins, cytoskeleton-altering toxins, and toxins with neural activity. Similarly, the complexity of the action of *C. difficile* toxin A is clear from a comparison of the results of *in vivo* and *in vitro* studies, discussed below. In addition, new data on the pathogenesis of EPEC infections suggest a broader framework for designating bacterial proteins as toxins. Second, certain enteric toxins have been "misnamed" and are commonly referred to as enterotoxins when in fact the data indicate that an alternative classification may be more appropriate. Third, several toxins produced by enteric bacteria can be classified as hemolysins based on the ability of the toxin

TABLE 7.3. ENTERIC BACTERIA STUDIED IN VOLUNTEERS

Bacteria	Inoculum[a]	Outcome	Reference
Vibrio cholerae[b]			
O1 (CT+)	10^3* (10^3)	Diarrhea	184
O139	10^4* (10^4)	Diarrhea	185
Non-O1/non-O139 (ST+)	10^6 (10^6)	Diarrhea	186
Non-O1/non-O139 (ST–)	10^9	No diarrhea	186
Shigella species			
dysenteriae	10^1* (2×10^2)	Diarrhea/dysentery	187
flexneri	10^2* (10^4)	Diarrhea/dysentery	187
sonnei	5×10^2* (5×10^2)	Diarrhea/dysentery	187
Escherichia coli			
enterotoxigenic	10^6* (10^6)	Diarrhea	188
enteropathogenic	10^6* (10^{10})	Diarrhea	40
enteroinvasive	10^8 (10^8)	Diarrhea/dysentery	189
enteroaggregative	7×10^8 (–)	Diarrhea	190
diffusely adherent	10^{10}	No diarrhea	191
Salmonella typhimurium	2×10^9	Diarrhea	192
Salmonella typhi	10^5 (10^7)	Typhoid fever	193
Campylobacter jejuni	8×10^2* (10^8)	Diarrhea	194
Vibrio parahaemolyticus	3×10^7 (10^8)	Diarrhea	195
Aeromonas hydrophila	10^{10}	No diarrhea	196
Plesiomonas shigelloides	4×10^9	No diarrhea	197

[a]Lowest inoculum in colony-forming units causing diarrhea in one or more subjects is shown; *indicates that this inoculum was the smallest one studied. The inoculum in parentheses is the smallest one causing diarrhea in 50% or more of subjects receiving that inoculum; (–) indicates that no inoculum tested caused diarrhea in 50% or more of subjects. Most but not all studies have administered sodium bicarbonate before the inoculum to neutralize stomach acidity.
[b]*V. cholerae* O1 lacking both cholera toxin (CT) and the TCP intestinal colonization factor have been fed to volunteers and did not cause diarrhea at inocula of 10^8. Genetically engineered *V. cholerae* O1 strains deleted of CT have caused diarrhea in volunteers at inocula of 10^4 (2). *V. cholerae* non-O1/non-O139 are strains belonging to serogroups other than O1 or O139; one such strain expressed a toxin similar to the *E. coli* heat-stable enterotoxin (ST).

to lyse erythrocytes of one or more species, but only in limited instances has this activity been correlated with the pathogenesis of intestinal secretion.

Potential Complexity of Enteric Bacterial Toxin Action: Cholera Toxin, *Escherichia coli* STa, *Clostridium difficile* Toxin A, and Enteropathogenic *Escherichia coli*

The disease cholera, characterized by rapidly dehydrating noninflammatory diarrhea, is caused by *V. cholerae.* Although recent data have identified other toxins produced by *V. cholerae* (26,43–46), the secretion observed in cholera is largely ascribed to the ability of the organism to produce CT. CT is a classic enterotoxin and does not injure intestinal epithelial cells. The first recognized and most ubiquitous activity of CT is to stimulate the intracellular production of cAMP via activation of adenylate cyclase (reviewed in references 27 and 47). *In vitro* studies indicate that cAMP stimulates chloride secretion and inhibits the absorption of sodium chloride (19,48). The chloride secretion is most likely mediated by the activation of A kinase with phosphorylation of the cystic fibrosis transmembrane regulator (CFTR), a major chloride channel present in intestinal epithelia (49). However, a combination of *in vivo* and *in vitro* observations suggest that the origin of secretion in response to CT is more complex. Most likely, the additional mechanisms described below by which CT may stimulate intestinal secretion augment and supplement (but do not supplant) cAMP-mediated intestinal secretion.

First, secretion stimulated by CT may utilize the intestinal epithelial cell cytoskeleton. Immobilization of F-actin in intestinal epithelial monolayers inhibits the chloride secretory response to agonists known to increase intracellular cAMP, which suggests that the modulation of intestinal epithelial cell F-actin may be necessary for CT to stimulate maximal epithelial cell chloride secretion (50). Subsequent data have indicated that the Na/K/2Cl co-transporter, which is key to the transepithelial secretion of chloride, is also functionally linked to the cytoskeleton (51). These data suggest that toxins that increase intracellular cAMP may also be classified as cytoskeleton-altering toxins. Second, *in vitro* and *in vivo* data implicate prostaglandins of the E series (PGE_1 and PGE_2) (52) and platelet-activating factor (53–55) in the pathogenesis of intestinal secretion stimulated by CT. Third, part of the secretory response to CT may be the consequence of an effect on the enteric nervous system, possibly through the stimulation of peptide hormone release (e.g., serotonin, vasoactive intestinal peptide) by intestinal enterochromaffin cells or through an increase in the smooth-muscle activity of the small bowel (reviewed in reference 55). Together, these data indicate that CT can be classified as a toxin with neural activity.

Enterotoxigenic *E. coli* organisms producing an 18- or 19-amino acid peptide with a molecular weight of about 2 kd (56) are an important cause of traveler's diarrhea and dehydrating diarrheal illnesses in children of the developing world. A 13-amino acid "toxic domain" or "core sequence" of STa, which includes a critical six cysteine residues, confers full binding and enterotoxic activities. This region of STa shares a striking identity with heat-stable enterotoxins secreted by other enteric pathogens, including *Y. enterocolitica* and *V. cholerae* non-O1 among others (56–58). The only definitive *E. coli* STa receptor identified to date is guanylate cyclase type C (GC-C) (59). However, both high- and low-molecular-weight STa-binding proteins have been identified in native intestine and intestinal epithelial cell lines (55,60,61). Available data suggest that binding of STa to GC-C may promote both internal dimerization and proteolytic cleavage of GC-C, which would account for the reported variable molecular weights of identified STa receptors. STa binding activates particulate intestinal guanylate cyclase or GC-C, thereby producing elevated cellular levels of cyclic guanosine monophosphate (cGMP) and activation of intracellular cyclic nucleotide-dependent kinases that stimulate chloride secretion and inhibit sodium chloride absorption; the result is net intestinal fluid secretion (17,20,21,62). Chloride secretion appears to be mediated by the stimulation of CFTR (63–65). The endogenous agonist for GC-C is a 15-amino acid hormone, guanylin, that contains four cysteines and is less potent than STa in activating GC-C and in stimulating chloride secretion (66,67). Guanylin presumably plays a role in basal gut homeostasis, and STa opportunistically utilizes GC-C to alter ion transport in the gut. Although STa is a classic enterotoxin without *in vivo* or *in vitro* evidence of histological damage, the secretory response to STa *in vitro* in T84 cells (human intestinal epithelial cells) has been reported to involve microfilament (F-actin) rearrangement only at the basal pole of these polarized cells (68), so that this toxin may also be classified as a cytoskeleton-altering toxin. Whether cGMP alone accounts for the full secretory response to STa is controversial (reviewed in reference 55). In rat jejunum, the secretory response to STa has been completely abrogated by 5-hydroxytryptamine (5-HT, or serotonin) receptor antagonists without any alteration in the cGMP response to STa. These results suggest that serotonin mediates STa secretion possibly through an effect on prostaglandin synthesis (HT_2 receptors) or neurons (HT_3 receptors). Additional *in vitro* studies in isolated rat intestinal epithelial cells suggest that STa may increase intracellular calcium and activate protein kinase C, but correlation of these data with a secretory response is not yet available. Lastly, a role for the enteric nervous system in STa-stimulated secretion has been suggested by studies of myoelectric activity in STa-treated rabbit small intestine and by studies of neuronal inhibitors that diminished the STa secretory response *in vivo.* These data suggest that *E. coli* STa may also be regarded as a toxin with neural activity.

Strains of *C. difficile* involved in antibiotic-associated diarrhea or, in its most severe clinical expression, pseudomembranous colitis produce two toxins, often designated as the "enterotoxin" (toxin A) and the cytotoxin (toxin B). In *in vivo* animal studies, toxin A induces hemorrhagic fluid secretion and markedly damages ileal and colonic epithelium; these observations indicate that toxin A is not an "enterotoxin." In guinea pig and rabbit ileal tissues mounted in Ussing chambers, toxin A stimulates chloride secretion, increases intestinal epithelial permeability, and alters epithelial cell structure (69,70). In contrast, although toxin B is a potent cytotoxin when tested in cultured cells *in vitro,* no cytotoxic or enterotoxic activity was detected in rodent or rabbit intestine (71). However, recent experiments examining the activity of toxins A and B on human colon in Ussing chambers revealed a similar pathophysiologic response to both toxins; in addition, and surprisingly, toxin B was more potent than toxin A in diminishing barrier function and inducing cytotoxic pathologic changes (72). In monolayers of human colonic epithelial cells (T84 cells) studied *in vitro,* both toxins A and B markedly diminished monolayer resistance (indicative of diminished barrier function) over time, but without evidence of cellular damage (73,74). However, the time course of the resistance changes and the patterns of staining of F-actin differ between toxins A and B. Both toxin A and toxin B have been shown to act identically to monoglucosylate members of the Rho family, small guanosine triphosphate (GTP)-binding proteins that play a central role in the regulation of the cellular cytoskeleton (75–77). Thus, the different responses to toxins A and B *in vivo* and *in vitro* suggest not only that the toxins bind to distinct receptors but also that either signaling from these receptors or the subsequent processing and intracellular transport of each toxin result in both distinct and overlapping pathophysiologic responses. Additional data on the mechanism of action of toxin A from *in vitro* and *in vivo* studies suggest it incites a complex array of responses that account for its ability to stimulate striking intestinal inflammation (71). Within minutes of binding to cells, toxin A both localizes to mitochondria, causing the generation of reactive oxygen species, and activates submucosal proinflammatory primary sensory neurons that utilize substance P and calcitonin gene-related peptide as neurotransmitters. The fact that these actions occur before the onset of Rho glucosylation (which takes 15 to 30 minutes) strongly suggests that Rho glucosylation is unable to account for the entire spectrum of pathophysiologic effects incited by toxin A, particularly those actions contributing to the inflammatory response to the toxin. Toxin A also activates nuclear factor-κβ, known to mediate the transcriptional up-regulation of, for example, the proinflammatory cytokine interleukin 8 (IL-8). In addition to IL-8, toxin A stimulates the release of other proinflammatory mediators, including macrophage inflammatory protein 2, leukotriene B_4, prostaglandin E_2, and tumor necrosis factor-α. Neutropenic rats and mice genetically deficient in mast cells exhibit attenuated intestinal inflammation and fluid secretion in response to toxin A. Furthermore, inhibitors of cytokine synthesis, neutrophil migration, mast cells, and primary sensory neurons all profoundly inhibit the inflammatory and secretory response to toxin A, which indicates the importance of these mediators and cells in the inflammatory response to toxin A. Together, these data indicate that toxin A stimulates secretion and inflammation most likely by direct effects on intestinal epithelial cells and indirect effects via activation of submucosal immune effector cells and the enteric nervous system. Thus, in this review, *C. difficile* toxin A has been classified as a cytotoxin with neural and immune activity based on the *in vivo* data, and as a cytoskeleton-altering toxin based on its effects on intestinal epithelial cells *in vitro.*

Both extensive epidemiologic data and human volunteer data have defined EPEC as an important human pathogen (78). Unlike most enteric pathogens, EPEC is essentially noninvasive, and until recently, it has not been shown to produce classic extracellular toxins. However, EPEC, an enteroadherent organism, produces in the intestinal mucosa and in tissue culture cells a unique morphologic change termed the *attaching and effacing lesion* (A/E lesion). The pathophysiologic effects of EPEC appear to be a consequence of its ability to deliver to the host cell through the A/E lesion several proteins—EspB (EPEC-secreted protein B), EspC, and EspF—that current data suggest may contribute to disease. Deletion of the *espB* gene yielded mutant organisms that did not cause diarrhea in human volunteers, which suggests that EspB is essential to virulence (41). Cell-free EspC, a member of the autotransporter family of proteins and so related to, for example, the EAEC plasma-encoded toxin (Pet) (Table 7.1), has recently been shown to stimulate an I_{sc} response in rat jejunum consistent with enterotoxic activity (79). EspF, delivered to intestinal cells by EPEC infection, disrupts intestinal barrier function without altering A/E lesion formation (80). These observations suggest that EPEC delivers proteins with toxic activities to cells and that enteric bacterial proteins acting as toxins need not always be detectable in the supernatants of bacterial cultures.

Enteric Bacterial Toxins: When the Name May Not Fit

The experimental, but not the clinical, data available for four enteric bacterial toxins suggest that these toxins are "misnamed." These are the *B. cereus* "diarrheal toxin," BFT, *C. difficile* toxin A (the "enterotoxin"), and *Clostridium perfringens* enterotoxin (CPE). The clinical illnesses associated with infection with each of these bacteria are most often characterized by watery diarrhea, not dysentery. One exception is pseudomembranous enterocolitis, which is the extreme clinical expression of infection with strains of *C.*

difficile producing toxin A. It is important to note that the histopathology of human intestinal tissue in these infections is generally not known, nor are detailed clinical evaluations examining for an intestinal inflammatory response typically available. Thus, a ready explanation for the discrepancy between the clinical presentation of these infections and the experimental data on the activity of the toxins as delineated below is not obvious at present.

The diarrheal toxin of *B. cereus,* frequently referred to as an enterotoxin in the literature, consists of a two- to three-component protein complex with possible hemolytic activity (81–83). Individual components of this toxin complex are biologically inactive until they are combined. The toxin stimulates secretion and necrosis in ligated ileal segments in rabbit and is cytotoxic for Vero cells, indications that it is a secretory cytotoxin, not an enterotoxin. BFT stimulates secretion in ligated intestinal segments in lamb, rat, rabbit, and calf (13,84). In intestinal epithelial cells treated with purified toxin, dramatic morphologic changes develop, such as gross changes in tight junctional complexes and loss of intestinal microvilli without cytotoxicity (85). Similar findings are observed in native intestine (including human colon) treated with purified toxin or ETBF; in addition, inflammation and frank hemorrhage may be seen (84,86). Thus, *in vitro* data suggest that this toxin is best classified at present as a secretory cytoskeleton-altering toxin, whereas *in vivo* data suggest a cytotoxic intestinal response.

C. difficile toxin A is commonly referred to as an enterotoxin. However, as delineated in the data discussed above, no evidence has been found of secretion stimulated by this toxin *in vivo* in the absence of histological damage and inflammation. Although chloride secretion (i.e., increased I_{sc}) in response to this toxin has not been identified in studies examining the toxin in an intestinal epithelial cell line (T84) or human colon, toxin A reduces barrier function, which is thought likely to contribute to secretion (72–74). These data suggest that *C. difficile* toxin A is best classified as a secretory cytotoxin with neural and immune activity.

Lastly, secretion stimulated by CPE is always associated with histologic damage in, for example, ligated ileal segments in rat and rabbit (87,88). In addition, detailed studies of the mode of action of CPE in rabbit brush border membranes and lipid bilayers suggest that this toxin binds irreversibly to cells and interacts with several eukaryotic proteins to form a large complex, thereby creating an ion-permeable pore (87). The resulting membrane permeability changes are rapidly lethal for eukaryotic cells. Most recently, a carboxyl terminus fragment of CPE has been shown in polarized renal epithelial cells to cleave claudins 3 and 4, key proteins of the zonula occludens or tight junction; the result is diminished barrier function without cytotoxicity (89). Overall, *in vivo* data indicate that CPE is a secretory cytotoxin, not an enterotoxin. However, the recent discovery that CPE can cleave certain claudin proteins has provided the first indication of the physiologic importance of these proteins in the barrier function of tight junctions and marked CPE as a useful tool to investigate eukaryotic cell functions.

Relationship of Enteric Bacterial Hemolysins to Intestinal Secretion

In the past, much of the literature on bacterial toxins has focused on toxins capable of lysing erythrocytes. Hemolytic toxins have been incriminated in extraintestinal diseases in addition to diarrheal diseases; in the latter, the linkage between lysis of erythrocytes and a secretory response in intestinal epithelial cells is not intuitive. Many hemolysins are known that play no role in intestinal disease, but several toxins that are linked to secretory diarrhea were first discovered on the basis of hemolytic activity.

One such toxin is the TDH, or Kanagawa phenomenon hemolysin, of *V. parahaemolyticus.* This toxin was first discovered and characterized on the basis of lysis of erythrocytes. Despite the lack of a mechanistic linkage between hemolysis and secretion, a striking epidemiologic linkage with diarrheal disease was noted wherein TDH+ strains were isolated almost exclusively from diarrheal stools and TDH− strains were isolated almost exclusively from nonclinical specimens. An isogenic mutant of *V. parahaemolyticus* was constructed in which the genes encoding TDH were specifically mutated (16). The TDH+ strain caused fluid accumulation in ligated loops in rabbit, whereas the TDH− strain did not. Furthermore, culture supernatants from the TDH+ strain increased I_{sc} in Ussing chambers, whereas supernatants from the TDH− strain did not. Histologic examination of rabbit intestine exposed to TDH in these experiments showed no evidence of cell damage (16). Further work with purified TDH in Ussing chambers suggested that TDH stimulates chloride secretion and that calcium is the intracellular mediator of secretion (90,91).

Another example of a hemolytic toxin for which a linkage to secretion has been established is the cytolytic enterotoxin (Table 7.1) or aerolysin of *Aeromonas hydrophila* and *Aeromonas sobria.* This toxin, also known as β-hemolysin or "cholera toxin cross-reactive cytolytic enterotoxin," lyses rabbit erythrocytes in addition to a wide variety of nonintestinal cells, such as CHO cells (92–94). The purified hemolysin also causes fluid accumulation in rabbit ileal loops and infant mouse intestines (92,93). Furthermore, culture filtrates of *A. sobria* produce enterotoxic activity in a rat jejunal perfusion system that is neutralized by monoclonal antibody against the aerolysin (95). In the rat perfusion system, the culture filtrates induce net water, potassium, and sodium loss rapidly (within <5 minutes) without changes in intestinal histology.

These examples, in addition to recent data implicating α-hemolysin as a virulence factor in strains of *E. coli* termed *diarrhea-associated hemolytic E. coli* (96), illustrate that toxins cytotoxic to erythrocytes may also be relevant to intestinal secretion. However, the use of hemolytic assays in studying such toxins should be limited to toxin purification studies or similar applications, and mechanistic studies should be conducted on relevant intestinal cells and tissues.

MECHANISMS BY WHICH ENTERIC BACTERIAL TOXINS STIMULATE INTESTINAL SECRETION

Two approaches are used to analyze how enteric bacterial toxins act to stimulate intestinal secretion. First, the relationship between the general mode of activity of a toxin (e.g., enterotoxin, cytotoxin) and mechanisms of secretion is discussed. Second, as detailed in Table 7.2, the enteric bacterial toxins are classified according to how clearly their mechanisms of action have been established. Of note, most of these toxins exhibit one or more activities for which mechanisms are incompletely established (possible or postulated mechanism of action) or not known at all.

Relationship between General Mode of Activity of Enteric Bacterial Toxins and Mechanisms of Secretion

The primary mechanism of action documented for unequivocal enterotoxins such as CT, the heat-labile and heat-stable enterotoxins of *E. coli* (LTI, LTII, STa), and EAST-1, is activation of either adenylate cyclase or GC-C with subsequent elevation of intracellular cyclic nucleotide levels (cAMP, cGMP). As discussed earlier in this chapter, one note of caution is that with certain toxins, such as CT and *E. coli* STa, alternative mechanisms (e.g., neural activity, change in intracellular calcium) (Table 7.2) may also contribute to the secretory response. For example, elevation of intracellular calcium by *V. cholerae* zonula occludens toxin (Zot) (97) or *V. parahaemolyticus* TDH (90,91) is an alternative mechanism by which enterotoxins may stimulate intestinal secretion.

With most of the cytoskeleton-altering toxins, the cytoskeletal protein(s) involved in a cellular morphologic change in response to toxin treatment is unknown. Of the three major cytoskeletal proteins—actin, tubulin, and keratin—only F-actin has repeatedly been shown to be altered by enteric bacterial toxins [e.g., BFT, *E. coli* STa, *C. difficile* toxins A and B, C2 toxin of *C. botulinum,* RTX ("repeats-in-toxin") of *V. cholerae* O1]. Many details of how these toxins modulate the microfilament (or F-actin) structure of cells are unknown. However, three mechanisms have been identified. First, the C2 toxin of *C. botulinum* adenosine diphosphate (ADP)-ribosylates arginine 177 of (monomeric) G-actin, thereby preventing the polymerization of G-actin to F-actin (98,99). Second, data suggest that four enteric bacterial toxins, *E. coli* CNF-1 and CNF-2 and *C. difficile* toxins A and B, catalytically modify (either monoglucosylation or deamidation) members of the Rho GTP-binding protein family that modulate microfilament structure in eukaryotic cells (75,76,100–103). Third, BFT cleaves the zonula adherens protein E-cadherin; the result is release of F-actin from its protein linkages to trigger cell shape changes with redistribution of F-actin (104). Potential mechanisms accounting for how a toxin that alters the cellular cytoskeleton stimulates secretion include regulation of the Na/K/2Cl co-transporter, a key protein in transepithelial chloride transport that is functionally linked to the cytoskeleton (51), and a reduction in barrier function, noted with several toxins that alter cellular F-actin structure (105). Of note, chloride secretion stimulated by *E. coli* STa (68) and cyclic AMP-dependent agonists (50,51) is also reduced when F-actin is immobilized in monolayers of intestinal epithelial cells studied in Ussing chambers.

The best-established mechanism of action for any of the enteric bacterial cytotoxins is inhibition of protein synthesis. This has been studied in detail only for Shiga toxins possessing *N*-glycosidase activity, in which adenine 4,324 is cleaved from the 3′ end of the 28S ribosomal RNA component of the eukaryotic ribosomal complex; the result is inhibition of peptide elongation and termination of protein synthesis (5,33,106). One postulated mechanism by which Shiga toxins affect intestinal secretion relates to the observation that in rabbits, the concentration of Gb3 receptor for Shiga toxin is greater in the absorptive villous cells than in the secretory crypt cells, so that the preferential killing of the villous cells leads to decreased fluid absorption (25). An alternative mechanism by which a cytotoxin may stimulate intestinal secretion is exemplified by CPE, which is lethal to eukaryotic cells, presumably by creating an ion-permeable membrane pore. Secretion stimulated by CPE is always linked to its cytotoxicity (87). The C2 toxin of *C. botulinum* is also ultimately lethal to eukaryotic cells (98). How ADP-ribosylation of G-actin by the C2 toxin of *C. botulinum* results in cell lethality is unknown.

Precise mechanisms of how enteric bacterial toxins such as CT and *E. coli* STa stimulate secretion through neural activity are not available. In contrast, antagonist studies have implicated submucosal primary sensory neurons in the secretion and inflammation stimulated by *C. difficile* toxin A (71,107). Certain bacterial toxins (Table 7.2) have been noted to stimulate cytokine production or alter polymorphonuclear neutrophil transmigration through intestinal epithelial cell monolayers. These immune responses are likely contributors to intestinal secretion stimulated by these proteins.

Enteric Bacterial Toxins with Established, Possible/Postulated, or Unknown Mechanisms of Action

Table 7.3 lists enteric bacterial toxins by degree of certainty regarding their mechanism of action. Toxins are considered to have an established mechanism of action if the molecular mechanism of action has been identified and the activity of the toxin has been linked to intestinal secretion. Within the established mechanisms of action, three general categories are as follows: (a) toxins that bind to a receptor to stimulate the release of a second messenger (e.g., cyclic nucleotides or calcium); (b) toxins with an A/B structure in which the B subunit mediates cell binding and the enzymatically active A subunit (with or without the B subunit) is translocated across the eukaryotic cell membrane to its cytosolic substrate; and (c) toxins that insert directly into the cell membrane to create an ion-permeable pore (55). Among the established mechanisms of action, the best-understood at the molecular level are the ADP-ribosyltransferase activity of CT and the *E. coli* LTs (27,30), the *N*-glycosidase activity of Shiga toxins (106), and the ADP-ribosyltransferase activity of the *C. botulinum* C2 toxin (99). In each of these examples, the specific residue modified by the enzymatic activity of the toxin has been identified. In certain cases—namely, toxins acting via calcium/calmodulin/protein kinase C signaling or the relatively new class of toxins demonstrating protease activity (Table 7.1)—the data establishing these mechanisms of action are less definitive than, for example, those for the toxins that stimulate adenylate or guanylate cyclase or inhibit protein synthesis, as described above. The documented ability of cyclic nucleotides to stimulate the chloride channel CFTR by activating protein kinases in the intestinal epithelial cell serves as perhaps the best direct evidence that this molecular mechanism of action can activate one or more intestinal epithelial cell ion transporters (49,63–65). Two toxins appear to act via a calcium-dependent mechanism. First, the *V. parahaemolyticus* TDH has been shown to trigger a calcium-dependent chloride current (90,91). Second, *V. cholerae* Zot, which decreases barrier function and stimulates secretion in rabbit small bowel (108), transiently activates protein kinase C-α in the membranes of intestinal epithelial cells, and protein kinase C inhibitors abolish the effect of Zot on barrier function (97). Modification of Rho by, for example, the *C. difficile* toxins A and B alters intestinal epithelial barrier function and potentially contributes to secretion (72–74,78,109). In contrast, stimulation of intestinal secretion by pore formation is less secure.

Toxins with possible or postulated mechanisms of action have been included in this category based on one of several criteria. First, the mechanism of action of the toxin has been inferred by the identification of a biologic activity specific for another toxin with a known mechanism of action. For example, like CT, the LT of *P. shigelloides* causes CHO cell elongation that can be neutralized by antisera against CT, which suggests that this toxin elevates intracellular cAMP (110). Second, the possible mechanism of action has been demonstrated only in nonintestinal cells. For example, in addition to its ability to form an ion-permeable channel in lipid bilayers (111), the δ toxin of *S. aureus* has been reported to stimulate a eukaryotic cell phospholipase A_2, which suggests that stimulation of arachidonic acid metabolism may contribute to the secretory response to this toxin (112). Third, the toxin has been shown to elevate a second messenger in intestinal epithelial cells, but the relevance to secretion has not yet been demonstrated. This criterion applies to the increases in intracellular calcium reported for the *E. coli* STa and STb toxins. *E. coli* STa has been reported to elevate intracellular calcium and stimulate the release of diacylglycerol in isolated rat intestinal epithelial cells (55,56,113). However, the relevance of these observations to secretion has not been demonstrated. The *E. coli* STb toxin has also been shown to elevate intracellular calcium in several cell types, including human intestinal epithelial cells HT29/C1 (114). This appears to occur through activation of a calcium channel regulated by a GTP-binding protein. As in the case of *E. coli* STa, experiments to demonstrate a secretory response correlating with the increase in intracellular calcium stimulated by *E. coli* STb have not yet been performed. Fourth, the mechanism of action of the toxin has been suggested by experiments with inhibitors or chelators of protein kinases or calcium, but direct data demonstrating kinase activation or increases in intracellular calcium are lacking. For example, secretion stimulated by the *V. cholerae* O1 Ace is nearly abrogated by inhibitors of intracellular or extracellular calcium (26). These data suggest, but do not prove, a role for calcium in the secretory activity of this toxin. Fifth, the mechanism of action of the toxin is based on computer modeling of the structure of the toxin deduced from its DNA sequence. For example, the potential pore-forming toxin *V. cholerae* O1 Ace toxin is predicted to be amphipathic, which suggests that polymers of the toxin molecules could insert into the intestinal epithelial cell membrane to create an ion-permeable channel (44). Direct data to support or refute this hypothesis are not yet available. Lastly, several toxins, including CT (52–54), *C. difficile* toxin A (71,115,116), *E. coli* STb (117), and the *Salmonella typhimurium* heat-labile enterotoxin (28,118), stimulate the release of arachidonic acid metabolites in the intestine. Furthermore, each of these toxins has been linked to secretion in one or more experimental intestinal models. However, the mechanistic steps between binding of the toxin to its intestinal epithelial cell receptor and the ultimate release of arachidonic acid metabolites are likely to be multiple and have not been fully delineated for any of these toxins.

Recent data have indicated that toxins about which a great deal is known in fact have unanticipated effects on intestinal epithelial cells that likely contribute to the secretory process. The observation that Shiga toxins induce IL-8 secretion by intestinal epithelial cells *in vitro* is an example of how toxins well-known to inhibit protein synthesis paradoxically also stimulate new protein synthesis by intestinal epithelial cells (119,120). For example, although IL-8 secretion by intestinal epithelial cells does not directly alter ion transport, IL-8 secretion is likely to contribute to the secretory process via induction of an inflammatory response and neutrophil infiltration in the gut.

The last category of enteric bacterial toxins comprises those with unknown mechanisms of action. Most enteric bacterial toxins have been classified according to various biologic activities demonstrated in one or more experimental systems. However, many biologic activities have been identified for which precise mechanistic explanations do not exist at present. Even among the best-studied toxins, the mechanism(s) for certain biologic activities are unknown. For example, the mechanism by which *E. coli* STa alters the appearance of F-actin in intestinal epithelial cells *in vitro* is unknown (68).

CONCLUSIONS

Although our understanding of the mechanisms of action of enteric bacterial toxins is expanding, our knowledge remains incomplete. The known enteric bacterial toxins comprise a wide spectrum ranging from recently discovered and unpurified toxins to toxins for which exquisite molecular detail has been revealed. Even in the case of toxins that have been studied intensively and whose mechanisms of action were thought to be known, recent data indicate that our previous mechanistic schemes were too simplistic and that specific toxins may in fact be acting in multiple ways that contribute to the intestinal secretory process. Modern molecular experimental approaches and accruing information about eukaryotic signal transduction pathways provide unprecedented opportunities for improving our understanding of how enteric bacterial toxins contribute to disease.

REFERENCES

1. Levine MM, Kaper JB, Black RE, et al. New knowledge on pathogenesis of bacterial enteric infections as applied to vaccine development. *Microbiol Rev* 1983;47:510–550.
2. Levine MM, Kaper JB, Herrington D, et al. Volunteer studies of deletion mutants of *Vibrio cholerae* O1 prepared by recombinant techniques. *Infect Immun* 1988;56:161–167.
3. Kelly CP, Pothoulakis C, LaMont JT. *Clostridium difficile* colitis. *N Engl J Med* 1994;330:257–262.
4. Lopez EL, Diaz M, Grinstein S, et al. Hemolytic uremic syndrome and diarrhea in Argentine children: the role of Shiga-like toxins. *J Infect Dis* 1989;160:469–475.
5. Paton JC, Paton AW. Pathogenesis and diagnosis of Shiga toxin-producing *Escherichia coli* infections. *Clin Microbiol Rev* 1998; 11:450–479.
6. Nair GB, Takeda Y. Detection of toxins of *Vibrio cholerae* O1 and non-O1. In: Wachsmuth IK, Blake PA, Olsvik, eds. Vibrio cholerae *and cholera: molecular to global perspectives.* Washington, DC: American Society for Microbiology Press, 1994:53–67.
7. Merson MH, Yolken RH, Sack RB, et al. Detection of *Escherichia coli* enterotoxins in stools. *Infect Immun* 1980;29:108–113.
8. Cohen A, Madrid Marina V, Estrov Z, et al. Expression of glycolipid receptors to Shiga-like toxin on human B lymphocytes: a mechanism for the failure of long-lived antibody response to dysenteric disease. *Int Immunol* 1990;2:1–8.
9. Azim T, Rashid A, Qadri F, et al. Antibodies to Shiga toxin in the serum of children with *Shigella*-associated haemolytic uremic syndrome. *J Med Microbiol* 1999;48:11–16.
10. Ludwig K, Karmali MA, Sarkim V, et al. Antibody response to Shiga toxins Stx2 and Stx1 in children with enteropathic hemolytic-uremic syndrome. *J Clin Microbiol* 2001;39: 2272–2279.
11. Merson MH, Morris GK, Sack DA, et al. Travelers' diarrhea in Mexico: a prospective study of physicians and family members attending a congress. *N Engl J Med* 1976;294:1299–1305.
12. Guerrant RL, Moore RA, Kirschenfeld PM, et al. Role of toxigenic and invasive bacteria in acute diarrhea of childhood. *N Engl J Med* 1975;293:567–573.
13. Sears CL. The *Bacteriodes fragilis* toxins. *Toxicon* 2001;39: 1737–1746.
14. De SN. Enterotoxicity of bacteria-free culture filtrate of *Vibrio cholerae. Nature* 1959;183:1533–1534.
15. Delor I, Cornelis GR. Role of *Yersinia enterocolitica* Yst toxin in experimental infection in young rabbits. *Infect Immun* 1992; 60:4269–4277.
16. Nishibuchi M, Fasano A, Russell RG, et al. Enterotoxigenicity of *Vibrio parahaemolyticus* with and without genes encoding thermostable direct hemolysin. *Infect Immun* 1992;60:3539–3545.
17. Hughes JM, Murad F, Chang B, et al. Role of cyclic GMP in the action of heat-stable enterotoxin of *Escherichia coli. Nature* 1978;2;71:755–756.
18. Richardson SH, Giles JC, Kruger KS. Sealed adult mice: new model for enterotoxin evaluation. *Infect Immun* 1984;43: 482–486.
19. Field M, Fromm D, Al-Awqati Q, et al. Effect of cholera enterotoxin on ion transport across isolated ileal mucosa. *J Clin Invest* 1972;51:796–804.
20. Field M, Graf LH, Laird WJ, et al. Heat-stable enterotoxin of *Escherichia coli*: *in vitro* effects on guanylate cyclase activity, cyclic GMP concentration, and ion transport in small intestine. *Proc Natl Acad Sci U S A* 1978;75:2800–2804.
21. Guandalini S, Rao MC, Smith PL, et al. cGMP modulation of ileal ion transport: *in vitro* effects of *Escherichia coli* heat-stable enterotoxin. *Am J Physiol* 1982;243:G36–G41.
22. Weikel CS, Nellans HN, Guerrant RL. *In vivo* and *in vitro* effects of a novel enterotoxin, STb, produced by *Escherichia coli. J Infect Dis* 1986;153:893–901.
23. Savarino SJ, Fasano A, Watson J, et al. Enteroaggregative *Escherichia coli* heat-stable enterotoxin 1 represents another subfamily of *E. coli* heat-stable toxin. *Proc Natl Acad Sci U S A* 1993;90:3093–3097.
24. Savarino SJ, Fasano A, Robertson DC, et al. Enteroaggregative *Escherichia coli* elaborate a heat-stable enterotoxin demonstrable in an *in vitro* rabbit intestinal model. *J Clin Invest* 1991;87: 1450–1455.
25. Kandel G, Donohue-Rolfe A, Donowitz M, et al. Pathogenesis of *Shigella* diarrhea. Selective targeting of Shiga toxin to villus cells of rabbit jejunum explains the effect of the toxin on intestinal electrolyte transport. *J Clin Invest* 1989;84:1509–1517.
26. Trucksis M, Conn TL, Wasserman SS, et al. *Vibrio cholerae* ACE stimulates Ca^{2+}-dependent Cl^-/CHO_3^- secretion in T84 cells *in vitro. Am J Physiol Cell Physiol* 2000;279:C567–C577.
27. Kaper JB, Morris JG Jr, Levine MM. Cholera. *Clin Microbiol Rev* 1995;8:48–86.
28. Peterson JW. *Salmonella* toxin. *Pharmacol Ther* 1980;11: 719–724.
29. Peterson JW, Molina NC, Houston CW, et al. Elevated cAMP in intestinal epithelial cells during experimental cholera and salmonellosis. *Toxicon* 1983;21:761–775.

30. Spangler BD. Structure and function of cholera toxin and the related *Escherichia coli* heat-labile enterotoxin. *Microbiol Rev* 1992;56:622–647.
31. Guerrant RL, Brunton LL, Schnaitman TC, et al. Cyclic adenosine monophosphate and alteration of Chinese hamster ovary cell morphology: a rapid, sensitive *in vitro* assay for the enterotoxins of *Vibrio cholerae* and *Escherichia coli*. *Infect Immun* 1974;10:320–327.
32. Donta ST, Moon HW, Whipp SC. Detection of heat-labile *Escherichia coli* enterotoxin with the use of adrenal cells in tissue culture. *Science* 1974;183:334–336.
33. Acheson DWK, Keusch GT. The family of Shiga toxins. In: Alouf SE, Freer JH, eds. *The comprehensive sourcebook of bacterial protein toxins.* London: Academic Press, 1999:229–242.
34. Terranova W, Blake PA. *Bacillus cereus* food poisoning. *N Engl J Med* 1978;298:143–144.
35. Tranter HS. Foodborne staphylococcal illness. *Lancet* 1990; 336:1044–1046.
36. Ohishi I. Response of mouse intestinal loop to botulinum C2 toxin: enterotoxic activity induced by cooperation of nonlinked protein components. *Infect Immun* 1983;40:691–695.
37. Ohishi I, Iwasaki M, Sakaguchi G. Purification and characterization of two components of botulinum C2 toxin. *Infect Immun* 1980;30:668–673.
38. Okeke IN, Lamikanra A, Steinruck H, et al. Characterization of *Escherichia coli* strains from cases of childhood diarrhea in provincial southwestern Nigeria. *J Clin Microbiol* 2000;38:7–12.
39. Albert MJ, Faruque SM, Faruque ASG, et al. Controlled study of cytolethal distending toxin-producing *Escherichia coli* infections in Bangladeshi children. *J Clin Microbiol* 1996;34:717–719.
40. Levine MM, Bergquist EJ, Nalin DR, et al. *Escherichia coli* strains that cause diarrhoea but do not produce heat-labile or heat-stable enterotoxins and are non-invasive. *Lancet* 1978;1: 1119–1122.
41. Tacket CO, Sztein MB, Losonsky G, et al. Role of EspB in experimental human enteropathogenic *Escherichia coli* infection. *Infect Immun* 2000;68:3689–3695.
42. Albert MJ, Faruque AS, Farque SM, et al. Case–control study of enteropathogens associated with childhood diarrhea in Dhaka, Bangladesh. *J Clin Microbiol* 1999;37:3458–3464.
43. Fasano A, Baudry B, Pumplin DW, et al. *Vibrio cholerae* produces a second enterotoxin, which affects intestinal tight junctions. *Proc Natl Acad Sci U S A* 1991;88:5242–5246.
44. Trucksis M, Galen JE, Michalski J, et al. Accessory cholera enterotoxin (Ace), the third toxin of a *Vibrio cholerae* virulence cassette. *Proc Natl Acad Sci U S A* 1993;90:5267–5271.
45. Lin W, Fullner KJ, Clayton R, et al. Identification of a *Vibrio cholerae* RTX toxin gene cluster that is tightly linked to the cholera toxin prophage. *Proc Natl Acad Sci U S A* 1999;96: 1071–1076.
46. Wu Z, Milton D, Nybom P, Sjo A, et al. *Vibrio cholerae* hemagglutinin/protease causes morphological changes in cultured epithelial cells and perturbs their paracellular barrier function. *Microb Pathog* 1996;21:111–123.
47. Lencer WI. Microbes and microbial toxins: paradigms for microbial–mucosal interactions. *V. cholerae*: invasion of the intestinal epithelial barrier by a stably folded protein toxin. *Am J Physiol Gastrointest Liver Physiol* 2001;280:G781–G786.
48. Field M. Ion transport in rabbit ileal mucosa. II. Effects of cyclic 3′,5′-AMP. *Am J Physiol* 1971;221:992–997.
49. Kartner N, Hanrahan JW, Jensen TJ, et al. Expression of the cystic fibrosis gene in non-epithelial invertebrate cells produces a regulated anion conductance. *Cell* 1991;64:681–691.
50. Shapiro M, Matthews J, Hecht G, et al. Stabilization of F-actin prevents cAMP-elicited Cl^- secretion in T84 cells. *J Clin Invest* 1991;87:1903–1909.
51. Matthew JB, Awtrey CS, Madara JL. Microfilament-dependent activation of $Na^+/K^+/2Cl^-$ cotransport by cAMP in intestinal epithelial monolayers. *J Clin Invest* 1992;90:1608–1613.
52. Peterson JW, Ochoa LG. Role of prostaglandins and cAMP in the secretory effects of cholera toxin. *Science* 1989;245:857–859.
53. Guerrant RL, Fang GD, Thielman NM, et al. Role of platelet activating factor (PAF) in the intestinal epithelial secretory and Chinese hamster ovary (CHO) cell cytoskeletal responses to cholera toxin. *Proc Natl Acad Sci U S A* 1994;91:9655–9658.
54. Thielman NM, Marcinkiewicz M, Sarosiek J, et al. Role of platelet-activating factor in Chinese hamster ovary cell responses to cholera toxin. *J Clin Invest* 1997;15:1999–2004.
55. Sears CL, Kaper JB. Enteric bacterial toxins: mechanisms of action and linkage to intestinal secretion. *Microbiol Rev* 1996; 60:167–215.
56. Nair GB, Takeda Y. The heat-stable enterotoxins. *Microb Pathog* 1998;24:123–131.
57. Yoshimura S, Ikemura H, Watanabe H, et al. Essential structure for full enterotoxigenic activity of heat-stable enterotoxin produced by enterotoxigenic *Escherichia coli*. *FEBS Lett* 1985;181: 138–141.
58. Shimonishi Y, Kidaka Y, Kaiumi. Metal mode of disulphide bond formation of a heat-stable enterotoxin (STh) produced by a human strain of enterotoxigenic *Escherichia coli*. *FEBS Lett* 1987;215:165–170.
59. Schulz S, Green CK, Yuen PST, et al. Guanylyl cyclase is a heat-stable enterotoxin receptor. *Cell* 1990;63:941–948.
60. Cohen MBN, Jensen NJ, Hawkins EA, et al. Receptors for *Escherichia coli* heat-stable enterotoxin in human intestine and in a human intestinal cell line (Caco-2). *J Cell Physiol* 1993; 156:138–144.
61. Vaandrager AB, Schulz S, de Jonge HR, et al. Guanylyl cyclase C is an *N*-linked glycoprotein receptor that accounts for multiple heat-stable enterotoxin binding proteins in the intestine. *J Biol Chem* 1993;268:2174–2179.
62. Huott PA, Liu W, McRoberts JA, et al. Mechanism of action of *Escherichia coli* heat stable enterotoxin in a human colonic cell line. *J Clin Invest* 1988;82:514–523.
63. Lin M, Nairn AC, Guggino SE. cGMP-dependent protein kinase regulation of a chloride channel in T84 cells. *Am J Physiol (Cell Physiol)* 1992;262:C1304–C1312.
64. Forte LR, Thorne PK, Eber SL, et al. Stimulation of intestinal Cl^- transport by heat-stable enterotoxin: activation of cAMP-dependent protein kinase by cGMP. *Am J Physiol (Cell Physiol)* 1992;263:C607–C615.
65. Tien X-Y, Brasitus TA, Kaetzel MA, et al. Activation of the cystic fibrosis transmembrane conductance regulator by cGMP in the human colonic cancer cell line, Caco-2. *J Biol Chem* 1994; 269:51–54.
66. Currie MG, Fok KF, Kato J, et al. Guanylin: an endogenous activator of intestinal guanylate cyclase. *Proc Natl Acad Sci U S A* 1992;89:947–951.
67. Forte LR, Eber SL, Turner JT, et al. Guanylin stimulation of Cl^- secretion in human intestinal T84 cells via cyclic guanosine monophosphate. *J Clin Invest* 1993;91:2423–2428.
68. Matthews JB, Awtrey CS, Thompson R, et al. Na^+-K^+-$2Cl^-$ cotransport and Cl^- secretion evoked by heat-stable enterotoxin is microfilament-dependent in T84 cells. *Am J Physiol* 1993; 265:G370–G378.
69. Mitchell TJ, Ketley JM, Burdon DW, et al. The effects of *Clostridium difficile* crude toxins and purified toxin A on stripped rabbit ileal mucosa in Ussing chambers. *J Med Microbiol* 1987;23:199–204.
70. Moore R, Pothoulakis C, LaMont JT, et al. *C. difficile* toxin A increases intestinal permeability and induces Cl^- secretion. *Am J Physiol* 1990;259:G165–G172.

71. Pouthoulakis C, LaMont TJ. Microbes and microbial toxins: paradigms for microbial mucosal interactions. II. The integrated response of the intestine to *Clostridium difficile* toxins. *Am J Physiol Gastrointest Liver Physiol* 280:G178–G183.
72. Riegler M, Sedivy R, Pothoulakis C, et al. *Clostridium difficile* toxin B is more potent that toxin A in damaging human colonic epithelium *in vitro. J Clin Invest* 1995;95:2004–2011.
73. Hecht G, Pothoulakis C, LaMont JT, et al. *Clostridium difficile* toxin A perturbs cytoskeletal structure and tight junction permeability of the cultured human intestinal epithelial monolayers. *J Clin Invest* 1988;82:1516–1524.
74. Hecht G, Koutsouris A, Pothoulakis C, et al. *Clostridium difficile* toxin B disrupts the barrier function of T 84 monolayers. *Gastroenterology* 1992;102:416–423.
75. Just I, Selzer J, Wilm M, et al. Glucosylation of Rho proteins by *Clostridium difficile* toxin B. *Nature* 1995;375:500–503.
76. Just I, Wilm M, Selzer J, et al. The enterotoxin gene from *Clostridium difficile* (ToxA) monoglucosylates the Rho proteins. *J Biol Chem* 1995;270:13932–13936.
77. Hall A. Rho GTPases and the actin cytoskeleton. *Science* 1998; 279:509–514
78. Hecht G. Microbes and microbial toxins: paradigms for microbial mucosal interactions. VII. Enteropathogenic *Escherichia coli* physiological alterations from an extracellular position. *Am J Physiol Gastrointest Liver Physiol* 2001;281:G1–G7.
79. Mellies JL, Navarro-Garcia F, Okeke I, et al. *EspC* pathogenicity island of enteropathogenic *Escherchia coli* encodes an enterotoxin. *Infect Immun* 2001;69:315–324.
80. McNamara BP, Koustsouris A, O'Connell CB, et al. Translocated EspF protein from enteropathogenic *Escherichia coli* disrupts host intestinal barrier function. *J Clin Invest* 2001; 107:621–629.
81. Turnbull PCB. *Bacillus cereus* toxins. *Pharmacol Ther* 1981;13: 453–505.
82. Thompson NE, Ketterhagen MJ, Bergdoll MS, et al. Isolation and some properties of an enterotoxin produced by *Bacillus cereus. Infect Immun* 1984;43:887–894.
83. Beecher DJ, Macmillan JD. A novel biocomponent hemolysin from *Bacillus cereus. Infect Immun* 1990;58:2220–2227.
84. Obiso RJ Jr, Lyerly DM, Van Tassell RL, et al. Proteolytic activity of the *Bacteroides fragilis* enterotoxin causes fluid secretion and intestinal damage *in vivo. Infect Immun* 1995;63:3820–3826.
85. Chambers FG, Koshy SS, Saidi RF, et al. *Bacteroides fragilis* toxin exhibits polar activity on monolayers of human intestinal epithelial cells (T 84 cells) *in vitro. Infect Immun* 1997;65: 3561–3570.
86. Riegler M, Lotz M, Sears C, et al. *Bacteroides fragilis* toxin 2 damages human colonic mucosa *in vitro. Gut* 1999;44:504–510.
87. McClane BA. *Clostridium perfringens* enterotoxin and intestinal tight junctions. *Trends Microbiol* 2000;8:145–146.
88. Sarker MR, Carman RJ, McClane BA. Inactivation of the gene (*cpe*) encoding *Clostridium perfringens* enterotoxin eliminates the ability of two cpe-positive *C. perfringens* type A human gastrointestinal disease isolates to affect rabbit ileal loops. *Mol Microbiol* 1999;33:946–958.
89. Sonoda N, Furuse M, Sasaki H, et al. *Clostridium perfringens* enterotoxin fragment removes specific claudins from tight junction strands: evidence for direct involvement of claudins in tight junction barrier. *J Cell Biol* 1999;147:195–204.118.
90. Raimondi F, Kao JPY, Kaper JB, et al. Calcium-dependent intestinal chloride secretion by *Vibrio parahaemolyticus* thermostable direct hemolysin in a rabbit model. *Gastroenterology* 1995;109:381–386.
91. Raimondi F, Kano JP, Fiorentini C, et al. Enterotoxicity and cytotoxicity of *Vibrio parahaemolyticus* thermostable direct hemolysin in *in vitro* systems. *Infect Immun* 2000;68:3180–3185.
92. Asao T, Kinoshita Y, Kozaki S, et al. Purification and some properties of *Aeromonas hydrophila* hemolysin. *Infect Immun* 1984;46:122–127.
93. Rose JM, Houston CW, Kurosky A. Bioactivity and immunological characterization of a cholera toxin cross-reactive cytolytic enterotoxin from *Aeromonas hydrophila. Infect Immun* 1989; 57:1170–1176.
94. Chopra AK, Houston CW. Enterotoxins in *Aeromonas*-associated gastroenteritis. *Microbes Infect* 1999;1:1129–1137.
95. Millership SE, Barer MR, Mulla RJ, et al. Enterotoxic effects of *Aeromonas sobria* haemolysin in a rat jejunal perfusion system identified by specific neutralization with a monoclonal antibody. *J Gen Microbiol* 1992;138:261–267.
96. Elliott SJ, Srinivas S, Albert MJ, et al. Characterization of the roles of hemolysin and other toxins in enteropathy caused by alpha-hemolytic *Escherichia coli* linked to human diarrhea. *Infect Immun* 1998;66:2040–2051.
97. Fasano A, Fiorentini C, Donelli G, et al. Zonular occludens toxin modulates tight junctions through protein kinase C-dependent actin reorganization *in vitro. J Clin Invest* 1995;96: 710–720.
98. Aktories K, Wegner A. Mechanisms of the cytopathic action of actin-ADP-ribosylating toxins. *Mol Microbiol* 1992;6: 2905–2908.
99. Vandekerckhove J, Schering B, Barmann M, et al. Botulinum C2 toxin ADP-ribosylates cytoplasmic beta/gamma-actin in arginine 177. *J Biol Chem* 1988;263:696–700.
100. Oswald E, Sugai M, Labigne A, et al. Cytotoxic necrotizing factor type 2 produced by virulent *Escherichia coli* modifies the small GTP-binding proteins Rho involved in assembly of actin stress fibers. *Proc Natl Acad Sci U S A* 1994;91:3814–3818.
101. Fiorentini C, Falzano L, Donelli G, et al. *E. coli* cytotoxic necrotizing factor I (CNF1) and its effects on cells. *Toxicon* 1993; 31:501.
102. Just I, Fritz G, Aktories K, et al. *Clostridium difficile* toxin B acts on the GTP-binding protein Rho. *J Biol Chem* 1994;269: 10706–10712.
103. Sugai M, Hatazaki K, Mogami A, et al. Cytotoxic necrotizing factor type 2 produced by pathogenic *Escherichia coli* deamidates a Gln residue in the conserved G-3 domain of the Rho family and preferentially inhibits the GTPase of RhoA and Rac1. *Infect Immun* 1999;67:6550–6557.
104. Wu S, Lim K-C, Huang J, et al. *Bacteroides fragilis* enterotoxin cleaves the zonular adherens protein, E-cadherin. *Proc Natl Acad Sci U S A* 1998;95:14979–14984.
105. Sears CL. Molecular physiology and pathophysiology of tight junctions V. Assault of the tight junctions by enteric pathogens. *Am J Physiol Gastrointest Liver Physiol* 2000;279:G1129–G1134.
106. Endo Y, Tsurugi K, Yutsudo T, et al. The site of action of a verotoxin (VT2) from *Escherichia coli* O157:H7 and of Shiga toxin on eukaryotic ribosomes: RNA *N*-glycosidase activity of the toxins. *Eur J Biochem* 1988;171:45–50.
107. Pothoulakis C, Castagliuolo I, LaMont JT, et al. CP-96,345, a substance P antagonist, inhibits rat intestinal responses to *Clostridium difficile* toxin A but not cholera toxin. *Proc Natl Acad Sci U S A* 1994;91:947–951.
108. Fasano A, Uzzau S, Fiore C, et al. The enterotoxic effect of zonula occludens toxin on rabbit small intestine involves the paracellular pathway. *Gastroenterology* 1997;112:839–846.
109. Nusrat A, Giry M, Turner JR, et al. Rho protein regulates tight junctions and perijunctional actin organization in polarized epithelia. *Proc Natl Acad Sci U S A* 1995;92:10629–10633.
110. Gardner SE, Fowlston SE, George WL. Effect of iron on production of a possible virulence factor by *Plesiomonas shigelloides. J Clin Microbiol* 1990;28:811–813.
111. Mellor IR, Thomas DH, Sansom MSP. Properties of ion chan-

nels formed by *Staphylococcus aureus. Biochim Biophys Acta* 1988;942:280–294.
112. Bernheimer AW, Rudy B. Interactions between membranes and cytolytic peptides. *Biochim Biophys Acta* 1986;864:123–141.
113. Bhattacharya J, Chakrabarti MK. Rise of intracellular free calcium levels with activation of inositol triphosphate in a human colonic carcinoma cell line (COLO 205) by heat-stable enterotoxin of *Escherichia coli. Biochim Biophys Acta* 1998;1403:1–4.
114. Dreyfus LA, Harville B, Howard DE, et al. Calcium influx mediated by the *Escherichia coli* heat-stable enterotoxin B (STB). *Proc Natl Acad Sci U S A* 1993;90:3202–3206.
115. Fonteles MC, Fang GD, Thielman NM, et al. Role of platelet activating factor in the inflammatory and secretory effects of *Clostridium difficile* toxin A. *J Lipid Mediat Cell Signal* 1995; 11:133–143.
116. Alcantara C, Stenson WF, Steiner TS, et al. Role of inducible cyclooxygenase and prostaglandins in *Clostridium difficile* toxin A-induced secretion and inflammation in an animal model. *J Infect Dis* 2001;184:648–652.
117. Harville BA, Dreyfus LA. Involvement of 5-hydroxytryptamine and prostaglandin E_2 in the intestinal secretory action of *Escherichia coli* heat-stable enterotoxin B (STb). *Infect Immun* 1995;63:745–750.
118. Giannella RA, Gots RE, Charney AN, et al. Pathogenesis of *Salmonella*-mediated intestinal fluid secretion: activation of adenylate cyclase and inhibition by indomethacin. *Gastroenterology* 1975;69:1238–1245.
119. Thorpe CM, Hurley BP, Lincicome LL, et al. Shiga toxins stimulate secretion of interleukin 8 from intestinal epithelial cells. *Infect Immun* 1999;67:5985–5993.
120. Yamasaki C, Natori Y, Zeng XT, et al. Induction of cytokines in a human colon epithelial cell line by Shiga toxin 1 (Stx1) and Stx 2 but not by non-toxic mutant Stx1, which lacks *N*-glycosidase activity. *FEBS Lett* 1999;442:231–234.
121. Turnbull PCB, Kramer JM, Jorgensen K, et al. Properties and production characteristics of vomiting, diarrheal, and necrotizing toxins of *Bacillus cereus. Am J Clin Nutr* 1979;32:219–228.
122. Lund T, De Buyser ML, Granum PE. A new cytotoxin from *Bacillus cereus* that may cause necrotic enteritis. *Mol Microbiol* 2000;38:254–261.
123. Obiso RJ Jr, Azghani AO, Wilkins TD. The *Bacteroides fragilis* toxin fragilysin disrupts the paracellular barrier of epithelial cells. *Infect Immun* 1997;65:1431–1439.
124. Wells CL, Van De Westerloo EMA, Jechorek RP, et al. *Bacteroides fragilis* enterotoxin modulates epithelial permeability and bacterial internalization by HT-29 enterocytes. *Gastroenterology* 1996;110:1429–1437.
125. Sears C, Myers LL, Lazenby A, et al. Enterotoxigenic *Bacteroides fragilis. Clin Infect Dis* 1995;20[Suppl 2]:S142–S148.
126. Guerrant RL, Wanke CA, Pennie RA, et al. Production of a unique cytotoxin by *Campylobacter jejuni. Infect Immun* 1987; 55:2526–2530.
127. Lee A, Smith SC, Coloe PJ. Detection of a novel *Campylobacter* cytotoxin. *J Appl Microbiol* 2000;89:719–725.
128. Johnson WM, Lior H. A new heat-labile cytolethal distending toxin (CLDT) produced by *Campylobacter* spp. *Microb Pathog* 1988;4:115–126.
129. Lara-Tejero M, Galan JE. A bacterial toxin that controls cell cycle progression as a deoxyribonuclease I-like protein. *Science* 2000;290:354–357.
130. Ohishi I, Miyake M, Ogura H, et al. Cytopathic effect of botulinum C2 toxin on tissue-culture cells. *FEMS Microbiol Lett* 1984;23:281–284.
131. Just I, Wille M, Chaponnier C, et al. Gelsolin–actin complex is target for ADP-ribosylation by *Clostridium botulinum* C2 toxin in intact human neutrophils. *Eur J Pharmacol* 1994;246: 293–297.
132. Hunter SE, Brown JE, Oyston PCF, et al. Molecular genetic analysis of beta-toxin of *Clostridium perfringens* reveals sequence homology with alpha-toxin, gamma-toxin, and leukocidin of *Staphylococcus aureus. Infect Immun* 1993;61:3958–3965.
133. Shatursky O, Bayles R, Rogers M, et al. *Clostridium perfringens* beta-toxin forms potential-dependent, cation-sensitive channels in lipid bilayers. *Infect Immun* 2000;68:5546–5551.
134. Titball RW, Leslie DL, Harvey S, et al. Hemolytic and sphingomyelinase activities of *Clostridium perfringens* alpha-toxin are dependent on a domain homologous to that of an enzyme from the human arachidonic acid pathway. *Infect Immun* 1991;59: 1872–1874.
135. Diener M, Egleme C, Rummel W. Phospholipase C-induced anion secretion and its interaction with carbachol in the rat colonic mucosa. *Eur J Pharmacol* 1991;299:267–276.
136. Skjelkvale R, Duncan CL. Characterization of enterotoxin purified from *Clostridium perfringens* type C. *Infect Immun* 1975; 11:1061–1068.
137. Skjelkvale R, Duncan CL. Enterotoxin formation by different toxigenic types of *Clostridium perfringens. Infect Immun* 1975; 11:563–575.
138. Eslava C, Navarro-Garcia F, Czeczulin JR, et al. Pet, an autotransporter enterotoxin from enteroaggregative *Escherichia coli. Infect Immun* 1998;66:3155–3163.
139. Navarro-Garcia F, Sears C, Eslava C, et al. Cytoskeletal effects induced by pet, the serine protease enterotoxin of enteroaggregative *Escherichia coli. Infect Immun* 1999;67:2184–2192.
140. Henderson IR, Hicks S, Navarro-Garcia F, et al. Involvement of the enteroaggregative *Escherichia coli* plasmid-encoded toxin in causing human intestinal damage. *Infect Immun* 1999;67: 5338–5344.
141. Villaseca JM, Navarro-Garcia F, Mendoza-Hernandez G, et al. Pet toxin from enteroaggregative *Escherichia coli* produces cellular damage associated with fodrin disruption. *Infect Immun* 2000;68:5920–5927.
142. Navarro-Garcia F, Eslava C, Villaseca JM, et al. *In vitro* effects of a high-molecular-weight heat-labile enterotoxin from enteroaggregative *Escherichia coli. Infect Immun* 1998;66: 3149–3154.
143. Fasano A, Kay BA, Russell RG, et al. Enterotoxin and cytotoxin production by enteroinvasive *Escherichia coli. Infect Immun* 1990;58:3717–3723.
144. Nataro JP, Seriwatana J, Fasano A, et al. Identification and cloning of a novel plasmid-encoded enterotoxin of enteroinvasive *Escherichia coli* and *Shigella* strains. *Infect Immun* 1995;63: 4721–4728.
145. Buchrieser C, Glaser P, Rusnioik C, et al. The virulence plasmid pWR100 and the repertoire of proteins secreted by the type III secretion apparatus of *Shigella flexneri. Mol Microbiol* 2000;38: 760–771.
146. Whipp SC. Protease degradation of *Escherichia coli* heat-stable mouse-negative pig-positive enterotoxin. *Infect Immun* 1987; 55:2057–2060.
147. Whipp SC. Assay for enterotoxigenic *Escherichia coli* heat-stable toxin b in rats and mice. *Infect Immun* 1990;58:930–934.
148. Whipp SC, Kokue E, Morgan RW, et al. Functional significance of histologic alterations induced by *Escherichia coli* pig-specific, mouse-negative, heat-stable enterotoxin (STb). *Vet Res Commun* 1987;11:41–55.
149. Chang PP, Moss J, Twiddy EM, et al. Type II heat-labile enterotoxin of *Escherichia coli* activates adenylate cyclase in human fibroblasts by ADP ribosylation. *Infect Immun* 1987;55: 1854–1858.
150. Donta ST, Tomicic T, Holmes RK. Binding of class II

Escherichia coli enterotoxins to mouse Y1 and intestinal cells. *Infect Immun* 1992;60:2870–2873.
151. Lee CM, Chang PP, Tsai SC, et al. Activation of *Escherichia coli* heat-labile enterotoxins by native and recombinant adenosine diphosphate-ribosylation factors, 20-kd guanine nucleotide-binding proteins. *J Clin Invest* 1991;87:1780–1786.
152. Holmes RK, Twiddy EM, Pickett CL. Purification and characterization of type II heat-labile enterotoxin of *Escherichia coli. Infect Immun* 1986;53:464–473.
153. Scott DA, Kaper JB. Cloning and sequencing of the genes encoding *Escherichia coli* cytolethal distending toxin. *Infect Immun* 1994;62:244–251.
154. De Rycke J, Milon A, Oswald E. Necrotoxic *Escherichia coli* (NETC): two emerging categories of human and animal pathogens. *Vet Res* 1999;30:221–233.
155. De Rycke J, Gonzalez EA, Blanco J, et al. Evidence for two types of cytotoxic necrotizing factor in human and animal clinical isolates of *Escherichia coli. J Clin Microbiol* 1990;28: 694–699.
156. Gerhard R, Schmidt G, Hofman F, et al. Activation of Rho GTPases by *Escherichia coli* cytotoxic necrotizing factor 1 increases intestinal permeability in Caco-2 cells. *Infect Immun* 1998;66:5125–5131.
157. Hofman P, Flatau G, Selva E, et al. *Escherichia coli* cytotoxic necrotizing factor 1 effaces microvilli and decreases transmigration of polymorphonuclear leukocytes in intestinal T84 epithelial cell monolayers. *Infect Immun* 1998;66:2494–2500.
158. Saraswathi B, Agarwal RK, Sanyal SC. Further studies on enteropathogenicity of *Plesiomonas shigelloides. Ind J Med Res* 1983;78:12–18.
159. Matthews BG, Douglas H, Guiney DG. Production of a heat-stable enterotoxin by *Plesiomonas shigelloides. Microb Pathog* 1988;5:207–213.
160. Wallis TS, Wood M, Watson P, et al. Sips, Sops, and SPIs but not stn influences *Salmonella* enteropathogenesis. *Adv Exp Med Biol* 1999;473:275–280.
161. Chopra AK, Huang JH, Xu X, et al. Role of *Salmonella* enterotoxin in overall virulence of the organism. *Microb Pathog* 1999; 27:155–171.
162. Watson PR, Galyov EE, Paulin SM, et al. Mutation of *invH* but not *stn* reduces *Salmonella*-induced enteritis in cattle. *Infect Immun* 1998;66:1432–1438.
163. Reeves-Darby VG, Turner JA, Prasad R, et al. Effect of cloned *Salmonella typhimurium* enterotoxin on rabbit intestinal motility. *FEMS Microbiol Lett* 1995;134:239–244.
164. Okuda J, Fukumoto M, Takeda Y, et al. Examination of diarrheogenicity of cytolethal distending toxin: suckling mouse response to the products of the cdtABC genes of *Shigella dysenteriae. Infect Immun* 1997;65:428–433.
165. Fasano A, Noriega FR, Liao FM, et al. Effect of *Shigella* enterotoxin 1 (ShET1) on rabbit intestine *in vitro* and *in vivo. Gut* 1997;40:505–511.
166. Noriega FR, Liao FM, Formal SB, et al. Prevalence of *Shigella* enterotoxin 1 among *Shigella* clinical isolates of diverse serotypes. *J Infect Dis* 1995;172:1408–1410.
167. Fasano A, Noriega FR, Maneval DR, et al. *Shigella* enterotoxin 1: an enterotoxin of *Shigella flexneri* 2a active in rabbit intestine *in vivo* and *in vitro. J Clin Invest* 1995;95:2853–2861.
168. Al-Hasani K, Henderson IR, Sakellaris H, et al. The *sigA* gene which is borne on the *she* pathogenicity island of *Shigella flexneri* 2a encodes an exported cytopathic protease involved in intestinal fluid accumulation. *Infect Immun* 2000;68:2457–2463.
169. Sullivan R, Asano T. Effects of staphylococcal enterotoxin B on intestinal transport in the rat. *Am J Physiol* 1971;220:1793–1797.
170. Huang KC, Chen TST, Rout WR. Effect of staphylococcal enterotoxins A, B, and C, on ion transport and permeability across the flounder intestine. *Proc Soc Exp Biol Med* 1974;147: 250–254.
171. Elias J, Shields R. Influence of staphylococcal enterotoxin on water and electrolyte transport in the small intestine. *Gut* 1976;17:527–535.
172. Johnson HM, Russell JK, Pontzer CH. Staphylococcal enterotoxin microbial superantigens. *FASEB J* 1991;5:2706–2712.
173. Kapral FA. *Staphylococcus aureus* delta toxin as an enterotoxin. In: Evered D, Whelan J, eds. *Microbial toxins and diarrhoeal disease.* London: Pitman, 1985:215–229.
174. Kapral FA, O'Brien AD, Ruff PD, et al. Inhibition of water absorption in the intestine by *Staphylococcus aureus* delta-toxin. *Infect Immun* 1976;13:140–145.
175. O'Brien AD, McClung HJ, Kapral FA. Increased tissue conductance and ion transport in guinea pig ileum after exposure to *Staphylococcus aureus* delta-toxin *in vitro. Infect Immun* 1978;21:102–113.
176. O'Brien AD, Kapral FA. Increased cyclic adenosine 3′,5′-monophosphate content in guinea pig ileum after exposure to *Staphylococcus aureus* delta-toxin. *Infect Immun* 1976;13:152–162.
177. Wu Z, Nybom P, Magnusson K-E. Distinct effects of *Vibrio cholerae* haemagglutinin/protease on the structure and localization of the tight junction-associated protein occludin and ZO-1. *Cell Microbiol* 2000;2:11–17.
178. Mel SF, Fullner KJ, Wimer-Mackin S, et al. Association of protease activity in *Vibrio cholerae* vaccine strains and decreases in transcellular epithelial resistance of polarized T84 intestinal epithelial cells. *Infect Immun* 2000;68:6487–6492.
179. Fullner KJ, Mekalanos JJ. *In vivo* covalent cross-linking of cellular actin by the *Vibrio cholerae* RTX toxin. *EMBO J* 2000;19: 5315–5323.
180. Zitzer A, Wassenaar TM, Walev I, et al. Potent membrane-permeabilizing and cytocidal action of *Vibrio cholerae* cytolysin on human intestinal cells. *Infect Immun* 1997;65:1293–1298.
181. Pal S, Datta A, Nair GB, et al. Use of monoclonal antibodies to identify phospholipase C as the enterotoxin factor of the bifunctional hemolysin-phospholipase C molecule of *Vibrio cholerae* O139. *Infect Immun* 1998;66:3947–3977.
182. Takahashi A, Kenjyo Nm Imura K, Myonsun Y, et al. C1(-) secretion in colonic epithelial cells induced by the *Vibrio parahaemolyticus* haemolytic toxin related to thermostable direct hemolysin. *Infect Immun* 2000;68:5345–5458.
183. Fabbri A, Falzano L, Frank C, et al. *Vibrio parahaemolyticus* thermostable direct hemolysin modulates cytoskeletal organization and calcium homeostasis in intestinal cultured cells. *Infect Immun* 1999;67:1139–1148.
184. Levine MM, Black RE, Clements ML, et al. Volunteer studies in development of vaccines against cholera and enterotoxigenic *Escherichia coli*: a review. In: Holme T, Holmgren J, Merson MH, et al., eds. *Acute enteric infections in children. New prospects for treatment and prevention.* Amsterdam: Elsevier Science, 1981:443–459.
185. Morris JG, Losonsky GE, Johnos JA, et al. Clinical and immunologic characteristics of *Vibrio cholerae* O139 Bengal infection in North American volunteers. *J Infect Dis* 1995;171: 903–908.
186. Morris JG Jr, Takeda T, Tall BD, et al. Experimental non-O group 1 *Vibrio cholerae* gastroenteritis in humans. *J Clin Invest* 1990;85:697–705.
187. DuPont HL, Levine MM, Hornick RB, et al. Inoculum size in shigellosis and implications for expected mode of transmission. *J Infect Dis* 1989;159:1126–1128.
188. Levine MM, Nalin DR, Hoover DL, et al. Immunity to enterotoxigenic *Escherichia coli. Infect Immun* 1979;23:729–736.

189. DuPont HL, Formal SB, Hornick RB, et al. Pathogenesis of *Escherichia coli* diarrhea. *N Engl J Med* 1971;285:1–9.
190. Mathewson JJ, Johnson PC, DuPont HL, et al. Pathogenicity of enteroadherent *Escherichia coli* in adult volunteers. *J Infect Dis* 1986;154:524–527.
191. Tacket CO, Moseley SL, Kay B, et al. Challenge studies in volunteers using *Escherichia coli* strains with diffuse adherence to HEp-2 cells. *J Infect Dis* 1990;162:550–552.
192. Blaser MJ, Newman LS. A review of human salmonellosis: I. Infective dose. *Rev Infect Dis* 1982;4:1096–1106.
193. Hornick RB, Greisman SE, Woodward TE, et al. Typhoid fever: pathogenesis and immunological control. *N Engl J Med* 1970; 283:686–691.
194. Black RE, Levine MM, Clements ML, et al. Experimental *Campylobacter jejuni* infection in humans. *J Infect Dis* 1988; 157:472–479.
195. Sanyal SC, Sen PC. Human volunteer study on the pathogenicity of *Vibrio parahaemolyticus.* In: Fujino T, Sakaguchi G, Sakazaki R, et al., eds. *International symposium on* Vibrio parahaemolyticus. Tokyo: Saikon, 1974:227–230.
196. Morgan DR, Johnson PC, DuPont HL, et al. Lack of correlation between known virulence properties of *Aeromonas hydrophila* and enteropathogenicity for humans. *Infect Immun* 1985;50:62–65.
197. Herrington DA, Tzipori S, Robins-Browne RM, et al. *In vitro* and *in vivo* pathogenicity of *Plesiomonas shigelloides. Infect Immun* 1987;55:979–985.
198. Charney AN, Egnor RW, Alexander-Chacko JT, et al. Effect of *E. coli* heat-stable enterotoxin on colonic transport in guanylyl cyclase C receptor-deficient mice. *Am J Physiol Gastrointestinal Liver Physiol* 2001;280:G216–G221.
199. Hoque KM, Pal A, Nair GB, et al. Evidence of calcium influx across the plasma membrane depends upon the initial rise of cytosolic calcium with activation of IP(3) in rat enterocytes by heat-stable enterotoxin of *Vibrio cholerae* non-O1. *FEMS Microbiol Lett* 2001;196:45–50.
200. Hardy SP, Lund T, Granum PE. CytK toxin of *Bacillus cereus* forms pores in planar lipid bilayer and is cytotoxic to intestinal epithelial cells. *FEMS Microbiol Lett* 2001;197:47–51.
201. Sanfilippo L, Li CK, Seth R, et al. *Bacteroides fragilis* enterotoxin induces the expression of IL-8 and transforming factor-beta by human colonic epithelial cells. *Clin Exp Immunol* 2000; 119:456–463.
202. Kim JM, Oh JK, Kim YJ, et al. Polarized secretion of CXC chemokines by human intestinal epithelial cells in response to *Bacteroides fragilis* enterotoxin: NF-κβ plays a major role in the regulation of IL-8 expression. *Clin Exp Immunol* 2001;123: 421–427.
203. Lee CA, Silva M, Siber AM, et al. A secreted *Salmonella* protein induces a proinflammatory response in epithelial cells, which promotes neutrophil migration. *Proc Natl Acad Sci U S A* 2000;97:12283–12288.
204. Hickey TE, McVeigh AL, Scott DA, et al. *Campylobacter jejuni* cytolethal distending toxin mediates release of interleukin-8 from intestinal epithelial cells. *Infect Immun* 2000;68: 6535–6541.
205. Whitehouse CA, Balbo PB, Pesci EC, et al. *Campylobacter jejuni* cytolethal distending toxin causes G2-phase cell cycle block. *Infect Immun* 1998;66:1934–1940.
206. Elwell MR, Liu CT, Spertzel RO, et al. Mechanisms of oral staphylococcal enterotoxin B-induced emesis in the monkey. *Proc Soc Exp Biol Med* 1975;148:424–427.

8

INTRACELLULAR MEDIATORS AND MECHANISMS OF PATHOGEN-INDUCED ALTERATIONS IN INTESTINAL ELECTROLYTE AND FLUID TRANSPORT

BARBARA A. HENDRICKSON
EUGENE B. CHANG

Gastrointestinal pathogens cause diarrhea by a variety of mechanisms, with the common end result being an imbalance in the absorption or secretion of water and electrolytes and net accumulation of luminal fluid. Many pathogens cause direct or toxin-induced mucosal injury that globally reduces absorptive, barrier, and digestive functions. Others primarily perturb specific cellular signaling processes or functions, thereby profoundly affecting normal water and electrolyte transport and barrier functions. This chapter reviews several pathogenic pathways that contribute to the development of infectious diarrheal illnesses.

FLUID AND ELECTROLYTE TRANSPORT IN THE NORMAL INTESTINE

Most infectious agents that cause diarrhea target normal processes involved in intestinal water and electrolyte transport. Consequently, an understanding of the physiology of intestinal fluid and ion transport during in health is essential.

The average daily fluid load to the gastrointestinal tract is 9 L, which is derived from approximately 2 L of ingested fluids and 7 L of endogenous secretions originating from salivary, intestinal, pancreatic, and biliary sources. The intestine and colon normally absorb most of the fluid load such that less than 200 mL or 200 g of stool per day are generated on a typical Western culture diet. The net balance between daily input and output of fluid and electrolytes is tightly regulated by the gut, and, if perturbed, diarrhea results, with stool output exceeding 200 g or 200 mL per day.

B. A. Hendrickson: Sections of Infectious Diseases, Department of Pediatrics, Department of Medicine, University of Chicago, Chicago, Illinois

E. B. Chang: Pritzker School of Medicine; Department of Medicine, Section of Gastroenterology, University of Chicago, Chicago, Illinois

The movement of water and solutes across the intestinal epithelium involves both transcellular transport across the apical and basolateral membranes as well as paracellular transport between cells. Transcellular transport, like that of sodium and glucose, is an active process with a high degree of molecular specificity (1). In contrast, the passage of water between cells is a passive process following the osmotic gradient generated by the transport of nutrients and electrolytes. The paracellular pathway appears to be dynamic and physiologically regulated in concert with alterations in mucosal transport (2).

In regard to electrolyte transport, the small intestine typically absorbs large amounts of sodium, chloride, and bicarbonate, and it secretes hydrogen ions. To a lesser degree, bicarbonate and chloride also are secreted (Fig. 8.1). Secretion appears to occur predominantly in the subsurface

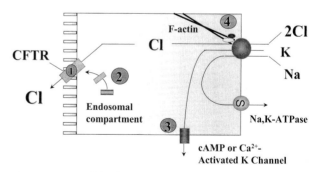

FIGURE 8.1. Model of intestinal chloride (Cl) secretion. Active secretion of Cl ion by intestinal epithelial cells requires (a) an apical membrane Cl-selective conductance, which probably involves cystic fibrosis transmembrane regulatory protein (CFTR) and other Cl channels that are regulated allosterically and by membrane trafficking; (b) Na/K/2Cl co-transporter in the basolateral membrane that allows Cl entry into the cell; (c) basolateral K channels that recycle K and maintain membrane potential favorable for Cl secretion; and (d) Na,K-ATPase, or Na pump, that creates favorable electrochemical gradients required for active Cl secretion.

crypts, whereas absorption takes place in the mature epithelial cells lining the mid and upper part of the villi (3). Under normal conditions, the absorptive capacity of the mature villous epithelial cells surpasses the secretory activity in the crypts such that the net result is absorption of water and electrolytes (3).

Sodium (NaCl) is the most important ion driving net nutrient and water absorption in the intestine (3,4). Sodium absorption, as shown in Figure 8.2, may be (a) coupled to glucose or amino acids, (b) through an ion (Na)-selective channel, or (c) by a process involving the coupled transport of sodium via an Na^+/H^+ cation exchanger and Cl^-/HCO_3^- anion exchanger. All of these pathways involve Na^+, K^+-ATPase pumps on the basolateral membrane of the epithelial cell, which create the necessary electrochemical gradients for vectorial transport of electrolytes (4). In addition to sodium absorption, anion secretion, particularly that of chloride, plays a critical role in fluid and electrolyte transport in the gut.

The absorptive and secretory functions of the intestine must be adaptable so that rapid compensations can be made in the face of large fluctuations in fluid and dietary intakes. Indeed, absorptive and secretory activities in the gut are tightly regulated by complex mechanisms including neural, paracrine, and humoral elements.

Agents that stimulate net secretion (secretagogues) inhibit active absorption of sodium or provoke active secretion of anions such as chloride (3). These include regulatory hormones such as vasoactive intestinal polypeptide, histamine, guanylin, and neurotransmitters such as acetylcholine and substance P. In contrast, proabsorptive agents stimulate active absorption of sodium or inhibit anion secretion. These include substances like norepinephrine, somatostatin, and neuropeptide Y, which have direct effects on intestinal epithelial cells or activate cellular or neural networks that promote net absorption.

GENERAL MECHANISMS OF PATHOGEN-INDUCED DIARRHEA

Diarrhea results from a disruption in the normal net absorptive state in the intestine. Many pathogens are cytotoxic and cause extensive mucosal destruction and inflammation. The loss of absorptive surface area and compromises in digestive and barrier functions of the mucosa contribute to the malabsorption of nutrients and fluid and significant protein-losing enteropathy. Nutrient maldigestion and malabsorption can add further to the diarrhea by creating luminal osmols that retain water and electrolytes. For example, patients often experience lactose malabsorption and osmotic diarrhea in conjunction with an episode of gastroenteritis due to depletion of the brush border hydrolase lactase. Because this enzyme is relatively inefficient and is not expressed in abundance, restitution of normal lactase activity takes time.

Additionally, pathogens can have selective effects on specific mucosal functions and processes. For example, pathogen-induced diarrhea is frequently a result of increases in intestinal secretion of ions such as chloride. Increased intestinal secretion can be the consequence of mucosal adherence and invasion of the organism or, alternatively, of toxins elaborated by the pathogen.

Secretory diarrhea is known to be associated with increased concentrations of the intracellular mediators

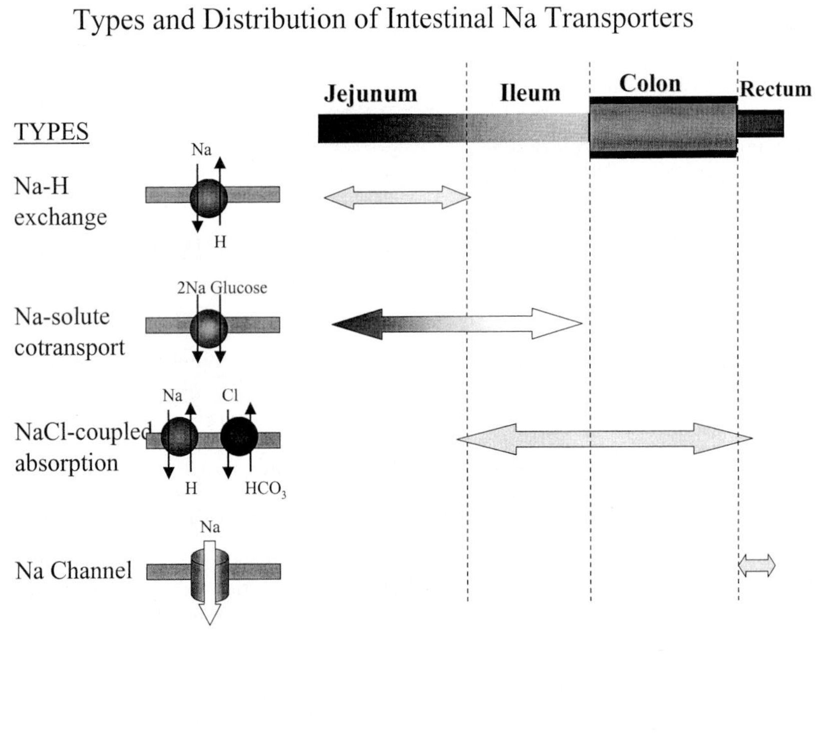

FIGURE 8.2. Many types of apical membrane transporters contribute to overall intestinal Na absorption. Their expression throughout the gut differs substantially.

cyclic adenosine monophosphate (cAMP), cyclic guanosine monophosphate (cGMP), nitric oxide, and calcium (3,4). Increases in these intracellular second messengers activate signaling pathways that lead to the inhibition of NaCl coupled transport and enhanced chloride secretion. Various secretagogues affect the concentrations of these intracellular mediators. In particular, a number of bacterial toxins, increase the intracellular concentrations of either cAMP (e.g., cholera toxin) or cGMP (e.g., *Escherichia coli* heat-stable enterotoxin). Both cAMP and cGMP are strong inhibitors of NaCl entry in the intestinal villi, whereas cAMP is a more potent stimulator of anion secretion from crypt cells than cGMP. The cystic fibrosis transmembrane regulatory protein (CFTR) appears to be the major anion channel targeted by these intracellular molecules, but other anion channels are likely involved as well (5–7). Finally, cytosolic calcium appears to be another intracellular mediator of intestinal ion transport, although the mechanisms involved are not well delineated. Increases in intracellular calcium levels in intestinal epithelial cells following infection have been described and may be a factor in the intestinal secretion stimulated by some pathogens, such as rotavirus.

Another important factor in diarrheal disease caused by several gastrointestinal pathogens appears to be changes in the actin cytoskeleton that occur during infection. The apical junctional complex of intestinal epithelial cells is composed of the tight junction, the adherens junction, and the desmosome (8). Both the adherens junction and the tight junction associate with the perijunctional actin ring. Tight junctions are the major barrier to the diffusion of solutes through the paracellular pathway, and they also function as a boundary between apical and basolateral membrane domains, which is important in the maintenance of epithelial cell polarity (1). Disruption of the tight junctions between cells by microbes or, alternatively, the host inflammatory response may lead to increased fluid secretion (see later discussion). Further remodeling of the cytoskeletal architecture leads to effacement of microvilli and loss of absorptive surface area. These changes may be associated with decreased brush border enzyme activity and the malabsorption of nutrients.

Secretagogues produced during the inflammatory response to the infection also may play a critical role in the diarrheal illness induced by some pathogens. For example, a number of studies have emphasized the significance of neurohumoral factors such as 5-hydroxytryptamine, vasoactive intestinal peptide, and substance P, which may act as intestinal secretagogues (4). Increased local prostaglandin production following gastrointestinal infection also may enhance the secretory activity of the intestine. Moreover, cytokines produced by responding immune cells such as interleukin-1 (IL-1) have been shown to have acute effects on intestinal barrier and transport function (9,10). Additionally, during gastrointestinal infection, reactive oxygen metabolites (ROM) including molecules such as superoxide (O^-), hydrogen peroxide (H_2O_2), monochloramines (NH_2Cl), and hydroxyl radical (OH−) are released by inflammatory cells and can cause significant tissue injury (11,12). The inflammatory cells also elaborate nitric oxide, which reacts with superoxide radical anion (O_2^-), resulting in the formation of peroxynitrite, a particularly toxic reactive anion that may be a major mediator of mucosal injury. Under acute or controlled situations, ROMs are rapidly metabolized by antioxidant mechanisms, preventing tissue injury (12). However, when these systems are overwhelmed, such as by excessive ROM production by inflammatory cells or tissue depletion of antioxidant mechanisms, substantial cellular injury may occur. ROMs injure tissue by causing oxidation of proteins, lipids, and nucleic acids, leading to denaturation, aggregation, and loss or altered function of these molecules. In addition, increased tyrosine phosphorylation of cellular proteins in several types of tissues has been observed, an effect possibly due to the inhibition of protein tyrosine phosphatases. This may be the mechanism by which oxidants decrease barrier function of intestinal epithelial cells. For instance, Rao and colleagues (12) observed that hydrogen peroxide rapidly reduces transepithelial electrical resistance (TER), a measure of barrier function, in Caco2 and T84 colonic cell monolayers. There was a concomitant increase in tyrosine phosphorylation of several proteins, and the effects of oxidants on TER and tyrosine protein phosphorylation were significantly blunted by inhibitors of tyrosine phosphorylation. Further evidence of the injurious role of ROMs in inflamed intestinal tissues is that iNOS, the inducible form of nitric oxide synthase which increases nitric oxide production, is abundantly expressed in inflamed colonic epithelium associated with ulcerative colitis, Crohn's disease, and diverticulitis, but is not detectable in normal tissues (13). Nitrotyrosine labeling, an indication of the formation and reaction with peroxynitrate, is also found near areas of iNOS staining, largely localized to lamina propria mononuclear cells and polymorphonuclear leukocytes (13).

In addition to their cytotoxic effects, ROMs have been shown to stimulate net intestinal secretion, at least in the acute setting, both *in vitro* and *in vivo* (14,15). However, the effects of sublethal oxidant concentrations on intestinal epithelial function may be dose- and time-dependent (15,16). Immediate pretreatment of T84 colon cell monolayers with monochloramine potentiates the secretory response to Ca-mediated agonists such as carbachol, but has no effect on cAMP-mediated secretion. In contrast, monochloramine treatment of T84 cells for greater than 24 hours selectively inhibits Ca-mediated secretion, but has no effect on baseline barrier function. The latter finding may be, in part, a basis for the enterocyte dysfunction observed in chronically inflamed intestinal mucosa.

There is little debate that loss of absorptive surface area due to mucosal injury or destruction is a major factor in the diarrhea accompanying gastrointestinal infections. However, diarrhea also is common in instances in which the mucosa appears endoscopically and histologically intact, albeit where the lamina propria may be expanded by infiltration of immune and inflammatory cells. As mentioned earlier, immune and inflammatory mediators such as prostaglandins, cytokines, chemotactic factors, and reactive oxygen metabolites have been implicated in causing net intestinal secretion, because many of these agents are potent stimuli of intestinal secretion *in vitro*. Because these agents also stimulate secretomotor enteric neurons, the secretory response can, in theory, be further amplified. However, increased anion secretion in inflamed bowel has not been observed in chronically inflamed mucosa (e.g., >24 hours), but rather there appears to be selective decreases in mucosal secretory, absorptive, and barrier functions and increases in antigen-presenting surface molecules. This is, in part, mediated by inflammatory mediators such as interferon-γ or tumor necrosis factor-α, the former causing decreased expression of key transport- and barrier-function related proteins (Fig. 8.3). These responses may represent a physiological adaptation of the mucosa to down-regulate metabolic processes not essential for cell survival. Alternatively, the mucosal cells may be undergoing a phenotypic shift aimed at augmenting their role in mucosal defense functions such as antigen presentation.

Another mechanism for enhancing intestinal secretion is mediated by the secretion of cryptdins from Paneth cells located at the crypt base. Cryptdins are cationic protein molecules that are antimicrobial. The antimicrobial activity of cryptdins results from their ability to form anion conductive pores in pathogen membranes, rendering the organisms permeable and susceptible to osmolar stress. However, cryptdins also may insert into the luminal membrane of intestinal epithelial cells and act as anion-selective channels, enhancing enterocyte secretory capacity, as illustrated in Figure 8.4 (17).

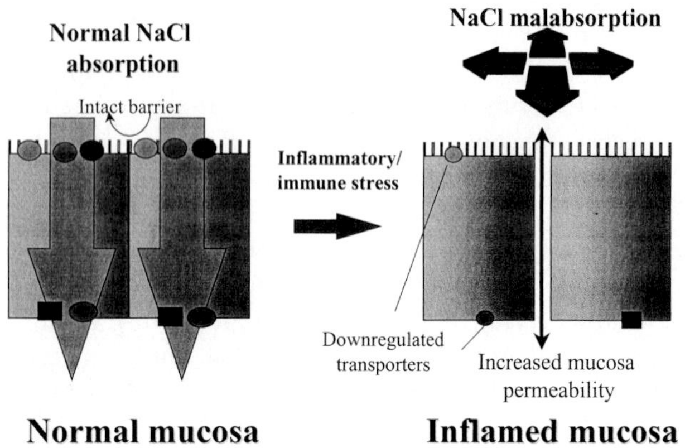

FIGURE 8.3. Chronic inflammation (>24 hours) caused by infectious pathogens can impair net NaCl and nutrient absorption and barrier function, contributing to the development of diarrhea.

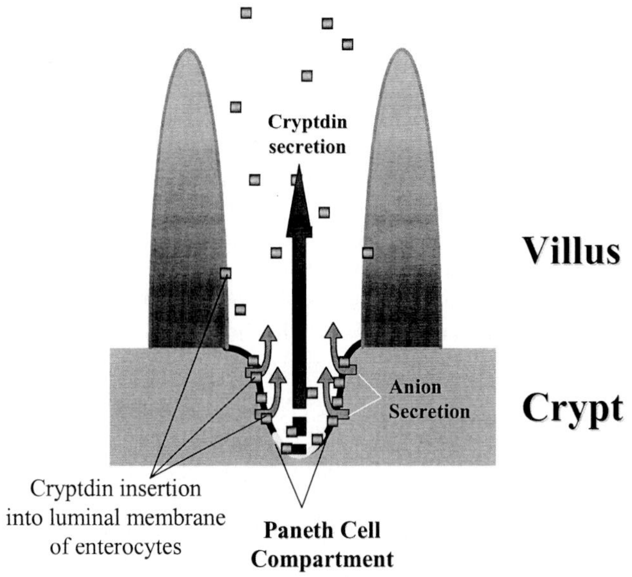

FIGURE 8.4. Cryptdins secreted by Paneth cells at the base of intestinal crypts have antimicrobial activity, but they may also contribute to the development of infectious diarrheas. They form anion-conductive pores in the luminal membrane of intestinal epithelial cells and act as anion-selective channels, enhancing enterocyte secretory capacity.

In addition to these mechanisms, net secretion of water and electrolytes can be facilitated by physiologically induced increases in mucosal permeability. For instance, in the inflamed mucosa, cytokines such as interferon-γ and growth factors including insulin-like growth factor 1 increase mucosal permeability, in part, by effects on perijunctional epithelial cytoskeletal proteins involved in the maintenance of intercellular tight junctions (18). Increases in mucosal permeability not only facilitate passive movement of counter ions and water during active anion secretion, but also make absorptive processes more inefficient by reducing the mucosal potential difference required for passive movement of many nutrients and electrolytes. The observation that other agents such as IL-10 stabilize cytokine-induced changes in mucosal permeability illustrates the interplay of immune and inflammatory mediators that affect tight junction permeability (19).

In summary, the ability of the infected host to correct perturbations in intestinal secretion and prevent life-threatening volume and metabolic disturbances is critical. Nonetheless, as described earlier, the host response clearly plays a role in the diarrhea that occurs during gastrointestinal infection. In fact, the diarrheal state may serve as an important host defense that purges the gut of harmful pathogens and enhances the luminal delivery of secretory immunoglobulin A or cryptdins. In addition to the host inflammatory response, the pathogens themselves may directly affect intestinal secretion.

SPECIFIC EXAMPLES OF PATHOGEN-INDUCED NET INTESTINAL SECRETION

Gastrointestinal pathogens that cause diarrhea appear to affect the regulation of both transcellular transport and paracellular transport pathways. Particular examples of the various mechanisms that have been described in this section are highlighted here.

Enterotoxin-Mediated Increases in Intracellular cAMP

Vibrio cholerae is the classic example of a noninvasive pathogen that produces a toxin that augments secretion by increasing intracellular cAMP concentrations in intestinal epithelial cells. Cholera toxin (CT) consists of five identical β subunits and a single α subunit composed of two functional domains known as α1 and α2. As shown in Figure 8.5, the β subunits bind to GM_1 ganglioside, which is expressed on the apical surface of the enterocyte. Subsequently, the α subunit translocates across the cell membrane into the host cell where it stimulates adenosine diphosphate ribosylation of an arginine residue on Gs, the stimulatory subunit of a heterotrimeric G protein located in the basolateral membrane of enterocytes. Binding of CT to Gs causes irreversible activation of Gs, resulting in significant increases in cytosolic cAMP (20–23). As noted earlier, increases in cAMP, possibly via activation of cAMP-dependent protein kinases, are associated with the inhibition of NaCl-coupled transport and enhanced chloride secretion.

Enterotoxin-Mediated Increases in Intracellular cGMP

E. coli heat-stable enterotoxin (Sta) induces watery diarrhea and increases intracellular cGMP but not cAMP or calcium. Sta binds to colonic guanylyl cyclase C, a transmembrane receptor on intestinal epithelial cells (24). The related epithelial receptors guanylyl cyclase A and B bind to atrial natriuretic peptides; however, the endogenous ligand for guanylyl cyclase C was unknown until 1992. At that time, Currie and colleagues (25) identified a peptide hormone homologous to Sta, which was named guanylin. Subsequently, guanylyl cyclase C also was reported to be the receptor for the peptide uroguanylin (26). However, Sta appears to bind to guanylyl cyclase C with greater affinity than guanylin or uroguanylin (25,26). Activation of guanylyl cyclase C by Sta, or its natural ligands guanylin or uroguanylin, results in the hydrolysis of guanosine triphosphate (GTP) and the generation of cGMP (Fig. 8.6). The second messenger cGMP exerts its physiological effects by interacting with various downstream targets including cGMP-sensitive anion channels, cGMP-dependent phosphodiesterases, or cGMP-regulated protein kinases. Intestinal epithelial cells express a specific isoform of cGMP-dependent kinase designated G kinase II (27). G kinase II appears to be involved in the regulation of fluid homeostasis in the intestine under basal conditions and has been implicated as one of the mediators of the effects of STa (28).

Pathogen-Induced Increases in Cytosolic Calcium

Rotavirus is an important cause of viral gastroenteritis in young children. Recently, the rotavirus nonstructural glycoprotein NSP4 has been shown to function as an enterotoxin (29). NSP4 appears to play an important role in the pathogenesis of rotaviral infections, and NSP4 mutations have been associated with an inability of the virus to induce diarrhea in mice (30). NSP4 is a transmembrane endoplasmic reticulum glycoprotein; however, a biologically active cleavage product of NSP4, which retains enterotoxin activity, also is secreted from rotavirus-infected cells (31). Current evidence suggests that NSP4 activates a signaling pathway

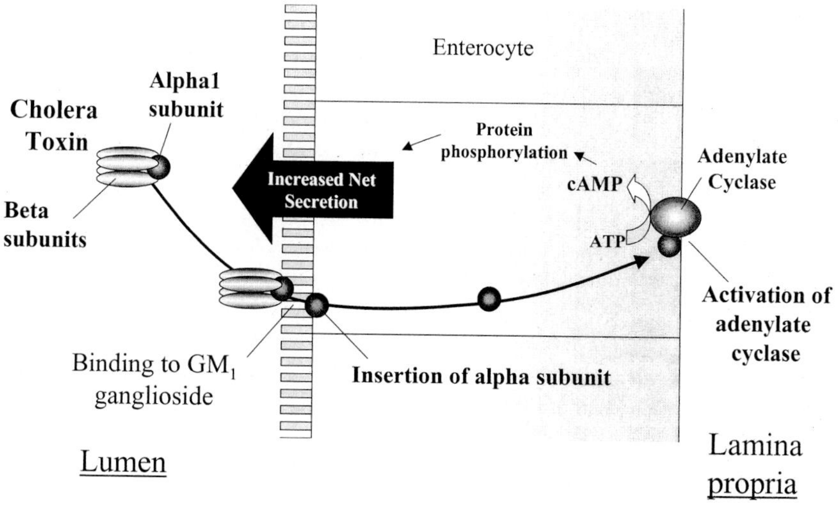

FIGURE 8.5. Cholera toxin (CT) consists of five identical β subunits and a single α subunit. The β subunits bind to GM_1 ganglioside expressed on the luminal surface of the enterocyte. Subsequently, the α subunit translocates across the cell membrane into the host cell where it stimulates ADP ribosylation of the GTP-binding protein, Gs. This action irreversibly activates basolateral membrane adenylate cyclase, resulting in significant increases in cytosolic cAMP and enhanced net secretion.

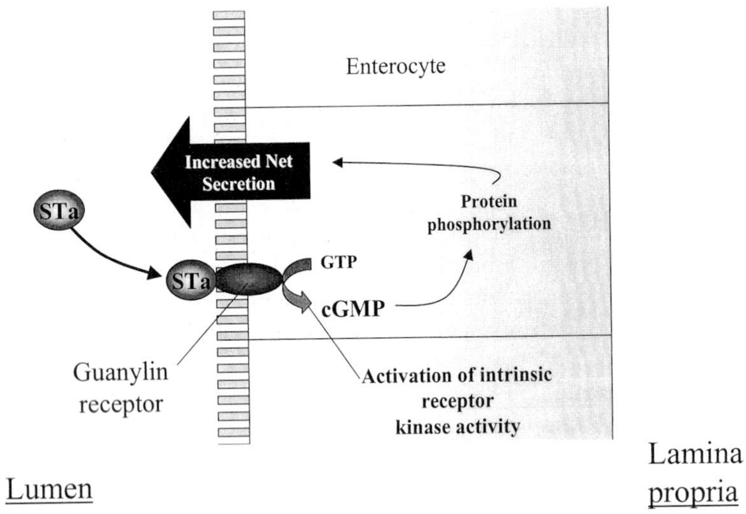

FIGURE 8.6. Mechanism of *Escherichia coli* heat-stable enterotoxin-induced net intestinal secretion. The *E. coli* heat stable enterotoxin, STa, appears to bind to guanylyl cyclase C receptor located on the luminal membrane of intestinal epithelial cells with greater affinity than the natural ligands, guanylin or uroguanylin. Activation of guanylyl cyclase C by STa (or by guanylin or uroguanylin) results in the hydrolysis of GTP and the generation of cGMP. This causes inhibition of neutral NaCl absorption and activation of active anion secretion, resulting in net intestinal secretion

that increases intracellular calcium levels by mobilizing calcium from the endoplasmic reticulum, thereby affecting an age-dependent, calcium-sensitive anion channel (29–32).

In addition to the effects of enterotoxins, infection-induced production of neurohumoral agents, such as serotonin, substance P, and acetylcholine, appears to be associated with increased epithelial cytosolic calcium levels. Stimulation of cholinergic, muscarinic, and serotonin receptors results in the activation of phospholipase C, which hydrolyzes the membrane phospholipid phosphatidylinositol 4,5-biphosphate to yield diacylglycerol, and inositol 1,4,5-triphosphate (IP_3) (33). IP_3 increases cytosolic calcium by binding to specific receptors located primarily on organelles such as the endoplasmic reticulum (34). This binding results in a conformational change in the tetrameric intracellular calcium channel, thereby releasing calcium into the cytosol. IP_3 also may regulate calcium influx across the plasma membrane of cells.

Furthermore, organisms such as *Salmonella typhimurium* appear to stimulate increases in cytosolic calcium that coincide with the organism's invasion of cultured intestinal epithelial cells (35,36). The entry of the *S. typhimurium* into cultured epithelial cells is coincident with tyrosine phosphorylation of the receptor for epidermal growth factor (35). Activation of the epidermal growth factor receptor results in downstream signaling events that lead to formation of leukotriene metabolites (37). Leukotriene metabolites, such as LTD4, may cause increased membrane permeability to calcium influx directly, or indirectly, through the activation of other intermediary processes (35).

Pathogen-Induced Effects on Cytoskeletal Elements

The perijunctional actomyosin ring is a beltlike cytoskeletal structure that is adjacent to the adherens junction and tight junction (8). Disruption of perijunctional actin leads to increases in tight junction permeability (8,38–40). Phosphorylation of myosin II regulatory light chain is associated with actomyosin contraction and is involved in the regulation of tight junction integrity (8,40). Perijunctional actomyosin ring contraction mediated by myosin light chain phosphorylation has been implicated in the alteration in intestinal epithelial cell barrier function that occurs after infection with enteropathogenic *E. coli* (41).

Several bacterial toxins have been shown to interfere with the activity of cellular Rho family GTPases, which are involved in cytoskeletal architecture and cell movement (42). For example, pathogenic strains of *Clostridium difficile* produce two exotoxins, toxin A and toxin B, that inactivate Rho family proteins. Both toxins bind to specific receptors on the luminal aspect of the colonic epithelium and then are transported into the cytoplasm (42). The NH2-terminal portion of the toxins carries an enzymatic domain that hydrolyzes uridine diphosphate (UDP)-glucose and transfers the glucose moiety to a conserved threonine residue of the Rho proteins (43). Monoglucosylation of the Rho proteins leads to disorganization of actin filaments and disruption of cellular tight junction integrity (42,44).

E. coli cytotoxic necrotizing factor 1 (CNF1) is another bacterial toxin that has been shown to modify the Rho family of GTPases is (38). CNF1 targets the low-molecular mass GTPase RhoA as well as Rho family members, Cdc42 and Rac. Unlike the *C. difficile* toxins, CNF1 activates RhoA by deamidation of Gln63, which inhibits both constitutive and GTPase-activating protein-induced GTP hydrolysis. CNF1 decreases the TER across human intestinal cell monolayers *in vitro* (45), likely altering barrier function. The mechanism of the TER changes is unclear. Conceivably, overactivation of RhoA results in a rigidity of the perijunctional actin ring and prevents tight junction sealing (38).

In addition to disorganization of apical and basal filamentous actin, pathogen-mediated increases in paracellular permeability have been linked to dissociation of the tight junction–associated proteins, occludin, ZO-1, ZO-2, from the lateral cellular membrane. For example, *C. difficile* toxin B–induced redistribution of occludin and ZO-1 from detergent-insoluble fractions constituting cholesterol-enriched "raftlike" membrane microdomains has been observed (44). Dephosphorylation of occludin occurs in association with its redistribution (44,46,47).

Some strains of *Bacteroides fragilis* produce a zinc-metalloproteinase toxin that has been implicated in diarrheal disease in animals and humans. In contrast to *C. difficile* toxin, *B. fragilis* toxin appears to affect paracellular permeability by cleaving the adherens junction protein E-cadherin (39).

Recent studies suggest that other mechanisms also may be involved in the ability of bacterial toxins to affect intestinal barrier function. For example, He and colleagues (48) have reported that *C. difficile* toxin A is associated with mitochondrial damage and a marked decrease in ATP levels in Chinese hamster ovary cells. In renal epithelial cells, ATP depletion resulted in reduced phosphorylation of ZO-1 and occludin and in alterations in tight junction integrity (49,50). Consequently, mitochondrial damage and the subsequent release of ROMs may play a role too in *C. difficile* toxin–mediated cell damage and cytoskeletal rearrangements of intestinal epithelial cells.

Moreover, host cell stress kinase pathways are activated by a wide variety of agents, including pathogenic bacteria (51). Three well-characterized stress kinase pathways have been identified: p44/p42 (ERK1/2), p38 MAP kinase, and stress-activated protein kinase/c-Jun terminal kinase (SAPK/JNK) (51). These pathways may play a role in epithelial barrier function. For instance, *C. difficile* toxin–mediated activation of p38 MAP kinase is associated with IL-8 production by monocytes (52). IL-8 is important for the recruitment of neutrophils to areas of inflammation. In animal models, blocking neutrophil extravasation prevented *C. difficile* toxin A–mediated enteritis and mucosal damage (52,53).

In summary, gastrointestinal pathogens affect a variety of different cellular processes involved in the transport of water and electrolytes. As evidenced by the example of *C. difficile* toxin, the pathogenesis of diarrhea caused by a particular pathogen is undoubtedly multifactorial, although one mechanism may predominate. Understanding the cellular and biochemical mechanisms of pathogen-induced fluid and electrolyte shifts in the gastrointestinal mucosa is the basis for effective therapeutic diarrheal strategies.

REFERENCES

1. Fanning AS, Mitic LL, Anderson JM. Transmembrane proteins in the tight junction barrier. *J Am Soc Nephrol* 1999;10:1337–1345.
2. Anderson JM, Van Itallie CM. Tight junctions and the molecular basis for regulation of paracellular permeability. *Am J Physiol* 1995;269(4 Pt 1):G467–G475.
3. Guandalini S. Acute diarrhea. In: Walker A, Durie P, Hamilton R, et al., eds. *Textbook of pediatric gastrointestinal diseases.* Chicago: Mosby, 2000:3.1–3.3.
4. Chang EB, Bookstein C. Mechanisms of intestinal absorption and secretion: an abbreviated review and update. In: Domschke W, Stoll R, eds. *Intestinal mucosa and its diseases—pathophysiology and clinics (Falk Symposium 110).* The Netherlands: Kluwer Academic Publishers, 1999.
5. Anderson MP, Sheppard DN, Berger HA, et al. Chloride channels in the apical membrane of normal and cystic fibrosis airway and intestinal epithelia. *Am J Physiol* 1992;263:L1–L14.
6. Anderson MP, Gregory RJ, Thompson S, et al. Demonstration that CFTR is a chloride channel by alteration of its anion selectivity. *Science* 1991;253:202–207.
7. Berger HA, Anderson MP, Gregory RJ, et al. Identification and regulation of the cystic fibrosis transmembrane conductance regulator-generated chloride channel. *J Clin Invest* 1991;88:1422–1431.
8. Turner JR. "Putting the squeeze" on the tight junction: understanding cytoskeletal regulation. *Semin Cell Dev Biol* 2000;11(4):301–308.
9. Field MJ, Rao MC, Chang EB. Intestinal electrolyte transport and diarrheal disease. *N Engl J Med* (2 part article) 1989;321:800–806, 879–883.
10. Chang EB, Musch MW, Mayer L. Interleukin 1 and 3 stimulate anion secretion in chicken intestine. *Gastroenterology* 1990;98:1518–1524.
11. Granger DN, Hollwarth ME, Parks DA. Ischemia-reperfusion injury: role of oxygen-derived free radicals. *Acta Physiol Scand* 1986;548:47–63.
12. Rao RK, Baker RD, Baker SS, et al. Oxidant-induced disruption of intestinal epithelial barrier function: role of protein tyrosine phosphorylation. *Am J Physiol* 1997;273:G812–G823.
13. Singer II, Kawka DW, Scott S, et al. Expression of inducible nitric oxide synthase and nitrotyrosine in colonic epithelium in inflammatory bowel disease. *Gastroenterology* 1996;111(4):871–885.
14. Tamai H, Gaginella TS, Kachur JF, et al. Ca-mediated stimulation of Cl secretion by reactive oxygen metabolites in human colonic T84 cells. *J Clin Invest* 1992;89:301–307.
15. Tamai H, Kachur JF, Baron DA, et al. Monochloramine, a neutrophil-derived oxidant stimulate rat colonic secretion. *J Pharmacol Exp Ther* 1990;257:884–894.
16. Sugi K, Musch MW, Chang EB. Acute and chronic effects of oxidant exposure on intestinal epithelial cell transport and barrier function. *Gastroenterology* 2001 *(in press).*
17. Lencer WI, Cheung G, Strohmeier GR, et al. Induction of epithelial chloride secretion by channel-forming cryptdins 2 and 3. *Proc Natl Acad Sci U S A* 1997;94:8585–8589.
18. McRoberts JA, Riley NE. Regulation of T84 cell monolayer permeability by insulin-like growth factors. *Am J Physiol* 1992;262(1 Pt 1):C207–C213.
19. Madsen KL, Lewis SA, Tavernini MM, et al. Interleukin 10 prevents cytokine-induced disruption of T84 monolayer barrier integrity and limits chloride secretion. *Gastroenterology* 1997;113:151–159.
20. Dominguez P, Barros F, Lazo PS. The activation of adenylate cyclase from small intestinal epithelium by cholera toxin. *Eur J Biochem* 1985;146:533–538.
21. Dominguez P, Velasco G, Barros F, et al. Intestinal brush border membranes contain regulatory subunits of adenylyl cyclase. *Proc Natl Acad Sci U S A* 1987;84:6965–6969.
22. Lynch CJ, Morbach L, Blackmore PF, et al. Alpha-subunits of N_s

are released from the plasma membrane following cholera toxin activation. *FEBS Lett* 1986;200:333–336.
23. Field M, Semrad CE. Toxigenic diarrheas, congenital diarrheas, and cystic fibrosis, disorders of intestinal ion transport. *Annu Rev Physiol* 1993;55:631–655.
24. Schulz S, Green CK, Yuen PST, et al. Guanylyl cyclase is a heat-stable enterotoxin receptor. *Cell* 1990;63:941–948.
25. Currie MG, Fok KF, Kato J, et al. Guanylin: an endogenous activator of intestinal guanylate cyclase. *Proc Natl Acad Sci U S A* 1992;89:947–951.
26. Hamra FK, Forte LR, Eber SL, et al. Uroguanylin: structure and activity of a second endogenous peptide that stimulates intestinal guanylate cyclase. *Proc Natl Acad Sci U S A* 1993;90: 10464–10468.
27. Edelman AM, Blumenthal DK, Krebs EG. Protein serine/threonine kinases. *Annu Rev Biochem* 1987;56:567–613.
28. Vaandrager AA, Bot AGM, Ruth P, et al. Differential role of cyclic GMP-dependent protein kinase II in ion transport in murine small intestine and colon. *Gastroenterology* 2000;118: 108–114.
29. Ball JM, Tian P, Zeng CQ, et al. Age-dependent diarrhea induced by a rotaviral nonstructural glycoprotein. *Science* 1996; 272:101–104.
30. Zhang M, Zeng CQ-Y, Dong Y, et al. Mutations in rotavirus nonstructural glycoprotein NSP4 are associated with altered virus virulence. *J Virol* 1998;72:3666–3672.
31. Zhang M, Zeng CQ-Y, Morris AP, et al. A functional NSP4 enterotoxin peptide secreted from rotavirus-infected cells. *J Virol* 2000;74:11663–11670.
32. Tian P, Hu Y, Schilling WP, et al. The nonstructural glycoprotein of rotavirus affects intracellular calcium levels. *J Virol* 1994;68: 251–257.
33. Matozaki T, Sakamoto C, Nagao M, et al. G protein in stimulation of PI hydrolysis by CCK in isolated rat pancreatic acinar cells. *Am J Physiol* 1988;255:E652–E659.
34. Meldolesi J, Villa A, Volpe P, et al. Cellular sites of IP_3 action. In: Putney JW Jr, ed. *Advances in second messenger and phosphoprotein research: inositol phosphates and calcium signaling,* vol 16. New York: Raven Press; 1993:187–208.
35. Pace J, Hayman MJ, Galan JE. Signal transduction and invasion of epithelial cells by *S. typhimurium*. *Cell* 1993;72:505–514.
36. Bliska JB, Galan JE, Falkow S. Signal transduction in the mammalian cell during bacterial attachment and entry. *Cell* 1993;73:903–920.
37. Hackel PO, Zwick E, Prenzel N, et al. Epidermal growth factor receptors: critical mediators of multiple receptor pathways. *Curr Opin Cell Biol* 1999;11:184–189.
38. Hopkins AM, Li D, Mrsny RJ, et al. Modulation of tight junction function by G protein-coupled events. *Adv Drug Deliv Rev* 2000;41:329–340.
39. Sears CL. Molecular physiology and pathophysiology of tight junctions V. Assault of the tight junction by enteric pathogens. *Am J Physiol Gastrointest Liver Physiol* 2000;279:G1129–G1134.
40. Nusrat A, Turner JR, Madara JL. Molecular physiology and pathophysiology of tight junctions. IV. Regulation of tight junctions by extracellular stimuli: nutrients, cytokines, and immune cells. *Am J Physiol Gastrointest Liver Physiol* 2000;279:G851–G857.
41. Yuhan R, Koutsouris A, Savkovic SD, et al. Enteropathogenic *Escherichia coli*-induced myosin light chain phosphorylation alters intestinal epithelial permeability. *Gastroenterology* 1997; 113:1873–1882.
42. Kelly CP, LaMont JT. *Clostridium difficile* infection. *Annu Rev Med* 1998;49:375–390.
43. Ciesla WP, Bobak DA. *Clostridium difficile* toxins A and B are cation-dependent UDP-glucose hydrolases with differing catalytic activities. *J Biol Chem* 1998;273 :16021–16026.
44. Nusrat A, von Eichel-Streiber C, Turner JR, et al. *Clostridium difficile* toxins disrupt epithelial barrier function by altering membrane microdomain localization of tight junction proteins. *Infect Immun* 2001;69:1329–1336.
45. Gerhard R, Schmidt G, Hofmann F, et al. Activation of Rho GTPases by *Escherichia coli* cytotoxic necrotizing factor 1 increases intestinal permeability in Caco-2 cells. *Infect Immun* 1998;66:5125–5131.
46. Simonovic I, Rosenberg J, Koutsouris A, et al. Enteropathogenic *Escherichia coli* dephosphorylates and dissociates occludin from intestinal epithelial tight junctions. *Cell Microbiol* 2000;2: 305–315.
47. McNamara BP, Koutsouris A, O'Connell CB, et al. Translocated EspF protein from enteropathogenic *Escherichia coli* disrupts host intestinal barrier function. *J Clin Invest* 2001;17:621–629.
48. He D, Hagen SJ, Pothoulakis C, et al. *Clostridium difficile* toxin A causes early damage to mitochondria in cultured cells. *Gastroenterology* 2000;119:138–150.
49. Tsukamoto T, Nigam SK. Tight junction proteins form large complexes and associate with the cytoskeleton in ATP depletion model for reversible junction assembly. *J Biol Chem* 1997;272: 16133–16139.
50. Gopalakrishnan S, Raman N, Atkinson SJ, et al. Rho GTPase signaling regulates tight junction assembly and protects tight junction during ATP depletion. *Am J Physiol* 1998;275:C798–C809.
51. Schafer C, Williams JA. Stress kinases and heat shock proteins in the pancreas: possible roles in normal function and disease. *J Gastroenterol* 2000;35:1–9.
52. Warny M, Keates AC, Keates S, et al. p38 MAP kinase activation by *Clostridium difficile* toxin A mediates monocyte necrosis, IL-8 production, and enteritis. *J Clin Invest* 2000;105:1147–1156.
53. Kelly CP, Becker S, Linevsky JK, et al. Neutrophil recruitment in *Clostridium difficile* toxin A enteritis in the rabbit. *J Clin Invest* 1994;93:1257–1265.

9

PHYSIOLOGIC DEFENSE MECHANISMS AGAINST GASTROINTESTINAL PATHOGENS

GLENN T. FURUTA
W. A. WALKER

NONIMMUNE MECHANISMS OF DEFENSE OF THE GASTROINTESTINAL TRACT

Despite daily exposure to microbes, the gastrointestinal tract maintains a healthy state of "physiologic inflammation." The oropharynx, esophagus, stomach, small intestine, and large intestine use a complex, intricate system of defenses composed of both immune and innate elements to protect the body from potentially deleterious effects of microbes. Typically, innate elements are described as lacking the specificity of the immune defense, but this is not always the case as evidenced by the antigen specificity of the enterocyte bacterial "receptors" or adherence factors. Physiologic mechanisms form the initial line of defense against microbes and function as both chemical and mechanical barriers that decrease the ability of microbes to attach to and invade the gastrointestinal mucosa (Fig. 9.1). This chapter describes the major forms of innate defenses. A description of mucus as it pertains to microbial infections is discussed in Chapter 5.

SALIVA

The parotid, submandibular, and sublingual glands contain mucus and serous cells, which secrete saliva. Saliva is a complex mixture of water, ions, enzymes, glycoproteins, amylase, immunoglobulins, lysozyme, lactoperoxidase, and lactoferrin (1,2). Saliva secretion is exclusively under neural control from the medulla and is secreted at a rate of 0.3 to .5 mL/min (3). Stimuli include dryness of the oral mucosa, chewing, and certain food textures.

G. T. Furuta and **W. A. Walker:** Department of Pediatrics, Harvard Medical School; Combined Program in Pediatric Gastroenterology and Nutrition, Children's Hospital; Mucosal Immunology Laboratory, Massachusetts General Hospital East, Boston, Massachusetts

Saliva is the initial line of innate defense of the intestinal tract. Several different components, in particular the peroxidase enzyme system, make saliva an effective chemical barrier. Peroxidase catalyzes the oxidation of thiocyanate (SCN^-) to hypothiocyanous acid (HOSCN) and hypothiocyanate ion ($OSCN^-$). These two chemicals inhibit bacterial growth and metabolism (4).

Saliva contains antigen-specific glycoproteins and immunoglobulins. Glycoproteins bind to human epithelial

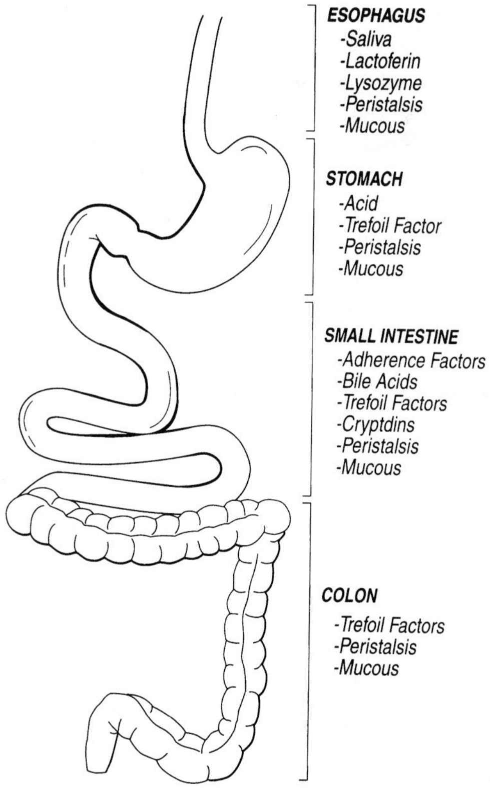

FIGURE 9.1. Innate mechanisms of gastrointestinal defense.

cell receptors for *Streptococcus sanguis* and *Streptococcus salivarius* and inhibit the attachment of these bacteria to epithelial cells and tooth enamel (5,6). This action facilitates bacterial removal and potentially desorbs preattached bacteria. Although they constitute only a minority of total body immunoglobulin (Ig) content, IgA, IgM, and IgG are secreted from the parotid gland (2).

Lactoferrin, found in saliva and in human breast milk and released by epithelial cells and neutrophils, has both bacteriostatic and bactericidal activities (7,8). By binding iron in the area of infection, lactoferrin decreases the pool of this nutrient necessary for bacterial growth. The bactericidal impact of lactoferrin rests in its abilities to form toxic hydroxyl radicals, increase bacterial membrane permeability, inhibit lipid peroxidation, and enhance the actions of lysozyme and sIgA (9–11). Lactoferrin has bactericidal effects on *Vibrio cholerae, Streptococcus mutans, Pseudomonas aeruginosa, Escherichia coli,* and *Candida albicans in vitro* (12).

Lysozyme is a ubiquitous salivary enzyme that splits muramic acid linkages in the cell wall, producing bacterial lysis and enhancing bacterial phagocytosis (13). It affects primarily gram-positive organisms but can also act synergistically with lactoferrin to kill gram-negative bacteria.

All of the effects of saliva may not be deleterious to oral bacteria. It contains binding proteins, which attach to several organisms including *C. albicans* (14,15) and some *Streptococcus* spp. (16). These proteins bind the organism to the buccal mucosa and tooth enamel, which can create a nidus for caries formation. Interestingly, *Helicobacter pylori* may acquire iron through the human lactoferrin system, thus enhancing the virulence of the bacteria (17).

Permanent damage to the salivary glands as a result of head and neck irradiation, Sjögren's syndrome, oral infections, and anticholinergic agents disturbs salivary flow, leading to xerostomia, increased dental caries, and, potentially, gastrointestinal infection. Some elderly individuals with xerostomia have an increased incidence of aspiration pneumonia when compared with those with normal salivary flow (18).

GASTRIC SECRETIONS

After passing through saliva, enteric pathogens encounter gastric juices. Gastric secretions contain pepsin, lysozyme, and mucus, but the main bactericidal component is acid. Hydrochloric acid is secreted from parietal cells following stimulation of histamine H_2, cholinergic receptors, or gastric receptors, with a basal acid output of 7.0 mmol/hr (19).

Bacteria do not survive in aspirates of gastric juice with a pH less than 4.0, and bacteria exposed to achlorhydric juices can live for hours (20). Gastric acid is bactericidal to *Salmonella* spp., *V. cholerae, Shigella* spp., *S. marcescens* and *E. coli.* Bacterial counts of *E. coli, Salmonella* spp., and *S. marcescens* are decreased by 99% after 15 minutes in gastric aspirates with a pH of 3.0. In contrast, gastric fluids from patients with achlorhydria and pernicious anemia have significantly higher bacterial counts (20). *Shigella sonnei* is killed within 10 minutes in gastric aspirates with a pH of 1.5 to 3.0 (21), but this finding is not confirmed in other *Shigella* spp. For instance, *Shigella* exposed to a media with a pH of 2.5 for 2 hours survived, but lost the ability to invade the epithelium (22).

Whether achlorhydria results from surgery or medication, it has been associated with an increased incidence of gastrointestinal infections in selected populations. After gastric resection, a higher incidence of *Salmonella* (23,24), *Giardia lamblia* (25), *V. cholerae* (26), and *Shigella* (27) infections has been observed. Critically ill patients treated with antacid or acid-suppressing medication are more susceptible to gram-negative nosocomial pneumonia and increased gastric colonization with pathogenic bacteria than patients who maintain gastric acidity (28,29). If acid production is normal, bacterial counts in the stomach are virtually nonexistent. If achlorhydria develops, gastric and small intestinal bacterial counts can increase significantly. The inoculating dose necessary to cause intestinal infection is higher in individuals with normal gastric acidity (30). After the ingestion of 10^8 *V. cholerae* organisms by normal individuals, clinical symptoms of cholera develop. After neutralization of gastric pH, only 10^4 organisms were required to create a similar clinical syndrome (31).

Although acid is effective in decreasing bacterial infections in selected patients, it is unclear whether common use of agents that inhibit acid production leads to increased infections in the normal host. The long-term use of proton pump inhibitors has not resulted in a significant increase in gastrointestinal infections (32).

ADHERENCE FACTORS

Adherence factors or receptors are expressed on the surface of epithelial cells and in the glycocalyx covering enterocytes. These molecules are composed of carbohydrates, phospholipids, or glycoproteins (33). A receptor consists of a hydrophobic end that is inserted into the epithelial lipid bilayer or glycocalyx and a hydrophilic end that is exposed to bacteria and its products. The attachment of bacteria or their products to tissue receptors is the initial event determining a the capacity of a microbe to colonize. If a host tissue does not express the receptor specific for the microbe or its products, the likelihood of infection is lessened. The presence of these receptors is genetically determined, but they are also subject to later modification or induction (34). One example of an intestinal epithelial receptor that may function in microbial attachment and epithelial activation is the toll-like receptor (TLR) (35,36). This family of proteins serves as potential binding sites on the host cell for microbes and their products. Originally, TLRs were identified in *Drosophila*; the ligation of these receptors set off a cascade of events leading to the production of antimicrobial peptides. Recent evidence suggests that TLRs show different expression in health and disease. For instance, TLR 3 is significantly down-regulated in the epithelium affected by Crohn disease but not ulcerative colitis, whereas TLR 4 is strongly up-regulated in both (37).

A variety of other domains have been identified as bacterial receptors. Fibronectin binds gram-positive bacteria, including *Staphylococcus aureus, Streptococcus pyogenes, S. mutans, S. salivarius,* and *S. mitior* but does not bind gram-negative bacteria as effectively (38). Three examples of bacteria or toxin with specific receptors are enteropathogenic *V. cholerae* toxin, *E. coli,* and *Clostridium difficile* toxin. The receptor for the cholera toxin has been studied extensively. The human receptor has a terminal sugar on the glycolipid receptor, *N*-acetylgalactosamine, along with a sialic acid residue. Three steps are involved in the series of events that produce clinical disease: (a) toxin binding, (b) signal transduction, and (c) chloride and water secretion. When toxins bind to intestinal surface receptors, they activate a cascade of transduction events resulting in ribosylation of G proteins. These proteins stimulate adenylate cyclase, producing an increase in intracellular cyclic adenosine monophosphate (cAMP) levels. Increases in cAMP stimulate fluid and electrolyte secretion into the intestinal lumen and decrease fluid and electrolyte absorption (39).

To produce intestinal disease in the pig, enteropathogenic *E. coli* requires the production of enterotoxin and K88 antigen, a fimbrial adhesin. If the glycolipid receptor for the K88 antigen is not present, clinical illness will not develop. For example, two porcine phenotypes differ in their susceptibility to enteropathogenic diarrheal syndrome. The infection-resistant phenotype is K88 antigen receptor negative and the infection-prone phenotype is receptor positive. Cross-breeding follows mendelian genetics and the receptor is coded by the autosomal dominant gene (34,40).

The glycoconjugate receptor for *C. difficile* toxin A has been identified in rat, rabbit, and human intestine (41,42). Age differences exist in the expression of these receptors. For instance, in rabbits, receptors are present in adulthood, whereas in hamsters, the receptors are present in both infancy and adulthood. The human intestine does not express the receptor during infancy, but it does appear during adulthood. This age-related difference in the human receptor may help explain the frequent detection of *C. difficile* toxin in the stools of healthy neonates.

BILE

After synthesis in the liver, the primary bile acids—cholic and chenodeoxycholic acid—are conjugated with taurine or glycine. These bile salts are released into the duodenum from the gallbladder and, after transit in the small intestine, are deconjugated by bacteria to form deoxycholic and lithocholic acid. These are largely reabsorbed in the terminal ileum and returned to the liver. One liter of bile is produced each day and secretion is stimulated by cholecystokinin (43).

The exact role of bile in gastrointestinal protection and mechanism of action is not clearly defined (44–48). *In vitro,* the unconjugated bile acids—chenodeoxycholic, cholic, and deoxycholic acid—inhibit the growth of stool isolates of *Clostridium* spp., *Bacteroides* spp., *Enterococcus* spp., and *Lactobacillus,* but they do not affect enteric aerobic organisms. Conjugated bile acids do not show this inhibitory effect. *In vitro,* the unconjugated bile salt sodium cholate kills *Giardia.*

Although bile acids may have bactericidal effects, other studies are less supportive. Concomitant measurements of bacterial counts and bile acid concentrations from intestinal luminal aspirates have shown that gram-negative anaerobes are abundant in areas with a high intraluminal concentration of deoxycholic acid. This would not be predicted because, *in vitro,* anaerobic bacteria are killed by this bile salt (49).

BLOOD GROUP FACTORS

The ABO blood group system is based on the expression of antigens on the erythrocyte cell surface. These carbohydrate antigens are determined by genetic pattern, and these particles can be released into saliva, mucus, and bile. People who release blood group antigens are secretors and those who do not are nonsecretors. The first association between blood groups and infectious diseases was made when similarities between blood group antigens and gram-negative bacteria antigens were noted (50,51). Then epidemiologic data showed an association between. blood group type and frequency of gastrointestinal and urinary tract infections (52,53).

Blood group carbohydrates share cross-reactivity with antigens expressed by bacteria and their toxins. *V. cholerae* O1 cell or toxin antigens share reactivity with blood type A or B carbohydrates. The blood group antigens can bind to the same intestinal receptors that bind *V. cholerae,* thus blocking the action of the bacteria or toxin (54). There is an increased frequency of nonsecretors among chronic *Salmonella typhi* carriers in Chile when compared with nonchronic carriers. This suggests that the lack of ABO carbohydrates in bile may allow adherence of *S. typhi* to the biliary tract (55).

Nonsecretors have a higher incidence of clinical intestinal illness. In endemic areas, individuals with group O blood type are at highest risk for development of cholera and group AB blood type are at lowest risk (56). Furthermore, individuals with blood group O have more severe cholera than those with blood group AB (53). Epidemiologic studies suggest that selective bias of cholera may account for the low prevalence of blood group O in people living in the Gangetic Delta, an endemic area for cholera (57). Lastly, nonsecretors have a higher incidence of oral candidiasis (58).

In contrast to findings that show a beneficial effect of secreting antigen, other studies present a different association. Epidemiologic studies have shown that individuals with blood group A have both a higher incidence and more severe illness with *G. lamblia* infection (59,60).

TREFOIL FACTORS

Trefoil factors (TFs), a family of peptides produced by intestinal goblet cells, lie in the viscoelastic mucous and are thought to participate in epithelial restitution (61). Although direct antimicrobial properties have not been identified, it is likely that these proteins participate in maintaining epithelial continuity.

The family of three trefoil peptides are defined by their regional specificity: (a) pS2 or TFF1 is located in the gastric mucosa, (b) spasmolytic polypeptide (SP) or TFF2 is located in the pancreaticobiliary ducts, and (c) intestinal trefoil factor (ITF) or TFF 3 is located in the goblet cells of the small and large intestine. The primary amino acid sequence demonstrates six cysteine residues that form three intrachain disulfide bonds. The loops created by these bonds resemble a shamrock, hence the name *trefoil.* This structure confers resistance to acid and protease degradation for the family.

Functionally, these peptides participate in the maintenance of epithelial integrity and restitution, thus potentially protecting the mucosa from bacterial invasion. For instance, when intestinal monolayers are injured with bile acids or *C. difficile* toxin A, the addition of exogenous trefoil peptides significantly reduces epithelial permeability (62). In animal models of gastric injury, TF expression is increased and administration of TFs protects the gastric mucosa from nonsteroidal antiinflammatory drug and ethanol-induced gastric mucosal injury (63–65). ITF-deficient mice have a normal phenotype but, when colitis is induced, they exhibit an increased morbidity and mortality when compared with their normal littermates (66). Treatment of these mice with recombinant ITF resulted in improvement in the colitis. Lastly, there is increased expression of TFs at sites of active inflammatory bowel disease and gastric ulcers, yet their role in these diseases is not yet certain (67,68).

ANTIMICROBIAL PEPTIDES

Numerous studies have identified innate antimicrobial peptides that are present in the human intestinal tract (69,70). Defensins, cathlicidens, salivary histatins, lipophilins, and lysins define a spectrum of specific proteins that possess bactericidal properties. These cationic proteins represent one of the earliest forms of innate host defense. Because of their broad spectrum of action, low host toxicity, and low level of microbial resistance, their therapeutic potential continues to be an area of active investigation.

Defensins are a family of low–molecular-weight peptides that have been isolated from human white blood cells. They possess a wide variety of antimicrobial activities against *E. coli, Listeria monocytogenes, Mycobacterium* spp., and *C. albicans* (71,72). Cryptdins are a type of defensin whose name is derived from their anatomic location in the crypts of Lieberkuhn. Cryptdins are produced in Paneth cells and are isolated from human and murine small intestine and from the intestinal lumen (73). The regulation of cryptdin synthesis and release is not well understood; they are present in the human fetal intestine and a noticeable increase in the cryptdin mRNA occurs in the murine model at the time of gut closure (74). Cryptdins are released into the intestinal lumen from the Paneth cell by exocytosis. They are produced in the intestinal tract of germ-free mice, suggesting that bacteria are not needed to induce expression, and are produced in mice who are void of T cells, suggesting independence from T-cell regulation (75,76). *In vitro,* cryptdins demonstrate antibacterial effects on phoP mutant strains of *S. typhimurium, L. monocytogenes,* and *E. coli* ML-35p. In addition, these peptides likely provide an antimicrobial barrier for the intestinal mucosa (77–80). Although the exact mechanism of action is not certain, these antimicrobial peptides create pore formation which leads to membrane instability, and induce chloride secretion, thus providing a flushing action of the intestinal crypt (81).

Mammals and insects possess other intestinal peptides with antibacterial properties. Initially, cecropins were found in the moth *Hyalophora cecropia* and recently were isolated from the pig intestine. They both kill gram-positive and gram-negative bacteria and exert their effects through lysis of the bacterial cell wall (82–85). Another antimicrobial protein termed *cathelicidins* have been identified in swine, sheep, cattle, mice, and humans (86). These proteins have been detected in the respiratory epithelium, neutrophils, and keratinocytes and, like the defensins, are thought to increase membrane permeability, bind LPS, or induce chemotaxis (86).

PERISTALSIS

Intestinal peristalsis provides a mechanical method for the removal of infectious particles. Migratory motor complexes (MMC) are the electric signals that drive this motility response. MMCs are initiated by a variety of stimuli, including cholinergic impulses; a variety of polypeptides such as histamine, motilin, somatostatin, gastrin, and cholecystokinin; and oxidative stress. When a peristaltic wave is initiated, it has been termed a *power propulsion.* Not only does peristalsis protect the small intestine but so does the ileocecal valve. In conjunction with peristalsis, this anatomic barrier helps prevent small intestinal bacterial overgrowth.

Peristalsis decreases the incidence of enteritis in murine models. For instance, rapid elimination of *V. cholerae* and *E. coli* occurs primarily as a result of intestinal peristaltic actions (87,88). In another model, direct cecal inoculation with *Shigella flexneri* following administration of opium resulted in significant inflammation of the ileal mucosa and increased mortality in subjects compared with untreated control subjects (89). Acute enteritis caused by *S. typhimurium* in opium-treated animals was histologically and clinically worse than in untreated control subjects (90). In humans receiving gastric inoculation of *Shigella* and treatment with Lomotil, systemic toxemia and prolonged carriage of the organism developed two to three times more often than in untreated control subjects. Although antiperistaltic medication decreased the amount of diarrhea that these patients experienced, they were still systemically ill (91). These findings advise against the use of antimotility agents in the treatment of certain cases of acute infectious diarrhea (92).

Peristalsis provides one of the main defenses against small bowel bacterial overgrowth. When intestinal stasis develops, whether secondary to medications, idiopathic pseudoobstruction, or systemic illness, such as scleroderma or diabetes mellitus, the normal anatomic populations of bacteria are disrupted, often resulting in bacterial overgrowth. Usually, the proximal small intestine contains less than 10^5 organisms/mL of primarily aerobic bacteria such as *Streptococcus* spp., the distal small intestine has greater than 10^8 organisms/mL of primarily anaerobic bacteria such as *Bacteroides* and *E. coli,* and the colon contains 10^{10} organisms/mL of predominately anaerobes. When peristalsis is pharmacologically altered, bacterial populations increase within hours. Proximal small intestine bacteria counts increase dramatically and the population of organisms assumes a character more like that of the lower small bowel (93,94). When the number of bacteria and the duration of contact time between bacteria and mucosa is prolonged, the likelihood of clinical illness increases (95). Morphine-induced peristaltic slowing results in increased bacterial translocation (96).

The sequelae of increased bacterial counts and mucosal contact time include not only the possibility of increased bacterial translocation but also the possibility of nutrient malabsorption and anemia. Malabsorption occurs because of bile salt depletion, disaccharide loss, and disruption of enterocytes. Anemia results from vitamin B_{12} malabsorption and intestinal blood loss.

CELLULAR ELEMENTS

A variety of cells participate in the innate defense of the intestinal tract. The epithelial layer, composed of five different cell types, comprise a mechanical and chemical barrier against infection. Enterocytes form tight junctions with adjacent cells to protect the immunologically potent lamina propria from antigen exposure. Enteroendocrine cells produce hormones and parietal cells secrete acid. Goblet cells secrete mucus and Paneth cells release cryptdins, lysozyme, tumor necrosis factor α and other bioactive mediators. The lamina propria, depending on its degree of inflammation, contain a number of immunologically active cells, including eosinophils and mast cells. In addition to producing multifunctional cytokines and lipid molecules, eosinophils produce highly charged cationic proteins. Two of these proteins, eosinophil major basic protein and eosinophil cationic protein, possess antibacterial properties (97). Mast cells in the lamina propria and submucosa can synthesize mediators, which affect nerve, endocrine, and other intestinal cells. After sensitization to *Trichinella spiralis* and secondary exposure to this parasite, mast cells release mediators, including histamine, serotonin, prostaglandins, leukotrienes, platelet-activating, factor, and cytokines. The regulated release of these factors signals the enteric nervous system to generate a sequence of power propulsions and epithelial cell fluid secretions. This coordinated response of diarrhea and expulsion of infection demonstrates the synergy linking the immune and the innate defenses of the bowel (98).

NUTRITION

The nutritional state of individuals can influence the development of infectious illnesses. In a like manner, infectious diseases can impact the host's nutritional status. Five hundred and sixty million people worldwide suffer from nutritional deficiencies (99). Twenty-four studies from underdeveloped countries have documented almost 1 billion cases/year of diarrhea (100). Numerous clinical and laboratory studies suggest a close association and complex relationship between nutrition, the immune system, and the development of infectious disease. Evidence suggesting, that malnutrition predisposes to infectious illness is based on laboratory and clinical experiments in animals and humans, and on epidemiologic observations. For several reasons, these studies are controversial and difficult to interpret. First, malnutrition may be interpreted in several ways. Some investigators include patients with marasmus (from the Greek word *marasmos,* meaning *withering*) or protein and calorie deprivation, others have included patients with kwashiorkor (from Ghana, meaning *displaced child*) or protein insufficient diets, and some include both (101). Next, it is difficult to examine nutritional deficiencies independently and separate other confounding variables (e.g., hygiene) that may also predispose to infectious disease. Lastly, many epidemiologic studies have used inadequate numbers of patients to demonstrate statistical significance or lack the data to document specific nutritional deficiencies and infections. Even so, clinical and laboratory studies suggest that the malnourished patient is more predisposed to infectious disease. In a comprehensive review of clinical and laboratory studies, Scrimshaw (102) noted that the relationship between nutrition and infection is synergistic; the morbidity and mortality rates of infectious illnesses are likely to be greater in those with malnutrition, and infectious diseases can make the malnourished state worse.

When immune and nonimmune defense mechanisms of normal individuals are compared with those of malnourished individuals, obvious differences are demonstrated. As starvation occurs, the epithelial layer atrophies, lymphoid tissue involutes, and antibody production decreases. Gross and histologic samples of malnourished human thymus, lymph nodes, spleen, and gut-associated lymphoid aggregates weigh less and have fewer lymphocytes than normal (103). Significant depletion of intraepithelial lymphocytes and decreased antibody formation develop in protein-malnourished rats when compared with their fed counterparts (104,105). Functional studies in humans demonstrate impaired cell-mediated immunity, decreased secretory antibody production, decreased IgA-producing plasma cells, altered intracellular killing, reduced complement activation, reduction in total number of intraepithelial lymphocytes, and lymphocyte responsiveness to interleukin (IL)-1 (106–108). The nonimmune mechanisms of defense are also affected. Gastric acidity and lysozyme secretion in individuals with marasmus or kwashiorkor are reduced (109).

Young, old, and immunocompromised malnourished individuals have more frequent and more severe gastrointestinal illness. The incidence and duration of diarrhea is increased twofold in children with protein–calorie malnutrition. In large epidemiologic studies, the highest morbidity and mortality rates from diarrheal illness is seen in children younger than 1 year of age (100). Small-for-gestational-age infants have reduced sIgA response to poliovirus vaccine, fewer circulating lymphocytes, decreased opsonization, and decreased neutrophil oxidative metabolism (105). In protein-malnourished rodents and their offspring, qualitative and quantitative IgA responses are impaired, which is reversed after refeeding (110–112). In some patients older than 60 years, cell-mediated immunity is impaired but is improved after nutritional supplementation (113–115). Although extensive prospective trials are incomplete, aggressive nutritional therapy may benefit AIDS patients, the newest population of malnourished individuals (103).

Not only is it important to receive sufficient protein and calories but also the route of intake of the calories is seemingly important. When rats are given the same quantities of nutrients either exclusively parenterally or enterally, intestinal atrophy develops in the group nourished parenterally (116). Functional studies in animals and human volunteers receiving all calories from parenteral nutrition show increased intestinal permeability when compared with their fed counterparts (116–118). Recent interest in omega-3 fatty acids, nucleotides, prebiotics, and probiotics provides new alternatives to prevent or treat infectious and inflammatory diseases of the intestinal tract.

SUMMARY AND CONCLUSIONS

This chapter reviews the nonimmune components of intestinal host defense against microorganisms. The synergy that exists between the nonimmune elements collectively protects the intestine from infectious disease. Microbial attachment is inhibited by glycoproteins and the gastric acid kills sIgA and organisms. Those microbes or microbial products that survive passage through the stomach are swept into the small intestine and are exposed to the antimicrobial actions of bile and cryptdins, and their attachment can be impeded by blood group factors or peristalsis. If they penetrate the mucosa, microbes encounter the potent milieu of the lamina propria with its T cells, eosinophils, and mast cells. When a part of the intestinal tract is excised or diseased, or when protein or calorie deprivation ensues, these defenses are impaired, making the host more susceptible to infectious diseases.

REFERENCES

1. Cole MF, et al. Specific and nonspecific immune factors in dental plaque fluid and saliva from young and old populations. *Infect Immun* 1981;31:998–1002.
2. Bowen WH. Defense mechanisms in the mouth and their possible role in the prevention of dental caries: a review. *J Oral Pathol* 1974;3:266–278.
3. Helm JF, et al. Acid neutralizing capacity of human saliva. *Gastroenterology* 1982;83:69.
4. Pruitt KM. The salivary peroxidase system: thermodynamic, kinetic and antibacterial properties. *J Oral Pathol* 1987;16: 417–420.
5. Prakobphol A, et al. Salivary agglutinin, which binds *Streptococcus mutans* and *Helicobacter pylori,* is the lung scavenger receptor cysteine-rich protein GP-340. J Biol Chem 2000;275: 39860–39866.
6. Williams RC, Gibbons RJ. Inhibition of streptococcal attachment to receptors on human buccal epithelial cells by antigenically similar salivary glycoproteins. *Infect Immun* 1975;11: 711–718.
7. Kruzel ML, et al. The gut. A key metabolic organ protected lactoferrin during experimental systemic inflammation in mice. *Adv Exp Med Biol* 1998;443:167–173.
8. Florey H. The relative amounts of lysozyme present in the tissues of some mammals. *Br J Exp Path* 1930:251–261.
9. Weinberg ED. Iron withholding: a defense against infection and neoplasia. *Physiol Rev* 1984;64:65–103.
10. Ellison RT, Glehl TJ. Killing of gram negative bacteria by lactoferrin and lysozyme. *J Clin Invest* 1991;88:1080–1091.
11. Yamauchi K, et al. Antibacterial activity of lactoferrin and a pepsin derived lactoferrin peptide fragment. *Infect Immun* 1993;61:719–728.
12. Arnold RR, Cole MF, McGhee JR. A bactericidal effect for human lactoferrin. *Science* 1977;197:263–265.

13. Clamp JR, Creeth JM. Some non-mucin components of mucus and their possible roles. In: *Mucus and mucosa.* London: Pitman, 1984:121–136.
14. Hoffman MP, Haidaris CG. Analysis of *Candida albicans* adhesion to salivary mucin. *Infect Immun* 1993;61:1940–1949.
15. Edgarton M., et al. Human submandibular-sublingual saliva promotes adhesion of *Candida albicans* to polymethylmethacrylate. *Infect Immun* 1993;61:2644–2652.
16. Orstavik D, Kraus FW, Henshaw LC. *In vitro* attachment of streptococci to the tooth surface. *Infect Immun* 1974;9:794–800.
17. Husson M, et al. Iron acquisition by *Helicobacter pylori:* importance of human lactoferrin. *Infect Immun* 1993;61:2694–2697.
18. Terpenning M., et al. Bacterial colonization of saliva and plaque in the elderly. *Clin Infect Dis* 1993;16[Suppl 4]:314–316.
19. Wise L, Ballinger WF. Gastric defense mechanisms. *Am J Surg* 1970;119:537–541.
20. Giannella R, Broitman SA, Zamcheck N. Influence of gastric acidity on bacterial and parasitic enteric infections. *Ann Intern Med* 1973;78:271–276.
21. Dare R, Macree JT, Mathison GE. *In vitro* studies on the bactericidal properties of natural and synthetic gastric juices. *J Med Microbiol* 1972;5:395–406.
22. Gorden J, Small PLC. Acid resistance in enteric bacteria. *Infect Immun* 1993;61:364–367.
23. Nordbring F. Contraction of salmonella gastroenteritis following previous operation on the stomach. *Acta Med Scand* 1956;171:783–790.
24. Gray JA, Trueman AM. Severe salmonella gastroenteritis associated with hypochlorhydria. *Scott Med J* 1971;16:255–258.
25. Roberts -Thomson IC. Genetic studies of human and murine giardiasis. *J Infect Dis* 1993;16[Suppl 2]:S98–S104.
26. Gitelson S. Gastrectomy, achlorhydria, and cholera. *Israel J Med Sci* 1971;7:663–667.
27. Dupont HL, et al. Immunity in shigellosis. I. Response of man to attenuated strains of shigella. *J Infect Dis* 1972;125:5–11.
28. Dirks MR, et al. Nosocomial pneumonia in intubated patients given sucralfate as compared with antacids or histamine type 2 blockers. *N Engl J Med* 1987;317:1376–1382.
29. Heyland DK, et al. The effect of acidified enteral feeds on gastric colonization in critically ill patient: results of a multicenter randomized trial. Canadian Critical Care Trials Group. *Crit Care Med* 1999;27:2399–2406.
30. Draser BS, Shiner M, McLeod GM. Studies on the intestinal flora. I. The bacterial flora of the gastrointestinal tract in healthy and achlorhydric persons.*Gastroenterology* 1969;56:71–79.
31. Hornick RB, et al. The Broad Street pump revisited: response of volunteers to ingested cholera vibrios. *Bull N Y Acad Med* 1971; 47:1181–1191.
32. Laine L, et al. Review articles: potential gastrointestinal effects of long-term acid suppression with proton pump inhibitors. *Aliment Pharmacol Ther* 2000;14:651–668.
33. Elbein AD, et al. Effect of inhibitors on glycoprotein biosynthesis and bacterial adhesion. In: *Adhesion and microorganism pathogenicity.* Pitman: Tunbridge Wells, 1981:270–287.
34. Warner L, Kim YS. Intestinal receptors for microbial attachment. In: Farthing MJG, Keusch GT, eds. *Enteric infection: mechanisms, manifestations and management.* New York: Raven Press, 1989:31–40.
35. Aderem A, Ulevitch RJ. Toll like receptors in the induction of the innate immune response. *Nature* 2000;406:782–787.
36. Kaisho T, Akira S. Critical roles of toll-like receptors in host defense. *Crit Rev Immunol* 2000;20:393–405.
37. Carlo E, Podolsky DK. Differential alteration in intestinal epithelial cell expression of toll-like receptor 3 and TLR4 in inflammatory bowel disease. *Infect Immun* 2000;68:7010–7017.
38. Baddour LM, et al. Microbial adherence. In: Mandell GL, Douglas RG, Bennet JE, eds. *Principles and practice of infectious diseases.* New York: Churchill-Livingstone, 1990:9–22.
39. Chu SW, Walker WA. Bacterial toxin interaction with the developing intestine. *Gastroenterology* 1993;104:916–925.
40. Sellwood R, et al. Adhesion of enteropathogenic *Escherichia coli* to pig intestinal brush borders: the existence of two pig phenotypes. *J Med Microbiol* 1975;8:405–411.
41. Rolfe RD, Song W. Purification of a functional receptor receptor for *Clostridium difficile* toxin A from intestinal brush border membranes of infant hamsters. *Clin Infect Dis* 1993;16[Suppl 4]:219–227.
42. Pothoulakis C, et al. The human colonic *Clostridium difficile* toxin A receptor is a trypsin sensitive glycoprotein. *Gastroenterology* 1992;103:2046.
43. West JB. Gallbladder. In: West JB, ed. *Physiological basis of medical practice.* Baltimore: Williams & Wilkins, 1985:643.
44. Jackson SLO. Antibacterial action of bile. *Br Med J* 1972;4:300.
45. Binder HJ, Filburn B, Floch M. Bile acid inhibition of intestinal anaerobic organisms. *Am J Clin Nutr* 1975;28:119–125.
46. Floch MH, et al. Bile acid inhibition of the intestinal microflora—a function for simple bile acids. *Gastroenterology* 1971;61:228–233.
47. Percy-Robb IW, Collee JG. Bile acids: a pH dependent antibacterial system in the gut.*BMJ* 1972;3:813–815.
48. Gillin FD, Das S, Reiner DS. Nonspecific defenses against human Giardia. In: Ruitenberg EJ, MacInnis AJ, eds. *Human parasitic diseases.* Amsterdam: Elsevier, 1990:199–213.
49. Mallory A, et al. Patterns of bile acids and microflora in the human small intestine.*Gastroenterology* 1973;64:26–42.
50. Muschel LH, Osawa E. Human blood group substance B and *Escherichia coli* 086. *Proc Soc Exp Biol Med* 1959;101: 614–617.
51. Springer GF, Williamson P, Brandes WC. Blood group activity of gram-negative bacteria. *J Exp Med* 1961;113:1077–1093.
52. Sheinfeld J, et al. Association of the Lewis blood group phenotype with recurrent urinary tract infections in women. *N Engl J Med* 1989;320:773–737.
53. Chaudhuri A, DasAdhikary CR. Possible role of blood group secretory substances in the aetiology of cholera. *Trans R Soc Trop Med Hyg* 1978;72:664–665.
54. Clemens JD, et al. ABO blood groups and cholera: new observations on specificity of risk and modification of vaccine efficacy. *J Infect Dis* 1989;159:770–773.
55. Hoffmann E, et al. Blood group antigen secretion and gallstone disease in the *Salmonella typhimurium* chronic carrier state. *J Infect Dis* 1993;167:993–994.
56. Barua D, Paauio AS. ABO blood groups and cholera. *Ann Hum Biol* 1977;4:489–493.
57. Glass RI, et al. Predisposition for cholera of individuals with O blood group. *Am J Epidemiol* 1985;121:791–796.
58. Burford-Mason A., Willoughby JMT, Weber JCP. Association between gastrointestinal tract carriage of *Candida,* blood group O and nonsecretion of blood group antigens in patients with peptic ulcer. *Dig Dis Sci* 1993;38:1453–1458.
59. Barnes GL, Kay R. Blood groups in giardiasis. *Lancet* 1976;2: 808.
60. Zisman M. Blood group A and giardiasis. *Lancet* 1977;l:1285.
61. Podolsky DK, et al. Identification of human intestinal trefoil factor. Goblet cell-specific expression of a peptide targeted for apical secretion. *J Biol Chem* 1993;268:6694–6702.
62. Kindon H, et al. Trefoil peptide protection of intestinal epithelial barrier function: cooperative interaction with mucin glycoprotein. *Gastroenterology* 1995;109:516–523.
63. Babyatsky MW. et al. Oral trefoil peptides protect against ethanol- and indomethacin-induced gastric injury in rats. *Gastroenterology* 1996;110:89–97.

64. McKenzie C, Thim L, Parsons ME. Topical and intravenous administration of trefoil factors protect the gastric mucosa from ethanol-induced injury in the rat. *Aliment Pharmacol Ther* 2000;14:1033–1040.
65. Cook GA, Yeomans ND, Giraud AS. Temporal expression of trefoil peptides in the TGF alpha knockout mouse after gastric ulceration. *Am J Physiol* 1997;272:G1540–G1549.
66. Mashimo H, et al. Impaired defense of intestinal mucosa in mice lacking intestinal trefoil factor. *Science* 1996;274:262–265.
67. Wright NA,et al. Trefoil peptide gene expression in gastrointestinal epithelial cells in inflammatory bowel disease. *Gastroenterology* 1993;104:12–20.
68. Lonaman RJ. Coordinated localisation of mucins and trefoil peptides in the ulcer associated cell lineage and the gastrointestinal mucosa. *Gut* 2000;47:792–800.
69. Huttner KM, Bevins CL. Antimicrobial peptides as mediators of epithelial host defense. *Pediatr Res* 1999;45:785–794.
70. Cole AM, Ganz T. Human antimicrobial peptides: analysis and application. *Biotechniques* 2000;29: 822–831.
71. Ogata K, et al. Activity of defensin from human neutrophilic granulocytes against *Mycobacterium avium–Mycobacterium intracellulare. Infect Immun* 1992;60:4720–4725.
72. Lehrer RI, et al. Modulation of the *in vitro* candidacidal activity of human neutrophil defensins by target cell metabolism and divalent cations. *J Clin Invest* 1988;81:1829–1835.
73. Lin MY, Munshi IA, Ouellette AT. The defensin related murine CRSI C gene: expression in Paneth cells and linkage to Defcr, the cryptdin locus. *Genomics* 1992;14:363–368.
74. Eisenhauer PB, Harwig SSSL, Lehrer RI. Cryptdins: antimicrobial defensins of the murine small intestine. *Infect Immun* 1992; 60:3556–3565.
75. Ouellette AJ, et al. Developmental regulation of cryptdin, a corticostatin/defensin precursor mRNA in mouse small intestinal crypt epithelium. J Cell Biol 1989;108:1687–1695.
76. Putsep K, et al. Germ-free and colonized mice generate the same products from enteric prodefensins. *J Biol Chem* 2000; 275:40478–40482.
77. Selsted ME, et al. Enteric defensins: antibiotic peptide components of intestinal host defense. *J Cell Biol* 1992;118:929–936.
78. Miller SI, et al. Characterization of defensin resistance phenotypes associated with mutations in the phoP virulence regulon of *Salmonella typhimurium. Infect Immun* 1990;58:3706–3710.
79. Jones DE, Bevins CL. Paneth cells of the human small intestine express an antimicrobial peptide gene. *J Biol Chem* 1992;267: 23216–23225.
80. Jones DE, Bevins CL. Defensin 6 mRNA in human Paneth cells: implications for antimicrobial peptides in host defense of the human bowel. *FEBS Lett* 1993;315:187–192.
81. Lencer WL, et al. Induction of epithelial chloride secretion by channel-forming cryptdins 2 and 3. *Proc Natl Acad Sci U S A* 1997;94:8585–8589.
82. Boman HG, Agerberth B, Boman A. Mechanisms of action on *Escherichia coli* of cecropin PI and PR-39, two antibacterial peptides from pig intestine. *Infect Immun* 1993;61:2978–2984.
83. Christensen B, et al. Channel forming properties of cecropins and related model compounds incorporated into planar lipid membranes. *Proc Natl Acad Sci U S A* 1988;85:5072–5076.
84. Lee J, et al. Antibacterial peptides from pig intestine: isolation of a mammalian cecropin. *Proc Natl Acad Sci U S A* 1989;86: 9159–9162.
85. Steiner S, Andreu D, Merrifield RB. Binding and action of cecropin and cecropin analogues: antibacterial peptides from insects. *Biochim Biophys Acta* 1988;939:260–266.
86. De Yang, et al. LL-37, the neutrophil granule- and epithelial cell-derived cathelicidin, utilizes formyl peptide receptor-like 1 (FPRL1) as a receptor to chemoattract human peripheral blood neutrophils, monocytes, and T cells. *J Exp Med* 2000;192: 1069–1074.
87. Knop J, Rowley D. Antibacterial mechanism in the intestine—elimination of *V. cholerae* from the gastrointestinal tract of adult mice. *Aust J Exp Biol Med Sci* 1975;53:137–146.
88. Dixon JMS. The fate of bacteria in the small intestine. *J Pathol Bact* 1960;79:131–140.
89. Formal SB, et al. Experimental *Shigella* infections IV. Role of the small intestine in an experimental infection in guinea pigs. *J Bacteriol* 1963;85:119–125.
90. Kent TH, Formal SB, Labrec EH. Acute enteritis due to *Salmonella typhimurium* in opium treated guinea pigs. *Arch Pathol* 1966;81:501–508.
91. Dupont HL, Hornick RB. Adverse effect of Lomotil therapy in shigellosis. *JAMA* 1973;226:1525–1528.
92. Vantrappen G, et al. The interdigestive motor complex of normal subjects and patients with bacterial overgrowth of the small intestine. *J Clin Invest* 1977;59:1158–1166.
93. Scott LD, Cahall DL. Influence of the interdigestive myoelectric complex on enteric flora in the rat digestive system. *Gastroenterology* 1982;82:737–745.
94. Hamilton I., et al. Simultaneous culture of salvia and jejunal aspirate in the investigation of small bowel bacterial overgrowth. *Gut* 1982;23:847–853.
95. Sprinz H. Pathogenesis of intestinal infection. *Arch Pathol* 1969; 87:556.
96. Runkel NSF, et al. Alterations in rat intestinal transit by morphine promote bacterial translocation. *Dig Dis Sci* 1993;38: 1530–1536.
97. Lehrer RI, et al. Antibacterial properties of eosinophil major basic protein and eosinophil cationic protein. *J Immunol* 1989;142:4428–4434.
98. Boedeker EC, McQueen CE. Intestinal immunity to bacterial and parasitic infections. *Immunol All Clin NA* 1988;8:393–421.
99. Chandra RK. Nutritional regulation of immunity and infection in the gastrointestinal tract. *J Pediatr Gastroenterol Nutr* 1983;2 [Suppl 1]:S181–S187.
100. Snyder JD, Merson MH. The magnitude of the global problem of acute diarrhoeal disease: a review of active surveillance data. *Bull WHO* 1982;60:605–613.
101. Chandra RK. Nutritional deficiency and susceptibility to infection. *Bull WHO* 1979;57:167–177.
102. Scrimshaw NS, Taylor CE, Gordon JE. *Interactions of nutrition and infection,* vol 57. Geneva: World Health Organization 1968:329.
103. Hickey HS, Weaver KE. Nutritional management of patients with ARC or AIDS. *Gastroenterol Clin North Am* 1988;17: 545–561.
104. Maffei HVL, et al. Intraepithelial lymphocytes in the jejunal mucosa of malnourished rats. *Gut* 1980;21:32–36.
105. Chandra RK. Antibody formation in first and second generation offspring of nutritionally deprived rats. *Science* 1975;190: 288–289.
106. Chandra RK, Newberne PM. *Nutrition, immunity, and infection—mechanisms of interactions.* New York: Plenum, 1977:246.
107. Watson RR, et al. Effect of age, malnutrition and renutrition on free secretory component and IgA in secretions. *Am J Clin Nutr* 1985;42:281–288.
108. Ulijaszek ST. Nutritional status and susceptibility to infectious disease. In: Harrison GA, Waterlow JC, eds. *Diet and disease.* Cambridge: Cambridge University Press, 1990:137–154.
109. Chandra RK. Fetal malnutrition and postnatal immunocompetence. *Am J Dis Child* 1975;129:450–454.
110. Barry WS, Pierce NF. Protein deprivation causes reversible impairment of mucosal immune response to cholera toxoid/ toxin in rat gut. *Nature* 1979;281:64–65.

111. Lim TS, Messiha N, Watson RR. Immune components of the intestinal mucosae of ageing and protein deficient mice. *Immunology* 1981;43:401–407.
112. McGee DW, McMurray DN. The effect of protein malnutrition on the IgA immune response in mice. *Immunology* 1988;63:25–29.
113. Chandra RK, et al. Nutrition and immunocompetence of the elderly: effect of short term nutritional supplementation on cell mediated immunity and lymphocyte subsets. *Nutr Res* 1982;2:223–232.
114. Chandra RK. Nutritional regulation of immunity and risk of infection in old age. *Immunology* 1989;67:141–147.
115. Sullivan DA, Vaerman JP, Soo C. Influence of severe protein malnutrition on rat lacrimal, salivary and gastrointestinal immune expression during development, adulthood and ageing. *Immunology* 1993;78:308–317.
116. Johnson LR, et al. Structural and hormonal alteration in the gastrointestinal tract of parenterally fed rats. *Gastroenterology* 1975;68:1177–1183.
117. McNeil LK, Hamilton JR. The effect of fasting on disaccharidase activity in the rat small intestine. *Pediatrics* 1971;47:65–72.
118. Buchman AL, et al. Intestinal permeability increases in normal volunteers receiving total parenteral nutrition. *Gut* 1993; [Suppl]:29.

10

THE MUCOSAL IMMUNE SYSTEM

CHARLES O. ELSON
JIRI F. MESTECKY

Mucosal surfaces represent the major interface between the host and the environment. Thus, it is not surprising that most pathogens invade through or infect mucosal surfaces (1). A number of defense mechanisms have clearly evolved in the host to deal with microbes in general and pathogens in particular. One of the most important of these is the mucosal immune system. This compartment of the immune system, quantitatively the largest, is marked by a number of distinguishing features that are unique to its specialized role. One of these features is the preferential production, transport, and secretion of IgA at all mucosal surfaces; IgA limits the absorption of protein antigens, inhibits the attachment of bacteria, and neutralizes a broad spectrum of viruses (2).

Mucosal IgA-producing plasma cells originate in organized lymphoepithelial structures that are present in the gastrointestinal tract (gut-associated lymphoepithelial tissue, or GALT) and respiratory tract (bronchus-associated lymphoepithelial tissue, or BALT). The discovery that antigen-stimulated GALT and BALT are the source of antigen-sensitized and IgA-committed plasma cell precursors that populate remote mucosal tissues and glands has led to the concept of a common mucosal immune system (3), in which an antigen exposure at one mucosal surface contributes cells that help protect remote mucosal sites as well (Fig. 10.1). For example, intestinal immunization can generate a mucosal response in the lung or in the vagina. This has led to a renewed interest in the development of oral vaccines to protect nonintestinal mucosal sites (4). Priming for a mucosal response via the intestine is convenient and effective, but optimal immunity at distant mucosal sites seems to require local exposure of that mucosal surface to the antigen. In fact, the common mucosal immune system may contain certain subcompartments such that optimal upper respiratory immune responses occur after nasopharyngeal or BALT immunization, whereas optimal vaginal immune responses occur after rectal or intranasal immunization (5).

In regard to the intestine, lymphoid cells constitute approximately 25% of the cells present in the intestine; therefore the intestine is a major lymphoid organ (6). The mucosal immune system of the gut is organized into several interconnecting compartments representing either inductive or effector sites. Inductive sites consist of Peyer's patches (PPs) and isolated lymphoid follicles, i.e., GALT; effector sites consist of the lamina propria and intraepithelial lymphocytes (IELs) (Fig. 10.1). The mesenteric lymph nodes, although outside the intestine proper, are frequently considered a fourth compartment. These different cell compartments are distinguished not only by differences in physical location and structure but by the types and functions of cells present within them.

The antigenic challenge to the intestinal immune system is enormous (Fig. 10.2). It has been estimated that the number of microbial cells in the body, most of them in the large intestine, exceeds the total number of cells in the body (7). One can add to these bacterial antigens the abundant antigens present in food and drink. Exactly how the intestinal mucosal system deals with this challenge is not yet known; however, it is apparent that the mucosal immune system is in a constant state of response, as witnessed by the large number of plasma cells present throughout the intestine and by studies on germ-free animals in which mucosal lymphoid tissue is poorly developed (8). These observations have led to the concept of "physiological inflammation," in which the "normal" intestine is viewed as being in a state of mild inflammation (9) due to the massive antigenic challenge. Physiological inflammation may represent an important aspect of host defense against pathogens, many of which are likely to have antigens cross-reactive with those of the enteric flora. In this view, the normal stimulation of the intestinal immune system by the enteric flora "arms" or "primes" the system for accelerated or more effective immune responses to pathogenic microbes.

C. O. Elson: Department of Medicine, University of Alabama at Birmingham and University Hospital, Birmingham, Alabama

J. F. Mestecky: Departments of Microbiology and Medicine, University of Alabama at Birmingham, Birmingham, Alabama

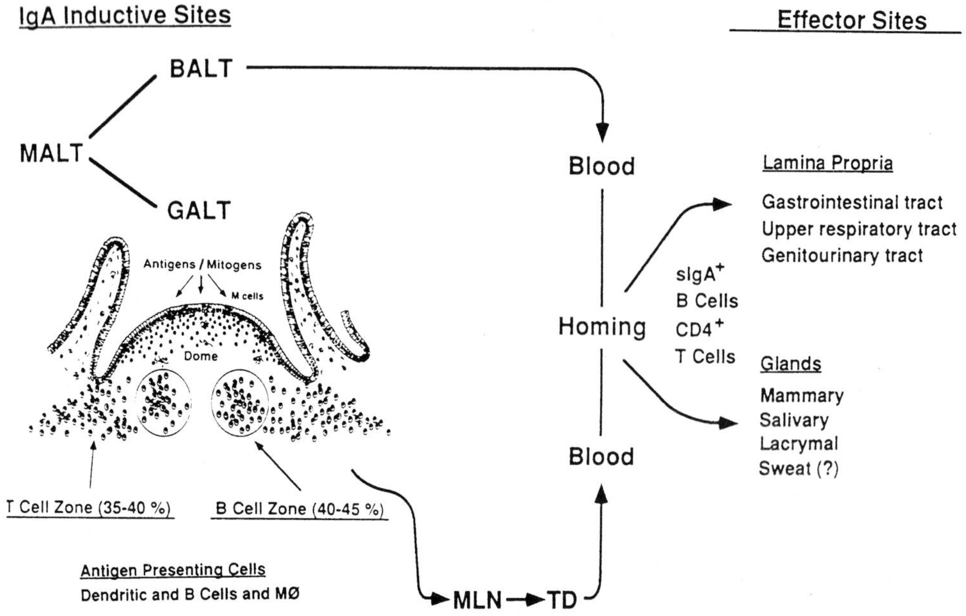

FIGURE 10.1. Schematic diagram of the common mucosal immune system in humans. The intestine contains organized lymphoid structures known as Peyer's patches as well as isolated lymphoid follicles. Luminal antigen enters these organized lymphoid tissues through a specialized epithelium containing pinocytotic and phagocytic M cells. Within the follicle, antigens interact with resident antigen-presenting cells, T cells, and B cells to generate immunoglobulin A (IgA)-committed and antigen-sensitized B cells and T cells. Once activated, cells leave the follicle and enter regional lymph nodes, such as mesenteric lymph nodes (MLN), then travel through the thoracic duct to the circulation, from which they populate various exocrine glands and mucosa-associated tissues in the salivary glands, respiratory tract, genitourinary tract, and lactating breast. Terminal differentiation into IgA-secreting plasma cells occurs in these mucosal tissues.

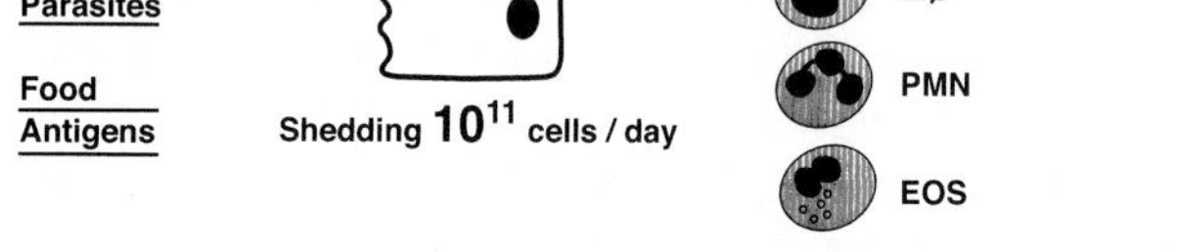

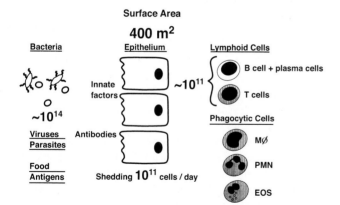

FIGURE 10.2. Defense mechanisms of mucosal membranes. Vast surfaces (approximately 400 m^2) of mucosal membranes, particularly of the gastrointestinal tract, are continuously exposed to enormous numbers of various bacteria (approximately 10^{14} in the colon) and ingested or inhaled antigens of microbial and food origin. The intestinal tract contains the largest accumulation of B and T lymphocytes and plasma cells (approximately 10^{11}) and macrophages in the body. The mucosal surface and lymphoid-macrophage compartments are separated by a single layer of highly active and dynamic epithelial cells.

In the following sections, each compartment of the intestinal immune system is considered separately, but, in reality, the compartments represent a dynamic and integrated system of host defense.

PEYER'S PATCHES AND LYMPHOID FOLLICLES

PPs are organized lymphoepithelial aggregates with one or more lymphoid follicles that extend from the epithelial layer into the lamina propria, and sometimes the submucosa. Although PPs are visible macroscopic structures clustered in certain regions, such as the ileum and appendix in humans, analogous small lymphoid follicles are dispersed abundantly throughout the intestine in humans and some other species (10). PPs and these small follicles together comprise GALT. PPs differ from other peripheral lymphoid tissues by their lack of afferent lymphatics, but they do have efferent lymphatics. Instead of afferent lymphatics, they have a specialized epithelium that actively pinocytoses material present in the intestinal lumen and delivers it via transcytosis and exocytosis into the follicle (Fig. 10.1) (11). Distinguishing features of this specialized follicle-associated epithelium include a relative lack of goblet cells and the presence of membrane, or M, cells that lack the polyimmunoglobulin receptor and alkaline phosphatase (see Chapter 11). The M cell serves as an important first step in the induction of intestinal immune responses, but relatively little is known about the factors determining its generation or function. Recent *in vitro* studies suggest that the direct interaction of epithelial cells with lymphocytes is essential for the differentiation of human epithelial cell lines into cells functionally and morphologically analogous to PP M cells (12). At present, it is unclear whether any selectivity other than size of particles is exerted by the M cell in the material that it will pinocytose or phagocytose. Soluble proteins, viruses, bacteria, protozoa, lysosomes, and microspheres are all capable of being taken up by M cells. Some organisms such as *Salmonella* exploit this feature, using M cells as a portal of entry into the body. M-cell uptake of *Salmonella* and particles such as microcapsules is being exploited to deliver vaccine antigens into GALT. No direct evidence of antigen presentation by M cells exists.

Consistent with this active antigen uptake by the specialized dome epithelium, PPs and related lymphoid follicles serve as sites for the induction of mucosal immune responses. GALT contains all the cells needed for immune induction, that is, B cells, T cells, and antigen-presenting cells (dendritic cells, macrophages). These cell types are structured in B-cell–dependent and T-cell–dependent areas similar to other peripheral lymphoid tissues. B cells predominate in the lymphoid follicles, whereas T cells predominate in the interfollicular areas and beneath the dome epithelium. Dendritic cells (DCs) appear to form a layer beneath the dome epithelium and extend into the follicles; DCs are present in interfollicular T-cell areas of the PP as well (13). DCs are potent antigen-presenting cells, particularly for the priming of naïve T cells, and DCs from the PP have this functional ability. However, PP DCs may have distinctive properties compared with DCs at other sites; for example, they produce high amounts of interleukin (IL)-10 and may favor a regulatory/Th2 pathway for CD4 T-cell differentiation (14). Antigen-loaded DCs that can prime naïve T cells have been identified in small intestinal lymph after oral antigen feeding, supporting a crucial role for these cells in the induction of mucosal immune responses (15). DC numbers can be markedly increased in GALT and other lymphoid tissues by the parenteral administration of flt3 ligand, a hematopoietic factor, raising the possibility that mucosal immune responses might be manipulated in the future by altering the number or function of this cell (16).

Quantitatively, B cells predominate in the PPs of adult animals, constituting some 60% to 70% of the total cells, whereas T cells, including both CD4+ and CD8+ cells, comprise about 20% of the total (6). Although T cells are present in smaller numbers, the rudimentary PPs and the deficient IgA responses found in T-cell–deficient mice indicate that PP function is highly dependent on T cells (17). An important feature of PP cells is that they consist of precursor rather than effector cells. For example, although the PPs contain many B cells, very few plasma cells are present, even after extensive immunization, because differentiating B cells and T cells appear to leave PPs and migrate to the gut and other lymphoid tissues (18). A second important feature of PPs is that the induction of immune responses there is highly dependent on the route of antigen exposure. PPs respond predominantly, if not exclusively, to antigen presented via the intestinal lumen, that is, antigen transported via M cells.

Although PPs are important sites of mucosal immune induction, there are some additional sites that can contribute as well. Mice that lack PPs (PP null mice) but have normally developed mesenteric lymph nodes have IgA-producing plasma cells in the intestinal lamina propria, and such animals produce mucosal IgA and serum IgG antibodies after oral immunization (19). Thus, it appears that organized PPs are not an absolute requirement for induction of mucosal IgA responses, perhaps because small lymphoid follicles or mesenteric lymph nodes can serve as an alternative or additional source of IgA precursor cells.

In mice, the peritoneal cavity is another source of intestinal IgA-producing cells. A special population of peritoneal B lymphocytes, known as B1 cells, contribute half or more of the B cells in the lamina propria (20–22). Removal of peritoneal B1 cells by peritoneal lavage with osmotic shock results in reduced numbers of IgA-producing cells in the lamina propria of the gut and decreased levels of secretory IgA (S-IgA). B1 cells display properties that differ from conventional (B2) B cells of bone marrow or PP origin. They appear early in ontogeny, have a capacity of self-renewal, are present in the peritoneal cavity, express different cell surface markers (e.g., high IgM^+, low IgD^+, $CD5^+$ on most cells), and produce low-affinity IgM, IgA, and IgG3 antibodies with broad specificity for some autoantigens and to common bacterial antigens such as phosphorylcholine, dextrans, lipopolysaccharides, certain bacterial toxins, and surface antigens of anaerobic intestinal microbiota (21,22). Thus, this has been termed *natural* IgA. Intestinal bacteria in mice are coated *in vivo* with IgA derived primarily from the peritoneal B1 lymphocytes, and it appears that these antibodies may substantially alter the composition of the intestinal microbiota (20). Recent studies (23) suggest that, in contrast to PP B cells, the production of IgA antibodies by intestinal B1-derived plasma cells is not strictly T-cell dependent. The B1 subset differs from conventional B cells in its cytokine response, that is, IL-15 and IL-15 receptor expressed on B1 lymphocytes selectively regulate their differentiation into IgA-producing cells (24). The importance of the peritoneal B1 cell population as a source of mucosal IgA precursor cells in humans is at present unknown. Limited studies of patients on peritoneal dialysis suggest that extensive flushing (three times per day for 1 year or more) does not lead to reduced levels of S-IgA and that intraperitoneal immunization with tetanus toxoid induces systemic IgM and IgG immune responses (25).

GALT, BALT, and related tissues are sites where there is preferential induction of IgA responses, an important activity considering that IgA is the major immunoglobulin at mucosal surfaces. PP cells are enriched for IgA B-cell precursors relative to other lymphoid tissues (26), particularly for IgA B-cell precursors recognizing antigens present in the intestine (27). The mechanism for this preferential expression of IgA by PP B cells is not clear, but microenvironment–B-cell interactions (27), the effects of a specialized DC (28), and the local expression of cytokines such as transforming growth factor-β (TGF-β) in PPs (29) are possible explanations. A cytokine-independent factor, activation-induced cytidine deaminase (AID), has been implicated also as a regulator of switching from IgM to IgA (30,31). T cells that regulate B-cell differentiation by secreting a variety of cytokines (Fig. 10.3) are present in the PPs as well (32,33).

The contribution of nonintestinal inductive sites, such as nasal-, bronchus-, and larynx-associated lymphoid tissues (NALT, BALT, and LALT, respectively) to cells populating the intestinal lamina propria in humans has not been adequately evaluated. Limited data based on intranasal immunization suggest that human oropharyngeal lymphoid tissues in Waldeyer's ring and nasal mucosa generate IgA-producing cells that localize in the upper respiratory and digestive tract (6). In animal models, intranasal immunization induces IgG responses in serum and IgA responses in nasal washes, saliva, genital tract secretions, and, to a lessor extent, in intestinal secretions (34,35). There appear to be marked differences among species in the presence and development of these different inductive sites, particularly in the respiratory tract, as well as differences in the role they play in the induction of intestinal immune responses.

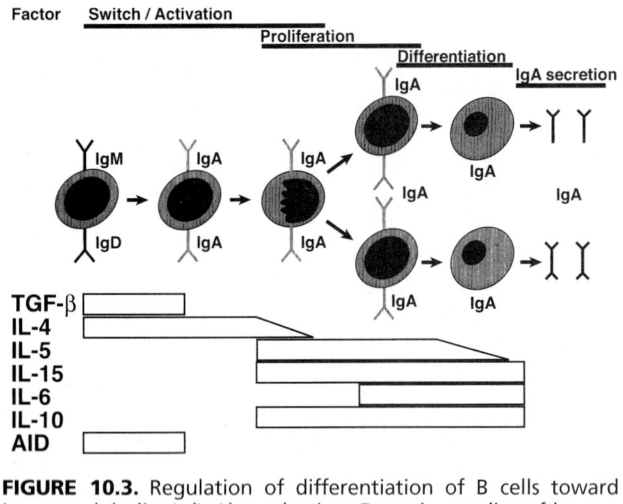

FIGURE 10.3. Regulation of differentiation of B cells toward immunoglobulin A (IgA) production. Extensive studies of human and murine B lymphocytes have revealed that several cytokines are involved in the regulation of switching of sIgM⁺ to sIgA⁺ cells (e.g., TGF-β in humans), their subsequent proliferation [e.g., interleukin (IL)-5 and IL-15], and terminal differentiation (e.g., IL-6 and IL-10). Thus, as currently proposed, a succession of cytokines drives B cells from their early stages through plasma cell differentiation. The mechanisms involved in the regulation of differentiation of human cells to IgA1 or IgA2 production have not been elucidated.

A cytokine-independent pathway of switching of $sIgM^+$ to $sIgA^+$ cells is mediated by a potential RNA editing enzyme, activation-induced cytidine deaminase (AID) (30,31); its overexpression in B cells augments isotype switching from $sIgM^+$ to $sIgA^+$ cells without participation of cytokines. Deficiency of AID in humans is characterized by the hyper-IgM syndrome, with a lack of IgM to IgA switching, a lack of immunoglobulin somatic hypermutation, and lymph node hyperplasia.

MUCOSAL LYMPHOCYTE TRAFFICKING

Lymphocytes stimulated in inductive sites (e.g., PPs) exit via efferent lymphatics and enter mesenteric lymph nodes where they may undergo further division and differentiation (Fig. 10.1) (3,36,37). From there the cells travel via the thoracic duct into the circulation and are dispersed widely in the body. However, these cells selectively accumulate back (or "home") to the intestine and other mucosal sites such as the lactating breast, salivary gland, lacrimal gland, and perhaps genitourinary tissues (38,39), that is, tissue of the common mucosal immune system (Fig. 10.1). However, there is a considerable degree of regionalization or compartmentalization with respect to stimulation at certain inductive sites and migration of sensitized B and T cells to a given effector site (6). For example, intranasal immunization with bacterial products (such as recombinant cholera toxin B subunit) or attenuated viruses not only induce local responses in nasal secretions and in saliva but also in secretions of the female genital tract in both humans and animals (40). The dose and type of antigen, the use of mucosal adjuvants, and the species all influence the magnitude and quality of the ensuing immune response. In humans, the migration of IgA-producing cells from GALT to the lactating breast is an important mechanism that provides specific sIgA antibodies in mothers' milk to protect suckling newborns against the microbes with which the infant is most likely to be colonized (41,42).

This dissemination of antigen-sensitized and IgA-committed cells from inductive sites to remote effector sites has important implications for the design of vaccines that could provide protective immunity at mucosal surfaces, the most frequent portals of entry of infectious agents. In order to populate the lamina propria of the intestine or remote secretory glands, such cells must exit the circulation. Numerous studies suggest that specific interactions between receptors on lymphocytes and their ligands on the endothelial cells of specialized high endothelial venules (HEVs) regulate the selective distribution of lymphocytes to secondary lymphoid tissues (38). The molecular mechanisms of cell trafficking is an area of active research. A number of molecules important in cell migration into mucosae have been identified to date. These lymphocyte molecules and their respective endothelial cell ligands include LFA-1 (CD18/CD11a) binding to ICAM-

1/ICAM-2, VLA-4 binding to VCAM-1, and CD44 binding to a 58- to 66-kDa molecule (43). Recent biochemical characterization of one mucosal vascular addressin receptor, designated the mucosal addressin cell-adhesion molecule (MAdCAM1), which is selectively expressed on HEV of mucosal lymphoid organs and on lamina propria venules, reveals that this receptor displays features common to members of the immunoglobulin gene superfamily (44). MAdCAM1 is composed of three immunoglobulin domains and a 37–amino acid region, localized between the second and third domains, that is rich in serine and threonine, which are potential glycosylation sites for *O*-linked carbohydrates. Interestingly, the first and the second domains display sequences homologous to the human VCAM-1 molecule and the third domain sequences homologous to the CH2 domain of human IgA1. The intervening serine/threonine-rich region exhibits structural features characteristic of mucins and may play a role in lymphocyte binding and migration. MAdCAM1 binds lymphocytes that display on their surfaces $\alpha4\beta7$ integrin. Indeed, peripheral blood lymphocytes including T cells and B cells, particularly of the IgA isotype, from volunteers immunized orally, rectally, or nasally express $\alpha4\beta7$ integrin (45,46). Such lymphocytes are present in peripheral blood 6 to 10 days after immunization, preceding the appearance of specific antibodies in external secretions. The mechanisms involved in preferential homing to selected effector sites (e.g., gut versus genital tract) have not been elucidated, but it is likely that additional homing receptors or chemotactic factors play a decisive role.

The entry of cells into a tissue such as the intestine is a critical component of mucosal immunity as well as of mucosal inflammation. In regard to the latter, inflammatory cytokines increase the expression of endothelial cell ICAM-1 and ELAM-1 during intestinal inflammation (47,48), thus facilitating entry of larger numbers of cells into inflammatory sites. The entry of nonspecific inflammatory cells into the intestine via these molecules is another important element of host defense against infectious pathogens, particularly during early infection before specific immunity has been triggered.

LAMINA PROPRIA CELLS

The intestinal lamina propria contains an abundance of B cells, plasma cells, T cells, and macrophages as well as a lesser number of other cell types such as eosinophils, mast cells, and dendritic cells (6). The intestinal lamina propria is the major site in the body where large numbers of plasma cells are present continuously. Approximately 70% to 90% of the plasma cells in the intestine produce IgA (6,49). The next most common isotype produced is IgM, representing 5% to 15%, followed by IgG, representing only 3% to 5%. IgE and IgD plasma cells are uncommon. Plasma cells are terminally differentiated end-stage cells whose half-life is approximately 5 days (50), indicating that there must be a dynamic, continuous repopulation of lamina propria B cells. The proliferation and differentiation of B cells appear to be regulated by cytokines produced by a broad spectrum of resident cell types, particularly T cells, but also including macrophages and epithelial cells (Fig. 10.3) (32,33,51,52). With respect to differentiation of mucosal B cells into IgA plasma cells, IL-5, IL-6, IL-10, and TGF-β play prominent roles (6,32,53,54), and these cytokines may be derived not only from T cells but also from epithelial cells, which can produce IL-6, IL-10, and TGF-β (52).

Cells isolated from human lamina propria include B cells, T cells, macrophages, and small numbers of mast cells, null cells, and natural killer (NK) cells. The proportions of the cells in such isolates may be different from what is present *in situ*, e.g., plasma cells are typically lost during the isolation procedure. Approximately two-thirds of isolated LP T cells are CD4+ and one-third are CD8+, which is similar to their ratio in peripheral blood. However, LP T cells differ in substantial ways from peripheral blood T cells. Most of the LP T cells have the CD45RO+ CD45RA– phenotype characteristic of memory cells, whereas the converse is true for peripheral blood T cells. Lamina propria T cells are in a higher state of activation based on expression of IL-2Rα chain, HLA-DR molecules, and transferrin receptors. Upon activation, LP T cells produce greater amounts of cytokines such as IL-2, IL-4, IL-5, and interferon-γ (IFN-γ), which is consistent with their increased helper activity for B-cell responses (55). The antigens stimulating this very large T-cell response are unknown, but the dearth of LP T cells in germ-free animals argues strongly that the majority of this response is directed toward antigens of the bacterial flora. Support for this idea has come from studies in T-cell receptor transgenic mice, whose LP T cells remain naïve in the absence of the relevant antigen, despite the presence of a normal bacterial flora (56).

The LP T-cell response to the enteric flora is complex and both effector and regulatory T cells are generated (discussed later). The effects of regulatory cells may explain the report that an individual's LP T cells are immunologically tolerant to the same individual's bacterial flora but respond to the bacterial flora obtained from other individuals (57). The presence of regulatory cells or their mediators may explain also the altered signaling pathways evident in human LP T-cell isolates, which is manifested by diminished responses to signaling via the TCR/CD3 complex, but the normal responses to signaling through CD2 or CD28 (58,59). T cells with markers consistent with cytolytic T-cell function are present in the lamina propria, and functional cytolytic activity has been demonstrated in intestinal lymphocytes by redirected lysis assays (60). Whether such cytolytic activity is brought into play during normal intestinal immune responses is unclear, but such cells could be important in host defense against certain pathogens.

INTRAEPITHELIAL LYMPHOCYTES

Lymphocytes that are physically located within the epithelial layer, or IELs, comprise one of every six to ten cells in the epithelium (61). The cellular composition of this compartment is different from that in either the PP or the lamina propria. Plasma cells and macrophages are not present, and B cells are absent or infrequent. The predominant cell type in small intestinal IEL is the CD8+ T cell, and in most mouse strains, about one-half bear αβ T-cell receptors (TCRs) and the other half γδ TCRs. In mice, IEL are quite heterogeneous based on expression of CD8 isoforms, Thy1, CD5, and cell density (61). Whether similar heterogeneity exists in human IEL is unclear. Analysis of human IEL TCR gene expression shows evidence of oligoclonality (62). In contrast to mice or chickens, human Tγδ cells are a minor component in human IELs, most of which are TCRαβ+, CD8+, CD45RO+. Most existing data on IEL come from studies done on small intestinal isolates. It is interesting, therefore, that mouse colon IELs have been found to consist mainly of CD4+, TCRαβ+ T cells, revealing previously unsuspected regional differences within the intestinal immune system (63,64). Whether similar regional differences exist for the lamina propria compartment is unknown. The environment in the small bowel and colon is dramatically different and so it should not be surprising that the mucosal immune system of these two sites is also different. It is quite possible that these regional differences in mucosal lymphoid populations are an important aspect of host defense against the enteric flora and against pathogens, but no direct evidence of this exists at present.

IEL TCRαβ cells appear to originate in the PP and traffic to the epithelium via the lamina propria (65), but there is also evidence for a thymic-independent lineage of T cells in small intestinal IELs, which bear the CD8αα isoform and are CD5– (61). Thymic-independent CD8αα$^+$ T cells in the IEL originate in cryptopatches, which are small lymphoid tissues in the crypt region of the murine small and large intestine. These lymphoid tissues are characterized by the presence of ckit$^+$, IL-7R+, T-helper-1 (Th1+) lymphoid progenitors (66). In many species, a large proportion of the IELs contain granules that stain metachromatically and resemble mast cell granules, but contain little or no histamine (67).

Multiple functions of IELs in host defense have been proposed. First, IELs have full cytotoxic capabilities including NK, ADCC, and T-cell cytotoxicity. Because IELs increase in number after parasitic infestations, they might serve a cytotoxic function directed primarily at parasites (68). Second, IELs are increased in experimental graft versus host disease, prompting the suggestion that an increase in IELs may be a marker for cell-mediated immune responses in the intestine. Third, IELs very likely defend the epithelium against viral infections by local secretion of IFN-γ and perhaps by direct cytotoxicity (69). They may also produce other cytokines that could influence enterocyte functions. Although little is known about their precise function *in vivo*, IELs are situated in a site that would render them exposed to a variety of antigenic stimuli and thus they likely play an important role in mucosal host defense. Fourth, IELs may play an important role in immune regulation, particularly in mucosal tolerance (69,70).

SECRETORY IgA AND ITS TRANSPORT SYSTEM

The appearance of large amounts of IgA in external secretions, particularly in the intestinal tract, is the result of complex molecular and cellular interactions that have been studied in great detail (for reviews, see references 71 and 72, and see Chapter 12). Most plasma cells at mucosal sites produce IgA in its polymeric (dimeric and tetrameric) form. Intracellular polymerization of monomers and the incorporation of an additional small glycoprotein known as *J chain* within the plasma cell results in the secretion of IgA molecules that can interact with a receptor specific for polymeric immunoglobulins of the IgA and IgM isotypes (6,72). This polyimmunoglobulin receptor (pIgR), whose extracellular part is called *secretory component* (SC), is expressed on the surface of epithelial cells and, in some species, on hepatocytes, and plays a key role in the selective epithelial transport of IgA. After pIgR is synthesized in the rough endoplasmic reticulum and heavily glycosylated in the Golgi complex, it reaches and is inserted into the basolateral membrane of the enterocyte, where it acts as a receptor. Biochemical studies reveal that pIgR belongs to the immunoglobulin superfamily and consists of five immunoglobulin domains (72–74). After the initial interactions of polymeric IgA with pIgR on epithelial cells through noncovalent binding, the first domain of pIgR binds to the Cα3 domain, and the fifth domain binds covalently to the Cα2 domain (75). J chain is essential for polymeric IgA to interact with pIgR, probably by inducing conformational changes in IgA that permit SC binding (76). Following these molecular events, the membrane pIgR/polymeric IgA complex is internalized and transported in vesicles toward the apical surface of the epithelial cells. Once there, these vesicles fuse with the apical membrane. Proteolytic cleavage of pIgR releases the assembled molecule of S-IgA into external secretions. pIgR-mediated transport of polymeric IgA represents a unique system of interaction between a receptor and its ligand: pIgR is produced by epithelial cells regardless of the presence of its ligand and is not recycled. SC remains permanently attached to polymeric IgA, conferring increased resistance on the S-IgA molecule to proteolytic enzymes in the intestinal tract. The importance of J chain for polymerization and pIgR for transport of IgA was convincingly demonstrated in mice with a disrupted J chain gene (76–79). The magnitude of such IgA transport is enormous, comprising 3 to 5 g S-IgA produced and transported each day into the human intestine.

The synthesis and expression of both J chain and pIgR is regulated by cytokines and hormones (72): IL-5, IL-2, and possibly IL-6 up-regulate J-chain synthesis, whereas IL-4, IFN-γ, tumor necrosis factor-α (TNF-α), and TGF-β significantly enhance pIgR expression. Thus, the synthesis of all component chains of S-IgA is regulated by cytokines that are locally produced in the intestinal microenvironment (Fig.10.4).

S-IgA in human external secretions is represented by molecules that are heterogenous with respect to their form and subclass, thereby enhancing S-IgA function (80). Although S-IgA antibodies can have lower affinities for antigens than IgG antibodies, the presence of four antigen-binding sites in a dimeric and eight sites in tetrameric S-IgA molecule endows them with high avidity due to the bonus effect of multivalency. Mucosal Ig and S-IgA in particular contain polyreactive antibodies with respect to microbes, with shared specificities to autoantigens that serve to protect the mucosa (81–83). IgA antibodies are able to interfere with IgG-mediated complement activation and thus provide an antiinflammatory activity, which may contribute to mucosal homeostasis in the face of the abundant and potentially inflammatory microbiota in the gut (2). In addition to its specific binding, S-IgA may prevent the adherence and penetration of intestinal bacteria by nonspecific binding of its heavy chain–associated glycan moieties, particularly those with high mannose content, to bacterial ligands (e.g., type I fimbriae). In this way, S-IgA may also prevent the interaction between bacterial ligands and their corresponding receptors expressed on intestinal epithelial cells (84).

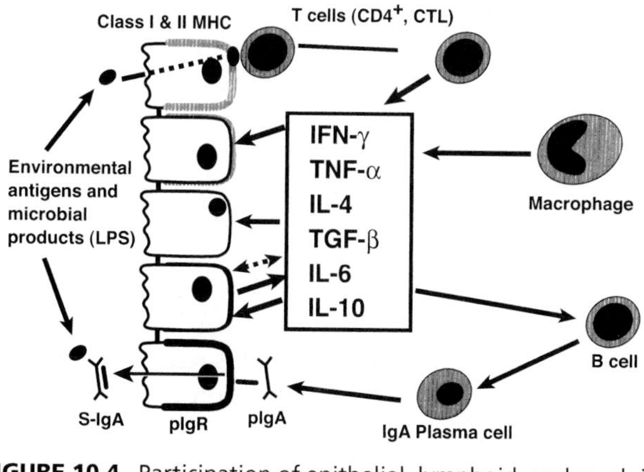

FIGURE 10.4. Participation of epithelial, lymphoid, and myeloid cells in cytokine networks of mucosal tissues. Epithelial cells are in constant contact with the antigens and bioactive products of microbes, which activate epithelial cells to produce a variety of cytokines that can interact with mucosal immune cells. Epithelial cells also can express class II major histocompatibility complex (MHC) molecules and thus potentially act as antigen-presenting cells to induce either immunity or tolerance. In turn, mucosal immune cells produce local cytokines that act on epithelial cells. The physiologic consequences for epithelial cell function are still being defined, but these cytokines can increase expression of certain molecules such as MHC class II molecules and polyimmunoglobulin receptor secretory components, as well as further enhance epithelial cell cytokine production.

In humans, there are two subclasses of IgA: IgA1 and IgA2 (80,85). Plasma cells producing IgA1 and IgA2 molecules are unequally distributed in systemic and mucosal lymphoid compartments (6,85,86). IgA1-producing cells predominate in the bone marrow, spleen, lymph nodes, respiratory tract, and gastric, jejunal, and ileal mucosae, whereas equal proportions of IgA1-and IgA2-producing cells are present in the large intestine and female genital tract. This distribution of IgA1- and IgA2-producing cells may be the result of clonal expansion induced by certain types of antigens. Most of the S-IgA antibodies with specificity to bacterial lipopolysaccharides (endotoxin), lipoteichoic acid, and polysaccharides are of the IgA2 subclass, whereas S-IgA antibodies to proteins and glycoproteins are predominantly of the IgA1 subclass (80,85). Thus, the preponderance of IgA2-producing cells in the large intestine is more likely due to the clonal expansion of cells producing antibodies to bacterial antigens rather than to differences in the expression of homing receptors on B cells that produce IgA1 rather than IgA2.

The liver can also transport IgA (71,72,87–89) as well as IgA immune complexes (90,91). This pathway is particularly important in certain rodents (e.g., the rat, in which 90% of intestinal sIgA is transported through the liver) (89). In humans, this pathway appears to be of minor importance (92); moreover, IgA transport occurs in humans through bile ductular cells rather than through the hepatocyte (93,94).

In contrast to some common species of laboratory animals (e.g., rats, rabbits, and mice), human external secretions, including those of the gastrointestinal tract, contain only small amounts of antibodies of plasma origin (71,72,92). Apparently, intravascular pIgA has limited access to the polymeric IgA receptor (pIgR), partly because of competition with pIgA produced locally in the gut by abundant subepithelial plasma cells. It is estimated that only 1% to 2% of intestinal immunoglobulin originates from plasma (92).

IMMUNOLOGIC FUNCTIONS OF INTESTINAL EPITHELIAL CELLS

Mucosal surfaces of the gastrointestinal tract, which represent by far the largest area of the contact with the external environment, are lined by enormous numbers of various types of epithelial cells. In addition to their mechanical barrier function, epithelial cells play an essential role in the innate as well as specific mucosal immune defense (24,51,52,95–101). In regard to innate defense, various populations of mucosal epithelial cells produce inorganic (HCl) and organic acids, mucins, lysozyme, lactoferrin, and antibacterial peptides (102), which all serve to protect the host against microbes

(Fig. 10.5). Furthermore, epithelial cells secrete complement factors C3, C4, and factor B, which are involved in classic, alternate, and lectin pathways of activation (103). Intestinal epithelial cells have on their surface a number of bacterial-specific receptors, such as members of the toll-like receptor family. Thus, epithelial cells can sense the presence and the composition of the luminal flora. The details of the epithelial cell response to such signals are being defined, but it is clear that epithelial cells are in "dialogue" with luminal bacteria and that such communication can alter gene expression in the epithelial layer (104).

Epithelial cells express many cytokine receptors and are also a source of cytokines that mediate biologically important functions in the intestinal tract (Fig. 10.6). Production of inflammatory (e.g., IL-1, IL-8) and regulatory (e.g., IL-6, IL-7, IL-10, IL-15) cytokines and chemokines (e.g., IL-8, RANTES, MIP-1β) have been observed in various human epithelial cell lines *in vitro* as well as in primary epithelial cells from normal jejunum. The production of cytokines and chemokines can be stimulated by certain viruses, bacteria, and bacterial products (95,96,100,101) and appears to be regulated by resident T cells. Thus, the exposure to invasive strains of Salmonellae profoundly up-regulates NFκB, which, in turn, activates genes that encode proinflammatory cytokines and chemokines, such as IL-8. In an interesting twist to this result, noninvasive *Salmonella* spp., which do not up-regulate NFκB in epithelial cells, appear to prevent the degradation of IκB, the major inhibitor of NFκB and thereby provide an antiinflammatory signal to the epithelial cell (106). It will be of great interest to learn whether products of commensal bacteria can do the same. As mentioned earlier, epithelial cells produce cytokines involved in the differentiation of B cells toward IgA-producing lymphoblast and plasma cells, including TGF-β, IL-10, and IL-6. Considering the enormous numbers of epithelial cells lining the gastrointestinal tract and other mucosal membranes, they may be one of the most important sources of cytokines in the body.

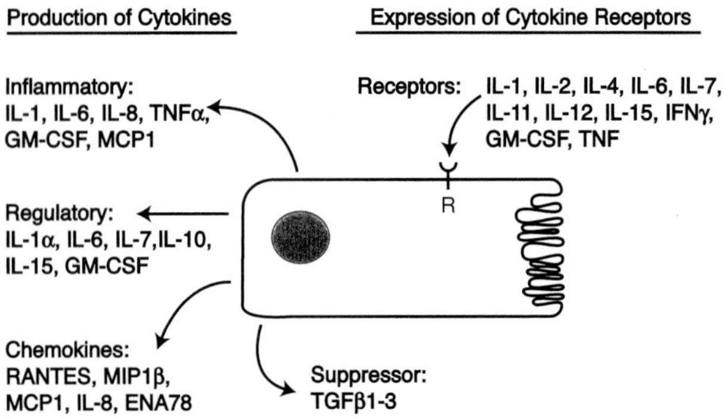

FIGURE 10.6. Production of cytokines and expression of cytokine receptors by epithelial cells. Compilation of data generated in human and animal primary epithelial cells and epithelial cell lines convincingly demonstrate that unstimulated and stimulated epithelial cells are capable of producing a broad array of proinflammatory and regulatory cytokines, which, in turn, influence local mucosal events, including influx of cells, differentiation, activation, or suppression of lymphocyte functions and other activities.

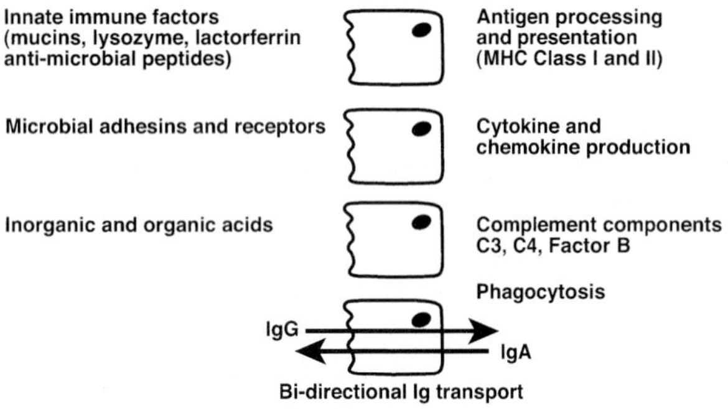

FIGURE 10.5. Immunologic functions of mucosal epithelial cells. Many recent studies have convincingly demonstrated that mucosal epithelial cells play essential roles in defense mechanisms, including the production of innate immune factors, cytokines and chemokines, and the transport of Ig of the three major isotypes from intestinal lumen into the circulation [milk immunoglobulin (Ig)G in certain animal species] and locally produced polymeric IgA (and IgM) into the external secretions.

Depending on the species, epithelial cells are involved in a bidirectional transport of immunoglobulins of all major isotypes (42). In species with nonexistent transplacental transport of maternal antibodies (e.g., pigs, cows, horses), ingestion of antibody-containing colostrum and milk is essential for the survival of the offspring, because IgG antibodies are absorbed from the gut of the suckling newborn into the circulation. However, even nonabsorbed antibodies delivered into the intestinal lumen after the closure of the temporarily permeable epithelial barrier exhibit a protective effect (42). Although immunoglobulins are not absorbed in significant quantities from the gut lumen of other neonates, including humans, the protective effects of breast-feeding or of passively administered antibodies prepared from human or bovine milk and serum or from eggs of immunized hens have proved effective in the prevention and treatment of gastrointestinal infections (42). A novel receptor capable of binding monomeric IgA has been recently described on human epithelial cell lines; its function in mucosal immunity remains to be explored (97).

A number of *in vitro* studies have demonstrated that intestinal epithelial cells can present antigen to primed T cells (99). Intestinal epithelial cells in the small intestine and, to a lesser extent, in the colon express functional class II MHC molecules, and their level of expression in intestinal cell lines can be up-regulated by IFN-γ treatment. On the other hand, epithelial cells lack costimulatory molecules such as B7-1 and B7-2. Whether epithelial cells actually present antigen to T cells *in vivo* remains an open question. Reports from several laboratories indicate that epithelial cells express nonclassic class I MHC molecules (CD1) that can interact with the T-cell receptor of $CD8^+$ T cells and can result in T-cell activation when costimulated by the interaction of CD8 with an epithelial cell 180-kD glycoprotein (99). The importance of these findings to *in vivo* antigen presentation and activation of $CD8^+$ T cells in the intraepithelial and lamina propria compartments awaits further experimentation.

Epithelial cells change their phenotype and function during the process of differentiation and migration from crypt to the tip of the villi. During this upward movement toward the gut lumen, which takes 2 to 3 days (107), columnar epithelial cells alter their gene expression. Crypt epithelial cells express pIgR and efficiently transport pIgA, but they do not express class II MHC antigens (6). Villus epithelial cells no longer express pIgR and therefore do not transport IgA; rather, they express class II MHC and perhaps function as antigen-presenting cells. Dynamic studies of the production of cytokines and expression of other immunologically important cell surface markers during the differentiation of epithelial cells from crypt to villus are rather limited.

As mentioned previously, epithelial cells interact with bacteria in the lumen. The bacterial flora represents not only a large mass of microbes but also an extraordinary diverse array of species, many of which have never been cultured *ex vivo* (7). Some of these microbes can bind to the epithelial cell surface via specific cell surface molecules. Such binding, particularly if it leads to microbial invasion, triggers the epithelial cell to produce cytokines, which, in turn, have effects on mucosal lymphoid cells (108). The response of the lymphoid cells to this cytokine signaling very likely modulates the bacterial flora. Thus, the bacterial flora, epithelium, and mucosal lymphoid cells can be viewed as an interacting circuit, with signals passing in both directions. This communication may contribute to the known protective effects of the commensal flora against mucosal pathogens (110).

REGULATION OF THE INTESTINAL MUCOSAL IMMUNE SYSTEM

Immunity to antigens after intestinal exposure is well documented following natural infections in humans and oral immunization regimens in experimental animals. For example, the large quantity of IgA produced in the intestine reflects a continuous and active mucosal immune response to antigens in the environment. The mechanisms by which this response is regulated are currently being defined, but T cells likely play a major role. Murine CD4+ T cells can be subdivided into two effector types based on the cytokines that they secrete and thus the functions that they serve (Fig. 10.7). Th1 CD4+ cells produce IL-2 and IFN-γ and medi-

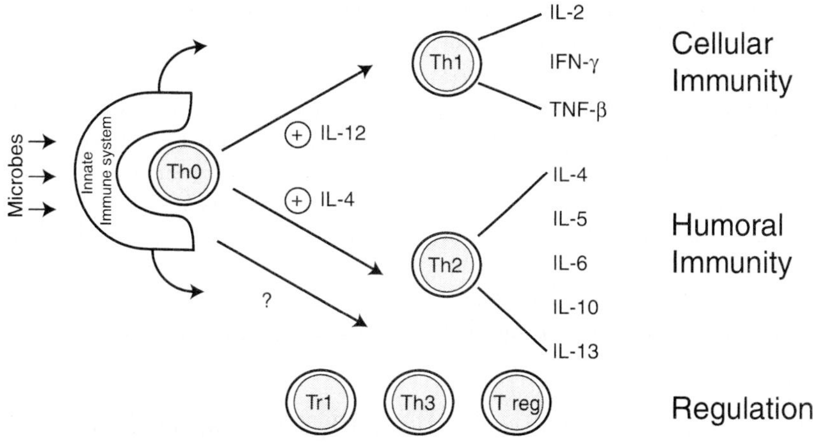

FIGURE 10.7. T-cell differentiation pathways induced by microbes. The initial encounter of microbes is with cells of the innate immune system (antigen-presenting cells, mast cells, granulocytes, stromal cells). This system provides a rapid but nonspecific response. Specific responses are generated by the presentation of microbial antigens by cells of the innate immune system to naive CD4+ T cells. Depending on the cytokine milieu in the microenvironment and other factors, CD4+ T-helper (Th) cells differentiate along one of several pathways, that is, into Th1 effector cells that mediate cellular immune responses or into Th2 effector cells that mediate humoral immunity. Th1 and Th2 cells are distinguished by their production of certain cytokines as shown. For a given microbe, the predominant effector pathway stimulated can determine whether the infection results in disease or recovery. CD4+ T cells can differentiate also into T-regulatory cells, such as T-regulatory-1 (Tr1) or T-helper-3 cells (Th3), which produce the inhibitory cytokines interleukin (IL)-10 or transforming growth factor (TGF)-β1, respectively. Other regulatory subsets (T reg) have been described, but whether they play a role in the mucosal immune system is unclear. T regulatory cells inhibit both the Th1 and Th2 subsets. Th1 and Th2 subsets can regulate one another in some systems, but this has not been demonstrated as yet at mucosal surfaces.

ate delayed hypersensitivity responses; Th2 CD4+ T cells produce IL-4, IL-5, IL-6, and IL-10 and serve as helper cells for B-cell responses (Fig. 10.4) (111). A number of other CD4 T-cell subsets have been identified that serve to regulate these T-effector subsets (111). Two of these—T-regulatory-1 (Tr1) cells and T-helper-3 (Th3) cells—produce the inhibitory cytokines IL-10 and TGF-β1, respectively, and have been found to be important in the intestinal mucosa. The balance between effector and regulatory T-cell subsets is very important in maintaining mucosal homeostasis and host defense (112). The factors that determine whether Th1, Th2, or T regulatory cells will predominate in the response to a given antigen are important but as yet not understood. The current notion is that the initial encounter of the microbe with cells of the innate immune system (e.g., macrophages, granulocytes, mast cells, epithelial cells) stimulates the production of certain cytokines (e.g., IL-12 or IL-4), which induce differentiation down the Th1 or Th2 pathway, respectively (Fig. 10.7). The cytokines that are important in induction of T regulatory cells are unknown.

The importance of the balance of T-effector and T-regulatory cells in the maintenance of mucosal homeostasis is illustrated by a number of experimental models in which this balance is perturbed and chronic intestinal inflammation results (113). For example, deletion of certain genes of the immune system in mice (e.g., IL-2, IL-10, or TGF-β1, among others) results in chronic intestinal inflammation in the absence of any further manipulation. Such experiments are defining the critical cells and molecules that are essential for the proper regulation of the mucosal immune response. In virtually every instance where it has been tested, the bacterial flora drives the disease, highlighting once again the immunologic challenge that the enteric flora represents to the host. Most of these experimental models appear to be due to defective immune regulation of the T-cell response to the enteric flora; this is the leading hypothesis to explain the pathogenesis of chronic inflammatory bowel disease in humans as well (113). The induction of T-effector versus T-regulatory cell responses to mucosal pathogens is likely also a critical factor in host response to infection, but one that has not yet been studied.

The presence of regulatory cells and other regulatory mechanisms in the mucosa is likely involved not only in the induction of humoral and cell-mediated immunity but also in the phenomenon of oral tolerance, in which the feeding of an antigen before parenteral immunization can induce a state of systemic unresponsiveness instead of immunity (Fig. 10.8) (114). Oral tolerance has been demonstrated in animals after the feeding of a variety of antigens, including proteins, contact allergens, heterologous erythrocytes, and viral hemagglutinin. Multiple mechanisms of tolerance have been demonstrated, including clonal deletion, clonal anergy, and the generation of regulatory T cells in GALT. An example of the latter is the Th3 regulatory cell, which secretes TGF-β1, an inhibitory cytokine (115). Feeding

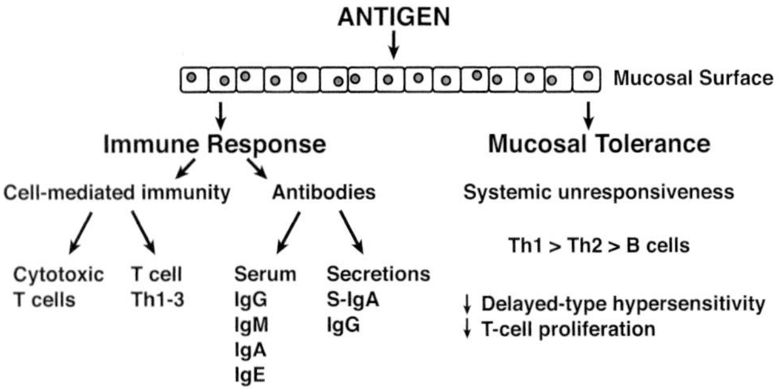

FIGURE 10.8. Immunologic consequences and types of responses induced by the exposure of mucosal surfaces to antigens. Concomitant induction of cellular and humoral immune responses on one hand and mucosal tolerance (*systemic* unresponsiveness to mucosally encountered antigen) on the other are the most important features. Many factors, including the dose, type, frequency, and site of antigen stimulation, and the age and species of the host influence the outcome of a response to favor induction of immunity or tolerance

autoantigens has been used to abrogate or treat experimental autoimmune diseases, but, thus far, trials in humans have had limited success. The feeding of a protein antigen to human volunteers did result in T-cell tolerance, establishing that oral tolerance does exist in humans (116). Whether protein antigens of bacterial origin can induce oral tolerance is unclear. Bacterial LPS given together with a nonbacterial antigen increased the degree of oral tolerance to the latter (117), so that the presence of highly stimulatory adjuvant molecules in microbes does not necessarily shift the mucosal response away from a tolerizing one. There have been very few studies in which enteric bacteria or their antigens have been tested for their ability to induce oral tolerance, but data suggest that individuals are immunologically tolerant to antigens of their own bacterial flora (57). The factors that determine whether tolerance or immunity occurs after a mucosal encounter with microbial antigens need to be defined. This is clearly an important consideration both for the outcome of any encounter with an intestinal pathogen as well as for the development of oral vaccines against such infectious agents.

ACKNOWLEDGMENTS

This work was supported by NIH grants DK44240, and AI35999, and AI28147.

REFERENCES

1. McGhee JR, Mestecky J. In defense of mucosal surfaces. Development of novel vaccines for IgA responses protective at the portals of entry of microbial pathogens. *Infect Dis Clin North Am* 1990;4:315–341.
2. Russell MW, Kilian M, Lamm ME. Biological activities of IgA. In: Ogra PL, Mestecky J, Lamm ME, et al., eds. *Mucosal*

immunology, second edition. New York: Academic Press, 1999: 225–240.

3. Mestecky J, Abram R, Ogra PL. Common mucosal immune system and strategies for the development of vaccines effective at the mucosal surfaces. In: Ogra PL, Mestecky J, Lamm M, et al., eds. *Handbook of mucosal immunology.* San Diego: Academic Press, 1994:357–372.
4. McGhee JR, Czerkinsky C, Mestecky J. Mucosal vaccines: an overview. In: Ogra PL, Mestecky J, Lamm ME, et al., eds. *Mucosal immunology,* second edition. New York: Academic Press, 1999:741–758.
5. Mestecky J, Fultz PN. Mucosal immune system of the human genital tract. *J Infect Dis* 1999;179[Suppl 3]:S470–S474.
6. Brandtzaeg P, Farstad IN, Johansen FE, et al. The B-cell system of human mucosae and exocrine glands. *Immunol Rev* 1999; 171:45–87.
7. Savage DC. Mucosal microbiota. In: Ogra PL, Mestecky J, Lamm ME, et al., eds. *Mucosal immunology,* second edition. New York: Academic Press, 1999:19–30.
8. Crabbe PA, Bazin H, Eyssen H, et al. The normal microbial flora as a major stimulus for proliferation of plasma cells synthesizing IgA in the gut. The germ-free intestinal tract. *Int Arch Allergy Appl Immunol* 1968;34:362–375.
9. Abrams GD, Bauer H, Sprinz H. Influence of the normal flora on mucosal morphology and cellular renewal in the ileum. *Lab Invest* 1963;12:355–364.
10. Cornes JS. Number, size, and distribution of Peyer's patches in the human small intestine. I. The development of Peyer's patches. *Gut* 1965;6:225–233.
11. Neutra MR, Kraehenbuhl J-P. Cellular and molecular basis for antigen transport across epithelial barriers. In: Ogra PL, Mestecky J, Lamm ME, et al., eds. *Mucosal immunology,* second edition. New York: Academic Press, 1999:101–114.
12. Kerneis S, Bogdanova A, Kraehenbuhl JP, et al. Conversion by Peyer's patch lymphocytes of human enterocytes into M cells that transport bacteria. *Science* 1997;277:949–952.
13. Kelsall BL, Strober W. Distinct populations of dendritic cells are present in the subepithelial dome and T cell regions of the murine Peyer's patch. *J Exp Med* 1996;183:237–247.
14. Iwasaki A, Kelsall BL. Freshly isolated Peyer's patch, but not spleen, dendritic cells produce interleukin 10 and induce the differentiation of T helper type 2 cells. *J Exp Med* 1999;190: 229–239.
15. Liu LM, MacPherson GG. Antigen acquisition by dendritic cells: intestinal dendritic cells acquire antigen administered orally and can prime naive T cells *in vivo. J Exp Med* 1993;177:1299–1307.
16. Viney JL, Mowat AM, O'Malley JM, et al. Expanding dendritic cells *in vivo* enhances the induction of oral tolerance. *J Immunol* 1998;160:5815–5825.
17. Guy-Grand D, Griscelli C, Vassalli P. Peyer's patches, gut IgA plasma cells and thymic function: study in nude mice bearing thymic grafts. *J Immunol* 1975;115:361–364.
18. Kagnoff MF. Functional characteristics of Peyer's patch cells. IV. Effect of antigen feeding on the frequency of antigen-specific B cells. *J Immunol* 1977;118:992–997.
19. Yamamoto M, Rennert P, McGhee JR, et al. Alternate mucosal immune system: organized Peyer's patches are not required for IgA responses in the gastrointestinal tract. *J Immunol* 2000;164: 5184–5191.
20. Kroese FGM, Bos NA. Peritoneal B-1 cells switch *in vivo* to IgA and these IgA antibodies can bind to bacteria of the normal intestinal microflora. *Curr Top Microbiol Immunol* 1999;246: 343–349.
21. Murakami M, Honjo T. Involvement of B-1 cells in mucosal immunity and autoimmunity. *Immunol Today* 1995;16:534–539.
22. Kroese FGM, Kantor AB, Herzenberg LA. The role of B-1 cells in mucosal immune responses. In: Ogra PL, Mestecky J, Lamm ME, et al., eds. *Handbook of mucosal immunology.* San Diego: Academic Press, 1994:217–224.
23. Macpherson AJ, Gatto D, Sainsbury E, et al. A primitive T cell-independent mechanism of intestinal mucosal IgA responses to commensal bacteria. *Science* 2000;288:2222–2226.
24. Booth C, Potten CS. Gut instincts: thoughts on intestinal epithelial stem cells. *J Clin Invest* 2000;105:1493–1499.
25. Donze HH, Lue C, Julian BA, et al. Human peritoneal B-1 cells and the influence of continuous ambulatory peritoneal dialysis on peritoneal and peripheral blood mononuclear cell (PBMC) composition and immunoglobulin levels. *Clin Exp Immunol* 1997;109:356–361.
26. Craig SW, Cebra JJ. Peyer's patches: an enriched source of precursors for IgA-producing immunocytes in the rabbit. *J Exp Med* 1971;134:188–200.
27. Gearhart PJ, Cebra JJ. Differentiated B lymphocytes. Potential to express particular antibody variable and constant regions depends on site of lymphoid tissue and antigen load. *J Exp Med* 1979;149:216–227.
28. Spalding DM, Williamson SI, Koopman WJ, et al. Preferential induction of polyclonal IgA secretion by murine Peyer's patch dendritic cell-T cell mixtures. *J Exp Med* 1984;160:941–946.
29. Coffman RL, Lebman DA, Shrader B. Transforming growth factor beta specifically enhances IgA production by lipopolysaccharide-stimulated murine B lymphocytes. *J Exp Med* 1989; 170:1039–1044.
30. Muramatsu M, Kinoshita K, Fagarasan S, et al. Class switch recombination and hypermutation require activation-induced cytidine deaminase (AID), a potential RNA editing enzyme *Cell* 2000;102:553–563.
31. Revy P, Muto T, Levy Y, et al. Activation-induced cytidine deaminase (AID) deficiency causes the autosomal recessive form of the hyper-IgM syndrome (HIGM2). *Cell* 2000;102:565–575.
32. Kelsall B, Strober W. Gut-associated lymphoid tissue: antigen handling and T-lymphocyte responses. In: Ogra PL, Mestecky J, Lamm ME, et al., eds. *Mucosal immunology,* second edition. New York: Academic Press, 1999:293–317.
33. McIntyre TM, Strober W. Gut-associated lymphoid tissue: regulation of IgA B-cell development. In: Ogra PL, Mestecky J, Lamm ME, et al., eds. *Mucosal immunology,* second edition. New York: Academic Press, 1999:319–356.
34. Coste A, Sirard JC, Johansen K, et al. Nasal immunization of mice with virus-like particles protects offspring against rotavirus diarrhea. *J Virol* 2000;74:8966–8977.
35. Wu H-Y, Abdu S, Stinson D, et al. Generation of female genital tract antibody responses by local or central (common) mucosal immunization. *Infect Immun* 2000;68:5539–5545.
36. Scicchitano R, Stanisz A, Ernst P, et al. A common mucosal immune system revisited. In: Husband AJ, ed. *Migration and homing of lymphoic cells,* vol 2. Boca Raton: CRC Press, 1988:1–35.
37. Phillips-Quagliata JM, Lamm ME. Lymphocyte homing to mucosal effector sites. In: Ogra PL, Mestecky J, Lamm ME, et al., eds. *Handbook of mucosal immunology.* San Diego: Academic Press, 1994;225–234.
38. Butcher EC. Lymphocyte homing and intestinal immunity. In: Ogra PL, Mestecky J, Lamm ME, et al., eds. *Mucosal immunology,* second edition. New York: Academic Press, 1999:507–522.
39. Rothkotter HJ, Hriesik C, Barman NN, et al. B and also T lymphocytes migrate via gut lymph to all lymphoid organs and the gut wall, but only IgA+ cells accumulate in the lamina propria of the intestinal mucosa. *Eur J Immunol* 1999;29:327–333.
40. Russell MW, Moldoveanu Z, White PL, et al. Salivary, nasal, genital, and systemic antibody responses in monkeys immunized intranasally with a bacterial protein antigen and the cholera toxin B subunit. *Infect Immun* 1996;64:1272–1283.

41. Goldblum RM, Ahlstedt S, Carlsson B, et al. Antibody forming cells in human colostrum after oral immunization. *Nature* 1975;257:797–799.
42. Mestecky J, Russell MW. Passive and active protection against disorders of the gut. *Vet Q* 1998;20:S83–S87.
43. Salmi M, Jalkanen S. Regulation of lymphocyte traffic to mucosa-associated lymphatic tissues. *Gastroenterol Clin North Am* 1991;20:495–510.
44. Brisken MJ, McEvoy LM, Butcher EC. MAdCAM-1 has homology to immunoglobulin and mucin-like adhesion receptors and to IgA1. *Nature* 1993;363:461–464.
45. Kantele A, Hakkinen M, Moldoveanu Z, et al. Differences in immune responses induced by oral and rectal immunizations with *Salmonella typhi* Ty21a: evidence for compartmentalization within the common mucosal immune system in humans. *Infect Immun* 1998;66:5630–5635.
46. Kantele A, Zivny J, Hakkinen M, et al. Differential homing commitments of antigen-specific T cells after oral or parenteral immunization in humans. *J Immunol* 1999;162:5173–5177.
47. Koizumi M, King N, Lobb R, et al. Expression of vascular adhesion molecules in inflammatory bowel disease. *Gastroenterology* 1992;103:840–847.
48. Nakamura S, Ohtani H, Watanabe Y, et al. *In situ* expression of the cell adhesion molecules in inflammatory bowel disease. Evidence of immunologic activation of vascular endothelial cells. *Lab Invest* 1993;69:77–85.
49. McGhee JR, Lamm ME, Strober W. Mucosal immune responses. In: Ogra PL, Mestecky J, Lamm ME, et al., eds. *Mucosal immunology,* second edition. New York: Academic Press, 1999:485–506.
50. Mattioli CA, Tomasi TBJ. The life span of IgA plasma cells from the mouse intestine. *J Exp Med* 1973;138:452–460.
51. Goodrich ME, McGee DW. Preferential enhancement of B cell IgA secretion by intestinal epithelial cell-derived cytokines and interleukin-2. *Immunol Invest* 1999;28:67–75.
52. Goodrich ME, McGee DW. Effect of intestinal epithelial cell cytokines on mucosal B-cell IgA secretion: enhancing effect of epithelial-derived IL-6 but not TGF-beta on IgA+ B cells. *Immunol Letters* 1999;67:11–14.
53. Lebman DA, Lee FD, Coffman RL. Mechanism for transforming growth factor beta and IL-2 enhancement of IgA expression in lipopolysaccharide-stimulated B cell cultures. *J Immunol* 1990;144:952–959.
54. Banchereau J, de Paoli P, Valle A, et al. Long-term human B cell lines dependent on interleukin-4 and antibody to CD40. *Science* 1991;251:70–72.
55. Zeitz M, Quinn TC, Graeff AS, et al. Mucosal T cells provide helper function but do not proliferate when stimulated by specific antigen in lymphogranuloma venereum proctitis in nonhuman primates. *Gastroenterology* 1988;94:353–366.
56. Saparov A, Kraus LA, Cong Y, et al. Memory/effector T cells in TCR transgenic mice develop via recognition of enteric antigens by a second, endogenous TCR. *Int Immunol* 1999;11:1253–1264.
57. Duchmann R, Kaiser I, Hermann E, et al. Tolerance exists towards resident intestinal flora but is broken in active inflammatory bowel disease (IBD). *Clin Exp Immunol* 1995;102:448–455.
58. Qiao L, Schurmann G, Betzler M, et al. Activation and signaling status of human lamina propria T lymphocytes. *Gastroenterology* 1991;101:1529–1536.
59. James SP, Kiyono H. Gastrointestinal lamina propria T cells. In: Ogra PL, Mestecky J, Lamm ME, et al., eds. *Mucosal immunology,* second edition. New York: Academic Press, 1999:381–396.
60. London SD, Rubin DH. Functional role of mucosal cytotoxic lymphocytes. In: Ogra PL, Mestecky J, Lamm ME, et al., eds. *Mucosal immunology,* second edition. New York: Academic Press, 1999:643–656.
61. Lefrancois L, Puddington L. Basic aspects of intraepithelial lymphocyte biology. In: Ogra PL, Mestecky J, Lamm ME, et al., eds. *Mucosal immunology,* second edition. New York: Academic Press, 1999:413–428.
62. Blumberg RS, Yockey CE, Gross GG, et al. Human intestinal intraepithelial lymphocytes are derived from a limited number of T cell clones that utilize multiple V beta T cell receptor genes. *J Immunol* 1993;150:5144–5153.
63. Beagley KW, Fujihashi K, Lagoo AS, et al. Differences in intraepithelial lymphocyte T cell subsets isolated from murine small versus large intestine. *J Immunol* 1995;154:5611–5619.
64. Camerini V, Panwala C, Kronenberg M. Regional specialization of the mucosal immune system. Intraepithelial lymphocytes of the large intestine have a different phenotype and function than those of the small intestine. *J Immunol* 1993;151:1765–1776.
65. Guy-Grand D, Griscelli C, Vassalli P. The mouse gut T lymphocyte, a novel type of T cell. Nature, origin, and traffic in mice in normal and graft-versus-host conditions. *J Exp Med* 1978;148:1661–1667.
66. Saito H, Kanamori Y, Takemori T, et al. Generation of intestinal T cells from progenitors residing in gut cryptopatches. *Science* 1998;280:275–278.
67. Cerf-Bensussan N, Guy-Grand D, Griscelli C. Intraepithelial lymphocytes of human gut: isolation, characterization and study of natural killer activity. *Gut* 1985;26:81–88.
68. Findly RC, Roberts SJ, Hayday AC. Dynamic response of murine gut intraepithelial T cells after infection by the coccidian parasite Eimeria. *Eur J Immunol* 1993;23:2557–2564.
69. Aranda R, Sydora BC, Kronenberg M. Intraepithelial lymphocytes: function. In: Ogra PL, Mestecky J, Lamm ME, et al., eds. *Mucosal immunology,* second edition. New York: Academic Press, 1999:429–438.
70. Vezys V, Olson S, Lefrancois L. Expression of intestine-specific antigen reveals novel pathways of CD8 T cell tolerance induction. *Immunity* 2000;12:505–514.
71. Mestecky J, Lue C, Russell MW. Selective transport of IgA. Cellular and molecular aspects. *Gastroenterol Clin North Am* 1991; 20:441–471.
72. Mostov K, Kaetzel CS. Immunoglobulin transport and the polymeric immunoglobulin receptor. In: Ogra PL, Mestecky J, Lamm ME, et al., eds. *Mucosal immunology,* second edition. New York: Academic Press, 1999:181–211.
73. Mostov KE, Friedlander M, Blobel G. The receptor for transepithelial transport of IgA and IgM contains multiple immunoglobulin-like domains. *Nature* 1984;308:37–43.
74. Eiffert H, Quentin E, Wiederhold M, et al. Determination of the molecular structure of the human free secretory component. *Biol Chem Hoppe Seyler* 1991;372:119–128.
75. Hexham JM, White KD, Carayannopoulos LN, et al. A human immunoglobulin (Ig)A Ca3 domain motif directs polymeric Ig receptor-mediated secretion. *J Exp Med* 1999;189:747–752.
76. Johansen FE, Braathen R, Brandtzaeg P. Role of J chain in secretory immunoglobulin formation. *Scand J Immunol* 2000;52: 240–248.
77. Johansen FE, Pekna M, Norderhaug IN, et al. Absence of epithelial immunoglobulin A transport, with increased mucosal leakiness, in polymeric immunoglobulin receptor/secretory component-deficient mice. *J Exp Med* 1999;190:915–922.
78. Hendrickson BA, Rindisbacher L, Corthesy B, et al. Lack of association of secretory component with IgA in J chain-deficient mice. *J Immunol* 1996;157:750–754.
79. Shimada S, Kawaguchi-Miyashita M, Kushiro A, et al. Generation of polymeric immunoglobulin receptor-deficient mouse with marked reduction of secretory IgA. *J Immunol* 1999;163: 5367–5373.
80. Mestecky J, Moro I, Underdown BJ. Mucosal immunoglobu-

lins. In: Ogra PL, Mestecky J, Lamm ME, et al., eds. *Mucosal immunology,* second edition. New York: Academic Press, 1999: 133–152.

81. Bouvet JP, Dighiero G. From natural polyreactive autoantibodies to a la carte monoreactive antibodies to infectious agents: is it a small world after all? *Infect Immun* 1998;66:1–4.
82. Bouvet JP, Fischetti VA. Diversity of antibody-mediated immunity at the mucosal barrier. *Infect Immun* 1999;67:2687–2691.
83. Quan CP, Berneman A, Pires R, et al. Natural polyreactive secretory immunoglobulin A autoantibodies as a possible barrier to infection in humans. *Infect Immun* 1997;65:3997–4004.
84. Wold AE, Mestecky J, Tomana M, et al. Secretory immunoglobulin A carries oligosaccharide receptors for *Escherichia coli* type 1 fimbrial lectin. *Infect Immun* 1990;58:3073–3077.
85. Mestecky J, Russell MW. IgA subclasses. In: Shakib F, ed. *Basic and clinical aspects of IgG subclasses,* vol 19. Basel: S Karger, 1986:277–301.
86. Crago SS, Kutteh WH, Moro I, et al. Distribution of IgA1-, IgA2-, and J chain-containing cells in human tissues. *J Immunol* 1984;132:16–18.
87. Peppard JV, Russell MW. Phylogenetic development and comparative physiology of IgA. In: Ogra PL, Mestecky J, Lamm ME, et al., eds. *Mucosal Immunology,* second edition. New York: Academic Press, 1999:163–179.
88. Lemaitre-Coelho I, Jackson GD, Vaerman JP. High levels of secretory IgA and free secretory component in the serum of rats with bile duct obstruction. *J Exp Med* 1978;147:934–939.
89. Jackson GD, Lemaitre-Coelho I, Vaerman JP, et al. Rapid disappearance from serum of intravenously injected rat myeloma IgA and its secretion into bile. *Eur J Immunol* 1978;8:123–126.
90. Peppard J, Orlans E, Payne AWR, et al. The elimination of circulating complexes containing polymeric IgA by excretion into the bile. *Immunology* 1981;42:83–89.
91. Russell MW, Brown TA, Mestecky J. Role of serum IgA. Hepatobiliary transport of circulating antigens. *J Exp Med* 1981;153: 968–976.
92. Delacroix DL, Hodgson HJ, McPherson A, et al. Selective transport of polymeric immunoglobulin A in bile. Quantitative relationships of monomeric and polymeric immunoglobulin A, immunoglobulin M, and other proteins in serum, bile, and saliva. *J Clin Invest* 1982;70:230–241.
93. Smith PD, Nagura H, Nakane PK, et al. IgA in human hepatic bile and liver. *J Immunol* 1981;80:1476–1480.
94. Brown WR. Ultrastructural studies on the translocation of polymeric immunoglobulins by intestinal epithelium and liver. In: Strober W, Hanson LA, Sell KW, eds. *Recent advances in mucosal immunity.* New York: Raven Press, 1982:251–266.
95. Elewaut D, DiDonato JA, Kim JM, et al. NF-kappa B is a central regulator of the intestinal epithelial cell innate immune response induced by infection with enteroinvasive bacteria. *J Immunol* 1999;163:1457–1466.
96. Gewirtz AT, Rao AS, Simon PO Jr, et al. *Salmonella typhimurium* induces epithelial IL-8 expression via Ca(2+)-mediated activation of the NF-kappaB pathway. *J Clin Invest* 2000;105:79–92.
97. Kitamura T, Garofalo RP, Kamijo A, et al. Human intestinal epithelial cells express a novel receptor for IgA. *J Immunol* 2000; 164:5029–5034.
98. Lorenzen DR, Dux F, Wolk U, et al. Immunoglobulin A1 protease, an exoenzyme of pathogenic neisseriae is a potent inducer of proinflammatory cytokines. *J Exp Med* 1999;190:1049–1058.
99. Mayer L. Current concepts in mucosal immunity. I. Antigen presentation in the intestine: new rules and regulations. *Am J Physiol* 1998;274:G7–G9.
100. Philpott DJ, Yamaoka S, Israel A, et al. Invasive *Shigella flexneri* activates NF-kappa B through a lipopolysaccharide-dependent innate intracellular response and leads to IL-8 expression in epithelial cells. *J Immunol* 2000;165:903–914.
101. Steiner TS, Nataro JP, Poteet-Smith CE, et al. Enteroaggregative *Escherichia coli* expresses a novel flagellin that causes IL-8 release from intestinal epithelial cells. *J Clin Invest* 2000;105:1769–1777.
102. Lehrer RI, Bevins CL, Ganz T. Defensins and other antimicrobial peptides. In: Ogra PL, Mestecky J, Lamm ME, et al., eds. *Mucosal immunology,* second edition. New York: Academic Press, 1999:89–99.
103. Christ AD, Blumberg RS. The intestinal epithelial cell: immunological aspects. *Springer Semin Immunopath* 1997;18: 449–461.
104. Bry L, Falk PG, Midtvedt T, et al. A model of host-microbial interactions in an open mammalian ecosystem. *Science* 1996; 273:1380–1383.
105. Mayer L, Blumberg RS. Antigen-presenting cells: epithelial cells. In: Ogra PL, Mestecky J, Lamm ME, et al., eds. *Mucosal immunology,* second edition. New York: Academic Press, 1999; 365–379.
106. Neish AS, Gewirtz AT, Zeng H, et al. Prokaryotic regulation of epithelial responses by inhibition of IκBα ubiquitination. *Science* 2000;289:1560–1563.
107. Potten CS, Morris RJ. Epithelial stem cells *in vivo. J Cell Sci Suppl* 1988;10:45–62.
108. Eckmann L, Kagnoff MF, Fierer J. Epithelial cells secrete the chemokine interleukin-8 in response to bacterial entry. *Infect Immun* 1993;61:4569–4674.
109. Henderson B, Poole B, Wilson M. Microbial/host interactions in health and disease: who controls the cytokine network? *Immunopharmacology* 1996;35:1–21.
110. O'Garra A. Cytokines induce the development of functionally heterogeneous T helper cell subsets. *Immunity* 1998;8:275–283.
111. Heinzel F, Sadick M, Holoday B, et al. Reciprocal expression of interferon gamma or interleukin 4 during the resolution or progression of murine leishmaniasis. Evidence for expansion of distinct helper T cell subsets. *J Exp Med* 1989;169:59–72.
112. Elson CO. Experimental models of intestinal inflammation: new insights into mechanisms of mucosal homeostasis. In: Ogra PL, Mestecky J, Lamm ME, et al., eds. *Mucosal immunology,* second edition. New York: Academic Press, 1999:1007–1024.
113. Mowat AM, Weiner HL. Oral tolerance—physiological basis and clinical applications. In: Ogra PL, Mestecky J, Lamm ME, et al., eds. *Mucosal immunology,* second edition. San Diego: Academic Press, 1999:587–618.
114. Miller A, Lider O, Roberts AB, et al. Suppressor T cells generated by oral tolerization to myelin basic protein suppress both *in vitro* and *in vivo* immune responses by the release of transforming growth factor beta after antigen-specific triggering. *Proc Nat Acad Sci U S A* 1992;89:421–425.
115. Husby S, Mestecky J, Moldoveanu Z, et al. Oral tolerance in humans. T cell but not B cell tolerance after antigen feeding. *J Immunol* 1994;152:4663–4670.
116. Khoury SJ, Lider O, al-Sabbagh A, et al. Suppression of experimental autoimmune encephalomyelitis by oral administration of myelin basic protein. III. Synergistic effect of lipopolysaccharide. *Cell Immunol* 1990;131:302–310.

11

INTERACTIONS OF MICROBIAL PATHOGENS WITH INTESTINAL M CELLS

MARIAN R. NEUTRA
PHILIPPE SANSONETTI
JEAN-PIERRE KRAEHENBUHL

INTRODUCTION

The Intestinal Epithelial Barrier

The intestinal mucosa represents a vast surface area, covered by a single layer of epithelial cells that provides a barrier against the contents of the intestinal lumen. Luminal microorganisms are generally excluded from close contact with epithelial cell surfaces by the interplay of mucous and fluid secretions, secretory antibodies, secreted antibacterial proteins, and other nonspecific defense mechanisms. In addition, the epithelium is sealed by continuous tight junctions that permit charge-selective passage of certain ions, water, and some small organic molecules, but effectively exclude peptides, macromolecules, and microorganisms (1). The major cell type responsible for maintaining this crucial barrier, the absorptive cell or enterocyte, is well equipped to face the microorganism-rich environment of the lumen. Apical plasma membranes of enterocytes are highly differentiated structures with rigid, closely packed microvilli (2) coated with an array of highly glycosylated stalked glycoprotein enzymes (3) and a thick layer of membrane-associated mucins called the filamentous brush border glycocalyx (4). In other cell types, membrane mucins have been shown to inhibit adherence to other cells and matrix (5). In the intestine, the apical coat serves as a diffusion barrier that prevents contact of most microorganisms with integral components of the enterocyte plasma membrane and impedes access to the small membrane domains between microvilli that are involved in endocytosis (6). The glycocalyx thus serves a protective function, preventing the uptake of antigens and pathogens while providing a highly degradative microenvironment that promotes the digestion and absorption of nutrients.

Despite its protective function, the epithelium provides the mucosal immune system with a continuous stream of information about the external environment of the lumen. For effective immune surveillance of potential pathogens in the intestinal lumen, antigens and microorganisms must be transported across the epithelial barrier to cells of the mucosal immune system located on its basolateral surface and in the lamina propria. In enterocytes, transepithelial vesicular transport of macromolecules is limited and involves complex, tightly regulated intracellular pathways that have been reviewed elsewhere (7). Transport of intact antigens and microorganisms in the intestine is concentrated at sites containing organized mucosal lymphoid follicles where the collaboration of epithelial cells with antigen-presenting and lymphoid cells is highly developed (8). In the follicle-associated epithelium (FAE), specialized epithelial M cells deliver samples of foreign material through active transepithelial vesicular transport from the lumen directly to intraepithelial lymphoid cells and to subepithelial organized mucosal lymphoid tissues that are designed to process antigens and initiate mucosal immune responses (8–10). Thus, the M cell transport system is crucial for induction of protective mucosal immune responses, but it also provides an entry route into the mucosa and thus plays a key role in the pathogenesis of certain bacterial and viral diseases (11–13). The M cell pathway not only serves as a portal of entry for invasive microorganisms but also transports noninvasive bacteria, including commensals, into organized mucosal lymphoid tissues. Mucosal immune responses against commensals, which involves T-cell–independent immunoglobulin A (IgA) antibody responses (14) may play a role in regulating endogenous microbial popula-

M. R. Neutra: Department of Pediatrics, Harvard Medical School and GI Cell Biology Laboratory, Children's Hospital, Boston, Massachusetts
P. Sansonetti: Department of Bacteriology and Mycology, Institut Pasteur, Paris, France
J-P Kraehenbuhl: Swiss Institute for Experimental Cancer Research and Institute of Biochemistry, University of Lausanne, Epalinges, Switzerland

tions in the lumen or in eliminating and inactivating bacteria that have crossed the mucosal epithelium.

Follicle-Associated Epithelium

The FAE overlying each mucosal lymphoid follicle in the intestine is formed by convergence of migrating cells from 12 or more follicle-associated crypts (15–17). Gene expression in cells of the follicle-associated crypts is distinct from that of villus-associated crypts and appears to be influenced by the lymphoid cells of the underlying follicle. Indeed, in a recent study using transgenic mice, a single gene was shown to be up-regulated specifically in the FAE (El Bahi S, Kraehenbuhl JP, Pringault E, unpublished data). There are other indications that the entire FAE differs from the epithelium of surrounding villi, and that the FAE presents a biochemical "face" to the lumen that is distinct. For example, FAE cells differ from villus cells in their glycosylation patterns (18–21) and follicle-associated enterocytes produce low levels of brush border hydrolases (17,22). Because of the paucity of goblet cells in the FAE, there is relatively little mucus production at these sites (23), and follicle-associated crypts have fewer defensin- and lysozyme-producing Paneth cells (24). Furthermore, the entire FAE is devoid of polymeric immunoglobulin receptors and therefore does not secrete IgA (25). All of these features of the FAE would tend to promote local contact of pathogens with the FAE surface.

There is indirect functional evidence for other differences in the surface chemistry of the FAE: for example, hydrophobic particles adhere more readily to the FAE than to villi (6,26). This may reflect subtle differences in surface charge, perhaps related to the composition and architecture of FAE cell surface glycoconjugates. In rabbits, a specific carbohydrate epitope containing α(2-3)-linked sialic acid and recognized by the lectin MAL II was accessible to lectin-coated microparticles on the FAE but not on villi (27). In addition, there is evidence that a subpopulation of FAE cells are not terminally or irreversibly differentiated and retain the ability to convert to M cells under conditions of microbial challenge or immune stimulation, as described later.

It has recently been shown that intestinal epithelial cells express chemokines that promote selective homing of lymphocyte subpopulations into the epithelium. The CC chemokine TECK (thymus-expressed chemokine) is expressed in villus epithelial cells of the small intestine but not colon and attracts T cells expressing the TECK receptor CCR9 (28). One of the authors (Kraehenbuhl J-P, unpublished data) recently observed that TECK is also produced by FAE epithelial cells. In the gut, TECK mediates chemotaxis of memory $\alpha4\beta7^{high}$ or $\alpha E\beta7$ intestinal CD4+ and CD8+ lymphocytes that carry CCR9 receptors, and may promote movement of lymphocytes into the lamina propria and epithelium of both the villi and FAE. Proinflammatory chemokines can be produced by intestinal enterocytes in response to danger signals (29). In contrast, FAE enterocytes constitutively express the CC chemokine MIP 3α (macrophage inhibitory protein), also known as LARC (liver and activation-regulated chemokine). In normal intestines of both humans and mice, MIP 3α is produced by intestinal FAE epithelial cells but not villus cells (30,31) and thus is the first marker of FAE epithelial cells. The fact that MIP 3α has selective chemotactic activity for naïve B and T lymphocytes and dendritic cells that express CCR6 receptors suggests that it may be involved in constitutive formation or maintenance of organized mucosal lymphoid tissues. However, MIP3α expression in epithelial cells is transiently induced *in vitro* by lipopolysaccharide (LPS), but not by cytokines such as tumor necrosis factor (TNF)-α, interferon (IFN)-γ, interleukin (IL)-1β, or IL-4 (31). Thus, this chemokine could play a key role in the induction of new lymphoid follicles that has been observed in response to luminal gram-negative enterobacteria. In mice lacking the chemokine receptor CCR6, dendritic cells expressing CD11c and CD11b are absent from the subepithelial dome of Peyer patches. These mice have an impaired humoral immune response to orally administered antigen and to enteropathogenic rotavirus (32).

Induction of the M Cell Phenotype

Differentiation of FAE and M cells involves a complex interaction between cells of organized lymphoid tissues and epithelial cells, and the luminal microbial flora plays an important role in this interaction. The extracellular matrix may also be involved in this complex cross-talk. It was recently shown that the composition of the basal lamina underlying the FAE is distinct from that of the villus epithelium. There is no laminin 2 in the basal lamina of the FAE or the crypts facing mucosal follicles, and myofibroblasts are absent under these epithelia (33). Lymphoid follicles and M cells have been documented in fetal animals and humans (reviews: 9,34) but after birth, microorganisms are crucial for full development of organized mucosal lymphoid tissues. For example, lymphoid follicles and M cells rapidly increase in number after transfer of germ-free mice to a normal animal house environment (35) or after exposure to a single bacterial species (36,37). Microorganisms may act by inducing epithelial and subepithelial cells to release cytokines and chemokines (29,30) that could play an indirect role in FAE differentiation by promoting the assembly of lymphoid follicles. Cells of the mucosal follicles can clearly play an inductive role in the differentiation of the specialized FAE and M cells. Experimental induction of follicles by injection of Peyer patch lymphocytes into the circulation of SCID mice (17) or into the submucosa of syngeneic normal mice (38) resulted in local assembly of new lymphoid follicles and the *de novo* appearance of FAE with typical M cells. Initial evidence that B cells play a crucial role in this phenomenon was obtained in adoptive transfer experiments using immunodeficient SCID mice, in which injection of fractions enriched in B cells were most effective in reconstituting mucosal fol-

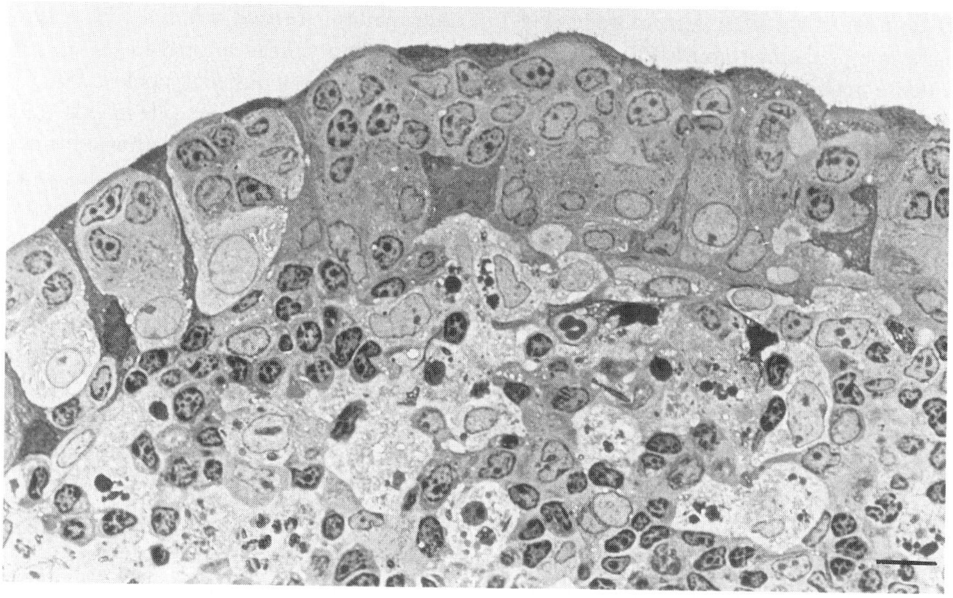

FIGURE 11.1. Follicle-associated epithelium of rabbit appendix. The epithelium contains numerous M cells. Large, pale M-cell nuclei lie at the bases of the cells, while densely staining lymphocyte nuclei are seen in the intraepithelial pockets. Large phagocytic cells as well as many lymphocytes occupy the region under the epithelium. Bar, 10 μm.

licles (17). B lymphocytes appear to participate in induction of FAE enterocytes because, in B-lymphocyte–deficient mice, the size of the epithelium associated with organized mucosal lymphoid tissues is dramatically reduced. The presence of B cells is not an absolute requirement for M-cell differentiation, however, because in these epithelia a few M cells are still present (39).

Differentiating M cells have been identified in the follicle-associated crypts by lectin and vimentin labeling and electron microscope (EM) studies (15,16,24,40,41). As they emerge from the crypts, M cells begin endocytic activity (40), fail to assemble typical brush borders (42), and acquire lymphocytes in their characteristic intraepithelial pocket (16,40). These observations suggest that inductive factors from the follicle act early in the differentiation pathway, inducing crypt cells to commit to FAE phenotypes. However, such factors may also act later to convert FAE enterocyte-like or uncommitted cells to antigen-transporting M cells. Cells with both enterocyte and M cell features are present in the FAE and M-cell numbers can increase rapidly after bacterial challenge (36). In addition, migration of B cells into an intestinal epithelial cell monolayer in culture resulted in appearance of cells with M-cell features (38).

The likelihood that a luminal microorganism will come into contact with an M-cell surface is determined in part by its motility and tropism, but also by intrinsic host factors such as the distribution and frequency of mucosal follicles and the frequency of M cells in each FAE. These parameters vary widely among species and in different intestinal regions (23,34). In mice, for example, patches of aggregated follicles are distributed throughout the small intestine as well as occurring in the cecum, colon, and rectum (23,43). In humans, large lymphoid follicle aggregates (Peyer patches) are restricted to the ileum, but isolated lymphoid follicles occur throughout the large intestine with highest frequency in the rectum (44–48). In both mice and humans, small intestinal FAE are visible from the lumen as domes covering mucosal follicles. The FAE in distal large intestine is sometimes sequestered at the base of a cryptlike epithelial invagination to form a "lymphoglandular complex" with a follicle deep in the mucosa (43,44,48,49). M-cell numbers in the FAE vary widely: whereas they represent only about 10% of the FAE in mice, they comprise 50% of the FAE in rabbit Peyer patch and appendix, often alternating with other cells (Fig. 11.1). In humans, 10% or less of ileal FAE cells are M cells, and these tend to lie on the lateral margins of the dome epithelium (45). In any case, the proportion of the intestinal mucosa represented by FAE is extremely small and M cells represent a tiny fraction of the epithelial surface area. The fact that microbial pathogens use M cells as entry points underscores the specificity of microbial-host cell interactions.

M-CELL BIOLOGY

M-Cell Architecture and Membrane Traffic

M cells form tight junctions with their epithelial neighbors that prevent paracellular passage of macromolecules (50,51) but they have a highly developed vesicular transport pathway (11,52). The basolateral cell surface is modified by a deep invagination that forms a large intraepithelial "pocket" lined by a distinct domain of the plasma membrane (Fig. 11.2). The unusual shape of the mature M cell appears to be supported by a dense network of intermediate filaments (IF) that surround the nucleus and course through the cytoplasm around the pocket (41). In some species these filaments contain vimentin, an IF protein not found in other normal intestinal epithelial cell types, in addition to conventional epithelial cytokeratins (41,53,54).

Between the short, irregular microvilli or microfolds on M-cell apical surfaces are many microdomains from which endocytosis occurs (55). Nonadherent, soluble proteins are endocytosed by M cells and delivered into the intraepithelial pocket (56,57), but macromolecules, particles, or microorganisms that can adhere to the apical plasma membranes of M cells are endocytosed or phagocytosed much more efficiently (55). M cells take up macromolecules, particles, and microorganisms by any or all of the endocytic mechanisms used by other cell types. These include adsorptive endocytosis via clathrin-coated pits and vesicles (6,40, 55,58,59), fluid-phase endocytosis (56,57), macropinocytosis (60), and phagocytosis involving extension of cellular processes and reorganization of submembrane actin assemblies (61,62). All of these uptake mechanisms result in transport of foreign material into a system of endosomal tubules and vesicles located in the apical cytoplasmic layer above the intraepithelial pocket (55,57,63). M cells are unique among epithelial cells in that transepithelial vesicular transport is the major pathway for endocytosed materials. Macromolecules and particles taken up at the apical surface of M cells are delivered to endosomes in the apical cytoplasm and these acidify their content and contain endosomal proteases (63,64). However, transport and release into the basolateral pocket is rapid, and to what extent antigens or microorganisms delivered into the pocket are altered in transit is not known.

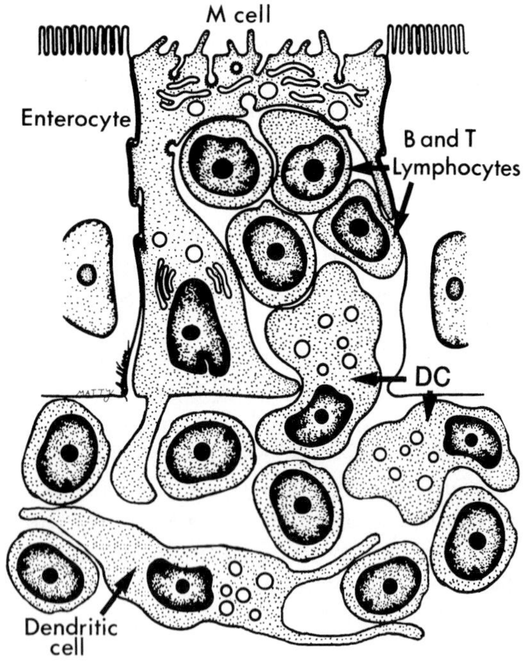

FIGURE 11.2. Diagram of an M cell. The M-cell basolateral surface is modified to form an intraepithelial pocket into which lymphocytes (and occasionally phagocytes) migrate. Antigens, microorganisms, and particles that adhere to the M-cell apical membrane are efficiently endocytosed and transported into the pocket, and hence to the subepithelial dome region of the organized mucosal lymphoid tissue where dendritic cells (DCs) and lymphocytes are abundant. (Adapted from Neutra MR, Frey A, Kraehenbuhl JP. Epithelial M cells: gateways for mucosal infection and immunization. *Cell* 1996;86:345–348.).

Apical Membrane Features that Promote Microbial Adherence

Apical membranes of M cells in Peyer patches show distinct features that may promote microbial contact and adherence (review: 65). Their microvilli are usually irregular and dispersed among membrane domains that are active in endocytosis, as described earlier. In addition, M cells generally lack the thick glycocalyx that coats brush border membranes of enterocytes (6). Nevertheless, M-cell apical membrane glycoproteins form a variable cell surface coat that is capable of preventing access of particles of 100 nm or more to the lipid bilayer (6,27). M-cell surface glycoconjugates clearly do not prevent microbial binding, however; indeed, they may allow pathogens to "recognize" M-cell surfaces. Studies from several laboratories using lectins or anticarbohydrate antibodies have shown that the glycosylation patterns of M-cell membrane glycoconjugates differ from those of enterocytes. In Peyer patches of BALB/c mice, for example, the lectin UEA-1 that is specific for certain carbohydrate structures containing α(1-2)-fucose, selectively stained all M cells in the FAE (24,66). Other lectins revealed variations in the glycosylation patterns of individual M cells within a single FAE (24). The functional significance of this heterogeneity is unproven, but we have suggested that this might allow the FAE to "sample" a variety of microorganisms. M-cell–specific carbohydrate structures exist in other species, including rabbits, but these structures differ among species and vary in intestinal regions, as shown in mice (24) and rabbits (18,67,68). Thus, to date, there is no single, universal lectin that can serve to identify all M cells. In a limited number of human samples analyzed, M cells displayed the sialyl Lewis A antigen, defined as Neu5Ac α(2-3) Gal β(1-3) GlcNAc [Fuc α(1-4)], whereas neighboring enterocytes did not (20). Several groups have shown that lectin conjugation of proteins, or lectin coating of particles or liposomes can enhance M-cell transport and subsequent mucosal immune responses in experimental animals (19,69,70). The practicality of this approach for vaccine targeting is not clear because most lectins also bind to the heterogeneous oligosaccharide side chains of secreted mucins. Lectin-carbohydrate interactions may allow the M cell to "sample" entire subclasses of luminal organisms. After transcytosis, most bacteria and viruses are readily released from the membrane into the intraepithelial pocket, which suggests multiple, low-affinity interactions with M-cell membrane components.

M-cell apical membranes also appear to have receptors for IgA. The FAE does not participate in IgA secretion, because it does not express basolateral polymeric immunoglobulin receptors (25). However, IgA that has been secreted into the lumen adheres selectively to the apical membranes of M cells, resulting in local accumulation of IgA on M cells of Peyer patches (59,68,71). In adult rabbits and mice, exogenous monoclonal IgA, monoclonal IgA-antigen complexes, and polyclonal secretory IgA adhered to apical membranes of M cells and were transported into the intraepithelial pocket (59). The mechanism and purpose of the IgA–M-cell interaction are unknown. One hypothesis for which there is some evidence is that uptake of specific IgA-antigen complexes by M cells could boost a preexisting secretory immune response (72,73). On the other hand, M-cell–associated IgA might sterically hinder binding of certain pathogens. An additional possibility is that the IgA–M-cell interaction may promote uptake of IgA-opsonized commensal microorganisms, promoting the maintenance of anticommensal immune responses that could control the luminal microflora and clear microorganisms from the mucosa. The recently identified novel Fc alpha/mu receptor on macrophages, B cells, and dendritic cells might play a role in this process (74).

M CELLS AS GATEWAYS TO THE MUCOSAL IMMUNE SYSTEM

Immediately under the FAE in the so-called dome region that caps the underlying lymphoid follicle is an extensive network of dendritic cells intermingled with CD4+ T cells and B cells that appear to be derived from the underlying B-cell follicle (8,75–77). Dendritic cells in the dome region appear to be immature (30), and thus would be competent for endocytosis of incoming pathogens. M-cell–transported lectins, cholera toxin conjugates, protein tracers, and particles have been detected in cells of the dome. A recent confocal light microscopic study detected live, attenuated *Salmonella typhimurium* in dendritic cells of the dome region after oral administration (78). However, the behavior of antigen- or pathogen-containing dendritic cells and their patterns of migration out of the dome region are in need of further investigation. Because of the importance of dendritic cells in processing and presentation of antigens to T cells, it was predicted that subepithelial dendritic cells would move to adjacent T-cell areas where presentation of antigens would occur (77). Indeed, subepithelial dendritic cells were recently shown to migrate to adjacent T-cell areas in response to an injected parasite antigen (30), but the possibility remains that they also enter the follicle or leave the mucosa to enter the T-cell areas of draining lymph nodes (77,79). Dendritic cell movements and accompanying cellular interactions are likely to be important determinants of mucosal immune responses (80–82). However, they may also facilitate microbial dissemination (83).

Antigens and pathogens released into the M-cell pocket would first contact the cellular inhabitants of the pocket, but almost nothing is known about the interactions that occur in this intraepithelial space. Pocket B and T cells display characteristic phenotypic markers as shown by immunocytochemistry in experimental animals (84,85) and humans (86). M-cell pocket T cells are distinct from villus intraepithelial lymphocytes: they are mostly CD4+ and in humans they display the antigen CD45RO typical of memory cells (75). Most of the B cells in the pocket express major histocompatibility complex class II and IgM but not IgG or IgA, suggesting that these cells are B memory cells that are capable of antigen presentation. The presence of such phenotypes suggests that pocket B cells have positioned themselves for reexposure to incoming antigen and efficient presentation of antigen to cognate T cells and that lymphoblast traffic into the M-cell pocket may allow amplification and diversification of the immune response (8). Interactions of pathogens with cells in the pocket might occur in the absence of circulating antibodies. This is suggested by the observation that injected immunoglobulins do not freely diffuse into the organized mucosal lymphoid tissues (87) and protein tracers injected intravenously percolated into the mucosa but did not readily enter the M-cell pockets (Weltzin R and Neutra MR, unpublished observation). Indeed, passively transferred neutralizing IgG antibodies failed to protect the Peyer patches of mice against M-cell-mediated entry and local infection by reovirus (88). On the other hand, some serum IgG clearly enters the Peyer patch because B-cell infection by mouse mammary tumor virus (MMTV) in Peyer patches or nasal associated lymphoid tissue was prevented by passive transfer of MMTV-specific antibodies (89).

The events in organized lymphoid tissues that immediately follow M-cell transport of pathogens reflect the differing pathogenic strategies of the incoming microorganisms (12). The tissue is organized for immunologic processing and presentation of macromolecules, particles, microbes, and mucosal vaccines. However, some pathogens disrupt these processes by inducing cytokine and chemokine release from epithelial cells, attracting neutrophils and monocytes, and setting in motion an inflammatory response that results in breakdown of the epithelial barrier. Other pathogens enter subepithelial antigen-presenting cells and use the migration of these cells to reach local and distant targets. However, in most cases M-cell–mediated uptake of microorganisms probably results in immune responses that are beneficial to the host.

ROLE OF M CELLS IN PROTECTION AGAINST COLONIZATION OF MUCOSAL SURFACES

The role of M cells in mucosal defense is clear in the case of noninvasive microorganisms that cause disease by colonizing mucosal surfaces. For example, M-cell binding and uptake of *Vibrio cholerae* and certain strains of *Escherichia coli* results in efficient sampling by the mucosal immune system and secretion of antimicrobial sIgA antibodies that play a major role in limiting the duration of mucosal disease and preventing reinfection.

Vibrio cholerae

V. cholerae organisms are motile, uniflagellate, gram-negative bacteria that cause severe enterotoxin-induced secretory diarrhea. Within the small intestine, *V. cholerae* expresses a group of coregulated proteins, including pili and adhesins, which allow them to adhere to epithelia of the proximal small intestine and form colonies on the mucosal surface, and cholera toxin (CT), which is endocytosed and induces secretion of chloride ions from intestinal epithelial cells (90–92). Expression of toxin-coregulated pili (tcp) was recently shown to occur in two stages. When vibrios are introduced into the small intestine of neonatal mice, tcp is initially expressed at low levels, resulting in initial adherence, and then at higher levels, along with CT, resulting in stabilization of colonies and induction of diarrhea (93). Colonization of the intestine by *V. cholerae* evokes a vigorous mucosal immune response that includes secretion of sIgA directed primarily against CT and LPS . Studies in various species, including humans, showed that secretion of IgA directed against LPS and CT is associated with protection against subsequent oral challenge (94,95). Studies in which monoclonal IgA antibodies were secreted from "backpack" tumors in suckling mice demonstrated that sIgA directed against LPS alone can protect against disease, presumably by preventing colonization (96,97). Although secretory IgAs against CT play a role in protection against disease in humans, monoclonal anti-CT IgA alone was unable to prevent disease in mice, presumably because colonization was not prevented and secreted IgA was not able to intercept CT produced on epithelial surfaces by colonies of adherent vibrios (96).

V. cholerae organisms inoculated into ligated intestinal loops containing Peyer patches in adult rabbits or mice interact closely with apical membranes of M cells and adhere to the glycocalyx of enterocytes without making close membrane contact (Fig. 11.3) (62,96,97). In adult mice that are not natural hosts, the intestine is poorly colonized and M-cell adherence is sporadic. In neonatal mice, however, more consistent adherence to M cells occurs, reflecting efficient mucosal colonization that results in disease. Nevertheless, M-cell transport of vibrio and cholera toxin occurs in adult mice and results in induction of specific IgA lymphoblasts in Peyer

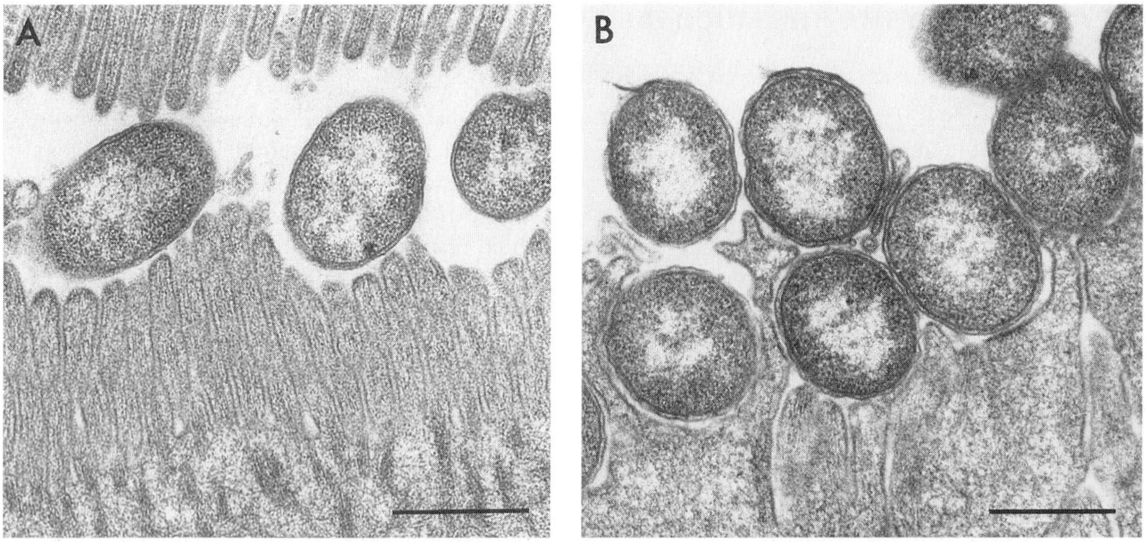

FIGURE 11.3. Interaction of *Vibrio cholerae* with apical surfaces of M cells and enterocytes in mouse Peyer patch epithelium. After injection into a ligated intestinal loop, *V. cholerae* adhered to the apical surface of a villus enterocyte **(A)** but did not directly contact the enterocyte membrane because of the thick glycoprotein coat on these cells, which is not visible in this EM preparation. In contrast, *V. cholerae* that adhered to an M cell **(B)** made close contact with the M-cell apical membrane. (From Apter FM, Michetti P, Winner LS III, et al. Analysis of the roles of anti-lipopolysaccharide and anti-cholera toxin IgA antibodies in protection against *Vibrio cholerae* and cholera toxin using monoclonal IgA antibodies *in vivo*. *Infect Immun* 1993;61:5279–5285, with permission.) Bar, 1 μm.

patches that have been recovered and used for generation of IgA hybridomas (97,98). Rabbit and mouse M-cell–vibrio interactions observed by EM are characterized by areas of close membrane apposition and assembly of local cytoskeletal specializations (61,96). Owen and colleagues (62) observed that, after binding of *V. cholerae*, rabbit M cells formed pseudopod-like cell surface processes surrounding the organisms, which were then transported in phagocytic vesicles and released, apparently unaltered, into the M-cell pocket below (62). The binding and uptake of vibrios in rabbits was shown to be dependent on bacterial viability (62), but live host cells were not required. Binding of *Vibrio cholerae* as well as *Vibrio parahaemolyticus* to the surfaces of M cells and other intestinal epithelial cells in formalin-fixed human mucosal tissue was documented, and these studies identified a vibrio hemagglutinin as a potential adherence factor (98–100). *Vibrio cholerae* adhered to the surfaces of M cells with greater efficiency than to other epithelial cells, but it is not known whether the same vibrio adhesins that mediate intestinal colonization are involved in M-cell adherence. Taken together, these observations underscore the value of vaccines based on live, genetically engineered *V. cholerae* organisms that are capable of interacting with intestinal M cells (101).

Escherichia coli

Most types of *Escherichia coli* found in the intestine do not selectively adhere to epithelial cell surfaces. Certain pathogenic strains do adhere and colonize or invade the mucosa, however, and these also interact with M cells. The interaction of two such strains with M cells has been analyzed ultrastructurally, and dramatic differences were observed. Within 1 hour of inoculation into ligated rabbit appendices, *E. coli* strain O:124 associated with the surfaces of rabbit M cells and were taken up into phagosome-like vesicles and later released into the intraepithelial pocket (102). In contrast, the rabbit pathogen *E. coli* RDEC-1, which causes diarrheal disease analogous to enteropathogenic *E. coli* (EPEC) in humans, engages in a complex interaction with both M cells and other epithelial cell types including enterocytes. When RDEC-1 was administered orally to rabbits, the bacteria initially bound preferentially to the surfaces of M cells, but later adhered to enterocytes (103). This difference in timing may reflect the relative accessibility of appropriate binding sites on M cells. Initial attachment of these *E. coli* strains to M cells is mediated by a plasmid-encoded AF/R1 pilus (104,105). Purified AF/R1 pili bound a sialoglycoprotein complex isolated from rabbit brush border preparations (106), but the exact epitope involved and whether the same component is present on the apical surfaces of M cells is unknown.

RDEC-1 initially associated with peripheral components of M-cell surfaces but later, M-cell microvilli/microfolds were effaced and the bacterium formed intimate adherence sites characterized by the presence of submembrane actin assemblies and formation of stable "pedestals" (103), the so-called attaching/effacing lesions that have been characterized in detail on other cell types, including absorptive enterocytes (107). Attaching/effacing lesions on the M-cell apical surface are ultrastructurally identical to those formed on enterocytes and cultured epithelial cells (103). The EPEC-epithelial cell interaction involves a complex sequence of events orchestrated by the bacterium from a chromosomal pathogenicity island (108,109). These events were demonstrated in cultured cells, but they presumably occur in enterocytes and M cells *in vivo* as well. After initial adherence to cell surface carbohydrates, the bacterium uses a type III secretion system to insert a bacterial product (Tir) into the host cell membrane. Tir is phosphorylated and then serves as receptor for the bacterial ligand (intimin). The subsequent cascade of host cell signal transduction events results in formation of an actin-supported pedestal that supports the bacterium (110). Although pedestal formation is thought to prevent transcytosis by M cells, some uptake nevertheless occurs and infection of humans with EPEC evokes a vigorous immune response (111).

EXPLOITATION OF M CELLS BY INVASIVE BACTERIAL PATHOGENS

Enteroinvasive bacterial pathogens such as *Salmonella, Shigella,* and *Yersinia* penetrate the intestinal epithelial barrier not simply by invading the general epithelial lining of the small intestinal villi or colonic surface. The earliest stage of infection involves bacterial translocation through FAE, even though, collectively, FAE represent only a tiny fraction—perhaps 1/10,000 or less—of the mucosal surface. M cells in the FAE appear to be responsible for transport of these bacteria into the mucosa. This invasion strategy makes translocation across the epithelium relatively easy but bacterial survival in the mucosa especially challenging in that, after the crossing, bacteria find themselves facing a dense network of phagocytic cells in the subepithelial dome region of the mucosal follicle (76,77). The process of intestinal infection by these pathogens includes three major steps: (a) translocation through the FAE via M cells, (b) survival in the dome region by various strategies including evasion of innate defense mechanisms, and (c) establishment of infection. Infection remains essentially local in the case of shigella, local and regional in the case of yersinia, and systemic in the case of salmonella (112). These pathogens represent three paradigms of intestinal invasion that have been extensively studied at the molecular and cellular level.

Shigella: Enteroinvasive Bacteria that Remain Localized in the Intestinal Mucosa

Infection by *Shigella* causes bacillary dysentery, an acute infectious rectocolitis characterized by the triad of fever, intestinal cramps, and bloody diarrhea with mucopurulent stools (113). The four *Shigella* species—*S. flexneri, S. sonnei, S. dysenteriae,* and *S. boydii*—all express a plasmid-encoded invasive phenotype that drives efficient invasion of the colonic and rectal mucosae after oral ingestion of a bacterial inoculum as low as 10 to 100 colony-forming units (114). *In vitro* assays have revealed a complex process of epithelial cell invasion in which shigellae are taken up at the basolateral (but not the apical) pole of epithelial cells (115) through a macropinocytic process that is induced by bacterial secretion of effector proteins (Ipa) through a type III secretory apparatus. Once in an intracellular compartment, shigellae lyse the membrane of their phagocytic vacuole, escape into the cytoplasm, and initiate an actin-based motility process that involves the polar nucleation and assembly of actin filaments on the bacterial surface mediated by IcsA, an outer membrane protein (116). Shigellae then spread from cell to cell by exploiting the actin networks and adhesion molecules associated with the zonula adherens of epithelial junctional complexes (117). These events represent a highly efficient and unique process of intracellular colonization. In addition, intracellular shigellae induce a proinflammatory program initiated primarily by LPS and involving activation of NFκB, resulting in massive production of IL-8 (118,119). As a result, polymorphonuclear leukocytes are strongly attracted toward the epithelium and the factors that they release cause epithelial rupture and severe mucosal destruction. *In vitro* assays left a key question unanswered, however: If *Shigella* invades the basolateral surfaces of colonic epithelial cells, what is the initial site of *Shigella* translocation across the epithelium?

Within 2 days of *Shigella* infection in patients, small inflammatory lesions resembling aphthoid ulcers are observed in the sigmoid colon and rectum (120). Inflammation then spreads to the surrounding mucosa and causes hemorrhagic and purulent destruction of the tissues. Histopathologic analysis of early lesions showed that they often correspond to lymphoid follicles, suggesting that M cells of the overlying FAE are the site of initial *Shigella* entry (120). Histopathologic analysis of colonic tissues from macaque monkeys following intragastric inoculation and rabbit intestinal tissues after experimental infection of ligated intestinal loops have confirmed that the FAE is indeed the initial site of *Shigella* entry (121–123). The limited number of M cells available for *Shigella* entry is difficult to reconcile with the low bacterial inoculum required to cause the disease. So far, no chemotactic or adherence system has been identified in *Shigella* that could account for specific targeting to the M-cell apical surface. Passage through M cells occurs without rupture of the endocytic vacuole membrane and thus bacteria are rapidly delivered to the intraepithelial pocket and subepithelial space where they immediately encounter resident macrophages and dendritic cells. Once phagocytosed, the survival strategy of *Shigella* is to cause the rapid death of macrophages by apoptosis (124). The *Shigella* invasion protein IpaB triggers apoptosis by activating the cysteine protease caspase-1 (125). This is likely to facilitate bacterial survival in the mucosa and allow *Shigella* access to the basolateral side of epithelial cells where they can initiate the cycle of epithelial colonization described earlier. However, activation of caspase-1 also initiates inflammation by causing maturation of IL-1β and IL-18, two potent proinflammatory cytokines. The inflammatory process leads to rapid disruption of the epithelial barrier, thereby facilitating further *Shigella* invasion (126). Thus, M cells play a strategic role in the first stage of *Shigella* invasion, initiating a process that eventually leads to rupture of the intestinal epithelium. *Shigella* has a remarkable capacity to spread from cell to cell in epithelial tissues and remains confined to the mucosa where it causes severe lesions, but does not spread regionally or systemically.

Yersinia: Enteroinvasive Bacteria that Achieve Local and Regional Colonization

Yersinia enterocolitica causes diarrheal disease, whereas *Yersinia pseudotuberculosis* causes mild or inapparent intestinal infection but may cause subsequent mesenteric lymphadenitis that sometimes leads to bacteremia or septicemia. Enteric *Yersinia* spp., like *Shigella,* are primarily targeted to the FAE although their major site of entry is the terminal ileum instead of the colon and rectum. In experimental mice and rabbits, *Y. enterocolitica* and *Y. pseudotuberculosis* have both been shown to cross the intestinal epithelial barrier through M cells and to cause subsequent destruction of the Peyer patches (127–130). Adherence of *Yersinia* to M cells appears to be mediated in part by invasin, an entry-associated outer membrane protein initially described in *Y. pseudotuberculosis* that binds β1 integrins with high affinity (131,132). Invasin-negative mutants of *Yersinia* can still adhere to and invade M cells but at a much lower level than the wild type strain, and their colonization potential for Peyer patches is strongly reduced (130,133,134). β1 integrins have been detected on the apical surfaces of M cells (133), unlike conventional epithelial cells where they are exclusively basolateral (135), and it is likely that these adhesion molecules act as receptors for *Yersinia in vivo.*

Like other enteroinvasive pathogens that cross the intestinal epithelium through the FAE, *Yersinia* organisms face phagocytosis by resident macrophages or dendritic cells in the dome region of mucosal lymphoid follicles and again in mesenteric lymph nodes. Unlike *Shigella* and *Salmonella, Yersinia* spp., including the plague bacillus *Yersinia pestis,* have developed a strategy for inhibiting phagocytosis. Their spectacular antiphagocytic strategy is based on the expression of a plasmid-encoded type III secretion system, which, upon contact with macrophages, secretes a set of Yop proteins into the target cell cytoplasm that disrupts the cytoskeleton, thereby blocking the phagocytic machinery (136) and eventually causing apoptosis of the macrophage (137–139). As a result, the bacteria are essentially extracellular in infected Peyer patches and mesenteric lymph nodes.

Salmonella: Enteroinvasive Bacteria that Achieve Systemic Dissemination

After oral administration in mice, *S. typhimurium* crosses the intestinal barrier and causes a lethal septicemia that closely mimics typhoid fever caused by *S. typhi* in humans. Following injection into ligated intestinal loops in mice, *S. typhimurium*, like *Shigella* and *Yersinia*, shows clear selectivity for M cells of the FAE (60,140). M cells are a site of rapid entry, but may not represent the exclusive route by which the bacteria enter the mucosa and dissemination systemically; there is evidence that *Salmonella* can also enter via the villus epithelium (141,142). *Salmonella* is cytotoxic to the M cells that take the bacteria up by macropinocytosis, which results in destruction of the FAE as well as severe inflammatory lesions in Peyer patches (60,143). Among the three adherence systems so far identified in *S. typhimurium* (i.e., Pef, Lpf, and Fim), only the long Lpf fimbriae seem to mediate somewhat specific adherence to M cells of the murine FAE (144). It is likely, however, that M-cell adherence involves multiple systems in that *lpf* mutants show reduced but still significant colonization of murine Peyer patches, and although the *lpf* operon is absent in *S. typhi*, it retains the capacity to invade and have cytopathic effects on murine M cells (143). A carbohydrate epitope containing galactose linked β(1-3) to galactosamine serves as receptor for *S. typhimurium* on Caco-2 cells (145) but it is not known whether this same structure mediates attachment to M cells *in vivo*. Adherence of *S. typhimurium* to the apical surfaces of M cells is followed by ruffling of the cell membrane, reflecting massive reorganization of the cell cytoskeleton and leading to an entry process that resembles the macropinocytic event observed in *in vitro* assays (146). The invasion machinery encoded by the *Salmonella* pathogenicity island 1 (SPI1), particularly the type III secretion system that allows delivery of *Salmonella* invasion proteins (Sip), contributes to invasion of M cells. SPI1 mutants are neither toxic for M cells nor destructive for the FAE (60,147). SPI1 is likely to be a pathogenicity island (PAI) that is primarily dedicated to the crossing of the intestinal barrier by *Salmonella* because SPI1 mutants conserve full virulence when administered intravenously (IV) or intraperitoneally (IP) instead of orally.

After crossing the FAE, *Salmonella* are captured by resident or recruited macrophages and dendritic cells (78). Expression of SPI1 is associated with the SipB-dependent apoptotic killing of infected phagocytes (148). This would indicate that the interactions of *Salmonella* with mucosal phagocytes are similar to those observed with *Shigella* and *Yersinia*. However, current evidence indicates that *Salmonella* has instead evolved a strategy of survival inside phagocytes (149) and that migration of these cells out of the mucosa facilitates its systemic dissemination (142). SPI2, another major PAI encoding an alternative type III secretion system and its dedicated effector proteins (150), as well as a battery of phoP/phoQ-regulated genes (*pag*) (149) are key factors responsible for *Salmonella* survival and growth inside macrophages. SPI2 and *pho*P/*pho*Q mutants retain the ability to cross the intestinal barrier but are severely impaired in virulence when administered IV or IP.

Summary

There is clear evidence that most enteroinvasive bacterial pathogens invade the intestinal mucosa via M cells of the FAE. In addition to the examples described, *Campylobacter jejuni* has been shown to selectively associate with and be transported through the FAE of Peyer patches in a rabbit model of infection (151). Mycobacteria also exhibit selective M-cell adherence and transcytosis. *Mycobacterium paratuberculosis*, inoculated into ligated ileal loops of calves, entered organized mucosal lymphoid tissues where they accumulated in macrophages (152). An EM study demonstrated that rabbit M cells efficiently transport BCG (Bacillus Calmette-Guerin) into mucosal lymphoid tissue (153). The "classic" view according to which pathogens are able to invade directly through the villous epithelium may still play a role in pathogenesis of certain bacteria and should not be ruled out. Nevertheless, the FAE pathway appears to play a central role in intestinal invasion by many enteropathogens. In addition, new information about the strategies used by bacteria to deal with phagocytic cells have elucidated the early events after M-cell transport that bear heavily on the course of disease. M-cell transport of bacteria has important potential applications. Genetically attenuated enteroinvasive bacteria may be delivered via M cells directly to the inductive sites of the mucosal immune system and thus are excellent candidate vaccines and vectors for mucosal immunization.

INTERACTION OF INVASIVE VIRUSES WITH M CELLS

Although there is evidence for enzymatic activity in viral surface proteins (154,155), viruses are relatively simple structures that generally depend on adherence to enter endocytic pathways of host epithelial cells. Two closely related viral pathogens—reovirus in mice and poliovirus in humans—have been shown to use selective adherence to M cells as an invasion strategy (58,156). Several other animal viruses have also been seen to be transported by M cells (review: 13). Under experimental conditions, HIV-1 adhered to rabbit and mouse M cells (157), but whether M-cell transport plays a role in human transmission is unknown.

Reovirus

The best-known example of M-cell-specific viral adherence is provided by the mouse pathogen, reovirus (156). Processing of reovirus by proteases in the intestinal lumen increases viral infectivity (158,159). Using type 1 reovirus in adult mice, we showed that proteolytic processing of the outer capsid is also required for M-cell adherence: neither unprocessed virus (administered with protease inhibitors) nor capsid-less cores can bind (160). Reovirus selectively binds to mouse M cells in the Peyer patches (156,160,161), colon (162), and airways (163). When reovirus is ingested orally, proteases in the intestinal lumen remove the outermost capsid protein (sigma 3), modify a second outer capsid protein (μ1c) and induce a conformational change in the sigma 1 protein that results in its extension up to 45 nm from the viral surface (164–166). Sigma 1, the adhesin used by the virus to bind to target neurons and fibroblasts in culture, is known to contain at least one lectin-like domain, which is sialic acid–specific in type 3 reovirus (167,168). Recent studies in this laboratory have shown that reovirus type 1 binding to M cells is likely to be mediated by interaction of the extended sigma 1 with a specific sialic acid–containing determinant on the M-cell apical surface. This determinant is present on all epithelial cells but appears to be more accessible on M cells where it is able to "reach" its M-cell–binding site only in the extended conformation (Silvey K, Mantis NJ, and Neutra MR, unpublished observations). Adherent reovirus is endocytosed by M cells in clathrin-coated pits (Fig. 11.4) and transcytosed to the intraepithelial pocket and subepithelial tissue where it can infect multiple cell types, primarily phagocytes (166). The fact that reovirus is unable to adhere to the apical membranes of enterocytes but can infect the entire epithelium from the basolateral side (161) underscores the importance of the brush border glycocalyx in protection of enterocytes against luminal pathogens.

The transepithelial transport pathway of M cells provides reovirus with multiple opportunities to infect both epithelial and lamina propria cells of the host. The virus may infect the M cell itself, either by fusing directly with the membrane of the transport vesicle or by reentering the cell by endocytosis from the intraepithelial pocket. This would explain the cytoplasmic viral factories observed in M cells within hours after M-cell uptake of virus *in vivo* and the fact that M cells are selectively lost during reovirus infection of suckling mice (161). M-cell destruction would cause loss of epithelial barrier function or impaired sampling of luminal antigens by the mucosal immune system.

Poliovirus

The pathogenesis of poliovirus in humans shows some intriguing parallels with reovirus in mice: poliovirus enters the body by the oral route and proliferates in Peyer patches

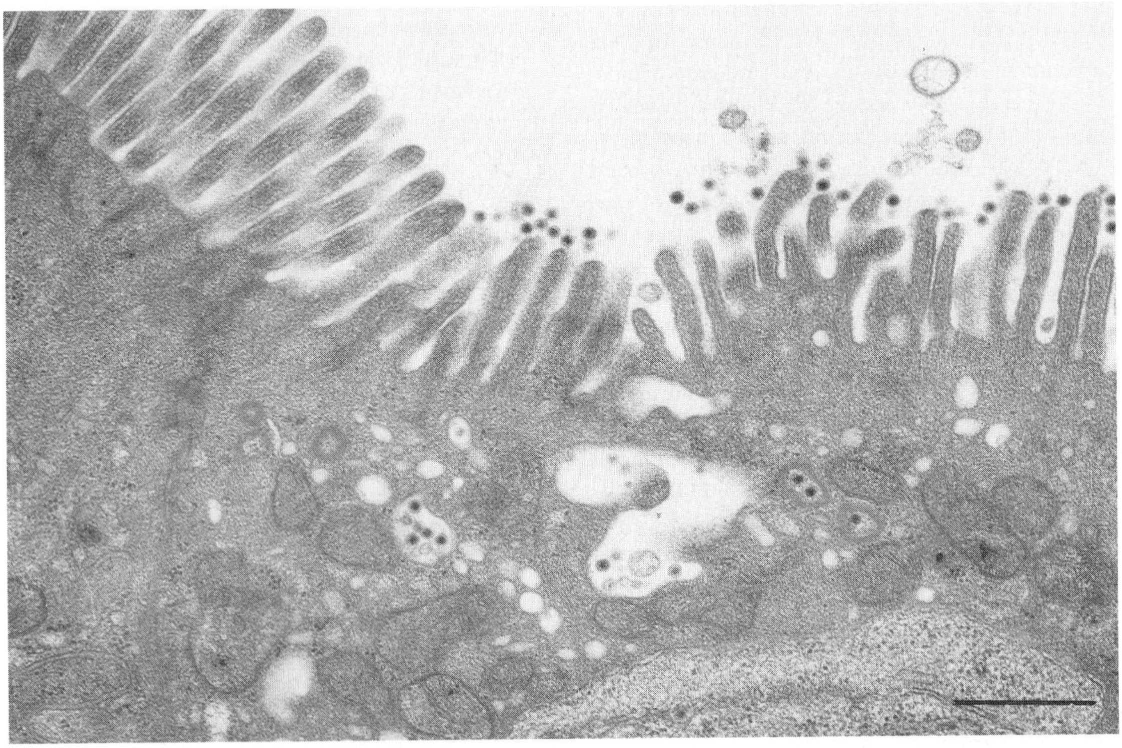

FIGURE 11.4. Interaction of reovirus with an M cell in mouse Peyer patch epithelium. Reovirus (type 1) was injected into the ileum of an adult mouse, and Peyer patch tissue was collected 1 hour later. Reovirus particles are associated with the apical surface of an M cell but not with the microvilli of neighboring enterocytes. (Micrograph by Dr. Richard Weltzin.) Bar, 1 μm

before spreading systemically (169). The efficacy of mucosal immunization with live, attenuated poliovirus was established decades ago and the mucosal immune response to polio vaccine was documented (170,171) long before the ultrastructure and antigen-transporting activity of M cells was first described (56). The mechanism of entry of poliovirus into the mucosa was revealed when small explants of human Peyer patches were exposed *in vitro* to wild poliovirus type 1 or to the attenuated Sabin strain, and were then examined by EM (58). Both viruses adhered to M cells and were endocytosed, whereas neither appeared to interact with enterocytes. The receptor for poliovirus on neuronal target cell membranes has been identified as a member of the immunoglobulin superfamily, and the cloned gene has been used to create transgenic mice that can be infected by injection of virus (172). When these mice were challenged orally, viral replication was not detected in the intestinal mucosa, perhaps because the transgene was not expressed in this site, but the nasal mucosa was infected and paralytic disease developed in the mice (169). It is not known whether the binding site that poliovirus uses to adhere to M cells is the same or different from that used on target neurons. Nevertheless, the ability of poliovirus to exploit M-cell transport for penetration of the epithelial barrier makes it a candidate oral vaccine vector for delivery of foreign antigens, either in recombinant viral particles or as empty pseudovirus particles (173).

Human Immunodeficiency Virus

Rectal exposure to infected semen is a major risk factor for HIV transmission (174). Entry of virus presumably occurs when epithelial barriers are damaged, but studies of simian immunodeficiency virus (SIV) transmission in monkeys have shown that free SIV can infect via intact rectal mucosa (175–177). The exact cellular and molecular events involved in HIV entry and mucosal infection in the rectum are not known, but there is evidence that M cells may be involved. Using mouse and rabbit mucosal explants in organ culture, we showed that HIV-1 can adhere to M cells and that these cells can transport HIV across the epithelial barrier (157). M cells of different species are functionally similar and mucosal lymphoid follicles covered by FAE containing M cells are abundant in human rectum (48). If HIV transport occurs at M-cell–containing sites, the virus would have rapid access to organized mucosal lymphoid tissues rich in target T cells, macrophages, and dendritic cells.

Intestinal epithelial cells of humans and monkeys *in vivo* do not express CD4 but their membranes do contain an alternate receptor, galactosylceramide (178,179), a glycosphingolipid that can mediate HIV infection of neoplastic intestinal epithelial cell lines such as HT29 and Caco-2 cells in culture (180,181). HIV infection of intestinal or rectal epithelial cells has not been detected in infected humans, however (182). When HIV-infected cells were applied to epithelial monolayers in culture, virus crossed the epithelium, presumably by a transcytotic vesicular pathway (183). Recently, one of our laboratories confirmed that free or cell-associated HIV-1 can infect, and cross by transcytosis, poorly differentiated Caco-2 cell monolayers and that transcytosis results in infection of mononuclear target cells on the serosal side of the epithelium. We further demonstrated that CCR5 or CXCR4 chemokine receptors together with galactosylceramide are required for infection of these epithelial cells by nonsyncytium-inducing (NSI) or syncytium-inducing (SI) HIV-1, respectively, and for transcytosis to occur (Fotopoulos G, Harari A, Trono D, Pantaleo G, Kraehenbuhl JP, unpublished data). M cells obtained by coculture of Caco-2 cells and B cells *in vitro* showed no difference from control Caco-2 cells in their ability to transmit the virus, as long as they expressed galactosylceramide and the appropriate chemokine receptor. These results suggest that transcytosis of HIV-1 across M cells *in vivo* may be receptor mediated. It is not clear how HIV particles or HIV-infected cells would gain access to glycolipids in human enterocyte membranes *in vivo* because enterocytes in the human rectum, like enterocytes throughout the intestine, have brush borders coated with a continuous, 400- to 500-nm thick glycocalyx. When applied to mouse and rabbit Peyer patch mucosa, HIV particles failed to penetrate the FBBG of enterocytes but did adhere to M-cell membranes (157). Further studies are needed to establish whether HIV actually enters the human rectal mucosa via the M-cell route.

Future design of mucosal vaccines against HIV and other sexually transmitted diseases must take into account mounting evidence that the location in which M-cell transport and inductive events occur has a profound influence on the subsequent regional distribution of specific IgA plasma cells and IgA secretion. A secretory immune response against poliovirus, for example, was demonstrated in colon but not in nasopharynx following immunization of distal colon (171). Similarly, secretory immune responses to Sendai virus in mice were concentrated in either the digestive tract or the airways, but not both, when administration of antigen was carefully restricted either to the stomach or the trachea (184). Studies using wicks or sponges made of an absorbent filter material for direct retrieval of secretions associated with mucosal surfaces of the gastrointestinal tract and vagina of mice (185) and humans (186,187) have shown that immunization via the rectum is the only route that induces high levels of specific sIgA in the mucus coating the rectum and distal colon. This is consistent with the fact that inductive sites (lymphoid follicles with M cells) are numerous in the distal colonic and rectal mucosa as well as the distal small intestine of humans.

CONCLUSION

The importance of M cells in invasion of the intestinal mucosa by pathogenic microorganisms and induction of mucosal immune responses has become widely recognized. However, much remains to be learned about the specific molecular recognition systems and nonspecific adherence mechanisms that underlie these phenomena. The same molecular mechanisms that allow M cells to selectively transport microorganisms to inductive sites of the mucosal immune system are presumably exploited by microbial pathogens to target themselves to these convenient invasion sites. A clearer understanding of these mechanisms could lead to design of more effective mucosal vaccines.

ACKNOWLEDGMENTS

We are grateful to current and former members of our laboratories who have contributed to the work summarized in this review. The authors are supported by NIH Research Grants HD17557, AI34757, AI35365 and NIH Center Grant DK34854 to the Harvard Digestive Diseases Center (MRN); The Howard Hughes Medical Institute and European Union Grant CEE QLK2-CT-1999.00973 (PJS); Swiss National Science Foundation Grant 31-56936-99; and Swiss League against Cancer Grant SKL 635-2-1998 (JPK).

REFERENCES

1. Madara JL, Nash S, Moore R, et al. Structure and function of the intestinal epithelial barrier in health and disease. *Monogr Pathol* 1990;31:306–324.
2. Mooseker M. Organization, chemistry and assembly of the cytoskeletal apparatus of the intestinal brush border. *Ann Rev Cell Biol* 1985;1:209–241.
3. Semenza G. Anchoring and biosynthesis of stalked brush border membrane glycoproteins. *Annu Rev Cell Biol* 1986;2:255–314.
4. Maury J, Nicoletti C, Guzzo-Chambraud L, et al. The filamentous brush border glycocalyx, a mucin-like marker of enterocyte hyper-polarization. *Eur J Biochem* 1995;228:323–331.
5. Wessling J, van der Valk SW, Vos HL, et al. Episialin (MUC 1) overexpression inhibits integrin-mediated cell adhesion to extracellular matrix components. *J Cell Biol* 1995;129:255–265.
6. Frey A, Lencer WI, Weltzin R, et al. Role of the glycocalyx in regulating access of microparticles to apical plasma membranes of intestinal epithelial cells: implications for microbial attachment and oral vaccine targeting. J Exp Med 1996;184:1045–1060.
7. Matter K, Mellman I. Mechanisms of cell polarity: sorting and transport in epithelial cells. *Curr Opin Cell Biol* 1994;6:545–554.
8. Brandtzaeg P, Baekkevold ES, Farstad IN, et al. Regional specialization in the mucosal immune system: what happens in the microcompartments? *Immunol Today* 1999;20:141–151.
9. Kraehenbuhl JP, Neutra MR. Epithelial M cells: differentiation and function. *Annu Rev Cell Dev Biol* 2000;16:301–332.
10. McGhee JR, Lamm ME, Strober W. Mucosal immune responses. In: Ogra R, Mestecky J, McGhee J, et al., eds. *Mucosal immunology,* second edition. New York: Academic Press; 1999:485–506.
11. Neutra MR, Frey A, Kraehenbuhl JP. Epithelial M cells: gateways for mucosal infection and immunization. *Cell* 1996;86: 345–348.
12. Phalipon A, Sansonetti PJ. Microbial-host interactions at mucosal sites. Host response to pathogenic bacteria at mucosal sites. *Curr Top Microbiol Immunol* 1999;236:163–190.
13. Siebers A, Finlay BB. M cells and the pathogenesis of mucosal and systemic infections. *Trends Microbiol* 1996;4:22–29.
14. MacPherson AJ, Gatto D, Sainsbury E, et al. A primitive T cell-independent mechanism of intestinal mucosal IgA responses to commensal bacteria. *Science* 2000;288:2222–2226.
15. Gebert A, Fassbender S, Werner K, et al. The development of M cells in Peyer's patches is restricted to specialized dome-associated crypts. *Am J Pathol* 1999;154:1573–1582.
16. Gebert A, Rothkötter H-J, Pabst R. M cells in Peyer's patches of the intestine. *Int Rev Cytol* 1996;167:91–159.
17. Savidge TC, Smith MW. Evidence that membranous (M) cell genesis is immunoregulated. *Adv Exp Med Biol* 1995;371:239–241.
18. Gebert A, Hach G. Differential binding of lectins to M cells and enterocytes in the rabbit cecum. *Gastroenterology* 1993;105: 1350–1361.
19. Giannasca PJ, Boden JA, Monath TP. Targeted delivery of antigen to hamster nasal lymphoid tissue with M-cell-directed lectins. *Infect Immun* 1997;65:4288–4298.
20. Giannasca PJ, Giannasca KT, Leichtner AM, et al. Human intestinal M cells display the sialyl Lewis A antigen *Infect. Immun* 1999;67:946–953.
21. Sharma R, Van Damme EJM, Peumans WJ, et al. Lectin binding reveals divergent carbohydrate expression in human and mouse Peyer's patches. *Histochem Cell Biol* 1996;105: 459–465.
22. Owen RL, Bhalla DK. Cytochemical analysis of alkaline phosphatase and esterase activities and of lectin-binding and anionic sites in rat and mouse Peyer's patch M cells. *Am J Anat* 1983; 168:199–212.
23. Owen R. Uptake and transport of intestinal macromolecules and microorganisms by M cells in Peyer's patches—a personal and historic perspective. *Semin Immunol* 1999;11:1–7.
24. Giannasca PJ, Giannasca KT, Falk P, et al. Regional differences in glycoconjugates of intestinal M cells in mice: potential targets for mucosal vaccines. *Am J Physiol* 1994;267:G1108–G1121.
25. Pappo J, Owen RL. Absence of secretory component expression by epithelial cells overlying rabbit gut-associated lymphoid tissue. *Gastroenterology* 1988;95:1173–1177.
26. Pappo J, Ermak TH. Uptake and translocation of fluorescent latex particles by rabbit Peyer's patch follicle epithelium: a quantitative model for M cell uptake. *Clin Exp Immunol* 1989;76: 144–148.
27. Mantis NJ, Frey A, Neutra MR. Accessibility of glycolipid and oligosaccharide epitopes on rabbit villus and follicle-associated epithelium. *Am J Physiol (Gastrointest Liver Physiol)* 2000;278: G915–G923.
28. Wurbel MA, Phillipe JM, Nguyen C, et al. The chemokine TECK is expressed by thymic and intestinal epithelial cells and attracts double- and single-positive thymocytes expressing the TECK receptor CCR9. *Eur J Immunol* 2000;30, 262–271.
29. Kagnoff MF, Eckmann L. Epithelial cells as sensors for microbial infection. *J Clin Invest* 1997;100:S51–S55.
30. Iwasaki A, Kelsall BL. Localization of distinct Peyer's patch dendritic cell subsets and their recruitment by chemokines macrophage inflammatory protein (MIP)-3a, MIP-3b, and secondary lymphoid organ chemokine. *J Exp Med* 2000;191: 1381–1393.
31. Tanaka Y, Imai T, Baba M, et al. Selective expression of liver and activation-regulated chemokine (LARC) in intestinal epithelium in mice and humans. *Eur J Immunol* 1999;29: 633–642.
32. Cook DN, Prosser DM, Forster R, et al. CCR6 mediates dendritic cell localization, lymphocyte homeostasis, and immune responses in mucosal tissue. *Immunity* 2000;12:495–503.
33. Sierro F, Pringault E, Simon Assman P, et al. Transient expression of M cell phenotype by enterocyte-like cells of the follicle-

associated epithelium of mouse Peyer's patches. *Gastroenterology* 2000;119:734–743.
34. Hein WR. Organization of mucosal lymphoid tissue. *Curr Top Microbiol Immunol* 1999;236:1–15.
35. Smith MW, James PS, Tivey DR. M cell numbers increase after transfer of SPF mice to a normal animal house environment. *Am J Pathol* 1987;128:385–389.
36. Borghesi C, Taussig MJ, Nicoletti C. Rapid appearance of M cells after microbial challenge is restricted at the periphery of the follicle-associated epithelium of Peyer's patch. *Lab Invest* 1999;79:1393–1401.
37. Savidge TC, Smith MW, James PS, et al. *Salmonella*-induced M-cell formation in germ-free mouse Peyer's patch tissue. *Am J Pathol* 1991;139:177–184.
38. Kernéis S, Bogdanova A, Kraehenbuhl JP, et al. Conversion by Peyer's patch lymphocytes of human enterocytes into M cells that transport bacteria. *Science* 1997;277:948–952.
39. Debard N, Sierro F, Browning J, et al. Effect of mature lymphocytes and lymphotoxin on the development of the follicle-associated epithelium and M cells in mouse Peyer's patches. *Gastroenterology* 2001;120:1173–1182.
40. Bye WA, Allan CH, Trier JS. Structure, distribution and origin of M cells in Peyer's patches of mouse ileum. *Gastroenterology* 1984;86:789–801.
41. Gebert A, Hach G, Bartels H. Co-localization of vimentin and cytokeratins in M-cells of rabbit gut-associated lymphoid tissue (GALT). *Cell Tissue Res* 1992;269:331–340.
42. Kernéis S, Bogdanova A, Colucci-Guyon E, et al. Cytosolic distribution of villin in M cells from mouse Peyer's patches correlates with the absence of a brush border. *Gastroenterology* 1996; 110:515–521.
43. Owen RL, Piazza AJ, Ermak TH. Ultrastructural and cytoarchitectural features of lymphoreticular organs in the colon and rectum of adult BALB/c mice. *Am J Anat* 1991;190:10–18.
44. Fujimura Y, Hosobe M, Kihara T. Ultrastructural study of M cells from colonic lymphoid nodules obtained by colonoscopic biopsy. *Dig Dis Sci* 1992;37:1089–1098.
45. Fujimura Y, Kihara T, Ohtani K, et al. Distribution of microfold cells (M cells) in human follicle-associated epithelium. *Gastroenterol Jpn* 1990;25:130.
46. Jacob E, Backer SJ, Swaminathan SP. M cells in the follicle-associated epithelium of the human colon. *Histopathology* 1987;11: 941–952.
47. Langman JM, Rowland R. The number and distribution of lymphoid follicles in the human large intestine. *J Anat* 1986; 194:189–194.
48. O'Leary AD, Sweeney EC. Lymphoglandular complexes of the colon: structure and distribution. *Histopathology* 1986;10: 267–283.
49. Kealy WF. Colonic lymphoid-glandular complex (microbursa): nature and morphology. *J Clin Pathol* 1976;29:241–244.
50. Gebert A, Bartels H. Occluding junctions in the epithelia of the gut-associated lymphoid tissue (GALT) of the rabbit ileum and cecum. *Cell Tissue Res* 1991;266:301–314.
51. Madara JL, Bye WA, Trier JS. Structural features of and cholesterol distribution in M-cell membranes in guinea pig, rat and mouse Peyer's patches. *Gastroenterology* 1984;87:1091–1103.
52. Neutra MR, Pringault E, Kraehenbuhl JP. Antigen sampling across epithelial barriers and induction of mucosal immune responses. *Annu Rev Immunol* 1996;14:275–300.
53. Gebert A, Rothkötter H-J, Pabst R. 1994. Cytokeratin 18 is an M cell marker in porcine Peyer's patches. *Cell Tissue Res* 1994; 276:213–221.
54. Jepson MA, Mason CM, Bennett MK, et al. Co-expression of vimentin and cytokeratins in M cells of rabbit intestinal follicle-associated epithelium. *Histochem J* 1992;24:33–39.
55. Neutra MR, Phillips TL, Mayer EL, et al. Transport of membrane-bound macromolecules by M cells in follicle-associated epithelium of rabbit Peyer's patch. *Cell Tissue Res* 1987;247: 537–546.
56. Bockman DE, Cooper MD. Pinocytosis by epithelium associated with lymphoid follicles in the bursa of Fabricius, appendix, and Peyer's patches. An electron microscopic study. *Am J Anat* 1973;136:455–478.
57. Owen RL. Sequential uptake of horseradish peroxidase by lymphoid follicle epithelium of Peyer's patches in the normal unobstructed mouse intestine: an ultrastructural study. *Gastroenterology* 1977;72:440–451.
58. Sicinski P, Rowinski J, Warchol JB, et al. Poliovirus type 1 enters the human host through intestinal M cells. *Gastroenterology* 1990;98:56–58.
59. Weltzin RA, Lucia Jandris P, Michetti P, et al. Binding and transepithelial transport of immunoglobulins by intestinal M cells: demonstration using monoclonal IgA antibodies against enteric viral proteins. *J Cell Biol* 1989;108:1673–1685.
60. Jones BD, Ghori N, Falkow S. *Salmonella typhimurium* initiates murine infection by penetrating and destroying the specialized epithelial M cells of the Peyer's patches. *J Exp Med* 1994;180: 15–23.
61. Neutra MR, Giannasca PJ, Giannasca KT, et al. M cells and microbial pathogens. In: Blaser M, Smith PD, Ravdin JI, et al., eds. *Infections of the gastrointestinal tract.*. New York: Raven Press, 1995:163–178.
62. Owen RL, Pierce NF, Apple RT, et al. M cell transport of *Vibrio cholerae* from the intestinal lumen into Peyer's patches: a mechanism for antigen sampling and for microbial transepithelial migration. *J Infect Dis* 1986;153:1108–1118.
63. Allan CH, Mendrick DL, Trier JS. Rat intestinal M cells contain acidic endosomal-lysosomal compartments and express class II major histocompatibility complex determinants. *Gastroenterology* 1993;104:698–708.
64. Finzi G, Cornaggia M, Capella C, et al. Cathepsin E in follicle associated epithelium of intestine and tonsils: localization to M cells and possible role in antigen processing. *Histochemistry* 1993;99:201–211.
65. Neutra MR, Mantis NJ, Frey A, et al. The composition and function of M cell apical membranes: implications for microbial pathogenesis. *Semin Immunol* 1999;11:171–181.
66. Clark MA, Jepson MA, Simmons NL, et al. Differential expression of lectin-binding sites defines mouse intestinal M-cells. *J Histochem Cytochem* 1993;41:1679–1687.
67. Jepson MA, Clark MA, Simmons NL, et al. Epithelial M cells in the rabbit caecal lymphoid patch display distinctive surface characteristics. *Histochemistry* 1993;100:441–447.
68. Lelouard H, Reggio H, Mangeat P, et al. Mucin related epitopes distinguish M cells and enterocytes in rabbit appendix and Peyer's patches. *Infect Immun* 1999;67:357–367.
69. Chen H, Torchilin V, Langer R. Lectin-bearing polymerized liposomes as potential oral vaccine carriers. *Pharm Res* 1996;13: 1378–1383.
70. Jepson MA, Clark MA, Foster N, et al. Targeting to intestinal M cells. *J Anat* 1996;189:507–516.
71. Roy MJ, Varvayanis M. Development of dome epithelium in gut-associated lymphoid tissues: association of IgA with M cells. *Cell Tissue Res* 1987;248:645–651.
72. Corthesy B, Kaufmann M, Phalipon A, et al. A pathogen-specific epitope inserted into recombinant secretory immunoglobulin is immunogenic by the oral route. *J Biol Chem* 1996;52: 33670–33677.
73. Zhou F, Kraehenbuhl JP, Neutra MR. Mucosal IgA response to rectally administered antigen formulated in IgA-coated liposomes. *Vaccine* 1995;13:637–644.

74. Shibuya A, Sakamoto N, Shimizu Y, et al. Fc alpha/mu receptor mediates endocytosis of IgM-coated microbes. *Nat Immun* 2000;1:441–446.
75. Brandtzaeg P, Farstad IN. The human mucosal B cell system. In: Ogra R, Mestecky J, McGhee J, et al., eds. *Mucosal immunology,* second edition. New York: Academic Press, 1999:439–468.
76. Kelsall BL, Strober W. Distinct populations of dendritic cells are present in the subepithelial dome and T cell regions of murine Peyer's patches. *J Exp Med* 1996;183:237–247.
77. Kelsall BL, Strober W. Gut-associated lymphoid tissue: antigen handling and T cell responses. In: Ogra R, Mestecky J, McGhee J, et al., eds. *Mucosal immunology,* second edition. New York: Academic Press, 1999:293–318.
78. Hopkins SA, Niedergang F, Corthesy-Theulaz IE, et al. A recombinant *Salmonella typhimurium* vaccine strain is taken up and survives within murine Peyer's patch dendritic cells. *Cellular Microbiol* 2000;2:59–68.
79. MacPherson GG, Jenkins CD, Stein MJ, et al. Endotoxin-mediated dendritic cell release from the intestine. Characterization of released dendritic cells and TNF dependence. *J Immunol* 1995;154:1317–1322.
80. Maldonado-Lopez R, De Smedt T, Michel P, et al. CD8a+ and CD8a– subclasses of dendritic cells direct the development of distinct T helper cells *in vivo*. *J Exp Med* 1999;189:587–592.
81. Rissoan MC, Soumelis V, Kadowaki N, et al. Reciprocal control of T helper cell and dendritic cell differentiation. *Science* 1999; 283:1183–1186.
82. Steinman RM. DC-SIGN: a guide to some mysteries of dendritic cells. *Cell* 2000;100:491–494.
83. Masurier C, Salomon B, Guettari N, et al. Dendritic cells route human immunodeficiency virus to lymph nodes after vaginal or intravenous administration to mice. *J Virol* 1998;72:7822–7829.
84. Ermak TH, Steger HJ, Pappo J. Phenotypically distinct subpopulations of T cells in domes and M-cell pockets of rabbit gut-associated lymphoid tissues. *Immunology* 1990;71:530–537.
85. Ermak TH, Bhagat HR, Pappo J. Lymphocyte compartments in antigen-sampling regions of rabbit mucosal lymphoid organs. *Am J Trop Med Hyg* 1994;50:S14–S28.
86. Farstad IN, Halstensen TS, Fausa O, et al. Heterogeneity of M cell-associated B and T cells in human Peyer's patches. *Immunology* 1994;83:457–464.
87. Allan CH, Trier JS. Structure and permeability differ in subepithelial villus and Peyer's patch follicle capillaries. *Gastroenterology* 1991;100:1172–1179.
88. Tyler KL, Virgin DH, Bassel-Duby R, et al. Antibody inhibits defined stages in the pathogenesis of reovirus serotype 3 infection of the nervous central system. *J Exp Med* 1989;170: 887–8959.
89. Velin D, Fotopoulos G, Kraehenbuhl JP, et al. Systemic antibodies can inhibit MMTV driven superantigen response in mucosal associated lymphoid tissues. *J Virol* 1999;73:1729–1733.
90. Herrington DA, Hall RH, Losonsky G, Mekalanos JJ, et al. Toxin, toxin-coregulated pili, and the toxR regulon are essential for *Vibrio cholerae* pathogenesis in humans. *J Exp Med* 1988; 168:1487–1492.
91. Lencer WI, Hirst TR, Holmes RK. Membrane traffic and the cellular uptake of cholera toxin. *Biochim Biophys Acta* 1999; 1450:177–190.
92. Miller JF, Mekalanos JJ, Falkow S. Coordinate regulation and sensory transduction in the control of bacterial virulence. *Science* 1989;243:916–921.
93. Lee SH, Hava DL, Waldor MK, et al. Regulation and temporal expression patterns of *Vibrio cholerae* virulence genes during infection. *Cell* 1999;99:625–634.
94. Jertborn M, Svennerholm AM, Holmgren J. Saliva, breast milk, and serum antibody responses as indirect measures of intestinal immunity after oral cholera vaccination or natural disease. *J Clin Microbiol* 1986;24:203–209.
95. Levine MM, Nalin DR, Craig JP, et al. Immunity to cholera in man: relative role of antibacterial verus antitoxic immunity. *Trans R Soc Trop Med Hyg* 1988;73:3–9.
96. Apter FM, Michetti P, Winner LS III, et al. Analysis of the roles of anti-lipopolysaccharide and anti-cholera toxin IgA antibodies in protection against *Vibrio cholerae* and cholera toxin using monoclonal IgA antibodies *in vivo*. *Infect Immun* 1993;61: 5279–5285.
97. Winner LS III, Mack J, Weltzin RA, et al. New model for analysis of mucosal immunity: intestinal secretion of specific monoclonal immunoglobulin A from hybridoma tumors protects against *Vibrio cholerae* infection. *Infect Immun* 1991;59: 977–982.
98. Apter FM, Lencer WI, Finkelstein RA, et al. Monoclonal immunoglobulin A antibodies directed against cholera toxin B subunit prevent the toxin-induced chloride secretory response and block toxin binding to epithelial cells *in vitro*. *Infect Immun* 1993;61:5271–5278.
98. Yamamoto T, Kamano T, Uchimura M, et al. *Vibrio cholerae* O1 adherence to villi and lymphoid follicle epithelium: *in vitro* model using formalin-treated human small intestine and correlation between adherence and cell-associated hemagglutinin levels. *Infect Immun* 1988;56:3241–3250.
99. Yamamoto T, Yokota T. Adherence targets of *Vibrio parahaemolyticus* in human small intestines. *Infect Immun* 1989;57: 2410–2419.
100. Yamamoto T, Yokota T. *Vibrio cholerae* O1 adherence to human small intestinal M cells *in vitro*. *J Infect Dis* 1989;160:168–169.
101. Killeen K, Spriggs D, Mekalanos JJ. Bacterial mucosal vaccines: *Vibrio cholerae* as a live attenuated vaccine/vector paradigm. *Curr Top Microbiol Immunol* 1999;236:237–254.
102. Uchida J. An ultrastructural study on active uptake and transport of bacteria by microfold cells (M cells) to the lymphoid follicles in the rabbit appendix. *J Clin Electron Microsc* 1987;20: 379–394.
103. Inman LR, Cantey JR. Specific adherence of *Escherichia coli* (strain RDEC-1) to membranous (M) cells of the Peyer's patch in *Escherichia coli* diarrhea in the rabbit. *J Clin Invest* 1983;71: 1–8.
104. Inman LR, Cantey JR. Peyer's patch lymphoid follicle epithelial adherence of a rabbit enteropathogenic *Escherichia coli* (strain RDEC-1). Role of plasmid-mediated pili in initial adherence. *J Clin Invest* 1984;74:90–95.
105. Sansonetti PJ, Arondel J, Cantey RJ, et al. Infection of rabbit Peyer's patches by *Shigella flexneri*: effect of adhesive and invasive bacterial phenotypes on follicular-associated epithelium. *Infect Immun* 1996;64:2752–2764.
106. Rafiee P, Leffler H, Byrd JC, et al. A sialoglycoprotein complex linked to the microvillus cytoskeleton acts as a receptor for pilus (AF/R1) mediated adhesion of enteropathogenic *Escherichia coli* (RDEC-1) in rabbit small intestine. *J Cell Biol* 1991;115: 1021–1029.
107. Knutton S, Lloyd DR, McNeish AS. Adhesion of enteropathogenic *Escherichia coli* to human intestinal enterocytes and cultured human intestinal mucosa. *Infect Immun* 1987;55:69–77.
108. Donnenberg MS, Kaper JB, Finlay BB. Interactions between enteropathogenic *Escherichia coli* and host epithelial cells. *Trends Microbiol* 1997;5:109–114.
109. Raupach B, Mecsas J, Heczko U, et al. Bacterial epithelial cell cross talk. *Curr Top Microbiol Immunol* 1999;236:137–162.
110. DeVinney R, Knoechel DG, Finlay BB. Enteropathogenic *Escherichia coli*: cellular harassment. *Curr Opin Microbiol* 1999; 2:83–88.
111. Karch H, Heesemann J, Laufs R, et al. Serological response to

type 1-like somatic fimbriae in diarrheal infection due to classical enteropathogenic *Escherichia coli. Microb Pathogen* 1987;2:425–434.
112. Sansonetti PJ, Phalipon A. M cells as ports of entry for enteroinvasive pathogens: mechanisms of interaction, consequences for the disease process. *Semin Immunol* 1999;11:193–203.
113. Hale TL. Bacillary dysentery. In: Hausler WJ, Sussman M, eds. *Topley and Wilson's microbiology and microbial infections. Bacterial infections,* vol 3. London: Arnold, 1998.
114. Dupont HL, Levine MM, Hornick RB, et al. Inoculum size in shigellosis and implications for expected mode of transmission. *J Infect Dis* 1989;159:1126–1128.
115. Mounier J, Vasselon T, Hellio R, et al. *Shigella flexneri* enters human colonic Caco-2 cells through the basolateral pole. *Infect Immun* 1992;60:237–248.
116. Bourdet-Sicard R, Egile C, Sansonetti PJ, et al. Diversion of cytoskeletal processes by *Shigella* during invasion of epithelial cells. *Microbes and Infection* 2000;2:813–819.
117. Sansonetti PJ, Mounier J, Prevost MC, et al. Cadherin expression is required for the spread of *Shigella flexneri* between epithelial cells. *Cell* 1994;76:829–839.
118. Elewaut D, DiDonato JA, Kim JM, et al. NFkB is a central regulator of the intestinal epithelial cell innate response induced by infection with enteroinvasive bacteria. *J Immunol* 1999;163:1457–1466.
119. Philpott DJ, Yamaoka S, Israël A, et al. Invasive *Shigella flexneri* activates NFkB through an LPS-dependent innate intracellular response and leads to IL-8 expression in epithelial cells. *J Immunol* 2000;165:903–914.
120. Mathan MM, Mathan VI. Morphology of rectal mucosa of patients with shigellosis. *Rev Infect Dis* 1991;13[Suppl.4:S314–S318.
121. Sansonetti PJ, Arondel J, Cantey JR, et al. Infection of rabbit Peyer's patches by *Shigella flexneri*: effect of adhesive or invasive bacterial phenotypes on follicle-associated epithelium. *Infect Immun* 1996;64:2752–2764.
122. Sansonetti PJ. Genetic and molecular basis of epithelial cell invasion by *Shigella* species. *Rev Infect Dis* 1991;13:S285–S292.
123. Wassef JS, Keren DF, Mailloux JL. Role of M cells in initial antigen uptake and in ulcer formation in the rabbit intestinal loop model of *Shigellosis. Infect Immun* 1989;57:858–863.
124. Zychlinsky A, Prévost MC, Sansonetti PJ. *Shigella flexneri* induces apoptosis in infected macrophages. *Nature*1992;358:167–169.
125. Hilbi H, Moss,JE, Hersh D, et al. Shigella-induced apoptosis is dependent on caspase-1 which binds to IpaB. *J Biol Chem* 1998;273:32895–32900.
126. Sansonetti PJ, Phalipon A, Arondel J, et al. Caspase-1 activation of IL-1b and IL-18 are essential for *Shigella flexneri-* induced inflammation. *Immunity* 2000;12:581–590.
127. Autenrieth, IB, Firsching R. Penetration of M cells and destruction of Peyer's patches by *Yersinia enterocolitica*: an ultrastructural and histological study. *J Med Microbiol* 1996;44:285–294.
128. Fujimura Y, Kihara T, Mine H. Membranous cells as a portal of *Yersinia pseudotuberculosis* entry into rabbit ileum. *J Clin Electron Microsc* 1992;25:35–45.
129. Grutzkau A, Hanski C, Hahn H, et al. Involvement of M cells in the bacterial invasion of Peyer's patches: a common mechanism shared by *Yersinia enterocolitica* and other enteroinvasive bacteria. *Gut* 1990;31:1011–1015.
130. Marra A, Isberg RR. Invasin-dependent and invasin-independent pathways for translocation of *Yersinia pseudotuberculosis* across the Peyer's patch intestinal epithelium. *Infect Immun* 1997;65:3412–3421.
131. Isberg, RR, Leong JM. Multiple b1 chain integrins are receptors for invasin, a protein that promotes bacterial penetration into mammalian cells. *Cell* 1990;60:861–871.
132. Isberg RR, Voorhis DL. Identification of invasin, a protein that allows enteric bacteria to penetrate mammalian cells. *Cell* 1987;50:769–778.
133. Clark MA, Hirst BH, Jepson MA. M-cell surface b1 integrin expression and invasin-mediated targeting of *Yersinia pseudotuberculosis* to mouse Peyer's patch M cells. *Infect Immun* 1998;66:1237–1244.
134. Pepe JC, Miller VL. *Yersinia enterocolitica* invasin: a primary role in the initiation of infection. *Proc Natl Acad Sci U S A* 1993;90:6473–6477.
135. Hynes RO. Integrins: versatility, modulation and signaling in cell adhesion. *Cell* 1992;69:11–25.
136. Fällmann M, Persson C, Wolf-Watz H. *Yersinia* proteins that target host-cell signaling pathways. *J Clin Invest* 1997;99:1153–1157.
137. Mills S, Boland A, Sory MP, et al. *Yersinia enterocolitica* induces apoptosis in macrophages by a process requiring functional type III secretion and translocation mechanism and involving YopP presumably acting as an effector protein. *Proc Natl Acad Sci U S A* 1997;94:12638–12643.
138. Monack DM, Mecsas J, Ghori N, et al. *Yersinia* signals macrophages to undergo apoptosis and Yop J is necessary for the cell death. *Proc Natl Acad Sci U S A* 1997;94:10385–10390.
139. Ruckdeschel K, Roggenkamp A, Lafont V, et al. Interaction of *Yersinia enterocolitica* with macrophages leads to macrophage cell death through apoptosis. *Infect Immun* 1997;65:4813–4821.
140. Clark MA., Jepson MA, Simmons NL, et al. Preferential interaction of *Salmonella typhimurium* with mouse Peyer's patch M cells. *Res Microbiol* 1994;145:543–552.
141. Takeuchi A. Electron microscope studies of experimental *Salmonella* infection. I. Penetration into the intestinal epithelium by *Salmonella typhimurium. Am J Pathol* 1967;50:109–136.
142. Vasquez-Torres A, Jones-Carson J, Baumler AJ, et al. Extraintestinal dissemination of Salmonella by CD18-expressing phagocytes. *Nature* 1999;401:804–808.
143. Kohbata S, Yokobata H, Yabuuchi E. Cytopathogenic effect of *Salmonella typhi* GIFU 10007 on M cells of murine ileal Peyer's patches in ligated ileal loops: an ultrastructural study. *Microbiol Immunol* 1986;30:1225–1237.
144. Baumler AJ, Tsolis RM, Heffron F. The *lpf* fimbrial operon mediates adhesion of *Salmonella typhimurium* to murine Peyer's patch. *Proc.Natl.Acad Sci.U S A* 1996;93:279–283.
145. Giannasca KT, Giannasca PJ, Neutra MR. Role of apical membrane glycoconjugates in adherence of *Salmonella typhimurium* to intestinal epithelial cells. *Infect Immun* 1996;64:135–145.
146. Finlay BB, Falkow S. *Salmonella* interactions with polarized human intestinal Caco-2 epithelial cells. *J Infect Dis* 1990;162:1096–1106.
147. Penheiter KL, Mathur N, Giles D, et al. Non-invasive *Salmonella typhimurium* mutants are avirulent because of an inability to enter and destroy M cells of ileal Peyer's patches. *Mol Microbiol* 1997;24:697–709.
148. Hersh D, Monack DM, Smith MR, et al. The *Salmonella* invasin SipB induces macrophage apoptosis by binding to caspase-1. *Proc Natl Acad Sci U S A* 1999;96:2396–2401.
149. Miller SI. PhoP/PhoQ: macrophage-specific modulator of *Salmonella* virulence? *Mol Microbiol* 1991;5:2073–2078.
150. Shea J, Hensel M, Gleeson C, et al. Identification of a virulence locus encoding a second type III secretion system in *Salmonella typhimurium Proc Natl Acad Sci U S A* 1996;93:2593–2597.
151. Walker RI, Schauder-Chock EA, Parker JL. Selective association and transport of *Campylobacter jejuni* through M cells of rabbit Peyer's patches. *Can J Microbiol* 1988;34:1142–1147.
152. Momotani E, Whipple DL, Thiermann AB, et al. Role of M cells and macrophages in the entrance of *Mycobacterium paratuberculosis* into domes of ileal Peyer's patches in calves. *Vet Pathol* 1988;25:131–137.

153. Fujimura Y. Functional morphology of microfold cells (M cells) in Peyer's patches. Phagocytosis and transport of BCG by M cells into rabbit Peyer's patches. *Gastroenterol Jpn* 1986;21:325–335.
154. Bisaillon M, Bernier L, Sénéchal S, et al. A glycosyl hydrolase activity of mammalian reovirus sigma1 protein can contribute to viral infection through a mucus layer. *J Mol Biol* 1999;286: 759–773.
155. Colman PM, Varghese JN, Laver WG. Structure of the catalytic and antigenic sites in influenza virus neuraminidase *Nature (London)* 1983;303:41–47.
156. Wolf JL, Rubin DH, Finberg RS, et al. Intestinal M cells: a pathway for entry of reovirus into the host. *Science* 1981;212: 471–472.
157. Amerongen HM, Weltzin RA, Farnet CM, et al. Transepithelial transport of HIV-1 by intestinal M cells: a mechanism for transmission of AIDS. *J Acquir Immune Defic Syndr* 1991;4: 760–765.
158. Bass DM, Bodkin D, Dambrauskas R, et al. Intraluminal proteolytic activation plays an important role in replication of type 1 reovirus in the intestines of neonatal mice. *J Virol* 1990;64: 1830–1833.
159. Bodkin DK, Nibert ML, Fields BN. Proteolytic digestion of reovirus in the intestinal lumen of neonatal mice. *J Virol* 1989; 63:4676–4681.
160. Amerongen HM, Wilson G, Fields BN, et al. Proteolytic processing of reovirus is required for adherence to intestinal M cells. *J Virol* 1994;68:8428–8432.
161. Bass DM, Trier JS, Dambrauskas R, et al. Reovirus type 1 infection of small intestinal epithelium in suckling mice and its effect on M cells. *Lab Invest* 1988;55:226–235.
162. Owen RL, Bass DM, Piazza AJ. Colonic lymphoid patches. A portal of entry in mice for type I reovirus administered anally. *Gastroenterology* 1990;98:A468
163. Morin MJ, Warner A, Fields BN. A pathway for entry of reoviruses into the host through M cells of the respiratory tract. *J Exp Med* 1994;180:1523–1527.
164. Dryden KA, Wang G, Yeager M, et al. Early steps in reovirus infection are associated with dramatic changes in supramolecular structure and protein conformation: analysis of virions and subviral particles by cryoelectron microscopy and image reconstruction. *J Cell Biol* 1993;122:1023–1041.
165. Lee PWK, Gilmore R. Reovirus cell attachment protein s1: structure-function relationships and biogenesis. In: Tyler KL, Oldstone MBA, eds. *Reoviruses. I: Structure, proteins, and genetics.* Berlin: Springer-Verlaag; 1998:137–153.
166. Nibert ML, Furlong DB, Fields BN. Mechanisms of viral pathogenesis. *J Clin Invest*1991;88:727–734.
167. Chappell JD, Duong JL, Wright BA, et al. Identification of carbohydrate-binding domains in the attachment proteins of type 1 and type 3 reoviruses. *J Virol* 2000;74:8472–8479.
168. Chappell JD, Gunn VL, Wetzel JD, et al. Mutations in type 3 reovirus that determine binding to sialic acid are contained in the fibrous tail domain of viral attachment protein s1. *J Virol* 1997;71:1834–1841.
169. Racaniello VR, Ren R. Poliovirus biology and pathogenesis. *Curr Top Microbiol Immunol* 1996;206:305–325.
170. Koprowski H. Immunization of man against poliomyelitis with attenuated preparations of living virus. *Ann N Y Acad Sci* 1955; 61:1039–1049.
171. Ogra PL, Karzon DT. Distribution of poliovirus antibody in serum, nasopharynx and alimentary tract following segmental immunization of lower alimentary tract with poliovaccine. *J Immunol* 1969;102:1423–1430.
172. Mendelsohn CL, Wimmer E, Racaniello VR. Cellular receptor for poliovirus: molecular cloning, nucleotide sequence, and expression of a new member of the immunoglobulin superfamily. *Cell* 1989;56:855–865.
173. Morrow CD, Novak MJ, Ansardi DC, et al. Recombinant viruses as vectors for mucosal immunity. *Curr Top Microbiol Immunol* 1998;236:255–274.
174. Milman G, Sharma O. Mechanisms of HIV/SIV mucosal transmission. *AIDS Res Human Retrovir*1994;10:1305–1312.
175. Clerici M, Clark EA, Polacino P, et al. T-cell proliferation to subinfectious SIV correlates with lack of infection after challenge of macaques. *AIDS* 1994;8:1391–1395.
176. Lehner T, Bergmeier L, Tao L, et al. Mucosal receptors and T- and B-cell immunity. In: Giraldo G, Bolognesi DP, Salvatore M, et al., eds. *Development and applications of vaccines and gene therapy in AIDS. Antibiot Chemother,* vol 4. Basel: Karger; 1996:21–29.
177. Pauza CD, Emau P, Salvato MS, et al. Pathogenesis of SIV mac51 after atraumatic inoculation of the rectal mucosa in rhesus monkeys. *J Med Primatol* 1993;22:154–161.
178. Butor C, Couedel-Courteille A, Guilet JG, et al. Differential distribution of galactosylceramide, H antigen, and carcinoembryonic antigen in rhesus macaque digestive mucosa. *J Histochem Cytochem* 1996;44:1021–1031.
179. Holgersson J, Stromberg N, Breimer ME. Glycolipids of human large intestine: differences in glycolipid expression related to anatomical localization, epithelial/non-epithelial tissue and the ABO, Le and Se phenotypes of the donors. *Biochimie* 1988;70:1565–1574.
180. Fantini J, Cook DG, Nathanson N, et al. Infection of colonic epithelial cell lines by type 1 human immunodeficiency virus (HIV-1) is associated with cell surface expression of galactosyl ceramide, a potential alternative gp120 receptor. *Proc Natl Acad Sci U S A* 1993;90:2700–2704.
181. Furuta Y, Erikkson K, Svennerholm B, et al. Infection of vaginal and colonic epithelial cells by the human immunodeficiency virus type 1 is neutralized by antibodies raised against conserved epitopes in the envelope glycoprotein gp120. *Proc Natl Acad Sci U S A* 1994;91:12559–12563.
182. Fox CH, Kotler D, Tierney A, et al. Detection of HIV-1 RNA in the lamina propria of patients with AIDS and gastrointestinal disease. *J Infect Dis* 1989;159:467–471.
183. Bomsel M. Transcytosis of infectious human immunodeficiency virus across a tight epithelial cell line barrier. *Nat Med* 1997; 3:42–47.
184. Nedrud JG, Liang XP, Hague N, et al. Combined oral/nasal immunization protects mice from Sendai virus infection. *J Immunol* 1987;139:3484–3492.
185. Haneberg B, Kendall D, Amerongen HM, et al. Induction of specific immunoglobulin A in the small intestine, colon-rectum, and vagina measured by a new method for collection of secretions from local mucosal surfaces. *Infect Immun* 1994;62:15–23.
186. Kozlowski PA, Cu-Uvin S, Neutra MR, et al. Comparison of the oral, rectal, and vaginal immunization routes for induction of antibodies in rectal and genital tract secretions of women. *Infect Immun*1997;65:1387–1394.
187. Kozlowski PA, Lynch RM, Patterson RR, et al. A modified wick method utilizing Weck-Cel sponges for collection of human rectal secretions and analysis of mucosal HIV antibody. *J AIDS* 2000;24:297–309.

12

STRUCTURE AND FUNCTION OF MUCOSAL IMMUNOGLOBULIN A

MICHAEL E. LAMM

Historically, the field of immunology, in particular the study of humoral immunity, developed in the context of resistance to infectious diseases. For almost a century, it has been recognized that the humoral immune system is compartmentalized in that antibodies in the mucosal secretions, as in the gastrointestinal tract, differ from those in the serum (1). Initially, these differences were studied in terms of the kinetics of appearance of antibody and the time for peak responses after exposure to antigen. It was observed that after intestinal infection and immunization, specific antibodies appeared sooner in the intestinal secretions and peaked earlier than did antibodies in the serum (2,3). Furthermore, resistance to challenge by virulent organisms correlated better with the titer of antibodies in the intestinal secretions than with the titer of serum antibodies.

It was only much later that the various classes of antibody were defined, with subsequent investigation showing that the immunoglobulin A (IgA) isotype, although only a minor component of the immunoglobulins in serum, is the major class of antibody in the mucosal secretions throughout the body, including the intestinal tract (4). Moreover, mucosal IgA antibodies are synthesized locally by plasma cells situated in the lamina propria; in fact, the intestinal lamina propria contains the highest tissue density of plasma cells in the body, and 90% of them make IgA (5). After secretion by these plasma cells, the IgA passes directly through the overlying epithelium to enter the mucosal fluids. In the course of its epithelial passage, IgA forms complexes with an epithelial cell receptor, part of which remains chemically bound to the IgA as it enters the luminal secretions (6); this extra polypeptide chain in secretory IgA is known as the *secretory component* (SC).

Thus, the relatively low concentration of IgA in serum does not reflect the amount of IgA actually being synthesized by the body. On a daily basis, the body synthesizes far more IgA, 66 mg/kg of body weight, than all other immunoglobulin classes combined (7). Most of this IgA is produced in the mucous membranes, much of it in the intestine, where it acts as the body's first line of immunologic defense, serving at the interface between the internal milieu and the external environment (8). Some 40 mg of secretory IgA per kilogram of body weight enters the intestinal secretions daily (9).

This chapter considers the structure, transport, and function of mucosal IgA and develops the thesis that it functions not only in the luminal secretions as a protective barrier but also in two other locations—namely, within the intestinal epithelium and in the mucosal lamina propria.

STRUCTURE OF IMMUNOGLOBULIN A

The IgA in serum is synthesized to a great extent in the bone marrow. It occurs mostly with a molecular weight of 160 kd in monomeric form—that is, the classic immunoglobulin structure of two heavy (H) α chains and two light (L) chains, either κ or λ in a given molecule (10) (Fig. 12.1). The two subclasses of IgA, IgA1 and IgA2, are defined by differences in the α chain, mostly the consequence of a deletion in the hinge region at the midpoint of the $\alpha 2$ chain (11). Within the α chains of the IgA2 subclass are two allotypic variants, IgA2m(1) and IgA2m(2), and possibly a third, IgA2(n) (12). As mediators of immune function, however, the two subclasses have not been assigned any major differences, although their ratio can vary in the local population of plasma cells in different parts of the body, in different body fluids and secretions, in the antibody response to different kinds of antigens, and in certain diseases (13). The IgA1 subclass is uniquely susceptible to proteolysis by IgA proteases, a family of enzymes produced by certain pathogenic bacteria, that manifest unusual substrate specificity for the hinge region of the $\alpha 1$ chain, which is lacking in IgA2 (14–16). The IgA1 subclass thus appears to be at somewhat of a disadvantage in resisting infections caused by such pathogens.

M.E. Lamm: Institute of Pathology, Case Western Reserve University, Cleveland, Ohio

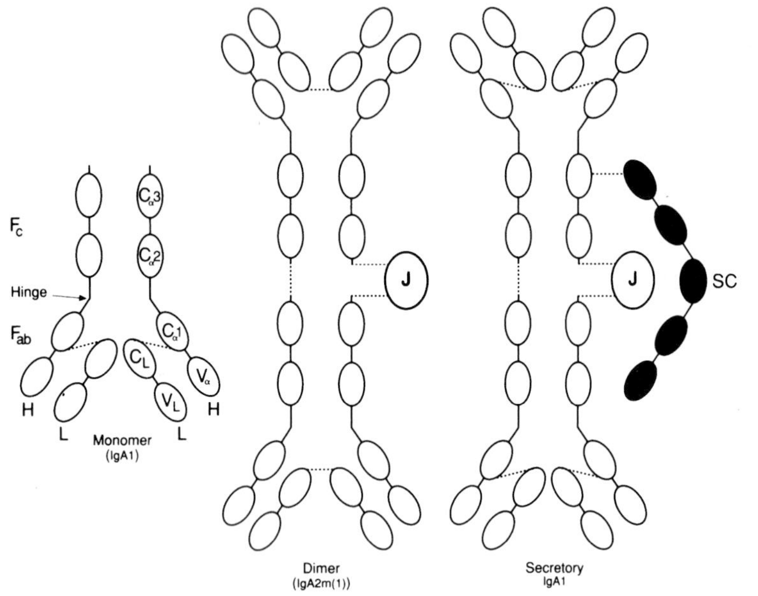

FIGURE 12.1. Structure of immunoglobulin A (IgA) monomer, IgA dimer, and secretory IgA. The domains of the component polypeptide chains are indicated by *ellipses*, *V* for variable amino acid sequence domains and *C* for constant sequence domains. Selected interchain disulfide bonds are indicated by *dashed lines*. The monomer (*left*) is composed of two heavy (H) α and two light (L) chains. In the IgA1 subclass (illustrated) and the IgA2m(2) allotype of the IgA2 subclass, the H and L chains are conventionally covalently linked by disulfide bonds. The IgA1 subclass has an extended hinge region, which is susceptible to IgA proteases. Dimeric IgA is shown in the middle. In the IgA2m(1) allotypic variant (shown), but not the IgA2m(2) variant, the L chains are linked by disulfide bonds to each other instead of to the H chains. Dimeric IgA also contains a J chain, which is disulfide-bonded to C-terminal penultimate half-cystines in the two IgA monomer subunits. In secretory IgA (*right*), the dimer additionally contains a secretory component (SC) chain; its C-terminal domain is disulfide-bonded to the Cα2 domain of one of the IgA monomer subunits. The SC chain is formed during the release of secretory IgA from the epithelial cell when the external, IgA-binding portion of the polymeric immunoglobulin receptor is cleaved by proteolysis from the membrane-spanning segment.

In contrast to the IgA in serum, which is mostly monomeric IgA1, the IgA produced by mucosal plasma cells that enters the local secretions is relatively enriched in IgA2 (17), the extent of increase varying in different mucous membranes. For example, the relative amount of IgA2 increases along the intestinal tract with the distance from the stomach (13). Furthermore, mucosal IgA is mostly dimeric (i.e., composed of two of the basic four-chain immunoglobulin subunits, so that the dimer possesses four α and four L polypeptide chains) (Fig. 12.1). The two subunits of the dimer are joined covalently end to end by a disulfide bridge between the penultimate cysteine residues at the C-termini of two of the α chains and by disulfide bridges from the analogous residues on the other two α chains to a third type of polypeptide chain, the 17-kd J chain (18–20). J chains, like immunoglobulin H and L chains, are synthesized by plasma cells and are present in all oligomeric immunoglobulins (i.e., all antibody molecules having more than one basic four-chain subunit, such as dimeric IgA and pentameric IgM). The J chain is thought to play a role in initiating or stabilizing the oligomeric structure and in providing a conformation for IgA that enhances binding to the epithelial polymeric immunoglobulin receptor (pIgR) (12,21,22).

As mentioned, the externally secreted form of IgA contains a fourth kind of polypeptide chain, SC, derived by cleavage of a parent molecule, the pIgR; it is incorporated into dimeric IgA as it binds to and passes through the epithelial cell on its way to the secretions. This SC, an 80-kd subunit containing five domains, is a member of the immunoglobulin superfamily (23–25). It is disulfide-bonded to dimeric IgA when a labile intrachain disulfide bridge in the pIgR rearranges to enable bridging to an α chain of one of the two monomer subunits of the IgA dimer during epithelial transcytosis (26–28). Fig. 12.1 shows the structure of the 420-kd secretory IgA molecule.

The SC portion of secretory IgA serves two important functions. One, actually performed by its parent molecule, the pIgR, is to promote binding of dimeric IgA to the mucosal epithelial cell and its transport through the cell into the secretions (25). The second function of SC, after secretion, is to stabilize and protect secretory IgA from proteolytic digestion by the enzymes present in the gastrointestinal fluids, both those secreted to aid in the digestion of food and those produced by the intestinal microflora (29–31).

BIOLOGIC PROPERTIES OF IMMUNOGLOBULIN A

The secretory form of IgA, containing an IgA dimer, has four combining sites for antigen in the Fab regions. These multiple combining sites, in comparison with the two in IgG, the principal immunoglobulin in serum, make secretory IgA a much more effective agglutinator of antigens (a property that is even more pronounced in IgM, which contains five four-chain immunoglobulin subunits and therefore 10 antibody combining sites). The biologic properties of antibodies, on the other hand, embrace those properties of antibodies that are mediated by their Fc regions, such as activation of complement and binding to receptors on phagocytic cells. The biologic properties of IgA have been reviewed (13,32).

Although some species variations may exist in the most biologically relevant systems, human IgA appears to be incapable of activating either the classic or alternative complement pathways; in fact, IgA antibodies can even diminish complement activation by IgG or IgM antibodies in the same immune complex (12,33,34). Furthermore, it is by no means clear that the intestinal secretions have a fully functional complement system capable of activation by antibody, or, if such activation is possible, what significance it may have *in vivo*.

An analogous situation holds with respect to binding to leukocyte Fc receptors (in this case, the Fcα receptor CD89), which alone or in concert with cell surface complement receptors may activate such functions as phagocytosis and degranulation. Although Fcα receptors have been described and may be significant within the mucosa (35–37), it is not clear to what extent binding to such receptors in the milieu of the mucosal secretions, which normally lack leukocytes, may be biologically significant. Interestingly, the Fcα receptor on Kupffer cells can be up-regulated to promote phagocytosis of IgA-coated bacteria; this may be an important mechanism to remove bacteria that have entered the portal circulation (38).

It is noteworthy that the well-characterized effector functions of antibodies in general relate to their functions within the body proper, including serum, not in the external secretions. In the author's view, even though IgA in internal body fluids may be capable of exerting some effector function, IgA is not particularly important within the body. It is clear that IgA, in comparison with IgG, IgE, and IgM, is certainly less potent (13,39). Also, no compelling evidence suggests, and perhaps there is no good reason to think so, that effector functions mediated by the Fc portion of antibodies are important in mucosal secretions. What is important for an exocrine immunoglobulin such as IgA is that it be able to reach the secretions, which it does via a selective transepithelial pathway mediated by the pIgR, and that within the secretions, like antibodies generically, it be able to bind to antigen. As discussed later, in the section entitled "Functions of Immunoglobulin A in Mucosal Defense," it should become evident that the usual effector functions of antibodies may not even be needed. Indeed, it is possible that during the course of evolution, IgA was selected not to mediate the typical effector functions of antibodies because it must operate in parts of the body where foreign substances are ever present, the best example being the gastrointestinal tract with its content of food and microbial flora. Thus, the abundantly available IgA antibodies are constantly interacting with antigen, and if the resulting immune complexes were capable of activating inflammatory mediators, the intestine would be subject to a chronic state of immunologically mediated inflammation, clearly an undesirable situation. In fact, IgA antibodies may be able to dampen the proinflammatory properties of the other classes of immunoglobulins (32). Therefore, it seems appropriate to consider that although the ability to bind antigens is important for IgA, the ability to trigger Fc effector functions may not be as important.

TRANSEPITHELIAL TRANSPORT OF IMMUNOGLOBULIN A

Only dimers and higher polymers of IgA are actively transported across epithelia because monomeric IgA cannot effectively bind to the pIgR. The transport of IgA and pIgR across epithelial cells has been studied mainly in intestinal epithelium and hepatocytes and in model systems with the use of polarized epithelial monolayers (6,8,25). Initially, dimeric IgA secreted by plasma cells in the intestinal lamina propria diffuses across the epithelial basement membrane to be able to bind noncovalently to pIgR on the basolateral surface of columnar epithelial cells, where it is especially prominent in intestinal crypts (Fig. 12.2). Following endocytosis, the complex enters a transcytotic vesicular system and the apical recycling compartment, through which it reaches the apical (microvillous) surface (25). Close to the time of secretion from the epithelial cell, the noncovalent binding between IgA and pIgR is stabilized by the formation of a disulfide bond

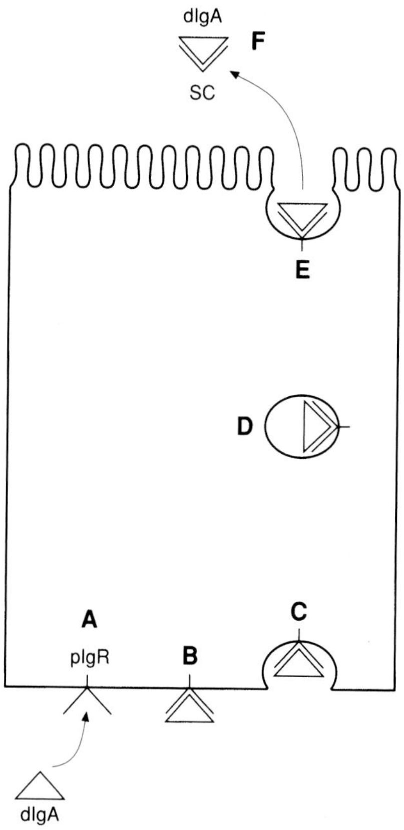

FIGURE 12.2. Epithelial transcytosis of immunoglobulin A (IgA). The cellular events associated with the transport of IgA across mucosal epithelia are illustrated. After synthesis in the rough endoplasmic reticulum, the polymeric immunoglobulin receptor (pIgR) passes through the Golgi apparatus, the trans-Golgi network, and vesicles that allow it to be inserted as a transmembrane protein into the basolateral plasma membrane of the cell (**A**), with its IgA-binding portion on the outside and its cytoplasmic tail containing cell-sorting signals on the inside. A molecule of dimeric IgA, after secretion by a local plasma cell, binds noncovalently to the pIgR (**B**), and the complex undergoes endocytosis (**C**). The complex enters a transcytotic system of vesicles (**D**) and via the apical recycling compartment reaches the apical (microvillous) plasma membrane (**E**), where a cell surface protease cleaves the external, IgA-binding portion of the pIgR, now termed *secretory component* (SC), from the transmembrane segment, releasing the complex of dimeric IgA and SC (i.e., secretory IgA) into the lumen (**F**). Near the time of release, the original noncovalent bonding of IgA to pIgR is stabilized by the formation of disulfide bonds.

between the fifth domain of pIgR and the Cα2 domain of IgA (26,28,40). Finally, an enzyme thought to be present in the apical plasma membrane (41,42) cleaves the pIgR between its external and transmembrane portions so that the complex of dimeric IgA and the external segment of the pIgR (i.e., SC) is secreted into the lumen. Although IgA is very much the dominant secretory immunoglobulin, it should be kept in mind that IgM (also oligomeric, containing a J chain, and capable of binding to pIgR, but present in smaller amounts in the lamina propria) is transported across the epithelium by the same mechanism (43).

The possible role of the liver in transporting IgA into the intestinal contents should be considered. In rodents, this is an important pathway because the hepatocyte expresses pIgR on its sinusoidal surface and the serum contains an appreciable amount of dimeric IgA, which can accordingly be transported into the bile (44–46). In humans, however, most of the IgA in serum is monomeric and hence incapable of binding to pIgR, and the hepatocyte does not express pIgR (47). The epithelium in the bile ducts and gallbladder in humans, on the other hand, does express pIgR and appears to be capable of transporting into bile small amounts of IgA, in part secreted by adjacent plasma cells.

FUNCTIONS OF IMMUNOGLOBULIN A IN MUCOSAL DEFENSE

Initial concepts of local immunity were based on observations that in response to immunization or challenge, the kinetics of intestinal antibody production do not mirror those in serum, and intestinal antibodies cannot therefore be mere transudates from the serum. In the more modern era of immunology, studies of the genesis of mucosal plasma cells and of the synthesis, structure, and transport of mucosal IgA have clarified many aspects of the origin of local humoral immunity. It is generally agreed that the role of mucosal IgA antibodies is to protect against infectious microorganisms (and other foreign matter), most of which either afflict mucous membranes or invade the body through a mucosal portal of entry. The concept that IgA offers such protection is supported by studies of oral (Sabin) vaccination against poliomyelitis, which induces the formation of intestinal IgA antibodies (48), and by studies of resistance to a variety of other mucosal infections, which have amply demonstrated that among the various immunologic parameters, resistance best correlates with the content of IgA antibodies in the local secretions (49–51). In addition, it is well established that patients with IgA deficiency manifest an increased incidence of mucosal infections and other disorders involving mucous membranes (52). This general background underlies modern efforts to develop oral immunization regimens for intestinal pathogens (53,54).

In addition to clinical studies, experiments in animals with monoclonal antibodies have now provided good evidence that IgA antibodies as the sole immunologic effector are able to prevent viral and bacterial infections in the respiratory (55–57) and intestinal tracts (58–60). Thus, the immunologic barrier/immune exclusion role for IgA, in which IgA antibodies in the luminal secretions defend against infection, is now well established. To mediate this protection, IgA antibodies bind to the surface of microorganisms and interfere with their motility and ability to bind to and penetrate the epithelial lining (61–64). In addition, IgA antibodies can neutralize bacterial toxins. As mentioned, IgA appears to be suited for this immune exclusion role more by virtue of having a selective mechanism for transport into the secretions than by having any special abilities as an antibody *per se.* In addition to being able to mediate exclusion via antigen-specific binding, the oligosaccharide side chains of IgA may bind to lectin-like bacterial fimbrial adhesins and thereby prevent bacteria from binding to glycan receptors on the intestinal epithelium (65).

It was long believed that immune exclusion is the only major function of mucosal IgA and its *raison d'être.* Recently, however, experiments *in vitro* and *in vivo* have led to the proposal that IgA antibodies function importantly in host defense in two other locales—namely, within epithelial cells during the transport of IgA into the secretions and within the mucosal lamina propria before epithelial transport (8).

The original experiments underlying these two newly proposed functions were carried out with cultures of epithelial cell monolayers. In this system, cells are polarized and attached to one another by tight junctions, which prevent passive diffusion of macromolecules between cells and across the monolayer. The epithelial cells used express pIgR on their basolateral surface and are thus able to transport dimeric IgA (66). To test the hypothesis that during transepithelial cell transport specific IgA antibodies have the potential to neutralize intracellular pathogens, cell monolayers were infected at the apical surface with virus and exposed to monoclonal IgA antibody at the basal surface. In this model, it was demonstrated by morphologic techniques that IgA antibody co-localizes with viral protein within the epithelial cells and, even more significantly, can inhibit production of virus (67–69). Moreover, IgA antibody *in vivo* appears to be able to neutralize virus intraepithelially (70) and to block the transcytosis of virus across epithelial cells (71).

The second hypothesis, that immune complexes containing dimeric IgA antibodies are transported by the same mechanism and route as free dimeric IgA, was also tested in the polarized epithelial monolayer system. Accordingly, soluble immune complexes of protein antigens and dimeric monoclonal IgA antibodies were shown to be transported from the basal to apical surface and into the medium above the monolayer (72). Transport depended on cellular expression of the pIgR, and the IgA antibody had to be polymeric. Moreover, intact immune complexes were transported, with no evidence of intracellular degradation. Even particles as large as a virus can be transported across epithelial cells by this mechanism (73). It was also demonstrated that immune complexes containing IgG (or monomeric IgA) and dimeric IgA antibodies bound in the same molecular complex to multivalent antigen are transported in like manner (74). Therefore, in principle, any immune complex in the mucosal lamina propria that contains a molecule of dimeric IgA is capable of being transported across the mucosal epithelium into the luminal secretions. Evidence for such transport of IgA immune complexes *in vivo* has recently been obtained (75). Thus, it is envisioned that IgA can function as an excretory immune system capable of excreting antigen from the mucosa, thereby ridding the body of potentially harmful immune complexes and minimizing the load of circulating immune complexes. However, the untoward possibility also exists that viruses in mucosal tissues can be complexed by IgA antibodies and thereby selectively introduced into epithelial cells (76).

These newly proposed functions of IgA may be important in mucosal defense. Certainly, mucous membranes are a common site of invasion by infectious agents, which can pass through or replicate in the lining epithelial cells. Therefore, the potential of IgA antibodies to encounter microbial pathogens within cells during their normal route of transport across the epithelium and to neutralize or excrete them is likely to be significant. However, even if the epithelial barrier were breached by microorganisms, IgA antibodies secreted by local plasma cells would have the opportunity to bind and eliminate them and their products across the epithelium, either as intact microorganisms coated by IgA antibody or as soluble immune complexes.

Thus, mucosal IgA can now be envisioned as functioning in any of three tiers to protect the host (Fig. 12.3). The innermost tier is the lamina propria, into which the abundant plasma cells secrete dimeric IgA. If IgA antibody binds antigen in the lamina propria, the complex can be directly excreted. The middle tier is the epithelial lining of the mucous membrane; if IgA antibody in transit to the secretions should meet an infectious pathogen inside an epithelial cell, it can neutralize or excrete it. The outermost tier, the place where secretory IgA has traditionally been thought to function, is within the intestinal lumen, where IgA antibody can bind to microbes or their toxins and prevent attachment to and penetration through the mucosal epithelium.

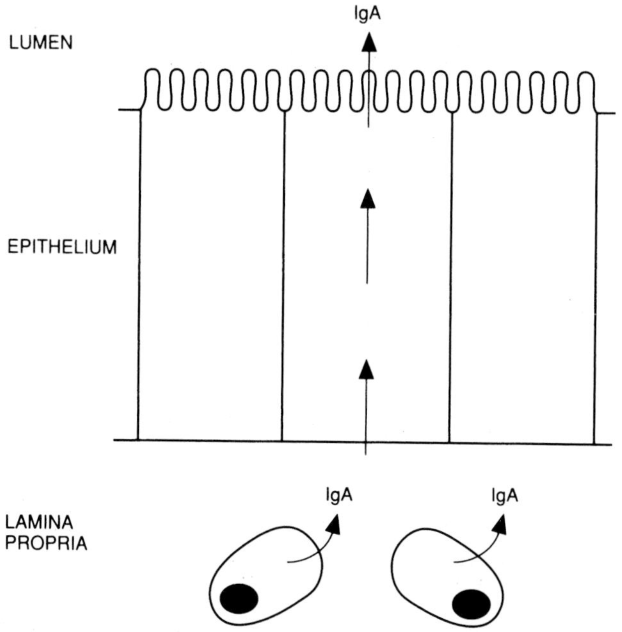

FIGURE 12.3. Three tiers of mucosal immunoglobulin A (IgA) function in host defense. Intestinal IgA is thought to be capable of functioning at three different levels. First, dimeric IgA antibodies secreted from plasma cells in the lamina propria have an opportunity to combine with antigens, including infectious agents and their products, that may be present in the lamina propria. Such immune complexes can then bind to and be transported into the intestinal lumen by the polymeric immunoglobulin receptor in the same manner as free dimeric IgA, an excretory function. Second, during their transepithelial transport, IgA antibodies have an opportunity to encounter intracellular microbes or their components within epithelial cells. In this way, they may be neutralized or excreted. Third, after epithelial transcytosis, secretory IgA antibodies may first encounter antigens within the intestinal lumen, where IgA can perform its immune exclusion function.

REFERENCES

1. Besredka A. *Local immunization.* Baltimore: Williams & Wilkins, 1927.
2. Burrows W, Deupree NG, Moore DE. The effect of X-irradiation on experimental enteric cholera in the guinea pig. *J Infect Dis* 1950;87:158–168.
3. Burrows W, Deupree NG, Moore DE. The effect of X-irradiation on fecal and urinary antibody response. *J Infect Dis* 1950;87: 169–183.
4. Tomasi TB. The discovery of secretory IgA and the mucosal immune system. *Immunol Today* 1992;13:416–418.
5. Lamm ME. Cellular aspects of immunoglobulin A. *Adv Immunol* 1976;22:223–290.
6. Brandtzaeg P. Role of J chain and secretory component in receptor-mediated glandular and hepatic transport of immunoglobulins in man. *Scand J Immunol* 1985;22:111–146.
7. Mestecky J, McGhee JR. Immunoglobulin A (IgA): molecular and cellular interactions involved in IgA biosynthesis and immune response. *Adv Immunol* 1987;40:153–245.
8. Lamm ME. Interaction of antigens and antibodies at mucosal surfaces. *Annu Rev Microbiol* 1997;51:311–340.
9. Conley ME, Delacroix DL. Intravascular and mucosal immunoglobulin A: two separate but related systems of immune defense *Ann Intern Med* 1987;106:892–899.
10. Kutteh WH, Prince SJ, Mestecky J. Tissue origins of human polymeric and monomeric IgA. *J Immunol* 1982;128:990–995.
11. Kerr MA. The structure and function of human IgA. *Biochem J* 1990;271:285–296.
12. Chintalacharuvu KR, Morrison SL. Production and characterization of recombinant IgA. *Immunotechnology* 1999;4:165–174.
13. Mestecky J, Lue C, Tarkowski A, et al. Comparative studies of the biological properties of human IgA subclasses. *Protides Biol Fluids* 1989;36:173–182.
14. Plaut AG. The IgA1 proteases of pathogenic bacteria. *Annu Rev Microbiol* 1983;37:603–622.

15. Kilian M, Reinholdt J, Lomholt H, et al. Biological significance of IgA1 proteases in bacterial colonization and pathogenesis: critical evaluation of experimental evidence. *APMIS* 1996;104:321–338.
16. Kilian M, Russell MW. Microbial evasion of IgA functions. In: Ogra PL, Mestecky J, Lamm ME, et al., eds. *Mucosal immunology,* second edition. San Diego: Academic Press, 1999:241–251.
17. Kett K, Brandtzaeg P, Radl J, et al. Different subclass distribution of IgA-producing cells in human lymphoid organs and various secretory tissues. *J Immunol* 1986;136:3631–3635.
18. Garcia-Pardo A, Lamm ME, Plaut AG, et al. J chain is covalently bound to both monomer subunits in human secretory IgA. *J Biol Chem* 1981;256:11734–11738.
19. Bastian A, Kratzin H, Eckart K, et al. Intra- and interchain disulfide bridges of the human J chain in secretory immunoglobulin A. *Biol Chem Hoppe Seyler* 1992;373:1255–1263.
20. Krugmann S, Pleass RJ, Atkin JD, et al. Structural requirements for assembly of dimeric IgA probed by site-directed mutagenesis of J chain and a cysteine residue of the α-chain CH2 domain. *J Immunol* 1997;159:244–249.
21. Brandtzaeg P, Prydz H. Direct evidence for an integrated function of J chain and secretory component in epithelial transport of immunoglobulins. *Nature* 1984;311:71–73.
22. Hendrickson BA, Conner DA, Ladd DJ, et al. Altered hepatic transport of immunoglobulin A in mice lacking the J chain. *J Exp Med* 1995;182:1905–1911.
23. Eiffert H, Quentin E, Decker J, et al. The primary structure of the human free secretory component and the arrangement of the disulfide bonds. *Hoppe Seylers Z Physiol Chem* 1984;365:1489–1495.
24. Krajci P, Kvale D, Tasken K, et al. Molecular cloning and exon–intron mapping of the gene encoding human transmembrane secretory component (the poly-Ig receptor). *Eur J Immunol* 1992;22:2309–2315.
25. Mostov K, Kaetzel CS. Immunoglobulin transport and the polymeric immunoglobulin receptor. In: Ogra PL, Mestecky J, Lamm ME, et al., eds. *Mucosal immunology,* second edition. San Diego: Academic Press, 1999:181–211.
26. Cunningham-Rundles C, Lamm ME. Reactive half-cystine peptides of the secretory component of human exocrine immunoglobulin A. *J Biol Chem* 1975;250:1987–1991.
27. Garcia-Pardo A, Lamm ME, Plaut AG, et al. Secretory component is covalently bound to a single subunit in human secretory IgA. *Mol Immunol* 1979;16:477–482.
28. Fallgreen-Gebauer E, Gebauer W, Bastian A, et al. The covalent linkage of secretory component to IgA. Structure of sIgA. *Biol Chem Hoppe Seyler* 1993;374:1023–1028.
29. Brown WR, Newcomb RW, Ishizaka K. Proteolytic degradation of exocrine and serum immunoglobulins. *J Clin Invest* 1970;49:1374–1380.
30. Underdown BJ, Dorrington KJ. Studies of the structural and conformational basis for the relative resistance of serum and secretory immunoglobulin A to proteolysis. *J Immunol* 1974;112:949–959.
31. Lindh E. Increased resistance of immunoglobulin A dimers to proteolytic degradation after binding of secretory component. *J Immunol* 1975;114:284–286.
32. Russell MW, Kilian M, Lamm ME. Biological activities of IgA. In: Ogra PL, Mestecky J, Lamm ME, et al., eds. *Mucosal immunology,* second edition. San Diego: Academic Press, 1999:225–240.
33. Jarvis GA, Griffiss JM. IgA1 blockade of IgG-initiated lysis of *Neisseria meningitidis* is a function of antigen-binding fragment binding to the polysaccharide capsule. *J Immunol* 1991;147:1962–1967.
34. Nikolova EB, Tomana M, Russell MW. All forms of human IgA antibodies bound to antigen interfere with complement (C3) fixation induced by IgG or by antigen alone. *Scand J Immunol* 1994;39:275–280.
35. Mazengera RL, Kerr MA. The specificity of the IgA receptor purified from human neutrophils. *Biochem J* 1990;272:159–165.
36. Monteiro RC, Cooper MD, Kubagawa H. Molecular heterogeneity of Fcα receptors detected by receptor-specific monoclonal antibodies. *J Immunol* 1992;148:1764–1770.
37. Kerr MA, Woof JM. Fcα receptors. In: Ogra PL, Mestecky J, Lamm ME, et al., eds. *Mucosal immunology,* second edition. San Diego: Academic Press, 1999:213–224.
38. van Egmond M, van Garderen E, van Spriel AB, et al. FcαRI-positive liver Kupffer cells: reappraisal of the function of immunoglobulin A in immunity. *Nat Med* 2000;6:680–685.
39. Emancipator SE, Lamm ME. Pathways of tissue injury initiated by humoral immune mechanisms. *Lab Invest* 1986;54:475–478.
40. Chintalacharuvu KR, Tavill AS, Louis LN, et al. Disulfide bond formation between dimeric immunoglobulin A and the polymeric immunoglobulin receptor during hepatic transcytosis. *Hepatology* 1994;19:162–173.
41. Musil LS, Baenziger JU. Proteolytic processing of rat liver membrane secretory component. Cleavage activity is localized to bile canalicular membranes. *J Biol Chem* 1988;263:15799–15808.
42. Solari R, Schaerer E, Tallichet C, et al. Cellular location of the cleavage event of the polymeric immunoglobulin receptor and fate of its anchoring domain in the rat hepatocyte. *Biochem J* 1989;257:759–768.
43. Natvig IB, Johansen F-E, Nordeng TW, et al. Mechanism for enhanced external transfer of dimeric IgA over pentameric IgM. Studies of diffusion, binding to the human polymeric Ig receptor, and epithelial transcytosis. *J Immunol* 1997;159:4330–4340.
44. Jackson GDF, Lemaitre-Coelho I, Vaerman J-P, et al. Rapid disappearance from serum of intravenously injected rat myeloma IgA and its secretion into bile. *Eur J Immunol* 1978;8:123–126.
45. Orlans E, Peppard J, Fry JF, et al. Secretory component as the receptor for polymeric IgA on rat hepatocytes. *J Exp Med* 1979;150:1577–1581.
46. Fisher MM, Nagy B, Bazin H, et al. Biliary transport of IgA: role of secretory component. *Proc Natl Acad Sci U S A* 1979;76:2008–2012.
47. Brown WR, Kloppel TM. The liver and IgA: immunological, cell biological and clinical implications. *Hepatology* 1989;9:763–784.
48. Ogra PL, Karzon DT. Formation and function of poliovirus antibody in different tissues. *Prog Med Virol* 1971;13:156–193.
49. Mills J, Van Kirk JE, Wright PF, et al. Experimental respiratory syncytial virus infection of adults. Possible mechanisms of resistance to infection and illness. *J Immunol* 1971;107:123–130.
50. Liew FY, Russell SM, Appleyard G, et al. Cross-protection in mice infected with influenza A virus by the respiratory route is correlated with local IgA antibody rather than serum antibody or cytotoxic T cell reactivity. *Eur J Immunol* 1984;14:350–356.
51. Offit PA, Clark HF. Protection against rotavirus-induced gastroenteritis in a murine model by passively acquired gastrointestinal but not circulating antibodies. *J Virol* 1985;54:58–64.
52. Burrows PD, Cooper MD. IgA deficiency. *Adv Immunol* 1997;65:245–276.
53. Nataro JP, Levine MM. Enteric bacterial vaccines: *Salmonella, Shigella, Cholera, Escherichia coli.* In: Ogra PL, Mestecky J, Lamm ME, et al., eds. *Mucosal immunology,* second edition. San Diego: Academic Press, 1999:851– 865.
54. Ward RL, Greenberg HB, Estes MK. Viral gastroenteritis vaccines. In: Ogra PL, Mestecky J, Lamm ME, et al., eds. *Mucosal immunology,* second edition. San Diego: Academic Press, 1999:867–880.
55. Mazanec MB, Nedrud JG, Lamm ME. Immunoglobulin A monoclonal antibodies protect against Sendai virus. *J Virol* 1987;61:2624–2626.
56. Renegar KB, Small Jr PA. Passive transfer of local immunity to influenza virus infection by IgA antibody. *J Immunol* 1991;146:1972–1978.

57. Weltzin R, Traina-Dorge V, Soike K, et al. Intranasal monoclonal IgA antibody to respiratory syncytial virus protects rhesus monkeys against upper and lower respiratory tract infection. *J Infect Dis* 1996;174:256–261.
58. Winner III L, Mack J, Weltzin R, et al. New model for analysis of mucosal immunity: intestinal secretion of specific monoclonal immunoglobulin A from hybridoma tumors protects against *Vibrio cholerae* infection. *Infect Immun* 1991;59:977–982.
59. Michetti P, Mahan MJ, Slauch JM, et al. Monoclonal secretory immunoglobulin A protects mice against oral challenge with the invasive pathogen *Salmonella typhimurium. Infect Immun* 1992; 60:1786–1792.
60. Blanchard TG, Czinn SJ, Maurer R, et al. Urease-specific monoclonal antibodies prevent *Helicobacter felis* infection in mice. *Infect Immun* 1995;63:1394–1399.
61. Williams RC, Gibbons RJ. Inhibition of bacterial adherence by secretory immunoglobulin A: a mechanism of antigen disposal. *Science* 1972;177:697–699.
62. Fubara ES, Freter R. Protection against bacterial infection by secretory IgA antibodies. *J Immunol* 1973;111:395–403.
63. Svanborg-Eden C, Svennerholm A-M. Secretory immunoglobulin A and G antibodies prevent adhesion of *Escherichia coli* to human urinary tract epithelial cells. *Infect Immun* 1978;22: 790–797.
64. Outlaw MC, Dimmock NJ. Mechanisms of neutralization of influenza virus on mouse tracheal epithelial cells by mouse monoclonal polymeric IgA and polyclonal IgM directed against the viral haemagglutinin. *J Gen Virol* 1990;71:69–76.
65. Wold A, Mestecky J, Tomana M, et al. Secretory immunoglobulin A carries oligosaccharide receptors for *Escherichia coli* type 1 fimbrial lectin. *Infect Immun* 1990;58:3073–3077.
66. Mostov KE, Deitcher DL. Polymeric immunoglobulin receptor expressed in MDCK cells transcytoses IgA. *Cell* 1986;46:613–621.
67. Mazanec MB, Kaetzel CS, Lamm ME, et al. Intracellular neutralization of virus by immunoglobulin A antibodies. *Proc Natl Acad Sci U S A* 1992;89:6901–6905.
68. Mazanec MB, Coudret CL, Fletcher DR. Intracellular neutralization of influenza virus by IgA anti-HA monoclonal antibodies. *J Virol* 1995;69:1339–1343.
69. Fujioka H, Emancipator SN, Aikawa M, et al. Immunocytochemical colocalization of specific immunoglobulin A with Sendai virus protein in infected polarized epithelium. *J Exp Med* 1998;188:1223–1229.
70. Burns JW, Siadat-Pajouh M, Krishnaney AA, et al. Protective effect of rotavirus VP6-specific IgA monoclonal antibodies that lack neutralizing activity. *Science* 1996;272:104–107.
71. Bomsel M, Heyman M, Hocini H, et al. Intracellular neutralization of HIV transcytosis across tight epithelial barriers by anti-HIV envelope protein dIgA or IgM. *Immunity* 1998;9:277–287.
72. Kaetzel CS, Robinson JK, Chintalacharuvu KR, et al. The polymeric immunoglobulin receptor (secretory component) mediates transport of immune complexes across epithelial cells: a local defense function for IgA. *Proc Natl Acad Sci U S A* 1991;88: 8796–8800.
73. Gan YJ, Chodosh J, Morgan A, et al. Epithelial cell polarization is a determinant in the infectious outcome of immunoglobulin A-mediated entry by Epstein-Barr virus. *J Virol* 1997;71:519–526.
74. Kaetzel CS, Robinson JK, Lamm ME. Epithelial transcytosis of monomeric IgA and IgG cross-linked through antigen to polymeric IgA. A role for monomeric antibodies in the mucosal immune system. *J Immunol* 1994;152:72–76.
75. Robinson JK, Blanchard TG, Levine AD, et al. A mucosal IgA-mediated excretory immune system *in vivo. J Immunol* 2001;166: 3688–3692.
76. Sixbey JW, Yao Q-Y. Immunoglobulin A-induced shift of Epstein-Barr virus tissue tropism. *Science* 1992;255:1578–1580.

13

SYSTEMIC AND MUCOSAL ANTIBODY RESPONSE TO ENTERIC PATHOGENS

EDWARD N. JANOFF

An elaborate array of host- and pathogen-specific factors affects whether an enteric pathogen causes acute or chronic infection and whether the infection is symptomatic. Certain enteric pathogens inhabit the bowel exclusively as superficial mucosal infections, eliciting either minimal inflammation (e.g., *Giardia lamblia, Vibrio cholerae*) or an appreciable acute local inflammatory response (e.g., *Clostridium difficile, Campylobacter jejuni*). Other pathogens may produce a locally invasive (e.g., *Shigella* species, non-*typhi* salmonellae, *Cryptosporidium parvum*) or a bacteremic (e.g., *Salmonella typhi, Campylobacter fetus*) phase. Independently of the extent of anatomic invasion or degree of associated inflammation, most pathogen-associated surface antigens and toxins elicit a systemic immune response (1–12), and, although it is less well characterized, a local humoral response (5,13–21). These responses are manifested by the presence of circulating antibodies to the organisms in serum and in mucosal secretions.

The presence of enteric pathogen-specific antibodies in serum supports the diagnosis of acute enteric infection (6,11,12,22–27) and epidemiologic investigations of outbreaks of enteric infection (28–34). Serologic investigations also serve to define the ecologic niche (e.g., age, race, sex, geographic distribution) of newly described pathogens and routine pathogens in new populations (35–42). Finally, systemic antibody responses to mucosal infections have been examined as indirect markers of immunity to enteric infection and protection against its associated symptoms (9,11,12,27,43–48). These data have been used to assess the risk for infection in a population and the efficacy of new vaccines (49–51). Moreover, analysis of the immunologic reactivity of sera and mucosal fluids from patients with enteric infections allows the characterization of immunogenic epitopes, virulence factors, and potential antigens for protective vaccines (1,6,47,52–54). This chapter examines the relationship between mucosal infections and the humoral responses they elicit so that the mechanisms, diagnostic value, and functional activities of these systemic and local antibody responses can be understood.

E. N. Janoff: Mucosal and Vaccine Research Center, Infectious Disease Section, Veterans Affairs Medical Center; Department of Medicine, University of Minnesota School of Medicine, Minneapolis, Minnesota

INDUCTION OF MUCOSAL AND SYSTEMIC IMMUNITY BY ENTERIC ANTIGENS

The primary goal of mucosal immunity is "immune exclusion"—the process of keeping harmful elements out of the body (55–59). The intestine is constantly exposed to high concentrations of foreign antigens, bacteria, and viruses and their proinflammatory components (e.g., toxins, lipopolysaccharide, polysaccharides). The mucosal immune system must minimize the local inflammatory response and the damage it provokes (60–62), and it must also recognize and respond to the antigens. A versatile system has evolved to serve these two potentially conflicting needs. The intestine comprises three distinct but interactive immunologic compartments: the lumen, the epithelium, and the subepithelial mucosa (Fig. 13.1). The latter includes an organized inductive compartment (lymphoid nodules and Peyer patches) and a compartment of diffuse effector cells, predominantly activated T cells and activated, differentiated plasma cells that produce antibody, primarily immunoglobulin A (IgA). The unique sequence of events, from the sampling of luminal antigens and transport across the epithelium to the development of systemic and local responses to enteric pathogens, is summarized in Fig. 13.1; the nontoxic but mucosally immunogenic B subunit of cholera toxin is used as a model antigen (63).

After being ingested into the small bowel lumen, antigens can traverse the epithelium in three ways. First, they may bind to epithelial cells (the B subunit of cholera toxin binds to the abundant ganglioside GM_1), which can process antigens by unique mechanisms (64). Second, luminal antigens can be sampled by modified membranous epithelial cells, M cells, that transport antigens and organisms intact across the epithelial surface to organized mucosal lymphoid tissue below (65–67). The density of M cells and associated

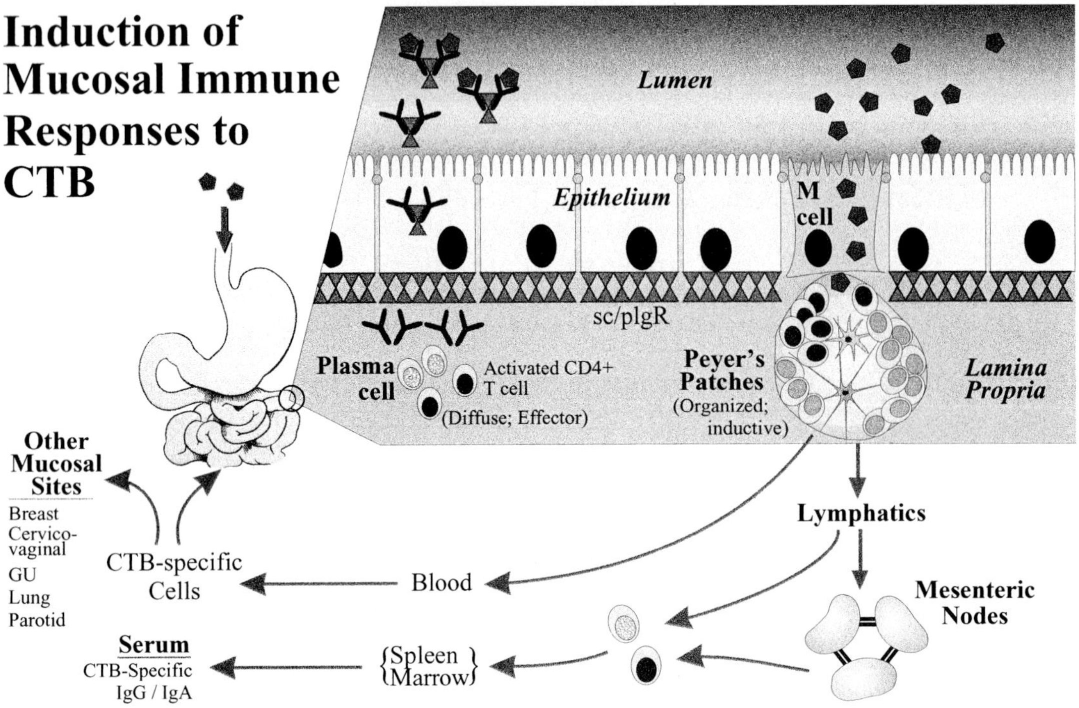

FIGURE 13.1. Pathways for induction of mucosal and systemic humoral immune response to cholera toxin B subunit (*pentagons*) after oral immunization or infection. Ingested free cholera toxin B subunit is shown in lumen of the duodenum in the upper right of the figure, and protective secretory immunoglobulin A bound to cholera toxin B subunit in the upper left of the lumen. In the model, Peyer patch nuclei of T cells are red, those of B cells are solid green, and those of plasmablasts and plasma cells are stippled green; a dendritic cell is shown as a blue stellate cell and a follicular dendritic cell as a green cell with long, slender stellate processes. *CTB,* cholera toxin B subunit; *sc/pIgR,* secretory component/polymeric Ig receptor; *GU,* genitourinary tract.

lymphoid follicles is greatest at the distal end of the gastrointestinal tract (i.e., terminal ileum, colon, and rectum) (68). Third, immature intraepithelial dendritic cells can also take up and transport antigen to lymphoid follicles and can serve as antigen-presenting cells as the dendritic cells mature in the follicles (69–72). These lymphoid follicles (Peyer patches) contain the dendritic cells, macrophages, T and B cells, and follicular dendritic cell network that support and generate the primary response to foreign antigens (73).

This primary response involves the activation and proliferation of antigen-specific lymphocytes in a germinal center reaction (74). Peyer patches are distinct in that antigen is acquired directly from the adjacent mucosal epithelial surface rather than from afferent lymphatics or arterioles, as in the peripheral nodes and spleen. However, unlike the B and T lymphocytes in peripheral sites, activated B and T lymphocytes from antigen-driven mucosal lymphoid follicles do not differentiate into antibody-secreting plasma cells in the organized mucosal compartment. Rather, these activated cells are carried through the blood and return (or home) to the lamina propria of the intestine (75), guided by complementary vascular and cellular receptors. In the lamina propria, under the influence of T cells and Th2 cytokines (e.g., transforming growth factor-β and interleukins 5, 6, and 10), antigen-stimulated B cells proliferate and differentiate into predominantly IgA-producing cells. These antibody-secreting cells are present at high densities in both the upper and lower bowel; IgG-secreting cells represent a small minority of cells in both sites (Fig. 13.2).

Immunoglobulin A is produced by plasma cells in both monomeric and polymeric (two or more molecules of IgA bound by a J chain) forms, but only polymeric IgA (pIgA) is transported into the lumen. The pIgA (and IgM) produced in the lamina propria bind the polymeric immunoglobulin receptor (pIgR), a protein distributed on the basolateral surface of epithelial cells (55). Just as M cells transport antigens intact from the lumen to the lamina propria, pIgR binds to IgA and transports it intact through the epithelial cells in the opposite direction, from the lamina propria to the lumen. Once secreted into the lumen from the apical epithelial surface, the modified pIgR (now called *secretory component,* or SC) serves to protect bound secretory IgA (sIgA = pIgA + SC) from enzymatic degradation in the bowel.

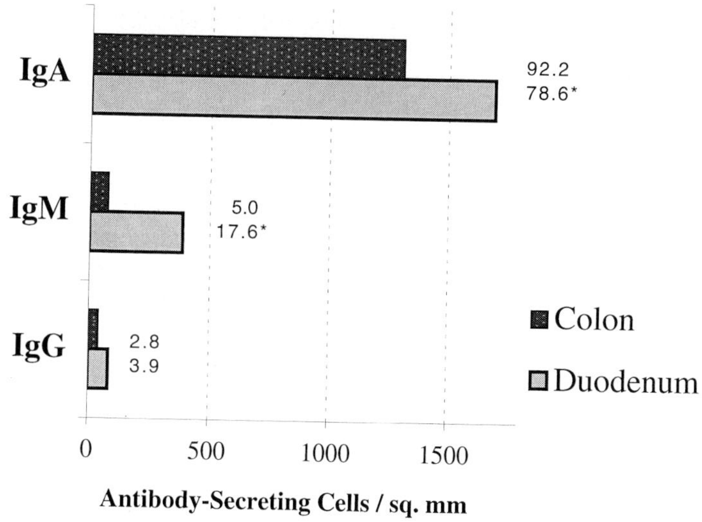

FIGURE 13.2. Distribution of immunoglobulin A (IgA)-, IgM-, and IgG-secreting plasma cells in duodenal (n = 12) and colon (n = 10) biopsy specimens from healthy adults in the United States. Results are shown by density (antibody-secreting cells per square millimeter) in lamina propria tissue (excluding epithelial cells). Numbers to the right of each bar represent the percentage of cells of that isotype as a proportion of all antibody-secreting cells in that tissue. Cells were stained with simultaneous triple immunofluorescence, one fluorochrome for each isotype, and analyzed with hand and digital counting. [From Scamurra RW, Lin XM, Janoff EN. (*submitted*).]

Specific sIgA performs many protective functions (Table 13.1), which include prevention of binding of enteric pathogens or toxins to the epithelial surface (immune exclusion) (e.g., cholera toxin, toxin A of *C. difficile*), neutralization of toxins and viruses, killing of organisms, and extrusion of antigens that have entered the lamina propria (16,76–84). Additionally, sIgA may inhibit complement activation and the associated inflammation (85,86) or support the killing of bacteria (87). These data highlight why the lymphoid follicles are considered to be the inductive sites of the mucosal immune system, and the lamina propria the functional or effector compartment (88).

Activated lymphocytes from lymphoid follicles also home to other mucosal sites (e.g., breast, genitourinary tract, salivary glands, lungs) (55,75,79,89–91). The presence of antigen-specific B cells in blood within 1 week after mucosal exposure (92,93), the subsequent appearance of these cells in distal mucosal sites, and the production at these sites of specific IgA are evidence for a common mucosal immune system (55,92,94). The clinical importance of this broadly deployed common mucosal system is exemplified by the protection afforded by breast milk to infants against intestinal infections (e.g., with *V. cholerae, Shigella* species, *Giardia,* rotavirus) (95–100), particularly breast milk from mothers with prior enteric exposure to the organism, which contains pathogen-specific sIgA.

In addition to stimulating *mucosal* IgA, mucosal antigens also may induce *systemic* antibody responses. Once transported below the epithelial surface, antigens can spread beyond the lymphoid follicles through lymphatics to regional mesenteric lymph nodes, where pathogen-specific immunoglobulin (particularly IgA) can be produced and released into the serum (77,101). Activated cells and persistent antigen from these nodes also can be carried by blood to spleen and bone marrow to stimulate the production of systemic (serum) immunoglobulin, including IgG in addition to IgA (55). Thus, the successful induction of humoral responses to luminal antigens in the organized mucosal lymphoid compartment initiates a broad and multifunctional fluid system that defends vulnerable portals of entry.

TABLE 13.1. CHARACTERIZATION OF MUCOSAL AND SYSTEMIC IMMUNOGLOBULIN A BY SUBCLASS AND MOLECULAR FORM

Subclass	Source of Ig: Intestine	Source of Ig: Serum
	% Total Ig	
IgG	3–5	75–80
IgM	6–18	12–15
IgA	80–90	8–10
	% IgA	
IgA1	40–60	80–90
IgA2	40–60[a]	10–20
Monomeric	<10	80–95
Polymeric	>90	5–20[b]
Bound to secretory component[c]	>95	<5

[a]The proportion of IgA2 increases from the proximal small bowel to the colon.
[b]Polymeric IgA may be increased in patients with liver disease.
[c]Only the polymeric form of IgA may contain secretory component, to which it binds at the basolateral surface of mucosal epithelial cells.

ROLE OF SYSTEMIC ANTIBODY IN THE DIAGNOSIS OF MUCOSAL INFECTIONS

Immunologic assays complement microbiologic tests in the diagnosis of enteric infections. Cultures and visual examination are often sensitive and specific for determining the presence of an organism in stool, but significant expertise and resources may be required. Antigen detection methods may circumvent these obstacles, but as with culture- and microscope-based methods, stool samples must be obtained at the time of interest (e.g., symptoms or survey). Serologic tests can be useful in the acute setting or allow diagnoses to be made retrospectively. In some cases, serology may help distinguish between invasive and asymptomatic infections, or between infection with invasive and noninvasive isolates (e.g., *Entamoeba histolytica* vs. *Entamoeba dispar*) (102), with the use of small amounts of more readily accessible and stable serum samples. A representative summary of reported assays is shown in Table 13.2.

The serologic response to enteric infections is influenced by the timing of the sample relative to the infection, age of the patient, and extent of the host's previous exposure to the organism. In neonates with rotavirus infection who were less than 3 weeks of age, specific IgG, IgM, and IgA in serum was of no diagnostic value (103). During primary rotavirus infection in older infants, rotavirus-specific IgM was present within a week of the onset of symptoms in most cases, whereas IgA and IgG were not (104). By 1 and 4 months, however, the prevalence of IgM had decreased (only 14%), whereas specific IgG or IgA was detected in almost all children. Among adults, particularly those in areas of endemicity, specific IgM responses to most enteric pathogens are of considerably less diagnostic value than are IgG or IgA responses (e.g., *Shigella* species in Israel, *C. difficile* in elderly Americans, *G. lamblia* in Colorado residents) (5,6,105).

Enteric protozoan infections also often elicit circulating antibody responses. *Toxoplasma gondii* is transmitted through the ingestion of infective cysts, which break down in the intestine and subsequently disseminate throughout the body. Whereas the presence of anti-*T. gondii* IgG or a reactive Sabin–Feldman dye test is a reliable marker of either acute or chronic infection (106), the detection of specific IgM and IgA, neither of which is present in chronic latent infection, suggests more recent infection (107–109) (Table 13.2). During acute symptomatic infections with *G. lamblia,* a noninvasive parasite of the upper small bowel, parasite-specific IgG and IgA were more sensitive indicators of infection than was IgM (6) (Fig. 13.3). The level of parasite-specific antibody may be most reliable as infections evolve with *Cryptosporidium* and *E. histolytica*; the sensitivity of enzyme-linked immunosorbent assay (ELISA) is approximately 75% with amebic colitis and more than 90% with liver abscess.

In these settings, antibody isotype may be helpful as an adjunct to the serologic diagnosis of enteric infections. However, usefulness depends on the organism, the assay, and the setting. IgG is typically the most sensitive indicator of *Cryptosporidium* and *E. histolytica* infections, but asymptomatic infections with either pathogen can elicit these antibodies, so that the serologic diagnosis is compromised in areas of high endemicity. The serologic diagnosis of *S. typhi* infections (typhoid fever) may be most sensitive and specific with immunoassays that detect either IgG or IgM (110). These assays compare favorably with the Widal test (bacterial agglutination), which depends primarily on IgM. Although widely used, the Widal test may lack specificity and reproducibility (11,111); these are most often improved with sensitive ELISA systems (10,22). As in *G. lamblia* infections, mentioned above, IgG and particularly IgA were more sensitive and more specific markers of acute *C. jejuni* enteritis than was IgM (1,4). Following this acute infection, levels of specific IgA declined more rapidly than did those of IgG or IgM. In an outbreak of *C. jejuni*-associated enteritis, levels of specific IgG and IgM, but not of IgA, rose in subjects exposed to the raw milk vector, whereas no rise was seen in unexposed persons. Baseline levels of IgG and IgM to *C. jejuni* were also increased in farm residents who continually ingested raw milk. In contrast, during a waterborne outbreak of giardiasis, only parasite-specific IgA, not IgG or IgM, correlated with rates of exposure, infection, and symptoms (32).

In contrast to the antibody responses to *S. typhi* and *C. jejuni,* specific IgG and IgA were both present at high levels in patients with chronic *Helicobacter pylori* infections, whereas IgM was not (7). The presence of circulating antibodies is a very sensitive indicator of ongoing *H. pylori* infection but does not predict the presence of *H. pylori*-associated ulcer disease. A decrease in titers may accompany resolution of the infection following antimicrobial therapy. Detection of *H. pylori*-specific antibodies has also been used with banked sera to suggest a link between an increased incidence of both gastric adenocarcinoma and lymphoma and long-term *H. pylori* infection (112,113). Just as specific antibodies in serum may persist during chronic *H. pylori* infection, serum IgG and IgA to toxin A of *C. difficile* may be present in the sera of healthy adults. However, these levels are not a marker of chronic infection, but they may reflect subclinical infections, and asymptomatic infection elicits acute changes in antibody levels (46).

Serologic responses may accompany symptomatic, but not asymptomatic, infections with certain bacteria [e.g., with enterotoxigenic *E. coli* (LT+) and *C. difficile*] (5,114). Serologic responses were also thought to be clinically useful in differentiating invasive *E. histolytica* infection from asymptomatic colonization. IgG responses to the parasite were routinely reactive within 1 to 2 weeks of the onset of colitis and liver abscess (102,115–119). In contrast, antibodies did not typically develop in the serum of persons asymptomatically infected with noninvasive strains. However, the differences in serologic response are now ascribed to antigenic and immunogenic differences in parasitologically identical *Entoamoebae* species. As noted above, asymptomatic infections with *E. dispar* do not stimulate systemic antibody responses, whereas both asymptomatic and invasive *E. histolytica* infections do. Therefore, in areas where *E. histolytica* is not endemic, a reactive serologic test result in a patient with appropriate symptoms is highly predictive of invasive infection. However, in areas where it is highly endemic, such as South Africa, Mexico, and India, positive

TABLE 13.2. SERUM RESPONSES TO ENTERIC INFECTIONS BY ANTIBODY CLASS

Infection	No. Subjects	Percentage Positive: IgG	IgM	IgA	Ref.
Bacteria					
■ Acute *C. jejuni* enteritis	111	—	—	88[a]	[4]
Controls: 0–9 years old	—	—	—	4	
≥40 years old	—	—	—	54	
■ Acute *C. jejuni* enteritis (ill for 21 days)	51	59	74	76	[1]
■ Chronic *H. pylori* gastritis	59	97	Low	97	[7]
- Healthy adults	96	50	—	40–55	
■ Enterotoxigenic *E. coli* diarrhea					
Antigen: LT	10	70	—	80	[158]
CFA	10	70	—	100	
LPS	15	73	—	80	
■ Children (Malaysia)					
- *S. typhi* (typhoid fever)	42	(95)[b]	(95)[b]	—	[110]
- Nontyphoid fever	49	(0)[b]	(0)[b]	—	
■ *E. coli* O157:H7 hemorrhagic colitis (days 5–62)					
- (ELISA) LPS	26	96	92	65	
- SLT I	—	23	—	—	
- SLT II	—	0	—	—	
■ *C. difficile* (toxin A neutralization)					[77]
- Acute symptomatic	18	0	—	6	
- Convalescent-symptomatic	18	0	—	33	
- Asymptomatic colonized	10	0	—	10	
Protozoa					
■ Acute *G. lamblia* diarrhea	27	67	41	78	[6]
- Healthy adults	66	6	2	2	
■ Acute toxoplasmosis (seroconversion and/or lymphadenitis)	22	(100)[c]	100	100	[107]
- Chronic latent *T. gondii* infection	20	(100)[c]	0	0	
■ *E. histolytica*					
- Liver abscess (S. Africa)	83	99	—	—	
- Nonpathogenic strains (S. Africa)	69	25	—	—	
- Uninfected controls (S. Africa)	32	25	—	—	
- Healthy controls (U.S.)	40	0	—	—	
■ *Cryptosporidium* diarrhea					[225]
- Acute—otherwise healthy adults	15	67[d]	80[d]	—	
- Chronic—patients with AIDS	26	100	15	—	
- Uninfected controls	42	5	—	—	
Viruses					
■ Rotavirus gastroenteritis					
- Infants >3 weeks old					[104]
- Acute	44	7	—	—	
- One month	44	91	100	68[e]	
- Four months	43	100	14	93[e]	
■ Rotavirus gastroenteritis					
- Neonates (India)					[103]
- Infected	37	8[f]	5	0	
- Uninfected	18	0	0	0	
■ Rotavirus gastroenteritis					[226]
- Acute	8	—	—	0	
- Convalescent	8	—	—	75	

[a]Specific IgA was predominantly polymeric in patients compared with that in control subjects (median 90% vs. 17% polymeric, respectively).
[b]A positive test result recorded if IgG and/or IgM positive. Either isotype alone was less sensitive, but percentages not noted.
[c]100% positive by Sabin–Feldman dye test.
[d]IgG positive in 87% and IgM in 93% by 2 weeks after diagnosis.
[e]Specific serum secretory IgA was only rarely detected (14% and 0% in acute and convalescent sera, respectively).
[f]Rise in IgG level in three neonates; specific IgG detectable in all neonates in cord sera. Salivary IgA to rotavirus detectable in 62% of infected neonates and 5.5% of uninfected neonates.
LT, labile toxin; CFA, colonization factor antigen; LPS, lipopolysaccharide; ELISA, enzyme-linked immunosorbent assay; SLT, Shiga-like toxin.

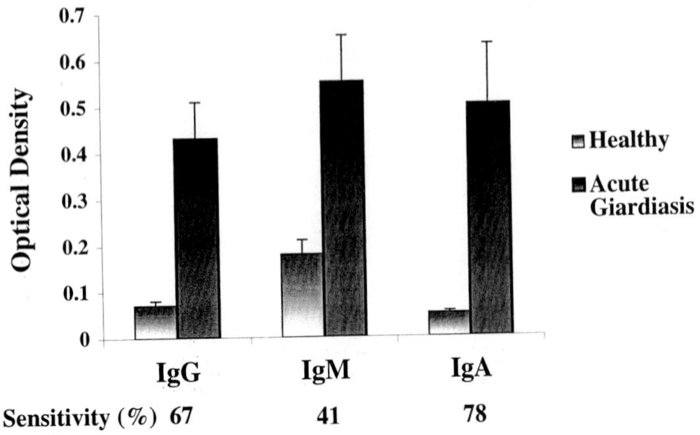

FIGURE 13.3. *Giardia lamblia*-specific antibodies in serum in acutely infected immunocompetent adults at the time of presentation and in healthy age-matched control subjects, Denver, Colorado. (Adapted from Janoff EN, Smith PD, Blaser MJ. Acute antibody responses to *Giardia lamblia* are depressed in patients with AIDS. *J Infect Dis* 1988;157:798–804, with permission.)

test results are frequent in the general population (102, 119). These findings may be a consequence of persistence of IgG antibodies, which may last for years after acute invasive infection, or of asymptomatic infection with invasive strains (102). In an endemic setting, the detection of *E. histolytica*-specific IgM may distinguish between active and previous infection in an symptomatic patient with detectable serum levels of specific IgG (119).

The serologic diagnosis of enteric pathogens is also useful in epidemiologic studies in which microbiologic specimens are not available or diagnostic facilities are inadequate. In a retrospective evaluation of an outbreak of amebic colitis in the United States in which six patients died, "therapeutic" colonic irrigation was confirmed as the source of infection (120). Evidence of *E. histolytica* infection was more often confirmed epidemiologically in patients who received irrigation (20 of 54 persons, or 37%) than in those who did not (1 of 42, or 2%). Positive results of indirect hemagglutination tests of sera yielded the diagnosis in 19 of 20 cases, whereas the organism was detected in only seven of these patients. In other settings, the detection of IgG, but not IgM, to *Cryptosporidium* in sera helped establish the organism as a cause of large waterborne outbreaks of gastroenteritis (29,30,34), and in yet another, it alerted clinicians to the risk of person-to-person transmission in the hospital setting (31). In the largest recognized outbreak of *Cryptosporidium* infection, preferentially high rates of seroconversion to two immunodominant antigens (increasing from ~15% to ~85% in the period around the outbreak) among children in one region confirmed the specific water treatment plant responsible (34).

In summary, the presence and pattern of antibodies to enteric pathogens in serum may suggest prior exposure to a specific organism, acute or chronic infection, or infection with invasive or noninvasive strains. In epidemiologic studies, serology is useful in establishing exposure rates in the community, risk factors for infection, and routes of transmission. International standardization of assay performance will help to elucidate the contribution of many variables on determinations of seropositivity rates of specific antibodies in different syndromes. These variables include the effects of isotype, age of the patient (114), biology of the organism (3), antigens being detected (1,6,52,121), endemicity of the infection in the population studied, and interaction of the organism with the mucosal immune system.

IMMUNOGLOBULIN A SUBCLASSES AND MOLECULAR FORMS

In addition to pathogen-specific antibodies of the IgA class, investigators have sought more specific and predictive markers in serum that indicate a mucosal origin for infections and antibodies (122). Defining the origin of the antibodies in serum would also clarify the physiologic interaction of systemic and mucosal immune responses. Of greatest biologic relevance is the predictive value of distinct antibodies in serum that reliably correlate with protection against pathogen-associated illness. Such antibodies may serve as markers of protection or represent the mechanisms of protection, as suggested for serum IgG responses to non-*typhi* salmonellae, *Shigellae,* and other gram-negative enteric pathogens (123).

The subclasses and molecular forms of IgA are distinct in mucosal and systemic sites (Table 13.1). The IgA1 and IgA2 subclasses are distinguished by minor variations in the sequence and length of the heavy chain hinge region (124). Of the IgA in serum, 80% to 90% or more is IgA1; the distribution of the two subclasses is more equal in mucosal fluids (125–129). The moderate predominance of IgA1 in the upper intestinal tract is reversed in the colon. A more distinct anatomic disparity in IgA distribution is seen between the monomeric and polymeric molecular forms of the antibody. In serum, the predominance of monomeric IgA is similar to that of IgA1 (130). Thus, most IgA in serum is monomeric and of the IgA1 subclass.

In contrast to the IgA in serum, virtually all the IgA in mucosal fluids is pIgA (Table 13.1), in which two or more complete IgA1 or IgA2 molecules are joined by a J chain (4,126,129–132). The union of IgA (or IgM) with the J chain occurs intracellularly before the antibody is secreted

(133–135). In both mucosal and systemic sites, both polymeric and monomeric IgA can be produced by the same cell (136), but only the transport of J chain-containing pIgA (and IgM) can be facilitated across the epithelial cell by pIgR/SC into luminal secretions (137). Thus, pIgA in serum may derive from cells in systemic or mucosal sites, but the low levels of sIgA (the complex of pIgA with SC) occasionally identified in serum can originate only in the mucosal lumen.

Limited numbers of studies have measured antigen-specific sIgA in serum. Gransfors and Toivanen (138) reported that levels of *Yersinia enterocolitica*-specific IgA2, pIgA, and sIgA in serum were increased in patients with postinfectious arthritis in comparison with values in patients without arthritis. These results suggest persistent mucosal antigenic stimulation, but no chronic intestinal infection was documented. Other investigators have shown that although serum IgA may be a sensitive indicator of rotavirus infection (Table 13.2), specific sIgA is only rarely detected in serum (104).

Although intestinal IgA is roughly half IgA1 and half IgA2, serum IgA specific for enteric organisms or mucosal vaccine antigens is most often of the IgA1 class (4,77), similar to the subclass pattern that follows parenteral antigenic exposure. Although the anatomic location of antigenic stimulation may not influence the IgA subclass response, the composition of the antigen, whether protein or polysaccharide, may. IgA to protein antigens (1,5,6,139–141) is predominantly IgA1 (4,77). However, IgA2 may represent a larger proportion of the serum response to surface polysaccharide or lipopolysaccharide antigens, which comprise important targets in intestinal pathogens, such as *Salmonellae* and *Shigellae* species, and mucosal respiratory pathogens (142).

A teleologic explanation for the preferential IgA2 response to certain polysaccharides is that an enzyme (IgA1 protease) produced by several encapsulated mucosal pathogens (*Streptococcus pneumoniae, Haemophilus influenzae, Neisseria meningitidis*) cleaves IgA1, but not IgA2, at the hinge sequence that distinguishes these subclasses. The cysteine proteinase of *E. histolytica* may also cleave IgA. Adherence of the resultant antigen-binding F(ab′)2 fragment to the surface polysaccharide without its associated Fc effector end may block binding by other antibodies and antibody-mediated clearance of the organism, so that invasion across the mucosal barrier is facilitated (79). However, the prominence of polysaccharide-specific IgA2 very early in the systemic response (143) may change with time to a predominance of IgA1 (144). Thus, although IgA subclasses may not predict a mucosal or systemic origin of infection, they may reflect, in part, the chemical composition of the antigen or the timing of the response.

Akin to IgA subclass expression, the molecular form of specific serum IgA appears to be influenced by the temporal sequence of humoral responses. The early acute IgA response to a range of bacterial and viral mucosal pathogens and vaccines is primarily polymeric; the structure typically switches to monomeric IgA during convalescence (4,84, 144) (Fig. 13.4). This switch in molecular form has been shown for viruses acquired through the respiratory mucosa (rubella, mumps, and varicella) (141) and genital mucosa (herpes simplex) (145). Consistent with these findings, reactivations of both varicella (herpes zoster) and genital herpes elicit monomeric IgA more often than the virus-specific polymeric IgA detected during acute primary infections. In sera from patients with acute *C. jejuni* enteritis, pIgA comprised most of the specific IgA within 1 to 2 weeks of presentation (median, 90%) (4). The high proportion of pIgA in acute sera decreased with time after resolution of infection and approached that of specific IgA in healthy control subjects (median, 17%).

Thus, the detection of polymeric or monomeric IgA reactive with mucosal pathogens may help to distinguish acute from previous infection and primary from reactivated infection, but both mucosal and parenteral stimulation with either polysaccharide or protein antigens can

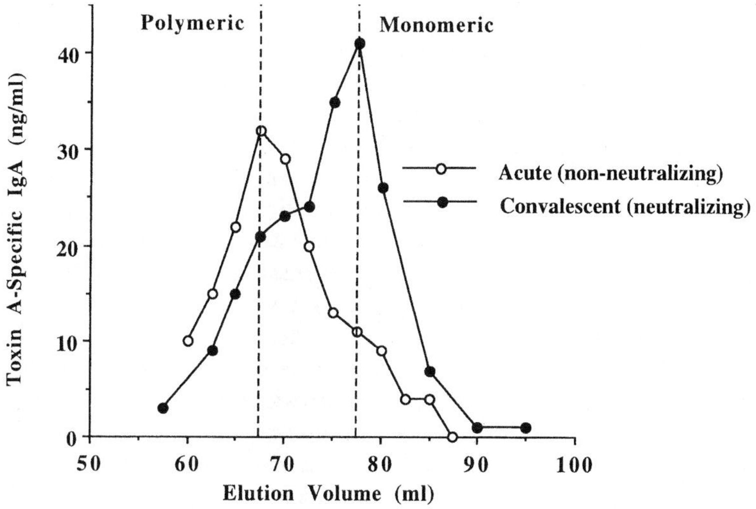

FIGURE 13.4. Serum immunoglobulin A (IgA) response to toxin A of *Clostridium difficile* in association with antibiotic-associated colitis. The change in molecular form of specific IgA from polymeric in the acute sample to primarily monomeric in the convalescent sample was associated with the ability of IgA to neutralize the cytotoxic activity of toxin A. (Adapted from Johnson S, Sypura WD, Gerding DN, et al. Selective neutralization of a bacterial enterotoxin by serum immunoglobulin A in response to mucosal disease. *Infect Immun* 1995;63:3166–3173, with permission.)

elicit specific pIgA in serum (4,77,122,142,144,146,147). Despite the consistency with which the transition from pathogen-specific polymeric to monomeric IgA has been shown, the immunologic mechanism underlying this progression has not been demonstrated (3,147). The advancing predominance of specific monomeric IgA may reflect clonal maturation and, ultimately, memory responses (3,148). Very early in the course of infection, as IgG and cellular responses are evolving, the multivalence of pIgA, similar to that of IgM, may enhance its functional activity in serum and at the mucosal interface (87,149).

MUCOSAL RESPONSES TO ENTERIC INFECTIONS

The intestinal mucosa has adapted to the remarkable challenge of coexisting peacefully with an enormous and persistent inoculum of foreign antigens and organisms, located but a cell or two away from the internal milieu. IgA comprises up to 90% of mucosal immunoglobulin in the healthy intestine (Fig. 13.2), but the total levels of immunoglobulins are much lower at the mucosal surfaces than in serum (10- to 20-fold lower for IgA, 50- to 500-fold for IgG). In conjunction with the activities of mucins and other innate immune factors (e.g., lysozyme, trefoil peptides, cryptins, defensins, nitric oxide), mucosal antibodies must play a critical role in maintaining the "immune exclusion" of potentially harmful and inflammatory agents. Neonates and germ-free animals have few intestinal antibody-producing cells, but the number of these cells increases with the bacterial population, likely under the influence of early colonizing bacteria (150–152). The body expends tremendous resources to maintain the production of mucosal antibodies, producing more than 3 g of mucosal IgA per day, more than the amount produced of all other immunoglobulins combined (58,131). Despite these associations, and the high rates and persistence of selected mucosal infections among persons with hypogammaglobulinemia (*G. lamblia, C. jejuni, Salmonella* species, and *C. difficile*) (153–155), efforts to determine the presence of pathogen-specific mucosal antibodies have been erratic, and defining their specific functional role has been challenging.

Many obstacles have limited the evaluation of intestinal antibodies, particularly in humans. The collection of intestinal fluids may require invasive or uncomfortable procedures, so that serial sampling is limited. The standardization of results is inconsistent because of undefined dilution factors. Often, only limited quantities of fluid and purified antibodies are available for the careful characterization of antibody structure, specificity, and function. In addition, mucosal antibodies may be difficult to purify, and specific functional studies may be confounded by interference from the activity of other mucosal factors that are present and may be purified along with antibodies. Finally, heretofore limited access to sufficient and appropriate mucosal tissues in humans has restricted our ability to induce local immune responses effectively and evaluate their effects clinically and *in vitro.* Approaches that have been used to evaluate intestinal mucosal responses include direct duodenal aspiration (limited volume), extraction of antibodies from stool samples (appreciable contamination and protease activity), intestinal lavage with saline solution or a nonabsorbable agent (e.g., polyethylene glycol), and the use of surrogate markers such as IgA (or IgG) in saliva, breast milk, or blood. Perhaps the most innovative approach was that of Ogra and Karzon (18), who monitored the effects of live attenuated oral polio vaccine on mucosal antibody responses in children with surgical colostomies. More recently, the use of fiberoptic endoscopy has allowed direct sampling of intestinal tissue from patients with intact intestinal tracts. These advances have facilitated the direct evaluation of antigen-specific antibody-secreting cells in the diffuse effector compartment of the lamina propria and the characterization of organized Peyer patch morphology and cells in humans.

Intestinal fluids from patients with bacterial dysentery, but not with amebic disease, were first shown to have activity against the organism. Since that time, intestinal antibodies, particularly sIgA, to a number of enteric bacteria have been identified (13,156) (Table 13.3). Specific antibodies, most often eluted from fecal samples, are present at rates above those in controls, and when tested, they increase with time (21,101). These data indicate the specificity of the local response. Most reports do not discriminate between sIgA and non-sIgA, but the infrequent detection of pathogen-specific IgG in these mucosal samples suggests that the antibodies are produced locally rather than passed from serum through an inflamed mucosa. As shown in Table 13.3, intestinal antibodies have been detected to *V. cholerae, C. jejuni,* Shigella species, enterotoxigenic *E. coli* and *E. coli* O157:H7 (13,20,21,101,156–158), related vaccines (2,93,159–163), and viral pathogens.

In children with acute rotavirus infection, simultaneous sequential measurements of antiviral antibodies in serum, duodenum, feces, and saliva indicated that IgM in serum and duodenal fluids best predicts acute infection (104). At 1 month, fecal IgA levels correlated well with duodenal fluid levels, so that direct intestinal sampling was not needed. The attenuation of early rotavirus infection in low-birth-weight infants in association with the administration of oral gamma globulin suggested a potential protective role for mucosal antibodies (164). In a prospective study of patients in whom *C. difficile* infection developed, measurement of toxin A-specific IgA in feces provided no advantage over measurement of specific IgG in serum in regard to sensitivity of diagnosis and predicting clinical response to acute infection (46). Although a relationship between the presence of pathogen-specific IgA in mucosal fluids and IgG or IgA in serum can often

TABLE 13.3. HUMAN MUCOSAL ANTIBODY RESPONSES TO ENTERIC INFECTIONS AND VACCINES

				Percentage Positive			
Organism and Clinical Setting	**Antigen/Assay**	**Source**	**No. Subjects**	**IgG**	**IgA**	**Comment**	**Ref.**
■ *V. cholerae* diarrhea	Vibriocidal	Feces	(25)	—	28[a]	No activity in 9 controls	[101]
		Small intestine	(12)	—	16[a]		
■ *V. cholerae* diarrhea		GI lavage					
(9–28 days)	CT		(9)	—	89		[168]
	LPS			—	89		
WC-BS vaccine	CT		(13–15)	—	87		
	LPS			—	92		
■ *Shigella sonnei* diarrhea (5 days)	LPS; Immunoblot	Serum	(9)	33	—		[21]
		Feces	(13)	—	77		
■ *C. jejuni* diarrhea (10–11 days)	OMP; Immunoblot	Feces	(8)	—	71		[20]
Controls			(5)	—	0		
■ *E. coli* O157							
Hemorrhagic colitis		Feces	(93)	—	63		[227]
Controls			(47)	—	21		
■ *C. difficile*	Toxin A	Serum	(35)	60	57	Toxin A biosassy inhibited by sIgA	[15]
	(ELISA)	Colon	(35)	—	57		
		Duodenum	(10)	—	10		
■ *C. difficile*	Toxin A	GI lavage					[5]
Acute	(ELISA)		(10)	—	70		
Convalescent			(6)	—	80		
Asymptomatic			(6)	—	16		
Controls			(9)	—	22		
■ *S. typhi*	LPS; Flagella	Feces					[159]
Ty21 vaccine							
Before			(11)	—	0		
Day 25			(11)	—	91–100		
24 months			(5)	—	0		
■ Polio vaccine	Neutralization	Duodenum					[26]
Inactivated (IM)			(3)	—	0		
Live (oral)			(3)	—	100	sIgA present for ≥300 days	
Rotavirus (1 month)		Duodenum	(19)	26	58	Significant rises from day 5–1 month;	[104]
		Feces	(44)	0	66	IgM most sensitive	
		Serum	(44)	91	68		

[a]Isotype not performed.
CT, cholera toxin; LPS, lipopolysaccharide; WC-BS, fixed *V. cholerae* whole cell + purified cholera toxin B subunit; OMP, outer membrane proteins; ELISA, enzyme-linked immunosorbent assay; sIgA, secretory immunoglobulin A.

be determined, most analyses suggest that the responses in the two compartments are independently regulated

RELATIONSHIP OF LOCAL AND CIRCULATING PATHOGEN-SPECIFIC ANTIBODIES

The detection of enteric pathogen-specific antibodies in serum often predicts their presence at mucosal sites. In studies of humoral responses to infection and immunization (*V. cholerae,* enterotoxigenic *E. coli, S. typhi,* rotavirus), the presence of specific IgG and IgA in serum showed a 70% to 80% correlation with organism-specific IgA in intestinal fluids; specific IgM showed the best correlation during acute primary infection (3,20,44,104,158). Extraintestinal fluids, particularly breast milk, contain antibodies to many bacterial, viral, and parasitic enteric pathogens (95–100,165). The prevalence of *G. lamblia*-specific IgG in serum correlated with that of specific sIgA in breast milk among women in Texas and Mexico (42). Similarly, saliva often contains specific antibodies after mucosal antigenic exposure. However, these relationships are not consistent, and specific antibodies to different antigens (e.g., lipopolysaccharides, toxin, adherence factors) may be present in one site and not another and may vary among patients. Overall, the antibodies in serum and breast milk may be more predictive of intestinal responses than those in saliva, but none consistently predicts protection.

Several general principles and caveats can be proposed about the interaction between mucosal and systemic immunity. First, oral immunization with non–pathogen-associated proteins, which elicit no intestinal damage or inflammation, is unlikely to provoke a systemic immune response (166,167). The immunogenicity of the nontoxic B subunit of cholera toxin given orally represents a striking exception to this principle. Second, parenteral immunization may not routinely elicit an appreciable mucosal response (26,146, 166,168,169). Nevertheless, parenteral immunization may be effective in preventing enteric disease (e.g., polio, *S. typhi* infection) (169–171). Third, parenteral immunization stimulates a mucosal response (e.g., sIgA) in subjects with prior mucosal exposure to the organism (2,162,163,169). This concept is consistent with the observation that parenterally administered killed cholera vaccines elicited an intestinal sIgA response in Pakistani women, among whom *V. cholerae* infection is endemic, but little local response among Swedish women, in whom these infections are absent (161). Thus, a positive correlation between the presence of specific antibodies in serum and in intestinal fluids depends on the initiation of a systemic immune response by mucosal stimulation.

Finally, the circulating antibody, particularly IgA, detected after mucosal infection or immunization does not originate in the mucosal lumen. Although total levels of sIgA in serum may be elevated in certain pathologic conditions, such as advanced HIV-1 infection and liver disease (172,173), suggestions of a mucosal source for significant proportions of the specific IgA in serum are generally unfounded (131). However, analysis of pathogen-specific IgA in serum may provide other clinically useful information about the character and kinetics of systemic responses to mucosal infections.

HUMORAL CORRELATES OF PROTECTION AGAINST ENTERIC DISEASE

Protection against specific acute symptomatic enteric infection may be related to previous or recurrent exposure to the organism. Persons exposed to *G. lamblia* organisms episodically, such as backpackers, travelers, and case contacts, exhibit high rates of symptomatic infection (174,175), whereas persons living in areas of endemicity and those with recurrent exposure to the organism, such as homosexual men and toddlers in day care centers, show low rates of symptomatic infection (36,176–178). Although differences in the virulence of individual *G. lamblia* strains may account for some of these clinical differences (179), the data suggest that immunity is acquired following recurrent exposure. In this regard, during waterborne outbreaks of *G. lamblia* infection in Colorado mountain towns, recently arrived tourists and short-term residents had significantly higher rates of illness than did long-term community residents (180,181). Similarly, 86% of infants in Bangladesh newly infected with *G. lamblia* had symptoms, but only 4% of infected mothers (182). The high rates of exposure and asymptomatic infection in regions where *G. lamblia* is endemic are most often associated with high rates of seropositivity and increased levels of *G. lamblia*-specific antibodies in serum (6,183–186), particularly IgA (187).

These observations of infection with *G. lamblia* are consistent with those of infection with bacterial (e.g., enterotoxigenic *E. coli, V. cholerae, C. jejuni*) (35,158,188), viral (e.g., rotavirus, calicivirus) (9,189), and protozoan (e.g., *Cryptosporidium* species) pathogens (190). In each instance, lower rates of infection or higher rates of asymptomatic infection in specific populations correlated with increased levels of pathogen-specific antibodies in their sera. Consistent with these results, levels of specific IgG and IgM were associated with a degree of protection against *Cryptosporidium* in a human experimental challenge system (191). In this study, the presence of antibodies in serum correlated with decreased numbers of excreted oocysts during infection, and increased levels were associated with a lower rate of symptomatic infection. Similarly, protective immunity develops in children exposed to rotavirus after sequential infections. The number of antibody-secreting cells reactive with rotavirus in blood by ELISPOT may correlate more closely with the number of these cells in the small-bowel mucosa than does the level specific IgA in serum (192). However, elevated levels of antiviral IgG and IgA were associated with protection against rotavirus infections, and elevated levels of IgA with decreased rates of moderate to severe disease in children (193). Among Israeli soldiers, elevated levels of IgG1 antibodies to lipopolysaccharide of *Shigella sonnei* and *Shigella flexneri* were associated with a decreased subsequent risk for symptomatic infection (194). Responses to lipopolysaccharide are most predictive of exposure to and infection with *Shigella* species and the related verotoxin-producing *E. coli* O157:H7 because the Shiga-like toxins (SLT I and II) are poorly immunogenic (195). These impaired responses may be related to the ability of the toxins to bind to IgG- and IgA-bearing B cells, so that B cell proliferation and immunoglobulin production are inhibited (196).

That increased levels of specific antibodies are associated with clinical protection does not confirm that these antibodies are the agents of such protection. In Bangladeshi children, higher titers of serum IgG to rotavirus by ELISA correlated with protection against both moderate and severe disease (9). However, further analysis of the neutralizing activity of antibodies to rotavirus in this population revealed that protection was not serotype-specific; protection against each of the four serotypes was more closely related to titers of heterotypic rather than of homotypic neutralizing antibodies (8). Thus, in some settings, antibodies in serum to enteric pathogens may be markers of immunity rather than the agents of direct functional mechanisms of protective immunity.

Recurrent exposure to *V. cholerae* is also closely associated with protection against subsequent infection (48,197). Specific IgG and IgA have been detected in both serum and intestinal fluids following both natural infection and immunization (162,163,168). Two classic virulence-associated antigens have been identified: cholera toxin, which mediates intestinal fluid secretion, and lipopolysaccharide, which is the target of vibriocidal antibodies. Despite the obvious pathogenic role of cholera toxin and its unique immunogenicity in the intestine, direct evidence linking protection against *V. cholerae*-induced diarrhea with levels of cholera toxin-specific IgG or IgA in blood or mucosa is inconsistent. Resistance to infection appears to correlate most closely with vibriocidal activity in serum (48,197). *V. cholerae* causes noninflammatory infection restricted to the intestinal surface. Cholera toxin can elicit robust local humoral responses (93), and evidence that breast milk from immune mothers protects against disease (100) supports a functional protective role for mucosal antibodies. The ability to provide such protection with a range of vaccines in the clinical setting has been more challenging.

MECHANISMS OF ANTIBODY-MEDIATED PROTECTION AGAINST MUCOSAL PATHOGENS

The rapidly expanding repertoire of immunodominant and functionally defined antigens on enteric pathogens, characterized in related chapters, is advancing our ability to diagnose and potentially prevent serious enteric infections. However, specific data that reliably define and predict functional mucosal mechanisms of protection have remained elusive. Such markers would facilitate the evaluation of new vaccines in volunteers and might limit the need for direct challenge studies and difficult field trials. The detection of circulating antigen-specific antibody-secreting cells by ELISPOT remains, to date, a promising but uncertain indicator of effective local responses (93,198,199). Optimal indicators would reflect a biologically plausible mechanism of activity and predict protection against illness rather than against infection (200).

Patients who recover from invasive infection with *E. histolytica* (hepatic abscess and colitis) show resistance to recurrent invasive disease in association with both pathogen-specific cellular and humoral responses. Antibodies to a 170-kd adherence lectin prominently recognized by such immune sera inhibit the ability of the organisms to adhere to target cells (201), to resist immune lysis by disrupting terminal complement pathway activation (202), and to cause amebic liver abscess in immunodeficient mice (203). sIgA reactive with this lectin has been detected in both saliva and fecal extracts from symptomatically infected patients (204) and abrogates, in part, adherence of the organism (205). sIgA from saliva also inhibits a virulence-associated amebic cysteine protease (206).

In approximately a third of patients with acute *C. difficile* colitis, antibodies develop in convalescent sera that neutralize the activity of the principal enterotoxin, toxin A (5, 77,207). Although neutralizing activity correlated with levels of both toxin A-specific IgG and IgA, this functional activity resided almost exclusively in the IgA, not the IgG, fraction of the convalescent sera. Thus, in this setting, a unique and selective relationship exists between the mucosal site of infection and the functional IgA response in serum. Moreover, as after exposure to *C. jejuni, V. cholerae,* and *S. typhi* organisms, the molecular form of the IgA response to *C. difficile* toxin A showed a transition with time (77). However, the transition from polymeric to monomeric toxin A-specific IgA with time did not occur in all patients; only those patients in whom neutralizing activity developed produced predominantly monomeric IgA, whereas those who showed no neutralizing activity retained the polymeric form of specific IgA, which more typically accompanies acute or immature responses (Fig. 13.3). Therefore, the evolution in the molecular form of the IgA response from polymeric in acute sera to primarily monomeric in convalescent sera may correlate with distinct changes in the functional activity of these antibodies to limit damage to the host. At mucosal sites, the polymeric configuration of IgA may confer distinct functional advantages over the monomeric form for the prevention and control of infection, such as enhanced binding avidity in the presence of comparable or lower intrinsic affinity (149) or more efficient complement activation (87). However, purified intestinal IgA from patients convalescent from *C. difficile* colitis showed no toxin A-neutralizing activity at the concentrations tested.

Specific IgA may also serve a more active role in systemic defense. Although IgA binding is not typically associated with complement activation, deposition, and bacterial lysis, recent data confirm that two mucosal pathogens—*N. meningitidis* and *H. influenzae*—are susceptible to IgA-driven complement-mediated lysis (208). The unique feature of these observations is that the lytic activity of IgA could be identified only in the absence of IgG, which reacted with capsular polysaccharides; the IgA reacted with other surface proteins. Thus, circulating IgG and IgA may have distinct activities and antigen specificities. In a similar context, both IgG and IgA, particularly polymeric IgA, from sera of adults infected *S. pneumoniae* or immunized with pneumococcal capsular polysaccharides support the ability of phagocytes to kill the organism in the presence of complement (87). sIgA from the breast milk of immunized women shows similar activity (A. Finn and E. N. Janoff, *unpublished data*).

Circulating IgA may also facilitate non–complement-mediated cellular immune responses. IgA in adult sera that reacted with *S. typhi* showed antibody-dependent cell-mediated antibacterial activity. The IgA was obtained from the sera of adults immunized orally with the live *S. typhi* mutant strain Ty21A or from normal sera (209–211). The effector cells in these assays were CD4+ lymphocytes, whereas IgA-driven complement-independent cellular activity against *N. meningitidis* type C was mediated by monocytes (212). Related mechanisms of complement-independent antibacterial activity have been proposed against *S. flexneri* in which Fc-bearing lymphocytes and phagocytes serve as the effector cells (213). An intriguing alternative for complement-independent killing of mucosal pathogens was recently proposed (87). Preliminary data suggest that neutrophils activated by inflammatory products, such as tumor necrosis factor-α and C5a, may support IgA-dependent killing of a gram-positive organism in the absence of hemolytic complement. The data also suggest that in the mucosal lumen, where complement levels are extremely low, phagocytes activated by the chemotactic factors that attracted them may phagocytize and kill pathogens in the presence of specific IgA and inflammation. In the absence of inflammation, IgA may perform its better-accepted functions, such as inhibition of adherence. Thus, experimental evidence in humans suggests that circulating IgA has both complement-mediated and complement-independent cell-mediated activity against mucosal pathogens. Moreover, IgA may protect in an IgA-rich and IgG-poor environment, such as intestinal and other mucosal tissues, where CD4+ T cells or phagocytes are also present, in the presence or absence of complement (208–212).

Mucosal antibodies have clearly been shown to have functional activity against enteric pathogens. Early experimental models offered evidence of mucosal protection against cholera toxin-mediated effects in animals (214). Among children between 1 and 13 years of age with past exposure to either polio vaccine or natural infection, 12 of 19 (63%) with detectable IgA in fecal samples showed neutralizing activity against at least one of three polio serotypes, as did samples from 3 of 12 adults (16). Neutralizing activity was absent in newborn infants but developed after immunization (17). sIgA from the saliva of patients with intestinal amebiasis inhibited adherence of the organisms *in vitro,* activity related in part to inhibition of the organism's galactose-binding lectin (205).

ROLE OF "NATURAL" ANTIBODIES

The ability of gram-negative enteric pathogens to evade the mucosal barrier and invade the systemic circulation is related to the bactericidal activity of normal human serum (215–218). Thus, *C. fetus* is relatively serum-resistant and often causes invasive infection with bacteremia, whereas *C. jejuni* is typically serum-sensitive and causes primarily mucosal infections and little bacteremia (217,218). The bactericidal activity of normal human serum involves both complement and antibody. Complement may bind to enteric gram-negative organisms without causing lysis; the specificity of the antibodies present may direct the location of complement deposition to lytic or nonlytic sites (219, 220). Enteric organisms have developed mechanisms to subvert activation of the lytic terminal complement membrane attack complex after activation by antibody (217, 218,221). The source of these "natural" antibodies in normal human serum is uncertain.

Natural antibodies are those present in serum in the absence of obvious prior symptomatic infection or immunization. They may derive from subclinical infection or colonization, represent cross-reactivity with related antigens, or be polyreactive antibodies (222). The first two situations may elicit IgG responses, whereas polyreactive antibodies are typically IgM; IgA may be elicited in each context. Asymptomatic colonization with enteric organisms such as *C. difficile* is reported to stimulate the production of serum IgG to toxin A, toxin B, and nontoxin antigens (46). In experimental models, natural antibodies localize viral and bacterial infections in regional secondary lymphoid tissues, limiting dissemination to other organs (46). Natural antibodies, particularly IgA, may also derive from T-independent mechanisms in response to intestinal commensal bacteria (150), particularly *Bacteroides* species (151,152). Such stimulation may occur via canonic pathogen-associated antigen patterns, such as lipopolysaccharide and peptidoglycans, which are recognized by receptors such as CD14 and the family of toll-like receptors (223). Polyreactive antibodies from CD5+ B cells react with low affinity but broad specificity. Characterization of the mutation rates and patterns in human intestinal plasma cells suggests that most mucosal antibodies are not akin to polyreactive antibodies with limited mutations; rather, they are highly mutated products of chronic antigenic stimulation (224). The ability of such "natural" antibodies, independent of their source, to clear organisms from the circulation by complement- or Fc-mediated mechanisms may serve as a first line of defense against systemic infection. The local counterparts of these natural antibodies may also limit mucosal adherence and disease.

SUMMARY

Enteric infections may be confined to the intestinal lumen, extend into local tissues or invade into the blood, with variable degrees of associated inflammation. The majority of these mucosal infections elicit detectable humoral responses to a range of antigens in blood and, as increasingly recognized, at the mucosa as well. The presence of pathogen-specific antibodies can be used for diagnosis of acute infection, for epidemiologic studies, or to predict protection against disease. To date, the most reliable data correlate the presence of specific IgG in serum with clinical and epidemiologic evidence of protective immunity. These relationships are most predictive when the antibodies detected recognized virulence-related antigens. Technical difficulties and a paucity of data preclude predictions about the role of mucosal antibodies in effecting immunity (from the Latin word for "exemption") from disease. The distinction of whether systemic antibodies reflect but do or do not mediate mucosal protection is key to our approach to characterizing pathogenic mechanisms employed by enteric pathogens. This distinction is also pivotal in decisions about whether to develop local and/or systemically active vaccines to prevent these common and morbid infections.

ACKNOWLEDGMENTS

This work was sponsored by the Mucosal and Vaccine Research Center, Veterans Affairs Research Service, Public Health Service/National Institutes of Health Grant AI-48796 and contract DE-72621. The author thanks Ronald W. Scamurra, Stuart Johnson, and David N. Taylor for thoughtful discussions, and Ann Emery for excellent secretarial support.

REFERENCES

1. Blaser MJ Duncan DJ. Human serum antibody response to *Campylobacter jejuni* infection as measured in an enzyme-linked immunosorbent assay. *Infect Immun* 1984;44:292–298.
2. Svennerholm A-M, Holmgren J, Hanson LÅ, et al. Boosting of secretory IgA antibody responses in man by parenteral cholera vaccination. *Scand J Immunol* 1977;6:1345–1349.
3. Mascart-Lemone F, Carlsson B, Jalil F, et al. Polymeric and monomeric IgA response in serum and milk after parenteral cholera and oral typhoid vaccination. *Scand J Immunol* 1988; 28:443–448.
4. Mascart-Lemone FO, Duchateau JR, Oosterom J, et al. Kinetics of anti-*Campylobacter jejuni* monomeric and polymeric immunoglobulin A1 and A2 responses in serum during acute enteritis. *J Clin Microbiol* 1987;25:1253–1257.
5. Johnson S, Gerding DN, Janoff EN. Systemic and mucosal antibody responses to toxin A in patients infected with *Clostridium difficile. J Infect Dis* 1992;166:1287–1294.
6. Janoff EN, Smith PD, Blaser MJ. Acute antibody responses to *Giardia lamblia* are depressed in patients with AIDS. *J Infect Dis* 1988;157:798–804.
7. Perez-Perez GI, Dworkin BM, Chodos JE, et al. *Campylobacter pylori* antibodies in humans. *Ann Intern Med* 1988;109:11–17.
8. Ward RL, Clemens JD, Knowlton DR, et al. Evidence that protection against rotavirus diarrhea after natural infection is not dependent on serotype-specific neutralizing antibody. *J Infect Dis* 1992;166:1251–1257.
9. Clemens JD, Ward RL, Rao MR, et al. Seroepidemiologic evaluation of antibodies to rotavirus as correlates of the risk of clinically significant rotavirus diarrhea in rural Bangladesh. *J Infect Dis* 1992;165:161–165.
10. Sarasombath S, Banchuin N, Sukosol T, et al. Systemic and intestinal immunities after natural typhoid infection. *J Clin Microbiol* 1987;25:1088–1093.
11. Brodie J. Antibodies and the Aberdeen typhoid outbreak of 1964. I. The Widal reaction. *J Hyg* 1977;79:161–180.
12. Brodie J. Antibodies and the Aberdeen typhoid outbreak of 1964. II. Coombs', complement fixation and fimbrial agglutination tests. *J Hyg* 1977;79:181–192.
13. Brown WR. Secretory antibody responses to enteric pathogens. In: Blaser MJ, Smith PD, Ravdin JI, et al., eds. *Infections of the gastrointestinal tract.* New York: Raven Press, 1995:87–197.
14. Corthesy B, Kraehenbuhl JP. Antibody-mediated protection of mucosal surfaces. *Curr Top Microbiol Immunol* 1999;236: 93–111.
15. Kelly CP, Pothoulakis C, Orellana J, et al. Human colonic aspirates containing immunoglobulin A antibody to *Clostridium difficile* toxin A inhibit toxin A-receptor binding. *Gastroenterology* 1992;102:35–40.
16. Keller R Dwyer JE. Neutralization of poliovirus by IgA coproantibodies. *J Immunol* 1968;101:192–202.
17. Keller R, Dwyer J, Oh W, et al. Intestinal IgA neutralizing antibodies in newborn infants following poliovirus immunization. *Pediatrics* 1969;43:330–338.
18. Ogra PL, Karzon DT. Distribution of poliovirus antibody in serum, nasopharynx, and alimentary tract following segmental immunization of lower alimentary tract with poliovaccine. *J Immunol* 1969;102:1423–1430.
19. Davies A. An investigation into the serological properties of dysentery stools. *Lancet* 1922;2:1009–1012.
20. Winsor DK Jr, Mathewson JJ, DuPont HL. Western blot analysis of intestinal secretory immunoglobulin A response to *Campylobacter jejuni* antigens in patients with naturally acquired *Campylobacter* enteritis. *Gastroenterology* 1986;90: 1217–1222.
21. Winsor DK Jr, Mathewson JJ, DuPont HL. Comparison of serum and fecal antibody responses of patients with naturally acquired *Shigella sonnei* infection. *J Infect Dis* 1988;158:1108–1112.
22. Beasley WJ, Joseph SW, Weiss E. Improved serodiagnosis of *Salmonella* enteric fevers by an enzyme-linked immunosorbent assay. *J Clin Microbiol* 1981;13:106–114.
23. Gary GW, Anderson LJ, Keswick BH, et al. Norwalk virus antigen and antibody response in an adult volunteer study. *J Clin Microbiol* 1987;25:2001–2003.
24. Christensen ML. Human viral gastroenteritis. *Clin Microbiol Rev* 1989;2:51–89.
25. Blacklow NR, Greenberg HB. Viral gastroenteritis. *N Engl J Med* 1991;325:252–264.
26. Ogra PL, Karzon DT, Righthand R, et al. Immunoglobulin response in serum and secretions after immunization with live and inactivated poliovaccine and natural infection. *N Engl J Med* 1968;279:893–900.
27. Kyne L, Warny M, Qamar A, et al. Association between antibody response to toxin A and protection against recurrent *Clostridium difficile* diarrhoea. *Lancet* 2001;357:189–193.
28. Kaplan JE, Gary GW, Baron RC, et al. Epidemiology of Norwalk gastroenteritis and the role of Norwalk virus in outbreaks of acute nonbacterial gastroenteritis. *Ann Intern Med* 1982;96: 756–761.
29. Hayes EB, Matte TD, O'Brien TR, et al. Large community outbreak of cryptosporidiosis due to contamination of a filtered public water supply. *N Engl J Med* 1989;320:1372–1376.
30. D'Antonio RG, Winn RE, Taylor JP, et al. A waterborne outbreak of cryptosporidiosis in normal hosts. *Ann Intern Med* 1985; 103:886–888.

31. Koch KL, Phillips DJ, Aber RC, et al. Cryptosporidiosis in hospital personnel. *Ann Intern Med* 1985;102:593–596.
32. Birkhead G, Janoff EN, Vogt RL, et al. Elevated levels of immunoglobulin A to *Giardia lamblia* during a waterborne outbreak of gastroenteritis. *J Clin Microbiol* 1989;27:1707–1710.
33. Ungar BLP, Mulligan M, Nuttman TB. Serologic evidence of *Cryptosporidium* infection in U.S. volunteers before and during Peace Corps Service in Africa. *Arch Intern Med* 1989;149:894–897.
34. McDonald AC, MacKenzie WR, Addiss DG, et al. *Cryptosporidium parvum*-specific antibody responses among children residing in Milwaukee during the 1993 waterborne outbreak. *J Infect Dis* 2001;183:1373–1379.
35. Echeverria P, Burke DS, Blacklow NR, et al. Age-specific prevalence of antibody to rotavirus, *Escherichia coli,* heat-labile enterotoxin, Norwalk virus, and hepatitis A virus in a rural community in Thailand. *J Clin Microbiol* 1983;17:923–925.
36. Gilman RH, Brown KH, Visvesvara GS, et al. Epidemiology and serology of *Giardia lamblia* in a developing country: Bangladesh. *Trans R Soc Trop Med Hyg* 1985;79:469–473.
37. Lengerich EJ, Addiss DG, Marx JJ, et al. Increased exposure to cryptosporidia among dairy farmers in Wisconsin. *J Infect Dis* 1993;167:1252–1255.
38. Ungar BLP, Gilman RH, Lanata CF, et al. Seroepidemiology of *Cryptosporidium* infection in two Latin American populations. *J Infect Dis* 1988;157:551–556.
39. Janoff EN, Reller LB. *Cryptosporidium* species, a protean protozoan. *J Clin Microbiol* 1987;25:967–975.
40. Current WL, Garcia LS. Cryptosporidiosis. *Clin Microbiol Rev* 1991;4:325–358.
41. Blaser MJ, Black RE, Duncan DJ, et al. *Campylobacter jejuni*-specific serum antibodies are elevated in healthy Bangladeshi children. *J Clin Microbiol* 1985;21:164–167.
42. Miotti PG, Gilman RH, Pickering LK, et al. Prevalence of serum and milk antibodies to *Giardia lamblia* in different populations of lactating women. *J Infect Dis* 1985;152:1025–1031.
43. Kapikian AZ, Wyatt RG, Levine MM, et al. Oral administration of human rotavirus to volunteers: induction of illness and correlates of resistance. *J Infect Dis* 1983;147:95–106.
44. Jertborn M, Svennerholm A-M, Holmgren J. Saliva, breast milk, and serum antibody responses as indirect measures of intestinal immunity after oral cholera vaccination or natural disease. *J Clin Microbiol* 1986;24:203–209.
45. Parrino TA, Schreiber DS, Trier JS, et al. Clinical immunity in acute gastroenteritis caused by Norwalk agent. *N Engl J Med* 1977;2:86–89.
46. Kyne L, Warny M, Qamar A, et al. Asymptomatic carriage of *Clostridium difficile* and serum levels of IgG antibody against toxin A. *N Engl J Med* 2000;342:390–397.
47. Cash RA, Music SI, Libonati JP, et al. Response of man to infection with *Vibrio cholerae.* II. Protection from illness afforded by previous disease and vaccine. *J Infect Dis* 1974;130:325–333.
48. Mosley WH. Vaccines and somatic antigens. The role of immunity in cholera: a review of epidemiological and serological studies. *Tex Rep Biol Med* 1969;27:228–241.
49. Clemens JD, Harris JR, Khan MR, et al. Field trial of oral cholera vaccines in Bangladesh. *Lancet* 1986;2:124–389.
50. Clemens JD, Sack DA, Harris JR, et al. Cross-protection by B subunit-whole cell cholera vaccine against diarrhea associated with heat-labile toxin-producing enterotoxigenic *Escherichia coli*: results of a large-scale field trial. *J Infect Dis* 1988;158:372–377.
51. Simanjuntak CH, O'Hanley P, Punjabi NH, et al. Safety, immunogenicity, and transmissibility of single-dose live oral cholera vaccine strain CVD 103-HgR in 24- to 59-month-old Indonesian children. *J Infect Dis* 1993;168:1169–1176.
52. Osek J, Jonson G, Svennerholm A-M, et al. Role of antibodies against biotype-specific *Vibrio cholerae* pili in protection against experimental classical and El Tor cholera. *Infect Immun* 1994;62:2901–2907.
53. Clemens JD, van Loon F, Sack DA, et al. Field trial of oral cholera vaccines in Bangladesh: serum vibriocidal and antitoxic antibodies as markers of the risk of cholera. *J Infect Dis* 1991;163:1235–1242.
54. Alfsen A, Iniguez P, Bouguyon E, et al. Secretory IgA specific for a conserved epitope on gp41 envelope glycoprotein inhibits epithelial transcytosis of HIV-1. *J Immunol* 2001;166:6257–6265.
55. Mestecky J, McGhee J. Immunoglobulin A (IgA): molecular and cellular interactions involved in IgA biosynthesis and immune response. *Adv Immunol* 1987;40:153–245.
56. Brandtzaeg P, Berstad AE, Farstad IN, et al. Mucosal immunity—a major adaptive defence mechanism. *Behring Inst Mitt* 1997;1–23.
57. Brandtzaeg P, Farstad IN, Johansen FE, et al. The B-cell system of human mucosae and exocrine glands. *Immunol Rev* 1999;171:45–87.
58. Mestecky J, Russell MW. Mucosal immunoglobulins and their contribution to defence mechanisms: an overview. *Biochem Soc Trans* 1997;25:457–462.
59. Mestecky J, Fultz PN. Mucosal immune system of the human genital tract. *J Infect Dis* 1999;179:S470–S474.
60. Ferretti M, Casini-Raggi V, Pizarro T, et al. Neutralization of endogenous IL-1 receptor antagonist exacerbates and prolongs inflammation in rabbit immune colitis. *J Clin Invest* 1994;94:449–453.
61. Cominelli F, Nast CC, Clark BD, et al. Interleukin 1 (IL-1) gene expression, synthesis, and effect of specific IL-1 receptor blockade in rabbit immune complex colitis. *J Clin Invest* 1990;86:972–980.
62. Kagnoff MF. A question of balance: ups and downs of mucosal inflammation. *J Clin Invest* 1994;94:1.
63. Lycke N, Holmgren J. Strong adjuvant properties of cholera toxin on gut mucosal immune responses to orally presented antigens. *Immunology* 1986;59:301–308.
64. Mayer L, Schlien R. Evidence for function of Ia molecules on gut epithelial cells in man. *J Exp Med* 1987;166:1471.
65. Yamanaka T, Straumfors A, Morton H, et al. M cell pockets of human Peyer's patches are specialized extensions of germinal centers. *Eur J Immunol* 2001;31:107–117.
66. Neutra MR. Interactions of viruses and microparticles with apical plasma membranes of M cells: implications for human immunodeficiency virus transmission. *J Infect Dis* 1999;179:S441–S443.
67. Wolf JL, Bye WA. The membranous epithelial (M) cell and the mucosal immune system. *Annu Rev Med* 1984;35:95–112.
68. O'Leary AD, Sweeney EC. Lymphoglandular complexes of the colon: structure and distribution. *Histopathology* 1986;10:267–283.
69. Coffin SE, Clark SL, Bos NA, et al. Migration of antigen-presenting B cells from peripheral to mucosal lymphoid tissues may induce intestinal antigen-specific IgA following parenteral immunization. *J Immunol* 1999;163:3064–3070.
70. Banchereau J, Steinman RM. Dendritic cells and the control of immunity. *Nature* 1998;392:245–252.
71. Bell SJ, Rigby R, English N, et al. Migration and maturation of human colonic dendritic cells. *J Immunol* 2001;166:4958–4967.
72. Pavli L, Hume D, Van de Pol E, et al. Dendritic cells, the major antigen-presenting cells of the human colonic lamina propria. *Immunology* 1993;78:132–141.
73. Kelsall BL, Strober W. Peyer's patch dendritic cells and the induction of mucosal immune responses. *Res Immunol* 1997;148:490–498.

74. Liu YJ, Arpin C. Germinal center development. *Immunol Rev* 1997;156:111–126.
75. Williams MB, Butcher EC. Homing of naïve and memory T lymphocyte subsets to Peyer's patches, lymph nodes, and spleen. *J Immunol* 1997;159:1746–1752.
76. Winner III L, Mack J, Weltzin R, et al. New model for analysis of mucosal immunity: intestinal secretion of specific monoclonal immunoglobulin A from hybridoma tumors protects against *Vibrio cholerae* infection. *Infect Immun* 1991;59: 977–982.
77. Johnson S, Sypura WD, Gerding DN, et al. Selective neutralization of a bacterial enterotoxin by serum immunoglobulin A in response to mucosal disease. *Infect Immun* 1995;63: 3166–3173.
78. Stokes CR, Soothill JF, Turner MW. Immune exclusion is a function of IgA [Letter]. *Nature* 1975;255:745–746.
79. Kilian M, Mestecky J, Russell MW. Defense mechanisms involving Fc-dependent functions of immunoglobulin A and their subversion by bacterial immunoglobulin A proteases. *Microbiol Rev* 1988;52:296–303.
80. Andre C, Lambert R, Bazin H, et al. Interference of oral immunization with the intestinal absorption of heterologous albumin. *Eur J Immunol* 1974;4:701.
81. Walker WA, Isselbacher KJ, Bloch KJ. Intestinal uptake of macromolecules: effect of oral immunization. *Science* 1972;177: 608.
82. Mazanec MB, Nedrud JG, Lamm ME. Immunoglobulin A monoclonal antibodies protect against Sendai virus. *J Virol* 1987; 61:2624–2626.
83. Mazanec MB, Kaetzel CS, Lamm ME, et al. Intracellular neutralization of virus by immunoglobulin A antibodies. *Proc Natl Acad Sci U S A* 1992;89:6901–6905.
84. Johnson S, Sypura WD, Gerding DN, et al. Neutralization of a bacterial enterotoxin by systemic IgA in response to mucosal infection. *J Immunol* 1993;150:117A(abst).
85. Imai H, Chen A, Wyatt RJ, et al. Lack of complement activation by human IgA immune complexes. *Clin Exp Immunol* 1988;73:479–483.
86. Russell MW, Mansa B. Complement-fixing properties of human IgA antibodies. Alternative pathway complement activation by plastic-bound, but not specific antigen-bound, IgA. *Scand J Immunol* 1989;30:175–183.
87. Janoff EN, Fasching C, Orenstein JM, et al. Killing of *Streptococcus pneumoniae* by capsular polysaccharide-specific polymeric IgA, complement, and phagocytes. *J Clin Invest* 1999;104: 1139–1147.
88. McGhee JR, Mestecky J, Dertzbaugh MT, et al. The mucosal immune system: from fundamental concepts to vaccine development. *Vaccine* 1992;10:75–88.
89. Farstad IN, Halstensen TS, Lazarovits AI, et al. Human intestinal B-cell blasts and plasma cells express the mucosal homing receptor integrin alpha 4 beta 7. *Scand J Immunol* 1995;42: 662–672.
90. Farstad IN, Halstensen TS, Kvale D, et al. Topographic distribution of homing receptors on B and T cells in human gut-associated lymphoid tissue: relation of L-selectin and integrin alpha 4 beta 7 to naïve and memory phenotypes. *Am J Pathol* 1997; 150:187–199.
91. Williams MB, Rose JR, Rott LS, et al. The memory B cell subset responsible for the secretory IgA response and protective humoral immunity to rotavirus expresses the intestinal homing receptor, alpha4beta7. *J Immunol* 1998;161:4227–4235.
92. Czerkinsky C, Prince SJ, Michalek SM, et al. IgA antibody-producing cells in peripheral blood after antigen ingestion: evidence for a common mucosal immune system in humans. *Proc Natl Acad Sci U S A* 1987;84:2449–2453.
93. Quiding M, Nordström I, Kilander A, et al. Intestinal immune responses in humans. *J Clin Invest* 1991;88:143–148.
94. McDermott MR, Bienenstock J. Evidence for a common mucosal immunologic system. I. Migration of B immunoblasts into intestinal, respiratory, and genital tissues. *J Immunol* 1979; 122:1892–1898.
95. Nayak N, Ganguly NK, Walia BN, et al. Specific secretory IgA in the milk of *Giardia lamblia*-infected and uninfected women. *J Infect Dis* 1987;155:724–727.
96. Hayani KC, Guerrero ML, Ruiz-Palacios GM, et al. Evidence for long-term memory of the mucosal immune system: milk secretory immunoglobulin A against *Shigella* lipopolysaccharides. *J Clin Microbiol* 1991;29:2599–2603.
97. Hanson LA, Björkander J, Carlsson B, et al. The heterogeneity of IgA deficiency. *J Clin Immunol* 1988;8:159–162.
98. Clemens JD, Sack DA, Harris JR, et al. Breast feeding and the risk of severe cholera in rural Bangladeshi children. *Am J Epidemiol* 1990;131:400–411.
99. France GL, Marmer DJ, Steele RW. Breast-feeding and *Salmonella* infection. *Am J Dis Child* 1980;134:147–152.
100. Glass RI, Svennerholm A-M, Stoll BJ, et al. Protection against cholera in breast-fed children by antibodies in breast milk. *N Engl J Med* 1983;308:1389–1392.
101. Waldman RH, Benzic Z, Deb BC, et al. Cholera immunology. II. Serum and intestinal antibody response after naturally occurring cholera. *J Infect Dis* 1972;126:401–407.
102. Ravdin JI, Jackson TFHG, Petri WA Jr, et al. Association of serum antibodies to adherence lectin with invasive amebiasis and asymptomatic infection with pathogenic *Entamoeba histolytica. J Infect Dis* 1990;162:768–772.
103. Jayashree S, Bhan MK, Kumar R, et al. Serum and salivary antibodies as indicators of rotavirus infection in neonates. *J Infect Dis* 1988;158:1117–1120.
104. Grimwood K, Lund JCS, Coulson BS, et al. Comparison of serum and mucosal antibody responses follow severe acute rotavirus gastroenteritis in young children. *J Clin Microbiol* 1988;26:732–738.
105. Cohen D, Block C, Green MS, et al. Immunoglobulin M, A, and G antibody response to lipopolysaccharide O antigen in symptomatic and asymptomatic *Shigella* infections. *J Clin Microbiol* 1989;27:162–167.
106. Brooks RG, McCabe RE, Remington JS. Role of serology in the diagnosis of toxoplasmic lymphadenopathy. *Rev Infect Dis* 1987; 9:1055–1062.
107. Stepick-Biek P, Thulliez P, Araujo FG, et al. IgA antibodies for diagnosis of acute congenital and acquired toxoplasmosis. *J Infect Dis* 1990;162:270–273.
108. Partanen P, Turunen HJ, Paasivuo RA, et al. Immunoblot analysis of *Toxoplasma gondii* antigens by human immunoglobulins G, M, and A antibodies at different stages of infection. *J Clin Microbiol* 1984;20:133–135.
109. Decoster A, Darcy F, Caron A, et al. IgA antibodies against P30 as markers of congenital and acute toxoplasmosis. *Lancet* 1988; 2:1104–1107.
110. Choo KE, Oppenheimer SJ, Ismail AB, et al. Rapid serodiagnosis of typhoid fever by dot enzyme immunoassay in an endemic area. *Clin Infect Dis* 1994;19:172–176.
111. Schroeder SA. Interpretation of serologic tests for typhoid fever. *JAMA* 1968;206:839–840.
112. Parsonnet J, Friedman GD, Vandersteen DP, et al. *Helicobacter pylori* infection and the risk of gastric carcinoma. *N Engl J Med* 1991;325:1127–1131.
113. Parsonnet J, Hansen S, Rodriguez L, et al. *Helicobacter pylori* infection and gastric lymphoma. *N Engl J Med* 1994;330: 1267–1271.
114. Cushing AH, Smart J. Gastrointestinal carriage of toxigenic

bacteria: relation to diarrhea and to serum immune response. *J Infect Dis* 1985;151:114–123.
115. Salata RA, Ravdin JI. Review of the human immune mechanisms directed against *Entamoeba histolytica. Rev Infect Dis* 1986;8:261–272.
116. Trissl D. Immunology of *Entamoeba histolytica* in human and animal hosts. *Rev Infect Dis* 1982;4:1154–1184.
117. Krupp IM. Antibody response in intestinal and extraintestinal amebiasis. *Am J Trop Med* 1970;19:57–62.
118. Katzenstein D, Rickerson V, Braude A. New concepts of amebic liver abscess derived from hepatic imaging, serodiagnosis, and hepatic enzymes in 67 consecutive cases in San Diego. *Medicine* 1982;61:237–246.
119. Jackson TFHG, Anderson CB, Simjee AE. Serological differentiation between past and present infection in hepatic amoebiasis. *Trans R Soc Trop Med Hyg* 1984;78:342–345.
120. Istre GR, Kreiss K, Hopkins RS, et al. An outbreak of amebiasis spread by colonic irrigation at a chiropractic clinic. *N Engl J Med* 1982;307:339–342.
121. Taylor GD, Wenman WM. Human immune responses to *Giardia lamblia* infection. *J Infect Dis* 1987;155:137–140.
122. Layward L, Allen AC, Harper SJ, et al. Increased and prolonged production of specific polymeric IgA after systemic immunization with tetanus toxoid in IgA nephropathy. *Clin Exp Immunol* 1992;88:394–398.
123. Robbins JB, Schneerson R, Szu SC. Perspective: hypothesis: serum IgG antibody is sufficient to confer protection against infectious diseases by inactivating the inoculum. *J Infect Dis* 1995;171:1387–1398.
124. Mestecky J, Russell MW. IgA subclasses. In: Shakib Fe, ed. *Basic and clinical aspects of IgG subclasses.* Basel: S Karger, 1986: 277–301.
125. Delacroix DL, Dive C, Rambaud JC, et al. IgA subclasses in various secretions and in serum. *Immunology* 1982;47:383–385.
126. Brandtzaeg P. Humoral immune response patterns of human mucosae: induction and relation to bacterial respiratory tract infections. *J Infect Dis* 1992;165[Suppl 1]:S167–S176.
127. Brandtzaeg P, Kett K, Rognum TO, et al. Distribution of mucosal IgA and IgG subclass-producing immunocytes and alterations in various disorders. *Monogr Allergy* 1986;20:179–194.
128. Kett K, Brandtzaeg P, Radl J, et al. Different subclass distribution of IgA-producing cells in human lymphoid organs and various secretory tissues. *J Immunol* 1986;136:3631–3635.
129. Crago SS, Kutteh WH, Moror I, et al. Distribution of IgA1, IgA2, and J-chain containing cells in human tissues. *J Immunol* 1984;132:16–18.
130. Jonard PP, Rambaud JC, Dive C, et al. Secretion of immunoglobulins and plasma proteins from the jejunal mucosa. *J Clin Invest* 1984;74:525–535.
131. Conley ME, Delacroix DL. Intravascular and mucosal immunoglobulin A: two separate but related systems of immune defense? *Ann Intern Med* 1987;106:892–901.
132. Underdown BJ, Schiff JM. Immunoglobulin A: strategic defense initiative at the mucosal surface. *Ann Rev Immunol* 1986;4: 389–417.
133. Brandtzaeg P. Immunohistochemical characterization of intracellular J-chain and binding site for secretory component (SC) in human immunoglobulin (Ig)-producing cells. *Mol Immunol* 1983;20:941–966.
134. Brandtzaeg P. Presence of J chain in human immunocytes containing various immunoglobulin classes. *Nature* 1974;252: 418–420.
135. Moro I, Iwase T, Komiyama K, et al. Immunoglobulin A (IgA) polymerization sites in human immunocytes: immunoelectron microscopic study. *Cell Struct Funct* 1990;15:85–91.
136. Kutteh WH, Prince SJ, Mestecky J. Tissue origins of human polymeric and monomeric IgA. *J Immunol* 1982;128:990–995.
137. South MA, Cooper MD, Wollheim FA, et al. The IgA system. I. Studies of the transport and immunochemistry of IgA in the saliva. *J Exp Med* 1966;123:615–627.
138. Granfors K, Toivanen A. IgA-anti-*Yersinia* antibodies in *Yersinia*-triggered reactive arthritis. *Ann Rheum Dis* 1986;45: 561–565.
139. Conley ME, Kearney JF, Lawton AR, et al. Differentiation of human B cells expressing the IgA subclass as demonstrated by monoclonal antibodies. *J Immunol* 1980;125:2311–2316.
140. Warny M, Vaerman JP, Avesani V, et al. Human antibody response to *Clostridium difficile* toxin A in relation to clinical course of infection. *Infect Immun* 1994;62:384–389.
141. Ponzi AN, Merlino C, Angerette A, et al. Virus-specific polymeric immunoglobulin A antibodies in serum from patients with rubella, measles, varicella, and herpes zoster virus infections. *J Clin Microbiol* 1985;22:505–509.
142. Tarkowski A, Lue C, Moldoveanu Z, et al. Immunization of humans with polysaccharide vaccines induces systemic, predominantly polymeric IgA2-subclass antibody responses. *J Immunol* 1990;144:3770–3778.
143. Carson PJ, Schut RL, Simpson ML, et al. Antibody class and subclass responses to pneumococcal polysaccharides following immunization of human immunodeficiency virus-infected patients. *J Infect Dis* 1995;172:340–345.
144. Johnson S, Opstad NL, Douglas JM Jr, et al. Prolonged and preferential production of polymeric immunoglobulin A in response to *Streptococcus pneumoniae* capsular polysaccharides. *Infect Immun* 1996;64:4339–4344.
145. Hashido M, Kawana T, Inouye S. Differentiation of primary from nonprimary genital herpesvirus infections by detection of polymeric immunoglobulin A activity. *J Clin Microbiol* 1989; 27:2609–2611.
146. Bartholomeusz RCA, Forrest BD, Labrooy JT, et al. The serum polymeric IgA antibody response to typhoid vaccination: its relationship to the intestinal IgA response. *Immunology* 1990; 69:190–194.
147. Mascart-Lemone F, Duchateau J, Conley ME, et al. A polymeric IgA response in serum can be produced by parenteral immunization. *Immunology* 1987;61:409–413.
148. Moldoveanu Z, Egan ML, Mestecky J. Cellular origin of human polymeric and monomeric IgA: intracellular and secreted forms of IgA. *J Immunol* 1984;133:3156–3162.
149. Renegar KB, Jackson GDF, Mestecky J. *In vitro* comparison of the biologic activities of monoclonal monomeric IgA, polymeric IgA, and secretory IgA. *J Immunol* 1998;160:1219–1223.
150. Macpherson AJ, Gatto D, Sainsbury E, et al. A primitive T cell-independent mechanism of intestinal mucosal IgA responses to commensal bacteria. *Science* 2000;288:2222–2226.
151. Gronlund MM, Arvilommi H, Kero P, et al. Importance of intestinal colonisation in the maturation of humoral immunity in early infancy: a prospective follow-up study of healthy infants aged 0-6 months. *Arch Dis Child Fetal Neonatal Ed* 2000;83: F186–F192.
152. Lanning D, Sethupathi P, Rhee KJ, et al. Intestinal microflora and diversification of the rabbit antibody repertoire. *J Immunol* 2000;165:2012–2019.
153. Ahnen DJ, Brown WR. *Campylobacter* enteritis in immune-deficient patients. *Ann Intern Med* 1982;96:187–188.
154. Brown WR, Butterfield D, Savage D, et al. Clinical, microbiological, and immunological studies in patients with immunoglobulin deficiencies and gastrointestinal disorders. *Gut* 1972;13:441–449.
155. Janoff EN, Smith PD. Gastrointestinal infections in the

immunocompromised host. *Curr Opin Gastroenterol* 1996;12: 95–101.
156. Bloom PD, Boedeker EC. Mucosal immune responses to intestinal bacterial pathogens. *Semin Gastrointest Dis* 1996;7:151–166.
157. Dinari G, Hale TL, Austin SW, et al. Local and systemic antibody responses to *Shigella* infection in Rhesus monkeys. *J Infect Dis* 1987;155:1065–1069.
158. Stoll BJ, Svennerholm A-M, Gothefors L, et al. Local and systemic antibody responses to naturally acquired enterotoxigenic *Escherichia coli* diarrhea in an endemic area. *J Infect Dis* 1986; 153:527–534.
159. Cancellieri V, Fara GM. Demonstration of specific IgA in human feces after immunization with live Ty21a *Salmonella typhi* vaccine. *J Infect Dis* 1985;151:482–484.
160. Langevin-Perriat A, Lafont S, Vincent C, et al. Intestinal secretory antibody response induced by an oral cholera vaccine in human volunteers. *Vaccine* 1988;6:509–512.
161. Svennerholm A-M, Hanson LÅ, Holmgren J, et al. Different secretory IgA antibody response to cholera vaccination in Swedish and Pakistani women. *Infect Immunol* 1980;30:427–430.
162. Svennerholm A-M, Holmgren J, Sack DA, et al. Intestinal antibody responses after immunisation with cholera B subunit. *Lancet* 1982;1:305–307.
163. Svennerholm A-M, Gothefors L, Sack DA, et al. Local and systemic antibody responses and immunological memory in humans after immunization with cholera B subunit by different routes. *Bull World Health Organ* 1984;62:909–918.
164. Barnes GL, Doyle LW, Hewson PH, et al. A randomised trial of oral gammaglobulin in low-birth-weight infants infected with rotavirus. *Lancet* 1982;1:1371–1373.
165. Yolken RH, Wyatt RG, Mata L, et al. Secretory antibody directed against rotavirus in human milk—measurement by means of enzyme-linked immunosorbent assay. *J Pediatr* 1978; 93:916–921.
166. Kaplan ME, Zalusky R, Remington J, et al. Immunologic studies with intrinsic factor in man. *J Clin Invest* 1963;42:368–382.
167. Husby S, Mestecky J, Moldoveanu Z, et al. Oral tolerance in humans. *J Immunol* 1994;152:4663–4670.
168. Svennerholm A-M, Jertborn M, Gothefors L, et al. Mucosal antitoxic and antibacterial immunity after cholera disease and after immunization with a combined B subunit-whole cell vaccine. *J Infect Dis* 1984;149:884–893.
169. Hone D, Hackett J. Vaccination against enteric bacterial diseases. *Rev Infect Dis* 1989;11:853–877.
170. Ashcroft MT, Ritchie JM, Nicholson CC. Controlled field trail in British Guiana school children of heat-killed phenolized and acetone-killed lyophilized typhoid vaccines. *Am J Hyg* 1964;79: 196–206.
171. Robbins JB, Chu C, Schneerson R. Hypothesis for vaccine development: protective immunity to enteric diseases caused by nontyphoidal salmonellae and shigellae may be conferred by serum IgG antibodies to the O-specific polysaccharide of their lipopolysaccharides. *Clin Infect Dis* 1992;15:346–361.
172. Vincent C, Cozon G, Zittoun M, et al. Secretory immunoglobulins in serum from human immunodeficiency virus (HIV)-infected patients. *J Clin Immunol* 1992;12:381–388.
173. Delacroix DL, Elkon KB, Geubel AP, et al. Changes in size, subclass, and metabolic properties of serum immunoglobulin A in liver diseases in other diseases with high serum immunoglobulin A. *J Clin Invest* 1983;71:358–367.
174. Steffen R, Rickenbach M, Wilhelm U, et al. Health problems after travel to developing countries. *J Infect Dis* 1987;156:84–91.
175. Barbour AG, Nichols CR Fukushima T. An outbreak of giardiasis in a group of campers. *Am J Trop Med Hyg* 1976;25:384–389.
176. Phillips SC, Mildvan D, Williams DC, et al. Sexual transmission of enteric protozoa and helminths in a venereal-disease clinic population. *N Engl J Med* 1981;305:603–606.
177. Pickering LK, Woodward WE, DuPont HL et al. Occurrence of *Giardia lamblia* in children in day-care centers. *J Pediatr* 1984; 104:522–526.
178. Zaki AM, DuPont HL, Elalamy MA, et al. The detection of enteropathogens in acute diarrhea in a family cohort population in rural Egypt. *Am J Trop Med Hyg* 1986;35:1013–1022.
179. Nash TE, Herrington DA, Losonsky GA, et al. Experimental human infections with *Giardia lamblia. J Infect Dis* 1987;156: 974–984.
180. Istre GR, Dunlop TS, Gaspard B, et al. Waterborne giardiasis at a mountain resort: evidence for acquired immunity. *Am J Publ Health* 1984;74:602–604.
181. Moore GT, Cross WM, McGuire D, et al. Epidemic giardiasis at a ski resort. *N Engl J Med* 1969;281:402–407.
182. Islam A, Stoll BJ, Ljungstrom I, et al. *Giardia lamblia* infections in a cohort of Bangladeshi mothers and infants followed for one year. *J Pediatr* 1983;103:996–1000.
183. Gilman RH, Marquis GS, Miranda E, et al. Rapid reinfection by *Giardia lamblia* after treatment in a hyperendemic third world community. *Lancet* 1988;1:343–345.
184. Hossain MM, Ljungstrom I, Glass RI, et al. Amoebiasis and giardiasis in Bangladesh: parasitological and serological studies. *Trans R Soc Trop Med Hyg* 1983;77:552–554.
185. Miotti PG, Gilman RN, Santosham M, et al. Age-related rate of seropositivity of antibody to *Giardia lamblia* in four diverse populations. *J Clin Microbiol* 1986;24:972–975.
186. Janoff EN, Smith PD. The role of immunity in *Giardia* infections. In: Meyer EAM, ed. *Giardiasis.* Amsterdam: Elsevier Science, 1990:215–233.
187. Janoff EN, Taylor DN, Echeverria P, et al. Serum antibodies to *Giardia lamblia* by age in populations in Colorado and Thailand. *West J Med* 1990;152:253–256.
188. Blaser MJ, Sazie E, Williams LP Jr. The influence of immunity on raw milk-associated *Campylobacter* infection. *JAMA* 1987; 257:43–46.
189. Nakata S, Chiba S, Terashima H, et al. Humoral immunity in infants with gastroenteritis caused by human calicivirus. *J Infect Dis* 1985;152:274–279.
190. Janoff EN, Mead P, Mead J, et al. Clinical, nutritional, and immunologic response to *Giardia lamblia* and *Cryptosporidium* infections in Thai orphans. *Am J Trop Med Hyg* 1990;43: 248–256.
191. Moss DM, Chappell CL, Okhuysen PC, et al. The antibody response to 27-, 17-, and 15-kDa *Cryptosporidium* antigens following experimental infection in humans. *J Infect Dis* 1998; 178:827–833.
192. Brown KA, Kriss JA, Moser CA, et al. Circulating rotavirus-specific antibody-secreting cells (ASCs) predict the presence of rotavirus-specific ASCs in the human small intestinal lamina propria. *J Infect Dis* 2000;182:1039–1043.
193. Velázquez FR, Matson DO, Guerrero ML, et al. Serum antibody as a marker of protection against natural rotavirus infection and disease. *J Infect Dis* 2000;182:1602–1609.
194. Robin G, Cohen D, Orr N, et al. Characterization and quantitative analysis of serum IgG class and subclass response to *Shigella sonnei* and *Shigella flexneri* 2a lipopolysaccharide following natural *Shigella* infection. *J Infect Dis* 1997;175: 1128–1133.
195. Barrett TJ, Green JH, Griffin PM, et al. Enzyme-linked immunosorbent assays for detecting antibodies to Shiga-like toxin I, Shiga-like toxin II, and *Escherichia coli* O157:H7 lipopolysaccharide in human serum. *Curr Microbiol* 1991;23: 189–195.

196. Cohen A, Madrid-Marina V, Estrov Z, et al. Expression of glycolipid receptors to Shiga-like toxin on human B lymphocytes: a mechanism for the failure of long-lived antibody response to dysenteric disease. *Int Immunol* 1990;2:1–8.
197. Svennerholm A-M, Jonson G, Holmgren J. Immunity to *Vibrio cholerae* infection. In: Wachsmuth IK, Blake PA, Olsvik O, eds. Vibrio cholerae *and cholera: molecular to global perspectives.* Washington, DC: American Society for Microbiology Press, 1994:257–271.
198. Kantele A, Arvilommi H, Jokinen I. Specific immunoglobulin-secreting human blood cells after peroral vaccination against *Salmonella typhi. J Infect Dis* 1986;153:1126–1131.
199. Forrest BD. Identification of an intestinal immune response using peripheral blood lymphocytes. *Lancet* 1988;8:81–83.
200. Clemens JD, Sack DA, Harris JR, et al. Field trials of oral cholera vaccines in Bangladesh: results from three-year follow-up. *Lancet* 1990;1:270–273.
201. Petri WA Jr, Joyce MP, Broman J, et al. Recognition of the galactose- or *N*-acetylgalactosamine-binding lectin of *Entamoeba histolytica* by human immune sera. *Infect Immun* 1987; 55:2327–2331.
202. Braga LL, Ninomiya H, McCoy JJ, et al. Inhibition of the complement membrane attack complex by the galactose-specific adhesion of *Entamoeba histolytica. J Clin Invest* 1992;90: 1131–1137.
203. Seydel KB, Braun KL, Zhang T, et al. Protection against amebic liver abscess formation in the severe combined immunodeficient mouse by human anti-amebic antibodies. *Am J Trop Med Hyg* 1996;55:330–332.
204. Abou-el-Magd I, Soong CJ, el-Hawey AM, et al. Humoral and mucosal IgA antibody response to a recombinant 52-kDa cysteine-rich portion of the *Entamoeba histolytica* galactose-inhibitable lectin correlates with detection of native 170-kDa lectin antigen in serum of patients with amebic colitis. *J Infect Dis* 1996;174:157–162.
205. Carrero JC, Diaz MY, Viveros M, et al. Human secretory immunoglobulin A anti-*Entamoeba histolytica* antibodies inhibit adherence of amebae to MDCK cells. *Infect Immun* 1994;62:764–767.
206. Guerrero-Manriquez GG, Sanchez-Ibarra F Avila EE. Inhibition of *Entamoeba histolytica* proteolytic activity by human salivary IgA antibodies. *APMIS* 1998;106:1088–1094.
207. Lyerly DM, Saum KE, Macdonald DK, et al. Effects of *Clostridium difficile* toxins given intragastrically to animals. *Infect Immun* 1985;47:349–352.
208. Jarvis GA, Griffiss JM. Human IgA1 initiates complement-mediated killing of *Neisseria meningitidis. J Immunol* 1989;143: 1703–1709.
209. Tagliabue A, Villa L, Boraschi D, et al. Natural anti-bacterial activity against *Salmonella typhi* by human T4+ lymphocytes armed with IgA antibodies. *J Immunol* 1985;135:4178–4182.
210. Tagliabue A, Villa L, De Magistris MT, et al. IgA-driven T cell-mediated anti-bacterial immunity in man after live oral Ty 21a vaccine. *J Immunol* 1986;137:1504–1510.
211. Tagliabue A, Nencioni L, Mantovani A, et al. Impairment of *in vitro* natural antibacterial activity in HIV-infected patients. *J Immunol* 1988;141:2607–2611.
212. Lowell GH, Smith LF, Grifiss JM, et al. IgA-dependent, monocyte-mediated antibacterial activity. *J Exp Med* 1980;152: 452–457.
213. Lowell GH, MacDermott RP, Summers PL, et al. Antibody-dependent cell-mediated antibacterial activity: K lymphocytes, monocytes, and granulocytes are effective against *Shigella. J Immunol* 1980;125:2778–2784.
214. Freter R, De SP, Mondal A, et al. Coproantibody and serum antibody in cholera patients. *J Infect Dis* 1965;115:83–87.
215. Roantree RJ, Pappas NC. The survival of strains of enteric bacilli in the blood stream is related to their sensitivity to the bactericidal effect of serum. *J Clin Invest* 1960;39:82–88.
216. Schoolnik GK, Buchanan TM, Holmes KK. Gonococci causing disseminated gonococcal infection are resistant to the bactericidal action of normal human sera. *J Clin Invest* 1976;58: 1163–1173.
217. Blaser MJ, Smith PF, Kohler PF. Susceptibility of *Campylobacter* isolates to the bactericidal activity of human serum. *J Infect Dis* 1985;151:227–235.
218. Blaser MJ, Smith PF, Repin JE, et al. Pathogenesis of *Campylobacter fetus* infections. II. Failure of encapsulated *Campylobacter fetus* to bind C3b explains serum and phagocytosis resistance. *J Clin Invest* 1988;81:1434–1444.
219. Joiner KA, Hammer CH, Brown EJ, et al. Studies on the mechanism of bacterial resistance to complement-mediated killing. I. Terminal complement components are deposited and released from *Salmonella minnesota* S218 without causing bacterial death. *J Exp Med* 1982;155:797–808.
220. Frank MM, Joiner K, Hammer C. The function of antibody and complement in the lysis of bacteria. *Rev Infect Dis* 1987;9: S537–S545.
221. Joiner KA. Complement evasion by bacteria and parasites. *Annu Rev Microbiol* 1988;42:201–230.
222. Casali P, Notkins AL. Probing the human B cell repertoire with EBV: polyreactive antibodies and CD5+ B lymphocytes. *Annu Rev Immunol* 1989;7:513–535.
223. Hoffmann JA, Kafatos FC, Janeway CA, et al. Phylogenetic perspectives in innate immunity. *Science* 1999;284:1313–1318.
224. Dunn-Walters DK, Boursier L, Spencer J. Hypermutation, diversity and dissemination of human intestinal lamina propria plasma cells. *Eur J Immunol* 1997;27:2959–2964.
225. Ungar BLP, Soave R, Fayer R, et al. Enzyme immunoassay detection of immunoglobulin M and G antibodies to *Cryptosporidium* in immunocompetent and immunocompromised persons. *J Infect Dis* 1986;153:57–58.
226. Offit PA, Hoffenberg EJ, Santos N, et al. Rotavirus-specific humoral and cellular immune response after primary, symptomatic infection. *J Infect Dis* 1993;167:1436–1440.
227. Siddons CA, Chapman PA. Detection of serum and faecal antibodies in haemorrhagic colitis caused by *Escherichia coli* O157. *J Med Microbiol* 1993;39:408–415.

14

CELLULAR IMMUNE MECHANISMS OF DEFENSE IN THE GASTROINTESTINAL TRACT (INCLUDING MAST CELLS)

STEPHEN P. JAMES

The mucosal immune system of the gastrointestinal tract comprises specialized structures, including Peyer's patches, mesenteric lymph nodes, and the intestinal lamina propria. A complex mixture of cells within these structures continually undergo activation, migration and homing, and terminal differentiation and perform effector functions, including the release of antibodies and numerous mediators of cytotoxic function. This complicated system, the organization of which is reviewed in Chapter 10, provides the host with mechanisms of protection against invasion by potential pathogens, and at the same time it allows the potentially immunogenic products of digestion and the resident normal intestinal microbial flora to be tolerated. The balance between the mechanisms that control protective immune responses and inflammation and those that generate tolerance or nonresponsiveness determine the nature of the host response and the type of pathophysiology observed in response to different immunologic stimuli. The fundamental differences between tolerance and immunity in the gut are also central to understanding the pathogenesis of autoimmunity and the development of oral vaccines. The aim of this chapter is to review the cellular immune mechanisms of the gastrointestinal system. The major humoral immune function of the gastrointestinal tract, the production of immunoglobulin A (IgA), is reviewed in Chapter 12. Although "cellular" and "humoral" immune mechanisms have historically been viewed as separate categories of immune function, this distinction is artificial because they are closely intertwined.

S. P. James: Division of Digestive Diseases and Nutrition, National Institute of Diabetes and Digestive and Kidney Diseases, National Institutes of Health, Bethesda, Maryland

MECHANISMS OF IMMUNITY AND INFLAMMATION

The mucosal host defense system contains an array of specialized cells that interact with other, nonimmune cells and mediators to generate complex, overlapping, innate nonspecific inflammatory and specific immune responses. The coordinated effect of these responses is to generate immediate inflammatory responses that contain invading pathogens, generate specific T-lymphocyte effector and antibody responses, and elicit long-term immunologic memory. The actions of the immune and inflammatory responses are closely related to the mechanisms of wound healing. Finally, the immune and inflammatory mechanisms are integrated with those of nonimmunologic systems to produce physiologic responses, such as the secretion of water and electrolytes by the intestinal epithelium and the neurologically controlled motor activity of the gut, that also are important in protecting the host from pathogens.

The effector mechanisms evoked by immune and inflammatory mechanisms are classified into several categories. Specific antibodies can mediate neutralization, in which the injurious effects of toxins and certain microorganisms are inhibited by binding to secretory antibodies. In the gastrointestinal tract, IgA promotes neutralization without generating potentially injurious inflammatory responses. Activated cells of the immune system also mediate cytotoxicity, in which target cells and microorganisms are killed by nonspecific or specific mechanisms. Many of the effects of the immune system are mediated by cytokines, which play numerous critical roles in cell proliferation, differentiation, effector function, and wound healing. Finally, the combined functions of the immune system are critical in generating inflammation, characterized by a cascade of cellular responses: recruitment of macrophages, neutrophils, and lymphocytes and triggering of mast cell and eosinophil mediator release; alteration of the vascular endothelium;

release of inflammatory cytokines; and activation of various humoral factors (complement, kinin, coagulation factors). A unique feature of the gastrointestinal tract is a continuous low-grade or "physiologic" state of inflammation, presumably caused by the presence of nonpathogenic microflora in the gastrointestinal lumen. In contrast, pathologic inflammation, such as that associated with invasive gastrointestinal bacterial pathogens, is characterized by an increased influx of inflammatory cells and lymphocytes and activation of cells with subsequent tissue injury.

INNATE IMMUNITY IN THE GASTROINTESTINAL TRACT

In recent years, it has become increasingly clear that the innate and adaptive arms of the immune system both play critical and complementary roles in protecting the host from microbial pathogens (Fig. 14.1). The innate immune system is evolutionarily primitive, and elements of innate immunity are found in all multicellular organisms, including plants, invertebrates, and vertebrates (1). The innate immune system is critical in providing the first line of defense and early warning to the host of invasion by infectious pathogens. A variety of mechanisms have evolved in the innate immune system to resist pathogens. These include resistance to the entry of pathogens across surface epithelia; secretion of antimicrobial peptides such as cryptidins, produced by Paneth cells in the intestinal crypts; activation of antimicrobial defense by polymorphonuclear leukocytes and monocytes; and activation of complex intracellular signaling pathways, such as cytokine production and activation of cell death, that serve to remove infected cells through central mediators such as nuclear factor -κβ (NF-κβ). The adaptive immune system, based on the actions of T and B lymphocytes, is fundamentally different from the innate immune system in that it involves a very complex series of events. These include somatic mutation and multiple rounds of both negative and positive selection to expand populations of cells with high-affinity receptors that recognize unique determinants, called *antigens*, in the context of self molecules; the result is an array of cellular cytotoxic, cytokine, and humoral antibody responses. In addition, the adaptive immune response, unlike the innate response, is capable of generating immunologic memory, the basis of protective adaptation to repeated infection and of vaccination. Although the triggers and effectors of innate and adaptive immune responses are distinct, the innate immune system is critical for triggering adaptive immune responses (2), and innate immunity provides the pathways for the action of vaccine adjuvants.

Considerable progress has been made in understanding the molecular basis of innate immunity (3). The system by which the innate immune system recognizes foreign invading microbes is based on receptors that, unlike the highly specific receptors of T and B cells, are not clonally derived; they recognize determinants expressed by microbial pathogens, but not the host (Table 14.1). Additional signaling molecules are being described in microbial pathogens, but the best described thus far include a variety of lipids, carbohydrates, and nucleic acids, such as lipopolysaccharide (LPS) in the cell walls of gram-negative bacteria, proteoglycans and lipoteichoic acid in gram-positive bacteria and other organisms, CpG DNA in bacteria, mannans in yeast cell walls, and formylated peptides. The molecular structures that trigger innate responses have been called *pathogen-asso-*

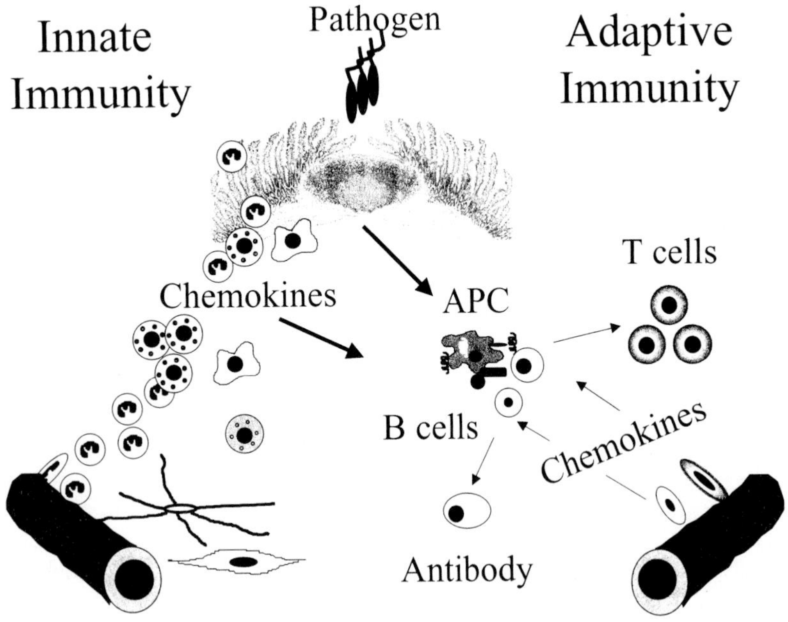

FIGURE 14.1. Role of the innate and adaptive arms of host defense in the gastrointestinal tract. Innate immune defense mechanisms in response to pathogens elicit the production of chemokines and cytokines; these cause inflammation, with an influx of neutrophils, monocytes, and lymphocytes, activation of mast cells and eosinophils, and triggering of neuromuscular responses. The innate signals trigger activation of the adaptive immune system, primarily by activating specialized antigen-presenting cells, which in turn activate T- and B-cell pathways.

TABLE 14.1. PATHOGEN-ASSOCIATED MOLECULAR PATTERN LIGANDS AND RECEPTORS THAT TRIGGER INNATE IMMUNE RESPONSES

PAMP	Pathogen	Pattern Recognition Receptor	Response
Lipoteichoic acid	Gram-positive bacteria	TLR2	Initiation of inflammation
LPS	Gram-negative bacteria	TLR4, CD14	"
Flagellin	Bacteria	TLR5	"
CpG	Many prokaryotes	TLR9	"
Lipoarabinomannan	Mycobacteria	TLR2, CD1	"
N-formyl-Met	Prokaryotes	f-Met receptors	Activation of myeloid cells
Mannan	Yeast	Mannose receptor, MBP	Phagocytosis
Zymosan	Yeast	Mannose, β-glucan receptors, TLR2	Phagocytosis, inflammation
Heat shock proteins	Prokaryotes and eukaryotes	Unknown	Inflammation

PAMP, pathogen-associated molecular pattern; LPS, lipopolysaccharide; TLR, toll-like receptor; CD, cluster of differentiation; Met, methionine.

ciated molecular patterns, and the receptors of the innate immune system have been called *pattern recognition receptors.* The receptors generally fall into two well-described classes: those that lead to activation of proinflammatory pathways and those that lead to activation of phagocytic cells.

The best-studied paradigm of innate immunity involves the responses triggered by endotoxin (LPS) from gram-negative bacteria (3). LPS is the central mediator of the bacterial septic shock syndrome, which, although studied for decades, has only recently been understood at the molecular level in terms of initial triggering events of the innate immune system. Although earlier studies demonstrated that the effects of LPS depended on a cell surface receptor, LPS-binding protein (CD14), it also became clear that CD14 could not account for signal transduction in responding cells. The major advance in this field was the discovery of the role of toll-like receptors (TLRs) in *Drosophila* and the identification of TLR homologues in mice as the genes responsible for LPS responses (4,5). In particular, it was found that the receptor TLR4 is mutated in the spontaneously LPS-hyporesponsive mouse strain C3H/HeJ. TLR4 was subsequently shown to mediate the signaling of LPS bound to CD14 by activating the adaptor protein MyD88 and the serine kinase IRAK, leading to activation of a kinase cascade and ultimately to activation of the central mediators of the immune and inflammatory responses, NF-κβ and AP-1, both critical in cytokine production (3).

To date, at least 10 different mammalian TLRs have been reported, and it will not be surprising if more related molecules are discovered (6–10). TLR2 appears to play an important role in signaling by molecules produced by gram-positive bacteria, such as lipoteichoic acid (6). Flagellin transduces cell signals through TLR5 (7,8). TLR9 was recently shown to be the receptor for methylated CpG present in bacteria, which is capable of activating innate responses (10). TLRs are currently being studied intensively, but one of the fundamental messages emerging is that these pathways lead to the activation of host responses through direct recognition of microbial structures by means of receptors that are invariant and do not involve recognition of self. The resultant responses in which myeloid lineage cells and nonimmune cells contain and kill microbial invaders are preprogrammed responses.

Another critical characteristic of the innate immune system is that it appears to be fundamental to the activation of adaptive T- and B-cell specific immune responses (3). Among the many innate responses are the elaboration of chemotactic cytokines and the up-regulation of co-stimulatory molecules such as CD80 and CD86 (B7.1 and B7.2, respectively). In recent years, it has become clear that the activation of T- and B-cell pathways requires cognate interactions, particularly with dendritic cells, which present not only the first, antigenic signal for activation but also the required second signaling molecules, such as CD80 and CD86. On a larger scale, it appears that one of the critical factors allowing the gastrointestinal mucosal host defense system to distinguish between normal flora within the lumen and potential pathogens is that the normal microbial flora do not interact intimately with host epithelial cells or invade the submucosa, whereas pathogens do; in so doing, they trigger both innate responses and subsequent adaptive immune responses.

Although defects of the innate immune response appear to be uncommon in humans, it is possible that subtle differences in innate responsiveness have not yet been identified in this relatively new field of investigation. Allelic differences in innate response genes may contribute to differences in host responses to infectious agents. In addition, defects in the innate host response may contribute to idiopathic diseases of the gastrointestinal tract. As an example, it has been shown that some patients with Crohn disease, an idiopathic inflammatory disorder of the gastrointestinal tract that has been suggested to involve an altered response to enteric flora (discussed in Chapter 28), have mutations in *Nod2,* a gene encoding a putative intracellular LPS-binding protein that may play a role in NF-κβ signaling (11–13).

DENDRITIC CELLS

When a microbe enters the host, it appears that one of the cell types that is key in determining the nature of the innate immune response and whether an adaptive immune response is triggered is the dendritic cell (DC). As indicated in the section on mucosal immunity, oral exposure to antigens may result in tolerance, either through the generation of regulatory Tr1 or Th3 suppressor cells or by the induction of lymphocyte apoptosis or anergy. Alternatively, certain intracellular pathogens, such as viruses or invasive bacteria, trigger a CD4+ T-cell Th1 response, characterized by the expression of interleukin 12 (IL-12) and interferon-γ (IFN-γ). In contrast, some extracellular pathogens, such as helminths, induce the expansion of CD4+ T cells of the Th2 phenotype, which express IL-4, IL-5, and IL-10. Generating the right type of response may determine whether the host successfully interacts with the antigen or microbe in the gastrointestinal environment. It appears that the initial instructions to T and B cells in the host response are determined at the level of the initial interaction of the antigen or microbe with DCs (14,15).

Dendritic cells are a family of professional antigen-presenting cells found in low numbers in many body tissues, including the gastrointestinal tract. They are heterogeneous in both phenotype and function. It is thought that DCs arise from distinct myeloid or lymphoid precursors, the former expressing high levels of CD11b and the latter expressing CD8α,α. DCs differentiate from an immature stage with a considerable potential for antigen uptake to more mature phenotypes, characterized by a decline in antigen-processing ability and an increased expression of major histocompatibility complex (MHC), co-stimulatory molecules, adhesion molecules, and cytokine receptors, which allows them to migrate to lymphoid organs and efficiently induce T-cell activation (14,15).

Recently, the murine Peyer's patch has been shown to contain DCs with three distinct phenotypes: myeloid DCs, lymphoid DCs, and DCs lacking both phenotypic markers (double negative) (16,17). Only myeloid DCs of the Peyer's patch produce high levels of IL-10 on stimulation, whereas the latter two produce high levels of IL-12p70. These findings suggest that the DCs of distinct lineages in the patch play an important role in tolerance versus a polarized Th1 or Th2 immune response. It appears that DCs sense microbes by means of the same pattern recognition molecules discussed above. The amplification of a Th1 or Th2 T-cell response appears to be circular in that the cytokines produced by T cells affect DCs to alter their function. Thus, IL-10 or transforming growth factor-β (TGF-β) activates Th2-inducing DCs, whereas DCs stimulated by IFN-γ enhance Th1 responses. Unrestrained activation of the immune system can obviously be deleterious to the host. DCs also possess mechanisms to down-regulate responses, including engagement of CTLA-4 on activated T cells via B7 molecules and expression of IL-10 and TGF-β. Interestingly, Peyer's patch DCs are capable of capturing apoptotic cells, and it is thought that the function of these cells is immune-inhibitory (18).

Although most investigations of gastrointestinal DCs have focused on the murine Peyer's patch for experimental reasons, it is likely that this is not the only site for important interactions between DCs and gastrointestinal microbes. Recently, it has been shown that DCs can send dendrites outside the epithelium directly between tight junctions of epithelial cells (19). DCs can maintain the integrity of the tight junction in this process by expressing tight junction proteins themselves. This potentially allows DCs to sample the luminal contents directly for antigens and pathogens and may provide a direct site of entry for pathogens.

ADAPTIVE IMMUNE RESPONSES

As indicated above, the innate immune response is particularly adapted to providing an immediate and early defense against microbial invasion. One of the important roles of innate signals is to trigger the adaptive immune system, characterized by the specific responses of T and B cells (reviewed in other chapters) against pathogens. In fact, the function of the innate immune system may be very important in determining whether the outcome of an antigenic exposure results in tolerance or an immune response. The reason for this is that the adaptive immune system plays the complex role of responding to foreign antigens that are recognized in the context of self antigens, and as such, the adaptive immune system must include mechanisms to prevent autoimmune destruction. Whereas formerly much research concentrated on the fundamental and intrinsic mechanisms by which T cells undergo positive and negative selection in the thymus to differentiate between self and non-self through interaction with MHC molecules, studies of immune responses to infectious pathogens suggest that the expression of co-stimulatory molecules and mediators such as cytokines may be more important in determining subsequent T- and B-cell responses in the periphery than are intrinsic factors such as MHC avidity. Furthermore, studies of the role of infectious agents in autoimmunity, such as *Campylobacter jejuni* in Guillain-Barré syndrome and reactive arthritis, may provide further insights into the factors that suppress autoimmunity.

GASTROINTESTINAL MUCOSAL T CELLS

T cells in the gastrointestinal tract are thought to play a central role in host defense and the regulation of gastrointestinal function (Fig. 14.2). Cells in organized lymphoid

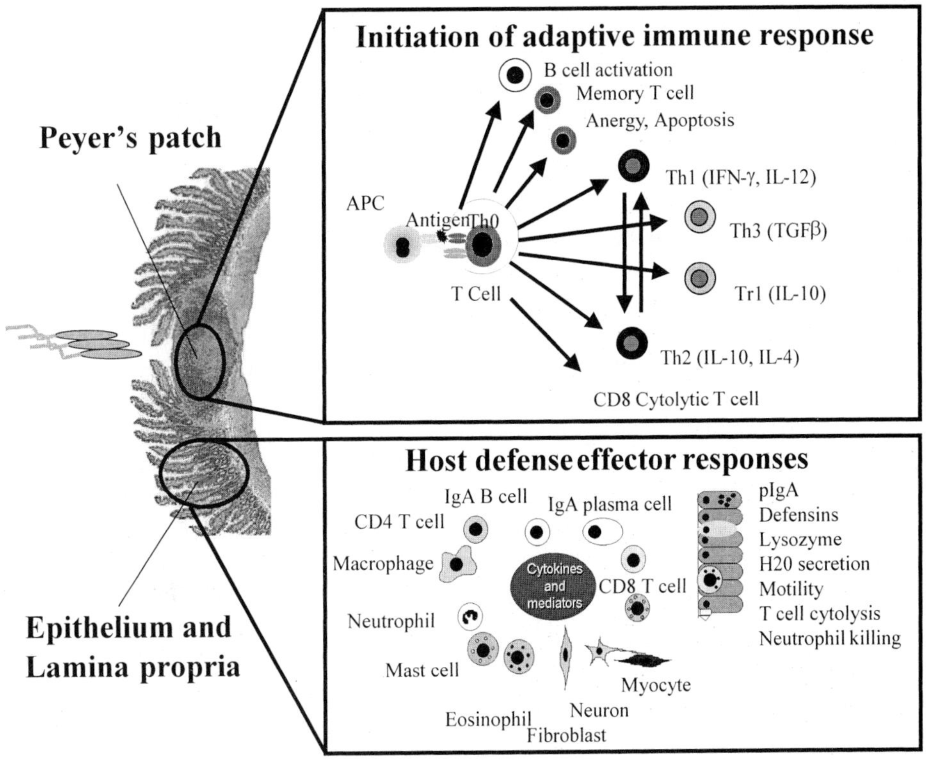

FIGURE 14.2. The Peyer's patch is an organized site specialized to initiate immune responses, whereas the diffuse epithelial and lamina propria compartments of the gut are adapted to host defense effector responses. Specialized cells in the Peyer's patch present antigens to T cells, which may differentiate along multiple pathways. B cells may be activated by T cell-dependent or T cell-independent mechanisms and differentiate into antibody-secreting plasma cells. These activated cells recirculate to the lamina propria and epithelium, where they carry out effector functions; these consist of cytokine production, helper T-cell function, and cytolytic T-cell function. The epithelium and lamina propria are rich in mast cells, eosinophils, and macrophages, and under conditions of activation, neutrophil transmigration occurs.

sites, such as the Peyer's patches, mesenteric lymph nodes, and appendix, are thought to carry out specialized tasks necessary for initiating responses to antigens in the intestinal lumen. After activation, the cells leave these sites and enter the systemic circulation, from which they reach the diffuse lamina propria compartment of the mucosa. In the epithelial compartment, which contains intraepithelial lymphocytes (IELs), are a mixture of cells, some of which may originate in the epithelium. The intestinal lamina propria and epithelium comprise the largest single site of T cells in humans. A number of important species differences are found between humans and mice; the Peyer's patches are much less prominent in humans than in rodents. In addition, the lamina propria of the colon in humans normally contains large numbers of lymphocytes, whereas in rodents it contains few lymphocytes. Substantial evidence indicates that the T lymphocytes associated with the gastrointestinal tract have unique characteristics reflecting their specialized roles in host defense in the mucosa. Some of these functional characteristics also vary between mice and humans.

LAMINA PROPRIA T LYMPHOCYTES

Many of the characteristics of mucosal lymphocytes are probably the result of prior activation in response to antigens and mitogens in the gastrointestinal lumen. Lymphocytes in the intestinal mucosa first interact with antigens in the organized lymphoid tissues (Peyer's patches and lymphoid follicles in the colon) and further differentiate and mature in the germinal centers of the lymphoid follicles. Thereafter, they rapidly leave the mucosa and migrate through the mesenteric lymph nodes and thoracic duct to reach the systemic circulation. From the blood, these antigen-activated lymphocytes migrate back to the mucosa by means of cell surface "homing" determinants, such as L-selectin and α4,β7 (see Chapter 10), and they extravasate preferentially into the lamina propria and intraepithelial compartment above the basement membrane. Thus, it is likely that many of the lymphocytes that enter the diffuse compartments of the gastrointestinal tract have previously been activated by antigen and are likely to be memory cells.

Memory T cells are by definition cells that have already been in contact with antigens; they adapt to their new tasks by the expression of various surface antigens that are absent or expressed to a lower degree on naïve cells, by an altered pattern of lymphokine secretion, by different functional capacities, and by changes in their proliferative responses to different stimuli (20). Previously, it has been shown that the *in vitro* activation of CD45RA+, CD29− peripheral blood T lymphocytes by antigen leads to a transition to CD45RA−, CD29+ T cells (21,22). This finding and functional studies have led to the conclusion that naïve (or virgin) T cells can be distinguished from memory T cells by their expression of different antigen specificities of the CD45 cell surface glycoprotein complex or CD29, the β1 chain of the integrin family (20). The transition from naïve to memory T-cell function is accompanied by a shift from the 205/220-kd determinant to the 180-kd form of the CD45 cell surface glycoprotein complex. These different molecules represent cell type-specific alternative splicing from a common precursor gene (21,23). Other markers have been described that are coexpressed with CD45 or CD29 after the transition from naïve to memory T cells (20). Naïve T cells can be characterized as follows: CD45RA-high, LFA-3-low, CD2-low, LFA-1-low, CD45RO-low, and CD29-low; memory T cells represent the reciprocal subset. CD4+ and CD8+ T cells are present in the lamina propria in a similar proportion as in the peripheral blood (24–26). However, only a small proportion of lamina propria lymphocytes express CD45RA, and the majority of cells are CD45RO+ (25). In contrast, in peripheral blood, approximately 30% of T cells are CD45RA+, and 30% to 50% are CD45RO+. Thus, the CD45 phenotype of lamina propria lymphocytes resembles that of memory T cells.

In addition to an increased expression of the CD45RO glycoprotein, it has been shown that circulating memory lymphocytes show an increased expression of a number of molecules that have been implicated in cell adhesion and cell interactions, including CD2, LFA-1, LFA-3, CD29, and CD44 (20). As indicated above, both CD29 (β chain of VLA-4) and CD44 (27) may play a role in the localization of lymphoid cells to the mucosal endothelium, and therefore CD29 and CD44 may be important in intestinal homing. VLA-4 (α4,β1) and CD44 are found on more than 80% of both lamina propria lymphocytes and IELs (28).

More than 95% of normal intestinal lamina propria T cells express the α,β T-cell receptor (TCR) heterodimer (29). Whereas γ,δ T cells are found in the human epithelium (IELs), as in the mouse, in humans only about 10% of small-bowel IELs (range, 5% to 20%) express this receptor. In the colon, a much higher proportion of IELs express γ,δ receptors (30,31). Thus, in humans, the majority of T cells in the mucosa express the α,β TCRs that predominate in the periphery. A number of studies have addressed the diversity of the T-cell repertoire in human mucosa with the use of polymerase chain reaction techniques. It has been shown that only a few Vβ families predominate in human IELs (32–34). Furthermore, sequences of V-D-J-C showed evidence of the oligoclonality of T-cell clones from human IELs. Although results for lamina propria T lymphocytes also showed skewing toward particular families, the level of heterogeneity was intermediate between that in peripheral blood and that in IELs, and the diversity of the human lamina propria TCR repertoire may approach that of the peripheral blood. Interestingly, with microdissection techniques, it has been shown that small areas of colon mucosa may contain clonally related T cells that are not found at distant sites (35). These interesting results suggest that certain factors in the intestinal epithelium, such as bacterial antigens, exogenous antigens, or superantigens, perhaps in combination with unique MHC determinants expressed in the epithelium, drive the selective expansion of specific families of T cells

T-cell activation is followed by early expression of the IL-2 receptor on the cell surface, and the interaction of the IL-2 receptor with IL-2 is a critical event in T-cell proliferation, differentiation, and function (36). Intestinal T cells are in close proximity to a large number of antigens and substances with mitogenic properties. Therefore, the question arises of whether the state of activation of lamina propria T cells differs from that of T cells in other sites of the immune system. With the use of Northern blot analysis in nonhuman primates to study the transcription of the gene for the IL-2 receptor α chain (CD25), it has been shown that messenger RNA (mRNA) for the IL-2 receptor α chain is clearly detectable in freshly isolated lymphocytes from the intestinal lamina propria, whereas in other populations, from the spleen, mesenteric lymph nodes, or peripheral blood, IL-2 receptor mRNA is found only after activation *in vitro* (37). The increased expression of CD25 on mucosal T cells may represent the presence of a specialized class of T regulatory cells with suppressor cell function (see below). Interestingly, although lamina propria lymphocytes display activation markers, in the normal lamina propria, dividing T lymphocytes are very infrequent (38), based on the virtual absence of Ki67+ lymphocytes. This suggests that lamina propria lymphocytes may be in a different state of activation or differentiation than are activated peripheral blood lymphocytes, which normally progress through the cell cycle following activation. This difference may be related to the special activation requirements of mucosal lymphocytes, described below.

Many of the functions carried out by T cells in the gastrointestinal immune system are thought to be mediated at least in part by their secreted lymphokines. Therefore, a detailed understanding of the lymphokines produced by mucosal T cells is necessary to understand their function. Furthermore, alterations in the patterns of cytokines produced by mucosal cells may be important in the pathogenesis of intestinal diseases. It should be noted at the outset that significant species differences exist in the expression of lymphokines in the gut, with murine cells displaying predominantly a Th2 phenotype and human cells displaying predominantly a Th1 phenotype. When conventional Northern blots were used, no specific hybridization with different lymphokine probes was detected in unactivated human lymphocytes obtained from any site. When lymphocytes from different sites were activated with a combination of ionomycin and PMA, both mesenteric lymph node and lamina propria T cells were found to express high levels of mRNA for IL-4 and IL-5 in comparison with cells from peripheral blood, spleen, and peripheral lymph nodes. Lamina propria lymphocytes also had the highest levels of IL-2 mRNA; mesenteric lymph node levels of IL-2 mRNA were lower. In contrast, levels of IFN-γ mRNA were low in mesenteric lymph nodes in comparison with those in all other sites. Thus, intestinal lamina propria lymphocytes have a large capacity to express IL-2, IFN-γ, IL-4, and IL-5 mRNA, whereas mesenteric lymph node cells have a much smaller capacity to express IL-2 and IFN-γ but a large capacity to express IL-4 and IL-5 mRNA after activation. The greater potential for expression of IL-2 was confirmed at the level of secreted proteins in studies of isolated primate lamina propria lymphocytes, in which it was shown that activated intestinal T cells have a high level of IL-2 bioactivity (37). These studies indicate that mucosal T cells may be substantially different from T cells in other sites in regard to their potential for modulating immune responses; further evidence that this is the case is presented below. T cells from the human intestinal lamina propria were shown to be large producers of IL-10 in comparison with peripheral blood T cells when the TCR was engaged and cells were co-stimulated through CD2 (39). Resting lamina propria T lymphocytes had no detectable IL-10 production. IL-7, which may be produced by the gastrointestinal epithelium, supports the proliferation of lamina propria in the absence of other activation, but not the proliferation of peripheral blood lymphocytes (40). In addition, the proliferation induced by IL-7 appears to depend on IL-2, which supports the critical role of IL-2 in lamina propria T-cell function.

Considerable evidence indicates that TCR-triggered activation of lamina propria lymphocytes differs from that of circulating T cells, and that co-stimulation through other pathways may be required for optimal activation. Anti-CD3-mediated activation of lamina propria lymphocytes is markedly lower than that of peripheral blood lymphocytes, but activation through the CD2 alternative pathway is normal in lamina propria lymphocytes (41). Other studies have indicated that optimal activation of lamina propria lymphocytes requires activation through the CD28 or a combination of the CD2 and CD28 pathways (28,42). Others have suggested that co-stimulatory molecules may be specifically expressed on gastrointestinal epithelial cells (43), which lamina propria lymphocytes can contact directly through endothelial cell fenestrations. The observation that lamina propria lymphocytes have special co-stimulatory requirements may explain why lamina propria lymphocytes are often unresponsive to specific antigens; this characteristic may be a protective adaptation of the gut in regard to harmless luminal antigens. A number of explanations have been proposed for why lamina propria cells are hyporesponsive. One is that the antigen-presenting cells of the lamina propria may not express the appropriate co-stimulatory molecules. Thus, lamina propria monocytes, in contrast to peripheral blood monocytes, exhibit a low level of expression of the ligands CD54, CD58, and CD80 for the corresponding counter-receptors on T cells CD11/18, CD2, and CD28 (44). Lamina propria T lymphocytes have been shown to have higher basal Ca^{2+} levels in comparison with peripheral blood lymphocytes (45), again consistent with the observations described above indicating a special state of partial activation of these cells. Impaired activation by CD3 can be reversed by 24 hours of culture of lamina propria lymphocytes in calcium-containing medium, which indicates that the state of hyporesponsiveness may be transient and reversible following removal of tissue-specific factors, which may include TGF-β.

Many of the functional studies described above have relied on the use of polyclonal activation of lymphoid cells to study their function. In a model of *Chlamydia trachomatis* rectal infection in nonhuman primates (46,47), as expected, T cells from peripheral blood, spleen, mesenteric lymph nodes, and particularly draining lymph nodes showed a significant proliferative response when exposed to *C. trachomatis* antigens. However, T cells isolated from either the involved rectum or distant sites in the lamina propria did not exhibit a proliferative response when challenged with chlamydial antigens, although they did proliferate in response to mitogens such as concanavalin A. This failure of lamina propria T cells to exhibit antigen-specific proliferative responses in lymphogranuloma venereum is not caused by the absence of functional antigen-presenting cells or the presence of suppressor cells. Furthermore, this finding may be a more general aspect of T-cell function in the lamina propria, as similar results were obtained in studies of animals rectally immunized with bacille Calmette-Guérin. An interesting aspect of these studies is that although T cells from the lamina propria did not proliferate in response to antigens, antigen-specific T cells are present in this site. Thus, antigen-specific T cells are present in the intestinal lamina propria, but at least in certain circumstances they have lost the capacity for proliferation. Consistent with the above observations, T cells from the intestinal lamina propria proliferate poorly *in vitro* in response to specific microbial and recall antigens (48).

Murine models of intestinal lamina propria T-cell function have taken advantage of transgenic TCR models to evaluate the function of mucosal cells. In the DO11.10 TCR transgenic mouse, in which antigen-specific responses to a protein analogue of a food antigen could be evaluated, lamina propria T cells did demonstrate the ability to proliferate in response to their nominal antigen and expressed IL-2, IL-4, and IFN-γ (49). The capacity for lamina propria cells to proliferate was confirmed *in vivo* with the systemic administration of antigen; it was observed that relatively low doses of antigen could trigger the uptake of BrdU, consistent with the thesis that lamina propria cells have a memory phenotype.

INTRAEPITHELIAL LYMPHOCYTES

Intestinal IELs are a specialized and heterogeneous population of lymphocytes in the gastrointestinal epithelium and the epithelium of other mucosal surfaces; they are thought to carry out specialized functions in immune regulation and host defense. Because of their location at mucosal surfaces, it is thought that they play an important role in interactions with the microbial environment of the gut. These cells are defined by their location within the epithelial cell layer of the mucosa, on the luminal side the lamina propria basement membrane and in intimate contact with intestinal epithelial cells. The population of IELs is large; one is found among every 8 to 12 epithelial cells in histologic sections of the gut, and they have long been recognized by a characteristic histologic appearance of abundant cytoplasm and cytoplasmic granules.

Important differences in these populations of cells have been noted between species, and the most information is available for murine IELs. IELs comprise two main subpopulations. One is either CD4 or CD8α/β and TCRα/β and has a T-cell repertoire consistent with selection by a thymic pathway. These cells are absent in athymic mice (50). A second population of lymphocytes expresses CD8α/α molecules and either TCRγ/δ or TCRα/β and is present in athymic animals. In addition, the cells express markers of both T cells and natural killer (NK) cells and represent a gut-specific population of NK T cells (51). Further evidence of the divergence of the two subpopulations of IELs is that although both have oligoclonal TCRs, the clonality of the two is markedly different (52). Based on clonal analysis, it has been shown that both the CD4 and CD8α/β IELs likely have a similar origin as conventional lamina propria T cells (53). Further, it is likely that these more conventional T cells arise via antigenic stimulation in Peyer's patches or other organized sites in the gut and recirculate to populate the gut via homing mechanisms. Although the oligoclonality of IELs has not been completely explained, it is probably related to exposure to common antigens in flora of the gut. In comparison with normal mice, mice raised in a germ-free environment have markedly fewer IELs. CD8α/α IELs, on the other hand, are thought potentially to originate in ontogeny in the gut and mature without influence of the thymus or a recirculating pathway.

All intestinal IELs express the αEβ7 integrin that binds E-cadherin and mediates adherence to epithelial cells (54). This potential interaction with epithelial cells may serve to anchor IELs within the epithelium and facilitate intimate interactions. It is less clear whether this interaction serves as a homing function, but intestinal epithelial cells also express chemokines for IELs, such as IP-10 and MIG (55). IELs are capable of producing Th1 cytokines IL-2 and IFN-γ (56). In addition, IELs have been shown to express IL-3, IL-5, IL-6, and TGF-β, but not IL-4, which suggests a potential immunoregulatory role for these cells. Interestingly, it has been suggested that IELs play a negative, down-regulatory immunomodulatory role based on the observation that susceptibility to inflammatory bowel diseases is increased in mice with γ,δ T-cell abnormalities (57). The development of IELs appears to depend on IL-7 and IL-15, which are abundantly expressed in the gut by epithelial cells (58). This latter property of IELs may link their development to the innate immune response properties of intestinal epithelial cells. Invasion of intestinal epithelial cells by pathogens such as *Listeria monocytogenes* activates the NF-κβ cascade, which coordinates up-regulation of IL-15 mRNA expression by epithelial cells (59).

Consistent with their potential role as a first line of defense against pathogens in the gut, IELs express perforin and granzymes and exhibit a variety of cytotoxic activities, including alloreactive and virus-specific cytotoxic lymphocyte activity, NK activity, and spontaneous cytotoxicity (60). Despite their observed functions *in vitro,* the antigenic targets of the markedly clonal IEL populations remain unclear at the present time. One current thesis is that a role of IELs is actually to recognize and kill infected epithelial cell neighbors in the gut, as demonstrated in an LCM virus infection model (61). It has also been suggested that IELs do not recognize their cytotoxic targets with conventional MHC, but rather with unconventional MHC-related molecules, such as MICA and MICB, which are up-regulated on intestinal epithelial cells by heat shock and can activate IELs (62).

IMMUNOREGULATORY FUNCTION OF MUCOSAL LYMPHOCYTES IN HOST DEFENSE AND ORAL IMMUNITY

As noted above, one of the principal challenges to the innate and adaptive immune systems in the complex microbial and antigen environment of the gut is to distinguish between harmless normal flora and antigens in food and pathogens (Fig. 14.3). This is in large part accomplished by the physical barrier function of the epithelium, as noted above. Normal flora and their products that gain access to the subepithelium presumably are recognized as pathogenic by the innate immune system, so that a continuous level of immune activity is maintained in the lamina propria that is recognized histologically as "physiologic" inflammation. However, evidence indicates that the barrier function of the epithelium is not the sole mechanism that protects against the potential for runaway immune responses and inflam-

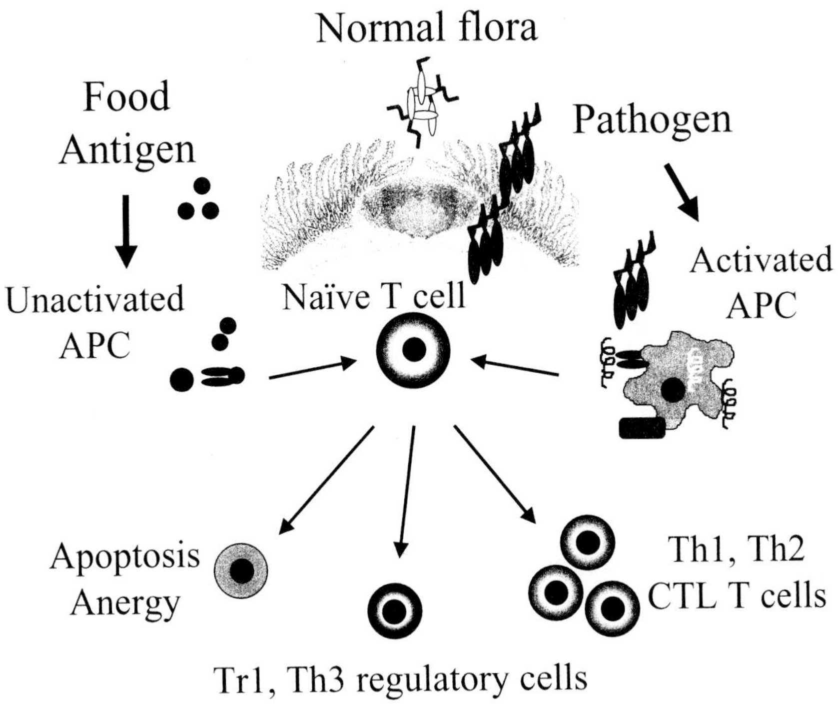

FIGURE 14.3. Differences in T-cell responses of the mucosal host defense system in response to food antigens, normal enteric flora, and pathogens. Harmless products of digestion do not activate antigen-presenting cells (APCs), and their interaction with naïve T cells results in apoptosis, anergy, or activation of suppressor T cells (Tr1, Th3 regulatory T cells). The normal flora appears to activate all mechanisms to a limited extent; such activation is seen as "physiologic inflammation," normally found in the gastrointestinal mucosa. Pathogens activate innate host defense mechanisms and APCs, eliciting a greater preponderance of Th1, Th2, or cytolytic T-cell responses.

mation triggered by the normal components of the gut lumen. One of the important functions of mucosal T cells is regulation, in particular negative regulation or suppression of these responses. The history of research on suppressor T cells is long; from being in the mainstream, such research was relegated to a position of ignominy in immunology after the advent of molecular techniques and the study of cytokines and receptors. However, research on suppressor T cells is again prominent, largely because of the need to understand the control of immune responses in the gut. It appears that recent research on regulatory T cells in the gut may provide not only insight into host defense and oral tolerance in the gut but also fundamental insight into the pathogenesis of autoimmune disease.

One of the areas of research that has led to an understanding of regulatory T cells in the gut has been the study of responses of DO11.10 TCR transgenic mice with large numbers of T cells recognizing antigenic determinants of ovalbumin. Mucosal CD4+ T cells from these animals, even in the absence of ovalbumin feeding, have an activated phenotype, and when challenged with antigen, they frequently have a phenotype of increased IL-10 and IFN-γ expression. It has also been shown that the mucosal lymphocytes of these animals are activated by a second, endogenous TCR that presumably recognizes antigens in the intestinal flora; this finding suggests that microbial antigen recognition by gut T cells is a common occurrence (63). Despite the frequent recognition of microbial antigens by mucosal T cells, it appears that proliferative responses to self bacterial antigens are small (64). The mechanisms that hold T-cell responses in check in the intestinal environment are beginning to unfold through several lines of evidence. Studies of mutant mice of various types, reviewed elsewhere in this book, suggest that immunologic defects interfering with the normal down-regulation of mucosal immune responses can result in unrestrained intestinal inflammation in response to intestinal microbial flora, recognizable as a phenotype of "inflammatory bowel disease." Studies of the CD45Rbhi transfer model of inflammatory bowel disease, in particular, have revealed the presence of a subset of T cells, functionally defined as regulatory T cells (Tr1 cells); these have the ability to produce IL-10, but not the prototypic Th2 cytokine IL-4, and they are capable of suppressing T-cell activation and proliferation and suppressing Th1 cytokine production (65). Another functionally defined subset of T cells has been identified in models with the use of oral antigen feeding. This subset of cells, Th3 cells, is characterized by the production of high levels of TGF-β and of lower levels of IL-10 and IL-4, so that their phenotype differs from that of Tr1 cells (66). Similar cells are thought to be present in humans (67). These cells are of great interest, not only because they are providing new insights into the control of normal immune responses in the gut, but also because they may increase our understanding of pathogenesis and make possible novel therapeutic approaches to autoimmune diseases.

MAST CELLS

Mast cells are widely distributed throughout the body and are abundant in mucosal surfaces, including those of the gastrointestinal tract, where they play an important role in host defense and mucosal inflammation. All differentiated mast cells bear high-affinity receptors for IgE (FcεRI), and when triggered, they release a variety of mediators, including histamine, proteinases, proteoglycans, arachidonic acid metabolites, and cytokines; these vary according to tissue site. Murine mucosal mast cells are histochemically different from murine mast cells in connective tissues, so that a simple classification is possible, described below. Mast cells in humans do not display these histochemical differences. Both human and rodent mast cells originate from pluripotent hematopoietic stem cells in bone marrow, where they undergo lineage commitment; they then enter the circulation and reside in an immature state in tissues, where they complete their differentiation (68,69). Human peripheral blood mast cell progenitors have the surface phenotype c-*kit*+, CD34+, CD13+, FcεRI–. In adult mice, the gastrointestinal tract contains the largest pool of committed mast cell progenitors. Based on differences in histochemical staining, mast cells in the gastrointestinal mucosa are known as *intestinal mucosal mast cells* (IMMCs), and those in the connective tissue, such as the skin, are called *connective tissue-type mast cells* (CTMCs). The final maturation of mast cells into tissue-specific mast cells is thought to depend on multiple factors expressed in the local microenvironment. All mast cell precursors and mast cells express c-*kit* (CD117), the ligand for stem cell factor, which is necessary for the proliferation and differentiation of mast cells. W/Wv mice and Ws/Ws rats have mutations in c-*kit* and are deficient in both CTMCs and IMMCs, and studies of these animals have provided a great deal of information about mast cell development and function. Multiple cofactors are necessary for mast cell development, including IL-3, IL-4, and IL-10 (70). Many differences have been identified between IMMCs and CTMCs, including lower levels of heparin glycosaminoglycans, higher levels of chondroitin sulfate glycosaminoglycans, low levels of histamine, high levels of activation-induced cysteinyl leukotrienes, and low levels of prostaglandin D_2 in IMMCs versus CTMCs. In addition to these factors, secretory granules of mast cells contain multiple proteases. Mice deficient in murine mast cell protease 1 lack the ability to expel *Trichinella spiralis,* which indicates a role for mast cell proteases in host defense (71). Mast cells also secrete a wide variety of cytokines and chemokines (72). Conversely, mast cell function can be regulated by secreted cytokines. Secreted cytokines are thought to play an important role in the overall proinflammatory response in the mucosa.

It is thought that differences in tissue-specific factors, including the cytokine products of T cells, account for the phenotypic differences in mast cells. This conclusion is based on multiple lines of evidence; for example, Ws/Ws rats infected with *Nippostrongylus brasiliensis* have IMMCs but not CTMCs, which suggests an important additional role of mucosal T cells in mucosal mast cell differentiation (73). In addition, disruption of cytokine genes in mice is associated with delayed clearance of intestinal parasite infections (74,75).

Mucosal mast cells are closely related to enteric nerves, and mast cell-derived proteinases can degrade numerous neuropeptides, such as vasoactive intestinal peptide and substance P. Neuropeptides such as substance P can stimulate histamine secretion by mast cells and the production of tumor necrosis factor-α (TNF-α). Mast cells may play a important role in diseases in which neurotransmitter function is critical, such as mucosal disease induced by *Clostridium difficile* toxin. Injury in models of this toxic injury is inhibited by agents that stabilize mast cell degranulation. (76). On the other hand, mast cell activity may be necessary for normal mucosal integrity, as the incidence of spontaneous gastric ulcers in W/Wv mice is increased.

EOSINOPHILS

Eosinophils are specialized proinflammatory leukocytes that play a role in innate regulatory and inflammatory immune responses. Interestingly, they are found in large numbers in the normal host, particularly in the gastrointestinal tract (77). Their presence there has been attributed to the chemokine eotaxin, which is widely expressed in the gut. A distinctive feature of eosinophils that allows them to be identified readily is the presence of granules that stain avidly with a variety of dyes. During Th2 antigenic or microbial challenges, the number of eosinophils in the gut increases markedly; this has been attributed to an increase in chemokine production and the effects of IL-5. Eosinophil granule components such as major basic protein and eosinophil cationic protein are cytotoxic not only in microbes but also in intestinal epithelium, which may account in part for pathologic injury characterized by an increased influx of eosinophils in the gut. Eosinophils also release an array of other mediators, such as neuromediators and leukotrienes. Eosinophil degranulation can be triggered by the FcγR and by IgA via the FcαR. Eosinophils interact with mucosal mast cells by means of secreted products such as major basic protein and eosinophil cationic protein, which can stimulate histamine secretion by mast cells. The interaction of T cells and eosinophils is likely bidirectional because multiple cytokines and chemokines are secreted by both cell types.

EPITHELIAL CELLS IN MUCOSAL IMMUNE RESPONSES

The primary defense of the host from the microbial flora of the gastrointestinal tract is the one-cell layer of intestinal epithelial cells, which on the one hand form a highly effective barrier to microbial entry but on the other provide a highly efficient site for the uptake of nutrients.

Intestinal epithelial cells maintain a barrier by forming intercellular tight junctions that prevent paracellular migration of macromolecules larger than 2 kd and bacteria. In the normal gastrointestinal environment, it is thought that intestinal epithelial cells play an important modulatory role in mucosal immune defense by communicating with underlying IELs and lamina propria lymphocytes. Various microbial pathogens have developed mechanisms with which to evade this host defense system: attaching intimately to intestinal epithelial cells, directly invading intestinal epithelial cells, disrupting tight junctions, entering the host through the specialized M cells, and entering through dendritic processes that extend through tight junctions into the gastrointestinal lumen. The immune response to microbial pathogens may also modify the barrier function of intestinal epithelial cells in that cytokines such as IL-4 and TNF-α may disrupt tight junctions. Adherence to or invasion of epithelial cells by pathogens may trigger a potent innate response, such as release of cytokines and chemokines, that activates the inflammatory and immune cascade.

The potential role of intestinal epithelial cells as antigen-presenting cells is a subject of considerable interest (78). Epithelial cells are also capable of antigen uptake by fluid phase pinocytosis and processing. They express MHC class I and class II molecules and nonclassic MHC 1b molecules. Whereas the classic pathways may be involved in the presentation of microbial antigens, the nonpolymorphic Cd1 family of molecules may be important in the presentation of carbohydrate or glycolipid antigens. Other receptors that may be involved in the transport of microbial antigens include the polymeric immunoglobulin receptor, which is capable of transporting antigens bound to IgA. Microbial factors may also act on epithelial cells through non–receptor-mediated mechanisms. The most important example of this phenomenon is the potent mucosal adjuvant effect of cholera toxin, which binds to GM1 ganglioside on the surface of epithelial cells. Finally, one of the intriguing aspects of intestinal epithelial cells as potential antigen-presenting cells is the near absence of critical co-stimulatory molecules such as CD80 and CD40. This important fact has suggested that one of the normal outcomes of antigen presentation by intestinal epithelial cells is anergy, and this rationale has been used to explain why antigen feeding is often a pathway to tolerance. On the other hand, intestinal epithelial cells may express CD58 (LFA-3) under pathologic conditions, and this molecule has been shown to act as a co-stimulator of mucosal T cells via interactions with CD2 expressed on the lymphocyte.

The likely targets in any antigen-presenting role of intestinal epithelial cells are likely to be IELs, with which they are in intimate contact, and lamina propria lymphocytes, with which they may have contact through fenestrations normally present in the lamina propria basement membrane. Intestinal epithelial cells have been shown to be capable of activating CD4+ T cells *in vitro*; however, the outcome of the potential interactions of intestinal epithelial cells with resident mucosal T cells *in vivo* is a difficult question to address experimentally and remains largely a matter of speculation

One of the characteristic features of many gastrointestinal mucosal infections and inflammatory diseases, such as inflammatory bowel disease, is the transepithelial migration of neutrophils, which presumably are recruited by the epithelial release of chemokines. In the mucosa and lumen, neutrophils are thought to contribute to host defense through phagocytosis and killing mechanisms, as they do elsewhere. Interestingly, although much of the cytokine secretion by intestinal epithelial cells is basolateral, directed at cytokine-responsive elements in the mucosa, intestinal epithelial cells secrete IL-6 apically into the lumen, where it may play a role in Ca^{2+}-mediated signaling to neutrophils (79).

An interesting and important observation about the gastrointestinal mucosa is that the germ-free animal, although on a diet rich in potentially antigenic materials, has a relatively underdeveloped mucosal immune system, with very few lymphocytes and myeloid or lymphoid cells and underdeveloped Peyer's patches. On introduction of a normal microbial flora, the gastrointestinal tract assumes its typical appearance, characterized by substantial numbers of immune and inflammatory cells, so-called physiologic inflammation. It is thought that this response largely represents the innate response of the intestinal epithelium to microbial flora and their products, with the release of chemokines. During infectious processes in the gastrointestinal tract, chemokine-initiated immune and inflammatory responses are thought to be greatly accentuated. Following the early demonstration of IL-8 production by intestinal epithelial cells, numerous cytokines produced by intestinal epithelial cells, including both type I chemokines, such as ENA-78 and gro-α, and type II chemokines, such as MIP-1α, MCP-1, and RANTES. In addition, other cytokines, such as IL-1, IL-6, IL-15, IL-17, and MDC, as Th2 T-cell chemokines, are expressed by intestinal epithelial cells. This complex mix of mediators is thought to play an important role in mobilizing the typical immune and inflammatory cell influx into the mucosa, both in normal physiologic interactions with the normal flora and in pathogenic infections of the gastrointestinal mucosa. Some of the cytokines produced by the epithelium are thought to have counter-regulatory roles; for example, IL-15 produced by the epithelium may inhibit the production of chemokines (80). Conversely, it is thought that cytokines produced by immune and nonimmune cells of the mucosa have important regulatory functions in the epithelium, including cell growth and differentiation, modulation of the tight junction barrier, and restitution and repair of the epithelium (81), and on the immune functions of epithelial cells.

MODIFICATION OF MUCOSAL HOST DEFENSE BY ENTERIC FLORA

As outlined above, the gastrointestinal mucosal immune system develops in large measure because of the presence of a resident microbial flora, which stimulates both innate and adaptive immune mechanisms that lead to "physiologic" inflammation. Innate mechanisms—in which TLRs are used, for example—may account in part for the development of the mucosal immune system. In addition, as noted above, evidence indicates that T cells develop in part because of reactivity to flora in the gastrointestinal tract, although the specific antigenic determinants recognized are largely unknown. At the present time, the detailed mechanisms of how the resident flora of the gastrointestinal tract interact symbiotically with the host is not well defined. One approach to the study of this phenomenon has been to colonize germ-free animals with defined flora. In this way, it has been shown that the interaction of commensal *Bacteroides* species with the host epithelium results in the mutual regulation of genes involved in the production of a substrate necessary for the flora, L-fucose (82). The physiologic significance of colonization of the gut with a normal flora is illustrated by studies in which the colonization of germ-free mice with *Escherichia coli* dramatically increased their survival after subsequent infection with the pathogen *Salmonella typhimurium* (83). Because of the very large number of potential pathways for the interaction of microbial flora and host, until recently it has been very difficult to address experimentally the mechanisms involved in microbe–host interaction in the gut on a comprehensive scale. However, the advent of gene chip technology has made possible initial attempts to characterize these interactions. In one study, in which germ-free mice were colonized with a nonpathogenic *Bacteroides* strain derived from commensal flora, a combination of laser capture microdissection of the gut microenvironment, gene array expression analysis, and real-time polymerase chain reaction for validation allowed an initial characterization of the induction of gene expression in the host intestine at the mRNA level (84). The bacterial colonization of young mice resulted in the expression of genes involved in several important gastrointestinal functions, including nutrient absorption, mucosal barrier fortification, xenobiotic metabolism, angiogenesis, and postnatal intestinal maturation. This report provides an initial glimpse of what happens early during colonization, and the approach would allow for an analysis of how microbes modify the host during a longer period of time. Similar approaches can be used to identify host alterations that occur as a result of the interaction of pathogens with the gastrointestinal tract. The interpretation of this type of data will require an understanding of the baseline interactions of the host with the normal resident flora.

The enteric flora may interact with host defense mechanisms via several other pathways. It is known that bacteria grown at high densities, as may occur in the gastrointestinal environment, secrete metabolic factors, quorum-sensing factors, that are not just waste products of metabolism but have the potential to regulate cassettes of genes that control important bacterial functions (85). The regulatory signals that have been identified to date are small, diffusible molecules, and multiple additional signaling molecules are clearly likely to be discovered. Although the effects of these signaling molecules on bacterial physiology have been studied extensively, relatively little attention has been given to the potential effects of quorum-sensing molecules on the eukaryotic host cells in the gastrointestinal environment. *Pseudomonas aeruginosa,* an important respiratory pathogen, has been shown to secrete a quorum factor, *N*-(3-oxododecanoyl)-L-homoserine lactone (OdDHL), which is capable of inducing IL-8 secretion by respiratory epithelial cells (86). In a more extensive study in which various immune assays were performed *in vitro* in both murine and human cells, OdDHL had multiple effects on immune function; OdDHL inhibited lymphocyte proliferation and TNF-α production by LPS-stimulated macrophages and down-regulated the production of IL-12, a Th-1-supportive cytokine. At high concentrations, it inhibited antibody production by keyhole limpet hemocyanin-stimulated spleen cells, but at lower concentrations it stimulated antibody production; it also promoted IgE production by IL-4-stimulated human peripheral blood mononuclear cells (87). These experimental findings obtained *in vitro* demonstrate that OdDHL may potentially influence the Th1–Th2 balance during infection by *P. aeruginosa.* Furthermore, the more general implications of these observations are that other quorum-sensing factors may have important effects on the function of cells of the mucosal immune system *in vivo,* but this possibility remains unexplored at the present time.

Another potential mechanism by which the resident flora may modulate the immune system of the gastrointestinal tract is direct modulation of the innate immune response of epithelial cells. In studies of the interaction of nonpathogenic *Salmonella* strains with epithelial cell monolayers, the interaction resulted in down-modulation of NF-κβ activation, which is one of the central pathways of innate responses. Furthermore, this down-regulation was shown to be targeted to a unique mechanism involving stabilization of the inhibitor of NF-κβ translocation, IKB, by preventing ubquitination and degradation of the inhibitor (88). This novel observation may illustrate one mechanism by which the apparently nonpathogenic flora of the gastrointestinal tract raises the threshold for the activation of innate responses.

The effects of the normal microbial flora on the mucosal barrier and host defense mechanisms of the gut are the basis of the potential clinical therapeutic uses of beneficial bacteria, so-called probiotics, administered in various situations in an effort to improve the health of the host. This approach has been beneficial in both animal models and in humans with inflammatory bowel disease; however, the mechanisms of action of the probiotic agents are largely unknown (89–91).

PARADIGMS OF MUCOSAL HOST DEFENSE RESPONSES IN GASTROINTESTINAL INFECTIONS

The most important insights that have been gained regarding gastrointestinal host defense mechanisms have probably come from studies of specific gastrointestinal pathogens; the various responses to specific pathogens have in fact served to define the considerable plasticity and wide diversity of host defense responses. The following brief description is only a summary of the types of responses observed, intended to illustrate their diversity. The details of many of the pathogenic features of these agents are discussed in considerable detail in the individual chapters devoted to each infectious agent.

One of the paradigms of gastrointestinal response is that elicited by enterotoxigenic bacteria and their toxins, the classic examples being enterotoxigenic *E. coli* and *Vibrio cholerae.* These pathogens are similar in that they express specific surface colonization factors that permit them to colonize the host, and produce very potent toxins, LT and cholera toxin, respectively, that cause disease, largely without invasion of the host. These toxins not only mediate profuse secretory diarrhea through direct effects on epithelial cells but also invoke an extraordinarily potent immune response, manifested by the production of circulating memory B cells and antibodies that provide effective protection from subsequent infection. Cholera elicits both a Th1 and in particular a potent Th2 immune response, particularly in the mouse (92). This latter feature of the toxins has led to extensive studies of their properties in an effort to develop adjuvants for oral vaccines (93).

An altogether different pattern of response is elicited by adherent bacteria, best exemplified by enteropathogenic *E. coli* (EPEC) and related species and by *Helicobacter pylori* in the stomach. The characteristic features of EPEC infection are an intimate interaction of the membranes of the bacteria with host epithelial cells and subsequent cytoskeletal rearrangements of the epithelial cells; many of the molecular mechanisms have been defined (94). Although relatively little is known about the mucosal immune response to this acute infection in humans, the closely related murine infection caused by *Citrobacter rodentium* elicits an intense Th1 immune and inflammatory response that presumably is triggered initially by the innate response of epithelial cells (95). In addition, EPEC organisms contain a novel gene, *lifA*; this is thought to encode a toxin, related to the large clostridial toxins, that inhibits lymphokine production by activated mononuclear cells *in vitro* (96). This latter property of EPEC may provide an additional mechanism of modulation of the host immune response. *H. pylori* infection of the stomach, unlike the other prototypic bacterial infections described here, is lifelong and associated with colonization of the host, more typical of normal flora. However, because the host response leads to the diseases associated with *H. pylori* infection [gastritis, peptic ulcer, adenocarcinoma, and MALT (mucosa-associated lymphoid tissue) lymphoma], the infection can hardly be considered commensal. The superficial interactions of *H. pylori* organisms with the epithelium, like those of EPEC organisms, elicit a potent Th1 immune response and antibody production. However, unlike EPEC infection, chronic *H. pylori* infection results in a symbiosis, in which the chronic immune response down-regulates colonization but does not eliminate infection; the reasons for this are not clear but probably include the tenacious adaptation of the microbes to the gastric microenvironment and the relative inefficiency of host defense mechanisms in eliminating luminal colonization. This aspect of *H. pylori* immunology presents a significant obstacle to the development of vaccines to prevent infection (97).

In *Salmonella* and *Shigella* infections, the molecular mechanisms of host invasion are distinctly different; these are classic paradigms of invasive bacterial infection of the gastrointestinal tract, and extensive information regarding the mechanisms of pathogenesis is available (98). Both types of infection elicit an exuberant immune response and in particular an inflammatory response characterized by a massive influx of neutrophils. The latter response is thought to be elicited by intense stimulation of innate chemotaxis in infected epithelial cells. Both infections also elicit substantial T- and B-cell antibody responses; these result in protective immunity, so that it is possible to develop protective vaccines.

The host defense response of the gastrointestinal tract to viral infections, exemplified by rotavirus infection, parallels the response to intracellular bacterial infections, and protective immune responses are elicited. Interestingly, the pathogenesis of rotavirus infection appears to involve an enterotoxin (99). However, for reasons not entirely clear, the host response in humans does not appear to result in durable immunity (100).

The final category of host response in the gastrointestinal tract is exemplified by responses to parasitic infections, which are distinctly different from those outlined above. The unique and important elements of the response to gastrointestinal parasitic infection that have emerged from an extensive body of literature are an integrated response of innate immunity, particularly involving mast cells, an integrated neuroimmune and secretory response, and a tendency for profound Th2 cytokine deviation of the response (101). Extensive studies of helminthic infections in murine models have shown convincingly that an immune response dominated by the production of IL-4, IL-5, IL-9, and IL-13 is associated with resistance to persistent infection, whereas interventions that promote Th1 responses, such as treatment with IL-12 or IL-18 or blockade of Th2 cytokines, is associated with persistent chronic infection (102). Interestingly, these properties of gastrointestinal parasitic infections have been shown to be able to modulate infection by a second agent in the gastrointestinal tract, such as *Helicobacter* in the stomach (103). This finding has profound implications for understanding the impact of the normal complex microflora of the gut in health and disease.

This very brief overview of the diversity of host responses to different types of gastrointestinal infections illustrates the considerable complexity of microbial host responses in the gut and emphasizes the need for further research to elucidate in detail the basis for the different types of response.

REFERENCES

1. Hoffmann JA, Kafatos FC, Janeway CA, et al. Phylogenetic perspectives in innate immunity. *Science* 1999;284(5418): 1313–1318.
2. Medzhitov R, Janeway CA Jr. Innate immune induction of the adaptive immune response. *Cold Spring Harb Symp Quant Biol* 1999;64:429–435.
3. Aderem A, Ulevitch RJ. Toll-like receptors in the induction of the innate immune response. *Nature* 2000;406:782–787.
4. Qureshi ST, Lariviere L, Leveque G, et al. Endotoxin-tolerant mice have mutations in Toll-like receptor 4 (Tlr4). *J Exp Med* 1999;189:615–625.
5. Hoshino K, Takeuchi O, Kawai T, et al. Cutting edge: toll-like receptor 4 (TLR4)-deficient mice are hyporesponsive to lipopolysaccharide: evidence for TLR4 as the *Lps* gene product. *J Immunol* 1999;162:3749–3752.
6. Takeuchi O, Hoshino K, Kawai T, et al. Differential roles of TLR2 and TLR4 in recognition of gram-negative and gram-positive bacterial cell wall components. *Immunity* 1999;11:443–451.
7. Gewirtz AT, Navas TA, Lyons S, et al. Cutting edge: bacterial flagellin activates basolaterally expressed tlr5 to induce epithelial proinflammatory gene expression. *J Immunol* 2001;167: 1882–1885.
8. Hayashi F, Smith KD, Ozinsky A, et al. The innate immune response to bacterial flagellin is mediated by Toll-like receptor 5. *Nature* 2001;410:1099–1103.
9. Chuang T, Ulevitch RJ. Identification of hTLR10: a novel human Toll-like receptor preferentially expressed in immune cells. *Biochim Biophys Acta* 2001;1518:157–161.
10. Hemmi H, Takeuchi O, Kawai T, et al. A Toll-like receptor recognizes bacterial DNA. *Nature* 2000;408:740–745.
11. Ogura Y, Bonen DK, Inohara N, et al. A frameshift mutation in *NOD2* associated with susceptibility to Crohn's disease. *Nature* 2001;411:603–606.
12. Hugot JP, Chamaillard M, Zouali H, et al. Association of *NOD2* leucine-rich repeat variants with susceptibility to Crohn's disease. *Nature* 2001;411:599–603.
13. Hampe J, Cuthbert A, Croucher PJP, et al. Association between insertion mutation in *NOD2* gene and Crohn's disease in German and British populations. *Lancet* 2001;357:1925–1928.
14. Pulendran B, Palucka K, Banchereau J. Sensing pathogens and tuning immune responses. *Science* 2001;293:253–256.
15. Cutler CW, Jotwani R, Pulendran B. Dendritic cells: immune saviors or Achilles' heel? *Infect Immun* 2001;69:4703–4708
16. Iwasaki A, Kelsall BL. Localization of distinct Peyer's patch dendritic cell subsets and their recruitment by chemokines macrophage inflammatory protein (MIP)-3alpha, MIP-3beta, and secondary lymphoid organ chemokine. *J Exp Med* 2000; 191:1381–1394.
17. Iwasaki A, Kelsall BL. Unique functions of CD11b+, CD8 alpha+, and double-negative Peyer's patch dendritic cells. *J Immunol* 2001;166:4884–4890.
18. Huang FP, Platt N, Wykes M, et al. A discrete subpopulation of dendritic cells transports apoptotic intestinal epithelial cells to T-cell areas of mesenteric lymph nodes. *J Exp Med* 2000;191: 435–444.
19. Rescigno M, Urbano M, Valzasina B, et al. Dendritic cells express tight junction proteins and penetrate gut epithelial monolayers to sample bacteria. *Nat Immunol* 2001;2:361–367.
20. Sanders ME, Makgoba MW, Sharrow SO, et al. Human memory T lymphocytes express increased levels of three cell adhesion molecules (LFA-3, CD2, and LFA-1) and three other molecules (UCHL1, CDw29, and Pgp-1) and have enhanced IFN-gamma production. *J Immunol* 1988;140;1401–1407.
21. Akbar AN, Terry L, Timms A, et al. Loss of CD45R and gain of UCHL1 reactivity is a feature of primed T cells. *J Immunol* 1988;140;2171–2178.
22. Clement LT, Yamashita N, Martin AM. The functionally distinct subpopulations of human CD4+ helper/inducer T lymphocytes defined by anti-CD45R antibodies derive sequentially from a differentiation pathway that is regulated by activation-dependent post-thymic differentiation. *J Immunol* 1988;141: 1464–1470.
23. Streuli M, Hall LR, Saga Y, et al. Differential usage of three exons generate at least five different mRNAs encoding human leukocyte common antigens. *J Exp Med* 1987;166:1548–1566.
24. Selby HL, Janossy G, Bofill M, et al. Lymphocyte subpopulations in the human small intestine. The findings in normal mucosa and in the mucosa of patients with adult coeliac disease. *Clin Exp Immunol* 1993;52:219–228.
25. Schieferdecker HL, Ullrich R, WeiB-Breckwoldt AN, et al. The HML-1 antigen of intestinal lymphocytes is an activation antigen. *J Immunol* 1990;144:2511–2519.
26. James SP, Fiocchi C, Graeff AS, et al. Phenotypic analysis of lamina propria lymphocytes: predominance of helper-inducer and cytolytic T-cell phenotypes and deficiency of suppressor-inducer phenotypes in Crohn's disease and control patients. *Gastroenterology* 1986;91:1483–1489.
27. Willerford DM, Hoffman PA, Gallatin WM. Expression of lymphocyte adhesion receptors for high endothelium in primates. Anatomic partitioning and linkage to activation. *J Immunol* 1989;142:3416–3422.
28. Ebert EC, Roberts AI. Costimulation of the CD3 pathway by CD28 ligation in human intestinal lymphocytes. *Cell Immunol* 1996;171:211–216.
29. Ullrich R, Schieferdecker HL, Ziegler K, et al. CD8 T cells in the human intestine express surface markers of activation and are preferentially located in the epithelium. *Cell Immunol* 1990; 128:619–627.
30. Porcelli S, Brenner MB, Band H. Biology of human T-cell receptor. *Immunol Rev* 1991;120:137–183.
31. Deusch K, Luling F, Reich K, et al. A major fraction of human intraepithelial lymphocytes simultaneously expresses the T-cell receptor, the CD8 accessory molecule and preferentially uses the V1 gene segment. *Eur J Immunol* 1991;21:1053–1059.
32. Balk SP, Ebert EC, Blumenthal RL, et al. Oligoclonal expansion and CD1 recognition by human intestinal intraepithelial lymphocytes. *Science* 1991;253:1411–1415.
33. Blumberg RS, Yockey CE, Gross GG, et al. Human intestinal intraepithelial lymphocytes are derived from a limited number of T-cell clones that utilize multiple V beta T cell receptor genes. *J Immunol* 1993;150:5144–5153.

34. Van Kerckhove C, Russell GJ, Deusch K, et al. Oligoclonality of human intestinal intraepithelial T cells. *J Exp Med* 1992;175: 57–63.
35. Dogan A, Dunn-Walters DK, MacDonald TT, et al. Demonstration of local clonality of mucosal T cells in human colon using DNA obtained by microdissection of immunohistochemically stained tissue sections. *Eur J Immunol* 1996;26:1240–1245.
36. Greene WC, Leonard WJ, Depper JM. Growth of human T lymphocytes: an analysis of interleukin 2 and its cellular receptor. *Prog Hematol* 1986;14:283–301.
37. Zeitz M, Green WC, Peffer NJ, et al. Lymphocytes isolated from the intestinal lamina propria of normal non-human primates have increased expression of genes associated with T-cell activation. *Gastroenterology* 1988;94:647–655.
38. Fell JM, Walker-Smith JA, Spencer J, et al. The distribution of dividing T cells throughout the intestinal wall in inflammatory bowel disease (IBD). *Clin Exp Immunol* 1996;104:280–285.
39. Braunstein J, Qiao L, Autschbach F, et al. T cells of the human intestinal lamina propria are high producers of interleukin-10. *Gut* 1997;41:215–220.
40. Watanabe M, Ueno Y, Yajima T, et al. Interleukin 7 is produced by human intestinal epithelial cells and regulates the proliferation of intestinal mucosal lymphocytes. *J Clin Invest* 1995; 95:2945–2953.
41. Qiao L, Schürman G, Betzler M, et al. Functional properties of human lamina propria T lymphocytes assessed with mitogenic monoclonal antibodies. *Immunol Res* 1991;10:218–225.
42. Fuss IJ, Neurath M, Boirivant M, et al. Disparate CD4+ lamina propria (LP) lymphokine secretion profiles in inflammatory bowel disease. Crohn's disease LP cells manifest increased secretion of IFN-gamma, whereas ulcerative colitis LP cells manifest increased secretion of IL-5. *J Immunol* 1996;157:1261–1270.
43. Panja A, Barone A, Mayer L. Stimulation of lamina propria lymphocytes by intestinal epithelial cells: evidence for recognition of nonclassical restriction elements. *J Exp Med* 1994;179: 943–950.
44. Qiao L, Braunstein J, Golling M, et al. Differential regulation of human T-cell responsiveness by mucosal versus blood monocytes. *Eur J Immunol* 1996;26:922–927.
45. De Maria R, Fais S, Silvestri M, et al. Continuous *in vivo* activation and transient hyporesponsiveness to TcR/CD3 triggering of human gut lamina propria lymphocytes. *Eur J Immunol* 1993;23:3104–3108.
46. James SP, Graeff AS, Zeitz M. Predominance of helper-induced T cells in mesenteric lymph nodes and intestinal lamina propria of normal non-human primates. *Cell Immunol* 1987;107: 372–383.
47. Zeitz M, Quinn TC, Graeff AS, et al. Mucosal T cells provide helper function but do not proliferate when stimulated by specific antigen in lymphogranuloma venereum proctitis in non-human primates. *Gastroenterology* 1988;94:353–366.
48. Khoo UY, Proctor IE, Macpherson AJ. CD4+ T-cell down-regulation in human intestinal mucosa: evidence for intestinal tolerance to luminal bacterial antigens. *J Immunol* 1997;158: 3626–3634.
49. Hurst SD, Cooper CJ, Sitterding SM, et al. The differentiated state of intestinal lamina propria CD4+ T cells results in altered cytokine production, activation threshold, and costimulatory requirements. *J Immunol* 1999;163:5937–5945
50. Rocha B, Guy-Grand D, Vassalli P. Extrathymic T-cell differentiation. *Curr Opin Immunol* 1995;7:235–242
51. Guy-Grand D, Cuenod-Jabri B, Malassis-Seris M, et al. Complexity of the mouse gut T-cell immune system: identification of two distinct natural killer T-cell intraepithelial lineages. *Eur J Immunol* 1996;26:2246–2258.
52. Regnault A, Cumano A, Vassalli P, et al. Oligoclonal repertoire of the CD8/α and the CD8/β TCR–/β murine intestinal intraepithelial T lymphocytes: evidence for the random emergence of T cells. *J Exp Med* 1994;180:1345–1358.
53. Arstila T, Arstila TP, Calbo S, et al. Identical T-cell clones are located within the mouse gut epithelium and lamina propria and circulate in the thoracic duct lymph. *J Exp Med* 2000;191: 823–834.
54. Cepek KL, Shaw SK, Parker CM, et al. Adhesion between epithelial cells and T lymphocytes mediated by E-cadherin and the E7 integrin. *Nature* 1994;372:190–193.
55. Shibahara T, Wilcox JN, Couse T, et al. Characterization of epithelial chemoattractants for human intestinal intraepithelial lymphocytes. *Gastroenterology* 2001;120:291–294.
56. Barrett TA, Gajewski TF, Danielpour D, et al. Differential function of intestinal intraepithelial lymphocyte subsets. *J Immunol* 1992;149:1124–1130.
57. Poussier P, Ning T, Chen J, et al. Intestinal inflammation observed in IL-2R/IL-2 mutant mice is associated with impaired intestinal T lymphopoiesis. *Gastroenterology* 2000; 118:880–891.
58. Lodolce JP, Boone DL, Chai S, et al. IL-15 receptor maintains lymphoid homeostasis by supporting lymphocyte homing and proliferation. *Immunity* 1998;9:669–676.
59. Yoshikai Y. The interaction of intestinal epithelial cells and intraepithelial lymphocytes in host defense. *Immunol Res* 1999;20:219–235.
60. Beagley KW, Husband AJ. Intraepithelial lymphocytes: origins, distribution and function. *Crit Rev Immunol* 1998;13:237–254.
61. Muller S, Buhler-Jungo M, Mueller C. Intestinal intraepithelial lymphocytes exert potent protective cytotoxic activity during an acute virus infection. *J Immunol* 2000;164:1986–1994.
62. Bauer S, Groh V, Wu J, et al. Activation of NK cells and T cells by NKG2D, a receptor for stress-inducible MICA. *Science* 1999;285:727–729.
63. Saparov A, Kraus LA, Cong Y, et al. Memory/effector T cells in TCR transgenic mice develop via recognition of enteric antigens by a second, endogenous TCR. *Int Immunol* 1999;11: 1253–1264.
64. Duchmann R, Neurath MF, Meyer zum Buschenfelde KH. Responses to self and non-self intestinal microflora in health and inflammatory bowel disease. *Res Immunol* 1997;148: 589–594.
65. Asseman C, Mauze S, Leach MW, et al. An essential role for interleukin 10 in the function of regulatory T cells that inhibit intestinal inflammation. *J Exp Med* 1999;190:995–1004.
66. Roncarolo MG, Levings MK. The role of different subsets of T regulatory cells in controlling autoimmunity. *Curr Opin Immunol* 2000;12:676–683.
67. Roncarolo MG, Levings MK. The role of different subsets of T regulatory cells in controlling autoimmunity. *Curr Opin Immunol* 2000;12:676–683.
68. Rottem M, Metcalfe DD. Development and maturation of mast cells and basophils. In: Busse WW, Holgate ST, eds. *Asthma and rhinitis.* Boston: Blackwell Science, 1995:167–181.
69. Gurish MF, Austen KF. The diverse roles of mast cells. *J Exp Med* 2001;194:F1–F5.
70. Renneck D, Hunte B, Holland G, et al. Co-factors are essential for stem cell factor-dependent growth and maturation of mast cell progenitors: comparative effects of interleukin-3 (IL-3), IL-4, IL-10 and fibroblasts. *Blood* 1995;85:57–65.
71. Knight PA, Wright SH, Lawrence CE, et al. Delayed expulsion of the nematode *Trichinella spiralis* in mice lacking the mucosal mast cell-specific granule chymase, mouse mast cell protease-1. *J Exp Med* 2000;192:1849–1856.
72. Lin T-J, Befus D. Mast cells and eosinophils in mucosal defenses and pathogenesis. In: Ogra PL, Mestecky J, Lamm ME, et al.,

eds. *Mucosal immunology,* second edition. San Diego: Academic Press, 1999:469–482.
73. Arizono N, Kasugai T, Yamada M, et al. Infection of *Nippostrongylus brasiliensis* induces development of mucosal-type but not connective tissue-type mast cells in genetically mast cell-deficient Ws/Ws rats. *Blood* 1993;81:2572–2579.
74. Lawrence CE, Paterson JC, Higgins LM, et al. IL-4-regulated enteropathy in an intestinal nematode infection. *Eur J Immunol* 1998;28:2672–2684.
75. Lantz CS, Boesiger J, Song CH, et al. Role for interleukin-3 in mast cell and basophil development and in immunity to parasites. *Nature* 1998;392:90–93.
76. Riegler M, Castagliuolo I, So PT, et al. Effects of substance P on human colonic mucosa *in vitro. Am J Physiol* 1999;276: G1473–G1483.
77. Rothenberg ME, Mishra A, Brandt EB, et al. Gastrointestinal eosinophils. *Immunol Rev* 2001;179:139–155.
78. Shao L, Serrano D, Mayer L. The role of epithelial cells in immune regulation in the gut. *Semin Immunol* 2001;13:163–176.
79. Sitaraman SV, Merlin D, Wang L, et al. Neutrophil–epithelial crosstalk at the intestinal luminal surface mediated by reciprocal secretion of adenosine and IL-6. *J Clin Invest* 2001;107: 861–869.
80. Lugering N, Kucharzik T, Maaser C, et al. Interleukin-15 strongly inhibits interleukin-8 and monocyte chemoattractant protein-1 production in human colonic epithelial cells. *Immunology* 1999;98:504–509.
81. Podolsky DK. Healing the epithelium: solving the problem from two sides. *J Gastroenterol* 1997;32:122–126.
82. Hooper LV, Xu J, Falk PG, et al. A molecular sensor that allows a gut commensal to control its nutrient foundation in a competitive ecosystem. *Proc Natl Acad Sci U S A* 1999;96: 9833–9838.
83. Hudault S, Guignot J, Servin AL. *Escherichia coli* strains colonising the gastrointestinal tract protect germ-free mice against *Salmonella typhimurium* infection. Gut 2001;49:47–55.
84. Hooper LV, Wong MH, Thelin A, et al. Molecular analysis of commensal host–microbial relationships in the intestine. *Science* 2001;291:881–884.
85. Withers H, Swift S, Williams P. Quorum sensing as an integral component of gene regulatory networks in gram-negative bacteria. *Curr Opin Microbiol* 2001;4:186–193.
86. Dimango E, Zar HJ, Bryan R, et al. Diverse *Pseudomonas aeruginosa* gene products stimulate respiratory epithelial cells to produce interleukin-8. *J Clin Invest* 1995;5:2204–2210.
87. Telford G, Wheeler D, Williams P, et al. The *Pseudomonas aeruginosa* quorum-sensing signal molecule *N*-(3-oxododecanoyl)-L-homoserine lactone has immunomodulatory activity. *Infect Immun* 1998;66:36–42.
88. Neish AS, Gewirtz AT, Zeng H, et al. Prokaryotic regulation of epithelial responses by inhibition of I-kappa-B-alpha ubiquitination. *Science* 2000;289:1560–1563.
89. Madsen KL, Doyle JS, Tavernini MM, et al. Antibiotic therapy attenuates colitis in interleukin 10 gene-deficient mice. *Gastroenterology* 2000;118:1094–1105.
90. Gionchetti P, Rizzello F, Venturi A, et al. Oral bacteriotherapy as maintenance treatment in patients with chronic pouchitis: a double-blind, placebo-controlled trial. *Gastroenterology* 2000; 119:305–309.
91. Rembacken BJ, Snelling AM, Hawkey PM, et al. Non-pathogenic *Escherichia coli* versus mesalazine for the treatment of ulcerative colitis: a randomised trial. *Lancet* 1999;354:635–639.
92. Walia K, Vohra H, Singh H, et al. Spectrum of gut immunologic reactions: selective induction of distinct responses to *Vibrio cholerae* WO7 and its toxin. *Microbiol Immunol* 2000;44: 931–940.
93. Pizza M, Giuliani MM, Fontana MR, et al. Mucosal vaccines: nontoxic derivatives of LT and CT as mucosal adjuvants. *Vaccine* 2001;19:2534–2541.
94. Donnenberg MS, Whittam TS. Pathogenesis and evolution of virulence in enteropathogenic and enterohemorrhagic *Escherichia coli. J Clin Invest* 2001;107:539–548.
95. Higgins LM, Frankel G, Connerton I, et al. Role of bacterial intimin in colonic hyperplasia and inflammation. *Science* 1999; 285:588–591.
96. Klapproth JM, Scaletsky IC, McNamara BP, et al. A large toxin from pathogenic *Escherichia coli* strains that inhibits lymphocyte activation. *Infect Immun* 2000;68:2148–2155.
97. Del Giudice G, Covacci A, Telford JL, et al. The design of vaccines against *Helicobacter pylori* and their development. *Annu Rev Immunol* 2001;19:523–563.
98. Donnenberg MS. Pathogenic strategies of enteric bacteria. *Nature* 2000;406:768–774.
99. Ciarlet M, Estes MK. Interactions between rotavirus and gastrointestinal cells. *Curr Opin Microbiol* 2001;4:435–441.
100. Franco MA, Greenberg HB. Challenges for rotavirus vaccines. *Virology* 2001;281:153–155.
101. Shi HN, Ingui CJ, Dodge I, et al. A helminth-induced mucosal Th2 response alters nonresponsiveness to oral administration of a soluble antigen. *J Immunol* 1998;160:2449–2455.
102. Helmby H, Takeda K, Akira S, et al. Interleukin (il)-18 promotes the development of chronic gastrointestinal helminth infection by downregulating il-13. *J Exp Med* 2001;194: 355–364.
103. Fox JG, Beck P, Dangler CA, et al. Concurrent enteric helminth infection modulates inflammation and gastric immune responses and reduces *Helicobacter*-induced gastric atrophy. *Nat Med* 2000;6:536–542.

15

FOOD POISONING

SONJA J. OLSEN
JOHN N. AUCOTT
DAVID L. SWERDLOW

Foodborne disease results from ingestion of either food or water contaminated with pathogenic microorganisms, microbial toxins, or chemicals, or from consumption of naturally occurring plant and animal toxins. More than 250 foodborne diseases have been described. The diversity of microorganisms and toxins that can be involved in foodborne disease results in a wide spectrum of clinical syndromes. This chapter focuses on foodborne disease with gastrointestinal symptoms occurring within 24 hours after ingestion. However, many serious foodborne illnesses such as hepatitis A (1,2), brucellosis (3), listeriosis (4,5), botulism (6), and diphylobrothium (7) do not have prominent gastrointestinal symptoms. In addition, foodborne illnesses may have prominent neurologic symptoms in addition to gastrointestinal symptoms. This chapter briefly discusses acute syndromes with neurologic features such as fish-related toxins (see Chapter 16) and botulism. Foodborne infections with longer incubation periods, such as those due to *Salmonella, Shigella* species *Escherichia coli, Campylobacter* spp., and *Yersinia* spp. are discussed in depth elsewhere (Part X).

Among foodborne disease outbreaks reported to the Centers for Disease Control and Prevention (CDC), bacterial agents are the most frequently recognized etiologic cause, causing 75% of the outbreaks and 86% of the individual cases in which a specific agent is eventually identified (8) (Table 15.1). Chemical, parasitic, and viral agents are less common, accounting for 17%, 2%, and 6% of the identified outbreaks, respectively. In 68% of outbreaks an etiologic agent cannot be determined. Although bacterial agents are the leading cause of recognized foodborne outbreaks with a known etiology, viral agents such as "Norwalk-like viruses" (NLVs) are suspected to play a much larger role (9); however, they are less likely to be diagnosed. Parasitic agents continue to play a major role in waterborne outbreaks (10).

S. J. Olsen: Foodborne and Diarrheal Diseases Branch, National Center for Infectious Diseases, Centers for Disease Control and Prevention, Atlanta, Georgia

J. N. Aucott: Department of Internal Medicine, Johns Hopkins at Green Spring Station, Maryland

D. L. Swerdlow: Clinical Outcomes Section, Surveillance Branch, Division of HIV/AIDS Prevention, Atlanta, Georgia

VEHICLES OF FOODBORNE ILLNESS

Foodborne disease can be caused by contaminated food and water (8,10), and outbreak investigations provide important clues to the epidemiology of foodborne illness. Raw foods of animal origin, such as raw meat and poultry, raw eggs, unpasteurized milk, and raw shellfish, are most likely to be contaminated with foodborne pathogens. Outbreak investigations have revealed an association between raw or undercooked pork, lamb, and wild game meat and toxoplasmosis (11), raw or undercooked ground beef and Shiga toxin–producing *E. coli* (12,13), and undercooked pork or bear meat and trichinosis (14). The increasing popularity of raw fish in sushi has increased the awareness of marine worm ingestions such as *Anisakis* (15,16). Bivalve molluscs such as oysters, clams, and mussels are particularly suspect because of their ability to transmit a variety of pathogens, including hepatitis A (17), NLVs (18,19), *Vibrio* species (20–23), *Salmonella* Typhi (24), and *Campylobacter* species. Raw fruits and vegetables are also a particular concern. From the 1970s to the 1990s, the number of fresh produce–associated outbreaks reported to CDC has increased nearly threefold. Water used for washing and chilling produce after it is harvested (25) and fresh manure used to fertilize vegetables are potential sources of contamination. Alfalfa sprouts and other raw sprouts pose a particular challenge, because the conditions under which they are sprouted are ideal for growing microbes as well as sprouts, and they are eaten without further cooking (26).

Chemical intoxication can be due to naturally occurring plant and animal toxins or by contamination of food with heavy metals, insecticides, or toxic oils. Fish and shellfish that are normally safe can accumulate toxins naturally present in the food chain (e.g., paralytic shellfish poisoning

TABLE 15.1. FOODBORNE-DISEASE OUTBREAKS AND OUTBREAK-ASSOCIATED CASES BY ETIOLOGY, REPORTED TO THE CENTERS FOR DISEASE CONTROL AND PREVENTION, 1993–1997

Etiologic Agent	No. Outbreaks (%)	No. Cases (%)
Bacterial		
Bacillus cereus	14 (0.5)	691 (0.8)
Brucella	1 (0.0)	19 (0.0)
Campylobacter	25 (0.9)	539 (0.6)
Clostridium botulinum	13 (0.5)	56 (0.1)
Clostridium perfringens	57 (2.1)	2,772 (3.2)
Escherichia coli	84 (3.1)	3,260 (3.8)
Listeria monocytogenes	3 (0.1)	100 (0.1)
Salmonella	357 (13.0)	32,610 (37.9)
Shigella	43 (1.6)	1,555 (1.8)
Staphylococcus aureus	42 (1.5)	1,413 (1.6)
Streptococcus, group A	1 (0.0)	122 (0.1)
Streptococcus, other	1 (0.0)	6 (0.0)
Vibrio cholerae	1 (0.0)	2 (0.0)
Vibrio parahaemolyticus	5 (0.2)	40 (0.0)
Yersinia enterocoliticus	2 (0.1)	27 (0.0)
Other bacterial	6 (0.2)	609 (0.7)
Total bacterial	655 (23.8)	43,821 (50.9)
Chemical		
Ciguatoxin	60 (2.2)	205 (0.2)
Heavy metals	4 (0.1)	17 (0.0)
Monosodium glutamate	1 (0.0)	2 (0.0)
Mushroom poisoning	7 (0.3)	21 (0.0)
Scrobotoxin	69 (2.5)	297 (0.3)
Shellfish	1 (0.0)	3 (0.0)
Other chemical	6 (0.2)	31 (0.0)
Total chemical	148 (5.4)	576 (0.7)
Parasitic		
Giardia lamblia	4 (0.1)	45 (0.1)
Trichinella spiralis	2 (0.1)	19 (0.0)
Other parasitic	13 (0.5)	2,261 (2.6)
Total parasitic	19 (0.7)	2,325 (2.7)
Viral		
Hepatitis A	23 (0.8)	729 (0.8)
Norwalk	9 (0.3)	1,233 (1.4)
Other viral	24 (0.9)	2,104 (2.4)
Total virus	56 (2.0)	4,066 (4.7)
Confirmed etiology	878 (31.9)	50,788 (59.0)
Unknown etiology	1,873 (68.1)	35,270 (41.0)
Total 1993–1997	2,751 (100.0)	86,058 (100.0)

and ciguatera) or can be contaminated with bacteria that produce toxic-level compounds when the fish is improperly stored (scombroid or histamine fish poisoning) (27–36). Some "foods" are intrinsically toxic to humans, and ingestion may result from faulty identification of edible species, such as mushrooms (37) and ornamental and wild plants (38,39). Illness resulting from ingestion of Chinese-style food may suggest intoxication due to monosodium glutamate (MSG) or fried rice may be contaminated with *Bacillus cereus* (40,41).

Other factors that contribute to foodborne outbreaks include improper holding temperature of food, inadequate cooking of food, contaminated equipment used to process food, using food from an unsafe source, and poor personal hygiene in a food handler. Among outbreaks reported to CDC between 1993 and 1997, the most commonly reported food preparation practice that contributed to foodborne disease was improper holding temperature, followed by inadequate cooking of food (8).

Waterborne diseases may be caused by bacterial pathogens, especially Shiga-toxin-producing *E. coli* or *Shigella,* viral pathogens such as hepatitis A, hepatitis E, or NLVs, and parasites such as *Giardia intestinalis* or *Cryptosporidium parvum* (10,42). Waterborne outbreaks may involve community water systems, well water, surface water, or bottled water (10).

MAGNITUDE AND SIGNIFICANCE OF PROBLEM

An estimated 76 million cases of foodborne disease occur each year in the United States (9). The majority of these cases are mild and cause symptoms for only a day or two. However, some cases are more serious: there are an estimated 323,000 hospitalizations and 5,000 deaths related to foodborne diseases each year (9). Most illness occurs as sporadic infection, that is, not part of a recognized outbreak; illnesses linked to outbreaks represent only a small fraction of the illnesses that actually occur. For example, in 1997, a total of 60 *Salmonella* outbreaks causing 1,731 infections were reported to CDC through the Foodborne Disease Outbreak Surveillance System (8). In contrast, during the same year, 34,608 infections were reported through the National *Salmonella* Surveillance System, a passive, laboratory-based system (43). Although many sporadic infections are captured through routine surveillance, because of marked underdiagnosis and underreporting, the true number of infections is larger than any surveillance numbers suggest. As mentioned, for most foodborne outbreaks, no etiology is identified (8). The inability to identify a specific causative agent may result from an incomplete epidemiologic investigation, inadequate specimen collection, or limited laboratory capability to assays for toxins, chemicals, viral agents, parasites, and certain disease-causing strains of bacteria, such as *E. coli* O157:H7.

Although foodborne disease may be mild, a large outbreak of foodborne disease may have significant economic impact and result in closure of hospitals and schools. Cost estimates for all foodborne illness in the United States, including the medical expenses and lost productivity of those affected as well as lost revenues and legal fees incurred by the food supplier, range from $7.7 to $23 billion per year (44). Bacterial illness accounts for approximately 80% of this cost, with salmonellosis accounting for 47% of the total (45).

ETIOLOGIC AGENTS

Foodborne Viral Disease

Although bacterial foodborne illnesses are most commonly reported, most foodborne illness in the United States is actually caused by viral agents; however, these illnesses frequently go undiagnosed (9). Unlike bacteria, viruses do not multiply or produce toxins in food. Food merely acts as a vehicle for their transfer. Most reported incidents of viral food- or waterborne illness are due to hepatitis A virus and NLVs (8,46). Hepatitis E should also be considered when a patient has traveled abroad and serologic markers are negative for hepatitis A, B, and C (42).

Recent studies suggest that most gastroenteritis outbreaks are caused by NLVs and that these viruses may also be the most common cause of foodborne disease outbreaks in the United States (46–49). NLVs, which belong to the family *Caliciviridae*, are single-stranded RNA viruses that are difficult to study because of their inability to be cultivated in cell culture. Current methods to diagnose NLVs, including reverse transcription-polymerase chain reaction, are not routine in clinical or public health laboratories. Several clinical and epidemiologic characteristics of NLVs, including low infectious dose (<100 organisms), prolonged asymptomatic shedding (up to 2 weeks), environmental stability, and lack of durable immunity, make prevention a challenge (48). Outbreaks of NLV infections have been linked to ill food handlers, contaminated water and ice, contaminated oysters, and person-to-person contact (49–51). Infection is spread by the fecal-oral route and droplet transmission, and the average incubation period is 12 to 48 hours. The size of an NLV outbreak can range from a few to thousands of ill persons, and all age groups are susceptible to infection (49).

Foodborne Bacterial Disease

Many different bacteria cause foodborne disease; however, here we focus on those causing gastrointestinal symptoms within 24 hours after ingestion (i.e., *Staphylococcus aureus*, *Clostridium perfringens*, and *B. cereus)*. Staphylococcal food poisoning causes a rapid-onset gastrointestinal illness that usually resolves within a day (52). Recently, the percentage of bacterial foodborne disease outbreaks due to *S. aureus* has been decreasing over time (53). From 1993 to 1997, *S. aureus* caused 6.4% of recognized bacterial foodborne disease outbreaks (8). More than 99% of cases of staphylococcal food poisoning are due to *S. aureus.* Other coagulase-positive staphylococci, including *Staphylococcus hyicus* and *Staphylococcus intermedius,* produce small amounts of enterotoxin but have not been the cause of outbreaks of foodborne illness (54). Rarely are cases traced to coagulase-negative *Staphylococcus* species (55).

S. aureus is capable of causing large outbreaks of illness, some of which have involved more than 1,000 individuals. Staphylococci exist in air, dust, sewage, water, milk, and food or on food equipment, environmental surfaces, humans, and animals. Humans and animals are reservoirs. Certain strains of *S. aureus* produce a toxin that can lead to acute gastrointestinal illness. The toxin can survive cooking. Multiplication of the organism with resultant toxin production occurs when contaminated food is not kept hot enough (60°C greater) or cold enough (7.2°C or less). Staphylococcal food poisoning has resulted from the ingestion of a number of foods, including custard-filled bakery goods, salad dressings, canned food, processed meat, potato salad, inadequately processed cheese, and ice cream. Contaminated food is normal in appearance, odor, and taste. Staphylococcal food poisoning rarely results from commercially prepared food (56); it is usually due to contamination of foods by handlers in food service establishments or in the home (54). Contamination from humans occurs through an infected wound on the hands or occasionally from coughing or sneezing. It is estimated that 20% to 50% of healthy individuals carry *S. aureus,* most often on the skin or in the nose or feces (54). Animals with mastitis can also transmit disease through infected milk (57).

Disease results from ingestion of one or more of the seven serologically distinct extracellular enterotoxins (A, B, C1, C2, C3, D, and E) produced by *Staphylococcus* (58,59). The majority of enterotoxigenic staphylococci involved in outbreaks of foodborne illness produce type A enterotoxin alone or in combination with type D toxin (52,60). Staphylococcal enterotoxins are resistant to heat, irradiation, pH extremes, and proteolysis (61–63) (Table 15.2). The puri-

TABLE 15.2. PATHOGENIC MECHANISMS IN BACTERIAL FOODBORNE ILLNESS

Preformed Toxin	Toxin Production *in vivo*	Tissue Invasion	Toxin Production and/or Tissue Invasion
Staphylococcus aureus	*Clostridium perfringens*	*Campylobacter jejuni*	*Vibrio parahaemolyticus*
Bacillus cereus (short incubation)	*B. cereus* (long incubation)	*Salmonella*	*Yersinia enterocolitica*
Clostridium botulinum	*C. botulinum* (infant botulism)	*Shigella*	
	Enterotoxigenic *Escherichia coli*	Invasive *E. coli*	
	Vibrio cholerae O1 or O139		
	V. cholerae non-O1		
	Shiga toxin-producing *E. coli*		

fied toxins are small, single-chain polypeptides (27 to 30 kd) whose emetic activity may be related to a conserved histidine domain at the active site (64,65). As little as 100 to 200 ng produces illness in humans. Assay for the presence of enterotoxin in food and its production *in vitro* provides an important epidemiologic tool. Phage typing of isolates is also useful for epidemiologic investigations to trace the source of infection (66). Enterotoxigenic *S. aureus* phage type III is most often associated with outbreaks of foodborne disease. Phage type I is less often involved in foodborne illness but can be found either alone or in combination with type III (54). Foods often implicated with outbreaks include dairy products, salads, and meats (especially ham). High-protein foods favor the growth of *Staphylococcus* and present an especially high risk for food poisoning. Although a pH of less than 5.0 inhibits the growth of the bacteria, semipreserved products packaged with salt or sugar may still support growth of *Staphylococcus.*

C. perfringens typically causes a mild gastrointestinal illness, but in rare instances it can be severe (67). Approximately 6.4% of recognized bacterial foodborne outbreaks reported to CDC from 1993 to 1997 were due to the mild form of *Clostridium* food poisoning (8). Like for *S. aureus*, the percentage of these outbreaks also appears to be decreasing over time (53). *C. perfringens* type C causes rare cases of necrotic enteritis (pigbel) that are still reported from isolated regions of the world such as Papua, New Guinea (68). This rare illness is due to production of the toxin, which is usually inactivated by proteolytic enzymes in the intestine. Susceptible individuals are either malnourished and lack these proteolytic enzymes, or their enzymes are inhibited by other substances in their diet (69). The majority of the typical cases of the mild diarrheal illness caused by *C. perfringens* seen in developed countries are due to type A strains that are present in soil throughout the world and in the intestinal tracts of virtually all vertebrate animals studied. *Clostridium* types B, C, D, and E are found only in animals and not in soil. Spores are heat resistant and survive cooking to germinate. The organism grows rapidly at temperatures of 15°C to 50°C, with an optimum growth temperature of 43°C to 45°C. The organism can double in number in as little as 10 minutes (70). *C. perfringens* type A produces a 35-kd enterotoxin protein during sporulation (Table 15.2). The enterotoxin alters the membrane ion permeability of intestinal epithelial cells and acts as a superantigen reactive with human T cells (71,72). The resultant illness only occurs after ingestion of heavily contaminated food with greater than 100 million bacteria per gram. Meats, meat products, and poultry are the foods most commonly implicated with outbreaks of food poisoning. High numbers of vegetative bacteria may be present while the food is palatable. Outbreaks are usually associated with foods left out at room temperature for prolonged periods, allowing rapid multiplication of the organism and production of enterotoxin. Outbreaks typically occur in food service establishments or homes. Commercially prepared, processed food is rarely the cause of foodborne disease due to *C. perfringens* (73).

B. cereus is a less common source of foodborne illness in the United States, accounting for approximately 2% of recognized bacterial foodborne outbreaks in the United States from 1973 to 1997 (8). *B. cereus* is a ubiquitous, aerobic, spore-forming, gram-positive rod that causes two forms of toxin-mediated food poisoning: a short incubation (1 to 6 hours) emetic syndrome and a long incubation (8 to 16 hours) diarrheal syndrome (41,74). *B. cereus* is present in soil and water sources throughout the world and in most raw foods (69). In addition, 10% to 40% of humans are colonized with these bacteria. Illness occurs from ingestion of preformed toxin in contaminated food; the bacteria multiply and produce toxin in food left at room temperature. The spores of *Bacillus* are heat resistant. The organism is capable of producing either the emetic or the diarrheal toxin, depending on the food on which it grows (75,76). There is evidence that the emetic syndrome is caused by a preformed toxin with a molecular weight of 5,000 to 10,000 kd, which is unaffected by heat, trypsin, pepsin, and pH extremes (Table 15.2). The emetic syndrome is frequently associated with eating fried rice. In contrast, the diarrheal syndrome is associated with proteinaceous foods, including vegetables, sauces, and pudding (69). The diarrheal enterotoxin is a heat-labile protein of molecular weight 38 to 46 kd (77). There is no consistent relationship between the strain of *Bacillus* and the toxin produced. Outbreaks of foodborne illness resulting from *B. subtilis*, *B. licheniformis*, and *B. pumilus* have been reported (69).

Foodborne Fungal Disease

Fungal mycotoxins are synthesized by numerous species of fungi, including *Aspergillus flavus, Aspergillus parasiticus,* and *Fusarium* species. Contamination of food, especially cereals and nuts, can occur in the field or during storage. Conditions of poor storage that favor growth of the fungi result in the production of these potent toxins, which can contaminate meat, eggs, and milk when animals are fed contaminated grain. Historically, dramatic episodes of mycotoxin poisoning have included gangrenous ergotism and alimentary toxic aleukia resulting from *Fusarium*-contaminated cereals in the former Soviet Union (78). Aflatoxin from *A. flavus* is a potent carcinogen in certain animals but the relationship to human illness is unclear (79).

Food and Waterborne Parasitic Disease

Although parasitic disease is more common in developing countries, recent estimates suggest that each year 2.5 million cases occur in the United States, although only approximately 14% of these can be attributed to foodborne transmission (9). Cases of trichinosis and giardiasis, which are usually transmitted through food- or waterborne routes, are reported to CDC almost every year (8,80), and within the last 2 decades, *Cyclospora cayetanensis* and *C. parvum* have emerged as important food- and waterborne pathogens (81,82). Most parasites that are transmitted by contaminated food and water do not cause recognized outbreaks of acute foodborne illness (83). This may seem surprising given the wide prevalence of protozoans and helminths, but may be explained by several factors. These include the inability of parasites to multiply in food, the high rate of asymptomatic infection with these organisms, the difficulty with diagnosis, and the long delay (often years) before clinical presentation of many infections such as helminthic infections. Outbreaks of protozoal disease that are identified in the United States are more frequently associated with water than food. Transmission of *G. intestinalis* and *C. parvum* by means of public water supplies has become a recognized public health problem in developed countries. In the United States, *G. intestinalis* was implicated as the etiologic agent in 4 of 17 waterborne outbreaks between 1997 and 1998 in which an agent was identified (10). *G. intestinalis* is commonly found in surface water throughout the world and is a hazard for outdoorsmen and campers. Because the cysts involved in the transmission of *G. intestinalis* and *C. parvum* are relatively chlorine resistant, public water supplies are a potential source of outbreaks as well. *C. parvum* may contaminate water supplies that are exposed to livestock excreta. Waterborne outbreaks of cryptosporidiosis have been reported with increasing frequency in North America, possibly exposing large numbers of individuals and resulting in significant morbidity in immunocompromised hosts (84). In 1993, a massive waterborne outbreak of *Cyptosporidium* infections occurred in Milwaukee after oocysts entered the city's public water system (85). Although uncommon, waterborne outbreaks of *Entamoeba histolytica* have occurred in both the United States and the United Kingdom (83).

Foodborne parasitic disease can be due to contaminated foods or contamination of foods from infected food handlers. Between 1993 and 1997, 19 reported foodborne outbreaks in the United States had a parasitic etiology (8). Nine outbreaks were due to *C. cayetanensis*, four to *C. parvum*, four to *G. intestinalis*, and two to *Trichinella spiralis. C. cayetanensis* was not a recognized cause of human illness until the late 1970s. In the 1990s, *C. cayetanensis* caused 14 recognized outbreaks; water, raspberries, and other raw produce were implicated vehicles in these cases (81). A massive, international outbreak that occurred in 1996 was associated with Guatemalan raspberries (86). Outbreaks of *C. parvum* infection have been epidemiologically linked to ingestion of contaminated food as well as water, and contamination by an ill food handler excreting oocysts was recently documented (82,83,87). *C. parvum* infection can be life threatening in persons with HIV (82). Giardiasis usually occurs as sporadic infection (80), although foodborne outbreaks have been reported (88,89). In foodborne outbreaks of giardiasis, food handlers were frequently found to have had recent contact with children who were excreting *G. intestinalis* in their stool. Transmission of *E. histolytica* has also been traced to contamination by food handlers (83).

The increased popularity of sushi in North America has brought attention to foodborne illness due to *Anisakis*, eustrongylides, and other fish tapeworms (15,16). These worms can be found in both fresh- and saltwater fish. Anecdotal evidence suggests that humans are usually exposed to these worms through the consumption of raw fish in sushi; occasionally illness has followed eating minnows or bait fish as a "stunt."

Foodborne Chemical Ingestions

Foodborne chemical ingestions may be the result of exogenous toxins contaminating foods or naturally occurring toxins found in animals, plants, and fungi (90). Pesticides used in agriculture that contain potent cholinesterase inhibitors have caused foodborne outbreaks of serious illness (91). Addition of drugs to animal feed has been reported to result in β-agonist food poisoning from ingestion of contaminated beef liver (92). Heavy metal ingestion has accounted for up to two outbreaks reported to CDC each year between 1993 and 1997 (8). These episodes are often related to beverages that are stored in improper containers such as galvanized metal cans. The beverages are usually acidic and have included fruit punch, limeade, and tomato juice. Outbreaks have been reported from schools, restaurants, and homes. Other rare mechanisms of heavy metal ingestion have included cadmium from a refrigerator shelf used as an improvised barbecue grill and copper from a corroded water heater (93,94).

Contamination of water with a wide variety of toxic chemicals can result in acute poisoning. Two of the 17 reported waterborne outbreaks between 1997 and 1998 in the United States were due to copper poisoning (10). Chemicals can be introduced into public water systems through back-siphoning; one case involved concentrated sodium hydroxide (51). Faulty water treatment with water-softening agents can result in excessive alkalinity or acidity of water. Contact of copper pipes with acidic water results in elevated copper levels and abdominal toxicity. Acute fluoride poisoning has been reported at least seven times in the United States. Fluoride and hydrogen ions in the stomach combine to form hydrofluoric acid, which is a gastric irritant. Outbreaks have affected hundreds of individuals and occasionally result in death, especially among patients with renal failure (95). Cross-connection of water systems with heating systems has resulted in the introduction of toxic levels of ethylene glycol into the water supply (51). In one episode, well water was contaminated with nitrates, resulting in fatal methemoglobinemia in an infant (51). When chemical toxins are suspected, testing urine samples may be diagnostic.

Food additives and substitutes can result in a variety of types of food poisoning. MSG has been implicated in the "Chinese restaurant syndrome" in which patients experience a burning sensation or pressure in the chest, lacrimation, and diaphoresis. Won ton soup is frequently identified as the offending food, possibly because the effects of MSG are accentuated when it is consumed on an empty stomach. Large outbreaks of delayed neurologic syndromes have been traced to the inadvertent ingestion of toxic oils, including industrial denatured rapeseed oil and a hydraulic fluid component, triorthocresyl phosphate. These industrial compounds have been found in olive oil, mustard oil, Jamaican ginger, and cooking oil. The delayed neurologic syndromes they produce are similar to those seen in eosinophilia-myalgia syndrome associated with L-tryptophan ingestion (96). In 1989 and 1990, the first epidemic of eosinophilia-myalgia syndrome occurred in the United States (97), with more than 1,500 cases reported to CDC. Epidemiologic studies implicated ingestion of L-tryptophan–containing products sold as dietary supplements (98,99). As a result, the U.S. Food and Drug Administration recalled dietary supplements containing L-tryptophan (99).

Animal toxins are primarily seen with ingestion of fish and shellfish (27,79,100). Fish and shellfish are associated with distinct food poisoning syndromes including ciguatera, scombroid, tetradotoxin, and paralytic and neurotoxic shellfish poisoning, which are discussed in separate chapters.

Poisoning with plant toxins can be the result of ingestion of inedible plants as well as plants thought to be edible (79). Toxicity may result from improper preparation of the foods (e.g., cassava), misidentification of toxic species for edible species (e.g., mushrooms), or genetic susceptibility of the host to normally innocuous components of food (e.g., favism). Susceptibility to favism is associated with a sex-linked gene; eating fava, horse, or broad beans, or inhaling the pollen causes an allergic response. The seeds of certain plants, including bitter almonds, cassava, various cherries, and lima beans, can cause cyanide poisoning. Unintentional overdoses of herbal remedies containing plant toxins may result in a variety of syndromes including neurologic disease and hepatitis (101).

Edible plants may occasionally cause food poisoning under specific circumstances (79). Potato glycoalkaloids are produced under conditions of stress, including exposure of potatoes to light, fungal, mechanical, or insect damage. Commercial blemish-free potato tubers generally contain low levels of toxic glycoalkaloids, which are further reduced by peeling the potatoes. However, poor quality or damaged potatoes can contain higher levels of the toxin. This results in acute potato poisoning, which manifests with neurologic symptoms, including apathy, restlessness, drowsiness, and visual disturbance. Legumes contain a variety of biologically active compounds including estrogenic isoflavones and coumestans, hemagglutinins, tannins, and glycosides. Fava beans contain plant glycosides vicine and convicine, which are broken down to oxidants that cause favism in G6PD-deficient individuals of Mediterranean descent.

Ornamental and wild plants are common sources of potential food poisoning, especially in children (102). Most ingestions involve house plants and ornamental plants, and fewer than 0.04% of reported cases result in major toxicity (103). Highly toxic wild plants are occasionally mistaken for edible species and have resulted in at least 58 fatalities in the United States between 1979 and 1988. For example, water hemlock, a highly toxic species, may be mistaken for a wild edible plant. When ingested, it results in gastrointestinal symptoms, seizures, and respiratory distress, with an overall mortality rate of 30% (38).

Mushroom poisoning can cause a variety of clinical syndromes ranging from a benign, self-limited gastrointestinal illness to major systemic syndromes including liver and renal failure, hemolysis, disulfiram-like reactions, cholinergic symptoms, and psychoactive central nervous system (CNS) effects (104). A large number of poisonous mushroom species grow abundantly, and species identification can be exceedingly difficult even for expert mycologists. Mushrooms known to be edible in one location may be poisonous in a different geographic location. Several types of mushrooms cause illness only when consumed with alcohol, causing a syndrome known as mushroom alcohol intolerance. Mushroom poisonings occur more frequently in the fall when the reproductive part of the fungus is most easily harvested. More than 80% of mushroom exposures reported to the American Association of Poison Control Centers were among children younger than 6 years of age.

CLINICAL DIAGNOSIS OF FOOD POISONING SYNDROMES

The diagnostic approach to food poisoning should consider a combination of the specific symptoms, including the presence of neurologic or systemic symptoms, the likely incubation period, the duration of the illness, and the food associated with the illness (Table 15.3). This chapter discusses illnesses that occur in the first 24 hours after exposure to a foodborne disease. However, many bacterial diseases that require replication in the host have incubation periods of 3 to 5 days (see Chapters 42, 44, and 46). Other foodborne illnesses have even longer incubation periods. Botulism may not manifest for up to 8 days after ingestion of toxin. The incubation period for trichinosis may range from 5 to 45 days, and *G. intestinalis* has an incubation period of 3 to 25 days or longer.

Searching for key historical clues and symptoms of food poisoning is essential to making the diagnosis and recognizing persons at risk for significant morbidity and mortality. The evaluation of gastrointestinal illness should focus on

TABLE 15.3. CLINICAL DIAGNOSIS OF FOODBORNE ILLNESS BY INCUBATION PERIOD AND SYMPTOM

	Incubation Period			
Predominant Symptoms	**<2 hr**	**1–7 hr**	**8–14 hr**	**>14 hr**
Upper interstinal, nausea/vomiting	Heavy metals, chemicals mushrooms	*Staphylococcus aureus, Bacillus cereus, Anisakis*	*Anisakis*	Norwalk-like viruses
Noninflammatory, diarrhea, few or no fecal leukocytes			*Clostridium perfringens, B. cereus*	*Cryptosporidium parvum,* Enterotoxigenic Escherichia *coli, Giardia intestinalis,* Norwalk-like viruses, *Vibrio cholerae,*
Inflammatory ileocolitis				*Salmonella, Shigella, Campylobacter, E. coli, Vibrio parahaemolyticus, Entamoeba histolytica, Yersinia enterocolitica,*
Extragastrointestinal, neurologic	Insecticides, mushroom and plant toxins, monosodium glutamate, shellfish, scombroid	Shellfish, ciguatera		Botulism

the presence or absence of vomiting and the differentiation of inflammatory from noninflammatory diarrhea. Diarrhea can be characterized as inflammatory by the presence of fecal leukocytes, heme-positive stool, fever, or leukocytosis. Such characterization of diarrheal illness may not always be clear-cut, in that certain bacteria such as *Vibrio parahaemolyticus* may manifest with inflammatory or noninflammatory syndromes. Recognizing neurologic symptoms of food poisoning is critical to diagnosing the rare life-threatening case of botulism and the unusual fish toxin–mediated syndromes such as ciguatera poisoning (see Chapter 16). Other important systemic symptoms include signs of cholinergic excess in ingestion of a cholinesterase inhibitor insecticide or anticholinergic symptoms resulting from ingesting mushrooms containing ibotenic acid and muscimol. Symptoms of histamine excess occur in scombroid fish poisoning, and cutaneous burning and tightness is seen with monosodium glutamate ingestion in the Chinese restaurant syndrome.

The specific pathogenic mechanism by which these agents produce disease helps explain the difference in incubation periods observed with different foodborne diseases. Foodborne bacterial disease is often toxin mediated. Toxins may be preformed in the food before ingestion or produced *in vivo* as the result of replication of the bacteria in the gastrointestinal tract. Foodborne illness caused by preformed toxins (*S. aureus* and some *B. cereus*) results in a short incubation illness with the rapid onset of toxin-mediated symptoms such as vomiting. In contrast, toxins that are produced by bacteria in the gastrointestinal tract, such as *C. perfringens* and long incubation *B. cereus*, result in a longer incubation period. These toxins typically result in noninflammatory, watery diarrhea without evidence of tissue invasion or fecal leukocytes. Organisms capable of tissue invasion include *Salmonella*, *Shigella*, invasive *E. coli*, and *Campylobacter*. Diseases resulting from these agents exhibit even longer incubation periods and produce inflammatory colitis.

Acute Upper Gastrointestinal Symptoms: Nausea, Vomiting within 0 to 6 Hours

The occurrence of acute gastrointestinal symptoms within 1 to 6 hours after the ingestion of food suggests the presence of a preformed toxin or a chemical irritant. Both *S. aureus* and *B. cereus* produce toxin under conditions of improper food storage. The main noninfectious consideration with this presentation is direct chemical irritation of the gastric mucosa by heavy metals or other direct toxins such as fluoride ion. Acute gastrointestinal symptoms are rarely produced by direct invasion of the gastric mucosa by parasitic worms ingested in raw fish. The clinical features that these etiologies share in common include prominent nausea and vomiting. *S. aureus* and *B. cereus* syndromes can include headache but should not include any motor or sensory neurologic features.

Staphylococcal toxin-mediated disease is the prototype for preformed toxin-mediated acute gastrointestinal disease. Two conditions are necessary for staphylococcal food poisoning. First, food must be contaminated with an enterotoxin-producing strain of the bacteria. Second, suitable time and temperature conditions for growth of the organism and toxin production must be present. Cooking food contaminated with *S. aureus* kills the bacteria but does not destroy the heat-stable toxin that has been produced. The mechanism of action of staphylococcal enterotoxins is not completely understood but may include stimulation of interleukin-1, interferon, and tumor necrosis factor (105,106). Animal studies suggest that the enterotoxins produce the emetic response after stimulation of neural receptors and vagus and sympathetic nerves. In turn, these activate the vomiting center in the CNS (107,108). Individuals have varied sensitivity to staphylococcal enterotoxin, and, in an outbreak, symptoms may be present in only a portion of the population exposed to the same dose of toxin. However, when concentration of the toxin is high, the attack rate approaches 100%. The diarrhea is not due to stimulation of adenylate cyclase activity and may be due to inhibition of water and sodium absorption in the small intestine by the enterotoxin (109,110).

Outbreaks of *S. aureus* toxin-mediated gastrointestinal disease can potentially affect large numbers of individuals. The amount of toxin consumed affects the amount of time to onset and severity of symptoms. Symptoms begin with nausea. Severe abdominal cramps develop that are followed by forceful continuous vomiting at 5- to 20-minute intervals. Emesis may occasionally be blood-streaked and blood may be seen in the stool in rare severe cases. Diarrhea is seen in 77% of cases, is usually mild (111), and only rarely occurs in the absence of vomiting. Abdominal pain, if present, is moderate and diffuse and there is no tenesmus. Mild, transient headache and muscular cramps of the flexors of the legs as well as sweating are common. Fever is not characteristic but can occur in up to 23% of cases (111). Individuals may be quite disabled because of the extremely rapid onset of severe vomiting. Extreme vomiting has the potential to lead to severe metabolic alkalosis and, rarely, hypotension. Acute symptoms are self-limited, usually lasting 5 to 8 hours. Symptoms are almost completely resolved by 12 hours, although prostration may remain for up to 24 to 48 hours. Morbidity and mortality are limited to individuals at risk for severe dehydration, including children, the elderly, and those with severe underlying medical conditions.

The diagnosis of staphylococcal food poisoning is made on the basis of the characteristic clinical syndrome. More than 10^5 colony-forming units of *Staphylococcus* per gram of food may be cultured. If *Staphylococcus* is cultured from the vomitus or feces of affected individuals or if food handlers are involved, the phage type should be the same as that in the food. Immunologically based assays, including enzyme-linked immunosorbent assay for enterotoxin, can detect as little as 0.1 to 1.0 ng of toxin per gram of food and may be useful for diagnosis in cases where the organisms have been killed by food processing (112–114). Antimicrobial therapy is not indicated because a preformed toxin causes the illness.

B. cereus causes an emetic syndrome with a short 1- to 6-hour incubation period that is similar to that caused by *S. aureus*. In a small percentage of episodes, incubation periods that are shorter (15 to 30 minutes) or longer (6 to 12 hours) have been reported. Symptoms include vomiting (100%), abdominal cramps (100%), and, often, diarrhea (33% to 80%) (41,74,115–116). Fever is not associated with this syndrome. Recovery is usually rapid, taking from 6 to 24 hours, although affected individuals often seek medical care in emergency departments (117). Severe dehydration in infants, the elderly, or debilitated persons is a theoretical possibility, but rarely is hospitalization needed. The syndrome is probably due to a distinct enterotoxin different from that involved in the diarrheal form of *B. cereus* food poisoning. The toxin produces vomiting when fed to rhesus monkeys; however, the mechanism of action of the toxin is unknown (74,75). The diagnosis of outbreaks resulting from *B. cereus* infection can be documented by isolation of $>10^5$ organisms per gram of suspected food, but if the food was reheated before serving, the organism are eliminated without decreasing the activity of the heat-stable toxin (117). Organisms may be cultured from the vomitus or stool of affected individuals. Serotyping of *B. cereus* can be helpful in linking isolates to a common source, because 14% of individuals may be transiently colonized in their gastrointestinal tract (118). Plasmid analysis may also play a role in epidemiologic investigations (118). As in *S. aureus* foodborne disease, antimicrobial therapy is not indicated.

B. subtilis has also been implicated in a short incubation emetic syndrome. Vomiting is the major symptom, followed by diarrhea, which occurs in 50% of cases. Additional symptoms include headache (10%), flushing sensation, and sweating (69).

Heavy metal poisoning should be considered when the incubation period is less than 1 hour (8). In a report of zinc poisoning, illness onset occurred 5 minutes to 2 hours after ingestion of an acidic beverage that had been stored in a galvanized metal container (119). Zinc is a major constituent of galvanized metal and is converted to readily absorbable zinc salts on contact with acidic beverages. The emetic dose of zinc is 225 to 450 mg for adults, a level that can be achieved from storage in galvanized containers. Symptoms include nausea (approximately 80%), abdominal cramps (approximately 60%), metallic taste (approximately 33%), headache (approximately 33%), dizziness (approximately 20%), and chills (approximately 10%). Vomiting is less frequent with heavy metal poisoning than with bacterial toxin-mediated syndromes. Symptoms usually subside within 2 to 3 hours after emesis of the offending agent. In an outbreak of fluoride poisoning caused by faulty fluoridation in a municipal water plant, the median interval between consumption and vomiting was 7 minutes and the median duration of symptoms was 24 hours. Ninety percent of patients had nausea, 80% vomiting, 52% abdominal pain, and 23% diarrhea. Fluoride ingestion resulted in profound hyperkalemia and hypocalcemia, which may result in cardiac dysrhythmias and death (95). When chemical toxins are suspected, collecting urine samples for laboratory testing may be critical to making the diagnosis.

A major consideration in the differential diagnosis of these emetic syndromes is viral gastroenteritis. Viral gastroenteritis due to NLV shares many of the features of bacterial toxin-mediated disease. The sudden and widespread involvement in NLV outbreaks often suggests a common-source outbreak that can be related to a foodborne source of infection, although many isolated cases occur as well (47). In addition, the onset of illness due to NLV is abrupt with explosive vomiting, watery diarrhea, or both. Stools are loose and watery without blood, mucus, or fecal leukocytes. Associated symptoms include anorexia, nausea, abdominal cramping, malaise, headache, and myalgias. Fever may be present in as many as 40% of patients (120). There are important differences between NLV infection and bacterial toxin-mediated disease. The incubation period for NLV is longer, ranging from 10 to 51 hours, and the secondary attack rates are high, resulting in recognition of an ongoing community-wide illness. The diagnosis of viral outbreaks is significantly limited by the current laboratory techniques for detecting these infections. Symptoms of NLV last 1 to 5 days, unlike the short duration of vomiting in staphylococcal disease. Carbohydrate and fat malabsorption may occur and last for 2 to 3 weeks after the initial onset of the illness. The diagnosis of viral gastroenteritis has depended on detection of viral particles in fecal specimens by electron microscopy. New polymerase chain reaction–based assays have been developed and have been used successfully to investigate outbreaks (48,49). Samples need to be collected within 48 hours after onset of symptoms and should be stored without freezing.

Gastrointestinal symptoms can occur after the ingestion of raw fish containing nematode larvae from the anisakis or eustrongylides family (15,16). Infection may localize acutely in the stomach or may be delayed with small intestine disease. In acute gastric anisakiasis, severe epigastric pain, nausea, and vomiting occur 1 to 12 hours after the ingestion of raw infected fish. Frequently, the episode terminates when the worm is regurgitated. The worm can be visualized and removed during fiberoptic endoscopy. Occasionally, invasion of the gastric mucosa occurs, which has been reported to cause perforation of the stomach or intestine. Invasion may also result in chronic gastrointestinal symptoms with a granulomatous response in the gastric mucosa.

Many types of mushrooms cause nonspecific gastrointestinal symptoms of nausea, vomiting, diarrhea, and abdominal cramping. In benign mushroom poisoning, the onset of symptoms ranges from a few minutes to 2 to 3 hours. The early onset distinguishes benign mushroom poisoning from the late-onset gastrointestinal symptoms that accompany the more serious mushroom poisoning syndromes. The onset of gastrointestinal symptoms is 6 to 12 hours in poisonings resulting from to amatoxins or monomethylhydrazine-containing mushrooms. These gastrointestinal symptoms subside before the onset of life-threatening hepatic or renal disease in the second phase of these syndromes. Ingestion of mushrooms often involves multiple species, making the presence of early symptoms an unreliable indicator of a benign course.

Upper Small Bowel Symptoms: Noninflammatory Watery Diarrhea within 8 to 16 Hours

The onset of abdominal cramps and diarrhea within 8 to 16 hours after food ingestion suggests toxin-mediated disease caused by *C. perfringens* or *B. cereus* infection. The toxins produced by these organisms are heat-labile proteins that cause intestinal fluid secretion. The toxins are produced *in vivo*, accounting for the longer incubation period compared with that seen with preformed toxins associated with *S. aureus* and the *B. cereus* emetic syndrome. Vomiting is not a prominent feature of these toxins, and the presence of vomiting in more than one third of affected patients should suggest that these organisms are not involved. The diarrhea in this syndrome is typically noninflammatory and is usually accompanied by abdominal cramping and nausea. This is in contrast to the inflammatory diarrhea and fever that are often seen with invasive pathogens such as *Salmonella, Shigella,* and *Campylobacter.*

The usual symptoms of foodborne disease caused by *C. perfringens* pathogens include severe abdominal cramps and diarrhea (67). Vomiting is unusual in these cases (69). The symptoms are due to toxin-mediated secretion of sodium and fluid and inhibition of chloride and glucose absorption throughout the small intestine (121,122). The enterotoxin is destroyed at 60°C after 10 minutes (123). The diagnosis of disease resulting from *C. perfringens* infection is difficult because more than 50% of healthy individuals have the organism in their bowels and antibody to the enterotoxin in their serum. In addition, serotyping is not generally available. Etiologic confirmation is provided by finding 10^6 *C. perfringens* spores per gram of feces in samples from two or more ill persons or 10^5 organisms per gram of epidemiologically implicated food. Demonstration of enterotoxin in the stool or a fourfold increase in antitoxin serum titers by reverse passive hemagglutination may be helpful (124).

B. cereus causes a diarrheal syndrome distinct from the emetic syndrome described earlier. The duration of illness is usually less than 24 hours, but has been reported to last several days in at least one outbreak (117). *B. cereus* causes a diarrheal syndrome very similar to that of *C. perfringens.* Vomiting is seen in up to 30% of cases. This syndrome is due to a 50,000-kd heat-labile protein that activates intestinal adenylate cyclase and results in ileal fluid secretion (76). This toxin may also have cytotoxic activity in rabbit small intestine and guinea pig skin (76). The diagnosis of diarrheal illness caused by *B. cereus* infection is based on culturing the organism from the stools of two or more ill persons and not from the stool of control subjects, or by isolation of 10^5 organisms per gram of implicated food.

The differential diagnosis of noninflammatory diarrhea includes infection with other infectious agents, ingestion of mushrooms and other toxins, and primary gastrointestinal disorders. Many of these disorders, including infections with enterotoxigenic *E. coli* and viral agents, are difficult to diagnose without specialized laboratory facilities (125). Bacterial pathogens to consider include enterotoxigenic *E. coli, V. parahaemolyticus,* and, occasionally, *Campylobacter jejuni, Salmonella,* and *Shigella.* These organisms typically have a median incubation period of 1 to 3 days, which is longer than that seen with *B. cereus* and *C. perfringens.* Shorter incubation periods are seen, however, presenting some potential for confusing these syndromes (125). The symptoms are similar, consisting of abdominal cramps and watery diarrhea and the absence of fever and vomiting. In contrast to infection with *B. cereus* and *C. perfringens,* illness caused by *E. coli* often lasts for 72 to 96 hours, which distinguishes these organisms. Viral gastroenteritis can mimic these syndromes, although vomiting is usually prominent and the occurrence of secondary cases in persons not exposed to the suspected food is an important clue. Mushroom poisoning resulting from infection with *Amanita* species manifests with a biphasic disease that begins with self-limited abdominal cramps and diarrhea for less than 24 hours. This is followed by hepatic and renal failure 1 to 2 days later, which has a mortality rate of 30% to 50%.

Inflammatory or Bloody Diarrhea within 16 or More Hours

Organisms causing inflammatory or bloody diarrhea include *Salmonella, Shigella, C. jejuni, V. parahaemolyticus, Yersinia enterocolitica*, and invasive *E. coli.* Fever, abdominal cramps, and inflammatory diarrhea with fecal leukocytes and fecal blood are common with these organisms. The illnesses last 2 to 7 days and vomiting occurs in 35% to 80% of cases. *Y. enterocolitica* is a common cause of foodborne disease in northern Europe and Canada and is notable for causing a syndrome of abdominal pain and fever resembling acute appendicitis (see Chapter 45).

Hemorrhagic colitis, sometimes complicated by hemolytic uremic syndrome, has been traced to infection with *E. coli* O157:H7 and other Shiga toxin–producing *E. coli* (see Chapter 42) (12,126). These organisms can produce watery diarrhea or frankly bloody diarrhea, without signs of inflammation. Fever is typically absent, and few white cells are present in stools.

Neurologic or Systemic Symptoms with or without Gastrointestinal Symptoms

Recognition of the occurrence of neurologic symptoms is critically important when evaluating possible food poisoning episodes. Important diseases that manifest with neurologic symptoms include botulism, several distinct fish- and shellfish-related syndromes, several types of mushroom poisoning, and chemical and pesticide poisoning. Muscular symptoms with eosinophilia should alert one to the possibility of trichinosis.

Mushroom-associated syndromes include several defined syndromes with characteristic systemic features. Cyclopeptides found in *Amanita* mushrooms interfere with RNA metabolism and cause hepatic and renal necrosis, often requiring eventual transplantation. Mushrooms containing ibotenic acid and muscimol mimic alcohol intoxication. Species containing muscarine cause parasympathetic symptoms. Hallucinogenic mushrooms containing psilocybin and psilocin cause acute psychotic reactions with hallucinations and inappropriate behavior. Coprinus mushrooms contain a disulfiram-like substance that causes an Antabuse-like reaction after ingestion of alcohol. *Gyromitra* species contain methylhydrazine, which may result in hepatic dysfunction, hemolysis, seizures, and coma. The treatment of mushroom poisoning is based on limited data and differs depending on the type of mushroom ingested (37).

The acute onset of abdominal pain, nausea, vomiting, and diarrhea in conjunction with peripheral and CNS symptoms and skeletal muscle symptoms should suggest the ingestion of a cholinesterase inhibitor (91). Symptoms of cholinergic excess can occur within 5 minutes of ingestion and include profuse sweating and salivation, blurred vision, pinpoint pupils, and excessive tearing. Muscle fasciculations and weakness, bradycardia and seizures, disorientation, and excitement also can occur. Both carbamate and organophosphate pesticides can cause this syndrome; however, because carbamates are reversible inhibitors of cholinesterases, poisoning with these compounds is less severe. Treatment is with atropine and supportive therapy.

The Chinese restaurant syndrome manifests with a burning in the neck, chest, abdomen, or arms and a sense of tightness over the face and chest. Headache, flushing, diaphoresis, lacrimation, nausea, abdominal cramps, and thirst also frequently occur (127). Symptoms are often due to ingestion of MSG in won ton soup when it is eaten on an empty stomach.

The differential diagnosis of foodborne illness with neurologic symptoms includes several fish and shellfish toxin syndromes and botulism. A history of fish ingestion should suggest either histamine fish poisoning or ciguatera fish poisoning. Shellfish may be associated with either a paralytic syndrome including paralysis and respiratory insufficiency or a neurotoxic syndrome without paralysis.

DIAGNOSTIC MEASURES AND EPIDEMIOLOGIC ASSESSMENT

The diagnosis of foodborne illness can be important in establishing an etiology and devising a therapeutic plan for a patient as well as for public health surveillance of an outbreak. Diagnostic tests available for each etiologic agent are listed in Table 15.4. The diagnostic approach to an individual patient may consider both the importance of establishing a definitive diagnosis and the cost of the evaluation (130). Ordering stool cultures and stool ova and parasite examinations only for selected patients, especially those with prolonged or inflammatory symptoms, can reduce the cost of the evaluation significantly. When a specific diagnosis of foodborne illness is sought, the clinician must anticipate that some diagnostic tests will not be routinely available. Tests that are not usually routine but that must be specifically requested include those used for identification of pathogenic *E. coli, C. perfringens, Vibrio* species, *Yersinia* species, NLVs, *Cryptosporidium* species, *C. cayetanensis,* and most bacterial, plant, or animal toxins. Consultation with local experts in the hospital or health department may be helpful in facilitating the evaluation.

Foodborne disease outbreaks are investigated by public health officials at the local, state, and federal levels, depending on availability of resources and expertise. CDC recently designed a Web-based training guide on foodborne disease outbreak investigations to aid public health practitioners (*http://www.phppo.cdc.gov/phtn/casestudies/*). Once investigated, health officials report foodborne disease outbreaks to CDC through the Foodborne Disease Outbreak Surveillance System. Surveillance for foodborne disease outbreaks serves three main purposes: disease prevention and control, knowledge of disease causation, and administrative guidance for food protection and public health programs (8).

TABLE 15.4. DIAGNOSIS OF FOODBORNE ILLNESS

Etiologic Agent	Patient-Based Test	Food
Bacterial		
Bacillus cereus	Culture stool, vomitus	Culture 10^5 organisms/g
Brucella	Culture blood, bone marrow; serology	
Campylobacter	Culture stool	Culture
Clostridium botulium	Culture stool, vomitus Toxin serum, stool, gastric contents[a]	Toxin[a]
Clostridium perfringens	Culture stool, >10^5 organisms/g Enterotoxin stool	Culture >10^5 organisms/g
Escherichia coli	Culture stool; toxin serum, stool	
Listeria monocytogenes	Culture sterile site	Culture
Salmonella	Culture stool, blood, CFS, urine	Culture
Shigella	Culture stool	Culture
Staphylococcus aureus	Culture stool, vomitus	Enterotoxin; culture >10^5 organisms/g
Streptococcus, group A	Culture throat	Culture
Vibrio cholerae	Culture stool, vomitus	Culture
Vibrio parahaemolyticus	Culture stool	Culture 10^5 organisms/g
Yersinia enterocoliticus	Culture	Culture
Chemical		
Ciguatoxin	Clinical syndrome	Ciguatoxin in fish[a]
Heavy metals	Clinical syndrome	High concentration of metal[a]
Monosodium glutamate	Clinical syndrome	
Mushroom poisoning	Clinical syndrome	Toxin in mushroom[a]
Paralytic shellfish poisoning	Clinical syndrome	Toxin,[a], dinoflagellates in water[a]
Puffer fish, tetrodotoxin	Clinical syndrome	Tetrodotoxin in fish[a]
Scrobotoxin	Clinical syndrome	Histamine in fish[a]
Parasitic		
Giardia intestinalis	Antigen in stool; organism in stool, duodenal contents or small-bowel biopsy	
Trichinella spiralis	Serology;[a] larvae in muscle biopsy	
Cryptosporidium	Acid-fast stain stool; FA; antigen in stool	
Anasakiasis	Gastroscopy	
Viral		
Hepatitis A	IgM anti-Hep A in serum	
Norwalk-like viruses	RT-PCR stool, vomitus;[a] immune electron microscopy;[a] >4-fold increase in antibody titer[a]	
Astrovirus	Enzyme immunoassay;[a] RT-PCR stool, vomitus;[a] electron microscopy[a]	

[a]Test may not be routinely available in some laboratories
CFS, cerebrospinal fluid

MANAGEMENT

Management of foodborne disease is based on recognizing that the majority of illnesses are self-limited and therapy is nonspecific and supportive (129). Initial management focuses on rehydration while identifying those cases requiring urgent diagnosis and intervention because of the potential for serious neurologic or systemic involvement (Fig. 15.1). For low-risk patients with isolated gastrointestinal disease, management is based on the expectation of rapid recovery. Treatment is directed at replacing gastrointestinal fluid losses with oral or parenteral electrolyte solutions. When toxin ingestion is recognized early, emesis may be induced if it has not occurred spontaneously. Antiemetics are contraindicated because they may allow further systemic absorption. Antiperistaltic agents should be avoided for patients with fever or fecal leukocytes, which suggest the presence of an invasive pathogen. The majority of the acute gastrointestinal illnesses discussed in this chapter resolve within 12 to 24 hours. The clinical course is not shortened by antibiotic therapy, and rarely do these illnesses result in significant morbidity or mortality. The diagnosis in these patients with self-limited illness can be inferred from the clinical presentation (Table 15.3). Identification of a specific etiology is usually not necessary for the management of individual patients. In contrast, diagnostic evaluation is indicated for patients who have either symptoms for more than 1 to 2 days' duration, severe dehydration, fever, bloody diarrhea, or unexplained abdominal pain or weight loss. For these patients, further evaluation may identify a bacterial or par-

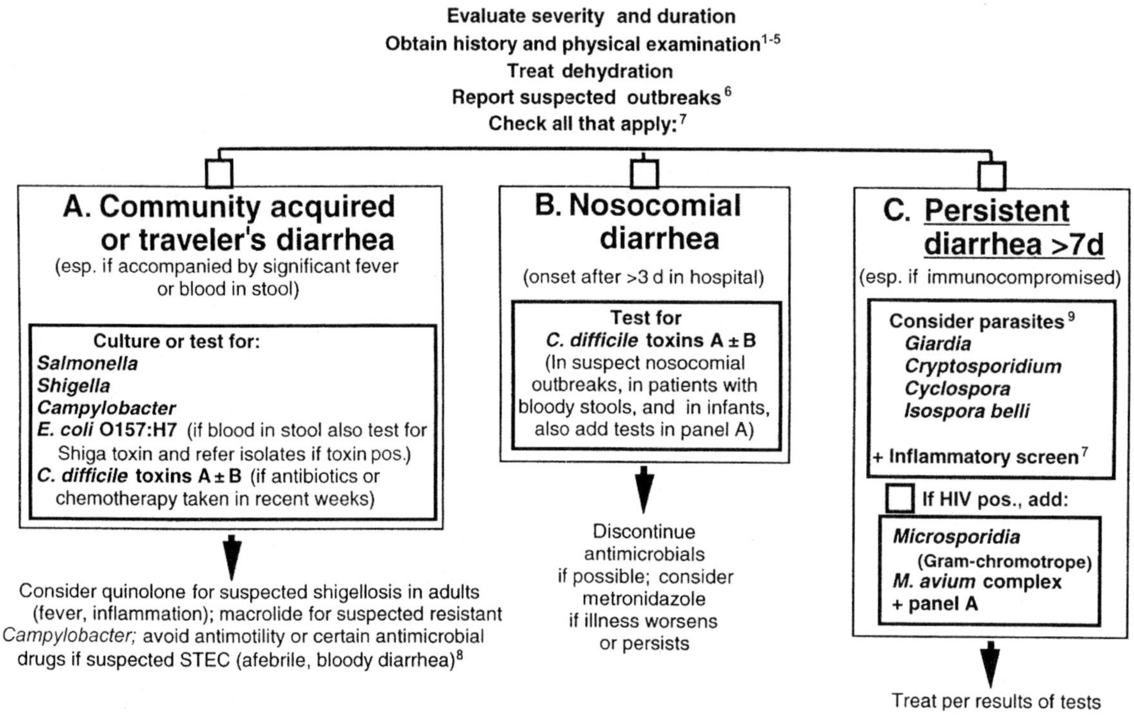

FIGURE 15.1. Recommendations for the diagnosis and management of diarrheal illnesses. Pos., positive. *1* Seafood or seacoast exposure should prompt culture for *Vibrio* species. *2* Traveler's diarrheal illnesses that have not responded to empirical therapy with a quinolone or trimethoprim-sulfamethoxazole should be managed with the above approach. *3* Persistent abdominal pain and fever should prompt culture for *Yersinia enterocolitica* and cold enrichment. Right-side abdominal pain without high fever but with bloody or non-bloody diarrhea should prompt culture for *Shiga* toxin-producing *Escherichia coli* (STEC) O157. *4* Proctitis in symptomatic homosexual men can be diagnosed with sigmoidoscopy. Involvement in only the distal 15 cm suggests herpesvirus, gonococcal, chlamydial, or syphilitic infection; colitis extending more proximally suggests *Campylobacter*, *Shigella*, *Clostridium difficile*, or chlamydial (LGV serotype) infection, and noninflammatory diarrhea suggests giardiasis. *5* Post diarrheal hemolytic uremic syndrome (HUS) should prompt testing of stools for STEC O157 and for *Shiga* toxin (send isolates to reference laboratory if toxin-positive but STEC-negative). *6* Outbreaks should prompt reporting to health department. Consider saving culture plates and isolates and freeze whole stools or swabs at -70°C. *7* Fecal lactoferrin testing or microscopy for leukocytes can help document inflammation, which is often present in invasive colitis with *Salmonella*, *Shigella*, or *Campylobacter*, with more severe *C. difficile* colitis, and with inflammatory bowel disease. *8* Some experts recommend avoiding administration of antimicrobial agents to persons in the United States with bloody diarrhea. *9* Commonly used tests for parasitic causes of diarrhea include fluorescence and EIA for *Giardia* and *Cryptosporidium*; acid-fast stains for *Cryptosporidium*, *Cyclospora*, *Isospora*, or *Mycobacterium* species (as well as culture for *Mycobacterium* avium complex); and special chromotrope or other stains for microsporidia.

asitic agent that requires antimicrobial therapy. Even so, most patients with prolonged symptoms have benign and self-limited viral or bacterial disease for which antimicrobial agents are not indicated. The possibility that Shiga toxin–producing *E. coli* infections may be made worse by antibiotic therapy should be considered before beginning empirical therapy of bloody diarrheal illness, especially if there is no fever.

PREVENTION

Foodborne diseases are largely preventable through the practice of proper food hygiene in combination with laws governing domestic and imported foods (129). In most outbreaks caused by bacterial pathogens such as staphylococci, *B. cereus,* and *C. perfringens,* the disease occurred because food was stored at improper holding temperatures. Growth of pathogens can be prevented if cold food is cooled rapidly and kept adequately refrigerated (<40°F) and if hot food is held at temperatures greater than 140°F before serving (54). Poor personal hygiene of food handlers also plays a role in bacterial as well as NLV and hepatitis A outbreaks. Cooking of food before serving eliminates the risk of disease for some agents, but not for staphylococcal toxins and disease caused by other organisms capable of producing heat-stable toxins. Inadequate cooking is usually an important factor in outbreaks of trichinosis and shellfish-borne disease. Shellfish meat should be heated to a temperature of 85°C to 90°C for 1.5 minutes in order to inactivate hepatitis A and other viruses (130). Contamination of food after cooking may result from poor food handling practices. Chlorine-based compounds should be used to disinfect contaminated cooking surfaces.

Investigations of outbreaks suggest that food handlers may be unaware of even the most common hazards associated with foodborne disease such as fried rice (40). Outbreaks of potential hepatitis A need to be investigated rapidly to allow early administration of immunoglobulin to exposed individuals, including other food handlers (1). High-risk patients, such as patients with liver cirrhosis and immunocompromised individuals, should be aware that foods such as raw oysters present a risk of fatal septicemia caused by *Vibrio vulnificus;* however, fewer than 15% of high-risk patients are aware of the risks associated with raw oyster consumption (20). These findings emphasize the need for education about basic practices for safe food handling and consumption.

Selection of foods plays an increasingly important role in preventing foodborne disease because food is transported worldwide and exotic foods are increasingly consumed. Raw or undercooked foods including milk, poultry, beef, pork, shellfish, fish, and eggs are important sources of foodborne pathogens. Application of polluted water or sewage sludge to fruit and vegetable crops can lead to transmission of bacterial, parasitic, and viral agents. Many foodborne illnesses can be prevented by good agricultural practices, careful slaughter hygiene, and sanitary preparation. For some foods, additional critical processing steps are needed such as pasteurization of milk and juice, high temperature canning, and irradiation of meat and poultry. Expertise in identification of safe food sources is necessary to prevent outbreaks of ciguatera and mushroom poisoning. Many chemical food poisonings result from use of defective storage containers, introduction of insecticides and other compounds into foods, or contamination of water supplies. Cysts of *G. intestinalis* and *C. parvum* are chlorine-resistant and require highly effective filtration to prevent their spread. Because suspected foodborne or waterborne illnesses may represent a threat to large numbers of people, these outbreaks should be recognized and promptly reported to local and state health departments and CDC.

REFERENCES

1. Centers for Disease Control and Prevention. Prevention of hepatitis A through active or passive immunization: recommendations of the advisory committee on immunization practices (ACIP). *MMWR Morb Mortal Wkly Rep* 1999;48:1–37.
2. Koff RS. Hepatitis A. *Lancet* 1998;341:1643–1649.
3. Wise RI. Brucellosis in the United States—past, present, and future. *JAMA* 1980;244:2318–2322.
4. Schuchat A, Swaminathan B, Broome CV. Epidemiology of human listeriosis. *Clin Microbiol Rev* 1991;4:169–183.
5. Slutsker L, Schuchat A. Listeriosis in humans. In: Ryser ET, Marth EH, eds. *Listeria, listeriosis, and food safety.* New York: Marcel Dekker, 1999:75–95.
6. Hughes JM, Blumenthal JR, Merson MH, et al: Clinical features of types A and B food-borne botulism. *Ann Intern Med* 1981;95:442–445.
7. Ishizuka T, Ishizuka A. A case of diphyllobothriasis due to eating masou-sushi. *Med J Aust* 1986;145:114.
8. Olsen SJ, MacKinnon LC, Goulding JS, et al. Surveillance for foodborne-disease outbreaks—United States, 1993-1997. *MMWR Morb Mortal Wkly Rep CDC Surveillance Summaries* 2000;49(No. SS-1):1–63.
9. Mead PS, Slutsker L, Dietz V, et al. Food-related illness and death in the United States. *Emerg Infect Dis* 1999;5:607–625.
10. Barwick RS, Levy DA, Craun GF, et al. Surveillance for waterborne-disease outbreaks—United States, 1997-1998. *MMWR Morb Mortal Wkly Rep CDC Surveillance Summaries* 2000; 49(No. SS-4):1–21.
11. Choi WY, Nam HW, Kwak NH, et al. Foodborne outbreaks of human toxoplasmosis. J Infect Dis 1997;175:1280–1282.
12. Riley LW, Remis RS, Helgerson SD, et al. Hemorrhagic colitis associated with a rare *Escherichia coli* serotype. *N Engl J Med* 1983;308:681–685.
13. Mead PS, Griffin PM. *Escherichia coli* 0157:H7. *Lancet* 1998;352:1207–1212.
14. Bailey TM, Schantz PM. Trichinosis surveillance, 1985. *MMWR Morb Mortal Wkly Rep* 1986;36(SS-2):1–5.
15. Wittner M, Turner JW, Jacquette G, et al. Eustrongylidiasis—a parasitic infection acquired by eating sushi. *N Engl J Med* 1989; 320:1124–1126.
16. Schantz PM. The dangers of eating raw fish. *N Engl J Med* 1989;320:1143–1145.

17. O'Mahony MC, Gooch CD, Smyth DA, et al. Epidemic hepatitis A from cockles. *Lancet* 1983;1:518–520.
18. Morse DI, Guzewich JJ, Hanrahan JP, et al. Widespread outbreaks of clam- and oyster-associated gastroenteritis. Role of Norwalk virus. *N Engl J Med* 1986;314:678–681.
19. Appleton H, Pereira MS. A possible virus aetiology in outbreaks of food poisoning from cockles. *Lancet* 1977;1:780–781.
20. Centers for Disease Control and Prevention. *Vibrio vulnificus* infections associated with raw oyster consumption—Florida, 1981–1992. *MMWR Morb Mortal Wkly Rep* 1993;42: 405–407.
21. Wilson R, Lieb S, Roberts A, et al. Non-O group 1 *Vibrio cholerae* gastroenteritis associated with eating raw oysters. *Am J Epidemiol* 1981;114:293–298.
22. Blake P, Merson H, Weaver R, et al. Disease caused by a marine vibrio. *N Engl J Med* 1979;300:1–4.
23. Centers for Disease Control and Prevention. Isolation of *Vibrio cholerae* O1 from oysters—Mobile Bay, 1991-1992. *MMWR Morb Mortal Wkly Rep* 1993;42:91–93.
24. Rippey SR. Infectious diseases associated with molluscan shellfish consumption. *Clin Microbiol Rev* 1994;7:419–425
25. Centers for Disease Control and Prevention. Outbreaks of *Shigella sonnei* infection associated with eating fresh parsley—United States and Canada, July-August 1998. *MMWR Morb Mortal Wkly Rep* 1999;48:285–289.
26. Taormina PJ, Beuchat LR, Slutsker L. Infections associated with eating seed sprouts: an international concern. *Emerg Infect Dis* 1999;5:626–634.
27. Eastaugh J, Shepherd S. Infectious and toxic syndromes from fish and shellfish consumption. *Arch Intern Med* 1989;149: 1735–1740.
28. Engleberg N, Morris J, Lewis J, et al. Ciguatera fish poisoning: a major common-source outbreak in the US Virgin Islands. *Ann Intern Med* 1983;98:336–337.
29. Frenette C, MacLean JD, Gyorkos TW. A large common-source outbreak of ciguatera fish poisoning. *J Infect Dis* 1988;158: 1128–1131.
30. Chretien J, Fermaglich J, Garagusi V. Ciguatera poisoning presentation as a neurological disorder. *Arch Neurol* 1981;15: 1225–1228.
31. Morrow JD, Margolies GR, Rowland J, et al. Evidence that histamine is the causative toxin of scombroid-fish poisoning. *N Engl J Med* 1991;324:716–720.
32. Kim R. Flushing syndrome due to mahimahi (scombroid fish) poisoning. *Arch Dermatol* 1979;115:963–965.
33. Etkind P, Wilson M, Gallagher K, et al. Bluefish-associated scombroid poisoning. *JAMA* 1987;258:3409–3410.
34. Sims J, Ostman D. Puffer fish poisoning: emergency diagnosis and management of mild human tetrodotoxication. *Ann Emerg Med* 1986;15:1094–1098.
35. Popkiss M, Horstman D, Harpur D. Paralytic shellfish poisoning: a report of 17 cases in Capetown. *South Afr Med J* 1979; 55:1017–1022.
36. Acres J, Gray J. Paralytic shellfish poisoning. *Can Med Assoc J* 1978;119:1195–1197.
37. Anonymous. Mushroom poisoning. *Med Lett Drug Ther* 1984; 26:67–69.
38. Centers for Disease Control. Water hemlock poisoning—Maine, 1992. *MMWR Morb Mortal Wkly Rep* 1994;43:229–231.
39. Litovitz TL. 1992 annual report of the American Association of Poison Control Centers Toxic Exposure Surveillance System. *Am J Emerg Med* 1993;11:494–555.
40. Centers for Disease Control and Prevention. *Bacillus cereus* food poisoning associated with fried rice at two child day care centers—Virginia, 1993. *MMWR Morb Mortal Wkly Rep* 1994;43: 177–178.
41. Mortimer PR, McCann G. Food-poisoning episodes associated with *Bacillus cereus* in fried rice. *Lancet* 1974;1:1043.
42. Centers for Disease Control and Prevention. Hepatitis E among U.S. travelers, 1989-1992. *MMWR Morb Mortal Wkly Rep* 1993;42:1–4.
43. Centers for Disease Control and Prevention. *Salmonella* surveillance: annual tabulation summary, 1997. Atlanta: US Department of Health and Human Services, CDC, 1998.
44. Todd E. Epidemiology of foodborne illness: North America. *Lancet* 1990;336:788–790.
45. Waites WM, Arbuthnott JP. Foodborne illness: an overview. *Lancet* 1990;336:722–725.
46. Appleton H. Small round viruses: classification and role in foodborne infections. In: Bock J, Whelan J, eds. *Novel diarrhoea viruses* (*CIBA Foundation Symposium* 128). Chichester: Wiley, 1987:108–125.
47. Hedberg CW, Osterholm MT. Outbreaks of food-borne and waterborne viral gastroenteritis. *Clin Microbiol Rev* 1993;6: 199–210.
48. Glass RI, Noel J, Ando T, et al. The epidemiology of enteric caliciviruses from humans: a reassessment using new diagnostics. *J Infect Dis* 2000;181:S254–S261.
49. Fankhauser RL, Noel JS, Monroe SS, et al. Molecular epidemiology of "Norwalk-like viruses" in outbreaks of gastroenteritis in the United States. *J Infect Dis* 1998;178:1571–1578.
50. Daniels NA, Bergmire-Sweat DA, Schwab KJ, et al. A foodborne outbreak of gastroenteritis associated with Norwalk-like viruses: first molecular traceback to deli sandwiches contaminated during preparation. *J Infect Dis* 2000;181:1467–1470.
51. Levine WC, Stephenson WT, Craun GF. Waterborne disease outbreaks, 1986-1988. *MMWR Morb Mortal Wkly Rep* 1990;39(SS-1):1–13.
52. Holmberg SD, Blake PA. Staphylococcal food poisoning in the United States. New facts and old misconceptions. *JAMA* 1984;251:487–489.
53. Bean NH, Griffin PM. Foodborne disease outbreaks in the United States, 1973-1987: pathogens, vehicles, and trends. *J Food Protect* 1990;53:804–817.
54. Tranter HS. Foodborne staphylococcal illness. *Lancet* 1990; 336:1044–1046.
55. Breckinridge JC, Bergdoll MS. Outbreak of foodborne gastroenteritis due to a coagulase-negative enterotoxin-producing staphylococcus. *N Engl J Med* 1971;284:541.
56. Centers for Disease Control. Multiple outbreaks of staphylococcal food poisoning caused by canned mushrooms. *MMWR Morb Mortal Wkly Rep* 1989;38:417–418.
57. dos Santos EC, Genigeorgis C, Farver TB. Prevalence of *Staphylococcus aureus* in raw and pasteurized milk used for commercial manufacturing of Brazilian Minas cheese. *J Food Protect* 1981; 44:172–176.
58. Merson MH. The epidemiology of staphylococcal foodborne disease. *Proceedings of the Staphylococcus in Foods Conference.* University Park, PA: Pennsylvania State University; 1973:20.
59. Marrack P, Kappler J. The staphylococcal enterotoxins and their relatives. *Science* 1990;248:705–711.
60. Bergdoll MS. *Staphylococcus aureus.* In: Doyle MP, ed. *Bacterial foodborne pathogens.* New York: Marcel Dekker; 1989:464–523.
61. Tatini Sr. Thermal stability of enterotoxins in food. *J Milk Food Technol* 1976;39:432–438.
62. Schwabe M, Notermans S, Boot R, et al. Inactivation of staphylococcal enterotoxins by heat and reactivation by high pH treatment. *Int Food Microbiol* 1990;10:33–42.
63. Spero L, Morlock BA. Biological activities of the peptides of staphylococcal enterotoxin C formed by limited tryptic hydrolysis. *J Biol Chem* 1978;253:8787–8791.
64. Stelma GN, Bergdoll MS. Inactivation of staphylococcal

enterotoxin A by chemical modification. *Biochem Biophys Res Commun* 1982;105:121–126.
65. Scheuber PH, Golecki JR, Kickhofen F, et al. Skin reactivity of unsensitized monkeys upon challenge with staphylococcal enterotoxin B: a new approach for investigating the site of toxic action. *Infect Immun* 1985;50:869–876.
66. De Saxe M, Coe AW, Wieneke AA. The use of phage typing in the investigation of food poisoning caused by *Staphylococcus aureus* enterotoxins. *Soc Appl Bacteriol Tech Ser* 1982;17:173–197.
67. Shandera WX, Tacket CO, Blake PA. Food poisoning due to *Clostridium perfringens* in the United States. *J Infect Dis* 1983; 147:167.
68. Murrell TG, Walker PD. The pigbel story of Papua New Guinea. *Trans R Soc Trop Med Hyg* 1991;85:119–122.
69. Lund BM. Foodborne disease due to *Bacillus* and *Clostridium* species. *Lancet* 1990;336:982–986.
70. Labbe R. *Clostridium perfringens.* In: Doyle MP, ed. *Foodborne bacterial pathogens.* New York: Marcel Dekker, 1989:191–234.
71. McClane B, Hanna P, Wnek A. *Clostridium perfringens* enterotoxin. *Microb Pathol* 1988;4:317–323.
72. Bowness P, Moss PA, Tranter H, et al. *Clostridium perfringens* enterotoxin is a superantigen reactive with human T cell receptors V beta 6.9 and V beta 22. *J Exp Med* 1992;176:893–896.
73. Loewenstein MS. Epidemiology of *Clostridium perfringens* food poisoning. *N Engl J Med* 1972;286:1026.
74. Terranova W, Blake PA. *Bacillus cereus* food poisoning. *N Engl J Med* 1978;298:143.
75. Turnbull PCB, Kramer JM, Jorgensen K. Properties and production characteristics of vomiting, diarrheal, and necrotizing toxins of *Bacillus cereus*. *Am J Clin Nutr* 1979;32:219.
76. Melling J, Capel BJ, Turnbull PCB, et al. Identification of a novel enterotoxigenic activity associated with *Bacillus cereus*. *J Clin Pathol* 1976;29:938.
77. Spira WM, Goepfert JM. Biological characteristics of an enterotoxin produced by *Bacillus cereus*. *Can J Microbiol* 1975;21: 1236–1246.
78. Morgan MRA, Fenwick GR. Natural foodborne toxicants. *Lancet* 1990;336:1492–1495.
79. Stoloff L. Carcinogenicity of aflatoxins. *Science* 1987;237: 1283–1284.
80. Furness BW, Beach MJ, Roberts JM. Giardiasis surveillance—United States, 1992-1997. *MMWR Morb Mortal Wkly Rep CDC Surveillance Summaries* 2000;49(SS-7):1–13.
81. Herwaldt BL. *Cyclospora cayetanensis:* A review, focusing on the outbreaks of cyclosporiasis in the 1990s. *Clin Infect Dis* 2000;31:1040–1057.
82. Juranek DD. Cryptosporidiosis: sources of infection and guidelines for prevention. *Clin Infect Dis* 1995;21:S57–S61.
83. Casemore DP. Foodborne protozoal infection. *Lancet* 1990; 336:1427–1432.
84. Smith JV, Rose JB. Waterborne cryptosporidiosis. *Parasitol Today* 1990;6:8–12.
85. Mac Kenzie WR, Hoxie NJ, Proctor ME, et al. A massive outbreak in Milwaukee of cryptosporidium infection transmitted through the public water supply. *N Engl J Med* 1994;331: 161–167.
86. Herwaldt BL, Ackers ML. An outbreak in 1996 of cyclosporiasis associated with imported raspberries. The Cyclospora Working Group. *N Engl J Med* 1997;336:1548–1556.
87. Quiroz ES, Bern C, MacArthur JR, et al. An outbreak of cryptosporidiosis linked to a foodhandler. *J Infect Dis* 2000;181: 695–700.
88. Osterholm MT, Forfang JC, Ristinen TL, et al. An outbreak of foodborne giardiasis. *N Engl J Med* 1981;304:24.
89. Petersen LR, Cartter ML, Hadler JL. A foodborne outbreak of *Giardia lamblia*. *J Infect Dis* 1988;157:846–848.
90. Huxtable RJ. The toxicology of alkaloids in foods and herbs. In Tu AT, ed. *Handbook of natural toxins, vol 7. Food Poisoning.* New York: Marcel Dekker, 1992:238–262.
91. Centers for Disease Control. Aldicarb food poisoning from contaminated melons—California. *MMWR Morb Mortal Wkly Rep* 1986;35:254–258.
92. Martinez-Navarro JF. Food poisoning related to consumption of illicit B-agonist in liver. *Lancet* 1989;336:1311.
93. Baker TD, Hafner WG. Cadmium poisoning from a refrigerator shelf used as an improvised barbecue grill. *Public Health Rep* 1961;76:543.
94. Semple AB, Parry WH, Phillips DE. Acute copper poisoning: an outbreak traced to contaminated water from a corroded geyser. *Lancet* 1960;2:700.
95. Gessner BD, Beller M, Middaugh JP, et al. Acute fluoride poisoning from a public water system. *N Engl J Med* 1994;330: 95–99.
96. Kibourne EM, Rigau-Perez JG, Heath CW Jr, et al. Clinical epidemiology of toxic-oil syndrome: manifestations of a new illness. *N Engl J Med* 1983;309:1408–1410.
97. Centers for Disease Control. Eosinophilia-myalgia syndrome—New Mexico. *MMWR Morb Mortal Wkly Rep* 1989;38:765–767.
98. Centers for Disease Control. Eosinophilia-myalgia syndrome and L-tryptophan-containing products—New Mexico, Minnesota, Oregon, and New York, 1989. *MMWR Morb Mortal Wkly Rep* 1989;38:785–788.
99. Centers for Disease Control. Update: eosinophilia-myalgia syndrome associated with ingestion of L-tryptophan—United States, through August 24, 1990. *MMWR Morb Mortal Wkly Rep* 1990;39:587–589.
100. Hughes J, Merson M. Fish and shellfish poisoning. *N Engl J Med* 1976;295:1117–1120.
101. Centers for Disease Control and Prevention. Jin Bu Huan toxicity in adults—Los Angeles, 1993. *MMWR Morb Mortal Wkly Rep* 1993;42:920–922.
102. Kingsbury JM. *Poisonous plants of the United States and Canada.* Englewood Cliffs, NJ: Prentice-Hall, 1964.
103. Litovitz TL. 1992 annual report of the American Association of Poison Control Centers Toxic exposure surveillance system. *Am J Emerg Med* 1993;11:494–555.
104. Hall AH, Spoerke DG, Rumack BH. Mushroom poisoning: identification, diagnosis, and treatment. *Pediatr Rev* 1987;8: 291–298.
105. Marrack P, Kappler J. The staphylococcal enterotoxins and their relatives. *Science* 1990;248:705–711.
106. Yaqoob M, McClelland P, Murray AE, et al. Staphylococcal enterotoxins A and C causing toxic shock syndrome. *J Infect* 1990;20:176–177.
107. Sugiyama H, Hayama T. Abdominal viscera as site of emetic action for staphylococcal enterotoxin in the monkey. *J Infect Dis* 1965;115:330.
108. Clark WG, Vanderhooft GF, Borison HL. Emetic effect of purified staphylococcal enterotoxin in cats. *Proc Soc Exp Biol Med* 1962;111:205.
109. Elias J, Shields R. Influence of staphylococcal enterotoxin on water and electrolyte transport in the small intestine. *Gut* 1976;17:527.
110. Beery JT, Taylor SL, Schlunz LR, et al. Effects of staphylococcal enterotoxin A on the rat gastrointestinal tract. *Infect Immun* 1984;44:234–240.
111. Feig M. Staphylococcal food poisoning. A report of two related outbreaks, and a discussion of the data presented. *Am J Public Health* 1950;40:279.
112. Tranter HS, Brehm RD. Production, purification and identification of the staphylococcal enterotoxins. *Soc Appl Bacteriol Symp Ser* 1990;19:109S–122S.

113. Fey H. Staphylococcal enterotoxins. In: Kohler RB, ed. *Antigen to diagnose bacterial infection,* vol 2. Boca Raton, FL: CRC Press, 1986:211–238.
114. Berry PR, Rodhouse JC, Wieneke AA, et al. Use of commercial kits for the detection of *Clostridium perfringens* and *Staphylococcus aureus* enterotoxins. *Soc Appl Bacteriol Tech* Ser 1987;24: 245–254.
115. Giannella RA, Brasile L. A hospital food-borne outbreak of diarrhea caused by *Bacillus cereus.* Clinical epidemiologic, and microbiologic studies. *J Infect Dis* 1979;139:366.
116. Midura T, Gerber M, Wood R, et al. Outbreak of food poisoning caused by *Bacillus cereus. Public Health Rep* 1970;85:45.
117. Centers for Disease Control. *Bacillus cereus*—Maine. *MMWR Morb Mortal Wkly Rep* 1986;35:408–410.
118. Ghosh AC. Prevalence of *Bacillus cereus* in the faeces of healthy adults. *J Hyg* 1978;80:233.
119. Centers for Disease Control. Illness associated with elevated levels of zinc in fruit punch—New Mexico. *MMWR Morb Mortal Wkly Rep* 1983;32:257–258.
120. Centers for Disease Control and Prevention. Multistate outbreak of viral gastroenteritis related to consumption of oysters—Louisiana, Maryland, Mississippi, and North Carolina, 1993. *MMWR Morb Mortal Wkly Rep* 1993;42:945–948.
121. McDonel JL, Duncan CL. Regional localization of activity of *Clostridium perfringens* type A enterotoxin in the rabbit ileum, jejunum and duodenum. *J Infect Dis* 1977;136:661.
122. McDonel JL. The molecular mode of action of *Clostridium perfringens* enterotoxin. *Am J Clin Nutr* 1979;32:210.
123. Stark RL, Duncan CL. Purification and biochemical properties of *Clostridium perfringens* type A enterotoxin. *Infect Immun* 1972;6:662.
124. Skjelkvale R, Uemura T. Detection of enterotoxin in faeces and anti-enterotoxin in serum after *Clostridium perfringens* food poisoning. *J Appl Bacteriol* 1977;42:355–358.
125. Dalton CB, Mintz ED, Wells JG, et al. Outbreaks of enterotoxigenic *Escherichia coli* infection in American adults: a clinical and epidemiologic profile. *Epidemiol Infect* 1999;123:9–16.
126. Centers for Disease Control and Prevention. Update: multistate outbreak of *Escherichia coli* O157:H7 infections from hamburgers—Western United States, 1992-1993. *MMWR Morb Mortal Wkly Rep* 1993;42:258–263.
127. Schaumburg HH, Byck R, Gerstl R, et al. Monosodium L-glutamate: its pharmacology and role in the Chinese restaurant syndrome. *Science* 1969;163:826.
128. Guerrant RL, Van Gilder T, Steiner TS, et al. Practice guidelines for the management of infectious diarrhea. *Clin Infect Dis* 2001;32:331–351.
129. Thompson P, Salsbury PA, Adams C, et al. US Food legislation. *Lancet* 1990;336:1557–1559.
130. Millard J, Appleton H, Parry JV. Studies on heat inactivation of hepatitis A virus with special reference to shellfish. *Epidemiol Infect* 1987;98:397–414.

16

NATURAL TOXINS ASSOCIATED WITH FISH AND SHELLFISH

J. GLENN MORRIS, JR.

Fish and shellfish can sometimes carry natural toxins or toxic substances that cause human disease (1–4). Ciguatera fish poisoning is the most common of these intoxications, causing a unique clinical syndrome characterized by a combination of gastrointestinal and neurologic symptoms (5–9); other syndromes include paralytic shellfish poisoning (PSP), neurotoxic shellfish poisoning, diarrhetic shellfish poisoning, and amnesic shellfish poisoning. In contrast to these entities, which are associated with toxins accumulated while fish or shellfish are alive, scombroid fish poisoning (10,11) results from mishandling of scombroid (tuna, mackerel, bonito) and related fish after capture. Bacterial decomposition of the fish leads to release of histamine, which, in turn, causes "histamine poisoning." Each of these clinical syndromes is considered in this chapter.

CIGUATERA FISH POISONING

Ciguatera fish poisoning is a clinical syndrome with characteristic gastrointestinal and neurologic symptoms that occur after the ingestion of tropical reef fish (5–9). The toxins that cause the syndrome originate in the dinoflagellate *Gambierdiscus toxicus* and other benthic algae that grow on reefs (12,13). Fish that eat the algae become toxic, and the effect is magnified through the food chain so that large predatory fish become the most toxic.

Pathogenesis

There appear to be multiple toxins responsible (either alone or in combination) for the clinical manifestations of ciguatera (13–19). These vary among geographic areas, among fish species, and across time (8). Vernoux and Lewis (15) have recently suggested adoption of a standard nomenclature: *CTX* is used to indicate toxins that accumulate in fish to levels likely to cause ciguatera symptoms in humans; a letter code is used to indicate source (**P**acific Ocean, **I**ndian Ocean, **A**tlantic Ocean, **C**aribbean Sea); and a numbering system is used to indicate the chronologic order of identification of the compound. Pacific ciguatoxins have been best characterized to date. P-CTX-1 (18) is a small, lipid-soluble polyether with a molecular weight of 1,112 and a molecular formula of $C_{60}H_{88}O_{19}$. Two other distinct but closely related toxins, P-CTX-2 and P-CTX-3 (16,19), have also been identified in ciguatoxic fish, together with a number of minor P-CTX congeners (8,9,18). Vernoux and Lewis (15) have identified toxic compounds present in Caribbean *Caranx latus*; these toxins, which differ from the Pacific family of ciguatoxins, were designated C-CTX-1 and C-CTX-2. Other toxins associated with ciguatera include scaritoxin, maitotoxin (20), and palytoxin (21).

While recognizing the diversity of toxins that may be present in ciguatoxic fish, there are certain general pathophysiologic responses that have been associated with ciguatera toxins and toxic fish extracts. The gastrointestinal symptoms (diarrhea) seen in patients with ciguatera appear to result from direct stimulation of mucosal ion transport, without accompanying damage to the intestinal mucosa. Extracts from toxic fish cause a striking increase in transepithelial electrical potential difference and short circuit current in Ussing chambers, with secretion apparently mediated by calcium (22). Neurologic symptoms appear to be related to the direct effect of toxin on mammalian nerves, associated with prolongation of sodium channel activation (18,23,24). Patients may have slowing of sensory conduction velocity and prolongation of the absolute refractory, relative refractory, and supernormal periods (25). In animal models, low doses of ciguatoxin cause mild hypotension and bradycardia. Higher doses give a biphasic response with an initial hypotension/bradycardia followed by hypertension/tachycardia; very high doses produce a phrenic nerve block with respiratory arrest (7).

J. G. Morris, Jr: Department of Epidemiology and Preventive Medicine, University of Maryland School of Medicine, Baltimore, Maryland

Epidemiology

Ciguatera-associated toxins, produced by dinoflagellates and algae on tropical reefs, are concentrated as they are passed up the food chain. More than 400 fish species are said to have the potential for becoming toxic (26). However, the risk of toxicity is greatest for carnivorous, predatory fish, such as barracuda (more than 70% of which may be toxic). Other fish that are commonly implicated in cases of ciguatera include amberjack (*Seriola* species), snappers (Lutjanidae), groupers (Serranidae), goatfish (Mullidae), and reef fish belonging to the family Carrangidae (1,27). Toxicity is associated with fish size; viscera also tend to have higher concentrations of toxin than fish flesh. The occurrence of toxic fish tends to be localized, but localization is not consistent and toxic fish may occur sporadically anywhere in a reef or island location (1,28,29). Data suggest that disruption of the reef environment by construction, military activities, storms, and the like, can result in an increase in the incidence of ciguatoxic fish, due presumably to increases in toxic dinoflagellate and algal populations (8,30–32). Worldwide coral bleaching is well documented, and there is a strong association between global warming and the bleaching and death of coral (8). Rougerie and Bagnis (33), working in Tahiti, have proposed a model in which reef disruptions/coral death result in seepages of nutrient-rich endo-upwelling interstitial waters (33); because these nutrients cannot be used by the stressed algal-coral ecosystem, they are taken up by epibenthic organisms such as *G. toxicus*, with a corresponding sharp increase in population density (and toxicity).

Ciguatera is a significant cause of morbidity in areas in which consumption of reef fish is common, including the Caribbean, southern Florida, Hawaii, the South Pacific, and Australia. The average incidence in the South Pacific from 1973 to 1983 was estimated in the range of 500 cases per 100,000 population per year (34), with some island groups having rates many times higher; the average incidence for 1960 to 1984 for the Gambier Archipelago was reported as 22,700 cases per 100,000 population per year (31). In a randomized, stratified community survey conducted in the U.S. Virgin Islands, the calculated incidence rate was 730 cases per 100,000 population per year (27). In Miami, on the edge of an endemic area, 129 cases of ciguatera were reported to the Dade County Health Department between 1972 and 1976, for an annual incidence of 5 cases per 100,000 population; the actual incidence was estimated to be 10 to 100 times this figure (i.e., 50 to 500 cases per 100,000 population per year) (35). In Reunion Island in the Indian Ocean, reported incidence between 1986 and 1994 was 7.8 cases per 100,000 population per year (36).

Clinical Features

Ciguatera fish poisoning is a clinical diagnosis based on a characteristic sequence of gastrointestinal and neurologic symptoms (5–7,28,35,37). As outlined in Table 16.1, gas-

TABLE 16.1. CLINICAL SYNDROMES ASSOCIATED WITH NATURAL TOXINS IN FISH AND SHELLFISH

Clinical Syndrome	Toxin Acquired before Harvest	Toxin Source	Most Common Fish	Clinical Presentation
Ciguatera fish poisoning	Yes	*Gambierdiscus toxicus*	Large, predacious reef fish, including barracuda, grouper amberjack, snapper	Initial gastrointestinal symptoms, followed by neurologic manifestations (paresthesias, pain and weakness in lower extremities)
Paralytic shellfish poisoning	Yes	*Alexandrium* species	Shellfish	Paresthesias, unsteady gait, difficulty swallowing, hypertension, respiratory paralysis
Neurotoxic shellfish poisoning	Yes	*Gymnodinium breve*	Shellfish	Paresthesias, gastrointestinal (GI) symptoms; respiratory symptoms may be triggered by aerosolization of toxin
Diarrhetic shellfish poisoning	Yes	*Dinophysis* species	Shellfish	GI symptoms
Amnesic shellfish poisoning	Yes	*Pseudo-nitzschia pungens*	Shellfish	GI symptoms, memory deficits, neuronal necrosis/loss
Scombroid fish poisoning	No	Associated with high levels of free histamine in fish flesh, related to bacterial decomposition	Fish in families Scombridae and Scomberesocidae (tuna, mackerel, skipjack, bonito) and some non-scombroid fish (mahi-mahi and others)	Perioral tingling and burning, facial flushing, GI symptoms, headache

trointestinal symptoms include diarrhea, vomiting, and abdominal pain and occur first, usually within 24 hours of eating an implicated fish. In severe cases, patients may also be hypotensive with a paradoxical bradycardia (6,28). These acute symptoms are accompanied or followed by neurologic manifestations, which may persist for weeks or months. Neurologic symptoms include pain and weakness in the lower extremities, a very characteristic symptom of patients in the Caribbean (6,28), and circumoral and peripheral paresthesias (Table 16.1). More bizarre symptoms such as temperature reversal (ice cream tastes hot, hot coffee seems cold) and "aching teeth" are frequently reported (5,6,35,38) and may prompt psychiatric referrals among physicians unacquainted with the disease. In severe cases, particularly in the South Pacific, neurologic symptoms may progress to coma and respiratory arrest within the first 24 hours of illness (39).

Toxicity can apparently be transmitted by breast milk (40) and by sexual intercourse (41). Maternal exposure at term may also result in symptoms in the newborn infant, although maternal intoxication during pregnancy does not appear to have a long-term effect on the fetus (42). Immunity does not occur after an initial intoxication; in contrast, intoxication may increase sensitivity to subsequent episodes of illness.

Within this general constellation of symptoms, the clinical syndrome may vary widely from patient to patient and from geographic area to geographic area. Variations in the symptom complex have also been associated with the type of fish eaten. In a Hawaiian study, circumoral paresthesias were reported in 75.7% of patients who had eaten *Ctenochaetus strigosus* (surgeon fish or kole), 68.4% of patients who had eaten *Seriola dumerili* (amberjack or kahala), and 28.4% of patients who had eaten *Caranx* species (ulua/papio or jack). Bradycardia, in contrast, was reported in 47.4% of patients who had eaten *S. dumerili,* but in only 5.3% of patients who had eaten *Caranx* species and in none of those who had consumed *S. dumerili* (43).

Although most patients recover completely within a few weeks, intermittent recrudescence of symptoms over a period of months to years can occur. These recrudescences can be triggered by a number of factors, including consumption of fish and alcohol (27). There is also a subset of patients who have long-term, chronic symptoms of fatigue and paresthesias that last for months or years. These symptoms can be severe, resulting in almost total disability. Development of chronicity is more likely in persons who had severe initial symptoms, a long interval to severe symptoms, or a long absolute duration of peak symptoms (37).

Diagnostic Measures

Ciguatera is a clinical diagnosis. There is no confirmatory test, such as a serologic assay, that establishes the diagnosis. Standard laboratory tests are usually within normal limits, although there is a report of elevated creatine phosphokinase (to 41,000 U/L) in one patient who ate fish containing palytoxin (21). As noted earlier, patients may have characteristic electrophysiologic findings (25).

Management

Intravenous mannitol (1 g/kg of 20% solution, infused over 45 minutes) may have a dramatic effect on acute symptoms of ciguatera fish poisoning, particularly in severe cases (39,44,45). Mannitol has the most pronounced effect on neurologic symptoms and may be life saving in severe cases that progressed to coma. Most of the data on mannitol have come from the South Pacific; efficacy of therapy may be less in other geographic areas, such as the Caribbean, because of the possible differences in the toxins responsible for the observed clinical syndromes.

Treatment of chronic manifestations is more difficult. In one small study (37), amitriptyline showed considerable benefit in two of nine patients and some benefit in an additional four patients. In this same study, tocainide demonstrated some benefit in three of four patients; the fourth reported worsening of symptoms. Benefit has also been reported with imipramine, nifedipine, and alprazolam. Mannitol outside of the acute setting does not appear to be of benefit, and there are no data to support the use of a variety of other proposed therapies, including vitamin B complex, ascorbic acid, and steroids (6,37). As is true for chronic pain syndromes, therapy in chronic cases needs to be individualized, with physician and patient working together to develop a rational, long-term plan of care.

Prevention

Ciguatoxic fish look and taste completely normal, and toxicity is not affected by cooking. Toxic fish have traditionally been identified by one of a number of bioassays, including feeding of suspect fish to the family cat (27). Hokama and colleagues (46,47) in Hawaii have developed a series of commercially available rapid ciguatera assays for toxic fish (Cigua-check, Oceanit Test Systems, Inc., Honolulu; www.cigua.com), and, in endemic areas, it may be possible to reduce the risk of illness by screening all large, "high-risk" fish before their consumption. However, these assays lack specificity, and questions have been raised about their utility in areas outside of Hawaii. In general, illness is best avoided by not eating large predacious reef fish; barracuda, in particular, should never be eaten. A household cat may also be useful.

PARALYTIC SHELLFISH POISONING

PSP results from eating bivalve molluscs (mussels, clams, oysters, scallops) that contain saxitoxins produced by *Alexandrium* species and other dinoflagellates (1–3,48). Saxitoxins (at least 12 of which have been identified) are thought to block the propagation of nerve and muscle action potentials by acting at the metal cation binding site in the sodium channels of the nerve membrane and interfering with changes in sodium permeability (48,49). The responsible dinoflagellates develop characteristic toxin profiles that usually contain six to eight saxitoxins; shellfish feeding on dinoflagellate blooms ingest all toxins but may selectively retain or biologically modify some derivatives.

PSP has been reported from both hemispheres, with cases concentrated in temperate coastal regions. In the United States, PSP is primarily a problem in New England, Alaska, California, and Washington (1–3,50,51). Blooms of the toxic dinoflagellates ("red tides") occur several times each year, primarily from April through October. It is currently not possible to predict occurrence of blooms. When blooms occur, shellfish become toxic and remain toxic for several weeks after the bloom subsides; in some instances, persistent toxicity may be observed (i.e., among butter clams in parts of Washington State and Alaska).

Symptoms of PSP are primarily neurologic (circumoral paresthesias and paresthesias of the hands and feet) and usually appear within an hour of eating toxic shellfish (50,51). In more severe illness, there may be unsteady gait, difficulty swallowing, and mental status changes. Hypertension may be seen, with blood pressure measurements corresponding with ingested toxin dose (52). In the most severe cases, respiratory paralysis occurs (generally within the first 24 hours of illness), leading to death if respiratory support is not available. In a retrospective review of PSP outbreaks occurring in Alaska between 1973 and 1992, a total of 29 (25%) of 117 ill persons required an emergency flight to a hospital, four (3%) required intubation, and one died (51). Recovery is complete, with symptoms usually resolving within hours to days after shellfish ingestion.

The diagnosis of PSP is based on clinical presentation and a history of having eaten potentially toxic shellfish immediately before onset of symptoms. Limited neurophysiologic data suggest that patients have prolonged distal motor and sensory latencies, slowed conduction velocities, and moderately diminished amplitudes, compatible with incomplete sodium channel blockade (53). On an experimental basis, it has been possible to demonstrate saxitoxins in serum during acute illness and in urine after acute symptom resolution (52). Measurement of toxicity in shellfish is based on a standard mouse bioassay. Alternative assays, such as a recently described receptor binding assay (54), are under active development. Treatment of PSP is symptomatic. In severe cases, it has been suggested that treatment should include administration of a cathartic, gastric lavage, or enema to remove unabsorbed toxin from the intestinal tract.

Prevention is based on avoiding shellfish harvested from areas known to be toxic or to have had recent dinoflagellate blooms. However, not all blooms are toxic, and toxicity can occur in the absence of a visible bloom. Surveillance of "high risk" harvest areas in the United States is routinely conducted by state health departments. Areas are closed to harvesting when toxin levels in shellfish exceed 80 μg/100 g, with warnings about toxic conditions posted in the media and at harvest sites (50). When cases occur, they are often associated with noncommercial harvesting of shellfish in closed areas.

NEUROTOXIC SHELLFISH POISONING

Neurotoxic shellfish poisoning is associated with blooms of *Gymnodinium breve,* which produce brevotoxin (1–3). Red tides caused by this organism occur sporadically in the Gulf of Mexico and off the coast of Florida; there has been at least one bloom with associated human illnesses reported from North Carolina (55). Symptoms after eating toxic shellfish include circumoral paresthesias and paresthesias of the extremities, dizziness and ataxia, muscle aches, and gastrointestinal symptoms, including nausea, abdominal pain, vomiting, and diarrhea. Respiratory symptoms have also been reported, associated with aerosolization of the toxin by wind and wave action (56).

DIARRHETIC SHELLFISH POISONING

Diarrhetic shellfish poisoning is caused by eating mussels, scallops, or clams that have been feeding on *Dinophysis fortii* or *Dinophysis acuminata* (1–3). In addition to diarrhea, symptoms of diarrhetic shellfish poisoning include nausea, vomiting, and abdominal pain. Okadaic acid and dinophysistoxin-1 have been implicated as the primary toxins responsible for the associated clinical syndrome (57,58). Cases are concentrated in Japan, with recent reports coming from Europe (59). No cases have been reported yet in the United States, although the organism has been identified in U.S. coastal waters (2,3).

AMNESIC SHELLFISH POISONING

Amnesic shellfish poisoning results from ingestion of shellfish containing domoic acid, produced by the diatom *Pseudo-nitzschia pungens* (2,3,60). A series of cases attributed to this toxin were reported in the Atlantic provinces of Canada in 1987. Symptoms included vomiting, abdominal cramps, diarrhea, headache, and loss of short-term memory (60). On neuropsychologic testing several months after the acute intoxication, patients were found to have severe anterograde memory deficits with relative preservation of other cognitive functions; patients also had clinical and electromyographic evidence of pure motor or sensorimotor neuropathy or axonopathy. Neuropathologic studies in four patients who died demonstrated neuronal necrosis and loss, predominantly in the hippocampus and amygdala (61). Canadian authorities analyze mussels and clams for domoic acid, and shellfish beds are closed to harvesting when levels exceed 20 μg/g (1).

Domoic acid has also been shown to be produced by *Pseudo-nitzschia* species, including *Pseudo-nitzschia australis, Pseudo-nitzschia multiseries,* and *Pseudo-nitzschia pungens,* on the west coast of the United States (3). In 1991, domoic acid was identified in razor clams and Dungeness crabs on the Oregon and Washington coast (3). There were anecdotal reports of associated human illness, although none were confirmed (59). Toxin-producing blooms have been documented from the Maine and Texas coasts, and low levels of domoic acid produced by *Pseudo-nitzschia pseudodelicatissima* have been reported from the Bay of Fundy and Danish and Norwegian waters (59). Even though no clear-cut human cases of amnesic shellfish poisoning have been identified outside of the original Canadian outbreaks, the clinical significance of ingestion of low levels of domoic acid (as may be occurring in persons eating shellfish and anchovies from areas where *Pseudo-nitzschia* is present) is unknown.

SCOMBROID FISH POISONING

Scombroid fish poisoning results from the eating of fish containing high levels of free histamine. The syndrome was initially associated with fish in the families Scombridae and Scomberesocidae (tuna, mackerel, skipjack, and bonito). However, nonscombroid fish, such as mahi mahi (dolphin), bluefish, and salmon, are commonly associated with illness (1,10,11,62–65).

In contrast to ciguatera and shellfish poisoning, which are caused by a preformed toxin derived from dinoflagellates or algae, scombroid is the result of bacterial decomposition of fish flesh after capture. Scombroid fish in particular contain substantial amounts of free histidine that can be decarboxylated to form histamine by enteric bacteria during spoilage (10,66). Illness may occur when free histamine levels exceed 20 mg/100 g of fish, levels that may be reached without overt evidence of spoilage. The U.S. Food and Drug Administration "action level" (i.e., the level at which further shipment or sale is prohibited) is 50 mg/100 g of fish. Controversy continues regarding the specific pathophysiologic mechanisms involved in the observed illness (10), with some recent suggestions that urocanic acid (like histamine, an imidazole compound derived from histidine in spoiling fish) contributes to the clinical syndrome (11). The number of reported outbreaks of scombroid fish poisoning in the United States approaches that of ciguatera (1). However, while ciguatera cases are concentrated in certain high-risk locations (i.e., areas with high levels of consumption of reef fish), scombroid tends to occur at low levels throughout the country.

Symptoms of scombroid fish poisoning typically occur within a few hours of eating the implicated fish and can last for up to 12 hours. Typical symptoms include tingling and burning sensations around the mouth, facial flushing and sweating, nausea and vomiting, headache, palpitations, dizziness, rash, and, occasionally, swelling of the face and tongue (10,11,62,67). Symptoms resolve spontaneously, but antihistamine drugs are effective and may be useful in more severe cases (10); there is one case report suggesting prompt resolution of symptoms with intravenous cimetidine (68). There are no long-term sequelae. Although essentially a clinical diagnosis, the diagnosis can be confirmed by demonstrating high histamine levels in the fish that was eaten or in the patient's urine (10).

Prevention of scombroid fish poisoning is dependent on preventing spoilage of fish after capture. This is accomplished by rapid cool-down of large fish, such as tuna, and maintenance of a cold chain from the time of harvest until the fish is eaten. This is of particular concern for fish imported from tropical or semitropical areas and for fish caught by recreational fishermen (69). If suspected, toxicity can be confirmed by assaying fish for histamine, although toxicity may vary from one part of a large fish to another. Toxic fish have been noted to have a "peppery" taste. Recognition of such a taste while eating suspect fish should be a warning not to proceed further with dinner.

REFERENCES

1. Institute of Medicine. *Seafood safety.* Washington, DC: National Academy Press, 1991.
2. Anderson DM, ed. *ECOHAB, The ecology and oceanography of harmful algal blooms: a national research agenda.* Woods Hole, MA: Woods Hole Oceanographic Institution, 1995.
3. Boesch DE, Anderson DM, Horner RA, et al. Harmful algal blooms in coastal waters: options for prevention, control, and mitigation. Silver Spring, MD: NOAA Coastal Oceans Program Decision Analysis Series No. 10. NOAA Coastal Oceans Office, 1996.
4. Morris JG Jr. Harmful algal blooms: an emerging public health problem with possible links to human stress on the environment. *Ann Rev Energy Environ* 1999;24:367–390.
5. Bagnis R, Kuberski T, Laugier S. Clinical observations on 3009 cases of ciguatera (fish poisoning) in the South Pacific. *Am J Trop Med Hyg* 1979;28:1067–1073.
6. Morris JG JR, Lewin P, Hargrett NT, et al. Clinical features of ciguatera fish poisoning: a study of the disease in the US Virgin Islands. *Arch Intern Med* 1982;142:1090–1092.
7. Gillespie NC, Lewis RJ, Pearn JH, et al. Ciguatera in Australia: occurrence, clinical features, pathophysiology and management. *Med J Aust* 1986;145:584–590.
8. Lehane L, Lewis RJ. Ciguatera: recent advances but the risk remains. *Int J Food Microbiol* 2000;61:91–125.
9. Lewis RJ. The changing face of ciguatera. *Toxicon* 2001;39:97–106.
10. Morrow JD, Margolies GR, Rowland J, et al. Evidence that histamine is the causative toxin of scombroid-fish poisoning. *N Engl J Med* 1991;324:716–720.
11. Lehane L, Olley J. Histamine fish poisoning revisited. *Int J Food Microbiol* 2000;58:1–37.
12. Bagnis R, Chanteau S, Chungue E, et al. Origins of ciguatera fish poisoning: a new dinoflagellate *Gambierdiscus toxicus* Adachi and Fukuyo definitely identified as a causal agent. *Toxicon* 1980;18: 199–208.

13. Holmes MJ, Lewis RJ, Poli MA, et al. Strain dependent production of ciguatoxin precursors (gambiertoxins) by *Gambierdiscus toxicus* (*Dinophyceae*) in culture. *Toxicon* 1991;29:761–775.
14. Hahn ST, Capra MF. The cyanobacterium *Oscillatoria erythraea* —a potential source of toxin in the ciguatera food chain. *Food Addit Contam* 1992:9:351–355.
15. Vernoux J-P, Lewis RJ. Isolation and characterization of Caribbean ciguatoxins from the horse-eye jack (*Caranx latus*). *Toxicon* 1997:35:889–900.
16. Lewis RJ, Sellin M. Multiple ciguatoxins in the flesh of fish. *Toxicon* 1992;30:915–919.
17. Lewis RJ, Jones A. Characterization of ciguatoxins and ciguatoxin congeners present in ciguateric fish by gradient reverse-phase high-performance liquid chromatography/mass spectrometry. *Toxicon* 1997:35:159–168.
18. Lewis RJ, Sellin M, Poli MA, et al. Purification and characterization of ciguatoxins from moray eel (*Lycodontis javanicus*, Muraenidae). *Toxicon* 1991;29:1115–1127.
19. Lewis RJ, Norton RS, Brereton IM, et al. Ciguatoxin-2 is a diastereomer of ciguatoxin-3. *Toxicon* 1993:31:637–643.
20. Takahashi M, Ohizumi Y, Yasumoto T. Maitotoxin, a Ca^{2+} channel activator candidate. *J Biol Chem* 1982;257:7287–7289.
21. Kodama AM, Hokama Y, Yasumoto T, et al. Clinical and laboratory findings implicating palytoxin as cause of ciguatera poisoning due to *Decapterus macrosoma* (mackerel). *Toxicon* 1989;27: 1051–1053.
22. Fasano A, Hokama Y, Russel R, et al. Diarrhea in ciguatera fish poisoning: preliminary evaluation of pathophysiological mechanisms. *Gastroenterology* 1991;100:471–476.
23. Bidard J-N, Vijverberg HPM, Frelin C, et al. Ciguatoxin is a novel type of Na+ channel toxin. *J Biol Chem* 1984;259:8353–8357.
24. Cameron J, Flowers AE, Capra MF. Effects of ciguatoxin on nerve excitability in rats. I. *J Neurol Sci* 1991;101:87–92.
25. Cameron J, Flowers AE, Capra MF. Electrophysiological studies on ciguatera poisoning in man. II. *J Neurol Sci* 1991;101:93–97.
26. Representative list of fishes reported as ciguatoxic. In: Halstead BW. *Poisonous and venomous marine animals of the world.* Princeton, NJ: Darwin Press, 1978:326–348.
27. Morris JG Jr, Lewin P, Smith CW, et al. Ciguatera fish poisoning: epidemiology of the disease on St. Thomas, U.S. Virgin Islands. *Am J Trop Med Hyg* 1982;31:574–578.
28. Engleberg NC, Moris JG Jr, Lewis J, et al. Ciguatera fish poisoning: a major common source outbreak in the U.S. Virgin Islands. *Ann Intern Med* 1983;98:336–337.
29. Hokama Y, Asahina AY, Titus E, et al. A survey of ciguatera: assessment of Puako, Hawaii, associated with ciguatera toxin epidemics in humans. *J Clin Lab Anal* 1993;7:147–154.
30. Anderson BS, Sims JK, Wiebenga N, et al. The epidemiology of ciguatera fish poisoning in Hawaii 1975-1982. *Hawaii Med J* 1983;42:326–334.
31. Ruff TA. Ciguatera in the Pacific: a link with military activities. *Lancet* 1989;1:201–205.
32. Thomassin BA, Ali Halidi ME, Quod JP, et al. Evolution of *Gambierdiscus toxicus* populations in the coral reef complex of Mayotte Island (SW Indian Ocean) during the 1985-1991 period. *Bull Soc Pathol Exot* 1992;85:449–452.
33. Rougerie F, Bagnis R. Bursts of ciguatera and endo-upwelling process on coral reefs. *Bull Soc Pathol Exot* 1992;85:464–466.
34. Lewis ND. Disease and development: ciguatera fish poisoning. *Soc Sci Med* 1986;10:983–993.
35. Lawrence DW, Enriquez MB, Lumish RM, et al. Ciguatera fish poisoning in Miami. *JAMA* 1980;244:254–258.
36. Quod JP, Turquet J. Ciguatera in Reunion Island (SW Indian Ocean): epidemiology and clinical patterns. *Toxicon* 1996;4: 779–785.
37. Lange WR, Snyder FR, Fudala PJ. Travel and ciguatera fish poisoning. *Arch Intern Med* 1992;152:2049–2053.
38. Deichmann WB, MacDonald WE, Cubit DA, et al. Pain in jawbones and teeth in ciguatera intoxications. *Florida Scientist* 1977; 40:227–237.
39. Palafox NA, Jain LG, Pinano AZ, et al. Successful treatment of ciguatera fish poisoning with intravenous mannitol. *JAMA* 1988; 259:2740–2742.
40. Blythe DG, deSylva DP. Mother's milk turns toxic following fish feast. *JAMA* 1990;264:2074.
41. Lange WR, Lipkin KM, Yang GC. Can ciguatera be a sexually transmitted disease? *J Toxicol Clin Toxicol* 1989;27:193–197.
42. Senecal PE, Osterloh JD. Normal fetal outcome after maternal ciguatera toxin exposure in the second trimester. *J Toxicol Clin Toxicol* 1991;29:473–478.
43. Kodama AM, Hokama Y. Variations in symptomatology of ciguatera poisoning. *Toxicon* 1989;27:593–595.
44. Pearn JH, Lewis RJ, Ruff T, et al. Ciguatera and mannitol: experience with a new treatment regimen. *Med J Aust* 1989;151: 77–80.
45. Stewart MP. Ciguatera fish poisoning: treatment with intravenous mannitol. *Trop Doctor* 1991;21:54–55.
46. Hokama Y. A rapid, simplified enzyme immunoassay stick test for the detection of ciguatoxin and related polys/ethers from fish tissue. *Toxicon* 1985;23:939–946.
47. Hokama Y, Asahina AY, Shang ES, et al. Evaluation of the Hawaiian reef fishes with the solid phase immunobead assay. *J Clin Lab Anal* 1993;7:26–30.
48. Schantz E. Chemistry and biology of saxitoxins and related toxins. *Ann N Y Acad Sci* 1986;479:15–23.
49. Henderson R, Ritchie JM, Strichartz GR. Evidence that tetrodotoxin and saxitoxin act as a metal cation binding site in the sodium channels of nerve membranes. *Proc Natl Acad Sci U S A* 1974;71:3936–3940.
50. Centers for Disease Control. Paralytic shellfish poisoning—Massachusetts and Alaska, 1990. *MMWR Morb Mortal Wkly Rep* 1991;40:157–161.
51. Gessner BD, Middaugh JP. Paralytic shellfish poisoning in Alaska: a 20-year retrospective analysis. Am J Epidemiol 1995; 141:766–770.
52. Gessner BD, Bell P, Doucette GJ, et al. Hypertension and identification of toxin in human urine and serum following a cluster of mussel-associated paralytic shellfish poisoning outbreaks. *Toxicon* 1997;35:711–722.
53. Long RR, Sargent JC, Hammer K. Paralytic shellfish poisoning: a case report and serial electrophysiologic observations. *Neurology* 1990;40:1310–1312.
54. Doucette GJ, Logan MM, Ramsdell JS, et al. Development and preliminary validation of a microtiter plate-based receptor binding assay for paralytic shellfish poisoning toxins. *Toxicon* 1997; 35:625–636.
55. Morris PD, Campbell DS, Taylor TH, et al. Clinical and epidemiological features of neurotoxic shellfish poisoning in North Carolina. *Am J Public Health* 1991;81:471–474.
56. Music SI, Howell JT, Brumback CL. Red tide: its public health implications. *J Fla Med Assoc* 1973;60:27–29.
57. Pleasance S, Quilliam MA, Marr JC. Ionspray mass spectrometry of marine toxins. IV. Determination of diarrhetic shellfish poisoning toxins in mussel tissue by liquid chromatography/mass spectroscopy. *Rapid Commun Mass Spectrom* 1992;6: 121–127.
58. Marr JC, Hu T, Pleasance S, et al. Detection of new 7-O-acyl derivatives of diarrhetic shellfish poisoning toxins by liquid chromatography-mass spectrometry. *Toxicon* 1992;30:1621–1630.
59. Todd ECD. Emerging diseases associated with seafood toxins

and other water-borne agents. Ann N Y Acad Sci 1994;740: 77–94.
60. Perl TM, Bedard L, Kosatsky T, et al. An outbreak of toxic encephalopathy caused by eating mussels contaminated with domoic acid. *N Engl J Med* 1990;322:1775–1780.
61. Teitelbaum JS, Zatorre RJ, Carpenter S, et al. Neurologic sequelae of domoic acid intoxication due to ingestion of contaminated mussels. *N Engl J Med* 1990;322:1781–1787.
62. Smart DR. Scombroid poisoning. A report of seven cases involving the Western Australian salmon, *Arripis truttaceus. Med J Aust* 1992;157:748–751.
63. Etkind P, Wilson ME, Gallagher K, et al. Bluefish-associated scombroid poisoning: an example of the expanding spectrum of food poisoning from seafood. *JAMA* 1987;258:3409–3410.
64. Kim R. Flushing syndrome due to mahimahi (scombroid fish) poisoning. *Arch Dermatol* 1979;115:963–965.
65. Centers for Disease Control. Scombroid fish poisoning—New Mexico, 1987. *MMWR Morb Mortal Wkly Rep* 1988;37:451.
66. Taylor SL. Histamine food poisoning: toxicology and clinical aspects. *CRC Crit Rev Toxicol* 1986;17:91–128.
67. Gilbert RJ, Hobbs G, Murray CK, et al. Scombrotoxic fish poisoning: features of the first 50 incidents to be reported in Britain (1976-9). *BMJ* 1980;281:71–72.
68. Guss DA. Scombroid fish poisoning: successful treatment with cimetidine. *Undersea Hyperb Med*1998;25:123–125.
69. Gellert GA, Ralls J, Brown C, et al. Scombroid fish poisoning. Underreporting and prevention among noncommercial recreational fishers. *West J Med* 1992;157:645–647.

17

ACUTE WATERY DIARRHEA

JOHN K. CRANE
RICHARD L. GUERRANT

And so it was proven, by an insidious questioning, that the symptoms of love are the same as the symptoms of cholera.

Gabriel Garcia Marquez
Love in the Time of Cholera

The syndrome of acute watery diarrhea is so common, so much a part of the universal human experience, that all readers, unless they have spent their life in a sterile, protective bubble, have experienced it firsthand. Perhaps it was the lightheadedness and the rapid heart rate caused by dehydration that inspired Garcia Marquez's comparison of cholera and the emotion of love. Indeed, for intestinal pathogens that cause watery diarrhea without invading the gut mucosa, dehydration is the most life-threatening aspect of the illness.

Features of a diarrheal illness that are important in making a clinical assessment include the volume and frequency of the diarrhea, the character of the diarrhea (especially the presence or absence of blood or mucus in the stools), the presence of fever, and associated gastrointestinal symptoms such as vomiting and abdominal cramps. As opposed to watery diarrhea, *dysentery* consists of frequent but smaller stools, often with a gelatinous appearance containing blood and mucus, and frequently accompanied by fever and abdominal cramps. Acute inflammatory diarrheal illness such as dysentery is discussed in Chapter 18. However, even disease caused by invasive pathogens (such as *Shigella* and *Entamoeba histolytica*) usually begins with watery diarrhea and gradually evolves toward the more classic dysenteric features as the illness progresses. For example, Ericsson and DuPont (1) report that, in their studies in Mexico where travelers had convenient access to medical care, approximately 90% of patients with *Shigella* infection initially presented with watery diarrhea. This illustrates the need for reevaluation of the patient with watery diarrhea if the patient worsens, if the character of the diarrhea changes, or if diarrhea persists for more than a few days.

J. K. Crane: Department of Medicine, University at Buffalo; Division of Infectious Diseases, Erie County Medical Center, Buffalo, New York

R. L. Guerrant: Division of International Medicine, University of Virginia School of Medicine; Division of Geographic Medicine, University of Virginia Hospital Charlottesville, Virginia

MICROBIOLOGY

The causes of acute watery diarrhea are varied and include toxic, noninfectious as well as infectious etiologies (Table 17.1) (Fig. 17.1). Noninfectious causes include various kinds of toxic ingestions (e.g., poison mushrooms, heavy metals, diarrheic shellfish poisoning, scombroid fish poisoning.) Among travelers to developing countries, the most common causes of diarrhea are, in approximate descending order: *Escherichia coli* (primarily toxigenic strains), *Campylobacter jejuni*, *Salmonella*, *Shigella*, viruses (Norwalk, Norwalk-like viruses, and rotavirus), and parasites (especially *Giardia* and *Cryptosporidium*).

Among children in developing countries, the most common causes of diarrhea include rotaviruses, enteropathogenic *E. coli*, toxigenic *E. coli*, enteroaggregative *E. coli*, *Shigella*, and *Campylobacter* (2–5). In studies of infants, a large proportion of cases (>50%) may show no known pathogen.

Among children in industrialized countries, the predominant diarrheal pathogens include rotaviruses, *Giardia lamblia*, *Salmonella*, and diarrheagenic *E. coli*, including Shiga-toxin producing *E. coli* (STEC), which is also called enterohemorrhagic *E. coli* (EHEC) (6,7).

PATHOGENESIS

All of the causes of watery diarrhea have in common an imbalance between the amount of fluid secreted into the gastrointestinal tract (estimated to be at least 10 L/day in a

TABLE 17.1 COMMON MICROBIAL CAUSES OF ACUTE WATERY DIARRHEA

Category	Common Examples	Associated Symptoms, Comments	Settings	Reference
Preformed bacterial toxins	Staphylococcal food poisoning, *Bacillus cereus* food poisoning	Nausea and vomiting predominate	Foodborne outbreaks	45
Viruses	Rotavirus	Fever common; 5- to 7-day duration	Increased incidence in winter in temperate climates	46, 47
	Adenovirus	Fever and respiratory symptoms common; 10- to 12-day duration of vomiting and diarrhea; mustard yellow or tan watery stools	Children; advanced AIDS	48, 49
	Norwalk virus	Prominent vomiting; headache; fever	Outbreaks, including shipboard outbreaks; associated with raw shellfish	50
	Norwalk-like viruses	Similar to Norwalk virus		51
Bacteria	Enterotoxigenic *Escherichia coli* (ETEC)	3- to 5-day duration; children often have fever	Travelers, infants in developing countries	52, 53
	Enteropathogenic *E. coli* (EPEC)	May be associated with fever and vomiting; "fishy odor"; may have longer duration than ETEC	Infants, urban areas of developing countries	4, 53, 54
	Campylobacter jejuni	Fever and bloody stools common; propensity to relapse	Developed and developing countries; increased incidence in winter	55
	Vibrio cholerae	Massive watery diarrhea; "rice water stools"; fishy odor	Epidemics	21
	Salmonella species	May also cause inflammatory diarrhea; fever common	Foodborne outbreaks	
	Many other enteric bacteria	*Aeromonas, Plesiomonas, Klebsiella, Citrobacter,* and others have been implicated		56, 57
Parasites	*Giardia lamblia*	Malabsorption syndrome; bloating; flatulence; foul-smelling stools; may produce persistent diarrhea	Travelers; backpackers; day care centers	6
	Cryptosporidium parvum	Watery diarrhea; persistent infections in immunocompromised patients	Travelers to St. Petersburg; outbreaks	20
	Isospora belli	Malabsorption; eosinophilia	Developing countries; AIDS	29
	Cyclospora cayetanensis (formerly CLOs, or cyanobacteria-like organisms)	Flulike onset with relapsing, remitting watery diarrhea lasting up to 2 months; stool examination shows nonrefractile spheres 8–10 μm in diameter	Travelers to Nepal; developing countries; waterborne outbreaks	58

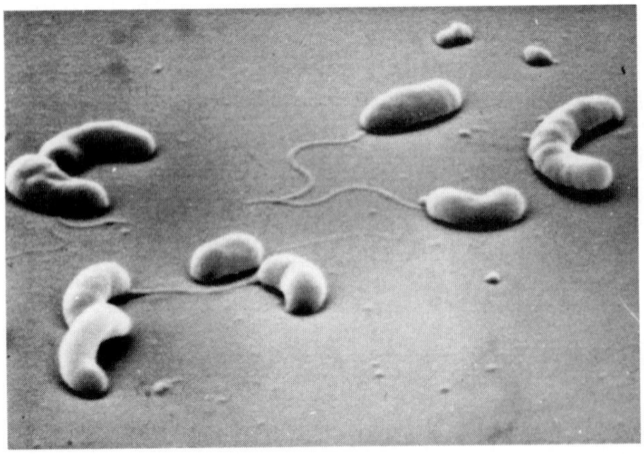

FIGURE 17.1. Scanning electron micrograph of *Vibrio cholerae.* Note the presence of polar flagella. From Banerjee D. *Microbiology of infectious diseases.* London: Gower Medical, 1990, with permission.

normal adult) and the ability of the intestinal epithelium to reabsorb that fluid. Viral enteric pathogens such as rotavirus preferentially infect and kill villous tip enterocytes over large areas of the small intestine, markedly impairing absorptive capacity (Fig. 17.2). The traditional view of rotavirus diarrhea is that the spared, normal crypt cells continue to secrete ions and fluid, and in the absence of adequate absorption, the amount of fluid presented to the colon overwhelms its reabsorptive capacity, resulting in diarrhea. This explanation is too simplistic, however, given recent findings about rotavirus. For example, the rotavirus nonstructural glycoprotein NP4 acts as an enterotoxin (8), and the diarrheal response to rotavirus depends on the enteric nervous system (9).

Many cases of diarrhea may be considered a pathologic exaggeration of what is normally a host protective response

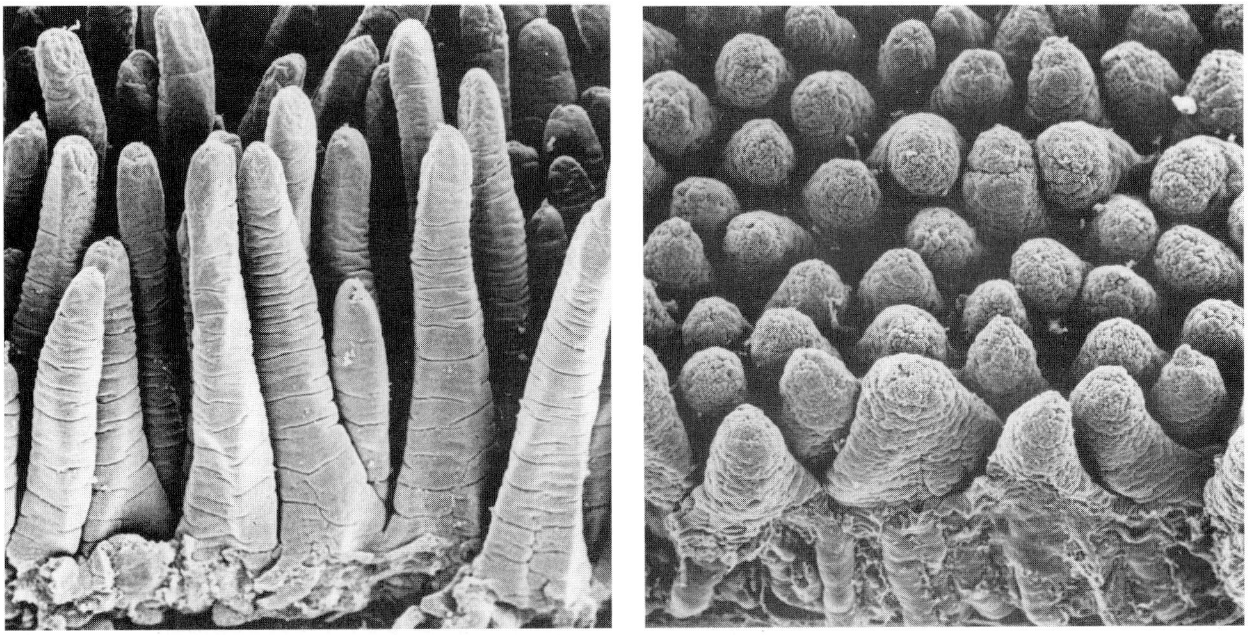

FIGURE 17.2. Scanning electron micrograph of normal and rotavirus-damaged intestinal villi. Small intestinal mucosa is shown from normal, uninfected (left) and rotavirus-infected gnotobiotic calf (right) 6 days after infection. In the infected calf, the villi are markedly shortened, some villi are fused together, and the surface enterocytes are swollen and abnormally arranged. Depth of the crypts is markedly increased in the infected tissue as a result of compensatory hyperplasia at this stage of the infection. (Photographs courtesy of Dr. Graham A. Hall, Public Health Laboratory Service, Salisbury, Wiltshire, U.K.)

to proliferation, attachment, or invasion by enteric microbes. For example, neutrophils infiltrating the intestinal mucosa in response to pathogens such as *Salmonella* release 5′-adenosine monophosphate (AMP), which acts as a secretagogue (10,11). Guanylin and uroguanylin are naturally occurring gut peptides that can stimulate fluid secretion via guanylyl cyclase C (12,13). Whether guanylin and uroguanylin are mediators of diarrhea in response to enteric infections is not known.

Study of the secretory pathways stimulated by microbial toxins has enhanced our understanding of the regulation of the normal secretory and absorptive apparatus of the intestinal cell. For example, cholera toxin and *E. coli* heat-labile toxin (LT) activate adenylyl cyclase. Cyclic AMP (cAMP) acts via cAMP-dependent protein kinase to phosphorylate and open the cystic fibrosis transmembrane regulator, which is a major chloride channel in the intestine.

The role of protein kinases other than the cyclic nucleotide-dependent protein kinases in intestinal fluid secretion remains unclear. An inhibitor of calmodulin kinases, zaldaride, reduces the severity of travelers' diarrhea (14). Protein kinase C may play a role in the secretory response to EPEC infection (15).

An important variable in the pathogenesis of diarrheal diseases is the infectious dose or the inoculum required to produce symptomatic disease in normal individuals. Table 17.2 lists the infectious dose for several enteric pathogens. The concept of the infectious dose has been criticized because it emphasizes the virulent characteristics of the pathogenic organism without taking into account the wide variability of host defenses. Indeed, the infectious dose of many bacterial pathogens is lowered markedly in individuals with decreased gastric acidity, patients already receiving

TABLE 17.2 INFECTIOUS DOSES OF VARIOUS DIARRHEAL PATHOGENS[a]

Pathogen	Infectious Dose
Low inoculum	
Shigella[b]	10^1–10^2
Enterohemorrhagic *Escherichia coli* (EHEC; STEC)	~10^2
Giardia lamblia	10^1–10^2 cysts
Entamoeba histolytica[b]	10^1–10^2 cysts
Rotavirus	10^1 plaque-forming units[c]
Intermediate inoculum	
Campylobacter jejuni	10^2–10^6
High inoculum	
Vibrio cholerae	10^8
Salmonella	10^5
E. coli (other than EHEC)	10^8

[a]Modified from reference 59.
[b]Classically assciated with dysenteric rather than watery diarrhea.
[c]From reference 60.

antibiotics, or patients with impaired intestinal motility or receiving antimotility drugs. In natural populations, behavioral factors such as food preferences, cooking methods, and hygienic practices are probably even more important than the aforementioned "biologic" factors in determining who becomes ill and who remains well after exposure to enteric pathogens. With these caveats in mind, the infectious dose can nevertheless be helpful in understanding the mode of transmission of disease and the approaches needed to interrupt transmission. "Low-inoculum" agents such as *Giardia, Cryptosporidium*, rotavirus, and *Shigella* are easily spread from person to person, whereas "high-inoculum" agents such as *Vibrio cholerae, Salmonella,* and toxigenic *E. coli* are usually acquired by ingesting larger numbers of organisms via contaminated food or water.

EPIDEMIOLOGY

The modes of transmission and epidemiologic features of the pathogens that cause acute watery diarrhea are varied, as emphasized by Tables 17.2 and 17.3. All of these infections are acquired by the inadvertent ingestion of organisms ultimately derived from feces (fecal-oral route). This statement, however, belies a great deal of ignorance in some cases about how enteric pathogens are actually spread.

Water

One of the most common adages heard by the traveler is "Don't drink the water." The pioneering sleuthing that allowed Dr. John Snow to link the Broad Street water pump with the spread of cholera in London in 1854 remains a classic in medical history. The incidence of diarrheal disease is markedly increased in some areas in the rainy season (16), strongly suggesting contamination of water from runoff. Water has been implicated in cholera outbreaks in various continents (17,18). Furthermore, evidence for direct acquisition of *Giardia* and *Cryptosporidium* from surface water or inadequately filtered municipal water supplies is well documented (19,20). However, solid evidence incriminating drinking water is lacking for many common pathogens such as toxigenic *E. coli* (1).

Food

For many pathogens, food is probably just as important, or more important, than water as a mode of transmission. Fish and shellfish have been incriminated in the spread of *V. cholerae*, noncholera *Vibrio, Vibrio parahaemolyticus*, and Norwalk virus (21). Eggs, including intact eggs, are a source of Salmonella, as are poultry and beef. The association between ground beef and *E. coli* O157:H7 is so strong that this infection has been nicknamed the "hamburger disease." However, many other vehicles for transmission of EHEC (O157:H7 as well as other serotypes) have been recognized, including unpasteurized cider and fruit juices, fresh produce, bean sprouts, and radish sprouts.

Vomitus and Other Modes of Transmission

Vomitus has been identified as the likely agent of transmission of Norwalk virus and other viral agents of gastroenteritis in outbreaks on cruise ships (22). Investigation of an outbreak of a Norwalk-like viral agent in a nursing home identified at least nine ill employees without any contact with patients or patients' body fluids, suggesting the possibility of airborne spread of virus (23).

Person-to-Person Contact

Secondary spread among close household contacts is common for low-inoculum pathogens (Table 17.2).

Insects

Flies and cockroaches have been blamed for contamination of food with enteric pathogens, but their role has not been conclusively proven. Cultures of microbes from the feet or digestive tracts of insects have been conducted and yielded

TABLE 17.3 ASSESSMENT OF DEHYDRATION

Symptoms or Signs	Mild or No Dehydration (<5%)	Moderate Dehydration (5–10%)	Severe Dehydration (>10%)
General condition	Well, alert	Restless, irritable	Lethargic or unconscious, floppy
Eyes	Normal	Sunken	Very sunken and dry
Tears	Present	Absent	Absent
Mouth and tongue	Moist	Dry	Very dry
Thirst	Drinks normally, not thirsty	Thirsty, drinks eagerly	Drinks poorly or not able to drink
Skin	Pinch retracts immediately	Pinch retracts slowly (2 sec)	Pinch retracts very slowly (3–5 sec)
Estimated fluid deficit	<50 mL/kg	50–100 mL/kg	>100 mL/kg
Appropriate type of fluid therapy	Maintenance fluid with increased intake of home fluids such as fruit juice, soups, or ORS		

From references 31 and 35.

pathogens such as *Salmonella* in a low percentage of individual insects (24).

CLINICAL FEATURES AND DIFFERENTIAL DIAGNOSIS

The clinical setting of a diarrheal illness provides information as important to the clinician as that from the physical examination or inspection of the diarrheal fecal specimen. Is the patient an adult or a child? Has the patient traveled? What is known about the patient's immune system? Does the patient have a decrease in gastric acidity? Was the patient taking antibiotics before the onset of illness?

The history of the diarrheal illness itself is the next crucial part of the assessment. The character of the diarrhea (consistency, color, odor, volume, and frequency) is critical in determining subsequent management. Diarrhea associated with blood or mucus in the stools suggests an inflammatory cause (see Chapter 18) and stool culture is usually indicated. Very high-volume diarrhea suggests rotavirus or, in the appropriate geographic setting, toxigenic *E. coli,* cholera or *Cryptosporidium.* Rotavirus and adenoviruses usually produce watery tan or yellowish stools. Cholera classically is associated with clear watery diarrhea containing light-colored flecks of mucus ("rice water" stools). *Giardia*-induced diarrhea is often watery and greenish with bits of undigested food and is associated with a foul odor. If the patient is unable to supply a fecal specimen at the time of the encounter, the appearance and odor of the stool must be elicited from the patient by direct questioning.

Prominent vomiting is often seen in infection with rotavirus, adenovirus, EPEC, Norwalk virus, and the Norwalk-like viruses.

Abdominal cramps are common in most diarrheal diseases and usually do not help distinguish one causative agent from another. Tenesmus, or painful rectal spasms, is an indication of proctitis and is an important clue toward invasive pathogens, such as *Shigella* or *E. histolytica.* Elevated temperature (>39°C) can be seen with these invasive pathogens but also with rotavirus and adenovirus (especially the classic, nonenteric serotypes) (25). Sexually transmitted causes of proctitis, including herpes simplex and cytomegalovirus, must be suspected if the patient has AIDS or is homosexually active. These patients may have rectal pain and mucoid rectal discharge but little actual diarrhea.

Physical examination of the patient with diarrhea is important to assess the patient's nutritional status, degree of dehydration (Table 17.3), and signs of poisoning (cholinesterase inhibitors cause constricted pupils; botulism causes dilated pupils) and to rule out signs, such as splenomegaly, of multisystem disease. The degree of dehydration usually is determined by physical examination, because it is difficult for the patient and physician to quantify the amount of diarrhea by history alone. In addition, the patient should be examined for physical signs of immune dysfunction, such as oral thrush, seborrheic dermatitis of the face, or lymphadenopathy, because the diagnostic approach is often different in the patient immunocompromised by HIV or AIDS. A rectal examination is important in assessing proctitis and to determine whether hemorrhoids are a confounding source of blood.

In this era in which patients' body fluids are whisked to the laboratory in sealed biohazard bags, the importance to the clinician of actually inspecting the patient's diarrhea specimen for blood and mucus cannot be overemphasized. In many cases, this affords the opportunity to perform a wet mount of the fecal specimen for leukocytes immediately, before spontaneous lysis of neutrophils occurs after prolonged standing at room temperature. Olfactory clues can be helpful in assessing diarrhea during inspection of the stool specimen. Frankly dysenteric stools resulting from infection with *Shigella* are usually almost odorless. *V. cholerae* and EPEC have been said to impart a fishy odor to the diarrhea they produce. *Giardia* infections are associated with foul-smelling stools and flatulence. *Salmonella* infections have been reported anecdotally to give a hydrogen sulfide or "rotten egg" odor in the feces, correlating with the ability of nontyphoidal *Salmonella* to produce H_2S *in vitro.*

DIFFERENTIAL DIAGNOSIS

Usually, the patient suspects an infectious etiology of acute diarrhea before seeking medical attention. Occasionally, however, physicians are confronted with patients whose illness is not due to an enteric pathogen but rather to a toxic exposure (Table 17.1), a systemic illness, or noninfectious causes. Malaria in the returning traveler can manifest with a predominance of abdominal symptoms, including diarrhea or circulatory collapse and abdominal pain (so-called algid malaria). A significant minority of malaria patients present with acute, watery diarrhea and fever. Harries and colleagues (26) reported that acute watery diarrhea was the second most common symptom (in 23%) in a series of 150 consecutive adult patients with *Plasmodium falciparum* malaria in Malawi. A similar study in Uganda showed that acute diarrhea, vomiting, or both were observed in a high percentage of children and adults with malaria (27). In typhoid fever, patients may be constipated early in their illness, but diarrhea may develop later. In both malaria and typhoid, the presence of persistent high temperature is a clue to ongoing systemic illness. Persistent diarrhea in a returning traveler occasionally leads to a gastroenterologic evaluation and a diagnosis of inflammatory bowel disease or intestinal parasite. Even more commonly, patients with a history of inflammatory bowel disease may suffer a flare-up after an intercurrent bout of traveler's diarrhea owing to the usual pathogens. In addition, patients may have their first episode of inflammatory bowel disease after foreign travel (28).

SPECIFIC DIAGNOSTIC MEASURES AND MANAGEMENT

Just as the usual impulse of the patient with diarrhea is to request antimotility medication to stop the diarrhea, the usual impulse of the physician is to send a stool culture. Although there are some situations in which these reflex actions are acceptable, in general, the physician should resist them and instead apply critical thinking. Stool cultures obtained from otherwise healthy adults and children suffering from acute watery diarrhea in developed countries have such a low rate of positivity as to make them economically contraindicated, especially because most important therapeutic decisions are made before the results of the cultures are known. Stool cultures in this setting may have a positivity rate as low as 2% or less and the cost per case detected may be $950 to $1,200, making the stool culture the "most expensive and least valuable microbiologic test in the hospital" (29–31). Stool examinations for ova and parasites in the same population, or in patients hospitalized for other reasons in whom diarrhea develops while in the hospital, almost never yield a diagnosis relevant to the management of the diarrheal illness. (A review of the patient's medication list and a test for *Clostridium difficile* or its toxin may be more helpful in the inpatient.) A test for fecal leukocytes or lactoterin can help suggest an inflammatory enteritis if this is uncertain by clinical presentation (Fig. 17.3). The value of the stool smear for fecal leukocytes has been evaluated in several studies and continues to be debated (32,33). One limitation of this test is that fecal leukocytes

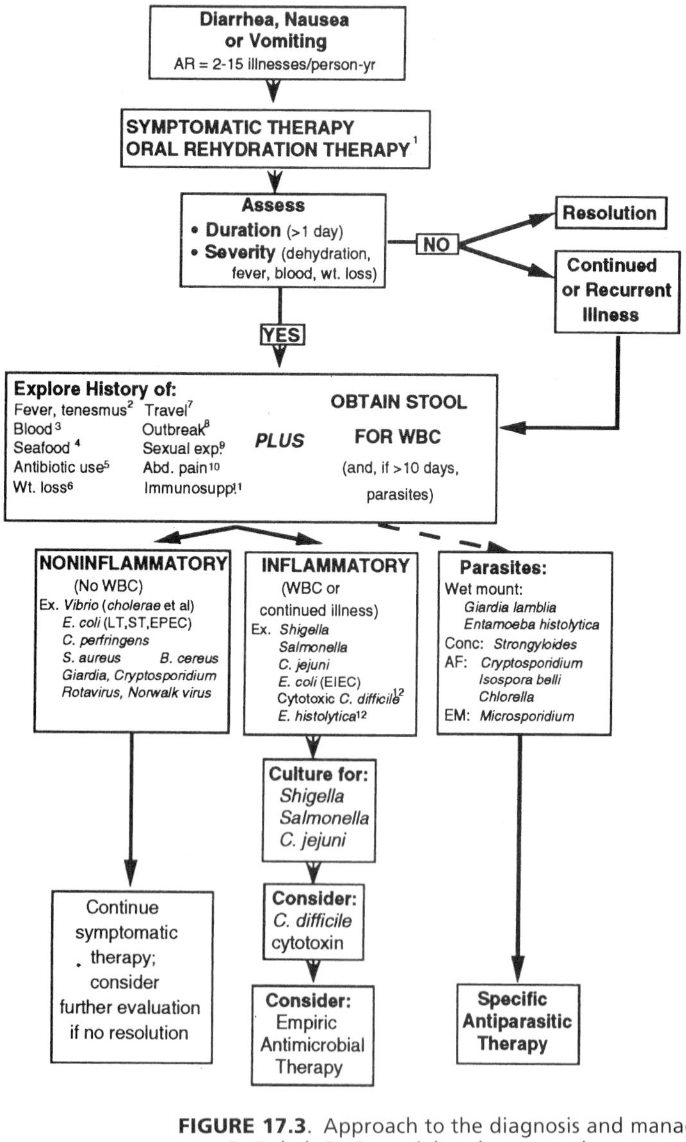

1. ORS can be prepared by adding 3.5g NaCl, 2.5g $NaHCO_3$ (or 2.9g Na citrate), 1.5g KCl and 20g glucose or glucose polymer (ex. 40g sucrose or 4 tablespoons sugar or 50-60g cereal flour such as rice, maize, sorghum, millet, wheat or potato) per liter (1.05qt.) of clean water. This makes approximately Na 90, K 20, Cl 80, HCO_3 30, glucose 111 mmol/L.
   One level teaspoon table salt and 8 level teaspoons table sugar per liter makes about 86 mmol Na and 30g sucrose/L to which one could add 1 cup orange juice or 2 bananas for potassium.

2. Fever or tenesmus suggest an inflammatory proctocolitis.

3. Diarrhea with blood, especially without fecal leukocytes, suggests enterohemorrhagic (Shiga-like-toxin-producing) E. coli O157 or amebiasis (in which leukocytes are destroyed by the parasite).

4. Ingestion of inadequately cooked seafood should prompt consideration of infections with Vibrio or Norwalk-like viruses.

5. Antibiotics should be stopped if possible and cytotoxigenic C. difficile considered. Antibiotics may also predispose to other infections such as salmonellosis.

6. Persistence (>10 days) with weight loss should prompt consideration of giardiasis or cryptosporidiosis.

7. Travel to tropical areas increases the chance of developing enterotoxigenic E. coli, as well as viral (Norwalk-like or rotaviral), parasite (Giardia, Entamoeba, Strongyloides, Cryptosporidium), and, if fecal leukocytes are present, invasive bacterial infections as noted in the algorithm.

8. Outbreaks should prompt consideration of S. aureus, B. cereus, anisakiasis (incubation period <6 hours), C. perfringens, ETEC, Vibrio, Salmonella, Campylobacter, Shigella, or EIEC infection. Consider saving E. coli for LT, ST, invasiveness, adherence testing, serotyping, and stool for rotavirus, and stool plus paired sera for Norwalk-like virus or toxin testing.

9. Sigmoidoscopy in symptomatic homosexual men should distinguish proctitis in the distal 15cm only (caused by herpesvirus, gonococcal, chlamydial, or syphilitic infection) from colitis (Campylobacter, Shigella, C. difficile, or chlamydial [LGV serotypes] infections) or noninflammatory diarrhea (due to giardiasis).

10. If unexplained abdominal pain and fever persist or suggest an appendicitis-like syndrome, culture for Y. enterocolitica with cold enrichment.

11. In immunocompromised hosts, a wide range of viral (cytomegalovirus, herpes simplex virus, coxsackievirus, rotavirus), bacterial (Salmonella, M. avium-intracellulare), and parasitic (Cryptosporidium, Isospora, Strongyloides, Entamoeba, and Giardia) agents should be considered.

12. Some inflammatory, colonic pathogens, such as, cytotoxigenic C. difficile or Entamoeba histolytica may destroy fecal leukocyte morphology, so a reliable leukocyte marker would provide a better screening test.

FIGURE 17.3. Approach to the diagnosis and management of infectious diarrhea. From Guerrant R, Bobak D. Bacterial and protozoal gastroenteritis. *N Engl J Med* 1991;325(5):327–340, with permission.

deteriorate after the specimen is collected, so the value of the test declines with a delay in examination. The test for fecal lactoferrin (a marker of fecal leukocytes) is not time-sensitive, however, and is more sensitive (34). The fecal lactoferrin test is commercially available in latex agglutination and enzyme-linked immunosorbent assay formats, and should soon be available as a dipstick (Leukotest, Leuko-ELISA, and Leuko-stick tests, Techlab, Inc., Blacksburg, VA). An examination for fecal leukocytes or the fecal lactoferrin test can aid in pointing to an inflammatory etiology of diarrhea such as that due to *Shigella, Salmonella, Campylobacter*, or *C. difficile*, or due to inflammatory bowel disease (Fig. 17.3). Such patients should have a stool culture, *C. difficile* toxin testing, or both.

Stool cultures may also be indicated at the time of presentation (or later if symptoms suggestive of dysentery develop) if the patient is immunocompromised, is suspected of having cholera, or appears to be part of an outbreak. If cholera is suspected, cultures for *Vibrio* must be specifically requested. When patients are hospitalized for diarrhea, the economic calculations change somewhat. For instance, although there is no specific therapy for rotavirus, an enzyme immunoassay (EIA) for rotavirus is probably indicated in the child hospitalized with diarrhea, because a confirmed diagnosis requires isolation and a confirmed diagnosis may spare the patient more expensive and even invasive diagnostic tests.

REHYDRATION THERAPY

Rehydration of the dehydrated patient and maintenance of adequate hydration in the patient not yet dehydrated are the cornerstone of therapy for all patients with diarrhea. For adults and children without clinical signs of dehydration, maintenance of good hydration can be accomplished by increased intake of typical home fluids including water, fruit juices, sport beverages, and non–caffeine-containing carbonated beverages (35–37). Oral rehydration solutions, such as Pedialyte and Rehydralyte, may also be used for maintenance hydration or mild dehydration. For the patient with moderate to severe dehydration, however, the common home fluids are not optimal (35,37). Fruit juices and soft drinks contain too much sugar (which results in too high an osmolarity) and too little salt to be useful in severe diarrhea. The osmolarity of Gatorade and similar sports or performance beverages, approximately 330 mmol/L, is close to physiologic but the concentration of sodium (20 mmol/L) is still too low. The same criticism applies to Pedialyte, with a sodium concentration of 45 mmol/L, which is far below the value of 75 to 90 mmol/L recommended by the American Academy of Pediatrics and World Health Organization (WHO). Rehydralyte, with a sodium concentration of 75 mmol/L, provides a commercially available product in the United States with a sodium concentration optimal for oral treatment of severe dehydration. Packets of WHO rehydration salts, available in remote locations around the world, are paradoxically not readily available in the United States. However, hospitals and clinics in North America may purchase packets of WHO rehydration salts in lots of 125 or more (Jianas Brothers, Kansas City, MO 64108). The cost is less than 60 cents per packet, which may significantly increase compliance in low-income populations (38); by comparison, the cost of the commercially available premixed liquids is $6 to $7 per liter. A more detailed discussion of the theory and practice of oral rehydration therapy is found in the Chapter 79.

ANTIMICROBIAL THERAPY OF DIARRHEA

While oral rehydration is the cornerstone of antidiarrheal therapy, recent progress has shown that antimicrobial therapy may be a useful adjunct to oral rehydration. The best studied of these situations is that of traveler's diarrhea, in which antibacterial agents such as the fluoroquinolones can markedly shorten the duration of illness (39). Details of the use of antibiotics for traveler's diarrhea is found in Chapter 19. A more controversial area is whether empirical antibiotic therapy (with quinolones or other antibiotics) has any role in the treatment of acute, nontraveler's diarrhea in adults (40). The high cost of the quinolones and the lower incidence of bacterial pathogens in developed countries in adults have prevented the widespread use of antibiotics for what is usually a short-lived illness.

The role of bismuth compounds, such as bismuth subsalicylate, in the treatment or prevention of acute diarrhea has attracted attention and investigation over the past decade. Bismuth subsalicylate is effective in both prophylaxis and treatment of traveler's diarrhea (41,42). In a study of children hospitalized with acute watery diarrhea in Peru, bismuth subsalicylate therapy resulted in a modest decrease in the severity and duration of illness that was evident by the third treatment day (43). It is unclear whether the modest benefits of bismuth subsalicylate warrant the trouble and cost of administering the drug to all of the potential recipients (44).

PREVENTION

Diarrheal disease caused by "high-inoculum" pathogens such as *E. coli, Salmonella*, and *Vibrio cholerae* is theoretically easier to prevent than that attributable to "low-inoculum" organisms, in that the former are usually spread through contamination of water distribution systems and violations of hygienic practices in the collection, storage, distribution, and preparation of food. In special situations such as in child day care centers, measures to isolate diapering areas and personnel from food preparation, and to exclude children with diarrhea from attendance can decrease but probably not eliminate transmission of enteric pathogens. Low-inoculum agents such as rotavirus and *Shigella* may spread easily among members of family and household; transmission may be decreased by careful personal hygiene measures such as handwashing.

ACKNOWLEDGMENT

Dr. Guerrant developed and licensed the fecal lactoferrin test to Techlab, Inc., Blacksburg, VA.

REFERENCES

1. Ericsson C, DuPont H. Travelers' diarrhea: approaches to prevention and treatment. *Clin Infect Dis* 1993;16:616–626.
2. Cama RI, Parashar UD, Taylor DN, et al. Enteropathogens and other factors associated with severe disease in children with acute watery diarrhea in Lima, Peru. *J Infect Dis* 1999;179(5):1139–1144.
3. Youssef M, Shurman A, Bougnoux M, et al. Bacterial, viral and parasitic enteric pathogens associated with acute diarrhea in hospitalized children from northern Jordan. *FEMS Immunol Med Microbiol* 2000;28(3):257–263.
4. Rosa AC, Mariano AT, Pereira AM, et al. Enteropathogenicity markers in *Escherichia coli* isolated from infants with acute diarrhoea and healthy controls in Rio de Janeiro, Brazil. *J Med Microbiol* 1998;47(9):781–790.
5. Dutta S, Pal S, Chakrabarti S, et al. Use of PCR to identify enteroaggregative *Escherichia coli* as an important cause of acute diarrhoea among children living in Calcutta, India. *J Med Microbiol* 1999;48:1011–1016.
6. Caeiro JP, Mathewson JJ, Smith MA, et al. Etiology of outpatient pediatric nondysenteric diarrhea: a multicenter study in the United States. *Pediatr Infect Dis J* 1999;18(2):94–97.
7. Huppertz H-I, Busch D, Schmidt H, et al. Diarrhea in young children associated with *Escherichia coli* non-O157 organisms that produce Shiga-like toxin. *J Pediatr* 1996;128:341–346.
8. Ball J, Tian P, Zeng C, et al. Age-dependent diarrhea induced by a rotavirus nonstructural glycoprotein. *Science* 1996;272:101–104.
9. Lundgren O, Peregrin A, Persson K, et al. Role of the enteric nervous system in the fluid and electrolyte secretion of rotavirus diarrhea. *Science* 2000;287:491–495.
10. Nash S, Parkos C, Nusrat A, et al. *In vitro* model of intestinal crypt abscess: a novel neutrophil derived secretagogue activity. *J Clin Invest* 1991;87:1474–1477.
11. Madara J, Patapoff T, Gillece-Castro B, et al. 5′-adenosine monophosphate is the neutrophil-derived paracrine factor that elicits chloride secretion from T84 intestinal epithelial monolayers. *J Clin Invest* 1993;91:2320–2325.
12. Currie M, Fok K, Kato J, et al. Guanylin: an endogenous activator of intestinal guanylate cyclase. *Proc Natl Acad Sci U S A* 1992;89:947–951.
13. Forte L, Currie M. Guanylin: a peptide regulator of epithelial transport. *FASEB J* 1995;9:643–650.
14. Okhuysen P, DuPont H, Ericsson C, et al. Zaldaride maleate (a new calmodulin antagonist) versus loperamide in the treatment of traveler's diarrhea: randomized, placebo-controlled trial. *Clin Infect Dis* 1995;21:341–344.
15. Crane JK, Oh JS. Activation of host cell protein kinase C by enteropathogenic *Escherichia coli*. *Infect Immun* 1997;65:3277–3285.
16. Giron J, Jones T, Millan-Velasco F, et al. Diffuse-adhering *Escherichia coli* (DAEC) as a putative cause of diarrhea in Mayan children in Mexico. *J Infect Dis* 1991;163:507–513.
17. Swerdlow D, Mintz E, Rodriguez M, et al. Waterborne transmission of cholera in Trujillo, Peru: lessons for a continent at risk. *Lancet* 1992;340:28–33.
18. Epidemic cholera—Burundi and Zimbabwe, 1992-1993. *MMWR Morbid Mortal. Wkly Rep* 1993;42:407–416.
19. Herwaldt B, Craun G, Stokes S, et al. Waterborne-disease outbreaks, 1989-1990. CDC Surveillance Summaries, Dec. 1991. *MMWR Morbid Mortal Wkly Rep* 1991;40:SS1–SS22.
20. Hayes E, Matte T, O'Brien T, et al. Large community outbreak of cryptosporidiosis due to contamination of a filtered public water supply. *N Engl J Med* 1989;320:1372–1376.
21. Update: Cholera—Western hemisphere, 1992. *MMWR Morbid Mortal Wkly Rep* 1992;41:667–668.
22. Ho M, Glass R, Monroe S, et al. Viral gastroenteritis aboard a cruise ship. *Lancet* 1989;2:961–964.
23. Gellert G, Waterman S, Ewert D, et al. An outbreak of acute gastroenteritis caused by a small round structured virus in a geriatric convalescent facility. *Infect Control Hosp Epidemiol* 1990;11:459–464.
24. Devi S, Murray C. Cockroaches (*Blatta* and *Periplaneta* species) as reservoirs of drug-resistant salmonellas. *Epidemiol Infect* 1991;107:357–361.
25. Svensson L, Uhnoo I, Wadell G. Enteric adenoviruses of man. In: Saif LJ, Theil KW, eds. *Viral diarrheas of man and animals.* Boca Raton, FL: CRC Press, 1990:97–111.
26. Harries A, Speare R, Wirima J. Symptoms and responses to chemotherapy in adult Malawians admitted to hospital with *Plasmodium falciparum* malaria. *Ann Trop Med Parisitol* 1985;82:511–512.
27. Muller O, Moser R. The clinical and parasitological presentation of *Plasmodium falciparum* malaria in Uganda is unaffected by HIV-1 infection. *Trans R Soc Trop Med Hyg* 1990;84:336–338.
28. Schumacher G, Kollberg B, Ljungh A. Inflammatory bowel disease presenting as travellers' diarrhea. *Lancet* 1993;341:241–242.
29. Guerrant R, Bobak D. Bacterial and protozoal gastroenteritis. *N Engl J Med* 1991;325(5):327–340.
30. Guerrant R, Shields D, Thorson S, et al. Evaluation and diagnosis of acute infectious diarrhea. *Am J Med* 1985;78:91–98.
31. Richards L, Claeson M, Pierce NF. Management of acute diarrhea in children: lessons learned. *Pediatr Infect Dis J* 1993;12:5–9.
32. Huicho L, Campos M, Rivera J, et al. Fecal screening tests in the approach to acute infectious diarrhea: a scientific overview. *Pediatr Infect Dis J* 1996;15:486–494.
33. Herbert ME. Medical myth: measuring white blood cells in the stools is useful in the management of acute diarrhea. *West J Med* 2000;172(6):414.
34. Guerrant R, Araujo V, Soares E, et al. Measurement of fecal lactoferrin as a marker of fecal leukocytes. *J Clin Microbiol* 1992;30:1238–1242.
35. Duggan C, Santosham M, Glass R. The management of acute diarrhea in children: oral rehydration, maintenance, and nutritional therapy. *MMWR Morbid Mortal Wkly Rep* 1992;41:RR1–RR20.
36. Avery M, Snyder J. Oral therapy for acute diarrhea. *N Engl J Med* 1990;323:891–894.
37. Snyder J. Oral therapy for diarrhea. *Hosp Pract* 1991;26:86–88.
38. Duggan C, Lasche J, McCarty M, et al. Oral rehydration solution for acute diarrhea prevents subsequent unscheduled follow-up visits. *Pediatrics* 1999;104(3):e29.
39. DuPont H, Ericsson C. Prevention and treatment of traveler's diarrhea. *N Engl J Med* 1993;328:1821–1827.
40. Editorial. Quinolones in acute non-travellers' diarrhea. *Lancet* 1990;336:282.

41. DuPont H, Sullivan P, Pickering L, et al. Symptomatic treatment of diarrhea with bismuth subsalicylate among students attending a Mexican university. *Gastroenterology* 1977;73:715–718.
42. DuPont H, Sullivan P, Evans D, et al. Prevention of travelers' diarrhea (emporiatric enteritis). Prophylactic administration of subsalicylate bismuth. *JAMA* 1980;243:237–241.
43. Figueroa-Quintanilla D, Salazar-Lindo E, Sack R, et al. A controlled trial of bismuth subsalicylate in infants with acute watery diarrheal disease. *N Engl J Med* 1993;328:1654–1658.
44. Snyder J. Can bismuth improve the simple solution for diarrhea? *N Engl J Med* 1993;328:1705–1706.
45. Crane J. Preformed bacterial toxins. *Clin Lab Med* 1999;19: 583–599.
46. Theil KW. Group A rotaviruses. In: Saif LJ, Theil KW, eds. *Viral diarrheas of man and animals.* Boca Raton, FL: CRC Press, 1990: 35–51.
47. Blacklow N, Cukor G. Viral gastroenteritis. *N Engl J Med* 1981; 304:397–406.
48. Uhnoo I, Olding-Stenkvist E, Kreuger A. Clinical features of acute gastroenteritis associated with rotavirus, enteric adenoviruses, and bacteria. *Arch Dis Child* 1986;61:732–738.
49. Van R, Wun CC, O'Ryan M, et al. Outbreaks of human enteric adenovirus types 40 and 41 in Houston day care centers. *J Pediatr* 1992;120:516–521.
50. Oyofo BA, Soderquist R, Lesmana M, et al. Norwalk-like virus and bacterial pathogens associated with cases of gastroenteritis onboard a US Navy ship. *Am J Trop Med Hyg* 1999;61(6):904–948.
51. Centers for Disease Control and Prevention. Outbreaks of Norwalk-like viral gastroenteritis—Alaska and Wisconsin, 1999. *MMWR Morbid Mortal Wkly Rep* 2000;49:207–211.
52. Guerrant RL, Kirchhoff LV, Shields DS, et al. Prospective study of diarrheal illnesses in northeastern Brazil: patterns of disease, nutritional impact, etiologies, and risk factors. *J Infect Dis* 1983; 148:986–997.
53. Cravioto A, Reyes RE, Trujillo F, et al. Risk of diarrhea during the first year of life associated with initial and subsequent colonization by specific enteropathogens. *Am J Epidemiol* 1990;131: 886–904.
54. Tardelli Gomes TA, Rassi V, MacDonald KL, et al. Enteropathogens associated with acute diarrheal disease in urban infants in Sao Paulo, Brazil. *J Infect Dis* 1991;164:331–337.
55. Blaser MJ, Reller LB. *Campylobacter* enteritis. *N Engl J Med* 1981;305:1444–1452.
56. Holmberg S, Schell W, Fanning G, et al. Aeromonas intestinal infections in the United States. *Ann Intern Med* 1986;105:683–689.
57. Holmberg S, Wachsmuth I, Hickman-Brenner F, et al. Plesiomonas enteric infections in the United States. *Ann Intern Med* 1986;105:690–694.
58. Ortega YR, Sterling CR, Gilman RH, et al. *Cyclospora* species—a new protozoan pathogen of humans. *N Engl J Med* 1993;328: 1308–1312.
59. Guerrant R. Principles and syndromes of enteric infection. In: Mandel G, Bennett J, Dolin R, eds. *Principles and practice of infectious diseases,* third edition. New York: Churchill Livingstone, 1995:946.
60. Ward RL, Bernstein DI, Young EC, et al. Human rotavirus studies in volunteers: determination of infectious dose and serological response to infection. *J Infect Dis* 1986;154:871–880.
61. Banerjee D. *Microbiology of infectious diseases.* London: Gower Medical, 1990.

18

ACUTE INFLAMMATORY DIARRHEA (DYSENTERY)

LEE W. RILEY

Oral rehydration therapy (ORT) is considered the cornerstone of global diarrheal disease control strategies. However, much of the life-saving benefits of ORT have applied to secretory and not to inflammatory diarrhea or dysentery. ORT has limited effect on mortality from inflammatory diarrhea, because deaths from inflammatory diarrhea are not caused by dehydration alone. In addition, inflammatory diarrhea is an important risk factor for persistent diarrhea—another manifestation of diarrhea associated with increased childhood mortality. Substantial progress has been made in developing countries in reducing the number of hospitalizations and deaths resulting from secretory diarrhea. In many countries, however, this has caused a relative increase in the proportion of diarrheal diseases caused by invasive pathogens, which, in turn, has created new concerns, including the emergence and spread of multidrug-resistant invasive bacterial organisms. The morbidity from inflammatory diarrhea is not limited to cases in developing countries. In developed countries or highly industrialized sectors of middle-income countries, bacterial agents of inflammatory diarrhea have intimately established themselves in the complex food distribution networks as well as in highly specialized nosocomial practices. This chapter highlights the pathogenesis, epidemiology, clinical features, and management of this syndrome.

DEFINITIONS

Inflammatory diarrhea is an acute enteric illness manifesting as diarrhea accompanied by fever and evidence in stool of an inflammatory process affecting the intestinal mucosa, such as pus, mucus, or blood. Dysentery is a severe manifestation of inflammatory diarrhea with blood or mucus in stool, accompanied by fever, crampy abdominal pain, and rectal tenesmus.

L. W. Riley: Infectious Diseases Unit, School of Public Health, University of California, Berkley, California

CLASSIFICATION

Syndromes that meet the definition of inflammatory diarrhea fall into two categories—those that are associated with recognized infectious agents and those that have no clearly identified infectious etiology (Table 18.1). Infectious agents that cause inflammatory diarrhea can be further divided into two subgroups—those organisms that elicit an inflammatory process by penetrating the intestinal mucosa and those that elaborate cytotoxins without invading the cells.

MICROBIOLOGY

Worldwide, invasive bacterial agents constitute the most important subgroup of etiologic agents of inflammatory diarrhea (1–24). Within the family Enterobacteriaceae, *Shigella* species (serogroups A–D: *dysenteriae, flexneri, sonnei,* and *boydii*), *Salmonella enterica*, enteroinvasive *Escherichia coli* (EIEC), and *Yersinia enterocolitica* cause inflammatory diarrhea. Among *Campylobacter* species, *Campylobacter jejuni* is the most common cause of inflammatory diarrhea. *Campylobacter coli* causes diarrhea in human hosts, but because most laboratories do not distinguish *C. coli* from *C. jejuni,* its true incidence is not known (25). In the United States, 5% to 10% of cases reported as *C. jejuni* may be caused by *C. coli* (26). Other species including *Campylobacter lari* (formerly *Campylobacter laridis*) and *Campylobacter hyointestinalis,* as well as *Helicobacter cindaedi* (formerly *Campylobacter cinaedi*) and *Helicobacter fenneliae* (formerly *Campylobacter fenneliae*), have been isolated from immunodeficient patients and homosexual men with enteritis and proctitis (27,28).

In patients with advanced AIDS, one of the many causes of acute diarrhea may include *Mycobacterium avium* complex (MAC), which can invade the intestinal mucosa (29,30).

Noninvasive bacterial pathogens can elicit inflammatory response in the intestine. The most common cause, espe-

TABLE 18.1. CLASSIFICATION OF INFLAMMATORY DIARRHEA

Diseases with recognized infectious etiology (pathogen) affecting all hosts:
Invasive pathogen diseases:
Amebic dysentery (*Entamoeba histolytica*)
Bacillary dysentery, shigellosis (*Shigella* species)
Balantidial dysentery (*Balantidium coli*)
Bilharzial dysentery (*Schistosoma japonicum, mansoni*)
Campylobacteriosis (*Campylobacter jejuni, coli*)
Invasive *E. coli* diarrhea (enteroinvasive *E. coli*)
Salmonellosis (*Salmonella* species)
Typhoid fever (*Salmonella typhi*)
Yersiniosis (*Yersinia enterocolitica*)
Cytotoxin-producing pathogen diseases:
Pseudomembranous colitis (*Clostridium difficile*)
Vibriosis (*Vibrio parahemolyticus*)
Diseases with recognized infectious etiology affecting predominantly hosts with underlying disease or immunodeficiency:
Persistent diarrhea (Enteroaggregative *E. coli*)
Cytomegalovirus colitis (cytomegalovirus)
Herpes virus colitis (herpes simplex)
Intestinal mycobacteriosis (*Mycobacterium avium*)
Isosporiasis (*Isospora belli*)
Phycomycosis (*Mucor, Rhizopus, Absidia*)
Strongylodiasis (*Strongyloides stercoralis*)
Diseases not recognized to be associated with specific infectious etiology:
Ulcerative colitis
Crohn's disease
Ischemic colitis
Neutropenic enterocolitis (typhlitis)
Chemical or metal poisonings (thallium sulfate, barium carbonate, arsenic, lead)
Other inflammatory diarrhea syndromes (associated pathogens):
Adult necrotizing entercolitis (*Clostridium perfringens* type C, others)
Neonatal necrotizing enterocolitis (polymicrobial etiology)

cially in nosocomial settings, is *Clostridium difficile,* a gram-positive, spore-forming obligate anaerobe. Other agents include *Vibrio parahaemolyticus* and *Clostridium perfringens* (31,32). *C. perfringens* type C is rarely associated with necrotizing enteritis in adults with poor nutrition or atypical dietary habits (33,34). A variety of bacterial agents have been implicated in necrotizing enterocolitis (NEC) in the newborn, including *Pseudomonas*, *Klebsiella*, *Clostridium butyricum*, *Salmonella*, and noninvasive *E. coli* strains (35–38). More recently, children infected with enteroaggregative *E. coli* (EaggEC) have been found to exhibit intestinal inflammatory response, and Caco cells infected with the organism elicit proinflammatory cytokines (39).

E. coli strains belonging to the enterohemorrhagic *E. coli* (EHEC) group cause a distinct syndrome called hemorrhagic colitis (40–42). Although this cytoxin-producing organism causes bloody diarrhea referred to as *hemorrhagic colitis,* this clinical manifestation is usually not considered part of the syndromes of inflammatory diarrhea (see later discussion). A detailed discussion of this pathogen is presented in Chapter 42.

The most common parasitic cause of inflammatory diarrhea is *Entamoeba histolytica.* A ciliate protozoan *Balantidium coli* can penetrate with its rotary boring action the mucosa of the cecum and terminal ileum, and cause a dysenteric syndrome (balantidial dysentery) (43). The coccidian parasite *Isospora belli* can penetrate colonic mucosal cells in AIDS patients and elicit diarrhea (44,45). Eggs deposited by adult trematodes *Schistosoma mansoni* and *Schistosoma japonicum* in the intestinal venules can rupture the wall of the venules, thus eliciting focal inflammation, bleeding, and diarrhea (46). Heavy intestinal infestation by *Strongyloides stercoralis* can cause dysentery, often associated with secondary bacterial infection (47).

Viral and fungal agents generally do not cause inflammatory diarrhea in immunocompetent hosts. Cytomegalovirus has been associated with colitis and bloody diarrhea in some patients with ulcerative colitis (48,49), AIDS (50,51), and other immunosuppressive disorders (52). A patient with AIDS often has several concurrent causes of diarrhea, and Herpes simplex and adenovirus have been attributed to some cases of colitis (53). Agents of phycomycosis have been rarely implicated in bloody diarrhea in diabetic patients (54,55).

Crohn's disease and ulcerative colitis are two major syndromes of chronic, relapsing inflammatory bowel disease for which infectious etiologies have not been demonstrated. Several recent studies have reported the possible association of *Mycobacterium paratuberculosis* in Crohn's disease (56,57). Using oligonucleotide primers based on *M. paratuberculosis* DNA sequences, several investigators have reported detecting *M. paratuberculosis* DNA sequences significantly more often from patients with than without Crohn's disease.

PATHOGENESIS

A traditional but rarely used method to demonstrate the capacity of bacteria to produce dysentery relies on the ability of the organism to elicit keratoconjunctivitis in guinea pigs (Sereny test) (58). Invasive bacterial organisms that cause inflammatory diarrhea have evolved a complex and highly regulated set of proteins to enter intestinal nonphagocytic and phagocytic cells, resist, subvert, or escape the antimicrobial machinery of the intracellular environment of host cells, and alter the host's immune response to the advantage of the pathogens themselves. The ability of the organism to enter cells, multiply, and spread from cell to cell is usually studied *in vitro* by infection of monolayers of cultured mammalian cells, such as HeLa, HEp-2, Henle, and Caco-2 cells, among others. Noninvasive, cytotoxin-elaborating bacterial organisms are studied by the demonstration of morphologic changes and cytopathic effects elicited by organisms in cultured cells, such as Vero, HeLa,

Chinese hamster ovary (CHO) cells, and human foreskin fibroblasts. These tissue culture models have greatly contributed to the identification and understanding of the molecular basis of cell invasion, host proinflammatory response, and diarrhea pathogenesis associated with the agents of inflammatory diarrhea.

Invasive Pathogens

Invasive bacterial pathogens enter mammalian cells via one of two major mechanisms (59). One is receptor-mediated phagocytosis or the "zipper" mechanism, in which bacteria express a surface ligand that binds tightly to a specific mammalian receptor that allows the plasma membrane of the cell to wrap around the entire organism as the organism is engulfed. The other is macropinocytosis or the "trigger" mechanism, in which the bacteria secrete a set of effector proteins into a mammalian cell upon contact and induce massive cytoskeletal rearrangement that leads to membrane ruffling (59). *Shigella* and *Salmonella* organisms initiate their association with intestinal cells by first entering nonphagocytic cells by macropinocytosis. *Yersinia* species, on the other hand, enter nonphagocytic cells by a receptor-mediated process, in which a surface protein called invasin binds to the β1 integrin on the enterocyte surface (60–62).

Invasive bacterial agents associated with inflammatory diarrhea elicit distinct clinical manifestations in human hosts, and these manifestations are ultimately determined by the characteristic interaction that these pathogens establish with host intestinal cells. *Shigella* organisms produce intense, acute inflammatory response in the colon with massive infiltration of neutrophils that leads to ulceration and abscess formation. Despite the intensity of this inflammatory response, *Shigella* rarely causes bacteremia; much of the infectious process is confined to the colon. Shigellae are believed to invade the colonic mucosa via the basolateral surface of enterocytes accessed by the organism through the opening of intercellular junctions (63). *Shigella* and EIEC carry several genes (*ipa* genes) clustered on a virulence plasmid of molecular mass between 180 and 230 kb that are required for mammalian cell invasion (64,65). After gaining entry into cells, Shigellae and EIEC have devised a mechanism to escape the membrane-bound vacuole or phagosome to enter the cytoplasm. This escape from the phagosome is facilitated by pore-forming proteins, belonging to a family of hemolysins also encoded by the *ipa* genes (66). IpaB is the major protein associated with vacuole lysis, but IpaC may also be involved (67). Once in the cytoplasm, the organism can proliferate and spread to adjacent cells by actin-dependent movement (68). A 120-kd outer membrane protein IcsA (also named VirG), encoded by the large plasmid, is necessary for F-actin comet tail formation, which facilitates this cell-to-cell spread (68). Expression of a cell adhesion molecule cadherin by the enterocyte is required for this spread (69).

In vivo, shigellae that escape the enterocytes may be taken up by lamina propria macrophages. *In vitro* as well as animal studies suggest that *Shigella flexneri* induces apoptosis in macrophages (70–72). Rectal biopsy studies of shigellosis in humans have demonstrated evidence of lamina propria macrophage apoptosis (73). *Shigella* IpaB, which in the enterocyte is required by the bacteria to escape the vacuole, binds to a cysteine protease caspase-1 inside macrophages to activate the apoptotic cascade (74). Caspase-1 is required by *Shigella* to activate IL-1β and IL-18 (75). IL-1β attracts neutrophils to the site of infection, which leads to the characteristic dysenteric inflammatory response observed with shigellosis. IL-18 may be involved in the induction of interferon (IFN) -γ, which facilitates elimination of the bacteria (75).

Yersinia species invade intestinal cells, presumably through the M cells located in lymphoid follicles (Peyer patch) of the intestine, and induce inflammation that leads to gastroenteritis, mesenteric lymphadenitis, and bacteremia. *Yersinia pseudotuberculosis* and *Yersinia enterocolitica* express a single 103-kd chromosomally encoded protein product called *invasin*, which mediates both attachment and invasion of the organism into cultured epithelial cells (60,61). Invasin interacts with the β1 subunit of heterodimeric proteins belonging to an integrin subfamily (VLA proteins) of cell adhesion molecules (62). Integrins are transmembrane proteins that mediate cell attachment by linking extracellular matrix proteins with intracellular cytoskeletal elements. During entry, actin and actin-associated proteins, such as filamin and talin, accumulate around an invading bacillus (76). Integrin binding by invasin presumably triggers a signal transduction that leads to cytoskeletal reorganization (76).

Yersinia organisms also express a set of virulence plasmid-encoded proteins called *Yersinia* outer membrane proteins (Yops), which are associated with phosphatase and kinase activities, microfilament disruption, G-protein–linked receptor stimulation, and cysteine protease activity that inhibits mitogen-activated protein kinase (MAPK) and nuclear factor κB (NF-κB) signal pathways in animal cells (77–81). The characteristic feature of *Yersinia* species is their ability to inactivate macrophages from the extracellular location, such that the organism is not engulfed by the cell, or, if the organism does enter the cell, it is not killed by the macrophage. This inactivation is accomplished by a unique set of effector Yops that are injected into macrophages by a specialized protein secretion mechanism that is shared by all of the invasive bacterial pathogens discussed in this section.

S. enterica species presumably enter the M cells via the apical surface by macropinocytosis. Like *Yersinia* organisms, they spread to mesenteric lymph nodes and blood to cause systemic infections. Like *Shigella*, the entry of *Salmonella* is accompanied by membrane ruffling (82). The different clinical manifestations of salmonellosis—gastroenteritis, bacteremia, systemic infections, or persistent asymptomatic carriage—may be determined by the differential and coordinate expression of a set of *Salmonella* genes located in specialized segments of the chromosome called *Salmonella* pathogenicity islands (SPI) (83,84). These SPIs encode a variety of proteins that allow the organism to initiate nonphagocytic cell invasion in the intestine, to survive and replicate inside the vacuolar compartment of these cells, to induce apoptosis in intestinal macrophages, to mediate inflammation and fluid secretion by the intestinal mucosa, and to persist *in vivo*. These proteins are described in detail in Chapter 44.

The invasive bacterial organisms described earlier have all evolved a common, general theme in their strategy to enter and survive the antimicrobial machinery of host cells. Moreover, the specificity of the proteins that comprise this strategy appears to determine the unique clinical features elicited in the host by these agents of inflammatory diarrhea. Many of the pathogenic features of these organisms have come to be attributed to a complex set of genes located in virulence plasmids or in chromosomal pathogenicity islands arranged to deliver virulence factors to mammalian cells; they are collectively termed *type III protein secretion systems* (85–87). The components of type III secretion systems, comprising more than 20 proteins, have been identified in animal and plant pathogens, and are related to some of the proteins involved in bacterial flagellar assembly (85,86). In *Shigella*, *Yersinia*, and *Salmonella* species, this protein export machinery is designed to deliver proteins (referred to *as effector proteins* or *translocated proteins*) that can subvert normal host cell signaling pathway by facilitating (in the case of *Shigella* and *Salmonella*) or inhibiting (in the case of *Yersinia*) cell uptake of the bacteria, allowing the intracellular organism to survive, triggering an apoptotic cascade in macrophages, or inducing a proinflammatory response *in vivo* that elicits the characteristic clinical manifestation associated with the organism. In addition to the translocated proteins, type III secretion systems are comprised of proteins that form a supramolecular structure known as the *needle complex* that spans the inner and outer membranes of gram-negative organisms to direct the effector proteins to mammalian cells (88). The effector proteins also require other proteins (chaperones) that prevent degradation or improper folding of the effector proteins as they are delivered to the mammalian cell. Finally, the expression of these proteins are highly regulated by the other gene products of this secretion system, where the regulation may be determined by environmental cues sensed by the organism as it enters different stages of its infection of the host. Many of the type III secretion system proteins contain sequence domains that are conserved across species, but, in general, the effector proteins themselves appear to be specific to a particular species. This specificity may determine the differences in disease manifestations associated with these enteric pathogens.

The pathogenicity islands contain other genes in addition to those belonging to the type III secretion system. To date, at least five SPIs have been identified in *S. enterica* serotype typhimurium (*S. typhimurium*) (84). The relatively low GC content (37% to 47%) of these regions compared with the rest of the chromosome (about 52%) suggests that *S. typhimurium* may have gained these large gene cassettes by horizontal transfer from phage or plasmids (84). SopB, a protein that is translocated into a mammalian cell cytoplasm, is encoded by SPI5, but it uses the SPI1 type III secretion apparatus to be exported (89). SopB has been identified as an inositol phosphate phosphatase that may be needed to activate a pathway that leads to chloride secretion and hence fluid influx by enterocytes (90).

Some of the genes in these other SPIs are, in turn, regulated by global regulators, such as the two-component regulatory system PhoP/PhoQ, which appears to be repressed by magnesium and calcium, at least *in vitro* (91,92). Furthermore, PhoP-activated genes in *S. typhimurium* have been recently shown to alter the cell envelope through changes in lipid A component of its lipopolysaccharide, which has been suggested to facilitate intracellular survival by allowing the organism to gain increased resistance to host cationic antimicrobial peptides (93–95). Thus, it is becoming clear that pathogenesis of invasive enteric bacterial pathogens involves a coordinate regulation of a complex set of proteins that are required by the organism at different stages of its infection and that these pathogens appear to have evolved by sampling cassettes of genes from elsewhere to assure their survival among a community of mammalian hosts.

A eukaryotic organism *E. histolytica* causes amebic dysentery and its pathogenesis is dependent on both organism and host factors. After excystation in the lumen of the intestines, *E. histolytica* trophozoites invade the colonic epithelium at the sites of their attachment mediated by a 260-kd galactose-specific lectin (96,97). The lectin confers some protection against amebic liver abscess, a complication of amebic dysentery, in lectin-immunized gerbils, suggesting that this adhesin is an important virulence factor of the organism (98). The amebas characteristically produce cytolysis and tissue destruction at the site of attachment, and these effects are contact- and temperature- (37°C) dependent (99). Ravdin and colleagues (100) reported that CHO cell lysis by *E. histolytica* trophozoites can be inhibited by antagonists of calcium-dependent phospholipase A activity. An antilectin monoclonal antibody that blocks the cytotoxic effect after adherence of the trophozoite has been identified, suggesting that the lectin itself may play a role in cytolysis (101). A number of other potential amebic cytolethal substances have been identified, but their role in pathogenesis has not been defined. Trophozoites lyse infiltrating neutrophils at the site of infection, and the released neutrophil enzymes are believed to contribute to some of the tissue pathology (102). *In vitro* as well as SCID mouse-human intestinal xenograft studies have shown that incubation of *E. histolytica* trophozoites with epithelial cell lines or with the mouse is associated with the production of proinflammatory cytokines, including IL-1 and IL-8 (103,104).

In the mouse model, the human xenograft cells were demonstrated to be the source of IL-8 (104).

Cytotoxin-Producing Pathogens

The invasive pathogen *S. dysenteriae* type 1, the cause of bacillary dysentery pandemics, produces a potent exotoxin called *Shiga toxin* (ST), which is cytotoxic to certain cultured cells and enterotoxic to ligated segments of rabbit ileum (105,106). It inhibits mammalian cell protein synthesis by depurinating ribosomal RNA (107). After the recent discovery of related cytotoxins elaborated by *E. coli* strains associated with diarrhea, ST has come to be considered a prototype of a family of toxins called Shiga-like toxins (108,109). The toxin consists of one A subunit linked to five B subunits. The B subunit is believed to bind the toxin to cellular neutral glycolipid Gb3 on the rabbit microvillus membrane, which is thought to inhibit the villus cell Na^+ absorption and hence elicit net fluid secretion (110). More recently, another exotoxin called *Shigella* exotoxin 2 (ShET-2) has been identified in *S. flexneri* (111). Encoded by the large *Shigella* plasmid, its role in pathogenesis is not yet clear.

An *S. dysenteriae* 1 strain deleted in the ST gene can produce cell death and diarrhea with pus in rhesus monkeys (112). Strains belonging to *Shigella* serogroups that elaborate only low levels of ST can produce severe dysentery. Although direct cytotoxic effects of ST on vascular endothelial cells have been demonstrated (113) and hence the toxin could conceivably produce the vascular damage that elicits bleeding, the aforementioned observations suggest that the inflammatory response may not be all related to the toxin effect.

C. difficile, the etiologic agent of pseudomembranous colitis and antibiotic-associated diarrhea, produces at least two toxins—an enterotoxin called toxin A (TxA) and a cytotoxin called toxin B (TxB) (114,115). TxA is a potent chemoattractant of neutrophils, which, in a rat model, was found to be dependent on macrophage-derived cytokines, including TNF-α and IL-1β (116). It can elicit inflammation and fluid accumulation in ligated rabbit ileal loops. Inhibitors of platelet-activating factor and phospholipase D can block these secretory and inflammatory responses. The role of TxB in diarrhea production has not been clearly demonstrated, but it is speculated that the toxin may require TxA to express its full biologic effect. Recently, both TxA and TxB have been shown to monoglucosylate members of small GTPases, including Rho, Rac, and Cdc42 (117,118). The glucosylation of these proteins would disrupt a variety of cellular functions, including cytoskeletal rearrangement, motility, adhesion, phagocytosis, NADPH oxidase activity, and other cell signaling processes. How these effects lead to the characteristic clinical manifestation of diarrhea and pseudomembranous colitis is not yet clear.

Most clinical isolates of *V. parahaemolyticus* induce β-hemolysis (Kanagawa phenomenon, or KP) in Wagatsuma blood agar medium, whereas only 1% to 2% of environmental isolates exhibit this reaction (119,120). Hence, the KP is epidemiologically associated with diarrhea caused by *V. parahaemolyticus.* The KP is mediated by thermostable direct hemolysin (TDH), which has cytotoxic and enterotoxic activities. It can stimulate fluid accumulation in ligated rabbit ileal loop (121). A wild-type *V. parahaemolyticus* strain but not its isogenic TDH mutant was shown to produce fluid accumulation in rabbit ileal loop (122). Invasion of the colonic mucosa by *V. parahaemolyticus* has also been reported (123).

Recently, children in Brazil infected with EaggEC have been shown to have significantly elevated lactoferrin, a marker of inflammation, as well as cytokines IL-8 and IL-1β in their stools (39). An *in vitro* study showed that clinical isolates of EaggEC elicited IL-8 release from Caco-2 cells and that this release was apparently mediated by a heat-stable, high-molecular-weight protein that appears to be a novel flagellin present in the culture filtrates (124).

Other Dysenteric Syndromes

Dysentery can be a component of syndromes in which infections result from a secondary complication of a primary disease process. These include NEC, ischemic colitis, and neutropenic enterocolitis.

The most important risk factor for NEC is premature birth. A variety of infectious agents have been associated with neonatal NEC, including *Klebsiella, Salmonella, E. coli, Pseudomonas,* and *Clostridium butyricum* (35–38). The intestinal pathology of NEC resembles that observed in ischemic injury (see later text), in which the areas of necrosis may become superinfected with intestinal flora. NEC in the newborn often follows episodes of asphyxia, apnea, respiratory distress syndrome, or hypothermia, which can contribute to the intestinal ischemia and devitalization. Others have suggested that the disease is promoted by a Schwartzman reaction following an infectious process (125). Neonatal NEC probably has a variety of causes, triggered by unknown factors that initially affect the gut mucosa, which is then secondarily infected with the gut flora; some of these organisms may produce gas and cause dissection through the friable bowel wall, and others may produce peritonitis or septicemia. Recent studies suggest that hematopoietic cytokines may play important roles in the intestinal inflammatory response, including regulation of nitric oxide (NO) production affecting the progression of NEC (126).

Neutropenic enterocolitis (typhlitis, ileocecal syndrome) has been described in patients treated for lymphoma and leukemia (127,128), transplant patients (129), and in patients with AIDS (130). Most of the cases were described before the association of *C. difficile* with pseudomembranous colitis was recognized and hence could represent antibiotic-associated or cancer chemotherapy–associated pseudomembranous colitis.

A patchy necrotizing small bowel disease progressing to segmental gangrene with pockets of gas occurs in adults in association with poor nutrition or certain dietary habits (33,34). *C. perfringens* type C β toxin may play a role in its pathogenesis (131).

EPIDEMIOLOGY

Worldwide, the etiologic agents of inflammatory diarrhea are isolated from 10% to more than 50% of children with diarrhea younger than 6 years of age, or from 15% to 75% of all diarrhea specimens in which a recognized enteric pathogen is identified (Table 18.2) (1–24). These differences result from variable study designs (geography, age, or socioeconomic groups examined, community versus institution-based study, and the types of organisms sought).

The most common cause of diarrhea among travelers to Latin America, Africa, and Asia is enterotoxigenic *E. coli* (ETEC). However, *Shigella, Salmonella,* and *Campylobacter* organisms are important causes of traveler's diarrhea in Nepal, Morocco, Saudi Arabia, Hong Kong, and Thailand, varying according to season and place of travel (11–24). Among American troops living in Saudi Arabia during Operation Desert Shield in 1990, agents of inflammatory diarrhea composed 50% of all diarrhea cases in which a pathogen was identified (Table 18.2), and *Shigella* was isolated more frequently than any other pathogen except ETEC (11). *Y. enterocolitica* infections are rare in tropical countries.

According to the U.S. Public Health Service surveillance system, the reported incidence (per 100,000 population) of salmonellosis, excluding typhoid fever, was between 10 and 15 in the 1970s, 15 to more than 25 in the 1980s, and between 12 and 18 in the 1990s (132). Shigellosis has also shown an increasing trend in incidence in the late 1980s through the 1990s, fluctuating between 7 to 12 per 100,000 population (132). These reported isolation rates probably represent only 1% to 5% of the infections that actually occur each year in the United States (133). In January 1996, the U.S. Public Health Service initiated the Foodborne Diseases Active Surveillance Network (Food-

TABLE 18.2. ETIOLOGIC STUDIES OF ACUTE DIARRHEA, 1984–1997

			Invasive Bacteria			
Study Site (Ref.)	Population Studied	Period of Study	No.	(%)[a]	(%)[b]	*Entamoeba histolytica* %[d]
Bangkok, Thailand[c] (1)	Children <5 yr	1988–1989	119	(31)	(52)	<1
Hong Kong[2] (2)	All ages with diarrhea	1984–1990	2004	(10)	(61)	NR
Sao Paulo, Brazil[c] (3)	Infants <12 mo	1985–1986	87	(19)	(24)	NR
Western Australia[c] (4)	Aboriginal children <5 yr	1985–1988	38	(NR)	(22)	0
Chiapas, Mexico[c] (5)	Children <6 yr	Summer 1987	19	(36)	(66)	NR
Anapur-Palla, India (6)	Children <3 yr	1985–1986	18	(10)	(25)	0
Djibouti, Djibouti (7)	All ages with diarrhea	February 1989	29	(14)	(30)	NR
Manila, Philippines[c] (8)	All ages with diarrhea	1984	466	(25)	(36)	0.1
Dhaka, Bangladesh[c] (9)	Children <6 yr	1984–1986	29	(13)	(53)	<1
Aswan, Egypt[c] (10)	Children <5 yr	July 86	30	(20)	(22)	<1
Saudi Arabia (11)	U.S. troops in Desert Shield	September to December 1990	125	(29)	(50)	NR
Kathmandu, Nepal[c] (12)	Travelers and US Peace Corps	1986–1987	114	(35)	(75)	5
Morocco (13)	Travelers from Finland	1989	64	(37)	(63)	NR
Bogota, Columbia[c] (14)	Infants and children	1997	31	(6)	(15)	15
Kansai Airport, Japan (15)	Returning travelers	1979–1995	3,478	(12)	(36)	NR
Rio de Janeiro, Brazil[c] (16)	Children 0–3 yr	1987–1988	48	(12)	(19)	NR
Lagos, Nigeria[c] (17)	Children <5 yr	1989–1990	21	(10)	(13)	0.5
Guinea-Bissau[c] (18)	Children <5 yr	1987–1988	134	(11)	(22)	2
Western Thailand[c] (19)	All ages with diarrhea	1991	125	(24)	(57)	NR
Hong Kong[c] (20)	Children <5 yr	1994–1995	117	(30)	(50)	NR
Melbourne, Australia[c] (21)	Children 0–14 yr	1980–1993	360	(10)	(17)	NR
Vientienne, Laos[c] (22)	All ages with diarrhea	1996–1997	229	(26)	(60)	NR
Jamaica[c] (23)	Travelers to Jamaica	1996–1997	44	(14)	(36)	1
Dhaka, Bangladesh[c] (24)	Children <5 yr	1993–1994	232	(29)	(39)	1

NR, not reported.
[a]Proportion of all cases of acute diarrhea.
[b]Proportion of all cases of diarrhea with specific diagnosis; invasive bacterial pathogens sought for included *Shigella, Salmonella, Campylobacter,* enteroinvasive *Escherichia coli, Yersinia,* and *Entamoeba histolytica*.
[c]Studies in which rotavirus was sought.
[d]Proportion of all microbiologically diagnosed cases.

Net) for culture-confirmed cases of *Campylobacter*, *Salmonella*, *Shigella*, *Yersinia*, *Vibrio*, and *E. coli* O157:H7. Between 1996 and 1999, three invasive bacterial pathogens—*Campylobacter*, *Salmonella*, and *Shigella*—accounted for more than 90% of these causes of foodborne diseases in the United States. (134).

In the United States, the peak isolation rates for *Salmonella* are observed in infants between 2 and 3 months of age, and for *Shigella,* in children between 2 and 3 years of age. The isolation rate for *Campylobacter* remains constant through the first year of life and peaks in the young adult age group (20 to 40 years of age). With *Y. enterocolitica,* age-specific attack rates are highest for children between 1 and 3 years of age.

Globally (excluding China), *E. histolytica* is estimated to infect about 500 million persons (135). Diarrhea develops in 8% to 10% of these cases. In contrast to invasive bacterial pathogens, the rate of infection with *E. histolytica* increases with age. Disease manifestation also varies geographically. Invasive disease develops in one of every five infected persons in Mexico compared with one of every 100 to 1,000 infections in the temperate areas (135).

Primates are the only reservoir of *Shigella* organisms, whereas *Salmonella* organisms have entrenched themselves into a variety of reservoirs, some of which are serotype (serovar)-specific. For example, humans are the only reservoir for *S. enterica* serovar Typhi. Poultry has become a major reservoir for the serotype *S. enterica* serovar Enteritidis in the United States; between 1993 and 1997, this one serotype was responsible for more cases, outbreaks, and deaths than any other *Salmonella* serotype (136). In industrialized countries, through their extensive food distribution network, a single contaminated food product can become a vehicle for infections in geographically widespread areas, and a single clone of *Salmonella* can be responsible for such epidemics (137,138).

C. jejuni is associated with the drinking of raw milk, but it is also commonly found in poultry products. In Japan, *V. parahaemolyticus* is the major cause of diarrhea in summer and is associated with eating uncooked fish (sushi, sashimi) or shellfish (31). In northern Europe, the main reservoir for *Y. enterocolitica* is the swine (139); in the United States, yersiniosis outbreaks have been attributed to contaminated pasteurized milk (140), pig intestines (chitterlings) (141), and homemade tofu (142).

Humans are the main reservoir of *E. histolytica,* but natural infections in macaque monkeys and pigs have been observed (143,144). Domesticated animals such as dogs and cattle may be secondarily infected from human feces. Pigs are the major reservoir of *B. coli* (43).

Shigella infections are predominantly transmitted person-to-person and are a common cause of day care center outbreaks (145,146). However, large outbreaks of shigellosis caused by contaminated foods are occasionally reported (147,148). As mentioned, animal food products are the major vehicles of *Salmonella* infections, but person-to-person transmission is also common. Often, *Salmonella* is introduced into a household through a contaminated food product and the infection is sustained thereafter via person-to-person transmission (149). Now rare in the United States, nosocomial outbreaks of salmonellosis, particularly with drug-resistant strains, pose a serious problem in some middle-income countries (150). *Y. enterocolitica,* which often causes bacteremia, can be enriched in phosphate buffer solution at 4 to 7°C. Hence, this organism may be transmitted by transfusion of contaminated blood (151,152). *E. histolytica* and *B. coli* are transmitted person-to-person. One form of NEC called *pig-bel,* associated with *C. perfringens* type C β toxin, is associated with a large pork feast in the highlands of New Guinea (33).

C. difficile is the most common cause of diarrhea in hospital settings, accounting for up to 45% of nosocomial diarrhea with a recognized cause (153). Widespread use of broad-spectrum antibiotics as well as antineoplastic agents contribute to its increasing incidence in hospitals.

Neonatal NEC is associated with low birth weight (35). Other reported associations include exchange transfusions, congenital deficiency of the bowel wall, trauma to the fetus in utero, use of umbilical catheters, the toxic effect of polyvinylchloride blood bags, and the infectious agents mentioned earlier (154–159).

CLINICAL FEATURES

As with all enteric pathogens, the agents of inflammatory diarrhea cause a wide spectrum of clinical manifestations, including asymptomatic carriage, explosive watery diarrhea, mucus- and blood-containing diarrhea, and extraintestinal or systemic complications. Disease manifestations and incubation periods are influenced by factors such as inoculum size, vehicles of infection, virulence properties of the organism, and host factors.

Factors that Influence Disease Manifestation

Information regarding minimum infective doses of organisms is usually derived from volunteer studies. One such study showed that approximately 10^5 *S. typhi* organisms caused symptoms in 28% of volunteers (160). These volunteer studies, however, are limited by the choice of strains used, the homogeneous age group of the volunteers (usually young males), and the choice of vehicle used to infect the volunteers (usually water). In natural settings, organisms can be introduced into the host via vehicles that buffer the organism from gastric acidity (fatty food items such as milk, cheese, chocolate). Thus, a lower inoculum dose can reach the intestines to cause symptomatic disease (161). In typhoid outbreaks traced to foods, the minimal infective dose of *S. typhi* was estimated to be less than 10^3 organisms (161). Organisms adapted to the human host, such as *Shigella* and *S. typhi,* are known to produce disease with lower infective doses. *Shigella* organisms can cause symptomatic disease with infective dose as low as 10 organisms (162).

Virulence determinants of an organism affect disease expression. *S. typhi* organisms possessing the Vi antigen cause a higher attack rate and shorter incubation periods among volunteers (160). In general, *S. sonnei* causes milder disease than *S. flexneri* or *S. dysenteriae* 1. The isoenzyme patterns of *E. histolytica* strains that produce asymptomatic disease are distinct from those that produce symptomatic disease (163), and the avirulent genotype is now distinguished as *E. dispar* (see Chapter 60).

Finally, it is well recognized that persons with underlying diseases such as malignancies, sickle cell anemia, schistosomiasis, gastrectomy, achlorhydria, and AIDS, and persons taking antacids or antibiotics have increased susceptibility to symptomatic illness after *Salmonella* infection (164–171). Penicillins, in particular, increase the chance of symptomatic infection due to multidrug-resistant strains of *Salmonella* (172). The variable age-specific attack rates of shigellosis, salmonellosis, and campylobacteriosis suggest age-dependent susceptibility to symptomatic disease. Disease manifestation varies with age also. *Salmonella* bacteremia is more common in infants and the elderly (173). During a multistate outbreak in 1982, *Y. enterocolitica* was isolated from 14 persons with pharyngitis; all 14 were adults and enteritis occurred only in children (174). Host immunity influenced by the frequency of background exposures to pathogens affects disease manifestation. In two separate diarrhea outbreaks, the attack rate after *C. jejuni* infection was lower among farmers who regularly drank raw milk than among persons who were not previously exposed (175).

Asymptomatic Carriage

Asymptomatic convalescent carriage (excretion of organism in stool for longer than a year) of *Shigella*, *Campylobacter*, or *Yersinia* is rare, occurs in less than 1% with nontyphi *Salmonella,* and is 1% to 3% with *S. typhi* infections (176). The median duration of excretion of nontyphi *Salmonella* after salmonellosis (convalescent carriage) has been estimated to be 5 weeks and is longer in children. In Norway, 47% of the patients with *Y. enterocolitica* illness had prolonged shedding of the organism (mean 50.4 days) (177). Asymptomatic chronic carriage of *E. histolytica* varies geographically but is lower when *E. dispar* infections are excluded (see Chapter 60) (135). Approximately 40% of healthy neonates colonized with *C. difficile* have high fecal toxin titers (178). High titers of fecal toxin are rarely detected in older children colonized with *C. difficile*, and although diarrhea may develop in a few, pseudomembranous colitis rarely develops (153).

Symptomatic Infections

Although *S. dysenteriae* 1 usually produces a more severe dysenteric illness than other *Shigella* serotypes, in Bangladesh the highest mortality rate attributed to shigellosis was associated with infection with *S. sonnei* (case fatality rate of 10.3%) (179). In developed countries, such as the United States, *S. sonnei* generally causes mild, self-limited illness. However, in the preantibiotic era, *S. sonnei* was associated with severe dysenteric syndrome with systemic complications such as seizures (180,181). These geographic or temporal differences in clinical manifestations may relate to the differences in background infectious inoculum size or pathogenicity of predominant clonal strains in the community.

S. typhi is associated with a clinical syndrome, distinct from typical salmonellosis, called *typhoid* or *enteric fever* in which enteritis is one component of a systemic illness. The incubation period is usually longer (7 to 14 days) than in nontyphoidal *Salmonella* infections (24 to 72 hours), and the first clinical manifestation is fever rather than gastrointestinal symptoms. Diarrhea is seen only in approximately one-half of the patients. Extraintestinal involvement such as splenomegaly and hepatomegaly occurs in approximately one-third of patients, and erythematous maculopapular lesions (rose spots) on the abdomen are seen in about one-half. The systemic involvement results from bacteremia. The illness may last 2 to 3 weeks. In the preantibiotic era, intestinal hemorrhage developed in 5% to 20% of the patients and intestinal perforation developed in 2% to 5%. With appropriate antimicrobial therapy and supportive care, the mortality rate attributed to typhoid fever is less than 1%, and the complications of intestinal perforation and hemorrhage are rare (<1%) (182).

Nontyphoidal salmonellosis is characteristically accompanied by fever, nausea, anorexia, vomiting, crampy abdominal pain, and frequent loose bowel movements—manifestations clinically indistinguishable from the typical manifestations of other invasive or cytotoxin-producing bacterial or invasive protozoal infections. Bloody diarrhea occurs with similar frequency (13% to 27%) as in *Campylobacter* enteritis, but with less frequency compared to shigellosis, and it occurs more often in children (1–24).

Some cases of salmonellosis, especially during the early phase of the illness, can be mistaken for secretory diarrhea. Explosive, watery diarrhea may resemble cholera-like illness with mild fever, and profound dehydration may develop. Such a presentation may depend on the serotype of the organism. A "choleriform syndrome" with *Salmonella infantis* and *Salmonella haardt* infections has been reported (183), and a possible role of an enterotoxin in some strains of *Salmonella* for this syndrome has been suggested (184).

Initially, watery diarrhea followed by blood-streaked stools develop in most patients with *C. jejuni* enteritis, but severe dehydration is rare. In advanced disease, colitis or proctitis with crypt abscess formation resembling severe shigellosis, amebiasis, or ulcerative colitis can develop (185).

Bloody diarrhea with yersiniosis occurs mostly in children. In addition to enteritis in infected patients, mesenteric adenitis and terminal ileitis, which can be mistaken for appendicitis, may develop. Furthermore, suppuration of the appendix itself from *Y. enterocolitica* infection can occur (186,187).

Bloody diarrhea is seen in 5% to 10% of patients with *C. difficile*-associated diarrhea. Most patients have brown or clear watery diarrhea, but 85% of patients with pseudomembranous colitis have mucus in the stool (188).

The characteristic symptomatic illness produced by *E. histolytica* is rectocolitis. Nearly all patients have heme-positive stool, but, unlike shigellosis, stool leukocytes may not be abundant because of their lysis by the organism (102,189,190). Also, in contrast to colitis from invasive bacterial pathogens, fever occurs in only approximately one-third of the symptomatic patients.

Liver abscess caused by *E. histolytica* often is not preceded by any symptomatic intestinal disease (up to 50%) and develops within 2 to 5 months after exposure (189). It can manifest acutely with abdominal pain, fever, and diarrhea, or subacutely with vague abdominal pain without diarrhea and accompanied only by weight loss. Hepatomegaly occurs in less than half of cases, and jaundice is not a feature of this disease.

Cytomegalovirus (CMV) can cause severe gastrointestinal illness in patients receiving solid organ or bone marrow transplants, in patients taking immunosuppressive drugs, or in persons with AIDS or ulcerative colitis (48–52). The symptoms may include malaise, anorexia, nausea, vomiting, fever, abdominal pain, and diarrhea with blood. The disease can involve the entire gastrointestinal tract, which is quite distinct from dysenteric disease caused by other pathogens. Hence, a patient may have bright red blood per rectum or melena, depending on the site of involvement. Bleeding results from ulcerations of the gut mucosa. Colon appears to be more commonly involved in kidney transplant patients, as opposed to the esophagus in heart or heart-lung transplant patients (52).

Complications

In Bangladesh, during 1 year of active surveillance in 1984, 39% of 46,607 cases of diarrhea were found to be bloody, but deaths from bloody diarrhea accounted for 62% of all diarrhea deaths (191). Watery diarrhea was responsible for 41% of all diarrhea cases but 36% of all deaths. *Shigella* was identified from 64% of cultured bloody stool samples. Hence, in places like Bangladesh, bloody diarrhea and, in particular, shigellosis is a major cause of mortality. Worldwide, *Shigella* is estimated to cause 200 million cases of diarrhea and 650,000 deaths each year (192).

Severe dehydration (>10% body weight) is not a prominent feature of most inflammatory diarrheal syndromes but can occur as a complication of these illnesses. In Bangladesh, patients with shigellosis rarely lost fluid of more than 30 mL/kg/day (193). In one study in Egypt, moderate to severe dehydration was most frequently seen with salmonellosis (91%), followed by *C. jejuni* diarrhea (10%), but not in shigellosis (10). A large study in Bangladesh showed that 12% of patients who died but only 1% of discharged patients had severe dehydration (179). However, a multivariate analysis showed that this association between dehydration and death was not apparent. Instead death was associated with age younger than 1 year, decreased serum protein, altered consciousness, and thrombocytopenia.

Other reported complications of shigellosis include seizures, ileus, intestinal perforation, toxic megacolon, rectal prolapse, hypoglycemia, hyponatremia, hemolytic-uremic syndrome (HUS), pneumonia, and bacteremia (194–197). Hypoglycemia is seen more often with *S. flexneri* than with *S. dysenteriae* type 1 dysentery (197). Toxic megacolon and bowel perforation are rare complications observed in many severe inflammatory conditions of the colon, including *C. difficile* pseudomembranous colitis, amebiasis, other invasive enteric bacterial infections, and ulcerative colitis.

Malnutrition and AIDS are risk factors for *Shigella* and *Salmonella* bacteremia (168,169,198,199). Shigellosis itself can provoke malnutrition in previously well-nourished children. In developing countries, invasive diarrhea can be a risk factor for persistent diarrhea (diarrhea lasting more than 2 weeks), itself associated with high rates of mortality and malnutrition (200). In Brazilian children with EAggEC infection with evidence in stool of inflammation, even without overt diarrhea, significant growth impairment has been observed (39).

In the United States, nontyphi *Salmonella* bacteremia occurs most commonly with *Salmonella cholerasuis* (62%), *Salmonella dublin* (40%), and *Salmonella paratyphi* A (59%) intestinal infections (201). Other serotypes can cause bacteremia (0.8% with *Salmonella newport* to 7.8% with *S. paratyphi* B), which is in contrast to *Shigella* or *C. jejuni* infections, which rarely cause bacteremia. The complications of salmonellosis, including rapid dehydration, convulsions, and septicemia, are more frequently seen in infants and elderly patients.

E. histolytica dysentery can be complicated by bowel perforation and peritonitis (1% to 4%). Pregnancy, malnutrition, and corticosteroid therapy are associated with fulminant colitis, which can be complicated by bowel necrosis, perforation, toxic megacolon, or liver abscess (202,203). An annular colonic mass, called *ameboma*, may develop in some patients. In addition to the hepatic abscess, other extraintestinal complications of amebiasis include direct or metastatic extension of the liver abscess into pleural or pericardial spaces, or, rarely, to the brain, kidneys, and lungs (189,190).

Patients with CMV enteritis may develop deep focal ulcerations extending to the submucosa into the muscularis. Such lesions may cause massive bleed, perforation, and shock. Gastrointestinal CMV disease is often a manifestation of systemic CMV infection and hence could be accompanied by CMV pneumonitis, hepatitis, or other organ involvement. CMV infection in patients with ulcerative colitis may develop as an infection superimposed on the inflamed mucosa or as a complication of the frequent use of immunosuppressive drugs. Mortality rate attributed to CMV enteritis exceeded 80% before the availability of ganciclovir; currently, though, death is relatively rare (52).

Complications of NEC include shock secondary to septicemia, fluid loss, or hemorrhage, and other features associated with the underlying illness. Many of the patients with NEC undergo surgery because of their signs of acute abdomen, and intraoperative or postoperative complications may develop.

Reactive arthritis and Reiter syndrome may follow infections with *Shigella* (204), *Salmonella* (205), *Yersinia* (206,207), or *Campylobacter* (208). In a cohort involved in a common source *S. flexneri* outbreak, probable reactive arthritis developed in less than 3% of the infected persons (207). The susceptibility to reactive arthritis is associated with but not limited to persons belonging to the HLA-B27 histocompatibility group (207,209). Reactive arthritis following *Yersinia* infection is more common in northern Europe than in the United States, suggesting that there may be geographic differences in the prevalence of "arthrogenic" strains (206).

Differential Diagnosis

Except for some unusual but characteristic complications of inflammatory diarrhea, it is difficult to clinically distinguish among the different causes of inflammatory diarrhea. Patient history and epidemiologic knowledge of the disease and pathogens help to narrow the possibilities. They can also be distinguished by their predilection to occur as sporadic illnesses only, as outbreaks, or as pandemics.

In North America or Europe, bloody diarrhea may be a manifestation of hemorrhagic colitis caused by a pathogen not considered to produce inflammatory diarrhea—*E. coli* O157:H7. The organism is not invasive and can produce an asymptomatic infection, watery diarrhea without blood, or grossly bloody diarrhea, with systemic complications that overlap the symptoms of inflammatory diarrhea (40–42). However, unlike dysentery, fever is either low grade or absent, even with profuse bloody diarrhea. However, fever may develop in more advanced disease, especially in the elderly (210), or in children in whom the complication HUS develops (211). HUS is a major complication of hemorrhagic colitis, but it also occurs as a complication of shigellosis, especially after *S. dysenteriae* type 1 infection (212).

Only approximately one-third of the patients with hemorrhagic colitis have fecal leukocytes. As mentioned, *E. histolytica* amebiasis can manifest with low-grade fever and dysenteric stool lacking fecal leukocytes. However, in North America or Europe, amebiasis is unusual among persons without a recent travel or homosexual history, and it rarely occurs as outbreaks. On the other hand, like campylobacteriosis, yersiniosis, shigellosis, and salmonellosis, hemorrhagic colitis can occur sporadically or as part of an outbreak in community or institutional settings.

A distinct form of enterocolitis called *ischemic colitis*, characterized by an abrupt onset of abdominal pain followed by diarrhea and bloody discharge, was described by Wilson and Qualheim in 1954 (213) and was further detailed by others (214,215). At necropsy, the bowel is characteristically edematous with hemorrhage and scattered shallow ulcers affecting the entire intestinal tract in varying proportions. Leukocyte infiltration and necrosis of the mucosa accompany bacterial colonization and invasion. These lesions are believed to result from vascular insufficiency resulting from underlying cardiovascular disease, particularly following episodes of hypotension. Transient episodes as well as fulminant, gangrenous forms of ischemic colitis have been reported (216,218). Hemorrhagic colitis in the elderly can be mistaken for ischemic colitis, and a barium enema test in both may show a characteristic "thumbprinting" pattern, indicating submucosal edema or hemorrhage (40,217). A bloody diarrhea in the elderly that occurs as part of an outbreak is unlikely to be ischemic colitis.

NEC associated with neonates, neutropenic patients, or bowel ischemia occurs with clinical manifestations that reflect their underlying disease. Symptoms include abdominal discomfort and severe pain with signs of acute abdomen (obstruction, perforation, or peritonitis) accompanied by fever and diarrhea that may be bloody. In patients with ileocecal involvement, abdominal pain localizes to the right lower quadrant, which may be mistaken for acute appendicitis or *Yersinia* enteritis. Features of the acute abdomen are more frequently observed in NEC than in diseases associated with invasive bacterial pathogens described earlier. Bacteremia with organisms normally associated with the gut flora in a patient with dysentery is highly suggestive of NEC.

Neonatal NEC can occur as a nosocomial outbreak (37,219), and adult forms of NEC have occurred as outbreaks in communities with atypical food habits, such as the pork feast in New Guinea (33), or in postwar Germany, where poor nutrition was shown to be associated with a form of enterocolitis called *Darmbrand* (34).

An acute exacerbation or the first manifestation of an inflammatory bowel disease may be difficult to distinguish from infectious inflammatory diarrhea. The possible role of an infectious agent, such as *M. paratuberculosis,* which causes Johne disease in ruminants, has been considered for Crohn's disease, but is not certain (56,57). Both Crohn's disease and ulcerative colitis produce diarrhea with blood accompanied by fever. Ulcerative colitis characteristically involves the entire colon, including the rectum, whereas Crohn's disease affects the colon and small intestine in a segmental fashion, sparing the rectum (220). The microabscesses in the superficial mucosa of the colon in ulcerative colitis may resemble those produced by severe amebiasis from *E. histolytica, Shigella,* or *Campylobacter.* However, in Crohn's disease, inflammation extends deeper into the bowel wall, and the macrophage predominance leads to the formation of noncaseating granulomas.

The arthritis of the spine and sacroiliac joints of inflammatory bowel disease resembles the reactive arthritis of shigellosis and yersiniosis, and is associated with the HLA-B27 histocompatibility type in all of these diseases. However, other manifestations such as uveitis and extraintestinal extension of fistulas may sway the diagnosis away from bacterial causes of inflammatory diarrhea. The chronic, relapsing pattern of the illness is also atypical for infectious inflammatory diarrhea, especially in adults.

Bloody diarrhea can be a manifestation of chemical or metal poisonings. Food items accidentally contaminated with the rodenticide thallium sulfate or barium carbonate produce acute watery or bloody diarrhea with nausea and vomiting, accompanied by neurologic symptoms (221,222). Acute arsenic poisoning may produce bloody diarrhea, tenesmus, severe dehydration, and shock (223). Lead poisoning is associated with burning of the pharynx, abdominal pain, vomiting, and bloody diarrhea (223). All of these chemical poisonings can be distinguished from the infectious causes of bloody diarrhea by their extremely short incubation periods—from minutes to 12 hours.

DIAGNOSTIC APPROACH

The initial approach to the diagnosis of inflammatory diarrhea involves careful history and physical examination, as well as familiarity with the epidemiology of the potential pathogens. These considerations influence the choice of laboratory tests.

Clinical and Epidemiologic History

History and physical examination may help to distinguish inflammatory from secretory diarrhea, but the previous discussions show that the positive predictive values of symptoms and signs to distinguish specific causes of inflammatory diarrhea, especially in low-prevalence areas, would be unsatisfactorily low. The most discriminating features of the agents of inflammatory diarrhea, as described earlier, are their epidemiologic and host characteristics.

Laboratory Tests

In developed countries, laboratory tests are usually performed to aid the clinical management of patients. However, in most parts of the world, such applications are not readily available or affordable. In such areas, diagnostic tests are instead used to characterize the epidemiology of an infectious agent, and it is this epidemiologic information that is used to manage patients with diarrhea. In Bangladesh, the presence of bloody diarrhea in children had a positive predictive value of 50% for shigellosis (191). Hence, this single microbiologic survey helped to establish a simple diarrhea management strategy that does not rely on stool culture from every patient: community health care workers are instructed to initiate antibiotics in all children in whom acute bloody diarrhea develops.

Some experts recommend microscopic examination of stool for leukocytes (224,225). The presence of fecal leukocytes indicates inflammatory process. A fresh fecal specimen is stained with methylene blue and examined for stained leukocytes. However, this method requires a microscope and a skilled microscopist. Leukocytes may be mistaken for amebas, such as *E. histolytica.* A latex agglutination method to detect lactoferrin, an iron-binding glycoprotein concentrated in secondary granules of leukocytes, has been found to be a useful test to discriminate inflammatory from secretory diarrhea (226–228). The advantage of this test is that it does not require any trained personnel, and the test can be performed on specimens containing leukocytes that may have been lysed as a result of prolonged storage or transport. The absence of fecal leukocytes or their surrogates does not rule out agents of inflammatory diarrhea.

The specific microbiologic diagnosis of inflammatory diarrhea pathogens is discussed in detail in the organism chapters. To ensure detection of a pathogen, stool specimens should be plated within 2 hours of collection. *Shigella* is especially susceptible to acid pH that develops in unprocessed stool. If specimens cannot be processed immediately, such as in field situations, transport medium such as Cary-Blair or buffered glycerol saline should be used.

Agents belonging to the family Enterobacteriaceae are isolated by a combination of selective, differential, and enrichment media. Selective media (MacConkey, eosin-methylene blue agar) are used to inhibit the growth of normal stool flora organisms, and differential media (xylose-lysine-deoxycholate, *Salmonella-Shigella,* Hektoen enteric, *Yersinia* enteric agars) are used to allow isolation of colonies that can be further characterized for final identification. Enrichment broth media (gram-negative broth, selenite broth) are used to allow growth of organisms that may be present in low numbers (such as in specimens collected in later phase of an acute illness, or from convalescent or chronic carriers). Cold enrichment in phosphate-buffered saline is used to increase the recovery of *Y. enterocolitica.*

Campylobacter species require other differential media as well as selective growth temperatures and atmosphere (42°C at 4% to 6% oxygen, 6% to 10% carbon dioxide for *C. jejuni*). Patients residing at or traveling to the seacoast in whom dysentery develops should be cultured for *V. para-*

haemolyticus, which is isolated on thiosulfate citrate bile salt sucrose agar.

Suspected organisms isolated from the selective or differential media are further characterized morphologically, biochemically, serologically, genetically, or for their pathogenicity for final identification. Because of increased risk of mortality, in endemic areas or during epidemics of *Shigella dysenteriae* type 1, it is important to rapidly examine suspected *Shigella* isolates with a slide agglutination test using antiserum against O antigens A-D. Although other serotypes of *S. dysenteriae* exist, agglutination in A antiserum would be highly suspicious of the pandemic-prone type 1.

Absence in bloody stool samples of *Shigella*, *Salmonella*, *Campylobacter*, *Yersinia*, or *E. histolytica* from a patient with no known underlying disease in North America, Europe, or Japan requires further examination of the *E. coli* for enterohemorrhagic strain, especially *E. coli* O157:H7. Most *E. coli* strains in the United States ferment sorbitol rapidly, whereas *E. coli* O157:H7 strains ferment sorbitol slowly or not at all (229,230). Therefore, MacConkey-sorbitol agar (available commercially) is used to select sorbitol-negative colonies, which are then tested for agglutination in O157 antiserum (230). Because *E. coli* O157 strains that have H antigens other than H7 are not associated with diarrhea, confirmatory diagnosis requires agglutination in H7 antiserum.

Blood cultures may be preferable to stool cultures in the diagnosis of typhoid fever. A variety of organisms may be detected in blood of patients with suspected NEC or ischemic colitis.

The diagnosis of *Salmonella*, *Shigella*, and *Campylobacter* species, as well as *E. coli* O157:H7, should not end with their final isolation. They should be reported immediately to the local county or state public health laboratories. It is likely that an isolation of these pathogens represents occurrence of an unrecognized outbreak, and it is critical that outbreaks be "diagnosed" just as rapidly as the cause of dysentery in an individual patient.

C. difficile can be isolated in differential and selective media, such as CCFA medium that contains cycloserine, cefoxitin, fructose, and egg yolk (231). Identification may be made with biochemical tests or gas-liquid chromatography (232). However, in hospitalized patients, the asymptomatic carriage can be as high as 21%; hence, the isolation of the organism per se does not confirm an etiologic diagnosis. Therefore, cytotoxicity assays on filtered fecal specimen should be performed. Specificity of the cytotoxicity is confirmed by neutralization of the effect by *C. difficile* or *Clostridium sordellii* antitoxin. Several kits for these assays are commercially available.

In general, the serologic diagnoses of bacterial inflammatory diarrhea are not helpful for acute management of the disease but may provide useful information for epidemiologic studies, such as assessing asymptomatic carriage status or prevalence of infection in a community.

Pathogens identified at the genus or species level can be further subtyped. Subtyping information may help to distinguish pathogenic from nonpathogenic or other pathogenic variety of strains (e.g., EIEC versus other *E. coli* strains). *Salmonella*, *Shigella* species, EIEC, and *Y. enterocolitica* are traditionally typed according to their O and flagellar antigens and their antibiotic susceptibility patterns. Molecular microbiologic methods, such as plasmid profile analysis, restriction fragment length polymorphism analysis, and "ribotyping" provide additional subtyping information to assist epidemiologic analyses (149,233–236).

The radiologic diagnosis of inflammatory diarrhea is discussed elsewhere. The definitive diagnosis of inflammatory bowel disease involves endoscopy and mucosal biopsy histologic examination. The mainstay of management of this syndrome is control of the inflammatory process, which requires antiinflammatory agents and immunosuppressive drugs—drugs that would not be indicated in infectious causes of inflammatory diarrhea. Hence, the definitive diagnosis is critical.

MANAGEMENT

Fluid and Electrolyte Balance

Oral glucose-electrolyte solutions were originally developed and evaluated in the treatment of cholera and subsequently in the treatment of other secretory diarrheas resulting form organisms such as ETEC and rotavirus (237,239). Because the principal cause of death from secretory diarrhea is severe dehydration, the World Health Organization advocates ORT to prevent diarrhea mortality. The agents of dysentery can cause fluid loss but rarely produce the profound dehydration associated with agents of secretory diarrhea. However, electrolyte and glucose imbalance can be complications of dysentery associated with increased mortality rates (195). Therefore, ORT may play a role in the prevention of such complications. Investigators in Thailand and Bangladesh have shown that ORT alone was effective for watery diarrhea from shigellosis manifesting predominantly as watery diarrhea instead of as dysentery (240,241).

Antimicrobial Therapy

WHO developed separate guidelines for the management of invasive diarrheas, emphasizing the use of specific antimicrobial agents (242). The choice of antibiotics depends on drug susceptibility data of the local agents of dysentery, cost, safety for children, and availability as an oral formulation. Resistance to ampicillin and trimethoprim-sulfamethoxazole, considered the drugs of choice for the treatment of shigellosis, has been observed with pandemic strains of *S. dysenteriae* 1 as well as other *Shigella* species in Asia and Africa (7,243,244). In the United States, 32% and 7% of the *Shigella* isolates were resistant to ampicillin and trimethoprim-sulfamethoxazole, respectively (245). In the United States, for shigellosis not associated with foreign travel, trimethoprim-sulfamethoxazole is considered the drug of choice. Fluoroquinolones are effective for shigellosis acquired abroad but are not approved for pediatric use.

In places such as the United States, where diagnosis can be readily made, the empirical use of antimicrobial agents for inflammatory diarrhea must take clinical, host, and epidemiologic factors into consideration. The use of ampicillin or ciprofloxacin in a patient with *Salmonella* gastroenteritis in an immunocompetent person may prolong the convalescent carriage state (246,247). On the other hand, treating mild diarrhea in a child with fever attending a day care center, where agents of inflammatory diarrhea have been implicated in outbreaks, may accelerate the clearance of organisms like *Shigella* and interrupt transmission.

The drug of choice for the treatment of *C. difficile* colitis is metronidazole. However, in severe or relapse cases, or in patients who cannot tolerate metronidazole, oral vancomycin can be used (153). The choice, however, may also be influenced by the prevalence in the hospital of vancomycin-resistant gram-positive bacterial nosocomial infections, such as *Staphylococcus* or *Enterococcus* species infections. Intravenous vancomycin is not indicated in *C. difficile* colitis treatment because the drug may not be excreted into the intestinal lumen.

The therapy for amebiasis caused by *E. histolytica* is dependent on the sites of infection (lumen, bowel wall, or extraintestinal) and is reviewed in detail in Chapter 59. The management of diarrhea resulting from other parasitic causes is also discussed elsewhere in this book.

Antiperistaltic agents such as diphenoxylate hydrochloride with atropine sulfate should never be used in dysenteric syndromes.

In developing countries, and in inner cities and rural areas of developed countries, nutritional management of inflammatory diarrhea is important. As mentioned earlier, hypoglycemia is a severe complication of dysentery associated with a high mortality rate. Hypoglycemia may result from failure of gluconeogenesis resulting from deficiencies in protein or fat substrates for gluconeogenesis; thus, hypoglycemia is more likely to develop in malnourished children (195). Infants and small children should continue to be fed breast milk or weaning foods during their illness.

PREVENTION

The general approach to the prevention of dysentery is similar to that for prevention of all types of diarrhea—improving sanitation and hygiene. However, these improvements in hygiene can be focused if the local epidemiology of the pathogens of dysentery is known. Improved inspection and efficient regulation by the dairy, poultry, and meat industries in developed countries will contribute substantially to the control of salmonellosis, campylobacteriosis, and yersiniosis, as well as disease caused by *E. coli* O157:H7. Proper food handling practices, including cooking at the recommended temperature and time of meat products and eggs at restaurants (especially fast food establishments) and at home, will significantly reduce the incidence of inflammatory diarrhea in the United States and Europe. Limiting the use of antimicrobial agents can prevent not only the emergence of drug-resistant *Salmonella,* especially in hospitals in middle-income countries, but also *C. difficile* colitis in all hospitals. Chronic care facilities as well as day care centers should be aware of the potential for transmission of *C. difficile* and *Shigella* in their settings.

Handwashing with soap is an effective method to reduce shigellosis among inhabitants of developing countries (248) and to reduce *C. difficile* colitis in hospitals in all countries (153). During epidemics of *S. dysenteriae* 1, provision of large volumes of clean water can reduce the spread of disease. Availability of large volumes of water encourages handwashing. Water sources used for drinking should be separated from sources used for bathing and washing, and defecation should not be allowed or latrines should not be located within 10 m of these water sources (242). The supply of chlorinated water or other chemicals for water treatment and of narrow-mouthed earthen jars with covers for storage will help to reduce transmission of enteric pathogens within families. Severe shigellosis occurs during or after measles in developing countries, so immunization against measles should be promoted. Bottle feeding is a recognized risk factor for death from shigellosis in infants, and early weaning in areas with poor sanitation is especially dangerous. Breast-feeding should be actively encouraged.

Travelers from developed countries to developing countries should avoid uncooked vegetables and untreated water. Data supporting the efficacy of antibiotic prophylaxis exist for causes of secretory diarrhea such as ETEC, but not for the agents of dysentery. Because dysentery is most likely to be treated with an antibiotic in travelers, the prophylactic use of antibiotics is discouraged; the potential emergence of drug-resistant infection limits the choice of the drugs to use in such situations.

Vaccine Development

Mucosal immunity and systemic immunity (either humoral or cell mediated) have been proposed to be important for protection against invasive pathogens such as *Shigella* and *Salmonella* (249). Therefore, antidysentery vaccine development efforts are directed at ways to promote these host responses. Currently, the only vaccines available for use against inflammatory diarrhea are typhoid vaccines. The parenteral, killed whole-cell vaccine offers 60% to 70% protection but is associated with many side effects. Multiple oral doses (three to four) of the enteric-coated, gal-epimerase-deficient, nonpathogenic strain of *S.*

typhi (Ty21a) have been shown to offer protection varying from 25% in a trial in Indonesian to 66% in Chilean children (250,251). Another injectable vaccine based on a single dose of purified Vi polysaccharide antigen has been licensed. It was shown to exhibit efficacy of about 65% over 18 to 21 months in trials in Nepal and South Africa (252,253).

The WHO Global Program for Vaccines and Immunization has proposed *Shigella* vaccine development to be a major priority. Experimental parenteral killed *Shigella* whole-cell vaccine has not shown any protection and is associated with severe side effects (254). Therefore, efforts have been directed at developing attenuated oral vaccines. These approaches have included constructions of (a) nonpathogenic *E. coli* strains or attenuated *Salmonella* strains expressing *S. flexneri* invasion-protein antigens, as well as genes encoding O-polysaccharides (255,256), (b) deletion mutants, rendering *Shigella* auxotrophic for metabolites unavailable in mammalian cells (257,258), and (c) live, genetically attenuated mutant strains of *Shigella* (259,260). Some of these constructs have shown protection in animal studies (258,261). A genetically attenuated *S. flexneri* 2a strain SC602 has been tested for safety and immunogenicity among adult volunteers (262). This strain, which has deletions in the plasmid-borne gene *icsA* which mediates intracellular spread, was shown to be partially protective for volunteers challenged with a virulent *S. flexneri* 2a strain (262). Vaccines against nontyphoidal *Salmonella* and other agents of dysentery are still under development.

In the developed world, despite their advanced technologies, diseases caused by agents of inflammatory diarrhea stubbornly remain unabated and actually continue to increase in incidence. In many developing countries, dysentery has replaced secretory diarrhea as a major cause of diarrheal mortality. It is clear that control efforts for inflammatory diarrhea worldwide require a multifaceted approach, which includes increasing our understanding of their epidemiology and pathogenesis, and a commitment to basic public health intervention strategies.

REFERENCES

1. Varavithya W, Vathanophas K, Bodhidatta L, et al. Importance of salmonellae and *Campylobacter jejuni* in the etiology of diarrheal disease among children less than 5 years of age in a community in Bangkok, Thailand. *J Clin Microbiol* 1990;28:2507–2510.
2. Ling JM, Cheng AF. Infectious diarrhoea in Hong Kong. *J Trop Med Hyg* 1993;96:107–112.
3. Gomes TAT, Rassi V, MacDonald KL, et al. Enteropathogens associated with acute diarrheal disease in urban infants in Sao Paulo, Brazil. *J Infect Dis* 1991;164:331–337.
4. Gunzburg S, Gracey M, Burke V, et al. Epidemiology and microbiology of diarrhoea in young aboriginal children in the Kimberley region of Western Australia. *Epidemiol Infect* 1992;108:67–76.
5. Giron JA, Jones T, Millan-Velasco F, et al. Diffuse-adhering *Escherichia coli* (DAEC) as a putative cause of diarrhea in Mayan children in Mexico. *J Infect Dis* 1991;163:507–513.
6. Bhan MK, Raj P, Levine MM, et al. Enteroaggregative *Escherichia coli* associated with persistent diarrhea in a cohort of rural children in India. *J Infect Dis* 1989;159:1061–1064.
7. Mikail IA, Fox E, Habergerger RL Jr, et al. Epidemiology of bacterial pathogens associated with infectious diarrhea in Djibouti. *J Clin Microbiol* 1990;956–961.
8. Adkins HJ, Escamilla J, Santiago LT, et al. Two-year survey of etiologic agents of diarrhea disease at San Lazaro Hospital, Manila, Republic of the Philippines. *J Clin Microbiol* 1987;25:1143–1147.
9. Stanton B, Silimperi DR, Khatun K, et al. Parasitic, bacterial and viral pathogens isolated from diarrhoeal and routine stool specimens of urban Bangladesh children. *J Trop Med Hyg* 1989;92:46–55.
10. Mikhail IA, Hyams KC, Podgore JK, et al. Microbiologic and clinical study of acute diarrhea in children in Aswan, Egypt. *Scand J Infect Dis* 1989;21:59–65.
11. Hyams KC, Bourgeois AL, Merrell BR, et al. Diarrheal disease during operation Desert Shield. *N Engl J Med* 1991;325:1423–1428.
12. Taylor DN, Houston R, Shlim DR, et al. Etiology of diarrhea among travelers and foreign residents in Nepal. *JAMA* 1988;260:1245–1248.
13. Mattila L, Siitonen A, Kyronseppa H, et al. Seasonal variation in etiology of travelers' diarrhea. *J Infect Dis* 1992;165:385–388.
14. Ruiz-Pelaez JG, Mattar S. Accuracy of fecal lactoferrin and other stool tests for diagnosis of invasive diarrhea at a Colombian pediatric hospital. *Pediatr Infect Dis* 1999;18:342–346.
15. Ueda Y, Suzuki N, Miyagi K, et al. Studies on bacillary dysentery cases of overseas travelers: during 1979 to 1995. *Japanese J Bacteriol* 1997;52:735–746.
16. Mangia AHR, Duarte AN, Duarte R, et al. Aetiology of acute diarrhea in hospitalized children in Rio de Janeiro City, Brazil. *J Trop Pediatr* 1993;39:365–367.
17. Ogunsanya TI, Rotimi VO, Adenuga A. A study of the aetiological agents of childhood diarrhoea in Lagos, Nigeria. *J Med Microbiol* 1994;40:10–14.
18. Molbak K, Wested N, Hojlyng N, et al. The etiology of early childhood diarrhea: a community study from Guinea-Bissau. *J Infect Dis* 1994;169:581–587.
19. Escheverria P, Hoge CW, Bodhidatta L, et al. Etiology of diarrhea in a rural community in Western Thailand: importance of enteric viruses and enterovirulent *Escherichia coli*. *J Infect Dis* 1994;169:916–919.
20. Biswas R, Lyon DJ, Nelson EAS, et al. Aetiology of acute diarrhoea in hospitalized children in Hong Kong. *Trop Med Int Health* 1996;1:679–683.
21. Barnes GL, Uren E, Stevens KB, et al. Etiology of acute gastroenteritis in hospitalized children in Melbourne, Australia, from April 1980 to March 1993. *J Clin Microbiol* 1998;36:133–138.
22. Yamashiro T, Nakasone N, Higa N, et al. Etiological study of diarrheal patients in Vientiane, Lao People's Democratic Republic. *J Clin Microbiol* 1998;36:2195–2199.
23. Steffen R, Collard F, Tornieporth N, et al. Epidemiology, etiology, and impact of traveler's diarrhea in Jamaica. *JAMA* 1999;281:811–817.
24. Albert MJ, Faruque ASG, Faruque SM, et al. Case-control study of enteropathogens associated with childhood diarrhea in Dhaka, Bangladesh. *J Clin Microbiol* 1999;37:3458–3464.
25. Riley LW, Finch MJ. Results of the first year of national surveillance of *Campylobacter* in the United States. *J Infect Dis* 1985;151:956–959.
26. Tauxe RV, Patton CM, Edmonds P, Barrett TJ, et al. Illness associated with *Campylobacter laridis,* a newly recognized *Campylobacter* species. *J Clin Microbiol* 1985;21:222–225.

27. Fennell CL, Totten PA, Quinn TC, et al. Characterization of *Campylobacter*-like organisms isolated from homosexual men. *J Infect Dis* 1984;149:58–66.
28. Edmonds P, Patton CM, Griffin PM, et al. *Campylobacter hyointestinalis* associated with human gastrointestinal disease in the United States. *J Clin Microbiol* 1987;25:685–691.
29. Hellyer TJ, Brown IN, Taylor NB, et al. Gastrointestinal involvement in *Mycobacterium avium-intracellulare* infection of patients with HIV. *J Infect* 1993;26:55–66.
30. Horsburgh CR Jr. *Mycobacterium avium* complex infection in the acquired immunodeficiency syndrome. *N Engl J Med* 1991; 324:1332–1338.
31. Kudoh Y, Sakai S. Current status of bacterial diarrheal diseases in Japan. In: Takeda Y, Miwatani T, eds. *Bacterial diarrheal diseases.* Tokyo: KTK; 1985.
32. Blake PA, Weaver RE, Hollis DG. Disease of humans (other than cholera) caused by vibrios. *Annu Rev Microbiol* 1980;34: 341–367.
33. Murrell TGC, Roth L, Egerton J, et al. Pig-bel: enteritis necroticans. *Lancet* 1966;1:217.
34. Hansen K, Jeckeln E, Jochims J, et al. *Dambrand-enteritis necroticanss.* Stuttgart: Georg Thiem Verlag, 1949.
35. Stein H, Beck J, Solomon, et al. Gastroenteritis with necrotizing enterocolitis in premature babies. *BMJ* 1972;2:616–619.
36. Olarte J, Ferguson WW, Henderson NI, et al. *Klebsiella* strains isolated from diarrheal infants. *Am J Dis Child* 1961;101:763–770.
37. Howard FM, Flynn DM, Bradley JM, et al. Outbreak of necrotising enterocolitis caused by *Clostridium butyricum. Lancet* 1977;2:1099–1102.
38. Santulli TY, Schullinger JN, Heird WC, et al. Acute necrotizing enterocolitis in infancy: a review of 64 cases. *Pediatrics* 1975;55: 376–387.
39. Steiner TS, Lima AAM, Nataro JP, et al. Enteroaggregative *Escherichia coli* produce intestinal inflammation and growth impairment and cause interleukin-8 release from intestinal epithelial cells. *J Infect Dis* 1998;177:88–96.
40. Riley LW, Remis RS, Helgerson SD, et al. Hemorrhagic colitis associated with a rare *Escherichia coli* serotype. *N Engl J Med* 1983;308:681–685.
41. Griffin PM, Ostroff SM, Tauxe RV, et al. Illnesses associated with *Escherichia coli* O157:H7 infections: a broad clinical spectrum. *Ann Intern Med* 1988;109:705–712.
42. Griffin PM, Tauxe RV. The epidemiology of infections caused by *Escherichia coli* O157:H7, other enterohemorrhagic *E. coli,* and the associated hemolytic uremic syndrome. *Epidemiol Rev* 1991;13:60–98.
43. Brown HW, Neva FA, eds. *Basic clinical parasitology,* fifth edition. Norwalk: Appleton-Century-Crofts, 1983.
44. DeHovitz JA, Pape JW, Boncy M, et al. Clinical manifestations and therapy of *Isospora belli* infection in patients with acquired immunodeficiency syndrome. *N Engl J Med* 1986;315:87–90.
45. Forthal DN, Guest SS. *Isospora belli* enteritis in homosexual men. *Am J Trop Med Hyg* 1984;33:1060–1064.
46. Sanguino J, Peixe R, Guerra J, et al. Schistosomiasis and vascular alterations of the colonic mucosa. *Hepatogastroenterology* 1993;40:184–187.
47. Boyajian T. Strongyloidiasis on the Thai-Cambodian border. *Trans R Soc Trop Med Hyg* 1992;86:661–662.
48. Tamura H. Acute ulcerative colitis associated with cytomegalic inclusion virus. *Arch Pathol Lab Med* 1973;96:164–167.
49. Wolfe M, Cherry JD. Hemorrhage from cecal ulcers of cytomegalovirus infection: report of a case. *Ann Surg* 1971;177: 490–494.
50. Jacobsen MA, Mills J. Serious cytomegalovirus disease in the acquired immunodeficiency syndrome (AIDS). *Ann Intern Med* 1988;108:585–594.
51. Frager HH, Frager JD, Wolf EL, et al. Cytomegalovirus colitis in acquired immunodeficiency syndrome: radiologic spectrum. *Gastroenterol Radiol* 1986;11:241–246.
52. Buckner FS, Pomeroy C. Cytomegalovirus disease of the gastrointestinal tract in patients without AIDS. *Clin Infect Dis* 1993;17:644–656.
53. Janoff EN, Orenstein JM, Manischewitz JF, et al. Adenovirus colitis in the acquired immunodeficiency syndrome. *Gastroenterology* 1991;100:976–979.
54. Smith JMB. Mycoses of the alimentary tract. *Gut* 1969;10: 1035–1040.
55. Centers for Disease Control. Diseases transmitted by foods. US Public Health Publication No. (CDC) 81-8237, 1979.
56. McFadden JJ, Butcher PD, Chiodini R, et al. Crohn's disease-isolated mycobacteria are identical to *Mycobacterium paratuberculosis,* as determined by DNA probes that distinguish between mycobacterial species. *J Clin Microbiol* 1987;25:796–801.
57. Sanderson JD, Moss MT, Tizard ML, et al. *Mycobacterium paratuberculosis* DNA in Crohn's disease tissue. *Gut* 1992;33: 890–896.
58. Sereny B. Experimental *Shigella* keratoconjunctivitis. *Acta Microbiol Acad Sci Hung* 1955;2:293–295.
59. Isberg R. Discrimination between intracellular uptake and surface adhesion of bacterial pathogens. Science. 1991;252:934–938.
60. Isberg RR, Falkow R. A single genetic locus encoded by *Yersinia pseudotuberculosis* permits invasion of cultured animal cells by *E. coli* K12. *Nature* 1985;317:262–264.
61. Isberg RR, Voorhis DL, Falkow S. Identification of invasin: a protein that allows enteric bacteria to penetrate cultured mammalian cells. *Cell* 1987;50:769–778.
62. Isberg RR, Leong JM. Multiple β_1 chain integrins are receptors for invasin, a protein that promotes bacterial penetration into mammalian cells. *Cell* 1990;60:861–871.
63. Goldberg MB, Sansonetti PJ. *Shigella* subversion of the cellular cytoskeleton: a strategy for epithelial colonization. *Infect Immun* 1993;61:4941–4946.
64. Hale TL, Oaks EV, Formal SB. Identification and antigenic characterization of virulence-associated, plasmid-coded proteins of *Shigella* spp. and enteroinvasive *Escherichia coli. Infect Immun* 1985;50:620–629.
65. Sansonetti PJ, Ryter A, Clerc P, et al. Multiplication of *Shigella flexneri* within HeLa cells: lysis of the phagocytic vacuole and plasmid-mediated contact hemolysis. *Infect Immun* 1986;1: 461–469.
66. High N, Mounier J, Prevost MC, et al. IpaB of Shigella flexneri causes entry into epithelial cells and escape from the phagocytic vacuole. *EMBO J* 1992;11:1991–1999.
67. Menard R, Dehio C, Sansonetti PJ. Bacterial entry into epithelial cells: the paradigm of *Shigella. Trends Microbiol.* 1996;4: 220–226.
68. Bernadini ML, Mounier J, d'Hauteville H, et al. Identification of icsA, a plasmid locus of *Shigella flexneri* which governs bacterial intra- and intercellular spread through interaction with F-actin. Proc Natl Acad Sci U S A 1989;86:3867–3871.
69. Sansonetti PJ, Mounier J, Prevost MC, et al. Cadherin expression is required for the spread of *Shigella flexneri* between epithelial cells. *Cell* 1994;76:829–839.
70. Zychlinsky A, Prevost MC, Sansonetti PJ. *Shigella flexneri* induces apoptosis in infected macrophages. *Nature* 1992;358: 167–168.
71. Zychlinsky A, Thirumalai K, Arondel J, et al. In vivo apoptosis in *Shigella flexneri* infection. *Infect Immun* 1996;64:5357–5365.
72. Hilbi H, Moss JE, Hersh D, et al. Shigella-induced apoptosis is dependent on caspase-1 which binds to IpaB. *J Biol Chem* 1998; 273:32895–32900.
73. Islam D, Veress B, Bardhan PK, et al. In situ characterization of

inflammatory responses in the rectal mucosae of patients with Shigellosis. *Infect Immun* 1997;65:739–749.
74. Chen Y, Smith MR, Thirumalai K, et al. A bacterial invasin induces macrophage apoptosis by binding directly to ICE. *EMBO J* 1996;15:3853–3860.
75. Sansonetti PJ, Phalipon A, Arondel J, et al. Caspase-1 activation of IL-1β and IL-18 are essential for *Shigella flexneri*-induced inflammation. *Immunity*2000;12:581–590.
76. Young VB, Falkow S, Schoolnik GK. The invasin protein of *Yersinia enterocolitica:* internalization of invasin-bearing bacteria by eukaryotic cells is associated with reorganization of the cytoskeleton. *J Cell Biol* 1992;116:197–207.
77. Guan K, Dixon JE. Protein tyrosine phosphatase activity of an essential virulence determinant in *Yersinia. Science* 1990;249: 553–556.
78. Leung KY, Straley SC. The *yop*M gene of *Yersinia pestis* GP1b alpha. *J Bacteriol* 1989;171:4623–4632.
79. Rosqvist R, Forsberg A, Wolf-Watz H. Intracellular targeting of the *Yersinia* YopE cytotoxin in mammalian cells induces actin microfilament disruption. *Infect Immun* 1992;59:4562–4569.
80. Palmer LE, Hobbie S, Galan J, et al. YopJ of *Yersinia pseudotuberculosis* is required for the inhibition of macrophage TNF-alpha production and downregulation of the MAP kinases p38 and JNK. *Molec Microbiol* 1998;27:953–965.
81. Orth K, Xu Z, Mudgett MB, et al. Disruption of signaling by *Yersinia* effector YopJ, a ubiquitin-like protein protease. *Science* 2000;290:1594–1597.
82. Francis CL, Ryan TA, Jones BD, et al. Ruffles induced by *Salmonella* and other stimuli direct macropinocytosis of bacteria. *Nature.* 1993;364:639–642.
83. Groisman EA, Ochman H. Pathogenicity islands: bacterial evolution in quantum leaps. *Cell* 1996;87:791–794.
84. Marcus SL, Brumell JH, Pfeifer CG, Finlay BB. *Salmonella* pathogenicity islands: big virulence in small packages. *Microbes Infect* 2000;2:145–156.
85. Hueck CJ. Type III protein secretion systems in bacterial pathogens of animals and plants. *Microbiol Mol Biol Rev* 1998; 62:379–433.
86. Lee VT, Schneewind O. Type III secretion machines and the pathogenesis of enteric infections caused by *Yersinia* and *Salmonella* spp. *Immunol Rev* 1999;168:241–255.
87. Collazo CM, Galan JE. The invasion-associated type-III protein secretion system in *Salmonella*—a review. *Gene* 1997;192:51–59.
88. Kubori T, Sukhan A, Aizawa S, et al. Molecular characterization and assembly of the needle complex of the *Salmonella typhimurium* type III protein secretion system. *Proc Natl Acad Sci U S A* 2000;97:10225–10230.
89. Galyov EE, Wood MW, Rosqvist R, et al. A secreted effector protein of *Salmonella dublin* is translocated into eukaryotic cells and mediates inflammation and fluid secretion in infected ileal mucosa. *Mol Microbiol* 1997;25:903–912.
90. Norris FA, Wilson MP, Wallis TS, et al. SopB, a protein required for virulence of *Salmonella dublin,* is an inositol phosphate phosphatase. *Proc Natl Acad Sci U S A* 1998;95:14057–14059.
91. Miller SI, Kukrai AM, Mekalanos JJ. A two-component regulatory system (phoP-phoQ) controls *Salmonella typhimurium* virulence. *Proc Natl Acad Sci U S A* 1989;86:5054–5058.
92. Deiwick J, Nikolaus T, Erdogan S, et al. Environmental regulation of *Salmonella* pathogenicity island 2 gene expression. *Molec Microbiol* 1999;31:1759–1773.
93. Guo L, Lim KB, Gunn JS, et al. Regulation of lipid A modification by *Salmonella typhimurium* virulence genes *phoP-phoQ. Science* 1997;276:250–253.
94. Gunn JS, Miller SI. PhoP-PhoQ activates transcription of pmrAB, encoding a two-component regulatory system involved in *Salmonella typhimurium* antimicrobial peptide resistance. *J Bacteriol* 1996;178:6857–6864.
95. Guo L, Lim KB, Poduje CM, et al. Lipid A acylation and bacterial resistance against vertebrate antimicrobial peptides. *Cell* 1998;95:189–198.
96. Ravdin JI. Pathogenesis of disease caused by *Entamoeba histolytica:* studies of adherence, secreted toxins, and contact-dependent cytolysis. *Rev Infect Dis* 1986;8:247–260.
97. Saffer LD, Petri WA Jr. *Entamoeba histolytica:* recognition of alpha- and beta-galactose by the 260-kDa adherence lectin. *Exp Parasitol* 1991;72:106–108.
98. Petri WA Jr, Ravdin JI. Protection of gerbils from amebic liver abscess by immunization with the galactose-specific adherence lectin of *Entamoeba histolytica. Infect Immun* 1991;59:97–101.
99. Ravdin JI, Guerrant RL. Role of adherence in cytopathogenic mechanisms of *Entamoeba histolytica:* study with mammalian tissue culture cells and human erythrocytes. *J Clin Invest* 1981; 68:1305–1313.
100. Ravdin JI, Murphy CF, Guerrant RL, et al. Effect of calcium and phospholipase A antagonists in the cytopathogenicity of *Entamoeba histolytica. J Infect Dis* 1985;152:542–549.
101. Saffer LD, Petri WA Jr. Role of the galactose lectin of *Entamoeba histolytica* in adherence-dependent killing of mammalian cells. *Infect Immun* 1991;59:4681–4683.
102. Guerrant RL, Brush J, Ravdin JI, et al. Interaction between *Entamoeba histolytica* and human polymorphonuclear neutrophils. *J Infect Dis* 1981;143:83–93.
103. Eckmann L, Reed SL, Smith JR. *Entamoeba histolytica* trophozoites induce an inflammatory cytokine response by cultured human cells through the paracrine action of cytolytically released interleukin-1-alpha. *J Clin Invest* 1995;96:1269–1279.
104. Seydel KB, Li E, Swanson PE, et al. Human intestinal epithelial cells produce proinflammatory cytokines in response to infection in SCID mouse-human intestinal xenograft model of amebiasis. *Infect Immun* 1997;65:1631–1639.
105. O'Brien AD, Holmes RK. Shiga and Shiga-like toxins. *Microbiol Rev* 1987;51:206–220.
106. Donohue-Rolfe A, Acheson DWK, Keusch GT. Shiga toxin: purification, structure, and function. *Rev Infect Dis* 1991;13 [Suppl 4]:S293–297.
107. Reisbig R, Olsnes S, Eiklid K. The cytotoxic activity of *Shigella* toxin. Evidence for catalytic inactivation of the 60 S ribosomal subunit. *J Biol Chem* 1981;256:8739-8744.
108. Knowalchuk J, Speirs JI, Stavric S. Vero response to a cytotoxin of *Escherichia coli. Infect Immun* 1977;18:775–779.
109. Karmali MA, Petric M, Lim C, et al. The association between idiopathic hemolytic uremic syndrome and infection by verotoxin-producing *Escherichia coli. J Infect Dis* 1985;151:775–782.
110. Jacewicz M, Clausen H, Nudelman E, et al. Pathogenesis of shigella diarrhea. XI. Isolation of a shigella toxin-binding glycolipid from rabbit jejunum and HeLa cells and its identification as globotriaosylceramide. *J Exp Med* 1986;163:1391–1404.
111. Vargas M, Gascon J, De Anta MTJ, et al. Prevalence of *Shigella* enterotoxins 1 and 2 among Shigella strains isolated from patients with traveler's diarrhea. *J Clin Microbiol.* 1999;37: 3608–3611.
112. Fontaine A, Arondel J, Sansonetti PJ. Role of Shiga toxin in the pathogenesis of bacillary dysentery studied using Tox⁻ mutant of *Shigella dysenteriae* 1. *Infect Immun* 1988;56:3099–3109.
113. Obrig TG, DelVecchi PJ, Brown JE, et al. Direct cytotoxic action of Shiga toxin on human vascular endothelial cells. *Infect Immun* 1988;56:2373–2378.
114. Lyerly DM, Lockwood DE, Richardson SH, et al. Biological activities of toxins A and B of *Clostridium difficile.* 1982;35:1147–1150.
115. Lyerly DM, Krivan HC, Wilkins TD. *Clostridium difficile:* its disease and toxins. *Clin Microbiol Rev* 1988;1:1–18.

116. Rocha MFG, Maia MET, Bezerra LRPS, et al. *Clostridium difficile* toxin A induces the release of neutrophil chemotactic factors from rat peritoneal macrophages: role of interleukin-1β, tumor necrosis factor alpha, and leukotrienes. *Infect Immun.* 1997;65:2740–2746.
117. Just I, Selzer J, Wilm M, et al. Glucosylation of Rho proteins by *Clostridium difficile* toxin B. *Nature* 1995;375:500–503.
118. Just I, Wilm M, Selzer J, et al. The enterotoxin from *Clostridium difficile* (ToxA) monoglucosylates the Rho proteins. *J Biol Chem* 1995;270:13932–13936.
119. Sakazaki R, Tamura K, Kato T, et al. Studies on the enteropathogenic facultatively halophilic bacteria, *Vibrio parahaemolyticus.* III. Enteropathogenicity. *Jpn J Med Sci Biol* 1968;21:325–331.
120. Miyamoto Y, Kato T, Obara Y, et al. *In vitro* hemolytic characteristics of *Vibrio parahaemolyticus:* its close correlation with human pathogenicity. *J Bacteriol* 1969;100:1147–1149.
121. Takeda Y. Thermostable direct hemolysin of *Vibrio parahaemolyticus. Pharmacol Ther* 1983;19:123–146.
122. Nishibuchi M, Fasano A. Russell RG, et al. Enterotoxigenicity of *Vibrio parahaemolyticus* with and without genes encoding thermostable direct hemolysin. *Infect Immun* 1992;60:3539–3545.
123. Chatterjee BD. Enteroinvasiveness model of *Vibrio parahaemolyticus. Indian J Med Res* 1984;79:151–158.
124. Steiner TS, Nataro JP, Poteet-Smith JA, et al. Enteroaggregative *Escherichia coli* expresses a novel flagellin that causes IL-8 release from intestinal epithelial cells. *J Clin Invest* 2000;105(12): 1769–1777.
125. Hermann RE. Perforation of the colon from necrotizing colitis in the newborn: report of a survival and new etiological concept. *Surgery* 1965;58:436–441.
126. Ledbetter DJ, Juul SE. Necrotizing enterocolitis and hematopoietic cytokines. *Neonatal Hematol* 2000;27:697–716.
127. Steinberg D, Gold J, Brodin A. Necrotizing enterocolitis in leukemia. *Arch Intern Med* 1973;131:538–544.
128. Mower MJ, Hawkins JA, Nelson EW. Neutropenic enterocolitis in adults with acute leukemia. *Arch Surg* 1986;121:571–574.
129. Frankel AH, Barker F, Williams G, et al. Neutropenic enterocolitis in a renal transplant patient. *Transplantation* 1991;52: 913–914.
130. Cutrona AF, Blinkhorn RJ, Crass J, et al. Probable neutropenic enterocolitis in patients with AIDS. *Rev Infect Dis* 1991;13: 828–831.
131. Lawrence G, Shann F, Frestone DS, et al. Prevention of necrotizing enteritis in Papua New Guinea by active immunization. *Lancet* 1979;1:227–230.
132. Centers for Disease Control and Prevention. Summary of notifiable diseases, United States 1998. *MMWR Morb Mortal Wkly Rep* 1999;47:1–85.
133. Chalker RB, Blaser MJ. A review of human salmonellosis: III. Magnitude of *Salmonella* infection in the United States. *Rev Infect Dis* 1988;10:111–124.
134. Centers for Disease Control and Prevention. Preliminary FoodNet data on the incidence of foodborne illnesses—selected sites, United States, 1999. *MMWR Morb Mortal Wkly Rep* 2000;49: 201–205.
135. Guerrant RL. The global problem of amebiasis: current status, research needs, and opportunities for progress. *Rev Infect Dis* 1986;8:218–227.
136. Centers for Disease Control and Prevention. Surveillance for foodborne-disease outbreaks, United States, 1993–1997. *MMWR Morb Mortal Wkly Rep* 2000;49 (SS-1).
137. Ryan CA, Nickels MK, Hargrett-Bean NT, et al. Massive outbreak of antimicrobial resistant salmonellosis traced to pasteurized milk. *JAMA* 1987;258:3268–3274.
138. Spika JS, Waterman SH, Soo Hoo G, et al. Chloramphenicol-resistant *Salmonella newport* traced through hamburger to dairy farms: a major persisting source of human salmonellosis in California. *N Engl J Med* 1987;316:565–570.
139. Tauxe RV, Vandepitte J, Wauters G, et al. *Yersinia enterocolitica* infections and pork: the missing link. *Lancet* 1987;1:1129–1132.
140. Tacket CO, Narain JP, Sattin R, et al. A multistate outbreak of infections caused by *Yersinia enterocolitica* transmitted by pasteurized milk. *JAMA* 1984;251:483–486.
141. Lee LA, Gerber AR, Lonsway DR, et al. *Yersinia enterocolitica* O:3 infections in infants and children, associated with the household preparation of chitterlings. *N Engl J Med* 1990;322:984–987.
142. Tacket CO, Ballard J, Harris N, et al. An outbreak of *Yersinia enterocolitica* infections caused by contaminated tofu (soybean curd). *Am J Epidemiol* 1985;121:705–711.
143. Hoare CA. Reservoir hosts and natural foci of human protozoal infection. *Acta Trop* 1962;19:281–317.
144. Dobell C. Researches on the intestinal protozoa of monkeys and man IV. An experimental study of the *histolytica*-like species of *Entamoeba* living naturally in macaques. *Parasitology* 1931;23:1–72.
145. Weissman JB, Schmerler A, Weiler P, et al. The role of preschool children and day-care centers in the spread of shigellosis in urban communities. *J Pediatr* 1974;84:797–802.
146. Black RE, Craun GF, Blake PA. Epidemiology of common-source outbreaks of shigellosis in the United States, 1961-1975. *Am J Epidemiol* 1978;108:47–52.
147. Lee LA, Ostroff SM, McGee HG, et al. An outbreak of shigellosis at an outdoor music festival. *Am J Epidemiol* 1991;133: 608–615.
148. Lew JF, Swerdlow DL, Dance ME, et al. An outbreak of shigellosis aboard a cruise ship caused by a multiple-antibiotic-resistant strain of *Shigella flexneri. Am J Epidemiol* 1991;134: 413–420.
149. Riley LW, DiFerdinando G, DeMelfi TM, et al. Evaluation of isolated cases of salmonellosis by plasmid profile analysis: introduction and transmission of a bacterial clone by precooked roast beef. *J Infect Dis* 1983;148:12–17.
150. Riley LW, Ceballos BSO, Trabulsi LR, et al. The significance of hospitals as reservoirs for endemic multiresistant *Salmonella typhimurium* causing infection in urban Brazilian children. *J Infect Dis* 1984;150:236–241.
151. Tipple MA, Bland JJ, Murphy MJ, et al. Sepsis associated with transfusion of red cells contaminated with *Yersinia enterocolitica. Transfusion* 1990;30:207–213.
152. Jacobs J, Jamaer D, Vandeven J, et al. *Yersinia enterocolitica* in donor blood: a case report and review. *J Clin Microbiol* 1989;27: 1119–1121.
153. Knoop FC, Owens M, Crocker IC. *Clostridium difficile:* clinical disease and diagnosis. *Clin Microbiol Rev* 1993;6:251–265.
154. Stein H, Kavin I, Faerber EN. Colonic strictures following non-operative management of necrotizing enterocolitis. *J Pediatr Surg* 1975;10:943–947.
155. Touloukian RJ, Kadar A, Spencer RP. The gastrointestinal complications of neonatal umbilical venous exchange transfusions: a clinical and experimental study. *Pediatrics* 1973;52:36–43.
156. Nienhuis L. Colon perforations in the newborn. *Am Surg* 1963; 29:835–840.
157. Stevenson JK, Graham CB, Oliver TK Jr, Goldenberg YE. Neonatal necrotizing enterocolitis. A report of 21 cases with 14 survivors. *Am J Surg* 1969;118:260–272.
158. Rogers AF, Dunn PM. Intestinal perforation, exchange transfusion and PVC. *Lancet* 1969;2:1203–1204.
159. Jaeger RJ, Rubin RJ. Migration of a phthalate ester plasticizer from polyvinyl chloride blood bags into stored human blood and its localization in human tissues. *N Engl J Med* 1972;287: 1114–1118.

160. Hornick RB, Greisman SE, Woodward TE, et al. Typhoid fever: pathogenesis and immunologic control. *N Engl J Med* 1970; 283:686–691.
161. Blaser MJ, Newman LS. A review of human salmonellosis: I. Infective dose. *Rev Infect Dis* 1982;4:1096–1106.
162. DuPont HL, Levine MM, Hornick RB, et al. Inoculum size in shigellosis and implications for expected mode of transmission. *J Infect Dis* 1989;159:1126–1128.
163. Sargeaunt PG, Williams JE. Electrophoretic isoenzyme patterns of the pathogenic and nonpathogenic intestinal amoebae of man. *Trans R Soc Trop Med Hyg* 1979;73:225–227.
164. Giannella RA, Broitman SA, Zamcheck N. Influence of gastric acidity on bacterial and parasitic enteric infections: a perspective. *Ann Intern Med* 1973;78:271–276.
165. Waddell WR, Kunz LJ. Association of salmonella enteritis with operation on the stomach. *N Engl J Med* 1956;255:555–559.
166. Han T, Sokal JE, Neter E. Salmonellosis in disseminated malignant diseases. *N Engl J Med* 1967;276:1045–1052.
167. Wolfe MS, Armstrong D, Louria DB, et al. Salmonellosis in patients with neoplastic disease. A review of 100 episodes at Memorial Cancer Center over a 13-year period. *Arch Intern Med* 1971;128:546–554.
168. Celum CL, Chaisson RE, Rutherford GW, et al. Incidence of salmonellosis in patients with AIDS. *J Infect Dis* 1987;156: 998–1002.
169. Jacobs JL, Gold JW, Murray HW, et al. *Salmonella* infections in patients with the acquired immunodeficiency syndrome. *Ann Intern Med* 1985;103:186–188.
170. Barret-Connor E. Bacterial infection and sickle cell anemia: an analysis of 250 infections in 166 patients and a review of the literature. *Medicine* 1971;50:97–112.
171. Black PH, Kunz LJ, Swartz MN. Salmonellosis—a review of some unusual aspects. *N Engl J Med* 1960;262:811–816, 846–870, 921–927.
172. Riley LW, Cohen ML, Seals JE, et al. Importance of host factors in human salmonellosis caused by multiresistant strains of *Salmonella*. *J Infect Dis* 1984;149:878–883.
173. Hook EW. Salmonellosis: certain factors influencing the interaction of *Salmonella* and the human host. *Bull N Y Acad Med* 1961;37:499–512.
174. Tacket CO, Davis BR, Carter GP, et al. *Yersinia enterocolitica* pharyngitis. *Ann Intern Med* 1983;99:40–42.
175. Blaser MJ, Duncan DJ, Osterholm MT, et al. Serologic study of two clusters of infection due to *Campylobacter jejuni*. *J Infect Dis* 1983;147:820–823.
176. Buchwald DS, Blaser MJ. A review of human salmonellosis: II. Duration of excretion following infection with nontyphi *Salmonella*. *Rev Infect Dis* 1984;6:345–356.
177. Ostroff SM, Kapperud G, Lassen J, et al. Clinical features of sporadic *Yersinia enterocolitica* infections in Norway. *J Infect Dis* 1992;166:812–817.
178. Cooperstock M, Riegle L, Fabacher D, et al. *Clostridium difficile* in formula-fed infants and sudden infant death syndrome. *Pediatrics* 1982;70:91–95.
179. Bennish ML, Harris JR, Wojtyniak BJ, et al. Death in shigellosis: incidence and risk factors in hospitalized patients. *J Infect Dis* 1990;161:500–506.
180. Blatt ML, Shaw NG. Bacillary dysentery in children. A study of three hundred and fifty-six cases from the children's division in the Cook County Hospital, Chicago. *Arch Pathol Lab Med* 1938;26:216–239.
181. Dodd K, Buddingh GJ, Rapoport S. The etiology of ekiri, a highly fatal disease of Japanese children. *Pediatrics* 1949;3:9–19.
182. Riley LW, Pape JW, Johnson WD Jr. Infections caused by *Salmonella* and *Shigella* species. In: Stein JH, ed. *Internal Medicine,* fourth edition. St. Louis: Mosby–Year Book, 1994:2140–2147.
183. Aguero J, Faundez G, Nunez M, et al. Choleriform syndrome and production of labile enterotoxin (CT/LT1)-like antigen by species of *Salmonella infantis* and *Salmonella haardt* isolated from the same patient. *Rev Infect Dis* 1991;13:420–423.
184. Giannella RA, Gots RE, Charney AN, et al. Pathogenesis of *Salmonella*-mediated intestinal fluid secretion. *Gastroenterology* 1975;69:1238–1245.
185. Blaser MJ, Parsons RB, Wang WL. Acute colitis caused by *Campylobacter fetus* ss *jejuni*. *Gastroenterology* 1980;78:448–453.
186. Snyder JD, Christenson E, Feldman RA. Human *Yersinia enterocolitica* infections in Wisconsin. Clinical, laboratory, and epidemiologic features. *Am J Med* 1982;72:768–774.
187. Black RE, Jackson RJ, Tsai T, et al. Epidemic *Yersinia enterocolitica* infection due to contaminated chocolate milk. *N Engl J Med* 1978;298:76–79.
188. Tedesco FJ, Barton RW, Alpers DH. Clindamycin-associated colitis. A prospective study. *Ann Intern Med* 1974;81:429–433.
189. Adams EB, MacLeod IN. Invasive amebiasis. II. Amebic liver abscess and its complications. *Medicine* 1977;56:325–334.
190. Juniper K. Parasitic diseases of the intestinal tract. In: Paulson M, ed. *Gastroenterologic medicine.* Philadelphia: Lea & Febiger, 1969:172.
191. Ronsmans C, Bennish ML, Wierzba T. Diagnosis and management of dysentery by community health workers. *Lancet* 1988; 2:552–555.
192. World Health Organization. Research priorities for diarrhoeal disease vaccines: memorandum from a WHO meeting. *Bull WHO* 1991;69:667–676.
193. Rabbani GH, Gilman RH, Spira WM. Intestinal fluid loss in *Shigella* dysentery: role of oral rehydration therapy. *Lancet* 1983;1:654.
194. Bennish ML. Potentially lethal complications of shigellosis. *Rev Infect Dis* 1991;13[Suppl 4]:S319–324.
195. Bennish ML, Azad AK, Rahman O, et al. Hypoglycemia during diarrhea in childhood. *N Engl J Med* 1990;322:1357–1363.
196. Ashkenazi S, Dinari G, Zevulunov A, et al. Convulsions in childhood shigellosis. Clinical and laboratory features in 153 children. *Am J Dis Child* 1987;141:208–210.
197. Struelens MJ, Patte D, Kabir I, et al. *Shigella* septicemia: prevalence, presentation, risk factors, and outcome. *J Infect Dis* 1985; 152:784–790.
198. Bhandari N, Bhan MK, Sazawal S. Mortality associated with acute watery diarrhea, dysentery and persistent diarrhea in rural north India. *Acta Paediatr Suppl* 1992;381:3–6.
199. Nelson MR, Shanson DC, Hawkins DA, Gazzard BG. *Salmonella, Campylobacter,* and *Shigella* in HIV-seropositive patients. *AIDS J* 1992;6:1495–1498.
200. Shahid NS, Sack DA, Rahman M, et al. Risk factors for persistent diarrhea. *BMJ* 1988;297:1036–1038.
201. Blaser MJ, Feldman RA. *Salmonella* bacteremia: reports to the Centers for Disease Control, 1968-1979. *J Infect Dis* 1981;143: 743–746.
202. Wagner VP, Smale LE, Lischke JH. Amebic abscess of the liver and spleen in pregnancy and the puerperium. *Obstet Gynecol* 1975;45:562–565.
203. Kanani SR, Knight R. Relapsing amoebic colitis of 12 years' standing exacerbated by corticosteroids. *BMJ* 1969;2:613–614.
204. Simon DG, Kaslow RA, Rosenbaum J, et al. Reiter's syndrome following epidemic shigellosis. *J Rheumatol* 1981;8: 969–973.
205. Warren CPW. Arthritis associated with salmonella infections. *Ann Rheum Dis* 1970;29:483–487.
206. Olson DN, Finch WR. Reactive arthritis associated with *Yersinia enterocolitica* gastroenteritis. *Am J Gastroenterol* 1981;76:524–546.
207. Finch M, Rodey G, Lawrence D, et al. Epidemic Reiter's syn-

drome following an outbreak of shigellosis. *Eur J Epidemiol* 1986;2:26–30.
208. Van de Putte LBA, Berden JHM, Boerbooms AMT, et al. Reactive arthritis after *Campylobacter jejuni* enteritis. *J Rheumatol* 1980;7:531–535.
209. Laitinen O, Leirisalo M, Skylv G. Relation between HLA-B27 and clinical features in patients with *Yersinia* arthritis. *Arthritis Rheum* 1977;20:1121–1124.
210. Ryan CA, Tauxe RV, Hosek GW, et al. *Escherichia coli* O157:H7 diarrhea in a nursing home: clinical, epidemiological, and pathological findings. *J Infect Dis* 1986;154:631–638.
211. Martin DL, MacDonald KL, White KE, et al. Epidemiology and clinical aspects of the hemolytic-uremic syndrome in Minnesota. *N Engl J Med* 1990;323:1161–1167.
212. Koster F, Levin J, Walker L, et al. Hemolytic-uremic syndrome after shigellosis. Relation to endotoxemia and circulating immune complexes. *N Engl J Med* 1978;298:927–933.
213. Wilson R, Qualheim RE. A form of acute hemorrhagic enterocolitis afflicting chronically ill individuals. *Gastroenterology* 1954;27:431–444.
214. Marston A, Pheils MT, Thomas ML, et al. Ischemic colitis. *Gut* 1966;7:1–15.
215. McGovern VJ, Goulston JM. Ischaemic enterocolitis. *Gut* 1965;6:213–220.
216. Clark AW, Lloyd-Mostyn RH, Sadler MR de C. "Ischaemic" colitis in young adults. *BMJ* 1972;4:70–72.
217. Miller WE, DePoto DW, Scholl HW, et al. Evanescent colitis in the young adult: a new entity? *Radiology* 1971;100:71–78.
218. Grossman H, Berdon WE, Baker DH. Reversible gastrointestinal signs of hemorrhage and edema in the pediatric age group. *Radiology* 1965;84:33–39.
219. Virnig NL, Reynolds JW. Epidemiological aspects of neonatal necrotizing enterocolitis. *Am J Dis Child* 1974;128:186–190.
220. Podolsky DK. Inflammatory bowel disease. 1 and 2. *N Engl J Med* 1991;325:928–937, 1008–1016.
221. Banks WJ, Pleasure DE, Suzuki K. Thallium poisoning. *Arch Neurol* 1972;26:456–464.
222. Ogen S, Rosenbluth S, Eisenberg A. Food poisoning due to barium carbonate in sausage. *Isr J Med Sci* 1967;3:565–568.
223. Hammond PR, Beliles RP. Metals. In: Doull J, Klaassen CD, Amdur MO, eds. *Casarett and Doull's toxicology. The basic science of poisoning,* second ed. New York: Macmillan,1980.
224. Harris JC, DuPont HL, Hornick RB. Fecal leukocytes in diarrheal illness. *Ann Intern Med* 1972;76:697–703.
225. Korzeniowski OM, Barada FA, Rouse JD, et al. Value of examination for fecal leukocytes in the early diagnosis of shigellosis. *Am J Trop Med Hyg* 1979;28:1031–1035.
226. Guerrant RL, Araujo V, Soares E, et al. Measurement of fecal lactoferrin as a marker of fecal leukocytes. *J Clin Microbiol* 1992;30:1238–1242.
227. Miller JR, Barrett LJ, Kotloff K, et al. A rapid test for infectious and inflammatory enteritis. *Arch Intern Med* 1994;154: 2660–2664.
228. Choi SW, Park CH, Silva TMJ, et al. To culture or not to culture: fecal lactoferrin screening for inflammatory bacterial diarrhea. J Clin Microbiol. 1996;34:928–932.
229. Wells JG, Davis BR, Wachsmuth IK, et al. Laboratory investigation of hemorrhagic colitis outbreaks associated with a rare *Escherichia coli* serotype. *J Clin Microbiol* 1983;18:512–520.
230. Farmer JJ, Davis BR. H7 antiserum-sorbitol fermentation medium: a single tube screening medium for detecting *Escherichia coli* O157:H7 associated with hemorrhagic colitis. *J Clin Microbiol* 1985;22:620–625.
231. George WL, Sutter VL, Citron D, et al. Selective and differential medium for isolation of *Clostridium difficile. J Clin Microbiol* 1979;9:214–219.
232. Gopill S, Sims HV. Presumptive identification of *Clostridium difficile* by detection of p-cresol in prepared peptone yeast glucose broth supplemented with p-hydroxyphenylacetic acid. *J Clin Microbiol* 1990;28:1851–1853.
233. Litwin CM, Storm AL, Chipowsky S, et al. Molecular epidemiology of *Shigella* infections: plasmid profiles, serotype correlation, and restriction endonuclease analysis. *J Clin Microbiol* 1991;29:104–108.
234. Wachsmuth IK. Molecular epidemiology of bacterial infections. Examples of methodology and investigations of outbreaks. *Rev Infect Dis* 1986;8:682–692.
235. Strockbine NA, Parsonnet J, Greene K, et al. Molecular epidemiologic techniques in analysis of epidemic and endemic *Shigella dysenteriae* type 1 strains. *J Infect Dis* 1991;163: 406–409.
236. Faruque SM, Haider K, Rahman MM, et al. Differentiation of *Shigella flexneri* strains by rRNA gene restriction patterns. *J Clin Microbiol* 1992;30:2996–2999.
237. Pierce NF, Sack RB, Mitra RC, et al. Replacement of water and electrolyte losses in cholera by an oral glucose electrolyte solution. *Ann Intern Med* 1969;70:1173–1181.
238. Nalin DR, Cash RA. Oral or nasogastric maintenance therapy for diarrhoea of unknown aetiology resembling cholera. *Trans R Soc Trop Med Hyg* 1970;64:769–771.
239. Black RE, Merson M, Taylor PR, et al. Glucose vs sucrose in oral rehydration solutions for infants and young children with rotavirus-associated diarrhea. *Pediatrics* 1981;67:79–83.
240. Nalin DR, Levine MM, Mata L, et al. Oral rehydration and maintenance of children with rotavirus and bacterial diarrhoeas. *Bull WHO* 1979;57:453–459.
241. Varavithya W, Sunthornkachit R, Eampokalap B. Oral rehydration therapy for invasive diarrhea. *Rev Infect Dis* 1991;13[Suppl 4]:S325–S331.
242. World Health Organization. A manual for the treatment of acute diarrhoea. *WHO/CDD/SER* 1984;80(2)Rev. 1.
243. Pal SC. Epidemic bacillary dysentery in West Bengal, India, 1984 [Letter]. *Lancet* 1984;1:1462.
244. Frost JA, Willshaw GA, Barclay EA, et al. Plasmid characterization of drug-resistant *Shigella dysenteriae* 1 from an epidemic in Central Africa. *J Hyg* 1985;94:163–172.
245. Tauxe RV, Puhr ND, Wells JG, et al. Antimicrobial resistance of *Shigella* isolates in the USA: the importance of international travelers. *J Infect Dis* 1990;162:1107–1111.
246. Aserkoff B, Bennett JV. Effect of antibiotic therapy in acute salmonellosis on the fecal excretion salmonellae. *N Engl J Med* 1969;281:636–640.
247. Neill MA, Opal SM, Heelan J, et al. Failure of ciprofloxacin to eradicate convalescent fecal excretion after acute salmonellosis: experience during an outbreak in health care workers. *Ann Intern Med* 1991;114:195–199.
248. Aung MH, Thein H. Prevention of diarrhoea and dysentery by hand washing. *Trans R Soc Trop Med Hyg* 1989;83:128–131.
249. Tagliabue A, Boraschi D, Villa DF, et al. Ig-A-dependent cell-mediated activity against enteropathogenic bacteria: distribution, specificity, and characterization of the effector cells. *J Immunol* 1984;133:988–992.
250. Levine MM. Development of vaccines against bacteria. In: Farthing MJG, Eeusch GT, eds. *Enteric infection: mechanisms, manifestations, and management.* London: Chapman and Hall, 1989:495.
251. World Health Organization. Annual report, Diarrheal Disease Control Programme. Geneva, World Health Organization, 1988.
252. Acharya IL, Lowe CU, Thapa R, et al. Prevention of typhoid fever in Nepal with the Vi capsular polysaccharide of *Salmonella typhi.* A preliminary report. *N Engl J Med* 1987;317:1101–1104.
253. Klugman KP, Gilbertson IT, Koornhof HJ, et al. Vaccination

Advisory Committee. Protective efficacy of Vi capsular polysaccharide against typhoid fever. *Lancet* 1987;2:1165–1169.
254. Shaugnessey HJ, Olsson RC, Bass K, et al. Experimental human bacillary dysentery: polyvalent dysentery vaccine in its prevention. *JAMA* 1946;132:362–368.
255. Baron LS, Kopecko DJ, Formal SB, et al. Introduction of *Shigella flexneri* 2a type and group antigen genes into oral typhoid vaccine strain *Salmonella typhi* Ty21a. *Infect Immun* 1987;55:2797–2801.
256. Formal SB, Hall TL, Kapfer C, et al. Oral vaccination of monkeys with an invasive *Escherichia coli* K12 hybrid expressing *Shigella flexneri* 2a somatic antigen. *Infect Immun* 1984;46:465–469.
257. Lindberg A, Karnell A, Pal T, et al. Construction of an auxotrophic *Shigella flexneri* strain for use as a live vaccine. *Microb Pathog* 1990;8:433–440.
258. Ahmed AU, Sarker MR, Sack DA. Protection of adult rabbits and monkeys from lethal shigellosis by oral immunization with a thymine-requiring and temperature-sensitive mutant of *Shigella flexneri* Y. *Vaccine* 1990;8:153–158.
259. Sansonetti PJ, Arondel J. Construction and evaluation of a double mutant of *Shigella flexneri* as a candidate for oral vaccination against shigellosis. *Vaccine* 1989;7:443–450.
260. Sansonetti PJ, Arondel J, Fontaine A, et al. OmpB (osmo-regulation) and icsA (cell-to-cell spread) mutants of *Shigella flexneri:* vaccine candidates and progress to study the pathogenesis of shigellosis. *Vaccine* 1991;9:416–422.
261. Karnell A, Stocker BAD, Katakura S, et al. An auxotrophic live oral *Shigella flexneri* vaccine: development and testing. *Rev Infect Dis* 1991;13[Suppl 4]:S357–361.
262. Coster TS, Hoge CW, VanDeVerg LL, et al. Vaccination against shigellosis with attenuated *Shigella flexneri* 2a strain SC602. *Infect Immun* 1999;67:3437–3443.

19

TRAVELER'S DIARRHEA

HERBERT L. DUPONT

Traveler's diarrhea is most often narrowly defined as a clinically important illness (i.e., the passage of three or four unformed stools in 24 hours with an additional symptom of enteric infection, such as abdominal pain and cramps) occurring in a person who comes from a highly industrialized region during travel to a developing tropical region. It may be more broadly defined to include diarrhea occurring in a person from any country who is away from the home region. The causes may differ in a person from the United States who is visiting Mexico and in a Mexican who is visiting the United States; however, in both cases, the temporary relocation is usually responsible.

IMPORTANCE

Approximately 600 million persons cross international boundaries each year (1). Of these, 50 million or more venture into developing regions, where enteric pathogens are hyperendemic and diarrhea is an important threat (2). Whether the travel is for business or pleasure, diarrhea is an important health matter for the traveler. For the host country, the stakes may even be higher, however. Undoubtedly, many persons elect not to venture into high-risk areas for pleasure or to stimulate business opportunities because of a realistic fear of experiencing enteric disease with an uncertain prospect of prevention and adequate therapy. If one considers that more than $400 billion is spent annually to support international travel and that only 20% of this money finds its way into developing regions (1), anything that can be done to promote additional tourism and business travel will result in important economic benefits for the regions that most require financial support.

Although traveler's diarrhea represents an important factor in decreased tourism and lost revenue to developing regions, the problem, which reflects inadequate general hygienic conditions, also translates into high local rates of infant gastroenteritis and enterocolitis and potentially preventable infant mortality. Thus, the health and economic burdens of low levels of hygiene and sanitation are enormous for the countries affected.

EPIDEMIOLOGY

Association of Travel with Diarrhea

Travel by its very nature leads to diarrhea in a percentage of persons, regardless of the regions of origin and destination. Persons leaving their own mini-environment must rely on food prepared and served by others that may contain microbes not found at home. Foods and beverages may contain nonmicrobial nonabsorbable materials that encourage the passage of unformed stools. Travelers are subjected to increased levels of stress, often keeping a chaotic schedule and consuming more alcohol than when at home. Not surprisingly, when persons from high-risk countries (e.g., Mexico) visit low-risk regions (e.g., United States), or when persons from one low-risk region (e.g., Switzerland) visit another low-risk region (e.g., United States, the Caribbean), acute diarrhea occurs in approximately 2% to 4% of cases (3–5). This can be considered the background rate of illness attributed to travel that is independent of the special problem of travel to developing tropical regions.

Host Factors

When persons travel to a high-risk area from a highly industrialized country, their chance of experiencing diarrhea depends on their underlying health (6,7), whether they have previously visited or lived in another high-risk area (8), and where they elect to have most of their meals (9,10). The overall risk for illness among persons from the industrialized world is about 40%. This was the rate of illness seen in U.S. students in Mexico by Kean (11) nearly four decades ago. When persons from one developing tropical area visit another, their rates of diarrhea are reduced in comparison with those of persons from industrialized

H. L. DuPont: Internal Medicine Service, St. Luke's Episcopal Hospital, Houston, Texas regions; however, they are not negligible (8). In Table 19.1, the rates of illness among groups of students coming to one school and living in the same dormitories, student housing, or nearby apartments differ by region of origin and time in the country. Newly arrived U.S. students had a 40% rate of illness. It was reduced to 20% in U.S. students who had been at the school for a semester or longer and to 12% in Latin American students. It did not matter whether the Latin American students were from Mexico or another region, or whether they were newly arrived or established students (8). Although it is clear that natural immunity does occur through exposure, it is also clear that immunity is not solid and that a substantial risk remains even for those previously exposed.

Individuals differ importantly in their susceptibility to diarrhea when traveling to a high-risk area. Some known related factors include gastric hypochlorhydria (7), apparent lack of the intestinal receptors required for pathogenesis (12,13), age (rates of illness are higher in the young) (11), and immunologic memory from previous exposure (14). Host genetics is an important area for future study. It is relevant that cholera is more severe in persons of blood group O (15) and that they more frequently experience shigellosis (University of Texas, *unpublished data*), whereas infection with enterotoxigenic *Escherichia coli* does not appear to be more common in persons of certain blood groups (16).

Geographic Considerations

The world can be divided into three general regions in terms of risk for acquiring diarrhea: low, intermediate, and high. The low-risk areas include the United States, Canada, northwestern Europe, South Africa, Japan, New Zealand, and Australia. The intermediate areas are southern Europe and the northern Mediterranean countries, the Middle East, China, Russia, and parts of southern Africa (Zambia, Zimbabwe, and Botswana). The high-risk areas include most parts of Latin America, southern Asia, and Africa. The risk for acquiring diarrhea of nonimmune persons traveling from low-risk to high-risk regions averages 40%. When the same persons venture into intermediate-risk areas, their chance of acquiring diarrhea is about 10% (3). When these people move from one low-risk area to another, even within the same country, their chance of experiencing diarrhea is probably in the range of the 2% to 4% background rate. Some small regions within the larger areas do not fit into the expected risk pattern. Examples include Haiti and the Dominican Republic, which are high-risk countries within a low-risk region, whereas Singapore and Hong Kong are low-risk areas within high-risk settings.

TABLE 19.1. OCCURRENCE OF DIARRHEA AMONG STUDENTS, JULY 1975, UNIVERSIDAD DE LAS AMERICAS, CHOLULA, PUEBLA, MEXICO

Student Group	No.	No. Ill (%)
U.S. newly arrived	55	22 (40)
U.S. established[a]	142	28 (20)
Latin American	95	11 (12)

[a]Present at the school for at least one semester.
From DuPont NL, Haynes GA, Pickering LK, et al. Diarrhea of travelers in Mexico. Relative susceptibility of United States and Latin American students attending a Mexican university. *Am J Epidemiol* 1977;105:37–41, with permission.

Sources

Most travelers to high-risk areas will tell you that the problem is the water, possibly the food. However, food is undoubtedly the major source of diarrhea among persons traveling to the larger cities of the developing world (9,10,17). For adventure travelers to more remote rural areas, water may also be an important problem. Furthermore, even in urban areas of the developing world, water may become contaminated during rainy seasons by fecal coliforms and pathogenic viruses (18) and so be an important cause of diarrhea. In many tropical regions, crops are raised in soil fertilized with human excreta. This ensures contamination with pathogenic microbes. Further errors occur. Foods frequently are not washed thoroughly when they reach retail stores and restaurants, they are not properly refrigerated after preparation when not immediately consumed, and workers who may harbor enteric organisms without having diarrhea (19) often do not adhere to optimal standards of personal hygiene. Such errors ensure an exposure to enteric pathogens (10). Also, foods contain antibiotic-resistant coliforms (20), which may explain the frequent acquisition of antimicrobial-resistant flora during a stay in a region where traveler's diarrhea is prevalent (21).

CLINICAL FEATURES

Traveler's diarrhea characteristically begins within a week after arrival in a foreign locale. It may occur during the 7 to 10 days after the return home. The diarrheal illness characteristically consists of the passage of 3 to 10 unformed stools daily for 3 to 5 days without curative therapy (8,11). Most travelers experience abdominal pain or cramps, and 10% to 20% of patients have one or more of the following: fever, vomiting, and dysentery, defined as the passage of small volumes of stool that contain gross blood and mucus (8,11,22). In 10% of affected persons, the diarrhea lasts more than a week, and in 2% it persists for a month or longer (23). During a bout of diarrhea, one-fifth of patients are confined to bed for 1 to 2 days (3,22,24). Except in classic syndromes (i.e., febrile dysentery), it is not possible to determine the cause of diarrhea based on clinical features (25).

ETIOLOGY

Bacterial agents cause approximately 85% of cases of traveler's diarrhea (26,27), which explains the remarkable value of antibacterial drugs in both preventing and treating the illness (to be discussed later). The specific agents responsible vary according to region and season. The accepted enteropathogenic agents, in order of occurrence, include enterotoxigenic *E. coli* (ETEC), *Shigella* species, *Campylobacter jejuni, Aeromonas* species, *Plesiomonas shigelloides, Salmonella* species, and noncholera vibrios (Table 19.2). ETEC is more common in the summer months in Mexico and Morocco, and in these areas during the autumn and winter, *C. jejuni* is the most important agent identified (28,29). *Aeromonas* species occur more commonly in Thailand and may rival ETEC in importance (30). *Vibrio cholerae* infection occurs only very rarely in travelers to areas of endemicity (22), and then only in persons who consume heavily contaminated food, usually poorly cooked or inadequately handled seafood (31). Noncholera vibrios may infect travelers to coastal areas of southeastern Asia (32).

We have been interested in determining the cause of diarrhea in the one-fifth of persons with traveler's diarrhea in whom an agent cannot be identified. One potentially important cause is *E. coli* with virulence properties other than conventional enterotoxin production. In studies performed in Mexico, in approximately 20% of patients with traveler's diarrhea and in one-third of pathogen-negative cases, HEp-2-adherent *E. coli* exhibiting enteroaggregative attachment to tissue culture cells (33) could be detected in stool (34). These enteroaggregative *E. coli* organisms appear to be a major cause of traveler's diarrhea (35). In other studies, carried out during two summers, we identified *Shigella*-like invasive *E. coli* in approximately 6% of cases (36).

In Mexico, rotavirus and Norwalk virus are important causes of enteric illness among travelers (37–40). When vomiting is the major clinical manifestation of enteric disease in travelers, viral gastroenteritis or food-borne intoxication caused by preformed toxin of either *Staphylococcus aureus* or *Bacillus cereus* should be suspected. *Giardia lamblia* is an important cause of diarrhea among travelers to mountainous areas of North America (41) and to St. Petersburg, Russia (42). In the latter setting, *Cryptosporidium* is also an important cause of traveler's diarrhea (42). *Entamoeba histolytica* infection is an unusual cause of illness among short-term travelers to developing regions (43). *Cyclospora* species have been shown to cause protracted diarrhea in immunocompetent travelers to developing countries, including Nepal, Mexico, and Haiti, and in patients with AIDS (44,45).

It is not possible to offer a complete list of pathogens and their relative importance in geographic areas, given the lack of available data. However, the available studies suggest a remarkable similarity of responsible pathogens, regardless of the developing region concerned (46,47). Most disease is bacterial in origin, and the common pattern of agents, regardless of specific geographic area, justifies use of the term *traveler's diarrhea* to denote a specific entity when treatment and prevention are being considered, despite the wide variation in potential etiologic agents. Traveler's diarrhea and pediatric diarrhea in any local country, with the possible exception of disease caused

TABLE 19.2. EPIDEMIOLOGY OF TRAVELER'S DIARRHEA: APPROXIMATE FREQUENCY OF ETIOLOGIC AGENTS

Etiologic Agent	Approximate Percentage	Comment
Enterotoxigenic *E. coli* (ETEC)	5–40	Single most important agent, particularly in summertime, at least in semitropical areas.
Enteroaggregative *E. coli* (EAEC)	10–20	May explain one-third of "culture-negative" cases of traveler's diarrhea.
Shigella and enteroinvasive *E. coli* (EIEC)	10–25	Major cause of fever and dysentery in travelers.
Salmonella	5–10	Resembles *Shigella* and EIEC diarrhea.
C. jejuni	3–15	More important in wintertime, at least in semitropical areas (more common in Asia).
Aeromonas	5	Particularly important in Thailand.
Plesiomonas	5	Statistically related to travel to tropical areas and consumption of seafood.
Vibrio	0–10	Cholera is unusual in travelers; non-cholera vibriones cause seafood-related diarrhea in travelers to coastal areas of southern Asia.
Rotavirus and Norwalk virus	10	Rotavirus is particularly important in Mexico.
G. lamblia	<2	Particularly common in travelers to mountainous regions and to St. Petersburg, Russia.
Cryptosporidium	2	Particularly common in travelers to St. Petersburg, Russia.
Cyclospora	<1	Occurs in travelers to Nepal, Haiti, and Peru.
Unknown	20	Most of these patients have bacterial diarrhea; the illness improves with antibacterial therapy.

by rotavirus infection, are similar in terms of incidence and etiology (48–51). Both affect highly susceptible nonimmune subjects who commonly become ill after infection by endemic enteropathogens.

As discussed in the section on "Clinical Features," traveler's diarrhea may be protracted in some patients, lasting weeks to months. The cause of such illness is highly variable, but the differential diagnosis includes infection by a protozoal pathogen, such as *G. lamblia, Cryptosporidium,* or *Cyclospora,* and, in patients with diarrhea lasting 1 to 3 weeks, infection by an invasive bacterial pathogen, including *Shigella, Salmonella,* and *Campylobacter.* Other diagnoses to be considered are disaccharidase deficiency secondary to small-bowel injury by an infecting organism, small-bowel overgrowth syndrome caused by small-bowel stasis (again, a result of small-bowel infection), and small-bowel injury produced by repeated exposures to enteric pathogens or toxic substances that results in a "tropical sprue"-like picture. A fairly well-characterized form of chronic diarrhea is known as *Brainerd diarrhea* after the initially reported outbreak in Brainerd, Minnesota (52). In this disease, protracted diarrhea may last years. It can usually be traced to the consumption of raw (unpasteurized) milk or untreated surface water (52,53). The etiology is uncertain; however, it appears to be an as yet undiscovered infectious agent. It does not respond to antibacterial therapy but characteristically has a benign outcome, as do most cases of prolonged diarrhea in travelers (54). The chronic diarrhea of travelers without detectable etiology after complete workup may best be classified as Brainerd diarrhea (55).

DIAGNOSIS

A history of travel is essential in making the diagnosis. Travel to a specific region may suggest the cause (see "Etiology"). The clinical presentation often is important in leading to the proper diagnosis (see "Clinical Features" and "Etiology"). Because most patients with acute traveler's diarrhea have a bacterial enteric infection, it is reasonable to initiate antibacterial therapy without a microbiologic evaluation. Laboratory study for parasites is largely reserved for patients with protracted illness.

PREVENTION AND CONTROL

In the attempt to prevent traveler's diarrhea, the three main general considerations are the following: decreased exposure through modification and improvement of hygiene levels in the environment and education of travelers regarding how to obtain the safest foods and beverages; chemoprophylaxis; and immunoprophylaxis.

Environmental and Educational Approaches

Unfortunately, physicians have not been effective in changing the way people eat while in high-risk areas. More attention to effective education of travelers is needed. Foods and beverages can be categorized as high-risk and low-risk based on a few basic principles. Table 19.3 lists the usually safe and unsafe foods. The most important principle is that heat kills microbes. The temperature of a food should be raised to approximately 59°C to ensure that pathogens are killed (56). Food that just reaches the point of being too hot to touch is at a temperature of 50°C. The careful traveler should warn the person serving food at a restaurant that all cooked food must be brought to the table steaming hot or it will be returned to the kitchen. It would not be entirely unreasonable for the most cautious traveler to check the internal temperature of a served item with a clinical thermometer before consuming it to be certain of its safety. Other safe foods include those that are dry (bread and crackers); those with high sugar content (jellies and syrups); citrus fruits with a low pH; fruits and vegetables that have been peeled; peanut butter; self-prepared foods of all sorts that have been thoroughly washed with clean, previously boiled water before consumption; and bottled carbonated beverages. Items that are often sources of enteric infection include moist food served at room temperature (often as part of a buffet); fruits and vegetables with intact skins (tomatoes, strawberries, grapes); salads; milk (unless powdered milk is reconstituted with previously boiled water or boxed irradiated milk is used and refrigerated after preparation/opening); and tap water. Ice cubes should be considered contaminated because they are often made with

TABLE 19.3. SAFE AND UNSAFE FOODS IN DEVELOPING TROPICAL REGIONS

Low-risk Foods and Beverages	High-risk Foods and Beverages
Any item served steaming hot (>59°C)	Foods that are moist and served at room temperature, especially those at a buffet
Foods that are dry (i.e., bread and crackers)	Fruits and vegetables with skin intact—strawberries, tomatoes, grapes
Items with very high sugar content (syrups and jellies)	Salads and other uncooked vegetables
Fruits and vegetables that have been peeled	Sauces and dressings in open containers on the table
Peanut butter	Milk (other than powdered milk that is constituted with previously boiled water or irradiated milk and kept refrigerated after being prepared or opened)
Any fresh food item properly washed and prepared by the traveler	
Bottled carbonated drinks, including mineral water, soft drinks, and beer	Tap water or ice

tap water. It is not practical to attempt to disinfect ice cubes with alcoholic beverages (57). With attention to dietary and beverage restriction, it is possible to reduce rates of diarrhea that occurs during travel to high-risk areas (58).

Chemoprophylaxis

It has been known for nearly four decades that antimicrobial drugs decrease the risk for diarrhea during travel to high-risk regions (11). Contemporary data providing evidence of the value of chemoprophylaxis can be dated back to the studies confirming ETEC as the major cause of disease (26). Soon thereafter, doxycycline (59) and trimethoprim-sulfamethoxazole (TMP-SMX) (60) were shown to prevent 80% to 90% of cases of disease that would have occurred without their use provided that the prevalent enteropathogenic bacteria were susceptible to the drugs (61). Because resistance to doxycycline and TMP is now frequent, these drugs are of limited value. Currently, the most predictably active of the antibacterial drugs are the fluoroquinolones. Both norfloxacin (62,63) and ciprofloxacin (64) have been used for prophylaxis of traveler's diarrhea with protection rates near 90%. Amdinocillin, a drug with *in vitro* activity against the more resistant enteropathogens, has also been shown to be an effective chemoprophylactic agent (65). With a protection rate of 90%, and a 40% chance of the development of diarrhea in untreated subjects during a period of risk, illness will occur in 4% of persons with antimicrobial prophylaxis.

Other approaches to chemoprophylaxis have been utilized. *Lactobacillus* preparations have been examined as prophylactic agents (66,67). The concept makes sense; the organism induces the fermentation of intraluminal carbohydrates, which results in the formation of bactericidal organic acids. *Lactobacillus* GG has been shown to be modestly effective in preventing diarrhea, probably because of the potential of the organisms to adhere to the intestinal lining. Bismuth subsalicylate (BSS) has produced more impressive results (68–71). The prophylactic value of BSS probably relates to its antimicrobial property and to the intestinal reaction products that form after it is ingested (72). BSS must be taken with meals, when the challenge by bacterial agents occurs, and at bedtime to be effective (69–71). The optimal dose is two 262-mg tablets, chewed well, taken four times a day with meals and at bedtime (69). At this dose, the protection rate is about 65%, which translates into a rate of diarrhea of about 14% when the frequency of illness in untreated subjects is 40%.

In a consideration of how prophylaxis may be used, the pros and cons of the approach must be thoroughly understood (6,24). Problems of prophylaxis include side effects of the drugs, a false sense of security on the part of the traveler, and difficulty in treating the diarrhea that results. Adverse effects of the drugs may be considered minor (skin rash, insomnia, vaginitis in the case of antimicrobials, and black tongue and stools and tinnitus in the case of BSS) or major (anaphylaxis, antibiotic-associated colitis, Stevens–Johnson syndrome). Minor reactions to the antibacterial drugs occur in about 3% of cases, and major reactions in about 1 in 10,000 (73). BSS commonly causes minor reactions in reasonably healthy persons, but severe reactions should not occur. In patients taking excessive doses, especially in those with underlying medical impairment, bismuth encephalopathy may occur (74). A potential complication of antimicrobial chemoprophylaxis is the development in antibiotic-resistant flora during the time the drug is taken (75).

The decision to recommend or approve the use of chemoprophylaxis is complex and revolves around a number of issues (6,76). Table 19.4 outlines one approach, which is based on the underlying health of the future traveler, the importance of the trip and of remaining disease-free, the traveler's willingness to follow dietary and beverage restrictions, and the traveler's orientation toward prophylaxis after acquiring an understanding of its limitations and risks. Most travelers should not be given antibacterial

TABLE 19.4. FACTORS USED TO DETERMINE WHETHER TO GIVE CHEMOPROPHYLAXIS TO A TRAVELER PLANNING A TRIP TO A HIGH-RISK AREA

Host Factor Used in Deciding About Prophylaxis	Prophylaxis May Be Considered
Important underlying disease: patient on proton pump inhibitor (e.g., omeprazole); diabetic on insulin; patient with heart disease, cancer, active inflammatory bowel disease, or AIDS; patient taking corticosteroids.	Antibacterial agent can be considered (see Table 19.5 for specific agents recommended and doses).
Importance of trip: mission could be ruined by illness rendered short-term by effective therapy.	Bismuth subsalicylate or an antibacterial drug can be considered (see Table 19.5 for doses).
Restrictions on food and beverages: is not willing to exercise care in choosing food and drink.	Bismuth subsalicylate can be considered (see Table 19.5 for dose).
Interest in prophylaxis: traveler wants prophylaxis after pros and cons are thoroughly explained and understood.	Bismuth subsalicylate is appropriate (see Table 19.5 for dose).

Adapted from DuPont NL, Ericsson CD. Prevention and treatment of traveler's diarrhea. *N Engl J Med* 1993;328:1821–1827, and from Farthing MJG, DuPont NL, Guandalini S, et al. Treatment and prevention of traveller's diarrhoea. *Gastroenterol Int* 1992;5:162–175, with permission.

chemoprophylaxis. The drugs used, with their indications and doses, are given in Table 19.5. This approach is only for short-term travel. The longer the trip, the less valuable the chemoprophylaxis. When the time to be spent in a high-risk area exceeds 3 weeks, chemoprophylaxis should not be used. The drugs are begun on the day of arrival in the high-risk area and continued for 2 days after the return home. Chemoprophylaxis is not appropriate for young infants or pregnant women. When the approach is desired for older children, BSS is recommended. Even persons electing chemoprophylaxis must take care in choosing food and drink if the lowest rates of illness are to be achieved (77).

Immunoprophylaxis

Great interest has been shown in immunoprophylactic approaches to preventing acute infectious diarrhea. Because traveler's diarrhea and endemic diarrhea in children living in the developing world are similar, a vaccine against one should have great utility in the other situation. Two approaches currently are being explored. The first is passive immunization with antibodies directed to enteropathogenic organisms or their purified virulence properties (78). The obvious limitation to this approach is that the preparation must be taken daily during the period of risk, possibly with each meal. Protection ends when the preparation is discontinued. The advantage of passive immunoprophylaxis is that antibodies can be easily and cheaply produced in cows with the purification of multivalent antibody preparations that can be tailored to the region to be visited.

Probably of greater potential value is the development of active vaccines made of the organisms or selected immunogenic properties that can be administered to subjects well in advance of their travels. A vaccine directed to ETEC and the prevalent types of *Shigella* could be of great value in limiting illness. With time in the region, natural immunity to ETEC develops (79,80). Immunity correlates with the occurrence of *E. coli* anti–heat-labile enterotoxin antibodies in the serum (81). An interesting preparation currently being evaluated as an anti-ETEC vaccine is a whole-cell killed *V. cholerae* or ETEC strains combined with the binding subunit of cholera; this is taken as two oral doses (82). The preparation should be effective in preventing cholera (82) and ETEC diarrhea (83), in view of the similarity of the two related heat-labile enterotoxins produced. This immunizing agent will be refined. Clearly, because of the multitude of etiologic agents that cause traveler's diarrhea, immunoprophylaxis, despite its valuable effect of reducing the frequency of illness, will not eliminate the problem.

MANAGEMENT

Regardless of the approach used, it is not possible to prevent all illness among travelers. This, plus the fact that by definition most cases of the diarrhea occur while a person is out of town and away from medical care, underscores the need for empiric self-therapy in most cases of illness. All travelers to high-risk areas should be armed with therapeutic agents to treat any illness that may occur. As with other forms of diarrhea, three different types of therapy are available: fluids and electrolytes, nonspecific symptomatic therapy, and antimicrobial therapy. These are considered separately.

During a bout of diarrhea, patients should be instructed to eat to acquire the calories (energy) needed to facilitate enterocyte renewal. Boiled starches, cereals, crackers, bananas, yogurt, soup, and boiled vegetables should be consumed.

Fluids and Electrolytes

Fluids and electrolytes represent the standard and most fundamental form of treatment for all cases of diarrhea. In travelers with good underlying health, severe dehydration is unusual. For this reason, it is recommended that most previously healthy older children and adults consume flavored mineral water (hypotonic solutions containing glucose) along with soups, broths, and saltine crackers to meet fluid and salt losses. For young infants and elderly persons, particularly when severe diarrhea and vomiting complicate the illness, more aggressive measures may rarely be needed. The parents of children under 2 years of age are advised to take

TABLE 19.5. DRUGS AND DOSAGES USED FOR PROPHYLAXIS OF TRAVELER'S DIARRHEA[a]

Chemoprophylactic Agent	Dose	Comment
Fluoroquinolones: norfloxacin (NF); ciprofloxacin (CF); levofloxacin (LF); fleroxacin (FO)	NF 400 mg; CF 500 mg; LF 500 mg; or FO 400 mg once daily	The most effective drugs available for adults for travel to all regions (except Thailand) during all seasons
Bismuth subsalicylate	Two 262-mg tablets chewed well four times a day (with meals and at bedtime)	Not as effective, but fewer side effects and probably effective in all regions and seasons

[a]All drugs are begun the day the destination is reached and continued for 2 days after the return home (not to be used for trips that exceed 3 weeks). This approach should be followed by a minority of travelers, only after they thoroughly understand the pros and cons of prophylaxis.

with them a supply of Pedialyte or Lytren should diarrhea occur. No therapy other than an electrolyte solution should be given to young infants.

Nonspecific Therapy

Three types of drugs play a role in relieving the symptoms of diarrhea. This approach is important because drugs that provide symptomatic relief may allow a traveler to function while out of town. The preparations used to treat the symptoms of traveler's diarrhea include antisecretory agents, antimotility drugs, and water-absorbing agents. Each has been shown to modify diarrheal illness. The major value of the drugs that relieve symptoms is in the treatment of mild forms of traveler's diarrhea. The course of illness in some travelers who pass only one or two unformed stools is nonprogressive, and antimicrobial agents may not be necessary. These patients may benefit from symptomatic therapy alone. Also, antimotility drugs can be combined with antimicrobial agents for patients with more intense illness, provided no fever or dysentery is present. Table 19.6 lists the doses and indications of the drugs used to treat the symptoms of traveler's diarrhea.

Antisecretory Agents

The most useful antisecretory agent available currently is BSS. For adults, the dosage of BSS is 524 mg (two tablets or 30 mL) taken every 30 minutes eight times; the same dose can be repeated in 24 hours (84). BSS at this dosage reduces diarrhea (number of stools, duration of illness) by about 50% in comparison with a placebo preparation (84). BSS exerts antisecretory effects against bacterial enterotoxins (85,86). It apparently works though salicylate-dependent antisecretory mechanisms (87) other than prostaglandin inhibition, and the preparation is entirely safe in terms of gastric effects. Aspirin is an effective antidiarrheal compound (88), but because of its gastric toxicity, it is not acceptable to use acetylsalicylic acid routinely to treat diarrhea. Interestingly, BSS can be used to treat aspirin-induced gastritis in experimental animals (89). It is not known whether the antimicrobial effects of the drug have any role in its antidiarrheal effects. BSS is probably the treatment of choice for enteric illness in travelers whose major clinical symptom is vomiting (90).

With information available to indicate that intestinal secretion is the most important pathophysiologic mechanism leading to diarrheal disease, novel antisecretory agents are currently being developed. Enterotoxin-mediated diarrhea, such as ETEC diarrhea, involves cyclic nucleotides, calmodulin, and intracellular calcium (91). A drug that inhibits intestinal calmodulin was shown to be an effective form of antisecretory therapy for traveler's diarrhea (92). Also, a drug that blocks chloride channels was shown by us to treat traveler's diarrhea effectively (*unpublished data*). This drug is probably the most effective of the antisecretory drugs available. It is marketed as SB-Normal Stool Formula (1-800-987-9920).

TABLE 19.6. THERAPY OF TRAVELER'S DIARRHEA ACCORDING TO SYMPTOMS

Clinical Symptoms/Signs	Suggested Therapy
Passage of 1–2 unformed stools /24 h without distressing enteric symptoms	Flavored mineral water and saltine crackers, no therapy.
Passage of 1–2 unformed stools with distressing enteric symptoms	Symptomatic therapy in adults: BSS 30 mL or two tablets every 30 min for 8 doses; or, loperamide 4 mg initially followed by 2 mg after passage of each unformed stool, not to exceed 8 tablets/d (prescription dose) or 4 caplets/d (OTC dose); drugs can be taken for 2 d.
Vomiting without important diarrhea	BSS therapy (dose above).
Passage of >2 unformed stools in 24 h, no fever, no dysentery or distressing abdominal pain/ cramps with fewer stools	Antimicrobial drug (see Table 19.7) plus loperamide (dose above).
Fever and or dysentery (diarrhea with passage of bloody stools)	Antimicrobial alone (see Table 19.7).

BSS, bismuth subsalicylate.

Antimotility Agents

The most effective of the drugs used to treat symptoms are the antimotility agents, including paregoric, tincture of opium, codeine, diphenoxylate, and loperamide. The first of the useful synthetic opiates was diphenoxylate with atropine. Although effective in treating diarrhea, this preparation is associated with two problems. First, it can cause central opiate effects in children who inadvertently take an overdose of their parents' medication. Second, atropine is added to the preparation to prevent overdose. Like other anticholinergic drugs, atropine can cause additional objectionable symptoms, such as dry mouth and blurred vision, and it has no antidiarrheal properties (93). The most useful of the antimotility drugs is loperamide, which is as effective as diphenoxylate but with lessened central opiate effects, and atropine is not added. While taken, loperamide reduces by 60% the number of stools passed and the duration of diarrheal illness, and it is more effective than BSS in treating traveler's diarrhea (94,95). The dose administered to adults is 4 mg (two capsules or two caplets) initially, followed by 2 mg (one capsule or one caplet) after each unformed stool; the dose is not to exceed eight capsules (16 mg) in 24 hours (prescription dose) or four caplets (8 mg) in 24 hours (over-the-counter dose), nor is the drug to be used for more than

48 hours. Other antimotility drugs, such as codeine, tincture of opium, and paregoric, probably exert antidiarrheal effects equivalent to those of loperamide, although they have a greater potential to cause central toxicity.

The mechanism of action of this class of drugs is slowing of intestinal transit of the intraluminal column, so that reabsorption is increased (96). Also, the drugs have an antisecretory effect, which may play a role (97). Three problems are associated with the use of loperamide. Overdose is a potential problem in young children, although the risk is less than with diphenoxylate. Second, loperamide does not cure all cases of traveler's diarrhea, and posttreatment clinical relapses are common (94). Finally, with highly invasive bacterial enteropathogens, such as *Shigella, Salmonella,* and *Campylobacter,* intestinal invasion may be facilitated by a greater contact time between the infecting strain and the gut mucosa (98). For this reason, patients with fever or dysentery should not be given the drug.

Water-Absorbing Agents

The water-absorbing agents are the least effective in reducing diarrhea. However, they are the safest of the available drugs because their effects are strictly intraluminal. Attapulgite is the most important example in this group (99). Because it remains unabsorbed, it can be given to patients who cannot tolerate the other preparations. It should be possible to treat young children and pregnant women who have acute traveler's diarrhea with attapulgite. The major result is the passage of more formed stools with some relief of the associated symptoms of enteric infection.

Antimicrobial Therapy

Because traveler's diarrhea is most often a bacterial infection, antibacterial agents are the most important drugs for therapy of the illness. The indications for antibacterial therapy are the passage of three or more unformed stools in 24 hours, diarrhea associated with distressing abdominal cramps or pain, the presence of fever, and the passage of bloody stools (dysentery). Antimicrobial agents shorten the duration of posttreatment diarrhea from approximately 59 to 93 hours without therapy to 16 to 30 hours provided that the prevalent organisms are susceptible to the drug used (100–102). The standard and U.S. Food and Drug Administration-approved antimicrobial for the treatment of traveler's diarrhea is TMP-SMX (100). TMP-SMX is no longer active against most enteropathogens in many regions of the developing world. For areas of the world where quinolone-resistant *C. jejuni* is not known to be an important cause of traveler's diarrhea, the quinolones are preferred for empiric antimicrobial therapy (Tables 19.6 and 19.7). The quinolones do not appear to differ in terms of therapeutic effect, and currently norfloxacin (103), ciprofloxacin (101), ofloxacin (104), fleroxacin (105), and levofloxacin (*unpublished data*) all appear to be equivalent. Unfortunately, children with traveler's diarrhea cannot be given one of the newer quinolones in view of their potential to damage growing articular cartilage (106). For children with diarrhea, optimal antimicrobial therapy for more severe disease includes either azithromycin or furazolidone (Table 19.7). When traveler's diarrhea develops in an area where quinolone-resistant *C. jejuni* is a major pathogen (e.g., Thailand), azithromycin is probably the treatment of choice (107).

Antimicrobials shorten the diarrheal illness associated with bacterial enteropathogens, including ETEC and *Shigella* species, the two major causes of illness. Also, the drugs shorten illness that is not associated with a definable pathogen, which is further evidence that bacterial agents are responsible for this form of the disease (100,104,108).

The optimal duration of antimicrobial therapy for patients with traveler's diarrhea has not been established.

TABLE 19.7. ANTIMICROBIAL THERAPY OF TRAVELER'S DIARRHEA

	Antimicrobial Therapy	
Indications	**Recommended Therapy**	**Alternative Therapy**
Travel to high-risk country other than Thailand*		
Adults	CF 500 mg bid or LF 500 mg once on day 1, repeat on days 2 and 3 if diarrhea continues	Azithromycin 500 mg on day 1, 250 mg on days 2 and 3 if diarrhea continues
Children	Azithromycin 10 mg/kg on day 1, 5 mg/kg on days 2 and 3 if diarrhea continues	Furazolidone 7.5 mg/kg per day in four divided doses for 5 days
Travel to Thailand		
Adults	Azithromycin (see above dose) for adults	CF or LF (see above dose for adults)
Children	Same as for children traveling to other areas	Same as for children traveling to other areas

CF, ciprofloxacin; LF, levofloxacin; other fluoroquinolones are equivalent in efficacy.
*Fluoroquinolone-resistant campylobacter frequently causes travelers diarrhea in Thailand.

The approved duration of therapy is 5 days (100). Evidence suggests that 3 days of therapy is sufficient for all cases (102,104), and single-dose treatment may be adequate for most (102,109,110). In all probability, treatment of this infection of the mucosal surface is similar to that of urinary tract infection. In both situations, drug concentrations at the site of infection reach very high levels (111,112). Until further definitive evidence is available, it may be reasonable to give single-dose therapy to patients with milder forms of illness and more prolonged treatment (3 to 5 days) to those with severe illness, including those with febrile dysenteric diseases (113).

The importance of the absorption of antibacterial drugs in cases of traveler's diarrhea has not been established. In children with shigellosis, oral ampicillin (an absorbed drug) was more effective than oral neomycin (a poorly absorbed drug) (114). Absorption of drug was assumed to be important in treating the mucosal infection. An alternative possibility is that oral aminoglycosides are not effective in the treatment of shigellosis despite *in vitro* activity against strains of *Shigella* (115).

Evidence suggests that the drugs bicozamycin and aztreonam, which are not absorbed and have *in vitro* activity against the prevalent bacterial agents, are effective in the treatment of traveler's diarrhea when taken orally (108,116). Furthermore, bicozamycin has been found effective in preventing illness when employed as a prophylactic agent (117). Neither preparation is available currently. Rifaximin, a poorly absorbed drug, is safe and effective in treating traveler's diarrhea (118). The drug has been shown to be more effective than TMP-SMX (118) and equivalent to ciprofloxacin (119) in treating traveler's diarrhea. Rifaximin is currently available in a few countries, including Mexico and Italy. It is hoped that it will soon be licensed in the United States.

Combination Therapy

In studies conducted in U.S. and Swiss travelers, drugs that relieved symptoms were more rapidly effective than antimicrobial drugs in treating diarrhea (120,121). Given the rapid response to the agents that relieve symptoms and the curative effects of the antimicrobials, it was logical to attempt combined therapy (102,110,120,122–124). Loperamide was selected as the drug to relieve symptoms in most of the trials because BSS may bind to the antimicrobial and prevent absorption (125).

EVALUATION OF PATIENTS WITH A HISTORY OF RECENT TRAVEL

Diarrheal illness in a person recently returned from a high-risk region is a common problem seen by physicians in practice. Three common forms of illness require evaluation: acute diarrhea, persistent or chronic diarrhea, and fever and toxicity. Each clinical presentation suggests special problems that should be approached in a different manner.

Acute Diarrhea

It is recommended that patients who present for medical evaluation with diarrhea after recent travel to a high- or intermediate-risk area be divided into two groups: those with acute diarrhea and those with persistent diarrhea. The stools of patients with acute diarrhea following travel to mountainous areas of North America or to Russia should be examined for protozoal pathogens, including *Giardia* and *Cryptosporidium*. Other patients can be given a course of antimicrobial therapy, according to the region visited, without laboratory evaluation (Table 19.7).

Prolonged Diarrhea

The stools of most patients with persistent illness (>14 days' duration) should be examined for routinely encountered enteric pathogens (see "Etiology" for a discussion of causative agents). If a potential agent is identified, it should be treated specifically. Patients with negative results after etiologic assessment should be given a short course of antibacterial therapy (Table 19.7). For those who fail this treatment, a 7-day course of metronidazole can be given for empiric treatment of giardiasis or small-bowel bacterial overgrowth. For those who fail the empiric treatment, a full workup by a gastroenterologist is indicated. It is not wise to treat patients with prolonged diarrhea continuously with antimicrobial drugs as the intestinal ecology will be severely disturbed; intermittent cycles of diarrhea and treatment, often with temporary improvement in symptoms early in the course of treatment, may be the result. Symptomatic treatment of these patients is warranted after evaluation if a cause is not identified. Fortunately, most patients with protracted diarrhea following travel have a benign course, and most cases eventually resolve (54).

Fever and Toxicity

When a previous traveler presents with fever and toxicity, an invasive bacterial infection should be considered. The list of possible etiologic agents includes *Shigella, Salmonella typhi, Salmonella enteritidis, C. jejuni, Brucella, Francisella tularensis, Leptospira,* and *Yersinia enterocolitica.* Stool and blood cultures are indicated, along with a serologic evaluation for brucellosis, tularemia, and leptospirosis. The patient is treated for the etiologic agent identified. If diarrhea is a prevalent part of the picture, shigellosis, campylobacteriosis, and salmonellosis are the most likely diagnoses. If a diagnosis is not made rapidly, a 7-day course of fluoroquinolone is not unreasonable for empiric treatment of the more easily treated infections.

THE FUTURE

We need to improve our approach to educating travelers about risks and the ways to minimize exposures to enteric pathogens. Travelers should demand safe foods! For example, if most travelers insisted that all foods served in a public eating establishment be steaming hot, the restaurants would soon learn that this is a minimum requirement. Also, research should be continued in an attempt to reduce the threat of illness through strategies of chemoprophylaxis and immunoprophylaxis. Both these approaches should play a role in dealing with the problem by reducing the threat of illness. However, they will not eliminate it.

The most feasible approach to reducing the threat of traveler's diarrhea is to do whatever is needed to make safer the environment in which translocated persons move. The requirements are easily understood and not impossible to achieve. Two ways to improve hygiene are the following: First, the host countries must increase ascribe greater importance to general health in their planning and tackle problems on a full-scale basis by improving water supplies, sewage removal, and general education, and by monitoring and enforcing standards of hygiene in public restaurants. Investigators in industrialized regions have taken the lead in research in the area of traveler's diarrhea, but the countries where the disease occurs should increasingly be involved. They have the most to gain. They should find it appalling that rates of traveler's diarrhea have not been reduced after four decades. They must realize not only that their economy depends on ensuring the good health of their visitors but also that the real payoff of the changes would be the improved health of their own population.

If these countries are unwilling to do what is needed, then the second way to reduce the threat of traveler's diarrhea is for the travel industry and research community to implement hygienic improvements to ensure a safer mini-environment for travelers. Club Med has attempted to do this. Although data are not available to show how successful the approach has been, it is a wonderful idea. Making genuinely safe water and food available to persons temporarily living in a resort or hotel will go a long way toward stimulating travel and ensuring good health and satisfaction with the experience. Some regions of the developing countries are among the most interesting and beautiful in the world, and persons who wish to visit should be able to do so in good health.

REFERENCES

1. Handszuh H. Tourism patterns and trends. In: DuPont HL, Steffen R, eds. *Textbook of travel medicine and health,* second edition. Hamilton, Ontario: BC Decker, 2001:34–36.
2. World Tourism Organization. *Tourism highlights 1999.* Madrid: World Tourism Organization Publication Unit, 1999.
3. Steffen R, Rickenbach M, Wilhelm U, et al. Health problems after travel to developing countries. *J Infect Dis* 1987;156:84–91.
4. Dandoy S. The diarrhea of travelers: incidence in foreign students in the United States. *Calif Med* 1966;104:458–462.
5. Ryder RW, Wells JG, Gangarosa EJ. A study of travelers' diarrhea in foreign visitors to the United States. *J Infect Dis* 1977;136:605–607.
6. DuPont HL, Ericsson CD. Prevention and treatment of traveler's diarrhea. *N Engl J Med* 1993;328:1821–1827.
7. Wingate DL. Acid reduction and recurrent enteritis. *Lancet* 1990;335:222.
8. DuPont HL, Haynes GA, Pickering LK, et al. Diarrhea of travelers in Mexico. Relative susceptibility of United States and Latin American students attending a Mexican university. *Am J Epidemiol* 1977;105:37–41.
9. Tjoa W, DuPont HL, Sullivan P, et al. Location of food consumption and travelers' diarrhea. *Am J Epidemiol* 1977;106: 61–66.
10. Wood LV, Ferguson LE, Hogan P, et al. Incidence of bacterial enteropathogens in foods from Mexico. *Appl Environ Microbiol* 1983;46:328–332.
11. Kean BH. The diarrhea of travelers to Mexico: summary of five-year study. *Ann Intern Med* 1963;59:605–614.
12. Parrino TA, Schreiber DS, Trier JS, et al. Clinical immunity in acute gastroenteritis caused by the Norwalk agent. *N Engl J Med* 1977;297:86–89.
13. Rutter JM, Burrows MR, Sellwood R, et al. A genetic basis for resistance to enteric disease caused by *E. coli. Nature* 1975;257: 135–136.
14. DuPont HL, Olarte J, Evans DG, et al. Comparative susceptibility of Latin American and United States students to enteric pathogens. *N Engl J Med* 1976;295:1520–1521.
15. Glass RI, Holmgren J, Haley CE, et al. Predisposition for cholera of individuals with O blood group. Possible evolutionary significance. *Am J Epidemiol* 1985;121:791–796.
16. van Loon FPL, Clemens JD, Sack DA, et al. ABO blood groups and the risk of diarrhea due to enterotoxigenic *Escherichia coli. J Infect Dis* 1991;163:1243–1246.
17. Merson MH, Morris GK, Sack DA, et al. Travelers' diarrhea in Mexico: a prospective study of physicians and family members attending a congress. *N Engl J Med* 1976;294:1299–1305.
18. Deetz TR, Smith EM, Goyal SM, et al. Occurrence of rota- and enteroviruses in drinking and environmental water in a developing nation. *J Infect Dis* 1984;18:567–571.
19. Pickering LK, DuPont HL, Evans DG, et al. Isolation of enteric pathogens from asymptomatic students from the United States and Latin America. *J Infect Dis* 1977;135:1003–1005.
20. Wood LV, Jansen DM, DuPont HL. Antimicrobial resistance of gram-negative bacteria isolated from foods in Mexico. *J Infect Dis* 1983;148:766.
21. Murray BE, Mathewson JJ, DuPont HL, et al. Emergence of resistant fecal *Escherichia coli* in travelers not taking prophylactic antimicrobial agents. *Antimicrob Agents Chemother* 1990;34: 515–518.
22. Steffen R. Epidemiologic studies of travelers' diarrhea, severe gastrointestinal infections, and cholera. *Rev Infect Dis* 1986;8 [Suppl 2]:S122–S130.
23. DuPont HL, Capsuto EG. Persistent diarrhea in travelers. *Clin Infect Dis* 1996;22:124–128.
24. Gorbach SL, Edelman R, eds. Travelers' diarrhea: National Institutes of Health Consensus Development Conference. *Rev Infect Dis* 1986;8[Suppl 2]:S109–S233.
25. Ericsson CD, Patterson TF, DuPont HL. Clinical presentation as a guide to therapy for travelers' diarrhea. *Am J Med Sci* 1987; 294:91–96.
26. Gorbach SL, Kean BH, Evans DG, et al. Travelers' diarrhea and toxigenic *Escherichia coli. N Engl J Med* 1975;292:933–936.
27. DuPont HL, Ericsson CD, DuPont MW. Emporiatric enteritis:

lessons learned from U.S. students in Mexico. *Trans Am Clin Climatol Assoc* 1985;97:32–42.
28. Mattila L, Siitonen A, Kyronseppa H, et al. Seasonal variation in etiology of travelers' diarrhea. *J Infect Dis* 1992;165:385–388.
29. Ericsson CD, DuPont HL. Travelers' diarrhea: approaches to prevention and treatment. *Clin Infect Dis* 1993;16:616–626.
30. Echeverria P, Sack RB, Blacklow NR, et al. Prophylactic doxycycline for travelers' diarrhea in Thailand: further supportive evidence of *Aeromonas hydrophila* as an enteric pathogen. *Am J Epidemiol* 1984;120:912–921.
31. Pan American Health Organization. *Epidemiol Bull* 1991;12: 1–24.
32. Sriratanaban A, Reinprayoon S. *Vibrio parahaemolyticus*: a major cause of travelers' diarrhea in Bangkok. *Am J Trop Med Hyg* 1982;31:128–130.
33. Vial PA, Mathewson JJ, DuPont HL, et al. Comparison of two assay methods for patterns of adherence to HEp-2 cells of *Escherichia coli* from patients with diarrhea. *J Clin Microbiol* 1990;28:882–885.
34. Mathewson JJ, Johnson PC, DuPont HL, et al. A newly recognized cause of travelers' diarrhea: enteroadherent *Escherichia coli*. *J Infect Dis* 1985;151:471–475.
35. Adachi JA, Jiang Z-D, Mathewson JJ, et al. Enteroaggregative *Escherichia coli* as a major etiologic agent in traveler's diarrhea in 3 regions of the world. *Clin Infect Dis* 2001;32:1706–1709.
36. Wanger AR, Murray BE, Echeverria P, et al. Enteroinvasive *Escherichia coli* in travelers' diarrhea. *J Infect Dis* 1988;158: 640–642.
37. Bolivar R, Conklin RH, Vollet JJ, et al. Rotavirus in travelers' diarrhea: study of an adult student population in Mexico. *J Infect Dis* 1978;137:324–327.
38. Vollet JJ, Ericsson CD, Gibson G, et al. Human rotavirus in an adult population with travelers' diarrhea and its relationship to location of food consumption. *J Med Virol* 1979;4:81–87.
39. Ryder RW, Oquist CA, Greenberg H. Traveler's diarrhea in Panamanian tourists in Mexico. *J Infect Dis* 1981;144:442–448.
40. Johnson PC, Hoy J, Mathewson JJ, et al. Occurrence of Norwalk virus infections among adults in Mexico. *J Infect Dis* 1990;162:389–393.
41. Wright RA, Spencer H, Brodsky RE, et al. Giardiasis in Colorado: an epidemiologic study. *Am J Epidemiol* 1977;105: 330–336.
42. Jokipii L, Pohjola S, Jokipii AMM. Cryptosporidiosis associated with traveling and giardiasis. *Gastroenterology* 1985;89:838–842.
43. Frachtman RL, Ericsson CD, DuPont HL. Seroconversion to *Entamoeba histolytica* among short-term travelers to Mexico. *Arch Intern Med* 1982;142:1299.
44. Shlim DR, Cohen MT, Eaton M, et al. An algae-like organism associated with an outbreak of prolonged diarrhea among foreigners in Nepal. *Am J Trop Med Hyg* 1991;45:383–389.
45. Ortega YR, Sterling CR, Gilman RH, et al. *Cyclospora* species—a new protozoan pathogen of humans. *N Engl J Med* 1993;328:1308–1312.
46. Taylor DN, Echeverria P. Etiology and epidemiology of travelers' diarrhea in Asia. *Rev Infect Dis* 1986;8[Suppl 2]:S136–S141.
47. Steffen R, Mathewson JJ, Ericsson CD, et al. Travelers' diarrhea in West Africa and in Mexico: fecal transport systems and liquid bismuth subsalicylate for self-therapy. *J Infect Dis* 1988;157:1008–1013.
48. Evans DG, Olarte J, DuPont HL, et al. Enteropathogens associated with pediatric diarrhea in Mexico City. *J Pediatr* 1977; 91:65–68.
49. Mathewson JJ, Oberhelman RA, DuPont HL, et al. Enteroadherent *Escherichia coli* as a cause of diarrhea among children in Mexico. *J Clin Microbiol* 1987;25:1917–1919.
50. Okhuysen PC, DuPont HL, Lopez JFF, et al. A comparative study of furazolidone and placebo in addition to oral rehydration in the treatment of acute infantile diarrhea. *Scand J Gastroenterol* 1989;24[Suppl 169]:39–46.
51. Bandres JC, Mathewson JJ, Ericsson CD, et al. Trimethoprim/sulfamethoxazole remains active against enterotoxigenic *Escherichia coli* and *Shigella* spp in Guadalajara, Mexico. *Am J Med Sci* 1992;303:289–291.
52. Osterholm MT, MacDonald KL, White KE, et al. An outbreak of a newly recognized chronic diarrhea syndrome associated with raw milk consumption. *JAMA* 1986;256:484–490.
53. Parsonnet J, Trock SC, Bopp CA, et al. Chronic diarrhea associated with drinking untreated water. *Ann Intern Med* 1989; 110:985–991.
54. Afzalpurkar RG, Schiller LR, Little KH, et al. The self-limited nature of chronic idiopathic diarrhea. *N Engl J Med* 1992; 327:1849–1852.
55. Mintz ED, Weber JT, Guris D, et al. An outbreak of Brainerd diarrhea among travelers to the Galapagos Islands. *J Infect Dis* 1998;177:1041–1045.
56. Bandres JC, Mathewson JJ, DuPont HL. Heat susceptibility of bacterial enteropathogens. Implications for the prevention of travelers' diarrhea. *Arch Intern Med* 1988;148:2261–2263.
57. Dickens DL, DuPont HL, Johnson PC. Survival of bacterial enteropathogens in the ice of popular drinks. *JAMA* 1985;253: 3141–3143.
58. Kozicki M, Steffen R, Schar J. "Boil it, cook it, peel it or forget it"; does this rule prevent travellers' diarrhoea? *Int J Epidemiol* 1985;14:169–172.
59. Sack DA, Kaminsky DC, Sack RB, et al. Prophylactic doxycycline for travelers' diarrhea: results of a prospective double-blind study of Peace Corps volunteers in Kenya. *N Engl J Med* 1978; 298:758–763.
60. DuPont HL, Galindo E, Evans DG, et al. Prevention of travelers' diarrhea with trimethoprim/sulfamethoxazole and trimethoprim alone. *Gastroenterology* 1983;84:75–80.
61. Sack RB, Santosham M, Froehlich JL, et al. Doxycycline prophylaxis of travelers' diarrhea in Honduras, an area where resistance to doxycycline is common among enterotoxigenic *Escherichia coli*. *Am J Trop Med Hyg* 1984;33:460–466.
62. Johnson PC, Ericsson CD, Morgan DR, et al. Lack of emergence of resistant fecal flora during successful prophylaxis of travelers' diarrhea with norfloxacin. *Antimicrob Agents Chemother* 1986;30:671–674.
63. Wistrom J, Norrby SR, Burman LG, et al. Norfloxacin versus placebo for prophylaxis against travellers' diarrhoea. *J Antimicrob Chemother* 1987;20:563–574.
64. Rademaker CM, Hoepelman IM, Wolfhagen MJ, et al. Results of a double-blind placebo-controlled study using ciprofloxacin for prevention of travelers' diarrhea. *Eur J Clin Microbiol Infect Dis* 1989;8:690–694.
65. Black FT, Gaarslev K, Ørskov F, et al. Mecillinam, a new prophylactic for travellers' diarrhoea: a prospective double-blind study in tourists traveling to Egypt and the Far East. *Scand J Infect Dis* 1983;13:189–193.
66. Oksanen PJ, Salminen S, Saxelin M, et al. Prevention of travellers' diarrhea by *Lactobacillus* GG. *Ann Intern Med* 1990;22: 53–56.
67. Hilton E, Kolakowski P, Singer C, et al. Efficacy of *Lactobacillus* GG as a diarrheal preventative in travelers. *J Travel Med* 1997;1:41–43.
68. DuPont HL, Sullivan P, Evans DG, et al. Prevention of travelers' diarrhea (emporiatric enteritis): prophylactic administration of subsalicylate bismuth. *JAMA* 1980;243:237–241.
69. DuPont HL, Ericsson CD, Johnson PC, et al. Prevention of travelers' diarrhea by the tablet formulation of bismuth subsalicylate. *JAMA* 1987;257:1347–1350.

70. Steffen R, DuPont HL, Heusser R, et al. Prevention of travelers' diarrhea by the tablet form of bismuth subsalicylate. *Antimicrob Agents Chemother* 1986;29:625–627.
71. Steffen R, Heusser R, DuPont HL. Prevention of travelers' diarrhea by non-antibiotic drugs. *Rev Infect Dis* 1986;8[Suppl]: S151–S159.
72. Graham DY, Estes MK, Gentry LO. Double-blind comparison of bismuth subsalicylate and placebo in the prevention and treatment of enterotoxigenic *Escherichia coli. Gastroenterology* 1983;85:1017–1022.
73. Reves RR, Johnson PC, Ericsson CD, et al. A cost-effectiveness comparison of the use of antimicrobial agents for treatment or prophylaxis of travelers' diarrhea. *Arch Intern Med* 1988;148: 2421–2427.
74. Mendelowitz PC, Hoffman RS, Weber S. Bismuth absorption and myoclonic encephalopathy during bismuth subsalicylate therapy. *Ann Intern Med* 1990;112:140–141.
75. Murray BE, Rensimer ER, DuPont HL. Emergence of high-level trimethoprim resistance in fecal *Escherichia coli* during oral administration of trimethoprim or trimethoprim/sulfamethoxazole. *N Engl J Med* 1982;306:130–135.
76. Farthing MJG, DuPont HL, Guandalini S, et al. Treatment and prevention of travellers' diarrhoea. *Gastroenterol Int* 1992;5: 162–175.
77. Ericsson CD, Pickering LK, Sullivan P, et al. The role of location of food consumption in the prevention of travelers' diarrhea in Mexico. *Gastroenterology* 1980;79:812–816.
78. Tacket CO, Losonsky G, Link H, et al. Protection by milk immunoglobulin concentrate against oral challenge with enterotoxigenic *Escherichia coli. N Engl J Med* 1988;318:1240–1243.
79. DuPont HL, Olarte J, Evans DG, et al. Comparative susceptibility of Latin American and United States students to enteric pathogens. *N Engl J Med* 1976;295:1520–1521.
80. Brown MR, DuPont HL, Sullivan PS. Effect of duration of exposure on diarrhea due to enterotoxigenic *Escherichia coli* in travelers from the United States to Mexico. *J Infect Dis* 1982; 145:582.
81. Evans DJ Jr, Ruiz-Palacios G, Evans DG, et al. Humoral immune response to the heat-labile enterotoxin of *Escherichia coli* in naturally acquired diarrhea and antitoxin determination by passive immune hemolysis. *Infect Immun* 1977;16:781–788.
82. Clemens JD, Harris JR, Sack DA, et al. Field trial of oral cholera vaccines in Bangladesh: results of one year of follow-up. *J Infect Dis* 1988;158:60–69.
83. Peltola H, Siitonen A, Kyronseppa H, et al. Prevention of travellers' diarrhoea by oral B-subunit/whole-cell cholera vaccine. *Lancet* 1991;338:1285–1289.
84. DuPont HL, Sullivan P, Pickering LK, et al. Symptomatic treatment of diarrhea with bismuth subsalicylate among students attending a Mexican university. *Gastroenterology* 1977;73: 715–718.
85. Ericsson CD, Evans DG, DuPont HL, et al. Bismuth subsalicylate inhibits activity of crude toxins of *Escherichia coli* and *Vibrio cholerae. J Infect Dis* 1977;136:693–696.
86. Gyles CL, Zigler M. The effect of adsorbent and anti-inflammatory drugs on secretion in ligated segments of pig intestine infected with *Escherichia coli. Can J Comp Med* 1978;42: 260–268.
87. Powell DW, Tapper EJ, Morris SM. Aspirin-stimulated intestinal electrolyte transport in rabbit ileum *in vitro. Gastroenterology* 1979;76:1429–1437.
88. Burke V, Gracey M. Reduction by aspirin of intestinal fluid loss in acute childhood gastroenteritis. *Lancet* 1980;1:1329–1330.
89. Goldenberg MM, Honkomp LJ, Burrous SE, et al. Protective effect of Pepto-Bismol liquid on the gastric mucosa of rats. *Gastroenterology* 1975;69:636–640.
90. Steinhoff MC, Douglas RG Jr, Greenberg HB, et al. Bismuth subsalicylate therapy of viral gastroenteritis. *Gastroenterology* 1980;78:1495–1499.
91. Stoclet JC, Gerard D, Kilhoffer MC, et al. Calmodulin and its role in intracellular calcium regulation. *Progr Neurobiol* 1987; 29:321–364.
92. DuPont HL, Ericsson CD, Mathewson JJ, et al. Zaldaride maleate (Zm), an intestinal calmodulin inhibitor, in the therapy of travelers' diarrhea. *Gastroenterology* 1993;104:709–715.
93. Reves RR, Bass P, DuPont HL, et al. Failure to demonstrate effectiveness of an anticholinergic drug in the symptomatic treatment of acute travelers' diarrhea. *J Clin Gastroenterol* 1983; 5:223–227.
94. Johnson PC, Ericsson CD, DuPont HL, et al. Comparison of loperamide with bismuth subsalicylate for the treatment of acute travelers' diarrhea. *JAMA* 1986;225:757–760.
95. DuPont HL, Sanchez JF, Ericsson CD, et al. Comparative efficacy of loperamide hydrochloride and bismuth subsalicylate in the management of acute diarrhea. *Am J Med* 1990;88[Suppl 6A]:15S–19S.
96. Schiller LR, Santa Ana CA, Morawski SG, et al. Mechanism of the antidiarrheal effect of loperamide. *Gastroenterology* 1984;86: 1475–1480.
97. Merritt JE, Brown BL, Tomlinson S. Loperamide and calmodulin. *Lancet* 1982;1:283.
98. DuPont HL, Hornick RB. Adverse effect of Lomotil therapy in shigellosis. *JAMA* 1973;226:1525–1528.
99. DuPont HL, Ericsson CD, DuPont MW, et al. A randomized, open-label comparison of nonprescription loperamide and attapulgite in the symptomatic treatment of acute diarrhea. *Am J Med* 1990;88[Suppl 6A]:20S–23S.
100. DuPont HL, Reves RR, Galindo E, et al. Treatment of travelers' diarrhea with trimethoprim/sulfamethoxazole and with trimethoprim alone. *N Engl J Med* 1982;307:841–844.
101. Ericsson CD, Johnson PC, DuPont HL, et al. Ciprofloxacin and trimethoprim/sulfamethoxazole as initial therapy for acute travelers' diarrhea. A placebo-controlled randomized trial. *Ann Intern Med* 1987;106:216–220.
102. Ericsson CD, DuPont HL, Mathewson JJ, et al. Treatment of travelers' diarrhea with sulfamethoxazole and trimethoprim and loperamide. *JAMA* 1990;263:257–261.
103. Wistrom J, Jertborn M, Hedstrom SA, et al. Short-term self-treatment of travellers' diarrhoea with norfloxacin: a placebo-controlled study. *J Antimicrob Chemother* 1989;23:905–913.
104. DuPont HL, Ericsson CD, Mathewson JJ, et al. Five versus three days of ofloxacin therapy for traveler's diarrhea: a placebo-controlled study. *Antimicrob Agents Chemother* 1992;36:87–91.
105. Steffen R, Jori R, DuPont HL, et al. Fleroxacin, a long-acting fluoroquinolone, as effective therapy for travelers' diarrhea. *Rev Infect Dis* 1989;11[Suppl 5]:S1154–S1155.
106. Gough A, Barsoum NJ, Mitchell L, et al. Juvenile canine drug-induced arthropathy: clinicopathological studies on articular lesions caused by oxolonic acid and pipemidic acids. *Toxicol Appl Pharmacol* 1979;51:177–187.
107. Kuschner RA, Trofa AF, Thomas RJ, et al. Use of azithromycin for the treatment of *Campylobacter* enteritis in travelers to Thailand, an area where ciprofloxacin resistance is prevalent. *Clin Infect Dis* 1995; 21:536–541.
108. DuPont HL, Ericsson CD, Mathewson JJ, et al. Oral aztreonam, a poorly absorbed yet effective therapy for bacterial diarrhea in US travelers to Mexico. *JAMA* 1992;267:1932–1935.
109. Salam I, Katelaris P, Leigh-Smith S, et al. Randomised trial of single-dose ciprofloxacin for travellers' diarrhoea. *Lancet* 1994; 344:1537–1539.
110. Ericsson CD, DuPont HL, Mathewson JJ. Single-dose ofloxacin plus loperamide compared with single dose or three

days of ofloxacin in the treatment of traveler's diarrhea. *J Travel Med* 1997;4:3–7.

111. Cofsky RD, DeBouchet L, Landesman SH. Recovery of norfloxacin in feces after administration of a single oral dose to human volunteers. *Antimicrob Agents Chemother* 1984;26:110–111.
112. DuPont HL, Ericsson CD, Robinson A, et al. Current problems in antimicrobial therapy for bacterial enteric infection. *Am J Med* 1987;82[Suppl 4A]:324–328.
113. Bennish ML, Abdus Salam M, Khan WA, et al. Treatment of shigellosis: III. Comparison of one- or two-dose ciprofloxacin with standard 5-day therapy A randomized, blinded trial. *Ann Intern Med* 1992;117:727–734.
114. Haltalin KC, Nelson JD, Hinton LV, et al. Comparison of orally absorbable and nonabsorbable antibiotics in shigellosis: a double-blind study with ampicillin and neomycin. *J Pediatr* 1968;72:708–720.
115. Nishida M, Mine Y, Nonoyama S, et al. Therapeutic efficacy of bicyclomycin for shigellosis experimentally induced in Rhesus monkeys. *J Antibiot* 1974;27:976–983.
116. Ericsson CD, DuPont HL, Sullivan P, et al. Bicozamycin, a poorly absorbable antibiotic, effectively treats travelers' diarrhea. *Ann Intern Med* 1983;98:20–25.
117. Ericsson CD, DuPont HL, Galindo E, et al. Efficacy of bicozamycin in preventing travelers' diarrhea. *Gastroenterology* 1985; 88:473–477.
118. DuPont HL, Ericsson CD, Mathewson JJ, et al. Rifaximin: a nonabsorbed antimicrobial in the therapy of travelers' diarrhea. *Digestion* 1998;59:708–714.
119. DuPont HL, Jiang Z-D, Ericsson CD, et al. Rifaximin versus ciprofloxacin for the treatment of traveler's diarrhea: a randomized, double-blind clinical trial. *Clin Infect Dis* 2001;33:1807–1815.
120. Ericsson CD, Johnson PC, DuPont HL, et al. Role of a novel antidiarrheal agent, BW942C, alone or in combination with trimethoprim/sulfamethoxazole in the treatment of traveler's diarrhea. *Antimicrob Agents Chemother* 1986;29:1040–1046.
121. Steffen R, Heusser R, Tschopp A, et al. Efficacy and side effects of six agents in the self-treatment of travellers' diarrhoea. *Travel Med Int* 1988;6:153–157.
122. Ericsson CD, Nicholls-Vasquez I, DuPont HL, et al. Optimal dosing of trimethoprim/sulfamethoxazole when used with loperamide to treat travelers' diarrhea. *Antimicrob Agents Chemother* 1992;36:2821–2824.
123. Taylor DN, Sanchez JL, Chandler W, et al. Treatment of travelers' diarrhea: ciprofloxacin plus loperamide compared with ciprofloxacin alone: a placebo-controlled, randomized trial. *Ann Intern Med* 1991;114:731–734.
124. Petruccelli BP, Murphy GS, Sanchez JL, et al. Treatment of traveler's diarrhea with ciprofloxacin and loperamide. *J Infect Dis* 1992;165:557–560.
125. Ericsson CD, Feldman S, Pickering LK, et al. Influence of subsalicylate bismuth on absorption of doxycycline. *JAMA* 1982; 247:2266–2267.

20

IDIOPATHIC CHRONIC DIARRHEA

JULIE PARSONNET
ERIC D. MINTZ
CHRISTINE A. WANKE

Chronic diarrhea is commonly defined as the passage of three or more loose or watery stools daily for 30 days or longer (14 days for persistent diarrhea in children). Myriad illnesses may present with persistent loose stools as a primary or secondary manifestation of disease. Predominant in the differential diagnosis are noninfectious processes, including inflammatory bowel diseases, endocrinopathies, malignancies, eating disorders, and somatoform illnesses (1). Only a small minority of chronic diarrheal illnesses are directly caused by infections. This is because infectious diarrheas typically are acute and self-limited, and when they do persist, they are diagnosed and treated long before the 30-day period that defines the chronic diarrhea syndrome has elapsed. Despite these caveats, many organisms ranging from viruses to parasites have been reported to cause chronic diarrhea (Table 20.1). With few exceptions (most notably giardiasis), however, these infections either rarely progress to chronicity or are found only in immunocompromised hosts.

This chapter does not focus on the many microorganisms that can occasionally cause sustained illness. These are discussed extensively in the chapters devoted to the specific infectious agents. Although HIV-associated diarrheal illness may well become the most common persistent diarrheal illness syndrome seen in the United States and throughout the world, that syndrome is also covered elsewhere in this text. Instead, this chapter focuses on three chronic diarrhea syndromes that present diagnostic

TABLE 20.1. INFECTIOUS CAUSES OF CHRONIC DIARRHEA IN INDUSTRIALIZED NATIONS[a]

	Pathogens	References
Viruses		
	Rotavirus	85
	Cytomegalovirus	86–88
	Adenovirus	89
	Astrovirus	90
	Picobirnavirus	90
Bacteria		
	Aeromonas hydrophila	91–94
	Campylobacter jejuni	95–99
	Clostridium difficile	100,101
	Dysgonic fermenter 3	102
	Enteropathogenic *E. coli*[b]	103,104
	Enteroadherent *E. coli*[b]	105,106
	Mycobacterium tuberculosis	107
	Atypical *mycobacteria*	108
	Plesiomonas	109
	Salmonella	110
	Tropheryma whippelii	
	Yersinia	111–114
Fungi		
	Candida	115
Protozoa		
	***Blastocystis hominis*[c]**	116,117
	Cryptosporidium	118,119
	Cyclospora	120,121
	Entamoeba histolytica	122,123
	Giardia lamblia	124,125
	Isospora belli	119,126,127
	Microsporidia	128–130
Helminths		
	Strongyloides	124
	Hookworm	124

[a]The organisms in bold represent infections that not uncommonly persist and cause chronic diarrhea in normal hosts. The remaining organisms either rarely result in chronic diarrhea in normal hosts (although they may commonly cause acute disease) or are exclusively pathogens in immunosuppressed patients.
[b]Reported as a cause of chronic diarrhea only in children.
[c]Remains a controversial cause of chronic diarrhea.

J. Parsonnet: Division of Infectious Diseases and Geographic Medicine, Department of Medicine, and Division of Epidemiology, Department of Health Research and Policy, Stanford University School of Medicine, Stanford, California

E. D. Mintz: Diarrheal Diseases Epidemiology Section, Foodborne and Diarrheal Diseases Branch, Division of Bacterial and Mycotic Diseases, National Center for Infectious Diseases, Centers for Disease Control and Prevention, Atlanta, Georgia

C. A. Wanke: Department of Medicine, Tufts University School of Medicine; Department of Infectious Disease, New England Medical Center, Boston, Massachusetts and treatment dilemmas to the gastroenterology and infectious disease specialist: Brainerd diarrhea, chronic sporadic diarrhea of adults, and chronic diarrhea of children in developing countries.

BRAINERD DIARRHEA

In 1983, an outbreak of a debilitating, chronic diarrheal illness occurred in rural Brainerd, Minnesota (2). One hundred twenty-two patients complained of the sudden onset of watery diarrhea with up to 20 bowel movements per day. Extreme fecal urgency with fecal incontinence was common. Illness lasted for longer than 1 year in the majority of cases, but no etiologic agent was identified. Since the Minnesota outbreak, eight other outbreaks of chronic diarrhea affecting 288 persons have been recognized (Table 20.2). The uniform clinical and epidemiologic features of these outbreaks suggest a common underlying disease process. Thus, the syndrome has taken on the name *Brainerd diarrhea.*

Clinical Features

Brainerd diarrhea is an impressive illness that causes marked disability and entails extensive medical costs. In the first weeks of illness, patients describe the sudden onset of frequent watery diarrhea accompanied by gas, borborygmi, and mild abdominal cramps (Table 20.3). Some patients describe up to 40 stools per day, although 10 to 20 stools is more typical. Except for mild weight loss, patients usually have no constitutional symptoms. Incontinence is the most debilitating feature; patients state that although they feel well, they try to be no more than 1 minute away from a bathroom. In the outbreak in Henderson County, Illinois, affected truck drivers described wearing diapers to work and running into fields to defecate so that they could complete their daily routes (J. Parsonnet, *unpublished data*).

As Brainerd diarrhea persists, stools decrease in frequency and volume. Body weight stabilizes. Because stool frequency varies from day to day during the natural course of illness, treatment efficacy has been difficult to assess. No therapy (not antibiotics, steroids, antiinflammatory drugs, fiber, bismuth, or cholestyramine) is consistently effective, although opiate antimotility agents appear to provide temporary relief of symptoms in a subset of patients (2–4; Oklahoma State Health Department and Centers for Disease Control, *unpublished data*). Anecdotally, patients often claim to control their symptoms by adjusting their diet, although no specific dietary changes are uniformly effective. Symptoms of loose stools persist for more than a year in the

TABLE 20.2. EPIDEMIOLOGY OF BRAINERD DIARRHEA OUTBREAKS

Location	Year	No. Cases	Median Age	Percentage Female	Source	Incubation Period	Secondary Transmission	Reference
Baca County, CO	1977	20	54[a]	50	Unknown	Unknown	NR	Centers for Disease Control, *unpublished data*
Brainerd, MN	1983–84	122	41	49	Unpasteurized milk	15 days	Possibly two cases in one household	2
Iva, SC	1984	4	62	75	Unknown	Unknown	NR	Centers for Disease Control, *unpublished data*
San Antonio, TX	1984–85	10	NR	NR	Restaurant	20 to 30 days	NR	6
Henderson County, IL	1987	72	56	50	Untreated water, restaurant	10 days	None	3
Mountain View, OK	1988–89	22	60[b]	64	Probably water	NR	None	Oklahoma State Health Department, *unpublished data*
Cruise ship, Galapagos Islands	1992	58	66[c]	50	Probably water	11 days	None	4
Fannin County, TX	1996	99	63	60	Restaurant[d]			Centers for Disease Control, *unpublished data*
Humboldt County, CA	1998	23	64	49	Restaurant	4–20 days	None	7

NR, not reported.
[a]Estimated from reported data.
[b]Mean age.
[c]Based on 52 subjects.
[d]Contaminated water was considered the most likely vehicle in the restaurant.

TABLE 20.3. CLINICAL FEATURES OF CASES OF BRAINERD DIARRHEA FROM SIX OUTBREAKS AND OF SPORADIC IDIOPATHIC CHRONIC DIARRHEA FROM 17 CASES

Symptom or Clinical Finding	Brainerd Diarrhea[a] Number	Brainerd Diarrhea[a] Percentage (range)	Sporadic Idiopathic Chronic Diarrhea[b] Number	Sporadic Idiopathic Chronic Diarrhea[b] Percentage (range)
Urgency	340/391	87 (75–100)	5/17	29
Fatigue	118/150	79 (71–83)	NA	NA
Weight loss	179/258	68 (55–76)	12/17	71
Incontinence	216/360	60 (51–81)	6/17	35
Cramps	209/381	55 (25–64)	5/17	29
Nausea	54/269	20 (14–28)	NA	NA
Fever or feverishness	14/289	5 (0–12)	2/17	12
Vomiting	13/289	5 (0–18)	1/17	5.9
Mean maximum number of stools per day	11		10	
Median duration of illness	12 to 16.5 months		12 months	

[a]From references 2–4, 6, and 8 and the Oklahoma State Health Department, *unpublished data*.
[b]From Afzalpurkar RG, Schiller LR, Little KH, et al. The self-limited nature of chronic idiopathic diarrhea. *N Engl J Med* 1992;327:1849–1852.

majority of subjects. Eventually, however, symptoms subside. In the two studies with the longest follow-up, all persons interviewed after 3 years were symptom-free (5; Centers for Disease Control, *unpublished data*).

Brainerd diarrhea is costly to the health care system. More than 80% of patients in the described outbreaks sought medical attention, and 20% were hospitalized for extensive diagnostic tests and rehydration. Subjects with Brainerd diarrhea are as likely to be female as male, although women have been more likely to seek medical attention and be hospitalized (3). Brainerd diarrhea has been reported in relatively few children, and when it does occur, the duration of illness may be shorter than in adults (2,3).

Epidemiology

Of the nine outbreaks of Brainerd diarrhea, four have been reported in the medical literature (2–4,6); four outbreaks investigated by state and federal public health departments remain unpublished (7; Centers for Disease Control, *unpublished data*) (Table 20.2). Eight outbreaks occurred in the United States, seven in rural settings. One outbreak occurred on a South American cruise ship.

Extensive epidemiologic investigations were conducted in all outbreaks. In Brainerd, unpasteurized milk was identified as the vehicle for disease transmission. In a case–control study, the odds ratio for cases drinking milk from one particular dairy was 28.3. The investigators also reported the occurrence of similar milk-related outbreaks in other settings, although details of these outbreaks have not been presented. Cases of chronic diarrhea were subsequently sought among drinkers of raw milk in South Carolina. Although a relatively high attack rate was identified among raw milk drinkers (4 of 26 exposed, or 15%), raw milk could not be named a risk factor for disease because no one without the exposure was interviewed (Centers for Disease Control, *unpublished data*).

Water has also been identified as a potential source for Brainerd diarrhea. In Henderson County, Illinois, illness was strongly linked to drinking untreated well water from a local restaurant (3). The well of the restaurant had many construction deficiencies and contained unacceptable levels of fecal coliforms, a marker for contamination with human or animal waste. Similarly, water was identified as a possible vehicle in one Texas outbreak, although in this instance, the implicated restaurant used community water, not its own well. Because no other water users in the community reported disease, contamination was presumed to have occurred in the plumbing of the restaurant (8). In Oklahoma, the outbreak was tentatively linked to a community water source (Oklahoma State Health Department, *unpublished data*). In this case, the water was not found to be contaminated with coliforms despite many deficiencies in the system. Water was also identified as the likely vehicle for disease on a Galapagos Islands cruise ship (4). Again, marked deficiencies in the water system were found, including intermittent lapses in chlorination, but the water was not contaminated at the time of inspection. In this outbreak, and in the waterborne outbreaks in Henderson County and Texas, illness was not associated with beverages prepared with water that had been boiled. This finding is consistent with an infectious etiology.

As with transmissible diseases in general, exposure does not invariably cause illness. Only 8% of raw milk drinkers in Brainerd became ill (2). Although all residents of Mountain View, Oklahoma, were exposed to community water, only 1.6% became ill (5). In Henderson County, Illinois, three men who drank more than 30 glasses of restaurant water during the outbreak period were among 15 (65%) of 23 exposed persons in whom diarrhea did not develop (4). Common to each of these outbreaks, however, was a dose–response relationship between exposure and disease: the greater the exposure, the higher the risk. In all outbreaks, the attack rate was also consistently higher among the elderly than among the young. In persons age 65 years and older, the likelihood of acquiring disease was twofold to threefold higher than in persons younger than 65 years (2,3; Oklahoma State Health Department and Centers for Disease Control, *unpublished data*).

One possible case of household transmission was described in the original Brainerd outbreak. Although person-to-person spread would corroborate an infectious etiology, no secondary cases were confirmed in any of the other outbreaks.

Laboratory Investigations

Extensive clinical and laboratory studies have been conducted in selected patients. Hematologic parameters and blood chemistries typically have been normal, although hypokalemia was reported with severe volume loss (3; Oklahoma State Health Department and Centers for Disease Control, *unpublished data*). The diarrhea causes moderate increases in stool volume (300 to 800 g/d). As with other secretory diarrheas, stool volume does not decrease with fasting (9,10). Serum levels of hormones that cause secretory diarrhea (i.e., gastrin, thyroxin, vasoactive intestinal polypeptide, pancreatic polypeptide, calcitonin) have been within the normal range (10). No evidence of malabsorption has been found. In a handful of subjects, however, small-bowel motility was abnormal, with unusual, prolonged, rapidly propagated, high-pressure waves noted in the jejunum (9).

Stool examinations have been unhelpful in identifying a cause for Brainerd diarrhea. A small number of fecal leukocytes may be observed in fewer than 20% of cases (2–4). Stool cultures, tests for bacterial toxins, and examinations for ova and parasites (including Microsporidia) have revealed no consistent pathogen. In the outbreak in Baca County, Colorado, *Klebsiella pneumoniae* was isolated from stool in 6 of 18 cases and in none of the controls (Centers for Disease Control, *unpublished data*). This finding has not been reproduced in other outbreaks. Other pathogens, such as *Blastocystis hominis, Giardia lamblia, Campylobacter,* and *Salmonella,* have each been isolated from one or two cases, although eradication of these organisms did not relieve symptoms (2–4). Cultures of implicated milk and water have yielded no likely pathogens. No viral agents have been identified by electron microscopy of stool or implicated water.

The only feature that may distinguish Brainerd diarrhea from other forms of chronic diarrhea has been found on colonoscopy (see Color Figure 20.1). Grossly, the bowel in Brainerd diarrhea looks either normal (>50% of cases) or mildly inflamed with nonspecific, patchy erythema, hyperemia, or punctate hemorrhages (2,10,11). Histopathologically, Janda et al. (10) identified an unusual inflammatory process that they termed *multifocal colitis.* In four of five subjects, biopsy specimens showed patchy areas of inflammation in the lamina propria just beneath the surface epithelium. This inflammatory process included a predominance of lymphocytes but also a large number of neutrophils and eosinophils, the latter extending into a flattened surface epithelium; crypt abscesses were occasionally observed. Subsequently, Bryant and colleagues (11) reviewed all previously collected biopsies from outbreaks and all upper and lower gastrointestinal endoscopy reports and specimens from 22 subjects in the Galapagos Island outbreak. In colonic biopsy specimens from 20 Galapagos outbreak patients, they reported increased numbers of surface epithelial lymphocytes without concomitant increases in crypt lymphocytes. These findings were confirmed on review of the biopsies from Henderson County and Brainerd. The investigators termed this finding *colonic epithelial lymphocytosis* and thought it might overlap with a sporadically occurring entity—lymphocytic colitis (described more fully below) (12).

The cause of Brainerd diarrhea remains a matter of speculation. Minimal data (the one case of person-to-person transmission, and the apparent protective effect of boiling implicated water) support an infectious etiology. On the other hand, the fact that antibiotics have had no effect on disease course does not favor a bacterial etiology. Attempts have been made in the laboratory to develop an animal model for the disease. Although Myers et al. (13) reported transmitting severe diarrheal illness to rabbits after inoculating them with stools from three Brainerd outbreak cases, stools from two additional Brainerd cases did not cause disease. Furthermore, stools from other outbreaks did not yield similar results. Thus, few conclusions can yet be made from this work.

After all the extensive investigations that have been conducted on Brainerd diarrhea, it is humbling to recognize that a cause of this serious, debilitating disease has escaped detection despite noble efforts. One reason the agent for Brainerd may be so elusive is that it may exist only transiently in the gut. In the first stages of illness, the causative agent could permanently damage the gastrointestinal tract and then be eliminated before extensive workup has begun. Several types of insults might fit this scenario. For example, if stem cells or nonregenerative cells such as endocrine or neural cells were damaged, even a short-term insult could result in long-term disability. Such damage could be instigated by an infection or a toxin. Similarly, an infection-induced autoimmune response could be a "hit-and-run" cause of disease. The hope for solving the problem of this disease rests in the expeditious investigation of outbreaks of chronic diarrhea in which new, ongoing cases can be identified in the early stages of illness.

CHRONIC IDIOPATHIC SECRETORY DIARRHEA OF ADULTS

Even in the absence of an outbreak, chronic diarrhea is a relatively common complaint among the patients of general practitioners and gastroenterologists. It has been estimated that between 3% and 5% of the U.S. population suffers from chronic diarrhea at any given time (14). The syndrome is frequently debilitating, restricting lifestyle and causing lost productivity at work. Before arriving at the specialist's office, patients with chronic diarrhea have often seen many doctors, undergone numerous diagnostic tests, and tried multiple home remedies and physician-prescribed therapies without success. In the majority of these patients, however, a cause for chronic diarrhea can eventually be identified. Usually, the cause is not infectious (1). Among 27 intensively studied patients with chronic diarrhea reported in 1980, 9 were found to have used laxatives or diuretics surreptitiously, 8 had irritable bowel syndrome, 2 inflammatory bowel disease, 2 anal sphincter dysfunction, and 1 beef allergy. Only one subject had diarrhea with an infectious etiology: bacterial overgrowth of the small bowel. However, the illness of four subjects (three with documented secretory diarrhea) remained undiagnosed. These undiagnosed cases are now classified by syndrome as chronic idiopathic secretory diarrhea (CISD).

Clinical Disease and Investigation

Although data are extremely limited, the clinical features of CISD appear to be similar to those of Brainerd diarrhea (5) (Table 20.3). In the only systematic study performed thus far, 17 patients with CISD described the sudden onset of watery diarrhea, accompanied rarely by nausea, vomiting, or feverishness (15). Bowel movements remained abnormal for months; patients not infrequently complained of nocturnal or early morning bowel movements, fecal incontinence, and abdominal cramps. Seventy-one percent of patients lost weight, with a median weight loss of 5 lb.

As with Brainerd diarrhea, many therapies were tried in an attempt to relieve the symptoms of CISD. Fifteen (88%) of the 17 patients described by Afzalpukar and colleagues (15) had been unsuccessfully treated with metronidazole before referral to the tertiary care center. Other antibiotics also provided no relief. Of the subjects who received opiate antimotility agents, however, approximately 40% experienced some symptomatic relief. The efficacy of loperamide in relieving CISD has similarly been observed in other studies (14,16). Other agents that were unsuccessfully tried in a few subjects included steroids, sulfasalazine, and cholestyramine. Despite the limited success of the treatments, the chronic diarrheal illness eventually resolved in all patients; the mean duration of diarrhea was 15 months (range, 7 to 31 months). In subsequent follow-up, patients had regained lost weight and described themselves as healthy.

The physical examination findings and results of routine blood tests in the patients described by Afzalpurkar et al. (15) were normal except for occasional hypokalemia. Stool cultures and tests for ova and parasites revealed no pathogens. No white cells were seen on Wright stain of the stools. The diarrhea was secretory in nature, with fecal fat increased in only one subject. Four subjects had excessive bacterial colonization of the jejunum, but appropriate treatment with antibiotics did not relieve symptoms. In physiologic studies of eight patients with CISD, evidence of bile acid malabsorption was found that did not correct with cholestyramine therapy (17). This suggested an ileal defect and was interpreted to indicate either an intestinal motility disorder or an underlying absorptive abnormality. The normal Shilling test results in these subjects, however, made the latter alternative somewhat less likely.

In CISD, the gross appearance on upper and lower gastrointestinal endoscopy and biopsy is typically normal. Microscopically, however, the findings in some sporadic cases are consistent with lymphocytic colitis, which suggests an overlap between this pathologic diagnosis and the clinical syndromes of Brainerd diarrhea and CISD (1,18). Moreover, natural history studies of lymphocytic colitis and colonic epithelial lymphocytosis suggest heterogeneous etiologies, some of which are consistent with CISD and Brainerd diarrhea (19–21).

Epidemiology

The epidemiology of CISD is largely undefined. To document disease prevalence, Mintz et al. (22) surveyed 8,000 members of the two largest professional gastroenterology societies in the United States. Members were asked to report the cases of idiopathic chronic diarrhea with an acute onset (symptoms for >2 months in a person older than 2 years) that had been seen in April 1991. HIV patients were excluded from the case definition. Although only 9% of gastroenterologists responded to the survey, a sampling of nonrespondents suggested that this group represented the overall population of specialists.

One hundred and sixty-five (28%) of the 589 respondents reported seeing 438 cases of chronic diarrhea in the preceding month. The median age of subjects was 47 years (range, 9 to 88 years), and 58% were female. Despite the rural location of many outbreaks of Brainerd diarrhea, rural residence did not appear to increase the risk for sporadic Brainerd-like diarrhea. Because many cases had not undergone extensive clinical evaluation (only one-third had undergone colonoscopy), it is possible that a substantial proportion of the reported cases did not represent true "idiopathic" disease. The epidemiologic findings, however, did corroborate the observations of Afzalpurkar et al. (15). The median age of their 17 CISD subjects was 54 years, and 41% of the subjects were female; only one patient was from a rural location. Overall, Mintz et al. (22) estimated that 5,000 to 8,000 patients with Brainerd-like chronic diarrhea visit U.S. gastroenterologists on a monthly basis.

It is thought that CISD is most common in travelers. In the study of Afzalpurkar et al. (15), 59% of 17 patients had a history of recent travel before disease onset. The travel was usually local rather than international. Unfortunately, no information is available on the frequency of travel in a comparison control population, and it is possible that the rate of local travel is equal in both ill and well populations. Among travelers, chronic symptoms develop in 2% to 11% of those with acute diarrhea (23,24); in most persons in this group, no cause is diagnosed despite extensive workup. In another study, a very high incidence of chronic diarrhea was found in Peace Corps volunteers who had served in the late 1980s (25). According to Peace Corps medical officers, 9 of 1,000 volunteers experienced CISD. CISD appeared to be particularly likely in persons stationed in Haiti (one-third of volunteers). Other high-risk areas included Nepal (31 of 1,000 volunteers) and Tunisia (28 of 1,000 volunteers). Illness among the Peace Corps volunteers was not thought to be related to residing in a rural area or drinking untreated water. However, the medical officers reported that drinking unpasteurized milk was a more common practice in countries where the risk for CISD was high. Among U.S. Gulf War veterans, 16% reported chronic idiopathic diarrhea lasting longer than 6 months; in comparison, the rate was 3% in military personnel who had not been deployed (26). Extensive workup for this diarrhea has not yielded an etiologic agent.

Some of the cases of CISD previously reported in the literature may represent infection with now-recognized pathogens (i.e., *Cryptosporidium*, Microsporidia, *Isospora, Cyclospora*). Rarely, cases among travelers may be tropical sprue, an illness of unknown etiology characterized by malabsorption and aerobic bacterial overgrowth of the small bowel (23). Some speculate that the increased incidence of chronic diarrhea among travelers indicates replacement of the host's normal flora with alien "normal" flora. This hypothesis remains unproven.

Comparison with Brainerd Diarrhea

It is not known whether outbreak-related Brainerd diarrhea and CISD represent one or many diseases. During investigations of outbreaks of Brainerd diarrhea, cases of chronic diarrhea were identified that appeared to be unrelated to the outbreak (i.e., the onset was not during the outbreak period). These cases were clinically indistinguishable from Brainerd diarrhea (J. Parsonnet, *unpublished data*). After extensive questioning of cases, it appeared possible that the sporadic cases were part of very small, unrecognized clusters of disease (Oklahoma State Health Department, *unpublished data*). Certainly the similarities between Brainerd and CISD are striking. Both begin with the sudden onset of watery diarrhea and cause few constitutional symptoms except for mild weight loss. Although outbreak-related cases describe more severe urgency and incontinence, this may be a consequence of the timing of the interview; outbreak cases tend to be evaluated earlier in the course of illness, when symptoms are most severe. Laboratory findings are minimal in both outbreak-related and sporadic disease. The finding of multifocal colitis, although unreported in sporadic chronic diarrhea, also requires substantiation in outbreak-related disease. Until the causative agent(s) are identified, however, the relationship between sporadic and outbreak-related diseases will remain uncertain (27).

PERSISTENT DIARRHEA IN CHILDREN IN DEVELOPING COUNTRIES

Diarrheal disease and malnutrition are widely accepted as two of the leading causes of morbidity and mortality in children in the developing world (28). It has become increasingly clear in the last decade that prolonged diarrheal illnesses and dysenteric diarrheal illnesses play a more prominent role in diarrheal morbidity and mortality than was previously suspected (29). For children in the developing world, prolonged or persistent diarrhea is defined as any diarrheal illness that lasts longer than 14 days. In children with chronic, recurrent diarrheal illnesses, a 3-day interval free of diarrhea is generally required before it can be said that they have new rather than persistent diarrheal illness. Prolonged diarrhea is likely to become an increasingly important issue as the epidemic of AIDS advances rapidly in children as well as in adults in the developing world (30,31).

Significant progress has been made in the last 10 years in understanding the epidemiology, natural history, etiologic agents, pathogenesis, and therapy of persistent diarrhea. As with acute diarrheal illness, it is difficult to generalize about persistent diarrhea. By definition, the term *persistent diarrhea* comprises a spectrum of illnesses ranging from simple diarrheal illnesses that last 15 days to wasting diarrheal illnesses that persist for months; persistent diarrhea may be a watery or mucoid diarrheal illness or it may be a dysenteric illness. In this population of children, an intestinal injury inflicted by an infectious agent cannot be differentiated from an intestinal injury caused by malnutrition, food allergy, or the complications of systemic disease. The cumulative effect of all these injuries is likely to be important in attempts to define the true etiology of persistent diarrheas (32). The physiologic parameters are also likely complicated further by the socioeconomic and cultural environments in which children live. The complex interactions of intestinal physiology and social science have been difficult to study and have hindered the understanding of persistent diarrhea.

Epidemiology

Data from mostly retrospective studies suggest that between 3% and 27% of all cases of childhood diarrhea are prolonged beyond 14 days in Indonesia, Bangladesh, and Guatemala (33–35). In a recent prospective study, 7.5% of all diarrheal illnesses were prolonged in children under the age of 5 years in rural Bangladesh, although the overall diarrheal incidence was particularly low in this population (36). In a 2-year prospective study performed in an urban slum in northeastern Brazil (37), 11% of all diarrheal episodes in children under the age of 5 years were prolonged beyond 14 days; the overall incidence of diarrhea was high in this population. Of all the diarrheal episodes in this community, 5% lasted longer than 21 days, and 50% of the days on which children had diarrheal disease were during episodes of persistent diarrhea. Eleven percent of all diarrheal illnesses were prolonged in a prospective study in Guatemala, and 23% were prolonged in a study in a rural community in Bangladesh (38,39). In Brazil, the peak incidence of persistent diarrhea was between the ages of 12 and 18 months (37). In the other studies, persistent diarrhea was seen most frequently in children under the age of 6 months in Guatemala and the rural wetlands of Bangladesh, and between 6 and 12 months in the rural community in Bangladesh (36,38,39).

The disease burden in these populations is not evenly spread among all children, however. In rural Bangladesh, 16% of the children followed prospectively had eight or more episodes of diarrhea per year, and 11% of the children had diarrhea for more than 21% of the study days (36). In the Brazilian slum, children with one episode of persistent diarrhea had diarrhea for an average of 135 days per year, whereas the children who did not have an episode of persistent diarrhea had diarrhea for an average of 15 days per year (37).

Diarrheal disease mortality is also not evenly spread among these populations. In northern India, 12% of diarrheal deaths were associated with nondysenteric persistent diarrhea (40). In Bangladesh, 49% of diarrheal deaths were associated with persistent wasting diarrhea, and 62% of all diarrheal deaths were associated with persistent diarrhea in southern Brazil (41,42).

Natural History and Clinical Course

The spectrum of persistent diarrheal illness in children of developing countries is so broad that it is difficult to develop an understanding of the natural history of the syndrome or predict outcome. Few studies examine the total duration of diarrheal illnesses in these cases, and diarrheal illnesses are classified as either acute or persistent. However, a few natural history data can be extracted from some of the studies. In the urban slums in northeastern Brazil, the average duration of the persistent diarrheal episodes was 26 to 27 days, and diarrhea remitted spontaneously in all these children without hospitalization and without any deaths (37). In 20% of the children, an infectious pathogen was identified on day 14 of their illness. In rural Bangladesh, when 7.5% of all diarrheal illnesses were persistent, 5% of all diarrheal illnesses also lasted longer than 22 days; disease was more severe in these children as measured by dehydration, decreased activity, vomiting, and the need to seek care at a health facility (36). The children with persistent diarrhea were also more likely to present with bloody or mucoid stool than with watery diarrhea. In many studies, malnutrition and skin test anergy serve as markers to identify children with prolonged diarrheal illness, but from the available literature, it is difficult to predict which children will go on to have prolonged diarrhea for 60% to 62% of days each year (Fig. 20.2).

Etiology

Bacteria

Small-bowel overgrowth with aerobic and anaerobic bacteria has been postulated to be a cause or contributory factor in persistent diarrheal disease in children in the developing world for the last two decades (43–47). The studies that

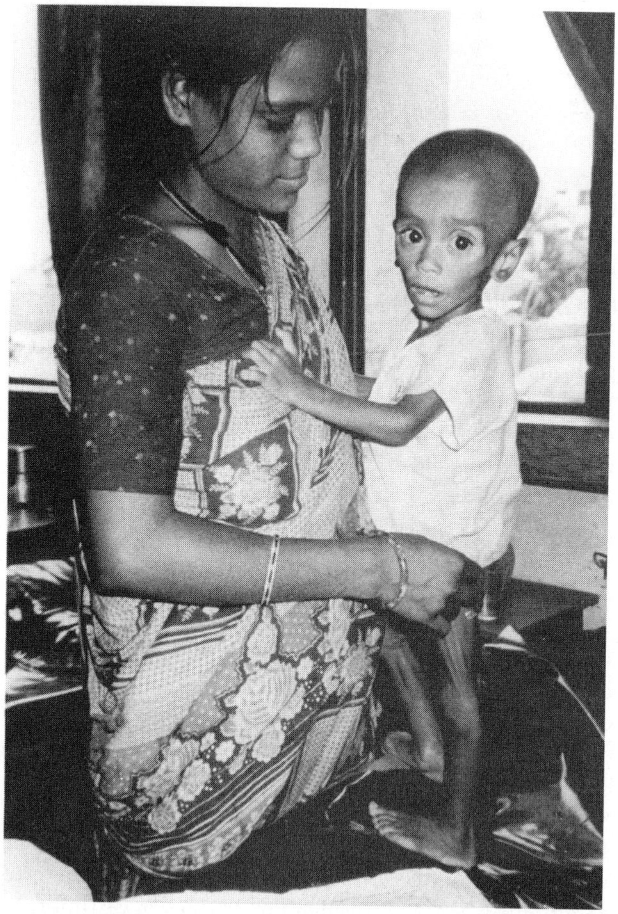

FIGURE 20.2. An 18-month-old child hospitalized in Dhaka, Bangladesh, for evaluation of chronic diarrhea. At admission at 18 months of age, this child weighed 6.2 kg and had had diarrheal illness for longer than 10 months. No etiologic agent was identified, although the child did have small-bowel overgrowth with gram-negative rods. (Courtesy of C. A. Wanke.)

have attempted to examine this question have been problematic and difficult to compare because of either small numbers, lack of appropriate controls, or differences in intubation technique and microbiologic evaluation. Most recently, reviews and results of carefully performed studies in Peru and India have suggested that nutritional status, age, and socioeconomic environment are more important in determining the number of bacteria within the small bowel than is the clinical presence of acute or persistent diarrhea (48,49). Although an animal model provides supporting data that small-bowel overgrowth with nonvirulent *Escherichia coli* organisms can produce watery and persistent diarrheal illness, it has not been possible to confirm the association of overgrowth with persistent diarrhea in the absence of a recognized pathogen in studies in children in the developing world (50,51). Additionally, data that examine chronic diarrheal disease in HIV-positive patients have not shown an association between small-bowel overgrowth and persistent diarrhea in this population (52; C. A. Wanke, *unpublished data*). However, new molecular techniques that more accurately identify and quantify all bacteria present in the small bowel may assist in clarifying these issues.

E. coli organisms are one of the most common causes of acute diarrheal disease in children in the developing world. Although *E. coli* organisms are more classically associated with acute, watery diarrheal disease, some of them have been associated with persistent diarrheal illness. Although the average duration of illness with enterotoxigenic *E. coli* (ETEC) is 4 to 5 days, 7% to 8% of diarrheal illnesses in rural Bangladesh associated with ETEC lasted longer than 20 days (35). In a northeastern Brazilian slum, ETEC was detected 20% of children with persistent diarrhea when cultures were performed after the fourteenth day of their illness (37). In Lima, Peru, ETEC was isolated in 42% of children with persistent diarrhea during the first week of their illness; ETEC was isolated in 34% of children in a different group with persistent diarrhea in Lima during the second and third weeks of illness (53). ETEC was present in culture in 14% of children during the fourth week of illness. Whether children remain infected with organisms such as ETEC throughout the entire duration of a persistent diarrheal illness is more difficult to say; the study from Lima suggests that only 30% of the children with ETEC were infected throughout the first and second week of the diarrheal illness with the same ETEC and could not document the persistence of any ETEC in the same child for longer than 2 weeks.

In the developed world, enteropathogenic *E. coli* (EPEC) organisms have routinely been associated with chronic diarrhea of childhood, but in the developing world they are not common pathogens, causing only 2% to 5% of childhood diarrheal illnesses. The burden of persistent diarrheal disease caused by EPEC may therefore be smaller than that caused by ETEC. EPEC organisms were associated with 8% of persistent diarrheal illnesses in Brazil and 4% in Lima, Peru, and rural Bangladesh. In these studies, the rates of occurrence of EPEC in persistent diarrhea were not significantly different from those seen in acute diarrheal disease. However, these studies did not examine the small bowel of the children with persistent diarrhea. It is possible that because of the tight attachment of EPEC organisms to the effaced small-bowel mucosa, small-bowel aspirates would have been more sensitive than stool cultures in identifying them (54). In a study from Brazil that did examine the small-bowel fluid of children with persistent diarrhea, EPEC organisms were identified in only 2 of 12 children studied, and then in small concentrations (55). In studies from India, EPEC was more frequently cultured from the stool than from the small-bowel fluid of children with persistent diarrhea (49)

Enteroaggregative *E. coli* (EAEC) organisms were recently identified as potential pathogens associated with diarrheal illness, in particular persistent diarrheal illness (56). To date, these organisms have been identified more often in children with persistent diarrhea than in those with acute diarrhea or those without diarrhea in Mexico, Brazil, India, and a rural community in Bangladesh (39,57–60). EAEC bacteria have also been associated with persistent diarrhea in adult patients with advanced HIV disease (61). In the studies among children, EAEC bacteria were associated with 19% to 53% of all episodes of persistent diarrhea and with 8% to 24% of episodes of acute diarrhea; they were identified in 5% to 19% of stools from matched control children without diarrhea. Conversely, the organisms were not associated with persistent diarrhea in other studies performed in Matlab, Bangladesh, in Peru, and in aboriginal children in Australia (53,62,63). Little is known about the clinical illness caused by EAEC organisms, but they were associated with bloody stool and the presence of inflammatory markers in stool in studies carried out in Mexico and Brazil (64). Laboratory studies have also suggested that some percentage of EAEC bacteria may be invasive, a feature that would correlate with the clinical finding of inflammatory markers and blood (57,65). An additional study has suggested that colonization with EAEC bacteria in children who do not have diarrhea may still be associated with malnutrition (64). Studies to date have suggested that EAEC organisms are a heterogeneous group with the same adherence phenotype, and that strains from various geographic locales may harbor different virulence traits.

Another group of *E. coli* bacteria, which adhere diffusely to cells in tissue culture rather than in the localized pattern of the EPEC or the stacked-brick pattern of the EAEC bacteria, has been less consistently associated with diarrheal disease. These diffusely adherent organisms were associated more frequently with persistent diarrhea in one study in Bangladesh and in older aboriginal children in Australia (62,63). The significance of these associations is not known.

The agents of dysenteric diarrheal illnesses have been associated with severe and complicated diarrheal illnesses, but these have not been consistently documented to be prolonged illnesses. The incidence of shigellosis varies widely by geographic area, so that studies of the pathogen have been complicated in many parts of the developing world. The incidence of shigellosis is particularly high in Bangladesh, but in community studies of persistent diarrhea, *Shigella* organisms were isolated in 5% to 9% of cases of persistent diarrhea (39,62), rates that were not higher than those seen with acute diarrheal illness. Many diarrheal disease treatment regimens for children in the developing world suggest empiric antibiotics at presentation for bloody diarrheal disease, which may explain the low incidence of *Shigella* infection in some studies of persistent diarrhea. Because illnesses caused by *Shigella* organisms may be more severe, studies of persistent diarrhea in patients requiring hospitalization might be of assistance in determining the role of *Shigella* in persistent diarrhea.

Other bacterial agents associated with dysentery include nontyphoidal salmonellae, which were isolated more often from children with persistent diarrhea than from control children without diarrhea in a study performed in northern India (59). *Campylobacter* organisms have also been associated with persistent and relapsing diarrheal disease in both the developed and developing world. Although these illnesses may be protracted in immunocompromised patients in the developed world, few data are available to establish a connection between severe malnutrition or cutaneous anergy and prolonged *Campylobacter* diarrhea in children in the developing world (66). Additionally, data regarding *Campylobacter* as a cause of persistent diarrhea are complicated by an extremely high asymptomatic carriage rate in children in parts of the developing world, with as many as 16% of children in South Africa, 25% of children in southern India, and 39% of 1-year-old children in Bangladesh found to harbor *Campylobacter* while free of diarrhea (67–69). In a study of persistent diarrhea carried out in a rural community in Bangladesh, *Campylobacter* organisms were isolated in 8% of children with persistent diarrhea when they were cultured on day 14 of the persistent illness, but in only 1% to 2% of children when they were cultured at the onset of illness. *Campylobacter* organisms were isolated at the same frequency of 8% in stools from nondiarrheal control children (39). In a recent study from Lima, Peru, *Campylobacter* organisms were isolated consistently from the stools of children with persistent diarrhea during a 3-week period; however, the numbers of children with *Campylobacter* in this group were very small.

Viral Agents

Rotavirus is the only viral agent that has been included in routine studies of etiologic agents in diarrheal illness in children in the developing world. Although rotavirus has been documented as a cause of persistent diarrheal disease, its true role in causation of disease is as complicated as that of *Campylobacter,* discussed above. Rotavirus has not been consistently identified more frequently in the stools of children with prolonged diarrhea than in the stools of children with acute diarrhea, although it can cause diarrhea that may persist for longer than 14 days. In diarrhea in the rural community in Bangladesh, rotavirus was identified more frequently on day 14 of the persistent illnesses than it was at the onset of the diarrheal illnesses. However, it was no more common in persistent than in acute cases. In an earlier study from Bangladesh, 3% of all rotavirus illnesses were prolonged beyond 20 days (35).

Parasitic Agents

Giardia lamblia is one of the most commonly recognized intestinal protozoa and may routinely and asymptomatically colonize the intestines of up to 20% of children under the age of 5 years (70). As with Campylobacter and rotavirus, discussed above, it becomes extremely difficult to discern the true contribution of such highly endemic potential pathogens. A child from Costa Rica in whom diarrhea developed at the age of 14 months and persisted for the following 2 years was consistently found to carry and excrete *Giardia* organisms during that period; *Giardia* organisms were found in 18 of the 22 stools examined during the 2-year period (71). Two pieces of intriguing data that may be pertinent to understanding the role of *Giardia* in prolonged diarrheal illnesses were recently reported. Various clones of *Giardia* have been identified, each of which has a distinctive phenotype. The clones vary in regard to response to serum cytotoxicity, ability to initiate infection in the intestine of an animal model, clinical severity of infection, and time required for infection to be cleared from the intestine (72). Additionally, it has been reported that a *Giardia*-specific immunoglobulin A antibody to a 57-kd heat shock antigen did not develop in children in Gambia with persistent diarrhea and giardiasis, whereas those children who cleared *Giardia* from their intestine showed a clear response to the same heat shock antigen (73).

Chronic, nondysenteric amebiasis was originally described in West Pakistan as a syndrome of intermittent diarrhea with mucus, flatus, weight loss, food intolerance, and abdominal pain for months to years (74). In a retrospective study of amebiasis in Bangladesh, cases of amebic dysentery had a longer duration of symptoms and more severe malnutrition than cases of nonamebic diarrheal illnesses seen at the same hospital; this syndrome occurred in persons of all ages, including children, but was not seen in infants under the age of 1 year (75).

As techniques for identifying *Cryptosporidium* in stool have improved, the ability to recognize the association of *Cryptosporidium* with persistent diarrheal disease in children in the developing world has also increased. Although *Cryptosporidium* had been recognized as a diarrheal pathogen since the turn of the century, it came to attention as a cause of severe watery diarrheal disease in HIV-positive patients early in the 1980s. Only recently has it been included in studies of etiologic agents of persistent diarrhea in the developing world. It was recognized as a sole pathogen in 13% of stools from children with persistent diarrhea in an urban slum in northeastern Brazil (55), and in 6% of stools from children with persistent diarrhea in rural Bangladesh (62). In this later study, *Cryptosporidium* was the only recognized pathogen associated specifically with persistent diarrhea but not acute diarrhea; it was also present significantly less frequently in the stools of children with acute diarrhea in the Brazilian study. Early infection with *Cryptosporidium* has been found to be a strong predictor of the subsequent persistence of diarrhea in children in Brazil (76,77).

APPROACH TO THE PATIENT WITH CHRONIC DIARRHEA

The differential diagnosis for chronic diarrhea in the immunocompetent host is substantial, and the workup can be extensive. Two excellent reviews outline algorithms for evaluating this syndrome in the United States (78,79). Essential components of both algorithms are a careful history and physical examination. Clinicians should obtain a detailed history of the diarrhea, including the appearance, consistency, and frequency of the stools and any associated weight loss or abdominal symptoms. With this information, the clinician can categorize the stools as bloody, fatty, or watery (80); this simple categorization narrows the differential diagnosis substantially. It is also useful to investigate the epidemiologic context of the illness. Inquiries should be made about other affected people in the patient's family, work environment, and community. A history of other medical problems, medications, allergies, recent travel, exposure to animals (including pets), use of well water, exposure to raw milk, and risk factors for HIV infection should also be elicited.

After a complete history and physical have been obtained, most algorithms for the workup of chronic diarrhea recommend a microbiologic evaluation of three stools (including enzyme-linked immunosorbent assay for *Giardia* and concentration of stools for *Cyclospora*) and blood tests (complete blood cell count and chemistry screen). Often, these have already been performed before the physician is consulted for chronic diarrhea (i.e., during the acute illness); if that is the case, the tests need not be repeated again unless metabolic derangement (e.g., hypokalemia) is suspected. Empiric therapy with antibacterial or antiparasitic agents or both can then be tried. If the patient shows no response to these trials, a 24-hour stool analysis for weight, electrolytes and osmotic gap, pH, stool fat, red cells, and white cells should be conducted (78,79). Because the assessment of white cells can be inaccurate if the technician is inexperienced or the stool sample is not tested within 24 to 48 hours, a latex agglutination test for lactoferrin may be preferable (81). With this series of tests, diarrhea can be definitively classified as inflammatory, secretory, osmotic, or malabsorptive. More specific evaluations—including endoscopic studies, tests for malabsorption, and assays for gastrointestinal peptide hormones—can then be based on these classifications. Once a diagnosis has been established, treatment should be directed at the specific cause of the diarrheal disease. If the results of the studies outlined above are all negative and diarrhea persists, a diagnosis of CISD can be made.

However, the algorithms described above are not necessarily appropriate for the majority of cases of chronic diarrhea worldwide. Health care workers treating children in developing countries do not have access to many of the suggested assays. In treating these children, the only recourse is a good history and physical examination followed by empiric therapy with antibacterial or antiparasitic agents. Even in the United States and other industrialized countries, if the results of routine stool and blood tests are negative, the approach to chronic diarrhea may best be empiric or symptomatic. For many patients with CISD—particularly travelers and patients who are part of an outbreak—it has been our experience that an extensive workup is rarely helpful. In no instance of Brainerd diarrhea has a complete gastrointestinal evaluation altered case management. In cases of chronic diarrhea in travelers, if the results of stool examinations are negative and malabsorption is not evident, it is also unusual to find a cause by endoscopic methods (23,82). Even patients who are not travelers seldom benefit from a colonoscopic evaluation. In one study of 809 patients with unexplained nonbloody chronic diarrhea, only 122 (15%) had histopathologic abnormalities in the colon (83), and 80 of these, a large majority, were categorized as microscopic colitis, an entity usually treated symptomatically with over-the-counter agents such as bismuth subsalicylate or opiate antidiarrheal preparations (80,84). Of the remaining 42 patients, 29 (3.5% of the total group) had lesions requiring specific treatment (Crohn's disease in 23, ulcerative colitis in 5, and tuberculosis in 1). Whether the $1.3 million spent to make these few diagnoses was cost-effective has yet to be thoroughly assessed (83).

If no definitive cause of chronic diarrhea can be identified, the typical scenario for CISD and Brainerd diarrhea, treatment options are limited. The patient's diet can be investigated and potentially problematic items (i.e., caffeine, gluten, milk products) restricted. Self-adjustment of diet often provides the patient with a sense of control over this disease. Opiate antimotility agents and bismuth subsalicylate can be expected to provide symptomatic relief in half of the cases. Most importantly, however, patients should be reassured that although the disease is unpleasant, it is not life-threatening. Furthermore, they can be heartened by the knowledge that the illness is almost always self-limited.

REFERENCES

1. Read NW, Krejs GJ, Read MG, et al. Chronic diarrhea of unknown origin. *Gastroenterology* 1980;78:264–271.

2. Osterholm MT, MacDonald KL, White KE, et al. An outbreak of a newly recognized chronic diarrhea syndrome associated with raw milk consumption. *JAMA* 1986;256:484–490.
3. Parsonnet J, Trock SC, Bopp CA, et al. Chronic diarrhea associated with drinking untreated water. *Ann Intern Med* 1989; 110:985–991.
4. Mintz ED, Weber JT, Guris D, et al. An outbreak of Brainerd diarrhea among travelers to the Galapagos Islands. *J Infect Dis* 1998;177:1041–1945.
5. Mintz ED, Parsonnet J, Osterholm MT. Chronic idiopathic diarrhea [Letter]. *N Engl J Med* 1993;328:1713–1714.
6. Martin DL, Hoberman LJ. A point source outbreak of chronic diarrhea in Texas: no known exposure to raw milk. *JAMA* 1986; 256:469.
7. Tsang T, Abbot S, Richmond J, et al. Brainerd diarrhea outbreak in California—role of *Campylobacter curvis*? Abstract presented at the 49th annual EIS Conference, Atlanta, April 2000.
8. Kimura AC, Mead P, Walsh B, et al., and the Chronic Diarrhea Working Group. Restaurant-associated outbreak of Brainerd diarrhea in the Red River Valley, Texas, 1996. Abstract presented at the 46th annual EIS Conference, Atlanta, 1997.
9. Kellow J, Phillips S, Miller L et al. Abnormalities of motility and absorption in an outbreak of chronic diarrhea. *Gastroenterology* 1985;88:1442.
10. Janda RC, Conklin JL, Mitros FA, et al. Multifocal colitis associated with an epidemic of chronic diarrhea. *Gastroenterology* 1991;100:458–464.
11. Bryant DA, Mintz ED, Puhr ND, et al. Colonic epithelial lymphocytosis associated with an epidemic of chronic diarrhea. *Am J Surg Pathol* 1996;20:1102–1109.
12. Lazenby AF, Yardley JH, Giardello FM, et al. Lymphocytic "microscopic" colitis: a comparative histopathologic study with particular reference to collagenous colitis. *Hum Pathol* 1989;20: 18–28.
13. Myers LL, Shoop DS, Potter ME, et al. Enteric disease in rabbits inoculated with stool filtrates from persons with chronic diarrhea. *J Infect Dis* 1989;159:133–135.
14. Fine KD, Schiller LR. AGA technical review on the evaluation and management of chronic diarrhea. *Gastroenterology* 1999; 116:1464–1486.
15. Afzalpurkar RG, Schiller LR, Little KH, et al. The self-limited nature of chronic idiopathic diarrhea. *N Engl J Med* 1992;327: 1849–1852.
16. Palmer KR, Corbett CL, Holdsworth CD. Double-blind crossover study comparing loperamide codeine and diphenoxylate in the treatment of chronic diarrhea. *Gastroenterology* 1980;79: 1272–1275.
17. Schiller LR, Hogan RB, Morawski SG, et al. Studies of the prevalence and significance of radiolabeled bile acid malabsorption in a group of patients with idiopathic chronic diarrhea. *Gastroenterology* 1987;92:151–160.
18. Perk G, Ackerman Z, Cohen P, et al. Lymphocytic colitis: a clue to an infectious trigger. *Scand J Gastroenterol* 1999;34:110–112.
19. Mullhaupt B, Guller U, Anabitarte M, et al. Lymphocytic colitis: clinical presentation and long-term course. *Gut* 1998;43: 629–633.
20. Wang N, Dumot JA, Achkar E, et al. Colonic epithelial lymphocytosis without a thickened subepithelial collagen table. *Am J Surg Pathol* 1999;23:1068–1074.
21. Baert F, Wouters K, D'Haens G, et al. Lymphocytic colitis: a distinct clinical entity? A clinicopathological confrontation of lymphocytic and collagenous colitis. *Gut* 1999;45:375–381.
22. Mintz ED, Mishu B, Guris D, et al. Prevalence of Brainerd-type chronic diarrhea among patients of AGA and ACG members. *Gastroenterology* 1993;104:A747(abst).
23. Taylor DN, Connor BA, Shlim DR. Chronic diarrhea in the returned traveler. *Med Clin North Am* 1999;83:1033–1052.
24. Steffan R, van der Linde F, Gyr IC, et al. Epidemiology of diarrhea in travelers. *JAMA* 1983;249:1176.
25. Addiss DG, Tauxe RV, Bernard KW. Chronic diarrhoeal illness in US Peace Corps volunteers. *Int J Epidemiol* 1990;19:217–218.
26. Fukuda K, Nisenbaum R, Stewart G. Chronic multisymptom illness affecting Air Force veterans of the Gulf War. *JAMA* 1998; 280:981.
27. Afzalpurkar RG, Schiller LR, Fordtran JS. Chronic idiopathic diarrhea [Letter]. *N Engl J Med* 1993;328:1714.
28. Snyder JD, Merson MH. The magnitude of the global problem of acute diarrhoeal disease: a review of active surveillance data. *Bull World Health Organ* 1982;60:605–613.
29. McAuliffe JF, Shields DS, de Souza MA, et al. Prolonged and recurring diarrhea in the northeast of Brazil: examination of cases from a community-based study. *J Pediatr Gastroenterol Nutr* 1986;5:902–906.
30. Prazuck T, Tall F, Nacro B, et al. HIV infection and severe malnutrition: a clinical and epidemiological study in Burkina Faso. *AIDS* 1993;7:103–108.
31. Keusch GT, Thea DM, Kamenga M, et al. Persistent diarrhea associated with AIDS. *Acta Paediatr Suppl* 1992;381:45–48.
32. Wanke CA. Infectious etiologies of prolonged diarrhea. In: Kallus G, ed. *Balliere's clinical tropical medicine and communicable disease.* England: Balliere and Tindall, 1988:567–590.
33. Joe LK, Rukmono B, Oemijati S, et al. Diarrhoea among infants in a crowded area of Djakarta, Indonesia. A longitudinal study from birth to two years. *Bull World Health Organ* 1966; 34:197–210.
34. Gordon JE, Ascoli W, Mata LJ, et al. Nutrition and infection field study in Guatemalan villages, 1959–1964. *Arch Environ Health* 1968;16:424–437.
35. Black RE, Merson MH, Rahman AS, et al. A two-year study of bacterial, viral, and parasitic agents associated with diarrhea in rural Bangladesh. *J Infect Dis* 1980;142:660–664.
36. Baqui AH, Black RE, Sack RB, et al. Epidemiological and clinical characteristics of acute and persistent diarrhoea in rural Bangladeshi children. *Acta Paediatr* 1992;81[Suppl 381]:15–21.
37. Schorling JB, Wanke CA, Schorling SK, et al. A prospective study of persistent diarrhea among children in an urban Brazilian slum: patterns of occurrence and etiologic agents. *Am J Epidemiol* 1990;132:144–156.
38. Cruz JR, Bartlett AV, Mendez H, et al. Epidemiology of persistent diarrhea among Guatemalan rural children. *Acta Paediatr* 1992;81[Suppl 381]:22–26.
39. Henry FJ, Udoy AS, Wanke CA, et al. Epidemiology of persistent diarrhea and etiologic agents in Mirzapur, Bangladesh. *Acta Paediatr* 1992;81[Suppl 381]:27–31.
40. Bhandari N, Bhan MK, Sazawal S. Mortality associated with acute watery diarrhea, dysentery and persistent diarrhea in rural north India. *Acta Paediatr* 1992;81[Suppl 381]:3–6.
41. Fauveau V, Henry FJ, Briend A, et al. Persistent diarrhea as a cause of childhood mortality in rural Bangladesh. *Acta Paediatr* 1992;81[Suppl 381]:12–14.
42. Victora CG, Huttly SR, Fuchs SC, et al. Deaths due to dysentery, acute and persistent diarrhoea among Brazilian infants. *Acta Paediatr* 2000;81[Suppl 381]:7–11.
43. Gracey M, Stone DE. Small-intestinal microflora in Australian aboriginal children with chronic diarrhoea. *Aust N Z J Med* 1972;2:215–219.
44. Coehlo-Ramirez P, Litshitz F. Enteric microflora and carbohydrate intolerance in infants with diarrhea. *Pediatrics* 1982;49:233–238.
45. Challacombe DN, Richardson JM, Rowe B, et al. Bacterial microflora of the upper gastrointestinal tract in infants with protracted diarrhoea. *Arch Dis Child* 1974;49:270–277.

46. Rowland MG, Cole TJ, McCollum JP. Weanling diarrhoea in the Gambia: implications of a jejunal intubation study. *Trans R Soc Trop Med Hyg* 1981;75:215–218.
47. Heyworth B, Browh J. Jejunal microflora in malnourished Gambian children. *Arch Dis Child* 1975;50:27–33.
48. Penny ME. The role of the duodenal microflora as a determinant of persistent diarrhoea. *Acta Paediatr* 1992;81[Suppl 381]: 114–120.
49. Bhatnagar S, Bhan MK, George C, et al. Is small bowel bacterial overgrowth of pathogenic significance in persistent diarrhea? *Acta Paediatr Suppl* 1992;381:108–113.
50. Wanke CA, Guerrant RL. Small bowel colonization alone is a cause of diarrhea. *Infect Immun* 1987;55:1924–1926.
51. Schlager TA, Wanke CA, Guerrant RL. Net fluid secretion and impaired villous function induced by colonization of the small intestine by non-toxigenic colonizing *Escherichia coli. Infect Immun* 1990;58:1337–1343.
52. Belitsos PC, Greenson JK, Yardley JH, et al. Association of gastric hypoacidity with opportunistic enteric infections in patients with AIDS. *J Infect Dis* 1992;166:277–284.
53. Lanata CF, Black RE, Maurtua D, et al. Etiologic agents in acute vs persistent diarrhea in children under three years of age in peri-urban Lima, Peru. *Acta Paediatr Suppl* 1992;381:32–38.
54. Ulshen MH, Rollo JL. Pathogenesis of *Escherichia coli* gastroenteritis in man—another mechanism. *N Engl J Med* 1980;302: 99–101.
55. Lima AA, Fang G, Schorling JB, et al. Persistent diarrhea in northeast Brazil: etiologies and interactions with malnutrition. *Acta Paediatr Suppl* 1992;381:39–44.
56. Vial PA, Robins-Browne R, Lior H, et al. Characterization of enteroadherent-aggregative *Escherichia coli,* a putative agent of diarrheal disease. *J Infect Dis* 1988;158:70–79.
57. Cravioto A, Tello A, Navarro A, et al. Association of *Escherichia coli* HEp-2 adherence patterns with type and duration of diarrhoea. *Lancet* 1991;337:262–264.
58. Wanke CA, Schorling JB, Barrett LJ, et al. Potential role of adherence traits of *Escherichia coli* in persistent diarrhea in an urban Brazilian slum. *Pediatr Infect Dis J* 1991;10:746–751.
59. Bhan MK, Khoshoo V, Sommerfelt H, et al. Enteroaggregative *Escherichia coli* and *Salmonella* associated with nondysenteric persistent diarrhea. *Pediatr Infect Dis J* 1989;8:499–502.
60. Bhan MK, Raj P, Levine MM, et al. Enteroaggregative *Escherichia coli* associated with persistent diarrhea in a cohort of rural children in India. *J Infect Dis* 1989;159:1061–1064.
61. Wanke CA, Mayer H, Weber R, et al. Enteraggregative *E. coli* as a potential cause of diarrheal disease in adults infected with HIV. *J Infect Dis* 1998;178:185–190.
62. Baqui AH, Sack RB, Black RE, et al. Enteropathogens associated with acute and persistent diarrhea in Bangladeshi children less than 5 years of age. *J Infect Dis* 1992;166:792–796.
63. Gunzburg ST, Chang BJ, Elliott SJ, et al. Diffuse and enteroaggregative patterns of adherence of enteric *Escherichia coli* isolated from aboriginal children from the Kimberley region of Western Australia. *J Infect Dis* 1993;167:755–758.
64. Steiner TS, Lima AA, Nataro JP, et al. Enteraggregative *E. coli* produce inflammation and growth impairment and cause IL-8 release from intestinal epithelial cells. *J Infect Dis* 1998;177: 88–96.
65. Benjamin P, Federman M, Wanke CA. Characterization of an invasive phenotype associated with enteroaggregative *Escherichia coli. Infect Immun* 1995;63:3417–3421.
66. Lloyd-Evans N, Drasar BS, Tomkins AM. A comparison of the prevalence of *Campylobacter, Shigella,* and *Salmonella* in faeces of malnourished and well-nourished children in the Gambia and northern Nigeria. *Trans R Soc Trop Med Hyg* 1983;77:245–247.
67. Bokkenheuser VD, Richardson NJ, Bryner JH, et al. Detection of enteric campylobacteriosis in children. *J Clin Microbiol* 1979; 9:227–232.
68. Mathan VI, Rajan DP, Klipstein FA, et al. Enterotoxigenic *Campylobacter jejuni* among children in South India [Letter]. *Lancet* 1984;2:981.
69. Blaser MJ, Glass RI, Huq MI, et al. Isolation of *Campylobacter fetus* subsp. *jejuni* from Bangladeshi children. *J Clin Microbiol* 1980;12:744–747.
70. WHO Scientific Working Group. Parasite-related diarrheas. *Bull World Health Organ* 1980;53:819–830.
71. Mata LJ, Urrutia JJ, Simmon A. Infectious agents in acute and chronic diarrhea of childhood. In: Lebenthal E, ed. *Chronic diarrhea in children.* New York: Raven Press, 1984:237–257.
72. Udezulu IA, Visvesvara GS, Moss DM, et al. Isolation of two *Giardia lamblia* (WB strain) clones with distinct surface protein and antigenic profiles and differing infectivity and virulence. *Infect Immun* 1992;60:2274–2280.
73. Char S, Cevallos AM, Yamson P, et al. Impaired IgA response to *Giardia* heat shock antigen in children with persistent diarrhoea and giardiasis. *Gut* 1993;34:38–40.
74. Haider Z, Rasul A. Chronic non-dysenteric intestinal amoebiasis—a review of 159 cases. *JPMA J Pak Med Assoc* 1975;25:75–78.
75. Wanke C, Butler T, Islam M. Epidemiologic and clinical features of invasive amebiasis in Bangladesh: a case–control comparison with other diarrheal diseases and postmortem findings. *Am J Trop Med Hyg* 1988;38:335–341.
76. Agnew DC, Lima AA, Newman RD, et al. *Cryptosporidium* in Northeastern Brazilian children associated with increased diarrheal morbidity. *J Infect Dis* 1998;177:754–760.
77. Lima AA, Moore SR, Barboza MS, et al. Persistent diarrhea signals a critical period of increased diarrheal burden and nutritional shortfall: a prospective cohort study in children in Northeastern Brazil. *J Infect Dis* 2000;181:1643–1651.
78. Donowitz M, Kokke FT, Saidi R. Evaluation of patients with chronic diarrhea. *N Engl J Med* 1995;332:725–729.
79. Clinical Practice and Practice Economics Committee, AGA Governing Board. American Gastroenterological Association Medical Position Statement: Guidelines for the evaluation and management of chronic diarrhea. *Gastroenterology* 1999;116:1461–1463.
80. Schiller LR. Microscopic colitis syndrome: lymphocytic colitis and collagenous colitis. *Semin Gastrointest Dis* 1999;10:145–155.
81. Fine KD, Ogunji F, George J, et al. Utility of a rapid fecal latex agglutination test detecting the neutrophil protein, lactoferrin, for diagnosing inflammatory causes of chronic diarrhea. *Am J Gastroenterol* 1998;93:1300–1305.
82. DuPont HL, Capsuto EG. Persistent diarrhea in travelers. *Clin Infect Dis* 1996;22:124–128.
83. Fine KD, Seidel RH, Do K. The prevalence, anatomic distribution, and diagnosis of colonic causes of chronic diarrhea. *Gastrointest Endosc* 2000;51:318–326.
84. Tremaine WJ. Collagenous colitis and lymphocytic colitis. *J Clin Gastroenterol* 2000;30:245–249.
85. Oishi I, Kimura T, Murakami T, et al. Serial observations of chronic rotavirus infection in an immunodeficient child. *Microbiol Immunol* 1991;35:953–961.
86. Buckner FS, Pomeroy C. Cytomegalovirus disease of the gastrointestinal tract in patients without AIDS. *Clin Infect Dis* 1993;17:644–656.
87. Meiselman MS, Cello JP, Margaretten W. Cytomegalovirus colitis. Report of the clinical, endoscopic, and pathologic findings in two patients with the acquired immune deficiency syndrome. *Gastroenterology* 1985;88:171–175.
88. Simon D, Brandt LJ. Diarrhea in patients with the acquired immunodeficiency syndrome. *Gastroenterology* 1993;105: 1238–1242.
89. Janoff EN, Orenstein JM, Manischewitz JF, et al. Adenovirus

colitis in the acquired immunodeficiency syndrome. *Gastroenterology* 1991;100:976–979.
90. Grohmann GS, Glass RI, Pereira HG, et al. Enteric viruses and diarrhea in HIV-infected patients. Enteric Opportunistic Infections Working Group. *N Engl J Med* 1993;329:14–20.
91. King GE, Werner SB, Kizer KW. Epidemiology of *Aeromonas* infections in California. *Clin Infect Dis* 1992;15:449–452.
92. San Joaquin VH, Pickett DA. *Aeromonas*-associated gastroenteritis in children. *Pediatr Infect Dis J* 1988;7:53–57.
93. Holmberg SD, Schell WL, Fanning GR, et al. *Aeromonas* intestinal infections in the United States. *Ann Intern Med* 1986; 105:683–689.
94. Rautelin H, Hanninen ML, Sivonen A, et al. Chronic diarrhea due to a single strain of *Aeromonas caviae. Eur J Clin Microbiol Infect Dis* 1995;14:51–53.
95. Blaser MJ, Wells JG, Feldman RA, et al. *Campylobacter* enteritis in the United States. A multicenter study. *Ann Intern Med* 1983;98:360–365.
96. Smalley JR, Klish WJ, Brown MR, et al. Chronic diarrhea associated with *Campylobacter. Clin Pediatr (Phila)* 1982;21:220.
97. Darbas H, Pelous C, Jean A, et al. Chronic diarrhea caused by *Campylobacter jejuni* in a patient with AIDS. *Pathol Biol (Paris)* 1988;36:888–890.
98. Perlman DM, Ampel NM, Schifman RB, et al. Persistent *Campylobacter jejuni* infections in patients infected with the human immunodeficiency virus (HIV). *Ann Intern Med* 1988; 108:540–546.
99. San Joaquin VH, Welch DF. *Campylobacter* enteritis. A 3-year experience. *Clin Pediatr (Phila)* 1984;23:311–316.
100. Bartlett JG. Antibiotic-associated pseudomembranous colitis. *Rev Infect Dis* 1979;1:530–539.
101. Schwan A, Sjolin S, Trottestam U, et al. Relapsing *Clostridium difficile* enterocolitis cured by rectal infusion of normal faeces. *Scand J Infect Dis* 1984;16:211–215.
102. Heiner AM, DiSario JA, Carroll K, et al. Dysgonic fermenter-3: a bacterium associated with diarrhea in immunocompromised hosts. *Am J Gastroenterol* 1992;87:1629–1630.
103. Hill SM, Phillips AD, Walker-Smith JA. Enteropathogenic *Escherichia coli* and life-threatening chronic diarrhoea. *Gut* 1991;32:154–158.
104. Clausen CR, Christie DL. Chronic diarrhea in infants caused by adherent enteropathogenic *Escherichia coli. J Pediatr* 1982; 100:358–361.
105. Lacroix J, Delage G, Gosselin F, et al. Severe protracted diarrhea due to multiresistant adherent *Escherichia coli. Am J Dis Child* 1984;138:693–696.
106. Rothbaum R, McAdams AJ, Giannella R, et al. A clinicopathologic study of enterocyte-adherent *Escherichia coli*: a cause of protracted diarrhea in infants. *Gastroenterology* 1982;83: 441–454.
107. Klimach OE, Ormerod LP. Gastrointestinal tuberculosis: a retrospective review of 109 cases in a district general hospital. *Q J Med* 1985;56:569–578.
108. Gillin JS, Urmacher C, West R, et al. Disseminated *Mycobacterium avium-intracellulare* infection in acquired immunodeficiency syndrome mimicking Whipple's disease. *Gastroenterology* 1983;85:1187–1191.
109. Penn RG, Giger DK, Knoop FC, et al. *Plesiomonas shigelloides* overgrowth in the small intestine. *J Clin Microbiol* 1982;15: 869–872.
110. Glynn JR, Palmer SR. Incubation period, severity of disease, and infecting dose: evidence from a *Salmonella* outbreak. *Am J Epidemiol* 1992;136:1369–1377.
111. Ostroff SM, Kapperud G, Lassen J, et al. Clinical features of sporadic *Yersinia enterocolitica* infections in Norway. *J Infect Dis* 1992;166:812–817.
112. Mollee T, Tilse M. *Yersinia enterocolitica.* Isolation from faeces of adults and children in Queensland. *Med J Aust* 1985;143: 488–489.
113. Saebo A, Lassen J. Acute and chronic gastrointestinal manifestations associated with *Yersinia enterocolitica* infection. A Norwegian 10-year follow-up study on 458 hospitalized patients. *Ann Surg* 1992;215:250–255.
114. Saebo A, Lassen J. A survey of acute and chronic disease associated with *Yersinia enterocolitica* infection. A Norwegian 10-year follow-up study on 458 hospitalized patients. *Scand J Infect Dis* 1991;23:517–527.
115. Gupta TP, Ehrinpreis MN. *Candida*-associated diarrhea in hospitalized patients. *Gastroenterology* 1990;98:780–785.
116. Kain KC, Noble MA, Freeman HJ, et al. Epidemiology and clinical features associated with *Blastocystis hominis* infection. *Diagn Microbiol Infect Dis* 1987;8:235–244.
117. Doyle PW, Helgason MM, Mathias RG, et al. Epidemiology and pathogenicity of *Blastocystis hominis. J Clin Microbiol* 1990; 28:116–121.
118. Wolfson JS, Richter JM, Waldron MA, et al. Cryptosporidiosis in immunocompetent patients. *N Engl J Med* 1985;312:1278–1282.
119. Soave R, Johnson WD Jr. *Cryptosporidium* and *Isospora belli* infections. *J Infect Dis* 1988;157:225–229.
120. Smith PM. Traveller's diarrhoea associated with a *Cyanobacterium*-like body [Letter]. *Med J Aust* 1993;158:724.
121. Long EG, Ebrahimzadeh A, White EH, et al. Alga associated with diarrhea in patients with acquired immunodeficiency syndrome and in travelers. *J Clin Microbiol* 1990;28:1101–1104.
122. Matseshe JW, Phillips SF. Chronic diarrhea. A practical approach. *Med Clin North Am* 1978;62:141–154.
123. Adams EB, MacLeod IN. Invasive amebiasis. I. Amebic dysentery and its complications. *Medicine (Baltimore)* 1977;56:315–323.
124. Butler T, Middleton FG, Earnest DL, et al. Chronic and recurrent diarrhea in American servicemen in Vietnam. An evaluation of etiology and small bowel structure and function. *Arch Intern Med* 1973;132:373–377.
125. Birkhead G, Vogt RL. Epidemiologic surveillance for endemic *Giardia lamblia* infection in Vermont. The roles of waterborne and person-to-person transmission. *Am J Epidemiol* 1989;129: 762–768.
126. Shaffer N, Moore L. Chronic travelers' diarrhea in a normal host due to *Isospora belli* [Letter]. *J Infect Dis* 1989;159:596–597.
127. DeHovitz JA, Pape JW, Boncy M, et al. Clinical manifestations and therapy of *Isospora belli* infection in patients with the acquired immunodeficiency syndrome. *N Engl J Med* 1986; 315:87–90.
128. Pol S, Romana CA, Richard S, et al. Microsporidia infection in patients with the human immunodeficiency virus and unexplained cholangitis. *N Engl J Med* 1993;328:95–99.
129. Eeftinck Schattenkerk JK, van Gool T, van Ketel RJ, et al. Clinical significance of small-intestinal microsporidiosis in HIV-1-infected individuals. *Lancet* 1991;337:895–898.
130. Orenstein JM, Chiang J, Steinberg W, et al. Intestinal microsporidiosis as a cause of diarrhea in human immunodeficiency virus-infected patients: a report of 20 cases. *Hum Pathol* 1990;21:475–481.

21

TROPICAL SPRUE: CHRONIC INTESTINAL MALABSORPTION IN THE TROPICS

GARY M. GRAY

Tropical sprue is a chronic malady of the small intestine manifested by the malabsorption of nutrients and vitamins; it occurs in persons residing in certain tropical locales. The essential features of the disease are an increased volume and number of stools, malabsorption of nutrients, and consequent weight loss in persons residing in a tropical region (1). It is uncertain when the disease was first recognized, but it may have been described as early as between 600 and 1300 B.C. in Indian writings on the disorders of assimilation of food. Before 1800 in Barbados, Hillary (2) provided a typical clinical description of what is now thought to be tropical sprue. In 1880, Manson (3) adopted a Dutch term, *sprouw,* that had been used to describe an illness involving buccal aphthous ulcers in children who had what is now known to be nontropical sprue (synonyms: celiac sprue, gluten-sensitive enteropathy). Although tropical sprue involves primarily the small intestine (4–7), folic acid and vitamin B_{12} deficiency and megaloblastic anemia are commonly present at the outset of the disease and almost always occur when it becomes well established (8,9). Tropical sprue appears to compromise tissues that replicate rapidly and have a life span of only a few days. When patients with such tropical malabsorption respond dramatically to treatment with oral folic acid and broad-spectrum antibiotics, the diagnosis becomes secure.

EPIDEMIOLOGY

Tropical sprue is endemic in numerous tropical locales between slightly more than 30 degrees north and south latitude; these include the Caribbean, India, and southern Africa (6). The disease is particularly prevalent in Cuba, the Dominican Republic, Haiti (10), and Puerto Rico (6) but has not been observed in Jamaica. It has also been well described in Colombia and Venezuela and probably occurs in Mexico (11). Perhaps the most extensive documentation of tropical sprue has been in India (7,12). The disease has also been observed in Africa (13), Borneo, Burma, China, Hong Kong (14), Indonesia, Malaysia, Singapore, Vietnam, Sri Lanka (15), the Philippines (16), and Tanzania (17)..

Besides occurring in indigenous populations, tropical sprue is contracted by those who visit the tropics for a month or longer. Typical tropical sprue developed in 10% of English military personnel who were in the India–Burma region (18,19) during World War II, and in those stationed in Malaya (20,21) and Hong Kong (14). Tropical sprue developed in a similar proportion of the United States military serving in Puerto Rico (21), and more recently, the disease was found to be common in Vietnam among visitors from the United States, including both military personnel (22) and a medical professional team (11% after only 3 months of exposure, and 28% after a year) (23). The incubation period for North American expatriates traveling in these tropical lands may be a year or more (24,25). Malabsorption and abnormal intestinal morphology developed within 6 months in nearly half of Peace Corps volunteers from the United States residing in Pakistan (25). Subsequent recovery of absorptive function required 1 to 2 years after the return to the United States (26). The prevalence of intestinal malabsorption in Indians and Pakistanis who immigrate to the New York City area is high, and the conversion to normal parameters usually requires a full year and sometimes as long as 2 or 3 years (27). The first symptoms of tropical sprue may emerge months or even years after expatriates have returned to their native temperate environments (28). It is rarely seen in short-term visitors to the tropics, probably because a prolonged exposure to a causative agent appears to be necessary and perhaps because antibiotics that may prevent intestinal infestations are now used extensively by travelers.

G. M. Gray: Division of Gastroenterology and Hepatology, Stanford University Medical Center, Stanford, California

Although most cases of tropical sprue appear to arise sporadically in endemic form, a significant proportion of persons in tropical regions (5% to 10%) may contract the disease. Epidemics of tropical sprue have been reported, particularly in India (29,30). The maximal attack rate of tropical sprue in the slowly developing Indian epidemics is as high as 10 to 25 cases per 100 persons per annum in adults. The frequency increases somewhat at about age 25 and may be even higher after age 40 (31–33). The attack rate in children is only about half that in adults, but the disease may be particularly severe and is not infrequently lethal in young children (see below). Typically, the onset and spread among family members of a household are gradual, with new cases cropping up on a month-by-month basis during a period of a year or more. The incubation period within a household usually is more than a month, and although the disease initially affects mainly adults, it is contracted by children as the epidemic evolves. Subsequent epidemics within the same community usually occur approximately every 5 to 6 years. The prevalence of symptomatic malabsorptive illness increases in children born after the first epidemic, which suggests that some immunity may be conferred on those who have contracted the disease (7). Perhaps because of the relatively slow evolution of such epidemics of tropical sprue and the fact that family members have become more mobile in recent years, the epidemic nature of the disease has not been established in tropical countries other than India. Furthermore, some features of Indian epidemic tropical sprue are not observed in sporadic endemic sprue. For instance, an acute enteritis, presumably infectious in nature and classically described as the first stage in Indian tropical sprue (33), is observed much less frequently in sprue elsewhere. Nevertheless, some experts consider an acute enteric episode to be an essential feature of the tropical sprue syndrome (34,35). Even though diarrheal syndromes, presumably caused by infectious organisms, are common and recurrent in many of these tropical locales, they usually do not herald the onset of the chronic sprue condition. Also, the dramatic response to antibiotic therapy usually reported in cases of tropical sprue, which is used to support the putative bacterial etiology of the disease, seems to be muted or absent in southern India (7,36). Hence, the question lingers of whether the tropical malabsorption observed in India is a different disease than that seen in other tropical regions.

PATHOGENESIS

The Case for an Infectious Cause

Because of the endemic nature of the disease and the fact that epidemics of tropical sprue have been repeatedly observed, an infectious agent has long been sought as the predominant or final eventual cause of chronic tropical sprue. Unfortunately, no unique organism has been identified, and no animal model of the human tropical malabsorption syndrome is available. Nonetheless, numerous studies have demonstrated an overgrowth of coliform organisms in the small intestine (37–40). In normal persons, the upper jejunum harbors very few organisms, and these are mainly gram-positive streptococci and lactobacilli. Streptococci and fungi are present in high titers in the more distal bowel. Facultative anaerobic coliforms are present in the distal ileum in small numbers and are the normal inhabitants of the colon. Although the recovery of small-intestinal samples is fraught with error because of contamination with nasopharyngeal organisms, studies of patients with tropical sprue have demonstrated facultative anaerobes in the upper small bowel, including *Klebsiella pneumoniae, Escherichia coli,* and *Enterobacter cloacae* (38). A high proportion (~50% to >90%) of patients with untreated tropical sprue from southern India (39) and Puerto Rico (40) and of Europeans traveling in Asia (34) were shown to harbor coliform bacteria in small-intestinal aspirates. In southern India, coliforms were demonstrated in the vast majority of patients with tropical sprue, but they were similarly frequent in healthy controls (39,41). Such enterobacteria have been shown to cause changes in the mucosal structure of animals with intestinal stasis produced by experimental blind loops (42). Although toxins from coliforms can produce a secretory diarrhea, they do not produce significant chronic intestinal histologic changes such as those seen in topical sprue.

Klipstein (6) noted three features of the tropical sprue syndrome that led to the opinion that the disease is caused by a bacterium: (a) Coliform overgrowth does not usually develop in other small-intestine maladies, such as celiac sprue; (b) coliform enterotoxins cause intestinal structural and functional alterations in experimental animals; and (c) antibiotic therapy both eradicates the coliform overgrowth and heals the intestinal lesion. However, the overgrowth of coliforms may be only an epiphenomenon. Although these organisms are capable of emitting toxins and producing a secretory diarrhea, it has not been established that they cause chronic pathologic changes in the human small intestine or chronic malabsorption. Furthermore, as estimated from the time required for orally ingested lactulose to be metabolized and expired as hydrogen, intestinal transit is prolonged in patients with tropical sprue (43); the long retention of nutrients and vitamins sets the stage for bacterial overgrowth and consequent interference with nutrient assimilation. Admittedly, the organisms that overgrow in the small intestine in tropical sprue are facultative anaerobes rather than the anaerobes commonly seen in classic stasis or small-intestinal overgrowth syndrome. However, factors other than stasis may allow the overgrowth of coliforms. Because of the higher ambient temperature in tropical regions, the level of bacterial contamination in ingested food is likely to be higher. Control subjects in the tropics who do not have malabsorption have not often been examined in parallel for possible bacterial overgrowth, but jejunal culture of coliforms has been observed in some control subjects from the same tropical environment who do not have malabsorption (39,41). Although coliform overgrowth in the small intestine may set the stage for the chronic malabsorptive condition in tropical regions of endemicity, rapid elimination of the organism by antibiotics does not lead to a prompt reversal of the malabsorptive syndrome. Instead, the reversal of malabsorption and malnutrition induced by folic acid and antibiotics in tropical sprue often requires several weeks or even months (44,45). In essence, the case for a bacterial cause of tropical sprue is circumstantial, the coliform organisms that proliferate in the tropics not having been shown to produce a chronic malabsorptive condition. The isolation of a putative bacterial agent that is capable of causing the chronic tropical sprue syndrome remains elusive.

Viral infestations have been considered as a possible cause of tropical sprue, but cultures of rectal swabs from patients have been negative (46). Culture of excreted enteric viruses is commonly unsuccessful, although virus-like particles have been observed in the stools of persons affected by tropical sprue in Indian epidemics (47). Corona-like virus particles were reported to be continuously present in the stools of a patient with tropical sprue (48), but the following features of the case make it less than compelling: (a) No antibodies against the virus were found in serum, and (b) the patient had undergone a vagotomy and a gastrojejunostomy for peptic disease, which might have permitted a chronic enteric viral infestation. Certainly, a more thorough analysis of a possible role of infection with one or more viruses in chronic tropical sprue is indicated.

Other Causative Considerations

In addition to intestinal stasis and coliform overgrowth, alterations in plasma concentrations of gastrointestinal hormones, including enteroglucagon, motilin, and peptide YY, have been demonstrated in tropical sprue (34,49). Although only moderately elevated in acute infectious diarrhea, peptide YY levels were 10 times higher than normal in patients with tropical sprue (49). This dramatic finding deserves further study.

Although it has been suggested that poor hygiene and low socioeconomic status may predispose persons in the tropics to development of the disease, no comprehensive studies have documented the role of altered nutrition or contaminated food in the etiology of tropical sprue.

The observations from India that the onset of tropical sprue is manifested by an acute enteritis that sets the stage for the chronic symptoms of the disease has prompted the hypothesis that tropical sprue is actually a postinfective tropical malabsorption (34,50). An enteritis produced by a variety of organisms is common in many tropical and subtropical regions and not infrequently produces a bloody colitis. In most instances of endemic tropical sprue, a discrete history of a preceding severe acute episode is lacking. Indeed, the acute episode itself, when it does occur, does not appear to be caused by a single or unique enteric pathogen. With the possible exception of Indian tropical sprue, it seems unlikely that an acute predisposing episode is an essential component of the chronic malabsorption syndrome typical of tropical sprue.

Whipple Disease

Can an analogy be made with Whipple disease? In many ways, the evolution of illness in tropical sprue seems analogous to the chronic intestinal malabsorption of Whipple disease, in which a specific bacterial cause was recently documented by the presence of a unique bacterial messenger RNA in intestinal tissues (51,52). Even though it is still not possible to cultivate the bacteria in Whipple disease, the indolent onset, the plodding but relentless progression to chronic weight loss and malnutrition, and the requirement for months of antibiotic therapy to ensure a complete remission are similar to what is observed in tropical sprue. However, Whipple disease is certainly distinct from tropical sprue because a unique bacterium is found not only in the intestine but also in numerous lymph node groups, on heart valves (53), and in the brain (54). Whipple disease is more common in temperate zones, and biopsy reveals in the intestinal tissue macrophages that stain with periodic acid–Schiff and contain bacterial bodies (55). Nevertheless, a comprehensive analysis of intestinal tissue with the method used successfully to define the organism responsible for Whipple disease may prove useful in determining whether a unique bacterium is present beneath the enterocyte layer in the intestinal mucosa of patients with tropical sprue. Certainly the epidemiologic features are most compatible with a permissive, chronic intestinal infection, primarily of the small intestine. Although the infectious agents remain to be identified, the dramatic, if somewhat delayed, response to antibiotic therapy strengthens this concept. It seems most likely that a fastidious organism, indigenous to the tropical climate, will be identified as the causative agent of chronic tropical sprue, just as the Whipple bacillus appears to be ubiquitous in the soils of temperate regions. In diseases such as those caused by chronically harbored fastidious bacteria, it remains to be established whether the putative organism itself alters the intestine by chronic infestation or whether bioactive toxic products are released that produce the ultimate damage.

For the present, the primary etiology of the chronic malabsorption syndrome in the tropics must be said to be undiscovered. Certainly tropical sprue is not an acute disease; a person must reside in the tropics for a year or longer before contracting the chronic syndrome. Even in the studies of epidemics of tropical sprue in India (see above), the incubation period was 1 month or longer. Perhaps the stage must first be set in the tropics for development of the illness in persons with a permissive constitution.

CLINICAL ILLNESS

Despite the report of acute diarrheal episodes preceding the onset of sprue in cases from southern India, the onset of tropical sprue in recent years in most locales within 30 degrees of the equator often has been very subtle. Although fatigue and malaise have not been emphasized as early symptoms, the author observed a series of U.S. Army recruits in Puerto Rico in whom the development of midday fatigue, lack of interest in work, and sleepiness often prevented the accomplishment of even the most sedentary tasks. The symptoms of lassitude and weakness are often more disturbing than the increased number (between 3 and 10) and volume (≥1,000 mL) of stools per day. Understandably, some of these people are initially reprimanded by their superiors until evidence appears that they have a systemic disease causing an obvious anemia or weight loss. The vitamin deficiencies are manifested by erythema and stinging pain of the tongue margins and painful cracking at the corners of the mouth. Although it is generally believed that folate and vitamin B_{12} deficiency are late manifestations of the disease (6), a megaloblastic anemia is often the first abnormality noted by general physicians. The extent of fat malabsorption may be mild or moderate (15 to 25 g/d), probably because caloric intake is often reduced appreciably as a consequence of severe anorexia and premature satiety associated with intestinal stasis and postprandial abdominal distention. However, some patients excrete more than 50 g/d. At least 90% of patients experience most of these abdominal symptoms and weight loss by the first month of the disease.

The disease may be particularly severe in childhood. Fevers, high-volume watery diarrhea (not infrequently bloody), and malnutrition are common (56,57). Death rates without medical intervention are higher than 30%. However, mortality can be uniformly reduced to a negligible incidence with appropriate medical therapy (57).

Physical examination reveals apathy, appreciable weight loss, relatively retarded physical movement, loss of tongue papillae, cracking at the corners of the mouth, a paradoxically protuberant abdomen despite the loss of body weight, muscle wasting in the extremities, and an associated prominence of bowel sounds, which often are audible without the aid of a stethoscope. About 25% to 30% of patients may have low-grade fevers at the beginning of the constitutional symptoms (58). After a few weeks of systemic manifestations, patients usually show a striking pallor, reflecting the associated anemia; an associated skin hyperpigmentation has been noted in the Indian studies (59). Systolic blood pressures of less than 100 mm Hg and paradoxically slow pulse rates of less than 80/min are common and may produce orthostasis. Pedal edema is usually present after a month of illness and may be severe. In well-established disease, anasarca often develops.

Laboratory Findings

Megaloblastic anemia (hematocrit, <30 mL/dL; mean corpuscular volume, >105 μ^3), much more severe than that seen in nontropical enteropathies, often causes more dominant symptoms than the intestinal lesion and is a hallmark of tropical sprue (9,60). Hypoalbuminemia (<3 g/dL) can be expected in patients who have been ill for a month or longer because of the combination of malabsorption of dietary amino acids and peptides and loss of serum proteins secondary to an increased effective pore size in the diseased intestinal membrane (61). The reduction in the capacity to absorb vitamin B_{12} is marked, and bone marrow analysis almost always reveals severe megaloblastosis. Steatorrhea (stool fat excretion, 15 to 50 g/d; normal, 6 g/d) and reduced xylose absorption (urine excretion, <4.0 g/5 h after ingestion of the 25-g dose) are uniformly found. Brush border disaccharidases and hydrolysis of disaccharides at the intestinal surface are markedly impaired in tropical sprue (62). These tend to return to the normal range after treatment, but the depression of lactase may be more severe than that of the other disaccharidases, and the recovery time may be delayed for months or years (63). Malabsorption of fat-soluble vitamins is common, and vitamin D deficiency may produce hypocalcemia. In severe cases, hyperparathyroidism secondary to protracted calcium malabsorption can be manifested by an elevated serum parathyroid hormone level. Although no evidence has been found that the disease has an immunologic basis, in the Puerto Rican population, HLA-Aw19 and especially HLA-Aw31 appear to be highly associated with tropical sprue (64).

Barium Contrast Radiography and Endoscopy

An upper small-bowel radiographic series reveals prominent folds with an irregular contour from the jejunum through the distal ileum, and retained intraintestinal contents dilute the barium contrast material. The radiologist may question whether the patient has fasted for the examination, but the findings are caused by substantial stasis related to altered motility (65,66). The important finding of ileal involvement is characteristic in tropical sprue and rare in nontropical sprue, Whipple disease, and other small-intestinal enteropathies.

Upper gastrointestinal endoscopy frequently reveals a diminished prominence of the transverse duodenal folds, and close examination may demonstrate a scalloped or "moth-eaten" appearance when the edge of the folds is scrutinized (67). In addition, a patchy mosaic pattern of pale regions with prominent vessels, presumably representing atrophied areas of mucosa, may be visualized. This finding may assist the operator in selecting the most seriously involved regions for endoscopic biopsy (67). Other enteropathies, including eosinophilic gastroenteritis, HIV-related enteritis, giardiasis, and especially celiac sprue (nontropical sprue), may also exhibit a moth-eaten appearance on endoscopic examination (68).

PATHOLOGY

Hematologic Changes

Although the megaloblastic anemia seen in established tropical sprue is often said to be a consequence of chronic malabsorption and malnutrition, it is more severe than the anemias that develop in other small-intestinal diseases associated with malabsorption. In part, this can be attributed to the involvement of the entire small intestine, including the ileum. However, severe megaloblastosis not infrequently develops early in the course of the disease, and the symptoms of anemia may be even more prominent than those of malabsorption (9,60). In addition, the prompt and often dramatic response to folic acid supplementation lends support to the theory that vitamin B deficiencies may be pivotal in the pathogenesis of tropical sprue.

Small Intestine

When symptomatic small-intestinal malabsorption with increased fat excretion and reduced D-xylose absorption occurs in an appropriate tropical locale, the definitive diagnosis of tropical sprue can be made from the characteristic histologic findings on the small-intestinal biopsy specimen. The hallmark of the disease is a generalized alteration in the small-intestinal mucosa (67,69). In contrast to the normal small intestine, which displays tall villi with a scalloped or "saw-toothed" epithelial layer (Fig. 21.1), peroral biopsy specimens from patients with tropical sprue show substantial blunting and broadening of the intestinal villi and deepening of the intestinal crypt epithelium (Fig. 21.2). Typical villus-to-crypt ratios are decreased from normal values of between 3:1 and 5:1 to 1:1 or less. The lamina propria is heavily infiltrated with chronic inflammatory cells, particularly lymphocytes, but an increase in plasma cells and histiocytes may also be seen. In severe disease, enterocytes become foreshortened from their normal, classic columnar shape to a cuboidal configuration, and the height and numbers of luminal membrane microvilli are reduced on electron micrographs. Often, a prominent infiltration of the single epithelial layer by migrating mononuclear cells from the underlying lamina propria is seen. Although it is not generally realized, histologic changes in untreated tropical sprue are distinctly characteristic and easily distinguished from those of untreated celiac sprue (gluten-sensitive enteropathy, nontropical sprue), a disease that occurs more commonly in temperate zones. Even though the villi are markedly altered in tropical sprue, identifiable villi and crypt units are almost always preserved (12,69,70). In contrast, untreated celiac sprue is usually associated with a virtual absence of villi, marked elongation of crypts, and infiltration of plasma-type mononuclear cells rather than lymphocytes (71). In addition, an accumulation of fat at the basilar membrane underlying the enterocyte layer may be seen in tropical sprue, but not in other enteropathies (72). Interestingly enough, reduction in villus height and elongation of crypts producing a villus-to-crypt ratio of approximately 1:1 are often seen in AIDS patients infected with HIV who have watery diarrhea, even in the absence of intestinal malabsorption (73,74). Indeed, the intestinal histology in AIDS may be very similar to that in tropical sprue (Fig. 21.3), and, in locales where AIDS is endemic, it is a more prevalent cause of intestinal injury than is tropical sprue. Differentiation from Whipple disease is relatively simple because of the macrophages that stain with periodic acid–Schiff, the presence of bacillary bodies on electron microscopy, and positive results of polymerase chain reaction analysis of the intestine for the responsible bacterium, *Tropheryma whippelii,* in Whipple disease (75). In primary intestinal lymphoma (Mediterranean lymphoma), the paucity of intestinal crypts and dense infiltration with mononuclear cells, tightly packed in the lamina propria, serve to distinguish that disease from tropical sprue, even though malignant cells are uncommonly identified in primary lymphoma (76). Unlike celiac sprue, which is most severe in the upper small intestine and usually spares the ileum, tropical sprue involves the entire small intestine, the ileal mucosa fre-

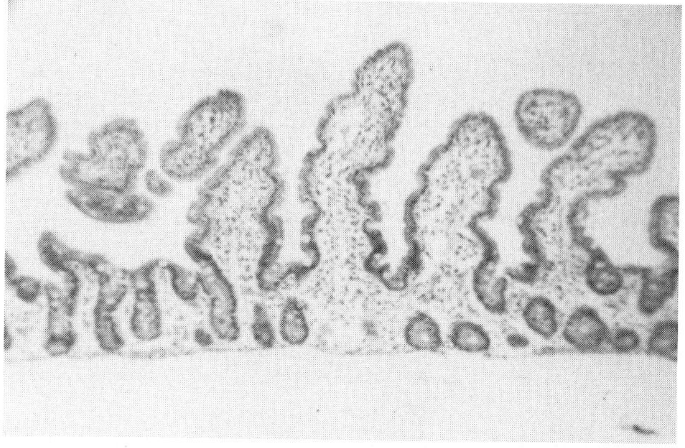

FIGURE 21.1. Normal jejunal mucosa obtained by peroral biopsy. The tall, finger-like villi have a scalloped epithelial layer, and the villus-to-crypt ratio is 3:1 or higher. Moderate numbers of lymphocytes and plasma cells in the lamina propria are seen as small dots at this magnification. ×100.

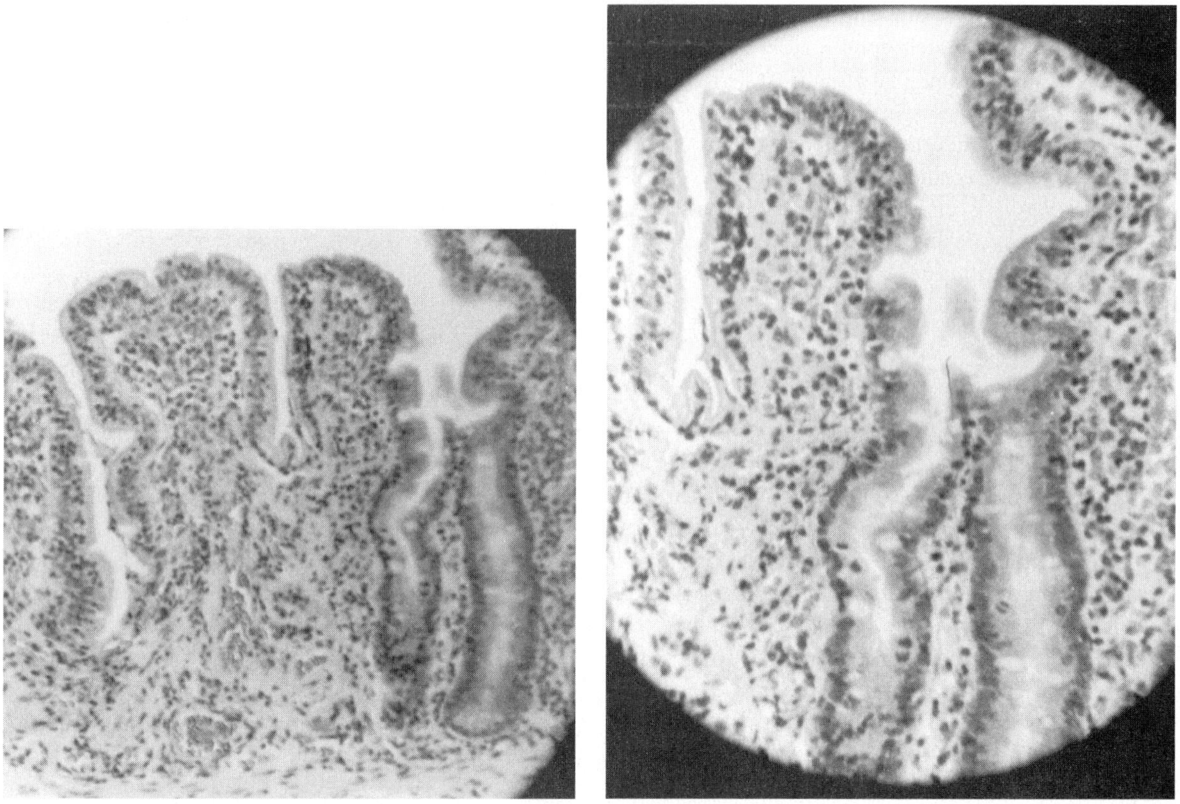

A B

FIGURE 21.2. Jejunal biopsy specimen from a patient with tropical sprue. **A:** Villi are widened by increased numbers of inflammatory cells infiltrating the lamina propria; the inflammatory cells have also migrated into the surface epithelial layer. ××100. **B:** At higher magnification, increased numbers of inflammatory cells, elongated crypts, and shortened villi are seen. The villus-to-crypt ratio is 1:1. ×400.

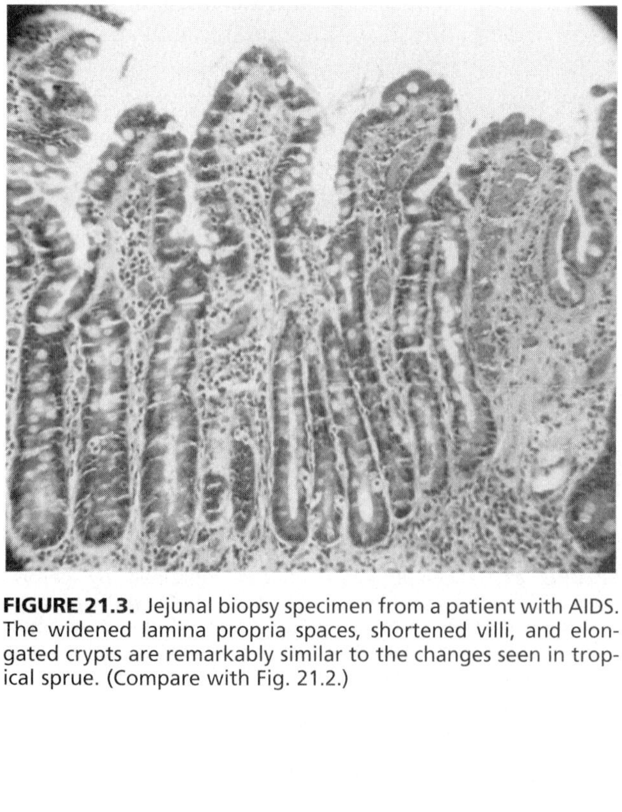

FIGURE 21.3. Jejunal biopsy specimen from a patient with AIDS. The widened lamina propria spaces, shortened villi, and elongated crypts are remarkably similar to the changes seen in tropical sprue. (Compare with Fig. 21.2.)

quently being at least as damaged as the jejunum. The more severe malabsorption of vitamin B_{12} in tropical sprue than in celiac sprue can be explained by the fact this vitamin can be absorbed only at specific sites in the ileum.

DIFFERENTIAL DIAGNOSIS: OTHER ENTEROPATHIES

In temperate climates, the most common gastrointestinal enteropathy, *celiac sprue,* may present similarly to tropical sprue, and it can also be seen in the tropics (77). Besides the more severe histologic abnormalities of the small intestine in celiac sprue, patients frequently know of family members who have had similar symptoms. Because in celiac sprue the ileum is minimally involved, if at all, vitamin B_{12} absorption is likely to be normal. Furthermore, the dramatic response to a gluten-free diet confirms the diagnosis of celiac sprue. The occasional response to gluten exclusion seen in tropical sprue is relatively muted by comparison. Diffuse *primary intestinal lymphoma* usually presents with chronic diarrhea that is often accompanied by bothersome abdominal pain, and malabsorption may not develop for months or even years. The paucity of crypts in the intestinal biopsy specimen in primary lymphoma is also a clue (76). Extensive small-intestinal *Crohn disease* may produce severe malabsorption, but intervening regions of normal mucosa and strictures are not seen in tropical sprue. *Intestinal tuberculosis* may be observed in some tropical countries and may mimic tropical sprue, but it is much less common; 100 patients with tropical sprue are seen for each one with intestinal tuberculosis (7). *AIDS* is manifested by watery diarrhea with some malabsorption and alterations in the small-intestinal histology that are very similar to those seen in tropical sprue (73,74) (compare Figs. 21.2 and 21.3). Although an enteric infection can be identified in some AIDS patients, no infectious cause can be detected in about half of them. Hence, in persons at risk for AIDS, appropriate diagnostic tests for AIDS are indicated. Small-intestinal *parasitic infestations* by *Cryptosporidium, Giardia,* and *Strongyloides* may cause diarrhea, and malabsorption may be intermittently manifested for many months or years. In Egypt, several cases of *Capillaria philippinensis* infection had severe malabsorption and intestinal changes similar to those of tropical sprue (78). However, the malabsorption secondary to parasitoses is usually mild and has little effect on the patient's nutritional status and body weight. The diagnosis can be made by appropriate stool examination for ova and parasites. Notably, vitamin B_{12} deficiency secondary to the relatively severe involvement in tropical sprue is rarely observed in parasitoses. The *intestinal stasis syndrome* (*blind loop syndrome*), in which bacterial overgrowth is caused by slowed intestinal transit, is usually a consequence of the presence of numerous small-intestinal diverticula or previous extensive gastric or intestinal surgery. Bacterial overgrowth may also occur in patients with achlorhydria, such as those with pernicious anemia (79) or the elderly (80,81), and may be associated with anorexia, diarrhea, mild malabsorption, and weight loss (82). Bacterial overgrowth may also develop in diseases that markedly alter the normal peristaltic activity in the small intestine, such as amyloidosis, pseudoobstruction, scleroderma, and extensive injury of the small intestine. Bacterial overgrowth can usually be distinguished from tropical sprue by minimal findings on small-intestinal radiography, the presence of anaerobes rather than the coliforms seen in tropical sprue, and mild and nonspecific findings on the small-intestinal biopsy specimen (83). Severe histologic lesions are occasionally seen in the intestinal stasis syndrome, and a single biopsy specimen may be insufficient to distinguish intestinal stasis syndrome from tropical sprue. However, analysis of several specimens from the same region usually reveals minimal changes in most samples in the stasis syndrome (71,83). Finally, tropical sprue frequently develops in a community setting in which an entity often called *tropical enteropathy* is highly prevalent (33,84). Such persons are healthy and their bowel habits are not altered, but intestinal biopsy may demonstrate nonspecific changes in the mucosal histology, such as a slight to moderate increase in mononuclear cellular infiltration of the lamina propria below the epithelium. The normal villus-to-crypt ratio of 3:1 to 5:1 is maintained in tropical enteropathy, and persons with this subclinical condition do not appear to be at greater risk for the development of tropical sprue than are those with normal intestinal histology.

THERAPY

Because of the apparent vitamin deficiencies in tropical sprue, yeast and liver extracts were used in the 1930s to achieve dramatic reversals of severe and often fatal anemia and malabsorption (85,86). Folic acid became available in the late 1940s (87,88) and was very effective orally as the sole therapy, especially when given to patients who had had the disease for only a few weeks. This vitamin relieves the megaloblastic anemia within days (21,22) and, during the ensuing weeks, induces a dramatic reversal of anorexia, an increase in caloric intake, and weight gain (44). The discrete response to therapy clinches the diagnosis of tropical sprue (6). A transient accentuation of pedal edema is common in the first week or so of therapy (44), but the edema subsides as nutrition improves and the serum albumin levels increase. Although it is not necessary in the acute phase of treatment, vitamin B_{12} (1,000 μg/IM weekly ×4, then monthly ×12) should also be given because a deficiency of this vitamin contributes to malabsorption. However, some intestinal malabsorption and altered histology often persist after vitamin therapy alone. When the disease has been well established for many months before the diagnosis is made, about 35% to 50% of patients may continue to have intestinal symptoms if treated only with folic acid, with or without vitamin B_{12} (21,22,44). For many of these patients, antibiotics are required to induce a complete remission. Antibacterial agents were first used in earnest during World War II, when poorly absorbed oral sulfonamides were found to be successful therapy in British military patients in the India–Burma region (18,89). Since then, both poorly absorbed sulfonamides (90) and particularly tetracycline have been given along with folic acid to achieve complete remission in the vast majority of patients with tropical sprue (45,91,92). Although the initial response may begin in only a few days, for continued improvement with reversal of all aspects of the malabsorptive enteric syndrome and the prevention of recurrence, 6 months of therapy may be required with 5 mg of oral folic acid and 250 mg of tetracycline given four times daily (45,93). Even then, intestinal biopsies may still demonstrate crypt hyperplasia and mild villus shortening for many years, and relapses requiring additional courses of therapy occur in 10% to 20% of patients who continue to reside in tropical regions where the disease is endemic (94).

THE FUTURE

Despite the intense interest shown in tropical sprue during the latter half of the twentieth century, less has been written about the malady in the last few years. Certainly it remains a formidable chronic condition causing malnutrition in many countries near the equator, where general nutrition in the local seemingly healthy population is known frequently to be borderline. It seems paradoxical that interest in this disease may be waning, even though several highly potent molecular techniques are now available for the analysis of secretions and tissues. The time is ripe for a renewed examination of microenvironmental factors in the intestinal cavity, intestinal tissue, and bone marrow, where a key to the etiology of tropical sprue seems sure to be found.

ACKNOWLEDGMENTS

Work of the author related to this chapter was supported by a research grant (DK 11270) and a Digestive Disease Center grant (DK 38707) from the National Institutes of Health, National Institute of Diabetes, Digestive and Kidney Diseases.

REFERENCES

1. Klipstein FA, Baker SJ. Regarding the definition of tropical sprue. *Gastroenterology* 1970;58:717–721.
2. Hillary W. *Observations on the changes of the air and concomitant epidemical diseases in the Island of Barbados.* London: Hitch and Hawes, 1759:277.
3. Manson P. China maritime customs II—special series No. 2. Medical reports for the half-year ended 31st March 1880, 19th issue. Shanghai: Statistical Department of the Inspectorate General, 1880:33.
4. Cook CG. Aetiology and pathogenesis of tropical sprue: do viruses play a role? *Trop Gastroenterol* 1985;6:1–3.
5. Klipstein FA, Short HB, Engert RF, et al. Contamination of the small intestine by enterotoxigenic coliform bacteria among the rural population of Haiti. *Gastroenterology* 1976;70:1035–1041.
6. Klipstein FA. Tropical sprue in travelers and expatriates living abroad. *Gastroenterology* 1981;80:590–600.
7. Mathan VI. Tropical sprue in southern India. *Trans R Soc Trop Med Hyg* 1988;82:10–14.
8. Stefanini M. Clinical features and pathogenesis of tropical sprue: observations on a series of cases among Italian prisoners of war in India. *Medicine* 1948;27:379–427.
9. Gardner FH. A malabsorption syndrome in military personnel in Puerto Rico. *Arch Intern Med* 1956;98:44–60.
10. Klipstein FA, Samloff IM, Schenk EA. Tropical sprue in Haiti. *Ann Intern Med* 1966;64:575–593.
11. Garcia S. Malabsorption and malnutrition in Mexico. *Am J Clin Nutr* 1968;21:1066–1076.
12. Mathan M, Mathan VI, Baker SJ. An electron-microscopic study of jejunal mucosal morphology in control subjects and in patients with tropical sprue in southern India. *Gastroenterology* 1975;68:17–32.
13. Moshal MG. Tropical sprue in Africa. *Lancet* 1970;2:827.
14. Webb JF, Simpson F. Tropical sprue in Hong Kong. *Br Med J* 1966;2:1162–1166.
15. O'Brien W. Historical survey of tropical sprue affecting Europeans in southeast Asia. In: *Tropical sprue and megaloblastic anaemia: Wellcome Trust Collaborative Study 1961–1969.* London: Churchill Livingstone, 1971:13–24.
16. Sparberg M, Knudson KB, Frank S. Tropical sprue from the Philippines: report of three cases. *Mil Med* 1967;132:809–815.
17. Peetermans WE, Vonck A. Tropical sprue after travel to Tanzania *J Travel Med* 2000;7:33–34.
18. Keele KD, Bound JP. Sprue in India: clinical survey of 600 cases. *Br Med J* 1946;1:77–81.
19. Ayrey F. Outbreaks of sprue during the Burma campaign. *Trans R Soc Trop Med Hyg* 1948;41:377–406.
20. O'Brien W, England NWJ. Military tropical sprue from south-east Asia. *Br Med J* 1966;2:1157–1162.
21. O'Brien W, England NWJ. Tropical sprue amongst British servicemen and their families in south-east Asia. In: *Tropical sprue and megaloblastic anaemia: Wellcome Trust Collaborative Study 1961–1969.* London: Churchill Livingstone, 1971:25–60.
22. Pittman FE, Pittman JC. Tropical sprue in American servicemen following return from Vietnam. *Am J Dig Dis* 1976;21:393–398.
23. Catino D, Proctor RF, Colwell EJ, et al. Tropical sprue. Prospective studies on incidence, early manifestations, and association with abnormal bacterial flora and intestinal parasitemia, January 1967–March 1968. Annual Progress Report, U.S. Army Medical Research Team (WRAIR), Vietnam and Institute Pasteur, Vietnam, 1 Sept 1967–30 June 1968.
24. Sheehy TW, Cohen WC, Wallace DK, et al. Tropical sprue in North Americans. *JAMA* 1965;194:1069–1076.
25. Lindenbaum J, Kent TH, Sprinz H. Malabsorption and jejunitis in American Peace Corps volunteers in Pakistan. *Ann Intern Med* 1966;65:2101–1208.
26. Lindenbaum J, Gerson CD, Kent TH. Recovery of small-intestinal structure and function after residence in the tropics. *Ann Intern Med* 1971;74:218–222.
27. Gerson CD, Kent TH, Saha JR, et al. Recovery of small-intestinal structure and function after residence in the tropics. II. Studies in Indians and Pakistanis living in New York City. *Ann Intern Med* 1971;75:41–48.
28. Klipstein FA, Falaiye JM. Tropical sprue in expatriates from the tropics living in the continental United States. *Medicine* 1969; 48:475–491.
29. Mathan VI, Baker SJ. Epidemic tropical sprue and other epidemics of diarrhea in South Indian villages. *Am J Clin Nutr* 1968;21:1077–1087.
30. Baker SJ, Mathan VI. An epidemic of tropical sprue in southern India. II Epidemiology. *Ann Trop Med Parasitol* 1970;64:453–467.
31. Mathan VI, Joseph S, Baker SJ. Tropical sprue in children. *Gastroenterology* 1969;56:556–569.
32. Santiago-Borrero PJ, Maldonado N, Horta E. Tropical sprue in children. *J Pediatr* 1970;76:470–479.
33. Baker SJ, Mathan VI. Tropical enteropathy and tropical sprue. *Am J Clin Nutr* 1972;25:1047–1055.
34. Cook GC. Aetiology and pathogenesis of postinfective tropical malabsorption (tropical sprue). *Lancet* 1984;1:721–723.
35. Glynn J. Tropical sprue—its aetiology and pathogenesis. *Trans R Soc Trop Med Hyg* 1986;79:599–606.
36. Baker SJ, Mathan VI. Tropical sprue in southern India. In: *Tropical sprue and megaloblastic anaemia: Wellcome Trust Collaborative Study 1961–1969.* London: Churchill Livingstone, 1971:189.
37. Tomkins AM, Drasar BS, James WPT. Bacterial colonization of jejunal mucosa in acute tropical sprue. *Lancet* 1975;1:59–62.
38. Gorbach SL, Banwell JG, Jacobs B, et al. Tropical sprue and malnutrition in West Bengal. I. Intestinal microflora and absorption. *Am J Clin Nutr* 1970;23:1545–1558.
39. Bhat P, Shantakumari S, Rajan D, et al. Bacterial flora of the gas-

trointestinal tract in southern Indian control subjects and patients with tropical sprue. *Gastroenterology* 1972;62:11–21.
40. Klipstein FA, Holdeman LV, Corcino JJ, et al. Enterotoxigenic intestinal bacteria in tropical sprue. *Ann Intern Med* 1973;79:632–641.
41. Appelbaum PC, Moshal MG, Hift W, et al. Intestinal bacteria in patients with tropical sprue. *S Afr Med J* 1980;57:1081–1083.
42. Toskes PP, Giannella RA, Jervis HR, et al. Small intestinal mucosal injury in the experimental blind loop syndrome: light- and electron-microscopic and histochemical studies. *Gastroenterology* 1975;68:193–203.
43. Read NW. Small bowel transit time of food in man: measurement, regulation and possible importance. *Scand J Gastroenterol* 1984;96[Suppl]:77–85.
44. Sheehy TW, Baggs B, Perez-Santiago E, et al. Prognosis of tropical sprue. A study of the effect of folic acid on the intestinal aspects of acute and chronic sprue. *Ann Intern Med* 1962;57:892–908.
45. Guerra R, Wheby MS, Bayless TM. Long-term antibiotic therapy in tropical sprue. *Ann Intern Med* 1965;63:619–634.
46. Bayless TM, Guardiola-Rotger A, Wheby MS. Tropical sprue: viral cultures of rectal swabs. *Gastroenterology* 1966;51:32–35.
47. Mathan M, Mathan VI, Swaminathan SP, et al. Pleomorphic virus-like particles in human feces. *Lancet* 1975;1:1068–1069.
48. Baker SJ, Mathan M, Mathan VI, et al. Chronic enterocyte infection with coronavirus. One possible cause of the syndrome of tropical sprue? *Dig Dis Sci* 1982;27:1039–1043.
49. Adrian TE, Savage AP, Bacarese-Hamilton AJ, et al. Peptide YY abnormalities in gastrointestinal diseases. *Gastroenterology* 1986;90:379–384.
50. Baker SJ, Mathan VI. Syndrome of tropical sprue in south India. *Am J Clin Nutr* 1968;21:984–993.
51. Wilson KH, Blitchington R, Frothingham R, et al. Phylogeny of the Whipple's disease-associated bacterium. *Lancet* 1991;338:474–475.
52. Relman DA, Schmidt TM, MacDermott RP, et al. Identification of the uncultured bacillus of Whipple's disease. *N Engl J Med* 1992;327:293–301.
53. Ratliff NB, McMahon JT, Naab TJ, et al. Whipple's disease in the porcine leaflets of a Carpentier–Edwards prosthetic mitral valve. *N Engl J Med* 1984;311:902–903.
54. Bayless TM, Knox DL. Whipple's disease: a multisystem infection. *N Engl J Med* 1979;300:920–921.
55. Dobbins WO, Kawanishi H. Bacillary characteristics in Whipple's disease: an electron microscopic study. *Gastroenterology* 1981;80:1468–1475.
56. Santiago-Borrero PJ, Maldonado N, Horta E. Tropical sprue in children. *J Pediatr* 1970;76:470–479.
57. Mathan VI, Joseph S, Baker SJ. Tropical sprue in children. A syndrome of idiopathic malabsorption. *Gastroenterology* 1969;56:556–569.
58. Trier JS. Case 15-1990. Case records of the Massachusetts General Hospital. Weekly clinicopathological exercises. *N Engl J Med* 1990;322:1067–1075.
59. Baker SJ. The recognition of vitamin B_{12} and folate deficiency. *N Z Med J* 1966;65:884–892.
60. Sparberg M, Knudson KB, Frank S. Tropical sprue from the Philippines: report of three cases. *Mil Med* 1967;809–815.
61. Vaish SK, Ignatius M, Baker SJ. Albumin metabolism in tropical sprue. *Q J Med* 1965;34:15–32.
62. Gray GM, Santiago NA. Disaccharide absorption in normal and diseased human intestine. *Gastroenterology* 1966;51:489–498.
63. Gray GM, Walter WM Jr, Colver EH. Persistent deficiency of intestinal lactase in apparently cured tropical sprue. *Gastroenterology* 1968;54:552–558.
64. Menendez-Corrada R, Nettleship E, Santiago-Delpin EA. HLA and tropical sprue. *Lancet* 1986;2:1183–1185.
65. Jayanthi V, Chacko A, Gani IK, et al. Intestinal transit in healthy southern Indian subjects in patients and tropical sprue. *Gut* 1989;30:35–38.
66. Cook GC. Delayed small-intestinal transit in tropical malabsorption. *Br Med J* 1978;2:238–240.
67. Tawil SC, Brandt LJ, Bernstein LH. Mosaic mucosa in tropical sprue. *Endoscopy* 1991;37:365–366.
68. Shah VH, Rotterdam H, Kotler DP, et al. All that scallops is not celiac disease. *Gastrointest Endosc* 2000;51:717–720.
69. Swanson VL, Wheby MS, Bayless TM. Morphologic effects of folic acid and vitamin B_{12} on the jejunal lesion of tropical sprue. *Am J Pathol* 1966;49:167–197.
70. Swanson VL, Thomassen RW. Pathology of the jejunal mucosa in tropical sprue. *Am J Pathol* 1965;46:511–551.
71. Perera DR, Weinstein WM, Rubin CE. Small intestinal biopsy. *Hum Pathol* 1975;6:157–217.
72. Schenk EA, Samloff IM, Klipstein FA. Morphologic characteristics of jejunal biopsy in celiac disease and tropical sprue. *Am J Pathol* 1965;47:765–781.
73. Kotler DP, Gaetz HP, Lange M, et al. Enteropathy associated with the acquired immunodeficiency syndrome. *Ann Intern Med* 1984;101:421–428.
74. Madi K, Trajman A, da Silver CF, et al. Jejunal biopsy in HIV-infected patients. *J AIDS* 1991;4:930–937.
75. Maiwald M, Relman DA. Whipple's disease and *Tropheryma whippelii*: secrets slowly revealed. *Clin Infect Dis* 2001;32:457–463.
76. Gray GM, Rosenberg SA, Cooper AD, et al. Lymphomas involving the gastrointestinal tract. *Gastroenterology* 1982;82:143–152.
77. Misra RC, Kasthuri D, Chuttani HK. Adult coeliac disease in tropics. *Br Med J* 1966;2:1230–1232.
78. Ahmed L, el-Dib NA, el-Boraey Y, et al. *Capillaria philippinensis*: an emerging parasite causing severe diarrhoea in Egypt. *J Egypt Soc Parasitol* 1999;29:483–493.
79. Lindenbaum J, Pezzimenti JF, Shea N. Small-intestinal function in vitamin B_{12} deficiency. *Ann Intern Med* 1974;80:326–331.
80. Roberts SH, James O, Jarvis EH. Bacterial overgrowth syndrome without "blind loop": a cause for malnutrition in the elderly. *Lancet* 1977;2:1193–1195.
81. McEvoy A, Dutton J, James OFW. Bacterial contamination of the small intestine is an important cause of occult malabsorption in the elderly. *Br Med J* 1983;287:789–793.
82. King CE, Toskes PP. Small intestine bacterial overgrowth. *Gastroenterology* 1979;76:1035–1055.
83. Ament ME, Shimoda SS, Saunders DR, et al. Pathogenesis of steatorrhea in three cases of small intestinal stasis syndrome. *Gastroenterology* 1972;63:728–747.
84. Chaves FJZC, Veloso FT, Cruz I, et al. Subclinical tropical enteropathy in Angola: peroral jejunal biopsies and absorption studies in asymptomatic healthy men. *Mt Sinai J Med* 1981;48:47–52.
85. Wills L. Treatment of "pernicious anaemia of pregnancy" and "tropical anaemia" with special reference to yeast extract as a curative agent. *Br Med J* 1931;1:1059–1064.
86. Rhoads CP, Miller DK. Intensive liver extract therapy of sprue. *JAMA* 1934;103:387–391.
87. Spies TD, Milanes F, Menendez A, et al. Observations on treatment of tropical sprue with folic acid. *J Lab Clin Med* 1946;31:227–241.
88. Suarez RM, Spies TD, Suarez RM Jr. Use of folic acid in sprue. *Ann Intern Med* 1947;26:643–677.

89. Keele KD, Bound JP. Sprue in India: a clinical survey of 600 cases. *Br Med J* 1946;1:77–81.
90. Maldonado N, Horta E, Guerra R, et al. Poorly absorbed sulfonamides in the treatment of tropical sprue. *Gastroenterology* 1969; 57:559–568.
91. French JM, Gaddie R, Smith NM. Tropical sprue: a study of seven cases and their response to combined chemotherapy. *Q J Med* 1956;25:333–351.
92. Sheehy TW, Perez-Santiago E. Antibiotic therapy in tropical sprue. *Gastroenterology* 1961;41:208–213.
93. Klipstein FA, Falaiye J. Tropical sprue in expatriates from the tropics living in the continental United States. *Medicine (Baltimore)* 1969;48:475–492.
94. Rickles FR, Klipstein FA, Tomasini J, et al. Long-term follow-up of antibiotic-treated tropical sprue. *Ann Intern Med* 1972;76: 203–210.

22

SMALL INTESTINE BACTERIAL OVERGROWTH, INCLUDING BLIND LOOP SYNDROME

PHILLIP P. TOSKES

The development of malabsorption in a patient with overgrowth of bacteria within the small intestine is known as the blind loop, stagnant loop, stasis, or bacterial overgrowth syndrome. In this condition, the bacterial flora of the proximal small intestine resembles that of the healthy colon. The qualitative and quantitative changes in flora that occur wreak havoc with the nutritional status of the human host. The overgrowth flora successfully competes with the human host for the ingested nutrients. What ensues is a complex array of clinical problems resulting from intraluminal bacterial catabolism of nutrients, often with production of toxic metabolites, and direct injury to the small-intestine enterocyte (1,2).

DESCRIPTION OF NORMAL ENTERIC FLORA

Normally the stomach and small intestine harbor relatively few bacteria. The qualitative and quantitative aspects of the flora of the normal human gastrointestinal (GI) tract are described in Table 22.1. The kinds of bacteria found in the normal upper small intestine (the jejunum is the standard reference site for intestinal aspirates) consist of gram-positive aerobes or facultative anaerobes in concentrations of up to 10^4 organisms per milliliter of jejunal secretions. The jejunum of a healthy subject may contain coliforms transiently, with concentrations rarely exceeding 10^3 bacteria per milliliter of secretions. The upper small intestine of healthy subjects does not contain anaerobic bacteroides.

The ileum appears to represent a zone of transition from the sparse populations of aerobic flora found in the stomach and proximal bowel and the very dense bacterial populations of anaerobic microorganisms found in the colon. In the ileum, the concentrations of microorganisms increase to levels of 10^5 to 10^9 organisms per gram of contents. Enterobacteria, including coliforms, occur only transiently and in small numbers in the proximal bowel but are regularly found in substantial numbers in the ileum. Strict anaerobes, which normally cannot survive in the jejunum, frequently colonize the ileum.

The most dramatic change in the enteric flora occurs across the ileocecal valve. The number of microorganisms increases up to one million fold and approximately 10^9 to 10^{12} microorganisms per gram of colonic contents. The large-bowel flora is dominated by fastidious anaerobic organisms such as bacteroides, anaerobic lactobacilli, and clostridia. These microorganisms, although difficult to culture, actually outnumber aerobic and facultative organisms by as many as 10,000 : 1 within the lumen of the colon. When the ileocecal valve is resected, the populations of the most distal portions of the ileum tend to resemble those of the cecum.

Table 22.2 lists, in order of decreasing frequency, those factors that normally prevent the development of bacterial overgrowth.

Undoubtedly, the major factor responsible for limiting bacterial proliferation in the small bowel is the cleansing

TABLE 22.1. NORMAL BACTERIAL FLORA WITHIN THE GASTROINTESTINAL TRACT

	Stomach	Jejunum	Ileum	Cecum
Total bacterial counts[a]	0–3	0–4	5–8	10–12
Aerobes and facultative anaerobes	0–3	0–4	2–5	2–9
Anaerobes	0	0	3–7	9–12

[a]Log10 of the number of viable microorganisms per gram of contents.
From Toskes P. Bacterial overgrowth of the gastrointestinal tract. *Adv Intern Med* 1993;38:387–407, with permission.

P.P. Toskes: Department of Medicine, University of Florida and Shands Hospital at the Univeristy of Florida, Gainesville, Florida

TABLE 22.2. ENDOGENOUS DEFENSE MECHANISMS FOR PREVENTING BACTERIAL OVERGROWTH

- Intestinal motility
- Gastric acid secretion
- Intact ileocecal sphincter
- Immunoglobulins within intestinal secretions
- Ill-defined mucosal factors
- Bacteriostatic properties of pancreatic–biliary secretion

action of normal propulsive motility of the intestinal tract. In the relatively stagnant contents of the large bowel, bacterial growth is luxuriant, whereas microorganisms are rapidly cleared from the small intestine. Of particular importance in this regard is the interdigestive migrating motor complex (MMC), which is responsible for sweeping the bowel clean. Mucus may aid in this mechanical process for removing bacteria, a possibility that is supported by the fact that microorganisms tend to concentrate in the mucous layer that lines the GI mucosa. The crucial importance of normal small-bowel peristalsis is emphasized because whenever normal motility is slowed or interrupted, bacterial overgrowth ($>10^4$ microorganisms per milliliter of jejunal contents) rapidly ensues.

Bacterial interactions within the gut lumen represent an important, if still poorly understood, determinant of the bacterial populations inhabiting the alimentary canal.

It is important to recognize, for example, that without the oxygen-using aerobes such as coliforms and enterococci, the colon would not be sufficiently anaerobic to maintain the large populations of fastidious anaerobes such as the bacteroides. Anaerobes stabilize the enteric flora, thereby preventing overgrowth with pathogens. In patients with bacterial overgrowth, the flora closely resembles that of the normal colon. Quantitative counts may reach 10^{10} viable bacteria per milliliter of secretions. Bacteroides and anaerobic lactobacilli usually predominate, but enterobacteria, enterococci, clostridia, and diphtheroids may also be present in high concentrations (1,2).

CLINICAL CONDITIONS ASSOCIATED WITH BACTERIAL OVERGROWTH

The recognized clinical conditions associated with bacterial overgrowth are listed in Table 22.3. In the past when much more aggressive GI tract surgery was performed on a more regular basis, anatomic abnormalities (e.g., Billroth II anastomosis and surgery for Crohn's disease) were the most common causes of clinically significant bacterial overgrowth. Blind pouches of the small intestine formed surgically by the creation of an end-to-side enteroenteric anastomosis frequently produce bacterial overgrowth. Similarly, stagnant loops of intestine resulting from fistulas or surgical enterostomies allow for continuous recirculation of small-intestine contents and consequent bacterial overgrowth. After partial gastrectomy and Billroth II anastomosis, dysfunction and stasis in the afferent loop may result in marked intraluminal proliferation of bacteria and consequent seeding of the remainder of the small intestine (3). Duodenal and jejunal diverticula may result in overgrowth, particularly in the setting of hypochlorhydria or achlorhydria (Fig. 22.1) (4). Obstruction of the small intestine due to Crohn's disease (Fig. 22.2), adhesions, radiation damage, lymphoma, or tuberculosis may cause bacterial overgrowth (5–8). Patients with gastrocolic or gastrojejunocolic fistulas with colonic contents passing into the stomach and small intestine may develop a massive bacterial seeding of the small intestine and devastating malabsorption (9). Patients with Kock distal ileal pouches (continent ileostomy) may experience malabsorption secondary to bacterial overgrowth (10).

TABLE 22.3. CLINICAL CONDITIONS ASSOCIATED WITH BACTERIAL OVERGROWTH

Gastric proliferation
- Hypochlorhydria or achlorhydria, especially when combined with motor or anatomic disturbances
- Sustained hypochlorhydria induced by omeprazole

Small intestinal stagnation

Anatomic
- Afferent loop of Billroth II partial gastrectomy
- Duodenal–jejunal diverticulosis
- Surgical blind loop (end-to-side anastomosis)
- Surgical recirculating loop (end-to-side anastomosis)
- Obstruction (stricture, adhesion, inflammation, neoplasm)

Motor
- Scleroderma
- Idiopathic intestinal pseudoobstruction
- Absent or disordered migrating motor complex
- Diabetic autonomic neuropathy

Abnormal communication between proximal and distal gastrointestinal tract
- Gastrocolic or jejunocolic fistula
- Resection of diseased ileocecal valve

Miscellaneous
- Chronic pancreatitis
- Immunodeficiency syndromes
- Cirrhosis

Modified from Toskes P, Kumar K. Enteric bacterial flora and bacterial overgrowth syndrome. In: Feldman M, Scharschmidt B, Sleisenger M, eds. Gastrointestinal and liver disease, sixth edition, Philadelphia, WB Saunders, 1998:1523–1535, with permission.

Abnormalities in intestinal motility, often combined with decreased gastric acid secretion, favor bacterial proliferation and subsequent malabsorption. Patients with scleroderma (11) (Fig. 22.3), intestinal pseudoobstruction (12), and diabetic autonomic neuropathy (13) are examples of such. Patients with an absent or disordered MMC may develop bacterial overgrowth and malabsorption (14); such patients may have no radiographic abnormalities.

Elderly patients may develop malabsorption secondary to bacterial overgrowth; indeed it has been suggested that

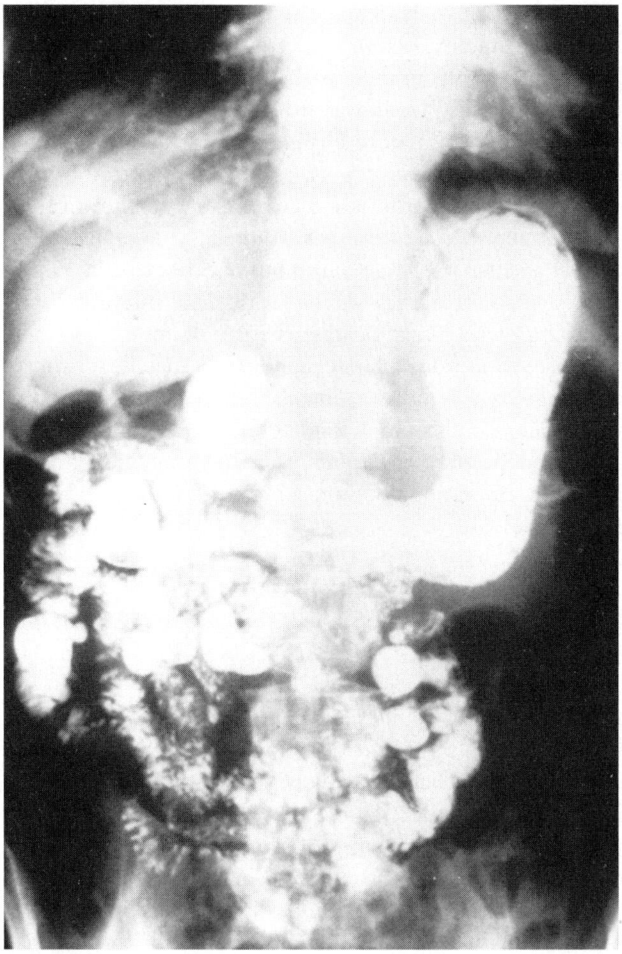

FIGURE 22.1. Multiple duodenal and jejunal diverticula in a patient with malabsorption secondary to bacterial overgrowth. (From Toskes PP. Bacterial overgrowth of the gastrointestinal tract. *Adv Intern Med* 1993;38:387–407, with permission.)

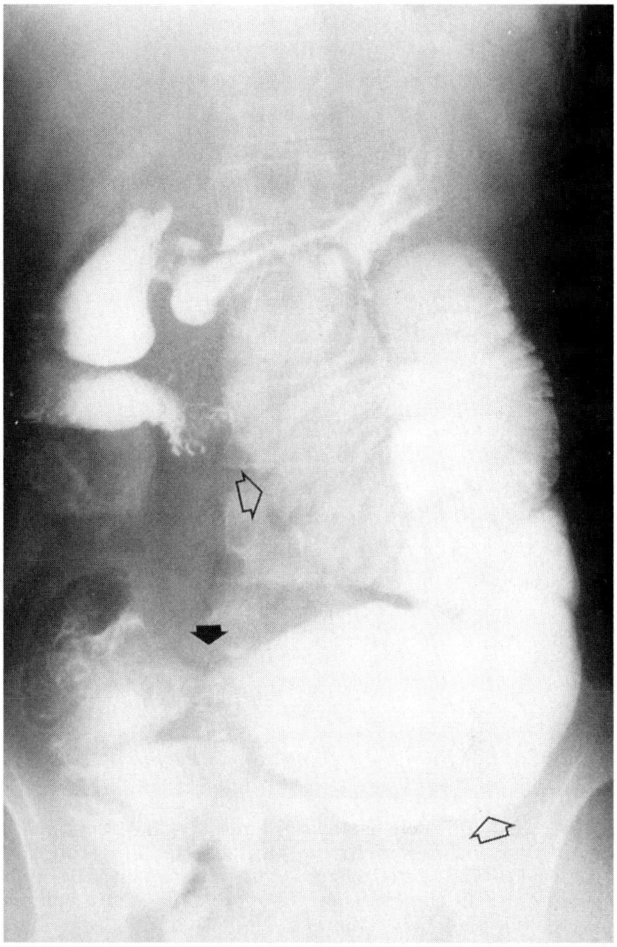

FIGURE 22.2. Stricture in proximal ileum (*solid arrow*) with proximal dilated small-bowel loops (*open arrows*) in a patient with Crohn's disease and clinically important malabsorption due to bacterial overgrowth. (From Toskes PP. Bacterial overgrowth syndromes. In: Haubricher W, Schaffner F, eds. *Bockus gastroenterology,* fifth edition. Philadelphia: 1995:1174–1182, with permission.)

bacterial overgrowth is the most common cause of clinically significant malabsorption in the elderly (15–18). The elderly may have motor disorders (often induced by prior GI tract surgery) of the small intestine and decreased acid secretion. Some studies have demonstrated correction of the "failure to thrive syndrome" in elderly subjects after treatment with antibiotics. Other studies in healthy elderly subjects demonstrated a high frequency of bacterial overgrowth, but it appeared to be of little clinical significance (19,20). Most of such individuals had normal absorption of nutrients despite significant overgrowth of the proximal small intestine. Such a condition has been called "simple colonization." It may very well be a different situation if elderly subjects are ill or have associated hypomotility of the small intestine or anatomic abnormalities such as duodenal diverticula or previous GI tract surgery.

Intestinal bacteria may metabolize a number of endogenous substances such as bile acids, cholesterol, and unabsorbed lipids, as well as proteins and carbohydrates. The byproducts of this metabolism may be of benefit or harm to the normal host. An exaggeration of this metabolism occurs in the bacterial overgrowth syndrome. It is important to point out that the normal bacterial flora also is important in the metabolism of some drugs and other xenobiotics. Medications metabolized by intestinal bacteria include digoxin, L-dopa, colchicine, morphine, conjugated estrogens, chloramphenicol, rifampin, and sulfasalazine. Just how important the excessive metabolism of medications is, which may occur in the bacterial overgrowth condition, is yet to be defined. This is particularly important when the many medications that the healthy and the unhealthy elderly subject consumes are taken into consideration. Perhaps this relatively frequent overgrowth condition in the elderly may lead to ineffective dosing schedules for the elderly and adverse clinical consequences.

The importance of both normal intestinal motility and normal gastric acid secretion to the prevention of clinically

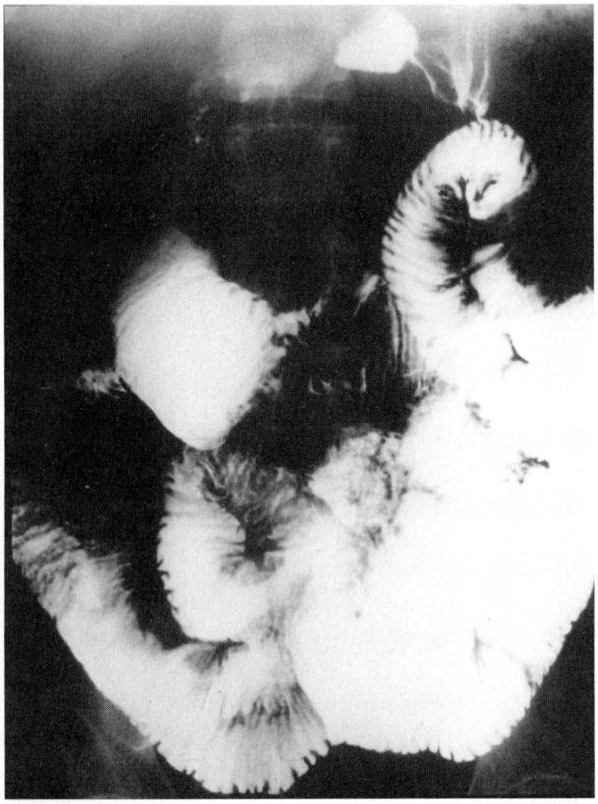

FIGURE 22.3. Diffusely dilated small intestine in a patient with scleroderma and malabsorption due to bacterial overgrowth. (From Toskes PP. Bacterial overgrowth syndromes. In: Haubricher W, Schaffner F, eds. *Bockus gastroenterology,* fifth edition. Philadelphia: 1995:1174–1182, with permission.)

significant bacterial overgrowth is underscored by recent clinical experiences wherein patients with scleroderma and reflux esophagitis doing relatively well on H_2 receptor antagonists or antacid therapy developed marked malabsorption (diarrhea, steatorrhea) after the institution of omeprazole. Omeprazole decreased markedly the remaining acid secretion in these patients, thus allowing bacterial overgrowth to occur. Bacterial overgrowth has been documented in 56% of 25 outpatients with reflux esophagitis and/or peptic ulcer disease who had received 40 mg of omeprazole for about 5 weeks (21). Whether this development of bacterial overgrowth in these types of ambulatory patients will have any clinical consequences remains to be determined. It appears that the bacterial overgrowth related to omeprazole treatment is similar to the simple colonization observed in the healthy elderly patient. Another study failed to show any effect of omeprazole therapy on fat or carbohydrate absorption despite the induction of bacterial overgrowth (20). In both of these studies, the use of omeprazole was short term. Perhaps long-term use of proton pump inhibitors might lead to clinically significant overgrowth, particularly if there is an associated abnormality (functional or structural) of the small intestine, as discussed above.

Up to 40% of patients with chronic pancreatitis may have concomitant bacterial overgrowth (22). Bacterial overgrowth may occur in these patients because of a decrease in intestinal motility resulting from pain, fever, use of narcotics, and inflammatory changes or obstruction from the enlarged inflamed pancreas or may be due to previous pancreatic surgery. Appropriate therapy of steatorrhea in these patients may require both pancreatic enzymes and antimicrobial agents. There are a number of other clinical conditions that seem to be associated with small-intestine bacterial overgrowth, but the pathogenesis is ill understood in all of these conditions. These conditions include cirrhosis, end-stage renal disease, myotonic muscular dystrophy, fibromyalgia, chronic fatigue syndrome, and various immunodeficiency syndromes such as chronic lymphocytic leukemia, immunoglobulin deficiencies, and selected T-cell deficiencies.

CLINICAL MANIFESTATIONS OF BACTERIAL OVERGROWTH

Although clinical manifestations vary greatly and depend, at least in part, on the nature of the small-intestine abnormality causing the bacterial overgrowth, certain clinical features are hallmarks of the bacterial overgrowth syndrome. These features are pointed out in Table 22.4. Patients with bacterial overgrowth may demonstrate some or all of these features.

Patients with strictures, surgically formed blind pouches of the small intestine, or functional dysmotility of the small intestine may note abdominal discomfort, bloating, and crampy periumbilical pain before diarrhea, steatorrhea, and the symptoms of anemia develop. When patients have strictures or fistulas caused by Crohn's disease of the small intestine or hypomotility caused by scleroderma or intestinal pseudoobstruction, the clinical features of the primary disease may completely overshadow any manifestations of intraluminal microbial proliferation. Furthermore, it may be difficult to determine in patients with Crohn's disease, radiation enteritis, short-bowel syndrome, or lymphoma the extent to which malabsorption is due to primary intestinal disease or secondary bacterial overgrowth.

Whatever the cause of the abnormal proliferation of microorganisms within the small-intestine lumen, the con-

TABLE 22.4. CLINICAL FEATURES OF BACTERIAL OVERGROWTH

- Cobalamin (vitamin B_{12}) malabsorption and deficiency
- Bloating
- Abdominal pain
- Steatorrhea
- Diarrhea
- Decreased urinary xylose excretion
- Hypoalbuminemia

sequences for the patient are the same. Weight loss associated with clinically apparent steatorrhea has been observed in about one third of patients with small-intestine bacterial overgrowth severe enough to cause cobalamin deficiency (23). Osteomalacia, vitamin K deficiency, night blindness, and even hypocalcemic tetany have been known to develop as a consequence of lipid malabsorption in patients with this disorder. Appropriate therapy or surgical correction of the small-intestine lesion conducive to stasis promptly reduced fecal fat excretion to normal or near normal levels.

The clinical features of small-intestine bacterial overgrowth are changing (24). Conditions previously noted to be commonly associated with bacterial overgrowth such as various surgically induced conditions are now encountered much less frequently. Dysmotility syndromes such as gastroparesis and irritable bowel syndrome, in addition to chronic pancreatitis, account for the majority of patients who are now found to have documented evidence of bacterial overgrowth. Patients with these conditions can have the same symptoms they would have with superimposed bacterial overgrowth. It is important to suspect and document superimposed bacterial overgrowth in patients with these conditions so the proper diagnosis and management can be accomplished. The most common symptoms in these patients are diarrhea, weight loss, bloating, and excess flatulence. Abdominal pain, nausea, and steatorrhea are also noted but somewhat less frequently.

PATHOGENESIS OF NUTRIENT MALABSORPTION AND DEFICIENCY DUE TO BACTERIAL OVERGROWTH

Ample evidence indicates that the anemia that develops in patients with blind loop syndrome is largely due to cobalamin (vitamin B_{12}) deficiency. The anemia is usually megaloblastic and macrocytic, and serum cobalamin levels are low. Furthermore, neurologic changes indistinguishable from those of pernicious anemia may develop, and the anemia can be corrected by physiologic doses of the vitamin. Cobalamin malabsorption, which cannot be corrected by intrinsic factor, is a hallmark of clinically significant small-bowel bacterial overgrowth. Competitive uptake of the vitamin is particularly characteristic of gram-negative aerobes and various anaerobes that proliferate in the small bowel during stasis. Intrinsic factor effectively inhibits aerobic microbial uptake of cobalamin but has no effect on cobalamin uptake by gram-negative anaerobes (*Bacteroides*) (25). Because *in vivo* intrinsic factor binds cobalamin before the vitamin comes in contact with intestinal bacteria, gram-negative anaerobes appear to be the bacteria responsible for the cobalamin malabsorption associated with bacterial overgrowth.

In the experimental blind loop syndrome and in some patients with overgrowth, iron deficiency is secondary to blood lost through the GI tract, perhaps secondary to ulcerated areas within stagnant loops (26). Under these circumstances, the patient may have guaiac-positive stools, together with a microcytic and hypochromic anemia, or in some instances anemia with two populations of red blood cells: microcytic and macrocytic. Folate deficiency is not a common occurrence in blind loop syndrome. Unlike the situation with cobalamin, folate synthesized by microorganisms in the small intestine appears to be available for the host, and in patients with small-intestine bacterial overgrowth, serum folate levels tend to be high, rather than low (27).

Bloating and abdominal pain often result from an action of the overgrowth flora on fat and carbohydrate substrates within the lumen of the small intestine. Because of a decreased transport of nutrients across the damaged small intestine, more unabsorbed nutrients are presented to the distal intestine, where further metabolism and production of toxic byproducts are produced, leading to abdominal distention, pain, diarrhea, or steatorrhea.

Fat malabsorption associated with small-bowel bacterial overgrowth results from bacterial alteration of bile salts (28). When bacteria proliferate in the small bowel, they deconjugate bile salts to form free bile acids, which are present in small-bowel contents as protonated bile acids, and which are readily reabsorbed from the jejunum. If bacterial hydrolysis of conjugated bile salts is sufficiently rapid, bile salt micelle formation is impaired because of low bile acid concentration, and fat is poorly absorbed.

Deficiency of bile salt unquestionably limits intestinal transport of monoglyceride and fatty acids, but bile salt deficiency is probably not the only factor responsible for steatorrhea in bacterial overgrowth. Accumulation of "toxic" concentrations of free bile acids may also contribute to steatorrhea in bacterial overgrowth, and the patchy intestinal mucosal lesion noted in blind loop syndrome almost certainly plays a role in fat malabsorption.

Diarrhea may result from bacterial production of organic acids, thereby increasing the osmolarity of small-intestine contents and decreasing the intraluminal pH level. Also, bacterial metabolites such as free bile acids, hydroxylated fatty acids, and organic acids stimulate secretion of water and electrolytes into the bowel lumen (28).

Experimental bacterial overgrowth in rats leads to small-intestine motility disturbances, which can be reversed with antibiotic therapy (29).

Decreased urinary xylose excretion is frequently seen in both the clinical and the experimental blind loop syndrome. Although studies employing carbon-14 (^{14}C)–xylose in the experimental blind loop syndrome have shown that the decreased urinary xylose excretion was due primarily to intraluminal catabolism of xylose to carbon dioxide, the decreased absorption of xylose in the setting of bacterial overgrowth may be secondary to both intraluminal catabolism of xylose by bacteria and diminished absorption due to small-intestine mucosal dysfunction (30).

Hypoproteinemia is a frequent manifestation of blind loop syndrome and is occasionally severe enough to cause edema. The etiology of the hypoproteinemia is multifactorial and may result from decreased uptake of amino acids by the damaged small intestine, intraluminal breakdown of protein and protein precursors by bacteria, and antibiotic-reversible protein-losing enteropathy (31).

In general, malabsorption can be attributed to intraluminal effects of proliferating bacteria, combined with damage to the enterocyte itself. A patchy small-bowel mucosal lesion of uncertain pathogenesis can be readily identified in experimental animals and in patients with bacterial overgrowth (31).

Moderate blunting of villi, loss of structural integrity of some of the surface epithelial cells, and increased cellular infiltration of the lamina propria are characteristic.

DIAGNOSIS OF BACTERIAL OVERGROWTH

Overgrowth of bacteria within the small intestine should be considered in the differential diagnosis of any patient who presents with diarrhea, steatorrhea, weight loss, or macrocytic anemia, particularly if the patient is elderly or has had abdominal surgery. The presence of dysphagia should suggest the diagnosis of scleroderma, or repeated bouts of intestinal obstruction without obvious organic cause suggest intestinal pseudoobstruction. The presence of small-intestine bacterial overgrowth should be strongly suspected in a patient with excessive bloating, abdominal distention, and flatulence, particularly if there may be an associated dysmotility condition.

When the clinical presentation suggests that proliferation of microorganisms in the small-intestine lumen may cause or contribute to malabsorption, further evaluation is necessary for optimal management. The presence of steatorrhea should be documented. If the patient has clinically significant bacterial overgrowth, cobalamin absorption is frequently impaired, even though the patient may not yet have become cobalamin deficient. Intrinsic factor will not improve cobalamin absorption in these patients. The urinary excretion of xylose may be decreased and the serum folate increased in some, but not all, patients with blind loop syndrome.

A small-intestine biopsy is of value in excluding primary mucosal disease as the cause of the malabsorption. Although striking histologic abnormalities of jejunal mucosa are not usually seen in patients with bacterial overgrowth, the biopsy results are often abnormal. A patchy lesion of variable severity may be observed. Increased infiltration of the lamina propria with lymphocytes, plasma cells, and polymorphonuclear leukocytes, together with thickening and blunting of villi, may be seen. However, one does not find the diffuse alterations of the surface absorptive cells regularly present in celiac sprue. Although in some cases, the biopsy specimen from a patient with blind loop syndrome may show changes suggestive of tropical sprue, the history and intestinal culture should differentiate these two disorders.

The sine qua non for the diagnosis of bacterial overgrowth is a properly collected and appropriately cultured aspirate from the proximal small intestine. The specimen should be obtained under anaerobic conditions, serially diluted, and cultured on several selective media. In patients with clinically significant bacterial overgrowth, a number of different species are found, and the total concentration of bacteria generally exceeds 10^5 organisms per milliliter. Bacteroides, anaerobic lactobacilli, coliforms, and enterococci are all likely to be present in varying numbers. Although in most patients the intraluminal microbial proliferation can be documented in the proximal jejunum, it is important to recognize that pockets of overgrowth may be missed by a single culture, and that bacterial overgrowth may occur only in the more distal portions of the small intestine. An intestinal culture requires intubation of the small intestine and time-consuming microbiologic analyses.

Another approach to diagnosing bacterial overgrowth is the timed analysis of breath excretion of volatile metabolites produced by intraluminal bacteria. Both measurement of expired labeled CO_2 after oral administration of ^{14}C or ^{13}C-labeled substrates and breath hydrogen after administration of nonlabeled fermentable substrate have been employed.

The bile acid or ^{14}C–cholylglycine breath test was the first ^{14}C breath test used to diagnose bacterial overgrowth. Although frequently able to detect bacterial overgrowth, the bile acid breath test does not differentiate bacterial overgrowth from ileal damage or resection with excessive breath $^{14}CO_2$ production due to bacterial deconjugation within the colon of unabsorbed ^{14}C bile salt. In addition, false-negative results have been described in 30% to 40% of patients with culture-proven overgrowth (32,33).

A 1-g ^{14}C–xylose breath test appears to be a sensitive and specific test to detect the presence of bacterial overgrowth (34). Elevated $^{14}CO_2$ levels appear within the breath in 85% of patients within the first 60 minutes of the test, with the 30-minute breath sample being the most reliable. Xylose is attractive as a substrate because (a) xylose is catabolized by gram-negative aerobes, which are always part of the overgrowth flora, (b) xylose is predominantly absorbed in the proximal small bowel as contrasted to the predominant ileal absorption of bile salts, leading to virtually no "dumping" of xylose into the colon, and (c) xylose is metabolized substantially less than other proximally absorbed substrates, such as glucose.

A number of laboratories throughout the world have evaluated the ^{14}C–xylose breath test and have documented its reliability in detecting small-intestine bacterial overgrowth (35,36). In those studies that used the intestinal culture as the gold standard and evaluated shorter sampling intervals, particularly the 30-minute time point, the sensitivity and specificity approximated 90%. Some recent studies have raised doubts concerning the reliability of the xylose breath test, but those studies evaluated patients with severe disorders of motility such that it is quite possible that the xylose never left the stomach appropriately to come in contact with the overgrowth flora in the proximal small intestine (37). In addition, there must be an overgrowth of gram-negative coliforms for the xylose test result to be positive. In at least one of the recent studies, failing to confirm the reliability of the xylose breath test, the culture seems to be lacking a significant amount of gram-negative coliforms (38). Others have suggested that refinement of the xylose breath test include a transit marker for intestinal motility, which may enhance the specificity (39).

Because it has been recommended that ^{14}C-labeled xylose not be used in the diagnosis of bacterial overgrowth in children or fertile women, ^{13}C-labeled substrates have been shown in preliminary studies to be quite effective in diagnosing this condition. Studies with both ^{13}C-labeled xylose or ^{13}C-labeled sorbitol have been reported.

Breath hydrogen analysis allows a distinct separation of metabolic activities of the overgrowth flora from that of the human host because hydrogen is not produced to any great significance in mammalian tissue. Excessive breath hydrogen production has been noted in patients with bacterial overgrowth after the administration of 50 to 80 g of glucose or 10 to 12 g of lactulose. A fasting elevation of breath hydrogen is an excellent test for detecting small-intestine bacterial overgrowth, but approximately only one-third of subjects with culture-proven overgrowth will have elevated fasting levels of breath hydrogen (40).

The sensitivity and specificity of the hydrogen breath test are disappointing when used to detect bacterial overgrowth (41). The nonradioactive nature and the ease of performance of hydrogen breath tests make them quite attractive. However, the preponderance of studies indicate that these tests have an unacceptable sensitivity and specificity for clinical use.

TREATMENT OF BACTERIAL OVERGROWTH

The aim of therapy for small-intestine bacterial overgrowth is to correct, when feasible, the cause of this condition, but surgery is often impractical (e.g., with scleroderma, multiple diverticula, diabetes, and intestinal pseudoobstruction) and unacceptable to the patient. Thus, medical management of patients with bacterial overgrowth is lifelong. Antibiotic therapy is the cornerstone of treatment and remarkable improvement in symptoms can be achieved in most patients. It is important to emphasize once again that bacterial overgrowth may be a treatable component of the malabsorption seen in patients with diseases such as Crohn's disease, intestinal lymphoma, radiation enteritis, gastroparesis, irritable bowel syndrome, and chronic pancreatitis. The deterioration in absorption in such patients may not be caused by their primary disease process but by the associated bacterial overgrowth. Clinicians also must be aware that bacterial overgrowth may be present without causing any disease. Not all patients who have a pathologic flora in the proximal small intestine develop clinically important symptoms. An abnormal breath test result similar to a pathologic culture must be put into perspective by the clinician before therapeutic decisions are made.

It would seem attractive to select the appropriate antibiotic by evaluation of the sensitivity of the bacteria present in the lumen of the small bowel. However, this approach is very problematic because many different bacterial species are present, often with very different sensitivities. It is important to select an antibiotic agent that is effective against both aerobic and anaerobic enteric bacteria. Although it is true that most patients with clinically significant malabsorption secondary to the bacterial overgrowth have a flora that is largely overgrown with anaerobes, there are patients with malabsorption associated predominantly with the overgrowth of gram-negative aerobes such as *Escherichia coli, Klebsiella, or Pseudomonas* (42). Table 22.5 lists antimicrobial agents that have been effective in treating bacterial overgrowth whether in controlled clinical trials or extensive clinical practice. The activities of antibiotics largely limited to anaerobes and antibiotics such as metronidazole or clindamycin have not been effective when used as monotherapy. Antibiotics that are known to have poor activity against anaerobes should not be used in treating bacterial overgrowth. Such antibiotics include penicillin, ampicillin, the oral aminoglycosides, kanamycin, and neomycin.

In most patients, a single course of therapy (10 days) markedly improves symptoms and the patient may remain symptom free for months; in others, symptoms recur quickly and acceptable results can only be obtained with cyclic therapy (1 week out of every 4 weeks); and in still others, continuous therapy may be needed for 1 or 2 months. If the

TABLE 22.5. EFFECTIVE ANTIMICROBIAL AGENTS FOR TREATING BACTERIAL OVERGROWTH

Agent	Dose (10-Day Course)
1. Tetracycline	250/mg qid
2. Doxycycline	100/mg bid
3. Minocycline	100/mg bid
4. Amoxicillin-Clavulanic acid	850/mg bid
5. Cephalexin + Mitronidazole	250/mg qid 250/mg tid
6. Colistin + Metronidazole	250,000 IU/kg/day 250/mg tid
7. Trimethroprim-sulfamethoxazole	One DS tab bid
8. Ciprofloxacin	500/mg bid
9. Norfloxacin	400/mg bid
10. Chloramphenicol	250/mg qid

bid, twice a day; qid, four times a day; tid, three times a day.

antimicrobial agent is effective, there will be a resolution of marked diminution of symptoms within several days of initiating therapy. Diarrhea will decrease, steatorrhea will decrease, and cobalamin malabsorption will be corrected. Prolonged antibiotic therapy does pose potential clinical problems including diarrhea, enterocolitis, patient intolerance, and bacterial resistance. A prokinetic agent that could help clear the small intestine of the overgrowth flora will be an attractive therapy. Experimental animal studies suggest that bacterial overgrowth might be favorably influenced by prokinetic agents. There have been two small studies of bacterial overgrowth in patients: one using octreotide and one using cisapride (43,44). Both agents led to clearing of the bacterial overgrowth. Large controlled trials of prokinetic therapy in patients with bacterial overgrowth have yet to be fully performed. It has long been thought by some that one can manipulate intestinal flora by giving live probiotic microbial supplements that would change the balance in the overgrowth flora. Studies to date with probiotic therapy in subjects with bacterial overgrowth have been disappointing. A recent placebo-controlled, randomized, crossover trial compared norfloxacin with amoxicillin–clavulanic acid and *Saccharomyces boulardii* in 10 symptomatic patients with bacterial overgrowth (45). Both antibiotic programs led to a significant decrease in symptoms and a substantial improvement in the results of hydrogen breath testing. The probiotic treatment with *S. boulardii* did not result in any improvement in these parameters.

Nutritional support is an important part of the treatment of bacterial overgrowth. This therapy may be needed despite maximally obtainable control of the overgrowth by antimicrobial agents. This is particularly true because there may be incompletely reversible damage to the small-intestine enterocyte. Therefore, a lactose-free diet, and substitution of a large part of dietary fat by medium-chain triglycerides may be necessary. Patients with cobalamin malabsorption should receive monthly injections of cobalamin (100 μg). Deficiencies of other nutrients such as calcium and vitamin K should be corrected.

Finally, it should be stressed that clinicians should have a low threshold for suspecting bacterial overgrowth as the cause of malabsorption in a given patient, because the entity is rather common and readily treatable. Figure 22.4 presents a cost-effective efficient algorithm for evaluating patients with malabsorption. The algorithm emphasizes the performance of non-invasive tests (breath tests for bacterial overgrowth, serum trypsin, and fecal elastase for pancreatic exocrine insufficiency) for the more common etiologies of malabsorption.

It behooves the clinician to be aware of what normal and abnormal floras (both qualitative and quantitative) are within the GI tract. The consequences of bacterial overgrowth within the small intestine can be serious malabsorption, resulting in clinically important deficiencies of several nutrients. Alterations in gastric acid secretion and intestinal motility provide the setting for the development of bacterial overgrowth. The elderly, in particular, appear to be at risk for malabsorption secondary to bacterial overgrowth. Bacterial overgrowth can be easily diagnosed and readily treated if the clinician's index of suspicion for this entity is high.

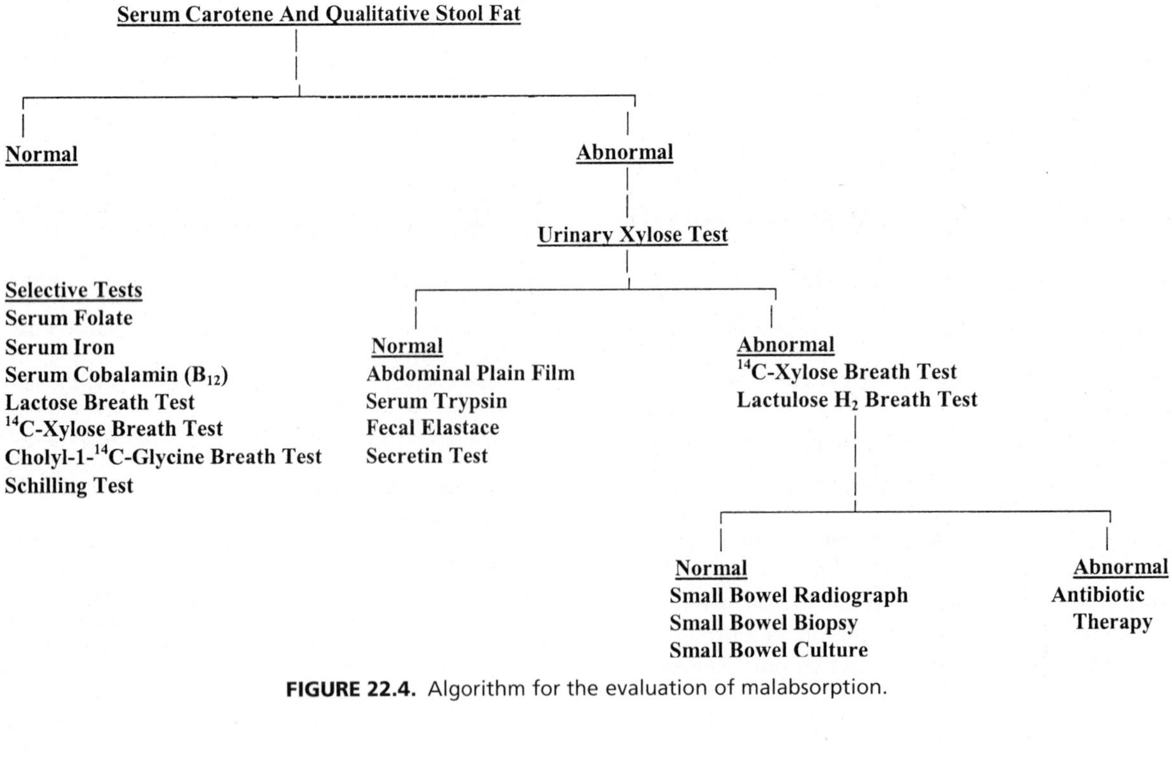

FIGURE 22.4. Algorithm for the evaluation of malabsorption.

REFERENCES

1. Toskes PP, Kumar A. Enteric bacterial flora and bacterial overgrowth syndrome. In: Feldman M, Scharschmidt BF, Sleisenger MH, eds. *Sleisenger & Fordtran's gastrointestinal and liver disease,* sixth edition. Philadelphia: WB Saunders, 1998:1523–1535.
2. Hanson LA, Dahlman-Hoglund A, Jarlsson M, et al. Normal microbial flora of the gut and the immune system. In: Hanson LA, Yolken RH, eds. *Probiotics, other nutritional factors and intestinal microflora.* Philadelphia: Lippincott–Raven Publishers, 1999:217–229.
3. Goldstein F, Wirts CW, Kramer S. The relationship of afferent limb stasis and bacterial flora to the production of post-gastrectomy steatorrhea. *Gastroenterology* 1961;40:47–55.
4. Doig A, Girdwood RG. The absorption of folic acid and labeled cyanocobalamin in intestinal malabsorption with observations on the fecal excretion of fat and nitrogen and the absorption of glucose and xylose. *Q J Med* 1960;29:333–374.
5. Beeken WL, Kanish RE. Microbial flora of the upper small bowel in Crohn's disease. *Gastroenterology* 1973;65:390–397.
6. Bishop RF, Anderson CM. Bacterial flora of stomach and small intestine in children with intestinal obstruction. *Arch Dis Child* 1960;35:487–492.
7. Swan RW. Stagnant loop syndrome resulting from small bowel irradiation injury and intestinal bypass. *Gynecol Oncol* 1974;8: 441–445.
8. Russell RM, Abadi P, Ismail-Beigi F. Role of bacterial overgrowth on the malabsorption syndrome of the primary small intestinal lymphoma. *Cancer* 1977;89:8579–8583.
9. Atwater JS, Butt HR, Priestley JT. Gastrojejunocolic fistulae with special reference to associated nutritional deficiencies and certain surgical aspects. *Ann Surg* 1943;117:414–419.
10. Kelly DG, Phillips SF, Kelly KA, et al. Dysfunction of the continent ileostomy: clinical features and bacteriology. *Gut* 1983;24: 193–198.
11. Kahn I, Jeffries GH, Sleisenger MH. Malabsorption in intestinal scleroderma. Correction by antibiotics. *N Engl J Med* 1966;274: 1339–1344.
12. Pearson AJ, Brzechwa-Adjukiewicz A, McCarthy CF. Intestinal pseudo-obstruction with bacterial overgrowth in the small intestine. *Am J Dig Dis* 1969;14:200–205.
13. Goldstein F, Wirts EC, Kowlessar OD. Diabetic diarrhea and steatorrhea. Microbiologic and clinical observations. *Ann Intern Med* 1970;72:215–218.
14. Vantrappen G, Janssens J, Hellemans J, et al. The interdigestive motor complex of normal subjects and patients with bacterial overgrowth of the small intestine. *J Clin Invest* 1977;59: 1158–1166.
15. Roberts SH, James O, Jarvis EH. Bacterial overgrowth syndrome without "blind loop:" a cause for malnutrition in the elderly. *Lancet* 1977;2:1193–95.
16. McEvoy A, Dutton J, James OF. Bacterial contamination of the small intestine is an important cause of occult malabsorption in the elderly. *Br Med J* 1983;287:789–793.
17. Montgomery RD, Haboubi NY, Mike NH, et al. Causes of malabsorption in the elderly. *Age Ageing* 1986;15:235–240.
18. Haboudi N, Montgomery R. Small bowel bacterial overgrowth in elderly people: clinical significance and response to treatment. *Age Ageing* 1992;21:13–19.
19. Lipski P, Jelly P, James F. Bacterial contamination of the small bowel in elderly people: is it necessary pathological. *Age Ageing* 1992;21:13–19.
20. Saltzman J, Kowdley K, Pedrosa M, et al. Bacterial overgrowth without clinical malabsorption in elderly hypochlorhydric subjects. *Gastroenterology* 1994;106:615–623.
21. Fried M, Slegrish H, Frei R, et al. Duodenal bacterial overgrowth during treatment with omeprazole in outpatients. *Gut* 1996;35: 23–27.
22. Lembeke B, Kraus B, Lankisch PG. Small intestinal function in chronic relapsing pancreatitis. *Hepatogastroenterology* 1985;32: 149–155.
23. Tabaquchali S. The pathophysiological role of the small intestinal bacterial flora. *Scand J Gastroenterol* 1970;Suppl 6: 139–163.
24. Toskes PP. The changing nature of small intestine bacterial overgrowth. *Curr Gastroenterol Rep* 1999;1:267–268.
25. Welkos SA, Toskes PP, Baer H, et al. Importance of anaerobic bacteria in the cobalamin malabsorption of experimental rat blind loop syndrome. *Gastroenterology* 1981;80:313–320.
26. Giannella RA, Toskes PP. Gastrointestinal bleeding and iron absorption in the experimental blind loop syndrome. *Am J Clin Nutr* 1976;29:754–757.
27. Hoffbrand AV, Tabaqchali S, Moilin, DL. High serum folate levels in intestinal blind loop syndrome. *Lancet* 1966;1: 1339–1342.
28. Kim YS, Spritz N, Blum M, et al. The role of altered bile acid metabolism in the steatorrhea of experimental blind loop syndrome. *J Clin Invest* 1966;45:956–962.
29. Justus PG, Fernandez A, Martin JL, et al. Altered myoelectric activity in the experimental blind loop syndrome. *J Clin Invest* 1983;72:1064–1071.
30. Toskes PP, King CE, Spivey JC, et al. Xylose catabolism in experimental rat blind loop syndrome: studies including newly developed D-(^{14}C) xylose breath test. *Gastroenterology* 1978;74: 691–697.
31. King CE, Toskes PP. Protein-losing enteropathy in the human and experimental rat blind loop syndrome. *Gastroenterology* 1981;80:504–509.
32. King CE, Toskes PP, Guilarte TR, et al. Comparison of the one gram ^{14}C-xylose breath test to the ^{14}C-bile acid breath test in patients with small intestine bacterial overgrowth. *Dig Dis Sci* 1980;25:53–58.
33. Ferguson J, Walker K, Thomson AB. Limitations in the use of ^{14}C-glycocholate breath and stool bile acid determinations in patients with chronic diarrhea. *J Clin Gastroenterol* 1986;8: 258–263.
34. King CE, Toskes PP, Spivey JC, et al. Detection of small intestine overgrowth by means of a ^{14}C-D-xylose breath test. *Gastroenterology* 1979;79:75–82.
35. Schneider A, Novis B, Chen V, et al. Value of the ^{14}C-D-xylose breath test in patients with intestinal bacterial overgrowth. *Digestion* 1985;32:86–91.
36. Pruthi HS, Mehta SK, Pathak CM. Evaluation of ^{14}C-D-xylose breath test in the diagnosis of small intestinal bacterial overgrowth. *Ind J Med Res* 1984;80:598–600.
37. Valdovinos M, Camilleri M, Thomforde G, et al. Reduced accuracy of 14-C-D-xylose breath test for detecting bacterial overgrowth in gastrointestinal motility disorders. *Scand J Gastroenterol* 1993;28:963–968.
38. Riordan S, McIver C, Duncombe V, et al. Factors influencing the 1-gram 14-C-D-xylose breath test for bacterial overgrowth. *Am J Gastroenterol* 1995;90:1455–1460.
39. Lewis SJ, Young G, Mann M, et al. Improvement in specificity of 14-C-D-xylose breath test for bacterial overgrowth. *Dig Dis Sci* 1997;42:1587–1591.
40. Perman JA, Modler S, Barr RG, et al. Fasting breath hydrogen concentration: normal values and clinical application. *Gastroenterology* 1984;87:1358–1363.
41. Corazza GR, Menozzi MG, Strocchi A, et al. The diagnosis of small bowel bacterial overgrowth. *Gastroenterology* 1990;98: 302–305.
42. Kocoshis SA, Schletewitz K, Lovelace G, et al. Duodenal bile

acids among children: keto derivatives and aerobic small bowel bacterial overgrowth. *J Pediatr Gastroenterol Nutr* 1987;6: 686–696.
43. Soudah HC, Hasler WL, Owyang C. Effect of octreotide on intestinal motility and bacterial overgrowth in scleroderma. *N Engl J Med* 1991;325:1461–1467.
44. Pardo A, Bartoli R, Lorenzo-Zuniga V, et al. Effect of cisapride on intestinal bacterial overgrowth and bacterial translocation in cirrhosis. *Hepatology* 2000;31:858–862.
45. Stotzer PO, Blomberg L, Conway PL, et al. Probiotic treatment of small intestinal bacterial overgrowth by *Lactobacillus fermentum* KLD. *Scand J Infect Dis* 1996;28:615–620.

23

APPENDICITIS

CHRISTINA M. SURAWICZ

Appendicitis is defined histopathologically as inflammation of the vermiform appendix. It is caused by obstruction of the appendix and is associated with a characteristic clinical syndrome. The first report of appendicitis in 1886 remains a classic description of the clinical presentation (1). Occasionally, however, presentation may be atypical, making the diagnosis less obvious. When appendicitis is treated promptly by appendectomy, morbidity and mortality rates are low. However, missed diagnosis and improperly treated appendicitis may result in perforation with abscess formation.

MICROBIOLOGY

Most cases of appendicitis are idiopathic. Histopathology of appendixes removed from persons with idiopathic appendicitis show inflammation but usually no identifiable pathogen. Nevertheless, a variety of infections can cause appendicitis. In addition, inflammation of contiguous organs or tissue can mimic appendicitis.

Bacteria

Yersinia enterocolitica has been reported to cause up to 6% of appendicitis in patients in northern European countries and Canada (2). Since 1981, additional strains have been reported to be associated with appendicitis, including the more invasive serotypes O3 and O9. In a prospective study of appendicitis in the United States, *Y. enterocolitica* was cultured from 9% (4 of 44) of inflamed appendixes and from none of 6 normal appendixes (2). In a retrospective study of nearly 3,000 patients, *Y. enterocolitica* O3 and O9 were the most common pathogens (3.6%) isolated from resected appendixes (3) (See Color Figure 23.1).

Other bacteria that cause infections that can mimic appendicitis include *Escherichia coli* O157:H7, *Campylobacter* species, *Salmonella* species., *Aspergillus,* and *Mycobacterium tuberculosis.* Like *Yersinia*, many of these invasive pathogens favor the ileocolic areas (4). *E. coli* O157:H7 is an enterohemorrhagic *E. coli* that typically causes hemorrhagic colitis, resulting in bloody diarrhea. *Campylobacter* species can cause a pseudoappendicitis in which mesenteric lymph nodes are inflamed but the appendix is usually normal. *Salmonella enteritis* can be associated with abdominal pain that mimics appendicitis, but diarrhea eventually becomes the predominant symptom. Tuberculosis of the gastrointestinal tract has a predilection for the ileocecal area, causing a chronic pain syndrome that contrasts with the acute pain of appendicitis. *M. tuberculosis* may rarely cause appendicitis (5). A study of *E. coli* isolates from appendicitis cases and control subjects suggested that virulent *E. coli* may play a role in pathogenesis (6), but these studies have apparently not been replicated. An early report (1911) documented the presence of spirochetes in the feces of patients with acute appendicitis (7). In the 1930s, a study showed that 10% of appendixes from individuals with appendicitis-like symptoms had spirochetes (8). A large review of hundreds of appendectomy specimens found that spirochetosis was present in 12% of uninflamed appendixes compared to 0.7% from inflamed appendixes (9). The spirochetes, classified as *Brachyspira aalborgi,* are 2 to 4.8 μm long and 0.2 μm wide. A more recent review of 109 cases found spirochetosis in only four persons, none of whom were children (10). Thus, the role of spirochetosis in the pathogenesis of appendicitis or pseudoappendicitis remains uncertain, but is not likely to be of major clinical significance.

Viruses

Viral causes of appendicitis and pseudoappendicitis are uncommon but include measles, adenovirus, and cytomegalovirus. Specimens from measles appendicitis have large multinucleate giant lymphoreticular cells. Adenovirus infection is characterized by intranuclear inclusions with viral particles identified by electron microscopy. Cytomegalovirus infection causes characteristic cytomegalic changes, typically in endothelial cells.

C. M. Surawicz: Department of Medicine, Division of Gastroenterology, University of Washington School of Medicine and Harborview Medical Center, Seattle, Washington

Parasites

Enterobius vermicularis, or pinworm, is the most common parasite found in appendectomy specimens, but the worms or eggs found in the lumen of the appendix are probably an incidental finding. Other parasites rarely associated with appendicitis include *Ascaris lumbricoides* (11), *Entamoeba histolytica, Schistosoma mansoni, Balantidium coli, Trichuris trichiura,* and *Strongyloides stercoralis* (Table 23.1). *Angiostrongylus costaricensis,* a nematode found in Central America, can also cause an appendicitis-like syndrome characterized by the presence of right lower quadrant mass with pain, fever, anorexia, and eosinophilia (12).

Fungi

Histoplasma capsulatum is the most common fungus associated with appendicitis, occurring in 9% of cases. Other fungi are rarely associated with appendicitis except in immunosuppressed persons. *Actinomyces* species have a predilection for the ileocecal area, causing a mass or sinus tracts. Actinomycosis should be considered in persons in whom a fistula develops following appendectomy. *Aspergillus* has been reported to cause appendicitis in patients with leukemia (13,14) and rarely in others (15).

TABLE 23.1. INFECTIOUS CAUSES OF APPENDICITIS

Bacteria
Yersinia enterocolitica
Campylobacter
Escherichia coli O157:H7
Salmonella
Shigella
Mycobacterium tuberculosis
Non-*T. pallidum* spirochetes
Brucella
Viruses
Measles
Adenovirus
Cytomelagovirus
Parasites
Enterobius vermicularis
Ascaris lumbricoides
Entamoeba histolytica
Schistosoma mansoni
Angiostrongylus
Balantidium coli
Trichuris trichiura, vulpis
Strongyloides stercoralis
Fasciola
Toxocara
Capillaria hepatica
Fungi
Histoplasma
Actinomycosis israelii, A. turicensis
Aspergillus

Granulomatous Appendicitis

Recent evidence suggests that granulomatous appendicitis, initially thought to be Crohn's disease of the appendix, is probably a distinct clinical entity caused by an unknown infectious etiology (16–18) (see Color Figure 23.2). Other specific causes of appendiceal granulomas include Crohn's disease, sarcoidosis, tuberculosis, and yersiniosis. One woman with leukemia had granulomatosis appendicitis in the setting of invasive candidiasis.(19)

Appendicitis in AIDS

Appendicitis develops infrequently in patients with AIDS. A high index of suspicion is required in such patients because leukocytosis and fever may be absent in up to one-third of cases. The differential diagnosis of appendicitis in such patients includes cytomegalovirus colitis, cryptosporidial and mycobacterial infections, as well as typhlitis and obstruction resulting from Kaposi sarcoma. A case of cytomegalovirus-associated ileal perforation in a patient with AIDS demonstrated the usefulness of *in situ* hybridization and immunohistochemical analysis for detecting cytomegalovirus nucleic acids and proteins in tissue specimens (20). Early use of diagnostic tests such as ultrasound and computed tomography (CT) scan may facilitate the diagnosis. Appendicitis does not appear to increase the morbidity in AIDS (21).

PATHOGENESIS

Appendicitis results when the lumen of the appendix becomes obstructed by objects such as a stone (fecalith) or parasite or by physical factors such as torsion. Less common causes of obstruction include tumor, foreign body, and lymphoid hyperplasia. Obstruction causes increased pressure within the appendix as secretions accumulate; the resulting decrease in blood flow causes ischemia, which may progress to necrosis and perforation with peritonitis. A walled-off perforation results in a periappendiceal abscess.

Pseudoappendicitis occurs when an adjacent tissue or organ becomes inflamed, causing symptoms that simulate appendicitis, although the appendix is not involved. Periappendicitis is caused by inflammation of the serosa of the appendix. This results from intraabdominal inflammation of other causes, such as pelvic inflammatory disease or diverticulitis.

EPIDEMIOLOGY

Even though appendicitis can occur at any age, it is most common in children, although rare in children younger than 2 years of age. Appendicitis is more common in Western than Eastern countries, leading to speculation that a diet high in fiber is associated with a decreased incidence.

CLINICAL FEATURES

The most common presenting symptom of acute appendicitis is abdominal pain, which typically begins as a diffuse periumbilical pain that subsequently localizes to the right lower quadrant. The pain is constant and increases in severity. Such pain is present in 95% of patients with appendicitis. There is usually associated anorexia, nausea, vomiting, and low-grade fever.

On physical examination, right lower quadrant tenderness is present. Guarding and rebound tenderness at the McBurney point are present in 80% of cases. The McBurney point is 1.5 to 2 inches from the anterior superior iliac spine on a line from the spine to the umbilicus. Other findings on physical examination include the psoas, obturator, and Rovsing signs, which are present in 80% to 90% of cases. A psoas sign is present if extending the thigh at the hip to stretch the peritoneum over the psoas muscle causes pain. The obturator sign, which is elicited when the obturator fascia is stretched by internal rotation of the thigh with the knee flexed, may be present in appendicitis, an inflamed retrocecal appendix, or a psoas muscle abscess. Rovsing sign is elicited when pressing on the left iliac fossa causes referred right lower quadrant pain. Tenderness with digital examination of the rectum is elicited in more than half (65%) of cases. In older patients, abdominal distention seen on CT scan may be common.

Laboratory evaluation usually reveals an elevated white blood cell count (>10,000 cells/mm^3) with an increase in the percentage of polymorphonuclear neutrophils. Urinalysis can show the presence of red or white blood cells in the absence of urinary tract infection. A urine sample for human chorionic gonadotropin (HCG) should be considered in sexually active females of childbearing age.

A history, physical examination, evaluation of blood studies, and radiographic examination of the abdomen are sufficient to make the diagnosis in most patients. Overall, clinical accuracy is 70% to 80%, decreasing to 30% to 50% in children and women of childbearing age. Missed diagnoses are more common in children because of the difficulty children have in communicating symptoms and in women, especially during pregnancy, because of confounding gynecologic pathology. The rate of perforation is highest in preschool age children. The rate of appendectomy for an inflamed appendix (40%) is highest in young women with regular menses and right lower quadrant pain. Surgeons should be involved early in the evaluation of patients with suspected appendicitis. When the diagnosis is unclear, additional tests such as ultrasound or CT scan may be helpful.

In a study of 150 children referred for possible appendicitis (22), half had immediate surgery. The most useful criteria to determine the need for immediate surgery were a history of epigastric pain localizing to the right lower quadrant, guarding, peritonitis, fever, and an elevated white blood cell count. When the diagnosis was unclear, close observation was the best approach to management. Of the 76 children who were observed, one-third ultimately had an appendectomy for histologically confirmed appendicitis, three of which had already perforated. The other two-thirds of the children improved and were discharged. These children were less likely to have had peritoneal signs, right lower quadrant tenderness, and guarding. A more recent study evaluated delay in diagnosis of appendicitis in children (23). The most common alternative diagnosis was gastroenteritis because diarrhea is a common early symptom in both. In gastroenteritis, however, there is profuse watery diarrhea in contrast to the severe progressive abdominal pain of appendicitis.

The diagnosis of appendicitis may be especially difficult in children with leukemia. In one study (24), the incidence of acute abdomen in this population was 4% to 5% and appendicitis 0.5%. Common symptoms were nausea, vomiting, and localized abdominal pain, but in children in whom diagnosis was delayed, symptoms were vague abdominal pain, abdominal distention, fever, dehydration, and diarrhea; guarding was absent, even when the appendix had ruptured. A specific diagnosis in children with leukemia is typhlitis. This inflammation of the terminal ileum and cecum is related to chemotherapy, neutropenia, and bacterial overgrowth, and is present in 10% of leukemic patients at autopsy. Unlike appendicitis, it may improve with medical therapy (24).

The diagnosis of appendicitis in pregnancy is difficult, in part because the position of the appendix changes as the uterus enlarges. The loss of elasticity of the abdominal wall muscles may also change the presenting signs. In the fifth month of pregnancy, pain caused by appendicitis may be present above the umbilicus. As the appendix becomes higher in location, signs and symptoms are different. In addition, the appendix is less likely to be contained by the omentum, and perforation may more frequently lead to generalized peritonitis. Appendicitis is the most common cause of acute abdomen in the pregnant patient and, accordingly, is the most common surgical emergency in any trimester. In one study, delayed diagnosis led to complication rates of the pregnancy of those in the first trimester (25). However, no complications occurred in those in the third trimester. Right lower quadrant tenderness is still the most common presenting symptom (26). Because of the difficulty in diagnosis, a higher false-negative rate at surgery of 30% is thought to be acceptable. In some studies, perforation rates can be high (up to 68%) (27). Appendicitis may be associated with premature labor and fetal distress. Prophylactic antibiotics and tocolytic drugs are often recommended.

The reliability of the classic symptoms of acute appendicitis is often assessed. The diagnosis is less likely in the absence of nausea, vomiting, right iliac fossa tenderness, or the presence of symptoms for longer than 72 hours without evidence of perforation. In women, pelvic inflammatory disease should be considered if symptoms occur near menses or if cervical or adnexal tenderness is present.

A specific scoring system with five clinical criteria has been developed to reduce the rate of appendectomy for inflamed appendixes (28). The criteria used by this system include abdominal pain, vomiting, right lower quadrant pain, low-grade fever, and either white blood cell count greater than 10,000 cells/mm^3 or polymorphonuclear neutrophils greater than 75%. The clinicians who developed the system recommend immediate laparotomy when four criteria are present and admission and observation when three criteria are present (28).

DIFFERENTIAL DIAGNOSIS

The most common differential diagnosis is infection or inflammation of adjacent tissues. Infections that involve the terminal ileum and cecum cause right lower quadrant tenderness. Similarly, Crohn's ileocolitis usually causes right lower quadrant pain. The most common other diagnoses in a group of 150 children who were incorrectly suspected of having appendicitis were gastroenteritis, mesenteric adenitis, ovarian cyst, pneumonia, and constipation (29). Infectious ileocolitis resulting from infection with *Yersinia, Campylobacter* and *Salmonella* can mimic appendicitis (4). *Y. enterocolitica* was the most common bacterial cause of appendicitis (see earlier text). This bacterium may also cause right-sided colitis with terminal ileitis as well as acute mesenteric adenitis or terminal ileitis, which may be mistaken for appendicitis. *Yersinia pseudotuberculosis* also can cause a pseudoappendicitis syndrome as well as appendicitis (see color Figure 23.1). *Campylobacter* species and nontyphoidal *Salmonella* species are the second and third most common bacterial causes of appendicitis after *Yersinia. Brucella* has also caused acute abdomen mimicking appendicitis (30). Shigellosis has been reported to cause perforated appendicitis (31). These infections involve the terminal ileum and cecum. When stool cultures are positive for one of these pathogens, acute appendicitis is less likely. Other bacterial, viral, fungal, and parasitic causes of appendicitis are described above.

In persons older than 50 years of age, neoplasms should be considered among the differential diagnoses. Cecal tumor can present as appendicitis. Adenoma and adenocarcinoma occurring in the right colon occasionally mimics appendicitis or, when involving the appendix itself, can cause appendicitis (32,33) as can lymphoma (34). Ultrasound or CT scan of the abdomen facilitates differentiation between neoplasm and appendicitis. Right-sided diverticulitis should also be considered in older persons. Elderly patients may also have an atypical presentation without fever or leukocytosis, increasing their rate of complications. In women, pathology of the ovary, fallopian tubes, or uterus may cause right lower quadrant pain. This is most often due to pelvic inflammatory disease, but a ruptured ovarian cyst or ectopic pregnancy should also be considered. Rare causes of right lower quadrant pain include osteomyelitis of the iliac bones (35) and abscess of the psoas or gluteal muscles. Invagination of the appendix is unusual, but it also can cause symptoms such as recurrent right lower quadrant pain with nausea and vomiting (36).

DIAGNOSTIC MEASURES

As discussed earlier, appendicitis is easily diagnosed on the basis of history, physical examination, blood studies, and abdominal radiography. The abdominal radiograph is abnormal in only 10% of patients with an acute abdomen, a fecalith being the most common finding. Because diagnostic yield is so low in diagnosis of appendicitis, some clinicians discourage its routine use (37). A barium enema may be helpful when colonic disease is considered. Nonfilling of the appendix, which is suggestive of appendicitis, has a diagnostic accuracy of 80% to 98%. However, 10% of normal appendixes may not fill, and 20% of acutely inflamed appendixes may fill. Thus, barium enema has a limited role as an ancillary diagnostic test. Upper gastrointestinal radiograph series may be helpful in the presence of ileal disease resulting from infection or Crohn's disease.

Abdominal ultrasound is useful when diagnosis is uncertain. In several series of patients in whom appendicitis was suspected but uncertain, ultrasound abnormalities were predictive of appendicitis in 80% to 90% of cases (38–40). When ultrasound is normal, the chance of appendicitis is very low. Ultrasound in one series reduced the rate of negative laparotomies from 23% to 13% and was especially useful in evaluating women of childbearing age (38). However, it altered clinical management in only 18%, confirming the importance of clinical evaluation and judgment.

Ultrasound also may indicate that perforation has occurred when loculated pericecal fluid, prominent pericecal fat, or circumferential loss of the submucosal layer of the appendix is present. The presence of periappendiceal fluid is specific for appendicitis (100%); however, because it is not always present, the sensitivity is only 40% (41). In children, loculated fluid and the absence of the echogenic submucosal layer was highly predictive of perforation, but the presence of free fluid or appendicoliths was not (42,43).

Ultrasound is especially useful in pregnant patients. However, it may be less helpful later in pregnancy (>35 weeks) when the appendix may not be visualized (44). In this circumstance, changes in patient positioning may be helpful.

Interest in CT diagnosis of appendicitis has been increasing. An important prospective study of helical CT with rectal contrast evaluated 100 consecutive patients in an emergency department for suspected appendicitis (45). CT results were correlated with surgery or with 2-month follow-up in those not operated. All 53 patients with appendicitis had a positive CT scan. Overall, 86 (86%) of patients had a specific diagnosis; appendiceal CT revealed the correct diagnosis in 81 (94%). Other diagnoses included biliary colic, endometriosis, and urinary tract infection. In this study, CT had a positive and negative predictive value of 98%. Cost savings overall was estimated to be $447.00 per patient.

Subsequent studies comparing ultrasound and unenhanced CT show better diagnostic accuracy for CT compared with ultrasonography (46–48). Advantages of unenhanced helical CT include the ability to scan immediately without patient preparation, no need for intravenous contrast although rectal contrast is given and its lower cost compared to standard abdominal CT scan. It is also more likely to detect other conditions that mimic appendicitis such as cecal diverticulitis, urinary tract infection, adnexal pathology, sigmoid diverticulitis, and other right lower quadrant lesions (47).

CT is more expensive than ultrasound. In one study of children with suspected appendicitis, ultrasound was performed first and limited CT was done if ultrasound was negative or inconclusive. In this setting, its accuracy was 94% (49).

In short, helical CT has a very good diagnostic accuracy, in the range of 95% to 98%. False-positive findings are rare. When results are normal, appendicitis is unlikely. It is more expensive than ultrasound, but less dependent on operator skill. Perhaps it is reasonable to screen suspected appendicitis with ultrasound in children, young women, or pregnant women. In older individuals, helical CT may be a more productive first test (or if ultrasound was negative) (50).

The most common CT sign of appendicitis is a large appendix with periappendiceal fat stranding; less common signs are changes in the apex of the cecum and appendicolitis.

Technetium-99 scan to identify inflammation is rarely useful in the diagnosis of acute appendicitis because it has a high false-negative rate, is expensive, and is often not available (51).

Laparoscopy has been used as a diagnostic test, but it has an 18% technical failure rate, is invasive, and requires a general anesthetic. Moreover, the appendix may not always be visualized.

TREATMENT

When the diagnosis is obvious, acute appendicitis should be treated by immediate appendectomy. Although diagnostic accuracy increases with observation, the risk of perforation also increases with time. Perforation is associated with a threefold increase in wound infection, a 15-fold increase in intraabdominal abscess, a 50-fold increase in mortality rate, and, in women, tubal scarring that may contribute to infertility. Recently, appendectomy is more likely to be performed by laparoscopic abdominal surgery. Controlled trials of laparoscopic appendectomy compared with open appendectomy show that laparoscopic surgery is safe and patients recover more rapidly (52). Laparoscopic appendectomy can even be performed in many cases of perforated appendix (53). Moreover, patients preferred the smaller scar.

The role of antibiotics in surgery for acute appendicitis has been debated, but when the appendix has perforated, they are clearly indicated.

REFERENCES

1. McBurney C. Experience with early operative interference in cases of disease of the vermiform appendix. *N Y Med J* 1989; 676–684.
2. Bennion RS, Thompson JE, Gil J, et al. The role of *Yersinia enterocolitica* in appendicitis in the southwestern United States. *Am Surgeon* 1991;57:766–768.
3. Van Noyen R, Selderslaghs R, Bekkaert J, et al. Causative role of *Yersinia* and other enteric pathogens in the appendicular syndrome. *Eur J Clin Microbiol Infect Dis* 1991;10:735–741.
4. Puylaert JB, Van der Zant FM, Mutsaers JA. Infectious ileocecitis caused by *Yersinia, Campylobacter,* and *Salmonella*: clinical, radiological and US findings. *Eur Radiol* 1997;7:3–9.
5. al-Hilaly MA, Abu-Zidan FM, Zayed FF, et al. Tuberculous appendicitis with perforation. Department of Surgery, Al Adan Hospital, Ministry of Public Health Kuwait. *Br J Clin Prac* 1990;44(12):632–633.
6. Saxen H, Tarkka E, Hannikainen P, et al. *Escherichia coli* and appendicitis: phenotypic characteristics of *E. coli* isolates from inflamed and noninflamed appendices. *Clin Infec Dis* 1996; 23:1038–1042.
7. Thiroloix J, Durand A. Spirochetemie au cours d'une appendicite aigue. Hemo et seroculture. Isolament et culture du parasite. Emploi du 606. Arreet de la septiciemie. *Bull Mem Soc Med Hosp III* 1911;31:653–662.
8. Mazza S. Espiroquetosis apendiculares. *Pren Med Argent* 1930; 17:464–468.
9. Henrik-Nielsen R, Lundbeck FA, Teglbjaerg PS, et al. Intestinal spirochetosis of the vermiform appendix. *Gastroenterology* 1985;88:971–977.
10. Yang M, Lapham R. Appendiceal spirochetosis. *South Med J* 1997;90:30–32.
11. Chrungoo RK, Hangloo VK, Faroqui MM, et al. Surgical manifestations and management of ascariasis in Kashmir. Department of Surgery, Government Medical College, Srinagar. *J Indian Med Assoc* 1992;90(7):171–174.
12. Hulbert TV, Larsen RA, Chandrasoma PT. Abdominal angiostrongyliasis mimicking acute appendicitis and Meckel's diverticulum: report of a case in the United States and review. *Clin Infect Dis* 1992;14:836–840.
13. Rogers S, Potter MN, Slade RR. *Aspergillus* appendicitis in acute myeloid leukemia. Department of Haematology, Southmead Hospital, Westbury-on-Trym, Bristol. *Clin-Lab Haematol* 1990; 12(4):471–476.
14. Bomelburg T, Roos N, von Lengerke HJ, et al. Invasive aspergillosis complicating induction chemotherapy of childhood leukemia. Kinderklinik, University at Munster, Federal Republic of Germany. *Eur J Pediatr* 1992;151(7):485–487.

15. Sabbe LJ, Van De Merwe D, Schouls L, et al. Clinical spectrum of infections due to the newly described *Actinomyces* species *A. turicensis, A. radingae*, and *A. europaeus*. *J Clin Microbiol* 1999; 37:8–13.
16. Dudley TH, Dean PJ. Idiopathic granulomatous appendicitis, or Crohn's disease of the appendix revisited. *Hum Pathol* 1993;24: 595–601.
17. Naschitz JE, Yeshurun D, Rosner I, et al. Idiopathic granulomatous appendicitis. Report of five cases, one of which presented as migratory arthritis. *J Clin Gastroenterol* 1995;21:290–294.
18. Richards ML, Aberger FJ, Landercasper J. Granulomatous appendicitis: Crohn's disease, atypical Crohn's or not Crohn's at all? *J Am Coll Surg* 1997;185:13–17.
19. Moyana TN, Kulaga A, Xiang J. Granulomatous appendicitis in acute myeloblastic leukemia: expanding the clinicopathologic spectrum of invasive candidiasis. *Arch Pathol Lab Med* 1996;120: 203–205.
20. Genta RM, Bleyzer I, Cate TR, et al. In situ hybridization and immunohistochemical analysis of cytomegalovirus-associated ileal perforation. *Gastroenterology* 1993;104:1822–1827.
21. Bova R, Meagher A. Appendicitis in HIV-positive patients. *Aust N Z J Surg* 1998;68:337–339.
22. Rasmussen OO, Hoffman J. Assessment of reliability of symptoms and signs of acute appendicitis. *J R Coll Surg Edinb* 1991; 36:372–377.
23. Cappendijk VC, Hazebroek FW. The impact of diagnostic delay on the course of acute appendicitis. *Arch Dis Child* 2000;83: 64–66.
24. Angel CA, Rao BN, Wrenn E Jr, et al. Acute appendicitis in children with leukemia and other malignancies: still a diagnostic dilemma. *J Pediatr Surg* 1992;27:476–479.
25. Andersen B, Nielsen TF. Appendicitis in pregnancy: diagnosis, management and complications. *Acta Obstet Gynecol Scand* 1999; 78:758–762.
26. Mourad J, Elliott JP, Erickson L, et al. Appendicitis in pregnancy: new information that contradicts long-held clinical beliefs. *Am J Obstet Gynecol* 2000;182:1027–1029.
27. Tracey M, Fletcher HS. Appendicitis in pregnancy. *Am Surg* 2000;66:555–559.
28. Christian F, Christian GP. A simple scoring system to reduce the negative appendectomy rate. *Ann R Coll Surg Engl* 1992;74: 281–285.
29. Dolgin SE, Beck AR, Tartter PI. The risk of perforation when children with possible appendicitis are observed in the hospital. *Surg Gynecol Obstet* 1992;175:320–324.
30. Fernandez MD, Garcia JL, Garcia FD, et al. Brucella acute abdomen mimicking appendicitis. *Am J Med* 2000;108:599–600.
31. Sukhotnik I, Miron D, Kawar B, et al. Perforated appendicitis in shigellosis. *Isr Med Assoc J* 1999;1:124–125.
32. Vander SA, Mandell GH. Villous adenoma of the appendix. Report of a case. *Arch Surg* 1968;97:562–564.
33. Munk JF. Villous adenoma causing acute appendicitis. *Br J Surg* 1977;64:593–595.
34. Huh J, Hong SM, Kim SS, et al. Angiocentric lymphoma masquerading as acute appendicitis. *Histopathology* 1999;34:378–380.
35. Ofiaeli O. Abnormal syndrome of iliac osteomyelitis presenting as acute appendicitis. Division of Orthopaedics and Traumatology, University Teaching Hospital, Anambra State, Nigeria. *Centr Afr J Med* 1992;38(4):171–173.
36. Lauwers GY, Prendergast NC, Wahl SJ, et al. Invagination of vermiform appendix. Case Report. *Dig Dis Sci* 1993;38:565–568.
37. Rao PM, Rhea JT, Rao JA, et al. Plain abdominal radiography in clinically suspected appendicitis: diagnostic yield, resource use, and comparison with CT. *Am J Emerg Med* 1999;17:325–328.
38. Schwerk WB, Wichtrup B, Rothmund M, et al. Ultrasonography in the diagnosis of acute appendicitis: a prospective study. *Gastroenterology* 1989;97:630–639.
39. Larson JM, Pierce JC, Ellinger DM, et al. The validity and utility of sonography in the diagnosis of appendicitis in the community setting. *AJR Am J Roentgenol* 1989;153:687–691.
40. Fa EM, Cronan JJ. Compression ultrasonography as an aid in the differential diagnosis of appendicitis. *Surg Gynecol Obstet* 1989; 169:290–298.
41. Borushok KF, Jeffrey RB, Laing FC, et al. Sonographic diagnosis of perforation in patients with acute appendicitis. *AJR Am J Roentgenol* 1990;154:275–278.
42. Quillin SP, Siegel MJ, Coffin CM. Acute appendicitis in children: value of sonography in detecting perforation. *AJR Am J Roentgenol* 1992;159:1265–1268.
43. Sivit CJ, Newman KD, Boenning DA, et al. Appendicitis: usefulness of US in diagnosis in a pediatric population. *Radiology* 1992;185:549–552.
44. Lim HK, Bae SH, Seo GS. Diagnosis of acute appendicitis in pregnant women: value of sonography. *AJR Am J Roentgenol* 1992;159:539–542.
45. Rao PM, Rhea JT, Novelline RA, et al. Effect of computed tomography of the appendix on treatment of patients and use of hospital resources. *N Engl J Med* 1998;338:141–146.
46. Pickuth D, Heywang-Kobrunner SH, Spielmann RP. Suspected acute appendicitis: is ultrasonography or computed tomography the preferred imaging technique? *Eur J Surg* 2000;166:315–319.
47. Lane MJ, Katz DS, Ross BA, et al. Unenhanced helical CT for suspected acute appendicitis. *AJR Am J Roentgenol* 1997;168: 405–409.
48. Choi YH, Fischer E, Hoda SA, et al. Appendiceal CT in 140 cases. Diagnostic criteria for acute and necrotizing appendicits. *Clin Imaging* 1998;22:252–271.
49. Garcia Pena BM, Mandl KD, Kraus SJ, et al. Ultrasonography and limited computed tomography in the diagnosis and management of appendicitis in children. JAMA 1999;282:1041–1046.
50. Birnbaum BA, Wilson SR. Appendicitis at the millennium. *Radiology* 2000;215:337–348.
51. Foley CR, Latimer RG, Rimkus DS. Detection of acute appendicitis by technetium 99 HMPAO scanning. *Am Surgeon* 1992; 58:761–765.
52. Hellberg A, Rudberg C, Kullman E, et al. Prospective randomized multicentre study of laparoscopic versus open appendectomy. *Br J Surg* 1999;86:48–53.
53. Khalili TM, Hiatt JR, Savar A, et al. Perforated appendicitis is not a contraindication to laparoscopy. *Am Surgeon* 1999;65:965–967.

24

DIVERTICULITIS

GABRIEL GARCIA

Colonic diverticula are saccular outpouches that protrude through the wall of the colon. The diverticula can be any in number, can be variable in size (although generally smaller than 1 cm), and can occur anywhere along the length of the colon, but are most common in the sigmoid colon.

Diverticular disease is the general term that encompasses the wide variety of clinical conditions that arise from the presence of diverticula within the colon, a condition known as *diverticulosis.* Approximately 70% to 80% of persons affected with diverticulosis are either completely asymptomatic or have uncomplicated courses characterized by pain and altered bowel habits. These latter symptoms can be similar in quality to those of irritable bowel syndrome. Complications can be seen in a sizable minority of those with diverticulosis and are most notable for (a) lower gastrointestinal bleeding that can range from a minor, self-limited process to one that is massive and life threatening, and (b) diverticulitis and its associated complications.

Diverticulitis is an inflammatory process that originates within a diverticulum and gives rise to a wide spectrum of clinical presentations. It is the most common significant complication of diverticular disease, affecting approximately 10% to 25% of those with colonic diverticula (1,2). This chapter focuses primarily on the pathogenesis, clinical syndromes, and approaches to the diagnosis and treatment of diverticulitis. Refer to two recently published practice guidelines for additional information (3,4).

PATHOGENESIS OF DIVERTICULOSIS

Colonic diverticula are an acquired deformity that generally are not present at birth and increase in number with aging. Strictly speaking, they are pseudodiverticula because they lack the muscular layer of the colonic wall; the mucosa and submucosa herniate through the muscularis propria, acquire a serosal coat, and give rise to the formation of these diverticula (5,6). Histologic sections reveal that the most likely sites of these herniations are at the point where the vasa recta, the colonic nutrient arteries, penetrate through the circular muscle bundles on either side of the mesenteric taenia and on the mesenteric side of the lateral taeniae (7,8). These sites are thought to be areas of relative weakness and thus predisposed to herniation (9,10).

What gives rise to the formation of diverticula? Multiple factors play a role. The key factors are the following:

1. A low-fiber diet
2. The aging process
3. Motility disorders
4. Connective tissue disorders, for example, Marfan and Ehlers-Danlos syndromes

Both epidemiologic and clinical data help in our understanding of this process and support the etiologic association with the factors listed. Foremost, this process has greatly different prevalences throughout the world (11–13). For example, in Africa and most of Asia, less than 1% of adults have diverticula, whereas in most industrialized nations, up to 50% of adults are affected. It has been postulated, but not proven, that low-fiber content is the primary culprit in this disparity (13,14). By increasing stool volume and thus luminal radius (see later text) and by decreasing intestinal transit time, fiber leads to a decreased intraluminal pressure (15). Milling of grains, which results in a refined, low-fiber product, became increasingly common in the Western world beginning in the late nineteenth century. At that time, diverticula were an uncommon curiosity and the incidence of diverticulosis was only 5% to 7% in autopsy series published in the United States in the 1930s and 1940s (16,17). As the Western diet has become fiber-deficient, the prevalence of diverticulosis has greatly increased (14). Support for the dietary fiber hypothesis is found in the lower frequency of diverticulosis in vegetarians on higher fiber diets compared with case-matched control subjects (1,18). In the study by Gear, 12% of vegetarians (mean daily fiber intake of 41.5 g) compared with 33% of nonvegetarians (mean fiber intake of 21 g) had diverticulosis by barium enema examination (19). Additional data arise from the observations that the preva-

G. Garcia: Department of Medicine, Stanford University Medical Center, Palo Alto, California lence of diverticulosis increases with time when people emigrate from low- to high-prevalence communities and when the diet changes from predominantly vegetarian to one that resembles a Western diet (20,21). Finally, in an animal model of diverticular disease, diverticula developed in rats fed a very low-fiber diet five times more frequently (45% versus 9%) than in rats fed a high-fiber diet (22). Even so, it has been difficult to show that Western populations with or without diverticula have different stool volumes and intestinal transit times, the expected outcome of changes in the fiber content of the diet.

In Western industrialized countries, the prevalence of diverticula clearly increases with age (2,16). Diverticula are rare before age 40 years, can be seen in 30% to 50% of those who are 50 years old, and are found in up to 67% of people by age 80 years (2). Increased elastin deposition, as opposed to decreased or abnormal collagen formation or muscular hypertrophy, occurs with aging, and is presently believed to be the underlying pathologic process that gives rise to diverticula formation (23). Elastin deposition leads to foreshortening and contraction of the colonic wall, giving it a thickened and corrugated appearance that has been termed *mychosis.* Similarly, congenital abnormalities in connective tissue formation have been implicated in the frequent and early appearance of diverticulosis in patients with connective tissue disorders (24).

Motility disorders have been implicated as a cause of diverticulosis based primarily on extrapolations from limited human data and principles of physics (25). It appears that the sigmoid colon is the most common site for diverticula because it is the site of the highest pressure gradient between the colonic lumen and the peritoneal space. Intraluminal pressure is proportional to the wall tension and inversely proportional to the luminal diameter (25). This principle is derived from the Laplace law. Wall tension is greatest in areas of increased muscle activity and mass, such as the sigmoid colon, and luminal diameter is also the smallest in the mychotic sigmoid colon. In addition, Painter hypothesized, based on manometric and radiographic data, prominent contractions of the circular smooth muscles of the sigmoid colon can effectively close off afferent and efferent loops of colon within a short segment of sigmoid colon ("segmentation") and thus lead to closed spaced compartments of focally high intraluminal pressure (26).

The location of colonic diverticula in the U.S. population is summarized as follows (27–29):

1. Ninety-six percent of patients with diverticula have sigmoid involvement.
2. Sixty percent have the diverticula confined to the sigmoid colon.
3. Eighty percent have the diverticula confined to the left colon.
4. Fifteen percent have the diverticula diffusely throughout the colon.
5. Four percent have the diverticula limited to the nonsigmoid colon, most commonly in the cecum.
6. Rectal involvement with diverticula is rare. In part, this is probably because the taeniae coli fan out and form a completely circumferential muscle layer.

The incidence of diverticulitis parallels the distribution of colonic diverticula, and more than 90% of all cases of diverticulitis involve the sigmoid colon (30). This distribution is not universal. In some Asian populations, diverticula are less common, tend to be right sided, and appear to occur about 10 years earlier (31,32). The reasons for these differences are not fully understood.

PATHOGENESIS OF DIVERTICULITIS

Obstruction at the mouth of the diverticulum secondary to impaction of fecal material (i.e., fecalith) is thought to be the initial common pathway in diverticulitis (33,34). Obstruction leads to a compromised blood supply to the diverticulum, which subsequently becomes ischemic and more susceptible to bacterial invasion. What then takes place is a progressive series of developments whose course is determined by host systemic and local factors and by the timing of the initiation of medical treatment.

The earliest stage has been termed *pericolitis* or *peridiverticulitis,* which reflects the development of a focal area of inflammation at the apex of the diverticulum. This is thought to be secondary to a "microperforation" of the colonic wall with focal extravasation of luminal contents into the adjacent serosa. This subsequently leads to a localized inflammatory mass within the colonic wall, that is, a pericolic phlegmon. Over a short period of time, tissue necrosis occurs and a pericolic abscess, which is confined by the colonic mesentery, is formed. A pericolic abscess can enlarge and perforate and thus form a pelvic abscess (35). If this inflammatory process is not contained or walled off by host factors or by the early initiation of medical treatment, a pelvic abscess can rupture and lead to generalized peritonitis with possible fecal soiling. Although free perforation is considered the most dreaded consequence of diverticulitis, numerous other complications can arise, including (a) localized abscess formation, (b) obstruction of either the colon or small bowel as a result of mass effect, and (c) fistula formation. Fibrosis and strictures may eventually result. Frank bleeding, more commonly arising from a right-sided diverticulum, is an unusual manifestation of diverticulitis. Conversely, most patients with diverticular hemorrhage have a minimal or absent inflammatory reaction at the bleeding site (36).

NATURAL HISTORY

Most patients with diverticulosis are asymptomatic. The overall incidence of diverticulitis is approximately 25% to 30% in those patients with known diverticulosis (1,37,38). The mean age at presentation with diverticulitis is between 60 and 70 years (30,39). A number of studies have reported a gradual increase in the incidence of diverticulitis with known longer duration of diverticulosis. Horner (27) followed up a group of 503 patients with radiologic evidence of diverticulosis. The incidence of diverticulitis was 10% by 5 years, 25% by 10 years, and 37% by 20 years. Boles (37) reported an incidence of approximately 30% in a group of 294 patients followed up for a mean of 15 years. The true incidence of diverticulitis as a complication of diverticulosis, however, is unknown. Most studies likely overestimate the true percentage because many patients with diverticulosis are asymptomatic and are never identified or included in the published studies.

Recurrent attacks, 27% to 45%, are not uncommon in patients who experienced a prior bout of diverticulitis. In those patients whose first episode is managed solely medically, the likelihood of relapse is approximately 15% to 40% (2,37–39). For those who underwent operative resection, recurrence rates are on the order of 3% to 12% depending on the extent of colonic resection (37,40–42).

Certain groups of patients, however, need to be managed with specialized attention. The following sections deal with the immunocompromised patient, the patient who uses nonsteroidal antiinflammatory drugs (NSAIDs), the patient with right-sided diverticulitis, and the patient younger than 40 years of age.

Immunocompromised patients, that is, those who are on long-term steroid therapy (43), have renal insufficiency (44), or have received a transplant (44–46), have an increased rate of morbidity and mortality with their attacks of diverticulitis. Current literature suggests that the incidence of diverticulitis in these populations is not increased, yet the impact of each event is magnified (47). This is thought to be the consequence of a delay in the development of classic symptoms, the difficulty in sorting through the broadened differential diagnosis, and the subsequent delay in definitive diagnosis and institution of medical treatment. Additionally, immunocompromised patients do not appear to "wall off" the inflammatory process as effectively. They more commonly have a free perforation, often with gross fecal soiling of the peritoneum, at first presentation. Tyau and co-workers (48) retrospectively reviewed 209 cases of diverticulitis, 40 of which were considered to involve immunocompromised patients. During the index hospitalization course, there was a 14% incidence of perforation in the immunocompetent group and a 43% incidence of perforation in the immunocompromised group. Surgical intervention was also more frequently required in the immunocompromised group. Mortality data from this study revealed significant differences with a death rate of 0.6% in the immunocompetent group and 25% in those who were immunocompromised.

Consensus favors an earlier consideration of definitive surgical intervention in the immunocompromised patient (43,45,47–49). Perkins and associates (47) noted a 100% failure rate for medical management in a small cohort of immunocompromised patients. Surgical intervention was ultimately required for progressive sepsis, peritonitis, perforation, obstruction, or abscess formation. The role of percutaneous drainage of an abscess in immunocompromised patients has not been studied, yet those centers with the greatest published experience with these techniques generally avoid it in this setting and also recommend early surgical intervention (50,51).

Concurrent use of NSAIDs has also been implicated in increased morbidity in patients with diverticular disease. A number of case reports and case–control studies have shown an increased rate of serious complications, including perforation and fistula formation, in patients presenting with diverticulitis who were on NSAIDs (52). A direct cause-and-effect relationship remains to be established.

Right-sided diverticulitis is an uncommon event in Western countries (53). In large part, this is because diverticula are much less common in the right colon. Right-sided diverticulitis appears to have a predilection for younger patients (mean age is 41 years) (54,55). The average age is approximately 10 to 15 years less than in patients with left-sided diverticula (41). The diagnosis is often confused with appendicitis, tubal or ovarian disorders, malignancy, Crohn disease, or infectious processes resulting from tuberculosis, amebiasis, or actinomycosis (56). Clinically, a variety of reports reveal that patients with right-sided diverticulitis usually have less nausea and vomiting and a longer duration of symptoms at presentation than those with appendicitis (57). Imaging studies such as barium enema or computed tomography (CT) scanning can be helpful yet may not be diagnostic (58), and even intraoperatively malignancy can be difficult to exclude.

In an uncomplicated case in which the diagnosis of diverticulitis has been confidently made noninvasively, a trial of medical management, with or without a drainage procedure, has been shown to be effective (54,57,59). However, most authorities recommend surgical management in any patient with complications associated with right-sided diverticulitis with a diverticulotomy, local excision, or partial right hemicolectomy (60). In addition, surgery needs to be considered when a right-sided inflammatory mass cannot be distinguished from a neoplasm or when there are recurrent episodes of diverticulitis (56,61). Although right-sided diverticulitis occurs more commonly in younger patients, most young patients have the expected distribution of colonic diverticula (left-sided) and present with diverticulitis of the sigmoid colon. However, young patients, that is, those younger than 40 years of age, appear to have a different natural history than older patients. In a number of large series, patients younger than 40 years old account for 2% to 6% of the reported cases of diverticulosis (29,62–64). Although the prevalence of diverticula in young patients is low, less than 5% to 10% (2), the incidence of diverticulitis and its associated complications appears to be modestly increased (63–67).

Acosta and associates (62) reviewed 285 cases of patients admitted to a hospital for management of diverticular disease (diverticulosis and diverticulitis). Of the total cohort, 6% were younger than 40 years of age, whereas in the subgroup with diverticulitis, 20% were younger than 40 years old. In the younger group, there was a male-to-female ratio of 3:1, which was not seen in the group as a whole (62). Ouriel and Schwartz (64) reported on 115 young patients who accounted for 2% of all the cases of diverticular disease seen at the University of Rochester Medical Center from 1961 through 1981 (64). In their series, 92 patients presented with diverticulitis; 17% needed urgent operations, 10% had elective surgery after a cooling-off period, and the rest were initially managed medically. Follow-up data over an average of 22 months showed that, of the group initially managed successfully with medical therapy (67 patients), 55% required rehospitalization for diverticular disease, 23% had serious complications, and ultimately 45% required operative management. Freischlag and co-workers (66) similarly reported that younger patients frequently presented with severe initial attacks and required surgery more frequently. In this series, 88% of young patients (compared with 42% of patients older than age 40 years) required urgent operations for complications of diverticulitis. All of these series reported a strong male predominance, and more than 80% of the episodes of diverticulitis involved the sigmoid colon. It appears that either elective or (if needed) urgent operative resection should be considered in all young patients with an episode of diverticulitis at the time of their initial presentation.

CLINICAL FEATURES

Presenting signs and symptoms of diverticulitis are consistent with the underlying stage of illness. The earliest symptoms are acute onset of pain, most commonly in the left lower quadrant, followed by fever, anorexia, nausea, vomiting, and altered bowel habits, usually constipation. Patients with a redundant sigmoid colon or diverticula at sites other than the sigmoid colon may localize their pain anywhere in the abdomen. Dysuria, urinary urgency, and frequency may indicate the presence of an inflammatory mass near the bladder wall.

Physical examination at this time generally reveals a patient in moderate distress, with depressed bowel sounds and with localized tenderness and often a palpable fullness in the left lower quadrant. Signs of local or diffuse peritoneal inflammation may be present. Digital rectal examination may reveal a tender mass in patients with a pelvic abscess.

Laboratory evaluation is notable for an increased peripheral white blood cell count with a left shift in more than 55% of patients; frequently there is an abnormal urinalysis, especially if the colonic inflammatory process is adjacent to the genitourinary system. If the inflammatory process fails to be confined to the immediate pericolonic space, signs of diffuse peritoneal irritation (abdominal rigidity) or bacteremia (tachycardia, hypotension, and eventual circulatory collapse) may predominate.

DIAGNOSIS

The diagnosis of diverticulitis is generally made on history and physical examination. Symptoms of left lower quadrant pain, fever, and decreased frequency and caliber of stools are significant. A tender, left lower quadrant abdominal mass with signs of local peritoneal irritation should be sought. Radiographic and endoscopic confirmation may be required, yet generally play a more useful role in recognizing the complications that can be associated with diverticulitis. Plain films of the abdomen are generally nondiagnostic; they may be normal, or reveal an ileus or evidence of obstruction or pneumoperitoneum. Barium or water-soluble contrast enemas can be administered cautiously during the acute phase if the diagnosis is uncertain (5,68,69), yet they are often deferred until later in the course. These studies may be diagnostic if contrast is seen outside the colonic lumen adjacent to a diverticulum. In addition, strictures, fistulas, or soft tissue inflammatory masses may be appreciated. Flexible sigmoidoscopy, like barium enemas, is also generally deferred during the acute setting because of the potential for converting a confined colonic perforation to a free peritoneal rupture and, as a consequence, causes fecal spoiling of the abdominal cavity. However, it can be employed if the diagnosis is uncertain and especially if one needs to rule out the possibility of malignancy, not diverticulitis, as the etiologic factor of either stricture formation or colonic obstruction in a patient without localized signs of inflammation. The presence of pus exuding from a diverticular opening can be diagnostic but is rarely seen.

More recently, CT scanning has become the test of choice in the acute phase of diverticulitis, when barium enema and flexible sigmoidoscopy can lead to complications such as free perforation, increased severity of obstruction, and spillage of barium sulfate into the peritoneal cavity (70–73). CT is extremely sensitive in confirming the diagnosis of diverticulitis by visualizing both the colonic and pericolonic regions, because most significant events in diverticulitis take place outside the colonic lumen. CT is also the ideal, noninvasive test for the critically ill patient when one is concerned about abscess or fistula formation or impending free perforation (71,74,75). CT effectively stratifies patients with diverticulitis according to severity of illness and helps to define subsequent treatment plans (76, 77). The use of rectal contrast (500 cm^3 of water-soluble contrast medium) has been recommended to improve the sensitivity and specificity of CT images when evaluating a patient with clinically suspected diverticulitis (78). Use of a helical CT scan and administration of only rectal contrast was highly accurate, detected unsuspected additional conditions in 58% of patients studied, and avoided the costs and risks of oral and intravenous contrast administration (79).

Ultrasound can also be used to help establish the diagnosis of diverticulitis (80–83). More importantly, ultrasound can be used to assess the abdomen for abscesses and screen for appendicitis or ovarian and tubal disorders, especially in a young patient with a clinical picture suggestive of right-sided diverticulitis. The sensitivity and specificity of ultrasound for diverticulitis are estimated to be 80% to 98% and, in expert hands, are similar to those of the CT scan (84–88).

DIFFERENTIAL DIAGNOSIS

See Table 24.1.

1. *Irritable bowel syndrome (89).* This syndrome is characterized by altered bowel habits associated with pain. The clinical presentation and management are similar to that of uncomplicated diverticulosis, except that diarrhea is frequent in irritable bowel syndrome.
2. *Appendicitis.* The most likely diagnosis in a young patient with right lower quadrant pain and fever is appendicitis. However, presentation can be identical to that of right-sided (cecal and ascending colon) diverticulitis or redundant sigmoid colon.
3. *Colonic carcinoma.* Colorectal cancer has epidemiologic features similar to those of diverticular disease and, at times, its presentation (e.g., obstructive symptoms) may overlap. Colonoscopy may be necessary to exclude colon cancer, but should be performed after the inflammatory process has ended.
4. *Inflammatory bowel disease (90).* Crohn disease in particular may mimic diverticulitis, because both can manifest with fever, lower abdominal pain, and abscess.
5. *Ischemic, infectious, or radiation-induced colitis.* In a patient at risk, a limited flexible sigmoidoscopy may be necessary to differentiate these conditions.
6. *Pelvic lesions.* Pelvic pathology, especially ovarian, tubo-ovarian, and uterine lesions, needs to be considered in any woman presenting with abdominal complaints.

TREATMENT

For uncomplicated diverticulosis, no specific treatment is required. For patients with uncomplicated diverticulosis

TABLE 24.1. DIVERTICULITIS: DIFFERENTIAL DIAGNOSIS

Diagnosis	Prevalence	Clinical Features	Diagnostic Tests	Treatment
Diverticulosis	Female = male; increases with age	Often asymptomatic; can lead to pain, altered bowel habits, lack of systemic signs	Barium enema; colonoscopy	Fiber, fluids
Diverticulitis	Female = male; increases with age	Constellation of abdominal pain, altered bowel habits	CT scan; plain films; barium enema; colonoscopy	Hydration, antibiotics, may need surgery
Irritable bowel syndrome	Female > male; most present by age 50	Abdominal pain; altered bowel habits; lack of systemic signs. Lifelong condition with recurrent symptoms	Sigmoidoscopy; barium enema	Fiber, antidiarrheal agents, laxatives, antispasmodics; psychological support
Appendicitis	Male > female; peak incidence 2nd–3rd decade	Pain followed by anorexia, nausea, vomiting, and fever	Ultrasound; CT scan; surgery	Appendectomy
Colon cancer	Increases with age	Often asymptomatic; can lead to GI bleeding, pain, vomiting, and fever	Barium enema; colonoscopy; surgery	Colonoscopic polypectomy or surgical resection
Pelvic lesions				
(A) Acute salpingitis	Most common in sexually active young women	High fever; subacute onset of bilateral lower abdominal pain; variable vomiting	Ultrasound; pelvic exam	Hydration, antibiotics
(B) Ruptured ectopic pregnancy	Most common in sexually active young women	Acute onset of lower abdominal pain; can rapidly lead into shock	Ultrasound; pelvic exam	Hydration, antibiotics, emergent surgery
Ischemic colitis	Increases with age	Crampy abdominal pain; GI bleeding; low-grade fever; often with symptomatic coexisting vascular disease	Plain films; barium enema; colonoscopy	Generally medical. Hydration, antibiotics; surgical resection in selected cases of transmural disease
Inflammatory bowel disease	Any age yet usually by age 30 (bimodal age of onset)	Pain; fever; altered bowel habits common; lifelong condition with recurrent symptoms	Barium enema; colonoscopy; small bowel X-rays	Medical if possible: Steroids, asulfidine derivatives, immuno suppressives; selective surgical resection

who complain of chronic abdominal discomfort or altered bowel habits, current recommendations parallel those for irritable bowel, that is, fiber (dietary or supplemental), fluids, antispasmodics such as dicyclomine, and, rarely, analgesics. The only therapy that has been validated by controlled trials is increased fiber intake, generally 10 to 25 g daily (91,92). Fiber supplementation may lead initially to bloating or worsening of symptoms; thus, beginning at a low dose and gradually increasing daily fiber intake is recommended.

Treatment for diverticulitis needs to be tailored to the medical condition at the time of presentation (34,35,73, 93,94). All patients with fever and leukocytosis in association with abdominal pain and evidence of local peritoneal irritation should be admitted to the hospital. Initial management includes bowel rest (with nasogastric decompression if nausea and vomiting are present, or there is evidence of bowel obstruction), intravenous hydration, and parenteral antibiotics. Empirical antibiotic coverage is directed at the likely organisms predictably involved. The spectrum of bacteria that complicates diverticulitis is the same as that found in the normal flora of the colon or feces. These include the enteric anaerobes (*Bacteroides fragilis*), the gram-negative aerobic bacilli (*Escherichia coli*), and the gram-positive coliforms (*Streptococcus faecalis*).

Common choices for antibiotic coverage include "triple coverage" with ampicillin, gentamicin, and metronidazole. Recently, the use of broad-spectrum cephalosporins (cefoxitin or cefotetan), extended spectrum penicillins (combined with a β-lactamase inhibitor) and quinolones have been advocated. Duma and Kellum (95) reviewed the efficacy of a wide variety of antibiotic regimens in patients with intraabdominal sepsis (95). They noted that aminoglycosides, broad-spectrum penicillins (96), cephalosporins (97,98), monobactams, and carbapenems (99) are all effective drugs in treating patients with gram-negative bacilli. Although some of these drugs have anaerobic coverage, drugs such as clindamycin and metronidazole are often added for additional anaerobic coverage (98). However, Kellum and colleagues (97), in a randomized prospective study of 51 patients with diverticulitis, compared the efficacy of cefoxitin to a combination of gentamicin and clindamycin. Both regimens had similar "cure rates" (greater than 85%) and were similarly well tolerated. On balance, these investigators favored the use of cefoxitin as a single agent, given its reduced risk of nephrotoxicity in an elderly population and its narrower spectrum, thus avoiding the emergence of highly resistant organisms (97).

When diverticulitis is recognized and treated promptly, the course is often uncomplicated and successfully managed with medical therapy, as is true in 70% to 85% of patients (38,39,100). A favorable response is generally seen within 2 to 4 days, with resolution of the signs and symptoms of the underlying illness. At this point, one can return to an oral diet. Antibiotics should be continued for a total of 7 to 10 days. Radiographic or endoscopic evaluation of the colon and abdomen should be performed after the acute inflammatory process has subsided.

In those patients who fail to respond to medical management and who remain with systemic or localized complaints, additional timely interventions are required. Workup may include the following:

1. Plain abdominal films—looking for free air or obstruction
2. Abdominal/pelvic CT scan—looking for abscess or fistula formation
3. "Gentle" lower gastrointestinal series (barium or, more commonly, a water-soluble agent)—looking for fistula or stricture formation, localizing the site of inflammation
4. Colonoscopy—ruling out malignancy and evaluation of a stricture (101), generally reserved for those patients in which radiographic studies are not helpful
5. Ultrasound—used to look for abscess, tuboovarian abscesses, ovarian cysts, or appendicitis (81,102,103)

CT scanning is becoming the primary diagnostic tool for evaluating patients in whom the diagnosis is uncertain or who are failing to respond to initial medical management. CT is regarded as a safe and highly sensitive tool. CT is useful in confirming the diagnosis as well as revealing the extent and nature of complications, including abscesses and fistulas (Fig. 24.1).

When a patient is failing medical therapy, a combination of the aforementioned tests is often required. The patient's clinical course as well as the physician's clinical judgment and local expertise are critical factors. The most likely interventions that may need to be considered are surgical intervention and percutaneous drainage of an abscess. Surgical treatment is generally divided into four categories: (a) emergent, (b) urgent, (c) abscess drainage, and (d) elective. Approximately 15% to 30% of patients may require surgical intervention during their initial hospitalization (103)

For the patient with frank peritoneal signs and free air on a plain film, indicative of free perforation into the abdominal cavity, attempts at stabilization should immediately be followed by operative intervention. In general, indications for immediate or urgent surgery include (a) progressive symptoms or sepsis despite antibiotics, (b) uncontained perforation, (c) large or small bowel obstruction not responsive to nasoenteral decompression, and (d) the persistence or progression of an abscess despite attempts at percutaneous drainage (30,104).

When a patient requires emergency surgery because of perforation or the inability to effectively stabilize with medical therapy, a two-stage operation is generally indicated. In this setting, the surgeon is usually managing an unstable patient with an unprepped colon. The risks of performing a primary anastomosis at the time of colonic resection are high and include anastomotic breakdown, fistula formation, and increased operative mortality rate (30,104,105). Currently, a two-stage operation is recommended (30,41).

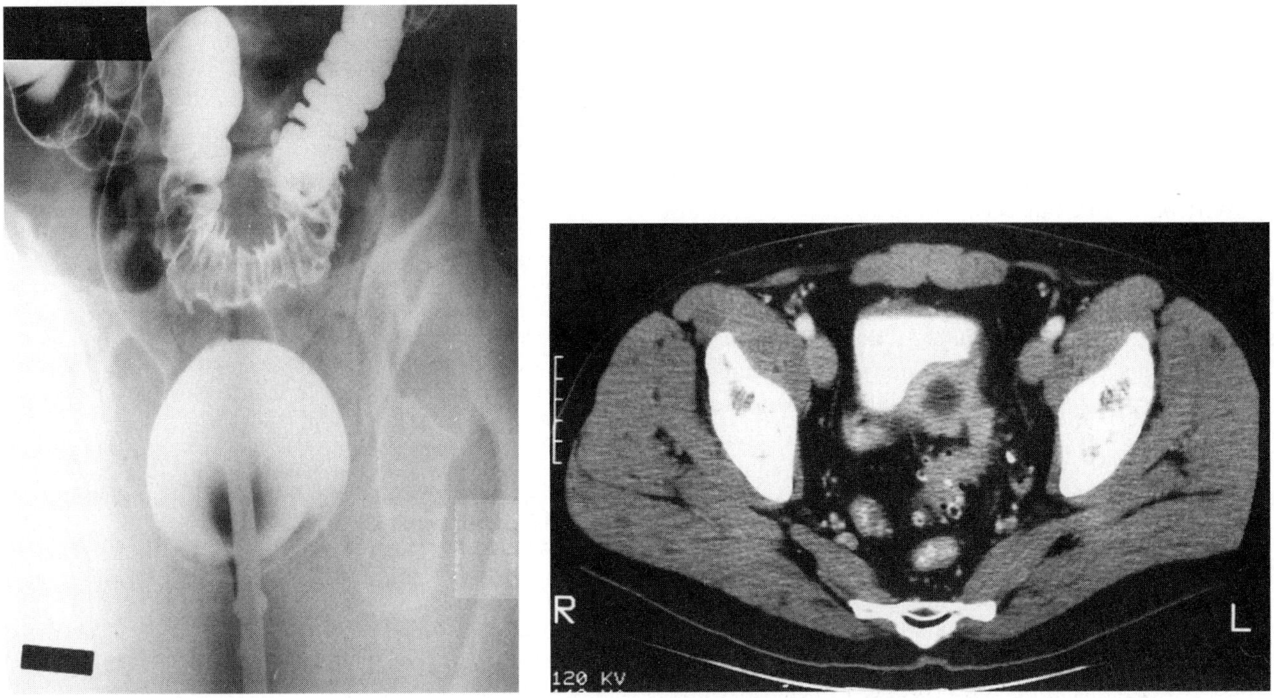

FIGURE 24.1. A 47-year-old man presented with fever, left lower quadrant pain, and absence of stools for 4 days. A barium enema *(left)* showed diverticula and narrowing of the sigmoid colon. A subsequent abdominal computed tomography scan *(right)* showed a pericolonic abscess at the site of the diverticula in the sigmoid colon.

During the first stage, the involved area of the colon is resected, the proximal loop is brought up as an end colostomy, the distal loop is either closed off (Hartmann pouch) or made into a mucous fistula, and the peritoneum is aggressively lavaged. At the time of the second stage, performed approximately 3 months later, restoration of colonic continuity can be accomplished.

For patients who can be stabilized with initial medical management yet who go on to abscess formation, the surgical approach often can be done in a single stage. This is true for abscesses that are generally small and contiguous with the colonic mesentery (mesocolic abscess) as well as for pelvic abscesses. Small mesocolic abscesses have a better prognosis and often can be managed with a single-stage operative procedure with en bloc removal of the abscess cavity and the diseased segment of the colon (106). In fact, surgery is not always required in this setting, because a small mesocolic abscess can respond to medical treatment with antibiotics without a drainage procedure (107).

A number of recent reports have shown that the optimal treatment of a larger (>5 cm) pelvic or paracolic abscess generally includes preoperative percutaneous placement of a drainage catheter into the abscess cavity (51,106,108–111). Percutaneous drainage is generally done under CT guidance and can be done in almost all patients with an abscess as long as the abscess cavity is readily accessible and the patient is without signs of generalized peritonitis. Percutaneous drainage has been shown to effectively resolve the acute inflammatory process in most patients. Review of most series reveals an approximately 70% success rate in converting an anticipated multistage to a one-stage surgical procedure by preoperative percutaneous drainage (51,106). The one-stage operation includes a full bowel prep and subsequent resection of the involved area with primary colonic closure. In Stabile and colleagues' (51) series, 14 of 17 patients, and in Mueller and colleagues' series (106), 13 of 21 patients were successfully managed with preoperative percutaneous drainage followed by a one-stage procedure. Operative mortality rate is thus thought to be reduced in a patient who has been stabilized, hydrated, and prepped and who requires only a one-stage surgical procedure.

In a small minority of patients with large abscesses who were successfully managed with percutaneous drainage, a definitive operative procedure was deferred for a variety of reasons, including patient refusal. Despite initial success, however, preliminary data reveal a high incidence of recurrent abscess formation and signs and symptoms of diverticulitis over the ensuing months (48,97). Elective resection of the involved colon is generally recommended to the one-third of patients who have at least two attacks of uncomplicated diverticulitis (107–111).

Surgery for diverticulitis may be performed using minimally invasive surgical techniques. This may be performed using a total laparoscopic approach, an assisted laparoscopic approach, or a dissection-facilitated laparoscopic resection. These alternative surgical approaches may benefit the patient and surgeon regarding degree of postoperative pain, length of hospitalization, and time to recovery of gut function (112–114).

Fistula formation is also a well-recognized complication of diverticulitis and can occur in up to 20% of patients reported in surgical series, yet the true incidence is likely to be much lower if one includes all cases of diverticulitis (115–118). The fistula usually forms after an abscess extends and subsequently ruptures into a nearby structure. The signs and symptoms of fistula are often subacute and can manifest after the acute colonic inflammatory process has resolved. The most common site is a colovesical fistula, which accounts for approximately two-thirds of all fistulas; others extend to the vagina, or less likely to other parts of the colon, the small intestine, the uterus, or the skin. Treatment of a fistula tract is surgical with complete excision of the fistula tract.

Fistulas as well as strictures and partial obstructions can also frequently be dealt with in a one-stage procedure as long as bowel preparation can be done. In general, when surgical intervention is performed, the proximal line of resection should be at a site above the inflamed or involved area that is focally free of diverticula (more proximal segments that harbor diverticula may remain), and the distal line should be carried beyond the point of the most distal diverticulum, usually the proximal rectum (40).

CONCLUSION

Diverticulitis, which occurs in up to 30% of individuals with diverticulosis, is the most common complication of diverticular disease. Most patients with diverticulitis can be treated medically, yet a variety of diagnostic and therapeutic options are available for those with complicated courses. Although the classic scenario is left lower quadrant abdominal pain and fever in a middle-aged to elderly person, one must be aware of the different presentations of diverticulitis in other subgroups of patients, such as the immunocompromised.

REFERENCES

1. Almy TP, Howell DA. Medical progress. Diverticular disease of the colon. *N Engl J Med* 1980;302:324–331.
2. Parks TG. Natural history of diverticular disease of the colon. *Clin Gastroenterol* 1975;4:53–69.
3. Stollman NH, Raskin JB. Diagnosis and management of diverticular disease of the colon in adults. *Am J Gastroenterol* 1999; 94:3110–3121.
4. Wong DW, Wexner SD, Lowry A, et al. Practice parameters for the treatment of sigmoid diverticulitis. *Dis Colon Rectum* 2000; 43:289–297.
5. Fleischner FG. Diverticular disease of the colon. New observations and revised concepts. *Gastroenterology* 1971;60:316–324.
6. Morson BC. Pathology of diverticular disease of the colon. *Clin Gastroenterol* 1975;4:37–52.
7. Drummond H. Sacculi of the large intestine, with special reference to their relations to the blood vessels of the bowel wall. *Br J Surg* 1916;4:407.
8. Meyers MA, Volberg F, Katzen B, et al. The angioarchitecture of colonic diverticula. Significance in bleeding diverticulosis. *Radiology* 1973;108(2):249–261.
9. Noer RJ. Hemorrhage as a complication of diverticulitis. *Ann Surg* 1955;141:674–685.
10. Slack WW. The anatomy, pathology, and some clinical features of diverticulitis of the colon. *Br J Surg* 1962;50:185.
11. Kyle J, Adesola AO, Tinckler LF, et al. Incidence of diverticulitis. *Scand J Gastroenterol* 1967;2:77–80.
12. Mendeloff Al. Thoughts on the epidemiology of diverticular disease. *Clin Gastroenterol* 1986;15:855–877.
13. Painter NS, Burkitt DP. Diverticular disease of the colon: a deficiency disease of western civilization. *BMJ* 1971;2:450–454.
14. Connell AM. Pathogenesis of diverticular disease of the colon. *Adv Intern Med* 1977;22:377–395.
15. Findlay JM, Smith AN, Mitchell WD, et al. Effects of unprocessed bran on colon function in normal subjects and in diverticular disease. *Lancet* 1974;1:146–149.
16. Painter NS, Burkitt DP. Diverticular disease of the colon, a 20th century problem. *Clin Gastroenterol* 1975;4:3–21.
17. Rankin FW, Brown PW. Diverticulitis of the colon. *Surg Gynecol Obstet* 1930;50:836.
18. Brodribb AJ, Humphreys DM. Diverticular disease: three studies. Part I—Relation to other disorders and fibre intake. *BMJ* 1976;1:424–425.
19. Gear JS, Ware A, Fursdon P, et al. Symptomless diverticular disease and intake of dietary fibre. *Lancet* 1979;1:511–514.
20. Segal I, Solomon A, Hunt JA. Emergence of diverticular disease in the urban South African black. *Gastroenterology* 1977;72: 215–219.
21. Mermann GN, Yatani R. Diverticulosis and polyps of the large intestine. A necropsy study of Hawaii Japanese. *Cancer* 1973; 31:1260–1270.
22. Fisher N, Berry CS, Fearn T, et al. Cereal dietary fiber consumption and diverticular disease: a lifespan study in rats. *Am J Clin Nutr* 1985;43:788–804.
23. Whiteway J, Morson BC. Elastosis in diverticular disease of the sigmoid colon. *Gut* 1985;26:258–266.
24. Beighton PH, Murdoch JL, Votteler T. Gastrointestinal complications of the Ehlers-Danlos syndrome. *Gut* 1969;10:1004–1008.
25. Eastwood MA, Watters DA, Smith AN. Diverticular disease—is it a motility disorder? *Clin Gastroenterol* 1982;11:545–561.
26. Painter NS, Turelove SC, Ardran GM, et al. Segmentation and the localization of intraluminal pressures in the human colon, with special reference to the pathogenesis of colonic diverticula. *Gastroenterology* 1965;49:169.
27. Horner JL. Natural history of diverticulosis of the colon. *Am J Dig Dis* 1958;3:343.
28. Hughes LE. Postmortem survey of diverticular disease of the colon. I. Diverticulosis and diverticulitis. II. The muscular abnormality of the sigmoid colon. *Gut* 1969;10:336–351.
29. Parks TG. Natural history of diverticular disease of the colon: a review of 521 cases. *BMJ* 1969;4:639–642.
30. Rodkey GV, Welch CE. Changing patterns in the surgical treatment of diverticular disease. *Ann Surg* 1984;200:466–478.
31. Sugihara K, Muto T, Morioka Y, et al. Diverticular disease of the colon in Japan. A review of 615 cases. *Dis Colon Rectum* 1984; 27:531–537.
32. Vajrabukka T, Saksornchai K, Jimakorn P. Diverticular disease of the colon in a far-eastern community. *Dis Colon Rectum* 1980;23:151–154.

33. Ming S-C, Fleischner FG. Diverticulitis of the sigmoid colon: reappraisal of the pathology and pathogenesis. *Surgery* 1965;58: 627.
34. Morson BC. The muscle abnormality in diverticular disease of the sigmoid colon. *Br J Radiol* 1963;36:385.
35. Hinchey EJ, Schaal PG, Richards GK. Treatment of perforated diverticular disease of the colon. *Adv Surg* 1978;12:85–109.
36. Meyers MA, Alonso DR, Gray GF, Baer JW. Pathogenesis of bleeding colonic diverticulosis. *Gastroenterology* 1976;71: 577–583.
37. Boles RS, Jordan SM. The clinical significance of diverticulosis. *Gastroenterology* 1958;35:579.
38. Colcock BP. Surgical management of complicated diverticulitis. *N Engl J Med* 1958;259:570–573.
39. Larson DM, Masters SS, Spiro HM. Medical and surgical therapy in diverticular disease: a comparative study. *Gastroenterology* 1976;71:734–737.
40. Benn PL, Wolff BG, Ilstrup DM. Level of anastomosis and recurrent colonic diverticulitis. *Am J Surg* 1986;151:269–271.
41. Chappuis CW, Cohn IJ. Acute colonic diverticulitis. *Surg Clin North Am* 1988;68:301–313.
42. Wolff BG, Ready RL, MacCarty RL, et al. Influence of sigmoid resection on progression of diverticular disease of the colon. *Dis Colon Rectum* 1984;27:645–647.
43. ReMine SG, McIlrath DC. Bowel perforation in steroid-treated patients. *Ann Surg* 1980;192:581–586.
44. Starnes HJ, Lazarus JM, Vineyard G. Surgery for diverticulitis in renal failure. *Dis Colon Rectum* 1985;28:827–831.
45. Guice K, Rattazzi LC, Marchioro TL. Colon perforation in renal transplant patients. *Am J Surg* 1979;138:43–48.
46. Lao A, Bach D. Colonic complications in renal transplant recipients. *Dis Colon Rectum* 1988;31:130–133.
47. Perkins JD, Shield C, Chang FC, et al. Acute diverticulitis. Comparison of treatment in immunocompromised and nonimmunocompromised patients. *Am J Surg* 1984;148:745–748.
48. Tyau ES, Prystowsky JB, Joehl RJ, et al. Acute diverticulitis. A complicated problem in the immunocompromised patient. *Arch Surg* 1991;126:855–859; discussion 858–859.
49. Alexander P, Schuman E, Vetto RM. Perforation of the colon in the immunocompromised patient. *Am J Surg* 1986;151:557–561.
50. Rodkey GV. Letter. *Am J Surg* 1990;159:104.
51. Stabile BE, Puccio E, vanSonnenberg E, et al. Preoperative percutaneous drainage of diverticular abscesses. *Am J Surg* 1990; 159:99–104; discussion.
52. Bjarnason I, Hayllar J, MacPherson AJ, et al. Side effects of nonsteroidal anti-inflammatory drugs on the small and large intestine in humans. *Gastroenterology* 1993;104:1832–1847.
53. Williams KL. Acute solitary ulcers and acute diverticulitis of the caecum and ascending colon. *Br J Surg* 1960;47:351–358.
54. Bova JG, Hopens TA, Goldstein HM. Diverticulitis of the right colon. *Dig Dis Sci* 1984;29:150–156.
55. Wagner D, Zollinger R. Diverticulitis of the cecum and ascending colon. *Arch Surg* 1961;83:436–442.
56. Wyble EJ, Lee WC. Cecal diverticulitis: changing trends in management. *South Med J* 1988;81:313–316.
57. Fischer MG, Farkas AM. Diverticulitis of the cecum and ascending colon. *Dis Colon Rectum* 1984;27:454–458.
58. Balthazar EJ, Megibow AJ, Gordon RB, et al. Cecal diverticulitis: evaluation with CT. *Radiology* 1987;162:79–81.
59. Morris J, Stellato TA, Lieberman J, et al. The utility of computed tomography in colonic diverticulitis. *Ann Surg* 1986;204: 128–132.
60. Arrington P, Judd CJ. Cecal diverticulitis. *Am J Surg* 1981;142: 56–59.
61. Schmit PJ, Bennion RS, Thompson JJ. Cecal diverticulitis: a continuing diagnostic dilemma. *World J Surg* 1991;15:367–371.
62. Acosta JA, Grebenc ML, Doberneck RC, et al. Colonic diverticular disease in patients 40 years old or younger. *Am Surg* 1992;58:605–607.
63. Eusebio EB, Eisenberg MM. Natural history of diverticular disease of the colon in young patients. *Am J Surg* 1973;125: 308–311.
64. Ouriel K, Schwartz SI. Diverticular disease in the young patient. *Surg Gynecol Obstet* 1983;156:1–5.
65. Feczko PJ, Nish AD, Craig BM, et al. Acute diverticulitis in patients under 40 years of age: radiologic diagnosis. *AJR Am J Roentgenol* 1988;150:1311–1314.
66. Freischlag J, Bennion RS, Thompson JJ. Complications of diverticular disease of the colon in young people. *Dis Colon Rectum* 1986;29:639–643.
67. Hannan CE, Knightly JJ, Coffey RJ. Diverticular disease of the colon in the younger age group. *Dis Colon Rectum* 1961;4: 419–423.
68. Hiltunen JN, Kolehmainen H, Vuorinen T, et al. Early water-soluble contrast enema in the diagnosis of acute colonic diverticulitis. *Int J Colorect Dis* 1991;6:190–192.
69. Nicholas GG, Miller WT, Fitts WT, et al. Diagnosis of diverticulitis of the colon: role of the barium enema in defining pericolic inflammation. *Ann Surg* 1972;176(2):205–209.
70. Ertan A. Colonic diverticulitis. Recognizing and managing its presentations and complications [see comments]. *Postgrad Med* 1990;88:67–72, 77.
71. Hulnick DH, Megibow AJ, Balthazar EJ, et al. Computed tomography in the evaluation of diverticulitis. *Radiology* 1984; 152:491–495.
72. Lieberman JM, Haaga JR. Computed tomography of diverticulitis. *J Comput Assist Tomogr* 1983;7:431–443.
73. Pohlman T. Diverticulitis. *Gastroenterol Clin North Am* 1988; 17:357–385.
74. Doringer E. Computerized tomography of colonic diverticulitis. *Crit Rev Diagn Imaging* 1992;33:421–435.
75. Pillari G, Greenspan B, Vernace FM, et al. Computed tomography of diverticulitis. *Gastrointest Radiol* 1984;9:263–268.
76. Hachigian MP, Honickman S, Eisenstat TE, et al. Computed tomography in the initial management of acute left-sided diverticulitis. *Dis Colon Rectum* 1992;35:1123–1129.
77. Ambrosetti P, Gossholz M, Becker C, et al. Computed tomography in acute left colonic diverticulitis. *Br J Surg* 1997;84:532–534.
78. Raval B, Lamki N, St Ville E. Role of computed tomography in diverticulitis. *J Comput Tomogr* 1987;11:144–150.
79. Rao PM, Rhea JT, Novelline RA, et al. Helical CT with only colonic contrast material for diagnosing diverticulitis: prospective evaluation of 150 patients. *AJR Am J Roentgenol* 1998;170: 1445–1450.
80. Parulekar SG. Sonography of colonic diverticulitis. *J Ultrasound Med* 1985;4:659–666.
81. Schwerk WB, Schwarz S, Rothmund M. Sonography in acute colonic diverticulitis. A prospective study. *Dis Colon Rectum* 1992;35:1077–1084.
82. Wada M, Kikuchi Y, Doy M. Uncomplicated acute diverticulitis of the cecum and ascending colon: sonographic findings in 18 patients. *AJR Am J Roentgenol* 1990;155:283–287.
83. Wilson SR, Toi A. The value of sonography in the diagnosis of acute diverticulitis of the colon. *AJR Am J Roentgenol* 1990; 154:1199–1202.
84. Verbanck J, Lambrecht S, Rutgeerts L, et al. Can sonography diagnose acute colonic diverticulitis in patients with acute intestinal inflammation? A prospective study. *J Clin Ultrasound* 1989;17:661–666.
85. Schwerk WB, Schwartz S, Rothmund M. Sonography in acute colonic diverticulitis: a prospective study. *Dis Colon Rectum* 1992;35:1077–1084.

86. Zielke A, Hasse C, Nies C, et al. Prospective evaluation of ultrasonography in acute colonic diverticulitis. *Br J Surg* 1997;84: 385-388.
87. Pradel JA, Adell J-F, Taourel P, et al. Acute colonic diverticulitis: prospective comparative evaluation with US and CT. *Radiology* 1997;205:503–512.
88. Eggesbo HB, Jacobsen R, Kolmannskog F, et al. Diagnosis of acute left-sided colonic diverticulitis by three radiological modalities. *Acta Radiol* 1998;39:315–321.
89. Otte JJ, Larsen L, Andersen JR. Irritable bowel syndrome and symptomatic diverticular disease—different diseases? *Am J Gastroenterol* 1986;81:529–531.
90. Schmidt GT, Lennard JJ, Morson BC, et al. Crohn's disease of the colon and its distinction from diverticulitis. *Gut* 1968;9: 7–16.
91. Brodribb AJ. Treatment of symptomatic diverticular disease with a high-fibre diet. *Lancet* 1977;1:664–666.
92. Weinreich J. Controlled studies with dietary fibre in the therapy of diverticular disease and irritable bowel syndrome. In: *Colon and nutrition. Proceedings of Falk Symposium #32.* Lancaster, England: MTP Press, 1981:239.
93. Hughes LE. Complications of diverticular disease: inflammation, obstruction and bleeding. *Clin Gastroenterol* 1975;4:147–170.
94. Ulin AW, Pearce AE, Weinstein SF. Diverticular disease of the colon: surgical perspectives in the past decade. *Dis Colon Rectum* 1981;24:276–281.
95. Duma RJ, Kellum JM. Colonic diverticulitis: microbiologic, diagnostic, and therapeutic considerations. *Curr Clin Top Infect Dis* 1991;11:218–247.
96. Najem AZ, Kaminski ZC, Spillert CR, et al. Comparative study of parenteral piperacillin and cefoxitin in the treatment of surgical infections of the abdomen. *Surg Gynecol Obstet* 1983;157: 423–425.
97. Kellum JM, Sugerman HJ, Coppa GF, et al. Randomized, prospective comparison of cefoxitin and gentamicin-clindamycin in the treatment of acute colonic diverticulitis. *Clin Ther* 1992;14:376–384.
98. Tally FP, Ho JL. Management of patients with intraabdominal infection due to colonic perforation. *Curr Clin Top Infect Dis* 1987;8:266–295.
99. Jones RN. Review of the in vitro spectrum of activity of imipenem. *Am J Med* 1985;78:22–32.
100. Konsten J, Gouma DJ, Obertop H, et al. Effect of preoperative risk factors on the outcome after surgery for complicated diverticular disease. *Neth J Surg* 1990;42:101–104.
101. Forde KA, Treat MR. Colonoscopy in the evaluation of strictures. *Dis Colon Rectum* 1985;28:699–701.
102. Jeffrey RJ, Laing FC, Townsend RR. Acute appendicitis: sonographic criteria based on 250 cases. *Radiology* 1988;167: 327–329.
103. Puylaert JB, Rutgers PH, Lalisang RI, et al. A prospective study of ultrasonography in the diagnosis of appendicitis. *N Engl J Med* 1987;317:666–669.
104. Lambert ME, Knox RA, Schofield PF, et al. Management of the septic complications of diverticular disease. *Br J Surg* 1986;73: 576–579.
105. Colcock BP. Diverticular disease: proven surgical management. *Clin Gastroenterol* 1975;4:99–119.
106. Mueller PR, Saini S, Wittenburg J, et al. Sigmoid diverticular abscesses: percutaneous drainage as an adjunct to surgical resection in 24 cases. *Radiology* 1987;164:321–325.
107. Ambrosetti P, Robert J, Witzig JA, et al. Incidence, outcome, and proposed management of isolated abscesses complicating acute left-sided colonic diverticulitis. A prospective study of 140 patients. *Dis Colon Rectum* 1992;35:1072–1076.
108. Neff CC, vanSonnenberg E, Casola G, et al. Diverticular abscesses: percutaneous drainage. *Radiology* 1987;163:15–18.
109. Saini S, Mueller PR, Wittenberg J, et al. Percutaneous drainage of diverticular abscess. An adjunct to surgical therapy. *Arch Surg* 1986;121:475–478.
110. Sparks FC, Strauss EB, Corey JM. Percutaneous drainage of a diverticular abscess can make colostomy unnecessary in selected cases. *Conn Med* 1990;54:305–307.
111. Sonnenberg E, Mueller PR, Ferrucci JJ. Percutaneous drainage of 250 abdominal abscesses and fluid collections. Part I., results, failures, and complications. *Radiology* 1984;151:337–341.
112. Bouillot JL, Aouad K, Badawy A, et al. Elective laparoscopic assisted colectomy for diverticular disease: a prospective study in 50 patients. *Surg Endosc* 1998;12:1393–1396.
113. Stevenson AR, Stitz RW, Lumley JW, et al. Laparoscopically assisted anterior resection for diverticular disease: Follow-up of 100 consecutive patients. *Ann Surg* 1998;227:335–342.
114. Carbajo Caballero MA, Martin del Olmo JC, Blanco JI, et al. The laparoscopic approach in the treatment of diverticular colon disease. *J Soc Laparoendosc Surg* 1998;2:159–161.
115. McConnell DB, Sasaki TM, Vetto RM. Experience with colovesical fistula. *Am J Surg* 1980;140:80–84.
116. Small WP, Smith AN. Fistula and conditions associated with diverticular disease of the colon. *Clin Gastroenterol* 1975;4: 171–199.
117. Steele M, Deveney C, Burchell M. Diagnosis and management of colovesical fistulas. *Dis Colon Rectum* 1979;22:27–30.
118. Woods RJ, Lavery IC, Fazio VW, et al. Internal fistulas in diverticular disease. *Dis Colon Rectum* 1988;31:591–596.

25

PERITONITIS AND INTRAABDOMINAL ABSCESS

DAVID W. HECHT
SYDNEY M. FINEGOLD

PERITONITIS

Peritonitis is inflammation of the serous lining of the peritoneal cavity. It represents a response to a variety of factors including microbial agents and chemical irritants. It is clearly much more of a problem than was appreciated by Stewardson (1), who wrote in 1844 in Elliotson's *Practice of Medicine:*

> The treatment of peritonitis is easy enough, it consists of a general bleeding, followed by an abundance of local bleeding (by means of leeches), a rapid affection of the mouth by mercury and keeping the bowels well purged the whole time.

The surface area of the peritoneum approximates that of the skin. Normally, the peritoneal cavity is lubricated with approximately 20 to 50 mL of clear yellow fluid with characteristics of a transudate; there are fewer than 300 cells/mm^3 (mostly macrophages and lymphocytes), the specific gravity is low (<1.016), and the protein (chiefly albumin) content is low (<3 g/dL). In bacterial peritonitis, there may be inflow of 300 to 500 mL of fluid/h into the peritoneal cavity (2).

Nonmicrobial peritonitis may follow the introduction into the peritoneal cavity of irritants such as blood, bile, pancreatic juice, other gastroduodenal juices, meconium, and starch or other foreign bodies. Peritonitis may occur in the course of sarcoidosis and familial Mediterranean fever (as part of familial paroxysmal polyserositis). Acute chylous peritonitis may have a sudden onset with crampy abdominal pain; the turbid ascitic fluid is typically sterile. On occasion, chemical peritonitis may be related to intraperitoneal administration of antimicrobial agents, such as vancomycin (3).

Infectious causes of peritonitis are considered in the following categories: primary or spontaneous peritonitis, secondary peritonitis, peritonitis relating to peritoneal dialysis, and miscellaneous types of peritonitis (including actinomycotic, fungal, parasitic, and tuberculous).

D. W. Hecht: Departments of Medicine and Infectious Diseases, Loyola University Medical Center, Maywood, Illinois
S. M. Finegold: Department of Medicine, VA West Los Angeles Medical Center, Los Angeles, California

Primary or Spontaneous Peritonitis

This syndrome is best defined as peritonitis without an evident gastrointestinal (GI) tract source (e.g., perforated viscus). For the most part, no local source is evident. It may, however, be related to female genital tract infection on occasion. There are variants. Cases with positive ascitic fluid culture but no clinical findings of peritonitis have been designated as *bacterascites*. These cases may represent early colonization but their associated mortality rate is comparable to that of classic cases of spontaneous bacterial peritonitis (SBP). Conversely, there are patients with clinical evidence of peritonitis and increased white blood cell counts in ascitic fluid, but with negative cultures. These have been called *culture-negative neutrocytic ascites.*

Background Factors

SBP in children is seen much less frequently than was true in the pre-antibiotic era; it presently accounts for only 1% to 2% of pediatric abdominal emergencies. In children, it is seen particularly in association with postnecrotic cirrhosis and with the nephrotic syndrome. There may be an association with urinary tract infection.

In adults, the major underlying factor is cirrhosis with ascites. The prevalence of SBP in such patients is approximately 15% (4). If culture-negative cases are included, the prevalence of SBP in cirrhotic patients with ascites is 19%. Although alcoholic cirrhosis is the principal background illness, SBP has been seen in patients with ascites due to postnecrotic cirrhosis, chronic active hepatitis, acute viral hepatitis, congestive heart failure, malignancy, systemic lupus erythematosus, rheumatoid arthritis, lymphedema, nephrotic syndrome, gonococcal perihepatitis, and Budd-Chiari syndrome. Rarely, there is no apparent underlying disease.

Andreu and associates (5) prospectively studied 110 patients with cirrhosis and ascites and found an incidence of first-episode SBP of 25%. There were a number of risk factors that would predict the occurrence of SBP, but for clinical purposes the two that served well were ascitic fluid protein level (>1 g/dL) and serum bilirubin level (>2.5 mg/dL). The follow-up was 46 plus or minus 3.5 weeks, with a range of 4 to 120 weeks. Runyon demonstrated that patients with low ascitic fluid total protein had a 10-fold higher incidence of SBP compared with those with a protein level of more than 1g/dL (6).

Etiology

Before the availability of antimicrobial agents, *Streptococcus pneumoniae* and group A streptococci were important agents in SBP in children; these organisms are much less frequent, having been replaced by predominantly gram-negative bacilli and occasionally staphylococci. In adults, gram-negative bacilli also dominate, followed by streptococci and other gram-positive cocci. Garcia-Tsao (4) tabulated 806 organisms recovered from 746 cases of SBP in 27 reported series of cases; only 8% had a polymicrobial flora. Gram-negative bacilli were found in 72% of cases; included were *Escherichia coli* (in 47%), *Klebsiella* species (13%), and others. Roughly one-fourth of cases had gram-positive cocci present; included were *S. pneumoniae,* other streptococci (primarily the viridans group), *Enterococcus,* and *Staphylococcus* (both *Staphylococcus aureus* and coagulase-negative forms). Anaerobes and microaerophiles were only seen in 5% of cases. A similar tabulation by Richardet and Beaugrand (7), involving 25 series published since 1978 and 532 patients, yielded similar results but with even fewer anaerobes. Boixeda and co-workers (8) found 49% gram-negative aerobes or facultative organisms, 10% *S. pneumoniae,* and 17% other aerobic gram-positive cocci. The remaining organisms listed were yeast or polymicrobial, with only 0.9% anaerobes. Targan and colleagues (9) found a 6% incidence of anaerobes or microaerophiles. Anaerobes may be uncommon in SBP because of the relatively high oxygen content of ascitic fluid, which is comparable to that of venous blood (10). In general, recovery of anaerobes from ascitic fluid, particularly in polymicrobial cases, should raise the possibility of secondary peritonitis. Cases of *Listeria monocytogenes* peritonitis with underlying ascites are rare (< 30 cases), but it is an important pathogen to recognize (3). Group A streptococci can also cause primary peritonitis in the absence of underlying disease or ascites, although it is rare (15 cases worldwide); it presents clinically as shock predominantly in women (11). Specific organisms that have been reported in SBP are listed in Table 25.1.

Pathogenesis and Pathology

The frequency with which bowel organisms are found in SBP suggests that the gut is the major source of the infection. However, other sources are evident as well. The urinary tract may be important as indicated by a study that found the same organism in urine and in ascitic fluid in

TABLE 25.1. ORGANISMS RECOVERED FROM SPONTANEOUS BACTERIAL PERITONITIS

Gram-negative bacilli
- *Citrobacter amalonaticus* (17)
- *Enterobacter aerogenes* (331)
- *Enterobacter cloacae*
- *Escherichia coli*
- *Klebsiella pneumoniae*
- *Proteus*
- *Providencia*
- *Salmonella*
- *Serratia*
- *Yersinia enterocolitica* (332)

Other
- *Acinetobacter*
- *Aeromonas hydrophila*
- *Aeromonas sobria* (333)

Brucella melitensis (334)

Campylobacter fetus
- *Flavobacterium meningosepticum*
- *Haemophilus*
- *Moraxella*
- *Pasteurella multocida* (335)
- *Pseudomonas aeruginosa*

Gram-negative cocci
- *Neisseria meningitidis* (336)
- *Neisseria gonorrheae*

Gram-positive cocci
- *Enterococcus faecium* (337)
- *Enterococcus faecalis* (338)
- *Streptococcus,* group A (339)
- *Streptococcus,* group B (340)
- *Streptococcus,* group D (nonenterococcal)
- *Streptococcus* (viridans group)
- *Streptococcus,* hemolytic
- *Streptococcus pneumoniae*
- *Staphylococcus aureus*
- Other staphylococci

Gram-positive bacilli
- *Bacillus*
- *Corynebacterium* (331)
- *Listeria monocytogenes*

Anaerobes
- *Bacteroides fragilis* (9)
- *Bacteroides* species
- *Clostridium perfringens* (9,341)
- *Clostridium cadaveris* (342)
- *Lactobacillus* (343)
- Microaerophilic streptococci[a]
- *Peptostreptococcus anaerobius*
- *Peptostreptococcus* species
- *Propionibacterium*

Other
- *Candida*
- *Chlamydia trachomatis*
- *Cytomegalovirus* (344)
- ECHO virus, type 4 (345)
- Measles virus (346)
- Rubella virus (345)
- *Mycobacterium tuberculosis*
- Mycoplasma

[a]These organisms are not true anaerobes.

44% of patients with SBP (12). The genital tract may also be the source in women; transfallopian spread is probably particularly important for pneumonococcus (13,14). Seeding of ascitic fluid during bacteremia is often a common denominator for these various organisms. A major pathogenic mechanism is likely to be impaired clearance of bacteria from blood. The reticuloendothelial system, which normally removes a major portion of blood-borne organisms, exhibits decreased phagocytic activity in cirrhotic patients, probably the result of shunting of blood via portosystemic shunts rather than because of inadequate intrinsic function (15). The severity of liver insufficiency is probably the main predisposing factor for development of SBP (6). Although ascites is a near prerequisite to development of SBP, the risk is not the same in all cirrhotic patients and depends on the capacity of ascitic fluid to eliminate bacteria (16). Peripheral destruction of microorganisms by neutrophils is impaired in patients with liver disease. In patients with cirrhosis, there has been demonstration of low serum complement (17,18), decreased serum opsonic activity (19), defective neutrophil chemotaxis (6,20), impaired immunoglobulin M antibody activity (21), and decreased intracellular killing of phagocytized organisms (22). Both opsonic activity (17) and bactericidal activity of ascitic fluid (23) are reduced. Levels of interleukin-6 (IL-6) and tumor necrosis factor-α (TNF-α) are markedly increased in the ascitic fluid of patients with SBP (24). These cytokines have been implicated in the pathogenesis of septic shock and in the cytopathic effects noted in infections; their marked overproduction in ascitic fluid may be a factor in the severity of SBP and the poor prognosis related to liver decompensation.

Clinical Picture

The clinical features of spontaneous bacterial peritonitis are variable. In children, there may be fever (often low-grade), abdominal pain, nausea, vomiting, diarrhea, diffuse abdominal tenderness, rebound tenderness, and hypoactive to absent bowel sounds suggestive of acute appendicitis. Adult patients with cirrhosis have preexisting ascites. Ten percent of cases are totally asymptomatic, whereas most patients have fever, chills, abdominal tenderness and rebound, or decreased to absent bowel sounds. Patients most often have only one or two of the typical presenting symptoms and signs of peritonitis; fever and abdominal pain are the most common. Atypical manifestations such as hypothermia, hypotension, diarrhea, refractoriness to diuretics, or unexplained decrease in renal function may be clues to SBP. Unexplained encephalopathy, hepatorenal syndrome, variceal bleeding, or other deterioration in a cirrhotic patient should raise the suspicion of asymptomatic SBP. It should also be appreciated that the amount of ascites may be so small as to be clinically undetectable. Aside from the complications noted earlier, the bacteremia that often accompanies SBP may be complicated by shock, renal failure, and disseminated intravascular coagulation. Spontaneous bacterial empyema may occur as a complication of SBP (25).

Diagnosis

The diagnosis of SBP requires ruling out the possibility of an intraabdominal source of infection. A high degree of suspicion is required. Accordingly, paracentesis should be performed on any patient with new onset of ascites, any cirrhotic patient with ascites in whom symptoms compatible with the diagnosis (including unexplained encephalopathy) develop, and any cirrhotic patient whose condition suddenly deteriorates. The principal indicator of SBP is the polymorphonuclear (PMN) count in ascitic fluid; counts less than 250/mm^3 essentially rules out SBP and counts greater than 500/mm^3 confirm it. PMN counts greater than 500/mm^3 have a diagnostic sensitivity of 80%, a specificity of 97%, and a diagnostic accuracy of 92% (4). Counts between 250/mm^3 and 500/mm^3 indicate infection only in patients with a compatible clinical picture. In the asymptomatic patient, such a count probably means absence of infection, but a follow-up paracentesis should be performed in the next 12 to 24 hours. Measurements of ascitic fluid pH, lactate concentration, glucose, protein, and lactate dehydrogenase are not useful diagnostically (26). Bacteriologic culture of ascitic fluid has had two problems—poor sensitivity and a relatively long delay for a result; both problems are decreased by culturing 10 mL of ascitic fluid in blood culture bottles at the patient's bedside (27). With this technique, cultures are positive in 63% to 93% of cases; this technique is superior to the lysis-centrifugation blood culture technique (28). Gram stains of ascitic fluid are often negative. Blood cultures should always be obtained in SBP patients before therapy is initiated. In HIV-infected individuals, ascitic fluid should be routinely sent for mycobacterial and mycologic stains and cultures, because there is an increased incidence of tuberculosis (8%) and fungal peritonitis (4%) in these patients (29).

The culture-negative variety of SBP, also called culture-negative neutrocytic ascites and probable SBP, is characterized by a negative culture in the presence of increased PMN leukocytes and no local source of infection or inflammation. The incidence of culture-negative SBP in cirrhotic patients with ascites is 4%. Among patients with elevated PMN counts in ascitic fluid, the percentage who are culture-negative (with culture in blood culture bottles) is 7% (27). Patients with positive ascitic fluid culture but neutrophil counts of less than 250/mm^3 are seen with relative frequency; Runyon (19a) calls these *monomicrobial nonneutrocytic bacterascites*. Two-thirds of such cases were found to have resolved spontaneously (negative cultures of ascitic

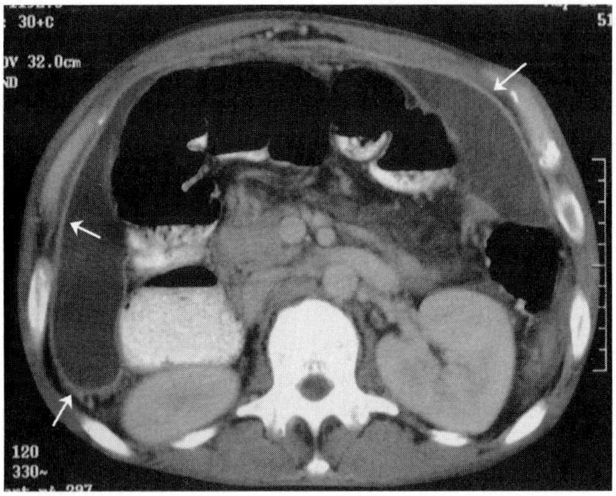

FIGURE 25.1. Primary peritonitis demonstrating inflamed peritoneum.

fluid on recheck, without treatment) and one-third progressed to SBP. Although radiographic visualization is rarely used to diagnose SBP, the appearance of an inflamed or enhanced peritoneum by computed tomography (CT) scan may be seen (Fig. 25.1).

The principle entity in the differential diagnosis of SBP is secondary peritonitis in which there is a local source of infection (usually perforation of the bowel or an abscess). Symptoms and physical findings are not adequate means for distinction between the two entities. Ascitic fluid indicative of secondary peritonitis is highly suspected with two of the following three findings: protein greater than 1 g/dL, glucose less than 50 mg/dL, and lactate dehydrogenase higher than the upper limits of normal for serum. After 48 hours of treatment, the number of ascitic fluid neutrophils is typically back to the pretreatment level in all patients with spontaneous peritonitis, but this is true in only two-thirds of patients with secondary peritonitis (30,31). A lack of response after 48 hours or the finding of two or more organisms cultured from fluid also suggests secondary peritonitis (31).

Therapy

Early institution of appropriate therapy is important for better survival risks. Initial therapy is empirical. Because more than 90% of cases of SBP are caused by enteric gram-negative bacilli (chiefly *E. coli*) and gram-positive cocci (predominantly streptococci, including enterococci), empirical therapy should be directed against these organisms. Some clinicians believe that cefotaxime is the first drug of choice for initiating empirical therapy based on a comparative study in which cefotaxime led to a cure rate of 85% whereas ampicillin plus tobramycin had a cure rate of only 56% (32). There were no side effects, no nephrotoxicity, and no superinfections noted in patients treated with cefotaxime. Other regimens that should be entirely satisfactory include ampicillin/sulbactam, ticarcillin/clavulanate, piperacillin/tazobactam, ticarcillin or piperacillin alone, ceftizoxime, cefoperazone, ceftriaxone, cefonicid (33), ceftazidime (34), and carbapenems. Aminoglycosides are best avoided because of potential renal toxicity and because of unpredictable and relatively slow penetration into ascitic fluid. Among fluoroquinolones, levofloxacin demonstrated similar results when compared with cefotaxime (35). A randomized study comparing short (5 days) and long (10 days) duration therapy concluded that both treatment regimens were equally effective and had similar recurrence rates (36). It has been suggested that measurements of TNF-α and IL-6 in ascitic fluid may be useful for monitoring response to therapy (37).

Prognosis

During the early 1970s, mortality rate attributable to SBP ranged near 90% (4,6). Over the past decade, this percentage has decreased significantly. Currently, short-term survival rates range from 60% to 80%, with nearly all deaths occurring in patients presenting with more severe or advanced SBP, which is associated with shock and renal failure.

Prevention

All cirrhotic patients with upper GI bleeding, with or without ascites, are at high risk for development of severe bacterial infections, including SBP, within the first few days of the bleed. Previous prophylactic antibiotic studies demonstrated reduced infection rates but not mortality rates. However, in three studies to date, the use of ofloxacin, intravenously (IV) and by mouth (PO) plus amoxicillin-clavulanic acid (IV form not available in the United States) before endoscopy, ciprofloxacin plus amoxicillin (IV and PO), or oral ciprofloxacin resulted in significantly lower infection rates than comparator control groups that did not use antibiotics (38–40). All three antibiotic arms demonstrated improved survival rates. Based on this evidence, a consensus panel has recently given a study recommendation for prophylaxis, recommending oral norfloxacin 400 mg every 12 hours for at least 7 days in cirrhotic patients with GI bleeding. The consensus panel also recommended prophylaxis of cirrhotic patients recovering from an episode of SBP, based on a meta-analysis (41) demonstrating a slight survival advantage among patients with ascites. However, this latter study included patients both with and without prior SBP. Use of prophylactic antibiotics has also been shown to decrease overall costs compared with diagnosis and treatment strategy (42). However, in patients with high ascitic protein (>10 g/Ll), long-term prophylaxis is not necessary (except for bleeding, as noted earlier). For patients with less than 10g/L protein, studies are not conclusive to identify subsets other than bleeding that benefit from this therapy (31).

Secondary Peritonitis

By definition, secondary peritonitis is associated with a predisposing GI lesion or event and involves GI flora.

Background Factors

Numerous intraabdominal processes may give rise to peritonitis. Disease, trauma, or surgery involving any part of the GI tract or genitourinary tract may be responsible. The process may involve the stomach, small bowel, large bowel, gallbladder or biliary tract, liver, spleen, pancreas, urinary bladder, uterus, or vagina. A variety of disease processes may be implicated, including infection, inflammation resulting from other causes, vascular disease, low-flow states, malignancy, spontaneous perforation, and congenital disease or a foreign body. Liver transplantation may be a background factor. Any type of microorganism may be responsible for underlying infections—bacterial, parasitic, viral, and fungal. Aside from the microbial agents, certain adjuvant substances such as bile, gastric juice, blood, and necrotic tissue play a role in the pathogenesis of peritonitis.

Etiology

The normal alimentary tract microflora is discussed in more detail elsewhere in this book. The stomach has a sparse flora, less than 10^3 organisms/mL, consisting chiefly of viridans group streptococci, anaerobic cocci, lactobacilli, and yeasts, which are transient flora from the oropharynx (43, 44). Bacterial counts in the upper small intestine are less than 10^7 and the organisms recovered include streptococci, staphylococci, lactobacilli, and yeasts among the nonanaerobes and anaerobic streptococci and lactobacilli (45). In the distal ileum, however, counts are much higher (roughly 10^4 to 10^7) and the flora begins to resemble colonic flora, with coliforms, *Bacteroides* and *Bifidobacterium.* Enterococci outnumber viridans streptococci in this location (45). Counts and diversity of the flora both increase as one traverses the large bowel; counts in the distal colon or feces are approximately 10^{12} per gram of dry weight (46). Anaerobes outnumber nonanaerobes by a factor of approximately 1000:1. Predominant anaerobes are the *Bacteroides fragilis* group, *Anaerobic cocci, Eubacterium, Bifidobacterium, Clostridium,* and *Bilophila wadsworthia* (47). Both anaerobic and facultative lactobacilli are found in relatively large numbers. Among the facultative anaerobes, *E. coli* predominates, followed by various streptococci and *Enterococcus.*

Various factors may influence the bacteriology of the GI tract and thus of infections whose flora is derived from it. There is a direct relationship between pH and quantity of gastric flora (48); the lower the pH, the lower the counts of microorganisms. In patients with bleeding or obstructing duodenal ulcer and those with gastric ulcer or malignancy, counts of gastric organisms are much higher than normal and many types are represented that are not seen normally (49). Patients receiving H_2 blockers, proton pump inhibitors, or antacids have greater numbers of facultative gram-negative bacilli and other organisms in their stomachs. The most profound influence on GI flora is exerted by antimicrobial agents (50). Organisms typically associated with nosocomial infections (e.g, *S. aureus, Staphylococcus epidermidis,* the *Klebsiella-Enterobacter-Serratia* group, *Pseudomonas aeruginosa, Enterococcus,* and *Candida*) may colonize the GI tract during hospitalization and by this means, or by direct introduction during surgery, become involved in postoperative infections following GI surgery. Marshall and co-workers (51) carried out a very important study in which they documented, by quantitative culture of gastric, duodenal, and proximal jejunal contents, that *Candida, S. epidermidis,* and *Pseudomonas* were the most common isolates and that counts at times exceeded 10^8 organisms/mL. All but one of the patients demonstrating these organisms in the upper GI tract had invasive infection with the same organisms. (The GI tract cultures were obtained via gastric or jejunal tubes that had been placed for therapeutic reasons; this may have facilitated entry of organisms into the upper GI tract from the external environment).

Anaerobes outnumber facultative bacteria by a ratio of 10:1 in the normal vaginal flora, anaerobic counts averaging $10^{8 \text{ to }} 10^9$/mL. The organisms most commonly encountered in relatively high counts are anaerobic and facultative lactobacilli, streptococci, *Anaerobic cocci, Prevotella bivia, P. disiens,* other *Prevotella,* pigmented anaerobic gram-negative bacilli, *Gardnerella,* diphtheroids, and *Staphylococcus epidermidis* (52–54). During menstruation, total bacterial counts decrease and the concentration of lactobacilli declines (55). In 1991, Mardh (56), found increased numbers of aciduric organisms such as lactobacilli and yeasts during pregnancy. By far the most comprehensive analysis of vaginal flora in pregnant women (with and without bacterial vaginosis) was performed by Hillier and associates (57). The most striking finding of this group was that hydrogen peroxide–producing lactobacilli were found in only 5% of women with bacterial vaginosis compared with 61% of women with a normal flora. The presence of a number of organisms was inversely related to vaginal colonization by H_2O_2-producing lactobacilli; included were *Gardnerella, Mycoplasma, Ureaplasma,* viridans streptococci, and seven different anaerobes. Oral contraceptives have little effect on vaginal flora, but long-term use of intrauterine contraceptive devices increases the numbers of anaerobes isolated from the cervix (56). Finally, sexual exposure may lead to colonization or infection with *Neisseria gonorrhoeae* and *Chlamydia.*

Infections of the stomach per se are rare. Shinagawa and colleagues (58) reported on the bacteriology of 63 cases of perforated duodenal ulcer (44% positive cultures) and 13 cases of perforated gastric ulcer or carcinoma (11 cases of gastric ulcer), with 39% having positive cultures in comparison with perforations of the small bowel (72%

positive), appendix (95% positive), colon (100% positive), and biliary tract (86% positive). Bacteria isolated, according to the site of perforation, are listed in Table 25.2. This is a unique and important study although it appears that anaerobic transport and culture techniques were not optimal. Mosdell and co-workers (59) described 480 patients with peritonitis associated with perforation of the appendix, 281 cases; a diverticulum, 98; colon other than diverticulum, 32; peptic ulcer, 26; gallbladder, 13; and other sites, 30. Specimens were cultured from approximately two-thirds of the patients and yielded an average of 2.6 isolates per culture. The most common isolates by far were *E. coli* and *B. fragilis*. Nonanaerobes also encountered relatively frequently included nonenterococcal streptococci, *Pseudomonas*, and *Klebsiella*; the other anaerobe encountered relatively often was *Peptostreptococcus* species. Table 25.3 summarizes the results from a recent clinical trial by Solomkin and associates (60) for 529 patients with secondary peritonitis using appropriate culture technique for identification of anaerobes. These results were similar to those recently published by Laroche and colleagues (35) for six other studies from the past decade. The predominant facultative bacteria recovered were *E. coli*, streptococci, *Klebsiella/Enterobacter*, staphylococci, pseudomonas, and enterococci. The predominant anaerobes were *B. fragilis*, other *Bacteroides*, anaerobic gram-positive cocci, *Peptostreptococcus*, *Clostridium*, and anaerobic gram-positive rods. Details of the bacteriologic results of these studies are listed in Table 25.2.

Enterococci are seen more frequently in intraabdominal infection and in associated bacteremia when patients have been treated with cephalosporins (61). Nichols and Muzik (61) also noted that enterococci were isolated much more frequently postoperatively from patients with perforation of the GI tract (in 56% of postoperative infections in this group).

Tertiary peritonitis may be defined as the persistence or recurrence of intraabdominal infection after apparently adequate therapy for primary or secondary peritonitis. In a study by Nathens and co-workers (62), ICU patients with uncomplicated secondary peritonitis (defined as clinical or bacteriologic infection following a single operation or drainage procedure) were compared with those with culture-proven intraabdominal infections persisting or recurring at least 48 hours after apparent adequate treatment. In contrast to patients with secondary peritonitis, patients with tertiary peritonitis grew *Enterococcus*, *Candida* species, *Enterobacter*, and *S. epidermidis*. Typically patients with tertiary peritonitis had poorly localized collections of fluid rather than abscesses. Thus, the number of surgical or reexploratory procedures did not affect outcome. Most deaths were associated with or caused by multiorgan dysfunction. This syndrome most frequently follows postoperative peritonitis (30%), pancreatitis (27%), necrotic bowel (20%),

TABLE 25.2. ISOLATED BACTERIA ACCORDING TO THE SITE OF PERFORATION

	Duodenum	Small Intestine	Appendix	Colon	Others	Total
No. of Cases	63	18	115	20	22	238
No. of Positive Cases	28	13	109	20	13	183
Gram-positive aerobes or facultatives						
Staphylococcus aureus	3		5		2	10
Coagulase-negative staphylococci	2	1	1	1	1	6
Streptococcus species	11		5	4	2	22
Enterococcus species	6	3	12	9	2	32
Subtotal	22	4	23	14	7	70
Gram-negative aerobes or facultatives						
Escherichia coli	2	4	78	15	3	102
Klebsiella species	1	7	18	7	2	35
Enterobacter species	1	3	7	1		12
Citrobacter species		1	9	3		13
Pseudomonas aeruginosa			10	2	1	13
Others			2	1	4	7
Subtotal	4	15	124	29	10	182
Gram-positive anaerobes						
Anaerobic streptococci	5		10	2	1	18
Peptostreptococcus species	4	5	16	7	3	35
Others	1	2	2	2		7
Subtotal	10	7	28	11	4	60
Gram-negative anaerobes						
B. fragilis group	2	5	64	13	6	90
Others		1	1	2	2	6
Subtotal	2	6	65	15	8	96
TOTAL	38	32	240	69	29	408

Modified from Shinagawa N, Muramoto M, Sakurai S, et al. A bacteriological study of perforated duodenal ulcers. Jpn J Surg 1991;21:1–7.

TABLE 25.3. MICROBIOLOGY OF PATIENTS WITH SECONDARY PERITONITIS

Patients with	Total	Patients with	Total
Gram-negative	262	Anaerobic organisms	208
Anaerobes	208	*Bacteroides fragilis*	100
Gram-positive cocci	210	*Bacteroides thetaiotaomicron*	59
Gram-negatives + anaerobes	178	*Bacteroides uniformis*	45
Gram-negatives + gram-positives + anaerobes	130	*Bacteroides vulgatus*	27
Gram-negatives + gram positives	171	*Bacteroides distasonis*	25
Gram-positives + anaerobes	149	Other *Bacteroides*	41
Organism		*Clostridium* species	62
Escherichia coli	212	*Prevotella* species	43
Pseudomonas aeruginosa	48	*Peptostreptococcus* species	56
Klebsiella species	49	*Fusobacterium* species	34
Citrobacter species	14	*Eubacterium* species	46
Enterobacter species	10	Others	74
Proteus species	20	Gram-positive organisms	
Other gram-negatives	25	Streptococcal species	180
		Enterococcus faecalis	39
		Enterococcus avium	18
		Enterococcus faecium	12
		Enterococcus species	7
		Staphylococcus aureus	17

Adapted from Solomkin JS, Wilson SE, Christov NV, et al. Results of a clinical trial of clinafloxacin versus imipenem/cilastatin for intraabdominal infections. Ann Surg 2001;233:79–87.

perforated ulcer (16%), and, occasionally, appendicitis or diverticulitis. It is associated with a significantly higher mortality rate than secondary peritonitis (64% versus 33%).

Mortality rate correlated highly with infection with *S. epidermidis* or *Candida* and poorly with infection with *Pseudomonas* or *E. coli.* Significant foci of invasive infection or of undrained abscesses were often absent at autopsy or exploration. Nathan and colleagues speculate on the importance of efforts to decrease gastric acidity in permitting the overgrowth of organisms demonstrated in the upper GI tract. They point out that translocation of organisms across the gut mucosal barrier might account for the invasive infection and that this proximal GI tract flora might alter normal systemic immune response, both antigen-specific and global immunity. In another study carried out in a surgical intensive care unit population, Rotstein and colleagues (62a) documented a unique flora in peritoneal fluid collections and bacteremia. Twenty-five patients had undergone at least two surgical procedures for abdominal sepsis and 23 had failure of at least three organ systems. The most common organisms from peritoneal cultures were *S. epidermidis, Candida albicans, P. aeruginosa, Enterobacter,* and *Enterococcus; E. coli* and *B. fragilis* were recovered relatively infrequently. In accompanying bacteremia, the most prevalent isolates were *S. epidermidis, Enterobacter, B. fragilis,* and *C. albicans.*

Neonatal peritonitis also has a unique infecting flora (63). *E. coli* was found in only 21% of such patients as compared with 69% of a control group of children with perforated appendicitis. In neonatal peritonitis, the most common gram-negative isolates were *Klebsiella* and *Enterobacter* and more than half of the cultures yielded gram-positive cocci (most often coagulase-negative staphylococci and enterococci). Anaerobes were seldom recovered from neonatal peritonitis cases and from only 50% of appendicitis cases. *Candida* was found in 10% of neonatal peritonitis patients.

The bacteriology of intraabdominal infection complicating female genital tract infection is very much like that seen in peritonitis resulting from a GI source. Differences include a higher incidence of *Anaerobic cocci* and of *Prevotella bivia* and *P. disiens* and a lower incidence of *B. fragilis.* In addition, the occurrence of gonococci, *Chlamydia trachomatis* (64), and actinomycosis related to intrauterine contraceptive devices (65) are unique. The latter infection may involve *Eubacterium nodatum* as well as various *Actinomyces* and *Propionibacterium propionicus.*

Bacteremia may be seen in 20% to 30% of patients with intraabdominal infection; organisms recovered have been chiefly *B. fragilis* and *E. coli* (66–70).

Pathogenesis and Pathology

Two major factors contribute to the establishment of peritonitis: (a) a continuing source of infection and (b) foreign material (e.g., intestinal contents, bile, gastric juice, or necrotic tissue) that protects bacteria from host defense mechanisms. Spillage of pancreatic enzymes results in enzymatic digestion and widespread necrosis. Bile in the peritoneal cavity is a serious problem and is associated with a poor prognosis. Free hemoglobin also facilitates peritonitis by enhancing bacterial virulence, perhaps by the capacity of red blood cells and hemoglobin to reduce nitric oxide (71). Bacteria gain access to the peritoneal cavity through perforations in the GI tract or gallbladder or by translocation from an intact bowel in response to serosal inflammation.

Plaques of fibrinous material accumulate on the inflamed peritoneum and cause loops of bowel to adhere to one another and to the parietal peritoneum. There is an outpouring of leukocyte-containing serous fluid. The greater omentum tends to localize infection by adhering to areas of peritonitis; ileus also plays a role in localization of the process. The ratio of bacteria to leukocytes is an important factor determining the outcome of peritonitis. Ischemia, surgical or other trauma, malignancy, and other factors lead to devitalized tissue, which lowers the oxidation-reduction potential so that obligate anaerobes may grow well. Bacterial factors play an important role in peritonitis; included are such entities as endotoxin, collagenase, other proteolytic enzymes (72), deoxyribonuclease, heparinase, leukocidin, and urease (73). Various host factors such as removal and killing of bacteria by macrophages and PMN leukocytes (74), fibrin deposition to localize peritoneal infection (75), TNF, other interleukins, interferons, arachidonic acid metabolism and its products, platelet-activating factor, coagulation abnormalities (76), nitric oxide, and macrophage procoagulant activity (77) play an important role in peritonitis and its complications. Synergy between various organisms appears to be a very important factor; this has been studied extensively with black-pigmented anaerobic gram-negative bacilli (78). In an animal model, both the *Enterococcus* (79) as well as *Candida* and *E. coli* have also been demonstrated as synergistic (80).

Clinical Picture

The mode of onset of peritonitis varies according to the precipitating event. Perforated peptic ulcer with spillage of gastric contents may produce severe epigastric pain that spreads to involve the entire abdomen in minutes, whereas pain from a perforated appendix is much more gradual. The usual findings are pain, abdominal distention, anorexia, nausea and vomiting, absence of abdominal respiratory movement, abdominal and rebound tenderness, diffuse muscle spasm and guarding, tenderness on rectal or vaginal examination, and fever. Patients characteristically lie quietly in bed with knees flexed; early in the course of the illness, the patient is alert, restless, and irritable, but later the patient may be apathetic or delirious. There may be inability to pass feces or flatus and there may be more serious signs such as toxemia and shock. The very young or old, patients with lax abdominal musculature (postpartum patients or cirrhotics with ascites), patients in shock, and patients on corticosteroids may not manifest pain and muscle spasm. A high index of suspicion is necessary in such patients; early in the course of peritonitis, there may be only an unexplained increase in pulse rate or hypotension; the most important physical finding is a completely silent abdomen on auscultation. The signs of peritonitis may be completely overshadowed by the manifestations of the underlying process. Complications include bacteremia, shock, intraabdominal or retroperitoneal abscess, respiratory failure, adhesions, and GI fistula.

Diagnosis

The diagnosis of secondary peritonitis is primarily a clinical one. Specific information regarding the pain of peritonitis—the site of origin, the site of the most intense pain, and the character and radiation pattern of the pain—is crucial in differentiating peritonitis from myocardial infarction, sickle cell anemia, herpes zoster, tabetic crisis, lupus erythematosus, arachnidism, porphyria, diabetic ketoacidosis, plumbism, familial Mediterranean fever, pulmonary disease, and renal disease. The peripheral white blood cell (WBC) count is usually greater than 12,000 but counts greater than 20,000 cells/mm^3 are rare in patients with an acute surgical abdomen. There is typically an increase in the percentage of PMN leukocytes and a moderate to marked shift to immature forms. Glycosuria and hyperglycemia may be seen in diabetic acidosis and in acute pancreatitis, but they are not typical in peritonitis. Hematuria and pyuria usually indicate primary involvement of the genitourinary tract, but they may reflect inflammatory disease such as appendicitis or diverticulitis adjacent to the ureter or bladder. Dehydration may lead to elevated hematocrit and blood urea nitrogen level. Very high levels of serum amylase are consistent with acute pancreatitis but lower levels may occur in peritonitis from any cause, intestinal obstruction, perforated viscus, uremia, and after injection of opiates. Both metabolic and respiratory acidosis are seen in severe or late peritonitis.

Supine, upright, or lateral decubitus radiographic films of the abdomen or CT may reveal free gas in the peritoneal cavity, encapsulated gas in an abscess, features of ileus or obstruction, peritoneal fluid, volvulus, intussusception, vascular occlusion, calcification within the gallbladder or elsewhere, or obliteration of the psoas shadows or other peritoneal lines. Chest radiographs may also be helpful in detecting or ruling out pulmonary disease and in detecting free gas under the diaphragm. Ultrasound examination and radionuclide scanning may also aid in diagnosis.

Needle aspiration of peritoneal fluid is often helpful. The fluid may be purulent, bloody, or turbid, or it may contain fat globules (pathognomonic of fat digestion), bile, or fecal material. Negative findings are not useful diagnostically. If fluid cannot be obtained directly, peritoneal lavage with 1 L of saline may be considered; the presence of more than 500 WBC/mm^3 correlates best with the presence of intraabdominal pathology (81). When pus or other fluid is obtained, Gram stain and aerobic and anaerobic cultures should be obtained. Blood cultures should always be obtained before initiating antimicrobial therapy. Peritoneoscopy or needle biopsy of the peritoneum may occasionally be useful.

Therapy

The principles of therapy are (a) to eliminate the primary source of infection by means of closure, excision, or isolation; (b) to aspirate as much of the infected peritoneal exudate as possible and to drain the site of the primary lesion; (c) to treat local or distant complications as needed; (d) to combat the effects of bacteria and their toxic metabolites; (e) to improve vascular perfusion by correcting fluid and electrolyte deficits; and (f) to reduce paralytic ileus (decompression of the gut by nasogastric tube, long intestinal tube, or enterostomy).

In most cases of secondary peritonitis, surgery is required for management of the underlying problem, for drainage of pus, and for excision of necrotic tissue. Surgery should be performed at the earliest possible time. Rotstein and Meakins (81) provide an excellent discussion of surgical principles and practices. For colonic pathology, surgery usually involves resecting the perforated segment of bowel and exteriorizing the proximal end as an end-colostomy; the distal end is either oversewn or a mucous fistula is created. A primary anastomosis in this setting creates a high risk of dehiscence and should be avoided. The risks associated with primary anastomosis of the small bowel are much lower; however, if there has been extensive peritoneal soiling or if there is concern about the viability of the intestine, resection with proximal and distal enterostomy may be indicated. Duodenal perforation related to peptic ulcer may be patched with a piece of omentum but perforated gastric ulcer requires local excision with primary closure or distal gastric resection with subsequent gastroduodenal or gastrojejunal anastomosis. Appendectomy is carried out for appendicitis.

At surgery, purulent exudates should be aspirated and loculations in the subphrenic spaces, paracolic gutters, and pelvis should be gently opened and debrided. Particulate debris such as feces or barium should be removed, but radical peritoneal debridement has not proven to be worthwhile and may lead to excessive bleeding. Intraoperative peritoneal lavage is standard practice during surgery for peritonitis but its efficacy is not well documented. However, there is no evidence that it is harmful and it reduces numbers of bacteria and removes substances such as blood, feces, and necrotic material. It is imperative to aspirate all fluid instilled and all collections of fluid before closure. The use of drains in patients with diffuse peritonitis is indicated only for drainage of abscess cavities and to establish a controlled fistula. Drains left in place can be a hazard in that they may erode into bowel or blood vessels and may provide access to the peritoneal cavity for exogenous organisms.

Abdominal wall closure is effected with a single fascial layer of interrupted monofilament suture. In high-risk patients (elderly, malnourished, or immunocompromised), retention sutures through the full thickness of the abdominal wall may be used in addition. Delayed primary closure of the skin and subcutaneous tissues may be used. In such a case, if the wound appears clean and granulating on the third or fourth postoperative day, skin edges can be apposed with skin tapes or fine sutures. Some surgeons have used an absorbable mesh or a mesh-plus-zipper-technique as temporary closures in patients for whom primary closure is not considered desirable (82).

Detailed discussion of the management of appendicitis and diverticulitis and their complications is given in Chapters 23 and 24. In general, it appears that primary closure is essentially always reasonable in appendicitis. Laparoscopic appendectomy is used by some (93). For diverticulitis, medical therapy is adequate for about 75% of patients. Surgical intervention is reserved for those who fail medical management and those with recurrent acute attacks, diffuse peritonitis, abscess, persistent obstruction, or fistula formation. Abdominal CT scans allow guided percutaneous drainage of selected patients with large abscesses. With this approach, a single elective operation without a temporary colostomy is possible for most patients. For patients requiring emergency surgery, the two-stage approach with resection of the diseased colon at the initial operation is much preferred over the old three-stage approach (83).

Antimicrobial therapy is a second major approach to management of secondary peritonitis and its complications. Systemic antimicrobial therapy should be used before and after surgical therapy. The choice of antimicrobial agents depends on the microorganisms involved and the usual susceptibility patterns in the hospital being used. In complex bacterial mixtures, it is reasonable to target only pathogens known to be problems in terms of virulence and antimicrobial resistance as well as organisms present in large numbers, in blood cultures, and on repeated culture.

When *S. aureus* is involved, one may use a penicillinase-resistant penicillin such as nafcillin or an antistaphylococcal cephalosporin such as cefazolin. In the case of methicillin-resistant *S. aureus* or *S. epidermidis,* vancomycin is the drug of choice. In the case of enterococci, many clinicians (84–86) believe that it is not necessary to provide antimicrobial coverage in non–intensive care unit (ICU) patients with the initial onset of secondary peritonitis unless these organisms are recovered from blood cultures. Patients in whom enterococcal infection develops later in the course of illness, following cephalosporin therapy, or in ICUs should have antimicrobial regimens that include coverage for enterococci. Ampicillin plus an aminoglycoside is often effective, but resistance is an increasingly serious problem with *Enterococcus.* Vancomycin plus an aminoglycoside is active against a number of strains resistant to ampicillin plus an aminoglycoside, but strains may be resistant to both of these agents as well (VRE). Agents that have been proven effective against VRE include quinupristin/dalfopristin and linezolid. Other streptococci (e.g, viridans streptococci, group A or B streptococci) are usually susceptible to penicillin or ampicillin, although resistance among some viridans streptococci is increasing.

For gram-negative non-anaerobic bacilli, many clinicians dealing with fairly sick patients use an aminoglycoside such as gentamicin or amikacin (at least initially, until the patient's condition improves) along with a β-lactam agent such as ticarcillin/clavulanic acid or piperacillin/tazobactam, or cefoxitin/cefoperazone/ceftazidime, or aztreonam or imipenem, depending on the particular gram-negative bacilli isolated, their likely susceptibility patterns, and the seriousness of the patient's condition. Some clinicians avoid aminoglycosides as initial empirical therapy because of their toxicity; in lieu of these agents, one may use combinations such as clindamycin plus aztreonam (87–89) or clindamycin plus ceftazidime (101). Trimethoprim-sulfamethoxazole, the fluoroquinolones (90), and chloramphenicol are other options that may be considered for gram-negative coverage. Gorbach (84) recommends reserving aminoglycosides for organisms resistant to other agents, for patients who have received other antibiotics within the past month, in association with reoperation or recurrence of infection, and for patients with prolonged hospitalization or nursing home residence preoperatively. Again, the usual susceptibility patterns of various gram-negative bacilli from the hospital in which the patient is being cared for and specific susceptibilities on the patient's isolates are important considerations in devising initial regimens and revising them if necessary.

Among the anaerobes, the *B. fragilis* group is the most commonly encountered and is relatively resistant to antimicrobials. *Bacteroides thetaiotaomicron,* a member of the *B. fragilis* group, is encountered fairly often and is much more resistant to antimicrobials than *B. fragilis.* Other species in this group may also be quite resistant. Among the agents listed, those with the greatest activity against the *B. fragilis* group and other anaerobes are the β-lactam/β-lactamase inhibitor combinations, imipenem and other penems, and chloramphenicol. The other drug with major activity against the anaerobes is metronidazole. Cefoxitin has moderately good activity against the *B. fragilis* group and many other anaerobes, as does clindamycin and broad-spectrum penicillins such as piperacillin or ticarcillin. Patterns of resistance for anaerobes, especially *B. fragilis,* vary by hospital (91). Few hospitals test anaerobic isolates for susceptibility, predominantly because automated methods are not available. Recently, additional testing has been recommended by the National Committee for Clinical Laboratory Standards and based upon clinical studies (70,92). For now, surveys are published periodically updating susceptibility pattern changes (91,93). Agents with poor or no activity against anaerobes include aminoglycosides, trimethoprim-sulfamethoxazole, older quinolones, aztreonam, and some of the newer cephalosporins.

For *C. albicans,* both fluconazole and amphotericin B are active. However, an increasing number of *Candida* species other than *C. albicans* have been isolated that demonstrate intermediate or high-level resistance to fluconazole while remaining susceptible to amphotericin B.

In considering different empirical regimens with which to initiate therapy of secondary peritonitis, it should be appreciated that there are major problems of interpretation and comparability between various studies (94,95). The major problems in interpretation relate to variable diagnostic criteria, unmeasured severity of disease, wide differences in the quality of bacteriologic studies, and unclear outcome measures. To address these deficiencies, a consistent system of definitions with minimum rules has been developed by a Joint Working Party of the Surgical Infection Societies of North America and Europe (96). Intraabdominal infection is defined as clinical peritonitis requiring both operative and microbiologic confirmation of infection. The APACHE II system is proposed for grading severity of infection and for stratification of risk of mortality. The main outcome measures, both independently and positively defined, are mortality and time until death on the one hand and recovery and time until recovery on the other. Table 25.4 lists appropriate agents determined to be effective in clinical trials as either monotherapy or in combination.

It is generally agreed that it is important to have activity against both facultative gram-negative rods and anaerobes in initiating empirical therapy. Clindamycin plus gentamicin has been a popular initial regimen because clindamycin has given good coverage against anaerobes and most gram-positive organisms other than enterococci and the aminoglycoside covers most gram-negative non-anaerobic bacilli. This remains a much used regimen, but resistance of the *B. fragilis* group and other anaerobes such as some peptostreptococci in some centers has led some clinicians to seek other regimens (92). Cefoxitin, with or without an aminoglycoside, has also been used widely (85,97–99). As noted earlier, a number of clinicians avoid the use of aminoglycosides, substituting various other agents with good activity against gram-negative non-anaerobic bacilli. Piperacillin (100,101) and ticarcillin have been used effectively in intraabdominal infection, as have β-lactam/β-lactamase inhibitor combinations such as ampicillin/sulbactam (102) and ticarcillin/clavulanate (103,104). However, resistance to piperacillin and ticarcillin has increased significantly since 1990 (91,93). Regimens using metronidazole for the anaerobic coverage, along with one or more additional agents with activity against other categories of organisms that may be encountered, have been very effective. Imipenem has also been used effectively as a single agent (86,105,106). For less severe peritonitis such as may be encountered with gangrenous or perforated appendicitis (localized rather than generalized

TABLE 25.4. COMPARATIVE ANTIMICROBIAL TRIALS FOR TREATMENT OF INTRAABDOMINAL AND PELVIC INFECTIONS

Intraabdominal	Ref
Cefoxitin ± aminoglycoside vs clindamycin + aminoglycoside	(347,348,349)
Ceftizoxime vs cefoxitin	(350)
Piperacillin vs cefoxitin	(351)
Ampicillin/sulbactam vs clindamycin + aminoglycoside	(352)
Imipenem vs. clindamycin + aminoglycoside	(353,86)
Aztreonam + clindamycin vs clindamycin + aminoglycoside	(354,355)
Aztreonam + clindamycin vs imipenem	(356)
Ticarcillin/clavulanate vs clindamycin aminoglycoside	(357)
Piperacillin/tazobactam vs imipenem	(358)
Piperacillin/tazobactam vs clindamycin + aminoglycoside	(359)
Meropenem vs clindamycin + tobramycin	(360)
Meropenem vs ceftizoxime + metronidazole	(361)
Ciprofloxacin + metronidazole vs imipenem	(362)
Clinafloxacin vs imipenem	(60)
Meropenem vs imipenem	(363)

Adapted from Hecht DW. *Bacteroides fragilis* group. In: Yu VL, Merigan TC Jr, Barriere SL, eds. Antimicrobial therapy and vaccines. Baltimore: Williams & Wilkins, 1999:44–52.

peritonitis), ceftizoxime and cefotetan have been used as single agents to good effect (107).

The problem of antimicrobial therapy of persistent peritonitis in ICU patients is grim. The organisms isolated (*S. epidermidis, Pseudomonas, Candida,* and enterococci) are relatively antimicrobial resistant, but even when appropriate antimicrobial agents are administered, these organisms tend to persist (108). This probably reflects impaired host defenses with multiple organ failure rather than failure of the antimicrobial agents. Mortality rate increases with increasing organ system failure (51,62).

Prognosis

The mortality rate in diffuse peritonitis has declined remarkably with the introduction of antimicrobials, but there may still be significant risk of death, depending on the underlying cause of the peritonitis and the presence of certain factors. The prognosis is poorer in the very old or very young; with prolonged contamination of the peritoneal cavity; with the presence of bile, pancreatic enzymes, or barium; with a serious underlying problem such as carcinoma; with significant associated problems (such as cardiovascular, respiratory, or renal disease); with certain organisms; and with associated bacteremia (109). The highest mortality rate, in terms of anatomic area involved, is associated with the pancreas and large bowel, with small intestine not far behind. Postoperative peritonitis carries a relatively high mortality rate. Septic shock and multisystem organ failure are major factors that affect mortality rate, which is essentially 100% in tertiary peritonitis (110,111). The most frequent causes of death are respiratory, hepatic, and renal failure. In a recent study of patients in whom peritonitis developed after elective intraabdominal surgery, inadequate antimicrobial therapy was associated with mortality in 45%, whereas there was only a 16% mortality rate in patients who received appropriate antibiotics. This difference in mortality rate was not affected by changes in therapy as a result of cultures (111).

Prevention

Postoperative peritonitis may be avoided by preventing contamination of the peritoneal cavity with GI or vaginal secretions. Good surgical technique and antimicrobial prophylaxis are important. For surgery on the stomach or duodenum at high risk for infection due to decreased gastric acidity or motility, parenteral prophylactic antimicrobial therapy is indicated. The *Medical Letter* (112) recommends cefazolin. Oral preoperative neomycin plus erythromycin "bowel prep" is clearly effective in reducing the amount of bowel flora and minimizing postoperative infection following colonic surgery (113). A short dosing period helps avoid colonization or overgrowth with resistant organisms. Whether parenteral therapy in addition would further improve results has not been determined definitively. (A study by Schoetz and colleagues [114] showed that addition of parenteral cefoxitin significantly reduced the incidence of postoperative wound infection; however, it did not reduce the incidence of intraabdominal infection). Mechanical cleansing with a low-residue diet followed by a liquid diet, cathartics, and enemas is very important. For vaginal hysterectomy, cefazolin, cefoxitin or cefotetan prophylaxis is recommended (112).

The early use of appropriate antimicrobials is efficacious in preventing infection following penetrating wounds of the abdomen that involve the bowel. The East Practice Management Working Group recommends systemic prophylaxis for up to 24 hours with a perforation of a hollow viscous (115). Current evidence does not support its continued use beyond 24 hours.

Peritonitis Complicating Peritoneal Dialysis

Background Factors

Since its development in the late 1970s, peritoneal dialysis has revolutionized the treatment of end-stage renal disease, providing a safe, cost-effective alternative to hemodialysis and transplantation (116). Despite extensive experience with this form of dialysis, peritonitis remains the most common complication and often limits its long-term utility. Peritonitis is the primary reason for discontinuing continuous ambulatory peritoneal dialysis (CAPD) due to method failure (117).

The incidence of peritonitis complicating CAPD varies considerably among individual patients and centers. The rates tend to reflect the experience of the center, the specific technology used, and the participants' susceptibility to infection and ability to comply with procedures (118). Historically, the average incidence of peritonitis is 1.3 to 1.4 episodes per patient per year of dialysis (120), although recent studies demonstrate rates as low as 0.55% episodes per patient year (119). More than half of all episodes are experienced by only 25% of patients (133), and many CAPD patients remain free of peritonitis for years. Men and women have equal risk for development of peritonitis, but African-Americans, diabetics older than 60 years of age, and persons with less education are at increased risk (117,121,122). Children also seem to have a higher incidence of peritonitis (one episode per 7.7 months versus one per 11.1 months) (123); however, in children whose parents perform the dialysate exchanges, the incidence of peritonitis approaches the rate seen in adults (124,125).

Etiology

In patients undergoing CAPD, peritonitis is usually caused by a single pathogen that originates from the normal flora of the skin or upper respiratory tract. Approximately 60% to 70% of cases are caused by gram-positive cocci, 20% to 30% by gram-negative bacilli, and the remainder by various anaerobic bacteria, fungi, and mycobacteria (119). Table 25.5 compares results by Zelenitsky and colleagues (119) for the period 1991 to 1998 with two studies predominantly from the 1980s. Coagulase-negative *Staphylococcus* is the single most commonly encountered pathogen in most series, followed by *S. aureus* and species of streptococci. Among the gram-negative organisms, most Enterobacteriaceae have been associated with CAPD peritonitis but no single species predominates in all series. Nonfermentative gram-negative bacilli also occur sporadically, sometimes in

TABLE 25.5. PERCENTAGE OF ISOLATES FROM PATIENTS WITH PERITONEAL DIALYSIS-RELATED PERITONITIS

Organism	Ref 119	Refs 142,131
Staphylococcus epidermidis	22.2%	30–45%[a]
Other coagulase-negative *Staphylococcus* species (*S. hominis, S. capitis, S. warneri, S. hemolyticus*)	10.8%	—
Staphylococcus aureus	14.6%	10–20%
Streptococcus species	14.7%	10–15%
Other	4.5%	1–2%
Gram-negative anaerobes		
Pseudomonas aeruginosa	6.2%	5–10%
Escherichia coli	5.4%	10–20%[b]
Klebsiella species	3.9%	—
Other	12.5%	2–3%
Other		
Yeasts	2.6%	5–15%
Anaerobes	2.6%	0–10%
Mycobacterium	—	0–3%

[a]Includes other coagulase-negative staphylococci.
[b]Includes *Klebsiella* species.

association with environmental contamination (126). Although a rare pathogen in other types of peritonitis, *P. aeruginosa* occurs with relative frequency in CAPD peritonitis (5% to 10% of cases). It warrants special note because of its association with significant morbidity and late complications (127–129).

Fungi have become an important cause of CAPD-related peritonitis in recent years because of their increasing frequency and problematic management. Many different fungi have been isolated, including *Aspergillus* species, *Mucor, Rhizopus, Alternaria, Fusarium, Penicillium, Drechslera, Cryptococcus, Acremonium, Trichosporin* species, and *Candida* species. In a recent report by Wang and associates (130), *Candida* species account for 70% of cases of fungal peritonitis, with *C. albicans* accounting for 14% and nonalbicans species 56%. *C. parapsilosis* was the most frequently isolated nonalbicans species (118,131–133). Risk factors for acquisition of fungal peritonitis are bacterial peritonitis within the preceding month, recent hospitalization, presence of extraperitoneal infection, use of immunosuppressive agents, lupus, and concomitant HIV infection; diabetes mellitus, age, sex, and education do not pose a special risk (132–134). *Mycobacterium* has been described as a pathogen in fewer than 3% of cases of CAPD-related peritonitis, but may also account for a portion of cases labeled as culture-negative (135). Overall, 86% of mycobacterial isolates reported in the literature are group IV (rapid growers), such as *M. fortuitum* and *M. chelonae* (136). One particularly large outbreak involved 17 patients in whom infection with *M. chelonae* developed following treatment with contaminated intermittent peritoneal dialysis machines (137). Other rare causes of peritonitis in patients undergoing CAPD are viruses (138), algae (139), *Stenotrophomonas maltophilia* (129), and *Pasteurella multocida* (140).

Pathogenesis

There are several potential routes of infection for development of peritonitis in CAPD patients. The two most important are (a) transluminal, resulting from a break in sterile technique during dialysate exchange, and (b) contiguous spread, in which microorganisms access the peritoneum along the tract of the dialysis catheter. In a review of factors leading to peritonitis at a single CAPD center, 36% of cases were due to suspected poor technique (transluminal contamination), 7% were attributed to known contamination, 20% to complicated exit site or tunnel infections, and 18% were of unknown origin (141). Less common portals of entry are hematogenous spread from a distant site of infection or direct contamination from the GI tract (142). Diverticular disease of the nonsigmoid colon appears to be a risk factor for acquisition of infection of intestinal origin, presumably through occult microperforations (143). Kim and Korbet (144) reported polymicrobial infections involving only gram-positive organisms in 21% of 43 patients, a mixture of gram-positive and gram-negative organisms in 44%, gram-negative only in 16%, and a combination with fungal organisms in 19%. Only 7% of polymicrobial infections were associated with an intraabdominal source. Furthermore, an increase in gram-positive organisms in mixed infections was noted from 1995 to 1997, attributed to a decrease in proportion of catheters removed. However, isolation of multiple enteric pathogens from peritoneal fluid, especially anaerobic bacteria, suggests fecal contamination from gross colonic perforations (118).

Factors that may contribute to microbial pathogenicity include production of extracellular slime (biofilm) and ability to grow in dialysis fluids such as for staphylococci, *C. albicans*, and *Pseudomonas* (145–147). Surrounding biofilm serves to anchor the organisms and protect them from host defenses and antibiotic activity; thus it may play a role both in the initiation and relapse of CAPD-associated peritonitis (148). Once organisms gain access to the peritoneal cavity, further growth may depend on their survival in the presence of dialysis fluid. Fresh dialysate solutions are capable of supporting growth of *E. coli* but not staphylococci. However, after instillation into the peritoneal cavity, dialysis effluent supports growth of both organisms (149). Further studies have shown that the growth of *P. aeruginosa* and *E. coli* are enhanced 1,000-fold in dialysis fluids from patients with peritonitis compared with uninfected control subjects (150). Accordingly, survival of bacteria contaminating the peritoneal cavity depends on timing of inoculation as well as the nature of the organism. Allen and associates (151) have suggested a possible role of iron dextran infusions with an incurred incidence of peritonitis in CAPD patients.

Another consideration in the pathogenesis of dialysis-associated peritonitis is the activity of host defenses (152). When used for dialysis, the peritoneal cavity does not provide a supportive milieu for operation of host defense mechanisms. The low pH (5.5 to 6.0), high osmolarity (300 to 400 mOsmol/kg), and dilution effects of the dialysate volume (2 L) act to diminish normal phagocytic function (152–154). Furthermore, dialysis has been shown to decrease the levels of immunoglobulin G (IgG) and complement (C3) in the peritoneum to approximately 1% of their normal levels (131). The significance of this observation is unclear because IgG levels in the dialysate do not correlate with occurrence of peritonitis (155). It is likely that the collective abnormalities in host defenses contribute to the pathogenesis of this infection. Renal transplant is also associated with an increased incidence of peritonitis in CAPD patients within 30 days following transplantation, resulting in increased hospital stays by an average of 3 days compared with patients on hemodialysis (156).

Clinical Manifestations

Criteria for the diagnosis of CAPD-associated peritonitis are (a) signs and symptoms of peritoneal irritation, (b) cloudy dialysate effluent with a leukocyte count greater than $100/mm^3$, and (c) a positive culture of dialysate fluid. Any two of these criteria may be adequate to establish the diagnosis (146). Signs and symptoms of peritonitis vary from mild to severe, depending largely on the virulence of the pathogen and the time course of the infection (118). Infections caused by coagulase-negative staphylococci tend to be indolent and mild, whereas those caused by *S. aureus* and gram-negative bacilli are more fulminant (157). Generally, turbid dialysate is the first and most common symptom to appear, followed shortly thereafter by abdominal pain and tenderness. Localized findings should suggest specific organ pathology such as cholecystitis or appendicitis. Other clinical manifestations of CAPD-related peritonitis are listed in Table 25.6.

TABLE 25.6. CLINICAL MANIFESTATIONS OF PERITONITIS IN PATIENTS RECEIVING CONTINUOUS AMBULATORY PERITONEAL DIALYSIS

Manifestation	%
Cloudy dialysate	90–100
Abdominal pain	70–80
Fever	35–60
Nausea, vomiting	25–35
Diarrhea	<10
Abdominal tenderness	50–80
Drainage problems	15
Peripheral leukocytes	30–45

Diagnosis

Laboratory evaluation of dialysate effluent is critical to the diagnosis. Fluid should be sent for total cell count, differential leukocyte count, Gram stain, and culture. Although a leukocyte count of greater than 100/mm^3 is a traditional cutoff for diagnosis, the value is not specific. In some cases of CAPD-associated peritonitis, WBC counts are less than 100/mm^3; moreover, counts greater than that (100 to 500/mm^3) have been observed in the absence of infection (158,159). The differential cell count of dialysate may have a better predictive value. In one study, PMN leukocytes composed greater than 50% of the total count (mean, 85%) in infected patients, whereas uninfected patients had less than 40% PMN leukocytes (mean, 12%) (160). On occasion, a preponderance of eosinophils may be noted in the fluid. This self-limited condition, eosinophilic peritonitis, often follows placement of the Tenckhoff catheter and may represent allergy to the tubing (161,162). Peritoneal eosinophilia also occurs with fungal peritonitis, intraperitoneal administration of antibiotics, and possibly with *Mycobacterium tuberculosis* (131,163).

Gram stain of dialysis fluid is of low sensitivity, detecting only 20% to 30% of peritonitis episodes. Gram-positive organisms, especially *S. aureus,* are more likely to be detected than are gram-negative ones (158,164). Culture has a greater yield than Gram stain, although the precise method influences its sensitivity. Because there is a relatively small number of organisms contained in a large volume, optimal culturing techniques rely on some form of concentration, such as centrifugation, filtration, or lysis-centrifugation (165). Even with these specialized methods, 3% to 30% of peritonitis episodes are culture-negative. Presumably, most are due to fastidious, low-virulence organisms or coagulase-negative staphylococci that survive less well in dialysis fluid (118,150). Cases of culture-negative peritonitis that do not respond to empirical antibiotic treatment should be further investigated by obtaining dialysate fluid cultures for mycobacteria and fungi. Blood cultures are usually negative regardless of the etiologic agent.

Therapy

Many patients with dialysis-related peritonitis can be managed on an ambulatory basis. Hospitalization is indicated for those patients who are severely ill or who are unable to manage administration of intraperitoneal antibiotics at home. A variety of antimicrobial agents have been used successfully for treatment, including penicillins, cephalosporins, aztreonam, imipenem, aminoglycosides, fluoroquinolones, and macrolide and glycopeptide antibiotics (166–170). Initial therapy is guided by results of the dialysis fluid Gram stain. If gram-positive bacteria are seen, a cephalosporin or vancomycin may be selected. Because of the high incidence of methicillin-resistant staphylococci in many centers, vancomycin is often preferred (171). For gram-negative types, an aminoglycoside is usually administered. When no organism is seen on the Gram stain, empirical treatment with a cephalosporin or vancomycin plus aminoglycoside is initiated. Alternatively, in relatively mild episodes of peritonitis, a single agent with antistaphylococcal activity may be suitable. Ultimately, empirical antibiotic selections are adjusted when the results of culture and sensitivity tests are known. A single specific agent is adequate treatment in most cases of bacterial peritonitis. *P. aeruginosa,* however, has been associated with a high therapeutic failure rate and frequent relapses (172,173). A synergistic combination of antibiotics, such as an antipseudomonal β-lactam plus an aminoglycoside, has been recommended in addition to removal of the dialysis catheter. Intraperitoneal administration of antibiotics is the preferred method for drug delivery in CAPD-associated peritonitis because it achieves high local concentrations and permits self-treatment by the patient (174). Therapy is usually continued for 10 to 14 days, but it may need to be extended with unusually severe or slow to respond infections. Recommendations for specific drug doses and routes of administration have been published elsewhere (146,174).

Treatment of fungal peritonitis is controversial because of the lack of controlled studies and the small numbers of cases seen at any single center. Although there are reports of successful treatment with intraperitoneal or systemic antifungal agents alone (175–177), removal of the dialysis catheter appears to be indicated, because risk of mortality is significantly higher when it remains *in situ* (130). A course of systemic amphotericin B totalling 250 to 500 mg is often given following catheter removal. Mycobacterial peritonitis also requires removal of the dialysis catheter for cure. Most of these organisms are resistant to conventional antituberculous agents, and susceptibilities vary greatly between the species. Antibiotic selections should be guided by either *in vitro* susceptibility tests or published recommendations (135–137,178).

Prognosis

CAPD-associated peritonitis is accompanied by reduction in ultrafiltration and protein loss in dialysis effluent. Rarely is it necessary to abandon use of the peritoneum for dialysis, but more frequent exchanges or hypertonic dialysate may be needed to prevent volume overload. The functional capacity of the peritoneal cavity returns to baseline in 7 to 10 days (179). After appropriate treatment of an episode of peritonitis, long-term resumption of CAPD is generally successful. Particularly severe or prolonged episodes of peritonitis may lead to formation of adhesions and an increased risk of peritoneal sclerosis but the same is not true of patients with repetitive bouts of infection (179). Mortality rate is 2% to 3% in younger patients (mean age, 45 years) but higher in elderly patients (7%) and those with fungal, mycobacterial, and polymicrobial infections (130,180,181). Required removal of the catheter is a major sequela of dialysis-related peritonitis. Relative indications for this are tunnel infection, catheter malfunction, relapse, bowel perforation, or fungal, mycobacterial, or *P. aeruginosa* infection (182). *S. aureus* is also associated with shorter time to peritoneal dialysis catheter removal and change to hemodialysis (182,183). In general, catheters can be reinserted upon adequate resolution of the primary infection (184). Some evidence suggests that resumption of CAPD after a single episode of *Pseudomonas* peritonitis is often unsuccessful even with replacement of the catheter (173).

Prevention

Critical to prevention of peritonitis is careful patient selection with intensive education regarding aseptic technique and catheter care. Efforts to reduce the incidence of peritonitis by using oral or intraperitoneal antibiotics have largely been unsuccessful (185–187). Although a decrease in the number of random positive dialysate culture results has been observed in clinical studies, occurrence of clinical peritonitis was unaffected by prophylactic antibiotics. In cases of known contamination, such as documented breaks in asepsis or contaminated dialysate fluid or tubing, use of appropriate antibiotics for prophylaxis, or "early presumptive treatment," is probably judicious (188,189). More recent preventive measures have addressed specific reduction of *S. aureus* infections because evidence suggests that pre-CAPD nasal carriers are at high risk for subsequent exit site infection and peritonitis (190). Use of topical mupirocin eliminates colonization but has not yet been shown to significantly impact the incidence of peritonitis (191). Oral trimethoprim-sulfamethoxazole also decreases colonization and the number of episodes of staphylococcal peritonitis but not the overall incidence of peritonitis (192). Staphylococcal vaccines have also been used in CAPD patients, but studies show conflicting results as to efficacy (193). A recent study by Gadallah and associates (194) has shown that administration of a single dose of vancomycin at the time of catheter placement does significantly decrease the incidence of peritonitis within 14 days after placement compared with treatment with cefazolin and no antibiotics.

The most significant advances in the prevention of dialysis-related peritonitis involve instrumentation changes, which are categorized as follows: (a) devices that facilitate connection of tubing, such as titanium adapters; (b) devices that help maintain field sterility during exchanges, such as ultraviolet light systems and in-line filters (195,196); and (c) devices that protect intraluminal sterility during exchanges, such as connector systems with disinfectant (Y-connector, O-set) (197,198). Most such devices have been shown to favorably impact the rate of peritonitis but add appreciably to the overall cost of CAPD.

Other Types of Peritonitis

Tuberculous Peritonitis

See Chapter 51. Although tuberculosis of the peritoneum is an uncommon disease, cases continue to occur in the United States, especially in the elderly, the urban poor, and those with HIV infection, cirrhosis, or debility (199). Currently, peritonitis is the sixth most common site of extrapulmonary tuberculosis (200). Most cases are thought to arise from reactivation of a latent focus of infection in the peritoneum or in an abdominal lymph node. Less commonly, it arises from contiguous spread from the intestines or fallopian tubes (201). Concomitant active pulmonary tuberculosis occurs in 4% to 21% of patients, although abnormal chest radiographs are reported in nearly half of cases (202). The clinical manifestations of tuberculous peritonitis begin insidiously, with most patients having had symptoms for weeks to months before presentation (203). Fever, chills, weight loss, and abdominal pain are common complaints. Ascites is present in virtually all patients, although it is not always detectable by clinical examination. The fluid is exudative (protein >2.5 g/dL) with a WBC count of 150 to 4,000/mm^3 (203). Mononuclear cells predominate in most cases, but as many as 10% of patients have an initial neutrophilic response (204). In cirrhotic patients, the diagnosis of tuberculous peritonitis is often difficult because lymphocytes also do not predominate in all cases and the ascitic fluid may not be exudative because of low serum albumin levels (205).

Acid-fast smears of ascitic fluid are rarely positive in tuberculous peritonitis, and conventional cultures yield the pathogen in only 25% of cases. Concentrated ascitic fluid produces a higher yield on culture (66%), but requires large volumes of fluid and delays of 4 to 8 weeks before growth of the organism is recognized on solid media (206). CT scan may reveal omental infiltration (Fig. 25.2). At present,

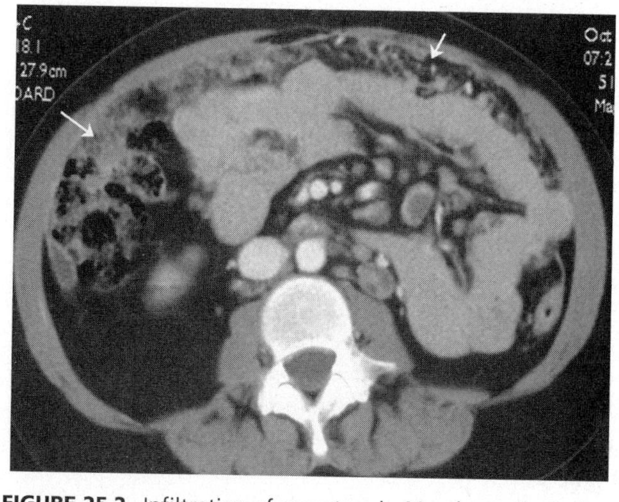

FIGURE 25.2. Infiltration of omentum in *Mycobacterium tuberculosis* peritonitis.

laparoscopy with directed peritoneal biopsy is the best way to make a rapid specific diagnosis (202). Determination of ascitic fluid adenosine deaminase activity has also proven to be a useful test in the diagnosis of peritoneal tuberculosis. Several studies have demonstrated that levels greater than 33 U/L are 100% sensitive and 95% specific to the diagnosis (207). Sumi and colleagues (208) reported the use of gallium-67scintigraphy of their patients with features that may optimize diagnosis of this disease (208).

Drug regimens used for treatment of pulmonary tuberculosis are similarly efficacious in the treatment of peritoneal infection. Drugs with bactericidal activity, such as isoniazid and rifampin, are preferred first-line agents to be given for a period of 9 months. Addition of pyrazinamide may permit shortening of the duration of treatment to 6 months but requires careful monitoring. Because of the recent emergence of drug resistance in HIV-infected patients, therapy of suspected tuberculosis in these patients is usually initiated with a minimum of four agents. Therapy is readjusted in accordance with clinical response and results of susceptibility tests. Even with appropriate therapy, overall mortality rate is in the range of 7% to 13% (205,209). Early recognition is probably the key to improving survival rates.

Fungal Peritonitis

See Chapter 53. With increasing numbers of immunosuppressed patients and advances in medical technology (e.g., organ transplantation), opportunistic fungal infections of the peritoneum have emerged as a significant clinical problem. By far, *Candida* species are the most important of the fungal pathogens producing peritonitis. In non-CAPD patients, *Candida* peritonitis occurs as a complication of perforated abdominal organs or GI surgery (210). Recent antibiotic use is an important predisposing factor (211). Although *Candida* is the sole pathogen in some cases, most infections are polymicrobial, involving other endogenous flora of the GI tract.

The significance of *Candida* growing on culture of peritoneal fluid has been debated, even when it was found in the presence of gross peritoneal contamination. Many clinicians have argued that it is nonpathogenic and requires no specific antifungal therapy (212,213). However, development of intraperitoneal abscesses, systemic fungemia, and late mortality in some cases left untreated defines a definite pathogenic role (214,215). Therapy for *Candida* peritonitis usually consists of a specific antifungal antibiotic and surgical intervention to drain suppurative collections and repair perforations. Amphotericin B in low doses of 0.3 mg/kg/d for a total of 350 to 500 mg is recommended, as long as there is no evidence of dissemination (210). In the case of polymicrobial infection, appropriate antibacterials are also administered. The role of fluconazole and other new azole antifungal agents in treatment of fungal peritonitis remains uncertain. Mortality rate is low in adequately treated patients, but exceeds 50% in those in whom specific antifungal therapy is delayed or withheld (214) and in those acquiring disease as a complication of liver transplantation (216).

On rare occasions, fungi such as *Coccidioides, Histoplasma, Blastomyces,* and *Cryptococcus* may involve the peritoneum as part of a syndrome of dissemination. Clinical manifestations are similar to those produced by bacterial peritonitis. Therapy is as required for the disseminated infection.

INTRAABDOMINAL ABSCESS

Intraperitoneal Abscess

Abscesses are well-defined purulent collections walled off from the rest of the peritoneal cavity by inflammatory adhesions, loops of bowel and their mesentery, the greater omentum, and other abdominal viscera. Abscesses represent successful intervention by host defenses in the peritoneal cavity because the infection has been localized and prevented from entering the bloodstream. The chief anatomic sites of abscess within the abdomen are the subphrenic areas (including subhepatic and subdiaphragmatic abscesses), the pelvis, the lumbar gutters, and the intermesenteric folds. Subphrenic abscesses are divided into three groups: right and left subdiaphragmatic abscesses and subhepatic abscesses. The large spaces above and below the liver are typically subdivided about their midpoints by pyogenic membranes, leading to the designations of anterior and posterior spaces. Subdiaphragmatic abscesses remain a special problem. There are three subdiaphragmatic areas on each side: two intraperitoneal areas (anterior and posterior) and one extraperitoneal area, which lies even further posteriorly. On the right, the extraperitoneal abscesses are in the layer of the crus of the diaphragm and coronary ligament; on the left, they arise above the superior pole of the left kidney. Abscesses may occur within abdominal viscera also; these are usually due to hematogenous or lymphatic spread of microorganisms to the affected organ.

Etiology

The specific etiology relates to the underlying process and the flora of the GI, biliary, or female genital tract area that gave rise to the problem. (Refer to the extensive discussion of the normal flora of some of these areas in the Secondary Peritonitis section.) The major pathogens are ordinarily various Enterobacteriaceae, other gram-negative non-anaerobic bacilli, the *B. fragilis* group, other anaerobic gram-negative rods, clostridia, and anaerobic cocci. Many other organisms may become involved, as detailed in the earlier section. *Salmonella* may be involved in intraabdominal abscess in relation to prior gastroenteritis or biliary tract infection (217). Psoas abscess occurs primarily in children and typically is due to *S. aureus,* but mycobacteria are also important causes and other organisms may be found (218, 219). A recent review by Brook and Frazier (220) include cumulative bacterial etiology for subphrenic abscesses average a 14-year period. *Clostridium septicum,* which is known for septicemia and a rapidly progressing course in association with colon malignancy, may also produce asymptomatic or minimally symptomatic abscesses in solid organs such as the liver and in the retroperitoneum (221). These may also be associated with colonic carcinoma, leukemia involving the bowel, and neutropenia, and there may be accompanying asymptomatic bacteremia. Aggressive search for underlying pathology and aggressive treatment may prevent progression to fulminant toxemia.

Pathogenesis and Pathology

Refer to the earlier section on Secondary Peritonitis. The underlying lesion in subphrenic abscess is almost always within the abdomen. Most recent cases have been related to the stomach or duodenum or the biliary tract, with relatively fewer cases of appendicitis than previously. A primary source in the lower intestinal tract or in the female genital tract is not uncommon. Abdominal surgery or trauma is also a relatively common cause of subphrenic abscess. The major route of infection is by direct extension or by way of lymphatic drainage. The suprahepatic space is much more likely to be infected than the infrahepatic space because the former is a closed space and has a negative pressure that is enhanced during inspiration. Left-sided subphrenic abscess is seen primarily after upper abdominal surgery or lesions of the stomach or duodenum.

The most common precursors of pelvic abscess are perforated appendix (usually the right lower quadrant), colonic diverticulitis (usually the left lower quadrant), and pelvic inflammatory disease. Pancreatitis is associated with lesser sac abscesses; perforation of the stomach or duodenum may also lead to lesser sac abscess. Acute diffuse peritonitis may also localize as a pelvic abscess. Paracolic abscess is more frequent on the right side.

Although host defenses may effectively localize infection by means of abscess formation, complete resolution of the abscess cannot usually be effected by host defense mechanisms because of local factors that impair these defense mechanisms or otherwise interfere with management (75, 81). These include local hypoxia and low pH (which interfere with leukocyte migration and killing and with the antimicrobial activity of aminoglycosides), large numbers of stationary phase bacteria (interfering with antimicrobial efficacy), large concentrations of microbial by-products and toxins (which impair phagocytic cell function, produce local tissue damage, and deplete complement), presence of necrotic debris (interferes with neutrophils and depletes complement), presence of hemoglobin (impairs phagocyte function), presence of fibrin (reduces access of host cells to bacteria), and sometimes the presence of barium sulfate (which impairs neutrophil function).

Clinical Picture

Many patients have an acute response with high intermittent fever, chills, abdominal pain, and tenderness. However, intraabdominal abscess, especially subphrenic abscess, may be an insidious process; manifestations may be nonexistent, nonspecific, or misleading. Most patients have fever. The findings are not uncommonly those of an intrathoracic rather than an intraabdominal process. Pain, when present, is referred to the lower chest almost as often as to the upper abdomen. Hiccups may be present and persistent. Dyspnea, cough, chest or shoulder pain, and dullness or rales over the lung base may be noted. There may be tenderness and even local edema localized directly above the abscess, particularly at the costal margin. In subhepatic abscess, pain and tenderness are much less common. Prior therapy or prophylaxis may suppress the process sufficiently to further minimize findings and even contribute to a considerable delay between the time of the inciting event and the overt manifestations of intraabdominal abscess.

Pelvic abscess may be characterized by pain, deep tenderness in one or both lower quadrants, fever, urinary frequency, dysuria, and diarrhea. There may be mucus in the stools. There may be tenderness of the pelvic peritoneum and bulging of the anterior rectal wall on rectal or vaginal examination. Paracolic abscess results in fever and a tender, enlarging mass that may be difficult to palpate. Abscesses that have formed between or below the folds of the jejunoileal mesentery are characteristically small, multiple, and difficult to diagnose. They may result in fever, anorexia, vague pains, or partial small bowel obstruction.

Complications include bacteremia, fistulas (including external fistulas) (222), and mesenteric vein thrombosis (223).

Diagnosis

A high index of suspicion may be necessary in cases with minimal findings. Most patients exhibit leukocytosis with a left shift. Roentgenographic studies are usually helpful. As with the clinical findings, the roentgenographic signs of subphrenic abscess may be chiefly thoracic: elevation and decreased mobility of the diaphragm, lower lobe infiltrates, atelectasis, and obliteration of a costophrenic angle or larger pleural effusions. In a postoperative patient, these findings may lead to a mistaken diagnosis of pneumonia. Gas under the diaphragm, gas bubbles or a gas-fluid level outside of the bowel, and displacement of intraabdominal organs are all important findings.

Ultrasonography, CT, and, occasionally, magnetic resonance imaging are much more powerful tools than conventional radiography, although the latter technique is still use-

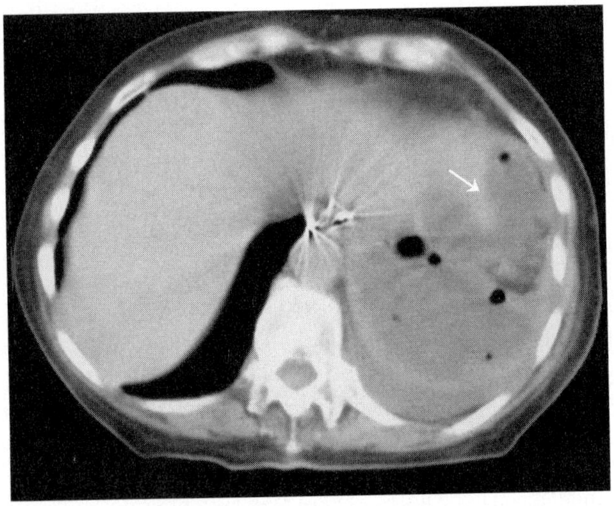

FIGURE 25.3. Subphrenic abscess.

ful (Figs. 25.3 and 25.4) (224). CT is generally the most widely utilized diagnostic tool with a sensitivity and specificity of 97% (225). One may see a low-density mass with a definable capsule that may be enhanced by intravenously administered contrast material. Contrast material is also administered orally and, at times, also rectally. With the bowel outlined in this manner, it is usually easy to determine that bubbles of gas or gas-fluid levels are extraluminal and therefore highly indicative of an abscess. CT can even detect the subtle thickening and edema of the colon wall and mesentery indicative of diverticulitis (83). Radionuclide scans (using technetium, gallium, or indium) may also be useful with a high degree of suspicion and a negative CT scan.

Blood cultures should always be obtained in cases of suspected intraabdominal abscess. The presence of a member of the *B. fragilis* group or two or more enteric non-anaerobes in a blood culture is indicative of intraabdominal infection. If an abscess is drained surgically or percutaneously, both aerobic and anaerobic cultures and appropriate direct smears should be obtained.

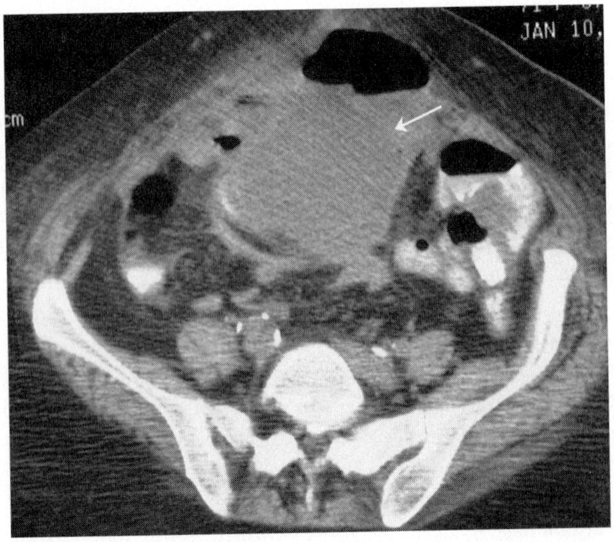

FIGURE 25.4. Pelvic abscess.

Ultimately, laparoscopy (226) or even exploratory laparotomy may be required in very difficult cases, but this has become rare because there are excellent diagnostic techniques available.

Therapy

Clearly, the principal approach to management of intraabdominal abscess is drainage. Most often this is best accomplished surgically, although percutaneous drainage or laparoscopic drainage (226) can be used successfully in many cases. The transperitoneal approach, rather than the posterior extraperitoneal approach, is used almost exclusively because it permits the complete exploration and drainage of the subdiaphragmatic space while enabling visualization and drainage of the subhepatic space (many subphrenic abscesses have subhepatic extensions or separate collections of pus). Pelvic abscesses may be drained by incision through the rectum (227,228) or vagina. Paracolic abscesses can be drained retroperitoneally through an incision lateral to the abscess. Intermesenteric abscesses are drained by evacuation after gentle separation of the mesenteric folds.

When CT or ultrasound examination reveals a unilocular abscess that is accessible, percutaneous drainage under CT or ultrasound guidance is typically effective; usually, insertion of a drainage catheter is desirable. Haaga (224) reported an overall success rate of 80.8% in a number of series reported in the literature. Aside from accessibility and unilocular nature, important requirements for effective percutaneous drainage are that (a) the abscess should not be vascular, (b) the patient should not have coagulopathy, (c) concomitant surgical evaluation and surgical backup for complications or failure should be available, and (d) there should be the possibility of dependent drainage via a catheter placed percutaneously. Percutaneous drainage has been effective in many multiple or complex abscesses; it may be necessary to insert multiple catheters. Brolin and co-workers (229) reported that 76% of 119 patients had successful drainage of abscesses percutaneously; the overall mortality rate was 16%, with a 75% mortality rate in the failure group. Failure with the percutaneous drainage procedure was greater in patients 60 years of age or older, in patients with pancreatic abscess, and patients with abscesses with large volumes (drainage persisting 3 days or longer). One should avoid traversing the pleural space for drainage of subphrenic abscesses (230) and it is best to avoid using a transhepatic or transsplenic approach for drainage of lesser sac abscesses (224). Percutaneous drainage in properly selected patients results in lower morbidity and mortality rates than surgical drainage. Percutaneous drainage and surgical drainage should be considered complementary rather than competitive. Whatever technique is used, patients should be improved within 24 to 48 hours after drainage (231); if a patient is not improved following percutaneous drainage, he or she should be reevaluated with CT, and the surgeon and radiologist should review the case together to agree on an appropriate course of action. Surgical treatment should not be avoided because the patient is considered "too ill."

Even patients with enteric fistulas may be managed successfully with the aid of percutaneous drainage of abdominal abscesses. Schuster and colleagues (232) found that various types of fistulas in 21 of 24 patients healed without surgical intervention (over periods of up to 3 months). Percutaneous drainage has also been used successfully as the initial therapy of intraabdominal abscess associated with a perforated viscus, thus avoiding the first stage of the traditional two-stage surgical approach (233). Stabile and associates (234) found that percutaneous drainage obviated the need for colostomy and multiple-stage surgery in approximately 75% of patients with large diverticular abscesses. Percutaneous drainage has also been used in immunocompromised patients, although the cure rate (53%) was lower than in nonimmunocompromised patients (73%) (235). Drainage of intraabdominal abscess with fistula formation has been effected via fistuloscopy in several patients in whom percutaneous drainage failed (236). Serial imaging may be important for evaluating response to therapy.

Antimicrobial agents are useful adjuncts to drainage procedures, but certainly are not a substitute. (See Secondary Peritonitis for details on indications for various antimicrobial agents.) The low pH and low Eh environment in abscesses may impair the effectiveness of a number of antimicrobial agents (e.g., aminoglycosides).

Prognosis

Mortality rate with subphrenic abscess is still relatively high. Mortality is associated particularly with failure to detect and drain the abscess, delay in drainage, old age, and concomitant serious underlying diseases.

The most frequent complications of subphrenic abscess are intrathoracic—serous effusion, empyema, necrotizing pneumonia, bronchial or bronchopleural fistula, pericarditis, and mediastinal abscess. Other complications include generalized peritonitis, and internal and external fistulas.

Prevention

Appropriate medical and surgical therapy of predisposing conditions should lower the incidence of intraabdominal abscess. Avoidance of postoperative drainage following splenectomy lowers the incidence of local complications, including abscess. Aseptic surgical technique is important in the prevention of postoperative infection.

The use of prophylactic antimicrobial agents in connection with abdominal surgery is discussed under Secondary Peritonitis.

Pancreatic Abscess

Etiology

Pancreatic abscess develops primarily as a complication of pancreatitis of any origin (alcoholic, biliary, postoperative, or related to trauma). It occurs in 3% to 4% of cases of acute pancreatitis (237–239), more often in severe pancreatitis (240). Infected pancreatic necrosis develops in 3% to 6% of patients with acute pancreatitis (239). Less common causes are a complication of endoscopic retrograde cholangiopancreatography (241), a posterior penetrating peptic ulcer, or a secondary infection of a pseudocyst. Pancreatic abscess has also followed pancreatic and liver transplantation (242,243). In a recent study by Knight and associeates (244), pancreatic abscess developed in 4 of 34 patients (12%) following pancreas transplantation, particularly in obese donors and possibly due to ischemic reperfusion injuries (244). Cytomegalovirus pancreatitis apparently may also predispose to pancreatic abscess (245). Men predominate over women in the incidence of pancreatic abscess by a ratio of approximately 2.5:1 and the peak incidence is in the 40- to 50-year age group (246).

Bacteriology

Enteric organisms are the organisms described most often from pancreatic abscess, with approximately half of cases showing a polymicrobial flora (239,247). *E. coli* is found most often (35% of abscesses) with enterococci, viridans streptococci, and *Klebsiella* each found in approximately 20% of cases (239,248). *S. aureus, Enterobacter, Pseudomonas,* and *Proteus* are seen in less than 10% of cases (246,249). *Candida* is seen occasionally. The flora of infected pancreatic necrosis and of infected pancreatic pseudocyst is similar (239,250). The role of anaerobes is undoubtedly underestimated because optimal anaerobic techniques have often not been used, but a number of studies have documented the presence of anaerobes (237–239,246,249–259). The incidence of anaerobes in various studies has been listed as 6% (246), 9% (239), 14% (249), and 16% (251). In a retrospective analysis using optimal anaerobe isolation techniques over a 15-year period, Brook and Frazier reported aerobic or facultative organisms in only 37% of 446 patients, anaerobes alone in 22%, and mixed in 41%. Predominant anaerobes included *Peptostreptococcus, B. fragilis* group, *Clostridium* species *Prevotella* species, *Veillonella* species, and *Fusobacterium* species (248). Anaerobes, including *B. fragilis,* have been recovered from bacteremia accompanying pancreatic abscess (258,259). Other anaerobes recovered from pancreatic abscesses include *Clostridium difficile, Clostridium cadaveris,* "anaerobic streptococci," and *Streptococcus milleri* (this group includes *S. anginosus, S. constellatus,* and *S. intermedius*). *Eikenella corrodens* and *Haemophilus influenzae* have been isolated from a pancreatic abscess (260) and *Eikenella* has been isolated from additional abscesses either in pure culture or together with other organisms (261). *M. tuberculosis* has also been found.

Pathogenesis and Pathology

The bacteriology of the infected pancreas suggests an enteric origin. However, animal studies have shown that bacteria may reach the pancreas from many sources, including colon, gallbladder, and urinary tract. Bacteria may reach the pancreas by various routes including the circulation and the main pancreatic duct as well as transperitoneally or by bacterial translocation (262). In animals, infection develops only in those with inflamed glands and the rate of infection is proportional to the extent of the pancreatic necrosis. There is also some evidence for reduced host resistance to infection in patients with acute pancreatitis. Pancreatic abscesses consist of a collection of pus or necrotic material enclosed by a capsule or pseudocapsule. There may be adjacent areas of necrotic tissue, hemorrhage, and fat necrosis. Approximately two-thirds of abscesses are multiple; they may be either unilocular or multilocular (239). Approximately 25% involve the entire gland and the rest are relatively evenly distributed among the head, body, and tail of the pancreas, although this varies in different reported series.

Clinical Picture

Persistence of fever, ileus, and tenderness or, more commonly, deterioration of the patient's condition 1 to 4 weeks after initial improvement in a patient with pancreatitis should raise the question of abscess. Most cases involve abdominal pain (usually epigastric in location and not uncommonly radiating to the back or flank), nausea and vomiting, and tenderness over the area of the abscess. There may also be guarding or rebound on examination. Low-grade fever to 40.6°C is common. About half the time, either a mass or fullness is palpable. Leukocytosis (15,000 to 20,000 WBC/mm^3) is usual but elevation of the serum amylase and lipase are irregular (21% to 66%) and elevation of serum bilirubin uncommon. Hypoalbuminemia and elevated serum alkaline phosphatase are commonly seen. The clinical picture of pancreatic abscess is nonspecific; one cannot reliably distinguish between pancreatic abscess, sterile or infected pancreatic necrosis, and sterile or infected pancreatic pseudocysts.

Most cases are diagnosed 2 to 3 weeks after the onset of acute pancreatitis, but onset may be considerably later; it appears that the later the onset, the more favorable the prognosis.

Complications include perforation into the peritoneal cavity or into the stomach, bowel, biliary tree, or a bronchus; hemorrhage into the abscess cavity; GI bleeding; empyema; bacteremia; and diabetes mellitus.

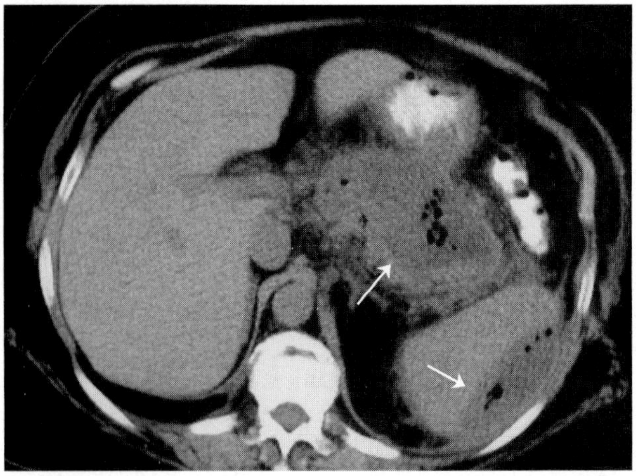

FIGURE 25.5. Pancreatic abscess with extension to the spleen.

Diagnosis

Chest roentgenograms may show abnormalities but findings are nonspecific. Abdominal films may show displacement of the gastric air bubble, retrogastric gas, or the classic "soap bubble" sign, all of which are suggestive of pancreatic infection. Sonograms often detect phlegmon or pseudocyst but are rarely diagnostic of an abscess; however, CT scanning (Fig. 25.5) can detect secondary pancreatic infection in more than 75% to 90% of patients (224,246). In addition, CT provides information on the site and size of the collection. High-dose intravenous contrast infusion in combination with CT scanning is said to be helpful in predicting pancreatic necrosis.

Percutaneous CT-guided aspiration of material for Gram stain and culture is the most reliable method for differentiating secondary pancreatic infection from pancreatic inflammation. Several reports confirm the reliability and safety of this approach (246). Blood cultures should always be done both aerobically and anaerobically.

Therapy

The principal therapeutic approaches to pancreatic abscess are surgical debridement and drainage, percutaneous drainage, and antimicrobial therapy. Many clinicians believe that finding bacteria in material obtained by percutaneous CT-guided drainage mandates surgical intervention. Others would reserve surgery for patients with clinical evidence of sepsis together with demonstration on CT scan of a nonresolving pancreatic collection. In a recent study by Baril and associates (263), aspiration of a suspected infected pancreas was positive in 42 of 82 patients. Twenty-five of the 42 patients had percutaneous catheter drainage, of which six required subsequent surgical therapy. This compared with 11 patients that had primary surgery of which five required subsequent surgery. Six received only antibiotics. The authors concluded that initial therapy for culture-positive patients should be percutaneous catheter drainage, with surgery reserved for failure. The goals of surgical therapy are to remove devitalized pancreatic and peripancreatic tissue, to drain purulent collections, and to provide continuous drainage. Local debridement and drainage may have significantly higher mortality risks than retroperitoneal exploration; extensive unroofing of the superior retroperitoneum is needed because of the tendency of these infections to spread widely. Specific surgical approaches are discussed by Lumsden and Bradley (246). For infected pancreatic pseudocyst, operative or transcutaneous external drainage is done (264). For more effective and safer surgery, intraoperative ultrasound has been recommended to localize fluid collections and the course of the pancreatic duct (265). When surgical debridement is required, external drainage is effected by the use of multiple sumps and stuffed Penrose drains brought out through several separate sites. Sumps and drains should remain in the abscess cavity for at least a week. Evaluation of literature reports is rendered difficult because many authors fail to adequately distinguish between the three types of pancreatic infection.

Antimicrobial therapy should always be used but plays only an adjunctive role. Ideally, information from Gram stain and culture should guide the choice of antimicrobial agents; empirical therapy follows the guidelines provided in the section on treatment of secondary peritonitis, because the flora of pancreatic abscess is typical of bowel flora. Antimicrobials that reach therapeutic levels in the pancreas include ceftazidime, cefotaxime, clindamycin, ciprofloxacin, rifampin, trimethoprim-sulfamethoxazole, and metronidazole (239, 266). Buchler and co-workers (251) ranked drugs in three classes. Included in a class with low tissue levels were netilmicin and tobramycin; in a class with levels adequate to inhibit some, but not all, bacteria found in pancreatic infection were mezlocillin, piperacillin, ceftizoxime, and cefotaxime; in a class with high pancreatic tissue levels and high bactericidal activity were ciprofloxacin, ofloxacin, levofloxacin, and imipenem.

Prognosis

Stanten and Frey (255) summarized the mortality risk in 582 patients with pancreatic abscess from 10 different series; mortality rates ranged from 9% to 38% with an average overall of 23%. Lumsden and Bradley (246) noted that death is rare in infected pseudocyst of the pancreas but that mortality rate is 15% to 20% in pancreatic abscess and 20% to 50% in infected pancreatic necrosis. Baril and colleagues (263) reported death rates of 12% for culture-positive patients, but included infected pancreas and abscess. In addition to impressive mortality rates, there is a high incidence of serious complications; fistulas may form between the abscess and the stomach, duodenum, or transverse colon. Septicemia with multiple organ failure is a common event terminally. Respiratory failure occurs in 9% to 61%, renal failure in 5% to 30%, hepatic failure in 6% to 12%, GI tract hemorrhage in 5% to 60%, peritonitis in 12% to 17%, and intestinal obstruction in 25% to 30%. Gastric outlet obstruction is also not uncommon.

Prevention

Early feeding after the onset of experimental pancreatitis results in an increased infection rate but there is no definite evidence that this occurs in humans. The value of early pancreatic resection or debridement requires further study; this may decrease or actually increase the incidence of subsequent infection. The early use of antibiotics in acute pancreatitis is supported to decrease the septic complications (12.2% versus 30.3%), but with only a trend toward decreased mortality in one study using imipenem (267). A more recent report comparing cefuroxime to no antibiotic in patients with acute pancreatitis demonstrated lower infectious complications and mortality rate in those receiving antibiotics (268).

Pyogenic Liver Abscess

Etiology and Pathogenesis

The incidence of pyogenic liver abscess ranges from 8 to 20 cases per 100,000 hospital admissions (269). Multiple routes of hepatic invasion are described and include the biliary tree, portal vein, direct extension from a focus of infection, hepatic artery, and penetrating trauma. Cryptogenic abscesses, for which no direct cause can be found, are the most common and are most often singular lesions (270) (58.9%) versus multiple abscesses, which are usually from biliary origin (45%). Systemic illnesses, including cirrhosis, diabetes, malignancy, and hemochromatosis, are common predisposing factors (271).

Bacteriology

In the pre-antimicrobial era, *E. coli* and streptococci (particularly members of the viridans group and enterococci) predominated as etiologic agents of liver abscess. Subsequently, other gram-negative bacilli such as *Klebsiella, Enterobacter, Proteus,* and *Pseudomonas* have been found with increasing frequency. Organisms encountered occasionally include *Listeria* (272), *Bartonella* (*Rochalimaea*) (273), *Aeromonas* (274), *Nocardia brasiliensis* (275), *Yersinia enterocolitica* (276), *Haemophilus* species (277), *Pediococcus* (278), *Chromobacterium* (279), *Edwardsiella* (280), *P. pseudomallei* (281), *Salmonella* (282), *Brucella* (283), *M. tuberculosis* (284), and *Aspergillus* (285). The exact incidence of anaerobes is uncertain because many studies have not used optimum anaerobic transport and culture techniques, and there has not been a proper prospective study. It appears, however, that if optimum techniques are used, anaerobes would be found in at least 50% of liver abscesses, often in the absence of other organisms (286). A literature survey published in 1977 found 379 anaerobic isolates from liver abscess patients (287). The most commonly encountered anaerobes currently are gram-negative rods (especially the *B. fragilis* group and other *Bacteroides* species, most of which would now be in *Prevotella* or *Porphyromonas*), anaerobic streptococci, *Fusobacterium, Clostridium,* and microaerophilic streptococci (*S. milleri*).

Hepatosplenic candidiasis (chronic disseminated candidiasis) is a major cause of morbidity and mortality in patients with hematologic malignancies, particularly following arabinosyl cytosine (ara-C) in high doses in combination with anthracycline, leading to prolonged neutropenia (288,289).

Clinical Picture

The most common clinical finding in liver abscess is fever, which may be accompanied by chills or sweats. The next most common finding is right upper quadrant pain. The pain is aching in character and tends to localize over the liver or the epigastrium; it may radiate to the right shoulder and be aggravated by inspiration. Percussion over the liver is painful. A mass may be localized beneath the costal margin or there may be fullness and tenderness of an intercostal space. Localized edema of the right lateral thoracic wall or the adjacent abdominal wall occurs at times. Nausea and vomiting are relatively uncommon. Upward enlargement of the liver may be detected in two-thirds of cases. Abscesses high in the right lobe may lead to cough, splinting of the chest, dyspnea, pleural effusion, and atelectasis. Jaundice is uncommon. The course is most often indolent. In a recent study, Seeto and Rockey (290) described acute presentations (3 days) more often associated with a hematogenous source of a liver abscess compared with a prolonged course associated with pylephlebitis (42 days).

Diagnosis

There is usually considerable leukocytosis (>20,000 WBC/mm^3) with a left shift. The serum alkaline phosphatase level is almost always elevated but liver function tests can be normal or slightly elevated but with a normal albumin and prothrombin time. Blood cultures may be helpful because they are positive in one-third to one-half of patients (290). Roentgenographic studies may show elevation of the diaphragm with reduced mobility and a change in contour; there may be pressure deformities or displacement of the stomach and duodenum. Occasionally there may be a gas-fluid level within the liver. CT, ultrasound (Fig. 25.6), and radionuclide studies are the most valuable procedures for diagnosing liver abscess and determining its location. Percutaneous aspiration may be undertaken for diagnostic purposes and to obtain material for Gram stain and aerobic and anaerobic culture. The principal entities to be considered in the differential diagnosis are amebic liver abscess (distinguished by epidemiologic factors, by the finding of amebae in the stools, or by serologic testing) and subphrenic abscess.

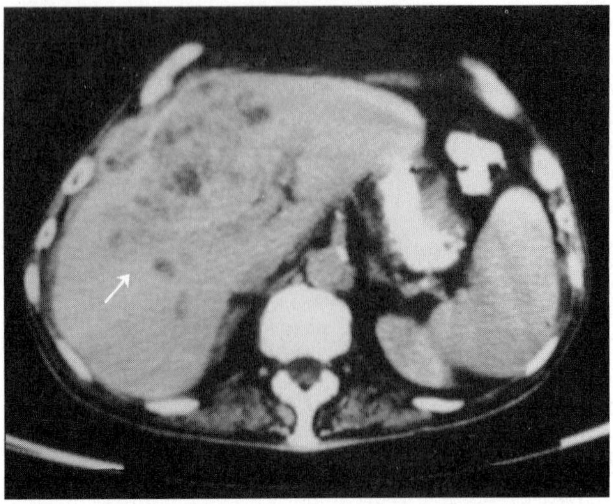

FIGURE 25.6. Multiloculated hepatic abscess.

Therapy

Most cases can be managed with percutaneous drainage under ultrasound or CT guidance, augmented by antimicrobial therapy (231,235,291). A review of 252 patients treated with percutaneous drainage and antimicrobial therapy from 14 series in the literature through 1990 showed an overall success rate of 77% (292). Additional studies demonstrate a success rate of 69% to 90% (290,293). The success rate of percutaneous aspiration without external drains is somewhat lower at 58% to 88% (293,294). Surgical therapy is required for some cases (295); some surgeons favor open drainage as the primary approach (296). Patients with multiple abscesses usually require an open drainage procedure (285,297). Antibiotic therapy alone may be successful, but is generally employed only in unusual circumstances (290,298). Ultrasound and CT scans are also important modalities for monitoring resolution of liver abscesses treated medically. Antimicrobial agents should be given for an extended period, depending on the speed of response as judged both clinically and by follow-up imaging procedures. The choice of agents depends on the specific infecting flora, as outlined in the treatment section under Secondary Peritonitis. Metronidazole supplemented with ampicillin and, at times, other coverage for gram-negative bacilli is one good choice; metronidazole is also effective against amebic liver abscess.

Prognosis

The prognosis of liver abscess is relatively good, although patients with multiple liver abscesses still represent a serious problem. The prognosis depends primarily on the nature of the underlying disease. Complications of liver abscess include bacteremia, empyema, pneumonia, lung abscess, hepatobronchial fistula, rupture into the pericardium, peritonitis, subphrenic abscess, and metastatic abscesses in other organs.

Prevention

Appropriate medical and surgical therapy of infections and other conditions that predispose to liver abscess lower the incidence of this problem.

Splenic Abscess

Etiology

Splenic abscesses are uncommon. They usually are secondary to hematogenous dissemination of microorganisms. The original focus can be anywhere in the body. On occasion, there may be direct inoculation related to surgery or trauma or spread of infection from nearby organs.

Bacteriology

Splenic abscesses secondary to endocarditis usually involve *S. aureus* or various streptococci. In a recent review by Brook and Frazier (299), aerobes were found in 23 of 56 cultures from 29 cases, with 31 specimens containing anaerobes or microaerophilic streptococci. Two specimens contained candidal organisms. Aerobic bacteria only were isolated from 31% and anaerobes only from 28%, with microaerophilic and anaerobic bacteria from 34%. Polymicrobial infections were found in 55%. Predominant aerobic facultative bacteria included *E. coli, P. mirabilis,* group D enterococci, *Klebsiella pneumoniae,* and *S. aureus.* The predominant anaerobes included *Peptostreptococcus, Bacteroides* species, *Fusobacterium* species, and *Clostridium* species. Other anaerobic bacteria reported include *Prevotella melanogenica* (300,301,302), *Actinomyces* (303), *Eubacterium* species (304,305), *Propionibacterium acnes* (306), and various *Clostridium* species (including *C. difficile*) (221,300,307–310). Salmonella in HIV-infected individuals has also been reported (311). Tuberculous splenic abscess is rare (284). Fungi, *Candida* species in particular, have been recovered from splenic abscesses in immunocompromised hosts; fungal splenic abscess is a part of the syndrome of hepatosplenic candidiasis. Blood cultures are positive in two-thirds of patients with multiple splenic abscesses but in only a small percentage of those with solitary abscesses.

Pathogenesis

In addition to the background factors mentioned previously, splenic infarction is a relatively common underlying feature. The spleen may be seeded at the time of the infarction (e.g, with underlying endocarditis) or organisms may seed an area that had undergone infarction earlier. Patients with sickle cell disease may be predisposed on this basis. Hematoma may also predispose to splenic abscess. An enlarged spleen itself may develop subcapsular infarcts that may subsequently become infected and lead to abscess of the spleen.

Clinical Picture

Onset of illness associated with splenic abscess is often sudden, with chills and fever and left upper quadrant pain. When the upper pole of the spleen is involved, there is commonly left pleuritic pain radiating to the shoulder, elevation of the left diaphragm, and left pleural effusion. With lower pole abscess, there may be signs of peritoneal inflammation. In less than half of patients, the spleen is palpable and tender; rarely, a friction rub may be heard over the organ. Before the availability of modern imaging techniques, the diagnosis was frequently made late in the course of the illness or at autopsy. Because bacteremia is a common background for abscess of the spleen, many patients have abscesses in other organs such as the liver, kidneys, and brain. As noted earlier, endocarditis is a common underlying problem. Other complications include thoracic empyema, subphrenic abscess, generalized peritonitis, and discharge of abscess contents into an adjacent viscus such as the colon or stomach.

Diagnosis

A high index of suspicion may be required. Splenic abscess should be considered in any patient with bacteremia and left upper quadrant symptoms or findings. Blood cultures, both aerobic and anaerobic, should be obtained; as noted earlier, bacteremia is relatively common. Leukocytosis is typically present but is not particularly helpful. Thrombocytosis is also commonly found (312), but this may be found in bacteremia and in various chronic bacterial infections. Roentgenograms may show compression of the gastric air shadow, displacement of other viscera, extraluminal gas or a gas-fluid level, elevation of the left diaphragm or left pleural effusion, left lower lung parenchymal infiltrates or atelectasis. CT scan is the most useful diagnostic procedure (Fig. 25.5).

Therapy

Surgery must be considered the procedure of choice presently (231), although increasing experience with percutaneous drainage suggests that there is a role for this procedure (313), particularly for smaller solitary abscesses. Splenectomy is generally the surgical procedure of choice. Previously, when the spleen was grossly enlarged, surrounded by dense adhesions, and disrupted by extensive suppuration, patients were managed by splenotomy and drainage of the abscess. With the early diagnosis that is the rule with the current available imaging techniques, however, splenotomy is rarely necessary (294). Percutaneous drainage carries the potential risk of bleeding and of damage to neighboring organs. Adjunctive antimicrobial therapy plays an important role also. The specific agents depend on the nature of the organisms involved and their antimicrobial susceptibility. There is one report of successful treatment of a 5-cm solitary splenic abscess with antibiotics alone (305).

Prognosis

The ultimate prognosis of splenic abscess depends on the underlying process (300). Delay in diagnosis and definitive surgical therapy leads to higher mortality risk. Higher mortality rates are also associated with the older age group, diabetes mellitus, alcoholism, and immunosuppressive disease or therapy (319). In two-thirds of patients with abscess of the spleen, the infection is a terminal manifestation of uncontrolled disease of other organs, but often these patients have multiple small abscesses that produce no special clinical manifestations (314). Overall mortality rates may still be as high as 40% in unselected series (315).

Abdominal Actinomycosis

Etiology

The three major types of actinomycosis are cervicofacial, thoracic, and abdominal. Cervicofacial is clearly the most commonly encountered form; the other two varieties account for roughly 20% of cases each. The disease appears in a variety of forms from localized intraabdominal disease, to disease localized to the liver, to widespread involvement within the abdomen, to widely disseminated disease. Hepatic involvement may be in the form of a small nodule (316), a pyogenic liver abscess (317), or multiple liver abscesses (318,319); involvement of the liver occurs in 15% of cases of abdominal actinomycosis. Yegüez and colleagues presented one case of pelvic actinomycosis and reviewed 38 other reports in the literature, describing a total of 505 cases of abdominal actinomycosis from 1938 to 1998 (320). The ileocecal region of the intestine (and the appendix in particular) is the site most frequently involved in abdominal actinomycosis, but there are reports of involvement of the stomach, small bowel, rectum, sigmoid and transverse colon, liver, gallbladder, pancreas, pelvis (typically associated with intrauterine contraceptive devices) (321), and abdominal wall (322). Most often, disease is limited to a single organ; disseminated infection is rare. It may be associated with an underlying disease such as neoplasm, appendicitis (323), or diverticulitis (324). The disease may originate in the thorax and extend through the diaphragm to involve the abdomen (325). A most unusual case of ruptured actinomycotic aneurysm of the splenic artery has been described (326).

Bacteriology

Any species of *Actinomyces* (*israelii, odontolyticus, naeslundii, viscosus, meyeri, georgiae,* or *gerencseriae*) may be involved, as may *Propionibacterium propionicus* (formerly *Arachnia propionica*). Hill and co-workers (327) reported that *Eubacterium nodatum* may also be involved in pelvic infection in women using intrauterine contraceptive devices and that a clinical and pathologic picture of actinomycosis may result. A variety of other anaerobic or microaerophilic bacteria may be found concurrently with the agents of actinomycosis, particularly pigmented anaerobic gram-negative bacilli and *Actinobacillus actinomycetemcomitans.*

Pathogenesis and Pathology

The causative agents of actinomycosis are part of the indigenous flora of the body. These agents may set up infection when some process such as surgery, trauma, or disease disrupts the mucosal barrier and lowers the oxidation-reduction potential so as to favor growth of anaerobic bacteria. In the case of abdominal actinomycosis, the Eh is normally low at the sites of normal carriage; furthermore, a number of *Actinomyces* are somewhat aerotolerant. Other predisposing factors are malignancy, the use of corticosteroids, and diabetes mellitus.

The disease typically spreads by direct extension, without regard for tissue planes, often producing sinus tracts or fistulas. The process classically involves suppuration, necrosis, acute and chronic inflammation, fibrosis, stricture formation, and obstruction.

Involvement of the liver in abdominal actinomycosis is usually due to spread via the portal vein from an intestinal source. However, it may occur by direct extension or via the hepatic artery during disseminated infection. It is not rare for no primary focus to be found (317).

Clinical Picture

The disease may be manifested by firm, indurated masses or abscesses within the abdomen; sinus tracts and fistulas are relatively common. These classic findings may not be apparent, particularly early in the course of illness, and presentation may be insidious. The most common symptoms are pain, weight loss, and fever. Anorexia and chills may also be present, particularly with visceral involvement.

Hepatic actinomycosis has a nonspecific presentation and should be considered in the differential diagnosis of liver abscess and other space-occupying lesions of the liver.

Diagnosis

Diagnosis of abdominal actinomycosis is difficult and is usually not made without the aid of surgery or needle biopsy. Because this disease shows a predilection for the right iliac fossa, the diagnosis should be entertained in appropriate clinical settings. The classic findings of fibrotic induration, sinus tract and fistula formation, or abscess formation, when present, are very helpful in suggesting the possibility of actinomycosis, although these findings are nonspecific. Among considerations in the differential diagnosis are carcinoma of the cecum, Crohn's disease, tuberculosis, and amebiasis. The presence of sulfur granules grossly visible in the pus from a draining sinus strongly enhances the possibility of actinomycosis.

Leukocytosis, elevated sedimentation rate, and elevated C-reactive protein are present but nonspecific. Elevation of the serum alkaline phosphatase is commonly present in liver abscess involving *Actinomyces* and related organisms but does not point to the specific etiology of the abscess. Conventional roentgenograms, ultrasound (328), and CT (329) are helpful in delineating masses, sinus tracts, and so forth, but definitive diagnosis depends on demonstrating the characteristic pathology and, specifically, sulfur granules on biopsy of appropriate materials (323,330). The sulfur granules are actually microcolonies of the organism, with the eosinophilic, clubbed material at the edges of the granule in tissue sections representing the host response to the organism. On Gram stain, the organism is shown to be gram-positive with branching filaments. It is non–acid-fast, in contrast to *Nocardia,* which is weakly acid-fast. The organisms of actinomycosis also show up well on Gomori methenamine-silver stain. Sulfur granules from pus should be cultured anaerobically and aerobically and crushed on a slide for Gram and acid-fast staining with a weak decolorizer. Cultures of pus or biopsy material for the agents of actinomycosis are positive in only 25% to 50% of cases that prove to be actinomycosis. The organisms are fastidious, even those that are relatively aerotolerant. Anaerobic blood cultures should be obtained.

Treatment

Most cases of intraabdominal actinomycosis require both surgical and antimicrobial therapy. The surgical approach depends on the exact nature and location of the disease process. The basic principles are incision and drainage of loculated pus, debridement, and excision of sinus tracts. Percutaneous drainage of abscesses may be adequate in selected cases (323), particularly in the case of isolated or even multiple liver abscesses (317,318). Intrauterine contraceptive devices should be removed in cases in which they served as the focus of the infection. Hyperbaric oxygen therapy failed in one patient in whom it was tried (322). Antimicrobial agents that are effective in actinomycosis include penicillin G, ampicillin, tetracycline, erythromycin, clindamycin, chloramphenicol, and imipenem. Penicillin G is the drug of choice for initiation of therapy and during periods of hospitalization. It should be given in high dosage—ordinarily 12 to 15 million units daily by the intravenous route in normal size adults with normal renal function. Certain of the agents may not be active against accompanying flora; for example, clindamycin is not active against *A. actinomycetemcomitans.* Therapy, regardless of the agent used, must be prolonged. The exact length of therapy depends on the extent and location of disease and the speed of response, but ordinarily should not be for less than 6 to 9 months and often is for a year or longer. CT is valuable for follow-up of patients on therapy (325).

Prognosis

Depending on the nature of any underlying disease (e.g., malignancy), most cases are amenable to cure, but it is often necessary to do repeated surgeries or percutaneous drainage procedures and, as indicated above, antimicrobial therapy must be given for extended periods. Raz and Lev (322) described a patient who had multiple relapses over a 7-year period despite long courses of several different antimicrobial agents, repeated surgical interventions, and even a course of hyperbaric oxygenation; this patient finally refused further therapy.

ACKNOWLEDGMENTS

We wish to thank Terrence C. Demos, M.D, for providing the radiographs used as figures in this chapter.

REFERENCES

1. Stewardson. Treatment of peritonitis. In: Elliotson J, ed. *Practice of medicine.* London: Carey & Hart, 1844:874.
2. Ahrenholz DH, Simmons RL. Peritonitis and other intraabdominal infections. In: Howard R , Simmons RL, eds. *Surgical Infectious Diseases,* second edition. Norwalk, CT: Appleton & Lange, 1988.
3. Charney DI, Gouge SF. Chemical peritonitis secondary to intraperitoneal vancomycin. *Am J Kidney Dis* 1991;17:76–79.
4. Garcia-Tsao G. Spontaneous bacterial peritonitis. *Gastroenterol Clin North Am* 1992;21:257–275.
5. Andreu M, Sola R, Sitges-Serra A, et al. Risk factors for spontaneous bacterial peritonitis in cirrhotic patients with ascites. *Gastroenterology* 1993;104:1133–1138.
6. Runyon BA. Low-protein-concentration ascitic fluid is predisposed to spontaneous bacterial peritonitis. *Gastroenterology* 1986;91:1343–1346.
7. Richardet JP, Beaugrand M. [Spontaneous bacterial peritonitis in cirrhotic patients]. *Gastroenterol Clin Biol* 1991;15:239–249.
8. Boixeda D, De Luis DA, Aller R, et al. Spontaneous bacterial peritonitis. Clinical and microbiological study of 233 episodes. *J Clin Gastroenterol* 1996;23:275–279.
9. Targan SR, Chow AW, Guze LB. Role of anaerobic bacteria in spontaneous peritonitis of cirrhosis: report of two cases and review of the literature. *Am J Med* 1977;62:397–403.
10. Sheckman P, Onderdonk AB, Bartlett JG. Anaerobes in spontaneous peritonitis. *Lancet* 1977;2:1223.
11. Moskovitz M, Ehrenberg E, Grieco R, et al. Primary peritonitis due to group A streptococcus. *J Clin Gastroenterol* 2000;30: 332–335.

12. Ho H, Guerra LG, Zuckerman MJ, et al. Urinary tract infection: a predisposing factor for spontaneous bacterial peritonitis. *Gastroenterology* 1990;98:A593.
13. Bruyn GA. Spontaneous pneumococcal peritonitis in young women. *Clin Infect Dis* 1993;16:728–729.
14. Hemsley C, Eykyn SJ. Pneumococcal peritonitis in previously healthy adults: case report and review. *Clin Infect Dis* 1998;27:376–379.
15. Rimola A, Soto R, Bory F, et al. Reticuloendothelial system phagocytic activity in cirrhosis and its relation to bacterial infections and prognosis. *Hepatology* 1984;4:53–58.
16. Runyon BA. Patients with deficient ascitic fluid opsonic activity are predisposed to spontaneous bacterial peritonitis. *Hepatology* 1988;8:632–635.
17. Runyon BA, Morrissey RL, Hoefs JC, et al. Opsonic activity of human ascitic fluid: a potentially important protective mechanism against spontaneous bacterial peritonitis. *Hepatology* 1985;5:634–637.
18. Bird G, Senaldi G, Panos M, et al. Activation of the classical complement pathway in spontaneous bacterial peritonitis. *Gut* 1992;33:307–311.
19. Wyke RJ, Rajkovic IA, Williams R. Impaired opsonization by serum from patients with chronic liver disease. *Clin Exp Immunol* 1983;51:91–98.
19a. Runyon BA. Monomicrobial nonneatrocytic bacterascites: a variant of spontaneous bacterial peritonitis. *Hepatology* 1990;12:710–715.
20. DeMeo AN, Anderson BR. Defective chemotaxis associated with a serum inhibitor in cirrhotic patients. *N Engl J Med* 1982;286:635–640.
21. Fierer J, Finley F. Deficient serum bactericidal activity against *Escherichia coli* in patients with cirrhosis of the liver. *J Clin Invest* 1979;63:912–921.
22. Rajkovic IA, Williams R. Abnormalities of neutrophil phagocytosis, intracellular killing and metabolic activity in alcoholic cirrhosis and hepatitis. *Hepatology* 1986;6:252–262.
23. Fromkes JJ, Thomas FB, Mekhjian HS, et al. Antimicrobial activity of human ascitic fluid. *Gastroenterology* 1977;73:668–672.
24. Deviere J, Content J, Crusiaux A, et al. IL-6 and TNF alpha in ascitic fluid during spontaneous bacterial peritonitis. *Dig Dis Sci* 1991;36:123–124.
25. Xiol X, Castellote J, Baliellas C, et al. Spontaneous bacterial empyema in cirrhotic patients: analysis of eleven cases. *Hepatology* 1990;11:365–370.
26. Runyon BA, Antillon MR. Ascitic fluid pH and lactate: insensitive and nonspecific tests in detecting ascitic fluid infection. *Hepatology* 1991;13:929–935.
27. Runyon BA, Antillon MR, Akriviadis EA, et al. Bedside inoculation of blood culture bottles with ascitic fluid is superior to delayed inoculation in the detection of spontaneous bacterial peritonitis. *J Clin Microbiol* 1990;28:2811–2812.
28. Siersema PD, de Marie S, van Zeijl JH, et al. Blood culture bottles are superior to lysis-centrifugation tubes for bacteriological diagnosis of spontaneous bacterial peritonitis. *J Clin Microbiol* 1992;30:667–669.
29. Such J, Runyon BA. Spontaneous bacterial peritonitis. *Clin Infect Dis* 1998;27:669–674.
30. Akriviadis EA, Runyon BA. Utility of an algorithm in differentiating spontaneous from secondary bacterial peritonitis. *Gastroenterology* 1990;98:127–333.
31. Rimola A, Garcia-Tsao G, Navasa M, et al. Diagnosis, treatment and prophylaxis of spontaneous bacterial peritonitis: a consensus document. International Ascites Club. *J Hepatol* 2000;32:142–153.
32. Felisart J, Rimola A, Arroyo V, et al. Cefotaxime is more effective than is ampicillin-tobramycin in cirrhotics with severe infections. *Hepatology* 1985;5:457–462.
33. Gomez-Jimenez J, Ribera E, Gasser I, et al. Randomized trial comparing ceftriaxone with cefonicid for treatment of spontaneous bacterial peritonitis in cirrhotic patients. *Antimicrob Agents Chemother* 1993;37:1587–1592.
34. McCormick PA, Greenslade L, Kibbler CC, et al. A prospective randomized trial of ceftazidime versus netilmicin plus mezlocillin in the empirical therapy of presumed sepsis in cirrhotic patients. *Hepatology* 1997;25:833–836.
35. Laroche M, Harding G. Primary and secondary peritonitis: an update. *Eur J Clin Microbiol Infect Dis* 1998;17:542–550.
36. Runyon BA, McHutchison JG, Antillon MR, et al. Short-course versus long-course antibiotic treatment of spontaneous bacterial peritonitis. A randomized controlled study of 100 patients. *Gastroenterology* 1991;100:1737–1742.
37. Zeni F, Tardy B, Vindimian M, et al. High levels of tumor necrosis factor-alpha and interleukin-6 in the ascitic fluid of cirrhotic patients with spontaneous bacterial peritonitis. *Clin Infect Dis* 1993;17:218–223.
38. Soriano G, Guarner C, Tomas A, et al. Norfloxacin prevents bacterial infection in cirrhotics with gastrointestinal hemorrhage. *Gastroenterology* 1992;103:1267–1272.
39. Bernard B, Cadranel JF, Valla D, et al. Prognostic significance of bacterial infection in bleeding cirrhotic patients: a prospective study. *Gastroenterology* 1995;108:1828–1834.
40. Pauwels A, Mostefa-Kara N, Debenes B, et al. Systemic antibiotic prophylaxis after gastrointestinal hemorrhage in cirrhotic patients with a high risk of infection. *Hepatology* 1996;24:802–806.
41. Bernard B, Grange JD, Khac EN, et al. Antibiotic prophylaxis for the prevention of bacterial infections in cirrhotic patients with ascites: a meta-analysis. *Digestion* 1998;59(Suppl. 2):54–57.
42. Inadomi J, Sonnenberg A. Cost-analysis of prophylactic antibiotics in spontaneous bacterial peritonitis. *Gastroenterology* 1997;113:1289–1294.
43. Giannella RA, Broitman SA, Zamcheck N. Gastric acid barrier to ingested microorganisms in man: studies *in vivo* and *in vitro*. *Gut* 1993;13:256.
44. Franklin MA, Skoryna SC. Studies on natural gastric flora. I. Bacterial flora of fasting human subjects. *Can Med Assoc J* 1966;95:1349–1355.
45. Gorbach SL, Nahas L, Lerner PI, et al. Studies of intestinal microflora. I. Effects of diet, age, and periodic sampling on numbers of fecal microorganisms in man. *Gastroenterology* 1967;53:845–655.
46. Finegold SM, Sutter VL, Mathisen GE. Normal indigenous intestinal flora. In: Hentges, DJ, ed. *Human intestinal microflora in health and disease.* New York: Academic Press, 1983:3–31.
47. Summanen PH, Jousimies-Somer H, Manley S, et al. *Bilophila wadsworthia* isolates from clinical specimens. *Clin Infect Dis* 1995;20 (Suppl. 2) S210–S211.
48. Draser BS, Hill MJ. *Human intestinal flora.* New York: Academic Press, 1974:1–263.
49. Nichols RL, Smith JW. Intragastric microbial colonization in common disease states of the stomach and duodenum. *Ann Surg* 1975;182:557–561.
50. Finegold SM, Mathisen GE, George WL. Changes in Human Intestinal Flora Related to the Administration of Antimicrobial Agents. In: Hentges DJ, ed. *Human intestinal microflora in health and disease.* New York: Academic Press, 1983;355–446.
51. Marshall JC, Christou NV, Horn R, et al. The microbiology of multiple organ failure. The proximal gastrointestinal tract as an occult reservoir of pathogens. *Arch Surg* 1988;123:309–315.
52. Bartlett JG, Onderdonk AB, Drude E, et al. Quantitative bacteriology of the vaginal flora. *J Infect Dis* 1977;136:271–277.
53. Levison ME, Corman LC, Carrington ER, et al. Quantitative microflora of the vagina. *Am J Obstet Gynecol* 1977;127:80–85.
54. Levison ME, Trestman I, Quach R, et al. Quantitative bacteri-

ology of the vaginal flora in vaginitis. *Am J Obstet Gynecol* 1979; 133:139–144.
55. Onderdonk AB, Zamarchi GR, Walsh JA, et al. Methods for quantitative and qualitative evaluation of vaginal microflora during menstruation. *Appl Environ Microbiol* 1986;51:333–339.
56. Mårdh PA. The vaginal ecosystem. *Am J Obstet Gynecol* 1991; 165:1163–1168.
57. Hillier SL, Krohn MA, Rabe LK, et al. The normal vaginal flora, H2O2-producing lactobacilli, and bacterial vaginosis in pregnant women. *Clin Infect Dis* 1993;16 (Suppl 4):S273–S281.
58. Shinagawa N, Muramoto M, Sakurai S, et al. A bacteriological study of perforated duodenal ulcers. *Jpn J Surg* 1991;21:1–7.
59. Mosdell DM, Morris DM, Voltura A, et al. Antibiotic treatment for surgical peritonitis. *Ann Surg* 1991;214:543–549.
60. Solomkin JS, Wilson SE, Christou NV, et al. Results of a clinical trial of clinafloxacin versus imipenem/cilastatin for intraabdominal infections. *Ann Surg* 2001;233:79–87.
61. Nichols RL, Muzik AC. Enterococcal infections in surgical patients: the mystery continues. *Clin Infect Dis* 1992;15:72–76.
62. Nathens AB, Rotstein OD, Marshall JC. Tertiary peritonitis: clinical features of a complex nosocomial infection. *World J Surg* 1998;22:158–163.
62a. Rotstein OD, Pruett TL, Simmons RL. Microbiologic features and treatment of persistent peritonitis in patients in the intensive care unit. *Can J Surg* 1986;29:247–250.
63. Mollitt DL, Tepas JJ, Talbert JL. The microbiology of neonatal peritonitis. *Arch Surg* 1988;123:176–179.
64. Yanagisawa N, Tomiyasu H, Hada T, et al. *Chlamydia trachomatis* peritonitis: report of a patient presenting spontaneous regression of ascites. *Intern Med* 1992;31:835–839.
65. Dawson JM, O'Riordan B, Chopra S. Ovarian actinomycosis presenting as acute peritonitis. *Aust N Z J Surg* 1992;62:161–163.
66. Chow AW, Guze LB. Bacteroidaceae bacteremia: clinical experience with 112 patients. *Medicine (Baltimore)* 1974;53:93–126.
67. Fry DE, Garrison RN, Polk HC. Clinical implications in *Bacteroides* bacteremia. *Surg Gynecol Obstet* 1979;149:189–192.
68. Bodner SJ, Koenig MG, Goodman JS. Bacteremic *Bacteroides* infections. *Ann Intern Med* 1970;73:537–544.
69. Gelb AF, Seligman SJ. Bacteroidaceae bacteremia. Effect of age and focus of infection upon clinical course. *JAMA* 1970;212: 1038–1041.
70. Nguyen MH, Yu VL, Morris AJ, et al. Antimicrobial resistance and clinical outcome of *Bacteroides* bacteremia: findings of a multicenter prospective observational trial. *Clin Infect Dis* 2000; 30:870–876.
71. Johnson ML, Billiar TR. Roles of nitric oxide in surgical infection and sepsis. *World J Surg* 1998;22:187–196.
72. Gharbia SE, Shah HN. Hydrolytic enzymes liberated by black-pigmented gram-negative anaerobes. *FEMS Immunol Med Microbiol* 1993;6:139–145.
73. Niederman R, Brunkhorst B, Smith S, et al. Ammonia as a potential mediator of adult human periodontal infection: inhibition of neutrophil function. *Arch Oral Biol* 1990;35 (Suppl): 205S–209S.
74. Dunn DL, Barke RA, Knight NB, et al. Role of resident macrophages, peripheral neutrophils, and translymphatic absorption in bacterial clearance from the peritoneal cavity. *Infect Immun* 1985;49:257–264.
75. Rotstein OD. Role of fibrin deposition in the pathogenesis of intraabdominal infection. *Eur J Clin Microbiol Infect Dis* 1992; 11:1064–1068.
76. Hau T. Bacteria, toxins, and the peritoneum. *World J Surg* 1990; 14:167–175.
77. Sawyer RG, Pruett TL. Cellular mechanisms of abscess formation: macrophage procoagulant activity and major histocompatibility complex recognition. *Surgery* 1996;120:488–495.
78. Gharbia SE, Shah HN. Interactions between black-pigmented gram-negative anaerobes and other species which may be important in disease development. *FEMS Immunol Med Microbiol* 1993;6:173–177.
79. Montravers P, Mohler J, Saint Julien L, et al. Evidence of the proinflammatory role of *Enterococcus faecalis* in polymicrobial peritonitis in rats. *Infect.Immun* 1997;65:144–149.
80. Klaerner HG, Uknis ME, Acton RD, et al. *Candida albicans* and *Escherichia coli* are synergistic pathogens during experimental microbial peritonitis. *J Surg Res* 1997;70:161–165.
81. Rotstein OD, Meakins JL. Diagnostic and therapeutic challenges of intraabdominal infections. *World J Surg* 1990;14: 159–166.
82. Farthmann EH, Schoffel U. Principles and limitations of operative management of intraabdominal infections. *World J Surg* 1990;14:210–217.
83. Stabile BE. Therapeutic options in acute diverticulitis. *Compr Ther* 1991;17:26–33.
84. Gorbach SL. Treatment of intra-abdominal infections. *J Antimicrob Chemother* 1993;31 (Suppl A):67–78.
85. Nichols RL, Smith JW, Klein DB, et al. Risk of infection after penetrating abdominal trauma. *N Engl J Med* 1984;311: 1065–1070.
86. Solomkin JS, Dellinger EP, Christou NV, et al. Results of a multicenter trial comparing imipenem/cilastatin to tobramycin/ clindamycin for intra-abdominal infections. *Ann Surg* 1990; 212:581–591.
87. Henry SA. Overall clinical experience with aztreonam in the treatment of intraabdominal infections. *Rev Infect Dis* 1985;7: S729–S733.
88. Berne TV, Yellin AE, Appleman MD, et al. Surgically treated gangrenous or perforated appendicitis. A comparison of aztreonam and clindamycin versus gentamicin and clindamycin. *Ann Surg* 1987;205:133–137.
89. Williams RR, Hotchkin D. Aztreonam plus clindamycin versus tobramycin plus clindamycin in the treatment of intraabdominal infections. *Rev Infect Dis* 1991;13 (Suppl 7):S629–S633.
90. Smith JA. Treatment of intra-abdominal infections with quinolones. *Eur J Clin Microbiol Infect Dis* 1991;10:330–333.
91. Snydman DR, Jacobus NV, McDermott LA, et al. Multicenter study of *in vitro* susceptibility of the *Bacteroides fragilis* group, 1995 to 1996, with comparison of resistance trends from 1990 to 1996. *Antimicrob Agents Chemother* 1999;43:2417–2422.
92. National Committee for Clinical Laboratory Standards. Methods for antimicrobial susceptibility testing of anaerobic bacteria. Approved standard M11-A5. 2001.
93. Hecht DW, Vedantam G, Osmolski JR. Antibiotic resistance among anaerobes: what does it mean? *Anaerobe* 1999;421–429.
94. Solomkin JS, Meakins JL, Allo MD, et al. Antibiotic trials in intra-abdominal infections. A critical evaluation of study design and outcome reporting. *Ann Surg* 1984;200:29–39.
95. Dellinger EP. Design and evaluation of clinical trials of antimicrobial agents in surgery. *Surg Gynecol Obstet* 1991;172 (Suppl): 65–72.
96. Nystrom PO, Bax R, Dellinger EP, et al. Proposed definitions for diagnosis, severity scoring, stratification, and outcome for trials on intraabdominal infection. Joint Working Party of SIS North America and Europe. *World J Surg* 1990;14:148–158.
97. Corder AP, Bates T, Prior JE, et al. Metronidazole v. cefoxitin in severe appendicitis—a trial to compare a single intraoperative dose of two antibiotics given intravenously. *Postgrad Med J* 1983;59:720–723.
98. Oh SJ, Halsey JH, Briggs DD. Guanidine in type B botulism. *Arch Intern Med* 1975;135:726–728.
99. Wilson SE, Boswick JA, Duma RJ, et al. Cephalosporin therapy in intraabdominal infections. A multicenter randomized, comparative study of cefotetan, moxalactam, and cefoxitin. *Am J Surg* 1988;155:61–66.

100. Najem AZ, Kaminski ZC, Spillert CR, et al. Comparative study of parenteral piperacillin and cefoxitin in the treatment of surgical infections of the abdomen. *Surg Gynecol Obstet* 1983;157: 423–425.
101. Paakkonen M, Alhava EM, Huttunen R, et al. Piperacillin compared with cefuroxime plus metronidazole in diffuse peritonitis. *Eur J Surg* 1991;157:535–537.
102. Foster MC, Kapila L, Morris DL, et al. A randomized comparative study of sulbactam plus ampicillin vs. metronidazole plus cefotaxime in the management of acute appendicitis in children. *Rev Infect Dis* 1986;8:S634–S638.
103. Fink MP, Helsmoortel CM, Arous EJ, et al. Comparison of the safety and efficacy of parenteral ticarcillin/clavulanate and clindamycin/gentamicin in serious intra-abdominal infections. *J Antimicrob Chemother* 1989;24 (Suppl B):147–156.
104. Sirinek KR, Levine BA. A randomized trial of ticarcillin and clavulanate versus gentamicin and clindamycin in patients with complicated appendicitis. *Surg Gynecol Obstet* 1991;172 (Suppl): 30–35.
105. Solomkin JS, Fant WK, Rivera JO, et al. Randomized trial of imipenem/cilastatin versus gentamicin and clindamycin in mixed flora infections. *Am J Med* 1985;78:85–91.
106. Scandinavian Study Group. Imipenem/cilastin versus gentamicin/clindamycin for treatment of serious bacterial infections. *Lancet* 1984;1:868–871.
107. Bennion RS, Thompson JE Jr, Baron EJ, et al. The use of single agent antibacterial regimens int he treatment of advanced appendicitis with peritonitis. *Drug Invest* 1992;4(Suppl 1):7–12.
108. Rotstein OD, Pruett TL, Simmons RL. Microbiologic features and treatment of persistent peritonitis in patients in the intensive care unit. *Can J Surg* 1986;29:247–250.
109. Pine RW, Wertz MJ, Lennard ES, et al. Determinants of organ malfunction or death in patients with intra-abdominal sepsis. A discriminant analysis. *Arch Surg* 1983;118:242–249.
110. Meakins JL, Wicklund B, Forse RA, et al. The surgical intensive care unit: current concepts in infection. *Surg Clin North Am* 1980;60:117–132.
111. Montravers P, Gauzit R, Muller C, et al. Emergence of antibiotic-resistant bacteria in cases of peritonitis after intraabdominal surgery affects the efficacy of empirical antimicrobial therapy. *Clin Infect Dis* 1996;23:486–494.
112. Antimicrobial prophylaxis in surgery *Med Lett* 1999;4175:75–80.
113. Condon RE, Bartlett JG, Greenlee H, et al. Efficacy of oral and systemic antibiotic prophylaxis in colorectal operations. *Arch Surg* 1983;118:496–502.
114. Schoetz DJ, Roberts PL, Murray JJ, et al. Addition of parenteral cefoxitin to regimen of oral antibiotics for elective colorectal operations. A randomized prospective study. *Ann Surg* 1990; 212:209–212.
115. Luchette FA, Borzotta AP, Croce MA, et al. Practice management guidelines for prophylactic antibiotic use in penetrating abdominal trauma: the EAST Practice Management Guidelines Work Group. *J Trauma* 2000;48:508–518.
116. Popovich RP, Moncrief JW, Nolph KD, et al. Continuous ambulatory peritoneal dialysis. *Ann Intern Med* 1978;88:449–456.
117. Korbet SM, Vonesh EF, Firanek CA. A retrospective assessment of risk factors for peritonitis among an urban CAPD population. *Perit Dial Int* 1993;13:126–131.
118. Saklayen MG. CAPD peritonitis. Incidence, pathogens, diagnosis, and management. *Med Clin North Am* 1990;74:997–1010.
119. Zelenitsky S, Barns L, Findlay I, et al. Analysis of microbiological trends in peritoneal dialysis-related peritonitis from 1991 to 1998. *Am J Kidney Dis* 2000;36:1009–1013.
120. Linblad AS, Novak JW, Nolph KD, et al. The 1987 USA National CAPD Registry report. *Trans Am Soc Artif Intern Organs* 1988;34:150–156.
121. Rubin J, Ray R, Barnes T, et al. Peritonitis in continuous ambulatory peritoneal dialysis patients. *Am J Kidney Dis* 1983;11:602–607.
122. Steinberg SM, Cutler SJ, Novak JK, et al. Report of the National CAPD registry of the National Institutes of Health: characteristics of participants and selected outcome measures for the period January 1, 1981 through August 31, 1984. National CAPD registry of the National Institute of Arthritis, Diabetes, and Digestive Kidney Diseases. Washington, DC: US Public Health Service, 1985.
123. Howard RL, Millspaugh J, Teitelbaum I. Adult and pediatric peritonitis rates in a home dialysis program: comparison of continuous ambulatory and continuous cycling peritoneal dialysis. *Am J Kidney Dis* 1990;16:469–472.
124. Powell D, San Louis E, Calvin S, et al. Peritonitis in children undergoing continuous ambulatory peritoneal dialysis. *Am J Dis Child* 1985;139:29–32.
125. McClung MR. Peritonitis in children receiving continuous ambulatory peritoneal dialysis. *Pediatr Infect Dis* 1983;2:328–332.
126. Ashline V, Stevens A, Carter MJ. Nosocomial peritonitis related to contaminated dialysate warming water. *Am J Infect Control* 1981;9:50–52.
127. Krotrapelli R, Duffy WB, Lacke C, et al. *Pseudomonas* peritonitis and continuous ambulatory peritoneal dialysis. *Arch Intern Med* 1982;142:1862–1863.
128. Kaczmarski EB, Tooth JA, Anastassiades E, et al. *Pseudomonas* peritonitis with continuous ambulatory peritoneal dialysis: six year study. *Am J Kidney Dis* 1988;14:413–417.
129. Szabo T, Siccion Z, Izatt S, et al. Outcome of *Pseudomonas aeruginosa* exit-site and tunnel infections: a single center's experience. *Adv Perit Dial* 1999;15:209–212.
130. Wang AY, Yu AW, Li PK, et al. Factors predicting outcome of fungal peritonitis in peritoneal dialysis: analysis of a 9-year experience of fungal peritonitis in a single center. *Am J Kidney Dis* 2000;36:1183–1192.
131. von Graevenitz A, Amsterdam D. Microbiological aspects of peritonitis associated with continuous ambulatory peritoneal dialysis. *Clin Microbiol Rev* 1992;5:36–48.
132. Eisenberg ES, Leviton I, Soeiro R. Fungal peritonitis in patients receiving peritoneal dialysis: experience with 11 patients and review of the literature. *Rev Infect Dis* 1986;8:309–321.
133. Huang JW, Hung KY, Wu KD, et al. Clinical features of and risk factors for fungal peritonitis in peritoneal dialysis patients. *J Formos Med Assoc* 2000;99:544–548.
134. Dressler R, Peters AT, Lynn RI. Pseudomonal and candidal peritonitis as a complication of continuous ambulatory peritoneal dialysis in human immunodeficiency virus-infected patients. *Am J Med* 1989;86:787–790.
135. Dunmire RB, Breyer JA. Nontuberculous mycobacterial peritonitis during continuous ambulatory peritoneal dialysis: case report and review of diagnostic and therapeutic strategies. *Am J Kidney Dis* 1991;18:126–130.
136. Hakim A, Hisam N, Reuman PD. Environmental mycobacterial peritonitis complicating peritoneal dialysis: three cases and review. *Clin Infect Dis* 1993;16:426–431.
137. Band JD, Ward JI, Fraser DW, et al. Peritonitis due to a mycobacterium chelonei-like organism associated with intermittent chronic peritoneal dialysis. *J Infect Dis* 1982;145:9–17.
138. Struijk DG, van Ketel RJ, Krediet RT, et al. Viral peritonitis in a continuous ambulatory peritoneal dialysis patient. *Nephron* 1986;44:384.
139. Gibb AO, Aggarwal R, Sainson CO. Successful treatment of *Prototheca* peritonitis complicating continuous ambulatory peritoneal dialysis. *J Infect* 1991;22:183–185.
140. Van Langenhove G, Daelemans R, Zachee P, et al. *Pasteurella multocida* as a rare cause of peritonitis in peritoneal dialysis. *Nephron* 2000;85:283–284.

141. Prowant B, Nolph K, Ryan L, et al. Peritonitis in continuous ambulatory peritoneal dialysis: analysis of an 8-year experience. *Nephron* 1986;43:105–109.
142. Horton MW, Deeter RG, Sherman RA. Treatment of peritonitis in patients undergoing continuous ambulatory peritoneal dialysis. *Clin Pharm* 1990;9:102–118.
143. Tranaeus A, Heimburger O, Granqvist S. Diverticular disease of the colon: a risk factor for peritonitis in continuous peritoneal dialysis. *Nephrol Dial Transplant* 1990;5:141–147.
144. Kim GC, Korbet SM. Polymicrobial peritonitis in continuous ambulatory peritoneal dialysis patients. *Am J Kidney Dis* 2000; 36:1000–1008.
145. Marrie TJ, Noble MA, Costerton JW. Examination of the morphology of bacteria adhering to peritoneal dialysis catheters by scanning and transmission electron microscopy. *J Clin Microbiol* 1983;18:1388–1398.
146. Peterson PK, Matzke G, Keane WF. Current concepts in the management of peritonitis in patients undergoing continuous ambulatory peritoneal dialysis. *Rev Infect Dis* 1987;9:604–612.
147. Gorman SP, Adair CG, Mawhinney WM. Incidence and nature of peritoneal catheter biofilm determined by electron and confocal laser scanning microscopy. *Epidemiol Infect* 1994;112: 551–559.
148. Holmes CJ, Evands R. Biofilm and foreign body infection—the significance of CAPD associated peritonitis. *Perit Dial Bull* 1986;6:168–177.
149. Verbrugh HA, Keane WF, Conroy WE, et al. Bacterial growth and killing in chronic ambulatory peritoneal dialysis fluids. *J Clin Microbiol* 1984;20:199–203.
150. Sheth NK, Bartell CA, Roth DA. *In vitro* study of bacterial growth in continuous ambulatory peritoneal dialysis fluids. *J Clin Microbiol* 1986;23:1096–1098.
151. Allen JR, Troidle LK, Juergensen PH, et al. Incidence of peritonitis in chronic peritoneal dialysis patients infused with intravenous iron dextran. *Perit Dial Int* 2000;20:674–678.
152. Lewis S, Holmes C. Host defense mechanisms in the peritoneal cavity of continuous ambulatory peritoneal dialysis patients. *Perit Dial Int* 1991;11:14–21.
153. Duwe AK, Vas SI, Weatherhead JW. Effects of the composition of peritoneal dialysis fluid on chemiluminescence, phagocytosis, and bactericidal activity *in vitro*. *Infect Immun* 1981;33: 130–135.
154. Gordon DL, Rice JL, Avery VM. Surface phagocytosis and host defence in the peritoneal cavity during continuous ambulatory peritoneal dialysis. *Eur J Clin Microbiol Infect Dis* 1990;9: 191–197.
155. De Vechi AF, Kopple JD, Young GA, et al. Plasma and dialysate immunoglobulin G in continuous ambulatory peritoneal dialysis patients: a multicenter study. *Am J Nephrol* 1990;10:451–456.
156. Passalacqua JA, Wiland AM, Fink JC, et al. Increased incidence of postoperative infections associated with peritoneal dialysis in renal transplant recipients. *Transplantation* 1999;68:535–540.
157. Tranaeus A, Heimburger O, Lindholm B. Peritonitis in continuous ambulatory peritoneal dialysis (CAPD): diagnostic findings, therapeutic outcome and complications. *Perit Dial Int* 1989;9:179–190.
158. Males BM, Walshe JJ, Amsterdam D. Laboratory indices of clinical peritonitis: total leukocyte count, microscopy, and microbiologic culture of peritoneal dialysis effluent. *J Clin Microbiol* 1987;25:2367–2371.
159. Korzets Z, Korzets A, Golan E, et al. CAPD peritonitis—initial presentation as an acute abdomen with a clear peritoneal effluent. *Clin Nephrol* 1992;37:155–157.
160. Flanigan MJ, Freeman RM, Lim VS. Cellular response to peritonitis among peritoneal dialysis patients. *Am J Kidney Dis* 1985; 6:420–424.
161. Digenis GE, Khanna K, Panatlony D. Eosinophilia after implantation of the peritoneal catheter. *Perit Dial Bull* 1982;2: 98–99.
162. Gokal R, Ramos JM, Ward MK, et al. "Eosinophilic" peritonitis in continuous ambulatory peritoneal dialysis (CAPD). *Clin Nephrol* 1981;15:328–330.
163. Hsu SC, Lan RR, Tseng CC, et al. Extrapulmonary tuberculous infection manifested as peritoneal fluid eosinophilia in a continuous ambulatory peritoneal dialysis patient. *Nephrol Dial Transplant* 2000;15:284–285.
164. Ludlam HA, Price TN, Berry AJ, et al. Laboratory diagnosis of peritonitis in patients on continuous ambulatory peritoneal dialysis. *J Clin Microbiol* 1988;26:1757–1762.
165. Bailie GR, Eisele G. Continuous ambulatory peritoneal dialysis: a review of its mechanics, advantages, complications, and areas of controversy. *Ann Pharmacother* 1992;26:1409–1420.
166. Bailie GR, Morton R, Ganguli L, et al. Intravenous or intraperitoneal vancomycin for the treatment of continuous ambulatory peritoneal dialysis associated gram-positive peritonitis? *Nephron* 1987;46:316–318.
167. Merchant MR, Anwar N, Were A, et al. Imipenem versus netilmicin and vancomycin in the treatment of CAPD peritonitis. *Adv Perit Dial* 1992;8:234–237.
168. Cheng IK, Chan CY, Wong WT. A randomised prospective comparison of oral ofloxacin and intraperitoneal vancomycin plus aztreonam in the treatment of bacterial peritonitis complicating continuous ambulatory peritoneal dialysis (CAPD). *Perit Dial Int* 1991;11:27–30.
169. Nikolaidis P. Newer quinolones in the treatment of continuous ambulatory peritoneal dialysis (CAPD) related infections. *Perit Dial Int* 1990;10:127–133.
170. Dratwa M, Glupczynski Y, Lameire N, et al. Treatment of gram-negative peritonitis with aztreonam in patients undergoing continuous ambulatory peritoneal dialysis. *Rev Infect Dis* 1991;13 (Suppl 7):S645–S647.
171. Flanigan MJ, Lim VS. Initial treatment of dialysis associated peritonitis: a controlled trial of vancomycin versus cefazolin. *Perit Dial Int* 1991;11:31–37.
172. Golper TA, Hartstein AI. Analysis of the causative pathogens in uncomplicated CAPD- associated peritonitis: duration of therapy, relapses, and prognosis. *Am J Kidney Dis* 1986;7: 141–145.
173. Juergensen PH, Finkelstein FO, Brennan R, et al. *Pseudomonas* peritonitis associated with continuous ambulatory peritoneal dialysis: a six-year study. *Am J Kidney Dis* 1988;11:413–417.
174. Keane WF, Alexander SR, Bailie GR, et al. Peritoneal dialysis-related peritonitis treatment recommendations: 1996 update. *Perit Dial Int* 1996;16:557–573.
175. Rubin J, Kirchner K, Walsh D, et al. Fungal peritonitis during continuous ambulatory peritoneal dialysis: a report of 17 cases. *Am J Kidney Dis* 1987;10:361–368.
176. Eisenberg ES. Intraperitoneal flucytosine in the management of fungal peritonitis in patients on continuous ambulatory peritoneal dialysis. *Am J Kidney Dis* 1988;11:465–467.
177. Venning MC, Ford M, Gould F K. Successful treatment of fungal peritonitis in CAPD using oral fluconazole. *Nephrol Dial Transplant* 1990;5:555.
178. Talwani R, Horvath JA. Tuberculous peritonitis in patients undergoing continuous ambulatory peritoneal dialysis: case report and review. *Clin Infect Dis* 2000;31:70–75.
179. Rubin J, Nolph K, Arfania D, et al. Follow-up of peritoneal clearances in patients undergoing continuous ambulatory peritoneal dialysis. *Kidney Int* 1979;16:619–623.
180. Smith JL, Flanigan MJ. Peritoneal dialysis catheter sepsis: a medical and surgical dilemma. *Am J Surg* 1987;154:602–607.
181. Valente J, Rappapport W. Continuous ambulatory peritoneal

dialysis associated with peritonitis in older patients. *Am J Surg* 1990;159:579–581.
182. Bayston R, Andrews M, Rigg K, et al. Recurrent infection and catheter loss in patients on continuous ambulatory peritoneal dialysis. *Perit Dial Int* 1999;19:550–555.
183. Peacock SJ, Howe PA, Day NP, et al. Outcome following staphylococcal peritonitis. *Perit Dial Int* 2000;20:215–219.
184. Swartz RD, Messana JM. Simultaneous catheter removal and replacement in peritoneal dialysis infections: update and current recommendations. *Adv Perit Dial* 1999;15:205–208.
185. Sharma BK, Rodriguez H, Gandhi VC, et al. Trial of oral neomycin during peritoneal dialysis. *Am J Med Sci* 1971;262: 175–178.
186. Axelrod J, Meyers BR, Hirschman SZ, et al. Prophylaxis with cephalothin in peritoneal dialysis. *Arch Intern Med* 1973;132: 368–371.
187. Churchill DN, Taylor DW, Vas SI, et al. Peritonitis in continuous ambulatory peritoneal dialysis patients: a randomized clinical trial of co-trimoxazole prophylaxis. *Perit Dial Bull* 1988;8: 125–128.
188. Rubin J, McElroy R. Peritonitis secondary to dialysis tubing contamination among patients undergoing continuous ambulatory peritoneal dialysis. *Am J Kidney Dis* 1989;14:92–95.
189. Usha K, Ponferrada L, Prowant BF, et al. Repair of chronic peritoneal dialysis catheter. *Perit Dial Int* 1998;18:419–423.
190. Luzar MA. Peritonitis prevention in continuous ambulatory peritoneal dialysis. *Nephrologie* 1992;13:171–177.
191. Perez-Fontan M, Rosales M, Rodriguez-Carmona A, et al. Treatment of *Staphylococcus aureus* nasal carriers in CAPD with mupirocin. *Adv Perit Dial* 1992;8:242–245.
192. Swartz R, Messana J, Starmann B, et al. Preventing *Staphylococcus aureus* infection during chronic peritoneal dialysis. *J Am Soc Nephrol* 1991;2:1085–1091.
193. Poole-Warren LA, Hallett MD, Hone PW, et al. Vaccination for prevention of CAPD associated staphylococcal infection: results of a prospective multicentre clinical trial. *Clin Nephrol* 1991;35: 198–206.
194. Gadallah MF, Ramdeen G, Torres C, et al. Preoperative vancomycin prophylaxis for newly placed peritoneal dialysis catheters prevents postoperative peritonitis. *Adv Perit Dial* 2000; 16:199–203.
195. Nakamura Y, Hara Y, Ishida H, et al. A randomized multicenter trial to evaluate the effects of UV-flash system on peritonitis rates in CAPD population. *Adv Perit Dial* 1992;8:313–315.
196. Stegmayr BG, Granbom L, Tranaeus A, et al. Reduced risk for peritonitis in CAPD with the use of a UV connector box. *Perit Dial Int* 1991;11:128–130.
197. Maiorca R, Cantaluppi A, Cancarini GC, et al. Prospective controlled trial of a Y-connector and disinfectant to prevent peritonitis in continuous ambulatory peritoneal dialysis. *Lancet* 1983; 1:642–644.
198. Dryden MS, McCann M, Wing AJ, et al. Controlled trial of a Y-set dialysis delivery system to prevent peritonitis in patients receiving continuous ambulatory peritoneal dialysis. *J Hosp Infect* 1992;20:185–192.
199. Goth AA, Kim U. The reappearance of abdominal tuberculosis. *Surg Gynecol Obstet* 1991;172:432–436.
200. Mehta JB, Dutt A, Harvill L, et al. Epidemiology of extrapulmonary tuberculosis. A comparative analysis with pre-AIDS era. *Chest* 1991;99:1134–1138.
201. Singh MM, Bhargava AN, Jain KP. Tuberculous peritonitis. An evaluation of pathogenetic mechanisms, diagnostic procedures and therapeutic measures. *N Engl J Med* 1969;281:1091–1094.
202. Marshall JB. Tuberculosis of the gastrointestinal tract and peritoneum. *Am J Gastroenterol* 1993;88:989–999.
203. Sochocky S. Tuberculous peritonitis. A review of 100 cases. *Am Rev Respir Dis* 1967;95:398–401.
204. Karney WW, O'Donoghue JM, Ostrow JH, et al. The spectrum of tuberculous peritonitis. *Chest* 1977;72:310–315.
205. Aguado JM, Pons F, Casafont F, et al. Tuberculous peritonitis: a study comparing cirrhotic and noncirrhotic patients. *J Clin Gastroenterol* 1990;12:550–554.
206. Menzies RI, Fitzgerald JM, Mulpeter K. Laparoscopic diagnosis of ascites in Lesotho. *BMJ (Clin Res Ed)* 1985;291:473–475.
207. Dwivedi M, Misra SP, Misra V, et al. Value of adenosine deaminase estimation in the diagnosis of tuberculous ascites. *Am J Gastroenterol* 1990;85:1123–1125.
208. Sumi Y, Ozaki Y, Hasegawa H, et al. Tuberculosis peritonitis: gallium-67 scintigraphic appearance. *Ann Nucl Med* 1999;13: 185–189.
209. Arend P, Valizadeh A, Dryjski J, et al. [Tuberculous peritonitis. Description of 2 cases associated with another infection and literature review]. *Acta Gastroenterol Belg* 1990;53:307–314.
210. Sobel JD, Vazquez J. Candidemia and systemic candidiasis. *Semin Respir Infect* 1990;5:123–137.
211. Bayer AS, Blumenkrantz MJ, Montgomerie JZ, et al. Candida peritonitis. Report of 22 cases and review of the English literature. *Am J Med* 1976;61:832–840.
212. Peoples JB. Candida and perforated peptic ulcers. *Surgery* 1986; 100:758–764.
213. Rutledge R, Mandel SR, Wild RE. *Candida* species. Insignificant contaminant or pathogenic species. *Am Surg* 1986;52:299–302.
214. Solomkin JS, Flohr AB, Quie PG, et al. The role of *Candida* in intraperitoneal infections. *Surgery* 1980;88:524–530.
215. Marsh PK, Tally FP, Kellum J, et al. Candida infections in surgical patients. *Ann Surg* 1983;198:42–47.
216. Castaldo P, Stratta RJ, Wood RP, et al. Clinical spectrum of fungal infections after orthotopic liver transplantation. *Arch Surg* 1991;126:149–156.
217. Nathwani D, Morris AJ, Laing RB, et al. Salmonella Virchow: abscess former amongst the contemporary invasive salmonellae? *Scand J Infect Dis* 1991;23:467–471.
218. Gruenwald I, Abrahamson J, Cohen O. Psoas abscess: case report and review of the literature. *J Urol* 1992;147:624–626.
219. Ibanez Perez de la Blanca MA, Mediavilla Garcia JD, Martinez R, et al. Primary abscess of the psoas muscle caused by *Streptococcus milleri* [Letter]. *Clin Infect Dis* 1992;15:883–884.
220. Brook I, Frazier EH. Microbiology of subphrenic abscesses: a 14-year experience. *Am Surg*, 1999;65:1049–1053.
221. Kolbeinsson ME, Holder WD, Aziz S. Recognition, management, and prevention of *Clostridium septicum* abscess in immunosuppressed patients. *Arch Surg* 1991;126:642–645.
222. Prickett D, Montgomery R, Cheadle WG. External fistulas arising from the digestive tract. *South Med J* 1991;84:736–739.
223. Yu JS, Bennett WF, Bova JG. CT of superior mesenteric vein thrombosis complicating periappendiceal abscess. *J Comput Assist Tomogr* 1993;17:309–312.
224. Haaga JR. Imaging intraabdominal abscesses and nonoperative drainage procedures. *World J Surg* 1990;14:204–209.
225. Sirinek KR. Management of intraabdominal infections. *Pharmacotherapy* 1991;11:99S–104S.
226. MacFayden BV, Wolfe BM, McKernan JB. Laparoscopic management of the acute abdomen, appendix, and small and large bowel. *Surg Clin North Am* 1992;72:1169–1183.
227. Bennett JD, Kozak RI, Taylor BM, et al. Deep pelvic abscesses: transrectal drainage with radiologic guidance. *Radiology* 1992; 185:825–828.
228. Gazelle GS, Haaga JR, Stellato TA, et al. Pelvic abscesses: CT-guided transrectal drainage. *Radiology* 1991;181:49–51.
229. Brolin RE, Flancbaum L, Ercoli FR, et al. Limitations of per-

cutaneous catheter drainage of abdominal abscesses. *Surg Gynecol Obstet* 1991;173:203–210.

230. Samelson SL, Ferguson MK. Empyema following percutaneous catheter drainage of upper abdominal abscess. *Chest* 1992;102: 1612–1614.
231. Levison MA. Percutaneous versus open operative drainage of intra-abdominal abscesses. *Infect Dis Clin North Am* 1992;6: 525–544.
232. Schuster MR, Crummy AB, Wojtowycz MM, et al. Abdominal abscesses associated with enteric fistulas: percutaneous management. *J Vasc Interv Radiol* 1992;3:359–363.
233. Flancbaum L, Nosher JL, Brolin RE. Percutaneous catheter drainage of abdominal abscesses associated with perforated viscus. *Am Surg* 1990;56:52–56.
234. Stabile BE, Puccio E, van Sonnenberg E, et al. Preoperative percutaneous drainage of diverticular abscesses. *Am J Surg* 1990;159:99–104; discussion.
235. Lambiase RE, Deyoe L, Cronan JJ, et al. Percutaneous drainage of 335 consecutive abscesses: results of primary drainage with 1-year follow-up. *Radiology* 1992;184:167–179.
236. Yamakawa T, Suzuki T, Kobayashi S, et al. Fistuloscopy for the management of postoperative intra-abdominal abscesses. *Endoscopy* 1992;24:218–221.
237. Becker JM, Pemberton JH, DiMagno EP, et al. Prognostic factors in pancreatic abscess. *Surgery* 1984;96:455–461.
238. Shi EC, Yeo BW, Ham JM. Pancreatic abscesses. *Br J Surg* 1984;71:689–691.
239. Widdison AL, Karanjia ND. Pancreatic infection complicating acute pancreatitis. *Br J Surg* 1993;80:148–154.
240. Gloor B, Uhl W, Muller CA, et al. The role of surgery in the management of acute pancreatitis. *Can J Gastroenterol* 2000;14 (Suppl D):136D–140D.
241. Hurley JE, Vargish T. Early diagnosis and outcome of pancreatic abscesses in pancreatitis. *Am Surg* 1987;53:29–33.
242. Patel BK, Garvin PJ, Aridge DL, et al. Fluid collections developing after pancreatic transplantation: radiologic evaluation and intervention. *Radiology* 1991;181:215–220.
243. Dupuy D, Costello P, Lewis D, et al. Abdominal CT findings after liver transplantation in 66 patients. *AJR Am J Roentgenol* 1991;156:1167–1170.
244. Knight RJ, Bodian C, Rodriguez-Laiz G, et al. Risk factors for intra-abdominal infection after pancreas transplantation. *Am J Surg* 2000;179:99–102.
245. Backman L, Brattstrom C, Reinholt FP, et al. Development of intrapancreatic abscess—a consequence of CMV pancreatitis? *Transpl Int* 1991;4:116–121.
246. Lumsden A, Bradley EL. Secondary pancreatic infections. *Surg Gynecol Obstet* 1990;170:459–467.
247. Altemeier WA, Alexander JW. Pancreatic abscess. A study of 32 cases. *Arch Surg* 1963;87:80–89.
248. Brook I, Frazier EH. Microbiological analysis of pancreatic abscess. *Clin Infect Dis* 1996;22:384–385.
249. Bassi C, Vesentini S, Nifosi F, et al. Pancreatic abscess and other pus-harboring collections related to pancreatitis: a review of 108 cases. *World J Surg* 1990;14:505–511; discussion 511–512.
250. Fedorak IJ, Ko TC, Djuricin G, et al. Secondary pancreatic infections: are they distinct clinical entities? *Surgery* 1992;112: 824–830; discussion 830–831.
251. Buchler M, Malfertheiner P, Friess H, et al. Human pancreatic tissue concentration of bactericidal antibiotics. *Gastroenterology* 1992;103:1902–1908.
252. Aranha GV, Prinz RA, Greenlee HB. Pancreatic abscess: an unresolved surgical problem. *Am J Surg* 1982;144:534–538.
253. Bradley EL, Fulenwider JT. Open treatment of pancreatic abscess. *Surg Gynecol Obstet* 1984;159:509–513.
254. Ammann R, Munch R, Largiader F, et al. Pancreatic and hepatic abscesses: a late complication in 10 patients with chronic pancreatitis. *Gastroenterology* 1992;103:560–565.
255. Stanten R, Frey CF. Comprehensive management of acute necrotizing pancreatitis and pancreatic abscess. *Arch Surg* 1990;125:1269–1274; discussion 1274.
256. Sofianou DC. Pancreatic abscess caused by *Clostridium difficile. Eur J Clin Microbiol Infect Dis* 1988;7:528–529.
257. Rotman N, Mathieu D, Anglade MC, et al. Failure of percutaneous drainage of pancreatic abscesses complicating severe acute pancreatitis. *Surg Gynecol Obstet* 1992; 714:141–144.
258. Jones CE, Polk HC, Fulton RL. Pancreatic abscess. *Am J Surg* 1975;129:44–47.
259. Vazquez F, Mendez FJ, Perez F, et al. Anaerobic bacteremia in a general hospital: retrospective five-year analysis. *Rev Infect Dis* 1987;9:1038–1143.
260. Lutwick LI. Pancreatic abscess with *Haemophilus influenzae* and *Eikenella corrodens. JAMA* 1976;236:2091–2092.
261. Stein A, Teysseire N, Capobianco C, et al. *Eikenella corrodens*, a rare cause of pancreatic abscess: two case reports and review. *Clin Infect Dis* 1993;17:273–275.
262. Troy MG, Dong QS, Dobrin PB, et al. Do topical antibiotics provide improved prophylaxis against bacterial growth in the presence of polypropylene mesh? *Am J Surg* 1996;171:391–393.
263. Baril NB, Ralls PW, Wren SM, et al. Does an infected peripancreatic fluid collection or abscess mandate operation? *Ann Surg* 2000;231:361–367.
264. Schoenberg MH, Rau B, Beger HG. New approaches in surgical management of severe acute pancreatitis. *Digestion* 1999;60 (Suppl 1):22–26.
265. Printz H, Klotter HJ, Nies C, et al. Intraoperative ultrasonography in surgery for chronic pancreatitis. *Int J Pancreatol* 1992; 12:233–237.
266. Drewelow B, Koch K, Otto C, et al. Penetration of ceftazidime into human pancreas. *Infection* 1993;21:229–234.
267. Pederzoli P, Bassi C, Vesentini S, et al. A randomized multicenter clinical trial of antibiotic prophylaxis of septic complications in acute necrotizing pancreatitis with imipenem. *Surg Gynecol Obstet* 1993;176:480–483.
268. Sainio V, Kemppainen E, Puolakkainen P, et al. Early antibiotic treatment in acute necrotising pancreatitis. *Lancet* 1995;346: 663–667.
269. Johannsen EC, Sifri CD, Madoff LC. Pyogenic liver abscesses. *Infect Dis Clin North Am* 2000;14:547–563.
270. Chou FF, Sheen-Chen SM, Chen YS, et al. Single and multiple pyogenic liver abscesses: clinical course, etiology, and results of treatment. *World J Surg* 1997;21:384–388.
271. Vadillo M, Corbella X, Pac V, et al. Multiple liver abscesses due to *Yersinia enterocolitica* discloses primary hemochromatosis: three cases reports and review. *Clin Infect Dis* 1994;18:938–941.
272. Braun TI, Travis D, Dee RR, et al. Liver abscess due to *Listeria monocytogenes*: case report and review. *Clin Infect Dis* 1993;17: 267–269.
273. Guerra LG, Neira CJ, Boman D, et al. Rapid response of AIDS-related bacillary angiomatosis to azithromycin. *Clin Infect Dis* 1993;17:264–266.
274. Karatassas A, Williams JA. Review of pyogenic liver abscess at the Royal Adelaide Hospital 1980-1987. *Aust N Z J Surg* 1990; 60:893–897.
275. Ramseyer LT, Nguyen DL. *Nocardia brasiliensis* liver abscesses in an AIDS patient: imaging findings. *AJR Am J Roentgenol* 1993;160:898–899.
276. Nemoto H, Murabayashi K, Kawamura Y, et al. Multiple liver abscesses secondary to *Yersinia enterocolitica. Intern Med* 1992; 31:1125–1127.

277. O'Bryan TA, Whitener CJ, Katzman M, et al. Hepatobiliary infections caused by *Haemophilus* species. *Clin Infect Dis* 1992; 15:716–719.
278. Sire JM, Donnio PY, Mesnard R, et al. Septicemia and hepatic abscess caused by *Pediococcus acidilactici. Eur J Clin Microbiol Infect Dis* 1992;11:623–625.
279. Martin J. *Chromobacterium violaceum* septicaemiae: the intensive care management of two cases. *Anaesth Intensive Care* 1992; 20:88–90.
280. Zighelboim J, Williams TW, Bradshaw MW, et al. Successful medical management of a patient with multiple hepatic abscesses due to *Edwardsiella tarda. Clin Infect Dis* 1992;14: 117–120.
281. Vatcharapreechasakul T, Suputtamongkol Y, Dance DA, et al. *Pseudomonas pseudomallei* liver abscesses: a clinical, laboratory, and ultrasonographic study. *Clin Infect Dis* 1992;14:412–417.
282. Collazos J, Egurbide V, de Miguel J, et al. Liver abscess due to *Salmonella enteritidis* 19 months after an episode of gastroenteritis in a man who underwent a cholecystectomy. *Rev Infect Dis* 1991;13:1027–1028.
283. Vargas V, Comas P, Llatzer R, et al. Brucellar hepatic abscess. *J Clin Gastroenterol* 1991;13:477–478.
284. Wilde CC, Kueh YK. Case report: tuberculous hepatic and splenic abscess. *Clin Radiol* 1991;43:215–216.
285. Swallow CJ, Rotstein OD. Management of pyogenic liver abscess in the era of computed tomography. *Can J Surg* 1990; 33:355–362.
286. Sabbaj J, Sutter VL, Finegold SM. Anaerobic pyogenic liver abscess. *Ann Intern Med* 1972;77:627–638.
287. Finegold SM. *Anaerobic bacteria in human disease.* New York: Academic Press, 1977.
288. Sobel JD, Vazquez J. Candidemia and systemic candidiasis. *Semin Respir Infect* 1990;5:123–137.
289. Bodey GP, Luna MA. Disseminated candidiasis in patients with acute leukemia: two diseases? *Clin Infect Dis* 1998;27:238.
290. Seeto RK, Rockey DC. Pyogenic liver abscess. Changes in etiology, management, and outcome. *Medicine (Baltimore)* 1996; 75:99–113.
291. Stain SC, Yellin AE, Donovan AJ, et al. Pyogenic liver abscess. Modern treatment. *Arch Surg* 1991;126:991–996.
292. Dondelinger RF, Kurdziel JC, Gathy C. Percutaneous treatment of pyogenic liver abscess: a critical analysis of results. *Cardiovasc Intervent Radiol* 1990;13:174–182.
293. Chu KM, Fan ST, Lai EC, et al. Pyogenic liver abscess. An audit of experience over the past decade. *Arch Surg* 1996;131: 148–152.
294. Livraghi T, Giorgio A, Marin G, et al. Hepatocellular carcinoma and cirrhosis in 746 patients: long-term results of percutaneous ethanol injection. *Radiology* 1995;197:101–108.
295. Pitt HA. Surgical management of hepatic abscesses. *World J Surg* 1990;14:498–504.
296. Hansen N, Vargish T. Pyogenic hepatic abscess: a case for open drainage. *Am Surg* 1993;59:219–222.
297. Barakate MS, Stephen MS, Waugh RC, et al. Pyogenic liver abscess: a review of 10 years' experience in management. *Aust N Z J Surg* 1999;69:205–209.
298. Huang CJ, Pitt HA, Lipsett PA, et al. Pyogenic hepatic abscess. Changing trends over 42 years. *Ann Surg* 1996;223:600–607.
299. Brook I, Frazier EH. Microbiology of liver and spleen abscesses. *J Med Microbiol* 1998;47:1075–1080.
300. Sarr MG, Zuidema GD. Splenic abscess—presentation, diagnosis, and treatment. *Surgery* 1982;92:480–485.
301. Oehring H, Schulz H, Kramer B, et al. [Bacteroides melaninogenicus as the cause of multiple brain abscesses]. *Med Klin* 1967;62:1347–1349.
302. Linos DA, Nagorney DM, McIlrath DC. Splenic abscess—the importance of early diagnosis. *Mayo Clin Proc* 1983;58: 261–264.
303. Garduno E, Rebollo M, Asencio MA, et al. Splenic abscesses caused by *Actinomyces meyeri* in a patient with autoimmune hepatitis. *Diagn Microbiol Infect Dis* 2000;37:213–214.
304. Berkman WA, Harris SA, Bernardino ME. Nonsurgical drainage of splenic abscess. *AJR Am J Roentgenol* 1983;141: 395–396.
305. Dylewski J, Portnoy J, Mendelson J. Antibiotic treatment of splenic abscess. *Ann Intern Med* 1979;91:493–494.
306. Dunne WM, Kurschenbaum HA, Deshur WR, et al. *Propionibacterium avidum* as the etiologic agent of splenic abscess. *Diagn Microbiol Infect Dis* 1986;5:87–92.
307. Radulescu D. [Surgical infections with anaerobic bacteria (splenic abscess ruptured into the peritoneum]. *Rev Chir Oncol Radiol O R L Oftalmol Stomatol Chir*, 979;28:129–136.
308. Gangahar DM, Delany HM. Intrasplenic abscess: two case reports and review of the literature. *Am Surg* 1981;47:488–491.
309. Studemeister AE, Beilke MA, Kirmani N. Splenic abscess due to *Clostridium difficile* and *Pseudomonas paucimobilis. Am J Gastroenterol* 1987;82:389–390.
310. Kinnaird DW, Melo JC, McKeown JM. Splenic abscess due to *Clostridium septicum* in a patient with multiple myeloma. *South Med J* 1987;80:1318–1320.
311. Torres JR, Rodriguez Casas J, Balda E, et al. Multifocal *Salmonella* splenic abscess in a HIV-infected patient. *Trop Geogr Med* 1992;44:66–68.
312. Sridharan GV, Wilkinson SP, Primrose WR. Pyogenic liver abscess in the elderly. *Age Ageing* 1990;19:199–203.
313. Chou YH, Hsu CC, Tiu CM, et al. Splenic abscess: sonographic diagnosis and percutaneous drainage or aspiration. *Gastrointest Radiol* 1992;17:262–266.
314. Gadacz T, Way LW, Dunphy JE. Changing clinical spectrum of splenic abscess. *Am J Surg* 1974;128:182–187.
315. Chun CH, Raff MJ, Contreras L, et al. Splenic abscess. *Medicine (Baltimore)* 1980;59:50–65.
316. Hisaoka M, Nakamura T, Haratake J, et al. Primary actinomycosis in the liver. *Sangyo Ika Daigaku Zasshi* 1991;13:29–34.
317. Miyamoto MI, Fang FC. Pyogenic liver abscess involving *Actinomyces*: case report and review. *Clin Infect Dis* 1993;16: 303–309.
318. Bhatt BD, Zuckerman MJ, Ho H, et al. Multiple actinomycotic abscesses of the liver. *Am J Gastroenterol* 1990;85:309–310.
319. Granger JK, Houn HY. Diagnosis of hepatic actinomycosis by fine-needle aspiration. *Diagn Cytopathol* 1991;7:95–97.
320. Yeguez JF, Martinez SA, Sands LR, et al. Pelvic actinomycosis presenting as malignant large bowel obstruction: a case report and a review of the literature. *Am.Surg* 2000;66:85–90.
321. Muller-Holzner E, Gschwendtner A, Abfalter E, et al. Actinomycosis and long-term use of intrauterine devices. *Lancet* 1990; 336:939.
322. Raz R, Lev A. Primary abdominal actinomycosis in a diabetic woman—an intractable disease. *J Infect* 1992;25:303–306.
323. Goldwag S, Abbitt PL, Watts B. Case report: percutaneous drainage of periappendiceal actinomycosis. *Clin Radiol* 1991; 44:422–424.
324. Samuel I, Dixon MF, Benson EA. Actinomycosis complicating chronic diverticulitis of the sigmoid colon: a missed association? *Postgrad Med J* 1992;68:57–58.
325. Lockhart GR, Williams GP, Gilbert-Barness E. Pathological case of the month. Thoracic and abdominal actinomycosis. *Am J Dis Child* 1993;147:317–318.
326. Kakkasseril J, Cabanas V, Saba K. Ruptured actinomycotic aneurysm of the splenic artery: a case report of successful resection. *Surgery* 1983;93:595–597.
327. Hill GB, Ayers OM, Kohan AP. Characteristics and sites of

infection of *Eubacterium nodatum, Eubacterium timidum, Eubacterium brachy,* and other asaccharolytic eubacteria. *J Clin Microbiol* 1987;25:1540–1545.
328. Evans TN, Fitzgerald EJ. Abdominal actinomycosis. *Br J Clin Pract* 1990;44:499–500.
329. Manoussakis CA, Triantafillidis JK, Dadioti P, et al. The role of computed tomography in the assessment of patients with abdominal actinomycosis. *Am J Gastroenterol* 1990;85:213–214.
330. Morrow JD, Neuzil KM. Primary hepatic actinomycosis—diagnosis by percutaneous transhepatic needle aspiration. *J Tenn Med Assoc* 1993;8699–101.
331. McDougal WS, Izant RJ, Zollinger RM. Primary peritonitis in infancy and childhood. *Ann Surg* 1975;181:310–313.
332. Flament-Saillour M, deTruchis P, Risbourg M, et al. *Yersinia enterocolitica* peritonitis in an HIV-infected patient. *Clin Infect Dis* 1994;655–656.
333. Garcia M, Sanroman AL, Gisbert JP, et al. *Aeromonas sobria* spontaneous bacterial peritonitis. *Am J Gastroenterol* 1992;87: 1890–1891.
334. Demirkan F, Akalin HE, Simsek H, et al. Spontaneous peritonitis due to *Brucella melitensis* in a patient with cirrhosis [letter]. *Eur J Clin Microbiol Infect Dis* 1993;12:66–67.
335. Gerding DN, Khan MY, Ewing JW, et al. *Pasteurella multocida* peritonitis in hepatic cirrhosis with ascites. *Gastroenterology* 1976;70:413–415.
336. Leggiadro RJ, Lazar LF. Spontaneous bacterial peritonitis due to *Neisseria meningitidis* serogroup Z in an infant with liver failure. *Clin Pediatr (Phila)* 1991;30:350–352.
337. Pascual J, Sureda A, Lopez-San Roman A, et al. Spontaneous peritonitis caused by *Enterococcus faecium. J Clin Microbiol* 1990;28:1484–1486.
338. Toledo C, Salmeron JM, Rimola A, et al. Spontaneous bacterial peritonitis in cirrhosis: predictive factors of infection resolution and survival in patients treated with cefotaxime. *Hepatology* 1993;17:251–257.
339. Christen RD, Moser R, Schlup P, et al. Fulminant group A streptococcal infections. Report of two cases. *Klin Wochenschr* 1990;68:427–430.
340. Runyon BA. Monomicrobial nonneutrocytic bacterascites: a variant of spontaneous bacterial peritonitis. *Hepatology* 1990; 12:710–715.
341. Tsurumi H, Tani K, Tajika K, et al. Spontaneous bacterial peritonitis due to *Clostridium perfringens* in a patient with liver cirrhosis and pure red cell aplasia. *Gastroenterol Jpn* 1992;27: 662–667.
342. Herman R, Goldman IS, Bronzo R, et al. *Clostridium cadaveris*: an unusual cause of spontaneous bacterial peritonitis. *Am J Gastroenterol* 1992;87:140–142.
343. Propst T, Propst A, Schauer G, et al. [Spontaneous bacterial peritonitis in chronic liver disease with ascites]. *Dtsch Med Wochenschr* 1993;118:943–946.
344. Wilcox CM, Forsmark CE, Darragh TM, et al. Cytomegalovirus peritonitis in a patient with the acquired immunodeficiency syndrome. *Dig Dis Sci* 1992;37:1288–1291.
345. Fowler R. Primary peritonitis: changing aspects 1956-1970. *Aust Paediatr J* 1971;7:73–83.
346. Armitage TG, Williamson RC. Primary peritonitis in children and adults. *Postgrad Med J* 1983;59:21–24.
347. Drusano GL, Warren JW, Saah AJ, et al. A prospective randomized controlled trial of cefoxitin versus clindamycin-aminoglycoside in mixed anaerobic-aerobic infections. *Surg Gynecol Obstet* 1982;154:715–720.
348. Nichols RL, Smith JW, Klein DB, et al. Risk of infection after penetrating abdominal trauma. *N Engl J Med* 1984;311: 1065–1070.
349. Tally FP, McGowan K, Kellum JM, et al. A randomized comparison of cefoxitin with or without amikacin and clindamycin plus amikacin in surgical sepsis. *Ann Surg* 1981;193:318–323.
350. Bennion RS, Thompson JE, Baron EJ, et al. Gangrenous and perforated appendicitis with peritonitis: treatment and bacteriology. *Clin Ther* 1990;12(Suppl C):31–44.
351. Najem AZ, Kaminski ZC, Spillert CR, et al. Comparative study of parenteral piperacillin and cefoxitin in the treatment of surgical infections of the abdomen. *Surg Gynecol Obstet* 1983;157: 423–425.
352. Study Group of Intra-Abdominal Infections. A randomized controlled trial of ampicillin plus sulbactam vs gentamicin plus clindamycin in the treatment of intra-abdominal infections. *Rev Infect Dis* 1986;8(Suppl 5):S533–S538.
353. Scandinavian Study Group. Imipenem-cilastin versus gentamicin-clindamycin for treatment of serious bacterial infections. *Lancet* 1983;868–871.
354. Birolini D, Moraes MF, de Souza OS. Comparison of aztreonam plus clindamycin with tobramycin plus clindamycin in the treatment of intra-abdominal infections. *Chemotherapy* 1989;35 (Suppl 1):49–57.
355. Williams RR, Hotchkin D. Aztreonam plus clindamycin versus tobramycin plus clindamycin in the treatment of intraabdominal infections. *Rev Infect Dis* 1991;13(Suppl 7):S629–S633.
356. de Groot HG, Hustinx PA, Lampe AS, et al. Comparison of imipenem/cilastatin with the combination of aztreonam and clindamycin in the treatment of intra-abdominal infections. *J Antimicrob Chemother* 1993;32:491–500.
357. Fink MP, Helsmoortel CM, Arous EJ, et al. Comparison of the safety and efficacy of parenteral ticarcillin/clavulanate and clindamycin/gentamicin in serious intra-abdominal infections. *J Antimicrob Chemother* 1989;24(Suppl B):147–156.
358. Brismar B, Malmborg AS, Tunevall G, et al. Piperacillin-tazobactam versus imipenem-cilastatin for treatment of intra-abdominal infections. *Antimicrob Agents Chemother* 1992;36: 2766–2773.
359. Polk HC, Fink MP, Laverdiere M, et al. Prospective randomized study of piperacillin/tazobactam therapy of surgically treated intra-abdominal infection. The Piperacillin/Tazobactam Intra-Abdominal Infection Study Group. *Am Surg* 1993;59:598–605.
360. Condon RE, Walker AP, Sirinek KR, et al. Meropenem versus tobramycin plus clindamycin for treatment of intraabdominal infections: results of a prospective, randomized, double-blind clinical trial. *Clin Infect Dis* 1995;21:544–550.
361. Kempf P, Bauernfeind A, Muller A, et al. Meropenem monotherapy versus cefotaxime plus metronidazole combination treatment for serious intra-abdominal infections. *Infection* 1996;24:473–479.
362. Solomkin JS, Reinhart HH, Dellinger EP, et al. Results of a randomized trial comparing sequential intravenous/oral treatment with ciprofloxacin plus metronidazole to imipenem/cilastatin for intra-abdominal infections. The Intra-Abdominal Infection Study Group. *Ann Surg* 1996;223:303–315.
363. Brismar B, Malmborg AS, Tunevall G, et al. Meropenem versus imipenem/cilastatin in the treatment of intra-abdominal infections. *J Antimicrob Chemother* 1995;35:139–148.
364. Hecht DW. *Bacteroides fragilis* group. In: Yu VL, Merigan TC Jr, Barriere SL, ed. *Antimicrobial therapy and vaccines.* Baltimore, MD: Williams & Wilkins, 1999: 44–52.

26

EXTRAINTESTINAL MANIFESTATIONS OF ENTERIC INFECTIONS

JAMES K. ROCHE

In addition to the gastrointestinal (GI) manifestations of enteric infections, various extraintestinal syndromes can occur, either simultaneously or at a later time, after detection of the enteric pathogen. These include nonseptic and septic arthritis, hemolytic–uremic syndrome, Guillain–Barré syndrome, and symptoms of disseminated infection. Each is described separately in this chapter, and evidence concerning mechanisms is discussed in instances in which data exist.

NONSEPTIC ARTHRITIS

Nonseptic arthritis is seen in patients as two separate syndromes, in association with enteric infection with several organisms (primarily *Yersinia enterocolitica, Yersinia pseudotuberculosis, Salmonella typhimurium, Salmonella enteritidis, Shigella flexneri, Shigella sonnei,* and *Campylobacter jejuni*). The first syndrome has been named reactive arthritis and postinfectious arthritis because it is usually seen after the onset of diarrhea but is present only in a few cases (e.g., 1.9% of all cases of *Salmonella* colitis) (1). Joint symptoms are usually asymmetric and migratory, with small-joint involvement predominating. Swelling, tenderness, and erythema of a joint may be associated with malaise, intermittent fever, and weight loss (2). After the onset of arthritis, joint fluid is usually serous, with cultures uniformly negative, as are blood cultures (3). Anecdotal evidence indicates that neither antibiotics nor corticosteroids affect the natural history of the arthritis, although one report suggests that indomethacin in high doses is effective (4). A remarkable feature of this arthritis is its long duration, averaging 5 months in 2 reports and more than 10 months in 9 of 13 cases reported in another series (1,3,5). In this syndrome, white blood cells (WBCs) in the joint fluid are present (average of 23,000 WBCs/mm^3), but not in the septic range, and there is eventual recovery in all cases for which long-term follow-up is available. Most patients (>70%) are positive for the human leukocyte antigen B27 (HLA-B27) (6). Carriage of the HLA-B27 antigen also strongly predisposes to spondylitis and acute anterior uveitis (7). Other features of reactive arthritis associated with *Salmonella, Campylobacter, Shigella,* or *Yersinia* are a male-to-female ratio approximately 1 : 1, a higher incidence of postinfectious arthritis after yersiniosis, and a recurrence one or more times in a substantial minority of patients (7).

A second syndrome, occurring as a postinfective event of an intestinal pathogen, is nonseptic arthritis associated with one or more other extraintestinal manifestations. The latter is most commonly an inflammatory eye disorder (iritis or conjunctivitis), occurring in 88% of patients with arthritis and shigellosis and in 2.3% to 26.5% of patients after *Salmonella, Campylobacter,* or *Yersinia* infections. The incidence of ocular lesions is said to vary with the location, stage, and severity of arthritis, as well as with the diligence with which lesions are sought. Uveitis is associated particularly with severe or recurrent arthritis and with sacroiliitis (8,9). Intraocular hemorrhage has been reported in severe cases, while corneal ulceration, keratitis, optic neuritis, and posterior uveitis are less frequent (7). The second most common extraintestinal manifestation associated with arthritis as a postinfectious syndrome is genital lesions, occurring in almost 70% of patients with arthritis after *Shigella* infection, including a 24% incidence of circinate balanitis; 12.5% to 23.8% of arthritis patients infected with *Yersinia, Campylobacter,* or *Salmonella* have genital lesions as well (7). The term Reiter's syndrome is reserved for the classic triad, consisting of arthritis, urethritis, and conjunctivitis. *Shigella, Salmonella, Yersinia,* and *Campylobacter* species have all been implicated as enteric pathogens preceding Reiter's syndrome (10). Of these, *S. flexneri* and *S. typhimurium* are most closely associated with this clinical syndrome. Extraintestinal manifestations of *Yersinia, Salmonella,* and *Shigella* infections have all been linked to individuals

J. K. Roche: Department Of Internal Medicine, University Of Virginia Health System, Charlottesville, Virginia with the HLA-B27 antigen and who tended to have a more chronic and aggressive course than HLA-B27–negative subjects, as well as a more frequent incidence of fever, weight loss, and eye involvement (11). For example, among 50 surviving patients with Reiter's syndrome from a 1944 *Shigella* epidemic, 39 were found to be HLA-B27 positive, compared with a frequency of 10% HLA-B27 positivity in the general population (12). It has been calculated that a HLA-B27–positive person with dysentery has a 19% to 32% chance of developing Reiter's syndrome. The occasional occurrence of Reiter's syndrome in HLA-B27–negative persons indicates either that an environmental insult may be able to override genetic factors or that additional host susceptibility factors exist besides HLA-B27 (11). Studies of long-term follow-up indicate that morbidity may continue after the first episode of Reiter's syndrome. Disease persisted in 4 of 10 patients 13 years after symptom onset in one study (11) in which the recurrence rate for Reiter's syndrome was estimated to be 15% per patient per year. However, a prospective study in an unselected white adult population indicated that Reiter's syndrome complicates only 1% to 3% of infections due to *S. flexneri* (13), a number that would be expected if Reiter's syndrome complicated 19% to 32% of the 10% of the population who are HLA-B27 positive.

That spondylitis occurs in higher frequency in patients with Reiter's syndrome is recognized and may relate to its association with the genetic marker HLA-B27 (14). For patients with short-lived disease of the mild variety, symptoms are reported in about 9%, with sacroiliitis detected by radiograph in 5% to 9% in retrospective studies. In patients with severe, chronic, or more recurrent Reiter's syndrome, an incidence of low back pain of 31% to 92% has been recorded, with abnormalities of the sacroiliac joint found by x-ray film in 73% of 33 patients.

Mechanism

The pathology of acute reactive arthritis may give some clue to etiology. Patchy, nonspecific changes are seen by microscopy of synovium, with infiltration by inflammatory cells, particularly polymorphonuclear (PMN) leukocytes. The presence of microbial products, either as an antigen in an immune complex or as a substance that elicits immune complexes for deposition in tissue, has been established in specific syndromes: Arthritis that follows meningococcal infection and that associated with the prodromal phase of hepatitis B infection does show, in some instances, deposition of immune complexes containing microbial antigen in the joint (15,16). These latter arthritides are different in their features in that they occur during or shortly after widespread antigen dissemination, are generally short-lived, and rarely recur.

Evidence for mechanisms linking an enteric infectious agent with arthritis comes from more recent studies. In one study, more advanced techniques were used to detect microbial antigens in 15 patients with reactive arthritis after *Yersinia* infection in which synovial fluid was culture negative. Synovial fluid cells, mostly PMN leukocytes, from 10 of the 15 patients stained positively on immunofluorescence with both a polyspecific and a monoclonal antibody elicited by *Yersinia* antigens. Only 1% to 10% of cells stained, but results in six of ten patients were confirmed using Western blotting with the same antibodies. None of the synovial cells from ten control patients with rheumatoid arthritis showed *Yersinia* antigens (17). Together with evidence that patients with *Yersinia* enteritis who develop reactive arthritis have a characteristically high and persisting immunoglobulin A (IgA)–anti-*Yersinia* antibody response (18), the doctor suggests that polysaccharides belonging to the *Yersinia* organism may be resistant to digestion and persist within phagocytic cells for long periods, providing a strong antigenic stimulus in patients destined to have arthritis. Studies in the last several years have been focused on identifying the epitopes within bacterial antigen and the type of host response that triggers reactive arthritis. Mertz et al. (19) isolated T-cell clones from the synovial fluid of affected patients and confirmed the importance of 12mer core epitopes of *Yersinia*-derived heat shock protein 60, using single alanine substitutions within the epitopes to gauge T-cell reactivity by cytokine release and cellular proliferation. Overall, ineffective elimination and therefore persistence of bacterial antigen was proposed as driving a local Th2 immune response, but cross-reactivity of their *Yersinia* antigen with human heat shock protein was not found (19). Others using similar human synovial T-cell clones from patients with reactive arthritis have detected strong proliferative responses to recombinant *Yersinia* antigens (20) and found the presence of HLA-B27 does not increase the invasive potential of bacteria but may confer a defect in intracellular elimination of the organism, allowing it to persist (21,22).

SEPTIC ARTHRITIS AT THE TIME OF ENTERIC INFECTION

Purulent synovitis occurring during enteric infection is relatively rare, with an incidence ranging from 0.2% to 2.5% after *Salmonella* infections, for example (23,24). As expected, most cases are monoarticular, generally involving large joints (knee, shoulder, and hip). Symptoms generally occur within 2 weeks but may occur as late as 7 weeks after GI symptoms begin, with peripheral leukocytosis, purulent joint fluid, and positive Gram stain in at least 50% of reported cases. Fewer than 30% of reported cases had a positive stool culture for an enteric pathogen at the time of septic arthritis despite that the arthritis was thought to represent hematogenous spread of organisms from the GI tract (2). Relatively minor damage to the joints is reported in *Salmonella* and other enteric infections and is generally of less than 3 months' duration. Association with the HLA-B27 antigen is not reported. Therapy with ampicillin, chloramphenicol, and trimethoprim-sulfamethoxazole in association with joint drainage has lead to successful outcomes (25,26).

HEMOLYTIC–UREMIC SYNDROME

Although many agents (drugs, chemicals, toxins, microbes) have been associated with individual cases of hemolytic–uremic syndrome, the most common form occurs in infancy and childhood, characteristically a few days after an acute diarrheal illness. Many microbes have been associated with this condition including *Shigella dysenteriae, Salmonella typhi, C. jejuni,* and *Y. pseudotuberculosis* (27). The triad of features characteristic of the syndrome includes acute renal failure, thrombocytopenia, and microangiopathic hemolytic anemia. In a series of 40 pediatric patients reported with idiopathic hemolytic–uremic syndrome, the most common clinical features were lethargy (34 patients), anuria (13 patients), oliguria (11 patients), disorientation or seizures (10 patients), peripheral edema (9 patients), temperature higher than 38°C (7 patients), and purpuric rash (6 patients). The mean WBC count was 20,200, and illness ranged in severity from mild to fulminant, with the latter culminating in death. Thirty-four patients fully recovered (85%), three (7.5%) had residual neurologic deficits, two died, and one had chronic renal impairment (27). Strain O157:H7 has been the most frequently reported species of *Escherichia coli* to be associated with hemolytic–uremic syndrome in the adult; both laparotomy and barium enema studies suggest that the right side of the colon is the site of most severe involvement for infection with this enteric organism; and culture of stool should be performed soon after presentation, because stool cultures have been found to be negative in most cases when taken more than 5 days after the onset of illness (28,29). Antibiotic administration was a risk factor for the development of hemolytic–uremic syndrome in a recent study of 71 children with diarrhea caused by *E. coli* O157:H7 (30), perhaps because several antimicrobial drugs (quinolones, trimethoprim, fumzolidone) increase the bacterial expression of the Shiga toxin gene. Antibiotics should be withheld until stool culture confirms *E. coli* O157:H7 is not present. Recent advances in diagnosis and therapy of these patients include a rapid (30-minute) test for detecting Shiga toxin–producing *E. coli* and Shiga toxin itself in the stool (Meridian Diagnostics, Cincinnati, OH) (31). The use of these silicon dioxide particles that bind with high-avidity Shiga toxin (Synsorb Pk) has been shown to reduce the risk of developing hemolytic–uremic syndromes by 54% if used within 3 days of the onset of diarrhea (32).

Mechanism

Although the pathogenesis of hemolytic–uremic syndrome is not well understood, it has been speculated that the primary event is injury to the endothelial cells of the glomerular capillaries, associated with local intravascular coagulation in the renal glomeruli, as well as thrombotic microangiopathy (33). Two factors have been suggested as the cause of endothelial cell damage. Because of their ability to damage vascular endothelium of renal glomeruli, as in the endotoxic shock syndrome (34), endotoxins have been implicated as an initiating mediator of injury. On the other hand, because immunoglobulin and complement have been detected in renal biopsy specimens of patients with hemolytic–uremic syndrome (35), an immunologic etiology has also been postulated. Direct support for both postulated mechanisms was reported by Koster et al. (36), in which circulating immune complexes by the Raji cell immunoassay and the C1q solid-phase assay were found in 10 of 20 patients with uncomplicated shigellosis and in 4 of 6 with severe hemolytic–uremic syndrome; and the limulus assay for endotoxemia was positive in 9 of 18 patients with hemolysis and in 3 of 61 patients with uncomplicated shigellosis. These authors suggested that endotoxin is the mediator of renal cortical thrombosis and that intestinal pathogens may produce mucosal inflammation resulting in the release of endotoxin and other mediators from the GI tract into the circulation. Measurement of circulating concentrations of cytokines has not revealed a clear and consistent pattern (37,38). Unanswered was why only certain patients develop the hemolytic–uremic syndrome despite the presence of endotoxin and immune complexes in the circulation.

Karmali et al. (27) identified a Shiga-like verocytotoxin (SLT) from *E. coli,* belonging to at least six different O serogroups that are now called enterohemorrhagic *E. coli* because of the hemorrhagic colitis they characteristically cause (see Chapter 42). Karmali et al. (27) detected SLT verotoxin in the stools of 24 (60%) of 40 pediatric patients with idiopathic hemolytic–uremic syndrome, with 75% of patients showing some evidence of renal involvement. The verotoxin was the only factor common to all strains associated with hemolytic–uremic syndrome in their study, and detection of free fecal verotoxin was regarded as the test most indicated for the early diagnosis of that infection (27). Some have gone on to suggest that vascular damage in the colon by verotoxin may allow entry into the circulation of inflammatory mediators that initiate hemolytic–uremic syndrome (39).

OTHER EXTRAINTESTINAL MANIFESTATIONS

Involvement of skin and mucous membranes has been reported with some enteric pathogens. Pharyngitis, sometimes in association with cervical adenopathy, has been reported in adults with *Yersinia* enterocolitis, as has erythema nodosum (40). Individual case reports of *Campylobacter* enteritis with erythema nodosum also exist (41). *Vibrio* infections of many species can cause direct cutaneous infections or severe hemorrhagic bullae as a manifestation of sepsis, the latter characteristically seen with fulminant *Vibrio vulnificus* infection, most often in patients with underlying liver disease who consume raw oysters.

NERVOUS SYSTEM INVOLVEMENT

The Guillain–Barré syndrome, the most common form of acute neuromuscular paralysis in persons in developed countries, succeeds a GI or respiratory tract infection in many cases. As a peripheral neuropathy with acute and chronic weakness of two limbs or more, and variants involving respiratory muscles and facial, bulbar, or ocular nerves, serologic studies have associated this syndrome with infection by *C. jejuni* (32%), cytomegalovirus (13%), or Epstein–Barr virus (10%) (42). Positive serologic responses were greatest in the months of September through November, male patients predominated by a ratio of 3 : 1, and the association was more marked with increasing age (43).

Host factors, particularly the immune response to *C. jejuni,* are speculated to predispose patients to the development of Guillain–Barré syndrome after intestinal infection. To explain how individuals with Guillain-Barré syndrome can be pathologically and clinically heterogeneous, studies have initially demonstrated that the immune system can selectively attack both functional and regional components of the peripheral nervous system. The autoantibody to GQ_{1b} has been associated with the occurrence of ophthalmoplegia (44). The more classic cases of Guillain–Barré syndrome without bulbar involvement are associated with the autoantibodies against gangliosides GM_1 and GD_{1b}. Further, evidence suggests that qualitative features of the antiglycosides humoral immune response (class of immunoglobulin and titer) may also determine the clinical features at onset (45,46).

Regarding the mechanism of peripheral nerve injury, recent studies suggest molecular mimicry between nerve tissue and an infectious agent. Thus, the oligosaccharide (Gal β1-3 Gal/NAc β1-4 [NeuAc α2-3] Gal β) on the lipopolysaccharide of the PEN 19 strain of *C. jejuni* has been shown by biochemical and physicochemical means to be identical to the terminal tetrasaccharide of the GM_1 ganglioside, a cell surface molecule on nervous tissue (47). Others have shown *in vitro* that antibody to the oligosaccharide GM_1 and gangliosides interferes with the function of the Na^+ channels at the node of Ranvier: firing, endplate potentials and muscle contractions are suppressed (48).

EXTRAINTESTINAL MANIFESTATIONS ASSOCIATED WITH DISSEMINATED INFECTION

Of the organisms highlighted in this review, the mucosa-invasive pathogens *Salmonella* and rarely *Shigella* are best recognized for their ability to be simultaneously present in blood, with potential for infecting distant sites. *Yersinia, Vibrio,* or *Campylobacter* can cause a similar "sepsis" syndrome. In *Yersinia* septicemia, patients generally have one of two presentations. In acute septicemia, symptoms of pyrexia, headache, malaise, abdominal pain, and diarrhea predominate, similar to that found with systemic salmonellosis. Prognosis largely depends on early diagnosis and the natural history of the underlying diseases, discussed below. The second form, described as subacute, is found in patients who are chronically ill, in which a bacteremic episode may even go unnoticed. Localizing symptoms may be due to metastatic foci of infection, such as liver or splenic abscess. Prognosis in this case is much more guarded, with a reported mortality rate of up to 50% (49,50). The importance of the liver in resistance of the host to *Y. enterocolitica* infection, particularly septicemia, has been suggested by the frequency of cirrhosis and conditions of iron overload in the reported series (50). Two mechanisms have been proposed for this. Data in mice indicate that injection of ferric ammonium citrate increases the mortality of animals infected with *Y. enterocolitica,* and iron excess may be present in those with hemolytic anemia, hemochromatosis, and other chronic liver diseases. A second mechanism, suggested by Conn (51), proposes that cirrhotic livers may be less effective in reducing the number of bacteria in the portal bloodstream, since some blood flow bypasses the reticuloendothelial system of the liver through shunts, allowing the microorganism to spread to peripheral tissues. Other conditions apparently predisposing to bacteremia with *Yersinia* include transfusion-dependent blood dyscrasias, immunosuppressive therapy, diabetes mellitus, alcoholism, and malnutrition (52). A wide array of abnormalities in extraintestinal sites have been recorded after bacteremic spread of this organism. In addition to hepatic and splenic abscesses (which were noted above), endocarditis, mycotic aneurysm, meningitis, peritonitis, osteomyelitis, septic arthritis, pulmonary infiltrates, lung abscess, renal abscess, and cutaneous pustules have all been reported in association with *Y. enterocolitica* bacteremia (52).

With regard to *Campylobacter, Campylobacter fetus* subspecies *fetus* is regarded as the most common etiologic agent for septicemia, and pure septicemia without metastatic infectious foci is the most common presentation. Complications at a distance reported with septicemia due to this organism include carditis, phlebitis, meningitis, other pyogenic processes, and abortion (53,54). Because several series have shown septicemia with *Campylobacter* primarily limited to debilitated patients, it has been considered an opportunist by investigators who have studied it. Most commonly associated conditions are cirrhosis, carcinoma, Hodgkin disease, agammaglobulinemia, chronic leukemia, and lymphoma (53,54). The incidence of fetal loss is high among infected mothers, with a fetal/neonatal mortality rate of 50%. Bacteremia is speculated to originate from the bowel, with seeding of organisms accounting for fetoplacental involvement. Mechanisms suggested to account for this latter phenomenon include the finding that the organism localizes in the placenta *in vivo* after parenteral inoculation and grows preferentially in placental tissue extracts *in vitro* (54). Further, the known depression of cell-mediated immunity during pregnancy may also account for the occurrence of some cases (55). Another subspecies, *C. jejuni,* although commonly causing enteritis, relatively infrequently seeds the bloodstream, occurring predominantly in immunocompromised patients.

CONCLUSION

The extraintestinal manifestations of enteric infections reflect a wide range of infections and immunologic consequences. Although still poorly understood, the immunologic mechanisms proposed raise intriguing hypotheses regarding microbial and host antigenicity, as well as their roles in acute and chronic extraintestinal inflammatory processes. Knowledge of the precise pathogenesis of these bacterial antigen-driven disorders may shed light on important idiopathic intestinal diseases with manifestations outside the intestinal tract such as ulcerative colitis and Crohn's disease.

REFERENCES

1. Vartianinen J, Hurri L. Arthritis due to *Salmonella typhimurium. Acta Med Scand* 1964;175:771–776.
2. Carroll WL, Balistreri WF, Brilli R, et al. Spectrum of *Salmonella*-associated arthritis. *Pediatrics* 1981;68:717–720.
3. Berglof FE. Arthritis and intestinal infection. *Acta Rheumatol Scand* 1963;9:141–149.
4. Stein HB, Abdullah A, Robinson HS, et al. *Salmonella* reactive arthritis in British Columbia. *Arthritis Rheum* 1980;23:206–210.
5. Warren CP. Arthritis associated with *Salmonella* infections. *Ann Rheum Dis* 1970;29:483–487.
6. Hakensson U, Eitrem R, Low B, et al. HLA antigen B27 in cases with joint infection in an outbreak of salmonellosis. *Scand J Infect Dis* 1976;8:245–248.
7. Keat A. Reiter's syndrome and reactive arthritis in perspective. *N Engl J Med* 1983;309:1606–1615.
8. Ford DK. Arthritis and venereal urethritis. *Br J Vener Dis* 1953; 29:123–133.
9. Oates JK, Young AC. Sacroiliitis and Reiter's disease. *Br Med J* 1959;1:1013–1015.
10. Leung F, Littlejohn GO, Bombardier C. Reiter's syndrome after *Campylobacter jejuni* enteritis. *Arthritis Rheum* 1980;23:948–950.
11. Calin A, Fries JF. An experimental epidemic of Reiter's syndrome revisited. *Ann Intern Med* 1976;84:564–566.
12. Sairanen E, Tilikainen A. HLA 27 in Reiter's disease following shigellosis. *Scand J Rheumatol* 1975;4[Suppl 8]:30–41.
13. Zsonka GW. Recurrent attacks in Reiter's disease. *Arthritis Rheum* 1960;3:164–169.
14. Schlosstein L, Terasaki PI, Bluestone R, et al. High association of an HLA antigen, B27, with ankylosing spondylitis. *N Engl J Med* 1973;288:704–706.
15. Herrick WW, Parkhurst GM. Meningococcal arthritis. *Am J Med Sci* 1919;158:473–481.
16. Schumacher HR, Gall EP. Arthritis in acute hepatitis and chronic active hepatitis: pathology of the synovial membrane with evidence for the presence of Australia antigen in synovial membranes. *Am J Med Sci* 1974;57:655–664.
17. Granfors K, Jalkanen S, von Essen R, et al. *Yersinia* antigens in synovial-fluid cells from patients with reactive arthritis. *N Engl J Med* 1989;320:216–221.
18. Granfors K, Toivanen A. IgA–anti-*Yersinia* antibodies in *Yersinia* triggered reactive arthritis. *Ann Rheum Dis* 1986;45:561–565.
19. Mertz AKH, Wu P, Sturniolo T, et al. Multispecific CD4+ T-cell response to a single 12-mer epitope of the immune-dominant heat shock protein 60 of *Yersinia enterocolitica* in *Yersinia*-triggered reactive arthritis: overlap with the B27-restricted CD8 epitope, functional properties, and epitope presentation by multiple DR alleles. *J Immunol* 2000;164:1529–1537.
20. Mertz AK, Ugrinovic S, Lauster R, et al. Characterization of the synovial T cell response to various recombinant *Yersinia* antigens in *Yersinia enterocolitica*-triggered reactive arthritis. *Arthritis Rheum* 1998;41:315–326.
21. Laito P, Virtala M, Salmi M, et al. HLA-B27 modulates intra-cellular survival of *Salmonella enteritidis* on human monocytic cells. *Eur J Immunol* 1997;27:1331–1338.
22. Ortiz-Alvarez O, Yu DT, Petty RE, et al. HLA B27 does not affect invasion of arthritogenic bacteria into human cells. *J Rheumatol* 1998;25:1765–1771.
23. Saphra I, Winter JW. Clinical manifestations in salmonellosis in man. *N Engl J Med* 1957;256:1128–1134.
24. Saphra I, Wussermann M. *Salmonella choleraesuis.* A clinical and epidemiological evaluation of 329 infections identified between 1940 and 1954 in the New York *Salmonella* Center. *Am J Med Sci* 1954;228:525–533.
25. Ortiz-Neu C, Marr JS, Cherubin CE, et al. Bone and joint infections due to *Salmonella. J Infect Dis* 1978;138:820–828.
26. Goldenberg DL, Cohen AS. Acute infectious arthritis. A review of patients with nongonococcal joint infections (with emphasis on therapy and prognosis). *Am J Med* 1976;60:369–377.
27. Karmali MA, Petric M, Lim C, et al. The association between idiopathic hemolytic uremic syndrome and infection by verotoxin-producing *Escherichia coli. J Infect Dis* 1985;151:775–782.
28. Spika JS, Parsons JE, Nordenberg D, et al. Hemolytic uremic syndrome and diarrhea associated with *Escherichia coli* O157:H7 in a day care center. *J Pediatr* 1986;109:287–291.
29. Riley LW, Renis RS, Helgerson SD, et al. Hemorrhagic colitis associated with a rare *Escherichia coli* serotype. *N Engl J Med* 1983;308:681–685. [Update from Sporadic hemorrhagic colitis. *MMWR Morb Mortal Wkly Rep* 1984;33:28–29.]
30. Wong CS, Jelacic S, Habeeb RL, et al. The risk of the hemolytic–uremic syndrome after antibiotic treatment of *Escherichia coli* O157:H7 infections. *N Engl J Med* 2000;342: 1930–1936.
31. MacKenzie AMR, Lebel P, Orrbine E, et al. Sensitivities and specificity of premier *E. coli* O157 and premier EHEC enzyme immunoassays for diagnosis of infection with verotoxin-producing *E. coli. J Clin Microbiol* 1998;36:1608–1611.
32. Rowe DC, Milner R, Orrbine E, et al. A phase II randomized controlled trial of Synsorb Pk for the prevention of hemolytic uremic syndrome in children with verotoxin-producing *E. coli* gastroenteritis. *Pediatr Res* 1997;41:283A.
33. Delans RJ, Biuso JD, Saba SR, et al. Hemolytic uremic syndrome after *Campylobacter*-induced diarrhea in an adult. *Arch Intern Med* 1984;144:1074–1076.
34. Thomas L, Good RA. Studies on the generalized Shwartzman reactions: general observation concerning the phenomena. *J Exp Med* 1952;96:605–624.

35. McCoy RC, Abramowsky CR, Krueger R. The hemolytic uremic syndrome with positive immunofluorescence studies. *J Pediatr* 1974;85:170–174.
36. Koster F, Levin J, Walker L, et al. Hemolytic uremic syndrome after shigellosis. *N Engl J Med* 1978;298:927–933.
37. Proulx F, Litalien C, Turgea JP, et al. Circulating levels of TGFβ1 and lymphokines among children with hemolytic uremic syndrome. *Am J Kidney Dis* 2000;30:29–34.
38. Proulx F, Thurgeon JP, Litalien C, et al. Inflammatory mediators in *Escherichia coli* O157:H7 hemorrhagic colitis and hemolytic–uremic syndrome. *Pediatr Inf Dis J* 1998;17:899–909.
39. Besser RE, Griffin PM, Slutsker L. *Escherichia coli* O157:H7 gastroenteritis and the hemolytic uremic syndrome. *Annu Rev Med* 1999;50:355–367.
40. Cover TL, Aber RC. *Yersinia* enterocolitica—medical progress. *N Engl J Med* 1989;321:16–23.
41. Lambert M, Marion E, Coche E, et al. *Campylobacter* enteritis and erythema nodosum. *Lancet* 1982;1:1409.
42. Jacobs BC, Rothbarth PH, van der Meché FGA, et al. The spectrum of antecedent infection in Guillain–Barré syndrome: a case control study. *Neurology* 1998;51:1110–1115.
43. Mishu B, Ilyas AA, Koski CL, et al. Serologic evidence of previous *Campylobacter jejuni* infection in patients with the Guillain–Barré syndrome. *Ann Intern Med* 1993;118:947–953.
44. Yuki N, Taki T, Takahashi M, et al. Molecular mimicry between G_{Q1b} ganglioside and lipopolysaccharides of *C. jejuni* isolated from patients with Fisher's syndrome. *Ann Neurol* 1994;36: 791–793.
45. Kaida K, Kusunoki S, Kamakura K, et al. Guillain–Barré syndrome with antibody to a ganglioside, *N*-acetylgalactosaminyl GD_{1a}. *Brain* 2000;123:116–124.
46. Schwerer B, Neisser A, Bernheimer H. Distinct immunoglobulin class and immunoglobulin G subclass patterns against ganglioside GQ_{16} in Miller Fisher syndrome following different types of infection. *Inf Immun* 1999;67:2414–2420.
47. Yuki N, Taki T, Inagaki F, et al. A bacterium lipopolysaccharide that elicits Guillain–Barré syndrome has a GM_1 ganglioside–like structure. *J Exp Med* 1993;178:1771–1775.
48. Takigawa T, Yasuda H, Kikkawa R, et al. Antibodies against G_{M1} ganglioside affect K^+ and Na^+ currents in isolated rat myelinated nerve fibers. *Ann Neurol* 1995;37:436–442.
49. Rabson AR, Hallett AF, Koornhof HJ. Generalized *Yersinia enterocolitica* infection. *J Infect Dis* 1975;131:447–451.
50. Bouza E, Dominguez A, Meseguer M, et al. *Yersinia enterocolitica* septicemia. *Am J Clin Pathol* 1980;74:404–409.
51. Conn HO. Spontaneous peritonitis and bacteremia in Laennec's cirrhosis caused by enteric organisms. *Ann Intern Med* 1964;60: 568–580.
52. Cover TL, Aber RC. *Yersinia enterocolitica. N Engl J Med* 1989; 321:16–24.
53. Walder M, Lindberg A, Schalen C, et al. Five cases of *Campylobacter jejunicoli* bacteremia. *Scand J Infect Dis* 1982;14:201–205.
54. Lowrie DB, Pearce JH. The placental localization of *Vibrio fetus. J Gen Microbiol* 1969;59:607–614.
55. Weinberg ED. Pregnancy-associated depression of cell-mediated immunity. *Rev Infect Dis* 1984;6:814–831.

27

SEXUALLY TRANSMITTED INFECTIONS OF THE ANUS AND RECTUM

JANICE R. VERLEY
THOMAS C. QUINN

Infections of the anus and rectum are frequently sexually transmitted and occur primarily in homosexual men and heterosexual women who engage in anorectal intercourse. The most common anorectal infections observed in heterosexual women are caused by the classic venereal pathogens *Treponema pallidum, Neisseria gonorrhoeae,* and *Chlamydia trachomatis.* These pathogens also cause infections in homosexual men, who are additionally at high risk for infection with other bacterial, viral, and protozoan organisms, including herpes simplex virus (HSV), human papillomavirus (HPV), and *Entamoeba histolytica.* These infections are endemic in the male homosexual population and may cause perianal lesions, proctitis, or proctocolitis.

An epidemic of anorectal infections was first recognized in homosexual men in the 1970s (1,2). In the study by Sohn and Robilotti (2), infections with *N. gonorrhoeae, T. pallidum, E. histolytica,* and *C. trachomatis* accounted for fewer than 20% of the anorectal infections in their patients. The majority had condyloma acuminatum infections and "nonspecific proctitis" that included hemorrhoids, fissures, and trauma caused by foreign bodies. However, in a later study, Quinn et al. (3) identified specific pathogens in more than 80% of symptomatic cases of proctitis and in 39% of asymptomatic homosexual men. Multiple pathogens were found in 22% of symptomatic and 4% of asymptomatic cases. The high prevalence of anorectal infection in this population was related to high-risk behaviors, such as anogenital and oral–anal intercourse (anilingus) and oral–genital sex (fellatio) following anal intercourse, that allow pathogens to be ingested or inoculated onto the anorectal mucosa.

During the early 1980s, the number of cases of many sexually transmitted diseases (STDs) declined in homosexual men, who were motivated to adopt safer sex practices because of the AIDS epidemic. The decrease in new HIV infections that followed the adoption of safer sex practices in the 1980s, the decrease in morbidity and mortality associated with highly active antiretroviral therapy (HAART), and the increased availability of HIV post-exposure prophylaxis have led to a more relaxed attitude about contracting HIV and a subsequent increase in unsafe sexual behavior. Multiple studies performed in the late 1990s indicated an increase in unprotected anal intercourse with multiple sexual partners in homosexual men. Between 23% and 58% of homosexual men now report unprotected sex (4–9). Forty-five percent of them do not know the HIV serostatus of their partner (4). This situation has been associated with increased rates of gonorrhea and outbreaks of syphilis in homosexual men. In the HIV-infected population, evidence suggests that persons on HAART with undetectable HIV viral loads are at increased risk for acquiring incident STDs, in part because of an increased sense of well-being, a renewed interest in sex, and decreased concerns about HIV infectivity (10,11). It is well documented that STDs increase the HIV viral load in local secretions, and it is therefore likely that the current trend toward unprotected anal intercourse will lead to an increase in the transmission of STDs, including HIV infection.

Among heterosexual women, anorectal intercourse and cervical infections are associated with anorectal infections. Early studies may have underestimated the number of women practicing anorectal sex (12). In a recent survey of 1,268 U.S. women, 32% reported engaging in anal sex in the previous 6 months. Anal sex was reported by a higher proportion of women whose partners did not always use condoms (13). Similarly, 44% of women attending an STD clinic in Denmark reported practicing anorectal sex (14). In women who do not practice anal intercourse, anorectal infections develop when cervicovaginal fluid from an infected cervix contaminates the anorectal area. Control of these infections has been complicated by the practice of having anonymous sex with large numbers of infected heterosexual or homosexual partners, an activity that enhances the spread

J. R. Verley and **T. C. Quinn:** Department of Medicine, Johns Hopkins University, Baltimore, Maryland

TABLE 27.1. COMPARISON OF ANATOMIC CHARACTERISTICS OF THE ANUS AND RECTUM

Characteristic	Anus	Rectum
Epithelium	Stratified squamous/cuboidal	Columnar
Nerve supply	Somatic sensory nerves	Autonomic nerves
Lymphatic drainage	Inguinal nodes	Pelvic nodes
Venous drainage	Inferior hemorrhoidal plexus/inferior vena cava	Superior hemorrhoidal plexus/portal vein
Common symptoms	Pruritus, discharge, pain	Hematochezia, discharge, tenesmus

of anorectal infections and impedes the tracing of contacts. Additionally, failure on the part of physicians to recognize these infections and delays in medical evaluation because of their sometimes asymptomatic nature perpetuate the human reservoir of infection. This chapter reviews the common infections of the anorectal region of the gastrointestinal tract. Because the more traditional gastrointestinal pathogens are discussed in detail in other chapters, this chapter focuses primarily on sexually transmitted pathogens.

ANATOMY AND CLINICAL SYMPTOMS

The epithelium of the skin and mucosa is an important barrier to infection of the perianal area, anus, and rectum (Fig. 27.1). Consequently, traumatic breaks in the epithelium caused by anal intercourse or the insertion of foreign bodies promote local infection. The anal canal extends 2 cm internally from the anal verge to the anorectal (pectinate or dentate) line separating the anal canal from the rectum. The cell lining, nervous supply, and lymphatic and venous drainage are different in the anus and rectum (Table 27.1). Stretching the rectum produces pain, but the area is otherwise insensitive, and infections of the rectum that spare the anus are relatively painless. Proctitis, which is an inflammation of the anorectal mucosa, can lead to spasms of the underlying anal sphincter muscles, which result in constipation and tenesmus (unproductive straining at stool), pain, hematochezia, and mucopurulent rectal discharge (15). Visual inspection of the rectal mucosa in a patient

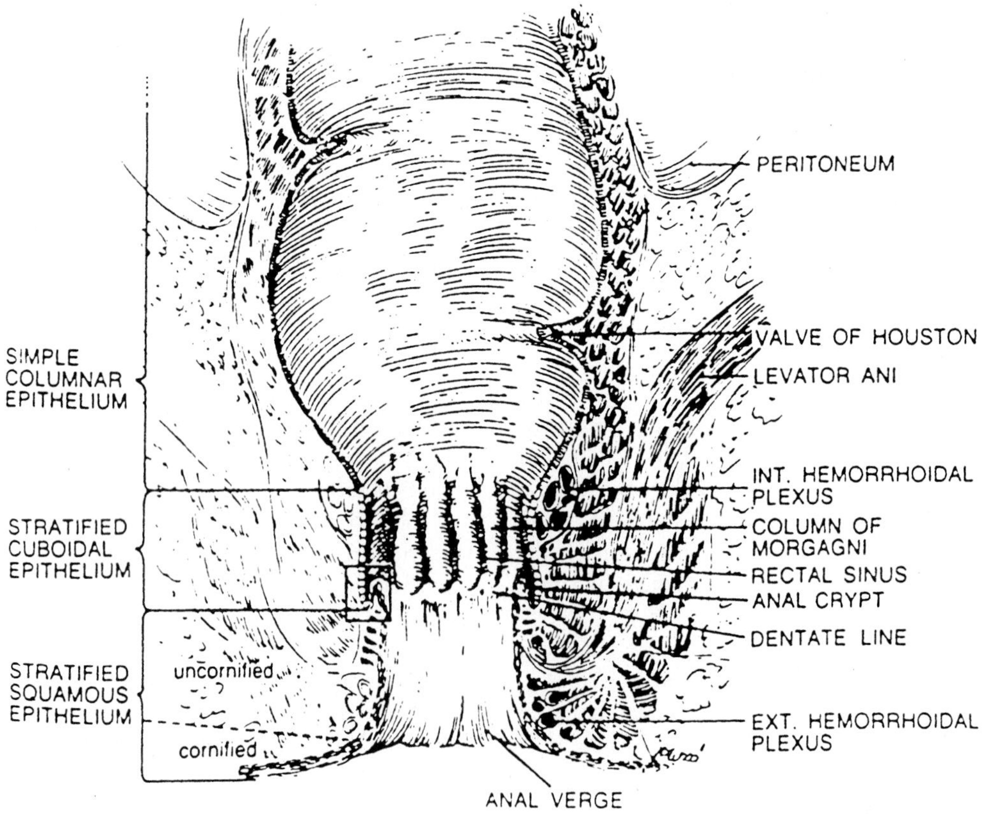

FIGURE 27.1. The normal anatomy of the rectum and anus. (From Hook EW III, Mara CM. Acquired syphilis in adults. *N Engl J Med* 1992;326:1060–1069, with permission.)

TABLE 27.2. CAUSES OF PROCTOCOLITIS

Infectious	Non-infectious
Chlamydia trachomatis	Ulcerative colitis
Treponema pallidum	Crohn disease
Neisseria gonorrhoeae	Hemorrhoids
Haemophilus ducreyi	Polyps
Mycobacterium tuberculosis	Carcinoma
Campylobacter jejuni	Lymphoma
Salmonella species	Hidradenitis suppurativa
Shigella species	Kaposi sarcoma
Herpes simplex virus	
Human papilloma virus	
Cytomegalovirus	
Entamoeba histolytica	
Enterobius vermicularis	
Candida albicans	

with symptoms of proctitis may reveal a normal mucosa or inflammation and ulcerations.

The spectrum of symptoms associated with anorectal infections is wide. Some infections are asymptomatic, whereas others cause severe proctocolitis with rectal pain, constipation, tenesmus, hematochezia, mucoid rectal discharge, fever, and inguinal lymphadenopathy. Whether or not symptoms develop and how severe they are depend on the infecting organism, virulence of the strain, size of the inoculum, and immunity of the host. HSV infections are more often symptomatic than asymptomatic, whereas *N. gonorrhoeae, T. pallidum,* and *E. histolytica* infections are more often asymptomatic. Non-lymphogranuloma venereum (LGV) strains of *C. trachomatis* often cause asymptomatic infection, whereas LGV strains may cause severe granulomatous proctitis simulating Crohn's disease (Table 27.2).

HERPES SIMPLEX VIRUS

Microbiology

Anorectal herpetic infection is caused by HSV-2 in 90% of cases and HSV-1 in 10% of cases. HSV is a member of the herpesvirus group, which includes varicella-zoster virus, cytomegalovirus, Epstein–Barr virus, and human herpesvirus 6. These enveloped viruses are approximately 120 to 300 nm in size and have double-stranded DNA comprising 125,000 to 250,000 base pairs contained within an icosahedral capsid (16–18). Base sequence homology between HSV-1 and HSV-2 is approximately 50%, and typing of isolates is generally performed with monoclonal antibodies (17). HSV attaches to the host cell surface via at least three different classes of cell surface receptors, one of which has been identified as a heparan sulfate-like receptor (19). Eight viral glycoproteins are known (B through I); three of the seven glycoproteins in the virus envelope (gpB, gpD, and gpH) are essential for infectivity (20). The virus can infect a wide range of cells, but infection in the immunocompetent human host is usually limited to mucocutaneous sites.

After entry into the cell, viral DNA is transcribed by host cell DNA polymerase under viral regulatory control. The HSV genome encodes at least 84 different polypeptides, each with several functions (19). Viral proteins are synthesized in the cytoplasm that are then transported to the nucleus, where the nucleocapsid is assembled. The viral envelope is acquired by budding through areas of the nuclear membrane that contain virus-specific glycoproteins. HSV infection ultimately kills cells by inhibiting cellular DNA replication, RNA processing, and protein synthesis. The neuron appears to be unique because production of the virion is not associated with cell lysis. Following replication in the dermis and epidermis, viral particles are transported to sensory neuronal ganglia, where latency is established. Animal studies indicate that this occurs within 48 hours of infection (21). During latency, the viral genome is maintained in an episomal state, and no viral genes that are necessary for lytic infection are expressed (22). The nondividing neuronal cells provide an environment in which the virus is sequestered from the host immune system. Triggers for reactivation include fever, ultraviolet light, physical or emotional stress, and tissue damage (19). Reactivation of viral replication is associated with recurrent disease, and the neuronal axon serves as a conduit for viral dissemination.

Pathogenesis and Immunity

Humoral immunity is important in controlling HSV infections (23,24). The major viral proteins that elicit antibody responses are surface glycoproteins (gpC, gpD, gpAB), major capsid protein (VP5), and a group of low-molecular-weight proteins (23). Antibody-dependent cellular cytotoxicity is detectable within the first week of HSV infection. This mechanism of protection acts by destroying infected cells before the release of progeny virus (24). In contrast, neutralizing antibody to HSV, which develops after 2 weeks of infection, appears to inhibit viral binding or penetration of target cells (23,25). The best evidence of protection by HSV-specific serum antibodies has been found in studies of neonatal exposure to HSV-2. Placental transfer of maternal antibodies appears to protect newborns from HSV infection because infants born to seronegative mothers with primary genital HSV-2 infection at the time of delivery are at a 10-fold higher risk for infection than are infants of seropositive mothers with recurrent HSV-2 infection (26,27). Both neutralizing and antibody-dependent cellular cytotoxicity (ADCC) antibodies are higher in the mothers of exposed infants without infection than in the mothers of infected infants. Local antibodies are also protective, as reflected in the inverse correlation between local HSV-specific immunoglobulin A (IgA) levels and isolation of HSV-2 from cervical samples (28). In addition, local antibody to

HSV-1 appears to play a role in modulating HSV-2 infection in patients seropositive for HSV-1 (23). Programmed cell death is another host defense against viral infection. At least three viral proteins appear to play a role in blocking this host defense mechanism (19).

More severe HSV infections occur in persons who are immunosuppressed because of organ transplantation, cancer chemotherapy, or HIV infection and in neonates (29–32). In immunosuppressed persons, impaired cytotoxic lymphocyte activity and reduced levels of interferon-γ (IFN-γ) may contribute to the severity and recurrence of HSV infections (23,33–35).

Epidemiology

In the United States, 44 million people are infected with HSV. Approximately 500,000 persons acquire primary genital herpes each year, and an additional 10 million present with recurrent genital infection (22,36). HSV infection accounts for 70% to 80% of cases of genital ulcer disease in Europe and North America (37). In the United States, HSV-2 seroprevalence has increased 34%, from 16.4% in 1980 to 22% in 1988 (38,39). Seroprevalence increases from about 20% to 30% at ages 15 through 29 to 35% to 60% by the age of 60 years (19). In addition to age, other risk factors for the acquisition of HSV include African-American race, female sex, urban residence, and lower socioeconomic status (40–42). Serologic studies show that 30% to 50% of persons from higher socioeconomic groups and 80% to 100% from lower socioeconomic groups have been exposed to HSV (40–42). In addition to socioeconomic status, sexual activity is a risk factor for acquisition of HSV. The seroprevalence of HSV-2 is 70% in prostitutes versus 3% in nuns and increases between the ages of 14 and 29, when sexual activity is increased (42). Symptoms occur in only a small percentage of cases, as only one-third of people with HSV-2 antibodies have a history of infection (40).

Humans are the only known reservoir of HSV. Transmission occurs by direct contact with a symptomatic or asymptomatic person actively shedding virus. Male-to-female transmission is more effective, and the annual rate of viral acquisition is higher in susceptible female partners without antibody to HSV-1 or HSV-2 (31.8%) than in female partners with antibody to HSV-1 (9.1%). In 70% of cases, transmission appears to result from sexual contact during periods of asymptomatic viral shedding (43). HIV infection, especially when associated with low CD4+ T-cell counts, is a risk factor for asymptomatic shedding of HSV-2.

The proportion of cases of proctitis caused by HSV has increased since the 1980s. Whereas safer sex practices have decreased the number of newly acquired herpetic infections, recurrent anorectal herpes infections have increased markedly in HIV-infected patients. Interestingly, several studies have shown an increased rate of acquisition of HIV-1 among persons with HSV infection (44–46). HSV disrupts the mucosa, thereby facilitating cell-associated and cell-free transfer of HIV-1 between sexual partners (46). HIV-1 RNA was detected on 67% of the days during which HSV-2 genital lesions were noted, and the HIV-1 RNA titers in the lesion exceeded 10,000 copies per milliliter in 75% of samples (47). Activation of HIV-1 infection from latency by co-infection with HSV-2 has also been postulated to have a direct effect on viral replication of HIV and disease progression (48).

Clinical Illness

The manifestations of HSV infection range from asymptomatic viral shedding to severe anal pain with ulcerative proctitis. Symptoms generally develop 4 to 21 days after exposure. The primary infection is self-limited and generally resolves within 3 weeks. Bacterial superinfection is more common in anorectal than in genital lesions and may prolong the course. Symptomatic recurrences tend to be less severe and shorter than the primary infection. The frequency of recurrence is approximately four times greater with HSV-2 than with HSV-1 infection (18,49,50).

Symptoms commonly associated with HSV proctitis include anorectal pain (100%), tenesmus (100%), constipation (78%), anal pruritus (80%), sacral paresthesia (26%), posterior thigh pain (26%), difficulty urinating (48%), perianal lesions (70%), inguinal adenopathy (57%), impotence (9%), and fever (48%) (51). The triad of constipation, anorectal pain, and urinary retention are strongly suggestive of herpetic proctitis. The constipation and urinary retention have been attributed to either a pain-induced reflex spasm of the anal and vesicular sphincters or a sacral radiculomyelopathy (52).

The presence of HIV-1 infection can adversely affect the clinical course of HSV proctitis. Unlike immunocompetent hosts, in whom lesions resolve spontaneously within 2 to 3 weeks, patients infected with HIV-1 tend to have chronic, progressive disease with the development of large, destructive perianal ulcers (53). Chronic mucocutaneous HSV infection in a person with a positive HIV serology is diagnostic of AIDS (54).

On physical examination, HSV proctitis is characterized by discrete vesicles, pustules, or shallow ulcers around the anus or in the anal canal and rectum. The lesions may be atypical in appearance and can be mistaken for fissures. Anoscopic examination is often necessary to diagnose the lesions. In a study of Quinn et al. (55), only 4 (27%) of 15 homosexual men with HSV anorectal infection had visible perirectal lesions. In a study of Koutsky et al. (56), 5 (19%) of 26 women with anorectal HSV-2 infection had perirectal lesions, and 8 (31%) of 26 lesions were restricted to the anus or rectum. On anoscopic examination, diffuse friability of the distal 10 cm of the rectal mucosa is likely to be noted in patients with HSV proctitis.

Diagnosis

The diagnosis of HSV proctitis is based on the presence of vesiculo-ulcerative lesions and characteristic symptoms. Viral culture of external lesions, a rectal swab, or a rectal biopsy specimen may be used to confirm the diagnosis. The sensitivity of culture for the detection of HSV infection depends on the clinical stage of the lesion, immune status of the host, and site of infection. Immunofluorescent staining for HSV antigens in tissue biopsy specimens may also be performed. A cytologic scraping or Tzanck preparation for typical intranuclear inclusion bodies or multinucleated giant cells may be helpful.

Histologic examination of rectal biopsy samples from patients with HSV proctitis usually shows acute, nonspecific inflammation. The characteristic findings of a perivascular mononuclear cell infiltrate, intranuclear inclusion bodies, and multinucleated giant cells may be present but are not unique to HSV infection. HSV serology can be used to confirm infection when paired serum samples demonstrate either seroconversion or a fourfold rise in titer (57). Commercially available enzyme immunoassays do not distinguish well between antibody subtypes (58). Recently, a type-specific glycoprotein, gpG, was identified, and a serologic assay in which this protein is used to distinguish antibody to viral subtypes is highly specific (59). Additionally, western blot has been used to detect HSV-specific antibodies (59). Although isolation of HSV is the most specific means of confirming a primary episode of infection, detection of HSV-2-specific antibody is the most sensitive way to confirm symptomatic reactivation and to detect asymptomatic infection (55).

Polymerase chain reaction (PCR) is now being used to detect HSV infection. In a study comparing PCR with culture, PCR detected HSV DNA from all culture-positive samples (60). In addition, HSV DNA was detected in ulcerative lesions on 15 of 17 days by PCR, but on only 3 of 17 days by viral isolation. The results of PCR detection became negative only after reepithelialization of the lesions. Although PCR does not differentiate between viable and nonviable HSV, it is more sensitive than culture for the detection of infection.

Treatment

The decision to treat HSV proctitis depends on the severity of symptoms because the infection is usually self-limited in immunocompetent persons. Conservative therapy with sitz baths, stool softeners, and analgesics is used for mild proctitis. Antiviral therapy for initial infection consists of 400 to 800 mg of oral acyclovir taken five times per day for 10 days, which decreases the duration of symptoms and viral shedding (61,62) (Table 27.3). For severe mucocutaneous disease, such as that associated with immunosuppression, intravenous acyclovir (5 to 10 mg/kg every 8 hours) should be used until the mucosal surface is healed (62–66). Because the discontinuation of therapy is generally associated with recurrent disease, 200 mg of oral acyclovir three to five times per day or 400 mg two times per day may be used to suppress clinical disease in immunosuppressed patients and in immunocompetent persons who have more than six episodes of symptomatic HSV infection per year (62). The safety of daily dosing of acyclovir has been demonstrated in patients treated for up to 6 years; therapy should be stopped after 1 year to determine recurrence (62,67). The severity and duration of recurrences may be decreased if 200 mg of oral acyclovir five times per day or 400 mg three times per day or 800 mg twice a day is initiated within 24 hours of onset of the lesion (62). Valacyclovir, the valine ester of acyclovir, and famciclovir, a prodrug of penciclovir, both have a high oral bioavailability and should be effective; however, no specific dosing guidelines are available for HSV proctitis. All acyclovir-resistant strains are also resistant to valcyclovir, and most are resistant to famciclovir, which requires viral thymidine kinase for phosphorylation to the active drug (68,69). A syndrome resembling hemolytic–uremic syndrome or thrombotic thrombocytopenic purpura developed in immunocompromised persons given 8 g of valacyclovir per day, but this has not been described in persons given the doses recommended for genital infection (62).

Mutants of HSV resistant to acyclovir have been isolated from immunocompetent and immunocompromised patients after prolonged use of the drug (70–74). Deficiency of thymidine kinase, which prevents the phosphorylation of acyclovir to its active form, is the most common mechanism of resistance (71,75); altered DNA polymerase occurs less frequently (72,76). Severe progressive mucocutaneous disease in HIV-infected patients can be associated with acyclovir-resistant HSV-2 (76). Foscarnet (phosphonoformic acid) in a dosage of 40 to 60 mg/kg every 8 to 12 hours can produce clinical and microbiologic cure in these patients (74,77). HSV disease generally recurs after the discontinuation of foscarnet, and these first recurrences are usually with an acyclovir-susceptible strain phenotypically similar to the one that established the initial infection (78). Foscarnet-resistant HSV strains have also been isolated from lesions that developed while patients were being treated with foscarnet. In several cases, these isolates were sensitive to acyclovir and responded to therapy with acyclovir, either alone or in combination with ganciclovir (79–81). Cidofovir is an acyclic nucleoside phosphonate that is phosphorylated by cellular enzymes and is therefore active against HSV strains with deficient or altered thymidine kinase levels (82,69). Acyclovir-resistant HSV strains may respond to intravenous cidofovir or to topical cidofovir 1% gel applied once daily to the lesion for 5 days consecutively (82,69).

TABLE 27.3. DIAGNOSIS AND TREATMENT OF INFECTIOUS CAUSES OF PROCTOCOLITIS

Organism	Symptoms of Proctitis	Histology	Diagnosis	Treatment	Anoscopy/ Physical Examination	Special Considerations
C. trachomatis (non-LGV)	May be Asx	Follicles; neutrophil infiltrate of lamina propria/crypts	Culture; DFA	Doxycycline 100 mg PO bid × 7 d; or azithromycin 1 g	Normal or erythema; erosion or rectal discharge	
C. trachomatis (LGV)	Usually Sx	Diffuse inflammation; crypt abscesses; granulomas; giant cells	Culture; DFA; serology	Doxycycline 100 mg × 21 d	Purulent discharge; hematochezia; adenopathy; diffusely friable mucosa	Histology similar to Crohn disease
N. gonorrhoeae	May be Asx	Nonspecific cellular infiltrate	Culture; Gram stain	Ciprofloxacin 500 mg; ofloxacin 400 mg	Normal or purulent discharge; erythema/ erosion; able to express mucopus	Possible disseminated gonococcal infection
T. pallidum	May be Asx	Nonspecific obliterative endarteritis; mononuclear cell infiltrate; granulomas; crypt abscesses	Dark-field microscopy; immunohistochemical stain; serology	1°/2° PCN 2.4 million U IM; latent—PCN 2.4 million U q wk × 3	Chancre; polypoid mass; condylomata lata; irregular mucosa; adenopathy	Treatment may be inadequate with HIV
Herpes simplex virus	Often Sx; recurrence possible	Nonspecific inflammation; mononuclear infiltrate; intranuclear inclusions; multinucleated giant cells	Clinical syndrome (sacral radiculomyelopathy); viral culture; Tzarck prep; serology (WB, IgG immunoassay)	ACV 400–800 mg 5×/d × 10d; suppression: ACV 400 mg 2×/d; ACV resistance; foscarnet	Discrete vesicles/ pustules; ulcers; erosion	
Human papillomavirus	May be Asx	Irregular epithelium; koilocytes; hyperkeratosis/ dyskeratosis; carcinoma	Clinical appearance; Papanicolaou smear; biopsy; PCR/Southern blot	Cryotherapy; TCA; surgical excision	Exophytic lesion; erosion ulcer	Increased risk of anal carcinoma
E. histolytica	Often Asx	Nonspecific	Serology (invasive disease); stool exam for O&P (3–6 samples); erythrophagocytosis; zymodeme analysis	Metronidazole plus iodoquinol (invasive disease); or iodoquinol; or paromomycin; or diloxanide furoate (colonization)	May be normal	

LGV, lymphogranuloma venereum; Asx, asymptomatic; Sx, symptomatic; DFA, direct fluorescent antibody; WB, Western blot; PCR, polymerase chain reaction; O&P, ova and parasites; PCN, penicillin; ACV, acyclovir; TCA, trichloracetic acid.

HUMAN PAPILLOMAVIRUS

Microbiology

The HPV is a member of the papovavirus family, which includes papillomaviruses, simian virus 40, and polyomaviruses (83). It is a non-enveloped, double-stranded DNA virus of approximately 7,900 base pairs encased in an icosahedral capsid. The genome is divided into early (E) and late (L) and control regions. The E regions code for eight regulatory gene products (E1 through E8), and the L region codes for a 53-kd protein that constitutes approximately 80% of the viral capsid proteins and a 70-kd minor capsid protein. The outer protein coat consists of two proteins, the major and minor capsid proteins. Capsid proteins appear to mediate viral attachment to susceptible cells, host range, and neutralization (84,85). The E-region gene products are differentially expressed in different HPV strains; the E6 and E7 regions code for proteins important in malignant transformation (86,87). Infection with HPV is initiated by entry and multiplication of the virus within the nucleus of cells of the basal germinal epithelium. Viral infection causes an acceleration of cell growth, which leads to an irregularly thickened epithelium with foci of koilocytic cells containing perinuclear cavitation and nuclear atypia. Skin and mucosal lesions occur 3 weeks to 2 years following infection, most typically within 3 to 4 months. Because only early gene products are expressed in the basal layers, viral particles and viral capsid proteins are absent in these cells but can be identified in the nondividing superficial cell layers. Viral transmission occurs when viral particles are shed with the superficial epithelial cells (84).

Pathogenesis and Immunity

Infection with HPV disrupts the normal skin morphology and causes an excess proliferation of all epidermal layers except the basal layer. As a consequence of these changes, acanthosis, parakeratosis, and sometimes hyperkeratosis develop (88). In some infected cells, koilocytic transformation occurs, with characteristic shrinking of the nucleus. Certain HPVs are associated with exophytic and neoplastic lesions (89,90). The molecular basis of the difference in oncogenic potential of the HPVs is unclear, but duration of infection and cofactors such as sunlight and radiation may contribute to malignant transformation (91,92). Integration of HPV DNA is a key factor in malignant transformation. In nonmalignant HPV lesions, viral DNA is located extrachromosomally, whereas in HPV-associated neoplasia, it is generally integrated. Integration may occur at any site in the host cell chromosome but only at a specific site, the E1–E2 region, in the viral genome (84). The undisturbed E2 gene product suppresses expression of E6 and E7. Interruption of E2 during integration into the host genome prevents the production of its protein, so that the E6–E7 region is left unregulated. Interaction of the E6 and E7 gene products with tumor suppressor genes *p53* and *Rb* (retinoblastoma), respectively, leads to cellular transformation (93,94).

Humoral and cell-mediated immunity to HPV is poorly understood. The lack of an *in vitro* system to support replication of the virus has limited the ability to study responses to immunologically important antigens. However, observations of the natural history of HPV infection suggest that host immunity plays an important role in the pathogenesis of HPV infection. Warts are less common in adults than in children, presumably because of immunity acquired in childhood. HPV-associated disease is more severe in conditions associated with impaired cell-mediated immunity, such as pregnancy (95), immunosuppressive therapy for organ transplantation (96), HIV infection, and lymphoproliferative disorders (97).

Persons infected with HPV produce antibodies to various HPV components. Antibodies are not effective in eradicating the infection; rather, IgG L1 serves as a marker of previous or ongoing HPV infection (94). Antibody to HPV-6b L1 fusion protein is reported to be present in 10% of children less than 5 years old and 60% of women attending a colposcopy clinic (98). Additional seroprevalence studies have shown that these antibodies are present in 44% of children, 39% of students from a university health service, and 56% of STD clinic patients, whereas 63% of patients with dysplasia, 67% of patients with vulvar carcinoma, and 66% patients with warts have such antibodies (98–100). Antibody reactivity to HPV-11 virions has been reported in 33% of patients with condylomata, but not in control subjects (101). Taken together, these data indicate that antibodies to HPV proteins are common in the general population. Antibodies to certain specific gene products are even more common in women with HPV-associated neoplasia (101–105). In particular, IgA antibodies to an E2 peptide of HPV-16 (peptide 245) may be up to threefold more common in women with carcinoma of the cervix than in control subjects (101). Serum antibodies to HPV-16 and HPV-18 E7 proteins also are more common in patients with invasive cervical cancer (104,105). Although antibodies to the E2 and E7 proteins have been suggested as markers for cervical or even anal cancer, their functional significance is still unknown.

Cell-mediated immunity is also involved in the pathogenesis of HPV infection (96,97). It is well established that cell-mediated immunity plays an important role in wart regression. Examination of spontaneously regressing warts shows mononuclear cell infiltrates with natural killer cells and activated CD4+ T cells (94). Evidence indicates that the recognition of HPV-infected cells by natural killer cells is defective in patients with anogenital tumors, and that the natural killer cells are unresponsive to the stimulatory effects of cytokines such as interleukin 2 (IL-2) and IL-6 (106). Evidence also suggests an important role for cytokines in mediating HPV expression in neoplastic cells (107). At least one mechanism appears to be suppression of the transcription of messenger RNA (mRNA) for transforming proteins (E6 and E7) by IFN-γ and leukoregulin (108). Another mechanism appears to be involved in HPV-associated neoplasia in patients with HIV, suggested by the ability of the HIV-1 tat protein to increase the transcription of E2-dependent HPV-16 (109).

Epidemiology

The lack of an accurate and reliable serologic assay to test large numbers of people for HPV infection makes it difficult to determine its prevalence in the general population. It is currently estimated that 5.5 million persons in the United States become infected with HPV each year, and 20 million are currently infected (110). HPV prevalence rates are estimated to vary from 9% in unselected women undergoing cytologic screening to 82% in repeatedly sampled prostitutes (111,112) and 51.5% in homosexual men (2). Genital warts probably represent only 10% of the total spectrum of genital HPV infection (113). Approximately 1% of sexually active persons in the United States have genital warts (114). Anal warts are common in homosexual men and heterosexual women practicing anal intercourse. Between 46% and 90% of patients with anal warts have a history of engaging in anal sex.

Eighty-three HPV types have been characterized; an additional 150 types have been identified through PCR products, but their complete genomes have not been fully characterized (114). Approximately 20% are detected in the anogenital tract, with HPV-6, -11, -16, -18, -31, -33, and -35 being the most common. HPV-6 and HPV-11 are found in most exophytic anal condylomata and have little oncogenic potential (89). HPV-16 and HPV-18 are found in 50% and 20%, respectively, of cervical cancers, and 56% and 5%, respectively, of anal cancers (89,90,115).

The annual incidence of anal squamous cell cancer is 0.7 per 100,000 men, but this increases to 35 per 100,000 in homosexual men (116). The rate in homosexual men approximates the rate of cervical cancer in women before cytologic screening. Although the association of HPV and cervical cancer has long been recognized, awareness of the role of HPV in anal cancer is increasing (117–120). The prevalence of HPV DNA in anal squamous cell cancer is 78% to 85% by PCR, 56% to 85% by Southern blot/dot-blot hybridization, and 50% to 100% by *in situ* hybridization (121). Several recent studies have examined the interaction of HPV and HIV and reported an increased risk for progression of HPV disease in HIV-infected persons (120–123). HIV-infected persons appear to be at increased risk for persistence of HPV infection, including infection with the oncogenic types HPV-16 and HPV-18, which increases the risk for malignant progression. In a prospective study of persons with no lesions at baseline followed for 2 years, anal squamous intraepithelial lesions developed in 52% of HIV-infected persons and in 17% of uninfected persons, and high-grade squamous intraepithelial lesions developed in 20% of those with HIV infection versus 8% of those without HIV infection. Risk factors for anal squamous intraepithelial lesions in persons with HPV infection include HIV infection, a decreased CD4+ T-cell count, increased levels of HPV in tissues, and increased numbers of HPV types, especially of types 16 and 18 (124). It is possible that as HIV-infected persons live longer because of HAART, an increase in the number of deaths from anal cancer will be seen. The recognition of the association of HPV with anal cancer is leading to recommendations for more aggressive diagnosis and therapy of dysplastic lesions. Although data do indicate that screening of HIV-infected homosexual men for anal malignancy may be cost-effective, no well-accepted guidelines are available in this area (125).

Clinical Illness

Anal warts appear as white, pink, or gray flat or heaped-up lesions that vary in extent and number. They may be mistaken for condylomata lata, which are generally more moist and smooth in appearance. Anal warts can resolve spontaneously, likely because of an effective immune system (126). It is estimated HPV infection resolves in 70% of teenage girls within 30 months (94). Patients with anorectal warts may be asymptomatic or complain of pruritus ani, rectal discharge, and bleeding. The warts are located in the perianal area or inside the anal canal (2). In cases in which perianal lesions are detected, an anoscopic examination should be performed to rule out the presence of lesions within the canal.

Diagnosis

The diagnosis of anorectal HPV infection is based on clinical observation. Other lesions that may have a similar appearance include condylomata lata and squamous cell carcinoma. The distinction between benign and malignant lesions can be made only by histologic examination of biopsy material, which should be performed for any lesion that has an atypical appearance or responds poorly to therapy. A Papanicolaou smear may reveal dyskeratosis and koilocytosis, classic signs of HPV infection, but this technique may be insensitive if only classic criteria are used, and DNA hybridization is more likely to detect latent HPV infection without cellular abnormality (127,128). Southern blot analysis has been considered the gold standard for the detection of HPV DNA. However, it is technically difficult to perform. Other DNA hybridization techniques, such as dot-blot and filter *in situ* hybridization, are simpler to perform but less sensitive and specific (95). PCR is now being developed for the diagnosis of HPV infection (129–132). The amplified DNA can be subjected to hybridization with the use of specific probes or restriction fragment length polymorphism for typing the isolates (133).

Treatment

Effective curative therapy for HPV infection is not currently available. Therefore, current treatment is aimed at symptomatic relief. It is unclear whether treatment alters the natural history of the infection or decreases infectivity. Several treatment options are available for external genital and perianal warts. The choice of treatment is based on the size, number, and location of lesions. Provider-administered therapies include cryotherapy with a cryoprobe or liquid nitrogen, which is effective in clearing 63% to 91% of lesions without scarring (134,135) (Table 27.3). Weekly application of 10%

to 20% podophyllin solution (<0.5 mL) in tincture of benzoin has been effective in removing up to 77% of lesions (136). Because the agent is caustic, it cannot be used within the anus, and because of its oncogenic and teratogenic potential, it is contraindicated in pregnancy. Additional caustic agents that are effective in removing external lesions are 80% to 90% solutions of trichloracetic acid and bichloracetic acid. An evaluation of the efficacy of trichloracetic acid versus cryotherapy in the treatment of external genital warts performed in 86 patients found a 70% rate of complete clearance with trichloracetic acid versus an 86% rate with cryotherapy (137). Patient-administered treatment options include podofilox, a less concentrated (0.5%) solution of podophyllin, or 5% imiquimod cream. Imiquimod presumptively works by inducing local responses of cytokines, including IFN-α and tumor necrosis factor-α, against HPV. Placebo-controlled studies indicate that warts are cleared in 45% to 82% of patients treated with podofilox and in 37% to 85% of patients treated with imiquimod (138).

Alternative treatments for persons not responding to other modalities include intralesional IFN. Intralesional IFN-α appear more effective than placebo for the treatment of condyloma acuminatum, and patients whose lesions contain detectable levels of HPV nucleic acid or papillomavirus antigens or in whom koilocytes are observed seem more likely to respond to this treatment (139). Utilization of this method is limited by its cost and systemic toxicity, which includes fever, chills, and myalgias. Carbon dioxide laser therapy and surgery are particularly useful for large lesions, but the requirement for local or general anesthesia limits their usefulness. In one study comparing podophyllin and surgery, surgery resulted in 93% clearance and 29% recurrence at 12 months, in comparison with 77% clearance and 65% recurrence for podophyllin (140). Because the recurrence rates with all these modalities are ultimately equivalent, their long-term efficacy rates do not differ.

Recommended therapies for anal warts include cryotherapy with liquid nitrogen, trichloracetic acid, or bichloracetic acid, or surgical excision. Sex partners should be counseled and advised that treatment of warts does not eliminate infectivity and that condoms reduce but do not eliminate the risk for transmission (62). HIV-infected persons may be less likely to respond to therapy and more likely to have clinical recurrences. Current guidelines do not recommend treatment of subclinical HPV infection. In the presence of squamous intraepithelial neoplasia, management should be based on the grade of dysplasia.

T. PALLIDUM

Microbiology

T. pallidum, a member of the Spirochaetaceae family, is a unicellular, helical, tightly coiled organism approximately 6 to 15 μm long and 0.15 μm wide. The size of the organism is below the level of resolution by light microscopy, so dark-field light-microscopic examination is necessary for visualization. The spirochete is surrounded by an amorphous outer layer composed of mucopolysaccharides, an outer membrane, a mucopeptide layer or periplast, a peptidoglycan layer, and a cytoplasmic membrane. Three fibrils that arise from each end of the organism and insert in the opposite end contract to propel the organism in a characteristic rotary flexing motion. *T. pallidum* cannot be cultivated *in vitro* but can remain motile for up to 7 days if kept at 35°C in a highly enriched environment with elevated levels of carbon dioxide (141).

Pathogenesis and Immunity

T. pallidum is able to infect skin or mucosa in which the epithelial layer is broken. The incubation period between exposure and development of a lesion depends on the size of the inoculum. In rabbits, 10^7 organisms produce a lesion in 5 to 7 days, but as few as four organisms can establish infection. Because the organism divides slowly (30 to 33 hours per division), the establishment of infection requires successful evasion of host immunity (141,142).

Although the clinical course of syphilis has been well described, the mechanisms of pathogenesis and immunity have not been fully elucidated. Early infection is associated with the development of a lesion (chancre) after an average of 21 days (range, 10 to 90 days). After several weeks, the lesion heals spontaneously. The primary chancre contains spirochetes within a mucoid material consisting of hyaluronic acid and chondroitin sulfate; this is rimmed by a cellular infiltrate composed primarily of neutrophils and macrophages known to phagocytose *T. pallidum* and lymphocytes (141–146). The origin of the mucoid material is uncertain, but it may contribute to the organism's ability to evade host immune responses.

During secondary syphilis, *T. pallidum* disseminates to the skin, mucosa, and organs despite the presence of *T. pallidum*-specific antibodies. In addition, immune complexes are deposited in various tissues during secondary syphilis. Dissemination at this stage has been attributed to impaired cell-mediated immunity (147), evidenced by the rapid and severe progression of disease in patients who are infected with HIV-1 or malnourished (148–150).

During the next stage of disease, referred to as *latency,* infection is effectively suppressed so that lesions are no longer apparent. It has been postulated that the organism is "disguised" during latency by the concealment of *T. pallidum* antigens from host defense mechanisms, referred to as the *immunoprotective niche* (151,152). However, relapses with secondary syphilis, and subsequent development of neurosyphilis, indicate that viable organisms are still present.

Tertiary syphilis becomes clinically apparent 1 to 20 years after disseminated infection. Late manifestations of the disease develop in only one-third of untreated patients.

It has been postulated that failure to mount an effective delayed-type hypersensitivity response early in infection permits further disease progression. Cell-mediated immune responses likely contribute to host protection but may also play a pathologic role because the development of large granulomatous lesions (gummas) during tertiary syphilis appears to represent a host-mediated hypersensitivity response to *T. pallidum* (153). These lesions often appear at sites prone to trauma (141).

Epidemiology

Between 1950 and 1978, the number of cases of syphilis increased from 19,000 to 26,000 per year (154). The incidence continued to increase in the late 1970s and early 1980s, largely because of an increased number of cases in homosexual men (154,155). By the mid-1980s, however, the incidence of syphilis in homosexual men began to decrease in association with behavioral changes adopted in response to the HIV epidemic. In 1985, as the rate in homosexual men decreased, the incidence of syphilis in urban heterosexuals began to increase (156). Between 1985 and 1990, the rate of syphilis increased 126% in black men and 231% in black women (156,157), likely reflecting limited access to health care and promiscuous sexual activity related to the epidemic of illicit drug use. Rates of primary and secondary syphilis have been declining in the United States since 1990. In 1999, 6,657 cases of primary and secondary syphilis (2.5 per 100,000 population) were recorded. This represents a 22% decrease from 1997 and an approximately 90% decrease from 1990. During the 1990s, heterosexual blacks and persons in the South had the highest rates of syphilis. However, recent outbreaks have been documented in homosexual men (158). During January to July of 2000, the proportion of cases of early syphilis in homosexual men in Southern California doubled (159). This statistic is further evidence of the resurgence of high-risk sexual behavior in homosexual men. Unfortunately, the same behavior patterns that place this population at risk for syphilis also enhance the acquisition of HIV infection (154,160–162).

Anorectal syphilis occurs primarily in homosexual men. In inner city STD clinics in the United Kingdom, 30% of cases of primary and secondary syphilis in homosexual men involved the anus and rectum (163). Among homosexual men attending one STD clinic in the United States, 12% had anorectal syphilis (55).

Clinical Illness

The gastrointestinal lesions of syphilis occur most commonly during the primary and secondary stages of *T. pallidum* infection. The presence and type of symptoms depend on the form of the lesion. The primary lesion, which usually develops 2 to 6 weeks after exposure, has a variable appearance, which accounts for the high rate of misdiagnosis. The anal chancre is the most common presentation; it may be single and eccentrically placed or multiple, forming mirror images ("kissing chancres"). The chancres occur anywhere in the anus or rectum (164,165). Because chancres are often asymptomatic, painful lesions may be attributed to trauma or anal fissures. Superinfection of the chancre is often associated with the development of symptoms. Inguinal lymphadenopathy is often associated with anorectal syphilis and helps to distinguish it from fissure. Primary anorectal syphilis may also present as ulcerated masses that are typically located on the anterior wall of the rectum (166).

Secondary syphilis is associated with spirochetemia and typically develops 6 weeks to 6 months after the initial infection. Condylomata lata are the most common anorectal lesions associated with secondary syphilis. They are smooth, warty masses located in or near the rectum and must be differentiated from the more highly keratinized condylomata acuminata. Condylomata lata are often pruritic and produce a foul discharge that is highly infectious. Other presentations include proctitis without a clear ulcer, polypoid growth, pseudotumor, mucosal ulceration and erythema, or submucosal irregularities with rubbery nodes suggesting lymphoma. Constitutional symptoms, skin rashes, and mucous patches can also occur (167–169). Inflammation of the gastrointestinal tract resulting from syphilis is usually limited to the distal 15 cm of the colon but may reach the distal 20 cm in secondary syphilis. The anorectal lesions of primary and secondary syphilis may also coexist (167). Untreated, syphilitic proctitis spontaneously resolves within 3 to 4 weeks. If the patient is not treated in the primary or secondary stage, a latent period ensues, during which the patient is infected but asymptomatic. Some of these patients progress to tertiary syphilis. Although gastrointestinal lesions are unusual at this stage, rectal gummas may occur and can be mistaken for malignancy. During tertiary syphilis, anal sphincter paralysis and severe anal pain may develop in association with tabes dorsalis.

Although the biopsy findings in syphilitic anal lesions are often nonspecific, histology may show an obliterative endarteritis with capillary proliferation; infiltration of the lamina propria by plasma cells, histiocytes, and lymphocytes; and occasionally granulomas (170,171).

Diagnosis

The diagnosis of primary or secondary syphilis is made by identifying the organisms in a lesion. The detection of typical organisms on dark-field microscopy is useful for perianal lesions, but the presence of nonpathogenic treponemes makes the test less helpful for lesions in the rectum (172). Immunohistochemical staining of exudate from a lesion may be useful when the dark-field examination result is negative (173). However, silver-stained treponemes may be mistaken for tissue components, especially reticulin fibers (171). Routine histologic examination is not useful because the findings are generally nonspecific and may be confused with those of other conditions, such as inflammatory bowel disease. Newer diagnostic techniques that utilize PCR are being developed but are not yet available for clinical use.

The serologic diagnosis of syphilis is based on the presence of antibodies to nontreponemal and treponemal antigens. Nontreponemal tests [Venereal Disease Research Laboratory (VDRL) and rapid plasma reagin (RPR)] are based on the detection of antibodies to a cardiolipin antigen that is produced during infection. The VDRL test result generally becomes positive 2 weeks after the development of a chancre. In untreated patients, titers peak during secondary syphilis and subsequently decline. The sensitivity of the VDRL test depends on the stage of infection. The test detects approximately 50% to 70% of cases of primary syphilis, 100% of cases of secondary syphilis, and 85% to 100% of cases of tertiary syphilis. A positive VDRL or RPR test result must be corroborated by a positive result of a test specific for antibody to *T. pallidum* antigens, such as the fluorescent treponemal antibody absorption (FTA-ABS) test or the microhemagglutination (MHATP) test. The specificity of the VDRL test varies with the population tested and is higher in healthy than in sick persons (141,154). The FTA-ABS test is the first serologic test to yield a positive result, and a positive result is present in 70% to 90% of patients with a chancre. This test is generally 100% sensitive in secondary and tertiary syphilis. Treponemal antibody titers do not correlate with disease activity and usually remain positive after infection.

Concomitant infection with HIV-1 may impair antibody responses to *T. pallidum.* Delayed or absent serologic test reactivity for syphilis occurs predominantly during the later stages of HIV infection (174–176). Higher RPR titers may occur in HIV-1–seropositive patients with secondary syphilis than in HIV-1–seronegative patients (177). Serologic false-positive test results, such as RPR-positive and FTA-ABS–negative results, which occur in a wide variety of infectious and noninfectious conditions, have been associated with HIV infection (154,178). Because of the association between HIV and *T. pallidum* infections, HIV testing is recommended for all patients with syphilis.

Treatment

Penicillin is the treatment of choice for syphilis. The administration of 2.4 million U of benzathine penicillin intramuscularly is effective for primary, secondary, and early latent syphilis of less than 1 year. In latent syphilis of more than 1 year and tertiary syphilis other than neurosyphilis, 2.4 million U of benzathine penicillin intramuscularly once a week for 3 weeks is recommended (62) (Table 27.3). For patients who cannot tolerate penicillin, 100 mg of doxycycline orally twice a day or 500 mg of tetracycline four times a day should be given for 2 weeks for early syphilis and for 4 weeks for latent or tertiary syphilis.

All patients with syphilis should be reexamined at 6, 12, and 24 months because failure to eradicate syphilis can occur with any regimen. Nontreponemal antibody titers should decline fourfold by 6 months in primary and secondary syphilis, and by 12 to 24 months in early or latent syphilis. Lack of an appropriate decline in antibody titer or the persistence of clinical signs or symptoms suggests treatment failure or reinfection, in which case the cerebrospinal fluid should be evaluated and re-treatment started. Sexual contacts should be evaluated clinically and serologically. Because a partner can be infected yet be seronegative within 90 days of exposure, treatment is indicated during this period (62).

Several reports have documented poor responses to standard therapy for syphilis in patients with HIV infection (179–182). Syphilis may have a more aggressive course in these patients, and single-dose therapy with benzathine penicillin for early syphilis has been associated with the subsequent development of neurosyphilis. In addition, the serologic titer may decrease more slowly after treatment in HIV-infected patients (182). Because patients with syphilis and HIV infection are at higher risk for failure of initial therapy, additional doses of benzathine penicillin may be considered, and more frequent follow-up is recommended. HIV-infected patients with syphilis should be evaluated at 3, 6, 9, 12, and 24 months following treatment, so that lack of a clinical or serologic relapse can be identified (62).

N. GONORRHOEAE

Microbiology

N. gonorrhoeae is a nonmotile, non–spore-forming, gram-negative diplococcus. The bacterium has a cytoplasmic membrane, peptidoglycan layer, and outer membrane. Unlike meningococci, gonococci lack a polysaccharide capsule. *In vivo,* the outer cell surface of most *N. gonorrhoeae* organisms is covered by pili, which are individual fibrils or fibrillar aggregates involved in organism attachment and invasion. Pili also serve as markers of pathogenicity; piliated strains are more pathogenic than nonpiliated strains. Nonreciprocal recombinational events involving the pilus gene lead to antigenic variations of the pili and also to alternation between piliated and nonpiliated morphologies (183).

Several gonococcal plasmids have been identified, some of which mediate antibiotic resistance. For instance, derivatives of a 36-kd plasmid confer tetracycline resistance (184), and several plasmids encode β-lactamases (185). Most gonococci also contain a 4.2-kilobase cryptic plasmid (186). The proportion of gonococcal infections caused by β-lactamase–producing *N. gonorrhoeae* increased significantly during the 1980s and early 1990s. By 1994, more than 30.5% of isolates exhibited chromosome- or plasmid-mediated resistance to penicillin or tetracycline (187). During 1990 through 1995 in the Americas, high-level plasmid-mediated resistance of *N. gonorrhoeae* to tetracycline and chromosomal resistance to penicillin and tetracycline increased while the incidence of penicillinase-producing *N. gonorrhoeae* decreased. Data from the Centers for Disease Control and Prevention for 1991 through 1994 indicate that although 99.9% of *N. gonorrhoeae* isolates remained highly susceptible to the broad-spectrum cephalosporins, resistance rates to ciprofloxacin increased from 0.4% to 1.3%. In some parts of Asia, such as Hong Kong, rates of quinolone resistance in *N. gonorrhoeae* approximate 24% (187,188). Therefore, persons who contract infections in these areas should be treated with a regimen of drugs other than quinolones.

Pathogenesis and Immunity

N. gonorrhoeae organisms most commonly infect the columnar epithelial cells of the urethra and endocervix. However, other sites, including the fallopian tubes, ovaries, rectum, and prostate, also may be infected. After attachment to the epithelial cell, the organism is internalized by endocytosis and transported to the subepithelial space (189,190). Infection is associated with a vigorous neutrophil response, sloughing of epithelial cells, and the development of submucosal microabscesses.

A lack of good animal models has limited the study of pathogenesis and immune response in this infection. The common occurrence of reinfection in both men and women indicates that protective immunity does not develop following natural infection. However, partial protection against reinfection with the same serovar does develop. For example, in Nairobi prostitutes, the risk for reinfection with the same serovar is generally decreased twofold to 10-fold, and the risk for gonococcal infection is inversely related to the length of time in which prostitution has been practiced (191). The ability of the organism to cause recurrent infections is in part a consequence of antigenic variation and its ability to mask relevant antigens. The relevant antigens include outer membrane components such as lipopolysaccharide, protein I, protein II (opa proteins), and protein III (192).

Protein I functions as a porin in the outer membrane and is used as an antigen for serotyping gonococcal isolates (193). It is an important determinant of antibiotic susceptibility (194), serum resistance (195), and invasiveness (196). Gonococcal isolates that cause disseminated disease are typically IA and are resistant to the bactericidal effects of normal human serum, whereas isolates causing local disease are usually serum-sensitive (197,183). It appears that the bactericidal effect of normal human serum occurs primarily through the binding of IgM antibodies to complement and lipopolysaccharide (198,199). Protein III appears to contain epitopes for binding blocking antibodies and bactericidal antibodies (200).

Protein II, or the opa family of proteins, is important in the antigenic variation seen among gonococcal isolates. Gonococci undergo phase switching (on/off expression of opas), and switching from one opa to another also occurs (192). This antigenic variation likely contributes to the bacterial evasion of host immune responses. Opas function as adhesins, promoting adherence to epithelial cells (201) and neutrophils (202) and aggregation of organisms in a colony (203). They also stimulate the production of bactericidal antibodies (204).

Delayed-type hypersensitivity responses to a variety of bacterial fractions and culture filtrates occurs in most persons infected with *N. gonorrhoeae* (205). Additionally, lymphocytes from infected persons undergo transformation when stimulated with gonococcal antigens. However, by 5 weeks after treatment, antigen-specific proliferation declines to undetectable levels (206,207), and the relationship between cellular immune responses and protection from gonococcal infection has not been elucidated.

Epidemiology

The worldwide incidence of *N. gonorrhoeae* infections is estimated at 60 million cases per year (187). In the United States, *N. gonorrhoeae* infection rates peaked in the 1970s, with approximately 500 cases per 100,000 population. Following a 13-year decline, the number of cases of gonorrhea increased 9% in 1998 (133 per 100,000) over the number in 1997 (122 per 100,000). Rates increased 10.5% in women and 7.4% in men (208). Unlike the national rates of gonorrhea, the rates of male rectal gonorrhea declined to a nadir of 20 per 100,000 in 1993, and from 1994 to 1997, they increased from 21 per 100,000 to 38 per 100,000 (209). In Seattle and Portland, the rates of *N. gonorrhoeae* infection in homosexual men increased 125% and 124%, respectively, from 1994 to 1996 (210). The increased rates of *N. gonorrhoeae* infection since 1993 are likely related to the increased proportion of homosexual men who have multiple sex partners and practice unprotected anal intercourse. The percentage of homosexual men who reported having multiple sex partners and engaging in unprotected anal intercourse increased from 23.6% in 1994 to 33.3% in 1997 (209).

N. gonorrhoeae is also a common cause of anorectal infections in women. Between 1966 and 1977, anorectal involvement was noted in 26% to 63% of women with gonorrhea, and in up to 20%, the rectum was the only involved site (211). The role of rectal intercourse in the etiology of anorectal *N. gonorrhoeae* in women has been difficult to determine. Among homosexual men, *N. gonorrhoeae* is the most frequently identified sexually transmitted pathogen. Of the homosexual men attending STD clinics, 28% to 55% have gonorrhea, and the anus is the only site of infection in 40%. The rectum is more commonly involved than the urethra or pharynx (55,165,212). Homosexual men are more frequently infected with strains having the *mtr* mutation, which confers antibiotic susceptibility. This mutation is also associated with decreased membrane permeability, which is thought to enhance the ability of the strain to survive in the rectum (213). In a study from the United Kingdom that evaluated gonococcal isolates from 383 episodes of infection in women, one serovar, Bajk, was isolated significantly more frequently in rectal (27%) than in genital (17%) infections (214). These studies suggest that different strains preferentially infect specific host sites.

Clinical Illness

Asymptomatic infections are common in anorectal gonorrhea and occur more frequently than urethral infections in homosexual men (55,215,216). When symptoms occur, they develop 5 to 7 days after exposure and include pruritus ani, bloody or mucopurulent discharge, tenesmus, and constipation. Anorectal gonorrhea may be associated with complications such as fistula, abscess, stricture, and disseminated infection. Disseminated gonococcal infection is typically associated with the AHU auxotype and host deficiency of complement components, particularly the terminal components (217,218).

On sigmoidoscopic examination, the rectal mucosa may be normal or erythematous; fissures, superficial erosion, and friability may be seen, particularly at the anorectal junction (219,220). Mucus and pus are commonly present (168,221). Histologic findings are nonspecific and include patchy disorganization of the mucus-secreting cells, vascular engorgement, and infiltration of the lamina propria with neutrophils, lymphocytes, plasma cells, and monocytes (211).

Diagnosis

The diagnosis of anorectal gonorrhea is made by Gram stain or culture of the material obtained by swab of the rectum. In symptomatic patients, an anoscope should be used to perform the rectal swab because the diagnostic yield can be increased from 33% with a blind swab to 79% with a swab performed under direct visualization (221). In asymptomatic patients, material from a blind swab is adequate; direct visualization does not increase the yield. Because the sensitivity of Gram stain of rectal samples is relatively low, culture is the preferred method of diagnosis (55). A positive Gram stain should be confirmed by culture of the organism on selected media, such as Thayer–Martin, which contains vancomycin, colistin, and trimethoprim to inhibit overgrowth of the gonococci by endogenous intestinal bacteria. The nucleic acid amplification and hybridization assays used for genital samples are not approved by the Food and Drug Administration for rectal samples. However, small studies have evaluated DNA hybridization assays and found a sensitivity of 96.4% and specificity of 100% for rectal samples (222).

Treatment

Single doses of ceftriaxone (125 mg intramuscularly), cefixime (400 mg orally), ciprofloxacin (500 mg orally), or ofloxacin (400 mg orally) are recommended treatment regimens for anorectal *N. gonorrhoeae* infection (62) (Table 27.3). Of the isolates, 99.9% remain susceptible to broad-spectrum cephalosporins, and 98.3% remain susceptible to ciprofloxacin (188). Ceftriaxone may have efficacy in the treatment of incubating syphilis and therefore offer greater benefit than the quinolones in cases at particularly high risk for syphilis. Because of the high rate of co-infection with *Chlamydia,* all patients with *N. gonorrhoeae* infection should also receive a 7-day course of 100 mg of doxycycline twice per day (62). Rates of *Chlamydia* co-infection range from 8.4% in heterosexual men to 15.2% in homosexual men with gonococcal urethritis (223)

Recommended alternatives include spectinomycin (2 g intramuscularly), ceftizoxime (500 mg intramuscularly), cefotaxime (500 mg intramuscularly), cefotetan (1 g intramuscularly), cefoxitin (2.0 g intramuscularly) plus probenecid (1.0 g orally), norfloxacin (800 mg orally), enoxacin (400 mg orally), and lomefloxacin (400 mg orally) as single-dose regimens (62). Azithromycin (2 g orally) is effective against uncomplicated *N. gonorrhoeae* infection but causes gastrointestinal side effects in 35% of treated patients (224). All patients should be instructed to return for follow-up evaluation and repeated culture if symptoms persist. (62). All patients with *N. gonorrhoeae* infection should also have a serologic test for syphilis and be offered testing for HIV infection. In addition, the sexual partners of infected patients exposed within the preceding 60 days should be treated presumptively.

C. TRACHOMATIS

Microbiology

Chlamydiae are gram-negative, obligate intracellular bacteria. The genome of *C. trachomatis* has recently been sequenced and consists of a 1,042,519-base pair chromosome and a 7,493-base pair plasmid. In addition to genes for potential adenosine triphosphate (ATP)/adenosine diphosphate (ADP) translocases, which are consistent with its intracellular life cycle, the organism has genes that may allow it to generate some ATP of its own (225).

The organisms have a biphasic growth cycle and exist as two discrete entities that differ in structure and function (226). The elementary body (EB) (diameter, 300 to 400 nm) is the infectious form of chlamydiae. Although a specific host cell receptor has not been identified, inhibition of adherence of any *C. trachomatis* strain by a heterologous strain suggests that attachment involves a common host cell receptor that may be different for LGV and trachoma biovars (227). Following attachment, the EB enters the host cell by active endocytosis (228). In polymorphonuclear leukocytes, fusion of lysosomes with *C. trachomatis* leads to subsequent degradation of the organism. In infected epithelial cells, phagolysosomal fusion does not occur until very late in infection; rather, within 6 to 8 hours after entrance into the cell, the EB differentiates into a larger (800 to 1,000 nm) reticulate body (RB). The RB, which is the metabolically active form of *Chlamydia,* differs structurally and morphologically from the EB. The RB multiplies by binary fission 8 to 24 hours after infection, with expansion of the phagosome into the typical intracellular inclusion that displaces the cytoplasm. After 24 hours, progeny RBs condense into EBs, which become evident in the phagosome. Subsequently phagolysosomal fusion occurs, and by 48 to 72 hours after infection, the cell ruptures, releasing infectious EBs that initiate new infection.

C. trachomatis is divided into three biovars, based in part on host susceptibility and DNA homology. Two of these biovars, the trachoma biovar and the LGV biovar, cause human infection; the third biovar does not. The trachoma biovar replicates only in columnar epithelial cells, and the LGV strains are also able to replicate in macrophages (229). The LGV and trachoma biovars have been serotyped into 15 serovars—A through K and L1, L2, and L3—based on differences in monoclonal antibody reactivity to the major outer membrane protein (MOMP), which is a cysteine-rich protein constituting 60% of the outer membrane of chlamydiae (230). Serovars A, B, Ba, and C are primarily associated with trachoma, serovars D through K with urogenital infections, and serovars L1, L2, and L3 with LGV.

Pathogenesis and Immunity

Protective immunity to *C. trachomatis* is short-lived and appears to be serovar-specific. Seroepidemiologic studies indicate that the presence of antichlamydial antibodies is associated with a reduced rate of isolation of *C. trachomatis* and that the antibodies are partially protective, so that infection is less severe (231,232). Previous infection reduces the likelihood of reinfection and is associated with less severe local disease. Additionally, serum antibodies may play a role in preventing the spread of infection. For example, postabortion salpingitis occurs more frequently in women infected with *Chlamydia* who have a lower serum antichlamydial antibody titer before abortion (233). Neutralizing antibody directed against epitopes of the MOMP is the primary mechanism of protective humoral immunity (234–238). The mechanism of neutralization has been attributed to inhibition of attachment and also to inhibition of infection following entry into the host cell (228,239).

Whereas humoral immunity appears to have a protective role in chlamydial infection, cellular immunity appears to play a dual role, contributing to both protection and pathogenesis (240,241). In the monkey model of ocular *C. trachomatis* infection, a delayed-type hypersensitivity response is associated with trachoma, and in particular with recurrent exposure to a 57-kd protein that is a member of the heat shock family of proteins (242). Additionally, antibodies to the 57-kd protein are more prevalent in women with *C. trachomatis* infection in whom the scarring sequelae of infection, tubal factor infertility, and ectopic pregnancy develop (243,244). In humans, lymphocytes proliferate *in vitro* in response to *C. trachomatis* antigens after initial infection (245), but such proliferation may be impaired in chronic infections (246). Cytokines, in particular IFN-γ, may be important in *C. trachomatis* infection. Several studies have shown *in vitro* inhibition of the replication of *Chlamydia* by IFN-γ, and in a mouse model, depletion of IFN-γ resulted in exacerbation of infection (247–249).

Protection and pathogenesis in chlamydial infections are the result of different types of immune responses to different antigens. Protection seems to be mediated in part by neutralizing antibody responses to MOMP and IFN-γ suppression of chlamydial replication. Atypical persistent infections may be produced in response to low levels of IFN-γ (250), and scarring and fibrosis appear to be caused by recurrent infections eliciting a delayed-type hypersensitivity reaction to the 57-kd protein.

Epidemiology

C. trachomatis causes approximately 50 million new infections a year worldwide. It is the leading bacterial cause of STD in the United States, with an estimated 3 million infections in 2000. Teenagers account for 40% of these infections.(251,252). Since the first isolation of *C. trachomatis* from the rectum of a homosexual man (253), several studies have evaluated the rate of *C. trachomatis* infection of the urethra, cervix, and rectum in men and women (3,254–257). In one STD population, 5% of homosexual men and 14% of heterosexual men had *C. trachomatis* infections. Prevalence decreased in both groups in persons more than 19 years of age (258). A more recent evaluation of a population with STD found even higher rates of infection, with 18% of homosexual men and 20% of heterosexual men having *C. trachomatis* infection (223). Prevalence rates of anorectal infection are higher in both men and women with symptoms of proctitis than in asymptomatic patients. In women with anorectal *C. trachomatis* infection, rectal intercourse was associated with the presence of symptoms (256). Barnes et al. (259) compared serovars causing anorectal infection in homosexual and bisexual men with those causing cervical infections in heterosexual women in the same STD clinic. They demonstrated that 53% of rectal and 18% of cervical isolates were serovar D/D, whereas serovar E was present in 32% of cervical and 6% of rectal isolates. An update of this study reviewing 767 rectal *Chlamydia* isolates confirmed serovar D, which was detected in 41% of the isolates, as the predominant serovar in rectal infections in this population (260). The highly significant difference in serovar types from the two sites may be attributed to limited transmission between the two populations or to a decreased capability of certain serovars to survive at different mucosal sites.

Infections with the LGV biovar of *C. trachomatis* are endemic in eastern and western Africa, South America, and the Caribbean, but they occur only sporadically in the United States and Europe. In the United States, LGV infections are more common in homosexual than in heterosexual men. Anorectal LGV infections may occur as primary anorectal infections in homosexual men and heterosexual women practicing receptive anal intercourse, or they may be caused by spread from infected vaginal secretions in women or by lymphatic spread from genital infection.

Clinical Illness

The clinical presentation of anorectal *Chlamydia* infections ranges from asymptomatic to severe granulomatous proctitis, depending on the infecting immunotype, presence or absence of other rectal infection, size of the inoculum, and the patient's prior immunity to *C. trachomatis.* LGV serovars are more likely to cause severe disease than are non-LGV serovars. Quinn et al. (254) found that all asymptomatic homosexual men infected with *C. trachomatis* had non-LGV serovars (D/E, D/G, C/J), whereas all three patients with LGV serovars were symptomatic. The less invasive non-LGV serovars were associated with asymptomatic infection in 80% of cases. Certain non-LGV serovars may be more likely to cause symptomatic infection. Boisvert et al. (261) found that men with C-complex serovars were less likely than those with B-complex serovars to have symptomatic proctitis. On sigmoidoscopic examination of patients infected with non-LGV serovars, the mucosa may be normal or show focal areas of erythema, friability, and erosion. Corresponding histology shows neutrophil infiltration of the lamina propria and prominent follicles (254,262).

An LGV infection often causes severe proctocolitis with pruritus, purulent rectal discharge, diarrhea or constipation, hematochezia, fever, lymphadenopathy, and lower abdominal pain. The mucosa is usually friable or diffusely bloody with multiple ulcerations. Bauwens et al. (260) described five cases of proctitis with an L1 variant that appeared to be less virulent and associated with less severe clinical manifestations than an L2 infection. Typical histologic features of this lesion include diffuse inflammation with the presence of mononuclear cells, plasma cells, neutrophils, eosinophils, crypt abscesses, granulomas, and giant cells (254,255,263). The histopathology resembles that of Crohn disease, and misdiagnosis is possible.

If left untreated, anorectal LGV infection can progress to perirectal abscess with necrosis, fibrosis, stricture, stenosis, and fistula formation (264). The rectal strictures usually develop 2 to 5 cm above the anocutaneous margin, an area rich in lymphatics. The obstruction of lymphatic and venous drainage may cause perianal outgrowths of lymphatic tissue, called *lymphorrhoids* or *perianal condylomata,* to form (264).

Diagnosis

Rectal *Chlamydia* infection can be diagnosed by culture of rectal exudate in McCoy cells and identification of infected cells with a fluorescein-labeled monoclonal antibody to chlamydial antigens. Rompalo et al. (265) used the direct fluorescent antibody technique to evaluate rectal swab samples for *C. trachomatis* and found a 90% sensitivity and 100% specificity with this technique in comparison with culture. Immunoassays for chlamydial antigens are associated with high false-positive rates and are not helpful for rectal samples (266,267). Nucleic acid detection techniques, such as ligase chain reaction and PCR, have become widely available to identify *C. trachomatis* in genital and urine samples. These assays are 15% to 50% more sensitive than culture for genital samples; however, few studies have looked at the assays for anorectal samples, and they currently are not approved by the Food and Drug Administration for use on such samples (268).

The usefulness of serology for the diagnosis of rectal *Chlamydia* infection depends on the duration and extent of disease, previous exposure, and infecting serotype. The high percentage of adults with antibodies to *C. trachomatis* (80% to 90%) makes antibody detection in a single serum sample of little value in the diagnosis of non-LGV infections (262). In addition, the most specific serologic assay, the microimmunofluorescence test, is not widely available, is difficult to perform, and often detects cross-reactive antibodies with other chlamydial species (269–271). Seroconversion or more than a fourfold rise in the titer in acute and convalescent sera by microimmunofluorescence has been used as supportive evidence of infection.

Treatment

C. trachomatis infections have been effectively treated with tetracycline, doxycycline, and erythromycin. *C. trachomatis* isolates resistant to doxycycline, azithromycin, and ofloxacin and associated with clinical treatment failure have been described and raise concerns regarding the future efficacy of these drugs (272). Currently, uncomplicated rectal infections with non-LGV biovars should be treated with 100 mg of doxycycline twice daily for 7 to 10 days (Table 27.3). A single dose of 1 g of oral azithromycin is as effective as a 7-day course of doxycycline for genital infections and has been recommended for uncomplicated rectal infections (273,274) (Table 27.3). Additionally, the high tissue levels and long half-life of azithromycin may make it effective in treating incubating syphilis. In persons unable to tolerate doxycycline, other regimens used for *Chlamydia* genital infections would be recommended. In pregnant women,

500 mg of erythromycin base four times daily for 7 days is recommended. In patients with stricture, antibiotics may reduce associated edema and inflammation, but surgical resection is usually necessary. If an alternate regimen is used, a test of cure should be performed.

E. HISTOLYTICA/E. DISPAR

Microbiology

Entamoeba histolytica and *Entamoeba dispar* belong to a family of amebae that includes several nonpathogenic species, such as *Entamoeba coli, Entamoeba hartmanni,* and *Entamoeba gingivalis* (275). Infection can be initiated by the ingestion of as little as a single *E. histolytica* cyst by a susceptible host. Excystation occurs in the small bowel; a metacystic ameba with four cystic nuclei is produced, from which eight metacystic trophozoites form by cytoplasmic division (276). Trophozoites multiply by binary fission in the colon and may either exist as commensals or cause invasive disease. Invasion of the colonic mucosa produces amebic dysentery, whereas invasion of the portal vein and hepatic parenchyma produces hepatic abscesses. Trophozoites are classified as pathogenic or nonpathogenic based on their ability to cause invasive disease. Pathogenic trophozoites can be distinguished from nonpathogenic forms by trophozoite isoenzyme (hexokinase, glucophosphoisomerase, and phosphoglucomutase) mobility on starch gel electrophoresis, referred to as *zymodeme analysis* (277). Pathogenic forms can also be identified by the presence of erythrophagocytosis (ingestion of red blood cells), which is characteristic of pathogenic *E. histolytica* (276). Other techniques, such as typing by monoclonal antibodies to surface antigens (278), nucleotide probe, and restriction fragment length polymorphism analysis of amplified PCR products, have also been used to distinguish pathogenic and nonpathogenic forms (279).

Pathogenesis and Immunity

Non-immune host factors play an important role in preventing invasive *E. histolytica* infection. Pancreatic proteases, bile salts, and colonic mucins all impede protozoal adherence (280). Intestinal colonization does not induce protective immunity because serum antibodies to *E. histolytica* do not develop in the absence of tissue invasion (281,282). In contrast, invasive infection invariably induces *E. histolytica*-specific antibodies in the serum that are associated with resistance to subsequent invasive amebiasis (283). The ability of the trophozoite to adhere to host cells is one of the most important determinants of virulence. Adherence must be established for the trophozoite to be able to lyse target cells (284,285). A key mechanism of protective immunity appears to be inhibition of adherence of the trophozoites to host cells. Petri et al. (286) isolated a 170-kd lectin galactose/*N*-acetyl-D-galactosamine (Gal/Gal NAc) that mediates adherence of the trophozoite to host cells. The 170-kd lectin is a subunit of a 260-kd surface protein. Serum *E. histolytica*-specific antibodies from immune persons primarily recognize the galactose-inhibitable 170-kd lectin, and adherence of the trophozoite can be prevented by human immune sera (287,288). The purified lectin, when used to immunize gerbils, protected them from the development of amebic liver abscess after infection with *E. histolytica* (289). Although this lectin plays a key role, other surface membrane lectins are also important for adherence (290).

A role for complement in the resolution of infection has been demonstrated by the complement-mediated killing of trophozoite with serum from healthy controls and from patients infected with *E. histolytica* and with high titers of antibody to *E. histolytica.* However, trophozoites causing invasive disease are resistant to complement-mediated lysis because of the degradation of complement components C3a and C5a by amebic cysteine proteases and inhibition of the assembly of the C8 and C9 membrane attack complex by the 170-kd subunit of *E. histolytica* (291,292).

Regarding cellular responses, antigen-driven lymphocyte proliferation and lymphokine production can be detected *in vitro* in invasive *E. histolytica* infection, as evidenced by antigen-specific lymphocyte proliferation and lymphokine production (293,294). *In vitro* lymphokine production is associated with macrophage-induced killing of the organisms (295). In addition, *E. histolytica* induces cytotoxic T-cell activity in patients with invasive amebiasis (293). The importance of cell-mediated immunity in limiting the extent of invasive disease is evidenced by the fact that fulminant amebiasis is seen most often in persons with impaired cell-mediated immunity, such as young pregnant women and persons on corticosteroid therapy (291). This indicates that patients with AIDS who are infected with invasive strains may be at increased risk for more severe disease.

Epidemiology

More than 10% of the world's population is believed to be infected with *E. histolytica/E. dispar* (291. Humans are the only reservoir of infection. Transmission is primarily by the waterborne route in areas of poverty and poor sanitation, so that the infection is endemic in many developing countries. In the United States, where the overall prevalence of infection is estimated to be 4% (291), most infections occur in mentally retarded persons, residents in long-term care facilities with poor personal hygiene, immigrants from and travelers to areas of endemicity, and homosexual men. In the largest cohort ever evaluated for *E. histolytica/E. dispar* infection in a developed country, 34,063 HIV-infected Americans, the incidence of *E. histolytica/E. dispar* infection was 13.5 per 10,000 person-years, and 92% of the infections occurred in homosexual men (296).

E. histolytica/E. dispar infection in homosexual men without a history of foreign travel was first reported in 1968 (1). Subsequent studies in the mid-1970s to mid-1980s documented a 20% to 40% prevalence of amebiasis in homosexual men in New York and San Francisco (297–300). Quinn et al. (254) detected *E. histolytica/E. dispar* in the stools of 28% of homosexual men in Seattle in the early 1980s and noted no significant difference in the prevalence of *E. histolytica* in homosexual men with (28.6%) and without (25%) gastrointestinal symptoms; 60% of symptomatic men with *E. histolytica/E. dispar* had co-infection with other pathogens. More recent studies in homosexual men from Los Angeles, Germany, and the United Kingdom found similar prevalence rates of 16% to 27% (301–303). Asymptomatic infections in this population undoubtedly facilitate transmission of the parasite.

Clinical Illness

E. histolytica and *E. dispar* may cause very different clinical syndromes. *E. dispar* colonizes only the intestine and has never been reported to cause symptomatic or invasive disease. Of *E. histolytica* infections, 90% are asymptomatic; the remaining 10% produce variable symptoms of colitis and extraintestinal disease. Amebic colitis in the homosexual population is characterized by the insidious onset of mild diarrhea, often accompanied by a bloody mucoid discharge, alternating with constipation; lower abdominal cramping and tenesmus are other symptoms. Chronic amebic colitis may be indistinguishable from inflammatory bowel disease; however, 90% of persons have *E. histolytica* antibodies. Fulminant colitis with severe diarrhea and fever is much less common but occurs with increased frequency in patients who are malnourished, receiving steroids, or pregnant (291). This form of amebic intestinal disease may progress to toxic megacolon and intestinal perforation and has a 50% mortality rate (291). Concurrent liver abscess is not uncommon. *E. histolytica* can also cause a granulomatous thickening of the bowel wall, referred to as an *ameboma* (304). These masses occur in 1% of patients with *E. histolytica* infections and are generally found in the terminal colon. Amebic liver abscess is the most common extraintestinal infection of *E. histolytica.* Other syndromes of extraintestinal amebiasis include pleuropulmonary, pericardial, and cerebral amebiasis. Cerebral amebiasis is found in 1.2% to 2.5% of patients with amebiasis at autopsy, although clinically it is seen in fewer than 0.1% of cases (285). Cutaneous infection with perianal ulcers has also been described (291).

Multiple studies have shown that homosexual men and persons with HIV/AIDS in developed countries are usually infected with "nonpathogenic" amebae (*E. dispar*), and therefore infection is usually asymptomatic (305,306). Conversion from nonpathogenic to pathogenic zymodemes has been reported from *in vitro* studies but has never been seen in serial isolates from infected patients (307).

Allason-Jones et al. (306) followed 55 HIV-infected and uninfected homosexual men with untreated nonpathogenic amebic infection for an average of 22 months and found a benign clinical course in all. In fact, infection cleared spontaneously in 31%. Homosexual men are frequently infected with multiple intestinal protozoa; up to 68% have at least one other pathogen, and intestinal symptoms can generally be ascribed to the other pathogens, such as *Giardia* (296, 305).

Diagnosis

The diagnosis of *E. histolytica* infection is generally made by microscopic examination of a wet mount of fresh stool or a rectal swab. Because cyst shedding is intermittent, the diagnostic yield is increased by examining purged or multiple (three to six) samples of stool (308). It is important to distinguish *E. histolytica* cysts and trophozoites from those of the smaller, nonpathogenic *E. hartmanni* and from neutrophils (309). Stool microscopy is often insensitive, missing 50% to 66% of infections detected by culture (304).

Serology is helpful for diagnosing disease caused by invasive *E. histolytica. E. dispar* infections generally do not cause seroconversion. The indirect hemagglutination test is the most widely used serologic test, and the result is positive in 81% to 98% of patients with proctocolitis. A high titer (>1:512) is particularly suggestive of invasive disease (310). However, the result of this test can remain positive for more than 10 years after clinical and parasitologic cure. The agar gel diffusion, counterimmunoelectrophoresis, and enzyme immunoassay techniques are quite sensitive (positive results in 87% to 95% of patients with proctocolitis and 95% to 100% of patients with liver abscess), and they are more useful for identifying current infection because the results become negative 6 to 12 months after infection (311). Several stool antigen detection tests are currently commercially available that can detect both *E. histolytica* and *E. dispar* or specifically *E. histolytica* with better than 85% sensitivity and better than 90% specificity (304,310). These assays are now widely used in the diagnosis of this infection. Culture of the organism with zymodeme analysis remains the gold standard for diagnosis but is technically difficult, and a lack of wide availability limits the usefulness of this technique. PCR assays are being developed for use in stool samples, and studies indicate sensitivity and specificity similar to those of the antigen detection assays (311).

Treatment

Treatment for *E. dispar* infection is not recommended because it is always asymptomatic. Treatment of *E. histolytica* infection depends on the type of infection. Asymptomatic carriage of the organisms should be treated to prevent possible invasive disease and continued transmission of the infection. Three luminal amebicides are available to treat this type

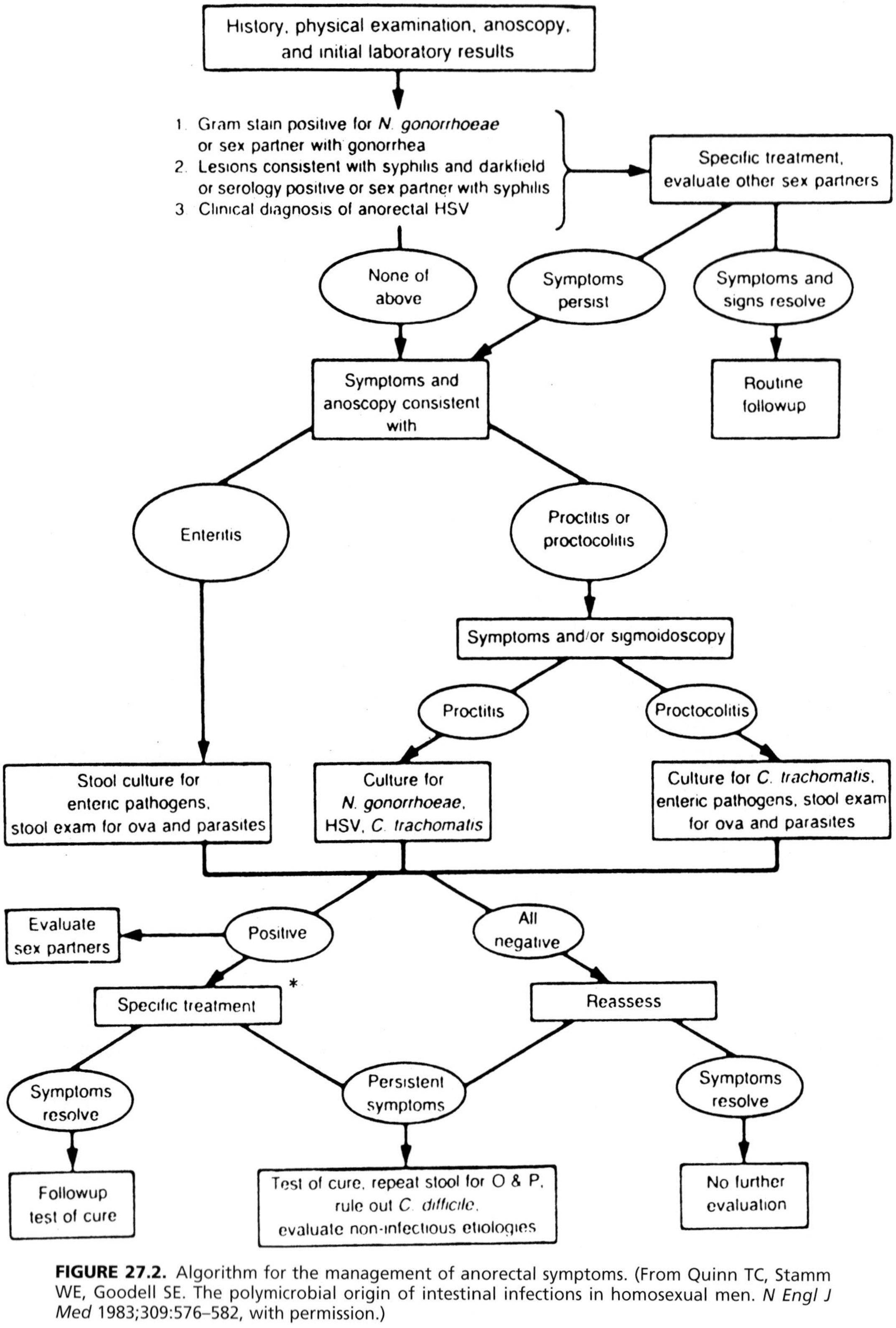

FIGURE 27.2. Algorithm for the management of anorectal symptoms. (From Quinn TC, Stamm WE, Goodell SE. The polymicrobial origin of intestinal infections in homosexual men. *N Engl J Med* 1983;309:576–582, with permission.)

of infection. Paromomycin (25 to 30 mg/kg per day in three doses for 7 days) is active in asymptomatic infections (312) (Table 27.3). Two cases of irreversible deafness caused by the use of paromomycin with neomycin have been reported. Iodoquinol (650 mg orally three times per day for 20 days) is generally well tolerated but should not be used in patients allergic to iodine. A few cases of optic atrophy, one leading to blindness, have been reported in patients given doses higher than those typically used for amebiasis (313,314). Diloxanide furoate (500 mg three times per day for 10 days) is widely used outside the United States for asymptomatic and mildly symptomatic infections and is available in the United States from the Centers for Disease Control and Prevention (304). Parasitologic cure with this agent approaches 90%, similar to the rates for iodoquinol and paromomycin; side effects include flatulence, diarrhea, abdominal cramping, nausea, and headache (315).

Invasive intestinal disease should be treated with metronidazole (750 mg three times per day for 10 days) (291,304). This drug is well absorbed and achieves good tissue levels but does not eradicate organisms in the lumen, so that paromomycin (500 mg orally three times per day for 7 days) or iodoquinol (650 mg three times per day for 20 days) should be given subsequently (316). Complete resolution of liver abscess may take up to 2 years. An alternate regimen for invasive disease is dihydroemetine (1.5 mg/kg per day intramuscularly for up to 5 days; maximum, 90 mg/d), or emetine (1 mg/kg per day intramuscularly for up to 5 days) followed by paromomycin or iodoquinol. These drugs also are available in the United States only from the Centers for Disease Control and Prevention. Metronidazole-resistant *E. histolytica* has never been reported. A lack of response in a patient with liver abscess is an indication for drainage and necessitates prolonged treatment with metronidazole (291,303).

CONCLUSION

Anorectal infections are common primarily in homosexual men and heterosexual women who practice receptive anal intercourse. The etiology is usually polymicrobial and the symptoms are variable depending on the pathogen and location of infection (anus vs. rectum). Because of the asymptomatic nature of some of these infections, levels of transmission and complication rates are high. A review of the sexual history and an anoscopic examination should be considered in a patient at risk for such infections and also in any patient with a relevant or suspect perianal lesion. Appropriate management, outlined in Fig. 27.2, should involve the treatment of partners and follow-up evaluation for persistent infection. It is important to remember that patients presenting with anorectal infections are at risk for HIV infection and that the presentation and response to therapy may be altered; additionally, associated conditions, such as malignancy, may develop.

REFERENCES

1. Most H. Manhattan: "a tropic isle"? *Am J Trop Med Hyg* 1968; 217:333–354.
2. Sohn N, Robilotti JG Jr. The gay bowel syndrome. *Am J Gastroenterol* 1977;67:478–484.
3. Quinn TC, Stamm WE, Goodell SE. The polymicrobial origin of intestinal infections in homosexual men. *N Engl J Med* 1983; 309:576–582.
4. Ekstrand ML, Stall RD, Paul JP, et al. Gay men report high rates of unprotected anal sex with partners of unknown or discordant HIV status. *AIDS* 1999;13:1525–1533.
5. Kim LS, Stansell J, Cello JP, et al. Discrepancy between sex and water-associated risk behaviors for cryptosporidiosis among HIV-infected patients in San Francisco. *J Acquir Immune Defic Syndr Hum Retrovirol* 1998;19:44–49.
6. Simon PA, Thometz E, et al. Prevalence of unprotected sex among men with AIDS in Los Angeles County, California, 1995–1997. *AIDS* 1999;13:987–990.
7. Centers for Disease Control and Prevention. Increases in unsafe sex and rectal gonorrhea among men who have sex with men—San Francisco, California, 1994–1997. *MMWR Morb Mortal Wkly Rep* 1999;48:45–48.
8. Ruiz J, Facer M, Sun RK. Risk factors for HIV and unprotected anal intercourse among young men who have sex with men. *Sex Transm Dis* 1998;25:100–107.
9. Katz MH, McFarland W, et al. Continuing high prevalence of HIV risk behaviors among young men who have sex with men: the young men's survey in San Francisco Bay Area in 1992–1993 and in 1994–1995. *J Acquir Immune Defic Syndr Hum Retrovirol* 1998;19:178–181.
10. Scheer S, Chu PL, et al. Effect of highly active antiretroviral therapy on diagnoses of sexually transmitted diseases in people with AIDS. *Lancet* 2001;357:432–435.
11. Medland N. Sexually transmitted diseases in HIV-1 infected patients. *Lancet* 2001;357:1533.
12. Bolling DR Jr. Prevalence, goals and complications of heterosexual anal intercourse in a gynecologic population. *J Reprod Med* 1977;19:120–124.
13. Gross M, Holt SE, Marmor M, et al. Anal sex among HIV-seronegative women at high risk for HV exposure. *J Acquir Immune Defic Syndr Hum Retrovirol* 2000;24:393–398.
14. Ostergaard L, Agner T, Krarup E, et al. PCR for detection of *Chlamydia trachomatis* in endocervical, urethral, rectal and pharyngeal swab samples obtained from patients attending an STD clinic. *Genitourin Med* 1997;73:493–497.
15. Spiro HM. *Clinical gastroenterology,* second edition. New York: Macmillan, 1977:881.
16. Roizman B. Herpesviridae: a brief introduction. In: Fields BN, ed. *Virology* 2nd ed. New York: Raven Press, 1990:1787–1789.
17. Spear GP. Biology of the herpesviruses. In: Holmes KK, ed. *Sexually transmitted diseases,* second edition. New York: McGraw-Hill, 1990:379–389.
18. Mertz GJ. Genital herpes simplex virus infections. *Med Clin North Am* 1990;74:1433–1454.
19. Whitley RJ, Roziman R. Herpes simplex virus infections. *Lancet* 2001;357:1513–1518.
20. Roizman BB. Herpes viruses and their replication. In: Fields BN, ed. *Virology* 2nd ed. New York: Raven Press, 1990:1795.

21. Mirdel A, ed. *Herpes simplex virus.* New York: Springer-Verlag, 1989:15–18.
22. Roizman B. Introduction: objectives of herpes simplex virus vaccines seen from a historical perspective. *Rev Infect Dis* 1991; 13[Suppl 11]:S892–S894.
23. Ashley R, Koelle DM. Immune responses to genital herpes infection. In: Quinn TC, ed. *Advances in host defense mechanisms,* vol 8. *Sexually transmitted diseases.* New York: Raven Press, 1992:201–331.
24. Shore SL, Cromeons TL, Romano JJ. Immune destruction of virus-infected cells early in the infection cycle. *Nature* 1976; 262:695–696.
25. Highlander SL, Cai W, Person S, et al. Monoclonal antibodies define a domain on herpes simplex virus glycoprotein B involved in virus penetration. *J Virol* 1988;62:1881–1888.
26. Prober CG, Sullender WM, Yasukawa LL, et al. Low risk of herpes simplex virus infections in neonates exposed to the virus at the time of vaginal delivery to mothers with recurrent genital herpes simplex virus infections. *N Engl J Med* 1987;316:240–244.
27. Brown ZA, Benedetti J, Ashley R, et al. Neonatal herpes simplex virus infection in relation to asymptomatic maternal infection at the time of labor. *N Engl J Med* 1991;324:1247–1252.
28. Merriman H, Woods S, Winter C, et al. Secretory IgA antibody in cervicovaginal secretions in women with genital herpes simplex virus infection. *J Infect Dis* 1984;149:505–510.
29. Pollard RB, Arvin AM, Gamberg P, et al. Specific cell-mediated immunity and infections with herpes viruses in cardiac transplant recipients. *Am J Med* 1982;73:679–687.
30. Meyers JD, Fluornoy N, Thomas ED. Infection with herpes simplex virus and cell-mediated immunity after marrow transplant. *J Infect Dis* 1980;142:338–346.
31. Quinnan GV, Masur H, Rook AH, et al. Herpesvirus infections in the acquired immune deficiency syndrome. *JAMA* 1984;252: 72–77.
32. Sullender WM, Miller JL, Yasukawa LL, et al. Humoral and cell-mediated immunity in neonates with herpes simplex virus infection. *J Infect Dis* 1987;155:28–37.
33. Toresth JW, Merigan TC. Significance of local gamma interferon in recurrent herpes simplex infection. *J Infect Dis* 1986; 153:979–983.
34. Linnavuori KH. History of recurrent mucocutaneous herpes correlates with relatively low interferon production by herpes simplex virus-exposed cultured monocytes. *J Med Virol* 1988; 25:61–68.
35. Cunningham AZ, Merigan TC. Gamma-interferon production appears to predict time of recurrence of herpes labialis. *J Immunol* 1983; 130:2397–2400.
36. Mertz GJ. Epidemiology of genital herpes infections. *Infect Dis Clin North Am* 1993;7:825–829.
37. Corey L, Holmes KK. Genital herpes simplex virus infections: current concepts in diagnosis, therapy and prevention. *Ann Intern Med* 1983;98:973–983.
38. Fleming DT, McQuillan GM, Johnson RE, et al. HSV-2 in the United States, 1976 to 1994. *N Engl J Med* 1997;337: 1105–1111.
39. Johnson RE, Nahmias AJ, et al. A seroepidemiologic survey of the prevalence of HSV-2 in the United States. *N Engl J Med* 1989;321:7–12.
40. Corey L. Genital herpes. In: Holmes KK, Mardh P, Sparling PF, et al., eds. *Sexually transmitted diseases,* second edition. New York: McGraw-Hill, 1990:391–414.
41. Guinan ME, Wolinsky SM, Reichman RC. Genital herpes simplex virus infection. *Epidemiol Rev* 1988;7:127.
42. Duenas A, Adam E, Melnick JZ, et al. Herpesvirus type 2 in a prostitute population. *Am J Epidemiol* 1972;95:483–489.
43. Mertz GJ, Benedetti J, Ashley R, et al. Risk factors for the sexual transmission of genital herpes. *Ann Intern Med* 1992;116: 197–202.
44. Holmberg SD, Stewart JA, Gerber AR, et al. Prior herpes simplex virus type 2 infection as a risk factor for HIV. *JAMA* 1988; 259:1048–1050.
45. Quinn TC. Epidemiology and serologic evidence for herpes simplex viruses in AIDS. In: Aurelian L, ed. *Herpes viruses, the immune system and AIDS.* Norwell, MA: Kluwer Academic Publishers, 1990:1–20.
46. Hook EW III, Cannon RO, Nahmias AJ, et al. Herpes simplex virus infection as a risk factor for human immunodeficiency virus infection in heterosexuals. *J Infect Dis* 1992;165:251–255.
47. Schacker T, Rynzarz AJ, et al. Frequent recovery of HIV-1 from genital HSV lesions in HIV-1 infected men. *JAMA* 1998;280: 61–66.
48. Golden MP, Kim S, Hammer SM, et al. Activation of human immunodeficiency virus by herpes simplex virus. *J Infect Dis* 1992;166:494–499.
49. Corey L, Adams HG, Brown ZA, et al. Genital herpes simplex virus infection: clinical manifestations, course and complications. *Ann Intern Med* 1983;98:958–972.
50. Corey L, Spear PG. Infections with herpes simplex viruses. Parts 1 and 2. *N Engl J Med* 1986;314:686–691, 749–757.
51. Goodell SE, Quinn TC, Mkrtichian E, et al. Herpes simplex virus proctitis in homosexual men: clinical, sigmoidoscopic, and histopathological features. *N Engl J Med* 1983;308:868–871.
52. Samarasinghe RL, Oates JK, Maclennan IPD. Herpetic proctitis and sacral radiculomyelopathy: a hazard for homosexual men. *Br Med J* 1979;2:365–366.
53. Siegal FP, Lopez C, Hammer GS, et al. Severe acquired immunodeficiency in male homosexuals, manifested by chronic perianal ulcerative herpes simplex lesions. *N Engl J Med* 1981;305: 1439–1444.
54. Centers for Disease Control and Prevention. Revision of the CDC surveillance case definition for acquired immunodeficiency syndrome. *MMWR Morb Mortal Wkly Rep* 1987;36 [Suppl]:1–15.
55. Quinn TC, Corey L, Chaffee RG, et al. The etiology of anorectal infections in homosexual men. *Am J Med* 1981;71:395–406.
56. Koutsky LA, Stevens CE, Holmes KK, et al. Underdiagnosis of genital herpes by current clinical and viral-isolation procedures. *N Engl J Med* 1992;326:1533–1539.
57. Stalder H, Oxman MN, Herman K. Herpes simplex virus microneutralization: a simplification of the test. *J Infect Dis* 1975;131:423–430.
58. Ashley R, Cent A, Maggs V, et al. Inability of enzyme immunoassays to discriminate between infections with herpes simplex virus types 1 and 2. *Ann Intern Med* 1991;115:520–526.
59. Ashley RL, Mitoni J, Lee F, et al. Comparison of Western blot (immunoblot) and glycoprotein G-specific immunodot enzyme assay for detecting antibodies to herpes simplex virus types 1 and 2 in human sera. *J Clin Microbiol* 1988;26:662–667.
60. Cone RW, Hobson AC, Palmer J, et al. Extended duration of herpes simplex virus DNA in genital lesions detected by the polymerase chain reaction. *J Infect Dis* 1991;164:757–760.
61. Rompalo AM, Mertz GJ, Davis LG, et al. Oral acyclovir for treatment of first-episode herpes simplex virus proctitis. *JAMA* 1988;259:2879–2881.
62. Centers for Disease Control and Prevention. Sexually transmitted diseases treatment guidelines, 1998. *MMWR Morb Mortal Wkly Rep* 1998;47:1–116.
63. Douglas JM, Critchlow C, Benedetti J, et al. A double-blind study of oral acyclovir for suppression of recurrences of genital herpes simplex virus infection. *N Engl J Med* 1984;310: 1551–1556.
64. Corey L, McCutchan JA, Ronald AR, et al. Evaluation of new

anti-infective drugs for the treatment of genital infections due to herpes simplex virus. Infectious Diseases Society of America and the Food and Drug Administration. *Clin Infect Dis* 1992;15 [Suppl 1]:S99–S107.

65. Fletcher CV. Treatment of herpes virus infections in HIV-infected individuals. *Ann Pharmacother* 1992;26:955–962.
66. Drugs for sexually transmitted diseases. *Med Lett* 1991;33: 119–124.
67. Goldberg LH, Kaufman RH, Kurtz TO, et al. Continuous five-year treatment of patients with frequently recurring genital herpes simplex virus infection with acyclovir. *J Med Virol* 1993; [Suppl 1]:45–50.
68. Schacker T., Hui-lin H., Koelle DM, et al. Famciclovir for the suppression of symptomatic and asymptomatic herpes simplex virus reactivation in HIV-infected men. *JAMA* 1998;280:61–66.
69. Geers TA, Isada CM. Update on antiviral therapy for genital herpes infection. *Cleve Clin J Med* 2000; 67:567–572.
70. Lehrman SN, Douglas JM, Corey L, et al. Recurrent genital herpes and suppressive oral acyclovir therapy: relation between clinical outcome and *in vitro* drug sensitivity. *Ann Intern Med* 1986;104:786–790.
71. Whitley RJ, Gnann JW Jr. Acyclovir: a decade later. *N Engl J Med* 1992;327:782–789.
72. Parker AC, Craig JIO, Collins P, et al. Acyclovir-resistant herpes simplex virus infection due to altered DNA polymerase. *Lancet* 1987;2:1461.
73. Wade JC, McLaren C, Meyers JD. Frequency and significance of acyclovir-resistant herpes simplex virus isolated from marrow transplant patients receiving multiple courses of treatment with acyclovir. *J Infect Dis* 1983;148:1077–1082.
74. Hardy WD. Foscarnet treatment of acyclovir-resistant herpes simplex virus infection in patients with acquired immunodeficiency syndrome: preliminary results of a controlled, randomized, regimen-comparative trial. *Am J Med* 1992;92[Suppl 2A]:30S–35S.
75. Oliver NM, Collins P, Van der Meer J, et al. Biological and biochemical characterization of clinical isolates of herpes simplex virus type 2 resistant to acyclovir. *Antimicrob Agents Chemother* 1989;33:635–640.
76. Collins P, Larder BA, Oliver NM, et al. Characterization of a DNA polymerase mutant of herpes simplex virus from a severely immunocompromised patient receiving acyclovir. *J Gen Virol* 1989;70:375–382.
77. Safrin S. Treatment of acyclovir-resistant herpes simplex virus infections in patients with AIDS. *J AIDS* 1992;5[Suppl 1]: S29–S32.
78. Svennerholm B, Vahlne A, Lowhagen GB, et al. Sensitivity of HSV strains isolated before and after treatment with acyclovir. *Scand J Infect Dis* 1985; [Suppl 47]:149–154.
79. Safrin S, Berger TG, Gilson I, et al. Foscarnet therapy in five patients with AIDS and acyclovir-resistant varicella-zoster virus infection. *Ann Intern Med* 1991;115:19–21.
80. Safrin S, Kemmerly S, Plotkin B. Foscarnet-resistant herpes simplex virus infection in patients with AIDS. *J Infect Dis* 1994; 169:193–196.
81. Cotte L. Herpes simplex virus infection during foscarnet therapy. *J Infect Dis* 1992;166:447–448.
82. Wald A. New therapies and prevention strategies for genital herpes. *Clin Infect Dis* 1999;28[Suppl 1]:S4–S13.
83. Shah KV, Howley PM. Papillomaviruses. In: Fields BN, et al., eds. *Virology.* New York: Raven Press, 1990:1651.
84. Shah KV. Biology of human genital tract papillomaviruses. In: Holmes KK, ed. *Sexually transmitted diseases,* second edition. New York: McGraw-Hill, 1990:425–431.
85. Viscidi RP, Shah KV. Immune response to genital tract infections with human papillomaviruses. In: Quinn TC, ed. *Advances in host defense mechanisms,* vol 8. *Sexually transmitted diseases.* New York: Raven Press, 1982:239–260.
86. Androphy EJ, Hubbert NL, Schiller JT, et al. Identification of the HPV-16 E6 protein from transformed mouse cells and human cervical carcinoma cell lines. *EMBO J* 1987;6:989–992.
87. Seedorf K, Oltersdorf T, Krammer G, et al. Identification of early proteins of the human papilloma viruses type 16 (HPV-16) and type 18 (HPV-18) in cervical carcinoma cells. *EMBO J* 1987;6:139–144.
88. Reichman RC, Bonnez W. Papillomaviruses. In: Mandell G, Douglas RG Jr, Bennett JE, eds. *Principles and practice of infectious diseases,* third edition. New York: Churchill Livingstone, 1990:1191–1199.
89. Lorincz AT, Temple GF, Kurman RJ, et al. Oncogenic association of specific human papillomavirus types with cervical neoplasia. *J Natl Cancer Inst* 1987;79:671–677.
90. Brown DR, Fife KH. Human papillomavirus infections of the genital tract. *Med Clin North Am* 1990;74:1455–1485.
91. Rabbett WF. Juvenile laryngeal papillomatosis: the relation of irradiation to malignant degeneration in this disease. *Ann Otol Rhinol Laryngol* 1965;74:1149–1163.
92. Sandberg JP. Papillomavirus infections in animals. In: Syrjanen K, et al., eds. *Papillomaviruses and human diseases.* Berlin: Springer-Verlag, 1987:240.
93. Shah KV. Human papillomaviruses and anogenital cancers. *N Engl J Med* 1997;337:1386–1388.
94. Sedlacek TV. Advances in the diagnosis and treatment of human papillomavirus infections. *Clin Obstet Gynecol* 1999;42: 206–220.
95. Schneider A, Holtz M, Gissmann L. Increased prevalence of human papillomaviruses in the lower genital tract of pregnant women. *Int J Cancer* 1987;40:198–201.
96. Rudlinger RM, Smith JW, Bunney MH, et al. Human papillomavirus infections in a group of renal transplant patients. *Br J Dermatol* 1986;115:681–692.
97. Bernard C, Mougin C, Madoz L, et al. Viral co-infections in human papillomavirus-associated anogenital lesions according to the serostatus for the human immunodeficiency virus. *Int J Cancer* 1992;52:731–737.
98. Li C-CH, Shah KV, Seth A, et al. Identification of the human papillomavirus type 6b L1 open reading frame protein in condylomas and corresponding antibodies in human sera. *J Virol* 1987;61:2684–2690.
99. Jenison SA, Yu X-P, Valentine JM, et al. Evidence of prevalent genital-type human papillomavirus infections in adults and children. *J Infect Dis* 1990;162:60–69.
100. Galloway DA, Jenison SA. Characterization of the humoral immune response to genital papillomaviruses. *Mol Biol Med* 1990;7:59–72.
101. Bonnez W, DaRin C, Rose RC, et al. Use of human papillomavirus type II virions in an ELISA to detect specific antibodies in humans with condylomata acuminata. *J Gen Virol* 1991; 72:1343–1347.
102. Dillner J. Mapping of linear epitopes of human papillomavirus type 16: the E_1, E_2, E_3, E_4, E_5, E_6, and E_7 open reading frames. *Int J Cancer* 1990;46:703–711.
103. Mann VM, Loud de Lao, Brenes M, et al. Occurrence of IgA and IgG antibodies to select peptides representing human papillomavirus type 16 among cervical cancer cases and controls. *Cancer Res* 1990;50:7815–7819.
104. Bleul C, Muller M, Frank R, et al. Human papillomavirus (HPV) type 18 E6 and E7 antibodies in human sera: increased anti-E7 prevalence in cervical cancer patients. *J Clin Microbiol* 1991;29:1579–1588.
105. Jochmus-Kudielka J, Schneider A, Braun R, et al. Antibodies against the human papillomavirus type 16 early proteins in

human sera: correlation of anti-E7 reactivity with cervical cancer. *J Natl Cancer Inst* 1989;81:1698–1704.

106. Malejczyk J, Malejczyk M, Majewski S, et al. NK-cell activity in patients with HPV 16-associated anogenital tumors: defective recognition of HPV 16-harboring keratinocytes and restricted unresponsiveness to immunostimulatory cytokines. *Int J Cancer* 1993;53:917–921.
107. Evans CH, Flugelman AA, DiPaolo JA. Cytokine modulation of immune defenses in cervical cancer. *Oncology* 1993;50:245–251.
108. Woodworth CD, Lichti U, Simpson S, et al. Leukoregulin and gamma-interferon inhibit human papillomavirus type 16 gene transcription in human papillomavirus-immortalized human cervical cells. *Cancer Res* 1992;52:456–463.
109. Vernon SD, Hart CE, Reeves WC, et al. The HIV-1 tat protein enhances E2-dependent human papillomavirus 16 transcription. *Virus Res* 1993;27:133–145.
110. Centers for Disease Control and Prevention. Biennial report. *Tracking the hidden epidemics: trends in STDs in the United States, December, 2000.* Atlanta, GA: Centers for Disease Control and Prevention, 2001.
111. de Villiers EM, Wagner D, Schneider A, et al. Human papillomavirus infections in women with and without abnormal cervical cytology. *Lancet* 1987;2:703–706.
112. Reeves WC, Arosemena JR, Garcia M, et al. Genital human papillomavirus infection in Panama City prostitutes. *J Infect Dis* 1989;160:599–603.
113. Koutsky LA, Galloway DA, Holmes KK. Epidemiology of genital human papillomavirus infection. *Epidemiol Rev* 199;10: 122–163.
114. Carr J, Gyorfi T. Human papillomavirus epidemiology, transmission, and pathogenesis. *Clin Lab Med* 2000; 20:235–255.
115. Lancaster WD, Jenson AB. Natural history of human papillomavirus infection of the anogenital tract. *Cancer Metastasis Rev* 1987;6:653–664.
116. Daling JR, Weiss NS, et al. Correlates of homosexual behavior and incidence of anal cancer. *JAMA* 1982;247:1988–1990.
117. Palefsky JM, Gonzalez J, et al. Anal intraepithelial neoplasia and anal papillomavirus infection among homosexual males with group IV HIV disease. *JAMA* 1990;263:2911–2916.
118. Scholefield JH, Sonnex C, Talbot IC, et al. Anal and cervical intraepithelial neoplasia: possible parallel. *Lancet* 1989;2: 765–769.
119. Critchlow CW, Sirawocz CM. Prospective study of high-grade anal squamous intraepithelial neoplasia in a cohort of homosexual men: influence of HIV infection, immunosuppression, and HPV infection. *AIDS* 1995;9:1255–1262.
120. Kiviat NB, Critchlow CW, Holmes KK, et al. Association of anal dysplasia and human papillomavirus with immunosuppression and HIV infection among homosexual men. *J AIDS* 1993;7:43–49.
121. Palefsky JM, Holly EA, Gonzales J, et al. Natural history of anal cytologic abnormalities and papillomavirus infection among homosexual men with group IV HIV disease. *J AIDS* 1992;5: 1258–1265.
122. Kiviat N, Rompalo A, Bowden R, et al. Anal human papillomavirus infection among human immunodeficiency virus-seropositive and -seronegative men. *J Infect Dis* 1990;163: 358–361.
123. Caussy D, Goedert JJ, Palefsky J, et al. Interaction of human immunodeficiency and papilloma viruses: association with anal epithelial abnormality in homosexual men. *Int J Cancer* 1990; 46:214–219.
124. Palefsky JM, Holly EA, et al. Virologic, immunologic, and clinical parameters in the incidence and progression of squamous intraepithelial lesions in HIV-positive and HIV-negative homosexual men. *J Acquir Immune Defic Syndr Hum Retrovirol* 1998; 17:314–319.
125. Goldie SJ, Kuntz KM, et al. Clinical effectiveness and cost effectiveness of screening for anal squamous intraepithelial lesion in homosexual and bisexual HIV-positive men. *JAMA* 1999;281:1822–1829.
126. Pyrohen S, Johansson E. Regression of warts: an immunological study. *Lancet* 1975;1:592–596.
127. Velasco J, Palacio V, Vazquez S, et al. Diagnostic accuracy of the cytologic diagnosis of anal human papillomavirus infection compared with DNA hybridization studies. *Sex Transm Dis* 1993;20:147–151.
128. Law CLH, Qassim M, Thompson CH, et al. Factors associated with clinical and subclinical anal human papillomavirus infection in homosexual men. *Genitourin Med* 1991;67:92–98.
129. Snijders PJF, Meijer CJLM, Walboomers JMM. Degenerate primers based on highly conserved regions of amino acid sequence in papillomaviruses can be used in a generalized polymerase chain reaction to detect productive human papillomavirus infections. *J Gen Virol* 1991;72:2781–2786.
130. Evander M, Wadell G. A general primer pair for amplification and detection of genital human papillomavirus types. *J Virol Methods* 1991;31:239–250.
131. Snijders PJF, Schulten EAJM, Mullink H. Detection of human papillomavirus and Epstein–Barr virus DNA sequences in oral mucosa of HIV-infected patients by the polymerase chain reaction. *Am J Pathol* 1990;137:659–666.
132. Kuyers JM, Critchlow CW, et al. Comparison of dot filter hybridization, southern transfer hybridization and PCR amplification for diagnosis of anal HPV infection. *J Clin Microbiol* 1993;31:1003–1006.
133. Pizzighella A, Rassu M, Piacentini I, et al. Polymerase chain reaction amplification and restriction enzyme typing as an accurate and simple way to detect and identify human papillomaviruses. *J Med Microbiol* 1993;39:33–38.
134. Bashi SA. Cryotherapy versus podophyllin in the treatment of genital warts. *Int J Dermatol* 1985;24:535–536.
135. Simmons PD, Langlet F, Thin RNT. Cryotherapy versus electrocautery in the treatment of genital warts. *Br J Vener Dis* 1981;57:273–274.
136. Simmons PD. Podophyllin 10% and 25% in the treatment of anogenital warts. *Br J Vener Dis* 1981;57:208–209.
137. Abdullah AN, Walzman M, Wade A. Treatment of external genital warts comparing cryotherapy (liquid nitrogen) and trichloracetic acid. *Sex Transm Dis* 1993;20:334.
138. Beutner KR, Wiley DJ, et al. Genital warts and their treatment. *Clin Infect Dis* 1999;28[Suppl 1]:S37–S56.
139. Reichman RC, Strike DG. Pathogenesis and treatment of human genital papillomavirus infections: a review. *Antiviral Res* 1989;11:109–118.
140. Jensen SL. Comparison of podophyllin application with simple surgical excision in clearance and recurrence of perinatal condylomata acuminata. *Lancet* 1985;12:1146–1147.
141. Musher DM. Biology of *Treponema pallidum.* In: Holmes KK, Mardh P, Sparling PF, et al., eds. *Sexually transmitted diseases,* second edition. New York: McGraw-Hill, 1990:205–209.
142. Tramont EC. *Treponema pallidum.* In: Mandell GL, Douglas RG Jr, Bennett JE, eds. *Principles and practice of infectious diseases,* third edition. New York: Churchill Livingstone, 1990: 1794–1807.
143. Baker-Zander SA, Lukehart SA. Macrophage-mediated killing of opsonized *Treponema pallidum. J Infect Dis* 1992;165:69–74.
144. Sell S, Hsu P-L. Delayed hypersensitivity, immune deviation, antigen processing and T-cell subset selection in syphilis pathogenesis and vaccine design. *Immunol Today* 1993;14:576–582.

145. Fitzgerald TJ. Pathogenesis and immunology of *Treponema pallidum. Annu Rev Microbiol* 1981;35:29–54.
146. Lukehart SA. Immunology and pathogenesis of syphilis. In: Gallin J, Fauci AS, eds. Quinn TC, guest ed. *Advances in host defense mechanisms.* New York: Raven Press, 1991:141–163.
147. Sell S, Norris SJ. The biology, pathology and immunology of syphilis. *Int Rev Exp Pathol* 1983;24:203–276.
148. Schell R, Marker D, eds. *Pathogenesis and immunology of treponemal infection.* New York: Marcel Dekker Inc, 1983.
149. Shulkin D, Trippoli L, Abell E. Lues maligna in a patient with human immunodeficiency virus infection. *Am J Med* 1988;85: 425–427.
150. Gregory N, Sanchez M, Buchness MR. The spectrum of syphilis in patients with human immunodeficiency virus infection. *J Am Acad Dermatol* 1990;22:1061–1067.
151. Goldmeier D, Hay P. A review and update on adult syphilis, with particular reference to its treatment. *Int J STD AIDS* 1993;4:70–83.
152. Medici MA. The immunoprotective niche: a new pathogenic mechanism for syphilis, the systemic mycoses and other infectious diseases. *J Theor Biol* 1972;36:617–625.
153. Marshak LC, Rothman S. Skin testing with purified suspension of *Treponema pallidum. Am J Syph* 1951;35:35–41.
154. Hook EW III, Mara CM. Acquired syphilis in adults. *N Engl J Med* 1992;326:1060–1069.
155. Centers for Disease Control and Prevention. Syphilis, United States. *MMWR Morb Mortal Wkly Rep* 1984;33:433–441.
156. Centers for Disease Control and Prevention. Primary and secondary syphilis—United States, 1981–1990. *MMWR Morb Mortal Wkly Rep* 1991;40:314–323.
157. Rolfs RT, Nakashima AK. Epidemiology of primary and secondary syphilis in the United States, 1981 through 1989. *JAMA* 1990;264:1432–1437.
158. Centers for Disease Control and Prevention. Primary and secondary syphilis—United States, 1999. *MMWR Morb Mortal Wkly Rep* 2001;50:113–116.
159. Centers for Disease Control and Prevention. Outbreak of syphilis among men who have sex with men—Southern California, 2000. *MMWR Morb Mortal Wkly Rep* 2001;50:117–119.
160. Stamm WE, Handsfield HH, Rompalo AM, et al. The association between genital ulcer disease and acquisition of HIV infection in homosexual men. *JAMA* 1988;260:1429–1433.
161. Quinn TC, Cannon RO, Glasser D, et al. The association of syphilis with risk of human immunodeficiency virus infection in patients attending STD clinics. *Arch Intern Med* 1990;150: 1297–1302.
162. Darrow WW, Echenberg DF, Jofee HW, et al. Risk factors for HIV infections in homosexual men. *Am J Public Health* 1987; 77:479–483.
163. British Cooperative Clinical Group. Homosexuality and venereal disease in the United Kingdom: a second study. *Br J Vener Dis* 1980;56:6–11.
164. Quinn TC, Stamm WE. Proctitis, proctocolitis, enteritis and esophagitis in homosexual men. In: Holmes KK, Mardh P, Sparling PF, et al., eds. *Sexually transmitted diseases,* second edition. New York: McGraw-Hill, 1990:663–684.
165. Mirdel A, Tovey SJ, Timmins DJ, et al. Primary and secondary syphilis: 20 years' experience. Clinical features. *Genitourin Med* 1989;65:1–3.
166. Bassi O, Cosa G, Colavolpe A, et al. Primary syphilis of the rectum—endoscopic and clinical features: report of a case. *Dis Colon Rectum* 1991;34:1024–1026.
167. Akdamar K, Martin RJ, Ichinose H. Syphilitic proctitis. *Dig Dis Sci* 1977;22:701–704.
168. Wexner SD. Sexually transmitted diseases of the colon, rectum, and anus. The challenge of the nineties. *Dis Colon Rectum* 1990; 33:1048–1062.
169. Quinn TC, Lukehart SA, Goodell SE, et al. Rectal mass caused by *Treponema pallidum*: confirmation by immunofluorescent staining. *Gastroenterology* 1982;82:135–139.
170. Hutchinson CM, Hook EW. Syphilis in adults. *Med Clin North Am* 1990;74:1389–1416.
171. Surawicz CM, Goodell SE, Quinn TC. Spectrum of rectal biopsy abnormalities in homosexual men with intestinal symptoms. *Gastroenterology* 1986;91:651–659.
172. Smibert RM. The spirochetes. In: Buchanan RE, Gibbons NE, eds. *Bergey's manual of determinative bacteriology,* eighth edition. Baltimore: Williams & Wilkins, 1974:167.
173. Hook EW III, Roddy RE, Lukehart SA, et al. Detection of *Treponema pallidum* in lesion exudate with a pathogen-specific monoclonal antibody. *J Clin Microbiol* 1985;22:241–244.
174. Hicks CB, Benson PM, Cupton GR, et al. Seronegative secondary syphilis in a patient infected with the human immunodeficiency virus (HIV) with Kaposi sarcoma: a diagnostic dilemma [published erratum appears in *Ann Intern Med* 1987;107:946]. *Ann Intern Med* 1987;107:492–495.
175. Gregory N, Sanchez M, Brehness MR. The spectrum of syphilis in patients with human immunodeficiency virus infection. *J Am Acad Dermatol* 1990;22:1061–1067.
176. Tikjoh G, Russel M, Petersen CS, et al. Seronegative secondary syphilis in a patient with AIDS: identification of *Treponema pallidum* in a biopsy specimen. *J Am Acad Dermatol* 1991;24: 506–508.
177. Hutchinson CM, Rompalo AM, Reichart CA, et al. Characteristics of patients with syphilis attending Baltimore STD clinics: multiple high-risk subgroups and interactions with human immunodeficiency virus infection. *Arch Intern Med* 1991;151: 511–516.
178. Rompalo AM, Cannon RO, Quinn TC, et al. Association of biologic false-positive reactions for syphilis with human immunodeficiency virus infection. *J Infect Dis* 1992;165:1124–1126.
179. Johns DR, Tierney M, Felsenstein D. Alteration in the natural history of neurosyphilis by concurrent infection with the human immunodeficiency virus. *N Engl J Med* 1987;316:1569–1572.
180. Berry CD, Hooten TM, Collier C, et al. Neurologic relapse after benzathine penicillin therapy for secondary syphilis in a patient with HIV infection. *N Engl J Med* 1987;316:1587–1589.
181. Musher DM, Hamill RJ, Baughn RE. Effect of human immunodeficiency virus (HIV) infection on the course of syphilis and the response to treatment. *Ann Intern Med* 1990;113:872–881.
182. Telzak EE, Greenberg MSZ, Harrison J, et al. Syphilis treatment response in HIV-infected individuals. *AIDS* 1991; 5:591–595.
183. Sparling PF. Biology of *Neisseria gonorrhoeae.* In: Holmes KK, Mardh P, Sparling PF, et al., eds. *Sexually transmitted diseases,* second edition. New York: McGraw-Hill, 1990:131–147.
184. Morse SA, Johnson SR, Biddle JW, et al. High-level tetracycline resistance in *Neisseria gonorrhoeae* is the result of acquisition of streptococcal tetM determinant. *Antimicrob Agents Chemother* 1986;30:664–670.
185. Perine PL, Thornsberry C, Schalla W, et al. Evidence for two distinct types of penicillinase-producing *Neisseria gonorrhoeae. Lancet* 1977;2:993–995.
186. Robert M, Piot P, Falkow S. The etiology of gonococcal plasmids. *J Gen Microbiol* 1979;114:491–494.
187. Ison CA, Dillon JR, Tapsall JW. Epidemiology of global antibiotic resistance among *Neisseria gonorrhoeae* and *Haemophilus ducreyi. Lancet* 1998;351[Suppl 111]:8–11.
188. Fox KK, Knapp JS, Holmes KK, et al. Antimicrobial resistance in *Neisseria gonorrhoeae* in the United States 1988–1994: the

emergence of decreased susceptibility to the fluoroquinolones. *J Infect Dis* 1997;175:1396–1403.

189. Sparling PF. Biology of *Neisseria gonorrhoeae.* In: Holmes KK, Mardh P, Sparling PF, et al., eds. *Sexually transmitted diseases,* second edition. New York: McGraw-Hill, 1990:131–148.
190. Handsfield HH. *Neisseria gonorrhoeae.* In: Mandell G, Douglas RG Jr, Bennett JE, eds. *Principles and practice of infectious diseases,* third edition. New York: Churchill Livingstone, 1990: 1613–1631.
191. Plummer FA, Simonsen JN, Chubb H, et al. Epidemiologic evidence for the development of serovar-specific immunity after gonococcal infection. *J Clin Invest* 1989;83:1472–1476.
192. Elkins C, Sparling PF. Immunobiology of *Neisseria gonorrhoeae.* In: Quinn TC, Cates W, eds. *Advances in host defense mechanisms,* vol 8. *Sexually transmitted diseases.* New York: Raven Press, 1992:113–139.
193. Knapp JS, et al. Serological classification of *Neisseria gonorrhoeae* with use of monoclonal antibodies to gonococcal outer membrane protein I. *J Infect Dis* 1984;150:44–48.
194. Carbonetti NC, Simnand VS, Elkin C, et al. Construction of isogenic gonococci with variable porin structures: effect on susceptibility to human serum and antibiotics. *Mol Microbiol* 1990;4:1009–1018.
195. Hildebrandt JF, Mayer LW, Wang SP, et al. *Neisseria gonorrhoeae* acquire a new principal outer membrane protein when transformed to resistance to serum bactericidal activity. *Infect Immun* 1978;20:267–272.
196. Virji M, Fletcher JN, Zak H, et al. The potential protective effect of monoclonal antibodies to gonococcal outer membrane protein IA. *J Gen Microbiol* 1987;133:2639–2646.
197. Eisenstein BI, Lee TJ, Sparling PF. Penicillin sensitivity and serum resistance of strains of *Neisseria gonorrhoeae* causing disseminated gonococcal infection. *Infect Immun* 1977;15:834–841.
198. Apicella MA, Westerink MA, Morse SA, et al. Bactericidal antibody response of normal human serum to the lipooligosaccharide of *Neisseria gonorrhoeae. J Infect Dis* 1986;153:520–525.
199. Rice PA, Kasper DL. Characterization of serum resistance of *Neisseria gonorrhoeae* that disseminate: roles of blocking and outer membrane proteins. *J Clin Invest* 1982;70:157–167.
200. Virji M, Heckels JE. Location of a blocking epitope on outer-membrane protein III of *Neisseria gonorrhoeae* by synthetic peptide analysis. *J Gen Microbiol* 1989;135:1895–1899.
201. Sugasawara RJ, Cannon JG, Black WJ, et al. Inhibition of *Neisseria gonorrhoeae* attachment to HeLa cells with monoclonal antibody directed against protein II. *Infect Immun* 1983;42:980–985.
202. Fischer SH, Rest RF. Gonococci possessing only certain PII outer membrane proteins stimulate and adhere to neutrophils. *Infect Immun* 1988;56:1574–1579.
203. Blake MS. Functions of the outer membrane proteins of *Neisseria gonorrhoeae.* In: Jackson GG, Thomas H, eds. *The pathogenesis of bacterial infections.* Berlin: Springer-Verlag, 1985:51–66.
204. Black WJ, Schwalbe RS, Nachamkin I, et al. Characterization of *Neisseria gonorrhoeae* protein II phase variation by use of monoclonal antibodies. *Infect Immun* 1984;45:453–457.
205. Corbus BC, Corbus BC Jr. The cutaneous diagnosis of gonococcal infection. *JAMA* 1941;116:113–115.
206. Cooper MD, Moticka EJ. Cellular immune responses during gonococcal and meningococcal infections. *Clin Microbiol Rev* 1989;2[Suppl]:S29–S34.
207. Wyle FA, Rowlett C, Blumenthal T. Cell-mediated immune response in gonococcal infections. *Br J Vener Dis* 1977;55:353–359.
208. Centers for Disease Control and Prevention. Gonorrhea—United States, 1998. *MMWR Morb Mortal Wkly Rep* 2000;49: 538–542.
209. Centers for Disease Control and Prevention. Increase in unsafe sex and rectal gonorrhea among men who have sex with men—San Francisco, California, 1994–1997. *MMWR Morb Mortal Wkly Rep* 1999;48:45–48.
210. Centers for Disease Control and Prevention. Gonorrhea among men who have sex with men. Selected sexually transmitted diseases clinics 1993–1996. *MMWR Morb Mortal Wkly Rep* 1997; 46:889–893.
211. Klein EJ, Fisher LS, Chow AW, et al. Anorectal gonococcal infection. *Ann Intern Med* 1977;86:340–346.
212. Judson FN, Miller KG, Schaffnet TM. Screening for gonorrhea and syphilis in the gay baths: Denver, Colorado. *Am J Public Health* 1977;67:740–742.
213. McFarland L, Mietzner TA, Knapp JS, et al. Gonococcal sensitivity to fecal lipids can be mediated by an MTR independent mechanism. *J Clin Microbiol* 1983;18:121–127.
214. Coghill DV, Young H. Genital gonorrhoea in women: a serovar correlation with concomitant rectal infection. *J Infect* 1989;18: 131–141.
215. Quinn TC. Clinical approach to intestinal infections in homosexual men. *Med Clin North Am* 1986;70:611–634.
216. Pariser H, Marino AF. Gonorrhea: frequency of unrecognized reservoirs. *South Med J* 1970;63:198–202.
217. Eisenstein BI, Masi AT. Disseminated gonococcal infection (DGI) and gonococcal arthritis (GCA): I. Bacteriology, epidemiology, host factors, pathogen factors, and pathology. *Semin Arthritis Rheum* 1981;10;155–172.
218. McWhinney PHM, Langhorne P, Love WC, et al. Disseminated gonococcal infection associated with deficiency of the second component of complement. *Postgrad Med J* 1991;67: 297–298.
219. Harkness A. The pathology of gonorrhea. *Br J Vener Dis* 1948; 24:132.
220. Darcel DC, Felman YM, Riccardi NB. The utility of anoscopy in the rapid diagnosis of symptomatic anorectal gonorrhea in men. *Sex Transm Dis* 1981;8:16–17.
221. Deherogada P. Diagnosis of rectal gonorrhea by blind anorectal swabs compared with direct vision swabs taken via proctoscope. *Br J Vener Dis* 1977;53:311–313.
222. Koumas EH, Johnson RE, et al. Laboratory testing for *N. gonorrhoeae* by recently introduced nonculture tests: a performance review with clinical and public health considerations. *Clin Infect Dis* 1998;27:1171–1180.
223. Ciemins EC, Flood J, et al. Re-examining the prevalence of *Chlamydia trachomatis* infection among gay men with urethritis. *Sex Transm Dis* 2000;27:249–255.
224. Handsfield HH, Daly ZA, et al. Multicenter trial of single-dose azithromycin vs. ceftriaxone in the treatment of uncomplicated gonorrhea. *Sex Transm Dis* 1994;21:107–111.
225. Stephens RS, Kalman S, et al. Genome sequence of an obligate intracellular pathogen of humans: *Chlamydia trachomatis. Science* 1998;282:754–759.
226. Ward ME. The chlamydial developmental cycle. In: Barron AL, ed. *Microbiology of* Chlamydia. Boca Raton: CRC Press, 1988: 71–96.
227. Su H, Watkins NG, Zhang YX, et al. *Chlamydia trachomatis* host cell interactions; role of the *Chlamydia* major outer membrane protein as an adhesin. *Infect Immun* 1990;58:1017–1025.
228. Lawn AM, Blyth WA, Tavern J. Interactions of TRIC agents with macrophages and BHK-21 cells observed by electron microscopy. *J Hyg (London)* 1973;72:515–528.
229. Kuo CC. Cultures of *Chlamydia trachomatis* in mouse peritoneal macrophages: factors affecting organism growth. *Infect Immun* 1978;20:439.
230. Schachter J. Biology of *Chlamydia trachomatis.* In: Holmes KK, Mardh P, Sparling PF, et al., eds. *Sexually transmitted diseases,* second edition. New York: McGraw-Hill, 1990:167–180.

231. Brunham RC, Kuo CC, Cles L, et al. Correlation of host immune response with quantitative recovery of *Chlamydia trachomatis* from the human endocervix. *Infect Immun* 1983;39:1491–1494.
232. Schachter J, Cles LD, Ray RM, et al. Is there immunity to chlamydial infections of the human genital tract? *Sex Transm Dis* 1983;10:123–125.
233. Brunham RC, Peeling R, Maclean I, et al. Postabortal *Chlamydia trachomatis* salpingitis: correlating risk with antigen-specific serological responses and with neutralization. *J Infect Dis* 1987;155:749–755.
234. Caldwell HD, Perry LJ. Neutralization of *Chlamydia trachomatis* infectivity with antibodies to the major outer membrane protein. *Infect Immun* 1982;38:745–754.
235. Peeling R, Maclean IW, Brunham RC. *In vitro* neutralization of *Chlamydia trachomatis* with monoclonal antibody to an epitope on the major outer membrane protein. *Infect Immun* 1984;46:484–488.
236. Qu Z, Cheng X, de la Maza LM, et al. Characterization of a neutralizing monoclonal antibody directed at variable domain I of the major outer membrane protein of *Chlamydia trachomatis* C-complex serovars. *Infect Immun* 1993;61:1365–1370.
237. Stephens RS, Tam MR, Kuo CC, et al. Monoclonal antibodies to *Chlamydia trachomatis*: antibody specificities and antigen characterization. *J Immunol* 1982;128:1083–1089.
238. Zhang YX, Stewart SJ, Caldwell HD. Protective monoclonal antibodies to *Chlamydia trachomatis* serovar- and serogroup-specific major outer membrane protein determinants. *Infect Immun* 1989;57:636–638.
239. Su H, Caldwell HD. *In vitro* neutralization of *Chlamydia trachomatis* by monovalent fab antibody specific to the major outer membrane protein. *Infect Immun* 1991;59:2843–2845.
240. Morrison RP, Lyng K, Caldwell HD. Chlamydial disease pathogenesis. Ocular hypersensitivity elicited by a genus-specific 57-kd protein. *J Exp Med* 1989;169:663–675.
241. Morrison RP. Immune responses to *Chlamydia* are protective and pathogenic. In: Bowie WR, Caldwell HD, Jones RP, et al., eds. *Chlamydial infections.* Cambridge, UK: Cambridge University Press, 1990:164–172.
242. Morrison RP, Manning DS, Caldwell HD. Immunology of *Chlamydia trachomatis* infections. Immunoprotective and immunopathogenic responses. In: Gallin JJ, Fauci AS, eds. Quinn TC, guest ed. *Advances in host defense mechanisms.* New York: Raven Press, 1992:57–84.
243. Brunham RC, Peeling R, Maclean I, et al. *Chlamydia trachomatis*-associated ectopic pregnancy: serologic and histologic correlates. *J Infect Dis* 1992;165:1076–1081.
244. Brunham RC, Maclean IW, Binns B, et al. *Chlamydia trachomatis*: its role in tubal infertility. *J Infect Dis* 1985;152:1275–1282.
245. Brunham RC, Martin DH, Kuo CC, et al. Cellular immune response during uncomplicated genital infection with *Chlamydia trachomatis* in humans. *Infect Immun* 1981;34:98–104.
246. Young E, Taylor HR. Immune mechanisms in chlamydial eye infection: cellular immune responses in chronic and acute disease. *J Infect Dis* 1984;150:745–751.
247. Rothermel CD, Byrne GI, Havell EA. Effect of interferon on the growth of *Chlamydia trachomatis* in mouse fibroblasts (L cells). *Infect Immun* 1983;39:362–370.
248. Byrne GI, Rothermel CD. Differential susceptibility of chlamydiae to exogenous fibroblast interferon. *Infect Immun* 1983;39:1004–1005.
249. Williams DM, Grubbs BG, Schachter J, et al. Gamma interferon levels during *Chlamydia trachomatis* pneumonia in mice. *Infect Immun* 1993;61:3556–3558.
250. Beatty WL, Byrne GI, Morrison RP. Morphologic and antigenic characterization of interferon gamma-mediated persistent *Chlamydia trachomatis* infection *in vitro. Proc Natl Acad Sci U S A* 1993;90:3998–4002.
251. Global Programme on AIDS, World Health Organization. *An overview of selected curable sexually transmitted diseases.* Geneva: World Health Organization, 1999.
252. Centers for Disease Control and Prevention. Recommendations for the prevention and management of *Chlamydia trachomatis* infections, 1993. *MMWR Morb Mortal Wkly Rep* 1993;42:1–39.
253. Goldmeier D, Darougar S. Isolation of *Chlamydia trachomatis* from throat and rectum of homosexual men. *Br J Vener Dis* 1977;53:184–185.
254. Quinn TC, Goodell SE, Mkritchian E. *Chlamydia trachomatis* proctitis. *N Engl J Med* 1981;305:195–200.
255. Stamm WE, Quinn TC, Mkrtichian EE, et al. *Chlamydia trachomatis* proctitis. In: Mardh P-A, et al., eds. *Chlamydial infections.* London: Elsevier Science, 1982:111–114.
256. Thompson CI, MacAulay AJ, Smith IW. *Chlamydia trachomatis* infections in the female rectum. *Genitourin Med* 1989;65:269–273.
257. McMillan A, Sommerville RG, McKie PMK. Chlamydial infection in homosexual men. Frequency of isolation of *Chlamydia trachomatis* from the urethra, ano-rectum, and pharynx. *Br J Vener Dis* 1981;57:47–49.
258. Stamm WE, Koutsky LA, Benedetti JK, et al. *Chlamydia trachomatis* urethral infections in men. Prevalence, risk factors, and clinical manifestations. *Ann Intern Med* 1984;100:47–51.
259. Barnes RC, Rompalo AM, Stamm WE. Comparison of *Chlamydia trachomatis* serovars causing rectal and cervical infections. *J Infect Dis* 1987;156:953–958.
260. Bauwens JE, Lampe MF, et al. Infection with *Chlamydia trachomatis* lymphogranuloma venereum serovar L1 in homosexual men with proctitis: molecular analysis of an unusual case cluster. *Clin Infect Dis* 1995;20:576–581.
261. Boisvert JF, Koutsky LA, et al. Clinical features of *Chlamydia trachomatis* rectal infection by serovar among homosexually active men. *Sex Transm Dis* 1999;26:392–398.
262. Mardh P, Paavonen J, Puolakkainen M. *Chlamydia.* New York: Plenum Press, 1989:15–55.
263. Levine JS, Smith PD, Bragge WR. Chronic proctitis in male homosexuals due to lymphogranuloma venereum. *Gastroenterology* 1980;79:563–565.
264. Perine PL, Osoba AO. Lymphogranuloma venereum. In: Holmes KK, Mardh P, Sparling PF, et al., eds. *Sexually transmitted diseases,* second edition. New York: McGraw-Hill, 1990:195–204.
265. Rompalo AM, Suchland RJ, Price CB, et al. Rapid diagnosis of *Chlamydia trachomatis* rectal infection by direct immunofluorescence staining. *J Infect Dis* 1987;155:1075–1076.
266. Pratt BC, Tait IA, Anyaegbunam WI. Rectal carriage of *Chlamydia trachomatis* in women. *J Clin Pathol* 1989;42:1309–1310.
267. Riordon T, Ellis DA, Mathews PI, et al. False-positive results with an ELISA for detection of chlamydial antigen. *J Clin Pathol* 1986;39:1276–1277.
268. Hammerschlag MR, Laraque D. Inappropriate use of nonculture tests for detection of *Chlamydia trachomatis* in suspected victims of child sexual abuse: a continuing problem. *Pediatrics* 1999;104(5 Pt 1):1137–1139.
269. Treharne JD, Forsey T, Thomas BJ. Chlamydial serology. *Br Med Bull* 1983;39:194–200.
270. Saikku P. Chlamydial serology. *Scand J Infect Dis Suppl* 1982;31:34–37.
271. Wang SP, Kuo CC, Grayston JT. Formalinized *Chlamydia trachomatis* organisms as antigen in the micro-immunofluorescence test. *J Clin Microbiol* 1979;10:259–261.

272. Somani J, Bhullar VB, et al. Multiple drug-resistant *Chlamydia trachomatis* associated with clinical treatment failure. *J Infect Dis* 2000;181:1421–1427.
273. Stamm WE, Hicks CB, et al. Azithromycin for empiric treatment of nongonococcal urethritis syndrome in men. *JAMA* 1995;274:545–549.
274. Rompalo AM. Diagnosis and treatment of sexually acquired proctitis and proctocolitis: update. *Clin Infect Dis* 1999;28 [Suppl 1]:S84–S90.
275. Ravdin JI, Petri WA. *Entamoeba histolytica* (amebiasis). In: Mandell GL, Douglas RG Jr, Bennett JE, eds. *Principles and practice of infectious diseases,* third edition. New York: Churchill Livingstone, 1990:2036–2049.
276. Manson PEC, Bell DR. *Manson's tropical diseases,* nineteenth edition. London: Bailliere-Tindall, 1987:1243–1249 (*Medical protozoology,* appendix 1).
277. Sargeaunt PG, Williams JE, Greene JD. The differentiation of invasive and noninvasive *Entamoeba histolytica* by isoenzyme electrophoresis. *Trans R Soc Trop Med Hyg* 1978;72:519–521.
278. Petri WA Jr, Jackson TFHG, Gathiram V, et al. Pathogenic and nonpathogenic strains of *Entamoeba histolytica* can be differentiated by monoclonal antibodies to the galactose-specific adherence lecithin. *Infect Immun* 1990;58:1802–1806.
279. Zannich E, Horstmann RD, Knoblock J, et al. Genomic DNA differences between pathogenic and nonpathogenic *Entamoeba histolytica. Proc Natl Acad Sci U S A* 1989;86:5118–5122.
280. Petri WA, Clark G, Diamond LS. Host–parasite relationships in amebiasis: conference report. *J Infect Dis* 1994;169:483–484.
281. Goldmeier D, Price AB, Billington O. Is *Entamoeba histolytica* in homosexual men a pathogen? *Lancet* 1986;1:641–644.
282. Law C. Sexually transmitted diseases and enteric infections in the male homosexual population. *Semin Dermatol* 1990;9:178–184.
283. Patterson M, Healy GR, Shabot JM. Serologic testing for amebiasis. *Gastroenterology* 1980;78:136–141.
284. Ravdin JI, Guerrant RL. The role of adherence in cytopathogenic mechanisms of *Entamoeba histolytica.* Study with mammalian tissue culture cells and human erythrocytes. *J Clin Invest* 1981;68:1305–1313.
285. Ravdin JI, Croft BY, Guerrant RL. Cytopathogenic mechanisms of *Entamoeba histolytica. J Exp Med* 1980;152:377–390.
286. Petri WA, et al. Isolation of the galactose-binding lectin which mediates the *in vitro* adherence of *Entamoeba histolytica. J Clin Invest* 1987;80:1238–1244.
287. Petri WA. Recognition of the galactose- or *N*-acetylgalactosamine-binding lectin of *Entamoeba histolytica* by human immune sera. *Infect Immun* 1987;55:2327–2331.
288. Petri WA, Ravdin JI. Cytopathogenicity of *Entamoeba histolytica. Eur J Epidemiol* 1987;3:123–126.
289. Petri WA Jr, Ravdin JI. Protection of gerbils from amebic liver abscess by immunization with the galactose-specific adherence lectin of *Entamoeba histolytica. J Clin Invest* 1991;59:97–101.
290. Kobiler D, Mirelman D. Lectin activity in *Entamoeba histolytica* trophozoites. *Infect Immun* 1980;29:221–225.
291. Ravdin JI. Amebiasis. *Clin Infect Dis* 1995;20:143–166.
292. Braga LL, Ninomiya H, McCoy JJ, et al. Inhibition of the complement membrane attack complex by galactose-specific adhesion of *Entamoeba histolytica. Proc Natl Acad Sci U S A* 1991; 88:1849–1853.
293. Salata RA, Martinez-Palomo A, Murray HW, et al. Patients treated for amebic liver abscess develop a cell-mediated immune response effective *in vitro* against *Entamoeba histolytica. J Immunol* 1986;136:2633–2639.
294. Salata RA, Pearson RD, Ravdin JI. Interaction of human leukocytes with *Entamoeba histolytica.* Killing of virulent amebae by the activated macrophage. *J Clin Invest* 1985;76:491–499.
295. Salata RA, Martinez-Palomo A, Murray HW, et al. Patients treated for amebic liver abscess develop cell-mediated immune responses effective *in vitro* against *Entamoeba histolytica. J Immunol* 1986;136:2633–2639.
296. Lowther SA, Dworkin MS, Hanson DL, et al. *Entamoeba histolytica/Entamoeba dispar* infections in HIV-infected patients in the United States. *Clin Infect Dis* 2000;30:955–959.
297. Schmerin MJ, Gelston A, Jones TC. Amebiasis: an increasing problem among homosexuals in New York City. *JAMA* 1977;238:1387–1389.
298. Pomerantz BM, Marr JS, Goldman WD. Amebiasis in New York City 1958–1978: identification of the male homosexual high-risk population. *Bull N Y Acad Med* 1980;56:232–244.
299. Dritz SK, Ainsworth TE, Back A, et al. Patterns of sexually transmitted enteric disease in a city. *Lancet* 1977;2:3–4.
300. Pearce RB. Intestinal protozoal infections and AIDS. *Lancet* 1983;2:51.
301. Allason-Jones E, Mindel A, et al. *Entamoeba histolytica* as a commensal intestinal parasite in homosexual men. *N Engl J Med* 1986;315:353–356.
302. Weinke T, Freidrich-Janicke B, et al. Prevalence and clinical importance of *Entamoeba histolytica* in two high-risk groups: travelers returning from the tropics and male homosexuals. *J Infect Dis* 1990;161:1029–1031.
303. Sorvillo FJ, Strassburg MA, et al. Amebic infections in asymptomatic homosexual men, lack of evidence of invasive disease. *Am J Public Health* 1986;76:1137–1139.
304. Petri WA, Singh W. Diagnosis and management of amebiasis. *Clin Infect Dis* 1999;29:1117–1125.
305. Reed SL, Wess DW. *Entamoeba histolytica* infection and AIDS. *Am J Med* 1991;90:269–270.
306. Allason-Jones E, Mindel A, Sargeaunt P, et al. Outcome of untreated infection with *Entamoeba histolytica* in homosexual men with and without HIV antibody. *Br Med J* 1988;297: 654–657.
307. Mirelman D, Bracha R, Wexler A, et al. Changes in isoenzyme patterns of a cloned culture of nonpathogenic *Entamoeba histolytica* during axenization. *Infect Immun* 1986;54:827–832.
308. William DC. Amebiasis. In: Ostrow DG, Sandholzer TA, Felman YM, eds. *Sexually transmitted diseases in homosexual men: diagnosis, treatment and research.* New York: Plenum Publishing, 1983:87–98.
309. Garcia LS. Parasitic infections in the compromised host. In: Isenberg HD, ed. *Clinical microbiology updates,* vol 3, No 1. Sommerville, NJ: Hoechst-Roussel, 1992.
310. Pillai R, Keystone JS, et al. *Entamoeba histolytica* and *Entamoeba dispar*: epidemiology and comparison of diagnostic methods in a setting of nonendemicity. *Clin Infect Dis* 1999;29:1315–1318.
311. Haque R, Akther KM, Petri W. Comparison of PCR, isoenzyme analysis, and antigen detection for diagnosis of *Entamoeba histolytica* infection. *J Clin Microbiol* 1998;36:449–452.
312. Sullam PM, Slutkin G, Gottlieb AB, et al. Paromomycin therapy of endemic amebiasis in homosexual men. *Sex Transm Dis* 1986;13:151–155.
313. American Academy of Pediatrics Committee on Drugs. Blindness and neuropathy from diiodohydroxygenin-like drugs. *Pediatrics* 1974;54:378–379.
314. Behress MM. Optic atrophy in children after diiodohydroxygen therapy. *JAMA* 1974;228:693–694.
315. McAuley JB, Herwaldt BL, Stokes SL, et al. Diloxanide furoate for treating asymptomatic *Entamoeba histolytica* cyst passers: 14 years' experience in the United States. *Clin Infect Dis* 1992;15: 464–468.
316. Irusen EM, Jackson TFHG, Simjee AE. Asymptomatic intestinal colonization by pathogenic *Entamoeba histolytica* in amebic liver abscess: prevalence, response to therapy, and pathogenic potential. *Clin Infect Dis* 1992;14:889–893.

28

MICROBIAL AGENTS IN THE PATHOGENESIS, DIFFERENTIAL DIAGNOSIS, AND COMPLICATIONS OF INFLAMMATORY BOWEL DISEASES

R. BALFOUR SARTOR

Ulcerative colitis and Crohn's disease, collectively termed idiopathic inflammatory bowel diseases (IBDs), are chronic spontaneously relapsing disorders that affect between 500,000 and 1 million persons in the United States (1). Microbial agents appear to be intimately involved in the pathogenesis of these disorders and contribute to some of their most frequent complications (2–6). Although it remains unclear whether specific infections initiate chronic relapsing inflammation, it is apparent that common pathogens can reactivate underlying intestinal inflammation and produce disease in normal hosts that closely mimics idiopathic IBD. Moreover, ubiquitous intestinal bacteria seem to be essential in perpetuating chronic inflammation and in causing the frequent suppurative complications of Crohn's disease. This chapter discusses current evidence that IBD is caused by a persistent pathogen or by an abnormal profile of resident bacteria, examines the role of resident luminal bacteria in its pathogenesis, outlines ways to distinguish intestinal inflammation caused by pathogens from idiopathic IBD, identifies pathogens that can reactivate or suprainfect established ulcerative colitis and Crohn's disease, and discusses ways to recognize and treat the frequent septic complications of IBD.

ETIOLOGIC CONSIDERATIONS: ARE CROHN'S DISEASE AND ULCERATIVE COLITIS CAUSED BY MICROBIAL AGENTS?

Ulcerative colitis and Crohn's disease are idiopathic disorders characterized by an unrestrained inflammatory response, but the factors initiating and perpetuating this chronic immune reaction remain unclear (7). Genetic and environmental contributions are evident. Microbial influences on the pathogenesis of these disorders are strongly supported by observations that IBD occurs in the distal intestine (the area of highest luminal bacterial concentrations), that patients with Crohn's disease clinically improve when luminal bacterial concentrations are decreased, and that ulcerative colitis and Crohn's disease closely resemble enterocolonic infections (2). Chronic IBD could be either a response to a specific pathogen or an inappropriate immunologic response to ubiquitous microbial constituents. Clinical and experimental data support six etiologic theories, as outlined in Table 28.1.

Persistent Pathogen

Because Crohn's disease closely resembles ileocecal tuberculosis (TB), *Yersinia* enteritis, and anorectal *Chlamydia* infections, and because ulcerative colitis mimics chronic *Campylobacter, Shigella,* and amebic colitis, investigators have diligently searched for specific pathogens in IBD. A number of organisms have been advanced as causes of ulcerative colitis and Crohn's disease (Table 28.2); most of these agents have not been confirmed by other investigators. Serum antibodies to various conventional pathogens are increased in IBD, particularly Crohn's disease (8,9) but may reflect an overly responsive immune reaction because antibody concentrations to a broad spectrum of commensal organisms are also increased (10–12). Sporadic reports of case clustering of Crohn's disease among family members, including spouses (13–15), and close friends (16) support an infectious origin of this disorder. Three pathogens are under active investigation as possible causes of Crohn's disease: *Mycobacterium paratuberculosis,* paramyxovirus (measles), and adherent/invasive *Escherichia coli.* Although

R. B. Sartor: Department of Medicine, Multidisciplinary Center for Inflammatory Bowel Disease Research and Treatment, University of North Carolina, Chapel Hill, North Carolina

TABLE 28.1. POSSIBLE MICROBIAL ETIOLOGIES OF INFLAMMATORY BOWEL DISEASE

1. Persistent infection with a pathogen (virulent pathogen or defective host clearance mechanisms)
2. Initiation of tissue injury by a transient pathogen, perpetuation by other mechanisms
3. Altered pathogenicity of endogenous enteric bacteria
4. Altered balance of beneficial and aggressive resident luminal bacteria
5. Abnormal host immune response to ubiquitous bacteria or bacterial components
6. Defective mucosal barrier function leading to enhanced uptake of luminal bacterial constituents

present data do not convincingly incriminate a single, persistent pathogen as a universal cause of Crohn's disease, this hypothesis must be considered in view of the possibility that Crohn's disease almost certainly represents a heterogeneous group of diseases with similar phenotypes and with the knowledge that all gastrointestinal (GI) pathogens have not yet been discovered.

Mycobacterium paratuberculosis

M. paratuberculosis is an extremely fastidious, slow-growing, mycobactin-dependent organism that causes Johne's disease (17), a chronic granulomatous enterocolitis in ruminants that does not respond to antimycobacterial therapy. In 1984, Chiodini et al. (18) recovered slow-growing *M. paratuberculosis* from tissues of three patients with Crohn's disease, and apparently identical isolates of *M. paratuberculosis* were cultured subsequently from Crohn's disease tissues by multiple centers (19).

Recovery of *M. paratuberculosis* from Crohn's disease tissue by culture is quite low (fewer than 15% of cases); even in the most experienced hands, the organism is rarely cultured from ulcerative colitis or control tissues. Slow-growing spheroplasts (cell wall-defective forms) have been recovered from 20% to 40% of patients with Crohn's disease and a small number of control subjects (20–22). Interest in this field was renewed by selective detection of *M. paratuberculosis* in patients with Crohn's disease using polymerase chain reaction (PCR) amplification based on a multicopy genomic DNA insertion element (IS-900) specific for *M. paratuberculosis* and more recently by positive serologic studies using defined proteins. Sanderson et al. (23) reported that 65% of Crohn's disease, 4% of ulcerative colitis, and 13% of control tissues had detectable IS-900 DNA. This observation has been confirmed in children (24). However, other groups have reported lower rates (0% to 8%) of detection (25,26), lack of specificity by PCR (27,28), or no evidence of *M. paratuberculosis* by 16S ribosomal DNA analysis (29). Collins et al. (28) reported that bacillus Calmette–Guérin vaccination decreased the recovery of tissue IS-900 in intestinal tissues fourfold. PCR technology has also been used to identify previously uncharacterized spheroplasts cultured from patients with IBD (21,22). In an intriguing case report, *M. paratuberculosis* was cultured from an enlarged cervical lymph node 5 years before the development of terminal ileitis similar to Crohn's disease (30).

Patients with Crohn's disease appear to have enhanced serologic responses to defined *M. paratuberculosis* proteins, including 35- and 36-kd antigens (31), a 14-kd protein (32), and a 32-kd mycobacterial protein homologous to human histone H_1, which is a possible target of human perinuclear antineutrophil cytoplasmic antibody (p-ANCA) (33). Because antibody responses to a wide variety of microbial pathogens and commensal bacteria are increased in active Crohn's disease (9,11,12), these results must be interpreted with caution.

Zoonotic transmission of *M. paratuberculosis* from cattle to humans has been suggested given the 20% to 30% prevalence rate of the organism in dairy herds in the United States (34–36). Whether routine pasteurization kills *M. paratuberculosis* in milk is not clear (37). *M. paratuberculosis* has been detected in breast milk of patients with Crohn's disease (38), although there is no evidence of increased frequency of Crohn's disease in the offspring of mothers with Crohn's disease. Waterborne transmission is also possible, as the organism has been isolated from the water supply of Los Angeles (27).

M. paratuberculosis is present in the environment and possibly commercial milk, meat, and water, but there is no convincing epidemiologic, immunologic, histochemical, or clinical evidence to support an etiologic role. The incidence of Crohn's disease is not increased in spouses of patients, health care workers attending patients with Crohn's disease, animals with Johne's disease, or farm residents associated with *M. paratuberculosis*-infected cattle. Diligent searches

TABLE 28.2. INFECTIOUS AGENTS SUGGESTED TO CAUSE INFLAMMATORY BOWEL DISEASES

Ulcerative colitis
- *Diplostreptococcus* (430)
- *Bacteroides necrophorum* (431)
- *Shigella* (432)
- RNA virus (433)
- Toxigenic/adherent *Escherichia coli* (72)

Crohn's disease
- *Chlamydia* (434)
- L forms of *Pseudomonas maltophilia* (93)
- Reovirus (435)
- *Mycobacterium kansasii* (436)
- *Mycobacterium paratuberculosis* (18)
- Paramyxovirus (measles) (45)
- *Listeria monocytogenes* (60)
- Adherent/invasive *E. coli* (77)
- *Pseudomonas fluorescens* (89,90)

Note: Numbers in parentheses indicate references.

for acid-fast bacilli and immunohistochemical evidence (39) of *M. paratuberculosis* antigen in IBD tissues have been negative or inconclusive (40). Although some patients have increased serologic responses to *M. paratuberculosis,* the absence of cell-mediated immune responses (32) eliminates the primary mechanism by which a paucibacillary infection could cause chronic granulomatous disease. Unfortunately, antibiotic trials remain nondefinitive, because they have not targeted patients with evidence of infection by PCR or serology, have not attempted to document clearance of the organism by molecular methods, and have used antibiotics that affect commensal bacteria rather than intracellular *M. paratuberculosis* (41–44). Thus, it is presently not possible to determine whether *M. paratuberculosis* causes Crohn's disease in a small subgroup of patients or whether this disease is an environmental contaminant that preferentially invades ulcerated tissue in patients with Crohn's disease.

Measles

Persistent measles infection of vascular endothelial cells has been suggested to cause Crohn's disease by inducing focal granulomatous vasculitis (45). Investigators have also postulated that live measles vaccines in early life lead to persistent viral infection that profoundly disrupts mucosal immune responses (46). Evidence for an etiologic role for measles include the following: paramyxovirus-like structures have been visualized by electron microscopy in the vascular endothelium of patients with Crohn's disease; measles antigen and RNA have been detected in granulomas and endothelial cells by immunohistochemistry and electron microscopy (45,47); and levels of anti-measles immunoglobulin M (IgM) antibody are increased in both patients with Crohn's disease and patients with ulcerative colitis (48). The authors of these studies postulate that measles infection induces focal vascular lesions that cause localized ischemia and ulceration (49). Epidemiologic evidence for an etiologic role for measles includes the development of Crohn's disease in some children born to mothers with measles infection during pregnancy (50), and increased incidences of Crohn's disease and ulcerative colitis in a British vaccinated cohort (51) and in persons born during measles epidemics in Sweden (50). Importantly, these observations have not been confirmed by other groups (52–56) and therefore must be viewed with caution. For example, Pardi et al. (57) found increased risks for Crohn's disease and ulcerative colitis in patients with documented measles infection before the age of 5 years but failed to find a risk with maternal infection during pregnancy (58). The selective immunohistochemical staining of Crohn's disease tissues with one (but not other) monoclonal antibodies to measles (59) has not been confirmed (60,61). Likewise, PCR (62,63) and serologic study results (64,65) for measles by independent investigators have been negative. Finally, large measles vaccination cohorts in the United States and Great Britain have not demonstrated an increased risk of Crohn's disease (54,66,67). Thus, serious questions remain regarding the role of measles infection in IBD.

Listeria monocytogenes

Listeria is a common environmental pathogen that frequently colonizes cheese and other foods. This organism selectively invades M cells overlying lymphoid aggregates and persists within the cytoplasm of macrophages. Liu et al. (60) demonstrated *Listeria monocytogenes* in 75% of Crohn's disease tissues by immunohistochemical staining and serology in 30% of patients with Crohn's disease compared with 8% of control subjects. However, these findings were limited to two multiplex families in rural France, and subsequent investigations have suggested secondary invasion of inflamed tissues, rather than a primary etiologic role for this ubiquitous pathogen. Also, the staining results have not been confirmed (68). Chen et al. (69) reported positive PCR results for *Listeria* in 13% of patients with Crohn's disease, 18% with ulcerative colitis, but 26% of control subjects, whereas Chiba et al. (70) detected *L. monocytogenes* DNA in 5% of patients with ulcerative colitis and 0% of patients with Crohn's disease by PCR (70). The latter group also has reported the absence of 16S ribosomal DNA sequences in intestinal lymphoid tissue from patients with IBD (29). Although suprainfection with *L. monocytogenes* can rarely lead to fulminant colitis in IBD (71), the organism appears not to have an etiologic role.

Adherent Invasive Escherichia coli

Several groups of investigators have described increased recovery of adherent or toxigenic *E. coli* from patients with ulcerative colitis and Crohn's disease. Burke and Axon(72) and Lobo et al. (73) demonstrated that patients with ulcerative colitis have an increased frequency of *E. coli* adherent to epithelial cells by mechanisms distinct from enteropathogenic *E. coli* (EPEC). Giaffer et al. (74) confirmed an increased frequency of adherent *E. coli* in patients with ulcerative colitis and those with Crohn's disease but found no correlation with disease activity. Others could not confirm an increased frequency of adherent *E. coli* in patients with ulcerative colitis (75,76). More recently, the Lille group reported the increased presence of mucosally associated enteroadherent *E. coli* in the ileum of patients with postoperative early recurrence of Crohn's disease (77). These *E. coli* secrete a novel cytokine, invade cells, and persist within macrophages (78). Molecular 16S ribosomal typing showed genetically linked *E. coli* in 79% of resected ileal tissues from patients with chronic Crohn's disease (79). Eighty percent of *E. coli* strains isolated from patients with active Crohn's disease adhered to Caco-2 cells (79). Whether these strains of *E. coli* can induce experimental inflammation in genetically susceptible rodents, activate

NFκB and chemokine expression in epithelial cells, and respond to ciprofloxacin therapy have not been determined.

Helicobacter *Species*

The ability of *Helicobacter pylori* to induce chronic active gastritis, relapsing peptic ulcer, and gastric cancer has raised suspicion that a similar organism causes IBD. However, *H. pylori* colonization is decreased in patients with IBD, perhaps due to the frequent use of antibiotics and sulfasalazine (80,81). In immunodeficient mice, multiple non-*pylori* intestinal *Helicobacter* species, including *Helicobacter hepaticus, Helicobacter bilis, Helicobacter typhlonicus,* and a novel urease-negative species isolated from interleukin 10 $(IL\text{-}10)^{-/-}$ mice, can cause cecal inflammation (typhlitis) (82,83). Whether *H. hepaticus* and related species can induce disease in immunocompetent hosts is controversial (84,85). Wood et al. (86) described a *Helicobacter*-like organism adherent to the mucosa of bypassed inflamed colonic segments in cotton-top tamarins. Suggested mechanisms of tissue injury include lack of organism clearance in T-cell deficient hosts, helper T-cell (Th1)-mediated immune responses in immunocompetent hosts (84), and production of a cytotoxin (87). To date, descriptions of the presence of these organisms in patients with IBD are limited, although *Helicobacter* species 16S ribosomal DNA sequences were identified in lymphoid tissues of 3 of 11 patients with Crohn's disease (88).

Pseudomonas fluorescens

A transcriptional regulation gene I_2 of *Pseudomonas fluorescens* (89) was recently detected in 43% of colonic tissues of patients with Crohn's disease but only 9% of ulcerative colitis and 5% control specimens (90). However, Chiba et al. (91) failed to detect *Pseudomonas* species 16S ribosomal RNA in the lymphoid follicles of patients with Crohn's disease. The organism probably represents invasion of ulcerated Crohn's disease tissues by a commensal organism, because approximately 50% of both patients and control subjects harbor this sequence in ileal samples (90). Subsequent studies have demonstrated that I_2 is a superantigen that reactivates T-cell receptor Vβ5 that induces IL-10 in CD4+ T cells in normal mice and interferon-γ (IFN-γ) in mice with colitis (92). Spheroplast forms of *Pseudomonas maltophilia* have been recovered from Crohn's disease tissues (93), but this finding is confounded by the use of antibiotic bowel preparations before surgery.

Transient Pathogenic Infection

Infection with a conventional pathogen can precede the onset of typical idiopathic IBD. A small percentage of patients involved in epidemics of *Shigella, Salmonella,* or *Yersinia* develop classic ulcerative colitis or Crohn's disease with no evidence of persistent bacterial infection (94). Other patients with acute enteric infections acquired either sporadically or by traveling have been reported to develop chronic IBD despite clearance of the initial pathogen (95–98). Self-limited tissue injury caused by these bacteria could initiate inflammation, which is subsequently perpetuated by separate mechanisms (Table 28.3), leading to chronic spontaneously relapsing IBD (2). Many infections and environmental insults can break the mucosal barrier or induce acute inflammation; therefore, the initiating event may be nonspecific. Thus, the induction of IBD may be analogous to the initiation of juvenile-onset diabetes mellitus by enteroviral Coxsackie and echo viral infections in human leukocyte antigen DR-3 (HLA-DR3), HLA-DR4, and/or HLA-DQ3 hosts (99) and the induction of reactive arthritis by enteric bacteria (*Yersinia, Shigella, Salmonella, Chlamydia*) in HLA-B27 patients (100). Alternatively, delayed exposure to common enteric pathogens because of improved hygiene can have potentially detrimental consequences, analogous to polio, where early childhood infection has only transient symptoms but adolescents or adults have devastating consequences (1).

Transient enteric infections could break the mucosal barrier by adhering to and invading epithelial cells (101), releasing enterotoxins, stimulating release of proinflammatory cytokines injurious to the epithelium or inducing production of chemotactic peptides (102,103). The induction of most proinflammatory molecules by bacterial pathogens in intestinal epithelial cells is mediated through stimulation of NFκB (104,105). The net result of each of these pathways is epithelial necrosis or disruption of tight junctions that enhance uptake of proinflammatory luminal bacteria and bacterial components (2). In susceptible hosts, transient inflammation could become self-sustaining due to defective down-regulation of the immune response or inefficient epithelial restitution (2). This is analogous to chronic inflammation in Lewis rats or $IL\text{-}10^{-/-}$ mice after short-term nonsteroidal antiinflammatory drug administration (106,107).

Alternatively, enteric infections could induce chronic intestinal inflammation by positively or negatively modulating the immune response. Enhanced activation of mucosal dendritic cells by bacterial adjuvants or induction of class II major histocompatibility complex antigens on

TABLE 28.3. MECHANISMS BY WHICH TRANSIENT INFECTIONS COULD INDUCE CHRONIC INFLAMMATION

1. Disrupted mucosal barrier leading to uptake of luminal antigens
2. Initiation of proinflammatory responses perpetuated by unrelated ubiquitous antigens
3. Modulation of host protective immune response
4. Autoimmune response (molecular mimicry)

epithelial cells may initiate pathologic immune responses to ubiquitous luminal antigens (loss of tolerance) or to host proteins (autoimmune responses). Cell wall polymers such as peptidoglycan–polysaccharide (PS-PG) complexes or lipopolysaccharide (LPS, endotoxin) from ubiquitous luminal bacteria and pathogens have potent adjuvant activities (108). Also, an array of infections can induce class II HLA antigens, adhesion molecules, and regulatory cytokines, such as IL-12, which can in turn enhance antigen-presenting cell function (103). Many of these innate immune responses to pathogens are mediated through NFκB (105). Recent evidence shows that microbial agents can secrete molecules that modulate host immune responsiveness. For example, Epstein–Barr virus (EBV) protein (BCRF1) shares structural homology and immunosuppressive activity with IL-10 (109) and EPEC secrete a large toxin that inhibits expression of IL-2, IL-4, and IL-5 by mitogen-stimulated mononuclear cells and suppresses lymphocyte activation (110). Of interest, patients with ulcerative colitis have decreased concentrations of IL-2 (111) and a 76% detection rate of EBV infection in one small series (112). Spontaneous colitis that develops in IL-2 and IL-10 knockout mice clearly illustrates the detrimental consequences of dysregulated mucosal lymphokines (113,114). Conversely, inflammatory mediators produced by activated immune cells can modulate bacterial function. For example, IL-1 can induce bacterial proliferation (115), and oxygen radicals can enhance bacterial production of formylated oligopeptides (f-met-leu-phe) (116).

A transient infection might induce chronic inflammation by initiating an autoimmune response, either by exposing intracellular "hidden" antigens or by molecular mimicry, that is, shared epitopes between microbial antigens and host proteins. Serum antibodies that react with both colonic epithelial cells and several *Enterobacteriaceae* have been demonstrated in ulcerative colitis (117,118). However, these antibodies are probably secondary responses to cellular damage, because there is no compelling evidence that the antibodies cause epithelial cell injury. A 40-kd colonic epithelial cell antigen, recently identified as the cytoskeletal protein tropomyosin, is specifically recognized by serum and mucosal-associated antibodies from patients with ulcerative colitis (119). Although no homologous epitope has been found in enteric bacteria, molecular mimicry is suggested by cross-reaction of tropomyosin with group A streptococcal M proteins (120). In contrast, p-ANCA, which is found in approximately 60% of patients with ulcerative colitis and 15% of patients with Crohn's disease (121,122), cross-reacts with enteric bacteria (123), including *Bacteroides caccae* and *E. coli* (124). The dominant epitope in human neutrophils is histone H_1, which exhibits homology with the 32-kd HupB mycobacterial protein (33). The close homology between bacterial (particularly mycobacterial) and mammalian heat shock proteins (Hsps) (125) raises the possibility that cross-reacting antibodies or cellular immune responses to these molecules could lead to chronic intestinal inflammation. Expression of these "stress proteins" is increased by a variety of stimuli, including inflammation and cytokines (126). These molecules protect the cell during stressful events and function as molecular chaperones for other cytoplasmic proteins. Hsp60 expression is increased in epithelial cells from patients with ulcerative colitis but does not correlate with disease activity (127), but Hsp immunoreactivity in Crohn's disease tissues is similar to that of control subjects (128). Similarly, Hsp70 immunoreactivity is enhanced in ulcerative colitis to a greater degree than Crohn's disease and self-limited infections (129), but Hsp90 expression is not up-regulated in IBD. Polymorphisms of Hsp70 have been related to clinical phenotypes in Crohn's disease (130). Serum antibodies to Hsp60 are increased in patients with Crohn's disease and those with ulcerative colitis (131,132), although responses are variable (132) and nonspecific in some patients (133). Similarly, cell mediated responses to Hsp60 are variable (128,134,135). The ability of these molecules to mediate inflammation is illustrated by the induction or inhibition of experimental arthritis by T-lymphocyte clones reacting to Hsp65 (136) and by the induction of mucosal inflammation in mice colonized or injected intraperitoneally with *E. coli* expressing *Yersinia enterocolitica* Hsp60 (137;138). Whether enhanced expression of mucosal Hsp and immune responsiveness is a consequence of the inflammatory response or involved in its pathogenesis remains to be determined, but the lack of consistent T-cell responses to this protein suggest a secondary, rather than a primary, etiologic role.

Altered Concentrations Of Luminal Bacteria

Subtle alterations in the composition of the "normal" bacteria (dysbiosis) of the intestinal constituents could lead to chronic stimulation of the mucosal immune system, resulting in chronic intestinal inflammation (2,139). These alterations may be a consequence of local environmental changes, such as exposure to antibiotics (140), diet (141, 142), genetic determinants (143), anatomic changes such as loss of the ileocecal valve, partial obstruction, and enterocolonic fistulas, or even a consequence of the host's inflammatory response (115,116). A number of investigators have described derangements of anaerobic bacterial constituents in Crohn's disease (2,143). A study of children of patients with Crohn's disease suggests that profiles of fecal anaerobes are genetically determined, and that abnormalities may precede clinical symptoms (143). Fecal concentrations of certain coccoid rods, such as eubacteria, *Peptostreptococcus,* and *Coprococcus,* are increased in patients with Crohn's disease (12,143–145). Fecal concentrations of *Bacteroides vulgatus* are also increased in active Crohn's disease (144,146) and therapeutic efficacy of metronidazole correlates with decreased *Bacteroides* concentrations (144). Further support

TABLE 28.4. BALANCE OF BENEFICIAL AND AGGRESSIVE COMMENSAL ENTERIC BACTERIA

Protective	Aggressive
Lactobacillus species	*Bacteroides* species
Bifidobacter species	*Enterococcus faecalis*
Streptococcus salivarius	*E. coli* (adherent/invasive/toxigenic)
Escherichia coli strains	Segmented filamentous species
	Fusobacterium varium
	Helicobacter hepaticus

for a role of anaerobic bacteria in the pathogenesis of Crohn's disease is provided by clinical responses to metronidazole (147); the preferential ability of *B. vulgatus* to induce colitis in guinea pigs fed carrageenan (148), in HLA-B27 transgenic rats (149), and in T-cell receptor-$\alpha^{-/-}$ mice (142); and the ability of cell wall polymers from certain *Eubacterium* species to induce chronic granulomatous arthritis in rats (108,150).

Similar alterations in the profile of luminal bacteria have not been detected in ulcerative colitis. However, nonspecific relative increases in aerobic bacteria, including enterococcal species, and decreases in anaerobic flora occur in this disorder and in patients with diarrhea of many etiologies (151,152). Recently, increased recovery of mucosally associated *B. vulgatus* and antibodies to this organism have been reported in patients with ulcerative colitis (153). Mucosal-associated bacterial species are increased in patients with IBD (154), and several studies document decreased luminal concentrations of lactic acid bacteria, including *Lactobacillus* and *Bifidobacterium,* in patients with active ulcerative colitis and Crohn's disease (151,155,156). Increased concentrations of streptococcal and clostridial species and decreased concentrations of lactobacilli in neonatal IL-$10^{-/-}$ mice before the onset of inflammation suggest an etiologic role for these bacteria (157). Together, these results support the concept that dysbiosis, caused by genetic, environmental, and/or dietary influences, participates in the pathogenesis of IBD (Table 28.4) (139) and opens the possibility of therapeutic manipulations by selective antibiotics, probiotic, or prebiotic approaches (158–161). This concept is supported by the therapeutic efficacy of administering *E. coli* Nissle strain to patients with ulcerative colitis (162), probiotic species to patients with recurrent pouchitis (163), and lactulose (164) or germinated barley (141) to animals with experimental colitis (141).

Abnormal Functional Properties Of Luminal Bacteria

Emerging data implicate functional alterations in commensal bacteria in ulcerative colitis and Crohn's disease. Abnormal bacterial metabolites or altered virulence factors could have profound effects on epithelial cell function and lead to chronic mucosal injury. Such metabolites and factors may not be detected by conventional microbiologic screening tests. As discussed earlier, functionally abnormal *E. coli* have been isolated from patients with Crohn's disease and those with ulcerative colitis (72,74,77–79). These strains display increased epithelial adherence and invasion, which can directly injure epithelial cells or stimulate secretion of chemotactic peptides, such as IL-8 (103), and enhanced neutrophil transmigration across epithelial monolayers (165). Other functional abnormalities of *E. coli* from patients with IBD have been described, including production of Vero toxin, Shiga-like toxin, necrotoxins, novel enterotoxins, and hemolysins (77,166,167). More recently, Giaffer et al. (74) found no Vero toxin production or hemolytic *E. coli* strains in patients with IBD but did find cytotoxin production in 10% of patients with Crohn's disease. Mucin-degrading enzymes are produced by *B. vulgatus* and group D streptococci (75,168), and enterococci from patients with ulcerative colitis can secrete hyaluronidase (169). Immunologically active products such as superantigens can be produced by luminal bacteria (92), although *Staphylococcal aureus* superantigens were detected in only 1 of 63 patients with IBD (170).

Roediger (171) proposed the novel hypothesis that ulcerative colitis is caused by defective metabolism of short-chain fatty acids (SCFAs), leading to epithelial cell starvation. SCFAs are produced by anaerobic bacterial fermentation of nonabsorbed carbohydrates and proteins. Colonocytes preferentially use luminal SCFAs, particularly butyrate, as fuel sources (172,173). Patients with ulcerative colitis have decreased luminal concentrations of SCFAs, although a selective defect in butyrate oxidation (171,173,174) and the therapeutic response to butyrate enemas is variable (175,176). Butyrate has important antiinflammatory effects, including blockade of NFκB activation (177) and IL-1β responses in epithelial cells (U. Boecker and R. B. Sartor, unpublished data). Hydrogen sulfide, which is produced by colonic bacteria, selectively inhibits epithelial cell butyrate metabolism, with the greatest effects in the distal colon; butyrate did not affect glucose metabolism (178). In addition to the inhibition of butyrate metabolism, hydrogen sulfide is toxic to colonic epithelial cells and mucus (179). Luminal hydrogen sulfide is increased in patients with ulcerative colitis (180), but sulfate-reducing bacteria, primarily *Desulfo Vibrio,* were not increased in patients with ulcerative colitis (179,181), and almost complete elimination of hydrogen sulfide by bismuth subsalicylate did not prevent acute experimental colitis (182).

Liberation of soluble immunoregulatory products by EPEC have been suggested to alter mucosal immune responses in patients with IBD (110), similar to that reported in IL-$2^{-/-}$ mice (113). Bacterial strains that affect NFκB activation by blocking IκBα ubiquination (183) or by inserting bioactive proteins that inhibit IκBα phosphorylation into the cytoplasm of intestinal epithelial cells (184) have not been searched for in IBD.

Abnormal Host Response To Ubiquitous Luminal Bacterial Constituents

Rodent models provide evidence that chronic, relapsing intestinal and systemic inflammation is a genetically determined, abnormal cell-mediated immune response to ubiquitous luminal bacterial constituents (2,5,7). In the normal host, potentially harmful inflammatory responses to luminal contents are prevented by the ability of an intact epithelial barrier, secretory antibodies, and mucus to exclude toxic macromolecules and the ability of immunosuppressive mediators and regulatory T lymphocytes to down-regulate the inflammatory responses. Ineffective barrier function or defective immunosuppression in the genetically susceptible host results in continuous stimulation of the mucosal immune system and consequently chronic inflammation.

Animal Models

Marked differences in the level of intestinal inflammation in genetically susceptible rodents raised under conventional versus sterile conditions support a role for commensal intestinal bacteria in the pathogenesis of IBD. In at least 11 separate animal models with induced, spontaneous, or genetically engineered disease (Table 28.5), chronic intestinal inflammation fails to develop in the absence of enteric bacteria, and the level of intestinal inflammation correlates with the concentrations of luminal bacteria and the presence of pathogens (2,3). For example, IL-$10^{-/-}$ mice raised under conventional conditions develop lethal small intestinal and colonic inflammation but in a sterile (germ-free) environment have no intestinal inflammation (185). Conventionally raised IL-$10^{-/-}$ mice exhibit a Th1-dominated immune response with increased IL-12 and IFN-γ and develop colonic adenocarcinomas with chronic inflammation (186,187). Importantly, specific pathogen-free (SPF) IL-$10^{-/-}$ mice develop inflammation in the colon only, whereas wild-type mice colonized with the same SPF organisms exhibit no intestinal inflammation or immune activation, demonstrating the nonpathogenic nature of the enteric bacteria causing disease in IL-$10^{-/-}$ mice. Colitis in SPF IL-$10^{-/-}$ mice is attenuated with broad-spectrum antibiotics; narrow-spectrum antibiotics such as metronidazole or gentamicin are effective in preventing, not treating, established disease (157,188). Finally, in HLA-B27 transgenic rats, cecal bacterial overgrowth enhances colitis, whereas cecal bypass decreases not only cecal inflammation but also distal colitis and gastritis (189), suggesting that activation of T lymphocytes by enteric bacteria preferentially occurs in the cecal tip. These results and a study (190) showing attenuation of colitis after amputation of the cecal tip ("appendectomy") in T-cell receptor-$\alpha^{-/-}$ mice are consistent with epidemiologic observations that appendectomy reduces the incidence of ulcerative colitis (1).

TABLE 28.5. ANIMAL MODELS IN WHICH INDUCED, SPONTANEOUS, OR GENETICALLY ENGINEERED INTESTINAL INFLAMMATION DOES NOT DEVELOP IN THE ABSENCE OF ENTERIC BACTERIA

Mice
IL-$2^{-/-}$ (113,437)
IL-$10^{-/-}$ (185)
T-cell receptor $\alpha^{-/-}$ (267)
$CD_3\varepsilon$ transgenic (194)
Samp-1/Yit (438)
$CD_{45}RB^{hi}$ T-cell transfer $\rightarrow$ SCID (439)
Multidrug resistance gene (440)
DSS-induced colitis (441)
Rats
HLA-B27 transgenic (149,197)
Indomethacin-induced enteritis (442)
Guinea pigs
Carrageenan-induced colitis (148)
Cotton-top tamarin
Thiry–Vella loop (86)

Note: Numbers in parentheses represent references.

The Th1-dominated immune response in most rodent models of intestinal inflammation (3,191) is directed toward luminal bacterial antigens. Serum antibodies recognize a broad array of commensal enteric bacterial species (192), and a pathogenic role for bacterial-responsive T lymphocytes (193) has been demonstrated in C_3H/HeJ Bir mice, which spontaneously develop colitis. The cell lines developed from these Th1 lymphocytes could transfer colitis to SPF T-cell-deficient (SCID) recipients (193). CD4+ T cells from bone marrow transplanted CD3ε transgenic mice with colitis secrete IFN-γ in response to cecal bacterial lysate but not to luminal food antigens or to colonic epithelial cells. An absence of pathologic cross-reactive responses to host antigens was confirmed by lack of colitis when activated mesenteric lymph node cells were transferred to germ-free CD3ε transgenic mice (194). It should be noted that B cells are not required for murine colitis (187,195), and that B-cell responses appear to be protective in T-cell receptor-$\alpha^{-/-}$ mice (196).

Enteric bacteria differ in their capacity to induce inflammation, and mice of different genetic backgrounds may respond selectively to these bacteria. For example, SPF HLA-B27/β_2 microglobulin transgenic rats develop colitis (149;197), mild/moderate colitis after colonization with *B. vulgatus* alone or in combination with five other bacterial species but no disease when monoassociated with *E. coli* or when colonized with the five bacteria without *B. vulgatus* (149,198). The concept that enteric bacteria have additive or synergistic activities is supported by the observation that colitis in SPF HLA-B27 transgenic rats is greater than rats monoassociated with *B. vulgatus* (149,198,199). Importantly, gnotobiotic IL-$10^{-/-}$ mice colonized with the same bacteria that cause colitis in HLA-B27 transgenic rats develop very mild inflammation (185), clearly demonstrating host species specificity of responses to bacterial stimuli.

Gnotobiotic IL-$10^{-/-}$ mice monoassociated with *Enterococcus faecalis* develop a predominantly distal moderate colitis with different kinetics and distribution than SPF IL-$10^{-/-}$ mice (185,200). IL-$10^{-/-}$ mice with colitis induced by *E. faecalis* monoassociation have selective *in vitro* T-cell responses to *E. faecalis* compared with *E. coli* and *B. vulgatus* (200). IL-$10^{-/-}$ mice selectively associated with viridans *Streptococcus* and *Clostridium* species have no evidence of colitis (201). The ability of *H. hepaticus* to induce colitis in immunocompetent mice is controversial (83–85,202).

Further support of the concept that various commensal bacteria have differential inflammatory capacities is the evidence that certain luminal bacterial constituents, mostly lactic acid species, can protect SPF IL-$10^{-/-}$ mice and HLA-B27 transgenic rats against intestinal inflammation (159, 160,164,203,204).

Enteric bacteria can profoundly influence the extraintestinal manifestations that may accompany intestinal inflammation (100). For example, small-intestinal bacterial overgrowth in susceptible rat strains leads to hepatobiliary inflammation, resembling sclerosing cholangitis, and can reactivate peripheral arthritis (205,206). This inflammation appears to be due to peptidoglycan–polysaccharide (PG-PS) complexes produced by luminal anaerobic bacteria and present in bile; hepatobiliary inflammation and arthritis are prevented when treated by metronidazole or mutanolysin, which selectively degrades PG-PS (205,207,208). In support of these results, intramural injection of PG-PS polymers into the ileum and cecum of susceptible Lewis rats induces chronic hepatic granulomas, arthritis, and anemia of chronic disease (209). Finally, SPF HLA-B27 transgenic rats develop peripheral and axial arthritis, which does not occur in the absence of intestinal bacteria (197).

Clinical Studies

Patients with Crohn's disease improve when luminal bacterial concentrations are decreased by antibiotics, bowel rest, and lavage therapy (2,160,210). Metronidazole (10 mg/kg of body weight per day) is superior to placebo (147) and equal to sulfasalazine (211) as primary therapy of Crohn's colitis and enterocolitis. In all studies to date, metronidazole alone or in combination with ciprofloxacin (212–214) is more effective in colonic or ileocolonic Crohn's disease than in isolated small-intestinal disease. Ciprofloxacin alone is equal to mesalamine in treating active Crohn's disease (215), and in a small open-labeled trial in patients with refractory Crohn's disease, clarithromycin was beneficial (42). High-dose metronidazole (20 mg/kg per day) begun at the time of surgery and continued for 3 months decreased the recurrence rate of symptomatic Crohn's disease at 1 year but had no long-lasting effects at 2 and 3 years postoperatively (216). Similarly, ornidazole, similar to metronidazole, has beneficial effects in preventing postoperative recurrence of Crohn's disease (217). Broad-spectrum antibiotics are routinely used by experienced investigators as primary treatment of Crohn's disease and are effective in uncontrolled trials (218,219) but have never been subjected to rigorously controlled trials. Although most antibiotics only transiently alter bacterial concentrations due to emergence of resistant strains, metronidazole (146) and ciprofloxacin (220) have been reported to eliminate *Bacteroides* species and gram-negative coliforms, respectively, during 6 months of treatment. Side effects include diarrhea in a subset of patients (214), candidiasis, and occasionally *C. difficile* suprainfection.

Chronic antibiotic administration is not routinely advocated for primary treatment of ulcerative colitis, although several studies suggest an adjunctive role for agents against gram-negative aerobes in addition to standard medical therapy (220–225). Most studies show that metronidazole has no effect in ulcerative colitis (160,226). However, antibiotics including metronidazole, ciprofloxacin, and rifaximin are effective in pouchitis (227–229). Thus, aerobes appear to be more important in the pathogenesis of ulcerative colitis and anaerobes in Crohn's disease.

Surgical diversion of the fecal stream decreases intestinal and colonic inflammation (230,231), and reanastomosis rapidly leads to recurrence of the inflammation (232,233). Filtration studies suggest that intact bacteria were the component necessary to reactivate inflammation.

Patients with active IBD have loss of tolerance to commensal bacteria and enhanced T-lymphocyte responses to autologous bacteria (234) and defined bacterial species (235). patients with IBD, particularly those with Crohn's disease, display exaggerated humoral responses to a wide variety of commensal and pathogenic enteric bacteria (2,11,12,153). Although probably not directly involved in tissue injury, serologic responses to defined bacterial epitopes, including *B. vulgatus, Pseudomonas fluorescens,* and *Mycobacterium* species, may be useful as diagnostic markers of IBD or of clinically useful patient subsets (33,90,153). Several bacterial antigens react with p-ANCA, including *B. caccae, E. coli,* and mycobacteria (33,124).

Probiotic Agents

Several probiotic agents appear to show therapeutic efficacy in IBD (158–160). Introduction of *E. coli* Nissle strain is equal to maintenance doses of mesalamine in preventing relapse of ulcerative colitis (162,236,237). Similarly, a cocktail of eight probiotic *Lactobacillus, Bifidobacterium,* and *Streptococcus* species (VSL-3) prevented relapse of recurrent pouchitis in a 9-month trial (15% recurrence rate in VSL-3 treated group versus 100% in the placebo group) (163). Although the mechanisms of protection are not yet defined, induction of tolerogenic T cells or dendritic cells is possible due to observed increases in tissue IL-10 concentrations in probiotic-treated patients (238). Additional novel approaches to IBD treatment with bacteria include genetic engineering to secrete immunosuppressive molecules, such as IL-10

(239); use of bacterial secretion mechanisms to insert proteins that block NFκB (183,240); and suppression of Th1 immune responses by helminthic colonization (241).

Defective Effector Cell Function

Defective neutrophil and macrophage cytotoxic activity for bacteria has been suggested to play a role in chronic granulomatous inflammation of Crohn's disease (242). This novel hypothesis is based on Crohn's-like lesions in children with neutrophil dysfunction (e.g., chronic granulomatous disease); typhlitis in patients with chemotherapy-induced neutropenia; and improvement of Crohn's disease with granulocyte colony-stimulating factor (G-CSF), which enhances microbicidal activity (243). This hypothesis is supported by defective phagocytosis and killing of *Candida albicans* by neutrophils and macrophages isolated from patients with ulcerative colitis and Crohn's disease, irrespective of disease activity and treatment (244). Similar functional responses have not been investigated in monocytes or macrophages from Crohn's disease patients with the recently described Nod-2 defect (245–247), but defective NFκB signaling to intracellular LPS in innate immune cells should lead to ineffective clearance of invading bacteria, such as enteroadherent/invasive *E. coli,* which block clearance by unknown mechanisms (78).

The mechanism by which luminal bacteria induce pathogenic immune responses is not known. Direct invasion (29,60,90,248) or the production of proinflammatory molecules that activate innate immune responses (2,108) may be involved. Bacterial cell wall polymers, such as LPS and PG-PS, and formylated oligopeptides can induce experimental enterocolitis (2,209,249–251). Purified, sterile PG-PS derived from certain bacterial strains, including group D streptococci (enterococci), can induce chronic, spontaneously relapsing granulomatous enterocolitis with extraintestinal manifestations in rats after intramural (subserosal) injection (209). Moreover, luminal PG-PS can potentiate acute indomethacin-induced enteritis (but not colitis) in germ-free rats (252) and has been implicated in hepatobiliary inflammation accompanying jejunal bacterial overgrowth in rats (207). Both PG-PS and LPS activate macrophages/monocytes and intestinal epithelial cells through toll-like receptor 2 (TLR-2) and TLR-4, respectively, which leads to NFκB translocation and transcription of a number of proinflammatory molecules (105,253). Thus, continuous absorption of toxic products of luminal bacteria could stimulate innate immune cells of the mucosa, leading to sustained intestinal inflammation in the susceptible host. Systemic distribution of bacterial cell wall polymers and antigens can occur (100,254,255), leading to extraintestinal manifestations. Finally, as discussed above, patients and rodents with IBD and experimental colitis have aggressive T-lymphocyte responses to a wide variety of commensal luminal bacteria (193,194,234,235), suggesting that absorbed bacterial antigens induce pathogenic responses.

Genetic Susceptibility

Increased host susceptibility to luminal bacteria or their components could be due to defects in the mucosal barrier, impairment of the normal down-regulation of inflammatory responses, an overly aggressive immune response to common stimuli, or defective clearance of pathogens. Defective barrier function or immunosuppression are likely genetically determined traits, reflected in the increased familial incidence of IBD, higher concordance rate of Crohn's disease in monozygotic than dizygotic twins, familial patterns of disease, chromosomal abnormalities in patients with Crohn's disease, and differential susceptibility of inbred rodents to experimental enterocolitis (246,256,257).

Mucosal permeability appears to be increased in active Crohn's disease. Most studies demonstrate a direct correlation between disease activity and mucosal permeability, suggesting an acquired defect (5,258). However, some studies indicate that a subset of family members of patients with Crohn's disease (10% to 35%) have a permeability defect (258,259), suggesting a genetic etiology. The demonstration by Podolsky and Isselbacher (260) of specific alterations in colonic mucin glycoprotein profiles in patients with ulcerative colitis, irrespective of disease activity, provides one explanation of defective barrier function. However, Pullan et al. (261) found that mucous gel thickness was normal in patients with mild ulcerative colitis, but that the gel was absent in patients with moderate to severe ulcerative colitis. Surprisingly, the mucous gel layer was intact in patients with active Crohn's disease. The importance of an intact mucous gel layer to barrier function and exclusion of luminal bacterial products is illustrated by a 50-fold increased uptake of chemotactic bacterial products after removal of surface mucus with dithiothreitol (262). Intestinal trefoil factor (ITF), which is produced by mucus-secreting goblet cells, contributes to mucosal barrier function by enhancing mucus viscosity and promoting epithelial restitution after injury (263). $ITF^{-/-}$ mice have increased mortality and increased colitis after dextran sodium sulfate administration; rectal administration of ITF enhanced healing of the experimental colitis (264). Epithelial tight junctions also contribute to mucosal barrier function, as evidenced by the focal enteritis that occurs in transgenic mice with defective N-cadherin (265). These rodent studies clearly indicate the potential contribution of genetic regulation of defective barrier function and restitution to IBD which is supported by observations of enhanced mucosal association with bacteria in IBD patients (450).

Genetic susceptibility to luminal bacteria and their components is demonstrated by differential progression of experimental inflammation in inbred rodent strains. Lewis rats, injected intramurally (subserosally) with PG-PS polymers, develop spontaneously relapsing granulomatous enterocolitis with fibrosis and extraintestinal inflammation (209). In contrast, Buffalo and Fischer F_{344} rats, the latter MHC matched with Lewis rats, exhibit self-limited intestinal inflammation, with no evidence of systemic manifestations (209). Lewis rats have selective activation of plasma kallikrein and a single base-pair polymorphism in the high-molecular-weight kininogen gene, leading to altered release of bradykinin (209; R. Colman and B. Sartor, unpublished observations). Similarly, Lewis rats injected subcutaneously with indomethacin develop chronic mid-small-bowel ulcerations with granulomas, periportal hepatic inflammation, anemia, and fibrosis. Low-responding Fischer rats develop similar degrees of acute enterocolitis, which quickly resolves without extraintestinal inflammation (266). In response to apparently identical luminal concentrations of anaerobic bacteria in the self-filling blind loop model, Lewis rats develop hepatobiliary inflammation within 2 to 4 weeks of jejunal bacterial overgrowth, Wistar rats display similar lesions after 8 to 12 weeks, but Fischer and Buffalo rats fail to develop inflammatory injury (206).

Genetic background is also a critical determinant of experimental colitis in mice. Knockout mice on the 129 background typically have more active colitis than those on the C57/Bl6 background (186,267), whereas various inbred strains have dramatically different responses to dextran sodium sulfate (268). A careful analysis of quantitative trait loci on IL-$10^{-/-}$ mice backcrossed on C3H/HeJ Bir and C57BL/6J backgrounds has lead to the identification of chromosomal regions associated with the activity and distribution of colitis (269). Of considerable interest, C3H/HeJ mice, which have defective LPS responses due to a spontaneous mutation in TLR-4, are consistent high responders in DSS-induced colitis (268). This is the parent strain for the C3H/HeJ Bir mouse strain, which spontaneously develops colitis (270). Consistent with this observation, C3H/HeJ mice infected with *Citrobacter freundii* develop chronic colitis, whereas DBA/2J mice similarly inoculated exhibit only transient inflammation (271). These models of dramatically different incidence, chronicity, and complications of experimental intestinal inflammation suggest that humans also may have differing genetic susceptibilities to noxious environmental stimuli. Supporting this hypothesis is the recent description of defects in the gene for Nod-2, an intracellular protein that transduces NFκB activation and apoptosis in monocytes/macrophages (272), in patients with Crohn's disease (245–247). The role that defects in this gene play in disease pathogenesis is under study.

CHRONIC ENTERIC INFECTIONS THAT MIMIC INFLAMMATORY BOWEL DISEASE

Several enteric infectious resemble ulcerative colitis and Crohn's disease (Table 28.6). These infections not only mimic the classic clinical features of IBD, including diarrhea (with or without blood), abdominal pain, and weight loss (273), they also have local complications and extraintestinal manifestations that resemble IBD. The local complications include toxic megacolon, perforation, abscesses, stricture, and fistula formation (274–278), and the extraintestinal manifestations include reactive arthritis, spondyloarthropathy, hepatobiliary inflammation, erythema nodosum, uveitis, and anemia (100).

TABLE 28.6. ENTERIC PATHOGENS THAT CAUSE INTESTINAL INFLAMMATION RESEMBLING INFLAMMATORY BOWEL DISEASE

Resemble Ulcerative Colitis	Resemble Crohn's Disease
Campylobacter jejuni	*Mycobacterium tuberculosis*
Salmonella species	*Mycobacterium avium* complex
Shigella species	*Yersinia enterocolitica*
Clostridium difficile	Cytomegalovirus
Escherichia coli O157:H7	*E. coli* O157:H7
Aeromonas species	*Entamoeba histolytica*
Plesiomonas species	*Chlamydia trachomatis*
Vibrio noncholera species	*Histoplasma capsulatum*
Neisseria gonorrhoeae	*Actinomyces* species
Legionella species	*Cryptococcus neoformans*
Treponema pallidum	
Herpes simplex virus type 2	
Blastocystis hominis	

Campylobacter jejuni

Campylobacter jejuni is a frequently isolated enteric pathogen, accounting for up to 31% of all pathogens recovered from patients with sporadic infectious diarrhea (279–281). Typically, patients present with acute fever, malaise, and headache, followed by abdominal pain and diarrhea that resolve in 3 to 5 days, with the peak incidence occurring in the summer months (282). A less common presentation is that of chronic bloody diarrhea and abdominal pain resembling ulcerative colitis and Crohn's disease (281,283,284). Toxic megacolon (285), erythema nodosum (286), and relapses with abscess (287) may complicate the infection. Rarely, *C. jejuni* can cause acute ileocolitis, mimicking appendicitis (288). *Campylobacter* colitis is characterized by abdominal pain more severe than anticipated from the sigmoidoscopic findings (283), which include mucosal edema, hyperemia, and shallow gray-based aphthous ulcers. In chronic *Campylobacter* colitis (>1 week's duration), the mucosa is granular and friable without ulceration, similar to ulcerative colitis. Histologic changes vary with the duration of infection (289). Predominant features of acute infection are superficial ulceration, cryptitis, mucus depletion, and an edematous lamina propria with neutrophil infiltration. Prolonged infection is accompanied by regenerating epithelia, mononuclear cell infiltration, edema restricted to the upper lamina propria, and lymphoid hyperplasia without distortion of the crypt architecture.

Salmonella Species

Salmonella typhimurium and *Salmonella enteritidis* are among the most frequently isolated bacterial pathogens in patients with acute diarrhea. The vast majority of infected patients have transient enteritis that resolves within a week. However, few patients develop colitis with an average duration of 3 weeks, although symptoms may persist for 3 months. Patients with colitis exhibit bloody diarrhea with fecal leukocytes, and complications include sepsis, toxic megacolon, and perforation (276,290). Sigmoidoscopic features include granularity, friability, and occasional ulceration; histology shows hemorrhage, mucosal ulceration, and crypt abscesses (291). Radiographic findings of granularity, fine ulceration, and loss of haustration are indistinguishable from ulcerative colitis, with the exception that rectal abnormalities may be absent (292). Segmental colitis with focal ulcers resembling Crohn's disease may rarely occur (293).

Shigella Species

In the United States, *Shigella sonnei* and *Shigella flexneri* account for 90% of reported cases of infectious colitis. *S. sonnei* is more common in patients younger than 15 years, whereas *S. flexneri* is more common in adolescents and adults. Mucosal invasion and enterotoxin production lead to colitis (294), which preferentially involves the distal colon, although the entire colon and terminal ileum may be inflamed (295). The most common clinical presentation is dysentery with bloody stools, mucus, and fever (296). Clinical symptoms usually persist for 5 to 7 days but may fluctuate over 2 to 3 weeks and rarely have a fulminant course leading to toxic megacolon and sepsis (278). *Shigells dysenteriae* type 1 has been reported to cause more virulent disease, possibly necessitating emergent colectomy (297). Histologic features are nonspecific acute mucosal inflammation (see below).

E. coli

Enteroinvasive *E. coli*, enterohemorrhagic strains, and *E. coli* O157:H7 can produce acute colitis with bloody stools. *E. coli* O157:H7 is now recognized as a frequent cause of acute diarrhea (279,298). Infection with *E. coli* O157:H7 may cause a spectrum of illness from nonbloody diarrhea to fulminant colitis complicated by the hemolytic–uremic syndrome and thrombotic thrombocytopenic purpura (299). Sporadic cases and outbreaks caused by the ingestion of unpasteurized milk and undercooked hamburger meat have been described (300). Bloody diarrhea is the most common symptom, and severe abdominal cramps, fever, and fecal leukocytes occur frequently. A segmental distribution within the colon, particularly the right colon (301) suggest Crohn's disease, but the typical rapid onset of symptoms more closely resembles ischemic colitis or *Clostridium difficile* toxin-induced colitis (302). Rarely, the distal ileum is involved (303). Histologic findings include focal necrosis with hemorrhage and acute inflammation in the superficial mucosa that resemble *C. difficile* toxin-mediated colitis (299,302). Of note, antibiotic therapy has not been shown to be beneficial.

Clostridium difficile

C. difficile is a nosocomially acquired bacterial pathogen in patients treated with broad-spectrum antibiotics; inflammation is mediated by the well-defined cytotoxins A and B (304). The clinical spectrum of disease ranges from asymptomatic carriers to pseudomembranous colitis. Patients complain of diarrhea, tenesmus, lower abdominal cramps, nausea, and occasionally fever beginning 1 to 3 weeks after antibiotic exposure. Rectal bleeding is unusual, but occult blood and fecal leukocytes in stool are common. Fulminant disease may result in toxic megacolon and perforation (305). Endoscopic examination shows 2- to 5-mm diameter yellow-white raised plaques that may become confluent. The diagnosis of *C. difficile*-associated colitis is more challenging when the rectum is spared (up to 30% of cases) and in early-onset disease before the appearance of pseudomembranes (306). In longstanding advanced cases, the correct diagnosis can usually be made by the detection of *C. difficile* toxin in stool and the presence of pseudomembranes (yellow plaques) on flexible sigmoidoscopy in a patient with a history of prior antibiotic exposure.

Aeromonas Species

Aeromonas hydrophilia and *Aeromonas sobria,* usually acquired from drinking untreated water, produce colitis in approximately 25% of infected patients (307,308). Symptoms usually resolve in a week, but 37% of children have symptoms for more than 2 weeks (307), and adults have diarrhea for an average of 6 weeks. Several cases have been described that have apparently progressed to typical ulcerative colitis (96,97).

Mycobacterium tuberculosis

Primary intestinal TB is rare in industrialized nations but is an important cause of ileocecal disease in some developing countries. The frequency of ileocecal infections, which occur in association with active pulmonary TB, is expected to increase, because the frequency of pulmonary infections in developed countries has recently risen (309). Intestinal infections have been documented in up to 28% of patients with smear-positive, cavitating pulmonary TB (310). Conversely, two-thirds of patients with ileocecal TB have evidence of pulmonary tuberculous lesions (311). Symptoms include abdominal pain (90%), weight loss (74%), anorexia (60%), and fever and diarrhea (56%) (312). An abdominal mass that is usually tender and located in the right lower quadrant is present in more than half of cases; ascites is detectable in 10%. Seventy-five percent of patients with GI TB have ileocecal involvement (312) and approximately 25% have segmental colonic disease without cecal involvement. Isolated ileal disease is quite rare, but isolated duodenal involvement has been reported (313).

Pathologic findings of ileocecal TB include transmural inflammation, large granulomas with frequent epithelioid cells, sharply defined mucosal ulcers with irregular margins, nodular mucosa, and serosal tubercles. Granulomas may be caseating, particularly in mesenteric lymph nodes. Complications include stricture formation, fistulas, perforation, and bleeding (309).

Definitive diagnosis is difficult with non-invasive tests. A high index of suspicion is based on the presence of pulmonary lesions, a positive skin test result, or emigration from endemic areas. Ileocecal TB can mimic Crohn's disease on barium contrast studies and colonoscopy (Fig. 28.1). Features that suggest TB rather than Crohn's colitis include the absence of rectal and perianal involvement, transverse or circumferential ulcers rather than longitudinal ulcers, and a patulous ileocecal valve (312). Small aphthous ulcers with normal surrounding mucosa, long strictures, and extraintestinal inflammation are more common in Crohn's disease. Histologic features of confluent or caseating granulomas suggest intestinal TB. Necrosis of massively enlarged mesenteric lymph nodes may be detected by computed tomography (CT) scan (314). Serodiagnosis using enzyme-linked immunosorbent assay has been reported to have a diagnostic accuracy of 84% (315). Definitive diagnosis is made by identification of the organism on mucosal biopsies or resected tissue using acid-fast stains, immunohistochemistry, or culture. However, acid-fast stains of mucosal biopsies are positive in an extremely low percentage of cases. When suspicion is high, a therapeutic trial of triple antimycobacterial drugs is warranted while waiting for culture results. Clinical improvement should occur within 3 to 4 weeks after initiating appropriate therapy.

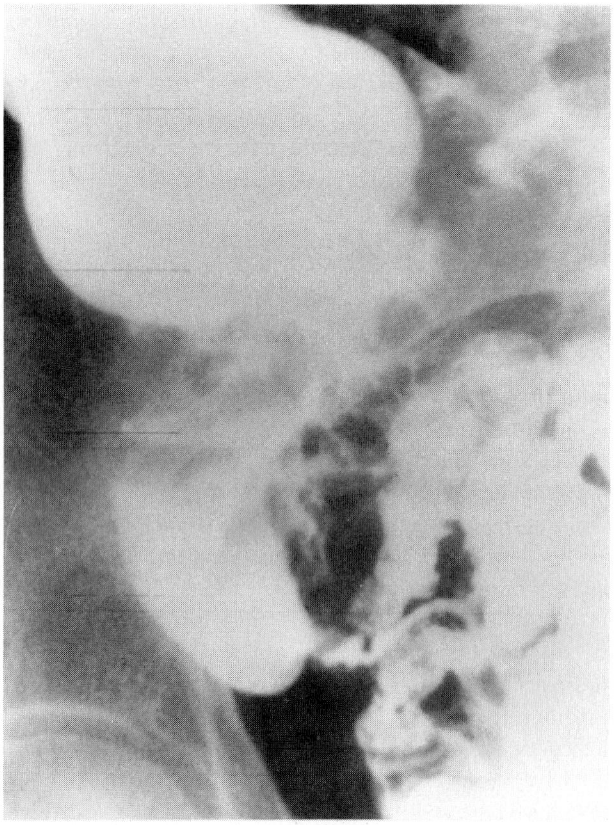

FIGURE 28.1. Cecal tuberculosis. A barium enema shows concentric, focal narrowing and ulceration of the cecum, near the ileocecal valve. The terminal ileum is not well visualized, but proximal ileal loops are normal. Patient's chest x-ray showed bilateral apical infiltration with probable cavitation, consistent with tuberculosis.

Yersinia Species

Y. enterocolitica and *Yersinia pseudotuberculosis* infections generally occur in persons younger than 25 years, usually during winter months, and commonly in Scandinavia. Children younger than 5 years typically develop acute gastroenteritis, whereas older persons usually have acute ileitis and mesenteric adenitis (316,317). Diarrhea and right lower quadrant abdominal pain are the most frequent symptoms; erythema nodosum, uveitis, and reactive arthritis may occur in HLA-B27-positive patients. Weight loss and vomiting are relatively rare, whereas tenesmus, fever, fecal leukocytes, occult bleeding, and peripheral blood leukocytosis are frequently present.

Most patients have a self-limited course that resolves within 2 weeks. However, 14% of patients in a long-term study were readmitted for abdominal pain or diarrhea, including two patients with ulcerative colitis, and 12% had

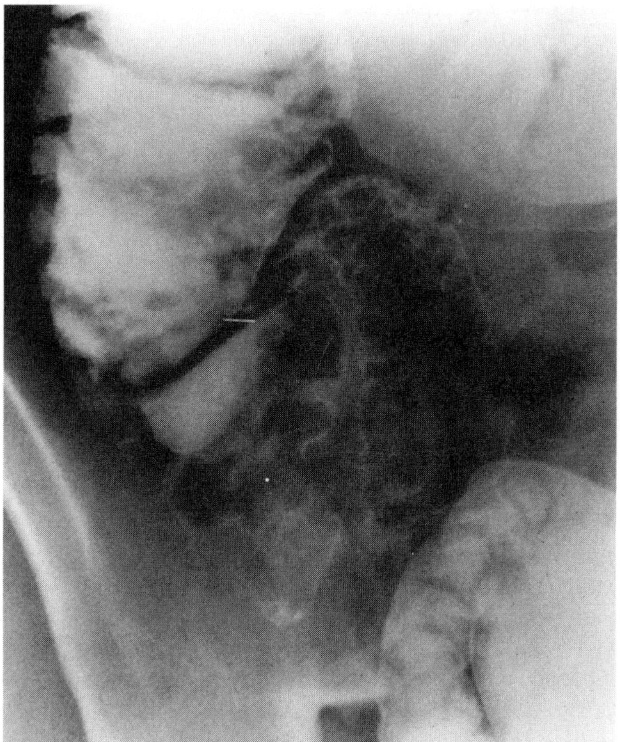

FIGURE 28.2. *Yersinia* ileitis. A small-bowel follow-through demonstrates nodularity of the distal ileum with no stenosis and minimal bowel wall thickening; stool grew *Yersinia enterocolitica*.

persistent arthritis, including ankylosing spondylitis (316). Rarely, patients have been reported to develop typical Crohn's disease after *Yersinia* infection (303). *Yersinia* bacteremia with focal abscesses is more common in patients with cirrhosis, hemolytic anemia, and diabetes.

Radiography and endoscopy of the ileum shows edema, ulceration, and lymphoid hyperplasia (Fig. 28.2). Aphthous ulcers may occur in the colon, but the rectum is usually spared (318,319). Pancolonic focal ulcers resembling Crohn's disease have been described in a child (320). Fistulas, abscesses, stenosis, and skip lesions are uncommon. Because of the right lower quadrant pain, patients with *Yersinia* infections often mistakenly undergo surgery for suspected appendicitis. Granulomas may be present in ileal biopsies and resected lymph nodes.

Entamoeba histolytica

Infection with *Entamoeba histolytica* is relatively unusual in developed countries. However, it should be considered in the differential diagnosis of IBD because of the risk of precipitating fulminant disease with corticosteroid therapy and complications such as hepatic abscess. High-risk persons include recent immigrants from endemic areas and institutionalized populations, particularly the mentally retarded (321). Patients with invasive colonic infections present with bloody, mucoid diarrhea, and abdominal pain. Fever, nausea, and vomiting are manifestations of fulminant disease (322). Radiographic and endoscopic features include flask-shaped ulcers that extend into the submucosa, loss of haustration, aphthoid ulcers, and marginal serration (323,324). Diagnosis is established by the identification of trophozoites in stool, adherent mucus, or mucosal biopsies (323). Serology is a valuable adjunct to the diagnosis of invasive amebiasis, because detection of trophozoites in stool is relatively insensitive (325).

Cytomegalovirus

Cytomegalovirus (CMV) colitis is rare in immunocompetent hosts but is an important cause of mucosal ulceration in immunosuppressed patients. In immunocompetent subjects or persons, the most common presentation is GI tract bleeding secondary to ulceration in the colon and duodenum (326). Anal intercourse is a risk factor with an apparent incubation period of 1 to 2 weeks. Approximately 10% of patients present with obstructive jaundice due to granulation tissue at the ampulla of Vater (326). CMV inclusion bodies were present in epithelial cells in areas of minimal inflammation and within endothelial cells in ulcerated areas (Fig. 28.3A), suggesting that ulceration is a result of

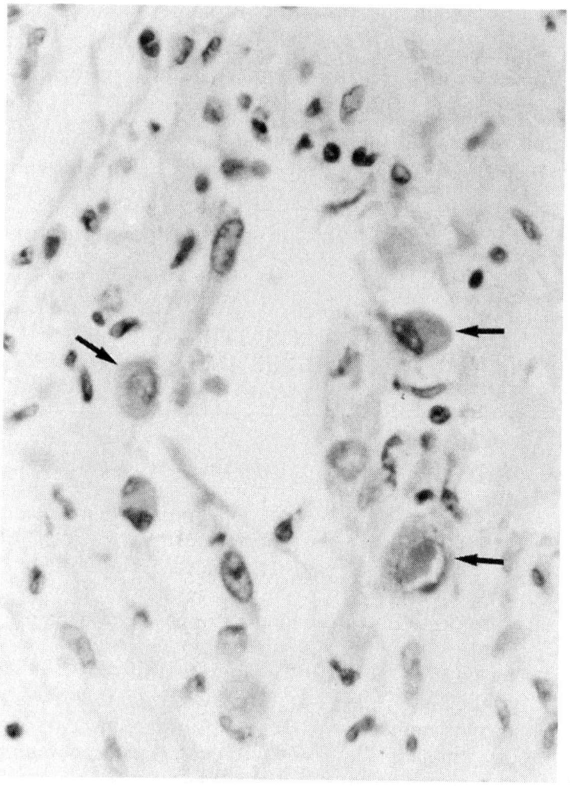
A

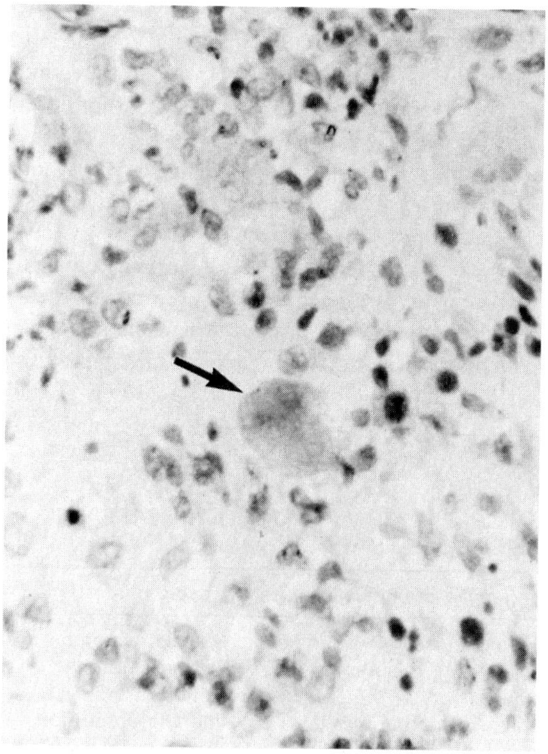
B

FIGURE 28.3. A: Cytomegalovirus (CMV) vasculitis. Viral inclusions are present within the cytoplasm and nucleus of endothelial cells in the ulcerated intestine of a patient with AIDS (*arrows*). **B:** CMV colitis. Cytoplasmic and intranuclear inclusions (*arrow*) in a mononuclear cell infiltrating the lamina propria of the colon. The overlying mucosa was ulcerated.

ischemia caused by virally induced vasculitis (326). In immunosuppressed patients, intestinal CMV infection can involve virtually any organ of the GI tract and take a fulminant course that includes toxic megacolon (299). Perforating ileocolitis, hemorrhagic proctocolitis, and toxic megacolon due to CMV can require emergent surgery in immunosuppressed patients (277,327).

Chlamydia trachomatis

Chlamydia trachomatis, particularly lymphogranuloma venereum (LGV) immunotypes, can cause chronic, granulomatous proctitis in homosexual men (328). Rectal disease may be complicated by strictures, fistulas, and abscesses (329). Non-LGV strains produce mild proctitis that mimics ulcerative colitis (328).

Clinical And Laboratory Criteria That Distinguish IBD From Infectious Enterocolitis

Crohn's disease and to a lesser extent ulcerative colitis typically have an indolent onset, averaging 3 years before diagnosis (330). However, some patients with IBD have an abrupt onset of symptoms similar to those of infectious enterocolitis, and some enteric infections have protracted courses. In all cases, infectious disorders must be excluded before the diagnosis of Crohn's disease or ulcerative colitis can be established.

A careful history, physical examination, and routine laboratory screen help distinguish IBD from an infection caused by a known pathogen (Table 28.7). An abrupt onset of symptoms, particularly with fever, in a previously healthy individual, favors an infectious origin. Between 15% and 25% of patients with IBD have a family history of these disorders (257), and up to 40% of patients with Crohn's disease will have associated perianal disease, particularly when colonic involvement is present. Exposure to untreated water, raw milk, undercooked ground beef, shellfish, other infected patients, travel, and oral or anal sex raise the possibility of an infectious etiology, as does suppression of the immune system by corticosteroids, immunosuppressive drugs, HIV-1 infection, cirrhosis, renal insufficiency, and diabetes. Abdominal cramps, fever, rectal bleeding, fecal leukocytes, and occult blood are nonspecific findings. A right lower quadrant mass strongly suggests Crohn's disease, but ileocecal TB and periappendiceal abscess must be considered. Chronic subclinical IBD is suggested by growth retardation in adolescents, unexplained weight loss, anemia, and hypoalbuminemia. In a retrospective study, approximately 60% of patients with IBD had white blood cell (WBC) counts of more than 10,000/mL, hemoglobin level of less than 12 g/dL (women) or less than 14 g/dL (men), and serum albumin level of less than 3.5 g/dL, in contrast to 14% to 25% of patients with infectious diarrhea (331). The best laboratory test to differentiate between an enteric infection and IBD was a platelet count of more than 450,000/mL, which occurred in 59% of patients with active IBD but only less than 2% of patients with an enteric infection (331).

Endoscopic features of infectious colitis overlap with those of idiopathic IBD. Patchy petechial hemorrhage, focal edema, and erythema in the rectosigmoid area are atypical findings in IBD and should suggest an infectious etiology (332). Rectal sparing, discontinuous disease, and focal ulcers are not found in ulcerative colitis; and circumferential ulcers are more typical of intestinal TB than Crohn's disease (312).

Histologic and immunohistologic examination of rectal biopsies help distinguish IBD from infectious enterocolitis. Seven histologic features with a predictive probability of 87% to 100% for IBD are listed in Table 28.8. The presence of distorted crypt architecture is the most useful finding and may appear within a month of the onset of symptoms (333). The discriminative value of these findings may be less for chronic infections. In a prospective study of new-onset coli-

TABLE 28.7. CLINICAL CRITERIA THAT DISTINGUISH INFLAMMATORY BOWEL DISEASE FROM INFECTIOUS DIARRHEA

Favoring Inflammatory Bowel Disease	Favoring Infection
Chronic course (>4 wk)	No prior symptoms
Spontaneous relapses	Exposure history
Family history	Antibiotic use
Perianal complications	Immunosuppression
Growth retardation	Acute course (<2 wk)
Anemia	
Albumin <3.5 mg/dL	
Platelets >450,000/mL	

TABLE 28.8. HISTOLOGIC FEATURES OF INFLAMMATORY BOWEL DISEASE VS. INFECTIOUS COLITIS

Inflammatory Bowel Disease	Specific Infectious Diseases
Distorted crypt architecture	Pseudomembranes (*Clostridium difficile, Escherichia coli* O157:H7, *Staphylococcus aureus*)
Crypt atrophy	
Basally located giant cells	Viral inclusions (Cytomegalovirus, herpes simplex virus 2)
Villous colonic epithelium	Caseating necrosis (*Mycobacterium tuberculosis*)
Mixed inflammatory cell population in lamina propria	Diagnostic organisms (*Entamoeba histolytica, Cryptosporidium*)
Noncaseating granulomas	Specific staining (*Mycobacterium, Histoplasma, Capsulatum*)
Lymphoid aggregates	

tis, basal plasmacytosis was the best indicator of IBD, followed by crypt branching, crypt distortion, villous mucosa, and mucosal atrophy (334). IBD tissue may also show an increase in IgG-secreting plasma cells in the lamina propria (280). Granulomas are not specific for Crohn's disease; they are also associated with *Mycobacterium, Chlamydia, Yersinia,* and syphilis infections. Acid-fast and silver stains are helpful for identifying mycobacterial and fungal infections. Immunohistochemical staining and *in situ* hybridization are used with increased frequency to detect CMV.

The most commonly used stool tests for the identification of infectious etiologies of intestinal inflammation are culture for bacteria, microscopic, and immunofluorescence examination for enteric parasites and immunoassay for *C. difficile* toxin. Tissue culture for mycobacteria and CMV is helpful for confirming histologic findings. Even in the best laboratories, stool cultures yield a diagnosis in only approximately 60% of cases of presumed infectious diarrhea. Serologic tests for *E. histolytica, Yersinia,* and *Chlamydia* improve the diagnostic yield.

Management Of Acute Colitis

Recent-onset diarrhea without accompanying fever, abdominal tenderness, fecal leukocytes, rectal bleeding, or leukocytosis should be conservatively evaluated and treated symptomatically. In contrast, diarrhea that does not resolve within 7 to 10 days or that is associated with rectal bleeding, fever, fecal red blood cells or leukocytes, abdominal tenderness, or leukocytosis should be more aggressively evaluated with flexible sigmoidoscopy, stool culture, and an ova and parasite examination. A *C. difficile* toxin assay should be performed if patients have been exposed to antibiotics or recently hospitalized. Immunocompetent patients with diarrhea for more than 4 weeks, particularly when accompanied by anemia, thrombocytosis, or hypoalbuminemia, as well as immunosuppressed patients with diarrhea of shorter duration should be thoroughly evaluated with stool culture and microscopy, colonoscopy with biopsies, and small-bowel follow-through x-ray. All patients with fulminant onset of symptoms or disease that does not respond to appropriate therapy should be evaluated for HIV-1, even if obvious risk factors are not present (334). Patients with appropriate exposure histories and compatible clinical symptoms should be further evaluated with a TB skin test, chest x-ray, special stains of biopsy, specimens, and appropriate serologies. Before beginning corticosteroid or Remicade therapy, patients should have a skin test for TB and a serologic assay for *E. histolytica* when indicated.

After a diagnosis of infectious enterocolitis is established, specific therapy is indicated unless the symptoms are already resolving. Exceptions to this approach include *Salmonella* gastroenteritis, for which antibiotic therapy may prolong the carrier state (335), and *E. coli* O157-H7 infection, because antibiotics may not shorten the clinical course but increase the risk of the hemolytic–uremic syndrome (337). The decision to begin empiric therapy for IBD with immunosuppressive therapy must be weighed against the risk of potentiating CMV, TB, and amebiasis (338,339). When emergent corticosteroid therapy is essential, empiric coverage for TB or amebiasis should be considered if there is a high risk of infection. Sulfasalazine and other 5-aminosalicylic acid compounds pose no risk of exacerbating infectious diseases, and metronidazole is effective as primary therapy of Crohn's colitis and certain infections, including amebiasis and *C. difficile.*

INFECTIONS THAT EXACERBATE INFLAMMATORY BOWEL DISEASE

Epidemiology

Between 40% and 60% of relapses of IBD are associated with a symptomatic respiratory tract infection (340,341), and up to one-third of patients are infected with an enteric bacterial or protozoal pathogen (342,343). *C. difficile* is the most common such pathogen, followed by *Salmonella, Shigella, Campylobacter,* and *Yersinia.* Rotavirus or Norwalk agents have been identified in 8% of patients with relapses of either ulcerative colitis or Crohn's disease.

Microbiology

An array of viral, bacterial, and parasitic pathogens have been associated with clinical relapses of IBD or recovered from tissues of patients with active disease (Table 28.9). *C. difficile* has been the most thoroughly studied agent, but the relationship between this organism and relapses of IBD remains controversial. *C. difficile* or its cytotoxin is present in up to 32% of patients with active IBD (342,344–346) and in 4% to 25% of patients with acutely relapsing disease (343,344). The presence of *C. difficile* is even higher (up to 50%) in hospitalized patients and patients with fulminant or refractory colitis (346,348). However, in nonhospitalized subjects, the recovery of *C. difficile* does not correlate with disease activity (345,346,349). Indeed, most patients with IBD undergoing relapses do not have associated *C. difficile* infections, indicating that it is not cost-effective to perform an assay for *C. difficile* toxin in the outpatient with a routine flare-up unless exposure to antibiotics is documented. In contrast, the risk of *C. difficile*-associated disease is substantially increased in hospitalized patients with IBD, particularly those with fulminant disease, and an assay for *C. difficile* toxin is indicated, particularly because undiagnosed infections can lead to serious complications such as toxic megacolon and perforation (347). The association between *C. difficile* infection and prior antibiotic use in patients with IBD is controversial (344,346).

Salmonella, Shigella, Campylobacter, and *Yersinia* have been detected in prospective studies in less than 2% of

TABLE 28.9. PATHOGENS ASSOCIATED WITH INFLAMMATORY BOWEL DISEASE RELAPSE

Viral	Bacterial	Parasitic
Cytomegalovirus (443)	*Clostridium difficile* (344)	*Entamoeba histolytica* (342)
Rotavirus (444)	*Salmonella* species (445)	
Norwalk agent (444)	*Shigella* species (343)	
Respiratory syncytial virus (341)	*Campylobacter jejuni* (287)	
Influenza A and B (341)	*Yersinia* species (446)	
Parainfluenza (341)	Enteropathogenic *Escherichia coli* (343)	
Rubella (341)	*Aeromonas* species (447)	
Epstein–Barr virus (341)	*Listeria monocytogenes* (71)	
Herpes simplex virus (443)		
Adenovirus (341)		

patients with relapsing IBD in industrialized countries (343) and in only 4% of such patients in developing countries (342). These studies, together with retrospective studies (350,351), suggest that routine culture for "enteric pathogens" is not indicated in uncomplicated flare-ups of IBD. However, PCR analysis revealed *Yersinia* DNA in resected specimens from 63% of Crohn's and 46% of patients with ulcerative colitis, as well as toxigenic *E. coli* in tissues from 21% of patients with ulcerative colitis (352), suggesting high carrier rates of pathogenic bacteria in refractory disease. These findings must be interpreted cautiously, because PCR may be overly sensitive, leading to false-positive results.

CMV is another potential cause of exacerbation of IBD (353,354) . CMV-induced GI tract inflammation occurs primarily in immunosuppressed patients (353,354) and rarely in steroid-naïve patients (355). Histologic review of colonic resections from 46 patients with ulcerative colitis revealed CMV in 6 patients (Fig. 28.3), all of whom were men with fulminant disease (356). Before the availability of CMV therapy, CMV suprainfection in IBD was associated with a severe clinical course and a high rate of mortality (357). In a recent series of patients with steroid-refractory IBD, 36% had evidence of CMV infection that improved after antiviral treatment (353). Diagnostic clues that suggest CMV include the presence of malaise, myalgias, fever, mild transaminase elevation, atypical lymphocytes, and steroid unresponsiveness. Diagnosis is based on the presence of viral inclusion bodies (Fig. 28.3) or a positive culture, buffy coat smears, plasma antigenemia, and serology. CMV infection can also occur in ileal pouches, mimicking idiopathic pouchitis (358,359). Increased titers of anti-CMV antibodies (360) and rates of CMV DNA in mucosal tissue in patients with ulcerative colitis and in those with Crohn's disease suggest increased exposure or reactivation of latent infection (361). The simultaneous presence of herpes simplex virus type 2 and CMV or EBV has been noted in some patients with ulcerative colitis, but whether the viruses act synergistically is unclear (361). A role for EBV and herpes virus type 6 in potentiating IBD was supported by improvement in intestinal and extraintestinal symptoms coincidental with the clearance of viral DNA from tissues after IFNα2a treatment (362).

Pathogenesis

The ability of antimicrobial therapy to induce resolution or improvement of relapsed IBD implicates a causative role for pathogens such as *C. difficile* and CMV in relapses of IBD (363). In some patients, however, active inflammation persists after clearance of the infecting agent (354), suggesting that idiopathic self-sustaining inflammation has been reactivated. Whether bacterial or viral suprainfection is a consequence of diminished resistance by an ulcerated mucosa, defective host immunologic clearance, relative immunosuppression due to drug therapy or malnutrition, decreased resistance to colonization due to antibiotic therapy, or increased exposure to nosocomial infections is unclear. Exacerbation of underlying IBD by upper respiratory tract infections (341) is more difficult to explain. Circulating cytokines liberated by inflammatory cells in the respiratory tract or viremia could preferentially activate intestinal lamina propria immune cells, which are in an enhanced (primed) state of responsiveness in patients with IBD (363,364).

INFECTIOUS COMPLICATIONS OF INFLAMMATORY BOWEL DISEASE

Extraluminal spread of ubiquitous enteric bacteria accounts for some of the most frequent complications of IBD (Table 28.10) (365), particularly in Crohn's disease where deep fis-

TABLE 28.10. INFECTIOUS COMPLICATIONS OF INFLAMMATORY BOWEL DISEASE

Abscess: intraabdominal, perianal, retroperitoneal, abdominal wall, hepatic
Fistula: enteroenteric, enterovesical, enterocutaneous, perianal
Postoperative infection: intraabdominal abscesses, wound infections
Hematogenous infection: sepsis, endocarditis
Opportunistic infection secondary to immunosuppressive therapy
Bacterial overgrowth: small bowel, pouchitis

sures, ulcers, and increased luminal pressures due to stenoses enhance the translocation of luminal bacteria. Chronic immunosuppressive therapy may inhibit the clearance of these organisms.

Intraabdominal Abscesses

Incidence

Abdominal abscess, one of the most common and dangerous complications of Crohn's disease, occurs in 10% to 20% of patients, and retroperitoneal abscesses occur in 3% to 4% of patients (366,367). Abscesses are extremely unusual in ulcerative colitis; perforation usually leads to peritonitis. Intraperitoneal abscesses occur with equal frequency in men and women, but retroperitoneal abscesses occur ninefold more commonly in men (367). A younger age at onset is characteristic of patients with Crohn's disease with abscesses (age 23 years) compared with those without abscesses (age 27 years). The distal ileum and sigmoid colon are the origin of most abscesses (366).

Pathogenesis And Microbiology

Abscesses can be spontaneous or postoperative. Abscesses that present spontaneously or more than 6 months after surgery are a consequence of localized perforation of a mucosal ulcer (Fig. 28.4). The thickened mesentery and adherent loops of intestine prevent free perforation in the vast majority of cases. Transmural extension of the ulcer leads to a localized abscess, which may drain spontaneously into adjacent bowel, bladder, psoas muscle, abdominal wall, or any adjacent structure. *E. coli, B. fragilis,* enterococci, and *Streptococcus viridans* are the principal bacteria isolated from intraabdominal abscesses (366), and *E. coli* and streptococci invade tissue adjacent to fistulas (351). These organisms are similar to those reported in intraabdominal abscesses in patients without IBD (368).

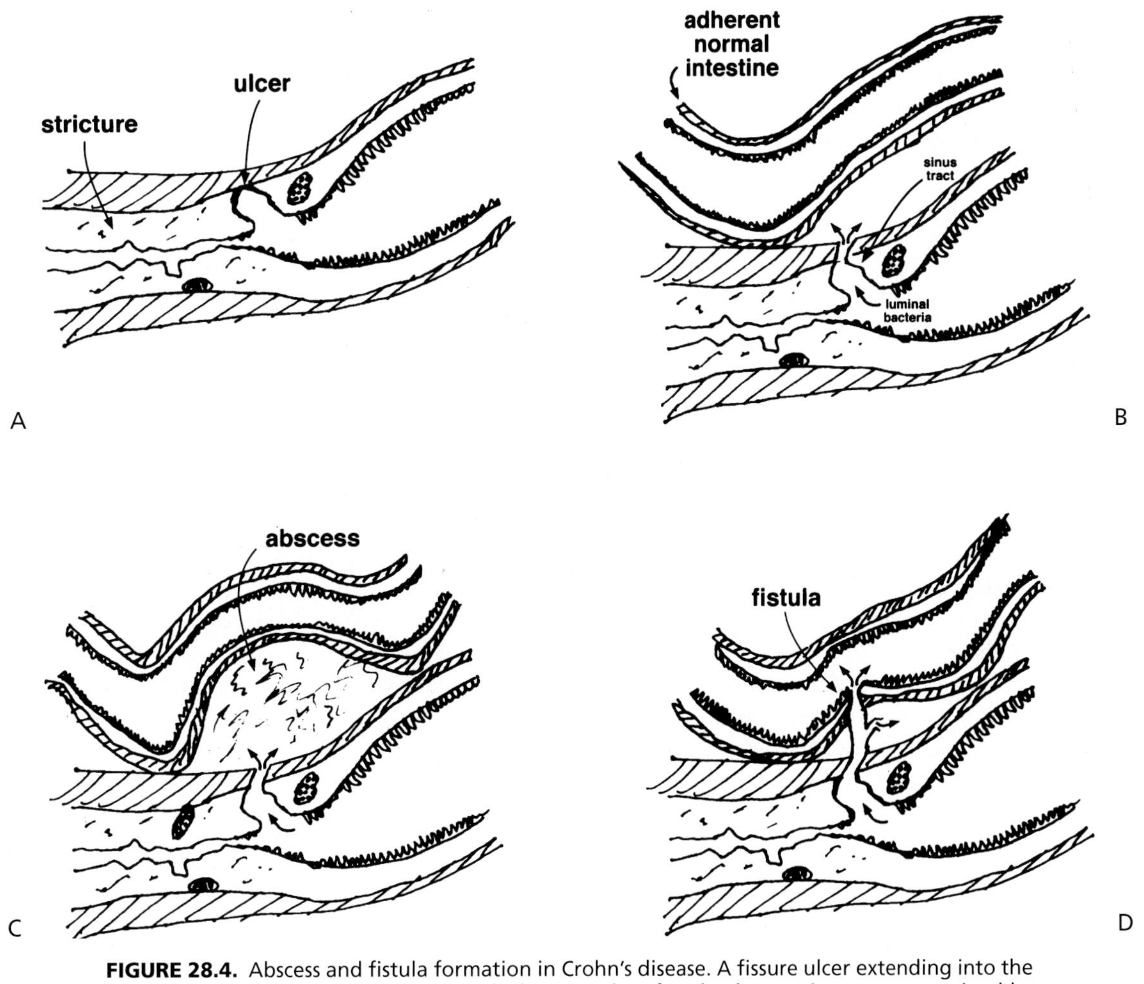

FIGURE 28.4. Abscess and fistula formation in Crohn's disease. A fissure ulcer extending into the submucosa **(A)** and penetrating through the serosal surface leads to a sinus tract contained by an adherent loop of intestine **(B).** Extravasation of luminal bacteria into the contained space forms an intraabdominal abscess **(C),** which perforates into the adjacent normal bowel to form an enteroenteric fistula **(D).**

Several factors may contribute to the high incidence of extramural extension of ulcers in Crohn's disease, including increased intramural pressures from obstruction, immunosuppression from medication or malnutrition, and secondary invasion of ulcers by luminal bacteria (368). Sinus tracts and perforations in the small intestine are associated with strictures (369,370). In the colon, the length of the stenosis is a higher risk factor for abscesses and fistulas than wall thickness (370). Crohn's disease can follow two distinct clinical courses, an aggressive form prone to abscesses and fistulas and a more indolent form that slowly strictures (371). The presence of these clinical patterns in families suggests a possible genetic predisposition to abscess formation (372).

Perioperative abscesses, which complicate up to 17% of operations for Crohn's disease, are a consequence of anastomotic breakdown and correlate strongly with surgery for intraabdominal abscesses or fistulas, preoperative steroid use, and low serum albumin levels (373,374). Similarly, the presence of preoperative abscesses increases the risk for postoperative abscesses, which complicate 8% of strictureplasties (375). Experimental studies show that extremely high doses of corticosteroids are necessary to interfere with anastomotic healing in normal hosts (376), suggesting that preoperative steroid use may be a marker of chronic aggressive disease, rather than a risk for anastomotic dehiscence.

Clinical Presentation

New-onset, continuous localized abdominal pain is the most common presenting symptom of an intraabdominal abscess (367). Two-thirds of patients with retroperitoneal abscesses have pain referred to the genitofemoral, lumbar, or other retroperitoneal nerves. GI tract bleeding occurs in 15% to 20% of patients with abscesses (367). The most frequent physical findings include intraabdominal mass, occurring in two-thirds of patients, and in the right lower quadrant in 80%, and fever, which may be spiking in nature. Eighty percent of patients with retroperitoneal abscesses have a positive psoas sign, fixed flexion of the hip, or limitation of hip extension, indicating irritation of the psoas muscle. Laboratory values may be nonspecific, with leukocytosis, mild anemia, hypoalbuminemia, and elevated alkaline phosphatase. A normal WBC count does not rule out an abscess (367). Importantly, more than half of abscesses detectable at the time of surgery were unsuspected (366).

Diagnosis

Distinguishing an intraabdominal abscess from active inflammatory Crohn's disease with an associated mass of inflamed mesentery, enlarged lymph nodes, and adherent bowel can be difficult and is best accomplished by radiographic imaging studies. Plain films of the abdomen showing extraluminal air and ultrasound scans may be diagnostic but have a relatively low yield because of difficulty in distinguishing intraintestinal and extraintestinal gas and fluid collections (377,378). Colonoscopy cannot visualize abscesses, although sinus tracts may be seen. Barium studies are relatively insensitive because the communication with the abscess may be intermittent; moreover, luminal barium has the disadvantage of delaying surgery and subsequent CT scans. Abdominal CT scan with luminal and intravenous contrast is a sensitive method of detecting abscesses and permits the best anatomic assessment of abscess versus underlying intestinal inflammation (Fig. 28.5) (377,378). However, CT is relatively expensive and exposes the patient to relatively high levels of radiation. Indium-11 or technetium-99m leukocyte scintigraphy offers the advantage of disease activity assessment and abscess detection (378,379) but is relatively insensitive and does not provide precise anatomic detail. Nuclear magnetic resonance imaging (MRI) with gadolinium can precisely localize abscesses and assess disease activity (380) but is quite expensive. Presently, CT scanning provides the most precise diagnostic approach and can be used to guide percutaneous drainage (see below).

Management

Intraabdominal abscesses large enough to be detected by CT scan require definitive therapy, as either a one-stage or a two-stage procedure. Definitive treatment includes resection of the diseased bowel, because simple drainage of the abscess cavity usually leads to a chronic fistula. In one study (367), only 16% of patients were cured by surgical incision and drainage compared with 76% who underwent *en bloc* resection. Alternatively, percutaneous drainage of the abscess under ultrasound or CT guidance, followed by elective surgical resection (381,382), may be appropriate for the extremely ill patient who can then undergo elective resection after antibiotic and nutritional support. Broad-spectrum antibiotic coverage is used to prevent hematogenous spread of bacteria during drainage and to improve local healing but is not effective as the sole approach. Definitive surgical resection is necessary in most cases to remove chronic obstructing stenotic segments and associated fistulas (382).

Fistulas

Enteric or colorectal fistulas occur (Fig. 28.6) in 20% to 40% of patients with Crohn's disease but are rare in ulcerative colitis (365). Fistulas are the result of a direct extension of an ulcer or spontaneous decompression or therapeutic drainage of an abscess (Fig. 28.4). In 639 patients with Crohn's disease undergoing abdominal surgery, 35% had at least one fistula: 69% between loops of intestine, 12% enterovesical, 16% enterocutaneous, 4% enterovaginal, and

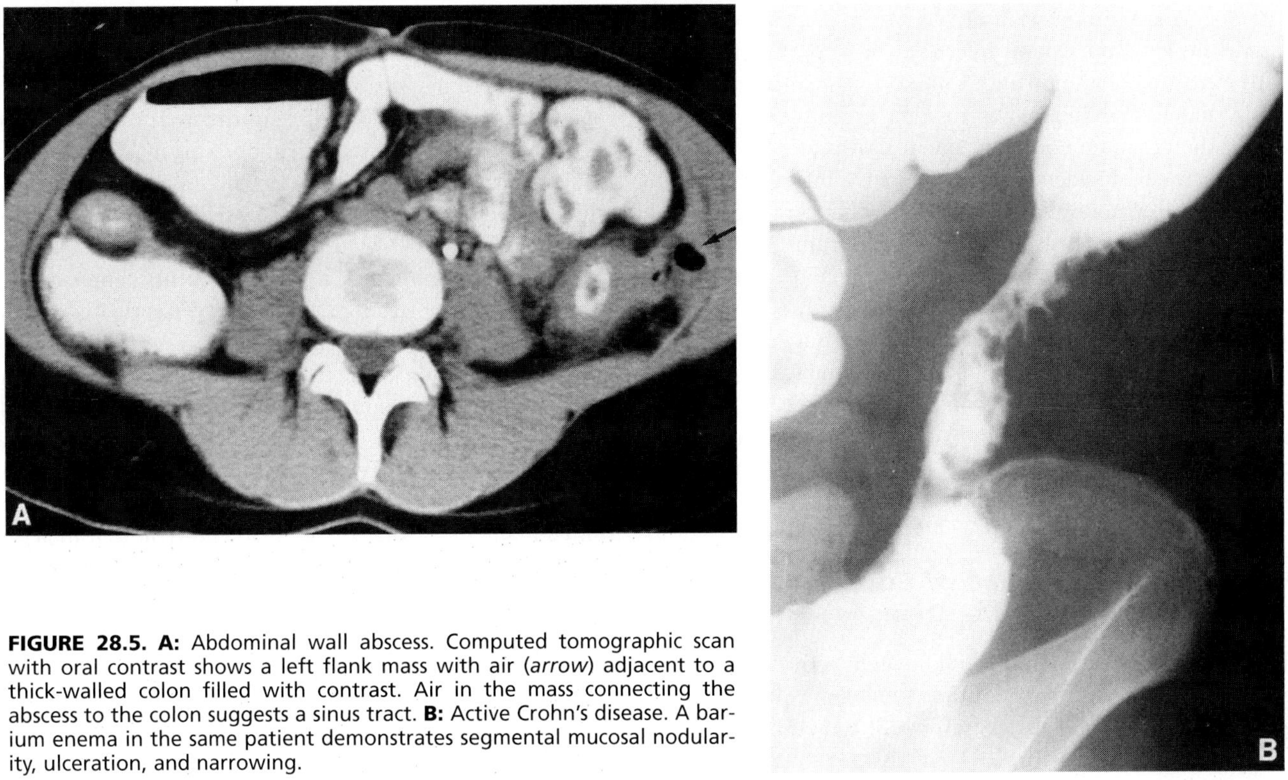

FIGURE 28.5. A: Abdominal wall abscess. Computed tomographic scan with oral contrast shows a left flank mass with air (*arrow*) adjacent to a thick-walled colon filled with contrast. Air in the mass connecting the abscess to the colon suggests a sinus tract. **B:** Active Crohn's disease. A barium enema in the same patient demonstrates segmental mucosal nodularity, ulceration, and narrowing.

95% originated from the ileum (383). Fistulous tracts in Crohn's disease can involve almost any organ, including the epidural space (384), salpinx, ureter, and urethra (383). Although the microbiology of fistulas has not been fully evaluated, luminal flora secondarily invade tissues (351) and provide a rationale for antibiotic therapy (160,385, 386). The clinical course and management of fistulas vary by location (383,387–391). Symptomatic enterocutaneous and rectovaginal fistulas usually require surgical management, although immunosuppressive therapy may be effective (392–395). Enterovesical fistulas frequently respond to combination treatment with antibiotics to sterilize the urine, infliximab, and 6-mercaptopurine (6-MP)–azathioprine (392,395). Perianal fistulas are particularly common in Crohn's disease. Diagnostic tests include an examination under anesthesia, combined with drainage of abscesses, CT scan or MRI to rule out deeper abscesses, and transrectal ultrasound. A comparison study indicated that anal endosonography with a linear probe is more accurate than MRI for detecting abscesses and the evaluation of complex perianal fistulas (396). Initial therapy is long-term metronidazole or ciprofloxacin (385,386), with approximately 50% of treatment-refractory patients responding to intravenous infliximab, oral 6-MP or azathioprine, or intravenous cyclosporine (392,394,395).

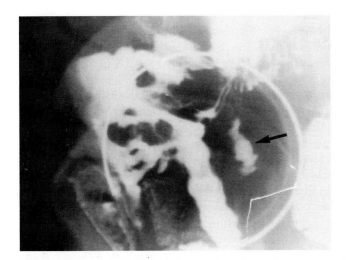

FIGURE 28.6. Complex ileocecal fistula. A small-bowel follow-through barium study demonstrates multiple fistulas between the distal ileum and cecum and a probable fistula from the distal ileum to the proximal small bowel. Extravasated barium medial to the ileum denotes an abscess (arrow).

Postoperative Infections

Perioperative infectious complications of IBD range from wound infections to peritonitis with sepsis (397). Septic complications after surgery are more common in emergent procedures when bowel preparation is incomplete and when the indication for surgery is intraabdominal sepsis. In one prospective study (398), septicemia occurred in 7% of patients, anastomotic leakage in 4%, intraabdominal abscess in 4%, and wound infections in 12%. Complications were more common with colonic disease, preoperative sepsis, and intraabdominal abscess. Emergent surgery and steroid therapy were not independent risk factors for infections. Increased incidence of postoperative infections after surgery for intraabdominal abscesses is common (366,367, 373,374); increased risk of septic complications related to corticosteroid therapy is less common (373,374). Creation of internal ileal pouches with anastomosis to the anorectal verge is a complex procedure associated with a 7% risk of infection (399) and 5% risk of perioperative abscess, which is associated with severe functional outcome (400). A relatively common complication of total proctocolectomy for ulcerative colitis is a persistent perineal wound, which occurs in up to 40% of operations (401).

Hematogenous Spread of Enteric Bacteria in Inflammatory Bowel Disease

The incidence of bacteremia is unknown in active IBD, but occasional sepsis (402), endocarditis (403–405), portal vein gas (406), and hepatic abscess (407,408) caused by enteric bacteria in patients with IBD clearly demonstrate that hematogenous dissemination of luminal bacteria must occur. Bacteremia in patients with IBD could be related to enhanced translocation of luminal bacteria across the inflamed mucosa into the lymphatic and portal circulations, overgrowth of luminal bacteria, immunosuppression due to medications or malnutrition, or increased frequency of colonoscopy with biopsy. Mucosal permeability is increased in active Crohn's disease and, to a lesser degree, in active ulcerative colitis (258). Bacteria have been cultured from the serosa or mesenteric lymph nodes of 56% of resected tissues from patients with Crohn's disease, compared with 17% of controls (248), and up to 27% of ulcerative colitis patients have portal vein bacteremia (409). Translocation of viable luminal bacteria to mesenteric lymph nodes occurs in a variety of animal models of intestinal inflammation (410,411) and small-bowel bacterial overgrowth (206) and is potentiated by obstruction (412), antibiotic use (413), and immunosuppression (414,415).

Opportunistic Infections

Patients with IBD have increased susceptibility to infection with enteric pathogens, possibly due to impaired mucosal host defense mechanisms. In addition, the use of increasingly potent immunosuppressive drugs to treat IBD is associated with the acquisition of opportunistic infections and potentiation of local septic complications. Chronic steroid use is frequently complicated by mucosal and systemic candidiasis but rarely by bacterial and viral infections (416). Steroid use was associated with a 27% risk of infection, including sepsis and liver abscess, compared with a 10% risk of infection in placebo-treated patients (417). In the European Crohn's disease study (418), no opportunistic infections were noted, but three of the five deaths occurred in steroid-treated patients with abdominal masses, although in the series by Felder et al. (419), no risks were associated with steroid therapy in patients with abdominal masses. Azathioprine and 6-MP at doses used in IBD are relatively safe, but surveys of large numbers of patients demonstrate a 7% incidence of infections, including disseminated CMV, herpes zoster encephalitis, and liver abscess (420). Use of cyclosporine in fulminant ulcerative colitis, usually in conjunction with intravenous corticosteroids, is associated with a substantial risk for infection, including *Pneumocystis* pneumonia, pulmonary abscess, mycotic aneurysm, and herpetic esophagitis (421–423). Prophylactic trimethoprim-sulfamethoxazole is used to prevent *Pneumocystis carinii* with cyclosporine and corticosteroid treatment. Infliximab (anti-tumor necrosis factor antibody) can potentiate abscesses (395) and has been associated with reactivation of quiescent TB and herpes zoster (424).

Bacterial Overgrowth

Approximately one-third of patients with Crohn's disease have increased luminal concentrations of predominantly aerobic bacteria in jejunal fluid; most of these patients have had resection of their ileocecal valve. Intestinal strictures and fistulas, particularly duodenal or jejunal fistulas to the colon, also predispose to proximal small-bowel overgrowth by anaerobes.

The ileal pouch–anal anastomosis procedure performed to preserve intestinal continuity after colectomy for ulcerative colitis can be complicated by intermittent pouch inflammation (pouchitis), which appears to be caused by an overgrowth of bacteria (229). A clinical response to metronidazole (425) or ciprofloxacin and increased luminal concentrations of either aerobic or anaerobic bacteria in symptomatic patients (426–428) suggest that both aerobes and anaerobes induce pouch inflammation. The number of adhesive *E. coli* in the pouch is increased but does not correlate with the level of inflammation (73). The pH level in the pouch also is increased, which enhances proteolytic enzyme activity and increases mucin degradation (427). The concept of an altered balance of beneficial versus detrimental bacteria in chronic pouchitis (139) is supported by the prevention of relapse in 85% of refractory patients with pouchitis treated with a cocktail of eight strains of probiotic lactobacteria, bifidobacteria, and streptococci (163). Of interest, clinical pouchitis occurs in at least 20% of patients with ulcerative colitis but is extremely rare in patients undergoing colectomy for familial polyposis (429), suggesting differential host susceptibility or perhaps a unique pathogenic flora in patients with ulcerative colitis.

CONCLUSION

The clinical and experimental information discussed in this chapter implicate microbial agents in the pathogenesis of chronic intestinal inflammation and its complications. Enteric pathogens induce inflammation that resembles the inflammatory responses of ulcerative colitis and Crohn's disease. It is possible that one or more enteric pathogens initiate IBD, which then is perpetuated by an independent cellular immune responses to certain components of the commensal luminal bacteria in genetically susceptible hosts, analogous to well-documented T-cell responses to bacteria in susceptible inbred rodents. Endogenous bacteria are also responsible for the most frequent complications of Crohn's disease. Careful attention to possible intestinal infections, judicious diagnostic evaluation, and appropriate treatment and prevention of suppurative complications of IBD should retard the progression of tissue damage in these disorders.

ACKNOWLEDGMENTS

The author gratefully acknowledges the expert secretarial assistance of Susie May. Original research described in this review was supported by National Institutes of Health grants DK40249, DK53347, DK47700, and DK34987, and the Crohn's and Colitis Foundation of America.

REFERENCES

1. Sandler RS, Eisen GM. Epidemiology of inflammatory bowel disease. In: Kirsner JB, ed. *Inflammatory bowel disease.* Chicago, IL: WB Saunders, 2000:89–112.
2. Sartor RB. Microbial factors in the pathogenesis of Crohn's disease, ulcerative colitis and experimental intestinal inflammation. In: Kirsner JB, ed. *Inflammatory bowel diseases,* fifth edition. Chicago, IL: WB Saunders, 1999:153–178.
3. Sartor RB. Intestinal microflora in human and experimental inflammatory bowel disease. *Curr Opin Gastroenterol* 2001;17: 324–330.
4. French N, Pettersson S. Microbe-host interactions in the alimentary tract: the gateway to understanding inflammatory bowel disease. *Gut* 2000;47:162–163.
5. Fiocchi C. Inflammatory bowel disease: etiology and pathogenesis. *Gastroenterology* 1998;115:182–205.
6. Elson CO, Cong Y, Iqbal N, Weaver CT. Immuno-bacterial homeostasis in the gut: new insights into an old enigma. *Semin Immunol* 2001;13:187–194.
7. Sartor RB. Pathogenesis and immune mechanisms of chronic inflammatory bowel diseases. *Am J Gastroenterol* 1997;92: 5S–11S.
8. Stainsby KJ, Lowes JR, Allan RN, et al. Antibodies to *Mycobacterium paratuberculosis* and nine species of environmental mycobacteria in Crohn's disease and control subjects. *Gut* 1993; 34:371–374.
9. Blaser MJ, Miller FA, Lacher J, et al. Patients with active Crohn's disease have elevated serum antibodies to antigens of seven enteric bacterial pathogens. *Gastroenterology* 1984;87: 888–894.
10. Tabaqchali S, O'Donoghue DP, Bettelheim KA. *Escherichia coli* antibodies in patients with inflammatory bowel disease. *Gut* 1978;19:108–113.
11. Macpherson A, Khoo UY, Forgacs I, et al. Mucosal antibodies in inflammatory bowel disease are directed against intestinal bacteria. *Gut* 1996;38:365–375.
12. Wensinck F, van de Merwe JP, Mayberry JF. An international study of agglutinins to *Eubacterium, Peptostreptococcus* and *Coprococcus* species in Crohn's disease, ulcerative colitis and control subjects. *Digestion* 1983;27:63–69.
13. Van Kruiningen HJ, Colombel JF, Cartun RW, et al. An in-depth study of Crohn's disease in two French families. *Gastroenterology* 1993;104:351–360.
14. Peeters M, Cortot A, Vermeire S, et al. Familial and sporadic inflammatory bowel disease: different entities? *Inflamm Bowel Dis* 2000;6:314–320.
15. Laharie D, Debeugny S, Peeters M, et al. Inflammatory bowel disease in spouses and their offspring. *Gastroenterology* 2001; 120:816–819.
16. Aisenberg J, Janowitz HD. Cluster of inflammatory bowel disease in three close college friends. *J Clin Gastroenterol* 1993;17: 18–20.
17. Chiodini RJ. Crohn's disease and the mycobacterioses: a review and comparison of two disease entities. *Clin Microbiol Rev* 1989;2:90–117.
18. Chiodini RJ, Van Kruiningen HJ, Thayer, et al. Possible role of mycobacteria in inflammatory bowel disease, I: an unclassified *Mycobacterium* species isolated from patients with Crohn's disease. *Dig Dis Sci* 1984;29:1073–1079.
19. Hermon-Taylor J, Bull TJ, Sheridan JM, et al. Causation of Crohn's disease by *Mycobacterium avium* subspecies paratuberculosis. *Can J Gastroenterol* 2000;14:521–539.
20. Graham DY. Mycobacteria and inflammatory bowel disease. *Gastroenterology* 1987;92:436–442.
21. Wall S, Kunze ZM, Saboor S. Identification of spheroplastlike agents isolated from tissues of patients with Crohn's disease and control tissues by polymerase chain reaction. *J Clin Microbiol* 1993;31:1241–1245.
22. Moss MT, Sanderson JD, Tizard ML, et al. Polymerase chain reaction detection of *Mycobacterium paratuberculosis* and *Mycobacterium avium* subsp *silvaticum* in long term cultures from Crohn's disease and control tissues. *Gut* 1992;33: 1209–1213.
23. Sanderson JD, Moss MT, Tizard ML, et al. *Mycobacterium paratuberculosis* DNA in Crohn's disease tissue. *Gut* 1992;33: 890–896.
24. Dell'Isola B, Poyart C, Goulet O, et al. Detection of *Mycobacterium paratuberculosis* by polymerase chain reaction in children with Crohn's disease. *J Infect Dis* 1994;169:449–451.
25. Kanazawa K, Haga Y, Funakoshi O, et al. Absence of *Mycobacterium paratuberculosis* DNA in intestinal tissues from Crohn's disease by nested polymerase chain reaction. *J Gastroenterol* 1999;34:200–206.
26. Fidler HM, Thurrel W, Johnson NM, et al. Specific detection of *Mycobacterium paratuberculosis* DNA associated with granulomatous tissue in Crohn's disease. *Gut* 1994;35:506–510.
27. Mishina D, Katsel P, Brown ST, et al. On the etiology of Crohn disease. *Proc Natl Acad Sci U S A* 1996;93:9816–9820.
28. Collins MT, Lisby G, Moser C, et al. Results of multiple diagnostic tests for *Mycobacterium avium* subsp. *paratuberculosis* in patients with inflammatory bowel disease and in controls. *J Clin Microbiol* 2000;38:4373–4381.
29. Chiba M, Kono M, Hoshina S, et al. Presence of bacterial 16S

ribosomal RNA gene segments in human intestinal lymph follicles. *Scand J Gastroenterol* 2000;35:824–831.
30. Hermon-Taylor J, Barnes N, Clarke C, et al. *Mycobacterium paratuberculosis* cervical lymphadenitis, followed five years later by terminal ileitis similar to Crohn's disease. *BMJ* 1998;316: 449–453.
31. Naser SA, Hulten K, Shafran I, et al. Specific seroreactivity of Crohn's disease patients against p35 and p36 antigens of *M. avium* subsp. paratuberculosis. *Vet Microbiol* 2000;77:497–504.
32. Olsen I, Wiker HG, Johnson E, et al. Elevated antibody responses in patients with Crohn's disease against a 14-kDa secreted protein purified from *Mycobacterium avium* subsp. *paratuberculosis*. *Scand J Immunol* 2001;53:198–203.
33. Cohavy O, Harth G, Horwitz M, et al. Identification of a novel mycobacterial histone H1 homologue (HupB) as an antigenic target of p-ANCA monoclonal antibody and serum immunoglobulin A from patients with Crohn's disease. *Infect Immun* 1999;67:6510–6517.
34. Chiodini RJ, Van Kruiningen HJ, Merkal, et al. Ruminant paratuberculosis (Johne's disease): the current status and future prospects. *Cornell Vet* 1984;74:218–262.
35. Sweeney RW, Whitlock RH, Rosenberger AE. *Mycobacterium paratuberculosis* cultured from milk and supramammary lymph nodes of infected asymptomatic cows. *J Clin Microbiol* 1992;30: 166–171.
36. Millar D, Ford J, Sanderson J, et al. IS900 PCR to detect *Mycobacterium paratuberculosis* in retail supplies of whole pasteurized cows' milk in England and Wales. *Appl Environ Microbiol* 1996;62:3446–3452.
37. Stabel JR, Steadham EM, Bolin CA. Heat inactivation of *Mycobacterium paratuberculosis* in raw milk: are current pasteurization conditions effective? *Appl Environ Microbiol* 1997;63: 4975–4977.
38. Naser SA, Schwartz D, Shafran I. Isolation of *Mycobacterium avium* subsp *paratuberculosis* from breast milk of Crohn's disease patients. *Am J Gastroenterol* 2000;95:1094–1095.
39. Kobayashi K, Blaser MJ, Brown WR. Immunohistochemical examination for mycobacteria in intestinal tissues from patients with Crohn's disease. *Gastroenterology* 1989;96:1009–1015.
40. Hulten K, Karttunen TJ, El-Zimaity HM, et al. In situ hybridization method for studies of cell wall deficient *M. paratuberculosis* in tissue samples. *Vet Microbiol* 2000;77: 513–518.
41. Thomas GA, Swift GL, Green JT, et al. Controlled trial of antituberculous chemotherapy in Crohn's disease: a five year follow up study. *Gut* 1998;42:497–500.
42. Prantera C, Kohn A, Mangiarotti R, et al. Antimycobacterial therapy in Crohn's disease: results of a controlled, double-blind trial with a multiple antibiotic regimen. *Am J Gastroenterol* 1994;89:513–518.
43. Gui GP, Thomas PR, Tizard ML, et al. Two-year-outcomes analysis of Crohn's disease treated with rifabutin and macrolide antibiotics. *J Antimicrob Chemother* 1997;39:393–400.
44. Leiper K, Morris AI, Rhodes JM. Open label trial of oral clarithromycin in active Crohn's disease. *Alimentary Pharmacol Ther* 2000;14:801–806.
45. Wakefield AJ, Pittilo RM, Sim R, et al. Evidence of persistent measles virus infection in Crohn's disease. *J Med Virol* 1993; 39:345–353.
46. Wakefield AJ, Montgomery SM, Pounder RE. Crohn's disease: the case for measles virus. *Italian J Gastroenterol Hepatol* 1999; 31:247–254.
47. Daszak P, Purcell M, Lewin J, et al. Detection and comparative analysis of persistent measles virus infection in Crohn's disease by immunogold electron microscopy. *J Clin Pathol* 1997;50: 299–304.
48. Balzola FA, Khan K, Pera A, et al. Measles IgM immunoreactivity in patients with inflammatory bowel disease. *Italian J Gastroenterol Hepatol* 1998;30:378–382.
49. Sankey EA, Dhillon AP, Anthony A. Early mucosal changes in Crohn's disease. *Gut* 1993;34:375–381.
50. Ekbom A, Daszak P, Kraaz W, et al. Crohn's disease after inutero measles virus exposure. *Lancet* 1996;348:515–517.
51. Thompson NP, Montgomery SM, Pounder RE, et al. Is measles vaccination a risk factor for inflammatory bowel disease? *Lancet* 1995;345:1071–1074.
52. Thompson NP, Pounder RE, Wakefield AJ. Perinatal and childhood risk factors for inflammatory bowel disease: a case–control study. *Eur J Gastroenterol Hepatol* 1995;7:385–390.
53. Thompson NP, Montgomery SM, Wadsworth ME, et al. Early determinants of inflammatory bowel disease: use of two national longitudinal birth cohorts. *Eur J Gastroenterol Hepatol* 2000;12:25–30.
54. Morris DL, Montgomery SM, Thompson NP, et al. Measles vaccination and inflammatory bowel disease: a national British Cohort Study. *Am J Gastroenterol* 2000;95:3507–3512.
55. Robertson DJ, Sandler RS. Measles virus and Crohn's disease: a critical appraisal of the current literature. *Inflamm Bowel Dis* 2001;7:51–57.
56. Ghosh S, Armitage E, Wilson D, et al. Detection of persistent measles virus infection in Crohn's disease: current status of experimental work. *Gut* 2001;48:748–752.
57. Pardi DS, Tremaine WJ, Sandborn WJ, et al. Early measles virus infection is associated with the development of inflammatory bowel disease. *Am J Gastroenterol* 2000;95:1480–1485.
58. Pardi DS, Tremaine WJ, Sandborn WJ, et al. Perinatal exposure to measles virus is not associated with the development of inflammatory bowel disease. *Inflamm Bowel Dis* 1999;5: 104–106.
59. Miyamoto H, Tanaka T, Kitamoto N, et al. Detection of immunoreactive antigen, with a monoclonal antibody to measles virus, in tissue from a patient with Crohn's disease. *J Gastroenterol* 1995;30:28–33.
60. Liu Y, Van Kruiningen HJ, West AB, et al. Immunocytochemical evidence of *Listeria, Escherichia coli,* and *Streptococcus* antigens in Crohn's disease. *Gastroenterology* 1995;108:1396–1404.
61. Iizuka M, Chiba M, Yukawa M, et al. Immunohistochemical analysis of the distribution of measles related antigen in the intestinal mucosa in inflammatory bowel disease. *Gut* 2000; 46:163–169.
62. Haga Y, Funakoshi O, Kuroe K, et al. Absence of measles viral genomic sequence in intestinal tissues from Crohn's disease by nested polymerase chain reaction. *Gut* 1996;38:211–215.
63. Afzal MA, Armitage E, Ghosh S, et al. Further evidence of the absence of measles virus genome sequence in full thickness intestinal specimens from patients with Crohn's disease. *J Med Virol* 2000;62:377–382.
64. Fisher NC, Yee L, Nightingale P, et al. Measles virus serology in Crohn's disease. *Gut* 1997;41:66–69.
65. Van Kruiningen HJ, Mayo DR, Vanopdenbosch E, et al. Virus serology in familial Crohn's disease. *Scand J Gastroenterol* 2000; 35:403–407.
66. Davis RL, Kramarz P, Bohlke K, et al. Measles-mumps-rubella and other measles-containing vaccines do not increase the risk for inflammatory bowel disease: a case–control study from the Vaccine Safety Datalink project. *Arch Pediatr Adolesc Med* 2001; 155:354–359.
67. Anonymous. WHO concludes that measles viruses are not associated with Crohn's disease. *Commun Dis Rep CDR Wkly* 1998:8.
68. Walmsley RS, Anthony A, Sim R, et al. Absence of *Escherichia coli, Listeria monocytogenes,* and *Klebsiella pneumoniae* antigens

within inflammatory bowel disease tissues. *J Clin Pathol* 1998; 51:657–661.

69. Chen W, Li D, Paulus B, et al. Detection of *Listeria monocytogenes* by polymerase chain reaction in intestinal mucosal biopsies from patients with inflammatory bowel disease and controls. *J Gastroenterol Hepatol* 2000;15:1145–1150.
70. Chiba M, Fukushima T, Inoue S, et al. *Listeria monocytogenes* in Crohn's disease. *Scand J Gastroenterol* 1998;33:430–434.
71. Chiba M, Fukushima T, Koganei K, et al. *Listeria monocytogenes* in the colon in a case of fulminant ulcerative colitis. *Scand J Gastroenterol* 1998;33:778–782.
72. Burke DA, Axon ATR. Adhesive *Escherichia coli* in inflammatory bowel disease and infective diarrhoea. *Br Med J* 1988;297: 102–104.
73. Lobo AJ, Sagar PM, Rothwell J, et al. Carriage of adhesive *Escherichia coli* after restorative proctocolectomy and pouch anal anastomosis: relation with functional outcome and inflammation. *Gut* 1993;34:1379–1383.
74. Giaffer MH, Holdsworth CD, Duerden BI. Virulence properties of *Escherichia coli* strains isolated from patients with inflammatory bowel disease. *Gut* 1992;33:646–650.
75. Hartley MG, Hudson MJ, Swarbrick ET, et al. Adhesive and hydrophobic properties of *Escherichia coli* from the rectal mucosa of patients with ulcerative colitis. *Gut* 1993;34:63–67.
76. Schultsz C, Moussa M, van Ketel R, et al. Frequency of pathogenic and enteroadherent *Escherichia coli* in patients with inflammatory bowel disease and controls. *J Clin Pathol* 1997; 50:573–579.
77. Darfeuille-Michaud A, Neut C, Barnich N, et al. Presence of adherent *Escherichia coli* strains in ileal mucosa of patients with Crohn's disease. *Gastroenterology* 1998;115:1405–1413.
78. Boudeau J, Glasser AL, Masseret E, et al. Invasive ability of an *Escherichia coli strain* isolated from the ileal mucosa of a patient with Crohn's disease. *Infect Immun* 1999;67:4499–4509.
79. Masseret E, Boudeau J, Colombel JF, et al. Genetically related *Escherichia coli* strains associated with Crohn's disease. *Gut* 2001;48:320–325.
80. Pearce CB, Duncan HD, Timmis L, et al. Assessment of the prevalence of infection with *Helicobacter pylori* in patients with inflammatory bowel disease. *Eur J Gastroenterol Hepatol* 2000; 12:439–443.
81. Puspok A, Dejaco C, Oberhuber G, et al. Influence of *Helicobacter pylori* infection on the phenotype of Crohn's disease. *Am J Gastroenterol* 1999;94:3239–3244.
82. Fox JG, Gorelick PL, Kullberg MC, et al. A novel urease-negative *Helicobacter* species associated with colitis and typhlitis in IL-10-deficient mice. *Infect Immun* 1999;64:1757–1762.
83. Franklin CL, Riley LK, Livingston RS, et al. Enteric lesions in SCID mice infected with "*Helicobacter typhlonicus,*" a novel urease-negative *Helicobacter species. Lab Anim Sci* 1999;49:496–505.
84. Kullberg MC, Ward JM, Gorelick P, et al. *Helicobacter hepaticus* triggers colitis in specific-pathogen-free interleukin-10 (IL-10)-deficient mice through an IL-12 and gamma interferon-dependent mechanism. *Infect Immun* 1998;66:5157–5166.
85. Dieleman LA, Arends A, Tonkonogy SL, et al. *Helicobacter hepaticus* does not induce or potentiate colitis in interleukin-10-deficient mice. *Infect Immun* 2000;68:5107–5113.
86. Wood JD, Peck OC, Tefend KS, et al. Evidence that colitis is initiated by environmental stress and sustained by fecal factors in the cotton-top tamarin (Saguinus oedipus). *Dig Dis Sci* 2000; 45:385–393.
87. Young VB, Knox KA, Schauer DB. Cytolethal distending toxin sequence and activity in the enterohepatic pathogen *Helicobacter hepaticus. Infect Immun* 2000;68:184–191.
88. Tiveljung A, Soderholm JD, Olaison G, et al. Presence of eubacteria in biopsies from Crohn's disease inflammatory lesions as determined by 16S rRNA gene-based PCR. *J Med Microbiol* 1999;48:263–268.
89. Wei B, Huang T, Dalwadi HN, et al. Identification of *Pseudomonas fluorescens* as the microorganism expressing the Crohn's disease-associated I2 gene. *Gastroenterology* 2001;120: A82(abst).
90. Sutton CL, Kim J, Yamane A, et al. Identification of a novel bacterial sequence associated with Crohn's disease. *Gastroenterology* 2000;119:23–31.
91. Chiba C, Nakamura T, Hoshina S, et al. Optimal cases and sites to search for primary microbial agents in Crohn's disease. *Gastroenterology* 2001;120:1066–1067.
92. Dalwadi H, Wei B, Kronenberg M, et al. The Crohn's disease-associated bacterial protein I2 is a novel enteric T cell superantigen. *Immunity* 2001;15:149–158.
93. Parent K, Mitchel P. Cell wall defective variants of *Pseudomonas* like (group Va) bacteria in Crohn's disease. *Gastroenterology* 1978;75:368–372.
94. Powell SJ, Wilmont AJ. Ulcerative postdysenteric colitis. *Gut* 1966;7:438–443.
95. Orvar K, Murray J, Carmen G, et al. Cytomegalovirus infection associated with onset of inflammatory bowel disease. *Dig Dis Sci* 1993;38:2307–2310.
96. Willoughby JM, Rahman AF, Gregory MM. Chronic colitis after *Aeromonas* infection. *Gut* 1989;30:686–690.
97. Leblanc M, Delage G, Rousseau E, et al. Prevalence of *Aeromonas* spp. pediatric gastroenteritis. *Can Med Assoc J* 1988; 138:714–717.
98. Saebo A, Lassen J. *Yersinia enterocolitica:* an inducer of chronic inflammation. *Int J Tissue React* 1994;16:51–57.
99. Fohlman J, Friman F. Is juvenile diabetes a viral disease? *Ann Med* 1993;25:569–574.
100. Sartor RB, Lichtman SN. Mechanisms of systemic inflammation associated with intestinal injury. In: Targan SR, Shanahan F, eds. *Inflammatory bowel disease: from bench to bedside.* Baltimore, MD: Williams & Wilkins, 1993:210–229.
101. Lu L, Walker WA. Pathologic and physiologic interactions of bacteria with the gastrointestinal epithelium. *Am J Clin Nutr* 2001;73:1124S–1130S.
102. Dwinell MB, Lugering N, Eckmann L, et al. Regulated production of interferon-inducible T-cell chemoattractants by human intestinal epithelial cells. *Gastroenterology* 2001;120: 49–59.
103. Kagnoff MF, Eckmann L. Epithelial cells as sensors for microbial infection. *J Clin Invest* 1997;100:6–10.
104. Elewaut D, DiDonato JA, Kim JM, et al. NF-kappa B is a central regulator of the intestinal epithelial cell innate immune response induced by infection with enteroinvasive bacteria. *J Immunol* 1999;163:1457–1466.
105. Jobin C, Sartor RB. The I kappa B/NF-kappa B system: a key determinant of mucosal inflammation and protection. *Am J Physiol Cell Physiol* 2000;278:C451–C462.
106. Han DS, Li F., Holt LC, et al. Keratinocyte growth factor-2 (fibroblast growth factor-10) promotes healing of indomethacin-induced small intestinal ulceration in rats and stimulates epithelial cell restitution and protective molecules. *Am J Physiol* 2000;279:G1011–G1022.
107. Berg DJ, Weinstock JV, Lynch R. Rapid induction of inflammatory bowel disease in NSAID-treated IL-10 –/– mice. *Gastroenterology* 2001;120:A685(abst).
108. Schwab JH. Phlogistic properties of peptidoglycan-polysaccharide polymers from cell walls of pathogenic and normal-flora bacteria which colonize humans. *Infect Immun* 1993;61: 4535–4539.
109. Hsu DH, de Waal Malefyt R, Fiorentino DF. Expression of

interleukin 10 activity by Epstein Barr virus protein BCRF1. *Science* 1990;250:830–832.
110. Klapproth JM, Scaletsky IC, McNamara BP, et al. A large toxin from pathogenic *Escherichia coli* strains that inhibits lymphocyte activation. *Infect Immun* 2000;68:2148–2155.
111. Mullin GE, Lazenby AJ, Harris ML, et al. Increased interleukin 2 messenger RNA in the intestinal mucosal lesions of Crohn's disease but not ulcerative colitis. *Gastroenterology* 1992;102: 1620–1627.
112. Wakefield AJ, Fox JD, Sawyerr AM, et al. Detection of herpes virus DNA in the large intestine of patients with ulcerative colitis and Crohn's disease using the nested polymerase chain reaction. *J Med Virol* 1992;38:183–190.
113. Sadlack B, Merz H, Schorle H, et al. Ulcerative colitis-like disease in mice with a disrupted interleukin-2 gene. *Cell* 1993;75: 253–261.
114. Kuhn R, Lohler J, Rennick D, et al. Interleukin-10-deficient mice develop chronic enterocolitis. *Cell* 1993;75:263–274.
115. Porat R, Clark BD, Wolff SM, et al. Enhancement of growth of virulent strains of *Escherichia coli* by interleukin 1. *Science* 1991;254:430–432.
116. Broom MF, Scherriff RM, Ferry DM, et al. Formyl-methionyl-leucyl-phenylalanine and the SOS operon in *Escherichia coli:* a model of host bacterial interactions. *Biochem J* 1993;291: 895–900.
117. Lagercrantz RS, Hammerstrom S, Perlmann P, et al. Immunological studies in ulcerative colitis, IV: origin of autoantibodies. *J Exp Med* 1968;128:1339–1352.
118. Thayer WR, Brown M, Sangree MH, et al. *Escherichia coli* O14 and colon hemagglutinating antibodies in inflammatory bowel disease. *Gastroenterology* 1969;57:311–318.
119. Geng X, Biancone L, Dai HH, et al. Tropomyosin isoforms in intestinal mucosa: production of autoantibodies to tropomyosin isoforms in ulcerative colitis. *Gastroenterology* 1998;114: 912–922.
120. Jones KF, Whitehead SS, Cunningham MW, et al. Reactivity of rheumatic fever and scarlet fever patients' sera with group A streptococcal M protein, cardiac myosin, and cardiac tropomyosin: a retrospective study. *Infect Immun* 2000;68:7132–7136.
121. Ruemmele FM, Targan SR, Levy G, et al. Diagnostic accuracy of serological assays in pediatric inflammatory bowel disease. *Gastroenterology* 1998;115:822–829.
122. Duerr RH, Targan SR, Landers CJ, et al. Anti-neutrophil cytoplasmic antibodies in ulcerative colitis. Comparison with other colitides/diarrheal illnesses. *Gastroenterology* 1991;100: 1590–1596.
123. Seibold F, Brandwein S, Simpson S, et al. pANCA represents a cross-reactivity to enteric bacterial antigens. *J Clin Immunol* 1998;18:153–160.
124. Cohavy O, Bruckner D, Gordon LK, et al. Colonic bacteria express an ulcerative colitis pANCA-related protein epitope. *Infect Immun* 2000;68:1542–1548.
125. el-Zaatari FA, Naser SA, Engstrand L, et al. Nucleotide sequence analysis and seroreactivities of the 65K heat shock protein from *Mycobacterium paratuberculosis. Clin Diagn Lab Immunol* 1995;2:657–664.
126. Heimbach JK, Reznikov LL, Calkins CM, et al. TNF receptor I is required for induction of macrophage heat shock protein 70. *Am J Physiol Cell Physiol* 2001;281:C241–C247.
127. Winrow VR, Mojdehi GM, Ryder SD, et al. Stress proteins in colorectal mucosa. Enhanced expression in ulcerative colitis. *Dig Dis Sci* 1993;38:1994–2000.
128. Baca-Estrada ME, Gupta RS, Stead RH, et al. Intestinal expression and cellular immune responses to human heat-shock protein 60 in Crohn's disease. *Dig Dis Sci* 1994;39:498–506.
129. Ludwig D, Stahl M, Ibrahim ET, et al. Enhanced intestinal expression of heat shock protein 70 in patients with inflammatory bowel diseases. *Dig Dis Sci* 1999;44:1440–1447.
130. Esaki M, Furuse M, Matsumoto T, et al. Polymorphism of heat-shock protein gene HSP70-2 in Crohn disease: possible genetic marker for two forms of Crohn's disease. *Scand J Gastroenterol* 1999;34:703–707.
131. Stevens TR, Winrow VR, Blake DR, et al. Circulating antibodies to heat shock protein 60 in Crohn's disease and ulcerative colitis. *Clin Exp Immunol* 1992;90:271–274.
132. Elsaghier A, Prantera C, Bothamley G, et al. Disease association of antibodies to human and mycobacterial hsp70 and hsp60 stress proteins. *Clin Exp Immunol* 1992;89:305–309.
133. el-Zaatari FA, Naser SA, Hulten K, et al. Characterization of *Mycobacterium paratuberculosis* p36 antigen and its seroreactivities in Crohn's disease. *Curr Microbiol* 1999;39:115–119.
134. Szewczuk MR, Depew WT. Evidence for T lymphocyte reactivity to the 65 kilodalton heat shock protein of mycobacterium in active Crohn's disease. *Clin Invest Med* 1992;15:494–505.
135. Spahn TW, Heimann H, Duchmann R, et al. Cellular and humoral immunity to the 60-kD heat shock protein in inflammatory bowel disease. *Digestion* 1997;58:469–475.
136. Van Eden W, van der Zee R. Cloning of the mycobacterial epitope recognized by T lymphocytes in adjuvant arthritis. *Nature* 1988;331:171–173.
137. Yagita A, Sukegawa Y, Maruyama S, et al. Mouse colitis induced by *Escherichia coli* producing *Yersinia enterocolitica* 60-kilodalton heat-shock protein: light and electron microscope study. *Dig Dis Sci* 1999;44:445–451.
138. Sukegawa Y, Kamiya S, Yagita A, et al. Induction of autoimmune colitis by *Yersinia enterocolitica* 60-kilodalton heat-shock protein. *Scand J Gastroenterol* 2000;35:1188–1193.
139. Sartor RB. Probiotics in chronic pouchitis: restoring luminal microbial balance. *Gastroenterology* 2000;119:584–587.
140. Wurzelmann JI, Lyles CM, Sandler RS. Childhood infections and the risk of inflammatory bowel disease. *Dig Dis Sci* 1994; 39:555–560.
141. Araki Y, Andoh A, Koyama S, et al. Effects of germinated barley foodstuff on microflora and short chain fatty acid production in dextran sulfate sodium-induced colitis in rats. *Biosci Biotechnol Biochem* 2000;64:1794–1800.
142. Kishi D, Takahashi I, Kai Y, et al. Alteration of V beta usage and cytokine production of CD4+ TCR beta beta homodimer T cells by elimination of *Bacteroides vulgatus* prevents colitis in TCR alpha-chain-deficient mice. *J Immunol* 2000;165: 5891–5899.
143. van de Merwe JP, Schroder AM, Wensinck F, et al. The obligate anaerobic faecal flora of patients with Crohn's disease and their first-degree relatives. *Scand J Gastroenterol* 1988;23:1125–1131.
144. Ruseler-van Embden JG, Both-Patoir HC. Anaerobic gram-negative faecal flora in patients with Crohn's disease and healthy subjects. *Antonie van Leeuwenhoek* 1983;49:125–132.
145. Auer IO, Roder A, Wensinck F, et al. Selected bacterial antibodies in Crohn's disease and ulcerative colitis. *Scand J Gastroenterol* 1983;18:217–223.
146. Krook A, Lindstrom B, Kjellander J, et al. Relation between concentrations of metronidazole and *Bacteroides* spp in faeces of patients with Crohn's disease and healthy individuals. *J Clin Pathol* 1981;34:645–650.
147. Sutherland L, Singleton J, Sessions J, et al. Double blind, placebo controlled trial of metronidazole in Crohn's disease. *Gut* 1991;32:1071–1075.
148. Onderdonk AB, Franklin ML, Cisneros RL. Production of experimental ulcerative colitis in gnotobiotic guinea pigs with simplified microflora. *Infect Immun* 1981;32:225–231.
149. Rath HC, Herfarth HH, Ikeda JS, et al. Normal luminal bacteria, especially *Bacteroides species,* mediate chronic colitis, gastri-

tis, and arthritis in HLA-B27/human beta2 microglobulin transgenic rats. *J Clin Invest* 1996;98:945–953.
150. Severijnen AJ, Hazenberg MP, van de M, et al. Induction of chronic arthritis in rats by cell wall fragments of anaerobic coccoid rods isolated from the faecal flora of patients with Crohn's disease. *Digestion* 1988;39:118–125.
151. Fabia R, Ar'Rajab A, Johansson ML, et al. Impairment of bacterial flora in human ulcerative colitis and experimental colitis in the rat. *Digestion* 1993;54:248–255.
152. Hartley MG, Hudson MJ, Swarbrick ET, et al. The rectal mucosa-associated microflora in patients with ulcerative colitis. *J Med Microbiol* 1992;36:96–103.
153. Matsuda H, Fujiyama Y, Andoh A, et al. Characterization of antibody responses against rectal mucosa-associated bacterial flora in patients with ulcerative colitis. *J Gastroenterol Hepatol* 2000;15:61–68.
154. Schultsz C, Van Den Berg FM, Ten Kate FW, et al. The intestinal mucus layer from patients with inflammatory bowel disease harbors high numbers of bacteria compared with controls. *Gastroenterology* 1999;117:1089–1097.
155. Giaffer MH, Holdsworth CD, Duerden BI. The assessment of faecal flora in patients with inflammatory bowel disease by a simplified bacteriological technique. *J Med Microbiol* 1991;35:238–243.
156. Favier C, Neut C, Mizon C, et al. Fecal beta-D-galactosidase production and *Bifidobacteria* are decreased in Crohn's disease. *Dig Dis Sci* 1997;42:817–822.
157. Madsen KL, Doyle JS, Tavernini MM, et al. Antibiotic therapy attenuates colitis in interleukin 10 gene-deficient mice. *Gastroenterology* 2000;118:1094–1055.
158. Shanahan F. Probiotics and inflammatory bowel disease: is there a scientific rationale? *Inflamm Bowel Dis* 2000;6:107–115.
159. Schultz M, Sartor RB. Probiotics and inflammatory bowel diseases. *Am J Gastroenterol* 2000;95:S19–S21
160. Gionchetti P, Rizzello F, Campieri M. Probiotics and antibiotics in inflammatory bowel diseases. *Curr Opin Gastroenterol* 2001;17:331–335.
161. Dunne C. Adaptation of bacteria to the intestinal niche: Probiotics and gut disorder. *Inflamm Bowel Dis* 2001;7:136–145.
162. Kruis W, Schutz E, Fric P, et al. Double-blind comparison of an oral *Escherichia coli* preparation and mesalazine in maintaining remission of ulcerative colitis. *Alimentary Pharmacol Ther* 1997;11:853–858.
163. Gionchetti P, Rizzello F, Venturi A, et al. Oral bacteriotherapy as maintenance treatment in patients with chronic pouchitis: a double-blind, placebo-controlled trial. *Gastroenterology* 2000;119:305–309.
164. Madsen KL, Doyle JS, Jewell LD, et al. *Lactobacillus species* prevents colitis in interleukin 10 gene-deficient mice. *Gastroenterology* 1999;116:1107–1114.
165. McCormick BA, Miller SI, Carnes D, et al. Transepithelial signaling to neutrophils by salmonellae: a novel virulence mechanism for gastroenteritis. *Infect Immun* 1995;63:2302–2309.
166. Cooke EM, Ewins SP, Hywel-Jones J, et al. Properties of strains of *Escherichia coli* carried in different phases of ulcerative colitis. *Gut* 1974;15:143–146.
167. von Wulffen H, Russmann H, Karch H, et al. Verocytotoxin-producing *Escherichia coli* O2:H5 isolated from patients with ulcerative colitis. *Lancet* 1989;1:1449–1450.
168. Ruseler-van Embden JG, van Der Helm R, der HR, et al. Degradation of intestinal glycoproteins by *Bacteroides vulgatus. FEMS Microbiol Lett* 1989;49:37–41.
169. van der Wiel-Korstanje JA, Winkler KC. The faecal flora in ulcerative colitis. *J Med Microbiol* 1975;8:491–501.
170. Chiba M, Hoshina S, Kono M, et al. Staphylococcus aureus in inflammatory bowel disease. *Scand J Gastroenterol* 2001;36:615–620.
171. Roediger WE. The colonic epithelium in ulcerative colitis: an energy-deficiency disease? *Lancet* 1980;2:712–715.
172. Harig JM, Soergel KH, Komorowski RA, et al. Treatment of diversion colitis with short-chain-fatty acid irrigation. *N Engl J Med* 1989;320:23–28.
173. Chapman MA, Grahn MF, Boyle MA, et al. Butyrate oxidation is impaired in the colonic mucosa of sufferers of quiescent ulcerative colitis. *Gut* 1994;35:73–76.
174. Allan ES, Winter S, Light AM, et al. Mucosal enzyme activity for butyrate oxidation; no defect in patients with ulcerative colitis. *Gut* 1996;38:886–893.
175. Scheppach W, Sommer H, Kirchner T, et al. Effect of butyrate enemas on the colonic mucosa in distal ulcerative colitis. *Gastroenterology* 1992;103:51–56.
176. Steinhart AH, Hiruki T, Brzezinski A, et al. Treatment of left-sided ulcerative colitis with butyrate enemas: a controlled trial. *Alimentary Pharmacol Ther* 1996;10:729–736.
177. Segain JP, Raingeard dlB, Bourreille A, et al. Butyrate inhibits inflammatory responses through NFkappaB inhibition: implications for Crohn's disease. *Gut* 2000;47:397–403.
178. Roediger WE, Duncan A, Kapaniris O, et al. Reducing sulfur compounds of the colon impair colonocyte nutrition: implications for ulcerative colitis. *Gastroenterology* 1993;104:802–809.
179. Pitcher MC, Gibson GR, Neale G, et al. Gentamicin kills multiple drug resistant sulfate reducing bacteria in patients with ulcerative colitis. *Gastroenterology* 1994;106:A753(abst).
180. Gibson GR, Cummings JH, Macfarlane GT. Growth and activities of sulphate-reducing bacteria in gut contents of healthy subjects and patients with ulcerative colitis. *FEMS Microbiol Ecol* 1991;86:103–111.
181. Pitcher MC, Beatty ER, Cummings JH. The contribution of sulphate reducing bacteria and 5-aminosalicylic acid to faecal sulphide in patients with ulcerative colitis. *Gut* January 2000;46:64–72.
182. Furne JK, Suarez FL, Ewing SL, et al. Binding of hydrogen sulfide by bismuth does not prevent dextran sulfate-induced colitis in rats. *Dig Dis Sci* 2000;45:1439–1443.
183. Neish AS, Gewirtz AT, Zeng H, et al. Prokaryotic regulation of epithelial responses by inhibition of IkappaB-alpha ubiquination. *Science* 2000;289:1560–1563.
184. Spiik AK, Meijer LK, Ridderstad A, et al. Interference of eukaryotic signaling pathways by the bacteria *Yersinia* outer protein YopJ. *Immunol Lett* 1999;68:199–203.
185. Sellon RK, Tonkonogy S, Schultz M, et al. Resident enteric bacteria are necessary for development of spontaneous colitis and immune system activation in interleukin-10-deficient mice. *Infect Immun* 1998;66:5224–5231.
186. Berg DJ, Davidson N, Kuhn R, et al. Enterocolitis and colon cancer in interleukin-10-deficient mice are associated with aberrant cytokine production and CD4(+) Th1-like responses. *J Clin Invest* 1996;98:1010–1020.
187. Davidson NJ, Leach MW, Fort MM, et al. T helper cell 1-type CD4+ T cells, but not B cells, mediate colitis in interleukin 10-deficient mice. *J Exp Med* 1996;184:241–251.
188. Dieleman LA, Hoentjen F, Ehre C, et al. Antibiotics with a selective aerobic and anaerobic spectrum have different therapeutic activities in various regions of the colon in IL-10 knockout mice. *Gastroenterology* 2001;120:A687(abst).
189. Rath HC, Ikeda JS, Linde HJ, et al. Varying cecal bacterial loads influences colitis and gastritis in HLA-B27 transgenic rats. *Gastroenterology* 1999;116:310–319.
190. Mizoguchi A, Mizoguchi E, Chiba C, et al. Role of appendix in the development of inflammatory bowel disease in TCR-alpha mutant mice. *J Exp Med* 1996;184:707–715.

191. Strober W, Ludviksson BR, Fuss IJ. The pathogenesis of mucosal inflammation in murine models of inflammatory bowel disease and Crohn's disease. *Ann Intern Med* 1998;128: 848–856.
192. Brandwein SL, McCabe RP, Cong Y, et al. Spontaneously colitic C3H/HeJBir mice demonstrate selective antibody reactivity to antigens of the enteric bacterial flora. *J Immunol* 1997; 159:44–52.
193. Cong Y, Brandwein SL, McCabe RP, et al. CD4+ T cells reactive to enteric bacterial antigens in spontaneously colitic C3H/HeJBir mice: increased T helper cell type 1 response and ability to transfer disease. *J Exp Med* 1998;187:855–864.
194. Veltkamp C, Tonkonogy SL, de Jong YP, et al. Continuous stimulation by normal luminal bacteria is essential for the development and perpetuation of colitis in Tg(epsilon26) mice. *Gastroenterology* 2001;120:900–913.
195. Ma A, Datta M, Margosian E, et al. T cells, but not B cells, are required for bowel inflammation in interleukin 2-deficient mice. *J Exp Med* 1995;182:1567–1572.
196. Mizoguchi A, Mizoguchi E, Smith RN, et al. Suppressive role of B cells in chronic colitis of T cell receptor alpha mutant mice. *J Exp Med* 1997;186:1749–1756.
197. Taurog JD, Richardson JA, Croft JT, et al. The germfree state prevents development of gut and joint inflammatory disease in HLA-B27 transgenic rats. *J Exp Med* 1994;180:2359–2364.
198. Rath HC, Wilson KH, Sartor RB. Differential induction of colitis and gastritis in HLA-B27 transgenic rats selectively colonized with *Bacteroides vulgatus* and *Escherichia coli. Infect Immun* 1999;67:2969–2974.
199. Rath HC, Schultz M, Freitag R, et al. Different subsets of enteric bacteria induce and perpetuate experimental colitis in rats and mice. *Infect Immun* 2001;69:2277–2285.
200. Kim SC, Tonkonogy SL, Balish E, et al. IL-10 deficient mice monoassociated with nonpathogenic *Enterococcus faecalis* develop chronic colitis. *Gastroenterology* 2001;120:A82(abst).
201. Sydora BC, Tavernini MM, Jewell LD, et al. Effect of bacterial monoassociation on tolerance and intestinal inflammation in IL-10 gene-deficient mice. *Gastroenterology* 2001;120:A517 (abst).
202. Kullberg MC, Jankovic D, Caspar P, et al. Bacteria-specific CD4+ T cell clones induce colitis in *Helicobacter hepaticus*-infected T cell deficient RAG-2 KO mice. *Gastroenterology* 2001;120:A519(abst).
203. Schultz M, Veltkamp C, Dieleman LA, et al. *Lactobacillus plantarum* 299v in the treatment and prevention of spontaneous colitis in IL-10 deficient mice. *Inflamm Bowel Dis* 2002;8: 71–80.
204. Dieleman LA, Goerres M, Arends A, et al. *Lactobacillus GG* prevents recurrence of colitis in HLA B27 transgenic rats after antibiotic treatment. *Gastroenterology* 2000;118:A814(abst).
205. Lichtman SN, Wang J, Sartor RB, et al. Reactivation of arthritis induced by small bowel bacterial overgrowth in rats: role of cytokines, bacteria, and bacterial polymers. *Infect Immun* 1995; 63:2295–2301.
206. Lichtman SN, Sartor RB, Keku J, et al. Hepatic inflammation in rats with experimental small intestinal bacterial overgrowth. *Gastroenterology* 1990;98:414–423.
207. Lichtman SN, Okoruwa EE, Keku J, et al. Degradation of endogenous bacterial cell wall polymers by the muralytic enzyme mutanolysin prevents hepatobiliary injury in genetically susceptible rats with experimental intestinal bacterial overgrowth. *J Clin Invest* 1992;90:1313–1322.
208. Lichtman SN, Keku J, Schwab JH, et al. Hepatic injury associated with small bowel bacterial overgrowth in rats is prevented by metronidazole and tetracycline. *Gastroenterology* 1991;100: 513–519.
209. Sartor RB, DeLa Cadena RA, Green KD, et al. Selective kallikrein-kinin system activation in inbred rats differentially susceptible to granulomatous enterocolitis. *Gastroenterology* 1996;110:1467–1481.
210. Colombel JF, Cortot A, Van Kruiningen HJ. Antibiotics in Crohn's disease. *Gut* 2001;48:647.
211. Ursing B, Alm T, Barany F, et al. A comparative study of metronidazole and sulfasalazine for active Crohn's disease: the cooperative Crohn's disease study in Sweden, II: result. *Gastroenterology* 1982;83:550–562.
212. Greenbloom SL, Steinhart AH, Greenberg GR. Combination ciprofloxacin and metronidazole for active Crohn's disease. *Can J Gastroenterol* 1998;12:53–56.
213. Prantera C, Zannoni F, Scribano ML, et al. An antibiotic regimen for the treatment of active Crohn's disease: a randomized, controlled clinical trial of metronidazole plus ciprofloxacin. *Am J Gastroenterol* 1996;91:328–332.
214. Steinhart AH, Feagan BG, Greenberg GR, et al. Combined budesonide and antibiotic therapy for active Crohn's disease: a randomized controlled trial. *Gastroenterology* 2001;120:A126 (abst).
215. Colombel JF, Lemann M, Cassagnou M, et al. A controlled trial comparing ciprofloxacin with mesalazine for the treatment of active Crohn's disease. Groupe d'Etudes Therapeutiques des Affections Inflammatoires Digestives (GETAID). *Am J Gastroenterol* 1999;94:674–678.
216. Rutgeerts P, Hiele M, Geboes K, et al. Controlled trial of metronidazole treatment for prevention of Crohn's recurrence after ileal resection. *Gastroenterology* 1995;108:1617–1621.
217. Rutgeerts PJ, D'Haens G, Baert F, et al. nitroimidazole antibiotics are efficacious for prophylaxis of postoperative recurrence of Crohn's disease: a placebo controlled trial. *Gastroenterology* 1999;116:G3506(abst).
218. Peppercorn MA. Antibiotics are effective therapy for Crohn's disease. *Inflamm Bowel Dis* 1997;3:318–319.
219. Moss AA, Carbone JV, Kressel HY. Radiologic and clinical assessment of broad-spectrum antibiotic therapy in Crohn's disease. *AJR Am J Roentgenol* 1978;131:787–790.
220. Turunen UM, Farkkila MA, Hakala K, et al. Long-term treatment of ulcerative colitis with ciprofloxacin: a prospective, double-blind, placebo-controlled study. *Gastroenterology* November 1998;115:1072–1078.
221. Mantzaris GJ, Archavlis E, Christoforidis P, et al. A prospective randomized controlled trial of oral ciprofloxacin in acute ulcerative colitis. *Am J Gastroenterol* 1997;92:454–456.
222. Burke DA, Axon AT, Clayden SA, et al. The efficacy of tobramycin in the treatment of ulcerative colitis. *Alimentary Pharmacol Ther* 1990;4:123–129.
223. Burke DA, Clayden SA, Dixon MF, et al. A follow up study of adjunctive oral tobramycin therapy in acute ulcerative colitis. *Gastroenterology* 1988;94:A55(abst).
224. Danzi JT. Trimethoprim-sulfamethoxazole therapy of inflammatory bowel disease. *Gastroenterology* 1989;96:A110(abst).
225. Peppercorn MA. Are antibiotics useful in the management of nontoxic severe ulcerative colitis? *J Clin Gastroenterol* 1993;17: 14–17.
226. Mantzaris GJ, Hatzis A, Kontogiannis P, et al. Intravenous tobramycin and metronidazole as an adjunct to corticosteroids in acute, severe ulcerative colitis. *Am J Gastroenterol* 1994;89: 43–46.
227. Nygaard K, Bergan T, Bjorneklett A, et al. Topical metronidazole treatment in pouchitis. *Scand J Gastroenterol* 1994;29: 462–467.
228. Gionchetti P, Rizzello F, Venturi A, et al. Antibiotic combination therapy in patients with chronic, treatment-resistant pouchitis. *Alimentary Pharmacol Ther* 1999;13:713–718.

229. Sandborn WJ. Pouchitis following ileal pouch-anal anastomosis: definition, pathogenesis, and treatment. *Gastroenterology* 1994;107:1856–1860.
230. Rutgeerts P, Goboes K, Peeters M, et al. Effect of faecal stream diversion on recurrence of Crohn's disease in the neoterminal ileum. *Lancet* 1991;338:771–774.
231. Harper PH, Truelove SC, Lee EC, et al. Split ileostomy and ileocolostomy for Crohn's disease of the colon and ulcerative colitis: a 20 year survey. *Gut* 1983;24:106–113.
232. D'Haens GR, Geboes K, Peeters M, et al. Early lesions of recurrent Crohn's disease caused by infusion of intestinal contents in excluded ileum. *Gastroenterology* 1998;114:262–267.
233. Harper PH, Lee EC, Kettlewell MG, et al. Role of the faecal stream in the maintenance of Crohn's colitis. *Gut* 1985;26:279–284.
234. Duchmann R, Kaiser I, Hermann E, et al. Tolerance exists towards resident intestinal flora but is broken in active inflammatory bowel disease (IBD). *Clin Exp Immunol* 1995;102:448–455.
235. Duchmann R, May E, Heike M, et al. T cell specificity and cross reactivity towards *Enterobacteria, Bacteroides, Bifidobacterium,* and antigens from resident intestinal flora in humans. *Gut* 1999;44:812–818.
236. Rembacken BJ, Snelling AM, Hawkey PM, et al. Non-pathogenic *Escherichia coli* versus mesalazine for the treatment of ulcerative colitis: a randomised trial. *Lancet* 1999;354:635–639.
237. Kruis W, Kalk EK, Fric P, et al. Maintenance of remission in ulcerative colitis is equally effective with *Escherichia coli* Nissle 1917 and with standard mesalamine. *Gastroenterology* 2001;120:A127(abst).
238. Helwig U, Rizzello F, Cifone G, et al. Elevated IL-10 levels in pouch-tissue after probiotic therapy. *Immunol Lett* 1999;69:159(abst).
239. Steidler L, Hans W, Schotte L, et al. Treatment of murine colitis by *Lactococcus lactis* secreting interleukin-10. *Science* 2000;289:1352–1355.
240. Schesser K, Spiik AK, Dukuzumuremyi JM, et al. The yopJ locus is required for *Yersinia*-mediated inhibition of NF-kappaB activation and cytokine expression: YopJ contains a eukaryotic SH2-like domain that is essential for its repressive activity. *Mol Microbiol* 1998;28:1067–1079.
241. Elliott DE, Li J, Crawford C, et al. Exposure to helminthic parasites protect mice from intestinal inflammation. *Gastroenterology* 1999;116:A706(abst).
242. Korzenik JR, Dieckgraefe BK. Is Crohn's disease an immunodeficiency? A hypothesis suggesting possible early events in the pathogenesis of Crohn's disease. *Dig Dis Sci* 2000;45:1121–1129.
243. Korzenik JR, Dieckgraefe BK. Immunostimulation in Crohn's disease: Results of a pilot study of G-CSF (R-Methug-CSF) in mucosal and fistulizing Crohn's disease. *Gastroenterology* 2000;118:A874(abst).
244. Caradonna L, Amati L, Lella P, et al. Phagocytosis, killing, lymphocyte-mediated antibacterial activity, serum autoantibodies, and plasma endotoxins in inflammatory bowel disease. *Am J Gastroenterol* 2000;95:1495–1502.
245. Hugot JP, Chamaillard M, Zouali H, et al. Association of NOD2 leucine-rich repeat variants with susceptibility to Crohn's disease. *Nature* 2001;411:599–603.
246. Ogura Y, Bonen DK, Inohara N, et al. A frameshift mutation in NOD2 associated with susceptibility to Crohn's disease. *Nature* 2001;411:603–606.
247. Hampe J, Cuthbert A, Croucher PJ, et al. Association between insertion mutation in NOD2 gene and Crohn's disease in German and British populations. *Lancet* 2001;357:1925–1928.
248. Ambrose NS, Johnson M, Burdon DW, et al. Incidence of pathogenic bacteria from mesenteric lymph nodes and ileal serosa during Crohn's disease surgery. *Br J Surg* 1984;71:623–625.
249. Von Ritter C, Sekizuka E, Grisham MB, et al. The chemotactic peptide N-formyl methionyl-leucyl-phenylalanine increases mucosal permeability in the distal ileum of the rat. *Gastroenterology* 1988;95:651–656.
250. Hsueh W, Gonzalez-Crussi F, Arroyave JL. Platelet-activating factor: an endogenous mediator for bowel necrosis in endotoxemia. *FASEB J* 1987;1:403–405.
251. Chester JF, Ross JS, Malt RA, et al. Acute colitis produced by chemotactic peptides in rats and mice. *Am J Pathol* 1985;121:284–290.
252. Davis SW, Holt LC, Sartor RB. Luminal bacterial and bacterial polymers potentiate indomethacin induced intestinal injury in the rat. *Gastroenterology* 1990;98:444A(abst).
253. Cario E, Rosenberg IM, Brandwein SL, et al. Lipopolysaccharide activates distinct signaling pathways in intestinal epithelial cell lines expressing toll-like receptors. *J Immunol* 2000;164:966–972.
254. Baker SJ, Jacob E, Bowden GH. Crohn disease arthropathy: antigens in synovial fluid share epitopes with strains of two species of viridans streptococci. *Scand J Gastroenterol* 2000;35:287–292.
255. Lichtman SN, Keku J, Schwab JH, et al. Evidence for peptidoglycan absorption in rats with experimental small bowel bacterial overgrowth. *Infect Immun* 1991;59:555–562.
256. Satsangi J, Jewell D, Parkes M, et al. Genetics of inflammatory bowel disease. A personal view on progress and prospects. *Dig Dis* 1998;16:370–374.
257. Peeters M, Nevens H, Baert F, et al. Familial aggregation in Crohn's disease: increased age-adjusted risk and concordance in clinical characteristics. *Gastroenterology* 1996;111:597–603.
258. May GR, Sutherland LR, Meddings JB. Is small intestinal permeability really increased in relatives of patients with Crohn's disease? *Gastroenterology* 1993;104:1627–1632.
259. Hilsden RJ, Meddings JB, Sutherland LR. Intestinal permeability changes in response to acetylsalicylic acid in relatives of patients with Crohn's disease. *Gastroenterology* 1996;110:1395–1403.
260. Podolsky DK, Isselbacher KJ. Composition of human colonic mucin. Selective alteration in inflammatory bowel disease. *J Clin Invest* 1983;72:142–153.
261. Pullan RD, Thomas GA, Rhodes M. Thickness of adherent mucus gel on colonic mucosa in humans and its relevance to colitis. *Gut* 1994;35:353–359.
262. Hobson CH, Butt TJ, Ferry DM, et al. Enterohepatic circulation of bacterial chemotactic peptide in rats with experimental colitis. *Gastroenterology* 1988;94:1006–1013.
263. Sands BE, Podolsky DK. The trefoil peptide family. *Annu Rev Physiol* 1996;58:253–273.
264. Mashimo H, Wu DC, Podolsky DK, et al. Impaired defense of intestinal mucosa in mice lacking intestinal trefoil factor. *Science* 1996;274:262–265.
265. Hermiston ML, Gordon JI. Inflammatory bowel disease and adenomas in mice expressing a dominant negative N-cadherin. *Science* 1995;270:1203–1207.
266. Sartor RB, Bender DE, Holt LC. Susceptibility of inbred rat strains to intestinal and extraintestinal inflammation induced by indomethacin. *Gastroenterology* 1992;102:A690(abst).
267. Mombaerts P, Mizoguchi E, Grusby MJ, et al. Spontaneous development of inflammatory bowel disease in T cell receptor mutant mice. *Cell* 1993;75:274–282.
268. Mahler M, Bristol IJ, Leiter EH, et al. Differential susceptibility of inbred mouse strains to dextran sulfate sodium-induced colitis. *Am J Physiol* 1998;274:G544–G551.
269. Farmer RG, Sundberg JP, Bristol IJ, et al. A major quantitative

trait locus on chromosome 3 controls colitis severity in IL-10 deficient mice. *Proc Natl Acad Sci U.S.A.* 2001;98:13820–13825.
270. Sundberg JP, Elson CO, Bedigian H, et al. Spontaneous, heritable colitis in a new substrain of C3H/HeJ mice. *Gastroenterology* 1994;107:1726–1735.
271. Barthold SW, Osbaldiston GW, Jonas AM. Dietary, bacterial and host genetic interactions in the pathogeneisis of transmissible murine colonic hyperplasia. *Lab Anim Sci* 1977;27: 938–945.
272. Ogura Y, Inohara N, Benito A, et al. Nod2, a Nod1/Apaf-1 family member that is restricted to monocytes and activates NF-kappaB. *J Biol Chem* 2001;276:4812–4818.
273. Farmer RG. Infectious causes of diarrhea in the differential diagnosis of inflammatory bowel disease. *Med Clin North Am* 1990;74:29–38.
274. Stuart RC, Leahy AL, Cafferkey MT, et al. *Yersinia enterocolitica* infection and toxic megacolon. *Br J Surg* 1986;73:590.
275. Moeller DD, Burger WE. Perforation of the ileum in *Yersinia enterocolitica* infection. *Am J Gastroenterol* 1985;80:19–20.
276. Raz R, Schonfeld S, Nasser F. Toxic megacolon in *Salmonella typhimurium* gastroenteritis. *Isr J Med Sci* 1988;24:719–720.
277. Orloff JJ, Saito R, Lasky S, et al. Toxic megacolon in cytomegalovirus colitis. *Am J Gastroenterol* 1989;84:794–797.
278. Christianson KA. Toxic megacolon complicating shigellosis. *J Royal Coll Surg Edinb* 1987;32:109–110.
279. Marshall WF, McLimans CA, Yu PK, et al. Results of a 6 month survey of stool cultures for *Escherichia coli* O157:H7. *Mayo Clin Proc* 1990;65:787–792.
280. Van Spreeuwel JP, Lindeman J, Meijer CJ. A quantitative study of immunoglobulin containing cells in the differential diagnosis of acute colitis. *J Clin Pathol* 1985;38:774–777.
281. Blaser MJ, Reller LB. *Campylobacter* enteritis. *N Engl J Med* 1981;305:1444–1452.
282. Steingrimsson O, Thorsteinsson SB, Hjalmarsdottir M, et al. *Campylobacter* ssp. infections in Iceland during a 24 month period in 1980–1982. Clinical and epidemiological characteristics. *Scand J Infect Dis* 1985;17:285–290.
283. Mee AS, Shield M, Burke M. *Campylobacter* colitis: differentiation from acute inflammatory bowel disease. *J Royal Soc Med* 1985;78:217–223.
284. Cooper R, Murphy S, Midlick D. *Campylobacter jejuni* enteritis mistaken for ulcerative colitis. *J Fam Pract* 1992;34:357–362.
285. Anderson JB, Tanner AH, Brodribb AJ. Toxic megacolon due to *Campylobacter* colitis. *Int J Colorectal Dis* 1986;1:58–59.
286. Frohli P, Hanselmann R, Koelz HR. Erythema nodosum in *Campylobacter jejuni* colitis. *Schweiz Med Wochenschr* 1990;120: 946–947.
287. Simson JN, Ayling R, Stoker TA. *Campylobacter jejuni* associated with acute relapse and abscess formation in Crohn's disease. *J Royal Coll Surg Edinb* 1985;30:397
288. Puylaert JB, Lalisan RI, Van der Werf SD, et al. *Campylobacter* ileocolitis mimicking acute appendicitis: differentiation with graded compression US. *Radiology* 1988;166:737–740.
289. Van Spreeuwel JP, Duursma GC, Meijer CJ, et al. *Campylobacter* colitis: histological immunohistochemical and ultrastructural findings. *Gut* 1985;26:945–951.
290. Gill KP, Feeley TM, Keane FB. Toxic megacolon and perforation caused by *Salmonella. Br J Surg* 1989;76:796.
291. Sarigol S, Wyllie R, Gramlich T, et al. Inflammatory bowel disease presenting as Salmonella colitis: the importance of early histologic examination in recognition and management. *Clin Pediatr* 1999;38:669–672.
292. Nakamura S, Iida M, Tominaga M, et al. *Salmonella* colitis: assessment with double contrast barium enema examination in seven patients. *Radiology* 1992;184:537–540.
293. Vender RJ, Marignani P. *Salmonella* colitis presenting as a segmental colitis resembling Crohn's disease. *Dig Dis Sci* 1983;28: 848–851.
294. Sansonetti PJ. Microbes and microbial toxins: paradigms for microbial-mucosal interactions, III: shigellosis: from symptoms to molecular pathogenesis. *Am J Physiol Gastrointest Liver Physiol* 2001;280:G319–G323.
295. Speelman P, Kabir I, Islam M. Distribution and spread of colonic lesions in shigellosis: a colonoscopic study. *J Infect Dis* 1984;150:899–903.
296. Halpern Z, Dan M, Giladi M, et al. Shigellosis in adults: epidemiologic, clinical, and laboratory features. *Medicine*1989;68: 210–217.
297. Caldwell GR, Reiss-Levy EA, De Carle DJ, et al. *Shigella dysenteriae* type 1 enterocolitis. *Aust N Z J Med* 1986;16:405–407.
298. Bokete TN, O'Callahan CM, Clausen CR, et al. Shiga-like toxin-producing *Escherichia coli* in Seattle children: a prospective study. *Gastroenterology*1993;105:1724–1731.
299. Griffin PM, Olmstead LC, Petras RE. *Escherichia coli* O157:H7-associated colitis. A clinical and histological study of 11 cases. *Gastroenterology* 1990;99:142–149.
300. O'Brien AD, Melton AR, Schmitt CK, et al. Profile of *Escherichia coli* O157:H7 pathogen responsible for hamburger-borne outbreak of hemorrhagic colitis and hemolytic uremic syndrome in Washington. *J Clin Microbiol* 1993;31: 2799–2801.
301. Ilnyckyj A, Greenberg H, Bernstein CN. *Escherichia coli* O157:H7 infection mimicking Crohn's disease. *Gastroenterology* 1997;112:995–999.
302. Gorbach SL, Graeme-Cook F, Smith RN. A 58-year-old woman with bloody diarrhea after chemotherapy for carcinoma of the tongue. *N Engl J Med* 1994;330:1811–1818.
303. Treacher DF, Jewell DP. *Yersinia* colitis associated with Crohn's disease. *Postgrad Med J* 1985;61:173–174.
304. Pothoulakis C, LaMont JT. Microbes and microbial toxins: paradigms for microbial-mucosal interactions, II: the integrated response of the intestine to Clostridium difficile toxins. *Am J Physiol Gastroint Liver Physiol* 2001;280:G178–G183.
305. Triadafilopoulos G, Hallstone AE. Acute abdomen as the first presentation of pseudomembranous colitis. *Gastroenterology* 199;101:685–691.
306. Tedesco FJ, Corless JK, Brownstein RE. Rectal sparing in antibiotic-associated pseudomembranous colitis: a prospective study. *Gastroenterology* 1982;83:1259–1260.
307. Gracey M, Burke V, Robinson J. *Aeromonas*-associated gastroenteritis. *Lancet* 1982;2:1304–1306.
308. Holmberg SD, Schell WL, Fanning GR, et al. Aeromonas intestinal infections in the United States. *Ann Intern Med* 1986;105:683–689.
309. Marshall JB. Tuberculosis of the gastrointestinal tract and peritoneum. *Am J Gastroenterol* 1993;88:989–999.
310. Pettengell KE, Larsen C, Garb M, et al. Gastrointestinal tuberculosis in patients with pulmonary tuberculosis. *Q J Med* 1990; 74:303–308.
311. Chen WS, Leu SY, Hsu H, et al. Trend of large bowel tuberculosis and the relation with pulmonary tuberculosis. *Dis Colon Rectum* 1992;35:189–192.
312. Shah S, Thomas V, Mathan M, et al. Colonoscopic study of 50 patients with colonic tuberculosis. *Gut* 1992;33:347–351.
313. Vijayraghavan M, Aruna BH, Sarda AK, et al. Duodenal tuberculosis: a review of the clinicopathologic features and management of twelve cases. *Jpn J Surg* 1990;20:526–529.
314. Balthazar EJ, Gordon R, Hulnick D. Ileocecal tuberculosis: CT and radiologic evaluation. *AJR Am J Roentgenol* 1990;154: 499–503.
315. Bhargava DK, Dasarathy S, Shriniwas MD, et al. Evaluation of enzyme-linked immunosorbent assay using mycobacterial

saline-extracted antigen for the serodiagnosis of abdominal tuberculosis. *Am J Gastroenterol* 1992;87:105–108.

316. Saebo A, Lassen J. Acute and chronic gastrointestinal manifestation associated with *Yersinia enterocolitica* infection. *Ann Surg* 1992;215:250–255.
317. Vantrappen G, Agg HO, Ponette E, et al. *Yersinia* enteritis and enterocolitis: gastrointestinal aspects. *Gastroenterology* 1977;72: 220–227.
318. Matsumoto T, Mitsuo I, Matsui T, et al. Endoscopic findings in *Yersinia enterocolitica* enterocolitis. *Gastrointest Endosc* 1990;36: 583–586.
319. Simmonds SD, Noble MA, Freeman HJ. Gastrointestinal features of culture-positive *Yersinia enterocolitica* infection. *Gastroenterology* 1987;92:112–117.
320. Tuohy AM, O'Gorman M, Byington C, et al. *Yersinia enterocolitis* mimicking Crohn's disease in a toddler. *Pediatrics* 1999;104:e36.
321. Ravdin JL. *Entamoeba histolytica*: from adherence to enteropathy. *J Infect Dis* 1989;159:420–429.
322. Aristizabal H, Acevedo J, Botero M. Fulminant amebic colitis. *World J Surg* 1991;15216–15221.
323. Matsui T, Iida M, Tada S, et al. The value of double-contrast barium enema in amebic colitis. *Gastrointest Radiol* 1989;14: 73–78.
324. Radhakrishnan S, Al Nakib B, Shaikh H, et al. The value of colonoscopy in schistosomal, tuberculous, and amebic colitis. Two-year experience. *Dis Col Rectum* 1986;29:891–895.
325. Patel AS, DeRidder PH. Amebic colitis masquerading as acute inflammatory bowel disease. *J Clin Gastroenterol* 1989;11: 407–410.
326. Cheung AN, Ng IO. Cytomegalovirus infection of the gastrointestinal tract in non-AIDS patients. *Am J Gastroenterol* 1993; 88:1882–1886.
327. Wexner SD, Smithy WB, Trillo C, et al. Emergency colectomy for cytomegalovirus ileocolitis in patients with the acquired immune deficiency syndrome. *Dis Col Rectum* 1988;31:755–761.
328. Quinn TC, Goodell SE, Mkrtichian E, et al. *Chlamydia trachomatis* proctitis. *N Engl J Med* 1981;305:195–200.
329. Mostafavi H, O'Donnell KF, Chong FK. Supralevator abscess due to chronic rectal lymphogranuloma venereum. *Am J Gastroenterol* 1990;85:602–606.
330. Sartor RB. Ulcerative colitis. *Consultant* May 1983:121–122.
331. Tedesco FJ, Hardin RD, Harper RN, et al. Infectious colitis endoscopically simulating inflammatory bowel disease: a prospective evaluation. *Gastrointest Endosc* 1983;29:195–197.
332. Surawicz CM, Belic L. Rectal biopsy helps to distinguish acute self-limited colitis from idiopathic inflammatory bowel disease. *Gastroenterology* 1984;86:104–113.
333. Schumacher G, Kollberg B, Sandstedt B. A prospective study of first attacks of inflammatory bowel disease and infectious colitis. Histologic course during the 1st year after presentation. *Scand J Gastroenterol* 1994;29:318–332.
334. Roskell DE, Hyde GM, Campbell AP, et al. HIV associated cytomegalovirus colitis as a mimic of inflammatory bowel disease. *Gut* 1995;37:148–150.
335. Askerkoff B, Bennett JV. Effect of antibiotic therapy in acute salmonellosis on the fecal excretion of salmonellae. *N Engl J Med* 1969;281:636–640.
336. Riley LW, Remis RS, Helgerson SD, et al. Hemorrhagic colitis associated with a rare *Escherichia coli* serotype. *N Engl J Med* 1983;308:681–685.
337. Butler T, Islam MR, Azad MA, et al. Risk factors for the development of hemolytic uremic syndrome during shigellosis. *J Pediatr* 1987;110:894–897.
338. Aukrust P, Moum B, Farstad IN, et al. Fatal cytomegalovirus (CMV) colitis in a patient receiving low dose prednisolone therapy. *Scand J Infect Dis* 1991;23:495–499.
339. Sands BE. Therapy of inflammatory bowel disease. *Gastroenterology* 2000;118:S68–S82
340. Mee AS, Jewell DP. Factors inducing relapse in inflammatory bowel disease. *Br Med J (Clin Res)* 1978;801–802.
341. Kangro HO, Chong SK, Hardiman A, et al. A prospective study of viral and mycoplasma infections in chronic inflammatory bowel disease. *Gastroenterology* 1990;98:549–553.
342. Kochhar R, Ayyagari A, Goenka MK, et al. Role of infectious agents in exacerbations of ulcerative colitis in India. *J Clin Gastroenterol* 1993;16:26–30.
343. Weber P, Koch M, Wolfgang RH, et al. Microbic superinfection in relapse of inflammatory bowel disease. *J Clin Gastroenterol* 1992;14:302–308.
344. Trnka YM, LaMont, JT. Association of *Clostridium difficile* toxin with symptomatic relapse of chronic inflammatory bowel disease. *Gastroenterology* 1981;80:693–696.
345. Greenfield C, Aguilar Ramirez JR, Pounder RE, et al. *Clostridium difficile* and inflammatory bowel disease. *Gut* 1983;24: 713–717.
346. Meyers S, Mayer E, Buttone F, et al. Occurrence of *Clostridium difficile* toxin during the course of inflammatory bowel disease. *Gastroenterology* 1981;80:697–700.
347. Farrell RJ, LaMont JT. Pathogenesis and clinical manifestations of *Clostridium difficile* diarrhea and colitis. *Curr Topics Microbiol Immunol* 2000;250:109–125.
348. Bolton RP, Sheriff RJ, Read AE. *Clostridium difficile* associated diarrhea: a role in inflammatory bowel disease? *Lancet* 1980;1: 383–384.
349. Tremaine WJ, Bille J, Huizenga KA, et al. Factors which influence the occurrence of *Clostridium difficile* infections in inflammatory bowel disease. *Gastroenterology* 1983;84:A1337.
350. Brown WJ, Hudson MJ, Patrick S, et al. Search for enteric microbial pathogens in patients with ulcerative colitis. *Digestion* 1992;53:121–128.
351. Cartun RW, Van Kruiningen HJ, Pedersen, et al. An immunocytochemical search for infectious agents in Crohn's disease. *Mod Pathol* 1993;6:212–219.
352. Kallinowski F, Wassmer A, Hofmann MA, et al. Prevalence of enteropathogenic bacteria in surgically treated chronic inflammatory bowel disease. *Hepatogastroenterology* 1998;45:1552–1558.
353. Cottone M, Pietrosi G, Martorana G, et al. Prevalence of cytomegalovirus infection in severe refractory ulcerative and Crohn's colitis. *Am J Gastroenterol* 2001;96:773–775.
354. Vega R, Bertran X, Menacho M, et al. Cytomegalovirus infection in patients with inflammatory bowel disease. *Am J Gastroenterol* 1999;94:1053–1056.
355. Pfau P, Kochman ML, Furth EE, et al. Cytomegalovirus colitis complicating ulcerative colitis in the steroid-naive patient. *Am J Gastroenterol* 2001;96:895–899.
356. Cooper HS, Raffensperger EC, Jonas L, et al. Cytomegalovirus inclusions in patients with ulcerative colitis and toxic dilation requiring colonic resection. *Gastroenterology* 1977;72: 1253–1256.
357. Berk T, Gordon SJ, Choi HY, et al. Cytomegalovirus infection of the colon: a possible in exacerbations of inflammatory bowel disease. *Am J Gastroenterol* 1985;80:355–360.
358. Munoz-Juarez M, Pemberton JH, Sandborn WJ, et al. Misdiagnosis of specific cytomegalovirus infection of the ileoanal pouch as refractory idiopathic chronic pouchitis: report of two cases. *Dis Colon Rectum* 1999;42:117–120.
359. Moonka D, Furth EE, MacDermott RP, et al. Pouchitis associated with primary cytomegalovirus infection. *Am J Gastroenterol* 1998;93:264–266.
360. Farmer GW, Vincent MM, Fuccillo DA, et al. Viral investigations in ulcerative colitis and regional enteritis. *Gastroenterology* 1973;65:8–18.

361. Wakefield AJ, Fox JD, Sawyer AM, et al. Detection of herpesvirus DNA in the large intestine of patients with ulcerative colitis and Crohn's disease using the nested polymerase chain reaction. *J Med Virol* 1992;38:183–190.
362. Ruther U, Nunnensiek C, Muller HA, et al. Interferon alpha (IFN alpha 2a) therapy for herpes virus-associated inflammatory bowel disease (ulcerative colitis and Crohn's disease). *Hepatogastroenterology* 1998;45:691–699.
363. Baldassano RN, Schreiber S, Johnston RBJ, et al. Crohn's disease monocytes are primed for accentuated release of toxic oxygen metabolites. *Gastroenterology* 1993;105:60–66.
364. Rogler G, Andus T, Aschenbrenner E, et al. Alterations of the phenotype of colonic macrophages in inflammatory bowel disease. *Eur J Gastroenterol Hepatol* 1997;9:893–899.
365. Huizenga KA, Schroeder KW. Gastrointestinal complications of ulcerative colitis and Crohn's disease. In: Kirsner JB, Shorter RG, eds. *Inflammatory bowel disease.* third edition. Philadelphia, PA: Lea & Febiger, 1988:257–279.
366. Keighley MR, Eastwood D, Ambrose NS, et al. Incidence and microbiology of abdominal and pelvic abscess in Crohn's disease. *Gastroenterology* 1982;83:1271–1275.
367. Ribeiro MB, Greenstein AJ, Yamazaki Y, et al. Intra-abdominal abscess in regional enteritis. *Ann Surg* 1991;213:32–36.
368. Lorber B, Swenson RM. The bacteriology of intraabdominal infections. *Surg Clin North Am* 1975;55:1349–1354.
369. Kelly JK, Siu TO. The strictures, sinuses, and fissures of Crohn's disease. *J Clin Gastroenterol* 1986;8:594–598.
370. Tonelli F, Ficari F. Pathological features of Crohn's disease determining perforation. *J Clin Gastroenterol* 1991;13:226–230.
371. Greenstein AJ, Lachman P, Sachar DB, et al. Perforating and non-perforating indications for repeated operations in Crohn's disease: evidence for two clinical forms. *Gut* 1988;29:588–592.
372. Bayless TM, Tokayer AZ, Polito JM, et al. Crohn's disease: concordance for site and clinical type in affected family members—potential hereditary influences. *Gastroenterology* 1996;111: 573–579.
373. Yamamoto T, Allan RN, Keighley MR. Risk factors for intra-abdominal sepsis after surgery in Crohn's disease. *Dis Colon Rectum* 2000;43:1141–1145.
374. Post S, Betzler M, Von Ditfurth B, et al. Risks of intestinal anastomoses in Crohn's disease. *Ann Surg* 1991;213:37–42.
375. Yamamoto T, Keighley MR. Factors affecting the incidence of postoperative septic complications and recurrence after strictureplasty for jejunoileal Crohn's disease. *Am J Surg* 1999;178: 240–245.
376. Aszodi A, Ponsky JL. Effects of corticosteroids on the healing bowel anastomosis. *Am Surg* 1984;50:546–548.
377. Knochel JQ, Koehler PR, Lee TG, et al. Diagnosis of abdominal abscesses with computed tomography, ultrasound, and 111-In leukocyte scans. *Radiology* 1980;137:425–432.
378. Wheeler JG, Slack NF, Duncan A, et al. The diagnosis of intraabdominal abscesses in patients with severe Crohn's disease. *Q J Med* 1992;82:159–167.
379. Weldon MJ, Joseph AE, French A, et al. Comparison of 99m technetium hexamethylpropylene-amine oxime labeled leucocyte with 111-indium tropolonate labeled granulocyte scanning and ultrasound in the diagnosis of intra-abdominal abscess. *Gut* 1995;37:557–564.
380. Shoenut JP, Semelka RC, Silverman R, et al. Magnetic resonance imaging in inflammatory bowel disease. *J Clin Gastroenterol* 1993;17:73–78.
381. Gerzof SG, Robbins AH, Johnson WC, et al. Percutaneous catheter drainage of abdominal abscesses. *N Engl Med* 1981; 305:653–657.
382. Jawhari A, Kamm MA, Ong C, et al. Intra-abdominal and pelvic abscess in Crohn's disease: results of noninvasive and surgical management. *Br J Surg* 1998;85:367–371.
383. Michelassi F, Stella M, Balestracci T, et al. Incidence, diagnosis, and treatment of enteric and colorectal fistulae in patients with Crohn's disease. *Ann Surg* 1993;218:660–666.
384. Piontek M, Hengels K, Hefter H, et al. Spinal abscess and bacterial meningitis in Crohn's disease. *Dig Dis Sci* 1992;37:1131–1135.
385. Bernstein LH, Frank MS, Brandt LJ, et al. Healing of perineal Crohn's disease with metronidazole. *Gastroenterology* 1980;79: 357–365.
386. Brandt LJ, Bernstein LH, Boley SJ, et al. Metronidazole therapy for perineal Crohn's disease: a follow-up study. *Gastroenterology* 1982;83:383–387.
387. Broe PJ, Bayless TM, Cameron JL. Crohn's disease: are enteroenteral fistulas an indication for surgery? *Surgery* 1982;91:249–253.
388. McIntyre PB, Ritchie JK, Hawley PR, et al. Management of enterocutaneous fistulas: a review of 132 cases. *Br J Surg* 1984; 71:293–296.
389. Margolin ML, Korelitz BI. Management of bladder fistulas in Crohn's disease. *J Clin Gastroenterol* 1989;11:399–402.
390. Heyen F, Winslet MC, Andrew H, et al. Vaginal fistulas in Crohn's disease. *Dis Colon Rectum* 1989;32:379–383.
391. Williams DR, Coller JA, Corman ML, et al. Anal complications in Crohn's disease. *Dis Colon Rectum* 1981;24:22–24.
392. Korelitz BI, Present DH. Favorable effect of 6-mercaptopurine on fistulae of Crohn's disease. *Dig Dis Sci* 1985;30:58–64.
393. Hanauer SB, Smith MB. Rapid closure of Crohn's disease fistulas with continuous intravenous cyclosporin A. *Am J Gastroenterol* 1993;88:646–649.
394. Present DH, Lichtiger S. Efficacy of cyclosporine in treatment of fistula of Crohn's disease. *Dig Dis Sci* 1994;39:374–380.
395. Present DH, Rutgeerts P, Targan S, et al. Infliximab for the treatment of fistulas in patients with Crohn's disease. *N Engl J Med* 1999;340:1398–1405.
396. Orsoni P, Barthet M, Portier F, et al. Prospective comparison of endosonography, magnetic resonance imaging and surgical findings in anorectal fistula and abscess complicating Crohn's disease. *Br J Surg* 1999;86:360–364.
397. Hurst RD. Complications of surgical treatment of ulcerative colitis and Crohn's disease. In: Kirsner JB, ed. *Inflammatory bowel disease.* Chicago, IL: WB Saunders, 2000:718–735.
398. Fasth S, Helleberg R, Hulten L, et al. Early complications after surgical treatment for Crohn's disease with particular reference to factors affecting their development. *Acta Chir Scand* 1980; 146:519–526.
399. Becker JM. Surgical management of ulcerative colitis. In: MacDermott RP, Stenson WF, eds. *Inflammatory bowel disease.* New York: Elsevier Science, 1992:599–614.
400. Farouk R, Dozois RR, Pemberton JH, et al. Incidence and subsequent impact of pelvic abscess after ileal pouch-anal anastomosis for chronic ulcerative colitis. *Dis Colon Rectum* 1998;41: 1239–1243.
401. Block GE, Schraut WH. Complications of the surgical treatment of ulcerative colitis and Crohn's disease. In: Kirsner JB, Shorter RG, eds. *Inflammatory bowel disease,* third edition. Philadelphia: Lea & Febiger, 1988:685–713.
402. Mellman RL, Spisak GM, Burakoff R. *Enterococcus avium* bacteremia in association with ulcerative colitis. *Am J Gastroenterol* 1992;87:375–378.
403. Kreuzpaintner G, Horstkotte D, Heyll A, et al. Increased risk of bacterial endocarditis in inflammatory bowel disease. *Am J Med* 1992;92:391–395.
404. Moshkowitz M, Arber N, Wajsman R, et al. *Streptococcus bovis* endocarditis as a presenting manifestation of idiopathic ulcerative colitis. *Postgrad Med J* 1992;68:930–931.
405. Tomomasa T, Itoh K, Matsui A. An infant with ulcerative coli-

tis complicated by endocarditis and cerebral infarction. *J Pediatr Gastroenterol Nutr* 1993;17:323–325.
406. Al-Jahdali H, Pon C, Thompson WG, et al. Nonfatal portal pyaemia complicating Crohn's disease of the terminal ileum. *Gut* 1994;35:560–561.
407. Vakil N, Hayne G, Sharma A, et al. Liver abscess in Crohn's disease. *Am J Gastroenterol* 1994;89:1090–1095.
408. Narayanan S, Madda JP, Johny M, et al. Crohn's disease presenting as pyogenic liver abscess with review of previous case reports. *Am J Gastroenterol* 1998;93:2607–2609.
409. Brooke BN, Dykes PW, Walker FC. A study of liver disorder in ulcerative colitis. *Postgrad Med J* 1961;37:245–251.
410. Yamada T, Deitch E, Specian RD, et al. Mechanisms of acute and chronic inflammation induced by indomethacin. *Inflammation* 1993;17:641–642.
411. Gardiner KR, Erwin PJ, Anderson NH, et al. Colonic bacteria and bacterial translocation in experimental colitis. *Br J Surg* 1993;80:512–516.
412. Schoeffel U, Jaeger D, Pelz K, et al. Effect of human bowel wall distension on translocation of indigenous bacteria and endotoxins. *Dig Dis Sci* 1994;39:490–493.
413. Berg RD. Promotions of the translocation from the gastrointestinal tracts of mice by oral treatment with penicillin, clindamycin or metronidazole. *Infect Immun* 1981;33:854–861.
414. Berg RD. Bacterial translocation from the gastrointestinal tracts of mice receiving immunosuppressive chemotherapeutic agents. *Curr Microbiol* 1983;8:285–292.
415. Gautreaux MD, Deitch EA, Berg RD. T lymphocytes in host defense against bacterial translocation from the gastrointestinal tract. *Infect Immun* 1994;62:2874–2884.
416. Seale JP, Compton MR. Side effects of corticosteroid agents. *Med J Aust* 1986;144:139–142.
417. Singleton JW, Law DH, Kelley ML Jr, et al. National Cooperative Crohn's Disease Study: adverse reactions to study drugs. *Gastroenterology* 1979;77:870–882.
418. Malchow H, Ewe K, Brandes JW. European Cooperative Crohn's Disease Study (ECCDS): results of drug treatment. *Gastroenterology* 1984;86:249–266.
419. Felder JB, Adler DJ, Korelitz BI. The safety of corticosteroid therapy in Crohn's disease with an abdominal mass. *Am J Gastroenterol* 1991;86:1450–1455.
420. Present DH, Meltzer SJ, Krumholz MP, et al. 6-Mercaptopurine in the management of inflammatory bowel disease: short- and long-term toxicity. *Ann Intern Med* 1989;111:641–649.
421. Smith MB, Hanauer SB. *Pneumocystis carinii* pneumonia during cyclosporine therapy for ulcerative colitis. *N Engl J Med* 1992;327:497–498.
422. Cohen RD, Stein R, Hanauer SB. Intravenous cyclosporin in ulcerative colitis: a five-year experience. *Am J Gastroenterol* 1999;94:1587–1592.
423. Kozarek R, Bedard C, Patterson D, et al. Cyclosporin use in the precolectomy chronic ulcerative colitis patient: a community experience and its relationship to prospective and controlled clinical trials. Pacific Northwest Gastroenterology Society. *Am J Gastroenterol* 1995;90:2093–2096.
424. Ricart E, Panaccione R, Loftus EV, et al. Infliximab for Crohn's disease in clinical practice at the Mayo Clinic: the first 100 patients. *Am J Gastroenterol* 2001;96:722–729.
425. Madden MV, McIntyre AS, Nicholls RJ. Double-blind crossover trial of metronidazole versus placebo in chronic unremitting pouchitis. *Dig Dis Sci* 1994;39:1193–1196.
426. Becker JM, Onderdonk AB. Bacterial dysbiosis in the pathogenesis of ileal pouchitis. *Gastroenterology* 1994;106:A650.
427. Ruseler-van Embden JH, Schoten WR, Lieshout LM. Pouchitis: result of microbial imbalance? *Gut* 1994;35:658–664.
428. McLeod RS, Antonioli D, Cullen J, et al. Histologic and microbiologic features of biopsy samples from patients with normal and inflamed pouches. *Dis Colon Rectum* 1994;37:26–31.
429. Becker JM, Raymond JL. Ileal pouch anal anastomosis. A single surgeon's experience with 100 consecutive cases. *Ann Surg* 1986;204:375–383.
430. Bargen JA. Experimental studies on etiology of chronic ulcerative colitis. *JAMA* 1924;83:332–336.
431. Dragsteadt IR, Dack GM, Kirsner JB. Chronic ulcerative colitis: a summary of evidence implicating *Bacterium necrophorum* as an etiologic agent. *Ann Surg* 1941;114:653
432. Macie TT. Ulcerative colitis due to chronic infection with flexnerbacillus. *JAMA* 1932;98:1706
433. Gitnick GL, Rosen VJ, Arthur MH, et al. Evidence for the isolation of a new virus from ulcerative colitis patients. *Dig Dis Sci* 1979;24:609–619.
434. Munro J, Mayberry JF, Matthews N, et al. *Chlamydia* and Crohn's disease. *Lancet* 1979;2:45–46.
435. Whorwell PJ, Phillips CA, Beeken WL, et al. Isolation of reoviruslike agents from patients with Crohn's disease. *Lancet* 1977;1:1169–1171.
436. Burnham WR, Lennard-Jones JE, Stanford JL, et al. Mycobacteria as a possible cause of inflammatory bowel disease. *Lancet* 1978;2:693–697.
437. Schultz M, Tonkonogy SL, Sellon RK, et al. IL-2-deficient mice raised under germfree conditions develop delayed mild focal intestinal inflammation. *Am J Physiol* 1999;276:G1461–G1472
438. Matsumoto S, Okabe Y, Setoyama H, et al. Inflammatory bowel disease-like enteritis and caecitis in a senescence accelerated mouse P1/Yit strain. *Gut* 1998;43:71–78.
439. Aranda R, Sydora BC, McAllister PL, et al. Analysis of intestinal lymphocytes in mouse colitis mediated by transfer of CD4+, CD45RBhigh T cells to SCID recipients. *J Immunol* 1997;158: 3464–3473.
440. Panwala CM, Jones JC, Viney JL. A novel model of inflammatory bowel disease: mice deficient for the multiple drug resistance gene, mdr1a, spontaneously develop colitis. *J Immunol* 1998;161:5733–5744.
441. Tlaskalova-Hogenova H, Stepankova R, Tuckova L, et al. Autoimmunity, immunodeficiency and mucosal infections: chronic intestinal inflammation as a sensitive indicator of immunoregulatory defects in response to normal luminal microflora. *Folia Microbiol* 1998;43:545–550.
442. Sartor RB, Bender DE, Grenther WB, et al. Absolute requirement for ubiquitous luminal bacteria in the pathogenesis of chronic intestinal inflammation. *Gastroenterology* 1994;106:A767.
443. Ruther U, Nunnensiek C, Muller HA, et al. Herpes simplex-associated exacerbation of Crohn's disease. Successful treatment with acyclovir. *Dtsch Med Wochenschr* 1992;117:46–50.
444. Gebhard RL, Greenberg HB, Singh N, et al. Acute viral enteritis and exacerbations of inflammatory bowel disease. *Gastroenterology* 1982;83:1207–1209.
445. Szilagyi A, Gerson M, Mendelson J, et al. *Salmonella* infections complicating inflammatory bowel disease. *J Clin Gastroenterol* 1985;7:251–255.
446. Payne M, Girdwood AH, Roost RW, et al. *Yersinia enterocolitica* and Crohn's disease. A case report. *South Afr Med J* 1987;72:53–55.
447. Bayerdorffer E, Schwarzkopf-Steinhauser G, Ottenjann R. New unusual forms of colitis. Report of four cases with known and unknown etiology. *Hepatogastroenterology* 1986;33:187–190.
448. Scheurlen C, Kruis W, Spengler U, et al. Crohn's disease is frequently complicated by giardiasis. *Scand J Gastroenterol* 1988; 23:833–839.
449. Nagler J, Brown M, Soave R. *Blastocystis hominis* in inflammatory bowel disease. *J Clin Gastroenterol* 1993;16:109–112.
450. Swidsinski A, Ladhoff A, Pernthaler A, et al. Mucosal flora in inflammatory bowel disease. *Gastroenterology* 2002;122:44–54.

29

GASTROINTESTINAL INFECTIONS IN HIV-1 DISEASE

PHILLIP D. SMITH
EDWARD N. JANOFF

Since its initial description in 1980, AIDS has become the greatest worldwide pandemic in history, eclipsing even the European-centered bubonic plague of the fourteenth century in magnitude and the number of deaths. Originating in chimpanzees in central Africa (1), AIDS first reached epidemic proportion in the 1980s in the United States and Europe, where most of the infections were acquired through homosexual contact. Subsequently, the epidemic spread to heterosexual populations, so by the end of 2001, 20 million people had died from AIDS and 40 million people were estimated to be infected with HIV-1, the causative agent of AIDS (2). In contrast to the initial focus of the epidemic in developed countries, currently more than 70% of infected persons, approximately 28 million, live in sub-Saharan Africa, where in some countries an astonishing 25% of the population is infected with HIV-1 (2). Today, the virus is transmitted by heterosexual contact in 75% to 85% of cases (3). As a consequence of the passage of HIV-1 to women of childbearing age, vertical transmission has become a devastating public health problem, particularly in developing countries, such as Botswana, where the prevalence of HIV-1 infection among pregnant women exceeds 30% (2).

Regardless of the route of HIV-1 transmission or whether the infected population is located in developed or developing countries, gastrointestinal (GI) infections are a major cause of morbidity and occasionally mortality in HIV-1-infected persons. Fungal, viral, bacterial, and parasitic pathogens are the most common causes of these infections. In this chapter, we review first the role of the GI tract mucosa in the transmission and immunobiology of HIV-1 infection, second the esophageal and intestinal infections responsible for most GI illnesses in HIV-1 disease, and third the effect of highly active antiretroviral therapy (HAART) on the epidemiology, morbidity, and treatment of those infections.

P. D. Smith: Division of Gastroenterology and Hepatology, Department of Medicine, University of Alabama and Veterans Affairs Medical Center, Birmingham, Alabama.

E. N. Janoff: Mucosal and Vaccine Research Center, Infectious Diseases Section, Department of Medicine, Veterans Affairs Medical Center and University of Minnesota School of Medicine, Minneapolis, Minnesota.

ROLE OF THE GI MUCOSA IN HIV-1 TRANSMISSION

Virtually all HIV-1 infections, excluding those acquired parenterally, are acquired via the mucosal surfaces of the genital and GI tracts (4). For heterosexual transmissions, the genital mucosa is the most common site of virus entry, whereas for vertical, orogenital, and anogenital transmissions, the GI mucosa is the portal of entry. In vertical transmission, HIV-1 enters the upper GI tract during the swallowing of infected amniotic fluid *in utero,* infected blood and cervical secretions intrapartum, and infected breast milk postpartum (5). In homosexual transmissions, orogenital contact may be more common than anogenital contact (6–8), implicating the upper and the lower GI tract mucosa in HIV-1 entry during homosexual contact.

Donor Infectiousness

Current concepts regarding the infectiousness of persons who carry HIV-1 are based largely on studies of heterosexual transmission. However, many factors that promote transmission across the genital mucosa likely enhance transmission across the GI mucosa as well (Table 29.1). The probability of transmitting HIV-1 is greatest when the index partner has primary HIV-1 infection, the period between virus exposure and the development of anti-HIV-1 antibodies (9), during which plasma levels of HIV-1 are the highest (10,11). Late-stage disease is also associated with increased levels of HIV-1 in blood and semen (12–14), as well as with an increased risk of HIV-1 transmission (15). The blood viral load, a key predictor of the risk of heterosexual transmission of HIV-1 (16,17), appears to correlate with the level in genital secretions and the amount of virus

TABLE 29.1. FACTORS THAT INCREASE HIV-1 TRANSMISSION ACROSS THE MUCOSA

- High viral load during primary HIV-1 infection in the index partner
- High viral load during end-stage HIV-1 disease in the index partner
- Mucosal trauma, inflammation, erosion, or ulcer in the recipient partner
- Mucosal infection in the recipient partner
- Increased frequency of sexual contacts
- Unprotected sexual contact
- Receptive anal intercourse
- Absence of circumcision in a male index partner

inoculated onto a mucosal surface. The presence of reproductive tract inflammation and infections further increases the infectiousness of the donor (18–20), likely due to increased HIV-1 shedding into semen.

Recipient Susceptibility

Trauma-induced disruption of the rectal mucosa provides inoculated virus direct access to the rectal microcirculation of the recipient and likely contributes to the high rate of HIV-1 transmission in receptive anal intercourse. Similarly, inflammation and erosions due to mucosal infections, such as herpes simplex proctitis and syphilis, provide inoculated virus access to lymphoid cells in the recipient's mucosa. In addition, certain mucosal infections enhance the susceptibility of mononuclear cells to HIV-1 infection. For example, *Mycobacterium avium* complex (MAC) enhances macrophage expression of CCR5, the chemokine co-receptor that serves as a receptor for macrophage-tropic HIV-1 (21). In certain populations, genetics also influences host susceptibility to HIV-1. Approximately 1% of whites have a 32-nucleotide deletion allele in the gene that encodes CCR5 (22,23), leading to the absence of functional CCR5 co-receptor and, consequently, mononuclear cell resistance to macrophage-tropic HIV-1 (22–25). Because the transmitted strains of HIV-1 are predominantly macrophage tropic, persons homozygous for the allele are not susceptible to infection with these strains. Finally, a spectrum of behavioral and sociologic factors, including increased frequency of sexual contacts (26), unprotected sexual contact (27), receptive anal intercourse, and the absence of circumcision in men (28), are associated with increased HIV-1 transmission (Table 29.1).

ROLE OF THE GI MUCOSA IN HIV-1 IMMUNOBIOLOGY

HIV-1 Entry

In the absence of mucosal trauma or infection, proposed cellular routes by which HIV-1 enters the mononuclear

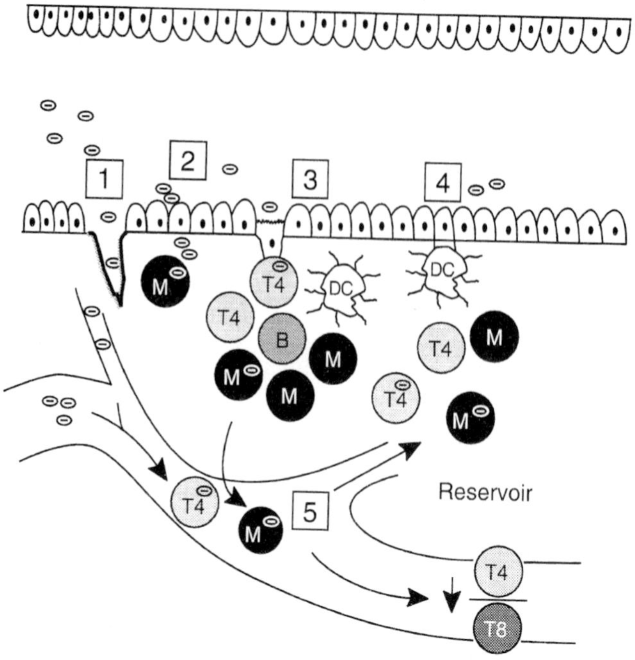

FIGURE 29.1. Schematic representation of the possible routes by which HIV-1 inoculated onto the mucosa can cross the epithelium to enter the lamina propria: **(1)** Mucosal erosion or tear; **(2)** epithelial cell; **(3)** M cell; and **(4)** dendritic cell. (From Smith PD, Wahl SM. Immunobiology of mucosal HIV-1 infection. In: Ogra PH, Mestecky J, Lamm ME, et al., eds. *Mucosal immunology,* second edition. San Diego: Academic Press, 1999:977–989, with permission.)

cell-rich lamina propria include M cells, dendritic cells, and epithelial cells (Fig. 29.1). M cells, specialized epithelial cells overlying Peyer patches in the small intestine and lymphoid follicles in the rectum, transport macromolecules and microorganisms by a non-degradative pathway to cells in the underlying lymphoid structure. Mouse and rabbit M cells are capable of transporting HIV-1 to mononuclear cells *in vitro* (29) and the inoculation of simian immunodeficiency virus (SIV) into the oral cavity of macaques leads to rapid infection of the M-cell-containing tonsils (30), suggesting M-cell uptake and transport of SIV (31). The high prevalence of M cells in human tonsils and rectum (32) strategically positions these cells for a potential role in HIV-1 entry. However, human M cells have not yet been reported to take up and transport HIV-1, probably due to the rapidity of the transport process and the unavailability of rectal tissue specimens shortly after virus inoculation.

Dendritic cells are highly efficient antigen-presenting cells that express CD4 and have been identified in rat small and large intestine (33), mouse Peyer patches (34), macaque cervicovaginal mucosa and foreskin (35), and human tonsil, adenoid, and colon (36,37). Tonsillar dendritic cells form conjugates with T cells, resulting in high levels of viral replication by HIV-1-infected T cells *in vitro* (36). Recent evidence indicates that dendritic cells bind HIV-1 envelope gp120 through a C-type lectin (38), allowing HIV-1 capture (but not infection) for subsequent delivery to T cells and dissemination to secondary lymphoid organs (38,39). Whether dendritic cells are involved in the pathogenesis of HIV-1 infection in the human small intestine or colon is not yet known.

As the most abundant cell type lining the mucosa of the intestine and colon, epithelial cells are an important potential route for HIV-1 entry. Epithelial cell lines can translocate HIV-1 from their apical to basolateral surface (40). We recently showed that freshly isolated intestinal epithelial cells express galactosylceramide (GalCer) (41), an alternative primary receptor for HIV-1 (42), and CCR5, the co-receptor for macrophage-tropic (R5) HIV-1 (41). In contrast, the cells do not express CXCR4, the chemokine co-receptor for lymphocyte-tropic (X4) HIV-1 or CD4, the primary receptor for HIV-1 on mononuclear cells (41). Consistent with their $GalCer^{+}CCR5^{+}CXCR4^{-}$ phenotype, intestinal epithelial cells selectively transfer R5 HIV-1 to CCR5-positive target cells (41).

Target Cells in the Intestinal Lamina Propria

HIV-1 that has crossed the epithelium and entered the lamina propria encounters the largest reservoir of macrophages and lymphocytes in the body. Surprisingly, lamina propria macrophages do not express CCR5 and are not permissive to R5 viruses (43,44), which may explain the very low prevalence of HIV-1-infected macrophages in the upper GI tract mucosa *in vivo* (45). Consequently, intestinal macrophages likely do not participate in the selection of R5 viruses in primary infection. Intestinal lymphocytes, on the other hand, express both CCR5 and CXCR4 and support replication by both R5 and X4 HIV-1 *in vitro* (44), indicating that intestinal lymphocytes also probably do not participate in the selective acquisition of R5 viruses during primary infection.

Local HIV-1 Replication and Depletion of Lamina Propria CD4+ T Cells

Consistent with the finding that human intestinal lymphocytes, not macrophages, are a target cell for HIV-1 infection *in vitro,* Veazey et al. (46) showed that during early SIV infection of macaques, infected macrophages are rare and infected T cells are more common in the intestinal mucosa than in the blood. Coincident with the early local accumulation of SIV-infected lymphocytes in the GI mucosa is the presence of a high viral load in the intestinal mucosa, which is associated with villous atrophy and malabsorption (47). Because HIV-1 replicates more efficiently in activated T cells, the abundance of activated CD4+ T cells in the intestinal lamina propria compared with the blood likely contributes to the initial higher frequency of virus-infected lymphocytes in the GI mucosa than in the blood. However, after 7 to 14 days of infection, CD4+ T cells in the intestinal and colonic mucosa become rapidly and profoundly depleted, probably due to cell lysis and apoptosis. This profound depletion of intestinal CD4+ T cells proceeds the depletion of such cells in the blood in both humans and macaques (46–49).

Sequence of Mucosal Events in Early HIV-1 Infection

The studies discussed above suggest the following sequence of events in the intestinal mucosa during early HIV-1 infection acquired by vertical transmission or homosexual contact. A mixture of R5 and X4 viruses, frequently present in the blood of chronically infected donors, are released into the milk or semen and then enter the recipient through inoculation into the oral cavity or rectum. After oral inoculation, virus that reaches the tonsils encounters M cells in the overlying epithelium, which deliver the virus to the dendritic cell-rich lymphoid tissue of the tonsils. Dendritic cells support HIV-1 replication through dendritic-cell–T-cell conjugates and disseminate HIV-1 to secondary lymphoid tissues. Local oral factors, such as secretory leukocyte protease, a potent inhibitor of HIV-1 infection (50), could limit local (tonsillar) infection, allowing swallowed virus to pass through the oral cavity. Passage through the stomach would be facilitated by the absence of gastric acid production in the fetus and neonate. In the adult, gastric acid could limit the amount of viable virus that reaches the intestine, but this issue requires further study. When a mixture of viruses reaches the recipient's upper GI tract mucosa, $GalCer^{+}CCR5^{+}CXCR4^{-}$ epithelial cells bind and selectively transfer R5 viruses from the cells' apical to basolateral surface, likely by microtubule-dependent, non-degradative transcytosis. Conceivably, virus inoculated onto the rectal mucosa enters the host via one of the above described cellular routes as well, but this awaits further study.

Virus translocated across the epithelium encounters lamina propria macrophages and T cells, but only the lymphocytes express CCR5, the co-receptor that mediates R5 HIV-1 entry. Because the lamina propria contains the largest reservoir of activated T cells in the body and because HIV-1 replicates most efficiently in activated T cells, the lamina propria becomes the initial major site of HIV-1 replication and amplification. Virus may then disseminate freely through the circulation. Alternatively, virus that infects activated T cells in the organized lymphoid structures could be disseminated to distant mucosal sites through mucosal receptor-mediated homing. HIV-1-induced T-cell death, presumably by cell lysis, apoptosis, and cytotoxic lymphocyte (CTL) killing, leads to rapid depletion of lamina propria CD4+ T cells, long before the decline in circulating CD4+ T cells.

Eventually, local and systemic T-cell depletion predisposes the GI mucosa to an array of opportunistic infections, leading to mucosal inflammation and the release of chemoattractant peptides. These peptides recruit to the mucosa co-receptor-positive blood mononuclear cells, which serve as new target cells for the perpetuation of local HIV-1 infection and replication. Thus, besides serving as a site of opportunistic infections in late-stage HIV-1 disease, the GI tract also plays a fundamental role in early HIV-1 disease by serving as the site for virus entry, the initial site of virus replication and amplification, and the initial site of CD4+ T-cell depletion.

ESOPHAGEAL INFECTIONS IN HIV-1 DISEASE

An array of infectious and non-infectious processes cause esophageal disease in HIV-1-infected persons (Table 29.2). The infectious processes are caused primarily by *Candida albicans,* cytomegalovirus (CMV), and herpes simplex virus (HSV); in approximately 20% of patients, two pathogens are present (51–53). Together, these infections cause esophageal symptoms in approximately 30% of HIV-1-infected patients (51) and represent the second most common GI manifestation of AIDS. Dysphagia (difficulty swallowing), odynophagia (painful swallowing), and, less frequently, substernal chest pain independent of deglutition are the most common symptoms, but no one symptom or combination of symptoms is specifically associated with a particular infection. Symptomatic esophagitis frequently causes a secondary reduction in oral nutrition and decrease in caloric intake. Reduced caloric intake exacerbates the weight loss and cachexia that characterizes HIV-1 infection, particularly when diarrhea and malabsorption are present.

Candida Oropharyngeal and Esophageal Infection

Description

C. albicans is a ubiquitous, dimorphic fungus that forms budding yeast, pseudohyphae, and occasionally true septate hyphae. The fungus is commonly present as a nonpathogenic commensal in the oral and GI tract flora of healthy adults. Among the potentially invasive *Candida* species (*C. albicans, Candida glabrata, Candida tropicalis, Candida parapsilosis*), *C. albicans* is the predominant species responsible for oropharyngeal and esophageal inflammatory disease in HIV-1-infected persons.

In the oral cavity, *Candida* infection has four presentations: (a) pseudomembranous candidiasis (thrush), exudative plaques on any tissue; (b) erythematous candidiasis, red and atrophic lesions on the palate and tongue; (c) hypertrophic candidiasis, adherent hyperplastic lesions; and (d) angular cheilitis, erythematous fissures at the corners of the mouth (54). The presence of oral candidiasis in persons at risk for AIDS is associated with the development of an AIDS-related infection or Kaposi sarcoma in 60% of patients within 2 years (55).

In the esophagus, *Candida* overgrowth occurs throughout the organ, although more frequently in the distal region, leading to mucosal keratinization and the raised white plaques containing exudate and fungal elements that are pathognomonic of *Candida* esophagitis (Fig. 29.2). Histologic examination of biopsy specimens from patients with esophageal candidiasis shows local invasion of the lamina propria but not into the submucosa. The absence of deep penetration and disseminated candidiasis in HIV-1-

TABLE 29.2. REPORTED CAUSES OF ESOPHAGEAL DISEASE OR INJURY IN HIV-1-INFECTED PERSONS

Infectious Agent	Neoplasm	Other
Fungal:	Kaposi sarcoma	Zidovudine pill injury
Candida albicans	Lymphoma	Zalcitabine pill injury
Torulopsis glabrata	Squamous cell carcinoma	Reflux esophagitis
Histoplasma capsulatum		
Viral:		
Cytomegalovirus		
Herpes simplex virus		
HIV-1		
Epstein–Barr virus		
Bacterial:		
Mycobacterium avium complex		
Mycobacterium tuberculosis		
Bacteriosis (unidentified)		
Protozoal:		
Cryptosporidium		
Pneumocystis carinii		
Leishmania species		

Source: From Adapted from Wilcox, CM. Esophageal disease in the acquired immunodeficiency syndrome: Etiology, diagnosis, and management. *Am J Med* 1992;92:412–421.

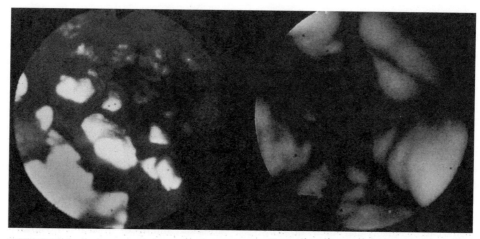

FIGURE 29.2. Endoscopic appearance of *Candida* esophagitis. **(Left)** Multiple exudative white plaques surrounded by inflamed erythematous mucosa. **(Right)** Circumferential inflammatory membrane covering inflamed mucosa in a patient with severe *Candida* esophagitis.

infected persons is likely due to the relatively intact function of polymorphonuclear neutrophils in patients with even late-stage HIV-1 disease.

The pathogenesis of *Candida* inflammation is likely multifactorial. The mechanical shearing forces of the esophagus have been suggested to tear the mucosa underlying *Candida* microabscesses, leading to ulceration (56). The similarity in phenotype and DNA characteristics among *C. albicans* isolated from AIDS patients and seronegative control subjects indicates that candidiasis in HIV-1-infected persons is due to common isolates that proliferate in the setting of impaired host defense mechanisms (57), such as reduced macrophage phagocytic and cytotoxic activities (58). The association between candidiasis and the severity of immune dysfunction (59), and the association between therapy-induced improvement in immune function and resolution of candidiasis (60), implicates immune dysfunction as a key factor in predisposing the mucosa to *C. albicans* infection.

Clinical Features

C. albicans is the most common cause of esophagitis in persons infected with HIV-1 (51–53). Indeed, among outpatient HIV-1-infected persons with CD4+ lymphocyte counts less than 300 cells/mm^3, *Candida* esophagitis is the most common opportunistic infection (61). Esophageal candidiasis is associated with both odynophagia and dysphagia. Although odynophagia may occur more frequently (62), neither symptom is predictive of *Candida* esophagitis (51–53). The symptoms occur with variable intensity, and the dysphagia may be associated with swallowing both solids and liquids. Occasionally, substernal chest pain is the primary symptom. Endoscopically, the pathognomonic lesion is a patchy or circumferential white "cheesy" plaque or membrane overlying inflamed mucosa (Fig. 29.2).

Oropharyngeal and esophageal candidiasis infection may occur independently, but both are frequently present in the same patient. In an early study (62), 100% of 10 AIDS patients with oropharyngeal candidiasis (thrush) with or without esophageal symptoms had esophageal candidiasis. Subsequent study (52,63) showed that the predictive value of thrush and esophageal symptoms as markers of esophageal candidiasis is less than originally thought (Table 29.3). Indeed, approximately 40% of patients with esophageal symptoms do not have thrush (52), and esophageal candidiasis may be asymptomatic (56,62). Nevertheless, the presence of thrush and esophageal symptoms in an HIV-1-infected person, particularly after AIDS has

TABLE 29.3. PREDICTIVE VALUE OF ORAL CANDIDIASIS AND ESOPHAGEAL SYMPTOMS FOR *CANDIDA* ESOPHAGITIS IN HIV-1-INFECTED PATIENTS

			Predictive Value (%)	
Condition	Sensitivity (%)	Specificity (%)	Positive	Negative
Oral candidiasis	88	81	81	88
Esophageal symptoms	60	100	100	73
Both	93	100	100	96

Source: From Porro GB, Parente F, Cernuschi M. The diagnosis of esophageal candidiasis in patients with acquired immune deficiency syndrome: is endoscopy always necessary? *Am J Gastroenterol* 1989;84:143–146, with permission.

developed, should alert the clinician to the possibility of concomitant esophageal candidiasis.

Diagnosis

Esophageal symptoms in HIV-1-infected persons should be thoroughly evaluated with an appropriate diagnostic test for the following reasons. First, a particular esophageal symptom is not diagnostic of a specific pathogen. Second, oropharyngeal candidiasis is not predictive of esophageal candidiasis. Third, *C. albicans* is the cause of the esophagitis in only about 50% to 60% of cases, and more than one pathogen may be present. Fourth, therapy is available for the major causes of infectious esophageal disease in HIV-1-infected persons.

Candida esophagitis can be reliably diagnosed endoscopically in more than 95% of patients by the presence of a white membrane or plaques overlying inflamed mucosa (64). Histologic identification of yeast and pseudohyphae in esophageal biopsies and cytologic identification of these forms in brush specimens confirm the endoscopic diagnosis but by themselves are not diagnostic, because they may be present when the esophageal mucosa is endoscopically normal (63). Double-contrast esophagography is only 25% as sensitive as endoscopy as a diagnostic procedure (64).

Treatment

C. albicans is one of the most readily treatable AIDS-defining opportunistic pathogens. Topical agents, including nystatin and clotrimazole; oral agents, including ketoconazole, itraconazole, and fluconazole; and the intravenous agent amphotericin B are currently used to treat mucosal (Table 29.4)

TABLE 29.4. THERAPY FOR ESOPHAGEAL AND INTESTINAL INFECTIONS IN HIV-1-INFECTED ADULTS

Pathogen	Treatment	Alternative
Protozoal:		
Cryptosporidium species	Paromomycin 500–750 mg PO qid	Paromomycin + azithromycin 600 mg qd for 4 wk
Microsporidia species	Albendazole 400 mg PO bid for 4 wk	Fumagillin (call 800-547-1392)
Isospora belli[a]	Trimethoprim-sulfamethoxazole 1 DS[b] tab PO qid for 10 d then bid for 3 wk	
Giardia lamblia	Metronidazole 250 mg PO tid for 10 d	Albendazole 400 mg PO qd for 5 d
Cyclospora[c]	Trimethoprim-sulfamethoxazole 1 DS tab PO qid for 10 d	
Viral:		
Cytomegalovirus[a,e,f]	Ganciclovir 5 mg/kg IV bid for 2–3 wk	Foscarnet 60 mg/kg IV or 90 mg IV bid for 2–3 wk
Herpes simplex virus[a,e,f]	Acyclovir 400 mg PO 5/d for 7–14 d	Famcilovir 500 mg PO bid for 7 d Valacyclovir 1,000 mg PO tid PO for 7 d
Adenovirus	NA	
Rotavirus[c]	NA	
Astrovirus[c]	NA	
Picobirnavirus[c]	NA	
Bacterial:		
Salmonella species	Ceftriaxone 1–2 g PO qd for 7 d	Amoxicillin 1 g PO tid for 7–14 d DS tab bid for 10–14 d
	Ciprofloxacin 500 mg PO bid for 7 d	Trimethoprim-sulfamethoxazole 1
Shigella flexneri[a,f]	Ciprofloxacin 500 mg PO bid for 7 d	Trimethoprim-sulfamethoxazole 1 DS tab bid for 10–14 d
	Ampicillin 500 mg PO qid for 5 d	Ceftriaxone 1–2 g PO qd for 7 d
Campylobacter jejuni[a,f]	Erythromycin 500 PO mg qid for 7 d Ciprofloxacin 500 PO mg bid for 7 d	Doxycycline 100 mg PO bid for 7 d Clarithromycin 500 mg PO qd for 7 d Azithromycin 500 mg PO qd for 7 d
Mycobacterium avium complex[a,f]	Clarithromycin 500 mg PO bid Azithromycin 500 mg PO qd Ethambutol 15–25 mg/kg PO qd Rifabutin 300 mg PO bid	Amikacin 25 mg/kg IV qd for 3 wk Ciprofloxacin 750 mg PO bid Ofloxacin 400 mg PO bid
Clostridium difficile	Metronidazole 500 mg PO tid for 10 d	Vancomycin 125 mg PO qid for 10 d
Bacteriosis[c]	Ciprofloxacin 500 mg PO bid for 4 wk[g]	
Fungal:		
Candida albicans	Fluconazole 100 mg PO qd for 14d	Itraconazole 200 mg qd for 14d
Histoplasma capsulatum	Amphotericin B 0.5–0.6 mg/kg IV qd for 4–8 wk	Itraconazole 200 mg bid

[a]Chronic suppression at reduced dosage may be necessary.
[b]Double strength.
[c]Pathogenicity in HIV-1 infection not established.
[d]Not available.
[e]Reduce dosage for decreased creatinine clearance.
[f]Resistance may develop; susceptibility testing necessessary.

Candida infections. For initial or uncomplicated recurrent oropharyngeal candidiasis in a patient without esophageal candidiasis and a CD4+ count higher than 50 cells/mm^3 on HAART, clotrimazole troches 10 mg five times daily for 7 to 14 days is effective (clinical cure in 90% and mycologic cure in most patients) and relatively inexpensive (65–69). However, multiple daily doses are inconvenient and treatment failures occur (70). For complicated (severe) oropharyngeal candidiasis or when esophageal candidiasis is present, the CD4+ count is less than 50 cells/mm^3, or HAART is not available, a systemic oral azole is recommended (65,66). The most commonly used such agent is fluconazole (100 mg daily), which is highly effective (more than 90% response rates) and is not dependent on a low pH level for absorption (71,72). However, drug interactions with rifamycin, warfarin, and phenytoin, as well as the emergence of resistance strains of *Candida* are potential problems.

For esophageal candidiasis, oral antifungal agents are used, because topical agents are ineffective. Currently, fluconazole (100 to 200 mg orally once a day for 2 to 3 weeks) is the drug of choice (69,73–76). In a multicenter, randomized, double-blinded trial comparing fluconazole with ketoconazole therapy for *Candida* esophagitis, endoscopic cure occurred in 91% of patients treated with fluconazole and 52% with ketoconazole, and symptomatic cure occurred in 85% of patients with fluconazole and 65% with ketoconazole (73). Both drugs are generally safe and well tolerated (73,74). The major side effects of fluconazole are nausea, skin rash, and increases in hepatic aminotransferase levels; hepatic necrosis has occurred in a few patients. Also, fluconazole can be absorbed in the absence of gastric acid, whereas ketoconazole absorption is acid-independent. When endoscopy is not available or the patient cannot tolerate the procedure, empiric therapy with fluconazole has been safe, efficacious, and cost-effective (77). For fluconazole-resistant *C. albicans,* amphotericin B (0.3 mg/kg intravenously daily for 7 days) is the treatment of choice. When severe oral or esophageal disease prevents swallowing tablets or capsules, a liquid formulation of itraconazole can be used in place of fluconazole; equal clinical response rates (more than 90%) and a higher mycologic cure rate (92% for itraconazole oral solution and 78% for fluconazole tablets) have been reported (78). The use of itraconazole oral solution also avoids the requirement for activating gastric acid, which limits the use of the pill form.

CMV Esophagitis

Description

CMV is a double-stranded DNA virus in the Herpesviridae family. The naked virus is a spherical DNA–protein complex core surrounded by an icosahedral capsid with 162 capsomeres. After infection of cells permissive to the virus, such as endothelial and mononuclear cells, viral particles accumulate in the nucleus and cytoplasm, enlarging the cells and producing the characteristic nuclear and cytoplasmic inclusions. The virus acquires a single or double membrane upon budding from the nuclear and cytoplasmic membrane. In immunocompetent persons, the virus enters a latent phase, during which it can be detected but not cultured from cells (79). Nonproductive latency can be interrupted when the host becomes immunosuppressed, such as during HIV-1 infection. As immunosuppression progresses, host antiviral mechanisms, including natural killer (NK) and CTL activities, decline (80) and infection becomes productive. CMV can then be cultured from a variety of cells, including circulating mononuclear and polymorphonuclear cells; body fluids, such as semen and cervical secretions; and tissues, including the alimentary tract mucosa.

The inflammation associated with CMV infection of the esophagus is characterized by the presence of cytomegalic inclusion cells, increased numbers of inflammatory cells, and frequently, although not invariably, vasculitis. The intimate relationship between CMV and ulcerative lesions of the esophagus implicates the virus in the pathogenesis of these lesions (81); increased numbers of CMV inclusion cells in the mucosa of the esophagus, as well as other regions of the GI tract, correlate directly with severity of inflammation (82). During severe intestinal disease, CMV has been identified in mucosal endothelial cells, enterocytes, fibroblasts, smooth muscle cells, and macrophages (83). Although previous reports suggested that CMV infection of endothelial cells and the associated vasculitis lead to vascular obstruction, ischemia, and tissue damage (84,85), the frequent absence of vasculitis in CMV-infected tissues suggests that CMV causes mucosal damage by a mechanism other than occlusive vasculitis. In this regard, we have shown that CMV can induce an array of pro-inflammatory cytokines, including interleukin 1, interleukin 6, interleukin 8, and tumor necrosis factor-α, by mononuclear phagocytes *in vitro* and in the esophageal mucosa (86–88); these cytokines likely play a key role in mediating CMV-induced inflammation.

Clinical Features

In the largest study to date, CMV was the second most common cause of esophageal disease among 110 HIV-1-infected persons with esophageal symptoms (52). Serious GI disease due to CMV occurs in approximately 3% of HIV-1-infected patients (89), and all organs of the GI tract can be involved (90). In the esophagus, the principal manifestation of CMV disease includes inflammation, ulcerations, and, infrequently, pseudotumor. The presenting symptoms include odynophagia and, less frequently, dysphagia (91). Although odynophagia is reportedly more common, it is not predictive of CMV disease because it commonly accompanies other causes of esophagitis. Endoscopically, ulceration is the characteristic feature of CMV

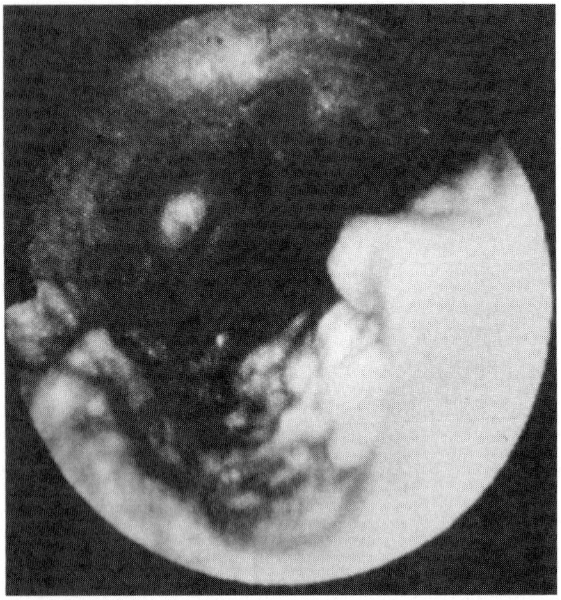

FIGURE 29.3. Endoscopic photograph of a large solitary ulcer caused by cytomegalovirus in the distal esophagus.

esophagitis (Fig. 29.3). The ulcers may be large (more than 5 cm^2), solitary, often hemorrhagic, well demarcated at the edges, and located predominantly, but not exclusively, in the distal esophagus. Smaller ulcers occur and are more commonly located in the mid and proximal regions of the esophagus. The mucosa between the ulcers usually appears normal. Erosive inflammation with or without ulceration is the second most frequent manifestation of CMV infection of esophageal mucosa (92,93). In contrast to the normal intervening mucosa associated with CMV ulcers, the mucosa in this setting is diffusely erythematous and friable. The least common manifestation of CMV esophageal disease is pseudotumor (93). This lesion resembles an exophytic mass, usually located in the distal esophagus that radiographically and endoscopically may be mistaken for carcinoma.

The differential for large, solitary esophageal ulcers includes CMV, HIV-1 (see "Idiopathic Esophageal Ulceration" below), and Epstein–Barr virus (94). *Mycobacterium tuberculosis* (95,96) and MAC (95) also may cause esophageal ulcerations, but usually when diffuse esophagitis or an inflammatory mass is also present. The fungus *Torulopsis glabrata* is a rare cause of esophageal ulcers (98). Noninfectious causes of esophageal ulcers include zidovudine (99) and zalcitabine (100) pill-induced injury.

The diffuse esophagitis associated with CMV infection can also accompany infection by most of the other pathogens listed in Table 29.2. *C. albicans,* however, causes esophagitis that is easily distinguished from diffuse CMV esophagitis by a raised white membrane of fungal elements and exudate overlying the inflammation. HSV esophagitis begins as vesicular lesions, but after the lesions erode and coalesce, an erosive esophagitis may be seen endoscopically. Novel causes of esophagitis include *Leishmania* species in endemic areas (101), cryptosporidiosis of the distal esophagus (102), and bacteriosis by unidentified bacteria (103).

The esophageal pseudotumor associated with CMV infection should be distinguished from processes with a potential for causing a mass-like effect, including Kaposi sarcoma (104), lymphoma (105), squamous cell carcinoma (106), and MAC (97). Although intestinal manifestations are more common, *Histoplasma capsulatum* has been reported to involve the esophagus in association with HIV-1 infection (107).

Diagnosis

The diagnosis of CMV esophageal disease is firmly established by the presence of endoscopic abnormality (ulcer and/or inflammation) and the histologic identification of cytomegalic inclusion cells with surrounding inflammation (108,109). Vasculitis may accompany the inflammation, but its presence is not required to diagnose CMV mucosal disease (81,83). Similarly, culture of CMV from a mucosal biopsy supports but is not required for the diagnosis.

Because the severity of inflammation correlates directly with the number of cells infected with CMV, it is reasonable to assume that the more severe the inflammation, the greater the likelihood of identifying the pathognomonic inclusion cell. When endoscopic and histologic evidence of inflammation is absent, the presence of CMV inclusion cells is consistent with the carrier state without CMV-associated disease. A problem arises, however, when ulcerative or inflammatory changes suggest CMV esophageal disease, but CMV inclusion cells are not identified (81). Although the false-negative rate for detecting CMV inclusions in CMV-diseased tissue is not known, one explanation for the inability to detect inclusion cells in this setting is sampling error. The development of more sensitive diagnostic techniques should address this problem.

The newer diagnostic techniques being evaluated for the detection of CMV in GI biopsies include immunocytochemical staining (110,111), *in situ* hybridization (111, 112), and polymerase chain reaction (PCR) (113). The utility of immunocytochemistry for confirming the histologic diagnosis was shown in a retrospective study in which inclusion cells were identified by staining in 92% of colon biopsies, whereas CMV was cultured in only 30% (109). In comparative studies (111), *in situ* hybridization for CMV DNA was more sensitive than immunostaining and more sensitive than routine staining with hematoxylin and eosin for the detection of CMV. The most promising and potentially sensitive and specific technique for detecting CMV GI biopsies appears to be amplification of CMV DNA by PCR, which has a sensitivity of 92% and a specificity of 93% to 100% for GI tract infection (113). These techniques may become more widely available after issues related to expense, the level of expertise required to perform the procedure, and the labor-intensive nature of performing the assays have been resolved.

Treatment

Ganciclovir [9-(1,3-dihydroxy-2-propoxymethyl)guanidine] is a nucleoside analogue that inhibits replication of CMV DNA through its triphosphate derivative, which is a substrate and potent inhibitor of CMV DNA polymerase. In early uncontrolled studies in HIV-1-infected patients (114–119), ganciclovir reduced or stabilized the signs and symptoms of esophageal and enteric CMV disease in 63% to 100% of cases and lowered or cleared CMV from available culture sites in 68% to 100%. However, in the only randomized, double-blinded, placebo-controlled study of ganciclovir therapy for CMV colitis, the drug reduced colonic inflammation, the number of colon cultures positive for CMV, and extracolonic disease but did not significantly reduce the diarrhea, abdominal pain, or fever (120). The current recommended dosage is 5 mg/kg intravenously twice daily for 14 to 21 days (Table 29.4); side effects include neutropenia and thrombocytopenia, which are usually reversed after withdrawal, as well as confusion, rash, fever, nausea, vomiting, and diarrhea (118,119). Toxicity may be increased when the drug is used with zidovudine. In addition to side effects, the emergence of resistance and recurrence after termination of therapy are important clinical problems. Approximately 8% of patients treated with ganciclovir secrete resistant strains after 3 months of therapy (121). Because the drug is virustatic and not virucidal, recurrence will occur in most patients after withdrawal of the drug. Thus, ganciclovir therapy should be individualized, with careful monitoring of patient improvement, potential side effects, and viral cultures. A tablet preparation awaits testing for GI CMV disease.

Foscarnet (trisodium phosphonoformate) was developed in response to the emergence of ganciclovir-resistant CMV strains and refractory CMV disease. Shown to be effective for the treatment of CMV disease of other organs, foscarnet therapy was reported to induce remission of CMV esophageal ulceration within 2 weeks in 83% of patients (122). In this uncontrolled study, only 20% of 15 patients had a recurrence during 9 months of follow-up. The recommended dosage of foscarnet is 60 mg/kg intravenously three times daily or 90 mg/kg intravenously twice daily for 14 to 21 days; side effects include renal dysfunction, seizures and other central nervous system disturbances, nausea, vomiting, and alterations in the levels of calcium, phosphate, potassium, and magnesium (123). Because recurrent disease is a potential problem, careful monitoring of the patient's clinical course is an important component of effective management.

The marked reduction in the incidence of CMV esophageal disease in association with HAART is discussed below.

HSV Esophagitis

Description

HSV is a member of the Herpesviridae family of viruses. Accordingly, its physical structure and replication cycle resemble that of other members of the group, such as that of CMV discussed above. Briefly, HSV is a double-stranded DNA virus composed of a DNA–protein core, an icosahedral capsid with 162 capsomeres, and a lipid-containing outer membrane. Key features of the life cycle include DNA replication in the host cell nucleus, assembly of the capsid in the cytoplasm, acquisition of the protein envelope upon budding from the nucleus, and lysis of the cell (except the neuron) with release of progeny virions. HSV establishes nonproductive latency in sensory nerve ganglia; reactivation of latent virus may occur in response to immunosuppression (HIV-1 infection), disruption of the skin (burns), and malnutrition (chronic hyperalimentation). Chronic HSV infection in homosexual men was one of the first infections to signal the emergence of AIDS (124). Since that initial description, HSV has remained one of the most prevalent opportunistic pathogens in persons infected with HIV-1.

As cell-mediated (NK and CTL) activity and humoral function deteriorates in response to HIV-1, HSV within sensory nerve ganglia is reactivated and the virus spreads peripherally along sensory nerve pathways. After reaching mucocutaneous sites, HSV spreads among epithelial cells by lysis and releases infectious virions that infect and lyse adjacent cells. Small superficial vesicular lesions with an inflammatory base develop in response to the infection and lysis of epithelial cells. As infection spreads, the resulting small foci of necrotic epithelium become progressively more confluent, resulting in the development of superficial erosions and ulcerations.

The prevalence of HSV infections among AIDS patients is approximately 30% (125). In most studies (52,53,56), HSV is the third most frequent cause of esophagitis among HIV-1-infected persons, accounting for 4% to 14% of cases. As discussed above, about 20% of patients with esophagitis are co-infected with two, and sometime three, opportunistic pathogens, including HSV.

Clinical Features

The symptoms of HSV esophagitis are similar to those of *C. albicans* and CMV. Odynophagia and dysphagia occur, although odynophagia is the predominant symptom. Three progressive stages of mucosal abnormality have been observed endoscopically: first, discrete raised vesicles; second, coalescence of the vesicles into larger 0.5- to 2-cm^2 lesions with raised borders; and third, diffuse mucosal erosions and ulcerative esophagitis (126). The areas of erosion and ulceration may be hemorrhagic.

The esophageal symptoms associated with HSV are nonspecific; consequently, the differential diagnosis is similar to those of *C. albicans* and CMV esophageal disease. The potential etiologies can be narrowed, however, when endoscopic visualization shows the characteristic mucosal changes described above (see Color Figure 29.4). Next to HSV, the most likely diagnosis is diffuse CMV esophagitis. Because advanced HSV lesions may have overlying plaques of exudate (126), *Candida* esophagitis is another, albeit less likely, consideration. Large solitary ulcers and inflammatory mass are not features of HSV esophagitis.

Diagnosis

The diagnostic procedure of choice is esophagoscopy. Visual inspection may strongly suggest HSV, but the diagnosis is based on cytologic identification of intranuclear (Cowdry type A) inclusions in multinucleated cells within a typical lesion and is confirmed by isolation of the virus.

Treatment

Acyclovir is the drug of choice for HSV esophagitis and is usually effective in reducing or clearing both symptoms and lesions. For primary or recurrent infection, acyclovir (200 mg orally five times per day for 14 days) is recommended (123). Acyclovir is generally well tolerated, and the major side effects are nausea, vomiting, headaches, and reversible renal dysfunction with high doses.

Because recurrent HSV is common, long-term suppressive therapy with acyclovir at 400 mg orally twice daily may be required (123). However, such therapy is associated with the emergence of resistant strains (127). Therefore, periodic monitoring of susceptibility to acyclovir is important for the early detection of resistance and individualization of therapy (128). Foscarnet at 40 mg/kg intravenously three times daily for 21 days is effective for acyclovir-resistant mucocutaneous HSV (122,129). The side effects are discussed above (see "CMV Esophagitis").

Idiopathic Esophageal Ulceration

Description

After opportunistic infections, idiopathic ulceration without detectable pathogens is the next most common esophageal complication of HIV-1 infection (130,131). Similar to the HAART-associated reduction in the incidence of esophageal infections, HAART has lead to a reduction in the incidence of idiopathic esophageal ulceration as well. Idiopathic esophageal ulceration is characterized by epithelial necrosis, accumulation of mononuclear and polymorphonuclear inflammatory cells, and collagen deposition. Histology and culture of biopsy specimens from the ulcer are negative for known pathogens, although *Candida* species may be present superficially, consistent with secondary infection. Electron microscopy (132), *in situ* hybridization (133,134), immunohistochemical staining (134), and coculture techniques (135) have revealed retrovirus-like particles or HIV-1 in association with the ulcers.

The pathogenesis of idiopathic esophageal ulceration in HIV-1-infected persons is likely multifactorial. During late-stage HIV-1 disease, the immunopathophysiology of alimentary tract mucosa is substantially altered, reflected in the dysregulation of local immune responses (136), enhanced cytokine production (137), and the presence of mild inflammation (138). These changes predispose the esophageal mucosa a 6- to 60-fold increase in the prevalence of HIV-1-infected mononuclear cells compared with peripheral lymph nodes (45) and possibly increased levels of pro-inflammatory cytokines. However, HIV-1 is commonly identified in nonidiopathic (i.e., CMV) ulcers as well (139), calling into question the direct etiologic role of HIV-1 in idiopathic esophageal ulceration.

Clinical Features

Esophageal ulceration may be the presenting manifestation of acute HIV-1 syndrome, occur during rapid progression of acute HIV-1 syndrome to AIDS, or (more commonly) herald accelerated progression of clinical latency to AIDS. Typically, patients with HIV-1-associated esophageal ulceration present with odynophagia and, less frequently, dysphagia, substernal chest pain, or a burning sensation independent of deglutition. Symptoms may limit the intake of food, exacerbating the weight loss that accompanies HIV-1 infection. As shown in Figure 29.5(see Color Figure 29.5), the ulcers have well-demarcated edges, vary in size (usually 1 to 5 cm^2), and occur throughout the esophagus as solitary or, more commonly, multiple lesions with normal intervening mucosa. The differential for isolated esophageal ulcers is discussed above (see "CMV Esophagitis").

Diagnosis

The definitive diagnostic procedure is esophagoscopy, which allows visual inspection and directed biopsy of abnormal mucosa (130,131). The diagnosis of HIV-1-associated ulceration is based on the absence of known pathogens in an esophageal ulcer in a patient with HIV-1 infection. The ability to identify esophageal opportunistic pathogens or pathologic processes in most AIDS patients with esophageal symptoms (53) indicates that a vigorous diagnostic evaluation should be pursued before the ulcer is diagnosed idiopathic.

Treatment

Although the esophageal ulcerations associated with HIV-1 infection may heal spontaneously, the administration of

TABLE 29.5. DIARRHEAL ILLNESSES ASSOCIATED WITH THE ACUTE, INTERMEDIATE, AND LATE HIV-1 INFECTION

Early	Intermediate	Late	
Acute HIV-1 syndrome	AIDS enteropathy	***Parasitic infections***	***Bacterial infections***
		Cryptosporidium	*Mycobacterium avium* complex
		Microsporidia	*Salmonella* species
		Isospora belli	*Shigella flexneri*
		Cyclospora	*Campylobacter jejuni*
		Viral infections	***Fungal infections***
		Cytomegalovirus	*Candida albicans*
		Herpes simplex virus	*Histoplasma capsulatum*
		Adenovirus	
		Picobirnavirus (?)	
		Astrovirus (?)	
		Rotavirus (?)	

high-dose steroids is effective therapy in many patients. Prednisone at 40 to 60 mg per day given orally or methylprednisolone given intravenously when swallowing is impaired usually provides rapid clinical and endoscopic improvement (140–143). Steroid therapy should be administered with caution, however, because immunosuppression may be potentiated, leading to increased HIV-1 expression and the acquisition or exacerbation of opportunistic infections. Recently, aphthous ulcers of the oral cavity and esophagus in HIV-1-infected persons were shown to respond to thalidomide (51,144). A prospective trial of thalidomide for esophageal ulcers is currently underway.

INTESTINAL INFECTIONS IN HIV-1 DISEASE

Evaluation

Although acute HIV-1 infection is associated with GI symptoms in approximately 30% of patients, here we focus on the opportunistic infections that occur predominantly during late-stage HIV-1 disease (Table 29.5). We use the three-phase protocol outlined in Table 29.6 to evaluate HIV-1-infected patients for an infectious etiology for diarrheal illness. This protocol was used for 10 years at the National Institutes of Health, yielding a specific pathogen in as many as 85% of patients with AIDS and diarrhea (145). Stool examination is the initial and most important diagnostic test. Based on only stool microbiologic evaluation and culture, enteric pathogens have been identified in 48% to 55% of HIV-1-infected patients with diarrhea (146,147). Steps 2 and 3 of the evaluation are performed successively when the microbiologic evaluation of at least two fresh stool specimens yields no identifiable pathogen or when the patient remains symptomatic despite therapy for an identified pathogen. These steps require the performance of an endoscopic procedure to obtain mucosal biopsy specimens. In this regard, esophagoduodenoscopy and sigmoidoscopy yielded a diagnosis in 50% of patients in whom no pathogen was detected by stool examination (148). Sigmoidoscopy is reportedly more sensitive than

TABLE 29.6. DIAGNOSTIC EVALUATION OF DIARRHEA IN HIV-1-INFECTED PERSONS

Step 1:
- Stool cultured for *Salmonella* species, *Shigella flexneri, Campylobacter jejuni,* and *Clostridium difficile* at least twice and assayed for *Clostridium difficile* toxin
- Stool specimens (direct, concentrated, or both) examined for parasites using saline, iodine, trichrome, acid-fast preparations and for mycobacteria

Step 2:
- Gastroduodenoscopy and colonoscopy performed to inspect tissue and obtain biopsy specimens and luminal material
- Biopsy specimens stained with hematoxylin eosin for protozoal and viral inclusion cells, with methenamine silver or Giemsa for fungi, and with Fite for mycobacteria
- Duodenal biopsy specimens cultured for mycobacteria (if present in the stool)
- Colonic biopsy specimens cultured for mycobacteria (if present in the stool) and for HSV (rectal tissue)
- Duodenal fluid specimens examined as above for parasites

Step 3:
- Biopsy specimens examined by electron microscopy for microsporidians (duodenal tissue) and adenovirus (colonic tissue)

Source: Adapted from Connolly GM, Forbes A, Bleeson JA, et al. The value of barium enema and colonoscopy in patients with infected with HIV. *AIDS* 1990;4:687–689, with permission.

colonoscopy (97% vs. 62%) in providing a diagnosis of an enteric pathogen in HIV-1-infected persons (149). Because small intestinal bacterial overgrowth is not a manifestation of HIV-1 infection (150), intestinal fluid is not routinely cultured for anaerobic and aerobic bacteria.

Management

Our approach to the management of diarrheal illness in HIV-1-infected persons is outlined in Table 29.7. The importance of identifying the infectious etiology is underscored by observations that specific antimicrobial therapy can reduce the volume and frequency of diarrhea in 50% to 69% of HIV-1-infected patients with diarrhea and an identifiable enteric pathogen (145,146). In the absence of detectable pathogens, supportive therapy with rehydration, electrolyte supplementation, and drugs that inhibit intestinal motility and secretion is associated with clinical improvement. Many patients may benefit symptomatically from therapy with loperamide, diphenoxylate, or paregoric. Some patients may also benefit from treatment with octreotide, a synthetic cyclic octapeptide analogue of somatostatin, which has been shown to reduce stool frequency and volume in as many as 60% of AIDS patients with refractory diarrhea and no detectable pathogen (151). In addition, HIV-1-infected patients with intestinal symptoms but no identifiable pathogens who received zidovudine have been reported to have higher levels of intestinal brush border enzymes than comparable patients who did not receive the drug (152), but the effect of this antiviral agent on intestinal symptoms is unclear. To date, the mainstay of management of HIV-1-infected persons with diarrhea but no detectable enteric pathogens remains symptomatic therapy.

TABLE 29.7. APPROACH TO THE MANAGEMENT OF INFECTIOUS DIARRHEA IN HIV-1-INFECTED PERSONS

1. Supportive therapy with fluids, electrolytes, and antimotility drugs is important.
2. Specific therapy is preferable to empiric therapy because the differential diagnosis is extensive and because drug intolerance and drug interactions are common.
3. Etiology may be multifactorial; consequently, therapy may be partially but not completely beneficial.
4. Microorganisms may be resistant to currently used agents or may develop resistance, necessitating repeated culture and drug sensitivity testing.
5. Many infectious syndromes recur; consequently, long-term suppressive therapy is often necessary.
6. Role of total parenteral nutrition, anabolic steroids, and appetite enhancers is uncertain.
7. Specific antimicrobial therapy and supportive care can enhance the quality of life and duration of survival.

Source: Adapted from Smith PD, Lane HC, Gill VJ, et al. Intestinal infections in patients with the acquired immunodeficiency syndrome (AIDS). Etiology and response to therapy. *Ann Intern Med* 1988;108:328–333, with permission.

Protozoal Infections

Cryptosporidium parvum

Description

Before the advent of HAART, *Cryptosporidium parvum* was present in approximately 20% of persons with AIDS and diarrhea in the United States (145,146,153,154) but as many as 55% of AIDS patients in developing countries such as Zaire and Haiti (155,156). A relatively common cause of self-limited watery diarrhea in immunocompetent persons (153,157,158), cryptosporidiosis causes debilitating diarrhea in patients with AIDS. Typically, the diarrhea is relentless, voluminous, nonbloody, and watery; abdominal cramps and weight loss are also prominent symptoms (159). Asymptomatic carriage has been reported (160), but symptoms of dehydration and wasting are more common. Malabsorption of both fat and carbohydrate is associated with cryptosporidiosis. Rarely, *Cryptosporidium* may spread to the biliary tract, leading to biliary tract obstruction (161,162), or the esophagus, causing esophagitis (163). The parasite has been identified throughout the length of the GI tract, developing within a parasitophorous vacuole beneath the epithelial cell membrane but outside the cytoplasm.

Diagnosis

Infection with *Cryptosporidium* is easily identified in stool microscopically with a modified acid-fast stain. Concentration of stool by zinc sulfate or sheather sucrose flotation enhances detection of rare or infrequent oocysts during intermittent shedding. Organisms may also be identified on small and large intestinal brush border by electron microscopy, but this technique is rarely necessary.

Treatment

Despite anecdotal reports of successful treatment of cryptosporidiosis in HIV-1-infected persons with spiramycin (164,165), paromomycin (166–168), bovine colostrum (169,170), transfer factor (171), somatostatin (151,172), and zidovudine (173), therapy with these agents has not been consistently effective and controlled clinical trials have not yet been performed. A course of paromomycin (Table 29.4), a nonabsorbable aminoglycoside, is reasonable based on preliminary studies reporting symptomatic improvement and oocyst clearance in some patients (166–169). Somatostatin may reduce the frequency and volume of *Cryptosporidium*-associated diarrhea (151,172), but therapy is complicated by requirements that the drug be given chronically several times daily and either intravenously or subcutaneously. HAART also appears to decrease the incidence of infection and enhance the resolution of *Cryptosporidium* infections.

Enterocytozoon bieneusi and *Septata intestinalis*

Description

Microsporidia are spore-forming, obligate intracellular protozoans that infect the small intestine (*Enterocytozoon bieneusi*) with dissemination (*Septata intestinalis*), liver (*Encephalitozoon cuniculi*), and cornea (*Encephalitozoon hellem*). The parasite has distinctive ultrastructural features; many organisms at different stages of development can be identified in the same enterocyte, causing cytopathic effect (174; see Chapter 64). *E. bieneusi* only infects enterocytes in the small intestine. *S. intestinalis,* which is ultrastructurally distinct from *E. bieneusi,* can penetrate into the lamina propria, infect macrophages, and disseminate to other organs such as the kidney (175–179). Until recently, microsporidia were identified exclusively in HIV-1-infected persons, but the parasite has now been diagnosed in immunosuppressed liver and renal transplant recipients without HIV-1 infection (180–182) and infrequently in immunocompetent persons (183–185).

Clinical Features

Infection with the parasite is associated with chronic, watery, nonbloody diarrhea of variable severity, frequently with substantial fluid and weight loss (186–188). Microsporidiosis has been reported to cause 40% to 50% of the cases of unexplained diarrhea in patients with HIV-1 infection (189,190), although in a single study (191), *E. bieneusi* was equally common in HIV-1-infected patients with and without diarrhea (191). The highest density of *E. bieneusi* is located in the jejunum (192), where the parasite infects enterocytes and may cause villous atrophy (193). The organism has been associated with AIDS-related biliary tract disease, including acalculous cholecystitis, cholecystitis with cholelithiasis, and cholangitis (194,195), presumably by ascending the proximal small intestine to infect the biliary tract. *S. intestinalis* also can cause biliary tract disease, including necrotizing cholangitis (196).

Diagnosis

Examination of small intestinal tissue or fluid obtained by endoscopy or biopsy capsule or tube is required for the diagnosis of microsporidiosis. Biopsies should be taken at the most distal site, where the parasite burden is the highest. Because of their small size, poor staining qualities, and minimal associated inflammation, microsporidia were formerly diagnosed exclusively by transmission electron microscopy. Today, trained observers can identify microsporidia by light microscopy in semithin plastic sections of small intestinal biopsies stained with methylene blue–azure II–basic fuchsin (181), touch preparations of mucosa stained with Giemsa (197,198), and stool specimens stained with a modified trichrome (chromotrope 2R) (199). Kotler et al. (200) compared these techniques and concluded that one light microscopic technique obviated the need for electron microscopy in more than 50% of cases and a combination of any two techniques obviated the need in more than 75% of cases. A rapid fluorescence technique based on uvitex 2B binding to chitin, a component of the spore wall, is reportedly effective for detecting microsporidia (190). However, because uvitex 2B binds to any chitin-containing microorganism, morphologic evaluation may be necessary to confirm the diagnosis. PCR was developed recently using primers for the rRNA gene of *E. bieneusi* and *S. intestinalis* to identify microsporidia in tissue specimens (201), but this diagnostic tool is not widely available.

Treatment

Curative therapy for microsporidiosis is not currently available. Albendazole, a benzimidazole derivative related to mebendazole, has been used to treat patients with both intestinal species of microsporidia (201) (Table 29.4). In open-label trials (202,203), albendazole (400 mg twice daily) was associated with resolution or improvement in diarrheal symptoms and weight gain or cessation of weight loss in HIV-1-infected patients with microsporidia-associated diarrhea. The agent appears to be more effective for *S. intestinalis* than *E. bieneusi* infections (204) and has been used successfully for disseminated *S. intestinalis* infections (178,179).

Isospora belli

Description And Clinical Features

I. belli is an obligate, intracellular coccidian parasite that resembles *Cryptosporidium* in its life cycle and small intestinal habitat. *I. belli* infection occurs in fewer than 3% of AIDS patients not on HAART in the United States but in as many as 15% of patients in developing nations such as Zambia and Haiti (205,206). Isosporosis is typically a chronic illness characterized by profuse, nonbloody, watery diarrhea that may be indistinguishable from the diarrheal illness associated with *Cryptosporidium* and Microsporidia infections. Weight loss of at least 10% may occur during the months before diagnosis (206,207). Nausea and abdominal cramps also typically accompany the illness; fever and vomiting are less frequent. In Haitian patients, dehydration requiring hospitalization has been reported in nearly 50% of patients (206). Steatorrhea and eosinophilia may also be present. Histology usually shows inflammation associated with some degree of villous atrophy; in contrast to *Cryptosporidium, I. belli* may invade the mucosa. Although concentrated in the small intestine, *I. belli* has been identified throughout the GI tract and has been associated with biliary disease, specifically acalculous cholecystitis (208). Rarely, the organism disseminates to extraintestinal sites, including mesenteric and tracheobronchial lymph nodes (209).

Diagnosis

The diagnosis of *I. belli* is established by the identification of the typical highly refractile, spherical oocysts (containing two sporoblasts) in stool using the modified Kinyoun acid-fast stain. Stool concentration may be necessary to detect infrequent or rare oocysts.

Treatment

The most effective therapeutic agent for *I. belli* is trimethoprim-sulfamethoxazole (160 mg of trimethoprim and 800 mg of sulfamethoxazole four times daily for 10 days then twice daily for 3 weeks) (Table 29.4). Because infection recurs in as many as 50% of cases after treatment, prolonged or repeated therapy with this agent may be required to suppress clinical illness.

Cyclospora cayetanensis

Description And Clinical Features

Cyclospora are obligate, intracellular coccidian parasites with morphologic and staining characteristics of a *Cyanobacteria*-like organism (210,211). Microscopically, the spherical cystlike organisms measure 8 to 10 μm in diameter and on modified acid-fast staining resemble *Cryptosporidium* (212). The *Cyclospora* oocyst has two sporocysts, each containing two sporozoites, distinguishing the structure of this coccidian parasite from that of the larger *I. belli* whose oocysts have two sporocysts, each containing four sporozoites (212). Both sexual and asexual forms have been identified in small intestinal epithelial cells, suggesting the organism can complete its life cycle in a single host (213). The organism has been identified in persons with diarrhea from Latin America (primarily Peru), the Caribbean, Southeast Asia, Eastern Europe, and the United States. In immunocompetent persons, the diarrhea is typically abrupt in onset, watery, and prolonged (lasting a mean of 6 weeks) but self-limited (214). The histopathology of the small intestine in patients with *Cyclospora*-associated diarrhea shows acute and chronic inflammation, surface epithelial disarray, and varying degrees of villous atrophy and crypt hyperplasia (215). *Cyclospora* infection in persons with AIDS is associated with prolonged or relapsing diarrhea and weight loss as great as 10% (216,217). Diffuse, cramping abdominal pain accompanies the diarrhea in more than half of patients and fever in one-third (217). *Cyclospora* outbreaks have been associated with contaminated drinking water and imported raspberries (218,219).

Diagnosis

Modified Kinyoun stain is used to identify *Cyclospora* oocysts in a concentrated fresh stool sample; oocysts appear as 8 to 9 μm, acid-fast, granular spheres.

Treatment

Trimethoprim-sulfamethoxazole (160 mg of trimethoprim and 800 mg of sulfamethoxazole twice daily) appears to be effective therapy for *Cyclospora* infection (217,220) (Table 29.4).

Giardia lamblia *And* Entamoeba histolytica

In immunosuppressed HIV-1-infected patients, *Giardia lamblia* does not cause more frequent or severe infection than in seronegative persons and responds appropriately to antimicrobial therapy with metronidazole (221). In addition, neither colitis nor liver abscess caused by *Entamoeba histolytica* infection appears to be more frequent or more severe in HIV-1-infected patients. The *Entamoeba* species usually detected in such patients is *E. dispar,* a nonpathogenic species (222).

Viral Infections

Cytomegalovirus

Description

See "CMV Esophagitis."

Clinical Features

The clinical manifestations of CMV disease in the GI tract include esophagitis (91), gastritis (223), small intestinal enteritis (223), and less frequently, acalculous cholecystitis (224), papillary stenosis (225,226), sclerosing cholangitis (226), pancreatitis (227), and appendicitis (228). Colitis appears to be the most common enteric manifestation of enteric CMV disease (90,229); among AIDS patients with colitis or enteritis, CMV has been identified in biopsies in 45% of patients (90). CMV colitis is characterized by diarrhea, fever, and weight loss. Abdominal pain and hematochezia are also frequently present and help distinguish CMV colitis from the protozoal diarrheal illnesses described above. The colon appears to be particularly susceptible to progression to ischemic necrosis and perforation during CMV infection (230). Regardless of whether diarrhea is present, CMV-associated disease of the biliary tract (usually without icterus or pruritus) should be included in the differential diagnosis of abdominal pain, nausea, and vomiting in patients with AIDS. Endoscopic findings that suggest CMV-induced disease range from localized hyperemia to hemorrhagic erythema to superficial or deep ulceration (Fig. 29.6). The pathogenesis of CMV-induced mucosal inflammation is discussed above (see "CMV Esophagitis").

Diagnosis

CMV should be suspected when endoscopic or colonoscopic visualization show discrete, often hemorrhagic, erosions or ulcerations with normal intervening mucosa in an HIV-1-infected patient. Colitis may be patchy in approximately 40% of cases and involve only the right colon or cecum in 18% (231), underscoring the importance of colonoscopy in the diagnostic evaluation of colitis in an HIV-1-infected patient. The diagnosis of CMV GI disease is established by the histopathologic identification of large (cytomegalic) mononuclear, endothelial or epithelial cells containing intranuclear and/or cytoplasmic inclusions with

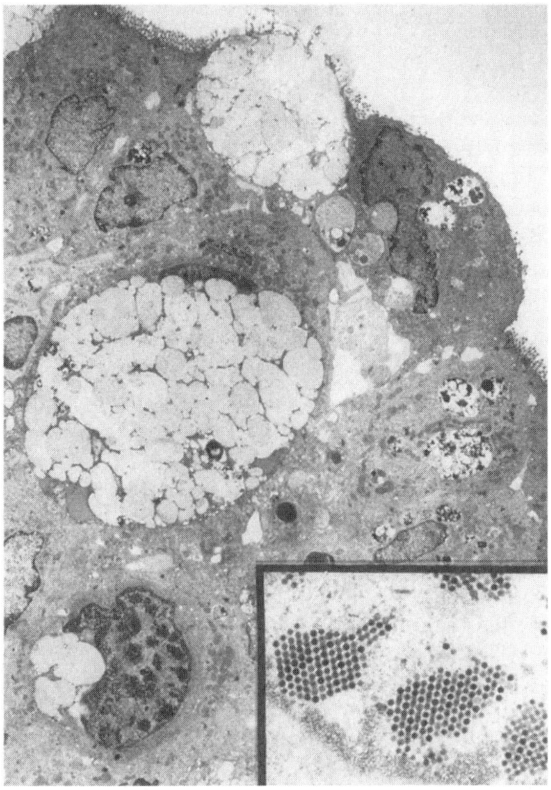

FIGURE 29.6. Transmission electron micrograph of colonic epithelium from an HIV-1-infected person with adenovirus colitis. The degenerating goblet cells show microvillous atrophy and a condensed nucleus containing a crystalline array of hexagonal nucleoids (*insert*) typical of adenovirus. ×5,390; *insert* ×33,600. (Courtesy of J. M. Orenstein.)

surrounding inflammation (Fig. 29.1B) (90,232) and confirmed by immunocytochemical staining, *in situ* hybridization or DNA amplification, as discussed above (see "CMV Esophagitis").

Treatment

The treatment is similar to that of CMV esophagitis.

Herpes Simplex Virus

Description

See "Herpes Simplex Virus Esophagitis."

Clinical Features

In contrast to the widespread GI involvement by CMV, GI HSV disease is confined to the perianal region, rectum, and esophagus. The perianal lesions are typically chronic cutaneous ulcers that cause localized pain but not diarrhea (124). Involvement of the rectum (proctitis) is often associated with perianal disease. Proctitis manifests as severe anorectal pain, tenesmus, constipation, inguinal lymphadenopathy, and less often, difficulty with urination and sacral paresthesias. Such symptoms may also be associated with proctitis in seronegative homosexual men (233). Diarrhea is not associated with typical proctitis, although the mucopurulent discharge may be misinterpreted as diarrhea. Proctocolitis, which occurs when the proctitis extends proximally into the distal sigmoid colon, can cause mild diarrhea associated with hematochezia, but the predominant symptoms are generally those of the proctitis. Overall, HSV proctocolitis is an infrequent cause of diarrhea in HIV-1-infected persons (90).

Diagnosis

Anoscopy and sigmoidoscopy are required to diagnose HSV proctitis and proctocolitis, respectively. Typical lesions begin as small vesicles and progress to erosions that often coalesce into diffuse ulcers. Diagnosis is predicated on the cytologic identification of intranuclear (Cowdry type A) inclusions in cells within the lesion and is confirmed by virus isolation.

Treatment

See "Herpes Simplex Virus Esophagitis."

Adenovirus

In HIV-1-infected patients, adenovirus has been isolated from various body sites and may induce hepatic necrosis (234,235), but intestinal involvement is rare. In the United States, adenovirus excretion is equally common in HIV-1-infected patients with and without diarrhea (146,236). In contrast, 23% of Australian HIV-1-infected patients with diarrhea reportedly excrete adenovirus, compared with 5.4% without diarrhea (237). Adenovirus has been identified with transmission electron microscopy and culture in inflamed colonic tissue of AIDS patients with chronic, watery, nonbloody, nonmucoid diarrhea (238,239). Weight loss was also a prominent symptom. Endoscopically, the colonic mucosa showed areas of discrete, often raised, erythematous lesions that were several millimeters in diameter. Light microscopy showed chronic inflammation surrounding epithelial cells containing large, amphophilic intranuclear, but not cytoplasmic, inclusions. Adenovirus appeared to infect only epithelial cells, particularly goblet cells, sparing lamina propria cells, which are frequent targets of CMV. At the ultrastructural level, adenovirus was associated with degeneration, death, and focal necrosis of infected epithelial cells, some of which had been extruded into the lumen (Fig. 29.6). Although adenovirus can cause pathogenic changes in the colonic mucosa, a causal relationship between adenovirus and diarrhea has not been established.

Astrovirus, Picobirnavirus, and Rotavirus

Prospective evaluation of chronic diarrhea in HIV-1-infected persons indicated an association between the presence of astrovirus and picobirnavirus and diarrhea in HIV-1-infected persons (240), but further epidemiologic and clinical studies are needed to define the role of these viruses in HIV-1 disease. Rotavirus is not associated with diarrhea in HIV-1-infected patients in the United States (90,146, 240,241) or Africa (Zaire) (242,243) but is the predominant virus detected in the stools of Australian HIV-1-infected homosexual men with diarrhea (244) and is present in the stool in approximately 14% of HIV-1-infected adults in Germany (245). These findings suggest geographic variation in the prevalence of rotavirus-associated diarrhea in HIV-1-infected persons, but additional studies are needed.

Bacterial Infections

Salmonella *Species,* Shigella flexneri, *and* Campylobacter jejuni

The diarrheal illnesses caused by *Salmonella* species (*Salmonella typhimurium* and less frequently, *Salmonella enteritidis*) (246–253), *Shigella flexneri* (253–257), and *Campylobacter jejuni* (258,259) are clinically similar. In HIV-1-infected persons, these bacteria cause recurrent or chronic diarrhea commonly associated with fever and abdominal cramps. During symptomatic infection, the stool often contains fecal leukocytes and grossly visible or microscopic blood. Compared with salmonellosis, shigellosis, and *C. jejuni* infection in seronegative people, these bacterial infections in AIDS patients occur substantially more frequently, cause a more prolonged or recurrent illness, and are more frequently associated with bacteremia and antibiotic resistance.

Diagnosis

These bacterial pathogens are diagnosed by culture of the stool.

Treatment

Appropriate antimicrobial therapy for these organisms is listed in Table 29.4. Because recurrence is common and antimicrobial resistance may develop, repeated cultures of stool and blood (when bacteremia is present) are required to monitor the response to antimicrobial therapy (Table 29.7).

Mycobacterium avium *Complex*

Description

MAC comprises two acid-fast, obligate, intracellular bacteria: *M. avium* and *Mycobacterium intracellulare.* Exposure is common, because the organisms are ubiquitous in the environment. In immunocompetent hosts, MAC is not pathogenic, but immunosuppressed HIV-1-infected persons (CD4+ lymphocyte count of less than 100 cells/mm^3) are highly susceptible to infection. Macrophages are an important reservoir for the bacteria, and during HIV-1 infection, macrophages appear able to phagocytose but not kill MAC. The organism up-regulates macrophage HIV-1 production in dual infected cells (260) and alters macrophage function (261). The GI tract is the likely portal of entry for MAC.

Clinical Features

MAC is the most common cause of systemic bacterial infection in HIV-1-infected persons in the United States. MAC is much less common in Africa and Haiti. End-organ involvement and bacteremia usually do not occur, however, until the number of CD4+ T cells declines to less than 100 cells/mm^3. Substantial GI tract disease, which is usually a manifestation of disseminated infection, may be associated with diarrhea, abdominal pain, malabsorption, weight loss, and fever, with or without night sweats (262,263). Concomitant hepatomegaly and splenomegaly due to MAC infection are often present. Evidence of numerous mycobacteria on histologic sections of biopsy or autopsy specimens suggests a causative or contributory role for MAC in the GI manifestations. Endoscopic abnormalities are nonspecific and include erythema, friability, erosions, and fine white nodules. Occasionally, an inflammatory mass, which can be mistaken for a tumor, is the major GI manifestation. The small intestine is reported to be involved more often than the colon (262), but this may reflect easier endoscopic access. Histologic examination shows diffuse infiltration of the lamina propria by macrophages filled with bacilli (Fig. 29.7). Granulomas are usually absent or poorly developed.

Diagnosis

The diagnosis of MAC is based on the identification of typical acid-fast organisms in stool or GI biopsy specimens (fixed and touch preparations) (262,263). Culture of GI tissue may increase the positivity rate compared with acid-fast staining alone (264). Isolation and speciation is achieved by culture of organisms from stool and biopsy specimens. Although the incidence of *M. tuberculosis* pulmonary infections has increased among HIV-1-infected persons, intestinal involvement is uncommon.

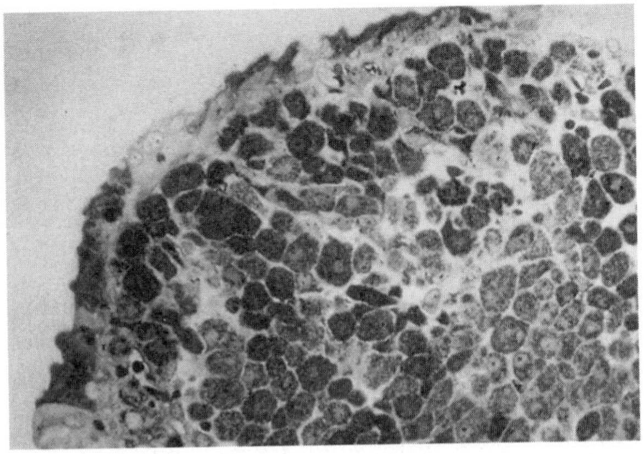

FIGURE 29.7. Light micrograph of colonic mucosa infected with *Mycobacterium avium* complex from a man with HIV-1 infection. Numerous lamina propria macrophages are filled with mycobacteria. Methylene blue–azure II, basic fuchsin stain; ×100. (Courtesy of J. M. Orenstein.)

Treatment

Although initial trials of antituberculosis agents proved disappointing, improved results with newer multidrug regimens provide reason for cautious optimism in treating MAC (265–267). Combination regimens have produced more sustained benefit, but such regimens are expensive, have adverse effects, and are often difficult to tolerate. The current recommended three-drug therapy is two antimycobacterial agents, including a macrolide/azole agent, and a third agent, such as ethambutol (268). For prophylaxis, when the CD4+ lymphocyte count falls to less than 50 cells/mm^3, clarithromycin or azithromycin are used hemoprophylaxis therapy. These agents are effective for reducing the development of MAC bacteremia and can reduce the frequency of disseminated MAC by 50% (269,270). Among patients on HAART who respond with an increase in the number of CD4+ lymphocytes to greater than 100 cells/mm^3 for more than 3 to 6 months with sustained suppression of HIV-1 plasma RNA for the same period, it is reasonable to discontinue prophylaxis therapy.

Clostridium difficile

C. difficile, a gram-positive bacterium, is one of the most important causes of nosocomial intestinal infection. *C. difficile* infection may be more common but not more severe in HIV-1-infected persons than in seronegative persons (270,271). Nevertheless, because of the frequent use of antimicrobial agents and frequent hospitalizations, HIV-1-infected patients with diarrhea should be evaluated for infection with *C. difficile* with stool culture and toxin assay.

Fungal Infection

Histoplasma capsulatum

Description

H. capsulatum is a dimorphic fungus that exists in two forms: (a) a mycelial form consisting of septate branching hyphae that contain infectious spores, which are readily airborne and transmit infection, and (b) a yeast form present in tissue (macrophages). The organism is endemic in the central region of the United States and in some tropical, subtropical, and temperate zone areas, where bird excrement provides microfoci of infection.

Clinical Features

Disseminated *H. capsulatum* is as an important opportunistic infection in HIV-1-infected persons who reside in endemic areas (272,273). GI involvement generally reflects disseminated disease, which is due primarily to reactivation of quiescent infection. Among persons with disseminated *H. capsulatum,* GI involvement has been detected in approximately 70% of cases by evaluation of biopsy specimens, but GI symptoms are present in only about 10% of patients (274). Symptoms include diarrhea, weight loss, fever, and abdominal pain. Similar to the infection with MAC, whether *H. capsulatum* itself causes these symptoms has not been proven. Most patients with GI manifestations of *H. capsulatum* have colonic involvement. Colonoscopy in such patients may show inflammation, ulcerations, or fungating mass lesions.

Diagnosis

The histologic examination of Giemsa-stained sections shows small yeastlike cells within macrophages or histiocytes. When infection is intense, the organism is not difficult to identify. However, the diagnosis of histoplasmosis is established by culture.

Treatment

Amphotericin B is the drug of choice for disseminated histoplasmosis (Table 29.4). The recommended initial course of therapy in HIV-1-infected persons is amphotericin B, 0.5 to 0.6 mg/kg intravenously daily for 4 to 8 weeks or longer, depending on the clinical response (275). Long-term therapy with amphotericin B (50 to 80 mg intravenously every 2 weeks) is also highly effective in suppressing relapses after initial treatment (273).

EFFECT OF HIGHLY ACTIVE ANTIRETROVIRAL THERAPY ON GI INFECTIONS

HAART

HAART combines reverse transcriptase inhibitor (RTI) and protease inhibitor (PI) drugs into a powerful and highly effective antiviral therapy. RTIs include nucleoside analogues, such as zidovudine, and nonnucleoside analogues, which inhibit the ability of HIV RNA to encode viral DNA. PIs block the cleavage of HIV-1 GagPol polyprotein precursor into structural core proteins and enzymes (reverse transcriptase, integrase, and protease), causing the production of abnormal viral proteins and non-infectious virions. Current HAART regimens typically include three or more agents, usually two RTI nucleoside analogues and one PI, to diminish or ablate viral replication, prevent the development of resistance, enhance recovery of immunologic competence, and improve clinical status (276–279).

Impact on Mortality

HAART has dramatically reduced the rate of death in patients with HIV-1. Among U.S. patients with advanced HIV-1 disease (CD4+ T-cells count less than 100 cells mm^3), mortality declined between 1995 and 1997 from 29.4 to 8.8 per 100 person-years (280). Concomitantly, the incidence of the three most common HIV-1-associated opportunistic infections (*Pneumocystis carinii* pneumonia, MAC disease, and CMV retinitis) declined more than 75% (Fig. 29.7) in the United States and Europe in response to

HAART (281–284). This decrease has been accompanied by decreased rates of GI infections as well, including esophageal candidiasis and enteric infections with MAC, CMV, cryptosporidia, and HSV.

The dramatic effects of HAART on mortality and HIV-1-related infections are most likely due to the inhibition of HIV-1 replication and the recovery of immune function, because most antiretroviral agents have little activity against other viruses or pathogens. Other than the activity of the PI amprenavir against *G. lamblia* (276) and adefovir dipivoxil against DNA viruses (HSV, CMV, and hepatitis B virus), most other antiretroviral agents have shown little activity against viral, bacterial, protozoal, or fungal pathogens. Thus, recovery from immune dysfunction underlies the clinical benefit that accompanies antiretroviral therapy-induced viral suppression. Because functional immunologic recovery takes several months, rates of HIV-1-related infections decline most prominently after 2 months of antiretroviral therapy (285). Thus, prophylactic therapy against many opportunistic infections may be discontinued in patients on HAART whose CD4+ lymphocytes have increased to 200 cells/mm^3 (or 14% of total lymphocytes) for more than 12 weeks (285–290).

Effect of HAART on the Natural History of GI Infections

HAART has three effects on the natural history of HIV-1-associated infections, including enteric infections. First, effective control of HIV-1 results in a decreased incidence of secondary infections and decreased rates of reactivation of latent infections. Second, an indirect benefit of the decreased rates of these infections is the discontinuation of chronic prophylactic antimicrobials, leading to fewer *C. difficile* infections (291,292) and drug reactions. A third consequence of HAART is the resolution of ongoing infections, likely due to repopulation of peripheral T cells. Recent reports indicate that as the viral load declines in the intestinal mucosa, CD4+ lymphocytes repopulate the mucosa (293,294); this repopulation occurs more rapidly in the intestinal mucosa than in the blood (294).

Early reports indicated that *Cryptosporidium* infection could improve clinically and microbiologically with zidovudine therapy (295,296). In a recent case–control study, antiretroviral therapy was associated with significant, but not absolute, protection against infection with *Cryptosporidium* (297). In an HIV-1-infected patient evaluated over time, persistent *C. parvum* infection resolved with HAART in association with decreases in viral RNA and dramatic and sustained increases in CD4+ lymphocyte cell number in blood and intestinal mucosa (298). In an open randomized trial in patients with previously diagnosed infections and persistent diarrhea, symptoms resolved and pathogens were undetectable in stools from three of six patients with microsporidiosis (*E. bieneusi*) and two patients with concomitant *Cryptosporidium* (299) after addition of the PI indinavir (298). Similarly, among nine patients with chronic diarrhea associated with microsporidiosis, cryptosporidiosis, or both (eight of whom had failed anti-parasitic therapy), HAART-induced resolution of symptoms, weight gain, parasitologic cure in most, and histologic improvement after 6 weeks of therapy (300). However, diarrhea recurred in four patients when they failed to respond to antiretroviral therapy.

Effect of HAART on AIDS Enteropathy

As discussed above, the number of HIV-1-infected persons with diarrheal illness in whom a pathogen cannot be detected has declined substantially. Nevertheless, some HIV-1-infected patients still have diarrhea without an identifiable pathogen. Consequently, a recent report that HAART induced sustained clinical improvement in eight AIDS patients with chronic diarrhea of unknown etiology suggests that HAART may also benefit patients with enteropathy syndrome (299).

Complications of HAART

A spectrum of toxicities are associated with antiretroviral and support drugs (301) (Table 29.8). In general, GI symptoms, such as nausea, vomiting, abdominal pain, and diarrhea, occur early in the course of therapy and may abate over time. GI toxicity significantly limits the initial tolerance to PIs, often requiring dose titration and sequential addition of other medications, such as RTI nucleoside analogues. Hepatic toxicity is more often associated with long-term therapy and is typically mild, although severe hepatic toxicity, particularly with the PI ritonavir, may require discontinuation of the medication (302). Pancreatitis is a more specific complication of individual drugs. Toxic reactions ascribed to each drug may be confounded by concomitant administration of two or more drugs. Increased rates of adverse events, such as pancreatitis or hepatic toxicity, may result from simultaneous administration of medications with overlapping toxicities. Moreover, differentiating the symptoms of drug toxicities from those of opportunistic infections may require careful evaluation of the timing of events and presence of comorbid findings.

HAART toxicities, which may occur more frequently in patients with advanced disease (CD4+ lymphocyte count of less than 200 cells/mm^3), may limit use of the antiretroviral drugs. Rates of specific intestinal complications for each agent are summarized in Table 29.8. In patients taking RTI nucleoside analogues, GI symptoms, including nausea, vomiting, abdominal pain, and diarrhea, occur in more than one-fourth of patients. The inhibition of cellular DNA polymerases with long-term therapy may result in mitochondrial toxicity and associated myopathic, neuropathic, hepatic, pancreatic, and hematologic complications (302–304). Among persons on RTI nonnucleoside analogues, GI and hepatic

TABLE 29.8. GI COMPLICATIONS OF ANTIRETROVIRAL THERAPY AND POTENTIAL INTERACTIONS WITH OTHER MEDICATIONS USED IN GI MEDICINE

Type of Medication	Medication	Trade Name	Primary GI Toxicity[a]	GI-associated Drug Interactions
Antiretroviral				
• Nucleoside analogue RTI (non-RTI)	Zidovudine (azidothymidine, ZDV)	Retrovir	Anorexia; nausea (4–26%); vomiting (3–8%) (rare hepatitis, steatosis, lactic acidosis)	Activity may be inhibited by ribavirin
	Didanosine (ddl)	Videx	Pancreatitis (4–8%); diarrhea (16%); ↑ ALT:AST (6–20%)	Potential increased rate of pancreatitis with pentamidine, azathioprine); buffers associated with ↓ absorption of itraconazole, ketoconazole, dapsone; tetracycline, ciprofloxacin; ddl levels ↑ with ranitidine, ganciclovir
	Zalcitabine (ddC)	HIVID	Stomatitis (self-limited) (2–17%); pancreatitis (0.5–9%)	Few; possible ↑ neuropathy with metronidazole, disulfuram
	Stavudine (d4T)	Zerit	Diarrhea (33%), nausea/vomiting (26%), abdominal pain (23%); ↑ ALT:AST (65%); significant GI symptoms and hepatic abnormalities in 4–10%	Few; possible ↑ neuropathy with ethanol; ribavirin may increase activity (in vitro data)
	Lamivudine (3TC)	Epivir	Limited; mild and transient diarrhea, nausea, abdominal pain	Few
	Abacavir (ABC)	Ziagen	Nausea (45%), diarrhea (25%), vomiting (15%), and abdominal pain (15%) may decrease over weeks of therapy; hypersensitivity reaction with fever ± rash, malaise, nausea, vomiting, ↑ ALT:AST in 2–5% within 1 mo	None reported
• Nucleotide analogue RTI	Adefovir dipivoxil	(Preveon)	Mild nausea and diarrhea, occassional vomiting (1–8%); ↑ ALT:AST (4%); (renal toxicity 38%)	None reported
	ZDV-3TC	Combivir	As above	
• Non–nucleoside RTI (NNRTI)	Nevirapine (NVP)	Viramune	Nausea; ↑ ALT:AST (1%); isolated ↑ GGT common; (rash most common)	
	Delavirdine (DLV)	Rescriptor	Nausea (7%); diarrhea (4%); ↑ ALT:AST (≤5%); (rash most common; usually transient)	Level ↓ with rifampin, rifabutin (P-450 system) and antacids (↑ gastric pH); level ↑ with clarithromycin, rifabutin, cisapride
	Efavirenz (EFV)	Sustiva	(Transient rash and CNS symptoms of headache, dizziness, impaired concentration)	Avoid cisapride; should not be taken within 2 hr of antacids; not recommended with clarithromycin; (interacts with other PIs)

(continued)

TABLE 29.8. *(continued)*

Type of Medication	Medication	Trade Name	Primary GI Toxicity[a]	GI-associated Drug Interactions
• Protease inhibitors (PIs)[b]	Saquinavir (SQC); saquinavir-SGC (soft-gel capsule)	Invirase; Fortovase	Nausea, diarrhea, abdominal pain, dyspepsia (5–10%)	Cisapride contraindicated; SQV level ↑ with ketoconazole, clarithromycin; SQV level ↓ with rifampin, rifabutin; clarithromycin level ↑ with SQV; (interacts with other PIs)
	Ritonavir (RTV)	Norvir	Nausea, diarrhea, vomiting, anorexia, abdominal pain (20–40%), particularly in first few weeks of therapy; taste perversion (10%); increased triglycerides (60%, but >1,500 mg/dL in 2–8%); ↑ ALT:AST (10–15%), particularly with NRTI	Cisapride contraindicated; caution with dronabinol, ondansetron, cimetidine, promethazine, corticosteroids; RTV level ↑ with ketoconazole, itraconazole; RTV level ↓ with rifampin; clarithromycin, erythromycin, rifampin, rifabutin levels increased with RTV; (interacts with other PIs)
	Indinavir (IDV)	Crixivan	Nausea, vomiting, diarrhea, abdominal pain (4–15%); increased indirect bilirubin (10%); (nephrolithiasis 5–10%)	Cisapride contraindicated; IDV level ↓ with rifabutin; IDV level ↑ with ketoconazole; rifabutin level ↑ with IDV; (interacts with other PIs)
	Nelfinavir (NLF)	Viracept	Diarrhea (usually mild) (2–19%)	Cisapride and rifabutin contraindicated; NLF levels ↓ with rifampin; rifabutin levels ↑ with NLF; (interacts with other PIs)
	Amprenavir	Agenerase	Diarrhea, nausea, vomiting (7–33%); (rash, 18%)	Cisapride and rifampin contraindicated; amprenavir levels ↓ with rifabutin; rifabutin levels ↑ with amprenavir; (interacts with other PIs)
	ABT 378 (lopinavir-ritonavir)	Kaletra	Diarrhea (10–20%); ↑ ALT:AST (8%)	Similar to other PIs
• Other	Interleukin 2	Proleukin	Diarrhea, abdominal pain, stomatitis (7%); nausea; vomiting; isolated ↑ bilirubin (8%); ↑ ALT:AST; acalculous cholecystitis; constitutional flulike symptoms (fever, chills, muscle/joint pain) (45%)	
	Hydroxyurea	Hydrea	Nausea (12%); ↑ ALT:AST (2%); stomatitis (8%); diarrhea; occassional anorexia, vomiting, diarrhea, constipation (myelosuppression; rash)	
• Alternative	Vitamin C			
	Allicin (garlic extract)			
	Malaleuca (Tea tree extract)			
	N-acetylcysteine (mucomyst)			

[a]Rates may vary among studies.
[b]As with other inhibitors of cytochrome P-50 system, specifically CYP 3A4, protease inhibitors should not be given with cisapride (Propulsid), astemizole (Hismanal), terfenadine (Seldane), midazolam (Versed), or triazolam (Halcion), or ergot derivatives.
RTI, reverse transcriptase inhibitors; ALT:AST, alanine/aspartate transaminase elevation >2.5–5-fold above normal values; GGT, γ-glutamyl transpeptidase.
Source: Adapted from Janoff EN, Smith PD. Emerging concepts in gastrointestinal aspects of HIV-pathogenesis and management. *Gastroenterology* 2001:120:607–621, with permission.

toxicities are not common. Mild rashes are the predominant side effect. Drug interactions with these agents are related primarily to their effects as inducers of and substrates for the cytochrome P-450 system. The most frequent dose-limiting toxicities with PIs are diarrhea, nausea, and abdominal discomfort. Hepatic toxicity is most often associated with ritonavir. The presence of chronic hepatitis B or hepatitis C may increase the rate but not necessarily the severity of hepatic effects (302); these infections should not limit the initiation of HAART.

Metabolic complications, particularly with any PI-containing regimen, and, less often with RTI nucleoside analogues, include glucose intolerance, elevations in triglyceride and cholesterol levels, and lipodystrophy syndrome. Patients with this latter syndrome may show one or more of the following: increased abdominal fat, loss of peripheral subcutaneous fat of the face, arms, legs, and buttocks, and the presence of a "buffalo hump." Women on therapy may experience breast enlargement. Rates of observed fat redistribution are 17% to 68% with PIs and 16% with dual RTI nucleoside analogues (299,303,306). Mitochondrial dysfunction has been invoked as one potential unifying mechanism underlying these syndromes in patients on PI-containing combination therapy (303,305). The first two conditions may be treated with standard medical management, but whether discontinuation of medications will reverse the potentially disfiguring effects of the lipodystrophy syndrome is currently unclear.

Management of HAART toxicity is complicated by the difficulty of identifying the causative agent in a multidrug regimen. Many of the toxic effects of antiretroviral medications are worse early in the course of treatment and are dose dependent; consequently, lowering the dose in this period may allow the continuation of therapy. However, optimal antiretroviral activity is usually dose dependent, particularly with PIs. Because the development of HIV-1 resistance may occur, clinical and virologic status should be monitored. Changing antiretroviral agents may be preferable to lowering doses. Evaluating the overlapping toxicities of different medications and their effects on drug metabolism may allow successful continuation of the most critical agents. Severe or prolonged complications require discontinuation of individual agents, as does the development of hypersensitivity reactions with abacavir. For GI side effects, antidiarrheal agents, such as loperamide or diphenoxylate atropine, may be useful for drug-related diarrhea, as may antiemetics for vomiting. Taking medications with or after eating, when appropriate, may limit nausea. Histamine receptor blockers and antacids, although commonly prescribed, may affect absorption of some drugs and usually do not alter symptoms.

Drug Interactions

Most of the drug interactions associated with PIs are related to their high affinity for, and thus inhibition of, several P-450 isoenzymes. Cisapride has potential life-threatening cardiotoxic effects in the presence of PIs, azole antifungals, and macrolides due to the ability of these agents to inhibit the hepatic metabolism of cisapride. Clinically significant interactions of PIs with rifampin/rifabutin, macrolides (erythromycin, clarithromycin, and azithromycin) and azole antifungals (ketoconazole, fluconazole, and itraconazole) are highlighted in Table 29.8 (and reviewed in reference 307). The chelating effects of didanosine, antacids, iron and calcium products, and sucralfate limit the absorption and levels of quinolone antibiotics, which are commonly used for the treatment of bacterial diarrhea.

In summary, the clinical care of HIV-1-infected patients has improved dramatically over the last decade due to a greater understanding of the pathogenesis of HIV-1 infection, more rapid diagnosis of HIV-1 disease and the associated GI infections, and the availability of potent antimicrobial and antiretroviral agents. Each advance has brought hope as well as new challenges for physicians caring for HIV-1-infected patients with GI infections.

ACKNOWLEDGMENT

This work was supported by National Institutes of Health grants and contract DK-47322, AI-41530, DE-72621, AI-39445, HD-41361 and the Research Service of the Department of Veterans Affairs.

REFERENCES

1. Gao F, Bailes E, Robertson DL, et al. Origin of HIV-1 in the chimpanzee Pan troglodytes. *Nature* 1999;397:436–441.
2. UNAIDS and WHO. AIDS epidemic update—December, 2001. Geneva: UNAIDS/WHO.
3. Royce RA, Sena A, Cates W Jr, et al. Sexual transmission of HIV. *N Engl J Med* 1997;336:1072–1078.
4. Smith PD, Wahl SM. Immunobiology of mucosal HIV-1 infection. In: Ogra PH, Mestecky J, Lamm ME, et al., eds. *Mucosal immunology,* second edition. San Diego: Academic Press, 1999: 977–989.
5. Newell M-L. Mechanisms and timing of mother-to-child transmission of HIV-1. *AIDS* 1998;12:831–837.
6. Maayan S, Soskoine V, Engelhard D, et al. Sexual behavior of homosexual and bisexual men attending an HIV testing clinic in Jerusalem. *Isr J Psychiatry Rel Sci* 1993;30:150–154.
7. Schwarcz SK, Kellogg TA, Kohn RP, et al. Temporal trends in human immunodeficiency virus seroprevalence and sexual behavior at the San Francisco municipal sexually transmitted disease clinic. *Am J Epidemiol* 1995;142:314–322.
8. Schacker T, Collier AC, Hughes J, et al. Clinical and epidemiologic features of primary HIV infection. *Ann Intern Med* 1996; 125:257–264.
9. Jacquez JA, Koopman SJ, Simon CP, et al. Role of the primary infection in epidemics of HIV infection in gay cohorts. *J Acquired Immune Defic Syndrome* 1994;7:1169–1184.
10. Kinloch-de Loes S, Hirschel BJ, Hoen B, et al. A controlled trial of zidovudine in primary human immunodeficiency virus infection. *N Engl J Med* 1995;333:408–413.

11. Daar ES, Moudgil T, Meyer RD, et al. Transient high levels of viremia in patients with primary human immunodeficiency virus type 1 infection. *N Engl J Med* 1991;324:961–964.
12. Vernazza PL, Eron JJ, Cohen MS, et al. Detection and biologic characterization of infectious HIV-1 in semen of seropositive men. *AIDS* 1994;8:1325–1329.
13. Mellors J, Rinaldo CR Jr, Gupta P, et al. Prognosis in HIV-1 infection predicted by the quantity of virus in plasma. *Science* 1996;272:1167–1170.
14. Anderson DJ, O'Brien TR, Politch JA, et al. Effects of disease stage and zidovudine therapy on the detection of human immunodeficiency virus type 1 in semen. *JAMA* 1992;267:2769–2774.
15. Nelson KE, Rungruengthanakit K, Margolick J, et al. High rates of transmission of subtype E human immunodeficiency virus type 1 among heterosexual couples in northern Thailand: role of sexually transmitted diseases and immune compromise. *J Infect Dis* 1999;180:337–343.
16. Quinn TC, Wawer MJ, Sewankambo N, et al. Viral load and heterosexual transmission of human immunodeficiency virus type 1. *N Engl J Med* 2000;342:921–929.
17. Fideli US, Allen SA, Musonda R, et al. Virologic and immunologic determinants of heterosexual transmission of human immunodeficiency virus type 1 (HIV-1) in Africa. *AIDS Res Hum Retrovirus* 2001;17:901–910.
18. Clemetson DB, Moss GB, Willerford DM. Detection of HIV DNA in cervical and vaginal secretions: prevalence and correlates among women in Nairobi, Kenya. *JAMA* 1993;269: 2860–2864.
19. Cohen MS, Hoffman IF, Royce RA, et al. Reduction of concentration of HIV-1 in semen after treatment of urethritis: implications for prevention of sexual transmission of HIV-1. *Lancet* 1997;349:1868–1873.
20. Fleming DT, Wasserheit JN. From epidemiologic synergy to public health policy and practice: the contribution of other sexually transmitted diseases to sexual transmission of HIV infection. *Sex Transm Infect* 1999;75:3–17.
21. Wahl SM, Greenwell-Wild T, Peng G, et al. Mycobacterium avium complex augments macrophage HIV-1 production and increases CCR5 expression. *Proc Natl Acad Sci U S A* 1998;5: 12574–12579.
22. Huang Y, Paxton WA, Wolinsky SM, et al. The role of a mutant CCR5 allele in HIV-1 transmission and disease progression. *Nature Med* 1996;2:1240–1243.
23. Dean M, Carrington M, Winkler C, et al. Genetic restriction of HIV-1 infection and progression to AIDS by a deletion allele of the CKR5 structural gene. *Science* 1996;273:1856–1862.
24. Liu R, Paxton WA, Choe S, et al. Homozygous defect in HIV-1 coreceptor accounts for resistance of some multiply-exposed individuals to HIV-1 infection. *Cell* 1996;86:367–377.
25. Samson M, Libert F, Doranz BJ, et al. Resistance to HIV-1 infection in Caucasian individuals bearing mutant alleles of the CCR-5 chemokine receptor gene. *Nature* 1996;382:722–725.
26. Vittinghoff E, Scheer S, O'Malley P, et al. Combination antiretroviral therapy and recent declines in AIDS incidence and mortality. *J Infect Dis* 1999;179:717–720.
27. Downs AM, De Vincenzi I. European Study Group in Heterosexual Transmission of HIV. Probability of heterosexual transmission of HIV: relationship to the number of unprotected sexual contacts. *J Acquir Immune Defic Syndrome Hum Retrovirol* 1996;11:388–395.
28. Halperin DT, Bailey RC. Male circumcision and HIV infection: 10 years and counting. *Lancet* 1999;354:1813–1815.
29. Amerongen HM, Weltzin R, Farnet CM, et al. Transepithelial transport of HIV-1 by intestinal M cells: a mechanism for transmission of AIDS. *J Acquired Immune Defic Syndrome* 1991;4: 760–765.
30. Baba TW, Trichel AM, An L, et al. Infection and AIDS in adults macaques after nontraumatic oral exposure to cell-free SIV. *Science* 1996;272:1486–1489.
31. Stahl-Hennig C, Steinman RM, Tenner-Racz K, et al. Rapid infection of oral mucosal-associated lymphoid tissue with simian immunodeficiency virus. *Science* 1999;285:1261–1265.
32. O'Leary AD, Sweeney EC. Lymphoglandular complexes of the colon: structure and distribution. *Histopathology* 1986;10: 267–283.
33. Maric I, Holt PG, Perdue MH, et al. Class II MHC antigen (Ia)-bearing dendritic cells in the epithelium of the rat intestine. *J Immunol* 1996;156:1408–1414.
34. Kelsall BL, Strober W. Distinct populations of dendritic cells are present in the subepithelial dome and T cell regions of the murine Peyer's patch. *J Exp Med* 1996;183:237–247.
35. Hussain LA, Lehner T. Comparative investigation of Langerhans' cells and potential receptors for HIV in oral, genitourinary and rectal epithelia. *Immunology* 1995;85:475–484.
36. Frankel SS, Wenig BM, Burke AP, et al. Replication of HIV-1 in dendritic cell-derived syncytia at the mucosal surface of the adenoid. *Science* 1996;272:115–117.
37. Pavli L, Hume D, Van de Pol E, et al. Dendritic cells, the major antigen-presenting cells of the human colonic lamina propria.*Clin Exp Immunol* 1993;78:132–141.
38. Geijtenbeek TBH, Kwon DS, Torensma R, et al. DC-SIGN, a dendritic cell-specific HIV-1-binding protein that enhances trans-infection of T cells. *Cell* 2000;100:587–597.
39. Cameron PU, Freudenthal PS, Barker JM, et al. Dendritic cells exposed to human immunodeficiency virus type-1 transmit a vigorous cytopathic infection to CD4+ T cells. *Science* 1992; 257:383–387.
40. Bomsel M. Transcytosis of infectious human immunodeficiency virus across a tight human epithelial cell line barrier. *Nature Med* 1997;3:42–47.
41. Meng G, Wei X, Wu X, et al. Primary intestinal epithelial cells transfer CCR5 R5 HIV-1 to CCR5+ cells. *Nature Med* 2002;8: 150–156.
42. Fantini J, Cook DG, Nathanson N, et al. Infection of colonic epithelial cell lines by type 1 human immunodeficiency virus is associated with cell surface expression of galactosylceramide, a potential alternative gp120 receptor. *Proc Natl Acad Sci U S A* 1993;90:2700–2704.
43. Li L, Meng G, Graham MF, et al. Intestinal macrophages display reduced permissiveness to human immunodeficiency virus 1 and decreased surface CCR5. *Gastroenterology* 1999;116:1043–1053.
44. Meng G, Sellers MT, Mosteller-Barnum M, et al. Lamina propria lymphocytes, not macrophages, express CCR5 and CXCR4 and are the likely target cell for human immunodeficiency virus type 1 in the intestinal mucosa. *J Infect Dis* 2000; 182:785–791.
45. Smith PD, Fox CH, Masur H, et al. Quantitative analysis of mononuclear cells expressing human immunodeficiency virus type 1 RNA in esophageal mucosa. *J Exp Med* 1994;180: 1541–1546.
46. Veazey RS, DeMaria M, Chalifoux LV, et al. Gastrointestinal tract as a major site of CD4+ T cell depletion and viral replication in SIV infection. *Science* 1998;280:427–431.
47. Kewenig S, Schneider T, Hohloch K, et al. Rapid mucosal CD4(+) T-cell depletion and enteropathy in simian immunodeficiency virus-infected rhesus macaques. *Gastroenterology* 1999;116:1115–1123.
48. Schneider T, Jahn HU, Schmidt W, et al. Loss of CD4 T lymphocytes in patients infected with immunodeficiency virus type 1 is more pronounced in the duodenal mucosa than in the peripheral blood. *Gut* 1995;37:524–529.
49. Clayton F, Snow G, Reka S, et al. Selective depletion of rectal

lamina propria rather than lymphoid aggregate CD4 lymphocytes in HIV infection. *Clin Exp Immunol* 1997;107:288–292.
50. McNeely TB, Dealy M, Dripps DJ, et al. Secretory leukocyte protease inhibitor: a human saliva protein exhibiting anti-human immunodeficiency virus 1 activity in vitro. *J Clin Invest* 1995;96:456–464.
51. Connolly GM, Hawkins D, Harcourt-Webster JN, et al. Esophageal symptoms, their causes, treatment, and prognosis in patients with acquired immunodeficiency syndrome. *Gut* 1989; 30:1033–1039.
52. Bonacini M, Young T, Laine L. The causes of esophageal symptoms in human immunodeficiency virus infection. A prospective study of 110 patients. *Arch Intern Med* 1991;151:1567–1562.
53. Smith PD, Eisner MS, Manischewitz JF, et al. Esophageal disease in AIDS is associated with pathologic processes rather than mucosal human immunodeficiency virus type 1. *J Infect Dis* 1993;167:547–552.
54. Klein RS, Harris CA, Small CB, et al. Oral candidiasis in high-risk patients as the initial manifestation of the acquired immunodeficiency syndrome. *N Engl J Med* 1984;311:354–358.
55. Sarmaranayake LP. Oral mycoses in HIV infection. *Oral Surg Oral Med Oral Pathol* 1992;73:171–180.
56. Gould E, Kory WP, Raskin JB, et al. Esophageal biopsy findings in the acquired immunodeficiency syndrome: clinicopathologic correlation in 20 patients. *South Med J* 1988;81:1392–1395.
57. Whelan WL, Kirsch DR, Kwon-Chung KJ, et al. *Candida albicans* in patients with the acquired immunodeficiency syndrome: absence of a novel or hypervirulent strain. *J Infect Dis* 1990;162: 513–518.
58. Baldwin GC, Fleischmann J, Chung Y, et al. Human immunodeficiency virus causes mononuclear phagocyte dysfunction. *Proc Natl Acad Sci U S A* 1990;87;3933–3937.
59. Darouiche RO. Oropharyngeal and esophageal candidiasis in immunocompromised patients: treatment issues. *Clin Infect Dis* 1998;26;259–274.
60. Kinlock-DeLose S, Hirschel B, Hoen B, et al. A controlled trial of zidovudine in primary human immunodeficiency virus infection. *N Engl J Med* 1995;333:408–413.
61. Moore RD, Chaisson RE. Natural history of opportunistic disease in an HIV-infected urban clinical cohort. *Ann Intern Med* 1996;124:633–642.
62. Tivitian A, Raufman JP, Rosenthal LE. Oral candidiasis as a marker for esophageal candidiasis in the acquired immunodeficiency syndrome. *Ann Intern Med* 1986;104:54–55.
63. Porro GB, Parente F, Cernuschi M. The diagnosis of esophageal candidiasis in patients with acquired immune deficiency syndrome: is endoscopy always necessary? *Am J Gastroenterol* 1989; 84:143–146.
64. Connolly GM, Forbes A, Gleeson JA, et al. Investigation of upper gastrointestinal symptoms in patients with AIDS. *AIDS* 1989;3:453–456.
65. Powderly WG, Mayer KH, Perfect JR. Diagnosis and treatment of oropharyngeal candidiasis in patients infected with HIV: a critical reassessment. *AIDS Res Hum Retroviruses* 1999;15:1405–1412.
66. Powderly WG, Gallant JE, Ghannoum MA, et al. Oropharyngeal candidiasis in patients with HIV: suggested guidelines for therapy. *AIDS Res Hum Retrovirus* 1999;15:1619–1623.
67. Kirkpatrich CH, Alling DW. Treatment of chronic oral candidiasis with clotrimazole troches. A controlled clinical trial. *N Engl J Med* 1978;299:1201–1204.
68. Drugs for AIDS and associated infections. *Med Lett* 1993;35: 79–86.
69. Systemic antifungal drugs. *Med Lett* 1994;36:16–18.
70. Lucatorio FM, Franker C, Hardy WD, et al. Treatment of refractory oral candidiasis with fluconazole. A case report. *Oral Surg* 1991;71:42–44.
71. Dewit S, Weerts D, Goossens H, et al. Comparison of fluconazole and ketoconazole for oropharyngeal candidiasis in AIDS. *Lancet* 1989;1:746–748.
72. De Wit S, Goossens H, Clumeck N. Single-dose versus 7 days of fluconazole treatment for oral candidiasis in human immunodeficiency virus-infected patients: a prospective, randomized pilot study. *J Infect Dis* 1993;168:1332–1333.
73. Laine L, Dretler RH, Conteas CN, et al. Fluconazole compared with ketoconazole for the treatment of *Candida* esophagitis in AIDS. A randomized trial. *Ann Intern Med* 1992;117:655–660.
74. Gil A, Lavilla P, Valencia E, et al. Safety and efficacy of fluconazole treatment for *Candida* esophagitis in AIDS. *Postgrad Med J* 1991;67:548–522.
75. Gritti FM, Raise E, Bonazzi L, et al. Fluconazole treatment for candidiasis and cryptococcosis in patients with AIDS and AIDS-related complex. *Curr Ther Res* 1990;47:1049–1062.
76. Powderly WG, Finkelstein DM, Feinbeerg J, et al. A randomized trial comparing fluconazole with clotrimazole troches for the prevention of fungal infections in patients with advanced human immunodeficiency virus infection. *N Engl J Med* 1995; 332:700–705.
77. Wilcox CM, Alexander LN, Clark WS, et al. Fluconazole compared with endoscopy for human immunodeficiency virus-infected patients with esophageal symptoms. *Gastroenterology* 1996;110:1803–1809.
78. Wilcox CM, Darouiche RO, Laine L, et al. A randomized, double-blind comparison of itraconazole oral solution and fluconazole tablets in the treatment of esophageal candidiasis. *J Infect Dis* 1997;176:227–232.
79. Rice GPA, Schrier RD, Oldstone MBA. Cytomegalovirus infects human lymphocytes and monocytes: virus expression is restricted to immediate-early gene products. *Proc Natl Acad Sci U S A* 1984;81:6134–6138.
80. Rook AH, Masur H, Lane HC, et al. Interleukin-2 enhances the depressed natural killer and cytomegalovirus-specific cytotoxic activities of lymphocytes from patients with acquired immune deficiency syndrome. *J Clin Invest* 1983;72:398–403.
81. Francis ND, Boylston AW, Roberts AHG, et al. Cytomegalovirus infection in gastrointestinal tracts of patients infected with HIV-1 or AIDS. *J Clin Pathol* 1989;42:1055–1064.
82. Hinnant KL, Rotterdam HZ, Bell ET, et al. Cytomegalovirus infection of the alimentary tract: a clinicopathological correlation. *Am J Gastroenterol* 1986;81:944–950.
83. Genta RM, Bleyzer I, Cate TR, et al. In situ hybridization and immunohistochemical analysis of cytomegalovirus-associated ileal perforation. *Gastroenterology* 1993;104:1822–1827.
84. Kyriazis AP, Mitra SK. Multiple cytomegalovirus-related intestinal perforations in patients with acquired immunodeficiency syndrome. Report of two cases and review of the literature. *Arch Pathol Lab Med* 1992;116:495–499.
85. Tatum ET, Sun PCJ, Cohn DL. Cytomegalovirus vasculitis and colon perforation in a patient with the acquired immunodeficiency syndrome. *Pathology* 1989;21:235–238.
86. Smith PD, Saini SS, Raffeld M, et al. Cytomegalovirus induction of tumor necrosis factor-α by human monocytes and mucosal macrophages. *J Clin Invest* 1992;90:1642–1648.
87. Wilcox CM, Harris PR, Redman TK, et al. High mucosal levels of tumor necrosis factor-α messenger RNA in AIDS-associated cytomegalovirus-induced esophagitis. *Gastroenterology* 1998;114: 77–82.
88. Redman TK, Britt WJ, Wilcox CM, et al. Human cytomegalovirus primes lamina propria macrophages for enhanced LPS-stimulated chemokine production. *J Infect Dis* 2002;185: 584–590.
89. Jacobson MA, Mills J. Serious cytomegalovirus disease in

acquired immunodeficiency syndrome (AIDS). Clinical findings, diagnosis, and treatment. *Ann Intern Med* 1988;108:585–594.
90. Smith PD, Quinn TC, Strober W, et al. Gastrointestinal infections in AIDS. *Ann Intern Med* 1992;116:63–77.
91. Wilcox CM, Diehl DL, Cello JP, et al. Cytomegalovirus esophagitis in patients with AIDS. A clinical, endoscopic and pathologic correlation. *Ann Intern Med* 1990;113:589–593.
92. Balthazar EJ, Megibow AJ, Hulnick DH. Cytomegalovirus esophagitis and gastritis in AIDS. *Am J Radiol* 1985;144: 1201–1204.
93. Laguna F, Garcia-Samaniego J, Alonso MJ, et al. Pseudotumoral appearance of cytomegalovirus esophagitis and gastritis in AIDS patients. *Am J Gastroenterol* 1993;88:1108–1111.
94. Kitchen VS, Helbert M, Francis ND, et al. Epstein-Barr virus associated esophageal ulcers in AIDS. *Gut* 1990;31:1223–1225.
95. Goodman P, Pinero SS, Rance RM, et al. Mycobacterial esophagitis in AIDS. *Gastrointest Radiol* 1989;14:103–105.
96. Mokoena T, Shama DM, Ngakane H, et al. Esophageal tuberculosis: a review of eleven cases. *Postgrad Med J* 1992;68:110–115.
97. Wall SD, Ominsky S, Altman DF, et al. Multifocal abnormalities of the gastrointestinal tract in AIDS. *Am J Radiol* 1986;146:1–5.
98. Tom W, Aaron JS. Esophageal ulcers caused by *Torulopsis glabrata* in a patient with acquired immune deficiency syndrome. *Am J Gastroenterol* 1987;82:766–768.
99. Edwards P, Turner J, Gold J, et al. Esophageal ulceration induced by zidovudine. *Ann Intern Med* 1990;112:65–66.
100. Indorf AS, Pegram PS. Esophageal ulceration related to zalcitabine (ddC). *Ann Intern Med* 1992;117:133–134.
101. Villaneuva JL, Torre-Cisnoeros J, Jurado R, et al. *Leishmania* esophagitis in an AIDS patient: an unusual form of visceral leishmaniasis. *Am J Gastroenterol* 1994;89:273–275.
102. Kazlow PG, Shah K, Benkov KJ, et al. Esophageal cryptosporidiosis in a child with acquired immune deficiency syndrome. *Gastroenterology* 1986;91:1301–1303.
103. Ezzell JH, Bremer J, Adamec TA. Bacterial esophagitis: an often forgotten cause of odynophagia. *Am J Gastroenterol* 1990;85: 296–298.
104. Friedman SL, Wright TL. Altman DF. Gastrointestinal Kaposi's sarcoma in patients with acquired immunodeficiency syndrome. Endoscopic and autopsy findings. *Gastroenterology* 1985;89:102–108.
105. Bernal Z, del Junco GW. Endoscopic and pathologic features of esophageal lymphoma: a report of four cases in patients with acquired immune deficiency syndrome. *Gastrointest Endosc* 1986;32:96–99.
106. Frager DH, Wolf EL, Competiello LS, et al. Squamous cell carcinoma of the esophagus in patients with acquired immunodeficiency syndrome. *Gastrointest Radiol* 1988;358–360.
107. Forsmark CE, Wilcox CM, Darragh T, et al. Disseminated histoplasmosis in AIDS: an unusual case of esophageal involvement and gastrointestinal bleeding. *Gastrointest Endosc* 1990;36:604–605.
108. Smith PD, Lane HC, Gill VJ, et al. Intestinal infections in patients with the acquired immunodeficiency syndrome. *Ann Intern Med* 1988;108:328–333.
109. Smith PD. Infectious diarrheas in patients with AIDS. *Gastroenterol Clin North Am* 1993;22:535–548.
110. Culpepper-Morgan JA, Cutler DP, Scholes JV, et al. Evaluation of diagnostic criteria for mucosal cytomegalic inclusion disease in the acquired immune deficiency syndrome. *Am J Gastroenterol* 1987;82:1264–1270.
111. Wu G-D, Shintaku IP, Chien K, et al. A comparison of routine light microscopy, immunohistochemistry, and in situ hybridization for the detection of cytomegalovirus in gastrointestinal biopsies. *Am J Gastroenterol* 1989;84:1517–1520.
112. Clayton F, Klein EB, Cutler DP. Correlation of in situ hybridization with histology and viral culture in patients with acquired immunodeficiency syndrome with cytomegalovirus colitis. *Arch Pathol Lab Med* 1989;113:1124–1126.
113. Cotte L, Drouet E, Bissuel F, et al. Diagnostic value of amplification of human cytomegalovirus DNA from gastrointestinal biopsies from human immunodeficiency virus-infected patients. *J Clin Microbiol* 1993;31:2066–2069.
114. Collaborative DHPG Treatment Study Group. Treatment of serious cytomegalovirus infections with 9-(1,3-dihydroxy-2-propoxymethyl)guanine in patients with AIDS and other immunodeficiencies. *N Engl J Med* 1986;314:801–805.
115. Chachoua A, Dieterich D, Krasinski K, et al. 9-(1,3-Dihydroxy-2-propoxymethyl)guanine (ganciclovir) in the treatment of cytomegalovirus gastrointestinal disease with the acquired immunodeficiency syndrome. *Ann Intern Med* 1987;107:133–137.
116. Laskin OL, Stahl-Bayliss CM, Kalman CM, et al. Use of ganciclovir to treat serious cytomegalovirus infections in patients with AIDS. *J Infect Dis* 1987;155:323–327.
117. Laskin OL, Cederberg DM, Mills J, et al. Ganciclovir for the treatment and suppression of serious infections caused by cytomegalovirus. *Am J Med* 1987;83:201–207.
118. Dieterich DT, Chachoua A, Lafleur F, et al. Ganciclovir treatment of gastrointestinal infections caused by cytomegalovirus in patients with AIDS. *Rev Infect Dis* 1988;10S:532–537.
119. Buhles WC, Mastre BJ, Tinker AJ, et al. Ganciclovir treatment of life- or sight-threatening cytomegalovirus infection: experience in 314 immunocompromised patients. *Rev Infect Dis* 1988;10S:495–504.
120. Dieterich DT, Cutler DP, Busch DF, et al. Ganciclovir treatment of cytomegalovirus colitis in AIDS: a randomized, double-blind, placebo-controlled multicenter study. *J Infect Dis* 1993;167: 278–282.
121. Drew WL, Miner RC, Busch DF, et al. Prevalence of resistance in patients receiving ganciclovir for serious cytomegalovirus infection. *J Infect Dis* 1991;163:716–719.
122. Nelson MR, Connolly GM, Hawkins DA, et al. Foscarnet in the treatment of cytomegalovirus infection of the esophagus and colon in patients with the acquired immune deficiency syndrome. *Am J Gastroenterol* 1991;86:876–881.
123. Drugs for non-HIV viral infections. *Med Lett* 1994;36:27–32.
124. Seigal FP, Lopez C, Hammer GS, et al. Severe acquired immunodeficiency in male homosexuals manifested by chronic herpes simplex lesions. *N Engl J Med* 1981;305:1439–1444.
125. Quinnan GV, Masur H, Rook AH, et al. Herpesvirus infections in the acquired immune deficiency syndrome. *JAMA* 1984;252: 72–77.
126. Agha FP, Lee HL, Nostrant TT. Herpetic esophagitis: a diagnostic challenge in immunocompromised patients. *Am J Gastroenterol* 1986;81:246–253.
127. Erlich DS, Mills J, Chatis P, et al. Acyclovir-resistant herpes simplex virus infections in patients with the acquired immunodeficiency syndrome. *N Engl J Med* 1989;320:293–296.
128. Englund JA, Zimmerman ME, Swierkosz EM, et al. Herpes simplex virus resistant to acyclovir. A study in a tertiary care center. *Ann Intern Med* 1990;112:416–422.
129. Safrin S, Crumpacker C, Chatis P, et al. A controlled trial comparing foscarnet with vidarabine for acyclovir-resistant mucocutaneous herpes simplex in the acquired immunodeficiency syndrome. *N Engl J Med* 1991;325:551–555.
130. Wilcox CM, Schwartz DA. Endoscopic characterization of idiopathic esophageal ulceration associated with human immunodeficiency virus infection. *J Clin Gastroenterol* 1993;16:251–256.
131. Wilcox CM, Schwartz DA, Clark WS. Esophageal ulceration in human immunodeficiency virus infection. Causes, response to therapy, and long-term outcome. *Ann Intern Med* 1995;122: 143–149.

132. Rabeneck L, Boyko WJ, McLean DM, et al. Unusual esophageal ulcers containing enveloped virus-like particles in homosexual men. *Gastroenterology* 1986;90:1882–1889.
133. Kotler DP, Wilson CS, Haroutiounian G, et al. Detection of human immunodeficiency virus-1 by ^{35}S-RNA *in situ* hybridization in solitary esophageal ulcers in two patients with the acquired immune deficiency syndrome. *Am J Gastroenterol* 1989;84:313–317.
134. Frager D, Kotler DP, Baer J. Idiopathic esophageal ulceration in the acquired immunodeficiency syndrome: radiologic reappraisal in 10 patients. *Abdom Imaging* 1994;19:2–5.
135. Rabeneck L, Popovic M, Gartner S, et al. Acute HIV infection presenting with painful swallowing and esophageal ulcers. *JAMA* 1990;263:2318–2322.
136. Janoff EN, Jackson S, Wahl SM, et al. Characterization of mucosal antibodies in persons with AIDS. *J Infect Dis* 1994; 170:299–307.
137. Wahl SM, Orenstein JM, Smith PD. Macrophage function in HIV-1 infection. In: Gupta SD, ed. *Immunology of human immunodeficiency virus type 1 infection.* Academic Press, San Diego, CA 1996:303–336.
138. Kotler DP, Reka S, Clayton F. Intestinal mucosal inflammation associated with human immunodeficiency virus infection. *Dig Dis Sci* 1993;38:1119–1127.
139. Wilcox CM, Zaki SR, Coffiedl LM, et al. Evaluation of idiopathic esophageal ulceration for human immunodeficiency virus. *Modern Pathol* 1995;8:568–572.
140. Bach MC, Valenti AJ, Howell DA, et al. Odynophagia from aphthous ulcers of the pharynx and esophagus in the acquired immunodeficiency syndrome. *Ann Intern Med* 1988;109: 338–339.
141. Bach MC, Howell DA, Valenti AJ, et al. Aphthous ulceration of the gastrointestinal tract in patients with the acquired immunodeficiency syndrome. *Ann Intern Med* 1990;112:465–467.
142. Wilcox CM, Schwartz DA. A pilot study of oral corticosteroid therapy for idiopathic esophageal ulcerations associated with human immunodeficiency virus infection. *Am J Med* 1992; 98:131–134.
143. Kotler DP, Reka S, Orenstein JM, et al. Chronic idiopathic esophageal ulceration in the acquired immunodeficiency syndrome. Characterization and treatment with steroids. *J Clin Gastroenterol* 1992;15:284–290.
144. Youle M, Clarbour J, Farthing C, et al. Treatment of resistant aphthous ulceration with thalidomide in patients positive for HIV antibody. *Br Med J* 1989;298:432.
145. Smith PD, Lane HC, Gill VJ, et al. Intestinal infections in patients with the acquired immunodeficiency syndrome (AIDS). Etiology and response to therapy. *Ann Intern Med* 1988;108:328–333.
146. Laughon BE, Druckman DA, Vernon A, et al. Prevalence of enteric pathogens in homosexual men with and without acquired immunodeficiency syndrome. *Gastroenterology* 1988; 94:984–993.
147. Dryden MS, Shanson DC. The microbial causes of diarrhea in patients infected with the human immunodeficiency virus. *J Infect* 1988;17:107–114.
148. Greenson JK, Belitsos PC, Yardley JH, et al. AIDS enteropathy: occult enteric infections and duodenal mucosal alterations in chronic diarrhea. *Ann Intern Med* 1991;114:366–372.
149. Connolly GM, Forbes A, Bleeson JA, et al. The value of barium enema and colonoscopy in patients with infected with HIV. *AIDS* 1990;4:687–689.
150. Wilcox CM, Waites KB, Smith PD. No relationship between gastric pH, small bowel bacterial colonisation and diarrhoea in HIV-1 infected patients. *Gut* 1999;44:101–105.
151. Cello JP, Grendell JH, Basuk P, et al. Effect of octreotide on refractory AIDS-associated diarrhea. A prospective, multicenter clinical trial. *Ann Intern Med* 1991;115:705–710.
152. Ullrich R, Heise W, Bergs C, et al. Effects of zidovudine treatment on the small intestinal mucosa in patients infected with the human immunodeficiency virus. *Gastroenterology* 1992;102: 1483–1492.
153. Janoff EN, Reller LB. *Cryptosporidium* species, a protean protozoan. *J Clin Microbiol* 1987;25:967–975.
154. Soave R, Armstrong D. *Cryptosporidium* and cryptosporidiosis in homosexual men. *Rev Infect Dis* 1986;8:1012–1023.
155. Colebunders R, Francis H, Mann JM, et al. Persistent diarrhea strongly associated with HIV infection in Kinshasa, Zaire. *Am J Gastroenterol* 1987;82:859–864.
156. Malebranche R, Arnoux E, Guerin JM, et al. Acquired immu nodeficiency syndrome with severe gastrointestinal manifestations in Haiti. *Lancet* 1983;2:873–878.
157. Wolfson JS, Richter JM, Waldron MA, et al. Cryptosporidiosis in immunocompetent patients. *N Engl J Med* 1985;312: 1278–1282.
158. MacKenzie WR, Hoxie NJ, Proctor ME, et al. A massive outbreak in Milwaukee of cryptosporidium infection transmitted through the public water supply. *N Engl J Med* 1994;331: 161–167.
159. Soave R, Danner RL, Honig CL, et al. Cryptosporidiosis in homosexual men. *Ann Intern Med* 1984;110:504–511.
160. Janoff EN, Limas C, Gebhard RL, et al. Cryptosporidial carriage without symptoms in the acquired immunodeficiency syndrome (AIDS). *Ann Intern Med* 1990;112:75–76.
161. Margulis SJ, Honig CL, Soave R, et al. Biliary tract obstruction in the acquired immunodeficiency syndrome. *Ann Intern Med* 1986;105:207–210.
162. Schneiderman DJ, Cello JP, Laing FC. Papillary stenosis and sclerosing cholangitis in the acquired immunodeficiency syndrome. *Ann Intern Med* 1987;106:546–549.
163. Kazlow PG, Shah K, Benkov KJ, et al. Esophageal cryptosporidiosis in a child with acquired immune deficiency syndrome. *Gastroenterology* 1986;91:1301–1303.
164. Portnoy D, Whiteside ME, Buckley E, et al. Treatment of intestinal cryptosporidiosis with spiramycin. *Ann Intern Med* 1984;101:202–204.
165. Moskovitz BL, Stanton TL, Kusmierek JJ. Spiramycin therapy for cryptosporidial diarrhea in immunocompromised patients. *J Antimicrob Chemother* 1988;22S:189–191.
166. Clezy K, Gold J, Blaze J, et al. Paromomycin for the treatment of cryptosporidial diarrhea in AIDS patients. *AIDS* 1991;5:12–13.
167. Armitage K, Flanigan T, Carey J, et al. Treatment of cryptosporidiosis with paromomycin. A report of five cases. *Arch Intern Med* 1992;152:2497–2499.
168. Danzinger LH, Kanyok TP, Novak RM. Treatment of cryptosporidial diarrhea in an AIDS patient with paromomycin. *Ann Pharmacother* 1993;27:1460–1462.
169. Ungar BP, Ward DJ, Fayer R, et al. Cessation of cryptosporidium-associated diarrhea in an acquired immunodeficiency syndrome patient after treatment with hyperimmune bovine colostrum. *Gastroenterology* 1990;98:486–489.
170. Shield J, Melville C, Novelli V, et al. Bovine colostrum immunoglobulin concentrate for cryptosporidiosis in AIDS. *Arch Dis Child* 1993;69:451–453.
171. Louie E, Borkowsky W, Klesius PH, et al. Treatment of *Cryptosporidium* with oral bovine transfer factor. *Clin Immunol Immunopathol* 1987;73:413–414.
172. Cook DJ, Kelton JG, Stanisz AM, et al. Somatostatin treatment for cryptosporidial diarrhea in a patient with the acquired immunodeficiency syndrome (AIDS). *Ann Intern Med* 1988; 108:708–709.
173. Greenberg RE, Mir R, Bank S, et al. Resolution of intestinal

cryptosporidiosis after treatment of AIDS with AZT. *Gastroenterology* 1989;97:1327–1330.
174. Cali A, Owen RL. Intracellular development of *Enterocytozoon,* a unique microsporidian found in the intestine of AIDS patients. *J Protozool* 1990;37:145–155.
175. Orenstein JM, Tenner M, Cali A, et al. A microsporidian previously undescribed in humans, infecting enterocytes and macrophages, and associated with diarrhea in an acquired immunodeficiency syndrome patient. *Hum Pathol* 1992;23:722–728.
176. Orenstein JM, Kietrich DT, Kotler D. Systemic dissemination by a newly recognized intestinal microsporidia species in AIDS. *AIDS* 1992;6:1143–1150.
177. Gunnarsson G, Hurbut D, DeGirolami PC, et al. Multiorgan microsporidiosis: report of five cases and review. *Clin Infect Dis* 1995;21:37–44.
178. Dore GJ, Marriott DJ, Hing MC, et al. Disseminated microsporidiosis due to *Septata intestinalis* in nine patients infected with human immunodeficiency virus: response to therapy with albendazole. *Clin Infect Dis* 1995;21:70–76.
179. Molina JM, Oksenhendler E, Beauvais B, et al. Disseminated microsporidiosis due to *Septata intestinalis* in patients with AIDS: clinical features and response to albendazole therapy. *J Infect Dis* 1995;171:245–249.
180. Gumbo T, Hobbs RE, Carlyn C, et al. Microsporidia infection in transplant patients. *Transplantation* 1999;67:482–484.
181. Guerard A, Rabodonirina M, Cotte L, et al. Intestinal microsporidiosis occurring in two renal transplant recipients treated with mycophenolate mofetil. *Transplantation* 1999;68:699–707.
182. Goetz M, Eichenlaub S, Pape GR, et al. Chronic diarrhea as a result of intestinal microsporidiosis in a liver transplant recipient. *Transplantation* 2001;71:334–447.
183. Desports-Livage I, Doumbo O, Pichard E, et al. Microsporidiosis in HIV-seronegative patients in Mali. *Trans Royal Soc Trop Med Hyg* 1998;92:423–424.
184. Gainzarain JC, Canut A, Lozano M, et al. Detection of *Enterocytozoon bieneusi* in two human immunodeficiency virus-negative patients with chronic diarrhea by polymerase chain reaction in duodenal biopsy specimens and review. *Clin Infect Dis* 1998; 27:394–398.
185. Muller A, Bialek R, Kamper A, et al. Detection of microsporidia in travelers with diarrhea. *J Clin Microbiol* 2001;39:1630–1632.
186. Desportes I, Le Charpentier Y, Galian A, et al. Occurrence of a new microsporidian: *Enterocytozoon bieneusi* n. g., n. sp., in the enterocytes of a human patient with AIDS. *J Protozool* 1985;32: 250–254.
187. Orenstein JM, Chang J, Steinberg W, et al. Intestinal microsporidiosis as a cause of diarrhea in human immunodeficiency virus-infected patients: a report of 20 cases. *Hum Pathol* 1990; 21:475–481.
188. Orenstein JM. Microsporidiosis in the acquired immunodeficiency syndrome. *J Parasitol* 1991;77:843–864.
189. Eeftinck Schattenkerk JKME, van Gool T, van Ketel RJ, et al. Clinical significance of small-intestinal microsporidiosis in HIV-1-infected individuals. *Lancet* 1991;1:895–898.
190. Molina J-M, Sarfati C, Beauvais B, et al. Intestinal microsporidiosis in human immunodeficiency virus-infected patients with chronic unexplained diarrhea: prevalence and clinical and biologic features. *J Infect Dis* 1993;167:217–221.
191. Rabeneck L, Gyorkey F, Genta R, et al. The role of microsporidia in the pathogenesis of HIV-related chronic diarrhea. *Ann Intern Med* 1993;119:895–899.
192. Orenstein JM, Tenner M, Kotler DP. Localization of infection by the microsporidian *Enterocytozoon bieneusi* in the gastrointestinal tract of AIDS patients with diarrhea. *AIDS* 1992;6:195–197.
193. Kotler DP, Rancisco A, Clayton F, et al. Small intestinal injury and parasitic diseases in AIDS. *Ann Intern Med* 1990;113:444–449.
194. Pol S, Romana CA, Richard S, et al. Microsporidia infection in patients with the human immunodeficiency virus and unexplained cholangitis. *N Engl J Med* 1993;328:95–99.
195. French AL, Beaudet LM, Benator DA, et al. Cholecystectomy in patients with AIDS: clinicopathologic correlations in 107 cases. *Clin Infect Dis* 1995;21:852–858.
196. Wilson R, Harrington R, Stewart B, et al. Human immunodeficiency virus 1-associated necrotizing cholangitis caused by infection with *Septata intestinalis. Gastroenterology* 1995;108:247–251.
197. Rijpstra AC, Canning EU, van Ketel, et al. Use of light microscopy to diagnose small-intestinal microsporidiosis in patients with AIDS. *J Infect Dis* 1988;157:827–831.
198. Simon D, Weiss LM, Tanowitz HB, et al. Light microscopic diagnosis and variable response to octreotide. *Gastroenterology* 1991;100:271–273.
199. Weber R, Bryan R, Owen RL, et al. Improved light-microscopical detection of microsporidia spores in stool and duodenal aspirates. *N Engl J Med* 1992;326:161–166.
200. Kotler DP, Giang TT, Garro ML, et al. Light microscopic diagnosis of microsporidiosis in patients with AIDS. *Am J Gastroenterol* 1994;89:540–544.
201. Coyle CM, Wittner M, Kotler DP, et al. Prevalence of microsporidiosis due to *Enterocytozoon bieneusi* and *Encephalitozoon (Septata) intestinalis* among patients with AIDS-related diarrhea: determination by polymerase chain reaction to the microsporidian small-subunit rTNA gene. *Clin Infect Dis* 1996;23: 1002–1006.
202. Dietrich D, Kotler D, Lew E, et al. Albendazole treatment of two species of microsporidial enteritis. *Am J Gastroenterol* 1992; 87:1312.
203. Banshard C, Ellis DS, Tovey DG, et al. Treatment of intestinal microsporidiosis with albendazole in patients with AIDS. *AIDS* 1992;6:311–313.
204. Molina JM, Chastang C, Goguel J, et al. Albendazole for treatment and prophylaxis of microsporidiosis due to Encephalitozoon intestinalis in patients with AIDS: a randomized double-blind controlled trial. *J Infect Dis* 1998;177:515–518.
205. Conlon CP, Pinching AJ, Perera CU, et al. HIV-related enteropathy in Zambia: a clinical, microbiological and histological study. *Am J Trop Med Hyg* 1990;42:83–88.
206. DeHovitz J, Pape JW, Boncy M, et al. Clinical manifestations and therapy of *Isospora belli* infection in patients with the acquired immunodeficiency syndrome. *N Engl J Med* 1986; 315:87–90.
207. Ng E, Markell EK, Fleming RL, et al. Demonstration of *Isospora belli* by acid-fast stain in a patient with acquired immune deficiency syndrome. *J Clin Microbiol* 1984;20:384–386.
208. Benator DA, French AL, Beaudet LM, et al. *Isospora belli* infection associated with acalculous cholecystitis in a patient with AIDS. *Ann Intern Med* 1994;121:663–664.
209. Restrepo C, Macher AM, Radany EH. Disseminated extraintestinal isosporiasis in a patient with acquired immune deficiency syndrome. *Am J Clin Pathol* 1987;87:536–542.
210. Outbreaks of diarrheal illness associated with Cyanobacteria (blue-green algae)-like bodies—Chicago and Nepal, 1989 and 1990. *MMWR Morb Mortal Wkly Rep* 1991;40:325–327.
211. Long EG, White EH, Carmichael WW, et al. Morphologic and staining characteristics of a cyanobacterium-like organism associated with diarrhea. *J Infect Dis* 1991;164:199–202.
212. Ortega YR, Sterling CR, Gilman RH, et al. *Cyclospora* species—a new protozoan pathogen of humans. *N Engl J Med* 1993;328: 1308–1312.
213. Ortega YR, Nagle R, Gilman RH, et al. Pathological and clinical findings in patients with cyclosporiasis and a description of intracellular parasite life-cycle stages. *J Infect Dis* 1997;176: 1584–1589.

214. Shlim DR, Cohen MT, Eaton M, et al. An alga-like organism associated with an outbreak of prolonged diarrhea among foreigners in Nepal. *Am J Trop Med* 1991;45:383–389.
215. Connor BA, Shlim DR, Scholes JV, et al. Pathologic changes in the small bowel in nine patients with diarrhea associated with a coccidia-like body. *Ann Intern Med* 1993;119:377–382.
216. Hart AS, Ridinger MT, Soundarajan R, et al. Novel organisms associated with chronic diarrhoea in AIDS. *Lancet* 1990;335: 169–179.
217. Pape JW, Verdier RI, Boncy M, et al. *Cyclospora* infection in adults infected with HIV. Clinical manifestations, treatment, and prophylaxis. *Ann Intern Med* 1994;121:654–657.
218. Huang P, Weber JT, Sosin DM, et al. The first reported outbreak of diarrheal illness associated with *Cyclospora* in the United States. *Ann Intern Med* 1995;123:409–414.
219. Herwaldt BL, Ackers M, and the Cyclospora Working Group. An outbreak in 1996 of cyclosporiasis associated with imported raspberries. *N Engl J Med* 1997;336:1548–1556.
220. Janoff EN, Smith PD, Blaser MJ. Acute antibody responses to *Giardia lamblia* are depressed in patients with AIDS. *J Infect Dis* 1988;157:798–804.
221. Ravdin JI. Amebiasis. *Clin Infect Dis* 1995;20:1453–1466.
222. Knapp AB, Horst DA, Eliopoulos G, et al. Widespread cytomegalovirus gastroenteritis in a patient with acquired immunodeficiency syndrome. *Gastroenterology* 1983;85:1399–1402.
223. Kavin Jones RB, Chowdhury L, Kabius S. Acalculous cholecystitis and cytomegalovirus infection in the acquired immunodeficiency syndrome. *Ann Intern Med* 1986;104:53–54.
224. Margulis SJ, Honig CL, Soave R, et al. Biliary tract obstruction in the acquired immunodeficiency syndrome. *Ann Intern Med* 1986;105:207–210.
225. Schneiderman DJ, Cello JP, Laing FC. Papillary stenosis and sclerosing cholangitis in the acquired immunodeficiency syndrome. *Ann Intern Med* 1987;106:546–549.
226. Wilcox CM, Forsmark CE, Grendell JH, et al. Cytomegalovirus-associated acute pancreatic disease in patients with the acquired immunodeficiency syndrome. Report of two patients. *Gastroenterology* 1990;99:263–267.
227. Valerdiz-Casasola S, Pardo-Mindan FJ. Cytomegalovirus infection of the appendix in a patient with the acquired immunodeficiency syndrome. *Gastroenterology* 1991;101:247–249.
228. Rene E, March C, Chevalier T, et al. Cytomegalovirus colitis in patients with acquired immunodeficiency syndrome. *Dig Dis Sci* 1988;33:171–175.
229. Meiselman MS, Cello JP, Margaretten W. Cytomegalovirus colitis. Report of the clinical, endoscopic, and pathologic findings in two patients with the acquired immune deficiency syndrome. *Gastroenterology* 1985;88:171–175.
230. Dieterich DT, Rahmin M. Cytomegalovirus colitis in AIDS: presentation in 44 patients and a review of the literature. *J Acquired Immun Defic Syndrome* 1991;4S:29–35.
231. Culpepper-Morgan JA, Kotler DP, Scholes JV, Tierney AR. Evolution of diagnostic criteria for mucosal cytomegalic inclusion disease in the acquired immune deficiency syndrome. *Am J Gastroenterol*1987;82:1264–1270.
232. Goodell SE, Quinn TC, Mkrtichian E, et al. Herpes simplex virus proctitis in homosexual men. Clinical, sigmoidoscopic, and histopathological features. *N Engl J Med* 1983;308:868–871.
233. Janoff EN, Orenstein JM, Manischewitz JF, Smith PD. Adenovirus colitis in the acquired immunodeficiency syndrome. *Gastroenterology* 1991;100:976–979.
234. de Jong PJ, Valderrama G, Spigland I, et al. Adenovirus isolates from urine of patients with acquired immunodeficiency syndrome. *Lancet* 1983;1:1293–1296.
235. Krilov LR, Rubin LG, Frogel M, et al. Disseminated adenovirus infection with hepatic necrosis in patients with human immunodeficiency virus infection and other immunodeficiency states. *J Infect Dis* 1990;12:303–307.
236. Kaljot KT, Ling JP, Gold JWM, et al. Prevalence of acute enteric viral pathogens in acquired immunodeficiency syndrome patients with diarrhea. *Gastroenterology* 1989;97:1031–1032.
237. Cunningham AL, Grohman GS, Harkness J, et al. Gastrointestinal viral infections in homosexual men who were symptomatic and seropositive for human immunodeficiency virus. *J Infect Dis* 1988;158:386–391.
238. Janoff EN, Orenstein JM, Manischeqitz JF, et al. Adenovirus colitis in the acquired immunodeficiency syndrome. *Gastroenterology* 1991;100:976–979.
239. Janoff EN. Diarrheal disease with viral enteric infections in immunocompromised patients. In: Owen R, Surawicz C, eds. *Gastrointestinal and hepatic infections.* Amsterdam: Elsevier Science, 1995.
240. Grohmann GS, Blass RI, Pereira HG, et al. Enteric viruses and diarrhea in HIV-infected patients. *N Engl J Med* 1993;329: 14–20.
241. Kaljot KT, Ling JP, Gold JWM, et al. Prevalence of acute enteric viral pathogens in acquired immunodeficiency syndrome patients with diarrhea. *Gastroenterology* 1989;97:1031–1032.
242. Thea DM, Glass R, Grohmann GS, et al. Prevalence of enteric viruses among hospital patients with AIDS in Kinshasa, Zaire. *Trans R Soc Trop Med Hyg* 1993;87:263–266.
243. Oshitani H, Kasolo FC, Mpabalwani M, et al. Association of rotavirus and human immunodeficiency virus infection in children hospitalized with acute diarrhea, Lusaka, Zambia. *J Infect Dis* 1994;169:897–900.
244. Cunningham AL, Grohmann GS, Harkness J, et al. Gastrointestinal viral infections in homosexual men who were symptomatic and seropositive for human immunodeficiency virus. *J Infect Dis* 1988;158:386–391.
245. Albrecht H, Stellbrink HJ, Fenske S, et al. Rotavirus antigen detection in patients with HIV infection and diarrhea. *Scand J Infect Dis* 1993;28:307–310.
246. Bottone EJ, Wormser GP, Duncanson FP. Nontyphoidal *Salmonella* bacteremia as an early infection in acquired immunodeficiency syndrome. *Diagn Microbiol Infect Dis* 1984;2:247–250.
247. Jacobs JL, Gold JWM, Murray HW, et al. *Salmonella* infections in patients with the acquired immunodeficiency syndrome. *Ann Intern Med* 1985;102:186–188.
248. Glaser JB, Morton-Kute L, Berger SR, et al. Recurrent *Salmonella typhimurium* bacteremia associated with the acquired immunodeficiency syndrome. *Ann Intern Med* 1985;102:189–193.
249. Fischl MA, Dickinson GM, Sinave C, et al. *Salmonella* bacteremia as a manifestation of acquired immunodeficiency syndrome. *Arch Intern Med* 1986;146:113–115.
250. Smith PD, Macher AM, Bookman MA, et al. *Salmonella typhimurium* enteritis and bacteremia in the acquired immunodeficiency syndrome. *Ann Intern Med* 1985;102:207–209.
251. Sperber SJ, Schleupner CJ. *Salmonella* during infection with human immunodeficiency virus. *Rev Infect Dis* 1987;9:925–934.
252. Celum CL, Chaisson RE, Rutherford GW, et al. Incidence of salmonellosis in patients with AIDS. *J Infect Dis* 1987;156: 998–1002.
253. Pithie AD, Malin AS, Robertson VJ. Salmonella and shigella bacteraemia in Zimbabwe. *Cent Afr J Med* 1993;39:110–112.
254. Baskin DH, Lax JD, Barenberg D. Shigella bacteremia in patients with the acquired immune deficiency syndrome. *Am J Gastroenterol* 1987;82:338–341.
255. Gander RM, LaRocco MT. Multiple drug-resistance in *Shigella flexneri* isolated from a patient with human immunodeficiency virus. *Diagn Microbiol Infect Dis* 1987;8:193–196.
256. Blaser MJ, Hale TL, Formal SB. Recurrent shigellosis complicating human immunodeficiency virus infection: failure of pre-

existing antibodies to confer protection. *Am J Med* 1989;86: 105–107.
257. Mandell W, Neu HC. *Shigella* bacteremia in adults. *JAMA* 1986;255:3116.
258. Dworkin B, Wormser GP, Abdoo RA, et al. Persistence of multiply antibiotic-resistant *Campylobacter jejuni* in a patient with the acquired immune deficiency syndrome. *Am J Med* 1986;80: 965–970.
259. Perlman DM, Ampel NM, Schifman RB, et al. Persistent *Campylobacter jejuni* infections in patients infected with human immunodeficiency virus (HIV). *Ann Intern Med* 1988;108: 540–546.
260. Orenstein JM, Fox C, Wahl SM. Macrophages as a source of HIV during opportunistic infections. *Science* 1997;276:1857–1861.
261. Newman GW, et al. concurrent infection of human macrophages with HIV-1 and *Mycobacterium avium* results in decreased cell viability, increased *M. avium* multiplication and altered cytokine production. *J Immunol* 1993;151:2261–2272.
262. Gray JR, Rabeneck L. Atypical mycobacterial infection of the gastrointestinal tract in AIDS patients. *Am J Gastroenterol* 1989; 84:1521–1524.
263. Horsburgh CR Jr. *Mycobacterium avium* complex in the acquired immunodeficiency syndrome. *N Engl J Med* 1991;324: 1332–1228.
264. Kiehn TE, Edwards FF, Brannon P, et al. Infections caused by *Mycobacterium avium* complex in immunocompromised patients: diagnosis by blood culture and fecal examination, antimicrobial susceptibility tests, and morphological and seroagglutination characteristics. *J Clin Microbiol* 1985;21:168–173.
265. Chaisson RE, Benson CA, Dube MP, et al. Clarithromycin therapy for bacteremic *Mycobacterium avium* complex disease. A randomized, double-blind, dose-ranging study in patients with AIDS. *Ann Intern Med* 1994;121:905–911.
266. Shafran SD, Singer J, Zarown DP, et al. A comparison of two regimens for the treatment of *Mycobacterium avium* complex bacteremia in AIDS: rifabutin, ethambutol, and clarithromycin versus rifampin, ethambutol, clofazimine, and ciprofloxacin. *N Engl J Med* 1996;335:377–383.
267. Centers for Disease Control and Prevention. 1999 USPHS/IDSA guidelines for the prevention of opportunistic infections in persons infected with human immunodeficiency virus: U.S. Public Health Service (USPHS) and Infectious Diseases Society of America (IDSA). *MMWR Morb Mortal Wkly Rep* 1999;48:1–66.
268. Pierce M, Crampton S, Henry D, et al. A randomized trial of clarithromycin as prophylaxis against disseminated *Mycobacterium avium* complex infection in patients with advanced acquired immunodeficiency syndrome. *N Engl J Med* 1996; 335:384–391.
269. Havlir DV, Dube MP, Sattler FR, et al. Prophylaxis against disseminated *Mycobacterium avium* complex with weekly azithromycin, daily rifabutin, or both. *N Engl J Med* 1996; 335:392–398.
270. Cozart JC, Kalangi SS, Clench MH, et al. *Clostridium difficile* diarrhea in patients with AIDS versus non-AIDS controls. *J Clin Gastroenterol* 1993;16:192–194.
271. Hutin Y, Molina J-M, Casin I, et al. Risk factors for *Clostridium difficile*-associated diarrhoea in HIV-infected patients. *AIDS* 1993;7:1441–1447.
272. Wheat LJ, Connolly-Stringfield P, Kohler RB, et al. *Histoplasma capsulatum* polysaccharide antigen detection in diagnosis and management of disseminated histoplasmosis in patients with acquired immunodeficiency syndrome. *Am J Med* 1989;87: 396–400.
273. McKinsey DS, Gupta MR, Riddler SA, et al. Long-term amphotericin B therapy for disseminated histoplasmosis in patients with the acquired immunodeficiency syndrome. *Ann Intern Med* 1989;111:655–659.
274. Driks MR, Gupta MR, McKinsey DS, et al. Gastrointestinal histoplasmosis in patients with the acquired immunodeficiency syndrome [Abstract]. *Proc 30th Intersci Conf Antimicrob Agents Chemother* 1990;A1272.
275. Drugs for AIDS and associated infections. *Med Lett* 1993;35: 7986.
276. Dolin R, Masur H, Saag MS. *AIDS therapy*. Philadelphia, PA: Churchill Livingstone, 1999:864.
277. Gulick RM, Mellors JW, Havlir D, et al. Treatment with indinavir, zidovudine, and lamivudine in adults with human immunodeficiency virus infection and prior antiretroviral therapy. *N Engl J Med* 1997;337:734–739.
278. Deeks SG, Smith M, Holodniy M, et al. HIV-1 protease inhibitors. A review for clinicians. *JAMA* 1997;277:145–153.
279. Gulick RM. Assessing the benefits of antiretroviral therapy [Editorial]. *Ann Intern Med* 2000;133:471–473.
280. Palella FJ Jr, Delaney KM, Moorman AC, et al. Declining morbidity and mortality among patients with advanced human immunodeficiency virus infection. *N Engl J Med* 1998;338: 853–860.
281. Vittinghoff E, Scheer S, O'Malley P, et al. Combination antiretroviral therapy and recent declines in AIDS incidence and mortality. *J Infect Dis* 1999;179:717–720.
282. Forrest DM, Seminari E, Hogg RS, et al. The incidence and spectrum of AIDS-defining illnesses in persons treated with antiretroviral drugs. *Clin Infect Dis* 1998;27:1379–1385.
283. Mocroft A, Katlama C, Johnson AM, et al. AIDS across Europe, 1994–98: the EuroSIDA Study. *Lancet* 2000;356:291–296.
284. Kaplan JE, Hanson D, Dworkin MS, et al. Epidemiology of human immunodeficiency virus-associated opportunistic infections in the United States in the era of highly active antiretroviral therapy. *Clin Infect Dis* 2000;30:S5–S14.
285. Michelet C, Arvieux C, Francois C, et al. Opportunistic infections occurring during highly active antiretroviral treatment. *AIDS* 1998;12:1815–1822.
286. Centers for Disease Control and Prevention. USPHS/IDSA guidelines for the prevention of opportunistic infections in persons infected with human immunodeficiency virus. *MMWR Morb Mortal Wkly Rep* 1999;48(RR-106).
287. Currier JS, Williams PL, Koletar SL, et al. Discontinuation of *Mycobacterium avium* complex prophylaxis in patients with antiretroviral therapy-induced increases in CD4+ cell count. *Ann Intern Med* 2000;133:493–503.
288. Furrer H, Egger M, Opravil M, et al. Discontinuation of primary prophylaxis against *Pneumocystis carinii* pneumonia in HIV-1-infected adults treated with combination antiretroviral therapy. *N Engl J Med* 1999;340:1301–1306.
289. Furrer H, Opravil M, Bernasconi E, et al., for the Swiss HIV Cohort Study. Stopping primary prophylaxis in HIV-1-infected patients at high risk of toxoplasma encephalitis. *Lancet* 2000; 355:2217–2218.
290. Mussini C, Pezzotti P, Govoni A, et al. Discontinuation of primary prophylaxis for *Pneumocystis carinii* pneumonia and toxoplasmic encephalitis in human immunodeficiency virus type 1-infected patients: the changes in opportunistic prophylaxis study. *J Infect Dis* 2000;181:1635–1642.
291. Hutin Y, Molina J-M, Casin I, et al. Risk factors for *Clostridium difficile*-associated diarrhoea in HIV-infected patients. *AIDS* 1993;7:1441–1447.
292. Tacconelli E, Tumbarello M, de Gaetano Donati K, et al. *Clostridium difficile*-associated diarrhea in human immunodeficiency virus infection—a changing scenario [Letter]. *Clin Infect Dis* 1999;28:936–937.
293. Mattapallil JJ, Smit-McBride Z, Dailey P, et al. Activated mem-

ory CD4(+) T helper cells repopulate the intestine early following antiretroviral therapy of simian immunodeficiency virus-infected rhesus macaques but exhibit a decreased potential to produce interleukin-2. *J Virol* 1999;73:6661–6669.

294. Kotler DP, Shimada T, Snow G, et al. Effect of combination antiretroviral therapy upon rectal mucosal HIV RNA burden and mononuclear cell apoptosis. *AIDS* 1998;12:597–604.
295. Greenberg RE, Mir R, Bank S, et al. Resolution of intestinal cryptosporidiosis after treatment of AIDS with AZT. *Gastroenterology* 1989;97:1327–1330.
296. Chandrasekar PH. "Cure" of chronic cryptosporidiosis during treatment with azidothymidine in a patient with the acquired immune deficiency syndrome [Letter]. *Am J Med* 1987;83:187.
297. Manabe YC, Clark DP, Moore RD, et al. Cryptosporidiosis in patients with AIDS: correlates of disease and survival. *Clin Infect Dis* 1998;27:536–542.
298. Schmidt W, Wahnschaffe U, Schäfer M, et al. Rapid increase of mucosal CD4 T-cells followed by clearance of intestinal cryptosporidiosis in an AIDS patient receiving highly active antiretroviral therapy indicating effective mucosal immune reconstitution. *Gastroenterology* 2001;128:984–987.
299. Foudraine NA, Weverling GJ, van Gool T, et al. Improvement of chronic diarrhoea in patients with advanced HIV-1 infection during potent antiretroviral therapy. *AIDS*1998;12:35–41.
300. Carr A, Marriott D, Field A, et al. Treatment of HIV-1-associated microsporidiosis and cryptosporidiosis with combination antiretroviral therapy. *Lancet* 1998;351:256–261.
301. Janoff EN, Smith PD. Emerging concepts in gastrointestinal aspects of HIV- pathogenesis and management. *Gastroenterology* 2001;120:607–621.
302. Sulkowski MS, Thomas DL, Chaisson RE, et al. Hepatotoxicity associated with antiretroviral therapy in adults infected with human immunodeficiency virus and the role of hepatitis C or B virus infection. *JAMA* 2000;283:74–80.
303. Max B, Sherer R. Management of the adverse effects of antiretroviral therapy and medication adherence. *Clin Infect Dis* 2000;30[Suppl 2]:S96–S116.
304. Brinkman K, ter Hofstede HJ, Burger DM, et al. Adverse effects of reverse transcriptase inhibitors: mitochondrial toxicity as common pathway. *AIDS* 1998;12:1735–1744.
305. Brinkman K, Smeitink JA, Romijn JA, et al. Mitochondrial toxicity induced by nucleoside-analogue reverse-transcriptase inhibitors is a key factor in the pathogenesis of antiretroviral-therapy-related lipodystrophy. *Lancet* 1999;354:1112–1115.
306. Carr A, Samaras K, Chisholm DJ, et al. Pathogenesis of HIV-1-protease inhibitor-associated peripheral lipodystrophy, hyperlipidaemia, and insulin resistance. *Lancet* 1998;351:1881–1883.
307. Burger DM, Hoetelmans RMW, Koopman PP, et al. Clinically relevant drug interactions with antiretroviral agents. *Antiviral Ther* 1997;2:149.

30

ENTERIC INFECTIONS IN HIV-1-INFECTED CHILDREN

HARLAND S. WINTER
TIEN-LAN CHANG

Infections of the gastrointestinal tract rank first among the worldwide causes of morbidity and mortality in children infected with HIV-1 (1). In the United States, such infections result in malnutrition and disability in HIV-1-infected children but are less frequently a cause of death. Although the diagnostic approach to enteric infections is similar for both children and adults, the spectrum and management of enteric infections in children infected with HIV-1 differ from those in HIV-1-infected adults. This chapter reviews the epidemiology of HIV-1 infection in children, the risk factors for enteric infections, the clinical features common to HIV-1-infected children, and the diagnostic and management issues involved in the treatment of opportunistic infections in HIV-1-infected children.

EPIDEMIOLOGY OF HIV-1 INFECTION IN CHILDREN

Modes of Infection

Children can acquire HIV-1 infection either perinatally from their mother (vertical transmission) or from contaminated blood or blood products. Since the institution of stringent screening procedures for blood donors in 1983 and specific HIV-1 testing of donated blood in 1985, the number of transfusion-acquired cases of AIDS in children in the United States has fallen dramatically. Only one case of HIV-1 infection, transmitted via blood transfusion from a seronegative donor to an infant, has been reported since screening procedures began (2,3).

The risk for receiving transfused blood from an HIV-1-infected person is estimated to be less than 1 in 40,000 (3). In the United States between 1981 and 1989, approximately 15% of children with HIV-1 infection acquired the infection from blood products, and 85% acquired it via perinatal transmission (4). In the 1990s, more than 95% of newly diagnosed cases of pediatric HIV-1 infection were associated with vertical transmission. In developing countries, HIV-1 transmission via blood transfusion remains a concern because the prevalence of HIV-1 disease in the general population is high and many nations do not routinely screen donors for HIV-1 (5). The rate of perinatal vertical transmission of HIV-1 infection from mothers to their infants ranges from 3% to 50%, depending on the resources available to pregnant women (6). Several factors may contribute to variations in the transmission rate. First, infection may be transmitted more frequently to infants born to women who are symptomatic and consequently have more advanced AIDS (7). Data have shown that giving zidovudine during pregnancy decreases the transmission rate to less than 10% (8). Studies reported at the World AIDS Conference in Durban, South Africa, describe how single doses of nevirapine given to mothers during labor and then to infants after birth dramatically decrease the vertical transmission of HIV-1. These observations suggest that viral replication and burden are important determinants of perinatal transmission. Second, the presence of maternal antibodies to specific epitopes of HIV-1 glycoprotein 120 may reduce the risk for transmission (9). Third, breast-feeding affects the rate of transmission because HIV-1 may be present in the milk of HIV-1-infected women (10). In a prospective study of 16 breast-fed infants born to African women who underwent seroconversion after delivery, the rate of postnatal transmission was estimated to be 36% to 53% (11). In Australia, the rate of perinatal transmission was 50% among breast-fed infants of HIV-1-infected women, 17% among the bottle-fed (12), and 27% among the breast-fed infants of women who underwent seroconversion post partum (13). The results of these and other studies suggest that breast-feeding is an additional risk for vertical transmission. Currently, because of the infant mortality associated with feeding formulas in unsanitary living conditions, the World Health Organization encourages the

H. S. Winter and **T.-L. Chang:** Division of Pediatric Gastroenterology and Nutrition, Department of Pediatrics, Massachusetts General Hospital for Children, Boston, Massachusetts practice of breast-feeding regardless of the mother's HIV-1 status (14). In countries where infant mortality from enteric infection is low, HIV-1-infected mothers should not breast-feed their infants. Furthermore, evidence suggests that the mortality of HIV-1-infected African mothers who breast-feed is increased in comparison with that of HIV-1-infected mothers who provide formula to their children (15,16). A reliable risk–benefit analysis considering the social aspects of each affected community, the health of the mother and infant, and the risk for HIV-1 transmission from breast-feeding is needed to provide guidance to governmental and other agencies involved in supporting programs for maternal and child health.

Prevalence

Based on seroprevalence studies and mathematical models, the World Health Organization estimates that 10 million persons have become infected with HIV-1 during the past decade, including 3 million women, primarily of childbearing age, and 500,000 children (14). Approximately 80% of these women and children live in sub-Saharan Africa (5). In developed countries, approximately 2% of reported patients with AIDS are under the age of 13 years. However, in developing countries, pediatric HIV-1-infected patients comprise 15% to 20% of all AIDS cases (5). Significantly, the number of HIV-1-infected children is almost 10 times the number of reported cases of AIDS in children.

Mortality and Morbidity

The mortality of children in the United States infected with HIV-1 is related to age at diagnosis, the presence or absence of opportunistic infection, and the CD4+ T-lymphocyte count or ratio of CD4+ to CD8+ lymphocytes. Children younger than 6 months with an AIDS-defining illness have a 1-year mortality rate of 45% to 55%, considerably higher than that of older children (15% to 28%) (17). Mortality is increased significantly in pediatric patients in whom certain opportunistic infections develop. For example, the median survival time is 4 to 10 months for children with disseminated nontuberculous mycobacterial infection (18–20), 9 months for those with *Pneumocystis carinii* pneumonia, and 63 months for those with pneumonia caused by *Haemophilus influenzae* or gram-positive organisms (17). Of children who acquired opportunistic infections, 92% had an abnormal ratio of CD4+ to CD8+ cells or a low CD4+ T-cell count; among those who died, 90% had a low CD4+ T-cell count (21).

Gastrointestinal infections are an important cause of morbidity in HIV-1-infected children. Diarrhea is present in 20% to 35% of children with AIDS, and malnutrition with growth failure is present in 45% to 60% (6,22–24). Gastrointestinal infections do not appear to shorten survival in HIV-1-infected children in developed countries (22). In contrast, in developing nations, diarrhea is the most common cause of death (1,25). The mortality rates attributed to diarrhea in Zairian infants followed from birth to the first 12 months of life were 132 per 1,000 live births for HIV-1-infected infants and 12 per 1,000 live births for uninfected infants (1). Persistent diarrhea lasting longer than 14 days occurred 4.8 times more often in HIV-1-infected Zairian children than in uninfected children (1). Moreover, 32% of all deaths in these HIV-1-infected children and 8% of deaths in HIV-1-uninfected children were attributed to persistent diarrhea (1).

In the United States and developed countries, morbidity and mortality from enteric infections may be more subtle (23–25). Diarrhea and malabsorption resulting from enteric infection may cause malnutrition, which in a growing child may impair T-cell function and increase the probability of opportunistic infection. Thus, in contrast to the rapid clinical deterioration observed in HIV-1-infected children with diarrhea in developing countries, the clinical presentation often is chronic disease with malnutrition and growth failure in developed countries.

PATHOBIOLOGY OF ENTERIC INFECTIONS IN HIV-1-INFECTED CHILDREN

Enteric infections in HIV-1-infected children affect gastrointestinal tract function, immune function, HIV-1 infection of the intestinal mucosa, maternal health, and malnutrition.

Gastrointestinal Function

Gastrointestinal function in the newborn and infant may facilitate the translocation of pathogens, including HIV-1, across the mucosal barrier. The secretion of gastric acid, an important barrier against enteric infection, is decreased in the first days of life and increases to adult levels by 1 to 3 months of age (26). Consequently, the neonate who swallows pathogenic organisms at birth may be at increased risk for infection because of an ineffective gastric acid barrier. The secretion of enzymes such as enterokinase, chymotrypsin, and carboxypeptidase is decreased in the first year of life, so that enteric pathogens and toxins, in theory, may not be inactivated effectively (27). The increased susceptibility to some enteric infections in infants may be explained by the higher number of receptor sites on intestinal epithelial cells for rotavirus and *Escherichia coli* heat-stable enterotoxin (28). In addition to differences in epithelial cell membrane proteins, intestinal permeability to carbohydrates and proteins is greater in infants than in adults (29). Thus, multiple nonimmunologic factors—secretion of gastric acid and proteolytic enzymes, binding of enteric pathogens to the mucosa, and intestinal permeability—may contribute to an enhanced translocation of pathogens across the mucosal barrier in children.

Immune Function

In newborn infants, the systemic immune responses to foreign antigens and infectious organisms are reduced (30), as are mucosal immune responses, reflected in reduced levels of fecal and salivary secretory immunoglobulin A (IgA) in the first month of life (31). In children with HIV-1 infection, particularly those with opportunistic infections, absolute numbers of CD4+ T cells and ratios of CD4+ to CD8+ T cells are reduced, antibody responses to immunization are impaired, and lymphocyte proliferative responses to vaccine antigens are abnormal (32,33). These alterations in systemic immune function are likely a consequence of HIV-1 infection or the accompanying malnutrition. Little is known about the effects of HIV-1 infection on the mucosal immune function of children.

In the normal newborn, maternal IgG acquired transplacentally and IgA in breast milk provide some mucosal immune function and reduce the severity and duration of intestinal symptoms during epidemics of enteric infection (34). Similarly, intravenous IgG (35) may protect the HIV-1-infected child from enteric infection.

HIV-1 Infection of the Intestinal Mucosa

HIV-1 messenger RNA can be identified in the small-intestinal mucosa of HIV-1-infected children (36), but as in adults, HIV-1 infects only lymphocytes macrophages in the lamina propria. Unlike the duodenal mucosa of HIV-1-infected adults, the duodenal mucosa of HIV-1-infected children frequently has a nodular appearance (Fig. 30.1), caused by the expansion of lymphoid elements in the lamina propria (Fig. 30.2). The cause of the proliferation of the cellular elements of the lamina propria is not known, but the proliferation may be analogous to the lymphoid interstitial pneumonia commonly observed in HIV-1-infected children but rarely in HIV-1-infected adults.

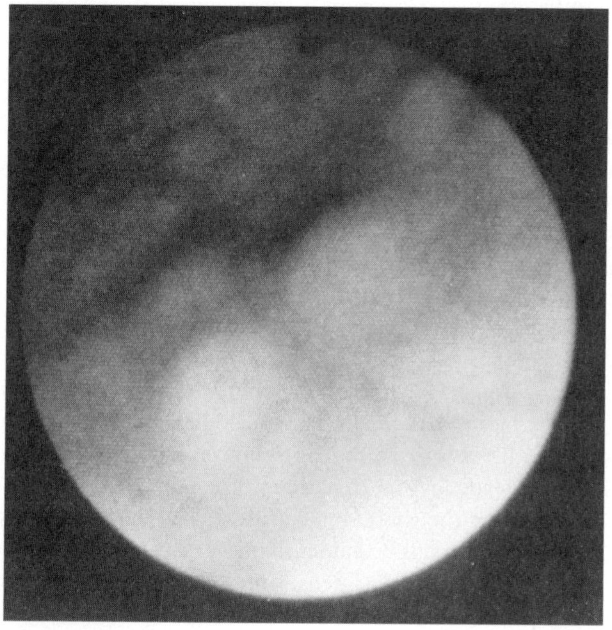

FIGURE 30.1. Nodular duodenal mucosa in an HIV-1-infected child with an identifiable enteric pathogen.

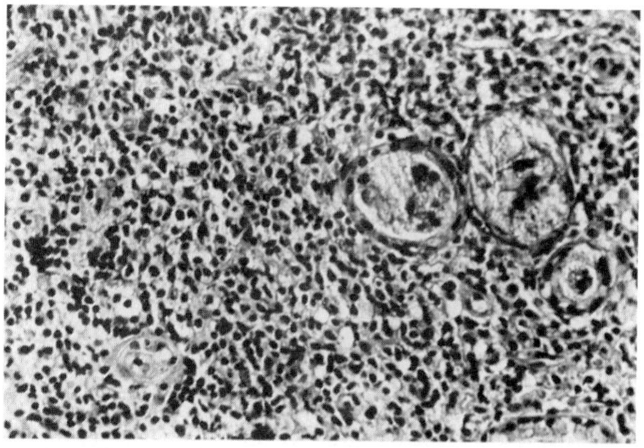

FIGURE 30.2. Lymphoid proliferation of the small-intestinal lamina propria in an HIV-1-infected child.

There is no solid evidence in adults or children that intestinal epithelial cells are infected with HIV-1 (37). However, the observation that lactose malabsorption develops earlier in HIV-1-infected children than would be predicted by normal genetic influences supports the hypothesis that maturation of the enterocytes is altered. The mechanism for this epithelial cell dysfunction and any possible relationship to lymphoid proliferation is not known. However, the specific activity of the brush border enzyme lactase is decreased. This observation correlates with impaired lactose absorption in HIV-1-infected infants. In HIV-1-infected children, lactase gene expression by *in situ* hybridization is decreased (38) (Figs. 30.3 and 30.4). A

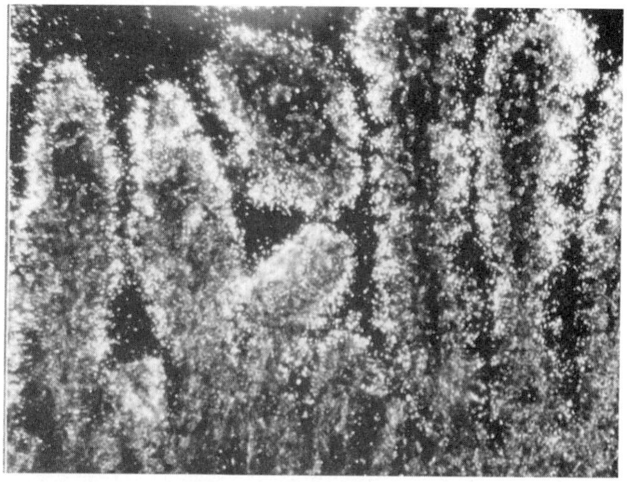

FIGURE 30.3. Lactase messenger RNA expression detected by *in situ* hybridization in the normal small intestine of a child. Detection of messenger RNA along the enteric villus.

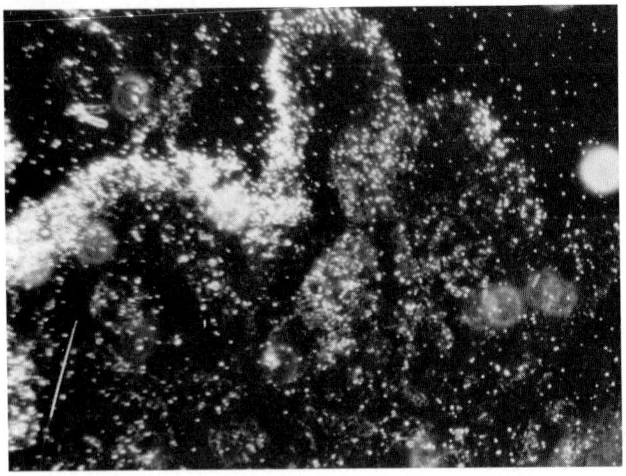

FIGURE 30.4. Lactase messenger RNA is decreased along the villus of an HIV-1-infected child.

mosaic pattern recently reported in normal adults with alactasia closely resembles the pattern of messenger RNA expression observed in HIV-1-infected children.

Maternal Health

An HIV-1-infected mother who becomes symptomatic with fever, weight loss, or diarrhea contributes to the illness of her child through at least two mechanisms. First, the mother may be a source of infectious agents for her child, either via placenta and breast milk (vertical transmission) or via the oral–fecal route (horizontal transmission). Second, a mother who is ill may be less able to care for an HIV-1-infected child for physical or psychological reasons. For infants not infected with HIV-1, the incidence of persistent diarrhea is nearly double if the HIV-1-infected mother is symptomatic; the risk is increased further if the mother dies (1). Regardless of the HIV-1 status of the child, the early introduction of either milk formula or solid food into the infant's diet correlates with the occurrence of acute diarrhea (1). Thus, in the management of an HIV-1-infected child, maternal health status must be considered.

Malnutrition

In developing nations where chronic diarrhea, enteric infections, and malnutrition are prevalent, severe malnutrition is a recognized risk factor for malabsorption and chronic diarrhea (39). Because of altered gastrointestinal function, increased nutritional requirements, reduced nutrient reserves, and poor maternal health, malnutrition is common in children infected with HIV-1. Protein-calorie malnutrition and deficiencies in micronutrients such as zinc and vitamin A (40) are associated with defects in cellular immunity and absorptive function. Vitamin A supplementation appears to decrease the risk for severe watery diarrhea but increases the risk for cough (41). These nutritional and immunologic deficiencies are also risk factors for diarrheal disease and enteric infection (42,43). Thus, a self-perpetuating cycle of malnutrition, malabsorption, immunodeficiency, and enteric infection occurs in HIV-1-infected children and is more severe in HIV-1-infected children than in adults.

CLINICAL ILLNESS

Viral Infections

Rotavirus usually causes diarrhea in children 3 months to 3 years of age, whereas newborns and older children tend to be asymptomatic or have minimal symptoms (44). In outbreaks of gastroenteritis in day care centers in the United States, rotavirus accounts for approximately half of cases with an identifiable cause, followed in frequency by adenovirus (4% to 9%) (45,46) and astrovirus (2% to 7%) (46,47). However, in malnourished or immunocompromised children, including those infected with HIV-1, rotavirus causes a protracted diarrhea (48), and in rare cases it can disseminate beyond the intestinal tract and cause acute hepatitis (49). In contrast, rotavirus does not appear to be a significant pathogen in adult patients with HIV-1 infection (50,51). The diagnosis of rotavirus infection is based on identification of the virus in the stool by an enzyme-linked immunoassay (52). Treatment of rotavirus-induced diarrhea consists of replacement of fluids and electrolytes. If the diarrhea persists for more than a week, nutritional support is necessary. Human serum immunoglobulin administered enterally may be beneficial for children with intractable diarrhea (53,54), but its effectiveness in HIV-1-infected children remains unproven.

Adenoviruses are common pathogens of the respiratory and gastrointestinal tracts. More than 40 different serotypes have been identified, but approximately 70% of adenovirus-associated enteric infections in normal children are attributable to serotypes 40 and 41 (55). The diarrhea in children caused by adenoviruses is related to injury of the small-intestinal mucosa. In one fatal case of adenovirus gastroenteritis, in a person not infected with HIV-1, virus was identified by electron microscopy in the intestinal epithelial cells (56). In children with HIV-1 infection and in other immunocompromised states, adenovirus can cause fulminant hepatitis as part of a disseminated infection that involves the lungs, liver, bone marrow, heart, and brain (57,58). Gastrointestinal hemorrhage has been reported to occur in 30% of immunocompromised patients with disseminated adenovirus infection (58). Adenovirus can be identified in the stool by culture or an enzyme-linked immunoassay. It has been identified by electron microscopy in colonic biopsy specimens from HIV-1-infected adult patients with adenovirus colitis (59) and in the stool of 15% of a group of adult men with HIV-1 who had diarrhea (vs. 5% of patients without diarrhea). The serotypes reported in HIV-1-infected patients have been serotypes other than types 40 and 41. Adenovirus is also a common pathogen in pharyngitis and respiratory infections, and a positive stool culture can be caused by virus shed from the tonsils and airway secretions and does not necessarily indicate enteric infection. Other than supportive measures, no specific treatment is known for adenovirus infection, although human serum globulin was used successfully in clearing adenovirus-induced pneumonia and hepatitis in a child with combined immunodeficiency (60). Ribavirin has potential as an experimental therapy.

The role of cytomegalovirus (CMV) as an enteric pathogen in immunocompetent children is unclear, except for its association with a protein-losing hypertrophic gastropathy (61). Children can acquire the infection vertically or horizontally. The risk for vertical transmission of CMV from a maternal carrier is approximately 1% in healthy infants. The majority of these infants are asymptomatic (62,63). In HIV-1-infected infants, however, the risk for infection is higher. In a group of children born to HIV-1-positive women and followed for 2 to 74 months, CMV was present in the urine in 46% of HIV-1-infected children and in 8% of children whose HIV-1 status was indeterminate (64). In patients infected with HIV-1, CMV can cause inflammatory lesions anywhere in the gastrointestinal tract, from the oral cavity to the rectum (65). Symptoms of CMV-induced disease include dysphagia, abdominal pain, vomiting, diarrhea, and upper or lower gastrointestinal bleeding; as in adults, hemorrhagic gastritis, ileitis, and colitis have all been reported in HIV-1-infected children with CMV infection (66,67).

Establishing CMV as the cause of enteric disease in a child is a diagnostic challenge. A urine culture positive for CMV, positive results of serology, and viral shedding in the gut can all be found in children with or without active disease. Consequently, the histopathologic identification of CMV in the presence of inflammation is the best way presently to confirm its pathogenic role (68). *In situ* hybridization with DNA probes complimentary for CMV has been proposed as an alternative or supportive diagnostic tool (69), but its utility remains to be established.

Treatment of CMV-induced gastrointestinal disease in HIV-1-infected adults with ganciclovir is generally effective in reducing disease activity (62,70). In a retrospective study of immunocompromised children (allograft recipients) with CMV disease involving different organs, 54% of patients improved after receiving 5 to 15 mg of ganciclovir per kilogram daily for 1 to 5 weeks (71). Foscarnet is an alternative drug for patients who fail to respond to ganciclovir (72,73). Both ganciclovir and foscarnet are associated with significant marrow suppression. Human immunoglobulin may have a beneficial effect when used in conjunction with ganciclovir in the treatment of CMV disease (74). The HIV-1-infected child with diarrhea, no focal or inflammatory enteric lesion, and CMV in the stool should not be treated for CMV-induced disease.

Other viruses have been detected by immunoassay or electron microscopy in the stools of HIV-1-infected adults with diarrhea. In HIV-1-infected children, astrovirus, picobirnavirus, and caliciviruses (75) have not been identified. Mucocutaneous herpes simplex virus infection has been reported in fewer than 1% of HIV-1-infected children (17).

Bacterial Infections

Bacterial infections, including those caused by *Salmonella, Shigella, Campylobacter, Yersinia, Clostridium difficile,* and *Escherichia coli* organisms, account for only a minor proportion of enteric infections in the general population in most developed countries. The exact incidence of enteric bacterial infections in HIV-1-infected children is unknown, but some studies suggest an increased risk for *Salmonella* infection in HIV-1-infected patients (76,77) in comparison with the general population. In HIV-1-infected children, enteric organisms (including *Salmonella, Enterococcus, E. coli, Lactobacillus, Enterobacter* species, and *Citrobacter*) accounted for almost half of the pathogens causing bacteremia (78). Because of the possibility of relapse and systemic dissemination, a longer course of antimicrobial treatment of enteric pathogens may be required in HIV-1-infected children than is recommended for immunocompetent hosts.

Strains of *E. coli* may be important causes of diarrhea in children in developing nations (1,22). In a study of Zairian children with an identifiable cause of diarrhea, pathogenic *E. coli* bacteria were isolated from the stool of 30% of HIV-1-negative children and 78% of HIV-1-infected children (22). These bacteria may be present in the colon or small intestine. *E. coli* and other bacteria, such as *Klebsiella,* have been found in high concentration in the small intestine of HIV-1-infected children with diarrhea (79,80). The frequency of bacterial overgrowth in HIV-1-infected children is not known, but overgrowth should be suspected in a child with elevated breath hydrogen or an early rise in breath hydrogen during a lactose breath test. The prevalence and importance of small-bowel bacterial overgrowth in the development of diarrhea in HIV-1-infected children are unknown.

C. difficile is present in the stool of 29% of normal neonates and 10% of children 4 months to 2 years of age (81). Consequently, the significance of comparable levels of *C. difficile* in the stool of HIV-1-infected children with diarrhea in these age groups is questionable. Certain serotypes of *C. difficile* appear to be associated with pathogenicity, even in infants (86). Although *C. difficile* colitis has been reported in infants and children (82,83), it has not been reported in HIV-1-infected children. Treatment of *C. difficile*-induced colitis with either vancomycin or metronidazole is effective in HIV-1-infected adults, but recurrence or treatment failure is possible (84).

Helicobacter pylori is recognized as an etiologic agent in peptic ulcer and gastritis in both adults and children. Serologic studies suggest a decreased incidence of *H. pylori* in both HIV-1-infected children and adults in comparison with the general population (85–87). Hypotheses to explain this decrease include an increased use of antibiotics and reduced acid production in HIV-1-infected patients (85).

Mycobacterial Infections

HIV-1-infected children infected with *Mycobacterium avium* complex (MAC) typically have multisystemic disease involving the bone marrow, lungs, liver, mesenteric lymph nodes, and gastrointestinal tract (18–20). The prevalence rate of disseminated MAC infection in children infected with HIV-1 is 11.4% (Pediatric Spectrum of Disease Project) (18). The gastrointestinal tract and respiratory system are thought to be potential sites of entry for MAC organisms (17), and a low CD4+ T-cell count is the major risk factor for disseminated MAC infection. MAC is identified in 18% of children with a CD4+ count below 50/mm^3 but only in 3% of children with a CD4+ count above 100/mm^3 (18). Abdominal pain and diarrhea are common in children with disseminated MAC infection, and the organism can be grown from the stool. Although acid-fast bacilli-laden macrophages are found in the jejunal mucosa, gastrointestinal injury by MAC organisms in HIV-1-infected children is rare. No effective treatment at present eradicates MAC from the gastrointestinal tract, but colony counts of MAC in blood cultures are decreased in response to single agents or combinations of drugs, such as azithromycin, clarithromycin, ethambutol, ciprofloxacin, amikacin, rifampin, and clofazimine (88). Clinical trials to evaluate the treatment of disseminated MAC infection in children are in progress.

In contrast to the high prevalence of MAC infection, few cases of *Mycobacterium tuberculosis* infection and no cases of gastrointestinal tuberculosis have been reported in HIV-1-infected children in the United States (89). Two cases of intestinal perforation associated with *M. tuberculosis* infection have been reported in HIV-1-infected adults (90). Because the demographic characteristics of the populations at risk for tuberculosis and for HIV-1 infection are similar, an increase in the number of HIV-1-infected children with tuberculosis is expected, and more cases with gastrointestinal tuberculosis likely will be identified.

Protozoan Infections

Giardia lamblia and *Cryptosporidium parvum* (91–93) are the most common protozoan pathogens identified in HIV-1-infected children, but *Isospora belli* and Microsporidia have been found in immunodeficient adults. *Isospora* is a rare pathogen even in HIV-1-infected adults, but Microsporidia is identified in as many as 50% of HIV-1-infected adults with chronic diarrhea in whom no pathogen can be identified by standard stool analysis (94–96). Although Microsporidia can be detected by light microscopy of touch preparations stained with Giemsa or paraffin-embedded sections of small intestine stained with hematoxylin and eosin, the diagnosis is enhanced by electron microscopy (94–96). Because the jejunum is a preferential site for Microsporidia infection (94), difficulty in obtaining tissue samples from this area may explain the absence of reported Microsporidia infection in children with HIV-1.

Giardia infection usually causes watery diarrhea, bloating, and abdominal pain, but the organisms can also be isolated from asymptomatic persons. It occurs more frequently in children than in adults, although its prevalence is not increased in HIV-1-infected children versus uninfected children with diarrhea (1,22,97). Giardiasis can be treated with 10 mg of metronidazole per kilogram three times daily for 10 to 14 days, or with furazolidone.

Cryptosporidium infection in HIV-1-infected children typically causes a chronic and debilitating secretory diarrhea. Only two cases were reported among 789 children with AIDS in New York from 1983 to 1990 (17). In contrast, *Cryptosporidium* infection was found in Tanzania in 13% of HIV-1-positive and 6% of HIV-1-negative children hospitalized for chronic diarrhea (97), and in Brazil in 7.1% of HIV-1-infected but only 0.4% of HIV-1-negative children (98). In addition to the small and large intestine, *Cryptosporidium* organisms can colonize gallbladder, bile duct, and pancreatic duct, and they have been implicated as a cause of cholangitis (91). Asymptomatic *Cryptosporidium* infection has been reported in HIV-1-infected adults (92), but its frequency is unknown. A retrospective study showed a 30% remission rate among 38 HIV-1-infected adults; those patients in clinical remission had a higher total lymphocyte count (99). Currently, no proven effective treatment is available for eradicating *Cryptosporidium* in HIV-1-infected patients. Anecdotal reports suggest some clinical benefit (reduction of diarrhea) from octreotide in adults; human immunoglobulin administered enterally to a child with leukemia led to resolution of the infection (93,100). A clinical trial with bovine hyperimmune colostrum in HIV-1-infected children is currently under way, based on encouraging results in case reports (101).

Blastocystis hominis is a protozoan found in asymptomatic children and adults; its role as an enteric pathogen is still debated. In one study, *B. hominis* was found more often in HIV-1-infected children (3 of 23) with diarrhea than in HIV-1-negative children (none of 36) (97). In contrast, the incidence of *B. hominis* infection in HIV-1-infected adults may be lower than that in the HIV-1-negative population (51). The discrepancy in these observations could be a consequence of the small sample size of reported studies or of the increased incidence of *Blastocystis* infection documented in children.

Fungal Infections

Fungal infections in HIV-1-infected children are mainly caused by *Candida* and *Histoplasma. Candida albicans* and other species can cause oral thrush in 15% to 40% of HIV-

1-infected children (102), esophagitis in 13% (7), and disseminated candidiasis in 7% (99). A retrospective review of 156 HIV-1-infected children in New York identified 11 cases of disseminated candidiasis during 7.5 years (99). Predisposing factors included central venous catheter placement, prolonged antibiotic use, oral thrush, and total parenteral nutrition. Neutropenia, defined as fewer than 200 cells per cubic millimeter, was present in only two patients and therefore was not a risk factor. *Candida* organisms were present in the esophagus in 45% of the 11 patients with candidiasis and in the gastrointestinal tract (location unspecified) in 18%. Other sites of *Candida* involvement included lungs, kidneys, brain, heart, liver, spleen, thyroid, skin, and bone. Coexistent enterococcal sepsis was present in 36% of patients, and mycobacterial disease in 27%. The mortality rate in this series, reported by Leibovitz et al. (99), was 90%. Four of the 11 cases were first diagnosed post mortem, which suggests that the presentation of disseminated candidiasis can be subtle. Treatment of *Candida* infection with fluconazole is effective for oral thrush and esophagitis (103), but for disseminated candidiasis, amphotericin B remains the treatment of choice in children.

Histoplasma capsulatum infection is endemic in the central United States. Disseminated histoplasmosis has been described in HIV-1-infected children and may be the AIDS-defining illness in as many as 8% of children and 25% of adults in the region where infection is endemic (104,105). Although gastrointestinal involvement in HIV-1-infected children has not been reported, 20% of other immunocompromised patients with systemic histoplasmosis have evidence of gastrointestinal involvement (106). Granuloma formation association with *Histoplasma* infection may mimic Crohn's disease radiologically, and intestinal obstruction and perforation are potential complications. Amphotericin B at a dosage of 1 mg/kg daily for 30 days is the recommended treatment for children with disseminated histoplasmosis (105).

DIAGNOSTIC EVALUATION

In HIV-1-infected children, rate of growth, fat-free mass, and energy intake are inversely related to viral load (107). Thus, any assessment of the nutritional status should begin with a determination of the activity of HIV-1 replication. In evaluating a child with a putative enteric infection, the treating physician should consider the following: First, the identification of some pathogens, including CMV, adenovirus, *Mycobacterium,* Microsporidia, and fungi, requires histologic examination of tissue biopsy specimens. Second, despite thorough investigation, infection will remain undiagnosed in up to 50% to 60% of children (1,23). Third, successful identification of a pathogen(s) may not reveal the cause of a patient's gastrointestinal symptoms. Many enteric pathogens can be found in the stool of asymptomatic persons, and multiple pathogens can be present in a single patient. Finally, a definite diagnosis does not guarantee an effective specific treatment. The vigor of the diagnostic investigation should be weighed against the severity of the symptoms. Some investigative procedures can be invasive and difficult for children. For adults, a staged evaluation has been proposed (108). A similar diagnostic algorithm, presented in Fig. 30.5, is based on a child's clinical status and ability to tolerate procedures that may help to make a diagnosis in the majority of patients (Fig. 30.2). According to this algorithm, the initial evaluation of a child with diarrhea should include stool cultures for bacterial pathogens, including *Salmonella, Shigella, Campylobacter, Yersinia,* and *C. difficile.* Culture for *E. coli* strain O157:H7 is now routine in many clinical laboratories in the United States and should be performed if blood is present in the stool. Parasites, including *G. lamblia, C. parvum,* and *I. belli,* can be identified in the stool by immunofluorescent techniques (e.g., *Giardia* antigen and *Cryptosporidium* antigen) or by histologic stains (e.g., Kinyoun stain for *Cryptosporidium* and *Isospora*) (109). Viruses such as rotavirus and adenovirus can be detected in the stool by enzyme-linked assays. These stool tests should be repeated at least once if no pathogen is isolated initially. Tests for enteroadherent factor-positive *E. coli* are not commonly available but may be performed at certain laboratories (e.g., Centers for Disease Control) if no other pathogens are isolated and the patient has a history of travel to regions where these bacteria are prevalent. Blood cultures should be obtained if fever is present to identify disseminated fungal infection, mycobacterial infection, or gastrointestinal bacterial infection, such as with *Salmonella* organisms, which tend to cause bacteremia.

Endoscopy in HIV-1-infected children is indicated to evaluate bleeding from the upper or lower gastrointestinal tract, dysphagia, and persistent diarrhea causing significant wasting and malnutrition. Endoscopic biopsy specimens should be obtained in saline solution for culture of fungi and mycobacteria, viral culture medium for culture of cytomegalovirus and adenovirus, formalin fixative for light microscopy, and glutaraldehyde fixative for electron microscopy to look for adenovirus, CMV, and microsporidians. In addition, if clinically indicated, endoscopic aspirates of the small-bowel fluid can be cultured quantitatively for aerobes and anaerobes to establish a diagnosis of bacterial overgrowth.

In addition to specific tests for pathogens and stool tests for fat or reducing substances, tests that evaluate absorptive function may be helpful in the management of diarrhea in children. Malabsorption of specific sugars can be assessed by breath hydrogen tests and are of particular value in children. However, the clinical significance of steatorrhea is unknown (110). In one study of 17 HIV-1-infected children, an abnormal lactose breath hydrogen test result correlated significantly with diarrheal disease (111), but in another study no such correlation was found (38). Nevertheless, if the breath test result is positive, the management

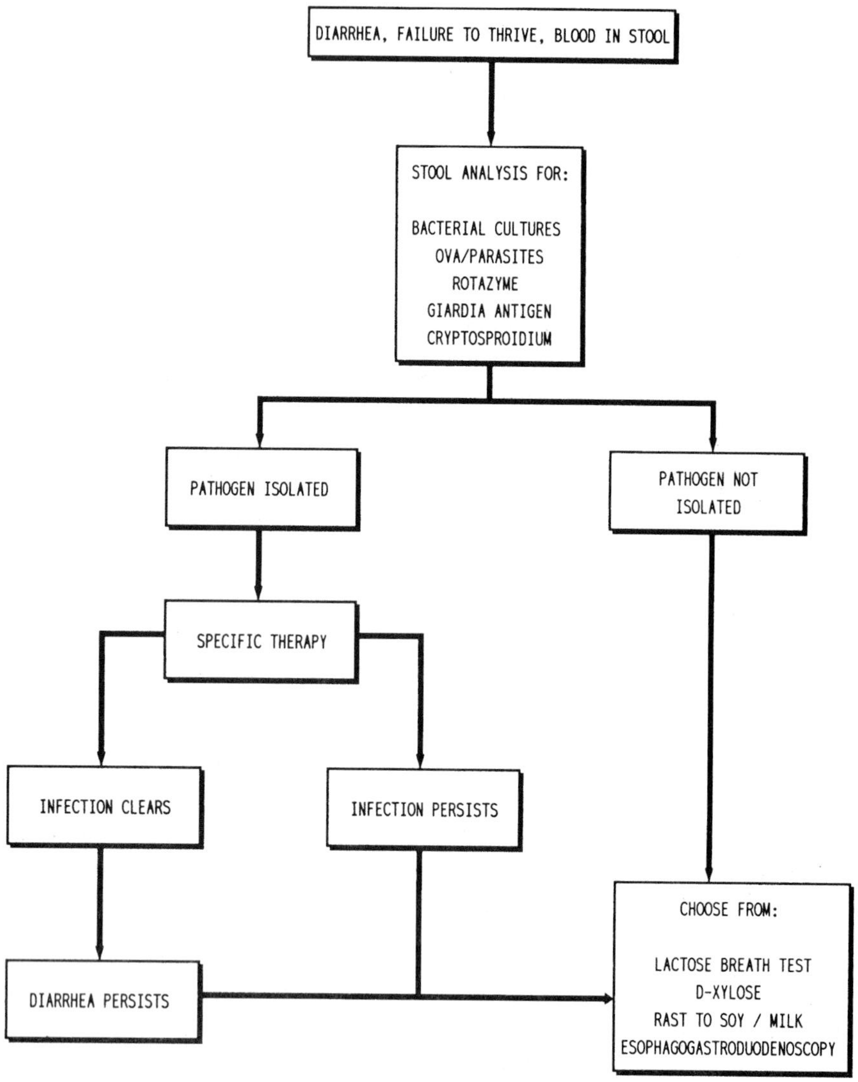

FIGURE 30.5. Algorithm for the diagnostic evaluation of a child suspected of having an enteric infection.

of a child with diarrhea may include a diet that avoids lactose. In addition, an early rise in the breath hydrogen concentration during a lactose breath test is an indication of small-bowel bacterial overgrowth (112). Therefore, breath hydrogen tests may be used as diagnostic tools in children with diarrhea in whom a pathogen is not identified and for whom a modified formula must be selected.

The serum levels of antibodies to food proteins are frequently elevated in children infected with HIV-1 (113). The presence of these antibodies may indicate only increased mucosal permeability rather than true allergy; however, increased numbers of eosinophils in the stool (determined by Wright or Giemsa stain), blood, or intestinal and rectal biopsy specimens provide additional evidence in support of an allergic cause.

MANAGEMENT OF PEDIATRIC HIV-1-RELATED ENTERIC INFECTION

If a specific treatable pathogen responsible for an HIV-1-related enteric infection is isolated from a child, medications can be administered according to the dosing schedules listed in Table 30.1. Because chronic carriage or prolonged fecal excretion of bacterial pathogens is common in the immunodeficient host, an extended course of treatment may be required. If no pathogen is found, an empiric course of antibiotic treatment may be considered if (a) it is suspected that a pathogen has been contracted during travel to a region where *E. coli* infection is endemic or (b) a positive breath hydrogen test result suggests small-bowel bacterial overgrowth.

TABLE 30.1. ANTIBIOTICS FOR ENTERIC INFECTIONS IN CHILDREN WITH HIV-1 INFECTION

Pathogen	Antibiotic	Dose/Duration
Salmonella	Ampicillin	100–200 mg/kg/d divided q6h for 10–14 days
	Ceftriaxone	100–150 mg/kg/d divided q12h for 10–14 days
	Chloramphenicol	80 mg/kg/d divided q6h for 10–14 days
	Ciprofloxacin	20–30 mg/kg/d divided q12h for 10–14 days
Campylobacter	Erythromycin	40 mg/kg/d divided q6h for 10 days
Shigella	TMP-SMX	10 mg/kg/d divided q12h for 5 days
	Ampicillin	100 mg/kg/d divided q6h for 5 days
	Ciprofloxacin	20–30 mg/kg/d divided q12h for 5 days
Clostridium difficile	Vancomycin	20 mg/kg/d divided q6h for 7 days
	Metronidazole	15–30 mg/kg/d divided q8h for 7 days
Giardia	Metronidazole	15–30 mg/kg/d divided q8h for 7 days
	Quinacrine HCl	6 mg/kg/d (maximum 300 mg/d) divided q8h for 7 days
	Furazolidone	6 mg/kg/d (maximum 400 mg/d) divided q6h for 7 days
Candida	Ketoconazole	5–10 mg/kg qd or divided q12h for 30 days
	Amphotericin B	0.5–1.5 mg/kg qd for 30 days
Histoplasma	Amphotericin B	0.5–1.5 mg/kg qd for 30 days

TMP-SMX, trimethoprim-sulfamethoxazole.

Beyond the acute phase of management, nutritional repletion has a key role in the overall medical care of children with HIV-1 and enteric infection. Repletion should begin with an assessment of the child's nutritional status and a determination of the number of calories and quantity of protein necessary to achieve appropriate weight gain. A determination of a child's caloric needs should take into account the following: nutritional status (ratio of weight-for-age to weight-for-height percentiles, midarm circumference, and triceps skinfold thickness), activity level, and severity of infection (fever and sepsis are known to increase energy demands). In HIV-1-infected girls, bone mineral content should be assessed (114). Measuring the serum total protein, albumin, prealbumin, and transferrin levels may help to assess the severity of protein deficiency. Deficiencies of micronutrients such as zinc, as previously mentioned, and selenium have been reported in children with HIV-1 infection (115,116), and levels should be monitored in the malnourished child. Selection of a formula or nutritional supplement for the HIV-1-infected child with an enteric infection depends on the severity of intestinal injury. If the infection cannot be eradicated and the mucosa restored to normal, special care should be taken to select a nutrient source that will sustain growth. Lactose-free formulas frequently are of benefit in HIV-1-infected children. For children with severe injury to the mucosa, hydrolyzed preparations with medium-chain triglyceride may be required. In children who are anorectic, a nasogastric catheter can be used temporarily (1 week to 1 month) for supplemental feedings to provide adequate nutrition. Because of the increased incidence of complications associated with a long-term indwelling nasogastric catheter (117,118), a gastrostomy may be preferable if supplemental feedings are required for more than a month. The supplemental feeding is best administered at night by a continuous drip, so that during the day the child can be orally stimulated with food. Daily monitoring of intake, output, and body weight will help to assess the adequacy of enteral feeding. Parenteral nutrition is indicated for children with chronic enteric infections, such as with MAC, for those who are unable to maintain or gain weight on enteral feedings, and for those who cannot be fed enterally because of vomiting, gastrointestinal bleeding, or pancreatitis. The relative risks and benefits of a central venous catheter for parenteral nutrition versus a gastrostomy should be considered carefully, especially when children are neutropenic or thrombocytopenic. This group appears to be at risk for complications such as infection, bleeding, and poor wound healing.

Recent advances in antiretroviral therapy have led to marked decreases in viral load. The use of protease inhibitor therapy has resulted in improved linear growth and weight gain (119,120). Whether these improvements in nutritional status will translate into a better quality of life and increase in longevity remains to be determined.

SUMMARY

The effect of enteric infections on the quality of life of children infected with HIV-1 is significant worldwide. Currently, only 40% to 50% of enteric infections in children infected with HIV-1 can be attributed to specific pathogens. The identification of new enteric pathogens in HIV-1-infected children has not resulted in the development of effective therapies. Medical interventions to treat infection with these pathogens are therefore mostly supportive. Optimal nutritional support and the provision of passive immunity may reduce morbidity and the frequency of enteric infection in HIV-1-infected children. However, to reduce morbidity and mortality in infants infected with HIV-1 globally, international public health efforts should be directed at providing appropriate nutrition for HIV-1-infected children and their families.

REFERENCES

1. Thea DM, St. Louis ME, Atido U, et al. A prospective study of diarrhea and HIV-1-1 infection among 429 Zairian infants. *N Engl J Med* 1983;329:1696–1702.
2. MacCarthy VP, Charles DL, Unger JL. Transfusion-associated HIV-1 infection in a neonate from a seronegative donor. *Am J Dis Child* 1987;2:84–87.
3. Ward JW, Holmberg SD, Allen JR, et al. Transmission of human immunodeficiency virus (HIV-1) by blood transfusions screened as negative for HIV-1 antibody. *N Engl J Med* 1988;318:473–478.
4. Jones DS, Byers RH, Bush TJ, et al. Epidemiology of transfusion-associated acquired immunodeficiency syndrome in children in the United States, 1981 through 1989. *Pediatrics* 1992; 89:123–127.
5. Quinn TC, Ruff A, Halsey N. Pediatric acquired immunodeficiency syndrome: special considerations for developing nations. *Pediatr Infect Dis J* 1992;11:558–568.
6. Oxtoby MJ. Perinatally acquired human immunodeficiency virus infection. *Pediatr Infect Dis J* 1990;9:609–619.
7. Ryder RW, Nsa E, Hassig SE, et al. Perinatal transmission of the human immunodeficiency virus type 1 to infants of seropositive women in Zaire. *N Engl J Med* 1989;320:1637–1642.
8. Centers for Disease Control. Zidovudine for the prevention of HIV-1 transmission from mother to infant. *MMWR Morb Mortal Wkly Rep* 1994;43:285–287.
90. Rossi P, Moschese V, Broliden PA, et al. Presence of maternal antibodies to human immunodeficiency virus 1 envelope glycoprotein gp120 epitopes correlates with the uninfected status of children born to seropositive mother. *Proc Natl Acad Sci U S A* 1989;86:8055–8058.
10. Michie CA, Gilmour J. Breast-feeding and the risks of viral transmission. *Arch Dis Child* 2001;84:381–382.
11. Van de Perre P, Simonon A, Msellati P, et al. Postnatal transmission of human immunodeficiency virus type 1 from mother to infant. A prospective cohort study in Kigali, Rwanda. *N Engl J Med* 1991;325:593–598.
12. Ziegler JB, Palasanthiran P, Cruickshank M, et al. Pediatric HIV-1: Australian perspective. *J AIDS* 1993;6[Suppl 1]: S20–S23.
13. Palasanthiran P, Ziegler JB, Stewart GJ, et al. Breast-feeding during primary maternal human immunodeficiency virus infection and risk of transmission from mother to infant. *J Infect Dis* 1983;167:441–444.
14. World Health Organization/United Nations Children's Fund. Statement on breast-feeding and HIV-1. WHO/UNICEF consultative meeting of April 30–May 1. *Wkly Epidemiol Rec* 1992;67:177–184.
15. Nduati R, Richardson BA, John G, et al. Effect of breast-feeding on mortality among HIV-1-1-infected women: a randomized trial. *Lancet* 2001;357:1651–1655.
16. Newell ML. Does breast-feeding really affect mortality among HIV-1-1-infected women? *Lancet* 2001;357:1634–1635.
17. Turner BJ, Denison M, Eppes SC, et al. Survival experience of 789 children with acquired immunodeficiency syndrome. *Pediatr Infect Dis J* 1993;12:310–320.
18. Horsburgh CR Jr, Caldwell B, Simonds RJ. Epidemiology of disseminated nontuberculous mycobacterial disease in children with acquired immunodeficiency syndrome. *Pediatr Infect Dis J* 1993;12:219–222.
19. Rutstein RM, Cobb P, McGowan KL, et al. *Mycobacterium avium–intracellulare* complex infection in HIV-1-infected children. *J AIDS* 1993;7:507–512.
20. Hoyt L, Oleske J, Holland B, et al. Nontuberculous mycobacteria in children with acquired immunodeficiency syndrome. *Pediatr Infect Dis J* 1992;11:354–360.
21. Duliege AM, Messiah A, Blanche S, et al. Natural history of human immunodeficiency virus type 1 infection in children: prognostic value of laboratory tests on the bimodal progression of the disease. *Pediatr Infect Dis J* 1992;11:630–635.
22. Pavia AT, Long EG, Ryder RW, et al. Diarrhea among African children born to human immunodeficiency virus-infected mothers: clinical, microbiologic and epidemiologic features. *Pediatr Infect Dis J* 1992;11:996–1003.
23. Italian Multicenter Study. Epidemiology, clinical features, and prognostic factors of paediatric HIV-1 infection. *Lancet* 1988;2: 1043–1046.
24. Pratt RD, Hatch R, Dankner WM, et al. Pediatric human immunodeficiency virus infection in a low seroprevalence area. *Pediatr Infect Dis J* 1993;12:304–310.
25. Pahwa S, Kaplan M, Fikrig S, et al. Spectrum of human T-cell lymphotropic virus type III infection in children. *JAMA* 1986; 255:2299–2305.
26. Grand RJ, Watkins JB, Torti FM. Development of the human gastrointestinal tract. *Gastroenterology* 1976;70:790–810.
27. Antonowicz I, Lebanthal E. Developmental pattern of small intestinal enterokinase and disaccharidase activities in the human fetus. *Gastroenterology* 1977;72:1299–1303.
28. Cohen MB, Guarino A, Shukla R, et al. Age-related differences in receptors for *Escherichia coli* heat-stable enterotoxin in the small and large intestine of children. *Gastroenterology* 1988;94:367–373.
29. Bezzara J, Thompson S, Dos Santos B, et al. Urinary lactose excretion of infants and adults following ingestion of disaccharide. *J Am Coll Nutr* 1988;7:417.
30. Madore DV, Johnson C, Phipps DC, et al. Safety and immune response to *Haemophilus influenzae* type b oligosaccharide-CRM197 conjugate vaccine in 1- to 6-month-old infants. *Pediatrics* 1990;85:331–337.
31. Selner JC, Merrill DAK, Clamen HN. Salivary immunoglobulin and albumin: development during the newborn period. *Pediatrics* 1968;72:685–689.
32. McKinney RE, Wilfert CM. Lymphocyte subsets in children younger than 2 years old: normal values in a population at risk for human immunodeficiency virus infection and diagnostic and prognostic application to infected children. *Pediatr Infect Dis J* 1992;11:639–644.
33. Borkowsky W, Rigaud M, Krasinski K, et al. Cell-mediated and humoral immune responses in children infected with human immunodeficiency virus during the first four years of life. *J Pediatr* 1992;120:371–375.
34. Ruiz-Palacios GM, Calva JJ, Pickering LK, et al. Protection of breast-fed infants against *Campylobacter* diarrhea by antibodies in human milk. *J Pediatr* 1990;116:707–713.
35. Ochs HD. Intravenous immunoglobulin in the treatment and prevention of acute infections in pediatric acquired immunodeficiency syndrome patients. *Pediatr Infect Dis J* 1987;6:509–511.
36. Poles MA. HIV-1 and the gut: feeding the enemy. *Physicians Res Network* (*www.prn.org*) 2000;5:15–18
37. Fox CH, Cottler-Fox M. The pathobiology of HIV-1 infection. *Immunol Today* 1992;13:353–356.
38. Miller TL, Orav EJ, Martin SR, et al. Malnutrition and carbohydrate malabsorption in children with vertically transmitted human immunodeficiency virus 1 infection. *Gastroenterology* 1991;100:1296–1302.

39. Berkowitz FE. Infections in children with severe protein-energy malnutrition. *Pediatr Infect Dis J* 1992;11:750–759.
40. Bogden JD, Kemp FW, Han S, et al. Status of selected nutrients and progression of human immunodeficiency virus type 1 infection. *Am J Clin Nutr* 2000;72:809–815.
41. Fawzi VW, Mbise R, Spiegelman D, et al. Vitamin A supplements and diarrheal and respiratory tract infections among children in Dar es Salaam, Tanzania. *Pediatrics* 2000;137: 660–667.
42. El Bushra HE, Ash L, Coulson AH, et al. Interrelationship between diarrhea and vitamin A deficiency: is vitamin A deficiency a risk factor for diarrhea? *Pediatr Infect Dis J* 1992;11: 380–384.
43. Keen CL, Gershwin ME. Zinc deficiency and immune function. *Annu Rev Nutr* 1990;10:415–431.
44. Bartlett AV III, Bednarz-Prashad J, DuPont HL, et al. Rotavirus gastroenteritis. *Annu Rev Med* 1987;38:399–415.
45. Van R, Wun CC, O'Ryan ML, et al. Outbreaks of human enteric adenovirus types 40 and 41 in Houston day care centers. *J Pediatr* 1992;120:516–521.
46. Mitchell DK, Van R, Morrow AL, Monroe SS, et al. Outbreaks of astrovirus gastroenteritis in day care centers. *J Pediatr* 1993; 123:725–732.
47. Kotloff KL, Herrmann JE, Blacklow NR, et al. The frequency of astrovirus as a cause of diarrhea in Baltimore children. *Pediatr Infect Dis J* 1992;11:587–589.
48. Oshitani H, Kasolo FC, Mpabalwani M. Association of rotavirus and human immunodeficiency virus infection in children hospitalized with acute diarrhea, Lusaka, Zambia. *J Infect Dis* 1994;169:897–900.
49. Gilger MA, Matson DO, Conner ME, et al. Extraintestinal rotavirus infections in children with immunodeficiency. *J Pediatr* 1992;120:912–917.
50. Smith PD, Lane HC, Gill VJ, et al. Intestinal infections in patients with the acquired immunodeficiency syndrome (AIDS). Etiology and response to therapy. *Ann Intern Med* 1988;108: 328–333.
51. Laughon BE, Druckman DA, Vernon AA, et al. Prevalence of enteric pathogens in homosexual men with and without AIDS. *Gastroenterology* 1988;94:984–993.
52. Knisley CV, Bednarz-Prashad AJ, Pickering LK. Detection of rotavirus in stool specimens using monoclonal and polyclonal based assay systems. *J Clin Microbiol* 1986;23:897–900.
53. Guarino A, Guandalini S, Albano F, et al. Enteral immunoglobulins for treatment of protracted rotaviral diarrhea. *Pediatr Infect Dis J* 1991;10:612–614.
54. Melamed I, Griffiths AM, Roifman CM. Benefit of oral immune globulin therapy in patients with immunodeficiency and chronic diarrhea. *J Pediatr* 1991;119:486–488.
55. Brandt CD, Kim HW, Rodrigues WJ, et al. Adenoviruses and pediatric gastroenteritis. *J Infect Dis* 1985;151:437.
56. Whitlaw A, Davies H. Electron microscopy of fatal adenovirus gastroenteritis. *Lancet* 1977;1:361.
57. Janner D, Petro AM, Belchis D, et al. Fatal adenovirus infection in a child with acquired immunodeficiency syndrome. *Pediatr Infect Dis J* 1990;9:434–436.
58. Krilov LR, Rubin LG, Frogel M, et al. Disseminated adenovirus infection with hepatic necrosis in patients with human immunodeficiency virus infection and other immunodeficiency states. *Rev Infect Dis* 1990;12:303–307.
59. Janoff EN, Orenstein JM, Manischewitz JF, et al. Adenovirus colitis in the acquired immunodeficiency syndrome. *Gastroenterology* 1991;100:976–979.
60. Dagan R, Schwartz RH, Insel RA, et al. Severe diffuse adenovirus 7a pneumonia in a child with combined immunodeficiency: possible therapeutic effect of human serum immunoglobulin containing a specific neutralizing antibody. *Pediatr Infect Dis J* 1984; 3:246–251.
61. Cieslak TJ, Mullett CT, Puntel RA, et al. Menetrier's disease associated with cytomegalovirus infection in children: report of two cases and review of the literature. *Pediatr Infect Dis J* 1993; 12:340–343.
62. Stagno S, Pass RF, Dworsky ME, et al. Maternal cytomegalovirus infection and perinatal transmission. *Clin Obstet Gynecol* 1982; 25:563–576.
63. Yow MD, Williamson DW, Leeds LJ, et al. Epidemiologic characteristics of cytomegalovirus infection in mothers and their infants. *Am J Obstet Gynecol* 1988;158:1189–1195.
64. Frenkel LD, Gaur S, Tsolia M, et al. Cytomegalovirus infection in children with AIDS. *Rev Infect Dis* 1990;12:S820–S826.
65. Schooley RT. Cytomegalovirus in the setting of infection with human immunodeficiency virus. *Rev Infect Dis* 1990;12: S811–S819.
66. Schwartz DL, So HB, Bungarz WR, et al. A case of life-threatening gastrointestinal hemorrhage in an infant with AIDS. *J Pediatr Surg* 1989;24:313–315.
67. Victoria MS, Nangia BS, Jindrak K. Cytomegalovirus pyloric obstruction in a child with acquired immunodeficiency syndrome. *Pediatr Infect Dis J* 1985;4:550–552.
68. Strano A. Light microscopy of selected viral diseases (morphology of viral inclusion bodies). *Pathol Annu* 1976;11:53–75.
69. Schwartz DA, Wilcox CM. Atypical cytomegalovirus inclusions in gastrointestinal biopsy specimens from patients with the acquired immunodeficiency syndrome: diagnostic role of *in situ* nucleic acid hybridization. *Hum Pathol* 1992;23:1019–1026.
70. Dietrich DT, Kotler DP, Busch DF, et al. Ganciclovir treatment of cytomegalovirus colitis in AIDS: a randomized, double-blind, placebo-controlled multicenter study. *J Infect Dis* 1993; 167:278–282.
71. Gudnason T, Belani KK, Balfour HH. Ganciclovir treatment of cytomegalovirus disease in immunocompromised children. *Pediatr Infect Dis J* 1989;8:436–440.
72. Dietrich DT, Poles MA, Dicker M, et al. Foscarnet treatment of cytomegalovirus gastrointestinal infections in acquired immunodeficiency syndrome patients who have failed ganciclovir induction. *Am J Gastroenterol* 1993;88:542–548.
73. Nelson MR, Connolly GM, Francis N, et al. Foscarnet in the treatment of cytomegalovirus infection of the esophagus and colon in patients with the acquired immunodeficiency syndrome. *Am J Gastroenterol* 1991;86:876–881.
74. Snydman DR. Cytomegalovirus immunoglobulins in the prevention and treatment of cytomegalovirus disease. *Rev Infect Dis* 1990;12[Suppl 7]:S839–S848.
75. Grohman GS, Glass RI, Pereira HG, et al. Enteric viruses and diarrhea in HIV-1-infected patients. *N Engl J Med* 1993;329: 14–20.
76. Sperber SJ, Schleupner CJ. Salmonellosis during infection with human immunodeficiency virus. *Rev Infect Dis* 1987;9:925–933.
77. Gotuzzo E, Frisancho O, Sanchez J, et al. Association between the acquired immunodeficiency syndrome and infection with *Salmonella typhi* or *Salmonella paratyphi* in an endemic typhoid area. *Arch Intern Med* 1991;151:381–382.
78. Bernstein LJ, Krieger BZ, Novick B, et al. Bacterial infection in the acquired immunodeficiency syndrome of children. *Pediatr Infect Dis J* 1985;4:472–475.
79. McLaughlin LC, Nord KS, Joshi VV, et al. Severe gastrointestinal involvement in children with the acquired immunodeficiency syndrome. *J Pediatr Gastroenterol Nutr* 1987;6:517–524.
80. Jain A, Reif S, O'Neil K, et al. Small intestinal bacterial overgrowth and protein-losing enteropathy in an infant with AIDS. *J Pediatr Gastroenterol Nutr* 1992;15:452–454.
81. Viscidi R, Willey S, Bartlett JG. Isolation rates and toxigenic

potential of *Clostridium difficile* isolates from various patient populations. *Gastroenterology* 1981;81:5–9.
82. Buts JP, Corthier G, Delmee M. *Saccharomyces boulardii* for *Clostridium difficile*-associated enteropathies in infants. *J Pediatr Gastroenterol Nutr* 1993;16:419–425.
83. Sutphen JL, Grand RJ, Flores A, et al. Chronic diarrhea associated with *Clostridium difficile* in children. *Am J Dis Child* 1983; 137:275–278.
84. Cozart JC, Kalangi SS, Clench MH, et al. *Clostridium difficile* diarrhea in patients with AIDS versus non-AIDS controls. Methods of treatment and clinical response to treatment. *Am J Gastroenterol* 1993;16:192–194.
85. Marano BJ Jr, Smith F, Bonano CA. *Helicobacter pylori* prevalence in acquired immunodeficiency syndrome. *Am J Gastroenterol* 1993;88:687–690.
86. Edwards PD, Carrick J, Turner J, et al. *Helicobacter pylori*-associated gastritis is rare in AIDS: antibiotic effect or a consequence of immunodeficiency? *Am J Gastroenterol* 1991;86:1761–1764.
87. Blecker U, Keymolen K, Souayah H, et al. *Helicobacter pylori* in children with acquired immunodeficiency syndrome. *Pediatrics* 1993;91:1217.
88. Masur H. Recommendations on prophylaxis and therapy for disseminated *Mycobacterium avium* complex disease in patients infected with the human immunodeficiency virus. *N Engl J Med* 1993;329:898–904.
89. Moss WJ, Dedyo T, Suarez M, et al. Tuberculosis in children infected with human immunodeficiency virus: a report of five cases. *Pediatr Infect Dis J* 1992;11:114–120.
90. Friedenberg KA, Draguesku JO, Kiyabu M, et al. Intestinal perforation due to *Mycobacterium tuberculosis* in HIV-1-infected individuals: report of two cases. *Am J Gastroenterol* 1993;88:604–607.
91. Teixidor HS, Godwin TA, Ramirez EA. Cryptosporidiosis of the biliary tract in AIDS. *Radiology* 1991;180:51–56.
92. McGowan I, Hawkins AS, Weller IVD. The natural history of cryptosporidial diarrhea in HIV-1-infected patients. *J AIDS* 1993;7:349–354.
93. Romeu J, Miro JM, Sirera G, et al. Efficacy of octreotide in the management of chronic diarrhea in AIDS. *J AIDS* 1991;5: 1495–1499.
94. Molina JM, Sarfati C, Beauvais B, et al. Intestinal microsporidiosis in human immunodeficiency virus-infected patients with chronic unexplained diarrhea: prevalence and clinical and biologic features. *J Infect Dis* 1993;167:217–221.
95. Kotler DP, Francisco A, Clayton F, et al. Small intestinal injury and parasitic diseases in AIDS. *Ann Intern Med* 1990;113: 444–449.
96. Greenson J, Belitsos P, Yardley J, et al. AIDS enteropathy: occult enteric infection and duodenal alterations in chronic diarrhea. *Ann Intern Med* 1991;114:366–372.
97. Cegielski JP, Msengi AE, Dukes CS, et al. Intestinal parasites and HIV-1 infection in Tanzanian children with chronic diarrhea. *J AIDS* 1993;7:213.
98. Santa Lucia MM, Ito HT, Castro M, et al. Diarrheal illness: comparative study between AIDS patients and non-infected children. Abstract presented at the seventh International Conference on AIDS, Florence, June 1991(abst WB2028).
99. Leibovitz E, Rigaud M, Chandwani S, et al. Disseminated fungal infections in children infected with human immunodeficiency virus. *Pediatr Infect Dis J* 1991;10:888–894.
100. Borowitz SM, Sausbury FT. Treatment of chronic cryptosporidial infection with orally administered human serum immune globulin. *J Pediatr* 1991;119:593–595.
101. Ungar BLP, Ward DJ, Fayer R, et al. Cessation of *Cryptosporidium*-associated diarrhea in an acquired immunodeficiency syndrome patient after treatment with hyperimmune bovine colostrum. *Gastroenterology* 1990;98:486–489.
102. Samaranayake LP, Holmstrup P. Oral candidiasis and human immunodeficiency virus infection. *J Oral Pathol Med* 1989;18: 554–564.
103. Laine L, Dretler RH, Conteas CN, et al. Fluconazole compared to ketoconazole for the treatment of *Candida* esophagitis in AIDS. A randomized trial. *Ann Intern Med* 1992;117: 655–660.
104. Schutze GE, Tucker NC, Jacobs RF. Histoplasmosis and perinatal human immunodeficiency virus. *Pediatr Infect Dis J* 1992; 11:501.
105. Byers M, Feldman S, Edwards J. Disseminated histoplasmosis as the acquired immunodeficiency syndrome-defining illness in an infant. *Pediatr Infect Dis J* 1992;11:127–128.
106. Shull HJ. Human histoplasmosis: disease with protean manifestations, often with digestive system involvement. *Gastroenterology* 1953;25:582.
107. Arpadi SM, Cuff PA, Kotler DP, et al. Growth velocity fat-free mass and energy intake are inversely related to viral load in HIV-1-infected children. *J Nutr* 2000;130:2498–2502.
108. Smith PD. Infectious diarrheas in patients with AIDS. *Gastroenterol Clin North Am* 1993;22:535–548.
109. Ma P, Soave R. Three-step stool examination for cryptosporidiosis in 10 homosexual men with protracted watery diarrhea. *J Infect Dis* 1983;147:824–828.
110. Sentongo TA, Rutstein RM, Stettler N, et al. Association between steatorrhea, growth, and immunologic status in children with perinatally acquired HIV-1 infection. *Arch Pediatr Adolesc Med* 2001;155:149–153.
111. Yolken RH, Hart W, Oung I, et al. Gastrointestinal dysfunction and disaccharide intolerance in children infected with human immunodeficiency virus. *J Pediatr* 1991;118:359–363.
112. Rhodes JM, Middleton P, Jewell DP. The lactulose hydrogen breath test as a diagnostic test for small-bowel bacterial overgrowth. *Scand J Gastroenterol* 1979;14:333–336.
113. Guarino A, Tarallo L, Guandalini S, et al. Impaired intestinal function in symptomatic HIV-1 infection. *J Pediatr Gastroenterol Nutr* 1991;12:453–458.
114. O'Brien KO, Rezavi M, Henderson RA, et al. Bone mineral content in girls perinatally infected with HIV-1. *Am J Clin Nutr* 2001;73:821–826.
115. Fabris N, Mocchigiani E, Galli M, et al. AIDS, zinc deficiency and thymic hormone failure. *JAMA* 1988;259:2850.
116. Kavanaugh-MacHugh A, Rowe S, Benjamin Y, et al. Selenium deficiency and cardiomyopathy in malnourished pediatric AIDS patients. Abstract presented at the fifth International Conference on AIDS, Montreal, 1989.
117. Mobarhan S, Trumbore LS. Enteral tube feeding: a clinical perspective on recent advances. *Nutr Rev* 1991;49:129–140.
118. Bussy V, Marechal F, Nasca S. Microbial contamination of enteral feeding tubes occurring during nutritional treatment. *JPEN J Parenter Enteral Nutr* 1992;16:552–557.
119. Dreimane D, Nielsen K, Deveikis A, et al. Effect of protease inhibitors combined with standard antiretroviral therapy on linear growth and weight gain in human immunodeficiency virus type 1-infected children. *Lancet* 2001;20:315–316.
120. Miller TL, Mawn BE, Oran EJ, et al. The effect of protease inhibitor therapy on growth and body composition in human immunodeficiency virus type 1-infected children. *Pediatrics* 2001; 107(5). URL: *http:www.pediatrics.org/cgi/content/full/107/5e77.*

31

GASTROINTESTINAL INFECTIONS IN TRANSPLANT RECIPIENTS

J. STEPHEN DUMMER
BAN MISHU ALLOS

The development of new, potent immunosuppressive medications during the last two decades, coupled with advances in basic science and expanding public awareness, has provided the impetus for rapid growth in clinical transplantation. From 1989 to 1998, the volume of solid organ transplants in the United States increased by 60%, with more than 20,000 transplants performed in 1998 (1). In the same year, the International Bone Marrow Transplant Registry recorded 23,000 transplants in North America, a third of which were allogeneic (2). This recent activity represented a 100% increase in allogeneic transplants and a 500% increase in autologous transplants during the previous decade. The tremendous growth in clinical transplantation, together with improving survival rates, guarantees that most physicians will encounter transplant patients in their daily practice.

Infections of the gastrointestinal tract frequently cause morbidity and mortality in transplant patients. Among 131 emergency department visits by patients who had undergone heart or lung transplantation, 10% were for gastrointestinal symptoms, including nausea, vomiting, and diarrhea (3). Gastrointestinal symptoms were the most common presenting complaint after fever and dyspnea. Eighty-three percent of children who had undergone bone marrow transplantation required workup for diarrhea during the first 21 months, and in a prospective study of 296 adult marrow recipients, significant diarrheal episodes occurred in 43% within the first 100 days after transplantation (4,5). The abdomen is the most frequent site of bacterial and fungal infections among patients with liver transplants, and serious colonic infections, such as diverticular abscesses, have also been described in up to 4% of renal transplant recipients (6–9).

The aim of this chapter is to provide a general approach to gastrointestinal infections in transplant patients. Detailed discussions of the pathogenesis, clinical presentation, and treatment of specific pathogens are available in other chapters. We review the overall importance of various enteric infections in transplant patients and try to place these in perspective along with other pathologic processes of the gastrointestinal tract, including the effects of immunosuppression and graft-versus-host-disease (GVHD).

MICROBIOLOGY

A broad range of organisms can produce disease in transplant recipients. Table 31.1 compares the morbidity caused by infectious pathogens in the gastrointestinal tract or abdomen in transplant patients with that in normal hosts.

Bacterial Infections

Listeria causes one of the classic infections seen in patients with defects in cell-mediated immunity (10). In experimental animal models, cytotoxic drugs, corticosteroids, and cyclosporine impair the development of immunity to this organism (11–13). Transplant patients account for 10% to 15% of cases of *Listeria* infection in large population-based surveys (14). These data suggest that the rate of *Listeria* infection in transplant patients is increased at least 1,000-fold over that in normal populations. *Listeria* was identified in the stools of 5.6% of renal transplant recipients followed for 1 year (15). Both carriage of organisms and clinical disease in transplant patients are more common during summer months. Not surprisingly, the greatest risk for listeriosis occurs in the first year after transplantation (15). *Listeria* organisms are highly susceptible to trimethoprim-sulfamethoxazole. The widespread use of this agent for *Pneumocystis* prophylaxis may have resulted in the decreased rate of *Listeria* infection in transplant recipients observed in recent years (16).

High rates of *Clostridium difficile*-associated colitis (14% to 15%) have been reported in some populations of patients undergoing bone marrow transplantation. These rates are likely associated with the prolonged use of antibiotics in

J. S. Dummer: Departments of Medicine and Surgery, Vanderbilt University School of Medicine and Vanderbilt Hospital, Nashville, Tennessee

B. M. Allos: Departments of Medicine and Preventive Medicine, Vanderbilt University School of Medicine, Nashville, Tennessee

TABLE 31.1. MORBIDITY CAUSED BY SELECTED ENTERIC PATHOGENS IN TRANSPLANT PATIENTS IN COMPARISON WITH THAT IN NORMAL HOSTS

Morbidity in Comparison with Normal Hosts	Pathogen			
	Bacteria	Viruses	Fungi	Parasites
Much greater	*Listeria*	Cytomegalovirus Adenovirus Epstein–Barr virus Herpes simplex virus	*Candida* *Aspergillus*	
Greater	*Salmonella* *Clostridium difficile*	Rotavirus Astrovirus	*Histoplasma*	*Strongyloides* *Cryptosporidium* *Giardia*
Equal	*Shigella* *Campylobacter* *Helicobacter*			
No data	*Escherichia coli* *Aeromonas* *Yersinia*	Norwalk agent		

neutropenic patients (4,17). However, a recent prospective study detected only six cases of *C. difficile* colitis in 296 marrow recipients (5). *C. difficile* colitis is also a problem in recipients of solid organs, especially livers, in whom rates of this illness are 3% to 6% (6,7). The institutional variation in the incidence of *C. difficile* colitis is wide, so that local knowledge is critical in evaluating the risk for patients (18). Substantial evidence supports the nosocomial spread of *C. difficile* infection (19,20).

The frequency of *Salmonella* infections is increased after renal transplantation. *Salmonella* infection developed in 20 of 592 renal transplant patients in Saudi Arabia; of these, 63% had bacteremia, 35% had focal abscesses outside the bowel, and 35% experienced relapse (21). High rates of salmonellosis in transplant patients have also been reported in a few European countries (22,23). Only sporadic cases of *Salmonella* infection have been reported from transplant centers in the United States (24,25).

Reports of *Shigella* infections among transplant patients are infrequent (26–28). Thus, it is not clear whether the incidence and clinical severity of *Shigella* infection are greater among transplant patients than in the general population, although bacteremia occurred in three of four reported cases. *Campylobacter* infections have been frequently identified in HIV-infected persons (29), but too few reports are available in transplant patients to determine the incidence accurately. Interestingly, some cases of Guillain-Barré syndrome have been associated with recent *Campylobacter* infection in transplant recipients (30,31). This post-infectious complication in normal hosts is apparently not prevented by immunosuppression. One case of bloody diarrhea caused by Shiga toxin-producing *Escherichia coli* was reported in a heart transplant recipient (32), but hemolytic–uremic syndrome did not develop; this complication occurs in 6% of cases but is more common in children than in adults.

Ulcer disease and gastritis have been frequently reported in transplant recipients, but studies of *Helicobacter pylori* infection are limited. In a single cross-sectional study of 202 renal transplant recipients, patients seropositive for *Helicobacter* were more likely to describe dyspeptic symptoms than were seronegative patients (33). In another study, *Helicobacter* organisms were identified in 16 (48%) of 33 renal transplant recipients who underwent upper gastrointestinal endoscopy for a variety of reasons; the presence of *Helicobacter* was associated with gastritis and dyspepsia (34). In contrast, endoscopic evaluation of 276 patients before and after bone marrow transplantation revealed only one documented *Helicobacter* infection (35). A seroepidemiologic study of 100 heart transplant recipients showed that 35% were seropositive before transplantation. Only 1 of 65 seronegative patients underwent seroconversion during 3 years of follow-up (36). Of the seropositive patients, 40% actually became seronegative during follow-up; these seroreversions were associated with the prolonged use of oral and intravenous antibiotics.

Infections caused by atypical mycobacteria have been described in case reports and small case series of transplant patients. Gastrointestinal involvement occurred in a few cases but is distinctly uncommon (37).

Viral Infections

Until recently, cytomegalovirus (CMV) was the most important pathogen in transplant recipients. After transplantation, cultures positive for CMV have been reported in 53% to 100% of solid organ transplant recipients and 32% to 52% of bone marrow recipients (38). The actual frequency with which CMV causes gastrointestinal disease is difficult to determine with certainty because endoscopy is required to confirm the diagnosis and involvement may be limited to areas, such as the small intestine, that are inaccessible to endoscopic examination. Gastrointestinal complaints are common in patients with CMV disease. In one series of heart and lung transplant recipients with symptomatic CMV disease, 41% experienced abdominal pain without another explanation (39). In recent years, the widespread use of antiviral prophylaxis has lessened the clinical impact of CMV infection (40).

Other herpesviruses are also important in transplant patients. Enteric infection with herpes simplex virus (HSV) is usually limited to the oral cavity and esophagus. Gastritis and colitis resulting from HSV infection are rare; the presence of either often indicates disseminated disease (41,42). Herpes zoster rarely involves the gastrointestinal tract, but the pain of prodromal shingles in an abdominal dermatome may be misinterpreted as bacterial peritonitis (43). Epstein–Barr virus (EBV) does not cause gastroenteritis *per se,* but EBV infection is a cause of B-cell lymphoproliferative disease after transplantation. Patients with EBV-induced B-cell tumors of the gastrointestinal tract may present with diarrhea, abdominal pain, or gastrointestinal hemorrhage (44).

Infections with adenovirus occur only sporadically in adults after solid organ transplantation (45). Such infections are more frequent (2% to 10%) after bone marrow transplantation and in children who receive liver transplants (5,45,46). Adenovirus infection may be disseminated or limited to the gastrointestinal tract or a single organ, such as the kidney. Disseminated disease is associated with high mortality rates.

Numerous reports document rotavirus infection in solid organ and bone marrow recipients. Infections occur in both adults and children (5,47–49), and nosocomial transmission has been documented (48,49). The disease is generally self-limited, although prolonged illness has been reported (47).

Coxsackievirus and astrovirus have also been reported to cause gastroenteritis in bone marrow recipients (5,17, 50,51). Information on coxsackievirus infections is limited, but in one reported outbreak, the infection was fatal in six of seven patients (50). In contrast, astrovirus infections are relatively common but rarely fatal, although they may cause prolonged symptoms of nausea and diarrhea (5,51). Astrovirus infections are seasonal, occurring most commonly in the winter and spring (5).

Fungal Infections

All transplant recipients are at risk for mucocutaneous candidiasis. *Candida* species, which are part of the normal gastrointestinal flora in immunocompetent persons, may become invasive under conditions of immunosuppression (52,53). Among cancer patients who did not receive antifungal prophylaxis, thrush developed in 60% within 2 weeks after a course of chemotherapy (54). Mucosal involvement with *Candida* infection is usually limited to the oral cavity and esophagus, but occasional cases of gastric or colonic candidiasis have been described (55). Peritonitis and abscesses caused by *Candida* organisms are reported in 3% to 19% of liver recipients and also may occur in other transplant patients after abdominal operations (56–58). The gut is thought to be the main portal of entry for systemic candidiasis.

The intestinal tract is also a common site for the secondary spread of *Aspergillus,* but primary infection of the bowel or abdominal cavity with *Aspergillus* is rare (59). However, wound and deep abdominal infection with *Aspergillus* has been described as a sequel of liver transplantation (60).

Disseminated histoplasmosis occurs in a small subset of transplant patients, most of whom reside in or have recently visited the midwestern and southeastern United States, where infection with *Histoplasma capsulatum* is endemic (61). Disseminated histoplasmosis can involve any region of the digestive tract, but the involvement is usually focal; in some cases, the digestive tract may be the only apparent site of infection (62). Clinical manifestations of intestinal tract histoplasmosis include chronic diarrhea, abdominal pain, gastrointestinal bleeding, and malabsorption.

Parasitic Infections

Immunocompromised hosts, including transplant recipients, are at risk for hyperinfection and disseminated infection with *Strongyloides stercoralis* (63,64). The migrating worms typically cause fever, abdominal pain, polymicrobial bacteremia, respiratory distress, and multilobar infiltrates. This disease was described in transplant patients in the 1970s and early 1980s, but the syndrome has now virtually disappeared. The reasons for its disappearance are unclear but may be related to changing demographics, the use of lower doses of corticosteroids, or inhibition of the parasite by cyclosporine (65).

Infection with *Cryptosporidium* has been infrequently described in transplant patients. The range of disease varies from asymptomatic carriage to intractable diarrhea (66,67). A nosocomial outbreak occurred in six patients in a bone marrow unit (67). Three cases of *Giardia lamblia* infection have been reported in bone marrow recipients (4,68). The diarrhea was fulminant in one case, but all patients responded to antibiotic therapy. Many cases of Microsporidia infection have been reported in patients with AIDS, but infection with the parasite was only recently described in transplant recipients (69). The usual symptoms are dyspepsia, weight loss, fatigue, and chronic diarrhea without fever. These symptoms may persist for many months or even more than a year.

PATHOGENESIS

Microorganisms that can establish latency and become reactivated during immunosuppression are an important source of enteric infections in transplant recipients. CMV and other herpesviruses are the most important examples of viruses that may become reactivated and subsequently cause enteric disease. CMV infection may represent reactivation of a latent infection or may be newly acquired from donated organs or blood transfusions (38). The site of CMV latency is not known but appears to be a tissue or cell common to all transplanted organs. HSV is latent in dorsal root ganglia and reaches the oral cavity by retrograde axonal spread from the trigeminal ganglion (70). Infection of the esophagus and stomach is thought to occur via simple mechanical spread from the mouth. Viral reactivation accounts for most cases of HSV disease in transplant patients, but rare cases of primary infection have been described (71,72). EBV is also associated with enteric disease in transplant recipients. B-cell lymphoproliferative tumors related to EBV infection develop in 1% to 4% of solid organ transplant recipients (73,74). One-half to two-thirds of these tumors occur in the first year after transplant and may arise in lymph nodes or various visceral sites, including the bowel. The tumors are more common in EBV-seronegative patients in whom primary EBV infection develops after transplantation (75,76).

Candida species normally colonize the gastrointestinal tract but may become pathogenic during immunosuppression, especially when the mucosa is injured by cytotoxic drugs or local defense mechanisms are impaired by corticosteroids (52,53). Bowel injury, which also predisposes a patient to candidiasis, may be caused by surgical trauma, radiation, cytotoxic chemotherapy, or GVHD. Disseminated candidiasis primarily occurs in patients who have one or more of these predisposing factors and also are neutropenic or receiving corticosteroids.

In contrast to enteric infections caused by endogenous pathogens, such as CMV and *Candida,* enteric infections acquired exogenously from food, water, animals, or other humans are not much more frequent in transplant populations. One exception is *Salmonella* infection, which is uncommon in transplant recipients in the United States but an important problem at transplant centers in developing countries (27). Pathogens transmitted in the nosocomial setting (e.g., *C. difficile,* rotavirus) have also caused outbreaks in transplant recipients.

For some important pathogens in transplant recipients, the mode of acquisition is not clear. Although adenovirus can latently infect cells and then become reactivated under conditions of immunosuppression, *de novo* acquisition of the virus has been described in hospitalized patients (77,78). In transplant recipients, adenovirus infections have not been thoroughly investigated because their incidence is low and type-specific antibody studies must be performed to investigate protective immunity and the frequency of prior infection.

The mechanical trauma of surgery is a major risk factor for infection in transplant patients. Liver transplant surgery is particularly lengthy and technically demanding, and the rate of bacterial and fungal infections following liver transplantation is strongly associated with the duration of surgery (6,7). In 30% to 40% of cases, the intestine is entered to create a Roux-en-Y loop for biliary drainage (79,80). In one large study of surgical complications associated with liver transplantation carried out at the University of Pittsburgh, 22% of patients required reoperation for bleeding or infection, and 17% required operative repair of biliary obstruction or leak (80). As a consequence of the technical complexity of liver transplant surgery, abdominal abscesses and peritonitis are common during the first 4 to 6 months after transplantation. The causative organisms include typical enteric bacteria (*Escherichia coli, Enterococcus, Bacteroides*) in addition to coagulase-negative and coagulase-positive *Staphylococcus* organisms. *Candida* infections occur in approximately one-third of cases, but *Aspergillus* infections are rare.

Intraabdominal infections may also complicate pancreas transplantation (81,82). These surgical infections are usually located in the vicinity of the pancreatic allograft, which is generally placed superior to the bladder. This enables pancreatic exocrine secretions to drain through a cuff of donor duodenum into the recipient's bladder. Intraabdominal infections are less common in heart, kidney, and lung transplant recipients and are usually associated with preexisting pathologic conditions, such as diverticulosis, cholelithiasis, or peptic ulcer disease. These infections occur both early and late after transplantation.

Immunosuppressive drugs increase the risk for infection. Additionally, some immunosuppressive drugs cause gastrointestinal symptoms, such as diarrhea, that may be confused with enteric infection. Corticosteroids remain a mainstay of transplant immunosuppression. Important pharmacologic actions of corticosteroids include reduction of vascular permeability, interference with neutrophil adherence, and inhibition of release of cytokines (83,84). The use of corticosteroids has been associated with the development of peptic ulcers and pancreatitis (85,86). With long-term use, corticosteroids may cause thinning of the bowel wall, which leads to an increased risk for perforation, especially from diverticulitis (87,88). Corticosteroids markedly decrease the signs and symptoms of intraabdominal inflammation, so that the diagnosis of significant infection may be delayed.

Azathioprine, an antimetabolite that blocks the replication of lymphocytes, was introduced in the early 1960s for the prevention of allograft rejection (89). Side effects of the drug include nausea and vomiting, which are more common during the initiation of therapy and the administration of high doses. Systemic signs, such as fever, rash, and diffuse myalgias, sometimes accompany these gastrointestinal symptoms. In long-term use and at lower doses, azathioprine is usually well tolerated.

Cyclosporine has been used in transplant patients since its introduction in the early 1980s. Cyclosporine blocks the antigen-stimulated release of interleukin 2 and interferon-γ from CD4+ T lymphocytes (90). Mild gastrointestinal intolerance, manifesting as bloating, anorexia, and nausea, is not uncommon during the introduction of cyclosporine.

These symptoms usually resolve with continued use (91). Cyclosporine has no known chronic effects on the gastrointestinal tract (92).

Tacrolimus (FK506) was approved by the U.S. Food and Drug Administration in 1994 for transplant immunosuppression. Like cyclosporine, tacrolimus inhibits the elaboration of key cytokines, such as interleukin 2 (93), but it is 10 to 100 times more potent than cyclosporine. Gastrointestinal side effects, such as diarrhea, are common after the initiation of therapy but generally abate with further use.

Mycophenolate mofetil, another recently introduced immunosuppressive agent, interferes with purine metabolism and has an antiproliferative effect on B and T lymphocytes. Designed to replace azathioprine in multidrug regimens, mycophenolate mofetil has been shown to be more effective than azathioprine in preventing rejection (94). However, it is associated with significant gastrointestinal side effects. Diarrhea occurs in up to 50% of patients and may not remit with continued use. The newest immunosuppressive agent is sirolimus (Rapamune). The mechanism of action of sirolimus is unique; it blocks cytokine-directed intracellular signaling in lymphocytes (95). It can cause nausea and diarrhea at high doses, but these side effects usually do not necessitate discontinuation.

A number of different preparations of antilymphocyte antibodies are used to prevent or treat organ rejection. These include the murine monoclonal antibody OKT3 (Muromonad-CD3), directed against the CD3 molecule on T cells, and a variety of polyclonal antithymocyte or antilymphocyte antibody preparations produced by immunizing rabbits, horses, and other animals with human lymphocytes or thymocytes (96,97). These preparations cause no direct toxic effects on the gastrointestinal tract, but associated increases in the frequency of serious infections with CMV, EBV, and fungi have been reported (7,98,99).

The pathogenesis of enteric and intraabdominal infections in bone marrow recipients is related to two major factors: (a) direct toxic effects of radiation and cytotoxic drugs on the gastrointestinal tract and (b) the consequences of GVHD, a condition that occurs in up to 70% to 80% of persons undergoing allogeneic marrow transplantation (100–102). Radiation and cytotoxic drugs cause direct injury to the gastrointestinal epithelium and may lead to frank ulceration (100,102). The gut-associated lymphoid tissue may be depleted of lymphoid cells, so that T-cell action and immunoglobulin production are restricted. Anorexia, odynophagia, nausea, vomiting, and diarrhea are common manifestations during the first 2 to 3 weeks after bone marrow transplantation. Although focal enteric and intraabdominal infections are uncommon during this interval, bloodstream infections with intestinal microorganisms are relatively frequent because of the enhanced ability of the microorganisms to invade the circulation via the injured mucosa (102,103). In patients undergoing autologous transplantation, the return of marrow function signals a marked improvement in immune function. Fatalities from infection are uncommon after autologous engraftment. In allogeneic transplantation, however, acute GVHD supervenes in 70% to 80% of cases and produces a secondary immunodeficiency. The gastrointestinal manifestations of acute GVHD include watery diarrhea, anorexia, nausea, and abdominal pain (102,104). Histologic examination of the mucosa during GVHD reveals dropout of crypts and foci of epithelial cell necrosis. Endoscopic examination may show edema, erythema, and mucosal ulceration. These changes can occur throughout the gastrointestinal tract but are most prominent in the distal small bowel and proximal colon. In parallel with mucosal injury, many components of the immune system are impaired, including local T- and B-cell responses (102,105,106). The immunosuppressive drugs used to treat GVHD add to the overall burden of immunosuppression. Consequently, the risk for serious local and systemic infection is substantially greater in patients with acute GVHD. When chronic GVHD follows acute GVHD, immunosuppression may persist for years (102,107).

A novel association between rejection and infection occurs in small-bowel transplantation (108). During severe acute rejection, the mucosa of the bowel may become disrupted and ulcerated; translocation of bacteria across the gut wall and bacterial sepsis follow. Effective management requires treatment for both infection and rejection. Recipients of small-bowel transplants also appear to have high rates of CMV enteritis (109). Additional studies are needed to delineate the role of other enteric pathogens in this small but unique group of patients.

EPIDEMIOLOGY

The predisposing factors for infection associated with transplantation and the temporal sequence of events have been elucidated (110–112). The most useful concept is that the type and frequency of infection vary over time (Table 31.2). The risk for infection is highest in the early post-transplant period and declines thereafter, although rates of infection among transplant recipients never decrease to those in the general population. For example, the risk for infection during the first month after liver transplantation is approximately 30 times greater than the risk 1 to 2 years after transplantation (7).

The nature of the infectious complications also varies with time (Table 31.2). During the first 3 to 4 weeks after transplantation, infections usually result from complications of the transplant operation or related procedures, such as intubation or line placement. In bone marrow transplant recipients, radiation and chemotherapy during this 3- to 4-week interval can cause profound depression of marrow function which is the main determinant of infection. The usual pathogens are nosocomially acquired bacteria and fungi in the more complex types of transplantation. HSV infections

TABLE 31.2. COMMON INFECTIOUS CAUSES OF ABDOMINAL SYMPTOMS IN TRANSPLANT RECIPIENTS ACCORDING TO TIME AFTER TRANSPLANTATION[a]

	Time After Transplantation		
Symptom	**0–30 Days**	**1–6 Months**	**>6 Months**
Esophageal symptoms	HSV *Candida*	CMV *Candida* HSV	Mostly noninfectious
Nausea and vomiting	Bacterial sepsis Cholangitis Abscess *Clostridium difficile*	CMV *C. difficile* Sepsis Abscess	Mostly noninfectious
Diarrhea	*C. difficile*	CMV *C. difficile* Other enteric pathogens	Common enteric pathogens
Upper abdominal pain	Cholangitis Abscess Peritonitis Wound infection HSV	CMV Adenovirus Cholangitis CMV Abscess EBV lymphoma	Cholangitis Peritonitis
Lower abdominal pain	Typhlitis *C. difficile* Diverticulitis Wound infection	CMV *C. difficile* Diverticulitis Cystitis	Diverticulitis Peritonitis Appendicitis Cystitis

CMV, cytomegalovirus; HSV, herpes simplex virus; EBV, Epstein–Barr virus.
[a]Cholangitis, abscess, peritonitis, and diverticulitis are seen primarily in solid organ transplant recipients. Typhlitis is restricted to bone marrow recipients.

become reactivated and also occur early after transplantation. During the second post-transplant interval, corresponding to 1 to 6 months after transplantation, the predominant infections are caused by opportunistic pathogens, such as CMV, EBV, adenovirus, *Pneumocystis, Nocardia, Aspergillus,* and *Mycobacterium tuberculosis.* Patients who receive augmented immunosuppression for acute rejection or treatment of GVHD are at even greater risk for the development of active infection with opportunistic pathogens during this interval (102,104). In bone marrow recipients who have significant chronic GVHD, the enhanced risk for infection with opportunistic pathogens may extend well beyond the 6-month period (102,107).

Beyond 6 months after transplantation, patients are still at increased risk for infection. Common bacterial processes, such as diverticulitis, sinusitis, or pneumonia, and infections with opportunistic pathogens, including *Cryptococcus, Listeria,* and *Nocardia,* may occur. Infection with community-acquired enteric pathogens, such as *Campylobacter,* are most often diagnosed during this late period.

CLINICAL FEATURES

The presentation of enteric and intraabdominal infections may not be the same in transplant recipients as in immunocompetent subjects. Abdominal symptoms, such as pain, are often milder in immunosuppressed patients receiving corticosteroids. Because the immunologic control of disease and the patients' perception of disease are both altered, the presentation of infection at a relatively advanced stage is common. For example, a large number of patients with *Salmonella* infection are bacteremic, and perforation has already developed in a large number of patients with diverticulitis at presentation (8,9,21). Pyogenic intraabdominal infections are more common in recipients of solid organ transplants than in recipients of bone marrow transplants. Peritonitis often occurs as a complication of abdominal surgery but also may result from underlying conditions such as ulcer disease, CMV infection, diverticulitis, lymphoproliferative disease, and ischemia.

In the interval between 1 and 6 months after transplantation, CMV has been the most important enteric pathogen (Table 31.2). Recently, however, the extensive use of antiviral prophylaxis has lessened the overall importance of CMV infection. Late after transplantation, abdominal symptoms are usually noninfectious in origin or caused by common infectious conditions, such as cholangitis and diverticulitis. Fever accompanies many enteric infections but may be absent in patients with localized mucocutaneous HSV infection, abdominal abscess, or peritonitis because some pathogens, such as *Candida,* are relatively avirulent; additionally, cases of CMV gastritis or enteritis and some cases of *C. difficile* colitis are mild and do not produce fever. Some enteric infections, such as giardiasis, never cause fever.

DIFFERENTIAL DIAGNOSIS

Many noninfectious conditions that occur in transplant recipients mimic infection. The radiation and chemotherapeutic conditioning regimens given to bone marrow recipients cause severe mucositis during the first 2 to 3 weeks after transplantation. Common symptoms of mucositis include diarrhea, which may be profuse and occasionally bloody, nausea, vomiting, and pain on swallowing (102,104). The conditioning regimens are also responsible for two distinct conditions that produce abdominal pain: neutropenic enterocolitis (typhlitis) and venoocclusive disease (VOD). Neutropenic enterocolitis, which is associated with profound neutropenia, is a severe inflammatory condition that usually involves the cecum and right side of the colon and is distinct from the pseudomembranous colitis related to antibiotic use (114,115). In one study, it was detected in 3 of 24 bone marrow transplant cases at autopsy (116). The cause of neutropenic enterocolitis has not been firmly established, but injury to the bowel from chemotherapy is thought to be a major factor (102,115). Such injury causes a breakdown of normal mucosal barriers and permits a necrotizing transmural infection with enteric organisms. Typical symptoms are fever, right lower quadrant pain, and abdominal distention.

Venoocclusive disease of the liver occurs most commonly in patients who receive high-dose chemotherapy and have underlying hepatic disease (117). In one large series, VOD developed in 15% of bone marrow recipients, and 98% of them died. Histologic examination of a liver with VOD reveals occlusion of the hepatic venules by reticulum, collagen, or cell fragments in association with necrosis of hepatocytes around the central vein (118). The clinical manifestations are right upper quadrant pain, hepatic tenderness, hepatomegaly, ascites, and weight gain resulting from fluid retention. Liver function tests show a cholestatic pattern, and the bilirubin is often markedly elevated. VOD can resemble cholecystitis, cholangitis, localized peritonitis, or intraabdominal abscess, but it is more common in bone marrow recipients than are these other conditions.

Graft-versus-host disease is the most important source of gastrointestinal symptoms during the interval from marrow engraftment until 3 to 4 months after transplantation (5,102). GVHD may cause virtually any gastrointestinal symptom. The concurrence of skin and liver disease with gastrointestinal symptoms is helpful in establishing a diagnosis of GVHD, but the presence of all three is not an absolute criterion for the diagnosis. Skin rashes may be caused by drug allergy, and liver injury may caused by residual VOD, drug toxicity, preexisting hepatitis B or C, or new infection with CMV or adenovirus. GVHD is a risk factor for CMV disease. Both CMV infection and acute GVHD may cause fever and leukopenia, but CMV infection usually does not cause rash or hyperbilirubinemia. Other noninfectious causes of abdominal symptoms occurring between 1 and 6 months after marrow transplantation include peptic disease, pancreatitis, and adverse effects of medications.

Chronic GVHD is the most common noninfectious cause of abdominal symptoms late after transplantation (102). Most patients with chronic GVHD have had acute GVHD, but in 20% to 30% of cases, chronic GVHD begins *de novo* 3 months or more after transplantation (101,102). Gastrointestinal involvement with chronic GVHD is frequently restricted to the esophagus. Fibrous bands, strictures, and mucosal desquamation may be seen on endoscopic examination. Patients typically complain of dysphagia, odynophagia, and weight loss. Esophageal dysfunction may cause recurrent aspiration pneumonia. Occasionally, chronic GVHD involves the intestine and leads to obstruction or malabsorption.

The differential diagnosis of gastrointestinal symptoms is less complex in recipients of solid organ transplants because chemotherapy is not used and GVHD is rare. Symptoms of gastritis or esophagitis are common in the early post-transplant period, and many centers routinely use agents to block gastric acid secretion. In kidney recipients, thrombosis of the renal artery anastomosis can mimic the clinical symptoms of an abdominal abscess; if surgical removal of the kidney is delayed, bacterial superinfection of the ischemic allograft may occur. Leaks at the ureteral anastomosis can produce abdominal discomfort and graft dysfunction and also may lead to localized infection (119).

Heart transplant recipients do not routinely undergo abdominal surgery; therefore, the differential diagnosis of abdominal complications is less extensive than after liver or renal transplantation. However, high rates of gastritis and esophagitis in the early post-transplant period have been reported from some centers (120,121). Persistent postprandial vomiting has been reported in some heart–lung recipients. This condition appears to be secondary to gastric atony resulting from incidental vagotomy during the transplant procedure. In severe cases, a drainage procedure, such as pyloroplasty, may be necessary to relieve the obstructive symptoms (122).

Noninfectious abdominal symptoms reported in liver recipients generally are related to complications of surgery, such as bile peritonitis and intraabdominal hemorrhage. These conditions pose a risk for superinfection with bacteria or fungi (7,57). Less severe complications, including medication-induced nausea or diarrhea, noninfectious gastritis, and esophagitis, also occur but have been overshadowed by the more severe complications.

DIAGNOSTIC APPROACH

Persistent gastrointestinal symptoms in a transplant recipient should lead to a prompt evaluation, especially when the symptoms are accompanied by fever or other evidence of systemic involvement. The diagnostic approach varies somewhat from that in immunocompetent hosts. Vague or nonspecific complaints may be the only indication of serious gastrointestinal infections. The physical findings are often subtle, even in catastrophic conditions, such as ischemic colitis (123). In a study of 23 heart and lung transplant patients with CMV disease, vague abdominal pain, gaseous distention, loss of appetite, and loose stools were frequently the only symptoms reported (124). It is often appropriate to proceed quickly to an invasive diagnostic workup. Endoscopic biopsy of the upper and lower gastrointestinal tract is the optimal method for the early diagnosis of opportunistic infection of the gastrointestinal tract (125,126). However, the benefits of endoscopic examination must be balanced against the risks of the procedure, particularly in bone marrow recipients, who may be predisposed to complications because of neutropenia or thrombocytopenia. In comparison with endoscopy, radiographic studies are considerably less sensitive for detecting gastrointestinal infections in transplant patients.

Serologic testing to diagnose infections of the gastrointestinal tract is of limited usefulness in transplant patients. Seroconversions may occur late in the course of infection, and in some patients, such as allogeneic bone marrow transplant recipients, a normal antibody response does not develop for a year or more after transplantation (127). Allogeneic bone marrow recipients also frequently receive intravenous immunoglobulin, which may result in false-positive results of serologic tests for CMV and other pathogens. Tests for *Cryptococcus* and *Histoplasma* antigens are well established and reliable (128), but tests for *Candida* antigen show poor sensitivity and specificity (129).

A major advance in the 1990s was the introduction of tests to measure CMV load. The two tests that have been validated and in which an increased viral load best correlates with patient outcome are an assay for whole blood antigenemia and quantitative polymerase chain reaction (PCR) (130,131). PCR testing for EBV has proved useful for monitoring children with intestinal transplants, who are at risk for lymphoproliferative disease (132). PCR testing may also be useful in the early detection of *Aspergillus* infection (133). The diagnostic use of PCR will likely be applied in the detection of many other infections during the next few years.

MANAGEMENT

The management of enteric infections in transplant patients is similar to the management in other hosts, and general guidelines are discussed in the chapters on specific infectious agents. A few important differences merit further discussion.

Therapy of Cytomegalovirus Infection

Ganciclovir was the first effective treatment for CMV infection (134). This drug inhibits CMV replication, and viral cultures are negative in 90% of infected persons after 7 to 10 days of treatment. The response of transplant recipients with CMV disease to ganciclovir therapy has been variable. In early studies of bone marrow recipients with CMV pneumonia, only 10% to 15% survived (135,136), but survival improved when intravenous immunoglobulin was administered with ganciclovir (137,138). Response rates in solid organ transplant patients with CMV disease have varied from 37% to 100% (138–141). Despite these disparate results, the consensus now is that ganciclovir therapy is beneficial (142,143), based on the results of prospective, randomized studies of ganciclovir prophylaxis (144–147) and retrospective studies showing less disease progression and viral dissemination after therapy (148).

After successful treatment of CMV disease, about 15% to 35% of transplant recipients relapse, usually within 3 to 6 weeks. Some relapses are mild and do not require retreatment. Foscarnet (trisodium phosphonoformate) is also active against CMV, but because of its associated renal toxicity, the drug has been used more sparingly than ganciclovir in transplant recipients (149). However, because less bone marrow toxicity is associated with foscarnet than with ganciclovir, foscarnet offers a significant advantage in bone marrow recipients with impaired marrow function. Foscarnet is also active against most ganciclovir-resistant strains of CMV (150).

Antifungal Therapy

Azole drugs, such as ketoconazole, fluconazole, and itraconazole, can be effective alternatives to amphotericin B for the treatment of susceptible fungi. All three agents interfere with the metabolism of cyclosporine and tacrolimus via a cytochrome P-450 mechanism and can lead to elevated levels of these drugs (151–154). The effect is most pronounced with ketoconazole, moderate with itraconazole, and usually mild with fluconazole (154). Fluconazole is well absorbed, but the absorption of ketoconazole and itraconazole is only optimal in the presence of food and gastric acid. An oral formulation of itraconazole in solution has recently been made available. It is well absorbed and is preferable in patients with absorption problems, such as bone marrow recipients (155).

Amphotericin B is the mainstay of antifungal therapy in seriously ill patients (156). However, patients receiving cyclosporine or tacrolimus are particularly susceptible to the nephrotoxic effects of amphotericin. Some centers preferentially use lipid-complexed formulations of amphotericin, which cause less toxicity (157,158). Neutropenic patients with invasive fungal disease should receive amphotericin after recovery of marrow function and should also complete a full course of amphotericin appropriate for the pathogen being treated (156,158). It is standard practice to administer systemic antifungal treatment (usually amphotericin B) to neutropenic patients with negative bacterial cultures and fever unresponsive to broad-spectrum antibacterial therapy (157,159). Empiric antifungal therapy may also be reasonable in solid organ transplant recipients with a high risk for occult fungal infection.

Antibacterial Therapy

The guidelines for the treatment of enteric and intraabdominal bacterial infections are similar in transplant recipients and immunocompetent patients. Neutropenic patients started on antibacterial treatment for infection with gram-negative rods should generally continue such therapy until their neutrophil counts return to normal. Because *Salmonella* infections often recur in transplant recipients, it may be advisable to administer a longer course of therapy and perform cultures to test for cure after therapy (21).

PREVENTION

At present, attention is focused on the prevention of enteric and intraabdominal infections in transplant patients. Inactivated vaccines are considered safe but may be less effective than in immunocompetent persons (160). Live attenuated vaccines are usually avoided despite a lack of evidence that they represent a risk to transplant recipients (161). An attenuated vaccine prepared from the Towne strain of CMV was developed in the late 1970s. Studies in renal transplant recipients showed that it was safe but provided only minor benefit (162). Environmental control to prevent infection is a common practice in bone marrow recipients and other neutropenic patients. When the use of laminar flow rooms was combined with other preventive measures, such as thoroughly cooking food and administering nonabsorbable antibiotics, infectious morbidity was reduced in some studies (163,164). In solid organ transplant recipients, however, evidence indicates that patients do not benefit from any infection control measure beyond simple hand washing (165).

Prophylactic antibiotics are widely used in transplant recipients to prevent infection. Intravenous antibiotics are used universally for surgical wound prophylaxis and are not discussed here. The oral administration of nonabsorbable antibiotics was the first form of prophylaxis to be investigated in neutropenic patients. This intervention can reduce the number of infectious episodes and fever, but it provides no consistent survival advantage (166,167). The regimens are also unpalatable and difficult to administer to patients with mucositis. Consequently, most bone marrow centers have abandoned them. A regimen of oral gentamicin, polymyxin B, and nystatin has been promoted to decrease gram-negative infections in liver transplant recipients (168), but the absence of controlled studies confirming benefit has limited the wider use of this regimen.

Sulfamethoxazole-trimethoprim (SMX-TMP) has also been extensively evaluated as a means to prevent infection in neutropenic patients. Most studies of oral SMX-TMP prophylaxis show a decrease in the rate of systemic infection but no definite impact on survival (168–173). Problems with the use of SMX-TMP included the development of drug resistance in gram-negative rods (172,174) and prolonged neutropenia in some patients (175,176). However, SMX-TMP is still widely used and very effective for the prevention of *Pneumocystis* infection in all types of transplantation (177). The doses required for *Pneumocystis* prophylaxis are low; a single-strength tablet daily or three double-strength tablets per week are sufficient. When used to prevent *Pneumocystis* infection, the drug is continued for a minimum of 6 to 12 months after transplantation. Many centers continue SMX-TMP for the life of the patient. SMX-TMP is also effective for the prevention of urinary infection after renal transplantation (178).

Fluoroquinolone antibiotics, such as ciprofloxacin and norfloxacin, are commonly used to prevent bacterial infections in neutropenic patients. Quinolone prophylaxis in such patients substantially decreases the rate of gram-negative infections but has not been shown, even in metaanalyses of multiple studies, to improve overall survival (179). Although quinolones are usually well tolerated, an increase in *Streptococcus viridans* sepsis and the potential for the development of resistance has made the routine use of quinolone prophylaxis controversial (156,180).

Antifungal prophylaxis for mucocutaneous *Candida* infection is a standard component of transplant care. The most commonly used regimen is an oral nystatin solution (500,000 units four times daily). This regimen is effective for the prevention of oral and esophageal candidiasis in solid organ and bone marrow recipients (181,182), but whether the regimen decreases the frequency of systemic candidiasis is unclear. Oral nystatin can be difficult or impossible to administer to patients who are intubated or have severe mucositis. Clotrimazole troches appear to work as well as nystatin and may be more palatable, but some *Candida* species are resistant to clotrimazole (182). In the past 10 years, additional regimens have been used to provide systemic in addition to topical protection. Ketoconazole prevents fungal mucositis, but this agent is poorly absorbed by some bone marrow recipients and dramatically decreases cyclosporine metabolism, so that drug dosing is difficult (154,183,184). Two large, randomized studies performed in bone marrow recipients have shown that prophylactic fluconazole (400 mg daily) decreases systemic and superficial *Candidia* infections in the early post-transplant period (185,186). One of these studies also demonstrated a decreased mortality in patients in the fluconazole arm (186). Despite its poor activity against molds, such as *Aspergillus,* fluconazole has proved to be a relatively effective prophylaxis for liver transplant recipients (187). Some *Candida* species, such as *C. krusei* and *C. glabrata,* are resistant to fluconazole (188), which has raised concern that the widespread prophylactic use of fluconazole will encourage the emergence of resistant species (189). Resistance of *C. albicans* to fluconazole is well documented in patients with AIDS but does not yet appear to be a significant problem in transplant populations (190). Itraconazole, another azole antifungal agent, is active against both *Candida* and *Aspergillus,* but the agent has not been well studied in transplant populations.

Low-dose intravenous amphotericin (0.1 to 0.2 mg/kg per day) has been used as parenteral prophylaxis for fungal disease in high-risk neutropenic patients (191,192). The efficacy of this regimen in preventing fungal infections is similar to that of fluconazole prophylaxis, but it is associated with significant nephrotoxicity in allogeneic transplant patients receiving cyclosporine.

Antiviral Prophylaxis

Acyclovir is effective prophylaxis for HSV infection. Divided doses of 600 to 800 mg/d administered orally prevent most oral, genital, and esophageal HSV infections in transplant patients (113). The toxicity of acyclovir is low, and apart from a small additional cost, its routine use entails no disadvantages in HSV-seropositive patients. Acyclovir prophylaxis should also prevent the occasional cases of tissue-invasive or systemic disease caused by HSV (71).

Prophylaxis of CMV infection is widely practiced but is a very complex topic. Although acyclovir is not an effective therapy for active CMV disease, prophylactic use of the drug can reduce the frequency of CMV disease in solid organ and bone marrow transplant populations (193–195). The regimens that have been shown to be effective for this purpose are high doses of intravenous (500 mg/M^2 every 8 hours) or oral (800 mg four times daily) medication (193–195). Valacyclovir, the prodrug of acyclovir, was remarkably effective in preventing CMV disease when given at high doses (2 g orally four times daily) for 3 months, but CMV disease developed in some patients after it was stopped (196).

Ganciclovir was the first potent drug to be investigated as prophylaxis against CMV disease. Placebo-controlled studies in bone marrow transplant patients have demonstrated significant reductions in CMV disease with the administration of ganciclovir, either prophylactically or as preemptive therapy in response to positive viral cultures (145,146). Neutropenia occurred in about 30% of treated patients and was associated with an increased risk for infection. Prophylaxis of CMV-seropositive solid organ transplant recipients for 28 days with intravenous ganciclovir reduced CMV disease, but a longer duration of prophylaxis appeared to be necessary to reduce CMV disease in CMV-seronegative patients transplanted with organs from seropositive donors (197). Oral ganciclovir (1 g three times daily for 12 weeks) was shown to be an effective CMV prophylaxis in liver recipients (198). Antiviral strategies employing close virologic monitoring and preemptive therapy with either oral or intravenous ganciclovir also appear to be effective and may be less expensive than universal prophylaxis (199).

The administration of CMV hyperimmunoglobulin also reduces the rate of CMV disease, at least in CMV seronegative kidney recipients with seropositive donors, and is used by some centers, either alone or with other antiviral medications (40,200).

CONCLUSION

In conclusion, the diagnosis and effective management of gastrointestinal infections in transplant patients require a knowledge of the unique defects induced in nonimmune and immune host defense mechanisms, the epidemiology of the infections, and the clinical syndromes. With such knowledge, therapies for the diseases caused by diverse viral, bacterial, and parasitic agents in transplant recipients can be implemented more effectively.

REFERENCES

1. United Network for Organ Sharing Web Site. *www.unos.org*
2. International Bone Marrow Transplant Registry. *www.ibmtr.org*
3. Sternbach GL, Varon J, Hunt SA. Emergency department presentation and care of heart and heart/lung transplant recipients. *Ann Emerg Med* 1992;21:1140–1144.
4. Blakey JL, Barnes GL, Bishop RF, et al. Infectious diarrhea in children undergoing bone-marrow transplantation. *Aust N Z J Med* 1989;19:31–36.
5. Cox GJ, Matsui SM, Lo RS, et al. Etiology and outcome of diarrhea after marrow transplantation: a prospective study. *Gastroenterology* 1994;107:1398–1407.
6. George DL, Arnow PM, Fox AS, et al. Bacterial infection as a complication of liver transplantation: epidemiology and risk factors. *Rev Infect Dis* 1991;13:387–396.
7. Kusne S, Dummer JS, Singh N, et al. Infections after liver transplantation: an analysis of 101 consecutive cases. *Medicine (Baltimore)* 1988;67:132–143.
8. Sawyer OI, Garvin PJ, Codd JE, et al. Colorectal complications of renal allograft transplantation. *Arch Surg* 1978;113:84–86.
9. Penn I, Brettschneider L, Simpson K, et al. Major colonic problems in human homotransplant recipients. *Arch Surg* 1970;100: 61–65.
10. Gellin BG, Broome CV. Listeriosis. *JAMA* 1989;261:1313–1320.
11. Tripathy SP, Mackaness GB. The effect of cytotoxic agents on the primary immune response to *Listeria monocytogenes. J Exp Med* 1969;130:1–16.
12. Miller JK, Hedberg M. Effects of cortisone on susceptibility of mice to *Listeria monocytogenes. Am J Clin Pathol* 1965;43: 248–250.
13. Hugin AW, Cerny A, Wrann M, et al. Effect of cyclosporin A on immunity to *Listeria monocytogenes. Infect Immun* 1986;52: 12–17.
14. Schuchat A, Deaver KA, Wenger JD, et al. Role of foods in sporadic listeriosis: case–control study of dietary risk factors. *JAMA* 1992;267:2041–2045.
15. MacGowan AP, Marshall RJ, MacKay IM, et al. *Listeria* faecal carriage by renal transplant recipients, haemodialysis patients and patients in general practice; its relation to season, drug ther-

apy, foreign travel, animal exposure and diet. *Epidemiol Infect* 1991;106:157–166.
16. Spitzer PG, Hammer SM, Karchmer AW. Treatment of *Listeria monocytogenes* infection with trimethoprim-sulfamethoxazole: case report and review of the literature. *Rev Infect Dis* 1986; 8:427–430.
17. Yolken RH, Bishop CA, Townsend TR, et al. Infectious gastroenteritis in bone-marrow-transplant recipients. *N Engl J Med* 1982;306:1009–1012.
18. Fekety R, Kyung-Hee K, Brown D, et al. Epidemiology of antibiotic-associated colitis: isolation of *Clostridium difficile* from the hospital environment. *Am J Med* 1981;70:906–908.
19. McFarland LV, Mulligan ME, Kwok RYY, et al. Nosocomial acquisition of *Clostridium difficile* infection. *N Engl J Med* 1989;320:204–210.
20. Wust J, Sullivan NM, Hardegger U, et al. Investigation of an outbreak of antibiotic-associated colitis by various typing methods. *J Clin Microbiol* 1982;16:1096–1101.
21. Dhar JM, Al-Khader AA, Al-Sulaiman M, et al. Non-typhoid *Salmonella* in renal transplant recipients: a report of twenty cases and review of the literature. *Q J Med* 1991;287:235–250.
22. Ocharan-Corcuera J, Montejo-Baranda M, Lampreabe-Gaztelu I, et al. Nontyphoid *Salmonella* infections after renal transplantation. *Transplantation* 1987;44:150–151.
23. Nielsen HE, Korsager B. Bacteremia after renal transplantation. *Scand J Infect Dis* 1977;9:111–117.
24. Anderson RJ, Schafer LA, Olin DB, et al. Septicemia in renal transplant recipients. *Arch Surg* 1973;106:692–694.
25. Smith EJ, Milligan SL, Filo RS. *Salmonella* mycotic aneurysm after renal transplantation. *South Med J* 1981;11:1399–1401.
26. Severn M, Michael J. *Shigella* septicemia following renal transplantation. *Postgrad Med J* 1980;56:852–853.
27. Gueco I, Daniel M, Mendoza M, et al. Tropical infections after renal transplantation. *Transplant Proc* 1989;21:2105–2107.
28. Neter E, Merrin G, Surgalla MJ, et al. *Shigella sonnei* bacteremia. *Urology* 1974;4:198–200.
29. Perlman DM, Ampel NM, Schifman RB, et al. Persistent *Campylobacter jejuni* infections in patients infected with human immunodeficiency virus (HIV). *Ann Intern Med* 1988;108:540–546.
30. Maccario M, Tarantino A, Nobile-Orazio C, et al. *Campylobacter jejuni* bacteremia and Guillain-Barré syndrome in a renal transplant recipient. *Transpl Int* 1998;11:439–442.
31. Hagensee ME, Benyunes M, Miller JA, et al. *Campylobacter jejuni* bacteremia and Guillain-Barré syndrome in a patient with GVHD after allogeneic BMT. *Bone Marrow Transplant* 1994; 13: 349–351.
32. Stock KJ, Scott MA, Davis SF, et al. Hemorrhagic colitis due to a novel *Escherichia coli* serotype (O121:H19) in a transplant recipient. *Transpl Int* 2001;14:44–47
33. Davenport A, Shallcross TM, Crabtree JE, et al. Prevalence of *Helicobacter pylori* in patients with end-stage renal failure and renal transplant recipients. *Nephron* 1991;59:597–601.
34. Teenan RP, Burgoyne M, Brown IL, et al. *Helicobacter pylori* in renal transplant recipients. *Transplantation* 1993;56:100–103.
35. Tobin A, Hackman RC, McDonald GB. *H. pylori* infection in the immunocompromised host: a prospective study of 276 patients. *Ir J Med Sci* 1992;161[Suppl 10]:64–65.
36. Dummer S, Perez-Perez G, Breinig MK, et al. Seroepidemiology of *H. pylori* infection in heart transplant (HTTX) recipients. *Clin Infect Dis* 1995;21:1303–1305.
37. Munoz RM, Alonso-Pulpon L, Yebra M, et al. Intestinal involvement by nontuberculous mycobacteria after heart transplantation. *Clin Infect Dis* 2000;30:603–605.
38. Ho M. Human cytomegalovirus infections in immunosuppressed patients. In: Ho M, ed. *Cytomegalovirus: biology and infection.* New York: Plenum Press, 1991:249–300.
39. Dummer JS, White LT, Ho M, et al. Morbidity of cytomegalovirus infection in recipients of heart or heart–lung transplants who received cyclosporine. *J Infect Dis* 1985;152:1182–1191.
40. Patel R, Snydman DR, Rubin RH, et al. Cytomegalovirus prophylaxis in solid organ transplant recipients. *Transplantation* 1996;61:1279–1289.
41. Adler M, Goldman M, Liesnard C, et al. Diffuse herpes simplex virus colitis in a kidney transplant recipient successfully treated with acyclovir. *Transplantation* 1987;43:919–921.
42. Buss DH, Scharyj M. Herpesvirus infection of the esophagus and other visceral organs in adults: incidence and clinical significance. *Am J Med* 1979;66:457–462.
43. Chang AE, Young NA, Reddick RL, et al. Small bowel obstruction as a complication of disseminated varicella-zoster infection. *Surgery* 1978;83:371–374.
44. Breinig MK, Zitelli B, Starzl TE, et al. Epstein–Barr virus, cytomegalovirus, and other viral infections in children after liver transplantation. *J Infect Dis* 1987;156:273–279.
45. Hierholzer JC. Adenoviruses in the immunocompromised host. *Clin Microbiol Rev* 1992;5:262–274.
46. Michaels MG, Green M, Wald ER, et al. Adenovirus infection in pediatric liver transplant recipients. *J Infect Dis* 1992;165: 170–174.
47. Willoughby RE, Wee SB, Yolken RH. Non-group A rotavirus infection associated with severe gastroenteritis in a bone marrow transplant patient. *Pediatr Infect Dis J* 1988;7:133–135.
48. Kruger W, Stockschlader M, Zander AR. Transmission of rotavirus diarrhea in a bone marrow transplantation unit by a hospital worker. *Bone Marrow Transplant* 1991;8:507–508.
49. Peigue-Lafeuille H, Henquell C, Chambon M, et al. Nosocomial rotavirus infections in adult renal transplant recipients. *J Hosp Infect* 1991;18:67–70.
50. Townsend TR, Bolyard EA, Yolken RH, et al. Outbreak of coxsackie A1 gastroenteritis: a complication of bone-marrow transplantation. *Lancet* 1982;1:820–823.
51. Cubitt WD, Mitchell DK, Carter MJ, et al. Application of electron microscopy, enzyme immunoassay, and RT-PCR to monitor an outbreak of astrovirus type 1 in a pediatric bone marrow transplant unit. *J Med Virol* 1999;57:313–321.
52. Mathieson R, Dutta SK. *Candida* esophagitis. *Dig Dis Sci* 1983;28:365–370.
53. Cohen R, Roth FJ, Delgado E, et al. Fungal flora of the normal human small and large intestine. *N Engl J Med* 1969;280: 638–641.
54. Samonis G, Rolston K, Karl C, et al. Prophylaxis of oropharyngeal candidiasis with fluconazole. *Rev Infect Dis* 1990;12: S369–S370.
55. Joshi SN, Garvin PJ, Sunwoo YC. Candidiasis of the duodenum and jejunum. *Gastroenterology* 1981;80:829–833.
56. Tollemar J, Ericzon BG, Barkholt L, et al. Risk factors for deep *Candida* infections in liver transplant recipients. *Transplant Proc* 1990;22:1826–1827.
57. Wajszczuk CP, Dummer JS, Ho M, et al. Fungal infections in liver transplant recipients. *Transplantation* 1985;40:347–353.
58. Hau T, Van Hook EJ, Simmons RL, et al. Prognostic factors of peritoneal infections in transplant patients. *Surgery* 1978;84: 403–416.
59. Young RC, Bennett JE, Vogel CL, et al. Aspergillosis: the spectrum of the disease in 98 patients. *Medicine (Baltimore)* 1970;0: 147–173.
60. Kusne S, Torre-Cisneros J, Manez R, et al. Factors associated with invasive lung aspergillosis and the significance of positive *Aspergillus* culture after liver transplantation. *J Infect Dis* 1992;166:1379–1383.
61. Wheat LJ, Smith EJ, Sathapatayavongs G, et al. Histoplasmosis in renal allograft recipients. *Arch Intern Med* 1983;143:703–707.

62. Brett MT, Kwan JTC, Bending MR. Caecal perforation in a renal transplant patient with disseminated histoplasmosis. *J Clin Pathol* 1988;41:992–995.
63. White JV, Garvey G, Hardy MA. Fatal strongyloidiasis after renal transplantation: a complication of immunosuppression. *Am Surg* 1982;48:39–41.
64. Stone WJ, Schaffner W. *Strongyloides* infections in transplant recipients. *Semin Respir Infect* 990;5:58–64.
65. Schad GA. Cyclosporine may eliminate the threat of overwhelming strongyloidiasis in immunosuppressed patients. *J Infect Dis* 1986;153:178.
66. Roncoroni AJ, Gomez MA, Mera J, et al. *Cryptosporidium* infection in renal transplant patients. *J Infect Dis* 1989;160:559.
67. Martino P, Gentile G, Caprioli A, et al. Hospital-acquired cryptosporidiosis in a bone marrow transplantation unit. *J Infect Dis* 1988;158:647–648.
68. Bromiker R, Korman SH, Or R, et al. Severe giardiasis in two patients undergoing bone marrow transplantation. *Bone Marrow Transplant* 1989;4:701–703.
69. Gumbo T, Hobbs RE, Carlyn C, et al. Microsporidial infection in transplant patients. *Transplantation* 1999;67:482–484.
70. Strauss SE, Rooney JF, Sever JL, et al. Herpes simplex virus infection: biology, treatment, and prevention. *Ann Intern Med* 1985;103:404–419.
71. Kusne S, Schwartz M, Breinig MK, et al. Herpes simplex virus hepatitis after solid organ transplantation in adults. *J Infect Dis* 1991;163:1001–1007.
72. Dummer JS, Armstrong J, Somers J, et al. Transmission of infection with herpes simplex virus by renal transplantation. *J Infect Dis* 1987;155:202–206.
73. Nalesnik MA. Lymphoproliferative disease in organ transplant recipients. *Springer Semin Immunopathol* 1991;13:199–216.
74. Hanto DW, Frizzera G, Gajl-Peczalska KJ, et al. Epstein–Barr virus, immunodeficiency, and B cell lymphoproliferation. *Transplantation* 1985;39:461–471.
75. Ho M, Jaffe R, Miller G, et al. The frequency of Epstein–Barr virus infection and associated lymphoproliferative syndrome after transplantation and its manifestations in children. *Transplantation* 1988;45:719–727.
76. Manez R, Breinig MC, Linden P, et al. Posttransplant lymphoproliferative disease in primary Epstein–Barr virus infection after liver transplantation: the role of cytomegalovirus disease. *J Infect Dis* 1997;176:1462–1467
77. Shields AF, Hackman RC, Fife KH, et al. Adenovirus infections in patients undergoing bone-marrow transplantation. *N Engl J Med* 1985;312:529–533.
78. Webb DH, Shields AF, Fife KH. Genomic variation of adenovirus type 5 isolates recovered from bone marrow transplant recipients. *J Clin Microbiol* 1987;25:305–308.
79. Starzl TE, Demetris AJ, Van Thiel D. Liver transplantation (first of two parts). *N Engl J Med* 1989;321:1014–1022.
80. Lebeau G, Yanaga K, Marsh JW, et al. Analysis of surgical complications after 397 transplantations. *Surg Gynecol Obstet* 1990;170:317–322.
81. Sollinger HW, Knechtle SJ, Reen A, et al. Experience with 100 consecutive simultaneous kidney–pancreas transplants with bladder drainage. *Ann Surg* 1991;214:703–711.
82. Ozaki CF, Stratta RJ, Taylor RJ, et al. Surgical complications in solitary pancreas and combined pancreas–kidney transplantations. *Am J Surg* 1992;164:546–551.
83. Swartz SL, Dluhy RG. Corticosteroids: clinical pharmacology and therapeutic use. *Drugs* 1978;16:238–255.
84. Wahl SM, Altman LC, Rosenstreich DL. Inhibition of *in vitro* lymphokine synthesis by glucocorticosteroids. *J Immunol* 1975;115:476–481.
85. Dayton MT, Kleckner SC, Brown DK. Peptic ulcer perforation associated with steroid use. *Arch Surg* 1987;122:376–380.
86. Fadul CE, Lemann W, Thaler HT, et al. Perforation of the gastrointestinal tract in patients receiving steroids for neurologic disease. *Neurology* 1988;38:348–352.
87. Alexander P, Schuman E, Vetto RM. Perforation of the colon in the immunocompromised patient. *Am J Surg* 1986;151:557–561.
88. Arsura EL. Corticosteroid-associated perforation of colonic diverticula. *Arch Intern Med* 1990;150:1337–1338.
89. Marsh JW, Vehe KL, White HM. Immunosuppressants. *Gastroenterol Clin North Am* 1992;21:679–693.
90. Bunjes D, Hardt C, Rollinghoff M, et al. Cyclosporin A mediates immunosuppression of primary cytotoxic T-cell responses by impairing the release of interleukin 1 and interleukin 2. *Eur J Immunol* 1981;11:657–661.
91. Kahan BD. Cyclosporine. *N Engl J Med* 1989;321:1725–1738.
92. Drewe J, Beglinger C, Kissel T. The absorption site of cyclosporin in the human gastrointestinal tract. *Br J Clin Pharmacol* 1992;33:39–43.
93. Peters DH, Fitton A, Plosker GL, et al. Tacrolimus. *Drugs* 1993;46:746–794.
94. Sollinger HW. Mycophenolate mofetil for the prevention of acute rejection in primary cadaveric renal allograft recipients. *Transplantation* 1995;60:225–232.
95. Vasquez EM. Sirolimus: a new agent for the prevention of renal allograft rejection. *Am J Health Syst Pharm* 2000;57:437–451.
96. Menkis AH, Powell AM, Novick RJ, et al. A prospective randomized controlled trial of initial immunosuppression with ALG versus OKT3 in recipients of cardiac allografts. *J Heart Lung Transplant* 1992;11:569–576.
97. Weir MR, Henry ML, Blackmore M, et al. Incidence and morbidity of cytomegalovirus disease associated with a seronegative recipient receiving seropositive donor-specific transfusion and living-related donor transplantation. *Transplantation* 1988;45:111–116.
98. Singh N, Dummer JS, Kusne S, et al. Infections with cytomegalovirus and other herpesviruses in 121 liver transplant recipients: transmission by donated organ and the effect of OKT3 antibodies. *J Infect Dis* 1988;158:124–131.
99. Swinnen LJ, Costanzo-Nordin MR, Fisher SG, et al. Increased incidence of lymphoproliferative disorder after immunosuppression with the monoclonal antibody OKT3 in cardiac-transplant recipients. *N Engl J Med* 1990;323:1723–1728.
100. Mitchell EP, Schein PS. Gastrointestinal toxicity of chemotherapeutic agents. *Semin Oncol* 1982;9:52–64.
101. Ferrara JLM, Deeg HJ. Graft-versus-host disease. *N Engl J Med* 1991;324:667–673.
102. McDonald GB, Shulman HM, Sullivan KM, et al. Intestinal and hepatic complications of human bone marrow transplantation. *Gastroenterology* 1986;90:460–484.
103. Winston DJ, Ho WG, Champlin RE, et al. Infectious complications of bone marrow transplantation. *Exp Hematol* 1984;12:205–215.
104. Tutschka PJ. Infections and immunodeficiency in bone marrow transplantation. *Pediatr Infect Dis* 1988;7:S22–S29.
105. Slavin RE, Santos GW. The graft versus host reaction in man after bone marrow transplantation: pathology, pathogenesis, clinical features, and implication. *Clin Immunol Immunopathol* 1973;1:472–498.
106. Beschorner WE, Yardley JH, Tutschka PJ, et al. Deficiency of intestinal immunity with graft-vs.-host disease in humans. *J Infect Dis* 1981;144:38–46.
107. Witherspoon RP, Storb R, Ochs HD, et al. Recovery of antibody production in human allogeneic marrow graft recipients: influence of time post-transplantation, the presence or absence of chronic graft-versus-host disease, and antithymocyte globulin treatment. *Blood* 1981;58:360–368.

108. Grant D, Hurlbut D, Zhong R, et al. Intestinal permeability and bacterial translocation following small bowel transplantation in the rat. *Transplantation* 1991;52:221–224.
109. Kusne S, Manez R, Frye BL, et al. Use of DNA amplification for diagnosis of cytomegalovirus enteritis after intestinal transplantation.. *Gastroenterology* 1997;112:1121–1128.
110. Deeg JH, Bowden RA. Introduction to marrow and stem cell transplantation. In: Bowden RA, Ljungman P, Paya CV eds. *Transplant infections.* New York, Lippincott–Raven Publishers, 1998:1–12.
111. Rubin RH. Infection in the renal and liver transplant patient. In: Rubin RH, Young LS, eds. *Clinical approach to infection in the compromised host.* New York: Plenum Press, 1988:557–621.
112. Dummer JS, Ho M. Infections in solid organ transplant patients. In: Mandell GL, Bennett JE, Dolin R. eds. *Mandell, Douglas and Bennett's principles and practice of infectious diseases,* fifth edition. New York: Churchill Livingstone, 2000:3148–3159.
113. Wade JC, Newton B, Flournoy N, et al. Oral acyclovir for prevention of herpes simplex virus reactivation after marrow transplantation. *Ann Intern Med* 1984;100:823–828.
114. Dworkin B, Winawer SJ, Lightdale CJ. Typhlitis: report of a case with long-term survival and a review of the recent literature. *Dig Dis Sci* 1981;26:1032–1037.
115. Dosik GM, Luna M, Valdivieso M, et al. Necrotizing colitis in patients with cancer. *Am J Med* 1979;67:646–656.
116. Bombi JA, Cardesa A, Llebaria C, et al. Main autopsy findings in bone marrow transplant patients. *Arch Pathol Lab Med* 1987; 111:125–129.
117. McDonald GB, Hinds MS, Fisher LD, et al. Veno-occlusive disease of the liver and multiorgan failure after bone marrow transplantation: a cohort study of 355 patients. *Ann Intern Med* 1993;118:255–267.
118. Shulman HM, McDonald GB, Matthews D, et al. An analysis of hepatic venoocclusive disease and centrilobular hepatic degeneration following bone marrow transplantation. *Gastroenterology* 1980;79:1178–1191.
119. Fine RN, Terasaki PI, Ettenger RB, et al. Renal transplantation update. *Ann Intern Med* 1984;100:246–257.
120. Villar HV, Neal DD, Levinson M, et al. Gastrointestinal complications after human transplantation and mechanical heart replacement. *Am J Surg* 1989;157:168–174.
121. Cates J, Chavez M, Laks H, et al. Gastrointestinal complications after cardiac transplantation: a spectrum of diseases. *Am J Gastroenterol* 1991;86:412–416.
122. Maurer JR. Therapeutic challenges following lung transplantation. *Clin Chest Med* 1990;11:279–290.
123. Flanigan RC, Reckard CR, Lucas BA. Colonic complications of renal transplantation. *J Urol* 1988;139:503–506.
124. Welch RW, Yokoyama Y, Cooper DKC, et al. The gastrointestinal management of patients undergoing heart transplantation. *J Okla State Med Assoc* 1991;84:557–562.
125. Lepinski SM, Hamilton JW. Isolated cytomegalovirus ileitis detected by colonoscopy. *Gastroenterology* 1990;98:1704–1706.
126. Steck TB, Durkin MG, Costanzo-Nordin MR, et al. Gastrointestinal complications and endoscopic findings in heart transplant patients. *J Heart Lung Transplant* 1993;12:244–251.
127. Lum LG The kinetics of immune reconstitution after human marrow transplantation. *Blood* 1987;69:369–380.
128. Wheat LJ, Kohler RB, Tewari RP. Diagnosis of disseminated histoplasmosis by detection of *Histoplasma capsulatum* antigen in serum and urine specimens. *N Engl J Med* 1986;314:83–88.
129. Bennett JE. Rapid diagnosis of candidiasis and aspergillosis. *Rev Infect Dis* 1987;9:398–402.
130. Boeckh M, Boivin G. Quantitation of cytomegalovirus: methodological aspects and clinical applications. *Clin Microbiol Rev* 1998;11:533–554.
131. Cope AV, Sabin C, Burroughs K, et al. Interrelationships among quantity of human cytomegalovirus (HCMV) DNA in blood, donor recipient serostatus and administration of methylprednisolone as risk factors for HCMV disease following liver transplantation. *J Infect Dis* 1997;176:1484–1490.
132. Green M, Burno J, Rowe D, et al. Predictive negative value of persistent low Epstein–Barr virus viral load after intestinal transplantation in children. *Transplantation* 2000;70:593–596.
133. Hebart H, Loffler J, Meisner C, et al. Early detection of *Aspergillus* infection after allogeneic stem cell transplantation by polymerase chain reaction. *J Infect Dis* 2000;181:173–179.
134. Buhles WC Jr, Mastre BJ, Tinker AJ, et al. Ganciclovir treatment of life- or sight-threatening cytomegalovirus infection: experience in 314 immunocompromised patients. *Rev Infect Dis* 1988;10[Suppl 3]:S495–S506.
135. Reed EC, Dandliker PS, Meyers JD. Treatment of cytomegalovirus pneumonia with 9-[2-hydroxy-*I*-(hydroxymethyl)ethoxymethyl]guanine and high-dose corticosteroids. *Ann Intern Med* 1986;105:214–215.
136. Shepp DH, Dandliker PS, de Miranda P, et al. Activity of 9-[2-hydroxy-*I*-(hydroxymethyl)ethoxymethyl]guanine in the treatment of cytomegalovirus pneumonia. *Ann Intern Med* 1985; 103:368–373.
137. Reed EC, Bowden RA, Dandliker PS, et al. Treatment of cytomegalovirus pneumonia with ganciclovir and intravenous cytomegalovirus immunoglobulin in patients with bone marrow transplants. *Ann Intern Med* 1988;109:783–788.
138. Emanuel D, Cunningham I, Jules-Elysee K, et al. Cytomegalovirus pneumonia after bone marrow transplantation successfully treated with the combination of ganciclovir and high-dose intravenous immune globulin. *Ann Intern Med* 1988;109:777–782.
139. Keay S, Petersen E, Icenogle T, et al. Ganciclovir treatment of serious cytomegalovirus infection in heart and heart–lung transplant recipients. *Rev Infect Dis* 1988;10[Suppl 3]:S563–S572.
140. Paya CV, Hermans PE, Smith TF, et al. Efficacy of ganciclovir in liver and kidney transplant recipients with severe cytomegalovirus infection. *Transplantation* 1988;46:229–234.
141. Hrebinko R, Jordan ML, Dummer JS, et al. Ganciclovir for invasive cytomegalovirus infection in renal allograft recipients. *Transplant Proc* 1991;23:1346–1347.
142. Snydman DR. Ganciclovir therapy for cytomegalovirus disease associated with renal transplants. *Rev Infect Dis* 1988;10[Suppl 3]:S554–S562.
143. Erice A, Jordan MC, Chace BA, et al. Ganciclovir treatment of cytomegalovirus disease in transplant recipients and other immunocompromised hosts. *JAMA* 1987;257:3082–3087.
144. Paul S, Dummer JS. Topics in clinical pharmacology: ganciclovir. *Am J Med Sci* 1992;304:272–277.
145. Goodrich JM, Mori M, Gleaves CA, et al. Early treatment with ganciclovir to prevent cytomegalovirus disease after allogeneic bone marrow transplantation. *N Engl J Med* 1991;325: 1601–1607.
146. Schmidt GM, Horak DA, Niland JC, et al. A randomized, controlled trial of prophylactic ganciclovir for cytomegalovirus pulmonary infection in recipients of allogeneic bone marrow transplants. *N Engl J Med* 1991;324:1005–1011.
147. Merigan TC, Renlund DG, Keay S, et al. A controlled trial of ganciclovir to prevent cytomegalovirus disease after heart transplantation. *N Engl J Med* 1992;326:1182–1186.
148. Fletcher CV, Balfour HH Jr. Evaluation of ganciclovir for cytomegalovirus disease. *DICP* 1989;23:5–11.
149. Ringden O, Lonngvist B, Paulin T, et al. Pharmacokinetics, safety and preliminary clinical experiences using foscarnet in the treatment of cytomegalovirus infections in bone marrow and renal transplant recipients. *J Antimicrob Chemother* 1986;17:373–387.
150. Chrisp P, Clissold SP. Foscarnet: a review of its antiviral activity,

pharmacokinetic properties and therapeutic use in immunocompromised patients with cytomegalovirus retinitis. *Drugs* 1991;41:104–129.
151. First MR, Schroeder TJ, Michael A, et al. Cyclosporine–ketoconazole interaction: long-term follow-up and preliminary results of a randomized trial. *Transplantation* 1993;55:1000–1004.
152. Kramer MR, Marshall SE, Denning DW, et al. Cyclosporine and itraconazole interaction in heart and lung transplant recipients. *Ann Intern Med* 1990;113:327–329.
153. Grant SM, Clissold SP. Fluconazole: a review of its pharmacodynamic and pharmacokinetic properties, and therapeutic potential in superficial and systemic mycoses. *Drugs* 1990;39:877–916.
154. Como JA, Dismukes WE. Oral azole drugs as systemic antifungal therapy. *N Engl J Med* 1994;330:263–272.
155. Michallet M, Persat F, Kranzhofer N, et al. Pharmacokinetics of itraconazole oral solution in allogeneic bone marrow transplant patients receiving total body radiation. *Transplantation* 1998;21:1239–1243.
156. Pizzo PA. Management of fever in patients with cancer and treatment-induced neutropenia. *N Engl J Med* 1993;328:1323–1332.
157. Walsh TJ, Lee J, Lecciones J, et al. Empiric therapy with amphotericin B in febrile granulocytopenic patients. *Rev Infect Dis* 1991;13:496–503.
158. Walsh TJ, Finberg RW, Arndt C, et al. Liposomal amphotericin B for empirical therapy in patients with persistent fever and neutropenia. *N Engl J Med* 1999;340:764–771.
159. EORTC International Antimicrobial Therapy Cooperative Group. Empiric antifungal therapy in febrile granulocytopenic patients. *Am J Med* 1989;86:668–672.
160. Burroughs M, Moscana A. Immunization of pediatric solid organ transplant candidates and recipients. *Clin Infect Dis* 2000;30:857–869.
161. Rand EB, McCarthy CA, Whitington PF. Measles vaccination after orthotopic liver transplantation. *J Pediatr* 1993;123:87–89.
162. Plotkin SA, Smiley ML, Friedman HM, et al. Towne-vaccine-induced prevention of cytomegalovirus disease after renal transplants. *Lancet* 1984;1:528–530.
163. Levine AS, Siegel SE, Schreiber AD, et al. Protected environments and prophylactic antibiotics: a prospective controlled study of their utility in the therapy of acute leukemia. *N Engl J Med* 1973;288:477–483.
164. Rodriguez V, Bodey GP, Freireich EJ, et al. Randomized trial of protected environment–prophylactic antibiotics in 145 adults with acute leukemia. *Medicine (Baltimore)* 1978;57:253–266.
165. Walsh TR, Guttenderf J, Dummer JS, et al. The value of isolation procedures in cardiac allograft recipients. *Ann Thorac Surg* 1989;47:1–5.
166. Schimpff SC, Greene WH, Young VM, et al. Infection prevention in acute nonlymphocytic leukemia: laminar air flow room reverse isolation with oral, nonabsorbable antibiotic prophylaxis. *Ann Intern Med* 1975;82:351–358.
167. Dankert J, Gaus W, Gaya H, et al. Protective isolation and antimicrobial decontamination in patients with high susceptibility to infection: a prospective cooperative study of gnotobiotic care in acute leukaemia patients III: the quality of isolation and decontamination. *Infection* 1978;6:175–191.
168. Wiesner RH. The incidence of gram-negative bacterial and fungal infections in liver transplant patients treated with selective decontamination. *Infection* 1990;18[Suppl 1]:S19–S21.
169. Enno A, Catovsky D, Darrell J, et al. Co-trimoxazole for prevention of infection in acute leukaemia. *Lancet* 1978;2:395–397.
170. Wade JC, Schimpff SC, Hargadon MT, et al. A comparison of trimethoprim-sulfamethoxazole plus nystatin with gentamicin plus nystatin in the prevention of infections in acute leukemia. *N Engl J Med* 1981;304:1057–1062.
171. Riben PD, Louie TJ, Lank BA, et al. Reduction in mortality from gram-negative sepsis in neutropenic patients receiving trimethoprim/sulfamethoxazole therapy. *Cancer* 1983;51:1587–1592.
172. Gualtieri RJ, Donowitz GR, Kaiser DL, et al. Double-blind randomized study of prophylactic trimethoprim/sulfamethoxazole in granulocytopenic patients with hematologic malignancies. *Am J Med* 1983;74:934–940.
173. Pizzo PA, Robichaud KJ, Edwards BK, et al. Oral antibiotic prophylaxis in patients with cancer: a double-blind randomized placebo-controlled trial. *J Pediatr* 1983;102:125–133.
174. Wilson JM, Guiney DG. Failure of oral trimethoprim-sulfamethoxazole prophylaxis in acute leukemia. *N Engl J Med* 1982;306:16–20.
175. Wade JC, de Jongh CA, Newman KA, et al. Selective antimicrobial modulation as prophylaxis against infection during granulocytopenia: trimethoprim-sulfamethoxazole vs. nalidixic acid. *J Infect Dis* 1983;147:624–634.
176. Dekker AW, Rozenberg-Arska M, Sixma JJ, et al. Prevention of infection by trimethoprim-sulfamethoxazole plus amphotericin B in patients with acute nonlymphocytic leukemia. *Ann Intern Med* 1981;95:555–559.
177. Dummer JS. *Pneumocystis carinii* infections in transplant recipients. *Semin Respir Infect* 1990;5:50–57.
178. Fox BC, Sollinger HW, Belzer FO, et al. A prospective, randomized, double-blind study of trimethoprim-sulfamethoxazole for prophylaxis of infection in renal transplantation: clinical efficacy, absorption of trimethoprim-sulfamethoxazole, effects on the microflora, and the cost–benefit ratio. *Am J Med* 1990;89:255–274.
179. Cruciani M, Rampazzo R, Malena M, et al. Prophylaxis with fluoroquinolones for bacterial infections in neutropenic patients. *Clin Infect Dis* 1996;23:795–805.
180. Elting LS, Bodey GP, Keefe BH. Septicemia and shock syndrome due to *viridans* streptococci: a case–control study of predisposing factors. *Clin Infect Dis* 1992;14:1201–1207.
181. Frick T, Fryd DS, Goodale RL, et al. Incidence and treatment of *Candida* esophagitis in patients undergoing renal transplantation: data from the Minnesota prospective randomized trial of cyclosporine versus antilymphocyte globulin–azathioprine. *Am J Surg* 1988;155:311–313.
182. Gombert ME, duBrucket L, Aulicino TM, et al. A comparative trial of clotrimazole troches and oral nystatin suspension in recipients of renal transplants. *JAMA* 1987;258:2553–2555.
183. Hann IM, Prentice HG, Corringham R, et al. Ketoconazole versus nystatin plus amphotericin B for fungal prophylaxis in severely immunocompromised patients. *Lancet* 1982;1:826–829.
184. Shepp DH, Klosterman A, Siegel MS, et al. Comparative trial of ketoconazole and nystatin for prevention of fungal infection in neutropenic patients treated in a protective environment. *J Infect Dis* 1985;152:1257–1263.
185. Goodman JL, Winston DJ, Greenfield RA, et al. A controlled trial of fluconazole to prevent fungal infections in patients undergoing bone marrow transplantation. *N Engl J Med* 1992;326:845–851.
186. Slavin MA, Osborne B, Adams R, et al. Efficacy and safety of fluconazole prophylaxis for fungal infections after marrow transplantation—a prospective, randomized, double-blind study. *J Infect Dis* 1995;171:1545–1552.
187. Winston DJ, Pakrasi A, Busuttil R. Prophylactic fluconazole in liver transplant recipients. *Ann Intern Med* 1999;131:729–737.
188. Rex JH, Pfaller MA, Galgiani, JN, et al. Development of interpretive breakpoints for antifungal susceptibility testing: conceptual framework and analysis of *in vitro–in vivo* correlation data for fluconazole, itraconazole, and *Candida* infections. *Clin Infect Dis* 1997;24:235–247.
189. Wingard JR, Merz WG, Rinaldi MG, et al. Increase in *Candida krusei* infections among patients with bone marrow transplan-

tation and neutropenia treated prophylactically with fluconazole. *N Engl J Med* 1991;325:1274–1277.
190. Troillet N, Durussel C, Bille J, et al. Correlation between *in vitro* susceptibility of *Candida albicans* and fluconazole-resistant oropharyngeal candidiasis in HIV-infected patients. *Eur J Clin Microbiol Infect Dis* 1993;12:911–915.
191. Wolff SN, Fay J, Stevens D, et al. Fluconazole versus low-dose amphotericin B for the prevention of fungal infections in patients undergoing bone marrow transplantation: a study of the North American Marrow Transplant Group. *Bone Marrow Transplant* 2000;25:853–859.
192. Perfect JR, Klotman ME, Gilbert CC, et al. Prophylactic intravenous amphotericin B in neutropenic autologous bone marrow transplant recipients. *J Infect Dis* 1992;165:891–897.
193. Meyers JD, Reed EC, Shepp DH, et al. Acyclovir for prevention of cytomegalovirus infection and disease after allogeneic marrow transplantation. *N Engl J Med* 1988;318:70–75.
194. Balfour HH Jr, Chace BA, Stapleton JT, et al. A randomized, placebo-controlled trial of oral acyclovir for the prevention of cytomegalovirus disease in recipients of renal allografts. *N Engl J Med* 1989;320:1381–1384.
195. Elkins CC, Frist WH, Dummer JS, et al. Cytomegalovirus disease after heart transplantation: is acyclovir prophylaxis indicated? *Ann Thorac Surg* 1993;56:1267–1272.
196. Lowance D, Neumayr HH, Legendre CM, et al. Valacyclovir for the prevention of cytomegalovirus disease after renal transplantation. *N Engl J Med* 1999;340:1462–1470.
197. Seu P, Winston DJ, Holt CD, et al. Long-term ganciclovir prophylaxis for successful prevention of primary cytomegalovirus (CMV) disease in CMV-seronegative liver transplant recipients with CMV seropositive donors. *Transplantation* 1997;64: 1614–1617.
198. Gane E, Saliba F, Valdecasas GJC, et al. Randomized trial of efficacy and safety of oral ganciclovir in the prevention of cytomegalovirus disease in liver transplant recipients. *Lancet* 1997;350:1729–1733.
199. Singh N, Paterson DL, Gayowski T, et al. Cytomegalovirus antigenemia-directed pre-emptive prophylaxis with oral versus I.V. ganciclovir for the prevention of cytomegalovirus disease in liver transplant recipients. *Tranplantation* 2000;70:717–722.
200. Snydman DR, Werner BG, Heinze-Lacey B, et al. Use of cytomegalovirus immune globulin to prevent cytomegalovirus disease in renal transplant recipients. *N Engl J Med* 1987;317: 1049–1054.

32

GASTROINTESTINAL INFECTIONS IN NEUTROPENIC PATIENTS

KENT A. SEPKOWITZ

The gastrointestinal tract is the most common source of systemic infection in the neutropenic patient. The majority of documented bacteremias derive from bowel flora that translocate into the bloodstream in the setting of chemotherapy-induced neutropenia and thrombocytopenia. In addition, fever or localized infection in several gastrointestinal sites, including the oral cavity, esophagus, intestine, cecum, and perianal area, may develop in the neutropenic patient. This chapter reviews the clinical syndromes associated with infections of the gastrointestinal tract in the neutropenic patient and presents a rational approach to managing these infections.

ORAL CAVITY

Overview

Oral complications develop in up to 40% of the 1 million new patients in whom cancer is diagnosed annually; these may be acute or chronic in nature (1). As the potency of treatment modalities intensifies, so too do the likelihood and severity of oral complications. Periodontal or mucosal infection may be limited locally or serve as a site of entry into the bloodstream for viruses, bacteria, or fungi.

Pathogenesis

Several factors contribute to the high rate of oral complications (2). First, the normal flora of the mouth routinely enter the bloodstream during simple everyday activities, such as chewing. Second, mucositis (stomatitis) is a common consequence of chemotherapy and radiation therapy to the head and neck. Third, control of local infection is severely compromised by neutropenia. Finally, the vast majority of adults have subclinical periodontal disease (3), which may worsen in the setting of neutropenia.

In various studies, the incidence of oral complications has ranged from 47% in patients with leukemia (including infection in 34%) (4), to 9.7% in patients with solid tumors (5), to 39% in patients with any type of cancer (6).

Presentation

Patients with periodontal infection or mucositis generally have pain on swallowing, talking, or chewing. Symptoms of other, concurrent medical problems, such as pneumonia, may make mouth discomfort of secondary importance to the patient, or the oral discomfort may predominate and obscure other, more potentially life-threatening problems. The inability to eat or swallow may sufficiently compromise nutrition and hydration such that parenteral feedings are required.

Almost any microbe may be recovered, including fungi, bacteria, and viruses. Attempts to define precisely which organism is causing local oral infection are confounded by the presence of normal oral flora that overgrow many cultures. In most series, fungi, particularly *Candida albicans* (in the presence or absence of thrush), predominate. Among patients with solid tumors, 67% of all oral infections were caused by *C. albicans,* versus about 50% of all infections among leukemic patients (5). In all series, commonly recovered bacteria included *Pseudomonas aeruginosa, Klebsiella* species, and *Escherichia coli* (4). Gram-positive cocci were seen in 4% of leukemic patients (4). Streptococcal species are common in some series (7,8). Anaerobes also have been recovered (3).

P. aeruginosa infection of the mouth may cause a specific clinical syndrome (5). *P. aeruginosa* is angiophilic and may invade gingival blood vessels, causing ischemia and necrosis of local tissue. Bacteremia may ensue. If the infection is controlled with antibiotics and the neutropenia resolves, the necrotic core of tissue will slough and normal granulation

K. A. Sepkowitz: Department of Medicine, Weill Medical College of Cornell University; Infectious Disease Service, Department of Medicine, Memorial Sloan-Kettering Cancer Center, New York, New York

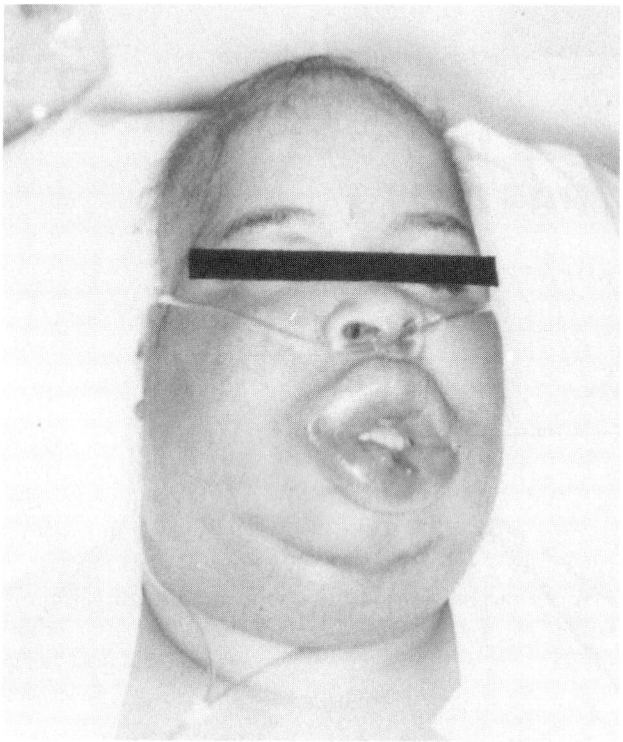

FIGURE 32.1. Diffuse facial cellulitis caused by *P. aeruginosa* infection in a 22-year-old woman with aplastic anemia. The infection was introduced when the patient pricked her gum with the tine of a fork while eating. Cellulitis spread despite treatment with antibiotics and the patient eventually died.

will begin (5). When the infection is not well controlled locally, it may spread rapidly to involve the face, neck, and mediastinum, with potentially catastrophic consequences (Fig. 32.1).

Herpes simplex is seen in about 10% of all patients with oral infection (4,5). Oral herpes simplex virus infection disrupts the integrity of the oral mucosa, thereby enhancing the opportunity for local bacterial flora to cause invasive or systemic disease. The identification and treatment of all oral herpes simplex infections is therefore crucial to the control of bacterial infections in the neutropenic cancer patient.

Treatment

Empiric antibiotic therapy directed at the usual bacteria anticipated in the febrile neutropenic patient, such as ticarcillin-clavulanic acid with an aminoglycoside, is adequate to cover empirically the organisms likely to cause periodontal disease in many hospitals. The empiric therapy should be determined by a knowledge of the susceptibility patterns at each specific hospital. For patients with severe disease from whom a specific organism is not recovered and who do not respond to standard antibiotics, metronidazole (500 mg administered intravenously every 6 to 8 hours) may be added. Increasing drug resistance of anaerobes has begun to limit the usefulness of metronidazole as an empiric agent for oral infection. In addition, control of pain with aggressive local care or systemically with narcotic analgesia is essential to allow the patient to eat, swallow, and speak.

ESOPHAGUS

Overview

Our appreciation of the spectrum of infectious esophageal diseases has increased in the wake of the AIDS epidemic. In cancer patients, esophageal infection with fungal, bacterial, or viral pathogens can be expected. The prompt institution of effective therapy is necessary to limit morbidity and prevent dissemination of an initially local infection.

Esophagitis, specifically caused by *C. albicans,* may be the presenting sign of an underlying malignancy. In two prospective endoscopic series comprising more than 3,500 patients, an underlying cancer was detected in 20 of 80 persons with *Candida* esophagitis (9).

Pathogenesis

Thoracic surgery, local radiation therapy, and chemotherapy all may predispose to esophageal disease by disrupting the integrity of the esophageal mucosa. Chemotherapy and immunosuppressive agents also impair cellular immunity.

Presentation

Patients who have esophagitis present typically with symptoms of dysphagia, odynophagia, or dull retrosternal ache. Three pathogens account for the majority of cases: *C. albicans,* herpes simplex virus, and cytomegalovirus (CMV). In AIDS, additional cases may occur secondary to aphthous ulcers, a syndrome without a clear cause. The frequency of this condition among cancer patients is not known but appears to be low. The pathogens do not each cause a distinct clinical syndrome, although in one series, nausea and vomiting were particularly common features of herpes simplex esophagitis in bone marrow transplant patients (10). Additional causes include infection with *Aspergillus* species (Fig. 32.2) and gram-positive and gram-negative bacteria (11) (see Color Figure 32.3).

Diagnosis is by endoscopic biopsy with culture. The practical algorithm developed for patients with HIV infection and esophagitis—initial treatment for fungal then herpetic disease, with endoscopy of nonresponders—may not be advisable for neutropenic patients who are already receiving antifungal and antiviral therapy. Biopsy, however, may be contraindicated because of thrombocytopenia. Even with endoscopic biopsy, the diagnosis of CMV infection may require an array of molecular diagnostic techniques (12).

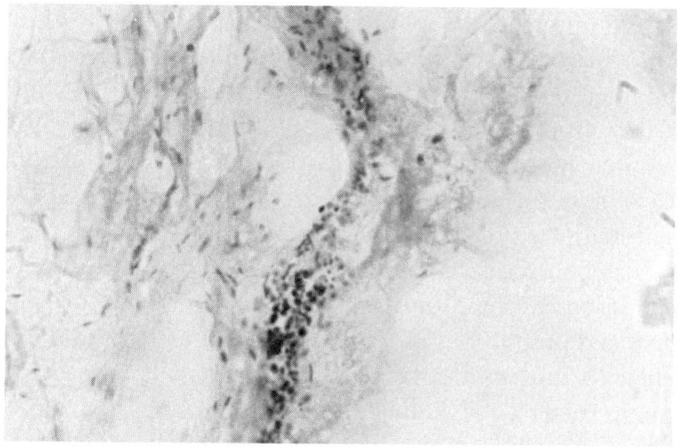

FIGURE 32.2. Fungal esophagitis caused by *Aspergillus flavus* infection in a bone marrow transplant patient. *Aspergillus* is a rare cause of esophagitis in the absence of other signs of aspergillosis.

Treatment

Treatment is directed at the recovered organism or empirically, as noted.

CECUM: TYPHLITIS

Overview

The term *typhlitis,* derived from the Greek *typhlon* ("blind pouch"), refers to the cecum, where most cases appear. Other names for this syndrome include *neutropenic enterocolitis, necrotizing enterocolitis,* and *ileocecal syndrome.*

Typhlitis is a necrotizing enterocolitis that usually affects the cecum. It carries a mortality rate that in some series exceeds 50%. After early reports (13), Wagner et al. (14), having reviewed the autopsies of children who died of leukemia, described the syndrome. They found an incidence of typhlitis of about 12%. Reviews have found children with acute leukemia to be the group at highest risk, although typhlitis has also been diagnosed in children and adults with organ transplants (15), drug-induced neutropenia (16), solid tumors (17), other hematologic neoplasms (17), sarcoma (17), aplastic anemia (18,19), cyclic neutropenia (20), AIDS (21), and other conditions. The disease is increasingly being diagnosed in adults (22,23) including solid organ transplant (24), and high-dose chemotherapy with stem cell rescue recipients (25).

Pathogenesis

The etiology of typhlitis is unknown. Anatomically, three types are recognized (18): confined to the cecum, involving the cecum plus the adjacent large and small bowel, and involving the cecum with scattered ulcers throughout the gastrointestinal tract.

Although chemotherapy and neutropenia appear to predispose patients to the development of typhlitis, but the occurrence of typhlitis in neutropenic patients who have not received chemotherapy, such as those with aplastic anemia or cyclic neutropenia, suggests that neutropenia is the more important risk factor. Importantly, cases have occurred among patients with normal white blood cell counts (21). In most cases, disease develops in the setting of chemotherapy-induced ulceration of the intestinal mucosa, combined with neutropenia and thrombocytopenia. Under these conditions, bacteria and fungi appear to invade into the cecal wall.

Why the disease occurs predominantly in the cecum is poorly understood. Peculiarities of the cecal blood supply, the motility, size, and distensibility of the cecum, or other factors may be pertinent.

Presentation

Most patients in whom typhlitis develops have received chemotherapeutic agents in the previous 30 days (17). Symptoms generally appear when neutropenia is most severe. The agents most commonly associated with the development of typhlitis include vincristine ara-C, and corticosteroids. Cases associated with taxanes (26) have also been described.

Common symptoms include fever, diarrhea, and right lower quadrant pain. Lower gastrointestinal bleeding is seen in up to 35% of patients. In one series (17), 62% of patients had a sore throat, reflecting diffuse chemotherapy-related mucositis and suggesting the important contribution of chemotherapeutic agents to the development of bowel mucositis. Nausea and vomiting are also commonly seen. In one study, typhlitis seldom presented without symptoms (17). In severe cases, intestinal perforation, often followed by shock, may occur. Pseudomembranous colitis resulting from *Clostridium difficile* infection must be considered in the differential diagnosis.

Up to 70% of patients with typhlitis have bacteremia (27). The frequent recovery of multiple organisms (35% of patients with typhlitis vs. 8% of those without typhlitis) (17) reflects a severely interrupted intestinal mucosa. Recovered organisms are predictable: aerobic intestinal flora, including *E. coli, Klebsiella* species, and *P. aeruginosa. Staphylococcus aureus* was noted in a pediatric series (18).

On gross examination of the cecum, bowel thickening and diffuse or discrete mucosal ulceration are seen. In addition, edema of the bowel wall, transmural hemorrhage, and necrosis occur. Microscopically, heavy invasion of bacteria into bowel wall with a scant inflammatory response is noted. Fungi are also sometimes seen. Leukemia cells are seldom found in the bowel wall. These findings further emphasize the contribution of chemotherapy-induced mucositis and neutropenia/thrombocytopenia.

Radiologic evaluation is essential (28–30), and specific abnormalities may predict a worse outcome (30). Abdominal plain films may reveal paralytic ileus; an absence of gas in the large intestine; a distended, fluid-filled cecum; or intramural air (pneumatosis intestinalis). Computed tomography and sonography similarly may show typical features, including ascites in the area of the cecum and thickening of the bowel wall and fascial planes. Barium enema and endoscopy are seldom performed, given their relative contraindication in the setting of neutropenia and accompanying thrombocytopenia.

Treatment

Consensus regarding the best therapy is lacking. Some experts recommend conservative management, including intravenous fluids, nasogastric suctioning, and broad-spectrum antibiotics. Antifungal antibiotics are added if no improvement is seen after 24 to 48 hours. This conservative approach is now commonly recommended (25,26,30). Some clinicians favor surgery, including right hemicolectomy, with suggestions of improved survival in some series. In a review of 22 cases of right hemicolectomy in the literature, Kunkel and Rosenthal (31) found 16 survivors versus 6 fatalities. Absolute indications for surgery include intractable gastrointestinal bleeding and cecal perforation.

Keidan et al. (23) suggested that elective right hemicolectomy be recommended for patients who survive the first episode but who must undergo additional chemotherapy, given the high risk for recurrence. The procedure would be performed after stabilization of the patient's condition and normalization of the white blood cell and platelet counts. This recommendation has not been adopted in all centers.

LARGE AND SMALL INTESTINE

Overview

The bowel flora is the source of most episodes of bacteremia in neutropenic patients (32). This is well demonstrated by the similar proportions of aerobic bacteria in the normal bowel flora and causing bacteremia in neutropenic hosts, in whom *E. coli, Klebsiella* species, and *P. aeruginosa* predominate (33). Thus, although it is never clinically evident, the bowel flora is the most common source of infection in the neutropenic host.

Pathogenesis

Enteric organisms may enter the bloodstream through chemotherapy-induced mucosal ulcerations, many of which are microscopic (32). Neutropenia, aggravated by thrombocytopenia, contributes to the poor healing of ulcers, enhancing further bacterial translocation. Systemic illnesses that are manifested in the gastrointestinal tract, including CMV infection and graft-versus-host disease (GVHD), also may compromise the normal mucosal barrier (32). In addition, patients who have received radiation therapy to the abdomen or pelvis may develop radiation enteritis, which further promotes the translocation of luminal bacteria into the circulation. The risk for radiation enteritis continues for years, if not decades, after radiation treatment has been delivered.

Many medical centers have published their experience with bacteremia and fungemia in neutropenic patients. The types and proportions of recovered organisms vary from one center to another, but at all medical centers, gram-negative enteric bacteria , including *E. coli, Klebsiella* species, and *P. aeruginosa,* are commonly recovered. In recent years, with the increasing use of central venous catheter devices, gram-positive organisms, including *Staphylococcus* species and *Streptococcus* species, have emerged.

Anaerobic bacteria account for fewer than 3% of recovered isolates. *Bacteroides* species and *Clostridium* species may be encountered, however, particularly when the bowel is necrotic and infiltrated with leukemia, lymphoma, or a solid tumor. As noted, anaerobes are increasingly resistant to various antibiotics. Awareness of the antibiotic resistance patterns of a hospital is essential for the selection of appropriate therapy.

Fungi, particularly *Candida* species, reside in normal bowel and may thrive when bacteria are suppressed by antibacterial therapy. Fungemia may ensue. *Trichosporon beigelii* is occurring more commonly as an opportunistic infection arising in the gastrointestinal tract of neutropenic patients. Molds, including *Aspergillus* species and the Mucorales, may rarely cause bowel infection and infarction, generally in the setting of overwhelming systemic infection.

Presentation

The diagnosis must be made from the clinical presentation—namely, fever in a neutropenic patient without localizing signs. The gastrointestinal source is usually not clinically evident. Abdominal signs are often minimal because the inflammatory response is dampened by the cytotoxic therapy. Blood cultures are positive in only 10% to 20% of episodes (34).

Treatment

The regimen for the empiric therapy of neutropenic fever should cover the bowel flora anticipated in the patient and is specific for a given hospital. Usually, two antimicrobial agents are administered, including an antipseudomonal semisynthetic penicillin and an aminoglycoside (34). Antifungal therapy to treat infection with *Candida* and *Aspergillus* species is added in persistently febrile persons. Guidelines for the management of this syndrome have been developed by the Infectious Disease Society of America and are revised frequently (34).

ANUS AND RECTUM

Overview

Anorectal disease complicates the course of 3% to 8% of patients hospitalized with malignant disease. An even higher proportion of patients with hematologic neoplasms, as many as 27% of those with nonlymphocytic leukemia and 8% of all those with leukemia, have anorectal disease (26,35). Grewal et al. (36) reviewed the MSKCC experience with anorectal disease in 2,618 patients hospitalized with leukemia from 1980 to 1990. Of these, 151 (5.8%) had symptomatic anorectal disease, including infection, anal fissure or fistula, and hemorrhoids.

Pathogenesis

Complications are more likely to develop in patients with preexisting conditions, such as fissures or hemorrhoids (36). The normal local trauma of defecation interrupts the mucosal surface promoting anorectal complications. Concurrent neutropenia and thrombocytopenia delay local healing, and infection may ensue.

Presentation

Common symptoms include fever, pain, and tenderness (27,36). Cellulitis and erythema are seen in fewer than half of patients, and purulence or fluctuance is seen in 13.5%. Bacteriologically, *P. aeruginosa* and *E. coli* predominate. Glenn et al. (37) demonstrated the importance of anaerobes and enterococci. In one series, *P. aeruginosa* alone predominated (35). In this series of 581 cancer patients, *P. aeruginosa* accounted for 15 of 22 abscesses and 12 episodes of resultant bacteremia. Several of these patients died.

Treatment

Treatment remains controversial, despite the advent of potent broad-spectrum antibiotics (38). Glenn et al. (37) reviewed 57 episodes in 44 patients with cancer. Overall, antibiotic therapy alone was adequate for half of the episodes; proper selection of antibiotics to include both specific anaerobic coverage (metronidazole or clindamycin) and an aminoglycoside, in addition to a broad-spectrum β-lactam antibiotic, resulted in an 88% response rate. In the review by Grewel et al. (36), 64% of the patients were treated conservatively and 36% operatively. Outcome was the same in the two groups and was more related to neutrophil count than to medical versus surgical management. This finding has been supported by others (37). In the series by Barnes et al. (38), surgical therapy resulted in high response rates with minimal surgical morbidity, so that the authors recommended that early incision and drainage be considered in all patients.

Local cellulitis with ischemia resulting from *P. aeruginosa* infection is a dreaded complication (Fig. 32.4). In one series, such patients did well with conservative therapy (39). The occurrence of this disease may have decreased, at least among children, when the practice of taking temperatures rectally was discontinued (39).

APPROACH TO THE PATIENT WITH NEUTROPENIA AND ABDOMINAL PAIN

Abdominal pain is a common symptom in neutropenic patients. The list of potential causes, which is considerable in normal hosts, is even more extensive in neutropenic patients. To complicate matters further, the physical examination findings may be less than dramatic because of the patient's diminished inflammatory response. Because the management of neutropenic patients leaves little margin for error, a prompt diagnosis and the institution of proper therapy are essential to limit morbidity and mortality. For patients without an obvious source of fever, immediate empiric therapy must be considered.

Diseases that are common in normal hosts, such as peptic ulcer disease, pancreatitis, and cholecystitis, also occur in neutropenic patients (Table 32.1). Peptic ulcer disease may be exacerbated by medications being taken, including corticosteroids. Gallbladder disease may be provoked by antibiotics, including ceftriaxone, and by the administration of total parenteral nutrition. Pancreatitis too may be provoked by numerous medications, including chemotherapy. Appendicitis may be particularly difficult to diagnose (40,41).

Diseases more specific to the immunocompromised host include typhlitis, a disease of the cecum that was discussed earlier. Sweet syndrome, also referred to as *neutrophilic*

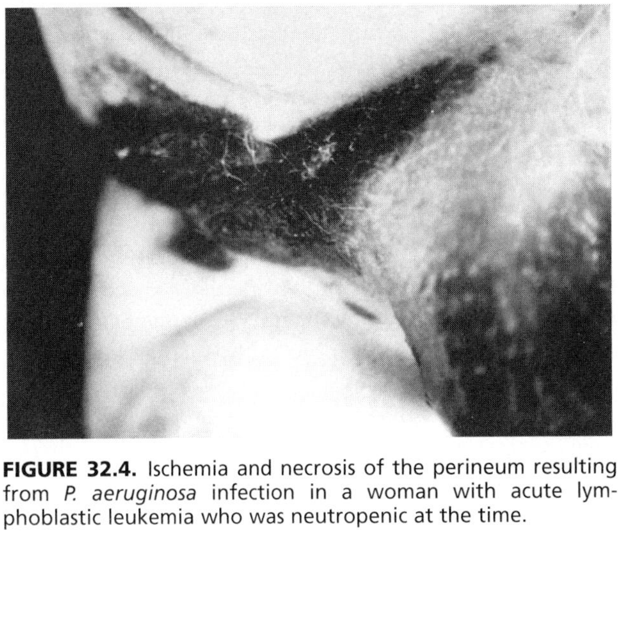

FIGURE 32.4. Ischemia and necrosis of the perineum resulting from *P. aeruginosa* infection in a woman with acute lymphoblastic leukemia who was neutropenic at the time.

TABLE 32.1. CAUSES OF ABDOMINAL PAIN IN NEUTROPENIC PATIENTS

Commonly seen in normal hosts (presentation may vary in neutropenic host)
Perforation
Appendicitis
Peptic ulcer disease
Pancreatitis
Cholecystitis
Gallbladder disease
Constipation
Specific to immunocompromised hosts
Infiltration by malignant cells
Hepatosplenic candidiasis
Typhlitis
Adynamic ileus
Sweet syndrome of bowel
Graft-versus-host disease
Cytomegalovirus

dermatosis, generally presents with one or several tender erythematous skin lesions and rarely may also cause abdominal pain and mucosal lesions of the gastrointestinal tract. GVHD, which occurs in some patients who have undergone allogeneic bone marrow transplantation, is a multisystem disease that particularly affects the skin, lungs, and gastrointestinal tract. Abdominal pain and bloody stool may develop. The diagnosis requires endoscopy with biopsy because the disease may mimic many conditions, particularly CMV colitis. CMV colitis may cause ulcers throughout the colon and present with pain and bleeding.

Also important to consider is infiltration by an aggressive tumor into visceral organs and lymph nodes. This may be seen in persons with either solid or hematologic neoplasm. Constipation and ileus should be considered, particularly in patients receiving large doses of narcotic analgesics for cancer-related pain. Vincristine commonly causes an ileus. Hepatosplenic candidiasis may also present with abdominal pain, often after the white blood cell count has returned to normal.

A comprehensive evaluation should be conducted quickly. After a routine history has been taken, a physical examination is performed, and blood for standard laboratory tests, including determination of amylase and lipase levels, is drawn. Abdominal radiographs should be obtained to exclude intestinal perforation. Wade et al. (42) have suggested that patients be divided according to distribution of pain; those with localizing pain should undergo an early radiographic study, such as sonography or computed tomography, whereas those with diffuse pain can be watched and treated conservatively. In all settings, surgical intervention is reserved for those with evidence of perforation, intraabdominal hemorrhage, or clinical worsening.

GUT DECONTAMINATION: PROS AND CONS

The use of oral antibiotics to "sterilize" or decontaminate the gut and therefore decrease the likelihood of neutropenia-associated bacteremia remains controversial (43–45). It has been a standard practice in many European medical centers, but less so in hospitals in the United States. Proponents point to fewer hospital days, less use of intravenous antibiotics, and lower rates of morbidity with improved "quality of life." Those against the routine use of antibiotics emphasize the failure of such decontaminating regimens to reduce mortality and the rate of hospital admissions for febrile neutropenic episodes (44). The most compelling argument against the routine use of gut sterilization is the inevitable emergence of resistant organisms. A study from the European Organization for Research and Treatment of Cancer (EORTC) emphasizes how rapidly resistance can emerge (45).

SUMMARY AND FUTURE CONCERNS

The gastrointestinal consequences of neutropenia include esophagitis, perirectal abcess and bacteremia and fungemia. The majority of bacteremic and fungemic episodes in neutropenic patients arise from the gastrointestinal tract. Micro-organisms from the mouth, esophagus, intestines, or perirectal area may enter the bloodstream when the mucosal barrier is disrupted by chemotherapy, surgery, or radiation therapy, particularly during neutropenia. Improved survival rates depend on a prompt diagnosis and the institution of effective therapy, including broad-spectrum antibiotics.

REFERENCES

1. National Institutes of Health Consensus Panel. Consensus statement: oral complications of cancer therapies. In: *Oral complications of cancer therapy. NCI Monogr* 1990;9:3–8.
2. Epstein JB, Chow AW. Oral complications associated with immunosuppression and cancer therapies. *Infect Dis Clin North Am* 1999;13:901–923.
3. Peterson DE, Minah GE, Overholser D, et al. Microbiology of acute periodontal infection in myelosuppressed cancer patients. *J Clin Oncol* 1987;5:1461–1468.
4. Dreizen S, McCredie KB, Bodey GP, et al. Quantitative analysis of the oral complications of antileukemia chemotherapy. *Oral Surg Oral Med Oral Pathol* 1986;62:650–653.
5. Dreizen S, Bodey GP, Valdivieso M. Chemotherapy-associated oral infections in adults with solid tumors. *Oral Surg Oral Med Oral Pathol* 1983;55:113–120.
6. Sonis ST, Sonis AL, Lieberman A. Oral complications in patients receiving treatment for malignancies other than of head and neck. *J Am Dent Assoc* 1978;97:468–472.
7. Winegard JR. Infectious and noninfectious systemic consequences. In: *Oral complications of cancer therapy. NCI Monogr* 1990;9:21–26.

8. Cohen J, Worsley AM, Goldman JM, et al. Septicaemia caused by *viridans* streptococci in neutropenic patients with leukaemia. *Lancet* 1983;2:1452–1454.
9. Baehr PH, McDonald GB. Esophageal infections: risk factors, presentation, diagnosis and treatment. *Gastroenterology* 1994; 106:509–532.
10. Spencer GD, Hackman RC, McDonald GB, et al. A prospective study of unexplained nausea and vomiting after bone marrow transplantation. *Transplantation* 1986;42:602–607.
11. Walsh TJ, Belitsos NJ, Hamilton SR. Bacterial esophagitis in immunocompromised patients. *Arch Intern Med* 1986;146: 1345–1348.
12. Hackman RC, Wolford JL, Cleaves CA, et al. Recognition and rapid diagnosis of upper gastrointestinal cytomegalovirus infection in marrow transplant recipients. *Transplantation* 1994;57: 231–237.
13. Amromin GD, Salomon RD. Necrotizing enteropathy. A complication of treated leukemia or lymphoma patients. *JAMA* 1962; 182:133–139.
14. Wagner ML, Rosenberg HS, Fernbacj DJ, et al. Typhlitis: a complication of leukemia in childhood. *Am J Roentgenol* 1970;109: 341–350.
15. Nagler A, Pavel L, Naparstek E, et al. Typhlitis occurring in autologous bone marrow transplantation. *Bone Marrow Transplant* 1992;9:63–64.
16. Clary RM, Wyatt SB, Henley RW, et al. Fatal typhlitis secondary to procainamide-induced agranulocytosis. *Va Med Q* 1984;3:697–698.
17. Dosik GM, Luna M, Valdivieso M, et al. Necrotizing colitis in patients with cancer. *Am J Med* 1979;67:646–656.
18. Katz JA, Wagner ML, Gresic MV, et al. Typhlitis: an 18-year experience and postmortem review. *Cancer* 1990;65:1041–1047.
19. Weinberger M, Hollingsworth H, Feuerstein IM, et al. Successful surgical management of neutropenic enterocolitis in two patients with severe aplastic anemia. *Arch Intern Med* 1994;153:107–113.
20. Geelhoed GW, Kane MA, Dale DC, et al. Colon ulceration and perforation in cyclic neutropenia. *J Pediatr Surg* 1973;8:379–382.
21. Till M, Lee N, Soper WD, et al. Typhlitis in patients with HIV-1 infection. *Ann Intern Med* 1992;116:998–1000.
22. Mower WJ, Hawkins JA, Nelson EW. Neutropenic enterocolitis in adults with acute leukemia. *Arch Surg* 1986;121:571–574.
23. Keidan RD, Fanning J, Gatenby RA, et al. Recurrent typhlitis: a disease resulting from aggressive chemotherapy. *Dis Colon Rectum* 1989;32:206–209.
24. Baerg J, Murphy JJ, Anderson R, et al. Neutropenic enteropathy: a 10-year review. *J Pediatr Surg* 1999;34:1068–1071.
25. Avigan D, Richardson P, Elias A, et al. Neutropenic enterocolitis as a complication of high-dose chemotherapy with stem cell rescue in patients with solid tumors: a case series with a review of the literature. *Cancer* 1998;83:409–414.
26. Kouroussis C, Samonis G, Androulakis N, et al. Successful conservative treatment of neutropenic enterocolitis complicating taxane-based chemotherapy: a report of five cases. *Am J Clin Oncol* 2000;23:309–313.
27. Bodey GP, Fainstein V, Guerrant R. Infections of the gastrointestinal tract in the immunocompromised patient. *Annu Rev Med* 1986;37:271–281.
28. Jones B, Wall SD. Gastrointestinal disease in the immunocompromised host. *Radiol Clin North Am* 1992;30:555–577.
29. Wall SD, Jones B. Gastrointestinal tract in the immunocompromised host: opportunistic infections and other complications. *Radiology* 1992;185:327–335.
30. Gomez L, Martino R, Rolston KV. Neutropenic enterocolitis: spectrum of the disease and comparison of definite and possible cases. *Clin Infect Dis* 1998;27:695–699.
31. Kunkel JM, Rosenthal D. Management of the ileocecal syndrome: neutropenic enterocolitis. *Dis Colon Rectum* 1986;29: 196–199.
32. Blijlevens NM, Donnelly JP, De Pauw BE. Mucosal barrier injury: biology, pathology, clinical counterparts and consequences of intensive treatment for haematological malignancy: an overview. *Bone Marrow Transplant* 2000;25:1269–1278.
33. Whimbey E, Kiehn TE, Brannon P, et al. Bacteremia and fungemia in patients with neoplastic disease. *Am J Med* 1987;82: 723–730.
34. Hughes W, Armstrong D, Bodey GP, et al. 1997 guidelines for the use of antimicrobial agents in neutropenic patients with unexplained fever. *Clin Infect Dis* 1997;25:551–573.
35. Schimpff SC, Wiernik PH, Block JB. Rectal abscesses in cancer patients. *Lancet* 1972;2:844–847.
36. Grewel H, Guillem JG, Quan SHQ, et al. Anorectal disease in neutropenic leukemics: operative versus non-operative management. *Dis Colon Rectum* 1994;37:1095–1099.
37. Glenn J, Cotton D, Wesley R, et al. Anorectal infections in patients with malignant disease. *Rev Infect Dis* 1988;10:42–52.
38. Barnes SG, Sattler FR, Ballard JO. Perirectal infections in acute leukemia: improved survival after incision and drainage. *Ann Intern Med* 1984;100:515–518.
39. Angel C, Patrick CC, Lobe T, et al. Management of anorectal/perineal infections caused by *Pseudomonas aeruginosa* in children with malignant disease. *J Pediatr Surg* 1991;26:487–493.
40. Wallace J, Schwaitzberg S, Miller K. Sometimes it really is appendicitis: case of a CML patient with acute appendicitis. *Ann Hematol* 1998;77:61–64.
41. Angel CA, Rao BN, Wrenn E, et al. Acute appendicitis in children with leukemia and other malignancies: still a diagnostic dilemma. *J Pediatr Surg* 1992;27:476–479.
42. Wade DS, Douglass H, Nava HR, et al. Abdominal pain in neutropenic patients. *Arch Surg* 1990;125:1119–1127.
43. Young LS. Antimicrobial prophylaxis in the neutropenic host: lessons of the past and perspective for the future. *Eur J Clin Microbiol Infect Dis* 1988;7:93–97.
44. Verhoef J. Prevention of infections in the neutropenic patient. *Clin Infect Dis* 1993;17[Suppl 2]:S359–S367.
45. Cometta A, Calandra T, Bille J, et al. *Escherichia coli* resistant to fluoroquinolones in patients with cancer and neutropenia. *N Engl J Med* 1994;330:1240–1241.

33

EPIDEMIOLOGY AND PATHOPHYSIOLOGY OF *HELICOBACTER PYLORI* GASTRIC COLONIZATION

JOHN C. ATHERTON
MARTIN J. BLASER

Helicobacter pylori is a gram-negative spiral flagellated bacterium that inhabits the mucous layer of the stomach (Fig. 33.1). Its association with gastric inflammation and hence its potential role in gastroduodenal disease were first described by Warren and Marshall in 1983 (1). It is now clear that the presence of *H. pylori* is the most important risk factor for peptic ulceration (2), distal gastric adenocarcinoma (3–5), and gastric lymphoma (6). Its medical importance has stimulated intense research during the last 20 years, including the publication of the complete genome sequence in 1997 (7). The description and characterization of *H. pylori* have led to the discovery of many other *Helicobacter* species in the stomach and elsewhere in the gastrointestinal tract of humans and animals. However, the only other significant colonizer of the human stomach is the incompletely classified "*Helicobacter heilmanii,*" a tight spiral that colonizes the gastric mucus of humans and other mammals and probably comprises about 2% of recognized human gastric *Helicobacter* colonizations (8,9). Although "*H. heilmanii*" has been described in association with gastroduodenal disease, it is not clear whether this is a chance association or whether it plays a causative role (10).

In this chapter, we focus first on the epidemiology of *H. pylori* colonization, including its changing worldwide incidence and prevalence and the implications for its mode of acquisition. We then describe how the organisms survive in the human stomach despite an active immune response and hostile acid environment. Next, we discuss the bacterial, host, and environmental factors that predispose to peptic ulceration and gastric adenocarcinoma and explain why disease develops in only a minority of people with *H. pylori* colonization. Finally, we describe the pathogenic mechanisms by which *H. pylori*-associated ulcers and cancer arise.

J. C. Atherton: Division of Gastroenterology and Institute of Infections and Immunity, University of Nottingham; Division of Gastroenterology, University Hospital, Nottingham, United Kingdom

M. J. Blaser: Departments of Medicine and Microbiology, New York University School of Medicine; Department of Internal Medicine, New York Harbor Veterans Affairs Medical Center, New York, New York

EPIDEMIOLOGY

Prevalence and Incidence of *H. pylori* Colonization

The prevalence of *H. pylori* colonization varies widely both between and within countries. In general, the prevalence in adults is around 40% in most developed countries but around 80% in most developing countries (11). Within countries, prevalence is associated most closely with older age and low socioeconomic status, and these associations offer insights into the modes of acquisition of *H. pylori* and risk factors for colonization.

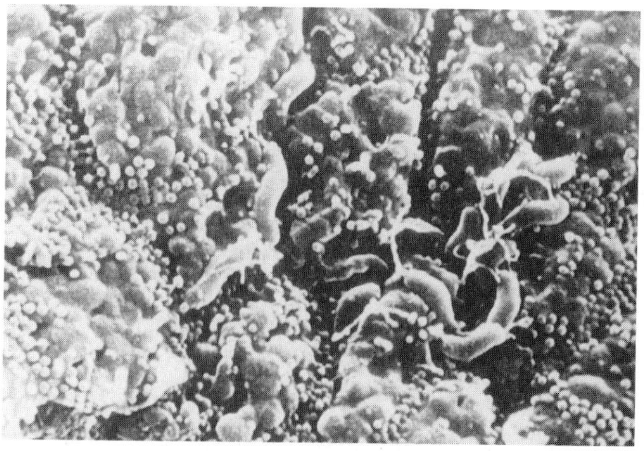

FIGURE 33.1. Scanning electron micrograph of *H. pylori* colonizing the gastric mucosa of a human volunteer days after experimental ingestion of the organisms. Note the close relationship of the organisms to the surface of the gastric mucosa, which *in vivo* would be deep within the mucous layer and thus partially protected from gastric acidity.

Rates of Acquisition and Loss of *H. pylori* in Adults

Through surveillance studies of populations carried out several years apart, rates of *H. pylori* acquisition and loss can be calculated. Such studies show that in the absence of specific treatment, most adults remain colonized or uncolonized over time (12–14). New colonization occurs only rarely and is balanced by a rare loss of colonization, perhaps partly a consequence of intercurrent antibiotic administration. The incidence of new colonization in adults appears to be about 0.4% per year (12,15), but because of the inaccuracy of diagnostic testing (some apparently initially uncolonized persons are in reality colonized), this figure is likely to be an overestimate.

Rates of Acquisition and Loss of *H. pylori* in Childhood

Prevalence rates in young children are high in developing countries and low in developed countries. Prevalence data suggest that *H. pylori* colonization is acquired throughout childhood, although mostly before the age of 5 years (16,17). Very young children may be transiently colonized (18), but why spontaneous clearance occurs only in this age group is unknown. Taken together with the data from studies in adults, the data from children show that *H. pylori* colonization is usually acquired in childhood and that, once established, it normally persists throughout life in the absence of specific antimicrobial treatment.

Age Associations and Trends in Prevalence

In developing countries, the prevalence of *H. pylori* is fairly constant across age groups in adults, but in developed countries, the prevalence is closely associated with age (Fig. 33.2). In the United States, it ranges from about 15% in 25-year-olds to 60% in persons aged 70 or older, with some regional variation (19–21). The age association in developed countries is thought mainly to be the consequence of an age cohort effect whereby, for example, the 65-year-old cohort would have been more commonly colonized in childhood than the 25-year-old cohort (14). The falling prevalence of *H. pylori* in developed countries is accompanied by a falling prevalence of peptic ulceration and gastric adenocarcinoma (14,22,23).

Socioeconomic Status, Marital Status, and Occupation

In both developing and developed countries, a strong inverse correlation is found between socioeconomic status and *H. pylori* prevalence (20,21,24,25). The closest association is with indicators of a relatively low socioeconomic status in childhood, such as crowding or absence of a fixed supply of hot water (26). Whether these factors are important themselves in childhood colonization, or merely markers for other unidentified factors, is not known. Being married to a positive partner is not a strong risk factor for acquisition, although data are contradictory and a weak effect is difficult to exclude (27,28). Data on occupation are also conflicting, with some suggesting a higher prevalence among certain groups of health care professionals, such as gastroenterologists and nurses (29,30), and others not (31). *H. pylori* colonization appears to be more common in adults living and working in crowded conditions, such as U.S. soldiers in the Gulf War (32). Together, these data suggest that children living in crowded conditions, with poor hygiene, are at highest risk for colonization, and that adults are at lower risk, even when cohabiting.

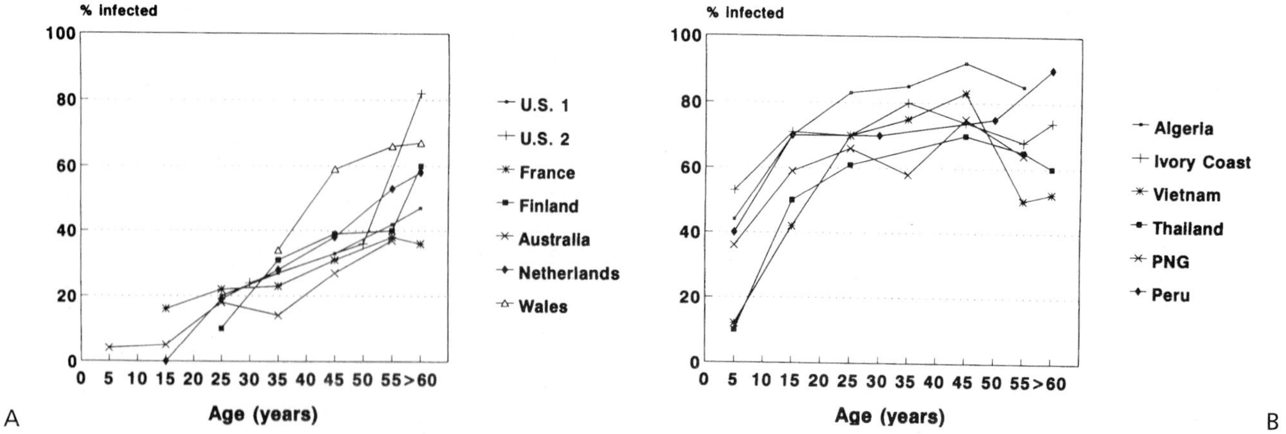

FIGURE 33.2. Panel A: Relationship between age and prevalence of *H. pylori* colonization among healthy persons in developed countries. U.S. 1 (*n* = 113), U.S. 2 (*n* = 53), France (*n* = 1,199), Finland (*n* = 500), Australia (*n* = 785), the Netherlands (*n* = 401), Wales (*n* = 1,175). (Data compiled by D. N. Taylor and J. Parsonnet.) **Panel B:** Relationship between age and prevalence of *H. pylori* colonization among healthy persons in developing countries. Algeria (*n* = 277), Ivory Coast (*n* = 374), Vietnam (*n* = 365), Thailand (*n* = 161), Papua New Guinea (*PNG*) (*n* = 157), Peru (*n* = 361). (Data compiled by D. N. Taylor and J. Parsonnet.)

Human Genetic Factors

In developing countries, where most of the population becomes colonized by *H. pylori,* host factors clearly do not greatly influence who becomes colonized. However, in developed countries, where *H. pylori* is not ubiquitous, host factors may be more important. Some studies suggest that the prevalence of *H. pylori* may be 10% to 20% higher in men than in women (33,34), although other studies show little or no effect of sex (24). Any association with sex could be a consequence of genetic or behavioral factors. The results of one study, a comparison of monozygotic and dizygotic twins, suggested that heritability may explain 57% of *H. pylori* prevalence (35). However, in a further study, of monozygotic twins reared apart, environmental factors in childhood were more important than genetic factors (36). A preliminary report has shown that polymorphisms affecting the production of the antiinflammatory and immunosuppressive cytokine interleukin 10 (IL-10) increase the risk for colonization (37), but little other work has been done in this area.

Transmission of *H. pylori* Infection

Evidence of Person-to-Person Spread

The association of *H. pylori* prevalence with direct markers of childhood crowding, such as bed sharing (26), and with surrogate markers, such as birth order and sibship size (34,38,39), suggests that the acquisition of *H. pylori* in childhood is through person-to-person spread. Outside the family, other situations in which childhood crowding occurs, such as in orphanages, are associated with a high prevalence of *H. pylori* (40). In adults, crowding appears less important. However, although epidemiologic evidence suggests that transmission between spouses is uncommon (27), definite evidence of identical strains in spouses derived from molecular typing implies that they can on occasion transmit to each other (41,42). Clustering of strains in families is well described, and family members in different generations are sometimes, although not always, colonized by the same strain (43–45).

Evidence for Nonhuman Sources of H. pylori

Many animals commonly carry *Helicobacter* species, and some of these (e.g., "*H. heilmanii*") can colonize humans (46). However, this species accounts for fewer than 5% of human helicobacters, and no clear evidence has been found that it causes disease despite occasional case reports (10). *H. pylori* itself has been described in a colony of laboratory cats (47), but pet cats have not been found to be widely colonized by *H. pylori,* and cat ownership is not a risk factor for human colonization (48). One possibility is that cats colonized with *H. pylori* have acquired the organism from humans, rather than vice versa. *H. pylori* has also been reported in monkeys (49), but here also, it may have been acquired from humans. *H. pylori* DNA has been detected in sheep milk by polymerase chain reaction (PCR) amplification (50), and prevalence is high in Sardinian shepherds (51), but these data could be explained by contamination of milk and socioeconomic confounding. Most experts do not accept that sheep are an important animal reservoir of *H. pylori.* Epidemiologic evidence from Peru suggests that the use of municipal water may be a risk factor for *H. pylori* colonization (52), and *H. pylori* DNA from water sources has been amplified by PCR (53). However, as with sheep milk, these findings could be explained by contamination and socioeconomic confounding. Furthermore, from what is known of *H. pylori* physiology, it appears unlikely that *H. pylori* organisms could survive in an infective form in the environment (54), and other studies have not shown any associations between *H. pylori* prevalence and water supply (39).

Route of Interpersonal Transmission of *H. pylori* Infection

Although the epidemiologic evidence points to person-to-person spread of *H. pylori,* the exact mode of transmission, in particular the dominant mode, is unclear.

Acquisition from Feces

Most enteric infections are spread by the fecal–oral route, and epidemiologic evidence indicates that *H. pylori* may be spread in this manner. Eating uncooked or raw vegetables in areas where hygiene is poor is a risk factor for *H. pylori* colonization, as it is for colonization with other enteric bacteria (34,55). *H. pylori* DNA (56) and antigens (57) are found reliably in stool, in the case of antigens with enough precision that the finding serves as a useful diagnostic test (58). On the other hand, viable *H. pylori* organisms have proved difficult to culture from feces, and successful culture has largely been confined to children and adults with diarrhea (59,60). However, diarrheal illness is common in childhood, and hygienic practices are less strict than in adults.

Acquisition from Saliva or Dental Plaque

H. pylori DNA from saliva and dental plaque has been amplified by PCR (61), but this does not prove that viable bacteria are present. Reports of successful culture are rare (62,63), and most workers do not consider the mouth to contain an important reservoir of *H. pylori.*

Acquisition from Vomitus and Gastric Juice

Unlike saliva, gastric juice contains large numbers of living *H. pylori* organisms. Moreover, they can remain viable in gastric juice for up to 24 hours and can be cultured from vomitus and even from the surrounding air (60,64). A physician who gave mouth-to-mouth resuscitation to a patient who had recently vomited became colonized with the patient's strain of *H. pylori* (65). Thus, *H. pylori* can be acquired from vomit, but no data are available on the importance of this mode of transmission.

Spread through Houseflies

Although *H. pylori* organisms in feces or vomitus could potentially be transmitted to the mouth by direct contact (especially in children), another possibility is that spread is indirect—for example, via houseflies. *H. pylori* DNA has been detected in houseflies (66), and experiments in which houseflies have been allowed access to cultured *H. pylori* organisms have shown that flies can spread the organisms to other surfaces (67). However, *H. pylori* is not recovered from houseflies exposed to feces containing the bacterium (68), and no epidemiologic evidence indicates that flies are important in *H. pylori* transmission.

Iatrogenic Transmission

In the past, *H. pylori* has been passed from stomach to stomach by inadequately disinfected endoscopes and by pH electrodes in physiologic studies (69). However, since the introduction of modern disinfectant regimens using 2% glutaraldehyde, this phenomenon has not been described.

Summary of Epidemiology of *H. pylori* Infection

H. pylori is acquired mainly in childhood through person-to-person spread, although it less commonly can be acquired in adult life. Once acquired, it usually persists for life in the absence of specific treatment. The main risk factors for acquisition are low socioeconomic status and crowding. Improvements in living conditions in developing countries are probably the main reason for the falling childhood incidence. *H. pylori* can be passed via the fecal–oral route or through contact with vomitus or refluxed gastric matter, but it is not clear which of these is the dominant route of transmission.

COLONIZATION AND SURVIVAL OF *H. PYLORI* IN THE STOMACH

H. pylori specifically colonizes gastric-type mucus, where most bacteria are free-living, although a few attach to the gastric epithelium. This gastric colonization, although superficial, provokes a vigorous local and systemic immune response. How *H. pylori,* uniquely among bacteria, permanently evade an active human immune response and survive the acid environment of the healthy human stomach has been the subject of much research.

Immune Response to *H. pylori*

Initially, *H. pylori* colonization provokes a rapid local inflammatory response consisting of neutrophil infiltration of the gastric mucosa, after which gradual infiltration by all classes of mononuclear cells takes place over several days (70–72). Both neutrophil and mononuclear cell infiltration of the gastric mucosa continues while *H. pylori* organisms remain in the stomach, and lymphoid follicles form in the submucosa (73). The inflammation is accompanied by minor epithelial damage and regenerative changes, and after long-term colonization gastric atrophy may develop, with parietal cell loss and intestinal metaplasia (74). Following treatment, the inflammatory cell infiltration resolves, except for a few scattered lymphoid follicles, but gastric atrophy, if present, persists (73). The inflammatory cell infiltration arises through *H. pylori*-induced stimulation of epithelial cells to release proinflammatory cytokines (75,76). *H. pylori* also induces an increased proliferation and apoptosis of epithelial cells, effects that are probably caused by a combination of direct bacterial stimulation, paracrine growth factors, and factors produced by inflammatory cells (77). After successful treatment, the local production of some cytokines, such as IL-8, falls rapidly, but up to 1 year is required for the production of others, such as IL-6, to fall to unstimulated levels (78).

Considerable interest has been shown in the type of T-cell response to *H. pylori* infection and whether this is primarily of the T helper (Th) 1 type (broadly proinflammatory with a cellular immune response) or Th2 type (broadly antiinflammatory with T helper promotion of humoral immunity). Although *H. pylori* provokes elements of both responses, the cytokine profile in the gastric mucosa suggests that the predominant response is of the Th1 proinflammatory type (79). Although the Th2 response is less pronounced, B-cell activation occurs along with an abundant antibody response, although clearly this is ineffective. A transient specific immunoglobulin M (IgM) response and delayed but persistent specific IgG and IgA responses are noted (80). Antibody levels fall only slowly after treatment (80,81). The detection of specific antibodies is useful in diagnosing *H. pylori* colonization, but because of the slow fall in levels, this is rather difficult to use for predicting treatment success (82).

Bacterial Factors Important for *H. pylori* Colonization and Survival

Motility and Chemotaxis

The spiral shape of helicobacters allows them to burrow efficiently through mucus in a corkscrew motion, which can be reversed so that they can move backward. Motility is accomplished through multiple sheathed flagella made up of two flagellum proteins, FlaA and FlaB (83). Sheaths at the bases of the flagella are thought to protect the flagella "motors" against gastric acid (84). The flagella "motors" are driven by the proton motive force, derived from membrane potential, and by pH differences across the bacterial membrane (85). A comparison of putative flagellum genes in the

H. pylori genome with homologues in other bacteria suggests that flagellum structure and mechanism are similar to those of *Salmonella,* although regulation may be different (86). Active motility is essential for colonization in animal models (87) and is probably important for persistence in the stomach during turnover of mucus and epithelial cells. Genome comparisons suggest that the chemotaxis system in *H. pylori* also is similar to that in *Salmonella* (86), and thus it probably has sensors for chemoattractants and chemorepellants that signal the flagellum motor to move forward or reverse. *In vitro, H. pylori* moves toward urea, bicarbonate, and mucin (88,89); this feature may help the bacteria evade acid exposure in the gastric lumen.

Acid Survival and Urease

The exact pH of the deep gastric mucus inhabited by *H. pylori* organisms is unknown, but is likely to be only mildly acidic. However, *H. pylori* organisms must also survive luminal stomach acid during host colonization and probably at times when the mucous layer thins or when the bacteria move away from the mucosal surface. Like acidophilic bacteria, *H. pylori* organisms are able to maintain a nearly neutral internal pH at external pH values ranging from 3 to 7 by changing their membrane potential (90). However, *H. pylori* bacteria can survive even lower pH values because of their abundant urease. Urease is primarily a cytoplasmic enzyme but is also found on the bacterial surface *in vivo* (91). It catalyzes the hydrolysis of urea to form ammonia and carbamate. Ammonia is a preferred nitrogen source for many bacteria, but *H. pylori* urease appears to have a dual action in that the ammonia produced is thought to form an "alkaline cloud" that neutralizes stomach acid around the bacteria. Recent evidence suggests that urea enters the bacterial cytoplasm through an H^+-gated channel that allows cytoplasmic urease activity to be regulated (92). Urease is essential for *H. pylori* colonization in animal models (93), and in human colonization, urease continues to be expressed at a high level throughout life, which suggests that it plays a continuing role in survival. This consistently high level of urease expression is the basis of the biopsy urease test, a major gastric biopsy-based test for *H. pylori* (95), and the urea breath test, a major noninvasive test (96). Being an abundant and surface-expressed protein, urease is a focus for the host immune response, which includes a specific anti-urease IgG response and a cell-mediated component.

Adhesion

During long-term *H. pylori* colonization, most bacteria are free-living in the gastric mucus, but a few adhere to the gastric mucosa. Whether any invade the mucosa is controversial, but most investigators agree that if invasion does occur, it is rare. Adhesion may be important in withstanding gastric acid [it is enhanced *in vitro* by a low pH, a possible adaptive mechanism (97)] and in avoiding bacterial shedding from the stomach. However, in addition to playing a role in survival, adhesion is important in the induction of inflammation and disease because *in vitro* it is a prerequisite for the production of proinflammatory cytokines by epithelial cells (98). Many putative *H. pylori* adhesins have been identified in laboratory experiments, but it remains unclear which ones, if any, are important *in vivo.* One adhesin, BabA, which binds to the Lewis b epitope on gastric epithelial cells, may be important in disease determination and is discussed later.

Metabolism and Nutrient Acquisition

The gastric mucus forms a barrier to help protect the mucosa from luminal acid and pepsin, and this is likely to block the delivery of gastric luminal nutrients to *H. pylori* organisms. Indeed, it has been suggested that *H. pylori*-induced inflammation is beneficial to the bacteria because it renders the mucosa leaky, thereby facilitating nutrient delivery from the serosal side (99). *H. pylori* organisms have specific mechanisms for acquiring micronutrients, such as iron (100) and trace elements. They are also adapted to the low oxygen and high carbon dioxide tension in the gastric mucus, in that they require carbon dioxide for survival and are microaerophilic. Genome information shows that glycolysis is likely to be the main pathway of energy production (8). A further striking feature noted on genome analysis is the presence of a single cytochrome oxidase, which implies that *H. pylori* is adapted for energetic metabolism in a rather narrow range of oxygen tensions. The restrictive metabolism of *H. pylori* suggests that the organisms are adapted for a specific niche (55) and supports epidemiologic evidence that is largely against the survival of *H. pylori* for significant periods outside the human stomach.

Lipopolysaccharide

In comparison with that of other bacteria, the lipopolysaccharide (LPS) coat of *H. pylori* exhibits relatively low immunogenicity (101) and biologic activity (102), which may contribute to the ability of the bacteria to evade the immune response and persist in the stomach. The low biologic activity of *H. pylori* LPS is at least in part the consequence of an unusual central lipid A moiety (103). Another unusual feature of *H. pylori* LPS is the presence of O-polysaccharide side chains; these mimic the Lewis X and Lewis Y blood group antigens found in human gastric mucosa (104). The role of these side chains is unclear, but one possibility is that they may camouflage *H. pylori* and help the bacteria to evade the immune response (105). A previously suggested role in pathogenesis, through the stimulation of cross-reactive autoantibodies to gastric mucosa and parietal cells, now appears unlikely because although Lewis-specific antibodies are observed, they are independent of *H. pylori* colonization (106).

Antibacterial Peptides

H. pylori has recently been shown to produce peptides with broad antibacterial properties (107). These could be important when the stomach is hypochlorhydric and so vulnerable to colonization by other, less specialized bacterial species (e.g., during initial colonization and late in human life when gastric atrophy occurs). However, at least in the atrophic stomach, they are incompletely effective, as other bacteria can readily be cultured.

PATHOPHYSIOLOGY OF *H. PYLORI*-ASSOCIATED DISEASE

In adults, acute *H. pylori* colonization causes variable upper gastrointestinal symptoms, such as nausea, vomiting, and abdominal pain, and also a temporary hypochlorhydria (71–73). Whether these features occur in acute childhood colonization is not known. Once the acute phase has resolved, most colonized people experience no *H. pylori*-related symptoms or clinical complications for the rest of their life despite an invariable continuing host response and persistent gastric inflammation. However, disease does occur in a small proportion; in developed countries, peptic ulceration affects up to 15% of colonized persons in their lifetime (108), gastric adenocarcinoma 0.5% to 1% (109), and primary gastric lymphoma a small fraction of a percentage. It is controversial whether upper gastrointestinal symptoms develop in a few persons with *H. pylori* colonization in the absence of these conditions, but it is clear that the great majority of cases of "non-ulcer dyspepsia" are not caused by *H. pylori* (see Chapter 34). Growing evidence suggests that *H. pylori* colonization may offer some protection against reflux esophagitis and its complications, including esophageal adenocarcinoma, and these controversial data are also discussed in Chapter 34. Here, we concentrate on the pathogenesis of diseases widely accepted as being attributable to *H. pylori*: peptic ulceration, distal gastric adenocarcinoma, and gastric lymphoma. A complex interaction of bacterial virulence factors, host genetic susceptibility, and environmental factors determines whether a person acquires one of these diseases.

H. pylori Virulence Factors

H. pylori strains are genetically diverse, and isolates from individual stomachs can easily be distinguished from one another by various DNA typing methods. *H. pylori* uses mutation as a system of gene regulation; genes are turned on and off by mutations occurring in specific hypermutable regions (8,110). However, the main reason for the detectable genetic diversity is the high level of DNA recombination between strains (111,112). Frequent recombination implies that individual genes or collections of genes in *H. pylori* that are disease-associated are not markers for clones, as they are in many other bacteria. Instead, such genes must be either involved directly in disease induction or functionally linked to genes important in pathogenesis. Several genes have been identified that are more common in *H. pylori* strains associated with disease than in non–disease-associated strains, and in some cases the mechanisms of pathogenicity are at least partly understood.

Cytotoxin-Associated Gene Island

About 70% of *H. pylori* strains in developed countries, and nearly all strains in developing countries, possess the cytotoxin-associated gene island (*cag* island). This is a group of about 30 genes, thought to have been acquired by some strains relatively late in *H. pylori* evolution from an unknown source (113). Nearly all strains associated with peptic ulceration or gastric adenocarcinoma possess the intact *cag* island, although such strains are common and many are not associated with disease (114–116). Some *cag* island genes encode proteins that constitute a type IV secretory system, a molecular syringe, through which another protein encoded on the island, CagA, is translocated into epithelial cells (117,118). Here, it is phosphorylated on tyrosine residues by the host cell, a common eukaryotic signaling mechanism, and stimulates signaling cascades that result in cytoskeletal reorganization and cellular proliferation (117,119,120). In addition to these functions, the type IV secretory system is important in increasing proinflammatory cytokine synthesis and release by epithelial cells (113,121,122), although it is unclear whether this is a consequence of the structure itself or of other translocated proteins. *In vivo, cag*-positive strains are associated with higher levels of gastric inflammation than are *cag*-negative strains, although all *H. pylori* strains are associated with some inflammation (77,115). Colonization with a *cag*-positive strain is more common in gastric adenocarcinoma, gastric ulceration, and duodenal ulceration (114–116), although gastric carcinoma only rarely develops later in patients with duodenal ulcers (123). The current view is that *cag*-positive *H. pylori* colonization increases the risk for associated disease through increased inflammation, but that other factors determine which disease develops (Fig. 33.3). The protein CagA is highly immunogenic, and antibodies to CagA are probably a reliable guide to colonization by a strain with an intact *cag* island (124). Such antibodies are easy to measure (115,125), and several commercial kits are available, although none are in clinical use. This is perhaps partly because although CagA-positive strains are more pathogenic, they are also very common, so that despite their enhanced pathogenicity, most carriage of CagA-positive strains does not result in disease.

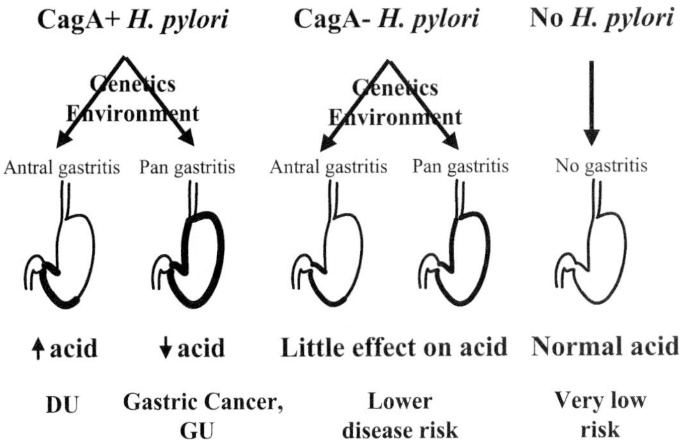

FIGURE 33.3. Pathogenic *H. pylori* organisms are thought to predispose to disease, but the pattern of gastric inflammation, and hence the pattern of disease development, is thought to depend on genetic or environmental factors. Some evidence indicates that the pangastritis pattern, which predisposes to gastric ulcers and gastric adenocarcinoma, may protect against acid-associated esophageal diseases, such as reflux esophagitis and esophageal adenocarcinoma.

Vacuolating Cytotoxin

The vacuolating cytotoxin VacA is a pore-forming toxin that induces vacuolation in cultured epithelial cells, leakiness in epithelial cell layers, and gastroduodenal damage in a mouse model (126–129). Nearly all *H. pylori* strains produce a VacA protein, but many do not cause vacuolation in cell lines (130). This is because the *vacA* gene is polymorphic; different forms are associated with different levels of VacA expression and different VacA amino acid sequences (130–132). One variable region of *vacA* encodes the start of the VacA protein and can be either of two types, s1 or s2. The s1 type of VacA is active, but the less common s2 type is nonvacuolating (131,133), and *vacA* s2 strains are usually *cag*-negative and rarely associated with disease (131,134). The second main variable region of *vacA,* the m region, encodes the last quarter of the secreted toxin, a region believed to be involved in toxin binding to cells (131,135). The m1 type of VacA is fully active, but the m2 type appears less active and causes vacuolation only in certain epithelial cell lines, which implies greater binding specificity (135). Both s1/m1 and s1/m2 types of VacA are associated with peptic ulceration (131), but s1/m1 types appear to have a closer association with gastric adenocarcinoma in some populations (136,137). VacA antibodies can be detected serologically (138), but the significance of a positive result is unclear because essentially all strains produce VacA. In commercial tests, the antigen used is type s1/m1 VacA, so the tests probably detect antibodies to this form more strongly than antibodies to other forms. Thus, although a weak association exists between VacA antibodies and gastric adenocarcinoma (139), VacA antibodies have no predictive accuracy.

Other Bacterial Factors

Several other bacterial factors either have been associated with disease or are thought to be important in enhancing inflammation and hence increasing risk for disease. The adhesin BabA is thought to mediate *H. pylori* binding to the gastric mucosa through the Lewis b antigen. It belongs to a family of outer membrane proteins, not all of which are expressed by any strain. Strains with one specific homologue of the *babA2* gene are most closely associated with peptic ulceration and gastric adenocarcinoma (140). Another protein, IceA (induced by contact with epithelium protein A) is encoded by a polymorphic gene, and one genotype, *iceA1,* is associated with disease in some populations (141). The significance of *iceA* as a virulence factor is unclear as it encodes a restriction endonuclease, although regulation of the downstream methylase gene may play a role. *H. pylori* organisms have also been shown to stimulate neutrophil activation directly *in vitro.* Strains that do this most intensely are more commonly isolated from patients with peptic ulcer disease (142,143). The mechanism underlying direct neutrophil activation remains unclear.

Host Genetic Susceptibility to *H. pylori*-Associated Disease

The cytokine IL-1β is central to the host inflammatory response to *H. pylori.* Several polymorphisms in the gene encoding IL-1β and its receptor antagonist affect levels of IL-1β production. Persons who carry polymorphisms associated with high-level IL-1β expression are at increased risk for the development of gastric adenocarcinoma (144). The mechanism may be through increased inflammation, which results from high levels of IL-1β, but IL-1β is also a powerful suppressor of gastric acid production, which is thought to be important in the pathogenesis of gastric adenocarcinoma. Much interest is now being shown in identifying other human gene polymorphisms that increase the risk for gastric adenocarcinoma and polymorphisms that increase the risk for duodenal ulceration.

Environmental Factors Contributing to *H. pylori*-Associated Disease

Many environmental factors previously thought to be important in the pathogenesis of gastroduodenal disease are now known to be significant only as markers for *H. pylori* colonization. Many have not been reexamined with *H. pylori* status taken into account. However, smoking is a strong risk factor for peptic ulceration among *H. pylori*-positive persons (145), and diet is an important modulator of the risk for gastric adenocarcinoma. Dietary antioxidants reduce the risk for gastric adenocarcinoma, but dietary salt increases the risk and may explain some of the regional differences in cancer prevalence (146). Aspirin and similar drugs reduce the risk for gastric adenocarcinoma, in addition to their better-known effect of reducing the risk for colonic carcinoma (147,148). Finally, age at colonization with *H. pylori* appears to affect the risk for gastric adenocarcinoma; people from large families or of high birth order (surrogate markers for young age at colonization) are at increased risk for the development of gastric cancer (149).

Pathogenesis of *H. pylori*-Associated Disease

Increased gastric inflammation is central in the pathogenesis of all *H. pylori*-associated diseases, but it is increasingly recognized that which disease arises is associated with the pattern of inflammation in the stomach and subsequent changes in acid secretion (Fig. 33.3). What determines the pattern of inflammation, and even whether this is determined by bacterial, host, or environmental factors, remains unclear.

Duodenal Ulceration

Duodenal ulcers occur in persons with antral-predominant gastritis (150,151) (Figs. 33.3 and 33.4). Antral inflammation causes a reduction in the numbers of somatostatin-producing D cells (152) and a reduction in somatostatin expression (153). Because somatostatin normally exerts a negative feedback on gastrin production by G cells (154), a reduction in levels of somatostatin results in hypergastrinemia (155). Whether *H. pylori* also directly affects G cells is unclear. Gastrin stimulates the healthy uninflamed corpus to secrete more acid (156), so that an increased acid load enters the duodenum. The duodenum is thought to adapt by developing a more stomach-like epithelium, so-called gastric metaplasia (157). *H. pylori* cannot colonize normal duodenum but colonizes areas of gastric metaplasia (158); such colonization results in duodenal ulceration, presumably caused by a combination of locally damaging agents released by *H. pylori* and increased acid exposure.

Gastric Ulceration and Distal Gastric Adenocarcinoma

Gastric ulcers and gastric cancer arise in persons with pangastritis, which is an inflammation of both the gastric antrum and the corpus (150,151) (Figs. 33.3 and 33.5). It is unclear why pangastritis develops in some persons, but one hypothesis is based on the observation that acid production is suppressed in individuals with genetic polymorphisms leading to the production of high levels of IL-1β in response to *H. pylori* colonization (144). This feature may allow the normally inhospitable gastric corpus to become colonized by *H. pylori.* Persons with pangastritis have hypergastrinemia through the same mechanism as those with antral-predominant gastritis. However, in pangastritis, the inflamed corpus

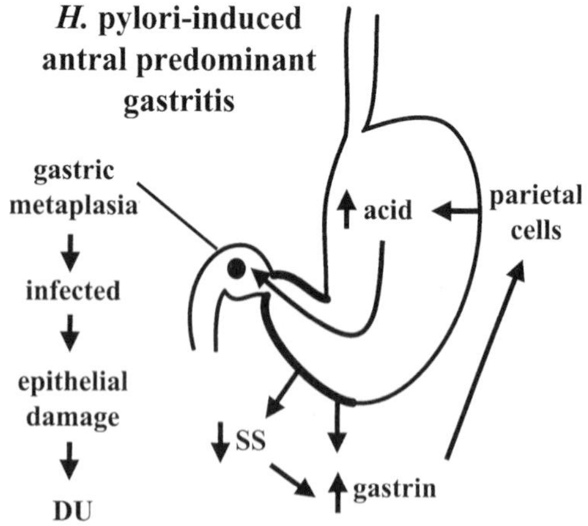

FIGURE 33.4. Pathogenesis of duodenal ulceration. Antral gastritis causes a reduced expression of somatostatin (*SS*). Somatostatin has a negative feedback effect on gastrin production, so that hypergastrinemia develops. The uninflamed corpus produces more acid, and the duodenal acid load increases. In response, gastric metaplasia develops in the duodenum, which can be colonized by *H. pylori.* The result is epithelial damage and ulceration.

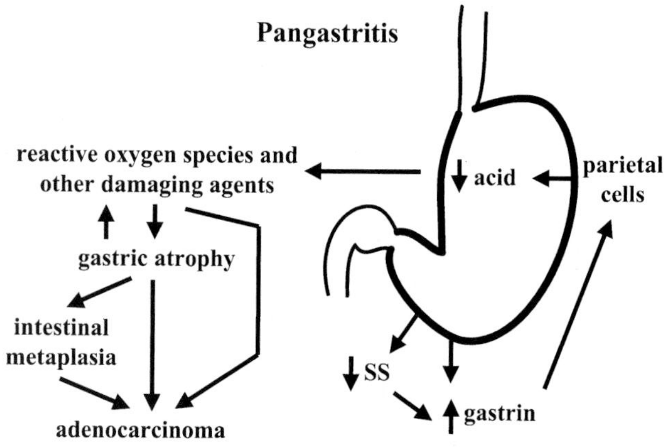

FIGURE 33.5. Pathogenesis of gastric adenocarcinoma. In pangastritis (either induced by *H. pylori* or autoimmune), levels of acid produced in the inflamed gastric corpus are low, so that DNA-damaging reactive oxygen and nitrogen species from inflammatory cells, *H. pylori* (if present), and other bacteria colonizing the hypochlorhydric stomach can survive. As a result, gastric atrophy develops, which in turn exacerbates the hypochlorhydria. The more common intestinal type of gastric cancer arises in areas of atrophy and usually intestinal metaplasia, but these intermediate steps generally do not occur in the diffuse type of gastric cancer.

produces little acid despite gastrin stimulation (159). The pathogenesis of gastric ulcers in this setting is poorly understood. They occur mostly in "junctional epithelium," where the gastric antrum meets the corpus, and these regions are heavily colonized and inflamed (160).

The two main *H. pylori*-associated types of gastric adenocarcinoma are a more common intestinal type, which appears to arise following a progression through gastric atrophy and intestinal metaplasia, and a less common diffuse type, which appears to arise *de novo* (146,161). The pathogenesis of both types is uncertain, although research has led to a suggested mechanism (Fig. 33.5). Epithelial proliferation is increased (78), both by the direct effect of bacteria on epithelial cells (119) and by the growth factor-life effects of gastrin, and this increased proliferation makes DNA-damaging events more likely. In the colonized and inflamed stomach, reactive oxygen and nitrogen species derived from neutrophils, and from *H. pylori* and other bacteria, cause an increase in oxidative DNA damage (162–164). The *H. pylori*-induced atrophy and hypochlorhydria enable other bacteria to survive and also would be expected to allow reactive oxygen and nitrogen species to survive longer. Intragastric levels of vitamin C, an important oxidant scavenger, are reduced in the atrophic stomach (165,166). Pangastritis and atrophy can also develop as an autoimmune condition, without *H. pylori* involvement, and pernicious anemia may develop in affected persons. People with *H. pylori*-associated pangastritis and atrophy are at increased risk for the development of gastric adenocarcinoma.

Primary Gastric Lymphoma

Lymphoma of the gastric mucosa-associated lymphoid tissue (MALT) develops when chronic antigenic stimulation of T helper cells by *H. pylori* leads to the clonal expansion of B cells in gastric lymphoid follicles (167). Although these lymphomas are low-grade, proliferation is still driven by *H. pylori,* and eradication of *H. pylori* alone can lead to complete regression (168,169). Higher-grade gastric MALT lymphomas are autonomous, and additional therapy is required

ACKNOWLEDGMENTS

John C. Atherton is funded by a Senior Clinical Fellowship from the Medical Research Council (U.K.). This work supported in part by RO1 DK 53707 and RO1 GM 63270 from the National Institute of Health.

REFERENCES

1. Warren J, Marshall B. Unidentified curved bacilli on gastric epithelium in active chronic gastritis. *Lancet* 1983;1:1273–1275.
2. Nomura A, Stemmermann GN, Chyou PH, et al. *Helicobacter pylori* infection and the risk for duodenal and gastric ulceration. *Ann Intern Med* 1995;120:977–981.
3. Forman D, Newell DG, Fullerton F, et al. Association between infection with *Helicobacter pylori* and risk of gastric cancer: evidence from a prospective investigation. *Br Med J* 1991;2: 377–380.
4. Nomura A, Stemmermann GN, Chyou PH, et al. *Helicobacter pylori* infection and gastric carcinoma among Japanese Americans in Hawaii. *N Engl J Med* 1991;325:1132–1136.
5. Parsonnet J, Friedman GD, Vandersteen DP, et al. *Helicobacter pylori* infection and the risk of gastric carcinoma. *N Engl J Med* 1991;325:1127–1131.
6. Parsonnet J, Hansen S, Rodriguez L, et al. *Helicobacter pylori* infection and gastric lymphoma. *N Engl J Med* 1994;330: 1267–1271.
7. Tomb JF, White O, Kerlavage AR, et al. The complete genome sequence of the gastric pathogen *Helicobacter pylori. Nature* 1997;388:539–547.
8. Dent JC, McNulty CAM, Uff JC, et al. Spiral organisms in the gastric antrum. *Lancet* 1987;2:96.
9. Solnick JV, O'Rourke J, Lee A, et al. An uncultured gastric spiral organism is a newly identified helicobacter in humans. *J Infect Dis* 1993;168:379–385.
10. Goddard AF, Logan RP, Atherton JC, et al. Healing of duodenal ulcer after eradication of *Helicobacter heilmannii. Lancet* 1997;349:1815–1816.
11. Pounder RE, Ng D. The prevalence of *Helicobacter pylori* infection in different countries. *Aliment Pharmacol Ther* 1995;9: 33–39.
12. Parsonnet J, Blaser MJ, Perez-Perez GI, et al. Symptoms and risk factors of *Helicobacter pylori* infection in a cohort of epidemiologists. *Gastroenterology* 1992;102:41–46.
13. Banatvala N, Mayo K, Megraud F, et al. The cohort effect and *Helicobacter pylori. J Infect Dis* 1993;168:219–221.
14. Kosunen TU, Aromaa A, Knekt P, et al. *Helicobacter* antibodies in 1983 and 1994 in the adult population of Vammala, Finland. *Epidemiol Infect* 1997;119:29–34.
15. Kuipers EJ, Pena AS, van Kamp G, et al. Seroconversion for *Helicobacter pylori. Lancet* 1993;342:328–331.
16. Oliveira AM, Queiroz DM, Rocha GA, et al. Seroprevalence of *Helicobacter pylori* infection in children of low socioeconomic level in Belo Horizonte, Brazil. *Am J Gastroenterol* 1994;89: 2201–2204.
17. Fiedorek SC, Malaty HM, Evans DL, et al. Factors influencing the epidemiology of *Helicobacter pylori* infection in children. *Pediatrics* 1991;88:578–582.
18. Klein PD, Gilman RH, Leonbarua R, et al. The epidemiology of *Helicobacter pylori* in Peruvian children between 6 and 30 months of age. *Am J Gastroenterol* 1994;89:2196–2200.
19. Dooley CP, Cohen H, Fitzgibbons PL, et al. Prevalence of *Helicobacter pylori* infection and histologic gastritis in asymptomatic persons. *N Engl J Med* 1989;321:1562–1566.
20. Graham DY, Malaty HM, Evans DG, et al. Epidemiology of *Helicobacter pylori* in an asymptomatic population in the United States. Effect of age, race, and socioeconomic status. *Gastroenterology* 1991;100:1495–1501.
21. Everhart JE, Kruszon-Moran D, Perez-Perez GI, et al. Seroprevalence and ethnic differences in *Helicobacter pylori* infection among adults in the United States. *J Infect Dis* 2000;181: 1359–1363.
22. Zheng T, Mayne ST, Holford TR, et al. The time trend and age–period–cohort effects on incidence of adenocarcinoma of the stomach in Connecticut from 1955–1989. *Cancer* 1993;72: 330–340.
23. Munnangi S, Sonnenberg A. Time trends of physician visits and treatment patterns of peptic ulcer disease in the United States. *Arch Intern Med* 1997;157:1489–1494.
24. The EUROGAST Study Group. Epidemiology of, and risk

factors for, *Helicobacter pylori* infection among 3,194 asymptomatic subjects in 17 populations. *Gut* 1993;34:1672–1676.

25. Louw JA, Jaskiewicz K, Girdwood AH, et al. *Helicobacter pylori* prevalence in non-ulcer dyspepsia—ethnic and socio-economic differences. *S Afr Med J* 1993;83:169–171.
26. Mendall MA, Goggin PM, Molineaux N, et al. Childhood living conditions and *Helicobacter pylori* seropositivity in adult life. *Lancet* 1992;339:896–897.
27. Perez-Perez GI, Witkin SS, Decker MD, et al. Seroprevalence of *Helicobacter pylori* infection in couples. *J Clin Microbiol* 1991; 29:642–644.
28. Ma JL, You WC, Gail MH, et al. *Helicobacter pylori* infection and mode of transmission in a population at high risk of stomach cancer. *Int J Epidemiol* 1998;27:570–573.
29. Mitchell HM, Lee A, Carrick J. Increased incidence of *Campylobacter pylori* infection in gastroenterologists: further evidence to support person-to-person transmission of *C. pylori. Scand J Gastroenterol* 1989;24:396–400.
30. Wilhoite SL, Ferguson DA, Soike DR, et al. Increased prevalence of *Helicobacter pylori* antibodies among nurses. *Arch Intern Med* 1993;153:708–712.
31. Pristautz H, Eherer A, Brezinschek R, et al. Prevalence of *Helicobacter pylori* antibodies in the serum of gastroenterologists in Austria. *Endoscopy* 1994;26:690–696.
32. Smoak BL, Kelley PW, Taylor DN. Seroprevalence of *Helicobacter pylori* infections in a cohort of U.S. Army recruits. *Am J Epidemiol* 1994;139:513–519.
33. Replogle ML, Glaser SL, Hiatt RA, et al. Biologic sex as a risk factor for *Helicobacter pylori* infection in healthy young adults. *Am J Epidemiol* 1995;142:856–863.
34. Goodman KJ, Correa P, Tengana Aux HJ, et al. *Helicobacter pylori* infection in the Colombian Andes: a population-based study of transmission pathways. *Am J Epidemiol* 1996;144:290–299.
35. Malaty HM, Engstrand L, Pedersen NL, et al. *Helicobacter pylori* infection: genetic and environmental influences. A study of twins. *Ann Intern Med* 1994;120:982–986.
36. Malaty HM, Graham DY, Isaksson I, et al. Co-twin study of the effect of environment and dietary elements on acquisition of *Helicobacter pylori* infection. *Am J Epidemiol* 1998;148:793–797.
37. El-Omar EM, Wang CD, McColl KE, et al. Interleukin-10 promoter polymorphisms influence risk of chronic *H. pylori* infection. *Gastroenterology* 2000;118:4922.
38. Goodman KG, Correa P. Transmission of *Helicobacter pylori* among siblings. *Lancet* 2000;355:358–362.
39. Teh BH, Lin JT, Pan WH, et al. Seroprevalence and associated risk factors of *Helicobacter pylori* infection in Taiwan. *Anticancer Res* 1994;14:1389–1392.
40. Vincent P, Gottrand F, Pernes P, et al. High prevalence of *Helicobacter pylori* infection in cohabiting children. Epidemiology of a cluster, with special emphasis on molecular typing. *Gut* 1994; 35:313–316.
41. Schutze K, Hentschel E, Dragosics B, et al. *Helicobacter pylori* reinfection with identical organisms: transmission by the patients' spouses. *Gut* 1995;36:831–833.
42. Georgopoulos SD, Mentis AF, Spiliadis CA, et al. *Helicobacter pylori* infection in spouses of patients with duodenal ulcers and comparison of ribosomal RNA gene patterns. *Gut* 1996;39: 634–638.
43. Nwokolo CU, Bickley J, Attard AR, et al. Evidence of clonal variants of *Helicobacter pylori* in three generations of a duodenal ulcer disease family. *Gut* 1992;33:1323–1327.
44. Bamford KB, Bickley J, Collins JS, et al. *Helicobacter pylori*: comparison of DNA fingerprints provides evidence for intrafamilial infection. *Gut* 1993;34:1348–1350.
45. VanderEnde A, Rauws EAJ, Feller M, et al. Heterogeneous *Helicobacter pylori* isolates from members of a family with a history of peptic ulcer disease. *Gastroenterology* 1996;111:638–647.
46. Stolte M, Wellens E, Bethke B, et al. *Helicobacter heilmannii* (formerly *Gastrospirillum hominis*) gastritis: an infection transmitted by animals? *Scand J Gastroenterol* 1994;29:1061–1064.
47. Handt LK, Fox JG, Dewhirst FE, et al. *Helicobacter pylori* isolated from the domestic cat: public health implications. *Infect Immun* 1994;62:2367–2374.
48. McIsaac WJ, Leung GM. Peptic ulcer disease and exposure to domestic pets. *Am J Public Health* 1999;89:81–84.
49. Dubois A, Fiala N, Heman-Ackah LM, et al. Natural gastric infection with *Helicobacter pylori* in monkeys: a model for spiral bacteria infection in humans. *Gastroenterology* 1994;106: 1405–1417.
50. Dore MP, Sepulveda AR, Osato MS, et al. *Helicobacter pylori* in sheep milk. High prevalence of *Helicobacter pylori* infection in shepherds. *Lancet* 1999;354:132.
51. Dore MP, Bilotta M, Vaira D, et al. High prevalence of *Helicobacter pylori* infection in shepherds. *Dig Dis Sci* 1999;44: 1161–1164.
52. Klein PD, Graham DY, Gaillour A, et al. Water source as risk factor for *Helicobacter pylori* infection in Peruvian children. Gastrointestinal Physiology Working Group. *Lancet* 1991;337: 1503–1506.
53. Hulten K, Han SW, Enroth H, et al. *Helicobacter pylori* in the drinking water in Peru. *Gastroenterology* 1996;110:1031–1035.
54. Marais A, Mendz GL, Hazell SL, et al. Metabolism and genetics of *Helicobacter pylori*: the genome era. *Microbiol Mol Biol Rev* 1999;63:642–674.
55. Hopkins RJ, Vial PA, Ferreccio C, et al. Seroprevalence of *Helicobacter pylori* in Chile: vegetables may serve as one route of transmission. *J Infect Dis* 1993;168:222–226.
56. Mapstone NP, Lynch DA, Lewis FA, et al. PCR identification of *Helicobacter pylori* in faeces from gastritis patients. *Lancet* 1993;341:447.
57. Makristathis A, Pasching E, Schutze K, et al. Detection of *Helicobacter pylori* in stool specimens by PCR and antigen enzyme immunoassay. *J Clin Microbiol* 1998;36:2772–2774.
58. Vaira D, Malfertheiner P, Megraud F, et al. Diagnosis of *Helicobacter pylori* infection by HpSA test. European *Helicobacter pylori* HpSA Study Group. *Lancet* 1999;354:1732.
59. Thomas JE, Gibson GR, Darboe MK, et al. Isolation of *Helicobacter pylori* from human faeces. *Lancet* 1992;340:1194–1195.
60. Parsonnet J, Shmuely H, Haggerty T. Fecal and oral shedding of *Helicobacter pylori* from healthy infected adults. *JAMA* 1999; 282:2240–2245.
61. Nguyen AM, Engstrand L, Genta RM, et al. Detection of *Helicobacter pylori* in dental plaque by reverse transcription-polymerase chain reaction. *J Clin Microbiol* 1993;31:783–787.
62. Krajden S, Fuksa M, Anderson J, et al. Examination of human stomach biopsies, saliva, and dental plaque for *Campylobacter pylori. J Clin Microbiol* 1989;27:1397–1398.
63. Ferguson DA, Li C, Patel NR, et al. Isolation of *Helicobacter pylori* from saliva. *J Clin Microbiol* 1993;31:2802–2804.
64. Galal G, Wharburton V, West A, et al. Isolation of *H. pylori* from gastric juice. *Gut* 1997;41:A40–A41.
65. Figura N. Mouth-to-mouth resuscitation and *Helicobacter pylori* infection. *Lancet* 1996;347:1342.
66. Grubel P, Huang L, Masubuchi N, et al. Detection of *Helicobacter pylori* DNA in houseflies (*Musca domestica*) on three continents. *Lancet* 1998;352:788–789.
67. Grubel P, Hoffman JS, Chong FK, et al. Vector potential of houseflies (*Musca domestica*) for *Helicobacter pylori. J Clin Microbiol* 1997;35:1300–1303.
68. Osato MS, Ayub K, Le HH, et al. Houseflies are an unlikely

reservoir or vector for *Helicobacter pylori. J Clin Microbiol* 1998; 36:2786–2788.
69. Langenberg W, Rauws EA, Oudbier JH, et al. Patient-to-patient transmission of *Campylobacter pylori* infection by fiberoptic gastroduodenoscopy and biopsy. *J Infect Dis* 1990;161:507–511.
70. Marshall BJ, Armstrong JA, McGechie DB, et al. Attempt to fulfill Koch's postulates for pyloric *Campylobacter. Med J Aust* 1985;142:436–439.
71. Morris A, Nicholson G. Ingestion of *Campylobacter pyloridis* causes gastritis and raised fasting gastric pH. *Am J Gastroenterol* 1987;82:192–199.
72. Sobala GM, Crabtree JE, Dixon MF, et al. Acute *Helicobacter pylori* infection: clinical features, local and systemic immune response, gastric mucosal histology, and gastric juice ascorbic acid concentrations. *Gut* 1991;32:1415–1418.
73. Genta RM, Hammer HW, Graham DY. Gastric lymphoid follicles in *Helicobacter pylori* infection: frequency, distribution, and response to triple therapy. *Hum Pathol* 1993;24:577–583.
74. Kuipers EJ, Uyterlinde AM, Pena AS, et al. Long-term sequelae of *Helicobacter pylori* gastritis. *Lancet* 1995;345:1525–1528.
75. Crabtree JE, Farmery SM, Lindley IJ, et al. CagA/cytotoxic strains of *Helicobacter pylori* and interleukin-8 in gastric epithelial cell lines. *J Clin Pathol* 1994;47:945–950.
76. Peek RM, Miller GG, Tham KT, et al. Heightened inflammatory response and cytokine expression *in vivo* to cagA(+) *Helicobacter pylori* strains. *Lab Invest* 1995;73:760–770.
77. Peek RM Jr, Moss SF, Tham KT, et al. Helicobacter pylori cagA+ strains and dissociation of gastric epithelial cell proliferation from apoptosis. *J Natl Cancer Inst* 1997;89:863–868.
78. Ando T, Kusugami K, Ohsuga M, et al. Differential normalization of mucosal interleukin-8 and interleukin-6 after *Helicobacter pylori* eradication. *Infect Immun* 1998;66:4742–4747.
79. Ermak TH, Giannasca PJ, Nichols R, et al. Immunization of mice with urease vaccine affords protection against *Helicobacter pylori* infection in the absence of antibodies and is mediated by MHC class II-restricted responses. *J Exp Med* 1998;188: 2277–2288.
80. Morris AJ, Ali MR, Nicholson GI, et al. Long-term follow-up of voluntary ingestion of *Helicobacter pylori. Ann Intern Med* 1991;114:662–663.
81. Veenendaal RA, Pena AS, Meijer JL, et al. Long-term serological surveillance after treatment of *Helicobacter pylori* infection. *Gut* 1991;32:1291–1294.
82. Kosunen TU, Seppala K, Sarna S, et al. Diagnostic value of decreasing IgG, IgA, and IgM antibody titres after eradication of *Helicobacter pylori. Lancet* 1992;339:893–895.
83. Suerbaum S, Josenhans C, Labigne A. Cloning and genetic characterization of the *Helicobacter pylori* and *Helicobacter mustelae flaB* flagellin genes and construction of *H. pylori flaA*- and *flaB*-negative mutants by electroporation-mediated allelic exchange. *J Bacteriol* 1993;175:3278–3288.
84. Geis G, Suerbaum S, Forsthoff B, et al. Ultrastructure and biochemical studies of the flagellar sheath of *Helicobacter pylori. J Med Microbiol* 1993;38:371–377.
85. Nakamura H, Yoshiyama H, Takeuchi H, et al. Urease plays an important role in the chemotactic motility of *Helicobacter pylori* in a viscous environment. *Infect Immun* 1998;66:4832–4837.
86. Josenhans C, Suerbaum S. *Helicobacter* and motility and chemotaxis. In: Helicobacter pylori*: molecular and cellular biology.* Wymondham, UK: Horizon Scientific Press, 2001.
87. Eaton KA, Suerbaum S, Josenhans C, et al. Colonization of gnotobiotic piglets by *Helicobacter pylori* deficient in two flagellin genes. *Infect Immun* 1996;64:2445–2448.
88. Mizote T, Yoshiyama H, Nakazawa T. Urease-independent chemotactic responses of *Helicobacter pylori* to urea, urease inhibitors, and sodium bicarbonate. *Infect Immun* 1997;65: 1519–1521.
89. Foynes S, Dorrell N, Ward SJ, et al. *Helicobacter pylori* possesses two CheY response regulators and a histidine kinase sensor, CheA, which are essential for chemotaxis and colonization of the gastric mucosa. *Infect Immun* 2000;68:2016–2023.
90. Meyer-Rosberg K, Scott DR, Rex D, et al. The effect of environmental pH on the proton motive force of *Helicobacter pylori. Gastroenterology* 1996;111:886–900.
91. Dunn BE, Vakil NB, Schneider BG, et al. Localization of *Helicobacter pylori* urease and heat shock protein in human gastric biopsies. *Infect Immun* 1997;65:1181–1188.
92. Weeks DL, Eskandari S, Scott DR, et al. An H^+-gated urea channel: The link between *Helicobacter pylori* urease and gastric colonization. *Science* 2000;287:482–485.
93. Eaton KA, Brooks CL, Morgan DR, et al. Essential role of urease in pathogenesis of gastritis induced by *Helicobacter pylori* in gnotobiotic piglets. *Infect Immun* 1991;59:2470–2475.
94. Dunn BE, Vakil NB, Schneider BG, et al. Localization of *Helicobacter pylori* urease and heat shock protein in human gastric biopsies. *Infect Immun* 1997;65:1181–1188.
95. Marshall BJ, Warren JR, Francis GJ, et al. Rapid urease test in the management of *Campylobacter pyloridis*-associated gastritis. *Am J Gastroenterol* 1987;82:200–210.
96. Graham DY, Klein PD, Evans DJ Jr, et al. *Campylobacter pylori* detected noninvasively by the ^{13}C-urea breath test. *Lancet* 1987; 1:1174–1177.
97. Corthesy-Theulaz I, Porta N, Pringault E, et al. Adhesion of *Helicobacter pylori* to polarized T84 human intestinal cell monolayers is pH-dependent. *Infect Immun* 1996;64:3827–3832.
98. Sharma SA, Tummuru MK, Miller GG, et al. Interleukin-8 response of gastric epithelial cell lines to *Helicobacter pylori* stimulation *in vitro. Infect Immun* 1995;63:1681–1687.
99. Blaser MJ. Hypotheses on the pathogenesis and natural history of *Helicobacter pylori*-induced inflammation. *Gastroenterology* 1992;102:720–727.
100. Dhaenens L, Szczebara F, Husson MO. Identification, characterization, and immunogenicity of the lactoferrin-binding protein from *Helicobacter pylori. Infect Immun* 1997;65:514–518.
101. Muotiala A, Helander IM, Pyhala L, et al. Low biological activity of *Helicobacter pylori* lipopolysaccharide. *Infect Immun* 1992;60:1714–1716.
102. Perez-Perez GI, Shepherd VL, Morrow JD, et al. Activation of human THP-1 cells and rat bone marrow-derived macrophages by *Helicobacter pylori* lipopolysaccharide. *Infect Immun* 1995; 63:1183–1187.
103. Moran AP, Lindner B, Walsh EJ. Structural characterization of the lipid A component of *Helicobacter pylori* rough- and smooth-form lipopolysaccharides. *J Bacteriol* 1997;179:6453–6463.
104. Aspinall GO, Monteiro MA, Pang H, et al. Lipopolysaccharide of the *Helicobacter pylori* type strain NCTC 11637 (ATCC 43504): structure of the O antigen chain and core oligosaccharide regions. *Biochemistry* 1996;35:2489–2497.
105. Wirth HP, Yang MQ, Peek RM, et al. *Helicobacter pylori* Lewis expression is related to the host Lewis phenotype. *Gastroenterology* 1997;113:1091–1098.
106. Claeys D, Faller G, Appelmelk BJ, et al. The gastric H^+,K^+-ATPase is a major autoantigen in chronic *Helicobacter pylori* gastritis with body mucosa atrophy. *Gastroenterology* 1998;115: 340–347.
107. Putsep K, Branden CI, Boman HG, et al. Antibacterial peptide from *H. pylori. Nature* 1999;398:671–672.
108. Feldman RA, James A, Eccersley P, et al. Epidemiology of *Helicobacter pylori*: acquisition, transmission, population prevalence and disease-to-infection ratio. *Br Med Bull* 1998;54:39–53.

109. Kuipers EJ. Review article: exploring the link between *Helicobacter pylori* and gastric cancer. *Aliment Pharmacol Ther* 1999; 13[Suppl 1]:3–11.
110. Josenhans C, Eaton KA, Thevenot T, et al. Switching of flagellar motility in *Helicobacter pylori* by reversible length variation of a short homopolymeric sequence repeat in *fliP,* a gene encoding a basal body protein. *Infect Immun* 2000;68:4598–4603.
111. Suerbaum S, Smith JM, Bapumia K, et al. Free recombination within *Helicobacter pylori. Proc Natl Acad Sci U S A* 1998;95: 12619–12624.
112. Achtman M, Azuma T, Berg DE, et al. Recombination and clonal groupings within *Helicobacter pylori* from different geographical regions. *Mol Microbiol* 1999;32:459–470.
113. Censini S, Lange C, Xiang Z, et al. cag, a pathogenicity island of *Helicobacter pylori,* encodes type I-specific and disease-associated virulence factors. *Proc Natl Acad Sci U S A* 1996;93: 14648–14653.
114. Cover TL, Dooley CP, Blaser MJ. Characterization of and human serologic response to proteins in *Helicobacter pylori* broth culture supernatants with vacuolizing cytotoxin activity. *Infect Immun* 1990;58:603–610.
115. Crabtree JE, Taylor JD, Wyatt JI, et al. Mucosal IgA recognition of *Helicobacter pylori* 120 kDa protein, peptic ulceration, and gastric pathology. *Lancet* 1991;338:332–335.
116. Blaser MJ, Perez-Perez GI, Kleanthous H, et al. Infection with *Helicobacter pylori* strains possessing cagA is associated with an increased risk of developing adenocarcinoma of the stomach. *Cancer Res* 1995;55:2111–2115.
117. Segal ED, Cha J, Lo J, et al. Altered states: involvement of phosphorylated CagA in the induction of host cellular growth changes by *Helicobacter pylori. Proc Natl Acad Sci U S A* 1999; 96:14559–14564.
118. Odenbreit S, Puls J, Sedlmaier B, et al. Translocation of *Helicobacter pylori* CagA into gastric epithelial cells by type IV secretion. *Science* 2000;287:1497–1500.
119. Naumann M, Wessler S, Bartsch C, et al. Activation of activator protein 1 and stress response kinases in epithelial cells colonized by *Helicobacter pylori* encoding the cag pathogenicity island. *J Biol Chem* 1999;274:31655–31662.
120. Asahi M, Azuma T, Ito S, et al. *Helicobacter pylori* CagA protein can be tyrosine phosphorylated in gastric epithelial cells. *J Exp Med* 2000;191:593–602.
121. Tummuru MK, Sharma SA, Blaser MJ. *Helicobacter pylori* picB, a homologue of the *Bordetella pertussis* toxin secretion protein, is required for induction of IL-8 in gastric epithelial cells. *Mol Microbiol* 1995;18:867–876.
122. Sharma SA, Tummuru MKR, Blaser MJ, et al. Activation of IL-8 gene expression by *Helicobacter pylori* is regulated by transcription factor nuclear factor-kappa B in gastric epithelial cells. *J Immunol* 1998;160:2401–2407.
123. Hansson LE, Nyren O, Hsing AW, et al. The risk of stomach cancer in patients with gastric or duodenal ulcer disease. *N Engl J Med* 1996;335:242–249.
124. Atherton JC. CagA, the cag pathogenicity island and *Helicobacter pylori* virulence. *Gut* 1999;44:307–308.
125. Cover TL, Glupczynski Y, Lage AP, et al. Serologic detection of infection with cagA+ *Helicobacter pylori* strains. *J Clin Microbiol* 1995;33:1496–1500.
126. Leunk RD, Johnson PT, David BC, et al. Cytotoxic activity in broth-culture filtrates of *Campylobacter pylori. J Med Microbiol* 1988;26:93–99.
127. Marchetti M, Arico B, Burroni D, et al. Development of a mouse model of *Helicobacter pylori* infection that mimics human disease. *Science* 1995;267:1655–1658.
128. Papini E, Satin B, Norais N, et al. Selective increase of the permeability of polarized epithelial cell monolayers by *Helicobacter pylori* vacuolating toxin. *J Clin Invest* 1998;102:813–820.
129. Tombola F, Carlesso C, Szabo I, et al. *Helicobacter pylori* vacuolating toxin forms anion-selective channels in planar lipid bilayers: possible implications for the mechanism of cellular vacuolation. *Biophys J* 1999;76:1401–1409.
130. Cover TL, Tummuru MK, Cao P, et al. Divergence of genetic sequences for the vacuolating cytotoxin among *Helicobacter pylori* strains. *J Biol Chem* 1994;269:10566–10573.
131. Atherton JC, Cao P, Peek RM Jr, et al. Mosaicism in vacuolating cytotoxin alleles of *Helicobacter pylori.* Association of specific vacA types with cytotoxin production and peptic ulceration. *J Biol Chem* 1995;270:17771–17777.
132. Forsyth MH, Atherton JC, Blaser MJ, et al. Heterogeneity in levels of vacuolating cytotoxin gene (*vacA*) transcription among *Helicobacter pylori* strains. *Infect Immun* 1998;66:3088–3094.
133. Letley DP, Atherton JC. Natural diversity in the N terminus of the mature vacuolating cytotoxin of *Helicobacter pylori* determines cytotoxin activity. *J Bacteriol* 2000;182:3278–3280.
134. Atherton JC, Peek RM Jr, Tham KT, et al. Clinical and pathological importance of heterogeneity in *vacA,* the vacuolating cytotoxin gene of *Helicobacter pylori. Gastroenterology* 1997;112: 92–99.
135. Pagliaccia C, de Bernard M, Lupetti P, et al. The m2 form of the *Helicobacter pylori* cytotoxin has cell type-specific vacuolating activity. *Proc Natl Acad Sci U S A* 1998;95:10212–10217.
136. van Doorn LJ, Figueiredo C, Sanna R, et al. Clinical relevance of the *cagA, vacA,* and *iceA* status of *Helicobacter pylori. Gastroenterology* 1998;115:58–66.
137. Kidd M, Lastovica AJ, Atherton JC, et al. Heterogeneity in the *Helicobacter pylori vacA* and *cagA* genes: association with gastroduodenal disease in South Africa? *Gut* 1999;45:499–502.
138. Cover TL, Cao P, Murphy UK, et al. Serum neutralizing antibody response to the vacuolating cytotoxin of *Helicobacter pylori. J Clin Invest* 1992;90:913–918.
139. Rudi J, Kolb C, Maiwald M, et al. Serum antibodies against *Helicobacter pylori* proteins VacA and CagA are associated with increased risk for gastric adenocarcinoma. *Dig Dis Sci* 1997;42: 1652–1659.
140. Gerhard M, Lehn N, Neumayer N, et al. Clinical relevance of the *Helicobacter pylori* gene for blood-group antigen-binding adhesin. *Proc Natl Acad Sci U S A* 1999;96:12778–12783.
141. Peek RM Jr, Thompson SA, Donahue JP, et al. Adherence to gastric epithelial cells induces expression of a *Helicobacter pylori* gene, *iceA,* that is associated with clinical outcome. *Proc Assoc Am Physicians* 1998;110:531–544.
142. Rautelin H, Blomberg B, Jarnerot G, et al. Nonopsonic activation of neutrophils and cytotoxin production by *Helicobacter pylori*: ulcerogenic markers. *Scand J Gastroenterol* 1994;29:128–132.
143. Zhang QB, Nakashabendi IM, Mokhashi MS, et al. Association of cytotoxin production and neutrophil activation by strains of *Helicobacter pylori* isolated from patients with peptic ulceration and chronic gastritis. *Gut* 1996;38:841–845.
144. El-Omar EM, Carrington M, Chow WH, et al. Interleukin-1 polymorphisms associated with increased risk of gastric cancer. *Nature* 2000;404:398–402.
145. Martin DF, Montgomery E, Dobek AS, et al. *Campylobacter pylori,* NSAIDs, and smoking: risk factors for peptic ulcer disease. *Am J Gastroenterol* 1989;84:1268–1272.
146. Correa P. Human gastric carcinogenesis: a multistep and multifactorial process—first American Cancer Society Award lecture on cancer epidemiology and prevention. *Cancer Res* 1992;52: 6735–6740.
147. Thun MJ, Namboodiri MM, Calle EE, et al. Aspirin use and risk of fatal cancer. *Cancer Res* 1993;53:1322–1327.

148. Langman MJS, Cheng KK, Gilman EA, et al. Effect of anti-inflammatory drugs on overall risk of common cancer: case–control study in general practice research database. *Br Med J* 2000;320:1642–1646.
149. Blaser MJ, Chyou PH, Nomura A. Age at establishment of *Helicobacter pylori* infection and gastric carcinoma, gastric ulcer, and duodenal ulcer risk. *Cancer Res* 1995;55:562–565.
150. Dixon MF, Genta RM, Yardley JH, et al. Classification and grading of gastritis. The updated Sydney System. International Workshop on the Histopathology of Gastritis, Houston 1994. *Am J Surg Pathol* 1996;20:1161–1181.
151. Schultze V, Hackelsberger A, Gunther T, et al. Differing patterns of *Helicobacter pylori* gastritis in patients with duodenal, prepyloric, and gastric ulcer disease. *Scand J Gastroenterol* 1998; 33:137–142.
152. Queiroz DM, Mendes EN, Rocha GA, et al. Effect of *Helicobacter pylori* eradication on antral gastrin- and somatostatin-immunoreactive cell density and gastrin and somatostatin concentrations. *Scand J Gastroenterol* 1993;28:858–864.
153. Moss SF, Legon S, Bishop AE, et al. Effect of *Helicobacter pylori* on gastric somatostatin in duodenal ulcer disease. *Lancet* 1992; 340:930–932.
154. Larsson LI, Goltermann N, de Magistris L, et al. Somatostatin cell processes as pathways for paracrine secretion. *Science* 1979; 205:1393–1395.
155. Levi S, Dollery CT, Bloom SR, et al. *Campylobacter pylori,* duodenal ulcer disease, and gastrin. *Br Med J* 1989;299: 1093–1094.
156. El-Omar EM, Penman ID, Ardill JE, et al. *Helicobacter pylori* infection and abnormalities of acid secretion in patients with duodenal ulcer disease. *Gastroenterology* 1995;109:681–691.
157. Khulusi S, Badve S, Patel P, et al. Pathogenesis of gastric metaplasia of the human duodenum: role of *Helicobacter pylori,* gastric acid, and ulceration. *Gastroenterology* 1996;110:452–458.
158. Wyatt JI, Rathbone BJ, Sobala GM, et al. Gastric epithelium in the duodenum: its association with *Helicobacter pylori* and inflammation. *J Clin Pathol* 1990;43:981–986.
159. El-Omar EM, Oien K, El-Nujumi A, et al. *Helicobacter pylori* infection and chronic gastric acid hyposecretion. *Gastroenterology* 1997;113:15–24.
160. Yoshimura T, Shimoyama T, Fukuda S, et al. Most gastric cancer occurs on the distal side of the endoscopic atrophic border. *Scand J Gastroenterol* 1999;34:1077–1081.
161. Lauren P. The two histological main types of gastric carcinoma: diffuse and so-called intestinal carcinoma. *Acta Pathol* 1965;64: 31–39.
162. Davies GR, Simmonds NJ, Stevens TR, et al. *Helicobacter pylori* stimulates antral mucosal reactive oxygen metabolite production *in vivo. Gut* 1994;35:179–185.
163. Baik SC, Youn HS, Chung MH, et al. Increased oxidative DNA damage in *Helicobacter pylori*-infected human gastric mucosa. *Cancer Res* 1996;56:1279–1282.
164. Farinati F, Cardin R, Degan P, et al. Oxidative DNA damage accumulation in gastric carcinogenesis. *Gut* 1998;42:351–356.
165. Sobala GM, Schorah CJ, Sanderson M, et al. Ascorbic acid in the human stomach. *Gastroenterology* 1989;97:357–363.
166. Ruiz B, Rood JC, Fontham ET, et al. Vitamin C concentration in gastric juice before and after anti-*Helicobacter pylori* treatment. *Am J Gastroenterol* 1994;89:533–539.
167. Hussell T, Isaacson PG, Crabtree JE, et al. The response of cells from low-grade B-cell gastric lymphomas of mucosa-associated lymphoid tissue to *Helicobacter pylori. Lancet* 1993;342:571–574.
168. Wotherspoon AC, Doglioni C, Diss TC, et al. Regression of primary low-grade B-cell gastric lymphoma of mucosa-associated lymphoid tissue type after eradication of *Helicobacter pylori. Lancet* 1993;342:575–577.
169. Weber DM, Dimopoulos MA, Anandu DP, et al. Regression of gastric lymphoma of mucosa-associated lymphoid tissue with antibiotic therapy for *Helicobacter pylori. Gastroenterology* 1994; 107:1835–1838.

34

CLINICAL APPROACH TO THE *HELICOBACTER PYLORI*-POSITIVE PATIENT

ERNST J. KUIPERS
JOHANNES G. KUSTERS
MARTIN J. BLASER

It was known from the late nineteenth century that the mucous layer of the human stomach often contains spiral bacteria (see Color Figure 34.1). Because their presence was generally considered to result from bacterial overgrowth—for example, in patients with delayed gastric emptying because of scarring following an ulcer or obstruction by a tumor—the bacteria were ignored until the early 1980s, when they were first isolated from biopsy specimens. Soon afterward, it became clear that the bacterium (*Helicobacter pylori*) causes "chronic active gastritis," which can be complicated by more serious conditions, such as peptic ulcer disease and the development of distal gastric adenocarcinomas and gastric lymphomas. This knowledge has had a significant impact on gastroenterologic practice in the past decade and has made the diagnosis and treatment of *H. pylori* colonization clinically relevant. In this chapter, we consider the various aspects of the diagnosis and treatment of *H. pylori* infection.

INDICATIONS FOR DIAGNOSIS AND TREATMENT

H. pylori colonization is not a disease but rather a circumstance that affects the risk for acquiring various clinical conditions of the upper gastrointestinal tract. *H. pylori* colonization thus parallels colonization with α-hemolytic streptococci in the upper respiratory tract and colonic colonization with certain *E. coli* strains. Therefore, in itself, a diagnosis of *H. pylori* colonization has no relevance, and testing for *H. pylori* should be performed either with the purpose of identifying the cause of a specific disorder, such as a duodenal ulcer or gastric MALT (mucosa-associated lymphoid tissue)-lymphoma, or with the thought of disease prevention, as in patients with an increased familial risk for gastric cancer. When testing is performed for either of these purposes, a positive result warrants treatment, and a negative result may indicate the need to search for other etiologic factors or preventive measures. To interpret these various aspects, a correct understanding of the clinical course of *H. pylori*-associated disorders and the effect of *H. pylori* eradication is needed.

Acute and Chronic Gastritis

Data on the acute phase of *H. pylori* colonization are scarce and largely come from adult subjects who deliberately or inadvertently ingested *H. pylori* organisms or underwent endoscopic procedures with contaminated equipment (1–6). Despite their limited number, these reports are generally consistent. It appears that colonization with *H. pylori* leads to intense infiltration of both the antrum and corpus of the stomach with neutrophilic and mononuclear cells. This is often accompanied by transient, nonspecific dyspeptic symptoms, such as fullness, nausea, and vomiting, which usually resolve within a few days. The inflammation of the mucosa of both the proximal and distal regions of the stomach, or pangastritis, is often associated with a considerable decrease in acid output, which can last for months. Seventeen volunteers became hypochlorhydric during studies with an *H. pylori*-contaminated pH electrode. The hypochlorhydria occurred 3 weeks after the studies and lasted a mean 4 months (7). These limited and nonspecific symptoms of early *H. pylori* colonization are rarely an indication for *H. pylori* diagnosis and treatment (4).

E.J. Kuipers and J.G. Kusters: Departments of Gastroenterology and Hepatology, Erasmus Medical Center, Rotterdam, the Netherlands
M.J. Blaser: Departments of Medicine and Microbiology, New York University School of Medicine; Department of Internal Medicine, New York Harbor Veterans Affairs Medical Center, New York, New York

The initial colonization may be transient or persistent *H. pylori* colonization becomes established, but the proportions are not known. In this chronic phase, a close correlation exists between the level of acid secretion and the distribution of gastritis. This correlation results from pH-related bacterial growth and from the effects of mucosal inflammation on acid-secretory capacity and regulation. In subjects with intact acid secretion, *H. pylori* most densely colonizes the gastric antrum, where few acid-secretory parietal cells are present. As a result, these subjects have an antrum-predominant gastritis. In subjects in whom acid secretion is hampered, regardless of the mechanism, the number of bacteria decreases in the antrum, whereas the bacteria in the corpus do not seem to increase in number but come into closer contact with the mucosa; such subjects thus have a corpus-predominant gastritis. Active inflammation of the corpus mucosa then augments hypochlorhydria (paralleling the acute phase of infection) because local inflammatory factors such as cytokines, including interleukin 1β (IL-1β), have a strong suppressive effect on parietal cell function.

The endoscopic macroscopic appearance of the gastric mucosa offers few clues to the presence of *H. pylori* gastritis. Signs such as reddening, edema, and nodularity are poor predictors of the presence of *H. pylori* gastritis. Chronic active gastritis is only a histologic diagnosis, in which mononuclear cells usually predominate but neutrophils often are present. The inflammation mostly affects the upper or foveolar layer and the deeper layer of the mucosa, which contains the gastric glands. In the earlier classifications of gastritis, infiltration of the foveolar layer was designated as *superficial gastritis,* whereas the presence of inflammatory cells in the glandular layer was believed to correspond to gland loss and was designated as *atrophic gastritis* (8). However, this concept was not pathophysiologically correct because the presence of inflammatory cells in the glandular mucosal layer is not synonymous with gland loss. Therefore, newer classification schema proposed that inflammation and gland loss or atrophy should be separately scored (9). The term *superficial gastritis,* although still widely used, has lost its meaning and been replaced by the term *chronic active gastritis,* which reflects a condition of mucosal inflammation of the foveolar and glandular layers. Gastritis and *H. pylori* colonization can be verified simultaneously in the same biopsy specimens. Although colonization with *H. pylori* is almost invariably associated with gastritis, and although gastritis is mostly a consequence of *H. pylori* colonization, other causes include infections, as with cytomegalovirus; chronic inflammatory and autoimmune disorders, such as Crohn's disease and pernicious anemia; and chemical damage, such as that caused by the use of alcohol or nonsteroidal antiinflammatory drugs (NSAIDs). *H. pylori* eradication leads to a complete resolution of inflammation, even though it can take more than a year before the mononuclear cell infiltrate disappears (10). An *H. pylori*-free gastric mucosa does not contain lymphoid tissue. However, gastritis *per se* is mostly asymptomatic and is not an indication for *H. pylori* treatment. Therefore, refraining from sampling gastric biopsy specimens in patients with normal endoscopic findings is justified. Physicians should prescribe eradication therapy to treat symptoms or to cure or prevent disease rather than merely treat a "positive" test result.

Peptic Ulcer Disease

Ulcers of the stomach or duodenum are defined as mucosal defects with a diameter of at least 0.5 cm penetrating through the muscularis mucosae. Smaller or more superficial defects are called *erosions.* Gastric ulcers occur mostly along the lesser curvature of the stomach, in particular at the transition from corpus to antrum mucosa. This transitional zone is usually located near the incisura of the stomach, but it can extend to an area close to the gastroesophageal junction. Gastric ulcers can be categorized by their localization into proximal ulcers (occurring in the corpus or cardia), ulcers at the incisura, and distal ulcers (occurring in the antrum). Duodenal ulcers usually occur in the bulb, the area most exposed to gastric acid.

Peptic ulcers occur frequently, although their incidence has been steadily decreasing in Western countries in past decades (11). This decrease is most likely the result of a decreasing prevalence of *H. pylori.* In Western countries, duodenal ulcers occur approximately four times more frequently than do gastric ulcers; elsewhere, gastric ulcers are more common. Duodenal ulcers are more common in younger adults, whereas elderly persons more often have gastric ulcers. The combined annual incidence of gastric and duodenal ulcers is estimated at 2 to 3 per 1,000 population, but exact data are lacking. The presence of *H. pylori* increases the risk for these ulcers. The recognition of the clinical relevance of this bacterium has had a major impact on the treatment and course of peptic ulcer disease. In earlier days, the disease was associated with a high rate of morbidity, and patients frequently required acid-suppressive maintenance therapy, surgery, or both. In the past decade, a considerable proportion of cases of ulcer disease have been treated with antibiotics, with a diminished chance of recurrence after eradication of *H. pylori* (Fig. 34.2). Soon after the first isolation of *H. pylori,* studies in different parts of the world reported an overall 84% prevalence of *H. pylori* among patients with gastric ulcers and a 95% prevalence among those with duodenal ulcers (12). The estimated lifetime risk for ulcer disease in *H. pylori*-positive subjects is 3 to 10 times higher than that in *H. pylori*-negative subjects (13). The cumulative long-term incidence of ulcer disease in *H. pylori*-positive subjects has been reported to vary between 10% and 15% (14,15), but it is unknown whether these data were influenced by selection of the study populations. The chance of ulcer development in the presence of *H. pylori* is influ-

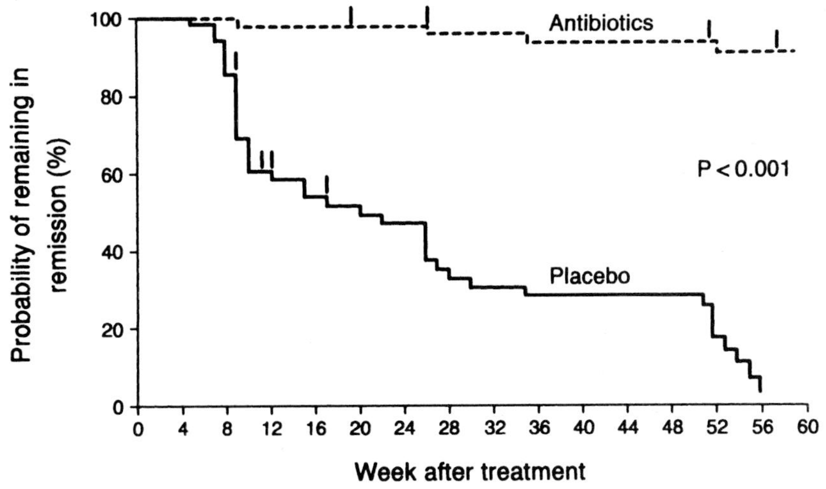

FIGURE 34.2. Influence of eradication therapy with ranitidine, metronidazole, and amoxicillin (n = 50) compared with ranitidine alone (n = 49) on duodenal ulcer relapse. Note that bismuth was not included in the treatment regimen, which indicates that the mucosal protective effects of bismuth are unlikely to explain the significantly lowered duodenal ulcer relapse rates identified by previous investigators. (From Hentschell E, Brandstätter G, Dragosics B, et al. Effect of ranitidine and amoxicillin plus metronidazole on the eradication of *Helicobacter pylori* and the recurrence of duodenal ulcer. *N Engl J Med* 1993;328:308–312, with permission.)

enced by a variety of host and bacterial factors (see Chapter 33). Ulcers mostly occur at the site where mucosal inflammation is most severe. In subjects with decreased acid output, this usually is the gastric transitional zone between corpus and antrum. If the rate of acid production is normal to high, the most severe inflammation is usually found in the distal stomach and proximal duodenum.

H. pylori-associated peptic ulcers tend to heal spontaneously, but 50% to 90% recur within 2 years. Healing is accelerated by acid-suppressive treatment with either histamine$_2$ (H_2) blockers or proton pump inhibitors (PPIs), but 20% to 30% of ulcers recur even during maintenance therapy. Prospective studies have shown that treatment of *H. pylori* significantly alters the course of peptic ulcer disease, reducing the ulcer recurrence rate to a small percentage per year (16). In one study with follow-up to 10 years, no recurrent ulcers were diagnosed among 141 patients with duodenal ulcers and 45 patients with gastric ulcers after successful *H. pylori* eradication (17). *H. pylori* eradication also significantly reduces the need for acid-suppressive drugs in patients with a history of ulcer disease (18). For these reasons, a diagnosis of gastroduodenal ulcer disease is a strong indication for *H. pylori* testing and treatment (Table 34.1). In practice, many clinicians disregard testing for *H. pylori* and simply start treating patients who have ulcers with antimicrobial therapy, reasoning that the prevalence of *H. pylori* among patients with ulcers is so high that a negative test result is more likely to be false rather than reflect a true absence of *H. pylori.* However, in Western countries, this policy is gradually becoming inadequate because of the diminishing prevalence of *H. pylori.* The proportion of *H. pylori*-negative ulcers is increasing. In the United States, several recent studies have shown a prevalence of *H. pylori* of 70% to 75% among patients with ulcers (19,20). The differential diagnosis of ulcer disease primarily includes NSAID use, but malignancy, Crohn's disease, ischemia, Zollinger–Ellison syndrome, stress and multiple organ failure, infection with other microbes (e.g., *Helicobacter heilmannii, Treponema pallidum,* cytomegalovirus, herpes simplex virus), and the use of medications such as doxycycline and alendronate all are involved.

Complicated Ulcer Disease

Ulcers can be complicated by bleeding, perforation, or stricture formation. An estimated 15% to 20% of gastroduodenal ulcers are complicated by bleeding (21). The risk for bleeding is higher if the patient is older, uses NSAIDs or aspirin, or has had a previous episode of bleeding. Each of these factors appears to increase the risk for bleeding approximately threefold. Bleeding is often severe; more than half of such patients present with signs of hypovolemic shock. In a Dutch survey, transfusion of a mean of 5 U of packed cells was required (22). After hemodynamic stabilization, endoscopy is required to establish a diagnosis and, if necessary, treat a persistently bleeding or visible vessel. Although in 80% of episodes bleeding from an ulcer stops spontaneously, the recurrence rate strongly depends on the appearance of the ulcer at endoscopy. In cases of persistent bleeding or visible vessel, the chance of recurrent bleeding is very high (23). Although endoscopic therapy can reduce the recurrence rate and need for transfusion, high-dose PPI therapy can do the same. After stabilization, patients with ulcers of unknown cause should be tested for *H. pylori,* and if the result is positive, they should be treated because treatment significantly reduces the chance of recurrent bleeding (24–26). This policy is also mandatory in patients with a perforated ulcer and those with benign gastric outlet obstruction resulting from stricture formation after recurrent peptic ulceration. In the latter group, *H. pylori* eradication leads to healing and prevention of ulcers and the gradual disappearance of edema (27). Thereafter, only a few patients require balloon dilation or surgery for persistent obstruction. In cases of perforation of an *H. pylori*-associated ulcer, the surgical procedure should be restricted to

TABLE 34.1. INTERNATIONAL GUIDELINES FOR *H. PYLORI* ERADICATION IN ADULTS

Condition	United States (295)	Canada (79,296)	Europe (78,297)	Asia-Pacific (298)	South America (299)	Japan (300)
Asymptomatic	No	No	Yes	No	—	—
Dyspepsia (NUD)	Consider	Yes	Yes	Consider	—	i.d.[c]
Gastritis	*m*[a]	Yes	Yes	—	Consider	—
Active or past ulcer	Yes	Yes	Yes	Yes	Yes	Yes
Erosive duodenitis	—	—	—	—	Yes	—
GERD/PPI therapy	No	No	Yes	—	—	No
NSAID use	—	No	Consider	Yes	—	No
Atrophic gastritis	—	—	Yes	—	—	i.d.
Gastric cancer[b]	No	—	Yes	Yes	—	i.d.
Cancer in relatives	—	Yes	Yes	No	Consider	—
MALT lymphoma	Yes	Yes	Yes	Yes	Consider	Yes
Hepatic encephalopathy	—	—	—	—	Consider	—

[a]Not addressed.
[b]Following resection of early gastric cancer.
[c]Addressed, but no conclusion because of insufficient data.
NUD, non-ulcer dyspepsia; GERD, gastroesophageal reflux disease; PPI, proton pump inhibitor; NSAID, nonsteroidal antiinflammatory drug; MALT, mucosa-associated lymphoid tissue.

ulcer closure without vagotomy. Eradication therapy after surgery adequately prevents ulcer recurrence and is not associated with the long-term side effects of vagotomy (28). Uncomplicated *H. pylori*-positive ulcers can be treated adequately with eradication therapy alone, without the need for further acid suppression (29). In complicated ulcer disease, clinicians may choose to be more conservative and continue with acid suppression until 1 week before tests to confirm eradication are performed to prevent early recurrence in those in whom therapy has failed. Continuation until the day of testing may interfere with the test result.

Non-ulcer Dyspepsia

Non-ulcer or functional dyspepsia is defined as symptoms of upper gastrointestinal distress without any identifiable structural abnormality. The symptoms may be typical of reflux, with heartburn and regurgitation as predominant signs, or of dysmotility, with early satiety and nausea, or of ulcer, with pain and vomiting (30). Such symptoms are experienced frequently by 20% to 40% of the adult population of the Western world (31). *H. pylori* is carried by 30% to 60% of patients with functional dyspepsia, but this prevalence is not much different from that in the unaffected population (32). A number of studies investigating the effect of *H. pylori* eradication on dyspeptic symptoms reported conflicting results; nearly all had design flaws (32). Four recent trials overcame the limitations of previous trials but reached opposite conclusions (33–36). In these studies, *H. pylori*-positive dyspeptic patients were randomly treated with either omeprazole and antibiotics to eradicate *H. pylori* or with omeprazole alone for 1 to 2 weeks. After 1 year, symptoms, *H. pylori* status, and quality of life were reassessed. In all four studies, *H. pylori* was eradicated in most (79% to 88%) of the patients treated with antibiotics and in only a few treated with omeprazole alone. In all studies, dyspepsia resolved in 21% to 28% of patients treated with antibiotics. However, in three studies, a similar improvement was noted in the patients treated with omeprazole alone (21% to 23%) (34–36), whereas the fourth study noted a significantly lower improvement rate (7%) in those treated with omeprazole alone (33). The studies differed with respect to exclusion criteria, scoring of dyspepsia, and number and geographic location of the study centers involved. The most likely explanation for the differences in outcome between these studies is the background prevalence of peptic ulcer disease in the respective populations. Prevalence is high in Scotland, where the study with the positive result originated (33), but low in the other populations. Importantly, all studies agreed that 70% to 80% of *H. pylori*-positive patients with functional dyspepsia do not improve after *H. pylori* eradication, and that any effect of such therapy is not much greater than that produced by 1 to 2 weeks of omeprazole alone. This lack of effect of *H. pylori* eradication on non-ulcer dyspepsia was confirmed in another recent study with a strict design (37). Data with follow-up considerably longer than 12 months are lacking.

What do these results mean in regard to the clinical approach to a patient with dyspepsia? A Canadian working group suggested a five-step approach (38), starting with a determination of whether the symptoms arise in the upper gastrointestinal tract or reflect another problem, such as coronary artery disease. Secondly, if a patient has "alarm" symptoms, such as weight loss, hematochezia, black stools, or an inability to pass food, or if the symptoms newly arise in a subject older than 50 to 55 years, endoscopy is indicated. The absence of abnormal findings is often reassuring and sufficient. In addition, advice on dietary, smoking, and drinking habits may prove helpful. Third, if the patient is using NSAIDs or aspirin, withdrawal of these drugs or the addition of acid suppressants is indicated. Fourth, if heartburn is the predominant symptom, a diagnosis of gastroesophageal reflux disease (GERD) should be made provisionally and acid suppressants started. For the remaining patients, the working group suggested a noninvasive *H. pylori* test (38), followed by eradication treatment for those with positive results. Non-ulcer dyspepsia is therefore not a generally accepted indication for *H. pylori* eradication (39). Nevertheless, many gastroenterologists routinely perform a biopsy to detect *H. pylori* if endoscopy is performed (40,41).

Atrophic Gastritis, Intestinal Metaplasia, and Gastric Cancer

Chronic *H. pylori*-induced inflammation can eventually lead to loss of the normal gastric mucosal architecture, with destruction of the gastric glands and replacement by fibrosis and intestinal-type epithelium (see Color Figure 34.3). These conditions, atrophic gastritis and intestinal metaplasia, occur in approximately half of the *H. pylori*-colonized population as a result of long-existing chronic gastritis, whereas they are rare in *H. pylori*-negative subjects (42). They first occur in those subjects and at those sites with the most severe inflammation. Thus, they are more common in persons colonized with *cagA*-positive strains than in those colonized with a *cagA*-negative strain (43) and are most common in the antrum. From there, the lesions extend with time multifocally, in particular along the smaller curvature. They do not give rise to any specific symptoms, and cobalamin absorption remains intact unless severe atrophy of the body mucosa occurs. However, these lesions increase the risk for gastric cancer fivefold to 90-fold, depending on the extent and severity of atrophy and possibly also on the type of metaplasia (44,45) (Fig. 34.4).

Evidence that *H. pylori* increases the risk for gastric cancer via the sequence of atrophy and metaplasia originates from various studies, in particular from a number of cohort follow-up studies (46–51). These studies showed that gastric cancer involving the distal stomach develops in *H. pylori*-positive subjects more often than in uninfected controls. This finding was supported by other data showing geographic associations

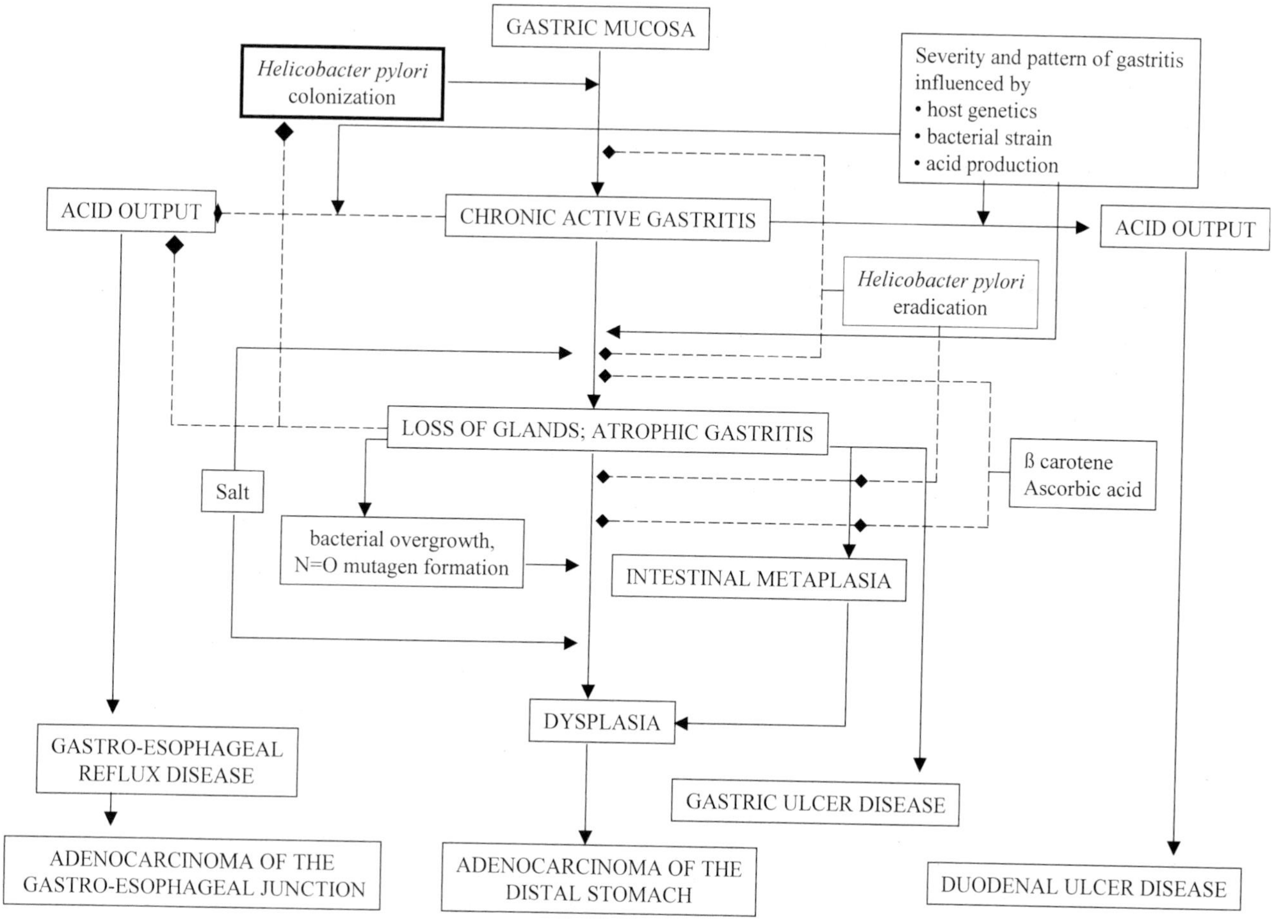

FIGURE 34.4. Hypothetical cascade leading to the development of adenocarcinoma of the distal stomach. *Square arrow heads* represent inhibition. (Adapted from Correa P, Haenszel W, Cuello C, et al. A model for gastric cancer epidemiology. *Lancet* 1975;2:58–59, with permission.)

between the prevalence of *H. pylori* and incidence of gastric cancer (52,53). Retrospective studies comparing the prevalence of *H. pylori* among patients with gastric cancer and controls did not always show a higher prevalence of *H. pylori* among the cancer patients (54). However, this discrepancy between prospective and retrospective data was explained by the gradual disappearance of *H. pylori* colonization during the development of atrophic gastritis and intestinal metaplasia (42,55,56). The explanation is supported by metaanalyses of prospective data showing that the calculated odds ratio for gastric cancer in the presence of *H. pylori* increases with a longer observation period (54,57).

On the basis of these findings, it is estimated that *H. pylori* colonization increases the risk for gastric cancer approximately 10-fold. In 1994, the International Agency for Research on Cancer, a department of the World Health Organization, classified *H. pylori* as a class I carcinogen, which means that the agency considered the evidence on the relation between *H. pylori* and gastric cancer conclusive (58). This conclusion was thereafter supported by experimental animal data. After 62 weeks of infection, intestinal-type adenocarcinoma developed in 37% of *H. pylori*-infected Mongolian gerbils but in none of the uninfected control animals (59). The risk for the development of atrophy and cancer in the presence of *H. pylori* is again related to host and bacterial factors, which influence the severity of the chronic inflammatory response. The risk is increased in subjects colonized with *cagA*-positive strains (60,61) and also in those with a genetic predisposition to a higher production of IL-1 in response to colonization (62). The lifetime risk for gastric cancer among *H. pylori*-positive subjects is estimated to approximate 1% to 2% in Western countries (63). In the developed world, 60% to 80% of gastric cancers are therefore related to the long-term presence of *H. pylori.* In certain regions, such as Japan, the risk for gastric cancer in *H. pylori*-positive subjects is estimated to be significantly higher, up to 5% during 10 years (64). For these reasons, large studies have begun to evaluate the effect of *H. pylori* eradication in the prevention and treatment of atrophic gastritis, and in the primary and secondary prevention of gastric cancer. Preliminary results suggest that *H. pylori* eradication stops the progression of atrophic gastritis and intestinal metaplasia and that regression of milder grades of atrophy can occur (65–67). Eradication treatment also eliminates gastritis, and previous cohort studies only rarely observed the development of atrophy and metaplasia in the absence of gastritis. It is likely that *H. pylori* eradication also prevents the development of atrophy and metaplasia, but this assumption has not been tested directly. In respect to the prevention of gastric cancer, Japanese investigators treated 132 *H. pylori*-positive patients with early gastric cancer by endoscopic resection of the tumor (68). Sixty-five of these patients were then treated to eradicate *H. pylori.* After a mean of 2 years of follow-up, 6 (9%) of the 67 persistently *H. pylori*-positive patients had a recurrence of cancer, versus none of the 65 patients in whom *H. pylori* had been eradicated. Secondary cancer prevention is feasible only if the primary lesion is detected at a very early stage. In most Western countries, fewer than 10% of gastric cancers are detected early. Primary prevention is therefore needed, but this entails large population screening programs. Epidemiologic calculations nevertheless suggest that such a strategy can be cost-effective in populations with a high prevalence of *H. pylori* and a high incidence of gastric cancer (69). Prospective studies are ongoing to test this hypothesis. The prevention of atrophy and cancer in the general population is not an indication for the widespread eradication of *H. pylori* until prospective studies have been concluded. Such a policy is supported by the shortage of data on the potential benefits of *H. pylori* colonization and the importance of bacterial and host heterogeneity (70). The incidence of gastric cancer has significantly decreased during the past decades in developed countries. In the United States, it decreased in the past 60 years from approximately 30 to 5 cases per 100,000 inhabitants per year. This decrease parallels the decrease in the prevalence of *H. pylori,* which is related to socioeconomic changes. The decrease, which is still ongoing, will significantly affect the incidence of *H. pylori*-associated conditions and the feasibility of potential population screening and treatment programs (69).

How then should a clinician approach the *H. pylori*-positive patient? In general, testing for *H. pylori* and treating the *H. pylori*-positive patient to prevent gastric cancer is at this moment not indicated. If asymptomatic *H. pylori*-positive subjects are treated with the intention to prevent cancer, there needs to be an awareness of the potential side effects of *H. pylori* eradication, the fact that the probability of gastric cancer in general is low, and the scarcity of data on the reduction of cancer risks at various stages of life and gastric histology. Exceptions for whom a policy of test and treat seems advisable include patients with marked signs of atrophy and metaplasia, in particular if these lesions occur at a younger age. Follow-up studies suggest that gastric cancer develops in approximately 5% to 10% of such patients within 10 to 15 years of follow-up (71–74). *H. pylori*-positive patients who have been successfully treated for early gastric cancer by local resection of the lesion may benefit from eradication treatment (68). Another category includes first-degree relatives of patients with gastric cancer, whose risk for gastric cancer is increased 1.5- to fourfold (75). In comparison with controls, they more often are colonized with *H. pylori* and have a higher prevalence of atrophic gastritis and hypochlorhydria (66,76,77). Eradication of *H. pylori* leads to a resolution of atrophy and hypochlorhydria in 50% of these subjects (66). It is therefore advisable to test and treat them for *H. pylori* (78,79).

Gastric MALT Lymphoma

Gastric mucosa that is not colonized with *H. pylori* does not contain lymphoid tissue, but MALT nearly always appears in response to colonization with *H. pylori*. In rare cases, a monoclonal population of B cells may arise from this tissue and slowly proliferate to form a MALT lymphoma. The histologic appearance of these usually low-grade lymphomas is often that of a dense lymphoid infiltrate of usually centrocyte-like cells that can invade and destroy epithelial structures, leading to so-called lymphoepithelial lesions (80). The endoscopic features of these lesions, which vary widely, include inapparent reddening of the mucosa or thickening of the gastric folds, ulceration, and tumorous lesions. The histologic criteria for the diagnosis of MALT lymphoma and its differentiation from polyclonal reactive infiltrates remain controversial. In particular, the diagnosis is based on the histologic appearance during routine microscopy and on the demonstration of clonality by immunohistochemistry or molecular techniques, such as polymerase chain reaction (PCR). Nearly all patients with MALT lymphoma are *H. pylori*-positive (81), and *H. pylori*-positive subjects have a significantly increased risk for the development of gastric MALT lymphoma (82). Because of the diagnostic controversies and the relative rarity of this disorder, the exact incidence in *H. pylori*-positive subjects is unknown, but MALT lymphomas occur in fewer than 1% of *H. pylori*-positive subjects. In a large German series from a third referral center, MALT lymphoma was diagnosed in 1,745 (0.66%) of 163,680 dyspeptic *H. pylori*-positive patients studied by gastric biopsy sampling, and in 8 (1.5%) of 543 *H. heilmannii*-positive patients (83). These high prevalence rates may be a consequence of case selection and changes in the diagnosis of MALT lymphoma. In the past, the incidence of gastric MALT lymphoma in Western countries approximated single cases per million inhabitants per annum. With the recognition of the association between *H. pylori* and MALT lymphoma, the effect of *H. pylori* eradication on MALT lymphoma was studied in series ranging from 6 to 120 patients. Eradication led to complete lymphoma remission in 60% to 100% of them. In the largest cohort, 120 patients were followed for a mean 38 months (range, 2 to 74 months) after *H. pylori* eradication. Complete and persistent remission occurred in 81%, 9% showed partial remission, and the remaining 10% showed no response (83). These results have established *H. pylori* eradication as first-line therapy for low-grade gastric MALT lymphoma. Once this disorder has been diagnosed in a patient, the usual approach for disease staging includes physical examination, bone marrow evaluation, chest roentgenography or thoracic computed tomography, and abdominal computed tomography for an assessment of distant disease. In addition, endoscopic ultrasonography allows an assessment of the depth of infiltration and the presence of perigastric lymph nodes. In the German series, the presence of such lymph nodes did not predict a failure to respond. Infiltration of the mucosa and submucosa without disease activity at distant locations can initially be treated with *H. pylori* eradication therapy alone, followed by confirmation of eradication after 1 month and follow-up examinations, preferably including endoscopy, histology, and endosonography, every 2 months until complete remission and then every 6 months. However, infiltration of lymphomas into the muscularis propria or serosa of the stomach and the presence of lymphoma at distant locations precludes complete remission with *H. pylori* eradication therapy alone. In these cases, additional treatment, such as chemotherapy, is needed. This is also the case for patients with high-grade lymphomas, although responses to *H. pylori* eradication have been described (83,84). In some cases, it is likely that benign lymphoid proliferation in the stomach is misdiagnosed as MALT lymphoma. The response of such patients to *H. pylori* eradication is usually remission of all pathologic lesions. Such overtreatment in part accounts for the high level of "success" of *H. pylori* eradication in what is diagnosed as MALT lymphoma.

Gastroesophageal Reflux Disease

H. pylori *and the Development of Gastroesophageal Reflux Disease*

For a long time, it was thought that GERD occurs independently of *H. pylori* colonization (i.e., occurs with the same frequency and severity in *H. pylori*-positive and *H. pylori*-negative subjects). This opinion was based on cross-sectional observations suggesting similar prevalence rates of *H. pylori* in patients with GERD and controls (85). However, further studies suggested that *H. pylori* may protect against the development of GERD and so be of benefit to the host. This slowly emerging concept came from repeated observations of a low prevalence of *H. pylori* among patients with GERD, opposing time and geographic trends for *H. pylori* prevalence in comparison with the incidence of GERD and its complications, a potentially increased incidence of GERD after *H. pylori* eradication, and the recognition that *H. pylori*-induced corpus gastritis reduces acid secretion.

Within both developing and developed countries, a lower prevalence of *H. pylori* has repeatedly been observed in patients with endoscopic signs of GERD versus controls with normal endoscopic findings. For example, in a Dutch study of 630 consecutive patients referred for upper gastrointestinal endoscopy, the prevalence rates of *H. pylori* were 29% and 23%, respectively, among patients with esophagitis and Barrett esophagus, versus 51% among patients without endoscopic abnormalities (85). Others reported similar results (86,87). In a metaanalysis of 26 case–control studies, 562 (39%) of 1,426 patients with GERD were *H. pylori*-positive, in comparison with 1,009 (50%) of 2,010 control subjects (88). GERD and *H. pylori* also show opposite geographic and time distributions. *H. pylori* is more common in developing countries; GERD is very common in Western countries, and its incidence is increasing in these countries while *H. pylori* prevalence is decreasing (11).

It has also been reported that the incidence of GERD in patients with duodenal ulcers within the 3 years following *H. pylori* eradication is increased in comparison with the incidence in persistently *H. pylori*-positive patients with ulcers (26% vs. 13%) (89). The risk for the development of GERD was particularly increased in patients who had previously had *H. pylori* corpus gastritis. However, because such gastritis is particularly frequently observed in *H. pylori*-positive patients who take acid-suppressive drugs (90), the discontinuation of these drugs rather than *H. pylori* eradication may have led to the appearance of GERD symptoms in some patients. Nevertheless, other reports have been published of a higher incidence of GERD or a worsening of preexistent GERD in patients after *H. pylori* eradication in comparison with persistently *H. pylori*-positive controls (91,92). Some studies have yielded contradictory results (93,94). In summary, the issue of whether *H. pylori* eradication increases the risk for subsequent development of GERD, or whether it is specific to particular subgroups, must be elucidated further.

Reflux disease results from the interaction between acid production, pressure in the lower esophageal sphincter, esophageal clearance, and gastric emptying. *H. pylori* may affect several of these factors, in particular acid production. Some people respond to *H. pylori* colonization with an exaggerated gastrin response, which leads to an increase in acid production (95). These subjects, an estimated 10% to 15% of all *H. pylori*-positive persons, are at risk for duodenal ulcer disease, and theoretically also for reflux disease. In others, however, gastric acidity is reduced by the release of substances such as the VacA protein, which may directly inhibit parietal cell function, and by bacterial urease activity, which generates acid-buffering ammonia. As a result of such factors, *H. pylori* gastritis extends into the gastric corpus, where mucosal inflammation may further impair acid production with the generation of IL-1, a potent suppressor of parietal cell function. The development of chronic atrophic gastritis is another step in lowering acid production in many *H. pylori*-positive subjects. The presence of factors that lead to a persistent decrease in acid production may explain the protective effect of *H. pylori* against GERD. This hypothesis is supported by observations of an inverse association between GERD and relatively severe corpus gastritis or atrophy (96,97). Further support for the hypothesis that severe corpus inflammation protects against reflux disease comes from studies evaluating the prevalence of *H. pylori* strains harboring the *cagA* gene. Subjects colonized with *cagA*-positive strains generally have more severe gastritis and an increased risk for the development of atrophic gastritis (43). Several cross-sectional studies have shown that patients with GERD in particular have a lower prevalence of *cagA*-positive *H. pylori* strains than do controls (98,99).

H. pylori *and Complications of Gastroesophageal Reflux Disease*

Gastroesophageal reflux disease predisposes to the development of Barrett esophagus and adenocarcinoma of the gastroesophageal junction (100). If *H. pylori* gastritis, in particular that induced by *cagA*-positive strains, protects against GERD, it may hypothetically also protect against these complications of chronic GERD. This hypothesis is supported by several recent studies showing a lower prevalence of *cagA*-positive *H. pylori* strains in patients with Barrett esophagus or proximal gastric cancer than in controls or patients with distal gastric cancer (101–103). A large serologic case–control study nested within a cohort of more than 100,000 Norwegians showed an inverse association between *H. pylori* and the development of proximal gastric cancer, with an odds ratio of 0.40 (95% confidence interval, 0.20 to 0.77) (51). These observations are persuasive indirect support for the hypothesis that severe inflammation of the corpus, in particular that resulting from colonization with *cagA*-positive *H. pylori* strains, protects against GERD and its complications through inhibition of acid secretion. The time trend observations of decreasing *H. pylori* prevalence and increasing incidence of cancers of the gastroesophageal junction provide additional support for the hypothesis. In Western countries, the incidence of GERD and its complications, including adenocarcinomas of the distal esophagus, has increased fourfold to sevenfold in the past decades, whereas the prevalence of *H. pylori* infection has decreased (11,104). Blot et al. (105) analyzed the incidence of adenocarcinomas of the esophagus and cardia according to sex and race in nine cancer registries accounting for 10% of the United States population. During the period from 1976 to 1987, the increase in annual incidence rates for adenocarcinomas of the esophagus and cardia exceeded that for esophageal squamous cell carcinoma and adenocarcinoma of the distal portion of the stomach by far. Similar trends have been observed in Europe (106). Thus, the decreasing prevalence of *H. pylori* appears to have led to both a decrease in the incidence of distal gastric cancer and an increase in the incidence of proximal gastric cancer.

H. pylori *and the Treatment of Gastroesophageal Reflux Disease*

Profound acid-suppressive therapy is the treatment of choice for many patients with GERD. During such therapy, usually with PPIs, active gastritis of the gastric corpus develops in *H. pylori*-positive subjects, which exaggerates the acid-suppressive effects of the drug (107,108). In a large clinical trial, *H. pylori*-positive patients with GERD responded significantly better to 40 mg of pantoprazole daily than did *H. pylori*-negative patients (109). The difference in endoscopic healing rates was 10% after 4 weeks and 4.6% after 8 weeks of treatment. Relief from heartburn and regurgitation also was significantly greater in *H. pylori*-positive patients after 4 weeks, but not after 8 weeks. More importantly, after withdrawal of PPI therapy, *H. pylori* corpus gastritis regresses only slowly, and as a result, acid secretion returns only slowly. In *H. pylori*-negative patients with GERD, however, a significant rebound hypersecretion of acid can occur after PPI withdrawal, but the data regarding the effect of this phenomenon on recurrence of symptoms are conflicting (110,111). *H. pylori*-positive and *H. pylori*-negative persons do not appear to differ with respect to recurrence rates or required PPI dose during maintenance therapy (112). However, such maintenance therapy is associated with persistent active corpus gastritis, which appears to accelerate the progression to atrophic body gastritis (113). After several years of PPI maintenance therapy, atrophic gastritis develops in 20% to 40% of *H. pylori*-positive patients with GERD; this does not happen in *H. pylori*-negative subjects (112,113). Smaller and more limited studies do not show this finding (114). In particular, atrophic gastritis occurs after the onset of therapy in those with moderate to severely active gastritis (112,113,115). This can be prevented by *H. pylori* eradication (116–118). In patients with GERD in whom atrophic gastritis has already developed, *H. pylori* eradication can also lead to a regression of atrophy (118).

Clinical Approach to H. pylori*-positive Patients with Gastroesophageal Reflux Disease*

How should the clinician then approach the *H. pylori*-positive patient with GERD? First, *H. pylori*-negative subjects appear to be at increased risk for the development of GERD and its complications. To what extent GERD can complicate *H. pylori* eradication is still unclear, so that this potential complication does not preclude eradication for sufficient clinical indications. In preexisting GERD, *H. pylori* eradication does not appear to increase the symptom recurrence rate or the need for medication. *H. pylori*-negative patients do not require higher PPI doses, although their initial response to therapy may be slightly slower. During maintenance treatment, atrophic gastritis can occur in *H. pylori*-positive patients. *H. pylori* testing and eradication should therefore be considered, particularly for younger patients with GERD if they require PPI maintenance therapy (78,113,119) (Table 34.1).

Other Conditions

Unusual Types of Gastritis

Hypertrophic (giant-fold) gastritis is a rare condition of unknown etiology for which few therapeutic options are available other than surgery. However, accumulating case data suggest that *H. pylori* eradication may yield an excellent clinical response in a high proportion of these patients (120–123). German investigators treated 47 *H. pylori*-positive patients with hypertrophic gastritis with omeprazole and amoxicillin (123). Of the 40 patients in whom *H. pylori* was eradicated, 36 showed complete normalization, one a partial regression, and three no response. Two of those three patients then appeared to have a misdiagnosed adenocarcinoma. In seven patients in whom eradication failed, no improvement was noted. Based on these data, *H. pylori* eradication should be the initial treatment of choice in patients with this disorder.

Autoimmune gastritis is a gastritis involving predominantly the corpus; it is characterized by diffuse periglandular lymphocytic infiltration of the corpus mucosa with destruction of glands and parietal cell hypertrophy. Although the disorder is associated with antiparietal cell and antiintrinsic factor antibodies, a considerable proportion of patients lack these antibodies. The inflammation can progress to atrophy of the corpus mucosa, with eventual impairment of cobalamin absorption and consequent pernicious anemia or neurologic complaints. Once the end stage of total atrophy of the corpus mucosa with cobalamin deficiency has developed, patients are usually *H. pylori*-negative, but some evidence suggests that the disorder can be triggered by *H. pylori* colonization and the development of cross-reacting antibodies (124,125). This is of no clinical consequence for patients with autoimmune atrophic gastritis unless signs of residual *H. pylori* colonization are present, in which case regression of histologic abnormalities after eradication therapy has been reported (126).

Lymphocytic gastritis and granulomatous gastritis are unusual histologic patterns that may have some relationship to *H. pylori* colonization. The former is characterized by large numbers of intraepithelial lymphocytes (>25 per 100 epithelial cells). Although histologic signs of *H. pylori* colonization often are absent, most lesions regress following *H. pylori* eradication (127,128). In a retrospective series of 98 patients, the condition of 89% of the 61 patients receiving eradication treatment improved, even though *H. pylori* was not visible in the pretreatment biopsy specimens of 32 (52%). In contrast, lymphocytic gastritis did not regress in any of the 37 patients who did not receive eradication treatment (128). The differential diagnosis of underlying disorders includes celiac disease; therefore, duodenal biopsy specimens should be obtained from these patients. Granulomatous gastritis also may regress slowly after *H. pylori* eradication (129). The differential diagnosis includes Crohn's disease and sarcoidosis. Finally, eosinophilic and collagenous gastritis and gastritis cystica profunda are rare types of gastric inflammation without any known relation to *H. pylori.* However, because these disorders are rare, it would be reasonable to test and treat affected patients to eradicate *H. pylori* in the hope of achieving a clinical response.

Extragastroduodenal Disorders

H. pylori has been linked to a variety of extragastroduodenal disorders. These include coronary heart disease, dermatologic disorders (e.g., rosacea and idiopathic urticaria), autoimmune thyroid disease, thrombocytopenic purpura, iron-deficiency anemia, Raynaud phenomenon, scleroderma, migraine, and Guillain-Barré syndrome. Underlying hypothetical mechanisms include chronic low-grade activation of the coagulation cascade, accelerating atherosclerosis, and antigenic mimicry between *H. pylori* and host epitopes, leading to autoimmune disorders. So far, none of these hypotheses and associations has been proved in adequate randomized trials, and at present, no indication to test and treat patients with these conditions for *H. pylori* has been established (130–132). Some studies indicate that *H. pylori*-positive persons are on average shorter than those who are *H. pylori*-negative (133,134). Whether early childhood eradication would affect this process is not known.

H. pylori *in Children*

In Western societies, the prevalence of *H. pylori* among native-born children is very low, but it is higher in ethnic minorities and immigrants from developing countries (135). Because of its low prevalence, this bacterium is an uncommon cause of upper gastrointestinal symptoms in native-born children. Also, *H. pylori*-positive children appear less susceptible to the development of peptic ulcers than *H. pylori*-positive adults, and those with non-ulcer dyspepsia respond poorly to *H. pylori* eradication (136). Finally, at least 20% of cases of duodenal ulcer disease in children are not induced by *H. pylori,* and the correlation between specific symptoms and the presence of ulcer disease or *H. pylori* is poor. Both Canadian and European pediatric guidelines advise that serology or breath tests not be performed in children with upper gastrointestinal symptoms, but recommend that endoscopy be performed and biopsy samples taken, if necessary. According to these guidelines, treatment should be limited to those in whom *H. pylori* has been identified during endoscopic investigation as a potential or very likely cause of symptoms (137,138) (Table 34.2). In developing countries, the prevalence of *H. pylori* among young children is high and in preliminary reports has been linked to iron deficiency and growth retardation (131,139), but thus far, no specific guidelines for testing and treatment are available.

TABLE 34.2. INTERNATIONAL GUIDELINES FOR *H. PYLORI* DIAGNOSIS AND TREATMENT IN CHILDREN[a]

Condition	Canada (137)	Europe (138)
Asymptomatic[a]	Yes	Yes
Abdominal pain	No	No
Gastritis	Consider	Consider
Active or past ulcer	Yes	Yes
MALT lymphoma	Yes	Yes

[a]Pediatric guidelines stress that testing is appropriate only when treatment is planned. Once the presence of *H. pylori* is established in a child, treatment should be offered irrespective of clinical symptoms.
MALT, mucosa-associated lymphoid tissue.

H. pylori and Nonsteroidal Antiinflammatory Drugs or Aspirin

H. pylori and NSAIDs are the main risk factors for peptic ulcer disease. In 1994, the National Institutes of Health Consensus Conference recommended that *H. pylori* be eradicated in patients in whom ulcer disease develops while they are taking NSAIDs (140). However, the possible interactions between these two factors remain poorly understood and controversial. Because of the controversy and the high prevalence of both *H. pylori* and NSAID/aspirin use, the approach to the *H. pylori*-positive patient using NSAIDs or aspirin remains a clinical problem. The data are conflicting and can be classified as either pertaining to the risk for development of ulcers during NSAID use or pertaining to the effects of treating ulcers during NSAID use.

Development of Ulcers during the Use of Nonsteroidal Antiinflammatory Drugs

The data on the development of ulcers can be divided into three categories. In the first are prevalence studies of the simultaneous occurrence of *H. pylori* colonization, NSAID use, and gastroduodenal ulceration. In a cross-sectional study of patients with rheumatoid arthritis who were using NSAIDs, 45 (44%) of 103 *H. pylori*-positive patients had ulcers, versus 18 (21%) of 87 *H. pylori*-negatives (141). A systematic review of 17 similar studies concluded that the presence of *H. pylori* in NSAID users increases the incidence of duodenal ulcers (odds ratio, 2.1; 95% confidence interval, 1.5 to 3.1), but not of gastric ulcers (odds ratio, 1.2; 95% confidence interval, 0.9 to 1.6) (142). In particular, this interaction is obvious in patients with bleeding ulcers. In one study, 60% of patients with bleeding peptic ulcers carried both risk factors, versus 25% of patients with nonbleeding ulcers (142). In the second category are follow-up studies in which subjects without ulcer disease were exposed to NSAIDs and studied for the incidence of ulceration in relation to their *H. pylori* status. Most of these studies had the disadvantages of a short follow-up (1 to 3 months) and baseline exclusion of subjects with past or present ulcer disease. Such studies did not report a significant association between *H. pylori* status and ulcer disease during NSAID use. However, one study with 6 months of follow-up reported that ulcers developed in 12 (40%) of 30 *H. pylori*-positive NSAID users, and in 3 (15%) of 20 *H. pylori*-negatives (143). In a second and larger study, the incidence rates of gastric ulcers were similar in *H. pylori*-positive and *H. pylori*-negative NSAID users, but the incidence of duodenal ulcers was significantly higher in the *H. pylori*-positives (18% vs. 5%; $p < .02$) (144,145). In another placebo-controlled prospective study, investigators observed a higher incidence of erosive gastritis in *H. pylori*-positive volunteers than in *H. pylori*-negatives during treatment with 81 or 325 mg of aspirin daily (146). The third category comprises randomized intervention trials that study the effect of *H. pylori* eradication on the incidence of ulcers during NSAID use. One small study reported that *H. pylori* eradication in healthy subjects could prevent the development of ulcers during subsequent NSAID use (147). However, this study showed an unexpectedly high incidence of ulcers in the control group with only 2 months of treatment. In addition, the results contrasted with those of the studies mentioned earlier. In summary, *H. pylori*-positive persons seem to be at increased risk for the development of duodenal ulcer disease during NSAID use in comparison with *H. pylori*-negatives, and they have a higher rate of ulcer bleeding. The effect is relatively small in comparison with the increased risk for ulcer disease and bleeding induced by NSAID use alone. Therefore, at present, *H. pylori* eradication is not generally accepted for the prevention of ulcers in NSAID users (Table 34.1). The incidence of gastric ulcers during NSAID use does not appear to differ between *H. pylori*-positives and *H. pylori*-negatives.

Treatment of Ulcers during the Use of Nonsteroidal Antiinflammatory Drugs

The data on the treatment of ulcers that occur during NSAID use contribute to the controversy and can also be divided into several categories. First, several studies have shown that in patients who continue to take NSAIDs, gastric ulcers heal faster during acid suppression if the patient is *H. pylori*-positive (144,148,149). This finding may be related to the fact that profound acid suppression in *H. pylori*-positives leads to active corpus gastritis (113), accompanied by increased mucosal prostaglandin synthesis and impaired parietal cell function. Thus, *H. pylori* enhances the acid-suppressive effect of PPIs (107). Eradication of *H. pylori* in patients with ulcers who continue to take NSAIDs not only fails to accelerate ulcer healing during acid suppression but may slow it (150–152). Also, *H. pylori* eradication does not prevent gastric ulcer recurrence in NSAID users (150,151,153).

Based on these findings, the current recommended clinical approach to a patient who starts NSAID therapy is to disregard the *H. pylori* status but to prescribe misoprostol or a PPI for patients at high risk for ulcer disease, such as elderly persons with severe concomitant disease. In patients in whom ulcer disease develops, the first step is to start PPI therapy and attempt to withdraw NSAIDs. After ulcer healing, *H. pylori* eradication does not provide an additional benefit to those who stop NSAIDs, nor does it prevent ulcer recurrence in those who continue NSAIDs. Therefore, PPI or misoprostol maintenance therapy is primarily indicated in the latter group.

Test and Treat, Test and Scope

The previous sections discussed the approach to the *Helicobacter*-positive patient with a specific clinical problem. However, in many cases, a clinical diagnosis is never established. Dyspeptic symptoms are common, endoscopic screening of dyspeptic patients requires considerable time and cost, and the diagnostic yield is often limited. Therefore, empiric approaches to certain categories of dyspeptic patients are commonly used. These categories include those who are below a threshold age (varying between 45 and 55 years in different populations), who do not have alarm symptoms, or who use specific medications, such as NSAIDs. The conventional empiric approach consists of a course of treatment with an acid-suppressive drug (154). However, with the increasing awareness of *H. pylori* prevalence and the gradual acceptance of multiple indications for treatment (Table 34.1), "test-and-treat" strategies have become common practice as a first-line empiric approach for patients with dyspepsia. These strategies consist of a non-invasive test for *H. pylori* (e.g., serology or a breath test) followed by antimicrobial therapy in the case of a positive test result. Patients whose test result is negative may either receive empiric acid-suppressive therapy or be referred for endoscopy. The validity of such a strategy, however, depends on various factors. The prevalence of *H. pylori* in the respective population and the accuracy of the test determine the predictive values of a positive test result. The prevalence rates of non-ulcer dyspepsia, peptic ulcer disease, and GERD determine the chance of eliminating symptoms with *H. pylori* eradication. These factors and the costs of endoscopy vary geographically and largely influence the impact of any test-and-treat strategy. In the United States, where endoscopy is associated with relatively high costs, it has been calculated that a test-and-treat strategy is cost-effective if the prevalence of *H. pylori*-associated ulcer disease is at least 10% or if symptom response following *H. pylori* eradication in non-ulcer dyspeptics is at least 8% (155). However, both premises often are not met. Finally, the age-related incidence of gastric cancer also affects the validity of test-and-treat regimens. In some European countries, gastric cancer presently is very rare below the age of 55 (156), whereas in Asia, gastric cancers occur even in persons younger than 45 years. In such cases, the opposite strategy of "test and scope" has been proposed (157). Non-invasive *H. pylori* testing is then followed by endoscopy for *H. pylori*-positives to screen for ulcers and gastric cancer, or empiric acid-suppressive therapy for *H. pylori*-negatives. European investigators evaluated patients referred for gastroscopy by their general practitioner (158). Patients who had alarm symptoms, used NSAIDs, or were *H. pylori*-positive underwent endoscopy, and the others were referred back for empiric treatment. Endoscopy was avoided in 36% of all dyspepsia referrals. After a 6-month follow-up, symptoms in both groups were similar, but the patients who had not undergone endoscopy used significantly less medication. Similar results were later obtained in studies involving general practice and an outpatient clinic (159,160).

In summary, noninvasive testing for *H. pylori* has been advocated as a primary approach to patients with dyspepsia but without alarm symptoms or other factors necessitating endoscopy. The preferred strategy following the detection of *H. pylori* depends on the prevalence of *H. pylori* in a community, the incidence of peptic ulcer disease, and the costs of endoscopy. However, the introduction of a strategy based on the local situation may be cost-effective in comparison with early endoscopy in all dyspeptic subjects.

DIAGNOSIS OF *H. PYLORI* INFECTION

Many tests to detect *H. pylori* have been developed, each with its own advantages and disadvantages. When their use is guided by the clinical setting in which they are requested (e.g., recent use of PPIs or antibiotics), local availability and experience, or economic considerations, most tests are reasonably accurate (see refs. 161–163 for review). Despite a somewhat lower specificity and sensitivity for certain assays, serology is inexpensive and easy to perform and so is ideal for the initial testing of large populations. However, for a primary diagnosis in individual patients, both the urea breath test (UBT) and direct detection methods (e.g., culture and histology) are the methods of choice. Direct detection methods require the availability of an endoscopic biopsy sample. Obtaining these samples is relatively simple because symptomatic patients often undergo an endoscopic examination to define the degree of inflammation and tissue damage accurately and test for the presence of gastric malignancies. Biopsy samples allow for rapid urease testing (RUT); because of its low cost, simplicity, accuracy, and rapidly available results, RUT is often used for initial diagnostic testing. Culture of the bacterium from biopsy samples permits antimicrobial susceptibility testing, which optimizes patient management. The best method for follow-up testing after treatment is less obvious. When performed more than 4 to 6 weeks after the completion of therapy, the UBT perform wells but because of its high cost and limited availability is not commonly used. Alternatives include the recently developed fecal antigen tests, although their diagnostic accuracy has not fully been established.

Non-invasive Tests

Non-invasive testing is recommended for the primary screening of healthy young persons and children who present with gastric complaints to spare them the high cost and risks associated with endoscopy. For similar reasons, non-invasive testing also is frequently considered for patients with previously diagnosed ulcer disease. A multitude of non-invasive tests are available, but serology and the UBT are both relatively standardized reliable tests, and for that reason they are frequently used in the follow-up evaluation of eradication therapy and in epidemiologic studies.

Urea Breath Tests

Urease is produced in large quantities by all *H. pylori* strains. This enzyme converts urea to ammonia and carbon dioxide, thereby raising the pH. The enzymatic activity, which allows the bacterium to survive in the acidic environment of the human stomach, forms the basis of the UBT (164). The UBT is a reliable test that has been validated in both adults and children, but unfortunately registration by health authorities and appropriate reimbursements for this test are often lacking, so that it is still not widely used (163). Another potential drawback of the UBT is that false-negative results are common in patients taking PPIs; they are somewhat less so in those who are taking H_2-receptor antagonists (165–167), have recently received antibiotic therapy, or have previously undergone gastric surgery. Both a ^{14}C-based test and a ^{13}C-based test are available, the disadvantage of the former being that it exposes the patient to a low dose of radioactivity. Its advantage is that the detection of ^{14}C requires only a simple scintillation counter, whereas the detection of ^{13}C requires a more expensive mass spectrometer. The high costs of ^{13}C detection by isotope ratio mass spectrometry of breath samples can be overcome by mailing samples to regional analytic centers or by using nondispersive isotope-selective infrared spectroscopy as a low-cost alternative for the detection of ^{13}C (168).

For patients, undergoing a UBT is simple. Patients must fast for about 6 hours and then consume a test meal followed by a small amount of either ^{14}C- or ^{13}C-labeled urea. The bacterial urease degrades the labeled urea molecules, thereby releasing labeled carbon dioxide. The labeled carbon dioxide then rapidly enters the bloodstream and is detected in a breath sample taken 20 to 40 minutes after ingestion of the labeled urea (Fig. 34.5). The detection of ^{13}C-bicarbonate in blood and the detection of ^{14}C-urea or ^{15}N-urea in urine have also been described as reliable methods to test for the presence of *H.pylori* (169–171), but these tests are more complicated than the breath test and hence less suitable for routine diagnostics.

Serology

Colonization by *H. pylori* induces a strong and polymorphic humoral immune response. The response is initially an immunoglobulin M (IgM) response, but IgA and IgG responses develop later that persist throughout the colonization and for months thereafter. The use of serum-based tests in the management of *H. pylori* has recently been reviewed (172). Serum antibodies against *H. pylori* can easily be detected by latex agglutination or by enzyme-linked immunosorbent assay (ELISA) (173,174). In general, the

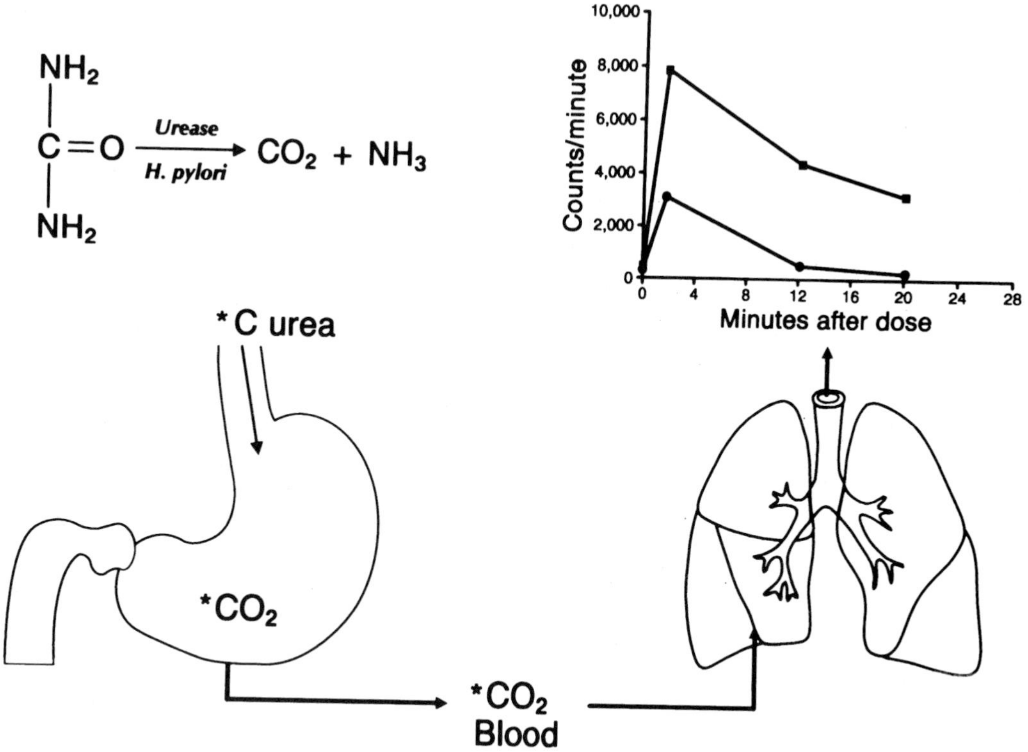

FIGURE 34.5. Schematic representation of the ^{14}C and ^{13}C breath tests. After labeled urea is ingested, it is metabolized by urease into ammonia and bicarbonate. Bicarbonate is exhaled as carbon dioxide through the lungs, and the concentration of labeled carbon atoms can be determined in the exhaled air. More than 1,000 counts per minute at 20 minutes defines a positive ^{14}C-urea breath test result (*upper curve*). An early peak can occur in both *H. pylori*-positive and *H. pylori*-negative cases if the mouth flora hydrolyzes urea.

detection of *H. pylori*-specific IgA antibodies is less sensitive than the detection of IgG antibodies. In addition to classic ELISA-based tests, a wide range of simplified latex agglutination and solid-phase ELISA tests are now commercially available for use as rapid near-to-the-patient tests. However, the accuracy of these rapid whole-blood tests is almost always inferior to that of classic laboratory-based ELISAs (175,176).

The main advantage of serology is its simplicity and cost-effectiveness. However, as a result of the prolonged period required for the decay of serologic titers present after the eradication of *H. pylori,* serology is not generally suitable for treatment monitoring (177) (Fig. 34.6). Also, because the antigenic properties of *H. pylori* strains vary somewhat between countries, these tests should be locally standardized. Ideally, antigens from local strains should be used, but at a minimum, cutoff values should be adjusted for each population tested. On the other hand, antibody tests are not affected by the recent use of antibiotics, bismuth compounds, or PPIs. In patients with atrophic gastritis, serology may perform better than histology or the UBT because bacterial densities tend to be low (178). Most immunologic tests are serum-based, but urine and saliva have also been used to detect IgG and IgA, respectively. These tests have not been extensively evaluated, are less accurate, and offer little benefit over serum-based tests.

Other Non-invasive Tests

Recently, a new type of non-invasive testing has been developed. These tests are not based on the detection of specific anti-*Helicobacter* antibodies; rather, they directly detect *H. pylori*-specific antigens (HpSAs) in diluted stool samples (161,179,180). Only a small stool sample is required, but samples must be processed directly, although they can be stored at 4°C for up to 3 days or for longer periods at 20°C without affecting test outcome (161). Initial studies indicate that the diagnostic performance of these tests is comparable with that of other non-invasive tests, such as serology and the UBT. In contrast to conventional serology, these tests can also be used in posttreatment control, in which they perform as well as UBTs but are less expensive (179–181). Although it has not been extensively evaluated, stool antigen detection is an attractive test for use in small children because obtaining breath or serum specimens can be difficult in very young patients.

Invasive Tests

Gastric biopsy material can be tested for the presence of *H. pylori* organisms, either directly by culture, histology, or

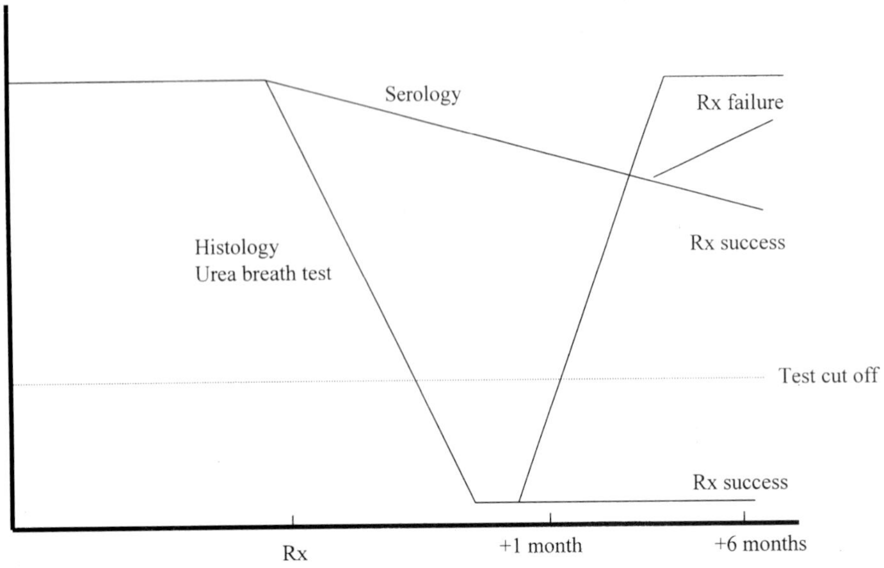

FIGURE 34.6. The effect of eradication therapy on the performance of diagnostic tests for *H. pylori*. Therapy failure may be associated with a temporary decrease in the density of *H. pylori* colonization. This affects the performance of histology and urea breath tests and may lead to false-negative results. Therefore, it is recommended that testing after therapy be delayed until at least 4 weeks after therapy has been completed. With serology, this interval is too short for an adequate prediction of the effect of therapy.

PCR or indirectly by the RUT. Because *H. pylori* may not be evenly distributed throughout the stomach, multiple samples obtained from various locations in the stomach are required for optimal sensitivity (182). The use of antibiotics or PPIs lowers the number of bacteria and induces a relative shift of *H. pylori* into the body of the stomach, thus affecting detection rates (182,183). Biopsy sampling of areas of apparent intestinal metaplasia may be relevant for establishing the severity of the dysplasia. However, *H. pylori* is seldom isolated from these areas, nor is it often detected during gastric bleeding (184,185). Most invasive testing involves an endoscopic procedure, but the recently developed string test may provide an inexpensive and patient-friendly alternative to endoscopy (186). The test involves swallowing a sampling device attached to a string, which can be pulled back after remaining in the stomach for some time and tested for *H. pylori* by culture, RUT, or PCR.

Endoscopy

Endoscopic signs of gastritis (diffuse reddening of the mucosa) or the lack thereof is of no diagnostic value in detecting *H. pylori* because actual histologic evidence of gastritis is only weakly correlated with such reddening (187,188). Gastroduodenal ulcerations and antral nodulation may be better indications of the presence of *H. pylori* but are not conclusive, and additional confirmation of the presence of *H. pylori* should always be obtained (189).

Culture

Originally, *H. pylori* was regarded as a difficult organism to grow because growth is slow and the organism requires specific media and an atmosphere low in oxygen. However, in experienced microbiologic laboratories, culture is very reliable, with a specificity of 100% and a sensitivity above 90%. Compared with other diagnostic techniques, culture is labor-intensive, but a benefit is that it permits antimicrobial susceptibility testing and genotyping of strains. The former is especially useful in populations with a high prevalence of antibiotic resistance or after failure of initial therapy.

For the best results, biopsy samples should immediately be transferred to broth or saline solution and cultured from these within several hours (190,191). Usually, 3 to 7 days of incubation at 37°C is required before visible colonies develop. When colonies grow for too long, or when they are exposed to unfavorable conditions, the bacterium loses its typical curved appearance and becomes rounded. This so-called coccoid form of the bacterium cannot be cultured *in vitro* and should be checked for during the preparation of standard inocula for use in antimicrobial sensitivity testing or of frozen stocks (192).

Histology

The reliability of histology is very much operator-dependent (193), but when performed by an experienced pathologist, histology is highly reliable and often considered the gold standard for the diagnosis of *H. pylori* colonization (187,188). Special stains, such as the Warthin–Starry stain, enhance detection of the bacterium, but experienced histopathologists easily recognize it in standard sections stained with hematoxylin and eosin (194,195). Bacteria appear as curved or *S*-shaped 3×0.5-µm rods and are usually present in large numbers in the mucus, close to the surface of the epithelial cells of the gastric antrum (Color Figure 34.1). Although the morphology alone does not prove that the organisms are *H. pylori,* the morphology is sufficiently typical that the diagnosis is fairly certain. The only similarly shaped gastric bacterium likely to be present in the human stomach is the related *Helicobacter heilmannii.* PCR or specific immunohistologic techniques are required for the definite histologic identification of *H. pylori,* but both are labor-intensive and therefore seldom used (196,197).

Rapid Urease Test

The RUT is probably the most widely used test (198,199). It is based on the ability of bacterial urease to convert urea into ammonia and carbon dioxide. This conversion is accompanied by an increase in pH that is detected by the color change of an indicator (usually phenol red). The RUT is reasonably specific because apart from *H. pylori,* urease-producing organisms are rarely observed in the human stomach. In adults, most false-positives are caused by bacterial overgrowth of the stomach, which is almost uniquely observed in patients with a low acid output (resulting from advanced atrophy or antacid use, or occurring in young children) (200). False-negatives are mostly the result of premature reading of the test (201) or low bacterial densities (e.g., following recent antibiotic therapy). The main advantages of the test are its simplicity and low cost and the rapid availability of results (some commercial tests can be read within the hour); however, it is less sensitive and less specific than most other direct tests.

Tests Based on Polymerase Chain Reaction

The PCR has become a common technique in many laboratories, but for the detection of *H. pylori* in gastric biopsy samples, it provides only marginal advantages over culture or histology (184,197). PCR techniques are still too expensive and labor-intensive for use in routine diagnostics. The advantages of the PCR are its easy standardization and the rapid availability of results, but its use in the routine diagnostic detection of *H. pylori* infection has not been extensively evaluated. It is used mostly in research settings, when the numbers of bacteria in diagnostic samples are extremely low (e.g., immediately after antibiotic treatment), or when only dead bacteria are present (e.g., in a paraffin-embedded histologic specimen). The diagnostic potential of PCR is rapidly increasing as the technique is being simplified by the use of colorimetric ELISA-like hybridization techniques for the specific detection of PCR products (202). These simplifications will soon result in the appearance of many commercial PCR tests based on the detection of genetic mutations associated with clarithromycin resistance and genes involved in pathogenicity (e.g., *cagA*) and the establishment of bacterial transmission routes.

Use of Specific Virulence Markers

Recent studies have indicated an association between disease outcome and specific virulence markers, such as the *cagA* and *vacA* genotypes of *H. pylori* (203–205). As a result, must interest has recently been shown in methods to test for the presence of these factors. Potential problems in such testing include the genetic variability of *H. pylori,* as a result of which tests may not work with all strains, and the colonization of subjects by two or more different *H. pylori* strains, a condition that is observed in more than 10% of *H. pylori*-positive subjects (206). Commercial kits and in-house protocols include Western blotting, ELISA and related immunologic assays, and PCR-based detection of *cagA, vacA,* and *iceA* alleles. Although all these genes have been associated with increased pathogenicity, the clinical value of the information obtained by such testing remains to be established (207–209).

TREATMENT OF THE *H. PYLORI*-POSITIVE PATIENT

Much effort has been expended in finding optimal treatment regimens for *H. pylori.* This effort was stimulated by the large numbers of subjects colonized with the bacterium, the proportion in whom disease develops, the expanding indications for *H. pylori* treatment, and the relative difficulty of eradicating the bacterium. The regimens used are generally categorized according to the number of drugs involved (Table 34.3).

TABLE 34.3. CURRENT THERAPIES FOR *H. PYLORI* ERADICATION

Medication[a]	Dose	Duration (ds)
Dual		
RBC + clarithromycin	400 mg bid / 500 mg bid	14
Triple		
Bismuth + metronidazole + tetracycline	120 mg qid / 400–500 mg tid / 500 mg qid	14
RBC + clarithromycin + amoxicillin	2 dd 400 mg / 2 dd 500 mg / 2 dd 1,000 mg	7–10
PPI + clarithromycin + amoxicillin	2 dd 20 mg / 2 dd 500 mg / 2 dd 1,000 mg	7–10
PPI + clarithromycin + metronidazole	2 dd 20 mg / 2 dd 250 mg/ 2 dd 500 mg	7–10
PPI + amoxicillin + metronidazole	2 dd 20 mg / 2 dd 1,000 mg/ 2 dd 500 mg	7–10
Quadruple		
PPI + bismuth + metronidazole + tetracycline	20 mg bid / 120 mg qid / 400–500 mg tid / 500 mg qid	4–7[b]

[a]Individual therapeutic choices depend on personal experience and the presence of antibiotic resistance and specific drug allergies. First-line therapy usually consists of a dual or triple regimen; second-line therapy after previous treatment failure often consists of quadruple therapy.
[b]Antibiotics given for 4 to 7 days; the PPI is usually started 3 days earlier.
RBC, ranitidine bismuth citrate; PPI, proton pump inhibitor; 2 dd, two daily doses.

Monotherapies

H. pylori is susceptible *in vitro* to many antimicrobial agents, with the exception of trimethoprim, nalidixic acid, the sulfonamides, and vancomycin, and to the PPIs. The first drugs to be used against *H. pylori* were bismuth compounds, in particular colloidal bismuth subcitrate and bismuth subsalicylate, which had been used in the nineteenth century to heal and prevent ulcers and to which *H. pylori* is susceptible *in vitro* (210). Although the underlying mechanisms are unknown, bismuth salts form complexes within the bacterial wall (211,212). However, although these compounds reduce the number of viable bacteria in the gastric mucus, they fail to eradicate *H. pylori in vivo* (213). Similar failures occur with other monotherapies. Only high-dose clarithromycin (2 g/d for 14 days) eradicates *H. pylori* in 50% of cases, an inadequate result.

In summary, monotherapy against *H. pylori* is not successful despite the excellent *in vitro* efficacy of both antimicrobials and PPIs. In the specific ecologic niche of the bacterium, the mucous layer of the gastric mucosa, the penetration of antimicrobials may be poor. Gastric motility and shape and thickness of the mucous layer all may contribute to the uneven distribution and concentration of therapeutic agents. Importantly, the local acidic conditions impair the efficacy of these drugs (214–216). Because *H. pylori* persists in the face of a host immune response, it is likely that any therapy must remove every last organism (as in bacterial endocarditis). The microscopic loci of bacteria where the agents do not penetrate can become sites of renewed colonization after treatment has ceased.

Dual Therapies

A number of strategies have been used to increase the efficacy of treatment to eradicate *H. pylori,* including combining multiple synergistic antibiotic drugs, combining antibiotics with an acid-suppressive drug, and prolonging drug administration. The earliest dual therapies included bismuth with either amoxicillin, metronidazole, or clarithromycin. The efficacy of these regimens was no higher than 30% to 70% (217,218), and the alternative combination of amoxicillin with a nitroimidazole compound was no more successful (219).

Newer dual therapies combined an acid suppressor with one antimicrobial drug, in particular amoxicillin or clarithromycin. These combinations have the advantages of quick symptom relief through acid suppression, a simple dosing schedule, and few side effects. However, although initial results with them were good (220,221), later studies were not able to confirm the findings. The overall eradication rate with the combination of a PPI plus clarithromycin or amoxicillin varies between 60% to 70% (222). The efficacy of the latter combination increases with higher doses of each drug and a longer duration of therapy (223,224) but does not depend on the frequency of PPI intake, and it significantly decreases when patients have been treated with acid suppression before amoxicillin is started. Overall, *H. pylori* eradication rates with the dual therapies are too low to justify clinical use. Importantly, the *H. pylori* strain in patients unsuccessfully treated with a regimen containing a macrolide or nitroimidazole should be considered to have become resistant to those drugs, so that further therapeutic possibilities are limited.

The limitations of dual therapy are partly overcome by ranitidine bismuth citrate, which combines the antimicrobial effect of bismuth with the acid-suppressive effect of ranitidine (225). A combination of 400 mg of ranitidine bismuth citrate twice daily for 4 weeks and 500 mg of clarithromycin two or three times daily during the first 2 weeks eradicates *H. pylori* in 82% to 92% of patients (226–228) and in effect mimics triple therapies.

Triple Therapies

Bismuth Triple Therapies

The first effective therapies against *H. pylori,* with eradication rates consistently over 80%, consisted of combinations of a bismuth compound and two antibiotics, in particular metronidazole and either amoxicillin or tetracycline. Various doses of these drugs were used in different studies, but it appears that combinations with tetracycline are slightly more effective than amoxicillin-containing regimens (229,230). The efficacy of these therapies depends on patient compliance, duration of treatment, and the prevalence of metronidazole resistance in the treated population. A combination of a bismuth compound four times daily, 500 mg of metronidazole three times daily, and 500 mg of tetracycline four times daily eradicates more than 90% of the metronidazole-sensitive strains of *H. pylori* if used for at least 7 days. It has been suggested that prolongation of treatment increases the success rate further (231), and administration of therapy for less than 7 days impairs efficacy (230). This triple therapy fails in at least 25% of patients infected with a metronidazole-resistant *H. pylori* strain, even when given for 14 days (232,233). The regimen of bismuth, tetracycline, and metronidazole is inexpensive and therefore very useful in subjects with a documented metronidazole-sensitive strain or in populations in which the prevalence of metronidazole resistance is low. Treatment for 7 days is sufficient in such cases.

Acid-suppressive Triple Therapy

The acidic environment in the stomach partially explains the discrepancy between the excellent *in vitro* susceptibility of *H. pylori* to most antibiotics and the poor results of *in vivo* therapy with the same drugs. To overcome this effect and accelerate ulcer healing, the bismuth compound in triple regimens can be replaced by an acid-suppressive drug. Usually, these regimens contain a PPI and two of the following antibiotics: a nitroimidazole (metronidazole or tinidazole), amoxicillin, and clarithromycin. Consistent eradication rates between 85% and 90% were obtained with a PPI in a dose equivalent to 20 mg of omeprazole in combination either with 1 g of amoxicillin and 500 mg of clarithromycin or with 400 to 500 mg of metronidazole or tinidazole and 250 mg of clarithromycin, with all drugs given twice daily for 7 days (222,234,235). In contrast to the efficacy of the PPI-based dual therapies, the efficacy of these triple therapies is not significantly affected by the dose of the PPI (e.g., 20 mg or 40 mg of omeprazole twice daily) (236) or the duration of treatment (7 vs. 14 days) (237–239), nor does any evidence indicate that pretreatment with a PPI affects the outcome of therapy. However, efficacy is impaired in patients colonized with a strain that is resistant to metronidazole, clarithromycin, or both (230,240,241); in such cases, longer treatment, for 10 to 14 days, is likely to be more effective. It is presently unknown whether the antibiotics should be taken before or after meals and whether the formulation of amoxicillin (tablets, capsules, or suspension) influences cure rates. Therapies with lansoprazole, pantoprazole, and rabeprazole are as effective as those with omeprazole (242–244). Omission of the PPI strongly reduces the efficacy of therapy (245). PPI triple therapies are presently most commonly used for *H. pylori* eradication. Overall, the combination therapies containing clarithromycin with either amoxicillin or a nitroimidazole appear to be slightly more effective than PPI triple therapies with amoxicillin and a nitroimidazole but without clarithromycin (234,246,247). Clarithromycin therapies with either amoxicillin or a nitroimidazole appear equally effective; only for nitroimidazole-resistant strains is the combination of clarithromycin with amoxicillin and a PPI more effective. Combinations with H_2-receptor antagonists, in particular ranitidine, are slightly less effective than those with omeprazole when they include amoxicillin and a nitroimidazole but appear equally effective when they include clarithromycin and a nitroimidazole (222,248, 249). Nevertheless, they are less commonly used. Triple therapies with ranitidine bismuth citrate and two antibiotics for 7 days are also effective for *H. pylori* eradication, with success rates between 87% and 95% (247,250).

Acid-suppressive triple therapy is generally considered as first-line treatment in both adults and children (Fig. 34.7). In the latter group, the most experience has been obtained

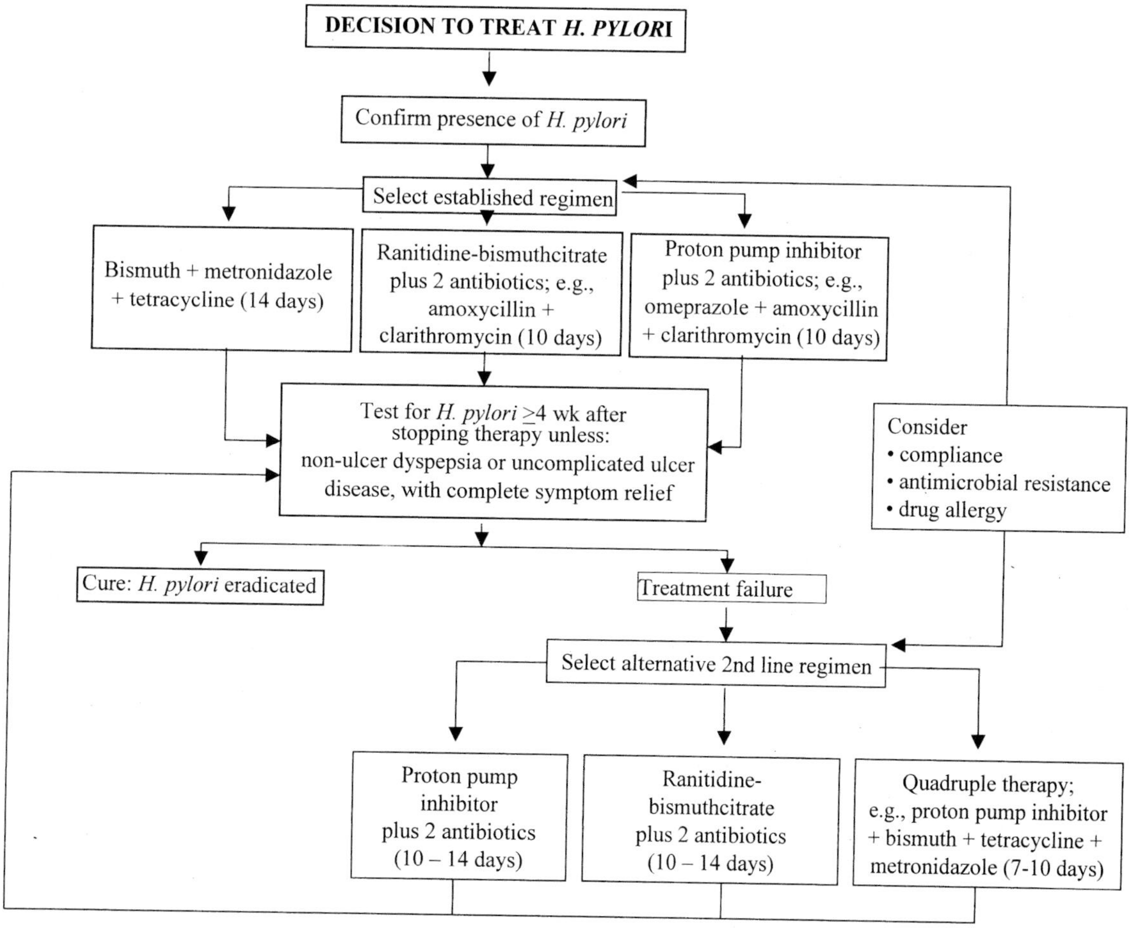

FIGURE 34.7. Strategy for the treatment of *H. pylori* colonization.

with omeprazole (1 to 2 mg/kg per day divided into two doses) in combination with clarithromycin and either amoxicillin or metronidazole in age-appropriate doses (251).

Quadruple Therapies

Quadruple therapy combines a PPI with a bismuth compound, tetracycline, and metronidazole. The standard quadruple regimen consists of a PPI in a dose equivalent to 20 mg of omeprazole twice daily, a bismuth compound four times daily, 500 mg of tetracycline mg four times daily, and 500 mg of metronidazole three times daily. The PPI is usually started 3 days before the antimicrobial drugs. This regimen eradicates *H. pylori* in at least 92% of cases when given for 7 to 14 days (230,252–258), and in contrast to previous therapies, it appears to be very effective in patients colonized with a metronidazole-resistant strain of *H. pylori* (255,256). Shortening the duration of therapy to 4 days affects efficacy only marginally (252,259), but 1- or 2-day quadruple therapy has a cure rate of 60% to 70% (259). Because of the considerable number of drugs involved, these therapies are generally reserved for secondary treatment after earlier failure with another regimen. However, some clinicians prefer quadruple therapy as first-line treatment because of its high rate of efficacy.

Side Effects

During treatment for *H. pylori* with multiple drugs, a considerate proportion of patients notice side effects. Bismuth compounds darken the stool. Nitroimidazoles often induce a metallic taste, nausea, and sometimes vomiting. In addition, patients must abstain from alcohol because these drugs have a disulfiram-like effect. Amoxicillin, tetracycline, and clarithromycin can lead to skin hypersensitivity reactions and diarrhea. Taste disturbances are common with clarithromycin and the nitroimidazoles. Pseudomembranous colitis is a rare but serious side effect of anti-*H. pylori* treatment. The use of acid suppressors may diminish the severity of side effects with a given regimen (257). A scoring system has been developed for use in clinical trials to evaluate the side effects of eradication treatment. This system distinguishes five grades of tolerance: no side effects, mild but not interfering with daily activities, moderate and interfering with daily activities, severe and requiring time lost from work, and severe requiring treatment cessation (233). The frequency of side effects with the different regimens listed above varies from approximately 10% to 40% (222). Side effects are more frequent in patients treated with clarithromycin or metronidazole than in those treated with amoxicillin and occur more often during triple than during dual therapy. Nevertheless, with all these regimens, only a few percentage of patients have to stop therapy because of severe side effects. Patients must be prospectively informed of the possible side effects of treatment to prevent noncompliance, which significantly lessens the efficacy of treatment (260).

Therapy Failure and Repeated Treatment

Despite the routine use of combinations of multiple drugs, therapy failures occur with all the different antibiotic regimens in at least 5% to 10% of treated patients, and usually more. Failure can be caused by a number of factors, in particular antimicrobial resistance and noncompliance. A metaanalysis of the results obtained in 4,823 patients treated in clinical trials with a nitroimidazole-containing regimen showed an overall eradication success rate of 93% in nitroimidazole-sensitive strains, versus 69% in nitroimidazole-resistant strains (odds ratio for the association between nitroimidazole resistance and therapy failure, 5.2; 95% confidence interval, 3.8 to 7.1) (261). Another metaanalysis noted a similar effect for clarithromycin resistance. The eradication success rate of PPI triple therapy with clarithromycin in combination with either amoxicillin or metronidazole was 31% in 51 patients with a clarithromycin-resistant strain, versus 88% in 966 with a clarithromycin-sensitive strain (246). Data on the effect of resistance for other antibiotics are too scarce to be interpreted. Other factors that have been suggested to increase the risk for therapy failure are smoking, age, and dense colonization with *cagA*-negative strains (262). Because antimicrobial resistance largely affects therapy outcome, clinicians should primarily base their choice of therapy on local prevalence rates of resistance. Routine pretreatment testing is currently not necessary but should be considered after therapy failure.

Other factors that influence outcome are compliance, which is related to both tolerability and cultural factors (231), method and frequency of dosing, duration of therapy, and potentially individual differences in drug metabolism (263). Posttreatment testing for *H. pylori* is not routine practice but should be performed in patients whose symptoms persist or recur after therapy, suggesting therapy failure, and is also recommended for patients with a history of ulcer disease complicated by bleeding, perforation, or stricture formation. In the latter group, it is essential that eradication be confirmed to prevent recurrence of complications. In cases of persistent *H. pylori* colonization, re-treatment can be targeted if results of antimicrobial resistance testing are available. If such information is lacking—for instance, because persistent colonization was demonstrated by means of a UBT—then triple therapy including ranitidine bismuth citrate or quadruple therapy including a PPI is preferred for optimal results (264). In patients remaining asymptomatic 1 year after treatment, follow-up serology should show markedly reduced antibody levels.

Antimicrobial Resistance

The widespread and increasing use of antibiotics has resulted in the development of antibiotic-resistant strains of

H. pylori. Spontaneous resistance to rifampicin, streptomycin, ciprofloxacin, tetracycline, clarithromycin, amoxicillin, and metronidazole have been reported; the mechanisms have been characterized in more detail for the latter five drugs. Although regional differences have been noted, the antibiotic resistance of *H. pylori* appears to be increasing globally. Resistance rates are highest for metronidazole, followed by clarithromycin. Resistance to tetracycline and resistance or tolerance to amoxicillin appear to be uncommon. Apart from patient compliance, *H. pylori* antibiotic resistance is currently believed to be the most important factor determining the outcome of antibiotic treatment (265). Given the large numbers of subjects colonized with *H. pylori,* the proportion in whom disease develops, and the relative difficulty of eradicating colonization, it is not surprising that much effort is being spent on understanding the mechanisms of antibiotic resistance. Understanding the mechanism may allow for the rapid determination of resistance and provide clues about how to delay its spread.

Comparison of the resistance rates between various countries, or even between national centers, is hampered by a lack of standardized methods to test susceptibility. The accurate determination of levels of resistance to an antimicrobial drug (usually expressed as minimal inhibitory concentration, or MIC) is important in assessing the susceptibility of strains. Although official testing guidelines are available, they often differ between countries. In addition, many laboratories prefer to use the commercially available E-test strips because these provide reproducible and reliable results for most antibiotics. Agar dilution and disk diffusion tests are the two other commonly used methods, but results with these three methods do not always correlate (266,267). In addition, factors such as inoculum size and conditions of bacterial growth affect the outcome. Regardless of testing methods, it is clear that the widespread use of antibiotics has resulted in a significant increase in the prevalence of antibiotic-resistant strains of *H. pylori* (268,269), and resistance to two commonly used drugs, metronidazole and clarithromycin, significantly reduces the efficacy of regimens containing either of them (246,261,270). *In vitro,* the spontaneous development of resistance to these two antibiotics occurs at a frequency of 10^{-5} to 10^{-9}, indicating that resistance most probably results from spontaneous point mutations, which has subsequently been confirmed. Resistance to clarithromycin was shown to result from mutations in the 23S ribosomal RNA genes that result in adenine-to-guanine substitutions in one of two adjacent adenosine residues, but occasionally an adenine-to-cytosine mutation is also observed (271,272). These mutations decrease the affinity of the macrolide drug for the ribosome and so result in an increased MIC. Some of the mutations have a negative effect on the growth rate of the bacterium (273,274), which may select for reversion to the sensitive wild-type sequence in the absence of clarithromycin (274,275). As expected, based on the resistance mechanisms, susceptibility and resistance to clarithromycin usually coincide with those for the related antibiotics azithromycin, erythromycin, clindamycin, and streptogramin type B (274, 276), so that these agents are rendered useless for the treatment of patients with clarithromycin-resistant isolates. Because resistance to clarithromycin seems to be based entirely on the mutation of two nucleotides, PCR-based detection methods have been proposed (272,277). These appear promising, and the tests can easily be automated and applied directly to biopsy specimens in combination with PCR-based detection of other relevant *H. pylori*-specific markers. Resistance to metronidazole has recently been shown to result from point mutations in a gene, *rdxA,* that encodes a nitroreductase responsible for reductive activation of the drug. A secondary mutation in the fumarate reductase gene, *frxA,* may further enhance the resistance levels of these *rdxA*-negative strains (278).

Although clinical isolates of *H. pylori* often contain small, cryptic plasmids, all mechanisms of antibiotic resistance in *H. pylori* thus far rely on mutations of genes located in chromosomes. Although most forms of antibiotic resistance of *H. pylori* are newly acquired, transfer from resistant to sensitive bacteria probably also occurs. Under laboratory conditions, natural transformation has been used to transfer markers of antibiotic resistance to other *H. pylori* strains (279–281), or to and from other (animal) *Helicobacter* species (282). It is currently unknown how often the exchange of genetic material plays a role in the acquisition of antibiotic resistance in *H. pylori.* The observation that antibiotic resistance is located on the chromosome of *H. pylori,* rather than on plasmids, combined with the lack of amoxicillin resistance in *H. pylori,* despite the fact that such resistance is easily acquired by other bacteria, makes extensive exchange of DNA with other bacterial species unlikely; however, it cannot be excluded because ample evidence indicates frequent genetic exchange within *H. pylori* (283).

Resistance seems to be generated *de novo* (284); therefore, monotherapy should never be used because it will promote the rapid induction and spread of resistance, and susceptibility testing should be performed whenever drugs are prescribed for which a high local rate of resistance has been reported. Nevertheless, most resistance in *H. pylori* probably arises from the use of antibiotics to treat unrelated infectious diseases involving the respiratory tract, skin, and other sites.

FUTURE PROSPECTS

Improved Diagnosis and Treatment

In the last 20 years of the twentieth century, enormous medical progress was made with the discovery of *H. pylori* as an important and treatable cause of a variety of gastroduodenal disorders. Nevertheless, many issues remain to be solved and new ones continue to arise, some of them as a result of the decreasing prevalence of *H. pylori* in developed countries. We have not solved the issue of the relationship between the considerable heterogeneity of *H. pylori* and clinical outcome, nor do we really know whether colonization with *H. pylori* has beneficial effects in the host. For these reasons and because of a lack of prospective data, the introduction of population-based screening and treatment of *H. pylori* is still unjustified. The outcome of a variety of studies presently ongoing will help to solve these issues. In the meantime, the decreasing prevalence of *H. pylori* means that diagnostic tests must be improved to lower the number of false-positive results. Also, current combination therapies are cumbersome and in clinical practice fail in 10% or more of the time. Therefore, other forms of therapy must be developed. Such developments first may come from the combination of several drugs within one formulation. Such an arrangement may improve therapy compliance but most likely will not reduce side effects or overcome antimicrobial resistance. Neither will it decrease the unwanted effects on non-*Helicobacter* microbial colonization. More promising treatment tools may therefore come from genetic research and the publication of *Helicobacter* genomes (285,286). This has, for instance, enabled the identification of the outer membrane-bound UreI protein, which is *H. pylori*-specific and controls the cellular influx of urea, thereby providing protection against a low environmental pH (287). Specific targeting of this protein with an inhibitor in theory would be an effective monotherapy for *H. pylori.*

Vaccine Development

Another approach, which may be particularly suitable in developing countries, is the development of a vaccine against *H. pylori.* In 1992, it was first shown that the administration of *Helicobacter felis* lysates in combination with cholera toxin protected mice against later infection with *H. felis* (288). Since then, much progress has been made, even though we still appear to be far from the clinical introduction of an effective vaccine. First of all, various animal models have been developed and applied in vaccine research, including models based on mice, gnotobiotic piglets, ferrets, squirrels, and Rhesus monkeys. In each of these experiments, adjuvants, in particular cholera or labile toxin, were used to stimulate the immune response. The effect of oral administration of antigenic proteins without an adjuvant appeared to be insufficient. The adjuvant not only elicits an immune response against itself, but also enhances the response against other proteins administered simultaneously. Unfortunately, these adjuvants are associated with significant side effects, especially diarrhea in humans, which is mainly caused by the adenosine diphosphate ribosylation site on the A subunit of these toxins. Detoxification of the adjuvant by modification of this site or use of the B subunit in most cases also led to a loss of adjuvant activity, but exceptions have been described (289,290). Parenteral administration of the B subunit and the use of other adjuvants may offer new solutions (291).

New approaches aim to bypass the need for adjuvants and also focus on other routes of administration. They include the use of live vectors, such as a modified strain of *Salmonella* expressing *H. pylori* urease subunits (292) or poliovirus replicons encoding the urease B subunit of *H. pylori,* and the use of microparticles to encapsulate bacterial antigens and so protect them from degradation in the stomach (291). Also, the mucosal injection of naked DNA particles may stimulate an immune response against proteins encoded by that DNA and is another method that may prove helpful in the development of *H. pylori* vaccines. With respect to other routes of administration, it has been shown in mice that administration via mucosal surfaces such as those of nose and rectum and subcutaneous injection may induce protective immunity against *H. pylori* (293).

Vaccination against *H. pylori* by the methods described offers various degrees of protection against subsequent challenges with *H. pylori* (prophylactic immunization) and also appears to decrease the density of colonization in animals already colonized (therapeutic immunization). In both cases, complete eradication is rarely achieved, but the severity of gastritis generally decreases, although challenges with *H. pylori* in previously uncolonized animals may lead to relatively more severe gastritis when administered immediately after vaccination (291). The mechanisms underlying these effects remain incompletely understood. Although the initial focus was the stimulation of a local antibody response, immunization also appears to develop in the complete absence of antibody production, as in a mouse model completely deficient in B lymphocytes (293). Cellular immunity therefore must play a role. This was supported by studies in which vaccination failed to protect mice lacking helper T (Th) cells against subsequent challenges with *H. pylori* (291,293). In most *H. pylori*-positive subjects, a predominantly Th1 response develops, with the production of interferon-γ, IL-2, and IL-12; nevertheless, *H. pylori* is not eradicated. If Th cells are important for immunization but Th1 cells fail to respond in clinical practice, this suggests that protective immunity may in particular result from the stimulation of Th2 cells and the production of other cytokines, such as IL-4, IL-5, and IL-13. Further studies, however, have shown that both Th1 and Th2 cells are capable of stimulating protective immunity (294). Which cytokines are most important and how immunity is actually established are questions that remain to be solved.

In summary, although many hurdles remain to be overcome, progress is being made in the development of a vaccine against *H. pylori.* Such a vaccine may potentially be used both for protection and therapy. It may be particularly useful in developing countries as a cost-effective alternative to expensive antimicrobial therapy. However, vaccine therapy may also become valuable in developed countries as antimicrobial resistance increases.

SUMMARY

The discovery of *H. pylori* as a causal factor in a variety of upper gastrointestinal disorders has had a major clinical impact and has in particular changed the management of patients with peptic ulcer disease. Colonization with *H. pylori* is common, but the mechanisms of transfer are incompletely understood. In Western populations, the prevalence of *H. pylori* is decreasing, but it remains high in developing countries. Colonization with *H. pylori* is an important etiologic factor in the development of ulcer disease, chronic gastritis, and gastric cancer, and it has been associated with a variety of other conditions. *H. pylori* can be diagnosed by a variety of invasive and non-invasive tests and can be successfully treated in the majority of patients with a single course of combination therapy. In the future, a vaccine may be developed, and intervention projects may be undertaken in high-risk areas to prevent gastric adenocarcinoma with screening and treatment for *H. pylori.*

REFERENCES

1. Marshall BJ, Armstrong JA, McGechie DB, et al. Attempt to fulfill Koch's postulates for pyloric *Campylobacter. Med J Austr* 1985;142:436–439.
2. Morris A, Nicholson G. Ingestion of *Campylobacter pyloridis* causes gastritis and raised fasting gastric pH. *Am J Gastroenterol* 1987;82:192–199.
3. Sobala GM, Crabtree JE, Dixon MF, et al. Acute *Helicobacter pylori* infection: clinical features, local and systemic immune response, gastric mucosal histology, and gastric juice ascorbic acid concentrations. *Gut* 1991;32:1415–1418.
4. Graham DY, Alpert LC, Smith JL, et al. Iatrogenic *Campylobacter pylori* infection is a cause of epidemic achlorhydria. *Am J Gastroenterol* 1988;83:974–980.
5. Figura N. Mouth-to-mouth resuscitation and *Helicobacter pylori* infection. *Lancet* 1996;347:1342.
6. Matysiak-Budnik T, Briet F, Heyman M, et al. Laboratory-acquired *Helicobacter pylori* infection. *Lancet* 1995;346: 1489–1490.
7. Harford WV, Barnett C, Lee E, et al. Acute gastritis with hypochlorhydria: report of 35 cases with long-term follow-up. *Gut* 2000;47:467–472.
8. Whitehead R, Truelove SC, Gear MWL. The histological diagnosis of chronic gastritis in fibreoptic gastroscope biopsy specimens. *J Clin Pathol* 1972;25:1–11.
9. Dixon MF, Genta RM, Yardley JH, et al. Classification and grading of gastritis. The updated Sydney system. *Am J Surg Pathol* 1996;20:1161–1181.
10. van der Hulst RWM, van der Ende A, Dekker FW, et al. Effect of *Helicobacter pylori* eradication on gastritis in relation to *cagA*: a prospective 1-year follow-up study. *Gastroenterology* 1997; 113:25–30.
11. El-Serag HB, Sonnenberg A. Opposing time trends of peptic ulcer and reflux disease. *Gut* 1997;43:327–333.
12. Kuipers EJ, Thijs JC, Festen HPM. The prevalence of *Helicobacter pylori* in peptic ulcer disease. *Aliment Pharmacol Ther* 1995;9S2:59–69.
13. Nomura A, Stemmermann GN, Chyou PH, et al. *Helicobacter pylori* infection and the risk for duodenal and gastric ulceration. *Ann Intern Med* 1994;120:977–981.
14. Sipponen P, Varis K, Fräki O, et al. Cumulative 10-year risk of symptomatic duodenal and gastric ulcer in patients with or without chronic gastritis. *Scand J Gastroenterol* 1990;25:966–973.
15. Cullen DJE, Collins J, Christiansen KJ, et al. Long-term risk of peptic ulcer disease in people with *Helicobacter pylori* infection—a community-based study. *Gastroenterology* 1993;104:A60(abst).
16. Treiber G, Lambert JR. The impact of *Helicobacter pylori* eradication on peptic ulcer healing. *Am J Gastroenterol* 1998;93: 1080–1084.
17. van der Hulst RWM, Rauws EAJ, Köycü B, et al. Prevention of ulcer recurrence after eradication of *Helicobacter pylori*: a prospective long-term follow-up study. *Gastroenterol* 1997;113: 1082–1086.
18. Hurenkamp GJ, Grundmeijer HG, van der Ende A, et al. Arrest of chronic acid suppressant drug use after successful *Helicobacter pylori* eradication in patients with peptic ulcer disease: a six-month follow-up study. *Aliment Pharmacol Ther* 2001;15: 1047–1054.
19. Sprung DJ, Apter MN. What is the role of *Helicobacter pylori* in peptic ulcer and gastric cancer outside the big cities? *J Clin Gastroenterol* 1998;26:60–63.
20. Ciociola AA, McSorley DJ, Turner K, et al. *Helicobacter pylori* infection rates in duodenal ulcer patients in the United States may be lower than previously estimated. *Am J Gastroenterol* 1999;94:1834–1840.
21. Hawkey CJ. Epidemiology and aetiology of upper gastrointestinal bleeding. In: Krasner N, ed. *Gastrointestinal bleeding.* London: BMJ Publishing Group, 1996:3–18.
22. Vreeburg EM, Snel P, de Bruijne HW, et al. Acute upper gastrointestinal bleeding in the Amsterdam area: incidence, diagnosis, and clinical outcome. *Am J Gastroenterol* 1997;92:236–243.
23. Forrest JAH, Finlayson NDC, Shearman DJC. Endoscopy in gastrointestinal bleeding. *Lancet* 1974;2:394–397.
24. Rokkas T, Karameris A, Mavrogeorgis A, et al. Eradication of *Helicobacter pylori* reduces the possibility of rebleeding in peptic ulcer disease. *Gastrointest Endosc* 1995;41:1–4.
25. Graham DY, Hepps KS, Ramirez FC, et al. Treatment of *Helicobacter pylori* reduces the rate of rebleeding in peptic ulcer disease. *Scand J Gastroenterol* 1993;28:939–942.
26. Laine LA. *Helicobacter pylori* and complicated ulcer disease. *Am J Med* 1996;100:52S–59S.
27. Brandimarte G, Tursi A, di Cesare L, et al. Antimicrobial treatment for peptic stenosis: a prospective study. *Eur J Gastroenterol Hepatol* 1999;11:731–734.
28. Ng EK, Lam YH, Sung JJ, et al. Eradication of *Helicobacter pylori* prevents recurrence of ulcer after simple closure of duodenal ulcer perforation: randomized controlled trial. *Ann Surg* 2000;231:153–158.
29. Tepes B, Krizman I, Gorensek M, et al. Is a one-week course of triple anti-*Helicobacter pylori* therapy sufficient to control active duodenal ulcer? *Aliment Pharmacol Ther* 2001;15:1037–1045.
30. Thompson WG, Longstreth GF, Drossman DA, et al. Functional bowel disorders and functional abdominal pain. *Gut* 1999;45:II43–II47.
31. Fisher RS, Parkman HP. Management of non-ulcer dyspepsia. *N Engl J Med* 1998;339:1376–1381.
32. Talley NJ, Hunt RH. What role does *Helicobacter pylori* play in dyspepsia and non-ulcer dyspepsia? Arguments for and against *H. pylori* being associated with dyspeptic symptoms. *Gastroenterology* 1997;113:S67–S77.
33. McColl KEL, Murray L, El-Omar E, et al. Symptomatic benefit from eradicating *Helicobacter pylori* infection in non-ulcer dyspepsia. *N Engl J Med* 1998;339:1869–1874.
34. Blum AL, Talley NJ, O'Morain C, et al. Lack of effect of treating *Helicobacter pylori* infection in patients with non-ulcer dyspepsia. *N Engl J Med* 1998;339:1875–1881.

35. Talley NJ, Janssens J, Lauritsen K, et al. Long-term follow-up of patients with non-ulcer dyspepsia after *Helicobacter pylori* eradication. A randomized double-blinded placebo-controlled trial. *BMJ* 1999;318:833–837.
36. Talley NJ, Vakil N, Ballard ED, et al. Absence of benefit of eradicating *Helicobacter pylori* in patients with non-ulcer dyspepsia. *N Engl J Med* 1999;341:1106–1111.
37. Greenberg PD, Cello JP. Lack of effect of treatment for *Helicobacter pylori* on symptoms of non-ulcer dyspepsia. *Arch Intern Med* 1999;159:2283–2288.
38. Veldhuyzen van Zanten SJO, Flook N, Chiba N, et al. Canadian Dyspepsia Working Group. *Can Med Assoc J* 2000;162: 513–523.
39. Veldhuyzen van Zanten SJO. Dyspepsia is no indication for *Helicobacter pylori* eradication. In: Hunt RH, Tytgat GNJ, eds. Helicobacter pylori. *Basic mechanisms to clinical cure 2000.* Dordrecht: Kluwer Academic Publishers, 2000:435–441.
40. Laine L, Schoenfeld P, Fennerty MB. Therapy for *Helicobacter pylori* in patients with non-ulcer dyspepsia. A meta-analysis of randomized, controlled trials. *Ann Intern Med* 2001;134: 361–369.
41. Moayyedi P, Soo S, Deeks J, et al. Systematic review and economic evaluation of *Helicobacter pylori* eradication treatment for non-ulcer dyspepsia. *BMJ* 2000;321:659–664.
42. Kuipers EJ, Uyterlinde AM, Peña AS, et al. Long-term sequelae of *Helicobacter pylori* gastritis. *Lancet* 1995;345:1525–1528.
43. Kuipers EJ, Pérez-Pérez GI, Meuwissen SGM, et al. *Helicobacter pylori* and atrophic gastritis; importance of the *cagA* status. *J Natl Cancer Inst* 1995;87:1777–1780.
44. Correa P, Haenszel W, Cuello C, et al. A model for gastric cancer epidemiology. *Lancet* 1975;2:58–59.
45. Sipponen P, Kekki M, Haapakoski J, et al. Gastric cancer risk in chronic atrophic gastritis: statistical calculations of cross-sectional data. *Int J Cancer* 1985;35:173–177.
46. Forman D, Newell DG, Fullerton F, et al. Association between infection with *Helicobacter pylori* and risk of gastric cancer: evidence from a prospective investigation. *Br Med J* 1991;302: 1302–1305.
47. Nomura A, Stemmermann GN, Chyou P, et al. *Helicobacter pylori* infection and gastric carcinoma among Japanese Americans in Hawaii. *N Engl J Med* 1991;325:1132–1136.
48. Parsonnet J, Friedman GD, Vandersteen DP, et al. *Helicobacter pylori* infection and the risk of gastric carcinoma. *N Engl J Med* 1991;325:1127–1131.
49. Lin JT, Wang LY, Wang JT, et al. A nested case–control study on the association between *Helicobacter pylori* infection and gastric cancer risk in a cohort of 9,775 men in Taiwan. *Anticancer Res* 1995;15:603–606.
50. Webb PM, Yu MC, Forman D, et al. An apparent lack of association between *Helicobacter pylori* infection and risk of gastric cancer in China. *Int J Cancer* 1996;67:603–607.
51. Hansen S, Melby KK, Aase S, et al. *Helicobacter pylori* infection and the risk of cardia cancer and non-cardia gastric cancer. *Scand J Gastroenterol* 1999;34:353–360.
52. Forman D, Sitas F, Newell DG, et al. Geographic association of *Helicobacter pylori* antibody prevalence and gastric cancer mortality in rural China. *Int J Cancer* 1990;46:608–611.
53. The Eurogast Study Group. An international association between *Helicobacter pylori* infection and gastric cancer. *Lancet* 1993;341:1359–1362.
54. Huang JQ, Sridhar S, Chen Y, et al. Meta-analysis of the relationship between *Helicobacter pylori* seropositivity and gastric cancer. *Gastroenterology* 1998;114:1169–1179.
55. Karnes WE, Samloff IM, Siurala M, et al. Positive serum antibody and negative tissue staining for *Helicobacter pylori* in subjects with atrophic gastritis. *Gastroenterology* 1991;101:167–174.
56. Valle J, Kekki M, Sipponen P, et al. Long-term course and consequences of *Helicobacter pylori* gastritis. *Scand J Gastroenterol* 1996;31:546–550.
57. Forman D, Webb P, Parsonnet J. *Helicobacter pylori* and gastric cancer. *Lancet* 1994;343:243–244.
58. International Agency for Research on Cancer. *Schistosomes, liver flukes and* Helicobacter pylori. Lyon: IARC, 1994 (*IARC monographs on the evaluation of carcinogenic risks to humans,* vol 61).
59. Watanabe T, Tada M, Nagai H, et al. *Helicobacter pylori* infection induces gastric cancer in Mongolian gerbils. *Gastroenterology* 1998;115:642–648.
60. Blaser MJ, Pérez-Pérez GI, Kleanthous H, et al. Infection with *Helicobacter pylori* strains possessing *cagA* is associated with an increased risk of developing adenocarcinoma of the stomach. *Cancer Res* 1995;55:2111–2115.
61. Parsonnet J, Friedman GD, Orentreich N, et al. Infection with the type I phenotype of *H. pylori* increases the risk for gastric cancer independent of corpus atrophy. *Gastroenterology* 1996; 110:A221(abst).
62. El-Omar EM, Carrington M, Chow WH, et al. Interleukin-1 polymorphisms associated with increased risk of gastric cancer. *Nature* 2000;404:398–402.
63. Kuipers EJ. Review article: exploring the link between *Helicobacter pylori* and gastric cancer. *Aliment Pharmacol Ther* 1999; 13:3–12.
64. Uemura N, Okamoto S, Yamamoto S, et al. *Helicobacter pylori* infection and the development of gastric cancer. *N Engl J Med* 2001;345:784–789.
65. Sung JJ, Lin SR, Ching JY, et al. Atrophy and intestinal metaplasia one year after cure of *H. pylori* infection: a prospective, randomized study. *Gastroenterology* 2000;119:7–14.
66. El-Omar E, Oien K, Murray L, et al. Increased prevalence of precancerous changes in relatives of gastric cancer patients: critical role of *H. pylori. Gastroenterology* 2000;118:22–30.
67. Ohkusa T, Fujiki K, Takashimizu I, et al. Improvement in atrophic gastritis and intestinal metaplasia in patients in whom *Helicobacter pylori* was eradicated. *Ann Intern Med* 2001;134: 380–386.
68. Uemura N, Mukai T, Okamoto S, et al. Effect of *Helicobacter pylori* eradication on subsequent development of cancer after endoscopic resection of early gastric cancer. *Cancer Epidemiol Biomarkers Prev* 1997;6:639–642.
69. Parsonnet J, Harris RA, Hack HM, et al. Modelling cost-effectiveness of *Helicobacter pylori* screening to prevent gastric cancer: a mandate for clinical trials. *Lancet* 1996;348:150–154.
70. Blaser MJ. All helicobacters are not created equal: should all be eliminated? *Lancet* 1997;349:1020–1022.
71. Siurala M, Varis K, Wiljasalo M. Studies of patients with atrophic gastritis: a ten- to fifteen-year follow-up. *Scand J Gastroenterol* 1966;1:40–48.
72. Walker IR, Strickland RG, Ungar B, et al. Simple atrophic gastritis and gastric carcinoma. *Gut* 1971;12:906–909.
73. Kuipers EJ. Review article: relationship between *Helicobacter pylori*, atrophic gastritis and gastric cancer. *Aliment Pharmacol Ther* 1998;12:25–36.
74. Kato I, Tominaga S, Ito Y, et al. A prospective study of atrophic gastritis and stomach cancer risk. *Jpn J Cancer Res* 1992;83: 1137–1142.
75. Parsonnet J. When heredity is infectious. *Gastroenterology* 2000;118:222–224.
76. Scott N, Diament R, Murday V, et al. *Helicobacter* gastritis and intestinal metaplasia in a gastric cancer family. *Lancet* 1990;335: 728.
77. Brenner H, Bode G, Boeing H. *Helicobacter pylori* among offspring of patients with stomach cancer. *Gastroenterology* 2000; 118:31–35.

78. Malfertheiner P. Current European concepts in the management of *Helicobacter pylori* infection: the Maastricht consensus report. *Gut* 1997;41:8–13.
79. Hunt R, Thompson ABR. Canadian *Helicobacter pylori* consensus conference. Canadian Association of Gastroenterology. *Can J Gastroenterol* 1998;12:31–41.
80. Wotherspoon AC. Criteria for the diagnosis of mucosa-associated lymphoid tissue lymphoma. In: Hunt RH, Tytgat GNJ, eds. Helicobacter pylori. *Basic mechanisms to clinical cure 1998.* Dordrecht: Kluwer Academic Publishers, 1998:362–372.
81. Eidt S, Stolte M, Fischer R. *Helicobacter pylori* gastritis and primary gastric non-Hodgkin's lymphomas. *J Clin Pathol* 1994;47:436–439.
82. Parsonnet J, Hansen S, Rodriguez L, et al. *Helicobacter pylori* infection and gastric lymphoma. *N Engl J Med* 1994;330:1267–1271.
83. Stolte M, Morgner A, Alpen B, et al. Evaluation of the long-term outcome of *Helicobacter pylori*-related gastric mucosa-associated lymphoid tissue (MALT) lymphoma. In: Hunt RH, Tytgat GNJ, eds. Helicobacter pylori. *Basic mechanisms to clinical cure 2000.* Dordrecht: Kluwer Academic Publishers, 2000:541–548.
84. Ng WW, Lam CP, Chau WK, et al. Regression of high-grade gastric mucosa-associated lymphoid tissue lymphoma with *Helicobacter pylori* after triple antibiotic therapy. *Gastrointest Endosc* 2000;51:93–96.
85. Werdmuller BFM, Loffeld RJLF. *Helicobacter pylori* has no role in the pathogenesis of reflux esophagitis. *Dig Dis Sci* 1997;42:103–105.
86. Varanasi RV, Fantry GT, Wilson KT. Decreased prevalence of *Helicobacter pylori* infection in gastroesophageal reflux disease. *Helicobacter* 1998;3:188–194.
87. Wu J, Sung J, Ng E, et al. Prevalence and distribution of *Helicobacter pylori* in gastroesophageal reflux disease: a study from the East. *Am J Gastroenterol* 1999;94:1790–1794.
88. O'Connor HJ. *Helicobacter pylori* and gastro-oesophageal reflux disease—clinical implications and management. *Aliment Pharmacol Ther* 1999;13:117–127.
89. Labenz J, Blum AL, Bayerdörffer E, et al. Curing *Helicobacter pylori* infection in patients with duodenal ulcer may provoke reflux esophagitis. *Gastroenterology* 1997;112:1442–1447.
90. Kuipers EJ, Uyterlinde AM, Peña AS, et al. Increase of *Helicobacter pylori*-associated corpus gastritis during acid suppressive therapy: implications for long-term safety. *Am J Gastroenterol* 1995;90:1401–1406.
91. Fallone CA, Barkun AN, Friedman G, et al. Is *Helicobacter pylori* eradication associated with gastroesophageal reflux disease? *Am J Gastroenterol* 2000;95:914–920.
92. McColl KE, Dickson A, El-Nujumi A, et al. Symptomatic benefit 1 to 3 years after *H. pylori* eradication in ulcer patients: impact of gastroesophageal reflux disease. *Am J Gastroenterol* 2000;95:101–105.
93. Tefera S, Hattlebak JG, Berstad A. The effect of *Helicobacter pylori* eradication on gastro-oesophageal reflux. *Aliment Pharmacol Ther* 1999;13:915–920.
94. Axon ATR, Bardhan K, Moayyedi P, et al. Does eradication of *Helicobacter pylori* influence the recurrence of symptoms in patients with symptomatic gastroesophageal reflux disease?—A randomized double-blinded study. *Gastroenterology* 1999;116:G0503.
95. Gillen D, El-Omar EM, Wirtz AA, et al. The acid response to gastrin distinguishes duodenal ulcer patients from *Helicobacter pylori*-infected healthy subjects. *Gastroenterology* 1998;114:50–57.
96. El-Serag HB, Sonnenberg A, Jamal MM, et al. Corpus gastritis is protective against reflux oesophagitis. *Gut* 1999;45:181–185.
97. Koike T, Ohara S, Sekine H, et al. *Helicobacter pylori* infection inhibits reflux esophagitis by inducing atrophic gastritis. *Am J Gastroenterol* 1999;94:3468–3472.
98. Loffeld RJLF, Werdmuller BFM, Kusters JG, et al. Colonization with *cagA*-positive *Helicobacter pylori* strains is inversely associated with reflux esophagitis and Barrett's esophagus. *Digestion* 2000;62:95–99.
99. Fallone CA, Barkun AN, Gottke MU, et al. Association of *Helicobacter pylori* genotype with gastroesophageal reflux disease and other upper gastrointestinal diseases. *Am J Gastroenterol* 2000;95:659–669.
100. Lagergren J, Bergström R, Lindgren A, et al. Symptomatic gastroesophageal reflux disease as a risk factor for esophageal adenocarcinoma. *N Engl J Med* 1999;340:825–831.
101. Chow WH, Blaser MJ, Blot WJ, et al. An inverse relation between *cagA*+ strains of *H. pylori* infection and risk of esophageal and gastric cardia adenocarcinoma. *Cancer Res* 1998;58:588–590.
102. Vicari JJ, Peek RM, Falk GW, et al. The seroprevalence of *cagA*-positive *Helicobacter pylori* strains in the spectrum of gastroesophageal reflux disease. *Gastroenterology* 1998;115:50–57.
103. Grimley CE, Holder RL, Loft DE, et al. *Helicobacter pylori*-associated antibodies in patients with duodenal ulcer, gastric and oesophageal adenocarcinoma. *Eur J Gastroenterol Hepatol* 1999;11:503–509.
104. Hesketh PJ, Clapp RW, Doos WG, et al. The increasing frequency of adenocarcinoma of the esophagus. *Cancer* 1989;64:526–530.
105. Blot WJ, Devesa SS, Kneller RW, et al. Rising incidence of adenocarcinoma of the esophagus and cardia. *JAMA* 1991;265:1287–1289.
106. Craanen ME, Dekker W, Blok P, et al. Time trends in gastric carcinoma: changing patterns of type and location. *Am J Gastroenterol* 1992;87:572–579.
107. Verdú EF, Armstrong D, Idström J-P, et al. Effect of curing *Helicobacter pylori* infection on intragastric pH during treatment with omeprazole. *Gut* 1995;37:743–748.
108. Labenz J, Tillenburg B, Peitz U, et al. Effect of curing *Helicobacter pylori* infection on intragastric acidity during treatment with ranitidine in patients with duodenal ulcer. *Gut* 1997;41:33–36.
109. Holtmann G, Cain C, Malfertheiner P. Gastric *Helicobacter pylori* infection accelerates healing of reflux esophagitis during treatment with the proton pump inhibitor pantoprazole. *Gastroenterology* 1999;117:11–16.
110. Gillen D, Wirz AA, Ardill JE, et al. Rebound hypersecretion post-omeprazole and its relation to on-treatment acid suppression and *Helicobacter pylori* status. *Gastroenterology* 1999;116:239–247.
111. Schwizer W, Thumshirn M, Dent J, et al. *Helicobacter pylori* and symptomatic relapse of gastro-oesophageal reflux disease: a randomised controlled trial. *Lancet* 2001;357:1738–1742.
112. Klinkenberg-Knol EC, Nelis F, Dent J, et al. Long-term omeprazole treatment in resistant gastroesophageal reflux disease: efficacy, safety and influence on gastric mucosa. *Gastroenterology* 2000;118:661–669.
113. Kuipers EJ, Lundell L, Klinkenberg-Knol EC, et al. Atrophic gastritis and *Helicobacter pylori* infection in patients with reflux esophagitis treated with omeprazole or fundoplication. *N Engl J Med* 1996;334:1018–1022.
114. Lundell L, Miettinen P, Myrvold HE, et al. Lack of effect of acid suppression therapy on gastric atrophy. *Gastroenterology* 1999;117:319–326.
115. Lundell L, Havu N, Miettinen P, et al. No effect of acid suppression therapy over five years on gastric glandular atrophy. Results of a randomised clinical study. *Gastroenterology* 1999;118:A214(abst).
116. Schenk BE, Kuipers EJ, Nelis GF, et al. Effect of *Helicobacter pylori* eradication on chronic gastritis during omeprazole therapy. *Gut* 2000;46:615–621.

117. Moayyedi P, Wason C, Peacock R, et al. Changing patterns of *Helicobacter pylori* gastritis in long-standing acid suppression. *Helicobacter* 2000;5:206–214.
118. Kuipers EJ, Nelis GF, Klinkenberg-Knol EC, et al. *Helicobacter pylori* eradication for the prevention of atrophic gastritis during omeprazole therapy; a prospective randomized trial. *Gastroenterology* 2001;120: (A14).
119. Graham DY. Therapy of *Helicobacter pylori*: current status and issues. *Gastroenterology* 2000;118:S2–S8.
120. Meuwissen SGM, Ridwan BU, Hasper HJ, et al. Hypertrophic protein-losing gastropathy. A retrospective analysis of 40 cases in the Netherlands. *Scand J Gastroenterol* 1992;27:1–7.
121. Groisman GM, George J, Berman D, et al. Resolution of protein-losing hypertrophic lymphocytic gastritis with therapeutic eradication of *Helicobacter pylori. Am J Gastroenterol* 1994;89: 1548–1551.
122. Yasunaga Y, Shinomura Y, Kanayama S, et al. Improved fold width and increased acid secretion after eradication of the organism in *Helicobacter pylori*-associated enlarged-fold gastritis. *Gut* 1994;35:1571–1574.
123. Stolte M, Batz CH, Bayerdorffer E, et al. *Helicobacter pylori* eradication in the treatment and differential diagnosis of giant folds in the corpus and fundus of the stomach. *Z Gastroenterol* 1995;33:198–201.
124. Varis O, Valle J, Siurala M. Is *Helicobacter pylori* involved in the pathogenesis of the gastritis characteristic of pernicious anemia? *Scand J Gastroenterol* 1993;28:705–708.
125. Faller G, Steininger H, Eck M, et al. Antigastric autoantibodies in *Helicobacter pylori* gastritis: prevalence, *in situ* binding sites and clues for clinical relevance. *Virchows Arch* 1996;427:483–486.
126. Stolte M, Meier E, Meining A. Cure of autoimmune gastritis by *Helicobacter pylori* eradication in a 21-year-old male. *Z Gastroenterol* 1998;36:641–643.
127. Hayat M, Arora DS, Dixon MF, et al. Effects of *Helicobacter pylori* eradication on the natural history of lymphocytic gastritis. *Gut* 1999;45:495–498.
128. Müller H, Volkholz H, Stolte M. Healing of lymphocytic gastritis by eradication of *Helicobacter pylori. Digestion* 2001;63:14–19.
129. Dixon MF. Unusual forms of gastric inflammation and their relationship to *Helicobacter pylori* infection. In: Hunt RH, Tytgat GNJ, eds. Helicobacter pylori. *Basic mechanisms to clinical cure 2000.* Dordrecht: Kluwer Academic Publishers; 2000:221–228.
130. Kusters JG, Kuipers EJ. *Helicobacter* and atherosclerosis. *Am Heart J* 1999;138:S523–S527.
131. Leontiades GI, Sharma VK, Howden CW. Non-gastrointestinal tract associations of *Helicobacter pylori* infection: what is the evidence? *Arch Intern Med* 1999;159:925–940.
132. Bamford JTM, Tilden RL, Blankush JL, et al. Effect of treatment of *Helicobacter pylori* infection on rosacea. *Arch Dermatol* 1999;135:659–663.
133. Sauve-Martin H, Kalach N, Raymond J, et al. The rate of *Helicobacter pylori* infection in children with growth retardation. *J Pediatr Gastroenterol Nutr* 1999;28:354–355.
134. Murray LJ, McCrum EE, Evans AE, et al. Epidemiology of *Helicobacter pylori* infection among 4,742 randomly selected subjects from Northern Ireland. *Int J Epidemiol* 1997;26:880–887.
135. Tindberg Y, Bengtsson C, Granath F, et al. *Helicobacter pylori* infection in Swedish school children: lack of evidence of child-to-child transmission outside the family. *Gastroenterology* 2001; 121:310–316.
136. Ashorn M, Ruuska T, Karikoski R, et al. *Helicobacter pylori* gastritis in dyspeptic children—a long-term follow-up after treatment with colloidal bismuth subcitrate and tinidazole. *Scand J Gastroenterol* 1994;29:203–208.
137. Sherman P, Hassall E, Hunt R, et al. Canadian *Helicobacter* Study Group consensus conference on the approach to *Helicobacter pylori* infection in children and adolescents. *Can J Gastroenterol* 1999;13:553–559.
138. Drumm B, Koletzko S, Oderda G, and the European Task Force on *Helicobacter pylori. Helicobacter pylori* infection in children: a consensus statement. *J Pediatr Gastroenterol Nutr* 2000; 30:207–213.
139. Choe YH, Kim SK, Hong YC. *Helicobacter pylori* infection with iron deficiency anemia and subnormal growth at puberty. *Arch Dis Child* 2000;82:136–140.
140. NIH Consensus Conference. *Helicobacter pylori* in peptic ulcer disease. *JAMA* 1994;272:65–69.
141. Taha AS, Dahill S, Sturrock RD, et al. Predicting NSAID-related ulcers—assessment of clinical and pathological risk factors and importance of differences in NSAID. *Gut* 1994;35: 891–895.
142. Huang JQ, Lad R, Hunt RH. Role of *Helicobacter pylori* infection in NSAID-associated gastropathy. In: Hunt RH, Tytgat GNJ, eds. Helicobacter pylori. *Basic mechanisms to clinical cure 2000.* Dordrecht: Kluwer Academic Publishers, 2000:443–451.
143. Taha AS, Sturrock RD, Russel RI. Mucosal erosions in long-term nonsteroidal antiinflammatory drug users: predisposition to ulceration and relation to *Helicobacter pylori. Gut* 1995;36: 334–336.
144. Hawkey CJ, Karrasch JA, Szczepanski L, et al. Omeprazole compared with misoprostol for ulcers associated with nonsteroidal antiinflammatory drugs. Omeprazole versus Misoprostol for NSAID-Induced Ulcer Management (OMNIUM) Study Group. *N Engl J Med* 1998;338:727–734.
145. Graham DY. Role of *Helicobacter pylori* in NSAID gastropathy: can *H. pylori* infection be beneficial? In: Hunt RH, Tytgat GNJ, eds. Helicobacter pylori. *Basic mechanisms to clinical cure 2000.* Dordrecht: Kluwer Academic Publishers, 2000:453–459.
146. Feldman M, Cryer B, Mallat D, et al. Role of *Helicobacter pylori* infection in gastroduodenal injury and gastric prostaglandin synthesis during long-term/low-dose aspirin therapy: a prospective placebo-controlled, double-blinded, randomized trial. *Am J Gastroenterol* 2001;96:1751–1757.
147. Chan FKL, Sung JJY, Chung SCS, et al. Randomised eradication of *H. pylori* before nonsteroidal antiinflammatory drug therapy to prevent peptic ulcer. *Lancet* 1997;350:975–979.
148. Cullen D, Bardhan KD, Eisner M, et al. Primary gastroduodenal prophylaxis with omeprazole for nonsteroidal antiinflammatory drug users. *Aliment Pharmacol Ther* 1998;12:135–140.
149. Yeomans ND, Tulassy Z, Juhasz L, et al. A comparison of omeprazole with ranitidine for ulcers associated with nonsteroidal antiinflammatory drugs. *N Engl J Med* 1998;338:719–726.
150. Bianchi Porro G, Parente F, Imbesi V, et al. Role of *Helicobacter pylori* in ulcer healing and recurrence of gastric and duodenal ulcers in long-term NSAID users. Response to omeprazole dual therapy. *Gut* 1996;39:22–26.
151. Hawkey CJ, Tulassay Z, Szczepansky L, et al. Randomised controlled trial of *Helicobacter pylori* eradication in patients on nonsteroidal antiinflammatory drugs: HELP NSAIDs Study. *Lancet* 1998;352:1016–1021.
152. Chan FK, Sung JJ, Suen R, et al. Does eradication of *Helicobacter pylori* impair healing of nonsteroidal antiinflammatory drug-associated bleeding peptic ulcers? A prospective randomized study. *Aliment Pharmacol Ther* 1998;12:1201–1205.
153. Chan FKL, Sung JY, Suen R, et al. Preventing recurrent upper gastrointestinal bleeding in patients with *Helicobacter pylori* infection who are taking low-dose aspirin or naproxen. *N Engl J Med* 2001;344:967–973.
154. Talley NJ, Silverstein MD, Agreus L, et al. AGA technical review: evaluation of dyspepsia. *Gastroenterology* 1998;114:582–595.
155. Sonnenberg A. Cost–benefit analysis of testing for *Helicobacter pylori* in dyspeptic patients. *Am J Gastroenterol* 1996;91:644–652.

156. Gillen D, McColl KEL. Does concern about missing malignancy justify endoscopy in uncomplicated dyspepsia in patients aged less than 55? *Am J Gastroenterol* 1999;94:75–79.
157. Sung JJY. The impact of the "test-and-treat" strategies for *Helicobacter pylori* infection—an Asian perspective? In: Hunt RH, Tytgat GNJ, eds. Helicobacter pylori. *Basic mechanisms to clinical cure 2000.* Dordrecht: Kluwer Academic Publishers, 2000: 483–486.
158. Patel P, Khulusi S, Mendall MA, et al. Prospective screening of dyspeptic patients by *Helicobacter pylori* serology. *Lancet* 1995; 346:1315–1318.
159. Joossen EAM, Reininga JHA, Manders JMW, et al. Costs and benefits of a test-and-treat strategy in *Helicobacter pylori*-infected subjects: a prospective intervention study in general practice. *Eur J Gastroenterol Hepatol* 2000;12:319–325.
160. Heaney A, Collins JSA, Watson RGP, et al. A prospective randomised trial of a "test and treat" policy versus endoscopy-based management in young *Helicobacter pylori*-positive patients with ulcer-like dyspepsia, referred to a hospital clinic. *Gut* 1999;45: 186–190.
161. Vaira D, Malfertheiner P, Megraud F, et al. Diagnosis of *Helicobacter pylori* infection with a new non-invasive antigen-based assay. HpSA European Study Group. *Lancet* 1999;354:30–33.
162. Zagari RM, Bazzoli F, Pozzato P, et al. Review article: non-invasive methods for the diagnosis of *Helicobacter pylori* infection. *Ital J Gastroenterol Hepatol* 1999;31:408–415.
163. Logan RP. Urea breath tests in the management of *Helicobacter pylori* infection. *Gut* 1998;43[Suppl 1]:S47–S50.
164. Graham DY, Klein PD, Evans DJ Jr, et al. *Campylobacter pylori* detected non-invasively by the ^{13}C-urea breath test. *Lancet* 1987;1:1174–1177.
165. Bazzoli F, Cecchini L, Corvaglia L, et al. Validation of the ^{13}C-urea breath test for the diagnosis of *Helicobacter pylori* infection in children: a multicenter study. *Am J Gastroenterol* 2000;95: 646–650.
166. Connor SJ, Seow F, Ngu MC, et al. The effect of dosing with omeprazole on the accuracy of the ^{13}C-urea breath test in *Helicobacter pylori*-infected subjects. *Aliment Pharmacol Ther* 1999; 13:1287–1293.
167. Connor SJ, Ngu MC, Katelaris PH. The impact of short-term ranitidine use on the precision of the ^{13}C-urea breath test in subjects infected with *Helicobacter pylori. Eur J Gastroenterol Hepatol* 1999;11:1135–1138.
168. Braden B, Schafer F, Caspary WF, et al. Nondispersive isotope-selective infrared spectroscopy: a new analytical method for ^{13}C-urea breath tests. *Scand J Gastroenterol* 1996;31:442–445.
169. Moulton-Barrett R, Triadafilopoulos G, Michener R, et al. Serum ^{13}C-bicarbonate in the assessment of gastric *Helicobacter pylori* urease activity. *Am J Gastroenterol* 1993;88:369–374.
170. Pathak CM, Panigrahi D, Bhasin DK, et al. Advantage of use of DPM for ^{14}C-urea breath test for the detection of *Helicobacter pylori. Am J Gastroenterol* 1992;87:1887–1888.
171. Pathak CM, Bhasin DK, Panigrahi D, et al. Evaluation of ^{14}C-urinary excretion and its comparison with $^{14}CO_2$ in breath after ^{14}C-urea administration in *Helicobacter pylori* infection. *Am J Gastroenterol* 1994;89:734–738.
172. Vaira D, Holton J, Menegatti M, et al. New immunological assays for the diagnosis of *Helicobacter pylori* infection. *Gut* 1999;45[Suppl 1]:I23–I27.
173. Kosunen TU, Seppälä K, Sarna S, et al. Diagnostic value of decreasing IgG, IgA and IgM antibody titres after eradication of *Helicobacter pylori. Lancet* 1992;339:893–895.
174. Laheij RJ, Straatman H, Jansen JB, et al. Evaluation of commercially available *Helicobacter pylori* serology kits: a review. *J Clin Microbiol* 1998;36:2803–2809.
175. Graham DY, Evans DJ Jr, Peacock J, et al. Comparison of rapid serological tests (FlexSure HP and QuickVue) with conventional ELISA for detection of *Helicobacter pylori* infection. *Am J Gastroenterol* 1996;91:942–948.
176. Hawthorne AB, Morgan S, Westmoreland D, et al. A comparison of two rapid whole-blood tests and laboratory serology in the diagnosis of *Helicobacter pylori* infection. *Eur J Gastroenterol Hepatol* 1999;11:863–865.
177. Lerang F, Haug JB, Moum B, et al. Accuracy of IgG serology and other tests in confirming *Helicobacter pylori* eradication. *Scand J Gastroenterol* 1998;33:710–715.
178. Kokkola A, Valle J, Haapiainen R, et al. *Helicobacter pylori* infection in young patients with gastric carcinoma. *Scand J Gastroenterol* 1996;31:643–647.
179. Braden B, Teuber G, Dietrich CF, et al. Comparison of new faecal antigen test with (13)C-urea breath test for detecting *Helicobacter pylori* infection and monitoring eradication treatment: prospective clinical evaluation. *BMJ* 2000;320:148.
180. Braden B, Posselt HG, Ahrens P, et al. New immunoassay in stool provides an accurate non-invasive diagnostic method for *Helicobacter pylori* screening in children. *Pediatrics* 2000;106: 115–117.
181. Vaira D, Holton J, Menegatti M, et al. Review article: invasive and non-invasive tests for *Helicobacter pylori* infection. *Aliment Pharmacol Ther* 2000;14[Suppl 3]:13–22.
182. Genta RM, Graham DY. Comparison of biopsy sites for the histopathologic diagnosis of *Helicobacter pylori*: a topographic study of *H. pylori* density and distribution. *Gastrointest Endosc* 1994;40:342–345.
183. Cutler AF. Diagnostic tests for *H. pylori*: a prospective evaluation of their accuracy, without selecting a single test as the gold standard. *Am J Gastroenterol* 1997;92:538–539.
184. Leung WK, Sung JJ, Siu KL, et al. False-negative biopsy urease test in bleeding ulcers caused by the buffering effects of blood. *Am J Gastroenterol* 1998;93:1914–1918.
185. Luthra GK, DiNuzzo AR, Gourley WK, et al. Comparison of biopsy and serological methods of diagnosis of *Helicobacter pylori* infection and the potential role of antibiotics. *Am J Gastroenterol* 1998;93:1291–1296.
186. Ferguson DA Jr, Jiang C, Chi DS, et al. Evaluation of two string tests for obtaining gastric juice for culture, nested-PCR detection, and combined single- and double-stranded conformational polymorphism discrimination of *Helicobacter pylori. Dig Dis Sci* 1999;44:2056–2062.
187. Maconi G, Vago L, Galletta G, et al. Is routine histological evaluation an accurate test for *Helicobacter pylori* infection? *Aliment Pharmacol Ther* 1999;13:327–331.
188. Calabrese C, Di Febo G, Brandi G, et al. Correlation between endoscopic features of gastric antrum, histology, and *Helicobacter pylori* infection in adults. *Ital J Gastroenterol Hepatol* 1999; 31:359–365.
189. Loffeld RJ. Diagnostic value of endoscopic signs of gastritis, with special emphasis on nodular antritis. *Neth J Med* 1999;54: 96–100.
190. Han SW, Flamm R, Hachem CY, et al. Transport and storage of *Helicobacter pylori* from gastric mucosal biopsies and clinical isolates. *Eur J Clin Microbiol Infect Dis* 1995;14:349–352.
191. Roosendaal R, Kuipers EJ, Peña AS, et al. Recovery of *Helicobacter pylori* from gastric biopsy specimens is not dependent on the transport medium used. *J Clin Microbiol* 1995;33: 2798–2800.
192. Kusters JG, Gerrits MM, Van Strijp JA, et al. Coccoid forms of *Helicobacter pylori* are the morphologic manifestation of cell death. *Infect Immun* 1997;65:3672–3679.
193. Chen XY, van der Hulst RW, Bruno MJ, et al. Interobserver variation in the histopathological scoring of *Helicobacter pylori*-related gastritis. *J Clin Pathol* 1999;52:612–615.

194. El Zimaity HM, Segura AM, Genta RM, et al. Histologic assessment of *Helicobacter pylori* status after therapy: comparison of Giemsa, Diff-Quik, and Genta stains. *Mod Pathol* 1998; 11:288–291.
195. El Zimaity HM. Modified triple stain (carbol fuchsin/alcian blue/hematoxylin–eosin) for the identification of *Helicobacter pylori. Arch Pathol Lab Med* 2000;124:1416–1417.
196. Marzio L, Angelucci D, Grossi L, et al. Anti-*Helicobacter pylori*–specific antibody immunohistochemistry improves the diagnostic accuracy of *Helicobacter pylori* in biopsy specimen from patients treated with triple therapy. *Am J Gastroenterol* 1998;93:223–226.
197. Lu JJ, Perng CL, Shyu RY, et al. Comparison of five PCR methods for detection of *Helicobacter pylori* DNA in gastric tissues. *J Clin Microbiol* 1999;37:772–774.
198. Chen YK, Godil A, Wat PJ. Comparison of two rapid urease tests for detection of *Helicobacter pylori* infection. *Dig Dis Sci* 1998;43:1636–1640.
199. Laine L, Lewin D, Naritoku W, et al. Prospective comparison of commercially available rapid urease tests for the diagnosis of *Helicobacter pylori. Gastrointest Endosc* 1996;44:523–526.
200. Van Der Wouden EJ, Thijs JC, Van Zwet AA, et al. Reliability of biopsy-based diagnostic tests for *Helicobacter pylori* after treatment aimed at its eradication. *Eur J Gastroenterol Hepatol* 1999;11:1255–1258.
201. Prince MI, Osborne JS, Ingoe L, et al. The CLO test in the UK: inappropriate reading and missed results. *Eur J Gastroenterol Hepatol* 1999;11:1251–1254.
202. Monteiro L, Cabrita J, Mégraud F. Evaluation of performances of three DNA enzyme immunoassays for detection of *Helicobacter pylori* PCR products from biopsy specimens. *J Clin Microbiol* 1997;35:2931–2936.
203. Rudi J, Rudy A, Maiwald M, et al. Direct determination of *Helicobacter pylori vacA* genotypes and *cagA* gene in gastric biopsies and relationship to gastrointestinal diseases. *Am J Gastroenterol* 1999;94:1525–1531.
204. van Doorn LJ, Figueiredo C, Sanna R, et al. Clinical relevance of the *cagA, vacA,* and *iceA* status of *Helicobacter pylori. Gastroenterology* 1998;115:58–66.
205. Yamaoka Y, Kodama T, Kita M, et al. Relation between clinical presentation, *Helicobacter pylori* density, interleukin 1-beta and 8 production, and *cagA* status. *Gut* 1999;45:804–811.
206. Hennig EE, Trzeciak L, Regula J, et al. *VacA* genotyping directly from gastric biopsy specimens and estimation of mixed *Helicobacter pylori* infections in patients with duodenal ulcer and gastritis. *Scand J Gastroenterol* 1999;34:743–749.
207. Fusconi M, Vaira D, Menegatti M, et al. Anti-CagA reactivity in *Helicobacter pylori*-negative subjects: a comparison of three different methods. *Dig Dis Sci* 1999;44:1691–1695.
208. Evans DG, Queiroz DM, Mendes EN, et al. *Helicobacter pylori cagA* status and s and m alleles of *vacA* in isolates from individuals with a variety of *H. pylori*-associated gastric diseases. *J Clin Microbiol* 1998;36:3435–3437.
209. Yamaoka Y, Kodama T, Kashima K, et al. Antibody against *Helicobacter pylori* CagA and VacA and the risk for gastric cancer. *J Clin Pathol* 1999;52:215–218.
210. Vogt K, Warrelmann M, Hahn H. The minimum inhibitory concentrations of various bismuth salts against *Campylobacter pylori. Zentralbl Bakt* 1989;271:304–308.
211. Armstrong JA, Wee SH, Goodwin CS, et al. Response of *Campylobacter pyloridis* to antibiotics, bismuth, and an acid-reducing agent *in vitro*—an ultrastructural study. *J Med Microbiol* 1987;24:343–350.
212. Lambert JR, Midolo P. The actions of bismuth in the treatment of *Helicobacter pylori* infection. *Aliment Pharmacol Ther* 1997; 11:27–33.
213. Marshall BJ, McGechie DA, Rogers PA, et al. Pyloric *Campylobacter* infection and gastroduodenal disease. *Med J Austr* 1985; 142:439–444.
214. Furuta T, Baba S, Takashima M, et al. Effect of *Helicobacter pylori* infection on gastric juice pH. *Scand J Gastroenterol* 1998; 33:357–363.
215. Greyson ML, Eliopoulos GM, Ferraro MJ, et al. Effect of varying pH on the susceptibility of *Camplylobacter pylori* to antimicrobial agents. *Eur J Clin Microbiol Infect Dis* 1989;8:888–889.
216. Debets-Ossenkopp YJ, Namavar F, Maclaren DM. Effects of an acidic environment on the susceptibility of *Helicobacter pylori* to trospectomycin and other antimicrobial agents. *Eur J Clin Microbiol Infect Dis* 1995;14:353–355.
217. O'Riordan T, Mathai E, Tobin E, et al. Adjuvant antibiotic therapy in duodenal ulcers treated with colloidal bismuth subcitrate. *Gut* 1990;31:999–1002.
218. Rubin CE. Are there three types of *Helicobacter pylori* gastritis? *Gastroenterology* 1997;112:2108–2110.
219. Glupczynski Y, Burrette A, de Koster E, et al. Metronidazole resistance in *Helicobacter pylori. Lancet* 1990;335:976–977.
220. Katelaris PH, Patchett SE, Zhang ZW, et al. A randomized prospective comparison of clarithromycin and amoxicillin in combination with omeprazole for eradication of *Helicobacter pylori. Aliment Pharmacol Ther* 1995;9:205–208.
221. Labenz J, Gyenes E, Ruhl GH, et al. Amoxicillin plus omeprazole versus triple therapy for eradication of *Helicobacter pylori* in duodenal ulcer disease: a prospective, randomized, and controlled study. *Gut* 1993;34:1167–1170.
222. Penston JG, McColl KEL. Eradication of *Helicobacter pylori*: an objective assessment of current therapies. *Br J Clin Pharmacol* 1997;43:223–243.
223. Labenz J, Gyenes E, Ruhl GH, et al. Omeprazole plus amoxicillin: efficacy of various treatment regimens to eradicate *Helicobacter pylori. Am J Gastroenterol* 1993;88:491–495.
224. van der Hulst RWM, Weel JFL, Verheul SB, et al. Treatment of *Helicobacter pylori* infection with low- or high-dose omeprazole combined with amoxicillin and the effect of early retreatment: a prospective randomised double-blinded study. *Aliment Pharmacol Ther* 1996;10:165–171.
225. Stables R, Campbell CJ, Clayton NM, et al. Gastric anti-secretory, mucosal-protective, anti-pepsin, and anti-*Helicobacter* properties of ranitidine bismuth citrate. *Aliment Pharmacol Ther* 1993;7:237–246.
226. Peterson WL, Ciociola AA, Sykes DL, et al. Ranitidine bismuth citrate plus clarithromycin is effective for healing duodenal ulcers, eradicating *H. pylori* and reducing ulcer recurrence. *Aliment Pharmacol Ther* 1996;10:251–261.
227. Axon ATR, Ireland A, Lancaster Smith MJ, et al. Ranitidine bismuth citrate and clarithromycin twice daily in the eradication of *Helicobacter pylori. Aliment Pharmacol Ther* 1997;11: 81–87.
228. Dobrilla G, Di Matteo G, Dodero M, et al. Ranitidine bismuth citrate with either clarithromycin 1 g/day or 1.5 g/day is equally effective in the eradication of *H. pylori* and healing of duodenal ulcer. *Aliment Pharmacol Ther* 1997;12:63–68.
229. Chiba N, Rao BV, Rademaker JW, et al. Meta-analysis of the efficacy of antibiotic therapy in eradicating *Helicobacter pylori. Am J Gastroenterol* 1992;87:1716–1727.
230. de Boer WA, Tytgat GNJ. How to treat *Helicobacter pylori* infection—should treatment strategies be based on testing bacterial susceptibility? A personal viewpoint. *Eur J Gastroenterol Hepatol* 1996;8:709–716.
231. Graham DY, Lew GM, Malaty HM, et al. Factors influencing the eradication of *Helicobacter pylori* with triple therapy. *Gastroenterology* 1992;102:493–496.
232. Bell GD, Powell K, Burridge SM, et al. Experience with triple

anti-*H. pylori* eradication therapy: side effects and the importance of testing the pretreatment bacterial isolate for metronidazole resistance. *Aliment Pharmacol Ther* 1992;6:427–435.
233. Thijs JC, van Zwet AA, Oey HB. Efficacy and side effects of a triple drug regimen for the eradication of *H. pylori. Scand J Gastroenterol* 1993;28:934–938.
234. Lind T, Veldhuyzen van Zanten SJO, Unge P, et al. The MACH-1 study: optimal one-week treatment for *H. pylori* defined? *Helicobacter* 1996;1:138–144.
235. van der Hulst RWM, Keller JJ, Rauws EAJ, et al. Treatment of *Helicobacter pylori* infection: a review of the world literature. *Helicobacter* 1996;1:6–19.
236. Moayyedi P, Sahay P, Tompkins DS, et al. Efficacy and optimum dose of omeprazole in a new 1-week triple-therapy regimen to eradicate *Helicobacter pylori. Eur J Gastroenterol Hepatol* 1995;7:835–840.
237. Laine L, Estrada R, Trujillo M, et al. Randomized comparison of differing periods of twice-a-day triple therapy for the eradication of *Helicobacter pylori. Aliment Pharmacol Ther* 1996;10:1029–1033.
238. Ogura K, Yoshida H, Maeda S, et al. Clarithromycin-based triple therapy for nonresistant *Helicobacter pylori* infection. How long should it be given? *Scand J Gastroenterol* 2001;36:548.
239. Calvet X, Gene E, Lopez T, et al. What is the optimal length of proton pump inhibitor-based triple therapies for *Helicobacter pylori*? A cost-effectiveness analysis. *Aliment Pharmacol Ther* 2001;15:1067–1076.
240. Bazzoli F, Zagari RM, Fossi S, et al. Short-term low-dose triple therapy for the eradication of *Helicobacter pylori. Eur J Gastroenterol Hepatol* 1994;6:773–777.
241. Lerang F, Moum B, Haug JB, et al. Highly effective twice-daily triple therapies for *Helicobacter pylori* infection and peptic ulcer disease: does *in vitro* metronidazole resistance have any clinical relevance? *Am J Gastroenterol* 1997;92:248–253.
242. Moayyedi P, Langworthy H, Shanahan K, et al. Comparison of one or two weeks of lansoprazole, amoxicillin, and clarithromycin in the treatment of *Helicobacter pylori. Helicobacter* 1996;1:71–74.
243. Harris AW, Price DI, Gabe SM, et al. Lansoprazole, clarithromycin and metronidazole for seven days in *Helicobacter pylori* infection. *Aliment Pharmacol Ther* 1996;10:1005–1008.
244. Labenz J, Tillenburg B, Weismüller J, et al. Efficacy and tolerability of a one-week triple therapy consisting of pantoprazole, clarithromycin and amoxicillin for cure of *Helicobacter pylori* infection in patients with duodenal ulcer. *Aliment Pharmacol Ther* 1997;11:95–100.
245. Lind T, Mégraud F, Unge P, et al. The MACH-2 study—the role of omeprazole in eradication of *Helicobacter pylori* with one-week triple therapies. *Gastroenterology* 1999;116:248–253.
246. Houben MHMG, van de Beek D, Hensen EF, et al. A systematic review of *Helicobacter pylori* eradication therapy: the impact of antimicrobial resistance on eradication rates. *Aliment Pharmacol Ther* 1999;13:1047–1055.
247. Janssen MJ, van Oijen AH, Verbeek AL, et al. A systematic comparison of triple therapies for treatment of *Helicobacter pylori* infection with proton pump inhibitor/ranitidine bismuth citrate plus clarithromycin and either amoxicillin or a nitroimidazole. *Aliment Pharmacol Ther* 2001;15:613–624.
248. Hentschell E, Brandstätter G, Dragosics B, et al. Effect of ranitidine and amoxicillin plus metronidazole on the eradication of *Helicobacter pylori* and the recurrence of duodenal ulcer. *N Engl J Med* 1993;328:308–312.
249. Spadaccini A, De Fanis C, Sciampa G, et al. Ranitidine vs. omeprazole: short-term triple therapy in patients with *Helicobacter pylori*-positive duodenal ulcer. *Gut* 1995;37:168.
250. Laine L, Estrada R, Trujillo M, et al. Randomized comparison of ranitidine bismuth citrate-based triple therapies for *Helicobacter pylori. Am J Gastroenterol* 1997;92:2213–2215.
251. Gold BD. Current therapy for *Helicobacter pylori* infection in children and adolescents. *Can J Gastroenterol* 1999;13:571–579.
252. de Boer WA, Driessen WMM, Tytgat GNJ. Only four days of quadruple therapy can effectively cure *Helicobacter pylori* infection. *Aliment Pharmacol Ther* 1995;9:633–638.
253. Hosking SW, Ling TKW, Chung SCS, et al. Duodenal ulcer healing by eradication of *H. pylori* without anti-acid treatment: randomised controlled trial. *Lancet* 1994;343:508–510.
254. Hosking SW, Ling TKW, Yung MY, et al. Randomised controlled trial of short-term treatment to eradicate *H. pylori* in patients with duodenal ulcer. *Br Med J* 1992;305:502–504.
255. de Boer W, Driessen W, Jansz A, et al. Effect of acid suppression on efficacy of treatment for *Helicobacter pylori* infection. *Lancet* 1995;345:817–820.
256. de Boer WA, Driessen WMM, Jansz AR, et al. Quadruple therapy compared with dual therapy for eradication of *Helicobacter pylori* in ulcer patients: results of a randomized prospective single-center study. *Eur J Gastroenterol Hepatol* 1995;7:1189–1194.
257. Borody TJ, Andrews P, Fracchia G, et al. Omeprazole enhances efficacy of triple therapy in eradicating *Helicobacter pylori. Gut* 1995;37:477–481.
258. Calvet X, Garcia N, Gene E, et al. Modified seven-day quadruple therapy as a first-line *Helicobacter pylori* treatment. *Aliment Pharmacol Ther* 2001;15:1061–1065.
259. Tucci A, Poli L, Paparo GF, et al. Weekend therapy for the treatment of *Helicobacter pylori* infection. *Am J Gastroenterol* 1998;93:737–742.
260. Graham DS, Malaty H, el-Zimaity HM, et al. Variability with omeprazole–amoxicillin combinations for treatment of *Helicobacter pylori* infection. *Am J Gastroenterol* 1995;90:1415–1418.
261. van der Wouden EJ, Thijs JC, van Zwet AA, et al. The influence of *in vitro* nitroimidazole resistance on the efficacy of nitroimidazole containing anti-*Helicobacter pylori* regimens: a meta-analysis. *Am J Gastroenterol* 1999;94:1751–1759.
262. Perri F, Villani MR, Festa V, et al. Predictors of failure of *Helicobacter pylori* eradication with the standard Maastricht triple therapy. *Aliment Pharmacol Ther* 2001;15:1023–1029.
263. Graham DY, Dore MP. Variability in the outcome of treatment of *Helicobacter pylori* infection: a critical analysis. In: Hunt RH, Tytgat GNJ, eds. Helicobacter pylori. *Basic mechanisms to clinical cure.* Dordrecht: Kluwer Academic Publishers, 1998:426–440.
264. Kearney DJ. Retreatment of *Helicobacter pylori* infection after initial treatment failure. *Am J Gastroenterol* 2001;96:1335–1339.
265. Graham DY. Antibiotic resistance in *Helicobacter pylori*: implications for therapy. *Gastroenterology* 1998;115:1272–1277.
266. Midolo PD, Bell JM, Lambert JR, et al. Antimicrobial resistance testing of *Helicobacter pylori*: a comparison of E-test and disk diffusion methods. *Pathology* 1997;29:411–414.
267. Alarcon T, Domingo D, Lopez-Brea M. Discrepancies between E-test and agar dilution methods for testing metronidazole susceptibility of *Helicobacter pylori. J Clin Microbiol* 1998;36:1165–1166.
268. van der Wouden EJ, van Zwet AA, Vosmaer GD, et al. Rapid increase in the prevalence of metronidazole-resistant *Helicobacter pylori* in the Netherlands. 1997;3:385–389.
269. Lopez-Brea M, Domingo D, Sanchez I, et al. Evolution of resistance to metronidazole and clarithromycin in *Helicobacter pylori* clinical isolates from Spain. *J Antimicrob Chemother* 1997;40:279–281.
270. Dore MP, Leandro G, Realdi G, et al. Effect of pretreatment antibiotic resistance to metronidazole and clarithromycin on outcome of *Helicobacter pylori* therapy: a meta-analytical approach. *Dig Dis Sci* 2000;45:68–76.
271. Debets-Ossenkopp YJ, Sparius M, Kusters JG, et al. Mecha-

nism of clarithromycin resistance in clinical isolates of *Helicobacter pylori. FEMS Microbiol Lett* 1996;142:37–42.
272. Stone GG, Shortridge D, Flamm RK, et al. Identification of a 23S rRNA gene mutation in clarithromycin-resistant *Helicobacter pylori. Helicobacter* 1996;1:227–228.
273. Wang G, Rahman MS, Humayun MZ, et al. Multiplex sequence analysis demonstrates the competitive growth advantage of the A-to-G mutants of clarithromycin-resistant *Helicobacter pylori. Antimicrob Agents Chemother* 1999;43:683–685.
274. Debets-Ossenkopp YJ, Brinkman AB, Kuipers EJ, et al. Explaining the bias in the 23S rRNA gene mutations associated with clarithromycin resistance in clinical isolates of *Helicobacter pylori. Antimicrob Agents Chemother* 1998;42:2749–2751.
275. Xia HX, Buckley M, Keane CT, et al. Clarithromycin resistance in *Helicobacter pylori*: prevalence in untreated dyspeptic patients and stability *in vitro. J Antimicrob Chemother* 1996;37:473–481.
276. Garcia-Arata MI, Baquero F, de Rafael L, et al. Mutations in 23S rRNA in *Helicobacter pylori* conferring resistance to erythromycin do not always confer resistance to clarithromycin. *Antimicrob Agents Chemother* 1999;43:374–376.
277. van Doorn LJ, Debets-Ossenkopp YJ, Marais A, et al. Rapid detection, by PCR and reverse hybridization, of mutations in the *Helicobacter pylori* 23S rRNA gene associated with macrolide resistance. *Antimicrob Agents Chemother* 1999;43:1779–1782.
278. Jeong JY, Mukhopadhyay AK, Akada JK, et al. Roles of FrxA and RdxA nitroreductases of *Helicobacter pylori* in susceptibility and resistance to metronidazole. *J Bacteriol* 2001;183:5155–5162.
279. Nedenskov-Sorensen P, Bukholm G, Bovre K. Natural competence for genetic transformation in *Campylobacter pylori. J Infect Dis* 1990;161:365–366.
280. Wang Y, Roos KP, Taylor DE. Transformation of *Helicobacter pylori* by chromosomal metronidazole resistance and by a plasmid with a selectable chloramphenicol resistance marker. *J Gen Microbiol* 1993;139:2485–2493.
281. Tsuda M, Karita M, Nakazawa T. Genetic transformation in *Helicobacter pylori. Microbiol Immunol* 1993;37:85–89.
282. Pot R, Kusters J, Smeets L, et al. Interspecies transfer of antibiotic resistance between *Helicobacter pylori* and *Helicobacter acinonychis. Antimicrob Agents Chemother* 2001;45:2975–2976.
283. Achtman M, Azuma T, Berg DE, et al. Recombination and clonal groupings within *Helicobacter pylori* from different geographical regions. *Mol Microbiol* 1999;32:459–470.
284. Covacci A, Falkow S, Berg DE, et al. Did the inheritance of a pathogenicity island modify the virulence of *Helicobacter pylori*? [see Comments]. *Trends Microbiol* 1997;5:205–208.
285. Alm RA, Ling LSL, Moir DT, et al. Genomic sequence comparison of two unrelated isolates of the human gastric pathogen *Helicobacter pylori. Nature* 1999;397:176–180.
286. Tomb JF, White O, Kerlavage AR, et al. The complete genome sequence of the gastric pathogen *Helicobacter pylori. Nature* 1997;388:539–547.
287. Weeks DL, Eskandari S, Scott DR, et al. An H^+-gated urea channel: the link between *Helicobacter pylori* urease and gastric colonization. *Science* 2000;287:482–485.
288. Chen M, Lee A, Hazell SL. Immunisation against *Helicobacter* infection in a mouse/*Helicobacter felis* model. *Lancet* 1992;339: 1120–1121.
289. Lee A, Chen MH. Successful immunization against gastric infection with *Helicobacter* species: use of a cholera toxin B-subunit whole-cell vaccine. *Infect Immun* 1994;62:3594–3597.
290. Marchetti M, Rossi M, Giannelli V, et al. Protection against *Helicobacter pylori* infection in mice by intragastric vaccination with *H. pylori* antigens is achieved using a nontoxic mutant of IX coli heat-labile (LT) as adjuvant. *Vaccine* 1998;16:33–37.
291. Sutton P, Lee A. Review article: *Helicobacter pylori* vaccines—the current status. *Aliment Pharmacol Ther* 2000;14:1107–1118.
292. Angelakopoulos H, Hohmann EL. Pilot study of *phoP/phoQ*-deleted *Salmonella enterica* serovar Typhimurium expressing *Helicobacter pylori* urease in adult volunteers. *Infect Immun* 2000;68:2135–2141.
293. Ermak TH, Giannasca PJ, Nichols R, et al. Immunization of mice with urease vaccine affords protection against *Helicobacter pylori* infection in the absence of antibodies and is mediated by MHC class II-restricted responses. *J Exp Med* 1998;188: 2277–2288.
294. Nedrud JG, Blanchard TG, Gottwein JM, et al. Systematic vaccination inducing either Th1 or Th2 immunity protects mice from challenge with *Helicobacter pylori. Immunol Lett* 1999; 69:52.
295. American Gastroenterological Association. Medical position statement: evaluation of dyspepsia. *Gastroenterology* 1998;114: 579–581.
296. Hunt R, Fallone CA, Thompson ABR. Canadian *Helicobacter pylori* consensus conference update: infection in adults. Canadian *Helicobacter pylori* Study Group. *Can J Gastroenterol* 1999; 13:213–217.
297. Rubin GP, Meineche-Schmidt V, Roberts AP, et al. The management of *Helicobacter pylori* infection in primary care. Guidelines from the ESPCG. *Eur J Gen Pract* 1999;5:98–104.
298. Lam SK, Talley NJ. Report of the 1997 Asia Pacific consensus conference on the management of *Helicobacter pylori* infection. *J Gastroenterol Hepatol* 1998;13:1–12.
299. de Paula las Rua L, Aleixo A. Brazilian consensus on *Helicobacter pylori* and associated diseases. *Acta Gastroenterol Latinoam* 1996;26:255–260.
300. Asaka M, Satoh K, Sugano K, et al. Guidelines in the management of *Helicobacter pylori* infection in Japan. *Helicobacter* 2001;6:177–186.

35

HELICOBACTER HEILMANNII AND OTHER GASTRIC INFECTIONS OF HUMANS

JANI L. O'ROURKE
ADRIAN LEE
JOHN E. KELLOW

Bacterial infections of the stomach have, until recently, been considered to be rare in humans, most commonly manifesting as secondary infections associated with disorders such as syphilis and tuberculosis (1). Our concepts of the stomach as an inhospitable environment for bacterial colonization, however, have been altered by the discovery that the bacterium *Helicobacter pylori* commonly colonizes the human stomach (2,3).

The observation of colonization of the gastric mucosa by large numbers of spiral-shaped bacteria is not new; for more than 100 years, these organisms have been reported in the stomachs of a wide range of animals (4–6). The data were much less definitive for humans. Scattered reports of spiral bacteria in human gastric samples appeared early in the past century (7), with the most systematic and accurate description of human gastric spiral-shaped bacteria coming from Doenges in 1939 (8). Doenges described four different types of bacteria in human gastric samples obtained at autopsy. The most prevalent organism, a "thick spirochaete with 2-3 turns," has come to be accepted as having been *H. pylori.* Moreover, in two cases, Doenges described a "spirochaete which showed sharp angulation, with 6-8 turns," which he had seen regularly in monkeys and which corresponded to earlier descriptions of the bacteria commonly seen in several other animal species (6). Similar bacteria were first described in 1987 by Dent and colleagues (9) in the post–*H. pylori* era when they described three cases of gastritis in humans associated with such an organism (9). *H. pylori* was not observed in any of these patients. The unofficial name *"Gastrospirillum hominis"* was originally assigned to this organism (10), but subsequent studies showed it belonged to the *Helicobacter* genus and the name *"Helicobacter heilmannii"* was proposed (11). The possibility arose that this represented another bacterium that could be associated with gastric disease in humans. This initial report alerted histopathologists to the existence of these organisms and, since then, more than 500 cases have appeared in the literature of the association of *H. heilmannii* with a variety of disease states in adults and children. The diagnoses in these patients have ranged from acute and chronic gastritis to peptic ulceration and gastric malignancy.

A third spiral bacterium has also been associated with human gastric disease. It is another *Helicobacter* species, *Helicobacter felis,* which was originally isolated from cats and dogs (12). It has been associated with three cases of gastritis in humans (13–15).

This chapter draws attention to the rare group of non–*H. pylori* gastric infections, including the newly discovered *Helicobacter* species as well as syphilis, tuberculosis, anthrax, and various mycotic infections. These infections not only result in serious illness in some instances, but they also can complicate diagnosis of more serious illnesses (e.g., gastric carcinoma) because they may mimic the symptoms of these diseases. Also discussed is the potential deleterious effect of bacterial overgrowth in the stomach, which accompanies the continual use of antimicrobial, immunosuppressive, and acid-suppressive therapies.

HELICOBACTER HEILMANNII (*GASTROSPIRILLUM HOMINIS*) AND OTHER GASTRIC *HELICOBACTER* INFECTIONS

Nomenclature

In this chapter, *"Gastrospirillum hominis"* and *"Helicobacter heilmannii"* are treated as the same organism. Other gastric

J. L. O'Rourke: Department of Microbiology and Immunology, University of New South Wales, Sydney, Australia

A. Lee: Department of Microbiology and Immunology, University of New South Wales, Sydney, Australia

J. E. Kellow: Department of Medicine, University of Sydney; Department of Gastroenterology, Royal North Shore Hospital, St. Leonard's, Sydney, Australia organisms that are morphologically identical to *H. heilmannii* include *Helicobacter bizzezeronii,* which has been successfully cultured from dog gastric mucosa (16), and *Candidatus Helicobacter suis,* which has yet to be cultured but is commonly found in pigs (17).

The original molecular studies of *H. heilmannii*–like bacteria showed the 16S ribosomal RNA sequences from two human samples (clones G1A1 and G2A9) were distinct (96.5% similarity), with both of them showing high degrees of homology with *H. felis* and *H. pylori* (97% to 98% and 95%, respectively) (11). The 16S rRNA gene has been a highly conserved gene over the course of bacterial evolution and is used to determine evolutionary differences among bacteria (18). Indeed, the 16S rRNA gene has been routinely used in identifying new members of the *Helicobacter* genus, which includes bacteria with a number of different morphologies located in a range of sites from a variety of hosts (19). Recent analysis of a number of *H. heilmannii*–like bacteria from humans and a number of animals has shown that the bacteria cluster into the two groups representing the two different human samples described earlier (20). These two groups are commonly referred to as *H. heilmannii* type I and type II. The basis for this differentiation is analysis of their 16S rRNA gene and urease gene. The type I strains comprise the majority of isolates found in humans, including *H. heilmannii* clone G1A1 (11) and those seen in pigs and a number of different primate species. Because this group is the dominant organism found in human infection, we are proposing that these organisms be referred to as *Helicobacter heilmannii* (in honor of the German histopathologist Konrad Heilmann [21]). None of these bacteria have as yet been cultured *in vitro*. The Type II strains include *H. heilmannii* clone G2A9 (11), a *H. heilmannii*–like organism (HHLO) cultured from human gastric mucosa (22,23) and isolates commonly found in cats and dogs (24). These bacteria also cluster closely with a number of the cultured species, including *H. bizzezeronii, H. salomonis,* and *H. felis.*

Description

H. heilmannii is a gram-negative, tightly spiraled or helical-shaped organism with between 4 and 20 turns (10,21,23, 25,26). These organisms are 4 to 10 μm in length and 0.5 to 1 μm in width, and they possess at least 12 to 14 sheathed flagella, 28 nm in diameter (Fig. 35.1*A*). Electron microscopic analysis has shown these bacteria to have truncated ends, an electron lucent area in the terminal region of the organism, and a *polar membrane*, similar to that found in other *Helicobacter* species and spiral-shaped bacteria (27).

H. felis is indistinguishable from *H. heilmannii* by light microscopy, with the major morphologic trait that differentiates these two organisms—the presence of periplasmic fibers—only observable by electron microscopy (Fig.

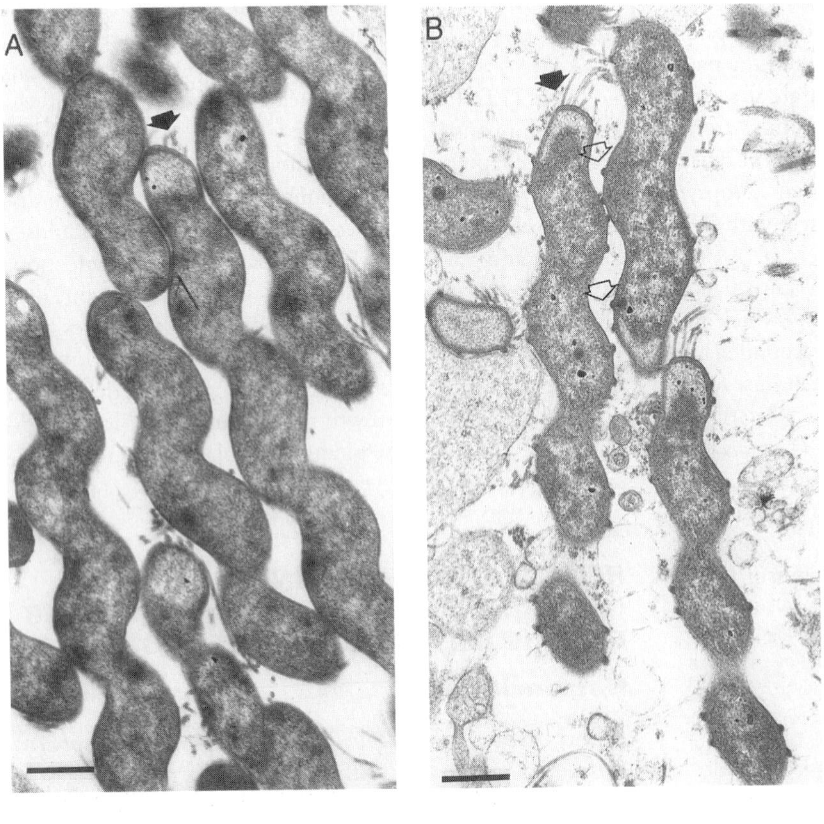

FIGURE 35.1. Transmission electron micrograph of *Helicobacter heilmannii* **(A)** and *Helicobacter felis* **(B)** showing the characteristic spiral/helical morphology of the bacteria and the tufts of flagella (*closed arrow*). The periplasmic fibers, characteristic of *H. felis*, are also indicated (*open arrow*). (Bars, 0.5 μm).

35.1*B*). *H. felis* is generally entwined by such periplasmic fibers; although the fibers usually are in pairs, their number can vary (12).

Microbiology

In addition to the standard methods used for the cultivation of other *Helicobacter* species, a variety of different types of enriched media and atmospheric conditions have been used in attempts to culture *H. heilmannii* type I strains from human gastric biopsies. None have been successful (10,25). By applying methods used by Salomon (6), we have been able to maintain human isolates of this bacterium *in vivo* (28,29). Specific pathogen-free mice were inoculated orally with gastric biopsy specimens obtained from human patients known to harbor *H. heilmannii*. The gastric mucosa of the mice was rapidly colonized with the helical organisms, which were kept alive by passage from mouse to mouse via oral administration of infected gastric homogenates.

H. felis was first cultured from the gastric mucosa of a cat, and, like *H. pylori*, it can be cultivated on blood agar plates containing Skirrow selective supplement (Oxoid, Basingstoke, United Kingdom) with microaerobic conditions and a high percentage of humidity (12). The HHLO was cultured from human biopsy specimens on nonselective lysed horse blood agar plates incubated under microaerobic conditions for at least 5 days (23). Both these organisms share many phenotypic traits with *H. pylori*, that is, they are urease, catalase, and oxidase positive and do not readily use carbohydrates (12, 23). In addition, sequence analysis of the urease genes of *H. heilmannii* and *H. felis* reveals that they share a high degree of homology with the urease genes of *H. pylori* (30).

Epidemiology

The prevalence of gastric infection with *H. heilmannii* is low, ranging from 0.2% to 0.6% in developed countries (10,13,21,31–33). Similar prevalence rates have been seen in asymptomatic patients (34) and in children (35). By comparison, higher prevalence rates (1.2% to 6.2%) have been reported in Eastern European countries (36) and Asian countries (37–40). Infection occurs at any age (range 2 to 79 years), is more commonly seen in male patients, and can be long term in nature (4 and 10 years) (21,41).

Even though the epidemiology of these infections is not completely understood, initial reports indicated that the infection could be a zoonoses (10,14,24,25,42). This concept was highlighted by Meining and co-workers (43) who showed in a large study of patients infected with *H. heilmannii* that, in comparison with *H. pylori*–infected individuals, contact with pigs, cats, and dogs led to a significant risk of *H. heilmannii* infection (odds ration, 4.99, 1.71, and 1.46 respectively) (43). Furthermore, successful eradication of *H. heilmannii* from a 12-year-old girl and her pet dog resulted in resolution of gastric disease in both the girl and her dog (44). Similar large helical-shaped bacteria are widespread in the animal kingdom, with hosts including domestic pets such as cats and dogs, farm animals such as pigs, and more exotic species including nonhuman primates and "big cats." Generally, in these hosts, the bacteria have been associated with a mild form of gastritis (45–49); however, in pigs, a strong association between gastric ulcer disease of the pars esophagus and the presence of *H. heilmannii* has been documented (50).

Given the ubiquity of *H. heilmannii* and *H. felis* infected animals, it is surprising that more humans are not infected with these bacteria. The bacteria appears to be relatively difficult to transmit, an observation consistent with the epidemiology of human *H. pylori* infection. Subtle differences between *H. pylori* and *H. heilmannii* may not allow the latter organism to readily colonize human gastric mucosa. It is unlikely that fecal-oral spread is involved; if this were the case, the infection rate in developing countries would be very high given the contamination of food and drinking water with animal excreta. Current evidence suggests an oral-oral route of transmission.

Pathogenesis and Immunity

The majority of reports of *H. heilmannii* infection are associated with a mild to moderate gastritis (Fig. 35.2*A* and *B*); however, there have been reports of duodenal ulceration (41,51,52), gastric ulceration (26,31,41,53,54), two cases of gastric carcinoma (38,55), and seven cases of mucosa-associated lymphoid tissue (MALT) lymphoma (Fig. 35.3) (33,41). The presence of these organisms is usually associated with an active chronic gastritis that tends to be less aggressive than *H. pylori* infections in humans (41). This is characterized by an infiltrate of polymorphonuclear leukocytes, lymphocytes, and plasma cells in the lamina propria. In some cases, superficial chronic gastritis, gastric neoplasia, or infiltration into the foveolar epithelium also has been present. An increasing number of acute infections are being reported in which the antral mucosa histologically shows acute erosions, congestion, and edema with severe infiltrates of polymorphonuclear neutrophil leukocytes in the lamina propria (Fig. 35.2*C*) (13,14,54,56).

H. heilmannii has been found to localize in the surface gastric mucosa and in the necks of and deep within the gastric glands (Fig. 35.4) (26). There does not appear to be evidence of direct attachment of the bacteria to the gastric epithelial cells, unlike infection with *H. pylori*. The colonization pattern is antral dominant (21, 41). Intracellular localization has only been rarely observed because of the small number of biopsy samples examined using electron microscopy (21,25). In these cases, the bacteria were seen in the cytoplasm and canniculi of parietal cells, and were associated with mitochondrial swelling and more severe degen-

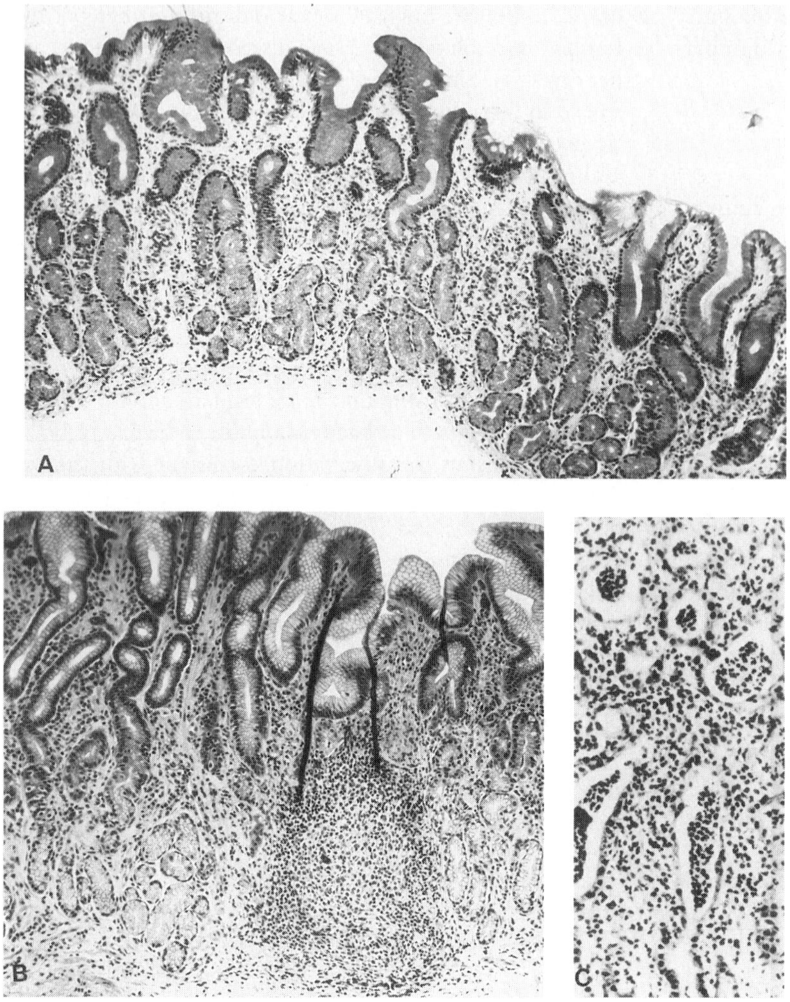

FIGURE 35.2. Gastric biopsies of patients colonized with *Helicobacter heilmannii* revealing mild chronic gastritis. **A:** Diffuse infiltrate of lymphoid cells as well as scattered eosinophils in the lamina propria of the mucosae (×450). **B:** As above, with a distinct lymphoid follicle abutting the muscularis mucosa (×450). **C:** A patient colonized with *Helicobacter felis* revealing acute diffuse gastritis (×200). (Micrograph courtesy of Wegmann W, Aschwanden M, Schaub N, et al. *Gastrospirillum hominis*-assoziierte gastritis - eine zoonose? *Schweiz Med Wochenschr* 1991;121:245–254.)

erative changes in cytoplasmic organelles. Heilmann suggested that a possible cytopathic effect may be indicated by the presence of lysozymes and vacuoles.

In their natural hosts, the presence of *H. heilmannii* is associated with a primary infiltration of mononuclear cells and lymphoid aggregates with little active inflammation with neutrophils. However, the mononuclear infiltration can be extensive and tissue damage does appear in some cases (45,47–49). In a foreign host, these animal *Helicobacter* organisms can induce significant pathology, which has been the basis of many small animal model studies. *H. felis* induces an aggressive active/chronic gastritis in germ-free mice (57). Long-term infection (more than 18 months) of conventional Swiss mice with these same organisms results in a progressively destructive atrophic gastritis (58) that is very similar to that seen in some patients with *H. pylori* infection. Lesions indicative of low-grade B-cell MALT lymphoma have also been observed in up to 25% of BABL/c mice infected long-term (18 to 26 months) with *H. heilmannii* or *H. felis* (59,60).

Clinical Features

In the majority of published reports of infection with *H. heilmannii* patients present with epigastric pain or discomfort. Other symptoms include nausea and, to a lesser extent, vomiting, anorexia, weight loss, diarrhea, and occasional gastrointestinal bleeding (32). According to the classification of functional dyspepsia proposed by Drossman and associates (61), most patients appear to fit the category of "ulcer-like" dyspepsia.

Diagnosis

Whereas macroscopically normal gastroduodenal mucosa is often seen at upper gastrointestinal panendoscopy, other findings have ranged from antral erythema to more severe antral gastritis, including erosions, gastric ulceration, edematous gastric mucosa with enlarged gastric folds, and duodenal erosions and ulceration (14,22,26,52–54,56,62). Ulcerated lesions were noted in the cases of gastric cancer (38,55), and

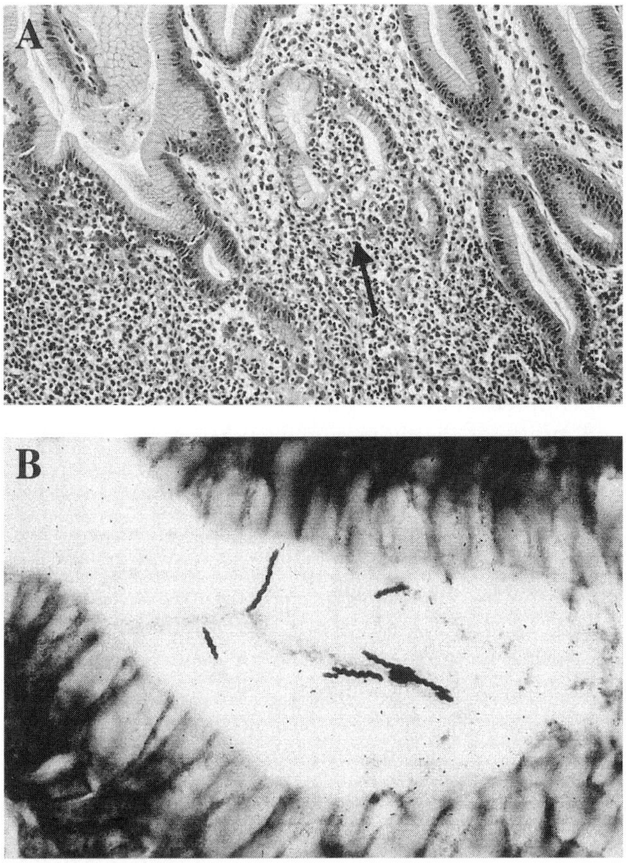

FIGURE 35.3. A: Histologic section of a low-grade mucosa associated lymphoid tissue lymphoma stained with hematoxylin and eosin showing mucosal infiltration with atypical lymphoid cells and lymphoepithelial destructions. **B:** Warthin-Starry stain showing *Helicobacter. heilmannii* on the surface of the epithelium. (Micrograph courtesy of 33. Morgner A, Lehn N, Andersen LP, et al. *Helicobacter heilmannii*-associated primary gastric low-grade MALT lymphoma: complete remission after curing the infection. *Gastroenterology* 2000;118:821–828.)

flat-polypoid tumors (1 to 4 cm) were seen in the patients with MALT lymphoma (33). Lymphoid nodules have been seen in a number of cases of *H. heilmannii* infection in children (35,44,53,63,64) (T. Bohane and J. Mitchell, personal communication), a feature rarely seen in adults.

The bacteria can be identified in gastric biopsy samples by observation of their distinct morphology (Figs. 35.3 and 35.4). Even though they can be seen in hematoxylin and eosin stained sections, they are more obvious when a Giemsa or silver stain is used. Alternatively, touch cytology of gastric smears appears to be a more sensitive method for detecting these bacteria (32).

Because *H. pylori* is associated with the majority of gastric infections, urease biopsy tests and serology have often been used to aid diagnosis. The rate of detected urease positivity appears lower than that for *H. pylori*. This may be misleading because a much slower change in the urease reaction than that commonly seen for *H. pylori* infections has been reported, probably due to lower numbers of bacteria colonizing the gastric mucosa (26). Serology results in which *H. pylori* is used as the primary antigen are not always reliable; studies have shown higher rates of seropositivity if *H. heilmannii* or *H. felis* are used as the primary antigen (33,65).

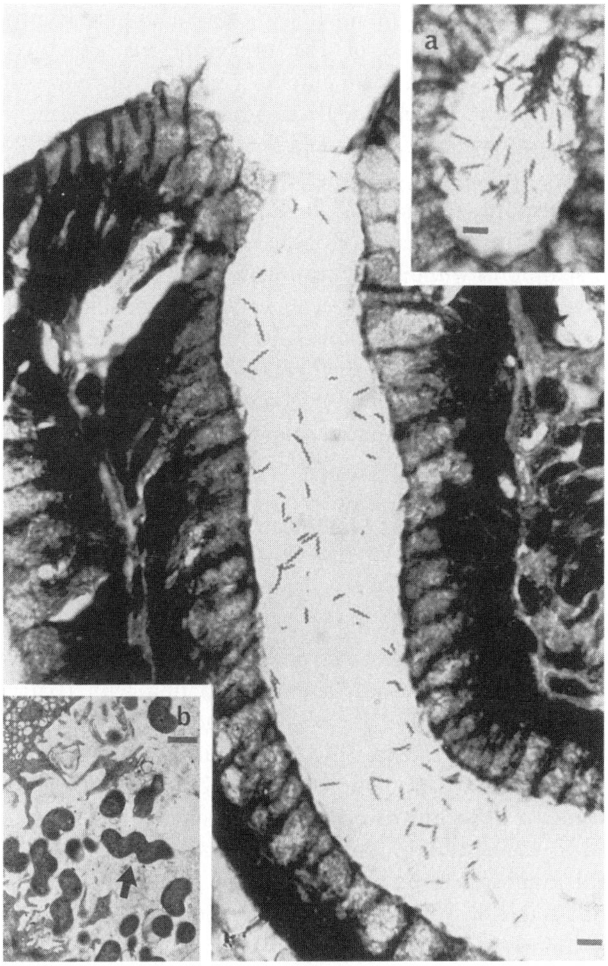

FIGURE 35.4. Gastric biopsy of a patient colonized with *Helicobacter heilmannii* showing the localization of the bacteria in the gastric lumen and deep into gastric glands **(A and B)** (bars, 5 μm) with higher magnification revealing the close association with microvilli **(C)** (bar, 1 μm). (Micrograph courtesy of Dick E, Lee A, Watson G, et al. Use of the mouse for the isolation and investigation of stomach-associated, spiral-helical shaped bacteria from man and other animals. *J Med Microbiol* 1989;29:55–62.

Mixed infection with both *H. pylori* and *H. heilmannii* has been reported in approximately 5% of cases, although monoinfection appears to be the norm (21,36,42,66).

Treatment

Treatment with bismuth, amoxicillin, metronidazole, H_2 blockers, and proton pump inhibitors in various combinations has been undertaken. Complete or near complete resolution of symptoms has occurred in the majority of patients to date (10,21,25,26,36,54,62). In the absence of placebo-controlled studies, however, it is difficult to gauge the significance of symptomatic improvement in functional dyspepsia. Clearance of the organism has also been obtained with such regimens. In a number of follow-up biopsy specimens, obtained 1 to 5 months after treatment, the characteristic bacteria could not be detected and the histologic appearance of the gastric tissue had improved or returned to normal (25,26,36,52,54). Several reports describe the disappearance of the bacterium and resolution of symptoms without any treatment being undertaken. Of more significance is the recent report of remission of primary gastric low-grade MALT lymphoma in five patients who had been cured of their *H. heilmannii* infection. Successful eradication of the bacteria was obtained by treating the patients with omeprazole and amoxicillin (33).

TREPONEMA PALLIDUM

Description

Changes in medical and social practices have recently altered our view on gastric syphilis. At the turn of the century, gastric syphilis was a rare association with tertiary syphilis (less than 1% of cases) with the incidence of these clinical identities decreasing as a result of the successful introduction of antibiotics (67). A recent increase in the incidence of syphilis associated with drug use, however, has led to an increasing number of reports of gastric syphilis, and it appears to be more commonly associated with the early stages of syphilis (68–70). In addition, the acceptance of *H. pylori* as a gastric pathogen and the large numbers of gastric biopsy specimens being examined increases the possibility of detecting other bacteria such as *T. pallidum.*

A history of untreated or inadequately treated syphilis usually has been regarded as a necessary criterion to establish a clinical diagnosis of gastric syphilis (67). The causative organism, *T. pallidum*, is a long slender spirochete (8 to15 μm × 0.2 μm), which is best visualized by dark-field microscopy or by the Warthin-Starry silver stain.

Clinical Features

Symptoms of gastric syphilis are nonspecific and depend on the stage of the illness (particularly for tertiary syphilis), the site of the gastric lesion (body or antrum), and the degree of associated deformity. The most common symptoms include ulcer-like abdominal pain, vomiting, gastrointestinal bleeding, weight loss, nausea, and early satiety (69,70).

Diagnosis

In its secondary or tertiary stage, syphilis can cause a wide range of gastric lesions, which can mimic other entities such as benign gastric ulceration, gastric carcinoma, or lymphoma. At upper gastrointestinal endoscopy or on contrast radiology, antral narrowing is the most frequent anatomic deformity seen, producing a funnel-shaped deformity or even a "linitis plastica" appearance, although ulceration with raised nodular edges or gumma within the gastric wall are also observed. An hourglass stomach may be produced if the predominant reaction has occurred in the fundus. In early secondary syphilis, edematous erythematous mucosa with scattered erosions can be present at endoscopy, whereas in late secondary syphilis, an erosive gastritis, particularly an edematous, friable, ulcerated antral mucosa, can be observed (68–71). Histologically, biopsies demonstrate a nonspecific chronic gastritis with an infiltrate of lymphocytes and plasma cells, variable degree of glandular destruction and reactive atypia, and a vasculitis without proliferative changes (68).

A survey of the more recent reports of gastric syphilis shows that concomitant infection with *H. pylori* is common (10 of 18 cases), which could influence treatment (68–73).

Definitive diagnosis of gastric syphilis can be confirmed by visualization of *T. pallidum* during examination of fresh biopsy material by dark-field microscopy or by positive staining of fixed tissue by specific fluorescent antibodies or by Warthin-Starry silver stain. As for many other bacterial infections, a polymerase chain reaction has been described that detects *T. pallidum* in fixed gastric specimens (73). Antibodies induced by *T. pallidum* infection also can be detected in patients' sera; the most commonly used technique is the VDRL (Venereal Disease Research Laboratory) slide flocculation test. The VDRL test also is useful for follow-up studies to determine whether treatment has been successful in eradicating the bacterium.

Treatment

Penicillin (e.g., benzathine penicillin G) remains the treatment of choice for gastric syphilis. The specific regimen depends on the stage and duration of the illness. The Centers for Disease Control and Prevention have outlined a recommended therapy. For early syphilis (primary, secondary, or latent infections of less than 1 year), 2.4 million units of penicillin G are given intramuscularly at a single session; the dosage is increased to three successive weekly intramuscular injections of 2.4 million units for syphilis of more than a 1-year duration (1). Alternative treatments using tetracycline have also been described for patients allergic to penicillin.

MYCOBACTERIUM TUBERCULOSIS

Description

Gastric tuberculosis is rarely encountered, although persons with primary pulmonary tuberculosis are at a higher risk of gastric infection. Older studies have shown prevalence levels ranging from 0.2% in normal necropsy specimens to 2.3% in necroscopy specimens obtained from patients with pulmonary tuberculosis (67). A number of case reports have appeared recently, possibly because of an increase in the worldwide incidence in pulmonary tuberculosis, which is especially prevalent in persons in developing countries, in migrants to developed countries, and in AIDS patients (74–78). The causative organism, *M. tuberculosis*, is a slender curved rod (2 to 4 μm × 0.2 to 0.5 μm) that exhibits properties of an intracellular parasite, primarily infecting macrophages. The organism is very slow growing but it can be cultured on specialized media and is most easily visualized by a Ziehl-Neelsen stain because of its acid-fast properties.

The bacteria can directly invade the gastric mucosa, enter via the bloodstream or lymphatic system, or invade by direct extension from adjacent structures. In patients with pulmonary tuberculosis, a gastric infection with *M. tuberculosis* can readily be superimposed on a preexisting, nonspecific lesion in the stomach (67) There also appears to be an association of gastric tuberculosis with gastric carcinoma.

Clinical Features

As with the other chronic gastric infections, the symptoms of gastric tuberculosis are nonspecific and include ulcer-like dyspepsia, weight loss, vomiting, and gastric bleeding. The majority of patients have symptoms and signs of tuberculosis at other sites in the body, including the intestine. Clinical features of gastric outlet obstruction may be present and a palpable abdominal mass occurs in approximately 50% of cases.

Diagnosis

Radiologic findings in the stomach are nonspecific. Thus, single or multiple gastric ulcerations are frequently present and may simulate benign gastric ulceration, gastric carcinoma, lymphoma, or Crohn's disease. There is often a continuity of ulceration from the duodenum into the antrum of the stomach. A hypertrophic response in the submucosa can produce gastric wall thickening and annular constriction of the lumen (79). Pyloric stenosis, or even fistula formation, also may occur (80,81). Endoscopically, the lesions are typically small, often multiple, shallow ulcerations that are more prominent in the distal stomach. Biopsies may demonstrate gastritis only; definitive diagnosis depends on the demonstration of tubercle bacilli or a caseating granuloma. Mycobacteria, however, can be demonstrated in tissue in only one-third of cases (82).

Treatment

Usually, treatment with three antituberculosis drugs is the appropriate management. The drugs of choice are isoniazid (300 mg/day), rifampicin (600 mg/day), and pyrazinamide (2 g/day) with ethambutol (1.2 g/day) and streptomycin (1 g/day) being used in some instances. Response to such chemotherapy is usually relatively rapid and effective, and various treatment regimens with periods of therapy of 6 to 9 or 18 to 24 months have been used. In the hypertrophic form of the disease, however, chemotherapy may not be as effective, necessitating surgical resection or bypass.

MYCOTIC INFECTIONS

Description

A number of systemic mycotic infections can involve the stomach in an invasive fashion, but these are exceedingly rare. Examples are *Candida*, *Mucor*, and *Rhizophus* species, *Histoplasma capsulatum* (83), *Torulopsis glabrata*, *Actinomyces israelii* (84), *Aspergillus fumigatus* (85) and *Basidiobolus ranarum* (86). *Candida albicans* has been the most frequently reported. Predisposing factors that result in increased frequency of gastric infection include diabetes, malignancies, burns, trauma, pregnancy, bone marrow transplantation, and immunodeficiency syndromes.

Clinical Features

Symptoms such as epigastric pain, anorexia, nausea, vomiting, and weight loss have been reported. However, symptoms are usually more pronounced if candidiasis is present in other areas of the gastrointestinal tract. Gastric candidiasis may be more prevalent in patients with previous partial gastrectomy.

Diagnosis

The radiologic appearance of gastric candidiasis reflects mucosal ulceration and submucosal invasion. Gastric spongelike semifluid masses appear to be typical of severe cases, in addition to filling defects, superficial ulceration, enlarged gastric folds, and a lack of gastric distensibility (87,88). At endoscopy, the presence of single or multiple whitish plaques, which are confluent and may form white or grey membranes, are characteristic of gastric candidiasis (89). Mucosal brushings of the lesions have a greater yield than biopsy specimens (90). Mucosal biopsies often demonstrate acute or chronic inflammation with absence of fungi.

Gastric infection with *H. capsulatum* can result in polypoid nodules that, by microscopy, are found to be submucosal focal aggregates of macrophages heavily infected with the fungi. Other mycotic infections manifest as necrotic lesions in which the causative organism often can be detected (83). Lately, however, *B. ranarum* was cultured from the gastric mucosa of a 37-year-old black woman who showed evidence of ulceration, necrosis and marked mural thickening (86).

A number of reports of gastric invasion by fungal agents in association with bone marrow transplantation and graft-versus-host disease have appeared in the literature. In one instance, the patient had a large gastric ulcer and necrotic ulceration in the distal esophagus with evidence of both fungal and cytomegalovirus infection. He showed an improvement in symptoms after therapy with amphotericin B, proton pump inhibitors, and ganciclovir (91). A second case involved a patient who died 10 days after presenting with severe diarrhea and diffuse abdominal pain. The postmortem findings included confluent bronchopneumonia and a 1.5-cm thick pseudomembrane covering the entire gastric mucosa, with both of these findings associated with the presence of *Aspergillus* species (85).

Treatment

Culture is required to determine the species and susceptibility to antifungal agents. For *C. albicans*, oral nystatin therapy is simple and often effective in cases that appear superficial as visualized by endoscopy. Amphotericin B or ketoconazole is useful in deeply invasive disease states. Yeast bezoars can usually be treated satisfactorily by mechanical disruption and oral nystatin.

OTHER GASTRIC INFECTIONS

The stomach is sometimes susceptible to infection by other microorganisms including *Bacillus anthracis*, protozoans, especially *Giardia lamblia*, and parasites such as *Strongyloides stercoralis* and *Anisakis* species.

Primary anthrax may develop in the stomach through the ingestion of contaminated foodstuffs. Infection can result in the invasion of the gastric mucosa and secondary ulceration, which then may disseminate to the bloodstream, possibly resulting in meningitis. Patients present with nonspecific symptoms; however, bleeding with hematemesis or melena may occur. The characteristic gram-positive spore-forming rod can be detected by culture or biopsy. Penicillin G remains the drug of choice for treatment (1).

G. lamblia has been reported in 0.3% of patients with upper gastrointestinal symptoms, usually in the presence of intestinal metaplasia or *H. pylori* infection (92). The protozoa can be found in the foveolar pits and in the overlying epithelium. Affected persons usually have moderate or severe chronic atrophic gastritis. The infection has been associated with a decrease in gastric acidity because some patients only become colonized with the protozoa after treatment with H_2 antagonists.

There have also been recent case reports of a *S. stercoralis* infection of the stomach (93, 94). The patients presented with symptoms of abdominal pain and distention, high temperature, diarrhea, and weight loss. Endoscopy of two patients revealed a large prepyloric ulcer with evidence of recent bleeding in one case and gastritis with linear erythema in the other case. In both cases, the lumen and mucosa were infiltrated by helminthic eggs and larvae, which were cleared with thiabendazole treatment, coinciding with resolution of symptoms.

Two cases of stomach granuloma have been associated with *Anisakis*-like nematodes (95). The worms penetrated into the stomach wall, causing severe diffuse inflammatory reactions, and were detected in submucosal granulomata associated with necrosis, extensive eosinophilic infiltration, and ulcerative lesions.

BACTERIAL OVERGROWTH IN THE STOMACH

Gastric acidity is of benefit to the human host in two major ways: as an aid to digestion and as a barrier to the entry of pathogens into the intestinal tract. If the acidity of the stomach is lowered, the gastric lumen may become colonized with large numbers of bacteria, which could result in clinical consequences. The two main predisposing factors that allow bacteria overgrowth are acid-suppressive therapy and increasing age.

There is a clear inverse relationship between the number of bacteria in gastric and duodenal secretions and the level of gastric acid. Drasar (96) showed that normal subjects with gastric pH less than 4 have fewer than 10^4 bacteria/mL in their fasting gastric juice (96). In contrast, patients on acid-suppressive therapy show a significant increase in the numbers of gastric bacteria that may occur after only 12 hours of acid suppression (97). Acid-suppressive therapy is commonly used in intensive care patients to prevent the development of stress ulcers, but it may also predispose patients to nosocomial pneumonia. This controversy has been excellently reviewed by Tryba (98), who concludes that drugs that increase the frequency of patients with gastric pH greater than 4 significantly increase the risk of pulmonary infection, at least among ventilated patients in the intensive care unit (98). Another source of nosocomial infection in critically ill patients may be translocation of intestinal bacteria across ischemic gastrointestinal epithelium (99).

Others claim a relationship between gastric acid secretion and advancing age (100). In a Norwegian study of 15 healthy older persons (mean age, 84 years), 12 (80%) were hypochlorhydric with a pH of 6.6 and a mean bacterial count of 10^8 colony forming units (CFU) per milliliter (range 10^5 to 10^{10}) in their fasting gastric aspirate (101). In contrast, Wormsley and Grossman (102) studied 75 control subjects, including 14 persons older than 60 years of age, and found no significant difference in acid secretion (102). The reason for these differences could probably be due to differences in rates of *H. pylori* infection or the degree of atrophic gastritis, the latter of which impairs acid secretion as a result of ablation of parietal cell function.

The origin of these overgrowing bacteria is also uncertain. In the group of healthy elderly persons with fasting hypochlorhydria described earlier, the microbial flora were dominated by viridans streptococci, coagulase-negative staphylococci, and *Haemophilus* species, indicating that the normal site of contamination is from the oral cavity (101). In another study of 108 patients, the majority were shown to have bacteria in the duodenum with a predominance of *E. coli* and *Enterococcus faecalis* (103). Thus, when duodenogastric reflux occurs, these fecal-type bacteria could seed the stomach. There are groups in which this phenomenon occurs with increased frequency (e.g., the severe atrophic gastritis associated with gastric cancer) (104), accounting for why patients with gastric carcinoma have a high rate of colonization with bacteria typical of the lower gastrointestinal tract (105).

CONCLUSION

H. pylori is the major pathogen infecting the human stomach. However, this chapter draws attention to a miscellany of other organisms that can, in certain circumstances, proliferate in the gastric mucosa with potentially deleterious effects to the host. These uncommon conditions should be considered when managing the small subsets of patients for whom a pathogen is suspected and *H. pylori* is not isolated or detected.

ACKNOWLEDGMENTS

This work is supported by the National Health and Medical Research Council of Australia. We would also like to thank the following for providing us with unpublished data relating to patients colonized with *H. heilmannii*: Dr. T. Bohane, Dr. J. Mitchell, Dr. T. Borody, Dr. C. Meredith, Dr. L. Hillman, Dr. W. Davies, Dr. G. Daskalopoulos, Dr. F. Bonar, Dr. R. Fischer, Dr. N. Figura, Prof. W. Wegmann, Dr. D. Queiroz, Dr. B. Marshall, Dr. A. Morris, Dr. H. Yang, and Dr. E. Ierardi.

REFERENCES

1. Manten HD , Harary AM. Chronic infections of the stomach. In: Berk JE, eds. *Bockus gastroenterology,* fourth edition. Philadelphia: WB Saunders, 1985:1328–1342.
2. Marshall BJ. Unidentified curved bacillus on gastric epithelium in active chronic gastritis. *Lancet* 1983;1:1273–1275.
3. Warren JR. Unidentified curved bacilli on gastric epithelium in active chronic gastritis. *Lancet* 1983;1:1273.
4. Rappin JP. Contr a l'etude de bacterium de la bouche a l'etat normal. Quoted. In: Breed RS, Murray EGD, Hitchens AP, eds. *Bergey's manual of determinative bacteriology,* sixth edition. Baltimore: Williams & Wilkins, 1881:68.
5. Bizzozero G. Ueber die schlauchfoermigen drusen des magendarmkanals und die beziehungen ihres epithels zu dem oberfachenepithel der schleimhaut. *Arch f Mikr Anat* 1892;42:82–152.
6. Salomon H. Uber das spirillum des saugetiermagens und sein verhalten zu den belegzellen. *Zentralb f Bakt* 1896;19:433–441.
7. Kreinitz W. Ueber das auftreten von spirochaeten verschiedener form im magenihalt bei carcinoma ventriculi. *Dsch Med Wochenschr* 1906;32:872.
8. Doenges JL. Spirochaetes in the gastric glands of *Macacus rhesus* and humans without definite history of related disease. *Arch Pathol* 1939;27:469–477.
9. Dent JC, McNulty CAM, Uff JC, et al. Spiral organisms in the gastric antrum. *Lancet* 1987;2:96.
10. McNulty CAM, Dent JC, Curry A, et al. New spiral bacterium in gastric mucosa. *J Clin Pathol* 1989;42:585–591.
11. Solnick JV, O'Rourke J, Lee A, et al. An uncultured gastric spiral organism is a newly identified *Helicobacter* in humans. *J Infect Dis* 1993;168:379–385.
12. Paster BJ, Lee A, Fox JG, et al. Phylogeny of *Helicobacter felis* sp. nov., *Helicobacter mustelae,* and related bacteria. *Int J Syst Bacteriol* 1991;41:31–38.
13. Wegmann W, Aschwanden M, Schaub N, et al. *Gastrospirillum hominis*-assoziierte gastritis - eine zoonose? *Schweiz Med Wochenschr*1991;121:245–254.
14. Lavelle JP, Landas S, Mitros FA, et al. Acute gastritis associated with spiral organisms from cats. *Dig Dis Sci* 1994;39:744–750.
15. Germani Y, Dauga C, Duval P, et al. Strategy for the detection of *Helicobacter* species by amplification of 16s rRNA genes and identification of *H. felis* in a human gastric biopsy. *Res Microbiol* 1997;148:315–326.
16. Hanninen ML, Happonen I, Saari S, et al. Culture and characteristics of *Helicobacter bizzezeronii,* a new canine gastric *Helicobacter* sp. *Int J System Bacteriol* 1996;46:160–166.
17. De Groote D, van Doorn LJ, Ducatelle R, et al. "*Candidatus* Helicobacter suis", a gastric *Helicobacter* from pigs, and its phylogenetic relatedness to other gastrospirilla. *Int J Syst Bacteriol* 1999;49:1769–1777.
18. Woese CR. Bacterial evolution. *Microbiol Rev* 1987;51:221–271.
19. On SL, Lee A, O'Rourke JL, et al. Genus *Helicobacter.* In: Garrity GM, Brenner DJ, eds. *Bergey's manual of systematic bacteriology,* 2nd ed. New York: Bergey's Manual Trust, 2001 *(in press).*
20. O'Rourke JL, Neilan BA, Lee A. Phylogenic relationship of *Helicobacter heilmannii*-like organisms originating from humans and animals. In: Mobley H, ed. *10th International Workshop on* Campylobacter, Helicobacter *and Related Organisms,* tenth edition. Baltimore: 1999.
21. Heilmann KL , Borchard F. Gastritis due to spiral shaped bacteria other than *Helicobacter pylori:* clinical, histological, and ultrastructural findings. *Gut* 1991;32:137–140.
22. Holck S, Ingeholm P, Blom J, et al. The histopathology of human gastric mucosa inhabited by *Helicobacter heilmannii*-like (*Gastrospirillum hominis*) organisms, including the first culturable case. *APMIS* 1997;105:746–756.
23. Andersen LP, Boye K, Blom J, et al. Characterization of a culturable "*Gastrospirillum hominis*" (*Helicobacter heilmannii)* strain isolated from human gastric mucosa. *J Clin Microbiol* 1999;37:1069–1076.
24. Dieterich C, Wiesel P, Neiger R, et al. Presence of multiple *Helicobacter heilmannii* strains in an individual suffering from ulcers and in his two cats. *J Clin Microbiol* 1998;36:1366-1370.
25. Dye KR, Marshall BJ, Frierson HFJ, et al. Ultrastructure of another spiral organism associated with human gastritis. *Dig Dis Sci* 1989;34:1787–1791.
26. Morris A, Ali MR, Thomsen L, et al. Tightly spiral shaped bacteria in the human stomach: another cause of active chronic gastritis? *Gut* 1990;31:139–143.
27. Lee A , O'Rourke JL. Ultrastructure of *Helicobacter* organisms and possible relevance for pathogenesis. In: Goodwin CS, Worsley BW, eds. Helicobacter pylori. *Biology and Clinical Practice.* Boca Raton: CRC Press, 1993:15–35.
28. Lee A, Eckstein RP, Fevre DI, et al. Non-*Campylobacter pylori* spiral organisms in the gastric antrum. *Aust N Z J Med* 1989; 19:156–158.
29. Dick E, Lee A, Watson G, et al. Use of the mouse for the isola-

tion and investigation of stomach-associated, spiral-helical shaped bacteria from man and other animals. *J Med Microbiol* 1989;29:55–62.
30. Solnick JV, O'Rourke J, Lee A, et al. Molecular analysis of urease genes from a newly identified uncultured species of *Helicobacter. Infect Immun* 1994;62:1631–1638.
31. Flejou JF, Diomande I, Molas G, et al. Human chronic gastritis associated with non-*Helicobacter pylori* spiral organisms (*Gastrospirillum hominis*). Four cases and review of the literature. *Gastroenterol Clin Biol* 1990;14:806–810.
32. Debongnie JC, Donnay M , Mairesse J. *Gastrospirillum hominis (Helicobacter heilmannii)*—a cause of gastritis, sometimes transient, better diagnosed by touch cytology. *Am J Gastroenterol* 1995;90:411–416.
33. Morgner A, Lehn N, Andersen LP, et al. *Helicobacter heilmannii*-associated primary gastric low-grade MALT lymphoma: complete remission after curing the infection. *Gastroenterology* 2000;118:821–828.
34. Mazzucchelli L, Wildersmith CH, Ruchti C, et al. *Gastrospirillum hominis* in asymptomatic, healthy individuals. *Dig Dis Sci* 1993;38:2087–2089.
35. Oliva MM, Lazenby AJ , Perman LA. Gastritis associated with *Gastrospirillum hominis* in children—comparison with *Helicobacter pylori* and review of the literature. *Mod Pathol* 1993;6: 513–515.
36. Kubonova K, Trupl J, Jancula L, et al. Presence of spiral bacteria (*"Gastrospirillum hominisi") in the gastric mucosa.* Eur J Clin Microb Infect Dis 1991;10:459–460.
37. Chen Z, Wang B , Xu H. Spiral shaped bacteria in the human gastric biopsy. *J West Chin Univ Med Sci* 1993;24:392–394.
38. Yang HT, Li XT, Xu ZM, et al. *"Helicobacter heilmannii"* infection in a patient with gastric cancer. *Dig Dis Sci* 1995;40:1013–1014.
39. Yang HT, Goliger JA, Song M, et al. High prevalence of *Helicobacter heilmannii* infection in China. *Dig Dis Sci* 1998;43: 1493.
40. Zhang YL, Yamada N, Wen M, et al. *Gastrospirillum hominis* and *Helicobacter pylori* infection in Thai individuals—comparison of histopathological changes of gastric mucosa. *Pathol Int* 1998;48:507–511.
41. Stolte M, Kroher G, Meining A, et al. Comparison of *Helicobacter pylori* and *H. heilmannii* gastritis—matched control study involving 404 patients. *Scand J Gastroenterol* 1997;32:28–33.
42. Stolte M, Wellens E, Bethke B, et al. *Helicobacter heilmannii* (formerly *Gastrospirillum hominis*) gastritis: an infection transmitted by animals? *Scand J Gastroenterol* 1994;29:1061–1064.
43. Meining A, Kroher G , Stolte M. Animal reservoirs in the transmission of *Helicobacter heilmannii* —results of a questionnaire-based study. *Scand J Gastroenterol* 1998;33:795–798.
44. Thomson MA, Storey P, Greer R, et al. Canine-human transmission of *Gastrospirillum hominis. Lancet* 1994;343:1605–1607.
45. Henry GA, Long PH, Burns JL, et al. Gastric spirillosis in beagles. *Am J Vet Res* 1987;48:831–836.
46. Dubois A, Tarnawski A, Newell DG, et al. Gastric injury and invasion of parietal cells by spiral bacteria in rhesus monkeys. Are gastritis and hyperchlorhydria infectious diseases? *Gastroenterology* 1991;100:884–891.
47. Eaton KA, Radin MJ, Kramer L, et al. Gastric spiral bacilli in captive cheetahs. *Scand J Gastroenterol* 1991;26:38–42.
48. Heilmann KL , Borchard F. Further observations on human spirobacteria. In: Menge H, Gregor M, Tytgat GNJ, et al., eds. Helicobacter pylori *1990.* Berlin: Springer-Verlag, 1991:63–70.
49. Geyer C, Colbatzky F, Lechner J, et al. Occurrence of spiral-shaped bacteria in gastric biopsies of dogs and cats. *Vet Record* 1993;133:18–19.
50. Queiroz DMD, Rocha GA, Mendes EN, et al. Association between *Helicobacter* and gastric ulcer disease of the pars esophagea in swine. *Gastroenterology* 1996;111:19–27.
51. Borody TJ, George LL, Brandl S, et al. *Helicobacter pylori*-negative duodenal ulcer. *Am J Gastroenterol* 1991;86:1154–1157.
52. Goddard AF, Logan R, Atherton JC, et al. Healing of duodenal ulcer after eradication of *Helicobacter helimannii. Lancet* 1997; 349:1815–1816.
53. Akin OY, Tsou VM , Werner AL. *Gastrospirillum hominis*-associated chronic active gastritis. *Pediatr Pathol Lab Med* 1995;15: 429–435.
54. Debongnie JC, Donnay M, Mairesse J, et al. Gastric ulcers and *Helicobacter heilmannii. Eur J Gastroenterol Hepatol* 1998;10: 251–254.
55. Morgner A, Bayerdorffer E, Meining A, et al. *Helicobacter heilmannii* and gastric cancer. *Lancet* 1995;346:511–512.
56. Al-Himyary AJS, Zabaneh RI, Zabaneh SS, et al. *Gastrospirillum hominis* in acute gastric erosion. *South Med J* 1994;87: 1147–1150.
57. Lee A, Fox JG, Otto G, et al. A small animal model of human *Helicobacter pylori* active chronic gastritis. *Gastroenterology* 1990; 99:1315–1323.
58. Lee A, Chen MH, Coltro N, et al. Long term infection of the gastric mucosa with *Helicobacter* species does induce atrophic gastritis in an animal model of *Helicobacter pylori* infection. *Zbl Bakt (Int J Med Microbiol)* 1993;280:38–50.
59. Enno A, O'Rourke JL, Howlett CR, et al. MALToma-like lesions in the murine gastric mucosa after long-term infection with *Helicobacter felis*—a mouse model of *Helicobacter pylori*-induced gastric lymphoma. *Am J Pathol* 1995;147:217–222.
60. O'Rourke JL, Enno A, Dixon MF, et al. Gastric B-cell MALT lymphoma and *Helicobacter heilmannii* infection. *Gut* 1999;45 [Suppl 111]:A69.
61. Drossman DA, Thompson WG, Talley NJ, et al. Identification of subgroups of functional gastrointestinal disorders. *Gastroenterol Int* 1990;3:159–172.
62. Nakshabendi IM, Peebles SE, Lee FD, et al. Spiral shaped microorganisms in the human duodenal mucosa. *Postgrad Med J* 1991;67:846–847.
63. Michaud L, Ategbo S, Gottrand F, et al. Nodular gastritis associated with *Helicobacter heilmannii* infection. *Lancet* 1995;346: 1499.
64. Drewitz DJ, Shub MD , Ramirez FC. *Gastrospirillum hominis* gastritis in a child with celiac sprue. *Dig Dis Sci* 1997;42: 1083–1086.
65. O'Rourke J , Lee A. The immune response in patients colonised with *"Helicobacter heilmannii" (Gastrospirillum hominis). Am J Gastroenterol* 1994;89:1334.
66. Queiroz DM, Cabral MM, Nogueira AM, et al. Mixed gastric infection by *"Gastrospirillum hominis"* and *Helicobacter pylori. Lancet* 1990;2:507–508.
67. Bockus HL. Syphilis and the stomach. In: Bockus HL, eds. *Gastroenterology,* third edition. Philadelphia: WB Saunders, 1974:1041–1059.
68. Fyfe B, Poppiti RJ, Lubin J, et al. Gastric syphilis—primary diagnosis by gastric biopsy—report of 4 cases. *Arch Pathol Lab Med* 1993;117:820–823.
69. Greenstein DB, Wilcox CM , Schwartz DA. Gastric syphilis—report of seven cases and review of the literature. *J Clin Gastroenterol* 1994;18:4–9.
70. Long BW, Johnston JH, Wetzel W, et al. Gastric syphilis—endoscopic and histological features mimicking lymphoma. *Am J Gastroenterol* 1995;90:1504–1507.
71. Kolb JC, Woodward LA. Gastric syphilis. *Am J Emerg Med* 1997;15:164–166.
72. Rank EL, Goldenberg SA, Hasson J, et al. *Treponema pallidum*

and *Helicobacter pylori* recovered in a case of chronic active gastritis. *Am J Clin Pathol* 1992;97:116–120.
73. Inagaki H, Kawai T, Miyata M, et al. Gastric syphilis—polymerase chain reaction detection of treponemal DNA in pseudolymphomatous lesions. *Hum Pathol* 1996;27:761–765.
74. Marshall JB. Tuberculosis of the gastrointestinal tract and peritoneum. *Am J Gastroenterol* 1993;88:989–999.
75. Singh B, Moodley J, Ramdial P, et al. Primary gastric tuberculosis—a report of 3 cases. *S Afr J Surg* 1996;34:29–32.
76. Quantrill SJ, Archer GJ , Hale RJ. Gastric tuberculosis presenting with massive hematemesis in association with acute myeloid leukemia. *Am J Gastroenterol* 1996;91:1259–1260.
77. Okoro EO, Komolafe OF. Gastric tuberculosis: unusual presentations in two patients. *Clin Radiol* 1999;54:257–259.
78. Lin OS, Wu SS, Yeh KT, et al. Case report: isolated gastric tuberculosis of the cardia. *J Gastroenterol Hepatol* 1999;14:258–261.
79. Abrams JS, Holden WD. Tuberculosis of the gastrointestinal tract. *Arch Surg* 1964;89:282–293.
80. Gaines W, Steinbach HL , Lowenhaupt E. Tuberculosis of the stomach. *Radiology* 1952;58:808–819.
81. Ackermann AJ. Roentgenological study of gastric tuberculosis. *AJR Am J Roentgenol* 1940;44:59.
82. Chazan B, Aitchison J. Gastric tuberculosis. *BMJ* 1960;2: 1288–1290.
83. Goodwin RA, Shapira JL, Thurman GH, et al. Disseminated histoplasmosis: clinical and pathologic correlations. *Medicine* 1980;59:1–33.
84. Fuller CC , Wood H. Actinomycotic granuloma of the stomach. *JAMA* 1945;129:1163.
85. Yong S, Attal H , Chejfec G. Pseudomembranous gastritis—a novel complication of *Aspergillus* infection in a patient with a bone marrow transplant and graft versus host disease. *Arch Pathol Lab Med* 2000;124:619–624.
86. Yousef OM, Smilack JD, Kerr DM, et al. Gastrointestinal basidiobolomycosis. Morphologic findings in a cluster of six cases. *Am J Clin Pathol* 1999;112:610–616.
87. Pugh TF, Fitch SJ. Invasive gastric candidiasis. *Pediatr Radiol* 1986;16:67–68.
88. Shanks SC, Kerley P. *A text book of X-ray diagnosis*. London: HK Lewis, 1958.
89. Minoli G, Terruzi V, Butti G, et al. Gastric candidiasis: An endoscopic histology study in 26 patients. *Gastrointest Endosc* 1982;28:59–61.
90. Knoke M, Bernhardt H. Endoscopic aspects of mycosis in the upper digestive tract. *Endoscopy* 1980;12:295–298.
91. Maertens J, Demuynck H, Verbeken EK, et al. Mucormycosis in allogeneic bone marrow transplant recipients: report of five cases and review of the role of iron overload in the pathogenesis. *Bone Marrow Transplant* 1999;24:307–312.
92. Doglioni C, De Boni M, Cielo R, et al. Gastric giardiasis. *J Clin Pathol* 1992;45:964–967.
93. Dees A, Batenburg PL, Umar HM, et al. *Strongyloides stercoralis* associated with a bleeding gastric ulcer. *Gut* 1990;31:1414–1415.
94. Wurtz R, Mirot M, Fronda G, et al. Short report—gastric infection by *Strongyloides stercoralis*. *Am J Trop Med Hyg* 1994;51: 339–340.
95. Asami K, Watanuki T, Sakai H, et al. Two cases of stomach granuloma caused by *Anisakis*-like larval nematodes in Japan. *Am J Trop Med Hyg* 1965;14:119–123.
96. Drasar BS. Other anaerobes-curved and spiral organisms. *Soc Appl Bacteriol Symp Ser* 1986;13:91–100.
97. Snepar R, Poporad GA, Romano JM, et al. Effect of cimetidine and antacid on gastric microbial flora. *Infect Immun* 1982;36:518–524.
98. Tryba M. The gastropulmonary route of infection—fact or fiction. *Am J Med* 1991;91[Suppl 2A]:135S–146S.
99. Fiddian-Green RG, Baker S. Nosocomial pneumonia in the critically ill: product of aspiration or translocation. *Crit Care Med* 1991;119:763–769.
100. Goldschmiedt M, Feldman M. Age-related changes in gastric acid secretion. In: Holt PR , Russell RM, eds. *Chronic gastritis and hypochlorhydria in the elderly*. Boca Raton, FL: CRC Press, 1993:13–30.
101. Husebye E, Skar V, Haverstad T, et al. Fasting hypochlorhydria with Gram positive gastric flora is highly prevalent in healthy elderly people. *Gut* 1992;33:1331–1337.
102. Wormsley KG , Grossman MI. Maximal Histalog test in control subjects and patients with peptic ulcer. *Gut* 1965;6:427–435.
103. Bach-Nielsen P, Amdrup E. Preoperative bacteriologic examination of the stomach and duodenum. *Acta Chir Scand* 1965;129:521–529.
104. Houghton PWJ, Mortensen NJ, Cooper MJ, et al. Intragastric bile acids and histological changes in gastric mucosa. *Br J Surg* 1986;73:354–356.
105. Sjostedt S, Kager L, Heimdahl A, et al. Microbial colonisation in tumors in relation to the upper gastrointestinal tract in patients with gastric carcinoma. *Ann Surg* 1988;207:341–346.

36

VIBRIO CHOLERAE O1 AND O139

JOAN R. BUTTERTON
STEPHEN B. CALDERWOOD

Vibrio cholerae O1 and O139 are gram-negative bacteria that cause a severe, dehydrating, and occasionally fatal diarrhea in humans. There are an estimated 5.5 million cases worldwide of cholera each year, resulting in more than 100,000 deaths. Over the second half of the twentieth century, cholera has been considered to occur primarily in developing countries of Asia and Africa, but during the 1990s, it also reached epidemic proportions in regions of South and Central America (1,2). The molecular mechanisms underlying the pathogenesis of *V. cholerae* infection have been intensively studied and provide outstanding paradigms for advancing modern understanding of bacterial virulence.

TAXONOMY

The genus *Vibrio* is a member of the family Vibrionaceae and is closely related to members of the Enterobacteriaceae. Although vibrios were originally distinguished from the Enterobacteriaceae by biochemical characteristics, more recent studies of the amino acid sequence divergence of enzymes (3), ribosomal RNA homologies (4), and the complete genomic sequence (5) have confirmed the ancestral relationship between the genus *Vibrio* and the family Enterobacteriaceae. At present, 34 *Vibrio* species are recognized, one-third of which are known to be pathogenic in humans (6).

Vibrio cholerae is currently divided into more than 190 serotypes on the basis of the O antigen of the cell surface lipopolysaccharide (LPS). The dominant part of the O1 antigen is a homopolymer containing the amino sugar D-perosamine substituted with 3-deoxy-L-glycerotetronic acid (7). Only *V. cholerae* of the O1 and O139 serotypes are responsible for epidemic cholera in humans; all other serotypes are referred to as non-O1. The non-O1 group has been associated with occasional cases of gastroenteritis and extraintestinal infections (see Chapter 37).

Biotypes and Serotypes

V. cholerae O1 is divided into two biotypes: classical and El Tor. The El Tor strains were first isolated in 1905 from returning Mecca pilgrims at the quarantine camp of El Tor in the Sinai Peninsula of Egypt (8). These strains agglutinated in O1 typing antiserum and produced typical cases of cholera, but they differed from previously isolated strains by producing hemolysins. In addition, the El Tor biotype differs from the classical biotype in agglutination of chicken red blood cells, in its resistance to polymyxin B, and in its production of a positive Voges-Proskauer reaction (9).

Both classical and El Tor biotypes can be further divided according to the antigenic subspecificity of the O1 antigen into three serotypes, named Ogawa, Inaba, and Hikojima. The *V. cholerae* O1 antigen is synthesized by genes in the *rfb* gene cluster; the product of the *rfbT* gene is required for determining the Ogawa serotype specificity, whereas Inaba strains are *rfbT* mutants (10).

Species identification is rapidly confirmed by slide agglutination tests with polyvalent O1 or O139 antiserum and type-specific Inaba and Ogawa antisera. No serotypes have been identified in the O139 serogroup (11). Biotyping is performed as described earlier.

MICROBIOLOGY

Cell Morphology

V. cholerae cells are single, short (1.5 to 3.0 by 0.5 μm), slightly curved gram-negative rods. Cells may rarely appear straight, spherical, or as spirilla; they may appear S- or C-shaped if joined (12). Bacilli may lie parallel to each other in smears from mucus in rice water stool. Cells have a single, long polar flagellum (Fig. 36.1) and show a characteristic rapid linear motility.

J. R. Butterton: Harvard Medical School, Division of Infectious Diseases, Massachusetts General Hospital, Boston, Massachusetts
S. B. Calderwood: Department of Medicine, Harvard Medical School; Division of Infectious Diseases, Massachusetts General Hospital, Boston, Massachusetts

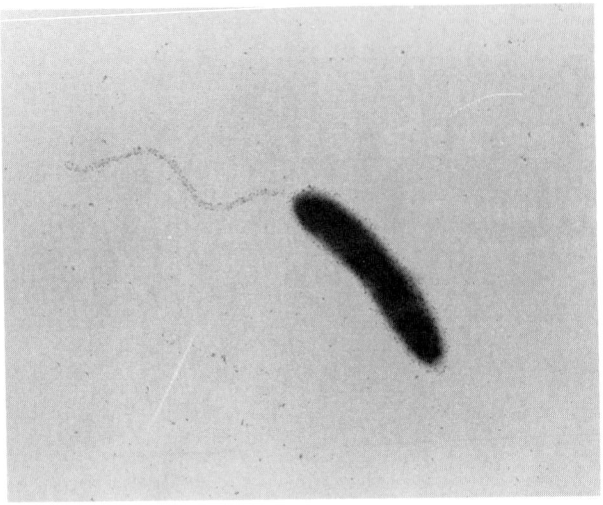

FIGURE 36.1. Electron micrograph of *Vibrio cholerae*, stained with immunogold antilipopolysaccharide antibodies. (Courtesy of Dr. John J. Mekalanos and Dr. Marian R. Neutra.)

Colonial Morphology and Pigmentation

After primary isolation in bile salt agar, *V. cholerae* form clear, translucent colonies with a sharp, round margin and a flat top; these are easily distinguished from the opaque, convex, grayish white colonies of enteric bacteria (12). The bile salts inhibit the growth of aerobic gram-positive bacilli and add to the translucency of the colonies. Colony morphology may undergo variations, appearing opaque, rugose, or dwarf (12).

Thiosulfate-citrate-bile salts-sucrose agar (TCBS) agar is the most extensively used selective medium for the isolation of *V. cholerae;* the growth of most enteric bacteria is inhibited. The sucrose-fermenting colonies of *V. cholerae* on TCBS appear large, yellow, smooth, and opaque (11). Colonies cultured on TCBS are sticky and cannot be used for direct slide agglutination; first they must be subcultured on nutrient agar.

Biochemical Characteristics

Cholera vibrios are facultative anaerobes that are characterized by their positive oxidase, catalase, and nitrate reduction tests. The positive oxidase reaction differentiates them from the oxidase-negative Enterobacteriaceae; their fermentative metabolism distinguishes them from the oxidase-positive *Pseudomonas* species. *Aeromonas* species are resistant to the vibriostatic compound O/129, to which most *V. cholerae* are susceptible (11). *V. cholerae* is lysine decarboxylase-positive and arginine dihydrolase-negative, grows in nutrient broth without added NaCl, and ferments sucrose (13).

Genomic Sequence

The genomic sequence of *V. cholerae* El Tor strain N16961 was completed in 2000 (5). The genome consists of two circular chromosomes (14) of 2,961,146 bp and 1,072,314 bp (chromosome 1 and chromosome 2), which encode 3,885 open reading frames. The average G + C content of the two chromosomes is 46.9% and 47.7%, respectively. The majority of essential genes and those critical for pathogenicity are located on the large chromosome; the small chromosome contains a larger fraction of hypothetical genes and those of unknown function. Whether the small chromosome originated as a megaplasmid captured by an ancestral *Vibrio* species (5) or arose by excision from a single large genome (15) remains a subject of debate.

EPIDEMIOLOGY

Pandemics

Ancient medical texts from India, Asia, and Europe contain descriptions of severe diarrheal diseases with vomiting that resemble cholera caused by *V. cholerae* O1 (16). The enormous impact that cholera has had throughout history contributed to the sanitary revolutions of North America and Europe, to the evolution of health care systems, and to many scientific discoveries. The history of cholera is discussed in detail in Chapter 1.

In the nineteenth century, six pandemics of cholera spread throughout the world, beginning in Asia, spreading to Europe, and then to the Americas (16). Three waves of cholera entered the United States in 1832, 1849, and 1866, causing heavy casualties (17). During the epidemic in London in 1849, John Snow demonstrated that transmission was linked to fecal contamination of water at the infamous Broad Street pump (18). Curved organisms were isolated from cholera victims in 1854 by Filippo Pacini and again by Robert Koch in 1883, who demonstrated the etiologic relationship of the comma-shaped organisms with the disease (19).

Throughout the early part of the twentieth century, cholera was a seasonal endemic disease in Asia. The current seventh pandemic began in 1961, spreading from an endemic focus in Sulawesi (Celebes), Indonesia (20) to the Pacific Islands, southeast Asia, and the Middle East. In 1970, cholera reached Africa (21) and Europe (22). Although the classical biotype of *V. cholerae* O1 caused the fifth and sixth pandemics, the seventh pandemic has been caused by the El Tor biotype. Biologic factors allowing the El Tor strain to replace the classical strain are discussed herein. However, 6 years after the El Tor strain replaced classical cholera in Bangladesh, the classical strain reappeared in 1979 (23). Reasons for its reappearance and current coexistence with El Tor strains are poorly understood (24).

In late January 1991, *V. cholerae* O1, serotype Inaba, biotype El Tor, appeared with explosive intensity in several coastal Peruvian cities (25), making its first appearance in South America since 1895. The epidemic spread quickly to other urban areas and then to neighboring countries, jumping southward to Santiago, Chile, and northward to Central America within months (1). The strain was related to the seventh pandemic *V. cholerae* O1 strains present in Africa and Asia, but could be clearly distinguished by microbiological and genetic markers (26,27).

Cholera rapidly spread through Latin America in 1991, causing nearly 400,000 reported cases and more than 4000 reported deaths in 16 countries (28). By the end of 1996, cholera had been reported from 21 countries, causing more than 1 million cases and nearly 12,000 deaths (29). Although epidemic levels rapidly decreased from the peak in 1991 and 1992 because of active surveillance, prevention, and disease control, another resurgence was detected in 1998, with the total number of reported cases increasing from 17,760 in 1997 to 57,106 in 1998 (30). This increase has been attributed to the effects of Hurricane Mitch and climactic changes caused by the El Nino phenomenon (30). The total number of cases in the Americas dropped by 86% from 1998 to 1999, with 8,126 cases and 103 deaths reported to the World Health Organization (WHO) (31).

Before the introduction of the seventh pandemic strain into Latin America in 1991, cholera was rarely imported into the United States. From 1961 to 1990, 41 cases of cholera were imported by travelers returning to the United States from countries with cholera (2), representing an estimated rate of less than 1 per 500,000 travelers to affected areas (32). In addition, in 1973, an endemic focus was identified in the Gulf of Mexico (33). Through 1992, a total of 65 cases associated with this focus was reported (33–35). Most of the cases associated with the endemic focus followed consumption of raw shellfish; in 1988 raw oysters from the Gulf of Mexico caused single cases in six states (36).

Significantly more cases occurred in the United States following the Latin American epidemic in 1991. From 1991 through March 1993, a total of 30 cases of cholera were reported in U.S. residents who had traveled to South America (37–39). Another 11 cases occurred in U.S. residents who ate crabs brought back from Ecuador by other travelers (37,38), and 75 cases were associated with food served aboard a 1992 airline flight from Peru (40). In 1998 and 1999, 15 and 6 cases, respectively, of imported cholera were detected in the United States (30,31).

An epidemic outbreak of cholera began in southern and eastern India in October 1992 (41) and in Bangladesh in January 1993 (42), and rapidly spread (43–45). The strains isolated during this outbreak did not agglutinate with O1 antiserum or with monoclonal antibodies against the A, B, or C antigens of *V. cholerae* O1, and were thus identified as non-O1 strains. These strains did not react with a panel of the then 137 known non-O1 antisera and so were designated as a new serogroup, O139, with the suggested name of "Bengal" (46). Genetic analysis suggested that the initial isolates of *V. cholerae* O139 Bengal were O-antigen mutants of a toxigenic El Tor strain, rather than evolving from a non-O1 strain that acquired virulence genes (41,42 44,47–49). Studies revealed that these strains had an insertion of a large genomic region encoding the O139-specific genes, along with simultaneous deletion of most of the O1 antigen-specific genes (50). Studies of the rapidly expanding clonal diversity of the O139 serogroup suggest that the O139-specific DNA is being acquired by different progenitor strains, which may have differing epidemic potential (51).

Initial O139 isolates were resistant to sulfamethoxazole, trimethoprim, chloramphenicol, and streptomycin (41). These resistances were found to be encoded by a 62-kb self-transmissible, conjugative, chromosomally integrating element designated the SXT element (52,53). After its initial spread throughout Bangladesh, *V. cholerae* O139 was transiently displaced by a new clone of El Tor vibrios, but then recurred in 1995. The new outbreak strains were predominantly susceptible to the aforementioned antibiotics, and molecular analysis revealed a deletion of a region of the SXT element in these strains (54). Recent surveys of *V. cholerae* O139 strains from 1992 to 1998 in Calcutta, India, have also demonstrated pan-susceptibility to chloramphenicol and trimethoprim-sulfamethoxazole (55).

The spread of *V. cholerae* O139 Bengal was the first time a non-O1 strain had been found to be responsible for epidemic cholera. Many of the cases were in adults, suggesting that immunity to *V. cholerae* O1 did not protect against the O139 serotype (44). *V. cholerae* O139 initially displaced *V. cholerae* O1 from the environment in areas in which it was causing disease, suggesting that *V. cholerae* O139 could have an intrinsic survival advantage over *V. cholerae* O1 (56,57), or that the lack of immunity to *V. cholerae* O139 allowed its niche to expand from infected persons into the environment through sewage contamination. The rapid spread of *V. cholerae* O139 raised concern that the appearance of this organism could signal the beginning of the eighth cholera pandemic (58). However, although 11 countries have officially reported cases of *V. cholerae* O139 through 1998 (29), outbreaks of this serotype have remained confined to Asia. In endemic countries in Asia in 1999, *V. cholerae* O139 accounted for approximately 17% of confirmed cholera cases (31). Because the rate of spread has slowed after the initial outbreaks, the concern that this strain might cause another pandemic has lessened (30).

The seventh pandemic is still ongoing, with cases being reported to the WHO from all regions of the world (31). An increasing number of areas are becoming endemic for cholera (59). In particular, the burden of cholera is greatest in Africa, with 206,746 cases reported to the WHO in 1999, accounting for 81% of the global total (31). With a reported 8,728 deaths, the case-fatality rate for Africa in 1999 was 4.2%, compared with less than 1% for the rest of the world (31). Natural and political disasters continue to provide potent examples of explosive cholera outbreaks when disease control cannot be maintained. In 1994 in a refugee camp in Goma, Democratic Republic of the Congo, 58,000 to 80,000 cases of cholera with 23,800 deaths occurred in 1 month (60).

Natural Reservoirs

V. cholerae O1 is a free-living inhabitant of brackish water and estuarine systems (61). Many studies have investigated the ability of *V. cholerae* O1 to be cultured from stool, sewage, water, and other environments (62). Survival is prolonged in cold, saline conditions (62). *V. cholerae* O1 is sensitive to desiccation; cells only survive several hours on dry surfaces (63).

The presence of *V. cholerae* O1 in the environment, perhaps serving as a reservoir between epidemics of human disease, was questioned because organisms could not be cultured from water sources uncontaminated by active cholera cases. However, *V. cholerae* O1 can change from a viable, culturable form to a nonculturable form under certain environmental conditions. Nonculturable forms do not grow on routine laboratory media but can be detected by fluorescent antibody staining or gene probes; they remain responsive to nalidixic acid and continue to take up radiolabeled substrate (64–66). Under starvation conditions, *V. cholerae* O1 cells become small and ovoid: such cells can survive, perhaps for years, in the culturable state in the environment (61). When starved cells are placed in a cold, saline environment, such as seawater, they become nonculturable, but viability can be demonstrated when they are introduced into rabbit ileal loops (64). *V. cholerae* O1, therefore, appear able to survive through cold seasons in a dormant state but remain potentially pathogenic.

Plankton and shellfish may serve as reservoirs of *V. cholerae* O1 in the environment. At least 10^4 to 10^5 organisms may attach to a single copepod. During a copepod bloom, the number of *V. cholerae* O1 may increase to the number needed to cause human disease (67). *V. cholerae* O1 may also adhere to water plants (68) and algae (69). Raw bivalves (clams, oysters, and mussels) and undercooked shellfish (shrimp, crabs) have been documented as important vehicles of transmission (34,36). Genes important in biofilm formation have been identified (70, 1), and may play a critical role in survival of *V. cholerae* in the environment. In addition, genes involved in cell density-dependent regulatory functions (quorum sensing), have been detected on both the large and the small chromosomes (72). Genes required for the autoinducer-2 quorum-sensing mechanism are divided, with *luxOSU* on chromosome 1 and *luxPQ* on chromosome 2 (5).

Transmission

V. cholerae O1 is transmitted by the fecal-oral route and is spread primarily through contaminated food and water. Since the classical observations by John Snow during the cholera epidemic in London in 1854 (18), water has been considered a major vehicle for cholera transmission. During the outbreak in Peru in the 1990s, fecal contamination of the municipal water supplies of large urban areas was associated with the majority of cases (73,74). Storage of water has also been associated with transmission of *V. cholerae* O1. In Peru, illness was strongly associated with drinking water into which others had introduced their hands (73). Contaminated noncarbonated bottled water (75) and contaminated ice (74) have been implicated in other outbreaks. Use of contaminated surface water for cooking, bathing, and washing also may lead to illness (76).

Food-borne transmission plays an important role in many cholera outbreaks (62). The duration of survival of *V. cholerae* O1 in various foods is influenced by the pH, humidity, temperature, and inoculum size (62,77–79). Organisms can survive on vegetables for 1 to 2 days at room temperature, or longer if moist or cooler (78); survival is also enhanced in alkaline foods (79). Cases of cholera have been associated with crops irrigated with sewage, with lettuce, millet gruel, rice, raw and cooked seafood, pickled or dried fish, and frozen coconut milk.

During active cholera outbreaks, human carriers provide a large reservoir of infection. Although asymptomatic carriers can be an important source of transmission during outbreaks (24), chronic carriage appears rare (80). Excretion of organisms rarely lasts longer than 2 weeks (62), although a few patients have been documented to excrete vibrios for months (81) or, in the case of cholera Dolores, for years (82). Direct person-to-person spread, rather than through contamination of food or water, is not usually an important route of transmission. Direct spread has been implicated in outbreaks in hospitals (83,84), during burial ceremonies in which intestinal contents are removed from the dead body (85), through sweat (86), and from ill children to their mothers (87), but in some of these cases contamination of food or water may have occurred.

Risk Factors

The previous exposure of a population is an important factor in the risk of contracting cholera. Patients who recover from *V. cholerae* O1 infection have long-lasting, perhaps lifelong, immunity to reinfection (88). In endemic areas such as eastern India and Bangladesh, cholera primarily affects nonimmune children 2 to 15 years of age (87), whereas in areas with little preexisting immunity, such as in Latin America or in regions newly affected by *V. cholerae* O139 Bengal, cholera is a disease affecting persons of all ages (44,73,74).

Persons with low gastric acidity, due to malnutrition, gastritis, surgery, or drugs such as antacids, H_2 receptor antagonists, and marijuana, are at increased risk for cholera infection (89–91). *V. cholerae* O1 is killed rapidly in gastric acid of pH less than 2.4 (89). Ingesting organisms with sodium bicarbonate or food reduces the infectious dose from 10^{11} organisms to 10^4 to 10^6 organisms (92). Infection with *Helicobacter pylori,* common in Latin American countries, has been proposed as a factor increasing the risk of *V. cholerae* O1 infection during the Latin American epidemic in the early 1990s (1,93).

Blood group O is associated with an increased risk of severe cholera, although the reasons for this association are unknown (94,95). The population of the Ganges Delta has the lowest prevalence of O blood group genes in the world. Only 30% of Bangladeshis but at least 75% of Peruvians are of blood group O, suggesting not only that cholera has selected against persons of the O blood group in the Ganges Delta (94) but also that Latin American populations may be predisposed to particularly severe clinical infection (1).

Bottle-feeding of infants is associated with a greater risk of cholera, whereas breast-feeding appears protective (96,97). Breast milk antibodies against cholera do not appear to protect children from colonization with *V. cholerae* O1 but do protect against disease in those who are colonized (97). Maternal vaccination may provide protection to their nonvaccinated breast-fed children (96). The reduced risk of cholera in breast-fed children could be a result of decreased ingestion of contaminated food or water, the antibacterial effect of lactoferrin in breast milk, a protective effect of breast milk antibodies, or improved nutrition. However, children with chronic malnutrition have not been demonstrated to have an increased risk of infection or disease with *V. cholerae* O1 (98).

The biotype of the infecting *V. cholerae* O1 strain may have an influence on the risk of infection. The El Tor biotype may be less immunogenic than the classical biotype (99) and produces higher rates of asymptomatic or mildly symptomatic infections (one clinical case per 30 to 100 infections with the El Tor biotype versus one case for each two to four infections with classical strains) (100,101). Duration of carriage following infection is longer with the El Tor biotype (102). The El Tor biotype may also survive longer in the environment (such as in water, feces, and sewage) and on food than the classical biotype (77).

PATHOGENESIS AND IMMUNITY

Pathogenesis

Colonization

After ingestion, *V. cholerae* O1 must pass through the gastric acid barrier of the stomach to colonize the small intestine. There the organism penetrates the mucous gel, adheres to the brush border of intestinal epithelial cells via specific adhesins, and produces a number of extracellular secreted proteins. Full virulence of *V. cholerae* depends on the coordinate regulation of many of these virulence factors.

Vibrios that survive passage through the gastric acid barrier of the stomach—due to a large inoculum size, a hypochlorhydric host, protection within a bolus of food, or a rapid gastric emptying time—must colonize the small intestine in order to produce disease. Adherence to the brush border of the intestinal epithelium is the initial step in colonization.

Pili play an important role in adherence. The best studied pilus, the toxin–coregulated pilus (TCP), is necessary for human colonization (103,104). A large gene cluster encodes the proteins required for the synthesis and function of TCP. The *tcp* gene cluster is located next to other virulence gene clusters, all of which are found on a 45.3 kb *Vibrio* pathogenicity island (VPI) on the large chromosome (5,105). Antibodies to the 20.5-kd major structural subunit of the pilus, TcpA, inhibit attachment of bacteria to epithelial cells *in vitro* and are protective in an animal model (106–108). In volunteer studies, mutant strains lacking pili fail to colonize the intestine or produce an immune response (104). Although both classical and El Tor biotypes possess the *tcpA* gene (108,109), the ability of the two biotypes to express pili in response to environmental conditions differs. It is not known whether this variation is an important factor in human disease.

Two additional types of fimbriae, types B and C, have been identified as morphologically distinct from TCP (110), but the genes encoding their structural subunits have not been defined. Conversely, another type IV pilus has been identified by genome sequencing but has not been visualized (111). The 5.4-kb *pil* gene cluster consists of five open reading frames, *pilABCD* and *yacE*. Deletion of *pilA* neither reduces colonization in the infant mouse model nor alters adherence to cells in culture (111). However, the *pilD* gene product is a type IV prepilin peptidase, which processes the amino-terminal signal sequences of a number of proteins in the EPS, MSHA, and TCP gene clusters (see later text) (111,112), and thus plays a critical role in virulence.

Other factors have been demonstrated to be important for the colonization of the small intestine by *V. cholerae* O1. Protease production may allow degradation of the mucus gel (113). An accessory colonization factor is encoded by the clustered *acfA, B, C,* and *D* genes, which lie next to the *tcp* gene cluster within the VPI (105). Mutations in any of these genes reduce the ability of vibrios to colonize the intestine of suckling mice (114–116).

A number of hemagglutinins (HA) are produced by *V. cholerae* and may function as adherence factors. Both cholera biotypes produce a soluble HA protease (HA/P) (117,118), which is a zinc-dependent metalloprotease (119,120) that cleaves mucin, fibronectin, and lactoferrin (121), and nicks and activates the A subunit of cholera toxin (122). HA/P appears not to play a primary role in virulence (118,123), but may act in the detachment of *V. cholerae* from the intestinal epithelium (123), in the disruption of proteins involved in maintaining epithelial tight junctions (124), and in the inactivation of the filamentous phage CTXϕ (see later text) (125).

Besides the soluble HA protease, several cell-associated HAs have been described. The D-mannose-D-fructose-sensitive HA (MSHA) is expressed by El Tor strains; it is a member of the type IV family of pili. Sixteen genes encoding the MSHA biogenesis and structural proteins are clustered on chromosome 1 (5,126). The role of MSHA in human disease is not clear; this pilus is not required for colonization of the intestine (127–129), but it is important in biofilm formation (70,71) and thus may play a role in the survival of El Tor *V. cholerae* in its aquatic environment outside a human host (126). In addition, MSHA acts as a receptor for the *V. cholerae* O139 filamentous bacteriophage 493 (130). The D-mannose-, L-fucose-resistant HA (MFRHA) is expressed by both *V. cholerae* biotypes. MFRHA activity has been associated with two genes, *mrhA* and *mrhB* (131); mutations in these genes reduced virulence in a mouse model (131).

A variety of outer membrane proteins have been characterized that appear to play a role in the intestinal colonization of vibrios. Antibodies to several porin-like outer membrane proteins have been demonstrated to protect against infection by inhibiting intestinal colonization (132). The LPS biosynthetic enzymes of *V. cholerae* are encoded by the *rfb* genes; deleting one of these genes, *rfbB,* produced a mutant with a severe colonization defect (133).

Motility appears to be an important factor in colonization by *V. cholerae* (134). Although flagellar antigens may play a role (135), they are less important (134). Motility combined with chemotaxis (136) may allow organisms to avoid clearance by peristalsis.

Cholera toxin itself may contribute to *V. cholerae* virulence by enhancing mucosal colonization. Mutant nontoxinogenic organisms show decreased colonization of rabbit intestinal mucosa compared to parent toxinogenic strains; when purified toxin is added to the nontoxinogenic strain, colonization increases to the level of the parent strain (137). Other investigators, however, have not detected a colonization defect in toxin-negative strains (138).

Cholera Toxin

The major virulence factor for *V. cholerae* O1 is cholera toxin (CT). The structure, mechanism of action, and genetic regulation of this toxin have been the focus of intense scientific activity over the past several decades.

CT is a multimeric protein composed of one A subunit (molecular weight 27,215) noncovalently attached to five B subunits (molecular weight 11,677) (139). The A subunit undergoes proteolytic nicking to produce A1 and A2 fragments linked by a disulfide bond. The A1 fragment (approximate molecular weight 22,500) contains the enzymatic activity of the toxin (140). The A2 fragment (approximate molecular weight 5500) attaches the A subunit to the B-subunit pentamer (139).

The B-subunit pentamer binds holotoxin to the enterocyte surface receptor, the ganglioside GM1 (141). *V. cholerae* produces a neuraminidase, which catalyzes conversion of gangliosides to GM1 (142). The role of neuraminidase in cholera pathogenesis is still unclear; it has been postulated that this enzyme may produce locally high concentrations of GM1 receptor for cholera toxin, thereby increasing the binding and uptake of CT by enterocytes (143).

Following binding of holotoxin, the A1 fragment catalyzes the adenosine diphosphate ribosylation of a guanosine triphosphate-binding protein and causes persistent activation of adenylate cyclase (144,145). The end result is an increase of cyclic adenosine monophosphate (cAMP) within the intestinal mucosa, stimulating chloride secretion and decreasing sodium absorption, leading to loss of fluid and electrolytes and the production of diarrhea (Fig. 36.2) (146).

The heat-labile enterotoxin (LT) produced by some enterotoxigenic strains of *Escherichia coli* shares an identical mode of action with cholera toxin. CT and LT have structural, antigenic, and DNA sequence homology (147), suggesting a common evolutionary origin (148).

cAMP may not be the sole mediator of intestinal water and electrolyte transport in cholera. Cholera toxin may lead to increased production of prostaglandins, which may independently contribute to the massive loss of water and electrolytes. A role for prostaglandins is suggested by the observation that drugs that inhibit prostaglandin synthesis reduce the effects of cholera toxin on fluid secretion in experimental animals (149,150), whereas patients with active disease have elevated prostaglandin E_2 concentrations in jejunal aspirates (151). In a rabbit model, treatment with cholera toxin caused a dose-dependent synthesis and release of prostaglandin E that correlated better than cAMP levels with fluid accumulation in the intestinal lumen (152).

The factors influencing cholera toxin production in the human intestine are not known. *In vitro* conditions that

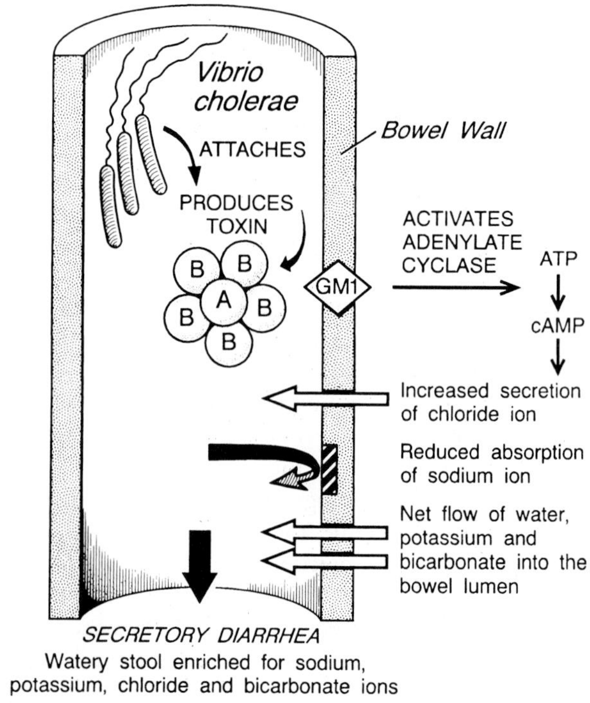

FIGURE 36.2. Pathophysiology of *Vibrio cholerae* infection. See text for details.

enhance production are low temperature (25 to 30°C), osmolarity (NaCl concentration of 50 to 60 mM), rich media, high aeration, a slightly acidic pH (6.5), and the presence of certain amino acids (asparagine, serine, glutamate, and arginine), phosphate, and trace elements (103,153,154). Different strains also show differing levels of toxin production. The observation that cholera toxin expression was regulated by environmental conditions led to the identification of other similarly regulated *V. cholerae* virulence factors (discussed later) (103,114).

The cholera toxin structural genes (*ctxAB*) were originally cloned with the use of homologous *E. coli* LT gene probes (155,156). Cholera toxin genes are poorly expressed in *E. coli* (156,157); the A subunit is not proteolytically nicked and the assembled holotoxin remains in the periplasm and is not secreted extracellularly (156). The DNA sequence of *ctxAB* has been determined for both El Tor (148,158–160) and classical (148,161) strains. Minor differences in the amino acid sequences of the various strains exist. *ctxB* lies immediately downstream of *ctxA*, overlapping by four nucleotides. The predicted length of CtxA is 258 amino acids, with the first 18 residues serving as a likely signal sequence; CtxB is 124 amino acids in length, with a 21-residue signal sequence. *ctxA* and *ctxB* are transcribed as an operon; consistent with the 5:1 ratio of B subunit to A subunit in holotoxin, the B subunit is more highly expressed, likely due to translational control (148).

The cholera toxin subunits are first transported across the bacterial inner membrane through the Sec pathway. After folding and assembly in the periplasm, the toxin is transported extracellularly by the products of the EPS (extracellular protein secretion) gene cluster, which encode a type II secretion system. The organization of the EPS apparatus has been the focus of a number of studies (162–164). In addition to transporting CTX, protease (162), and chitinase (165), the EPS mechanism also plays a role in rugose polysaccharide production (166). Intriguingly, the outer membrane component of the EPS system, EpsD, has been demonstrated to be required for secretion of the CTXϕ as well, thus providing a fascinating convergence of the secretion system in both pathogenicity and in horizontal transfer of a key virulence gene (167).

CTXϕ

The cholera toxin genes were originally described as lying within a transposon-like genetic element (168), composed of a 4.5-kilobase pair (kbp) core region containing the genes *cep, orfU, ace, zot,* and *ctxAB,* flanked by one or more copies of a 2.7- or 2.4-kbp directly repeated region called, respectively, RS1 or RS2 (169,170). It is now clear that the genes encoding *ctxAB* are located on the genome of a lysogenic filamentous bacteriophage, called CTXΦ (171). The 4.5-kbp core region and the 2.4-kbp RS2 region comprise the 6.9 kbp CTXΦ genome. The genes in the core region, other than *ctxAB,* are required for the formation of CTXΦ (171). The integration, replication, regulation, and biotype-specific immunity of CTXΦ depends on the genes *rstR, rstA2,* and *rstB2,* which lie within RS2 (172,173). Extracellular CTXΦ particles are produced from toxigenic *V. cholerae* under appropriate conditions. *V. cholerae* contains a specific 18-bp chromosomal integration site for the CTXΦ, called *attRS* (170). The previously described 2.7-kbp RS1 regions are similar to the RS2 regions but also encode another gene, *rstC* and are often found flanking the prophage on the chromosome of CTXϕ lysogens (172).

Approximately 70%< of El Tor strains have a single copy of the CTXϕ prophage on chromosome 1; the rest carry two or more tandemly repeated copies (5,169,174). The presence of multiple copies loosely correlates with increased toxin production (169). Strains of the classical biotype contain a single copy of the prophage on chromosome 1 and a second copy on chromosome 2 (5,14); both express active cholera toxin (148).

Of considerable interest is the fact that TCP is the bacterial cell receptor for infection of *V. cholerae* by CTXΦ (171). Therefore, the expression of TCP, a virulence factor for infection, which itself was acquired by *V. cholerae* by horizontal transmission of the VPI, is required for *V. cholerae* to acquire an additional virulence factor, CTXΦ. It has been suggested that the VPI is itself encoded by a filamentous bacteriophage, which uses the TCP pilin as a coat protein (175). Three genes flank the VPI, which encode phage-related proteins: a helicase, a transcriptional activator, and an integrase (105), but no other genes have been identified that encode proteins with homology to phage structural products (5).

Regulation of Virulence

Many *V. cholerae* virulence genes have been found to be coordinately regulated in response to the environmental signals that were initially identified as regulating the expression of the cholera toxin genes *in vitro*. The regulatory cascade controlling many of the known virulence genes in *V. cholerae* is shown in Fig. 36.3. Such regulatory cascades controlling virulence factors have likely evolved to allow pathogens to control precisely when virulence genes will be expressed, thus conferring a survival advantage by allowing organisms to adapt to varying environmental conditions (176).

Expression of virulence genes in *V. cholerae* was initially believed to be controlled by a single 32.5-kd transmembrane protein, ToxR (157), and thus was named the ToxR regulon (see refs. 177 and 178 for reviews). ToxR does not directly activate the *ctxAB* promoter, but affects toxin expression by activating another transcriptional activator, ToxT (see later text) (179). ToxR is a transmembrane protein (153); the amino terminus is a DNA-binding region that is similar to the activator class of proteins in the family of prokaryotic two-component regulators (180). The periplasmic carboxy

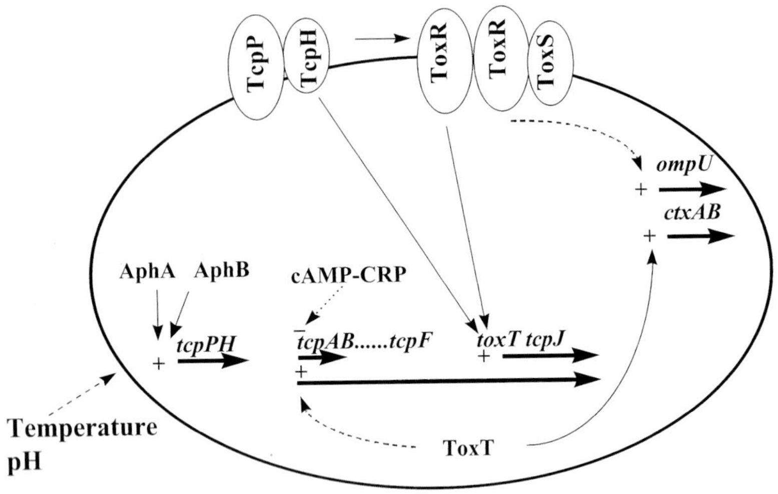

FIGURE 36.3. Model for the virulence regulatory cascade of *Vibrio cholerae*. See text for details. (Adapted from Murley YM, Carroll PA, Skorupski K, et al. Differential transcription of the *tcpPH* operon confers biotype-specific control of the *Vibrio cholerae* ToxR virulence regulon. *Infect Immun* 1999;67:5117–5123, with permission.)

terminus of ToxR senses environmental changes, leading to conformational changes in the DNA-binding amino terminus and altered gene transcription (180).

A second gene in the *toxR* operon is *toxS,* which lies immediately downstream of *toxR* and is part of the same transcriptional unit (181,182). *toxS* encodes a 19-kd protein that is located in the periplasm (182). ToxS is necessary for ToxR activation, perhaps by facilitating dimerization (181,182).

Two other regulatory proteins, TcpP and TcpH, whose genes lie on the TCP pathogenicity island within the *tcp* gene cluster, work in concert with ToxR and ToxS to regulate transcription of yet another member of the *tcp* gene cluster, *toxT* (183,184). ToxT is a 32-kd protein belonging to the AraC family of transcriptional activators (185,186). ToxT activates *ctxAB* and also activates the *tcp* operon encoding the TCP (103,114), the *acf* genes encoding an accessory colonization factor (114), and the *aldA* gene encoding the enzyme aldehyde dehydrogenase (187). However, some ToxR-regulated genes are independent of ToxT (179,188), such as the genes encoding two major outer membrane proteins, OmpT and OmpU, and genes involved in motility and chemotaxis.

It is not yet known which proteins sense the environmental changes that regulate gene expression. Temperature and pH changes can alter the production of TcpP and TcpH; transcription of the *tcpPH* genes is controlled by these factors independently of ToxR (183). In an environment with a high concentration of NaCl, TcpPH is less able to activate ToxT (189). Two additional regulatory proteins, AphA and AphB, have been identified as being necessary for activation of *tcpPH,* and may regulate *tcpPH* expression in response to changes in the environment (190,191). It is also possible that TcpPH and ToxR directly sense environmental changes, or perhaps other regulatory proteins will be identified that affect the expression of these known regulators. However, most environmental conditions do not appear to influence ToxR expression directly (153,192). One exception is that ToxR expression is reduced at high temperatures (37°C), perhaps because of preferential activation at high temperatures of the promoter of the heat shock gene, *htpG,* which lies directly upstream of and in the opposite orientation from *toxR* (192). The classical and El Tor biotypes of *V. cholerae* respond differently to environmental conditions. The molecular mechanisms underlying these biotype differences have been explored by a number of investigators and are due to variations in control over the expression of ToxT (193) and of TcpP and TcpH (194,195).

Additional regulatory mechanisms may play a role in the regulation of virulence. Many bacteria can respond to carbon sources by modulating their cAMP expression via the global regulator CRP; the cAMP-CRP system also influences the expression of ToxR-regulated virulence genes (196). A homologue of the conserved global regulatory gene *gacA,* whose protein product belongs to the family of two-component signal transducing molecules, has been identified in *V. cholerae.* Transcription of this gene is independent of ToxR and mutants in this gene produce less TCP and CT, and are attenuated in colonization (197). Expression of CT from the replicative form of CTXΦ has been demonstrated to be largely independent of ToxR and ToxT (198), suggesting that phage induction and replication may act as an additional mechanism for the regulation of CT production *in vivo.* Finally, recombinase-based *in vivo* expression technology has allowed investigators to begin to examine the complex regulation of temporal expression patterns of virulence genes during infection in an animal model (199).

Other Virulence Factors

Several other enterotoxins, besides cholera toxin, have been described in *V. cholerae* O1. The genes encoding two of these, *zot* and *ace,* lie upstream of *ctxAB* within the core region of the CTXΦ genome. Zot (zonula occludens toxin) increases the permeability of the small intestinal mucosa by affecting the structure of the intercellular tight junctions (200,201), whereas Ace (accessory cholera enterotoxin) (202) increases ion transport across rabbit ileal mucosa and causes fluid secretion in ligated rabbit ileal loops. The mechanism of action of Ace is unknown, but its predicted protein sequence is similar to eukaryotic ion-transporting ATPases, including the product of the cystic fibrosis gene (202). With the identification of Ace and Zot as structural proteins required in CTXϕ morphogenesis (171), the role of these proteins as toxins is being reexamined.

Adjacent to the CTXϕ prophage is the *rtx* gene cluster (*rtxACBD*) encoding an RTX toxin, its activator, and transporters (203). Nucleotide composition analysis suggests that these genes were horizontally acquired along with two downstream genes that encode a sensor histidine kinase and response regulator, suggesting that these regulators may play a role in the regulation of RTX toxin expression in response to environmental changes (5). This toxin causes the depolymerization of actin stress fibers and covalent cross-linking of cellular actin into multimers, leading to the rounding of epithelial cells (204).

Although the genome sequence of *V. cholerae* El Tor strain N16961 did not reveal genes encoding homologues of *E. coli* heat stable toxin (5), other strains of V. *cholerae* O1 produce four molecular species of heat-stable enterotoxins, all homologous to the heat-stable enterotoxin of some *V. cholerae* non-O1 strains (205). At the protein level, these toxins are homologous to the heat-stable enterotoxin of enterotoxigenic *E. coli,* although the genes encoding these proteins lack nucleotide similarity (205), suggesting convergent evolution. The relevance of these enterotoxins to human disease is not yet known. *V. cholerae* was postulated to produce a Shiga toxin, analogous to the Shiga toxins found in a variety of strains of enterohemorrhagic *E. coli* (206), but the genome sequence has not revealed an *stx* homologue.

A number of virulence genes in *V. cholerae* are expressed under low-iron conditions. Iron is an important signal for the regulation of many bacterial virulence factors, and *in vivo*–grown *V. cholerae* O1 expresses proteins that are similar to those seen following *in vitro* growth in low-iron conditions, suggesting that the organism may sense low-iron conditions in the intestine (207). The major 77-kd iron-regulated outer membrane protein of *V. cholerae* O1, IrgA, has been shown to be a virulence factor; a mutation in *irgA* produces a 100-fold defect in the virulence of *V. cholerae* O1 in a suckling mouse model and a 10-fold defect in colonization compared with the wild-type parent strain (208). Expression of *irgA* depends on a second iron-regulated gene, *irgB,* whose protein product acts as a transcriptional activator for *irgA* (209,210). The mechanism by which IrgA and IrgB affect the pathogenesis of *V. cholerae* O1 infection, however, remains undefined (211).

The *V. cholerae* hemolysin genes are also negatively regulated by iron concentration (212,213). The hemolysin, which distinguishes the usually hemolytic El Tor biotype from the nonhemolytic classical biotype, has been the subject of intensive investigations. All examined classical strains have an 11-bp deletion in the structural gene, *hlyA,* of the El Tor biotype (214). However, both hemolytic and nonhemolytic variants of one El Tor strain have identical *hlyA* sequences, suggesting that other genes may affect hemolysis (215). Another gene, *hlyB,* may contribute to expression of the hemolytic phenotype (216). Two potential regulatory loci, *hlyR* (217) and *hlyU* (213), have also been described. The *V. cholerae* O1 hemolysin also has enterotoxic and cytotoxic activity (218). Volunteer studies, however, have not revealed a difference in the ability of hemolytic and nonhemolytic strains to cause diarrhea (219), leaving unresolved the question of the role of hemolysin in the pathogenesis of disease.

Recent advances in molecular biology techniques have led to the identification of virulence genes that are expressed *in vivo*. Signature-tagged transposon mutagenesis has identified several novel genes critical for colonization in the suckling mouse model (220). Recombinase-based *in vivo* expression technology has been used to detect genes that are transcriptionally induced during infection (221), and has been used to monitor the temporal expression of specific virulence genes during the course of infection (199).

Immunity

Naturally Occurring Immunity

Patients who recover from cholera infection are believed to have long-lasting immunity to reinfection (88). In volunteer challenge studies, clinical infection with *V. cholerae* of the classical biotype provides complete protection against illness after rechallenge with classical Ogawa or Inaba strains; organisms cannot be recovered from stool after rechallenge (88,92,222). Protection lasts for at least 3 years (88). In contrast, infection with El Tor strains provides only 90% protection against rechallenge with El Tor Ogawa or Inaba strains (88,222) and organisms can be recovered from the stools of 30% of the rechallenged volunteers (222). Population studies in endemic areas give conflicting estimates of the protection provided by natural infection, ranging from none (223) to 90% (87). The protection conferred by an initial episode of cholera may be influenced by the biotype of the initial infection (99). In a large field study in Bangladesh, the overall incidence of cholera was 61% lower in persons who had been previously ill with cholera than in persons who had not had a known prior infection. In that study, initial episodes of classical cholera provided complete protection against subsequent cholera, whereas initial episodes of El Tor cholera were associated with negligible protection (99).

Mucosal Immunity

As a mucosal pathogen, *V. cholerae* adheres selectively to the M cells of the gastrointestinal tract (224) and is a strong stimulus to the common mucosal immune system; oral cholera vaccination in humans produces a strong secretory immune response, as judged by salivary IgA directed against cholera toxin B subunit (225). Secretory IgA by itself is sufficient to protect mice against subsequent intestinal disease from *V. cholerae* (226). Animal studies have demonstrated that prior colonization with *V. cholerae* produces substantial resistance to recolonization, suggesting that mucosal colonization is essential for immunizing efficiency (227). The observation that prior oral immunization with nontoxigenic strains interferes with stimulation of a mucosal antitoxin response by toxigenic strains also points to the importance of colonization in the induction of a mucosal immune response (228). However, cholera toxin clearly plays a role in enhancing mucosal colonization, as discussed earlier; in addition, cholera toxin is a strong adjuvant, enhancing mucosal secretory antibody responses to a variety of oral antigens (229).

Systemic Immunity

Intestinal antibodies are thought to provide the primary protection against disease caused by *V. cholerae;* serum antibodies are likely not protective but are used as markers for the presence of secretory IgA directed against relevant antigens. Both antibacterial and antitoxic immunity are important in the host response. Parenteral immunization of animals with cholera toxin, toxoids, or B subunit alone provides only brief protection in that serum antitoxin antibodies decrease rapidly (230–232). Oral B subunit alone, however, given with oral killed whole-cell vaccine, produces both serum and intestinal antitoxin antibody responses and leads to a greater protective effect than with whole-cell vaccine alone (233). Serum IgG antitoxic antibodies increase after clinical cholera and can persist for several years (234,235). However, epidemiologic studies have not demonstrated a correlation between the presence of serum antitoxic antibodies and protection against infection (236). The presence of secretory IgA antitoxic antibodies in breast milk, however, is correlated with protection of breast-fed children, suggesting that serum antitoxic antibody levels may not fully reflect intestinal secretory IgA protection (97).

Antibacterial immunity is an essential component to protection against cholera. Both parenteral and oral killed whole-cell vaccines, which produce no antitoxin response, can lead to protection against clinical disease, as can live oral vaccines that lack the genes for cholera toxin (237,238). The presence of serum vibriocidal antibodies, which are measured by their ability to kill bacteria in the presence of complement, clearly correlates with protection against disease; epidemiologic studies have shown a clear relationship between the vibriocidal antibody titer and protection against cholera (236,239). Most vibriocidal antibodies appear to be antilipopolysaccharide antibodies, although other components of the cell surface may play a role (240). Vibriocidal antibody titers are also used in cholera diagnosis. Titers peak 10 to 21 days after infection; a fourfold increase between acute (days 1 to 5) and early convalescent (days 10 to 21) sera, or a fourfold decline in antibody titers between early and late (>2 months) convalescent sera, is considered diagnostic.

CLINICAL ILLNESS

Incubation Period

The incubation period of cholera is usually 1 to 3 days, with a range of a few hours to 5 days (92,241). Human volunteer studies have demonstrated an inverse relationship between the incubation period and the ingested dose of organisms (92,241), as well as with the gastric pH (24).

Asymptomatic and Mild Disease

The majority of persons infected with *V. cholerae* O1 remain asymptomatic. Mild disease is indistinguishable from many other forms of infectious diarrhea, with no prodromal symptoms, a few episodes of watery stools without mucus or blood, rare nausea and vomiting, and no significant fluid loss (242). In areas experiencing an epidemic outbreak, however, most cases of diarrhea are likely to be a result of *V. cholerae* infection; during the 1992 epidemic in Peru, *V. cholerae* O1 was recovered from 79% of patients presenting with diarrhea (73).

Cholera Gravis

Severe disease, called *cholera gravis,* is characterized by severe watery diarrhea, vomiting, and dehydration (242). Clinical findings are due to rapid and massive fluid and electrolyte loss. Diarrhea may begin slowly or abruptly and is painless; stools quickly become watery and clear with flecks of mucus. Cholera stools are classicalally described as "rice water" stools, for their similarity to water in which uncooked rice has been washed. Stools characteristically have a mild "fishy" odor. Vomiting is common, often beginning after the onset of diarrhea but sometimes before (92). There is usually no abdominal pain or fever.

Severe cholera is distinguished by how rapidly a healthy person can become dramatically ill. Patients may present after only a few hours of illness and may look cadaveric in appearance. Fluid loss due to diarrhea and vomiting may be massive, between 500 mL and 1 L of fluid per hour, and can lead to the rapid loss of more than 10% of body weight (242). Diarrhea is most severe during the first 48 hours, then slows, ending after 4 to 6 days in patients treated with appropriate rehydration (243–245). Total volume loss during illness may reach 100% of body weight (244). Along with rapid fluid losses come large electrolyte losses; cholera stools contain high concentrations of sodium, potassium, chloride, and bicarbonate.

Patients with severe cholera present with signs of volume and electrolyte loss. Mild dehydration is indicated by thirst, dry mouth, decreased axillary sweat, and slight weight loss. Signs of moderate dehydration include tachycardia, an orthostatic decrease in blood pressure, skin tenting, and sunken eyes or fontanelle. Signs of severe dehydration are hypotension, anuria, and mental status changes. Rapid assessment of the degree of dehydration is essential for optimal rehydration therapy of patients with cholera (Table 36.1).

Complications of severe cholera are the result of sustained volume loss or electrolyte imbalances. Severe acidosis is the result of loss of bicarbonate in the stool, along with lactic acidemia from shock, hyperphosphatemia from renal failure, and hyperproteinemia from dehydration (246). Acidosis may be manifested as tachypnea, Kussmaul breathing, or, in end-stage cases, pulmonary edema (247). Loss of potassium in the stool may lead to hypokalemia, which can cause cardiac arrhythmias, paralytic ileus, and painful leg cramps. Renal failure follows acute tubular necrosis from hypovolemia (248). Hypoglycemia may be a complication of severe cholera, especially in children (249), and has been implicated in mental status changes and seizures seen in severe cholera. Cholera in pregnancy carries a high mortality rate, with a 50% risk of fetal death during the third trimester (250).

Mortality

The large, rapid volume losses in cholera gravis can lead to hypovolemic shock and death within 2 to 3 hours. More commonly, untreated patients progress to shock in 4 to 12 hours and death in 18 hours to several days (251). Mortality or "the mortality rate" in untreated patients may be as high as 50% to 70% (60,252), particularly in outbreak situations.

DIAGNOSIS

Clinical Diagnosis

Although cholera cannot be definitively distinguished clinically from other causes of severe watery diarrhea and vomiting, cholera should be considered in all such cases, particularly those with rapid progression and severe dehydration (2). Many infectious diseases cause severe diarrhea in children, but dehydrating diarrhea in an adult is uncommon and raises the suspicion of cholera (253). Clinical suspicion should be increased for travelers to areas with cholera in whom diarrhea develops within 5 days of leaving the area, or in persons who recently ingested raw or undercooked shellfish (2,253,254).

Laboratory Diagnosis

To confirm a case of cholera requires laboratory identification of toxinogenic *V. cholerae* O1 or *V. cholerae* O139 Bengal from a person with diarrhea (11). It is essential, however, not to wait for laboratory confirmation before treating patients who are suspected of having cholera because death by dehydration can occur quickly.

Stool specimens or rectal swabs should be collected soon after the start of illness and before antibiotic treatment, if possible. If specimens must be held or transported, they should be placed in transport medium; semisolid Cary-Blair medium is the one most extensively used (11). Swabs in holding medium can be kept at room temperature, whereas liquid stool should be refrigerated (255). Vibrios can survive for up to 5 weeks in stools placed on blotting paper and kept in sealed plastic bags (256). Several practical methods have been developed to isolate *V. cholerae* from water (257) or sewage (258) for use in surveillance.

TABLE 36.1. SIGNS AND SYMPTOMS OF DEHYDRATION AMONG PATIENTS WITH DIARRHEA

	Outcome		
Examination	**No Signs of Dehydration**	**Some Dehydration**	**Severe Dehydration**
Look at			
Mental status	Well, alert	Restless, irritable[a]	Lethargic or unconscious; floppy infant[a]
Eyes	Normal	Sunken	Very sunken and dry
Tears	Present	Absent	Absent
Mouth/tongue	Moist	Dry	Very dry
Thirst	Drinks normally, not thirsty	Thirsty, drinks eagerly[a]	Drinks poorly or not able to drink[a]
Feel			
Skin pinch	Goes back rapidly	Goes back slowly[a]	Goes back very slowly[a]
Pulse	Normal	Faster than normal[a]	Very fast, weak or nonpalpable[a]
Fontanelle	Normal	Sunken	Very sunken
Decide degree of dehydration	*No* signs of dehydration, <2.5% of body weight	If two or more of these signs exist, including at least one important sign, then there is *some* dehydration, from 2.5% to 10% of body weight	If two or more of these signs exist, including at least one important sign, then there is *severe* dehydration, >10% of body weight

[a]Important signs and symptoms for assessment of dehydration.

The stools of patients with acute, untreated cholera contain extremely large numbers of vibrios (10^6 to 10^8/mL) (259), so Gram's stain of such stools revealing sheets of vibrio forms may suggest the diagnosis. Vibrios can be rapidly detected in stool by dark field or phase contrast microscopy. The organisms are motile and appear like "shooting stars" (11). Specificity can be demonstrated by inhibiting motility with specific antisera (260). Other rapid diagnostic methods in use are monoclonal antibody–based stool tests (261) and detection via polymerase chain reaction (262). Direct plating of acute stool specimens on selective media, such as TCBS, is usually sufficient for the isolation of organisms. Enrichment in alkaline peptone water for 6 to 8 hours, which selects for vibrios because of their tolerance to high pH, increases the recovery of *V. cholerae* when bacterial numbers are low, as occurs in convalescent carriers (11,255).

Yellow colonies on TCBS are subcultured and biochemically confirmed as *V. cholerae. V. cholerae* O1 and O139 strains can be serotyped with specific antisera (11). Toxinogenic strains can be detected with the polymerase chain reaction, enzyme-linked immunosorbent assays, or a latex agglutination assay (263–265).

Vibriocidal and antitoxin antibody titers can be used retrospectively to confirm *V. cholerae* O1 infection. An increase in antitoxic antibody titers, which increase 2 to 4 weeks after the onset of disease and remain elevated, may be diagnostic.

Because epidemic strains of *V. cholerae* O1 and O139 can acquire plasmids carrying antibiotic resistance, it is important to determine the antimicrobial susceptibility of strains isolated in the laboratory. This can be done using disk diffusion methods or other standard techniques (266).

TREATMENT

Degree of Dehydration

The prime consideration in treatment of clinical cholera is rapid, appropriate volume replacement. Physicians should be aware that fluid losses may be greater than for most diarrheas usually seen and that aggressive rehydration with large volumes of fluid may be necessary (2). The rapid assessment of the degree of dehydration of an individual patient should guide the course of treatment. WHO guidelines for deciding whether patients have no (<2.5% body weight), some (2.5% to 10% body weight), or severe (>10% body weight) dehydration are shown in Table 36.1.

Oral Rehydration

The treatment of cholera was revolutionized by the promotion of oral rehydration solutions, which depend on the fact that glucose-facilitated sodium and water absorption in the small intestine remains intact in the presence of cholera toxin. The availability of oral rehydration solutions has reduced mortality rates from cholera from more than 50% to less than 1% (59). The WHO recommends a solution containing 3.5 g of sodium chloride, 2.5 g of sodium bicarbonate, 1.5 g of potassium chloride, and 20 g of glucose (or 40 g of sucrose) per liter of water (267). Alternatives to glucose have been widely studied, and are effective in reducing stool volume and shortening the duration of diarrhea (268,269). Guidelines for rehydration and maintenance therapy with oral rehydration solutions are reviewed in Chapter 79.

Intravenous Rehydration

Patients who are severely dehydrated (>10% of body weight) or in whom mental status changes or vomiting precludes the use of oral therapy should be treated with intravenous solutions such as Ringer's lactate, which is the only generally available solution in the United States with the appropriate electrolyte composition (270). Many developing countries have other appropriate intravenous replacement solutions. In the United States, if Ringer's lactate is not available, normal or half-normal saline solutions can be used, but they do not contain needed bicarbonate or potassium. Plain glucose in water is ineffective in replacing intravascular fluid and electrolyte losses in cholera (270). Oral rehydration solution should be given as soon as a patient can drink. Severely dehydrated patients need to have large volumes of fluid given rapidly. Patients must be monitored for complications of fluid overload, but if oral rehydration therapy is begun when initial rehydration is complete, this should be unusual; insufficient hydration is much more common than overhydration. Volumes of intravenous fluids to be given and rates of administration are listed in Table 36.2.

Antimicrobial Therapy

Rehydration therapy is the only treatment necessary for cholera patients. Use of antibiotics, however, can reduce the duration and thus the expense of treatment, an important consideration for cholera control. Antibiotics have been demonstrated to reduce the volume and duration of diarrhea by about half and reduce the duration of vibrio excretion to an average of 1 day (243,271). Oral antibiotics can be given when vomiting stops, usually about the time that initial rehydration is completed. Injectable antibiotics are unnecessary (267).

Antibiotics recommended for the treatment of cholera are listed in Table 36.3. Clinicians should determine the antibiotic susceptibility pattern in their area to guide therapy. Tetracycline has historically been the drug most commonly used. However, a single dose of doxycycline in adults has been found to be as effective clinically as multiple-dose tetracycline treatment, although doxycycline-treated patients excrete vibrios for longer (272). Doxycycline is

TABLE 36.2. GUIDELINES FOR INTRAVENOUS TREATMENT OF PATIENTS WITH SEVERE DEHYDRATION

Age	First Give 30 mL/kg	Then Give 70 mL/kg
Infants (younger than 12 mo)	1 h[a]	5 h
Children and adults	30 min[a]	2.5 h

[a]Repeat if radial pulse is still very weak or not detectable.
From Swerdlow DL, Ries AA. Cholera in the Americas. *JAMA* 1992;267:1495–1499.

therefore the preferred agent in the field to improve compliance and decrease cost.

V. cholerae O1 was originally found to be universally sensitive to tetracycline (271), but large outbreaks of multiply antibiotic-resistant organisms have been documented in many areas of the world (2,273). Because the majority of *V. cholerae* O139 strains are resistant to trimethoprim-sulfamethoxazole and furazolidone, as are many O1 El Tor strains in India and Bangladesh (274), these antibiotics, previously widely recommended, are no longer preferred. Fluoroquinolones have become the alternative of choice for treatment of adults in areas with a high frequency of antibiotic-resistant organisms. Multidose norfloxacin, multidose ciprofloxacin, and single-dose ciprofloxacin have all been found to be effective in the treatment of adults with cholera in clinical studies (275–277).

Erythromycin is the standard choice for treating cholera in children. Azithromycin may prove to be an attractive alternative, because it is highly active *in vitro* against both O139 and O1 strains (274). Tetracycline and doxycycline are not recommended for pregnant women and children younger than 8 years of age, because they may cause permanent tooth discoloration. Quinolones have not been recommended for use in children, because cartilage toxicity from these drugs were observed in animal studies; however, these recommendations may be revised as more experience with the use of quinolones in children accumulates.

Tetracycline treatment of family contacts of patients with cholera has been demonstrated to be effective in preventing illness (278,279). Because of the difficulties in determining who is a close contact (and limiting treatment to such persons), in treating before infection can spread, in isolating treated contacts to prevent reinfection, and in the cost of surveillance and treatment programs, the WHO only recommends the use of selective chemoprophylaxis if surveillance shows that an average of one household member in a family of five becomes ill after the first case (270). None of the cholera cases imported by the United States since 1961 have resulted in secondary transmission (32); chemoprophylaxis of family contacts in the United States is therefore not recommended (280). Families should be instructed in proper handwashing and in cleaning contaminated clothes and bedding with soap and chlorine bleach. Homes should be inspected to confirm that sewage treatment is sufficient to decontaminate feces (280). Mass chemoprophylaxis of an entire community has not been successful in limiting the spread of cholera, and such action draws resources away from effective control measures (270).

Other Therapies

Many antisecretory drugs have been tested in cholera patients; none have proven to be of benefit (281). The WHO recommends against the use of antidiarrheal, antiemetic, antispasmodic, cardiotonic, or corticosteroid medications in the treatment of cholera (270).

PREVENTION

Hygiene

Prevention of the spread of epidemic cholera requires interruption of fecal-oral transmission. Ensuring the safety of food and water depends on the availability of adequate sewage collection and disposal, the protection of clean water sources, and effective water treatment (282). Many develop-

TABLE 36.3. ANTIBIOTIC REGIMENS FOR TREATMENT OF CHOLERA ACCORDING TO AGE AND THE LIKELIHOOD OF TETRACYCLINE RESISTANCE

Tetracycline Resistance	Antibiotics	Regimen	Dose: Children	Dose: Adults
Uncommon	Doxycycline	One dose	6 mg/kg (only if older than age 8 yr, see text)	300 mg
	Tetracycline	Four times per day for 3 days	12.5 mg/kg (only if older than age 8 yr, see text)	500 mg
Common	Erythromycin	Adults: four times per day for 3 days; children: three times per day for 3 days	10 mg/kg	250 mg
	Ciprofloxacin	One dose	Not recommended (see text)	1000 mg
	Norfloxacin	Two times per day for 3 days	Not recommended (see text)	400 mg

Adapted with permission from Butterton JR. Approach to the patient with *Vibrio cholerae* infection. In: Rose BD, ed. UpToDate, Wellesley, MA, 2001. Copyright 2001 UpToDate, Inc. For more information visit *www.uptodate.com.*

ing countries do not possess the infrastructure to provide clean water and sewage treatment to their populations.

Measures that can be taken on a local level include the construction of latrines, education concerning the importance of handwashing after defecation, and education on how to make food and water safe at home (270). Water can be disinfected with chlorine or iodine, by filtration, or by bringing water to a rolling boil for 30 sec at sea level or for 3 min at higher altitudes (282). Carbonated bottled water may be safe, because *V. cholerae* will not survive in an acidic environment for more than 1 day (22). In emergencies, two drops of household bleach (5.25% chlorine) may be mixed well in a quart of water and allowed to stand for 10 min before consumption; such water should not be used for more than short periods (282). Food should be cooked until hot and eaten while hot. Utensils should be washed and thoroughly dried after use and hands should be washed before preparing and eating food (270).

Surveillance

Cholera is an internationally notifiable disease. In the United States, physicians must report cases of cholera to local and state health departments; isolates from presumed cases should be sent to state health departments and to the Centers for Disease Control and Prevention (CDC) for laboratory confirmation. The CDC investigates outbreaks, assisted by the U.S. Environmental Protection Agency if transmission appears to be by water (282). Confirmed cases are reported to the WHO, which is responsible for global surveillance.

Vaccines

The parenteral killed whole-cell vaccine preparation that is currently licensed for use in the United States provides less than 50% protection from disease, for a duration of only 3 to 6 months. The vaccine does not reduce the rate of asymptomatic infections and so does not prevent transmission of disease (283). The vaccine is no longer recommended for international travelers and should not be used in contacts of patients with cholera (283). Because of these limitations, the 26th World Health Assembly abolished the requirement in the International Health Regulations for a certificate of vaccination against cholera (270).

The development of improved vaccines is an area of intense research activity. In Europe, two additional vaccines are available: an oral killed whole cell–cholera toxin recombinant B subunit vaccine (WC-rBS) (284), and an oral live attenuated *V. cholerae* vaccine (CVD 103-HgR) (31,238,285). The potential use of oral cholera vaccines in emergency situations was the subject of a WHO meeting in May, 1999 (31,286). It was recommended that the oral WC-rBS vaccine should be considered among the tools to prevent cholera in populations believed to be at risk of a cholera epidemic within 6 months and not experiencing a current epidemic (286). See Chapter 80.

ACKNOWLEDGMENTS

This work was supported by Public Health Service Grants DK59010 from the National Institute of Diabetes and Digestive and Kidney Diseases and DK43351 from the Center for the Study of Inflammatory Bowel Diseases (to J.R.B.) and by Public Health Service Grants AI40725 and AI44487 from the National Institute of Allergy and Infectious Diseases and HD39165 from the National Institute of Child Health and Development (to S.B.C.).

REFERENCES

1. Tauxe RV, Blake PA. Epidemic cholera in Latin America. *JAMA* 1992;267:1388–1390.
2. Swerdlow DL, Ries AA. Cholera in the Americas. *JAMA* 1992; 267:1495–1499.
3. Baumann L, Bang SS, Baumann P. Study of relationship among species of *Vibrio, Photobacterium,* and terrestrial enterobacteria by an immunological comparison of glutamine synthetase and superoxide dismutase. *Curr Microbiol* 1980;4:133–138.
4. MacDonell MT, Swartz DG, Ortiz-Conde BA, et al. Ribosomal RNA phylogenies for the *Vibrio*-enteric group of eubacteria. *Microbiol Sci* 1986;3:172–178.
5. Heidelberg JF, Eisen JA, Nelson WC, et al. DNA sequence of both chromosomes of the cholera pathogen *Vibrio cholerae. Nature* 2000;406:477–483.
6. Janda JM, Powers C, Bryant RG, et al. Current perspectives on the epidemiology and pathogenesis of clinically significant *Vibrio* spp. *Clin Microbiol Rev* 1988;1:245–267.
7. Kenne L, Lindberg B, Unger P, et al. Structural studies of the *Vibrio cholerae* O-antigen. *Carbohydr Res* 1982;100:341–349.
8. Gotschlich T. Vibrios Choleriques isoles au compement de Tor. Retour du pelerinage de l'annee, 1905. Report adresse au President du Conseil quarante naine d'Egypt, Alexandria. *Bull Inst Louis Pasteur* 1905;3:726.
9. Sakazaki R. Bacteriology of *Vibrio* and related organisms. In: Barua D, Greenough WB III, eds. *Cholera.* New York: Plenum Press, 1992:37–55.
10. Stroeher UH, Karageorgos LE, Morona R, et al. Serotype conversion in *Vibrio cholerae* O1. *Proc Natl Acad Sci U S A* 1992; 89:2566–2570.
11. Centers for Disease Control and Prevention. Isolation and identification of *Vibrio cholerae* serogroups O1 and O139. *Laboratory methods for the diagnosis of epidemic dysentery and cholera.* Atlanta: Centers for Disease Control and Prevention, 1999:41–54.
12. Chatterjee BD. Vibrios and campylobacters. In: Braude AI, Davis CE, Fierer J, eds. *Infectious Diseases and Medical Microbiology,* 2nd ed. Philadelphia: W. B. Saunders, 1986:303–314.
13. Kelly MT, Hickman-Brenner FW, Farmer JJI. *Vibrio.* In: Balows A, Hausler WJ, Herrmann KL, et al., eds. *Manual of clinical microbiology,* fifth edition. Washington, DC: American Society for Microbiology, 1991:384–395.
14. Trucksis M, Michalski J, Deng YK, et al. The *Vibrio cholerae* genome contains two unique circular chromosomes. *Proc Natl Acad Sci U S A* 1998;95:14464–14469.
15. Waldor MK, RayChaudhuri D. Treasure trove for cholera research. *Nature* 2000;406:469–470.

16. Barua D. History of cholera. In: Barua D, Greenough WB III, eds. *Cholera.* New York: Plenum Press, 1992:1–36.
17. Duffy J. The history of Asiatic cholera in the United States. *Bull N Y Acad Med* 1971;47:1152–1168.
18. Snow J. *On the mode of communication of cholera.* London: John Churchill, 1849.
19. Koch R. An address on cholera and its bacillus. *BMJ* 1884;2: 403–407, 453–459.
20. Barua D. The global epidemiology of cholera in recent years. *Proc R Soc Med* 1972;65:423–428.
21. Goodgame RW, Greenough WB III. Cholera in Africa: a message for the West. *Ann Intern Med* 1975;82:101–106.
22. Blake PA, Rosenberg ML, Bandeira Costa J, et al. Cholera in Portugal, 1974. I. Modes of transmission. *Am J Epidemiol* 1977; 105:337–343.
23. Samadi AR, Huq MI, Shahid NS, et al. Classicalal *Vibrio cholerae* biotype displaced El Tor in Bangladesh. *Lancet* 1983;1:805–807.
24. Glass RI, Black RE. The epidemiology of cholera. In: Barua D, Greenough WB III, eds. *Cholera.* New York: Plenum Press, 1992:129–154.
25. Centers for Disease Control and Prevention. Cholera—Peru, 1991. *MMWR Morbid Mortal Wkly Rep* 1991;40:108–109.
26. Wachsmuth IK, Bopp CA, Fields PI. Difference between toxigenic *Vibrio cholerae* O1 from South America and US Gulf Coast. *Lancet* 1991;337:1097–1098.
27. Wachsmuth IK, Evins GM, Fields PI, et al. The molecular epidemiology of cholera in Latin America. *J Infect Dis* 1993;167: 621–626.
28. Centers for Disease Control and Prevention. Update: Cholera—Western hemisphere, 1992. *MMWR Morbid Mortal Wkly Rep* 1993;42:89–91.
29. Centers for Disease Control and Prevention. Etiology and epidemiology of cholera. *Laboratory methods for the diagnosis of epidemic dysentery and cholera.* Atlanta: Centers for Disease Control and Prevention, 1999:37–40.
30. World Health Organization. Cholera, 1998. *Wkly Epidemiol Rec* 1999;74:257–264.
31. World Health Organization. Cholera, 1999. *Wkly Epidemiol Rec* 2000;75:249–256.
32. Snyder JD, Blake PA. Is cholera a problem for US travelers? *JAMA* 1982;247:2268–2269.
33. Weissman JB, De Witt WE, Thompson J, et al. A case of cholera in Texas, 1973. *Am J Epidemiol* 1974;100:487–498.
34. Blake PA, Allegra DT, Snyder JD, et al. Cholera: a possible endemic focus in the United States. *N Engl J Med* 1980;302: 305–309.
35. Lowry PW, Pavia AT, McFarland LM, et al. Cholera in Louisiana: widening spectrum of seafood vehicles. *Arch Intern Med* 1989;149:2079–2084.
36. Pavia AT, Campbell JF, Blake PA, et al. Cholera from raw oysters shipped interstate. *JAMA* 1987;258:2374.
37. Centers for Disease Control and Prevention. Cholera—New Jersey and Florida. *MMWR Morbid Mortal Wkly Rep* 1991;40: 287–289.
38. Centers for Disease Control and Prevention. Cholera—New York, 1991. *MMWR Morbid Mortal Wkly Rep* 1991;40:516–518.
39. Centers for Disease Control and Prevention. Importation of cholera from Peru. *MMWR Morbid Mortal Wkly Rep* 1991;40: 258–259.
40. Centers for Disease Control and Prevention. Cholera associated with an international airline flight, 1992. *MMWR Morbid Mortal Wkly Rep* 1992;41:134–135.
41. Ramamurthy T, Garg S, Sharma R, et al. Emergence of novel strain of *Vibrio cholerae* with epidemic potential in southern and eastern India. *Lancet* 1993;341:703–704.
42. Albert MJ, Siddique AK, Islam MS, et al. Large outbreak of clinical cholera due to *Vibrio cholerae* non-O1 in Bangladesh. *Lancet* 1993;341:704.
43. Bhattacharya MK, Bhattacharya SK, Garg S, et al. Outbreak of *Vibrio cholerae* non-O1 in India and Bangladesh. *Lancet* 1993; 341:1346–1347.
44. Cholera Working Group, International Centre for Diarrhoeal Diseases Research, Bangladesh. Large epidemic of cholera-like disease in Bangladesh caused by *Vibrio cholerae* O139 synonym Bengal. *Lancet* 1993;342:387–390.
45. Chongsa-nguan M, Chaicumpa W, Moolasart P, et al. *Vibrio cholerae* O139 Bengal in Bangkok. *Lancet* 1993;342:430–431.
46. Shimada T, Nair GB, Deb BC, et al. Outbreak of *Vibrio cholerae* non-O1 in India and Bangladesh. *Lancet* 1993;341:1346.
47. Hall RH, Khambaty FM, Kothary M, et al. Non-O1 *Vibrio cholerae. Lancet* 1993;342:430.
48. Waldor M, Colwell R, Mekalanos J. The *Vibrio cholerae* O139 serogroup antigen includes an O-antigen capsule and lipopolysaccharide virulence determinants. *Proc Natl Acad Sci U S A* 1994;91:11388–11392.
49. Bik EM, Bunschoten AE, Gouw RD, et al. Genesis of the novel epidemic *Vibrio cholerae* O139 strain: evidence for horizontal transfer of genes involved in polysaccharide synthesis. *EMBO J* 1995;14:209–216.
50. Stroeher UH, Jedani KE, Dredge BK, et al. Genetic rearrangements in the *rfb* regions of *Vibrio cholerae* O1 and O139. *Proc Natl Acad Sci U S A* 1995;92:10374–10378.
51. Faruque SM, Saha MN, Asadulghani, et al. The O139 serogroup of *Vibrio cholerae* comprises diverse clones of epidemic and nonepidemic strains derived from multiple *V. cholerae* O1 or non-O1 progenitors. *J Infect Dis* 2000;182:1161–1168.
52. Waldor MK, Tschape H, Mekalanos JJ. A new type of conjugative transposon encodes resistance to sulfamethoxazole, trimethoprim, and streptomycin in *Vibrio cholerae* O139. *J Bacteriol* 1996;178:4157–4165.
53. Hochhut B, Waldor MK. Site-specific integration of the conjugal *Vibrio cholerae* SXT element into *prfC. Mol Microbiol* 1999;32:99–110.
54. Faruque SM, Siddique AK, Saha MN, et al. Molecular characterization of a new ribotype of *Vibrio cholerae* O139 Bengal associated with an outbreak of cholera in Bangladesh. *J Clin Microbiol* 1999;37:1313–1318.
55. Basu A, Garg P, Datta S, et al. *Vibrio cholerae* O139 in Calcutta, 1992–1998: incidence, antibiograms, and genotypes. *Emerg Infect Dis* 2000;6:139–147.
56. Islam MS, Hasan MK, Miah MA, et al. Isolation of *Vibrio cholerae* O139 Bengal from water in Bangladesh. *Lancet* 1993; 342:430.
57. Jesudason MV, John TJ. Major shift in prevalence of non-O1 *Vibrio cholerae. Lancet* 1993;341:1090–1091.
58. Swerdlow DL, Ries AA. *Vibrio cholerae* non-O1—the eighth pandemic? *Lancet* 1993;342:382–383.
59. World Health Organization. Cholera. WHO Report on Global Surveillance of Epidemic-Prone Infectious Diseases. 2000. Report No.: WHO/CDS/CSR/ISR/2000.1.
60. Goma Epidemiology Group. Public health impact of the Rwandan refugee crisis: What happened in Goma, Zaire in July 1994? *Lancet* 1995;345:359–361.
61. Colwell RR, Spria WM. The ecology of *Vibrio cholerae.* In: Barua D, Greenough WB III, eds. *Cholera.* New York: Plenum Press, 1992:107–128.
62. Feachem R, Miller C, Drasar B. Environmental aspects of cholera epidemiology. II. Occurrence and survival of *Vibrio cholerae* in the environment. *Trop Dis Bull* 1981;78:865–880.
63. Pesigan TP, Plantilla J, Rolda M. Applied studies on the viability of El Tor vibrios. *Bull WHO* 1967;37:779–786.
64. Colwell RR, Brayton PR, Grimes DJ, et al. Viable but noncul-

turable *Vibrio cholerae* and related pathogens in the environment: implications for release of genetically engineered microorganisms. *Biotechnology* 1985;3:817–820.
65. Huq A, Colwell RR, Rahman R, et al. Detection of *Vibrio cholerae* O1 in the aquatic environment by fluorescent-monoclonal antibody and culture methods. *Appl Environ Microbiol* 1990;56:2370–2373.
66. Xu H-S, Roberts N, Singleton FL, et al. Survival and viability of non-culturable *Escherichia coli* and *Vibrio cholerae* in the estuarine and marine environment. *Microb Ecol* 1982;8:313–323.
67. Tamplin ML, Gauzens AL, Huq A, et al. Attachment of *Vibrio cholerae* serogroup O1 to zooplankton and phytoplankton of Bangladesh waters. *Appl Environ Microbiol* 1990;56:1977–1980.
68. Spira WM, Huq A, Ahmed QS, et al. Uptake of *Vibrio cholerae* biotype El Tor from contaminated water by water hyacinth (*Eichornia crassipes*). *Appl Environ Microbiol* 1981;42:550–553.
69. Islam MS, Drasar BS, Bradley DJ. Long-term persistence of toxigenic *Vibrio cholerae* O1 in the mucilaginous sheath of a blue-green alga, *Anabaena variabilis. J Trop Med Hyg* 1990;193: 133–139.
70. Watnick PI, Kolter R. Steps in the development of a *Vibrio cholerae* El Tor biofilm. *Mol Microbiol* 1999;34:586–593.
71. Watnick PI, Fullner KJ, Kolter R. A role for the mannose-sensitive hemagglutinin in biofilm formation by *Vibrio cholerae* El Tor. *J Bacteriol* 1999;181:3606–3609.
72. Bassler BL, Greenberg EP, Stevens AM. Cross-species induction of luminescence in the quorum-sensing bacterium *Vibrio harveyi. J Bacteriol* 1997;179:4043–4045.
73. Swerdlow DL, Mintz ED, Rodriguez M, et al. Waterborne transmission of epidemic cholera in Trujillo, Peru: lessons for a continent at risk. *Lancet* 1992;340:28–33.
74. Ries AA, Vugia DJ, Beingolea L, et al. Cholera in Piura, Peru: a modern urban epidemic. *J Infect Dis* 1992;166:1429–1433.
75. Blake PA, Rosenberg ML, Florencia J, et al. Cholera in Portugal, 1974. II. Transmission by bottled mineral water. *Am J Epidemiol* 1977;105:344–348.
76. Hughes JM, Boyce JM, Levine RJ, et al. Epidemiology of El Tor cholera in rural Bangladesh: importance of surface water in transmission. *Bull WHO* 1982;60:395–404.
77. Kolvin JL, Roberts D. Studies on the growth of *Vibrio cholerae* biotype eltor and biotype classicalal in foods. *J Hyg* 1982;89: 243–252.
78. Gerichter CB, Sechter I, Gavish A, et al. Viability of *Vibrio cholerae* biotype El Tor and of cholera phage on vegetables. *Isr J Med Sci* 1975;11:889–895.
79. St. Louis ME, Porter JD, Helal A, et al. Epidemic cholera in West Africa: the role of food handling and high-risk foods. *Am J Epidemiol* 1990;131:719–728.
80. McCormack WM, Islam MS, Fahimuddin M, et al. A community study of inapparent cholera infections. *Am J Epidemiol* 1969;89:658–664.
81. Pierce NF, Banwell JG, Sack RB, et al. Convalescent carriers of *Vibrio cholerae:* detection and detailed investigation. *Ann Intern Med* 1970;72:357–364.
82. Azurin JC, Kobari K, Barua D, et al. A long-term carrier of cholera: cholera Dolores. *Bull WHO* 1967;37:745–749.
83. Mhalu FS, Mtango FDE, Msengi AE. Hospital outbreaks of cholera transmitted through close person-to-person contact. *Lancet* 1984;2:82–84.
84. Ryder RW, Mizanur Rahman ASM, Alim ARMA. An outbreak of nosocomial cholera in a rural Bangladesh hospital. *J Hosp Infect* 1986;8:275–282.
85. Mandar MP, Mhalu FS. Cholera control in an inaccessible district in Tanzania: importance of temporary rural centers. *Med J Zambia* 1980;15:10–13.
86. Isaacson M, Clarke KR, Ellacombe GH, et al. The recent cholera outbreak in the South African gold mining industry: a preliminary report. *S Afr Med J* 1974;48:2557–2560.
87. Glass RI, Becker S, Huq MI, et al. Endemic cholera in rural Bangladesh. *Am J Epidemiol* 1982;116:959–970.
88. Levine MM, Black RE, Clements ML, et al. Duration of infection-derived immunity to cholera. *J Infect Dis* 1981;143: 818–820.
89. Nalin DR, Levine RJ, Levine MM, et al. Cholera, non-vibrio cholera, and stomach acid. *Lancet* 1978;2:856–859.
90. Schiraldi O, Benvestito V, Di Bari C, et al. Gastric abnormalities in cholera: epidemiological and clinical considerations. *Bull WHO* 1974;51:349–352.
91. Nalin DR, Levine MM, Rhead J, et al. Cannabis, hypochlorhydria, and cholera. *Lancet* 1978;2:859–861.
92. Cash RA, Music SI, Libonati JP, et al. Response of man to infection with *Vibrio cholerae.* I. Clinical, serologic, and bacteriologic responses to a known inoculum. *J Infect Dis* 1974;129:45–52.
93. Shahinian ML, Passaro DJ, Swerdlow DL, et al. *Helicobacter pylori* and epidemic *Vibrio cholerae* O1 infection in Peru. *Lancet* 2000;355:377–378.
94. Glass RI, Holmgren J, Haley CE, et al. Predisposition for cholera of individuals with O blood group: possible evolutionary significance. *Am J Epidemiol* 1985;121:791–796.
95. Clemens JD, Sack DA, Harris JR, et al. ABO blood groups and cholera: new observations on specificity of risk and modification of vaccine efficacy. *J Infect Dis* 1989;159:770–773.
96. Clemens JD, Sack DA, Harris JR, et al. Breast feeding and the risk of severe cholera in rural Bangladeshi children. *Am J Epidemiol* 1990;131:400–411.
97. Glass RI, Svennerholm A-M, Stoll BJ, et al. Protection against cholera in breast-fed children by antibodies in breast milk. *N Engl J Med* 1983;308:1389–1392.
98. Glass RI, Svennerholm A-M, Stoll BJ, et al. Effects of undernutrition on infection with *Vibrio cholerae* O1 and on response to oral cholera vaccine. *Pediatr Infect Dis J* 1989;8:105–109.
99. Clemens JD, Van Loon F, Sack DA, et al. Biotype as determinant of natural immunising effect of cholera. *Lancet* 1991;337: 883–884.
100. Woodward WE, Moseley WH. The spectrum of cholera in rural Bangladesh. II. Comparison of El Tor, Ogawa and classicalal Inaba infection. *Am J Epidemiol* 1972;96:342–351.
101. Bart KJ, Huq Z, Khan M, et al. Seroepidemiologic studies during a simultaneous epidemic of infection with El Tor Ogawa and classicalal Inaba *Vibrio cholerae. J Infect Dis* 1970;121 [Suppl]:S17–S24.
102. Dizon JJ, Alvero MG, Joseph PR, et al. Studies on El Tor in the Philippines: 1. Characteristics of cholera El Tor in Negros Occidental Province, November 1961 to September 1962. *Bull WHO* 1965;33:627.
103. Taylor RK, Miller VL, Furlong DB, et al. Use of *phoA* gene fusions to identify a pilus colonization factor coordinately regulated with cholera toxin. *Proc Natl Acad Sci U S A* 1987;84: 2833–2837.
104. Herrington DA, Hall RH, Losonsky G, et al. Toxin, toxin-coregulated pili, and the *toxR* regulon are essential for *Vibrio cholerae* pathogenesis in humans. *J Exp Med* 1988;168:1487–1492.
105. Karaolis DKR, Johnson JA, Bailey CC, et al. A *Vibrio cholerae* pathogenicity island associated with epidemic and pandemic strains. *Proc Natl Acad Sci U S A* 1998;95:3134–3139.
106. Sun DX, Mekalanos JJ, Taylor RK. Antibodies directed against the toxin-coregulated pilus isolated from *Vibrio cholerae* provide protection in the infant mouse experimental cholera model. *J Infect Dis* 1990;161:1231–1236.
107. Sharma DP, Thomas C, Hall RH, et al. Significance of toxin-coregulated pili as protective antigens of *Vibrio cholerae* in the infant mouse model. *Vaccine* 1989;7:451–456.

108. Sharma DP, Stroeher UH, Thomas CJ, et al. The toxin-coregulated pilus (TCP) of *Vibrio cholerae:* molecular cloning of genes involved in pilus biosynthesis and evaluation of TCP as a protective antigen in the infant mouse model. *Microb Pathog* 1989; 7:437–448.
109. Taylor R, Shaw C, Peterson K, et al. Safe, live *Vibrio cholerae* vaccines? *Vaccine* 1988;6:151–154.
110. Hall RH, Vial PA, Kaper JB, et al. Morphological studies on fimbriae expressed by *Vibrio cholerae* O1. *Microb Pathog* 1988; 4:257–265.
111. Fullner KJ, Mekalanos JJ. Genetic characterization of a new type IV-A pilus gene cluster found in both classicalal and El Tor biotypes of *Vibrio cholerae. Infect Immun* 1999;67:1393–1404.
112. Marsh JW, Taylor RK. Identification of the *Vibrio cholerae* type 4 prepilin peptidase required for cholera toxin secretion and pilus formation. *Mol Microbiol* 1998;29:1481–1492.
113. Schneider DR, Parker CD. Isolation and characterization of protease-deficient mutants of *Vibrio cholerae. J Infect Dis* 1978; 138:143–151.
114. Peterson KM, Mekalanos JJ. Characterization of the *Vibrio cholerae* ToxR regulon: identification of novel genes involved in intestinal colonization. *Infect Immun* 1988;56:2822–2829.
115. Parsot C, Taxman E, Mekalanos JJ. ToxR regulates the production of lipoproteins and the expression of serum resistance in *Vibrio cholerae. Proc Natl Acad Sci U S A* 1991;88:1641–1645.
116. Parsot C, Mekalanos JJ. Structural analysis of the *acfA* and *acfD* genes of *Vibrio cholerae:* effects of DNA topology and transcriptional activators on expression. *J Bacteriol* 1992;174:5211–5218.
117. Finkelstein RA, Hanne LF. Purification and characterization of the soluble hemagglutinin (cholera lectin) produced by *Vibrio cholerae. Infect Immun* 1982;36:1199–1208.
118. Hase CC, Finkelstein RA. Cloning and nucleotide sequence of the *Vibrio cholerae* hemagglutinin/protease (HA/protease) gene and construction of an HA/protease-negative strain. *J Bacteriol* 1991;173:3311–3317.
119. Booth BA, Boesman-Finkelstein M, Finkelstein R. *Vibrio cholerae* soluble hemagglutinin/protease is a metalloenzyme. *Infect Immun* 1983;42:558–560.
120. Hase CC, Finkelstein RA. Comparison of the *Vibrio cholerae* hemagglutinin/protease and the *Pseudomonas aeruginosa* elastase. *Infect Immun* 1990:58:4011-4015.
121. Finkelstein RA, Boesman-Finkelstein M, Holt P. *Vibrio cholerae* hemagglutinin/lectin/protease hydrolyzes fibronectin and ovomucin: F. M. Burnet revisited. *Proc Natl Acad Sci U S A* 1983; 80:1092–1095.
122. Booth BA, Boesman-Finkelstein M, Finkelstein RA. *Vibrio cholerae* hemagglutinin/protease nicks cholera enterotoxin. *Infect Immun* 1984;45:558–560.
123. Finkelstein RA, Boesman-Finkelstein M, Chang Y, et al. *Vibrio cholerae* hemagglutinin/protease, colonial variation, virulence, and detachment. *Infect Immun* 1992;60:472–478.
124. Wu Z, Milton D, Nybom P, et al. *Vibrio cholerae* hemagglutinin/protease (HA/protease) causes morphological changes in cultured epithelial cells and perturbs their paracellular barrier function. *Microb Pathog* 1996;21:111–123.
125. Kimsey HH, Waldor MK. *Vibrio cholerae* hemagglutinin/protease inactivates CTXϕ. *Infect Immun* 1998;66:4025–4029.
126. Marsh JW, Taylor RK. Genetic and transcriptional analyses of the *Vibrio cholerae* mannose-sensitive hemagglutinin type 4 pilus gene locus. *J Bacteriol* 1999;181:1110–1117.
127. Attridge SR, Manning PA, Holmgren J, et al. Relative significance of mannose-sensitive hemagglutinin and toxin-coregulated pili in colonization of infant mice by *Vibrio cholerae* El Tor. *Infect Immun* 1996;64:3369–3373.
128. Tacket CO, Taylor RK, Losonsky G, et al. Investigation of the roles of toxin-coregulated pili and mannose-sensitive hemagglutinin pili in the pathogenesis of *Vibrio cholerae* O139 infection. *Infect Immun* 1998;66:692–695.
129. Thelin KH, Taylor RK. Toxin-coregulated pilus, but not mannose-sensitive hemagglutinin, is required for colonization by *Vibrio cholerae* O1 El Tor biotype and O139 strains. *Infect Immun* 1996;64:2853–2856.
130. Jouravleva EA, McDonald GA, Marsh JW, et al. The *Vibrio cholerae* mannose-sensitive hemagglutinin is the receptor for a filamentous bacteriophage from *V. cholerae* O139. *Infect Immun* 1998;66:2535–2539.
131. Franzon VF, Baker A, Manning PA. Nucleotide sequence and construction of a mutant in the mannose-fucose-resistant hemagglutinin (MFRHA) of *Vibrio cholerae* O1. *Infect Immun* 1993;61:3032–3037.
132. Sengupta DK, Sengupta TK, Ghose AC. Major outer membrane proteins of *Vibrio cholerae* and their role in induction of protective immunity through inhibition of intestinal colonization. *Infect Immun* 1992;60:4848–4855.
133. Chiang SL, Mekalanos JJ. *rfb* mutations in *Vibrio cholerae* do not affect surface production of toxin-coregulated pili but still inhibit intestinal colonization. *Infect Immun* 1999;67:976–980.
134. Richardson K. Roles of motility and flagellar structure in pathogenicity of *Vibrio cholerae:* analysis of motility mutants in three animal models. *Infect Immun* 1991;59:2727–2736.
135. Attridge SR, Rowley D. The role of the flagellum in the adherence of *Vibrio cholerae. J Infect Dis* 1983;147:864–872.
136. Freter R, O'Brien CM, Macsai MS. Role of chemotaxis in the association of motile bacteria with intestinal mucosa: *in vivo* studies. *Infect Immun* 1981;34:234–240.
137. Pierce NF, Kaper JB, Mekalanos JJ, et al. Role of cholera toxin in enteric colonization by *Vibrio cholerae* O1 in rabbits. *Infect Immun* 1985;50:813–816.
138. Finn TM, Reiser J, Germanier R, et al. Cell-associated hemagglutinin-deficient mutant of *Vibrio cholerae. Infect Immun* 1987; 55:942–946.
139. Gill DM. The arrangement of subunits in cholera toxin. *Biochemistry* 1976;15:1242–1248.
140. Gill DM, King CA. The mechanism of action of cholera toxin in pigeon erythrocyte lysates. *J Biol Chem* 1975;250:6224–6432.
141. van Heyningen WE, Carpenter CC, Pierce NF, et al. Deactivation of cholera toxin by ganglioside. *J Infect Dis* 1971;124: 415–418.
142. Holmgren J, Lonnroth I, Mansson J-E, et al. Interaction of cholera toxin and membrane GM1 ganglioside of small intestine. *Proc Natl Acad Sci U S A* 1975;72:2520–2524.
143. Galen JE, Ketley JM, Fasano A, et al. Role of *Vibrio cholerae* neuraminidase in the function of cholera toxin. *Infect Immun* 1992;60:406–415.
144. Cassel D, Pfeuffer T. Mechanism of cholera toxin action: covalent modification of the guanyl-binding protein of the adenylate cyclase system. *Proc Natl Acad Sci U S A* 1978;75:2669–2673.
145. Gill DM, Meren R. ADP-ribosylation of membrane proteins catalyzed by cholera toxin: basis of the activation of adenylate cyclase. *Proc Natl Acad Sci U S A* 1978;75:3050–3054.
146. Holmgren J. Actions of cholera toxin and the prevention and treatment of cholera. *Nature* 1981;292:413–417.
147. Dallas WS, Falkow S. Amino acid sequence homology between cholera toxin and *Escherichia coli* heat-labile toxin. *Nature* 1980;288:499–501.
148. Mekalanos JJ, Swartz DJ, Pearson GD, et al. Cholera toxin genes: nucleotide sequence, deletion analysis and vaccine development. *Nature* 1983;306:551–557.
149. Wald A, Gotterer GS, Rajendra GR, et al. Effect of indomethacin on cholera-induced fluid movement, unidirectional sodium fluxes, and intestinal cAMP. *Gastroenterology* 1977;72: 106–110.

150. Jacoby HI, Marshall CH. Antagonism of cholera enterotoxin by antiinflammatory agents in the rat. *Nature* 1972;235:163–165.
151. Speelman P, Rabbani GH, Bukhave K, et al. Increased jejunal prostaglandin E2 concentrations in patients with acute cholera. *Gut* 1985;26:188–193.
152. Peterson JW, Ochoa LG. Role of prostaglandins and cAMP in the secretory effects of cholera toxin. *Science* 1989;245:857–859.
153. Miller VL, Taylor RK, Mekalanos JJ. Cholera toxin transcriptional activator ToxR is a transmembrane DNA binding protein. *Cell* 1987;48:271–279.
154. Miller VL, Mekalanos JJ. A novel suicide vector and its use in construction of insertion mutations: osmoregulation of outer membrane proteins and virulence determinants in *Vibrio cholerae* requires *toxR*. *J Bacteriol* 1988;170:2575–2583.
155. Kaper JB, Levine MM. Cloned cholera enterotoxin genes in study and prevention of cholera. *Lancet* 1981;2:1162–1163.
156. Pearson GD, Mekalanos JJ. Molecular cloning of *Vibrio cholerae* enterotoxin genes in *Escherichia coli* K-12. *Proc Natl Acad Sci U S A* 1982;79:2976–2980.
157. Miller VL, Mekalanos JJ. Synthesis of cholera toxin is positively regulated at the transcriptional level by *toxR*. *Proc Natl Acad Sci U S A* 1984;81:3471–3475.
158. Lockman HA, Galen JE, Kaper JB. *Vibrio cholerae* enterotoxin genes: Nucleotide sequence analysis of DNA encoding ADP-ribosyltransferase. *J Bacteriol* 1984;159:1086–1089.
159. Lockman H, Kaper JB. Nucleotide sequence analysis of the A2 and B subunits of *Vibrio cholerae* enterotoxin. *J Biol Chem* 1983;258:13722–13726.
160. Gennaro ML, Greenaway PJ. Nucleotide sequences within the cholera toxin operon. *Nucleic Acids Res* 1983;1:3855–3861.
161. Sanchez J, Holmgren J. Recombinant system for overexpression of cholera toxin B subunit in *Vibrio cholerae* as a basis for vaccine development. *Proc Natl Acad Sci U S A* 1989;86:481–485.
162. Sandkvist M, Michel LO, Hough LP, et al. General secretion pathway (*eps*) genes required for toxin secretion and outer membrane biogenesis in *Vibrio cholerae. J Bacteriol* 1997;179: 6994–7003.
163. Sandkvist M, Hough LP, Bagdasarian MM, et al. Direct interaction of the EpsL and EpsM proteins of the general secretion apparatus in *Vibrio cholerae. J Bacteriol* 1999;181:3129–3135.
164. Sandkvist M, Bagdasarian M, Howard SP. Characterization of the multimeric Eps complex required for cholera toxin secretion. *Int J Med Microbiol* 2000;290:345–350.
165. Connell TD, Metzger DJ, Lynch J, et al. Endochitinase is transported to the extracellular milieu by the *eps*-encoded general secretory pathway of *Vibrio cholerae. J Bacteriol* 1998;180: 5591–5600.
166. Ali A, Johnson JA, Franco AA, et al. Mutations in the extracellular protein secretion pathway genes (*eps*) interfere with rugose polysaccharide production in and motility of *Vibrio cholerae. Infect Immun* 2000;68:1967–1974.
167. Davis BM, Lawson EH, Sandkvist M, et al. Convergence of the secretory pathways for cholera toxin and the filamentous phage, CTXϕ. *Science* 2000;288:333–335.
168. Goldberg I, Mekalanos JJ. Effect of a *recA* mutation on cholera toxin gene amplification and deletion events. *J Bacteriol* 1986; 165:723–731.
169. Mekalanos JJ. Duplication and amplification of toxin genes in *Vibrio cholerae. Cell* 1983;35:253–263.
170. Pearson GDN, Woods A, Chiang SL, et al. CTX genetic element encodes a site-specific recombination system and an intestinal colonization factor. *Proc Natl Acad Sci USA* 1993;90: 3750–3754.
171. Waldor MK, Mekalanos JJ. Lysogenic conversion by a filamentous bacteriophage encoding cholera toxin. *Science* 1996;272: 1910–1914.
172. Waldor MK, Rubin EJ, Pearson GDN, et al. Regulation, replication, and integration functions of the *Vibrio cholerae* CTXϕ are encoded by regions RS2. *Mol Microbiol* 1997;24:917–926.
173. Kimsey HH, Waldor MK. CTXΦ immunity: Application in the development of cholera vaccines. *Proc Natl Acad Sci U S A* 1998;95:7035–7039.
174. Davis BM, Kimsey HH, Chang W, et al. The *Vibrio cholerae* O139 Calcutta bacteriophage CTXϕ is infectious and encodes a novel repressor. *J Bacteriol* 1999;181:6779–6787.
175. Karaolis DK, Somara S, Maneval DRJ, et al. A bacteriophage encoding a pathogenicity island, a type-IV pilus and a phage receptor in cholera bacteria. *Nature* 1999;399:375–379.
176. DiRita VJ. Co-ordinate expression of virulence genes by ToxR in *Vibrio cholerae. Mol Microbiol* 1992;6:451–458.
177. Skorupski K, Taylor RK. Control of the ToxR virulence regulon in *Vibrio cholerae* by environmental stimuli. *Mol Microbiol* 1997;26:1003–1009.
178. Faruque SM, Albert MJ, Mekalanos JJ. Epidemiology, genetics, and ecology of toxigenic *Vibrio cholerae. Microbiol Molec Biol Rev* 1998;62:1301–1314.
179. Champion GA, Neely MN, Brennan MA, et al. A branch in the ToxR regulatory cascade of *Vibrio cholerae* revealed by characterization of *toxT* mutant strains. *Mol Microbiol* 1997;23:323–331.
180. Miller JF, Mekalanos JJ, Falkow S. Coordinate regulation and sensory transduction in the control of bacterial virulence. *Science* 1989;243:916–922.
181. Miller VL, DiRita VJ, Mekalanos JJ. Identification of *toxS*, a regulatory gene whose product enhances *toxR*-mediated activation of the cholera toxin promoter. *J Bacteriol* 1989;171:1288–1293.
182. DiRita VJ, Mekalanos JJ. Periplasmic interaction between two membrane regulatory proteins, ToxR and ToxS, results in signal transduction and transcriptional activation. *Cell* 1991;64:29–37.
183. Carroll PA, Tashima KT, Rogers MB, et al. Phase variation in *tcpH* modulates expression of the ToxR regulon in *Vibrio cholerae. Mol Microbiol* 1997;25:1099–1111.
184. Hase CC, Mekalanos JJ. TcpP protein is a positive regulator of virulence gene expression in *Vibrio cholerae. Proc Natl Acad Sci U S A* 1998;95:730–734.
185. DiRita VJ, Parsot C, Jander G, et al. Regulatory cascade controls virulence in *Vibrio cholerae. Proc Natl Acad Sci U S A* 1991; 88:5403–5407.
186. Higgins DE, Nazareno E, DiRita VJ. The virulence gene activator ToxT from *Vibrio cholerae* is a member of the AraC family of transcriptional activators. *J Bacteriol* 1992;174:6974–6980.
187. Parsot C, Mekalanos JJ. Expression of the *Vibrio cholerae* gene encoding aldehyde dehydrogenase is under control of ToxR, the cholera toxin transcriptional activator. *J Bacteriol* 1991;173: 2842–2851.
188. Crawford JA, Kaper JB, DiRita VJ. Analysis of ToxR-dependent transcription activation of *ompU,* the gene encoding a major envelope protein in *Vibrio cholerae. Mol Microbiol* 1998;29: 235–246.
189. Hase CC, Mekalanos JJ. Effects of changes in membrane sodium flux on virulence gene expression in *Vibrio cholerae. Proc Natl Acad Sci U S A* 1999;96:3183–3187.
190. Skorupski K, Taylor RK. A new level in the *Vibrio cholerae* ToxR virulence cascade: AphA is required for transcriptional activation of the *tcpPH* operon. *Mol Microbiol* 1999;31:763.
191. Kovacikova G, Skorupski K. A *Vibrio cholerae* LysR homolog, AphB, cooperates with AphA at the *tcpPH* promoter to activate expression of the ToxR virulence cascade. *J Bacteriol* 1999;181: 4250–4256.
192. Parsot C, Mekalanos JJ. Expression of ToxR, the transcriptional activator of the virulence factors in *Vibrio cholerae,* is modulated by the heat shock response. *Proc Natl Acad Sci U S A* 1990;87: 9898–9902.

193. DiRita VJ, Neely M, Taylor RK, et al. Differential expression of the ToxR regulon in classicalal and El Tor biotypes of *Vibrio cholerae* is due to biotype-specific control over *toxT* expression. *Proc Natl Acad Sci U S A* 1996;93:7991–7995.
194. Murley YM, Carroll PA, Skorupski K, et al. Differential transcription of the *tcpPH* operon confers biotype-specific control of the *Vibrio cholerae* ToxR virulence regulon. *Infect Immun* 1999;67:5117–5123.
195. Kovacikova G, Skorupski K. Differential activation of the *tcpPH* promoter by AphB determines biotype specificity of virulence gene expression in *Vibrio cholerae. J Bacteriol* 2000;182: 3228–3238.
196. Skorupski K, Taylor RK. Cyclic AMP and its receptor protein negatively regulate the coordinate expression of cholera toxin and toxin-coregulated pilus in *Vibrio cholerae. Proc Natl Acad Sci U S A* 1997;94:265–270.
197. Wong SM, Carroll PA, Rahme LG, et al. Modulation of expression of the ToxR regulon in *Vibrio cholerae* by a member of the two-component family of response regulators. *Infect Immun* 1998;66:5854–5861.
198. Lazar S, Waldor MK. ToxR-independent expression of cholera toxin from the replicative form of CTXϕ. *Infect Immun* 1998; 66:394–397.
199. Lee SH, Hava DL, Waldor MK, et al. Regulation and temporal expression patterns of *Vibrio cholerae* virulence genes during infection. *Cell* 1999;99:625–634.
200. Fasano A, Baudry B, Pumplin DW, et al. *Vibrio cholerae* produces a second enterotoxin, which affects intestinal tight junctions. *Proc Natl Acad Sci U S A* 1991;88:5242–5246.
201. Baudry B, Fasano A, Ketley J, et al. Cloning of a gene (*zot*) encoding a new toxin produced by *Vibrio cholerae. Infect Immun* 1992;60:428–434.
202. Trucksis M, Galen J, Michalski J, et al. Accessory cholera enterotoxin (Ace), the third toxin of a *Vibrio cholerae* virulence cassette. *Proc Natl Acad Sci U S A* 1993;90:5267–5271.
203. Lin W, Fullner KJ, Clayton R, et al. Identification of a *Vibrio cholerae* RTX toxin gene cluster that is tightly linked to the cholera toxin prophage. *Proc Natl Acad Sci U S A* 1999;96: 1071–1076.
204. Fullner KJ, Mekalanos JJ. *In vivo* covalent cross-linking of cellular actin by the *Vibrio cholerae* RTX toxin. *EMBO J* 2000;19: 5315–5323.
205. Yoshino K-I, Miyachi M, Takao T, et al. Purification and sequence determination of heat-stable enterotoxin elaborated by a cholera toxin-producing strain of *Vibrio cholerae* O1. *FEBS Lett* 1993;326:83–86.
206. O'Brien AD, Chen ME, Holmes RK, et al. Environmental and human isolates of *Vibrio cholerae* and *Vibrio parahaemolyticus* produce a *Shigella dysenteriae* 1 (Shiga)-like cytotoxin. *Lancet* 1985;1:77–78.
207. Sciortino CV, Finkelstein RA. *Vibrio cholerae* expresses iron-regulated outer membrane proteins in vivo. *Infect Immun* 1983;42: 990–996.
208. Goldberg MB, DiRita VJ, Calderwood SB. Identification of an iron-regulated virulence determinant in *Vibrio cholerae,* using Tn*phoA* mutagenesis. *Infect Immun* 1990;58:55–60.
209. Goldberg MB, Boyko SA, Calderwood SB. Transcriptional regulation by iron of a *Vibrio cholerae* virulence gene and homology of the gene to the *Escherichia coli* Fur system. *J Bacteriol* 1990;172:6863–6870.
210. Goldberg MB, Boyko SA, Calderwood SB. Positive transcriptional regulation of an iron-regulated virulence gene in *Vibrio cholerae. Proc Natl Acad Sci U S A* 1991;88:1125–1129.
211. Goldberg MB, Boyko SA, Butterton JR, et al. Characterization of a *Vibrio cholerae* virulence factor homologous to the family of TonB-dependent proteins. *Mol Microbiol* 1992;6:2407–2418.
212. Stoebner JA, Payne SM. Iron-regulated hemolysin production and utilization of heme and hemoglobin by *Vibrio cholerae. Infect Immun* 1988;56:2891–2895.
213. Williams SG, Manning PA. Transcription of the *Vibrio cholerae* haemolysin gene, *hlyA,* and cloning of a positive regulatory locus, *hlyU. Mol Microbiol* 1991;5:2031–2038.
214. Alm RA, Stroeher UH, Manning PA. Extracellular proteins of *Vibrio cholerae:* nucleotide sequence of the structural gene (*hlyA*) for the haemolysin of the haemolytic El Tor strain 017 and characterization of the *hlyA* mutation in the non-haemolytic classicalal strain 569B. *Mol Microbiol* 1988;2:481–488.
215. Rader AE, Murphy JR. Nucleotide sequences and comparison of the hemolysin determinants of *Vibrio cholerae* El Tor RV79(Hly+) and RV79(Hly–) and classicalal 569B(Hly–). *Infect Immun* 1988;56:1414–1419.
216. Alm RA, Manning PA. Characterization of the *hlyB* gene and its role in the production of the El Tor haemolysin of *Vibrio cholerae* O1. *Mol Microbiol* 1990;4:413–425.
217. von Mechow S, Vaidya AB, Bramucci MG. Mapping of a gene that regulates haemolysin production in *Vibrio cholerae. J Bacteriol* 1985;163:799–802.
218. Alm RA, Mayrhofer G, Kotlarski I, et al. Amino-terminal domain of the El Tor haemolysin of *Vibrio cholerae* O1 is expressed in classicalal strains and is cytotoxic. *Vaccine* 1991;9: 588–594.
219. Levine MM, Kaper JB, Herrington D, et al. Volunteer studies of deletion mutants of *Vibrio cholerae* O1 prepared by recombinant techniques. *Infect Immun* 1988;56:161–167.
220. Chiang SL, Mekalanos JJ. Use of signature-tagged transposon mutagenesis to identify *Vibrio cholerae* genes critical for colonization. *Mol Microbiol* 1998;27:797–805.
221. Lee SH, Angelichio MJ, Mekalanos JJ, et al. Nucleotide sequence and spatiotemporal expression of the *Vibrio cholerae vieSAB* genes during infection. *J Bacteriol* 1998;180:2298–2305.
222. Levine MM, Black RE, Clements ML, et al. Volunteer studies in development of vaccines against cholera and enterotoxigenic *Escherichia coli:* a review. In: Holme T, Holmgren J, Merson MH, et al., eds. *Acute enteric infections in children: new prospects for treatment and prevention.* Amsterdam: Elsevier, 1981:443–459.
223. Woodward W. Cholera reinfection in man. *J Infect Dis* 1971; 123:61–66.
224. Owen RL, Pierce NF, Apple RT, et al. M cell transport of *Vibrio cholerae* from the intestinal lumen into Peyer's patches: a mechanism for antigen sampling and for microbial transepithelial migration. *J Infect Dis* 1986;153:1108–1118.
225. Czerkinsky C, Svennerholm A-M, Quiding M, et al. Antibody-producing cells in peripheral blood and salivary glands after oral cholera vaccination of humans. *Infect Immun* 1991;59: 996–1001.
226. Winner III L, Mack J, Weltzin R, et al. New model for analysis of mucosal immunity: intestinal secretion of specific monoclonal immunoglobulin A from hybridoma tumors protects against *Vibrio cholerae* infection. *Infect Immun* 1991;59:977–982.
227. Cray WCJ, Tokunaga E, Pierce NF. Successful colonization and immunization of adult rabbits by oral inoculation with *Vibrio cholerae* O1. *Infect Immun* 1983;41:735–741.
228. Pierce NF, Kaper JB, Mekalanos JJ, et al. Determinants of the immunogenicity of live virulent and mutant *Vibrio cholerae* O1 in rabbit intestine. *Infect Immun* 1987;55:477–481.
229. Lycke N, Holmgren J. Strong adjuvant properties of cholera toxin on gut mucosal immune responses to orally presented antigens. *Immunology* 1986;59:301–308.
230. Fujita K, Finkelstein RA. Antitoxic immunity in experimental cholera: comparison of immunity induced perorally and parenterally in mice. *J Infect Dis* 1972;125:647–655.
231. Holmgren J, Svennerholm A-M, Ouchterlony O, et al. Anti-

toxic immunity in experimental cholera: protection and serum and local antibody responses in rabbits after enteric and parenteral immunization. *Infect Immun* 1975;12:463–470.
232. Pierce NF, Reynolds HY. Immunity to experimental cholera. I. Protective effect of humoral IgG antitoxin demonstrated by passive immunization. *J Immunol* 1974;113:1017–1023.
233. Clemens JD, Sack DA, Harris JR, et al. Field trial of oral cholera vaccines in Bangladesh. *Lancet* 1986;2:124–127.
234. Levine MM, Young CR, Hughes TP, et al. Duration of serum antitoxin response following *Vibrio cholerae* infection in North Americans: relevance for seroepidemiology. *Am J Epidemiol* 1981;114:348–354.
235. Svennerholm A-M, Jertborn M, Gothefors L, et al. Mucosal antitoxic and antibacterial immunity after cholera disease and after immunization with a combined B subunit whole cell vaccine. *J Infect Dis* 1984;149:884–893.
236. Glass RI, Svennerholm A-M, Khan RN, et al. Seroepidemiological studies of El Tor cholera in Bangladesh: association of serum antibody levels with protection. *J Infect Dis* 1985;151:236–242.
237. Levine MM, Pierce NF. Immunity and vaccine development. In: Barua D, Greenough WB III, eds. *Cholera.* New York: Plenum Press, 1992:285–328.
238. Ryan ET, Calderwood SB. Cholera vaccines. *Clin Infect Dis* 2000;31:561–565.
239. Mosley WH, Woodward WE, Azia KMS, et al. The 1968–1969 cholera vaccine field trial in rural East Pakistan. Effectiveness of monovalent Ogawa and Inaba vaccines and a purified Inaba antigen, with comparative results of serological and animal protection tests. *J Infect Dis* 1970;121:S1–S9.
240. Levine MM, Kaper JB, Black RE, et al. New knowledge on pathogenesis of bacterial enteric infections as applied to vaccine development. *Microbiol Rev* 1983;47:510–550.
241. Hornick RB, Music SI, Wenzel R, et al. The Broad Street pump revisited: response of volunteers to ingested cholera vibrios. *Bull N Y Acad Med* 1971;47:1181–1191.
242. Rabbani GH, Greenough WB III. Pathophysiology and clinical aspects of cholera. In: Barua D, Greenough WB III, eds. *Cholera.* New York: Plenum Press, 1992:209, 228.
243. Carpenter CCJ, Barua D, Wallace CK, et al. Clinical studies in Asiatic cholera. IV. Antibiotic therapy in cholera. *Bull Johns Hopkins Hosp* 1966;118:216–229.
244. Hirschhorn N, Kinzie JL, Sachar DB, et al. Decrease in net stool output in children during intestinal perfusion with glucose-containing solution. *N Engl J Med* 1968;279:176–181.
245. Pierce NF, Banwell JG, Mitra RC, et al. A controlled comparison of tetracycline and furazolidone in cholera. *BMJ* 1968;3: 277–280.
246. Wang F, Butler T, Rabbani GH, et al. The acidosis of cholera: contributions of hyperproteinemia, lactic acidemia, and hyperphosphatemia to an increased serum anion gap. *N Engl J Med* 1986;315:1591–1595.
247. Greenough WB III, Hirschhorn N, Gordon RSJ, et al. Pulmonary edema associated with acidosis in patients with cholera. *Trop Geogr Med* 1976;28:86–90.
248. Benyajati C, Keoplug M, Beisel WR, et al. Acute renal failure in Asiatic cholera: clinicopathologic correlations with acute tubular necrosis and hypokalemic nephropathy. *Ann Intern Med* 1960;52:960–975.
249. Bennish ML, Azad AK, Rahman O, et al. Hypoglycemia during diarrhea in childhood: prevalence, pathophysiology, and outcome. *N Engl J Med* 1990;322:1357–1363.
250. Hirschhorn N, Chaudhury AKMA, Lendenbaum J. Cholera in pregnant women. *Lancet* 1969;1:1230–1232.
251. Greenough WB. *Vibrio cholerae.* In: Mandell GL, Douglas GR, Bennet JE, eds. *Principles and practice of infectious diseases,* third edition. New York: Churchill Livingstone, 1990:1636–1646.
252. Lindenbaum J, Greenough WB III, Islam MR. Antibiotic therapy of cholera. *Bull WHO* 1967;36:871–833.
253. Centers for Disease Control and Prevention. Surveillance for epidemic cholera in the Americas: an assessment. In: CDC surveillance summaries, March 1992. *MMWR Morbid Mortal Wkly Rep* 1992;41(No. SS-1):27–34.
254. Centers for Disease Control and Prevention. Update: Cholera —Western hemisphere. *MMWR Morbid Mortal Wkly Rep* 1991; 40:860.
255. Pal SC. Laboratory diagnosis. In: Barua D, Greenough WB III, eds. *Cholera.* New York: Plenum Press, 1992:229–252.
256. Barua D, Gomez CZ. Blotting-paper strips for transportation of cholera stools. *Bull WHO* 1967;37:798.
257. Spira WM, Ahmed QS. Gauze filtration and enrichment procedures for recovery of *Vibrio cholerae* from contaminated waters. *Appl Environ Microbiol* 1981;42:730–733.
258. Barrett TJ, Blake PA, Morris GK, et al. Use of Moore swabs for isolating *Vibrio cholerae* from sewage. *J Clin Microbiol* 1980;11: 385–388.
259. Gorbach SI, Banwell JG, Jacob B, et al. Intestinal microflora in Asiatic cholera. I. Rice-water stool. *J Infect Dis* 1970;121:32–37.
260. Benenson AS, Islam MR, Greenough WB III. Rapid identification of *Vibrio cholerae* by darkfield microscopy. *Bull World Health Organ* 1964;30:827.
261. Qadri F, Hasan JA, Hosain J, et al. Evaluation of the monoclonal antibody-based kit Bengal SMART for rapid detection of *Vibrio cholerae* O139 synonym Bengal in stool samples. *J Clin Microbiol* 1995;33:732–734.
262. Albert MJ, Islam D, Nahar S, et al. Rapid detection of *Vibrio cholerae* O139 Bengal from stool specimens by PCR. *J Clin Microbiol* 1997;35:1633–1635.
263. Almeida RJ, Hickman-Brenner FW, Sowers EG, et al. Comparison of a latex agglutination assay and an enzyme-linked immunosorbent assay for detecting cholera toxin. *J Clin Microbiol* 1990;28:128–130.
264. Fields PI, Popovic T, Wachsmuth K, et al. Use of polymerase chain reaction for detection of toxigenic *Vibrio cholerae* O1 strains from the Latin American cholera epidemic. *J Clin Microbiol* 1992;30:2118–2121.
265. Keasler SP, Hall RH. Detecting and biotyping *Vibrio cholerae* O1 with multiplex polymerase chain reaction. *Lancet* 1993;341:1661.
266. Centers for Disease Control and Prevention. Antimicrobial susceptibility testing. *Laboratory methods for the diagnosis of epidemic dysentery and cholera.* Atlanta: Centers for Disease Control and Prevention, 1999:61–74.
267. World Health Organization. (Programme for Control of Diarrhoeal Diseases). A manual for the treatment of diarrhea. 1990. Report No.: WHO/CCD/SER/80.2 rev 2.
268. Molla AM, Adhmed SM, Greenough WB III. Rice-based oral rehydration solution decreases the stool volume in acute diarrhoea. *Bull World Health Org* 1985;63:751–756.
269. Ramakrishna BS, Venkataraman S, Srinivasan P, et al. Amylase-resistant starch plus oral rehydration solution for cholera. *N Engl J Med* 2000;342:308–313.
270. World Health Organization. (Programme for Control of Diarrhoeal Disease). Guidelines for cholera control. 1991. Report No.: WHO/CDD/SER/80.4 rev 2.
271. Greenough WB III, Rosenberg IS, Gordon RS, et al. Tetracycline in the treatment of cholera. *Lancet* 1964;1:355–357.
272. Alam AN, Alam NH, Sack DA. Randomised double blind trial of single dose doxycycline for treating cholera in adults. *BMJ* 1990;300:1619–1621.
273. Ouellette M, Gerbaud G, Courvalin P. Genetic, biochemical and molecular characterization of strains of *Vibrio cholerae* multiresistant to antibiotics. *Ann Inst Pasteur Microbiol* 1988;139: 105–113.

274. Yamamoto T, Nair G, Albert MJ, et al. Survey of *in vitro* susceptibilities of *Vibrio cholerae* O1 and O139 to antimicrobial agents. *Antimicrob Agents Chemother* 1995;39:241–244.
275. Dutta D, Bhattacharya SK, Bhattacharya MK, et al. Efficacy of norfloxacin and doxycycline for treatment of *Vibrio cholerae* O139 infection. *J Antimicrob Chemother* 1996;37:575–581.
276. Gotuzzo E, Seas C, Echevarria J, et al. Ciprofloxacin for the treatment of cholera: a randomized, double-blind, controlled clinical trial of a single daily dose in Peruvian adults. *Clin Infect Dis* 1995;20:1485–1490.
277. Khan WA, Bennish ML, Seas C, et al. Randomised controlled comparison of single-dose ciprofloxacin and doxycycline for cholera caused by *Vibrio cholerae* O1 or O139. *Lancet* 1996; 348:296–300.
278. McCormack WM, Chowdhury AM, Jahangir N, et al. Tetracycline prophylaxis in families of cholera patients. *Bull WHO* 1968;38:787–792.
279. Gupta PGS, Sircar BK, Mondal S, et al. Effect of doxycycline on transmission of *Vibrio cholerae* infection among family contacts of cholera patients in Calcutta. *Bull World Health Organ* 1978;56:323–326.
280. Centers for Disease Control and Prevention. Update: Cholera—Western hemisphere, and recommendations for treatment of cholera. *MMWR Morbid Mortal Wkly Rep* 1991; 40:562–565.
281. Mahalanabis D, Molla AM, Sack D. Clinical management of cholera. In: Barua D, Greenough WB III, eds. *Cholera.* New York: Plenum Press, 1992:253–284.
282. Craun G, Swerdlow D, Tauxe R, et al. Prevention of waterborne cholera in the United States. *J Am Waterworks Assoc* 1991; 83:40–46.
283. Centers for Disease Control and Prevention. ACIP: cholera vaccine. *MMWR Morbid Mortal Wkly Rep* 1988;37:617–624.
284. Holmgren J, Jertborn M, Svennerholm A-ML. New and improved vaccines against cholera: Part ii: Oral B subunit killed whole-cell cholera vaccine. In: Levine MM, Woodrow GC, Kaper JB, et al., eds. *New generation vaccines.* New York: Marcel Dekker, 1997:459–468.
285. Kaper JB, Tacket CO, Levine MM. New and improved vaccines against cholera: i: Attenuated *Vibrio cholerae* O1 and O139 strains as live oral cholera vaccines. In: Levine MM, Woodrow GC, Kaper JB, et al., eds. *New generation vaccines.* New York: Marcel Dekker, 1997.
286. World Health Organization. Potential use of oral cholera vaccines in emergency situations. Report of a WHO meeting. 12–13 May 1999. Report No.: WHO/CDS/CSR/EDC/99.4.

37

"NONCHOLERA" *VIBRIO* SPECIES

J. GLENN MORRIS, JR.

A major concern of early cholera investigators was the differentiation of epidemic-associated strains of *Vibrio cholerae* from other, "atypical" *Vibrio* strains. Work by Gardner and Venkatraman and others in the 1930s (1,2) led to the concept that *V. cholerae* strains could be divided into two groups: those in O group 1, which agglutinated with antisera directed against antigens present on strains isolated from cholera patients, and other "nonagglutinating" or "noncholera" *Vibrio* strains, which were regarded primarily as nonpathogenic, environmental isolates. Some early writers discussed the possibility that nonagglutinating isolates were responsible for "paracholera" or similar clinical syndromes (2). However, it was not until the 1950s and 1960s that investigators began to identify outbreaks of disease directly attributable to these strains (3–7).

As more attention was paid to nonagglutinating vibrios, it became increasingly obvious that these isolates were a heterogeneous group, including species besides *V. cholerae.* These observations have led, since the late 1970s, to the designation of a number of new *Vibrio* species. As shown in Table 37.1, there are 11 *Vibrio* species other than *V. cholerae* that have been associated with human illness (8,9). At the same time, there has been increasing recognition that *V. cholerae* strains in O groups other than 1 can cause both epidemic and endemic disease (10–16). *V. cholerae* in O groups 1 and 139 cause epidemic cholera; they are described separately in Chapter 36. Infections with *V. cholerae* in other O groups, as well as other *Vibrio* species that are acquired through the gastrointestinal tract (*V. parahaemolyticus, V. fluvialis, V. mimicus, V. hollisae, V. furnissii,* and *V. vulnificus*) are discussed in this chapter. *V. alginolyticus* and *V. damsela* (18) are generally acquired by exposure of wounds to seawater. Descriptions of infections with *V. cincinnatiensis* (18), *V. carchariae* (19), and *V. metschnikovii* (20,21) have been restricted to case reports, and the significance of their isolation from humans remains to be determined. Interestingly, *V. metschnikovii* DNA was identified in the colonic contents of the more than 5,000-year-old "Tyrolean Iceman" found frozen in an alpine glacier (22).

Vibrios are naturally occurring (autochthonous) bacteria in estuarine or marine environments. Aside from the 12 species cited, there are at least another 23 *Vibrio* species that have been isolated from environmental sources (8). It is likely that the actual number of *Vibrio* species is much greater, with isolates obtained during environmental surveys often belonging to as yet unidentified or unnamed *Vibrio* species.

VIBRIO CHOLERAE IN O GROUPS OTHER THAN 1 OR 139 (NONEPIDEMIC *VIBRIO CHOLERAE*)

V. cholerae is a highly diverse species that is widely distributed in aquatic environments. Epidemic cholera is associated with certain clonal groups within the species that are characterized by the presence of CTXΦ (a single-stranded DNA filamentous bacteriophage that encodes cholera toxin

TABLE 37.1. *VIBRIO* SPECIES IMPLICATED AS A CAUSE OF HUMAN DISEASE

	Clinical Presentation		
Species	Gastroenteritis	Wound/ Ear	Septicemia
V. cholerae			
Epidemic (O1, O139)	++	(+)	
Nonepidemic	++	+	+
V. mimicus	++	+	
V. parahaemolyticus	++	+	(+)
V. fluvialis	++	+	+
V. furnissii	++		
V. hollisae	++	+	(+)
V. vulnificus	+	++	++
V. alginolyticus		++	
V. damsela		++	
V. cincinnatiensis			(+)
V. carchariae		(+)	
V. metschnikovii	(+)		(+)

++, most common presentation; +, other clinical presentations; (+), very rare presentation.

J. G. Morris, Jr.: Department of Epidemiology and Preventive Medicine, University of Maryland School of Medicine, Baltimore, Maryland

[CT] [23]), and a 40-kb *Vibrio* pathogenicity island (VPI) that incorporates key colonization-associated genes (24). To date, all such isolates have been within serogroups O1 and O139, although recent data suggest that some clinical, outbreak-associated O37 strains also carry this gene combination (25). *V. cholerae* strains lacking the "epidemic" combination of virulence characteristics have been associated with sporadic illness, probably reflecting occasional introduction of environmental isolates into human populations (26).

Microbiology

All *V. cholerae* share essentially identical microbiologic and biochemical characteristics (8). Like other *Vibrio* species, *V. cholerae* is a facultatively anaerobic, asporogenous, gram-negative rod. *V. cholerae* is oxidase-positive, reduces nitrate, and is motile by a single polar, sheathed flagellum. Growth is stimulated by the addition of 1% NaCl; however, in contrast to other *Vibrio* species, *V. cholerae* grows in the absence of NaCl. Differentiation of epidemic and nonepidemic strains is based on serotyping (27) and molecular screening for the presence of CTX and VPI.

Epidemiology

The most common clinical manifestation of nonepidemic *V. cholerae* infections is gastroenteritis. However, nonepidemic *V. cholerae* strains are also routinely isolated from blood, wounds, and other sites (Table 37.2). Illness is most common during warm summer months, reflecting the increased *Vibrio* counts in the environment seen in association with increased water temperature.

Reservoirs

Nonepidemic *V. cholerae* organisms have been isolated from surface water in multiple sites in North America, Europe, Asia, and Australia, and it is likely that they are present in coastal and estuarine areas throughout the world (28–33). As would be expected with a naturally occurring estuarine organism, environmental studies have generally shown no correlation between isolation of non-O1 *V. cholerae* and the presence of fecal coliforms (29–32). Isolation rates are influenced by salinity (isolation generally occurs in water with a salinity of 2 to 20 ppt) and water temperature (optimally greater than 17°C) (30,33). However, isolation has been reported from freshwater (34), and infections have occurred after exposure to freshwater inland lakes (35,36).

Nonepidemic *V. cholerae* is a common isolate from shellfish, particularly from filter feeders such as oysters. In one study conducted by the U.S. Food and Drug Administration, nonepidemic *V. cholerae* was isolated from 111 (14%) of 790 samples of freshly harvested oyster shell stock (37), with isolation rates being highest during warm summer months. Nonepidemic *V. cholerae* has also been isolated from wild and domestic animals (31,38–41), and asymptomatic carriage by humans is known to occur (42,43).

Transmission

Virtually all cases of nonepidemic *V. cholerae* gastroenteritis acquired in the United States are associated with eating raw or undercooked shellfish, particularly raw oysters (15). Although the linkage is less strong (44), there is also a suggestion that septicemia can result from ingestion of the organism in seafood (45,46). Isolation from other sites (such as skin, ears, or sputum) can occur in association with exposure to estuarine environments (i.e., isolation from sputum in cases of near drowning).

Seafood remains an important vehicle of infection for sporadic nonepidemic *V. cholerae* disease outside of the United States. However, it is clear that transmission can also occur through other routes (3,26,47), including water (5)

TABLE 37.2. NONCHOLERA *VIBRIO* INFECTIONS REPORTED TO CDC BY SYNDROME AND COMPLICATIONS, 1999[a]

Species	Total	Syndrome: Gastroenteritis (%)	Septicemia (%)	Wound Infections (%)	Other/Unknown[b] (%)	Complications: Hospitalized[c] (%)	Deaths[c] (%)
Nonepidemic *V. cholerae*	46	31 (67%)	2 (4%)	5 (11%)	8 (17%)	13/43 (30%)	0
V. mimicus	10	7 (70%)	0	1 (10%)	2 (20%)	5/9 (55%)	0
V. parahaemolyticus	116	95 (81%)	0	16 (14%)	5 (4%)	21/105 (20%)	1/26 (4%)
V. fluvialis	19	12 (63%)	2 (10%)	4 (21%)	1 (5%)	4/17 (23%)	0
V. furnissii	1	1 (100%)	0	0	0	0	0
V. hollisae	13	11 (85%)	0	2 (15%)	0	8 (61%)	0
V. vulnificus	83	5 (6%)	41 (49%)	28 (34%)	9 (11%)	36/51 (71%)	11/48 (23%)
TOTAL	288						

[a]Data shown for species acquired primarily through the gastrointestinal tract. Data from 22 states; for many of these states, reporting of *Vibrio* infections is not routine, and consequently numbers may not reflect the true number of cases. Data kindly provided by Dr. Robert Tauxe, U.S. Centers for Disease Control and Prevention.
[b]Includes gallbladder, otitis, urine, eye, peritonitis, and unknown.
[c]Denominator shown represents number of cases for which data on hospitalization and death were known.

and a variety of other foods (48,49). In one recent study in Vellore, South India, nonepidemic *V. cholerae* strains were isolated from 41% of drinking water samples and 100% of untreated surface water samples (50).

Frequency of Isolation

There is wide variability in the reported frequency of isolation of nonepidemic *V. cholerae* from stool cultures of persons with diarrhea (26). In Cancun, Mexico, an isolation rate of 16% has been reported (48); in a comparable study conducted in Mexico City (at a high altitude and at some distance from the coast), no non-O1 strains were identified from patients with diarrhea (51). In Bangladesh, isolation rates of nonepidemic *V. cholerae* strains from persons with diarrhea at the Cholera Research Laboratory in Dhaka (6) and the Matlab Treatment Center (52) have been reported to be 3% and 7%, respectively. Among children with diarrhea in Bangkok, reported isolation rates are in the range of 1.0% to 1.3% (53).

Rates of isolation in the United States, based on cases reported to the Centers for Disease Control and Prevention (CDC) (Table 37.2), appear to be lower (although these numbers probably represent substantive underreporting of cases). In one population-based study, nonepidemic *V. cholerae* strains were isolated from 13 (2.7%) of 479 persons in a cohort of physicians attending a convention in New Orleans in late September (42); however, only 2 (15%) of the 13 culture-positive persons were symptomatic.

Pathophysiology

In volunteer studies, a strain of CT-negative, nonepidemic *V. cholerae* caused gastroenteritis in healthy young adults (16). However, in these same studies, illness was only seen in association with one of three strains tested, suggesting that many strains are nonpathogenic and may be isolated simply as a commensal from clinical specimens. This is supported by the observation that disease rates are relatively low, despite the high rate of isolation of the organism from the environment and seafood. At this point, no single virulence factor has been identified that can account for all reported cases. Analogous to our current understanding of diarrheogenic *E. coli* (and in keeping with the genetic diversity seen among nonepidemic *V. cholerae* strains), there may be several subgroups of strains that are able to cause disease, each through a different pathogenic mechanism. Possible mechanisms are discussed in the following paragraphs.

Production of Cholera Toxin. *V. cholerae* strains outside of epidemic lineages (i.e., not O1 or O139) can, at times, carry genes for cholera toxin production. These CT-positive, nonepidemic strains have generally been isolated in the Indian subcontinent, and, in patients, have been associated with increased severity of illness, compared with illness in persons infected with CT-negative strains (54–59). However, more recent data from India (60,61), as well as data from other geographic areas (15,62), suggest that such strains constitute a relatively small proportion of nonepidemic *V. cholerae* strains isolated from patients with diarrheal disease.

Production of NAG-ST. Some non-O1 strains produce a 17-amino-acid, heat-stable enterotoxin (designated NAG-ST) that closely resembles the heat-stable toxin produced by enterotoxigenic strains of *E. coli* and *Yersinia enterocolitica* (63,64). The strain that caused illness in the volunteer studies noted earlier produced NAG-ST (16); NAG-ST–producing strains have been associated with disease outbreaks (65), and strains producing this toxin have been shown to be closely related genetically, with a common capsular type (66).

Other Putative Toxins. A variety of other possible toxins have been proposed, including the El Tor hemolysin (67–72); a second hemolysin that is very closely related to the thermostable direct hemolysin of *V. parahaemolyticus* (see section on *V. parahaemolyticus*) (64,67); a Shiga-like toxin (67,73); and various cell-associated hemagglutinins (74). Clinical nonepidemic strains often have cytotoxic activity in tissue culture (60).

Colonization Factors. Nonepidemic *V. cholerae* strains from patients with diarrhea are significantly more likely to colonize and cause disease in rabbits than are environmental isolates (76). In the previously noted volunteer studies, a second strain that produced NAG-ST but did not colonize did not produce illness (16), suggesting that colonization is a necessary prerequisite for occurrence of disease.

A different set of pathogenic mechanisms appear to be involved in occurrence of nonepidemic *V. cholerae* sepsis. Greater than 90% of nonepidemic *V. cholerae* strains produce a polysaccharide capsule that confers resistance to serum bactericidal activity and is associated with increased virulence in mice (77,78). Heavily encapsulated strains are significantly more likely to be isolated from patients with septicemia than strains with minimal or no capsular polysaccharide (78). In contrast, strains of *V. cholerae* O1 are not encapsulated, and, with one or two possible exceptions, *V. cholerae* O1 has not been isolated from blood.

Clinical Syndromes

Gastroenteritis

Although it is generally mild, the gastroenteritis associated with nonepidemic *V. cholerae* can include profuse, watery diarrhea comparable to that seen in epidemic cholera (6,9,44,79). In a group of 14 U.S. cases (15), symptoms included diarrhea (100% of patients), abdominal cramps (93%), fever (71%), bloody diarrhea (25%), and nausea and vomiting (21%). Median duration of illness was 6.4

days, with 8 of the 14 patients requiring hospitalization; however, because these patients were identified on the basis of positive cultures, more severely ill patients were likely to have been overrepresented. Similar symptoms were reported in a case series from Taiwan (44); this latter study also noted that 7 of 8 patients had an elevated peripheral white blood cell count. The hospital course in the Taiwan cases ranged from 1 to 2 days. In an outbreak that occurred on an airplane flight to Australia (47), the mean incubation period was 11.5 hours (range 5.25 to 37.5 hours); illness was generally mild (with abdominal cramps again prominent), and resolved in a majority of cases in less than 24 hours.

In volunteer studies (16), the median incubation period before onset of gastroenteritis was 10 hours (range 5.5 to 96 hours). Diarrheal stool volumes ranged from 140 to 5,397 mL. The diarrheal illness tended to be short-lived, with a median duration of 21 hours (range 3.5 to 48 hours). Abdominal cramps were prominent, with one volunteer (who received 10^6 CFU) having only abdominal cramps and no diarrhea.

Septicemia

Most cases of nonepidemic *V. cholerae* sepsis have involved immunocompromised patients, particularly those with cirrhosis or hematologic malignancies (44,46). The case fatality rate in a recent case series from Taiwan was 47% (44); in older U.S. literature, the rate exceeds 60% (46).

Infections at Other Sites

Nonepidemic *V. cholerae* has been isolated from a variety of other sites, including skin (cellulitis, wounds), ears, sputum, urine, and cerebrospinal fluid (44,79–82).

Diagnosis

Methodology for isolation of *V. cholerae* is identical for epidemic and nonepidemic strains). For isolation from stool, a selective media such as TCBS (thiosulfate-citrate-bile salts-sucrose) is generally necessary. *V. cholerae* grows well on blood agar and other nonselective media that may be used for wound cultures and in standard blood culture media. Identification is based on standard biochemical tests (8).

Therapy

As with epidemic strains of *V. cholerae*, the mainstay of therapy of diarrheal disease is oral rehydration (83,84). There have been no controlled trials of antimicrobial therapy in persons infected with nonepidemic *V. cholerae* strains, and there are anecdotal data (44) suggesting that it does not influence the course of what is generally a mild, self-limited disease. For patients with a more prolonged course (>5 days of diarrhea), administration of tetracycline would appear to be reasonable, based on data from studies with epidemic *V. cholerae* (83–85). Nonepidemic *V. cholerae* is generally susceptible *in vitro* to a number of antibiotics, including tetracycline, chloramphenicol, trimethoprim-sulfamethoxazole, ciprofloxacin, aminoglycoside, and third-generation cephalosporins (8,44,86). Strains show variable resistance to ampicillin, and data suggest that ampicillin has reduced efficacy in the treatment of cholera (87); ampicillin is not recommended for therapy. When tetracycline cannot be used, ciprofloxacin would be a reasonable alternative. Recent problems with development of antibiotic resistance have been noted in Thailand (53), highlighting the need for susceptibility testing, particularly in dealing with infections acquired outside of the United States.

In cases of septicemia, supportive care and correction of shock is essential. Although no controlled studies are available, a combination of minocycline (100 mg every 12 hours orally) and cefotaxime (2.0 g every 8 hours intravenously) has been recommended for treatment of *V. vulnificus* sepsis (88,89) (see section on *V. vulnificus*) and appears to be reasonable in management of *V. cholerae* sepsis.

Prevention

In countries such as the United States, nonepidemic *V. cholerae* infections can be prevented by not eating raw or undercooked seafood, particularly during warm months in the late summer and early fall. For healthy adults, the risk of infection is low, and, if it does occur, the resultant gastroenteritis is generally mild. Persons who have underlying liver disease or who are immunosuppressed also are at risk for septicemia. Given the high fatality rates associated with septicemia, persons in these groups should not consume raw oysters. In developing countries, transmission of non-O1 *V. cholerae* appears to parallel that of other enteric pathogens, with the risk of illness minimized by making certain that food and water come from clean sources.

VIBRIO MIMICUS

Before 1981, strains now classified as *V. mimicus* were identified as sucrose-negative *V. cholerae.* DNA-DNA homology studies at that time demonstrated that these strains constituted a separate species (90); the name *mimicus* was proposed because of the similarity of these strains to *V. cholerae. V. mimicus* also has been isolated from a number of environmental sources, including oysters (90,91), and gastroenteritis is significantly associated with raw oyster consumption (92).

Between 10% and 16% of isolates (including environmental isolates) produce a heat-labile toxin that appears to be identical to cholera toxin (90,93–96). Some *V. mimicus* strains produce a heat-stable enterotoxin (Vm-ST) that is closely related to NAG-ST produced by nonepidemic *V. cholerae* (94,97). Strains also can produce a thermostable direct hemolysin-like hemolysin (Vm-TDH) that is virtually identical to the thermostable direct hemolysin of *V. parahaemolyticus* (98,99).

In a study of 19 cases identified retrospectively based on isolation of *V. mimicus* from stool (92), symptoms included diarrhea (94%), nausea, vomiting, and abdominal cramps (67%), fever (44%), and headache (39%). Three patients had bloody diarrhea. Diarrhea lasted a median of 6 days. Diagnosis is based on isolation of the organism from stool, with isolation facilitated by use of a selective media such as TCBS (8). *V. mimicus* has also been associated with wound and ear infections (Table 37.2).

As with other types of gastroenteritis, rehydration is the key element of therapy. Isolates are sensitive *in vitro* to tetracycline, trimethoprim-sulfamethoxazole, chloramphenicol, and ciprofloxacin (86), although development of antibiotic resistance has been noted (100).

VIBRIO PARAHAEMOLYTICUS

In the fall of 1950, there was an outbreak of food poisoning in Osaka, Japan; of 272 patients with acute gastroenteritis, 20 died. These deaths led to an intensive investigation of the outbreak and, ultimately, to the identification of an etiologic agent that was first named *Pasteurella parahaemolyticus,* with subsequent reclassification as *Vibrio parahaemolyticus* (101).

Even though *V. parahaemolyticus* has always been recognized as an important enteropathogen, there has been a striking increase in the incidence of infections since the mid-1990s. This increase has been noted in several countries, including Japan (Fig. 37.1) (102) and the United States (103), and appears to be associated with the appearance of a new clonal group with pandemic potential, including isolates in serotypes O3:K6, O4:K68, and O1:K untypeable (O1:KUT) (102–107).

Microbiology

V. parahaemolyticus is halophilic, or salt loving, and requires NaCl for growth. Traditionally, clinical isolates have been differentiated from environmental strains based on their hemolytic activity when grown on special media (Wagatsuma agar) (101,108,109); this is termed the Kanagawa reaction, named for the Japanese prefecture where the original study was done. Before the 1980s, most *V. parahaemolyticus* isolated were urease-negative (110). Since that time, however, urease-positive isolates have been seen with increasing frequency, particularly along the Pacific Coast of North America (111–113). In contrast to the traditional experience with urease-negative strains, urease-positive strains isolated from patients with gastroenteritis are often Kanagawa-negative (111,113–115).

Epidemiology

As with *V. cholerae, V. parahaemolyticus* is part of the naturally occurring bacterial flora in estuarine areas throughout the world. As a halophilic (salt-loving) bacterium, *V. parahaemolyticus* is a common isolate from estuarine and marine water, sediment, suspended particulates, plankton, fish, and shellfish (101,114–117); counts in oysters may exceed those in water by 100-fold (111). In temperate climates, isolation is seasonal, with *V. parahaemolyticus* apparently passing the winter in sediments and then proliferating as water temperatures increase (101,111).

As noted earlier, incidence rates internationally have shown a striking increase since 1995, associated with the appearance of strains within the O3:K6/O4:K68/O1:KUT group (102–107). In Japan, *V. parahaemolyticus* has long been one of the major causes of food-borne illness. However, from the 1950s through the early 1990s, incidence declined steadily, only to dramatically increase beginning in 1994 (Fig. 37.1). Similar increases have been seen in the

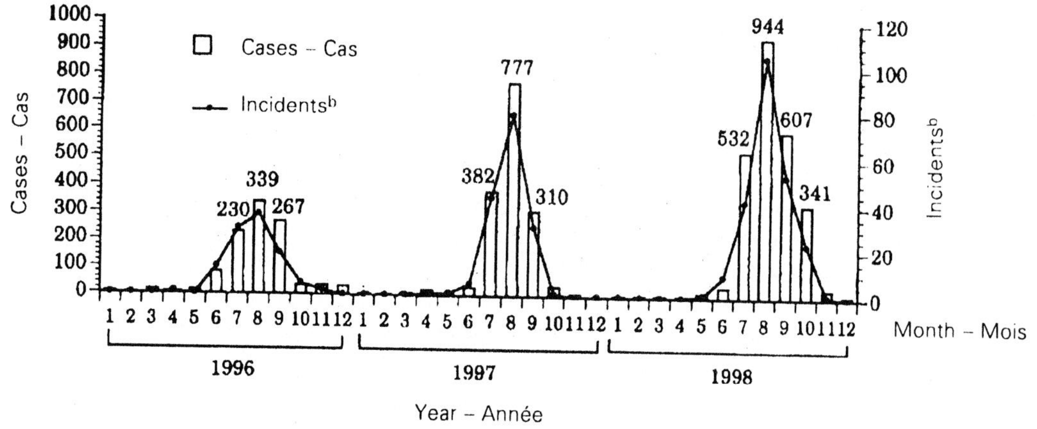

FIGURE 37.1. Monthly reports of isolation of *Vibrio parahaemolyticus*, Japan, 1996–1998

United States (103). In 1989, reported isolation rates of *V. parahaemolyticus* were comparable to those of nonepidemic *V. cholerae* (80); in 1999, as shown in Table 37.2, *V. parahaemolyticus* isolates reported to CDC outnumbered nonepidemic *V. cholerae* by almost 3 to 1. For U.S. cases, it has been suggested that increasing water temperatures in shellfish-growing areas served as a cofactor in the increasing isolation rates of *V. parahaemolyticus* (103,118); further work is needed to assess the relative impact of water temperature versus appearance of O3:K6 and related strains.

Before 1980, *V. parahaemolyticus* outbreaks in the United States reported to CDC had been associated with seafood, but not specifically consumption of raw oysters (103,119). In the 1990s, raw oysters were the vehicle of transmission in 11 (69%) of the 16 *V. parahaemolyticus* outbreaks reported to CDC (103). The increase in summer harvesting of oysters may have contributed, in part, to this change, with 10 (91%) of the 11 oyster-associated outbreaks in the past decade occurring during summer months.

Pathogenesis

The virulence of *V. parahaemolyticus* for humans has traditionally been correlated with hemolytic activity: more than 95% of strains isolated from patients with gastroenteritis in Japan are Kanagawa-positive, in contrast to 2% or less of environmental isolates (101,108,109,120). The association of a Kanagawa-positive reaction with clinical disease has been confirmed in volunteer studies. Volunteers fed up to 10^{10} CFU of *V. parahaemolyticus* strain 255/72 (a Kanagawa-negative strain) remained asymptomatic. In contrast, diarrheal illness was seen in two of four volunteers who ingested 3×10^7 CFU of *V. parahaemolyticus* strain 129/71 (a Kanagawa-positive strain), with one of four volunteers receiving 2×10^5 CFU of this strain reporting abdominal cramps (but no diarrhea) (121).

Hemolytic activity in Kanagawa-positive strains has been linked with production of thermostable direct hemolysin (Vp-TDH) (122,123). Thermostable direct hemolysin-related hemolysins (Vp-TRH) have also been identified that appear to have phenotypic activity similar to that of Vp-TDH and that share sequence homology with Vp-TDH (124–126). When tested by polymerase chain reaction (PCR), *V. parahaemolyticus* strains, which are urease-positive but Kanagawa-negative, can almost always be shown to carry the genes for Vp-TRH (127,128).

V. parahaemolyticus can cause a dysentery-like syndrome (129,130), suggesting that some strains have invasive capabilities. In limited studies, isolates have not given a positive reaction in the Sereny test (which tests for invasiveness in the guinea pig or rabbit eye) (129); however, it has been shown that Kanagawa-positive strains are able to penetrate the intestinal epithelium of infant rabbits (131).

Work is still underway to fully characterize the new O3:K6/O4:K68/O1:KUT *V. parahaemolyticus* clonal group. With rare exceptions, these strains carry *tdh* (104,132), and, on molecular characterization, strains in all three serogroups are closely related. There are preliminary data from Japan suggesting that strains within this group have a common insertion of a Vf33-like filamentous phage (133), which may indicate introduction of a common gene or gene cluster.

Clinical Manifestations

V. parahaemolyticus most commonly causes gastroenteritis. In a summary of clinical data from 337 patients with *V. parahaemolyticus* infections reported to CDC between 1988 and 1997 (103), manifestations included diarrhea (98%), abdominal cramps (89%), nausea (76%), vomiting (55%), and fever (52%); 29% of patients reported bloody diarrhea. In food-borne outbreaks, the median incubation period was 17 hours (range 4 to 90 hours); median reported duration of illness was 2.4 days (range 8 hours to 12 days). A frank dysentery-like syndrome associated with *V. parahaemolyticus* has been reported in India and Bangladesh (122); although such a syndrome is not as common in the United States, there is one report of a U.S. patient with blood and leukocytes in her stool, and superficial colonic ulcerations noted on sigmoidoscopy (130). There are anecdotal reports of cardiac arrhythmias and sudden death in persons infected with *V. parahaemolyticus.*

V. parahaemolyticus also is a cause of infection in seawater-associated wounds (79,80). Wound infections may progress to septicemia, particularly in persons with reduced host defenses. Whereas occasional cases of primary septicemia have been reported (i.e., septicemia without an obvious focus of infection), rates are much lower than those reported for nonepidemic *V. cholerae* or *V. vulnificus.*

Diagnosis

Blood agar and other nonselective media support the growth of *V. parahaemolyticus,* but isolation from feces generally requires the use of a selective medium such as TCBS. The colonies of *V. parahaemolyticus* on TCBS are blue-green (sucrose-negative). Species identification is based on standard biochemical tests. Unlike *V. cholerae, V. parahaemolyticus* does not grow in 0% NaCl but does grow in the relatively high concentrations of 6% to 8% NaCl. A positive Kanagawa reaction (as identified by hemolytic activity on Wagatsuma agar or hybridization with DNA probes for Vp-TDH) (134,135) may be useful in differentiating potentially pathogenic from nonpathogenic strains. As noted earlier, this distinction is not as useful for isolates from along the Pacific coast of North America where *V. parahaemolyticus* isolates from patients with gastroenteritis have been urease-positive and Kanagawa-negative (111,112).

Therapy

As in other diarrheal diseases (83), the key to management of patients with *V. parahaemolyticus* gastroenteritis is provision of adequate rehydration. *V. parahaemolyticus* is susceptible *in vitro* to tetracycline, chloramphenicol, trimethoprim-sulfamethoxazole, and the quinolones; the minimum inhibitory concentration 90% for gentamicin is 4 μg/mL and that of ampicillin greater than 128 μg/mL (25,84). Although there are no data regarding antimicrobial efficacy, patients with persistent diarrhea (>5 days) may benefit from treatment with tetracycline or a quinolone.

VIBRIO FLUVIALIS

Vibrio fluvialis includes strains previously designated as enteric group EF-6 or group F *Vibrio. Fluvialis* is from the Latin for "river," reflecting the early isolation of the organism from river and estuarine waters (136). Biochemically, *V. fluvialis* is similar to *Aeromonas*, and identification systems in common use in hospital microbiology laboratories in the United States may identify *V. fluvialis* as an *Aeromonas* species.

V. fluvialis has been isolated from estuarine environments and shellfish (136–138), with anecdotal U.S. reports suggesting that infections are associated with eating seafood (139,140). A major outbreak of *V. fluvialis*-associated gastroenteritis has been reported from Bangladesh (141).

Symptoms in the Bangladesh outbreak included diarrhea (100%), vomiting (97%), abdominal pain (75%), moderate to severe dehydration (67%), and fever (35%). Seventy-five percent of the patients had leukocytes and red blood cells in their stools. There are anecdotal reports of the organism being associated with intestinal ulceration. Diagnosis is based on stool culture results. No data are available on therapy, although based on antimicrobial susceptibility patterns and experience with other *Vibrio* species, treatment with tetracycline appears to be reasonable in gastroenteritis cases in which diarrhea has persisted for more than 5 days or in cases with bloody diarrhea.

VIBRIO FURNISSII

The species *V. furnissii* includes aerogenic strains (strains that produce gas from glucose) previously classified as biovar II of *V. fluvialis* (136,142). The organism is present in the marine environment (136), and there is a suggestion that gastroenteritis is associated with eating seafood.

An outbreak of gastroenteritis associated with an organism retrospectively identified as *V. furnissii* occurred in 1969 on a flight from Tokyo to Seattle (143,144). Patients' symptoms included diarrhea (91%), abdominal cramps (79%), nausea (65%), and vomiting (39%). One of 23 sick passengers died, and two others required hospitalization.

VIBRIO HOLLISAE

DNA hybridization studies conducted in 1982 determined that *Vibrio* strains previously designated as belonging to enteric group EF-13 constituted a separate species, which was subsequently designated *Vibrio hollisae* (145). Illness in the United States has been associated with eating raw seafood (17).

In a retrospective study of U.S. cases identified on the basis of stool isolates (17), symptoms associated with *V. hollisae* included diarrhea, vomiting (five of nine patients), and fever (five of nine patients). Septicemia may occur in patients with underlying liver disease (146,147). The diagnosis of *V. hollisae* infections is complicated by the organism's tendency to grow poorly on TCBS medium, which is normally used to screen for *Vibrio* species; isolation may require the identification of colonies on blood agar plates.

VIBRIO VULNIFICUS

V. vulnificus, initially identified simply as a halophilic lactose-positive marine *Vibrio,* received its present name in 1979 (148,149). The organism causes severe wound infections, septicemia, and gastroenteritis (148,150–153).

Microbiology

V. vulnificus is a facultatively anaerobic, asporogenous, halophilic gram-negative rod. Although initially classified based on its ability to ferment lactose, 10% to 15% of isolates are lactose-negative (8). Definitive identification of the organism may sometimes be difficult based on biochemical reactions alone; confirmation of species identity may require use of DNA probes (154) or 16s sequence analysis.

Two biotypes and one distinct serovar of *V. vulnificus* are currently recognized. The majority of clinical and environmental *V. vulnificus* isolates reported to date are in biotype 1. Strains initially classified as biotype 2 are responsible for sepsis in eels (155); they do not cause human disease. More recently, it has been recognized that the biotyping characteristics described for these strains lacked specificity; however, the eel pathogens are homogeneous in their lipopolysaccharide-based serogroup, leading to their reclassification as serovar E (156). Biotype 3 strains were described in association with wound infections related to handling of live fish (tilapia) from fish farms in Israel (157). As reported for non-O1 *V. cholerae, V. vulnificus* strains produce a polysaccharide capsule (158,159). Typing systems based on the capsule have not been developed, due in part to the great diversity seen in capsular types: in one study of 120 strains, 96 different capsular types ("carbotypes") were identified (160).

Epidemiology

As is true for other pathogenic vibrios, *V. vulnificus* is a naturally occurring (autochthonous) bacteria in estuarine or marine environments. Highest numbers are found in areas with intermediate salinities (5 to 25 ppt) and warmer temperatures (optimally, >20°C). Isolation has been reported from the U.S. Atlantic, Gulf, and Pacific coasts (161–163), as well as the Atlantic coast of Europe, the Mediterranean, the Indian Ocean, Malaysia, and the Pacific Coast of Asia (164–166). It is likely that the organism is present in virtually all estuarine areas with appropriate salinity and temperature ranges. Using a DNA probe, *V. vulnificus* was identified in 80% of Chesapeake Bay water samples collected during months in which water temperatures exceeded 8° C. Concentrations ranged from 3.0×10^1 to 2.1×10^2/CFU/mL, representing approximately 8% of the total culturable heterotrophic bacteria (161). However, none of the samples collected during February and March, when temperatures were less than 8°C, were positive for this organism. Concentrations in oysters tend to be 100-fold higher than those of the surrounding water (161). During warm summer months, virtually 100% of oysters carry the organism (161,167).

Bacteremia without an obvious focus of infection ("primary septicemia") occurs in persons who are alcoholic or who have chronic underlying illnesses, such as liver disease, cirrhosis, or hemochromatosis (Table 37.3) (148,150–153, 168). In one study, an increased risk of infection was associated with consumption of as little as 1 ounce of alcohol per day (168). Infection is thought to be acquired by eating oysters containing the organism. Wound infections occur after exposure to estuarine water. Typical exposures include wounds acquired while opening an oyster or in a boating accident. Wounds may become infected in normal hosts. However, the most severe manifestations are seen in persons with underlying defects in host defense mechanisms.

V. vulnificus is the most common cause of serious *Vibrio* infections in the United States (Table 37.2), with an incidence in community-based studies in coastal regions of approximately 0.5 cases per 100,000 population per year (79,150,168). Based on the number of cases reported to the Florida Health Department between 1981 and 1992, the annual rate of illness from *V. vulnificus* infection for adults with self-reported liver disease in Florida who ate raw oysters was 7.2 per 100,000 adults, 80 times the rate for adults without known liver disease who ate raw oysters (0.09 cases per 100,000 population) (169). Case series have been reported from Korea and Taiwan (151,153), and it is likely that *V. vulnificus* infections have a worldwide distribution.

TABLE 37.3. EPIDEMIOLOGIC FEATURES AND CLINICAL MANIFESTATIONS OF PATIENTS WITH PRIMARY SEPTICEMIA CAUSED BY *VIBRIO VULNIFICUS*

Feature	Gastroenteritis (n = 23)	Primary Septicemia (n = 181)	Wound Infections (n = 189)
Major Risk Factors[a]			
Liver Disease	14%	80%	22%
Alcoholism	14%	65%	32%
Diabetes	5%	35%	20%
Heart disease	10%	26%	34%
Hematologic disorder	0	18%	8%
Peptic ulcer disease	0	18%	10%
Malignancy	16%	17%	10%
Immunodeficiency	5%	10%	9%
Renal disease	5%	7%	7%
Gastrointestinal surgery	11%	7%	6%
Any of above	35%	97%	68%
Patient Characteristics			
Median age, years (range)	35 (0–84)	54 (24–92)	59 (4–91)
% Male	57	89	88
Symptoms/Signs			
Fever	59%	91%	76%
Diarrhea	100%	58%	—
Abdominal cramps	84%	53%	—
Nausea	71%	59%	—
Vomiting	68%	54%	—
Shock[b]	0	64%	30%
Localized cellulitis	—	—	91%
Bullous skin lesions	0	49%	—
Hospitalized	65%	97%	89%
Death	9%[c]	61%	17%

[a]Conditions are not mutually exclusive.
[b]Systolic blood pressure less than 90 mm Hg.
[c]Deaths occurred in two patients with underlying medical conditions (liver disease, alcohol abuse).
Data from Shapiro RL, Alkekruse S, Hulwagner L, et al. The role of Gulf Coast oysters harvested in warmer months in *Vibrio vulnificus* infections in the United States 1988–1996. *J Infect Dis* 1998;178:752–759.

Pathogenesis

V. vulnificus strains are encapsulated, with the capsule providing resistance to the bactericidal activity of normal human serum and to phagocytosis. Capsular material may also play a role in directly stimulating host cytokines, contributing to subsequent development of a shock syndrome (170). Loss of the capsule correlates with loss of virulence (171). There is a suggestion that certain capsular types are more common among clinical than environmental isolates (159). However, no one capsular type predominates among clinical isolates, and, at this point, it is not possible to differentiate clinical from environmental isolates on the basis of capsule structure or type.

V. vulnificus is also sensitive to the degree of binding of iron by transferrin in the host and serum ferritin concentration (172–174). *V. vulnificus* grows rapidly in serum with transferrin 70% saturated with iron, whereas growth is severely restricted at less than 70% (in normal adults, transferrin is approximately 30% saturated). These observations may explain the increased risk of disease in persons with hemochromatosis or in malnourished alcoholics with low concentrations of transferrin and correspondingly high saturation of transferrin (172).

V. vulnificus produces a variety of extracellular products, including a cytolysin, proteases, collagenase, and phospholipases (175–178), which have been implicated as possible virulence factors. These products have clear biologic activity (179,180) and may contribute to specific manifestations observed in patients infected with the organism; for example, the purified cytolysin has been shown to cause skin damage and skin lesions similar to those seen in patients with septicemia (179). At the same time, these products do not appear to be essential to the disease process. In studies with genetically engineered isogenic mutants, deletion or inactivation of the gene encoding the cytolysin or the protease had a minimal effect on virulence of the organism in animals (172,181).

Given the frequency of isolation of *V. vulnificus* from oysters, the incidence of disease is still much less than might be expected, even taking into account the need for an appropriate host (169). This may reflect the need for a high infectious dose (although no data are currently available to support this hypothesis). Alternatively, strains of *V. vulnificus* may differ in their ability to cause illness. Even though this latter hypothesis is attractive, there is no way to clearly differentiate strains with increased potential for causing human disease (if such strains exist) from less virulent environmental isolates.

Clinical Manifestations

Patients with primary septicemia present with fever and hypotension (Table 37.3). One-third have shock when first seen or become hypotensive within 12 hours of hospitalization (150). Depending on the study, 50% to 90% of patients have distinctive bullous skin lesions (Fig. 37.2). Thrombocytopenia is common, and there is often evidence of disseminated intravascular coagulation; gastrointestinal bleeding is not infrequent. More than 50% of patients with primary septicemia die; the mortality rate exceeds 90% for those who are hypotensive within 12 hours of initial presentation (150).

Wound infections range from mild, self-limited lesions to rapidly progressive cellulitis and myositis that mimics clostridial myonecrosis in rapidity of spread and destructiveness (182,183). Up to 35% of patients with wound infections may become bacteremic. Mortality rates as high as 25% have been reported, with deaths (and bacteremia) concentrated in the same populations that are at risk for primary septicemia.

Patients who survive severe *V. vulnificus* infections often have some degree of residual disability. This does not appear to be related to the actual infection, which clears readily with antibiotic therapy, but rather to the consequences of multiple organ system failure and the prolonged hospitalization associated with occurrence of a shock syndrome.

Diagnosis

Early diagnosis of *V. vulnificus* septicemia is essential, given its severity and the rapidity with which the disease progresses, and the possible benefit of early antimicrobial therapy (150). A presumptive clinical diagnosis can be made on the basis of (a) occurrence of shock or hypotension, or other signs suggesting sepsis (for wound infections, evidence of rapidly progressive cellulitis or myositis); (b) a history of cirrhosis, chronic alcoholism, immunosuppression, or hemochromatosis; (c) a history of recent consumption of raw oysters or exposure of wounds to estuarine water; and (d) the presence of characteristic bullous skin lesions.

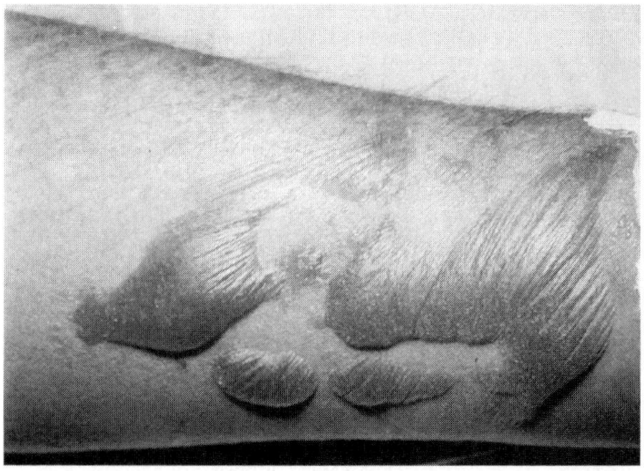

FIGURE 37.2. Bullous skin lesion of a patient with *Vibrios vulnificus* septicemia and hypotension. Photograph was taken approximately 48 hours after onset of symptoms.

A definitive diagnosis requires isolation of *V. vulnificus* from blood. In some instances, skin bullae may also harbor the organism. Blood agar and other nonselective media, including media used in commercial blood culture systems, are adequate for isolation. Because the organism is presumed to enter the body through the intestinal tract in cases of primary septicemia, stool cultures may be positive for *V. vulnificus* (184). TCBS is the preferred medium for isolation from feces; more than 90% of strains produce blue-green (sucrose-negative) colonies. In the proper clinical setting, isolation of *V. vulnificus* from stool is highly suggestive of the diagnosis (although there is a possibility that such isolation reflects incidental, asymptomatic intestinal carriage of the organism).

Presumptive identification of *V. vulnificus* from cultures is based on standard biochemical tests. The identity of individual bacterial colonies can be further evaluated by immunologic assays directed against various *V. vulnificus* surface antigens (185,186) or by PCR or with DNA probes (154,187).

Therapy

The early administration of antimicrobial agents is critical to successful treatment, with case fatality rates showing a significant increase with increasing time between onset of symptoms and initiation of therapy (150). *V. vulnificus* is susceptible to a wide range of agents *in vitro,* including ampicillin, tetracycline, chloramphenicol, trimethoprim-sulfamethoxazole, and ciprofloxacin; the minimum inhibitory concentration 90% to gentamicin is 8 μg/mL (86). Studies in mice indicate that tetracycline has the best efficacy against the organism (188), and there is a suggestion from a large series of cases from Florida that antimicrobial combinations that included tetracycline were more efficacious (150). Recent *in vitro* and animal studies from Taiwan indicate that there is synergism between minocycline and cefotaxime in treatment of serious *V. vulnificus* infections. In light of these latter studies, therapy with minocycline (100 mg every 12 hours orally) and cefotaxime (2.0 g every 8 hours intravenously), with doses appropriately adjusted for underlying renal or hepatic disease, is recommended for patients with septicemia or serious wound infections (88,89). As is true for any patient with gram-negative sepsis, persons in shock require careful monitoring and aggressive supportive care.

Prevention

As long as oysters and other shellfish are harvested from warm waters and eaten raw or with minimal cooking, there is risk of infection with *V. vulnificus.* Persons who are immunocompromised, have cirrhosis (or a history of heavy ingestion of ethanol), or have conditions predisposing them to increased saturation of their transferrin with iron should not eat raw oysters, particularly during the summer and early fall when water temperatures may exceed 20°C. Persons in these same risk groups also should try to minimize exposure of wounds to warmer estuarine or marine waters.

REFERENCES

1. Gardner AD, Venkatraman VK. The antigens of the cholera group of vibrios. *J Hyg* 1935;35:262–282.
2. Pollitzer R. *Cholera.* Geneva: WHO, 1959.
3. Aldova E, Laznickova K, Stepankova E, et al. Isolation of nonagglutinable vibrios from an enteritis outbreak in Czechoslovakia. *J Infect Dis* 1968;118:25–31.
4. El-Shawi N, Thewaini AJ. Non-agglutinable vibrios isolated in the 1966 epidemic of cholera in Iraq. *Bull WHO* 1969;40: 163–166.
5. Kamal AM. Outbreak of gastroenteritis by non-agglutinable (NAG) vibrios in the republic of the Sudan. *J Egypt Public Health Assoc* 1971;46:125–173.
6. McIntyre OR, Feeley JC, Greenough WB, et al. Diarrhea caused by non-cholera vibrios. *Am J Trop Med Hyg* 1965;14: 412–418.
7. Yajnik BS, Prasad BG. A note on vibrios isolated in Kumbh Fair, Allahbad, 1954. *Ind Med Gazette* 1954;89:341–349.
8. Tison DL. *Vibrio.* In: Murray PR, Baron EJ, Pfaller MA, et al., eds. *Manual of Clinical Microbiology,* seventh edition. Washington, DC: ASM Press, 2000:497–506.
9. Morris JG Jr, Black RE. Cholera and other vibrioses in the United States. *N Engl J Med* 1985;312:343–350.
10. International Center for Diarrheal Disease Research, Bangladesh, Cholera Working Group. Large epidemic of cholera-like disease in Bangladesh caused by *Vibrio cholerae* O139 synonym Bengal. *Lancet* 1993;342:387–390.
11. Ramamurthy T, Garg S, Sharma R, et al. Emergence of novel strain of *Vibrio cholerae* with epidemic potential in southern and eastern India. *Lancet* 1993;341:703–704.
12. Chongsa-nguan M, Chaicumpa W, Moolasart P, et al. *Vibrio cholerae* O139 Bengal in Bangkok. *Lancet* 1993;342:430–431.
13. Shehabi AA, Abu Rajab AB, Shaker AA. Observations on the emergence of non-cholera vibrios during an outbreak of cholera. *Jordan Med J* 1980;14:125–127.
14. Dutt AK, Alwi S, Velauthan T. A shellfish-borne cholera outbreak in Malaysia. *Trans R Soc Trop Med Hyg* 1971;65:815–818.
15. Morris JG Jr, Wilson R, Davis BR, et al. Non-O Group 1 *Vibrio cholerae* gastroenteritis in the United States. *Ann Intern Med* 1981;94:656–658.
16. Morris JG Jr, Takeda T, Tall BD, et al. Experimental non-O group 1 *Vibrio cholerae* gastroenteritis in humans. *J Clin Invest* 1990;85:697–705.
17. Morris JG JR, Miller HG, Wilson RA, et al. Illness caused by *Vibrio damsela* and *Vibrio hollisae. Lancet* 1982;1:1294–1297.
18. Bode RB, Brayton PR, Colwell RR, et al. A new *Vibrio* species, *Vibrio cincinnatiensis,* causing meningitis: successful treatment in an adult. *Ann Intern Med* 1986;104:55–56.
19. Pavia AT, Bryan JA, Maher KL, et al. *Vibrio carchariae* infection after a shark bite. *Ann Intern Med* 1989;111:85–86.
20. Jean-Jacques W, Rajashekaraiah KR, Farmer JJ III, et al. *Vibrio metschnikovii* bacteremia in a patient with cholecystitis. *J Clin Microbiol* 1981;14:711–712.
21. Farmer JJ III, Hickman-Brenner FW, Fanning GR, et al. Characterization of *Vibrio metschnikovii* and *Vibrio gazogenes* by DNA-DNA hybridization and phenotype. *J Clin Microbiol* 1988;26:1993–2000.
22. Cano RJ, Tiefenbrunner F, Ubaldi M, et al. Sequence analysis

of bacterial DNA in the colon and stomach of the Tyrolean Iceman. *Am J Phys Anthropol* 2000;112:297–309.
23. Waldor MK, Mekalanos JJ. Lysogenic conversion by a filamentous phage encoding cholera toxin. *Science* 1996;272: 1910–1914.
24. Karaolis DKR, Johnson JA, Bailey CC, et al. *Vibrio cholerae* pathogenicity island associated with epidemic and pandemic strains. *Proc Natl Acad Sci U S A* 1998;95:3134–3139.
25. Karaolis DKR, Sozhamannan S, Johnson JA, et al. Novel non-O1/non-O139 *Vibrio cholerae* containing the VPI and CTX. 98th General Meeting of the American Society for Microbiology, Atlanta, GA, 1988, Abstract B-179.
26. Morris JG Jr. Non-O group 1 *Vibrio cholerae:* a look at the epidemiology of an occasional pathogen. *Epidemiol Rev* 1990;12: 179–191.
27. Sakazaki R, Shimada T. Serovars of *Vibrio cholerae. Jpn J Med Sci Biol* 1977;30:279–282.
28. West PA, Brayton PR, Twilley RR, et al. Numerical taxonomy of nitrogen-fixing "decarboxylase-negative" *Vibrio* species isolated from aquatic environments. *Int J Sys Bacteriol* 1985;35:198–205.
29. Amaro C, Toranzo AE, Gonzalez EA, et al. Surface and virulence properties of environmental *Vibrio cholerae* non-O1 from Albufera Lake (Valencia, Spain). *Appl Environ Microbiol* 1990; 56:1140–1147.
30. Kaper JB, Lockman H, Colwell RR, et al. Ecology, serology, and enterotoxin production of *Vibrio cholerae* in Chesapeake Bay. *Appl Environ Microbiol* 1979;37:91–103.
31. Lee JV, Bashford DJ, Donovan TJ, et al. The incidence and distribution of *V. cholerae* in England. In: Colwell RR, ed. *Vibrios in the environment.* New York: John Wiley and Sons, 1984: 427–450.
32. Roberts NC, Seibeling RJ, Kaper JB, et al. Vibrios in the Louisiana Gulf Coast environment. *Microb Ecol* 1982;8:299–312.
33. Colwell RR, West PA, Maneval D, et al. Ecology of pathogenic *Vibrios* in Chesapeake Bay. In: Colwell RR, ed. *Vibrios in the environment.* New York: John Wiley and Sons, 1984:367–387.
34. Rhodes JB, Smith HL Jr, Ogg JE. Isolation of non-O1 *Vibrio cholerae* serovars from surface waters in western Colorado. *Appl Environ Microbiol* 1986;51:1216–1219.
35. Mulder GD, Reis TM, Beaver TR. Non-toxigenic *Vibrio cholerae* wound infection after exposure to contaminated lake water. *J Infect Dis* 1989;159:809–811.
36. Pitrak DL, Gindorf JD. Bacteremia cellulitis caused by non-serogroup O1 *Vibrio cholerae* acquired in a freshwater inland lake. *J Clin Microbiol* 1989;27:2874–2876.
37. Twedt RM, Madden JM, Hunt JM, et al. Characterization of *Vibrio cholerae* isolated from oysters. *Appl Environ Microbiol* 1981;41:1475–1478.
38. Sack RB. A search for canine carriers of *Vibrio. J Infect Dis* 1973;127:709–712.
39. Sanyal SC, Singh SJ, Tiwari IC, et al. Role of household animals in maintenance of cholera infection in a community. *J Infect Dis* 1974;130:575–579.
40. Bisgaard M, Sakazaki R, Shimada T. Prevalence of non-cholera vibrios in cavum nasi and pharynx of ducks. *Acta Pathol Microbiol Scand* Sect B 1978;86:261–266.
41. Rhodes JB, Schweitzer D, Ogg JE. Isolation of non-O1 *Vibrio cholerae* associated with enteric disease of herbivores in western Colorado. *J Clin Microbiol* 1985;22:572–575.
42. Lowry PW, McFarland LM, Peltier BH, et al. *Vibrio* gastroenteritis in Louisiana: a prospective study among attendees of a scientific congress in New Orleans. *J Infect Dis* 1989;160:978–984.
43. Zafari Y, Zarifi AZ, Rahmanzadeh S, et al. Diarrhea caused by non-agglutinable *Vibrio cholerae* (non-cholera *Vibrio*). *Lancet* 1973;2:429–430.
44. Ko W-C, Chuang Y-C, Huang G-C, et al. Infections due to non-O1 *Vibrio cholerae* in Southern Taiwan: predominance in cirrhotic patients. Clin Infect Dis 1998;27:774–780.
45. Klontz KC. Fatalities associated with *Vibrio parahaemolyticus* and *Vibrio cholerae* non-O1 infections in Florida (1981-1988). *South Med J* 1990;83:500–502.
46. Safrin S, Morris JG Jr, Adams M, et al. Non-O:1 *Vibrio cholerae* bacteremia: case report and review. *Rev Infect Dis* 1988;10: 1012–1017.
47. Dakin WPH, Howell DJ, Sutton RGA, et al. Gastroenteritis due to non-agglutinable (non-cholera) vibrios. *Med J Aust* 1974;2:487–490.
48. Finch MJ, Valdespino JL, Wells JG, et al. Non-O1 *Vibrio cholerae* infections in Cancun, Mexico. *Am J Trop Med Hyg* 1987;36:393–397.
49. Taylor DN, Echeverria P, Pitarangsi C, et al. Application of DNA hybridization techniques in the assessment of diarrheal disease among refugees in Thailand. *Am J Epidemiol* 1988;127: 179–187.
50. Thomson CJ, Jesudason MV, Balaji V, et al. The prevalence of *Vibrio* spp in drinking water and environmental samples in Vellore South India. Epidemiol Infect 1998;121:67–76.
51. Varlea G, Olarte J, Perez-Miravete A, et al. Failure to find cholera and non-cholera vibrios in diarrheal disease in Mexico City, 1966-7. *Am J Trop Med Hyg* 1971;20:925–926.
52. Black RE, Merson MH, Brown KH. Epidemiological aspects of diarrhea associated with known enteropathogens in rural Bangladesh. In: Chen LC, Scrimshaw NS, eds. *Diarrhea and malnutrition.* New York: Plenum Press, 1983:73–86.
53. Dalsgaard A, Forslund A, Bodhidatta L, et al. A high proportion of *Vibrio cholerae* strains isolated from children with diarrhoea in Bangkok, Thailand, are multiple antibiotic resistant and belong to heterogenous non-O1, non-O139 O-serotypes. *Epidemiol Infect* 1999;122:217–226.
54. Datta-Roy K, Banerjee K, De SP, et al. Comparative study of expression of hemagglutinins, hemolysins, and enterotoxins by clinical and environmental isolates of non-O1 *Vibrio cholerae* in relation to their enteropathogenicity. *Appl Environ Microbiol* 1986;52:875–879.
55. Spira WM, Daniel RR, Ahmed QS, et al. Clinical features and pathogenicity of O group 1 non-agglutinating *Vibrio cholerae* and other vibrios isolated from cases of diarrhea in Dacca, Bangladesh. In: Takeya J, Zinnaka Y, eds. *Symposium on cholera:* Karatsu 1978: Proceedings of the 14th Joint Conference U.S.-Japan Cooperative Medical Science Program Cholera Panel. Tokyo: Toho University, 1978:137–153.
56. Yamamoto K, Takeda Y, Miwatani T, et al. Evidence that a non-O1 *Vibrio cholerae* produces enterotoxin that is similar but not identical to cholera enterotoxin. *Infect Immun* 1983;41:896–901.
57. Hanchalay S, Seriwatana J, Echeverria P, et al. Non-O1 *Vibrio cholerae* in Thailand: homology with cloned cholera toxin genes. *J Clin Microbiol* 1985;21:288–289.
58. Kaper JB, Nataro JP, Roberts NC, et al. Molecular epidemiology of non-O1 *Vibrio cholerae* and *Vibrio mimicus* in the U.S. Gulf Coast region. *J Clin Microbiol* 1986;23:652–654.
59. Chakraborty S, Mukhopadhyay AK, Bhadra RK, et al. Virulence genes in environmental strains of *Vibrio cholerae. Appl Environ Microbiol* 2000;66:4022–4028.
60. Sharma C, Thungapathra M, Ghosh A, et al. Molecular analysis of non-O1, non-O139 *Vibrio cholerae* associated with an unusual upsurge in the incidence of cholera-like disease in Calcutta, India. *J Clin Microbiol* 1988;36:756–763.
61. Dalsgaard A, Albert MJ, Taylor DN, et al. Characterization of *Vibrio cholerae* non-O1 serogroup obtained from an outbreak of diarrhoea in Lima, Peru. *J Clin Microbiol* 1995;33:2715.
62. Ramamrthy T, Bag PK, Pal A, et al. Virulence patterns of *Vibrio cholerae* non-O1 strains isolated from hospitalized patients

with acute diarrhoea in Calcutta, India. *J Med Microbiol* 1993; 39:310.

63. Arita M, Takeda T, Honda T, et al. Purification and characterization of *Vibrio cholerae* non-O1 heat-stable enterotoxin. *Infect Immun* 1986;52:45–49.
64. Honda T, Arita M, Takeda T, et al. Non-O1 *Vibrio cholerae* produces two newly identified toxins related to *Vibrio parahaemolyticus* hemolysin and *Escherichia coli* heat-stable enterotoxin. *Lancet* 1985;2:163–164.
65. Bagchi K, Echeverria P, Arthur JD, et al. Epidemic of diarrhea caused by *Vibrio cholerae* non-O1 that produced heat-stable toxin among Khmers in a camp in Thailand. *J Clin Microbiol* 1993;31:1215–1217.
66. Johnson JA, Salles CA, Morris JG Jr. Correlation of heat-stable enterotoxin and capsule type of non-O1 *Vibrio cholerae.* 32nd Interscience Conference on Antimicrobial Agents and Chemotherapy, Anaheim, California, October 11–14, 1992.
67. Gyobu Y, Kodama H, Sato S. Studies on the enteropathogenic mechanism of non-O1 *Vibrio cholerae.* III. Production of enteroreactive toxins. *Kansenshogaku Zasshi* 1991;65:781–787.
68. Ichinose Y, Yamamoto K, Nakasone N, et al. Enterotoxicity of El Tor-like hemolysin of non-O1 *Vibrio cholerae. Infect Immun* 1987;55:1090–1093.
69. McCardell BA, Madden JM, Shah DB. Isolation and characterization of a cytolysin produced by *Vibrio cholerae* serogroup non-O1. *Can J Microbiol* 1985;31:711–720.
70. Yamamoto K, Ichinose Y, Nakasone N, et al. Identity of hemolysins produced by *Vibrio cholerae* non-O1 and *V. cholerae* O1, biotype El Tor. *Infect Immun* 1986;51:927–931.
71. Levine MM, Kaper JB, Herrington D, et al. Volunteer studies of deletion mutants of *Vibrio cholerae* O1 prepared by recombinant techniques. *Infect Immun* 1988;56:161–167.
72. Johnson JA, Panigrahi P, Russell RG, et al. Role of hemolysin in the pathogenesis of non-serogroup O1 *Vibrio cholerae.* 31st Interscience Conference on Antimicrobial Agents and Chemotherapy, Chicago, Illinois, September 29–October 2, 1991.
73. O'Brien AD, Chen ME, Holmes RK, et al. Environmental and human isolates of *Vibrio cholerae* and *Vibrio parahaemolyticus* produce a *Shigella dysenteriae* 1 (Shiga-like) cytotoxin. *Lancet* 1984;1:77–78.
74. Shehabi AA, Drexler H, Richardson SH. Virulence mechanisms associated with clinical isolates of non-O1 *Vibrio cholerae. Zentralbl Bakteriol Mikrobiol Hyg* 1986;A261:232–239.
76. Spira WM, Fedorka-Cray PJ, Pettebone P. Colonization of the rabbit small intestine by clinical and environmental isolates of non-O1 *Vibrio cholerae* and *Vibrio mimicus. Infect Immun* 1983; 41:1175–1183.
77. Johnson JA, Panigrahi P, Morris JG Jr. Non-O1 *Vibrio cholerae* NRT36S produces a polysaccharide capsule that determines colony morphology, serum resistance, and virulence in mice. *Infect Immun* 1992;60:684–689.
78. Johnson JA, Joseph A, Panigrahi P, et al. Frequency of encapsulated versus unencapsulated strains of non-O1 *Vibrio cholerae* isolated from patients with septicemia or diarrhea, or from environmental strains. American Society for Microbiology Annual Meeting, New Orleans, Louisiana, May 26–30, 1992.
79. Bhattachaya MK, Dutta D, Bhattacharya SK, et al. Association of a disease approximating cholera caused by *Vibrio cholerae* of serogroups other than O1 and O139. *Epidemiol Infect* 1998; 120:1–5.
80. Hoge CW, Watsky D, Peeler RN, et al. Epidemiology and spectrum of vibrio infections in a Chesapeake Bay community. *J Infect Dis* 1989;160:985–993.
81. Levine WC, Griffin PM, Gulf Coast *Vibrio* Working Group. *Vibrio* infections on the Gulf Coast: results of first year of regional surveillance. *J Infect Dis* 1993;167:479–483.
81. Bonner JR, Coker AS, Berryman CR, et al. Spectrum of *Vibrio* infections in a Gulf Coast community. *Ann Intern Med* 1983; 99:464–469.
82. Hughes JM, Hollis DG, Gangarosa EJ, et al. Non-cholera *Vibrio* infections in the United States: clinical, epidemiologic, and laboratory features. *Ann Intern Med* 1978;88:602–606.
83. Black RE. The prophylaxis and therapy of secretory diarrhea. *Med Clin North Am* 1982;66:611–621.
84. Swerdlow DL, Ries AA. Cholera in the Americas: guidelines for the clinician. *JAMA* 1992;267:1495–1499.
85. Wallace CK, Anderson PN, Brown TC, et al. Optimal antibiotic therapy in cholera. *Bull WHO* 1968;39:239–245.
86. Morris JG Jr, Tenney JH, Drusano GL. *In vitro* susceptibility of pathogenic *Vibrio* species to norfloxacin and six other antimicrobial agents. *Antimicrob Agents Chemother* 1985;28: 442–445.
87. Northrup RS. Antibiotics in cholera therapy. *J Pakistan Med Assoc* 1969;19:363–365.
88. Chuang YC, Liu JW, Ko WC, et al. *In vitro* synergism between cefotaxime and minocycline against *Vibrio vulnificus. Antimicrob Agents Chemother* 1997; 41:2214.
89. Chuang YC, Ko WC, Wang ST, et al. Minocycline and cefotaxime in the treatment of experimental murine *Vibrio vulnificus* infection. *Antimicrob Agents Chemother* 1998;42:1319.
90. Davis BR, Fanning GR, Madden JM, et al. Characterization of biochemically atypical *Vibrio cholerae* strains and designation of a new pathogenic species, *Vibrio mimicus. J Clin Microbiol* 1981;14:631–639.
91. Chowdhury MA, Yamanaka H, Miyoshi S, et al. Ecology of *Vibrio mimicus* in aquatic environments. *Appl Environ Microbiol* 1989;55:2073–2078.
92. Shandera WX, Johnston JM, Davis BR, et al. Disease from infection with *Vibrio mimicus,* a newly recognized *Vibrio* species. *Ann Intern Med* 1983;99:169–171.
93. Spira WM, Fedorka-Cray PJ. Production of cholera toxin-like toxin by *Vibrio mimicus* and non-O1 *Vibrio cholerae:* batch culture conditions for optimal yields and isolation of hypertoxigenic lincomycin-resistant mutants. *Infect Immun* 1983;42:501–509.
94. Gyobu Y, Isobe J, Kodama H, et al. Enteropathogenicity and enteropathogenic toxin production of *Vibrio mimicus. J Jpn Assoc Infect Dis* 1992;66:115–120.
95. Tamplin ML, Jalali R, Ahmed MK, et al. Variation in epitopes of the B subunit of *Vibrio cholerae* non-O1 and *Vibrio mimicus* cholera toxins. *Can J Microbiol* 1990;36:409–413.
96. Shi L, Miyoshi S, Hiura M, et al. Detection of genes encoding cholera toxin (CT), zonula occludens toxin (ZOT), accessory cholera enterotoxin (ACE) and heat-stable enterotoxin (ST) in *Vibrio mimicus* clinical strains. *Microbiol Immunol* 1998;42: 823–828.
97. Arita M, Honda T, Miwatani T, et al. Purification and characterization of a heat-stable enterotoxin of *Vibrio mimicus. FEMS Microbiol Lett* 1991;63:105–110.
98. Yoshida H, Honda T, Miwatani T. Purification and characterization of a hemolysin of *Vibrio mimicus* that relates to the therostable direct hemolysin of *Vibrio parahaemolyticus. FEMS Microbiol Lett* 1991;68:249–253.
99. Terai A, Shirai H, Yoshida O, et al. Nucleotide sequence of the thermostable direct hemolysin gene (tdh gene) of *Vibrio mimicus* and its evolutionary relationship with the tdh genes of *Vibrio parahaemolyticus. FEMS Microbiol Lett* 1990;59:319–323.
100. Ananthan S, Dhamodaran S. Toxigenicity and drug sensitivity of *Vibrio mimicus* isolated from patients with diarrhoea. *Indian J Med Res* 1996;104:336–341.
101. Joseph SW, Colwell RR, Kaper JB. *Vibrio parahaemolyticus* and related halophilic vibrios. *CRC Crit Rev Microbiol* 1983;10: 77–124.

102. World Health Organization. *Vibrio parahaemolyticus,* Japan, 1996-1998. *Wkly Epidemiol Rep* 1999;43:361–363.
103. Daniels NA, MacKinnon L, Bishop R, et al. *Vibrio parahaemolyticus* infections in the United States, 1973-1998. *J Infect Dis* 2000;181:1661–1666.
104. Chowdhury NR, Chakraborty S, Ramamurthy T, et al. Molecular evidence of clonal *Vibrio parahaemolyticus* pandemic strains. *Emerg Infect Dis* 2000;6:631–636.
105. Okuda J, Ishibashi M, Hayakawa E, et al. Emergence of a unique O3:K6 clone of *Vibrio parahaemolyticus* in Calcutta, India, and isolation of strains from the same clonal group from southeast Asian travellers arriving in Japan. *J Clin Microbiol* 1997;37:2354–2357.
106. Bag PK, Nandi S, Bhadra RK, et al. Clonal diversity among the recently emerged strains of *Vibrio parahaemolyticus* O3:K6 associated with pandemic spread. *J Clin Microbiol* 1999;37: 2354–2357.
107. Chiou CS, Hsu SY, Chiu SI, et al. *Vibrio parahaemolyticus* serovar O3:K6 as cause of unusually high incidence of foodborne disease outbreaks in Taiwan from 1996-1999. *J Clin Microbiol* 2000;38:4621–4625.
108. Sakazaki R, Tamura K, Kato T, et al. Studies on the enteropathogenic, facultatively halophilic bacteria, *Vibrio parahaemolyticus.* III. Enteropathogenicity. *Jpn J Med Sci Biol* 1968;21: 325–331.
109. Miyamoto Y, Kato T, Obara Y, et al. *In vitro* hemolytic characteristic of *Vibrio parahaemolyticus:* its close correlation with human pathogenicity. *J Bacteriol* 1969;100:1147–1149.
110. Fujino T, Sakazaki R, Tamura K. Designation of the type strain of *Vibrio parahamolyticus* and description of 200 strains of the species. *Int J Syst Bacteriol* 1974;24:447–449.
111. Kelly MT, Stroh EM. Urease-positive, Kanagawa-negative *Vibrio parahaemolyticus* from patients and the environment in the Pacific Northwest. *J Clin Microbiol* 1989;27:2820–2822.
112. Abbott SL, Powers C, Kaysner CA, et al. Emergence of a restricted bioserovar of *Vibrio parahaemolyticus* as the predominant cause of *Vibrio*-associated gastroenteritis on the west coast of the United States and Mexico. *J Clin Microbiol* 1989;27: 2891–2893.
113. Magalhaes M, Magalhaes V, Antas MG, et al. Isolation of urease-positive *Vibrio parahaemolyticus* from diarrheal patients in northeast Brazil. *Revista do Instituto de Medicina Tropical de Sao Paulo* 1991;33:263–265.
114. Kaysner CA, Abeyta C Jr, Stott RF, et al. Incidence of urea-hydrolyzing *Vibrio parahaemolyticus* in Willapa Bay, Washington. *Appl Environ Microbiol* 1990;56:904–907.
115. Honda S, Matsumoto S, Miwatani T, et al. A survey of urease-positive *Vibrio parahaemolyticus* strains isolated from traveller's diarrhea, sea water and imported frozen sea foods. *Eur J Epidemiol* 1992;8:861–864.
116. DePaola A, Hopkins LH, Peeler JT, et al. Incidence of *Vibrio parahaemolyticus* in U.S. coastal waters and oysters. *Appl Environ Microbiol* 1990;56:2299–2302.
117. Kumazawa NH, Fukuma N, Komoda Y. Attachment of *Vibrio parahaemolyticus* strains to estuarine algae. *J Vet Med Sci* 1991; 53:201–205.
118. Daniels NA, Ray B, Easton A, et al. Emergence of a new *Vibrio parahaemolyticus* serotype in raw oysters: A prevention quandary. *JAMA* 2000;284:1541–1545.
119. Barker WH Jr. *Vibrio parahaemolyticus* outbreaks in the United States. *Lancet*1974;1:551–554.
120. Thompson CA Jr, Vanderzant C, Ray SM. Serological and hemolytic characteristics of *Vibrio parahaemolyticus* from marine sources. *J Food Sci* 1976;41:204–205.
121. Sanyal SC, Sen PC. Human volunteer study on the pathogenicity of *Vibrio parahaemolyticus.* In: International Symposium on *Vibrio parahaemolyticus.* Tokyo, Japan, September 17–18, 1973. Tokyo: Saikon, 1973:227–230.
122. Kaper JB, Campen RK, Seidler RJ, et al. Cloning of the thermostable direct or Kanagawa phenomenon-associated hemolysin of *Vibrio parahaemolyticus. Infect Immun* 1984;45:290–292.
123. Nishibuchi M, Fasano A, Russell RG, et al. Enterotoxigenicity of *Vibrio parahaemolyticus* with and without genes encoding thermostable direct hemolysin. *Infect Immun* 1992;60:3539–3545.
124. Honda T, Ni YX, Hata A, et al. Properties of a hemolysin related to the thermostable direct hemolysin produced by a Kanagawa phenomenom negative, clinical isolate of *Vibrio parahaemolyticus. Can J Microbiol* 1990;36:395–399.
125. Yoh M, Miwatani T, Honda T. Comparison of *Vibrio parahaemolyticus* hemolysin (Vp-TRH) produced by clinical and environmental isolates. *FEMS Microbiol Lett* 1992;71:157–161.
126. Shirai H, Ito H, Hirayama T, et al. Molecular epidemiologic evidence for association of thermostable direct hemolysin (TDH) and TDH-related hemolysin of *Vibrio parahaemolyticus* with gastroenteritis. *Infect Immun* 1990;58:3568–3573.
127. Suthienkul O, Ishibashi M, Iida T, Nettip N, et al. Urease production correlates with possession of the *trh* gene in *Vibrio parahaemolyticus* strains isolated in Thailand. *J Infect Dis* 1995;172: 1405–1408.
128. Okuda J, Ishibashi M, Abbott SL, et al. Analysis of the thermostable direct hemolysin (*tdh*) gene and the tdh-related hemolysin (*trh*) genes in urease-positive strains of *Vibrio parahaemolyticus* isolated on the West Coast of the United States. *J Clin Microbiol* 1997;35:1965–1971.
129. Hughes JM, Boyce JM, Aleem ARMA, et al. *Vibrio parahaemolyticus* enterocolitis in Bangladesh: report of an outbreak. *Am J Trop Med Hyg* 1978;27:106–112.
130. Bolen JL, Zamiska SA, Greenough WB III. Clinical features in enteritis due to *Vibrio parahaemolyticus. Am J Med* 1974;57: 638–641.
131. Calia FM, Johnson DE. Bacteremia in suckling rabbits after oral challenge with *Vibrio parahaemolyticus. Infect Immun* 1975; 11:1222–1225.
132. Wong HC, Liu SH, Wang TK, et al. Characteristics of *Vibrio parahaemolyticus* O3:K6 from Asia. *Appl Environ Microbiol* 2000;66:3981–3986.
133. Chang B, Yoshida S, Miyamoto H, et al. A unique and common restriction fragment pattern of the nucleotide sequences homologous to the genome of Vf33, a filamentous bacteriophage, in pandemic strains of *Vibrio parahaemolyticus* O3:K6 O4:K68, and O1:K untypeable. *FEMS Microbiol Lett* 2000; 15:231–236.
134. Nishibuchi M, Ishibashi M, Takeda Y, et al. Detection of the thermostable direct hemolysin gene and related DNA sequences in *Vibrio parahaemolyticus* and other *Vibrio* species by the DNA colony hybridization test. *Infect Immun* 1985;49:481–486.
135. Nishibuchi M, Hill WE, Zon G, et al. Synthetic oligodeoxyribonucleotide probes to detect Kanagawa phenomenon-positive *Vibrio parahaemolyticus. J Clin Microbiol* 1986;23:1091–1095.
136. Lee JV, Shread P, Furniss AL, et al. Taxonomy and description of *Vibrio fluvialis* sp. nov. (synonym group F Vibrios, group EF-6). *J Appl Bacteriol* 1981;50:73–94.
137. Seidler RJ, Allen DA, Colwell RR, et al. Biochemical characteristics and virulence of environmental group F bacteria isolated in the United States. *Appl Environ Microbiol* 1980;40:715–720.
138. Maugeri TL, Caccamo D, Gugliandolo C. Potentially pathogenic vibrios in brackish waters and mussels. *J Appl Microbiol* 2000;89:261–266.
139. Klontz KC, Desenclos JC. Clinical and epidemiological features of sporadic infections with *Vibrio fluvialis* in Florida, USA. *J Diarrhoeal Dis Res* 1990;8:24–26.
140. Huq MI, Alam AKMJ, Brenner DJ, et al. Isolation of Vibrio-

like group, EF-6, from persons with diarrhea. *J Clin Microbiol* 1980;11:621–624.
141. Thekdi RJ, Lakhani AG, Rale VB, et al. An outbreak of food poisoning suspected to be caused by *Vibrio fluvialis*. *J Diarrhoeal Dis Res* 1990;8:163–165.
142. Brenner DJ, Hickman-Brenner FW, Lee JV, et al. *Vibrio furnissii* (formerly aerogenic biogroup of *Vibrio fluvialis*), a new species isolates from human feces and the environment. *J Clin Microbiol* 1983;18:816–824.
143. Centers for Disease Control. An outbreak of acute gastroenteritis during a tour of the orient—Alaska. *MMWR Morbid Mortal Wkly Rep* 1969;18:150.
144. Centers for Disease Control. Follow-up outbreak of gastroenteritis during a tour of the orient—Alaska. *MMWR Morbid MortalWkly Rep* 1969;18:168.
145. Hickman FW, Farmer JJ III, Hollis DG, et al. Identification of *Vibrio hollisae* sp. nov. from patients with diarrhea. *J Clin Microbiol* 1982;15:395–401.
146. Lowry PW, McFarland LM, Threefoot HK. *Vibrio hollisae* septicemia after consumption of catfish. *J Infect Dis* 1986;154: 730–731.
147. Rank EL, Smith IR, Langer M. Bacteremia caused by *Vibrio hollisae*. *J Clin Microbiol* 1988;26:375–376.
148. Blake PA, Merson MH, Weaver RE, et al. Disease caused by a marine *Vibrio:* clinical characteristics and epidemiology. *N Engl J Med* 1979;300:1–5.
149. Farmer JJ III. *Vibrio* (*Beneckea*) *vulnificus,* the bacterium associated with sepsis, septicemia, and the sea. *Lancet* 1979;2:903.
150. Klontz KC, Lieb S, Schreiber M, et al. Syndromes of *Vibrio vulnificus* infections: clinical and epidemiological features in Florida cases, 1981–1987. *Ann Intern Med* 1988;109:318–323.
151. Park SD, Shon HS, Joh NJ. *Vibrio vulnificus* septicemia in Korea: clinical and epidemiologic findings in seventy patients. *J Am Acad Dermatol* 1991;24:397–403.
152. Shapiro RL, Alkekruse S, Hutwagner L, et al. The role of Gulf Coast oysters harvested in warmer months in *Vibrio vulnificus* infections in the United States, 1988–1996. *J Infect Dis* 1998;178:752–759.
153. Chang JJ, Sheen IS, Peng SM, et al. *Vibrio vulnificus* infection –report of 8 cases and review of cases in Taiwan. *Changgeng Yi Xue Za Zhi* 1994;17:339–346.
154. Morris JG, Wright AC, Roberts DM, et al. Identification of environmental *Vibrio vulnificus* isolates with a DNA probe for the cytotoxin-hemolysin gene. *Appl Environ Microbiol* 1987;53: 193–195.
155. Tison DL, Nishibuchi M, Greenwood JD, et al. *Vibrio vulnificus* biogroup 2: new biogroup pathogenic for eels. *Appl Environ Microbiol* 1982;44:640–646.
156. Biosca EG, Amaro C, Larsen JL, et al. Phenotypic and genotypic characterization of *Vibrio vulnificus*: proposal for the substitution of the subspecific taxon biotype for serovar. *Appl Environ Microbiol* 1997;63:1460–1466.
157. Bisharat N, Agmon V, Finkelstein R, et al. Clinical, epidemiological, and microbiological features of *Vibrio vulnificus* biogroup 3 causing outbreaks of wound infection and bacteremia in Israel. *Lancet* 1999;354:1421–1424.
158. Reddy GP, Hayat U, Abeygunawardana C, et al. Purification and structure determination of *Vibrio vulnificus* capsular polysaccharide. *J Bacteriol* 1992;174:2620–2630.
159. Hayat U, Reddy GP, Bush CA, et al. Capsular types of *Vibrio vulnificus:* an analysis of strains from clinical and environmental sources. *J Infect Dis* 1993;168:758–762.
160. Bush CA, Patel P, Gunawardena S, et al. Classification of *Vibrio vulnificus* strains by the carbohydrate composition of their capsular polysaccharides. *Anal Biochem* 1997;250:186–195.
161. Wright AC, Hill RT, Johnson JA, et al. Distribution of *Vibrio vulnificus* in the Chesapeake Bay. *Appl Environ Microbiol* 1996; 62:717–724.
162. Oliver JD, Warner RA, Cleland DR. Distribution and ecology of *Vibrio vulnificus* and other lactose-fermenting marine vibrios in coastal waters of the southeastern United States. *Appl Environ Microbiol* 1982;44:1404–1414.
163. Kaysner CA, Abeyta C Jr, Wekell MM, et al. Virulent strains of *Vibrio vulnificus* isolated from estuaries of the United States West Coast. *Appl Environ Microbiol* 1987;53:1349–1351.
164. Barbieri E, Falzano L, Fiorentini C, et al. Occurrence, diversity, and pathogenicity of halophilic *Vibrio* spp. and non-O1 *Vibrio cholerae* from estuarine waters along the Italian Adriatic coast. *Appl Environ Microbiol* 1999;65:2748–2753.
165. Wu HS, Liu DP, Hwang CH, et al. Survey on the distribution of Vibrionaceae at the seaport areas in Taiwan, 1991–1994. *Zhonghua Min Guo Wei Sheng Wu Ji Mian Yi Xue Za Zhi* 1996; 29:197–209.
166. Ghinsberg RC, Dror R, Nitzan Y. Isolation of *Vibrio vulnificus* from sea water and sand along the Dan region coast of the Mediterranean. *Microbios* 1999;97:7–17.
167. Motes ML, DePaola A, Cook DW, et al. Influence of water temperature and salinity on *Vibrio vulnificus* in northern Gulf and Atlantic Coast oysters. *Appl Environ Microbiol* 1998;64:1459-65.
168. Johnston JM, Becker SF, McFarland LM. *Vibrio vulnificus*: man and the sea. *JAMA* 1985;253:2850–2852.
169. Centers for Disease Control. *Vibrio vulnificus* infections associated with raw oyster consumption—Florida, 1981–1992. *MMWR Morbid Mortal Wkly Rep* 1993;42:405–407.
170. Powell JL, Wright AC, Wasserman SS, et al. Release of TNF-α in response to *Vibrio vulnificus* capsular polysaccharide using *in vivo* and *in vitro* models. *Infect Immun* 1997;65:3713–3718.
171. Wright AC, Simpson LM, Oliver JD, et al. Phenotypic evaluation of acapsular transposon mutants of *Vibrio vulnificus*. *Infect Immun* 1990;58:1769–1773.
172. Brennt EC, Wright AC, Dutta SK, et al. Growth of *Vibrio vulnificus* in serum from alcoholics: association with high transferrin iron saturation [Letter]. *J Infect Dis* 1991;164: 1030–1032.
173. Morris JG Jr, Wright AC, Simpson LM, et al. Virulence of *Vibrio vulnificus:* association with utilization of transferrin-bound iron, and lack of correlation with levels of cytotoxin or protease production. *FEMS Microbiol Lett* 1987;40:55–59.
174. Hor L-I, Chang T-T, Wang S-T. Survival of *Vibrio vulnificus* in whole blood from patients with chronic liver diseases: association with phagocytosis by neutrophils and serum ferritin levels. *J Infect Dis* 1999;179:275–278.
175. Gray LD, Kreger AS. Purification and characterization of an extracellular cytolysin produced by *Vibrio vulnificus*. *Infect Immun* 1985;48:62–72.
176. Kothary MH, Kreger AS. Production and partial characterization of an elastolytic protease of *Vibrio vulnificus*. *Infect Immun* 1985;50:534–540.
177. Smith GC, Merkel JR. Collagenolytic activity of *Vibrio vulnificus:* potential contribution to its invasiveness. *Infect Immun* 1982;35:1155–1156.
178. Testa J, Daniel LW, Kreger AS. Extracellular phospholipase A_2 and lysophospholipase produced by *Vibrio vulnificus*. *Infect Immun* 1984;45:458–463.
179. Gray LD, Kreger AS. Mouseskin damage caused by cytolysin from *Vibrio vulnificus* and by *V. vulnificus* infection. *J Infect Dis* 1987;155:236–241.
180. Miyoshi N, Miyoshi S-I, Sugiyama K, et al. Activation of the plasma kallikrein-kinin system by *Vibrio vulnificus* protease. *Infect Immun* 1987;55:1936–1939.

181. Shao CP, Hor LI. Metalloprotease is not essential for *Vibrio vulnificus* virulence in mice. *Infect Immun* 2000;68: 3569–3573.
182. Kelly MT, McCormick WF. Acute bacterial myositis caused by *Vibrio vulnificus. JAMA* 1981;246:72–73.
183. Castillo LE, Winslow DL, Pankey GA. Wound infection and septic shock due to *Vibrio vulnificus. Am J Trop Med Hyg* 1981; 30:844–848.
184. Pollak SJ, Parrish EF III, Barrett TJ, et al. *Vibrio vulnificus* septicemia: isolation of organism from stool and demonstration of antibodies by indirect immunofluorescence. *Arch Intern Med* 1983;143:837–838.
185. Simonson J, Siebeling RJ. Rapid serological identification of *Vibrio vulnificus* by anti-H coagglutination. *Appl Environ Microbiol* 1986;52:1299–1304.
186. Tamplin ML, Martin AL, Ruple AD, et al. Enzyme immunoassay for identification of *Vibrio vulnificus* in seawater, sediment, and oysters. *Appl Environ Microbiol* 1991;57:1235–1240.
187. Cerda-Cuellar M, Jofre J, Blanch AR. A selective medium and a specific probe for detection of *Vibrio vulnificus. Appl Environ Microbiol* 2000;66:855–859.
188. Bowdre JH, Hull JH, Cocchetto DM. Antibiotic efficacy against *Vibrio vulnificus* in the mouse: superiority of tetracycline. *J Pharmacol Exp Ther* 1983;225:595–598.

38

TYPES OF *ESCHERICHIA COLI* ENTEROPATHOGENS

RICHARD L. GUERRANT
THEODORE S. STEINER
NATHAN M. THIELMAN

Within the versatile species of *E. coli* is practically the entire range of types of microbial enteropathogens and representative mechanisms by which microorganisms derange intestinal function to cause secretion or inflammation and thus diarrhea. As noted in Table 38.1, these include four different types of enterotoxigenic *E.coli*, or ETECs (LT/I, LT/II, STa, STb), SLT/I or SLT/II-producing enterohemorrhagic *E. coli* (EHEC), enteroinvasive *E. coli* (EIEC), classic (locally adherent) enteropathogenic *E. coli* (EPEC), enteroaggregative *E. coli* (EAEC), and diffusely adherent *E. coli* (DAEC), for a total of nine different types of potential *E. coli* enteropathogens. Of these, the six underlined in the table have their pathogenicity in humans established in either outbreaks or in volunteer studies. These include LT/I, STa, EHEC (SLTI/II), EIEC, EPEC, and EAEC. In addition, there are reported isolates that do not meet strict criteria for one of the aforementioned groups, but they may also be categorized based on phenotypes (such as enteric colonizing *E. coli,* cell-detaching *E. coli,* or CDEC, and chain-like-adherent *E. coli* or CLA-EC) (1,2). The roles of LT/II-, STb-, DAEC-, CLA, and enteric-colonizing *E. coli* remain to be definitively established as causes of diarrhea in humans (although STb-producing *E. coli* causes significant diarrhea in some animals).

Because the genetic codes for many of these virulence traits reside on plasmids or phages (or on chromosomal elements regulated by plasmid-encoded products), the capacity to be a pathogen consequently may be transferred from one serotype of *E. coli* to another. Moreover, there is some overlap among the different pathogenic types, for example, EAEC expressing SLT and EHEC expressing the enteroaggregative heat-stable toxin EAST-1 (3–5). Nevertheless, the serogroups listed in column 5 of Table 38.1 tend to predominate to a greater or lesser extent among the different types of *E. coli.* Indeed, for many years serotyping provided the only potential means to recognize classic "enteropathogenic serotypes" of *E. coli,* the specific virulence mechanisms of which are now being further distinguished by both biotype and DNA probe as local and aggregative adherence. Some clinicians suggest that we should move away from serotypical characterization of these organisms in favor of definition by virulence traits or by the presence of genetic elements that encode these traits.

Cholera-like LT/I-producing ETECs, which activate adenylate cyclase and may act through additional pathways such as those that involve prostaglandin synthesis and PAF production (6–8), are well established in both field and volunteer studies as enteropathogens. In contrast, the other well-established ETECs produce the heat-stable enterotoxin STa, which is much smaller (16 to 18 amino acids) and less antigenic, and which promptly and reversibly activates guanylate cyclase rather than adenylate cyclase to cause chloride-dependent net secretion by elevating cyclic guanylate monophosphate instead of cyclic adenosine monophosphate (9–15). A similar activity has been identified with EAST-1 (16,17). Furthermore, this guanylate cyclase–activating ST family of enterotoxins not only has been expanded to include STs produced by microorganisms other than *E. coli* but has also uncovered the ST-like mammalian tissue products from intestine or kidney such as guanylin (18).

The methanol-insoluble heat-stable toxin STb, recognized predominantly from animal isolates, is much larger and causes cyclic nucleotide-independent bicarbonate secretion in piglet loops (19,20). Although Whipp and col-

R. L. Guerrant: Divisions of Geographic and International Medicine and Infectious Diseases, Department of Medicine, University of Virginia School of Medicine; University of Virginia Hospital, Charlottesville, Virginia

N. M. Thielman: Division of Infectious Diseases and International Health, Duke University Medical Center, Durham, North Carolina

T. S. Steiner: Department of Medicine, University of British Columbia; Departments of Medicine and Infectious Diseases, Vancouver Hospital and Health Sciences Center, Vancouver, British Columbia

TABLE 38.1. TYPES OF *E. COLI* ENTEROPATHOGENS

	Genetic Code	Mechanism	Model	Predominant O Serogroups	Type of Diarrhea
Enterotoxigenic (ETEC):	Plasmid	CFA/I-V-colonize	MRHA		
LT	Plasmid/ chromosomal	Adenylate cyclase secretion	18th Rabbit ileal loop CHO/Y1 cells	1,6,7,8,9,11,15,20,25,27, 60,63,75,80,85,88,89,99, 101,109,114,128,139,153	Acute watery
STa	Plasmid	Guanylate cyclase secretion	4–8h Rabbit ileal loop suckling mice	11,12,15,20,25,27,60,63,75, 78,80,85,88,89,99,101, 109,114,115,139,148, 149,153,159,166,167	Acute watery
STb	Plasmid	Cyclic nucleotide-independent HCO_3 secretion	Piglet loop		
Enterohemorrhagic (EHEC) SLT	Phage/?plasmid (some also have eaeA; see below)	Glycosidase cleaves adenosine-4324 in 28SrRNA of 60S ribosomal subunits to halt protein synthesis	HeLa cell cytotoxicity	157,26,103,111,113 et al. 104,153,163	Bloody (±HUS)
Enteroinvasive (EIEC)	plasmid (140 Md) + chromosomal	Cell invasion and spread 58- to 80-kd EIET (chromosomal)	Sereny test	11,28,29,112,115,121,124, 138,143,144,147,152, 164,173	Acute dysenteric
Enteropathogenic (EPEC)	1. Plasmid (60 MDa;) EAF, bfpA	BFP-efficient localized adherence (LA)	LA to HEp-2 cells	18,26,44,55,86,111,114, 119,125,126,127,128, 142,157,158	Acute + persistent
	2. Chromosomal (cfm)	Tyrosine kinase and intracellular Ca^{2+}-dependent actin condensation	Fluorescence actin staining (FAS)		
	3. Chromosomal (*eaeA*)	94-kd intimin → intimate-effacing adherence			
Enteroaggregative (EAggEC)	Plasmid (60 Md;AA)	BFP-aggregative adherence (AA)	AA to HEp-2 cells	3(17-2), 15,44(042),51,77, 78,86,91,92(221)	Persistent (? Acute)
	Plasmid (60 Md;AA)	2- to 5-Kd EAST-1, guanylate cyclase, EALT pore-forming Ca^{2+} ionophore	Ussing chambers	111,113,126,141,146, ?(346)	
Diffusely adherent (DAEC)	Chromosoaml (daaC probe)	Fimbrial adhesion (F1845)	Diffuse adherence to HEp-2 cells	75(F1845), ?(189), 15 (57-1), 126(AIDA-I)	? Acute ?Persister
	Plasmid	Afimbrial adhesin (hemologeous to *Shigella* IcsA)			
Enteric Colonizing	Plasmid	CFA/I-V ?Hydrophobic	MRHA $(NH_4)_2SO_4$ hydrophobicity	—	?Persistent
GU/CNS/Normal flora	Chromosomal/ plasmid	type I pill P—fimbriae S-fimbriae AFA—I	MSHA bind P blood gp. Ag.	1,2,4,6,7,25,45,75,81	None

Underline signifies pathogenicity in humans established in outbreaks or volunteer studies.
HUS, hemolytic-uremic syndrome. BFP, bundle-forming pill; LT, heat labile toxin; ST, heat stable toxin; SLT, Shiga-like toxin.

leagues (21–23) demonstrated that rabbit and mouse loops were not responsive to STb because of protease degradation, which can be inhibited, an extensive search among *E. coli* isolates from Brazil and Bangladesh using a gene probe for STb as well as *in vitro* study of STb on human intestinal tissue in Ussing chambers failed to shown an effect of STb on human tissue or an association with diarrhea in humans (19,24).

EHEC that produces at least one or more of the Shiga-like toxins, or verocytotoxins (SLT/I or SLT/II), is associated with rare hamburger ingestion in several outbreaks as well as with ingestion of unpasteurized juices (25–28), and even contamination of a municipal water supply (Walkerton, ON) (29). The characteristic pathogenicity of EHEC depends on its ability to produce these Shiga-like toxins. Indeed, the toxin may be found more often than the organism is cultured in some fecal specimens in outbreaks. Many of the recognized EHEC outbreaks have involved *E. coli* O157:H7, which is often (albeit not always) sorbitol-negative and can therefore be suspected by routinely culturing fecal specimens on sorbitol MacConkey agar plates as recommended by the Centers for Disease Control and Prevention (30).

EIEC behave much like a fifth serogroup of *Shigella* to which *E. coli* is closely related, even to the point of sharing a similar 140-mDa plasmid and chromosomal elements responsible for cell invasion and spread as well as certain O-antigen cross-reactivity.

Besides ETEC, EHEC, and EIEC, a group of *E. coli* enteropathogens can be recognized by their ability to adhere in one of three or more characteristic patterns to HEp-2 (and other) cells in tissue culture. These include (a) the locally adherent, classically recognized EPEC, (b) enteroaggregative *E.coli* (EAggEC) which adhere in a "stacked-brick" pattern to both HEp-2 cells and glass slides, and (c) the DAEC, which adhere in a diffuse pattern to cells only. Additional patterns of adherence (chainlike adherence) have been reported, but larger-scale studies are lacking (1,2). The EPEC adherence factor (EAF), 60-mDa plasmid-encoded bundle forming pili (which cross-react with the bundle-forming toxin coregulated pili [TCP] on *Vibrio cholerae*), mediate the initial local adherence of EPEC seen *in vitro* as microcolonies on tissue culture cells. This is followed by an impressive pedestal formation by the host cell (HEp2 cells or intestinal epithelial cells), which requires injection of a bacterial protein, Tir, into the host cell via a type III secretion system and intimin-mediated intimate-effacing adherence encoded on a chromosomal pathogenicity island (31–35). A functionally homologous *pathogenicity island* in EHEC O157:H7 mediates pedestal formation also, but in a mechanism not requiring tyrosine phosphorylation of Tir (36). Thus, the events leading to the localized adherence and attachment and effacement by EPEC (and perhaps other *E. coli* such as EHEC as well) appear to involve the orchestration of at least three separable plasmid and chromosomally encoded traits.

EAggEC (EAEC) that exhibit stacked-brick adherence have become increasingly recognized in recent years in association with persistent diarrhea in studies in India, Brazil, Chile, and Mexico (37–41). Strain 221 (O92:H33) isolated from a patient with traveler's diarrhea in Mexico, initially thought to be a DAEC, was subsequently shown to exhibit the aggregative pattern of adherence and has variably caused diarrhea in volunteer studies in Houston but not in Maryland (43). The strongest evidence for pathogenicity lies with EAEC strain 042 (serotype O44:H18), which caused diarrhea or abdominal symptoms in four of five volunteers given this organism (43). Scotland and co-workers further found that certain O44, O111, and O126 serogroups have exhibited aggregative rather than localized adherence to HEp2 cells and, thus, at least some of these organisms probably belong in the EAEC group rather than EPEC (44). In addition, strain 34B has been shown to exhibit aggregative adherence. Potential virulence traits identified to date include aggregative adherence fimbriae AAF/I and AAF/II, EAST-1, Pet (a 104-kD serine protease autotransporter protein that cleaves host cytoskeletal elements), Pic (a mucinase), ShET-1 (a possible enterotoxin), heat-labile hemolysin, and FliC (the major flagellar subunit, which causes interleukin-8 secretion from epithelial cells). The only pathogenic feature statistically associated with diarrhea in epidemiologic surveys to this point is AAF/II.(45)

DAECs include well-characterized strains C1845 (O75:NM), 189 (O?:H33/35), and 57-1 (015:HM), which have all been identified and characterized, and are probe-positive for either fimbriate or afimbriate adhesins but have failed to cause diarrhea in volunteer studies to date. In addition, DAEC strain O126:H7 exhibits the AIDA-I adhesin, which was studied by Benz and Schmidt (46). The role of DAEC in acute or persistent disease has been questioned in some studies in which these organisms are found in control subjects as often as in cases (39), but suggested by others with an increasing association in children older than 18 months of age with acute or persistent diarrhea (47). The pathogenesis of DAEC diarrhea remains unknown, but may involve adherence of DAEC fimbriae to decay accelerating factor (DAF or CD55) with subsequent activation of host signaling cascades (48,49).

Enteric-colonizing *E. coli,* represented by strains such as 1392, which had previously been an ETEC but that now expresses only the colonization factor antigen (CFA/II) without recognized enterotoxins, has caused diarrhea in human volunteers as well as in the reversible ileal tie adult rabbit diarrhea model (RITARD). In this model, colonization by that organism was associated with an impairment of normal water and electrolyte absorption as well as impaired disaccharidase activity and diarrhea (50,51). The potential role for colonization, therefore, in causing persistent diarrhea in children in tropical developing areas (as well as possibly in diarrhea caused by genetically engineered colonizing live vaccine organisms) remains to be clarified, as does the mechanism by which these colonizing organisms may trigger diarrhea. A recent study documented elevated fecal lactoferrin and cytokines in patients receiving a diarrheogenic attenuated cholera vaccine strain (CVD 110), suggesting that adherence may trigger host responses, such as inflammation, which may contribute to diarrhea (52).

Finally, the "normal flora" *E. coli* tend to occur in yet a different range of serogroups and may sometimes include *E. coli* organisms that produce type 1 pili or those that produce P or S fimbriae or AFA and may be associated with genitourinary or central nervous system infections (53–56).

In summary, it is clear that, within the versatile species of *E. coli* are a range of lessons regarding virulence traits involved in the pathogenesis of bacterial diarrheas of many types, as reviewed in subsequent chapters.

REFERENCES

1. Gioppo NMR, Elias Jr, WP, Vidotto MC, et al. Prevalence of HEp-2 cell-adherent *Escherichia coli* and characterisation of enteroaggregative *E. coli* and chain-like adherent *E. coli* isolated from children with and without diarrhoea, in Londrina, Brazil. *FEMS Microbiol Let* 2000;190:293–298.
2. Gomes TAT, Suzart S, Guth BEC, et al. Distinctive pattern of adherence to HeLa cells. Abstracts of the 98th General Meeting of the American Society for Microbiology, Atlanta, GA, 1998:D-114.
3. Iyoda S, Tamura K, Itoh K, et al. Inducible stx2 phages are lysogenized in the enteroaggregative and other phenotypic *Escherichia coli* O86:NM isolated from patients. *FEMS Microbiol Lett* 2000;191:7–10.
4. Morabito S, Karch H, Mariani-Kurkdjian P, et al. Enteroaggregative, Shiga toxin-producing *Escherichia coli* O111:H2 associate with an outbreak of hemolytic-uremic syndrome. *J Clin Microbiol* 1998;36:840–842.
5. Savarino SJ, McVeigh A, Watson J, et al. Enteroaggregative *Escherichia coli* heat-stable enterotoxin is not restricted to enteroaggregative *Escherichia coli. J Infect Dis* 1996;173:1019–1022.
6. Peterson JW, Ochoa G. Role of prostaglandins and cAMP in the secretory effects of cholera toxin. *Science* 1989;245:857–859.
7. Peterson JW, Reitmeyer JC, Jackson CA, et al. Protein synthesis is required for cholera toxin-induced stimulation or arachidonic acid metabolism. *Biochim Biophys Acta* 1991;1092:79–84.
8. Thielman N, Fang GD, Barrett LJ, et al. Inhibition of cholera toxin effects on intestinal secretion and CHO cell elongation by platelet activating factor (PAF) antagonists. Proceedings of the 29th Joint Conference US-Japan Cholera Meeting, Monterey, CA 1993:172–176.
9. Hughes JM, Murad F, Chang B, et al. Role of cyclic GMP in the action of heat-stable enterotoxins of *Escherichia coli. Nature* 1978;271:755–756.
10. Field M, Graf LH Jr, Mata LJ. Heat stable enterotoxin of *E. coli. In vitro* effects on guanylate cyclase activity, cyclic GMP concentration, and ion transport in small intestine. *Proc Natl Acad Sci U S A* 1978;75:2800–2804.
11. Guerrant RL, Hughes JM, Chang B, et al. Activation of intestinal guanylate cyclase by heat-stable enterotoxin of *E. coli:* studies of tissue specificity, potential receptors and intermediates. *J Infect Dis* 1980;142:220–228.
12. Chen LC, Rohde JE, Sharp GWG. Intestinal adenyl-cyclase activity in human cholera. *Lancet* 1971;1:939–941.
13. Kimberg DV, Field M, Johnson J, et al. Stimulation of intestinal mucosal adenyl cyclase by cholera enterotoxin and prostaglandins. *J Clin Invest* 1971;50:1218–1230.
14. Guerrant RL, Chen LC, Sharp GWG. Intestinal adenyl-cyclase activity in canine cholera: Correlation with fluid accumulation. *J Infect Dis* 1972;125:377–381.
15. Guerrant RL, Ganguly U, Casper AGT, et al. Effect of *Escherichia coli* on fluid transport across canine small bowel: mechanism and time-course with enterotoxin and whole bacterial cells. *J Clin Invest* 1973;52:1707–1714.
16. Savarino SJ, Fasano A, Robertson DC, et al. Enteroaggregative *Escherichia coli* elaborate a heat-stable enterotoxin demonstrable in an *in vitro* rabbit intestinal model. *J Clin Invest* 1991;87: 1450–1455.
17. Savarino SJ, Fasano A, Watson J, et al. Enteroaggregative *Escherichia coli* heat-stable enterotoxin 1 represents another subfamily of *E. coli* heat-stable toxin. *Proc Nat Acad Sci U S A* 1993;90:3093–3097.
18. Currie MG, Fok KF, Kato J, et al. Guanylin: an endogenous activator of intestinal guanylate cyclase. *Proc Natl Acad Sci U S A* 1992;89:947–951.
19. Weikel CS, Nellans HN, Guerrant RL. The *in vivo* and *in vitro* effects of a novel enterotoxin, STb, produced by *Escherichia coli. J Infect Dis* 1986;153:893–901.
20. Kennedy DJ, Greenberg RN, Dunn JA, et al. Effects of *Escherichia coli* heat-stable enterotoxin STb on intestines of mice, rats, rabbits, and piglets. *Infect Immun* 1984;46:639–643.
21. Kupersztoch YM, Tachias K, Moomaw CR, et al. Secretion of methanol-insoluble heat-stable enterotoxin (ST_B): energy- and *secA*-dependent conversion of Pre-ST_B to an intermediate indistinguishable from the extracellular toxin. *J Bacteriol* 1990;172:2427–2432.
22. Whipp SC. Protease degradation of *Escherichia coli* heat stable, mouse negative, pig positive enterotoxin. *Infect Immun* 1987;55: 2057–2060.
23. Whipp S. Assay for enterotoxigenic *Escherichia coli* heat-stable toxin b in rats and mice. *Infect Immun* 1990;58:930–934.
24. Weikel CS, Tiemans K, Moseley S, et al. Species specificity and lack of production of sTb enterotoxin by *Escherichia coli* strains isolated from humans with diarrheal illness. *Infect Immun* 1986; 52:323–325.
25. Anonymous. Preliminary report: foodborne outbreak of *Escherichia coli* O157:H7 infections from hamburgers—western United States, 1993. *MMWR Morbid Mortal Wkly Rep* 1993;42:85–86.
26. Davis M, Osaki C, Gordon D, et al. Update: multistate outbreak of *E. coli* O157:H7 infections from hamburgers—W. U.S., 1992–1993. Centers for Disease Control. *MMWR Morbid Mortal Wkly Rep* 1993;42:258–263.
27. MacDonald KL, Osterholm MT. The emergence of *Escherichia coli* O157:H7 infection in the United States. The changing epidemiology of foodborne disease [editorial; comment]. *JAMA* 1993;269:2264–2266.
28. Besser RE, Lett SM, Weber JT. An outbreak of diarrhea and hemolytic uremic syndrome from *Escherichia coli* O157:H7 in fresh-pressed apple cider (see comments). *JAMA* 1993;269: 2217–2220.
29. Waterborne outbreak of gastroenteritis associated with a contaminated municipal water supply, Walkerton, Ontario, May-June 2000. *Can Commun Dis Rep* 2000;26:170–173.
30. Centers for Disease Control. Emerging infectious diseases. *MMWR Morbid Mortal Wkly Rep* 1993;42:257–263.
31. Donnenberg MS, Tackett CO, James JP. Role of the eaeA gene in experimental enteropathogenic *Escherichia coli* infection. *J Clin Invest* 1993;92:1412–1417.
32. Donnenberg MS, Tzipori S, McKee ML, et al. The role of *eae* gene and of enterohemorrhagic *Escherichia coli* in intimate attachment *in vitro* and in a porcine model. *J Clin Invest* 1993; 92:1418–1424.

33. Donnenberg MS, Kaper JB. Enteropathogenic *Escherichia coli. Infect Immun* 1992;60:3953–3961.
34. Schoolnik GK. Intimin and the intimate attachment of bacteria to human cells [editorial; comment]. *J Clin Invest* 1993;92: 1117–1118.
35. Kenny B, DeVinney R, Stein M, et al. Enteropathogenic *E. coli* (EPEC) transfers its receptor for intimate adherence into mammalian cells. Cell. 1997;91:511–520.
36. DeVinney R, Stein M, Reinscheid D, et al. Enterohemorrhagic *Escherichia coli* O157:H7 produces Tir, which is translocated to the host cell membrane but is not tyrosine phosphorylated. *Infect Immun* 1999;67:2389–2398.
37. Bhan MK, Raj P, Levine MM. Enteroaggregative *Escherichia coli* associated with persistent diarrhea in a cohort of rural children in India. *J Infect Dis* 1989;159:1061–1064.
38. Bhan MK, Khoshoo V, Sommerfelt H, et al. Enteroaggregative *Escherichia coli* and *Salmonella* associated with nondysenteric persistent diarrhea. *Pediatr Infect Dis J* 1989;8:499–502.
39. Wanke CA, Schorling JB, Barrett LJ, et al. Adherence traits of *Escherichia coli,* alone and in association with other stool pathogens: potential role in pathogenesis of persistent diarrhea in an urban Brazilian slum. *Pediatr J Infect Dis* 1991;10: 746–751.
40. Fang GD, Lima AM, Wanke CA, et al. HEp-2 cell-adherent *E. coli:* potential causes of persistent diarrhea of multiple genotypes and different adherence phenotypes. *Clin Res* 1991; 39:223A.
41. Cravioto A, Tello A, Navarro A, et al. Association of *Escherichia coli* HEp-2 adherence patterns with type and duration of diarrhoea. *Lancet* 1991;337:262–264.
42. Nataro JP, Yikang D, Giron JA, et al. Aggregative adherence fimbria I expression in enteroaggregative *Escherichia coli* requires two unlinked plasmid regions. *Infect Immun* 1993;61:1126–1131.
43. Nataro JP, Steiner T, Guerrant RL. Enteroaggregative *Escherichia coli. Emerg Infect Dis* 1998;4:251–261.
44. Scotland SM, Smith HR, Said B, et al. Identification of enteropathogenic *Escherichia coli* isolated in Britain as enteroaggregative or as members of a subclass of attaching-and-effacing *E. coli* not hybridising with the EPEC adherence-factor probe. *J Med Microbiol* 1991;35:278–283.
45. Okeke IN., Lamikanra A, Czeczulin J, et al. Heterogeneous virulence of enteroaggregative *Escherichia coli* strains isolated from children in Southwest Nigeria. *J Infect Dis* 2000;181:252–260.
46. Benz I, Schmidt MA. Isolation and serologic characterization of AIDA-I, the adhesin mediating the diffuse adherence phenotype of the diarrhea-associated *Escherichia coli* strain 2787 (O126: H27). *Infect Immun* 1992;60:13–18.
47. Baqui AH, Sack RB, Black RE, et al. Enteropathogens associated with acute and persistent diarrhea in Bangladeshi children <5 years of age. *J Infect Dis* 1992;166:792–796.
48. Bilge SS, Clausen CR, Lau W, et al. Molecular characterization of a fimbrial adhesin, F1845, mediating diffuse adherence of diarrhea-associated *Escherichia coli* to HEp-2 cells. *J Bacteriol* 1989;171:4281–4289.
49. Peiffer I, Servin AL, Bernet-Camard MF. Piracy of decay-accelerating factor (CD55) signal transduction by the diffusely adhering strain *Escherichia coli* C1845 promotes cytoskeletal F-actin rearrangements in cultured human intestinal INT407 cells. *Infect Immun* 1998;66:4036–4042.
50. Wanke C, Guerrant RL. Small bowel colonization alone is a cause of diarrhea: a rabbit model. *Infect Immun* 1987;55:1924–1926.
51. Schlager TA, Wanke CA, Guerrant RL. Net fluid secretion and impaired villous function induced by colonization of the small intestine by nontoxigenic colonizing *Escherichia coli. Infect Immun* 1990;58:1337–1343.
52. Silva TM, Schleupner MA, Tacket CO, et al. New evidence for an inflammatory component in diarrhea caused by selected new, live attenuated cholera vaccines and by El Tor and O139 *Vibrio cholerae. Infect Immun* 1996;64:2362–2364.
53. Svanborg C, Agace W, Hedges S, et al. Bacterial adherence and mucosal inflammation in the bowel and the urinary tract. *Scand J Urol Nephrol Suppl* 1992;142:54.
54. Svanborg Eden C, Engberg I, Hedges S. Consequences of bacterial attachment in the urinary tract. *Biochem Soc Trans* 1989;17: 464–466.
55. Svanborg-Eden C, Hausson S, Jodal U, et al. Host-parasite interaction in the urinary tract. *J Infect Dis* 1988;157:421–426.
56. Hedges S, Svensson M, Svanborg C. Interleukin-6 response of epithelial cell lines to bacterial stimulation *in vitro. Infect Immun* 1992;60:1295–1301.

39

ENTEROTOXIGENIC *ESCHERICHIA COLI*

MITCHELL B. COHEN
RALPH A. GIANNELLA

Enterotoxigenic strains of *Escherichia coli* (ETEC) are an important worldwide cause of diarrheal disease in humans and domestic animals. These organisms cause intestinal secretion by elaborating enterotoxins without invading or damaging intestinal epithelial cells. Characteristically, these organisms elaborate one or more enterotoxins that are either heat stable (ST) or heat labile (LT).

The ST group can be further subdivided into two categories. The first class of toxins is the STa (or STI) family. These are small methanol-soluble peptides that activate a transmembrane guanylate cyclase and lead to intestinal hypersecretion. STa can also be abbreviated STp or STh to indicate strains of porcine or human origin, respectively. The second subset is designated STb (or STII). These toxins are methanol insoluble and do not activate guanylate cyclase. However, they also mediate diarrheal disease, most commonly in pigs.

The LT group can also be further subdivided. LTI binds to a GM_1 ganglioside receptor, activates adenylate cyclase, and is neutralized by antiserum to cholera toxin (CT). LTI can also be designated LTp or LTh to indicate strains of porcine or human origin, respectively. LTII, which was originally isolated from water buffalo, does not bind to a GM_1 ganglioside and is not neutralized by CT antisera. The LTII toxins have been further categorized into LTIIa and LTIIb on the basis of chemical and antigenic properties.

ETEC organisms also possess fimbrial attachments that enable these organisms to come in close contact with intestinal receptors for the elaborated enterotoxins. These proteinaceous structures on the surface of ETEC are also called colonization factor antigens (CFAs) (Fig. 39.1); they are almost always encoded by plasmids that also encode for ST and/or LT.

M. B. Cohen: Department of Pediatrics, University of Cincinnati College of Medicine; Division of Pediatric Gastroenterology, Hepatology and Nutrition, Children's Hospital Medical Center, Cincinnati, Ohio

R. A. Giannella: Department of Internal Medicine, Division of Digestive Diseases, University of Cincinnati College of Medicine, Cincinnati, Ohio

In this chapter, we review the history, epidemiology, pathogenesis, clinical features, treatment, and prevention of ETEC infections.

HISTORY

The toxin-producing potential of *E. coli* was first discovered in the 1960s (2). Taylor et al. (2) reported that certain *E. coli* isolated from children with diarrhea caused secretion in a ligated rabbit intestinal loop model. This was in contrast to strains that were isolated from the stools of healthy infants and urinary tract isolates of *E. coli* that did not cause secretion.

The clinical importance of human infection with ETEC was outlined in the 1970s by investigators in Calcutta who

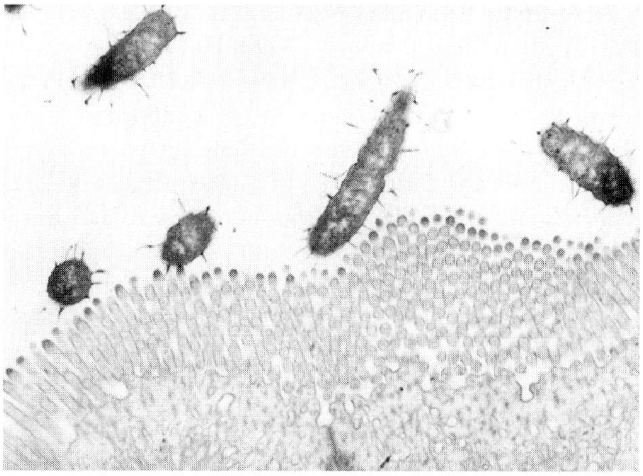

FIGURE 39.1. Attachment of enterotoxigenic *Escherichia coli* (ETEC). Electron micrograph of porcine small intestine. ETEC must express both virulence factors of adherence and toxin elaboration to be fully pathogenic. Specific attachment factors (Fimbriae or colonization factor antigens) permit colonization of the intestine by ETEC. Unlike enteropathogenic *E. coli*, ETEC organisms do not alter the architecture of the brush border membrane during attachment. (From Moon HW, Nagy B, Isaacson RE. Intestinal colonization and adhesion by enterotoxigenic *Escherichia coli:* ultrastructural observations on adherence to ileal epithelium of the pig. *J Infect Dis* 1977;136:S124–S129, with permission.)

identified these organisms as a major cause of endemic diarrhea (3–5). At approximately the same time, ETEC strains were also shown to be a major cause of diarrhea in swine (6,7).

EPIDEMIOLOGY

Although diarrheal disease caused by ETEC is usually less severe than that caused by cholera, ETEC-associated morbidity and mortality rates probably exceed those of cholera on a worldwide basis because of the high frequency of ETEC infection. The incidence of ETEC infection is greater than or comparable to that of rotavirus and these two organisms are among the predominant causes of dehydrating diarrheal disease throughout the developing world (8–11). In developing countries, children younger than 2 or 3 years experience two to three episodes of diarrhea a year due to infections with ETEC; this represents more than 25% of all diarrheal illnesses (10,11). The incidence of ETEC infections then declines rapidly to reach a constant lower level of infection seen in adults (10,11).

In Naples, Italy, where sanitation conditions may be intermediate between developed and developing countries, ETEC infection accounts for approximately 5.4% of episodes of acute diarrhea (12). In contrast, in the United States, despite initial reports that ETEC was responsible for a significant portion of severe childhood diarrheal disease in Chicago (13), ETEC organisms have not been isolated in prospective studies of urban childhood diarrhea in Boston, Baltimore, and Houston (14–16).

Several factors may explain the rarity of ETEC-mediated diarrhea in the United States: A large dose (10^8 organisms) is required for clinical illness (17,18), ETEC organisms are not excreted during convalescence (19–21), and they are not prevalent in the environment of developed countries (22,23). Host immunity probably does not play a significant factor in the rarity of ETEC infection in developed countries, because ETEC is a common cause of diarrhea in adults from developed areas who visit endemic areas (19,24,25). In fact, in many studies, ETEC strains are the leading cause of traveler's diarrhea. ETEC organisms can be isolated from 20% of travelers to endemic areas (26). In studies in Kenya (27) and Mexico City (24), approximately three-quarters of traveler's diarrhea cases in adults were due to ETEC infection. In addition, ETEC organisms have been identified as an important cause of traveler's diarrhea in soldiers deployed to the Middle East (28,29).

ETEC organisms are acquired by ingestion of contaminated water and food. In endemic areas, ETEC infection is more prominent in the wet season (30,31), possibly due to increased contamination of water sources due to runoff. ETEC organisms have been isolated from water supplies in endemic areas including the White River Apache Reservation (32) and both river (31) and tank water (33) in Bangladesh. Children are at increased risk for ETEC infection at the time of weaning. More than 40% of food (milk, rice, and water) fed to weaning children in Bangladesh has been shown to be contaminated with ETEC (30). In a prospective study involving physicians and their families attending a conference in Mexico, food and raw salad in particular were implicated in the transmission of disease (24). Although uncommon, food-borne and waterborne outbreaks have also been reported in the United States (20,34). From 1975 to 1995, there were 14 ETEC outbreaks in the United States and 7 on cruise ships, caused by 17 different serotypes and affecting 5,683 persons (35).

PATHOGENESIS

To be fully pathogenic, enterotoxigenic *E. coli* organisms must express both the virulence factors of adherence and enterotoxin elaboration. The bacteria first colonize the small intestine with the aid of specific CFA attachment factors. Unlike enteropathogenic *E. coli,* ETEC organisms do not alter the ultrastructure of the brush border membrane of the enterocyte during attachment (Fig. 39.1). Once these organisms colonize the small intestine, they elaborate ST and/or LT. Different combinations of these pathogenic factors probably account in part for the spectrum of illness associated with ETEC infection.

Adherence Factors And Serotypes

As is the case for the other categories of diarrheagenic *E. coli,* ETEC organisms generally belong to restricted serogroups (36). Moreover, much has been learned about the surface fimbriae, or pili, of these organisms that mediate the ability of these strains to adhere to intestinal mucosa. ETEC fimbriae confer species specificity. For example, ETEC strains expressing K99 are pathogenic for calves and pigs, whereas K88-expressing organisms are pathogenic only for pigs. Human ETEC strains possess colonization fimbriae, the CFAs. A large number of these fimbrial antigens have been identified and others are presumed to exist based on the properties of ETEC strains. The large number of these antigens has been a major obstacle in ETEC vaccine development.

The CFAs can be characterized on the basis of their morphology: rigid rods, bundle-forming flexible rods, and thin flexible wiry structures (37). CFA/I is the prototype of the rigid rod (38). CFA/III is a bundle-forming pilus. CFA/II and CFA/IV are comprised of multiple subunits. CFA/II producers express the thin flexible colony surface factor 3 (CS3) with or without the rod-shaped CS1 and CS2. CFA/IV producers express the nonfimbrial CS6 with rod-shaped CS4 or thin flexible CS5. Epidemiologic studies suggest that CFA/I, CFA/II, or CFA/IV are expressed by approximately 75% of clinical isolates of human ETEC strains (39). The more recently described bundle-forming fimbria designated *longus* has also been found on many ETEC strains (40,41). The plasmids that encode CFA/I and CFA/II often, but not always, encode ST and/or LT as well.

Enterotoxins

By definition, ETEC organisms elaborate ST and/or LT. Although many ETEC organisms elaborate both ST and LT, we discuss these two groups separately for purposes of clarity.

STa

Structure And Physicochemical Characteristics

The heat-stable toxins are of two major types: the STa (or STI) family and STb (or STII). The amino acid structure of the STa family of toxins is shown in Fig. 39.2. An 18–amino acid toxin, also found in pigs, is often described as STp. A 19–amino acid toxin of human origin is often described as STh. These STa enterotoxins are small (molecular weight of approximately 2,000) heat-stable and acid-stable toxins with no subunit structure containing three disulfide bonds that are important for biologic activity. The carboxyl terminal amino acids of these two toxins are highly conserved with differences between them occurring largely in the amino terminus. Biologic activity of these toxins is predominantly confined to the carboxyl terminus (42–45).

Although naturally occurring *E. coli* STa peptides are either 18 or 19 amino acids (42–48), the bacterial transposon that encodes for STa encodes a pre-propeptide of 72 amino acids (49). This gene product is shortened by post-translational removal of a hydrophobic leader sequence in the bacterial periplasm and extracellular processing of the propeptide to yield a smaller mature toxin (49–51). The family of STa peptides shares certain physicochemical properties engendered by their primary and secondary structures (52,53): (a) They retain full biologic activity when heated to 60°C for several hours or 100°C for 15 minutes; (b) they are stable in acid and not denatured by detergents; (c) they are soluble in water and, unlike STb, are soluble in methanol; (d) they are resistant to many proteases (pronase, trypsin, chymotrypsin) (54,55); and (e) disruption of disulfide bonds destroys their biologic activity (52). The disulfide bonds are between Cys5/Cys10, Cys6/Cys14, and Cys9/Cys17 (56,57). In addition, substitution of individual amino acids can have a dramatic effect on the biochemical and pharmacologic properties of STa, further illustrating the importance of the primary and secondary structure of this peptide (58,59).

Biologic Actions

STa, like CT and LT, causes fluid and electrolyte secretion. However, they differ in their mechanism of action. The biologic effect of CT and LT has a lag phase, is irreversible, and is mediated by activation of adenylate cyclase. In contrast, STa has an immediate onset of action, is reversible, and activates guanylate cyclase (54,60–65).

An overall schema of the mechanism of action of STa is shown in Fig. 39.3. There is strong evidence that the action of STa is mediated by increased concentration of cyclic guanosine monophosphate (cGMP). In both rabbit ileum and T84 cells mounted in the Ussing chamber, the time course for STa-induced elevation of cGMP concentration was identical to the onset of secretion measured by a rise in short-circuit current (Isc) (61,66). In the suckling mouse bioassay, the time course of intestinal fluid accumulation was also immediately preceded by an increase in tissue levels of cGMP (67,68).

Complementary DNAs (cDNAs) encoding a protein with STa-binding properties and guanylate cyclase activity have been cloned from rat (65) and human intestine (69–71). The receptor, a member of the guanylyl cyclase receptor–cyclase family, has been designated guanylate cyclase type C (GC-C) to indicate its similarity to the other

	Amino terminus — Carboxyl terminus
E. coli STp	N-T-F-Y-**C-C-E-L-C-C-N-P-A-C**-A-**G-C**-Y
E. coli STh	N-S-S-N-Y-**C-C-E-L-C-C-N-P-A-C**-T-**G-C**-Y
Citrobacter freundi ST	N-T-T-Y-**C-C-E-L-C-C-N-P-A-C**-A-**G-C**
Y. enterocolitica ST	.....-D-**C-C**-D-Y-**C-C-N-P-A-C**-A-**G-C**
V. cholerae non-01 ST	**-D-C-C-E**-I-**C-C-N-P-A-C**-F-**G-C**-L-N
E. coli EAST-1	....A-S-S-Y-A-S-**C**-I-W-**C**-T---T-**A-C**-A-S-**C**-H-G....
Guanylin$_{human}$	-E-D-P-G-T-**C-E**-I-**C**-A-Y-A-**A-C**-T-**G-C**
Uroguanylin$_{human}$	-N-D-D-----**C-E**-L-**C**-V-**N**-V-**A-C**-T-**G-C**-L

FIGURE 39.2. Comparison of the amino acid sequence of STp (porcine), STh (human), *Citrobacter freundii* ST, *Yersinia enterocolitica* ST, *Vibrio cholerae* non-O1 ST, enteroaggregative *Escherichia coli* heat-stable enterotoxin 1, guanylin, and uroguanylin. Conserved amino acid sequences are highlighted in bold. STp and STh are both forms of *E. coli* STa.

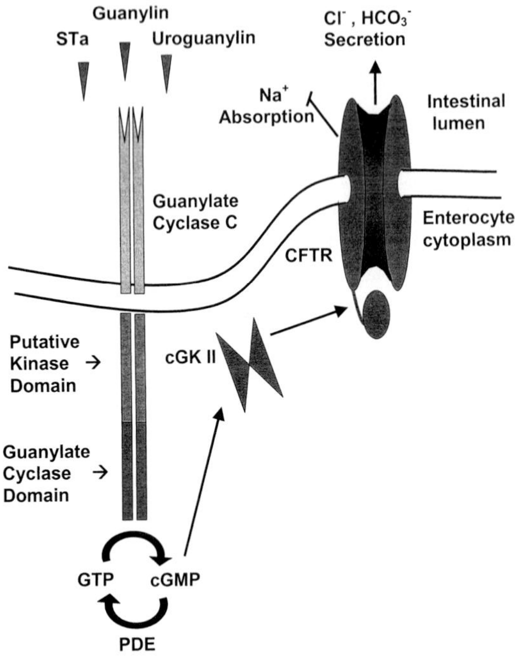

FIGURE 39.3. Outline of the overall schema of action of STa. STa, guanylin, or uroguanylin, the endogenous mammalian homologues, bind to a receptor (guanylate cyclase type C) that includes extracellular, transmembrane, putative kinase, and guanyl cyclase domains. This results in increased intracellular levels of cyclic guanosine monophosphate, which leads to increased chloride secretion via the cystic fibrosis transmembrane regulator and decreased sodium absorption.

particulate guanylate cyclases (guanylate cyclase types A and B) that bind atrial natriuretic peptides (65,72). Each GC-C cDNA encodes a 121-kd transmembrane protein containing three domains: an extracellular domain linked through a single transmembrane region to an intracellular protein kinase–like region and a guanylyl cyclase catalytic domain (65) (Fig. 39.3). The extracellular domain of GC-C binds STa, guanylin, and uroguanylin but does not bind the natriuretic peptide ligands (65). Incubation of STa with GC-C–transfected COS cells results in a dose-dependent increase in the level of intracellular cGMP (65,69,71,73).

Despite the persuasive evidence that STa activates guanylate cyclase, there is also good evidence that alternate pathways, including protein kinase C, intracellular calcium, and inositol triphosphate participate in the cGMP response engendered by STa (74–77). Carbachol, a cholinergic agent, also acts synergistically with STa to produce an Isc response in T84 cells, suggesting that multiple intracellular mediators may influence the ability of STa to cause intestinal secretion (78). Other cofactors, including adenine nucleotides, may potentiate the action of STa on GC-C (73,79–81). Adenosine triphosphate (ATP) may interact directly with GC-C, stabilizing its active conformation (82).

STa has a dual effect on chloride transport, both reducing the mucosal to serosal flux and increasing the serosal to mucosal flux of chloride (61). STa also reduces the mucosal to serosal flux of sodium (83). The observation that both sodium and chloride flux from mucosa to serosa are inhibited suggests that like theophylline, which increases cyclic adenosine monophosphate (cAMP), STa inhibits neutral Na^+Cl^- absorption. The effects of STa and theophylline on neutral Na^+Cl^- absorption are equal and not additive, suggesting a final common pathway. It is now clear that chloride secretion occurs via the major intestinal chloride channel, the cystic fibrosis transmembrane regulator (CFTR) (84). Animals and humans with cystic fibrosis, or a defect in the CFTR, are resistant to STa and to the endogenous mammalian ligand, guanylin (84,85). In addition to Cl^- secretion, STa also stimulated HCO_3 secretion, particularly in the duodenum. This HCO_3 isecretion also appears to occur via the CFTR (86).

Both the T84 and the Caco-2 human colonic carcinoma cell lines have proved useful in the study of the biologic actions of STa. ETEC organisms adhere to Caco-2 cells (87,88) and STa activates guanylate cyclase (GC-C) in both of these cell lines (55,71,89). T84 cells resemble small intestinal crypt epithelium and secrete Cl^- in response to various secretagogues (90–93). STa stimulates Cl^- secretion across T84 monolayers by elevating cGMP and activating apical Cl^- and basolateral K^+ channels (66). It is thought that this cGMP-mediated channel activation is similar to the cAMP-mediated channel activation of Cl^- secretion (66). However, in contrast to the similar magnitude of effect by STa and theophylline on neutral chloride absorption, STa is less potent than cAMP in stimulating electrogenic chloride secretion (66).

The intermediate steps by which cGMP leads to these transport alterations are not entirely clear and may vary regionally in the intestine. STa stimulates a membrane-bound cGMP-dependent protein kinase, PKG_2, which phosphorylates CFTR. It is very likely that PKG_2 is essential to STa-induced small intestinal secretion, since mice lacking PKG_2 are resistant to STa (94). Whether cAMP-dependent protein kinase also participates is uncertain. In the colon, however, a different intermediate mechanism may apply. Vaandrager et al. (95) have shown that in mice lacking PKG_2, STa continues to induce secretion probably via a cGMP-inhibitable phosphodiesterase. These intracellular signaling mechanisms are discussed in Chapter 8. Furthermore, although it is traditionally thought that enterotoxins do not alter the cytoskeletal architecture, exposure of T84 cells to STa results in functional rearrangement of basolateral filamentous actin filaments (96), which if inhibited results in STa-stimulated $Na^+/K^+/2Cl^-$ co-transport activity being reduced by approximately 60% (96). This suggests that the ability of STa to elicit a cytoskeletal rearrangement is an important intermediate in STa-induced electrogenic Cl^- secretion.

In addition to this classic pathway, STa also induces intestinal secretion via a mechanism involving the enteric nervous system. Briefly, after binding to enterocytes, STa causes the release of 5-hydroxytryptamine (serotonin) and prostaglandin E_2 (PGE_2), which activate one or more enteric neurogenic reflexes which induce secretion (97,98).

Interaction With Receptors

Kinetic measurements of STa binding to recombinant cell lines (293-STaR) gives an association constant of 10^8 L/mol (65,69,71). However, in all transfected cell lines studied, there appears to be a discrepancy between the dose of STa required for inhibition of radiolabeled STa binding and STa-induced stimulation of guanylate cyclase activity. Although the reasons for this discrepancy are not clear, it is probable that STa binding is necessary but not uniquely sufficient for guanylate cyclase activation and that some other events are required for full expression of guanylate cyclase activity. It has recently been shown that after STa binding, GC-C forms oligomers (99) and that GC-C is phosphorylated (100).

Although the biologic action of STa is rapidly and completely reversible (62,63), it has not been possible to demonstrate the reversibility of STa binding as clearly (54,55,64,101,102). This discrepancy could be due to a dynamic interaction between STa and its receptor after binding occurs.

In the rat and human, the number of STa receptors and their affinity for STa are similar in jejunum and ileum (54). In the small intestine, STa receptors are primarily if not exclusively localized to the brush border membrane, rather than the basolateral membrane (55). Although it is thought that the principal site of action of bacterial enterotoxins is in the small intestine, both STa binding activity and STa-responsive guanyl cyclase are present in the human colon as well (103,104). In the rat, the number of receptors per colonocyte is even greater than the number of receptors per small-bowel enterocyte (62). Furthermore, there may be site-specific effects of STa within the colon (105).

Immature humans and other animals are at increased risk for STa-mediated diarrheal disease. Immune mechanisms may play a major role in this increased susceptibility. In addition, there is increased age-specific colonization of the intestinal epithelium by piliated ETEC organisms in pigs, calves, and mice (106,107). The number of intestinal STa receptors also plays a role in the severity of STa-mediated diarrheal disease. For example, there is an absence of ST receptors in piglets that are refractory to the experimental induction of STa-mediated diarrhea (108). Some investigators have shown greater STa-receptor density in the immature compared with the adult intestine of the rat, pig, and human (103,109–111).

Recently, two laboratories have produced GC-C "knockout" mice, that is, mice lacking the GC-C receptor (112,113). These mice develop normally, live a normal life span, and are fully fertile. The intestine of these animals does not respond to STa or to guanylin (112–114). However, we have recently found that GC-C–deficient mice have impaired duodenal HCO_3 secretion (115) and are more susceptible to CCl_4-induced liver injury (116). The physiologic significance of these observations is unclear.

Extraintestinal Receptors For STa

Initially, binding studies of the tissue specificity of the STa receptor in the rat demonstrated no STa receptor activity in the lung, liver, brain, heart, pancreas, and gastric antrum (83,117). Recent data demonstrate low levels of GC-C expression in adrenal gland, testis, liver, placenta, tracheal epithelium, brain, and other sites (118–120). Maximal expression of GC-C in the rat liver occurs in the perinatal period. The presence of GC-C in multiple tissues is analogous to the tissue distribution of other members of the guanylate cyclase family. Surprisingly, there is no evidence of GC-C expression in the kidney (118,119), an organ with structural and enzymatic homology to the intestine and from which an endogenous ligand for GC-C has been isolated. The function of the STa receptor in these tissues is uncertain, although it is possible that guanylin and uroguanylin bind to these extraintestinal receptors to activate transport and other functions.

GC-C messenger RNA (mRNA) is expressed in the regenerating rat liver after either partial hepatectomy or CCl_4-induced hepatic necrosis (121). We have also shown that GC-C mRNA expression occurred in association with an acute-phase reaction (121). Coordinate with the expression of GC-C mRNA, there was up-regulation of radiolabeled STa binding to liver plasma membranes. Maximal binding occurred in preparations enriched for the canalicular domain (121). Although the function of GC-C in the liver is unknown, localization to the canalicular domain would be consistent with a role for GC-C in hepatic chloride secretion.

Related Bacterial Toxins

Other organisms that elaborate highly homologous ST enterotoxins include *Y. enterocolitica* (123), *Citrobacter freundii*, non-O1 vibrios (124,125), and other *Vibrio* species (126). These enterotoxins, whose structure is shown in Fig. 39.2, act in a manner similar to that of *E. coli* STa; that is, they bind to GC-C and stimulate production of cGMP. There is direct evidence of interspecies transfer of the ST plasmid to other non–*E. coli* bacterial strains (127).

In addition, enteroaggregative *E. coli* (EAEC) produce a low-molecular-weight ST enterotoxin designated EAEC heat-stable enterotoxin 1 (EAST-1) (128,129). EAEC strains have been epidemiologically associated with infantile diarrhea in rural Chile (130) and with persistent diarrhea in children in India (131), Mexico (132), and Brazil (133). Other studies have shown no difference in the colonization by EAEC from controls (134–137). The structural gene for EAST-1 shows significant homology with the enterotoxic domain of STa. However, unlike STa, which requires six cysteines and three disulfide linkages for full biologic activity, EAST-1 contains four cysteine residues. Interestingly, this is similar to guanylin and uroguanylin (vide infra), endogenous ligands for the STa receptor that also contain four cysteines (45).

Endogenous Mammalian Ligands

Endogenous mammalian ligands homologous to STa have been isolated from rat intestine and kidney—that is, guanylin and uroguanylin (45,138–140). Unlike STa, these peptides have only four cysteine residues and the peptides are only active when fully disulfide bonded. Both guanylin and uroguanylin bind to GC-C in the intestine, cause an increase in cGMP concentration, and stimulate Cl^- and HCO_3^- secretion (45,140–142). However, they are approximately 10-fold to 20-fold less potent than STa (143).

Guanylin, a 15–amino acid peptide, is produced in the intestine. Uroguanylin, a 16–amino acid peptide, is produced both in the intestine and in the kidney and appears in urine (138,139,141). In the intestine, guanylin expression is greatest in colon and ileum while uroguanylin expression is greatest in the duodenum (144). Both are secreted into the lumen of the intestine and into the bloodstream (145). Thus, both circulate in blood presumably to interact with receptors in various organs (146). Uroguanylin has been shown to stimulate Na^+, K^+, and cGMP excretion by the kidney (143,147). The extraintestinal function of guanylin is unknown.

It is likely that uroguanylin, released by the intestine in response to various signals, modulates renal Na^+ and K^+ handling by the kidney (148). Furthermore, it is possible that these ligands modulate other functions in the intestine as a result of increased intracellular levels of cGMP (146).

Assays

Three whole-animal models have been used to detect STa. Initially, a rabbit ileal loop assay was performed (149), but this was replaced by a standardized suckling mouse bioassay (150,151). The suckling mouse assay tests for fluid accumulation in the intestine of newborn (1 to 4 days old) Swiss CD4 mice after percutaneous injection of culture supernatants from *E. coli* colonies isolated from fecal specimens (151). Although this assay is reliable and reproducible, it is cumbersome and labor intensive and requires large numbers of suckling mice. A guinea pig ileal loop assay for ST was also described (152). This assay uses an intestinal dilation index to measure the secretory response, and compared with the suckling mouse assay, a much larger minimum effective dose is required for STa. Furthermore, both STa and STb cause a positive assay.

Another bioassay was described by Currie et al. (45). This assay relies on the observation that STa activates particulate guanylate cyclase in intestinal cell tissue culture lines. A 30,000- to 100,000-fold increase in cGMP concentrations was seen in the T84 cell line after the addition of STa.

A number of radioimmunoassays have been developed to detect STa-producing organisms (153,154). Several enzyme-linked immunosorbent assays (ELISA) using anti-STa antibody have shown complete correlation with the suckling mouse assay and radioimmunoassay (155–157). One of these assays is commercially available (157).

For mass screening approaches to detect STa-producing organisms, the best system has been the use of gene probe assays and the colony blot approach to detect one or more of the ST enterotoxins (158–160). These assays are based on the cloned genes for STh and STp. There is a positive predictive value of more than 95% when comparing alkaline phosphatase conjugated oligonucleotide probes, phosphorus-32 (^{32}P)–labeled oligonucleotide probes, and/or cloned digoxigenin or ^{32}P-labeled polynucleotide probes with the suckling mouse bioassay (161). Commercial DNA hybridization assay kits are available (161,162). Trivalent probes that detect both ST toxins and LT toxins have also been described (163,164). Lastly, a combination of immunomagnetic separation of pili-expressing *E. coli* and a nested colorimetric polymerase chain reaction (PCR) was shown to identify genes encoding the heat-stable enterotoxin in porcine fecal specimens (165).

STb

Moon and Whipp (166) identified a second type of ST enterotoxin elaborated by diarrheagenic *E. coli.* This toxin, termed STb or STII, causes secretion in weaned pigs. STb is unlike STa in that STb is methanol insoluble and is inactive in the suckling mouse assay (167). Although culture filtrates of STa cause no histologic lesions, culture filtrates of STb result in loss of villus absorptive cells and partial atrophy (168,169).

STb was initially thought to cause fluid secretion only in piglets (167,170,171). More recently, Whipp (172) demonstrated that the host response specificity of STb could be attributed to the susceptibility of STb to protease. Soybean trypsin inhibitor protected STb from proteolysis and resulted in positive responses of STb in intestinal segments of mice, rats, calves, and rabbits, demonstrating that the activity of STb is not species specific (172–174).

The gene for STb encodes a 71–amino acid prohormone with a 32–amino acid leader sequence (175,176). This is consistent with the observation that the toxin is found in the bacterial periplasm as an 8.1-kd precursor, which is converted to a 5.2-kd mature, active form that is secreted (177). Mature STb was recently purified and is composed of 48–amino acid residues that contain two disulfide bonds (178,179). However, there is no amino acid homology with STa; antisera raised against each of these toxins do not recognize the other (154,180).

Exposure of pig intestine mounted in an Ussing chamber to STb results in an increase in Isc (181), but unlike STa, there is no change in neutral sodium and chloride absorption or electrogenic chloride secretion (181). STb does effect the calculated net residual ion flux. This likely represents bicarbonate secretion and is consistent with the observation that STb raises luminal pH level and the bicarbonate content of intestinal secretion *in vivo* (181). STb does not change cAMP or cGMP levels (170,182). Although initial reports suggested that the action of a crude STb is not affected by the presence of calcium ions in the bathing solution (183), more recent data demonstrate that pure STb induces a dose-dependent increase in intracellular calcium concentrations that is entirely dependent on a source of extracellular calcium (184). STb-mediated intracellular calcium elevation is not inhibited by drugs that block voltage-gated calcium channels or agents that deplete and block internal calcium stores (184). These data suggest that STb opens a receptor-operated calcium channel in the plasma membrane. In addition, prostaglandins may play a role in the mechanism of STb action. The level of PGE_2 is increased in the secreted fluid accumulated as a result of STb, and the prostaglandin synthetase inhibitors aspirin and indomethacin significantly reduce the response to STb (171). Current data suggest that a lipid extract sulfatide present on the jejunal mucosa could represent a natural target binding molecule for STb (185,186).

Although STb is the most prevalent toxin associated with diarrheagenic *E. coli* of porcine origin (173), STb-producing *E. coli* are not thought to be a major cause of diarrheal illness in humans (187–189). However, STb-elaborating strains of *E. coli* have been isolated from humans with diarrhea in Canada and Japan (190,191).

Heat-labile Toxins (LTI, LTII)

LTI is actually a family of high-molecular-weight proteins that are structurally and functionally similar to CT. The LTI family includes the subtypes LThI and LTpI, which designate antigenic variants originally isolated from humans and pigs (192). There is also immunologic heterogeneity within the LThI subtype (193). Similar to CT, LTI consists of a single enzymatically active A subunit surrounded by five binding B subunits (194). The deduced amino acid sequences of the A and B subunits are approximately 80% homologous between LTII and CT (195–200) and the action of LTI is neutralized by antisera against CT. Similar to CT, LTI induces intestinal secretion by activating adenylate cyclase in an NAD-dependent reaction (201,202). This results in increased intracellular concentrations of cAMP. However, in contrast to CT, LTI binds not only to a GM_1 ganglioside receptor to initiate this pathway, but also to a 130- to 140-kd glycoprotein receptor present on the intestinal brush border membrane (203–208). This second binding site is 20 to 30 times more prevalent in intestinal brush border membranes than is the binding site for CT (206). Evidence for the full biologic effectiveness of this second receptor comes from the fact that saturation of the GM1 ganglioside receptor by CT does not inhibit the secretory response to LTI in the rabbit and only partially blocks the effect of LTI in humans (205,207).

The classic pathway of LT-mediated secretion involves increased levels of cAMP, resulting in activation of protein kinase A and phosphorylation of the CFTR. There is increasing evidence for a more complex pathway, particularly with respect to CT, although presumably the same pathways are potentially relevant for LT as well (reviewed in reference 209). One alternative pathway involves toxin-mediated release of arachidonic acid metabolites that affect intestinal ion secretion and motility. A second potential mechanism also involves the enteric nervous system and toxin-mediated release of serotonin and vasoactive intestinal peptide. A third mechanism involves the release of proinflammatory cytokines that in turn activate the enteric nervous system. The mechanisms of action of LTI and its relationship to CT is further discussed in Chapter 36.

Heat-labile toxins that are not neutralized by antisera against CT are designated LTII (210). LTIIa can be distinguished from LTIIb based on antigenic determinants and chemical properties (211) and the ability to inhibit the binding of other enterotoxins to Y1 adrenal cells (212). The gene encoding the A subunit of LTIIa is 50% to 60% homologous with the corresponding genes encoding the A subunits of LThI and CT (213). However, there is no homology between the B subunits of LTIIa and LThI or CT (213). Consequently, LTIIa demonstrates binding characteristics to the glycoprotein receptor that are dissimilar to LThI or CT (214).

A number of other bacteria elaborate LT-like toxins including *Klebsiella, Enterobacter, Aeromonas hydrophila, Plesiomonas shigelloides, Campylobacter, Salmonella typhimurium,* and *Salmonella enteritidis* (4,215–223).

LT Assays

The two standard assays for LT are immunologic assays (e.g., Biken test) and tissue culture assays (e.g., Y1 adrenal or CHO cells assays). In the Biken test, LT is detected by the appearance of a precipitin line between growth of the organism and antisera against LT (224,225). Although reagents for this test are commercially available, the test takes 5 days to complete (226). Standard LT tissue culture assays use Y1 adrenal or CHO cells (227–230). The amount of LT present in a culture supernatant is titered by serial dilution to detect rounding of at least 50% of Y1 (or stretches of CHO) cells. Several different tests for LT using immunologic methods including ELISA and passive hemagglutination have been described (231–233). However, the unavailability of reagents for these tests has limited their usefulness. More recently, an immunologic assay that uses latex bead agglutination (234–236), as well as a commercially available reversed passive latex agglutination test (VET-RPLA) (237) and a staphylococcal coagglutination test (Phadebact ETEC-LT) (238) have been described. Both of the commercial tests are highly accurate (237–240). Both PCR-based assays (241) and gene probe assays for LT-producing organisms are also available (158–160,242–244). At present, all of these tests are difficult to perform in the field and are not generally available in clinical laboratories.

CLINICAL ILLNESS

Illness caused by ETEC is characterized by watery diarrhea. The spectrum of illness ranges from very mild to dehydrating cholera-like purging. In travelers, ETEC disease often occurs between 5 and 15 days after arrival in an endemic area, with an incubation period of 14 to 50 hours (245). Infection with ST-producing organisms cannot be differentiated from infection with LT-producing organisms, although LT/ST disease is more severe than LT disease alone (246). Stools are watery, yellow, and devoid of mucus, pus, and fecal leukocytes. The illness is most often self-limited, lasting less than 5 days with few cases persisting more than 3 weeks (27,247). Abdominal pain is modest or absent and fever is usually absent.

Infection with ETEC has also been specifically associated with short- and long-term adverse nutritional consequences in infants and children. Infection with ETEC not only caused acute diarrheal disease and the interruption of normal feeding patterns but also resulted in diminished long-term linear growth (10,11).

DIAGNOSIS

Specific tests for ST or LT or polynucleotide probes for LT or ST genes are described above. ETEC strains are particularly useful to identify with stool blot hybridization assays because of the utility of the available probes and the large numbers of organisms shed in the stool of affected individuals. These tests are often used in batches to achieve economy of scale. However, although a positive test result for LT or ST defines an ETEC strain, full virulence requires the presence of CFAs specific for humans. Thus, simply screening for the presence of LT or ST genes may overestimate the true incidence of pathogenic organisms.

TREATMENT

Most diarrheal illness due to ETEC does not require antibiotic treatment, because the illness is short-lived and oral rehydration therapy is safe, effective, and commercially available. The use of oral rehydration solutions containing between 35 and 90 mEq of sodium per liter, with added glucose, potassium, and bicarbonate, has proven remarkably effective in underdeveloped countries and has prompted their use in developed countries (248). Three placebo-controlled studies have evaluated whether antibiotics are efficacious in the treatment of ETEC infection (246,249,250). Merson et al. (246) showed that tetracycline slightly shortened the duration of diarrhea in adults with naturally acquired infection. Black et al. (249) showed that early therapy (after the third loose stool) with trimethoprim-sulfamethoxazole (TMP-SMX) significantly decreased the duration of diarrhea and the fecal excretion of ETEC in young adult volunteers who were experimentally infected with an LT/ST-producing strain. DuPont et al. (250) demonstrated that TMP-SMX and trimethoprim alone significantly reduced the duration of diarrhea, the number of loose stools, and the fecal excretion of ETEC in college students from the United States with natural infection acquired while in Mexico (250). However, since these studies were reported, there has been increasing resistance of *E. coli* to antimicrobials in developing countries (251,252).

Pepto-Bismol and its active ingredient, bismuth subsalicylate (BSS), significantly inhibit fluid accumulation in experimental animals inoculated with *E. coli*-producing ST, LT, or both (253); clinical studies with Pepto-Bismol have also shown effectiveness in treating ETEC diarrhea (254). A number of studies have shown efficacy of BSS, TMP-SMX, and ciprofloxacin to prevent or treat traveler's diarrhea, which is commonly caused by ETEC (250,255,256).

Antidiarrheal drugs are generally not used in the treatment of infants with acute diarrhea. In adults, the use of antidiarrheal drugs such as loperamide decreases the stool volume and provides symptomatic relief. Therapy is more thoroughly discussed in Chapters 19, 78, and 79.

VACCINES

A number of approaches have been tried to develop effective vaccines against ETEC. These approaches have used nonliving oral antigens and live oral vaccines designed to stimulate anticolonization immunity and/or antitoxic immunity (257). The major problem associated with developing an efficacious vaccine against ETEC is the fact that ETEC organisms are antigenically diverse; that is, they are found in a number of O serogroups and they possess one of several possible CFAs. In addition, one of the important toxins they produce, ST, is not antigenic because of its small size.

One live oral vaccine approach involves the use of ETEC that express CFA but not ST or LT (257,258). A prototype vaccine was highly protective against experimental challenge with ETEC expressing the same CFA (259–261). This validates the concept but would provide immunity to only a fraction of ETEC. An ideal vaccine would contain all of the common CFAs and would contain the B subunit (immunogenic binding, nontoxic subunit) of LT and possibly an immunogenic nontoxic variant of ST and/or LT.

A better understanding of the common ETEC serotypes and CFA involved in clinical infections will provide a guide to more effective candidate vaccines (29,262).

Another live oral vaccine strategy uses attenuated *Salmonella typhi* strains that have been genetically engineered to produce the B subunit of LT and some CFAs; these vaccines have been shown to be immunogenic (263,264). Nonliving oral toxoid vaccines consisting of synthetic ST linked to the B subunit of LT have also shown an immune response (265,266). Purified fimbriae have been used as vaccines but to date have not been protective against clinical infection in people possibly because of antigenic degradation in the stomach (33,258,267). New approaches using fimbrial adhesin antigens include the use of CFA encapsulated in biodegradable microspheres of poly(lactide-co-glycolide) (268). These microspheres protect CFA from degradation and deliver antigen to the enteric immune system (268,269). Clinical studies using these vaccines are underway. Fimbrial vaccines are routinely given parenterally to pregnant cattle, sheep, and swine to protect suckling newborn calves, lambs, and pigs against ETEC infections (270). However, the efficacy of these vaccines and the effect of these vaccines in selecting for novel or previously low-prevalence fimbrial antigen types have not been well studied (270).

Alternative strategies include oral, inactivated ETEC composed of formalin-killed ETEC strains expressing various colonization factors (e.g., CFA/I, CFA/II, and CFA/IV together with 1 mg of recombinant CT B subunit). Such vaccines have been shown to be safe and immunogenic (271–273) and are being tested for protective efficacy.

Finally the use of food substances (eggs and milk) to deliver passive protection against enteropathogens was recently explored. Oral ingestion of egg yolk immunoglobulin from hens immunized with an ETEC strain prevented diarrhea in rabbits challenged with the same strain (274,275). This leads to the speculation that hens or cows immunized with appropriate antigens may have usefulness as a source of passive immunity against ETEC. In initial studies, milk-derived antibodies against CFAs alone were sufficient for protection against ETEC infection in human volunteer studies (276). In a subsequent study, orally administered bovine immunoglobulins with specific activity against colonization factors of ETEC (CFA/I, CS3, and CS6) were not sufficient to provide passive protection against ETEC challenge (277).

Probably of greatest excitement is the combination of food substances and vaccine strategies to provide active protection against enteropathogens. Such an approach was taken to design and construct a synthetic gene encoding the *E. coli* LTb, for use in transgenic plants as an edible vaccine against ETEC. Expression of the synthetic LTb gene in potato plants under the control of a constitutive promoter yielded increased accumulation of LTb in leaves and tubers, as compared with the bacterial LTb gene. The plant-derived LTb assembled into native pentameric structures, as evidenced by its ability to bind ganglioside. Mice fed the raw tubers were partially protected from intestinal secretion resulting from challenge with LT (278). This proof of principle has tremendous potential implications for improving the delivery of vaccines and administering booster doses in foodstuffs. Specific vaccine strategies are discussed more thoroughly in Chapter 80.

REFERENCES

1. Moon HW, Nagy B, Isaacson RE. Intestinal colonization and adhesion by enterotoxigenic *Escherichia coli:* ultrastructural observations on adherence to ileal epithelium of the pig. *J Infect Dis* 1977;136:S124–S129.
2. Taylor J, Wilkins MP, Payne JM. Relation of rabbit gut reaction to enteropathogenic *Escherichia coli. Br J Exp Pathol* 1961;42: 43–52.
3. Gorbach SL, Banwell JG, Chatterjee BD, et al. Acute undifferentiated human diarrhea in the tropics, I: alterations in intestinal microflora. *J Clin Invest* 1971;50:881–889.
4. Guerrant RL, Moore RA, Kirschenfeld BA, et al. Role of toxigenic and invasive bacteria in acute diarrhea of childhood. *N Engl J Med* 1975;293:567–573.
5. Sack RB. Enterotoxigenic *Escherichia coli:* identification and characterization. *J Infect Dis* 1980;142:279–286.
6. Whipp SC, Moon HW, Lyon NC. Heat-stable *Escherichia coli* enterotoxin production *in vivo. Infect Immun* 1975;12:240–244.
7. Gyles CL. Heat labile and heat stable forms of the enterotoxin from *Escherichia coli* strains enteropathogenic for pigs. *Ann N Y Acad Sci* 1971;176:314–322.
8. Sack RB. Human diarrheal disease caused by enterotoxigenic *Escherichia coli. Annu Rev Microbiol* 1975;29:333–353.
9. Lanata CF, Black RE, Gil A, et al. Etiologic agents in acute vs. persistent diarrhea in children under three years of age in peri-urban Lima, Peru. *Acta Paediatr* 1992;81[Suppl 381]:32–38.
10. Black RE, Merson HM, Huq I, et al. Incidence and severity of rotavirus and *Escherichia coli* in rural Bangladesh. *Lancet* 1981; 1:141–143.
11. Black RE, Brown KH, Becker S, et al. Longitudinal studies of infectious diseases and physical growth of children in rural Bangladesh, II: Incidence of diarrhea and association with known pathogens. *Am J Epidemiol* 1982;115:315–324.
12. Guarino A, Alessio M, Tarallo L, et al. Heat stable enterotoxin by *Escherichia coli* in acute diarrhea. *Arch Dis Child* 1989;64: 808–813.
13. Gorbach SL, Khurana CM. Toxigenic *Escherichia coli:* a cause of infantile diarrhea in Chicago. *N Engl J Med* 1972;287:791–796.
14. Echeverria P, Blacklow NR, Smith DH. Role of heat-labile toxigenic *Escherichia coli* and reovirus-like agent in diarrhea in Boston children. *Lancet* 1975;2:1113–1116.
15. Kotloff KL, Wasserman SS, Steciak JY, et al. Acute diarrhea in Baltimore children attending an outpatient clinic. *Pediatr Infect Dis J* 1988;7:753–759.
16. Caeiro JP, Mathewson JJ, Smith MA, et al. Etiology of outpatient pediatric nondysenteric diarrhea: a multicenter study in the United States. *Pediatr Infect Dis J* 1999;18:94–97.
17. DuPont HL, Formal SB, Hornick RB, et al. Pathogenesis of *Escherichia coli* diarrhea. *N Engl J Med* 1971;285:1–9.
18. Levine MM, Caplan ES, Watermann D, et al. Diarrhea caused by *Escherichia coli* that produce only heat-stable enterotoxin. *Infect Immun* 1977;17:78–82.
19. Gorbach SL, Kean BH, Evans DG, et al. Traveler's diarrhea and toxigenic *Escherichia coli. N Engl J Med* 1975;292:933–936.
20. Rosenberg ML, Koplan JP, Wachsmuth IK, et al. Epidemic diarrhea at Crater Lake from enterotoxigenic *Escherichia coli:* a large waterborne outbreak. *Ann Intern Med* 1977;86:714–718.
21. Levine MM, Rennels MB, Cisneros L, et al. Lack of person-to-person transmission of enterotoxigenic *Escherichia coli* despite close contact. *Am J Epidemiol* 1980;111:347–355.
22. Brunton J, Hinde D, Langston C, et al. Enterotoxigenic *Escherichia coli* in central Canada. *J Clin Microbiol* 1980;11: 343–438.
23. Bäck E, Blomberg S, Wadstrom T. Enterotoxigenic *Escherichia coli* in Sweden. *Infection* 1977;5:2–5.

24. Merson MH, Morris GK, Sack DA, et al. Traveler's diarrhea in Mexico. A prospective study of physicians and family members attending a congress. *N Engl J Med* 1976;294:1299–1305.
25. Consensus Conference. Traveler's diarrhea. *JAMA* 1985;253: 2700–2704.
26. Jiang ZD, Mathewson JJ, Ericsson CD, et al. Characterization of enterotoxigenic *Escherichia coli* strains in patients with travelers' diarrhea acquired in Guadalajara, Mexico, 1992–1997. *J Infect Dis* 2000;181:779–782.
27. Sack DA, Kaminsky DC, Sack RB, et al. Enterotoxigenic *Escherichia coli* diarrhea of travelers: a prospective study of American Peace Corps volunteers. *Johns Hopkins Med J* 1977; 141:63–70.
28. Hyams KC, Bourgeois AL, Merrell BR, et al. Diarrheal disease during Operation Desert Storm. *N Engl J Med* 1991;325: 1423–1428.
29. Wolf MK, Taylor DN, Boedeker EC. Characterization of enterotoxigenic *Escherichia coli* isolated from US troops deployed to the Middle East. *J Clin Microbiol* 1993;31:851–856.
30. Black RE, Merson MH, Rahman ASMM, et al. A two year study of bacterial viral and parasitic agents associated with diarrhea in rural Bangladesh. *J Infect Dis* 1980;142:660–665.
31. Guerrant RL, Kirchhoff LV, Nations MK, et al. Prospective study of diarrheal illness in northeastern Brazil. *J Infect Dis* 1983;148:986–997.
32. Sack RB, Hirschorn N, Brownlee I, et al. Enterotoxigenic *Escherichia coli* associated diarrheal illness in Apache children. *N Engl J Med* 1975;292:1041–1045.
33. Ryder RW, Sack DA, Kapikian AZ, et al. Enterotoxigenic *Escherichia coli* and reovirus-like agent in rural Bangladesh. *Lancet* 1976;1:659–662.
34. Taylor WR, Schell WL, Wells JG, et al. A foodborne outbreak of enterotoxigenic *Escherichia coli* diarrhea. *N Engl J Med* 1982; 306:1093–1095.
35. Dalton CB, Mintz ED, Wells JG, et al. Outbreaks of enterotoxigenic *Escherichia coli* infection in American adults: a clinical and epidemiologic profile. *Epidemiol Infect* 1999;123:9–16.
36. Levine MM. *Escherichia coli* that cause diarrhea: enterotoxigenic, enteropathogenic, enteroinvasive, enterohemorrhagic, enteroadherent. *J Infect Dis* 1987;155:377–389.
37. Nataro JP, Kaper JB. Diarrheogenic *Escherichia coli. Clin Microbiol Rev* 1998;11:142–201.
38. Jann K, Hoschutsky. Nature and organization of adhesins. *Curr Top Microbiol Immunol* 1991;151:55–85.
39. Wolf MK. Occurrence, distribution and association of O and H serogroups, colonization factor antigens and toxins of enterotoxigenic *Escherichia coli. Clin Microbiol Rev* 1997;10: 569–584.
40. Giron JA, Levine MM, Kaper JB. Longus: a long pilus ultrastructure produced by human enterotoxigenic *Escherichia coli. Mol Microbiol* 1994;12:71–82.
41. Giron JA, Viboud GI, Sperandio V, et al. Prevalence and association of the longus pilus structural gene (lngA) with colonization factor antigens, enterotoxin types and serotypes of enterotoxigenic *Escherichia coli. Infect Immun* 1995;63:4195–4198.
42. Takao T, Hitouji T, Aimoto S, et al. Amino acid sequence of a heat-stable enterotoxin isolated from enterotoxigenic *Escherichia coli* strain 18D. *FEBS Lett* 1983;152:1–5.
43. Chan S-K, Giannella RA. Amino acid sequence of heat-stable enterotoxin produced by *Escherichia coli* pathogenic for man. *J Biol Chem* 1981;256:7744–7746.
44. Thompson MR, Giannella RA. Revised amino acid sequence for a heat-stable enterotoxin produced by and *Escherichia coli* strain (18D) that is pathogenic for humans. *Infect Immun* 1985; 47:834–836.
45. Currie MG, Fok KF, Kato J, et al. Guanylin: an endogenous activator of intestinal guanylate cyclase. *Proc Natl Acad Sci U S A* 1992;89:947–951.
46. Giannella RA, Luttrell M. Characteristics of the binding of pure human *Escherichia coli* heat-stable enterotoxin to rat intestine. In: Kuwahara S, Pierce NF, eds. *Advances in research on cholera and related diseases.* Tokyo: KTK, 1983:259–268.
47. Yoshimura S, Ikemura H, Watanabe H, et al. Essential structure for full enterotoxigenic activity of heat-stable enterotoxin produced by enterotoxigenic *Escherichia coli. FEBS Lett* 1985;181: 138–142.
48. Waldman SA, O'Hanley P. Influence of a glycine or proline substitution on the functional properties of a 14–amino-acid analog of *Escherichia coli* heat-stable enterotoxin. *Infect Immun* 1989;57:2420–2424.
49. So M, McCarthy BJ. Nucleotide sequence of the bacterial transposon TN1681 encoding a heat-stable enterotoxin (ST) and its identification in enterotoxigenic *Escherichia coli* strains. *Proc Natl Acad Sci U S A* 1980;77:4011–4015.
50. Rasheed JK, Guzman-Verduzco LM, Kupersztoch YM. Two precursors of the heat-stable enterotoxin of *Escherichia coli:* evidence of extracellular processing. *Mol Microbiol* 1990;4:265–273.
51. Guzman-Verduzco LM, Kupersztoch YM. Export and processing of a fusion between the extracellular heat-stable enterotoxin and the periplasmic B subunit of the heat-labile enterotoxin in *Escherichia coli. Mol Microbiol* 1990;4:253–264.
52. Staples SJ, Asher SE, Giannella RA. Purification and characterization of heat-stable enterotoxin produced by a strain of *Escherichia coli* pathogenic for man. *J Biol Chem* 1980;255: 4716–4721.
53. Rao MC. Toxins which activate guanylate cyclase: heat-stable *Escherichia coli* enterotoxin. In: Evered D, Whelan J, eds. *Microbial toxins and diarrheal disease.* Ciba Foundation Symposium 112. London: Pitman, 1985:74–93.
54. Giannella RA, Luttrell M, Thompson M. Binding of *Escherichia coli* heat-stable enterotoxin to receptors on rat intestinal cells. *Am J Physiol* 1983;243:G36–G41.
55. Guarino A, Cohen MB, Overmann GJ, et al. Binding of *E. coli* heat-stable enterotoxin to rat brush border and basolateral membranes. *Dig Dis Sci* 1987;32:1017–1026.
56. Houghton RA, Ostresh JM, Klipstein FA. Chemical synthesis of an octadecapeptide with the biological and immunological properties of human heat-stable *Escherichia coli* enterotoxin. *Eur J Biochem* 1984;145:157–162.
57. Shimonshi Y, Hidaka Y, Koizumi M. Mode of disulfide bond formation by a heat-stable enterotoxin (STh) produced by a human strain of enterotoxigenic *Escherichia coli. FEBS Lett* 1987;215:165–170.
58. Kubota H, Hidaka Y, Ozaki H, et al. A long-acting heat-stable enterotoxin analogy of enterotoxigenic *Escherichia coli* with a single D-amino acid. *Biochem Biophys Res Commun* 1989;161: 229–235.
59. Okamoto K, Jukitake J, Kawamoto Y, et al. Substitutions of cysteine residues of *Escherichia coli* heat-stable enterotoxin by oligonucleotide-directed mutagenesis. *Infect Immun* 1987;55: 2121–2125.
60. Hughes JM, Murad F, Chang B, et al. Role of cyclic GMP in the action of heat-stable enterotoxin of *Escherichia coli. Nature* 1978;271:755–756.
61. Field M, Graf LH, Laird WJ, et al. Heat stable enterotoxin of *Escherichia coli: in vitro* effects on guanylate cyclase activity, cyclic GMP concentration, and ion transport in small intestine. *Proc Natl Acad Sci U S A* 1978;75:2800–2804.
62. Mezoff AG, Giannella RA, Eade MN, et al. *Escherichia coli* enterotoxin (STa) binds to receptors, stimulates guanyl cyclase and impairs absorption in rat colon. *Gastroenterology* 1992;102: 816–822.

63. Giannella RA, Walls D, Eade MN. Effect of pure *E. coli* heat-stable enterotoxin on small and large intestinal water and glucose absorption, mucosal histology and intestinal permeability. In: Kuwahara S, Pierce N, eds. *Advances in research on cholera and related diseases.* Tokyo: KTK, 1986;327–332.
64. Cohen MB, Thompson MR, Overmann GJ, et al. Association and dissociation of *Escherichia coli* heat-stable enterotoxin from rat brush border membrane receptors. *Infect Immun* 1987;55:329–334.
65. Schulz S, Green CK, Yuen PST, et al. Guanylyl cyclase is a heat-stable enterotoxin receptor. *Cell* 1990;63:941–948.
66. Huott PA, Liu W, McRoberts JA, et al. Mechanism of action of *Escherichia coli* heat stable enterotoxin in a human colonic cell line. *J Clin Invest* 1988;82:514–523.
67. Giannella RA, Drake KW. Effect of purified *Escherichia coli* heat-stable enterotoxin on intestinal cyclic nucleotide metabolism and fluid secretion. *Infect Immun* 1979;24:19–23.
68. Newsome PM, Burgess MN, Mullan NA. Effect of *Escherichia coli* heat-stable enterotoxin on cyclic GMP levels in mouse intestine. *Infect Immun* 1978;22:290–291.
69. deSauvage FJ, Camerato TR, Goeddel DV. Primary structure and functional expression of the human receptor for *Escherichia coli* heat-stable enterotoxin. *J Biol Chem* 1991;266:17912–17918.
70. Singh S, Singh G, Helm JM, et al. Isolation and expression of a guanylate cyclase-coupled heat stable enterotoxin receptor cDNA from a human colonic cell line. *Biochem Biophys Res Commun* 1991;179:1455–1463.
71. Mann EA, Cohen MB, Giannella RA. Comparison of receptors for *Escherichia coli* heat-stable enterotoxin: novel receptor present in IEC-6 cells. *Am J Physiol* 1993;264:G172–G178.
72. Schulz S, Singh S, Bellet RA, et al. The primary structure of a plasma membrane guanylate cyclase demonstrates diversity within this new receptor family. *Cell* 1989;58:1155–1162.
73. deSauvage FJ, Horuk R, Bennett G, et al. Characterization of the recombinant human receptor for *Escherichia coli* heat-stable enterotoxin. *J Biol Chem* 1992;267:6479–6482.
74. Bhattacharya J, Chakrabarti MK. Rise of intracellular free calcium levels with activation of inositol triphosphate in human colonic carcinoma cell line (COLO 205) by heat-stable enterotoxin of *E. coli. Biochem Biophys Acta* 1998;1403:1–4.
75. Weikel CS, Spann CL, Chambers CP, et al. Phorbol esters enhance the cyclic GMP response of T84 cells to the heat-stable enterotoxin of *Escherichia coli* (STa). *Infect Immun* 1990;58:1402–1407.
76. Crane JK, Burrell LL, Weikel CS, et al. Carbachol mimics phorbol esters in its ability to enhance cyclic GMP production by STa, the heat-stable enterotoxin of *Escherichia coli. FEBS Lett* 1990;274:199–202.
77. Crane JK, Wehner MS, Bolen EJ, et al. Regulation of intestinal guanylate cyclase by the heat stable enterotoxin of *Escherichia coli* (STa) and protein kinase C. *Infect Immun* 1992;60:5004–5012.
78. Levine SA, Donowitz M, Watson AJ, et al. Characterization of the synergistic interaction of *Escherichia coli* heat-stable toxin and carbachol. *Am J Physiol* 1991;261:G592–G601.
79. Gazzano H, Wu HI, Waldman SA. Activation of particulate guanylate-cyclase by *Escherichia coli* heat-stable enterotoxin is regulated by adenine nucleotides. *Infect Immun* 1991;59:1552–1557.
80. Katwa LC, Parker CD, Dybing JK, et al. Nucleotide regulation of heat-stable enterotoxin receptor binding and of guanylate cyclase activation. *Biochem J* 1992;283:727–735.
81. Hakki S, Crane M, Hugues M, et al. Solubilization and characterization of functionally coupled *Escherichia coli* heat-stable toxin receptors and particulate guanylate cyclase associated with the cytoskeleton compartment of intestinal membranes. *Int J Biochem* 1993;25:557–566.
82. Vaandrager AB, van der Wiel E, de Jonge HR. Heat-stable enterotoxin activation of immunopurified guanylyl cyclase C. Modulation by adenine nucleotides. *J Biol Chem* 1993;268:19598–19603.
83. Guandalini S, Rao MC, Smith PL, et al. cGMP modulation of ileal ion transport: in vitro effects of *Escherichia coli* heat-stable enterotoxin. *Am J Physiol* 1982;243:G36–G41.
84. Cuthbert AW, Hickman ME, MacVinish LJ, et al. Chloride secretion in response to guanylin in colonic epithelia from normal and transgenic cystic fibrosis mice. *Br J Pharmacol* 1994;112:31–36.
85. Goldstein JL, Sahi J, Bhuva M, et al. *E. coli* heat-stable enterotoxin-mediated colonic Cl– secretion in absent in cystic fibrosis. *Gastroenterology* 1994;107:950–956.
86. Guba M, Kuhn M, Forssmann WG, et al. Guanylin strongly stimulates rat duodenal HCO_3 secretion: proposed mechanism and comparison with other secretogogues. *Gastroenterology* 1996;111:1558–1568.
87. Darfeuille-Michaud A, Aubel D, Chauviere G, et al. Adhesion of enterotoxigenic *Escherichia coli* to the human colon carcinoma cell line Caco-2 in culture. *Infect Immun* 1990;58:893–902.
88. Kerneis S, Chauviere G, Darfeuille-Michaud A, et al. Expression of receptors for enterotoxigenic *Escherichia coli* during enterocytic differentiation of human polarized intestinal epithelial cells in culture. *Infect Immun* 1992;60:2572–2580.
89. Cohen MB, Jensen NJ, Hawkins JA, et al. Receptors for *Escherichia coli* heat stable enterotoxin in human intestine and in a human intestinal cell line (Caco-2). *J Cell Physiol* 1993;156:138–144.
90. Weymer A, Huott P, Liu W, et al. Chloride secretory mechanism induced by prostaglandin E_1 in a colonic epithelial cell line. *J Clin Invest* 1985;76:1828–1836.
91. Cartwright CA, McRoberts JA, Mandel KG, et al. Synergistic action of cyclic adenosine monophosphate- and calcium-mediated chloride secretion in a colonic cell line. *J Clin Invest* 1985;76:1837–1842.
92. Dharmsathaphorn K, Mandel KG, Masui H, et al. Vasoactive intestinal polypeptide-induced chloride secretion by a colonic epithelial cell line. Direct participation of a basolaterally localized Na^+, K^-, Cl^- cotransport system. *J Clin Invest* 1985;75:462–471.
93. Dharmsathaphorn K, Pandol SJ. Mechanism of chloride secretion induced by carbachol in a colonic cell line. *J Clin Invest* 1986;77:348–354.
94. Pfeifer A, Aszodi A, Seidler U, et al. Intestinal secretory defects and dwarfism in mice lacking cGMP-dependent protein kinase II. *Science* 1996;274:2082–2086.
95. Vaandrager AB, Bot AGM, Ruth P, et al. Differential role of cyclic GMP-dependent protein kinase II in ion transport in murine small intestine and colon. *Gastroenterology* 2000;118:108–114.
96. Matthews JB, Awtrey CS, Thompson R, et al. Na^+-K^+-$2Cl^-$ cotransport and Cl^- secretion evoked by heat-stable enterotoxin is microfilament dependent in T84 cells. *Am J Physiol* 1993;265:G370–G378.
97. Eklund S, Jodal M, Lundgren O. The enteric nervous system participates in the secretory response to the heat-stable enterotoxins of *E. coli* in rats and cats. *Neuroscience* 1985;14:673–681.
98. Beubler E, Badhri P, Schirgi-Degan A. 5HT receptor antagonists and heat-stable *E. coli* enterotoxin-induced effects in the rat. *Eur J Pharmacol* 1992;219:445–450.
99. Vaandrager A, van der Weil E, Hom ML, et al. Heat-stable enterotoxin/receptor/guanylyl cyclase C is an oligomer consisting of functionally distinct subunits, which are non-covalently linked in the intestine. *J Biol Chem* 1994;269:16409–16415.
100. Crane JK, Shanks KL. Phosphorylation and activation of the intestinal guanylyl cyclase receptor for *E. coli* heat-stable toxin by protein kinase C. *Mol Cell Biochem* 1996;165:111–120.

101. Matthews JB, Awtrey CS, Madara JL. Microfilament dependent activation of $Na^{+}/K^{+}/Cl^{-}$ cotransport by cAMP in intestinal epithelial monolayers. *J Clin Invest* 1992;90:1608–1613.
102. Gariepy J, Lane A, Frayman F, et al. Structure of the toxic domain of the *Escherichia coli* heat-stable enterotoxin ST1. *Biochemistry* 1986;25:7854–7866.
103. Cohen MB, Guarino A, Shukla R, et al. Age-related differences in receptors for *Escherichia coli* heat-stable enterotoxin in the small and large intestine of children. *Gastroenterology* 1988;94: 367–373.
104. Guarino A, Cohen MB, Giannella RA. Small and large intestinal guanylate cyclase activity in children: effect of age and stimulation by *Escherichia coli* heat-stable enterotoxin. *Pediatr Res* 1987;21:551–555.
105. Nobles M, Diener M, Rummel W. Segment-specific effects of the heat-stable enterotoxin of *E. coli* on electrolyte transport in the rat colon. *Eur J Pharmacol* 1991;202:201–211.
106. Dean EA, Whipp SC, Moon HW. Age-specific colonization of porcine intestinal epithelium by 987P-piliated enterotoxigenic *Escherichia coli. Infect Immun* 1989;57:82–87.
107. Runnels PL, Moon HW, Schneider RA. Development of resistance with host age to adhesion of K99+ *Escherichia coli* to isolated intestinal epithelial cells. *Infect Immun* 1980;28: 298–300.
108. Saeed AM, McMillan R, Huckelberry V, et al. Specific receptor for *Escherichia coli* heat-stable enterotoxin (STa) may determine susceptibility of piglets to diarrheal disease. *FEMS Microbiol Lett* 1987;43:247–251.
109. Cohen MB, Moyer MS, Luttrell M, et al. The immature rat small intestine exhibits an increased response and sensitivity to *Escherichia coli* heat-stable enterotoxin. *Pediatr Res* 1986;20: 555–560.
110. Guarino A, Cohen M, Thompson M, et al. T84 cell receptor binding and guanylate cyclase activation by *E. coli* heat stable toxin. *Am J Physiol* 1987;253:G775–G780.
111. Mezoff AG, Jensen NJ, Cohen MB. Mechanisms of increased susceptibility of immature and weaned pigs to *Escherichia coli* heat-stable enterotoxin. *Pediatr Res* 1991;29:424–428.
112. Mann EA, Jump ML, Wu J, et al. Mice lacking the guanylyl cyclase C receptor are resistant it STa-induced intestinal secretion. *Biochem Biophys Res Commun* 1997;239:463–466.
113. Schulz S, Lopez MJ, Kuhn M, et al. Disruption of the guanylyl cyclase C gene leads to a paradoxical phenotype of viable but heat-stable enterotoxin-resistant mice. *J Clin Invest* 1997;100: 1590–1595.
114. Charney AN, Egnor RW, Alexander-Chacko JT, et al. Effect of *E. coli* heat-stable enterotoxin on colonic transport in guanylyl cyclase C receptor-deficient mice. *Am J Physiol Gastrointest Liver Physiol* 2001;280:G216–221.
115. Zhou RH, Pratha VA, Hogan DL, et al. Guanylate cyclase C plays a major role in duodenal mucosal bicarbonate secretion. *Gastroenterology* 1999;116:890–891.
116. Mann EA, Sheil-Puopolo MP, Giannella RA. Guanylyl cyclase C deficient mice have more severe carbon tetrachloride induced liver injury that wild-type controls. *Gastroenterology* 2000;118:292.
117. Guerrant RL, Hughes JM, Chang B, et al. Activation of intestinal guanylate cyclase by heat-stable enterotoxin of *Escherichia coli:* studies of tissue specificity, potential receptors, and intermediates. *J Infect Dis* 1980;142:220–228.
118. Schulz S, Chrisman TD, Garbers DL. Cloning and expression of guanylin. Its existence in various mammalian tissues. *J Biol Chem* 1992;267:16019–16021.
119. Laney DW Jr, Mann EA, Dellon SC, et al. Novel sites for expression of *Escherichia coli* heat-stable enterotoxin receptor in the developing rat. *Am J Physiol* 1992;263:G816–G821.
120. Zhang ZH, Jow F, Numann R, et al. The airway epithelium: a novel site of action by guanylin. *Biochem Biophys Res Commun* 1998;244:50–56.
121. Laney DW Jr, Bezerra JA, Kosiba JL, et al. Upregulation of the *Escherichia coli* heat stable enterotoxin receptor in the regenerating rat liver. *Am J Physiol* 1994;29:G899–G906.
122. Takao T, Tominga N, Shimonshi Y. Primary structure of heat-stable enterotoxin produced by *Yersinia enterocolitica. Biochem Biophys Res Commun* 1984;125:845–851.
123. Rao MC, Guandalini S, Laird W, et al. Effects of heat stable enterotoxin of *Yersinia enterocolitica* on ion transport and cyclic guanosine 3',5'-monophosphate metabolism in rabbit ileum. *Infect Immun* 1979;26:875–879.
124. Takao T, Shimonishi Y, Kobayashi M, et al. Amino acid sequence of heat-stable enterotoxin produced by *Vibrio cholerae* non-O1. *FEBS Lett* 1985;193:250–254.
125. Arita M, Takeda T, Honda T, et al. Purification and characterization of *Vibrio cholerae* non-O1 heat-stable enterotoxin. *Infect Immun* 1986;52:45–49.
126. Nair GB, Takeda Y. The heat-stable enterotoxins. *Microb Pathog* 1998;24:123–131.
127. Alessio M, Albano F, Tarallo L, et al. Interspecific plasmid transfer and modification of heat-stable enterotoxin expression by *Klebsiella pneumoniae* for infants with diarrhea. *Pediatr Res* 1993;33:205–208.
128. Savarino SJ, Fasano A, Watson J, et al. Enteroaggregative *Escherichia coli* heat-stable enterotoxin 1 represents another subfamily of *E. coli* heat-stable toxin. *Proc Natl Acad Sci U S A* 1993;90:3093–3097.
129. Savarino SJ, Fasano A, Robertson DC, et al. Enteroaggregative *Escherichia coli* elaborate a heat-stable enterotoxin demonstrable in an in vitro rabbit intestinal model. *J Clin Invest* 1991;87: 1450–1455.
130. Levine MM, Prado V, Robins-Browne R, et al. Use of DNA probes and HEp-2 cell adherence assay to detect diarrheogenic *Escherichia coli. J Infect Dis* 1988;158:224–228.
131. Bhan MK, Raj P, Levine MM, et al. Enteroaggregative *Escherichia coli* associated with persistent diarrhea in cohort of rural children in India. *J Infect Dis* 1989;159:1601–1604.
132. Cravioto A, Tello A, Navarro A, et al. Association of *Escherichia coli* HEp-2 adherence patterns with type and duration of diarrhea. *Lancet* 1991;337:262–264.
133. Wanke CA, Shorling JB, Barrett LJ, et al. Potential role of adherence traits of *Escherichia coli* in persistent diarrhea in an urban Brazilian slum. *Pediatr Infect Dis* 1991;10:746–751.
134. Echeverria P, Serichantalerg S, Changchawalit S, et al. Tissue culture-adherent *Escherichia coli* in infantile diarrhea. *J Infect Dis* 1992;165:141–143.
135. Giron JA, Jones T, Millan-Velasco F, et al. Diffuse adhering *Escherichia coli* (DAEC) as a putative cause of diarrhea in Mayan children in Mexico. *J Infect Dis* 1991;163:507–513.
136. Gomes TAT, Blake PA, Tabulsi LR. Prevalence of *Escherichia coli* strains with localized, diffuse and aggregative adherence to HeLa cells in infants with diarrhea and matched controls. *J Clin Microbiol* 1989;27:266–269.
137. Cohen MB, Hawkins JA, Weckbach LS, et al. Colonization by enteroaggregative *Escherichia coli* in travelers with and without diarrhea. *J Clin Microbiol* 1993;31:351–353.
138. Forte LR, Hamra FK. Guanylin and uroguanylin: intestinal peptide hormones that regulate epithelial transport. *New Physiol Sci* 1996;11:17–24.
139. Forte LR. Guanylin regulatory peptides: structures, biological activities mediated by cyclic GMP and pathobiology. *Reg Peptides* 1999;81:25–39.
140. Hamra FK, Forte LR, Eber SL, et al. Uroguanylin: structure and activity of a second endogenous peptide that stimulates intestinal guanylate cyclase. *Proc Natl Acad Sci U S A* 1993;90:10464–10468.

141. Forte LR, Eber SL, Turner JT, et al. Guanylin stimulation of Cl^- secretion in human intestinal T84 cells via cyclic guanosine monophosphate. *J Clin Invest* 1993;91:2423–2428.
142. Joo NS, London RM, Kim HD, et al. Regulation of intestinal Cl^- and HCO_3 secretion by uroguanylin. *Am J Physiol* 1998; 274:G633–644.
143. Greenberg RN, Hill M, Crytzer J, et al. Comparison of effects of uroguanylin, guanylin, and *E. coli* heat-stable enterotoxin STa in mouse intestine and kidney: evidence that uroguanylin is an intestinal natriuretic hormone. *J Invest Med* 1997;45: 276–283.
144. Whitaker TL, Witte DP, Scott MC, et al. Uroguanylin and guanylin: distinct but overlapping patterns of expression in mouse intestine. *Gastroenterology* 1997;113:1000–1006.
145. Martin S, Adermann K, Forssmann WG, et al. Regulated, side-directed secretion of proguanylin from isolated rat colonic mucosa. *Endocrinology* 1999;140:5022–5029.
146. Garbers DL. Guanylyl cyclase receptors and their endocrine, paracrine and autocrine ligands. *Cell* 1992;71:1–4.
147. Forte LR, London RM, Freeman RH, et al. Guanylin peptides: renal actions mediated by cyclic GMP. *Am J Physiol* 2000;278: F180–F191.
148. Kita T, Kitamura K, Sakata J, et al. Marked increase of guanylin secretion in response to salt loading in the rat small intestine. *Am J Physiol* 1999;277:G960–G966.
149. Evans DG, Evans DJ Jr, Pierce NF. Differences in the response of rabbit small intestine to heat-labile and heat-stable enterotoxins of *Escherichia coli. Infect Immun* 1973;7:873–880.
150. Dean AG, Ching Y, Williams RG, et al. Test of *Escherichia coli* enterotoxin using infant mice: application in a study of diarrhea in children in Honolulu. *J Infect Dis* 1972;125:407–411.
151. Giannella RA. Suckling mouse model for detection of heat-stable *Escherichia coli* enterotoxin: characteristics of the model. *Infect Immun* 1976;14:95–99.
152. Choudry MA, Gupta S, Yadava JN. Guinea pig ileal loop assay: a better replacement of the suckling mouse assay for detection of heat-stable enterotoxins of *Escherichia coli. J Trop Med Hyg* 1991;94:234–240.
153. Giannella RA, Drake KW, Luttrell M. Development of a radioimmunoassay for *Escherichia coli* heat stable enterotoxin. *Infect Immun* 1981;33:186–192.
154. Frantz JC, Robertson DC. Immunological properties of *Escherichia coli* heat-stable enterotoxins: development of a radioimmunoassay specific for heat-stable enterotoxins with suckling mouse activity. *Infect Immun* 1981;33:193–198.
155. Thompson MR, Jordan RL, Luttrell MA, et al. Blinded, two-laboratory comparative analysis of *Escherichia coli* heat-stable enterotoxin production by using monoclonal antibody enzyme-linked immunosorbent assay, radioimmunoassay, suckling mouse assay and gene probes. *J Clin Microbiol* 1986;24: 753–758.
156. Cryan B. Comparison of three assay systems for detection of enterotoxigenic *Escherichia coli* heat-stable enterotoxin. *J Clin Microbiol* 1990;28:792–794.
157. Scotland SM, Willshaw GA, Said B, et al. Identification of *Escherichia coli* that produces heat-stable enterotoxin STa by a commercially available enzyme-linked immunoassay and comparison of the assay with infant mouse and DNA probe tests. *J Clin Microbiol* 1989;27:1697–1699.
158. Moseley SL, Echeverria P, Seriwatana J, et al. Identification of enterotoxigenic *Escherichia coli* by colony blot hybridization using three gene probes. *J Infect Dis* 1982;145:863–869.
159. Echeverria P, Taylor DN, Seriwatana J, et al. A comparative study of enterotoxin gene probes and tests for toxin production to detect enterotoxigenic *Escherichia coli. J Infect Dis* 1986; 153:255–260.
160. Gicquelais KG, Baldini MM, Martinez J, et al. Practical and economical method for using biotinylated DNA probes with bacterial colony blots to identify diarrhea-causing *Escherichia coli. J Clin Microbiol* 1990;28:2485–2490.
161. Bopp CA, Threatt VL, Moseley SL, et al. A comparison of alkaline phosphatase and radiolabeled gene probes with bioassays for enterotoxigenic *Escherichia coli. Mol Cell Probes* 1990;4:193–203.
162. Cryan B. Comparison of the synthetic oligonucleotide gene probe and infant mouse bioassay for detection of enterotoxigenic *Escherichia coli. Eur J Clin Microbiol Infect Dis* 1990;9: 229–232.
163. Abe A, Komase K, Bangtrakulnonth A, et al. Trivalent heat-labile and heat-stable enterotoxin probe conjugated with horseradish peroxidase for detection of enterotoxigenic *Escherichia coli* by hybridization. *J Clin Microbiol* 1990;28:2616–2620.
164. Saez-Llorens X, Guzman-Verduzco LM, Shelton S, et al. Simultaneous detection of *Escherichia coli* heat-stable and heat labile enterotoxin genes with a single RNA probe. *J Clin Microbiol* 1989;27:1684–1688.
165. Hornes E, Wasteson Y, Olsvik O. Detection of *Escherichia coli* heat-stable enterotoxin genes in pig stool specimens by immobilized, colorimetric, nested polymerase chain reaction. *J Clin Microbiol* 1991;29:2375–2379.
166. Moon HW, Whipp SC. Development of resistance with age by swine intestine to effects of enteropathogenic *Escherichia coli. J Infect Dis* 1970;122:220–223.
167. Burgess MN, Bywater RJ, Cowley CM, et al. Biological evaluation of a methanol-soluble, heat-stable *Escherichia coli* enterotoxin in infant mice, pigs, rabbits and calves. *Infect Immun* 1978;21:526–531.
168. Whipp SC, Moseley SL, Moon HW. Microscopic alterations in jejunal epithelium of 3-week old pigs induced by pig-specific, mouse-negative, heat-stable *Escherichia coli* enterotoxin. *Am J Vet Res* 1986;47:615–618.
169. Rose R, Whipp SC, Moon HW. Effects of *Escherichia coli* heat-stable enterotoxin b on small intestinal villi in pigs, rabbits and lambs. *Vet Pathol* 1987;24:71–79.
170. Kennedy DJ, Greenberg RN, Dunn JA, et al. Effects of *Escherichia coli* heat-stable enterotoxin STb on intestines of mice, rats, rabbits and piglets. *Infect Immun* 1984;46:639–643.
171. Hitotsubashi S, Fujii Y, Yamanaka H, et al. Some properties of purified *Escherichia coli* heat-stable enterotoxin II. *Infect Immun* 1992;60:4468–4474.
172. Whipp SC. Protease degradation of *Escherichia coli* heat-stable, mouse-negative, pig-positive enterotoxin. *Infect Immun* 1987; 55:2057–2060.
173. Whipp SC. Assay of enterotoxigenic *Escherichia coli* heat-stable toxin b in rats and mice. *Infect Immun* 1990;58:930–934.
174. Whipp SC. Intestinal responses to enterotoxigenic *Escherichia coli* heat-stable toxin b in non-porcine species. *Am J Vet Res* 1991;52:734–737.
175. Lee CH, Moseley SL, Moon HW, et al. Characterization of the gene encoding heat-stable toxin II and preliminary molecular epidemiological studies of enterotoxigenic *Escherichia coli* heat-stable toxin II producers. *Infect Immun* 1983;42:264–268.
176. Picken RN, Mazaitis AJ, Maas WK, et al. Nucleotide sequence of the gene for heat-stable enterotoxin II of *Escherichia coli. Infect Immun* 1983;42:269–275.
177. Kupersztoch YM, Tachias K, Mooman CR, et al. Secretion of methanol-insoluble heat-stable enterotoxin (STb): energy and secA dependent conversion of pre-STb to an intermediate indistinguishable from the extracellular toxin. *J Bacteriol* 1990;172: 2427–2432.
178. Fujii Y, Hayashi M, Hitotsubashi S, et al. Purification and characterization of *Escherichia coli* heat-stable enterotoxin II. *J Bacteriol* 1991;173:5516–5522.
179. Dreyfus LA, Urban RG, Whipp SC, et al. Purification of the

STb enterotoxin of *Escherichia coli* and the role of selected amino acids on its secretion, stability and toxicity. *Mol Microbiol* 1992;6:2397–2406.
180. Urban RG, Pipper EM, Dreyfus LA. Monoclonal antibodies specific for the *Escherichia coli* heat-stable enterotoxin STb. *J Clin Microbiol* 1991;29:1963–1968.
181. Weikel CS, Nellans HN, Guerrant RL. *In vivo* and *in vitro* effects of a novel enterotoxin, STb, produced by *Escherichia coli. J Infect Dis* 1986;153:893–901.
182. Greenberg RN, Chang B, Murad F, et al. Lack of effect of porcine *Escherichia coli* enterotoxin (STb) on cyclic nucleotide metabolism. *Clin Res* 1980;28:830.
183. Weikel S, Guerrant RL. STb enterotoxin of *Escherichia coli:* cyclic nucleotide independent secretion. In: Evered D, Whelan J, eds. *Microbial toxins and diarrhoeal disease.* Ciba Foundation Symposium 112. London: Pitman, 1985:94–115.
184. Dreyfus LA, Harville B, Howard DE, et al. Calcium influx mediated by the *Escherichia coli* heat-stable enterotoxin B (STB). *Proc Natl Acad Sci U S A* 1993;90:3202–3206.
185. Rousset E, Dubreuil JD. Evidence that *Escherichia coli* STb enterotoxin binds to lipidic components extracted from the pig jejunal mucosa. *Toxicon* 1999;37:1529–1537.
186. Rousset E, Harel J, Dubreuil JD. Sulfatide from the pig jejunum brush border epithelial cell surface is involved in binding of *Escherichia coli* enterotoxin b. *Infect Immun* 1998;66:5650–5658.
187. Weikel CS, Tiemens KM, Moseley SL, et al. Species specificity and lack of production of STb enterotoxin by *Escherichia coli* strains isolated from humans with diarrheal illness. *Infect Immun* 1986;52:323–325.
188. Echeverria P, Seriwatana J, Patamaroj U, et al. Prevalence of heat-stable II enterotoxigenic *Escherichia coli* in pigs, water, and people at farms in Thailand as determined by DNA hybridization. *J Clin Microbiol* 1984;19:489–491.
189. Echeverria P, Seriwatana J, Taylor DN, et al. Identification by DNA hybridization of enterotoxigenic *Escherichia coli* in a longitudinal study of villages in Thailand. *J Infect Dis* 1985;151: 124–130.
190. Lortie LA, Dubreuil JD, Harel J. Characterization of *Escherichia coli* strains producing heat-stable enterotoxin b (STb) isolated from humans with diarrhea. *J Clin Microbiol* 1991;29:656–659.
191. Okamoto K, Fujii Y, Akashi N, et al. Identification and characterization of heat-stable enterotoxin-II producing *Escherichia coli* from patients with diarrhea. *Microbiol Immunol* 1993;37: 411–414.
192. Honda T, Tsuji T, Takeda Y, et al. Immunological nonidentity of heat-labile enterotoxins from human and porcine enterotoxigenic *Escherichia coli. Infect Immun* 1981;33:677–682.
193. Qu Z-H, Boesman-Finkelstein M, Kazemi M, et al. Heterogeneity of immunotypes of heat-labile enterotoxins of enterotoxigenic *Escherichia coli* of human origin. *J Infect Dis* 1991; 164:796–799.
194. Gill DM, Clements JD, Robertson DC, et al. Subunit number and arrangement in *Escherichia coli* heat-labile enterotoxin. *Infect Immun* 1981;33:677–682.
195. Spicer EK, Kavanaugh WM, Dallas WS, et al. Sequence homologies between A subunits of *Escherichia coli* and *Vibrio cholerae* enterotoxins. *Proc Natl Acad Sci U S A* 1981;78:50–54.
196. Spicer EK, Noble JA. *Escherichia coli* heat-labile enterotoxin. Nucleotide sequence of the A subunit gene. *J Biol Chem* 1982; 257:5716–5721.
197. Dallas WS, Falkow S. Amino acid sequence homology between cholera toxin and *Escherichia coli* heat-labile toxin. *Nature* 1980; 288:499–501.
198. Lockman H, Kaper JB. Nucleotide sequence analysis of the A2 and B subunits of *Vibrio cholerae* enterotoxin. *J Biol Chem* 1983;258:13722–13726.
199. Mekalanos JJ, Swartz DJ, Pearson GD, et al. Cholera toxin genes; nucleotide sequence, deletion analysis and vaccine development. *Nature* 1983;306:551–557.
200. Yamamoto T, Nakazawa T, Miyata T, et al. Evolution and structure of two ADP-ribosylation enterotoxins: *Escherichia coli* heat-labile and cholera toxin. *FEBS Lett* 1984;169:241–246.
201. Evans DJ, Chen LC, Curlin GT, et al. Stimulation of adenyl cyclase by *Escherichia coli* enterotoxin. *Nature* 1972;236: 137–138.
202. Gill DM, Evans DJ Jr, Evans DG. Mechanism of activation of adenylate cyclase in vitro by polymyxin-released, heat-labile enterotoxin of *Escherichia coli. J Infect Dis* 1976;133: S103–S107.
203. Moss J, Garrison S, Fishman PH, et al. Gangliosides sensitize unresponsive fibroblasts to *Escherichia coli* heat-labile enterotoxin. *J Clin Invest* 1979;64:381–384.
204. Holmgren J. Comparison of the tissue receptors for *Vibrio cholerae* and *Escherichia coli* enterotoxins by means of gangliosides and natural cholera toxoid. *Infect Immun* 1973;8:851–859.
205. Holmgren J, Fredman P, Lindblad M, et al. Rabbit intestinal glycoprotein receptor for *Escherichia coli* heat-labile enterotoxin lacking affinity for cholera toxin. *Infect Immun* 1982;38:424–433.
206. Griffiths SL, Critchley DR. Characterisation of the binding sites for *Escherichia coli* heat-labile toxin type I in intestinal brush borders. *Biochem Biophys Acta* 1991;1075:154–161.
207. Holmgren J, Lindblad M, Fredman P, et al. Comparison of receptors for cholera and *Escherichia coli* enterotoxins in human intestine. *Gastroenterology* 1985;89:27–35.
208. Zemelman BV, Chu S-HW, Walker WA. Host response to *Escherichia coli* heat-labile enterotoxin via two microvillus membrane receptors in the rat intestine. *Infect Immun* 1989;57: 2947–2952.
209. Sears CL, Kaper JB. Enteric bacterial toxins: mechanisms of action and linkage to intestinal secretion. *Microbiol Rev* 1996; 60:167–215.
210. Green BA, Neill RJ, Ruyechan WT, et al. Evidence that a new enterotoxin of *Escherichia coli* which activates adenylate cyclase in eucaryotic target cells is not plasmid mediated. *Infect Immun* 1983;41:383–389.
211. Chang PP, Moss J, Twiddy EM, et al. Type II heat-labile enterotoxin of *Escherichia coli* activates adenylate cyclase in human fibroblasts by ADP ribosylation. *Infect Immun* 1987;55: 1854–1858.
212. Donta ST, Tomicic T, Holmes RK. Binding of class II *Escherichia coli* enterotoxins to mouse Y1 and intestinal cells. *Infect Immun* 1992;60:2870–2873.
213. Pickett CL, Weinstein DL, Holmes RK. Genetics of type IIa heat-labile enterotoxin of *Escherichia coli:* operon fusions, nucleotides sequence, and hybridization studies. *J Bacteriol* 1987;169:5180–5187.
214. Fukuta S, Magnani JL, Twiddy EM, et al. Comparison of the carbohydrate-binding specificities of cholera toxin and *Escherichia coli* heat-labile enterotoxins LTh-1 and LT-IIb. *Infect Immun* 1988;56:1748–1753.
215. Back E, Molby R, Kaijser B, et al. Enterotoxigenic *Escherichia coli* and other gram-negative bacteria of infantile diarrhea: surface antigens, hemagglutinins, colonization factor antigen, and loss of enterotoxigenicity. *J Infect Dis* 1980;142:318–326.
216. Schultz AJ, McCardell BA. DNA homology and immunological cross-reactivity between *Aeromonas hydrophila* cytotonic toxin and cholera toxin. *J Clin Microbiol* 1988;26:57–61.
217. Rose JM, Houston CW, Cappenhaver DH, et al. Purification and chemical characterization of cholera toxin: cross-reactive cytolytic enterotoxin produced by a human isolate of *Aeromonas hydrophila. Infect Immun* 1989;57:1165–1169.
218. Gardner SE, Fowiston SE, Geroge WL. In vitro production of

cholera toxin-like activity by *Plesiomonas shigelloides. J Infect Dis* 1987;156:720–722.
219. Ruiz-Palacios GM, Torres J, Torres NI, et al. Cholera-like enterotoxin produced by *Campylobacter jejuni:* characteristics and clinical significance. *Lancet* 1983;2:250–253.
220. Walker RI, Caldwell MB, Lee EC, et al. Pathophysiology of *Campylobacter* enteritis. *Microbiol Rev* 1986;50:81–94.
221. Jiwa SFH. Probing for enterotoxigenicity among the salmonellae. *J Clin Microbiol* 1981;14:463–472.
222. Finkelstein RA, Marchlewicz BA, McDonald RJ, et al. Isolation and characterization of a cholera-related enterotoxin from *Salmonella typhimurium. FEMS Microbiol Lett* 1983;17:239–241.
223. Baloda SB, Faris A, Krovacek K, et al. Cytotonic enterotoxins and cytotoxic factors produced by *Salmonella enteritidis* and *Salmonella typhimurium. Toxicon* 1983;21:785–796.
224. Honda T, Taga S, Takeda Y, et al. Modified Elek test for detection of heat-labile enterotoxin of enterotoxigenic *Escherichia coli. J Clin Microbiol* 1981;13:1–5.
225. Honda T, Arita M, Takeda Y, et al. Further evaluation of the Biken (modified Elek test) for detection of enterotoxigenic *Escherichia coli* producing heat-labile enterotoxin and application of the test to sampling of heat-stable enterotoxin. *J Clin Microbiol* 1982;16:60–62.
226. Sutton RGA, Merson M, Craig JP, et al. Evaluation of the Biken test for the detection of LT-producing *Escherichia coli.* In: Takeda Y, Miwatani T, eds. *Bacterial diarrheal diseases.* Tokyo: KTK, 1985:209–218.
227. Donta ST, Moon HW, Whipp SC. Detection of heat-labile *Escherichia coli* enterotoxin with the use of adrenal cells in tissue culture. *Science* 1974;183:334–336.
228. Scotland SM, Gross RJ, Rowe B. Laboratory tests for enterotoxin production, enteroinvasion and adhesion in diarrheogenic *Escherichia coli.* In: Sussman M, ed. *The virulence of* Escherichia coli. *Reviews and methods.* London: Academic Press, 1985: 395–405.
229. Guerrant RL, Brunton LL, Schnaitman TC, et al. Cyclic adenosine monophosphate and alteration of Chinese hamster ovary cell morphology: a rapid, sensitive, in vitro assay for the enterotoxins of *Vibrio cholerae* and *Escherichia coli. Infect Immun* 1974;10:320–327.
230. Guerrant RL, Brunton LL. Characterization of the Chinese hamster ovary cell assay for the enterotoxins of *Vibrio cholerae* and *Escherichia coli* and for antitoxins: differential inhibition by gangliosides, specific antisera and toxoid. *J Infect Dis* 1977;135: 720–728.
231. Bongaerts GPA, Bruggeman-Ogle KM, Mouton RP. Improvements in the microtire GM_1 ganglioside enzyme-linked immunosorbent assay for *Escherichia coli* heat-labile enterotoxin. *J Appl Bacteriol* 1985;59:443–449.
232. Evans DJ Jr, Evans DG. Direct serological assay for the heat-labile enterotoxin of *Escherichia coli* using passive immune homolysis. *Infect Immun* 1977;16:604–609.
233. Yolken RH, Greenberg HB, Merson MH, et al. Enzyme-linked immunosorbent assay for detection of *Escherichia coli* heat-labile enterotoxin. *J Clin Microbiol* 1977;5:439–444.
234. Finkelstein RA, Yang Z. Rapid test for identification of heat labile enterotoxin of *Escherichia coli* colonies. *J Clin Microbiol* 1983;18:1417–1418.
235. Finkelstein RA, Yang Z, Moseley LS, et al. Rapid latex particle agglutination test for *Escherichia coli* strains of porcine origin producing heat-labile enterotoxin. *J Clin Microbiol* 1983;18: 1417–1418.
236. Ito T, Kuwahara S, Yokota T. Automatic and manual latex agglutination tests for measurement of cholera toxin and heat-labile enterotoxin of *Escherichia coli. J Clin Microbiol* 1983;17:7–12.
237. Scotland SM, Flowmen RH, Rowe B. Evaluation of a reversed passive latex agglutination test for detection of *Escherichia coli* heat-labile toxin in culture supernatants. *J Clin Microbiol* 1989; 27:339–340.
238. Speirs J, Stavric S, Buchanan B. Assessment of two commercial agglutination kits for detecting *Escherichia coli* heat-labile enterotoxin. *Can J Microbiol* 1991;37:877–880.
239. Bettelheim KA, Hanna N, Smith DL, et al. Evaluation of the Phadebact ETEC-LT test for the heat-labile enterotoxin of *Escherichia coli. Int J Med Microbiol* 1989;271:70–76.
240. Chapman PA, Daly CM. Comparison of Y1 mouse adrenal cell and coagglutination assays for detection of *Escherichia coli* heat-labile enterotoxin. *J Clin Pathol* 1989;42:755–758.
241. Wernars K, Delfgou E, Soentoro PS, et al. Successful approach for detection of low numbers of enterotoxigenic *Escherichia coli* in minced meat by using the polymerase chain reaction. *Appl Environ Microbiol* 1991;57:1914–1919.
242. Moseley SL, Huq I, Alim ARMA, et al. Detection of enterotoxigenic *Escherichia coli* by DNA colony hybridization. *J Infect Dis* 1980;142892–142898.
243. Olive DM, Khalik DA, Sethi SK. Identification of enterotoxigenic *Escherichia coli* using alkaline phosphatase-labeled synthetic oligodeoxyribonucleotide probes. *Eur J Clin Microbiol Infect Dis* 1988;7:167–171.
244. Dallas WS, Gill DM, Falkow S. Cistrons encoding *Escherichia coli* heat-labile toxin. *J Bacteriol* 1979;139:850–858.
245. Nalin DR, McLaughlin JC, Rahaman M, et al. Enteropathogenic *Escherichia coli* and idiopathic diarrhea in Bangladesh. *Lancet* 1975;2:1116–1119.
246. Merson MH, Sack RB, Islam S, et al. Disease due to enterotoxigenic *Escherichia coli* in Bangladeshi adults: clinical aspects in a controlled trial of tetracycline. *J Infect Dis* 1980;141:702–708.
247. Echeverria P, Blacklow NR, Sanford LB, et al. Travelers diarrhea among peace corps volunteers in Thailand. *J Infect Dis* 1981; 143:767–771.
248. Santosham M, Burns B, Nadkarni V, et al. Oral rehydration therapy for acute diarrhea in ambulatory children in the United States: a double-blind comparison of four different solutions. *Pediatrics* 1985;76:159–164.
249. Black RE, Levine MM, Clements ML, et al. Treatment of experimentally induced enterotoxigenic *Escherichia coli* with trimethoprim-sulfamethoxazole or a placebo. *Rev Infect Dis* 1982;4:540–545.
250. DuPont HL, Reves RR, Galindo E, et al. Treatment of travelers' diarrhea with trimethoprim/sulfamethoxazole and with trimethoprim alone. *N Engl J Med* 1982;307:841–844.
251. Lester SC, de Pilar-Pla M, Perez-Schael I, et al. The carriage of *Escherichia coli* resistant to antimicrobial agents in healthy children in Boston, in Caracas and in Qin Pu, China. *N Engl J Med* 1990;323:285–289.
252. Murray BE, Rensimer ER, DuPont HL. Emergence of high-level trimethoprim resistance in fecal *Escherichia coli* during oral administration of trimethoprim or trimethoprim-sulfamethoxazole. *N Engl J Med* 1982;306:130–135.
253. Ericsson CD, Tannenbaum C, Charles TT. Antisecretory and antiinflammatory properties of bismuth subsalicylate. *Rev Infect Dis* 1990;12:S16–S20.
254. DuPont HL, Sullivan P, Pickering LK, et al. Symptomatic treatment of diarrhea with bismuth subsalicylate among students attending a Mexican University. *Gastroenterology* 1977;73: 715–718.
255. DuPont HL, Sullivan P, Evans DG, et al. Prevention of traveler's diarrhea: prophylactic administration of subsalicylate bismuth. *JAMA* 1980;243:237–241.
256. Ericsson CD, Johnson PL, DuPont HL, et al. Ciprofloxacin or trimethoprim-sulfamethoxazole as initial therapy for traveler's diarrhea. *Ann Intern Med* 1987;106:216–220.

257. Levine MM, Kaper JB, Black RE, et al. New knowledge on pathogenesis of bacterial infections as applied to vaccine development. *Microbiol Rev* 1983;47:510–550.
258. Levine MM, Morris JG, Losonsky G, et al. Fimbriae (pili) adhesins as vaccines. In: Lark D, Normak S, Brent-Uhiln E, eds. *Protein-carbohydrate interactions in biological systems.* London: Academic Press, 1986:143–145.
259. Levine MM. Development of vaccines against bacteria. In: Farthing MJG, Keusch GT, eds. *Enteric infection: mechanisms, manifestations and management.* New York: Raven Press, 1989: 495–508.
260. Levine MM, Kaper JB, Herrington D, et al. Volunteer studies of deletion mutants of *Vibrio cholerae* C1 prepared by recombinant techniques. *Infect Immun* 1987;56:161–167.
261. Sack RB, Kline RL, Spira WM. Oral immunization of rabbits with enterotoxigenic *Escherichia coli* protects against intraintestinal challenge. *Infect Immun* 1988;56:387–394.
262. Lopez-Vidal Y, Calva JJ, Trujillo A, et al. Enterotoxins and adhesins of enterotoxigenic *Escherichia coli:* are they risk factors for acute diarrhea in the community? *J Infect Dis* 1990;162: 442–447.
263. Clemens JD, El-Morshiday S. Construction of a potential live oral bivalent vaccine for typhoid fever and cholera—*Escherichia coli* related diarrheas. *Infect Immun* 1984;46:564–569.
264. Yamamoto T, Tamura Y, Yokota T. Enteroadhesion fimbriae and enterotoxin of *Escherichia coli:* genetic transfer to a streptomycin-resistant mutant of the *GalE* oral-route live-vaccine *Salmonella typhi* Ty21a. *Infect Immun* 1985;50:925–928.
265. Klipstein FA, Engert RF, Houghton RA. Immunization of volunteers with a synthetic peptide vaccine for enterotoxigenic *Escherichia coli. Lancet* 1986;1:471–473.
266. Houghton RA, Engert RF, Osteresh JM, et al. A completely synthetic toxoid vaccine containing *Escherichia coli* heat-stable toxin and antigenic determinants of the heat-labile toxin and antigenic determinants of the heat-labile toxin B subunit. *Infect Immun* 1985;48:735–740.
267. Evans DG, Graham DY, Evans DG. Administration of purified colonization factor antigens (CFA/I, CFA/II) of enterotoxigenic *Escherichia coli* to volunteers. *Gastroenterology* 1984;87: 934–940.
268. Edelman R, Russell RG, Losonsky G, et al. Immunization of rabbits with enterotoxigenic *Escherichia coli* colonization factor antigen (CFA/I) encapsulated in biodegradable microspheres of poly(lactide-co-glycolide). *Vaccine* 1993;11:155–158.
269. Reid RH, Boedeker EC, McQueen CE, et al. Preclinical evaluation of microencapsulated CFA/II oral vaccine against enterotoxigenic *Escherichia coli. Vaccine* 1993;11:159–193.
270. Moon HW, Bunn TO. Vaccines for preventing enterotoxigenic *Escherichia coli* infections in farm animals. *Vaccine* 1993;11: 213–220.
271. Jertborn M, Ahren C, Holmgren J, et al. Safety and immunogenicity of an oral inactivated enterotoxigenic *Escherichia coli* vaccine. *Vaccine* 1998;16:255–260.
272. Cohen D, Orr N, Haim M, et al. Safety and immunogenicity of two different lots of the oral, killed enterotoxigenic *Escherichia coli*-cholera toxin B subunit vaccine in Israeli young adults. *Infect Immun* 2000;68:4492–4497.
273. Savarino SJ, Hall ER, Bassily S, et al. Oral, inactivated, whole cell enterotoxigenic *Escherichia coli* plus cholera toxin B subunit vaccine: results of the initial evaluation in children. PRIDE Study Group. *J Infect Dis* 1999;179:107–114.
274. O'Farrelly C, Branton D, Wanke CA. Oral ingestion of egg yolk immunoglobulin from hens immunized with an enterotoxigenic *Escherichia coli* strain prevents diarrhea in rabbits challenged with the same strain. *Infect Immun* 1992;60:2593–2597.
275. Yokoyama H, Peralta RC, Diaz R, et al. Passive protective effect of chicken egg yolk immunoglobulins against experimental enterotoxigenic *Escherichia coli* infection in neonatal piglets. *Infect Immun* 1992;60:998–1007.
276. Freedman DJ, Tacket CO, Delehanty A, et al. Milk immunoglobulin with specific activity against purified colonization factor antigens can protect against oral challenge with enterotoxigenic *Escherichia coli. J Infect Dis* 1998;177:662–667.
277. Tacket CO, Losonsky G, Livio S, et al. Lack of prophylactic efficacy of an enteric-coated bovine hyperimmune milk product against enterotoxigenic *Escherichia coli* challenge administered during a standard meal. *J Infect Dis* 1999;180:2056–2059.
278. Mason HS, Haq TA, Clements JD, et al. Edible vaccine protects mice against Escherichia coli heat-labile enterotoxin (LT): potatoes expressing a synthetic LT-B gene. *Vaccine* 1998;16:1336–1343.

40

ENTEROPATHOGENIC *ESCHERICHIA COLI*

MICHAEL S. DONNENBERG

DESCRIPTION

Enteropathogenic *Escherichia coli* (EPEC) strains comprise a unique class of intestinal pathogens with remarkable characteristics. EPEC was the first group of *E. coli* shown to cause diarrhea and has been responsible for devastating outbreaks of nosocomial neonatal diarrhea with extraordinary mortality. EPEC strains have been implicated by epidemiologic studies as important etiologic agents of infant diarrhea in virtually every continent. The mechanism by which EPEC strains cause disease, totally enigmatic until recently, is now yielding to experimental investigation and is currently appreciated as among the most fascinating examples of the host–parasite relationship under study.

Controversy over the identity of this class of diarrheogenic *E. coli* existed for decades and was rooted in our ignorance of the pathogenic mechanisms by which EPEC strains cause diarrhea. However, recent advances (described below) allow a more precise categorization of the strains that make up this class of *E. coli.* EPEC strains have been defined as a class of diarrheogenic *E. coli* organisms, pathogenic for humans, which *attach* intimately to and *efface* the microvilli of enterocytes but do not produce high levels of Shiga-like toxins (1). The attaching and effacing effect is characterized by intimate adherence of the bacteria to epithelial cells, with destruction of microvilli and the formation of cuplike pedestals composed of actin and other cytoskeletal proteins beneath the adherent organisms (Fig. 40.1A). "Typical" EPEC strains are defined as those that display a pattern of localized adherence (defined below) to tissue culture cells or those that produce the bundle-forming pilus (BFP) responsible for this pattern of adherence.

An understanding of the role of EPEC in human diarrheal disease requires examination of these strains from a historical perspective. For greater detail than can be presented here, the reader is referred to excellent reviews of the subject (2,3). *E. coli* was first widely accepted as a cause of diarrhea on the basis of epidemiologic investigations of outbreaks of community-acquired and nosocomial infantile gastroenteritis in the United Kingdom in the 1940s (4–7). These outbreaks were characterized by their explosive nature and extraordinary mortality rates, sometimes exceeding 50% (4,6,8). Investigations of these outbreaks depended on the recognition that strains of *E. coli* cultured from infants with diarrhea could be agglutinated by specific antiserum raised against isolates from index cases, whereas *E. coli* isolated from well children could not. Soon a number of serologically distinct strains had been isolated from outbreaks (7). With the advent of the serologic typing system of Kauffmann and Dupont (9), it was recognized that these early outbreak strains belonged to certain serogroups (particularly O111 and O55) that are rarely found among *E. coli* isolated from healthy individuals (9). Neter (10) coined the term enteropathogenic to refer specifically to the strains associated with infantile gastroenteritis long before it was appreciated that *E. coli* can cause diarrhea by more than one mechanism. Thus, the term diarrheogenic is often used generically, and enteropathogenic is understood to refer specifically to strains that cause diarrhea by the mechanism common to the originally reported isolates. More recently, many of the isolates from the original investigations of infantile gastroenteritis have been resurrected and confirmed to possess the virulence genes that are characteristic of this group (see below), thus validating the relationship between classic EPEC strains and those used in recent genetic investigations (11).

During the 1950s, additional serogroups were added to the list of those epidemiologically incriminated as causing diarrhea (2,3). Also during this period, human challenge studies confirmed the hypothesis that EPEC strains were pathogenic (12–14). However, with the discovery of the heat-labile and heat-stable enterotoxins of enterotoxigenic *E. coli* (ETEC) (see Chapter 39) and of the invasive properties of enteroinvasive strains of *E. coli* (EIEC) (Chapter 43), there

M. S. Donnenberg: Division of Infectious Diseases, Department of Medicine, University of Maryland, Baltimore, Maryland

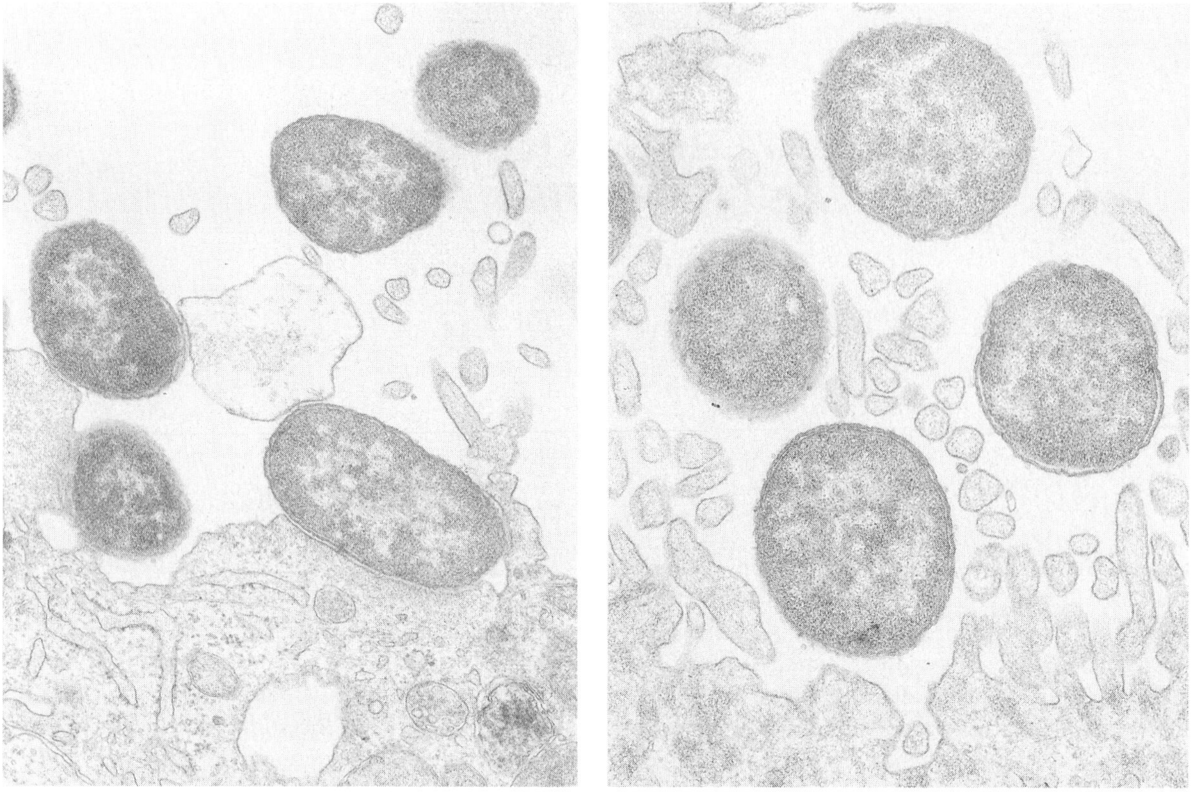

A B

FIGURE 40.1. Electron micrographs of Caco-2 intestinal tissue culture cells infected with **(A)** a wild type enteropathogenic *Escherichia coli* (EPEC) strain or **(B)** an isogenic mutant of that strain with an *eae* gene deletion. **A:** The attaching and effacing effect of EPEC on intestinal tissue culture cells; bacteria are found intimately attached to the epithelial cell, which responds by forming cuplike pedestals composed of cytoskeletal proteins. **B:** In contrast, the mutant adheres at a distance from the cells. (From Donnenberg MS, Kaper JB. Construction of an *eae* deletion mutant of enteropathogenic *Escherichia coli* by using a positive-selection suicide vector. *Infect Immun* 1991;59:4310–4317, with permission.)

ensued a period of confusion and doubt over the pathogenic potential of EPEC strains. Investigators soon realized that strains belonging to EPEC serogroups lacked the virulence characteristics associated with ETEC and EIEC (15,16). Some suggested that most strains belonging to EPEC serogroups were not pathogenic (16) while others speculated that, over the years, the original EPEC strains had lost plasmids necessary for virulence, accounting for their lack of definable virulence traits (17). These doubts were allayed when Levine et al. (18) reported that strains belonging to traditional EPEC serogroups, confirmed to lack features characteristic of ETEC and EIEC, maintained their pathogenicity in volunteer studies (18). Thus, new impetus was added to the search for pathogenic mechanisms of EPEC.

MICROBIOLOGY

EPEC Serotypes

EPEC organisms were originally distinguished from other *E. coli* organisms by serogroup (somatic lipopolysaccharide [LPS] O antigen testing) or serotype (flagellar H antigen and O antigen testing) (2,3,19). Some serotypes, such as O111:H2, O55:H6, and O119:H6, are quite common and exhibit an association with diarrhea worldwide (20–23). Others originally thought to represent EPEC, such as O18:H7 and O18:H14, have rarely been associated with diarrhea and appear not to be pathogenic (19). Still other serotypes consist of strains that lack the virulence characteristics that define EPEC strains and therefore should no longer be considered members of this category. Included among these are serotypes now considered to consist of strains that belong to other pathogenic classes. For example, O26:H11 is now considered an enterohemorrhagic *E. coli* (EHEC) serotype (24,25), and O44:H18 and O126:H27 strains often belong to the enteroaggregative *E. coli* category (26). Further complicating matters, strains from serotypes other than those commonly included among EPEC have been isolated from children with diarrhea and shown to possess the putative virulence properties characteristic of EPEC (27–29). Overall, the use of serotyping, a laborious procedure, no longer appears to be a useful method to define or diagnose EPEC infection.

Clonal Relatedness Of EPEC

From the point of view of the clinical microbiology laboratory, EPEC strains are similar in most respects to conventional *E. coli.* However, particular serotypes of EPEC tend to have certain biochemical idiosyncrasies, principally in their ability to ferment sugars (30–32). This observation and the observation that outer membrane protein profiles of EPEC correlate with serotyping led to the suggestion that the EPEC population structure is clonal (30). The results of multilocus enzyme electrophoresis analysis, a technique for quantifying the genetic relatedness of microorganisms on the basis of allelic variants of "housekeeping" enzymes, have confirmed this hypothesis (33). EPEC strains examined to date appear to comprise two great lineages (33,34). One group (arbitrarily EPEC1) includes serotypes O55:H6, O125:H6, O142:H6, and O86:H34. Also related was a single isolate of O127:H–, perhaps a nonmotile mutant of O127:H6. The other lineage (EPEC2) includes serotypes O111:H2 and O128:H2. It appears from these experiments that the flagellar H antigen is more indicative of relatedness than the O antigen (33). Strains from the two lineages appear to be only distantly related to each other. The relationships among many other serotypes of EPEC remain to be elucidated.

The EPEC strains share notable pathogenic features with the EHEC strains; the latter are distinguished by the production of high levels of Shiga-like toxins. The most important EHEC serotype, O157:H7, shares a common ancestor with EPEC serotype O55:H7, which in turn is related to the H6 EPEC lineage (34). Interestingly, many strains of the O55:H7 serotype, like EHEC, commonly lack the adherence plasmid found in most other EPEC strains (26). In contrast, EHEC strains of serotypes O26:H11 and O111:H8 are more closely related to the H2 EPEC lineage (35). These observations suggest that horizontal transfer of Shiga-like toxin genes encoded by bacteriophages was an important step in the divergent evolution of EPEC and EHEC strains.

EPIDEMIOLOGY

An understanding of the epidemiology of EPEC infection is hampered by the use in different studies of different criteria for the diagnosis of EPEC infections. Results may vary depending on whether EPEC strains were sought by serogroup, serotype, the results of DNA probe assays for virulence genes, or the results of a fluorescent assay used as a surrogate test for the attaching and effacing effect. Despite these limitations, the data clearly indicate that EPEC is an endemic diarrheal pathogen of considerable importance among infants in developing countries. Our knowledge of the incidence of EPEC in developed countries is less complete however, due to the abandonment by clinical microbiology laboratories in the 1970s of efforts to diagnose EPEC infection.

Transmission

The predominant mode of EPEC transmission is not firmly established, but strong evidence suggests that person-to-person spread by the fecal-oral route is most important (3,36). Several outbreaks of nosocomial EPEC infection have been traced to an index case (8,37,38). EPEC may be isolated from asymptomatic children, particularly those older than 6 months (39–41). Such carriers may represent the primary reservoir for infection. Occasionally, asymptomatic infection in an adult is implicated as the source of an outbreak or sporadic case (37,42). Contamination of the hands of caretakers has been documented and suggested to be a major mode of nosocomial transmission (3,37). Hand washing effectively eliminates the organism (37). There is no evidence of an animal reservoir for EPEC infection, as attaching and effacing bacteria of animals generally belong to serotypes not associated with human disease (43–47). Similarly, although environmental contamination occurs with EPEC (3,37), contaminated food and water is the cause of only rare EPEC outbreaks (29,48,49).

EPEC In The Developing World

The evidence that EPEC organisms are an important cause of infant diarrhea in underdeveloped countries is very convincing. Prospective studies performed on six continents have demonstrated a higher rate of isolation of EPEC strains from infants with diarrhea than from matched controls (Table 40.1). Studies showing an association between EPEC and diarrhea have included patients presenting to hospitals and to outpatient clinics, as well as community-based longitudinal studies. The association between EPEC and diarrhea is particularly strong among younger children (39,41) and strongest among infants younger than 6 months (23,40,50). In the youngest children, EPEC may be the most common identifiable bacterial cause of diarrhea and in several studies has exceeded even rotavirus in incidence (23,50–52).

The possibility that bottle-feeding is a risk factor for the development of EPEC infection has been suggested since the 1940s (6,8). More recent case–control studies have confirmed that breast-feeding is protective for the development of EPEC diarrhea (51,53). Both the immunoglobulin and the oligosaccharide fractions of breast milk have been shown to inhibit EPEC adherence to epithelial cells (54). Antibodies against several EPEC virulence factors have been demonstrated in breast milk (55–57). Recent hospitalization also appears to greatly increase the risk of EPEC infection (53).

EPEC In Developed Countries

A reexamination of 93 *E. coli* strains submitted to the Centers for Disease Control and Prevention between 1934 and 1987 from 50 outbreaks in the United States of diarrhea in

TABLE 40.1. SUMMARY OF PROSPECTIVE CONTROLLED STUDIES OF THE ROLE OF ENTEROPATHOGENIC *ESCHERICHIA COLI* IN CHILDHOOD DIARRHEA

Country	Year	Age-group	Setting	Reference
Mexico	1988	<2 y	Community	23
Mexico	1991	<2 y	Community	21
Peru	1985	<1 y	Community	180
Brazil	1983	<2 y	Outpatient Clinic	20
Brazil	1989	<1 y	Hospital	52
Brazil	1989	<1 y	Hospital	22
Brazil	1991	<1 y	Hospital	50
Brazil	1998	<2 y	Outpatient/Inpatient Hospital	214
Chile	1987	"Infants or young children"	Hospital	215
Venezuela	1997	<2 y	Hospital	216
Yugoslavia	1989	<6 y	Outpatient Clinic	39
South Africa	1980	<2 y	Hospital	51
Ethiopia	1982	<2 y (98%)	Hospital	173
Guinea-Bissau	1994	<4 y	Community	217
Thailand	1987	<5 y	Hospital	40
Thailand	1991	<6 mo	Hospital	196
China	1991	"Children" (median age 1 y)	Hospital	182
China (Hong Kong)	1996	≤15 y	Hospital	193
India	1989	<3 y	Community	218
India	1992	<6 mo	Hospital	219
New Caledonia	1993	<10 y	Hospital	183
New Caledonia	1996	<10 y	Not stated	220
Australia	1992	<5 y	Community	221

children younger than 2 years revealed that most of these strains were EPEC (58). Although two outbreaks were from 1983, most of the EPEC outbreaks were from the 1950s and 1960s.

It is generally accepted that EPEC strains are no longer a common cause of diarrhea in the United States and other developed nations. However, the validity of this assumption is subject to debate. In Manitoba, Canada, EPEC organisms were still an important cause of community-acquired diarrhea among infants in 1976 (42), and in a study conducted between 1983 and 1986 in the former West Germany, EPEC serotypes were found significantly more often in infants with diarrhea than controls (59). In a recent uncontrolled study from Washington, EPEC isolates (defined genotypically, see below) were identified from the stool of 5% of children with diarrhea (59a). On the other hand, EPEC was not significantly associated with diarrhea in recent studies from Italy and France (60,61). The abandonment in many hospitals of efforts to diagnose EPEC may have led to significant underappreciation of the prevalence of EPEC disease. The availability of improved methods for EPEC diagnosis based on virulence factors (see below) should prompt a reinvestigation of the role of EPEC in developed countries. Despite that EPEC organisms are not often sought, outbreaks and sporadic cases of EPEC infection in the United States, the United Kingdom, Finland, and Japan have been recently reported (29,36,38,48,62–66). Two severe outbreaks were associated with child day care centers, an increasingly popular environment with great potential for EPEC transmission (38,64). The AIDS epidemic may also provide a reservoir of susceptible hosts. Attaching and effacing bacteria, possibly EPEC, have been described in a patient with AIDS with persistent diarrhea (67). Further studies on patients with diarrhea and HIV infection appear warranted.

PATHOGENESIS AND IMMUNITY

Pathology

The histopathology of severe natural EPEC infection has been studied in detail. Gross examination of the intestines rarely reveals abnormalities, even in fatal cases (8,68). However, on microscopic inspection of the jejunum, there is severe villous atrophy, often accompanied by crypt hypertrophy (62,63,69,70). An inflammatory infiltrate is found in the lamina propria, which may be mononuclear (63,70) or composed of neutrophils, as well as lymphocytes, plasma cells, and macrophages (36,62). Similar changes can be found in ileal and rectal biopsies of severe cases, suggesting that in such cases the infection may involve virtually the entire gut (63,71). On ultrastructural examination, bacteria are found intimately attached to epithelial cells, microvilli are effaced, and the cytoskeleton is dramatically rearranged (see below). In addition, progressive loss of cytoplasmic organelles has been described (71), an observation consistent with cellular necrosis. The loss of microvilli is correlated with a loss of activity of enzymes associated with the brush border (70,72). Some reports describe invasion of epithelial cells (73,74).

Molecular Pathogenesis

There has been an explosion of information in the last decade that has helped clarify the pathogenesis of EPEC infection. The description and analysis of mutants deficient in various aspects of the EPEC–host interaction have been instrumental in advancing our understanding (75,76). The major virulence factors of EPEC are summarized in Table 40.2.

Localized Adherence

The first breakthrough in understanding the pathogenesis of EPEC infection was the observation by Cravioto et al. (77) that unlike most *E. coli* organisms, EPEC organisms adhere avidly to epithelial cells in tissue culture. Rather than covering the entire surface of the cells, EPEC organisms bind as tight microcolonies (Fig. 40.2) in a pattern termed localized adherence (78).

Pioneering work in the laboratory of James Kaper soon thereafter led to the realization that the localized adherence phenomenon is plasmid encoded. EPEC strains representing various serotypes were found to possess large highly conserved plasmids (79–81). Loss of the plasmid from one strain was associated with loss of the ability to perform localized adherence, while transfer of the plasmid to a laboratory *E. coli* strain led to gain of this function. Furthermore, the attack rate for diarrhea was lower in individuals fed a plasmid-cured EPEC strain than in those fed the parental plasmid-containing wild type strain (82).

The identification by Girón et al. (83) of a plasmid-associated fimbria in EPEC was the next breakthrough in understanding localized adherence. The fimbriae appear as flexible ropelike bundles that intertwine, linking individual bacteria. The *bfpA* gene encoding bundlin, the major structural subunit of this fimbriae in one EPEC strain, was soon described and a mutant with a disruption of this gene was reported to be deficient in localized adherence (84). These observations were soon confirmed in an unrelated EPEC strain (85). The DNA sequence of *bfpA* predicts a pilin protein of the type IV fimbriae family that includes the pili of *Vibrio cholerae, Pseudomonas aeruginosa, Neisseria gonorrhoeae,* and other pathogens and confirms the amino acid sequence obtained from the purified fimbria (83). There exists considerable variation in *bfpA*

TABLE 40.2. SUMMARY OF PROPOSED AND CONFIRMED VIRULENCE FACTORS OF *ESCHERICHIA COLI*

Feature	Description	Genetic Locus	Reference
BFP	Type IV fimbria required for localized adherence and auto-aggregation phenotypes of EPEC	EPEC adherence factor plasmid containing 14-gene *bfp* operon	
		The *bfpA* gene encoding bundlin, the major structural subunit of the pilus[a]	92
		The *bfpF* gene encoding a protein that is required for dis-aggregation and formation of higher order fimbrial bundles[a]	92
Attaching and effacing activity	Ability to attach intimately to enterocytes, efface microvilli, and induce the formation of actin-rich cuplike pedestals on which the bacteria sit	The LEE pathogenicity island containing 41 open reading frames including the genes for a type III secretion system	
		The *eae* gene encoding intimin, a 94-kda outer membrane adhesin protein required for intimate attachment[a]	129
		The *tir* gene encoding the Tir, which is inserted into the host cell membrane by the type III secretion system	
		The *espB* gene encoding a protein secreted and translocated into host cells by the type III system that is required for the translocation of Tir into host cells and for attaching and effacing activity[a]	125
Gene regulation	Activation of BFP and LEE expression	The *perA (bfpT)* gene encoding an AraC-like regulator	92

[a]Virulence factor confirmed in volunteer trial.
EPEC, enteropathic *Escherichia coli*; LEE; locus of enterocyte effacement; Tir, translocated intimin receptor; BFP, bundle-forming pilus.

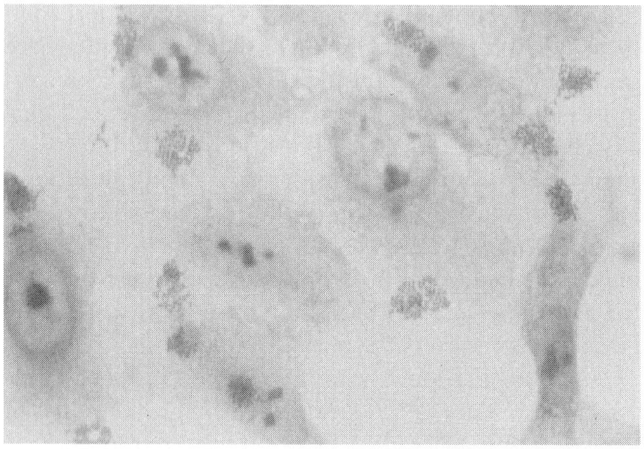

FIGURE 40.2. HEp-2 tissue culture cells infected with an enteropathogenic *Escherichia coli* strain and stained with Giemsa. Bacteria adhere in discrete microcolonies characteristic of localized adherence.

sequences among EPEC strains, particularly in residues encoding amino acids that are predicted to be exposed on the surface of the pili, suggesting selective pressure for antigenic diversity (86).

The *bfpA* gene is the first cistron in an operon of 14 genes. When this operon was expressed in a laboratory strain of *E. coli,* BFP were produced; the first time that a recombinant strain was constructed that could produce a type IV pilus (87). Further work has demonstrated that most of the genes in the cluster are required for BFP biogenesis (88–90). In addition, the ubiquitous *E. coli dsbA* locus, encoding a periplasmic oxidoreductase, is required for efficient formation of a disulfide bond in the pilin protein to prevent its degradation (91). The ability to produce BFP has been confirmed to be a virulence property of EPEC, as a mutant unable to do so because of mutations in *bfpA* is less pathogenic in a volunteer model than the wild type strain from which it was derived (92).

The ability of BFP to intertwine into bundles appears to be critical for the formation of microcolonies characteristic of localized adherence and is related to the ability of EPEC to form auto-aggregates under conditions favoring BFP expression. Mutants deficient in making BFP are always deficient in auto-aggregation and localized adherence (90). The BfpF protein appears to play a special role in BFP function. Inactivation of the *bfpF* gene does not block BFP formation. On the contrary, *bfpF* mutants produce more pili and are hyperadherent in comparison to wild type (88,92). Furthermore, auto-aggregates of *bfpF* mutants are irregular in contour and fail to disaggregate (92), and the pili produced by a *bfpF* mutant fail to form higher-order bundles of filaments during tissue culture infection (93). Surprisingly, a *bfpF* mutant is less virulent in adult volunteers than the wild type strain from which it was derived (92). Thus, aspects of BFP function, in addition to its presence and ability to mediate localized adherence and auto-aggregation, are important for infection.

Attaching and Effacing and the Locus of Enterocyte Effacement

The hallmark of EPEC infection is the ability of the organism to attach intimately to epithelial cells and efface microvilli (Fig. 40.1). This effect was first described by Staley et al. (94) in 1969, although the term "attaching and effacing" was coined by Moon et al. (95) in 1983. The attaching and effacing effect consists of bacteria near the plasma membrane of enterocytes, separated by a distance of only 10 nm. Microvilli vesiculate early in the interaction between bacterium and epithelial cell, are absent directly beneath intimately attached bacteria, and are elongated adjacent to the organisms (96). The epithelial cell responds by forming cuplike pedestals, on which the bacteria rest. Directly beneath adherent organisms, there is a reorganization of cytoskeletal elements including actin (97), a light chain of myosin (98), α-actinin, talin, and ezrin (99). These cytoskeletal elements are so sharply focused beneath the organisms that when viewed by fluorescence microscopy using probes for these eukaryotic proteins, it appears as though the bacteria themselves were stained.

Attaching and effacing activity has been observed with EPEC of classic serogroups (96) and with prototypic strains from the original outbreaks (11). The effect has been noted using animal models (94,95,100,101), tissue culture cells (75,102), and in pathologic tissue from human infections (62,63,70,72–74,103). Unlike localized adherence, attaching and effacing activity does not require the presence of the EPEC plasmid, although the plasmid facilitates this effect (96,101,102). It has recently been demonstrated that some strains originally reported to be *Hafnia alvei* that were isolated from humans with diarrhea and capable of attaching and effacing activity are actually *E. coli* and therefore EPEC (104). There exists a cadre of attaching and effacing *E. coli* strains that infect various animals including cattle, pigs, dogs, and psittacine birds (43,45–47,105–107). *Citrobacter rodentium* causes identical lesions in mice (108). Attaching and effacing activity has also been observed in animal models of EHEC infection (109,110).

Attaching and effacing activity is encoded on a 35,624-bp pathogenicity island called the locus of enterocyte effacement (LEE) (111,112). Similar LEE elements are present in all other attaching and effacing pathogens. The LEE from one EPEC strain is capable of conferring the ability to produce the attaching and effacing effect on nonpathogenic *E. coli* strains when introduced on an episomal element (113). The LEE has 41 open reading frames potentially encoding proteins that include the components of a type III secretion apparatus, proteins secreted via this apparatus, an adhesin and its cognate receptor, a regulator, and proteins of unknown function. Type III secretion systems are widespread in gram-negative bacterial species that interact closely with eukaryotic hosts (114,115). They function to export proteins, not only past the inner and outer membranes of the bacteria but also in some cases directly into the host cell membrane or cytoplasm. Proteins exported via type III systems may be effector molecules that are delivered to the host cell where they have specific functions or they may be components of the translocation apparatus, which is required for delivery of the effector proteins into the host cell.

The proteins secreted by the type III secretion system of EPEC include EspA, EspB (previously known as EaeB), EspD, EspF, and Tir. Mutations in the genes encoding EspA, EspB, and EspD abolish the ability of EPEC to produce the attaching and effacing effect (116–118). Antibodies raised against EspA decorate a surface structure that resembles a pilus, which seems to bridge the gap between the EPEC bacteria and host cells early in the course of incubations performed *in vitro* (119). Because EspA remains protease sensitive throughout such incubations (120), and an *espA* mutant is incapable of delivering the effector molecules Tir and EspF to host cells (see below), it appears that EspA is a major component of the translocation apparatus. The function of EspB is less well defined. Because EspB is a secreted protein required for translocation of Tir but not for secretion of any other secreted proteins, it is by definition part of the translocation apparatus. Furthermore, EspA and EspB bind each another and are localized in close proximity during infection of cells (121). However, EspB is protease resistant during incubations of bacteria and host cells (120) and is delivered to the cytoplasm and membrane of host cells (122,123). Furthermore, when EspB is expressed within cells, they lose their actin stress fibers and change shape dramatically, suggesting that EspB may play a role in actin dynamics within cells (124). EspB has also been shown to be an important virulence factor for EPEC as significantly fewer (1 of 10) volunteers who ingested an *espB* mutant strain had diarrhea than volunteers (9 of 10) who ingested the wild type strain from which it was derived (125). EspD has also been localized to host cell membranes (126). Mutants with disruptions of *espD* form EspA-containing surface appendages that are shorter than those of wild type bacteria, suggesting a role in translocation (119).

EPEC produce a 94-kd outer membrane protein called intimin that is encoded by the *eae* gene within the LEE (75,127). Mutants at the *eae* locus are incapable of attaching intimately to epithelial cells (Fig. 40.1B) (75,128) and are attenuated in experimental human EPEC infection (129). Intimin is similar in amino acid sequence and structure to the invasin protein of *Yersinia pseudotuberculosis* and *Yersinia enterocolitica.* This latter protein confers on normally noninvasive *E. coli* strains the ability to enter epithelial cells with high efficiency (130). Invasin binds tenaciously to members of the β_1 class of integrins, receptors normally involved in interactions between eukaryotic cells and extracellular substrates and ligands (131). Although intimin can bind *in vitro* to integrins (132), the affinity of this binding has not been measured and it is not clear that integrins serve as intimin receptors *in vivo.* Instead, the principal receptor for intimin appears to be a bacterially encoded protein called Tir, for translocated intimin receptor (133). Tir is encoded by the *tir* gene, located two cistrons upstream of *eae.* Tir is secreted via the type III secretion apparatus and translocated to the host cell membrane. The Tir protein of EPEC is modified within host cells by phosphorylation at a critical tyrosine residue and by serine and/or threonine phosphorylation (134). Purified intimin and EPEC that express intimin, but not *eae* mutant bacteria that cannot express intimin, bind to host cells that contain Tir. Thus, EPEC use a type III secretion apparatus to insert the receptor for intimate adherence into host cells.

Recently the global fold of the C-terminal, receptor-binding domain of intimin in solution and the crystal structure of this portion of intimin bound to the extracellular domain of Tir have been solved (135,136). Intimin consists of a series of three immunoglobulin-like domains that are postulated to protrude from the surface of the bacteria to form a relatively rigid rod (see Color Figure 40.3). A fourth domain at the extreme carboxyl terminus (C-terminus) of the protein has a lectin-like fold but lacks a calcium-binding fold, indicating that it is not likely to function as a lectin. Tir is a dimer, each molecule composed of antiparallel α helices joined by a hairpin loop. Together the Tir dimer forms a four-helix bundle, with the loops protruding from each end. The principle contacts between Tir and intimin occur between the Tir loops and one surface of the intimin lectin-like domain. The binding constant of this interaction has been estimated to be 3.2×10^6 M^{-1}. The contacts between intimin and Tir occur in a plane roughly parallel to the surface of both the bacteria and the host cells, thereby explaining the close approximation of bacteria and host cells observed by electron microscopy.

EPEC–Host Cell Signaling

The host cell proteins involved in the dramatic rearrangements of cytoskeletal proteins that occur as part of the attaching and effacing effect of EPEC are the subject of intensive investigation. Recent studies have demonstrated that the Arp2/3 complex is activated and localized to areas of intimate EPEC attachment (137). The Arp2/3 multiprotein complex is critical to the formation of filamentous actin in cells. Arp2/3 is activated by members of the Wiscott–Aldrich syndrome protein (WASP) family and N-WASP is also localized to and activated in areas of EPEC attaching and effacing bacteria. N-WASP in turn is usually activated by the small guanosine triphosphatases (GTPases), Rho, Rac, and Cdc42, but these proteins do not play a role in EPEC attaching and effacing activity (138). Therefore, it has been proposed that N-WASP is activated by EPEC through another mechanism. The extracellular domain of Tir is bounded by two membrane-spanning domains that place both the amino and C-terminals in the host cell cytoplasm. The current hypothesis states that phosphorylation of a critical tyrosine residue at the C-terminus of Tir and binding of intimin to Tir are important for subsequent activation of N-WASP and the attaching and effacing effect.

Several additional cellular responses to EPEC infection have been noted. Early reports of rises in intracellular calcium in response to EPEC infection have not been substantiated by more careful study (139). Elevations in inositol phosphate levels have been detected in cells infected with EPEC, indicating activation of phospholipase C (140,141). Additional work has shown that phospholipase Cγ is phosphorylated in response to EPEC infection (142). Careful study has also substantiated earlier suggestions that EPEC activates protein kinase C (143). The transcription factor nuclear factor-κβ is also activated in intestinal cells in response to EPEC infections (144), which in turn leads to secretion of interleukin 8 and may be involved in the transepithelial migration of neutrophils (145). EPEC infection leads to phosphorylation of a myosin light chain (98). Myosin light-chain kinase appears to be primarily responsible for this phosphorylation and phosphorylation of myosin light chain appears to result in alterations in tight junction permeability (146).

Other Potential Virulence Factors

Lysates from some EPEC and EHEC strains inhibit lymphocyte activation (147). In the presence of these lysates, the ability of lymphocytes to proliferate and produce interleukin 2, interleukin 4, interleukin 5, and interferon γ in response to phorbol esters, mitogens, antigen, or CD3 cross-linking is inhibited (147,148). The lymphocytes do not undergo apoptosis and they remain viable. The gene encoding this activity, *lifA* has been identified and a mutant with a disruption in the gene completely lacks the inhibitory activity (149). Lymphostatin, the product of *lifA* is a large protein (the largest ever described in *E. coli*) with homology near its amine terminus with the enzymatic portion of the large clostridial cytotoxins. The mechanism of action of lymphostatin is not yet known. The *lifA* gene is found in many, but not all, strains of EPEC. A similar gene is present on the large plasmid of EHEC strains of serotype O157:H7, but the EPEC gene is located on the chromosome.

BipA is a protein encoded by a gene found not only in EPEC, but in the nonpathogenic K12 *E. coli* strain as well. BipA appears to be a GTPase with similarity to ribosome-binding elongation factors. In EPEC, but not in *E. coli* K12, BipA is tyrosine phosphorylated (150). Although *bipA* is not part of the LEE, a *bipA* mutant is deficient in attaching and effacing activity and in flagella-mediated motility. The mechanism of action of BipA remains to be identified.

Gene Regulation

The virulence genes of EPEC are not expressed constitutively but are under the control of a complex hierarchy of regulatory elements. This network of regulation has not been fully dissected, but several elements have been described. Expression of the *bfpA* genes and the genes in the LEE is under the control of an AraC-like protein called PerA (plasmid-encoded regulator), which is also known as BfpT (151). In the LEE, PerA directly activates an operon, the first gene of which encodes the LEE-encoded regulator (Ler), which in turn activates expression of the other LEE operons (152). PerA also directly regulates its own expression and that of the *bfp* operon (153). A *perA* (*bfpT*) mutant is attenuated for virulence in the adult volunteer model (92). Expression of the genes of the LEE is also strictly dependent on integration host factor, a protein involved in regulation of many genes in *E. coli,* which binds upstream of *ler* (154). In addition, the genes of the LEE are under *luxS* quorum sensing control, a ubiquitous cross-species system that uses a common secreted factor to regulate expression of genes by cell density (155).

MECHANISM OF DIARRHEA IN EPEC INFECTION

Despite the progress in understanding EPEC interactions with host cells, the mechanisms by which these interactions lead to diarrhea remain to be clarified. Three mechanisms are potentially involved: loss of surface area leading to malabsorption and osmotic diarrhea, loss of intestinal barrier function leading to leakage of ions and water into the lumen, and stimulation of ion secretion or blockade of ion absorption leading to secretory diarrhea.

It has been proposed that the loss of microvilli that accompanies EPEC infection may result in malabsorption. In protracted cases of EPEC disease, both the small and the large intestine may be heavily involved, perhaps resulting in loss of enough of the absorptive surface to cause diarrhea by this mechanism (71). Furthermore, in severe cases diarrhea may decrease after institution of total parenteral nutrition (TPN), again suggesting that malabsorption is contributory (63). Yet diarrhea can persist despite TPN (70). Furthermore, in volunteer studies, EPEC diarrhea usually begins within 12 hours, and in some cases, the onset is less than 3 hours after ingestion, even though the volunteers are fasting during much of this period (129). This suggests that secretory mechanisms operate as well.

In a polarized tissue culture model, prolonged incubation of an intestinal epithelial cell line with EPEC results in an increase in transcellular tissue conductance (156–159). The increased conductance may be indicative of an increase in permeability that could contribute to diarrhea through loss of solute and water across the epithelial barrier. This increase in conductance is reversible after the bacteria are killed with antibiotics and is accompanied by phosphorylation of myosin light chain (146) and by decreased staining for the tight junction-associated protein ZO-1 (158). Mutants with defects either in the ability to adhere to cells (plasmid-cured and *bfpA* mutants) or in attaching and effacing activity (*eae, espA, espB*) are defective in the ability to produce this effect. However, the deficiencies of these mutants may be indirect, the result of an inability to deliver sufficient EspF to host cells. An *espF* mutant, although it remains fully adherent and capable of attaching and effacing activity, is deficient in the ability to increase tissue conductance (160). Complementation of the mutant with a wild type *espF* allele under the control of an inducible promoter leads to a dose–response relationship between the amount of EspF expressed and the degree to which tissue conductance increases. These observations, combined with evidence that EspF is translocated directly into host cells, suggest that EspF may be the factor that increases tissue conductance. It is not yet clear whether this effect is due to a specific effect on tight junctions or results more generally from damage to host cells as EspF has also been shown to cause host cell death resembling apoptosis (161).

Studies of fecal electrolytes in children with EPEC infection have also provided support for the concept that secretory mechanisms are responsible, at least in part, for EPEC-induced diarrhea (62). In *in vitro* models, EPEC can directly and indirectly cause changes in ion secretion and absorption in host cells. When EPEC organisms infect patch-clamped HeLa or Caco-2 cells, they induce a decrease in membrane depolarization that may be correlated with changes in ion secretion (162). EPEC organisms that have been grown under conditions that induce expression of BFP and LEE proteins cause a rapid and transient change in the short-circuit current in polarized monolayers (159). Such changes indicate a net change in the flow of ions across the monolayer. Mutants with disruptions in *eae, espA, espB,*and *espD* are defective in the ability to induce this effect (163). Finally, EPEC and other diarrheogenic *E. coli* have been shown to up-regulate the expression of the galanin-1 receptor, which in turn leads to increased secretion of chloride (164). Thus, various mechanisms by which EPEC strains may produce a secretory diarrhea have been described. In all probability, both secretory and osmotic mechanisms are operative in severe EPEC infection.

IMMUNE RESPONSE AND PROTECTION

EPEC disease is largely restricted to the very young. The highest incidence occurs in infants younger than 6 months, whereas infections in adults are rare. This observation may indicate that infants are exposed to EPEC early in life and develop protective immunity. Indeed, early studies demonstrated that volunteers convalescent from EPEC infection develop increases in strain-specific antibodies directed against the O antigen (13). The incidence of such antibodies increases with age; approximately 50% of children older than 1 year have hemagglutinating antibodies against O111, O55, and O26 LPS (10). More recent studies have demonstrated that infants convalescing from EPEC infection have serum antibodies against intimin, EspA, EspB, and bundlin (165). Furthermore, the titer of antibodies against bundlin rose from birth to age 6 months in a sample of infants from Mexico, suggesting exposure to antigen during this period (57). Volunteers infected with EPEC develop responses to LPS, intimin, EspB, bundlin, and type I fimbriae (12,82,125,129,166,167). Cell-mediated immune responses against EspB were also detected in some volunteers (125). The risk of diarrhea due to EPEC seems to decrease with previous infection. In a longitudinal study (168), 34 (64%) of 53 infants younger than 1 year had diarrhea when first colonized by an EPEC strain. In comparison, only two of eight infants had diarrhea during a second episode of EPEC colonization. The foregoing observations are consistent with the development of protective immunity against EPEC infection. On the other hand, infants may be inherently susceptible and older children and adults inherently resistant to EPEC infection, for example, because of the loss with age of specific receptors or the maturation of innate immune protective mechanisms. In a classic study, Mushin and Dubos (169) reported that infant mice were readily colonized and often died after oral or intragastric administration of a serogroup O26 strain of *E. coli*. In contrast, adult mice from the same colony were not colonized (169). Furthermore, colonized mice abruptly cleared their infection at 24 to 28 days of age, regardless of when they were infected. Although the O26 strain is no longer considered an EPEC serogroup, these studies clearly point to the possibility of age-specific differences in susceptibility. There is suggestive evidence that EPEC susceptibility also decreases with increasing age in humans. EPEC disease is not only more common, but also more severe during the first 6 months of life (168). Volunteer studies (13,18) and common source outbreaks (48,49) have clearly demonstrated that it is possible for adults to be infected with EPEC; however, it appears that the inoculum required to cause illness in adults is large. On the other hand, the propensity for person-to-person spread of EPEC in hospital neonatal units (37) and day care centers (38) strongly suggests that the inoculum required for natural infection in children may be lower than that needed for adults in experimental infection and common source outbreaks.

It has not been possible to demonstrate protective immunity to EPEC in experimental infection. In comparison to naive controls, volunteers previously given EPEC did not have a significant reduction in diarrheal attack rate when challenged with either a heterologous or the homologous strain, but the power to detect a difference in this study was low (167). Also, the model of high-inoculum adult experimental infection may not mimic natural infection in infants.

Interestingly, an influence of prior infection on disease severity was suggested by a significant inverse correlation between prechallenge serum anti-LPS immunoglobulin G (IgG) titer and total stool output. Furthermore, there was a correlation between prechallenge serum IgG titer against bundlin and the proportion of organisms from stool that had lost the adherence plasmid. This observation suggests that these antibodies may have selected for plasmid-cured (and less virulent) EPEC variants.

The association of EPEC infection with bottle-feeding suggests a protective role for breast milk. Antibodies against EPEC LPS and specific EPEC antigens have been detected in breast milk (54,57,170) and breast milk has been shown to inhibit localized adherence of EPEC to epithelial cells *in vitro* (54,171). Thus, passive immunity may have a role in protection against EPEC infection.

CLINICAL ILLNESS

It is ironic that with all of the progress that has recently been made in elucidating the molecular pathogenesis of EPEC infection, our knowledge of clinical aspects of the disease remains incomplete. There are no recent detailed descriptions of the clinical manifestations of EPEC infection. However, detailed reports from early outbreaks reveal that the disease as originally described was devastating. Infants with EPEC infection had profuse watery diarrhea. Vomiting and low-grade fever were common. Illness was often relentlessly progressive, and staggering mortality rates of 25% to 70% were reported (6–8,68). More recent descriptions of disease in the outbreak setting have been comparable. Four of thirteen infants infected with EPEC in a 1985 Kenyan preterm nursery outbreak died (172). In a 1987 outbreak in the United States involving infants in a day care center with secondary cases in hospital and home contacts, there was an average of 8 to 12 stools passed per day (38). All infants had low-grade fever and symptoms lasted for a mean of 18 days. Four of six infants infected as outpatients required hospitalization and one of four secondary nosocomial infections was fatal. In another outbreak in a child care center, 14 of 25 children developed watery diarrhea (64). Five of fourteen ill children had fever, two had vomiting, and two were hospitalized with dehydration. Rothbaum et al. (63) described 15 infants hospitalized in Cincinnati, Ohio, between 1979 and 1981 with severe EPEC infection and chronic diarrhea requiring TPN. Duration of hospitalization ranged from 25 to 120 days.

The foregoing studies are all retrospective and most are from developed countries and describe illness in the outbreak setting. These reports are therefore likely to overestimate the severity of EPEC infection. Unfortunately, there is little information regarding the clinical features of EPEC infection in developing countries. In a prospective study from São Paulo, Brazil, where EPEC is the most common identifiable cause of diarrhea in young infants, fever was present in 59%, vomiting in 80%, and dehydration in 71% of infants with EPEC (50). In this study, EPEC diarrhea was more severe than diarrhea due to rotavirus. In Ethiopia, EPEC infection was characterized by watery diarrhea and fever. Dehydration was present in 3 of 10 infants. The clinical features of EPEC in Ethiopia were not distinctive in comparison to other pathogens (173). In a longitudinal community study in Mexico, which should be subject to less reporting and selection bias than hospital-based studies, EPEC diarrhea lasted a mean of 8 days, was associated with fever in 63% and vomiting in 48% of infants, and was more severe in infants younger than 6 months than those between the ages of 6 months and 1 year (168).

EPEC can cause protracted diarrheal illness, an important factor in mortality due to diarrheal disease (174). In addition to numerous case reports of persistent diarrhea due to EPEC (36,38,62–64,69,70), case–control studies in some parts of the world (174,175), but not others (21,48), testify to the importance of EPEC in chronic diarrhea. Little is known regarding the proportion of EPEC infections that become chronic, but in one retrospective review of 26 children with EPEC admitted to Queen Elizabeth Hospital for Children in London between 1984 and 1987, six developed persistent diarrhea (62).

In experimental infections of adult volunteers in which a large inoculum is given, watery diarrhea ensues approximately 7 to 16 hours after inoculation and lasts on average less than 2 days (12,18,129). The incubation period may be as short as 3 hours. Diarrhea on occasion is voluminous and may exceed 3.5 kg. Abdominal cramps, nausea, vomiting, malaise, and fever are common. Fecal leukocytes are sometimes seen (129).

DIAGNOSIS

Serogrouping And Serotyping

The classic procedure for the diagnosis of EPEC infection is slide agglutination of suspected colonies using commercial polyvalent antisera recognizing O antigens considered to represent EPEC. The advantage of this method is that it is extremely easy to perform. The disadvantages are legion. First, a positive result can be due to low titer cross-reactivity between antigens. Second, some important EPEC serogroups are not included in the antisera. More importantly, some of the O antigens included in the sera, such as O18, O26, and O44, have a very low specificity, because most strains belonging to these serogroups are not EPEC (19,24,26). Even among serogroups that contain EPEC serotypes, many (e.g., O86) are also common among commensal *E. coli*. Thus, particularly in situations in which the prevalence of EPEC infection is low, such as sporadic cases of diarrhea in developed countries, the positive predictive value of commercial slide agglutination tests is low. Thus, serogrouping should be abandoned as an unreliable method for the diagnosis of EPEC. Unfortunately, despite such recommendations decades ago (176), serogrouping is still performed in some institutions and positive results are interpreted as evidence for EPEC.

The diagnostic accuracy of serologic testing for EPEC can be improved considerably by performing complete serotyping for all 173 O antigens and all 56 H antigens, with tube dilutions of the test antigens to confirm the specificity of the reaction (19). Obviously, this is an extremely laborious exercise that is performed in a handful of reference laboratories worldwide.

Identification of EPEC on the Basis of Putative Virulence Factors

Because of limitations in the predictive value of serogrouping, and because of impracticalities relating to the work required for serotyping, there is considerable interest in the use of markers for virulence factors for the diagnosis of EPEC infection. Such markers include tissue culture tests for adherence phenotypes, fluorescence microscopy with actin probes for cytoskeletal disruption, radioactive and nonradioactive DNA probes, and polymerase chain reaction (PCR). By definition, the use of these tests provides more accurate diagnosis of EPEC infection than serogrouping or serotyping.

The localized adherence phenotype is easily tested and highly conserved among EPEC from the most common serotypes (31,177,178). This method requires only tissue culture facilities and a light microscope, so it can be used in many microbiology laboratories. Transformed cell lines, such as HeLa or HEp-2 cells, are incubated with bacteria, fixed, stained, and examined for adherent microcolonies of bacteria. Virtually all *E. coli* strains that produce large microcolonies in this assay are EPEC. Problems associated with the use of this assay include the subjective nature of distinguishing localized adherence from other adherence patterns, the effect of incubation conditions on the pattern of adherence, the requirement for tissue culture facilities, and the fact that some serotypes such as O55:H7 that are considered EPEC often produce small microcolonies (26). Some of these problems can be overcome by performing the test under standard conditions and by establishing predefined objective criteria for localized adherence (179).

DNA probes provide a more objective method for EPEC diagnosis. The EPEC adherence factor (EAF) probe (180), the first of these to be described, is a 1-kb fragment of the EPEC adherence plasmid several kilobytes downstream of the *bfp* operon. The probe correlates very well with localized adherence and has been used to study the epidemiology of EPEC infections worldwide (21,22,41,52,58,172,180–183). Variations of the originally described probe include nonisotopic labeling to enhance its use in clinical laboratories (183,184) and the use of an oligonucleotide derived from within the EAF probe fragment to increase sensitivity and specificity and to reduce ambiguous results (185). Still, strains have been described that exhibit attaching and effacing activity, that do not produce high levels of Shiga-like toxins, and that produce at least modest localized adherence yet are negative with the EAF probe (21,65,186–188). Some of these strains are positive when tested with a *bfpA* DNA probe consisting of the gene for the major structural subunit of the BFP (189). The latter probe has been proposed as an improvement over the EAF probe, because it represents a known virulence factor, may have superior diagnostic accuracy, and is present on a higher copy number vector.

A fragment derived from within the *eae* coding sequences hybridizes with all EPEC and EHEC has also been widely used for the diagnosis of EPEC infection in conjunction with tests to exclude EHEC (60,61,190–195).

An alternative to the use of DNA probes for the diagnosis of EPEC infection is the application of fluorescence microscopy to identify the concentrated filamentous actin in epithelial cells beneath the sites of EPEC attachment as a surrogate marker for the attaching and effacing effect (97). This fluorescence–actin staining (FAS) test correlates perfectly with electron microscopy for attaching and effacing activity. The FAS test has been applied to epidemiologic studies with encouraging results (21,65,196,197). Some FAS-positive *E. coli,* of both EPEC-associated and non-EPEC–associated serotypes, are negative when tested with the EAF probe (21,65). The role of FAS-positive, EAF-negative strains needs to be further clarified, because in some studies these strains have not been significantly associated with diarrhea (196). Disadvantages of the FAS test include the need for relatively expensive fluorescent microscopes and reagents and the need to combine the test with assays for Shiga-like toxin genes or activity to distinguish EPEC from EHEC, which are also FAS positive.

The use of PCR to detect EPEC virulence determinants such as *eae* and *bfpA* is increasing (29,198,199). Strains that are positive for *eae* and *bfpA* or those that are positive for *eae* and negative for the genes for Shiga toxins are by definition EPEC. The numerous advantages to this approach, including ease, speed, and sensitivity, make PCR a very attractive method for diagnosing EPEC. When using PCR, the selection of primers that represent highly conserved areas of the genes being sought is a major consideration (86), and the possibility of cross-contamination must always be guarded against.

TREATMENT

Diarrhea due to EPEC is often severe and may be life threatening. The primary concern in caring for a patient with EPEC diarrhea is to prevent and correct fluid and electrolyte disturbances. This can be accomplished in most patients with oral rehydration therapy (see Chapter 79).

However, some patients with EPEC infection have severe vomiting or massive fluid losses that cannot be replaced by the oral route and require parenteral rehydration (62,63,200). In most cases of EPEC infection, early feeding should be instituted to prevent or reverse the rapid decline in nutritional status that can result from acute and chronic diarrhea. In young infants, breast milk or lactose-free formula should be reinstituted as soon as the fluid deficit is corrected. In older infants and children, high-calorie foods should be used. In some cases of EPEC diarrhea, reducing substances are present in the stool and the volume of diarrhea increases with enteral feeding, suggesting that malabsorption due to extensive microvillus effacement is contributing an osmotic component to the diarrhea (36,63). In these cases, TPN should be initiated if available to prevent and reverse severe nutritional depletion.

In addition to nonspecific measures to correct and prevent fluid, electrolyte, and nutritional imbalances, consideration should be given to therapeutic measures to ameliorate the diarrhea. In one randomized placebo-controlled trial, bismuth subsalicylate, at a dose of 100 mg/kg of body weight per day in divided doses every 4 hours, given in addition to oral rehydration and early feeding, reduced the duration of diarrhea, the duration of hospitalization, and the total stool output in infants and children younger than 5 years (201). The most common potential etiologic agents identified in this study were rotaviruses and *E. coli* of EPEC serogroups. Furthermore, this regimen appeared to be free of toxicity or adverse effects.

The role of antibiotics in the therapy of EPEC infection is not well defined. The apparent beneficial effects of the initiation of antibiotic therapy in patients with prolonged diarrhea due to EPEC have been noted (36,62), but controlled clinical trials are uncommon. In one study, conducted in Ethiopian children with diarrhea associated with EPEC serogroups, therapy for 5 days with trimethoprim-sulfamethoxazole or mecillinam resulted in a higher percentage of patients free of diarrhea at 3 days, compared with children given no antibiotics (202). However, resistance to multiple antibiotics is the rule for EPEC, greatly limiting the available therapeutic options (37,50,58,69, 195,203–206).

There is increasing interest in alternatives to antimicrobial therapy in the treatment of infectious diseases. Among the alternative approaches under investigation are therapeutic agents such as receptor and ligand analogues aimed at interfering with bacterial adhesion (see Chapter 6). As the ligands responsible for EPEC attachment are identified, this approach may become feasible. Another innovative strategy is passive immunotherapy. Preliminary data from a study of bovine milk immunoglobulin concentrate prepared from cows immunized with a mixture of formalin killed organisms representing 14 EPEC serogroups suggest that this approach may have beneficial effects (207). Clearly more studies of this sort are welcome.

PREVENTION

Strategies for the prevention of EPEC infection include efforts to improve social and economic conditions in developing countries, efforts to encourage breast-feeding, and efforts to prevent nosocomial transmission of infections. In addition to these laudable, but elusive goals, the possibility of preventing EPEC infection through immunization remains an attractive objective (208).

The impressive potential for protection against diarrheal disease by passive immunization was illustrated by the ability of a bovine milk immunoglobulin concentrate prepared by immunizing cows with a mixture of ETEC antigens to completely prevent diarrhea due to ETEC in a placebo-controlled volunteer trial (209). The inhibitory activity of human milk against EPEC adherence suggests that such an approach may be feasible for the protection of humans against this pathogen as well.

The evidence for the existence of protective immunity against EPEC infection has been summarized above. Attempts to develop an EPEC vaccine have met with limited success. A killed oral vaccine consisting of a mixture of *E. coli* of O111, O55, and O86 serogroups has been administered in multiple doses to hospitalized infants. The vaccine had a protective efficacy of 31% to 74%, depending on the age of the infant, in preventing nosocomial diarrhea due to *E. coli* (210). The protective effect lasted only 1 month. Efforts to produce conjugated polysaccharide vaccines using EPEC O antigens have also been reported, but these vaccines have not been tested in humans (211).

The prospect of longer lasting immunity may be realized by using alternative approaches including live attenuated EPEC strains and attenuated stains of other species that express EPEC antigens (208). Thus far, EPEC strains that have lost the ability to produce virulence factors such as *eae, espB, bfpA,* and *bfpF* mutants all retain some capacity to cause diarrhea in volunteers and are thus not fully attenuated (92,125,128). Furthermore, the *eae* and *espB* mutants produced less-robust immune responses in volunteers than the wild type strain and the *eae* mutant strain did not protect against challenge with the wild type strain (167). Thus, there are currently no promising candidates for a live attenuated EPEC vaccine. The approach of inserting EPEC virulence determinants into an attenuated strain of another species deserves consideration (212). The primary candidates for this approach would be bundlin and intimin, the products of the *bfpA* and *eae* genes. For bundlin, there are two major groups of allelic variants that induce immune responses with limited cross-reactivity against each other (86). For intimin, there are at least three such groups (213). Thus, it may be necessary to construct multivalent vaccines consisting of strains that express more than one variant of these proteins.

If the problems of developing an effective EPEC vaccine are overcome, the next issue would be identifying a population group to which the vaccine should be targeted. Because infants younger than 6 months suffer the brunt of the burden of EPEC infection, infants of this age-group in countries with high prevalence of EPEC infection would have the most to gain. An alternative strategy would be to immunize pregnant women to induce passive immunity in newborns conferred by both the transplacental and secretory (breast milk) routes. The goal of this approach would be to postpone EPEC infection beyond the period of greatest risk or to a time when active immunization by oral vaccination could be accomplished.

Progress in the elucidation of EPEC pathogenesis, agonizingly slow initially, has been accelerating exponentially. Further research will likely yield important insights into host–bacterium interactions in general and eventually will be translated into novel prophylactic and therapeutic interventions to reduce the affliction imposed by this common and serious pathogen.

ACKNOWLEDGMENT

This work was supported by Public Health Service awards AI32074 and AI37606 from the National Institutes of Health.

REFERENCES

1. Kaper JB. Defining EPEC. *Rev Microbiol Sao Paulo* 1996;27 [Suppl 1]:130–133.
2. Robins-Browne RM. Traditional enteropathogenic *Escherichia coli* of infantile diarrhea. *Rev Infect Dis* 1987;9:28–53.
3. Levine MM, Edelman R. Enteropathogenic *Escherichia coli* of classic serotypes associated with infant diarrhea: epidemiology and pathogenesis. *Epidemiol Rev* 1984;6:31–51.
4. Bray J. Isolation of antigenically homogeneous strains of *Bacterium coli neapolitanum* from summer diarrhea of infants. *J Pathol Bacteriol* 1945;57:239–247.
5. Giles C, Sangster G. An outbreak of infantile gastroenteritis in Aberdeen. *J Hyg* 1948;46:1–9.
6. Taylor J, Powell BW, Wright J. Infantile diarrhea and vomiting: a clinical and bacteriological investigation. *Br Med J* 1949;2:117–141.
7. Smith J. The association of certain types (a and b) of *Bacterium coli* with infantile gastro-enteritis. *J Hyg* 1949;47:221–226.
8. Giles C, Sangster G, Smith J. Epidemic gastroenteritis of infants in Aberdeen during 1947. *Arch Dis Child* 1949;24:45–53.
9. Kauffmann F, Dupont A. *Escherichia* strains from infantile epidemic gastroenteritis. *Acta Pathol* 1950;27:552–564.
10. Neter E, et al. Demonstration of antibodies against enteropathogenic *Escherichia coli* in sera of children of various ages. *Pediatrics* 1955;16:801–808.
11. Robins-Browne RM, et al. Examination of archetypal strains of enteropathogenic *Escherichia coli* for properties associated with bacterial virulence. *J Med Microbiol* 1993;38:222–226.
12. Ferguson WW, June RC. Experiments of feeding adult volunteers with *Escherichia coli* 111, B_4, a coliform organism associated with infant diarrhea. *Am J Hyg* 1952;55:155–169.
13. June RC, Ferguson WW, Worfel MT. Experiments in feeding adult volunteers with *Escherichia coli* 55, B_5, a coliform organism associated with infant diarrhea. *Am J Hyg* 1953;57:222–236.
14. Koya G, et al. Observations on the multiplication of *Escherichia coli* O-111 B4 in the intestinal tract of adult volunteers in feeding experiments: the intubation study with Miller–Abbott's double lumen tube. *Jpn J Med Sci Biol* 1954;7:197–203.
15. Goldschmidt MC, DuPont HL. Enteropathogenic *Escherichia coli:* lack of correlation of serotype with pathogenicity. *J Infect Dis* 1976;133:153–156.
16. Echeverria P, et al. Enterotoxigenicity and invasive capacity of "enteropathogenic" serotypes of *Escherichia coli. J Pediatr* 1976;89:8–10.
17. Sack RB. Human diarrheal disease caused by enterotoxigenic *Escherichia coli. Annu Rev Microbiol* 1975;29:333–353.
18. Levine MM, et al. *Escherichia coli* strains that cause diarrhea but do not produce heat-labile or heat-stable enterotoxins and are non-invasive. *Lancet* 1978;1:1119–1122.
19. Ørskov F, Ørskov I. *Escherichia coli* serotyping and disease in man and animals. *Can J Microbiol* 1992;38:699–674.
20. Toledo MR, et al. Enteropathogenic *Escherichia coli* serotypes and endemic diarrhea in infants. *Infect Immun* 1983;39:586–589.
21. Cravioto A, et al. Association of *Escherichia coli* HEp-2 adherence patterns with type and duration of diarrhea. *Lancet* 1991;337:262–264.
22. Gomes TAT, et al. Serotype-specific prevalence of *Escherichia coli* strains with EPEC adherence factor genes in infants with and without diarrhea in São Paulo, Brazil. *J Infect Dis* 1989;160:131–135.
23. Cravioto A, et al. Prospective study of diarrheal disease in a cohort of rural Mexican children: incidence and isolated pathogens during the first two years of life. *Epidemiol Infect* 1988;101:123–134.
24. Levine MM, et al. A DNA probe to identify enterohemorrhagic *Escherichia coli* of O157:H7 and other serotypes that cause hemorrhagic colitis and hemolytic uremic syndrome. *J Infect Dis* 1987;156:175–182.
25. Scotland SM, et al. Properties of strains of *Escherichia coli* O26:H11 in relation to their enteropathogenic or enterohemorrhagic classification. *J Infect Dis* 1990;162:1069–1074.
26. Scotland SM, et al. Identification of enteropathogenic *Escherichia coli* isolated in Britain as enteroaggregative or as members of a subclass of attaching-and-effacing *E. coli* not hybridizing with the EPEC adherence-factor probe. *J Med Microbiol* 1991;35:278–283.
27. Albert MJ, et al. Localized adherence and attaching-effacing properties of nonenteropathogenic serotypes of *Escherichia coli. Infect Immun* 1991;59:1864–1868.
28. Pedroso MZ, et al. Attaching-effacing lesions and intracellular penetration in HeLa cells and human duodenal mucosa by two *Escherichia coli* strains not belonging to the classical enteropathogenic *E. coli* serogroups. *Infect Immun* 1993;61:1152–1156.
29. Makino S, et al. Molecular epidemiological study of a mass outbreak caused by enteropathogenic *Escherichia coli* O157:H45. *Microbiol Immunol* 1999;43:381–384.
30. Stenderup J, Ørskov F. The clonal nature of enteropathogenic *Escherichia coli* strains. *J Infect Dis* 1983;148:1019–1024.
31. Scaletsky ICA, et al. Correlation between adherence to HeLa cells and serogroups, serotypes, and bioserotypes of *Escherichia coli. Infect Immun* 1985;49:528–532.
32. Katouli M, Kühn I, Möllby R. Biochemical phenotypes of enteropathogenic *Escherichia coli* common to Iran and Sweden. *J Med Microbiol* 1991;35:270–277.
33. Ørskov F, et al. Clonal relationships among classic enteropathogenic *Escherichia coli* (EPEC) belonging to different O groups. *J Infect Dis* 1990;162:76–81.
34. Whittam TS, et al. Clonal relationships among *Escherichia coli*

strains that cause hemorrhagic colitis and infantile diarrhea. *Infect Immun* 1993;61:1619–1629.
35. Campos LC, et al. *Escherichia coli* serogroup O111 includes several clones of diarrheogenic strains with different virulence properties. *Infect Immun* 1994;62:3282–3288.
36. Clausen CR, Christie DL. Chronic diarrhea in infants caused by adherent enteropathogenic *Escherichia coli. J Pediatr* 1982; 100:358–361.
37. Wu S-X, Peng R-Q. Studies on an outbreak of neonatal diarrhea caused by EPEC O127:H6 with plasmid analysis restriction analysis and outer membrane protein determination. *Acta Paediatr Scand* 1992;81:217–221.
38. Bower JR, et al. *Escherichia coli* O114:nonmotile as a pathogen in an outbreak of severe diarrhea associated with a day care center. *J Infect Dis* 1989;160:243–247.
39. Cobeljiać M, et al. The association of enterotoxigenic and enteropathogenic *Escherichia coli* and other enteric pathogens with childhood diarrhea in Yugoslavia. *Epidemiol Infect* 1989; 103:53–62.
40. Chatkaeomorakot A, et al. HeLa cell-adherent *Escherichia coli* in children with diarrhea in Thailand. *J Infect Dis* 1987;156: 669–672.
41. Gunzburg ST, et al. Virulence factors of enteric *Escherichia coli* in young Aboriginal children in north-west Australia. *Epidemiol Infect* 1992;109:283–289.
42. Gurwith M, et al. A prospective study of enteropathogenic *Escherichia coli* in endemic diarrheal disease. *J Infect Dis* 1978; 137:292–297.
43. Peeters JE, Geeroms R, Orskov F. Biotype, serotype, and pathogenicity of attaching and effacing enteropathogenic *Escherichia coli* strains isolated from diarrheic commercial rabbits. *Infect Immun* 1988;56:1442–1448.
44. Pohl PH, et al. Identification of *eae* sequences in enteropathogenic *Escherichia coli* strains from rabbits. *Infect Immun* 1993; 61:2203–2206.
45. Moxley RA, Francis DH. Natural and experimental infection with an attaching and effacing strain of *Escherichia coli* in calves. *Infect Immun* 1986;53:339–346.
46. Beaudry M, et al. Genotypic and phenotypic characterization of *Escherichia coli* isolates from dogs manifesting attaching and effacing lesions. *J Clin Microbiol* 1996;34:144–148.
47. Schremmer C, et al. Enteropathogenic *Escherichia coli* in *Psittaciformes. Avian Pathol* 1999;28:349–354.
48. Viljanen MK, et al. Outbreak of diarrhea due to *Escherichia coli* O111:B4 in schoolchildren and adults: association of Vi antigen-like reactivity. *Lancet* 1990;336:831–834.
49. Schtoeder SA, et al. A waterborne outbreak of gastroenteritis in adults associated with enteropathogenic *Escherichia coli. Lancet* 1968;1:737–740.
50. Gomes TAT, et al. Enteropathogens associated with acute diarrheal disease in urban infants in São Paulo, Brazil. *J Infect Dis* 1991;164:331–337.
51. Robins-Browne R, et al. Summer diarrhea in African infants and children. *Arch Dis Child* 1980;55:923–928.
52. Gomes TAT, Blake PA, Trabulsi LR. Prevalence of *Escherichia coli* strains with localized, diffuse, and aggregative adherence to HeLa cells in infants with diarrhea and matched controls. *J Clin Microbiol* 1989;27:266–269.
53. Blake PA, et al. Pathogen-specific risk factors and protective factors for acute diarrheal disease in urban Brazilian infants. *J Infect Dis* 1993;167:627–632.
54. Cravioto A, et al. Inhibition of localized adhesion of enteropathogenic *Escherichia coli* to HEp-2 cells by immunoglobulin and oligosaccharide fractions of human colostrum and breast milk. *J Infect Dis* 1991;163:1247–1255.
55. Camara LM, et al. Inhibition of enteropathogenic *Escherichia coli* (EPEC) adhesion to HeLa cells by human colostrum: detection of specific sIgA related to EPEC outer-membrane proteins. *Int Arch Allergy Immunol* 1994;103:307–310.
56. Loureiro I, et al. Human colostrum contains IgA antibodies reactive to enteropathogenic *Escherichia coli* virulence-associated proteins: intimin, BfpA, EspA, and EspB. *J Pediatr Gastroenterol Nutr* 1998;27:166–171.
57. Parissi-Crivelli A, Parissi-Crivelli JM, Girón JA. Recognition of enteropathogenic *Escherichia coli* virulence determinants by human colostrum and serum antibodies. *J Clin Microbiol* 2000; 38:2696–2700.
58. Moyenuddin M, et al. Serotype, antimicrobial resistance, and adherence properties of *Escherichia coli* strains associated with outbreaks of diarrheal illness in children in the United States. *J Clin Microbiol* 1989;27:2234–2239.
59. Karch H, Heesemann J, Laufs R. Phage-associated cytotoxin production by and enteroadhesiveness of enteropathogenic *Escherichia coli* isolated from infants with diarrhea in West Germany. *J Infect Dis* 1987;155:707–715.
59a. Bokete TN, et al. Genetic and phenotypic analysis of *Escherichia coli* with enteropathogenic characteristics isolated from Seattle children. *J Infect Dis* 1997;175:1382-1389.
60. Morelli R, et al. Detection of enteroadherent *Escherichia coli* associated with diarrhea in Italy. *J Med Microbiol* 1994;41: 399–404.
61. Forestier C, et al. Enteroadherent *Escherichia coli* and diarrhea in children: A prospective case–control study. *J Clin Microbiol* 1996;34:2897–2903.
62. Hill SM, Phillips AD, Walker-Smith JA. Enteropathogenic *Escherichia coli* and life threatening chronic diarrhea. *Gut* 1991;32:154–158.
63. Rothbaum R, et al. A clinicopathological study of enterocyte-adherent *Escherichia coli:* a cause of protracted diarrhea in infants. *Gastroenterology* 1982;83:441–454.
64. Paulozzi LJ, et al. Diarrhea associated with adherent enteropathogenic *Escherichia coli* in an infant and toddler center, Seattle, Washington. *Pediatrics* 1986;77:296–300.
65. Knutton S, et al. Screening for enteropathogenic *Escherichia coli* in infants with diarrhea by the fluorescent–actin staining test. *Infect Immun* 1991;59:365–371.
66. Hedberg CW, et al. An outbreak of foodborne illness caused by *Escherichia coli* O39:NM, an agent not fitting into the existing scheme for classifying diarrheogenic *E-coli. J Infect Dis* 1997; 176:1625–1628.
67. Kotler DP, Orenstein JM. Chronic diarrhea and malabsorption associated with enteropathogenic bacterial infection in a patient with AIDS. *Ann Intern Med* 1993;119:127–128.
68. Bray J, Beavan TED. Slide agglutination of *Bacterium coli* var. *neapolitanum* in summer diarrhea. *J Pathol Bacteriol* 1948;60: 395–401.
69. Khoshoo V, et al. A fatal severe enteropathy associated with enteropathogenic *E. coli. Indian Pediatr* 1988;25:308–309.
70. Ulshen MH, Rollo JL. Pathogenesis of *Escherichia coli* gastroenteritis in man—another mechanism. *N Engl J Med* 1980;302: 99–101.
71. Rothbaum RJ, et al. An ultrastructural study of enteropathogenic *Escherichia coli* infection in human infants. *Ultrastruct Pathol* 1983;4:291–304.
72. Taylor CJ, et al. Ultrastructural and biochemical changes in human jejunal mucosa associated with enteropathogenic *Escherichia coli* (O111) infection. *J Pediatr Gastroenterol Nutr* 1986;5:70–73.
73. Fagundes-Neto U, et al. Enteropathogenic *Escherichia coli* O111ab:H2 penetrates the small bowel epithelium in an infant with acute diarrhea. *Acta Paediatr* 1995;84:453–455.
74. Scaletsky ICA, Pedroso MZ, Fagundes-Neto U. Attaching and

effacing enteropathogenic *Escherichia coli* O18ab invades epithelial cells and causes persistent diarrhea. *Infect Immun* 1996;64:4876–4881.
75. Jerse AE, et al. A genetic locus of enteropathogenic *Escherichia coli* necessary for the production of attaching and effacing lesions on tissue culture cells. *Proc Natl Acad Sci U S A* 1990; 87:7839–7843.
76. Donnenberg MS, et al. Construction and analysis of Tn*phoA* mutants of enteropathogenic *Escherichia coli* unable to invade HEp-2 cells. *Infect Immun* 1990;58:1565–1571.
77. Cravioto A, et al. An adhesive factor found in strains of *Escherichia coli* belonging to the traditional infantile enteropathogenic serotypes. *Curr Microbiol* 1979;3:95–99.
78. Scaletsky ICA, Silva MLM, Trabulsi LR. Distinctive patterns of adherence of enteropathogenic *Escherichia coli* to HeLa cells. *Infect Immun* 1984;45:534–536.
79. Baldini MM, et al. Plasmid-mediated adhesion in enteropathogenic *Escherichia coli. J Pediatr Gastroenterol Nutr* 1983;2: 534–538.
80. Nataro JP, et al. Characterization of plasmids encoding the adherence factor of enteropathogenic *Escherichia coli. Infect Immun* 1987;55:2370–2377.
81. McConnell MM, et al. Properties of adherence factor plasmids of enteropathogenic *Escherichia coli* and the effect of host strain on expression of adherence to HEp-2 cells. *J Gen Microbiol* 1989;135:1123–1134.
82. Levine MM, et al. The diarrheal response of humans to some classic serotypes of enteropathogenic *Escherichia coli* is dependent on a plasmid encoding an enteroadhesiveness factor. *J Infect Dis* 1985;152:550–559.
83. Girón JA, Ho ASY, Schoolnik GK. An inducible bundle-forming pilus of enteropathogenic *Escherichia coli. Science* 1991;254: 710–713.
84. Donnenberg MS, et al. A plasmid-encoded type IV fimbrial gene of enteropathogenic *Escherichia coli* associated with localized adherence. *Mol Microbiol* 1992;6:3427–3437.
85. Sohel I, et al. Cloning and characterization of the bundle-forming pilin gene of enteropathogenic *Escherichia coli* and its distribution in *Salmonella* serotypes. *Mol Microbiol* 1993;7: 563–575.
86. Blank TE, et al. Molecular variation among type IV pilin (*bfpA*) genes from diverse enteropathogenic *Escherichia coli* strains. *Infect Immun* 2000;68:7028–7038.
87. Stone KD, et al. A cluster of fourteen genes from enteropathogenic *Escherichia coli* is sufficient for biogenesis of a type IV pilus. *Mol Microbiol* 1996;20:325–337.
88. Anantha RP, Stone KD, Donnenberg MS. The role of BfpF, a member of the PilT family of putative nucleotide-binding proteins, in type IV pilus biogenesis and in interactions between enteropathogenic *Escherichia coli* and host cells. *Infect Immun* 1998;66:122–131.
89. Ramer SW, Bieber D, Schoolnik GK. BfpB, an outer membrane lipoprotein required for the biogenesis of bundle-forming pili in enteropathogenic *Escherichia coli. J Bacteriol* 1996;178: 6555–6563.
90. Anantha RP, Stone KD, Donnenberg MS. Effects of *bfp* mutations on biogenesis of functional enteropathogenic *Escherichia coli* type IV pili. *J Bacteriol* 2000;182:2498–2506.
91. Zhang H-Z, Donnenberg MS. DsbA is required for stability of the type IV pilin of enteropathogenic *Escherichia coli. Mol Microbiol* 1996;21:787–797.
92. Bieber D, et al. Type IV pili, transient bacterial aggregates, and virulence of enteropathogenic *Escherichia coli. Science* 1998; 280:2114–2118.
93. Knutton S, et al. The type IV bundle-forming pilus of enteropathogenic *Escherichia coli* undergoes dramatic alterations in structure associated with bacterial adherence, aggregation and dispersal. *Mol Microbiol* 1999;33:499–509.
94. Staley TE, Jones EW, Corley LD. Attachment and penetration of *Escherichia coli* into intestinal epithelium of the ileum in newborn pigs. *Am J Pathol* 1969;56:371–392.
95. Moon HW, et al. Attaching and effacing activities of rabbit and human enteropathogenic *Escherichia coli* in pig and rabbit intestines. *Infect Immun* 1983;41:1340–1351.
96. Knutton S, Lloyd DR, McNeish AS. Adhesion of enteropathogenic *Escherichia coli* to human intestinal enterocytes and cultured human intestinal mucosa. *Infect Immun* 1987;55:69–77.
97. Knutton S, et al. Actin accumulation at sites of bacterial adhesion to tissue culture cells: basis of a new diagnostic test for enteropathogenic and enterohemorrhagic *Escherichia coli. Infect Immun* 1989;57:1290–1298.
98. Manjarrez-Hernandez HA, et al. Purification of a 20 kDa phosphoprotein from epithelial cells and identification as a myosin light chain: phosphorylation induced by enteropathogenic *Escherichia coli* and phorbol ester. *FEBS Lett* 1991;292:121–127.
99. Finlay BB, et al. Cytoskeletal composition of attaching and effacing lesions associated with enteropathogenic *Escherichia coli* adherence to HeLa cells. *Infect Immun* 1992;60:2541–2543.
100. Polotsky YE, et al. Pathogenic effect of enterotoxigenic *Escherichia coli* and *Escherichia coli* causing infantile diarrhea. *Acta Microbiol Acad Sci Hungaricae* 1977;24:221–236.
101. Tzipori S, Gibson R, Montanaro J. Nature and distribution of mucosal lesions associated with enteropathogenic and enterohemorrhagic *Escherichia coli* in piglets and the role of plasmid-mediated factors. *Infect Immun* 1989;57:1142–1150.
102. Knutton S, et al. Role of plasmid-encoded adherence factors in adhesion of enteropathogenic *Escherichia coli* to HEp-2 cells. *Infect Immun* 1987;55:78–85.
103. Sherman P, et al. Adherence of bacteria to the intestine in sporadic cases of enteropathogenic *Escherichia coli*–associated diarrhea in infants and young children: a prospective study. *Gastroenterology* 1989;96:86–94.
104. Janda JM, Abbott SL, Albert MJ. Prototypal diarrheogenic strains of *Hafnia alvei* are actually members of the genus *Escherichia. J Clin Microbiol* 1999;37:2399–2401.
105. Goffaux F, et al. Bovine attaching and effacing *Escherichia coli* possess a pathogenesis island related to the LEE of the human enteropathogenic *Escherichia coli* strain E2348/69. *FEMS Microbiol Lett* 1997;154:415–421.
106. Helie P, et al. Experimental infection of newborn pigs with an attaching and effacing *Escherichia coli* O45:K"E65" strain. *Infect Immun* 1991;59:814–821.
107. Licois D, et al. Scanning and transmission electron microscopic study of adherence of Escherichia coli O103 enteropathogenic and or enterohemorrhagic strain GV in enteric infection in rabbits. *Infect Immun* 1991;59:3796–3800.
108. Frankel G, et al. Intimin from enteropathogenic *Escherichia coli* restores murine virulence to a *Citrobacter rodentium eaeA* mutant: induction of an immunoglobulin A response to intimin and EspB. *Infect Immun* 1996;64:5315–5325.
109. Francis DH, Collins JE, Duimstra JR. Infection of gnotobiotic pigs with an *Escherichia coli* O157:H7 strain associated with an outbreak of hemorrhagic colitis. *Infect Immun* 1986;51:953–956.
110. Tzipori S, et al. The pathogenesis of hemorrhagic colitis caused by *Escherichia coli* O157:H7 in gnotobiotic pigs. *J Infect Dis* 1986;154:712–716.
111. McDaniel TK, et al. A genetic locus of enterocyte effacement conserved among diverse enterobacterial pathogens. *Proc Natl Acad Sci U S A* 1995;92:1664–1668.
112. Elliott SJ, et al. The complete sequence of the locus of enterocyte effacement (LEE) of enteropathogenic *E. coli* E2348/69. *Mol Microbiol* 1998;28:1–4.

113. McDaniel TK, Kaper JB. A cloned pathogenicity island from enteropathogenic *Escherichia coli* confers the attaching and effacing phenotype on K-12 *E. coli. Mol Microbiol* 1997;23:399–407.
114. Cornelis GR. The *Yersinia* deadly kiss. *J Bacteriol* 1998;180: 5495–5504.
115. Lee CA. Type III secretion systems: machines to deliver bacterial proteins into eukaryotic cells? *Trends Microbiol* 1997;5:148–156.
116. Donnenberg MS, Yu J, Kaper JB. A second chromosomal gene necessary for intimate attachment of enteropathogenic *Escherichia coli* to epithelial cells. *J Bacteriol* 1993;175:4670–4680.
117. Kenny B, et al. EspA, a protein secreted by enteropathogenic *Escherichia coli* (EPEC), is required to induce signals in epithelial cells. *Mol Microbiol* 1996;20:313–323.
118. Lai LC, et al. A third secreted protein that is encoded by the enteropathogenic *Escherichia coli* pathogenicity island is required for transduction of signals and for attaching and effacing activities in host cells. *Infect Immun* 1997;65:2211–2217.
119. Knutton S, et al. A novel EspA-associated surface organelle of enteropathogenic *Escherichia coli* involved in protein translocation into epithelial cells. *EMBO J* 1998;17:2166–2176.
120. Kenny B, Finlay BB. Protein secretion by enteropathogenic *Escherichia coli* is essential for transducing signals to epithelial cells. *Proc Natl Acad Sci U S A* 1995;92:7991–7995.
121. Hartland EL, et al. The type III protein translocation system of enteropathogenic *Escherichia coli* involves EspA–EspB protein interactions. *Mol Microbiol* 2000;35:1483–1492.
122. Wolff C, et al. Protein translocation into host epithelial cells by infecting enteropathogenic *Escherichia coli. Mol Microbiol* 1998; 28:143–155.
123. Taylor KA, et al. The EspB protein of enteropathogenic *Escherichia coli* is targeted to the cytoplasm of infected HeLa cells. *Infect Immun* 1998;66:5501–5507.
124. Taylor KA, Luther PW, Donnenberg MS. Expression of the EspB protein of enteropathogenic *Escherichia coli* within HeLa cells affects stress fibers and cellular morphology. *Infect Immun* 1999;67:120–125.
125. Tacket CO, et al. Role of EspB in experimental human enteropathogenic *Escherichia coli* infection. *Infect Immun* 2000; 68:3689–3695.
126. Wachter C, et al. Insertion of EspD into epithelial target cell membranes by infecting enteropathogenic *Escherichia coli. Mol Microbiol* 1999;31:1695–1707.
127. Jerse AE, Kaper JB. The *eae* gene of enteropathogenic *Escherichia coli* encodes a 94-kilodalton membrane protein, the expression of which is influenced by the EAF plasmid. *Infect Immun* 1991;59:4302–4309.
128. Donnenberg MS, Kaper JB. Construction of an *eae* deletion mutant of enteropathogenic *Escherichia coli* by using a positive-selection suicide vector. *Infect Immun* 1991;59:4310–4317.
129. Donnenberg MS, et al. The role of the *eaeA* gene in experimental enteropathogenic *Escherichia coli* infection. *J Clin Invest* 1993;92:1412–1417.
130. Isberg RR, Voorhis DL, Falkow S. Identification of invasin: a protein that allows enteric bacteria to penetrate cultured mammalian cells. *Cell* 1987;50:769–778.
131. Tran Van Nhieu G, Isberg RR. The *Yersinia pseudotuberculosis* invasin protein and human fibronectin bind to mutually exclusive sites on the a_5b_1 integrin receptor. *J Biol Chem* 1991;266: 24367–24375.
132. Frankel G, et al. The cell binding domain of intimin from enteropathogenic *Escherichia coli* binds to β_1 integrins. *J Biol Chem* 1996;271:20359–20364.
133. Kenny B, et al. Enteropathogenic *E. coli* (EPEC) transfers its receptor for intimate adherence into mammalian cells. *Cell* 1997; 91:511–520.
134. Kenny B. Phosphorylation of tyrosine 474 of the enteropathogenic *Escherichia coli* (EPEC) Tir receptor molecule is essential for actin nucleating activity and is preceded by additional host modifications. *Mol Microbiol* 1999;31:1229–1241.
135. Kelly G, et al. Structure of the cell-adhesion fragment of intimin from enteropathogenic *Escherichia coli. Nat Struct Biol* 1999;6:313–318.
136. Luo Y, et al. Crystal structure of enteropathogenic *Escherichia coli* intimin-receptor complex. *Nature* 2000;405:1073–1077.
137. Kalman D, et al. Enteropathogenic *E. coli* acts through WASP and Arp2/3 complex to form actin pedestals. *Nat Cell Biol* 1999;1:389–391.
138. Ben-Ami G, et al. Agents that inhibit Rho, Rac, and Cdc42 do not block formation of actin pedestals in HeLa cells infected with enteropathogenic *Escherichia coli. Infect Immun* 1998;66: 1755–1758.
139. Bain C, et al. Increased levels of intracellular calcium are not required for the formation of attaching and effacing lesions by enteropathogenic and enterohemorrhagic *Escherichia coli. Infect Immun* 1998;66:3900–3908.
140. Dytoc MT, Sherman PM, Fedorko L. Phospholipase C mediates attaching and effacing activities of gastrointestinal pathogens *in vitro. J Cell Biol* 1991;115:218a.
141. Foubister V, et al. The *eaeB* gene of enteropathogenic *Escherichia coli* is necessary for signal transduction in epithelial cells. *Infect Immun* 1994;62:3038–3040.
142. Kenny B, Finlay BB. Intimin-dependent binding of enteropathogenic *Escherichia coli* to host cells triggers novel signaling events, including tyrosine phosphorylation of phospholipase $C_{\gamma 1}$. *Infect Immun* 1997;65:2528–2536.
143. Crane JK, Oh JS. Activation of host cell protein kinase C by enteropathogenic *Escherichia coli. Infect Immun* 1997;65: 3277–3285.
144. Savkovic SD, Koutsouris A, Hecht G. Activation of NF-κβ in intestinal epithelial cells by enteropathogenic *Escherichia coli. Am J Physiol* 1997;273:C1160–C1167.
145. Savkovic SD, Koutsouris A, Hecht G. Attachment of a noninvasive enteric pathogen, enteropathogenic *Escherichia coli* to cultured human intestinal epithelial monolayers induces transmigration of neutrophils. *Infect Immun* 1996;64:4480–4487.
146. Yuhan R, et al. Enteropathogenic *Escherichia coli*–induced myosin light chain phosphorylation alters intestinal epithelial permeability. *Gastroenterology* 1997;113:1873–1882.
147. Klapproth J-M, et al. Products of enteropathogenic *Escherichia coli* inhibit lymphocyte activation and lymphokine production. *Infect Immun* 1995;63:2248–2254.
148. Malstrom C, James S. Inhibition of murine splenic and mucosal lymphocyte function by enteric bacterial products. *Infect Immun* 1998;66:3120–3127.
149. Klapproth J-M, et al. A large toxin from pathogenic *Escherichia coli* strains that inhibits lymphocyte activation. *Infect Immun* 2000;68:2148–2155.
150. Farris M, et al. BipA: a tyrosine-phosphorylated GTPase that mediates interactions between enteropathogenic *Escherichia coli* (EPEC) and epithelial cells. *Mol Microbiol* 1998;28:265–279.
151. Gómez-Duarte OG, Kaper JB. A plasmid-encoded regulatory region activates chromosomal *eaeA* expression in enteropathogenic *Escherichia coli. Infect Immun* 1995;63:1767–1776.
152. Mellies JL, et al. The Per regulon of enteropathogenic *Escherichia coli:* identification of a regulatory cascade and a novel transcriptional activator, the locus of enterocyte effacement (LEE)–encoded regulator (Ler). *Mol Microbiol* 1999;33:296-306.
153. Martínez-Laguna Y, Calva E, Puente JL. Autoactivation and environmental regulation of *bfpT* expression, the gene coding for the transcriptional activator of *bfpA* in enteropathogenic *Escherichia coli. Mol Microbiol* 1999;33:153–166.
154. Friedberg D, et al. Hierarchy in the expression of the locus of

enterocyte effacement genes of enteropathogenic *Escherichia coli. Mol Microbiol* 1999;34:941–952.
155. Sperandio V, et al. Quorum sensing controls expression of the type III secretion gene transcription and protein secretion in enterohemorrhagic and enteropathogenic *Escherichia coli. Proc Natl Acad Sci U S A* 1999;96:15196–15201.
156. Canil C, et al. Enteropathogenic *Escherichia coli* decreases the transepithelial electrical resistance of polarized epithelial monolayers. *Infect Immun* 1993;61:2755–2762.
157. Spitz J, et al. Enteropathogenic *Escherichia coli* adherence to intestinal epithelial monolayers diminishes barrier function. *Am J Physiol Gastrointest Liver Physiol* 1995;268:G374–G379.
158. Philpott DJ, et al. Infection of T84 cells with enteropathogenic *Escherichia coli* alters barrier and transport functions. *Am J Physiol Gastrointest Liver Physiol* 1996;270:G634–G645.
159. Collington GK, Booth IW, Knutton S. Rapid modulation of electrolyte transport in Caco-2 cell monolayers by enteropathogenic *Escherichia coli* (EPEC) infection. *Gut* 1998;42:200–207.
160. Hecht G, et al. Enteropathogenic *E. coli* secreted protein F is required for alteration of host intestinal barrier function. *Gastroenterology* 2000;118:A433–A433.
161. Crane JK, McNamara BP, Donnenberg MS. Role of EspF in host cell death induced by enteropathogenic *Escherichia coli. J Cell Microbiol* 2001;3:197–211.
162. Stein MA, et al. Enteropathogenic *Escherichia coli* (EPEC) markedly decreases the resting membrane potential of Caco-2 and HeLa human epithelial cells. *Infect Immun* 1996;64: 4820–4825.
163. Collington GK, et al. Enteropathogenic *Escherichia coli* virulence genes encoding secreted signaling proteins are essential for modulation of Caco-2 cell electrolyte transport. *Infect Immun* 1998;66:6049–6053.
164. Hecht G, et al. Pathogenic *Escherichia coli* increase Cl− secretion from intestinal epithelia by upregulating galanin-1 receptor expression. *J Clin Invest* 1999;104:253–262.
165. Martinez MB, et al. Antibody response of children with enteropathogenic *Escherichia coli* infection to the bundle-forming pilus and locus of enterocyte effacement-encoded virulence determinants. *J Infect Dis* 1999;179:269–274.
166. Karch H, et al. Serological response to type 1-like somatic fimbriae in diarrheal infection due to classical enteropathogenic *Escherichia coli. Microbial Pathogenesis* 1987;2:425–434.
167. Donnenberg MS, et al. Effect of prior experimental human enteropathogenic *Escherichia coli* infection on illness following homologous and heterologous rechallenge. *Infect Immun* 1998; 66:52–58.
168. Cravioto A, et al. Risk of diarrhea during the first year of life associated with initial and subsequent colonization by specific enteropathogens. *Am J Epidemiol* 1990;131:886–904.
169. Mushin R, Dubos R. Colonization of the mouse intestine with *Escherichia coli. J Exp Med* 1965;122:745–757.
170. Sussman S. The passive transfer of antibodies to *Escherichia coli* O111:B4 from mother to offspring. *Pediatrics* 1961;27:308–313.
171. Silva MLM, Giampaglia CMS. Colostrum and human milk inhibit localized adherence of enteropathogenic *Escherichia coli* to HeLa cells. *Acta Paediatr Scand* 1992;81:266–267.
172. Senerwa D, et al. Enteropathogenic *Escherichia coli* serotype O111:HNT isolated from preterm neonates in Nairobi, Kenya. *J Clin Microbiol* 1989;27:1307–1311.
173. Thorén A, et al. Aetiology and clinical features of severe infantile diarrhea in Addis Ababa, Ethiopia. *J Trop Pediatr* 1982;28: 127–131.
174. Lima AA, et al. Persistent diarrhea in northeast Brazil: etiologies and interactions with malnutrition. *Acta Paediatr Suppl* 1992; 381:39–44.
175. Fagundes Neto U, et al. Protracted diarrhea: the importance of the enteropathogenic *E. coli* (EPEC) strains and *Salmonella* in its genesis. *J Pediatr Gastroenterol Nutr* 1989;8:207–211.
176. Gangarosa E, Merson MH. Epidemiologic assessment of the relevance of the so-called enteropathogenic serogroups of *Escherichia coli* in diarrhea. *N Engl J Med* 1977;296:1210–1213.
177. Nataro JP, et al. Plasmid-mediated factors conferring diffuse and localized adherence of enteropathogenic *Escherichia coli. Infect Immun* 1985;48:378–383.
178. Levine MM, et al. Use of DNA probes and HEp-2 cell adherence assay to detect diarrheogenic *Escherichia coli. J Infect Dis* 1988;158:224–228.
179. Vial PA, et al. Comparison of two assay methods for patterns of adherence to HEp-2 cells of *Escherichia coli* from patients with diarrhea. *J Clin Microbiol* 1990;28:882–885.
180. Nataro JP, et al. Detection of an adherence factor of enteropathogenic *Escherichia coli* with a DNA probe. *J Infect Dis* 1985; 152:560–565.
181. Echeverria P, et al. HeLa cell-adherent enteropathogenic *Escherichia coli* in children under 1 year of age in Thailand. *J Clin Microbiol* 1987;25:1472–1475.
182. Kain KC, et al. Etiology of childhood diarrhea in Beijing, China. *J Clin Microbiol* 1991;29:90–95.
183. Begaud E, et al. Detection of diarrheogenic *Escherichia coli* in children less than ten years old with and without diarrhea in New Caledonia using seven acetylaminofluorene-labeled DNA probes. *Am J Trop Med Hyg* 1993;48:26–34.
184. Gicquelais KG, et al. Practical and economical method for using biotinylated DNA probes with bacterial colony blots to identify diarrhea-causing *Escherichia coli. J Clin Microbiol* 1990;28: 2485–2490.
185. Jerse AE, et al. Oligonucleotide probe for detection of the enteropathogenic *Escherichia coli* (EPEC) adherence factor of localized adherent EPEC. *J Clin Microbiol* 1990;28:2842–2844.
186. Senerwa D, et al. Colonization of neonates in a nursery ward with enteropathogenic *Escherichia coli* and correlation to the clinical histories of the children. *J Clin Microbiol* 1989;27:2539–2543.
187. Scotland SM, Smith HR, Rowe B. *Escherichia coli* O128 strains from infants with diarrhea commonly show localized adhesion and positivity in the fluorescent–actin staining test but do not hybridize with an enteropathogenic *E. coli* adherence factor probe. *Infect Immun* 1991;59:1569–1571.
188. Scotland SM, et al. Strains of *Escherichia coli* O157:H8 from human diarrhea belong to attaching and effacing class of *E coli. J Clin Pathol* 1992;45:1075–1078.
189. Girón JA, et al. Distribution of the bundle-forming pilus structural gene (*bfpA*) among enteropathogenic *Escherichia coli. J Infect Dis* 1993;168:1037–1041.
190. Jerse AE, Gicquelais KG, Kaper JB. Plasmid and chromosomal elements involved in the pathogenesis of attaching and effacing *Escherichia coli. Infect Immun* 1991;59:3869–3875.
191. Giammanco A, et al. Characteristics of *Escherichia coli* strains belonging to enteropathogenic *E coli* serogroups isolated in Italy from children with diarrhea. *J Clin Microbiol* 1996;34:689–694.
192. Scotland SM, et al. Use of gene probes and adhesion tests to characterize *Escherichia coli* belonging to enteropathogenic serogroups isolated in the United Kingdom. *J Med Microbiol* 1996;44:438–443.
193. Biswas R, et al. Mol epidemiology of *Escherichia coli* diarrhea in children in Hong Kong. *J Clin Microbiol* 1996;34:3233–3234.
194. Bokete TN, et al. Genetic and phenotypic analysis of *Escherichia coli* with enteropathogenic characteristics isolated from Seattle children. *J Infect Dis* 1997;175:1382–1389.
195. Vila J, et al. Antimicrobial resistance of diarrheogenic *Escherichia coli* isolated from children under the age of 5 years from Ifakara, Tanzania. *Antimicrob Agents Chemother* 1999;43:3022–3024.
196. Echeverria P, et al. Attaching and effacing enteropathogenic

Escherichia coli as a cause of infantile diarrhea in Bangkok. *J Infect Dis* 1991;164:550–554.
197. Shariff M, et al. Evaluation of the fluorescence actin staining test for detection of enteropathogenic *Escherichia coli. J Clin Microbiol* 1993;31:386–389.
198. Tornieporth NG, et al. Differentiation of pathogenic *Escherichia coli* strains in Brazilian children by PCR. *J Clin Microbiol* 1995;33:1371–1374.
199. Gunzburg ST, Tornieporth NG, Riley LW. Identification of enteropathogenic *Escherichia coli* by PCR-based detection of the bundle-forming pilus gene. *J Clin Microbiol* 1995;33:1375–1377.
200. Marin L, et al. Unsuccessful oral rehydration therapy in an infant with enteropathogenic *E. coli* diarrhea. Studies of fluid and electrolyte homeostasis. *Acta Paediatr Scand* 1985;74:477–479.
201. Figueroa-Quintanilla D, et al. A controlled trial of bismuth subsalicylate in infants with acute watery diarrheal disease. *N Engl J Med* 1993;328:1653–1658.
202. Thorén A, et al. Antibiotics in the treatment of gastroenteritis caused by enteropathogenic *Escherichia coli. J Infect Dis* 1980; 141:27–31.
203. Antai SP, Anozie SO. Incidence of infantile diarrhea due to enteropathogenic *Escherichia coli* in Port Harcourt metropolis. *J Appl Bacteriol* 1987;62:227–229.
204. Thorén A. Antibiotic sensitivity of enteropathogenic *Escherichia coli* to mecillinam, trimethoprim-sulfamethoxazole and other antibiotics. *Acta Pathol Microbiol Scand [B]* 1980;88:265–268.
205. Senerwa D, et al. Antimicrobial resistance of enteropathogenic *Escherichia coli* strains from a nosocomial outbreak in Kenya. *APMIS* 1991;99:728–734.
206. Lim YS, Ngan CCL, Tay L. Enteropathogenic *Escherichia coli* as a cause of diarrhea among children in Singapore. *J Trop Med Hyg* 1992;95:339–342.
207. Mietens C, et al. Treatment of infantile *E. coli* gastroenteritis with specific bovine anti–*E. coli* milk immunoglobulins. *Eur J Pediatr* 1979;132:239–252.
208. Levine MM. Vaccines against enteropathogenic *Escherichia coli. Rev Microbiol Sao Paulo* 1996;27:126–129.
209. Tacket CO, et al. Protection by milk immunoglobulin concentrate against oral challenge with enterotoxigenic *Escherichia coli. N Engl J Med* 1988;318:1240–1243.
210. Kubinyi L, Kiss I, Lendvai KG. Epidemiological-statistical evaluation of oral vaccination against infantile *Escherichia coli*enteritis. *Acta Microbiol Acad Sci Hungaricae* 1974;21:187–191.
211. Gupta RK, et al. Comparative immunogenicity of conjugates composed of *Escherichia coli* O111 O-specific polysaccharide, prepared by treatment with acetic acid or hydrazine, bound to tetanus toxoid by two synthetic schemes. *Infect Immun* 1995; 63:2805–2810.
212. Schriefer A, et al. Expression of a pilin subunit BfpA of the bundle-forming pilus of enteropathogenic *Escherichia coli* in an *aroA* live salmonella vaccine strain. *Vaccine* 1999;17:770–778.
213. Adu-Bobie J, et al. Identification of immunodominant regions within the C-terminal cell binding domain of intimin a and intimin b from enteropathogenic *Escherichia coli. Infect Immun* 1998;66:5643–5649.
214. Rosa ACP, et al. Enteropathogenicity markers in *Escherichia coli* isolated from infants with acute diarrhea and healthy controls in Rio de Janeiro, Brazil. *J Med Microbiol* 1998;47:781–790.
215. Nataro JP, et al. Patterns of adherence of diarrheogenic *Escherichia coli* to HEp-2 cells. *Pediatric Infectious Diseases Journal* 1987; 6:829–831.
216. González R, et al. Age-specific prevalence of *Escherichia coli* with localized and aggregative adherence in Venezuelan infants with acute diarrhea. *J Clin Microbiol* 1997;35:1103–1107.
217. Molbak K, et al. The etiology of early childhood diarrhea: A community study from Guinea-Bissau. *J Infect Dis* 1994;169: 581–587.
218. Bhan MK, et al. Enteroaggregative *Escherichia coli* associated with persistent diarrhea in a cohort of rural children in India. *J Infect Dis* 1989;159:1061–1064.
219. Ghosh AR, et al. Entero-adherent *Escherichia coli* is an important diarrheogenic agent in infants aged below 6 months in Calcutta, India. *J Med Microbiol* 1992;36:264–268.
220. Germani Y, et al. Prevalence of enteropathogenic, enteroaggregative, and diffusely adherent *Escherichia coli* among isolates from children with diarrhea in New Caledonia. *J Infect Dis* 1996;174:1124–1126.
221. Gunzburg S, et al. Epidemiology and microbiology of diarrhea in young Aboriginal children in the Kimberly region of Western Australia. *Epidemiol Infect* 1992;108:67–76.

41

ENTEROAGGREGATIVE AND DIFFUSELY ADHERENT *ESCHERICHIA COLI*

JAMES P. NATARO
THEODORE S. STEINER

BACKGROUND AND HISTORY

Escherichia coli strains were first recognized as diarrheal pathogens in 1898, when Lesage demonstrated that serum from patients with diarrhea agglutinated strains of *E. coli* isolated from other patients in the same outbreak, but not those of controls (1). In 1945, Bray discovered that *E. coli* strains of certain serogroups were the predominant cause of summer diarrhea in infants in the United Kingdom, coining the term enteropathogenic *E. coli* (EPEC) (1) (see Chapter 40). EPEC strains were recognized as important causes of infant diarrhea in the 1950s and 1960s in the developed world and subsequently have been shown to be common agents of gastroenteritis in the developing world (1–3).

In 1979, Cravioto et al. (4) observed that most EPEC isolates adhered to HEp-2 cells in cell culture. Baldini et al. (5) subsequently showed that this adherence trait was associated with the presence of a 60-MDa plasmid. Scaletsky et al. (6) and Nataro et al. (7) examined collections of *E. coli* from studies of diarrhea in the developing world and, like Cravioto (4), found that most EPEC organisms adhered to HEp-2 cells. However, these investigators also showed that many *E. coli* strains that were not of EPEC serogroups adhered to HEp-2 cells and that the adherence phenotype was clearly distinguishable from that of EPEC. The adherence pattern of EPEC was described as "localized adherence," denoting the presence of clusters or microcolonies on the surface of the HEp-2 cells (8). In contradistinction, non-EPEC strains did not adhere in the characteristic microcolonies, instead displaying a phenotype initially described as "diffuse adherence" (DA). A DNA probe specific for the 60-MDa adherence plasmid of EPEC (designated the EPEC adherence factor [EAF] probe) was shown to correlate closely with localized, EPEC-type adherence, whereas HEp-2–adherent *E. coli* strains of non-EPEC serogroups were generally EAF-probe negative (9). Nataro et al. (7) reported that in one "diffuse-adherent" non-EPEC and EAF-probe–negative strain, *E. coli* 042 (serotype 044:H18), HEp-2 adherence was associated with the presence of a 65-MDa plasmid (7). Thus, the "DA" factor was hypothesized to be plasmid mediated, yet to be genetically distinct from that conferring localized adherence. Moreover, DNA hybridization studies of the plasmid from strain 042 with the EAF plasmid of EPEC revealed no significant homology (7).

Mathewson et al. (10) concurrently observed that *E. coli* that adhered to HEp-2 cells but were not of EPEC serotypes were associated with diarrheal disease in adult travelers to Mexico. Furthermore, these investigators demonstrated that one such strain was capable of causing diarrhea in adult volunteers (11). In these reports, diarrheogenic *E. coli* organisms that adhered to HEp-2 cells but that were not of EPEC serotypes were termed enteroadherent *E. coli.*

Subsequently, Nataro et al. (8) examined the HEp-2 adherence properties of *E. coli* isolated from the stools of 154 children with diarrhea and 66 healthy controls in Santiago, Chile. In the course of this study, these investigators were able to divide the DA phenotype into two further categories: aggregative and (true) diffuse (Fig. 41.1). Aggregative adherence (AA) was defined by the prominent autoagglutination of the bacterial cells to each other; often this occurred on the surface of the cells and on the glass coverslip free from the HEp-2 cells. The sine qua non of AA was and remains the characteristic layering of the bacteria in a "stacked brick" configuration. In true DA, bacteria were seen dispersed over the surface of the HEp-2 cell, with little aggregation and little adherence to the glass coverslip free from the cells. Of 253 EAF-probe–negative *E. coli* from Chilean patients with diarrhea, 84 (33%) exhibited the AA pattern of adherence. In contrast, only 20 (15%) of 134 probe-negative strains from asymptomatic controls were AA positive ($p < .001$). Recognizing a new pathotype of diar-

J. P. Nataro: Center for Vaccine Development, University of Maryland; Department of Pediatrics, University of Maryland Hospital, Baltimore, Maryland

T. S. Steiner: Department of Medicine, University of British Columbia; Departments of Medicine and Infectious Diseases, Vancouver Hospital and Health Sciences Center, Vancouver, British Columbia

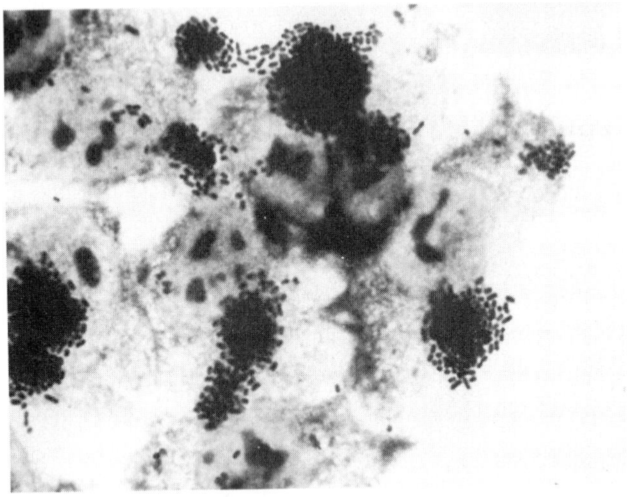
A

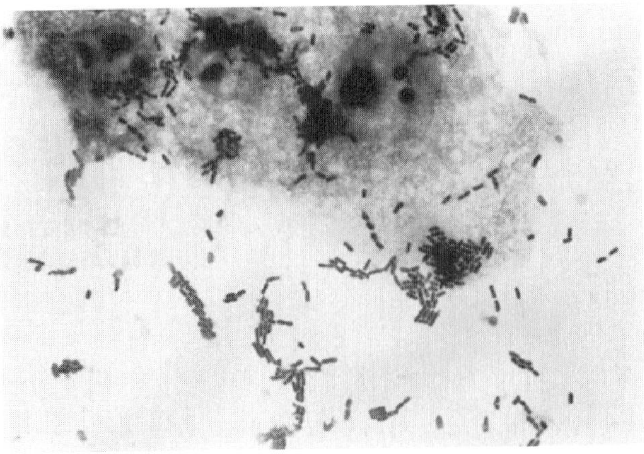
B

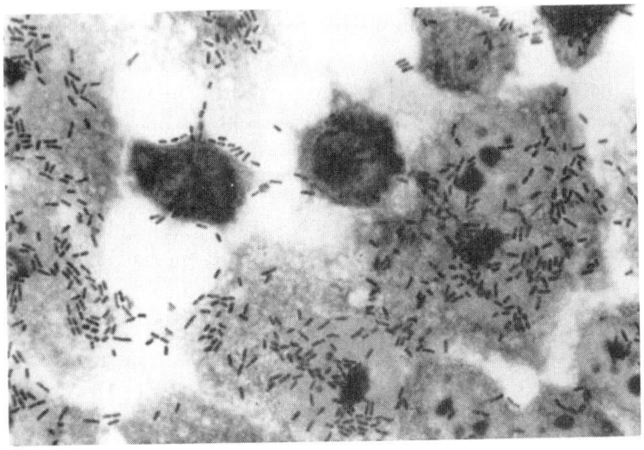
C

FIGURE 41.1. Adherence patterns of *Escherichia coli* to HEp-2 cells after 3-hour incubation according to the method of Cravioto et al. (4). **A:** Localized adherence: Note clusters or microcolonies of bacteria on the surface of the HEp-2 cells. This pattern is typical of enteropathogenic *E. coli*. **B:** Aggregative adherence: Note aggregation of bacteria in typical "stacked brick" pattern on the surface of the cell and free from the cell. **C:** Diffuse adherence: Bacteria are scattered over the surface of the cell with little aggregation or adherence to the glass background.

rheagenic *E. Coli*, these investigators coined the term enteroadherent-aggregative *E. coli*, later shortened to enteroaggregative *E. coli* (EAEC) to describe organisms expressing AA. Diffusely adherent *E. coli* (DAEC) were not associated with diarrhea in this study.

ENTEROAGGREGATIVE *E. COLI*

EAEC strains are currently defined as *E. coli* that do not secrete heat-labile (LT) or heat-stable (ST) enterotoxins and that adhere to HEp-2 cells in an aggregative pattern (3). It is likely that this definition encompasses both pathogenic and nonpathogenic clones which share a factor conferring a common phenotype. Much EAEC research involves the identification of factors that will define truly virulent strains.

Microbiology

Each pathotype of diarrheogenic *E. coli* comprises its own characteristic serotypes (3). Serotypic markers most likely correlate with clones expressing a particular package of virulence determinants, rather than the antigens themselves conferring virulence (the K1 antigen of systemic *E. coli* may be an exception). The serotypes characteristic of EAEC are not thoroughly described, although several serotypes are found consistently. Table 41.1 summarizes the serotypes of EAEC from all studies in which serotyping was performed. The table illustrates the heterogeneity of EAEC isolates, but notably, a few serotypes are isolated commonly from multiple locations. Also, as for EPEC, certain flagellar antigens are conserved across O serogroups and may signify a clonal relationship (3). The most frequently isolated serotypes may be the most virulent EAEC, and indeed, evidence for the pathogenicity of 044:H18 is compelling (see below). Table 41.1 also indicates that nontypeable *E. coli* may express the AA phenotype; interestingly, however, Vial et al. (12) found that most of these nontypeable strains were resistant to rough-specific phages.

EAEC Volunteer Studies

Several EAEC strains have been fed to adult volunteers to characterize the illness and to identify truly pathogenic strains. A summary of the studies reported to date is provided in Table 41.2.

TABLE 41.1. SEROTYPES OF ENTEROAGGREGATIVE *ESCHERICHIA COLI* COMPILED FROM PUBLISHED REPORTS

Serotype	Number Isolated	Site
O15:H18	21	Chile, Thailand
O44:H18	16	United Kingdom, Peru
O77:H18	15	India, Chile
O126:H27	14	United Kingdom
O3:H2	12	Chile
O111ab:H21	10	United Kingdom
O141:H49	7	Bangladesh
O51:H11	6	India
O?:H33	6	Chile, United Kingdom
O?:NM	6	Chile, India
O86:H2	6	Chile
O92:H33	4	India, United Kingdom
O113:NM	4	Bangladesh
Rough:H33	4	Chile
Rough:H2	3	Chile
O?:H21	3	Thailand, India

Mathewson et al. (11) fed two EAEC strains to two groups of volunteers. EAEC strain JM221, isolated from the stool of a diarrhea patient in Mexico, was fed to eight volunteers, each at doses of 7×10^8 or 1×10^{10}. Of the volunteers fed the higher dose, three experienced diarrhea and two others reported "enteric" symptoms including borborygmi and cramps.

Nataro et al. (13) conducted volunteer studies using four different EAEC strains isolated from different locations and representing different serotypes. As seen in Table 41.2, of five volunteers fed 10^{10} EAEC 042 (044:H18), three met the study definition of diarrhea (>200 mL of loose stool). One additional volunteer fed 042 developed enteric symptoms, including low-volume liquid stools and borborygmi. Of the 15 volunteers fed other EAEC strains (including JM221), none met the study definition of diarrhea and only one of the 15 had stools looser than normal. These data support strongly the pathogenicity of EAEC in humans and, moreover, suggest that the virulence of these strains varies according to as yet unknown properties.

Epidemiology of EAEC

EAEC Outbreaks

The pathogenicity of EAEC has been established incontrovertibly with the identification of EAEC outbreaks (Table 41.3). The first reported outbreak occurred in a Serbian nursery, in which 19 infants developed watery diarrhea (14). Three such infants developed persistent diarrhea; none died. Subsequently, several other outbreaks were reported, the largest of which involved nearly 2,700 Japanese children who developed watery diarrhea linked to consumption of a contaminated school lunch (15). Thirty of these children with persistent diarrhea yielded the offending pathogen, an EAEC of serotype 0?:H10. Outbreaks have occurred in adult populations as well (16).

EAEC In Endemic Diarrhea

The first description of EAEC implicated these organisms in diarrheal disease of children in Santiago, Chile (see above) (8). As shown in Table 41.3, subsequent studies have supported the association of EAEC with diarrhea in other developing populations, most prominently in association with persistent diarrhea (≥14 days).

Bhan et al. (17,18) conducted two separate studies in Indian children and first reported the association of EAEC with persistent diarrhea. These investigators performed weekly household surveillance on a cohort of 452 children (younger than 3 years) who lived in the rural village of Anapur-Palla in northern India (18). Fecal specimens were obtained from 240 episodes of diarrhea and from age-matched asymptomatic controls in the same population. EAEC organisms (defined by AA in the HEp-2 assay) were found in the stools of 10% and 13% of controls and acute diarrhea cases compared with 30% of persistent cases (18). Bhan et al. (17) subsequently studied 92 children (younger

TABLE 41.2. VOLUNTEER STUDIES WITH ENTEROAGGREGATIVE *ESCHERICHIA COLI*

Strain	Dose	Number of Volunteers	Number with Diarhea	Number with Enteric Symptoms[a]	Reference
JM221	7×10^8	8	2	1	11
JM221	1×10^{10}	8	3	5	11
JM221	1×10^{10}	5	0	0	13
189	7×10^8	4	1	3	11
189	1×10^{10}	4	0	0	11
17-2	1×10^{10}	24	1	1	13
042	1×10^{10}	5	3	4	13
34b	1×10^{10}	5	0	0	13

[a]Includes abdominal pain, borborygmi, nausea, and vomiting.

TABLE 41.3. EPIDEMIOLOGIC STUDIES IMPLICATING ENTEROAGGREGATIVE *ESCHERICHIA COLI* AS AN AGENT OF DIARRHEAL DISEASE

	Country	References
Endemic diarrhea	Chile	8
	India	17,18,77–79
	Bangladesh	80
	Brazil	20,21,81
	Venezuela	82
	Congo	83
	Nigeria	84
	Mexico	19
	Iran	85
	United Kingdom	22
	Germany	86
Growth retardation	Brazil	52
	Australia	Elliott and Nataro (*unpublished data*)
Traveler's diarrhea	Mexico	27
	Jamaica	Dupont et al. (in press)
	Spain	26
HIV-associated diarrhea	Germany	36
	United States	34,86
Outbreaks	Serbia	14
	Japan	15
	United Kingdom	16
	France	87
	Mexico	88

than 2 years) admitted to the All India Medical Institute with nondysenteric diarrhea for more than 14 days. Ninety-two children admitted for nondiarrheal diseases were selected as controls. Stools were collected from all subjects and tested for enteric pathogens, including analysis of five *E. coli* in the HEp-2 adherence assay. In patients, the most frequently isolated stool pathogen was EAEC (18 of 92 or 19.6%); EAEC organisms were isolated from the stools of only 6 (6.5%; p = .016) of 92 controls.

Cravioto et al. (19) followed a cohort of 75 infants and children younger than 2 years born in the Mexican village of Lugar Sobre la Tierra Blanca. Household visits were performed every 48 hours to assess children for the presence of diarrhea; when cases were detected, stool specimens were obtained from the patient and a matched control from the village. EAEC organisms were found in 29 (51%) of the 57 cases of diarrhea, which persisted for more than 14 days. In contrast, EAEC organisms were found in only 49 (8%) of 579 acute cases and 5 (5%) of 100 nondiarrheal controls (p <0.05).

Guerrant and co-workers have been conducting long-term surveillance of a cohort of infants and children (younger than 5 years) in Fortaleza, Brazil (20,21,81). A number of studies published by these investigators have consistently found a high rate of isolation of EAEC and have demonstrated a strong association between the presence of EAEC and persistence of diarrhea past 14 days. Wanke et al. (20) reported the results of 27 months of surveillance in this population. Household visits were conducted three times per week and specimens were collected from those with diarrhea and from asymptomatic controls. EAEC organisms were found in 2 (5%) of 28 asymptomatic controls, 4 (8%) of 50 acute diarrhea cases, and 8 (20%) of 40 persistent cases (p <0.05).

Subsequent studies have implicated EAEC as important endemic pathogens of pediatric diarrhea in many other countries in Asia, Africa, and South America (Table 41.3). EAEC in these studies is generally associated with acute or persistent watery diarrhea, usually without blood or mucus. Children of any age may be afflicted, although breast-fed infants may be at least partially protected.

EAEC In Industrialized Countries

EAEC are not confined to the developing world. A large prospective cohort study in England implicated EAEC with diarrhea among all age-groups; in this study, EAEC was the second most common cause of bacterial gastroenteritis after *Campylobacter* (22).

EAEC In Traveler's Diarrhea

HEp-2–adherent *E. coli* was first implicated in traveler's diarrhea (TD) in a report by Mathewson et al. (23) in 1983. These investigators isolated "enteroadherent" *E. coli* in 14 of 161 students presenting with diarrhea during study abroad in Guadalajara, Mexico. Only two of these isolates belonged to classic EPEC serogroups, including 044, which is now a common EAEC serogroup (Table 41.1). In a later report, they identified adherent *E. coli* in 30.4% of TD patients with no other identified pathogens, compared with only 7.6% of well travelers (10). Scotland et al. (24) in 1994 found EAEC, as defined by HEp-2 adherence and gene probe, in 10 of 43 patients with TD and found ETEC in only 7 of 43 (two of whom also carried EAEC). This was the first report of EAEC per se as a potential cause of TD.

Subsequent studies have strongly suggested a role for EAEC in TD, although a complete understanding of its epidemiology has been hampered by a lack of consistent methodology and both geographic and pathogenic variation. Several studies used only the AA probe (see below) or polymerase chain reaction (PCR) of the corresponding DNA to identify EAEC.

In 1993, Cohen et al. (25) screened 278 U.S. travelers for carriage of AA-probe–positive *E. coli* before and after travel to Latin America or the Caribbean. These travelers were part of a prospective trial comparing SXT and ciprofloxacin with placebo for prevention of TD. EAEC was found in 2.5% of subjects before travel and 27%, 33%, and 2% of patients after travel who received placebo, SXT, or ciprofloxacin, respectively. Despite these high colonization rates, only 12% of carriers in the placebo group and 13.8% in the SXT group developed diarrhea, while an additional 17.2% in the latter group had intestinal symptoms falling short of the strict definition of diarrhea. Although this study failed to demonstrate a significant association of EAEC carriage with TD, it confirmed the frequency of acquisition of EAEC and its high rate of antibiotic resistance.

In contrast, in 1998, Gascón et al. (26) found that 85% of returning Spanish travelers with EAEC (as defined by PCR of the AA-probe region) manifested diarrhea. Overall, 13.9% of diarrhea cases and only 2.4% of controls (matched travelers without diarrhea) carried EAEC (p = .0003). By comparison, 89.3% of ETEC shedders had diarrhea, and ETEC was present in 15.2% of cases and 1.8% of controls. Of note, the *astA* gene (encoding EAEC heat-stable enterotoxin 1 [EAST-1]) was present in only 6 of 23 EAEC strain cases and 2 of four EAEC from controls, suggesting that EAST-1 is not an important contributor to TD (see below). Finally, only 2 of 21 travelers to South America (compared with 6 of 37 to India) had EAEC detected by PCR; given the relatively high rate of AA-probe–negative EAEC in South America (authors' observations), the actual rates of EAEC infection may have been underestimated.

More direct evidence for a pathogenic role of EAEC in TD was demonstrated by Glandt et al. in 1999 (27). As part of a comparative trial of TD therapies, 354 U.S. travelers to Jamaica or Mexico who developed TD were screened for "conventional" pathogens (including ETEC, *Shigella, Giardia, Entamoeba histolytica,* and *Campylobacter*). Of 105 patients with no pathogens detected by these means, 64 were studied for the presence of EAEC by HEp-2 adherence and the response to ciprofloxacin or placebo. Overall, 29 (45.3%) of these 64 patients had EAEC. Among them, the identified symptoms were abdominal pain/cramps (89.7%), watery diarrhea (72.4%), urgency to defecate (86.2%), flatulence and nausea (72.4%), vomiting (24.1%), and tenesmus (20.7%). Only one patient reported fever. Of the stool samples obtained from 26 patients, 9 had fecal leukocytes, 10 had visible mucus, 6 had occult blood, and 2 had visible blood. Despite having a higher incidence of fecal leukocytes (50% versus 7.7%), the patients with EAEC who received ciprofloxacin had a significantly shortened duration of diarrhea (35.3 versus 55.5 hours; p = .049).

Adachi et al. (27a) examined 636 patients with TD for the presence of EAEC by HEp-2 adherence. Among travelers to Jamaica, Guadalajara, and Goa, EAEC and ETEC organisms were found in nearly equal numbers (25.5% versus 30.3%), with all other bacteria combined accounting for only 24%. There was no identified seasonal distribution of EAEC infections, and no consistent clonality demonstrated by PFGE. The authors calculated that EAEC was the cause of 16.3% to 53.3% of otherwise unexplained cases of TD. Together, these studies strongly implicate EAEC as a frequent cause of TD, with a prevalence rivaling that of ETEC.

Two more recent published studies failed to demonstrate an association of EAEC with TD. Schultsz et al. (28) examined 171 European patients with TD and 109 controls (patients presenting to a travel clinic with complaints other than TD) and found ETEC and EAEC in 10.7% and 9.5% of cases and 3.7% and 6.5% of controls, respectively. EAEC was associated with acute but not persistent diarrhea in a univariate analysis, but only ETEC remained significantly associated with TD in a multivariate model. However, the definition of an EAEC infection required both HEp-2 AA and hybridization with the AA probe, again likely underestimating the prevalence of EAEC. Likewise, a study of Swedish outpatients with diarrhea, of whom 50% had recently traveled, only identified EAEC in 14 of 394 patients (29). Here, PCR alone was used to define EAEC.

In summary, EAEC is likely an important cause of TD in many parts of the world, although the quantity of data has not reached that of ETEC, which is considered the leading cause of TD. Because outbreaks and volunteer studies suggest that EAEC is a pathogen in adults, at least some EAEC organisms are likely to be agents of TD, yet the epidemiologic picture may be influenced by opportunities for infection, method of detection, particular virulence traits, and the frequency of subclinical infections.

EAEC In HIV-infected Patients

Persistent or chronic diarrhea has been a common feature of AIDS since the beginning of the epidemic, with a prevalence ranging from 30% to 60% in developed areas to up to 90% in some parts of Africa. The list of pathogens causing AIDS-associated diarrhea is long, but often no pathogen is identified despite thorough evaluation.

In 1993, Kotler and Orenstein (30) reported adherent bacteria with attaching and effacing (A/E) lesions characteristic of EPEC infection in a colonic biopsy specimen from a patient with unexplained diarrhea and AIDS. They later expanded this finding to demonstrate a "chronic bacterial enteropathy" in 11 of 66 intestinal biopsy specimens from patients with AIDS (31). In addition to A/E lesions, they reported two more adherence patterns: intercalation of bacteria between microvilli and adherence of bacteria within the surface glycocalyx (the pattern typically associated with EAEC). All three types of adherence were associated with epithelial damage and inflammation, and the presence of adherent bacteria was significantly associated with weight loss. Only 12 of these biopsy specimens were cultured; of these, five had EAEC (including one whose histopathology showed A/E lesions). Interestingly, no isolates hybridized with the EPEC *eae* gene probe despite typical EPEC lesions.

In 1995, Mayer and Wanke (32) reported the first isolation of EAEC from a patient with AIDS and chronic diarrhea and wasting with no other identified pathogen. The patient responded transiently to treatment with ciprofloxacin. In a follow-up study, Wanke et al. (33) found EAEC in 30 of 68 patients with AIDS-associated diarrhea versus 18 of 60 without diarrhea (p = 0.05). The patients with EAEC and diarrhea had significantly lower CD4 counts than those with EAEC but no diarrhea (p <0.05).

The largest study to date of HEp-2–adherent *E. coli* in HIV-associated diarrhea involved 114 patients in Zambia, of whom 80 were HIV positive (35). HEp-2–adherent bacteria were significantly associated with HIV infection and diarrhea in this cohort. EAEC, DAEC, and EPEC were identified in 36%, 36%, and 26% of HIV-positive patients with diarrhea, respectively. As in previous studies, none of the strains hybridized with the EPEC EAF probe. Of these 80 patients, 32 underwent endoscopy because of chronic diarrhea. Eight patients had adherent bacteria in the colon, associated with a mixed inflammatory infiltrate, epithelial disruption, and mucus depletion.

The advent of highly active antiretroviral therapy (HAART) has complicated the study of HIV-associated diarrhea for several reasons. Most obvious is that many patients with previously fatal opportunistic infections (such as those causing chronic diarrhea) now recover thanks to immune reconstitution. At the same time, however, many patients on HAART regimens, particularly those containing a protease inhibitor, develop diarrhea or other intestinal complaints as a medication side effect. Finally, with reference to EAEC, it is not known what specific immune defects may predispose to persistent or chronic infection. Therefore, it may be difficult to formulate hypotheses about the impact of HAART on the outcomes of EAEC infection. The only study to date examining these issues involved patients in the Swiss HIV Cohort Study who presented with diarrhea (36). EAEC organisms (by HEp-2 assay) were isolated from stools of 24 of 111 patients with diarrhea and 21 of 68 controls (cohort patients without diarrhea), making EAEC the most prevalent diarrheal pathogen identified. The authors also screened isolates with PCR for the AA probe and found seven PCR-positive isolates from patients, versus only one from controls. The symptoms identified among these seven patients were watery diarrhea (86%), abdominal pain (43%), and fever (57%). In a multivariate model, however, the strongest predictor of diarrhea was being on antiretroviral therapy (p = .02), with a weaker association for PCR plus AA (p = .078).

These studies demonstrate that in various settings, EAEC and other HEp-2–adherent *E. coli* can be isolated in a substantial number of cases of diarrhea in patients with HIV. Based on the limited evidence from endoscopy specimens, it appears that colonic adherence of these bacteria and the resultant epithelial disruption and inflammation may be involved in producing the diarrhea or wasting in many of these patients. Because of the increased number of variables introduced by the use of HAART, chances are that much larger studies, with a particular emphasis on known or suspected virulence traits, will be needed to clarify the importance of EAEC in HIV-associated diarrhea.

Inconsistency of Epidemiologic Associations

Acceptance of EAEC as an enteric pathogen has been slowed because some epidemiologic studies have not found a statistically significant association between isolation of EAEC and diarrheal symptoms, leading many to doubt their pathogenicity. The full explanation for this observation is not clear, but several possible explanations can be offered. Indeed, EAEC is found commonly in virtually all intensively studied populations; asymptomatic excretion rates can be 30% or higher. This may represent prolonged excretion after a diarrheal episode or asymptomatic colonization in a previously exposed host. Moreover, it is likely that the definition of EAEC (AA in the HEp-2 assay) includes nonpathogenic *E. coli* that may be missing one or more necessary virulence determinants. This latter possibility is favored by volunteer and epidemiologic studies. Moreover, it may be that EAEC causes persistent, intermittent, or mild diarrhea, or even inflammation without diarrhea; conceivably, the traditional endpoints of classical diarrhea studies could miss some EAEC-induced clinical manifestations.

Pathogenesis of EAEC Diarrhea

The study of EAEC has been hampered by the fact that the virulence of strains is apparently heterogeneous and that observations made in nonpathogenic isolates may not be relevant to virulent EAEC. However, the identification of virulent strains in outbreaks and volunteer studies has

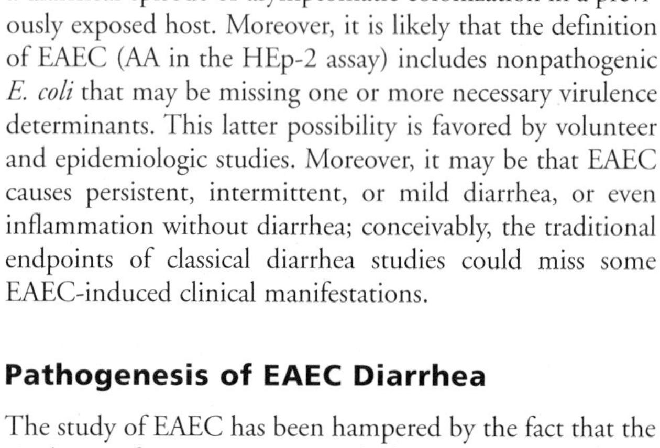

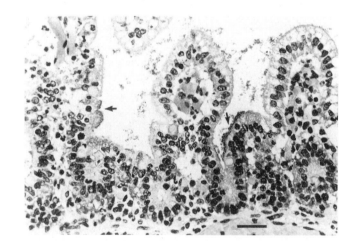

FIGURE 41.2. Histopathology of enteroaggregative *Escherichia coli* infection in the gnotobiotic piglet ileum. At 24 hours of age, piglets were fed a dose of 1×10^{10} colony-forming units of the inoculum strain 17-2 and observed for 3 days. The light photomicrograph is typical of the lesion seen in the ileum of piglets who experienced diarrhea. Enterocytes appear swollen; edema and vascular congestion are seen in the lamina propria, accompanied by coagulated erythrocytes. Aggregates of bacteria (*arrow*) on the mucosal surface (bar = 50 μm). (From Tzipori S, Montanaro J, Robins-Browne RM, et al. Studies with enteroaggregative *Escherichia coli* in the gnotobiotic piglet gastroenteritis model. *Infect Immun* 1992;60:5302–5306, with permission.)

added considerable weight to epidemiologic studies, and a picture of EAEC pathogenesis is beginning to emerge.

Histopathology

Vial et al. (12) studied the histopathology of infection with EAEC strains 042 and 17-2 in rabbit (Fig. 41.2) and rat ileal loop models. Both organisms elicited a destructive lesion on light microscopy, characterized by shortening of the villi, hemorrhagic necrosis of the villous tips, and a mild inflammatory response with edema and mononuclear infiltration of the submucosa. Transmission electron microscopy showed normal microvillar architecture without invasion of enterocytes. Both light and electron microscopy revealed prominent adherence of bacteria to the mucosal surface.

Tzipori et al. (37) fed JM221 and 17-2 to gnotobiotic piglets. Of six piglets fed strain 17-2, four developed severe enteric signs, two leading to death. Necropsy of all the piglets fed strain 17-2 revealed a histopathologic lesion of the ileum similar to that described by Vial et al. (12), but with more prominent edema and without necrosis of the villous tips. Bacteria adhered strongly to the mucosa in a stacked brick pattern. Two of six piglets fed strain JM221 became ill and three developed abnormalities of the ileal mucosa. Full description of the EAEC histopathologic lesion and site of infection awaits data from affected humans.

Adherence

The earliest work on EAEC pathogenesis fortuitously focused on the 044:H18 strain, 042. Both Nataro et al. (7) and Vial et al. (12) demonstrated that the AA property in this strain was associated with the presence of the 65-MDa plasmid. Upon acquisition of the 65-MDa plasmid, *E. coli* HB101 was found to adhere to HEp-2 cells an AA pattern and to express surface fimbriae. In addition, HB101, which was transformed with the 65-MDa plasmid, was found to have acquired a new LPS 0-antigen profile.

Vial et al. (12) examined the surface of several wild type EAEC strains using electron microscopy. Eight of the strains were found to express surface fimbriae of a rodlike morphology, 6 to 7 nm in diameter, despite being negative for type 1 fimbrial expression. Antiserum raised against purified fimbriae from one strain reacted on immunoblot with the other seven, suggesting that some EAEC share a common fimbria.

Knutton et al. (38) studied 44 strains producing characteristic AA to HEp-2 cells (organisms adhering to the glass coverslip but not the cells were excluded from analysis); all 44 were positive for the AA probe described below. These investigators found that all 44 strains possessed surface fimbriae, detectable by negative staining and transmission electron microscopy. The fimbrial structures were categorized according to four morphologies: hollow rod, rod, fibrillar, and fibrillar bundles. All of the strains expressed the fibrillar bundle morphology and most expressed at least one of the other morphologies. These investigators also studied the adherence of EAEC to cells in tissue culture and to human and animal intestinal sections (38). EAEC adherence to Caco-2 cell surfaces featured a distinct space between the bacterium and the cell, similar to that reported in animal models by Vial et al. (12), but in contrast to the intimate adherence seen with EPEC. In addition, it was shown that whereas EAEC strains did not adhere to cultured duodenal mucosa, all 44 strains adhered markedly to cultured colonic mucosa.

The mechanisms of HEp-2 adherence by EAEC strains have been studied in detail. Nataro et al. (39) identified a flexible bundle-forming fimbrial structure, designated AA fimbriae I (AAF/I) (39), which mediates HEp-2 adherence and human erythrocyte hemagglutination (Fig. 41.3). The genes for AAF/I are organized as two separate gene clusters on the AA plasmid of strain 17-2, separated by 9 kb of intervening DNA (40–42). Region 1 encodes a cluster of genes required for fimbrial synthesis and assembly, including the structural subunit of the fimbria itself (42). Region 2 encodes a transcriptional activator of AAF/I expression (called AggR), which shows homology to members of the AraC family of DNA-binding proteins (41). AAF/I fimbrial genes were found to be homologous to those of the Dr family of adhesins, which mediate adherence of uropathogenic *E. coli* and which typically mediate DA (see below). However, in a survey of EAEC strains, Czeczulin et al. (43) have found that only a minority of strains express AAF/I. These investigators identified a related adhesin, designated AAF/II, which is encoded on the AA plasmid of strain 042. AAF/II was shown to mediate adherence to human colonic mucosa sections *in vitro* (43). Like AAF/I, AAF/II is present in a minority of EAEC strains, so it appears that like ETEC, EAEC strains adhere to the mucosa by virtue of multiple surface adhesins (44).

Most EAEC strains harbor a chromosomal locus that comprises overlapping virulence-related genes (44). This locus encodes an auto-transporter mucinase called Pic and, on the opposite strand, the oligomeric enterotoxin called ShET1 (*Shigella* enterotoxin 1) (45). The mode of action of the latter toxin is not yet understood, but it may contribute to the secretory phase of EAEC illness.

Toxins

While studying the AA plasmid of strain 17-2, Savarino et al. (46) identified an open reading frame encoding a 4,100-kd homologue of the heat-stable enterotoxin (ST), designated EAST-1 (46). EAST-1 is a 38–amino acid protein that consists of four cysteine residues, unlike the six-characteristic *E. coli* ST. Of considerable interest is the observation that the eukaryotic membrane protein, guanylin, previously shown to have homology to ST, also contains four cysteine residues. The role of EAST-1 in secretion has not yet been determined, although EAST-1 clones yield net increases in the short-circuit current in the rabbit mucosal Ussing chamber model.

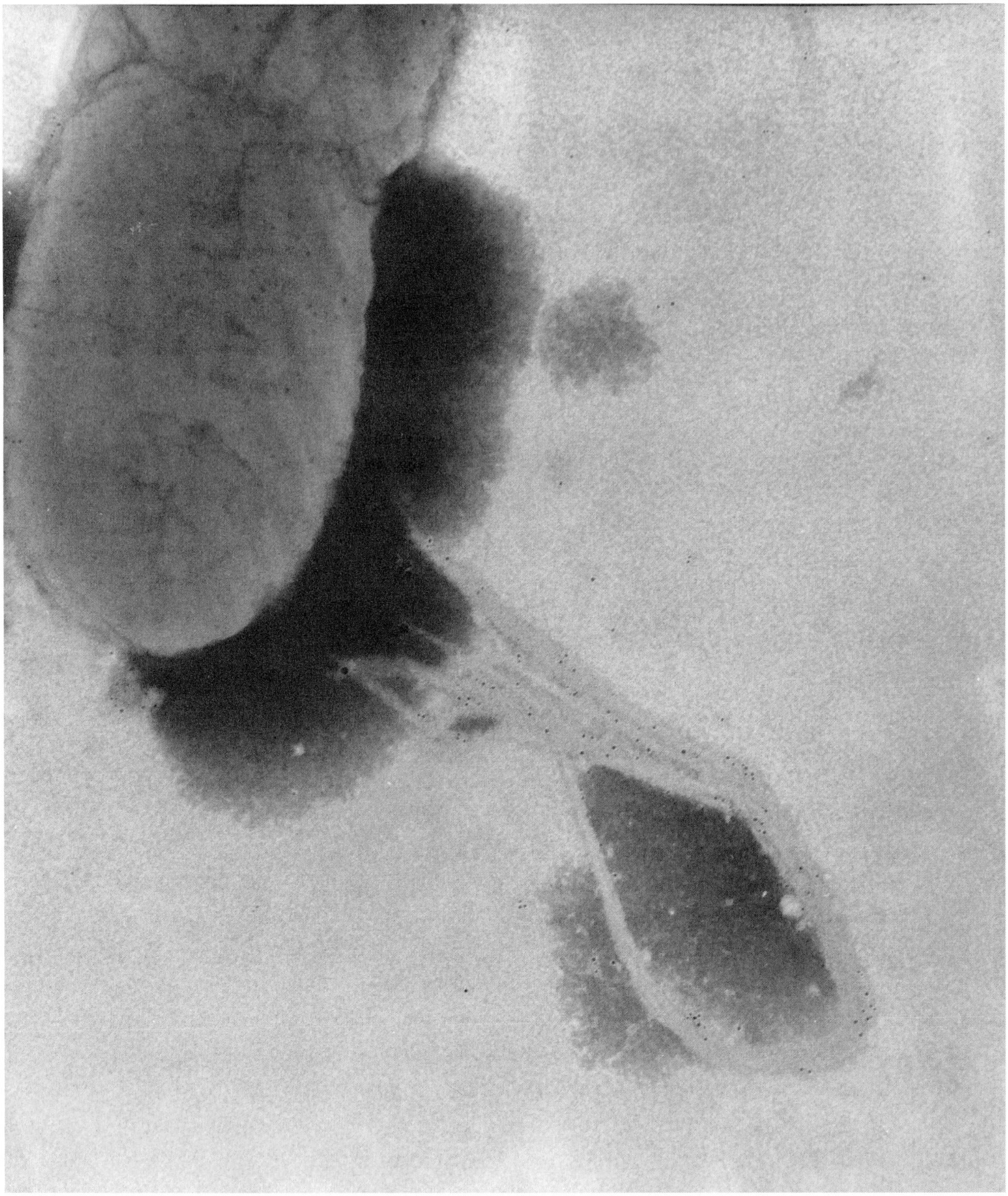

FIGURE 41.3. Aggregative adherence fimbriae I (AAF/I) on strain 17-2. Bacteria were harvested from a static L-broth culture grown overnight at 37°C then incubated with anti-AAF/I antiserum and secondary antibody labeled with 10-nm gold particles. Specimens were negative stained and visualized under transmission electron microscopy at ×25,000. Note flexible bundle-forming morphology of the fimbriae; individual filaments are 2 to 3 nm in diameter. (From Nataro JP, Deng Y, Maneval DR, et al. Aggregative adherence fimbriae I of enteroaggregative *Escherichia coli* mediate adherence to HEp-2 cells and hemagglutination of human erythrocytes. *Infect Immun* 1992;60:2297–2304, with permission.)

Recently, several investigators have identified a secreted protease toxin called plasma-encoded toxin (Pet), which elicits enterotoxic and cytopathic effects (47–49). The toxin has been shown to mediate mucosal toxicity in an *in vitro* organ culture model (50). A putative mode of action of this toxin has been suggested, which comprises entry into epithelial cells (50a), followed by proteolytic cleavage of an intracellular protein, which is thought to be the cytoskeletal protein fodrin (51).

Inflammation and Growth Impairment

Using samples obtained from the childhood diarrhea cohort in Fortaleza, Brazil, Steiner et al. (52) demonstrated elevated lactoferrin titers and concentrations of interleukin 8 (IL-8), interleukin-1β, and interleukin 1β/interleukin 1 receptor antagonist ratios in stool samples from children with persistent diarrhea due to EAEC infection. This inflammation distinguishes EAEC from other common persistent diarrheal pathogens (EPEC, *Cryptosporidium*) in which fecal lactoferrin titers are characteristically normal or only slightly elevated. Moreover, exclusive EAEC infection (defined as a HEp-2 or AA-probe diagnosis of EAEC with no other identified pathogens) was associated with elevated fecal inflammatory markers even among children with no diarrhea observed in prospective surveillance.

The potentially dramatic clinical importance of this finding was reinforced by the observation that EAEC infection itself, regardless of the presence of other pathogens or of diarrhea, was associated with shortfalls in "height for age" and "weight for age" among infected children (53). Moreover, early observations of children in the Fortaleza cohort have demonstrated that early childhood diarrhea correlates with long-term impairments in physical fitness and certain cognitive markers. The role of EAEC itself in producing these impairments is currently under investigation.

Based on these findings, Steiner et al. (53) demonstrated that culture filtrates of 042, 17-2, and several other EAEC isolates caused release of IL-8 from cultured intestinal epithelial cells. This IL-8 release was subsequently demonstrated to be due to expression of a flagellin protein homologous to a reportedly unexpressed flagellin encoded by *Shigella dysenteriae*. Several other strains with the H18 serotype also express IL-8–releasing flagella, as do several H10 isolates (including strain 101-1, the cause of the large Japanese diarrheal outbreak [15]).

The clinical importance of proinflammatory flagellar expression remains to be determined. However, neutrophil transmigration across the epithelium in response to IL-8 can itself lead to tissue disruption and fluid secretion, both of which could contribute to the clinical features of EAEC infections.

Pathogenetic Models

Available data do not permit a full description of EAEC pathogenesis, yet several hypotheses can be entertained. Colonization of the bowel is a highly conserved feature of enteric pathogenesis, and fimbrial adherence factors have been identified in most categories of diarrheogenic *E. coli* (3). AAF fimbriae are candidates for factors that may facilitate initial colonization. Several *in vivo* and *in vitro* models of EAEC infection suggest that adherence to the mucosa occurs as a thick biofilm, in which mucus may serve as an interbacterial matrix (12,37,54). However, the site of EAEC infection has not been established with certainty. EAEC organisms adhere most abundantly to the colonic mucosa *in vitro* (38,55), but in volunteer studies, duodenal string cultures were frequently positive for EAEC (13).

The association of EAEC with persistence deserves special attention. Severe damage to mucosal cells implies that a longer time would be needed for regeneration of functional epithelium than that required for secretory diarrheas alone; this regeneration would be further retarded in malnourished children in the developing world. Secondly, it is tempting to speculate that EAEC may directly affect the host immune response, which is normally responsible for elimination of enteric pathogens, yet experimental support for this hypothesis is lacking. A third viable hypothesis to explain EAEC persistence is that these organisms may act in concert with other pathogens, concurrently or perhaps sequentially.

Diagnosis Of EAEC Infection

EAEC infection is diagnosed by the isolation of *E. coli* from the stools of patients and the analysis of such isolates in the HEp-2 assay, by DNA probe or PCR. The AA probe (56) was empirically derived from the AA plasmid and does not correspond to any known virulence factor. The percentage of EAEC that hybridize with the AA probe varies among studies, and whether or not probe-positive strains are more virulent than probe-negative strains is still controversial, although some data suggest that this may be the case (36). Implication of specific virulence factors in diarrhea is also unresolved, although one study suggested that AAF/II-expressing strains may be more virulent than strains that do not express this adhesin (57).

The number of *E. coli* isolates per stool specimen that are tested in the HEp-2 assay has varied in published studies from two to five colonies. No formal data exist to suggest the minimum number of colonies needed for optimal diagnostic yield. However, analysis of data compounded in the author's laboratory (J. P. N.) suggests that in more than 70% of cases in which three colonies are selected from each patient, the same *E. coli* category is found in at least two of the three isolates. Thus, including more than three colonies per specimen is unlikely to provide substantially greater sensitivity.

AA in the HEp-2 assay still defines EAEC. The optimum method for performing this assay has been rigorously researched and includes a 3-hour incubation of bacteria with cells (58). HeLa cells may be used instead of HEp-2 cells with similar results.

Methods other than the HEp-2 and DNA-probe assays have been proposed. Albert et al. (59) reported that AA-probe–positive organisms display an unusual pellicle formation in Mueller–Hinton broth. Similarly, growing EAEC strains in polystyrene culture tubes or dishes at 37°C overnight without shaking produces a bacterial film on the polystyrene surface, easily visualized with Giemsa stain (60). Both phenotypes are likely due to high-surface hydrophobicity. Either one of these techniques is a convenient substitute for the DNA probe in identifying EAEC. However, until epidemiologic studies establish greater pathogenicity of probe-positive strains over probe-negative strains, the HEp-2 assay should remain the gold standard for EAEC detection.

The critical question in the management of patients from whom EAEC are isolated is whether or not the isolate is responsible for the patient's symptoms. It is wise to approach any such isolate with skepticism. Due to the prevalence of asymptomatic EAEC colonization, the authors currently accept an EAEC as a likely cause of the patient's diarrhea principally in three situations: (a) when the patient presents in the course of a documented EAEC outbreak, (b) when the patient's isolate can be shown to belong to one of the common EAEC serotypes associated with disease (e.g., O44:H18), and/or (c) when the patient's stools repeatedly yield a single EAEC as the predominant flora in the absence of another enteric pathogen. Other situations are possible and should be handled on a case-by-case basis.

Treatment

Yamamoto et al. (61) and Okeke et al. (57) suggested that most EAEC strains are resistant to antibiotics routinely used for the treatment of gastroenteritis, including amoxicillin and cotrimoxazole; most strains are sensitive to fluoroquinolones. Thus, any study evaluating antibiotic therapy for EAEC diarrhea would require the testing of antibiotic sensitivity patterns. The decision of whether to treat a patient from whom an EAEC is isolated depends on the considerations of causality listed above, the antibiotic susceptibility of the isolate and the severity of the patient's presentation. The studies of Glandt et al. (27) and Wanke et al. (34), as cited above, support efficacy of ciprofloxacin treatment in the amelioration of EAEC infection, although further studies are needed.

Prevention

The association of EAEC with persistent disease makes this syndrome less amenable to management with oral rehydration therapy alone, so the development of preventive strategies, including vaccination, would be a high priority for areas (such as India) in which this disease commonly occurs. Candidates under investigation as potential critical antigens include the AAF adhesins.

DIFFUSELY ADHERING *E. COLI*

Description

The first descriptions of DA failed to distinguish this phenotype from AA. Thus, early papers describing DAEC actually include EAEC strains (7). Little is known of the pathogenesis and clinical characteristics of what we now consider DAEC. No published reports allow characterization of characteristic serotypes, although the authors' experience suggests that nontypeable and roughlike strains are characteristic of DAEC as they are for EAEC.

Epidemiology

Initial studies in which DAEC organisms were clearly distinguished from EAEC failed to find an association between DAEC and diarrheal disease (8). However, more recent studies have occasionally demonstrated such an association (62–65). Of interest is that in such studies, the association is generally seen in children outside of infancy.

Giron et al. (62) performed a community-based case–control study in a southern Mexican village covering 3 weeks during the peak diarrhea season. Among the 24 of 58 cases from whom no recognized pathogen was identified, DAEC organisms were significantly associated with diarrhea. Gunzberg et al. (65) studied the adherence characteristics of 138 *E. coli* samples from the stools of Aboriginal children from whom no recognized pathogen had been isolated. Twenty-five (36.8%) of 68 children with diarrhea and 32 (45.7%) of 70 without diarrhea had diffusely adherent isolates (p >.25). After age stratification, however, DAEC strains were found to be significantly associated with diarrhea in children age 18 months or older.

Levine et al. (64) performed a prospective cohort study of children in Santiago, Chile. There were 360 children recruited from the village of Santa Julia, all younger than 4 years. From each year of age, 90 children were chosen. Each child was followed until age 60 months, at which time, they were dropped from the study and replaced by a child younger than 12 months. Observation was continued for 30 months. During this period, stool samples were obtained from 1,081 cases of diarrhea and from case-matched controls from the same population. Table 41.4 illustrates that the frequency of isolation of DAEC in cases varied between 12.3% and 19.7% among the age strata. The association between DAEC and diarrheal disease increased with each year of age, maximizing at a relative risk of 2.1 at 48 to 60 months. In this study, the seasonal pattern of DAEC infection was similar to that of ETEC, occurring more commonly in the warm season.

Baqui et al. (63) followed a cohort of 705 children younger than 5 years in rural Bangladesh, for 13 months. Age-matched controls from the same cohort were chosen for each case of diarrhea; cases that persisted for 14 days or more were matched with both asymptomatic and acute diarrheal

TABLE 41.4. ASSOCIATION OF DIFFUSELY ADHERENT *ESCHERICHIA COLI* WITH DIARRHEA BY AGE IN A COHORT OF CHILEAN CHILDREN

Age (mo)	Rate of DAEC Isolation in Cases (%)	Rate of DAEC Isolation in Controls (%)	Relative Risk
0–11	20/162 (12.3)	18/159 (11.3)	1.1
12–23	51/281 (18.1)	41/275 (14.9)	1.2
24–35	44/251 (17.5)	31/249 (12.4)	1.4
36–47	33/230 (14.3)	21/223 (9.4)	1.5
≥48	31/157 (19.7)	15/157 (9.6)	2.1
Total	179/1081 (16.6)	126/1063 (11.9)	1.4

Source: From Gascón J, Vargas M, Quinto L, et al. Enteroaggregative *Escherichia coli* strains as a cause of traveler's diarrhea: a case—control study. *J Infect Dis* 1998;177:1409–412, with permission.

cases. In this study, DAEC strains were found in 16.4% of 177 cases of persistent diarrhea, 10.3% of matched acute diarrheal cases, and 8.2% of asymptomatic matched controls. Jallat et al. (66) characterized 262 strains of *E. coli* isolated from diarrhea patients of all ages hospitalized in Clermont-Ferrand France. One-hundred strains (38.2%) exhibited the DA phenotype, compared with 8.9% (8 of 90) of *E. coli* isolated from asymptomatic patients (p<.0001). This study demonstrates that although DAEC prevalence may be very much dependent on geography, these organisms may be quite common in the developed world. Moreover, the high rate of isolation from hospitalized patients suggests a relatively severe clinical presentation.

Pathogenesis And Immunity

Several features of EAEC pathogenesis are beginning to emerge. Bilge et al. (67) cited preliminary evidence that strain C1845 is capable of inducing inflammatory lesions in the ileum of gnotobiotic piglets. These investigators have described the cloning and characterization of surface fimbriae in this strain, which mediates the DA phenotype (67). The genes encoding these fimbriae (designated *F1845*) can be found on either the bacterial chromosome or on a plasmid. The fimbrial genes show homology to members of the Dr group of bacterial adhesins, so called because they mediate adherence to the Dr blood group antigen. LeBouguenec et al. (68) found that the small protein designated AfaD in the AFA adhesins mediates binding to and internalization into epithelial cells (68). This may promote invasion by DAEC strains, although this has yet to be shown in infected patients or animals. A similar protein has also been found in EAEC adhesin gene clusters (68).

Benz et al. (69) described a 100-kd outer membrane protein that is associated with the DA phenotype in one strain of serotype O126:H27. The gene encoding this factor (designated AIDA-I) has been completely sequenced. Use of a DNA probe specific for AIDA-I suggests that this factor is expressed by a minority of DAEC isolates (authors' observations).

Servin et al. (70–72) and Cookson and Nataro (73) characterized a cytopathic effect that is unique to DAEC strains (Fig. 41.4). Infected epithelial cells develop long protrusions that wrap around the adherent bacteria. This effect may be due to binding and clustering of the DAF receptor by the Dr family fimbriae. Several signal transduction cascades are induced by DAEC binding and these may account at least in part for DAEC enteric disease.

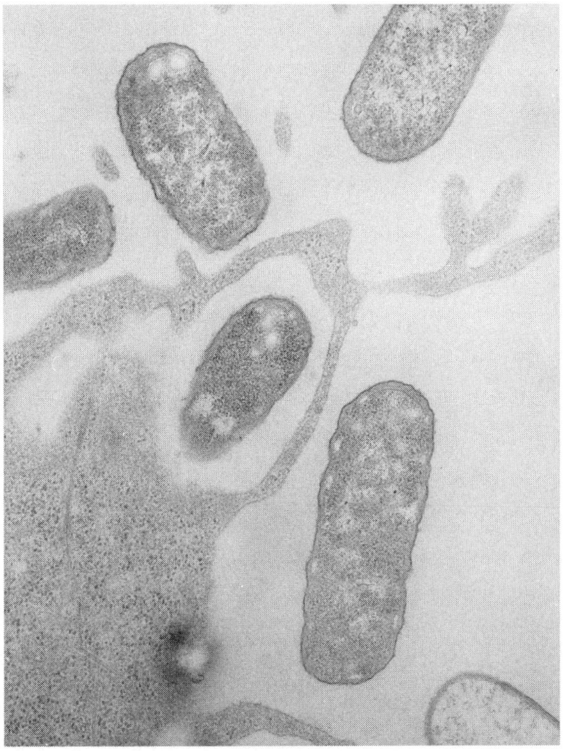

FIGURE 41.4. Cytopathic effect induced by binding of diffusely adherent *Escherichia coli* to epithelial cells. Note long plasma membrane projections that are seen to wrap around bacteria at the cell surface. (From Cookson ST, Nataro JP. Characterization of HEp-2 cell projection formation induced by diffusely adherent *Escherichia coli*. *Microb Pathog* 1996;21:421–434, with permission.)

DAEC Volunteer Studies

Tacket et al. (74) fed two different DAEC strains (57-1 and C1845) to two cohorts of volunteers at escalating doses as high as 10^{10} colony-forming units. Despite fecal shedding of the challenge organisms, none of the volunteers experienced diarrhea. There are several possible explanations for the failure of the DAEC strains to cause diarrhea. The most obvious is that neither of the two strains fed is a true pathogen. This does not preclude the possibility that other DAEC strains may be pathogenic, as was seen with the EAEC volunteer study. Another possible explanation could be that adults are resistant to DAEC diarrhea.

Diagnosis

Methods and considerations useful for diagnosing DAEC disease are similar to those used for EAEC. Presence of the DA pattern in the HEp-2 assay defines DAEC. A DAEC DNA probe is available, which consists of a part of the *daaC* gene, necessary for expression of the F1845 fimbriae (75). Other molecular probes and PCR assays have been developed for the adhesin subunits of the Dr adhesins, and these promise to improve diagnostics and epidemiologic understanding of DAEC (76).

Treatment

No studies have yet been reported describing treatment of DAEC infections. Antibiotic susceptibility data for large numbers of isolates have similarly not been reported.

REFERENCES

1. Levine MM. *Escherichia coli* that cause diarrhea: enterotoxigenic, enteropathogenic, enteroinvasive, enterohemorrhagic, and enteroadherent. *J Infect Dis* 1987;155:377–389.
2. Levine MM, Edelman R. Enteropathogenic *Escherichia coli* of classic serotypes associated with infant diarrhea: epidemiology and pathogenesis. *Epidemiol Rev* 1984;6:31–51.
3. Nataro JP, Kaper JB. Diarrheogenic *Escherichia coli. Clin Microbiol Rev* 1998;11:142–201.
4. Cravioto A, Gross RJ, Scotland SM, et al. An adhesive factor found in strains of *Escherichia coli* belonging to the traditional infantile enteropathogenic serotypes. *Curr Microbiol* 1979;3:95–99.
5. Baldini MM, Kaper JB, Levine MM, et al. Plasmid-mediated adhesion in enteropathogenic *Escherichia coli. J Pediatr Gastroenterol Nutr* 1983;2:534–538.
6. Scaletsky IC, Silva ML, Trabulsi LR. Distinctive patterns of adherence of enteropathogenic *Escherichia coli* to HeLa cells. *Infect Immun* 1984;45:534–536.
7. Nataro JP, Scaletsky IC, Kaper JB, et al. Plasmid-mediated factors conferring diffuse and localized adherence of enteropathogenic *Escherichia coli. Infect Immun* 1985;48:378–383.
8. Nataro JP, Kaper JB, Robins Browne R, et al. Patterns of adherence of diarrheogenic *Escherichia coli* to HEp-2 cells. *Pediatr Infect Dis J* 1987;6:829–831.
9. Nataro JP, Baldini MM, Kaper JB, et al. Detection of an adherence factor of enteropathogenic *Escherichia coli* with a DNA probe. *J Infect Dis* 1985;152:560–565.
10. Mathewson JJ, Johnson PC, DuPont HL, et al. A newly recognized cause of travelers' diarrhea: enteroadherent *Escherichia coli. J Infect Dis* 1985;151:471–475.
11. Mathewson JJ, Johnson PC, DuPont HL, et al. Pathogenicity of enteroadherent *Escherichia coli* in adult volunteers. *J Infect Dis* 1986;154:524–527.
12. Vial PA, Robins Browne R, Lior H, et al. Characterization of enteroadherent-aggregative *Escherichia coli*, a putative agent of diarrheal disease. *J Infect Dis* 1988;158:70–79.
13. Nataro JP, Yikang D, Cookson S, et al. Heterogeneity of enteroaggregative *Escherichia coli* virulence demonstrated in volunteers. *J Infect Dis* 1995;171:465–468.
14. Cobeljic M, Miljkovic-Selimovic B, Paunovic-Todosijevic D, et al. Enteroaggregative *Escherichia coli* associated with an outbreak of diarrhea in a neonatal nursery ward. *Epidemiol Infect* 1996; 117:11–16.
15. Itoh Y, Nagano I, Kunishima M, et al. Laboratory investigation of enteroaggregative *Escherichia coli* O untypeable:H10 associated with a massive outbreak of gastrointestinal illness. *J Clin Microbiol* 1997;35:2546–2550.
16. Spencer J, Smith HR, Chart H. Characterization of enteroaggregative *Escherichia coli* isolated from outbreaks of diarrheal disease in England. *Epidemiol Infect* 1999;123:413–421.
17. Bhan MK, Khoshoo V, Sommerfelt H, et al. Enteroaggregative *Escherichia coli* and Salmonella associated with nondysenteric persistent diarrhea. *Pediatr Infect Dis J* 1989;8:499–502.
18. Bhan MK, Raj P, Levine MM, et al. Enteroaggregative *Escherichia coli* associated with persistent diarrhea in a cohort of rural children in India. *J Infect Dis* 1989;159:1061–1064.
19. Cravioto A, Tello A, Navarro A, et al. Association of *Escherichia coli* HEp-2 adherence patterns with type and duration of diarrhea. *Lancet* 1991;337:262–264.
20. Wanke CA, Schorling JB, Barrett LJ, et al. Potential role of adherence traits of *Escherichia coli* in persistent diarrhea in an urban Brazilian slum. *Pediatr Infect Dis J* 1991;10:746–751.
21. Lima AA, Fang G, Schorling JB, et al. Persistent diarrhea in northeast Brazil: etiologies and interactions with malnutrition. *Acta Paediatr Suppl* 1992;381:39–44.

21a. Lima AA, Moore SR, Barboza MS Jr, et al. Persistent diarrhea signals a critical period of increased diarrhea burdens and nutritional shortfalls: A prospective cohort study among children in Northeastern Brazil. *J Infect Dis* 2000;181:1643–1651.

22. Tompkins DS, Hudson MJ, Smith HR, et al. A study of infectious intestinal disease in England: microbiological findings in cases and controls [see comments]. *Commun Dis Public Health* 1999;2:108–113.
23. Mathewson JJ, DuPont HL, Morgan DR, et al. Enteroadherent *Escherichia coli* associated with travellers' diarrhea [Letter]. *Lancet* 1983;1:1048.
24. Scotland SM, Willshaw GA, Cheasty T, et al. Association of enteroaggregative *Escherichia coli* with travellers' diarrhea [Letter]. *J Infect* 1994;29:115–116.
25. Cohen MB, Hawkins JA, Weckbach LS, et al. Colonization by enteroaggregative*Escherichia coli* in travelers with and without diarrhea. *J Clin Microbiol* 1993;31:351–353.
26. Gascón J, Vargas M, Quinto L, et al. Enteroaggregative *Escherichia coli* strains as a cause of traveler's diarrhea: a case–control study. *J Infect Dis* 1998;177:1409–412.
27. Glandt M, Adachi JA, Mathewson JJ, et al. Enteroaggregative *Escherichia coli* as a cause of traveler's diarrhea: clinical response to ciprofloxacin. *Clin Infect Dis* 1999;29:335–338.

27a. Adachi JA, Jiang ZD, Mathewson JJ, et al. Enteroaggregative *Escherichia coli* as a major etiologic agent in traveler's diarrhea in 3 regions of the world. *Clin Infect Dis* 2001;32:1706–1709.

28. Schultsz C, Ende JVD, Cobelens F, et al. Diarrheogenic *Escherichia coli* and acute and persistent diarrhea in returned travelers. *J Clin Microbiol* 2000;38:3550–3554.

29. Svenungsson B, Lagergren A, Ekwall E, et al. Enteropathogens in adult patients with diarrhea and healthy control subjects: a 1-year prospective study in a Swedish clinic for infectious diseases. *Clin Infect Dis* 2000;30:770–778.
30. Kotler DP, Reka S, Clayton F. Intestinal mucosal inflammation associated with human immunodeficiency virus infection. *Dig Dis Sci* 1993;38:1119–1127.
31. Kotler DP, Orenstein JM. Chronic diarrhea and malabsorption associated with enteropathogenic bacterial infection in a patient with AIDS. *Ann Intern Med* 1993;119:127–128.
32. Mayer HB, Wanke CA. Enteroaggregative *Escherichia coli* as a possible cause of diarrhea in an HIV-infected patient. *N Engl J Med* 1995;332:273–274.
33. Mayer H, Acheson D, Wanke C. *Enteroaggregative* Escherichia coli *are a potential cause of persistent diarrhea in adult HIV patients in the United States.* Kiawah Island, SC: Joint United States–Japan Cooperative Medical Sciences Program: Malnutrition and Cholera; 1995.
34. Wanke CA, Gerrior J, Blais V, et al. Successful treatment of diarrheal disease associated with enteroaggregative *Escherichia coli* in adults infected with human immunodeficiency virus. *J Infect Dis* 1998;178:1369–1372.
35. Mathewson JJ, Jiang ZD, Zumla A, et al. HEp-2 cell-adherent *Escherichia coli* in patients with human immunodeficiency virus–associated diarrhea. *J Infect Dis* 1995;171:1636–1639.
36. Durrer P, Zbinden R, Fleisch F, et al. Intestinal infection due to enteroaggregative *Escherichia coli* among human immunodeficiency virus–infected persons [In Process Citation]. *J Infect Dis* 2000;182:1540–1544.
37. Tzipori S, Montanaro J, Robins-Browne RM, et al. Studies with enteroaggregative *Escherichia coli* in the gnotobiotic piglet gastroenteritis model. *Infect Immun* 1992;60:5302–5306.
38. Knutton S, Shaw RK, Bhan MK, et al. Ability of enteroaggregative *Escherichia coli* strains to adhere in vitro to human intestinal mucosa. *Infect Immun* 1992;60:2083–2091.
39. Nataro JP, Deng Y, Maneval DR, et al. Aggregative adherence fimbriae I of enteroaggregative *Escherichia coli* mediate adherence to HEp-2 cells and hemagglutination of human erythrocytes. *Infect Immun* 1992;60:2297–2304.
40. Nataro JP, Yikang D, Giron JA, et al. Aggregative adherence fimbria I expression in enteroaggregative *Escherichia coli* requires two unlinked plasmid regions. *Infect Immun* 1993;61:1126–1131.
41. Nataro JP, Yikang D, Yingkang D, et al. AggR, a transcriptional activator of aggregative adherence fimbria I expression in enteroaggregative *Escherichia coli. J Bacteriol* 1994;176:4691–4699.
42. Savarino SJ, Fox P, Yikang D, et al. Identification and characterization of a gene cluster mediating enteroaggregative *Escherichia coli* aggregative adherence fimbria I biogenesis. *J Bacteriol* 1994;176:4949–4957.
43. Czeczulin JR, Balepur S, Hicks S, et al. Aggregative adherence fimbria II, a second fimbrial antigen mediating aggregative adherence in enteroaggregative *Escherichia coli. Infect Immun* 1997;65:4135–4145.
44. Czeczulin JR, Whittam TS, Henderson IR, et al. Phylogenetic analysis of enteroaggregative and diffusely adherent *Escherichia coli. Infect Immun* 1999;67:2692–2699.
45. Henderson IR, Czeczulin J, Eslava C, et al. Characterization of pic, a secreted protease of *Shigella flexneri* and enteroaggregative *Escherichia coli. Infect Immun* 1999;67:5587–5596.
46. Savarino SJ, Fasano A, Robertson DC, et al. Enteroaggregative *Escherichia coli* elaborate a heat-stable enterotoxin demonstrable in an in vitro rabbit intestinal model. *J Clin Invest* 1991;87:1450–1455.
47. Eslava CE, Navarro-Garcia F, Czeczulin JR, et al. Pet, an autotransporter enterotoxin from enteroaggregative *Escherichia coli. Infect Immun* 1998;66:3155–3163.
48. Navarro-Garcia F, Eslava CE, Villaseca JM, et al. *In vitro* effects of a high-molecular weight heat-labile enterotoxin from enteroaggregative *Escherichia coli. Infect Immun* 1998;66:349–354.
49. Navarro-Garcia F, Sears C, Eslava C, et al. Cytoskeletal effects induced by pet, the serine protease enterotoxin of enteroaggregative *Escherichia coli. Infect Immun* 1999;67:2184–2192.
50. Henderson IR, Hicks S, Navarro-Garcia F, et al. Involvement of the enteroaggregative *Escherichia coli* plasmid-encoded toxin in causing human intestinal damage. *Infect Immun* 1999;67:5338–5344.
50a. Navarro-Garcia F, Canizalez-Roman A, Luna J, et al. Plasmid-encoded toxin of enteroaggregative *Escherichia coli* is internalized by epithelial cells. *Infect Immun* 2001;69:1053–1060.
51. Villaseca JM, Navarro-Garcia F, Mendoza-Hernandez G, et al. Pet toxin from enteroaggregative *Escherichia coli* produces cellular damage associated with fodrin disruption [In Process Citation]. *Infect Immun* 2000;68:5920–5927.
52. Steiner TS, Lima AA, Nataro JP, et al. Enteroaggregative *Escherichia coli* produce intestinal inflammation and growth impairment and cause interleukin-8 release from intestinal epithelial cells. *J Infect Dis* 1998;177:88–96.
53. Steiner TS, Nataro JP, Poteet-Smith CE, et al. Enteroaggregative *Escherichia coli* expresses a novel flagellin that causes IL-8 release from intestinal epithelial cells. *J Clin Invest* 2000;105:1769–1777.
54. Nataro JP, Hicks S, Phillips AD, et al. T84 cells in culture as a model for enteroaggregative *Escherichia coli* pathogenesis. *Infect Immun* 1996;64:4761–4768.
55. Hicks S, Candy DC, Phillips AD. Adhesion of enteroaggregative *Escherichia coli* to formalin-fixed intestinal and ureteric epithelia from children. *J Med Microbiol* 1996;44:362–371.
56. Baudry B, Savarino SJ, Vial P, et al. A sensitive and specific DNA probe to identify enteroaggregative *Escherichia coli,* a recently discovered diarrheal pathogen. *J Infect Dis* 1990;161:1249–1251.
57. Okeke IN, Lamikanra A, Czeczulin J, et al. Heterogeneous virulence of enteroaggregative *Escherichia coli* strains isolated from children in Southwest Nigeria. *J Infect Dis* 2000;181:252–260.
58. Vial PA, Mathewson JJ, DuPont HL, et al. Comparison of two assay methods for patterns of adherence to HEp-2 cells of *Escherichia coli* from patients with diarrhea. *J Clin Microbiol* 1990;28:882–885.
59. Albert MJ, Qadri F, Haque A, et al. Bacterial clump formation at the surface of liquid culture as a rapid test for identification of enteroaggregative *Escherichia coli. J Clin Microbiol* 1993;31:1397–1399.
60. Yamamoto T, Koyama Y, Matsumoto M, et al. Localized, aggregative, and diffuse adherence to HeLa cells, plastic, and human small intestines by *Escherichia coli* isolated from patients with diarrhea. *J Infect Dis* 1992;166:1295–1310.
61. Yamamoto T, Echeverria P, Yokota T. Drug resistance and adherence to human intestines of enteroaggregative *Escherichia coli. J Infect Dis* 1992;165:744–749.
62. Giron JA, Jones T, Millan-Velasco F, et al. Diffuse-adhering *Escherichia coli* (DAEC) as a putative cause of diarrhea in Mayan children in Mexico. *J Infect Dis* 1991;163:507–513.
63. Baqui AH, Sack RB, Black RE, et al. Enteropathogens associated with acute and persistent diarrhea in Bangladeshi children less than 5 years of age. *J Infect Dis* 1992;166:792–896.
64. Levine MM, Ferreccio C, Prado V, et al. Epidemiologic studies of *Escherichia coli* diarrheal infections in a low socioeconomic level peri-urban community in Santiago, Chile. *Am J Epidemiol* 1993;138:849–869.
65. Gunzburg ST, Chang BJ, Elliott SJ, et al. Diffuse and enteroaggregative patterns of adherence of enteric *Escherichia coli* isolated from aboriginal children from the Kimberley region of Western Australia. *J Infect Dis* 1993;167:755–758.
66. Jallat C, Livrelli V, Darfeuille-Michaud A, et al. *Escherichia coli* strains involved in diarrhea in France: high prevalence and heterogeneity of diffusely adhering strains. *J Clin Microbiol* 1993;31:2031–2037.

67. Bilge SS, Clausen CR, Lau W, et al. Molecular characterization of a fimbrial adhesin, F1845, mediating diffuse adherence of diarrhea-associated *Escherichia coli* to HEp-2 cells. *J Bacteriol* 1989;171:4281–4289.
68. Garcia MI, Jouve M, Nataro JP, et al. Characterization of the AfaD-like family of invasins encoded by pathogenic *Escherichia coli* associated with intestinal and extra-intestinal infections. *FEBS Lett* 2000;479:111–117.
69. Benz I, Schmidt MA. Diffuse adherence of enteropathogenic *Escherichia coli* strains. *Res Microbiol* 1990;141:785–786.
70. Bernet-Camard MF, Coconnier MH, Hudault S, et al. Pathogenicity of the diffusely adhering strain *Escherichia coli* C1845: F1845 adhesin-decay accelerating factor interaction, brush border microvillus injury, and actin disassembly in cultured human intestinal epithelial cells. *Infect Immun* 1996;64: 1918–1928.
71. Peiffer I, Servin AL, Bernet-Camard MF. Piracy of decay-accelerating factor (CD55) signal transduction by the diffusely adhering strain *Escherichia coli* C1845 promotes cytoskeletal F-actin rearrangements in cultured human intestinal INT407 cells. *Infect Immun* 1998;66:4036–4042.
72. Peiffer I, Guignot J, Barbat A, et al. Structural and functional lesions in brush border of human polarized intestinal caco-2/TC7 cells infected by members of the Afa/Dr diffusely adhering family of *Escherichia coli. Infect Immun*i 2000;68:5979–5990.
73. Cookson ST, Nataro JP. Characterization of HEp-2 cell projection formation induced by diffusely adherent *Escherichia coli. Microb Pathog* 1996;21:421–434.
74. Tacket CO, Moseley SL, Kay B, et al. Challenge studies in volunteers using *Escherichia coli* strains with diffuse adherence to HEp-2 cells. *J Infect Dis* 1990;162:550–552.
75. Germani Y, Begaud E, Duval P, et al. Prevalence of enteropathogenic, enteroaggregative, and diffusely adherent *Escherichia coli* among isolates from children with diarrhea in new Caledonia. *J Infect Dis* 1996;174:1124–1126.
76. Le Bouguenec C, Archambaud M, Labigne A. Rapid and specific detection of the *pap, afa,* and *sfa* adhesin-encoding operons in uropathogenic *Escherichia coli* strains by polymerase chain reaction. *J Clin Microbiol* 1992;30:1189–1193.
77. Bhatnagar S, Bhan MK, Sommerfelt H, et al. Enteroaggregative *Escherichia coli* may be a new pathogen causing acute and persistent diarrhea. *Scand J Infect Dis* 1993;25:579–583.
78. Paul M, Tsukamoto T, Ghosh AR, et al. The significance of enteroaggregative *Escherichia coli* in the etiology of hospitalized diarrhea in Calcutta, India and the demonstration of a new honey-combed pattern of aggregative adherence. *FEMS Microbiol Lett* 1994;117:319–325.
79. Kang G, Mathan MM, Mathan VI. Evaluation of a simplified HEp-2 cell adherence assay for *Escherichia coli* isolated from south Indian children with acute diarrhea and controls. *J Clin Microbiol* 1995;33:2204–2205.
80. Henry FJ, Udoy AS, Wanke CA, et al. Epidemiology of persistent diarrhea and etiologic agents in Mirzapur, Bangladesh. *Acta Paediatr Suppl* 1992;381:27–31.
81. Fang GD, Lima AA, Martins CV, et al. Etiology and epidemiology of persistent diarrhea in northeastern Brazil: a hospital-based, prospective, case–control study. *J Pediatr Gastroenterol Nutr* 1995;21:137–144.
82. Gonzalez R, Diaz C, Marino M, et al. Age-specific prevalence of *Escherichia coli* with localized and aggregative adherence in Venezuelan infants with acute diarrhea. *J Clin Microbiol* 1997; 35:1103–1107.
83. Jalaluddin S, de Mol P, Hemelhof W, et al. Isolation and characterization of enteroaggregative *Escherichia coli* (EAggEC) by genotypic and phenotypic markers, isolated from diarrheal children in Congo. *Clin Microbiol Infect* 1998;4:213–219.
84. Okeke IN, Lamikanra A, Steinruck H, et al. Characterization of *Escherichia coli* strains from cases of childhood diarrhea in provincial southwestern Nigeria. *J Clin Microbiol* 2000;38:7–12.
85. Bouzari S, Jafari A, Farhoudi-Moghaddam AA, et al. Adherence of non-enteropathogenic *Escherichia coli* to HeLa cells. *J Med Microbiol* 1994;40:95–97.
86. Huppertz HI, Rutkowski S, Aleksic S, et al. Acute and chronic diarrhea and abdominal colic associated with enteroaggregative *Escherichia coli* in young children living in western Europe. *Lancet* 1997;349:1660–1662.
87. Wanke CA, Mayer H, Weber R, et al. Enteroaggregative *Escherichia coli* as a potential cause of diarrheal disease in adults infected with human immunodeficiency virus. *J Infect Dis* 1998; 178:185–190.
88. Morabito S, Karch H, Mariani-Kurkdjian P, et al. Enteroaggregative, Shiga toxin-producing *Escherichia coli* O111:H2 associated with an outbreak of hemolytic-uremic syndrome. *J Clin Microbiol* 1998;36:840–842.
89. Eslava C. Cytotoxic effects of enteroaggregative *E. coli.* 93rd Meeting of the American Society for Microbiology; 1993.

42

ESCHERICHIA COLI O157:H7 AND OTHER ENTEROHEMORRHAGIC *E. COLI*

PATRICIA M. GRIFFIN
PAUL S. MEAD
SUMATHI SIVAPALASINGAM

In 1982, two outbreaks of severe bloody diarrhea in the United States were linked to the same fast-food restaurant chain. The bacterium *Escherichia coli* was isolated from the stools of ill persons. The specific serotype, O157:H7, had not previously been recognized to cause human illness (1). That same year, an outbreak of bloody diarrhea occurred in a nursing home in Canada, and again *E. coli* O157:H7 was isolated from ill patients (2). These outbreak strains produced toxins active on Vero (green monkey kidney) cells (2,3). At the same time, investigators in Canada found that stools from children with hemolytic–uremic syndrome (HUS) contained *E. coli* strains that produced a toxin active on Vero cells (4).

Further investigation demonstrated that *E. coli* O157:H7 strains produce one or both of two toxins, one neutralized by antisera to Shiga toxin (Stx) produced by *Shigella dysenteriae* type 1 and the other not (3,5,6). This finding led to two parallel nomenclatures: Vero cytotoxin 1 or Stx1 for the toxin neutralized by antisera to Stx, and Vero cytotoxin 2 or Stx2 for the other (7). Any *E. coli* that produces either of these toxins is called an Stxproducing *E. coli* (STEC), or a verocytotoxin-producing *E. coli.* In this chapter, the terms Stx and STEC are generally used even if the original report used the parallel nomenclature.

Although *E. coli* O157:H7 is the most widely recognized STEC serotype, more than 200 other serotypes of *E. coli* produce Stxs. Many have been linked to human illness, but some are probably not human pathogens. In recognition of the unique clinical features of *E. coli* O157 infection—and as a means of distinguishing STEC strains that produce human illness from those that do not—a new class of pathogenic *E. coli* was defined, the enterohemorrhagic *E. coli* (EHEC). EHEC strains were originally defined as those serotypes that cause a clinical illness similar to that caused by *E. coli* O157:H7, produce one or more phage-encoded Stxs, possess a 60-megadalton (Md) virulence plasmid, and produce attaching and effacing (A/E) lesions in an animal model (8,9). The term EHEC is generally used to refer to those STEC organisms that can cause human illness. In this chapter, we often use the shortened term *E. coli* O157 to refer to *E. coli* O157:H7 or STEC O157:NM. (*NM* denotes a nonmotile isolate.)

MICROBIOLOGY

E. coli O157:H7 is similar to most other *E. coli* in that it ferments lactose, but unlike most *E. coli* in human stool, it typically does not ferment sorbitol rapidly (10) or produce β-glucuronidase (11). *E. coli* O157 strains that ferment sorbitol have been isolated principally in Germany and surrounding areas; they are also nonmotile (12). *E. coli* O157 does not grow well at 44°C to 45.5°C, the usual temperature for detecting *E. coli* in food and water (13,14). *E. coli* O157 also survives well in acid environments, such as apple cider and fermented sausage (15). Biochemical traits that would aid in screening have not been described for the other STEC strains. In the United States, surveillance in the year 2000 showed that among more than 400 strains of *E. coli* O157, 90% were susceptible to all of a standard panel of antimicrobial agents; the most common resistance pattern was to sulfamethoxazole, tetracycline, streptomycin, and chloramphenicol (Centers for Disease Control and Prevention [CDC], *unpublished data,* see *www.cdc.gov/ncidod/dbmd/narms/*).

The Stx family consists of Stx1, Stx2, and variants of Stx2, which are encoded on bacteriophages inserted into the chromosome (16). Stx1 is identical to Stx from *S. dysenteriae* type 1 (7) . Stx2 has 56% nucleotide sequence homology to Stx1. Stxs are composed of a single A subunit and five B subunits; the B pentamer binds the toxin to cells by interaction with a membrane glycolipid called globotriaosylceramide. The toxin is then endocytosed from coated pits to the Golgi apparatus, where the A subunit acts on the 60S ribosomal subunits to

P. M. Griffin, P. S. Mead, and **S. Sivapalasingam:** Foodborne and Diarrheal Diseases Branch, Division of Bacterial and Mycotic Diseases, National Center for Infectious Diseases, Centers for Disease Control and Prevention, Atlanta, Georgia inhibit protein synthesis (16). In most collections reported, most *E. coli* O157 strains produce Stx2, about 80% also produce Stx1, and few produce only Stx1. (17). The Stx produced varies by serotype; for example, the vast majority of STEC O26:H11 strains produce only Stx1 (18).

EPIDEMIOLOGY

Animal Reservoir

Healthy ruminants, including cattle, sheep, deer, and goats, carry *E. coli* O157:H7 and other STEC strains (19,20). Although the first reported isolation of *E. coli* O157:H7 from an animal was from a calf in Argentina with colibacillosis (21), *E. coli* O157:H7 is generally not a pathogen for cattle (22). Studies in the United Kingdom indicate that *E. coli* O157:H7 is found more frequently in cattle than in sheep or pigs at slaughter, is present in up to one-half of cattle herds, and is excreted by up to 10% of cattle intended for human consumption (23). More sensitive detection methods are likely to find even higher rates. Carriage appears to be similar in many other geographic locations, although variations in sampling and culturing methods make comparison between regions difficult. Fecal shedding is highest among young weaned cattle and in the warm season (24). Excretion by cattle herds seems to be characterized by short periods of high prevalence, separated by longer periods of reduced shedding (24); epidemics of shedding have been described (25). Non-O157 STEC strains are isolated from a higher proportion of cattle and other animals than *E. coli* O157:H7 (26,27).

Certain cattle production practices and conditions have been postulated to have contributed to the emergence of *E. coli* O157:H7 and to favor the persistence of this organism on farms; these include particular feed types (28), feed and water troughs that allow multiplication of organisms (29), crowding of animals, and use of manure on grazing land. It is possible but unproven that crowded conditions in feedlots, where cattle are fattened before slaughter, may result in higher carriage of STEC in the intestines or on the skin, facilitating the entry of organisms into meat. Research is needed to identify measures that will decrease the transmission and persistence of human STEC pathogens on farms and to determine whether transporting and holding cattle in crowded feedlots before slaughter increases the proportion infected with or carrying pathogenic STEC.

Modes Of Transmission And Risk Factors

STEC can be transmitted by food or water, directly from one person to another, and from animals to persons (17,30). In the United States, about 35 outbreaks of *E. coli* O157 infections are investigated each year, but only few outbreaks of non-O157 STEC have ever been identified (CDC, *unpublished data,* 2001). Between 1982 and 2000, contaminated food was responsible for 66% of U.S. *E. coli* O157 outbreaks, person-to-person spread (usually in child care centers) for 19%, water for 12%, and animal contact for 3% (Rangel, CDC, *unpublished data,* 2001).

Bovine products, mainly ground beef, have caused the highest proportion of U.S. food-borne outbreaks. Other bovine products that have caused outbreaks in various locations include roast beef, salami, steak, raw milk, yogurt, and cheese. A large outbreak in Scotland was traced to cooked meats that were probably cross-contaminated (31), and several outbreaks, including one due to *E. coli* O111, were caused by consumption of salami (17,32,33). In the 1990s, juice (e.g., apple cider and apple juice) and produce (e.g., alfalfa sprouts, lettuce, and cabbage) became important causes of outbreaks (17), including a massive outbreak in Japan in 1996 due to radish sprouts (34). In most produce-associated outbreaks, the contamination was thought to have occurred on the farm or in transport, most likely from contact with animal manure or contaminated water; in a few outbreaks, cross-contamination has occurred in the kitchen from beef or from an ill food handler (CDC, *unpublished data*).

Recreational water, including lakes (35), ponds, and inadequately chlorinated swimming pools (36), has also caused outbreaks of *E. coli* O157 infections. Drinking water outbreaks have been linked to municipal water (37), well water, and unregulated temporary-use water systems (38). A large municipal water outbreak in Canada in 2000 was linked to more than 1,000 illnesses and seven deaths (*www.publichealthbrucegrey.on.ca*).

Because of its low infectious dose, direct transmission of *E. coli* O157 from an ill person to a well person is responsible for many diarrheal illnesses (39) and for HUS (40). This often occurs in the home, where children age 1 to 4 years are at highest risk of contracting illness, usually from their siblings (41,42). Many outbreaks have occurred in child day care centers (43).

Human STEC infections are most common in rural areas, particularly those with high cattle density (44). Factors that may contribute to the higher incidence rate include direct contact with cattle or their environment (30,45) and drinking contaminated well water (46,47). Guidelines have been developed to decrease the risk of illness among children visiting farms (30).

Other factors affect the risk of infection. Several studies have reported that toddlers and the elderly population are at greatest risk of illness (26). One report found increased risk associated with receiving antimicrobial therapy before the onset of illness (48), and another found a trend in this direction (49). Previous gastrectomy was a risk factor in one outbreak (48). Nosocomial and laboratory-acquired infections also can occur (50).

Frequency And Geography Of Isolations

With human infection now documented in more than 30 countries on six continents, the distribution of *E. coli* O157:H7 can be considered global. Among countries with ongoing surveillance for STEC infections, rates of isolation vary widely, reflecting differences in both incidence and surveillance systems.

In the United States, surveillance in the sites included in the CDC Foodborne Diseases Active Surveillance Network (FoodNet) has yielded overall rates for *E. coli* O157 infection of two to three culture-confirmed cases per 100,000 population from 1996 to 1999 (51). Although based on active surveillance, these rates are still subject to underreporting. In 1999, only about 50% of clinical laboratories in FoodNet sites reported screening all stool specimens for *E. coli* O157:H7 (CDC, *unpublished data*). Rates across the nine FoodNet sites ranged from fewer than one to four cases per 100,000 population. The regional differences are unlikely to be fully explained by physician or laboratory culturing practices. Data from other studies suggest that higher rates of infection are seen among persons living in northern states (52) and in rural areas (53). Accounting for underreporting and regional variation, the CDC estimates that *E. coli* O157 strains cause 73,000 illnesses and 60 deaths in United States each year (54).

Rates of *E. coli* O157 infection in other industrialized nations are generally similar to those in the United States. In England and Wales, regional incidence rates ranged from 0.6 to 3.2 cases per 100,000 population between 1995 and 1998 (55), and in Japan, rates of symptomatic and asymptomatic infection ranged from about 0.5 to about 4 cases per 100,000 population in 2000 (56). To date, the highest reported rates of sporadic infection have come from Canada, where many clinical laboratories routinely culture stools for *E. coli* O157:H7. In 1989, rates of culture-confirmed infection per 100,000 population were 29 for Calgary, 18.5 for Saskatoon, and 4 for Toronto (52). High incidence rates have also been reported in regions of Scotland (57) and are likely in Argentina, where HUS is endemic (58).

Several studies provide information on the rate of *E. coli* O157:H7 isolation relative to other bacterial pathogens. The rate is similar to that of *Shigella,* with some studies reporting higher rates for *E. coli* O157:H7 (59,60) and others reporting lower rates (46,61). Bloody stool specimens are particularly likely to yield the organism. In one Canadian study, *E. coli* O157:H7 was isolated from 39% of bloody stools collected in Alberta during the warmer months (62), a rate threefold higher than that for any other bacterial pathogen. In a U.S. multicenter study, *E. coli* O157:H7 was the first or second most commonly isolated pathogen in 6 of 10 study sites and accounted for 39% of bloody specimens that yielded a bacterial pathogen (52). Such a high yield may not apply in all situations however, because in a smaller study of U.S. patients presenting to emergency departments, *E. coli* O157 was isolated less frequently from bloody stools than *Shigella, Salmonella,* or *Campylobacter* (61).

The identification of non-O157 STEC strains requires techniques not used routinely in many clinical laboratories. In a survey of clinical laboratories in FoodNet sites, only about 3% of laboratories reported ever screening stools using immunoassays for Stx (CDC, *unpublished data*). Because these organisms are rarely sought, most of what is known about the frequency of non-O157 STEC infections is based on special studies. Interpretation of isolation rates is further complicated by the possibility that some non-O157 STEC strains may be nonpathogenic and thus represent an incidental finding when recovered from stool.

Studies from North America suggest that diarrhea due to non-O157 STEC infection is anywhere from one-third as common to slightly more common than diarrhea due to O157 STEC (63,64). A study of stools from 5,415 persons in Alberta, Canada, which was conducted in the mid-1980s, yielded non-O157 STEC from 0.7% of stools, compared with 2.5% for O157 STEC and 0.5% for *Shigella* (65). Similarly, in a Seattle study of 445 ill children, non-O157 STEC organisms were isolated from 1.1% of stools, compared with 2.9% for O157 STEC and 0.2% for *Shigella* (59). More recently, studies of STEC infections in Minnesota (Besser, *personal communication,* 2001), Connecticut (66), and New Mexico (67) have yielded non-O157 and O157 STEC in nearly equal proportions. Non-O157 STEC serotypes most often associated with human illness in North America include O26:H11 or NM, O111:H8 or NM, O103:H2 or H11 or H2S, O121:H19, O45:H2, O145:NM, O165:H25 or NM, and O113:H21 (26,65,68). Studies outside North America have confirmed that non-O157 STEC are ubiquitous and in some regions may be more common than O157 STEC as a cause of diarrhea (63).

Seasonality

Human cases of *E. coli* O157:H7 infection generally peak during the summer months in both the Northern and Southern hemispheres (17). The reason for this seasonal variation is unknown. However, the fact that cattle shedding also peaks during the summer months (17) suggests that increased food contamination plays a role. This could be exacerbated by seasonal variations in ground beef consumption or cooking practices.

Infectious Dose

Although volunteer feeding studies of enteric pathogens are sometimes performed to determine the infectious dose, no such studies of STEC infection have been performed because of the severity of possible complications and lack of specific therapy. Two outbreaks, one implicating ground beef patties (69) and the other, dry fermented salami (70), provided evidence that the infectious dose for *E. coli* O157:H7 may be fewer than 700 organisms and as low as 2 to 45 organisms. Culture of implicated dry fermented sausage linked to an outbreak of *E. coli* O111:H^- infections in Australia suggested an infectious dose of about one organism per 10 g of sausage (71). The epidemiologic features of *E. coli* O157:H7 are typical of an organism with a low infectious dose, with person-to-person spread in child care centers (43) and transmission by water, a medium that dilutes organisms and restricts growth.

Carriage

Young children carry *E. coli* O157:H7 longer after resolution of symptoms than older children and adults. In a study of 24 children younger than 5 years in day care center outbreaks, the median duration of shedding after onset of symptoms was 17 days, and 38% shed *E. coli* O157:H7 for more than 20 days (43). A study of day care center-associated infections of *E. coli* O157:H7 in Germany showed that the median duration of shedding was 13 days (range, 2 to 62 days) for patients with diarrhea or hemorrhagic colitis but 21 days (range, 5 to 124 days) for patients who developed HUS (72). Shedding may be intermittent (43). By comparison, the duration of shedding of *E. coli* O157:H7 is much shorter than that for *Salmonella* in children and adults (73). Studies of carriage for other STEC strains are lacking.

Incubation Period

The usual incubation period for *E. coli* O157:H7 infections is 3 or 4 days (74); however, longer incubation periods of 5 to 9 days are not uncommon (75). Incubation periods for culture-confirmed illnesses as short as 1 or 2 days (74,76) have been reported. The incubation period for *E. coli* O111 infections appears to be similar (77).

Isolations From Food And Water

Investigations of human illnesses have led to isolation of *E. coli* O157:H7 from implicated ground beef (78), beef rounds (79), raw milk (80), veal chops (81), venison jerky (82), unpasteurized apple juice (75), well water used for drinking (38), and other products. A federal microbiologic survey of ground beef samples in retail stores in the year 2000 demonstrated that 17 (1%) of 1,292 samples contained *E. coli* O157:H7 (Phyllis Sparling, *personal communication*). *E. coli* O157:H7 has also been isolated from food samples that have not been linked to human illness, including lamb, chicken, turkey, pork, and veal kidneys (13,26,83).

Non-O157 STEC strains are more readily isolated from food than *E. coli* O157:H7. Surveys in the United States and Canada have isolated non-O157 STEC organisms from 15% to 40% of retail ground beef samples (63). Given roughly similar isolation rates from diarrheal stools, the far higher rate of isolation of non-O157 STEC organisms from food suggests that not all of these strains are pathogenic for humans.

PATHOGENESIS AND IMMUNITY

Virulence attributes of STEC include production of Stxs, adherence factors, and other factors. The variable presence of these virulence factors among different serotypes likely accounts for the predominance of certain serotypes in causing human illness. Host factors and immunity also affect the risk of illness.

Shiga Toxins

Stxs are cytotoxic for some cell lines; they are enterotoxic, mediating fluid accumulation in ligated ileal loops, and cause paralysis and death when injected intravenously in mice and rabbits (6). Many lines of evidence indicate that Stx production is the major virulence factor of STEC. The only other enteric pathogen recognized to cause HUS is *S. dysenteriae* type 1, which is the only *Shigella* species that produces Stx (84,85). Many different STEC strains have been isolated from patients with postdiarrheal HUS, suggesting that the common pathogenic mechanism is production of Stx. Stx1 and Stx2 are toxic for human endothelial cells *in vitro* (86,87), and glomerular capillary endothelial cell injury is the most consistent renal finding in patients with HUS (88). Histopathologic studies of patients with HUS have demonstrated microvascular angiopathy, and rabbits injected with Stx1 develop thrombotic microvascular angiopathy similar to that seen in humans with HUS (89). Finally, globotriaosylceramide, the receptor for Stx (90), is present in human renal tissue (91).

The data indicate that Stx acts locally on the gut mucosa and that circulating toxin may also affect the gut. The histologic pattern of human colonic injury in *E. coli* O157:H7 infection caused by strains producing Stx2 with or without Stx1 is similar to that of *Clostridium difficile* colitis, which is caused by a locally acting toxin (92). Free Stx can be identified in the stools of persons with STEC infection. Stx is cytotoxic to cultured epithelial cells from human colon and ileum (93). Studies of *S. dysenteriae* type 1 infection suggest that Stx damages the microvasculature of the large intestine, resulting in edema, local ischemia, and an influx of inflammatory cells into the mucosa. Animal models also indicate that circulating toxin can cause intestinal injury (89,94,95).

Although the simplest mechanism for HUS involves direct cytotoxic action on renal endothelial cells, the pathways for systemic disease are probably more complex. Stx and lipopolysaccharide (LPS) may elicit production of interleukin 1 (IL-1) and tumor necrosis factor (TNF) from macrophages (96,97). IL-1β, TNF-α, and LPS may then increase the sensitivity of endothelial cells to Stx by increasing expression of globotriaosylceramide on the cell surface (97–99). Stx inhibits protein synthesis (6), and affected endothelial cells may detach, exposing platelets to the subendothelium and initiating coagulation (97). Stx has never been demonstrated free in human sera; however, Stx2 was identified in circulating polymorphonuclear leukocytes of patients with HUS (100). In addition, Stx has been reported in the distal renal tubular epithelial cells of a child who died from *E. coli* O157-associated HUS (101).

Data on animals support human data suggesting that Stx2 is a more important virulence factor than Stx1. Streptomycin-treated mice fed *E. coli* K12 strains containing only Stx2 genes died, but those fed a strain containing only Stx1 genes did not die (102). Only strains that produced high levels of Stx2 killed mice. Streptomycin-treated mice fed an *E. coli* strain that produced both Stx1 and Stx2 were protected from renal tubular necrosis by passive transfer of antibodies to Stx2 but not Stx1 (102). The increased lethality of Stx2 compared with Stx1 in streptomycin-treated mice was also observed after injection of toxins (103). In another model, gnotobiotic piglets inoculated with *E. coli* O157:H7 strains that produced only Stx2 or both Stx1 and Stx2 developed brain lesions, and loss of ability to produce Stx2 resulted in loss of ability to cause brain lesions (104).

Adherence Factors

Adherence to mucosal surfaces prevents loss of bacteria into the environment and promotes the delivery of toxins to eukaryotic cell surfaces in a concentrated manner. The 94- to 97-kd outer membrane protein intimin, encoded by the *eae* gene, is the only factor that has been demonstrated to play a role in intestinal colonization of *E. coli* O157 *in vivo* in an animal model (16). In piglets and tissue culture cells, *E. coli* O157 strains produce attaching and effacing (A/E) adherence. This is characterized by intimate adherence with dissolution of the brush border at the site of attachment (105). Within the enterocyte, filamentous actin accumulates at the site of attachment and the enterocyte membrane may cup the bacteria, forming a pedestal-like structure that can be detected by fluorescence–actin staining (106). Although adherence of STEC to the human gastrointestinal mucosa has not been demonstrated, A/E lesions have been demonstrated in the gut of infants with diarrhea due to enteropathogenic *E. coli* strains, which have a similar adherence mechanism (107). STEC strains likely possess other intestinal adherence factors because *eae*-negative STEC strains can adhere to cultured epithelial cells (16) and can cause human illness (108).

Other Bacterial Factors

Animal models suggest that LPS may play an important role in pathogenesis. In rabbits and mice, the effects of Stx2 can be enhanced or inhibited by LPS, depending on the timing of its administration (109). The fact that most patients with severe illness develop an antibody response to the O157 LPS suggests that LPS is hematogenously disseminated from the gut (110).

STEC strains contain other possible virulence factors, some of which are mentioned here. Virtually all strains of *E. coli* O157:H7 and most other STEC organisms isolated from humans contain a 60-Md plasmid (pO157) that encodes enterohemolysin and a catalase peroxidase (16). One study demonstrated the enterohemolytic phenotype in 88% of *E. coli* O111 strains from patients with HUS but in only 22% of those from patients with only diarrhea (111). Enterohemolysin can lyse human erythrocytes, thus releasing heme and hemoglobin (112). These compounds stimulate the growth of *E. coli* O157, probably because this organism contains a specialized iron transport system that allows it to use heme or hemoglobin as an iron source. Of interest, the gene encoding this iron transport system has not been identified in other STEC strains (16).

Host Factors And Immunity

STEC strains have host specificity, the determinants of which are not well understood. For example, serotypes that cause edema disease in pigs have rarely been detected in humans. Cattle lack gut vascular receptors for Stx, which may explain why they are tolerant reservoir hosts for STEC (113).

The increased rates of infection and complications in children younger than 5 years and in the elderly (26) suggest some role for immunity. However, it is not known whether circulating antibody to O157 LPS or to Stx may decrease the likelihood of infection or severe illness. Repeated infections with *E. coli* O157, including HUS, have been described in children without evident immunologic abnormalities (114,115).

Animal Models

Although several animal models of STEC infection exist, none reproduce typical human colonic disease with progression to HUS. Edema disease of pigs, caused primarily by STEC serogroups O138, O139, and O141, is a naturally occurring model in which piglets develop edema of the eyelids, ataxia, and convulsions; diarrhea may occur but is not characteristic (116). The histologic lesion is microvascular angiopathy affecting many organs, most often the brain and intestine. A colonization factor and Stx2e are the major virulence factors (117).

CLINICAL ILLNESS

Diarrhea And Manifestations Other Than Hemolytic–Uremic Syndrome

E. coli *O157:H7*

The clinical spectrum of *E. coli* O157:H7 infection ranges from asymptomatic shedding to nonbloody diarrhea, bloody diarrhea (hemorrhagic colitis), HUS, thrombotic thrombocytopenic purpura (TTP), and death. *E. coli* O157:H7 has been isolated from persons with chronic diarrhea, but causality has not been proven (118).

Illness typically begins as nonbloody diarrhea accompanied by abdominal cramps. Among patients seeking medical care, stools frequently become bloody on the second or third day of illness, with the amount of blood observed ranging from small streaks to large quantities. Up to one-half of patients report vomiting, and abdominal tenderness may be prominent. Patients with *E. coli* O157:H7 infection have been mistakenly diagnosed with appendicitis, intussusception, primary inflammatory bowel disease, and ischemic colitis. As a result, some patients have undergone unnecessary surgical procedures (26). Evidence of right-sided colonic inflammation by barium enema or colonoscopy with histologic changes suggesting ischemia and/or infectious injury in a patient with a compatible clinical illness strongly suggests *E. coli* O157:H7 infection. Without stool cultures, *E. coli* O157:H7 infection may be difficult to differentiate from ischemic colitis or pseudomembranous colitis in elderly patients (119). The presence of similar illness in others, which suggests a common exposure, and right-sided colonic involvement should make one suspect *E. coli* O157:H7 infection. Although bloody diarrhea is generally recognized as a hallmark of *E. coli* O157:H7 infection, in some outbreaks, most patients have reported only nonbloody diarrhea (26).

Among persons in FoodNet surveillance sites with *E. coli* O157 infection severe enough to have a stool culture performed, the hospitalization rate is 39% and the death rate 1.4% (51). Most patients recover spontaneously in 7 to 10 days with no obvious sequelae. Intussusception (120), appendicitis (118), and inflammation of the small bowel, predominantly the terminal ileum (121), have been reported in patients with *E. coli* O157:H7 infection without HUS. Rarely, *E. coli* O157:H7 has been isolated from extraintestinal sites including urine (122) and blood (123) from persons with diarrhea.

Non-O157 Stx-producing E. coli

Some non-O157 STEC strains are capable of producing all the features of *E. coli* O157:H7 infection, including bloody diarrhea and HUS, whereas other strains appear to be nonpathogenic. This likely reflects the fact that Stx production alone is generally insufficient to cause disease and that a portion of non-O157 STEC strains lack one or more accessory virulence factors needed to cause human illness (16).

As a group, non-O157 STEC strains that cause human illness appear somewhat less virulent than *E. coli* O157:H7 (16,63). In a study of 113 cases of STEC infection in Canada, 42% of patients with non-O157 STEC reported bloody diarrhea, compared with 97% of patients infected with *E. coli* O157:H7 (65). Many sero groups have been isolated from patients with bloody diarrhea including O26, O111, and O103 (see also "Frequency and Geography of Isolations" section). Among patients who do not develop HUS, reported complications of non-O157 STEC infection include small bowel obstruction (124) and suppurative mesenteric lymphadenitis (59). When evaluating a patient whose stool has yielded a non-O157 STEC, it should be remembered that co-infection with *E. coli* O157:H7 has been reported (65) and that overall non-O157 STEC organisms may be recovered from approximately 1% stools of healthy persons (26). As with *E. coli* O157:H7, non-O157 STEC organisms are occasionally recovered from extraintestinal sites, particularly urine. In some instances, infection of these sites appears to have occurred in the absence of concomitant diarrheal illness (125,126). Non-O157 STEC organisms have been isolated from intestines of children with sudden infant death syndrome (127) and from patients with ulcerative colitis (128); however, a causal role in these conditions has not been established. Further studies are needed to determine which non-O157 STEC strains are human pathogens.

HUS And Thrombotic Thrombocytopenic Purpura

HUS is characterized by microangiopathic hemolytic anemia, thrombocytopenia, renal failure, and often central nervous system involvement (129). It was first well described in 1955 in Switzerland (130). About 90% of cases of HUS are preceded by diarrhea (131). Complications of HUS include bowel perforation, bowel necrosis, toxic megacolon, gastrointestinal tract stricture, anal abnormalities, myocardial dysfunction, pulmonary edema, pancreatitis, hepatitis, and neurologic abnormalities such as stroke, seizure, and coma. Among children with HUS, 3% to 5% die acutely (132–134), and 12% have severe sequelae of renal impairment, neurologic injury, or hypertension (131).

TTP includes all the clinical features of HUS (135). In general, nephrologists call the syndrome they see HUS, and hematologists call it TTP (129); children are generally diagnosed with HUS, adults with TTP. In case series of patients with TTP, diarrhea was not even mentioned as a preceding symptom (135,136). The rare patient with TTP whose illness was preceded by diarrhea is likely to have STEC infection (26). We use the term HUS for any illness with the features of HUS or TTP that is preceded by gastrointestinal illness or that has evidence of STEC infection, in a person of any age. Most studies of HUS have focused on children; studies of adults are needed.

Studies of patients with postdiarrheal HUS in Europe and North America indicate that most cases can be linked to STEC infection (137). Serologic data indicate that *E. coli* O157 causes most cases: Antibody responses to O157 LPS were identified in 73% of HUS patients in the United Kingdom (138), 73% in Central Europe (139), and 80% in the United States (137). However, far fewer persons have stools that yield STEC because HUS is typically diagnosed a week after the onset of diarrhea, when the numbers of pathogens in the stool is decreasing (140). Studies of HUS in which stool specimens were obtained within 6 days of the onset of diarrhea report high isolation rates for *E. coli* O157—96% in the United States (140) and 87% in Canada (141). Non-O157 STEC organisms have been isolated from some HUS patients in most studies. A worldwide questionnaire survey found that O111 and O26 were the non-O157 STEC serogroups most commonly isolated from persons with HUS (142).

In rare instances, nondiarrheal STEC infection may result in HUS. There are several reports of HUS in patients with STEC isolated from urine; most did not have a prodrome of diarrhea, and *E. coli* O157 was isolated from only one (126). *E. coli* O157 was isolated in a stool specimen from a man diagnosed with TTP who had abdominal pain and hemorrhagic gastroduodenitis without diarrhea (143).

Isolation of an enteric pathogen other than STEC from the stool of a patient with HUS does not confirm that pathogen as the cause of the illness. In one instance, a child with *E. coli* O157-associated HUS also had *Salmonella* and group A β-streptococcal bacteremia (144). In other reports, *Campylobacter, Salmonella* species, rotavirus, corona virus, respiratory syncytial virus, and *Cryptosporidium* were identified in HUS patients who also had evidence of STEC infection (133,139)

In a Canadian study among children with *E. coli* O157 diarrhea severe enough to have a stool specimen cultured, the risk of HUS was 8%; children younger than 5 years had the highest rate, with 13% developing HUS or hemolytic anemia (145). The rate of HUS in adults with *E. coli* O157 infection is not known. Among persons in U.S. outbreaks caused by *E. coli* O157, which included patients with mild illness who did not seek medical care, the rate of HUS was 4% (CDC, *unpublished data*). The relatively low proportion of HUS cases from which non-O157 STEC organisms are isolated, along with the similar isolation rates of O157 and non-O157 STEC from diarrhea, suggests that non-O157 STEC organisms as a group are less likely to cause HUS. However, infections with some serogroups, such as O111, may have a high rate of HUS.

Host and bacterial factors both influence the risk of HUS. Among children infected with one strain of *E. coli* O157, use of antimotility agents, initial leukocytosis, vomiting, young age, and a short diarrheal prodrome were associated with increased risk of HUS (146). Some of these findings have been confirmed by others (147). Other factors reported to increase the risk of HUS include very young or old age, female gender, bloody diarrhea, fever, and treatment with an antimicrobial agent (see "Treatment" section) (26). In retrospective analyses, persons infected with an *E. coli* O157:H7 strain that produced only Stx2 were more likely to develop HUS than those infected with strains that produce both toxins or only Stx1 (148–150).

Human Gut Endoscopic And Histologic Findings

On colonoscopy, the mucosa of patients with *E. coli* O157:H7 infection without HUS typically shows edema, erythema, and superficial ulceration, usually in a patchy distribution. Dusky-appearing mucosa or bleeding may also be observed. A gradient of severity of findings is typical, with the most severe disease in the cecum and right colon (92). Typical findings of pseudomembranous colitis are uncommon (151).

Colonic biopsy specimens from persons with bloody diarrhea due to *E. coli* O157:H7 may show only an ischemic pattern of injury, only an infectious pattern, both, or neither (92). In a series of patients with illness severe enough to warrant colonoscopy, most patients had hemorrhage and edema in the colonic lamina propria. Focal necrosis with hemorrhage and acute inflammation in the superficial mucosa, but preservation of the deep crypts, similar to the findings in acute ischemic colitis (Fig. 42.1A), was common. Specimens from some patients had fibrin/platelet thrombi within mucosal capillaries, and some had deep apoptosis of colonic

A

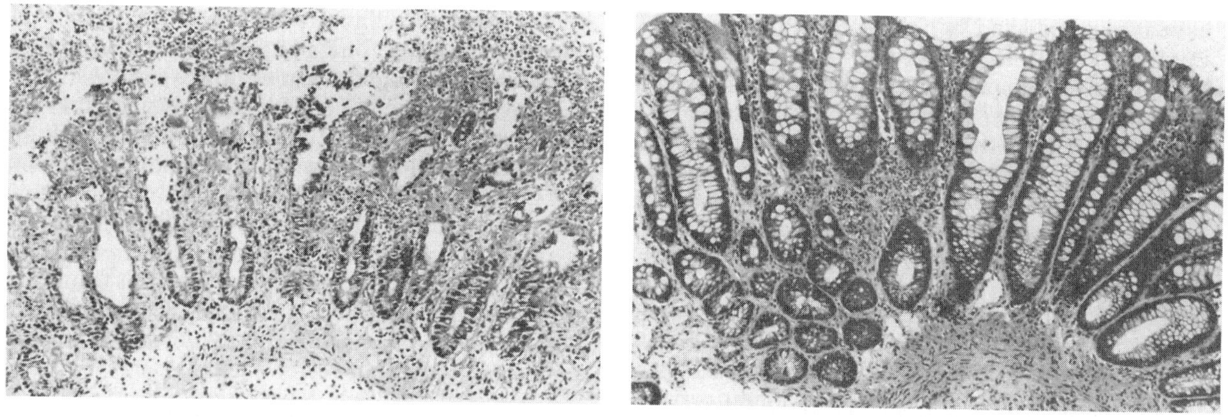

B

FIGURE 42.1. Endoscopic mucosal biopsy specimens from patients with *Escherichia coli* O157:H7 infection. **A:** The ischemic pattern of injury with superficial necrosis, mucosal hemorrhage, an overlying pseudomembrane, and relative preservation of deep crypts. **B:** The infectious pattern of injury with an area of focal infiltration of the lamina propria by neutrophils. (From Griffin PM, Olmstead LC, Petras RE. *Escherichia coli* O157:H7-associated colitis. A clinical and histological study of 11 cases. *Gastroenterology* 1990;99:142–149, with permission.)

crypts. Neutrophilic infiltration of the lamina propria and crypts, similar to the findings in infectious colitis (Fig. 42.1B), was also common. Poorly formed pseudomembranes were observed. Nonspecific changes and normal specimens have also been described; because the disease is often patchy, obtaining more than one biopsy specimen increases the likelihood of identifying an abnormality (92). In addition, because the gradient of injury is from the right side to the left side of the colon, rectal biopsy specimens are least likely to demonstrate abnormalities (92). Histologic features in patients who develop HUS are likely to be more severe. For example, hemorrhage and necrosis of the distal small bowel and distal esophagus were described in a patient with HUS associated with STEC O111 infection (152).

LABORATORY DIAGNOSIS

Stool

Stool characteristics are not good predictors of STEC infection. In a multicenter study, fecal leukocytes were identified in 71% of patients with *E. coli* O157:H7 infection, more than in persons with any other bacterial diarrheas, probably reflecting the higher proportion with bloody diarrhea. However, only 24% of persons with *E. coli* O157:H7 infection had more than 10 leukocytes per high-power field (52).

Clinical laboratory screening tests for *E. coli* O157:H7 take advantage of the fact that although it ferments lactose like most *E. coli,* it does not ferment sorbitol within 24 hours (153). Sorbitol-MacConkey (SMAC) agar, in which lactose is replaced by sorbitol, is commercially available and is the medium of choice for screening (10). Sorbitol-negative (clear) colonies should be selected from the SMAC plate and tested with commercially available O157 antiserum. Modifying SMAC medium by adding cefixime, rhamnose, and tellurite can improve detection (154). Sorbitol-fermenting Stx-producing *E. coli* O157 strains have been identified, principally from Germany (155).

Immunomagnetic separation as a selective enrichment step increases the yield of *E. coli* O157:H7 over direct plating. In this method, O157-specific antibodies attached to paramagnetic polystyrene beads are added to an enriched sample and then subjected to magnetic separation. *E. coli* O157:H7 organisms are removed along with the magnetic beads. This is most advantageous when examining specimens in which *E. coli* O157:H7 strains are present in small numbers, such as those from patients presenting a long time after the onset of illness (154).

Presumptive identification of *E. coli* O157:H7 can be reported for any organism that is sorbitol negative on SMAC agar, agglutinates in O157 antiserum, and is biochemically an *E. coli.* Confirmation requires the identification of the H7 flagellar antigen or determination that the strain produces Stx (154). Some *E. coli* O157 strains are nonmotile; most of these produce Stx, suggesting that they previously expressed the H7 antigen.

Toxin testing of sporadic *E. coli* O157:H7 isolates is generally not necessary because nontoxigenic strains are very rare (150). Toxin testing should be done on nonmotile *E. coli* O157 strains because only toxin-producing strains have been linked to human illness.

Several sensitive, specific, and rapid immunologic assays for detection of Stx are commercially available (156). These assays are easy to perform and helpful in differential diagnosis, in conducting treatment trials, and in selecting patients for close monitoring. A disadvantage to using these methods is that the isolate is not available for characterization. For example, it would be helpful to know that an Stx-positive specimen contains *E. coli* O157 because of the high virulence of this organism and its outbreak potential. Similarly, increased isolation and reporting of a particular non-O157 STEC serotype would merit public health interventions. Therefore, a positive reaction in an immunoassay should be confirmed by culture to isolate the organism (154).

Research laboratories use several other techniques for demonstrating the presence of genes encoding Stxs, including DNA probes and polymerase chain reaction (PCR). DNA probes for Stx genes, the 60-Md plasmid of *E. coli* O157:H7, and the *E. coli* A/E gene (*eae*) have been used to characterize STEC. Several PCR assays have been developed to characterize various genes present in STEC, including potential virulence or virulence-associated genes such as *eae,* the enterohemolysin gene EHEC-*hlyA,* and *katP,* a gene on the large plasmid of *E. coli* O157:H7 that encodes a novel catalase peroxidase (154). These assays have been important in identifying different pathogenic groups of STEC.

An immunoassay for detection of the O157 antigen is commercially available (157). Direct testing of stools by this method is rapid, but a negative test result does not exclude the possibility of *E. coli* O157 infection, and a positive test result should be followed up with culture. Unlike SMAC agar, this immunoassay can detect sorbitol-fermenting *E. coli* O157. However, other tests must be performed to distinguish nontoxigenic from toxigenic strains (154).

Subtyping of *E. coli* O157:H7 is useful in the detection and investigation of outbreaks. Methods include antibiograms, toxin typing, phage typing, and pulsed-field gel electrophoresis (PFGE) (158). Subtyping can link seemingly sporadic cases so a vehicle can be implicated epidemiologically. Subtyping by PFGE has been valuable in many outbreaks of *E. coli* O157:H7 infections, including a multistate outbreak from hamburgers (78), an outbreak from lettuce (159), and an international outbreak from commercial apple juice (75).

The CDC has established an international network of public health laboratories called PulseNet; participating laboratories perform subtyping using standardized methods on *E. coli* O157 and other enteric pathogens (158). The CDC requests that all *E. coli* O157:H7 strains isolated by clinical laboratories be submitted to public health laboratories for subtyping.

Serology

Measurement of antibodies to STEC is particularly useful in studies of patients who may not have had appropriate stool cultures performed early enough in their diarrheal illness to isolate a pathogen. Serologic assays include enzyme immunoassay (EIA) to detect antibodies to LPS, Stx, and secreted proteins; Western blot assays to detect antibodies against LPS, Stx, enterohemolysin, flagellar, and outer membrane and secreted proteins; cell culture assays to measure toxin-neutralizing antibodies; and indirect hemagglutination assays to detect antibodies against LPS (154). Currently, a sensitive immunologic assay for the diagnosis of all STEC infections is not available. Only 18% to 35% of patients with STEC infections develop antibodies to the toxins, mainly against Stx1, whereas most persons respond to the LPS of their infecting STEC strain. Therefore, assays that measure antibodies against these antigens, particularly EIAs, are the most widely used in the serodiagnosis of STEC infections (110,154). Intimin is produced by a large proportion of STEC organisms (160) and many patients with *E. coli* O157 infection develop an antibody response to intimin (161); this could be the basis of a diagnostic test applicable to many STEC infections. These serologic assays are not yet commercially available in the United States.

TREATMENT

There is no proven specific therapy for infection with *E. coli* O157:H7 or other STEC strains. Considerations for patient management include identification of patients at increased risk of complications, the administration of hydration and supportive care, and use of antidiarrheal and antimicrobial medications.

Children younger than 10 years, the elderly, and persons with fever, elevated leukocyte count, or bloody diarrhea should be followed closely for signs of hemolysis, thrombocytopenia, and renal dysfunction (146). Because of concern that hypovolemia may potentiate renal injury, some clinicians recommend prompt hospitalization and aggressive intravenous hydration for all patients with confirmed *E. coli* O157:H7 infection. As with other causes of bloody diarrhea, antimotility agents are not indicated for persons with *E. coli* O157:H7 infection. In some retrospective analyses, receiving an antimotility agent has been associated with increased risk of progression to HUS (146,162).

The use of antimicrobial agents to treat STEC infections remains controversial (163). Most *E. coli* O157:H7 strains are susceptible to commonly used antimicrobial agents (see "Microbiology" section); however, these agents have had no effect on the duration of diarrhea in some studies (164) and have been associated with prolonged bloody diarrhea in others (146). More importantly, there is debate over whether antimicrobial therapy increases or decreases the risk of developing HUS. *In vitro,* exposure of *E. coli* O157:H7 to sublethal doses of antimicrobial agents can induce Stx-encoding bacteriophage and increase Stx production, although the details of this effect vary from study to study (165–167). In a mouse model of *E. coli* O157:H7 infection, treatment with subtherapeutic doses of ciprofloxacin resulted in high mortality rates and increased levels of Stx in feces, despite decreased shedding of viable organisms (168). In contrast, neither fecal Stx levels nor mortality rates were increased among mice treated with fosfomycin, a cell wall synthesis inhibitor that does not induce bacteriophage (168).

These and other studies suggest that subtherapeutic dosing with certain antimicrobial agents may increase the risk of developing HUS, just as inappropriate antibiotic use increases the risk of HUS among patients infected with *S. dysenteriae* type 1 (84). It remains unresolved whether therapeutic doses of antimicrobial agents are harmful or may in fact be beneficial if given early in the course of infection. To date, most studies have been nonrandomized (Table 42.1) and are therefore confounded by the greater tendency of

TABLE 42.1. FREQUENCY OF HEMOLYTIC–UREMIC SYNDROME AMONG PATIENTS TREATED AND NOT TREATED WITH ANTIMICROBIAL AGENTS IN SELECTED PUBLISHED STUDIES

Reference	Total	Hemolytic–uremic Syndrome Treated (%)	Hemolytic–uremic syndrome Not Treated (%)	*p* Value
Nonrandomized, retrospective studies				
Riley et al., 1983 (1)	23	0/11 (0)	0/12 (0)	NS
Cimolai et al., 1994 (162)	118	13/64 (20)	15/54 (28)	NS
Bell et al., 1997 (146)	278	8/50 (16)	28/218 (13)	NS
Slutsker et al., 1998 (46)	93	4/39 (10)	3/54 (6)	NS
Gilbert et al., 2000 (185)	293	14/168 (8)	9/125 (7)	NS
Nonrandomized, prospective studies				
Pavia et al., 1990 (49)	17	6/8 (75)	2/7 (28)	NS
Wong et al., 2000 (169)	71	5/9 (56)	5/62 (8)	.002
Randomized, prospective				
Proulx et al., 1992 (171)	47	2/22 (9)	4/25 (16)	NS

NS, not significant.

severely ill patients to receive antimicrobial treatment. Despite this inherent bias, most nonrandomized studies do not suggest an increased risk of HUS among patients receiving antimicrobial agents (Table 42.1). One partially randomized study did find an increased risk of HUS among patients receiving sulfonamides (49), and a more recent nonrandomized study found a positive association with receiving antimicrobial agents in general (169). However, interpretation of these two studies is complicated by the extraordinarily high rates of HUS observed in treated patients, rates far higher than those in larger retrospective analyses (Table 42.1). Countering these studies is an evaluation of STEC cases identified during a large outbreak in Japan. In this study (170), patients treated with fosfomycin very early in the course of illness were less likely to develop HUS than those who received treatment later. The only randomized trial published found no difference in HUS rates among patients who did and did not receive antibiotics (171); however, this study is limited by the fact that many participants were not randomized until late in the course of illness.

Given the central role of Stxs in the development of HUS (172), several agents have been developed in hopes of binding the toxin in the gut, thus preventing its absorption into the body. The best studied of these investigational agents is Synsorb, a compound composed of Stx-binding glycosides covalently linked to diatomaceous earth. In a phase II clinical trial involving 347 patients with suspected or confirmed STEC infection, an intention-to-treat analysis showed no benefit to receiving Synsorb. However, in a subanalysis limited to patients who were enrolled early, who were compliant with the treatment, and who were not infected with other pathogens, treatment was associated with a nearly 40% decrease in the risk of HUS (173). Recently, Paton et al. (174) reported development of a recombinant bacterium that expresses Stx receptors with a binding affinity far higher than Synsorb. In a mouse model of infection with Stx2-producing STEC, oral administration of the recombinant strain was highly protective (174). Studies of edema disease in pigs suggest that anti-Stx immune globulin could also be a valuable treatment modality. In a study of 119 infected piglets, intraperitoneal administration of anti-Stx2e was highly protective, even when administered after the onset of symptoms (175). Further studies are needed to determined the clinical utility of this new agent. Additional information on general supportive and investigational treatment of patients with HUS is provided in reference 176.

PREVENTION

Because the primary therapeutic option for *E. coli* O157:H7 infection is supportive care, preventing infection is paramount. Several characteristics of the organism make prevention a particular challenge, including its widespread presence in healthy cattle and their environment, its ability to survive in food and water, its acid tolerance, and its low infectious dose.

Changing some farm management practices could reduce STEC carriage by animals and contamination of the environment. For example, decreasing contamination of feeds and water troughs and decreasing crowding may decrease transmission among cattle. Improved disposal of cattle manure could decrease contamination of groundwater, streams, and produce. Practices to reduce contamination of cattle hides during and after transport, holding in feedlots, and slaughtering should be investigated, because pathogens can be transferred from hides to meat. Attention to the condition of animals after transport, after holding in feedlots, and to the manner of slaughter could suggest methods to decrease the contamination of meat.

After a large outbreak from hamburger patties in 1993, the Food and Drug Administration (FDA) made changes in the Model Food Code for cooking temperatures of ground beef at retail, and the U.S. Department of Agriculture (USDA) required manufacturing plants to heat meat patties sold as fully cooked sufficiently to kill pathogenic microorganisms. In 1994, the USDA declared *E. coli* O157:H7 an adulterant in ground beef, and the sale of raw ground beef known to contain this pathogen was prohibited. The USDA also introduced the Pathogen Reduction/Hazard Analysis and Critical Control Points (HACCP) rule, which mandates requirements for federally inspected meat and poultry plants (178). The basic principle of HACCP is to identify critical control points in production, processing, transportation, and preparation of food products, and then to implement appropriate controls at these points to allow early detection and correction of problems.

Irradiation kills bacteria in ground beef and is approved for this purpose (179). The allowable doses of radiation will not make food radioactive or significantly alter its appearance or nutritional qualities (179). Unless beef is precooked or irradiated, a digital meat thermometer should be used after cooking hamburgers to ensure that the internal temperature reaches 160°F.

Procedures to ensure that fresh fruits and vegetables are kept free of contamination on the farm, in transport, in processing, and in the kitchen are important, particularly for items that are not cooked. Contamination can be reduced by protecting produce from contact with animals or animal feces and using disinfected processing water (159). The importance of prevention is illustrated by alfalfa, on which a few organisms on the seed can multiply to high levels during the sprouting process, and treatment of seeds and sprouts with very high concentrations of chlorine does not eliminate pathogens (180). As a result of outbreaks, the FDA now requires that apple juice and cider shipped interstate either be pasteurized or have a warning label (181). Pasteurization of milk and juices provides the best assurance of safety.

E. coli strains, including O157, are highly chlorine sensitive (182). Protection, purification, and disinfection of public water supplies are essential to prevent transmission through drinking water. Tighter regulation of temporary public drinking water systems for agricultural fairs and other events is needed (38). Swimming pools should be adequately chlorinated, and swimming areas in lakes should have convenient toilets.

Consumers and food preparers should be taught that raw foods of animal origin can harbor infectious agents. Ground beef that is not thoroughly cooked is a high-risk food because a single serving typically contains meat from many different animals that came from many different farms, and contaminants on the outside of meat can be mixed in when it is ground. "Safe handling" labels also help to educate consumers (183). Consumers should wash produce and prevent cross-contamination from raw or undercooked meat products.

Precautions should be taken to reduce the risk for transmission of STEC at petting zoos and other venues where direct contact between farm animals, particularly calves, and humans occurs. Venues should separate animal petting areas and eating areas, hand-washing facilities should be available, persons at high risk for serious illness (such as children younger than 5 years, the elderly, and the immunocompromised) should be supervised or exercise increased precaution, and raw milk should not be served (30).

Prevention of person-to-person spread of *E. coli* O157:H7 is a challenge because the infectious dose is low. An initial *E. coli* O157:H7 infection from contaminated food or water can cause a cascade of person-to-person spread, sometimes resulting in death (48). Infected patients and their families should be counseled to increase hand-washing practices with soap to prevent the spread of infection within the home (42). Exclusion of infected children from day care until two consecutive stool cultures are negative can prevent transmission (43), but keeping asymptomatic children at home is burdensome for parents who may instead send their children to other day care centers. This can lead to further dissemination of an outbreak. Medical personnel who care for persons with diarrhea or HUS and laboratory workers who deal with stool specimens should take special precautions to avoid contact with feces. Hand washing is the most important preventive measure to reduce the risk of person-to-person transmission.

CONCLUSION

Diagnosing STEC infections has important benefits for both the individual and the community. Diagnosis can be critical for individual patients who may be spared unnecessary and even life-threatening diagnostic and surgical procedures and therapies. Diagnosis of STEC infection can result in increased attention to hydration to prevent HUS and earlier initiation of dialysis, which may improve outcome (184). Detecting individual cases of STEC infection, particularly due to *E. coli* O157 and O111, is the first step in detecting outbreaks. Immediate steps to prevent further illnesses in an outbreak setting include measures such as removing contaminated food from the market, closing contaminated lakes, and improving hygiene in affected child care centers. Investigations of outbreaks is critical because the findings exert pressure on industry and government officials to develop and implement measures to increase the safety of food, drinking and swimming water, child day care centers, and venues where the public can have contact with cattle.

ACKNOWLEDGMENTS

The authors thank Joy Wells for assistance on the laboratory sections, Karyn Bourke for technical assistance, and Lynne McIntyre for editorial assistance.

REFERENCES

1. Riley LW, Remis RS, Helgerson SD, et al. Hemorrhagic colitis associated with a rare *Escherichia coli* serotype. *N Engl J Med* 1983;308:681–685.
2. Johnson WM, Lior H, Bezanson GS. Cytotoxic *Escherichia coli* O157:H7 associated with haemorrhagic colitis in Canada. *Lancet* 1983;1:76.
3. O'Brien AO, Lively TA, Chen ME, et al. *Escherichia coli* O157:H7 strains associated with haemorrhagic colitis in the United States produce a *Shigella dysenteriae* 1 (Shiga) like cytotoxin. *Lancet* 1983;1:702.
4. Karmali MA, Petric M, Lim C, et al. The association between idiopathic hemolytic uremic syndrome and infection by verotoxin-producing *Escherichia coli. J Infect Dis* 1985;151:775–782.
5. Strockbine NA, Marques LR, Newland JW, et al. Two toxin-converting phages from *Escherichia coli* O157:H7 strain 933 encode antigenically distinct toxins with similar biologic activities. *Infect Immun* 1986;53:135–140.
6. O'Brien AD, Holmes RK. Shiga and Shiga-like toxins. *Microbiol Rev* 1987;51:206–220.
7. Nataro JP, Kaper JB, Robins-Browne R, et al. Patterns of adherence of diarrheogenic *Escherichia coli* to HEp-2 cells. *Pediatr Infect Dis J* 1987;6:829–831.
8. Levine MM, Edelman R. Enteropathogenic *Escherichia coli* of classic serotypes associated with infant diarrhea: epidemiology and pathogenesis. *Epidemiol Rev* 1984;6:31–51.
9. Levine MM, Xu JG, Kaper JB, et al. A DNA probe to identify enterohemorrhagic *Escherichia coli* of O157:H7 and other serotypes that cause hemorrhagic colitis and hemolytic uremic syndrome. *J Infect Dis* 1987;156:175–182.
10. March SB, Ratnam S. Sorbitol-MacConkey medium for detection of *Escherichia coli* O157:H7 associated with hemorrhagic colitis. *J Clin Microbiol* 1986;23:869–872.
11. Thompson JS, Hodge DS, Borczyk AA. Rapid biochemical test to identify verocytotoxin-positive strains of *Escherichia coli* serotype O157. *J Clin Microbiol* 1990;28:2165–2168.
12. Karch H, Bohm H, Schmidt H, et al. Clonal structure and pathogenicity of Shiga-like toxin-producing, sorbitol-fermenting *Escherichia coli* O157:H7. *J Clin Microbiol* 1993;31:1200–1205.
13. Doyle MP. *Escherichia coli* O157:H7 and its significance in foods. *Int J Food Microbiol* 1991;12:289–301.

14. Raghubeer EV, Matches JR. Temperature range for growth of *Escherichia coli* serotype O157:H7 and selected coliforms in *E. coli* medium. *J Clin Microbiol* 1990;28:803–805.
15. Zhao T, Doyle MP, Besser RE. Fate of enterohemorrhagic *Escherichia coli* O157:H7 in apple cider with and without preservatives. *Appl Environ Microbiol* 1993;59:2526–2530.
16. Nataro JP, Kaper JB. Diarrheogenic *Escherichia coli* [published erratum appears in *Clin Microbiol Rev* April 1998;11(2):403]. *Clin Microbiol Rev* 1998;11:142–201.
17. Mead PS, Griffin PM. *Escherichia coli* O157:H7. *Lancet* 1998; 352:1207–1212.
18. Scotland SM, Willshaw GA, Smith HR, et al. Properties of strains of *Escherichia coli* O26:H11 in relation to their enteropathogenic or enterohemorrhagic classification. *J Infect Dis* 1990;162:1069–1074.
19. Trevena WB, Hooper RS, Wray C, et al. Vero cytotoxin–producing *Escherichia coli* O157 associated with companion animals [Letter]. *Veterinary Rec* 1996;138:400.
20. Sargeant JM, Hafer DJ, Gillespie JR, et al. Prevalence of *Escherichia coli* O157:H7 in white-tailed deer sharing rangeland with cattle. *J Am Veterinary Med Assoc* 1999;215:792–794.
21. Orskov F, Orskov I, Villar JA. Cattle as reservoir of verotoxin-producing *Escherichia coli* O157:H7 [Letter]. *Lancet* 1987;2:276.
22. Armstrong GL, Hollingsworth J, Morris JG Jr. Emerging foodborne pathogens: *Escherichia coli* O157:H7 as a model of entry of a new pathogen into the food supply of the developed world. *Epidemiol Rev* 1996;18:29–51.
23. Synge B, Paiba G. Verocytotoxin-producing*E coli* O157. *Veterinary Rec* 2000;147:27.
24. Hancock DD, Besser TE, Rice DH, et al. A longitudinal study of *Escherichia coli* O157 in fourteen cattle herds. *Epidemiol Infect* 1997;118:193–195.
25. Besser TE, Hancock DD, Pritchett LC, et al. Duration of detection of fecal excretion of *Escherichia coli* O157:H7 in cattle. *J Infect Dis* 1997;175:726–729.
26. Griffin PM, Tauxe RV. The epidemiology of infections caused by *Escherichia coli* O157:H7, other enterohemorrhagic *E. coli,* and the associated hemolytic uremic syndrome. *Epidemiol Rev* 1991;13:60–98.
27. Wilson JB, McEwen SA, Clarke RC, et al. Distribution and characteristics of verocytotoxigenic *Escherichia coli* isolated from Ontario dairy cattle. *Epidemiol Infect* 1992;108:423–439.
28. Russell JB, Diez-Gonzalez F, Jarvis GN. Invited review: effects of diet shifts on *Escherichia coli* in cattle. *J Dairy Sci* 2000; 83:863–873.
29. Hancock DD, Besser TE, Rice DH, et al. Multiple sources of *Escherichia coli* O157 in feedlots and dairy farms in the northwestern USA. *Prev Veterinary Med* 1998;35:11–19.
30. Centers for Disease Control and Prevention. Outbreaks of *Escherichia coli* O157:H7 infections among children associated with farm visits—Pennsylvania and Washington, 2000. *MMWR Morb Mortal Wkly Rep* 2001;50:293–297.
31. Stevenson J, Hanson S. Outbreak of *Escherichia coli* O157 phage type 2 infection associated with eating precooked meats. *Commun Dis Rep CDR Rev* 1996;6:R116–R118.
32. Dalton CB, Douglas RM. Great expectations: the coroner's report on the South Australian haemolytic–uraemic syndrome outbreak. *Med J Aust* 1996;164:175–177.
33. Ammon A, Petersen LR, Karch H. A large outbreak of hemolytic uremic syndrome caused by an unusual sorbitol-fermenting strain of *Escherichia coli* O157:H7. *J Infect Dis* 1999; 179:1274–1277.
34. Mermin JH, Griffin PM. Public health in crisis: outbreaks of *Escherichia coli* O157:H7 infections in Japan [see Comment]. *Am J Epidemiol* 1999;150:797–805.
35. Keene WE, McAnulty JM, Hoesly FC, et al. A swimming-associated outbreak of hemorrhagic colitis caused by *Escherichia coli* O157:H7 and *Shigella sonnei. N Engl J Med* 1994;331: 579–584.
36. Friedman MS, Roels T, Koehler JE, et al. *Escherichia coli* O157:H7 outbreak associated with an improperly chlorinated swimming pool. *Clin Infect Dis* 1999;29:298–303.
37. Swerdlow DL, Woodruff BA, Brady RC, et al. A waterborne outbreak in Missouri of *Escherichia coli* O157:H7 associated with bloody diarrhea and death [see Comments]. *Ann Intern Med* 1992;117:812–819.
38. Centers for Disease Control and Prevention. Outbreak of *Escherichia coli* O157:H7 and *Campylobacter* among attendees of the Washington County Fair—New York, 1999. *MMWR Morb Mortal Wkly Rep* 1999;48:803–805.
39. Parry SM, Salmon RL, Willshaw GA, et al. Risk factors for and prevention of sporadic infections with Vero cytotoxin (Shiga toxin) producing *Escherichia coli* O157 [see Comments]. *Lancet* 1998;351:1019–1022.
40. Rowe PC, Orrbine E, Lior H, et al, the CPKDRC co-investigators. Diarrhea in close contacts as a risk factor for childhood haemolytic uraemic syndrome. *Epidemiol Infect* 1993;110:9–16.
41. Parry SM, Salmon RL. Sporadic STEC O157 infection: secondary household transmission in Wales. *Emerg Infect Dis* 1998; 4:657–661.
42. Cieslak PR, Barrett TJ, Griffin PM, et al. *Escherichia coli* O157:H7 infection from a manured garden. *Lancet* 1993;342: 367.
43. Belongia EA, Osterholm MT, Soler JT, et al. Transmission of *Escherichia coli* O157:H7 infection in Minnesota child day-care facilities. *JAMA* 1993;269:883–888.
44. Michel P, Wilson JB, Martin SW, et al. Temporal and geographical distributions of reported cases of *Escherichia coli* O157:H7 infection in Ontario. *Epidemiol Infect* 1999;122: 193–200.
45. Shukla R, Slack R, George A, et al. *Escherichia coli* O157 infection associated with a farm visitor centre. *Commun Dis Rep CDR Rev* 1995;5:R86–R90.
46. Slutsker L, Ries AA, Maloney K, et al. A nationwide case–control study of *Escherichia coli* O157:H7 infection in the United States. *J Infect Dis* 1998;177:962–966.
47. Licence K, Oates KR, Synge BA, et al. An outbreak of *E. coli* O157 infection with evidence of spread from animals to man through contamination of a private water supply. *Epidemiol Infect* 2001;126:135–138.
48. Carter AO, Borczyk AA, Carlson JA, et al. A severe outbreak of *Escherichia coli* O157:H7-associated hemorrhagic colitis in a nursing home. *N Engl J Med* 1987;317:1496–1500.
49. Pavia AT, Nichols CR, Green DP, et al. Hemolytic–uremic syndrome during an outbreak of *Escherichia coli* O157:H7 infections in institutions for mentally retarded persons: clinical and epidemiologic observations. *J Pediatr* 1990;116:544–551.
50. Coia JE. Nosocomial and laboratory-acquired infection with *Escherichia coli* O157. *J Hosp Infect* 1998;40:107–113.
51. Centers for Disease Control and Prevention. *FoodNet surveillance report for 1999* [Final Report]. Atlanta, GA: Centers for Disease Control and Prevention, 2000.
52. Slutsker L, Ries AA, Greene KD, et al. *Escherichia coli* O157:H7 diarrhea in the United States: clinical and epidemiologic features. *Ann Intern Med* 1997;126:505–513.
53. Mead P, Slutsker L, Ivey C, et al. Laboratory-based surveillance for *Escherichia coli* O157:H7 infections in the United States. International Conference on Emerging Infectious Diseases; 1998; Atlanta, GA. Abstract P-3.5:82.
54. Mead PS, Slutsker L, Dietz V, et al. Food-related illness and death in the United States. *Emerg Infect Dis* 1999;5:607–625.
55. Willshaw GA, Cheasty T, Smith HR, et al. Verocytotoxin-pro-

ducing *Escherichia coli* (VTEC) O157 and other VTEC from human infections in England and Wales: 1995–1998. *J Med Microbiol* 2001;50:135–142.

56. Anonymous. Enterohemorrhagic *Escherichia coli* infection in Japan as of April 2001. *Infect Agents Surv Rep* 2001;22:135.
57. Reilly W. *E. coli* in Scotland—an overview. *Scottish Centre Infect Environ Health Wkly Rep* 1997;1[Suppl]:4–5.
58. Rivas M, Balbi L, Miliwebsky ES, et al. Hemolytic uremic syndrome in children of Mendoza, Argentina: association with Shiga toxin–producing *Escherichia coli* infection. *Medicina* 1998;58:1–7.
59. Bokete TN, O'Callahan CM, Clausen CR, et al. Shiga-like toxin-producing *Escherichia coli* in Seattle children: a prospective study [published erratum appears in *Gastroenterology* June 1997;112(6):2164]. *Gastroenterology* 1993;105:1724–1731.
60. Park CH, Gates KM, Vandel NM, Et al. Isolation of Shiga-like toxin producing *Escherichia coli* (O157 and non-O157) in a community hospital. *Diagn Microbiol Infect Dis* 1996;26:69–72.
61. Talan D, Moran G, Newdow M, et al. Etiology of bloody diarrhea among patients presenting to United States emergency departments: prevalence of *Escherichia coli* O157:H7 and other enteropathogens. *Clin Infect Dis* 2001;32:573–580.
62. Bryant HE, Athar MA, Pai CH. Risk factors for *Escherichia coli* O157:H7 infection in an urban community. *J Infect Dis* 1989;160:858–864.
63. Johnson R, Clarke R, Wilson J, et al. Growing concerns and recent outbreaks involving non-O157:H7 serotypes of verotoxigenic *Escherichia coli. J Food Protect* 1996;59:1112–1122.
64. Jaeger JL, Acheson DW. Shiga toxin–producing *Escherichia coli. Curr Infect Dis Rep* 2000;2:61–67.
65. Pai CH, Ahmed N, Lior H, et al. Epidemiology of sporadic diarrhea due to verocytotoxin-producing *Escherichia coli:* a two-year prospective study. *J Infect Dis* 1988;157:1054–1057.
66. Fiorentino T, Hurd, Howard. Emergence of nonculture methods for detecting Shiga toxin–producing *E. coli* (STEC) in Connecticut (CT) laboratories, 2000 [Abstract]. The American Society for Microbiology 101st General Meeting; Orlando, Florida. *Am Soc Microbiol* 2001:187.
67. Nims L, Horensky D, Buck L, et al. Isolation of Shiga toxin–producing *Escherichia coli* in New Mexico [Abstract]. The American Society for Microbiology 101st General Meeting; Orlando, Florida. *Am Soc Microbiol* 2001:187.
68. Brooks JT, Sowers EG, Wells JG, et al. Non-O157 Shiga toxin–producing *Escherichia coli* reported to CDC, 1983-2000. Program and abstracts of the 39th Annual Meeting of the Infectious Diseases Society of America. San Francisco, CA: Infectious Diseases Society of America, 2001 Abstract 856:185.
69. Tuttle J, Gomez T, Doyle MP, et al. Lessons from a large outbreak of *Escherichia coli* O157:H7 infections: insights into the infectious dose and method of widespread contamination of hamburger patties. *Epidemiol Infect* 1999;122:185–192.
70. Tilden J, Young W, McNamara AM, et al. A new route of transmission for *Escherichia coli:* infection from dry fermented salami. *Am J Public Health* 1996;86:1142–1145.
71. Paton AW, Ratcliff RM, Doyle RM, et al. Molecular microbiological investigation of an outbreak of hemolytic–uremic syndrome caused by dry fermented sausage contaminated with Shiga-like toxin-producing *Escherichia coli. J Clin Microbiol* 1996;34:1622–1627.
72. Karch H, Russmann H, Schmidt H, et al. Long-term shedding and clonal turnover of enterohemorrhagic *Escherichia coli* O157 in diarrheal diseases. *J Clin Microbiol* 1995;33:1602–1605.
73. Buchwald DS, Blaser MJ. A review of human salmonellosis: II. duration of excretion following infection with nontyphi *Salmonella. Rev Infect Dis* 1984;6:345–356.
74. Ostroff SM, Griffin PM, Tauxe RV, et al. A statewide outbreak of *Escherichia coli* O157:H7 infections in Washington State. *Am J Epidemiol* 1990;132:239–247.
75. Cody SH, Glynn MK, Farrar JA, et al. An outbreak of *Escherichia coli* O157:H7 infection from unpasteurized commercial apple juice. *Ann Intern Med* 1999;130:202–209.
76. Salmon RL, Farrell ID, Hutchison JG, et al. A christening party outbreak of haemorrhagic colitis and haemolytic uraemic syndrome associated with *Escherichia coli* O157:H7. *Epidemiol Infect* 1989;103:249–254.
77. Centers for Disease Control and Prevention. *Escherichia coli* O111:H8 outbreak among teenage campers—Texas, 1999. *MMWR Morb Mortal Wkly Rep* 2000;49:321–324.
78. Bell BP, Goldoft M, Griffin PM, et al. A multistate outbreak of *Escherichia coli* O157:H7-associated bloody diarrhea and hemolytic uremic syndrome from hamburgers. The Washington experience. *JAMA* 1994;272:1349–1353.
79. Rodrigue DC, Mast EE, Greene KD, et al. A university outbreak of *Escherichia coli* O157:H7 infections associated with roast beef and an unusually benign clinical course. *J Infect Dis* 1995;172:1122–1125.
80. Wells JG, Shipman LD, Greene KD, et al. Isolation of *Escherichia coli* serotype O157:H7 and other Shiga-like toxin-producing *E. coli* from dairy cattle. *J Clin Microbiol* 1991;29:985–989.
81. Lior H. Incidence of hemorrhagic colitis due to *Escherichia coli* in Canada. *Cmaj* 1988;139:1073–1074.
82. Keene WE, Sazie E, Kok J, et al. An outbreak of *Escherichia coli* O157:H7 infections traced to jerky made from deer meat. *JAMA* 1997;277:1229–1231.
83. Doyle MP, Schoeni JL. Isolation of *Escherichia coli* O157:H7 from retail fresh meats and poultry. *Appl Environ Microbiol* 1987;53:2394–2396.
84. Butler T, Islam MR, Azad MA, et al. Risk factors for development of hemolytic uremic syndrome during shigellosis. *J Pediatr* 1987;110:894–897.
85. Koster F, Levin J, Walker L, et al. Hemolytic–uremic syndrome after shigellosis. Relation to endotoxemia and circulating immune complexes. *N Engl J Med* 1978;298:927–933.
86. Obrig TG, Del Vecchio PJ, Brown JE, et al. Direct cytotoxic action of Shiga toxin on human vascular endothelial cells. *Infect Immun* 1988;56:2373–2378.
87. Tesh VL, Samuel JE, Perera LP, et al. Evaluation of the role of Shiga and Shiga-like toxins in mediating direct damage to human vascular endothelial cells. *J Infect Dis* 1991;164: 344–352.
88. Fong JS, de Chadarevian JP, Kaplan BS. Hemolytic–uremic syndrome. Current concepts and management. *Pediatr Clin North Am* 1982;29:835–856.
89. Richardson SE, Rotman TA, Jay V, et al. Experimental verocytotoxemia in rabbits. *Infect Immun* 1992;60:4154–4167.
90. Lingwood CA, Law H, Richardson S, et al. Glycolipid binding of purified and recombinant *Escherichia coli* produced verotoxin *in vitro. J Biol Chem* 1987;262:8834–8839.
91. Boyd B, Lingwood C. Verotoxin receptor glycolipid in human renal tissue [published erratum appears in *Nephron* 1989;51(4): 582]. *Nephron* 1989;51:207–210.
92. Griffin PM, Olmstead LC, Petras RE. *Escherichia coli* O157:H7-associated colitis. A clinical and histological study of 11 cases. *Gastroenterology* 1990;99:142–149.
93. Moyer MP, Dixon PS, Rothman SW, et al. Cytotoxicity of Shiga toxin for primary cultures of human colonic and ileal epithelial cells. *Infect Immun* 1987;55:1533–1535.
94. Barrett TJ, Potter ME, Wachsmuth IK. Continuous peritoneal infusion of Shiga-like toxin II (SLT II) as a model for SLT II–induced diseases. *J Infect Dis* 1989;159:774–777.
95. Padhye VV, Beery JT, Kittell FB, et al. Colonic hemorrhage produced in mice by a unique Vero cell cytotoxin from an

Escherichia coli strain that causes hemorrhagic colitis. *J Infect Dis* 1987;155:1249–1253.
96. Barrett TJ, Potter ME, Strockbine NA. Evidence for participation of the macrophage in Shiga-like toxin II–induced lethality in mice. *Microbial Pathogen* 1990;9:95–103.
97. Louise CB, Obrig TG. Shiga toxin-associated hemolytic–uremic syndrome: combined cytotoxic effects of Shiga toxin, interleukin-1 beta, and tumor necrosis factor alpha on human vascular endothelial cells *in vitro*. *Infect Immun* 1991;59:4173–4179.
98. van de Kar NC, Monnens LA, Karmali MA, et al. Tumor necrosis factor and interleukin-1 induce expression of the verocytotoxin receptor globotriaosylceramide on human endothelial cells: implications for the pathogenesis of the hemolytic uremic syndrome. *Blood* 1992;80:2755–2764.
99. Kaye SA, Louise CB, Boyd B, et al. Shiga toxin–associated hemolytic uremic syndrome: interleukin-1 beta enhancement of Shiga toxin cytotoxicity toward human vascular endothelial cells *in vitro*. *Infect Immun* 1993;61:3886–3891.
100. Te Loo DM, van Hinsbergh VW, van den Heuvel LP, et al. Detection of verocytotoxin bound to circulating polymorphonuclear leukocytes of patients with hemolytic uremic syndrome. *J Am Soc Nephrol* 2001;12:800–806.
101. Uchida H, Kiyokawa N, Horie H, et al. The detection of Shiga toxins in the kidney of a patient with hemolytic uremic syndrome. *Pediatr Res* 1999;45:133–137.
102. Wadolkowski EA, Sung LM, Burris JA, et al. Acute renal tubular necrosis and death of mice orally infected with *Escherichia coli* strains that produce Shiga-like toxin type II. *Infect Immun* 1990;58:3959–3965.
103. Tesh VL, Burris JA, Owens JW, et al. Comparison of the relative toxicities of Shiga-like toxins type I and type II for mice. *Infect Immun* 1993;61:3392–3402.
104. Francis DH, Moxley RA, Andraos CY. Edema disease–like brain lesions in gnotobiotic piglets infected with *Escherichia coli* serotype O157:H7. *Infect Immun* 1989;57:1339–1342.
105. Moon HW, Whipp SC, Argenzio RA, et al. Attaching and effacing activities of rabbit and human enteropathogenic *Escherichia coli* in pig and rabbit intestines. *Infect Immun* 1983; 41:1340–1351.
106. Knutton S, Baldwin T, Williams PH, et al. Actin accumulation at sites of bacterial adhesion to tissue culture cells: basis of a new diagnostic test for enteropathogenic and enterohemorrhagic *Escherichia coli*. *Infect Immun* 1989;57:1290–1298.
107. Jerse AE, Yu J, Tall BD, et al. A genetic locus of enteropathogenic *Escherichia coli* necessary for the production of attaching and effacing lesions on tissue culture cells. *Proc Natl Acad Sci U S A* 1990;87:7839–7843.
108. Paton AW, Woodrow MC, Doyle RM, et al. Molecular characterization of a Shiga toxigenic *Escherichia coli* O113:H21 strain lacking *eae* responsible for a cluster of cases of hemolytic–uremic syndrome. *J Clin Microbiol* 1999;37:3357–3361.
109. Barrett TJ, Potter ME, Wachsmuth IK. Bacterial endotoxin both enhances and inhibits the toxicity of Shiga-like toxin II in rabbits and mice. *Infect Immun* 1989;57:3434–3437.
110. Barrett TJ, Green JH, Griffin PM, et al. Enzyme-linked immunosorbent assays for detecting antibodies to Shiga-like toxin I, Shiga-like toxin II, and *Escherichia coli* O157:H7 lipopolysaccharide in human serum. *Curr Microbiol* 1991;23: 189–195.
111. Schmidt H, Karch H. Enterohemolytic phenotypes and genotypes of shiga toxin–producing *Escherichia coli* O111 strains from patients with diarrhea and hemolytic–uremic syndrome. *J Clin Microbiol* 1996;34:2364–2367.
112. Schmidt H, Maier E, Karch H, et al. Pore-forming properties of the plasmid-encoded hemolysin of enterohemorrhagic *Escherichia coli* O157:H7. *Eur J Biochem* 1996;241:594–601.
113. Pruimboom-Brees IM, Morgan TW, Ackermann MR, et al. Cattle lack vascular receptors for *Escherichia coli* O157:H7 Shiga toxins. *Proc Natl Acad Sci U S A* 2000;97:10325–10329.
114. Siegler RL, Griffin PM, Barrett TJ, et al. Recurrent hemolytic uremic syndrome secondary to *Escherichia coli* O157:H7 infection. *Pediatrics* 1993;91:666–668.
115. Robson WL, Leung AK, Miller-Hughes DJ. Recurrent hemorrhagic colitis caused by *Escherichia coli* O157:H7. *Pediatr Infect Dis J* 1993;12:699–701.
116. Kausche FM, Dean EA, Arp LH, et al. An experimental model for subclinical edema disease (*Escherichia coli* enterotoxemia) manifest as vascular necrosis in pigs. *Am J Veterinary Res* 1992; 53:281–287.
117. MacLeod DL, Gyles CL, Wilcock BP. Reproduction of edema disease of swine with purified Shiga-like toxin-II variant. *Veterinary Pathol* 1991;28:66–73.
118. Cimolai N, Anderson JD, Bhanji NM, et al. *Escherichia coli* O157:H7 infections associated with perforated appendicitis and chronic diarrhea. *Eur J Pediatr* 1990;149:259–260.
119. Ryan CA, Tauxe RV, Hosek GW, et al. *Escherichia coli* O157:H7 diarrhea in a nursing home: clinical, epidemiological, and pathological findings. *J Infect Dis* 1986;154:631–638.
120. Lopez EL, Devoto S, Woloj M, et al. Intussusception associated with *Escherichia coli* O157:H7. *Pediatr Infect Dis J* 1989;8: 471–473.
121. Tarr PI, Weinberger E, Hatch EI Jr, et al. Bacterial ileocecalis caused by*Escherichia coli* O157:H7. *J Pediatr Gastroenterol Nutr* 1992;14:261–263.
122. Grandsen WR, Damm MA, Anderson JD, et al. Haemorrhagic cystitis and balanitis associated with verotoxin-producing *Escherichia coli* O157:H7 [Letter]. *Lancet* 1985;2:150.
123. Krishnan C, Fitzgerald VA, Dakin SJ, et al. Laboratory investigation of outbreak of hemorrhagic colitis caused by *Escherichia coli* O157:H7. *J Clin Microbiol* 1987;25:1043–1047.
124. Rivas M, Miliwebsky E, Balbi L, et al. Intestinal bleeding and occlusion associated with Shiga toxin–producing *Escherichia coli* O127:H21. *Medicina* 2000;60:249–252.
125. Tarr PI, Fouser LS, Stapleton AE, et al. Hemolytic–uremic syndrome in a six-year-old girl after a urinary tract infection with Shiga-toxin–producing *Escherichia coli* O103:H2 [see Comments]. *N Engl J Med* 1996;335:635–638.
126. Starr M, Bennett-Wood V, Bigham AK, et al. Hemolytic–uremic syndrome following urinary tract infection with enterohemorrhagic *Escherichia coli:* case report and review. *Clin Infect Dis* 1998;27:310–315.
127. Bettelheim KA, Goldwater PN, Evangelidis H, et al. Distribution of toxigenic *Escherichia coli* serotypes in the intestines of infants. *Compar Immunol Microbiol Infect Dis* 1992;15:65–70.
128. Ljungh A, Eriksson M, Eriksson O, et al. Shiga-like toxin production and connective tissue protein binding of *Escherichia coli* isolated from a patient with ulcerative colitis. *Scand J Infect Dis* 1988;20:443–446.
129. Neild GH. Hemolytic uremic syndrome/thrombotic thrombocytopenic purpura: pathophysiology and treatment. *Kidney Int* 1998;64[Suppl]:S45–S49.
130. Gasser C, Gautier E, Steck A, et al. [Scientific raisins from 127 years SMW (Swiss Medical Weekly). Hemolytic–uremic syndrome: bilateral kidney cortex necrosis in acute acquired hemolytic anemia. 1925]. *Schweizerische Medizinische Wochenschrift. J Suisse Med* 1995;125:2528–2532.
131. Siegler RL, Pavia AT, Christofferson RD, et al. A 20-year population-based study of postdiarrheal hemolytic uremic syndrome in Utah. *Pediatrics* 1994;94:35–40.
132. Martin DL, MacDonald KL, White KE, et al. The epidemiology and clinical aspects of the hemolytic uremic syndrome in Minnesota. *N Engl J Med* 1990;323:1161–1167.

133. Milford DV, Taylor CM, Guttridge B, et al. Haemolytic uraemic syndromes in the British Isles 1985–8: association with verocytotoxin producing *Escherichia coli.* Part 1: clinical and epidemiological aspects. *Arch Dis Child* 1990;65:716–721.
134. Rowe PC, Orrbine E, Wells GA, et al, the Canadian Pediatric Kidney Disease Reference Centre. Epidemiology of hemolytic–uremic syndrome in Canadian children from 1986 to 1988. The Canadian Pediatric Kidney Disease Reference Centre. *J Pediatr* 1991;119:218–224.
135. Amorosi EL, Ultmann JE. Thrombotic thrombocytopenic purpura: report of 16 cases and review of the literature. *Medicine* 1966;45:139–159.
136. Ridolfi RL, Bell WR. Thrombotic thrombocytopenic purpura. Report of 25 cases and review of the literature. *Medicine* 1981; 60:413–428.
137. Banatvala N, Griffin PM, Greene KD, et al. The United States national prospective hemolytic uremic syndrome study: microbiologic, serologic, clinical, and epidemiologic findings. *J Infect Dis* 2001;183:1063–1070.
138. Chart H, Smith HR, Scotland SM, et al. Serological identification of *Escherichia coli* O157:H7 infection in haemolytic uraemic syndrome. *Lancet* 1991;337:138–140.
139. Bitzan M, Ludwig K, Klemt M, et al. The role of *Escherichia coli* O157 infections in the classical (enteropathic) haemolytic uraemic syndrome: results of a Central European, multicentre study. *Epidemiol Infect* 1993;110:183–196.
140. Tarr PI, Neill MA, Clausen CR, et al. *Escherichia coli* O157:H7 and the hemolytic uremic syndrome: importance of early cultures in establishing the etiology. *J Infect Dis* 1990;162:553–556.
141. Rowe PC, Orrbine E, Lior H, et al, CPKDRC co-investigators. A prospective study of exposure to verotoxin-producing *Escherichia coli* among Canadian children with haemolytic uraemic syndrome. *Epidemiol Infect* 1993;110:1–7.
142. Scheutz F, Beutin L, Smith HR. Characterisation of non-O157 verocytotoxigenic *E. coli* (VTEC) isolated from patients with haemolytic uraemic syndrome (HUS) world-wide from 1982 to 2000. Fourth International Symposium and Workshop on Shiga Toxin (Verocytotoxin)–producing *Escherichia coli* Infections. Kyoto, Japan: VTEC 2000 Organizing Committees; 2000:96.
143. Windler F, Weh HJ, Hossfeld DK, et al. Verotoxin in thrombotic thrombocytopenic purpura [Letter]. *Eur J Haematol* 1989;42:103.
144. Ornt DB, Griffin PM, Wells JG, et al. Hemolytic uremic syndrome due to *Escherichia coli* O157:H7 in a child with multiple infections. *Pediatr Nephrol* 1992;6:270–272.
145. Rowe PC, Orrbine E, Lior H, et al. Risk of hemolytic uremic syndrome after sporadic *Escherichia coli* O157:H7 infection: results of a Canadian collaborative study. [see Comments]. *J Pediatr* 1998;132:777–782.
146. Bell BP, Griffin PM, Lozano P, et al. Predictors of hemolytic uremic syndrome in children during a large outbreak of *Escherichia coli* O157:H7 infections. *Pediatrics* 1997;100:e12.
147. Buteau C, Proulx F, Chaibou M, et al. Leukocytosis in children with *Escherichia coli* O157:H7 enteritis developing the hemolytic–uremic syndrome. *Pediatr Infect Dis J* 2000;19:642–647.
148. Scotland SM, Willshaw GA, Smith HR, et al. Properties of strains of *Escherichia coli* belonging to serogroup O157 with special reference to production of Vero cytotoxins VT1 and VT2. *Epidemiol Infect* 1987;99:613–624.
149. Ostroff SM, Tarr PI, Neill MA, et al. Toxin genotypes and plasmid profiles as determinants of systemic sequelae in *Escherichia coli* O157:H7 infections. *J Infect Dis* 1989;160:994–998.
150. Thomas A, Chart H, Cheasty T, et al. Vero cytotoxin-producing *Escherichia coli,* particularly serogroup O157, associated with human infections in the United Kingdom: 1989–91. *Epidemiol Infect* 1993;110:591–600.
151. Hunt CM, Harvey JA, Youngs ER, et al. Clinical and pathological variability of infection by enterohaemorrhagic (Vero cytotoxin producing) *Escherichia coli* [see Comments]. *J Clin Pathol* 1989;42:847–852.
152. Richardson SE, Karmali MA, Becker LE, et al. The histopathology of the hemolytic uremic syndrome associated with verocytotoxin-producing *Escherichia coli* infections. *Hum Pathol* 1988;19:1102–1108.
153. Ratnam S, March SB, Ahmed R, et al. Characterization of *Escherichia coli* serotype O157:H7. *J Clin Microbiol* 1988;26: 2006–2012.
154. Strockbine NA, Wells JG, Bopp CA, et al. Overview of detection and subtyping methods. In: Kaper JB, O'Brien AD, eds. Escherichia coli *O157:H7 and other shiga toxin–producing* E. coli *strains.* Washington, DC: ASM Press, 1998:331–356.
155. Bielaszewska M, Schmidt H, Karmali MA, et al. Isolation and characterization of sorbitol-fermenting Shiga toxin (Verocytotoxin)–producing *Escherichia coli* O157:H– strains in the Czech Republic. *J Clin Microbiol* 1998;36:2135–2137.
156. Kehl KS, Havens P, Behnke CE, et al. Evaluation of the premier EHEC assay for detection of Shiga toxin–producing *Escherichia coli. J Clin Microbiol* 1997;35:2051–2054.
157. Stapp JR, Jelacic S, Yea YL, et al. Comparison of *Escherichia coli* O157:H7 antigen detection in stool and broth cultures to that in sorbitol-MacConkey agar stool cultures. *J Clin Microbiol* 2000;38:3404–3406.
158. Swaminathan B, Barrett TJ, Hunter SB, et al, CDC PulseNet Task Force. PulseNet: the molecular subtyping network for foodborne bacterial disease surveillance, United States. *Emerg Infect Dis* 2001;7:382–389.
159. Ackers ML, Mahon BE, Leahy E, et al. An outbreak of *Escherichia coli* O157:H7 infections associated with leaf lettuce consumption. *J Infect Dis* 1998;177:1588–1593.
160. Law D. Virulence factors of *Escherichia coli* O157 and other Shiga toxin–producing *E. coli. J Appl Microbiol* 2000;88:729–745.
161. Jenkins C, Chart H, Smith HR, et al. Antibody response of patients infected with verocytotoxin-producing *Escherichia coli* to protein antigens encoded on the LEE locus. *J Med Microbiol* 2000;49:97–101.
162. Cimolai N, Basalyga S, Mah DG, et al. A continuing assessment of risk factors for the development of *Escherichia coli* O157:H7-associated hemolytic uremic syndrome. *Clin Nephrol* 1994;42:85–89.
163. Proulx F, Seidman E. Is antibiotic therapy of mice and humans useful in *Escherichia coli* O157:H7 enteritis? *Eur J Clin Microbiol Infect Dis* 1999;18:533–534.
164. Cimolai N, Anderson JD, Morrison BJ. Antibiotics for *Escherichia coli* O157:H7 enteritis? *J Antimicrob Chemother* 1989;23:807–808.
165. Grif K, Dierich MP, Karch H, et al. Strain-specific differences in the amount of Shiga toxin released from enterohemorrhagic *Escherichia coli* O157 following exposure to subinhibitory concentrations of antimicrobial agents. *Eur J Clin Microbiol Infect Dis* 1998;17:761–766.
166. Walterspiel JN, Ashkenazi S, Morrow AL, et al. Effect of subinhibitory concentrations of antibiotics on extracellular Shiga-like toxin I. *Infection* 1992;20:25–29.
167. Murakami J, Kishi K, Hirai K, et al. Macrolides and clindamycin suppress the release of Shiga-like toxins from *Escherichia coli* O157:H7 *in vitro. Int J Antimicrob Agents* 2000; 15:103–109.
168. Zhang X, McDaniel AD, Wolf LE, et al. Quinolone antibiotics induce Shiga toxin–encoding bacteriophages, toxin production, and death in mice. *J Infect Dis* 2000;181:664–670.
169. Wong CS, Jelacic S, Habeeb RL, et al. The risk of the hemolytic–uremic syndrome after antibiotic treatment of *Escherichia*

coli O157:H7 infections [see Comments]. *N Engl J Med* 2000;342:1930–1936.

170. Ikeda K, Ida O, Kimoto K, et al. Effect of early fosfomycin treatment on prevention of hemolytic uremic syndrome accompanying *Escherichia coli* O157:H7 infection. *Clin Nephrol* 1999; 52:357–362.
171. Proulx F, Turgeon JP, Delage G, et al. Randomized, controlled trial of antibiotic therapy for *Escherichia coli* O157:H7 enteritis. *J Pediatr* 1992;121:299–303.
172. Cornick NA, Matise I, Samuel JE, et al. Shiga toxin–producing *Escherichia coli* infection: temporal and quantitative relationships among colonization, toxin production, and systemic disease. *J Infect Dis* 2000;181:242–251.
173. Armstrong GD, McLaine PN, Rowe PC. Clinical trials of Synsorb Pk in preventing hemolytic–uremic syndrome. In: Kaper JB, O'Brien AD, eds. Escherichia coli *O157:H7 and other Shiga toxin–producing* E. coli *strains.* Washington, DC: ASM Press, 1998:374–384.
174. Paton AW, Morona R, Paton JC. A new biological agent for treatment of Shiga toxigenic *Escherichia coli* infections and dysentery in humans [see Comments]. *Nat Med* 2000;6: 265–270.
175. Matise I, Cornick NA, Booher SL, et al. Intervention with Shiga toxin (Stx) antibody after infection by Stx-producing *Escherichia coli. J Infect Dis* 2001;183:347–350.
176. Trachtman H, Christen E. Pathogenesis, treatment, and therapeutic trials in hemolytic uremic syndrome. *Curr Opin Pediatr* 1999;11:162–168.
177. Thayer DW, Boyd G. Elimination of *Escherichia coli* O157:H7 in meats by gamma irradiation. *Appl Environ Microbiol* 1993; 59:1030–1034.
178. US Department of Agriculture. Pathogen reduction; hazard analysis and critical control point (HACCP) systems; final rule. *Federal Register* 1996;61:38806–38989.
179. Tauxe RV. Food safety and irradiation: protecting the public from foodborne infections. *Emerg Infect Dis* 2001;7:516–521.
180. Taormina PJ, Beuchat LR, Slutsker L. Infections associated with eating seed sprouts: an international concern. *Emerg Infect Dis* 1999;5:626–634.
181. US Food and Drug Administration. Hazard analysis and critical control point (HACCP); procedures for the safe and sanitary processing and importing of juice; food labeling: warning notice statements; labeling of juice products; proposed rules. *Federal Register* 1998;63:20449–20486.
182. Rice EW, Clark RM, Johnson CH. Chlorine inactivation of *Escherichia coli* O157:H7. *Emerg Infect Dis* 1999;5:461–463.
183. US Department of Agriculture. 9 CFR parts 317 and 381. Mandatory safe handling statements on labeling of raw meat and poultry products: final rule. *Federal Register* 1994;59: 14528–14540.
184. Kaplan BS, Katz J, Krawitz S, et al. An analysis of the results of therapy in 67 cases of the hemolytic–uremic syndrome. *J Pediatr* 1971;78:420–425.
185. Gilbert L, Mead P, Blake P, et al. Antimicrobial use is not a risk factor for hemolytic uremic syndrome after *E. coli* O157 infection: results of a 1996–1997 FoodNet study. Abstract of the International Conference on Emerging Infectious Diseases; Atlanta, Georgia; 2000:73.

43

SHIGELLA AND ENTEROINVASIVE *ESCHERICHIA COLI*

GERALD T. KEUSCH

The prototypic member of the genus *Shigella*, *S. dysenteriae* type 1, was identified by Kiyoshi Shiga (1) during an epidemic of severe dysentery in Japan in 1896 with nearly 90,000 cases and a mortality rate approaching 30%. Shiga's complete description of the distinctive gram-negative rod he isolated included the demonstration of a serologic response in the infected patents, thus superseding prior descriptions of what was probably the same organism. Other workers quickly confirmed that Shiga's bacillus was found in all parts of the world (2,3). Over the subsequent 40 years, related antigenically and biochemically distinctive organisms, now known as *S. flexneri*, *S. boydii*, and *S. sonnei*, were identified.

In 1900, Flexner reported that injections of killed *Shigella dysenteriae* cultures caused diarrhea and death in animals, suggesting that the disease was due to "a toxic agent rather than infection per se" (2). However, Flexner was undoubtedly observing the effects of lipopolysaccharide (LPS) endotoxin, and, for many years thereafter, unavoidable contamination of bacterial protein preparations with LPS continued to confuse interpretation of experiments to study this toxin. In 1903, Conradi (4) demonstrated that intravenous injection of rabbits with autolysates of 18-hour cultures of *S. dysenteriae* type 1 resulted in diarrhea, paralysis, and death within 48 to 72 hours. These neurologic manifestations were unique to this organism (5) and the toxic activity came to be known as Shiga neurotoxin.

Over the subsequent 50 years, the microbiology and epidemiology of *Shigella* species were clarified, culminating in the 1950 Congress of the International Association of Microbiologists designation of *Shigella* as the genus name (6). Since then, *Shigella* pathogenesis has been intensively investigated (7,8), especially during the past 2 decades. The resulting explosion in our understanding of the cellular biochemistry, cell biology, and genetic elements involved in *Shigella* virulence has led to the development of an entirely new paradigm of pathogenesis, described here. In addition, a group of enteroinvasive *Escherichia coli* (EIEC) has been identified and shown to share many common virulence genes with *Shigella*. EIEC is taxonomically more closely related to *Shigella* than to other *E. coli*; therefore, EIEC is briefly considered with *Shigella* in this chapter.

G. T. Keusch: Fogarty International Center, Department of Health and Human Services, Pubic Health Service, National Institutes of Health, Bethesda, Maryland

MICROBIOLOGY

Shigella belongs to the family Enterobacteriaceae, tribe Escherichiae, and genus *Shigella*. The organisms closely resemble *E. coli* at the genetic level, and if they were discovered today, they would be considered to be a distinctive group of virulent *E. coli* (9). Interestingly, although EIEC appears to have evolved from a different ancestral strain (10), the organisms are closely related to *Shigella* and possess similar genes present in their large virulence plasmids (11). There are four species of *Shigella* (*S. dysenteriae*, *S. flexneri*, *S. boydii*, *S. sonnei*), which are differentiated by group-specific polysaccharide antigens of LPS designated A, B, C, and D, respectively, and by biochemical properties (Table 43.1), supplemented with phage or colicin typing information. *Shigella* organisms do not possess flagella, are nonmotile, and express no H antigens useful for diagnosis or for use as candidate vaccine antigens. *S. dysenteriae* consists of 16 antigenic types, of which type 1, previously known as *S. shigae* or Shiga's bacillus, produces Shiga toxin. *S. flexneri* is divided into six types and 14 subtypes, each possessing type- and subtype-specific antigens. *S. boydii* includes eight serologic types, and, although there is only one *S. sonnei* serotype, there are at least 20 colicin types. *Shigella* organisms are gram-negative, nonencapsulated rod-shaped bacilli, typically non–lactose-fermenting, non–gas-producing (with rare exceptions), and lysine decarboxylase, acetate-, and mucate-negative, which serves to distinguish them from most *E. coli* forms. An important exception is *S. sonnei*, which is a delayed lactose fermenter and therefore could be misidentified as *E. coli*. In addition, *S. flexneri* 6

TABLE 43.1. COMPARISON OF BIOCHEMICAL CHARACTERISTICS OF *SHIGELLA* AND *ESCHERICHIA COLI*

Test or Substrate	Result for *Shigella* (% Positive)	Result for *E. coli* (% Positive)
Acetate	–	+ (84)
Adonitol	–	–
Argine decarboxylase	– (8)	Variable (17)
Citrate	–	Variable (24)
DNase	–	–
Esculin	–	Variable (31)
Gas from glucose[a]	– (<1–2)	+ (91)
Hydrogen sulfide on TSI agar	–	–
Indole	Variable (38)	+ (99)
Inositol	–	–
KCN	–	–
Lactose fermentation[b]	– (<1–2)	+ (91)
Lysine decarboxylase	–	+ (90)
Malonate	–	–
Mannitol	+ (except *S. dysenteriae*)	+
Methyl red	+	+
Motility	–	+ (80)
Mucate	–	+ (92)
Ornithine decarboxylase[c]	Variable (20–23)	+ (63)
Phenylalanine deaminase	–	–
Salicin	–	+ (40)
Sucrose	– (<1–2)	+ (50)
Urease	–	–
Voges-Proskauer	–	–
Xylose	– (2–5)	+ (95)

[a]Some *S. flexneri* 6 organisms produce gas from glucose.
[b]*S. sonnei* organisms usually ferment lactose or sucrose after several days in culture.
[c]Some *S. sonnei* organisms decarboxylate ornithine.
Adapted from Pupo GM, Karaolis DK, Lan R, et al. Evolutionary relationships among pathogenic and nonpathogenic *Escherichia coli* strains inferred from multilocus enzyme electrophoresis and mdh sequence studies. *Infect Immun* 1997;65:2685–2692.

and *S. boydii* 13 produce gas from glucose, a characteristic of avirulent *E. coli*. In practice, biochemical tests aside from lactose fermentation, are of limited utility for the identification of *Shigella* in the clinical microbiology laboratory. Rather, differentiation among species depends primarily on serologic methods using group- and type-specific antisera. Not all commercially available antisera are equally sensitive or specific, especially for detection of *S. flexneri* (12). In the future, more specific monoclonal antibody reagents will offer a more reliable alternative (13).

EIEC can be difficult to identify unless specifically sought. Most EIEC serogroups also share antigenic specificities with *Shigella* serovars (14), but these are not included in typing sera sets for enteropathogenic *E. coli*. Like *Shigella*, EIEC organisms are consistently lysine decarboxylase-negative, nonmotile (except for O124), and often lactose-negative (15) (Table 43.2), and therefore may easily be misclassified.

EPIDEMIOLOGY

Shigellosis occurs throughout the world, causing an estimated 1.3 million deaths per year, primarily in young infants and children (16). The organisms are highly host adapted and naturally infect only humans and some nonhuman primates. Although point source food- and water-associated outbreaks do occur, most transmission is via person-to-person contact (17). *S. flexneri* and *S. dysenteriae* type 1 are at present the predominant species in developing countries, whereas *S. sonnei* is the major isolate in developed countries, accounting for more than three-fourths of the isolates in the United States. The fourth species, *S. boydii*, is uncommon except in the Indian subcontinent, where it was first identified.

One of the most striking features of shigellosis, in contrast to other enteric pathogens, is the exceedingly small inoculum of organisms necessary to cause disease. As few as 10 to 100 *S. dysenteriae* type 1 organisms and a few thousand S. flexneri and *S. sonnei* are sufficient to cause clinical dysentery in an otherwise healthy adult (18). More recent experiments using a Shiga toxin-deletion mutant (Δ-*stxA*) of *S. dysenteriae* type 1 in a new experimental infection protocol demonstrated an enhanced attack rate but a greater inoculum size (19), suggesting a role for Shiga toxin in the special virulence of *S. dysenteriae* type 1. This inoculum is readily transmitted directly from anus to mouth by fecal contamination of the hands, or in food or water without the need for multiplication. As a consequence, approximately 20% of household contacts of cases acquire infection (20). For the same reason, person-to-person spread of shigellosis has been common in settings in which personal hygiene is difficult to maintain, such as day care settings for young children.

Although shigellosis is distributed worldwide, the prevalence of shigellosis differs from place to place (21). It is prominently associated with poverty, overcrowding, poor personal hygiene, inadequate water supplies, and malnutrition. These conditions characterize developing countries and disadvantaged populations of developed countries, and represent important social determinants of infection. The

TABLE 43.2. BIOCHEMICAL CHARACTERISTICS OF *SHIGELLA* AND EIEC

Characteristic	*E. coli*[a] (% Positive)	EIEC[b] (% Positive)	*Shigella*[a] (% Positive)
Lysine decarboxylase	89	0	0
Christensen citrate	95	8.3	0
Motility	69	7.2[c]	0
Lactose	90	30.9	0.3

[a]Data from reference 13.
[b]Data from reference 14.
[c]Primarily serotype O124.

relevance of these factors is shown by dramatic differences in the estimated incidence of shigellosis between developing countries (750 to 2,000 cases per 1,000 children per year) compared with industrialized nations (0.22 cases per 1,000 children per year in the United States, based on cases voluntarily reported to the Centers for Disease Control and Prevention). Although the U. S. data significantly underestimates the real incidence of shigellosis, because many cases are neither bacteriologically identified nor reported, even a 10- to 100-fold increase in the rate in the United States would still be substantially less than in developing countries. There are also settings in the United States in which the incidence is much higher, for example, in the southwestern states along the Mexican border and among Native American populations.

Endemic shigellosis is a pediatric disease; patients are generally younger than 10 years of age, and most are younger than 5 years old. The disease is uncommon in infants younger than 6 months of age, even in highly endemic settings. When severe shigellosis occurs in neonates, it is more frequent and more likely to be severe in non–breast-fed infants (22). Endemic shigellosis often exhibits seasonal peaks, although the specifics can vary from one country to another. For example, transmission peaks in the hot dry season in Bangladesh and Egypt but in the rainy season in Guatemala (21). These differences have been related to the use of contaminated water for consumption or decreased personal hygiene in times of water scarcity in the former and to water-washed transmission during heavy rains in the latter.

Major global sequential shifts in the predominant *Shigella* species have occurred in the past century and remain without adequate epidemiologic explanation (23). Before World War I, *S. dysenteriae* type 1 was the most common *Shigella* everywhere. In the period between World Wars I and II, however, *S. flexneri* emerged as the predominant isolate around the world, only to be replaced by *S. sonnei* after 1945 in industrialized nations but not developing countries. In 1969, epidemic *S. dysenteriae* type 1 infection reemerged in Mexico and Central America (24), followed by epidemics in central and southern Africa (including Zaire, Rwanda, Central African Republic, Zambia, Mozambique, and South Africa), Asia (including Myanmar, Viet Nam, and Thailand), and the Indian subcontinent (including India, Bangladesh, and Pakistan) (21). As might be expected when a serotype not in recent circulation in the community is introduced, acquired immunity is negligible and attack rates tend to be high across all age groups.

Two subpopulations in developed countries are at particular risk of *Shigella* infection. First, children in day care centers, among whom incidence rates are reported to be as high as 669 per 1,000 per year. This is attributable to the ease of person-to-person transmission of the organism and the laissez-faire attitude of young infants about feces and hygiene (25). In prospective studies, infection was introduced into the household in 26% of families with an affected child in day care. The second group at greater risk is homosexual males, in whom sexually transmitted shigellosis is well documented (26). Curiously, although *S. sonnei* is the predominant *Shigella* isolate in the U. S. population as a whole, *S. flexneri* is the most common isolate in male homosexuals (27). The incidence of *S. flexneri* in the United States has for the first time in recent decades been increasing significantly, and, whereas the rates in females and children have continued to decline, there has been an increase in young adult males. As a consequence, in the past 2 decades, the average age of patients with *S. flexneri* has risen from around 5 years to approximately 25 years (28).

Shigellosis, especially among young infants, is potentially life threatening. The resurgence of epidemic *S. dysenteriae* type 1 in Guatemala and Zaire was associated with minimum reported case-fatality rates of 7.4% and 2.5%, respectively (29,30). Although this already exceeds the death rate in the huge Latin America cholera epidemic of 1991, the estimate of the *Shigella* death rate is certainly too low due to incomplete case reporting. The *S. dysenteriae* type 1 epidemic in Bangladesh in 1984 was associated with a 42% increase in all-cause mortality among children age 1 to 4 years (31). The mortality rate among inpatients with documented shigellosis at the International Centre for Diarrhoeal Disease Research in Dhaka, Bangladesh, is approximately 10%. Malnutrition is an important conditioning factor for lethal infection and may account for the similarly high mortality rates due to all four *Shigella* species in Bangladesh, including *S. sonnei*, which does not ordinarily terminate fatally in developed nations. Dysentery mortality rate in Bangladesh is more than twice as high in female compared with male children, probably reflecting sociologic factors and cultural practices, such as parental preference for male children over female children, exemplified by preferential feeding and provision of medical care to males over females.

There is little published information on the epidemiology of EIEC. One of the first recognizable outbreaks probably occurred during World War II (32), long before EIEC was identified, when *S. dysenteriae* type 3 was identified as the cause of bloody diarrhea. However, this organism was subsequently found to be the enteroinvasive *E. coli* serogroup O124. In 1947 (33), an organism that later was determined to be an EIEC was isolated from a food-borne outbreak at an English school. These retrospectively diagnosed outbreaks serve to illustrate that EIEC has been around for decades. *E. coli* O124 has remained the most prevalent serogroup among the several EIEC serogroups now known. This organism was the cause of a 1973 outbreak in the United States associated with imported French camembert cheese (34) that brought attention to the distinctive illness caused by these organisms and identified their ability to invade mammalian cells much like *Shigella*. Whereas EIEC accounts for only 1% to 2% of endemic disease episodes where they have been sought, it is now being reported from an increasing number of countries.

CLINICAL FEATURES

Shigellosis usually begins with generalized constitutional symptoms, including fever, fatigue, anorexia, and malaise, followed soon thereafter by watery diarrhea. In some patients, in part depending on the infecting species, the diarrhea becomes bloody or progresses to dysentery within a few hours to a few days. In patients with dysentery, the watery phase may be brief or even absent altogether (21). Even though large-volume diarrhea leading to severe dehydration is not common during shigellosis, profound and prolonged hyponatremia can be a problem, likely due to inappropriate secretion of antidiuretic hormone (35). The classic dysenteric stool consists of a small amount of pus and mucus, sometimes appearing grossly purulent. However, more often, patients with shigellosis pass partially formed stools mixed with blood, pus, and mucus. Clinical dysentery is defined as the frequent passage of dysenteric or bloody stools associated with abdominal cramps and tenesmus (spasms of pain associated with straining to pass stool) due to proctitis. The intestinal mucosal inflammatory response characteristic of shigellosis can also result in rectal prolapse due to intense straining to pass stools, especially in the very young in whom the ligamentous support of the rectum is poorly developed (36).

Macroscopic and microscopic mucosal damage is most evident in the distal large bowel, becoming progressively milder in the transverse and ascending colon (37). Ulcerations occur as epithelial cells die and are sloughed. These may extend to the lamina propria, associated with an inflammatory infiltrate in the submucosa and exudates in the bowel lumen. Stool frequency is dramatically increased, typically at least 8 to 10 movements per day, but this can be as often as 100 times per day in an occasional unfortunate patient. But because stool volume is small—usually no more than 30 mL/kg/day—dehydration is mild and easily managed by oral rehydration (21). Anorexia, prominent at the outset, may persist well into the convalescent period and contribute in a major way to the adverse effects of shigellosis on nutritional status (38).

In developed countries, shigellosis is usually mild, self-limiting, and does not even precipitate a visit to a physician (21). In developing countries, however, shigellosis is frequently a severe disease that may persist for weeks to months unless appropriate antibiotic therapy is given (21,31). This is, in large part, related to the causative *Shigella* species. Progression to clinical dysentery is uncommon in *S. sonnei* infection, occurs more often in *S. boydii* infection, is common in *S. flexneri*, and occurs in most patients when *S. dysenteriae* type 1 is the cause (21).

Shigellosis can cause both local intestinal and systemic complications that can be severe and life threatening. In the United States and other industrialized countries, intestinal obstruction and toxic megacolon during shigellosis are rare events but in developing countries they occur regularly and are associated with a high mortality rate, especially if perforation of the dilated intestine occurs (39,40). The pathogenesis of toxic megacolon remains obscure but its increased association with *S. dysenteriae* type 1 infection supports the concept that it is a direct consequence of the intensity of the inflammatory reaction in the mucosa.

Mucosal inflammation in shigellosis results in a protein-losing enteropathy (41). This has been quantitatively assessed in some studies by measuring stool excretion of the serum enzyme, α_1-antitrypsin, as a marker of the escape of serum proteins into the gut lumen. Mean stool excretion of α_1-antitrypsin is 50% greater in *S. dysenteriae* type 1 compared with all other *Shigella* infections and correlates with the number of erythrocytes in the stool. Because protein losses are cumulative during infection, protein-losing enteropathy contributes to the generalized negative nitrogen balance during a febrile illness like shigellosis and increases the risk of acute protein-energy malnutrition. If uncorrected during convalescence, protein losses are manifested as growth retardation in children, which is associated with increased morbidity and mortality (21,31).

Documented *Shigella* bacteremia has been considered to be rare but when routinely looked for is not uncommon. For example, bacteremia due to the causative *Shigella* species was documented in 4% of a series of severely ill patients with shigellosis in Bangladesh, and an additional 4% were bacteremic with other Enterobacteriaceae (42). Bacteremic patients were more likely to die. Compared with a mortality rate of 10% in the absence of bacteremia, the mortality rate in *Shigella* sepsis was 21%, reaching 51% in patients with sepsis due to other gram-negative rods. Even without documented bacteremia, however, circulating endotoxin is commonly detected in hospitalized patients with *Shigella* infection in developing countries, with the highest levels recorded in *S. dysenteriae* type 1 infection.

Associated systemic complications are especially frequent in dysentery due to *S. dysenteriae* type 1, including toxic megacolon, leukemoid reactions with leukocyte counts in excess of 50,000/dL, and hemolytic-uremic syndrome (HUS) (21,31,43). HUS is a microangiopathic hemolytic process, resulting from damage to the small vessels in the kidney and elsewhere, leading to hemolytic anemia, thrombocytopenia (usually in the range of 30,000 to 100,000), and acute renal failure (44). Procoagulant activity is increased in HUS patients, including elevated circulating levels of von Willebrand factor multimers and plasminogen activator inhibitor-1 and reduced levels of prostacyclin (PGI_2), and elevated circulating and urinary levels of the vasoconstrictor factor endothelin. HUS usually becomes clinically apparent in the convalescent phase of the intestinal illness (45). This is consistent with the initiation of events early in the course of the illness, probably when both endotoxin (an important activator of endothelial cell synthesis of cytokines and other vasoactive mediators) and presumably Shiga toxin (which targets endothelial cells) are present. The hemolysis may be dramatic, for example, a decrease in hematocrit of 10% or more within a 24-hour period, often requiring immediate blood transfusion as a life-saving intervention. Uremia develops more slowly and can necessitate dialysis. In some patients, dialysis may be avoided because the increase in creatinine is gradual and more conservative management does not increase morbidity or mortality risks (46). Ironically, the preexisting total body potassium deficiency associated with malnutrition and diarrhea among children in developing countries often precludes clinically significant hyperkalemia from developing and may reduce the need for dialysis.

Neurologic complications, especially seizures, are also well documented in shigellosis. Seizures are commonly generalized, occur early in the course of disease caused by any *Shigella* species, are often associated with a rapidly rising temperature, usually do not recur, and are rarely associated with permanent sequelae (35). They resemble typical febrile seizures in children, except for the higher mean age in *Shigella* patients. Pathogenesis is unknown, and the suggestion that it may be due to Shiga toxin or other cytotoxins remains unproven (47). Encephalopathy independent of hypoglycemia may develop, especially during infection with *S. flexneri* (35,48). These manifestations contribute to the occasional overlap in clinical presentation between shigellosis and bacterial meningitis. Fatalities in HUS are often associated with central nervous system pathology and cerebral edema, or cerebral hemorrhages associated with acute hypertension (49).

Other recognized complications include post-*Shigella* reactive arthritis or full-blown Reiter's syndrome, particularly, it seems, with *S. flexneri* infection (50) but not *S. dysenteriae* type 1 infection (51). There is a strong correlation between reactive arthritis and expression of the HLA-B27 histocompatibility antigen, suggesting an immunologic basis for the joint manifestations. There is suggestive evidence that *S. flexneri* either alters the presentation of HLA-B27 molecules (52) or itself expresses proteins that cross-react with B27 epitopes (53), raising the possibility that molecular mimicry between organism and host may be the basis for the response.

PATHOGENESIS

The molecular basis of shigellosis is complex and the more this is studied the more complex it appears to be (7,8,54). In the past decade, the primary paradigm for pathogenesis has been dramatically revised. The new understanding of virulence mechanisms is based on considerable evidence that the organism enlists host inflammatory responses that are essential for clinical disease. This suggests that new strategies for disease control that are based on interrupting the host contribution to pathogenesis may be possible.

What remains unchanged is the understanding that virulence of *Shigella* is absolutely determined by the capacity of the organism to invade mammalian cells. The ability of a strain to invade epithelium has often been assessed by the Sereny test, which involves the inoculation of *Shigella* onto the cornea of a guinea pig or rabbit. Invasive strains cause a purulent conjunctivitis as a consequence of bacterial invasion and replication within the corneal epithelium. Now, invasive capacity is most often demonstrated *in vitro* in cell culture. The genetics and biochemical basis of invasion are discussed in detail below.

However, cellular invasion, which sequesters organisms away from host immune defenses, does not fully explain the most unique characteristic of *Shigella* pathogenesis, that is, the very small inoculum required to cause disease (18,19), and additional mechanisms must be involved. One such mechanism is likely to relate to the effect of gastric acid on organisms traversing the stomach. Infectivity of acid-susceptible *V. cholerae* and nontyphoidal *Salmonella* serovars is enhanced by factors that diminish acid secretion, such as prior gastrectomy or vagotomy, or the use of H_2 blockers for ulcer disease (55). However, systematic *in vitro* study of *S. flexneri* under controlled conditions of pH and time of exposure reveals significantly greater acid resistance than with *Salmonella* or *E. coli* (56). This property is strikingly dependent on growth phase. It develops during late exponential growth and becomes fully expressed in stationary phase. Genetic recombination experiments have implicated a global regulatory system involving a putative stationary phase σ factor encoded by the *rpo*^{s} gene, along with other still unidentified genes (57).

Acid-resistant organisms lose their ability to invade epithelial cells, and because invasion is clearly required for shigellae to cause disease, they are avirulent in this state. That there may be a tradeoff for the ability to survive low pH becomes apparent when these features are placed in an epidemiologic context. Acid resistance is most useful when the organisms initially enter the host, because this allows them to survive gastric acid. *Shigella* organisms reach stationary phase growth and are acid resistant as they exit the host and enter the environment. Once ingested and past the stomach, the organisms begin to multiply, acid resistance is suppressed, and other critical virulence traits associated with log phase growth are expressed, including the ability to invade host cells.

Although *Shigella* and EIEC share a number of virulence determinants, the infective dose for EIEC has been reported to be at least 1,000-fold higher (58). The explanation for this is not readily apparent but may account, in part, for the relative infrequency of EIEC infections.

The New Inflammatory Paradigm of Shigellosis

Although earlier models for *Shigella* pathogenesis involved direct invasion of intestinal epithelial cells from the lumen, leading to cell death and the initiation of an inflammatory response, work primarily by Sansonetti's group (59) have provided evidence for a new paradigm involving the host as an active participant in disease pathogenesis. First, the organisms do not invade at the apical (luminal) membrane of intestinal epithelial cells (60); rather, invasion initially occurs across M cells. These are specialized antigen sampling cells lacking a brush border and are part of the follicle-associated epithelium overlaying the mucosal lymphoid follicles scattered throughout the intestinal mucosa (61,62). Next, bacteria translocating across the mucosa are rapidly taken up by macrophages in the dome of the lymphoid follicles (63), resulting in apoptotic death of the macrophage. This occurs within 2 to 3 hours of incubation of organisms and macrophages *in vitro* (59), and appears to involve the binding of a microbial product, IpaB, to the cysteine protease caspase 1 (64), which activates signaling pathways for apoptosis (65,66). The next step is rather remarkable, because at the same time that apoptosis is initiated, *Shigella* activates the production and secretion by macrophages of proinflammatory cytokines such as interleukin (IL)-1β (67). One connection between the two processes is the requirement for caspase activation of proinflammatory cytokines, releasing mature IL-1β and IL-18 (68). This is clearly important in pathogenesis; for example, infusion of rabbits infected with *S. flexneri* with the IL-1 inhibitor IL-1RA prevents the development of disease in this experimental model (69). In the first few hours of this experimental model, IL-1RA production is inhibited, with a marked decrease in the IL-1RA/IL-1 ratio, which favors the expression of the proinflammatory effects of IL-1 at the outset of infection (70).

At the same time, epithelial cells are activated to produce the chemokine IL-8, which is a powerful attractant for neutrophils. The stimulus for IL-8 production may be the bacteria escaping the macrophage, which secondarily invade epithelial cells across their permissive basolateral membrane (71). In the case of *S. dysenteriae* type 1, Shiga toxin itself significantly activates the synthesis and secretion of IL-8 (72). Neutrophils, attracted to the lamina propria, transmigrate through the paracellular space between epithelial cells to the intestinal lumen. This serves to break down the interepithelial cell tight junctions, permitting a massive influx of organisms to the basal surface of the epithelium, significantly ratcheting up the invasion process of epithelial cells (73). A large deletion in the invasion plasmid, termed a "black hole," results in enhanced virulence of *Shigella* and EIEC (74). One of the genes in this black hole is *cadA*, which in ordinary *E. coli* encodes lysine decarboxylase. When this enzyme is restored to *S. flexneri* by the introduction of the cadA gene, the ability of the organism to induce neutrophil migration across the epithelial cell layer is diminished, attributed to the release of cadaverine produced in the decarboxylation of lysine (75). Inhibition of the migration of leukocytes with monoclonal antibodies directed toward neutrophil surface antigens, such as CD18, also blocks pathogenesis of shigellosis in experimental models (76), indicating the key role of cytokines in the initiation of an inflammatory cell infiltrate. These inflammatory cells form the exudates present in the lumen of the affected bowel and in the dysenteric stool. Evidence from clinical human cases of shigellosis in Bangladesh confirms that there is a strong proinflammatory cytokine response in both stool and serum (77), proportional to the severity of illness, with higher levels being recorded in stool (78).

Genetics of Invasion

Shigella is a dramatic example of the polygenic nature of virulence, with virulence genes present on both the chromosome and plasmids (6) (Fig. 43.1). The application of genetic methods over the past 2 decades have led to the identification of multiple chromosomal loci associated with *Shigella* virulence (Table 43.3). Although not yet well studied, it is likely that some of these loci may be missing or differently expressed in EIEC to account for the difference in pathogenicity. Hale (6) has classified these *Shigella* genes in three groups: (a) determinants such as siderophores, somatic antigens, and superoxide dismutase that affect survival of *Shigella* in the gastrointestinal lumen or in the mucosa; (b) cytotoxins; and (c) regulatory factors.

Siderophores

Pathogenic microorganisms including *Shigella* require iron for survival and therefore possess mechanisms for iron acquisition that will operate within their host. Biosynthetic and transport genes for aerobactin-type iron-binding proteins have been found in all *Shigella* species except *S. dysenteriae* type 1 and some strains of *S. sonnei* that instead express enterobactin siderophores. *S. flexneri* also possess enterobactin genes; however, these are usually cryptic (6). Siderophores operate *in vivo* where virtually all iron is protein-bound, and it is not surprising that tissue culture models, in which all requirements are supplied by the culture medium, fail to differentiate the virulence potential of siderophore phenotypes (79). However, subtle differences in the virulence of aerobactin mutants can be detected *in vivo*. For example, an *iuc* aerobactin mutant produces a delayed positive Sereny test (80). When the inoculum is increased, this difference disappears, suggesting that the role of the aerobactin gene is to facilitate the initial multiplication of *Shigella* when the inoculum is small (6).

Group-Specific Somatic Antigen

One of the earliest indications that O side chains of the somatic antigen involved conjugal transfer of the genes encoding *E. coli* somatic antigens 8 or 25 into *S. flexneri* 2a (81). These O serotypes were chosen because O-25 resembles *S. flexneri* 2a in having a high mannose content, whereas O-8 is chemically distinctive. All O-8 hybrids were avirulent, but some of the O-25 hybrids retained virulence

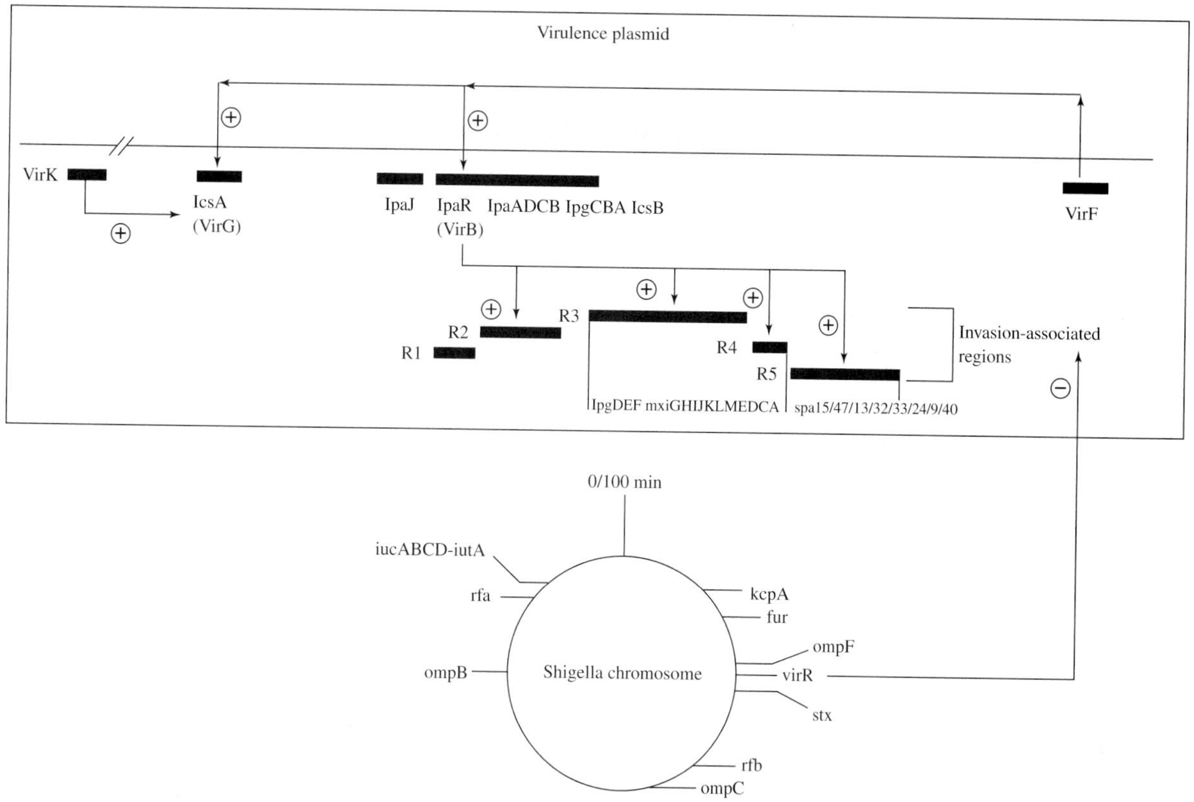

FIGURE 43.1. Composite map of the *Shigella* chromosomal and invasion plasmid virulence genes, indicating the positive regulatory pathways (*heavy line arrow*) and negative regulatory pathways (*fine line arrow*). R1 to R5 refer to regions in the invasion plasmid and constitute the 30-kb pathogenicity island discussed in the text and essential for cell invasion and apoptotic death of macrophages. (Courtesy of Dr. J. Buysse.)

TABLE 43.3. CHROMOSOMAL LOCI ASSOCIATED WITH VIRULENCE IN *S. FLEXNERI*

Locus	Virulence Phenotype of Mutants	Regulatory or Effector Function
T locus	Y variant expressing only group 3,4 somatic antigen may exhibit decreased virulence	Integration site for incorporation of lysogenic phage 4 encoding type specific somatic antigen
kcpA	Sereny-negative with limited intracellular and intercellular bacterial spread in tissue culture monolayers	Positive regulation of plasmid gene *virG (icsA)*
virR	Invasive in tissue culture when grown at 30°C	Repression of plasmid invasion loci, e.g., *ipaA,B,C,D,* in response to temperature
stx	Decrease in vascular damage in the colonic epithelium or orally challenged monkeys[a]	Synthesis of Shiga toxin
rfb	Sereny-negative, decreased intercellular spread in infected tissue culture monolayers	Synthesis of group-specific somatic antigen
ompR-envZ	Decreased invasion in tissue culture: Sereny-negative	Induction of plasmid invasion loci
rfa	Delayed or negative Sereny test, decreased intercellular spread in infected tissue culture monolayers	Synthesis of somatic antigen basal core
iucA,B,C,D-iutA	Delayed Sereny reaction, decreased mortality rate in orally challenged guinea pig; decreased histopathology and fluid response in ligated rabbit ileal loop; diminished virulence in orally challenged monkey model	Synthesis of aerobactin and 76-kDa aerobactin receptor protein
sodB	Sensitivity to oxygen-dependent killing by phagocytes; Sereny-negative; greatly decreased histopathology in ligated rabbit ileal loop	Superoxide dismutase inactivates superoxide radicals produced by phagocytes during respiratory burst

[a]The *stx* gene is only present in the chromosome of *S. dysenteriae* type 1.
Modified from Hale TL. Genetic basis of virulence in *Shigella* species. *Microbiol Rev* 1991;55:206–224, which should be consulted for a complete list of references.

by both Sereny test and oral challenge, suggesting that the chemical composition and structure of the O side chain affects *Shigella* virulence. Rough strains of *Shigella* lacking O side chains retain the ability to invade and multiply within tissue culture cells but are not able to spread to adjacent cells and are avirulent *in vivo* in animal models (82,83). They also do not cause infection in laboratory workers in contrast to smooth isolates that regularly result in laboratory acquired disease.

Together with the now extensive epidemiologic evidence of type-specific immunity to *Shigella* infection, these data indicate the importance of LPS antigens in the pathogenesis of shigellosis. A Tn5 transposon insertion into the *rfa* locus, necessary for the synthesis of the LPS basal core region, results in delayed plaque formation in cell culture and a delayed Sereny test reaction *in vivo*, indicating a diminished ability of the organism to invade and spread from cell to cell (82). It remains possible, however, that alterations in LPS core composition do not directly affect virulence but rather exert an indirect effect on the expression, insertion, or conformation of outer membrane proteins involved in virulence (6). In contrast to *S. flexneri*, plasmid-encoded enzymes are required for somatic antigen biosynthesis in both *S. dysenteriae* type 1 and *S. sonnei*. For example, the galactose transferase gene (*rfp*) is located on a 9-kb plasmid in the former (84,85). Although the precise role of LPS in virulence is not clear, it is possible to express O antigen biosynthesis genes from *Shigella* in various hosts, which may be useful for studying its role in virulence and potentially for developing vaccines (86).

Superoxide Dismutase

Superoxide dismutase (*sodB*) may enhance the survival of *Shigella in vivo* by inhibiting the bactericidal effect of host-derived reactive oxygen radicals (6,87). Allelic exchange of the unmapped *S. flexneri* superoxide dismutase gene has been accomplished and the resulting *sodB-Shigella* mutant is extremely sensitive to oxygen stress and killing by either mouse peritoneal macrophages or human polymorphonuclear leukocytes. When inoculated into ligated rabbit ileal loops, such mutants cause little histopathologic damage to the mucosa.

Shiga Toxin and Other *Shigella* Enterotoxins

More is known about Shiga toxin than other putative *Shigella* toxins. Nonetheless, and despite the description in 1972 of its ability to cause both a fluid secretory and inflammatory response in the rabbit ileal loop model (88), its role, if any, in the intestinal phase of shigellosis has remained uncertain to this day. However, the discovery that closely related Shiga toxins (also known as *verotoxins*) are made by certain *E. coli* associated with HUS, as is the Shiga toxin–producing *S. dysenteriae* type 1, has firmly implicated Shiga toxin in pathogenesis of HUS (89).

Shiga toxin consists of two noncovalently linked peptides, a 32-kd enzymatically active A subunit and five 7- to 8-kd B subunits responsible for toxin binding to its cell surface receptor, the glycolipid globotriaosylceramide (Gb3). The enzymatically active Shiga toxin A subunit is activated by proteolytic processing and reduction of an internal disulfide linkage, producing an amino terminal A1 fragment (27 kd) and a carboxy terminal A2 fragment (4 kd) (7). A1 possesses the identical N-glycosidase enzymatic activity present in the toxic plant lectin, ricin. Both irreversibly release adenine from a single specific residue in the 28S component of the 60S ribosomal subunit and block the ability to support peptide chain elongation. A single toxin molecule gaining entrance to a cell catalytically inactivates all ribosomes, ultimately stopping protein synthesis completely and resulting in cell death (90).

Certain amino acid residues have been shown to critically affect the enzymatic action of Shiga toxin. For example, glutamic acid$_{167}$ is a critical active site residue of *E. coli* Shiga toxin type 1 (Stx-1), which differs from Shiga toxin in one amino acid change in the A subunit (91). Even a conservative change of glutamic acid$_{167}$ to aspartic acid resulted in a 1,000-fold reduction in enzymatic activity. The B subunits of Shiga toxin and Stx-1 are identical. They have been purified to homogeneity by several groups (7,89) and their x-ray crystallographic structure solved (92). This reveals a pentameric folding of Stx-1B very similar to that of cholera toxin and the B oligomer of heat-labile enterotoxin from *E. coli*, which is composed of five noncovalently linked identical B subunits. Stein and co-workers (92) speculated that a conserved carbohydrate binding site may be formed by the β-sheet interaction between adjacent Stx B monomers, suggesting the presence of five potential binding sites per pentamer. Site-directed mutagenesis of Shiga toxin B subunit reveals that the aspartate residues at positions 16 and 17 are part of the receptor binding site (93). Aspartate$_{17}$ is one of the amino acids lining a potential binding cleft described by Stein and co-workers (92), consistent with the notion that this is an important functional residue.

Shiga toxin has been purified to homogeneity using a variety of techniques (7). The toxin is cytotoxic to certain tissue culture cell lines (HeLa, Vero, a number of intestinal villus-like epithelial cell lines, and low-passage primary vascular endothelial cell cultures, especially those derived from microvascular sources) but not others (CHO, WI-38). It also results in "neurotoxicity" (paralysis and delayed death) after parenteral inoculation in experimental animals, and it is an enterotoxin (i.e., it leads to intestinal fluid accumulation in ligated rabbit ileal loop model). The chromosomal *stx* gene is uniquely present in *S. dysenteriae* type 1, located at 28 minutes near *pyrF*, a known hot spot for chlorate mutagenesis. The genes for Shiga toxin and the closely related *E. coli* Shiga toxins, which are encoded on transforming phage, have been sequenced and show significant homology, ranging from 99% for Stx-1 to 55% for Stx-2 (89). The production of Shiga toxin is suppressed by anaerobiasis and by high levels of iron, due to the influence on the *stx* operon of the *fur* gene product. Fur is a DNA-binding protein that, when complexed with iron in the presence of high iron concentrations as in the intestinal lumen, binds to the *stx* promoter and blocks transcription (94). Low free iron conditions, as are present within the mucosa and within cells, thus releases the transcriptional block and synthesis of toxin proceeds.

The glycolipid receptor for Shiga toxin, Gb3, was independently identified by two groups using different approaches (95,96). The critical feature of the carbohydrate toxin-binding site is the presence of a galactose-$\alpha 1 \rightarrow 4$-galactose disaccharide. The binding is highly specific; for example, alteration of the galactose-galactose linkage to $\alpha 1 \rightarrow 3$ destroys its capacity to bind Shiga toxin.

That the glycolipid binding site is a functional receptor is demonstrated by the finding that infant rabbits do not respond to the enterotoxin activity of Shiga toxin inoculated into the intestinal lumen until day 16 when they first express the receptor in the intestinal microvillus membrane. In the following days, the sharp increase in expression of Gb3 in the microvillus membrane of intestinal epithelial cells (97) is accompanied by a progressive increase in the fluid response to toxin (98). Developmental regulation of Gb3 in rabbit small intestine correlates with increasing activity of the biosynthetic enzyme, UDP-galactose:lactosylceramide galactosyltransferase, and decreasing activity of the degradative enzyme, α-galactosidase after day 16 of life (99).

The necessary role of Gb3 in Shiga toxin action is readily demonstrated *in vitro* using cell cultures. Susceptibility to Shiga toxin is directly related to the cellular content and surface expression of Gb3 in various cell lines (100). Selection for Shiga toxin–resistant HeLa cells coselects for reduced activity of the synthetic Gb3-galactosyltransferase and diminished expression of Gb3 (101). Cellular Gb3 levels may be increased by blocking the degradative enzymatic pathway involving α-galactosidase or decreased by blocking the initial enzyme in neutral glycolipid synthesis, UDP-glucose:ceramide glucosyltransferase. These manipulations result in an increase or decrease in the cytotoxic activity of the toxin, respectively (101). Shiga toxin resistance in HeLa or Vero cells can be reversed by transfer of preformed Gb3 delivered via liposomes (101). Control cultures, in which other related glycolipids lacking the terminal galactose-$\alpha 1 \rightarrow 4$-galactose disaccharide are transferred, show no change in sensitivity to the toxin. In addition to expression of Gb3, other traits appear to be required to confer sensitivity to Shiga toxin. For example, CHO cells constitutively lack Gb3 synthetic enzymes, do not produce Gb3, and do not bind Shiga toxin. Insertion of Gb3 delivered by liposomes to the CHO cell membrane restores their ability to bind toxin; however, there is no subsequent biologic effect. This suggests that additional machinery is necessary to confer sensitivity to toxin action by altering the uptake, processing, or intracellular trafficking of the toxin.

Shiga toxin placed in the lumen of rabbit small bowel reduces sodium absorption without altering chloride secretion (102). This suggests that the physiologic effect of toxin on intestinal electrolyte transport is primarily on sodium absorptive villus cells. Villus cells isolated from rabbit small bowel preferentially express Gb3 and are susceptible to toxin *in vitro*, whereas crypt cells lack Gb3 and are toxin resistant. This is consistent with the finding that differentiated intestinal villus-like cell lines (CaCo-2 and HT-29) express Gb3 and respond to toxin, whereas less differentiated cryptlike lines (T-84) neither express Gb3 nor respond to toxin (103).

Following binding to its receptor, Shiga toxin is taken up by receptor-mediated endocytosis at clathrin-coated pits (104,105) and is transported within vesicles to the trans-Golgi network. There the toxin moves in retrograde fashion through the Golgi stack to the endoplasmic reticulum where the A1 subunit reaches its ribosomal target. Shiga toxin lacks the KDEL trafficking sequence (-Lys-Asp-Glu-Leu-) that determines intracellular pathways of other toxins, and instead the pathway for Shiga toxin appears to be determined by the composition of the fatty acids of Gb3 itself (106). The details of the transfer of the A chain across the vesicular membrane are not known; however, cell intoxication is blocked by brefeldin A, which disrupts the Golgi membrane (107). Cleavage of the Shiga toxin A subunit peptide increases its enzymatic activity. This event probably occurs in early endosomes or in the trans-Golgi network, mediated by a calcium-dependent serine protease, furin (108).

New evidence has suggested that Shiga toxin may act by mechanisms other than cytotoxicity in certain cells, such as leukocytes and endothelial cells, activating certain genes and increasing production of their protein products. A variety of cell signaling systems are implicated, including the nuclear factors NF-κβ and AP-1. These, in turn, mediate the superinduction of a set of early response genes, a process that in other systems is known to proceed through the combination of an activation stimulus together with the inhibition of protein synthesis. Among the genes activated are those for cytokines/chemokines such as IL-8, which may play a role in the induction of the inflammatory response to *Shigella* invasion, as well as genes for cell adhesins such as ICAM-1, VCAM-1, and E-selectin, procoagulants, and others. Shiga toxin stimulation of IL-8 secretion by Hct-8 intestinal epithelial cells is blocked by inhibitors of the p38/RK mitogen-activated kinase system (109), a component of the ribotoxic stress response involving the early activation of *c-jun* mRNA. Considerable work is currently devoted to working out the complex stimulatory and regulatory pathways involved, and to identify the sequence of gene activation and the nature of the products being made.

At the same time, there is clear *in vitro* evidence that

exposure of target endothelial cells to proinflammatory cytokines increases the expression of Gb3, which increases toxin binding and enhances the biologic effects of the toxin on these cells (110). It remains difficult, however, to put all of these observations into a clear and sequential schema of pathogenesis of either the intestinal events or the systemic complications associated with Shiga toxin–producing organisms, such as HUS.

The lack of Shiga toxin production by non-*dysenteriae* type 1 strains of *Shigella* has brought into question the role of the toxin in pathogenesis, except as an accessory virulence factor in *S. dysenteriae* type 1 and in the pathogenesis of HUS. There is, however, ample evidence that Shiga toxin has profound effects on intestinal cell lines *in vitro*, on isolated human colonic cells in primary culture, and on the epithelial cell layer of rabbit ileal mucosa *in vivo* (111). Construction of Shiga toxin–negative mutants has allowed the assessment of its role in pathogenesis. The original mutations were made by mutagenesis with chlorate because of the proximity of the chlorate sensitive site to the chromosomal *stx* operon. Chlorate resistant mutants, which turned out to be hypotoxigenic (112), and a specific toxin gene deletion *S. dysenteriae* type 1 strain (113) retained clinical virulence, although the clinical illness was less severe than disease due to wild-type organisms. Toxin-producing strains, however, caused more extensive inflammatory lesions and capillary destruction in the colonic mucosa in a Rhesus monkey oral infection-dysentery model (113).

Histopathology of dysenteric intestine and kidney tissue from patients with HUS suggests that microvascular endothelials cells are a target in shigellosis (114,115). Shiga toxin binds to many endothelial cell types and is cytotoxic to these cells (111). Human umbilical vein endothelial cells are far more sensitive to Shiga toxin when these cells are pretreated with LPS or proinflammatory cytokines such as tumor necrosis factor-α (TNF-α) or interleukin-1β). This is related to an increase in Gb3 expression and toxin binding (116). Induction of Gb3 synthesis by LPS and cyotkines may be vascular bed specific, reflecting the role of cytokines in the progression of pathophysiologic events *in vivo*. In view of the strong association of endotoxemia with systemic complications in shigellosis and the well-known effect of LPS to upregulate cytokine synthesis, endotoxemia early in *S. dysenteriae* type 1 infection may sensitize endothelial cell beds to the effects of Shiga toxin translocating from the gut lumen across the epithelial cell layer (117). Parenteral administration to young piglets of the related *E. coli*Shiga toxins, Stx-2 and porcine Stx-2e, produces damage to brain endothelial cells and reproduces central nervous system manifestations of porcine edema disease (118). These findings not only implicate Shiga toxin in pathogenesis of this syndrome but also localize its action to central nervous system endothelial cells.

Shigella species also produce enterotoxins distinct from Shiga toxin (119,120). These toxins, designated Shigella enterotoxin (ShET)-1 and ShET-2, alter ion transport across rabbit small bowel tissue *in vitro* and cause fluid secretion *in vivo* in ligated rabbit ileal loops (121). ShET-1, a 55-kd complex protein, is encoded by an iron-regulated chromosomal gene (*set1*) located within a 603-bp pathogenicity island called *she* (122), whereas *set2*, the structural gene for ShET-2, a 62.8-kd protein, is located on the large *Shigella* invasion plasmid and is highly homologous with a previously described EIEC enterotoxin (120). ShET-1 is essentially restricted to *S. flexneri* 2a, whereas the *set2* gene sequence is present in most isolates of all *Shigella* species and serotypes (123,124). Their role, if any, in the pathogenesis of the watery diarrhea phase of shigellosis and diarrhea due to EIEC is still uncertain.

Cellular Invasion by *Shigella* and Enteroinvasive *E. coli*

The full invasive process of *Shigella* and EIEC is highly intricate and dependent on multiple genes, present primarily on the large invasion plasmid present in these organisms (125,126). This plasmid has been completely sequenced (127), revealing the presence of coding sequences over the whole plasmid with intervening, often incomplete, insertion sequences (IS) (128). Of the 286 open reading frames identified, 53% were related to known IS elements, indicating that there have been multiple importations of genetic material in the development of virulence by *Shigella* spp. Of the putative protein coding sequences, 50 are previously unknown and 18 have a G+C content of less than 40%, similar to other known virulence genes on the plasmid. There is a large (30-kb) segment packed with the genes of the *ipa/mxi/spa* operons (described later). This region represents the major pathogenicity island of this plasmid, containing all of the genes necessary for cellular invasion. These genes encode a type III secretion system used by the organism to deliver microbial proteins directly into the host cell membrane or the cytoplasm. For convenience, the invasion process is arbitrarily divided into four stages for discussion: (a) initial entry into cells, (b) intracellular multiplication, (c) intra- and intercellular spread, and (d) host cell killing.

Initial Entry

Most studies have used *S. flexneri* as a model invasive organism, but it is likely that the process in other *Shigella* species as well as EIEC closely follows the *S. flexneri* model. Although *Shigella* was previously believed to invade intestinal epithelial cells from their apical (luminal) membrane, the present conceptualization is rather different, involving M cells, the antigen sampling cells scattered along the intestinal mucosa, and invasion plasmid gene products (129). Organisms in the lumen are translocated across the M cell to the lamina propria where they can subsequently efficiently invade intestinal epithelial cells across their invasion permissive basolateral membranes. This proceeds via a complex process beginning with actin polymerization at the site of contact of bacterium and host cell (130). This leads to the formation of long host cell pseudopods (Fig. 43.2) that ultimately engulf and internalize the organism within a vesicle (Fig. 43.3). This is an active energy-consuming process resembling phagocytosis, although it occurs in the normally nonphagocytic intestinal epithelial cell. This ingestion of the organisms is initiated and directed by bacterium-related factors. A critical event is the accumulation of aggregated actin filaments and myosin beneath the plasma membrane at the points of interaction between microbe and host cell surface (131).

These changes in cytoskeletal organization, revealed by the use of fluorescently labeled probes, are directed by Ipa (*i*nvasion *p*lasmid *a*ntigen) proteins, such as IpaC, and regulated by Rho GTPases (Cdc42, Rac, Rho) (132). Rho is also involved in the extension of actin structures via activation of

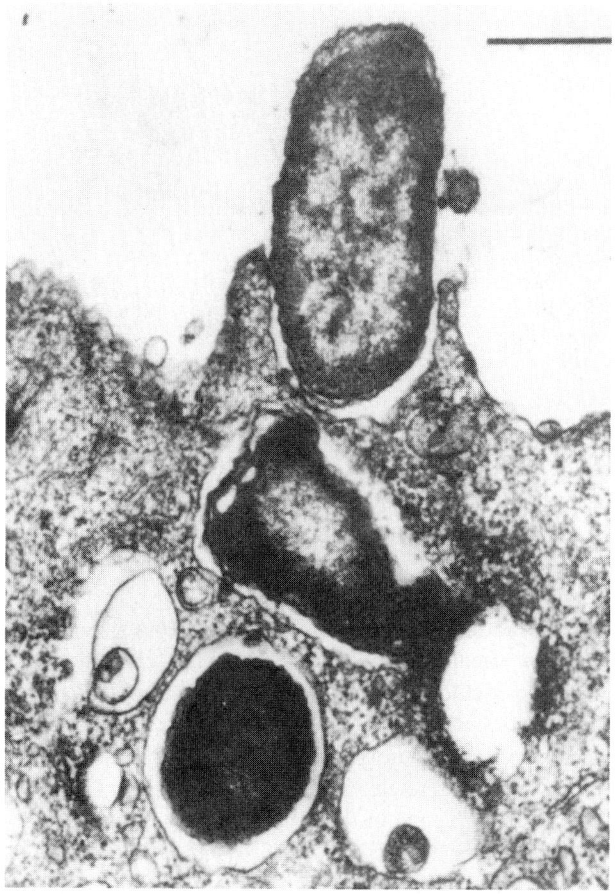

FIGURE 43.2. Shigella invasion. Phagocytosis of virulent *Shigella flexneri* 2a by HeLa cells in culture. Note the host cell pseudopods beginning to engulf the organism at the top of the figure; these will ultimately fuse to form a phagocytic vesicle within the cytoplasm. In addition, several internalized bacteria are present within this cell. Bar = 1 ?m. (From Jacewicz MS, Mobassaleh M, Acheson DWK, et al. Maturational regulation of globotriaosylceramide, the Shiga-like toxin 1 receptor, by butyrate in intestinal epithelial lines. *J Clin Invest* 1995;96:1328–1335, with permission.)

the protooncogene c-src leading to phosphorylation of cortactin, an actin-binding protein, and ezrin, which links the membrane and cytoskeleton and promotes further extensions of the pseuodopods (133,134). For efficient cell entry, IpaA must be injected into the host cell; IpaA mutants induce entry foci but have difficulty entering the cell (135). Activation of vinculin by IpaA opens up a binding site for α-actinin, which is associated with microbial entry as well.

A great deal is now known about the *Shigella* invasion plasmid (59). The process is complex and further complicated by the fact that the same gene has been identified by different investigators in several *Shigella* species and given different designations. For example, region 1 of the 30-kb pathogenicity island (Fig. 43.1) contains a positive regulatory gene named *virB* in *S. flexneri* 2a (136), *ipaR* in *S. flexneri* 5a (137), and *invE* in *S. sonnei* (138). Under control of a second positive regulatory gene, *virF*, *ipaR*/*virB* induces several invasion genes contained in other regions of the 30-kb element (139). Region 2 is the most extensively studied element, encoding the *ipa* genes mediating the synthesis of Ipa proteins. Regions 3 and 4 contain the *mxi* genes, encoding Mxi (***m***embrane e***x***pression of ***i***nvasion plasmid antigens) proteins required for export and insertion of the Ipa proteins into the host cell (140). Mxi proteins assemble into a structure containing a 60-nm "needle complex" through which IpA and other microbial proteins are transferred into the host cell (141).

Expression of the seven plasmid-encoded Ipa proteins (IpaA-G) in *S. flexneri* minicells (small anucleate cells resulting from aberrant cell division at the polar ends of the organism) enabled them to invade cultured HeLa cells, although new data indicate that only IpaB, C, and D are required (142). IpaA-D are antigenic in the host and induce antibodies that react with the same proteins in all *Shigella* species as well as EIEC (143). The Ipa genes cluster in the transcriptional order *ipaB*/*ipaC*/*ipaD*/*ipaA* (144) (Fig. 43.1). These operons are coordinately regulated by the *ipaR* gene product in a temperature-activated manner. A complex of IpaB/IpaC is inserted into the host cell membrane, forming a pore through which other microbial proteins enter the host cell (145). The IpaB/IpaD complex controls the flux of other proteins through the type III secretory system. The early events in actin polymerization and cytoskeletal reorganization are initiated by the C-terminal region of IpaC (146).

Secretion and surface presentation of IpaB and IpaC is abolished by transposon insertions in other loci, either *mxiA* or the nearby *spa* locus (*s*urface *p*resentation of invasion plasmid *a*ntigens), which is downstream from *mxiA* in region 5 of the 30-kb segment of the virulence plasmid (147,148). The *mxiD* and *mxiJ* regions, located between *ipa* and *mxiA*, also are required for secretion of Ipa proteins. Three additional *i*nvasion *p*lasmid *g*enes, *ipgD*, *ipgE*, and *ipgF*, located in the 5′ end of the *mxi-spa* locus, appear to belong to the same operon (149). *IpgD* encodes a secreted protein of approximately 58 to 60 kd, which is dependent on *mxi* gene products for secretion. Mutations in *ipgD* and *ipgF* do not

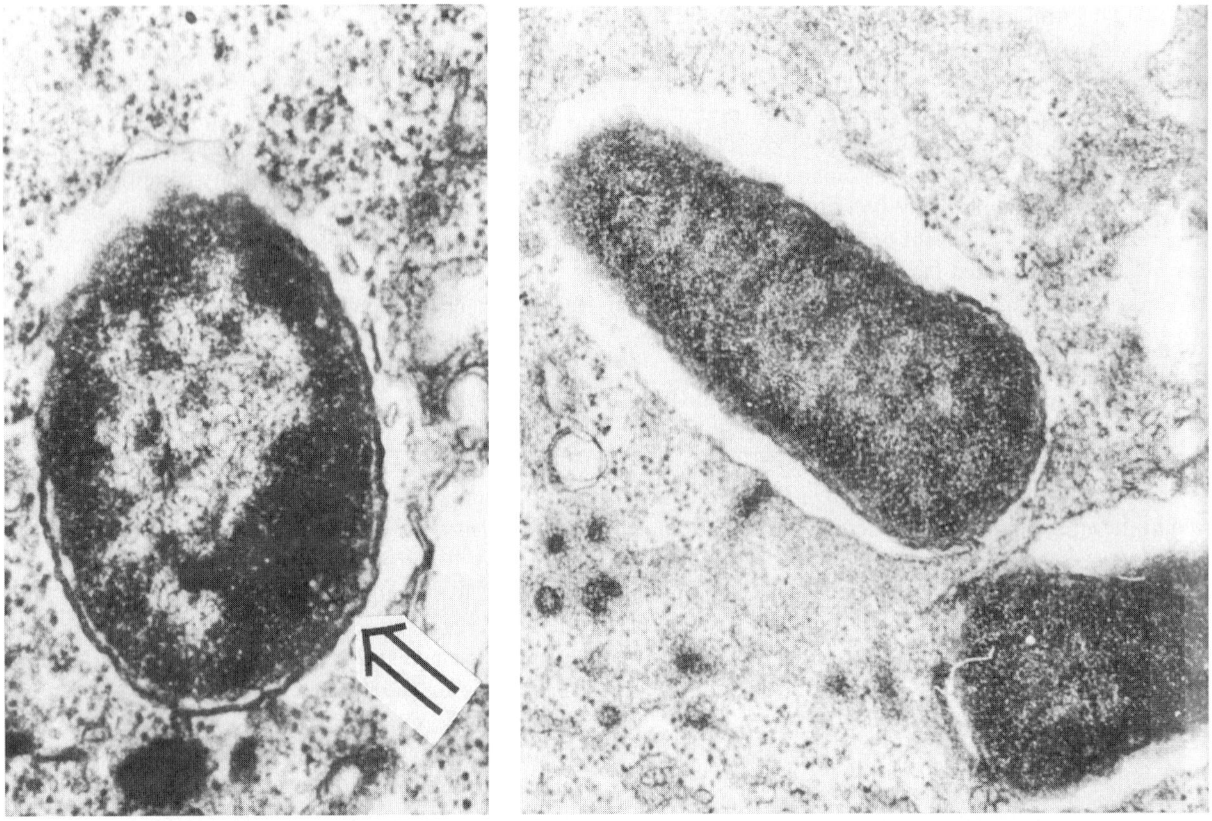

FIGURE 43.3. Escape from the phagosome. Dissolution of the phagosomal vesical membrane, which occurs soon after invasion of the cell, can be seen over the upper portion of the organism in the left panel (arrow points to the still intact portion of the phagosomal membrane). In the right panel, two organisms are lying free within the cytoplasm after the phagosomal membrane has completely disintegrated. (Courtesy of Dr. P. J. Sansonetti.)

affect invasion of cultured cells, however, and the precise role of these genes in virulence has yet to be determined.

It is not known whether there is a separate mechanism for adherence of *Shigella* to eukaryotic cells before invasion. Moreover, the molecular basis for selective invasion of the colon rather than small bowel is not understood.

Intracellular Multiplication

Following invasion of the epithelial cells, the organisms multiply intracellularly. HeLa cells have been a useful model to study, revealing lysis of the vesicle containing intracellular *S. flexneri* within minutes of its formation, allowing the organisms to enter into the cytoplasm (Fig. 43.3) where they multiply rapidly (150). Vesicle lysis is associated with the expression of a contact hemolytic activity necessary for virulence because hemolysin-negative strains are avirulent (151). Growth of virulent strains at 30°C inhibits expression of hemolysin and limits multiplication in host cells. The relevance of hemolysin is further suggested by the observation that hemolysin activity increases 100- to 1,000-fold because the pH decreases from neutral to the acidic pH present within the phagocytic vesicle. IpaC contributes to this process. The purified protein lyses lipid vesicles, which is also pH dependent (145). A role for IpA and IpaD also seems likely (152). Insertional IpaC mutants are defective in their ability to lyse membranes and escape from intracellular vesicles (153).

Mutations affecting intracellular growth are attenuating. Mutations in *aro* genes, blocking folic acid synthesis via the aromatic pathway, impairs intracellular growth, and such strains are attenuated *in vivo*. *aro* mutants are therefore candidates to include or develop into a live *Shigella* vaccine. Mutations of the porins OmpC and OmpF and deletion mutants in the regulatory gene *ompB* also inhibit intracellular growth and attenuate virulence. *ompB* and *ompC* deletion mutants are defective in their ability to spread from cell to cell and kill epithelial cells (154). The *ompB* deletion mutant was restored to virulence by introducing a recombinant plasmid carrying the cloned *E. coli ompC* gene, indicating the requirement for a functional OmpC protein in virulence.

Intracellular Spread

In the third phase of the invasion process, intracellular organisms move within the cytoplasm to reach the plasma membrane in order to invade adjacent cells using elements of the host cell cytoskeleton much as they did in the initial entry (155). The *IcsA/virG/*gene is necessary for this process (156). Because *Shigella* does not have flagella and is nonmotile, movement of organisms within the cytoplasm of the host cell, and from cell to cell, depends on their ability to coopt the host cell cytoskeleton. Within 2 hours of entry, *Shigella* becomes coated with polymerized actin, which is redistributed to one end of the bacterium (157) (Fig. 43.4). The continuous polar deposition of actin and myosin provides a propulsive force for the organisms to move toward the periphery of the cell. In cell culture they often cause a protrusion of the cytoplasm that reaches to the adjacent cell (Fig. 43.5), providing the cell-to-cell contact that facilitates cell-to-cell invasion.

TnphoA insertion mutants of *icsA* lose the ability to move within the cell, or from cell to cell, because the latter is presumably dependent on the former (158). These mutants do not produce IcsA, a 120-kd outer membrane protein, they do not induce actin polymerization, and they are attenuated in their ability to cause disease. In certain cells, *Shigella* also moves with the cell by binding to actin stress fibers in a very organized manner following the cytoskeletal architecture (159). The intracellular movement and cell-to-cell spread of *Shigella* has been divided into two phenotypes: Ics (intracellular and intercellular spread) and Olm (organelle-like movement). Movement of *S. flexneri* appears to result from the expression of both the Olm and Ics phenotypes. In the intestinal cell line, CaCo-2, Olm movement is associated with colonization of organisms in the actin filament ring of the perijunctional area, and Ics movement is related to cell-to-cell spread of infection. Together the two processes provide a mechanism for a single organism to gain entry to a cell, to multiply, and to spread in a contiguous fashion in a monolayer without ever exiting from the intracellular milieu during the process (160).

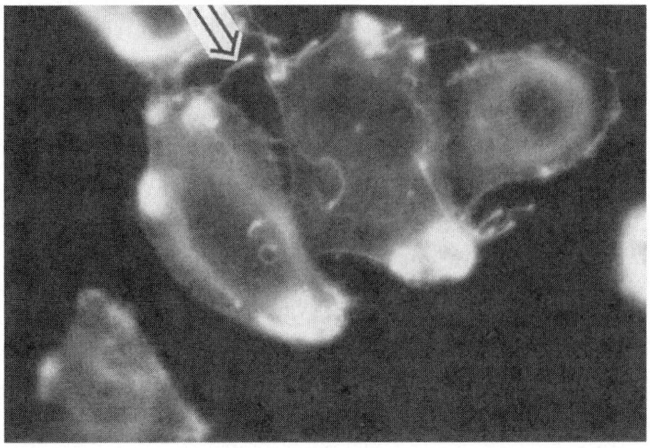

FIGURE 43.5. Intercellular spread. HeLa cells exposed to invasive, virulent *Shigella flexneri* 2a have been stained as in Figure 43.4 with fluorescein-conjugated phalloidin, a reagent that reacts with polymerized actin. The arrow points to an organism that has been propelled to the periphery of the cell where it is projecting beyond the plane of the cell membrane, thus approaching the adjacent cell, which will be invaded by this organism when the membrane of the projection fuses with the membrane of the second cell. In this manner, the organism can infect from cell to cell without ever leaving the protected intracellular environment. (From Venkatesan MM, Goldberg MB, Rose DJ, et al. Complete DNA sequence and analysis of the large virulence plasmid of *Shigella flexneri*. *Infect Immun* 2001;69:3271–3285, with permission.)

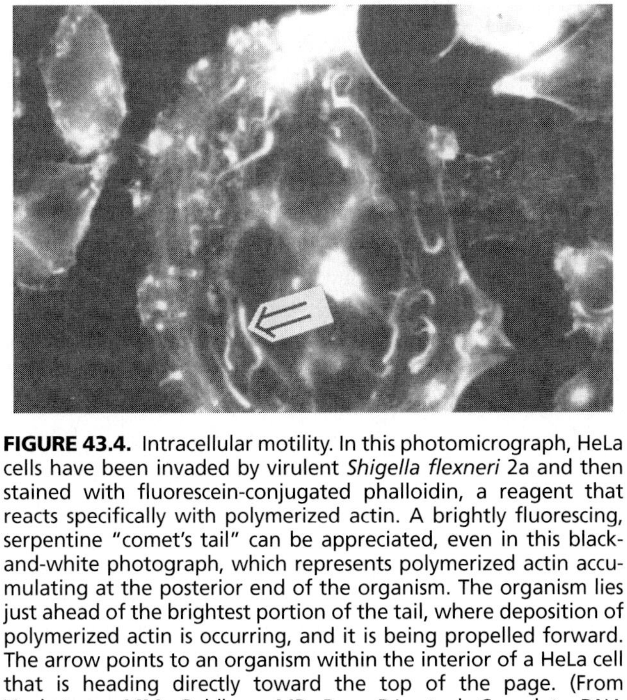

FIGURE 43.4. Intracellular motility. In this photomicrograph, HeLa cells have been invaded by virulent *Shigella flexneri* 2a and then stained with fluorescein-conjugated phalloidin, a reagent that reacts specifically with polymerized actin. A brightly fluorescing, serpentine "comet's tail" can be appreciated, even in this black-and-white photograph, which represents polymerized actin accumulating at the posterior end of the organism. The organism lies just ahead of the brightest portion of the tail, where deposition of polymerized actin is occurring, and it is being propelled forward. The arrow points to an organism within the interior of a HeLa cell that is heading directly toward the top of the page. (From Venkatesan MM, Goldberg MB, Rose DJ, et al. Complete DNA sequence and analysis of the large virulence plasmid of *Shigella flexneri*. *Infect Immun* 2001;69:3271–3285, with permission.)

IcsA is a major substrate for phosphorylation by cyclic nucleotide-dependent protein kinases from the host cell (161). Site-directed mutagenesis of a sequence encoding a phosphorylation consensus motif almost completely abolishes the ability of IcsA to be phosphorylated by protein kinase A. This mutant expressed a "super Ics" phenotype, characterized by an increased capacity to spread from cell to cell. Thus, host cell phosphorylation of microbial products may be an important defense mechanism against *Shigella*.

Cell Death

The mechanism whereby *Shigella* induces cell death is not entirely understood. Macrophages are rapidly killed by phagocytosed *Shigella* organisms, independent of their capacity to produce Shiga toxin. Considerable evidence already discussed implicates apoptosis as the underlying mechanism by which the organisms induce eukaryotic cell death in other cells as well, although the binding of isolated Shiga toxin B subunit to Gb3 induces apoptosis in Burkitt lymphoma cells, which express high levels of Gb3 (162). The relevance of the findings in these two cell types for events affecting intestinal epithelial cells or endothelial cells remains to be demonstrated.

Regulation of *Shigella* Virulence Genes

Regulation of virulence genes *in vivo* is critical to the success of pathogenic microorganisms surviving in their host and subsequent transmission to the next host. For example, like a number of other toxins, Shiga toxin transcription is iron-regulated via the *fur* gene system (7). Temperature and osmotic pressure also affect the expression of *Shigella* virulence (163). When grown at 30°C, virulent strains of *S. flexneri*, *S. sonnei*, and *S. dysenteriae* type 1 lose their ability to invade epithelial cells *in vitro* and *in vivo*. At temperatures below the critical level of 32°C, the H-NS protein (also known as virR) represses the expression of virF, inhibiting expression of the set of virulence genes controlled by virF (164). When the incubation temperature is shifted back to 37°C, virulence factors are once again made; however, this takes several generations of replication and is dependent on the synthesis of new proteins. Temperature-regulated proteins that are involved in virulence include the Shiga toxin, *ipaA-D* gene products, *mxi* gene products, contact hemolytic activity, expression of the positive regulators *virF* and *ipaR*, and the already mentioned *hns/virR*, a chromosomal gene located just in front of *stx* that serves as a negative regulator of the temperature-regulated genes for Ipa proteins and the *mxi/spa* gene products (Fig. 43.1).

Environmental osmolarity rapidly changes when *Shigella* is ingested and reaches the intestinal lumen of their mammalian host. Two classes of genes in *Shigella* respond to changes in osmolarity (165). The first includes genes whose expression is required for the actual physiologic adaption to osmotic stress, such as *proU, ompF, ompC,* and *kdp*. The second class includes genes not directly involved in physiologic adaptation but whose expression is clearly optimized under conditions of high osmolarity and, as such, may also play a role in pathogenesis. Regulation of *ompC-ompF* expression in *Shigella* is controlled by *ompR-envZ*, which constitutes the *ompB* locus. Regulation is similar to the system in *E. coli* in that high osmolarity favors the expression of OmpC in preference to OmpF. Deletion of *ompB* or an *envZ::*Tn10 mutation in *S. flexneri* 5a significantly inhibits the capability of the organism to invade HeLa cells and results in a delayed Sereny response *in vivo*.

DIAGNOSIS

There are at least three means to diagnose shigellosis or infection due to EIEC: clinical, microbiologic, and serologic.

Clinical Diagnosis

Patients presenting with a classic picture of dysentery, with frequent, small-volume, bloody stools, abdominal cramps, and tenesmus, especially associated with fever and the presence of large clumps of leukocytes in the stool, can be considered to have shigellosis or EIEC infection until proven otherwise (21). Examination of stool for leukocytes has been used as a simple and rapid method to differentiate shigellosis and other invasive bacterial diarrheas from amebiasis or secretory bacterial diarrhea such as cholera (166). Leukocytes are present not only in dysentery but also in the watery diarrhea associated with *S. sonnei* onfection, demonstrating that inflammation is a characteristic of all shigellosis and not just dysentery. In Bangladesh, 85% of patients with documented shigellosis had greater than 50 leukocytes per high-power field when stool was directly examined by light microscopy, compared with 28% of patients with diagnosed amebic dysentery, even though the latter is generally believed to be without much inflammatory exudates in stool because the parasite lyses neutrophils. This finding is not specific; in a study in Thailand, fecal leukocytes were detected not only in shigellosis but also as expected in patients with diarrhea due to EIEC, *Campylobacter*, and *Salmonella*, as well as in some patients with enteropathogenic or enterotoxigenic *E. coli* and even rotavirus (167). However, the number of leukocytes was low in the non-*Shigella* cases, whereas the presence of sheets of neutrophils in the stool remains a good clue to the diagnosis of *Shigella* infection.

Patients with shigellosis benefit from antimicrobial therapy and therefore etiologic diagnosis is useful. However, drug resistance remains a major problem. Therefore, even when antibiotic treatment is begun empirically, laboratory confirmation of the specific etiology is useful to guide continuing therapy. Microbiologic diagnosis is simple in principle but fraught with potential problems.

Laboratory Diagnosis

The first problem with microbiologic diagnosis is that *Shigella* organisms are fastidious and rapidly die off if the stool sample is not well handled. The best way to isolate them is to obtain both stool and rectal swabs, to rapidly inoculate specimens onto selective culture plates, preferably at the bedside, and to quickly incubate them at 37°C (168). If a delay in transporting specimens to the laboratory for processing is expected, they should be inoculated directly into transport medium such as buffered glycerol saline (BGS) or Carey-Blair transport medium (169). BGS serves as a true transport medium, and it should be refrigerated after inoculation and used to plate on selective media as rapidly as possible when the specimen reaches the laboratory. If *Shigella* is strongly suspected on clinical grounds, multiple separate cultures should be obtained to maximize chances of recovering the organism.

To optimize isolation of *Shigella*, more than one medium should be used for each culture (170). Ideally, these should include mildly selective media, such as MacConkey agar (considered to be the standard), deoxycholate, and eosin-methylene blue (EMB), and highly selective media, such as Hektoen-enteric (HE), *Salmonella-Shigella* (SS), and xylose-lysine-deoxycholate (XLD) agars. SS agar has the advantage of not requiring autoclaving in the field because it is so inhibitory to common contaminants; however, it is much better for isolation of *Salmonella* than *Shigella*, and is not very good at all for *S. dysenteriae* type 1. The choice of media is best determined by the experience of the microbiologist and the prevalent strains as well. For example, in the United States and United Kingdom, where *S. sonnei* accounts for most isolates, the optimal choice of media may be different from that in India where *S. flexneri* and *S. dysenteriae* type 1 strains abound. In one study (170), media for the isolation of *Shigella* from 645 children with diarrhea in Bangkok were compared. *Shigella* organisms were isolated from 98 (15%) of the children, equally divided between *S. sonnei* and *S. flexneri*. MacConkey was the best medium (Table 43.4). MacConkey supplemented with xylose (MacConkey-X medium) is reported to be superior to MacConkey itself (171). In the 1969 Guatemala epidemic, isolation of *S. dysenteriae* type 1 was facilitated by the use of tergitol-7-tetrazolium agar (172). Appropriate antibiotic therapy rapidly renders cultures negative.

EIEC is more difficult to identify than *Shigella* because the biochemical reactions are more variable, distinctive flags such as the inability to ferment lactose are lacking, and the organisms do not fall into classic EPEC serotypes for which many laboratories have typing sera. Even though plasmid analysis for the large invasion plasmid or the Sereny test or tissue culture assays can be used to screen *E. coli* isolates, neither is practical for the routine laboratory (168). EIEC organisms have usually been found to belong to a restricted number of O antigen serogroups, including O28, O29, O112, O124, O136, O143, O144, O147, O152, O164, and O167 (14,143), but typing sera are not usually found in clinical laboratories. In addition, fully 10% of EIEC isolates in Thailand belonged to other serogroups, including a new serogroup of *E. coli* (O171) identified in the same study (168).

The development of molecular techniques using DNA probes or the polymerase chain reaction (PCR) has enabled investigators to determine the prevalence of both *Shigella* and EIEC in the stool. Although use of DNA probes is both more specific and sensitive than conventional microbiologic techniques, this method is somewhat labor-intensive, time-consuming, and costly, whether radioactive or nonradioactive detection systems are used. PCR allows the detection of very small numbers of organisms, is more sensitive than either conventional microbiologic techniques or DNA probes, and is simple and quick (173). Direct PCR of stool using enzyme-linked immunosorbent assay (ELISA) to detect the PCR products appears to be superior to agarose gel electrophoresis and allows automation and scale up (174). At the same time, PCR results may be so sensitive that a true positive PCR resulting from a small number of transiting organisms provide a false-positive diagnosis. The use of molecular diagnostic techniques also requires expertise, equipment, and separate clean laboratory areas to avoid contamination with exogenous DNA, conditions that may be difficult to achieve in developing countries. One outstanding advantage of PCR-based diagnostics, however, is the potential to identify *Shigella* and EIEC in patients who have taken antibiotics, because amplification of bacterial DNA does not rely on microbial replication. PCR can also differentiate between *Shigella* and EIEC (175). In a practical sense, multiplex PCR can be developed to detect and distinguish several pathogens simultaneously in a diarrheal stool sample (176).

Examination for fecal leukocytes can be used also to guide the use of stool cultures for diagnosis. In the United States, the cost per positive stool culture can be markedly reduced if stools are first screened for leukocytes and cultured only if these cells are present (177). This increases the likelihood of isolating *Shigella*, *Salmonella*, and *Campylobacter* species. The presence of erythrocytes in stool is another useful criteria to prescreen stool samples for culture. The philosophy underlying prescreening is to target laboratory examinations to identify causes of diarrhea that require treatment other than rehydration and to reduce the costs of medical care.

TABLE 43.4. COMPARISON OF MEDIA FOR THE ISOLATION OF *SHIGELLA* SPECIES FROM 645 FECAL SPECIMENS IN BANGKOK

Culture Medium	Number of Isolates (% Positive)	
	S. flexneri	*S. sonnei*
McConkey	44 (6.8)	43 (6.7)
Teknaf enteric[a]	36 (5.6)	3 (0.4)
Hektoen	36 (5.6)	30 (4.6)
Salmonella-Shigella	34 (5.3)	40 (6.2)

[a]Teknaf enteric is MacConkey supplemented with 1 mg of potassium tellurite/mL.
Modified from Watanabe H, Arakawa E, Ito K, et al. Genetic analysis of an invasion region by use of a Tn3–lac transposon and identification of a second positive regulator gene, *invE* for cell invasion of *Shigella sonnei* significant homology of inv E with par B of plasmid P1. *Bacteriol* 1990;172:619–629.

Serologic Diagnosis

For epidemiologic studies, detection of antibodies to *Shigella* LPS is an alternative method for diagnosis of past *Shigella* infection (178). This technology has been further developed recently as a consequence of the increasing knowledge of the LPS structure in *Shigella* (179,180). The LPS of *S. dysenteriae* type 1 has a unique repeating unit that is thought to be shared only with *E. coli* O-antigenic groups 1 and 120, neither of which is a common bacterial pathogen. The LPS of *S. flexneri* types 1a to 5b, in contrast, is built by a repeating tetrasaccharide with extensive cross-reactions among the serotypes, whereas the LPS from *S. flexneri* type 6 is serologically distinctive. The O antigen of *S. sonnei* is a disaccharide of two unusual sugars, 2-acetamido-2-deoxy-L-alturonic acid linked 1→4 to 2 acetamido-4-amino-2,4,6-trideoxy-D-galactose, and is shared only with *Plesiomonas shigelloides*. Unfortunately, the quality of commercial antisera remains variable, with some performing poorly in the clinical laboratory (12).

An LPS-enzyme immunoassay (EIA) for *S. dysenteriae* type 1 has been developed and appears to provide sensitive and specific serodiagnosis when immunoglobulin class-specific IgG or IgA anti-LPS is assessed (178). Serotype-specific LPS-EIA for *S. flexneri* 1a to 5 is a problem because of the presence of one or more common epitopes, whereas a species-specific EIA works well for diagnosis of acute infection in countries where *S. flexneri* is uncommon and primary responses are expected in all patients regardless of age. In contrast, in *S. flexneri* endemic countries, the EIA may be useful only for children younger than 3 years of age. EIA for *S. sonnei* LPS appears to be specific and reasonably sensitive, but would probably not be clinically useful in the United States because the illness would be finished in most patients by the time the EIA became positive.

Differentiating EIEC from culture-negative shigellosis in the clinical microbiology laboratory can be difficult, because serotyping for invasive *E. coli* strains is generally unavailable, although this could be accomplished by PCR if the method was routinely used. However, in purely clinical terms, it is of little consequence because the manifestations of the two diseases overlap, with EIEC usually being the milder illness; clinical management is similar and can be guided by clinical features.

TREATMENT

Dysentery or bloody diarrhea due to *Shigella* or EIEC infection is generally not a severely dehydrating illness. Nonetheless, the first therapy for these infections is to replace lost fluids and electrolytes because this is simple, helpful, and usually can be done by the oral route except in severe dysentery in which anorexia may impede oral intake. In most patients in the United States, especially with infection due to *S. sonnei*, the disease is self-limited in a few days. In more severe *Shigella* infections, for example, in children in Bangladesh, the illness can be prolonged for weeks (181), and anorexia persists even into convalescence (182). Clinically significant hyponatremia occurs in many hospitalized patients infected with either *S. dysenteriae* type 1 or *S. flexneri*, with serum sodium levels decreasing to less than 120 mmol/L and resulting in central nervous system depression (183). Because these findings are associated with increased mortality rate, some authorities recommend the infusion of hypertonic (3%) saline, 12 mL/kg over 2 hours, to elevate the serum Na by approximately 10 mmol/L. This rapidly reverses the central nervous system manifestations. However, unless access to *ad libitum* water is restricted, hyponatremia may recur as a result of an inappropriate secretion of antidiuretic hormone (184).

Hypoglycemia, although not common in well-nourished patients with shigellosis or EIEC infection in the United States, can occur. It is quite frequent in children in developing countries, usually associated with *S. dysenteriae* type 1 or *S. flexneri* infections (185). Hypoglycemia appears to be related to an inadequate gluconeogenic response in relation to energy needs. Because the blood glucose levels may be less than 1 mmol/L, immediate correction is needed to prevent a fatal outcome. The rapid infusion of 1 g of glucose per kilogram body weight (5.6 mmol/kg) over 5 to 10 minutes, followed by continuous infusion of fluid containing 50 g glucose/L (278 mmol/L) until the infection is controlled has been recommended.

Shigellosis also represents a major nutritional insult, with anorexia and catabolic stress during the acute infection associated with fever and cytokine-mediated changes in host metabolism added onto a protein-losing enteropathy due to inflammatory intestinal damage. As a rule of thumb, it takes around four times as long to repair such deficits as it takes to incur them, assuming unrestricted access to food with adequate high-protein quality and energy density (186). Recent evidence suggests that an energy-dense diet early in the course of treatment with antibiotics improves weight gain and reduces the incidence of rectal prolapse, although it does not alter the resolution of fever, dysentery, stool frequency, or tenesmus (187). It is especially important to ensure that nutritional rehabilitation is continued during convalescence in children in developing countries until weight for age is normalized, although this is often difficult in the very patient population most affected because of poverty and inadequate health supervision.

Seizures associated with shigellosis are generally related to the sharp increase in body temperature early in the illness and usually do not recur; these rarely require anything more than antipyretics to reduce body temperature. Unfortunately, in developing countries, the commonly available, locally produced antipyretic acetaminophen can become adulterated with ethylene glycol due to poor quality control during manufacture. Epidemics of fatal acute renal failure have periodically resulted (188). Only rarely is there an indication for more targeted anticonvulsive therapy with barbiturates or diazepam.

Specific therapy in shigellosis requires the administration of effective antimicrobial agents, which is known to lower mortality rate and shorten the illness (190). Because *Shigella* acquires multiple antibiotic resistances with apparent ease, the most difficult aspect has been to find drugs that are effective, affordable, and safe, particularly in developing countries (190). Virtually all *Shigella* organisms now carry resistance for streptomycin, tetracycline, and chloramphenicol; many strains are resistant to ampicillin, and, depending on geographic locale, a varying proportion is also resistant to trimethoprim-sulfamethoxazole and nalidixic acid (191,192,193). In the United States and other developed countries, it is possible to use an oral (194) or parenteral (195) third-generation cephalosporin, oral azithromycin (196) or, in the case of adults, a new 4-fluoroquinolone (197) (Table 43.5). The quinolones remain unapproved by the Food and Drug Administration (FDA) for use in persons younger than 17 years of age because of the possibility of cartilage damage; however, there appears to be no clinical data to support this possibility (198) and ciprofloxacin is effective in children (199,200). Faced with the choice of cartilage damage or a severe or even fatal illness, the use of quinolones certainly appears to be justified.

Unless single-dose therapy is shown to be consistently effective and unlikely to select for resistance, the cost of these drugs currently precludes their routine use by the health services in developing countries. The cost factor has led to the extensive use of a first-generation quinolone, nalidixic acid (not an FDA approved use of this drug in the United States), which is effective, or inexpensive oral formulations of aminoglycosides or nitrofurantoins, although these are clinically useless (192,193).

There are no randomized clinical trials that clearly demonstrate that early treatment with an effective agent reduces the incidence of systemic complications, and some retrospective studies have suggested that antibiotic treatment may be a risk factor for HUS (201). This is difficult to prove, however, in that the most severely affected are the most likely to both receive antibiotics and to develop complications. In contrast, in disease due to Shiga toxin–producing *E. coli*, antibiotics that interact with DNA increase the proliferation of the transforming phage encoding the *E. coli* Shiga toxins associated with HUS, and increase toxin production (202) and perhaps the likelihood and severity of HUS (203).

There are no randomized comparative clinical trials of antibiotic treatment of EIEC. These infections generally behave as mild "culture-negative" shigellosis. Antibiotics are often not needed clinically, but should reduce the duration of illness as in shigellosis. Similar to *Shigella,* selection of an appropriate drug is problematic because resistance to commonly used agents may be common.

PREVENTION

Prevention of shigellosis falls under two headings: general preventive measures that apply to any disease transmitted by the fecal-oral route and the use of *Shigella*-specific vaccines. Common sense hygienic practices can reduce person-to-person transmission of *Shigella* infection. Simple measures such as separating food preparation and eating from the care of infected individuals and appropriate handling of objects potentially contaminated with feces can be very effective in the hospital setting, in day care centers, and at home. It has been shown under controlled conditions that handwashing with soap prevents transmission of shigellosis, even in a

TABLE 43.5. OPTIONS FOR ANTIMICROBIAL THERAPY OF SHIGELLOSIS

Drug	Cost/5 Days[a]	Dose: Children	Dose: Adult	Comments
First-line agents				
Ampicillin	0.48/kg; $3.00	100 mg/kg/day	500 mg qid	Resistance common in Sd, Sf, and Ss
TMP-SMZ	$0.15/kg; $1.40	10/50 mg/kg/day in two doses	1 ds tablet bid	Resistance common in Sd and Ss; variable for Sf
Ciprofloxacin	—; $29.23	Not recommended	500 mg bid	Resistance rare to date
Other new quinolones		Not recommended	Depends on the drug used	
Alternative agents				
Amdinocillin	Not available in the United States	80 mg/kg/day	400 mg qid[b]	Resistance rare to date
Cefixime	$1.15/kg; $24.00	8 mg/kg/day	400 mg/day[b]	Effective in TMP-SMZ resistance strains
Ceftriaxone	$8.84/kg; $157–305	50 mg/kg IV qd	1–2 g/day[b]	2 days as effective as 5 days
Alternative for developing countries				
Naladixic acid	$1.10/kg; $20.50	55 mg/kg/day	1 g qid	Widely used to treat ampicillin- and TMP-SMZ–resistant Sd and Sf in developing countries but not FDA-approved for use in the United States.

Sd, *S. dysenteriae* type 1; Sf, *S. flexneri;* Ss, *S. sonnei;* TMP, trimethoprim-sulfamoxazole.
[a]Based on *Redbook* listing for average drug cost (generic when available) for pediatric patients per kilogram body weight using suspension formulations and total dose for adults for a 5-day course of treatment (does not include the cost of drug administration, if any, and does not include pharmacist markup). Cost for pediatric patients is also an underestimate because pharmacists will ordinarily dispense and charge for an entire commercial package of suspension, which may exceed the need for that child.
[b]Use not reported in adults.

highly endemic area such as Bangladesh (204). The principal problem is how to motivate people to change age-old customs and wash hands adequately after defecation when access to clean water may be difficult. Moreover, in some cultures, concepts of cleanliness are not based on the germ theory of disease but rather are viewed in a socioreligious context in which handwashing serves physical and spiritual needs and is performed according to traditions that do not consider how to interrupt bacterial transmission routes (205).

Where flies are plentiful and have access to human feces, that is, wherever flush toilets or water seal privies and sewage systems do not exist, flies can transmit infectious inocula of *Shigella* from feces to food. Fly control can therefore reduce the incidence of infection (206,207).

Although much has been learned about pathogenesis and host immune responses in shigellosis (208), developing a satisfactory safe and effective vaccine has proven elusive. Even though it is likely that secretory IgA on mucosal surfaces and mucosal lymphocytes and cell-mediated immunity play a role in the immunologic defense against shigellosis, the most effective protective immune responses remain undefined. The only established principle is that protection in natural shigellosis is serotype-specific, presumably related to antibodies to antigenic LPS oligosaccharides. Thus, an individual convalescent after *S. flexneri* 2a infection is protected against reinfection only with the homologous serotype. To insure that protective antibodies would be present in the gut lumen, most vaccine developers have turned from killed parenteral to oral live vaccine approaches. However, the limited success with this approach using various *Shigella* virulence proteins as candidate vaccine antigens has led to a recent resurgence in interest in LPS antigens for immunization, even by the parenteral route (209).

The primary evidence that protective immunity to *Shigella* infection can be elicited is epidemiologic. For example, shigellosis is a pediatric disease in endemic countries, suggesting that protection follows infection early in life. Alternative explanations are possible, for example, behavioral changes may reduce exposure or improve personal hygiene practices, or age-related alterations in susceptibility may be due to developmentally regulated host factors. Early vaccine trials comparing two mixtures of live streptomycin-dependent vaccine strains, each containing a different group of several serotypes, demonstrated protection against the serotypes present in the administered vaccine but not against the serotypes in the other vaccine (210).

The original *Shigella* vaccines were, like other bacterial vaccines, heat- or acetone-killed whole-cell preparations for parenteral administration, designed to induce circulating IgG antibody. These failed to provide significant protection when administered either enterally or parenterally (211). With advances in understanding of mucosal immunity, attention turned to inducing secretory IgA and sensitizing mucosal lymphocytes. Secretory IgA bathing mucosal surfaces can prevent attachment of microorganisms to the mucosa and neutralize microbial products such as toxins. Neither mechanism has been shown to be relevant to shigellosis. Antibody-dependent cellular cytotoxicity responses develop during shigellosis (212,213). The nature of the antibody, however, is IgG, the antigens involved remain undetermined, and relevance to protection has not been shown. Classic cell-mediated immune responses to *Shigella* are just beginning to be investigated.

Contemporary vaccine development for shigellosis has concentrated on the use of living attenuated strains, broadly classified into three types: *Shigella* strains with attenuating chromosomal mutations, *Shigella* strains with attenuating plasmid mutations, and attenuated hybrid *Shigella/E. coli* strains expressing a limited set of *Shigella* virulence determinants (211). It is likely that a clinically useful and effective vaccine will need to induce immunity to several microbial antigens. The early genetic approach used *E. coli-S. flexneri* hybrid strains in which genes were moved back and forth to attenuate virulent *Shigella* or introduce genes for key *Shigella* antigens into *E. coli*. Although too reactogenic to use, a principle emerged from these experiments that noninvasive hybrids are unlikely to generate a protective immune response in contrast to invasive but metabolically attenuated strains such as *aroD*$^-$ *E. coli-S. flexneri* hybrids (214). A variety of attenuating chromosomal mutations have been studied, including spontaneous mutations such as streptomycin dependence (SmD), a combination of spontaneous and chemical mutagenesis (Pur$^-$/Rif), spontaneous and ultraviolet mutagenesis (TSF-21), or insertional mutagenesis (Sfl-114). Problems have arisen with each, including reversion to virulence, high rates of reactions including fever, tenesmus, and diarrhea, or limited protection. Sfl-114 is a genetically engineered strain with a precise mutation in the *aroD*gene (214). Insertions into *aroD* inhibit the biosynthesis of aromatic metabolites and subsequent synthesis of folic acid. These strains are able to invade host cells, but subsequent intracellular survival is very limited (215). Even though the immune response is reasonable, mild transient intestinal discomfort was reported in 12% of the volunteers given 10^9 and 54% given 10^{10} organisms. Such reactogenicity has been a common problem in live oral vaccine strains, and in this case led to its abandonment for further testing. More highly attenuated candidates are being produced by the introduction of multiple mutations, such as CVD1207, which has specific deletions in the *virG, sen, set* and *guaBA* genes (216). The concern is that too highly attenuated strains will not generate protective immunity and the problem is to find the right balance between attenuation and immunogenicity, and to ensure safety and minimal reactogenicity.

Various vaccines based on attenuating plasmid mutations continue to be made in the hope of overcoming the limited and disappointing level of protection obtained thus far and the need for multiple immunizations. A series of specifically designed *icsA* mutants have been produced by

Sansonetti et al. (217) that are invasive but fail to spread from cell to cell. Although they elicit significant serum immune responses in monkeys, they too are excessively reactogenic for use in humans.

The recent interest in vaccines that induce cell mediated immunity is based on new data in experimental models suggesting that IFN-γ and NK cells are involved in resistance to *Shigella* infection (218,219). Consistent with these data, increased IFN-γ production and expression of the IFN-γ receptor in the epithelium has been observed in rectal biopsy samples from infected humans in Bangladesh (220). More recent studies in humans experimentally infected with a virulent Shiga toxin negative mutant of *S. dysenteriae* type 1, support the idea that Th1 immune responses develop in shigellosis. Studies in infected human volunteers have shown that immunization increases the amount of IFN-γ and IL-10 produced by peripheral blood mononuclear cells in response to homogenates or particulate preparations of the immunizing organisms (221). Antibody and cell-mediated responses to IpaC and IpaD were detected. Although there is an innate IFN-γ response, it is stimulated still further during infection while activating macrophages to kill ingested organisms rather than suffer apoptotic death. The induction of IL-10 is interesting because this cytokine inhibits Th1 cytokines and NK cells but induces IL-1 production, which is involved in activating the inflammatory response so critical to *Shigella* pathogenesis. IL-10 also induces TGF-β, which inhibits the IL-1 driven inflammatory response and limits lymphocyte proliferation. This action, combined with the lack of induction of IL-2 and IL-15 in this model, suggests that T-cell help for B-cell proliferation and antibody production may be restricted during shigellosis. This immunologic feature seems to plague many of the vaccine candidates tested up to this time. *Shigella* also diminishes macrophage presentation of antigens and further subverts the host immune response in shigellosis (222). These data make it clear that *Shigella* induces a complex immune response, that immunity to this organism is not simple in concept, and that better understanding of immune responses to the organism and the nature of protective immunity induced by live attenuated *Shigella* strains is the key to developing a better and usable vaccine.

Other groups have continued to explore the use of killed vaccine preparations. For example, investigators, primarily in Russia, have been studying the use of ribosomal vaccines, with some limited experimental support for the approach (223). In a modern day throwback to the original LPS-based vaccines of the early twentieth century, purified O-specific side chains of *Shigella* LPS have been conjugated to carrier proteins for parenteral administration to elicit IgG antibodies (224,225). The goal is to use conjugates to immunize young children at risk, with the goal to produce IgG antibody in the lamina propria in sufficient titer to leak into the lumen during infection to kill organisms before they invade the host. The form of the antigen and the nature of the conjugate are critical for induction of a vigorous immune response. For example, recent data show that synthetic O-specific oligosaccharides of *S. dysenteriae* type 1 conjugated to a protein induce a significantly greater immune response than the natural antigen from the organism (226). Circulating bactericidal antibody could potentially be of value against organisms gaining entrance to the circulation by augmenting the serum bactericidal response to the more virulent *S. dysenteriae* type 1 and *S. flexneri* 2 (227). Some degree of success has been achieved in initial human trials in adults with vaccines of this sort (224) and further trials are underway.

Even though progress is being made, it is still unlikely that a safe, effective, affordable vaccine will become available in the near future that would reduce morbidity and mortality in the highly vulnerable infants and children in the developing world. On the other hand, a vaccine useful to protect better nourished populations against the milder infection due to *S. sonnei*, such as infants in day care or custodial care in the United States, or attenuate infection due to more virulent *Shigella* among the military and other travelers to endemic countries, may be possible. The need for *Shigella* vaccines is underscored by the unlikely probability that widespread implementation of protected water supplies and sanitary fecal disposal will happen soon in developing countries; this is simply unrealistic. The main *Shigella* vaccine developers are academic and government scientists supported primarily by public funds or the military. Pharmaceutical firms have not accorded a high enough priority to vaccines for shigellosis, because the major need is in the developing world. A major boost to the efforts to develop a vaccine has been the recent entry of the Bill and Melinda Gates Foundation into this area. Until there is a useful vaccine, preventive strategies must continue to involve teaching and reinforcing behavioral modifications (228) such as handwashing, protection of food and drinking water supplies from contamination, case containment and management, including appropriate and appropriately restricted use of antibiotics, and the encouragement of breast-feeding wherever HIV is not prevalent.

REFERENCES

1. Shiga K. Ueber den Dysenteriebacillus (*Bacillus dysenteriae*). *Zentbl Bakt ParasitKde Abt I Orig* 1898;24:817–824.
2. Flexner S. On the etiology of tropical dysentery. *Bull Johns Hopkins Hosp* 1900;11:231–242.
3. Kruse W. Ueber die Ruhr als Volkskrankheit und ihrer Erreger. *Deutsch Med Wschr* 1900;26:637–639.
4. Conradi H. Uber losliche, durch aseptische Autolyse erhlatene Giftstoffe von Ruhrund Typhus bazillen. *Deutsch Med Wschr* 1903;20:26–28.
5. Todd C. On a dysentery toxin and antitoxin. *J Hyg* 1904;4: 480–494.
6. Hale TL. Genetic basis of virulence in *Shigella* species. *Microbiol Rev* 1991;55:206–224.

7. Acheson DW, Kane AV, Keusch GT. Shiga toxins. *Methods Mol Biol* 2000;145:41–63.
8. Tran Van Nhieu G, Bourdet-Sicard R, Dumenil G, et al. Bacterial signals and cell responses during *Shigella* entry into epithelial cells. *Cell Microbiol* 2000;2:187–193.
9. Pupo GM, Karaolis DK, Lan R, et al. Evolutionary relationships among pathogenic and nonpathogenic *Escherichia coli* strains inferred from multilocus enzyme electrophoresis and mdh sequence studies. *Infect Immun* 1997;65:2685–2692.
10. Rolland K, Lambert-Zechovsky N, Picard B, et al. Shigella and enteroinvasive *Escherichia coli* strains are derived from distinct ancestral strains of *E. coli*. *Microbiology* 1998;144:2667–2672.
11. Lan R, Lumb B, Ryan D, et al. Molecular evolution of large virulence plasmid in *Shigella* clones and enteroinvasive *Escherichia coli*. *Infect Immun* 2001;69:6303–6309.
12. Lefebvre J, Gosselin F, Ismail J, et al. Evaluation of commercial antisera.for *Shigella* serogrouping. *J Clin Microbiol* 1995;33: 1997–2001.
13. Carlin NIA, Lindberg AA. Monoclonal antibodies specific for O-antigenic polysaccharides of *Shigella flexneri:* clones bind to II, II:3,4 and 7,8 epitopes. *J Clin Microbiol* 1983;18:1183–1189.
14. Cheasty T, Rowe B. Antigenic relationships between the enteroinvasive *Escherichia coli* O antigens O28ac, O112ac, O136, O143, O144, O152 and O164 and *Shigella* O antigens. *J Clin Microbiol* 1983;17:681–684.
15. Toledo MRF, Trabulsi LR. Correlation between biochemical and serological characteristics of *Escherichia coli* and results of the Sereny test. *J Clin Microbiol* 1983;17:419–421.
16. Kotloff KL, Winickoff JP, Ivanoff B, et al. Global burden of *Shigella* infections: implications for vaccine development and implementation of control strategies. *Bull WHO* 1999;77: 651–666.
17. Mosley WH, Adams B, Lyman ED. Epidemiological and sociologic features of a large urban outbreak of shigellosis. *JAMA* 1962;182:1307–1311.
18. DuPont HL, Levine MM, Hornick RB, et al. Inoculum size in shigellosis and implications for expected mode of transmission. *J Infect Dis* 1989;159:1126–1128.
19. Kotloff KL, Nataro JP, Losonsky GA, et al. A modified Shigella volunteer challenge model in which the inoculum is administered with bicarbonate buffer: clinical experience and implications for Shigella infectivity. *Vaccine* 1995;13:1488–1494.
20. Wilson R, Feldman RA, Davis J, et al. Family illness associated with *Shigella* infection: the interrelationship of age of the index patient and the age of household members in acquisition of illness. *J Infect Dis* 1981;143:130–132.
21. Keusch GT, Bennish ML. Shigellosis. In: Evans AS, Brachman PS, eds. *Bacterial infections of humans,* third edition. New York: Plenum, 1997:631–656.
22. Clemens JD, Stanton B, Stoll B, et al. Breast feeding as a determinant of severity in shigellosis. *Am J Epidemiol* 1986;123: 710–718.
23. Kostrewski J, Stypulkowska-Misiurewicz H. Changes in the epidemiology of dysentery in Poland and the situation in Europe. *Arch Immunol Ther Exp Med* 1968;20:608–615.
24. Mata LJ, Gangarosa EJ, Caceres A, et al. Epidemic Shiga bacillus dysentery in Central America. I. Etiologic investigations in Guatemala, 1969. *J Infect Dis* 1969;122:170–180.
25. Pickering LK, Bartlett AV, Woodward WE. Acute infectious diarrheas among children in day care: epidemiology and control. *Rev Infect Dis* 1986;8:539–547.
26. Dritz SK, Black AF. *Shigella* enteritis venereally transmitted. *N Engl J Med* 1974;291:1194.
27. Drusin LM, Genvert G, Topf-Olstein B, et al. Shigellosis: another sexually transmitted disease? *Br J Vener Dis* 1976;52: 348–350.
28. Tauxe RV, McDonald RC, Hargrett-Bean N, et al. The persistence of *Shigella flexneri* in the United States: the increased role of the adult male. *Am J Public Health* 1988;78:1432–1435.
29. Gangarosa EJ, Perera DR, Mata LJ, et al. Epidemic Shiga bacillus dysentery in Central America. II. Epidemiologic studies, 1969. *J Infect Dis* 1970;122:170–180.
30. Malengreau M, Molima-Kaba, Gillieaux M, et al. Outbreak of *Shigella* dysentery in Eastern Zaire, 1980–1982. *Ann Soc Belg Med Trop* 1983;63:59–67.
31. Bennish ML, Wojtyniak BJ. Mortality due to shigellosis: community and hospital data. *Rev Infect Dis* 1991;13:S245–S251.
32. Ewing WH, Gravatti JL. *Shigella* types encountered in the Mediterranean area. *J Bacteriol* 1947;53:191–195.
33. Hobbs BC, Thomas MEM. School outbreak of gastroenteritis associates with a pathogenic paracolon bacillus. *Lancet* 1949;2: 530–532.
34. Marier R, Wells JC, Swanson RC, et al. An outbreak of enteropathogenic *Escherichia coli* foodborne disease traced to imported French cheese. *Lancet* 1973;2:1376–1378.
35. Khan WA, Dhar U, Salam MA, et al. Central nervous system manifestations of childhood shigellosis: prevalence, risk factors, and outcome. *Pediatrics* 1999;103:E18
36. Eriksen CA, Hadley GP. Rectal prolapse in childhood—the role of infections and infestations. *S Afr Med J* 1985;68:790–791.
37. Speelman P, Kabir I, Islam M. Distribution and spread of colonic lesions in shigellosis: a colonoscopic study. *J Infect Dis* 1984;150:899–903.
38. Rahman MM, Kabir I, Mahalanabis D, et al. Decreased food intake in children with severe dysentery due to *Shigella dysenteriae* 1 infection. *Eur J Clin Nutr* 1992;46:833–838.
39. Azad MAK, Islam M, Butler T. Colonic perforation in *Shigella dysenteriae* type I infection. *Pediatr Infect Dis* 1986;5:103–104.
40. Bennish ML, Azad AK, Yousefzadeh D. Intestinal obstruction during shigellosis: incidence, clinical features, risk factors, and outcome. *Gastroenterology* 1991;101:626–634.
41. Bennish ML, Salam MA, Wahed MA. Enteric protein loss during shigellosis. *Am J Gastroenterol* 1993;88:53–57.
42. Struelens MJ, Pate D, Kabir I, et al. *Shigella* septicemia: prevalence, presentation, risk factors, and outcome. *J Infect Dis* 1985; 152:784–790.
43. Koster F, Levin J, Walker L, et al. Hemolytic-uremic syndrome after shigellosis: relation to endotoxemia and circulating immune complexes. *N Engl J Med* 1978;298:927–933.
44. Koster FT, Boonpucknavig V, Sujaho S, et al. Renal histopathology in the hemolytic-uremic syndrome following shigellosis. *Clin Nephrol* 1984;21:126–133.
45. Bhimma R, Rollins NC, Coovadia HM, et al. Post-dysenteric hemolytic uremic syndrome in children during an epidemic of *Shigella* dysentery in Kwazulu/Natal. *Pediatr Nephrol* 1997;11: 560–564.
46. Bhimma R, Coovadia HM, Adhikari M, et al. Re-evaluating criteria for peritoneal dialysis in "classical" (D+) hemolytic uremic syndrome. *Clin Nephrol* 2001;55:133–142.
47. Ashkenazi S, Cleary KR, Pickering LK, et al. The association of Shiga toxin and other cytotoxins with the neurologic manifestations of shigellosis. *J Infect Dis* 1990;161:961–965.
48. Mulligan K, Nelson S, Friedman HS, et al. Shigellosis-associated encephalopathy. *Pediatr Infect Dis J* 1992;11:889–890.
49. Kaplan BS, Meyers KE, Schulman SL. The pathogenesis and treatment of hemolytic uremic syndrome. *J Am Soc Nephrol* 1998;9:1126–1133.
50. Sieper J, Braun J, Wu P, et al. The possible role of *Shigella* in sporadic enteric reactive arthritis. *Br J Rheumatol* 1993;32:582–585.
51. Mazumder RN, Salam MA, Ali M, et al. Reactive arthritis associated with *Shigella dysenteriae* type 1 infection. *J Diarrhoeal Dis Res* 1997;15:21–24.

52. Boisgerault F, Mounier J, Tieng V, et al. Alteration of HLA-B27 peptide presentation after infection of transfected murine L cells by *Shigella flexneri. Infect Immun* 1998;66:4484–4490.
53. Raybourne RB, Williams KM. Monoclonal antibodies against an HLA-B27–derived peptide react with an epitope present on bacterial proteins. *J Immunol* 1990;145:2539–2544.
54. Yoshikawa M, Sasakawa C. Molecular pathogenesis of shigellosis: a review. *Microbiol Immunol* 1991;35:809–824.
55. Evans CA, Gilman RH, Rabbani GH, et al. Gastric acid secretion and enteric infection in Bangladesh. *Trans R Soc Trop Med Hyg* 1997;91:681–685.
56. Gorden J, Small PLC. Acid resistance in enteric bacteria. *Infect Immun* 1993;61:364–367.
57. Waterman SR, Small PL. Identification of sigma S-dependent genes associated with the stationary-phase acid-resistance phenotype of *Shigella flexneri. Mol Microbiol* 1996;21:925–940.
58. DuPont HL, Formal SB, Hornick RB, et al. Pathogenesis of *Escherichia coli. N Engl J Med* 1971;285:1–9.
59. Sansonetti PJ. Rupture, invasion and inflammatory destruction of the intestinal barrier by *Shigella*, making sense of prokaryote-eukaryote cross-talks. *FEMS Microbiol Rev* 2001;25:3–14.
60. Mounier J, Vasselon T, Hellio R, et al. *Shigella flexneri* enters human colonic Caco-2 epithelial cells through their basolateral pole. *Infect Immun* 1992;60:237–248.
61. Wassef J, Keren DF, Mailloux JL. Role of M cells in initial bacterial uptake and in ulcer formation in the rabbit intestinal loop model in shigellosis. *Infect Immun* 1989;57:858–863.
62. Sansonetti PJ, Arondel J, Cantey RJ, et al. Infection of rabbit Peyer's patches by *Shigella flexneri*: effect of adhesive or invasive bacterial phenotypes on follicular-associated epithelium. *Infect Immun* 1996;64:2752–2764.
63. Zychlinsky A, Prevost MC, Sansonetti PJ. *Shigella flexneri* induces apoptosis in infected macrophages. *Nature* 1992;358:167–169.
64. Zychlinsky A, Kenny B, Menard R, et al. IpaB mediates macrophage apoptosis induced by *Shigella flexneri. Mol Microbiol* 1994;11:619–627.
65. Chen Y, Smith MR, Thirumalai K, et al. A bacterial invasin induces macrophage apoptosis by binding directly to ICE. *EMBO J* 1996;15:3853–3860.
66. Guichon A, Hersh D, Smith MR, et al. Structure-function analysis of the *Shigella* virulence factor IpaB. *J Bacteriol* 2001;183:1269–1276.
67. Zychlinsky A, Fitting C, Cavaillon JM, et al. Interleukin 1 is released by macrophages during apoptosis induced by *Shigella flexneri. J Clin Invest* 1994;94::1328–1332.
68. Sansonetti PJ, Phalipon A, Arondel J, et al. Caspase-1 activation of IL-1β and IL-18 are essential for *Shigella flexneri*-induced inflammation. *Immunity* 2000;12:581–590.
69. Sansonetti PJ, Arondel J, Cavaillon JM, et al. Role of IL-1 in the pathogenesis of experimental shigellosis. *J Clin Invest* 1995;96:884–892.
70. Arondel J, Singer M, Matsukawa A, et al. Increased IL-1 and imbalance between IL-1 and IL-1 receptor antagonist during acute inflammation in experimental shigellosis. *Infect Immun* 1999;67:6056–6066.
71. Jung HC, Eckmann L, Yang S-K, et al. A distinct array of proinflammatory cytokines is expressed in human colonic epithelial cells in response to bacterial invasion. *J Clin Invest* 1995;95:55–65.
72. Thorpe CM, Hurley BP, Lincicome LL, et al. Shiga toxins stimulate secretion of interleukin-8 from intestinal epithelial cells. *Infect Immun* 1999;67:5985–5993.
73. Perdomo JJ, Gougnon P, Sansonetti PJ. Polymorphonuclear leukocyte transmigration promotes invasion of colonic epithelial monolayer by *Shigella flexneri. J Clin Invest* 1994;93:633–643.
74. Maurelli AT, Fernandez RE, Bloch CA, et al. "Black holes" and bacterial pathogenicity: a large genomic deletion that enhances the virulence of *Shigella* spp. And enteroinvasive *Escherichia coli. Proc Natl Acad Sci U S A* 1998;95:3943–3948.
75. McCormick BA, Fernandez MI, Siber AM, et al. Inhibition of *Shigella flexneri*-induced transepithelial migration of polymorphonuclear leucocytes by cadaverine. *Cell Microbiol* 1999;1:143–155.
76. Perdomo JJ, Cavaillon JM, Huerre M, et al. Acute inflammation causes epithelial invasion and mucosal destruction in experimental shigellosis. *J Exp Med* 1994;180:1307–1319.
77. Raqib R, Lindberg AA, Wretlind B, et al. Persistence of local cytokine production in shigellosis in acute and convalescent stages. *Infect Immun* 1995;63:289–296.
78. RaqibR, Wretlind B, Andersson J, et al. Cytokine secretion in acute shigellosis is correlated to disease activity and directed more to stool than to plasma. *J Infect Dis* 1995;171:376–384.
79. Payne SM. Iron and virulence. *Mol Microbiol* 1989;3:1301–1306.
80. Nassif X, Mazert MC, Mouniew J, et al. Evaluation with an *iuc*::Tn10 mutant of the role of aerobactin production in the virulence of *Shigella flexneri. Infect Immun* 1987;55:1963–1969.
81. Gemski P, Sheahan DG, Washington O, et al. Virulence of *Shigella flexneri* hybrids expressing *Escherichia coli* somatic antigens. *Infect Immun* 1972;6:104–111.
82. Okada N, Sasakawa C, Tobe T, et al. Virulence-associated chromosomal loci of *Shigella flexneri* identified by random Tn5 insertion mutagenesis. *Mol Microbiol* 1991;5:187–195.
83. Okamura N, Nagai T, Nakaya R, et al. HeLa cell invasiveness and O antigen of *Shigella flexneri* as separate and prerequisite attributes of virulence to evoke keratoconjunctivitis in guinea pigs. *Infect Immun* 1983;39:505–513.
84. Watanabe H, Nakamura A, Timmis KN. Small virulence plasmid of *Shigella dysenteriae* 1 strain W30864 encodes a 41,000 dalton protein involved in formation of specific lipopolysaccharide side chains of serotype 1 isolates. *Infect Immun* 1984;46:55–63.
85. Watanabe H, Timmis KN. A small plasmid in *Shigella dysenteriae* I specifies one or more functions essential for O antigen production and bacterial virulence. *Infect Immun* 1984;43:391–396.
86. Brahmbhatt HN, Lindberg AA, Timmis KN. *Shigella* lipopolysaccharide: structure, genetics and vaccine development. In: Sansonetti PJ, ed. *Pathogenesis of shigellosis. Current topics in microbiology and immunology.* Berlin: Springer-Verlag, 1992:45–64.
87. Franzon VL, Arondel J, Sansonetti PJ. Contribution of superoxide dismutase and catalase activities to *Shigella flexneri* pathogenesis. *Infect Immun* 1990;58:529–535.
88. Keusch GT, Grady GF, Mata LJ, et al. The pathogenesis of *Shigella* diarrhea I. Enterotoxin production by *Shigella dysenteriae* 1. *J Clin Invest* 1972;51:1212–1218.
89. O'Brien AD, Tesh VL, Donohue-Rolfe, et al. Shiga toxin: biochemistry, genetics, mode of action and role in pathogenesis. In: Sansonetti PJ, ed. *Pathogenesis of shigellosis. Current topics in microbiology and immunology.* Berlin: Springer-Verlag, 1992:65–94.
90. Endo Y, Tsurugi K, Yutsudo K, et al. Site of action of Vero toxin (VT2) from *Escherichia coli* O157:H7 and of Shiga toxin on eukaryotic ribosomes. RNA N-glycosidase activity of the toxins. *Eur J Biochem* 1988;171:45–50.
91. Endo Y, Tsurugi K, Yutsudo K, et al. Site of action of Vero toxin (VT2) from *Escherichia coli* O157:H7 and of Shiga toxin on eukaryotic ribosomes. RNA N-glycosidase activity of the toxins. *Eur J Biochem* 1988;171:45–50.
92. Stein PE, Boodhoo A, Tyrrell GJ, et al. Crystal structure of the cell-binding B oligomer of verotoxin-1 from *E. coli. Nature* 1992;355:748–750.

93. Jackson MP, Wadolkowski EA, Weinstein DL, et al. Functional analysis of the Shiga toxin and Shiga-like toxin type II variant binding subunits by using site-directed mutagenesis. *J Bacteriol* 1990;172:653–658.
94. Calderwood SB, Mekalanos JJ. Iron regulation of Shiga-like toxin expression in *Escherichia coli* is mediated by the fur locus. *J Bacteriol* 1987;169:4759–4764.
95. Jacewicz M, Clausen H, Nudelman E, et al. Pathogenesis of *Shigella* diarrhea XI. Isolation of shigella toxin-binding glycolipid from rabbit jejunum and HeLa cells and its identification as globotriaosylceramide. *J Exp Med* 1986;163:1391–1404.
96. Lindberg AA, Brown JE, Stromberg N, et al. Identification of the carbohydrate receptor for Shiga toxin produced by *Shigella dysenteriae* type 1. *J Biol Chem* 1987;262:1779–1785.
97. Mobassaleh M, Gross SK, McCluer RH, et al. Quantitation of the rabbit intestinal glycolipid receptor for Shiga toxin. Further evidence for the developmental regulation of globotriaosylceramide in microvillus membranes. *Gastroenterology* 1989;97:384–391.
98. Mobassaleh M, Donohue-Rolfe A, Jacewicz M, et al. Pathogenesis of *Shigella* diarrhea: evidence for a developmentally regulated glycolipid receptor for *Shigella* toxin involved in the fluid secretory response of rabbit small bowel. *J Infect Dis* 1988;157:1023–1031.
99. Mobassaleh M, Koul O, Mishra K, et al. Developmental regulation of intestinal Gb3 galactosyltransferase and -galactosidase control shiga toxin receptors. *Am J Physiol* 1994;267:G618–624.
100. Jacewicz M, Feldman HA, Donohue-Rolfe A, et al. Pathogenesis of *Shigella* diarrhea XIV. Analysis of Shiga toxin receptors on cloned HeLa cells. *J Infect Dis* 1989;159:881–889.
101. Jacewicz MS, Mobassaleh M, Gross SK, et al. Pathogenesis of *Shigella* diarrhea. XVII. A mammalian cell membrane glycolipid, Gb3, is required but not sufficient to confer sensitivity to Shiga toxin. *J Infect Dis* 1994;169:538–546.
102. Kandel G, Donohue-Rolfe A, Donowitz M, et al. Pathogenesis of *Shigella* diarrhea. XVI. Selective targeting of Shiga toxin to villus cells or rabbit jejunum explains the effect of the toxin on intestinal electrolyte transport. *J Clin Invest* 1989;84:1509–1517.
103. Jacewicz MS, Mobassaleh M, Acheson DWK, et al. Maturational regulation of globotriaosyl-ceramide, the Shiga-like toxin 1 receptor, by butyrate in intestinal epithelial lines. *J Clin Invest* 1995;96:1328–1335.
104. Jacewicz M, Keusch GT. Pathogenesis of *Shigella* diarrhea. VIII. Evidence for a translocation step in the cytotoxic action of Shiga toxin. *J Infect Dis* 1983;148:844–854.
105. Sandvig K, Olsnes S, Brown JE, et al. Endocytosis from coated pits of Shiga toxin: a glycolipid-binding protein from *Shigella dysenteriae* I. *J Cell Biol* 1989;108:1331–1343.
106. Sandvig K, van Deurs B. Endocytosis, intracellular transport and cytotoxic action of Shiga toxin and ricin. *Physiol Rev* 1996; 76:949–966.
107. Donta ST, Tomicic TK, Donohue-Rolfe A. Inhibition of Shiga-like toxins by brefeldin A. *J Infect Dis* 1995;171:721–724.
108. Garred O, Dubinina E, Holm PK, et al. Role of processing and intracellular transport for optimal toxicity of Shiga toxin and toxin mutants. *Exp Cell Res* 1995;218:39–49.
109. Thorpe CM, Smith WE, Hurley BP, et al. Shiga toxins induce, superinduce, and stabilize a variety of C-X-C chemokine mRNAs in intestinal epithelial cells, resulting in increased chemokine expression. *Infect Immun* 2001;69:6140–6147.
110. Keusch GT, Acheson DWK, Aaldering L, et al. Comparison of Shiga-like toxin 1 on cytokine and butyrate treated human umbilical and saphenous vein endothelial cells. *J Infect Dis* 1996;173:1164–1170.
111. O'Loughlin EV, Robins-Browne RM. Effect of Shiga toxin and Shiga-like toxins on eukaryotic cells. *Microbes Infect* 2001;3: 493–507.
112. Neill RJ, Gemski P, Formal SB, et al. Deletion of the Shiga toxin gene in a chlorate-resistant derivative of *Shigella dysenteriae* type I that retains virulence. *J Infect Dis* 1988;158:737–741.
113. Fontaine A, Arondel J, Sansonetti PJ. Role of Shiga toxin in the pathogenesis of bacillary dysentery studied using a Tox- mutant of *Shigella dysenteriae* I. *Infect Immun* 1988;56:3099–3109.
114. Islam MM, Azad AK, Bardhan PK, et al. Pathology of shigellosis and its complications. *Pediatr Res* 2001;49:413–416.
115. Inward CD, Howie AJ, Fitzpatrick MM, et al. Renal histopathology in fatal cases of diarrhoea-associated haemolytic uraemic syndrome. *Pediatr Nephrol* 1997;11:556–559.
116. van de Kar NC, Monnens LA, Karmali MA, et al. Tumor necrosis factor and interleukin-1 expression of the verocytotoxin receptor globotriaosylceramide on human endothelial cells: implications for the pathogenesis of the hemolytic uremic syndrome. *Blood* 1991;80:2755–2764.
117. Louise CB, Obrig TG. Shiga toxin-associated hemolytic uremic syndrome: combined cytotoxic effects of Shiga toxin and lipopolysaccharide (endotoxin) on human vascular endothelial cells *in vitro*. *Infect Immun* 1992;60:1536–1543.
118. MacLeod DL, Gyles CL, Wilcock BP. Reproduction of edema disease of swine with purified Shiga-like toxin-II variant. *Vet Pathol* 1991;28:66–73.
119. Fasano A, Guandalini S, Russell RG, et al. Enterotoxin production by *Shigella flexneri* 2a. *J Pediatr Gastroenterol Nutr* 1991;13:320.
120. Fasano A, Kay BA, Russell RG, et al. Enterotoxin and cytotoxin production by enteroinvasive *Escherichia coli. Infect Immun* 1990;58:3717–3723.
121. Fasano A, Noriega FR, Liao FM, et al. Effect of shigella enterotoxin (ShET1) on rabbit intestine *in vitro* and *in vivo*. *Gut* 1997;40:505–511.
122. Al-Hasani K, Rajakumar K, Bulach D, et al. Genetic organization of the she pathogenicity island in *Shigella flexneri* 2a. *Microb Pathog* 2001;30:1–8.
123. Noriega FR, Liao FM, Formal SB, et al. Prevalence of *Shigella flexneri* enterotoxin 1 among Shigella clinical isolates of diverse serotypes. *J Infect Dis* 1995;172:1408–1410.
124. Vargas M, Gascon J, Jimenez De Anta MT, et al. Prevalence of *Shigella* enterotoxins 1 and 2 among Shigella strains isolated from patients with traveler's diarrhea. *J Clin Microbiol* 1999;37: 3608–3611.
125. Sansonetti PJ, Kopecko DJ, Formal SB. Involvement of a plasmid in the invasive ability of *Shigella flexneri. Infect Immun* 1982;35:852–860.
126. Sansonetti PJ, Hale TL, Dammin GI, et al. Alterations in the pathogenesis of *Escherichia coli* K12 after transfer of plasmid and chromosomal genes from *Shigella flexneri. Infect Immun* 1983;39:1392–1402.
127. Venkatesan MM, Goldberg MB, Rose DJ, et al. Complete DNA sequence and analysis of the large virulence plasmid of *Shigella flexneri. Infect Immun* 2001;69:3271–3285.
128. Sansonetti PJ. Microbes and microbial toxins: paradigms for microbial-mucosal interactions. III. Shigellosis: from symptoms to molecular pathogenesis. *Am J Physiol Gastrointest Liver Physiol* 2001;280:G319–G323.
129. Sansonetti PH, Phalipon A. M cells as ports of entry for enteroinvasive pathogens: mechanisms of interaction, consequences for the disease process. *Semin Immunol* 1999;11:193–203.
130. Adam T, Arpin M, Prevost MC, et al. Cytoskeletal rearrangements and the functional role of T-plastin during entry of *Shigella flexneri* into HeLa cells. *J Cell Biol* 1995;129:367–381.
131. Clerc P, Sansonetti PJ. Entry of *Shigella flexneri* into HeLa cells: evidence for direct phagocytosis involving actin polymerization and myosin accumulation. *Infect Immun* 1987;55:2681–2688.
132. Mounier J, Laurent V, Hall A, et al. Rho family GTPases control entry of *S. flexneri* into epithelial cells but not intracellular motility. *J Cell Sci* 1999;112:2069–2080.

133. Dehio C, Prevost MC, Sansonetti PJ. Invasion of epithelial cells by *Shigella flexneri* induces tyrosine phosphorylation of cortactin by a pp60c-src mediated signaling pathway. *EMBO J* 1995;14:2471–2482.
134. Skoudy A, Tran Van Nhieu G, Mantis N, et al. A functional role for ezrin during *Shigella* entry into epithelial cells. *J Cell Sci* 1999;112:2059–2069.
135. Tran Van Nhieu G, Ben Ze'ev A, Sansonetti PH. Modulation of bacterial entry in epithelial cells by association between vinculin and the *Shigella* IpaA invasin. *EMBO J* 1997;16:2717–2729.
136. Sansonetti PJ. Rupture, invasion and inflammatory destruction of the intestinal barrier by *Shigella*, making sense of the prokaryote-eukaryote cross-talks. *FEMS Microbiol Rev* 2000;25:3–14.
137. Adler B, Sasakawa C, Tobe T, et al. A dual transcriptional activation system for the 230kb plasmid genes coding for virulence associated antigens of *Shigella flexneri. Mol Microbiol* 1989;3: 627–635.
138. Buysse JM, Venkatesan JA, Mills JA, et al. Molecular characterization of a trans-acting positive effector (*ipaR*) of invasion plasmid antigen synthesis in *Shigella flexneri* serotype 5. *Microb Pathog* 1990;8:197–211.
139. Watanabe H, Arakawa E, Ito K, et al. Genetic analysis of an invasion region by use of a Tn3–lac transposon and identification of a second positive regulator gene, *invE* for cell invasion of *Shigella sonnei:* significant homology of inv E with par B of plasmid Pl. *J Bacteriol* 1990;172:619–629.
140. Dorman CJ, Porter ME. The *Shigella* virulence gene regulatory cascade: a paradigm of bacterial gene control mechanisms. *Mol Microbiol* 1998;29:677–684.
141. Blocker A, Gounon P, Larquet E, et al. Role of Shigella's type III secretion system in insertion of IpaBand IpaC into the host membrane. *J Cell Biol* 1999;147:683–693.
142. Blocker A, Jouihri N, Larquet E, et al. Structure and composition of the *Shigella flexneri* "needle complex", a part of its type III secretion. *Mol Microbiol* 2001;39:652–663.
143. Gemski P, Griffin DE. Isolation and characterization of minicell-producing mutants of *Shigella* spp. *Infect Immun* 1980;30: 297–302.
144. Hale TL, Sansonetti PF, Schad PA, et al. Characterization of virulence plasmids and plasmid-associated outer membrane proteins in *Shigella flexneri, Shigella sonnei* and *Escherichia coli. Infect Immun* 1983;40:340–350.
145. Buysse JM, Stover CK, Oaks EV, et al. Molecular cloning of invasion plasmid antigen (ipa) genes from *Shigell flexneri:* analysis of *ipa* gene products and genetic mapping. *J Bacteriol* 1987; 169:2561–2569.
146. De Geyter C,Wattiez R, Sansonetti P, et al. Characterization of the interaction of IpaB and IpaD, proteins required for entry of *Shigella flexneri* into epithelial cells, with a lipid membrane. *Eur J Biochem* 2000 ;267:5769–5776.
147. Tran Van Nhieu G, Caron E, Hall A, et al. IpaC determines filopodia formation during *Shigella* entry into epithelial cells. *EMBO J* 1999;18:3249–3262.
148. Andrews GP, Hromockyj AE, Coker C, et al. Two novel virulence loci, *mxiA* and *mxiB,* in *Shigella flexneri* 2a facilitate excretion of invasion plasmid antigens. *Infect Immun* 1991;59: 1997–2005.
149. Venkatesan MM, Buysse JM, Oaks EV. Surface presentation of *Shigella flexneri* invasion plasmid antigens requires the products of the *spa* locus. *J Bacteriol* 1992;174:1900–2001.
150. Allaoui A, Menard R, Sansonetti PJ, et al. Characterization of the *Shigella flexneri ipgD* and *ipgF* genes, which are located in the proximal part of the *mxi* locus. *Infect Immun* 1993;61: 1707–1714.
151. Sansonetti PJ. Molecular and cellular biology of *Shigella flexneri* invasiveness: from cell assay systems to shigellosis. In: Sansonetti PJ, ed. *Pathogenesis of shigellosis. Current topics in microbiology and immunology.* Berlin: Springer-Verlag, 1992: 1–19.
152. Clerc P, Baudry B, Sansonetti PJ. Plasmid-mediated contact hemolytic activity in *Shigella* species: correlation with penetration into HeLa cells. *Ann Inst Pasteur Microbiol* 1986;137A:267–278.
153. de Geyter C, Wattiez R, Sansonetti P, et al. Characterization of the interaction of IpaB and IpaD, proteins required for entry of *Shigella flexneri* epithelial cells, with a lipid membrane. *Eur J Biochem* 2000;267:5769–5776.
154. Barzu S, Benjelloun-Touimi Z, Phalipon A, et al. Functional analysis of the *Shigella flexneri* IpaC invasin by insertional mutagenesis. *Infect Immun* 1997;65:1599–1605.
155. Bernardini ML, Sanna MG, Fontaine A, et al. OmpC is involved in invasion of epithelial cells by *Shigella flexneri. Infect Immun* 1993;61:3625–3635.
156. Goldberg MB, Sansonetti PJ. *Shigella* subversion of the cellular cytoskeleton: a strategy for epithelial colonization. *Infect Immun* 1993;61:4941–4946.
157. Makino S, Sasakawa C, Kamata K, et al. A genetic determinant required for continuous reinfection of adjacent cells on large plasmid in *Shigella flexneri* 2a. *Cell* 1986;46:551–555.
158. Bernardini ML, Mounier J, d'Hauteville H, et al. Identification of *icsA,* a plasmid locus of *Shigella flexneri* that governs intra- and intercellular spread through interaction with F-actin. *Proc Natl Acad Sci U S A* 1989;86:3867–3871.
159. Steinhauer J, Agha R, Pham T, et al. The unipolar *Shigella* surface protein IcsA is targeted directly to the bacterial old pole: IcsP cleavage of IcsA occurs over the entire bacterial surface. *Mol Microbiol* 1999;32:367–377.
160. Vasselon T, Mounier J, Prevost MC, et al. A stress fiber-based movement of *Shigella flexneri* within cells. *Infect Immun* 1991; 59:1723–1732.
161. Vasselon T, Mounier J, Hellio R, et al. Movement along actin filaments of the perijunctional area and de novo polymerization of cellular actin are required for *Shigella flexneri* colonization of epithelial Caco-2 cell monolayers. *Infect Immun* 1992;60: 1031–1040.
162. d'Hauteville H, Sansonetti PJ. Phosphorylation of IcsA by cAMP-dependent protein kinase and its effect on intercellular spread of *Shigella flexneri. Mol Microbiol* 1992;6:833–841.
163. Mangeney M, Lingwood CA, Taga S, et al. Apoptosis induced in Burkitt's lymphoma cells via Gb3/CD77, a glycolipid antigen. *Cancer Res* 1993;53:5314–5319.
164. Durand JM, Dagberg B, Uhlin BE, et al. Transfer RNA modification, temperature and DNA superhelicity have a common target in the regulatory network of *Shigella flexneri*: the expression of the virF gene. *Mol Microbiol* 2000;35:924–935.
165. Falconi M, Colonna B, Prosseda G, et al. Thermoregulation of *Shigella* and *Escherichia coli* EIEC pathogenicity. A temperature-dependent structural transition of DNA modulates accessibility of virF promoter to transcriptional repressor H-NS. *EMBO J* 1998;17:7033–7043.
166. Maurelli AT, Hromockyj AE, Bernardini ML. Environmental regulation of *Shigella* virulence. In: Sansonetti PJ, ed. *Pathogenesis of shigellosis. Current topics in microbiology and immunology.* Berlin: Springer-Verlag, 1992:85–116.
167. Speelman P, McGlaughlin R, Kabir I, et al. Differences in clinical features and stool findings in shigellosis and amebic dysentery. *Trans R Soc Trop Med Hyg* 1987;81:549–551.
168. Echeverria P, Sethabutr O, Pitarangsi C. Microbiology and diagnosis of infections with *Shigella* and enteroinvasive *E. coli. Rev Infect Dis* 1991;13:S220–S225.
169. Atkins HJ, Santiago LT. Increased recovery of enteric pathogens by use of both stool and rectal swab specimens. *J Clin Microbiol* 1987;25:158–159.

170. Wells JG, Morris GK. Evaluation of transport methods for isolating *Shigella* ssp. *J Clin Microbiol* 1981;13:789–790.
171. Pitarangsi C, Taylor DN, Echeverria P, et al. Media for the isolation of *Shigella. J Diarrh Dis Res* 1987;5:43.
172. Altwegg M, Buser J, von Graevenitz A. Stool cultures for *Shigella* spp: improved specificity by using MacConkey agar with xylose. *Diagn Microbiol Infect Dis* 1996;24:121–124.
173. Mata LJ, Gangarosa EJ, Caceres A, et al. Epidemic Shiga bacillus dysentery in Central America. I. Etiologic investigations in Guatemala. *J Infect Dis* 1969;123:25–38.
174. Dutta S, Chatterjee A, Dutta P, et al. Sensitivity and performance characteristics of a direct PCR with stool samples in comparison to conventional techniques for diagnosis of *Shigella* an enteroinvasive *Escherichia coli* infection in children with acute diarrhoea in Calcutta, India. *J Med Microbiol* 2001;50:667–674.
175. Sethabutr O, Venkatesan M, Yam S, et al. Detection of PCR products of the ipaH gene from *Shigella* and enteroinvasive *Escherichia coli* by enzyme linked immunosorbent assay. *Diagn Microbiol Infect Dis* 2000;37:11–16.
176. Houng HS, Sethaburt O, Echeverria P. A simple polymerase chain reaction technique to detect and differentiate *Shigella* and enteroinvasive *Escherichia coli* in human feces. *Diagn Microbiol Infect Dis* 1997;28:19–25.
177. Oyofo BA, Mohran ZS, el-Etr SH, et al. Detection of enterotoxigenic *Escherichia coli, Shigella* and *Campylobacter* spp. by multiplex PCR assay. *J Diarrhoeal Dis Res* 1996;14:207–210.
178. Guerrant RL, Shields DS, Thorson SM, et al. Evaluation and diagnosis of acute infectious diarrhea. *Am J Med* 1985;78: 91–98.
179. Lindberg AA, Cam PD, Chan N, et al. Shigellosis in Vietnam: seroepidemiologic studies with use of lipopolysaccharide antigens in enzyme immunoassays. *Rev Infect Dis* 1991;13:S231–S237.
180. Ewing WH, Lindberg AA. Serology of *Shigella.* In: Bergan T, ed. *Methods in microbiology.* London: Academic Press, 1984;14: 113–142.
181. Lindberg AA, Karnell A, Weintraub A. The lipopolysaccharide of *Shigella* bacteria as a virulence factor. *Rev Infect Dis* 1991;13 [Suppl 4]:S279–S284.
182. Ahmed F, Ansaruzzaman M, Haque E, et al. Epidemiology of postshigellosis persistent diarrhea in young children. *Pediatr Infect Dis J* 2001;20:525–530.
183. Rahman MM, Kabir I, Mahalanabis D, et al. Decreased food intake in children with severe dysentery due to *Shigella dysenteriae* 1 infection. *Eur J Clin Nutr* 1992;46:833–888.
184. Samadi AR, Wahed MA, Islam MR, et al. Consequences of hyponatremia and hypernatremia in children with acute diarrhoea in Bangladesh. *BMJ* 1983;286:671–673.
185. Bennish ML, Harris JR, Wojtyniak BJ, et al. Death in shigellosis: incidence and risk factors in hospitalized patients. *J Infect Dis* 1990:161:500–506.
186. Bennish ML, Azak AK, Rahman O, et al. Hypoglycemia during childhood diarrhea: prevalence, pathophysiology and outcome. *N Engl J Med* 1990;322:1357–1363.
187. Scrimshaw NS. Effect of infection on nutrient requirements. *Am J Clin Nutr* 1977;30:1536–1544.
188. Mazumber RN, Ashraf H, Hoque SS, et al. Effect of an energy-dense diet on the clinical course of acute shigellosis in undernourished children. *Br J Nutr* 2000;84:775–779.
189. Hanif M, Mobarak MR, Ronan A, et al. Fatal renal failure caused by diethylene glycol in paracetamol elixir: the Bangladesh epidemic. *BMJ* 1995;311:88–91.
190. Salam MA, Bennish ML. Antimicrobial therapy of shigellosis. *Rev Infect Dis* 1991;13:S332–S341.
191. Bennish ML, Salam MA. Rethinking options for the treatment of shigellosis. *J Antimicrob Chemother* 1992;30:243–247.
192. Mates A, Eyny D, Philo S. Antimicrobial resistance trends in *Shigella* serogroups isolated in Israel, 1990–1995. *Eur J Clin Microbiol Infect Dis* 2000;19:108–111.
193. Islam MR, Alam AN, Hossain MS, et al. Double-blind comparison of oral gentamicin and nalidixic acid treatment of acute shigellosis in children. *J Trop Pediatr* 1994;40:320–325.
194. Mudzamiri WS, L'Herminez M, Peterson DE, et al. Hospitalized dysentery cases during an outbreak of *Shigella dysenteriae* type 1: Ndanga District Hospital, Zimbabwe. *Cent Afr J Med* 1996;42:177–179.
195. Ashkenazi S, Amir J, Waisman Y, et al. A randomized double-blind study comparing cefixime and trimethoprim-sulfamethoxazole in the treatment of childhood shigellosis. *J Pediatr* 1993;123:817–821.
196. Eidlitz T, Cohen YH, Nussimovitch M, et al. Comparative efficacy of two- and five-day courses of ceftriaxone for treatment of severe shigellosis in children. *J Pediatr* 1993;123:822–824.
197. Khan WA, Seas C, Dhar U, et al. Treatment of shigellosis: V. Comparison of azithromycin and ciprofloxacin. A double-blind, randomized, controlled trial. *Ann Intern Med* 1997;126: 697–703.
198. Bennish ML, Salam MA, Khan WA, et al. Treatment of shigellosis. III. Randomized, blinded comparison of one- or two-dose ciprofloxacin with standard five day therapy. *Ann Intern Med* 1992;117:727–734.
199. Gendrel D, Moulin F. Fluoroquinolones in paediatrics. *Paediatr Drugs* 2001;3365–377.
200. Salam MA, Dhar U, Khan WA, et al. Randomised comparison of ciprofloxacin and pivmecillinam for childhood shigellosis. *Lancet* 1998;352:522–527.
201. Leibovitz E, Janco J, Piglansky L, et al. Oral ciprofloxacin vs. intramuscular ceftriaxone as empiric treatment of acute invasive diarrhea in children. *Pediatr Infect Dis J* 2000;19:1060–1067.
202. Butler T, Islam MR, Azad MAK, et al. Risk factors for development of hemolytic-uremic syndrome during shigellosis. *J Pediatr* 1987;100:894–897.
203. Zhang X, McDaniel AD, Wolf LE, et al. Quinolone antibiotics induce Shiga toxin-encoding bacteriophages, toxin production, and death in mice. *J Infect Dis* 2000;181:664–670.
204. Wong CS, Jelacic S, Habeeb RL, et al. The risk of the hemolytic-uremic syndrome after antibiotic treatment of *Escherichia coli* O157:H7 infections. *N Engl J Med* 2000;342: 1930–1936.
205. Khan MU. Interruption of shigellosis by hand washing. *Trans R Soc Trop Med Hyg* 1982;76:164–168.
206. Zeitlyn S, Islam F. The use of soap and water in two Bangladeshi communities: implications for the transmission of diarrhea. *Rev Infect Dis* 1991;13:S259–S264.
207. Levine OS, Levine MM. Houseflies (*Musca domestica*) as mechanical vectors of shigellosis. *Rev Infect Dis* 1991;13: 688–696.
208. Cohen D, Green M, Block C, et al. Reduction of transmission of shigellosis by control of houseflies (*Musca domestica*). *Lancet* 1991;337:993–997.
209. Autenrieth IB, Schmidt MA. Mucosal surfaces: implications for vaccine development. *Trends Microbiol* 2000;8:457–464.
210. Robbins JB, Chu C, Schneerson R. Hypothesis for vaccine development: protective immunity to enteric diseases caused by non-typhoidal *Salmonellae* and *Shigellae* may be conferred by serum IgG antibodies to the O-specific polysaccharide of their lipopolysaccharides. *Clin Infect Dis* 1992;15:346–361.
211. Mel DM, Arsic BL, Mikolic BD, et al. Studies on vaccination against bacillary dysentery. 4. Oral immunization with live monotypic and combined vaccines. *Bull WHO* 1968;39: 375–380.
212. Hale TL, Kern DF. Pathogenesis and immunology in shigellosis: applications for vaccine development. In: Sansonetti PJ,

ed. *Pathogenesis of shigellosis. Current topics in microbiology and immunology.* Berlin: Springer-Verlag, 1992:117–137.

213. Lowell GH, McDermott RP, Sommers PL, et al. Antibody-dependent cell-mediated antibacterial activity: K lymphocytes, monocytes, and granulocytes are effective against *Shigella. J Immunol* 1980;125:2778–2784.
214. Tagliabue A, Nencioni L, Villa L, et al. Antibody-dependent cell-mediated antibacterial activity of intestinal lymphocytes with secretory IgA. *Nature* 1983;306:184–186.
215. Lindberg AA, Karnell A, Pal T, et al. Construction of an auxotrophic *Shigella flexneri* strain for use as a live vaccine. *Microb Pathog* 1990;8:433–440.
216. Karnell A, Stocker BAD, Katakura S, et al. An auxotrophic live oral *Shigella flexneri* vaccine: development and testing. *Rev Infect Dis* 1991;13:S357–S361.
217. Kotloff KL, Noriega FR, Samandari T, et al. *Shigella flexneri* 2a strain CVD 1207, with specific deletions in virG, sen, set and guaBA, is highly attenuated in humans. *Infect Immun* 2000; 68:1034–1039.
218. Sansonetti PJ, Arondel J. Construction and evaluation of a double mutant of *Shigella flexneri* as a candidate for oral vaccination against shigellosis. *Vaccine* 1989;7:443–450.
219. Van de Verg LL, Maleett CP, Collins HH, et al. Antibody and cytokine responses in a mouse pulmonary model of *Shigella flexneri* serotype 2a infection. *Infect Immun* 1995;63:1947–1954.
220. Way SS, Borczuk AC, Dominitz R, et al. An essential role for γ-interferon in innate resistance to *Shigella flexneri* infection. *Infect Immun* 1998;66:1342–1348.
221. Raqib R, Ljungdalhl A, Lindberg AA, et al. Local entrapment of interferon γ in the recovery from *Shigella dysenteriae* type 1 infection. *Gut* 1996;38:328–336.
222. Samandari T, Kotloff KL, Losonsky GA, et al. Production of IFN-γ and IL-10 to *Shigella* invasions by mononuclear cells from volunteers orally inoculated with a Shiga toxin-deleted *Shigella dysenteriae* type 1 strain. *J Immunol* 2000;164: 2221–2232.
223. Schwan WR, Kopecko DJ. Uptake of pathogenic intracellular bacteria into human and murine macrophages downregulates the eukaryotic 26S protease complex ATPase gene. *Infect Immun* 1997;65:4754–4760.
224. Levenson VJ, Mallett CP, Hale TL. Protection against local *Shigella sonnei* infection in mice by parenteral immunization with a nucleoprotein subcellular vaccine. *Infect Immun* 1995; 63:2762–2765.
225. Cohen D, Ashkenazi S, Green MS, et al. Double-blind vaccine-controlled randomized efficacy trial of an investigational *Shigella sonnei* conjugate vaccine in young adults. *Lancet* 1997; 349:155–159.
226. Fries LF, Montemarano AD, Mallett CP, et al. Safety and immunogenicity of a proteosome-*Shigella flexneri* 2a lipopolysaccharide vaccine administered intranasally to healthy adults. *Infect Immun* 2001;69:4545–4553.
227. Pozgay V, Chu C, Pannell L, et al. Protein conjugates of synthetic saccharides elicit higher levels of serum IgG lipopolysaccharide antibodies in mice than do those of the O-specific polysaccharide from *S. dysenteriae* type 1. *Proc Natl Acad Sci U S A* 1999;96:5194–5197.
228. Okamura N, Nakaya R, Suzuki K, et al. Differences among *Shigella* spp. In susceptibility to the bactericidal activity of human serum. *J Gen Microbiol* 1988;134:2057–2065.
229. Kunstadter P. Social and behavioral factors in transmission and response to shigellosis. *Rev Infect Dis* 1991;13:S272–S278.

44

SALMONELLA, INCLUDING *SALMONELLA TYPHI*

DAVID A. PEGUES
MICHAEL E. OHL
SAMUEL I. MILLER

Salmonellae are named for the pathologist Salmon, who first isolated *S. choleraesuis* from porcine intestine (1). Salmonellae are effective commensals and pathogens that cause a spectrum of diseases in humans and animals, including domesticated and wild mammals, reptiles, birds, and insects (2). Some *Salmonella* serotypes, such as *S. typhi, S. paratyphi,* and *S. sendai,* are highly adapted to humans and have no other known natural hosts (3), whereas others, such as *S. typhimurium,* have a broad host range and can infect a wide variety of animals and humans (3). Some *Salmonella* serotypes, such as *S. dublin* (cattle) (4) and *S. arizonae* (reptiles) (5,6), are most adapted to an animal species and only occasionally infect humans. The widespread distribution of salmonellae in the environment, their increasing prevalence in the global food chain, and their virulence and adaptability have an enormous medical, public health, and economic impact worldwide.

HISTORY

Before the nineteenth century, typhus fever and typhoid fever were confused. Although various clinical distinctions were proposed, none reliably distinguished these syndromes. In Paris in 1829, P. Ch. A. Louis (7) separated typhoid from other fevers on the basis of intestinal lymph node and spleen pathology. He also described the clinical phenomena of rose spots, intestinal perforation, and hemorrhage. In the English literature, William Jenner in 1850 settled the question of whether typhus and typhoid were different diseases (8). He distinguished typhoid based on the pathologic evidence of enlargement of the Peyer's patches and mesenteric lymph nodes. Jenner also noted that prior attacks of typhoid protected against subsequent attacks; this was not the case for typhus. In 1869, the term *enteric fever* was proposed by Wilson as an alternative to *typhoid fever,* given the anatomic site of infection (9). Although *enteric fever* remains a more accurate term, use of the term *typhoid* persists today.

In 1873, Budd (10) demonstrated that food, water, and fomites could transmit typhoid fever. The typhoid bacillus was isolated by Gaffkey in Germany in 1884 from the spleens of infected patients (11,12). In 1896, Pfeiffer and Kalle made the first typhoid vaccine with heat-killed organisms (13). In the same year, Widal (14) and others demonstrated that convalescent sera from typhoid patients caused the organisms to "stick together in large balls and lose their motility." He coined the term *agglutinin* to describe this observation. The antigenic classification or serotyping of *Salmonella* used today is the result of years of study of antibody interactions with bacterial surface antigens by Kauffman and White during the 1920s to 1940s (15). In 1948, Theodore Woodward and colleagues (16) reported the successful treatment of Malaysian typhoid patients with chloramphenicol (Chloromycetin), and the modern age of antimicrobial therapy for typhoid fever began. In 1952, Zinder and Lederberg (17), using *S. typhimurium,* discovered genetic transduction, the transfer of genetic information from one cell to another by a virus particle, bacteriophage P22. Ames and co-workers in 1973 (18) reported the development of the Ames test, in which *S. typhimurium* auxotrophic mutants are used to test the mutagenic activity of chemical compounds. At present, *Salmonella* pathogenesis is widely studied in animal and tissue culture models of mammalian infection as an important model of host–parasite interactions.

CLASSIFICATION AND TAXONOMY

Salmonella is a genus of the family Enterobacteriaceae (19). Before 1983, the existence of multiple *Salmonella* species was taxonomically accepted. Currently, as a result of experiments indicating a high degree of DNA similarity, the genus *Salmonella* is divided into two species, each with mul-

D. A. Pegues: Department of Medicine, UCLA School of Medicine and UCLA Medical Center, Los Angeles, California

M. E. Ohl: Division of Infectious Diseases, University of Washington, Seattle, Washington

S. I. Miller: Departments of Medicine and Microbiology, University of Washington, Seattle, Washington

TABLE 44.1. *SALMONELLA* SPECIES, SUBSPECIES, SEROTYPES, AND THEIR USUAL HABITATS

Salmonella species and subspecies	No. serotypes within subspecies	Usual habitat
S. enterica subsp. *enterica* (I)	1,454	Warm-blooded animals
S. enterica subsp. *salamae* (II)	489	Cold-blooded animals and the environment[a]
S. enterica subsp. *arizonae* (IIIa)	84	Cold-blooded animals and the environment[a]
S. enterica subsp. *diarizonae* (IIIb)	324	Cold-blooded animals and the environment[a]
S. enterica subsp. *houtenae* (IV)	70	Cold-blooded animals and the environment[a]
S. enterica subsp. *indica* (VI)	12	Cold-blooded animals and the environment[a]
S. bongori (V)	20	Cold-blooded animals and the environment[a]
Total	2,463	

[a]Isolates of all species and subspecies have occurred in humans.
Adapted from Brenner FW, Villar RG, Angulo FJ, et al. *Salmonella* nomenclature. *J Clin Microbiol* 2000;38:2465–2467.

tiple subspecies and serotypes. The two species are *S. choleraesuis,* which contains six subspecies (I, II, IIIa, IIIb, IV, and VI), and *S. bongori,* which was formerly subspecies V (20). *S. choleraesuis* subspecies I contains almost all the serotypes pathogenic for humans, except for rare human infections with subspecies IIIa and IIIb, which were formerly designated by the genus *Arizonae.* Because *S. choleraesuis* refers to both a species and a serotype, the species designation *S. enterica* has been recommended and is widely adopted.

Members of the seven *Salmonella* subspecies can be serotyped into one of more than 2,400 serotypes (serovars) according to somatic O, surface Vi, and flagellar H antigens and habitats (20,21) (Table 44.1). The name usually refers to the location where the *Salmonella* serotype was first isolated. According to the current *Salmonella* nomenclature system in use at the U.S. Centers for Disease Control and Prevention and World Health Organization laboratories, the full taxonomic designation of *S. enterica* subspecies enterica serotype *typhimurium* can be shortened to *Salmonella* serotype *typhimurium* or *S. typhimurium* (21).

MICROBIOLOGY

Salmonellae are gram-negative, non–spore-forming, facultatively anaerobic bacilli that measure 2 to 3 by 0.4 to 0.6 μm in size. Like other Enterobacteriaceae, they produce acid on glucose fermentation, reduce nitrates, and do not produce cytochrome oxidase (19,22). All organisms except *S. gallinarum–pullorum* are motile, having peritrichous flagella, and most do not ferment lactose. However, approximately 1% of organisms are able to ferment lactose and therefore may not be detected if only MacConkey agar or another semiselective medium is used to identify *Salmonella* based on colorimetric assay for fermentation of lactose. The differential metabolism of sugars can be used to distinguish many *Salmonella* serotypes; serotype *typhi* is the only organism that does not produce gas on sugar fermentation (19).

Freshly passed stool is preferred for the isolation of *Salmonella* and should be plated directly onto agar plates. Media with low selectivity, such as MacConkey agar and deoxycholate agar, and intermediately selective media, such as *Salmonella–Shigella* xylose–lysine–deoxycholate, or Hektoen agar, are widely used to screen for both *Salmonella* and *Shigella* species. Media highly selective for *Salmonella,* such as selenite with brilliant green, should be reserved for use in stool cultures of suspected carriers and during special circumstances, such as outbreaks (23). *Salmonella* enrichment broths, such as tetrathionate broth with brilliant green, can be added to the primary medium to facilitate the recovery of low numbers of organisms (22). Bismuth sulfite agar, which contains an indicator of hydrogen sulfite production and does not contain lactose, is preferred for the isolation of *S. typhi* and can be used to detect the 1% of *Salmonella* strains (including most *Salmonella* serogroup C strains) that ferment lactose (24). After primary isolation, possible *Salmonella* isolates can be tested in commercial identification systems or inoculated into screening media such as triple sugar iron and lysine iron agar (22). Tests for the direct detection of *Salmonella* organisms, including virulence genes, from stool specimens by latex agglutination (25) and polymerase chain reaction (PCR)-based assays are under development and may be most useful to detect *Salmonella* in food samples (26–28).

Isolates with typical biochemical profiles for *Salmonella* should be serogrouped with commercially available polyvalent antisera or sent to a reference or public health laboratory for complete serogrouping. Three kinds of surface antigens determine the organisms' reaction to specific antisera (22). After treatment with formaldehyde, antibodies to the flagellar or H antigen can be used to agglutinate the organism. After heat, acid, or acetone treatment abolishes the labile flagellar antigen, antibodies to the somatic or polysaccharide O antigen can be used to agglutinate the bacteria. In *S. typhi* and *S. paratyphi C,* the polysaccharide Vi antigen can inhibit O antigen agglutination because it is so abundant. The Vi antigen is a homopolymer of *N*-acetylgalactosaminouronic acid and is identical to that of the closely related *Citrobacter freundii* (29–32). Most antigenic variability occurs in the O antigen, which is composed of chains of oligosaccharide attached to a core oligosaccharide linked covalently to lipid A.

Although serotyping of all surface antigens can be used for formal identification, most laboratories perform a few simple agglutination reactions that define specific O antigens into serogroups, designated groups A, B, C_1, C_2, D, and E of *Salmonella* (33). Strains in these serogroups cause approximately 99% of *Salmonella* infections in humans and warm-blooded animals. Although this grouping is useful in epidemiologic studies and can be used to confirm genus identification, it cannot predict whether an organism is likely to cause enteric fever, as considerable cross-reactivity occurs among serogroups. For example, *S. enteritidis,* which typically causes gastroenteritis, and *S. typhi,* which causes enteric fever, are both in group D. Similarly, another frequent cause of gastroenteritis, *S. typhimurium,* and some *S. paratyphi,* another cause of enteric fever, are both in group B.

Bacteriophage typing can be used to distinguish *Salmonella* organisms within serotypes and is most useful for characterizing outbreak-associated strains, especially *S. typhi* (34–37). Both lipopolysaccharide (LPS) content and gene products encoded on virulence plasmids are involved in phage type identity (38,39). Many strains of nontyphoidal *Salmonella,* especially *S. typhimurium, S. enteritidis,* and *S. dublin,* contain large, 34-kd to 160-kd plasmids that encode virulence factors and resistance determinants (40,41). Plasmid profile analysis has been used to characterize *Salmonella* strains associated with common-source outbreaks and also sporadic multidrug-resistant isolates (42–44). More discriminative genotyping techniques, including ribosomal RNA restriction fragment length polymorphism (i.e., ribotyping) (45–47), pulsed-field gel electrophoresis of chromosomal DNA (48,49), analysis of *Salmonella*-specific insertion sequences (50–52), RAPD (random amplified polymorphic DNA)-PCR and ERIC (enterobacterial repetitive intergenic consensus)-PCR of chromosomal DNA (53), and multiplex PCR of virulence genes (54), have been used in epidemiologic studies to differentiate strains within a given serotype. However, a lack of standardization and time requirements limit the widespread use of these genotyping techniques.

EPIDEMIOLOGY

S. typhi and *S. paratyphi*

S. typhi and *S. paratyphi* colonize only humans, and therefore disease can be acquired only through close contact with a person who has had typhoid fever or is a chronic carrier. Most often, infection is acquired by the ingestion of fecally contaminated food or water. Usually, waterborne transmission involves the ingestion of fewer microorganisms; as a result, the incubation period is longer and the attack rate lower than in food-borne transmission (55). Although direct person-to-person transmission is rare, anal–oral transmission of *S. typhi* has been demonstrated (56). Occasionally, health care workers can acquire the disease from infected patients as a result of poor hand-washing techniques or handling laboratory specimens (57–59). Sewage workers are not at higher risk for acquiring typhoid, although this is a theoretic concern (55).

Typhoid fever continues to be a global health problem, with an estimated 12 to 33 million cases occurring worldwide each year (12). The disease is endemic in many developing countries, particularly the Indian subcontinent, Southeast Asia, South and Central America, and Africa, with annual incidence rates estimated to be as high as 900 per 100,000 population in Asia (60). These countries share several characteristics, including rapid population growth, increasing urbanization, inadequate treatment of human waste, limited water supplies, and overburdened health care systems. Recent outbreaks of typhoid fever in eastern Europe and the newly independent states have followed political and social collapse (61,62).

In areas of endemicity, the incidence of *S. typhi* infection is highest among children older than 1 year of age and likely reflects their lack of acquired immunity (63). When children less than 1 year of age acquire typhoid, the disease is often more severe and associated with a higher rate of complications (64). In addition, patients with immunosuppression, biliary or urinary tract abnormalities, or reticuloendothelial system defects, such as hemoglobinopathies, malaria, schistosomiasis, bartonellosis, and histoplasmosis, are at increased risk for severe disease (3,65–68).

Outbreaks of typhoid fever in developing countries can result in high rates of morbidity and mortality, especially when caused by antimicrobial-resistant strains (69–71). Antimicrobial resistance in developing countries may be promoted by the widespread use of "over-the-counter" antibiotics, the presence of immigrant workers, and international travel (72). In the 1970s, epidemic typhoid fever caused by chloramphenicol-resistant strains emerged in Mexico and on the Indian subcontinent (73–75). Since 1989, multidrug-resistant strains of *S. typhi,* with plasmid-encoded resistance to chloramphenicol, ampicillin, and trimethoprim, have emerged on the Indian subcontinent, Southeast Asia, and Africa; they have caused numerous outbreaks and been associated with increased morbidity and mortality. Although these multidrug-resistant strains belong to different Vi phage types, they typically contain a 120-Md plasmid of the H_1 incompatibility type that often also encodes resistance to streptomycin, sulfonamides, and tetracyclines (49,74–76). More recently, chromosome- and plasmid-encoded resistance to ciprofloxacin has appeared among *S. typhi* isolates from the Indian subcontinent, Viet Nam, and Tajikistan in association with the widespread use of ciprofloxacin to control outbreaks of multidrug-resistant *S. typhi* infection (62,77–79).

In the United States, substantial progress has been made in the eradication of *S. typhi.* Since 1985, an average of 245 cases of typhoid fever have been reported each year, with an annual incidence below 0.2 per 100,000 population, in comparison with 35,994 cases of typhoid fever in 1920 (80,81). This progress clearly is related to improved food-handling practices and water treatment. Although food-borne outbreaks of typhoid fever are rare today in developed countries, the potential still exists for outbreaks related to food contamination by a chronic carrier, such as "typhoid Mary" Mallon (82–84). The financial costs of typhoid outbreaks in comparison with those of nontyphoidal *Salmonella* outbreaks are considerable. Estimates vary from approximately $2,500 to $4,500 per person for typhoid illness, versus $645 per person for nontyphoidal salmonellosis (83).

In the United States, typhoid fever increasingly is associated with international travel, especially to developing countries (81,85,86). Between 1985 and 1994, 72% of the 2,445 reported cases of typhoid in the United States were associated with recent international travel, including travel to the Indian subcontinent (India, 25%; Pakistan, 8%), Mexico (28%), the Philippines (10%), El Salvador (5%), and Haiti (4%) (81). The proportion of *S. typhi* isolates resistant to chloramphenicol, ampicillin, and trimethoprim-sulfamethoxazole (TMP-SMX) has increased dramatically—0.6% during 1985 to 1989, 12% during 1990 to 1994, and 17% during 1996 to 1997 (81,86). During 1996 to 1997, although no ciprofloxacin-resistant isolates were detected in the United States, 7% of *S. typhi* isolates were resistant to nalidixic acid (86).

Nontyphoidal Salmonellae

In many countries, the incidence of human *Salmonella* infections has increased markedly, although good national or hospital-based surveillance data are mostly lacking. In the United States, the incidence rate of nontyphoidal *Salmonella* infection has doubled in the last two decades, with an estimated 1.4 million cases occurring annually (86,87) (Fig. 44.1). In 1999, the incidence rate of salmonellosis (17.7 per 100,000 population) was highest among nine potentially food-borne diseases under active surveillance and varied little by geographic region (88) (Fig. 44.2). In 1998, *S. typhimurium* and *S. enteritidis* were the most common serotypes, together accounting for 44% of all laboratory-confirmed cases of human salmonellosis (89). Nontyphoidal *Salmonella* organisms cause a small but significant proportion of cases of diarrhea among travelers (90) and young children in developing countries (91,92). The highest incidence of salmonellosis occurs during the rainy season in tropical climates and during May through October in temperate climates, coinciding with the peak in food-borne outbreaks (93).

In humans, nontyphoidal *Salmonella* infections are most often associated with food products, and nontyphoidal salmonellae are the most frequently identified agents of outbreaks of food-borne disease (93,94). Food of animal origin, including meat, poultry, eggs, or dairy products, can become contaminated with *Salmonella.* Eating uncooked or inadequately cooked food or foods cross-contaminated with these products may lead to human infection. In the developed world, the acquisition of nontyphoidal salmonellosis most often is associated with the consumption of poultry and eggs (93–96), but a wide range of vehicles have been implicated in transmission to humans (93,94,97–99). Although food-borne outbreaks predominate, waterborne outbreaks of salmonellosis also have been reported (100,101).

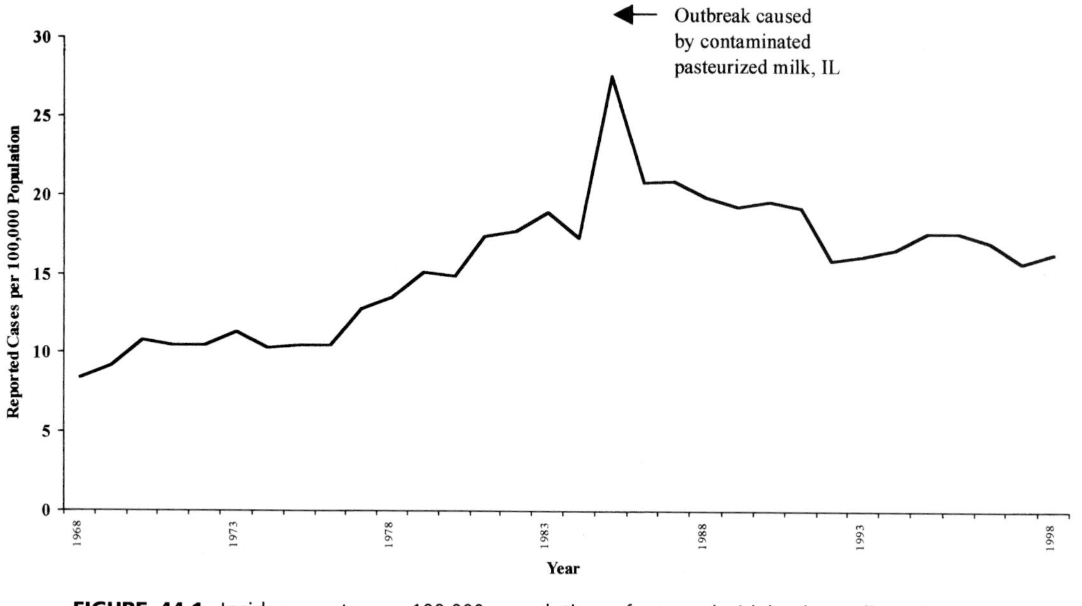

FIGURE 44.1. Incidence rate per 100,000 population of nontyphoidal salmonellosis by year, United States, 1968–1998. (From Centers for Disease Control and Prevention. Summary of notifiable diseases, United States, 1998. *MMWR Morb Mortal Wkly Rep* 1999;47:ii–92.)

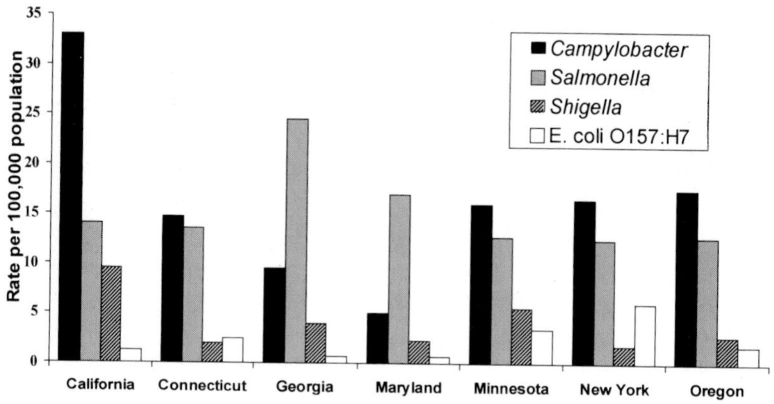

FIGURE 44.2. Incidence rate per 100,000 population of laboratory-confirmed infections with *Campylobacter, Salmonella, Shigella,* and *E. coli* O157:H7 by selected sites in the United States, Foodborne Diseases Active Surveillance Network, 1999. (From Centers for Disease Control and Prevention. Preliminary FoodNet data on the incidence of foodborne illnesses—selected sites, United States, 1999. *MMWR Morb Mortal Wkly Rep* 2000;49:201–205.)

Salmonellosis associated with exotic pets is a resurgent public health problem, with an estimated 3% to 5% of all cases of salmonellosis in humans associated with exposure to exotic pets, especially reptiles (97,99). As many as 90% of reptiles may be carriers of *Salmonella* (102). The recognition of pet turtle-associated salmonellosis led to a ban on the shipment of pet turtles in several countries but not to an elimination of the problem (99,103). Exposure to iguanas has been associated with infection with *Salmonella,* including *S. marina* and *S. chameleon,* especially among infants (104), and exposure to snakes has been associated with *S. arizonae* infection (105). Exposure to pet birds, pet rodents, dogs, and cats also is a potential source of salmonellosis (106,107).

During the 1980s and 1990s, *S. enteritidis* associated with shell eggs emerged as the predominant *Salmonella* serotype and source of food-borne disease in the United States and some other countries (95,96,108,109). In the United States, the rate of reported *S. enteritidis* isolates increased from 0.6 per 100,000 population in 1976 to a high of 3.6 per 100,000 in 1996 before declining to 2.2 per 100,000 in 1998 (110). During 1985 to 1998, *S. enteritidis* accounted for 796 reported outbreaks, 28,689 cases of illness, 2,839 hospitalizations, and 79 deaths (110).

Infection of egg-laying and broiler poultry flocks with *S. enteritidis* is widespread. It is postulated that the transmission of *S. enteritidis* from farm to farm may be facilitated by the ingestion of feed contaminated with mouse droppings (111); *S. enteritidis* strains cultured from the spleens of mice caught on farms show an enhanced ability to contaminate eggs (111,112). Infection localizes to the ovaries and upper oviduct tissue and is transmitted to the forming egg before the shell is deposited (113). An estimated 0.01% to more than 0.1% of shell eggs contain *S. enteritidis,* predominantly phage types 8 and 13a in the United States (96) and phage type 4 in Europe (108). Outbreaks of *S. enteritidis* infection have been associated with the ingestion of uncooked or lightly cooked eggs (e.g., sunny side up), egg-containing food products, and inadequately cooked poultry (96,110). Although cooking eggs until all liquid yolk is solidified kills *S. enteritidis* organisms, the use of pasteurized eggs products remains the safest alternative for institutions and the general public.

Changes in food consumption and the rapid growth of international trade in agricultural food products have facilitated the dissemination of new *Salmonella* serotypes associated with fresh fruits and vegetables (114). Human or animal feces may contaminate the surface of fruits and vegetables and may not be removed by washing. Recent food-borne outbreaks of salmonellosis have been associated with fresh produce such as cantaloupe (115), unpasteurized orange juice (116), and raw seed sprouts (117,118). Treating seeds and sprouts with chlorinated water or other disinfectant does not eliminate the risk for sprout-associated illness (118).

Manufactured food items pose an enormous potential hazard for food-borne salmonellosis in developed countries because of their centralized production and wide-scale distribution. In 1994, an estimated 224,000 cases of *S. enteritidis* gastroenteritis developed among persons in the United States who ate a nationally distributed ice cream product (119). The source of the *S. enteritidis* was most likely pasteurized ice cream premix contaminated during transport in tanker trailers that had previously carried unpasteurized liquid eggs. Other recent outbreaks have been associated with manufactured food products such as pasteurized milk (United States, *S. typhimurium*) (120), powdered milk products and infant formula (Canada and United States, *S. tennessee*) (121), unpasteurized goat milk cheese (France, *S. paratyphi*) (122), and ready-to-eat snacks (123,124).

Antimicrobial resistance among human nontyphoidal *Salmonella* isolates is increasing worldwide and is likely a consequence of the widespread use of antimicrobial agents for the empiric treatment of febrile syndromes (125) and as growth promoters in animal production (126,127). High rates of resistance (>50%) to chloramphenicol, TMP-SMX, and ampicillin have been reported from Africa, Asia, and South America (128–135). Multidrug-resistant nontyphoidal *Salmonella* isolates are now emerging in developed countries (136–140). Persons infected with resistant *Salmonella* isolates are more likely than those with susceptible ones to have a systemic infection, to be hospitalized, and to have been treated recently with an antimicrobial agent (140). A diversity of transferable resistance plasmids have been identified from multidrug-resistant nontyphoidal *Salmonella* istrains (135) and contribute to the intergeneric transfer of resistance between enteric bacterial species (141–143).

Of particular concern is the recent emergence of a distinct strain of multidrug-resistant *S. typhimurium,* characterized as definitive phage type 104 (DT104), that is resistant to five antimicrobials: ampicillin, chloramphenicol, streptomycin, sulfonamides, and tetracyclines. The DT104 strain has broad host reservoirs and is difficult to control in domestic livestock; as a result, widespread clonal dissemination has occurred among cattle and humans in Europe and the United States (144–146). In the United Kingdom, *S. typhimurium* DT104 is now the second most prevalent strain of *Salmonella* isolated from humans after *S. enteritidis* PT4 (147). In the United States, the prevalence of *S. typhimurium* isolates with the five-drug pattern of resistance increased from less than 1% during the years 1979 to 1980 to 34% in 1996, and most of these were a single clone of DT104 (145) (Fig. 44.3). Acquisition of DT104 strains has been associated with contact with ill farm animals and with consumption of a variety of meat products (148,149). Infection with DT104 may be associated with greater morbidity and mortality than that caused by susceptible *S. typhimurium* strains (148).

All DT104 strains contain a chromosome- and integron-encoded β-lactamase PSE-1 that appears to have been acquired from plasmids in *Pseudomonas* species (144). In the United Kingdom, *S. typhimurium* DT104 strains

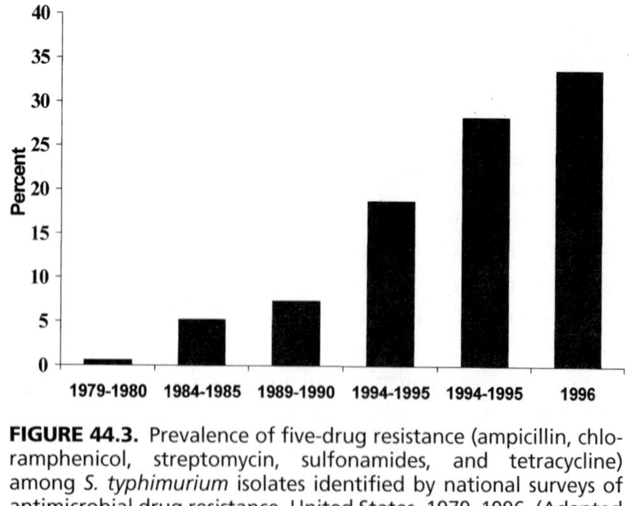

FIGURE 44.3. Prevalence of five-drug resistance (ampicillin, chloramphenicol, streptomycin, sulfonamides, and tetracycline) among *S. typhimurium* isolates identified by national surveys of antimicrobial drug resistance, United States, 1979–1996. (Adapted from Glynn MK, Bopp C, Dewitt W, et al. Emergence of multidrug-resistant *Salmonella enterica* serotype *typhimurium* DT104 infections in the United States. *N Engl J Med* 1998;338:1333–1338, with permission.)

increasingly also are resistant to trimethoprim and fluoroquinolones (150). Transmission from swine to humans of a DT104 strain that was resistant to nalidixic acid and had reduced susceptibility to ciprofloxacin has been reported from Denmark (151), which emphasizes the role of livestock in the evolution of multidrug-resistant *Salmonella* infection among humans.

Recently, outbreaks and sporadic cases of nontyphoidal *Salmonella* infection resistant to third-generation cephalosporins have been reported in both developed and developing countries, including the Argentina, Spain, Turkey, Algeria, and India (143,152–157). Resistance to third-generation cephalosporins is conferred by conjugative plasmid-encoded β-lactamases from functional groups 1 and 2 (154–156,158). The first reported case of ceftriaxone-resistant *Salmonella* infection acquired domestically in the United States occurred in a child in Nebraska and was associated with exposure to cattle on his family's ranch. The ceftriaxone-resistant *S. typhimurium* isolate from the child and that from the cattle were indistinguishable, and all but one of the 13 resistance determinants were encoded on a 160-kb plasmid (159). Carbapenem-resistant strains have been reported rarely (160).

Quinolone-resistant *Salmonella* strains have been emerging among humans and animals, and resistance is attributed to mutations of the intracellular targets of these agents, DNA gyrase (*gyrA* or *gyrB*) or topoisomerase IV, or to overproduction of efflux pumps (161–164). In the United States, of 4,008 *Salmonella* isolates tested in a national survey conducted between 1994 and 1995, 0.5% were resistant to nalidixic acid and 0.02% were ciprofloxacin-resistant (165). In comparison, in the United Kingdom, the incidence of quinolone resistance increased from zero in 1993 to 14% in 1996 and was highest among *S. hadar, S. virchow,* and *S. newport* isolates (166). This increase was concurrent with the licensing of the fluoroquinolone enrofloxacin for veterinary use in that country in 1993 (147), so that concern has been raised that the ongoing use of the fluoroquinolones as growth promoters in livestock may select for quinolone-resistant *Salmonella* among food animals and humans.

Although nosocomial salmonellosis is infrequent, such infections have been associated with substantial morbidity and mortality (57,167–170). Recurrent outbreaks of *Salmonella* wound infection among immunocompromised patients on burn wards have been associated with a high rate of secondary bacteremia (170). *Salmonella* resistance to silver may emerge in a clinical setting, such as burn units, where silver is used as a biocide and is mediated by a plasmid-encoded, silver-specific binding protein and efflux pumps (171).

Nosocomial transmission of *Salmonella* from patients to health care workers has been associated with handling soiled linen, noncompliance with barrier precautions, and fecally incontinent residents (172,173). However, the risk for transmission from health care workers to patients appears to be low if infection control measures are observed carefully (174). In contrast, the risk for nosocomial transmission to neonates and infants from acutely or chronically infected family members is high (175). Neonates are at high risk for fecal–oral transmission of *Salmonella* because of their relative gastric achlorhydria and the buffering capacity of ingested breast milk and formula (176). High-iron infant formula may further increase the risk for infant salmonellosis in comparison with breast-feeding (177). Outbreaks in day care centers also have been reported, and control may be difficult because of the need for frequent diaper changing and the higher rate and longer duration of convalescent carriage seen in the preschool age-group (178–180).

The elderly are at increased risk for *Salmonella* bacteremia and extraintestinal infection because of debility, underlying illnesses, and waning immunity (67,181,182). Residents of nursing homes may be at particular risk for salmonellosis because many of these institutions have only limited infection control programs (183–185). From 1975 through 1987, nontyphoidal *Salmonella* was the most common agent of food-borne outbreaks reported from U.S. nursing homes, accounting for 52% of outbreaks and 81% of outbreak-associated deaths (184).

PATHOGENESIS

Infectious Dose

Data on the number of *Salmonella* organisms required to cause disease come from volunteer studies and investigations of outbreaks in which the numbers of bacteria in contaminated foodstuffs are known. In volunteer studies performed with a variety of *Salmonella* serotypes, the attack rate increased with inoculum size and varied with the host specificity of the organism (186). However, it may not be possible to make generalizations based on the results of volunteer studies because usually few subjects are studied, laboratory-passaged bacterial strains may be attenuated in virulence, and higher doses of organisms are probably needed to infect healthy adult volunteers than persons at high risk for salmonellosis. Based on data from outbreaks of salmonellosis, small inocula (<100 organisms) may produce nontyphoidal *Salmonella* gastroenteritis, and the ingested dose is an important determinant of the incubation period, symptoms, and disease severity (186,187). The most important host factor in lowering the infectious dose appears to be decreased gastric acidity (188–190).

Gastrointestinal Tract Host–Pathogen Interactions

Ingested *Salmonella* organisms must transverse the acid barrier of the stomach—the first line of defense against enteric infections (186,189). Although salmonellae survive poorly at normal gastric pH (i.e., <1.5), the organisms survive well at a pH above 4.0 and have an adaptive acid tolerance response that may promote survival at a low pH (191,192). After leaving the stomach, salmonellae must traverse the mucous layer overlying the epithelium of the small intestine and evade secretory products of the intestine (e.g., antimicrobial defensin peptides and lysozyme secreted by Paneth cells), pancreas, and gallbladder (e.g., bile salts) to cause infection (193,194). Secretory immunoglobulin A (IgA) and intestinal mucus also may play a role in preventing salmonellae from penetrating to the enterocytes that line the intestinal wall (195).

After crossing the mucous layer overlying the small-intestinal epithelium, salmonellae interact with both enterocytes and microfold cells (M cells) that overlie the ileal Peyer's patches (196,197). On contact with the M cells, organisms are rapidly internalized and transported into the submucosal lymphoid tissue, where they may enter the systemic circulation. Salmonellae also have the ability to induce nonphagocytic cells, including enterocytes, to internalize them via a process termed *bacteria-mediated endocytosis.* This process involves the formation of large membrane ruffles around the organisms and cytoskeletal rearrangements similar to those induced by the exposure of cells to growth factors (198–202). Salmonellae are then internalized within membrane-bound vacuoles, in which the organisms travel from the apical to the basolateral surface in polarized tissue culture cells (203). Although the efficiency of transcytosis is low *in vitro,* it may be an important pathway for invasive salmonellae to reach deeper tissues *in vivo.* Salmonellae may also passively cross the intestinal barrier following ingestion by CD18+ phagocytes and subsequent phagocyte migration from the intestinal lumen to lymphoid tissues (204).

After salmonellae cross the intestinal epithelial barrier, the organisms rapidly interact with macrophages and lymphocytes in Peyer's patches and other lymphoid tissue located in the small-intestinal submucosa (205). Recruitment of additional mononuclear cells and lymphocytes can result in marked enlargement and necrosis of the Peyer's patches after several weeks of infection. This process likely is the cause of the abdominal pain that is characteristic of typhoid fever and the pseudoappendicitis that is infrequently associated with nontyphoidal *Salmonella* infection (3).

Interactions of Salmonellae with Phagocytes

The ability of salmonellae to survive within macrophages is probably essential to typhoid fever pathogenesis and the spread of organisms beyond the bowel to the systemic circulation. In patients with typhoid fever and positive blood cultures, almost all the organisms are contained in the mononuclear cell fraction (206). Eventually, organisms are taken up by tissue macrophages in the bone marrow, liver, spleen, and Peyer's patches (3,207,208). During the asymptomatic incubation phase of typhoid fever, most organisms are localized intracellularly within macrophages and possibly epithelial cells (209). The host innate immune system senses this bacterial colonization by means of receptors specific for conserved elements of gram-negative bacterial structure, including LPS, membrane lipoproteins, and flagella (210,211). Activation of these receptors stimulates cytokine production by macrophages, and persistent bacterial replication leads to ongoing cytokine production that ultimately contributes to the symptoms of typhoid fever (12,207). The characteristic enlargement of the liver and spleen is likely related to *S. typhi* survival or replication within reticuloendothelial cells, the pathologic recruitment of mononuclear cells, and the development of a cell-mediated immune response (3).

The morphology and cell biology of *S. typhimurium* infection of mouse macrophages have been studied. Salmonellae induce membrane ruffling in macrophages similar to that observed in epithelial cells. Unlike other enteric bacteria, such as *Yersinia enterocolitica,* salmonellae enter macrophages by the induction of generalized macropinocytosis rather than by receptor-mediated endocytosis, even when they are opsonized with complement (212). Salmonellae are internalized in 2- to 5-μm membrane-bound vacuoles with a large amount of extracellular fluid (termed *macropinosomes*) that are formed by fusion of the ends of membrane ruffles. After internalization, the fusion of macropinosomes can result in the formation of large vacuoles containing salmonellae, termed *spacious phagosomes* (213). Studies of the maturation of the *Salmonella*-containing vacuole (SCV) have yielded conflicting results. One study reveals rapid and complete fusion of the SCV with lysosomes (214), whereas other studies report novel trafficking of SCVs characterized by the exclusion of specific lysosomal hydrolases (215). These discrepancies may result from variations in the cell lines and growth states of bacteria used in the studies. In tissue culture models of infection, salmonellae also induce macrophage cell death by a caspase 1-dependent mechanism (216,217). This activity appears important in *Salmonella* colonization of intestinal lymphoid tissues (218). The ability to induce phagocytosis by macrophages and epithelial cells may also protect salmonellae from phagocytosis by neutrophils. Salmonellae are killed rapidly by neutrophils, with less than 10% of an initial inoculum surviving after phagocytosis (219).

Bacterial Factors

Multiple bacterial factors are important in the pathogenesis of salmonellosis. Many of the genes that are important to the virulence of *S. typhimurium* are located on two *Salmonella* "pathogenicity islands," SPI-1 and SPI-2, each consisting of 40 kb of DNA located at centrosomes 63 and 30 of the chromosome, respectively (220,221). Both of these regions encode specialized secretion systems, termed *type III systems,* and their targets. The targets of the secretion apparatus are translocated to the mammalian cytoplasm following bacterial contact with host cell membranes (222–225). Analogous systems are present in a wide variety of bacterial pathogens and are adapted to alter eukaryotic cell processes, including apoptosis, cytokine production, and cytoskeletal function. As such, these systems may play a role in cell death, inflammation, alteration of phagocytosis, and other essential innate immune responses. SPI-1 encodes proteins important in the induction of macropinocytosis by epithelial cells and neutrophil transmigration and thus may be important for pathogenic processes at the mucosal surface, including gastroenteritis. In contrast, the SPI-2 type III secretion system is expressed following *Salmonella* invasion of host cells and functions to translocate target proteins across the phagosomal membrane into the host cell cytoplasm (226). SPI-2 is required for *Salmonella* replication within macrophages and the establishment of systemic infection, although the functions of individual SPI-2 translocated proteins remain unknown.

Although residence in the macrophage shields *Salmonella* from elements of humoral immunity, it also exposes the bacterium to the nutrient-poor and microbicidal environment of the phagosome. Antimicrobial activities of the macrophage include the production of reactive oxygen and nitrogen species and also the antimicrobial peptides and hydrolytic enzymes that enrich the mature phagolysosome. Salmonellae must sense the phagosomal environment and activate virulence mechanisms that allow them to resist or evade these antimicrobial effectors. This principle is illustrated by the PhoP/PhoQ two-component response regulator. The PhoP/PhoQ system senses the phagosomal environment and activates the transcription of numerous *Salmonella* genes necessary for survival within the macrophage (227). Activation of the PhoP regulon leads to widespread modifications in the protein and LPS components of the bacterial envelope. These surface modifications, which promote *Salmonella* survival in the stressful environment of the phagosome, include the synthesis of novel transmembrane cation transporters and LPS with an altered lipid A structure (228,229). PhoP-regulated modifications of lipid A promote resistance to antimicrobial peptides and reduce the effect of LPS of stimulating macrophage production of proinflammatory cytokines, including tumor necrosis factor-α (228,230). PhoP/PhoQ mutants of *S. typhi* are avirulent in humans and are promising new live typhoid fever vaccine candidates (231).

Salmonellae also express several enzymes that directly inactivate reactive oxygen and nitrogen species produced by the macrophage. The resistance of salmonellae to nitric oxide (NO) and related reactive nitrogen compounds is mediated partly by the synthesis of homocysteine, an antagonist of NO (232). *Salmonella* mutants unable to synthesize homocysteine because of a mutation in the *metL* gene are hypersensitive to NO and are less virulent. In addition, salmonellae produce at least one superoxide dismutase that can inactivate reactive oxygen species, and inactivation of this enzyme leads to decreased survival in macrophages (233).

The major surface molecules of *Salmonella* appear to be important in systemic pathogenesis. The Vi antigen of *S. typhi* prevents antibody-mediated opsonization, increases resistance to peroxide, and confers resistance to complement activation by the alternate pathway and complement-mediated lysis (209). Vi antigen thus may function to inhibit phagocytosis of salmonellae by neutrophils while not interfering with the induction of phagocytosis by more permissive macrophages and epithelial cells. In addition, both deep rough (missing the core polysaccharide) and rough (missing the O polysaccharide side chain) LPS mutants are avirulent (234). Modification of the O side chains increases resistance to complement-mediated serum killing and phagocytosis (234).

Multiple other bacterial factors, including incompletely characterized cytotoxin genes (235), genes that encode the synthesis of essential nutrients (236), and the virulence plasmids found in many nontyphoidal *Salmonella* serotypes, also are important in *Salmonella* systemic pathogenesis (69,237). The virulence plasmids of *S. typhimurium, S. dublin, S. choleraesuis,* and *S. enteritidis* all contain an 8-kb region that appears to confer serum resistance and promote bacteremia in humans

Pathophysiology of Gastroenteritis

The mechanisms by which nontyphoidal salmonellae cause gastroenteritis remain obscure despite extensive study. Although a number of enterotoxins antigenically similar to cholera toxin and *Escherichia coli* heat-labile toxin have been described in *Salmonella* species, none has ever been purified or fully characterized biochemically (238–240). Because of the presence of multiple plasmids in *Salmonella* species, it is possible that the heat-labile toxin, which is carried on a plasmid, occasionally is transferred among *Salmonella* species. However, some enterotoxin-producing strains that cause fulminate watery diarrhea in humans produce this toxin activity after plasmid curing (238).

It seems more likely that diarrhea is caused by bacterial entry into enterocytes or by the induction of an immune response in the intestine. The entrance of salmonellae into epithelial cells is associated with a number of biochemical alterations, including phosphorylation of the mitogen-associated kinase and activation of leukotriene synthesis through phospholipase A_2, that results in increased vascular permeability and leukocyte chemotaxis (201,202). In human intestinal cell lines, *Salmonella* infection has been demonstrated to result in the production of D-myo-inositol-1,4,5,6-tetrakisphosphate [Ins(1,4,5,6)P_4], and this may promote chloride flux and subsequent diarrhea (240). Induction of Ins(1,4,5,6)P_4 synthesis is dependent on the inositol phosphate phosphatase activity of SopB, a *Salmonella* virulence protein translocated into the host intestinal epithelial cell by the SPI-1 type III secretion system (241).

Nontyphoidal *Salmonella* gastroenteritis in humans is characterized by massive neutrophil infiltration into both the large- and small-bowel mucosa, whereas typhoid fever is associated with infiltration of the small-bowel mucosa with mononuclear cells (3). In addition, only *Salmonella* serotypes that cause human gastroenteritis can induce intestinal epithelial cells to secrete interleukin 8 (IL-8), a potent neutrophil chemotactic factor (242). IL-8 secretion is mediated at least in part through nuclear factor-κβ and requires an intact SPI-1 type III secretion system (243). Degranulation and release of toxin substances by neutrophils may contribute to inflammation and result in tissue damage and fluid secretion or leakage across the intestinal mucosa via alterations in epithelial cell tight junctions.

Host Factors

The virulence of any microorganism involves a complex interaction between the microorganism and the host's ability to limit infection. In *Salmonella* infection, host specificity is extremely important to disease. For example, *S. typhi* causes potentially lethal typhoid fever in humans but is avirulent in mice (244). In contrast, *S. typhimurium,* the most common serotype to cause gastroenteritis in humans, causes lethal infection in mice. In inbred mice, susceptibility to *S. typhimurium, Mycobacterium,* and *Leishmania* segregates in a dominant mendelian pattern, and a locus (termed *Bcg, Lsh,* or *Ity*) identified on mouse chromosome 1 controls susceptibility to these infections through an alteration in macrophage function (245). A gene designated *Nramp* has been identified within the *Ity* locus (246); this gene encodes a divalent cation transporter that is recruited to the phagosomal membrane, which suggests that the Nramp protein may function to deplete the phagosome of divalent cations essential for bacterial metabolism (247–250). In addition, mice with a mutation in toll-like receptor 4 (TLR-4) show decreased macrophage activation in response to LPS and increased susceptibility to *Salmonella* infection (251).

In humans, the risk for invasive salmonellosis is increased in persons with defects of cell-mediated immunity, including those with AIDS, transplanted organs, and lymphoproliferative diseases (252–257). In persons deficient in the IL-12 receptor, the type 1 helper T-cell response and the production of interferon-γ are defective, and such people are extremely susceptible to mycobacterial and *Salmonella* infections (258). This finding demonstrates the importance of an intact cell-mediated immunity to control intracellular bacterial infections, such as salmonellosis. Morphine also may alter innate immune function and permit leakage of bacteria from the gastrointestinal tract; the risk for gastrointestinal infection is increased in injection drug users, especially those infected with HIV (259). In a mouse model, orally administered morphine markedly potentiated *S. typhimurium* infection of the gastrointestinal tract; disseminated infection and death ensued (259).

The incidence of salmonellosis is increased in persons at the extremes of age and with chronic granulomatous disease or diseases causing phagocytic overload, such as bartonellosis, malaria, schistosomiasis, histoplasmosis, and sickle cell disease (65,66,68,260,261). Susceptibility to salmonellosis can be increased by alterations in the gastrointestinal tract resulting from decreased gastric acidity (188,262), the effects of antimicrobial therapy on the endogenous flora (127), gastrointestinal surgery (67,188), and chronic gastrointestinal diseases such as inflammatory bowel disease and malignancy (253).

IMMUNITY

Immunity to *S. typhi* requires both cell-mediated and humoral immune responses and is achievable by vaccination (263). Although most persons are immune after typhoid infection, reinfection can rarely occur and is often associated with early institution of antimicrobial therapy (264). Little is known about the immune response to the more than 2,000 nontyphoidal *Salmonella* serotypes that infect humans, but the invasive nature of the bacteria and the histology of infection suggest that both cell-mediated and humoral mucosal and systemic immunity are important.

Although both serum and intestinal antibody responses have been documented after typhoid fever or vaccination (265), little is known about the protective antigens against which an immune response must be generated. Vaccine studies indicate that the Vi polysaccharide antigen should be an important immune target because parenteral immunization with this antigen leads to increased protection in endemic areas (266). No data are available on whether immunization with this antigen can protect previously unexposed persons. Chronic carriers of *S. typhi* are immune to active infection and have very high antibody titers to *Salmonella* surface proteins, including the Vi antigen (267). However, these high titers may reflect chronic exposure to the organism rather than provide protection against clinical disease. By extrapolation from animal studies, it seems likely that antibody to the O polysaccharide of LPS is also important (268). The importance of an intestinal immune response is suggested by an animal model of infection in which a single monoclonal IgA antibody against O antigen secreted into the intestinal lumen provided measurable protection against *Salmonella* infection (195).

In addition to the formation of antibodies directed against the *Salmonella* surface proteins, lymphocyte proliferation assays have documented that a cell-mediated immune response occurs after *S. typhi* infection (269). Consistent with this observation are data from studies with live vaccine indicating that a cell-mediated immune response against crude typhoid antigen is correlated with the development of immunity after vaccination. In addition, cytotoxic CD4+ T lymphocytes can be enhanced by vaccine-induced IgA antibodies (270).

CLINICAL MANIFESTATIONS

Specific *Salmonella* serotypes most often produce characteristic clinical manifestations that have been given the syndromic designations of *gastroenteritis, enteric fever, bacteremia and vascular infection, localized infection,* and *chronic carrier state.* Although these syndromic designations are clinically useful, they have neither pathogenic nor prognostic significance.

Gastroenteritis

Infection with nontyphoidal *Salmonella* most often results in a self-limited acute gastroenteritis that is indistinguishable from that caused by many other gastrointestinal bacterial pathogens. Within 6 to 48 hours after the ingestion of contaminated food or water, nausea, vomiting, and diarrhea occur (271). In most cases, the stools are loose, of moderate volume, and without blood. In rare cases, the stools may be watery and of large volume ("cholera-like") or of small volume and associated with tenesmus ("dysentery-like"). Fever (38°C to 39°C), abdominal cramping, nausea, vomiting, and chills are frequently reported. Headache, myalgias, and other systemic symptoms also may occur. Microscopic examination of stools shows neutrophils and, less frequently, red blood cells. Infrequently, *Salmonella* can cause a syndrome of pseudoappendicitis or mimic the intestinal changes of inflammatory bowel disease (271,272).

Diarrhea is usually self-limited, typically lasting for 3 to 7 days (271). Diarrhea that persists for more than10 days should suggest another diagnosis. If fever is present, it usually resolves within 48 to 72 hours. Occasionally, patients require hospitalization because of dehydration, and death occurs infrequently. In the United States, nontyphoidal *Salmonella* infections result in an estimated hospitalization rate of 2.2 per 1 million population and 582 deaths per year (87). A disproportionate number of these deaths occur among the elderly, especially those residing in long-term care facilities (96,184).

After gastroenteritis resolves, the mean duration of carriage of nontyphoidal *Salmonella* in the stool is 4 to 5 weeks and varies by *Salmonella* serotype (180). Some studies have demonstrated that antimicrobial therapy may increase the duration of carriage (180,273). In addition, the proportion of neonates with prolonged carriage is relatively high; in one study, 50% of neonates were still excreting *Salmonella* at 6 months (274). However, the delayed clearance of infection in neonates does not result in permanent carriage, as almost all chronic carriers are adults (180,274).

Enteric Fever

Human typhoid fever and paratyphoid fever are severe systemic illnesses characterized by fever and abdominal symptoms. In the pre-antibiotic era, approximately 15% of patients with typhoid fever died (16,275). More recently, mortality rates of up to 30% have been reported from developing countries in Asia and Africa, where infection with a multidrug-resistant strain and delayed antimicrobial therapy increase the risk for death (69–71,276–278). Currently in the United States, approximately 0.4% of persons with typhoid fever die (81).

The syndrome of enteric fever is most often caused by *S. typhi.* A similar but less severe syndrome is caused by *S. paratyphi A, S. paratyphi B* (*S. schottmuelleri*), and *S. typhi C* (*S. hirschfeldii*) (207,275). When enteric fever is caused by *S. typhi,* it is often referred to as *typhoid fever,* and when caused by *S. paratyphi,* it is referred to as *paratyphoid fever.* Although enteric fever classically is described as an acute illness with fever and abdominal tenderness, the symptoms are nonspecific and may be insidious in onset. The diagnosis of enteric fever should be considered strongly in the evaluation of any traveler who returns from a tropical or subtropical area with fever. The differential diagnosis of gradual onset of fever and abdominal pain with hepatosplenomegaly also includes malaria, amebic liver abscess, visceral leishmaniasis, and viral syndromes such as dengue fever.

The incubation period of *S. typhi* ranges from 5 to 21 days, depending on the inoculum ingested and the health and immune status of the patient. After the organism has been ingested, enterocolitis may develop with diarrhea lasting several days; these symptoms usually resolve before the onset of fever. Diarrhea is more common in certain geographic areas and among patients with AIDS and children under 1 year of age (64,279). Typically, fecal leukocytes are detected and stool protein is increased (64). Constipation is present in 10% to 38% of patients (64). Although fever is a classic sign of typhoid fever, it does not always develop, and the pattern of fever is not clinically useful. In addition, only 20% to 40% of patients have abdominal pain at presentation; the frequency of other abdominal symptoms varies widely (275,280).

Nonspecific symptoms, such as chills, diaphoresis, headache, anorexia, cough, weakness, sore throat, dizziness, and muscle pains, are frequently present before the onset of fever in cases of typhoid (281). Neuropsychiatric manifestations, including psychosis and confusion, occur in 5% to 10% of patients and may be related to cytokine release from *S. typhi*-infected macrophages (12,275,282,283). This so-called typhoid state has been described as "muttering delirium" and "coma vigil" (282). Picking at the bedclothes and imaginary objects and muscle twitching are characteristic. Seizures and coma are reported in fewer than 1% of cases, and seizures may represent febrile seizures of childhood. The cerebrospinal fluid is usually normal, and abnormal results of cerebrospinal fluid studies or recurrent seizures should suggest another diagnosis.

Patients with typhoid fever usually appear acutely ill, although those who previously have been exposed to *S. typhi* or who seek early medical attention can present with a milder illness. Relative bradycardia is neither a sensitive nor a specific sign of typhoid fever, occurring in fewer than 50% of patients (275,283). Approximately 30% of patients have rose spots—a faint, salmon-colored maculopapular rash on the trunk (283). Organisms can be cultured from punch biopsy specimens of these lesions, and a characteristic pathologic feature is a perivascular mononuclear cell infiltrate. The rash can be very subtle, especially in highly pigmented persons, and frequently fades to small macules that appear to be resolving skin hemorrhages. Cervical lymphadenopathy develops in some patients. Rales are infrequently noted, and chest radiographic findings are almost always normal (64,282). Examination of the abdomen usually reveals pain on deep palpation, and peristalsis frequently is increased. Approximately 50% of patients have hepatosplenomegaly. Pain may be localized to the right upper quadrant in the approximately 3% of adults with typhoid fever in whom necrotizing cholecystitis develops (275). Pancreatitis has been described rarely (284).

Among survivors, most symptoms resolve by the fourth week of infection without antimicrobial therapy. However, weakness, weight loss, and debilitation may persist for months, and 10% of patients relapse (207,275,281). In the pre-antibiotic era, two thirds of pregnancies complicated by typhoid fever resulted in fetal demise and miscarriage (285). Several sex-specific differences in the clinical manifestations, laboratory abnormalities, and complications of typhoid fever were found in one small retrospective study from South Africa, but prospective studies are needed to determine whether any differences in immune response underlie these findings (286).

Many of the complications of untreated enteric fever occur in the third or fourth week of infection (3). In as many as 3% to 10% of patients, intestinal perforation develops as a result of hyperplasia, ulceration, and necrosis of the ileocecal lymphoid tissue (12,64,84,278). In such cases, the patient's blood should be recultured and antimicrobial therapy broadened to cover aerobic and anaerobic enteric organisms. Other infectious complications include endocarditis and localized infections, such as pericarditis, orchitis, and liver abscesses. Splenic abscesses and spontaneous rupture have been reported (287).

Hematologic abnormalities associated with typhoid include leukopenia and anemia (288). Leukocytosis is seen most often in children and within the first 10 days of illness. Thrombocytopenia and clotting abnormalities develop in some patients; these usually resolve spontaneously. Moderately elevated levels of serum liver enzymes [e.g., aspartate aminotransferase (AST) and alanine aminotransferase (ALT) values of 300 to 500 U/dL] and muscle enzymes are common (289); liver biopsies demonstrate focal Kupffer cell hyperplasia and mononuclear cell infiltration of the portal space (290). Rarely, proteinuria and immune complex glomerulonephritis develop. Creatine clearance is usually normal, and irreversible loss of renal function has not been reported. Nonspecific ST-segment and T-wave electrocardiographic abnormalities are seen infrequently.

Diagnosis of Enteric Fever

The definitive diagnosis of enteric fever requires the isolation of *S. typhi* or *S. paratyphi* organisms from blood, bone marrow, another sterile site, rose spots, stool, or intestinal secretions (291–293). The duodenal string test is a useful noninvasive technique for sampling duodenal secretions (292,294,295). The sensitivity of blood culture alone is only 50% to 70% (296), probably because small quantities of *S. typhi* organisms (i.e., <15/mL) are typically present in the blood of patients with typhoid fever (206,297). However, the diagnosis is established in more than 90% of patients if blood, bone marrow, and intestinal secretions are all cultured (293,298). Oxgall media cultures may increase the sensitivity of blood but not of bone marrow cultures (12). Because almost all *S. typhi* organisms in blood are associated with the mononuclear cell–platelet fraction, centrifugation of blood and culture of the buffy coat fraction can reduce the time to isolation of the organism but do not increase sensitivity (206,299).

The sensitivity of bone marrow culture is 90% and, unlike that of blood culture, is not reduced by up to 5 days of prior antimicrobial therapy (293,298,300). In some patients with negative bone marrow cultures, duodenal string cultures have been positive (298). In one study, the combination of blood and duodenal string culture in children was as sensitive as bone marrow culture (295). The incidence of positive stool cultures is also higher in children than in adults (60% vs. 27%) (12). Therefore, in both adults and children, blood, bone marrow, stool, and duodenal string cultures ideally should all be performed.

A number of serologic tests, including the classic Widal test, have been developed to detect *S. typhi* antigen or antibody (12,301–306). None of these tests is sufficiently sensitive or specific to replace culture-based methods for the diagnosis of enteric fever in developed countries. However, in countries where resources are limited, rapid and simple tests to detect anti-*S. typhi* antibody against LPS or outer membrane protein may replace the less accurate Widal test (307,308). PCR methods to detect *S. typhi* in blood have been developed and appear to be more rapid and sensitive than standard culture, but they are not yet commercially available (309,310).

Bacteremia and Vascular Infection

Classically, *S. choleraesuis* and *S. dublin* produce a syndrome of sustained bacteremia with fever, but any *Salmonella* serotype can cause bacteremia (271,311). From 1% to 4% of immunocompetent persons with *Salmonella* gastroenteritis have positive blood cultures (67,180,311). The risk for bacteremia is greater in infants, the elderly, and the immunocompromised (65,66,252–256,260,312). Among children, nontyphoidal *Salmonella* bacteremia usually is associated with gastroenteritis, infrequently causes focal infections, and is fatal in fewer than 10% of cases (313–315). In contrast, adults are more likely to have primary bacteremia, and the incidence of secondary focal infections and death is high in adults (313).

Salmonellae tend to infect vascular sites, and high-grade or persistent bacteremia suggests an endovascular infection (316). The risk for endovascular infection complicating *Salmonella* bacteremia is estimated to be 25% in persons over 50 years of age and is most often associated with seeding of atherosclerotic plaques or aneurysms (285,316,317).

Salmonellosis and HIV Infection

In persons with HIV infection, the risk for salmonellosis is estimated to be 20- to 100-fold higher than that in the general population (256,318). *Salmonella* is more likely to cause severe invasive disease in patients with AIDS than in immunocompetent persons; fulminant diarrhea, acute enterocolitis, rectal ulceration, recurrent bacteremia, meningitis, and death occur despite antimicrobial therapy (257, 318–322). In contrast, the severity of *Salmonella* infection in persons with AIDS-related complex or asymptomatic HIV infection is similar to that in immunocompetent persons.

Among HIV-infected persons in Africa, *Salmonella* species are one of the most common causes of bacteremia; they are often multidrug-resistant and associated with a high mortality rate (24% to 80%) (323–327). Focal infections caused by nontyphoidal *Salmonella* are infrequent among HIV-infected persons, most often occurring among those with CD4+ counts below 100/mm^3 (322).

Recurrent nontyphoidal *Salmonella* bacteremia is an AIDS-defining illness (328); bacteremia apparently recurs because the primary infection is incompletely cleared as a consequence of impaired cell-mediated immunity. Without maintenance antimicrobial therapy, up to 45% of persons with HIV infection have recurrent bacteremia (255). Among persons with HIV infection, the incidence of recurrent nontyphoidal *Salmonella* bacteremia has declined in recent years (257), likely because of the direct bactericidal activity of zidovudine on *Salmonella* species and the use of TMP-SMX to prevent *Pneumocystis* pneumonia (257,329,330).

Localized Infection

Localized infections develop in approximately 5% to 10% of persons with *Salmonella* bacteremia, and the presentation may be delayed (311,331). The extraintestinal complications of salmonellosis are summarized in Table 44.2.

Chronic Carrier State

The chronic carrier state is defined as the persistence of *Salmonella* organisms in stool or urine for periods longer than

TABLE 44.2. EXTRAINTESTINAL INFECTIOUS COMPLICATIONS OF SALMONELLOSIS

Site (refs.)	Incidence	Risk Factors	Manifestations	Complications	Mortality	Diagnosis	Therapy
Endocarditis (285,431)	0.2–0.4%	Preexisting valvular heart disease	Valvular vegetation, infected mural thrombus	Valve perforation, relapse (20–25%), pericarditis	~70%	Blood culture, echocardiography	Early surgery + 6 wk P ceph 3 or P amp
Arteritis (317, 347,410,412, 432–435)	Rare	Atherosclerosis, prosthetic graft, aortic aneurysm, endocarditis, myelodysplasia	Prolonged fever; pain in back, chest, or abdomen	Mycotic aneurysm, aneurysm rupture, aortoenteric fistula, vertebral osteomyelitis	~45%	Blood culture, CT, or nuclear scan	Early surgical bypass + 6 wk P ceph 3 or P amp
Central nervous system (436–443)	0.1–0.9%	Infants (esp. neonates)	Meningitis, ventriculitis, cerebral abscess, subdural empyema	Seizures, mental retardation, hydrocephalus, brain infarction, relapse	~20–60%	CSF culture, CT, or MRI	≥3 wk P ceph 3, P amp, or carbapenem
Pulmonary (444,331)	Rare	Lung malignancy, pulmonary disease, sickle cell anemia	Pneumonia	Lung abscess empyema broncho-pleural fistula	~25–60%	Respiratory culture, chest radiograph	≥2 wk P/PO abx
Bone (445–447)	<1%	Sickle cell anemia, male gender, bone disease, immunosuppression	Femur, tibia, humerus, lumbar vertebrae	Relapse, chronic osteomyelitis	Very low	Bone radiograph	≥4 wk P ceph 3 or P amp + surgery for sequestra
Joint: reactive (448–452)	0.6%	HLA-B27	Three or more joints involved (esp. knee, ankle, wrist, and sacroiliac)	Prolonged symptoms (mean duration, 5.5 mo)	Negligible	Joint fluid examination and culture	Nonsteroidal anti-inflammatory agent
Joint: septic (453–455)	0.1–0.2%	Same as bone, joint disease	Knee, hip, shoulder	Joint destruction osteomyelitis	Very low	Joint fluid examination and culture	Repeated needle aspiration + ≥4 wk P/PO abx
Muscle/soft tissue (456,457)	Rare	Local trauma, male gender, diabetes, HIV infection	Abscess, pyomyositis	Osteomyelitis, endovascular infection, frequent relapse	~33%	Ultrasonography, aspiration	Drainage + ≥2 wk P abx
Hepatobiliary (458–460, 467,468)	Rare	Cholelithiasis, cirrhosis, amebic abscess, echinococcal cyst	Hepatomegaly, cholecystitis, hepatic abscess	Rupture w/2° peritonitis, subphrenic abscess, spontaneous bacterial peritonitis	~10%	Ultrasonography, aspiration	Drainage + ≥2 wk P abx
Splenic (461)	Rare	Sickle cell anemia, splenic cyst, splenic hematoma	Splenomegaly	Left-sided empyema, subphrenic abscess, rupture w/2° peritonitis	<10%	Ultrasonography, aspiration	≥2 wk P abx ± splenectomy
Urinary (254,462,463)	0.6%	Urolithiasis, malignancy, renal transplant	Cystitis, pyelonephritis	Renal abscess, interstitial nephritis, relapse	~20%	Urine culture, ultrasonography	Removal of structural abnormality + 1–2 wk abx + ≥6 wk PO quinolone or TMP-SMX
Genital (285,464)	Rare	Pregnancy, renal transplant	Ovarian abscess, testicular abscess, prostatitis, epididymitis	Abscess	Very low	Ultrasonography, aspiration	Drainage of collection + 1–2 wk P abx + ≥6 wk PO quinolone or TMP-SMX
Soft tissue (465,466)	<1%	Local trauma, immunosuppression	Pustular dermatitis, SQ abscess, wound infection	Septic thrombophlebitis, endophthalmitis	~15%	Drainage culture	≥2 wk P abx + drainage of collection

P ceph 3, parenteral third-generation cephalosporin; P amp, parenteral ampicillin; P/PO, parenteral or oral antimicrobial (e.g., quinolone, ampicillin, trimethoprim-sulfamethoxazole, chloramphenicol, or third-generation cephalosporin).

1 year. Chronic carriage develops in 0.2% to 0.6% of patients with nontyphoidal salmonellosis (332) and in 1% to 4% of patients with *S. typhi* infection (275,281,285). The frequency of chronic carriage is higher in women, persons with biliary abnormalities or concurrent bladder infection with *Schistosoma,* and infants (66,333). Chronic carriage of *S. typhi* and *S. paratyphi A* has been associated with an increased incidence of carcinoma of the gallbladder and other gastrointestinal malignancies (334,335). Serology for the Vi antigen can be useful in distinguishing chronic carriage from acute infection with *S. typhi*; chronic carriers often have a high antibody titer to this antigen (267).

IMMUNIZATION AGAINST *S. TYPHI*

Enteric fever can be prevented by immunization, and three commercially available vaccines are available in for use in the United States: an oral live-attenuated vaccine manufactured from the Ty21a strain of *S. typhi,* a parenteral heat-phenol–inactivated vaccine that has been widely used for many years, and a parenteral capsular polysaccharide vaccine (ViCPS) (336). These vaccines have been most extensively evaluated in endemic populations; they achieve approximately 50% to 80% efficacy, depending on prior exposure, and confer protection that lasts only for several years (336).

Typhoid vaccine is not required for international travel, but it is recommended for travelers to areas where exposure to *S. typhi* is a risk, especially persons traveling to the Indian subcontinent and other developing countries who will be exposed to potentially contaminated food and drink for a prolonged period of time (336). Vaccination is particularly recommended for those traveling to smaller cities, villages, and destinations off the usual tourist itineraries. In addition, laboratory workers who work with *S. typhi* and household contacts of known *S. typhi* carriers should be vaccinated (334). Because the protective efficacy of the vaccine can be overcome by high inocula, which are common in food-borne exposures, the most frequent exposures among travelers (207,336), it is controversial whether all travelers to areas with high rates of typhoid fever should be immunized (337). Immunization is an adjunct and not a substitute for avoiding high-risk foods and beverages or utilizing good laboratory technique. With all the currently available vaccines, documented cases of typhoid fever in vaccinated travelers have still occurred. Immunization is not recommended for adults residing in areas where typhoid is endemic or in the management of persons potentially exposed to a common source outbreak. However, immunization of school-age children should be considered in areas where typhoid is a public health problem and antimicrobial-resistant *S. typhi* strains are prevalent (79).

Since the nineteenth century, the heat-killed whole-organism *S. typhi* vaccine has been the mainstay of immunization against typhoid fever. The heat-phenol–inactivated *S. typhi* vaccine manufactured by Wyeth-Ayerst is from 51% to 77% effective in comparison with tetanus placebo in studies in endemic populations (335,338,339). An acetone-inactivated vaccine provided greater protection (range, 79% to 94%) in endemic populations (340,341); the higher efficacy was attributed to the preservation of Vi antigen in this preparation (337,342). However, the acetone-inactivated vaccine is associated with more frequent side effects, costs more than the heat-phenol–inactivated vaccine (336,339), and in the United States is available only to the military. Both preparations appear to result in equal protection in immunologically naïve persons.

Local and systemic adverse reactions occur frequently with the parenteral heat-phenol–inactivated vaccine, including fever (17% to 29%), severe headache (10%), and significant local pain at the site of administration (35% to 60%) (338,340). After vaccination, reactions occur within hours and can persist for up to 72 hours; approximately 25% of persons miss work or school. In general, reactions are milder with subsequent vaccine doses. Severe reactions to immunization can include anaphylaxis, chest pain, liver damage, neurologic problems, and reactive arthropathy (343,344).

Primary vaccination with heat-phenol–inactivated vaccine consists of two 0.5-mL subcutaneous injections separated by 4 weeks or more (336). For children between 6 months and 10 years of age, two 0.25-mL doses should be administered separated by 4 weeks or more. The manufacturer does not recommend the vaccine for use in children less than 6 months of age. Booster doses should be administered every 3 years and can be given subcutaneously (0.5 mL for those ages 10 years and older and 0.25 mL for those ages 6 months to 10 years) or intradermally (0.1 mL for those older than 6 months) (336).

A live-attenuated oral Ty21a vaccine (Vivotif Berna vaccine, Swiss Serum and Vaccine Institute) has been licensed in the United States since 1989. The molecular basis of attenuation of Ty21a is unknown and is not related to the *galE* mutation present in the vaccine strain (345). Side effects are markedly fewer with the oral Ty21a vaccine than with the parenteral vaccines (12,263,336). No serious adverse reactions have been observed in large-scale field trials or during postmarketing surveillance in Switzerland. Following the administration of three doses of Ty21a vaccine containing 10^9 organisms on alternate days, the protective efficacy ranged from 43% to 96% in endemic populations (346,347).

Primary vaccination consists of four oral doses of Ty21a vaccine in an enteric-coated capsule taken 1 hour before a meal with cool liquid on alternate days. The stored capsules must be refrigerated (336). Noncompliance with the multiple dose administration schedule and the requirement for home refrigeration has been reported (347). A booster series of four capsules is recommended every 5 years, although few data are available on the persistence of antibody titers against *S. typhi.* A four-dose series is recommended for boosting every 5 years.

Evidence for the efficacy of Ty21a in immunologically naïve persons is limited; in some studies in travelers, no efficacy was demonstrated (348,349). Nevertheless, based on studies in endemic populations, it is likely that Ty21a is as effective as the heat-phenol–inactivated vaccine if compliance is adequate. Because of the possibility of illness associated with the administration of a live-attenuated vaccine, Ty21a is not recommended for children less than 6 years of age, immunosuppressed persons, and those on antibiotic therapy (336). Ty21a can be administered simultaneously with immunoglobulin or viral vaccines. Some antimicrobial agents, including mefloquine but not chloroquine, may inhibit the growth of Ty21a *in vitro,* and vaccination with Ty21a should be delayed for more than 24 hours after the administration of any antibacterial agent or mefloquine. In addition, the administration of proguanil may diminish anti-*S. typhi* LPS antibody production.

A ViCPS (Typhim Vi, Pasteur Mérieux Connaught) is widely used, and protein conjugate Vi vaccine is under study. Primary vaccination with ViCPS consists of one 0.5-mL (25-µg) dose administered intramuscularly (336). It causes fewer side effects than heat-phenol–inactivated vaccine; these include fever (0 to 1%), headache (1.5% to 3%), and local erythema or induration at the injection site (7%) (350). ViCPS is not recommended for use among children less than 2 years of age. A single booster dose can be given every 2 years. Long-term clinical experience with ViCPS is mostly lacking, but the vaccine was 55% effective and high Vi antibody levels persisted during a 3-year period among South African children (351).

In summary, none of the currently available typhoid vaccines has been demonstrated to have sufficient efficacy in travelers to recommend their widespread use. Because of the low frequency of side effects, either oral Ty21a or parenteral ViCPS can be administered to travelers who will be spending a prolonged period in a high-risk area. Use of the parenteral heat-phenol–inactivated vaccine is limited by the high incidence of serious side effects and its failure to protect against large inocula. However, the heat-phenol–inactivated vaccine is the only available option for children less than 2 years old and may be used for immunosuppressed persons when prolonged exposure to *S. typhi* is anticipated (336). In light of the emergence of quinolone-resistant strains of *S. typhi* in developing countries, mass immunization may be useful for the control of prolonged epidemics of multidrug-resistant typhoid fever (79).

THERAPY FOR SALMONELLOSIS

Typhoid Fever

Chloramphenicol has been the treatment of choice for typhoid fever since its introduction in 1948 (16). Chloramphenicol is inexpensive and highly effective after oral administration, and it remains the standard with which newer antimicrobials must be compared. Treatment with chloramphenicol (500 mg orally four times daily) reduces typhoid fever mortality from approximately 20% to 1% and the duration of fever from 14 to 28 days to 3 to 5 days (16,352). However, chloramphenicol therapy has been associated with the emergence of resistance (16,70,74,353,354), a high relapse rate (10% to 25%) (207,352,355,356), a high rate of continued and chronic carriage (207), bone marrow toxicity (357,358), and high mortality rates in some recent series from the developing world (70,283,355). If intravenous therapy is required, chloramphenicol succinate should not be used because it is excreted in the urine before it is converted to chloramphenicol, so that much lower serum concentrations are achieved than with the equivalent oral dose (359,360). Although the results of *in vitro* studies have not always correlated with *in vivo* efficacy, chloramphenicol is bacteriostatic only against clinical isolates (361,362) and against *S. typhi* within cultured human macrophages. In contrast, ceftriaxone, ampicillin, and quinolones are highly bacteriocidal for intracellular *S. typhi* organisms (362).

The emergence of plasmid-mediated resistance to chloramphenicol in the 1970s (74,353,354,363,364) has prompted the use of amoxicillin (1 g orally every 6 hours) (365,366) and TMP-SMX (one double-strength tablet twice daily) (367,368) as alternatives for the treatment of typhoid fever. Despite several studies suggesting that ampicillin is inferior to chloramphenicol, these agents are probably equivalent to chloramphenicol when administered orally to treat infections caused by susceptible strains and may decrease the relapse rate (355). Because of the recent emergence of strains of *S. typhi* resistant to multiple drugs, including ampicillin and trimethoprim, the efficacy of these drugs has diminished (75,369,370).

In areas with a high prevalence of multidrug-resistant *Salmonella* infection (e.g., the Indian subcontinent, Southeast Asia, Africa), all patients suspected of having typhoid fever should be treated with an oral quinolone or parenteral third-generation cephalosporin until the results of culture sensitivities are available. Parenterally administered third-generation cephalosporins are effective in the treatment of typhoid fever (371–375). Ceftriaxone (1 to 2 g daily) administered either intravenously or intramuscularly for 10 to 14 days is equivalent to oral or intravenous chloramphenicol for the treatment of susceptible *S. typhi* strains (371,374,375). Excellent response rates have been reported with ceftriaxone when administered for 5 to 7 days, but the relapse rate remains incompletely defined (371). After initial control of the symptoms of typhoid fever with parenteral third-generation cephalosporins, many practitioners switch to an oral agent to complete 10 to 14 days of therapy. Oral cefixime (10 to 15 mg/kg twice daily for 14 days) and oral azithromycin (500 mg once daily for 7 days) warrant further study for the initial treatment of multidrug-resistant typhoid fever (376–378).

Several small studies have reported the successful treatment of typhoid fever with aztreonam (379,380). However, a prospective clinical trial in children in Malaysia was discontinued because of a high failure rate with aztreonam (381). First- and second-generation cephalosporins are clinically ineffective and should not be used to treat typhoid fever or nontyphoidal salmonellosis, despite adequate *in vitro* killing activity (382–385). In addition, aminoglycosides are clinically ineffective, perhaps because they lack activity against intracellular salmonellae (386).

Quinolones are highly active against *S. typhi in vitro* and reach high concentrations in macrophages and bile (387,388). Ciprofloxacin (500 mg orally twice daily for 10 days) is the drug of choice for the treatment of multidrug-resistant typhoid fever (76,277,335,389,390). Other quinolones, including ofloxacin, norfloxacin, fleroxacin, and perfloxacin, have been effective in small clinical trials (391–393). Short-course therapy with ofloxacin (10 to 15 mg/kg daily divided into two doses for 2 to 3 days) appears to be simple, safe, and effective in the treatment of uncomplicated multidrug-resistant typhoid fever when the strain is susceptible to nalidixic acid (77). However, in a small study from Viet Nam (77), when *S. typhi* strains were relatively quinolone-resistant (resistant to nalidixic acid and minimum inhibitory concentration of ciprofloxacin of 0.125 to 1 μg/mL), patients treated with short-course quinolone therapy (<5 days) had prolonged fever, and 33% required repeated treatment. All *S. typhi* isolates should be screened for nalidixic acid resistance and tested against a clinically appropriate quinolone (77). Patients with nalidixic acid-resistant strains should be treated with higher doses of ciprofloxacin (i.e., 10 mg/kg twice daily for 10 days) or ofloxacin (10 to 15 mg/kg daily divided into two doses for 7 to 10 days) (77,370,394–396). Patients with *S. typhi* strains for which the minimum inhibitory concentration of ciprofloxacin is 2 mg/mL or higher should be treated with a third-generation cephalosporin (397).

The preferred treatment of known or suspected multidrug-resistant typhoid in children is a parenteral third-generation cephalosporin, especially ceftriaxone (70,371,374). Quinolones are not recommended for children less than 10 years old or pregnant women because cartilage damage has been demonstrated in young animals (398). However, quinolones have been used to treat multidrug-resistant typhoid in children and pregnant patients without adverse effects (399–402).

The use of glucococorticosteroids has been advocated in the treatment of severe typhoid fever based on the results of a study in Jakarta showing a significant reduction in mortality among patients with severe typhoid fever (i.e., associated delirium, obtundation, stupor, coma, or shock) treated with chloramphenicol and dexamethasone versus chloramphenicol alone (case fatality rate, 10% vs. 56%) (64). Although the case fatality rate in the control group was high and the study has never been repeated, based on this study, dexamethasone (3 mg/kg intravenously followed by eight doses of 1 mg/kg every 6 hours) should be considered in the treatment of severe typhoid associated with altered mental status or shock. Steroid treatment beyond 48 hours may increase the relapse rate (403).

Nontyphoidal *Salmonella* Infection

Salmonella gastroenteritis is usually a self-limited disease, and therapy primarily should be directed to the replacement of fluid and electrolyte losses (404). In a large metaanalysis, antimicrobial therapy for uncomplicated nontyphoidal *Salmonella* gastroenteritis, including short-course or single-dose regimens of oral quinolones, amoxicillin, or TMP-SMX, did not significantly decrease the length of illness, including fever and diarrhea, and was associated with an increased risk for relapse, a positive culture after 3 weeks, and adverse drug reactions (405). Therefore, antimicrobials should not be used routinely to treat uncomplicated nontyphoidal *Salmonella* gastroenteritis or to reduce convalescent stool excretion.

Although bacteremia develops in fewer than 5% of all patients with *Salmonella* gastroenteritis, certain patients are at increased risk for invasive infection and may benefit from preemptive antimicrobial therapy. Antimicrobial therapy should be considered for neonates, persons older than 50 years, and patients who are immunosuppressed or have cardiac valvular or endovascular abnormalities or prosthetic vascular grafts. Treatment should consist of an oral or intravenous antimicrobial administered for 48 to 72 hours or until the patient becomes afebrile. Longer treatment may result in a higher rate of chronic carriage and relapse. With susceptible organisms, treatment with an oral quinolone, TMP-SMX, or amoxicillin is adequate. Occasionally, antimicrobial prophylaxis has been required to control institutional outbreaks, especially in long-term-care facilities and pediatric wards, where compliance with infection control measures may be difficult (406,407).

Although quinolones are not recommended for children under 10 years of age (398), they may have a role in treating severe nontyphoidal salmonellosis in this age-group. In one small study, seven children with severe typhoidal or nontyphoidal salmonellosis who failed conventional therapy improved rapidly when treated with oral perfloxacin (12 mg/kg daily for 7 days) (408). Furthermore, in a double-blinded, placebo-controlled trial from Turkey, intravenous immunoglobulin (500 mg/kg on days 1, 2, 3, and 8) in combination with cefoperazone, when administered to preterm neonates with *S. typhimurium* infection, reduced mortality, complications, and duration of antimicrobial therapy versus cefoperazone alone, a finding that merits further study (409).

Bacteremia

Because of the increasing prevalence of antimicrobial resistance, empiric therapy for life-threatening bacteremia or focal infection suspected to be caused by nontyphoidal *Salmonella* should include a third-generation cephalosporin and a quinolone until susceptibilities are known. It is also important to document whether the bacteremia is high-grade (i.e., >50% of three or more blood cultures positive) and, if so, to search for endovascular abnormalities by echocardiogram or other imaging techniques. Low-grade bacteremia not involving vascular structures should be treated with an intravenous antimicrobial for 7 to 14 days. Six weeks of intravenous therapy with a β-lactam antibiotic such as ampicillin or ceftriaxone is recommended to treat documented or suspected endovascular infection. Chloramphenicol should not be used to treat endovascular infection because failure rates are high (311,316). In addition, surgical resection of infected aneurysms or other infected endovascular sites is often required (410,411). Patients with infected prosthetic vascular grafts that could not be resected have been maintained successfully on long-term suppressive oral therapy (412).

Recurrent *Salmonella* Bacteremia in Persons with AIDS

Persons with AIDS and a first episode of *Salmonella* bacteremia should receive 1 to 2 weeks of intravenous antimicrobial therapy followed by 4 weeks of oral quinolone therapy (e.g., 500 to 750 mg of ciprofloxacin twice daily) in an attempt to eradicate the organism and decrease the risk for recurrent bacteremia (413). Persons who relapse following 6 weeks of antimicrobial therapy should receive long-term suppressive therapy with an oral quinolone or TMP-SMX. Quinolones and zidovudine have a synergistic antibacterial effect against *Salmonella*; administration of both drugs may dramatically decrease the risk for recurrent infection (414,415). Although data are lacking, TMP-SMX may be a good choice for the long-term suppressive therapy of salmonellosis if the organism is susceptible because TMP-SMX effectively prevents other opportunistic infections, including *Pneumocystis* pneumonia (416).

Focal Infections

Treatment recommendations for the management of focal infections are summarized in Table 44.2. Of note, quinolone treatment failure has been associated with low-dose oral therapy and with administration to patients who have undrained abscesses or osteomyelitis, in which antimicrobial penetration may be poor (394,395,417–419).

Chronic Carrier State

The management of chronic carriage of nontyphoidal *Salmonella* is similar to that of typhoid carriage. Amoxicillin and TMP-SMX are effective in eradicating chronic carriage, with cure rates of better than 80% after 6 weeks of therapy (420,421). Similar results have been obtained with the administration of ciprofloxacin or norfloxacin for 4 to 6 weeks, including the eradication of chronic carriage in a small number of patients with gallstones (387,422,423). The high concentration of amoxicillin and quinolones in bile and the superior intracellular penetration of quinolones are theoretic advantages over TMP-SMX. Cost considerations favor the use of amoxicillin to treat carriage of susceptible organisms. However, antimicrobial agents are infrequently effective in eradicating the carrier state if anatomic abnormalities, such as biliary or kidney stones, are present. In such cases, a combination of surgery and antimicrobial therapy is often required for eradication (332,424).

PREVENTION AND CONTROL

The prevention and control of salmonellosis require both an understanding of the complex cycles of transmission and ongoing surveillance to characterize trends in *Salmonella* occurrence and identify outbreaks. To control food-borne salmonellosis, barriers to the introduction and multiplication of *Salmonella* organisms must be implemented along the route from farm to table (126,425). To recognize food-borne outbreaks, clinicians must have a high index of suspicion, order appropriate laboratory tests, and promptly report positive cultures to public health departments. In the United States, active population-based surveillance for food-borne diseases has improved estimates of disease burden (110), and the application of computer algorithms to laboratory surveillance data has improved the ability to detect clusters and outbreaks of salmonellosis prospectively (88). The establishment of cooperative international surveillance systems has facilitated the rapid exchange of data to prevent human salmonellosis associated with widely distributed agricultural and manufactured foods (426,427).

Although most cases of *Salmonella* infection occur sporadically, large numbers of people may potentially become infected when commercial kitchens serve *Salmonella*-contaminated foods that have not been sufficiently cooked or that have been mishandled. Commercial food service establishments can reduce the risk for food-borne *S. enteritidis* illness if they substitute pasteurized eggs for pooled eggs whenever possible and do not serve food containing raw or undercooked eggs. It is recommended that all nursing homes and hospitals use pasteurized eggs in recipes that call for bulk pooled eggs (184).

The most cost-effective approach to the control of salmonellosis in food handlers is attention to good personal hygiene and the maintenance of time–temperature standards for food handling. It is a common practice to screen food handlers for carriage after gastroenteritis before they are allowed to return to work. However, this approach does not seem to be justified because few outbreaks are related to specific food handlers, prolonged carriage in food handlers after gastroenteritis is rare, and the number of organisms present is small. Therefore, it is reasonable to allow people to return to work after diarrhea resolves. Two consecutive negative stool samples should be required only for food handlers whose work involves touching unwrapped foods that are consumed raw or served without further cooking. Routine surveillance of food handlers for asymptomatic stool carriage of *Salmonella* is not recommended (428).

To limit the risk for nosocomial transmission to patients and health care workers, patients excreting *Salmonella* should be managed with standard precautions, including the use of barriers when direct patient care is performed or soiled articles are handled (429). Control of *Salmonella* outbreaks in long-term care facilities or neonatal care areas may be difficult because of poor compliance with isolation precautions and the increased susceptibility of these patients (172). Although *Salmonella* infection in newborns, the elderly, and immunocompromised persons can be severe, the risk for transmission of *Salmonella* from health care workers to patients appears to be very small (174). Once health care workers are asymptomatic and passing formed stool, they should be allowed to return to work if standard precautions are observed (430). However, local and state regulations should be followed; some require that health care workers who have salmonellosis stay away from work until two or more stool cultures obtained at least 24 hours apart are negative.

REFERENCES

1. Smith T. The hog-cholera group of bacteria. *US Bureau Animal Ind Bull* 1894;6:6–40.
2. Committee on *Salmonella. An evaluation of the* Salmonella *problem.* Washington, DC: National Academy of Science, 1969.
3. Rubin RH, Weinstein L. *Salmonellosis: microbiologic, pathologic, and clinical features.* New York: Stratton Intercontinental, 1977.
4. Fang FC, Fierer J. Human infection with *Salmonella dublin. Medicine* 1991;70:198–207.
5. Waterman SH, Juraez G, Carr SJ, et al. *Salmonella arizonae* infections in latinos associated with rattlesnake folk medicine. *Am J Public Health* 1990;80:286–289.
6. Bhatt BD, Zuckerman MJ, Foland JA, et al. Disseminated *Salmonella arizonae* infection associated with rattlesnake meat ingestions. *Am J Gastroenterol* 1989;84:433–435.
7. Louis PCA. *Recherches anatomiques, pathologiques et thérapeutiques sur la maladie connue sous les noms de gastroenterite, fièvre putride, adynamique, typhoïde, comparée avec les maladies aigues les plus ordinaires.* Paris: J-B Baillière, 1829.
8. Jenner W. *On the identity of typhoid and typhus fevers.* London: C. SJ. Adlard, 1850.
9. Wilson JC. *A treatise on the continued fevers.* New York: Wood Publishing, 1881.
10. Budd W. *Typhoid fever: its nature, mode of spreading, and prevention.* London: Longman's Publishing, 1873.
11. Schroeter J. *Kryptogamenflora von Schlesien Bd. 3.* Breslau: J. U. Kern, 1885.
12. Edelman R, Levine MM. Summary of an international workshop on typhoid fever. *Rev Infect Dis* 1986;8:329–349.
13. Pfeiffer R, Kalle W. Experimentelle untersuchunger zur Frage der Schitzimphung des Menschen geger thypus abdominalis. *Dtsch Med Wochenschr* 1896;22:735.
14. Widal F. Serodiagnostic de la fièvre typhoïde. *Bull Med Hop Paris* 1896;13:561–566.
15. Kauffman F. The diagnosis of *Salmonella* types. Springfield, IL: Charles C Thomas Publisher, 1950.
16. Woodward TE, Smadel JE, Ley HL, et al. Preliminary report on the beneficial effect of Chloromycetin in the treatment of typhoid fever. *Ann Intern Med* 1948;29:131–134.
17. Zinder ND, Lederberg J. Genetic exchange in *Salmonella. J Bacteriol* 1952;64:679–699.
18. Ames BN, Lee FD, Durston W. An improved bacterial test system for detection and classification of mutagens and carcinogens. *Proc Natl Acad Sci U S A* 1973;70:782–786.
19. Farmer JJ. Enterobacteriaceae: introduction and Identification. In: Murray PR, Baron EJ, Pfaller M, et al., eds. *Manual of clinical microbiology,* sixth edition. Washington, DC: American Society for Microbiology Press, 1995:438–449.
20. Popoff MY, Bockemühl J, Brenner FW. Supplement 1998 (No. 42) to the Kauffmann–White scheme. *Res Microbiol* 2000;151: 63–65.
21. Brenner FW, Villar RG, Angulo FJ, et al. *Salmonella* nomenclature. *J Clin Microbiol* 2000;38:2465–2467.
22. Gray LD. *Escherichia, Salmonella, Shigella,* and *Yersinia.* In: Murray PR, Baron EJ, Pfaller M, et al., eds. *Manual of clinical microbiology,* sixth edition. Washington, DC: American Society for Microbiology Press, 1995:450–456.
23. Forward KR, Rainnie BJ. Use of selenite enrichment broth for the detection of *Salmonella* from stool: a report of one year experience at a provincial public health laboratory. *Diagn Microbiol Infect Dis* 1997;29:215–217.
24. Ruiz J, Nunez ML, Diaz J, et al. Comparison of five plating media for isolation of *Salmonella* species from human stools. *J Clin Microbiol* 1996;34:686–688.
25. Banffer JRJ, van Zwol-Saaloos JA, Broere LJ. Evaluation of a commercial latex agglutination test for rapid detection of *Salmonella* in fecal samples. *Eur J Clin Microbiol Infect Dis* 1993; 12:633–636.
26. Chiu CH, Ou JT. Rapid identification of *Salmonella* serovars in feces by specific detection of virulence genes, *invA* and *spvC,* by an enrichment broth culture–multiplex PCR combination assay. *J Clin Microbiol* 1996;34:2619–2622.
27. Haedicke W, Wolf H, Ehret W, et al. Specific and sensitive two-step polymerase chain reaction assay for the detection of *Salmonella* species. *Eur J Clin Microbiol Infect Dis* 1996;15:603–607.
28. Makino S, Kurazono H, Chongsanguam M, et al. Establishment of the PCR system specific to *Salmonella* spp. and its application for the inspection of food and fecal samples. *J Vet Med Sci* 1999;61:1245–1247.
29. Felix A, Pitt RM. A new antigen of *B. typhosus. Lancet* 1934; 2:186–191.
30. Baker EE, Whiteside RE, Derow MA. The Vi antigen of the Enterobacteriaceae. II. Immunologic and biologic properties. *J Immunol* 1959;83:680–686.
31. Daniels EM, Schneerson R, Egan WE, et al. Characterization of the *Salmonella paratyphi C* Vi polysaccharide. *Infect Immun* 1989;57:3159–3164.
32. Heyns K, Kiessling G. Strukturaufklarung des Vi-antigens aus *Citrobacter freundii* and *E. coli* 5396/38. *Carbohydr Res* 1967;3: 340–352.
33. Gray PW, Flaggs G, Leong SR, et al. Cloning of a human neutrophil bactericidal protein. Structural and functional correlations. *J Biol Chem* 1989;264:9505–9509.
34. Anderson ES, Wand LR, De Saxe MJ, et al. Bacteriophage typing designations of *Salmonella typhimurium. J Hyg* 1977;78:297–300.
35. Gershman M. Single phage-typing set for differentiating salmonellae. *J Clin Microbiol* 1977;5:302–314.
36. Threlfall EJ, Chart H, Ward LR, et al. Interrelationships

between strains of *Salmonella enteritidis* belonging to phage types 4, 7, 7a, 8, 13, 13a, 23, 24, and 30. *J Appl Bacteriol* 1993; 75:43–48.
37. Altekruse S, Koehler J, Hickman-Brenner F, et al. A comparison of *Salmonella enteritidis* phage types from egg-associated outbreaks and implicated laying flocks. *Epidemiol Infect* 1993;110: 17–22.
38. Gulig PA, Danbara H, Guiney DG, et al. Molecular analysis of *spv* virulence genes of the *Salmonella* virulence plasmids. *Mol Microbiol* 1993;7:825–830.
39. Reeves MW, Evins GM, Heiba AA, et al. Clonal nature of *Salmonella typhi* and its genetic relatedness to other *Salmonella* as shown by multilocus enzyme electrophoresis, and proposal of *Salmonella bongori* comb. nov. *J Clin Microbiol* 1989;27:313–320.
40. Vatopoulos AC, Mainas E, Balis E, et al. Molecular epidemiology of ampicillin-resistant clinical isolates of *Salmonella enteritidis. J Clin Microbiol* 1994;32:1322–1325.
41. Saha SK, Talukder SY, Islam M, et al. A highly ceftriaxone-resistant *Salmonella typhi* in Bangladesh. *Pediatr Infect Dis J* 1999; 18:387.
42. O'Brien TF, Hopkins JD, Gilleece ES, et al. Molecular epidemiology of antibiotic resistance in *Salmonella* from animals and human beings in the United States. *N Engl J Med* 1982; 307:1–6.
43. Rodrigue DC, Cameron DN, Puhr ND, et al. Comparison of plasmid profile, phage types, and antimicrobial resistance patterns of *Salmonella enteritidis* isolates in the United States. *J Clin Microbiol* 1992;30:854–857.
44. Threlfall EJ, Hampton MD, Schofield SL, et al. Epidemiological application of differentiating multiresistant *Salmonella typhimurium* DT104 by plasmid profile. *Commun Dis Rep CDR Rev* 1996;6:R155–R159.
45. Esteban E, Snipes K, Hird D, et al. Use of ribotyping for characterization of *Salmonella* serotypes. *J Clin Microbiol* 1993;31: 233–237.
46. Guerra B, Landeras E, Gonzalez-Hevia MA, et al. A three-way ribotyping scheme for *Salmonella* serotype *typhimurium* and its usefulness for phylogenetic and epidemiological purposes. *J Med Microbiol* 1997;46:307–313.
47. Nastasi A, Mammina C, Fantasia M, et al. Epidemiological analysis of strains of *Salmonella enterica* serotype *enteritidis* from foodborne outbreaks occurring in Italy, 1980–1994. *J Med Microbiol* 1997;46:377–382.
48. Suzuki Y, Ishihara M, Matsumoto M, et al. Molecular epidemiology of *Salmonella enteritidis.* An outbreak and sporadic cases studied by means of pulsed-field gel electrophoresis. *J Infect* 1995;31:211–217.
49. Hampton MD, Ward LR, Rowe B, et al. Molecular fingerprinting of multidrug-resistant *Salmonella enterica* serotype *typhi. Emerging Infect Dis* 1998;4:317–320.
50. Threlfall EJ, Torre E, Ward LR, et al. Insertion sequence IS200 fingerprinting of *Salmonella typhi*: an assessment of epidemiological applicability. *Epidemiol Infect* 1994;112:253–261.
51. Pelkonen S, Romppanen EL, Siitonen A, et al. Differentiation of *Salmonella* serovar *infantis* isolates from human and animal sources by fingerprinting IS200 and 16S rrn loci. *J Clin Microbiol* 1994;32:2128–2133.
52. Millemann Y, Gaubert S, Remy D, et al. Evaluation of IS200-PCR and comparison with other molecular markers to trace *Salmonella enterica* subsp. *enterica* serotype *typhimurium* bovine isolates from farm to meat. *J Clin Microbiol* 2000;38:2204–2209.
53. Millemann Y, Lesage-Descauses MC, Lafont JP, et al. Comparison of random amplified polymorphic DNA analysis and enterobacterial repetitive intergenic consensus-PCR for epidemiological studies of *Salmonella. FEMS Immunol Med Microbiol* 1996;14:129–134.
54. Khan AA, Nawaz MS, Khan SA, et al. Detection of multidrug-resistant *Salmonella typhimurium* DT104 by multiplex polymerase chain reaction. *FEMS Microbiol Lett* 2000;182:355–360.
55. Ryan CA, Hargrett-Bean NT, Blake PA. *Salmonella typhi* infections in the United States, 1975–1984: increasing role of foreign travel. *Rev Infect Dis* 1989;11:1–8.
56. Dritz SK, Braff EH. Sexually transmitted typhoid fever. *N Engl J Med* 1977;296:1359–1360.
57. Weikel CS, Guerrant RL. Nosocomial salmonellosis [Editorial]. *Infect Control* 1985;6:218–220.
58. Blaser MJ, Hickman FW, Farmer JJD, et al. *Salmonella typhi*: the laboratory as a reservoir of infection. *J Infect Dis* 1980;142: 934–938.
59. Koay AS, Jegathesan M, Rohani MY, et al. Pulsed-field gel electrophoresis as an epidemiologic tool in the investigation of laboratory-acquired *Salmonella typhi* infection. *Southeast Asian J Trop Med Public Health* 1997;28:82–84.
60. Ivanoff B. *Typhoid fever: global situation and WHO recommendations.* Proceedings of the 2nd Asia–Pacific Symposium on Typhoid Fever and Other Salmonellosis. Bangkok: Infectious Disease Association of Thailand, 1994.
61. Bradaric N, Punda-Polic V, Milas I, et al. Two outbreaks of typhoid fever related to the war in Bosnia and Herzegovina. *Eur J Epidemiol* 1996;12:409–412.
62. Mermin JH, Villar R, Carpenter J, et al. A massive epidemic of multidrug-resistant typhoid fever in Tajikistan associated with consumption of municipal water. *J Infect Dis* 1999;179: 1416–1422.
63. Thikyakorn U, Mansuwan P, Taylor DN. Typhoid and paratyphoid fever in 192 children in Thailand. *Am J Dis Child* 1987;141:862–865.
64. Butler T, Islam A, Kabir I, et al. Patterns of morbidity and mortality in typhoid fever dependent on age and gender: review of 552 hospitalized patients with diarrhea. *Rev Infect Dis* 1991;13:85–90.
65. Barrett-Connor E. Bacterial infection and sickle cell anemia: an analysis of 250 infections in 166 patients and a review of the literature. *Medicine* 1971;50:97–112.
66. Neves J, Raso P, Marinko PP. Prolonged septicemic salmonellosis intercurrent with *Schistosomiasis mansoni* infection. *J Trop Med Hyg* 1971;74:9.
67. Black PH, Kunz KL, Swartz MN. Salmonellosis—a review of some unusual aspects. *N Engl J Med* 1960;262:864–870, 921–927.
68. Wheat LJ, Rubin RH, Harris NL, et al. Systemic salmonellosis in patients with disseminated histoplasmosis. Case for "macrophage blockade" caused by *Histoplasma capsulatum. Arch Intern Med* 1987;147:561–564.
69. Goldstein FW, Chumpitaz JC, Guevara JM, et al. Plasmid-mediated resistance to multiple antibiotics in *Salmonella typhi. J Infect Dis* 1986;153:261–266.
70. Bhutta ZA, Naqvi SH, Razzaq RA, et al. Multidrug-resistant typhoid in children: presentation and clinical features. *Rev Infect Dis* 1991;1991:832–836.
71. Vasquez V, Calderon E, Rodriquez R. Chloramphenicol- resistant strains of *Salmonella typhosa. N Engl J Med* 1972;286:1220.
72. Luby SP, Faizan MK, Fisher-Hoch SP, et al. Risk factors for typhoid fever in an endemic setting, Karachi, Pakistan. *Epidemiol Infect* 1998;120:129–138.
73. Threlfall EJ, Rowe B, Ward LR. Occurrence and treatment of multi-resistant *Salmonella typhi. Public Health Laboratory Service Microbiol Dig* 1991;8:56–59.
74. Paniker CK, Vimala KN. Transferable chloramphenicol resistance in *Salmonella typhi. Nature* 1972;239:109–110.
75. Anderson ES. The problem and implication of chloramphenicol resistance in the typhoid bacillus. *J Hyg* 1975;74:289–299.
76. Rowe B, Ward LR, Threlfall EJ. Multidrug-resistant *Salmonella*

typhi: a worldwide epidemic. *Clin Infect Dis* 1997;24[Suppl 1]: S106–S109.
77. Wain J, Hoa NT, Chinh NT, et al. Quinolone-resistant *Salmonella typhi* in Viet Nam: molecular basis of resistance and clinical response to treatment. *Clin Infect Dis* 1997;25:1404–1410.
78. Anand AC, Kataria VK, Singh W, et al. Epidemic multiresistant enteric fever in eastern India [Letter]. *Lancet* 1990;335:352.
79. Tarr PE, Kuppens L, Jones TC, et al. Considerations regarding mass vaccination against typhoid fever as an adjunct to sanitation and public health measures: potential use in an epidemic in Tajikistan. *Am J Trop Med Hyg* 1999;61:163–170.
80. Martin SM, Hardgrett-Bean N, Tauxe RV. *An atlas of Salmonella in the United States: serotype-specific surveillance 1968–1986.* Atlanta, GA: US Department of Health and Human Services, Public Health Services, Centers for Disease Control and Prevention, 1987.
81. Mermin JH, Townes JM, Gerber M, et al. Typhoid fever in the United States, 1985–1994: changing risks of international travel and increasing antimicrobial resistance. *Arch Intern Med* 1998;158:633–638.
82. Lin FYC, Becke JM, Groves C. Restaurant-associated outbreak of typhoid fever in Maryland: identification of carrier facilitated by measurement of serum Vi antibodies. *J Clin Microbiol* 1988; 26:1194–1197.
83. Shandera WX, Taylor JP, Betz TG, et al. An analysis of economic costs associated with an outbreak of typhoid fever. *Am J Public Health* 1985;75:71–73.
84. Birkhead GS, Morse DL, Levine WC, et al. Typhoid fever at a resort hotel in New York: a large outbreak with an unusual vehicle. *J Infect Dis* 1993;167:1228–1232.
85. Misra S, Diaz PS, Rowley AH. Characteristics of typhoid fever in children and adolescents in a major metropolitan area in the United States. *Clin Infect Dis* 1997;24:998–1000.
86. Ackers ML, Puhr ND, Tauxe RV, et al. Laboratory-based surveillance of *Salmonella* serotype *typhi* infections in the United States: antimicrobial resistance on the rise. *JAMA* 2000;283:2668–2673.
87. Mead PS, Slutsker L, Dietz V, et al. Food-related illness and death in the United States. *Emerging Infect Dis* 1999;5:607–625.
88. Centers for Disease Control and Prevention. Preliminary FoodNet data on the incidence of foodborne illnesses—selected sites, United States, 1999 [published erratum appears in *MMWR Morb Mortal Wkly Rep* 2000 Apr 7;49(13):286]. *MMWR Morb Mortal Wkly Rep* 2000;49:201–205.
89. Centers for Disease Control and Prevention. Summary of notifiable diseases, United States, 1998. *MMWR Morb Mortal Wkly Rep* 1999;47:ii–92.
90. Gorbach SL, Kean BH, Evans DG, et al. Travelers' diarrhea and toxigenic *Escherichia coli*. *N Engl J Med* 1975;292:933–936.
91. Mølbak K, Wested N, Højlyng N, et al. The etiology of early childhood diarrhea: a community study from Guinea-Bissau. *J Infect Dis* 1994;169:581–587.
92. Saidi SM, Iijima Y, Sang WK, et al. Epidemiological study on infectious diarrheal diseases in children in a coastal rural area of Kenya. *Microbiol Immunol* 1997;41:773–778.
93. Bean NH, Goulding JS, Lao C, et al. Surveillance for foodborne-disease outbreaks—United States, 1988–1992. *MMWR CDC Surveillance Summaries* 1996;45:1–66.
94. Todd EC. Epidemiology of foodborne diseases: a worldwide review. *World Health Stat Q* 1997;50:30–50.
95. St. Louis ME, Morse DL, Potter ME, et al. The emergence of grade A eggs as a major source of *Salmonella enteritidis* infections. New implications for the control of salmonellosis [see Comments]. *JAMA* 1988;259:2103–2107.
96. Mishu B, Koehler J, Lee LA, et al. Outbreaks of *Salmonella enteritidis* infections in the United States, 1985–1991. *J Infect Dis* 1994;169:547–552.
97. Centers for Disease Control and Prevention. Reptile-associated salmonellosis—selected states, 1996–1998. *MMWR Morb Mortal Wkly Rep* 1999;48:1009–1013.
98. Centers for Disease Control and Prevention. Outbreak of salmonellosis associated with beef jerky—New Mexico, 1995. *MMWR Morb Mortal Wkly Rep* 1995;44:785–788.
99. Woodward DL, Khakhria R, Johnson WM. Human salmonellosis associated with exotic pets. *J Clin Microbiol* 1997;35: 2786–2790.
100. Kramer MH, Herwaldt BL, Craun GF, et al. Surveillance for waterborne-disease outbreaks—United States, 1993–1994. *MMWR CDC Surveillance Summaries* 1996;45:1–33.
101. Angulo FJ, Tippen S, Sharp DJ, et al. A community waterborne outbreak of salmonellosis and the effectiveness of a boil water order. *Am J Public Health* 1997;87:580–584.
102. Chiodini RJ, Sundberg JP. Salmonellosis in reptiles: a review. *Am J Epidemiol* 1981;113:494–499.
103. Tauxe RV, Rigau-Perez JG, Wells JG, et al. Turtle-associated salmonellosis in Puerto Rico. Hazards of the global turtle trade. *JAMA* 1985;254:237–239.
104. Mermin J, Hoar B, Angulo FJ. Iguanas and *Salmonella marina* infection in children: a reflection of the increasing incidence of reptile-associated salmonellosis in the United States. *Pediatrics* 1997;99:399–402.
105. Sanyal D, Douglas T, Roberts R. *Salmonella* infection acquired from reptilian pets. *Arch Dis Child* 1997;77:345–346.
106. Centers for Disease Control and Prevention. *Salmonella* serotype *montevideo* infections associated with chicks— Idaho, Washington, and Oregon, spring 1995 and 1996. *MMWR Morb Mortal Wkly Rep* 1997;46:237–239.
107. Glaser CA, Angulo FJ, Rooney JA. Animal-associated opportunistic infections among persons infected with the human immunodeficiency virus [see Comments]. *Clin Infect Dis* 1994; 18:14–24.
108. Rodrigue DC, Tauxe RV, Rowe B. International increase in *Salmonella enteritidis*: a new pandemic? *Epidemiol Infect* 1990;105: 21–27.
109. Hedberg CW, David MJ, White KE, et al. Role of egg consumption in sporadic *Salmonella enteritidis* and *Salmonella typhimurium* infections in Minnesota. *J Infect Dis* 1993;167: 107–111.
110. Centers for Disease Control and Prevention. Outbreaks of *Salmonella* serotype *enteritidis* infection associated with eating raw or undercooked shell eggs—United States, 1996–1998. *MMWR Morb Mortal Wkly Rep* 2000;49:73–79.
111. Guard-Petter J, Henzler DJ, Rahman MM, et al. On-farm monitoring of mouse-invasive *Salmonella enterica* serovar *enteritidis* and a model for its association with the production of contaminated eggs. *Appl Environ Microbiol* 1997;63:1588–1593.
112. Guard-Petter J, Parker CT, Asokan K, et al. Clinical and veterinary isolates of *Salmonella enterica* serovar *enteritidis* defective in lipopolysaccharide O-chain polymerization. *Appl Environ Microbiol* 1999;65:2195–2201.
113. Keller LH, Benson CE, Krotec K, et al. *Salmonella enteritidis* colonization of the reproductive tract and forming and freshly laid eggs of chickens. *Infect Immun* 1995;63:2443–2449.
114. Altekruse SF, Cohen ML, Swerdlow DL. Emerging food-borne diseases. *Emerging Infect Dis* 1997;3:285–293.
115. Mohle-Boetani JC, Reporter R, Werner SB, et al. An outbreak of *Salmonella* serogroup *saphra* due to cantaloupes from Mexico. *J Infect Dis* 1999;180:1361–1364.
116. Centers for Disease Control and Prevention. Outbreak of *Salmonella* serotype *muenchen* infections associated with unpasteurized orange juice—United States and Canada, June 1999. *MMWR Morb Mortal Wkly Rep* 1999;48:582–585.
117. Mahon BE, Pönkä A, Hall WN, et al. An international out-

break of *Salmonella* infections caused by alfalfa sprouts grown from contaminated seeds. *J Infect Dis* 1997;175:876–882.
118. Taormina PJ, Beuchat LR, Slutsker L. Infections associated with eating seed sprouts: an international concern. *Emerging Infect Dis* 1999;5:626–634.
119. Hennessy TW, Hedberg CW, Slutsker L, et al. A national outbreak of *Salmonella enteritidis* infections from ice cream. *N Engl J Med* 1996;334:1281–1286.
120. Ryan CA, Nickels MK, Hargrett-Bean NT, et al. Massive outbreak of antimicrobial-resistant salmonellosis traced to pasteurized milk. *JAMA* 1987;258:3269–3274.
121. Centers for Disease Control and Prevention. *Salmonella* serotype *tennessee* in powdered milk products and infant formula—Canada and United States, 1993. *MMWR Morb Mortal Wkly Rep* 1993;42:516–517.
122. Desenclos JC, Bouvet P, Benz-Lemoine E, et al. Large outbreak of *Salmonella enterica* serotype *paratyphi B* infection caused by a goats' milk cheese, France, 1993: a case finding and epidemiological study [see Comments]. *BMJ* 1996;312:91–94.
123. Lehmacher A, Bockemuhl J, Aleksic S. Nationwide outbreak of human salmonellosis in Germany due to contaminated paprika and paprika-powdered potato chips. *Epidemiol Infect* 1995;115: 501–511.
124. Killalea D, Ward LR, Roberts D, et al. International epidemiological and microbiological study of outbreak of *Salmonella agona* infection from a ready to eat savoury snack—I: England and Wales and the United States [see Comments]. *BMJ (Clinical Research Ed)* 1996;313:1105–1107.
125. Pavia AT, Shipman LD, Wells JG, et al. Epidemiologic evidence that prior antimicrobial exposure decreases resistance to infection by antimicrobial-sensitive *Salmonella. J Infect Dis* 1990; 161:255–260.
126. World Health Organization. Control of *Salmonella* infections in animals and prevention of human foodborne *Salmonella* infections. *Bull World Health Organ* 1994;72:831.
127. Spika JS, Waterman SH, Hoo GW, et al. Chloramphenicol-resistant *Salmonella newport* traced through hamburger to dairy farms. A major persisting source of human salmonellosis in California. *N Engl J Med* 1987;316:565–570.
128. Zoukh K. Resistance to antibiotics of salmonellae other than *typhi* and *paratyphi* isolated in Algeria from 1979 to 1985 [in French]. *Pathologie Biologie* 1988;36:255–257.
129. Georges-Courbot MC, Wachsmuth IK, Bouquety JC, et al. Cluster of antibiotic-resistant *Salmonella enteritidis* infections in the Central African Republic. *J Clin Microbiol* 1990;28: 771–773.
130. Mirza NB, Wamola IA. *Salmonella typhimurium* outbreak at Kenyatta National Hospital (1985). *East Afr Med J* 1989;66: 453–457.
131. Lepage P, Bogaerts J, Van Goethem C, et al. Multiresistant *Salmonella typhimurium* systemic infection in Rwanda. Clinical features and treatment with cefotaxime. *J Antimicrob Chemother* 1990;26[Suppl A]:53–57.
132. Farhoudi-Moghaddam AA, Katouli M, Jafari A, et al. Antimicrobial drug resistance and resistance factor transfer among clinical isolates of salmonellae in Iran. *Scand J Infect Dis* 1990;22: 197–203.
133. Chowdhury MN. Antibiotic sensitivity pattern: experience at University Hospital, Riyadh, Saudi Arabia. *J Hyg Epidemiol Microbiol Immunol* 1991;35:289–301.
134. Shehabi AA. Extra-intestinal infections with multiply drug-resistant *Salmonella typhimurium* in hospitalized patients in Jordan. *Eur J Clin Microbiol Infect Dis* 1995;14:448–451.
135. Kariuki S, Gilks C, Corkill J, et al. Multi-drug resistant non-*typhi* salmonellae in Kenya. *J Antimicrob Chemother* 1996;38: 425–434.
136. Reina J, Gomez J. Decrease in resistance to ampicillin and co-trimoxazole in *Shigella* species isolated from faeces, 1983–1992 [Letter]. *J Antimicrob Chemother* 1994;33:1257–1258.
137. Munoz P, Diaz MD, Rodriquez-Creixems M, et al. Antimicrobial resistance of *Salmonella* isolates in a Spanish hospital. *Antimicrob Agents Chemother* 1993;37:1200.
138. Threlfall EJ, Rowe B, Ward LR. A comparison of multiple drug resistance in salmonellas from humans and food animals in England and Wales, 1981 and 1990. *Epidemiol Infect* 1993;111: 189–197.
139. MacDonald KL, Cohen ML, Hargrett-Bean NT, et al. Changes in antimicrobial resistance of *Salmonella* isolated from humans in the United States. *JAMA* 1987;258:1496–1499.
140. Lee LA, Puhr ND, Maloney EK, et al. Increase in antimicrobial-resistant *Salmonella* infections in the United States, 1989–1990. *J Infect Dis* 1994;170:128–134.
141. Kariuki S, Gilks C, Brindle R, et al. Antimicrobial susceptibility and presence of extrachromosomal deoxyribonucleic acid in *Salmonella* and *Shigella* isolates from patients with AIDS. *East Afr Med J* 1994;71:292–296.
142. Boyd EF, Hartl DL. Recent horizontal transmission of plasmids between natural populations of *Escherichia coli* and *Salmonella enterica. J Bacteriol* 1997;179:1622–1627.
143. Morosini MI, Blázquez J, Negri MC, et al. Characterization of a nosocomial outbreak involving an epidemic plasmid encoding for TEM-27 in *Salmonella enterica* subspecies *enterica* serotype *othmarschen. J Infect Dis* 1996;174:1015–1020.
144. Casin I, Breuil J, Brisabois A, et al. Multidrug-resistant human and animal *Salmonella typhimurium* isolates in France belong predominantly to a DT104 clone with the chromosome- and integron-encoded beta-lactamase PSE-1. *J Infect Dis* 1999;179: 1173–1182.
145. Glynn MK, Bopp C, Dewitt W, et al. Emergence of multidrug-resistant *Salmonella enterica* serotype *typhimurium* DT104 infections in the United States [see Comments]. *N Engl J Med* 1998;338:1333–1338.
146. Baggesen DL, Sandvang D, Aarestrup FM. Characterization of *Salmonella enterica* serovar *typhimurium* DT104 isolated from Denmark and comparison with isolates from Europe and the United States. *J Clin Microbiol* 2000;38:1581–1586.
147. Threlfall EJ, Frost JA, Ward LR, et al. Increasing spectrum of resistance in multiresistant *Salmonella typhimurium* [Letter]. *Lancet* 1996;347:1053–1054.
148. Wall PG, Morgan D, Lamden K, et al. A case–control study of infection with an epidemic strain of multiresistant *Salmonella typhimurium* DT104 in England and Wales. *Commun Dis Rep CDR Rev* 1994;4:R130–R135.
149. Wall PG, Morgan D, Lamden K, et al. Transmission of multiresistant strains of *Salmonella typhimurium* from cattle to man. *Vet Rec* 1995;136:591–592.
150. Threlfall EJ, Ward LR, Skinner JA, et al. Increase in multiple antibiotic resistance in nontyphoidal salmonellas from humans in England and Wales: a comparison of data for 1994 and 1996. *Microb Drug Resist* 1997;3:263–266.
151. Mølbak K, Baggesen DL, Aarestrup FM, et al. An outbreak of multidrug-resistant, quinolone-resistant *Salmonella enterica* serotype *typhimurium* DT104. *N Engl J Med* 1999;341: 1420–1425.
152. Bauernfeind A, Casellas JM, Goldberg M, et al. A new plasmidic cefotaximase from patients infected with *Salmonella typhimurium. Infection* 1992;20:158–163.
153. Poupart MC, Chanal C, Sirot D, et al. Identification of CTX-2, a novel cefotaximase from a *Salmonella mbandaka* isolate. *Antimicrob Agents Chemother* 1991;35:1498–1500.
154. Barguellil F, Burucoa C, Amor A, et al. *In vivo* acquisition of extended-spectrum beta-lactamase in *Salmonella enteritidis* dur-

ing antimicrobial therapy. *Eur J Clin Microbiol Infect Dis* 1995; 14:703–706.

155. Vahaboglu H, Hall LM, Mulazimoglu L, et al. Resistance to extended-spectrum cephalosporins, caused by PER-1 beta-lactamase, in *Salmonella typhimurium* from Istanbul, Turkey. *J Med Microbiol* 1995;43:294–299.
156. Bhatia R, Kaur P, John PC, et al. Transferable beta-lactam resistance against cephalosporins in *Salmonella typhimurium* strains in India. *Ind J Med Res* 1994;99:203–205.
157. Wattal C, Kaul V, Chugh TD, et al. An outbreak of multidrug resistant *Salmonella typhimurium* in Delhi (India). *Ind J Med Res* 1994;100:266–267.
158. Gaillot O, Clément C, Simonet M, et al. Novel transferable beta-lactam resistance with cephalosporinase characteristics in *Salmonella enteritidis. J Antimicrob Chemother* 1997;39:85–87.
159. Fey PD, Safranek TJ, Rupp ME, et al. Ceftriaxone-resistant *Salmonella* infection acquired by a child from cattle [see Comments]. *N Engl J Med* 2000;342:1242–1249.
160. Digranes A, Solberg CO, Sjursen H, et al. Antibiotic susceptibility of blood culture isolates of Enterobacteriaceae from six Norwegian hospitals 1991–1992. *APMIS* 1997;105:854–860.
161. Giraud E, Cloeckaert A, Kerboeuf D, et al. Evidence for active efflux as the primary mechanism of resistance to ciprofloxacin in *Salmonella enterica* serovar *typhimurium. Antimicrob Agents Chemother* 2000;44:1223–1228.
162. Heisig P. High-level fluoroquinolone resistance in a *Salmonella typhimurium* isolate due to alterations in both *gyrA* and *gyrB* genes. *J Antimicrob Chemother* 1993;32:367–377.
163. Reyna F, Huesca M, González V, et al. *Salmonella typhimurium gyrA* mutations associated with fluoroquinolone resistance. *Antimicrob Agents Chemother* 1995;39:1621–1623.
164. Griggs DJ, Gensberg K, Piddock LJ. Mutations in *gyrA* gene of quinolone-resistant *Salmonella* serotypes isolated from humans and animals. *Antimicrob Agents Chemother* 1996;40:1009–1013.
165. Herikstad H, Hayes P, Mokhtar M, et al. Emerging quinolone-resistant *Salmonella* in the United States. *Emerging Infect Dis* 1997;3:371–372.
166. Frost JA, Kelleher A, Rowe B. Increasing ciprofloxacin resistance in salmonellas in England and Wales 1991-1994. *J Antimicrob Chemother* 1996;37:85–91.
167. Maiorini E, Lopez EL, Morrow AL, et al. Multiply resistant nontyphoidal *Salmonella* gastroenteritis in children. *Pediatr Infect Dis J* 1993;12:139–145.
168. Roberts FJ. Nontyphoidal, nonparatyphoidal *Salmonella* septicemia in adults. *Eur J Clin Microbiol Infect Dis* 1993;12: 205–208.
169. Wall PG, Ryan MJ, Ward LR, et al. Outbreaks of salmonellosis in hospitals in England and Wales: 1992–1994. *J Hosp Infect* 1996;33:181–190.
170. Nair D, Gupta N, Kabra S, et al. *Salmonella senftenberg*: a new pathogen in the burns ward. *Burns* 1999;25:723–727.
171. Gupta A, Matsui K, Lo JF, et al. Molecular basis for resistance to silver cations in *Salmonella. Nat Med* 1999;5:183–188.
172. Standaert SM, Hutcheson RH, Schaffner W. Nosocomial transmission of *Salmonella* gastroenteritis to laundry workers in a nursing home. *Infect Control Hosp Epidemiol* 1994;15:22–26.
173. Wall PG, Ryan MJ. Faecal incontinence in hospitals and residential and nursing homes for elderly people [Letter; Comment]. *BMJ (Clin Res Ed)* 1996;312:378.
174. Tauxe RV, Hassan LF, Findeisen KO, et al. Salmonellosis in nurses: lack of transmission to patients. *J Infect Dis* 1988;157: 370–373.
175. Wilson R, Feldman RA, Davis J, et al. Salmonellosis in infants: the importance of intrafamilial transmission. *Pediatrics* 1982; 69:436–438.
176. Agunod M, Yamaguchi N, Lopez R, et al. Correlative study of hydrochloric acid, pepsin, and intrinsic factor secretion in newborns and infants. *Am J Dig Dis* 1969;14:400–414.
177. Haddock RL, Cousens SN, Guzman CC. Infant diet and salmonellosis. *Am J Public Health* 1991;81:997–1000.
178. Chorba TL, Meriwether RA, Jenkins BR, et al. Control of a non-foodborne outbreak of salmonellosis: day care in isolation. *Am J Public Health* 1987;77:979–981.
179. Evans HS, Maguire H. Outbreaks of infectious intestinal disease in schools and nurseries in England and Wales 1992 to 1994 [published erratum appears in *Commun Dis Rep CDR Rev* 1996 Aug 16;6(9):R128]. *Commun Dis Rep CDR Rev* 1996;6: R103–R108.
180. Buchwald DS, Blaser MJ. A review of human salmonellosis: II. Duration of excretion following infection with non-*typhi Salmonella. Rev Infect Dis* 1984;6:345–356.
181. Blaser MJ, Feldman RA. From the Centers for Disease Control. *Salmonella* bacteremia: reports to the Centers for Disease Control, 1968–1979. *J Infect Dis* 1981;143:743–746.
182. Riley LW, Cohen ML, Seals JE, et al. Importance of host factors in human salmonellosis caused by multiresistant strains of *Salmonella. J Infect Dis* 1984;149:878–883.
183. Taylor JL, Dwyer DM, Groves C, et al. Simultaneous outbreak of *Salmonella enteritidis* and *Salmonella schwarzengrund* in a nursing home: association of *S. enteritidis* with bacteremia and hospitalization [Letter]. *J Infect Dis* 1993;167:781–782.
184. Levine WC, Smart JF, Archer DL, et al. Foodborne disease outbreaks in nursing homes, 1975 through 1987. *JAMA* 1991;266: 2105–2109.
185. Smith PW. Consensus conference on nosocomial infections in long-term care facilities. *Am J Infect Control* 1987;15:97–100.
186. Blaser MJ, Neuman LS. A review of human salmonellosis: I. Infective dose. *Rev Infect Dis* 1982;4:1096.
187. Mintz ED, Cartter ML, Hadler JL, et al. Dose–response effects in an outbreak of *Salmonella enteritidis. Epidemiol Infect* 1994; 112:13–23.
188. Waddell WR, Kunz LJ. Association of *Salmonella enteritis* with operation of stomach. *N Engl J Med* 1956;255:555–559.
189. Gianella RA, Broitman SA, Zamcheck N. Gastric acid barrier to ingested microorganisms in man: studies *in vivo* and *in vitro. Gut* 1972;13:251–256.
190. McCullough NB, Eisele CW. Experimental human salmonellosis. IV. Pathogenicity of strains of *Salmonella pullorum* obtained from spray-dried whole egg. *J Infect Dis* 1951;89:1540–1545.
191. Gorden J, Small PL. Acid resistance in enteric bacteria. *Infect Immun* 1993;61:364–367.
192. Foster JW, Hall HK. Adaptive acidification tolerance response of *Salmonella typhimurium. J Bacteriol* 1990;172:771–778.
193. Selsted ME, Miller SI, Henschen AH, et al. Enteric defensins: antibiotic peptide components of intestinal host defense. *J Cell Biol* 1992;118:929–936.
194. Lehrer RI, Ganz T, Selsted ME. Defensins: endogenous antibiotic peptides of animal cells. *Cell* 1991;64:229–230.
195. Michetti P, Mahan MJ, Slauch JM, et al. Monoclonal secretory immunoglobulin A protects mice against oral challenge with the invasive pathogen *Salmonella typhimurium. Infect Immun* 1992;60:1786–1792.
196. Brandtzaeg P. Overview of the mucosal immune system. *Curr Top Microbiol Immunol* 1989;146:13–25.
197. Kohbata S, Yokoyama H, Yabuuchi E. Cytopathogenic effect of *Salmonella typhi* GIFU 10007 on M cells of murine ileal Peyer's patches in ligated ileal loops: an ultrastructural study. *Microbiol Immunol* 1986;30:1225–1237.
198. Takeuchi A. Electron microscopic studies of experimental *Salmonella* infection I. Penetration into the intestinal epithelium by *Salmonella typhimurium. Am J Pathol* 1967;50:109–136.
199. Francis CL, Starnbach. MN, Falkow S. Morphological and

cytoskeletal changes in epithelial cells occur immediately upon interaction with *Salmonella typhimurium* grown under low-oxygen conditions. *Mol Microbiol* 1992;6:3077–3087.
200. Finlay BB, Falkow S. Comparison of the invasion strategies used by *Salmonella cholerae-suis, Shigella flexneri* and *Yersinia enterocolitica* to enter cultured animal cells: endosome acidification is not required for bacterial invasion or intracellular replication. *Biochimie* 1988;70:1089–1099.
201. Pace J, Hayman MJ, Galán JE. Signal transduction and invasion of epithelial cells by *S. typhimurium. Cell* 1993;72:505–514.
202. Galan JE, Pace J, Hayman MJ. Involvement of the epidermal growth factor receptor in the invasion of cultured mammalian cells by *Salmonella typhimurium. Nature* 1992;357:588–589.
203. Finlay BB, Gumbiner B, Falkow S. Penetration of *Salmonella* through a polarized Madin-Darby canine kidney epithelial cell monolayer. *J Cell Biol* 1988;107:221–230.
204. Vazquez-Torres A, Jones-Carson J, Baumler AJ, et al. Extraintestinal dissemination of *Salmonella* by CD18-expressing phagocytes. *Nature* 1999;401:804–808.
205. Hackett J, Kotlarski I, Mathan V, et al. The colonization of Peyer's patches by a strain of *Salmonella typhimurium* cured of the cryptic plasmid. *J Infect Dis* 1986;153:1119–1125.
206. Rubin FA, McWhirter PD, Burr D, et al. Rapid diagnosis of typhoid fever through identification of *Salmonella typhi* within 18 hours of specimen acquisition by culture of the mononuclear cell-platelet fraction of blood. *J Clin Microbiol* 1990;28:825–827.
207. Hornick RB, Greisman SE, Woodward TE, et al. Typhoid fever: pathogenesis and immunologic control. *N Engl J Med* 1970; 283:686–691.
208. Greisman SE, Woodward TE, Hornick RB, et al. Typhoid fever: a study of pathogenesis and physiologic abnormalities. *Trans Am Clin Climatol Assoc* 1961;73:146–161.
209. Looney RJ, Steigbigel RT. Role of the Vi antigen of *Salmonella typhi* in resistance to host defense *in vitro. J Lab Clin Med* 1986;108:506–516.
210. Ciacci-Woolwine F, Blomfield IC, Richardson SH, et al. *Salmonella* flagellin induces tumor necrosis factor alpha in a human promonocytic cell line. *Infect Immun* 1998;66:1127–1134.
211. Medzhitov R, Janeway C Jr. Innate immune recognition: mechanisms and pathways. *Immunol Rev* 2000;173:89–97.
212. Alpuche-Aranda CM, Racoosin EL, Swanson JA, et al. *Salmonella* stimulate macrophage macropinocytosis and persist within spacious phagosomes. *J Exp Med* 1994;179:601–608.
213. Alpuche-Aranda CM, Swanson JA, Loomis WP, et al. *Salmonella typhimurium* activates virulence gene transcription within acidified macrophage phagosomes. *Proc Natl Acad Sci U S A* 1992;89:10079–10083.
214. Oh Y-K, Alpuche-Aranda CM, Berthiaume E, et al. Rapid and complete fusion of macrophage lysosomes with phagosomes containing *Salmonella typhimurium. Infect Immun* 1996;64: 3877–3883.
215. Rathman M, Barker LP, Falkow S. The unique trafficking pattern of *Salmonella typhimurium*-containing phagosomes in murine macrophages is independent of the mechanism of bacterial entry. *Infect Immun* 1997;65:1475–1485.
216. Chen LM, Kaniga K, Galán JE. *Salmonella* spp. are cytotoxic for cultured macrophages. *Mol Microbiol* 1996;21:1101–1115.
217. Monack DM, Raupach B, Hromockyj AE, et al. *Salmonella typhimurium* invasion induces apoptosis in infected macrophages. *Proc Natl Acad Sci U S A* 1996;93:9833–9838.
218. Monack DM, Hersh D, Ghori N, et al. *Salmonella* exploits caspase-1 to colonize Peyer's patches in a murine typhoid model. *J Exp Med* 2000;192:249–258.
219. Weiss J, Victor M, Stendhal O, et al. Killing of gram-negative bacteria by polymorphonuclear leukocytes: role of an O_2-independent bactericidal system. *J Clin Invest* 1982;69:959–970.
220. Mills DM, Bajaj V, Lee CA. A 40-kb chromosomal fragment encoding *Salmonella typhimurium* invasion genes is absent from the corresponding region of the *Escherichia coli* K-12 chromosome. *Mol Microbiol* 1995;15:749–759.
221. Shea JE, Hensel M, Gleeson C, et al. Identification of a virulence locus encoding a second type III secretion system in *Salmonella typhimurium. Proc Natl Acad Sci U S A* 1996;93:2593–2597.
222. Collazo CM, Galán JE. The invasion-associated type III system of *Salmonella typhimurium* directs the translocation of Sip proteins into the host cell. *Mol Microbiol* 1997;24:747–756.
223. Pegues DA, Hantman MJ, Behlau I, et al. PhoP/PhoQ transcriptional repression of *Salmonella typhimurium* invasion genes: evidence for a role in protein secretion. *Mol Microbiol* 1995;17:169–181.
224. McCormick BA, Miller SI, Delp-Archer C, et al. Transepithelial signaling to neutrophils by *Salmonella*: a novel virulence mechanism for gastroenteritis. *Infect Immun* 1995;63:2302–2309.
225. Hueck CJ, Hantman MJ, Bajaj V, et al. *Salmonella typhimurium*-secreted invasion determinants are homologous to *Shigella* Ipa proteins. *Mol Microbiol* 1995;18:479–490.
226. Miao EA, Miller SI. A conserved amino acid sequence directing intracellular type III secretion by *Salmonella typhimurium. Proc Natl Acad Sci U S A* 2000;97:7539–7544.
227. Miller SI, Kukral AM, Mekalanos JJ. A two-component regulatory system (*phoP phoQ*) controls *Salmonella typhimurium* virulence. *Proc Natl Acad Sci U S A* 1989;86:5054–5058.
228. Guo L, Lim K, Gunn JS, et al. Regulation of lipid A modifications by *Salmonella typhimurium* virulence genes *phoP-phoQ. Science* 1997;276:250–253.
229. Moncrief MB, Maguire ME. Magnesium and the role of MgtC in growth of *Salmonella typhimurium. Infect Immun* 1998;66: 3802–3809.
230. Guo L, Lim KB, Poduje CM, et al. Lipid A acylation and bacterial resistance against vertebrate antimicrobial peptides. *Cell* 1998;95:189–198.
231. Hohmann EL, Oletta CA, Killeen KP, et al. *phoP/phoQ*-deleted *Salmonella typhi* (TY800) is a safe and immunogenic single dose typhoid fever vaccine in volunteers. *J Infect Dis* 1996;173: 1408–1414.
232. De Groote MA, Testerman T, Xu Y, et al. Homocysteine antagonism of nitric oxide-related cytostasis in *Salmonella typhimurium. Science* 1996;272:414–417.
233. Fang FC, DeGroote MA, Foster JW, et al. Virulent *Salmonella typhimurium* has two periplasmic Cu, Zn-superoxide dismutases. *Proc Natl Acad Sci U S A* 1999;96:7502–7507.
234. Finlay BB, Falkow S. Virulence factors associated with *Salmonella* species. *Microbiol Sci* 1988;5:324–328.
235. Reitmeyer JC, Peterson JW, Wilson KJ. *Salmonella* cytotoxin: a component of the bacterial outer membrane. *Microb Pathog* 1986;1:503–510.
236. Tacket CO, Hone DM, Curtiss III R, et al. Comparison of the safety and immunogenicity of *ΔaroC ΔaroD* and *Δcya Δcrp Salmonella typhi* strains in adult volunteers. *Infect Immun* 1992;60: 536–541.
237. Levine MM, Herrington D, Murphy JR, et al. Safety, infectivity, immunogenicity, and *in vivo* stability of two attenuated auxotrophic mutant strains of *Salmonella typhi,* 541Ty and 543Ty, as live oral vaccines in humans. *J Clin Invest* 1987;79:888–902.
238. Aguero J, Faundez G, Nunez M, et al. Choleriform syndrome and production of labile enterotoxin (CT/LT1)-like antigen by species of *Salmonella infantis* and *Salmonella haardt* isolated from the same patient. *Rev Infect Dis* 1991;13:420–423.
239. Peterson NJ. *Salmonella* toxins. In: Dorner F, Drews J, eds. *Pharmacology of bacterial toxins.* New York: Pergamon Press, 1986:227–234.
240. Eckmann L, Rudolf MT, Ptasznik A, et al. D-Myo-inositol-

1,4,5,6-tetrakisphosphate produced in human intestinal epithelial cells in response to *Salmonella* invasion inhibits phosphoinositide-3-kinase signaling pathways. *Proc Natl Acad Sci U S A* 1997;94:14456–14460.
241. Norris FA, Wilson MP, Wallis TS, et al. SopB, a protein required for virulence of *Salmonella dublin,* is an inositol phosphate phosphatase [see Comments]. *Proc Natl Acad Sci U S A* 1998;95:14057–14059.
242. McCormick BA, Colgan SP, Delp-Archer C, et al. *Salmonella typhimurium* attachment to human intestinal epithelial monolayers: transcellular signalling to subepithelial neutrophils. *J Cell Biol* 1993;123:895–907.
243. Hobbie S, Chen LM, Davis RJ, et al. Involvement of mitogen-activated protein kinase pathways in the nuclear responses and cytokine production induced by *Salmonella typhimurium* in cultured intestinal epithelial cells. *J Immunol* 1997;159:5550–5559.
244. O'Brien AD. Innate resistance of mice to *Salmonella typhi* infection. *Infect Immun* 1982;38:948–952.
245. Lissner CR, Swanson R, O'Brien A. Genetic control of the innate resistance of mice to *Salmonella typhimurium*: expression of the *Ity* gene in peritoneal and splenic macrophages isolated *in vitro. J Immunol* 1983;131:3006–3013.
246. Vidal SM, Malo D, Vogan K, et al. Natural resistance to infection with intracellular parasites: isolation of a candidate for Bcg. *Cell* 1993;73:469–485.
247. Vidal SM, Pinner E, Lepage P, et al. Natural resistance to intracellular infections: *Nramp1* encodes a membrane phosphoglycoprotein absent in macrophages from susceptible (Nramp1D169) mouse strains. *J Immunol* 1996;157:3559–3568.
248. Gruenheid S, Pinner E, Desjardins M, et al. Natural resistance to infection with intracellular pathogens: the Nramp1 protein is recruited to the membrane of the phagosome. *J Exp Med* 1997; 185:717–730.
249. Gruenheid S, Canonne-Hergaux F, Gauthier S, et al. The iron transport protein NRAMP2 is an integral membrane glycoprotein that colocalizes with transferrin in recycling endosomes. *J Exp Med* 1999;189:831–841.
250. Jabado N, Jankowski A, Dougaparsad S, et al. Natural resistance to intracellular infections. Natural resistance-associated macrophage protein 1 (nramp1) functions as a pH-dependent manganese transporter at the phagosomal membrane [In Process Citation]. *J Exp Med* 2000;192:1237–1248.
251. Poltorak A, He X, Smirnova I, et al. Defective LPS signaling in C3H/HeJ and C57BL/10ScCr mice: mutations in *Tlr4* gene. *Science* 1998;282:2085–2088.
252. Han T, Sokal JE, Neter E. Salmonellosis in disseminated malignant diseases. A seven-year review (1959–1965). *N Engl J Med* 1967;276:1045–1052.
253. Wolfe MS, Louria DB, Armstrong D, et al. Salmonellosis in patients with neoplastic disease. A review of 100 episodes at Memorial Cancer Center over a 13-year period. *Arch Intern Med* 1971;128:546–554.
254. Mussche MM, Lameire NH, Ringoir SM. *Salmonella typhimurium* infections in renal transplant patients. Report of five cases. *Nephron* 1975;15:143–150.
255. Sperber SJ, Schleupner CJ. Salmonellosis during infection with human immunodeficiency virus. *Rev Infect Dis* 1987;9:925–934.
256. Celum CL, Chaisson RE, Rutherford GW, et al. Incidence of salmonellosis in patients with AIDS. *J Infect Dis* 1987;156: 998–1002.
257. Angulo FJ, Swerdlow DL. Bacterial enteric infections in persons infected with human immunodeficiency virus. *Clin Infect Dis* 1995;21[Suppl 1]:S84–S93.
258. de Jong R, Altare F, Haagen IA, et al. Severe mycobacterial and *Salmonella* infections in interleukin-12 receptor-deficient patients. *Science* 1998;280:1435–1438.
259. MacFarlane AS, Peng X, Meissler JJ Jr, et al. Morphine increases susceptibility to oral *Salmonella typhimurium* infection. *J Infect Dis* 2000;181:1350–1358.
260. Moellering RC Jr, Weinberg AN. Persistent *Salmonella* infection in a female carrier for chronic granulomatous disease. *Ann Intern Med* 1970;73:595–601.
261. Wright J, Thomas P, Serjeant GR. Septicemia caused by *Salmonella* infection: an overlooked complication of sickle cell disease [see Comments]. *J Pediatr* 1997;130:394–399.
262. Giannella RA, Broitman SA, Zamcheck N. Gastric acid barrier to ingested microorganisms in man: studies *in vivo* and *in vitro. Gut* 1972;13:251–256.
263. Levine MM, Ferreccio C, Black RE, et al. Progress in vaccines against typhoid fever. *Rev Infect Dis* 1989;11[Suppl 3]: S552–S567.
264. Marmion DE, Naylor GRE, Stewart IO. Second attacks of typhoid fever. *J Hyg* 1953;51:260–267.
265. Forrest BD, LaBrooy JT, Beyer L, et al. The human humoral immune response to *Salmonella typhi* Ty21a. *J Infect Dis* 1991; 163:336–345.
266. Acharya IL, Lowe CU, Thapa R, et al. Prevention of typhoid fever in Nepal with the Vi capsular polysaccharide of *Salmonella typhi.* A preliminary report. *N Engl J Med* 1987;317:1101–1104.
267. Lanata CF, Levine MM, Ristori C, et al. Vi serology in detection of chronic *Salmonella typhi* carriers in an endemic area. *Lancet* 1983;2:441–443.
268. Blanden RV, Mackaness GB, Collins FM. Mechanisms of acquired resistance in mouse typhoid. *J Exp Med* 1966;124: 585–600.
269. Murphy JR, Wasserman SS, Baqar S, et al. Immunity to *Salmonella typhi*: considerations relevant to measurement of cellular immunity in typhoid-endemic regions. *Clin Exp Immunol* 1989;75:228–233.
270. Nencioni L, Villa L, De Magistris MT, et al. Cellular immunity against *Salmonella typhi* after live oral vaccine. *Adv Exp Med Biol* 1987;216B:1669–1675.
271. Saphra I, Winter JW. Clinical manifestations of salmonellosis in man: an evaluation of 7,779 human infections identified at the New York Salmonella Center. *N Engl J Med* 1957;256:1128.
272. Dagash M, Hayek T, Gallimidi Z, et al. Transient radiological and colonoscopic features of inflammatory bowel disease in a patient with severe *Salmonella* gastroenteritis. *Am J Gastroenterol* 1997;92:349–351.
273. Askeroff B, Schroder SA. Salmonellosis in the United States—a 5-year review. *Am J Epidemiol* 1970;92:13.
274. Szanton VL. Epidemic salmonellosis. *Pediatrics* 1957;20: 794–808.
275. Stuart BM, Pullen RL. Typhoid: clinical analysis of three hundred and sixty cases. *Arch Intern Med* 1946;78:629–661.
276. Arand AC, Kataria VK, Singh W, et al. Epidemic multiresistant enteric fever in Eastern India. *Lancet* 1990;335:352.
277. Sugandhi Rao P, Rajashekar V, Varghese GK, et al. Emergence of multidrug-resistant *Salmonella typhi* in rural southern India. *Am J Trop Med Hyg* 1993;48:108–111.
278. Carmeli Y, Raz R, Schapiro JM, et al. Typhoid fever in Ethiopian immigrants to Israel and native-born Israelis: a comparative study. *Clin Infect Dis* 1993;16:213–215.
279. Gotuzzo E, Frisancho O, J. S, et al. Association between the acquired immunodeficiency syndrome and infection with *Salmonella typhi* or *Salmonella paratyphi* in an area endemic for typhoid fever. *Arch Intern Med* 1991;151:381–382.
280. Hoffman TA, Ruiz CJ, Counts GW. Water-borne typhoid fever in Dade County, FL: clinical and therapeutic evaluations of 105 bacteremic patients. *Am J Med* 1975;59:481.
281. Roland HAK. The complications of typhoid fever. *J Trop Med Hyg* 1961;64:143.

282. Verghese A. The "typhoid state" revisited. *Am J Med* 1985;79:370–372.
283. Hoffman SL, Punjabi NH, Kumala S, et al. Reduction of mortality in chloramphenicol-treated severe typhoid fever by high-dose dexamethasone. *N Engl J Med* 1984;310:82–88.
284. Hearne SE, Whigham TE, Brady CEI. Pancreatitis and typhoid fever. *Am J Med* 1989;86:471–473.
285. Cohen JI, Bartlett JA, Corey GR. Extra-intestinal manifestations of *Salmonella* infections. *Medicine* 1987;66:349–388.
286. Khan M, Coovadia YM, Connolly C, et al. Influence of sex on clinical features, laboratory findings, and complications of typhoid fever. *Am J Trop Med Hyg* 1999;61:41–46.
287. Julià J, Canet JJ, Lacasa XM, et al. Spontaneous spleen rupture during typhoid fever. *Int J Infect Dis* 2000;4:108–109.
288. Khan M, Coovadia YM, Connoly C, et al. The early diagnosis of typhoid fever prior to the Widal test and bacteriological culture results. *Acta Trop* 1998;69:165–173.
289. El-Newihi HM, Alamy ME, Reynolds TB. Salmonella hepatitis: analysis of 27 cases and comparison with acute viral hepatitis. *Hepatology* 1996;24:516–519.
290. Calva JJ, Ruiz-Palacios GM. *Salmonella* hepatitis: detection of *Salmonella* antigens in the liver of patients with typhoid fever [Letter]. *J Infect Dis* 1986;154:373–374.
291. Khourieh M, Schlesinger M, Tabachnik E, et al. Typhoid fever diagnosed by isolation of *S. typhi* from gastric aspirate. *Acta Pediatr Scand* 1989;78:653–655.
292. Avendano A, Herrera P, Horwitz I, et al. Duodenal string cultures: practicality and sensitivity for diagnosing enteric fever in children. *J Infect Dis* 1986;153:359–362.
293. Gilman RH, Terminel M, Hernandez-Mendoza P, et al. Relative efficacy of blood, urine, rectal swab, bone-marrow and rose-spot cultures for recovery of *Salmonella typhi* in typhoid fever. *Lancet* 1975;1:1211–1213.
294. Hoffman SL, Punjabi NH, Rockhill RC, et al. Duodenal string-capsule culture compared with bone-marrow, blood, and rectal-swab cultures for diagnosing typhoid and paratyphoid fever. *J Infect Dis* 1984;149:157–161.
295. Benavente L, Gotuzzo E, Guerra J, et al. Diagnosis of typhoid fever using a string capsule device. *Trans R Soc Trop Med Hyg* 1984;78:564–565.
296. Farooqui BJ, Khurshid M, Ashfaq MK, et al. Comparative yield of *Salmonella typhi* from blood and bone marrow cultures in patients with fever of unknown origin. *J Clin Pathol* 1991;44:258–259.
297. Watson K. Isolation of *Salmonella typhi* from the blood stream. *J Lab Clin Med* 1959;47:329–332.
298. Guerra-Caceres JG, Gotuzzo-Herencia E, Crosby-Dagnino E, et al. Diagnostic value of bone marrow culture in typhoid fever. *Trans R Soc Trop Med Hyg* 1979;73:680–683.
299. Wain J, Diep TS, Ho VA, et al. Quantitation of bacteria in blood of typhoid fever patients and relationship between counts and clinical features, transmissibility, and antibiotic resistance. *J Clin Microbiol* 1998;36:1683–1687.
300. Gasem MH, Dolmans WM, Isbandrio BB, et al. Culture of *Salmonella typhi* and *Salmonella paratyphi* from blood and bone marrow in suspected typhoid fever. *Trop Geogr Med* 1995;47:164–167.
301. Welch H, Mickle FL. A rapid slide test for the serological diagnosis of typhoid and paratyphoid fevers. *Am J Public Health* 1936;26:248–255.
302. Isomaki O, Vuento R, Granfors K. Serological diagnosis of *Salmonella* infections by enzyme immunoassay. *Lancet* 1989;1:1411–1414.
303. Coovadia YM, Singh V, Bhana RH, et al. Comparison of passive haemagglutination test with Widal agglutination test for serological diagnosis of typhoid fever in an endemic area. *J Clin Pathol* 1986;39:680–683.
304. Abraham G, Teklu B, Gedebu M, et al. Diagnostic value of the Widal test. *Trop Geogr Med* 1981;33:329–333.
305. Wicks ACB, Cruickshank JG, Musewe N. Observations on the diagnosis of typhoid fever in an endemic area. *S Afr Med J* 1974;48:1368–1370.
306. Shukla S, Patel B, Chitnis DS. One hundred years of Widal test and its reappraisal in an endemic area. *Ind J Med Res* 1997;105:53–57.
307. Lim PL, Tam FC, Cheong YM, et al. One-step 2-minute test to detect typhoid-specific antibodies based on particle separation in tubes. *J Clin Microbiol* 1998;36:2271–2278.
308. Bhutta ZA, Mansurali N. Rapid serologic diagnosis of pediatric typhoid fever in an endemic area: a prospective comparative evaluation of two dot-enzyme immunoassays and the Widal test. *Am J Trop Med Hyg* 1999;61:654–657.
309. Cocolin L, Manzano M, Astori G, et al. A highly sensitive and fast non-radioactive method for the detection of polymerase chain reaction products from *Salmonella* serovars, such as *Salmonella typhi,* in blood specimens. *FEMS Immunol Med Microbiol* 1998;22:233–239.
310. Chaudhry R, Laxmi BV, Nisar N, et al. Standardisation of polymerase chain reaction for the detection of *Salmonella typhi* in typhoid fever. *J Clin Pathol* 1997;50:437–439.
311. Cohen PS, O'Brien TF, Schoenbaum SC, et al. The risk of endothelial infection in adults with *Salmonella* bacteremia. *Ann Intern Med* 1978;89:931–932.
312. Levine WC, Buehler JW, Bean NH, et al. Epidemiology of non-typhoidal *Salmonella* bacteremia during the human immunodeficiency virus epidemic. *J Infect Dis* 1991;164:81–87.
313. Shimoni Z, Pitlik S, Leibovici L, et al. Nontyphoid *Salmonella* bacteremia: age-related differences in clinical presentation, bacteriology, and outcome. *Clin Infect Dis* 1999;28:822–827.
314. Zaidi E, Bachur R, Harper M. Non-*typhi Salmonella* bacteremia in children. *Pediatr Infect Dis J* 1999;18:1073–1077.
315. Sirinavin S, Jayanetra P, Thakkinstian A. Clinical and prognostic categorization of extraintestinal nontyphoidal *Salmonella* infections in infants and children. *Clin Infect Dis* 1999;29:1151–1156.
316. Parsons R, Gregory J, Palmer DL. *Salmonella* infections of the abdominal aorta. *Rev Infect Dis* 1983;5:227–231.
317. Gabbi E, Rossi G, Ghidoni I. *Salmonella typhimurium* infection of thoracic aorta aneurysm in immunocompetent subject. Case report and literature review. *Infection* 1989;17:306–308.
318. Tocalli L, Nardi G, Mammino A, et al. Salmonellosis diagnosed by the laboratory of the "L. Sacco" Hospital of Milan (Italy) in patients with HIV disease. *Eur J Epidemiol* 1991;7:690–695.
319. Ramos JM, Garcia-Corbeira P, Aguado JM, et al. Clinical significance of primary vs. secondary bacteremia due to nontyphoid *Salmonella* in patients without AIDS. *Clin Infect Dis* 1994;19:777–780.
320. Gilks CF, Ojoo SA. A practical approach to the clinical problems of the HIV-infected adult in the tropics. *Tropical Doctor* 1991;21:90–97.
321. Gutiérrez A, Teira R, Varona M, et al. Recurrent *Salmonella enteritidis* meningitis in a patient with AIDS. *Scand J Infect Dis* 1995;27:177–178.
322. Fernández Guerrero ML, Ramos JM, et al. Focal infections due to non-*typhi Salmonella* in patients with AIDS: report of 10 cases and review. *Clin Infect Dis* 1997;25:690–697.
323. Vugia DJ, Kiehlbauch JA, Yeboue K, et al. Pathogens and predictors of fatal septicemia associated with human immunodeficiency virus infection in Ivory Coast, West Africa. *J Infect Dis* 1993;168:564–570.
324. Gilks CF, Brindle RJ, Otieno LS, et al. Life-threatening bacteraemia in HIV-1 seropositive adults admitted to hospital in Nairobi, Kenya [see Comments]. *Lancet* 1990;336:545–549.

325. Archibald LK, den Dulk MO, Pallangyo KJ, et al. Fatal *Mycobacterium tuberculosis* bloodstream infections in febrile hospitalized adults in Dar es Salaam, Tanzania. *Clin Infect Dis* 1998;26:290–296.
326. Wolday D, Erge W. Antimicrobial sensitivity pattern of *Salmonella*: comparison of isolates from HIV-infected and HIV-uninfected patients. *Tropical Doctor* 1998;28:139–141.
327. Okome-Kouakou M, Bekale J, Kombila M. Salmonellosis in HIV infection in a hospital setting in Gabon [in French]. *Med Trop (Mars)* 1999;59:46–50.
328. Council of State and Territorial Epidemiologists, AIDS Program, Center for Infectious Disease. Revision of the CDC surveillance case definition for acquired immunodeficiency syndrome. *MMWR Morb Mortal Wkly Rep* 1987;36[Suppl 1]:1S.
329. Salmon D, Detruchis P, Leport C, et al. Efficacy of zidovudine in preventing relapses of *Salmonella* bacteremia in AIDS. *J Infect Dis* 1991;163:415–416.
330. Casado JL, Valdezate S, Calderon C, et al. Zidovudine therapy protects against *Salmonella* bacteremia recurrence in human immunodeficiency virus-infected patients. *J Infect Dis* 1999; 179:1553–1556.
331. Aguado JM, Ramos JM, Garcia-Corbeira P, et al. The clinical spectrum of focal infection due to nontyphoid *Salmonella*: 32 years' experience [in Spanish]. *Med Clin (Barc)* 1994;103: 293–298.
332. Musher DM, Rubenstein AD. Permanent carriers of nontyphosal salmonellae. *Public Health Rep* 1973;132:869.
333. Balfour AE, Lewis R, Ahmed S. Convalescent excretion of *Salmonella enteritidis* in infants. *J Infect* 1999;38:24–25.
334. Nath G, Singh H, Shukla VK. Chronic typhoid carriage and carcinoma of the gallbladder. *Eur J Cancer Prev* 1997;6: 557–559.
335. Agalar C, Usubütün S, Tütüncü E, et al. Comparison of two regimens for ciprofloxacin treatment of enteric infections. *Eur J Clin Microbiol Infect Dis* 1997;16:803–806.
336. Centers for Disease Control and Prevention. *Health information for international travel 1999–2000.* Atlanta, GA: Department of Health and Human Services, 1999.
337. Woodruff BA, Pavia AT, Blake PA. A new look at typhoid vaccination. *JAMA* 1991;265:756–759.
338. Comission YT. A controlled field trial of the effectiveness of acetone-dried and inactivated and heat phenol-inactivated typhoid vaccines in Yugoslavia. *Bull World Health Organ* 1964;30: 623–630.
339. Hejfec LB, Salmin LV, Lejtman MZ, et al. A controlled field trial and laboratory study of five typhoid vaccines in the USSR. *Bull World Health Organ* 1966;34:321–339.
340. Ashcroft MT, Morrison RJ, Nicholson CC. Controlled field trial in British Guiana school children of heat-killed phenolized and acetone-killed lyophilized typhoid vaccines. *Am J Hyg* 1964; 79:196–206.
341. Ashcroft MT, Singh B, Nicholson CC, et al. A seven-year field trial of two typhoid vaccines in Guyana. *Lancet* 1967;2: 1056–1059.
342. Typhoid vaccination: weighing the options [Editorial]. *Lancet* 1992;340:341–342.
343. Research WRAIo. Preparation of dried acetone-inactivated and heat-phenol-inactivated typhoid vaccines. Bull World Health Organ 1964:30.
344. Edwards EA, Johnson DP, Pierce WE, et al. Reactions and serologic responses to monovalent acetone-inactivated typhoid vaccine and heat-killed TAB when given by jet injection. *Bull World Health Organ* 1974;51:501–505.
345. Hone DM, Attridge SR, Forrest B, et al. A *galE* Via (Vi antigen)-negative mutant of *Salmonella typhi* Ty2 retains virulence in humans. *Infect Immun* 1988;56:1326–1333.
346. Black RE, Levine MM, Clements ML, et al. Prevention of shigellosis by a *Salmonella typhi-Shigella sonnei* bivalent vaccine. *J Infect Dis* 1987;155:1260–1265.
347. Levine MM, Ferreccio C, Black RE, et al. Large-scale field trial of Ty21a live oral typhoid vaccine in enteric-coated capsule formulation. *Lancet* 1987;1:1049–1052.
348. Simanjuntak CH, Paleologo FP, Punjabi NH, et al. Oral immunisation against typhoid fever in Indonesia with Ty21a vaccine [see Comments]. *Lancet* 1991;338:1055–1059.
349. Kaplan DT, Hill DR. Compliance with live oral Ty21a a typhoid vaccine. *JAMA* 1992;267:1074.
350. Hessel L, Debois H, Fletcher M, et al. Experience with *Salmonella typhi* Vi capsular polysaccharide vaccine. *Eur J Clin Microbiol Infect Dis* 1999;18:609–620.
351. Klugman KP, Koornhof HJ, Robbins JB, et al. Immunogenicity, efficacy and serological correlate of protection of *Salmonella typhi* Vi capsular polysaccharide vaccine three years after immunization. *Vaccine* 1996;14:435–438.
352. El Ramli A. Chloramphenicol in treatment of typhoid fever. *Lancet* 1950;1:618.
353. Olarte J, Galindo E. *S. typhi* resistant to chloramphenicol, ampicillin, and other antimicrobial agents: strains isolated and extensive typhoid fever epidemic in Mexico. *Antimicrob Agents Chemother* 1973;4:597–601.
354. Lampe PM, Mansuwan P, Duangmain C. Chloramphenicol-resistant typhoid. *Lancet* 1974;1:623–624.
355. Butler T, Rumans L, Arnold K. Response of typhoid-fever caused by chloramphenicol-susceptible and chloramphenicol-resistant strains of *Salmonella typhi* to treatment with trimethroprim-sulfamethoxazole. *Rev Infect Dis* 1982;4:551–561.
356. Bouquier Y, Hervonet D, Hilleritean H. Résultats du traitement par la chloromycétine de soixante fièvres typhoïdes. *Bull Mem Soc Med Hop Paris* 1949;32:1396.
357. Erselv A. Hematopoietic depression induced by Chloromycetin. *Blood* 1953;8:170–174.
358. Wallerstein RO, Condit PK, Kasper CK, et al. Statewide study of chloramphenicol therapy and fatal aplastic anemia. *JAMA* 1969;208:2045–2050.
359. Glazko AJ, Dill WA, Kinkel AW, et al. Absorption and excretion of parenteral doses of chloramphenicol sodium succinate (CMS) in comparison with peroral doses of chloramphenicol (CM). *Clin Pharmacol Ther* 1977;21:104.
360. Ti TT, Monteiro EH, Lam S, et al. Chloramphenicol concentrations in sera of patients with typhoid fever being treated with oral or intravenous preparation. *Antimicrob Agents Chemother* 1990;34:1809–1811.
361. Rahal JJJ, Simberkoff MS. Bactericidal and bacteriostatic action of chloramphenicol against meningeal pathogens. *Antimicrob Agents Chemother* 1979;16:13–18.
362. Chang HR, Vladoianu IR, Pechere JC. Effects of ampicillin, ceftriaxone, chloramphenicol, pefloxacin and trimethoprim-sulphamethoxazole on *Salmonella typhi* within human monocyte-derived macrophages. *J Antimicrob Chemother* 1990;26:689–694.
363. Brown JD, Mo DH, Rhoades ER. Chloramphenicol-resistant *Salmonella typhi* in Saigon. *JAMA* 1975;231:162–166.
364. Linh NN, Arnold K. Treatment of typhoid fever and typhoid carriers in South East Asia: viewpoint from South Vietnam. *Drugs* 1975;9:241–246.
365. Pillay N, Adams EB, North-Coobes D. Comparative trial of amoxicillin and chloramphenicol in treatment of typhoid fever in adults. *Lancet* 1975;2:332–334.
366. Scragg JN, Rubidge CJ. Amoxicillin in the treatment of typhoid fever in children. *Am J Trop Med Hyg* 1975;24:860–865.
367. Herzog C. Chemotherapy of typhoid fever. *Infection* 1976;4: 166–173.
368. Brodie J, MacQueen IA. Effect of trimethroprim-sulfamethox-

azole on typhoid and *Salmonella* carriers. *Br Med J* 1970;3: 318–319.
369. Vimala KN, Paniker CK. Resistance transfer between *E. coli* and *Salmonella* strains from Kerala. *Ind J Med Res* 1972;60:334–338.
370. Threlfall EJ, Graham A, Cheasty T, et al. Resistance to ciprofloxacin in pathogenic Enterobacteriaceae in England and Wales in 1996. *J Clin Pathol* 1997;50:1027–1028.
371. Moosa A, Rubidge CJ. Once daily ceftriaxone vs. chloramphenicol for treatment of typhoid fever in children. *Pediatr Infect Dis J* 1989;8:696–699.
372. Pape JW, Gerdes H, Oriol L, et al. Typhoid fever: successful therapy with cefoperazone. *J Infect Dis* 1986;153:272–276.
373. Islam A, Butler T, Nath SK, et al. Randomized treatment of patients with typhoid fever by using ceftriaxone or chloramphenicol. *J Infect Dis* 1988;158:742–747.
374. Bhutta ZA. Therapeutic aspects of typhoidal salmonellosis in childhood: the Karachi experience. *Ann Trop Paediatr* 1996;16: 299–306.
375. Soe GB, Overturf GD. Treatment of typhoid fever and other systemic salmonelloses with cefotaxime, ceftriaxone, cefoperazone, and other newer cephalosporins. *Rev Infect Dis* 1987;9:719.
376. Memon IA, Billoo AG, Memon HI. Cefixime: an oral option for the treatment of multidrug-resistant enteric fever in children. *South Med J* 1997;90:1204–1207.
377. Girgis NI, Tribble DR, Sultan Y, et al. Short-course chemotherapy with cefixime in children with multidrug-resistant *Salmonella typhi* septicaemia. *J Trop Pediatr* 1995;41:364–365.
378. Butler T, Sridhar CB, Daga MK, et al. Treatment of typhoid fever with azithromycin versus chloramphenicol in a randomized multicentre trial in India. *J Antimicrob Chemother* 1999;44: 243–250.
379. Tanaka Kido J, Ortega L, Santos JI. Comparative efficacies of aztreonam and chloramphenicol in children with typhoid fever. *J Pediatr Infect Dis* 1990;9:44–48.
380. Farid Z, Girgis NI, Kamal M, et al. Successful aztreonam treatment of acute typhoid fever after chloramphenicol failure. *Scand J Infect Dis* 1990;22:505–506.
381. Choo KE, Ariffin WA, Ong KH, et al. Aztreonam failure in typhoid fever. *Lancet* 1991;337:498.
382. Cherubin CE, Eng RHK, Smith SM, et al. Cephalosporin therapy for salmonellosis. *Arch Intern Med* 1986;146:2149–2152.
383. Preblud SR, Gill CJ, Campos JM. Bactericidal activities of chloramphenicol and eleven other antibiotics against *Salmonella* spp. *Antimicrob Agents Chemother* 1984;3:327–330.
384. Barros F, Korzeniowski OM, Sande MA, et al. *In vitro* antibiotic susceptibility of *Salmonellae. Antimicrob Agents Chemother* 1977;6:1071–1073.
385. De Carvalho EM, Martinelli R. Cefamandole treatment of *Salmonella* bacteremia. *Antimicrob Agents Chemother* 1982;21: 334–336.
386. Vaudaux P, Waldvogel FA. Gentamicin antibacterial activity in the presence of human polymorphonuclear leukocytes. *Antimicrob Agents Chemother* 1979;16:743–749.
387. Rodriguez-Noriega E, Andrade-Villaneuva J, Amaya-Tapia G. Quinolones in the treatment of *Salmonella* carriers. *Rev Infect Dis* 1989;11:S1179–S1187.
388. Easmon CSF, Crane JP, Blowers A. Effect of ciprofloxacin on intracellular organisms: *in vitro* and *in vivo* studies. *J Antimicrob Chemother* 1986;18:43–48.
389. Stanley PJ, Flegg PJ, Mandal B, et al. Open study of ciprofloxacin in enteric fever. *J Antimicrob Chem* 1989;23:789–791.
390. Mandal BK. Treatment of multiresistant typhoid fever [Letter; Comment]. *Lancet* 1990;336:1383.
391. Sabbour MS, Osman LM. Experience with ofloxacin in enteric fever. *J Chemother* 1990;2:113–115.
392. Sarma PS, Durairaj P. Randomized treatment of patients with typhoid and paratyphoid fevers using norfloxacin or chloramphenicol. *Trans R Soc Trop Med Hyg* 1991;85:670–671.
393. Arnold K, Hong CS, Nelwan R, et al. Randomized comparative study of fleroxacin and chloramphenicol in typhoid fever. *Am J Med* 1993;94:3A195S–3A200S.
394. Piddock LJ, Whale K, Wise R. Quinolone resistance in *Salmonella*: clinical experience [Letter]. *Lancet* 1990;335:1459.
395. Piddock LJ, Griggs DJ, Hall MC, et al. Ciprofloxacin resistance in clinical isolates of *Salmonella typhimurium* obtained from two patients. *Antimicrob Agents Chemother* 1993;37:662–666.
396. Lewin CS. Treatment of multiresistant *Salmonella* infection. *Lancet* 1991;337:47.
397. Threlfall EJ, Ward LR, Skinner JA, et al. Ciprofloxacin-resistant *Salmonella typhi* and treatment failure [Letter]. *Lancet* 1999; 353:1590–1591.
398. Christ W, Lehner T, Ulbrich B. Specific toxicologic aspects of the quinolones. *Rev Infect Dis* 1988;10[Suppl I]:141–146.
399. Cheesbrough JS, Mwema FI, Green SD, et al. Quinolones in children with invasive salmonellosis [Letter; Comment]. *Lancet* 1991;338:127.
400. Dawood ST, Uwaydah AK. Treatment of multiresistant *Salmonella typhi* with intravenous ciprofloxacin. *Pediatr Infect Dis* 1991;10:343.
401. Seçmeer G, Kanra G, Figen G, et al. Ofloxacin versus co-trimoxazole in the treatment of typhoid fever in children. *Acta Paediatr Jpn* 1997;39:218–221.
402. Thomsen LL, Paerregaard A. Treatment with ciprofloxacin in children with typhoid fever. *Scand J Infect Dis* 1998;30:355–357.
403. Cooles P. Adjuvant steroids and relapse of typhoid fever. *J Trop Med Hyg* 1986; :229——231.
404. Richards L, Claeson M, Pierce NF. Management of acute diarrhea in children: lessons learned. *Pediatr Infect Dis J* 1993;12:5.
405. Sirinavin S, Garner P. Antibiotics for treating *Salmonella* gut infections. *Cochrane Database Syst Rev* 2000;93:CD001167.
406. Kassis I, Dagan R, Chipman M, et al. The use of prophylactic furazolidone to control a nosocomial epidemic of multiply resistant *Salmonella typhimurium* in pediatric wards. *Pediatr Infect Dis J* 1990;9:551–555.
407. Lightfoot NF, Ahmad F, Cowden J. Management of institutional outbreaks of *Salmonella* gastroenteritis. *J Antimicrob Chemother* 1990;26:37–46.
408. Gendrel D, Raymond J, Legall MA, et al. Use of pefloxacin after failure of initial antibiotic treatment in children with severe salmonellosis. *Eur J Clin Microbiol Infect Dis* 1993;12:209–211.
409. Gokalp AS, Toksoy HB, Turkay S, et al. Intravenous immunoglobulin in the treatment of *Salmonella typhimurium* infections in preterm neonates. *Clin Pediatr (Phila)* 1994;33: 349–352.
410. Wang JH, Liu YC, Yen MY, et al. Mycotic aneurysm due to non-*typhi Salmonella*: report of 16 cases. *Clin Infect Dis* 1996; 23:743–747.
411. Meerkin D, Yinnon AM, Munter RG, et al. *Salmonella* mycotic aneurysm of the aortic arch: case report and review [see Comments]. *Clin Infect Dis* 1995;21:523–528.
412. Donabedian H. Long-term suppression of *Salmonella* aortitis with an oral antibiotic. *Arch Intern Med* 1989;149:1452–1453.
413. Jacobson MA, Hahn SM, Gerberding JL, et al. Ciprofloxacin for *Salmonella* bacteremia in the acquired immunodeficiency syndrome (AIDS). *Ann Intern Med* 1989;110:1027–1029.
414. Lewin CS, Allen RA, Amyes SG. Antibacterial activity of fluoroquinolones in combination with zidovudine. *J Med Microbiol* 1990;33:127–131.
415. Salmon-Ceron D, Detruchis P, Jaccard A, et al. Non-typhic *Salmonella* bacteremias in HIV infections. Clinical and therapeutic data, and course in 68 patients [in French]. *Presse Med* 1992;21: 847–851.

416. Centers for Disease Control and Prevention. Recommendations for prophylaxis against *Pneumocystis carinii* pneumonia for adults and adolescents infected with human immunodeficiency virus. *MMWR Morb Mortal Wkly Rep* 1992;41:1–11.
417. Gibb AP, Lewin CS, Garden OJ. Development of quinolone resistance and multiple antibiotic resistance in *Salmonella bovismorbificans* in a pancreatic abscess [Letter]. *J Antimicrob Chemother* 1991;28:318–321.
418. Workman MR, Philpott-Howard J, Bragman S, et al. Emergence of ciprofloxacin resistance during treatment of *Salmonella* osteomyelitis in three patients with sickle cell disease. *J Infect* 1996;32:27–32.
419. Pers C, Søgaard P, Pallesen L. Selection of multiple resistance in *Salmonella enteritidis* during treatment with ciprofloxacin. *Scand J Infect Dis* 1996;28:529–531.
420. Nolan CM, White PCJ. Treatment of typhoid carrier with amoxicillin. *JAMA* 1978;239:2352–2354.
421. Freerksen E, Rosenfield M, Freerksen REA. Treatment of chronic *Salmonella* carriers. *Chemotherapy* 1977;23:192.
422. Sammalkorpi K, Lahdevirta J, Makela R. Treatment of chronic *Salmonella* carriers with ciprofloxacin. *Lancet* 1987;2:164–165.
423. Ferreccio C, Morris JG Jr, Valdivieso C, et al. Efficacy of ciprofloxacin in the treatment of chronic typhoid carriers. *J Infect Dis* 1988;157:1235.
424. Freitag JL. Treatment of chronic typhoid carrier by cholecystectomy. *Public Health* 1973;32:869.
425. Hogue A, White P, Guard-Petter J, et al. Epidemiology and control of egg-associated *Salmonella enteritidis* in the United States of America. *Rev Sci Tech* 1997;16:542–553.
426. Fisher IST, Rowe B, Bartlett CLR, et al. "Salm-Net"-laboratory-based surveillance of human *Salmonella* infections in Europe. *PHLS Microbiol Dig* 1994;11:181.
427. Hastings L, Burnens A, de Jong B, et al. Salm-Net facilitates collaborative investigation of an outbreak of *Salmonella tosamanga* infection in Europe. *Commun Dis Rep CDR Rev* 1996;6:R100–R102.
428. Khuri-Bulos NA, Abu Khalaf M, Shehabi A, et al. Food handler-associated *Salmonella* outbreak in a university hospital despite routine surveillance cultures of kitchen employees. *Infect Control Hosp Epidemiol* 1994;15:311–314.
429. Garner JS. Guideline for isolation precautions in hospitals. The Hospital Infection Control Practices Advisory Committee [published erratum appears in *Infect Control Hosp Epidemiol* 1996 Apr;17(4):214]. *Infect Control Hosp Epidemiol* 1996;17:53–80.
430. Centers for Disease Control and Prevention. Draft guideline for infection control in health care personnel, 1997—CDC. Notice. *Federal Register* 1997;62:47276–47327.
431. Alvarez-Elcoro S, Soto-Ramirez L, Metos-Mora M. *Salmonella* bacteremia. *Am J Med* 1984;77:61–63.
432. Zak FG, Strauss L, Saphra I. Rupture of diseased large arteries in the course of enterobacterial (*Salmonella*) infection. *N Engl J Med* 1958;258:824–828.
433. Morrow C, Safi H, Beall AC Jr. Primary aortoduodenal fistula caused by *Salmonella* aortitis. *J Vasc Surg* 1987;6:415–418.
434. Jarrett F, Darling CR, Mundth E, et al. Experience with infected aneurysms of the abdominal aorta. *Arch Surg* 1975; 110:1281–1286.
435. Soravia-Dunand VA, Loo VG, Salit IE. Aortitis due to *Salmonella*: report of 10 cases and comprehensive review of the literature. *Clin Infect Dis* 1999;29:862–868.
436. Kinsella TR, Yogev R, Shulman ST, et al. Treatment of *Salmonella* meningitis and brain abscess with the new cephalosporins: two case reports and a review of literature. *Pediatr Infect Dis J* 1987;6:476–480.
437. Rabinowitz SG, MacLeod NR. *Salmonella* meningitis. A report of three cases and review of the literature. *Am J Dis Child* 1972; 123:529.
438. Dunn DW, McAllister J, Craft JC. Brain abscess and empyema caused by *Salmonella. Pediatr Infect Dis* 1984;4:394–398.
439. Bryan JP, Scheld WM. Therapy of experimental meningitis due to *Salmonella enteritidis. Antimicrob Agents Chemother* 1992;36: 949–954.
440. Huang LT, Ko SF, Lui CC. *Salmonella* meningitis: clinical experience of third-generation cephalosporins. *Acta Paediatr* 1997; 86:1056–1058.
441. Lee WS, Puthucheary SD, Omar A. *Salmonella* meningitis and its complications in infants. *J Paediatr Child Health* 1999;35: 379–382.
442. Chiu CH, Ou JT. Persistence of *Salmonella* species in cerebrospinal fluid of patients with meningitis following ceftriaxone therapy. *Clin Infect Dis* 1999;28:1174–1175.
443. Kumari P, Kan VL. *Salmonella typhimurium* brain abscess: post-operative complication. *Clin Infect Dis* 2000;30:621–622.
444. Aguado JM, Obeso G, Cabanillas JJ, et al. Pleuropulmonary infections due to nontyphoidal strains of *Salmonella. Arch Intern Med* 1990;150:54–56.
445. Diggs LW. Bone and joint lesions in sickle cell disease. *Clin Orthop* 1967;52:119–143.
446. Hook EW, Campbell CG, Weens HS, et al. *Salmonella* osteomyelitis in patients with sickle cell anemia. *N Engl J Med* 1957;257:403–407.
447. Santos EM, Sapico FL. Vertebral osteomyelitis due to salmonellae: report of two cases and review. *Clin Infect Dis* 1998;27:287–295.
448. Hakansson U, Eitrem R, Low B, et al. HLA-antigen B27 in cases with joint affections in an outbreak of salmonellosis. *Scand J Infect Dis* 1976;8:245–248.
449. Maki-Ikola O, Leirisalo-Repo M, Kantele A, et al. *Salmonella*-specific antibodies in reactive arthritis. *J Infect Dis* 1991;164: 1141–1148.
450. Thomson GT, DeRubeis DA, Hodge MA, et al. Post-*Salmonella* reactive arthritis: late clinical sequelae in a point source cohort. *Am J Med* 1995;98:13–21.
451. Leirisalo-Repo M, Helenius P, Hannu T, et al. Long-term prognosis of reactive *Salmonella* arthritis. *Ann Rheum Dis* 1997;56: 516–520.
452. Ekman P, Kirveskari J, Granfors K. Modification of disease outcome in *Salmonella*-infected patients by HLA-B27. *Arthritis Rheum* 2000;43:1527–1534.
453. Warren CPW. Arthritis associated with *Salmonella* infection. *Ann Rheum Dis* 1970;29:483–487.
454. Stein M, Houston S, Pozniak A, et al. HIV infection and *Salmonella* septic arthritis. *Clin Exp Rheumatol* 1993;11:187–189.
455. Chen JY, Luo SF, Wu YJ, et al. *Salmonella* septic arthritis in systemic lupus erythematosus and other systemic diseases. *Clin Rheumatol* 1998;17:282–287.
456. Collazos J, Mayo J, Martínez E, et al. Muscle infections caused by *Salmonella* species: case report and review. *Clin Infect Dis* 1999;29:673–677.
457. Neuwirth C, Francois C, Laurent N, et al. Myocarditis due to *Salmonella virchow* and sudden infant death [Letter]. *Lancet* 1999;354:1004.
458. Marr J, Haff R. Superinfection of an amoebic abscess by *Salmonella enteritidis. Arch Intern Med* 1971;128:291–294.
459. Matossian RM, Najjar F. Suppurative salmonellosis in human hepatic hydatid cysts. *Ann Trop Med Parasitol* 1968;62:143–146.
460. McConkey SJ, McCarthy ND, Keane CT. Primary peritonitis due to nonenteric salmonellae. *Clin Infect Dis* 1999;29:211–212.
461. Torres JR, Gatuzzo E, Isturiz R, et al. *Salmonella* splenic abscess in the antibiotic era: a Latin American perspective. *Clin Infect Dis* 1994;19:871.

462. Ramos JM, Aguado JM, García-Corbeira P, et al. Clinical spectrum of urinary tract infections due to nontyphoidal *Salmonella* species. *Clin Infect Dis* 1996;23:388–390.
463. Ozdemir S, Topaloglu R, Ecevit Z, et al. A rare cause of acute tubulointerstitial nephritis: *Salmonella typhimurium* infection [Letter]. *Nephrol Dial Transplant* 1997;12:1542–1543.
464. Burgmans JP, van Erp EJ, Brimicombe RW, et al. *Salmonella enteritidis* in an endometriotic ovarian cyst. *Eur J Obstet Gynecol Reprod Biol* 1997;72:207–211.
465. Behr MA, McDonald J. *Salmonella* neck abscess in a patient with beta-thalassemia major: case report and review. *Clin Infect Dis* 1996;23:404–405.
466. Carswell W, Magrath IT. Skin ulceration caused by *Salmonella dublin. Br Med J* 1973;1:331–332.
467. Hirchowitz B. Pyogenic liver abscess. A review with a case report of a solitary abscess caused by *Salmonella enteritidis. Gastroenterology* 1952;21:291–299.
468. de la Fuente-Aguado J, Bordón J, Esteban AR, Aguilar A, Moreno JA. Spontaneous non-typhoidal *Salmonella peritonitis* in patients with serious underlying disorders. *Infection* 1999;27:224–227.

45

YERSINIA ENTEROCOLITICA AND *YERSINIA PSEUDOTUBERCULOSIS*

TIMOTHY L. COVER
ROY M. ROBINS-BROWNE

DESCRIPTION

Infection of humans with *Yersinia enterocolitica* most frequently results in diarrheal illness, but may be associated with a wide spectrum of other clinical manifestations, including abdominal pain, septicemia, arthritis, and erythema nodosum (1–4). *Yersinia pseudotuberculosis* is an enteropathogen of wild and domestic animals that causes human disease less commonly than *Y. enterocolitica. Yersinia pestis,* the cause of bubonic plague, is not discussed in this chapter. Several other *Yersinia* species, including *Yersinia bercovieri, Yersinia mollaretii, Yersinia intermedia, Yersinia kristensenii, Yersinia frederiksenii, Yersinia aldovae,* and *Yersinia rohdei,* are widespread in the environment but are rarely human pathogens.

MICROBIOLOGY

Y. enterocolitica and *Y. pseudotuberculosis* are facultatively anaerobic gram-negative organisms that are classified in the family Enterobacteriaceae. Metabolic and nutritional requirements and synthetic functions of these organisms are regulated by temperature. At 25°C, the organisms are motile and have minimal nutritional requirements, whereas at 37°C, they are nonmotile, require additional nutrients for growth (4), and produce various plasmid-encoded proteins related to virulence. Like *Escherichia coli* and salmonellae, *Y. enterocolitica* is a heterogeneous species, comprised of more than 50 O antigen serotypes and several biotypes and phage types (4). However, only a few pathogenic *Y. enterocolitica* serotypes commonly cause human disease (1–4). *Y. pseudotuberculosis* and *Y. pestis* exhibit a high level of chromosomal DNA relatedness, whereas chromosomal DNA from *Y. enterocolitica* shows greater divergence (4).

EPIDEMIOLOGY

The frequency of *Y. enterocolitica* infection as a cause of diarrheal illness has been assessed in several studies in which stool cultures were collected from diarrheic persons. In Montreal, *Y. enterocolitica* organisms were isolated from 2.8% of 6,364 symptomatic children during a 15-month period (5). In similar studies in Finland, Belgium, the Netherlands, Italy, British Columbia, and Australia, the organism was cultured from 4.7%, 5.9%, 2.9%, 1.4%, 6.7%, and 0.7% of stool specimens, respectively (6–11). In most studies conducted in the United States, *Y. enterocolitica* organisms have been isolated from 1% or less of stool specimens (12–14). Seasonal clustering of cases in fall and winter months has been described in Europe and the United States (9,14,15). There is general agreement that the incidence of *Y. enterocolitica* infection is higher in several northern countries, including Scandinavia, the Netherlands, Belgium, and Canada, than elsewhere (15). However, during the past decade, there has been a gradual decrease in the incidence of *Y. enterocolitica* infections in Belgium (16).

The predominant serotypes of *Y. enterocolitica* isolated from symptomatic humans vary according to geographic location. In Europe and Japan, illness is most commonly caused by serotypes O:3 or O:9 (6–9,15,17), whereas serotypes O:8, O:4,32, O:13a,13b, O:18, O:20, and O:21 are isolated almost exclusively from American patients (18–21) and have been termed American serotypes. Serotype O:3 was rarely isolated from ill persons in the United States before 1980 but has been steadily increasing in prevalence in several regions of the United States (15,22–25). Outbreaks of *Y. enterocolitica* infection have

T. L. Cover: Departments of Medicine and Microbiology and Immunology, Vanderbilt University School of Medicine; and VA Medical Center, Nashville, Tennessee

R. M. Robins-Browne: Department of Microbiology and Immunology, University of Melbourne; Department of Microbiology and Infectious Diseases, Royal Children's Hospital, Parkeville, Victoria, Australia been reported commonly in the United States (2,25–34), whereas in European countries with a high incidence of *Y. enterocolitica* infection, outbreaks have rarely been reported and sporadic disease seems to predominate (2,15). These geographical differences may become less pronounced with time, in association with the introduction of American serotypes into Europe and Japan, and the dissemination of serotype O:3 in the United States (22–25).

Swine are a major reservoir for *Y. enterocolitica,* particularly the pathogenic serotypes O:3 and O:9 (35). *Y. enterocolitica* may be cultured from the tongue, throat, tonsils, cecal contents, and feces of swine, as well as from pork, ham, and butcher shop cutting boards (2,36). Serotype O:3 isolates from swine and symptomatic humans are indistinguishable by genetic analysis (37,38). In a Belgian case–control study, *Y. enterocolitica* infection with serotype O:3 or O:9 was strongly associated with consumption of raw pork in the 2 weeks before the onset of illness (15). Similarly, an outbreak of infection with serotype O:3 in Atlanta, Georgia, in 1988 was associated with consumption or preparation of chitterlings (raw pork intestines) (25). Thus, swine and the consumption of undercooked pork products play a major role in the epidemiology of human *Y. enterocolitica* infections.

Several outbreaks of *Y. enterocolitica* infection have been attributed to ingestion of contaminated milk products (26,27,30,31,34). *Y. enterocolitica* may commonly be cultured from cow feces (39), raw milk, and occasionally pasteurized milk or pasteurized milk products (40–42). The mechanisms whereby *Y. enterocolitica* organisms survive pasteurization or contaminate milk after pasteurization are unclear. However, *Y. enterocolitica* organisms can multiply in milk stored at 4°C (43,44), so small inocula potentially could proliferate during refrigerated storage.

In addition to isolation of *Y. enterocolitica* from swine and cows, the organism has been isolated from a wide array of other mammals, as well as birds, frogs, fish, flies, fleas, snails, crabs, and oysters (2,18,45). The organism also may be isolated from lakes, streams, well water, and soil (46,47), which presumably are seeded with fecally shed organisms. *Y. enterocolitica* occasionally has been transmitted from dogs to humans (28,48). In addition, the ingestion of unchlorinated water has resulted in sporadic cases and several outbreaks of *Y. enterocolitica* infection (49,50). However, *Y. enterocolitica* isolates from most animals and environmental sources typically belong to nonpathogenic serotypes (18,45), so most of these reservoirs have not been implicated commonly as sources of human infections.

Transmission of infection from person to person has been suggested by the sequential onset of illness in family members (5,17,28,51,52). In addition, there have been several reported incidents of nosocomial transmission of *Y. enterocolitica* infection (53–56). Although person-to-person transmission by a fecal-oral route probably occurs, it is likely that most human infections are acquired instead by consumption of contaminated food or beverages. In addition to fecal-oral transmission, person-to-person transmission occasionally occurs by transfusion of contaminated blood products (57–59).

Similar to *Y. enterocolitica* infections, human infections with *Y. pseudotuberculosis* occur as both sporadic and epidemic disease (60–75) and occur most frequently among children (71,72). In several countries, there has been a clustering of human infections during winter months (73). *Y. pseudotuberculosis* organisms have been isolated from many animal species, including cattle, horses, deer, sheep, goats, swine, hare, foxes, rodents, cats, dogs, and birds (60–65). In addition, *Y. pseudotuberculosis* organisms have been isolated from environmental sources such as streams and lakes (61). Transmission of infection to humans has been possibly associated with ingestion of water or sand contaminated by an infected cat (74), ingestion of unpasteurized goat's milk (75), and ingestion of mountain stream water (61). However, the sources of most human cases of *Y. pseudotuberculosis* infection have not been successfully determined.

PATHOGENESIS

Y. enterocolitica and *Y. pseudotuberculosis* cause a similar range of diseases by virtue of their large number of shared virulence determinants (76). However, not all strains are equally virulent (Table 45.1). *Y. enterocolitica* biovars 1B, 2, 3, 4, and 5 and *Y. pseudotuberculosis* invade cultured epithelial cells in large numbers and possess a panoply of interactive virulence determinants, including a chromosomally encoded invasin and 70-kb virulence plasmid, termed pYV (which stands for "plasmid for *Yersinia* virulence) (76). In addition, biovar 1B strains of *Y. enterocolitica* (which comprise the so-called American serotypes) and all strains of *Y. pseudotuberculosis* carry a pathogenicity island that is involved with the acquisition of iron and thus enhances virulence. In contrast, various other *Y. enterocolitica* strains (particularly biovar 1A) do not carry pYV and fail to invade epithelial cells in large numbers *in vitro* (77,78).

Until recently, weakly invasive, pYV-negative strains of *Y. enterocolitica* (most of which belong to biovar 1A) were regarded as avirulent. However, there is now persuasive evidence to indicate that at least some of these strains may cause gastrointestinal symptoms clinically indistinguishable

TABLE 45.1. CHARACTERISTICS OF THE PATHOGENIC SUBGROUPS OF *YERSINIA ENTEROCOLITICA*

Subgroup	Biovars	Virulence-associated Determinants
Classic	1B,2,3,4,5	Invasin, Ail, Myf, enterotoxin (Yst), pYV, high pathogenicity island (biovar 1B only)
Atypical	1A	Unknown

from those due to pYV-bearing strains (77,79–81). Because the mechanisms by which biovar 1A strains cause disease are unknown, this section focuses on the virulence determinants of the classic pathogenic, pYV-bearing strains of *Y. enterocolitica* and *Y. pseudotuberculosis.*

Pathologic Changes

Examination of surgical specimens from patients and experimental animals with yersiniosis has revealed that *Y. enterocolitica* and *Y. pseudotuberculosis* are invasive pathogens that display a tropism for lymphoid tissue. Ingestion of *Y. enterocolitica* or *Y. pseudotuberculosis* by human volunteers has not been encouraged because of concerns regarding possible autoimmune sequelae; therefore, most information regarding the pathogenesis of yersiniosis *in vivo* has been obtained from experimental animals, particularly mice and rabbits (82–84). These animals are not natural hosts of the serotypes of *Y. enterocolitica* that commonly infect humans, but they have provided valuable insights into the pathogenesis of human disease. Nevertheless, some data derived from animal studies should be interpreted with caution, particularly where death is used as the endpoint of infection, because this is not the usual outcome of human infection (85).

After oral inoculation of mice with a virulent strain of *Y. enterocolitica* serotype O:8, biovar 1B, most bacteria remain within the intestinal lumen, and a few adhere to the mucosal epithelium, showing no particular preference for any cell type (86). In contrast, invasion of the epithelium takes place almost exclusively through M cells (86). The latter are specialized epithelial cells that overlie intestinal lymphoid follicles (Peyer's patches), where they play a major role in antigen sampling (87). Studies in artificially inoculated rabbits and pigs have shown that after penetrating the epithelium, *Y. enterocolitica* traverses the basement membrane to reach the gut-associated lymphoid tissue and the lamina propria, where it causes localized tissue destruction and forms microabscesses (83,88,89). *Y. enterocolitica* and *Y. pseudotuberculosis* often spread via the lymphatic system to mesenteric lymph nodes, where they may also evoke microabscess formation. Although *Y. enterocolitica* and *Y. pseudotuberculosis* are generally regarded as facultative intracellular pathogens because of their innate resistance to killing by macrophages (90,91), most of the bacteria observed in histologic sections are located extracellularly (92,93). Nevertheless, macrophages containing viable bacteria may play an important role in the dissemination of Yersinia throughout the body (88,94).

Virulence Determinants

Adherence and Invasion

At least four different proteins including invasin (Inv), Ail, YadA, and Myf may mediate adhesion of *Y. enterocolitica* and *Y. pseudotuberculosis* to host cells. Binding of yersinia to these cells via Inv and YadA is associated with subsequent internalization. Thus, *Y. enterocolitica* and *Y. pseudotuberculosis* may adhere to and enter host cells via several different pathways.

The most efficient pathway for intracellular entry *in vitro* is mediated by Inv, a surface-expressed protein that is produced by *Y. pseudotuberculosis* and all classic pathogenic strains of *Y. enterocolitica.* Inv was first identified in *Y. pseudotuberculosis* as the product of the chromosomal *inv* gene (95). When introduced into an innocuous laboratory strain of *E. coli*, such as *E. coli* K12, *inv* confers the capacity to penetrate mammalian cells, including epithelial cells and macrophages (90,95). Despite the difference in size of Inv proteins from *Y. enterocolitica* (91 kd) and *Y. pseudotuberculosis* (102 kd), the two proteins are functionally highly conserved. The principal receptors for Inv are members of the β_1-integrin family, which occur on many cell types including epithelial cells, macrophages, T lymphocytes, and Peyer's patch M cells (96,97). Their physiologic role is to act as receptors for fibronectin, laminin, and related host proteins, which may bear conformational similarities to Inv (98). However, the affinity of Inv for several β_1-integrins is much greater than that of fibronectin. Accordingly, when Inv binds to these molecules, it causes them to cluster and initiate a sequence of events, including the activation of focal adhesion kinase, which results in reorganization of the host cell cytoskeleton and internalization of the bacteria (99,100). Inhibitors of actin polymerization and tyrosine kinases block Inv-mediated invasion (101,102), confirming that uptake of yersinia by eukaryotic cells requires both an intact cytoskeleton and signal transduction pathways involving tyrosine phosphorylation.

Although DNA sequences homologous to *inv* occur in all *Yersinia* species (except *Yersinia ruckeri*) this gene is functional only in *Y. pseudotuberculosis* and the classic pathogenic biovars (1B through 5) of *Y. enterocolitica,* suggesting that Inv plays a key role in virulence (103). In comparison to wild type strains, *inv* mutants of *Y. enterocolitica* and *Y. pseudotuberculosis* exhibit a pronounced reduction in the capacity to invade epithelial cells *in vitro* and diminished translocation into Peyer's patches of mice, but their virulence for orally inoculated mice is barely affected (85,104). This suggests that M cells may be able to ingest bacteria to some extent in the absence of a specific stimulus, or that alternative adhesins such as YadA (see below), can compensate for a lack of Inv.

Ail (attachment invasion locus) is another surface protein produced by the classic pathogenic strains of *Y. enterocolitica* that confers invasive ability on *E. coli in vitro* (103). This 17-kd peptide is unrelated to invasin and is specified by the chromosomal *ail* gene. In concert with YadA, Ail may also permit Yersinia to persist extracellularly in host tissues by inhibiting the binding of complement and protecting the bacteria from complement-mediated lysis (105). Surprisingly, an *ail* mutant of *Y. enterocolitica* showed no reduction in virulence for perorally inoculated mice when compared with the wild type strain, which indicates that Ail is not required to establish infection or even to cause systemic infection in these animals (106). Notably, *Y. enterocolitica* is innately susceptible to complement-mediated killing by human serum but resistant to complement-mediated killing by murine serum (107). This suggests that the mouse model may not be well suited for investigating the contribution of Yersinia anticomplement factors to virulence.

YadA, formerly known as *Yersinia* outer membrane protein type 1 (Yop-1) or P-1, is a 44- to 47-kd, pYV-encoded outer membrane protein. Early studies of the morphology of YadA suggested that it polymerized to form fibrils on the bacterial surface (108), but subsequent work revealed that it forms lollipop-shaped oligomers that envelop the entire outer membrane as a densely packed array (109). YadA mediates adhesion of *Y. enterocolitica* to intestinal mucus and to certain extracellular matrix proteins, including collagen, laminin, and cellular fibronectin (110). These proteins in turn may bind to β_1-integrins on epithelial cells and stimulate bacterial internalization in a manner similar to that mediated by Inv (110). YadA may also promote bacterial invasion by binding to integrins directly (111,112).

Apart from its role as an adhesin and invasin, YadA contributes to the virulence of *Y. enterocolitica* by conferring resistance to complement-mediated opsonization. It achieves this by binding factor H, thereby reducing deposition of C3b on the bacterial surface (113). As a consequence, expression of YadA is associated with the resistance of *Y. enterocolitica* to complement-mediated lysis and phagocytosis, as well as an ability to inhibit the respiratory burst of polymorphonuclear leukocytes (both of which require the bacteria to be preopsonized) (113,114). YadA mutants of *Y. enterocolitica* show markedly reduced virulence for mice when compared with wild type strains (115,116). In contrast, YadA mutants of *Y. pseudotuberculosis* show no attenuation, and *Y. pestis,* which is extremely virulent for mice, is naturally defective in YadA production due to a single-base-pair deletion resulting in a shift of the reading frame of the gene (117,118).

Apart from Inv, Ail, and YadA, the classic pathogenic varieties of *Y. enterocolitica* also produce a fimbrial adhesin, named Myf (mucoid *Yersinia* fibrillae), because it bestows a mucoid appearance on bacterial colonies that express it (119). Myf are narrow flexible fibrillae that resemble CS-3, a colonization factor of some human strains of enterotoxigenic *E. coli.* MyfA, the major structural subunit of Myf, shows some homology to the PapG protein of pyelonephritis-associated strains of *E. coli,* and is 44% identical at the DNA level to the pH6 antigen of *Y. pseudotuberculosis* and *Y. pestis,* which also has a fibrillar structure and mediates thermoinducible binding of *Y. pseudotuberculosis* to tissue culture cells (120,121). The main role of Myf in virulence, however, may relate to its ability to mediate binding of bacteria to intestinal mucus, before the bacteria make contact with epithelial cells (104).

Overcoming Host Defenses Via The Yersinia *Virulence Plasmid*

All fully virulent, highly invasive strains of *Y. enterocolitica* and *Y. pseudotuberculosis* carry a 70-kilobase plasmid, pYV, which is highly conserved among these species and *Y. pestis* (reviewed in reference 122). The factors encoded by pYV function primarily to enable the bacteria that carry it to resist phagocytosis and complement-mediated lysis, thereby allowing them to persist extracellularly in tissues. Yersinia that carry pYV exhibit a distinctive *in vitro* phenotype known as either calcium dependency or the low-calcium response, because it is manifested only when the bacteria are grown in media containing low concentrations of Ca^{2+}. The principal features of this phenotype are the cessation of bacterial growth after one or two generations and the appearance of at least 12 new proteins on the bacterial surface or in the culture medium. These proteins are termed Yops because they were once thought to be outer membrane proteins, but they are now known to be secreted by the bacteria via a type III secretory pathway. Yops exhibit no homology to each other, but they are grouped together because they are all encoded by pYV, share a common mode of secretion, and are subject to genetic co-regulation by a pYV-encoded regulator, known as VirF.

The genes carried by pYV include those that encode the following products: (a) YadA (discussed above); (b) a type III secretion apparatus (Ysc), which functions to transport Yops across the *Yersinia* inner and outer membranes; (c) at least six distinct antihost, effector Yops; (d) a translocation apparatus, which the effector Yops use to gain access to the cytosol of the host cell, and (e) factors for the regulation of Yop biosynthesis, secretion, and translocation. Genes for the effector Yops are scattered around pYV, whereas those required for Yop secretion and translocation are clustered together (Fig. 45.1). pYV also encodes YlpA, a 29-kd lipoprotein related to the TraT protein of various enterobacteria, and in *Y. enterocolitica* strains of biovars 2 to 5 (but not biovar 1B or *Y. pseudotuberculosis*), an operon that specifies resistance to arsenic (123).

Effector Yops

All six effector Yops of *Y. enterocolitica* and *Y. pseudotuberculosis* are translocated into the cytosol of host cells from bacteria that are bound to these cells (Fig. 45.1). Although each effector Yop has a distinct function, they act in coordinated fashion to disrupt cellular immune phagocytosis.

YopE is a 25-kd protein that disrupts actin microfilaments and leads to cytotoxic changes in host cells (124). YopE does not act on actin directly but appears to function as a guanosine triphosphatase (GTPase)-activating protein, which inhibits Rho GTPases that are required for actin integrity (125,126). YopT is a 35-kd protein that exerts an effect on actin microfilaments that is similar to that caused by YopE (127). The intracellular target of YopT appears to

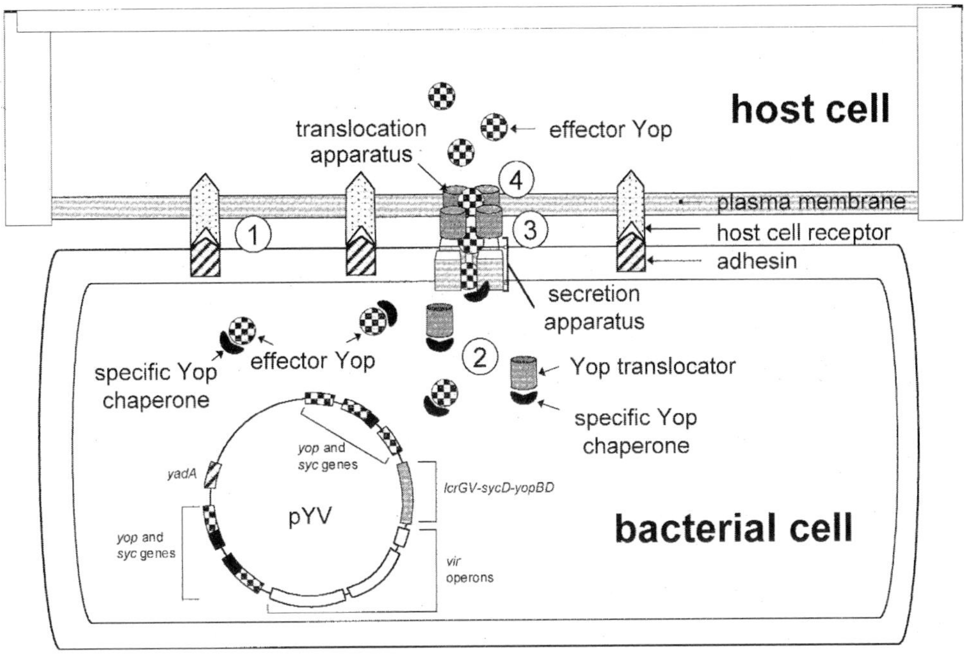

FIGURE 45.1. Depiction of the translocation of effector *Yersina* outer membrane proteins (Yops) across the eukaryotic cell membrane. Once bacteria have established contact with the **(1)** host cell, pYV-encoded effector Yops are synthesized together with their chaperones, **(2)** translocators, and the **(3)** components required for their secretion. Yops are secreted by the **(4)** bacteria and then transported across the eukaryotic plasma membrane by the translocators, **(5)** YopB and YopD. (Effector Yops are represented by checkered balls and the translocators by shaded cylinders. The Ysc secretion apparatus is shown as open cubes and the Yop chaperones as solid crescents. Striped arrows represent bacterial adhesins and dotted arrows depict eukaryotic cell receptors. The genes encoding the bacterial proteins are depicted on pYV with the corresponding pattern and shading.

be RhoA, a Rho GTPase (128). YopO is an 82-kd protein, known as *Yersinia* protein kinase A (YpkA) in *Y. pseudotuberculosis.* It is secreted by the bacteria in an inactive form, which is activated by actin within the target cell (129). The functional kinase then disrupts actin to retard phagocytosis.

YopP (known as YopJ in *Y. pseudotuberculosis*) is a 32-kd protein that is encoded by the same operon as YopO/YpkA. It induces apoptosis in macrophages by interfering with the mitogen-activated protein kinase activities of c-Jun N-terminal kinase, p38, and extracellular signal-regulated kinase (130). YopP also acts on various cell types to inhibit release of tumour necrosis factor α (TNF-α), possibly via an inhibitory action on nuclear factor-κB (NF-κB). TNF-α is a proinflammatory cytokine that plays a central role in inflammatory and immune responses (131). Accordingly, YopP may contribute to the establishment of Yersinia in tissues by eliminating macrophages while retarding inflammatory responses (132).

YopH is a 51-kd protein tyrosine phosphatase, which dephosphorylates several phosphotyrosine residues, including those on focal adhesion kinase and the focal adhesion proteins, paxillin and $p130^{cas}$ (133). Focal adhesions are sites where integrins act as transmembrane bridges between extracellular matrix proteins and intracellular signaling proteins. The fact that autophosphorylation of focal adhesion kinase contributes to invasin-mediated uptake of Yersinia by epithelial cells (99), provides an explanation for the antiphagocytic effects of YopH.

YopM is a 41-kd protein, which contains a succession of 12 repeated structures resembling leucine-rich repeat motifs (134). For this reason, YopM shows weak homology to a large number of proteins, including the α chain of membrane glycoprotein Ib (GPIbα), a platelet-specific receptor for thrombin and the von Willebrand factor (134). Although YopM is able to bind to thrombin *in vitro,* the finding that it is translocated into cells and traffics to the nucleus by means of a vesicle-associated, microtubule-dependent pathway (135) suggests that it may have another function that is unrelated to its antithrombin activity.

Yop Secretion And Translocation

Secretion of Yops across the inner and outer membranes of the *Yersinia* cell wall occurs via a type III pathway, which also functions to inject (translocate) proteins into the cytosol of host cells (136). The transport of Yops from the bacterial cytoplasm (via Ysc) into the host cell cytosol (via the translocation apparatus) is envisioned to occur in one step from bacteria that are closely bound to the host cell (via Inv and/or YadA) (Fig. 45.1) (137).

Protein secretion via the type III pathway is governed by the nucleotide sequence at the 5′ end of the messenger RNA and/or by the amino terminal sequence of the secreted protein (136). In contrast to proteins exported via the Sec-dependent (type II) pathway, the amino termini of type III-secreted proteins show no resemblance to each other and are not cleaved during export (reviewed in references 136 and 138). Another feature of type III secretion is the presence of structurally conserved chaperone proteins that bind to individual secreted proteins and guide them to the secretion apparatus while preventing their premature interaction with other proteins. Chaperone proteins for Yops are denoted by the prefix Syc (for specific Yop chaperone), and include SycE (for YopE), SycH (for YopH), SycD (for YopB and YopD), SycN (for YopN), and SycT (for YopT). The genes encoding these chaperones are located on pYV close to the corresponding *yop* genes. Although they show no significant homology to each other, all Yop chaperones identified to date are low-molecular-weight (14- to 19-kd) proteins with a C-terminal amphipathic α helix and a pI of around 4.5 (122). The Ysc secretion apparatus is encoded by 29 genes within four contiguous loci, called *virC, virG, virA,* and *virB* (Fig. 45.1) (139). Some components of Ysc have been localized to the bacterial cell envelope, where they are envisioned to form a channel that spans the inner and outer membranes (122).

The translocation of effector Yops into host cells also requires YopB (42 kd) and YopD (33 kd). These proteins have hydrophobic domains, which suggests that they could interact directly with host cell membranes (140,141). YopB resembles members of the RTX toxin family and can evidently form pores in the plasma membrane of eukaryotic cells (141). YopD associates with YopB and may contribute to the formation of pores (141). The observation that YopD is translocated into cells, however, suggests that it may also serve other functions (142).

YopB and YopD are encoded by the *lcrGV-sycD-yopBD* operon, which also encodes LcrV, LcrG, and SycD, the chaperone for YopB and YopD (Fig. 45.1). LcrV, also known as the V antigen, is a versatile Yop that acts as an essential component of the translocation apparatus, a regulator of Yop expression, and possibly as an effector Yop that inhibits neutrophil chemotaxis and cytokine production (143,144). Its key role in the virulence of *Y. pestis* is evidenced by the fact that antibodies to LcrV protect mice from infection with this species (145).

The production and secretion of Yops is tightly regulated. *In vitro,* Yops, their Syc chaperones, and the Ysc secretory apparatus are synthesized at 37°C (but not at temperatures less than 30°C) when the concentration of Ca^{2+} is sufficiently low to induce bacteriostasis. The mechanism of regulation by temperature involves VirF, a pYV-encoded, DNA-binding protein of the AraC family (which itself is regulated by temperature) and probably involves DNA supercoiling (146,147). VirF also controls the synthesis of YadA, production of which is regulated at the transcriptional level by temperature, but not by the concentration of Ca^{2+}.

Other Virulence Determinants

Heat-stable Enterotoxins

When first isolated from clinical specimens, most strains of *Y. enterocolitica* secrete a 30-amino acid heat-stable enterotoxin, known as Yst (148). The carboxyl terminus of Yst is homologous to heat-stable enterotoxins from enterotoxigenic *E. coli, Citrobacter freundii* and non-O1 serotypes of *Vibrio cholerae,* as well as to guanylin, an intestinal paracrine hormone (149–152). These polypeptides share a common mechanism of action, which involves binding to and activation of cell-associated guanylate cyclase, with subsequent elevation of intracellular concentrations of cyclic guanosine monophosphate (cGMP) (153). Yst is encoded by the chromosomal *yst* gene, which is present mainly in the classic pathogenic biovars of *Y. enterocolitica* (154). Its contribution to the pathogenesis of diarrhea is evidenced by the observation that a *yst* mutant of a serotype O:9 strain of *Y. enterocolitica* caused milder diarrhea in infant rabbits than did the wild type strain (155). Toxins that resemble Yst in terms of heat stability and reactivity in infant mice, but with a different structure, molecular weight, and/or mechanism of action, have been detected in biovar 1A strains of *Y. enterocolitica* and "avirulent" *Yersinia* species, such as *Y. bercovieri* and *Y. mollareti* (151,156–158). Because these bacteria may be responsible for diarrhea in some patients, it seems likely that these toxins contribute to bacterial virulence (159).

After repeated passage or prolonged storage, Yst-secreting strains of *Y. enterocolitica* frequently lose the capacity for toxin production. This phenomenon is not caused by mutation of the *yst* gene but is due to silencing of this gene by *Yersinia* modulator type A (YmoA). The latter is an 8-kd protein that resembles histones and evidently down-regulates gene expression in Yersinia by altering DNA topology (160). Expression of *yst* is also regulated by RpoS, an alternative sigma factor of RNA polymerase, which is involved in regulating the expression of a number of stationary-phase genes in enterobacteria (161).

Iron Acquisition

Iron is an essential micronutrient for almost all bacteria, but the availability of iron in many extracellular locations is limited (162). This is because most iron in tissues is bound to high-affinity glycoproteins such as transferrin and lactoferrin or is incorporated into organic molecules such as hemoglobin. The observation that a disproportionate number of patients with *Yersinia* septicemia suffer from iron overload suggests that the availability of iron in tissues may be a factor that helps to determine the outcome of yersiniosis (163). Yersinia use several different mechanisms to acquire iron from inorganic and organic sources (164,165). Most clinical isolates of *Y. enterocolitica* do not produce siderophores (i.e., low-molecular-weight, high-affinity iron chelators that are commonly released by pathogenic bacteria as a mechanism for iron acquisition), which accounts for their reliance on abnormally high concentrations of iron for growth in tissues. However, biovar 1B strains (which are intrinsically more virulent than strains of biovars 2 to 5), as well as *Y. pestis* and *Y. pseudotuberculosis,* carry genes for the biosynthesis, transport, and regulation of a catechol-containing siderophore, known as yersiniabactin. The 40-kilobase *ybt* locus that contains these genes has a higher G+C content (57.5 mol%) than that of the *Y. enterocolitica* chromosome (47 mol%), is flanked on one side by an *asn* tRNA gene, and carries the gene for a putative integrase (166). These features, which are typical of a pathogenicity island, have led to the designation of the *ybt* locus as "the *Yersinia* high pathogenicity island." The designation "high" alludes to the observation that bacteria that carry this locus are more virulent for mice infected perorally (median lethal dose less than 10^3 colony-forming units [CFU]) than are strains that lack it (median lethal dose typically more than 10^6 CFU). The complete nucleotide sequence of the high pathogenicity island of a serotype O:8 strain of *Y. enterocolitica* has been determined (166). It contains 22 open reading frames within 43.4 kilobases, approximately 30.5 kilobases of which is conserved among *Y. enterocolitica, Y. pestis,* and *Y. pseudotuberculosis.* The functions of several genes in the pathogenicity island have not yet been elucidated, but it is known that the synthesis of yersiniabactin requires *irp* (iron-regulated protein) genes *irp1* to *irp5,* as well as *ybtA,* which encodes an AraC-like regulator. The ortholog of *irp9* in *Y. pestis* may also be involved in the synthesis of yersiniabactin, whilst those of *irp6, irp7,* and *irp8* may contribute to the uptake of the ferriyersiniabactin complex. The major receptor for this complex is a 65-kd outer membrane protein, named FyuA, which also serves as a receptor for pesticin, a bacteriocin produced by *Y. pestis.* For this reason, strains of *Yersinia* species that carry the high pathogenicity island are susceptible to pesticin (167). Transport of ferriyersiniabactin complexes across the cell wall of *Y. enterocolitica* resembles the analogous pathway in *E. coli,* in that it is an energy-dependent process that requires TonB. The latter protein couples energy provided by inner membrane metabolism to outer membrane protein receptors, such as FyuA. TonB-, FyuA-, and yersiniabactin-deficient mutants of *Y. enterocolitica* all show reduced virulence for mice, presumably because of their limited capacity to acquire sufficient iron to grow in tissues (168). The fact that *aroA,* a gene required for the biosynthesis of aromatic amino acids, is also require to synthesize yersiniabactin may partly explain the reduced virulence of *aroA* mutants of *Y. enterocolitica* for mice (169).

Although biovars of *Y. enterocolitica* other than 1B do not produce yersiniabactin, they are able to acquire iron from a number of sources, including ferrisiderophore complexes in which the siderophore (such as desferrioxamine B) was synthesized by another microorganism (168–170). The resultant iron-desferrioxamine complex (known as ferrioxamine) binds to FoxA, a 76-kd outer membrane protein, which is homologous to FhuA, the high-affinity ferrichrome receptor of *E. coli* (171). The ability of *Y. enterocolitica* to acquire iron from ferrioxamine may have important clinical implications, because desferrioxamine B is used therapeutically to reduce iron overload in patients with hemosiderosis and other forms of iron intoxication. When administered to patients, desferrioxamine B forms a ferrisiderophore complex, which *Y. enterocolitica* can use as a growth factor (172). Accordingly, if patients undergoing iron chelation therapy with desferrioxamine B become infected with *Y. enterocolitica,* the bacteria may be able to proliferate in tissues where under normal circumstances the poor availability of iron would limit their growth. In addition to its effects on microbial iron metabolism, desferrioxamine B may also increase susceptibility to systemic yersiniosis by interfering with host immune responses (173).

Lipopolysaccharide

As with other enterobacteria, *Y. enterocolitica* can be classified as smooth or rough depending on the amount of O side-chain polysaccharide attached to the inner core region of the cell wall lipopolysaccharide (LPS). Synthesis of the O side chain by *Y. enterocolitica* is specified by the chromosomal *rfb* locus and is regulated by temperature, such that colonies are smooth when grown at temperatures less than 30°C, but rough at 37°C (174). *Y. enterocolitica* strains of serotypes O:3 and O:8 that carry a mutation in the *rfb* locus display reduced virulence for mice, indicating that the bacteria require smooth LPS for the full expression of virulence (174,175). The outer core region of LPS plays a role in maintaining outer membrane integrity and may contribute to the resistance of *Y. enterocolitica* to bactericidal peptides in host tissues (176).

Phospholipase

Some isolates of *Y. enterocolitica* are hemolytic due to the production of phospholipase A, encoded by *yplA.* A strain of *Y. enterocolitica* in which the *yplA* gene was deleted showed diminished virulence for perorally inoculated mice (177). Interestingly, this mutant induced less inflammation and necrosis in intestinal and lymphoid tissues than did the wild type, suggesting that phospholipase contributes to microabscess formation.

Urease

All enteric pathogens must negotiate the acid barrier of the stomach to cause disease. In *Y. enterocolitica,* acid resistance relies on the production of urease, which catalyses the release of ammonia from urea and allows the bacteria to resist a pH level as low as 2.5 (178,179). Urease also contributes to the survival of *Y. enterocolitica* in host tissues, but the mechanism by which this occurs is not known (180). Although *Y. pseudotuberculosis* also produces urease, it has a relatively low specific activity and evidently does not contribute to acid resistance in this species (181).

Coordinated Expression Of *Yersinia* Virulence Factors

Y. enterocolitica and *Y. pseudotuberculosis* are versatile foodborne pathogens with a remarkable ability to adapt to a wide range of environments inside and outside their mammalian hosts. These bacteria typically enter their mammalian hosts via food or water, in which bacterial growth will have occurred to stationary phase at ambient temperature. Under these circumstances, *Y. enterocolitica* expresses factors such as urease and smooth LPS, which facilitate bacterial passage through the stomach and the mucous layer of the small intestine. Bacteria in this state may also carry Myf fibrillae (pH6 antigen) and Inv, which may promote adherence to and penetration of M cells. Once *Y. enterocolitica* begins to replicate in the intestine at 37°C, LPS becomes rough, exposing Ail and YadA on the bacterial surface. These factors may promote further invasion while protecting the bacteria from complement-mediated opsonization. When yersinia make contact with host cells in lymphoid tissue, they are stimulated to synthesize, secrete, and translocate Yops, notably the effector Yops, YopE, YopT, YopH, YopO/YpkA, and Yop P/J, which retard the inflammatory response and impair the function of phagocytic cells. Subsequent bacterial replication may lead to tissue damage and the formation of microabscesses. If *Y. pseudotuberculosis* or strains of *Y. enterocolitica* that bear the high-pathogenicity island gain access to sites where iron supplies are growth limiting, they may produce yersiniabactin so replication can proceed. Eventually, the cycle is completed when the bacteria rupture through microabscesses in intestinal crypts to reenter the intestine and regain access to the environment. This well-defined life cycle of *Y. enterocolitica* and *Y. pseudotuberculosis,* with its distinctive temperature-induced phases, is reminiscent of the flea-rat-flea cycle of *Y. pestis.*

CLINICAL ILLNESS

Y. enterocolitica infection may be associated with various syndromes, which occur with differing frequency depending in part on the age and physical state of the host (Table 45.2). Overall, illness occurs most commonly among children (15,17,29,30). Enterocolitis, the most common presentation, is characterized by diarrhea, low-grade fever, and abdominal pain (10,15,17,24,182–184). In a prospective study of 181 Canadian children (median age, 24 months) with symptomatic *Y. enterocolitica* infection, diarrhea was present in 98%, fever in 88%, abdominal pain in 64%, and vomiting in 38% of cases (5). Grossly bloody stools are present in about one-fourth of patients (5,15,17,24) and seem to occur more commonly in young persons than adults (17). Fecal leukocytes and erythrocytes are present in 10% to 50% of cases (10,28). Leukocytosis is typically present, frequently accompanied by marked "left shifts" with immature to total neutrophil ratios more than 0.5 (17,25). The mean duration of illness is typically 14 to 22 days (5,15,17), but symptoms occasionally persist for several months (17, 185). The mean duration of excretion of organisms in stool is 6 to 7 weeks (5,17). Most infections are self-limited, but complications may include appendicitis, diffuse ulceration, and inflammation of the small intestine and colon (28), intestinal perforation (186), peritonitis (30), ileocolic intussusception, toxic megacolon, cholangitis, and mesenteric vein thrombosis (2).

The pseudoappendicular syndrome occurs primarily in older children and adults (5,27,185,187,188). The cardinal features of this syndrome are fever, abdominal pain, tenderness of the right lower quadrant, and leukocytosis, with or without diarrhea. Due to the clinical similarities between this syndrome and appendicitis, laparotomy is frequently performed. Among patients in Scandinavia with suspected appendicitis, stool cultures or operative specimens from 50 (3.6%) of 1,362 patients who underwent laparotomy yielded *Y. enterocolitica* (188). In other studies, *Y. enterocolitica* infec-

TABLE 45.2. CLINICAL MANIFESTATIONS OF *YERSINIA ENTEROCOLITICA* INFECTION

Syndrome	Typical Age of Patient	Predisposing Host Factors
Enterocolitis	Child or adult	Young age
Pseudoappendicular syndrome	Older child or adult	None
Septicemia	Child or adult	Iron overload; deferoxamine therapy; immunocompromise
Reactive arthritis	Adult	HLA-B27; residence in Scandinavia
Erythema nodosum	Adult	Residence in Scandinavia; female gender

tion has been detected in 1.9% to 5.4% of patients with suspected appendicitis (189–191). The operative findings in patients with this syndrome include marked mesenteric lymphadenopathy, terminal ileitis, and a normal or slightly inflamed appendix (27,182,187,188,192,193). Ultrasonography is potentially useful in distinguishing true appendicitis from *Y. enterocolitica* infection (193).

Pharyngitis, frequently associated with cervical adenopathy, may occur either in association with *Y. enterocolitica* enterocolitis or independent of gastrointestinal illness (15,17,28,30,185,194,195). Cutaneous infection also may occur and is manifested as cellulitis, abscesses, or wound infection (2,28,29,196–198). Other focal suppurative infections that have occurred in the absence of detectable bacteremia include suppurative conjunctivitis (199), urinary tract infections (30), renal abscesses, pneumonia (200,201), and lung abscess (2).

Y. enterocolitica septicemia is typically a severe illness with case-fatality rates of 7.5% to 50% (202–204). Pathologic conditions associated with an iron-overloaded state are well-recognized predisposing factors for severe systemic *Y. enterocolitica* infection; these include hemochromatosis, acute iron poisoning, and transfusion-dependent blood dyscrasias (202–205). Other predisposing factors for *Y. enterocolitica* septicemia include desferrioxamine therapy, cirrhosis, immunosuppressive therapy, diabetes mellitus, alcoholism, and malnutrition (202,203).

The bacteremic spread of *Y. enterocolitica* to extraintestinal sites may result in abscess formation in the liver, spleen, or other sites (202,205–207). Other complications of *Y. enterocolitica* bacteremia include endocarditis (208), mycotic aneurysm (209), meningitis, osteomyelitis (210), septic arthritis, lung abscess, empyema (211), renal abscess, panophthalmitis, cutaneous pustules, and bullous skin lesions (2,30, 208–211).

Y. enterocolitica septicemia occasionally results from the transfusion of contaminated blood products (57–59). This syndrome is characterized by the sudden onset of fever, hypotension, and generalized pain within 1 hour after the start of transfusion (57–59). Vomiting and explosive diarrhea may also occur. More than 50% of reported cases are fatal. The diagnosis may quickly be established by Gram stain of the untransfused blood. Donors of the implicated contaminated blood products have been healthy at the time of blood donation but typically have reported a history of diarrheal illness during the 4 weeks before giving the donation (57–59). The donors are presumed to have had asymptomatic bacteremia at the time of blood donation. The contaminated erythrocytes in these cases have typically been stored for longer than 25 days. After a lag phase of 10 to 20 days, low inocula of *Y. enterocolitica* can proliferate in blood stored at 4°C, resulting in bacterial counts of 10^7 to 10^8 CFU/mL (212). *Y. enterocolitica* is able to use hemin as an iron source (213), and therefore, progressive hemolysis of stored blood may be required for bacterial proliferation to occur.

Acute reactive arthritis accompanies *Y. enterocolitica* infection in 10% to 30% of cases in Scandinavia (182,214–219). Arthritis occurs predominantly in adults (17) and is associated with the presence of the human leukocyte antigen B27 (HLA-B27 antigen) (217–219). Arthritic symptoms may accompany acute illness (17) or may occur weeks to months after gastrointestinal illness (17). Arthritic symptoms typically persist for one to several months, but chronic arthritis may develop (182).

The pathogenesis of reactive arthritis after *Y. enterocolitica* infection is poorly understood. Possible explanations for the link between yersiniosis and this condition include antigen persistence, molecular mimicry, and infection-induced presentation of normally cryptic cell antigens (220,221). Viable organisms cannot be cultured from affected joints, but the synovial fluid generally contains bacterial antigens, including LPS and heat shock proteins (Hsps), within inflammatory cells (222,223). Although patients with reactive arthritis display higher levels of serum immunoglobulin A (IgA) antibodies to *Yersinia* antigens than individuals without arthritis, these antibodies are unlikely to contribute to the development of arthritis. Instead, they probably reflect enhanced stimulation of the mucosal immune system by persistent bacterial antigens in the intestine or other tissues (224).

The observation that rats transgenic for HLA-B27 show a weaker cytotoxic T-cell response to *Y. pseudotuberculosis* compared with nontransgenic syngeneic rats provides a potential link between prolonged bacterial infection, antigen persistence, and HLA-B27 (225). Moreover, Hermann et al. (226) have shown that T-cell clones derived from the synovial fluid of patients with *Yersinia*-triggered reactive arthritis are selectively cytotoxic for HLA-B27-bearing cells infected with *Y. enterocolitica*. This suggests that CD8+, major histocompatibility complex (MHC) class I-restricted cytotoxic T cells can recognize specific *Yersinia*-derived peptides when they are presented together with HLA-B27. The nature of these peptides is not known.

Support for the molecular mimicry hypothesis comes from the demonstration of auto-reactive T cells in the synovial tissue of patients with reactive arthritis (226). Among the bacterial antigens that may provoke auto-reactivity, Hsps have been proposed as possible candidates, based on the conservation of these proteins among bacteria and mammals. Accordingly, an immune response to *Yersinia* Hsps may lead to an autoimmune response at sites where bacterial antigens accumulate. In keeping with this suggestion, synovial fluid from patients with reactive arthritis may contain CD4+, MHC class II-restricted T lymphocytes that recognize epitopes that are shared by a 60-kd *Yersinia* Hsp and its human counterpart (226). In addition, Lo et al. (227) have shown that when an immunodominant epitope of GroEL (an Hsp of *Salmonella typhimurium,* which is almost identical to the homologous protein in *Y. enterocolitica*) is presented by a class I MHC molecule of mice, the complex can subsequently be recognized by CD8+ cytotoxic T cells that cross-react with a peptide derived from a Hsp of mice (227).

Other *Yersinia* antigens that have been claimed to contribute to autoimmunity via specific interactions with the immune system include YadA and the β subunit of urease (228,229). Early suggestions that YadA shared epitopes with the peptide-binding groove of the HLA-B27 antigen have been discounted (230). The β subunit of urease is a cationic protein that is recognized by CD4+ T cells from patients with *Yersinia*-induced reactive arthritis and produces arthritis when injected into the joints of rats (229). Nevertheless, the observation that a urease-deficient mutant of *Y. enterocolitica* retains its capacity to induce arthritis in a rat model casts doubt on the role of urease in this condition (180).

Y. enterocolitica and *Y. pseudotuberculosis* may also induce polyclonal T-cell stimulation by virtue of their ability to secrete toxins that resemble superantigens (231,232). YpmA and its variant, YpmB, are 14- to 15-kd proteins, produced by approximately 20% of *Y. pseudotuberculosis* strains, that activate human T cells of Vβ phenotypes 3, 9, 13.1, and 13.2 (233,234). The *Y. enterocolitica* superantigen is not as well characterized as that of *Y. pseudotuberculosis,* but evidently it can stimulate T cells with Vβ phenotypes 3, 7, 8.1, 9, and 11 (232). Yersinia may also provoke nonspecific immune stimulation when Inv binds to β_1-integrins on T lymphocytes, thus providing a co-stimulatory signal to these cells (235).

Uveitis (236) and Reiter's syndrome (218) occur commonly in Scandinavia in association with *Y. enterocolitica* infection (182), and the presence of the HLA-B27 antigen is a risk factor for these conditions. In addition, erythema nodosum is reported in up to 30% of cases of *Y. enterocolitica* infection in Finland, predominantly in adult women (182). In contrast to arthritis, there is no association between erythema nodosum and the presence of the HLA-B27 antigen (217).

Numerous studies have reported that *Y. enterocolitica* infection is associated with a high incidence of subsequent inflammatory diseases (237,238), including ankylosing spondylitis (237), myocarditis (182,216,239), glomerulonephritis (240,241), and thyroid disease (242–244). The known capacity of *Y. enterocolitica* to induce inflammatory joint disease suggests that individual cases of many of these other inflammatory syndromes may indeed be precipitated by *Y. enterocolitica* infection. Although a temporal association between *Y. enterocolitica* infection and various nonsuppurative complications supports a causal relationship, in many reports, preceding *Y. enterocolitica* infections have been documented only by serologic assays. False-positive serology results potentially could occur due to polyclonal immune activation in these inflammatory disorders and thus lead to erroneous conclusions. In addition, many studies that report a high prevalence of anti-*Yersinia* antibodies among patients with inflammatory diseases have not compared the prevalence of anti-*Yersinia* antibodies in properly matched healthy controls. The high prevalence in Scandinavia of both the HLA-B27 antigen and *Y. enterocolitica* infection makes it imperative that these variables be assessed independently. Notably, follow-up of patients many years after infection with *Y. enterocolitica* or *Y. pseudotuberculosis* has shown no increased frequency of thyroid disease, and there is no evidence that hyperthyroidism is exacerbated by infection with *Y. enterocolitica* (221). The relationship between *Y. enterocolitica* and the many diseases with which it is potentially associated will be further clarified as additional prospective, well-controlled studies of patients with culture-proven *Y. enterocolitica* infection are performed.

The clinical manifestations of *Y. pseudotuberculosis* infection closely resemble those of *Y. enterocolitica* infection (249,250). Diarrheal illness, abdominal pain, and fever are the most common clinical features in healthy hosts (182). At laparotomy, mesenteric lymphadenopathy is commonly noted (251). Complications of infection include sepsis (252), liver abscesses (253), erythema nodosum (67), and reactive arthritis (182,254,255). Several cases of hemolytic–uremic syndrome and nephritis have been attributed to *Y. pseudotuberculosis* (182,256,257).

Y. pseudotuberculosis infection in Japan has been associated with clinical features different from those observed in the United States and Europe. Infected Japanese children may develop a high fever, a desquamative rash, red or crusted lips, strawberry tongue, conjunctivitis, and lymphadenopathy (258,259). These symptoms are identical to those described in an epidemic Japanese illness known as Izumi fever (258). Thus, it is likely that *Y. pseudotuberculosis* infection is the cause of many cases formerly classified as Izumi fever. Production of antigens with superantigen activity (260,261) may be important in the pathogenesis of this syndrome. Despite the clinical similarities between this syndrome and Kawasaki disease, no cases of Kawasaki disease associated with *Y. pseudotuberculosis* have been identified in the United States or Europe.

DIAGNOSIS

Y. enterocolitica and *Y. pseudotuberculosis* may be isolated from stool on commonly used selective media, such as MacConkey agar, and appear as lactose-negative colonies after 48 hours of growth at 25°C to 28°C. The use of cefsulodin-irgasin-novobiocin agar (262) and cold-enrichment techniques (7,263) may increase the rate of recovery from stool cultures. Nonpathogenic *Y. enterocolitica* may occasionally be isolated from stools, particularly if cold-enrichment techniques are used (263), and therefore, rapid clinical tests to distinguish between pathogenic and nonpathogenic *Y. enterocolitica* isolates are useful.

Formerly, virulent strains of *Y. enterocolitica* were identified by their pathogenicity for animals or their ability to invade tissue culture cells in large numbers. More recently, these tests have been superseded by *in vitro* surrogate assays, such as the demonstration of calcium dependency or an ability to bind Congo red or crystal violet (264–267). Calcium dependency refers a characteristic growth restriction of certain *Y. enterocolitica* and *Y. pseudotuberculosis* strains (i.e., those that carry the pYV plasmid) at 37°C on media containing low concentrations of calcium. Media for detection of Congo red binding and calcium dependency concurrently can be used for the primary isolation of *Y. enterocolitica* to permit early tentative identification of pYV-bearing strains. More direct evidence of the presence of virulence-associated genes can be obtained by hybridization with labeled DNA probes or by polymerase chain reaction (PCR) amplification of selected pYV-borne genes (such as *virF* or *yadA*) or chromosomal genes (such as *ail* and *yst*), which are more or less restricted to highly invasive strains. PCR also can be used for the rapid detection of potentially pathogenic strains of *Y. enterocolitica* (268–270). Because of the inherent instability of pYV, particularly in cultures held at 37°C, caution is necessary in interpreting negative assays for the presence of pYV-borne determinants.

Because of the occasional difficulty in achieving a bacteriologic diagnosis of yersiniosis, particularly in patients with immune-mediated disorders, a number of investigators have turned to serologic assays to facilitate diagnosis. A wide range of serologic techniques are available to measure antibodies to *Y. enterocolitica* (1). These include enzyme-linked immunosorbent assay, radioimmunoassay, and complement-fixation tests, but most experience has been gained with whole-cell agglutination tests. Serum antibody titers ranging from 80 to more than 10,000 have been detected within 7 days of acute infection. Interpretation of these assays is fraught with difficulty; because sera from healthy individuals commonly contain low levels of antibodies to Yersinia, and sera from patients with yersiniosis may exhibit a prozone phenomenon (271). In addition, some *Y. enterocolitica* O antigens cross-react with antigens from unrelated bacteria (272). This poses a particular problem with the *Y. enterocolitica* serotype O:9 antigen, which can cross-react with antigens from *Brucella abortus, E. coli* O157, *Morganella morganii,* and *Salmonella* group N, among others (272–274).

Patients with uncomplicated yersiniosis often show a moderate elevation of antibody titers to the infecting strain compared with an uninfected population, and patients with systemic infections typically exhibit even higher titers. There is no consensus on what constitutes a diagnostic titer level, so a fourfold or greater rise in titer between acute and convalescent sera should be sought whenever possible (271,275). Because patients with reactive arthritis and other autoimmune complications of yersiniosis are often at a stage of the illness when bacteriologic cultures are likely to be negative, considerable reliance may be placed on serology to make a specific diagnosis. Such individuals typically have high titers of agglutinins to *Y. enterocolitica* (276) and differ from patients with uncomplicated infection by demonstrating selected and prolonged elevation of *Yersinia*-specific antibodies of the IgA or IgG2 isotypes (277,278). These can be demonstrated by enzyme immunoassay or immunoblotting using heat-killed bacteria or purified LPS as antigens (279,280). Enzyme immunoassay and immunoblotting using Yops as antigens are also useful for the serologic diagnosis of yersiniosis (281,282). An advantage of these tests is the elimination of any requirement for the separate O antigens needed for assays based on whole bacteria or purified LPSs. Yop-based serology is also subject to fewer cross-reactions than assays based on whole cells.

TREATMENT

Y. enterocolitica isolates are typically susceptible *in vitro* to tetracycline, chloramphenicol, aminoglycosides, trimethoprim-sulfamethoxazole (TMP-SMX), third-generation cephalosporins, ticarcillin clavulanate, imipenem, aztreonam, and fluoroquinolones (283,284). Resistance to ampicillin and first-generation cephalosporins is mediated by β-lactamases (285). Doxycycline, fluoroquinolones, and gentamicin are efficacious for treatment of yersiniosis in a mouse model of infection (286–288).

Uncomplicated cases of enterocolitis or pseudoappendicular syndrome due to *Y. enterocolitica* or *Y. pseudotuberculosis* typically resolve spontaneously without antibiotics, so antimicrobial therapy is usually not required. In a placebo-controlled, double-blinded evaluation of TMP-SMX for *Y. enterocolitica* infection in children, treatment did not shorten the clinical or bacteriologic course of the illness (289). However, in this study the mean duration of illness before the institution of therapy was 12 days. Similarly, in a randomized trial of treatment for *Y. pseudotuberculosis,* there was no clinical benefit associated with ampicillin treatment compared with placebo (290). This apparent lack of treatment efficacy may be attributable to delays in instituting therapy (17). Although antimicrobial therapy may reduce the period of postsymptomatic fecal shedding (17), this benefit is probably not clinically important. Localized suppurative infection, bacteremia in compromised hosts, and severe systemic infection in healthy hosts should be treated with antibiotics, but controlled clinical trials to determine optimal therapies have not been performed. Until the results of antimicrobial susceptibility tests are available, institution of therapy with combinations of gentamicin, cefotaxime, ciprofloxacin, or doxycycline is appropriate. Cessation of desferrioxamine therapy is also recommended.

PREVENTION

Prevention of yersiniosis relies chiefly on good hygienic practices, particularly with regard to food preparation. Because pork products are the most frequently identified source of human infections with *Y. enterocolitica* serotypes O:3 and O:9 (15), measures to reduce contamination and improve hygiene during all stages of pig and pork processing should reduce rates of infection with these bacteria (291). Pigs infected with *Y. enterocolitica* are asymptomatic, making the detection of infection during routine meat inspection impractical. However, serologic testing of herds can identify infected animals, which can then be separated from seronegative herds to reduce the overall rate of infection (292). Because contamination of meat usually occurs during slaughtering, particular attention should be paid to critical control points, such as excision of the tongue, pharynx, and tonsils; the deboning of head meat; and the removal of the intestine (291). Raw chitterlings should be handled with caution and not at all by children (25). Bacterial numbers in contaminated meat can be reduced by gamma irradiation, scalding, and thorough cooking (15). Contamination of milk can be controlled by adequate pasteurization (293). Because *Y. enterocolitica* is able to grow at temperatures approaching 0°C, chilling of food should not be viewed as an effective control measure.

Measures to reduce the risk of transmission of *Y. enterocolitica* by blood transfusion include excluding blood donors with a recent history of gastrointestinal illness, screening of blood products for *Yersinia* species by PCR, and specific strategies to minimize bacterial numbers by filtration, removal of the buffy coat, or storage of blood at 0°C (294–297).

Although natural infection with *Y. enterocolitica* and *Y. pseudotuberculosis* affords immunity to reinfection (not only with the autologous strain but to some extent with other *Yersinia* species) (298,299), there is no licensed vaccine for these species. Indeed, a vaccine for humans seems unlikely given the relatively low incidence of infections with these bacteria and the possibility that immunization may induce the autoimmune complications that vaccination is partly intended to prevent. On the other hand, immunization of food animals, particularly pigs, to reduce bacterial load is a worthwhile goal. Approaches to vaccine development include the development of live attenuated vaccines or recombinant protective antigens (such as LcrV) (145,300,301). Although some experimental vaccines have proved effective in laboratory animals, their usefulness for reducing the extent of bacterial colonization in food animals is not known.

REFERENCES

1. Bottone EJ. *Yersinia enterocolitica:* the charisma continues. *Clin Microbiol Rev* 1997;10:257–276.
2. Cover TL, Aber RC. *Yersinia enterocolitica. N Engl J Med* 1989; 321:16–24.
3. Black RE, Slome S. *Yersinia enterocolitica. Infect Dis Clin North Am* 1988;2:625–641.
4. Brubaker RR. Factors promoting acute and chronic diseases caused by yersiniae. *Clin Microbiol Rev* 1991;4:309–324.
5. Marks MI, Pai CH, Lafleur L, et al. *Yersinia enterocolitica* gastroenteritis: a prospective study of clinical, bacteriologic, and epidemiologic features. *J Pediatr* 1980;96:26–31.
6. Ahvonen P. Human yersiniosis in Finland: bacteriology and serology. *Ann Clin Res* 1972;4:30–38.
7. Van Noyen R, Vandepitte J, Wauters G, et al. *Yersinia enterocolitica:* its isolation by cold enrichment from patients and healthy subjects. *J Clin Pathol* 1981;34:1052–1056.
8. Hoogkamp-Korstanje JAA, de Koning J, Samsom JP. Incidence of human infection with *Yersinia enterocolitica* serotypes O3,O8, and O9 and the use of indirect immunofluorescence in diagnosis. *J Infect Dis* 1986;153:138–141.
9. Mingrone MG, Fantasia M, Figura N, et al. Characteristics of *Yersinia enterocolitica* isolated from children with diarrhea in Italy. *J Clin Microbiol* 1987;25:1301–1304.
10. Mollee T, Tilse M. *Yersinia enterocolitica*: isolation from faeces of adults and children in Queensland. *Med J Aust* 1985;143: 488–489.
11. Barteluk RL, Noble MA. Routine culturing of stool specimens for *Yersinia enterocolitica. J Clin Microbiol* 1988;26:1616–1617.
12. Marymont JH Jr, Durfee KK, Alexander H, et al. *Yersinia enterocolitica* in Kansas: attempted recovery from 1,212 patients. *Am J Clin Pathol* 1982;77:753–755.
13. Kachoris M, Ruoff KL, Welch K, et al. Routine culture of stool specimens for *Yersinia enterocolitica* is not a cost-effective procedure. *J Clin Microbiol* 1988;26:582–583
14. Metchock B, Lonsway DR, Carter GP, et al. *Yersinia enterocolitica:* a frequent seasonal stool isolate from children at an urban hospital in the Southeast United States. *J Clin Microbiol* 1991;29:2868–2869.
15. Tauxe RV, Vandepitte J, Wauters G, et al. *Yersinia enterocolitica* infections and pork: the missing link. *Lancet* 1987;1:1129–1132.
16. Verhaegen J, Charlier J, Lemmens P, et al. Surveillance of human *Yersinia enterocolitica* infections in Belgium: 1967–1996. *Clin Infect Dis* 1998;27:59–64.
17. Ostroff SM, Kapperud G, Lassen J, et al. Clinical features of sporadic *Yersinia enterocolitica* infections in Norway. *J Infect Dis* 1992;166:812–817.
18. Shayegani M, DeForge I, McGlynn DM, et al. Characteristics of *Yersinia enterocolitica* and related species isolated from human, animal, and environmental sources. *J Clin Microbiol* 1981;14:304–312.
19. Bissett ML. *Yersinia enterocolitica* isolates from humans in California, 1968–1975. *J Clin Microbiol* 1976;4:137–144.
20. Snyder JD, Christenson E, Feldman RA. Human *Yersinia enterocolitica* infections in Wisconsin: clinical, laboratory and epidemiologic features. *Am J Med* 1982;72:768–774.
21. Kay BA, Wachsmuth K, Gemski P, et al. Virulence and phenotypic characterization of *Yersinia enterocolitica* isolated from human in the United States. *J Clin Microbiol* 1983;17:128–138.
22. Bottone EJ. Current trends of *Yersinia enterocolitica* isolates in the New York City area. *J Clin Microbiol* 1983;17:63–67.
23. Bissett ML, Powers C, Abbott SL, et al. Epidemiologic investigations of *Yersinia enterocolitica* and related species: sources, frequency, and serogroup distribution. *J Clin Microbiol* 1990;28: 910–912.
24. Lee LA, Taylor J, Carter GP, et al. *Yersinia enterocolitica* O:3: an emerging cause of pediatric gastroenteritis in the United States. *J Infect Dis* 1991;163:660–663.
25. Lee LA, Gerber AR, Lonsway DR, et al. *Yersinia enterocolitica* O:3 infections in infants and children, associated with the household preparation of chitterlings. *N Engl J Med* 1990;322: 984–987
26. Shayegani M, Morse D, DeForge I, et al. Microbiology of a major foodborne outbreak of gastroenteritis caused by *Yersinia enterocolitica* serogroup O:8. *J Clin Microbiol* 1983;17:35–40.

27. Black RE, Jackson RJ, Tsai T, et al. Epidemic *Yersinia enterocolitica* infection due to contaminated chocolate milk. *N Engl J Med* 1978;298:76–79.
28. Gutman LT, Ottesen EA, Quan TJ, et al. An inter-familial outbreak of *Yersinia enterocolitica* enteritis. *N Engl J Med* 1973;288: 1372–1377.
29. Tacket CO, Ballard J, Harris N, et al. An outbreak of *Yersinia enterocolitica* infections caused by contaminated tofu (soybean curd). *Am J Epidemiol* 1985;121:705–711
30. Tacket CO, Narain JP, Sattin R, et al. A multistate outbreak of infections caused by *Yersinia enterocolitica* transmitted by pasteurized milk. *JAMA* 1984;251:483–486.
31. de Grace M, Laurin M-F, Belanger C, et al. *Yersinia enterocolitica* gastroenteritis outbreak-Montreal. *Canada Dis Wkly Rep* 1976;2:41–44.
32. Maruyama T. *Yersinia enterocolitica* infection in humans and isolation of the microorganism from pigs in Japan. *Contrib Microbiol Immunol* 1987;9:48–55.
33. Aber RC, McCarthy MA, Berman R, et al. An outbreak of *Yersinia enterocolitica* gastrointestinal illness among members of a Brownie troop in Centre County, Pennsylvania. Paper presented at: 22nd Interscience Conference on Antimicrobial Agents and Chemotherapy; October 4–6, 1982; Miami Beach, FL.
34. Ackers ML, Schoenfeld S, Markman J, et al. An outbreak of *Yersinia enterocolitica* O:8 infections associated with pasteurized milk. *J Infect Dis* 2000;181:1834–1837.
35. Toma S, Deidrick VR. Isolation of *Yersinia enterocolitica* from swine. *J Clin Microbiol* 1975;2:478–481.
36. Pedersen KB. Occurrence of *Yersinia enterocolitica* in the throat of swine. *Contrib Microbiol Immunol* 1979;5:253–256.
37. Kapperud G, Nesbakken T, Aleksic S, et al. Comparison of restriction endonuclease analysis and phenotypic typing methods for differentiation of *Yersinia enterocolitica* isolates. *J Clin Microbiol* 1990;28:1125–1131.
38. Blumberg HM, Kiehlbauch JA, Wachsmuth IK. Molecular epidemiology of *Yersinia enterocolitica* O:3 infections: use of chromosomal DNA restriction fragment length polymorphisms of rRNA genes. *J Clin Microbiol* 1991;29:2368–2374.
39. Davey GM, Bruce J, Drysdale EM. Isolation of *Yersinia enterocolitica* and related species from the faeces of cows. *J Appl Bacteriol* 1983;55:439–443.
40. Greenwood MH, Hooper WL. Excretion of *Yersinia* spp. associated with consumption of pasteurized milk. *Epidemiol Infect* 1990;104:345–350.
41. Greenwood MH, Hooper WL, Rodhouse JC. The source of *Yersinia* spp. in pasteurized milk: an investigation at a dairy. *Epidemiol Infect* 1990;104:351–360.
42. Hughes D. Repeated isolation of *Yersinia enterocolitica* from pasteurized milk in a holding vat at a dairy factory. *J Appl Bacteriol* 1980;48:383–385.
43. Schiemann DA. Association of *Yersinia enterocolitica* with the manufacture of cheese and occurrence in pasteurized milk. *Appl Environ Microbiol* 1978;36:274–277.
44. Olsvik O, Kapperud G. Enterotoxin production in milk at 22 and 4 degrees C by *Escherichia coli* and *Yersinia enterocolitica. Appl Environ Microbiol* 1982;43:997–1000.
45. Shayegani M, Stone WB, DeForge I, et al. *Yersinia enterocolitica* and related species isolated from wildlife in New York state. *Appl Environ Microbiol* 1986;52:420–424.
46. Harvey S, Greenwood JR, Pickett MJ, et al. Recovery of *Yersinia enterocolitica* from streams and lakes of California. *Appl Environ Microbiol* 1976;32:352–354.
47. Highsmith AK, Feeley JC, Skaliy P, et al. Isolation of *Yersinia enterocolitica* from well water and growth in distilled water. *Appl Environ Microbiol* 1977;34:745–750.
48. Wilson HD, McCormick JB, Feeley JC. *Yersinia enterocolitica* infection in a 4-month-old infant associated with infection in household dogs. *J Pediatr* 1976;89:767–769.
49. Thompson JS, Gravel MJ. Family outbreak of gastroenteritis due to *Yersinia enterocolitica* serotype O:3 from well water. *Can J Microbiol* 1986;32:700–701.
50. Keet EE. *Yersinia enterocolitica* septicemia: source of infection and incubation period identified. *N Y State J Med* 1974;74: 2226–2230.
51. Martin T, Kasian GF, Stead S. Family outbreak of yersiniosis. *J Clin Microbiol* 1982;16:622–626.
52. Rose FB, Camp CJ, Antes EJ. Family outbreak of fatal *Yersinia enterocolitica* pharyngitis. *Am J Med* 1987;82:636–637
53. McIntyre M, Nnochiri E. A case of hospital-acquired *Yersinia enterocolitica* gastroenteritis. *J Hosp Infect* 1986;7:299–301.
54. Cannon CG, Linnemann CC Jr. *Yersinia enterocolitica* infections in hospitalized patients: the problem of hospital-acquired infections. *Infect Control Hosp Epidemiol* 1992;13:139–143.
55. Ratnam S, Mercer E, Picco B, et al. A nosocomial outbreak of diarrheal disease due to *Yersinia enterocolitica* serotype O:5, biotype 1. *J Infect Dis* 1982;145:242–247.
56. Toivanen P, Toivanen A, Olkkonen L, et al. Hospital outbreak of *Yersinia enterocolitica* infection. *Lancet* 1973;1:801–803.
57. Tipple MA, Bland LA, Murphy JJ, et al. Sepsis associated with transfusion of red cells contaminated with *Yersinia enterocolitica. Transfusion* 1990;30:207–213
58. Bufill JA, Ritch PS. *Yersinia enterocolitica* serotype O:3 sepsis after blood transfusion. *N Engl J Med* 1989;320:810.
59. Woernle CH, Hoffman RE, Smith JD, et al. Update: *Yersinia enterocolitica* bacteremia and endotoxin shock associated with red blood cell transfusions—United States, 1991. *MMWR Morb Mortal Wkly Rep* 1991;40:176–178.
60. Hubbert WT. Yersiniosis in mammals and birds in the United States. *Am J Trop Med Hyg* 1972;21:458–463.
61. Fukushima H, Gomyoda M, Shiozawa K, et al. *Yersinia pseudotuberculosis* infection contracted through water contaminated by a wild animal. *J Clin Microbiol* 1988;26:584–585.
62. Fukushima H, Gomyoda M, Kaneko S. Mice and moles inhabiting mountainous areas of Shimane peninsula as sources of infection with *Yersinia pseudotuberculosis. J Clin Microbiol* 1990; 28:2448–2455.
63. Slee KJ, Skilbeck NW. Epidemiology of *Yersinia pseudotuberculosis* and *Yersinia enterocolitica* infections in sheep in Australia. *J Clin Microbiol* 1992;30:712–715.
64. Tsubokura M, Otsuki K, Sata K, et al. Special features of distribution of *Yersinia pseudotuberculosis* in Japan. *J Clin Microbiol* 1989;27:790–791.
65. Toma S. Human and nonhuman infections caused by *Yersinia pseudotuberculosis* in Canada from 1962 to 1985. *J Clin Microbiol* 1986;24:465–466.
66. Randall KJ. Family outbreak of *Pasteurella pseudotuberculosis* infection. *Lancet* 1962;1:1042–1043.
67. Nakano T, Kawaguchi H, Nakao K, et al. Two outbreaks of *Yersinia pseudotuberculosis* 5a infection in Japan. *Scan J Infect Dis* 1989;21:175–179.
68. Inoue M, Nakashima H, Ueba, et al. Community outbreak of *Yersinia pseudotuberculosis. Microbiol Immunol* 1984;28:883–891.
69. Tertti R, Granfors K, Lehtonen O-P, et al. An outbreak of *Yersinia pseudotuberculosis* infection. *J Infect Dis* 1984;149:245–250.
70. Stahlberg TH, Tertti R, Wolf-Watz H, et al. Antibody response in *Yersinia pseudotuberculosis* III infection: analysis of an outbreak. *J Infect Dis* 1987;156:388–391.
71. Saari TN, Triplett DA. *Yersinia pseudotuberculosis* mesenteric adenitis. *J Pediatr* 1974;85:656–659.
72. Knapp W. Mesenteric adenitis due to *Pasteurella pseudotuberculosis* in young people. *N Engl J Med* 1958;259:776–778.
73. deGroote G, Vandepitte J, Wauters G. Surveillance of human

Yersinia enterocolitica infections in Belgium: 1963–1978. *J Infect* 1982;4:189–197.
74. Fukushima H, Gomyoda M, Ishikura S, et al. Cat-contaminated environmental substances lead to *Yersinia pseudotuberculosis* infection in children. *J Clin Microbiol* 1989;27:2706–2709.
75. Prober CG, Tune B, Hoder L. *Yersinia pseudotuberculosis* septicemia. *Am J Dis Child* 1979;133:623–624.
76. Hartland EL, Robins-Browne RM. Infections with enteropathogenic *Yersinia* species: paradigms of bacterial pathogenesis. *Rev Med Microbiol* 1998;9:191–205.
77. Grant T, Bennett-Wood V, Robins-Browne RM. Identification of virulence-associated characteristics in clinical isolates of *Yersinia enterocolitica* lacking classical virulence markers. *Infect Immun* 1998;66:1113–1120.
78. Robins-Browne RM, Miliotis MD, Cianciosi S, et al. Evaluation of DNA colony hybridization and other techniques for detection of virulence in *Yersinia* species. *J Clin Microbiol* 1989; 27:644–650.
79. Burnens AP, Frey A, Nicolet J. Association between clinical presentation, biogroups and virulence attributes of *Yersinia enterocolitica* strains in human diarrheal disease. *Epidemiol Infect* 1996;116:27–34.
80. Grant T, Bennett-Wood V, Robins-Browne RM. Characterization of the interaction between *Yersinia enterocolitica* biotype 1A and phagocytes and epithelial cells in vitro. *Infect Immun* 1999;67:4367–4375.
81. Morris JG Jr, Prado V, Ferreccio C, et al. *Yersinia enterocolitica* isolated from two cohorts of young children in Santiago, Chile: incidence of and lack of correlation between illness and proposed virulence factors. *J Clin Microbiol* 1991;29:2784–2788.
82. Heesemann J, Gaede K, Autenrieth IB. Experimental *Yersinia enterocolitica* infection in rodents: a model for human yersiniosis. *Acta Pathol Microbiol Immun Scand* 1993;101:417–429.
83. Lian CJ, Hwang WS, Kelly JK, et al. Invasiveness of *Yersinia enterocolitica* lacking the virulence plasmid: an *in-vivo* study. *J Med Microbiol* 1987;24:219–226.
84. Une T. Studies on the pathogenicity of *Y. enterocolitica*. I. Experimental infection in rabbits. *Microbiol Immunol* 1977;21:349–363.
85. Pepe JC, Miller VL. *Yersinia enterocolitica* invasin: a primary role in the initiation of infection. *Proc Natl Acad Sci U S A* 1993;90:6473–6477.
86. Grützkau A, Hanski C, Hahn H, et al. Involvement of M cells in the bacterial invasion of Peyer's patches: a common mechanism shared by *Yersinia enterocolitica* and other enteroinvasive bacteria. *Gut* 1990;31:1011–1015.
87. Sansonetti PJ, Phalipon A. M cells as ports of entry for enteroinvasive pathogens: mechanisms of interaction, consequences for the disease process. *Semin Immunol* 1999;11:193–203.
88. Robins-Browne RM, Tzipori S, Gonis G, et al. The pathogenesis of *Yersinia enterocolitica* infection in gnotobiotic piglets. *J Med Microbiol* 1985;19:297–308.
89. Tzipori S, Robins-Browne R, Prpic JK. Studies on the role of virulence determinants of *Yersinia enterocolitica* in gnotobiotic piglets. *Contrib Microbiol Immunol* 1987;9:233–238.
90. de Koning-Ward TF, Grant T, Oppedisano F, et al. Effect of bacterial invasion of macrophages on the outcome of assays to assess bacterium-macrophage interactions. *J Immunol Methods* 1998;215:39–44.
91. Simonet M, Fauchere JL, Berche P. Role of virulence-associated plasmid in the uptake and killing of *Yersinia pseudotuberculosis* by resident macrophages. *Ann Instit Pasteur Microbiol* 1985; 136B:283–294.
92. Hanski C, Kutschka U, Schmoranzer HP, et al. Immunohistochemical and electron microscopic study of interaction of *Yersinia enterocolitica* serotype O8 with intestinal mucosa during experimental enteritis. *Infect Immun* 1989;57:673–678.
93. Simonet M, Richard S, Berche P. Electron microscopic evidence for in vivo extracellular localization of *Yersinia pseudotuberculosis* harboring the pYV plasmid. *Infect Immun* 1990;58:841–845.
94. Nikolova S, Najdenski H, Wesselinova D, et al. Immunological and electronmicroscopic studies in pigs infected with *Yersinia enterocolitica* O:3. *Zentralblatt Bakteriol* 1997;286:503–510.
95. Isberg RR, Falkow S. A single genetic locus encoded by *Yersinia pseudotuberculosis* permits invasion of cultured animal cells by *Escherichia coli* K-12. *Nature* 1985;317:262–264.
96. Saltman LH, Lu Y, Zaharias EM, et al. A region of the *Yersinia pseudotuberculosis* invasin protein that contributes to high affinity binding to integrin receptors. *J Biol Chem* 1996;271: 23438–23444.
97. Clark MA, Hirst BH, Jepson MA. M-cell surface $beta_1$ integrin expression and invasin-mediated targeting of *Yersinia pseudotuberculosis* to mouse Peyer's patch M cells. *Infect Immun* 1998; 66:1237–1243.
98. Hamburger ZA, Brown MS, Isberg RR, et al. Crystal structure of invasin: a bacterial integrin-binding protein. *Science* 1999; 286:291–295.
99. Alrutz MA, Isberg RR. Involvement of focal adhesion kinase in invasin-mediated uptake. *Proc Natl Acad Sci U S A* 1998;95: 13658–13663.
100. Dersch P, Isberg RR. A region of the *Yersinia pseudotuberculosis* invasin protein enhances integrin-mediated uptake into mammalian cells and promotes self-association. *EMBO J* 1999;18: 1199–1213.
101. Finlay BB, Falkow S. Comparison of the invasion strategies used by *Salmonella cholerae-suis, Shigella flexneri* and *Yersinia enterocolitica* to enter cultured animal cells: endosome acidification is not required for bacterial invasion or intracellular replication. *Biochimie* 1988;70:1089–1099.
102. Rosenshine I, Duronio V, Finlay BB. Tyrosine protein kinase inhibitors block invasin-promoted bacterial uptake by epithelial cells. *Infect Immun* 1992;60:2211–2217.
103. Miller VL, Falkow S. Evidence for two genetic loci in *Yersinia enterocolitica* that can promote invasion of epithelial cells. *Infect Immun* 1988;56:1242–1248.
104. Marra A, Isberg RR. Invasin-dependent and invasin-independent pathways for translocation of *Yersinia pseudotuberculosis* across the Peyer's patch intestinal epithelium. *Infect Immun* 1997;65:3412–3421.
105. Bliska JB, Falkow S. Bacterial resistance to complement killing mediated by the Ail protein of *Yersinia enterocolitica. Proc Natl Acad Sci U S A* 1992;89:3561–3565.
106. Wachtel MR, Miller VL. *In vitro* and *in vivo* characterization of an *ail* mutant of *Yersinia enterocolitica. Infect Immun* 1995; 63:2541–2548.
107. Pai CH, De Stephano L. Serum resistance associated with virulence in *Yersinia enterocolitica. Infect Immun* 1982;35:605–611.
108. Kapperud G, Namork E, Skarpeid HJ. Temperature-inducible surface fibrillae associated with the virulence plasmid of *Yersinia enterocolitica* and *Yersinia pseudotuberculosis. Infect Immun* 1985;47:561–566.
109. Aepfelbacher M, Zumbihl R, Ruckdeschel K, et al. The tranquilizing injection of *Yersinia* proteins: a pathogen's strategy to resist host defense. *Biol Chem* 1999;380:795–802.
110. Skurnik M, el Tahir Y, Saarinen M, et al. YadA mediates specific binding of enteropathogenic *Yersinia enterocolitica* to human intestinal submucosa. *Infect Immun* 1994;62:1252–1261.
111. Bliska JB, Copass MC, Falkow S. The *Yersinia pseudotuberculosis* adhesin YadA mediates intimate bacterial attachment to and entry into HEp-2 cells. *Infect Immun* 1993;61:3914–3921.
112. Yang Y, Isberg RR. Cellular internalization in the absence of invasin expression is promoted by the *Yersinia pseudotuberculosis yadA* product. *Infect Immun* 1993;61:3907–3913.

113. China B, Sory MP, N'Guyen BT, et al. Role of the YadA protein in prevention of opsonization of *Yersinia enterocolitica* by C3b molecules. *Infect Immun* 1993;61:3129–3136.
114. China B, N'Guyen BT, de Bruyere M, et al. Role of YadA in resistance of *Yersinia enterocolitica* to phagocytosis by human polymorphonuclear leukocytes. *Infect Immun* 1994;62:1275–1281.
115 Pepe JC, Wachtel MR, Wagar E, et al. Pathogenesis of defined invasion mutants of *Yersinia enterocolitica* in a BALB/c mouse model of infection. *Infect Immun* 1995;63:4837–4848.
116. Roggenkamp A, Neuberger H-R, Flugel A, et al. Substitution of two histidine residues in YadA protein of *Yersinia enterocolitica* abrogates collagen binding, cell adherence and mouse virulence. *Mol Microbiol* 1995;16:1207–1219.
117. Han YW, Miller VL. Reevaluation of the virulence phenotype of the *inv yadA* double mutants of *Yersinia pseudotuberculosis. Infect Immun* 1997;65:327–330.
118. Rosqvist R, Skurnik M, Wolf-Watz H. Increased virulence of *Yersinia pseudotuberculosis* by two independent mutations. *Nature* 1988;334:522–524.
119. Iriarte M, Vanooteghem JC, Delor I, et al. The Myf fibrillae of *Yersinia enterocolitica. Mol Microbiol* 1993;9:507–520.
120. Lindler LE, Tall BD. *Yersinia pestis* pH 6 antigen forms fimbriae and is induced by intracellular association with macrophages. *Mol Microbiol* 1993;8:311–324.
121. Yang Y, Isberg RR. Transcriptional regulation of the *Yersinia pseudotuberculosis* pH6 antigen adhesin by two envelope-associated components. *Mol Microbiol* 1997;24:499–510.
122. Cornelis GR, Boland A, Boyd AP, et al. The virulence plasmid of *Yersinia,* an antihost genome. *Microbiol Mol Biol Rev* 1998; 62:1315–1352.
123. Neyt C, Iriarte M, Thi VH, et al. Virulence and arsenic resistance in yersiniae. *J Bacteriol* 1997;179:612–619.
124. Rosqvist R, Forsberg A, Wolf-Watz H. Intracellular targeting of the *Yersinia* YopE cytotoxin in mammalian cells induces actin microfilament disruption. *Infect Immun* 1991;59:4562–4569.
125 Pederson KJ, Vallis AJ, Aktories K, et al. The amino-terminal domain of *Pseudomonas aeruginosa* ExoS disrupts actin filaments via small molecular weight GTP-binding proteins. *Mol Microbiol* 1999;32:393–401.
126. Pawel-Rammingen U, Telepnev MV, Schmidt G, et al. GAP activity of the *Yersinia* YopE cytotoxin specifically targets the Rho pathway: a mechanism for disruption of actin microfilament structure. *Mol Microbiol* 2000;36:737–748.
127. Iriarte M, Cornelis GR. YopT, a new *Yersinia* Yop effector protein, affects the cytoskeleton of host cells. *Mol Microbiol* 1998; 29:915–929.
128. Zumbihl R, Aepfelbacher M, Andor A, et al. The cytotoxin YopT of *Yersinia enterocolitica* induces modification and cellular redistribution of the small GTP-binding protein RhoA. *J Biol Chem* 1999;274:29289–29293.
129. Juris SJ, Rudolph AE, Huddler D, et al. A distinctive role for the *Yersinia* protein kinase: actin binding, kinase activation, and cytoskeleton disruption. *Proc Natl Acad Sci U S A* 2000;97: 9431–9436.
130. Ruckdeschel K, Machold J, Roggenkamp A, et al. *Yersinia enterocolitica* promotes deactivation of macrophage mitogen-activated protein kinases extracellular signal-regulated kinase-1/2, p38, and c-Jun NH2-terminal kinase. Correlation with its inhibitory effect on tumor necrosis factor-a production. *J Biol Chem* 1997;272:15920–15927.
131. Boland A, Cornelis GR. Role of YopP in suppression of tumor necrosis factor alpha release by macrophages during *Yersinia* infection. *Infect Immun* 1998;66:1878–1884.
132. Monack DM, Mecsas J, Bouley D, et al. *Yersinia*-induced apoptosis *in vivo* aids in the establishment of a systemic infection of mice. *J Exp Med* 1998;188:2127–2137.
133. Persson C, Carballeira N, Wolf-Watz H, et al. The PTPase YopH inhibits uptake of *Yersinia,* tyrosine phosphorylation of p130[Cas] and FAK, and the associated accumulation of these proteins in peripheral focal adhesions. *EMBO J* 1997;16:2307–2318.
134. Leung KY, Straley SC. The yopM gene of *Yersinia pestis* encodes a released protein having homology with the human platelet surface protein GPIb alpha. *J Bacteriol* 1989;171:4623–4632.
135. Skrzypek E, Cowan C, Straley SC. Targeting of the *Yersinia pestis* YopM protein into HeLa cells and intracellular trafficking to the nucleus. *Mol Microbiol* 1998;30:1051–1065.
136. Hueck CJ. Type III protein secretion systems in bacterial pathogens of animals and plants. *Microbiol Mol Biol Rev* 1998; 62:379–433.
137. Lee VT, Anderson DM, Schneewind O. Targeting of *Yersinia* Yop proteins into the cytosol of HeLa cells: one-step translocation of YopE across bacterial and eukaryotic membranes is dependent on SycE chaperone. *Mol Microbiol* 1998;28:593–601.
138. Pugsley AP. The complete general secretory pathway in gram-negative bacteria. *Microbiol Rev* 1993;57:50–108.
139. Iriarte M, Cornelis GR. Identification of SycN, YscX, and YscY, three new elements of the *Yersinia* Yop virulon. *J Bacteriol* 1999; 181:675–680.
140. Håkansson S, Bergman T, Vanooteghem JC, et al. YopB and YopD constitute a novel class of Yersinia Yop proteins. *Infect Immun* 1993;61:71–80.
141. Neyt C, Cornelis GR. Insertion of a Yop translocation pore into the macrophage plasma membrane by *Yersinia enterocolitica:* requirement for translocators YopB and YopD, but not LcrG. *Mol Microbiol* 1999;33:971–981.
142. Francis MS, Wolf-Watz H. YopD of Yersinia pseudotuberculosis is translocated into the cytosol of HeLa epithelial cells: evidence of a structural domain necessary for translocation. *Mol Microbiol* 1998;29:799–813.
143. Fields KA, Nilles ML, Cowan C, et al. Virulence role of V antigen of *Yersinia pestis* at the bacterial surface. *Infect Immun* 1999;67:5395–5408.
144. Welkos S, Friedlander A, McDowell D, et al. V antigen of *Yersinia pestis* inhibits neutrophil chemotaxis. *Microb Pathogenesis* 1998;24:185–196.
145. Une T, Brubaker RR. Roles of V antigen in promoting virulence and immunity in yersiniae. *J Immunol* 1984;133:2226–2230.
146. Cornelis G, Sluiters C, de Rouvroit CL, et al. Homology between *virF,* the transcriptional activator of the *Yersinia* virulence regulon, and AraC, the *Escherichia coli* arabinose operon regulator. *J Bacteriol* 1989;171:254–262.
147. Rohde JR, Fox JM, Minnich SA. Thermoregulation in *Yersinia enterocolitica* is coincident with changes in DNA supercoiling. *Mol Microbiol* 1994;12:187–199.
148. Pai CH, Mors V, Toma S. Prevalence of enterotoxigenicity in human and nonhuman isolates of *Yersinia enterocolitica. Infect Immun* 1978;22:334–338.
149. Currie MG, Fok KF, Kato J, et al. Guanylin: an endogenous activator of intestinal guanylate cyclase. *Proc Natl Acad Sci U S A* 1992;89:947–951.
150. Huang X, Yoshino K, Nakao H, et al. Nucleotide sequence of a gene encoding the novel *Yersinia enterocolitica* heat-stable enterotoxin that includes a pro-region- like sequence in its mature toxin molecule. *Microb Pathogenesis* 1997;22:89–97.
151. Ramamurthy T, Yoshino Ki, Huang X, et al. The novel heat-stable enterotoxin subtype gene (*ystB*) of *Yersinia enterocolitica:* nucleotide sequence and distribution of the *yst* genes. *Microb Pathogenesis* 1997;23:189–200.
152. Takao T, Tominaga N, Yoshimura S, et al. Isolation, primary structure and synthesis of heat-stable enterotoxin produced by *Yersinia enterocolitica. Eur J Biochem* 1985;152:199–206.
153. Robins-Browne RM, Still CS, Miliotis MD, et al. Mechanism

of action of *Yersinia enterocolitica* enterotoxin. *Infect Immun* 1979;25:680–684.
154. Delor I, Kaeckenbeeck A, Wauters G, et al. Nucleotide sequence of *yst,* the *Yersinia enterocolitica* gene encoding the heat-stable enterotoxin, and prevalence of the gene among pathogenic and nonpathogenic yersiniae. *Infect Immun* 1990;58:2983–2988.
155. Delor I, Cornelis GR. Role of *Yersinia enterocolitica* Yst toxin in experimental infection of young rabbits. *Infect Immun* 1992;60: 4269–4277.
156. Robins-Browne RM, Takeda T, Fasano A, et al. Assessment of enterotoxin production by *Yersinia enterocolitica* and identification of a novel heat-stable enterotoxin produced by a noninvasive *Y. enterocolitica* strain isolated from clinical material. *Infect Immun* 1993;61:764–767.
157. Sulakvelidze A, Kreger A, Joseph A, et al. Production of enterotoxin by *Yersinia bercovieri,* a recently identified *Yersinia enterocolitica*-like species. *Infect Immun* 1999;67:968–971.
158. Yoshino K, Takao T, Huang X, et al. Characterization of a highly toxic, large molecular size heat-stable enterotoxin produced by a clinical isolate of *Yersinia enterocolitica. FEBS Lett* 1995;362:319–322.
159. Sulakvelidze A. Yersiniae other than *Y. enterocolitica, Y. pseudotuberculosis,* and *Y. pestis:* the ignored species. *Microbes Infect* 2000;2:497–513.
160. Cornelis GR, Sluiters C, Delor I, et al. ymoA, a *Yersinia enterocolitica* chromosomal gene modulating the expression of virulence functions. *Mol Microbiol* 1991;5:1023–1034.
161. Iriarte M, Stainier I, Cornelis GR. The *rpoS* gene from *Yersinia enterocolitica* and its influence on expression of virulence factors. *Infect Immun* 1995;63:1840–1847.
162. Weinberg ED. Iron withholding: a defense against infection and neoplasia. *Physiol Rev* 1984;64:65–102.
163. Robins-Browne RM, Rabson AR, Koornhof HJ. Generalised infection with *Yersinia enterocolitica* and the role of iron. *Contrib Microbiol Immunol* 1979;5:277–282.
164. Perry RD. Acquisition and storage of inorganic iron and hemin by the yersiniae. *Trends Microbiol* 1993;1:142–147.
165 Perry RD, Fetherston JD. *Yersinia pestis*-etiologic agent of plague. *Cllin Mircrobiol Rev* 1997;10:35–66.
166. Rakin A, Noelting C, Schubert S, et al. Common and specific characteristics of the high-pathogenicity island of *Yersinia enterocolitica. Infect Immun* 1999;67:5265–5274.
167. Heesemann J, Hantke K, Vocke T, et al. Virulence of *Yersinia enterocolitica* is closely associated with siderophore production, expression of an iron-repressible outer membrane polypeptide of 65,000 Da and pesticin sensitivity. *Mol Microbiol* 1993;8: 397–408.
168. Baumler A, Koebnik R, Stojiljkovic I, et al. Survey on newly characterized iron uptake systems of *Yersinia enterocolitica. Int J Med Microbiol Virol Parasitol Infect Dis* 1993;278:416–424.
169. Bowe F, O'Gaora P, Maskell D, et al. Virulence, persistence, and immunogenicity of *Yersinia enterocolitica* O:8 *aroA* mutants. *Infect Immun* 1989;57:3234–3236.
170. Robins-Browne RM, Prpic JK, Stuart SJ. Yersiniae and iron. A study in host-parasite relationships. *Contrib Microbiol Immunol* 1987;9:254–258.
171. Baumler AJ, Hantke K. Ferrioxamine uptake in *Yersinia enterocolitica:* characterization of the receptor protein FoxA. *Mol Microbiol* 1992;6:1309–1321.
172. Robins-Browne RM, Prpic JK. Effects of iron and desferrioxamine on infections with *Yersinia enterocolitica. Infect Immun* 1985;47:774–779.
173. Autenrieth IB, Reissbrodt R, Saken E, et al. Desferrioxamine-promoted virulence of *Yersinia enterocolitica* in mice depends on both desferrioxamine type and mouse strain. *J Infect Dis* 1994; 169:562–567.
174. Skurnik M, Toivanen P. *Yersinia enterocolitica* lipopolysaccharide: genetics and virulence. *Trends Microbiol* 1993;1:148–152.
175. Zhang L, Radziejewska-Lebrecht J, Krajewska-Pietrasik D, et al. Molecular and chemical characterization of the lipopolysaccharide O-antigen and its role in the virulence of *Yersinia enterocolitica* serotype O:8. *Mol Microbiol* 1997;23:63–76.
176. Skurnik M, Venho R, Bengoechea JA, et al. The lipopolysaccharide outer core of *Yersinia enterocolitica* serotype O:3 is required for virulence and plays a role in outer membrane integrity. *Mol Microbiol* 1999;31:1443–1462.
177. Schmiel DH, Wagar E, Karamanou L, et al. Phospholipase A of *Yersinia enterocolitica* contributes to pathogenesis in a mouse model. *Infect Immun* 1998;66:3941–3951.
178. de Koning-Ward TF, Robins-Browne RM. Contribution of urease to acid tolerance in *Yersinia enterocolitica. Infect Immun* 1995;63:3790–3795.
179. Young GM, Amid D, Miller VL. A bifunctional urease enhances survival of pathogenic *Yersinia enterocolitica* and *Morganella morganii* at low pH. *J Bacteriol* 1996;178:6487–6495.
180. Gripenberg-Lerche C, Zhang L, Ahtonen P, et al. Construction of urease-negative mutants of *Yersinia enterocolitica* serotypes O:3 and O:8: role of urease in virulence and arthritogenicity. *Infect Immun* 2000;68:942–947.
181. Riot B, Berche P, Simonet M. Urease is not involved in the virulence of *Yersinia pseudotuberculosis* in mice. *Infect Immun* 1997;65:1985–1990.
182. Ahvonen P. Human yersiniosis in Finland: II. Clinical features. *Ann Clin Res* 1972;4:39–48.
183. Simmonds SD, Noble MA, Freeman HJ. Gastrointestinal features of culture-positive *Yersinia enterocolitica* infection. *Gastroenterology* 1987;92:112–117.
184. Vantrappen G, Agg HO, Ponette E, et al. *Yersinia* enteritis and enterocolitis: gastroenterological aspects. *Gastroenterology* 1977; 72:220–227.
185. Marriott DJE, Taylor S, Dorman DC. *Yersinia enterocolitica* infection in children. *Med J Aust* 1985;143:489–492.
186. Mazzoleni G, deSa D, Gately J, et al. *Yersinia enterocolitica* infection with ileal perforation associated with iron overload and deferoxamine therapy. *Dig Dis Sci* 1991;36:1154–1160.
187. Olinde AJ, Lucas JF Jr, Miller RC. Acute yersiniosis and its surgical significance. *South Med J* 1984;77:1539–1544.
188. Van Noyen R, Selderslaghs R, Bekaert J, et al. Causative role of *Yersinia* and other enteric pathogens in the appendicular syndrome. Eur J Clin Microbiol Infect Dis 1991;10:735–741.
189. Jepsen OB, Korner B, Lauritsen KB, et al. *Yersinia enterocolitica* infection in patients with acute surgical abdominal disease. A prospective study. Scand J Infect Dis 1976;8:189–194.
190. Nilehn B, Sjostrom B. Studies on *Yersinia enterocolitica*: occurrence in various groups of acute abdominal disease. *Acta Path Microbiol Scand* 1967;71:612–628.
191. Pai CH, Gillis F, Marks MI. Infection due to *Yersinia enterocolitica* in children with abdominal pain. *J Infect Dis* 1982;146: 705.
192. Bradford WD, Noce PS, Gutman LT. Pathologic features of enteric infection with *Yersinia enterocolitica. Arch Pathol* 1974; 98:17–22.
193. Puylaert JBCM, Vermeijden RJ, van der Werf SDJ, et al. Incidence and sonographic diagnosis of bacterial ileocaecitis masquerading as appendicitis. *Lancet* 1989;2:84–86.
194. Tacket CO, Davis BR, Carter GP, et al. *Yersinia enterocolitica* pharyngitis. *Ann Intern Med* 1983;99:40–42.
195. Jaffe KM, Smith AL. *Yersinia enterocolitica* cervical lymphadenitis. *J Pediatr* 1980;97:937–939.
196. Lewis JF, Alexander J. Facial abscess due to *Yersinia enterocolitica. Am J Clin Pathol* 1976;66:1016–1018.
197. Karmali MA, Toma S, Schiemann DA, et al. Infection caused

by *Yersinia enterocolitica* serotype O:21. *J Clin Microbiol* 1982; 15:596–598.
198. Krogstad P, Mendelman PM, Miller VL, et al. Clinical and microbiologic characteristics of cutaneous infection with *Yersinia enterocolitica. J Infect Dis* 1992;165:740–743.
199. Crichton EP. Suppurative conjunctivitis caused by *Yersinia enterocolitica. Can Med Assoc J* 1978;118:22–24.
200. Cropp AJ, Gaylord SF, Watanakunakorn C. Case report: cavitary pneumonia due to *Yersinia enterocolitica* in a healthy man. *Am J Med Sci* 1984;288:130–132.
201. Bigler RD, Atkins RR, Wing EJ. *Yersinia enterocolitica* lung infection. *Arch Intern Med* 1981;141:1529–1530.
202. Rabson AR, Hallett AF, Koornhof HJ. Generalized *Yersinia enterocolitica* infection. *J Infect Dis* 1975;131:447–451.
203. Bouza E, Dominguez A, Meseguer M, et al. *Yersinia enterocolitica* septicemia. *Am J Clin Pathol* 1980;74:404–409.
204. Gayraud M, Scavizzi MR, Mollaret HH, et al. Antibiotic treatment of *Yersinia enterocolitica* septicemia: a retrospective review of 43 cases. *Clin Infect Dis* 1993;17:405–410.
205. Mofenson HC, Caraccio TR, Sharieff N. Iron sepsis: *Yersinia enterocolitica* septicemia possibly caused by an overdose of iron. *N Engl J Med* 1987;316:1092–1093.
206. Viteri AL, Howard PH, May JL, et al. Hepatic abscess due to *Yersinia enterocolitica* without bacteremia. *Gastroenterology* 1981;81:592–593.
207. Leighton PM, MacSween HM. *Yersinia* hepatic abscesses subsequent to long-term iron therapy. *JAMA* 1987;257:964–965.
208. Appelbaum JS, Wilding G, Morse LJ. *Yersinia enterocolitica* endocarditis. *Arch Intern Med* 1983;143:2150–2151.
209. Plotkin GR, O'Rourke JN. Mycotic aneurysm due to *Yersinia enterocolitica. Am J Med Sci* 1981;281:35–42.
210. Thirumoorthi MC, Dajani AS. *Yersinia enterocolitica* osteomyelitis in a child. *Am J Dis Child* 1978;132:578–580.
211. Clarridge J, Roberts C, Peters J, et al. Sepsis and empyema caused by *Yersinia enterocolitica. J Clin Microbiol* 1983;17:936–938.
212. Arduino MJ, Bland LA, Tipple MA, et al. Growth and endotoxin production of *Yersinia enterocolitica* and *Enterobacter agglomerans* in packed erythrocytes. *J Clin Microbiol* 1989;27: 1483–1485.
213. Stojiljkovic I, Hantke K. Hemin uptake system of *Yersinia enterocolitica:* similarities with other TonB-dependent systems in Gram-negative bacteria. *EMBO J* 1992;11:4359–4367.
214. Kingsley G, Panayi G. Antigenic responses in reactive arthritis. *Rheum Dis Clin North Am* 1992;18:49–66.
215. Granfors K. Do bacterial antigens cause reactive arthritis? *Rheum Dis Clin North Am* 1992;18:37–48.
216. Leino R, Kalliomaki JL. Yersiniosis as an internal disease. *Ann Intern Med* 1974;81:458–461.
217. Laitinen O, Leirisalo M, Skylv G. Relation between HLA-B27 and clinical features in patients with *Yersinia* arthritis. *Arthritis Rheum* 1977;20:1121–1124.
218. Aho K, Ahvonen P, Lassus A, et al. HLA-B27 in reactive arthritis: a study of Yersinia arthritis and Reiter's disease. *Arthritis Rheum* 1974;17:521–526.
219. Dequeker J, Jamar R, Walravens M. HLA-B27, arthritis and *Yersinia enterocolitica* infection. *J Rheumatol* 1980;7:706–710.
220. Hermann E. T cells in reactive arthritis. *Acta Pathol Microbiol Immunol Scand* 1993;101:177–186.
221. Toivanen P, Toivanen A. Does *Yersinia* induce autoimmunity? *Int Arch Allergy Immunol* 1994;104:107–111.
222. Gaston JS, Cox C, Granfors K. Clinical and experimental evidence for persistent *Yersinia* infection in reactive arthritis. *Arthritis Rheum* 1999;42:2239–2242.
223. Granfors K, Jalkanen S, von Essen R, et al. *Yersinia* antigens in synovial-fluid cells from patients with reactive arthritis. *N Engl J Med* 1989;320:216–221.
224. de Koning J, Heesemann J, Hoogkamp-Korstanje JA, et al. *Yersinia* in intestinal biopsy specimens from patients with seronegative spondyloarthropathy: correlation with specific serum IgA antibodies. *J Infect Dis* 1989;159:109–112.
225. Falgarone G, Blanchard HS, Riot B, et al. Cytotoxic T-cell-mediated response against *Yersinia pseudotuberculosis* in HLA-B27 transgenic rat. *Infect Immun* 1999;67:3773–3779.
226. Hermann E, Yu DT, Meyer zum Buschenfelde KH, et al. HLA-B27-restricted CD8 T cells derived from synovial fluids of patients with reactive arthritis and ankylosing spondylitis. *Lancet* 1993;342:646–650.
227. Lo WF, Woods AS, DeCloux A, et al. Molecular mimicry mediated by MHC class Ib molecules after infection with gram-negative pathogens. *Nat Med* 2000;6:215–218.
228. Gripenberg-Lerche C, Skurnik M, Zhang L, et al. Role of YadA in arthritogenicity of *Yersinia enterocolitica* serotype O:8: Experimental studies with rats. *Infect Immun* 1994;62:5568–5575.
229. Skurnik M, Batsford S, Mertz A, et al. The putative arthritogenic cationic 19-kilodalton antigen of *Yersinia enterocolitica* is a urease beta-subunit. *Infect Immun* 1993;61:2498–2504.
230. Lahesmaa R, Skurnik M, Granfors K, et al. Molecular mimicry in the pathogenesis of spondyloarthropathies. A critical appraisal of cross-reactivity between microbial antigens and HLA-B27. *Br J Rheumatol* 1992;31:221–229.
231. Abe J, Onimaru M, Matsumoto S, et al. Clinical role for a superantigen in *Yersinia pseudotuberculosis* infection. *J Clin Invest* 1997;99:1823–1830.
232. Stuart PM, Woodward JG. *Yersinia enterocolitica* produces superantigenic activity. *J Immunol* 1992;148:225–233.
233. Carnoy C, Müeller-Alouf H, Haentjens S, et al. Polymorphism of *ypm, Yersinia pseudotuberculosis* superantigen encoding gene. *Zentralblatt Bakteriol* 1998;29[Suppl]:397–398.
234. Miyoshi-Akiyama T, Fujimaki W, Yan XJ, et al. Identification of murine T cells reactive with the bacterial superantigen *Yersinia pseudotuberculosis*-derived mitogen (YPM) and factors involved in YPM-induced toxicity in mice. *Microbiol Immunol* 1997;41: 345–352.
235. Brett SJ, Mazurov AV, Charles IG, et al. The invasin protein of *Yersinia* spp. provides co-stimulatory activity to human T cells through interaction with beta 1 integrins. *Eur J Immunol* 1993; 23:1608–1614.
236. Wakefield D, Stahlberg TH, Toivanen A, et al. Serologic evidence of *Yersinia* infection in patients with anterior uveitis. *Arch Ophthalmol* 1990;108:219–221.
237. Lindholm H, Visakorpi R. Late complications after a *Yersinia enterocolitica* epidemic: a follow up study. *Ann Rheum Dis* 1991; 50:694–696.
238. Saebo A, Lassen J. A survey of acute and chronic disease associated with *Yersinia enterocolitica* infection. *Scand J Infect Dis* 1991;23:517–527.
239. Agner E, Larsen JH, Leth A. *Yersinia enterocolitica* carditis as a differential diagnosis and the prognosis of this disease. *Scand J Rheumatol* 1978;7:26–28.
240. Friedberg M, Denneberg T, Brun C, et al. Glomerulonephritis in infections with *Yersinia enterocolitica* O-serotype 3. II. The incidence and immunological features of *Yersinia* infection in a consecutive glomerulonephritis population. *Acta Med Scand* 1981;209:103–110.
241. Denneberg T, Friedberg M, Samuelsson T, et al. Glomerulonephritis in infections with *Yersinia enterocolitica* O-serotype 3. I. Evidence for glomerular involvement in acute cases of yersiniosis. *Acta Med Scand* 1981;209:97–101.
242. Shenkman L, Bottone EJ. Antibodies to *Yersinia enterocolitica* in thyroid disease. *Ann Intern Med* 1976;85:735–739.
243. Bech K, Nerup J, Larsen JH. *Yersinia enterocolitica* infection and thyroid diseases. *Acta Endocrinol* 1977;84:87–92.

244. Tomer Y, Davies TF. Infection, thyroid disease, and autoimmunity. *Endocr Rev* 1993;14:107–120.
245. Stuart PM, Woodward JG. *Yersinia enterocolitica* produces superantigenic activity. *J Immunol* 1992;148:225–233.
246. Heyma P, Harrison LC, Robins-Browne R. Thyrotrophin (TSH) binding sites on *Yersinia enterocolitica* recognized by immunoglobulins from humans with Graves' disease. *Clin Exp Immunol* 1986;64:249–254.
247. Luo G, Fan JL, Seetharamaiah GS, et al. Immunization of mice with *Yersinia enterocolitica* leads to the induction of antithyrotropin receptor antibodies. *J Immunol* 1993;151:922–928.
248. Zhang H, Kaur I, Niesel DW, et al. Lipoprotein from *Yersinia enterocolitica* contains epitopes that cross-react with the human thyrotropin receptor. *J Immunol* 1997;158:1976–1983.
249. Weber J, Finlayson NB, Mark JBD. Mesenteric lymphadenitis and terminal ileitis due to *Yersinia pseudotuberculosis. N Engl J Med* 1970;283:172–174.
250. Hubbert WT, Petenyi CW, Glasgow LA, et al. *Yersinia pseudotuberculosis* infection in the United States. Septicemia, appendicitis, and mesenteric lymphadenitis. *Am J Trop Med Hyg* 1971;20:679–684.
251. El-Maraghi NRH, Mair NS. The histopathology of enteric infection with *Yersinia pseudotuberculosis. Am J Clin Pathol* 1979;71:631–639.
252. Boelaert JR, van Landuyt HW, Valcke YJ, et al. The role of iron overload in *Yersinia enterocolitica* and *Yersinia pseudotuberculosis* bacteremia in hemodialysis patients. *J Infect Dis* 1987;156: 384–387.
253. Farrer W, Kloser P, Ketyer S. Case report: *Yersinia pseudotuberculosis* sepsis presenting as multiple liver abscesses. *Am J Med Sci* 1988;295:129–132.
254. Chalmers A, Kaprove RE, Reynolds WJ, et al. Postdiarrheal arthropathy of *Yersinia pseudotuberculosis. Can Med Assoc J* 1978;118:515–516.
255. Bignardi GE. *Yersinia pseudotuberculosis* and arthritis. *Ann Rheum Dis* 1989;48:518–519.
256. Davenport A, Finn R. Haemolytic uraemic syndrome induced by *Yersinia pseudotuberculosis. Lancet* 1988;1:358–359.
257. Okada K, Yano I, Kagami S, et al. Acute tubulointerstitial nephritis associated with *Yersinia pseudotuberculosis* infection. *Clin Nephrol* 1991;35:105–109.
258. Sato K, Ouchi K, Taki M. *Yersinia pseudotuberculosis* infection in children, resembling Izumi fever and Kawasaki syndrome. *Pediatr Infect Dis* 1983;2:123–126.
259. Chiba S, Kaneko K, Hashimoto N, et al. *Yersinia pseudotuberculosis* and Kawasaki disease. *Pediatr Infect Dis* 1983;2:494.
260. Abe J, Takeda T, Watanbe Y, et al. Evidence for superantigen production by *Yersinia pseudotuberculosis. J Immunol* 1993;151:4183–4188.
261. Uchiyama T, Miyoshi-Akiyama T, Kato H, et al. Superantigenic properties of a novel mitogenic substance produced by *Yersinia pseudotuberculosis* isolated from patients manifesting acute and systemic symptoms. *J Immunol* 1993;151:4407–4413.
262. Head CB, Whitty DA, Ratnam S. Comparative study of selective media for recovery of *Yersinia enterocolitica. J Clin Microbiol* 1982;16:615–621.
263. Pai CH, Sorger S, Lafleur L, et al. Efficacy of cold enrichment techniques for recovery of *Yersinia enterocolitica* from human stools. *J Clin Microbiol* 1979;9:712–715.
264. Bhaduri S, Turner-Jones C, Lachica RV. Convenient agarose medium for simultaneous determination of the low-calcium response and congo red binding by virulent strains of *Yersinia enterocolitica. J Clin Microbiol* 1991;29:2341–2344.
265. Bhaduri S, Conway LK, Lachica RV. Assay of crystal violet binding for rapid identification of virulent plasmid-bearing clones of *Yersinia enterocolitica. J Clin Microbiol* 1987;25: 1039–1042.
266. Kandolo K, Wauters G. Pyrazinamidase activity in *Yersinia enterocolitica* and related organisms. *J Clin Microbiol* 1985;21: 980–982.
267. Riley G, Toma S. Detection of pathogenic *Yersinia enterocolitica* by using congo red-magnesium oxalate agar medium. *J Clin Microbiol* 1989;27:213–214.
268. Feng P. Identification of invasive *Yersinia* species using oligonucleotide probes. *Mol Cell Probes* 1992;6:291–297.
269. Ibrahim A, Liesack W, Griffiths MW, et al. Development of a highly specific assay for rapid identification of pathogenic strains of *Yersinia enterocolitica* based on PCR amplification of the *Yersinia* heat-stable enterotoxin gene (*yst*). *J Clin Microbiol* 1997;35:1636–1638.
270. Robins-Browne RM, Miliotis MD, Cianciosi S, et al. Evaluation of DNA colony hybridization and other techniques for detection of virulence in *Yersinia* species. *J Clin Microbiol* 1989; 27:644–650.
271. Bottone EJ, Sheehan DJ. *Yersinia enterocolitica*: guidelines for serologic diagnosis of human infections. *Rev Infect Dis* 1983;5: 898–906.
272. Corbel MJ, Stuart FA, Brewer RA. Observations on serological cross-reactions between smooth *Brucella* species and organisms of other genera. *Dev Biol Stand* 1984;56:341–348.
273. Chart H, Okubadejo OA, Rowe B. The serological relationship between *Escherichia coli* O157 and *Yersinia enterocolitica* O9 using sera from patients with brucellosis. *Epidemiol Infect* 1992; 108:77–85.
274. Perry MB, Bundle DR, MacLean L, et al. The structure of the antigenic lipopolysaccharide O-chains produced by *Salmonella urbana* and *Salmonella godesberg. Carbohydr Res* 1986;156: 107–122.
275. Lange S, Larsson P. What do serum antibodies to *Yersinia enterocolitica* indicate? *Rev Infect Dis* 1984;6:880–881.
276. Granfors K, Viljanen M, Tiilikainen A, et al. Persistence of IgM, IgG and IgA antibodies to *Yersinia* in *Yersinia* arthritis. *J Infect Dis* 1980;141:424–429.
277. Mattila PS, Valtonen V, Tuori MR, et al. Antibody responses in arthritic and uncomplicated *Yersinia enterocolitica* infections. *J Clin Immunol* 1985;5:404–411.
278. Toivanen A, Granfors K, Lahesmaa-Rantala R, et al. Pathogenesis of *Yersinia*-triggered reactive arthritis: immunological, microbiological and clinical aspects. *Immunol Rev* 1985;86: 47–70.
279. Granfors K, Isomäki H, von Essen R, et al. *Yersinia* antibodies in inflammatory joint disease. *Clin Exp Immunol* 1983;1: 215–218.
280. Gripenberg M, Nissenen A, Vaisanen E, et al. Demonstration of antibodies against *Yersinia enterocolitica* lipopolysaccharide in human sera by enzyme-linked immunosorbent assay. *J Clin Microbiol* 1979;10:279–284.
281. Mäki-Ikola O, Pulz M, Heesemann J, et al. Antibody response against 26 and 46 kilodalton released proteins of *Yersinia* in *Yersinia* triggered reactive arthritis. *Ann Rheum Dis* 1992;51: 1247–1249.
282. Stahlberg TH, Heesemann J, Granfors K, et al. Immunoblot analysis of IgM, IgG, and IgA responses to plasmid encoded released proteins of *Yersinia enterocolitica* in patients with or without *Yersinia* triggered reactive arthritis. *Ann Rheum Dis* 1989;48:577–581.
283. Pham JN, Bell SM, Lanzarone JYM. Biotype and antibiotic sensitivity of 100 clinical isolates of *Yersinia enterocolitica. J Antimicrob Chemother* 1991;28:13–18.
284. Segreti J, Nelson JA, Goodman LJ, et al. *In vitro* activities of

lomefloxacin and temafloxacin against pathogens causing diarrhea. *Antimicrob Agents Chemother* 1989;33:1385–1387.
285. Pham JN, Bell SM, Lanzarone JYM. A study of the beta-lactamases of 100 clinical isolates of *Yersinia enterocolitica. J Antimicrob Chemother* 1991;28:19–24.
286. Scavizzi MR, Alonso J-M, Philippon AM, et al. Failure of newer beta-lactam antibiotics for murine *Yersinia enterocolitica* infection. *Antimicrob Agents Chemother* 1987;31:523–526.
287. Lemaitre BC, Mazigh DA, Scavizzi MR. Failure of beta-lactam antibiotics and marked efficacy of fluoroquinolones in treatment of murine *Yersinia pseudotuberculosis* infection. *Antimicrob Agents Chemother* 1991;35:1785–1790.
288. Jimenez-Valera M, Gonzalez-Torres C, Moreno E, et al. Comparison of ceftriaxone, amikacin, and ciprofloxacin in treatment of experimental *Yersinia enterocolitica* O9 infection in mice. *Antimicrob Agents Chemother* 1998;42:3009–3011.
289. Pai CH, Gillis F, Tuomanen E, et al. Placebo-controlled double-blind evaluation of trimethoprim-sulfamethoxazole treatment of *Yersinia enterocolitica* gastroenteritis. *J Pediatr* 1984;104:308–311.
290. Sato K, Ouchi K, Komazawa M. Ampicillin vs. placebo for *Yersinia pseudotuberculosis* infection in children. *Pediatr Infect Dis J* 1988;7:686–689.
291. Kapperud G. *Yersinia enterocolitica* in food hygiene. *Int J Food Microbiol* 1991;12:53–65.
292. Skjerve E, Lium B, Nielsen B, et al. Control of *Yersinia enterocolitica* in pigs at herd level. *Int J Food Microbiol* 1998;45:195–203.
293. D'Aoust JY, Park CE, Szabo RA, et al. Thermal inactivation of *Campylobacter* species, *Yersinia enterocolitica,* and hemorrhagic *Escherichia coli* O157:H7 in fluid milk. *J Dairy Sci* 1988;71:3230–3236.
294. Bradley RM, Gander RM, Patel SK, et al. Inhibitory effect of 0°C storage on the proliferation of *Yersinia enterocolitica* in donated blood. *Transfusion* 1997;37:691–695.
295. Feng P, Keasler SP, Hill WE. Direct identification of *Yersinia enterocolitica* in blood by polymerase chain reaction amplification. *Transfusion* 1992;32:850–854.
296. Gong J, Hogman CF, Hambraeus A, et al. Transfusion-transmitted *Yersinia enterocolitica* infection. Protection through buffy coat removal and failure of the bacteria to grow in platelet-rich or platelet-poor plasma. *Vox Sanguis* 1993;65:42–46.
297. Wenz B, Burns ER, Freundlich LF. Prevention of growth of *Yersinia enterocolitica* in blood by polyester fiber filtration. *Transfusion* 1992;32:663–666.
298. Alonso JM, Hurtrel B, Mazigh D, et al. Temperature-modulated immunogenicity to *Yersinia pestis* from *Yersinia enterocolitica* O3. *Infect Immun* 1982;36:423–425.
299. Uchida I, Kaneko K, Hashimoto N. Cross-protection against fecal excretion of *Yersinia enterocolitica* and *Yersinia pseudotuberculosis* in mice by oral vaccination of viable cells. *Infect Immun* 1982;36:837–840.
300. Bowe F, O'Gaora P, Maskell D, et al. Virulence, persistence, and immunogenicity of *Yersinia enterocolitica* O:8 *aroA* mutants. *Infect Immun* 1989;57:3234–3236.
301. Igwe EI, Russmann H, Roggenkamp A, et al. Rational live oral carrier vaccine design by mutating virulence-associated genes of *Yersinia enterocolitica. Infect Immun* 1999;67:5500–5507.

46

CAMPYLOBACTER JEJUNI

MARTIN B. SKIRROW
MARTIN J. BLASER

It is perhaps surprising that *Campylobacter* enteritis, the most common form of acute infective diarrhea in developed countries, was not recognized until the mid-1970s. How *Campylobacter jejuni* came to be overlooked by bacteriologists for so long is a matter for debate, but a too rigid adherence to traditional methods of culture and a failure to pick up ideas from the rich field of veterinary microbiology were certainly factors. Yet there were several points in history when the discovery might have been made.

As long ago as 1886, Theodor Escherich described and sketched spiral organisms that with hindsight must have been campylobacters in colonic mucus of infants who died of "cholera infantum," but they could not be cultured and he did not attach any great importance to them (1). Campylobacters were first isolated in culture by McFadyean and Stockman in 1906 in the United Kingdom from aborted sheep fetuses, but these were *Campylobacter fetus* (2). *C. jejuni,* which can also cause abortion in sheep, was first distinguished in 1931 by Jones et al. (3) in the United States, but it was not until 1957 that King (4), also in the United States, described the group more fully (provisionally named related vibrio) and observed an association with human diarrhea. The isolates she studied were from blood, because at that time nobody knew how to isolate them from feces. That vital breakthrough was made some 15 years later by Butzler et al. (5) in Belgium, and it soon became apparent that campylobacters, far from being rare curiosities in humans, were a common cause of diarrhea (6).

MICROBIOLOGY

Campylobacters are small, spiral or S-shaped, non-spore-forming, gram-negative bacteria. They have single polar unsheathed flagella that give them a rapid darting motility reminiscent of vibrios. Indeed, they were initially placed in the genus *Vibrio,* but in 1963 they were assigned to a new genus *Campylobacter* (Greek, curved rod) (7).

Campylobacters belong to a distinct phylogenetic group of bacteria that includes *Arcobacter* (see Chapter 47) and *Helicobacter* (see Chapters 33 to 35) (8). Most of the bacteria in this group are microaerophilic, spiral in shape, and motile, features that facilitate their colonizing mucous membranes; many change into coccal forms when exposed to oxygen.

The genus *Campylobacter* currently contains 15 species. *C. jejuni* and *Campylobacter coli* together are the main cause of *Campylobacter* enteritis and form the subject of this chapter. The name *C. jejuni* is often used loosely to include *C. coli* and *C. jejuni,* because differentiation between the two species is seldom of clinical value, and in most regions, *C. coli* accounts for less than 10% of infections. Other species, such as *Campylobacter upsaliensis* and *Campylobacter lari,* usually are less commonly associated with diarrheal disease and are described in Chapter 47.

There are two subspecies of *C. jejuni:* subspecies *jejuni* and subspecies *doylei. C. jejuni* subspecies *doylei* is slow growing and much less common. In this chapter, the name *C. jejuni* is used to indicate *C. jejuni* subspecies *jejuni.*

Metabolism And Growth Requirements

Campylobacters are strict microaerophiles: They need oxygen for growth, yet the oxygen concentration in air is toxic, because they are vulnerable to superoxides and free radicals. *C. jejuni* grow best in an atmosphere containing 5% to 10% oxygen and 1% to 10% carbon dioxide, which means that plate cultures must be incubated in sealed containers charged with an appropriate gas mixture. *Campylobacter* culture media usually contain compounds that quench superoxides and free radicals, and isolation media also contain antimicrobial agents that suppress other fecal organisms. A notable feature of *C. jejuni, C. coli,* and *C. lari* is that they have an optimum growth temperature of 42°C to 43°C and have been called the thermophilic *Campylobacter* group. A landmark in

M. B. Skirrow: Public Health Laboratory Service, Gloucestershire Royal Hospital, Gloucester, United Kingdom

M. J. Blaser: Department of Medicine, New York University School of Medicine; Department of Internal Medicine, New York Harbor Veterans Affairs Medical Center, New York, New York the study of campylobacters was the sequencing of the entire genome of a strain of *C. jejuni* (14). The genome was unusual in that virtually no insertion sequences or phage-associated sequences were found, but there were hypervariable sequences in genes encoding the synthesis or modification of surface structures, which might permit antigenic variation.

Susceptibility To Physical And Chemical Agents.

Campylobacters are more susceptible to physical and chemical agents than most bacteria. They are killed by pasteurization ($D \leq 1$ minute at 60°C) and damaged by freezing and thawing, which causes a 1 to 2 $\log_{10}$ fall in numbers. They can survive in natural water for several weeks at 4°C but for only a few days at temperatures higher than 15°C (9), and they may be able to survive in a "nonculturable" form for much longer periods, particularly within biofilms (10). Although mice and chickens have been infected by drinking water from which campylobacters cannot be cultured in the laboratory (11,12), it is not certain whether this is due to a specific survival form or simply that culture is a less sensitive method of detection. Campylobacters are highly susceptible to drying and are at least as susceptible as salmonellae and other enterobacteria to ultraviolet light, gamma irradiation and disinfectants such as hypochlorites, phenols, iodophors, and quaternary ammonium compounds. Campylobacters are progressively inactivated at pH values outside the range of 5.0 to 9.0. However, they can survive in 6.5% NaCl for 3 weeks at 4°C, so it is likely that they could survive in salted, uncooked meats if initial contamination is heavy (13).

EPIDEMIOLOGY

Campylobacter enteritis is an infection of worldwide distribution, but the pattern of disease differs greatly between industrialized and developing countries.

Campylobacter Enteritis In Industrialized Countries

Incidence And Costs

Campylobacters are the most frequently identified bacterial cause of acute infective diarrhea in industrialized countries. Active surveillance, as measured by laboratory diagnosed cases, per 100,000 population, ranges from 23.5 in the United States to 106 in the United Kingdom to 318 in New Zealand. These figures represent only a fraction of all *Campylobacter* infections and are not strictly comparable due to differences in availability and use of diagnostic services. In the United States, the loss of cases at each step of the reporting chain has been placed at 37.7, which when applied as a multiplier to the rate of 23.5 laboratory-diagnosed cases gives a figure of 2.4 million *Campylobacter* infections annually (15). Estimates of mortality are imprecise because they depend on extrapolations, but in the United States, they have been placed in the range 50 to 150 deaths per year (15). In general the incidence is higher in rural than urban communities. The total cost of health care and lost productivity for *Campylobacter* enteritis in the United States is estimated at $1.5 to $8.0 billion annually (16).

Seasonal Variation

In temperate climates, *Campylobacter* enteritis shows a strikingly consistent seasonal pattern. Incidence rates rise sharply in early summer to about twice the mean and then decrease gradually to low winter levels (17). This seasonal variation becomes more pronounced with increasing latitude. A broadly similar pattern pertains in the United States, but there is sometimes a secondary peak in the fall; infections in the fall and in the spring tend to be associated with outbreaks (15).

Age And Sex Distribution

Population-based studies show that *Campylobacter* enteritis affects people of all ages, but the incidence has a unique bimodal age distribution, with peaks in children younger than 1 year and adults age 15 to 24 years (15,17). The high incidence in young children may be partly due to high sampling rates at that age (17), although a survey of children (median age, about 3 years) attending day nurseries in the United Kingdom gave an annual incidence of 169 per 1,000; half of the infections were asymptomatic and most illnesses were mild (18). The high incidences in young adults must reflect particular exposures. The incidence of infection is higher in males than females (average male-to-female ratio of 1.2 : 1), a trend that is most evident in young adults (1.7 : 1) and exaggerated during the summertime peak (2.1 : 1) (15,17).

Pattern Of Infection In The Community

Most infections are isolated sporadic cases; community outbreaks are uncommon. Clusters of two or three cases within a household are easily missed and are probably more frequent than reports suggest. In one study, other infected persons were found in the households of 40% of index cases; 15% of the infected contacts had no symptoms (6). In such instances, the timing of illness often suggests a common source, but secondary cases occur, particularly when the index case is a young child. The prevalence of symptomless *Campylobacter* excretion in the general population of industrialized countries is less than 1%. Although large community outbreaks of *Campylobacter* enteritis are rare, they can be of major significance. Such outbreaks are almost always waterborne or milk borne.

Campylobacter Enteritis In Developing Countries

Campylobacters are environmentally abundant in developing countries and infection is hyperendemic. Consequently, children are exposed to the organisms from infancy. Breast-fed infants are largely protected against infection until weaned, partly through ingesting antibodies in the mother's milk, but infections begin to appear in the second 6 months of life. Some of these infants have diarrhea, but as they progress through their second and third years, they develop immunity (19,20) and an increasing proportion of infections are asymptomatic (21).

Apart from a high frequency of asymptomatic infection, children with *Campylobacter* enteritis in developing countries tend to have watery, rather than inflammatory, diarrhea and infection with multiple pathogens, including multiple *Campylobacter* strains. Children older than 5 years (2 years in some areas) and adults are immune and untroubled by *Campylobacter* infection. In general, *Campylobacter* enteritis does not cause as much serious dehydrating diarrhea as rotavirus or pathogenic *E. coli* in developing countries, but it is still a major contributor to childhood morbidity from diarrhea (22). Visitors to developing countries are at increased risk of infection and campylobacters are a common cause of traveler's diarrhea. A history of recent foreign travel is given by 10% to 19% of patients with *Campylobacter* enteritis in the United Kingdom and 50% to 65% of patients in Scandinavia (15).

Sources Of Human Infection

C. jejuni and *C. coli* live as commensals in the intestinal tracts of a wide variety of birds and mammals, including domestic pets and animals used for food production, notably poultry (23). *C. coli* is the predominant species in swine, and there are areas where swine are believed to be the source of unusually high proportions of *C. coli* infection in humans (24). Both *C. jejuni* and *C. coli* can be pathogenic to lambs, calves, and puppies, and they are a common cause of epizootic abortion in ewes. Their optimum growth temperature of 42°C to 43°C reflects an adaptation to birds, indeed population genetics suggests that humans are an accidental and dead-end host for these species. *Campylobacter* enteritis is truly a zoonosis.

Transmission

Most *Campylobacter* infections are acquired by the consumption of contaminated food or water. However, infection also may be acquired from direct contact with infected animals or their products. Such contact is usually occupational, involving farmers, butchers, or workers in poultry processing plants, but acquisition from infected pets, usually a puppy or kitten with diarrhea, is well recognized. In one study, it was estimated that 6.3% of *Campylobacter* enteritis cases were attributable to exposure to animals with diarrhea (25). Person-to-person spread is infrequent but when occurring usually is from a young child to its mother or attendant. Conversely, babies born to mothers excreting campylobacters at the time of birth are at risk of infection. Homosexual men who engage in various sexual practices are at increased risk of infection from *C. jejuni* and other *Campylobacter* species (26). A rare form of spread is via blood transfusion (27).

Water And Milk

Virtually all surface waters contain campylobacters, even in remote regions where the source of contamination is wild birds. Waterborne outbreaks affecting as many as 3,000 people have arisen from the distribution of unchlorinated water (28,29). Sporadic infections from drinking untreated surface water in wilderness areas also occur, and *C. jejuni* may be a more common cause of "backpacker's" diarrhea than *Giardia* (30). Major outbreaks have also arisen from the consumption of raw or inadequately pasteurized milk (31,32). In the United States, children and college students have contracted *Campylobacter* enteritis after drinking raw milk while on educational visits to farms (33). An unusual source of sporadic milk-borne infection has been described in the United Kingdom, where milk is delivered to the doorsteps of houses in aluminium foil-topped bottles. In certain areas, magpies (*Pica pica*) and jackdaws (*Corvus monedula*) developed the habit of pecking through the foil bottle tops and contaminating the contents with campylobacters (34). Contaminated raw milk taken in tea or coffee can cause infection (35).

Raw Or Undercooked Meats

The contamination of abattoir carcasses with gut contents is universal and reflects on the bacterial quality of retailed raw meats (23). *Campylobacter* contamination rates averaging 3% have been found in raw red meats and 22% in offal, but in broiler chickens, rates average about 60%. Contamination often is heavy in chickens, with *Campylobacter* counts exceeding 10^6 per fresh bird and 2.4×10^7 in uneviscerated birds (36). Considering that nine billion birds are sold annually in the United States (about 36 per capita), it is thus not surprising that the consumption of broiler chickens accounted for 48% of all cases of *Campylobacter* enteritis in a Seattle study (37).

Infection can be acquired from raw meats in three ways. First, bacteria may be transferred to the mouth when handling meat; inexperienced food handlers (e.g., male college students) are particularly at risk. Second, the product may be consumed in the raw or undercooked state; undercooking is particularly likely with barbecue or fondue cooking. Third, other foods may become cross-contaminated from raw meats in the kitchen by means of hands or utensils. The latter is probably a frequent route, but it is the most difficult to substantiate, which may be why the source of many sporadic infections remains unknown (38). In contrast to salmonellosis, food-borne *Campylobacter* enteritis rarely takes the form of explosive outbreaks. This may be because campylobacters do not multiply in food, as salmonellae do; they are more fastidious, grow more slowly, and not below 30°C. Infections therefore tend to follow the chance cross-contamination of odd food items, resulting in sporadic cases or small family outbreaks.

PATHOGENESIS

Initial Events

Experimental *C. jejuni* infection has been induced with as few as 500 organisms (39). In volunteer studies, attack rates have been dose dependent (40). In these studies and in outbreaks, the incubation period to onset of symptoms has ranged from about 1 day to 1 week. *C. jejuni* are susceptible to the low pH level present in the gastric lumen (9), which is consistent with the dose effect. This phenomenon may help explain outbreaks involving vehicles such as milk and water, which may enhance survival through the gastric phase, by buffering or rapid wash-through, respectively. *C. jejuni* multiplies in the presence of bile, which may be a selective advantage in the bile-rich small intestine (9).

Intestinal Luminal Events

In animal models, motility of *C. jejuni* is critical for the establishment of colonization or infection (41). Spiral morphology undoubtedly contributes to the ability to move in the intestinal mucus gel. *C. jejuni* possess a single flagellum at one or both poles that is necessary for motility, and there is phase variation of expression of flagellation (42). The flagellar structural proteins are encoded by two highly related genes, *flaA* and *flaB* (with 98% homology) (43). In most strains, the product of both genes are expressed and the flagellar filament represents a complex of both proteins (44). However *flaA* mutants have only slight motility, whereas *flaB* mutants retain motility, indicating the dominant role of the *flaA* product in flagellar biosynthesis and function (44); nevertheless, the presence of both gene products is necessary for maximal motility. The two structural genes are under the independent control of two different promoters, sigma28 for *flaA* and sigma54 for *flaB* (44). As with other genes under the control of sigma54 promoters, *flaB* is subject to environmental regulation by pH level, temperature, and concentrations of certain inorganic salts and divalent cations (45). Another gene, *flbA,* a homologue of *lcr* genes in *Yersinia,* may be involved in flagellar assembly and export because mutants deficient in its product are not motile (46).

Adherence to epithelial cells also plays a role in *C. jejuni* pathogenesis; in general a pattern of diffuse adherence to tissue culture cells may be seen (47–49). The ability of *C. jejuni* strains to adhere to HeLa cells may be correlated with the severity of clinical infection (49). Flagellation appears to enhance adherence, perhaps only by bringing the bacterial cells in contact with the mucosa, or the flagella may be adhesins per se (47). Although it was believed that *C. jejuni* express pili, recent studies suggest that the finding was an artifact of *in vitro* growth.

PATHOLOGY

From biopsies and occasional autopsies, it is evident that *C. jejuni* causes an acute inflammatory enteritis (50). Both the colon and the small intestine may be involved (51,52). Involved tissue shows infiltration of the lamina propria with neutrophils and mononuclear cells; edema is common and eosinophils also may be present. The inflammatory lesions may cause a cryptitis; and the presence of crypt abscesses has been mistaken for ulcerative colitis (51,52). Occasionally, granulomas may be present and can mimic Crohn disease (53). The mucosal epithelium also is disrupted with decreased mucus production, abnormal architecture of the epithelial glands, and occasionally ulceration. The findings are nonspecific, but trained pathologists can distinguish infectious from idiopathic (inflammatory bowel disease [IBD]) colitis (53). After appropriate antibiotic therapy, the lesions usually resolve within several weeks. Considering the pathology, the finding of leukocytes and erythrocytes commonly in fecal specimens from affected persons is not surprising (54,55). In experimental infections of nonhuman primates, electron microscopy showed invasion of *C. jejuni* into epithelial cells (56). Other animal models generally support this notion, but due to the paucity of organisms, the issue is not completely resolved. In a rabbit model, the organisms are taken up by M cells, but whether this represents nonspecific antigenic sampling or the usual route of invasion is not known (57).

Toxins

A cholera-like enterotoxin produced by *C. jejuni* strains *in vitro* has been found by some investigators (58–60), but in other laboratories, this activity could not be reproduced (61,62). Furthermore, analysis of fecal specimens from persons with *C. jejuni* enteritis did not reveal enterotoxic activity (63) and affected persons do not produce serum antibodies to the putative toxin. Thus, more than 10 years after its initial description, there is uncertainty as to whether the cholera-like enterotoxin of *C. jejuni* actually exists. Because the predominant pathology is that of an inflammatory enteritis, the biologic relevance of an enterotoxin, if present, would be limited. Finally, the genome of *C. jejuni* does not include any genes homologous to that of cholera toxin (14). In contrast, a cytolethal distending toxin (CDT) has been well described (64,65), although its exact role in pathogenesis is uncertain. This toxin is a member of the CDT family, with three subunits, similar to *E. coli.* Intoxication with CDT causes cells to show nuclear and cytoplasmic enlargement with Gap2 (G_2) cell cycle arrest (66). Very recently, the *C. jejuni* CDT was shown to have genotoxic activity (67) in a model system. Cytotoxin activity is relevant to the pathology observed and several other candidates have been described (68,69). A minority of strains produce a cytolethal toxin that is specifically neutralized by antiserum to *E. coli,* Shiga-like toxin type 1 (SLT-1) (68). However, this activity is produced *in vitro* at low titers (68), and fecal filtrates from infected persons and controls show no great difference in cytotoxicity (63). Other cytotoxic activities may be present in *in vitro* culture supernatants, but their biologic relevance is uncertain. Recently, the presence of a HEp-2 elongating toxin was found to be associated with the development of a postinfectious irritable bowel syndrome (70).

Tissue Invasion

Although apparently less common than *Salmonella* enteritis, *C. jejuni* infection can result in bacteremia (71,72). This phenomenon suggests that at least for a subgroup of strains, tissue invasion represents a part of the pathogenetic mechanism. Studies of tissue culture cell lines *in vitro* indicate that invasion occurs (73–75), however, at a low level compared with other known enteroinvasive organisms. Because *C. jejuni* is a fastidious organism, lack of high-titer invasion *in vitro* is not surprising. This invasion of epithelial cells apparently requires either microtubule-dependent endocytosis mechanisms (76,77), a microfilament-dependent mechanism (74), or both (76). After invasion of epithelial cells or after passage of *C. jejuni* in ileal loops (73), proteins that are not expressed *in vitro* have been observed, and secreted proteins appear critical (78). Nevertheless, the ability of *C. jejuni* to invade cultured cells appears to be strain dependent (73,79).

Genetic Studies

The solving of the genomic sequence of *C. jejuni* strain 11-168 has opened new vistas for understanding pathogenesis (14). The presence of multiple homopolymeric and dinucleotide repeat tracts indicate that *C.jejuni* may use mutation and phase variation as a means for regulating phenotypic expression. The identification of a high-molecular plasmid in strain 81-176 appears critical for virulence (80). Much attention has turned to the role and genetics of the synthesis of the lipooligosaccharide (LOS) and capsular polysaccharide structures in the virulence of *C. jejuni* (81,82). In particular, *C.jejuni* surface molecules including proteins such as flagellin (83), and glycolipids frequently are sialylated (84,85). This sialylation recently has been shown to be critical in both serum resistance and virulence (80,82).

HOST RESPONSES

Antigens

After *C. jejuni* infections, there is a humoral response to various *C. jejuni* proteins and to its LOS. The response to the LOS is both species specific and type specific (86). The anti-LOS response is important because type O19 shows antigenic cross-reactivity with sialylated host glycolipids, such as GM_1 ganglioside; this may contribute to the pathogenesis of the Guillain–Barré syndrome (GBS) after O19 infections (84). Other important antigens include those of the flagellar proteins, the major outer membrane protein (a porin), and a group of antigens approximately 28 to 32 kd in size. One of these, Peb1, a conserved antigen among *C. jejuni* and *C. coli* strains to which most affected persons convert (87), has been identified as a major adhesin to epithelial cells (88). This molecule may be a vaccine candidate.

Humoral Responses

Persons infected with *C. jejuni* develop both serum (40) and intestinal antibodies (89). The serum responses are in immunoglobulin A (IgA), immunoglobulin G (IgG), and immunoglobulin M (IgM); they peak within 2 to 4 weeks and then rapidly decline (40). Hypogammaglobulinemic patients develop prolonged and severe infections, which they often cannot clear, a phenomenon illustrating the central role of the humoral response in controlling *C. jejuni* infections. In developing countries, where *C. jejuni* infections are hyperendemic and recurrent exposure occurs, specific serum IgA levels rise progressively in healthy persons (19,90). IgG responses rise in early childhood and then decline after high levels of IgA have been reached.

Cellular Responses

Little is known about the cellular immune response to *C. jejuni* infections. However, the increased frequency of this infection in persons infected with HIV (91) suggests that cell-mediated immunity is important in determining whether an infection is clinically apparent. In HIV-infected patients, *C. jejuni* infections also may be recurrent, but this phenomenon also may correlate with acquired hypogammaglobulinemia (92). In the presence of serum, *C. jejuni* induces a superoxide response by phagocytic cells (89), although intracellular survival has been reported (93).

Immunity

Most *C. jejuni* strains are relatively susceptible to the nonspecific complement-mediated bactericidal activity present in normal human serum (94). This may help to explain why bacteremia is uncommon except in immunodeficient hosts (95,96). Occasional strains are serum resistant and have been isolated from cerebrospinal fluid of patients with meningitis (97). Sialylation differences may partially explain variation in serum susceptibility (80,82).

There is increasing evidence that specific immunity to intestinal *C. jejuni* infection may be acquired.

Volunteer studies indicate that short-term immunity to homologous rechallenge occurs (40,89). In developing countries in which infection is common in early childhood, infection rates decline with age (22). The case-to-infection ratio (21), as well as the duration and magnitude of convalescent carriage (20), both inverse correlates of intestinal phase immunity, also decline with age. Studies of colony-raised nonhuman primates show similar phenomena (98). The basis of immunity is not known, but the serum IgA response may reflect this (19,90). Despite the marked heterogeneity of *C. jejuni* serotypes, the development of immunity under natural conditions implies that conserved antigens are present and that development of a vaccine is feasible.

CLINICAL ASPECTS

Incubation Period

In human volunteer studies, the mean incubation period from *C. jejuni* ingestion to the onset of fever and diarrhea was 68 hours and 88.5 hours, respectively (40). With a more infective strain, the reported means to the onset of diarrhea and fever were 53 hours and 67 hours, respectively. However, the range of incubation periods recorded in individual volunteers was 32 hours to 7 days. Analysis of reports of 17 point source outbreaks of *Campylobacter* enteritis involving about 1,700 individual victims showed mean incubation periods ranging from 1.5 to 5.0 days (mean, 3.2 days), with a range of 18 hours to 8 days.

Description Of Illness

Campylobacter enteritis is essentially an acute diarrheal disease (Fig. 46.1) that is clinically indistinguishable from that caused by *Salmonella* or *Shigella,* although some differences are evident when groups of patients are compared, notably the increased severity of abdominal pain in *Campylobacter* enteritis (99). The mean frequencies of the principal features of *Campylobacter* enteritis (Table 46.1) are derived from surveys of community outbreaks, which included patients who did not seek medical advice. Surveys of hospital patients show higher proportions with fever (63%), vomiting (28%), and blood in their stools (31%).

Prodrome

The illness usually starts abruptly with abdominal cramps and diarrhea, but about one-third of patients suffer a prodromal period of fever, headache, dizziness, myalgia, and other nonspecific influenza-like symptoms. Prodromal symptoms appear to be associated with more severe illness and have been reported in 50% of patients attending hospital (100) versus 30% in the community (101). Rigors were found in 22% of patients in three surveys (54,102,103). Temperatures exceeding 40°C have been observed in 4% of patients (104) and may be associated with delirium in adults or convulsions in children. Occasional patients exhibit meningismus (105). This "flulike" or "typhoidal" prodrome can be highly misleading in the absence of abdominal symptoms, which may not arise for 2 or even 3 days.

Acute Gastrointestinal Stage

Abdominal pain is usually the first gastrointestinal symptom to appear. It is usually colicky and periumbilical, but it may become continuous and radiate to the right iliac fossa, resulting in surgery for suspected appendicitis. In at least 10% of infected persons, the illness does not go beyond this stage, and diarrhea is absent or slight. This pattern of illness can be identified from outbreak investigations: 30% of cases in a British boarding school had pain without diarrhea (106), and in a Japanese school, 83% of children were reported as having fever, 63% abdominal pain, but only 27% diarrhea (107). Nevertheless, diarrhea is usually the main complaint that results in a stool culture, ranging from a few loose movements to profuse prostrating watery diarrhea. At least 50% of patients attending emergency rooms have 10 or more bowel actions per day (51,54,102,108,109). The presence of blood in the stools is more frequent in *Campylobacter* than in *Salmonella* or *Shigella* infection (55,110). Vomiting is not a

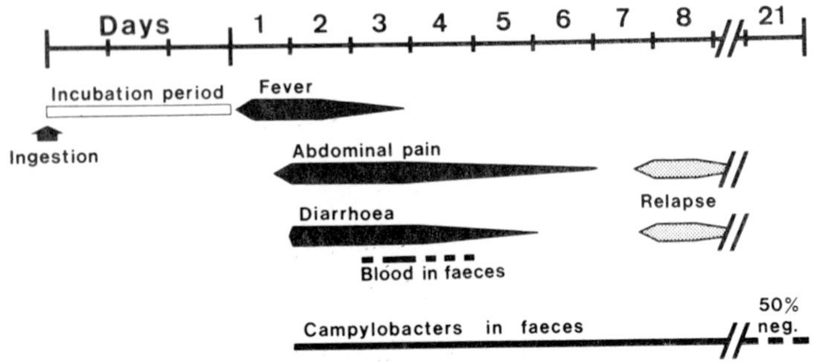

FIGURE 46.1. The typical course of *Campylobacter* enteritis. (From Greenwood D, Slack RCB, Peutherer JF, eds. *Medical microbiology. A guide to microbial infections: pathogenesis, immunity, laboratory diagnosis and control.* Edinburgh: Churchill Livingstone, 1997:291, with permission.

TABLE 46.1. FREQUENCY (PERCENTAGE) OF CLINICAL FEATURES OF *CAMPYLOBACTER* ENTERITIS DERIVED FROM SURVEYS OF COMMUNITY OUTBREAKS[a]

	Diarrhea (44)	Abdominal Pain (43)	Fever (42)	Headache (35)	Myalgia (8)	Vomiting (34)	Blood in Feces (11)
Mean	86	78	53	39	40	15[b]	14
Range	27–100	39–100[c]	6–90	0–72	27–59	0–44	0.5–32

[a]Numbers in parentheses are numbers of outbreaks from which data are taken.
[b]Excluding waterborne outbreaks, as excess vomiting in some suggested co-infection with Norwalk-like virus.
[c]The 39% was recorded in a nursery outbreak affecting children age 1 to 5 years; the lowest figure in patients old enough to complain of abdominal pain was 48%.

major symptom, although nausea is common. Resolution usually occurs within a few days, but abdominal pain or discomfort often persists longer, and short relapses of diarrhea have been reported in 15% to 25% of hospital patients (54,109,111). Any injudicious loading of the stomach during recovery is likely to precipitate a sharp return of symptoms. Weight loss of at least 5 kg is not unusual during the course of illness.

Skin rashes, notably urticaria, occur in association with *Campylobacter* enteritis (112–114); 10% of boys had urticaria toward the end of a large school outbreak (112), and rash was a feature in 2% of 148 victims in a milk-borne outbreak (115). Erythema nodosum is an uncommon late complication (see page 728).

Duration Of Illness And Morbidity

The mean duration of illness among 1,500 people affected in nine separate outbreaks of *Campylobacter* enteritis was 4.6 days, but in two of the outbreaks, 20% and 33% of victims were ill for more than 7 days (116,117). In a Norwegian study of 135 sporadic cases, the mean duration of symptoms was 14.6 days (range, 2 to 67 days) (104). The proportion of patients admitted to hospital in the nine outbreaks averaged 4.9% (range, 0.5% [118] to 22% [32]). In four studies of sporadic cases, the equivalent range was 9.4% to 32% (104,110,119,120). Chronic diarrhea due to *C. jejuni* is rare in the absence of immune deficiency, but there is an extraordinary case of an otherwise healthy young man who apparently had *C. jejuni* diarrhea for 17 years until treated with erythromycin (121). Death is rare and usually due as much to underlying disease as to *Campylobacter* infection (71,122). There is conflicting evidence as to the relative severity of symptoms due to *C. jejuni* and *C. coli* (123,124).

Convalescent Excretion Of Campylobacters

The proportion of patients excreting campylobacters in their feces after illness falls exponentially with time. Early studies showed that 50% to 85% of patients are culture negative after 3 weeks and 5 weeks, respectively. Culture methods have since improved, and in a more recent study, the mean excretion period was 38 days (maximum, 69 days) (104). Long-term carriage has only been reported in patients with immune deficiency. As discussed above, in developing countries, excretion is more brief (22).

Campylobacter Enteritis In Children

In general, children tolerate *Campylobacter* infection better than adults. In infants, abdominal pain and fever are often absent, whereas vomiting and the passage of blood in stools are more frequent. In one series, 92% of children (mostly infants younger than 1 year) admitted to a children's hospital with *Campylobacter* infection had frank blood in their stools (125). Very occasionally, the passage of blood via rectum is accompanied by severe constitutional symptoms that mimic necrotizing enterocolitis (126). In toddlers and older children, the pattern of infection resembles that in adults, but bloody stools remain more frequent. Children age 1 to 5 years may develop febrile convulsions. In a milk-borne outbreak affecting about 2,500 children, 9 were hospitalized due to grand mal seizures; 7 previously had suffered a febrile seizure (118,127). Acute encephalopathy has been associated with *Campylobacter* infection in a previously healthy 6-year-old boy (128).

Abortion And Perinatal Infection

The predilection of campylobacters for ovine placentas is not frequently paralleled in humans. About 30 fetal *Campylobacter* infections have been reported, half each due to *C. jejuni* or *C. coli*, or to *C. fetus* (129–131). The average stage of gestation for women infected with *C. jejuni* was 19 weeks (28 weeks for *C. fetus*), and none of the infants survived. Placentitis probably arises from hematogenous spread from the gut. Although septic abortion due to *Campylobacter* is apparently rare, this may be an underestimate because specific cultures are rarely performed. Nevertheless, most women who develop *Campylobacter* infection during pregnancy have no undue consequences (131,132). A woman with acquired agammaglobulinemia and *Campylobacter* diarrhea suffered recurrent early abortions (133).

Mothers who become infected near or at term pose a different problem, because their babies are at risk of becoming infected during delivery (134). Diagnosis may be difficult, because these mothers often do not provide a history of recent diarrhea and the only symptom in the baby may be hematochezia (135,136). This passage of blood in the absence of fever can mimic intussusception and result in unnecessary laparotomy. Bacteremia and occasionally meningitis has been reported in *Campylobacter*-infected neonates (134). Five nosocomial outbreaks in maternity units have been reported (137–139), and in one, 11 newborn infants developed meningitis due to a single strain of *C. jejuni* (138); all infants survived.

ACUTE-STAGE COMPLICATIONS

Colitis

Although the colon is usually involved in *Campylobacter* infection, in some patients, colitic symptoms dominate and mimic an acute attack of nonspecific IBD (51,52,100, 140–143), and the distinction from IBD is not easily made (53,144). Endoscopic appearances may be normal or show mild nonspecific colitis with intact epithelium, mucosal granularity, friability, spontaneous bleeding, or patchy aphthous-type ulceration. Active colitis has been observed as proximal as the splenic flexure and one patient had ulcers up to 3×5 cm and "cobblestone" mucosa, with "skip areas" of normal mucosa (142). The histologic appearance on colonic biopsy is indistinguishable from *Salmonella* or *Shigella* colitis but may be distinguished from IBD (53). However, there are difficulties, particularly in patients who have been ill for more than a week (100), and mistakes occur (53). *Campylobacter* antigens have been found in the mucosa of infected patients by immunohistochemical methods and IgG-containing plasma cells in the mucosa are increased in patients with IBD but not *Campylobacter* colitis (50). There is no evidence that *Campylobacter* colitis initiates IBD, although it may precipitate an exacerbation (145–146).

Toxic megacolon-complicating *Campylobacter* colitis has been reported in four patients (147,148); one had been treated with loperamide (148). Such cases are best treated conservatively with appropriate antibiotics unless there is bowel perforation. *Campylobacter* colitis has also been described in children (150,151), including pancolitis in a 14-year-old boy (141), fatal infection superimposed on Crohn disease in a 4-year-old girl (151), and bowel obstruction, colon distention and stasis, and aphthous ulceration in a 7-year-old boy (152).

Acute Appendicitis And Pseudoappendicitis

Although *Campylobacter*-associated appendicitis appears rare and possibly is a distinct disease, it is probably underreported, as surgically removed appendices are usually not cultured for campylobacters. Immunohistochemical and electron microscopical evidence of *Campylobacter* infection has been found in 3% of appendectomy specimens studied retrospectively (153), and campylobacters have been isolated from acutely inflamed appendices (154). Yet patients with genuine *Campylobacter* appendicitis are far outnumbered by patients with "pseudoappendicitis." In a survey of 533 children and adults admitted to hospital with signs of acute appendicitis, campylobacters were isolated from 15 (2.8%), but only one had histologic evidence of appendicitis; the others had ileocecitis and mesenteric adenitis diagnosed by ultrasonography (259). Nevertheless, in children, delayed diagnosis of appendicitis is common, so progressive abdominal pain or deterioration calls for rapid assessment by an experienced surgeon.

Other Intestinal And Abdominal Problems

Massive life-threatening hemorrhage from a terminal ileum ulcer occurred in a previously healthy 24-year-old nurse with *Campylobacter* enteritis necessitating emergency hemicolectomy (155). Two patients with long-established ileostomies suffered extensive stomach ulceration due to *Campylobacter* infection. Ulceration was believed due to partial strangulation, resulting from gross edema and congestion. Ulceration persisted for weeks, but eventual healing was complete. *C. jejuni* and *Citrobacter freundii* were isolated from a perirectal abscess in a 64-year-old woman 3 weeks after she had suffered from acute diarrhea (156). Spontaneous rupture of the spleen was reported in a 71-year-old man 7 days after the onset of acute *Campylobacter* enteritis (157).

Cholecystitis And Hepatitis

Acute, or acute on chronic, cholecystitis may be caused by *C. fetus* or *C. jejuni* (158). An acute diarrheal illness before cholecystitis was variably present. Campylobacters were not found in more than 280 cholecystectomy samples that were specifically cultured (159), so infection must be considered rare. Mildly elevated serum transaminase concentrations have been found in 14% to 25% of *Campylobacter* enteritis patients admitted to hospital (100,109,111), but clinical hepatitis appears rare (160,161). Experimental *C. jejuni* infections in mice suggest that some strains produce hepatotoxic factors, and in rhesus monkeys, experimentally infected with *C. jejuni,* the liver and gall bladder were the most consistently colonized sites (162).

Pancreatitis

Several cases of pancreatitis complicating *Campylobacter* enteritis have been described (163,164). In a Finnish study of hospital patients with *Campylobacter* enteritis, 11 (22%) of 50 patients were considered to have pancreatitis based on elevated serum amylase or lipase values (109), but in another series of patients, none had raised values (165).

Peritonitis

Campylobacter peritonitis, mostly due to *C. jejuni,* in patients on continuous ambulatory peritoneal dialysis (CAPD) has been well reported (166). Most patients are elderly, and the peritonitis is usually preceded by diarrhea but not by detectable bacteremia. In most cases, the infection is controlled by empiric antimicrobial treatment, such as an aminoglycoside or even vancomycin. It is unknown whether the bacteria seed the peritoneum from the bloodstream, from the gut by transluminal migration, or directly from the catheter site. *Campylobacter* peritonitis in patients on CAPD is probably underdiagnosed, because typical protocols for culturing CAPD fluid are not ideal for isolating campylobacters. Diarrhea should alert clinicians to the possibility of campylobacters in peritoneal fluid, particularly if no organisms are seen on Gram-stained smears. Spontaneous *Campylobacter* peritonitis is rare (Table 46.2).

Bacteremia And Focal Extraintestinal Infection

Transient bacteremia probably occurs more frequently than reports suggest, because blood cultures are seldom obtained from patients with acute diarrhea. In the United Kingdom, routine reporting of *Campylobacter* infections shows a bacteremia rate of 0.2%. However, if rigors signify bacteremia, then bacteremia occurs in about 2% of all patients with bacteriologically confirmed *Campylobacter* infection or about 20% of hospitalized *Campylobacter*-infected patients. In a United Kingdom study, bacteremia rates rose steeply in patients older than 55 years and were lowest in children age 1 to 4 years (71) (Fig. 46.2). Of the bacteremic patients, 29% had immunodeficiency or another underlying disease. Bacteremia rates were almost twice as high in males than females. *C. jejuni* strains belonging to serogroups O4 and O18 (Penner) were slightly more frequent among blood than fecal isolates. Bacteremia carries a risk of focal infection anywhere in the body, but in the case of campylobacters, this is rare. With the exception of septic abortion, focal infection is virtually limited to patients with immune deficiency or predisposing lesions (Table 46.2). Although acute cystitis (177) and prostatitis (178) due to *Campylobacter* have been described these are probably underdiagnosed.

Renal And Hemolytic Syndromes

Renal disease occurring days to weeks after acute *Campylobacter* enteritis includes mesangial IgA glomerulonephritis (179), acute glomerulonephritis (180), diffuse proliferative endocapillary glomerulonephritis (181), and self-limited tubulointerstitial nephritis (182). A 5-year-old girl developed pulmonary hemorrhage and anemia with progressive glomerulonephritis (Goodpasture's syndrome) 3 to 4 weeks after the onset of diarrhea (183). Renal biopsy showed immune complex-mediated crescentic glomerulonephritis, and *C. jejuni* antigen was identified in the glomeruli. Children, particularly younger than 5 years, may develop hemolytic–uremic syndrome (HUS) during the course of *Campylobacter* enterocolitis (184–185). The signs of HUS become apparent 3 to 10 days after the onset of the bowel infection. Most patients recover without apparent sequelae, but deaths occur. The possibility that some or all of these

TABLE 46.2. FOCAL INFECTIONS DUE TO *CAMPYLOBACTER JEJUNI*

Focus of Infection	Age (y)/ Sex of Patient	Predisposing Condition	Organism	References
Spontaneous peritonitis	56 M; 76 M	Alcoholic liver disease	*C. jejuni*	167–168
	46 M		*Campylobacter coli*	
	83 M	Liver cirrhosis from congestive cardiac failure	*C. jejuni/coli*	
Chest wall abscess	72 F	Mastectomy scar, postirradiation	*C. jejuni*	169
Osteitis of foot	57 M	Site of previously removed histiocytoma	*C. jejuni*	170
Prosthetic hip sepsis	60 M	AIDS	*C. jejuni*	171
Septic arthritis of knee	51 F	Rheumatoid arthritis	*C. jejuni*	172
Septic arthritis of shoulder	90 M	NK	*Campylobacter* species	Unpublished[a]
Acute bursitis	81 M	Chronic bursitis	*C. jejuni*	173
Meningitis (nonneonatal)	34 M	Longstanding ventricular shunt	*C. jejuni*	174
	41 M	Alcoholism and neurosurgery	*C. jejuni*	175
Subdural sepsis	2½ F	Previous hemispherectomy	*C. jejuni*	176
Empyema	70 M	NK	*C. jejuni*	Unpublished[a]
	52 M	NK	*C. coli*	Unpublished[a]

NK, not known; M, male; F, female.
[a]Public Health Laboratory Service, United Kingdom.

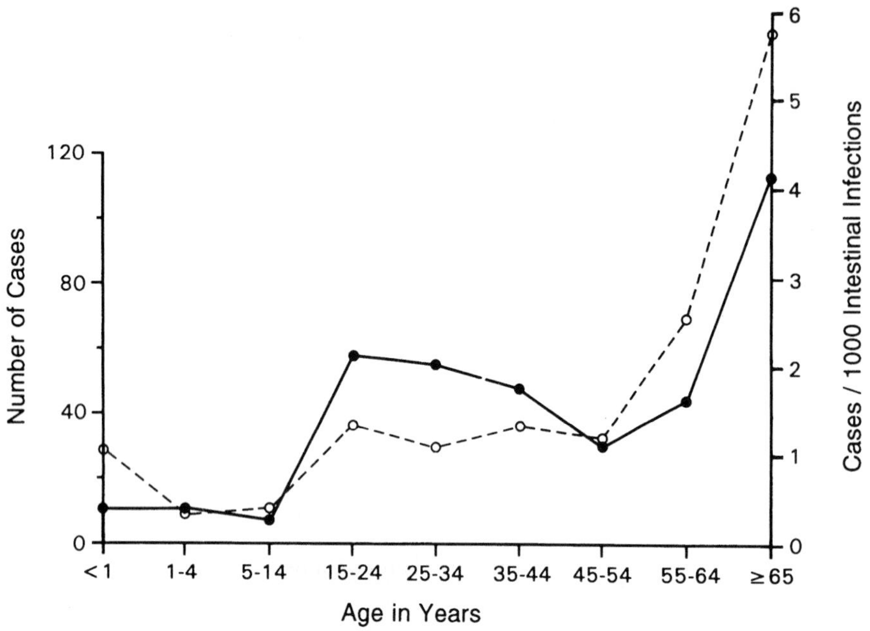

FIGURE 46.2. Distribution of *Campylobacter* bacteremia cases by age in England and Wales, 1981 to 1991. ●—●, number of cases (n = 374; ○—○ cases per 1,000 intestinal infections. (From Skirrow MB, Jones DM, Sutcliffe J, et al. *Campylobacter* bacteraemia in England and Wales, 1981–91. *Epidemiol Infect* 1993;110:567–573, with permission.)

cases were due to coincident infection with Vero toxin-producing *E. coli* cannot be excluded. Hemolytic anemia without apparent renal involvement can occur in patients with *Campylobacter* enteritis (186).

Cardiorespiratory Disease

Myocarditis has arisen 7 and 3 days after the onset of *C. jejuni* enteritis (187). Elderly patients with *Campylobacter* enteritis may develop transient atrial fibrillation (188). Pneumonia occurring during the acute stages of *Campylobacter* enteritis has been described in elderly patients, malnourished children, and splenectomized patients, but in none was there clear evidence of pulmonary *Campylobacter* infection (189,190).

LATE-ONSET COMPLICATIONS

Reactive Arthritis, Reiter Syndrome, and other Hypersensitivity Phenomena

Reactive (aseptic) arthritis is a well-recognized sequela of *Campylobacter* enteritis (191,192), and the syndrome appears no different from that following *Salmonella, Shigella,* or *Yersinia* enteritis. Pain and swelling of the joints typically appear 1 to 2 weeks (range, 3 to 42 days) after the onset of the bowel symptoms. Ankles, knees, wrists, and the small joints of the hands and feet are most commonly affected, often in a migratory fashion. The arthritis, which may be incapacitating, usually lasts 1 to 21 weeks, but occasionally for as long as a year, and complete resolution is the rule. Conjunctivitis is common and the full Reiter syndrome has been observed in about one-fifth of patients developing arthritis (191,193). Acute erosions of the hamate bone of the wrist and distal ends of the clavicles have been reported in one patient (194). Persons possessing the HLA-B27 antigen have a strong predisposition to reactive arthritis and are the majority of patients with this complication. A prevalence of reactive arthritis of 5% in patients coming to the hospital has been reported in Scandinavia, where about 14% of the population are HLA-B27 positive; however, prevalence ranging from 0% to 1.7% has been observed in community outbreaks of *Campylobacter* enteritis (28,117,118,195–197). A tenuous association between "irritable hip" and (symptomless) *Campylobacter* infection in young boys has been reported (198).

Uveitis without arthritis has been reported in two middle-age women with *Campylobacter* enteritis. One had hypogammaglobulinemia (199), but the other had previously been healthy, and conjunctivitis preceded the uveitis by several weeks (200). Evidence of *Campylobacter* infection in Behçet's disease has been reported from Turkey, but the link may not be significant (201).

Erythema nodosum associated with *Campylobacter* enteritis has been reported in five patients, all women (202–203). The lesions appeared within 1 to 2 weeks of onset of diarrhea and lasted 3 to 7 weeks. Immune complex vasculitis with thrombophlebitis has been described in a 51-year-old man with *Campylobacter* enteritis (204).

Guillain–Barré Syndrome

The first case report, in 1982 (205), linking *Campylobacter* infection with GBS had far-reaching consequences, as

Campylobacter infection has since emerged as the most frequently identified antecedent event in GBS (20% to 40% of cases) (206). Moreover, patients with *Campylobacter*-associated GBS have a worse prognosis than those with nonassociated disease. Fortunately, only a small proportion of *Campylobacter* enteritis patients develop GBS, yet it has been estimated that 526 to 3,830 patients suffer from *Campylobacter*-associated GBS in the United States each year, with costs totaling $0.2 to $1.8 billion (207). Neurologic symptoms appear 1 to 3 weeks after the onset of *Campylobacter* infection, which is usually manifested by diarrhea but may be silent. Males outnumber females by a ratio of 3 : 2, and the HLA-B35 haplotype may be particularly associated with *Campylobacter*-induced GBS (206).

The Miller–Fisher variant of GBS, characterized by external ophthalmoplegia, ataxia, and areflexia, also has followed *Campylobacter* infection (206,208,209), and a 12-year-old girl developed isolated bilateral abducens paresis a few days after *Campylobacter* diarrhea onset (210).

In classic GBS, the essential lesion is demyelinating polyneuropathy, but variants exist in which axonal damage predominates, notably acute motor axonal neuropathy (AMAN), which is common in China. AMAN is closely associated with antecedent *Campylobacter* infection (206).

Nerve damage in GBS is believed to be caused by an immunologic cross-reaction between antigens shared by *Campylobacter* and by peripheral nerve myelin, which trigger an autoimmune response. This theory of molecular mimicry is supported by the finding that certain *C. jejuni* strains are particularly associated with GBS, notably serotype O:19 (206). The critical factor seems to be specific ganglioside-like structures present in the LOS of certain strains (206).

Campylobacter Infection And Immune Deficiencies

Hypogammaglobulinemia and AIDS are forms of immune deficiency that are particularly liable to cause long-term intestinal carriage of campylobacters, sometimes with recurrent enteritis and bacteremia. In a survey of 41 patients with hypogammaglobulinemia, 5 were found to have experienced at least one episode of *C. jejuni* septicemia and three also had erysipelas-like cellulitis (211). In patients with symptomatic AIDS, the incidence of *Campylobacter* infection was found to be 40-fold higher than background in one study (91); moreover, it is often persistent and sometimes fatal (212). Antimicrobial therapy is liable to fail and resistance may develop in the infecting *Campylobacter* strain. However, in patients with hypogammaglobulinemia, good results have been obtained with a commercial IgM-containing preparation (Pentaglobin) given in conjunction with antimicrobial therapy (213). Maternal plasma also has been used successfully in this way to treat a 7-year-old boy with X-linked agammaglobulinemia (214).

LABORATORY DIAGNOSIS

A definitive diagnosis of *Campylobacter* enteritis can only be made by identifying campylobacters in a patient's stool (or blood). Therefore, the laboratory plays an essential role both in the diagnosis of individual patients and in the compilation of epidemiologic statistics. Feces should be examined for *Campylobacter* in all protocols involving patients with acute diarrhea; it is the most frequently identified pathogen in most populations.

Collection And Transport Of Specimens

Fecal samples in plain containers are satisfactory, provided they are examined within a few hours of collection or held in a refrigerator. If delays of more than a day are anticipated, Cary–Blair transport medium is recommended. Rectal swabs should only be used as a last resort and they must be placed in transport medium.

Microscopy And Direct Detection Methods

The detection of campylobacters in feces by direct microscopy is seldom used routinely, but it could be useful, for example, in patients in whom acute appendicitis or colitis is suspected. Sensitivity varies between 66% and 90% (215), depending on the freshness of the sample and the experience of the examiner. Feces voided within 2 hours can be examined wet by dark-field or phase-contrast microscopy for campylobacters showing their characteristic darting motility. Alternatively, their distinctive "gull-wing" S-shaped forms can be seen in dried smears stained with carbol fuchsin. Such methods could be useful in office laboratories where access to a full microbiologic laboratory service is difficult. The detection of *Campylobacter* species in feces by PCR-based methods is feasible (216) but is currently too costly and insensitive to replace culture as a routine method.

Culture

Dedicated media and cultural conditions are necessary for the isolation of campylobacters from feces; details are available elsewhere (215). In brief, fecal suspensions should be plated on a medium containing one or more selective antimicrobial agents and then incubated in sealed containers under increased CO_2 and reduced oxygen tension. Incubation at 42°C to 43°C favors the isolation of *C. jejuni* and *C. coli* (also *C. lari*), but when it is relevant to look for other *Campylobacter* species, incubation should be at 37°C. At 42°C to 43°C, growth of *C. jejuni* usually is visible by 2 days after incubation. Filtration, a means of selecting campylobacters from mixed bacterial flora is the method by which they were first isolated from human feces (5). Campylobacters are sufficiently small to pass through 0.45- to 0.65-μm pore-sized filters, whereas other enteric bacteria are retained. Filtrates can be cultured on media without antimicrobial agents, which is advantageous because occasional strains of *C. jejuni* and *C. coli* strains, as well as several other *Campylobacter* and related species, are inhibited by conventional selective media (see Chapter 47).

Identification And Typing Of Isolates

The recognition of campylobacters on a culture plate is simple and quick, but species identification by traditional methods takes 1 or 2 extra days, latex agglutination and PCR can be done much more rapidly (215,216). Because there is no clinical difference between *C. jejuni* and *C. coli,* it is customary to report the presence of *Campylobacter* species or *C. jejuni.* However, when clinical and epidemiologic circumstances require that isolates be speciated and typed, temperature tolerance, hippurate and indoxyl acetate hydrolysis, H_2S production, and susceptibility to nalidixic acid and cephalothin give presumptive speciation (215).

Serotyping is the most widely used method for typing campylobacters. Two complementary systems are in use: the Penner system based on heat-stable antigens, and the Lior system based on heat-labile antigens. In total, they recognize well over 100 serotypes. Serotyping is restricted to reference laboratories. Biotyping and phage typing are less discriminatory but are simpler and are adjuncts to serotyping. Typing methods based on molecular RNA or DNA analysis can be highly discriminatory, but they lack standardization between laboratories (217). Although strain typing is most commonly used for outbreak investigations, it can be used for sporadic cases to understand *Campylobacter* transmission (218), showing, for example, that patients may be infected with more than one strain.

Serodiagnosis

Serodiagnosis may occasionally be of value in patients with suspected late complications of infection, such as reactive arthritis or GBS, in whom stool cultures are negative because of antimicrobial treatment or the passage of time. Serodiagnostic tests provide a general screen for *Campylobacter* infection by detecting antibodies to *Campylobacter* antigens common to all *C. jejuni* and *C. coli* strains or can be used to screen for specific strains. Examples of the broad tests are the complement-fixation test (CFT) (219) and enzyme-linked immunosorbent assays (ELISA), which can detect different antibody classes (IgA, IgM, IgG). An example of a strain-specific test is the bactericidal assay (220), but ELISAs also can be adapted. In general, serologic tests for *Campylobacter* are available only in reference laboratories. Up to 20% of patients with *Campylobacter* enteritis may have serologic cross-reactions with *Legionella pneumophila* antigens (221).

SPECIAL INVESTIGATIONS

Hematology And Biochemistry

The erythrocyte sedimentation rate (ESR) and C-reactive protein level are usually raised (100). Mean ESR values of 25 to 30 mm per hour, with occasional values in excess of 100 mm per hour, have been reported in surveys of hospital inpatients. Leukocyte counts are usually normal or only mildly raised (102,108,109,222), but *Campylobacter* enteritis may be distinguished from other forms of acute diarrhea (except shigellosis) by a relatively high band form count (mean, 15.1%), particularly in the presence of a modest total leucocyte count (222). In the absence of dehydration, biochemical values in *Campylobacter* enteritis are normal, although in one study, metabolic acidosis was detected in 14 (32%) of 44 hospital patients (109). Mildly raised serum transaminase levels have been reported in 14% to 25% of hospital patients (100,109,111) and slightly raised alkaline phosphatase values were found in 10% (111).

Diagnostic Imaging

Plain radiographs of the abdomen in severely affected patients with *Campylobacter* enteritis may (223) or may not (102) show dilated intestinal loops with fluid levels. Computed tomography showed pronounced swelling of the distal ileum and colorectum in a 28-year-old man with severe abdominal pain and bloody diarrhea (224). Contrast radiography is usually normal, but gross changes have been observed in severe infections: pancolitis (52,141); multiple aphthous type ulceration, in one case highly suggestive of Crohn disease (152); right-sided colonic ulceration and dilation; nodular mucosal thickening of the terminal ileum. Barium enema may suggest colonic carcinoma due to an intrinsic mass (225) or narrowed colonic segments with mucosal irregularity (226); in one case (225), hemicolectomy was performed. Graded compression ultrasonography may be used to distinguish *Campylobacter* ileocolitis from acute appendicitis (227).

TREATMENT

General Measures

Most patients with *Campylobacter* enteritis require no more than oral rehydration and electrolyte replacement therapy (as described in Chapter 78). Patients in hospital need not have more than universal isolation precautions. The low infectivity of campylobacters is well illustrated by the case of a man who developed severe *Campylobacter* enteritis and infectious hepatitis after falling into a tank of concentrated sewage (229). Despite having profuse diarrhea for 19 days, there was no spread of *Campylobacter* infection to his attendant nurses, yet seven contracted hepatitis A (229).

Antimicrobial Therapy

Controlled trials of antimicrobial therapy given at the time of bacteriologic diagnosis, when patients have usually been ill for 4 to 6 days, show no clear shortening of illness, although fecal *Campylobacter* excretion is sharply reduced (230–233), a feature that has been used to control the spread of infection when there is special risk (234). However, trials in which antimicrobial agents such as erythromycin, ciprofloxacin, or norfloxacin were given empirically when patients first presented demonstrated a shortening of illness (235–238). There also are clear instances of clinical benefit from antimicrobial treatment, usually with erythromycin, in patients with severe or chronic illness, often where other measures have failed (52,140,152,226). Thus, antimicrobial therapy for *Campylobacter* enteritis can be given when the patient first presents with acute diarrhea, particularly in the setting of immunosuppression, or can be restricted to patients remaining acutely ill at the time of bacteriologic diagnosis, or who have complications, such as systemic infection.

Choice Of Antimicrobial Agent

Macrolides

For specific therapy for campylobacters, erythromycin is the agent of choice because it has low toxicity, a fairly narrow spectrum of activity, and a low cost, and it is usually active against fluoroquinolone-resistant strains (see below). Most *Campylobacter* strains are inhibited by 2.7 mg/L (Table 46.3). Although high-prevalence resistance can develop (239), resistance rates remain less than 5%. Erythromycin resistance is far more frequent in *C. coli* than *C. jejuni,* which probably reflects the use of the macrolide tylosin for growth promotion in pigs, which are principal hosts of *C. coli* (239). The resistance mechanisms of campylobacters to antimicrobials agents are extensively reviewed (240).

There are theoretic grounds for choosing erythromycin stearate as the best treatment for *Campylobacter* enteritis, but there is no clinical evidence of superiority to other forms of erythromycin. The stearate is acid resistant, stable, and incompletely absorbed and therefore exerts a contact effect throughout the bowel as well as a systemic effect. A suitable dosage is 500 mg twice daily for 5 days; higher doses should not be given because they are liable to cause nausea and acute abdominal pain (241). Enteric-coated pills are not recommended for patients with diarrhea because they are likely to be passed intact without having released their contents. For children, the recommended treatment is erythromycin ethylsuccinate (40 mg/kg of body weight per day in divided doses for 5 days).

Among other macrolides, clindamycin, clarithromycin, azithromycin, and rokitamycin have activities as good as or better than that of erythromycin but are ineffective against erythromycin-resistant strains (242). There is insufficient evidence of the superiority of these new macrolides over erythromycin to justify their cost for the treatment of *Campylobacter* enteritis.

Fluoroquinolones

Fluoroquinolones are the most widely used agents for the empiric treatment of patients with acute diarrhea before bacteriologic results are available. Although they are highly

TABLE 46.3. ACTIVITY OF COMMONLY USED ANTIMICROBIAL AGENTS AGAINST SUSCEPTIBLE *CAMPYLOBACTER JEJUNI* AND *CAMPYLOBACTER COLI* STRAINS

	MIC_{90} in Milligrams per Liter		
Agent	Number of Studies	Mean Value	Range
Erythromycin	23	2.7	0.5–8.0
Ciprofloxacin	9	0.5	0.2–1.0
Gentamicin	15	0.5	0.2–1.6
Chloramphenicol	16	5.8	1.8–12.5
Furazolidone	5	0.4	<0.1–0.8
Tetracycline	12	0.8[a]	0.1–2.0[a]
Doxycycline	12	0.4[a]	0.1–1.0[a]
Ampicillin	15	14.3	4.0–32
Cefotaxime	11	22.1	1.0–64
Other cephalosporins[b]		>125	
Trimethoprim		>125	

Data compiled from published studies. MIC, minimum inhibitory concentration.
[a]MIC_{50}.
[b]Most other cephalosporins.

active against most strains of *C. jejuni* and *C. coli,* resistance rates have risen sharply since the late 1980s. In the United States, fluoroquinolone resistance in *C. jejuni* has risen from 0% to 24% (215,243). In the United Kingdom, 12% of strains isolated in 1997 were found to be resistant (244), but in Spain the figure was 72% (245). A major factor in the aquisition of quinolone resistance by *C. jejuni* is believed to be the extensive use of enrofloxacin and related fluoroquinolones in poultry (243). Resistance is chromosomally mediated (242). Local resistance rates and a patient's travel history will influence decisions to give a fluoroquinolone. If one is given, we recommend ciprofloxacin (500 mg orally twice a day for 5 days), although shorter courses probably also are effective.

Other Antimicrobial Agents

Tetracycline and chloramphenicol are occasionally useful for the treatment of *Campylobacter* enteritis when other agents are contraindicated because of strain resistance or idiosyncratic responses in patients. Up to 25% of strains may have plasmid-mediated resistance to tetracyclines, but nearly all strains are sensitive to chloramphenicol. Furazolidone is highly active against campylobacters (Table 46.3) and resistance is rare, but anxieties concerning toxicity have inhibited its use. It has been used successfully to treat *Campylobacter* enteritis in Belgium. We emphasize that trimethoprim, which is sometimes recommended for the empiric treatment of traveler's diarrhea, is totally ineffective against campylobacters.

Gentamicin, related aminoglycosides, and imipenem are highly active against campylobacters, and resistance rates consistently remain less than 1% (243). Gentamicin—or imipenem in patients with renal damage—is the drug of choice for patients with systemic infection. Because campylobacters are inherently resistant to most cephalosporins, there agents should be avoided unless susceptibility has been demonstrated. Conversely, *Campylobacter* infection must be considered in patients who have persisting signs of infection while on empiric cephalosporin therapy.

PREVENTION

Campylobacter enteritis is a zoonosis, so prevention of human infection must focus on campylobacters in animals and their products. The wide distribution of campylobacters in nature ensures that there is a permanent reservoir of infection in domestic and food-producing animals. Prevention must be aimed at minimizing infection in these animals and interrupting transmission to humans. Direct transmission from animals can be prevented by basic hygiene and hand washing. This is of particular importance on school farm visits and in homes in which there are puppies or other pets with *Campylobacter* diarrhea (25). The importance of hand washing can hardly be overemphasized, applying equally to those caring for children with *Campylobacter* diarrhea and those handling food (see below). Because flies can carry campylobacters and are potential sources of food contamination (246), fly control is particularly important in warm climates.

Treatment Of Sewage And Water

The safe disposal of sewage and the purification of water supplies are fundamental control measures for all agents transmitted by the fecal-oral route. Conventional treatments remove nearly all campylobacters from sewage; less than 0.1% of the incoming campylobacters are likely to remain in the final effluent (247,248). Yet surface waters invariably contain campylobacters, mainly from the excreta of sheep, cattle, and wild birds. Thus, all surface water destined for drinking should be chlorinated, a process that reliably inactivates campylobacters (249). In 14 of 20 recorded waterborne outbreaks of *Campylobacter* enteritis, the implicated water was unchlorinated, in 2 it was only intermittently chlorinated, and in the remaining 4, there was a failure of chlorination or a fault in the distribution system.

Heat Treatment Of Milk

A basic and unequivocally effective preventive measure is the pasteurization or other approved heat treatment of all milk sold for human consumption. Outbreaks of *Campylobacter* enteritis regularly occur where the sale of raw milk is still allowed (31,33). Because no amount of care during milking can prevent contamination with campylobacters (250) (either from fecal contamination or from a cow with silent *Campylobacter* mastitis), heat treatment is the only answer. Milk that is delivered to doorsteps in foil-topped bottles should be protected in areas where birds have developed the habit of pecking through the tops and contaminating the contents (34).

Food Production And Handling

To prevent human infection from raw meats, particularly poultry, measures can be applied at three points: (a) on the farm to reduce colonization of the source animal; (b) in abattoirs and processing plants to minimize contamination of carcasses and meat products; (c) in the kitchen to prevent organisms on raw meats from contaminating other foods and to render meats safe by adequate cooking.

Although red meats are commonly contaminated with campylobacters, the frequency and extent of contamination is low relative to poultry, due to the heavy loss of campylobacters from surface drying during conventional forced air chilling of carcasses. In contrast, broiler flocks are not only nearly universally and more intensely colonized during life but also become heavily contaminated after processing (251); the high degree of mechanization used for processing birds causes massive cross-contamination of gut contents that is difficult to control (252). There are many approaches to controlling the colonization of broiler flocks (253): (a) the application of hygienic measures to prevent campylobacters entering into chicken sheds (the boots and clothing of attendants, small birds, animals, and insects are possible vectors); (b) the cleansing and redesign of water supplies to broiler houses; (c) the alteration of gut flora by competitive exclusion and probiotics; and (d) vaccination. Most of these approaches are experimental and require extensive collaboration between microbiologists, veterinarians, private industry, and government to research and implement. Such enterprises need to be considered in the light of the costs of poultry-borne *Campylobacter* enteritis, which is estimated to be half of all *Campylobacter* enteritis cases in the United States and costing $0.75 to $4.0 billion annually (207). Terminal irradiation of poultry carcasses, which kills other pathogens as well as campylobacters, is a promising solution, but there are problems with public acceptability (253). Hyperchloridation of chiller water appears to be reducing *Campylobacter* counts on poultry carcasses in the United States.

A frequent form of *Campylobacter* infection is the consumption of foods such as salads, bread, or cooked foods that have become cross-contaminated in the kitchen from raw meats. Campylobacters do not multiply in food such as salmonellae, but the infectious dose may be low. Good food-preparation hygiene requires separating the storage and handling of raw meats from all other foods, use separate utensils for each, and washing hands between handling each. In the home, surfaces and utensils should be scrupulously washed with hot water and detergent between use for meats and other foods. Public education lags; a United Kingdom, survey showed that only one-third of respondents appreciated the need to handle raw meats separately from other foods. Meats should be adequately cooked, which kills campylobacters (254), but barbecue and fondue cooking may not be sufficient.

Food handlers who have diarrhea (from whatever cause) should not be allowed to prepare food, but there is no evidence that symptomless *Campylobacter* excreters pose a risk to consumers. No infections were found among children at a day care center or members of a hospital who had eaten food prepared over 10 days by two cooks who were excreting *C. jejuni* (255). Responsible food handlers who happen to be excreting campylobacters should not be excluded from their work.

Surveillance

Active surveillance is particularly relevant to *Campylobacter* control by showing changing demographic patterns of infection, changes due to interventions, and warnings of outbreaks through sudden rises of incidence. Surveillance of *Campylobacter* enteritis must be laboratory based (because the diagnosis can only be made bacteriologically) such as in the U.S. Foodborne Diseases Active Surveillance Network (FoodNet) (256). The value of surveillance is much enhanced if a strain typing service is also available (257).

Vaccination

Vaccination would be an appropriate form of control for children in developing countries, and possibly for travelers to such countries, and possibly to lessen the incidence of GBS. An orally administered, formalin-inactivated, whole-cell vaccine containing modified *E. coli* heat-labile toxin is currently under development (258).

REFERENCES

1. Escherich T. Articles adding to the knowledge of intestinal bacteria, III. on the existence of vibrios in the intestines and feces of babies [in German]. *Münch Med Wochenschr* 1886;33:815–817.
2. McFadyean J, Stockman S. *Report of the Departmental Committee appointed by the Board of Agriculture and Fisheries to inquire into epizootic abortion. Part III: abortion in sheep.* London: His Majesty's Stationary Office, 1913.
3. Jones FS, Orcutt M, Little RB. Vibrios (*Vibrio jejuni* n. sp.) associated with intestinal disorders of cows and calves. *J Exp Med* 1931;53:853–863.
4. King EO. Human infections with *Vibrio fetus* and a closely related vibrio. *J Infect Dis* 1957;101:119–128.
5. Butzler JP, Dekeyser P, Detrain M, et al. Related vibrio in stools. *J Pediatr* 1973;82:493–495.
6. Skirrow MB. *Campylobacter* enteritis: a "new" disease. *Br Med J* 1977;2:9–11.
7. Sebald M, Véron M. Teneur en bases de l'ADN et classification des vibrions. *Ann Inst Pasteur* 1963;105:897–910.
8. Vandamme P, Falsen E, Rossau R, et al. Revision of *Campylobacter, Helicobacter* and *Wolinella* taxonomy: emendation of generic descriptions and proposal of *Arcobacter* gen. nov. *Int J Syst Bact* 1990;41:88–103.
9. Blaser MJ, Hardesty HL, Powers B, et al. Survival of *Campylobacter fetus* subsp. *jejuni* in biological milieus. *J Clin Microbiol* 1980;11:309–313.
10. Buswell CM, Herlihy YM, Lawrence LM, et al. Extended survival and persistence of *Campylobacter* spp. in water and aquatic biofilms and their detection by immunofluorescent-antibody and -rRNA staining. *Infect Immun* 1998;64:733–741.
11. Jones DM, Sutcliffe EM, Curry A. Recovery of viable but nonculturable *Campylobacter jejuni. J Gen Microbiol* 1991;137: 2477–2482.
12. Pearson AD, Greenwood M, Healing TD, et al. Colonization of broiler chickens by waterborne *Campylobacter jejuni. Appl Environ Microbiol* 1993;59:987–996.
13. Abram DD, Potter NN. Survival of *Campylobacter jejuni* at different temperatures in broth, beef, chicken and cod supplemented with sodium chloride. *J Food Protect* 1984;47:795–800.
14. Parkhill J, Wren BW, Mungall K, et al. The genome sequence of the food-borne pathogen *Campylobacter jejuni* reveals hypervariable sequences. *Nature* 2000;403:665–668.
15. Friedman CR, Neimann J, Wegener HC, et al. Epidemiology of *Campylobacter jejuni* infections in the United States and other industrialized nations. In: Nachamkin I, Blaser MJ, eds. *Campylobacter,* 2nd ed. Washington, DC: ASM Press, 2000:121–138.
16. Buzby JC, Mishu Allos B, Roberts T. The economic burden of *Campylobacter*-associated Guillain–Barré syndrome. *J Infect Dis* 1997;176:S192–S197.

17. Skirrow MB. A demographic survey of *Campylobacter, Salmonella* and *Shigella* infections in England. *Epidemiol Infect* 1987; 99:647–657.
18. Riordan T. Intestinal infection with *Campylobacter* in children. *Lancet* 1988;1:992.
19. Blaser MJ, Taylor DN, Echeverria P. Immune response to *Campylobacter jejuni* in a rural community in Thailand. *J Infect Dis* 1986;153:249–254.
20. Taylor DN, Perlman DM, Echeverria PD, et al. *Campylobacter* immunity and quantitative excretion rates in Thai children. *J Infect Dis* 1993;168:754–758.
21. Calva JJ, Ruiz-Palacios GM, Lopez-Vidal AB, et al. Cohort study of intestinal infection with *Campylobacter* in Mexican children. *Lancet* 1988;1:503–506.
22. Oberhelman RA, Taylor DN. *Campylobacter* infections in developing countries. In: Nachamkin I, Blaser MJ, eds. *Campylobacter,* 2nd ed. Washington, DC: ASM Press, 2000:139–153.
23. Jacobs-Reitsma W. *Campylobacter* in the food supply. In: Nachamkin I, Blaser MJ, eds. *Campylobacter,* 2nd ed. Washington, DC: ASM Press, 2000:467–481.
24. Popovic-Uroic T. *Campylobacter jejuni* and *Campylobacter coli* diarrhea in rural and urban populations in Yugoslavia. *Epidemiol Infect* 1989;102:59–67.
25. Saeed AM, Harris NV, DiGiacomo RF. The role of exposure to animals in the etiology of *Campylobacter jejunicoli* enteritis. *Am J Epidemiol* 1993;137:108–114.
26. Totten PA, Fennell CL, Tenover FC, et al. *Campylobacter cinaedi* (sp. nov.) and *Campylobacter fennelliae* (sp. nov.): two new *Campylobacter* species associated with enteric disease in homosexual men. *J Infect Dis* 1985;151:131–139.
27. Pepersack F, Prigogyne T, Butzler JP, et al. *Campylobacter jejuni* post-transfusional septicaemia. *Lancet* 1979;2:911.
28. Mentzing L-O. Waterborne outbreaks of *Campylobacter* enteritis in central Sweden. *Lancet* 1981;2:352–354.
29. Vogt RL, Sours HE, Barrett T, et al. *Campylobacter* enteritis associated with contaminated water. *Ann Intern Med* 1982;96: 292–296.
30. Taylor DN, McDermott KT, Little JR, et al. *Campylobacter* enteritis from untreated water in the Rocky Mountains. *Ann Intern Med* 1983;99:38–40.
31. Robinson DA, Jones DM. Milk-borne *Campylobacter* infection. *Br Med J* 1981;282:1374–1376.
32. Potter ME, Blaser MJ, Sikes RK, et al. Human *Campylobacter* infection associated with certified raw milk. *Am J Epidemiol* 1983;117:475–483.
33. Wood RC, MacDonald KL, Osterholm MT. *Campylobacter* enteritis outbreaks associated with drinking raw milk during youth activities. *JAMA* 1992;268:3228–3230.
34. Hudson SJ, Lightfoot NF, Coulson JC, et al. Jackdaws and magpies as vectors of milkborne human *Campylobacter* infection. *Epidemiol Infect* 1991;107:363–372.
35. Hudson PJ, Vogt RL, Brondum J, et al. Isolation of *Campylobacter jejuni* from milk during an outbreak of campylobacteriosis. *J Infect Dis* 1984;150:789.
36. Hood AM, Pearson AD, Shahamat M. The extent of surface contamination of retailed chickens with *Campylobacter jejuni* serogroups. *Epidemiol Infect* 1988;100:17–25.
37. Harris NV, Weiss NS, Nolan CM. The role of poultry and meats in the etiology of *Campylobacter jejunicoli* enteritis. *Am J Public Health* 1986;76:407–411.
38. Brown P, Kidd D, Riordan T, Barrell RA. An outbreak of food borne *Campylobacter jejuni* infection and the possible role of cross-contamination. *J Infect* 1988;17:171–176.
39. Robinson DA. Infective dose of *Campylobacter jejuni* in milk. *Br Med J* 1981;282:1584.
40. Black RE, Levine MM, Clements ML, et al. Experimental *Campylobacter jejuni* infection in humans. *J Infect Dis* 1988; 157:472–479.
41. Caldwell MB, Guerry P, Lee EC, et al. Reversible expression of flagella in *Campylobacter jejuni. Infect Immun* 1985;50:941–943
42. Harris LA, Logan SM, Guerry P, et al. Antigenic variation of *Campylobacter jejuni* flagella. *J Bacteriol* 1987;169:5066–5071.
43. Guerry P, Logan SM, Thornton S, et al. Genomic organization and expression of *Campylobacter* flagellin genes. *J Bacteriol* 1990;172:1853–1860.
44. Guerry P, Alm RA, Power ME, et al. Role of two flagellin genes in *Campylobacter* motility. *J Bacteriol* 1990;173:4757–4764.
45. Alm RA, Guerry P, Trust TJ. Distribution and polymorphism of the flagellin genes from isolates of *Campylobacter coli* and *Campylobacter jejuni. J Bacteriol* 1993;175:3051–3057.
46. Miller S, Pesci EC, Pickett CL. A *Campylobacter jejuni* homolog of the LcrD/FlbF family of proteins is necessary for flagellar biogenesis. *Infect Immun* 1993;61:2930–2936.
47. McSweegan E, Walker RI. Identification and characterization of two *Campylobacter jejuni* adhesins for cellular and mucous substrates. *Infect Immun* 1986;53:141–148.
48. Lindblom GB, Cervantes LE, Sjögren E, et al. Adherence, enterotoxigenicity, invasiveness, and sero-groups in *Campylobacter jejuni* and *Campylobacter coli* strains from adult humans with acute enterocolitis. *APMIS* 1990;98:179–184.
49. Fauchère JL, Kervella M, Rosenau A, et al. Adhesion to HeLa cells of *Campylobacter jejuni* and *C. coli* outer membrane components. *Res Microbiol* 1989;140:379–392.
50. Van Spreeuwel JP, Duursma GC, Meijer CJLM, et al. *Campylobacter* colitis: histological immunohistochemical and ultrastructural findings. *Gut* 1985;26:945–951.
51. Price AB, Jewkes J, Sanderson PJ. Acute diarrhea: *Campylobacter* colitis and the role of rectal biopsy. *J Clin Pathol* 1979;32: 990–997.
52. Blaser MJ, Parsons RB, Wang W-LL. Acute colitis caused by *Campylobacter fetus* ss. *jejuni. Gastroenterology* 1980;78:448–453.
53. Surawicz CM, Belic L. Rectal biopsy helps to distinguish acute self-limited colitis from idiopathic inflammatory bowel disease. *Gastroenterology* 1984;86:104–113.
54. Blaser MJ, Berkowitz ID, LaForce FM, et al. *Campylobacter* enteritis: clinical and epidemiologic features. *Ann Intern Med* 1979;91:179–185.
55. Blaser MJ, Wells JG, Feldman RA, et al. *Campylobacter* enteritis in the United States. A multicenter study. *Ann Intern Med* 1983;98:360–365.
56. Russell RG, O'Donnoghue M, Blake DC, et al. Early colonic damage and invasion of *Campylobacter jejuni* in experimentally challenged *Mucaca mulatta. J Infect Dis* 1993;168:210–215.
57. Walker RI, Schmauder-Chock A, Parker JL, et al. Selective association and transport of *Campylobacter jejuni* through M cells of rabbit Peyer's patches. *Can J Microbiol* 1988;34:1143–1147.
58. Ruiz-Palacios GM, Torres J, Torres NI, et al. Cholera-like enterotoxin produced by *Campylobacter jejuni. Lancet* 1983; 1:250–253.
59. Klipstein FA, Engert RF. Properties of crude *Campylobacter jejuni* heat-labile enterotoxin. *Infect Immun* 1984;45:314–319.
60. Klipstein FA, Engert RF. Purification of *Campylobacter jejuni* enterotoxin. *Lancet* 1985;1:1123–1124.
61. Olsvik O, Wachsmuth K, Morris G, et al. Genetic probing of *Campylobacter jejuni* for cholera toxin and *Escherichia coli* heat-labile enterotoxin. *Lancet* 1984;1:449.
62. Pérez-Pérez GI, Cohn DL, Guerrant RL, et al. Clinical and immunological significance of cholera-like toxin and cytotoxin production by *Campylobacter* species in patients with acute inflammatory diarrhea. *J Infect Dis* 1989;160:460–468.
63. Cover TL, Pérez-Pérez GI, Blaser MJ. Evaluation of cytotoxic activity in fecal filtrates from patients with *Campylobacter jejuni*

or *Campylobacter coli* enteritis. *FEMS Microbiol Lett* 1990;70: 301–304.
64. Johnson WM, Lior H. Cytotoxic cytotonic factor produced by *Campylobacter jejuni, Campylobacter coli,* and *Campylobacter laridis. J Clin Microbiol* 1986;24:275–281.
65. Johnson WM, Lior H. A new heat-labile cytolethal distending toxin (CLDT) produced by *Campylobacter* spp. *Microb Pathog* 1988; 4:103–113.
66. Whitehouse CA, Balbo PV, Pesci EC, et al. *Campylobacter jejuni* cytolethal distending toxin causes a G_2-phase cell cycle block. *Infect Immun* 2000;6:1934–1940.
67. Hassane DC, Lee RB, Mendenhall MD, et al. Cytolethal distending toxin demonstrates genotoxic activity in a yeast model. *Infect Immun* 2001;69:5752–5759.
68. Moore MA, Blaser MJ, Pérez-Pérez GI, et al. Production of a Shiga-like cytotoxin by *Campylobacter. Microb Pathog* 1988;4: 455–462.
69. Guerrant RL, Wanke CA, Pennie RA, et al. Production of a unique cytotoxin by *Campylobacter jejuni. Infect Immun* 1987; 55:2526–2530.
70. Thornley JP, Jnkins D, Neal K, et al. Relationship of *Campylobacter* toxigenicity *in vitro* to the development of post infectious irritable bowel syndrome. *J Infect Dis* 2001;184:606–609.
71. Skirrow MB, Jones DM, Sutcliffe J, et al. *Campylobacter* bacteraemia in England and Wales, 1981–91. *Epidemiol Infect* 1993; 110:567–573.
72. Guerrant RL, Lahita RG, Winn WC, et al. Campylobacteriosis in man: pathogenic mechanisms and review of 91 bloodstream infections. *Am J Med* 1978;65:584–592.
73. Konkel ME, Joens LA. Adhesion to and invasion of HEp-2 cells by *Campylobacter* spp. *Infect Immun* 1989;57:2984–2990.
74. De Melo MA, Gabbiani G, Pechère JC. Cellular events and intracellular survival of *Campylobacter jejuni* during infection of HEp-2 cells. *Infect Immun* 1989;57:2214–2222.
75. Fauchere JL, Rosenau M, Veron M, et al. Association with HeLa cells of *Campylobacter jejuni* and *C. coli* isolated from human feces. *Infect Immun* 1986;54:283–287.
76. Oelshlager TA, Guerry P, Kopecko DJ. Unusual microtubule dependent endocytosis mechanisms triggered by *Campylobacter jejuni* and *Citrobacter freundii. Proc Natl Acad Sci U S A* 1993; 90:6884–6888.
77. Hu L, Kopecko DL. *Campylobacter jejuni* 81-176 associates with microtubules and dynein during invasion into human intestinal cells. *Infect Immun* 1999;67:4171–4182.
78. Konkel ME, Kim BJ, Rivera-Amill V, et al. Bacterial secreted proteins are required for the internalization of *Campylobacter jejuni* into cultured mammalian cells. *Mol Microbiol* 1999;32: 691–702.
79. Konkel ME, Joens LA, Mixler PF. Molecular characterization of *Campylobacter jejuni* virulence determinants. In: Nachamkin I, Blaser MJ, eds. *Campylobacter,* 2nd ed. Washington, DC: ASM Press, 2000:217–240.
80. Bacon DJ, Alm RA, Burr DH, et al. Involvement of a plasmid in virulence of *Campylobacter jejuni* 81-176. *Infect Immun* 2000;68:4384–4390.
81. Fry BN, Oldfield NJ, Korolik V, et al. Genetics of *Campylobacter* lipopolysaccharide biosynthesis. In: Nachamkin I, Blaser MJ, eds. *Campylobacter,* 2nd ed. Washington, DC: ASM Press, 2000:381–403.
82. Bacon DJ, Szmanski CM, Burr DH, et al. A phase-variable capsule is involved in virulence of *Campylobacter jejuni* 81-176. *Mol Microbiol* 2001;40:769–777.
83. Doig P, Kinsella N, Guerry P, et al. Characterization of a post-translational modification of *Campylobacter* flagellin: identification of a sero specific glycosyl moiety. *Mol Microbiol* 1996;19: 379–387.
84. Yuki N, Taki T, Inagaki F, et al. A bacterium lipopolysaccharide that elicits Guillain–Barré syndrome has a GM_1 ganglioside-like structure. *J Exp Med* 1993;178:1771–1775.
85. Guerry P, Ewing CP, Hickey TE, et al. Sialylation of lipooligosaccharide cores affects immunogenicity and serum resistance of *Campylobacter jejuni. Infect Immun* 2000;68:6656–6662.
86. Blaser MJ, Pérez-Pérez GI. Humoral immune response to lipopolysaccharide antigens of *Campylobacter jejuni.* In: Nachamkin I, Blaser MJ, Tompkins LS, eds. *Campylobacter jejuni. Current status and future trends.* Washington, DC: American Society of Microbiology, 1992:230–235.
87. Pei Z, Ellison RT III, Blaser MJ. Identification, purification and characterization of major antigenic proteins of *Campylobacter jejuni. J Biol Chem* 1991;266:16363–16369.
88. Kervella M, Pagès J-M, Pei Z, et al. Isolation and characterization of two *Campylobacter* glycine-extracted proteins that bind to HeLa cell membranes. *Infect Immun* 1993;61:3440–3448.
89. Black RE, Perlman D, Clements ML, et al. Human volunteer studies with *Campylobacter jejuni.* In: Nachamkin I, Blaser MJ, Tompkins LS, eds. *Campylobacter jejuni. Current status and future trends.* Washington, DC: American Society of Microbiology, 1992:207–215.
90. Blaser MJ, Black RE, Duncan DJ. *Campylobacter jejuni*-specific serum antibodies are elevated in healthy Bangladeshi children. *J Clin Microbiol* 1985;21:164–167.
91. Sorvillo FJ, Lieb LE, Waterman SH. Incidence of campylobacteriosis among patients with AIDS in Los Angeles County. *J AIDS* 1991;4:598–602.
92. Perlman DM, Ampel NM, Schifman RB, et al. Persistent *Campylobacter jejuni* infections in patients infected with human immunodeficiency virus (HIV). *Ann Intern Med* 1988;108:540–546.
93. Kiehlbauch JA, Albach RA, Baum LL, et al. Phagocytosis of *Campylobacter jejuni* and its intracellular survival in mononuclear phagocytes. *Infect Immun* 1985;48:446–451.
94. Blaser MJ, Smith PF, Kohler PA. Susceptibility of *Campylobacter* isolates to the bactericidal activity in human serum. *J Infect Dis* 1985;151:227–235.
95. Johnson RJ, Wang SP, Shelton WR, et al. Persistent *Campylobacter jejuni* infection in an immunocompromised host. *Ann Intern Med* 1984;100:832–834.
96. Melamed A, Zakuth V, Schwartz D, et al. The immune system response to *Campylobacter* infection. *Microbiol Immunol* 1988; 32:75–82.
97. Blaser MJ, Pérez-Pérez GI, Smith PF, et al. Extraintestinal *Campylobacter jejuni* and *Campylobacter coli* infections: host factors and strain characteristics. *J Infect Dis* 1986;153:552–559.
98. Russell RG, Blaser MJ, Sarmiento I, et al. Experimental *Campylobacter jejuni* infection in *Macaca nemestrina. Infect Immun* 1989;57:1438–1444.
99. Jewkes J, Larson HE, Price AB, et al. Aetiology of acute diarrhea in adults. *Gut* 1981;22:388–392.
100. McKendrick MW, Geddes AM, Gearty J. *Campylobacter* enteritis: a study of clinical features and rectal mucosal changes. *Scand J Infect Dis* 1982;14:35–38.
101. Wallace JM. Milk-associated *Campylobacter* infection. *Health Bull (Edinb)* 1980;38:57–61.
102. Pentland B. *Campylobacter* enteritis: an in-patient study. *Scot Med J* 1979;24:299–301.
103. Pitkänen T, Pettersson T, Pönkä A, et al. Clinical and serological studies in patients with *Campylobacter fetus* ssp. *jejuni* infection: I. clinical findings. *Infection* 1981;9:274–278.
104. Kapperud G, Lassen J, Ostroff SM, et al. Clinical features of sporadic *Campylobacter* infections in Norway. *Scand J Infect Dis* 1992;24:741–749.
105. Wright EP. Meningism associated with *Campylobacter jejuni* enteritis. *Lancet* 1979;1:1092.

106. Wilson PG, Davies JR, Hoskins TW, et al. Epidemiology of an outbreak of milk-borne enteritis in a residential school. In: Pearson AD, Skirrow MB, Rowe B, et al, eds. *Campylobacter II: proceedings of the Second International Workshop on Campylobacter Infections.* London: Public Health Laboratory Service, 1983:143.
107. Matsusaki S, Katayama A. Studies on outbreaks of food poisoning due to *Campylobacter jejuni* between 1980 and 1982 in Yamaguchi prefecture, Japan. *Yamaguchi J Vet Med* 1984;11:53–56.
108. Svedhem Ä, Kaijser B. *Campylobacter fetus* subspecies *jejuni:* a common cause of diarrhea in Sweden. *J Infect Dis* 1980;142: 353–359.
109. Pitkänen T, Pönkä A, Pettersson T, et al. *Campylobacter* enteritis in 188 hospitalized patients. *Arch Intern Med* 1983;143: 215–219.
110. Rao GG, Fuller M. A review of hospitalized patients with bacterial gastroenteritis. *J Hosp Infect* 1992;20:105–111.
111. Drake AA, Gilchrist MJR, Washington JA, et al. Diarrhea due to *Campylobacter fetus* subspecies *jejuni. Mayo Clin Proc* 1981; 56:414–423.
112. Hoskins TW. *Campylobacter* enteritis and erythema nodosum. *Br Med J* 1982;285:1661.
113. Bretag AH, Archer RS, Atkinson HM, et al. Circadian urticaria: another *Campylobacter* association. *Lancet* 1984;1:954.
114. Lopez-Brea M, Fontelas PM, Baquero M, et al. Urticaria associated with *Campylobacter* enteritis. *Lancet* 1984;1:1354.
115. Porter IA, Reid TMS. A milk-borne outbreak of *Campylobacter* infection. *J Hyg (Lond)* 1980;84:415–419.
116. Blaser MJ, Checko P, Bopp C, et al. *Campylobacter* enteritis associated with foodborne transmission. *Am J Epidemiol* 1982; 116:886–894.
117. Millson M, Bokhout M, Carlson J, et al. An outbreak of *Campylobacter jejuni* gastroenteritis linked to meltwater contamination of a municipal well. *Can J Public Health* 1991;82:27–31.
118. Jones PH, Willis AT, Robinson DA, et al. *Campylobacter* enteritis associated with the consumption of free school milk. *J Hyg (Lond)* 1981;87:155–162.
119. Sockett PN, Pearson AD. Cost implications of human *Campylobacter* infections. In: Kaijser B, Falsen E, eds. Campylobacter *IV: Proceedings of the fourth international workshop on* Campylobacter *infections.* Göteborg: University of Göteborg, 1988: 261–264.
120. Steingrimsson O, Thorsteinsson SB, Hjalmarsdottir M, et al. *Campylobacter* ssp. infections in Iceland during a 24-month period in 1980–1982. *Scand J Infect Dis* 1985;17:285–290.
121. Paulet Ph, Coffernils M. Very long term diarrhea due to *Campylobacter jejuni. Postgrad Med J* 1990;66:410–411.
122. Smith GS, Blaser MJ. Fatalities associated with *Campylobacter jejuni* infections. *JAMA* 1985;253:2873–2875.
123. Popovic-Uroic T, Gmajnicki B, Kalenic S, et al. Clinical comparison of *Campylobacter jejuni* and *C. coli* diarrhea. *Lancet* 1988;1:176–177.
124. Figura N, Guglielmetti P. Clinical characteristics of *Campylobacter jejuni* and *C coli* enteritis. *Lancet* 1988;1:942–943.
125. Karmali MA, Fleming PC. *Campylobacter* enteritis in children. *J Pediatr* 1979;94:527–533.
126. Colver AF, Pedler SJ, Hawkey PM. Severe *Campylobacter* infection in children. *J Infect* 1985;11:217–220.
127. Havalad S, Chapple MJ, Kahakachchi M, et al. Convulsions associated with *Campylobacter* enteritis. *Br Med J* 1980;280: 984–985.
128. Levy I, Weissman Y, Sivan Y, et al. Acute encephalopathy associated with *Campylobacter* enteritis. *Br Med J* 1986;293:424.
129. Simor AE, Karmali MA, Jadavji T, et al. Abortion and perinatal sepsis associated with *Campylobacter* infection. *Rev Infect Dis* 1986;8:397–402.
130. Moscuna M, Gross Z, Korenblum R, et al. Septic abortion due to *Campylobacter jejuni. Eur J Clin Microbiol Infect Dis* 1989;8: 800–801.
131. Simor AE, Ferro S. *Campylobacter jejuni* infection occurring during pregnancy. *Eur J Clin Microbiol Infect Dis* 1990;9:141–144.
132. Youngs ER, Roberts C. *Campylobacter* carriage and pregnancy. *Br J Obstet Gynaecol* 1985;92:541–542.
133. Pines A, Goldhammer E, Bregman J, et al. *Campylobacter* enteritis associated with recurrent abortions in agammaglobulinemia. *Acta Obstet Gynecol Scand* 1983;62:279–280.
134. Wong S-K, Tam AY-C, Yuen K-Y. *Campylobacter* infection in the neonate: case report and review of the literature. *Pediatr Infect Dis* 1990;9:665–669.
135. Anders BJ, Lauer BA, Paisley JW. *Campylobacter* gastroenteritis in neonates. *Am J Dis Child* 1981;135:900–902.
136. Karmali MA, Norrish B, Lior H, et al. *Campylobacter* enterocolitis in a neonatal nursery. *J Infect Dis* 1984;149:874–877.
137. Terrier A, Altwegg M, Bader P, et al. Hospital epidemic of neonatal *Campylobacter jejuni* infection. *Lancet* 1985;2:1182.
138. Goossens H, Henocque G, Kremp L, et al. Nosocomial outbreak of *Campylobacter jejuni* meningitis in newborn infants. *Lancet* 1986;2:146–149.
139. Van Dijk WC, van der Straaten PJC. An outbreak of *Campylobacter jejuni* infection in a neonatal intensive care unit. *J Hosp Infect* 1988;11:91–99.
140. Newman A, Lambert JR. *Campylobacter* jejuni causing flare-up in inflammatory bowel disease. *Lancet* 1980;2:919.
141. Lambert ME, Schofield PF, Ironside AG, et al. *Campylobacter* colitis. *Br Med J* 1979;1:857–859.
142. Loss RW, Mangla JC, Pereira M. *Campylobacter* colitis presenting as inflammatory bowel disease with segmental colonic ulcerations. *Gastroenterology* 1980;79:138–140.
143. Rutgeerts P, Geboes K, Ponette E, et al. Acute infective colitis caused by endemic pathogens in western Europe. *Endoscopy* 1982;14:212–219.
144. Mee AS, Shield M, Burke M. *Campylobacter* colitis: differentiation from acute inflammatory bowel disease. *J Roy Soc Med* 1985;78:217–223.
145. Blaser MJ, Hoverson D, Ely IG, et al. Studies of *Campylobacter jejuni* in patients with inflammatory bowel disease. *Gastroenterology* 1984;86:33–38.
146. Blaser MJ, Miller RA, Lacher J, et al. Patients with active Crohn's disease have elevated serum antibodies to antigens of seven enteric bacterial pathogens. *Gastroenterology* 1984;87:888–894.
147. Stephenson TJ, Cotton DWK. Toxic megacolon complicating *Campylobacter* colitis. *Br Med J* 1985;291:1242.
148. Schneider A, Runzi M, Peitgen K, et al. *Campylobacter jejuni*-induced severe colitis—a rare cause of toxic megacolon. *Z Gastroenterol* 2000;38:307–309.
149. Guandalini S, Cucchiara S, de Ritis G, et al. *Campylobacter* colitis in infants. *J Pediatr* 1983;102:72–74.
150. Heyman MB, Paterno VI, Ament ME. *Campylobacter* colitis: a cause of chronic diarrhea in children. *West J Med* 1982;137: 243–245.
151. Coffin CM, L'Heureaux P, Dehner LP. *Campylobacter*-associated enterocolitis in childhood: report of a fatal case. *Am J Clin Pathol* 1982;78:117–123.
152. Bentley D, Lynn J, Laws JW. *Campylobacter* colitis with intestinal aphthous ulceration mimicking obstruction. *Br Med J* 1985; 291:634.
153. Meijer CJLM, Lindeman J, Elbers JRJ, et al. *Campylobacter* associated appendicitis: prevalence, clinical and histological features. *Pathol Res* 1985;180:295(abst).
154. Cappendijk VC, Hazebroek FWJ. The impact of diagnostic delay on the course of acute appendicitis. *Arch Dis Child* 2000; 83:64–66.
155. Michalak DM, Perrault J, Gilchrist MJ, et al. *Campylobacter*

fetus ss. *jejuni:* a cause of massive lower gastrointestinal hemorrhage. *Gastroenterology* 1980;79:742–745.
156. Krajden S, Burul CJ, Fuksa M. *Campylobacter jejuni* associated with a perirectal abscess. *Can J Surg* 1986;29:228.
157. Frizelle FA, Rietveld JA. Spontaneous splenic rupture associated with *Campylobacter jejuni* infection. *Br J Surg* 1994;81:718.
158. Van der Hoop AG, Veringa EM. Cholecystitis caused by *Campylobacter jejuni. Clin Infect Dis* 1993;17:133.
159. Darling WM, Peel RN, Skirrow MB, et al. *Campylobacter* cholecystitis. *Lancet* 1979;1:1302.
160. Ampelas M, Perez C, Jourdan J, et al. Hépatite à *Campylobacter coli. Nouv Presse Méd* 1982;11:593–595.
161. Korman TM, Varley CC, Spelman DW. Acute hepatitis associated with *Campylobacter jejuni* bacteraemia. *Eur J Clin Microbiol Infect Dis* 1997;16:678–681.
162. Fitzgeorge RB, Baskerville A, Lander KP. Experimental infection of Rhesus monkeys with a human strain of *Campylobacter jejuni. J Hyg (Lond)* 1981;86:343–351.
163. Ezpeleta C, Rojo de Ursua P, Obregon F, et al. Acute pancreatitis associated with *Campylobacter jejuni* bacteremia. *Clin Infect Dis* 1992;15:1050.
164. Dutronc Y, Duong M, Buisson M, et al. Pancréatite aiguë et infection à *Campylobacter jejuni. Méd Mal Infect* 1995;25: 1168–1169.
165. Murphy S, Beeching NJ, Rogerson SJ, et al. Pancreatitis associated with *Salmonella* enteritis. *Lancet* 1991;338:571.
166. Wood CJ, Fleming V, Turnidge J, et al. *Campylobacter* peritonitis in continuous peritoneal dialysis: a report of eight cases and a review of the literature. *Am J Kidney Dis* 1992;19:257–263.
167. Ho DD, Ault MJ, Ault MA, et al. *Campylobacter* enteritis. *Arch Intern Med* 1982;142:1858–1860.
168. Schmidt U, Chmel H, Kaminski Z, et al. The clinical spectrum of *Campylobacter fetus* infections: report of five cases and review of the literature. *Q J Med (New Series)* 1980;49:431–442.
169. Muytjens HL, Hoogenhout J. *Campylobacter jejuni* isolated from a chest wall abscess. *Clin Microbiol Newslett* 1982;4:166.
170. Pedler SJ, Bint AJ. Osteitis of the foot due to *Campylobacter jejuni. J Infect* 1984;8:85.
171. Peterson MC, Farr RW, Castiglia M. Prosthetic hip infection and bacteremia due to *Campylobacter jejuni* in a patient with AIDS. *Clin Infect Dis* 1993;16:439–440.
172. Pasticci MB, Baratta E, Del Favero A, et al. *Campylobacter jejuni:* an unusual cause of infectious arthritis. *Postgrad Med J* 1992;68:150–152.
173. Schieven BC, Baird D, Leatherdale CL, et al. *Campylobacter jejuni* infected bursitis. *Diagn Microbiol Infect Dis* 1991;14: 507–508.
174. Norrby R, McCloskey RV, Zackrisson G, et al. Meningitis caused by *Campylobacter fetus* ssp *jejuni. Br Med J* 1980;280:1164.
175. Burch KL, Saeed K, Sails AD, et al. Successful treatment by meropenem of *Campylobacter jejuni* in a chronic alcoholic following neurosurgery. *J Infect* 1999;39:241–243.
176. Ritchie PMA, Forbes JC, Steinbok P. Subdural space *Campylobacter* infection in a child. *Can Med Assoc J* 1987;137:45–46.
177. Feder HM, Rasoulpour M, Rodriquez AJ. *Campylobacter* urinary tract infection: value of the urine Gram's stain. *JAMA* 1986;256:2389.
178. Davies JS, Penfold JB. *Campylobacter* urinary infection. *Lancet* 1979;1:1091.
179. Carter JE, Cimolai N. IgA nephropathy associated with *Campylobacter jejuni* enteritis. *Nephron* 1991;58:101–102.
180. Menck H. *Campylobacter jejuni* enteritis complicated by glomerulonephritis. *Ugeskr Laeger* 1981;143:1020–1021.
181. Maidment CGH, Evans DB, Coulden RA, et al. *Campylobacter* enteritis complicated by glomerulonephritis. *J Infect* 1985;10: 177–178.
182. Rautelin HI, Outinen AV, Kosunen TU. Tubulointerstitial nephritis as a complication *Campylobacter jejuni* enteritis. *Scand J Urol Nephrol* 1987;21:151–152.
183. Andrews PI, Kainer G, Yong LCJ, et al. Glomerulonephritis, pulmonary hemorrhage and anemia associated with *Campylobacter jejuni* infection. *Aust N Z J Med* 1989;19:721–723.
184. Haq JA, Rahman KM, Akbar MS. Haemolytic–uraemic syndrome and *Campylobacter. Med J Aust* 1985;142:662–663.
185. May Th., Gerard A, Voiriot P, et al. Entérite à *Campylobacter jejuni* associée è un syndrome hémolytique et urémique. *Presse Med* 1986;15:803–804.
186. Damani NN, Humphrey CA, Bell B. Haemolytic anaemia in *Campylobacter* enteritis. *J Infect* 1993;26:109–110.
187. Florkowski CM, Ikram RB, Crozier IM, et al. *Campylobacter jejuni* myocarditis. *Clin Cardiol* 1984;7:558–560.
188. Kell RJA, Ellis ME. Transient atrial fibrillation in *Campylobacter jejuni* infection. *Br Med J* 1985;291:1542.
189. Tee W, Mijch A. *Campylobacter jejuni* bacteremia in human immunodeficiency virus (HIV)-infected and non-HIV-infected patients: comparison of clinical features and review. *Clin Infect Dis* 1998;26:91–96.
190. Sakran W, Raz R, Levi Y, et al. *Campylobacter* bacteremia and pneumonia in two splenectomized patients. *Eur J Clin Microbiol Infect Dis* 1999;18:496–498.
191. Schaad UB. Reactive arthritis associated with *Campylobacter* enteritis. *Pediatr Infect Dis* 1982;1:328–332.
192. Peterson MC. Rheumatic manifestations of *Campylobacter jejuni* and *C. fetus* infections in adults. *Scand J Rheumatol* 1994; 23:167–170.
193. Saari KM, Kauranen O. Ocular inflammation in Reiter's syndrome associated with *Campylobacter jejuni* enteritis. *Am J Ophthalmol* 1980;90:572–573.
194. Ebright JR, Ryan LM. Acute erosive reactive arthritis associated with *Campylobacter jejuni*-induced colitis. *Am J Med* 1984;76: 321–323.
195. Eastmond CJ, Rennie JAN, Reid TMS. An outbreak of *Campylobacter* enteritis: a rheumatological followup survey. *J Rheumatol* 1983;10:107–108.
196. Melby K, Dahl OP, Crisp L, et al. Clinical and serological manifestations in patients during a waterborne epidemic due to *Campylobacter jejuni. J Infect* 1990;21:309–316.
197. Rautelin H, Koota K, von Essen R, et al. Waterborne *Campylobacter jejuni* epidemic in a Finnish hospital for rheumatic diseases. *Scand J Infect Dis* 1990;22:321–326.
198. Jones DA. Irritable hip and *Campylobacter* infection. *J Bone Joint Surg* 1989;71B:227–228.
199. Lever AML, Dolby JM, Webster ADB, et al. Chronic *Campylobacter* colitis and uveitis in patient with hypogammaglobulinaemia. *Br Med J* 1984;288:531.
200. Howard RS, Sarkies NJC, Sanders MD. Anterior uveitis associated with *Campylobacter jejuni* infection. *J Infect* 1987;14:186–187.
201. Toivanen A, Lahesmaa-Rantala R, Meurman O, et al. Antibodies against *Yersinia, Campylobacter, Salmonella,* and *Chlamydia* in patients with Behçet's disease. *Arthritis Rheum* 1987;30: 1315–1316.
202. Eastmond CJ, Reid TMS. *Campylobacter* enteritis and erythema nodosum. *Br Med J* 1982;285:1421–1422.
203. Ashworth J, English JSC. Recurrent erythema nodosum and prolonged *Campylobacter jejuni* excretion. *Br Med J* 1984;288: 830.
204. Nagaratnam N, Goh TK, Ghoughassian D. *Campylobacter jejuni*-induced vasculitis. *Br J Clin Pract* 1990;44:636–637.
205. Rhodes KM, Tattersfield AE. Guillain–Barré syndrome associated with *Campylobacter* infection. *Br Med J* 1982;285:173–174.
206. Nachamkin I, Mishu Allos B, Ho T. *Campylobacter* species and Guillain–Barré syndrome. *Clin Microbiol Rev* 1998;11:555–567.

207. Buzby JC, Mishu Allos B, Roberts T. The economic burden of *Campylobacter*-associated Guillain–Barré syndrome. *J Infect Dis* 1997;176:S192–S197.
208. Roberts T, Shah A, Graham JG, et al. The Miller–Fisher syndrome following *Campylobacter* enteritis, report of two cases. *J Neurol Neurosurg Psychiatry* 1987;50:1557–1558.
209. Kohler A, de Torrenté A, Inderwildi B. Fisher's syndrome associated with *Campylobacter jejuni* infection. *Eur Neurol* 1988;28: 150–151.
210. Van der Kruijk RA, Lampe AS, Endtz H Ph. Bilateral abducens paresis following *Campylobacter jejuni* enteritis. *J Infect* 1992;24:215–216.
211. Kerstens PJSM, Endtz HP, Meis JFGM, et al. Erysipelas-like skin lesions associated with *Campylobacter jejuni* septicemia in patients with hypogammaglobulinemia. *Eur J Clin Microbiol Infect Dis* 1992;11:842–847
212. Manfredi R, Nanetti A, Ferri M, et al. Fatal *Campylobacter jejuni* bacteraemia in patients with AIDS. *J Med Microbiol* 1999;48:601–603.
213. Borleffs JCC, Schellekens JF, Brouwer E, et al. Use of an immunoglobulin M-containing preparation for treatment of two hypogammaglobulinemic patients with persistent *Campylobacter jejuni* infection. *Eur J Clin Microbiol Infect Dis* 1993;12: 772–775.
214. Autenrieth IB, Schuster V, Ewald J, et al. An unusual case of refractory *Campylobacter jejuni* infection in a patient with X-linked agammaglobulinemia: successful combined therapy with maternal plasma and ciprofloxacin. *Clin Infect Dis* 1996;23: 526–531.
215. Nachamkin I, Engberg J, Aarestrup FM. Diagnosis and antimicrobial susceptibility of *Campylobacter* species. In: Nachamkin I, Blaser MJ, eds. *Campylobacter,* 2nd ed. Washington, DC: ASM Press, 2000:45–66.
216. Lawson AJ, Logan JMJ, O'Neill GL, et al. Large-scale survey of *Campylobacter* species in human gastroenteritis by PCR and PCR-enzyme-linked immunosorbent assay. *J Clin Microbiol* 1999;37:3860–3864.
217. Wassenaar TM, Newell DG. Genotyping of *Campylobacter* spp. *Appl Environ Microbiol* 2000;66:1–9.
218. Newell DG, Frost JA, Duim B, et al. New development in the subtyping of *Campylobacter* species. In: Nachamkin I, Blaser MJ, eds. *Campylobacter,* 2nd ed. Washington, DC: ASM Press, 2000:27–44.
219. Van Duin JM, Bänffer JRJ, Nuyten PJM, et al. Comparison of Western blot, counterimmunoelectrophoresis, complement fixation and enzyme-linked immunosorbent assay for the diagnosis of *Campylobacter* infection. *Serodiagn Immunother Infect Dis* 1993;5:231–236.
220. Jones DM, Robinson DA, Eldridge J. Serological studies in two outbreaks of *Campylobacter jejuni* infection. *J Hyg (Lond)* 1981;87:163–170.
221. Boswell TCJ. Serological cross reaction between legionella and *Campylobacter* in the rapid microagglutination test. *J Clin Pathol* 1996;49:584–586.
222. De Witt TG, Humphrey KF, Doern GV. White blood cell counts in patients with *Campylobacter*-induced diarrhea and controls. *J Infect Dis* 1985;152:427–428.
223. Bradshaw MJ, Brown R, Swallow JH, et al. *Campylobacter* enteritis in Chelmsford. *Postgrad Med J* 1980;56:80–84.
224. Brown G, Bui A, Vrazas J. Florid computed tomographic appearance of acute *Campylobacter* enterocolitis. *Australas Radiol* 2000; 36:3567–3573.
225. Doberneck RC. *Campylobacter* colitis mimicking colonic cancer during barium enema examination. *Surgery* 1983;93:508–509.
226. Noble CJ, Hibbert DJ, Patel GJ. *Campylobacter* colitis: a case with unusual radiological features. *J Infect* 1982;5:199–200.
227. Puylaert JBCM, Lalisang RI, van der Werf SDJ, et al. *Campylobacter* ileocolitis mimicking acute appendicitis: differentiation with graded-compression US. *Radiology* 1988;166:737–740.
229. Sumathipala RW, Morrison GW. Campylobacter enteritis after falling into sewage. *Br Med J* 1983;286:1356.
230. Anders BJ, Lauer BA, Paisley JW, et al. Double-blind placebo controlled trial of erythromycin for treatment of *Campylobacter* enteritis. *Lancet* 1982;1:131–132.
231. Pitkänen T, Pettersson T, Pönkä A. Effect of erythromycin on the fecal excretion of *Campylobacter fetus* subspecies *jejuni. J Infect Dis* 1982;145:128.
232. Pai CH, Gillis F, Tuomanen E, et al. Erythromycin in treatment of *Campylobacter* enteritis in children. *Am J Dis Child* 1983; 137:286–288.
233. Mandal BK, Ellis ME, Dunbar EM, et al. Double-blind placebo-controlled trial of erythromycin in the treatment of clinical *Campylobacter* infection. *J Antimicrob Chemother* 1984; 13:619–623.
234. Ashkenazi S, Danziger Y, Varsano Y, et al. Treatment of *Campylobacter* gastroenteritis. *Arch Dis Child* 1987;62:84–85.
235. Salazar-Lindo E, Sack RB, Chea-Woo E, et al. Early treatment with erythromycin of *Campylobacter jejuni*-associated dysentery in children. *J Pediatr* 1986;109:355–360.
236. Pichler HET, Diridl G, Stickler K, et al. Clinical efficacy of ciprofloxacin compared with placebo in bacterial diarrhea. *Am J Med* 1987;82[Suppl 4A];329–332.
237. Goodman LJ, Trenholme GM, Kaplan RL, et al. Empiric antimicrobial therapy of domestically acquired acute diarrhea in urban adults. *Arch Intern Med* 1990;150:541–546.
238. Wiström J, Jertborn M, Ekwall E, et al. Empiric treatment of acute diarrheal disease with norfloxacin. *Ann Intern Med* 1992; 117:202–208.
239. Aarestrup FM, Nielsen EM, Madsen M, et al. Antimicrobial susceptibility pattern of thermophilic *Camylobacter* spp. from humans, pigs, cattle, and broilers in Denmark. *Antimicrob Agents Chemother* 1997;41:2244–2250.
240. Trieber CA, Taylor DE. Mechanisms of antibiotic resistance in *Campylobacter.* In: Nachamkin I, Blaser MJ, eds. *Campylobacter,* 2nd ed. Washington, DC: ASM Press, 2000:441–454.
241. Butzler JP, Vanhoof R, Clumeck N, et al. Clinical and pharmacological evaluation of different preparations of oral erythromycin. *Chemotherapy* 1979;25:367–372.
242. Taylor DE, Chang N. *In vitro* susceptibilities of *Campylobacter jejuni* and *Campylobacter coli* to azithromycin and erythromycin. *Antimicrob Agents Chemother* 1991;35:1917–1918.
243. Smith KE, Bender JB, Osterholm MT. Antimicrobial resistance in animals and relevance to human infections. In: Nachamkin I, Blaser MJ, eds. *Campylobacter,* 2nd ed. Washington, DC: ASM Press, 2000:483–495.
244. Thwaites RT, Frost JA. Drug resistance in *Campylobacter jejuni C. coli* and *C. lari* isolated from humans in North West England and Wales, 1997. *J Clin Pathol* 1999;52:812–814.
245. Saenz Y, Zarazaga M, Lantero M, et al. Antibiotic resistance in *Campylobacter* strains isolated from animals, foods, and humans in Spain in 1997–1998. *Antimicrob Agents Chemother* 2000;44:267–271.
246. Rosef O, Kapperud G. House flies (*Musca domestica*) as possible vectors of *Campylobacter fetus* subsp. *jejuni. Appl Environ Microbiol* 1983;45:381–383.
247. Arimi SM, Fricker CR, Park RWA. Occurrence of 'thermophilic' campylobacters in sewage and their removal by treatment processes. *Epidemiol Infect* 1988;101:279–286.
248. Stampi S, Varoli O, De Luca G, et al. Occurrence, removal and seasonal variation of "thermophilic" campylobacters in a sewage treatment plant in Italy. *Int J Med Microbiol* 1992;193: 199–210.

249. Blaser MJ, Smith PF, Wang W-LL, et al. Inactivation of *Campylobacter jejuni* by chlorine and monochloramine. *Appl Environ Microbiol* 1986;51:307–311.
250. Humphrey TJ, Beckett P. *Campylobacter jejuni* in dairy cows and raw milk. *Epidemiol Infect* 1987;98:263–269.
251. Newell DG, Wagenaar JA. Poultry infections and their control at farm level. In: Nachamkin I, Blaser MJ, eds. *Campylobacter,* 2nd ed. Washington, DC: ASM Press, 2000:497–509.
252. Humphrey TJ. *Salmonella, Campylobacter,* and poultry: possible control measures. Abstr. *Hyg Commun Dis* 1989;64:R1–R8.
253. Farkas J. Irradiation as a method for decontaminating food: a review. *Int J Food Microbiol* 1998;44:189–204.
254. Gill CO, Harris LM. Hamburgers and broiler chickens as potential sources of human *Campylobacter* enteritis. *J Food Protect* 1984;47:96–99.
255. Norkrans G, Svedhem Å. Epidemiological aspects of *Campylobacter jejuni* enteritis. *J Hyg*1982;89:163–170.
256. Ransom GM, Kaplan B, McNamara AM, et al. *Campylobacter* prevention and control: the USDA Food Safety and Inspection Service role and new food safety approaches. In: Nachamkin I, Blaser MJ, eds. *Campylobacter,* 2nd ed. Washington, DC: ASM Press, 2000:511–528.
257. Swaminathan B, Barrett TJ, and the CDC PulseNet Task Force. A national network for food-borne bacterial disease surveillance in the United States. In: Nachamkin I, Blaser MJ, eds. *Campylobacter,* 2nd ed. Washington, DC: ASM Press, 2000:529–535.
258. Scott DA, Tribble DR. Protection against *Campylobacter* infection and vaccine development. In: Nachamkin I, Blaser MJ, eds. *Campylobacter,* 2nd ed. Washington, DC: ASM Press, 2000:303–319.
259. Pulaert JBCM, Vermeijden RJ, van der Werf SDJ, Doornbos L, Koumans RKJ. Incidence and sonographic diagnosis of bacterial ileocaecitis masquerading as appendicitis. *Lancet* 1989;2: 84–86.

47

ATYPICAL *CAMPYLOBACTERS* AND RELATED MICROORGANISMS

ALBERT J. LASTOVICA
MARK E. ENGEL
MARTIN J. BLASER

Campylobacter species are the most frequently identified bacterial causative agents of diarrhea in humans, especially very young children, in both developed and developing countries. *Campylobacter* species have also been associated with other clinical conditions, such as bacteremia, Guillain-Barré syndrome, hemolytic–uremic syndrome, pancreatitis, and reactive arthritis. Traditionally, more than 95% of the *Campylobacter* strains isolated and identified in cases of human disease have been *C. jejuni* subsp *jejuni* or *C. coli.* However, the isolation procedures currently used in many diagnostic laboratories may not support the growth of other potentially pathogenic non-*jejunicoli Campylobacter* species. These organisms may be fastidious, requiring special atmospheric and temperature conditions, or unable to tolerate the antibiotics commonly included in selective media plates; alternatively, the incubation period may not be sufficiently long. The disease potential of these non-*jejunicoli Campylobacter* species is beginning to be appreciated, particularly in areas where they are frequently isolated.

These organisms are found in a variety of habitats and are implicated in a range of human and animal diseases (Table 47.1). This chapter describes the sources, microbiology, epidemiology, and clinical features of *Campylobacter* species other than *C. jejuni* subsp *jejuni* and *C. coli* that are associated with human disease. In the discussion, we refer to *C. jejuni* subsp *jejuni* and *C. coli* simply as *C. jejuni.*

A. J. Lastovica: Department of Medical Microbiology, University of Cape Town Medical School, Cape Town, South Africa

M. E. Engel: Department of Pathology, Red Cross Children's Hospital, Cape Town, South Africa

M. J. Blaser: Department of Medicine, New York University School of Medicine; Department of Internal Medicine, New York Harbor Veterans Affairs Medical Center, New York, New York

DETECTION OF ATYPICAL CAMPYLOBACTERS

Most strains of some atypical *Campylobacter* species (non-*C. jejuni* subsp *jejuni* or *C. coli*), such as *C. upsaliensis, C. lari,* and *C. jejuni* subsp *doylei,* can be isolated by the same protocols used for *C. jejuni.* Traditionally, because other components of the enteric flora in stool specimens grow more rapidly than campylobacters, media containing antibiotics have been used to suppress the growth of contaminating organisms. However, the isolation of *C. upsaliensis* and other non-*jejuni Campylobacter* species from stools may be unsuccessful when media containing cephalothin or other antibiotics, to which these organisms are susceptible, are used. Other species, such as *C. concisus,* require a hydrogen-enhanced microaerobic atmosphere for growth. Conventional isolation procedures generally used to isolate *C. jejuni* will fail to isolate these species (1–4). In an Australian study of 676 patients hospitalized with gastroenteritis, 75 strains of *Campylobacter* were isolated on blood-free medium with a selective supplement, but concurrent isolation onto antibiotic-free blood agar overlaid with a membrane filter yielded 213 *Campylobacter* strains (2). Some researchers have recommended both membrane filtration and selective media for the optimal isolation of *Campylobacter* organisms (2,3). However, an efficient procedure, the "Cape Town protocol" (4), for the isolation of campylobacters from stool specimens without the use of selective media has been developed. This method involves the filtration of stools through a membrane filter onto antibiotic-free blood agar plates *and* subsequent incubation in a hydrogen-enhanced microaerobic atmosphere (4,5). With the "Cape Town protocol," in use since 1990, stool cultures positive for campylobacters or related organisms have risen to 21.8% from the 7.1% previously obtained with Skirrow and other antibiotic-containing selective media and incubation under microaerobic conditions (4). Concurrently, the number of

TABLE 47.1. SOURCES AND DISEASE ASSOCIATIONS OF NON-*JEJUNI/COLI CAMPYLOBACTER* AND RELATED BACTERIA

Species/Subspecies	Known Sources	Human Disease Association	Animal Disease Association
C. fetus subsp *fetus*	Cattle, sheep	Septicemia, gastroenteritis, abortion, meningitis, vascular infections	Bovine, ovine spontaneous abortion
C. fetus subsp *venerealis*	Cattle	Septicemia	Bovine infectious infertility
C. upsaliensis	Cats, dogs, ducks, monkeys	Gastroenteritis, septicemia, abscesses	Canine, feline gastroenteritis
C. hyointestinalis subsp *hyointestinalis*	Cattle, hamsters, pigs, monkeys	Gastroenteritis, septicemia[c]	Porcine and bovine enteritis
C. lari	Cats, dogs, chickens, monkeys, horses, seals, mussels, oysters, river and sea water	Gastroenteritis, septicemia, colitis	Avian gastroenteritis
C. concisus[a]	Humans	Periodontal disease, gastroenteritis, septicemia[c]	Unknown
C. sputorum biovar sputorum[b]	Humans, cattle, pigs, sheep	Abscesses, gastroenteritis	Unknown
C. jejuni subsp *doylei*	Humans	Gastroenteritis, septicemia,[c] gastritis	Unknown
C. gracilis	Humans	Periodontal disease, soft tissue abcesses	Unknown
H. cinaedi	Humans, hamsters	Gastroenteritis, septicemia,[c] proctocolitis	Hamster enteritis
H. fennelliae	Humans	Gastroenteritis, septicemia,[c] proctocolitis	Unknown
H. pullorum	Poultry	Gastroenteritis	Avian hepatitis
A. butzleri	Pigs, bulls, horses, cattle, chickens, primates, ostriches, ducks, water, sewage	Gastroenteritis, septicemia	Porcine, bovine, primate gastroenteritis; porcine abortion
A. cryaerophilus	Pigs, bulls, poultry, sheep, sewage, horses	Gastroenteritis, septicemia	Bovine, porcine, ovine, equine abortion
"Flexispira rappini"	Humans, mice, sheep	Gastroenteritis	Ovine abortion

[a]Includes *C. curvus* and *C. rectus*.
[b]Includes biovar bubulus.
[c]Children and patients with HIV infection.
Data from references 11,12,93,96,127,131,141,183,190,193.

species or subspecies detected has increased from 5 to 17 (4). Antibiotic-containing selective plates have a limited shelf life and are expensive, and a selection of different media may be required to isolate all clinically relevant *Campylobacter, Helicobacter,* and *Arcobacter* species. Membrane filtration onto antibiotic-free media *and* incubation in a hydrogen-enhanced microaerobic atmosphere is a simple and efficient isolation protocol and the only method presently available for the isolation of some *Campylobacter* species (3,5).

C. FETUS

Early this century, McFaydean and Stockman (6) first recognized *Campylobacter* as a causative agent of fatal infection and abortion in sheep. The gram-negative rods were initially called *Vibrio fetus ovis* because of their curved shape. In 1919, Smith (7) reported that the organisms, then called *Vibrio fetus,* caused abortion in cattle. Evidence has suggested that these strains were *C. fetus,* which is now recognized as a major cause of septic abortions in domestic animals (8). Since 1947, *C. fetus* has been implicated as a causative agent of human intestinal and extraintestinal illness.

C. fetus is separated into two subspecies, *C. fetus* subsp *fetus* and *C. fetus* subsp *venerealis.* This division stems from the realization that two different disease entities can be attributed to two varieties of strains (9). One variety ("*Vibrio fetus*" var intestinalis) originates in the intestine and causes sporadic abortion in cattle; the other ("*Vibrio fetus*" var venerealis) originates in the prepuce of asymptomatic bulls, causing infertility and occasionally abortion in cows. Although the two groups of bacteria are distinct in their biologic properties, disease associations, and habitat, they were not considered separate species by Véron and Chatelain (10) because they do not form separate groups in DNA–DNA hybridization tests and have a similar G + C (guanine plus cytosine) content, and strains of both subspecies agglutinate in the same antiserum. DNA–DNA hybridization studies have confirmed that the two subspecies are closely related (11). In this chapter, the term *C. fetus* refers to *C. fetus* subsp *fetus* unless otherwise indicated.

Microbiology

C. fetus, like other campylobacters, grows in a microaerobic atmosphere of 6% to 12% carbon dioxide. The organisms are positive for catalase, oxidase, and nitrate reductase (Table 47.2) *C. fetus* strains grow well at 25°C and 37°C, but unlike *C. jejuni,* they do not usually grow at 42°C (12). *C. fetus* is resistant to nalidixic acid, susceptible to cephalothin, and lacks pyrazinamidase activity (13); these diagnostic characteristics are useful for distinguishing *C. fetus* from *C. jejuni.*

Although early investigators (14) reported that the isolation of *C. fetus* from stools was rare, its natural habitat is the intestine. The susceptibility of *C. fetus* to cephalothin and the fact that most strains do not grow at 42°C may explain why the organism is not isolated from stools more frequently. Many clinical laboratories incubate samples at 4°C and may use a medium that contains cephalothin or other inhibitory antibiotics (15). Laboratories may incubate blood cultures for only 7 days or less, which may be insufficient time for *C. fetus* to grow (16). Filtration of stools through 0.6-µm filters onto the surface of antibiotic-free blood agar plates allows the smaller *C. fetus* bacteria to be isolated from larger, contaminating microorganisms (17).

A polymerase chain reaction (PCR) assay based on 16S ribosomal RNA (rRNA) has proved useful for the identification of *C. fetus* (18). Hum and colleagues (19) have developed a PCR assay for the identification and differentiation of *C. fetus* subsp *fetus* and *C. fetus* subsp *venerealis.* This PCR technique, when compared with traditional phenotyping, indicates that the two *C. fetus* subspecies are often misidentified in diagnostic microbiology laboratories.

C. fetus subsp *fetus*

The major habitat of *C. fetus is* the intestine, and it is commonly isolated from healthy sheep and cattle (Table 47.1). The organism has been isolated from the genital tracts of cattle and sheep, cattle fetuses, and the placentas and stomachs of aborted sheep (8). In pregnant animals, ingestion of *C. fetus* leads to intestinal infection, followed by bacteremia and infection of the placenta and fetus (20). A similar mechanism of gastrointestinal colonization, with or without enteritis, followed by a hematogenous spread and then a placental infection, is likely to occur in women (21). *C. fetus* infection in pregnant women is usually recognized during the third trimester, and although the illness is mild in mothers, the outcome is often poor in their infants. Neonates may be infected transplacentally or during delivery. Even with appropriate antimicrobial therapy, the overall mortality of fetuses and neonates can be 80% (22,23). *C. fetus* may also cause premature labor and perinatal sepsis in humans (23). Fetal infection and abortion may follow maternal infection by several weeks. Infection is believed to arise from bacteria in the intestine acquired through food or water contaminated with *C. fetus.* During the course of a bacteremic phase, the organisms, which have a high affinity for placental tissue, invade the uterus and multiply in the immunologically immature fetus, which is generally aborted. Laboratory diagnosis depends on the isolation and identification of the organisms from the placenta or other organs where they can occur in large numbers (21).

Human infections caused by *C. fetus* are generally limited to septicemia in patients with predisposing conditions (24). Other clinical conditions include septic arthritis, meningitis, pericarditis, peritonitis, salpingitis, and abscesses (25–28). Previously, *C. fetus* was not thought to be involved in human enteritis, however, *C. fetus* has been isolated from the stools of patients with gastroenteritis (15,29). *C. fetus* is rarely involved in pediatric gastroenteritis; in a study of 4,212 *Campylobacter* stool isolates at a children's hospital, the organism was isolated only 7 (0.16%) times (Table 47.3). The clinical details of these pediatric isolates are given in Table 47.4. In a study of *Campylobacter* blood culture strains isolated at the same hospital, only 8 (3.6%) of 221 *Campylobacter* strains were *C. fetus* (30).

C. fetus subsp *venerealis*

C. fetus subsp *venerealis* has adapted to the bovine genital tract and is the major cause of bovine genital campylobacteriosis, an infectious disease of major concern to the cattle industry (8). The principal habitat of *C. fetus* subsp *venerealis* is prepuce of asymptomatic bull; the infection is transmitted to the cow, and infecting bacteria cause a chronic genital tract inflammation that leads to infertility. *C. fetus* subsp *venerealis* is not considered an important human pathogen, although infection among homosexual males (29) and women with vaginosis (31) has been reported.

Epidemiology

Of 66 *C. fetus* isolates reported to the Centers for Disease Control and Prevention (CDC), 18 were from blood, 41 from stool, and 7 from other sites (32). The incidence of *C. fetus* infection peaks in late summer and early autumn, similar to the incidence of *C. jejuni* infection. In 1995, the CDC, U.S. Department of Agriculture, and Food and Drug Administration developed FoodNet as an active surveillance system; it monitors 7.8% of the U.S. population (33). Data from more than 300 clinical laboratories routinely culturing stools for pathogens are transmitted electronically to the CDC. In 1998, *Campylobacter,* with an iso-

TABLE 47.2. BIOCHEMICAL AND PHENOTYPIC CHARACTERISTICS OF *CAMPYLOBACTER*, INTESTINAL *HELICOBACTER*, AND *ARCOBACTER* OF CLINICAL SIGNIFICANCE

Species/Subspecies	Cat[f]	Nit Red[g]	Arylsulf[h]	Pyrazin[i]	Hipp[j]	Nal[k]	Ceph[l]	Rapid H_2S[m]	Lead Ace[n]	TSI[o]	Growth at 25°C	Growth at 37°C	Growth at 42°C	Ind Ace[p]	H_2 Req[q]
C. jejuni subsp *jejuni* biotype 1[a]	+	+	–	+	+	S	R	–	++	–	–	+	+	+	–
C. jejuni subsp *jejuni* biotype 2[a]	+	+	+	+	+	S	R	+	++	–	–	+	+	+	–
C. jejuni subsp *doylei*	(+)	–	–	+	(+)	S	(S)	–	–	–	–	+	(+)	+	e
C. coli	+	+	–	+	–	S	R	–	++	–	–	+	+	+	–
C. fetus subsp *fetus*	+	+	–	–	–	R	S	–	+	–	+	+	(–)	–	–
C. upsaliensis	(+)	+	–	+	–	S	S	–	(+)	–	–	+	(+)	+	e
C. lari	+	+	–	+	–	R	R	+	+	–	(–)	+	+	–	e
C. hyointestinalis	+	+	–	–	–	R	S	–	5+	3+	(+)	+	+	–	e
C. sputorum biovar sputorum	–	+	+	+	–	R	S	+	5+	3+	–	+	+	–	–
C. sputorum biovar bubulus	–	+	+	–	–	R	S	+	5+	3+	–	+	(+)	–	–
C. concisus	–	+	+	+	–	(R)	(S)	–	3+	(+)	–	+	(–)	–	+
C. curvus	–	+	+	+	–	R	S	–	5+	+	–	+	+	+	+
C. rectus	–	+	+	+	–	S	R	–	3+	+	–	+	+	+	+
C. gracilis	–	+	ND	ND	–	S	R	ND	ND	+	ND	ND	ND	+	–
H. cinaedi[b]	+	+	–	–	–	S	(S)	–	(+)	–	–	+	–	–	–
H. fennelliae[b,c]	+	–	+	–	–	S	(S)	–	+	–	–	+	–	+	–
H. pullorum	(+)	+	ND	ND	–	S	R	ND	ND	+	ND	+	ND	–	ND
A. butzleri[d]	(+)	+	–	–	–	S	(R)	–	–	–	–	+	(+)	+	–
A. cryaerophilus[d]	(+)	+	–	–	–	S	(R)	–	–	–	+	+	–	+	–
"Flexispira rappini"	(+)	–	ND	ND	ND	R	R	ND	ND	–	–	+	+	ND	ND

[a]Biotypes 1 and 2 of Skirrow's scheme (101); [b]spreading, noncolonial growth; [c]hypochlorite odor; [d]aerobic growth at 30°C; [e]some strains grow better in H_2-enhanced microaerobic conditions; [f]catalase; [g]nitrate reduction; [h]arylsulfatase; [i]pyrazinamidase; [j]hippurate hydrolysis; [k]nalidixic acid resistance; [l]cephalothin resistance; [m]method of Skirrow and Benjamin (101); [n]lead acetate; [o]triple sugar iron; [p]indoxylacetate; [q]H_2-enhanced microaerobic conditions. Susceptibilities are based on 30-µg disks.

+, Positive; (+), most strains positive; –, negative; (–), most strains negative; R, resistant; (R), most strains resistant; S, susceptible; (S), most strains susceptible; ND, not done.

Data from references 5,13,60,93,97,110,116,137,193.

TABLE 47.3. DISTRIBUTION OF *CAMPYLOBACTER* AND RELATED SPECIES ISOLATED FROM 20,228 DIARRHETIC STOOLS OF PEDIATRIC PATIENTS AT THE RED CROSS CHILDREN'S HOSPITAL, CAPE TOWN, SOUTH AFRICA, FROM OCTOBER 1, 1990, TO JUNE 30, 2000

Species/Subspecies	No.	Percentage (%)
C. jejuni subsp *jejuni*[a]	1,299	30.85
C. concisus	999	23.72
C. upsaliensis	978	23.22
C. jejuni subsp *doylei*	384	9.11
H. fennelliae	266	6.32
C. coli	121	2.87
C. hyointestinalis	53	1.26
H. cinaedi	42	1.00
CLO/HLO	35	0.83
A. butzleri	16	0.37
C. fetus subsp *fetus*	7	0.16
C. sputorum biovar sputorum/ *C. lari*	4	0.10
C. curvus/C. rectus	4	0.10
"Flexispira rappini"	4	0.09
Total	4,212	100.00

[a]Biotypes 1 and 2 of Skirrow and Benjamin (101).
CLO/HLO, *Campylobacter*-like or *Helicobacter*-like organisms.
Data from Lastovica A, Le Roux E. Efficient isolation of campylobacteria from stools. *J Clin Microbiol* 2000;38:2798–2799, with permission, and from unpublished results.

lation rate of 21.7 per 100,000, was the most common bacterial enteric pathogen in the United States, surpassing *Salmonella* and *Shigella* (33). The vast majority of isolates reported were *C. jejuni* subsp *jejuni* or *C. coli,* with very few reports made of other *Campylobacter,* enteric *Helicobacter,* or *Arcobacter* species (33). These sparse reports may reflect the less than optimal isolation protocol for *Campylobacter* used by the various reporting laboratories. The source of *C. fetus* infections in humans is likely to be zoonotic. *C. fetus* has been isolated from sheep, cattle, poultry, swine, and reptiles (12) (Table 47.1). Feces from infected animals may contaminate soil, fresh water, and carcasses during abattoir processing (34), so that human infection probably results from the consumption of contaminated food or water. Consumption of raw calf's liver as a nutritional supplement caused a *C. fetus* infection in 10 people in California (35). The drinking of unpasteurized milk has initiated several outbreaks (36,37). The modes of transmission of *C. fetus* infection in humans are not well understood, despite evidence suggesting zoonotic transmission (14).

Clinical Features

Clinically, the diarrheal disease caused by *C. fetus* infection in healthy persons is similar to the diarrhea resulting from infection with *C. jejuni.* Sequelae are uncommon, and most patients do not require antibiotic treatment. *C. fetus* infection usually occurs in compromised patients, more than 75% of whom are men who have serious medical conditions, such as diabetes mellitus, atherosclerosis, hepatic cirrhosis, and chronic alcoholism, or are being treated with immunosuppressive agents (14,16,24). *C. fetus* accounts for more cases of bacteremia in adults than do other *Campylobacter* species, except for *C. jejuni* (30,38). Infections with *C. fetus* were previously considered primarily to cause bacteremia in elderly men with chronic underlying illness, but AIDS patients may now represent the most typical infected population (39). Prolonged relapsing illness, characterized by chills, fever, and myalgia and without an identified source of infection, may be caused by *C. fetus* (14,24). Occasionally, secondary seeding to an organ may occur, which can lead to complications and an occasionally fatal outcome (40).

Bacteremia caused by *C. fetus* can be primary, presumably arising from the gastrointestinal tract, or secondary, arising from infection at another site. *C. fetus* infection can occur as a direct result of invasion of the bloodstream through venipuncture or an intravenous line (24). Although the organism is rarely isolated from feces, diarrhea precedes or accompanies bacteremia in nearly half the cases (16,24,30). High fevers frequently occur and are usually well tolerated, but the mortality is approximately 20% (39,40). *C. fetus* exhibits an affinity for vascular tissue, and infections have been associated with thrombophlebitis, cellulitis, and mycotic aneurysms (24,41,42). Bär (43) reviewed 26 cases of *C. fetus*-associated endocarditis, and all the patients had some predisposing disorder, such as hepatic cirrhosis, rheumatic or ischemic heart disease, or alcoholism.

The central nervous system may be infected by *C. fetus,* and the most common presentation in both adults and children is meningoencephalitis (44–46). Subarachnoid hemorrhages, brain abscesses, and cerebral infarctions are possible, and although two-thirds of the patients survive, neurologic sequelae are frequent. In neonates, the prognosis is worse. The cerebrospinal fluid typically shows polymorphonuclear pleocytosis, and subdural effusion may be present (44).

C. fetus can remain latent after bacteremic seeding in a bony focus of an immunocompromised host, only to be reactivated years later (47). It has been responsible for infection in a postoperative prosthetic hip joint (48), chronic osteomyelitis of the ankle (49), and pyogenic vertebral osteomyelitis (50). *C. fetus* may be an unobtrusive inhabitant of the gut, but with decreased host immunity, the organism may invade the mucosa and cause generalized infection (51). Other signs of *C. fetus* infection are lung abscess, salpingitis, thrombophlebitis, cellulitis, and cholecystitis (52,53). Infection of the peritoneum by *C. fetus* has been reported in patients on peritoneal dialysis; direct contamination of the catheter has been postulated (54). *C. fetus*

TABLE 47.4. CLINICAL FEATURES OF SOUTH AFRICAN CHILDREN INFECTED WITH *CAMPYLOBACTER* AND RELATED ORGANISMS[a]

	Distribution of the Pathogen among Infected Patients								
Feature[b]	*C. jejuni subsp jejuni*[c]	*C. concisus*	*C. upsaliensis*	*C. jejuni subsp doylei*	*H. fennelliae*	*H. cinaedi*	*C. hyointestinalis*	*C. fetus subsp fetus*	*A. butzleri*
Number of isolates	1,013	759	617	214	104	34	21	9	9
	Percentage distribution of clinical features in patients								
Symptoms									
Diarrhea	68	66	62	64	64	53	71	22	56
Vomiting	1	2	2	3	1	6	0	0	0
Fever	2	3	1	2	2	0	0	22	0
Stool consistency									
Formed	5	4	10	3	10	6	16	0	0
Loose	82	75	72	72	72	82	68	100	100
Watery	13	21	18	25	18	12	16	0	0
Presence of blood in stools									
Leukocytes	33	35	23	28	27	18	14	11	22
Erythrocytes	21	22	13	16	19	12	14	0	0
Coexisting enteric pathogens									
Bacterial[d]	5	18	8	15	5	6	10	11	0
Parasitic[e]	9	16	26	26	33	15	43	0	0
Preexisting conditions									
Anemia/leukemia	2	1	5	2	4	0	0	0	0
HIV/immunocompromised	2	2	0.5	0	2	3	0	0	0
Respiratory-related[f]	0.3	0.3	0.5	0	0	0	5	0	0
Nutrition-related[g]	4	3	6	10	4	15	19	22	22

[a]Data from Table 47.3.
[b]Sole pathogen detected.
[c]*C. jejuni* subsp *jejuni* biotypes 1 and 2.
[d]*Salmonella* and *Shigella.*
[e]*Ascaris, Trichuris, Cryptosporidium* (others not stated).
[f]Tuberculosis, bronchopneumonia (others not stated)
[g]Kwashiorkor, marasmus, failure to thrive (others not stated).

peritonitis has occurred in patients with alcoholic cirrhosis (51), possibly because of impaired reticuloendothelial clearance of portal bacteremia. The prime virulence determinant of *C. fetus* is the proteinaceous surface layer (S layer), which forms a paracrystalline surface array that functions as a capsule and strongly inhibits the binding of C3b. Disruption of C3b binding explains the observed serum and phagocytosis resistance. *C. fetus* is able to change the antigenic characteristics of the particular S-layer protein expressed. This antigenic variation, which occurs frequently, favors long-term residence at mucosal sites. Additional aspects of the molecular biology of the S layer are covered in detail in the review article by Thompson and Blaser (55).

Treatment

Often, *C. fetus* infections are prolonged and relapsing, but most patients recover with appropriate antibiotic treatment and medical procedures. The prognosis depends on the severity of the underlying illness and the rapidity with which an antibiotic treatment is applied. Infection by *C. fetus* can be lethal in some debilitated persons and can hasten the demise of others. Immunocompetent patients with uncomplicated intestinal infections usually do not need antibiotics. However, patients with systemic *C. fetus* infection usually require parenteral therapy. Patients with *C. fetus* endocarditis may require up to a month of antibiotic therapy. Ampicillin or third-generation cephalosporins are usually effective against established *C. fetus* infections (47). Patients with serious infections caused by *C. fetus* have been treated successfully with aminoglycosides, ampicillin, chloramphenicol, or doxycycline (50). Patients with persistent bacteremia and hypogammaglobulinemia may require lifelong antibiotic therapy. Intravenous immunoglobulins are not effective in treating immunodeficient persons with *C. fetus* infection because the serum from normal persons usually does not contain opsonizing antibodies to *C. fetus* (47).

C. UPSALIENSIS

C. upsaliensis is a recognized human pathogen in both healthy and immunocompromised patients, causing both acute and chronic, recurrent diarrhea. This organism, originally described as a catalase-negative/catalase-weak (CNW) campylobacter, can cause bacteremia in debilitated and immunocompromised patients. It has been associated with hemolytic–uremic syndrome (56), Guillain-Barré syndrome (57), and spontaneous human abortion (58). *C. upsaliensis* was first isolated from the stools of healthy and diarrhetic dogs in 1983. DNA–DNA hybridization studies indicated that this organism was a new species, and the name *upsaliensis* was proposed after the Swedish town, Uppsala, where the organism was first isolated (59). A review by Bourke et al. (60) has summarized the data on *C. upsaliensis.*

Microbiology

C. upsaliensis is a thermotolerant *Campylobacter* species that usually grows well at 42°C but not at 25°C under microaerobic conditions. Some strains grow better in a hydrogen-enhanced microaerobic atmosphere. This organism is catalase-negative or only weakly catalase-positive (61); it is negative for hippurate and arylsulfatase but positive for nitrate reductase and indoxylacetate (Table 47.2). A striking and distinguishing characteristic of *C. upsaliensis* is its intense susceptibility to both nalidixic acid and cephalothin, with inhibitory zones of up to 80 mm for cephalothin (62). *C. upsaliensis* cannot be isolated with selective media containing cephalothin. This may account for suboptimal isolation of the organism in some laboratories. Based on differences in colony morphology on primary isolation and subsequent biochemical and serologic confirmation, multiple isolates of two to five species were found in 16.2% of the stools of South African pediatric patients with gastroenteritis (4). In this study, *C. upsaliensis* was frequently isolated together with other campylobacters, such as *C. jejuni* subsp *jejuni, C. jejuni* subsp *doylei,* and particularly *Helicobacter fennelliae* (4). If infection by more than one species is suspected, considerable care must be taken to separate the domed colonies of *C. upsaliensis* from the spreading, noncolonial growth of *H. fennelliae* or *Helicobacter cinaedi* before positive identification can be undertaken (Fig. 47.1).

Epidemiology

In a study of Sanstedt et al. (63), *C. upsaliensis* comprised 63 (64%) of 98 *Campylobacter* strains isolated from dog

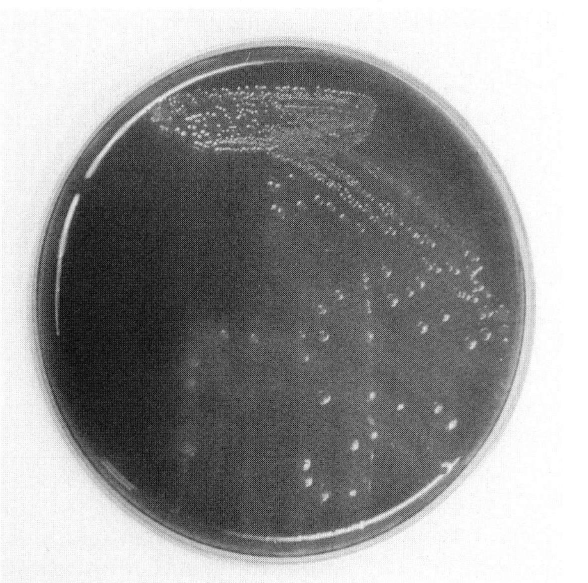

FIGURE 47.1. A culture plate showing the spreading, diffuse, noncolonial growth of *H. fennelliae* contrasted with the domed colonies of *C. upsaliensis.*

stools. *C. upsaliensis* has been isolated from a dog with chronic diarrhea (64), healthy puppies and kittens (65,66), and asymptomatic vervet monkeys (67). Although the exact source of *C. upsaliensis* infection in humans in unknown, zoonotic transmission is a distinct possibility. Four of seven patients with *C. upsaliensis* infection in one study reported animal contact (68). *C. upsaliensis* that appeared to be the same strain was cultured from the stools of a 53-year-old man with bloody diarrhea and his healthy 3-year-old dog (65). Gurgan and Diker (58) documented the isolation of *C. upsaliensis* in the blood and fetoplacental specimens of a woman who had had a spontaneous abortion at 18 weeks' gestation. A *C. upsaliensis* strain was isolated from her asymptomatic cat, and protein profile analysis indicated a strong similarity between the human and feline isolates (58). Although these observations are suggestive, animal-to-human transmission of *C. upsaliensis* remains to be proved unequivocally. Indirect evidence also suggests person-to-person transmission of *C. upsaliensis.* Goossens et al. (69) documented *C. upsaliensis* infection in 44 children in four day care centers in Brussels, Belgium. Multiple typing methods indicated that the outbreaks of *C. upsaliensis* infection in three of the four centers were caused by the same strain, which was closely related to the strain isolated from the fourth day care center (69).

C. upsaliensis infection occurs in all seasons, but in two separate studies at pediatric hospitals in Toronto and Cape Town, the majority of isolates were obtained in the respective autumns of the northern and southern hemispheres (4,70). Between 1990 and 2000, a pediatric hospital in South Africa isolated 978 strains of *C. upsaliensis,* which accounted for 23% of all the campylobacters isolated and identified (Table 47.3). This high isolation rate of *C. upsaliensis* is attributed to the isolation protocol used (4,5). In distinct contrast are the results of an Australian retrospective study of diarrhetic children admitted to a pediatric hospital between 1992 and 1999, in which 666 (3.6%) of 18,516 stools yielded *C. jejuni* and an additional 19 (0.1%) were *C. upsaliensis* (71). A Belgian study of 15,185 fecal samples yielded 802 *Campylobacter* strains, and 99 (12%) were identified as *C. upsaliensis* (1). Only a single *C. upsaliensis* strain was obtained in a study of 631 stools from Thai children (72). In a Canadian study of 915 *Campylobacter* stool isolates, only 7 (0.1%) were *C. upsaliensis* (73). In a survey of 394 *Campylobacter* blood culture strains isolated from patients in England and Wales, 2 (0.8%) were *C. upsaliensis* (38). By contrast, in a South African study of 221 *Campylobacter* isolates obtained from the blood cultures of pediatric patients, 39 (18%) were *C. upsaliensis* (30). Differences in the isolation and culture protocols used in various laboratories could account for part of the wide variation in the prevalence of *C. upsaliensis.* Alternatively, data from South Africa in comparison with those from other studies may reflect differences in prevalence and exposure to *C. upsaliensis,* or possibly differences in colonization and the nature of *C. upsaliensis* infection in different geographic areas.

Characterization of Isolates

C. upsaliensis has a plasmid carriage rate of about 90%, much higher than that of other species of *Campylobacter* (74,75), and fewer than 20% of the strains examined have been related (75). Although the serotyping of *C. upsaliensis* strains has been of limited value (62), sodium dodecyl sulfate-polyacrylamide gel electrophoresis (SDS-PAGE) protein profile analysis (76) has proved useful for the differentiation of individual *C. upsaliensis* isolates. Digestion of chromosomal DNA with *Hae*III (75) and pulsed-field gel electrophoresis (77) of *C. upsaliensis* have indicated considerable molecular heterogeneity among strains. *C. upsaliensis* can be identified by PCR techniques based on 16S rRNA or guanosine triphosphatase (GTPase) genes (78,79).

Clinical Features

The usual symptoms associated with *C. upsaliensis* infection are gastrointestinal and include watery diarrhea, abdominal cramps, vomiting, and low-grade fever (68,80,81). Although most patients recover quickly, others may be ill for several weeks (68,70,80,81). In a study of 99 patients with *C. upsaliensis* in their stools, in whom the onset of symptoms was abrupt, 92% had diarrhea, 14% had vomiting, and 0.6% presented with fever (1). Symptoms persisted for more than 1 week in 16% of these patients; 25% had blood in their stools, and 10% had fecal leukocytes. In a study of 619 pediatric patients from whom *C. upsaliensis* was the sole pathogen isolated, the median age was 18 months (range, 1 month to 10 years). Diarrheal symptoms were present in 62%, vomiting in 2%, and fever (>38°C) in 1% of these patients. Additional clinical details are given in Table 47.4. *C. upsaliensis* was almost equally found in the blood (21%) and stool (23%) cultures of pediatric patients (30) (Fig. 47.2). Most patients with *C. upsaliensis* bacteremia have other, serious underlying medical conditions, and bacteremia may be secondary to intestinal infections (62,68,82). *C. upsaliensis* has been isolated from the breast abscess of a patient who reported no animal contact or gastrointestinal symptoms (83), and has been linked to the hemolytic–uremic syndrome (56) and the Guillain-Barré syndrome (57).

Pathogenesis

The mechanisms of pathogenicity of *C. upsaliensis* are not fully understood. Sylvester et al. (84) demonstrated that *C. upsaliensis* is capable of binding to Chinese hamster ovary and HEp-2 cells in tissue culture. These authors also detected 50- to 90-kd surface proteins on *C. upsaliensis* isolates that were capable of binding to phosphatidylethanola-

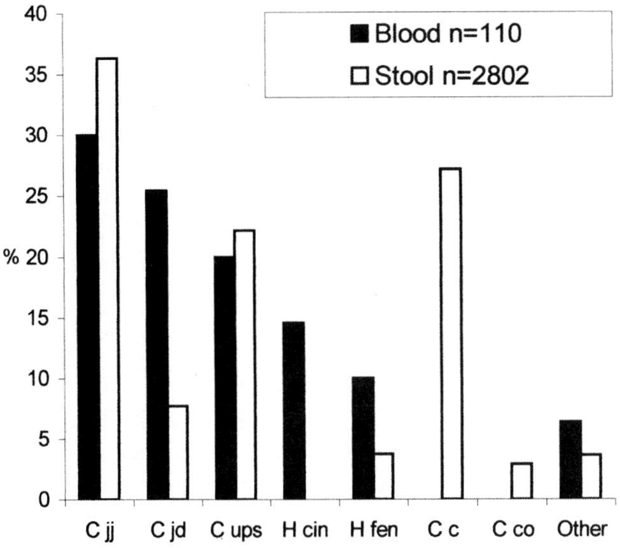

FIGURE 47.2. *Campylobacter* species isolated from pediatric blood and stool cultures in Cape Town, South Africa (1990–2000). *C jj, C. jejuni* subsp *jejuni; C jd,* C. jejuni subsp *doylei; C ups, C. upsaliensis; H cin, H. cinaedi; H fen, H. fennelliae; C c, C. concisus; C co, C. coli.* (Data from Lastovica AJ. *Campylobacter/Helicobacter* bacteremia in Cape Town, South Africa, 1977–1995. In: Newell DG, Ketley JM, Feldman RA, eds. *Campylobacters, helicobacters, and related organisms.* New York: Plenum Publishing, 1996:47–479, with permission.).

mine, a putative cell membrane receptor. Biotin-labeled *C. upsaliensis* strains bound in a concentration-dependent fashion to human small-intestinal mucin, which implies that *C. upsaliensis* organisms express adhesin(s) capable of recognizing specific mucin epitope(s) (84). Possibly, the binding of mucins may influence bacterial access to cell membrane receptors and thus influence host resistance to infection. *C. upsaliensis* sepsis in a boy with hypogammaglobulinemia (82) suggests that antibody-mediated killing of *C. upsaliensis* is important. Pickett et al. (85) confirmed the presence of a cytolethal distending toxin homologue on *C. upsaliensis.* However, the appropriate *cdt* gene(s) have yet to be cloned. Conclusive proof of *C. upsaliensis* as a human enteropathogen will require controlled studies, such as comparisons of isolation rates in asymptomatic and symptomatic subjects and animal challenge experiments, before *C. upsaliensis* can be unequivocally recognized as a causative agent of human disease.

Treatment

The most active antimicrobial agents available for the treatment of *C. upsaliensis* infection are the fluoroquinolones (86). Erythromycin was once the preferred treatment for *Campylobacter* infections, but 4% to 18% of *C. upsaliensis* isolates are resistant to erythromycin (1,68,74). Infections with *C. upsaliensis* have been treated successfully with augmentin, cefotaxime, and doxycycline (68,82).

C. HYOINTESTINALIS

C. hyointestinalis was identified in 1983, and Gebhart et al. (87) suggested that it might be a cause of proliferative enteritis in pigs. This organism was subsequently isolated from human stools and may be a cause of watery, nonbloody diarrhea in children. The term *hyointestinalis* is derived from the Latin *hyo* ("hog") and *intestinalis* ("pertaining to the intestine"). *C. hyointestinalis* subsp *lawsonii* subsp nov and *C. hyointestinalis* subsp *hyointestinalis* subsp nov have been described by On et al. (88,89).

Microbiology, Diagnosis, and Epidemiology

C. hyointestinalis is closely related to *C. fetus* and is catalase- and nitrate reductase-positive, indoxyl acetate-negative, susceptible to cephalothin, and resistant to nalidixic acid. *C. hyointestinalis* differs from *C. fetus* in its copious production of hydrogen sulfide in triple sugar iron (TSI) agar, which often entirely blackens lead acetate strips (Table 47.2). *C. hyointestinalis* grows under microaerobic conditions, but some strains require additional hydrogen (4,90). These isolates can be differentiated from other hydrogen-requiring isolates by the catalase and other tests (91) (Table 47.2). *C. hyointestinalis* is thermotolerant (not thermophilic); all strains grow at 37°C, but some strains will grow only at 42°C. Lack of aryl sulfatase activity and intolerance to 3.5% sodium chloride are useful diagnostic tests (13). Filtration onto antibiotic-free blood agar media and incubation under a hydrogen-enhanced microaerobic atmosphere at 37°C have proved to be extremely efficient for the isolation of *C. hyointestinalis* (4).

Pulsed-field gel electrophoresis and SDS-PAGE have been used to differentiate strains of *C. hyointestinalis* from one another and from other *Campylobacter* species (92,93). DNA probes have been useful for the detection of *C. hyointestinalis* in swine with proliferative enteritis (94). Oligodeoxynucleotide probes based on 16S rRNA sequence data (95) and a PCR assay based on the 16S rRNA gene (78) have been successfully used to detect *C. hyointestinalis.* *C. hyointestinalis* has been consistently isolated from the intestines of pigs with proliferative enteritis, but not from asymptomatic pigs or pigs with other enteric diseases (88). This organism has also been isolated from hamsters, cattle, and nonhuman primates (96,97).

Clinical Features and Treatment

In 1986, the first case of human illness was reported when a *C. hyointestinalis* strain was isolated as the sole pathogen from the stool of a homosexual man with proctitis. The patient's symptoms resolved and the organism disappeared after appropriate antibiotic treatment (98). Subsequently, *C. hyointestinalis* strains were isolated from the stool specimens of four patients, all of whom had nonbloody, watery diarrhea (90). An 8-month-old girl, the youngest patient, had drunk unpasteurized milk, and the oldest, a 78-year-old woman, exhibited fever and vomiting. No leukocytes were present in their stools, and both patients recovered with appropriate antibiotic therapy. The other two patients, both homosexual men, had abdominal cramps, and one was febrile. One patient recovered with trimethoprim-sulfamethoxazole. No antibiotic treatment was administered to the other patient, who continued to have intermittent diarrhea and cramps for several months (90). An additional case of *C. hyointestinalis*-associated diarrhea was reported in a 52-year-old woman who was immunodeficient because of an evolutive chronic myeloid leukemia (99). In a recent review, Breynaert et al. (100) examined the clinical features of nine adult and pediatric patients infected with *C. hyointestinalis.* Six patients experienced diarrhea, and five had abdominal pain. Two asymptomatic patients were the youngest, a 1-year-old girl with constipation, and the oldest, an 89-year-old woman with a myocardial infarction. No patient was seriously immunocompromised, but most of the adult patients had a history of neurologic or vascular disease (100).

Fifty-three (1.3%) strains of *C. hyointestinalis* were isolated in a study of 4,212 South African pediatric *Campylobacter* stool isolates (Table 47.3). The median age of these patients with *C. hyointestinalis* infection was 29 months (range, 1 month to 7 years). The clinical features are indicated in Table 47.4. The only known extraintestinal isolation of *C. hyointestinalis* was from the blood culture of a 22-year-old man after a bone marrow transplantation operation (30).

C. LARI

C. lari is a nalidixic acid-resistant, thermophilic *Campylobacter* organism first identified in 1980 by Skirrow and Benjamin (101). Initially, most strains were isolated from seagulls (genus *larus*); the name *C. laridis* was proposed, then later changed to *C. lari* in 1990 (102). Although the first human isolate was from an asymptomatic 6-year-old boy, *C. lari* can produce acute diarrheal illness in normal hosts and bacteremia in immunocompromised patients.

Microbiology and Epidemiology

C. lari organisms are microaerobic (some isolates grow better in hydrogen-enhanced microaerobic growth conditions), thermophilic campylobacters that grow at 42°C but not usually at 25°C. Most are oxidase- and nitrate reductase-positive and do not hydrolyze hippurate (103) (Table 47.2).

C. lari has been isolated from a variety of environmental sources (Table 47.1). Of 312 riverine samples collected in a U.K. study, 134 yielded campylobacters, and 7 (5%) of these were *C. lari* (104). In a survey of surface waters in Norway, 2 (2%) of 96 *Campylobacter* samples were *C. lari* (105). These isolations may be significant, as water is an established vehicle for the transmission of campylobacters to humans (91). *C. lari* isolation rates were up to 29% in seagulls (106) and 7% in crows (107). In a study of *Campylobacter* species in oysters and mussels in the Netherlands, Van Doorn et al. (108) found that of 44 *Campylobacter* isolates, 38 were *C. lari. C. lari* has been isolated from fresh vegetables (109), pigs (110), poultry (111), and dogs (112). *C. lari* is infrequently isolated from pediatric diarrheic stools (Table 47.3).

Diagnosis

Because the spectrum of clinical disease described in association with *C. lari* infection is similar to that seen with other campylobacters, the diagnosis of *C. lari* infection depends on the isolation and identification of the organism from cultured specimens. *C. lari* is distinct from *C. jejuni,* most notably in its resistance to nalidixic acid, to which *C. jejuni* is sensitive. The correct identification of *C. lari* may be difficult because some clinical microbiology laboratories do not routinely test isolates for resistance to nalidixic acid. Isolates of *C. lari* that are susceptible to nalidixic acid and strains of *C. jejuni* that are resistant to nalidixic acid have been described (70,104,113). The hippurate hydrolysis test result is negative with *C. lari* but positive with *C. jejuni* (Table 47.2), and *C. jejuni* strains hydrolyze indoxyl acetate, whereas *C. lari* does not (114). Linton et al. (78) have developed a PCR assay based on the nucleotide sequence for the 16S rRNA gene, specific for *C. lari.* Van Doorn and associates (79) proposed a PCR assay for *C. lari* based on a novel putative GTPase gene. In a study of 38 *C. lari* strains isolated from mussels and oysters by Van Doorn et al. (108), the *C. lari* isolates were a more heterogeneous group than was previously thought. Based on sequence information, a PCR assay was developed to permit the specific and rapid detection of *C. lari* variants (108).

Clinical Features

C. lari is an enteric pathogen in both immunocompetent and immunocompromised hosts. The first human isolates of *C. lari* were from asymptomatic persons (115,116), and the pathogenicity of *C. lari* was realized only in 1984 when a fatal case of *C. lari* bacteremia in a severely immunocompromised patient was described (117). Other bloodstream isolates have confirmed its pathogenic potential. *C. lari* induced colitis in a 32-year-old HIV-positive woman, who required extensive antimicrobial therapy before her symptoms were relieved (118). The blood cultures of another HIV-infected patient with *C. lari* bacteremia remained persistently positive despite aminoglycoside treatment (119). *C. lari* has been infrequently isolated from blood cultures (38).

C. lari was isolated from the diarrhetic stools of five immunocompetent persons, two of whom were hospitalized. Illness lasted from 1 week to 4 months (median, 2 weeks), and all patients recovered completely (103). None of these patients was febrile, but four had abdominal cramps, four had had contact with pets, and four had eaten chicken in the week before symptoms became apparent. Simor and Wilcox (120) reported a patient with *C. lari* enteritis and demonstrated specific serum antibodies to the isolated *C. lari* strain, which indicated an association between enteritis and *C. lari* infection. Urease-positive, nalidixic acid-susceptible variants of *C. lari* were isolated from the stools of two compromised adult patients (one had ovarian cancer and one was an alcoholic) with diarrhea in France and from the inflamed appendix of an immunocompetent 10-year-old boy (113). A urinary tract infection caused by a urease-positive, nalidixic acid-susceptible *C. lari* variant was reported in an alcoholic man with cirrhosis (121). *C. lari* has been identified in a permanent pacemaker infection associated with bacteremia (122) and in an 80-year-old debilitated patient with purulent pleurisy (123). In 1985, a common source waterborne outbreak of *C. lari* infection occurred in Ontario (124). Gastroenteritis developed among construction workers who had drunk water contaminated with surface water from Lake Ontario, which has a large population of sea gulls. Of 162 ill persons, 87% had diarrhea, 70% had abdominal pain, and 20% had fever; vomiting, nausea, and headaches were noted (124). Only one patient reported bloody stools, and the mean duration of illness was 4 days (range, 1 to 10 days). Of 125 stool samples cultured, 7 yielded *C. lari,* which is probably an underestimate because collection was delayed and specimens were transported in dry containers, so that the bacterial viability was reduced. *C. lari* strains are capable of producing both cytotoxic and cytotonic factors (125); however, the role of these factors in the disease process is still unknown.

Treatment

C. lari infections associated with uncomplicated diarrhea are self-limiting and generally do not require antibiotic intervention. With severe symptoms, aminoglycosides, erythromycin, and chloramphenicol have been successfully used (117,118,120). *C. lari* is resistant to third-generation cephalosporins, vancomycin, penicillin, and trimethoprim-sulfamethoxazole (118,120). Quinolone-resistant strains have been reported in HIV-infected persons (118).

H. CINAEDI AND *H. FENNELLIAE*

Initially, *Helicobacter cinaedi* and *Helicobacter fennelliae* were called *Campylobacter*-like organisms (CLOs) and were divided into three phenotypic groups: CLO1, CLO2, and CLO3. Subsequently, CLO1 was found to comprise two genetically distinct groups, CLO1A and CLO1B (126). CLO1A was initially called *C. cinaedi,* from the Latin word *cinaedi* ("of a homosexual"). CLO2 isolates were initially called *C. fennelliae* for Cynthia Fennell, the microbiologist who first isolated these organisms from the rectal swabs of homosexual men. The names of the organisms were subsequently amended to *H. cinaedi* and *H. fennelliae* (126).

Microbiology

H. cinaedi and *H. fennelliae* grow under microaerophilic conditions, but some strains require hydrogen-enhanced microaerophilic conditions for optimal growth. These bacteria grow at 37°C but grow poorly or not at all at 42°C (Table 47.2). *H. fennelliae* may be differentiated from *H. cinaedi* by differences in aryl sulfatase activity (13), SDS-PAGE profiles (127), and serology (128). A useful diagnostic test is the smell of a mature growth of *H. fennelliae,* which is similar to that of hypochlorite ("Clorox"); the odor is absent in *H. cinaedi* and campylobacters (129). Whereas *Campylobacter* and *Arcobacter* species form domed colonies on agar plates, both *H. cinaedi* and *H. fennelliae* exhibit flat, spreading growth, without discrete colonies, on freshly prepared agar plates (129). This growth may be missed on primary isolation plates, particularly if the domed colonies of a *Campylobacter* species are also present. *H. fennelliae* is often isolated together with *C. jejuni* subsp *jejuni, C. jejuni* subsp *doylei,* or *C. upsaliensis* (4,5). In cases of suspected mixed infection, extreme care must be taken to separate the noncolonial spreading growth of *H. fennelliae* or *H. cinaedi* from the domed colonies of other campylobacters (Fig. 47.1).

Characterization of Strains

Kiehlbauch et al. (130) characterized 34 human and animal strains of *H. cinaedi* and two animal and two human strains of *H. fennelliae.* In their studies, most isolates of *H. cinaedi* formed a single group, both phenotypically and by DNA–DNA hybridization studies, and subgroups were distinguishable by ribotyping. The two human *H. fennelliae* strains were related but had ribotyping patterns different from those of the two *H. fennelliae* animal strains.

Epidemiology and Clinical Features

Campylobacter-like organisms were first recognized as human pathogens when they were isolated from the stools of 26 of 158 homosexual men with gastroenteritis (131). These organisms were also isolated from 6 of 75 asymptomatic homosexual men but were not isolated from 150 heterosexual men and women (131). In a study of the diarrheal stools of homosexual or bisexual men in Baltimore and Washington, D.C., 9 (27%) of 33 patients had *Campylobacter* or *Helicobacter* in their stools, whereas 2 patients had *H. cinaedi* infections and 1 had a CLO3 strain (132). Two CLO3 strains have been isolated from the stools of homosexual men with proctitis (133,134). In descriptions of patients with gastroenteritis who had symptoms attributed to CLO infections, the clinical features, which included diarrhea, abdominal cramps, and hematochezia, were similar to those of patients with *C. jejuni* infection (131). CLO infections were also noted to produce fever, anal discharge, and pain (131). Sigmoidoscopic examinations of infected patients indicated mucosal bleeding and ulcers. Fecal leukocytes were present in most cases, and histologic examination revealed crypt abscesses and polymorphonuclear leukocytes scattered throughout the lamina propria. In a subsequent report, HIV-infected patients with *H. cinaedi* in their stools experienced chronic but mild diarrhea lasting several weeks (135); no blood or polymorphonuclear leukocytes were found in their stools.

H. cinaedi and *H. fennelliae* can cause bacteremia, particularly in HIV-positive patients (136,137). Chills, low-grade fevers, lethargy, and malaise are usually present in patients with *H. cinaedi* bacteremia, who often have had preceding gastrointestinal symptoms. Recurrent *H. cinaedi* bacteremia developed in a homosexual man with AIDS (138). This patient had had 2 months of intermittent diarrhea and fecal incontinence. His blood cultures yielded a second organism, which was identified as *H. fennelliae,* and cultures were consistently positive despite treatment with ciprofloxacin and trimethoprim-sulfamethoxazole. The patient died 4 months later, although the role of the *H. cinaedi* and *H. fennelliae* isolates was not clearly defined (138). In a survey of 394 blood culture *Campylobacter* isolates from patients in England and Wales, 2 (0.5%) of the isolates were *H. fennelliae* and 1 (0.25%) was *H. cinaedi* (38). In a study of 221 South African pediatric blood culture isolates, 7 (3.2%) of the strains were *H. fennelliae* and 5 (2.3%) were *H. cinaedi* (30). The same hospital isolated 4,212 *Campylobacter, Helicobacter,* or *Arcobacter* strains from 20,123 diarrhetic stools (Table 47.3). In this study, 266 (6.3%) of the detected strains were *H. fennelliae* and 42 (1.0%) were *H. cinaedi. H. cinaedi* and *H. fennelliae* are more likely to be associated with blood than with stool infection, which may imply an invasive role for these organisms (Fig. 47.2). The median age of the infected children was 19 months for those with *H. cinaedi* and 23 months for those with *H. fennelliae* (range, 2 weeks to 11 years). Of these patients, 64% had diarrhea, 1% had vomiting, and 2% had fever. Additional clinical details are given in Table 47.4. Hsueh et al. (139) reported a case of bacteremia and septic shock caused by *H. fennelliae* in a 48-year-old non–HIV-infected heterosexual man with diabetes mellitus and cirrhosis of the liver. Lasry et al. (140) documented *H. cinaedi* septic arthritis and bacteremia in an immunocompetent heterosexual 20-year-old man. These reports suggest that *H. cinaedi* and *H. fennelliae* infections may occur more frequently than previously thought in heterosexual and immunocompetent populations.

Gastroenteritis caused by *H. cinaedi* or *H. fennelliae* infection has been reported in heterosexual men and women and in children (135,141). The source of human infection by these organisms is not known; however, transmission from animals is a possibility. *H. cinaedi* was isolated from the cerebrospinal fluid and blood of a 5-day-old neonate whose mother had had a mild diarrheal illness during her third trimester of her pregnancy. The mother had cared for pet hamsters during the first two trimesters of her pregnancy (142). *H. cinaedi* has been isolated from 72% of commercially available hamsters (143) and from the stools of diarrheic dogs (144).

Pathogenesis

Evidence for the pathogenicity of *H. cinaedi* and *H. fennelliae* comes from several sources. The detection of these organisms in homosexual men with proctitis and enteritis, but not in asymptomatic men, suggests a causal relationship. The presence of fecal leukocytes and bacteremia in immunocompromised patients indicates a pathogenic role for these organisms. Flores et al. (145) studied the effects of experimental *H. cinaedi* and *H. fennelliae* infection in infant macaque monkeys. After four monkeys were challenged with *H. cinaedi,* diarrhea developed in two animals, and *H. cinaedi* was isolated from the stools and blood of all four monkeys. When challenged with *H. fennelliae,* all the monkeys became bacteremic, and diarrhea developed in two animals. *H. fennelliae* was isolated from their stools (145).

Treatment

Although *H. cinaedi* and *H. fennelliae* infections have not resulted in death, some patients have shown a slow clinical response to antimicrobial therapy. Antimicrobial agents that have demonstrated *in vitro* activity against *H. cinaedi* and *H. fennelliae* include ampicillin, tetracycline, rifampin, nalidixic acid, chloramphenicol, and gentamicin (133,139). However, 28% of the strains were resistant to erythromycin and clindamycin and 17% were resistant to sulfamethoxazole (133). Of *H. cinaedi* and *H. fennelliae* stool and blood culture isolates from South African pediatric patients, 13% were resistant to erythromycin (146). Oral fluoroquinolones may be the best treatment for severe or persistent *H. cinaedi* and *H. fennelliae* infection (136,140).

A. BUTZLERI AND *A. CRYAEROPHILUS*

The genus *Arcobacter* now comprises four species that were previously included in the genus *Campylobacter*: *A. cryaerophilus* group 1A and group 1B, *A. nitrofigilis, A. butzleri,* and *A. skirrowii* (93). These organisms, after DNA–DNA hybridization studies, were moved from the genus *Campylobacter* to the genus *Arcobacter* (91,126).

Arcobacters are morphologically similar to campylobacters, but unlike campylobacters, all arcobacters are able to grow in air. The type species, *A. nitrofigilis,* was originally isolated from the roots and associated sediment of salt marsh plants, where the organisms fix nitrogen, but it has not been isolated from humans or animals. The clinical significance of these organisms is limited, and the majority of human isolates described to date belong to the species *A. butzleri.*

Microbiology

Physiologically, *Arcobacter* species are aerotolerant bacteria, whereas *Campylobacter* species are microaerobic or hydrogen-enhanced microaerobic bacteria; differences in their biochemical characteristics are outlined in Table 47.3. Both *A. cryaerophilus* and *A. butzleri* grow poorly or not at all at 42°C on blood agar plates (146) (Table 47.3) but grow on MacConkey agar; they are generally resistant to cephalothin and are aerotolerant at 37°C. *A. butzleri* was identified by Kiehlbauch et al. (147) during a study of aerotolerant *Campylobacter* isolates. Genetic studies indicated that these aerotolerant bacteria belong to two groups. The group 2 strains were named *A. butzleri* in honor of Jean-Paul Butzler, a Belgian microbiologist.

Clinical Features

A. butzleri can produce diarrhea and associated gastrointestinal symptoms in humans (Table 47.4), and it has been isolated from patients' blood cultures (147). Most (>50%) of these patients experienced nausea, abdominal pain, chills, vomiting, and fever. On et al. (148) isolated a strain of *A. butzleri* from the blood culture of a neonate. Clinical details suggested that this infection was contracted *in utero,* and appropriate antibiotic therapy successfully resolved the infection in the preterm infant (148). Yan et al. (149) reported *A. butzleri* bacteremia in a 60-year-old man with liver cirrhosis who presented with fever and esophageal visceral bleeding. *A. butzleri* has been isolated and identified in the stools of diarrhetic children in Thailand (150) and South Africa (Table 47.3). An outbreak of *A. butzleri* infection occurred among 10 Italian children, 2 to 5 five years of age; none of them had diarrhea or fever, but all had episodes of recurrent abdominal cramps, lasting up to 2 hours, several times a day for up to 10 days (151). The children felt well between attacks, and the illness was self-limiting. Most of them underwent seroconversion, and all strains belonged to a single serogroup with an identical protein profile, which indicated a common source. The successive timing of these cases suggested person-to-person contact (151).

Dediste et al. (152) examined 16 strains of *A. butzleri* and two of *A. cryaerophilus* isolated from 14 symptomatic and four asymptomatic patients. An absence of fever was noted in the patients with *A. butzleri* infection; watery diarrhea occurred in 13 of 16 patients. No blood or inflammatory exudate was detected on microscopic examination of the stools. Vomiting and abdominal pain occurred in about half the patients, who were treated with amoxicillin and clavulanate and recovered rapidly. The remainder improved spontaneously with conservative management (152). In one case, in which *A. cryaerophilus* was the sole pathogen, the patient presented with symptoms of watery diarrhea, fever, and abdominal pain; the other case of *A. cryaerophilus* infection was asymptomatic (152). *A. cryaerophilus* has been isolated from the blood cultures of two patients and the stools of a patient with gastroenteritis (147). An *A. cryaerophilus* group 1B strain was isolated from the blood of a 72-year-old uremic woman with hematogenous pneumonia. This patient was successfully treated with ceftizoxime and tobramycin (153). In a study of 4,212 campylobacters isolated from the diarrhetic stools of pediatric patients (median age, 18 months), only 16 (0.38%) of the isolates were *A. butzleri* (Table 47.3). Additional clinical details of the patients are given in Table 47.4.

Epidemiology

One hundred strains of *A. butzleri* and 41 strains of *A. butzleri*-like or *Arcobacter* species were isolated recently from six drinking water plants in Germany (154). Two strains of *A. butzleri* were isolated from a contaminated well in Idaho (155). Survival studies, conducted at 5°C, a temperature typical of ground water, indicated that *A. butzleri* can remain viable for up to 16 days (155). *A. butzleri* infection was found in 14 (6%) of 222 nonhuman primates with diarrhea. Colonic specimens obtained at necropsy from three macaques with active colitis yielded *A. butzleri* (156). *A. butzleri* was isolated from the stools of 7 (39%) of 18 *Macata nemestrina* monkeys cultured weekly from birth to 1 year of age (96). *A. cryaerophilus* was first isolated from porcine, equine, and bovine feces and aborted porcine and bovine fetuses (157). An Australian traveler with gastroenteritis was thought to be the first human infected with *A. cryaerophilus,* but this organism was later correctly identified as *A. butzleri* (158). *A. cryaerophilus* has been found in urban sewage (159). In a study of 25 broiler chickens obtained from a poultry abattoir and a supermarket, all 25 carcasses yielded *A. butzleri,* 13 carcasses carried *A. cryaerophilus,* and 2 carcasses carried *A. skirrowii* (160). In a Canadian study (161), 121 of 125 broiler chicken carcasses examined were positive for *A. butzleri* after primary abattoir processing. *A. butzleri* was recovered from whole and ground chicken, turkey, and pork samples from retail stores (161,162).

Pathogenicity

Neonatal piglets have been used as models to determine relative pathogenicities (163). Cesarean-derived, colostrum-deprived 1-day-old piglets were infected *per os* with field and type strains of *A. butzleri, A. cryaerophilus,* and *A. skirrowii. Arcobacter* species were detected at least once in rectal swab samples of all but one of the experimentally infected piglets. At necroscopy, *Arcobacter* species were cultured from the liver, kidney, ileum, or brain tissue of two of four piglets infected with *A. butzleri*. However, no severe gross pathology was noted. These data suggest that *Arcobacter* species, particularly *A. butzleri,* can colonize neonatal pigs (163).

Characterization of Isolates

A multiplex PCR assay has been developed to identify *Arcobacter* isolates and distinguish *A. butzleri* from other arcobacters (164). Based on 23S rRNA gene polymorphisms, Hurtado and Owen (165) have proposed a PCR scheme for the rapid identification of *Campylobacter* and *Arcobacter* species. Digestion of the PCR amplicons with four restriction endonucleases (*Hae*III, *Cfo*I, *Hpa*II, *Hinf*I) enabled speciation at the genomic level of *Campylobacter* and *Arcobacter.* With this scheme, *A. butzleri* and *A. nitrofigilis* gave unique profiles; *A. cryaerophilus* and *A. skirrowii* produced identical profiles that were different from those of *A. butzleri* and *A. nitrofigilis* (165). Ribotyping and other molecular assays can distinguish between *A. cryaerophilus* and *A. butzleri* (166).

C. JEJUNI SUBSP *DOYLEI*

Based on DNA hybridization studies, *C. jejuni* has been divided into two subspecies: *C. jejuni* subsp *jejuni* and *C. jejuni* subsp *doylei* (167). *C. jejuni* subsp *doylei* was named after a microbiologist, L. P. Doyle (168). In the vast majority of human *Campylobacter* infections to date, *C. jejuni* subsp *jejuni* has been implicated. Although far fewer clinical isolates of *C. jejuni* subsp *doylei* have been documented, the pathogenic potential of this organism is beginning to be appreciated. Clinical and other aspects of *C. jejuni* subsp *jejuni* and *C. coli* are covered in detail elsewhere in this volume.

Microbiology and Diagnosis

The inability to reduce nitrate to nitrite (168) is the determining phenotypic characteristic distinguishing *C. jejuni* subsp *doylei* from *C. jejuni* subsp *jejuni* and all other campylobacters (Table 47.3). Although *H. fennelliae* is also nitrate reductase-negative, it has a spreading colony morphology on blood agar plates and a strong hypochlorite smell (130), and it is resistant to polymyxin B (13). These characteristics readily differentiate the two species. *C. jejuni* subsp *doylei* grows poorly at 42°C and is sensitive to nalidixic acid, but unlike *C. jejuni* subsp *jejuni,* it is also sensitive to cephalothin (Table 47.2). Filtration of stools onto antibiotic-free blood agar plates is a simple and efficient method for obtaining these microorganisms (4,5). Differences in colony morphology on primary isolation and subsequent characterization by biochemical and serologic tests indicate that *C. jejuni* subsp *doylei* can be co-isolated with *C. jejuni* subsp *jejuni, C. upsaliensis,* and *H. fennelliae* (4,62,146). Care must taken to separate the discrete, domed colonies of *C. jejuni* subsp *doylei* from the noncolonial spreading growth of *H. fennelliae* in suspected cases of mixed infection.

Epidemiology and Clinical Features

C. jejuni subsp *doylei* can be present in the upper gastrointestinal tract (169,170). Urease-negative CLOs, originally called GCLO2 *isolates* then subsequently *C. jejuni* subsp *doylei,* were identified in the gastric antral biopsy specimens of six patients (169,170). Four of the patients did not have *Helicobacter pylori* infection, yet all had gastric ulcers and active chronic gastritis. Identical microorganisms were found in the feces of young Australian children hospitalized with gastritis (171). Other studies have shown that this microorganism may be associated with pediatric diarrhea (4,146,172,173). In a study of 631 diarrhetic Thai children, campylobacters were isolated from the stool of 93 (15%), and of these, 1 (1.1%) was a strain of *C. jejuni* subsp *doylei* (150). In a Belgian investigation of 15,185 stools, *C. jejuni* subsp *doylei* accounted for 4 (0.5%) of 802 *Campylobacter* isolates cultured (1).

In a South African study, 384 (9.11%) strains of *C. jejuni* subsp *doylei* were isolated from a total of 4,212 *Campylobacter Helicobacter* isolates obtained from the diarrhetic stools of children (Table 47.3) whose median age was 18 months (range,1 month to 11 years). Seventy-two percent of the children had loose stools, and 25% had watery stools. Other clinical details are indicated in Table 47.4. In a separate study of South African pediatric *Campylobacter* blood cultures, 53 (24.0%) of 221 isolates were *C. jejuni* subsp *doylei* (30). Twenty-six of the 53 children had diarrhea, often chronic, which suggested that intestinal infection preceded systemic infection. Thirty of the 53 patients had severe protein deficiency diseases, such as marasmus and kwashiorkor. *C. jejuni* subsp *doylei* comprised fewer than 10% of the campylobacters found in stool (Table 47.3) but accounted for 24% of the *Campylobacter* blood cultures seen at the same pediatric hospital (Fig. 47.2). This observation suggests a pathogenic, possibly invasive role for *C. jejuni* subsp *doylei.*

CAMPYLOBACTERS REQUIRING HYDROGEN

Campylobacter species that have an essential growth requirement for hydrogen are beginning to be appreciated as potential human pathogenic agents. *C. concisus* (Latin *concisus,* "concise") (174), *C. curvus* (Latin *curvus,* "curved") (175), and *C. rectus* (Latin *rectus,* "straight") (176) are known to be implicated in human periodontal disease.

Microbiology

Six *Campylobacter* species are known to have an essential hydrogen requirement for growth: *C. concisus, C. mucosalis,*

C. gracilis, C. showae, C. rectus, and *C. curvus.* Many of these hydrogen-requiring species are susceptible to cephalothin and nalidixic acid, with an inhibitory zone up to 50 mm in diameter often seen (177). *C. curvus* may be difficult to differentiate from *C. concisus* because the indoxyl acetate assay is not infallible (178) and serologic (176) or other methods may be required. Figura et al. (179) reported two suspected cases of *C. mucosalis* enteritis in Italian school children. However, these isolates were characterized only by variable phenotypic criteria, such as colony color. Investigation of these presumptive *C. mucosalis* strains by other researchers with DNA–DNA hybridization indicated that these strains were misidentified *C. concisus* strains (177). Some isolates of *C. hyointestinalis, C. jejuni* subsp *doylei, C. upsaliensis,* or *C. lari* may require a hydrogen-enriched microaerobic atmosphere for growth. However, these strains can easily be differentiated from the above hydrogen-requiring species by different results of biochemical and phenotypic tests (Table 47.2).

Epidemiology and Clinical Features

C. rectus was isolated from 80% of 1,654 adults and children with periodontitis and patients with periodontitis and inflammatory bowel disease (180,181). Two isolates of *C. rectus* have been identified in the diarrhetic stools of South African children (Table 47.3). This organism has been recovered from patients with periodontitis and septicemia (175). *C. curvus* has been isolated from the diarrheal stools of children in Belgium (178) and South Africa (Table 47.3).

The association of *C. concisus* with human periodontal disease is well-known (174,176), but a direct causal role has not been established. *C. concisus* may have been responsible for osteomyelitis of the sacrum in a patient with a sacral decubitus ulcer (182). In a Belgian study, the range of clinical sites for *C. concisus* was expanded to include the feces, stomach, duodenum, esophagus, and blood of patients with gastroenteritis (183). In another Belgian study, comprising 174 children (184), no statistically significant difference was found between the *C. concisus* isolation rates of children with diarrhea (13.2%) and the rates of those without diarrhea (9%). These authors used arbitrary primer PCR DNA fingerprinting to demonstrate that 35 of 37 children attending the same day care center harbored different strains of *C. concisus* (184) and concluded that *C. concisus* is not pathogenic (184). Evidence that *C. concisus* is an enteric pathogen is accumulating. In a study of Zhi et al. (185), concentrations in serum of an antibody to a *C. concisus* antigen preparation were higher in infected patients than in control groups, but the differences were not large. Istivan et al. (186) presented data on a putative virulence factor, a membrane-bound thermolabile hemolysin that was present in all 21 *C concisus* strains studied. In another study, filtration onto antibiotic-free blood agar plates and incubation in a hydrogen-enriched microaerobic atmosphere were used to examine the stools of 3,165 children and 1,265 adults. Seventy-five (2.4%) and 19 (1.5%) of the *Campylobacter* isolates obtained from adults' and children's stools, respectively, were *C. concisus* (178). Fifty-four percent of the children infected with *C. concisus* were less than 1 year old; only 9% were more than 5 years old. Seventy-two percent of the children had gastrointestinal symptoms; 62% had diarrhea and 22% had vomiting. The mean age of the adults infected with *C. concisus* was 60 years (range, 21 to 87 years), and all but two had diarrhea. Five of the 19 patients had abdominal cramps, and five had signs of colitis. In a South African study of 1,519 *Campylobacter* isolates, 187 (12.3%) required hydrogen for growth (177). Of these, one was from an adult diarrheal stool, 184 were from pediatric diarrheal stools, one was from the blood culture of an 18-day-old infant, and one was from the duodenal biopsy specimen of an adult. All 187 hydrogen-requiring *Campylobacter* isolates were characterized as *C. concisus* based on phenotypic testing. Ninety-two of these isolates were chosen and confirmed as *C. concisus* by DNA–DNA hybridization studies (177). The median age of the patients with *C. concisus* gastroenteritis was 19 months (range, 4 days to 11 years). Twenty-one percent of the stools were watery, and 72% were loose. Sixty-four percent of the patients had diarrhea; additional details are given in Table 47.4. During a decade in a South African pediatric hospital, nearly 1,000 strains of *C. concisus* were isolated from the diarrhetic stools of children (Table 47.3). Only a single *C. concisus* pediatric blood culture isolate was obtained during this time (177), which suggests that *C. concisus* is not invasive from the intestine. Thirty pediatric *C. concisus* isolates were tested against eight antimicrobial agents (187). Ciprofloxacin was the most effective agent examined. All strains were susceptible to tetracycline, ampicillin, and gentamicin. All but one of the strains were resistant to erythromycin.

C. gracilis (formerly *Bacteroides gracilis*) organisms are oxidase-negative, nonmotile straight rods (174). Clinical isolates have been obtained from gingival crevices, soft-tissue abscesses, and infections of the viscera and neck and head. The association of *C. gracilis* with serious deep-tissue infection implies that this organism is an underrated pathogen. *C. showae* organisms are straight rods having bundles of up to five unsheathed flagella (188). Although isolated from human dental plaque and infected root canals, other aspects of the pathogenicity of this organism are unknown.

ADDITIONAL CAMPYLOBACTERS

Other campylobacters have been implicated as causative agents of human disease, but their role as pathogens remains to be established. *C. sputorum* has three biovars (subspecies) that may be clinically relevant. *C. sputorum* biovar sputorum is normally found in the human oral cavity and gastrointestinal tract, whereas *C. sputorum* biovar bubulus is normally found in the reproductive tract of cattle. Both organisms have been isolated from the human lung and from abscesses of the groin and perianal and axillary areas (189,190). Both are rarely isolated from cases of gastroenteritis (Table 47.3). Strains of *C. sputorum* biovar fecalis have been isolated from bovine semen and the vagina, but no evidence for a pathogenic role in humans is available at present. Stanley et al. (191) have described *Helicobacter pullorum,* a new species isolated from poultry liver, duodenum, and cecum and from humans with gastroenteritis (191). *Helicobacter canadensis* strains have been isolated from the diarrhetic stools of Canadian patients by Fox et al. (192). These organisms were originally designated as *H. pullorum,* but subsequent biochemical and 16S rRNA analysis revealed that the isolates were a new species. *"Flexispira rappini"* is the provisional name for a fusiform gram-negative bacterium with bipolar sheathed flagella. Bacteremia associated with *"Flexispira rappini"* has been reported in a child with pneumonia (193) and in an adult undergoing hemodialysis (194), which suggests that this organism may be an invasive pathogen in immunocompromised patients. Trivett-Moore et al. (195) have recently described *Helicobacter westmeadii* sp nov, isolated from the blood cultures of two Australian AIDS patients with fever and diarrhea. Weir et al. (196) isolated an unusual *Helicobacter* species from the blood of an HIV-infected patient. Phenotypic and 16S rRNA gene sequence analysis indicated that the isolate was a *Helicobacter* species, closely related to *H. westmeadii.* Because both these organisms have been isolated from the blood of HIV-infected patients, they, along with *H. cinaedi,* form a cluster of closely related species that may represent an emerging group of pathogens in immunocompromised patients. Possibly, these organisms are more widespread than commonly reported, as they are difficult to detect, and because of their morphology, they may be misidentified as *Campylobacter* species.

CONCLUSIONS

New species of the genus *Campylobacter* and related genera are being identified on a regular basis. Many of these "atypical" campylobacters may play a greater role in causing human and animal disease than has previously been recognized. Because methods originally formulated for the isolation of *C. jejuni* often fail to support the growth of non-*jejuni/coli Campylobacter* species, these fastidious organisms are most likely underdetected in clinical specimens. Appreciation and application of the correct protocol are essential for the isolation of non-*jejuni/coli Campylobacter* species in surveillance, epidemiologic, and other studies. Reservoirs of newly described non-*jejuni/coli Campylobacter* species have been found in animals such as pigs, cattle, dogs, foxes, and rodents. However, nonmammalian species such as birds and shellfish have recently been implicated as reservoirs for these organisms. Also, surface and ground water are known to harbor non-*jejuni/coli Campylobacter* species and related organisms At present, the role that these newly described *Campylobacter* species play in the disease process is not fully understood. The sources, incidence, and range of infection associated with these organisms are almost entirely unknown, and additional research is essential for elucidation.

REFERENCES

1. Goossens H, Pot B, Vlaes L, et al. Characterization and description of *Campylobacter upsaliensis* isolated from human feces. *J Clin Microbiol* 1990;28:1039–1046.
2. Albert MJ, Tee W, Leach A, et al. Comparison of a blood-free medium and a filtration technique for the isolation of *Campylobacter* spp. from diarrhoea stools of hospitalized patients in central Australia. *J Med Microbiol* 1992;37:176–179.
3. Engberg J, On SLW, Harrington CS, et al. Prevalence of *Campylobacter, Arcobacter, Helicobacter,* and *Sutterella* spp. in human fecal samples as estimated by a reevaluation of isolation methods for campylobacters. *J Clin Microbiol* 2000;38:286–291.
4. Le Roux E, Lastovica AJ. The Cape Town protocol: how to isolate the most campylobacters for your dollar, pound, franc, yen, etc. In: Lastovica AJ, Newell DG, Lastovica EE, eds. Campylobacter, Helicobacter *and related organisms.* Cape Town: Institute of Child Health, 1998:30–33.
5. Lastovica AJ, Le Roux E. Efficient isolation of campylobacteria from stools. *J Clin Microbiol* 2000;38:2798–2799.
6. McFaydean J, Stockman S. Report of the department of committee appointed by the Board of Agriculture and Fisheries to inquire into epizootic abortions (appendix to part III: abortion in sheep). 1913:1–29(abst).
7. Smith T. The etiological relationship of spirilla (*Vibrio fetus*) to bovine abortion. *J Exp Med* 1919;30:313–322.
8. Garcia MM, Eaglesome MD, Rigby C. Campylobacters important in veterinary medicine. *Vet Bull* 1983;53:793–818.
9. Florent A. Les deux vibriosis génitales: la vibriose due à *V. foetus venerealis* et la vibriose d'origine intestinale due à *V. foetus intestinalis. Meded Veeartsenijsch Rijksuniv Gent* 1959;3:1–60.
10. Véron M, Chatelain R. Taxonomic study of the genus *Campylobacter* Sebald and Véron and designation of the neotype strain for the type species *Campylobacter fetus* (Smith and Taylor) Sebald and Véron. *Int J Syst Bacteriol* 1973;23: 122–134.
11. Harvey SM, Greenwood JR. Relationships among catalase-positive campylobacters determined by deoxyribonucleic acid–deoxyribonucleic acid hybridization. *Int J Syst Bacteriol* 1983; 33:275–284.
12. Smibert RM. Genus *Campylobacter.* In: Krieg NR, Holt HG, eds. *Bergey's manual of systematic bacteriology,* vol 1. Baltimore: Williams & Wilkins, 1993:111–118.
13. Burnens AP, Nicolet J. Three supplementary diagnostic tests for *Campylobacter* species and related organisms. *J Clin Microbiol* 1993;31:708–710.
14. Bokkenheuser V. *Vibrio fetus* infection in man. I. Ten new cases and some epidemiologic observations. *Am J Epidemiol* 1970; 91:400–409.
15. Harvey SM, Greenwood JR. Probable *Campylobacter fetus* subsp *fetus* gastroenteritis. *J Clin Microbiol* 1983;18:1278–1279.
16. Francioli P, Herzstein J, Grob J-P, et al. *Campylobacter fetus* subspecies *fetus* bacteremia. *Arch Intern Med* 1985;145:289–292.
17. Steele TW, McDermott JN. Technical note: the use of membrane

filters applied directly to the surface of agar plates for the isolation of *Campylobacter jejuni* from feces. *Pathology* 1984;16:263–265.
18. Oyarzabal OA, Wesley IV, Harmon KM, et al. Specific identification of *Campylobacter fetus* by PCR targeting variable regions of the 16S rRNA. *Vet Microbiol* 1997;58:61–71.
19. Hum S, Quinn K, Brunne J, et al. Evaluation of a PCR assay for the identification and differentiation of *Campylobacter fetus* subspecies. *Aust Vet J* 1997;75:827–831.
20. Miller VA, Jenson R, Gilroy JJ. Bacteremia in pregnant sheep following oral administration of *Vibrio fetus. Am J Vet Res* 1959; 20:677–679.
21. Lowrie DB, Pearce JH, The placental localisation of *Vibrio fetus. J Med Microbiol* 1970;3:607–614.
22. Eden AH. Perinatal mortality caused by *Vibrio fetus.* Review and analysis. *J Pediatr* 1966;68:297.
23. Simor AE, Karmali MA, Jadavji T, et al. Abortion and perinatal sepsis associated with *Campylobacter* infection. *Rev Infect Dis* 1986;8:397–402.
24. Guerrant RL, Lahita RG, Winn EC Jr, et al. Campylobacteriosis in man: pathogenic mechanisms and review of 91 bloodstream infections. *Am J Med* 1978;65:584–592.
25. Kilo C, Hagemann PO, Maryi J. Septic arthritis and bacteremia due to *Vibrio fetus. Am J Med* 1965;38:962.
26. Lawrence R, Nibbe AF, Levin S. Lung abscess secondary to *Vibrio fetus* malabsorption and syndrome and acquired agammaglobulinemia. *Chest* 1971;60:191.
27. Brown WJ, Sautter R. *Campylobacter fetus* septicemia with concurrent salpingitis. *J Clin Microbiol* 1977;6:72–75.
28. Wens R, Dratwa M, Potvliege C, et al. *Campylobacter fetus* peritonitis followed by septicaemia in a patient on continuous ambulatory peritoneal dialysis. *J Infect* 1985;10:249–251.
29. Devlin HR, McIntyre L. *Campylobacter fetus* subspecies fetus in homosexual males. *J Clin Microbiol* 1983;18:999–1000.
30. Lastovica AJ. *CampylobacterHelicobacter* bacteremia in Cape Town, South Africa, 1977–1995. In: Newell DG, Ketley JM, Feldman RA, eds. *Campylobacters, helicobacters, and related organisms.* New York: Plenum Publishing, 1996:475–479.
31. Hoist E, Schalen C, Mardh P-A. Isolation of *Campylobacter* spp. from the vagina. In: Kaijser B, Falsen, E. eds. *Campylobacter IV.* Götenborg: University of Götenborg, 1988:167–168.
32. U.S. Department of Health and Human Services, Public Health Service. *Centers for Disease Control* Campylobacter *annual tabulation 1987–1989.* Washington, DC: U.S. Department of Health and Human Services, 1990:5–10.
33. Friedman CR, Neimann J, Wegener HC, et al. Epidemiology of *Campylobacter jejuni* infections in the United States and other industrialized nations. In: Nachamkin I, Blaser MJ, eds. *Campylobacter,* second edition. Washington, DC. American Society for Microbiology Press, 2000:121–138.
34. Blaser MJ, Taylor DN, Feldman RA. Epidemiology of *Campylobacter jejuni* infections. *Epidemiol Rev* 1983;5:157–176.
35. Centers for Disease Control and Prevention. *Campylobacter* sepsis associated with "nutritional therapy" in California. *MMWR Morb Mortal Wkly Rep* 1981;30:294–295.
36. Klein BS, Vergeront JM, Blaser MJ, et al. *Campylobacter* infection associated with raw milk: an outbreak of gastroenteritis due to *Campylobacter jejuni* and thermotolerant *Campylobacter fetus* subspecies *fetus. JAMA* 1986;255:361–364.
37. Taylor PR, Weinstein WM, Bryner JH. *Campylobacter fetus* infection in human subjects: association with raw milk. *Am J Med* 1979;66:779–783.
38. Skirrow, MB, Jones DM, Sutcliff E, et al. *Campylobacter* bacteraemia in England and Wales, 1981–91. *Epidemiol Infect* 1993;110:567–573.
39. Rao GG, Karim QN, Maddocks A, et al. *Campylobacter fetus* infections in two patients with AIDS. *J Infect* 1990;20:170–172.
40. Dickgiesser N, Kasper G, Kihm W. *Campylobacter fetus* ssp. *fetus* bacteremia: a patient with liver cirrhosis. *Infection* 1983;5:288.
41. Ichiyama S, Hirai S, Minami Y, et al. *Campylobacter fetus* subspecies *fetus* cellulitis associated with bacteraemia in debilitated hosts. *Clin Infect Dis* 1998;27:252–255.
42. Montera A, Corbella X, López M, et al. *Campylobacter fetus*-associated aneurysms: report of a case involving the popliteal artery and a review of the literature. *Clin Infect Dis* 1997;24:1019–1021.
43. Bär W, Mérquez de Bär G, Nitschke H-M, et al. Endocarditis associated with *Campylobacter fetus.* In: Lastovica AJ, Newell DG, Lastovica EE, eds. Campylobacter, helicobacter, *and related organisms.* Cape Town: Institute of Child Health, 1998:162–165.
44. Morooka T, Umeda A, Fujita M, et al. Epidemiological application of pulsed-field gel electrophoresis to an outbreak of *Campylobacter fetus* meningitis in a neonatal intensive care unit. *Scand J Infect Dis* 1996;28:269–270.
45. Dronda F, Garcia-Arata I, Navas L, et al. Meningitis in adults due to *Campylobacter fetus* subspecies *fetus. Clin Infect Dis* 1998;27:906–907.
46. Gunderson CH, Sack GE. Neurology of *Vibrio fetus. Neurology (New York)* 1971;21:307.
47. Neuzil K, Wang E, Haas D, et al. Persistence of *Campylobacter fetus* bacteremia associated with absence of opsonizing antibodies. *J Clin Microbiol* 1994;32:1718–1720.
48. Yao JDC, Ng HMC, Campbell I. Prosthetic hip joint infection due to *Campylobacter fetus. J Clin Microbiol* 1993;31:3323–3324.
49. Bracikowski JP, Hess IE, Rein MF. *Campylobacter* osteomyelitis. *South Med J* 1984;77:1611–1613.
50. Yamashita K, Aoki Y, Hiroshima K. Pyogenic vertebral osteomyelitis caused by *Campylobacter fetus* subspecies *fetus.* A case report. *Spine* 1999;24:582–584.
51. Targan SR, Chow AW, Guze LB. Spontaneous peritonitis of cirrhosis due to *Campylobacter fetus. Gastroenterology* 1976;71: 311–313.
52. Takatsu M, Ichiyama T, Nada T, et al. *Campylobacter fetus* subsp *fetus* cholecystitis in a patient with advanced hepatocellular carcinoma. *Scand J Infect Dis* 1997;29:197–198.
53. Carbone KM, Heinrich MC, Quinn TC. Thrombophlebitis and cellulitis due to *Campylobacter fetus* ssp. *fetus. Medicine* 1985; 64:244–250.
54. Wens R, Dratwa M, Potvliege C, et al. *Campylobacter fetus* peritonitis followed by septicaemia in a patient on continuous ambulatory peritoneal dialysis. *J Infect* 1985;10:249–251.
55. Thomson S A, Blaser, M J. Pathogenesis of *Campylobacter fetus* infections. In: Nachamkin I, Blaser MJ, eds. *Campylobacter,* second edition. Washington, DC: American Society for Microbiology Press, 2000:321–347.
56. Carter JE, Cimolai N. Hemolytic–uremic syndrome associated with acute *Campylobacter upsaliensis* gastroenteritis. *Nephron* 1996;74:489.
57. Lastovica AJ, Goddard EA, Argent AC. Guillain-Barré syndrome in South Africa associated with *Campylobacter jejuni* O:41 strains. *J Infect Dis* 1997;176[Suppl]:S139–S143.
58. Gurgan T, Diker KS. Abortion associated with *Campylobacter upsaliensis. J Clin Microbiol* 1994;32:93–94.
59. Sandstedt K, Ursing J, Walder M. Thermotolerant *Campylobacter* with no or weak catalase activity isolated from dogs. *Curr Microbiol* 1983;8:209–213.
60. Bourke B, Chan VL, Sherman P. *Campylobacter upsaliensis*: waiting in the wings. *Clin Microbiol Rev* 1998;11:440–449.
61. Sandstedt K, Ursing J. Description of *Campylobacter upsaliensis* sp. nov. previously known as the CNW group. *Syst Appl Microbiol* 1991;14:39–48.
62. Lastovica AJ, Le Roux E, Penner JL. *"Campylobacter upsaliensis"* isolated from blood cultures of pediatric patients. *J Clin Microbiol* 1989;27:657–659.

63. Sandstedt K, Ursing J, Walder M. Thermotolerant *Campylobacter* with no or weak catalase activity isolated from dogs. *Curr Microbiol* 1983;8:209–213.
64. Davies AP, Beghart CJ, Meric SA. *Campylobacter*-associated chronic diarrhea in a dog. *J Am Vet Med* 1984;184:469–471.
65. Goossens H, Vales L, Butzler JP, et al. *Campylobacter upsaliensis* enteritis associated with canine infections. *Lancet* 1991;337: 1486–1487.
66. Hald B, Madsen M. Healthy puppies and kittens as carriers of *Campylobacter* spp. with special reference to *Campylobacter upsaliensis. J Clin Microbiol* 1997;35:3351–3352.
67. Lastovica AJ, Le Roux E, Jooste M. *"Campylobacter upsaliensis"* isolated from vervet monkeys. *Microb Ecol Health Dis* 1991;4 [Suppl]:587.
68. Patton CM, Shaffer N, Edmonds T. Human disease associated with *"Campylobacter upsaliensis"* (catalase-negative or weakly positive *Campylobacter* species) in the United States. *J Clin Microbiol* 1989;27:66–73.
69. Goosens H, Giesendorf BAJ, Vandamme P, et al. Investigation of an outbreak of *Campylobacter upsaliensis* in day care centers in Brussels: analysis of relationships among isolates by phenotypic and genotypic typing methods.*J Infect Dis* 1995;172:1298–1305.
70. Walmsley SL, Karmali MA. Direct isolation of thermophilic *Campylobacter* species from human feces on selective agar medium. *J Clin Microbiol* 1989;27:668–670.
71. Jimenez SG, Heine RG, Ward PB, et al. *Campylobacter upsaliensis* gastroenteritis in childhood. *Pediatr Infect Dis* 1999;18:988–992.
72. Taylor DN, Kiehlbauch JA, Tee W, et al. Isolation of group 2 aerotolerant *Campylobacter* species from Thai children with diarrhea. *J Infect Dis* 1991;163:1062–1067.
73. Taylor DE, Hiratsuks K, Mueller L. Isolation and characterization of catalase-negative and catalase-weak strains of *Campylobacter* species, including *"Campylobacter upsaliensis,"* from humans with gastroenteritis. *J Clin Microbiol* 1987;27:2042–2045.
74. Da Silva-Tatley FM, Lastovica AJ, Steyn LM. Plasmid profiles of *"Campylobacter upsaliensis"* isolated from blood cultures and stools of pediatric patients. *J Med Microbiol* 1992;37:8–14.
75. Owen RJ, Hernandez J. Occurrence of plasmids in *"Campylobacter upsaliensis"* (catalase-negative or weak group) from geographically diverse patients with gastroenteritis or bacteremia. *Eur J Epidemiol* 1990;6:111–117.
76. Owen RJ, Morgan DD, Costas M, et al. Identification of *"Campylobacter upsaliensis"* and other catalase-negative campylobacters from pediatric blood cultures by numerical analysis of electrophoretic protein patterns. *FEMS Microbiol Lett* 1989;58: 145–150.
77. Bourke B, Sherman PM, Woodward H, et al. Pulsed-field gel electrophoresis indicates genotype heterogeneity among *Campylobacter upsaliensis* strains. *FEMS Microbiol Lett* 1996;143:57–61.
78. Linton D, Owen RJ, Stanley, J. Rapid identification by PCR of the genus *Campylobacter* and five *Campylobacter* species enteropathogenic for man and animals. *Res Microbiol* 1996;147: 707–718.
79. Van Doorn LJ, Giesendorf BA, Bax R, et al. Molecular discrimination between *Campylobacter jejuni, Campylobacter coli, Campylobacter lari,* and *Campylobacter upsaliensis* by polymerase chain reaction based on a novel putative GTPase gene. *Mol Cell Probes* 1997;11:177–185
80. Mégraud F, Bonnet F. Unusual campylobacters in human feces. *J Infect* 1986;12:275–276.
81. Taylor DN, McDermott KT, Little JR, et al. *Campylobacter* enteritis from untreated water in the Rocky Mountains. *Ann Intern Med* 1983;99:38–40.
82. Chusid MJ, Wortmann DW, Dunne WM. *"Campylobacter upsaliensis"* sepsis in a boy with acquired hypogammaglobulinemia. *Diagn Microbiol Infect Dis* 1990;13:367–369.
83. Gaudreau C, Lamonthe F. *Campylobacter upsaliensis* isolated from a breast abscess. *J Clin Microbiol* 1992;30:1354–1356.
84. Sylvester FA, Philpott D, Lastovica A, et al. Adherence to lipids and intestinal mucin by a recently recognized human pathogen, *Campylobacter upsaliensis. Infect Immun* 1996;64: 4060–4066.
85. Pickett CL, Pecsi EC, Cottle DL, et al. Prevalence of cytolethal distending toxin production in *Campylobacter jejuni* and relatedness of *Campylobacter* spp. *cdtB* genes. *Infect Immun* 1996;64: 2070–2078.
86. Preston MA, Simor AE, Walmsley SL, et al. *In vitro* susceptibility of *"Campylobacter upsaliensis"* to twenty-four antimicrobial agents. *Eur J Clin Microbiol Infect Dis* 1990;9:822–824.
87. Gebhart CJ, Edmonds P, Ward GE, et al. *"Campylobacter hyointestinalis"* sp. nov.: a new species of *Campylobacter* found in the intestines of pigs and other animals. *J Clin Microbiol* 1985;21: 715–720.
88. On SL, Bloch B, Holmes B, et al. *Campylobacter hyointestinalis* subspecies *lawsonii* subspecies nov., isolated from the porcine stomach, and an emended description of *Campylobacter hyointestinalis. Int J Syst Bacteriol* 1995;45:767–774.
89. On SLW. Identification methods for campylobacters, helicobacters, and arcobacters. *Clin Microbiol Rev* 1996;9:405–422.
90. Edmonds P, Patton CM, Griffin PM, et al. *Campylobacter hyointestinalis* associated with human gastrointestinal disease in the United States. *J Clin Microbiol* 1987;25:685–691.
91. Vandamme P, De Ley J. Proposals for a new family, Campylobacteriaceae. *Int J Syst Bacteriol* 1991;41:451–455.
92. Costas M, Owen RJ, Jackman PH. Classification of *Campylobacter sputorum* and allied campylobacters based on numerical analysis of electrophoretic patterns. *Syst Appl Microbiol* 1987;9: 125–131
93. Vandamme P, Pot B, Falsen E, et al. Intra- and interspecific relationships of veterinary campylobacters revealed by numerical analysis of electrophoretic protein profiles and DNA–DNA hybridizations. *Syst Appl Microbiol* 1990;13: 295–303.
94. Gebhardt CJ, Murtaugh MP, Lin GF, et al. Species-specific DNA probes for *Campylobacter* species isolated from pigs with proliferative enteritis. *Vet Microbiol* 1990;24:367–379.
95. Wesley IV, Wesley RD, Cardella FE, et al. Oligodeoxynucleotide probes for *Campylobacter fetus* and *Campylobacter hyointestinalis* based on 16S rRNA sequences. *J Clin Microbiol* 1991; 29:1812–1817.
96. Russell RG, Kiehlbauch JA, Gebhart CJ, et al. Uncommon *Campylobacter* species in infant *Macca nemestrina* monkeys housed in a nursery. *J Clin Microbiol* 1992;30:3024–3027.
97. Walder M, Sandstedt K, Ursing J. Phenotypic characteristics of thermotolerant *Campylobacter* from human and animal sources. *Curr Microbiol* 1983;9:291–296.
98. Fennell CL, Rompalo AM, Totten PA, et al. Isolation of *"Campylobacter hyointestinalis"* from a human. *J Clin Microbiol* 1986;24:146–148.
99. Minet J, Grosbois B, Megraud F. *Campylobacter hyointestinalis*: an opportunistic enteropathogen? *J Clin Microbiol* 1988;26: 2659–2660.
100. Breynaert J, Vandamme P, Lauwers S. Review of 9 cases of human infection with *Campylobacter hyointestinalis.* In : Lastovica, AJ, Newell, DG, Lastovica EE, eds. Campylobacter, helicobacter, *and related organisms.* Cape Town: Institute of Child Health, 1998:428–431.
101. Skirrow MB, Benjamin J. Differentiation of enteropathogenic *Campylobacter. J Clin Pathol* 1980;33:1122.
102. Von Graevenitz A. Revised nomenclature of *Campylobacter laridis, Enterobacter intermedium,* and *"Flavobacterium branchophilia." Int J Syst Bacteriol* 1990;40:211.

103. Tauxe RV, Patton CM, Edmonds P, et al. Illness associated with *Campylobacter laridis,* a newly recognized *Campylobacter* species. *J Clin Microbiol* 1985;21:222–225.
104. Bolton FJ, Coates D, Hutchinson N, et al. A study of thermophilic *Campylobacter* in a river system. *J Appl Bacteriol* 1987; 62:167–176.
105. Brennhoud O, Kapperud G, Langeland G. Survey of thermotolerant *Campylobacter* spp. and *Yersinia* spp. in three surface water sources in Norway. *Int J Food Microbiol* 1992;15:327–338.
106. Glunder G, Peterman S. The occurrence and characterisation of *Campylobacter* spp. in silver gulls (*Laurus argentatus*), three-toed gulls (*Rissa tridactyla*), and house sparrows (*Passer domesticus*). *Zenbl Veterinaemed Reihe B* 1989;36:123–130.
107. Maruyama M, Tanaka T, Katsube H, et al. Prevalence of thermophilic campylobacters in crows (*Corvus lavaillantii, Corvus corone*) and the serogroups of the isolates. *Jpn J Vet Sci* 1990; 52:1237–1244.
108. Van Doorn LJ, Verschuuren-VanHaperen A, Van Belkum A, et al. Rapid identification of diverse *Campylobacter lari* strains isolated from mussels and oysters using a reverse hybridization line probe assay. *J Appl Microbiol* 1998;84:545–550.
109. Park CE, Sanders GW. Occurrence of thermotolerant campylobacters in fresh vegetables sold at farmer's outdoor markets and supermarkets. *Can J Microbiol* 1992;38:313–316.
110. Lindblom GB, Johny M, Khalil K, et al. Enterotoxigenicity and frequency of *Campylobacter jejuni, C. coli,* and *C. laridis* in human and animal isolates from different countries. *FEMS Microbiol Lett* 1990;54:163–167.
111. Tresierra-Ayala A, Bendayan ME, Bermuy A, et al. Chicken as potential contamination source of *Campylobacter lari* in Iquitos, Peru. *Rev Inst Med Trop Sao Paulo* 1994;36:497–499.
112. Kakkar M, Dogra SC. Prevalence of *Campylobacter* infections in animals and children in Haryana, India. *J Diarrhoeal Dis Res* 1990;8:34–36.
113. Mégraud F, Chevrier D, Desplaces N, et al. Urease-positive thermophilic *Campylobacter* (*Campylobacter laridis* variant) isolated from an appendix and from human feces. *J Clin Microbiol* 1988;26:1050–1051.
114. Popovic-Uroic T, Patton CM, Nicholson MA, et al. Evaluation of indoxylacetate hydrolysis test for rapid differentiation of *Campylobacter, Helicobacter,* and *Wolinella* species. *J Clin Microbiol* 1990;28:2335–2339.
115. Benjamin J, Leaper S, Owen RJ, et al. Description of *Campylobacter laridis,* a new species comprising the nalidixic acid-resistant thermophilic *Campylobacter* (NARTC) group. *Curr Microbiol* 1983;8:231–238.
116. Skirrow MB, Benjamin J. "1001" campylobacters from man and animals. *J Hyg (Lond)* 1980;85:427–442.
117. Nachamkin I, Stowell C, Skalina A, et al. *Campylobacter laridis* causing bacteremia in an immunocompromised patient. *Ann Intern Med* 1984;101:55–57.
118. Evans TG, Riley D. *Campylobacter laridis* colitis in a human immunodeficiency virus-positive patient treated with a quinolone. *Clin Infect Dis* 1992;15:172–173.
119. Vargas J, Corzo JE, Perez MJ, et al. Bacteremia por *Campylobacter* e infection por HIV. *Enfern Infecc Microbiol Clin* 1992;10:155–157.
120. Simor AE, Wilcox L. Enteritis associated with *Campylobacter laridis. J Clin Microbiol* 1987 25:10–12
121. Bézian MC, Ribou G, Barberis-Giletti C, et al. Isolation of a urease-positive thermophilic variant of *Campylobacter lari* from a patient with urinary tract infection. *Eur J Clin Microbiol Infect Dis* 1990;9:895–897
122. Morris CN, Scully B, Garvey GJ. *Campylobacter lari* associated with permanent pacemaker infection and bacteremia. *Clin Infect Dis* 1998;27:220–221.
123. Bruneau B, Burc L, Bizet C, et al. Purulent pleurisy caused by *Campylobacter lari. Eur J Clin Microbiol Infect Dis* 1998;17: 185–88.
124. Borczyk A, Thompson S, Smith D, et al. Water-bourne outbreak of *Campylobacter laridis*-associated gastroenteritis. *Lancet* 1987;1:164–165.
125. Johnson WM, Lior H. Cytotoxic and cytotonic factors produced by *Campylobacter jejuni, Campylobacter coli,* and *Campylobacter laridis. J Clin Microbiol* 1986;24:275–281.
126. Vandamme P, Falsen E, Rossau B, et al. Revision of *Campylobacter, Helicobacter,* and *Wolinella* taxonomy: emendation of generic descriptions and proposal of *Arcobacter* gen. nov. *Int J Syst Bacteriol* 1991;41:88–103.
127. On SLW, Owen RJ, Lastovica AJ, et al. Taxonomic study of *Helicobacter* (*Campylobacter*) *fennelliae* from clinical material by numerical analysis of one-dimensional electrophoretic protein patterns. *Microb Ecol Health Dis* 1991;4[Suppl]:S103.
128. Flores BM, Fennell CL, Stamm WE. Characterization of *Campylobacter cinaedi* and *Campylobacter fennelliae* antigens and analysis of human immune response. *J Infect Dis* 1989; 159:635–640.
129. Fennell CL, Totten PA, Quinn TC, et al. Characterization of *Campylobacter*-like organisms isolated from homosexual men. *J Infect Dis* 1984;149:58–66.
130. Kiehlbauch JA, Brenner DJ, Cameron AG, et al. Genomic and phenotypic characterization of *Helicobacter cinaedi* and *Heliocobacter fennelliae* strains isolated from humans and animals. *J Clin Microbiol* 1995;33:2940–2947.
131. Quinn TC, Goodell SE, Fennell CL, et al. Infections with *Campylobacter jejuni* and *Campylobacter*-like organisms in homosexual men. *Ann Intern Med* 1984;101:187–192.
132. Laughton BE, Druckman DA, Vernon A, et al. Prevalence of enteric pathogens in homosexual men with and without acquired immunodeficiency syndrome. *Gastroenterology* 1988; 94:984–993.
133. Flores BM, Fennell CL, Holmes KK, et al. *In vitro* susceptibility of *Campylobacter*-like organisms to twenty antimicrobial agents. *Antimicrob Agents Chemother* 1985;28:188–191.
134. Totten PA, Fennell CL, Tenover FC, et al. *Campylobacter cinaedi* (sp. nov.) and *Campylobacter fennelliae* (sp. nov.): two new *Campylobacter* species associated with enteric disease in homosexual men. *J Infect Dis* 1985;151:131–139.
135. Grayson ML, Tee W, Dwyer B. Gastroenteritis associated with *Campylobacter cinaedi. Med J Aust* 1989;150:214.
136. Burman WJ, Cohn DL, Reeves R, et al. Multifocal cellulitis and monoarticular arthritis as manifestations of *Helicobacter cinaedi* bacteremia. *Clin Infect Dis* 1995;20:564–570.
137. Kemper CA, Mickelson P, Morton B, et al. *Helicobacter* (*Campylobacter*) *fennelliae*-like organisms as an important but occult phase of bacteraemia in a patient with AIDS. *J Infect* 1993;26:97–101.
138. Ng VL, Hadley WK, Fennell CL, et al. Successive bacteremias with *"Campylobacter cinaedi"* and *"Campylobacter fennelliae"* in a bisexual male. *J Clin Microbiol* 1987;25:2008–2009.
139. Hsueh P-R, Teng L-J, Hung C-C, et al. Septic shock due to *Helicobacter fennelliae* in a non–human immunodeficiency virus-infected heterosexual patient. *J Clin Microbiol* 1999; 37:2084–2086.
140. Lasry S, Simon J, Marais A, et al. *Helicobacter cinaedi* septic arthritis and bacteremia in an immunocompetent patient. *Clin Infect Dis* 2000;31:201–202.
141. Burnens AP, Stanley J, Schaad VB, et al. Novel *Campylobacter*-like organism resembling *Helicobacter fennelliae* isolated from a boy with gastroenteritis and from dogs. *J Clin Microbiol* 1993; 31:1916–1917.
142. Orlicek SL, Welch DF, Kuhls TL. Septicemia and meningitis

caused by *Helicobacter cinaedi* in a neonate. *J Clin Microbiol* 1993;31:569–571.

143. Gebhardt CJ, Fennell CL, Murtaugh MP, et al. *Campylobacter cinaedi* is the normal intestinal flora in hamsters. *J Clin Microbiol* 1989;27:1692–1694.
144. Burnens AP, Angeloy-Wick B, Nicolet J. Comparison of *Campylobacter* carriage rates in diarrheic and healthy pet animals. *J Vet Med Ser B* 1992; 39:175–180.
145. Flores BM, Fennell CL, Stamm WE, et al. Characterization of *Campylobacter cinaedi* and *Campylobacter fennelliae* antigens and analysis of human immune response. *J Infect Dis* 1989;159: 635–640.
146. Lastovica AJ, Le Roux E. Prevalence and distribution of *Campylobacter* spp. in the diarrhoetic stools and blood cultures of paediatric patients. *Acta Gastroenterol Blg* 1993;56[Suppl]:34.
147. Kiehlbauch JA, Brenner DJ, Nicholson MA, et al. *Campylobacter butzleri* sp. nov. isolated from humans and animals with diarrheal illness. *J Clin Microbiol* 1991;29:376–385.
148. On SLW, Stacey A, Smyth J. Isolation of *Arcobacter butzleri* from a neonate with bacteremia *Clin Microbiol Rev* 1996;31: 225–227.
149. Yan JJ, Ko WC, Huang AH, et al. *Arcobacter butzleri* bacteremia in a patient with liver cirrhosis. *J Formos Med Assoc* 2000;99: 166–169.
150. Taylor DN, Kiehlbauch JA, Tee W, et al. Isolation of group 2 aerotolerant *Campylobacter* species from Thai children with diarrhea. *J Infect Dis* 1991;163:1062–1067.
151. Vandamme P, Pugina P, Benzi G, et al. Outbreak of recurrent abdominal cramps associated with *Arcobacter butzleri* in an Italian school. *J Clin Microbiol* 1992;30:2335–2337.
152. Dediste A, Aeby A, Ebraert A. et al.*Arcobacter* in stools: clinical features, diagnosis and antibiotic susceptibility. In: Lastovica AJ, Newell DG, Lastovica EE, eds. Campylobacter, Helicobacter, *and related organisms.* Cape Town: Institute for Child Health, 1998:436–439.
153. Hsueh P-R, Teng L-J, Yang P-C, et al. Bacteremia caused by *Arcobacter cryaerophilus* 1B. *J Clin Microbiol* 1997;35:489–491.
154. Jacob JD, Woodward D, Feuerpfeil I, et al. Isolation of *Arcobacter butzleri* in raw water and drinking water treatment plants in Germany. *Zentbl Hyg Umweltmed* 1998;201:189–198.
155. Rice EW, Rodgers MR, Wesley IV. Isolation of *Arcobacter butzleri* from ground water. *Lett Appl Microbiol* 1999;28:31–35
156. Anderson FK, Kielhbauch JA, Anderson DC, et al. *Arcobacter (Campylobacter) butzleri* associated with diarrheal illness in a non-human primate. *Infect Immun* 1993;61:2220–2223.
157. Boudreau M, Higgins R, Mittal KR. Biochemical and serological characterization of *Campylobacter cryaerophila. J Clin Microbiol* 1991;29:54–58
158. Tee W, Baird R, Dyall-Smith M, et al. *Campylobacter cryaerophila* isolated from a human. *J Clin Microbiol* 1988;26: 2469–2473.
159. Stampi S, Varoli O, Zanetti F, et al. *Arcobacter cryaerophilus* and thermophilic campylobacters in a sewerage treatment plant in Italy: two secondary treatments compared. *Epidemiol Infect* 1993;110:633–639.
160. Atabay HI, Corry JE, On SL. Diversity and prevalence of *Arcobacter* spp. in broiler chickens. *J Appl Microbiol* 1998;84: 1007–1016.
161. Lammerding AM, Harris JE, Lior H, et al. Isolation method for the recovery of *Arcobacter butzleri* from fresh poultry and poultry products. In: Newell DG, Ketley JM, Feldman RA, eds. *Campylobacters, helicobacters, and related organisms.* New York: Plenum Publishing, 1996:329–233.
162. Zanetti F, Varoli O, Stampi S, et al. Prevalence of thermophilic *Campylobacter* and *Arcobacter butzleri* in food of animal origin. *Int J Food Microbiol* 1996;33:315–321.
163. Wesley IV, Baetz AL, Larson DJ. Infection of cesarean-derived colostrum-deprived 1-day-old piglets with *Arcobacter butzleri, Arcobacter cryaerophilus,* and *Arcobacter skirrowii. Infect Immun* 1996;64:2295–2299.
164. Harmon KM, Wesley IV. Multiplex PCR for the identification of *Arcobacter* and differentiation of *Arcobacter butzleri* from other arcobacters. *Vet Microbiol* 1997;58:215–218.
165. Hurtado A, Owen RJ. A molecular scheme based on 23S rRNA gene polymorphisms for rapid identification of *Campylobacter* and *Arcobacter* species. *J Clin Microbiol* 1997;35:2401–2404.
166. Kiehlbauch JA, Plikaytis BD, Swaminathan B, et al. Restriction fragment length polymorphisms in the ribosomal genes for specific identification and subtyping of aerotolerant *Campylobacter* species. *J Clin Microbiol* 1991;29:1670–1676.
167. Steele TW, Sangster N, Lanser JA. DNA relatedness and biochemical features of *Campylobacter* spp. isolated in central and south Australia. *J Clin Microbiol* 1985;22:71–74.
168. Steele TW, Owen RJ. *Campylobacter jejuni* subsp *doylei* (subspecies nov.) is a subspecies of gram-negative campylobacters isolated from clinical specimens. *Int J Syst Bacteriol* 1988;38: 316–318.
169. Kaspar G, Dickgiesser N. Isolation from the gastric epithelium of *Campylobacter*-like bacteria that are distinct from *Campylobacter pylori. Lancet* 1985;1:111–112.
170. Owen RJ, Beck A, Borman P. Restriction endonuclease digest patterns of chromosomal DNA from nitrate-negative *Campylobacter jejuni*-like organisms. *Eur J Epidemiol* 1985;1:281–287.
171. Steele TW, Lanser JA, Sangster N. Nitrate-negative *Campylobacter*-like organisms. *Lancet* 1988;1:294.
172. Férnandez H, Fagundes U, Ogatha S, et al. Acute diarrhoea associated with *Campylobacter jejuni* subsp *doylei* in Sao Paulo, Brazil. *Infect Dis J* 1997;16:1098–1099.
173. Morey F. Five years of *Campylobacter* bacteremias in Central Australia. In: Newell DG, Ketley JM, Feldman RA, eds. *Campylobacters, helicobacters, and related organisms.* New York: Plenum Publishing, 1996:491–494.
174. Tanner ACR, Badger S, Lai CH, et al. *Wolinella* gen. nov., *Wolinella succinogenes* (*Vibrio succinogenes* Wolin et al.) comb. nov., and description of *Bacteroides gracilis* sp. nov. , *Wolinella recta* sp. nov., *Campylobacter concisus* sp. nov., and *Eikenella corrodens* from humans with periodontal disease. *Int J Syst Bacteriol* 1981;31:432–435.
175. Tanner ACR, Listgarten, MA. Ebersole JL. *Wolinella curva* sp. nov.: *"Vibrio succinogenes"* of human origin. *Int J Syst Bacteriol* 1984;34:275–282.
176. Tanner ACR, Dzink JL, Ebersole JL, et al. *Wolinella recta, Campylobacter concisus, Bacteroides gracilis,* and *Eikenella corrodens* from periodontal lesions. *J Periodontal Res* 1987;22:327–330.
177. Lastovica AJ, Le Roux E, Warren R, et al. Clinical isolates of *Campylobacter mucosalis. J Clin Microbiol* 1993;31:2835–2836.
178. Lauwers S, Devreker R, Van Etterijck, et al. Isolation of *Campylobacter concisus* from human faeces. *Microb Ecol Health Dis* 1991;4[Suppl]:S91.
179. Figura N, Gugliemetti P, Zanchi N, et al. Two cases of *Campylobacter mucosalis* enteritis in children. *J Clin Microbiol* 1993; 31:727–728.
180. Rams TE, Feik D, Slots J. *Campylobacter rectus* in human periodontitis. *Oral Microbiol Immunol* 1993;8:230–235.
181. Van Dyke TE, Dowell VR, Offenbacher S, et al. Potential role of microorganisms isolated from periodontal lesions in the pathogenesis of inflammatory bowel disease. *Infect Immun* 1986;53:671–677.
182. Johnson CC, Finegold SM. Uncommonly encountered motile, anaerobic gram-negative bacilli associated with infection. *Rev Infect Dis* 1987;9:1150–1162.
183. Vandamme P, Falsen E, Pot B, et al. Identification of EF group

22 campylobacters from gastroenteritis cases as *Campylobacter concisus. J Clin Microbiol* 1989;27:1775–1781.

184. Van Etterijck R, Breynaert J, Revets H, et al. Isolation of *Campylobacter concisus* from feces of children with and without diarrhea. *J Clin Microbiol* 1996;34:2304–2306.
185. Zhi N, Revets H, Van Zeebroek A, et al. Serological response to *Campylobacter concisus* infection. In: Newell DG, Ketley JM, Feldman RA, eds. *Campylobacters, helicobacters, and related organisms.* New York: Plenum Publishing, 1996:673–678.
186. Istivan T S, Ward, P B, Lee A, et al. Haemolysins of *Campylobacter concisus.* In: Lastovica AJ, Newell DG, Lastovica EE, eds. Campylobacter, Helicobacter, *and related organisms.* Cape Town: Institute of Child Health, 1998:440–444.
187. Greig A, Hanslo D, Le Roux E, et al. *In vitro* activity of eight antimicrobial agents against pediatric isolates of *C. concisus* and *C. mucosalis. Acta Gastroenterol Belg* 1993;56[Suppl]:12.
188. Etoh Y, Dewhirst FE, Paster A, et al. *Campylobacter showae* sp. nov. isolated from the human oral cavity. *Int J Syst Bacteriol* 1993;43:631–639.
189. Borczyk A, Lior H, McKeown A, et al. Isolation of *Campylobacter sputorum* associated with human infection. In: Kaijser B, Falsen E, eds. *Campylobacter IV.* Göteborg: University of Göteborg, 1987:166–167.
190. On SL, Ridgewell F, Cryan B, et al. Isolation of *Campylobacter sputorum* biovar *sputorum* from an axillary abscess. *J Infect* 1992; 24:175–179.
191. Stanley J, Linton D, Burnens AP, et al. *Helicobacter pullorum* sp. nov.—genotype and phenotype of a new species isolated from poultry and human patients with gastroenteritis. *Microbiology* 1994;140:3441–3449.
192. Fox J, Chien CC, Dewhirst FE, et al. *Helicobacter canadensis* sp. nov. isolated from humans with diarrhea as an example of an emerging pathogen. *J Clin Microbiol* 2000;38:2546–2549.
193. Tee W, Leder K, Karroum E, et al. *"Flexispira rappini"* bacteremia in a child with pneumonia. *J Clin Microbiol* 1998;36: 1679–1682.
194. Sorlin P, Vandamme P, Nortier J, et al. Recurrent *"Flexispira rappini"* bacteremia in an adult patient undergoing hemodialysis: case report. *J Clin Microbiol* 1999;37:1319–1323.
195. Trivett-Moore NL, Rawlinson WD, Yuen M. *Helicobacter westmeadii* sp. nov., a new species isolated from blood cultures in two AIDS patients. *J Clin Microbiol* 1997;35:1144–1150.
196. Weir SC, Gibert CL, Gordin FM, et al. An uncommon *Helicobacter* isolate from blood: evidence of a group of *Helicobacter* spp. pathogenic in AIDS patients. *J Clin Microbiol* 1999;37: 2729–2733.

48

CLOSTRIDIUM DIFFICILE

DALE N. GERDING
STUART JOHNSON

HISTORICAL BACKGROUND

Historically, the road to linking the causative organism *Clostridium difficile* to pseudomembranous colitis (PMC) and to antimicrobial use has been a long and tortuous one. PMC was observed first in 1893 by surgeon J. M. T. Finney of Johns Hopkins University, who described "diphtheritic colitis" in a 22-year-old patient in whom diarrhea developed 10 days after surgery to remove a gastric pyloric tumor and who died 5 days later (1). Photographs of the histologic sections from the case, published by John Bartlett, show an intense cellular infiltration and inflammatory response, but not the pseudomembranes described grossly (2). PMC was reported infrequently in the preantibiotic era, most often following gastrointestinal surgery, and, early in the postantibiotic era (1954), an increased incidence of PMC was not appreciated (3).

With the advent of more widespread antibiotic use in the 1950s and 1960s, an entity termed *pseudomembranous enterocolitis* was increasingly observed and attributed to *Staphylococcus aureus.* Although the pathology and bacteriology of this disease are not well described, oral vancomycin was highly effective in treating this disease, whether caused by *S. aureus* or by *C. difficile* (4,5). Bartlett (2) has expressed skepticism that *S. aureus* caused many cases of PMC, largely because of the rather common observation of *S. aureus* in stool cultures in the presence or absence of enterocolitis. Nonetheless, the presence of pseudomembranes in both the large and small bowel with pseudomembranous enterocolitis is clearly different from the strictly colonic involvement of PMC attributed to *C. difficile* today, and remains an unexplained difference between the two diagnoses.

D. N. Gerding: Department of Medicine, Northwestern University; Medical Service, VA Medical Center–Lakeside Division, Chicago, Illinois

S. Johnson: Infectious Disease Section, VA Chicago–Lakeside Division, Northwestern University Medical School, Chicago, Illinois

C. difficile, first described by Hall and O'Toole in 1935 (6), was originally named *Bacillus difficilis* because of the difficulty in isolating the organism from the intestinal flora of infants. The same investigators also described the toxigenic properties of the organism (6). Subsequently, the organism was isolated from stools of normal infants, and the toxin was shown to be lethal if injected into cats, dogs, rats, guinea pigs, rabbits, or pigeons (7). Antitoxin prepared in rabbits and dogs prevented death in challenged guinea pigs, and nontoxigenic strains of *C. difficile* were discovered (7). In 1974, Hafiz, published his Ph.D. thesis on *C. difficile* and showed the organism to be widespread in soil as well as the stools of infants, cows, donkeys, and horses (2). He showed that *C. difficile* produced a lethal toxin, and he developed a neutralizing toxin antibody. However, the connection between *C. difficile* and human PMC or fatal disease in animals was not made at this time.

Further confounding the reports of human pseudomembranous enteritis were reports of acute toxicity and death following use of penicillin in the guinea pig in 1943 (8). Other antibiotics were also found to be fatal in guinea pigs and hamsters. The autopsy findings in animals showed a dilated cecum with liquid stool and pathologic lesions of the colon similar to PMC in humans. In the 1950s, the chinchilla fur industry was threatened by a fatal diarrheal illiness associated with contamination of the commercial chinchilla feed with oxytetracycline. The disease, mistakenly attributed to *S. aureus* based on Gram stains, was prevented by removal of oxytetracycline from the feed or by adding neomycin plus bacitracin to the drinking water of the animals (9).

In 1974, the focus on PMC in human disease was reinitiated by the report by Tedesco and co-workers (10) of a PMC incidence of 10% in patients who were given clindamycin. Following this report in which endoscopy was used to visualize the colonic pseudomembranes, the disease was referred to for many years as clindamycin-associated colitis. *S. aureus* could not be isolated from any colonic specimens from these patients, suggesting that the disease was not caused by *S. aureus* (10).

In 1968, Small (11) described fatal enterocolitis in Syrian hamsters following administration of lincomycin. This observation was extended to clindamycin as well, and in 1977, two investigator groups reported that oral vancomycin prolonged survival and prevented death as long as it was administered (12,13). At the same time, using tissue culture assay methods, the cytotoxic activity of filtered stool specimens from patients with antibiotic-associated PMC was also documented and shown to be neutralized first by polyvalent gas gangrene antitoxin, and later by *Clostridium sordellii* antitoxin (14–20). Bartlett and associates (21) and George and co-workers (22) showed that *C. difficile* could be isolated from stool specimens of patients with PMC. These human isolates produced a similar disease in antibiotic-treated hamsters, implicating *C. difficile* as the cause of the disease in both hamsters and humans. It has come to be known that the neutralization of the cytotoxic activity by *C. sordellii* antitoxin is a result of cross reactivity of these antibodies to similar *C. difficile* toxins.

C. difficile was initially believed to produce only a single toxin that caused the cytotoxic effect, but two toxins, designated A and B, were subsequently identified (23) (see "Microbiology"). Variant toxin-producing strains, however, that do not produce detectable toxin A, but produce a genetically altered toxin B, have been shown to cause disease in both hamsters and humans (24,25). Research in the 1980s and 1990s focused on the epidemiology of *C. difficile*-associated disease (CDAD) in hospital patients, studies that have been greatly aided by the development of molecular typing methods to distinguish specific strains (26–30). In addition, the basic cellular function of toxins A and B and their genetic sequence have been elucidated during this time (31–33).

MICROBIOLOGY

C. difficile is a large, anaerobic, gram-positive spore-forming rod. *C. difficile* has not been easy to grow because it requires good anaerobic technique and quality control of the selective growth media. The ease of transmission is explained by the ability of *C. difficile* to form spores and the low inoculum required for infection in susceptible hosts. Spores may persist on environmental surfaces for months or longer. In an animal model of *C. difficile* disease, fatal cecitis developed in hamsters rendered susceptible by treatment with clindamycin after the administration of only 10 spores (25).

C. difficile characteristically forms subterminal spores, and, unlike other clostridia, sporulation is not associated with toxin production. Toxin production is highest during the stationary growth phase. Sodium cholate and sodium taurocholate stimulate germination of spores and have been used to increase the sensitivity of culture, particularly when sampling environmental surfaces and when conducting patient surveillance with rectal swabs (34,35). Sodium thioglycolate and lysozyme treatment and alcohol-shock or heat-shock procedures can also be used to inhibit vegetative organisms or enhance sporulation and spore recovery (36,37).

Culture in the laboratory and vegetative growth of *C. difficile* requires anaerobic conditions. Although *C. difficile* is slightly more aerotolerant than strict anaerobes, such as *Clostridium tetani*, culture of *C. difficile* requires vigilance in maintaining the anaerobic environment whether using an anaerobic chamber or a jar/bag system with gas-generating kits. Colonies of *C. difficile* on selective CCFA (cycloserine-cefoxitin-fructose agar) media are flat, yellow, ground-glass appearing with a surrounding yellow halo. The colonies may also exhibit yellow fluorescence under long-wavelength ultraviolet light and exhibit a characteristic "horse-dung" odor. Presumptive identification of *C. difficile* can be made by observing the characteristic colony formation on CCFA and by Gram staining of the colonies. Spore formation is not typically seen on CCFA unless the medium is supplemented with sodium taurocholate. Further confirmation can be obtained by gas chromatography (GC) or by commercial identification kits such as the RapID ANA (Innovative Diagnostic Systems, Inc., Atlanta, GA) (38). Two relatively unusual metabolic products of *C. difficile* are isocaproic acid and *p*-cresol, which have been used for presumptive identification (39,40).

Virulence Factors

Disease due to *C. difficile* is primarily toxin-mediated and *C. difficile* produces two large, single-unit toxins: toxin A, an enterotoxin, and toxin B, a cytotoxin, which share significant homology (31). Toxin A has been implicated as the primary virulence determinant because of its potent enterotoxic activity and ability to produce disease in animal models (41). The enterotoxic effect of toxin A in the rabbit ileal loop assay, production of a viscous hemorrhagic fluid, is distinct from the pure secretory fluid response seen with cholera toxin in this assay, consistent with the toxins acting by different mechanisms. Although not active in the rabbit ileal loop assay, toxin B *in vitro* is 1,000-fold more active than toxin A on most eukaryotic cell lines and likely acts in concert with toxin A *in vivo*. For example, toxin B is lethal when it is administered to hamsters intragastrically with low, sublethal doses of toxin A or when it is given alone following manipulation or bruising of the intestinal tract (41). The effect of toxin B may be different on human colonic mucosa than on the intestinal mucosa of laboratory animals (42). In addition to toxigenic strains of *C. difficile*, nontoxigenic strains are frequently recovered from clinical and environmental specimens. These strains lack the genes for toxin A and B (43), and there is no evidence that they cause human disease.

Toxin A and toxin B are members of a family of large clostridial toxins that act by glycosylation of small GTP-binding proteins of the Rho subfamily, which are involved in the organization of the cell cytoskeleton (44). Despite a high degree of similarity by functional domain and amino acid sequence, the effects of these toxins are quite different, as noted earlier. The genes for the toxins (*tcdA* and *tcdB*) are located together on the chromosome along with three open reading frames (*tcdD, E, C*) in a specific genetic unit sometimes referred to as a pathogenicity island or locus (PaLoc) (45) (Fig. 48.1). These genes are coordinately regulated, and *tcdD* and *tcdC* are involved with transcription of the other *tcd* genes (33,46). In nontoxigenic strains of *C. difficile,* the entire PaLoc is replaced by a 115-bp sequence (47). The gene for each toxin has a series of repetitive sequences on the 3′ end that code for the ligand or receptor binding portion of the toxin and a region on the 5′ end that codes for the toxic domain by virtue of its glucosyltransferase activity (32); there is a putative translocation domain in the middle. The receptor binding region of toxin A is recognized by the monoclonal antibody PCG-4 that is used in most commercial enzyme immunoassays (EIAs) for toxin A detection (48). The difference in physiologic activity of toxin A and B may be due to differences in enzymatic activity, substrate targets, or differences in receptor binding and cell tropism (49).

C. difficile strains that differ from the standard toxin profile have been recovered from clinical specimens and partially characterized. One of the first toxin variant strains recognized (designated 8864) failed to produce toxin A as detected by immunoassay or column purification (50); the toxin A gene in this strain is severely truncated at the 3′ end (51,52) (Fig. 48.1). This unique variant strain, which has only been recovered from one clinical specimen, is pathogenic in hamsters (albeit less virulent than fully toxigenic strains), despite the apparent lack of toxin A production (53). Toxin B produced by strain 8864 has been suggested to cause disease by virtue of enhanced cytotoxicity and weak enterotoxicity.

Another *C. difficile* toxin variant strain is the reference strain for serogroup F, strain 1470 (54). The toxin A gene of strain 1470 also has a truncated 3′ end, but the truncation is not as great as that of strain 8864 (55) (Fig. 48.1). In contrast to strain 8864, strains similar to 1470 have been recovered from clinical specimens around the world. These variants correspond to toxinotype VIII (56) and REA group CF (57), in which a 1.8-Kb deletion in the toxin A gene and altered restriction sites in the toxin B gene are present. In addition, a point mutation at the 5′ end of *tcdA* in strain 1470 and other toxinotype VIII strains introduces a prema-

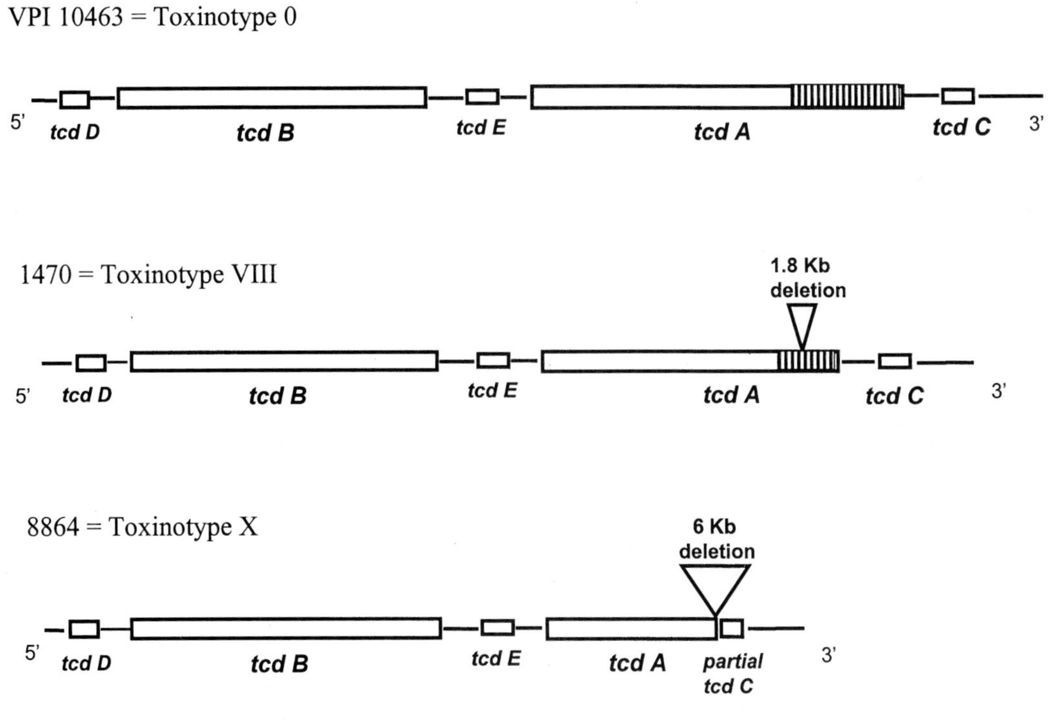

FIGURE 48.1. Schematic representation of the genes encoding the large toxins of *Clostridium difficile* located in the genetic unit referred to as the *pathogenesis locus* (PaLoc). The PaLoc for the standard toxigenic strain (prototype isolate, VPI 10463) is shown on top with PaLoc variations for the two best studied toxin variant strains shown below: strain 1470 (*middle*) and strain 8864 (*bottom*), representing toxinotypes VIII and X, respectively, as described by Rupnik and colleagues (56). The hatched bars designate the repetitive sequence region of the toxin A gene, which codes for the ligand or receptor binding portion of toxin A. See text for description of the open reading frames (tcdA through E).

ture stop codon and no functional toxin A is produced (57,58).

Until recently, most reports suggested toxinotype VIII strains were nonpathogenic, because they were recovered primarily from asymptomatic children in Belgium and Japan (54,59,60). More recent reports have documented recovery of toxinotype VIII strains from patients with CDAD (57) and fatal PMC (61). A nosocomial outbreak of CDAD caused by a toxinotype VIII variant *C. difficile* strain was also reported from a hospital in Winnipeg, Canada (24). It has become clear that these strains are capable of causing the full spectrum of CDAD syndromes. However, because the strains do not produce toxin A, they are not detected by EIA tests for toxin A. Toxin A EIA tests are the sole method of *C. difficile* detection used by nearly one-half of all clinical laboratories (61). The incidence of toxinotype VIII strains in any particular clinical setting is unknown at this time, but clinicians should be aware of the wide geographic distribution of these strains. Thus, no single laboratory test should be used to exclude the diagnosis of CDAD. REA Type CF2, a toxinotype VIII variant, is also pathogenic in hamsters (again, with decreased virulence compared with other, fully toxigenic strains) despite the lack of toxin A production (25), suggesting a role for other virulence factors in *C. difficile*.

In addition to the large clostridial toxins, some strains of *C. difficile* produce an ADP-ribosyltransferase (binary toxin), which also induces alterations in the actin cytoskeleton. This toxin has recently been shown to be present in approximately 6% of toxinogenic isolates (62). The presence of genes for binary toxin correlates with toxinotype strains that contain variations in the genes for toxins A and B but not with strain 1470 or other toxinotype VIII strains (62). The role of binary toxin in the pathogenesis of CDAD has not yet been determined. Some strains of *C. difficile* produce capsules and fimbriae-like structures, but their presence has no obvious association with virulence. *C. difficile* has also been shown to express S-layer glycoproteins on its outer surface similar to many other diverse bacteria (63). The S-layer in *C. difficile* is composed of two distinct layers and is highly immunogenic. Although no role has yet been assigned to the S-layer in *C. difficile*, this structure forms the major interface between the organism and the host and could potentially interfere with host defense mechanisms as has been shown in other bacteria (64).

Antibiotic Susceptibility

Antimicrobial susceptibility has potential relevance to both the precipitating agent and treatment of CDAD. The relationship between susceptibility of the *C. difficile* strain to the precipitating antimicrobial agent is not always obvious. Although *C. difficile* isolates are highly resistant to some agents commonly implicated in precipitating CDAD (e.g., cephalosporins), other antimicrobials (e.g., penicillins such as ampicillin) show marked activity against *C. difficile in vitro* (65). For other antimicrobial agents, *C. difficile* shows heterogeneity in susceptibility (e.g., clindamycin, erythromycin, tetracycline, and chloramphenicol). Therefore, factors other than antimicrobial susceptibility *in vitro* are important in determining the risk for *C. difficile* diarrhea. Recently, clindamycin use was shown to be a risk for infection with a highly clindamycin-resistant *C. difficile* strain with broad geographic distribution (66). The presence or absence of these strains in the hospital environment may partially explain differences in rates of CDAD following clindamycin use.

C. difficile isolates are typically susceptible to low concentrations of metronidazole and vancomycin, the two therapeutic agents most commonly used to treat CDAD. Almost all isolates are susceptible to metronidazole concentrations of 1 μg /mL or less with a typical MIC_{50} of 0.3 μg/mL (65,67). *C. difficile* isolates are somewhat less susceptible to vancomycin (compared with metronidazole), with a typical MIC_{50} of 1 μg/mL and occasional isolates are found with MICs of 8 or 16 μg/mL (65,68). However, fecal vancomycin concentrations are typically in the 100 to 1,000 μg/g range with oral therapy (69), and there is no evidence that isolates with the higher MIC values exhibit clinical resistance. Other potential therapeutic agents with high activity against *C. difficile* include rifampin and teicoplanin, whereas bacitracin and fusidic acid have slightly higher MIC values.

C. difficile isolates with elevated MIC values have been recovered from veterinary sources (70), or the isolates are mostly nontoxigenic strains (71) and their clinical relevance is not clear. One recent report, however, has documented recovery of an isolate with an MIC of greater than 64 μg/mL from a patient with CDAD (72) and surveillance for metronidazole resistance in *C. difficile* in other populations should be performed.

PATHOGENESIS

Antimicrobial therapy and hospitalization are well-established risk factors for CDAD. Nearly all affected patients have recently been treated with antimicrobials or, occasionally, cancer chemotherapeutic agents. The role of antimicrobial therapy in the pathogenesis of CDAD is in the disruption of the indigenous intestinal flora, which normally provides defense against infection with *C. difficile*. Hospitalization provides an opportunity for exposure to *C. difficile* spores, which may contaminate environmental surfaces throughout health care facilities as well as the hands of health care workers. In this regard, the risk of *C. difficile* acquisition increases in direct proportion to the length of hospital stay (Fig. 48.2) (73). Culture surveillance of hospitalized patients indicates that many patients infected with *C. difficile* are not symptomatic. Such patients may be at

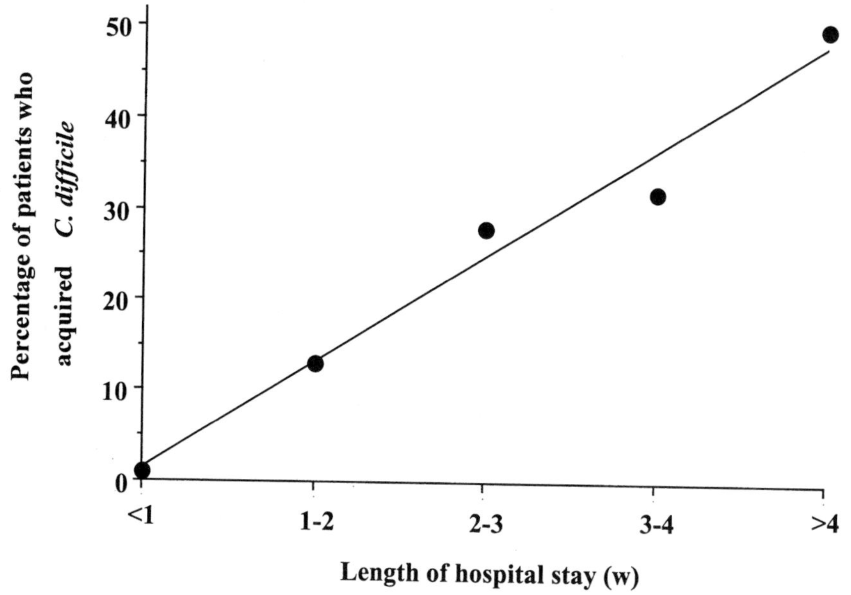

FIGURE 48.2. Rate of *Clostridium difficile* acquisition as a function of length of hospital stay. Data are from a prospective study of 557 hospitalized patients initially culture-negative for *C. difficile* who were monitored by weekly rectal swab cultures (73). For 323 patients whose hospital stay was less than 1 week, the rate of culture positivity was 1% (3 of 23), but the rate was 50% (10 of 20) for patients hospitalized for more than 4 weeks. From reference 206, which is in the public domain.

increased risk for CDAD when exposed to antimicrobials (Fig. 48.3*A*).

Contrary to the notion that colonized patients are at increased risk for CDAD, one prospective study of *C. difficile* acquisition and disease failed to show that asymptomatic carriers were at increased risk of CDAD (74). Data from four similar longitudinal studies were pooled in a random-effects analysis (75) and showed that colonized patients were actually at a reduced risk for subsequent CDAD (75). An explanation for this unexpected finding is

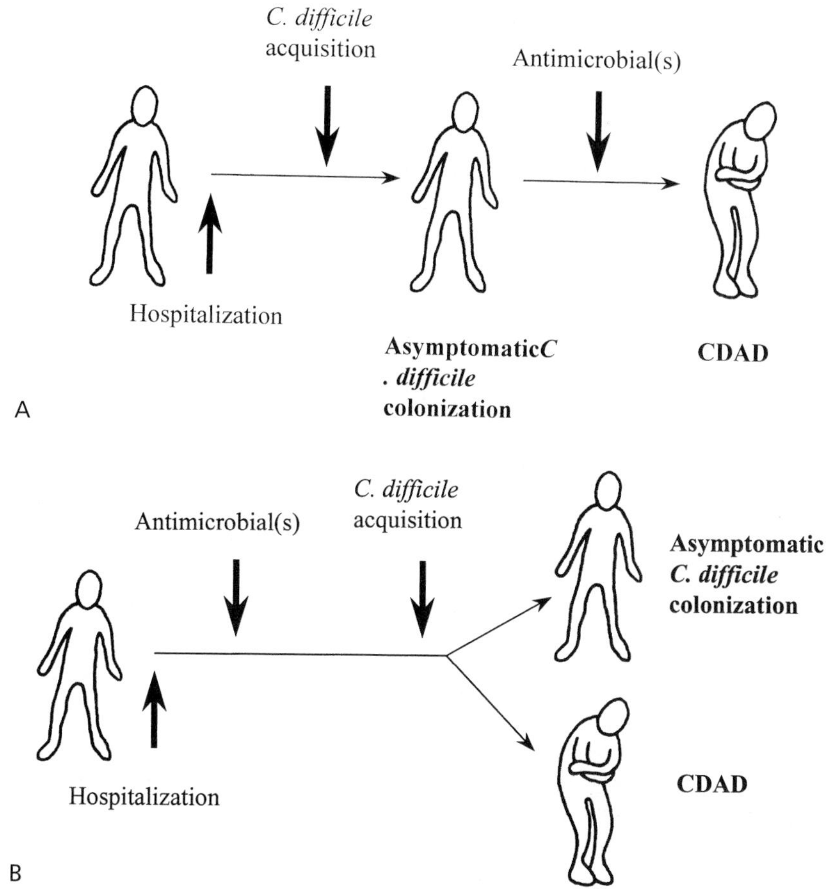

FIGURE 48.3. A: Initial hypothesis: *Clostridium difficile* acquisition and pathogenesis of *C. difficile*-associated disease (CDAD). According to this hypothesis, the patient acquires *C. difficile* during hospitalization and is at risk for CDAD if an antimicrobial is given. **B:** Revised hypothesis: In this hypothesis, the patient is at risk of CDAD or colonization by *C. difficile* only after exposure to antimicrobial therapy. After a short incubation period of a few days following infection, the clinical outcome is determined. Data supporting this hypothesis have been obtained by Shim and associates (75) and Kyne and colleagues (91). From reference 206, which is in the public domain.

summarized in Figure 48.3*B*. Accordingly, we suggest that a patient admitted to the hospital is at negligible risk for CDAD until he receives an antimicrobial agent. If during or after receiving antimicrobial(s) he is exposed to *C. difficile*, he will develop CDAD after a short incubation period of a few days or become colonized without diarrhea. Once established as an asymptomatic colonized carrier, the patient is at decreased risk for CDAD. Patients are likely exposed to *C. difficile* throughout their hospitalization (Fig 48.2) but become susceptible to infection only after they have been exposed to antimicrobials.

When susceptible individuals ingest spores of toxigenic *C. difficile* and these spores survive the acidity and other upper gastrointestinal defense mechanisms, the spores germinate and colonize the lower intestinal tract. Following toxin elaboration by vegetative *C. difficile* organisms, a number of intestinal responses ensue that are only partially understood. In addition to the enterotoxic and cytotoxic-effects of toxin A and toxin B, the toxins induce proinflammatory changes that may explain the classic pathologic findings of severe CDAD, pseudomembranes associated with CDAD. Toxin A is a potent chemoattractant for neutrophils *in vivo* (76), and both toxins induce cytokine release from monocytes (77).

Three factors influence the development of CDAD (78). The timing of these factors or "hits" appears to be essential. First, exposure to antimicrobials establishes susceptibility to *C. difficile*. Second, the host is exposed to toxigenic *C. difficile*. Without antimicrobial exposure, the host is not susceptible. Prospective observations have shown that the majority of patients do not become ill after the first two hits. A third factor appears to be necessary for CDAD to occur. This factor may be related to *C. difficile* virulence, the type and timing of the antimicrobial exposure, or the host immune response. Importantly, even the most virulent *C. difficile* organism produces asymptomatic colonization more often than CDAD, suggesting that, in addition to organism virulence, host factors, particularly the immune response, are important to the development of CDAD.

IMMUNITY

Circulating antibodies to toxin A and B (or only one) are common in *C. difficile*-infected persons (79). Antitoxin antibodies are typically acquired early in life (79), and low titer or low avidity serum antibodies to toxins A or B are detectable in greater than 70% of the adult population (79–82) and are corroborated by the high levels of antitoxin A and B antibody in pooled human IgG (83,84). High levels of serum antitoxin antibodies detected by enzyme-linked immunosorbent assay correlate with serum neutralization of the toxins in cell culture assays (79–81).

Systemic antibody responses to toxins A or B develop in 50% to 75% of patients with CDAD (79,81,82,85,86). Although systemic responses are somewhat more common to toxin B than to toxin A (79,85,86), most patients do not develop a fourfold increase in titer to either toxin following CDAD (79,81). In one-third of patients with CDAD, toxin A- or toxin B-neutralizing serum antibodies develop (81,85). Serum neutralization of toxin A in the convalescent phase sera from patients with diarrhea is typically mediated by IgA, not IgG (87). Serum IgA neutralizes both the cytotoxic and enterotoxic effects of toxin A and, characteristic of systemic-derived IgA, is predominately monomeric and of the IgA1 subclass (87). However, IgG antitoxin A neutralizing antibodies were detected in a patient with *C. difficile* splenic abscess, a rare systemic manifestation of *C. difficile* infection (88).

A role of antibody in the clinical manifestation of *C. difficile* disease has been documented in children with decreased antibody levels. Among children with chronic diarrhea, *C. difficile* has been isolated more often among those with hypogammaglobulinemia than in those with normal immunoglobulin levels (89). Moreover, children with hypogammaglobinemia (90) or low levels of antitoxin A IgG (83) appear to be predisposed to chronic relapsing CDAD.

The role of antitoxin antibodies in determining clinical outcome has been controversial (81,82). This issue has been partially resolved by two recent prospective studies (91,92). In the first study, baseline (precolonization) antibody levels were similar in those patients who later became colonized and those in whom CDAD developed. However, at the time of colonization, median antitoxin A IgG levels in the serum were significantly higher in asymptomatic carriers than in patients in whom CDAD developed (91). Antitoxin B levels were not significantly different among persons in these two groups. This study suggests that an anamnestic response to toxin A at the time of exposure to *C. difficile* is protective against diarrhea but not colonization, and supports the earlier observation that asymptomatic *C. difficile* carriers are at decreased risk of subsequent CDAD (75). The second study found that the early antibody response in those patients in whom CDAD developed also influenced the risk of diarrhea recurrence. Antitoxin A IgM levels on day 3 and antitoxin IgG levels on day 12 were significantly higher in those patients who only had a single episode of diarrhea (92). Additional support for the role of antitoxin antibodies in modifying the clinical course of infected patients comes from studies showing benefit of intravenous administration of immune globulin in patients with CDAD who have multiple relapses (83,93,94).

A mucosal immune response to *C. difficile* is reflected in the presence of antibodies to *C. difficile* toxins in colostrum and intestinal secretions (95,96). In patients with CDAD, intestinal IgA responses develop to toxin A that parallel serum IgG antitoxin responses (81). Toxin A–specific fecal IgA may also influence the risk of diarrhea recurrence (82).

EPIDEMIOLOGY

C. difficile is the major diagnosed cause of infectious diarrhea that develops in patients following hospital admission in the United States and developed countries around the world (97,98). The unique epidemiologic aspects of this enteric pathogen are the high-risk reservoirs of infection (e.g., hospitals and chronic care facilities) and the dependence of *C. difficile* infection on the disruption of the indigenous intestinal microflora by antimicrobial therapy.

Antimicrobial Agents

Almost all CDAD patients have recently been treated with antimicrobials or, occasionally, cancer chemotherapy agents that also possess antibiotic activity. Clindamycin, ampicillin, and cephalosporins were previously the antimicrobial agents most frequently associated with CDAD. More recently, the second- and third-generation cephalosporins, particularly cefotaxime, ceftriaxone, cefuroxime, and ceftazidime, have been the most frequently implicated agents, whereas penicillin plus beta-lactamase inhibitor combinations such as ticarcillin-clavulanate and piperacillin-tazobactam have significantly less risk (99–102). Some cephalosporin risks have been dramatic, for example, in a large outbreak in Great Britain, 76.3% of 169 patients infected with *C. difficile* had received cephalosporins (103). The use of third-generation cephalosporins for inpatient treatment of community-acquired pneumonia is thought to be a factor in the increasing rate of CDAD in the United Kingdom (104). The increased risk for CDAD with cephalosporin exposure may be related to the resistance of *C. difficile* to cephalosporins versus susceptibility to the beta-lactamase inhibitor combinations.

All antibiotics, including vancomycin and metronidazole, the most common treatment agents for CDAD, have been found to have risk of a subsequent episode of CDAD when administered to a patient. A metaanalysis of risk factors for *C. difficile* infection showed that the antimicrobial agents with the lowest risk (risk odds ratios 1.3 to 3.7) were tetracyclines, penicillin, first-generation cephalosporins, vancomycin, antistaphylococcal penicillins, trimethoprim-sulfamethoxazole, erythromycin, and ampicillin or amoxicillin (105). Intermediate risk antimicrobials (risk odds ratios 5.2 to 9.9) in ascending risk order were metronidazole, aminoglycosides, cefaclor, fluoroquinolones, clindamycin or lincomycin, antipseudomonal penicillins, and cefuroxime. Highest risk antimicrobials (risk ratios >10) were cefoxitin, amoxicillin-clavulanate, ceftazidime, and cefotaxime. Careful review of this list reveals some possible surprises: amoxicillin-clavulanate is high risk whereas ampicillin and amoxicillin are low-risk. Furthermore, single studies have shown other beta-lactamase inhibitor combinations (ticarcillin-clavulanate and piperacillin-tazobactam) are low-risk agents (99,102). Fluoroquinolones and aminoglycosides, generally thought to be low risk, have risk comparable to clindamycin and lincomycin. Multiple use of antimicrobials may be confounding these risks, in that only two of the reviewed studies separated multiple use from single use (105).

Clindamycin has been viewed as uniquely predisposing to CDAD as demonstrated by the initial description of the disease (10) and by several large hospital outbreaks in which removal of this agent from the hospital formulary was the single intervention responsible for stopping the outbreak (106,107). Clindamycin is highly active against most anaerobic bacteria and in the hamster model has a prolonged effect on the colonic flora that persists long after the drug is stopped. In the original report by Tedesco (10), symptoms developed in one-third of patients after clindamycin was stopped, a finding difficult to explain if CDAD was caused by the antibiotic itself. In retrospect, these patients likely demonstrated the prolonged carryover effect of clindamycin on bowel flora after the antibiotic had been stopped, coupled with the continued risk of exposure to *C. difficile* while hospitalized. One definite marker for *C. difficile* strains implicated in multiple U.S. epidemics has been clindamycin resistance (66). Outbreaks of CDAD in four hospitals of wide geographic distribution were attributed to an epidemic strain that carried the same *ermB* resistance gene for clindamycin (and macrolide and streptogramin antibiotics as well). Infection with the epidemic strain was associated with prior clindamycin use, and in one of the hospitals, the epidemic ended dramatically with control of clindamycin (106).

Asymptomatic Carriers

Surveillance cultures of stool or rectal swabs of patients on hospital wards identify asymptomatic *C. difficile* fecal excreters or carriers in institutions that have endemic or epidemic CDAD (27,74). In the hospital setting, asymptomatic carriers usually outnumber symptomatic patients by several-fold, whereas colonization of healthy, nonhospitalized adults by *C. difficile* is uncommon. The rate of colonization in hospitalized adults is often 20% or greater for patients hospitalized more than 1 week, compared with 1% to 3% of community residents. Some hospitalized patients are colonized on admission, especially if they have been hospitalized and received antibiotics recently, but for patients initially culture-negative, the risk of *C. difficile* acquisition increases in direct proportion to length of hospital stay (Fig. 48.2) (73). Asymptomatic fecal carriage of *C. difficile* in healthy neonates is common, often exceeding 50% in the first 6 months of life, but rates decrease markedly during the first year. Carriage rates in neonates vary significantly among different postnatal wards, most likely as a result of varying rates of nosocomial acquisition.

Sources of *C. difficile* in the institutional setting include environmental surfaces where the organism can persist for months in the spore form, and hospital personnel whose hands become transiently contaminated during patient care activities and are not decontaminated adequately between patients (27). Other than humans, reservoirs for *C. difficile* include numerous animal species and soil, water, and mud (108). Community-acquired cases of CDAD are reported, but the incidence (7.7 cases per 100,000 person-years of observation) is low (109). CDAD is diagnosed rarely in the outpatient setting, but there is concern that diagnostic testing is not being performed sufficiently in the proper patient group, those receiving antimicrobials. The diagnosis of *C. difficile* as the cause of community-acquired diarrhea increased from 2.6% to 10.7% after *C. difficile* testing was included in the evaluation of outpatients with diarrhea (110).

Reduced Risk of CDAD with *C. difficile* Colonization

With the known high prevalence of asymptomatic *C. difficile* carriers on hospital wards, it seemed intuitive to hypothesize that colonized patients would be at highest risk for CDAD, particularly when exposed to antimicrobial therapy (Fig. 48.3*A*). If this hypothesis were true, asymptomatic carriers would be a potential target for infection control interventions to prevent CDAD. Based on this hypothesis, eradication of *C. difficile* colonization was investigated in a controlled fashion (69). Asymptomatic carriers (fecal excreters) were treated with metronidazole, vancomycin, or placebo to eliminate the carrier state. Metronidazole treatment was comparable to placebo; this was likely because of the low or nonexistent fecal drug concentrations of metronidazole in the absence of diarrhea. Vancomycin treatment was temporarily effective, but vancomycin-treated patients were significantly more likely to have culture-positive stools at the end of the 70-day follow-up than those given placebo, despite fecal drug concentrations of 1,000 μg/g stool or higher during treatment. We presume this to be a result of continued exposure to *C. difficile* and increased susceptibility to *C. difficile* reinfection or relapse as a result of altered bowel flora from vancomycin treatment.

Our initial prospective study (74) and three additional similar longitudinal studies showed that colonized patients actually had a decreased risk of subsequent CDAD ($p < .021$) (75). Many of these patients were colonized with nontoxigenic strains (explaining their lack of clinical illness), but 56% were colonized with virulent, toxigenic strains that caused CDAD in other patients. These findings were totally contrary to our initial hypothesis and prompted us to hypothesize (Fig. 48.3*B*) that a newly hospitalized patient is at negligible risk for CDAD until administration of an antimicrobial agent. If during or after receiving antimicrobials the patient is exposed to *C. difficile*, one of the following may occur: (a) CDAD develops after a short incubation period of a few days, (b) colonization occurs without the development of diarrhea, or (c) the patient clears the organism without becoming infected or colonized. Patients appear to be continually at risk of exposure to *C. difficile* throughout their hospitalization (Fig. 48.2) but are susceptible to CDAD only after they have been exposed to antimicrobials.

Typing Systems Are Critical to Epidemiologic Investigation

Molecular typing studies using restriction endonuclease analysis (REA) of whole DNA indicate that even the most virulent of *C. difficile* organisms produces asymptomatic colonization more often than CDAD, suggesting that factors in addition to organism virulence are necessary for CDAD to occur (74). REA has also been used to show that recurrent CDAD is caused by both relapses from the original infecting strain and reinfection with a new strain of *C. difficile* (111). Outbreaks caused by a specific strain or type of *C. difficile* have frequently been reported in hospitals, as evidenced by pyrolysis mass spectrometry typing, which showed that 79% of strains in a large British outbreak were of one indistinguishable cluster that also heavily contaminated the environment (103). In the presence of an outbreak caused by one predominant strain of *C. difficile*, multiple other different strains will also be found. Genotypic typing systems such as REA, pulse-field gel electrophoresis, arbitrary-primed polymerase chain reaction (AP-PCR), and PCR ribotyping (of the 16S-23S rRNA intergenic spacer) have demonstrated a remarkable heterogeneity of *C. difficile* strains (28,112,113). More than 500 unique types of *C. difficile* organized into more than 100 distinct toxin-negative or toxin-positive groups have been identified in our laboratory by HindIII REA, suggesting wide organism diversity. PCR ribotyping has identified 116 different ribotypes (112). An additional genetic typing system that utilizes PCR of the 19-Kb region encompassing the pathogenicity locus of *C. difficile* has also been used to characterize strains by variations in the genes responsible for pathogenicity, including the toxin A and B genes, *tcdA* and *tcdB* (56,114). This typing method has identified 15 unique toxinotypes that represent typical and variant toxin types of *C. difficile* (114).

Phenotypic typing systems for *C. difficile* include serogrouping, sodium dodecyl sulphate polyacrylamide gel electrophoresis (SDS-PAGE) followed by radiolabeled methionine autoradiography, and immunoblotting of PAGE proteins (115). Phenotypic methods have generally identified fewer *C. difficile* strains than most genotypic methods. No universally accepted method of typing *C. difficile* has emerged. A unified nomenclature for *C. difficile* typing has been proposed, but collaborative comparative typing studies continue to be published (116,117).

The presence of multiple *C. difficile* strains in the same hospital in different patients with little obvious epidemiologic linkage has been interpreted by some as evidence that the infections result from endogenous carriage of *C. difficile.* On one hospital ward where rectal swab cultures were obtained weekly and the rate of *C. difficile* diarrhea was low, 19 distinct HindIII REA types of *C. difficile* were both introduced and acquired by different patients (73). Acquisition of a strain by a patient was preceded by a documented introduction of that strain to the ward by an asymptomatic carrier in 16 (84%) of 19 instances, implicating asymptomatic carriers rather than endogenous activation of the patient's own *C. difficile* as the source of infection for most patients.

Additional Risks for CDAD

In addition to antimicrobial use, environmental contamination by *C. difficile* spores, hand contamination of personnel, and the presence of patients infected with *C. difficile* (both symptomatic and asymptomatic), other risk factors for CDAD have been identified. Enteral feeding via a tube was shown in a cohort study to be a risk factor for *C. difficile* acquisition and for CDAD (118). Postpyloric placement of the tube was a highly significant risk factor (odds ratio, 11.4; 95% confidence interval, 1.3 to 103.7) suggesting that bypassing gastric acid defenses in the stomach may increases risk for both *C. difficile* acquisition and CDAD. Similarly, antacid treatment has been found to be a risk factor ($p < .001$) in a case–control study, although use of the H_2 blocker cimetidine was not a risk factor (26). Other risk factors include gastrointestinal surgery, older patient age, greater severity of illness, and use of electronic rectal thermometers (97,98,119–121).

The risk factors for infection with *C. difficile* and for vancomycin-resistant enterococci (VRE) are remarkably similar. Both infections are significantly associated with exposure to any antimicrobials, to multiple antimicrobials, and to increased days of antimicrobial treatment. Other risk factors in common are exposure to third-generation cephalosporins, clindamycin, metronidazole, and imipenem, as well as older patient age, greater severity of underlying illness, longer patient hospital stay, electronic rectal thermometer use, and enteral feedings (122). In addition, both infections are characterized by asymptomatic patient stool carriage, environmental contamination, and hand contamination of health care workers by the organism (122). *C. difficile* diarrhea may increase the risk for VRE transmission by disseminating VRE in the environment when patients with CDAD also are colonized with VRE (123,124).

CLINICAL ILLNESS

Clinical Findings

Most patients with clinical illness caused by *C. difficile* present with diarrhea. Diarrhea is almost never grossly bloody, stools range from soft and unformed to watery or mucoid in consistency (26), and stools have a characteristic odor. Stool frequency varies widely from 3 to 20 or more bowel movements per day. Associated clinical symptoms include abdominal pain and cramping (22% of one large series) and fever found in 28% of patients in the same series (26). Leukocytosis is found in 50% of patients, often to levels in excess of 40,000 white blood cells/mm^3 (26). Occult blood has been detected in 26% of patients (26).

Abdominal x-ray study revealed ileus in 21% of patients in one series, all of whom continued to have diarrhea (26). When ileus results in cessation of stools, the diagnosis of *C. difficile* disease is frequently overlooked, but if diagnosed, the absence of intestinal movement may prevent orally administered treatment from reaching the site of infection (125). Such patients are at high risk of complications of *C. difficile* infection, particularly toxic megacolon and colonic perforation. Toxic megacolon complicating *C. difficile* diarrhea occurred in 11 (3.1%) of patients in a Montreal hospital between 1992 and 1994 and 64% died (126). Overall, mortality rate associated with CDAD ranges from 0.6% of 908 patients in one hospital over 10 years to 3.5% of 208 patients at another hospital in a similar 10-year period (125,127).

Extracolonic manifestations of *C. difficile* infection are rare. Reactive arthritis, usually involving large joints and beginning 7 to 35 days after the onset of CDAD, has been described as a complication in 17 patients reported through 1993 (128). Ascites with low serum albumin to ascites albumin gradient has been reported in five patients with PMC, three of whom were also infected with the HIV-1 virus (129). *C. difficile* cultures from the ascitic fluid were negative, but the percent of polymorphonuclear neutrophils (58% to 88%) was increased in ascitic fluid with total white blood cell counts ranging from 287 to 3,560 cells/mm^3. Rarely, *C. difficile* has been isolated from body sites other than stool, including joint fluid, blood, peritoneal fluid, splenic abscess, and ascitic fluid (88).

Recurrent *C. difficile* Diarrhea

Recurrence of *C. difficile* diarrhea following treatment occurs in from 7% to 20% of patients. Recurrences may be either relapses from the same organism or reinfections with a new strain of *C. difficile.* Data from three studies suggest that approximately half of all recurrences are a result of relapse and half are due to reinfection (111,130,131). Relapses occurred earlier after treatment than reinfections (14.5 days versus 42.5 days) in our study (111). The real rate of reinfections may be higher than observed, because matching isolates have been assumed to be relapses, but they could also have caused reinfection.

Recurrence of clinical CDAD does not correlate with continued isolation of the organism from stool following treatment, which occurs commonly. Most patients respond to retreatment following the first recurrence and do not have further episodes, but as many as 26 recurrences have been reported in a single patient (125,133). The risk factors for recurrence are increased age, decreasing quality of life score, and failure to develop an anamnestic serum antibody response to toxin A (92,132). Severity of CDAD does not increase with the number of recurrent episodes (132).

C. difficile Diarrhea in Patients with Underlying Illnesses

C. difficile disease may complicate the diagnosis and management of patients with inflammatory bowel disease (IBD). An early study by LaMont and Trnka (134) demonstrated the presence of *C. difficile* toxin in six patients with chronic IBD. All six patients improved with the disappearance of toxin in the stool, although they continued to have diarrhea or proctoscopic evidence of chronic colitis. In another study, 13% of the stools from 109 patients with IBD were positive for *C. difficile* toxin, and the frequency of a positive stool was higher when the patients were in hospitals, suggesting nosocomial acquisition (135). Other studies (136,137) have found a higher incidence of *C. difficile* and toxin in stools from IBD patients; therefore, stool from patients with IBD should be tested for *C. difficile* toxin, especially during IBD exacerbation, poor response to standard treatment, or when there is a history of recent antibiotic use. Efforts to treat IBD with chronic courses of metronidazole on the assumption that the underlying disease might be caused by *C. difficile* have been unrewarding and have resulted in significant metronidazole neurotoxicity.

Patients with HIV-1 infection are at high risk for CDAD in that they have frequent antibiotic exposures and hospitalizations if disease is advanced. For HIV-1–infected patients in whom CDAD is diagnosed and treated promptly, there appears to be a good response to treatment, and the recurrence rate is similar to non–HIV-1–infected patients (138–140).

DIAGNOSIS AND PATHOLOGY

Clinical Definition of CDAD

The diagnosis of CDAD is based on a combination of clinical and laboratory criteria established by the Society for Healthcare Epidemiology of America and include the following clinical criteria: (a) diarrhea, defined by a range of criteria: six or more watery or unformed stools in a 36-hour period; three or more unformed stools per 24 hours for a minimum of 2 days; or 8 unformed stools in 48 hours; and (b) no other recognized cause for diarrhea. When this clinical definition is combined with (a) visualization of colonic pseudomembranes, (b) toxin A or B in the stool, or (c) stool culture positive for a toxin-producing *C. difficile* organism, then the diagnosis of CDAD can be made with confidence (98,141). Antimicrobial exposure in the prior 8 weeks is almost universally present but is not required for diagnosis. A response to treatment with oral metronidazole or vancomycin supports the diagnosis of CDAD.

Diagnostic Tests—Endoscopic Examination

Visualization of colonic pseudomembranes by sigmoidoscopy, colonoscopy, surgery, or autopsy is diagnostic of PMC (see Color Figure 48.4*A*). PMC is a more advanced form of CDAD and is visualized at endoscopy in only approximately 50% of patients who meet the clinical diarrhea requirements for CDAD and have a positive stool culture and toxin assay for *C. difficile* (26,142). Small pseudomembranes may be difficult to visualize because they

TABLE 48.1. SENSITIVITY AND SPECIFICITY OF TESTS FOR THE DIAGNOSIS OF *CLOSTRIDIUM DIFFICILE*-ASSOCIATED DISEASE[a]

Test	Sensitivity	Specificity	Utility of Test
Endoscopy	51%	~100%	Diagnostic of PMC and therefore CDAD
Culture for *C. difficile*	89–100%	84–100%	Most sensitive test; confirmation of organism toxicity necessary to improve specificity
Cell culture cytotoxin test	67–100%	85–100%	With clinical data is diagnostic of CDAD Highly specific but not as sensitive as culture
EIA toxin test	63–99%	75–100%	With clinical data is diagnostic of CDAD Rapid but not as sensitive as culture or cell culture cytotoxin test
Latex test for *C. difficile* antigen	58–92%	80–96%	Less sensitive and specific than other tests but gives rapid results
PCR toxin gene detection	Undetermined	Undetermined	Research test

Abbreviations: CDAD, *Clostridium difficile*-associated disease; EIA, enzyme immunossay; PCR, polymerase chain reaction; PMC, pseudomembranous colitis.
[a]Using both clinical and test-based criteria.
Adapted from Gerding DN, Johnson S, Peterson LR, et al. Society for Healthcare Epidemiology of America position paper or *Clostridium difficile*-associated diarrhea and colitis. *Infect Control Hosp Epidemiol* 1995;16:459–477, with permission.

may be only a few millimeters in size (see Color Figure 48.4*B*) (143). Biopsy and histologic examination of suspicious lesions is helpful to confirm the diagnosis. Endoscopy is used infrequently for the diagnosis of CDAD because various stool toxin and culture assays are more readily available; however, endoscopy remains a valuable and rapid diagnostic tool in seriously ill patients with an acute abdomen and suspected PMC. Visualization of pseudomembranes is diagnostic, but a negative examination does not rule out *C. difficile* disease because of the low sensitivity of endoscopy in clinically proven CDAD (Table 48.1).

Diagnostic Tests—Detection of *C. difficile* Toxins

Stool specimens for detection of *C. difficile* toxin or culture do not require anaerobic handling. The specimen should be collected and submitted to the laboratory in a clean, watertight container. Some laboratories analyze only watery or unformed stool specimens (i.e., specimens that retain the shape of the container), a practice that has been recommended by a position paper (98) to better assure the presence of diarrhea and meet the clinical definition of CDAD. Occasionally, semisolid and formed stools contain *C. difficile* toxin, but positive test results may not be indicative of *C. difficile* disease if diarrhea is absent. Best results are obtained when testing fresh stool specimens within 24 hours of collection. If testing cannot be performed immediately, the specimens should be held at refrigerator temperature until the assay is performed.

An array of methods and commercial tests are available for detection of *C. difficile* and its toxins (Table 48.1), but the ideal tests have not been developed. Cell cytotoxicity testing of stool is the most specific test for CDAD, but it takes 1 to 2 days for turnaround and it is not as sensitive as stool culture for *C. difficile*. For this reason, some clinical laboratories use two tests, often combining a specific test for toxin (cell cytotoxin or enzyme immunoassay) with stool culture to increase sensitivity; however, this approach is labor intensive and expensive (144). Some laboratory resources are saved by culturing only specimens that are negative by toxin testing. Another strategy used to overcome the relative insensitivity of stool toxin assays is to submit additional specimens if the original specimen is negative and diarrhea persists; this too is labor intensive but increases sensitivity (145).

Cell Culture Cytotoxicity Assay

A variety of cell lines are used to test for toxins A and B produced in stool by *C. difficile*. The tissue culture assay detects toxin B, which masks the weaker cytotoxic activity of toxin A in fecal specimens. The primary advantage of the test, which can detect as little as 1 pg of toxin B, is its sensitivity. Even so, positive cytotoxin test results correlate only 70% to 80% with results of stool culture for *C. difficile* performed in laboratories that are proficient at culturing the organism. The several cell lines most commonly used to determine cell cytotoxicity (WI-38, MRC-5, human foreskin, and Chinese hamster ovary cells) are comparable in sensitivity. Cell cytotoxicity is detected by a rounding of the cells and is confirmed to be caused by *C. difficile* when the cytotoxic effect is neutralized by mixing *C. difficile* or *C. sordelli* (which cross reacts with *C. difficile* toxin) antitoxin with the specimen. The specificity of the cell cytotoxicity assay (85% to 100%) is among the highest of available tests, but sensitivity is approximately 20% to 30% lower than that of stool culture, the most sensitive test (146). Results typically take 1 to 2 days or longer, limiting its utility when rapid diagnosis is desired.

Enzyme Immunoassays for Toxin A and B

EIAs use specific monoclonal or polyclonal antibodies to toxin A or toxin B (or both) to detect *C. difficile* toxin in stool specimens. These tests are generally much more rapid than the cell cytotoxicity assay, yielding results in 1 to 3 hours. Specificity for the best of the tests exceeds 95%, but sensitivity is somewhat lower, ranging from 63% to 99% when compared with stool culture (Table 48.1). EIA tests for toxin A do not detect strains of *C. difficile* that produce variant toxin A (or no toxin A) but are capable of causing human disease (24,61). Use of EIA tests that combine testing for toxin A and toxin B can theoretically circumvent the failure to detect toxin A variant strains by toxin A–specific EIAs. Clinical experience is limited, but one commercially available toxin A/B test did detect two stool specimens that were shown to contain toxin A–/B+ organisms (147). EIA tests are popular because they are rapid and relatively easy to perform (61). However, the sensitivity, including that of toxin A plus B EIAs, is not sufficient to rely on these tests alone without backup by stool culture (148,149). In addition, some EIA tests have a high percentage of indeterminate or uninterpretable results (150).

Diagnostic Tests—Isolation/Detection of the Organism

Stool Culture

Stool culture for *C. difficile* is performed using a selective antibiotic-containing media such as CCFA (151). The concentrations of cycloserine (500 μg/mL) and cefoxitin (16 μg/mL) originally described by George and colleagues (152) continue to provide the best balance between *C. difficile* isolation and inhibition of other stool flora (151). CCFA media should be anaerobically reduced for at least 4 hours before use to maximize *C. difficile* growth; incubation can be performed in an anaerobic chamber, jar, bag or pouch with equivalent yields (151). *C. difficile* grows as flat, yellow, ground-glass colonies surrounded by a yellow halo on CCFA. Careful quality control in the laboratory is essential because commercial CCFA media may vary considerably in recovery rates. Culture is more difficult to perform than for other *C. difficile* tests and demonstrates more results variability from laboratory to laboratory (153). *C. difficile* culture lacks specificity in diagnosing CDAD because nontoxigenic strains that do not cause CDAD may be isolated. Specificity can be increased by toxin testing of isolates recovered from cultures and reporting as positive only those specimens containing toxin-producing *C. difficile* (153).

Latex Agglutinaton

Latex agglutination (LA) tests are rapid and easy to use. They detect the enzyme glutamate dehydrogenase, a nontoxic protein produced by all toxigenic and nontoxigenic isolates of *C. difficile* and by some other clostridia and anaerobes, including *Clostridium sporogenes*, certain *Clostridium botulinum* organisms, and *Peptostreptococcus anaerobius* (154). The LA test was initially marketed as a test for toxin A (155). However, the glutamate dehydrogenase detected in the test has no relationship with either toxin A or toxin B, and the LA tests do not distinguish between toxigenic and nontoxigenic isolates. Sensitivity (68%) for the commercial LA test is comparable to the cell cytotoxicity assay, but well below that of *C. difficile* stool culture (146). Specificity was intermediate between that of culture and cell cytotoxicity assay (98). Additional testing must be done to detect the presence of toxin if the LA test is positive. Common antigen detection (glutamate dehydrogenase) and toxin A detection by EIA have been combined into a single test to increase the specificity of the common antigen test (156). This strategy has not been successful, in that the detection of toxin A was relatively insensitive when compared with the cell cytotoxin assay, detecting only 5 of 16 (31%) of cell cytotoxin positive specimens (156).

Diagnostic Tests—Other Methods

Polymerase Chain Reaction

Using PCR to amplify a 399-bp fragment of the toxin B gene, Gumerlock and colleagues (157,158) found that all the toxigenic strains studied were amplified with these primers and that DNA from *C. sordellii* and *Clostridium bifermentans* were not amplified. When applied to clinical specimens, all 18 that were positive by cell cytotoxicity assay were positive by this method. Selection of primers from within the toxin B gene makes the test attractive for the specific detection of toxigenic *C. difficile*. Others have used PCR to amplify portions of the toxin A gene (159–161). However, when Kato and colleagues (160) applied the procedure in the analysis of stool specimens, they found that factors in the stools inhibited the PCR amplication step. Ion exchange after phenol-chloroform extraction was required to remove the inhibitory activity, after which their results correlated 100% with cell cytotoxicity assays on 39 specimens. Boondeekhun and co-workers (161) found that PCR was more sensitive than culturing for the organism. PCR methods are encouraging, but, despite availability for more than 10 years, commercial clinical application has not occurred.

Fecal Leukocytes and Fecal Lactoferrin

Fecal leukocytes are present in the stool of 35% to 63% of patients with CDAD and 37% to 40% of patients with diarrhea from causes other than *C. difficile* (145,162). Fecal lactoferrin, an enzyme marker for degraded polymorphonuclear leukocytes (163), has a positivity rate in patients whose stool contains *C. difficile* toxin of 61% compared with a 31% positivity rate in patients whose stool is negative for *C. difficile* toxin (145). The presence of lactoferrin in stool increases with the cell cytotoxicity titer of the stool specimen, from 39% in cytotoxin-negative specimens to 79% in specimens with cytotoxin titer greater than or equal to 100 (164). These tests are not sufficiently sensitive or specific to be used as screening tests for CDAD.

Pathology

Macroscopic Appearance

The pseudomembrane found in association with antibiotic PMC is confined to the colon (3). Pseudomembranes initially appear as small (1 to 2 mm), whitish-yellow plaques along the colonic wall and are diagnostic for PMC. The intervening mucosa appears unremarkable. As the disease progresses, the pseudomembranes may coalesce to form larger plaques and in advanced cases become confluent over the entire colon wall (see Color Figure 48.5). The distribution of lesions typically involves the entire colon, but rectal sparing occurs in about 10% of patients (165,166). Disease is confined to the colon and stops abruptly at the ileocecal valve. Patients who have had prior colectomy have been found to have pseudomembranes in the small bowel.

Microscopic Appearance

Microscopically, the pseudomembranes contain necrotic leukocytes, fibrin, mucus, and cellular debris with a point of attachment to the underlying mucosa. The leukocytes likely contribute significantly to the tissue damage that occurs during the disease because of the tissue-damaging enzymes and substances they release. The infiltration of leukocytes is presumed to be from the tissue damage caused by toxin A and by the chemotactic properties of the toxin (76). The mucosa beneath the pseudomembrane is inflamed, with a predominantly neutrophil infiltration (see Color Figure 48.6). The changes are focal with unremarkable adjacent mucosa. The superficial epithelium is commonly eroded with superficial necrosis, but full-thickness ulceration is rare (167).

TREATMENT

During the past 2 decades, the major change in the treatment of *C. difficile* diarrhea has been the greater use of metronidazole rather than vancomycin because of the emergence of vancomycin-resistant organisms such as the enterococci (169). The major deficiencies in the treatment of CDAD are the high recurrence rates and the lack of effective treatments for complications such as ileus, toxic megacolon, and perforation. Biotherapeutic or probiotic approaches to the prevention and treatment of CDAD are receiving increased interest (170). At this time, only the yeast *Saccharomyces boulardii* has shown efficacy as adjunctive therapy for the treatment of recurrent *C. difficile* diarrhea (171).

Treatment of Uncomplicated First Episodes of CDAD

C. difficile-associated diarrhea resolves in 15% to 23% of patients within 2 to 3 days after discontinuing the precipitating antimicrobial (125,172). The risk of recurrence following cessation of the inciting antibiotic is assumed to be zero, but actual recurrence rates are not known (125,172). Withholding specific anti–*C. difficile* treatment may avoid the 10% to 42% risk of recurrence following specific treatment, but placebo treatment (or no treatment) is not as effective as specific treatment with vancomycin or metronidazole (173,174).

General treatment guidelines for *C. difficile*–associated diarrhea have been proposed (98,175). If possible, the offending antimicrobials should be discontinued. If antimicrobials must be continued, substitution of agents that are possibly less predisposing to *C. difficile* diarrhea (e.g., metronidazole, vancomycin, or an aminoglycoside) may be beneficial, but no specific data are available. Fluids and electrolytes should be given as supportive measures to maintain hydration. Antiperistaltic agents and opiates should probably be avoided to prevent (a) masking of symptoms, (b) possible worsening of disease by retaining toxin in the colon, and (c) increased absorption of metronidazole as diarrhea is reduced, potentially causing metronidazole treatment failure (176). That said, antimotility drugs have been used with vancomycin or metronidazole for treatment of CDAD of mild to moderate severity without demonstrable adverse effects (177). Finally, test-of-cure cultures or toxin assays following treatment are not recommended, because they are imperfect predictors of subsequent recurrence (178), and treatment of asymptomatic patients colonized with *C. difficile* has been ineffective (69).

The results of prospective randomized CDAD clinical treatment trials in humans are summarized in Table 48.2. The primary endpoint for evaluation has been clinical cessation of diarrhea, and treatment comparisons among antibiotics show no statistical differences; however, vancomycin has been shown to be superior to placebo, whereas colestipol has been shown to be no better than placebo and

TABLE 48.2. SUMMARY OF RANDOMIZED, COMPARATIVE TRIALS OF ORAL THERAPY FOR INITIAL EPIDSODES OF *CLOSTRIDIUM DIFFICILE*-ASSOCIATED DIARRHEA

Antibiotic	Regimen	Number of Patients	Resolution of Diarrhea (%)	Recurrence (%)	Mean Days to Resolution	References
Metronidazole	250 mg qid × 10 days	42	40 (95)	2 (5)	2.4	Teasley et al (172)
	500 mg tid × 10 days	31	29 (94)	5 (17)	3.2	Wenisch et al (182)
Vancomycin	500 mg tid × 10 days	31	29 (94)	5 (17)	3.1	Wenisch et al (182)
	500 mg qid × 10 days	87	87 (100)	13 (15)	2.6–3.6	Teasley et al (172) deLalla et al (183) Dudley et al (180)
	125 mg qid × 7 day	21	18 (86)	6 (33)	4.2	Young et al (181)
	125 mg qid × 5 day	12	9 (75)	?	<5	Keighley et al (173)
Teicoplanin	400 mg bid × 10 day	28	27 (96)	2 (7)	2.8	Wenisch et al (182)
	100 mg bid × 10 day	26	25 (96)	2 (8)	3.4	deLalla et al (183)
Bacitracin	25,000 U qid × 10 day	15	12 (80)	5 (42)	3.0	Dudley et al (180)
	20,000 U qid × 7 days	21	16 (76)	5 (31)	4.1	Young et al (181)
Colestipol	10 g qid	12	3 (25)	?	<5	Mogg et al (179)
Placebo		14	3 (21)	?	<5	Mogg et al (179)

Adapted from Peterson LR, Gerding DN. Antimicrobial agents in *Clostridium difficile*-associated intestinal disease. In: Rambaud J-C, Ducluzeau R, eds. Clostridium difficile*-associated intestinal disease.* Paris: Springer-Verlag, 1990:115–127, with permission.

inferior to antimicrobial treatment agents (173,179). Although not significant, the clinical response rate for bacitracin was 10% to 20% lower than for vancomycin, making bacitracin a third- or fourth-line CDAD agent in our view (180,181). Although they are highly effective treatment agents, neither fusidic acid nor teicoplanin are available clinically in the United States (182,183). Secondary endpoints evaluated have been (a) clinical recurrence of disease and (b) clearance of *C. difficile* or its toxin from stools following treatment. One randomized trial showed a significant reduction in recurrence rate for teicoplanin compared with fusidic acid (182).

Specific therapy, particularly with vancomycin, should be administered orally. Bactericidal fecal concentrations can be achieved in patients with acute diarrhea when using intravenous metronidazole (185,186), and anecdotal evidence supports such treatment for CDAD (186). However, in the presence of adynamic ileus, intravenous metronidazole has also failed to successfully treat PMC (187).

Nearly all patients with CDAD (95% to 100%) respond to specific therapy with oral vancomycin or metronidazole (125), including both high (500 mg) and low (125 mg) doses of vancomycin (188). Most patients show some improvement within the first 2 days of treatment, but the mean time to resolution of diarrhea ranges between 2 and 4 days in prospective studies (168,172,182). Time to resolution of diarrhea was found to be longer for metronidazole (4.6 days) than for vancomycin (3.0 days, $p < .01$) treatment in a retrospective study, but this has not been confirmed in any prospective trials (Table 48.2) (177). With vancomycin treatment, approximately 90% of patients respond within 7 days and 10% respond thereafter (188). Thus, patients should not be deemed therapeutic failures until at least 6 days of treatment have passed (168). Vancomycin given at a dosage of 125 mg four times daily for 5 to 7 days (Table 48.2) appears to be less efficacious than when given for at least 10 days (98). Our view is that treatment is more likely to be successful if given for 10 days, although no controlled comparisons are available.

Metronidazole is effective for *C. difficile* treatment although it does not have Food and Drug Administration (FDA) approval for this use. The safety of metronidazole in children has not been proven and it is a category B drug for use in pregnancy, factors that should be taken into account when selecting therapies for these patients (175). Although rare metronidazole-resistant isolates have been reported (70–72), treatment failure with metronidazole does not correlate with *in vitro* resistance (189). In addition, metronidazole is the least expensive antimicrobial agent for the treatment of CDAD (182).

Although vancomycin is highly effective for *C. difficile* treatment and is the drug against which all subsequent therapies have been compared (190), the increasing prevalence of vancomycin resistance among enterococci and staphylococci in the United States has caused the Hospital Infection Control Practices Advisory Committee to discourage the use of oral vancomycin for the treatment of *C. difficile* diarrhea except for metronidazole treatment failure or severe, potentially life-threatening illness (169).

Treatment of CDAD Recurrences

Most recurrences of CDAD (89% in our experience) resolve with retreatment (125). We routinely use metronidazole to treat first recurrences of CDAD. Vancomycin treatment of first recurrences does not appear to be necessary, given the resistance concerns and the higher cost (130). For patients with two or more recurrences, there is no standard approach supported by data. Treatment strategies invoking biotherapeutic agents include the following: (a) vancomycin or metronidazole followed by use of the yeast *S. boulardii* (171,191), (b) metronidazole or bacitracin followed by *Lactobacillus* GG (192), (c) vancomycin followed by synthetic fecal bacterial enema (193), and (d) administration of a nontoxigenic *C. difficile* strain (194,195). *S. boulardii* should be used with caution in debilitated or immunocompromised patients because invasive *S. boulardii* infections and fungemia have been reported in these patients (195). The aesthetics and safety of the bacterial rectal infusion methods are also a concern. *S. boulardii*, *Lactobacillus* GG, nontoxigenic *C. difficile*, and fecal enemas are not available as pharmaceuticals in the United States and do not have FDA approval for use in treating CDAD. Other approaches include vancomycin in tapering doses over 21 days followed by pulse dosing for 21 days (196), no treatment with careful observation, vancomycin followed by the anion-exchange binding resin cholestyramine (197), and combined treatment with vancomycin and rifampin for 7 days (198). Our approach is to administer 10 days of vancomycin (125 mg orally four times per day) and rifampin (600 mg orally twice daily) for multiple recurrences; this is a relatively simple approach and usually effective.

In children with recurrent *C. difficile* diarrhea and low levels of serum IgG antibodies to *C. difficile* toxin A, treatment with intravenous gamma globulin has resulted in clinical and bacteriologic improvement (83,84). These patients often have selective IgG1 deficiency. The high cost and restricted availability of intravenous immunoglobulin limit this approach to the few chronically infected children who have antibody deficiency.

Treatment of Complications

The most serious *C. difficile* treatment problem is in the rare patient with an acute abdomen, toxic megacolon, or ileus. These patients often present without diarrhea, mimicking an acute surgical abdomen (126,199,200). Sepsis syndrome is also a rare complication of severe CDAD (201,202). Acute abdomen may occur with or without toxic megacolon and may show signs of obstruction, ileus, bowel wall thickening, and ascites on abdominal computed tomography, accompanied by a marked peripheral blood leukocytosis (200–202). Thus, *C. difficile* infection should be included in the differential diagnosis of an acute abdomen, sepsis, or toxic megacolon if the patient has received antibiotics within the previous 2 months, whether diarrhea is present or not. Rapid diagnosis of *C. difficile* disease can best be achieved by performing cautious sigmoidoscopy or colonoscopy to document the presence of pseudomembranes.

There is no established effective treatment for patients with complicated CDAD. Management is difficult because of the inability to achieve effective concentrations of metronidazole or vancomycin in the colon by the oral route in the presence of ileus. Treatment with intravenous metronidazole or vancomycin at dosages greater than or equal to 2 g/day, instillation of vancomycin via intestinal catheter, or administration of vancomycin by enema has been proposed. We have successfully treated six patients with severe ileus with vancomycin by nasogastric tube and by retention enema plus intravenous metronidazole (125).

Patients with toxic megacolon or acute abdomen who do not respond to medical management or who are suspected of having colonic perforation are candidates for surgical intervention. Surgery is rarely required to treat CDAD. Lipsett and colleagues (203) reported 0.39% of patients with CDAD in one hospital required surgical intervention, but among critically ill patients in an intensive care unit, 20.3% of patients with *C. difficile* colitis had surgical intervention (204). Mortality rate is high in patients who require surgery, ranging from 32% to 50%, and is predictable from the severity of illness (200,203,205). The best surgical procedure is not clear, but Lipsett and colleagues (203), in an nonrandomized experience, reported a lower mortality rate (14%) for patients undergoing subtotal colectomy compared with those undergoing left hemicolectomy (100%).

PREVENTION AND CONTROL OF *C. DIFFICILE* INFECTION

Control and prevention strategies for *C. difficile* infections can be divided into two types: (a) barrier/isolation/disinfection procedures of various types to prevent transmission of the organism to the patient and (b) reduction of the risk of clinical illness if the patient does contact the organism (Table 48.3). One of the latter methods that has been remarkably successful is restriction of the use of certain antibiotics to reduce the risk of colonization and infection. Neither barrier precautions nor changes in antimicrobial use are easy to implement successfully, a factor that may

TABLE 48.3. INFECTION CONTROL MEASURES FOR THE PREVENTION OF HORIZONTAL TRANSMISSION OF *CLOSTRIDIUM DIFFICILE* AND FOR THE PREVENTION OF *CLOSTRIDIUM DIFFICILE*-ASSOCIATED DISEASE IF TRANSMISSION OCCURS

	Intervention Efficacy[a]
I. Prevention of horizontal transmission of *C. difficile*	
1. Barrier precautions	
a. Glove use	Proven
b. Handwashing	Probable
c. Private room or cohorting	Probable
d. Gowns	Untested
2. Environmental cleaning, disinfection, or use of disposables	
a. Rooms	Possible
b. Commodes	Untested
c. Rectal thermometers	Proven
d. Endoscopes	Probable
II. Prevention of disease if transmission occurs	
1. Antimicrobial usage restriction	Proven
2. Prophylactic treatment of patients receiving antimicrobials	
a. *Saccharomyces boulardii*	Possible
b. *Lactobacillus* species	Untested
c. Nontoxigenic *Clostridium difficile*	Untested

[a]Proven: Published efficacy in reducing incidence of CDAD when employed in the health care setting.
Probable: Accepted practice without specific published evidence of efficacy with CDAD.
Possible: Some published evidence of use, but efficacy inconclusive.
Untested: No published human efficacy data.
Adapted from Gerding DN, Johnson S, Peterson LR, et al. Society for Healthcare Epidemiology of America position paper on *Clostridium difficile*-associated diarrhea and colitis. *Infect Control Hosp Epidemiol* 1995;16:459–477, with permission.

account for the limited success of control and prevention measures to date. Two guidelines have been published with recommendations for prevention and control of *C. difficile* infection (98,175); the recommendations are summarized in Table 48.3 (206).

Prevention of Contact with the *C. difficile* Organism

Prevention and control of *C. difficile* infection is difficult to achieve because of high rates of environmental contamination with *C. difficile* spores, presence of asymptomatically colonized patients, carriage of the organism on employee hands, increased antimicrobial use, and increasing rates despite active infection control programs (26,27,73,125). Transmission prevention methods include barrier precautions, gloving, handwashing, environmental disinfection, replacement of electronic rectal thermometers, and treatment of asymptomatic carriers of *C. difficile* with vancomycin or metronidazole (98). Of these interventions, only discontinuation of the use of contaminated electronic thermometers and wearing of gloves by personnel as control measures have unequivocally reduced CDAD rates in actual hospital clinical practice (Table 48.3) (119,207).

Environmental disinfection with hypochlorite solutions reduces *C. difficile* contamination in the hospital environment, presumably because of the sporicidal properties of hypochlorite (208). However, because of odor and bleaching of surfaces by hypochlorite, there has not been widespread adaptation of these products in hospitals. Most U. S. hospitals use quaternary ammonium products as environmental disinfectants, whereas in the United Kingdom detergents are routinely used for environmental cleaning. Neither agent is sporicidal. Wilcox and Fawley (209) have grown *C. difficile* in fecal emulsions in the presence and absence of subinhibitory concentrations of detergents and chlorine-based disinfectants, and found that the major epidemic *C. difficile* strain in U. K. hospitals sporulated significantly more in the presence of the detergents than in the presence of the disinfectants. They speculate that this strain may be epidemic because of its ability to sporulate when exposed to detergents in the hospital. Whether changing to a chlorine-based disinfectant will reduce environmental spore contamination and lower CDAD rates remains to be determined. Overall, infection control requires ongoing personnel education and compliance to be effective; high turnover rates among hospital personnel may at least partially account for the sporadic efficacy of prevention measures in many hospitals (125,210).

Prevention of Clinical Illness if *C. difficile* Is Encountered

Because prevention of organism transmission has proved difficult, control measures have also focused on reducing clinical illness when transmission does occur. Control of antimicrobial use, initially clindamycin and subsequently second- and third-generation cephalosporins, has been the most effective prevention strategy (Table 48.3) (106,107,211–213). In the case of clindamycin, outbreaks of CDAD have correlated with *C. difficile* resistance to clindamycin and have resolved with restriction of the antibiotic (66,106). The risk with cephalosporin use may be similar to that for clindamycin, because *C. difficile* is also resistant to cephalosporins. It has been proposed that "herd immunity" may be an important concept in susceptibility to *C. difficile* infection (214). Thus, it is likely that the majority of patients are "immune" to *C. difficile* as long as they are not given antimicrobials, but herd immunity diminishes in proportion to the number of patients taking antibiotics, the number of patients with CDAD, and the number of patients colonized with *C. difficile*.

Biologic prophylaxis of patients receiving antimicrobials has also been used to prevent *C. difficile* illness. Administration of the yeast *S. boulardii* to patients taking antibiotics successfully reduced the incidence of diarrhea, but did not reduce the incidence of CDAD (215). *Lactobacillus* species have also been recommended for the prevention of antibiotic-associated diarrhea, but controlled trials for prevention of CDAD have not been done (216). *Lactobacillus*-containing yogurt given to clindamycin-treated hamsters did not prevent *C. difficile* disease (217). *C. difficile* antibody harvested from bovine colostrum and milk has been shown to protect hamsters from *C. difficile* diarrhea and mortality, but no human data are available (218).

Prevention Strategy for the Future

A vaccine to prevent CDAD has been successful in the hamster model using a formalin-inactivated culture filtrate preparation administered by a number of routes (intranasal, intragastric, rectal, subcutaneous, intraperitoneal). Maximal prevention required both intranasal and intraperitoneal administration (219). Toxin vaccine approaches are attractive but require multiple administrations of the antigens and several weeks to become effective, a major drawback if unvaccinated patients are placed at immediate risk by antibiotic treatment in the hospital.

Studies of *C. difficile* colonization prevention in the hamster model of CDAD published in the 1980s suggested that administration of a nontoxigenic strain of *C. difficile* following antibiotic treatment produces some protection from subsequent challenge with a toxigenic strain of *C. difficile* (220,221). We used nontoxigenic strains of *C. difficile* isolated from asymptomatic patients to colonize hamsters and prevent disease from toxigenic *C. difficile* (222). Deliberate colonization of humans with nontoxigenic *C. difficile* to prevent CDAD has not been reported, but our data from four human epidemiologic studies over the past 12 years suggest the validity of a colonization approach to prevention of CDAD (75). Before patient prevention trials can occur, further safety and efficacy of colonization studies in animals and in human volunteers must be demonstrated.

In summary, CDAD continues to be the major identified cause of nosocomial diarrhea. Rates appear to be increasing, possibly related to the increased use of antimicrobial agents in the community and hospital. The best strategies for prevention continue to be rigorous compliance with infection control measures to prevent transmission of *C. difficile* to the patient, but perhaps more promising are efforts directed at controlling and manipulating antimicrobial use to minimize the risk of CDAD if transmission does occur. Finally, the future for prevention strategies may be the development of a *C. difficile* vaccine or biotherapeutic approaches that will rapidly restore patient resistance to *C. difficile* infection following antimicrobial treatment.

ACKNOWLEDGMENTS

Dr. Gerding and Dr. Johnson are both supported by Department of Veterans Affairs Research Service Merit Review Grants for the study of *C. difficile* disease pathogenesis and prevention.

REFERENCES

1. Finney JMT. Gastro-enterostomy for cicatrizing ulcer of the pylorus. *Bull Johns Hopkins Hosp* 1893;4:53–55.
2. Bartlett JG. Introduction. In: Rolfe RE, Finegold SM, eds. Clostridium difficile: *its role in intestinal disease.* New York: Academic Press, 1988:1–13.
3. Pettet JD, Baggenstoss AH, Dearing WH, et al. Postoperative pseudomembranous colitis. *Surg Gynecol Obstet* 1954;98: 546–552.
4. Wallace JF. Oral vancomycin treatment of staphylococcal enterocolitis. *N Engl J Med* 1965;272:1014–1015.
5. Khan MY, Hall WH. Staphylococcal enterocolitis treatment with oral vancomycin. *Ann Intern Med* 1966;65:1–8.
6. Hall JC, O'Toole E. Intestinal flora in new-born infants with a description of a new pathogenic anaerobe, *Bacillus difficilis. Am J Dis Child* 1935;49:390–402.
7. Snyder ML. The normal fecal flora of infants between two weeks and one year of age. *J Infect Dis* 1940;66:1–16.
8. Hambre DM, Raki G, McKnee CM, et al. The toxicity of penicillin as prepared for clinical use. *Am J Med Sci* 1943;206: 642–653.
9. Wood JS, Bennet IL, Yardley JH. Staphylococcal enterocolitis in chinchillas. *Bull Johns Hopkins Hosp* 1956;98:454–463.
10. Tedesco FJ, Barton RW, Alpers DH. Clindamycin-associated colitis. *Ann Intern Med* 1974;81:429–433.
11. Small JD. Fatal enterocolitis in hamsters given lincomycin hydrochloride. *Lab Animal Care* 1968;18:411–420.
12. Bartlett JG, Onderdonk AB, Cisneros RL, et al. Clindamycin-associated colitis in hamsters: Protection with vancomycin. *Gastroenterology* 1977;73:772–776.
13. Browne RA, Fekety R, Silva J, et al. The protective effect of vancomycin on clindamycin-induced colitis in hamsters. 1977;141: 183–192.
14. Larson HE, Parry JV, Price AB, et al. Undescribed toxin in pseudomembranous colitis. *BMJ* 1977;1:1246–1248.
15. Larson HE, Price AB. Pseudomembranous colitis: presence of clostridial toxin. *Lancet* 1977;2:1312–1314.
16. Rifkin GD, Fekety FR, Silva J, et al. Antibiotic-induced colitis implication of a toxin neutralised by *Clostridium sordellii* antitoxin. *Lancet* 1977;2:1103–1106.
17. Bartlett JG, Gorbach SL. Pseudomembranous enterocolitis (antibiotic-related colitis). *Adv Intern Med* 1977;22:455–476.
18. Bartlett JG, Chang TW, Gurwith M, et al. Antibiotic-associated pseudomembranous colitis due to toxin-producing clostridia. *N Engl J Med* 1978;298:531–534.
19. Bartlett JG, Onderdonk AB, Cisneros RL, et al. Clindamycin associated colitis due to a toxin-producing species of *Clostridium* in hamsters. *J Infect Dis* 1977;136:701–705.
20. Rifkin GD, Silva J, Fekety R. Gastrointestinal and systemic toxicity of fecal extracts from hamsters with clindamycin-induced colitis. *Gastroenterology* 1978;74:52–57.
21. Bartlett JG, Chang TW, Gurwith M, et al. Antibiotic-associated pseudomembranous colitis due to toxin-producing clostridia. *N Engl J Med* 1978;298:531–534.
22. George RH, Symmonds JM, Dimmock F, et al. Identification of *Clostridium difficile* as a cause of pseudomembranous colitis. *BMJ* 1978;1:695.
23. Taylor NS, Thorne GM, Bartlett JG. Separation of an enterotoxin from the cytotoxin of *Clostridium difficile. Clin Res* 1980; 28:285.
24. Alfa MJ, Kabani A, Lyerly D, et al. Characterization of a toxin A-negative, toxin B-positive strain of *Clostridium difficile* responsible for a nosocomial outbreak of *Clostridium difficile*-associated diarrhea. *J Clin Microbiol* 2000;38:2706–2714.
25. Sambol, SP, Tang JK, Merrigan MM, et al. Infection of hamsters with epidemiologically important strains of *Clostridium difficile. J Infect Dis* 2001;183:1760–1766.
26. Gerding DN, Olson MM, Peterson LR, et al. *Clostridium difficile*-associated diarrhea and colitis in adults: A prospective case-controlled epidemiologic study. *Arch Intern Med* 1986;146: 95–100.
27. McFarland LV, Mulligan M, Kwok RYY, et al. Nosocomial acquisition of *Clostridium difficile* infection. *N Engl J Med* 1989;320:204–210.
28. Clabots CR, Johnson S, Bettin KM, et al. Development of a rapid and efficient restriction endonuclease analysis typing system for *Clostridium difficile* and correlation with other typing systems. *J Clin Microbiol* 1993;31:1870–1875.
29. Mulligan ME, Peterson LR, Kwok RYY, et al. Immunoblots and plasmid fingerprints compared with serotyping and polyacrylamide gel electrophoresis for typing *Clostridium difficile. J Clin Microbiol* 1988;26:41–46.
30. Tabaqchali S, O'Farrell S, Holland D, et al. Method for the typing of *Clostridium difficile* based on polyacrylamide gel electrophoresis of [35S]methionine-labeled proteins. *J Clin Microbiol* 1986;23:197–198.
31. von Eichel-Streiber C, Laufenberg-Feldmann R, Sartingen S, et al. Comparative sequence analysis of the *Clostridium difficile* toxins A and B. *Mol Gen Genet* 1992;233:260–268.
32. Hofmann F, Busch C, Prepens U, et al. Localization of the glycosyltransferase activity of *Clostridium difficile* toxin B to the N-terminal part of the holotoxin. *J Biol Chem* 1997;272: 11074–11078.
33. Hundsberger T, Braun V, Weidmann M, et al. Transcription analysis of the genes *tcdA - E* of the pathogenicity locus of *Clostridium difficile. Eur J Biochem* 1997;244:735–742.
34. Bliss DZ, Johnson S, Clabots CR, et al. Comparison of cycloserine-cefoxitin-fructose agar (CCFA) and taurocholate-CCFA for recovery of *Clostridium difficile* during surveillance

of hospitalized patients. *Diagn Microbiol Infect Dis* 1997;29: 1–4.
35. Wilson KH, Kennedy MJ, Fekety FR. Use of sodium taurocholate to enhance spore recovery on a medium selective for *Clostridium difficile. J Clin Microbiol* 1982;5:443–446.
36. Clabots CR, Gerding SJ, Olson MM, et al. Detection of asymptomatic *Clostridium difficile* carriage by an alcohol shock procedure. *J Clin Microbiol* 1989;27:2386–2387.
37. Wilcox MH, Fawley WN, Parnell P. Value of lysozyme agar incorporation and alkaline thioglycollate exposure for the environmental recovery of *Clostridium difficile. J Hosp Infect* 2000; 44:65–69.
38. Kelly PJ, Peterson LR. The role of the clinical microbiology laboratory in the management of *Clostridium difficile*-associated diarrhea. *Infect Dis Clin North Am* 1993;7:277–293.
39. Johnson LL, McFarland LV, Dearing P, et al. Identification of *Clostridium difficile* in stool specimens by culture-enhanced gas-liquid chromatography. *J Clin Microbiol* 1989;27:2218–2221.
40. Sivsammye G, Sims HV. Presumptive identification of *Clostridium difficile* by detection of p-cresol in prepared peptone yeast glucose broth supplemented with p-hydroxyphenylacetic acid. *J Clin Microbiol* 1990;28:1851–1853.
41. Lyerly DM, Saum KE, MacDonald D, et al. Effect of toxins A and B given intragastrically to animals. *Infect Immun* 1985;47: 349–352.
42. Riegler M, Sedivy R, Pothoulakis C, et al. *Clostridium difficile* toxin B is more potent than toxin A in damaging human colonic epithelium in vitro. *J Clin Invest* 1995;95:2004–11.
43. Fluit AC, Wolfhagen MJHM, Verdonk GPHT, et al. Nontoxigenic strains of *C. difficile* lack the genes for both toxin A and Toxin B. *J Clin Microbiol* 1991;29:2666–2667.
44. von Eichel-Streiber C, Boquet P, Sauerborn M, et al. Large clostridial cytotoxins—a family of glycosyltransferases modifying small GTP-binding proteins. *Trends Microbiol* 1996;4: 375–82.
45. Hammond GA, Johnson JL. The toxigenic element of *Clostridium difficile* strain VPI 10463. *Microb Pathogen* 1995;19: 203–213.
46. Hammond GA, Lyerly DM, Johnson JL. Transcriptional analysis of the toxigenic element of *Clostridium difficile. Microb Pathogen* 1997;22:143–154.
47. Braun V, Hundsberger T, Leukel P, et al. Definition of the single integration site of the pathogenicity locus in *Clostridium difficile. Gene* 1996;181:29–38.
48. Frey SM, Wilkins TD. Localization of two epitopes recognized by monoclonal antibody PCG-4 on *Clostridium difficile* toxin A. *Infect Immun* 1992;60:2488–2492.
49. Chaves-Olarte E, Weidmann M, Eichel-Streiber C, et al. Toxins A and B from *Clostridium difficile* differ with respect to enzymatic potencies, cellular substrate specificities, and surface binding to cultured cells. *J Clin Invest* 1997;100:1734–1741.
50. Torres JF. Purification and characterization of toxin B from a strain of *Clostridium difficile* that does not produce toxin A. *J Med Microbiol* 1991;35:40–44.
51. Lyerly DM, Barroso LA, Wilkins TD, et al. Characterization of a toxin A-negative, toxin B-positive strain of *Clostridium difficile. Infect Immun* 1992;60:4633–4639.
52. Soehn F, Wagenknecht-Wiesner A, Leukel P, et al. Genetic rearrangements in the pathogenicity locus of *Clostridium difficile* strain 8864—implications for transcription, expression and enzymatic activity of toxins A and B. *Mol Gen Genet* 1998; 258: 222–232.
53. Borriello SP, Wren BW, Hyde S, et al. Molecular, immunological, and biological characterization of a toxin A-negative, toxin B-positive strain of *Clostridium difficile. Infect Immun* 1992;60: 4192–4199.
54. Delmée M, Avesani V. Virulence of ten serogroups of *Clostridium difficile* in hamsters. *J Med Microbiol* 1990;33:85–90.
55. Rupnik M, Braun V, Soehn F, et al. Characterization of polymorphisms in the toxin A and B genes of *Clostridium difficile. FEMS Microbiol Lett* 1997;148:197–202.
56. Rupnik M, Avesani V, Janc M, et al. A novel toxinotyping scheme and correlation of toxinotypes with serogroups of *Clostridium difficile* isolates. *J Clin Microbiol* 1998;36:2240–2247.
57. Sambol SP, Merrigan MM, Lyerly DM, et al. Toxin gene analysis of a variant strain of *Clostridium difficile* that causes human clinical disease. *Infect Immun* 2000;68:5480–5487.
58. von Eichel-Streiber C, Zec-Pirnat I, Grabnar M, et al. A nonsense mutation abrogates production of a functional enterotoxin A in *Clostridium difficile* toxinotype VIII strains of serogroups F and X. *FEMS Micribiol Lett* 1999;178:163–168.
59. Depitre C, Delmée M, Avesani V, et al. Serogroup F strains of *Clostridium difficile* produce toxin B but not toxin A. *J Med Microbiol* 1993;38:434–441.
60. Kato H, Kato N, Watanabe K, et al. Identification of toxin A-negative, toxin B-positive *Clostridium difficile* by PCR. *J Clin Microbiol* 1998;36:2178–82.
61. Johnson S, Kent SA, O'Leary KJ, et al. Fatal pseudomembranous colitis associated with a variant *Clostridium difficile* strain not detected by toxin A immunoassay. *Ann Intern Med* 2001; 135:434–438.
62. Stubbs S, Rupnik M, Gibert M, et al. Production of actin-specific ADP-ribosyltransferase (binary toxin) by strains of *Clostridium difficile. FEMS Microbiol Lett* 2000;186:307–312.
63. Cerquetti M, Molinari A, Sebastianelli A. Characterization of surface layer proteins from different *Clostridium difficile* clinical isolates. *Microb Pathog* 2000;28:363–372.
64. Blaser MJ, Pei Z. Pathogenesis of *Campylobacter fetus* infections. Critical role of the high molecular weight S-layer proteins in virulence. *J Infect Dis* 1993;167:696–706.
65. Dzink J, Bartlett JG. *In vitro* susceptibility of *Clostridium difficile* isolates from patients with antibiotic-associated diarrhea or colitis. *Antimicrob Agents Chemother* 1980;17:695–698.
66. Johnson S, Samore MH, Farrow KA, et al. Epidemics of diarrhea caused by a clindamycin-resistant strain of *Clostridium difficile* in four hospitals. *N Engl J Med* 1999;341:1645–1651.
67. Clabots CR, Shanholtzer CJ, Peterson LR, et al. *In vitro* activity of efrotomycin, ciprofloxacin, and six other antimicrobials against *Clostridium difficile. Diagn Microbiol Infect Dis* 1987;6: 49–52.
68. Burdon DW, Brown DJ, Youngs DJ, et al. Antibiotic susceptibility of *Clostridium difficile. J Antimicrob Chemother* 1979;5: 307–10.
69. Johnson S, Homann SR, Bettin KM, et al. Treatment of asymptomatic *Clostridium difficile* carriers (fecal excretors) with vancomycin or metronidazole. *Ann Intern Med* 1992;117:297–302.
70. Jang SS, Hansen LM, Breher JE, et al. Antimicrobial susceptibilities of equine isolates of *Clostridium difficile* and molecular characterization of metronidazole-resistant strains. *Clin Infect Dis* 1997;25[Suppl 2]:S266–S267.
71. Barbut F, Decré D, Burghoffer B, et al. Antimicrobial susceptibilities and serogroups of clinical strains of *Clostridium difficile* isolated in France in 1991 and 1997. *Antimicrob Agent Chemother* 1999;43:2607–2611.
72. Wong SS, Woo PC, Luk WK, et al. Susceptibility testing of *Clostridium difficile* against metronidazole and vancomycin by disk diffusion and Etest. *Diagn Microbiol Infect Dis* 1999;34: 1–6.
73. Clabots CR, Johnson S, Olson MM, et al. Acquisition of *Clostridium difficile* by hospitalized patients: evidence for colonized new admissions as the source of infection. *J Infect Dis* 1992;166:561–7.

74. Johnson S, Clabots CR, Linn FV, Olson MM, Peterson LR, Gerding DN. Nosocomial *Clostridium difficile* colonization and disease. *Lancet* 1990;336:97–100.
75. Shim JK, Johnson S, Samore MH, Bliss DZ, Gerding DN. Primary asymptomatic colonization by *Clostridium difficile* is associated with a decreased risk of subsequent *C. difficile* diarrhea. *Lancet* 1998;351:633–6.
76. Pothoulakis C, Sullivan R, Melnik DA, et al. *Clostridium difficile* toxin A stimulates intracellular calcium release and chemotactic response in human granulocytes. *J Clin Invest* 1988;81: 1741–1745.
77. Miller PD, Pothoulakis C, Baeker TR, et al. Macrophage-dependent stimulation of T cell-depleted spleen cells by *Clostridium difficile* toxin A and calcium ionophore. *Cell Immunol* 1990;126:155–63.
78. Gerding DN. *Clostridium difficile*-associated disease: a persistently plaguing problem. *APUA Newsletter* 1996;14:1–6.
79. Viscidi R, Laughon BE, Yolken R, et al. Serum antibody response to toxins A and B of *Clostridium difficile. J Infect Dis* 1983;148:93–100.
80. Aronsson B, Granstrom M, Mollby R, et al. Enzyme-linked immunosorbent assay (ELISA) for antibodies to *Clostridium difficile* toxins in patients with pseudomembranous colitis and antibiotic-associated diarrhoea. *J Immunol Methods* 1983;60: 341–350.
81. Johnson S, Gerding DN, Janoff EN. Systemic and mucosal antibody responses to toxin A in patients infected with *Clostridium difficile. J Infect Dis* 1992;166:1287–1294.
82. Warny M, Vaerman J-P, Avesani V, et al. Human antibody response to *Clostridium difficile* toxin A in relation to clinical course of infection. *Infect Immun* 1994;62:384–389.
83. Leung DYM, Kelly CP, Boguniewicz M, et al. Treatment with intravenously administered gamma globulin of chronic relapsing colitis induced by *Clostridium difficile* toxin. *J Pediatr* 1991; 118:633–637.
84. Salcedo J, Keates S, Pothoulakis C, et al. Intravenous gammaglobulin for severe *Clostridium difficile* colitis. *Gut* 1997;41: 366–370.
85. Aronsson B, Granstrom M, Mollby R, et al. Serum antibody response to *Clostridium difficile* toxins in patients with *Clostridium difficile* diarrhoea. *Infection* 1985;13:97–101.
86. Bacon AE, Fekety R. Immunoglobulin G directed against toxins A and B of *Clostridium difficile* in the general population and patients with antibiotic-associated diarrhea. *Diagn Microbiol Infect Dis* 1994;18:205–209.
87. Johnson S, Sypura WD, Gerding DN, et al. Selective neutralization of a bacterial enterotoxin by serum immunoglobulin A in response to mucosal disease. *Infect Immun* 1995;63: 3166–3173.
88. Stieglbauer KT, Gruber SA, Johnson S. Elevated serum antibody response to toxin A following splenic abscess due to *Clostridium difficile. Clin Infect Dis* 1995;20:160–162.
89. Perlmutter DH, Leichtner AM, Goldman H, et al. Chronic diarrhea associated with hypogammaglobulinemia and enteropathy in infants and children. *Dig Dis Sci* 1985;30:1149–1155.
90. Gryboyski JD, Pellerano R, Young N, et al. Positive role of *Clostridium difficile* infection in diarrhea in infants and children. *Am J Gastroenterol* 1991;86:685–689.
91. Kyne L, Warny M, Qamar A, et al. Asymptomatic carriage of *Clostridium difficile* and serum levels of IgG antibody against toxin A. *N Engl J Med* 2000;342:390–397.
92. Kyne L, Warny M, Qamar A, et al. Association between antibody response to toxin A and protection against recurrent *Clostridium difficile* diarrhea. *Lancet* 2001;357:189–193.
93. Warny M, Denie C, Delmée M, et al. Gamma globulin administration in relapsing *Clostridium difficile*- induced pseudomembranous colitis with a defective antibody response to toxin A. *Acta Clin Belg* 1995;50:36–39.
94. Hassett J, Meyers S, McFarland L, et al. Recurrent *Clostridium difficile* infection in a patient with selective IgG1 deficiency treated with intravenous immune globulin and *Saccharomyces boulardii. Clin Infect Dis* 1995;20[Suppl 2]:S266–S268.
95. Kim K, Pickering LK, DuPont HL, et al. *In vitro* and *in vivo* neutralizing activity of human colostrum and milk against purified toxins A and B of *Clostridium difficile. J Infect Dis* 1984; 150:57–62.
96. Kelly CP, Pothoulakis C, Orellana J, et al. Human colonic aspirates containing immunoglobulin A antibody to *Clostridium difficile* toxin A inhibit toxin A-receptor binding. *Gastroenterology* 1992;102:35–40.
97. Barbut F, Corthier G, Charpak Y, et al. Prevalence and pathogenicity of *Clostridium difficile* in hospitalized patients. *Arch Intern Med* 1996;156:1449–1454.
98. Gerding DN, Johnson S, Peterson LR, et al. Society for Healthcare Epidemiology of America position paper on *Clostridium difficile*-associated diarrhea and colitis. *Infect Control Hosp Epidemiol* 1995;16:459–477.
99. Anand A, Bashey B, Mir T, et al. Epidemiology, clinical manifestations, and outcome of *Clostridium difficile*-associated diarrhea. *Am J Gastroenterol* 1994;89:519–523.
100. Zadik PM, Moore AP. Antimicrobial associations of an outbreak of diarrhoea due to *Clostridium difficile. J Hosp Infect* 1998;39:189–193.
101. Impallomeni M, Galletly NP, Wort SJ, et al. Increased risk of diarrhoea caused by *Clostridium difficile* in elderly patients receiving cefotaxime. *BMJ* 1995;311:1345–1346.
102. Settle CD, Wilcox MH, Fawley WN, et al. Prospective study of the risk of *Clostridium difficile* diarrhea in elderly patients following treatment with cefotaxime or piperacillin-tazobactam. *Aliment Pharmacol Ther* 1998;12:1217–1223.
103. Cartmill TDI, Panigrahi H, Worsley MA, et al. Management and control of a large outbreak of diarrhoea due to *Clostridium difficile. J Hosp Infect* 1994;27:1–15.
104. Wilcox MH. Respiratory antibiotic use and *Clostridium difficile* infection: is it the drugs or is it the doctors? *Thorax* 2000;55: 633–634.
105. Bignardi GE. Risk factors for *Clostridium difficile* infection. *J Hosp Infect* 1998;40:1–15.
106. Pear SM, Williamson TH, Bettin KM, et al. Decrease in nosocomial *Clostridium difficile*-associated diarrhea by restricting clindamycin use. *Ann Intern Med* 1994;120:272–277.
107. Climo MW, Israel DS, Wong ES, et al. Hospital-wide restriction of clindamycin: effect on the incidence of *Clostridium difficile*-associated diarrhea and cost. *Ann Intern Med* 1998;128: 989–995.
108. Riley TV, Adams JE, O'Neill GL, et al. Gastrointestinal carriage of *Clostridium difficile* in cats and dogs attending veterinary clinics. *Epidemiol Infect* 1991;107:659–665.
109. Hirschhorn LR, Trnka Y, Onderdonk A, et al. Epidemiology of community-acquired *Clostridium difficile*-associated diarrhea. *J Infect Dis* 1994;169:127–133.
110. Riley TV, Cooper M, Bell B, et al. Community-acquired *Clostridium difficile*-associated diarrhea. *Clin Infect Dis* 1995;20 [Suppl 2]:S263–S265.
111. Johnson S, Adelmann A, Clabots CR, et al. Recurrences of *Clostridium difficile* diarrhea not caused by the original infecting organism. *J Infect Dis* 1989;159:340–343.
112. Stubbs SLJ, Brazier JS, O'Neill GL, et al. PCR targeted to the 16S-23S rRNA gene intergenic spacer region of *Clostridium difficile* and construction of a library consisting of 116 different PCR ribotypes. *J Clin Microbiol* 1999;37:461–463.
113. Samore M, Killgore G, Johnson S, et al. Multicenter typing

comparison of sporadic and outbreak *Clostridium difficile* isolates from geographically diverse hospitals. *J Infect Dis* 1997; 176:1233–1238.
114. Rupnik M, Brazier JS, Duerden BI, et al. Comparison of toxinotyping and PCR ribotyping of *Clostridium difficile* strains and description of novel toxinotypes. *Microbiology* 2001; 147:439–447.
115. Jumaa P, Wren B, Tabaqchali S. Epidemiology and typing of *Clostridium difficile. Eur J Gastroenterol Hepatol* 1996;8: 1035–1040.
116. Brazier JS, Holland D, O'Farrel S, et al. Proposed unified nomenclature for *Clostridium difficile* typing. *Lancet* 1994;343:1578–1579.
117. Brazier JS, Mulligan ME, Delmee M, et al. Preliminary findings of the international typing study on *Clostridium difficile. Clin Infect Dis* 1997;25[Suppl 2]:S199–S201.
118. Bliss DZ, Johnson S, Savik K, et al. Acquisition of *Clostridium difficile* and *Clostridium difficile*-associated diarrhea in hospitalized patients receiving tube feeding. *Ann Intern Med* 1998;129: 1012–1019.
119. Brooks SE, Veal RO, Kramer M, et al. Reduction in incidence of *Clostridium difficile*-associated diarrhea in an acute care hospital and a skilled nursing facility following replacement of electronic thermometers with single-use disposables. *Infect Control Hosp Epidemiol* 1992;13:98–103.
120. Thibault A, Miller MA, Gaese C. Risk factors for the development of *Clostridium difficile*-associated diarrhea during a hospital outbreak. *Infect Control Hosp Epidemiol* 1991;12:345–348.
121. Pierce PF Jr, Wilson R, Silva J Jr, et al. Antibiotic-associated pseudomembranous colitis: an epidemiologic investigation of a cluster of cases. *J Infect Dis* 1982;145:269–274.
122. Gerding DN. Is there a relationship between vancomycin-resistant enterococcal infection and *Clostridium difficile* infection? *Clin Infect Dis* 1997;25[Suppl 2]:S206–S210.
123. Rafferty ME, McCormick MI, Bopp LH, et al. Vancomycin-resistant enterococci in stool specimens submitted for *Clostridium difficile* cytotoxin assay. *Infect Control Hosp Epidemiol* 1997; 18:342–344.
124. Garbutt JM, Littenberg B, Evanoff BA, et al. Enteric carriage of vancomycin-resistant *Enterococcus faecium* in patients tested for *Clostridium difficile. Infect Control Hosp Epidemiol* 1999;20: 664–670.
125. Olson MM, Shanholtzer CJ, Lee JT Jr, et al. Ten years of prospective *Clostridium difficile*-associated disease surveillance and treatment at the Minneapolis VA Medical Center, 1982–1991. *Infect Control Hosp Epidemiol* 1994;15:371–381.
126. Trudel JL, Deschenes M, Mayrand S, et al. Toxic megacolon complicating pseudomembranous enterocolitis. *Dis Colon Rectum* 1995;38:1033–1038.
127. Jobe BA, Grasley A, Deveney KE, et al. *Clostridium difficile* colitis: an increasing hospital-acquired illness. *Am J Surg* 1995;169: 480–483.
128. Putterman C, Rubinow A. Reactive arthritis associated with *Clostridium difficile* pseudomembranous colitis. *Semin Arthritis Rheum* 1993;22:420–426.
129. Zuckerman E, Kanel G, Chung H, et al. Low albumin gradient ascites complicating severe pseudomembranous colitis. *Gastroenterology* 1997;112:991–994.
130. Wilcox MH, Fawley WN, Settle CD, et al. Recurrence of symptoms in *Clostridium difficile* infection-relapse or reinfection? *J Hosp Infect* 1998;38:93–100.
131. O'Neill GL, Beaman MH, Riley TV. Relapse versus reinfection with *Clostridium difficile. Epidemiol Infect* 1991;107:627–635.
132. McFarland LV, Surawicz CM, Rubin M, et al. Recurrent *Clostridium difficile* disease: epidemiology and clinical characteristics. *Infect Control Hosp Epidemiol* 1999;20:43–50.
133. Gorbach SL. *Clostridium difficile*-associated diarrhea. *Infect Dis Clin Practice* 1996;5:84.
134. LaMont JT, Trnka YM. Therapeutic implications of *Clostridium difficile* toxin during relapse of chronic inflammatory bowel disease. *Lancet* 1980;1:381–383.
135. Greenfield C, Aguilar Ramirez JR, Pounder RE, et al. *Clostridium difficile* and inflammatory bowel disease. *Gut* 1983;24: 713–717.
136. Bolton RP, Sheriff RJ, Read AE. *Clostridium difficile* associated diarrhoea: a role in inflammatory bowel disease. *Lancet* 1980;1: 383–384.
137. Keighley MRB, Youngs D, Johnson M, et al. *Clostridium difficile* toxin in acute diarrhoea complicating inflammatory bowel disease. *Gut* 1982;23:410–414.
138. Willingham FF, Chavez ET, Taylor DN, et al. Diarrhea and *Clostridium difficile* infection in Latin American patients with AIDS. *Clin Infect Dis* 1998;27:487–493.
139. Lu SS, Schwartz JM, Simon DM, et al. *Clostridium difficile*-associated diarrhea in patients with HIV positivity and AIDS: a prospective controlled study. *Am J Gastroenterol* 1994;89: 1226–1229.
140. Barbut F, Depitre C, Delmee M, et al. Comparison of enterotoxin production, cytotoxin production, serogrouping, and antimicrobial susceptibilities to *Clostridium difficile* strains isolated from AIDS and human immunodeficiency virus-negative patients. *J Clin Microbiol* 1993:31:740–742.
141. Gerding D, Brazier JS. Optimal methods for identifying *Clostridium difficile* infections. *Clin Infect Dis* 1993;16: S439–S442.
142. Bergstein JM, Kramer A, Wittman DH, et al. Pseudomembranous colitis: how useful is endoscopy? *Surg Endosc* 1990;4: 217–219.
143. Gebhard RL, Gerding DN, Olson MM, et al. Clinical and endoscopic findings in patients early in the course of *Clostridium difficile*-associated pseudomembranous colitis. *Am J Med* 1985;78:45–48.
144. Gerding DN. Diagnosis of *Clostridium difficile*-associated disease: patient selection and test perfection. *Am J Med* 1996;100: 485–486.
145. Manabe YC, Vinetz JM, Moore RD, et al. *Clostridium difficile* colitis: an efficient clinical approach to diagnosis. *Ann Intern Med* 1995;123:835–840.
146. Peterson LR, Olson MM, Shanholtzer CJ, et al. Results of a prospective, 18-month clinical evaluation of culture, cytotoxin testing, and Culturette brand (CDT) latex testing in the diagnosis of *Clostridium difficile*-associated diarrhea. *Diagn Microbiol Infect Dis* 1988;10:85–91.
147. Lyerly DM, Neville LM, Evans DT, et al. Multicenter evaluation of the *Clostridium difficile* TOX A/B TEST. *J Clin Microbiol* 1998;36:184–190.
148. Lozniewski A, Rabaud C, Dotto E, et al. Laboratory diagnosis of *Clostridium difficile*-associated diarrhea and colitis: usefulness of Premier Cytoclone A+B enzyme immunoassay for combined detection of stool toxins and toxigenic *C. difficile* strains. *J Clin Microbiol* 2001;39:1996–1998.
149. Vargas SO, Horensky D, Onderdonk AB. Evaluation of a new enzyme immunoassay for *Clostridium difficile* toxin A. *J Clin Pathol* 197;50:996–1000.
150. Shanholtzer CJ, Willard KE, Holter JJ, et al. Comparison of VIDAS *C. difficile* toxin A immunoassay (CDA) with *C. difficile* culture, cytotoxin, and latex test. *J Clin Microbiol* 1992; 30:1837–1840.
151. Mundy LS, Shanholtzer CJ, Willard KE, et al. Laboratory detection of *Clostridium difficile*: a comparison of media and incubation systems. *Am J Clin Pathol* 1995;103:52–56.
152. George WL, Sutter VL, Citron D, et al. Selective and differen-

tial medium for isolation of *Clostridium difficile. J Clin Microbiol* 1979;9:214–219.
153. Staneck JL, Weckbach LS, Allen SD, et al. Multicenter evaluation of four methods for *Clostridium difficile* detection: ImmunoCard *C. difficile,* cytotoxin assay, culture, and latex agglutination. *J Clin Microbiol* 1996;34:2718–2721.
154. Lyerly DM, Barroso LA, Wilkins TD. Identification of the latex-reactive protein of *Clostridium difficile* as glutamate dehydrogenase. *J Clin Microbiol* 1991;29:2639–2642.
155. Lyerly DM, Wilkins TD. Commercial latex test for *Clostridium difficile* toxin A does not detect toxin A. *J Clin Microbiol* 1986; 23:622–623.
156. Landry ML, Topal J, Ferguson D, et al. Evaluation of Biosite Triage *Clostridium difficile* panel for rapid detection of *Clostridium difficile* in stool samples. *J Clin Microbiol* 2001;39: 1855–1858.
157. Gumerlock PH, Tang YJ, Meyers FJ, et al. Use of the polymerase chain reaction for the specific and direct detection of *Clostridium difficile* in human feces. *Rev Infect Dis* 1991; 13:1053–1060.
158. Gumerlock PH, Tang YJ, Weiss JB, et al. Specific detection of toxigenic strains of *Clostridium difficile* in stool specimens. *J Clin Microbiol* 1993;31:507–511.
159. Kato N, Ou CY, Kato H, et al. Identification of toxigenic *Clostridium difficile* by the polymerase chain reaction. *J Clin Microbiol* 1991;29:33–37.
160. Kato N, Ou CY, Kato H, et al. Detection of toxigenic *Clostridium difficile* in stool specimens by the polymerase chain reaction. *J Infect Dis* 1993;167:455–458.
161. Boondeekhun HS, Gurtler V, Odd ML, et al. Detection of *Clostridium difficile* enterotoxin gene in clinical specimens by the polymerase chain reaction. *J Med Microbiol* 1993;38: 384–387.
162. Shanholtzer CJ, Peterson LR, Olson MM, et al. Prospective study of Gram-stained stool smears in diagnosis of *Clostridium difficile* colitis. *J Clin Microbiol* 1983;17:906–908.
163. Guerrant RL, Araujo V, Soares E, et al. Measurement of fecal lactoferrin as a marker of fecal leukocytes. *J Clin Microbiol* 1992;30:1238–1242.
164. Schleupner MA, Garner DC, Sosnowski KM, et al. Concurrence of *Clostridium difficile* toxin A enzyme-linked immunosorbent assay, fecal lactoferrin assay, and clinical criteria with *C. difficile* cytotoxin titer in two patient cohorts. *J Clin Microbiol* 1995;33:1755–1759.
165. Pesce CM, Colacino R, Martelli M. Autopsy study of pseudomembranous colitis: characteristics of the affected population and antibiotic involved. *Acta Gastroenterol Bel* 1984;47: 58–63.
166. Tedesco FJ. Pseudomembranous colitis: pathogenesis and therapy. *Med Clin North Am* 1982;66:655–664.
167. Sumner HW, Tedesco FJ. Rectal biopsy in clindamycin-associated colitis: an analysis of 23 cases. *Arch Pathol* 1975;99: 237–241.
168. Peterson LR, Gerding DN. Antimicrobial agents in *Clostridium difficile*-associated intestinal disease. In: Rambaud J-C, Ducluzeau R, eds. Clostridium difficile-*associated intestinal diseases.* Paris: Springer-Verlag, 1990:115–127.
169. Hospital Infection Control Practices Advisory Committee (HICPAC) Recommendations for preventing the spread of vancomycin resistance. *Infect Control Hosp Epidemiol* 1995;16:105–113.
170. Elmer GW, Surawicz CM, McFarland LV. Biotherapeutic Agents. *JAMA* 1996;275:870–876.
171. McFarland LV, Surawicz CM, Greenberg RN, et al. Randomized placebo-controlled trial of *Saccharomyces boulardii* in combination with standard antibiotics for *Clostridium difficile* disease. *JAMA* 1994;271:1913–1918.
172. Teasley DG, Gerding DN, Olson MM, et al. Prospective randomized trial of metronidazole versus vancomycin for *Clostridium difficile*-associated diarrhea and colitis. *Lancet* 1983;2: 1043–1046.
173. Keighley MR, Burdon DW, Arabi Y, et al. Randomized controlled trial of vancomycin for pseudomembranous colitis and postoperative diarrhoea. *BMJ* 1978;2:1667–1669.
174. Zimmerman MJ, Bak A, Sutherland LR. Review article: treatment of *Clostridium difficile* infection. *Aliment Pharmacol Ther* 1997;11:1003–1012.
175. Fekety R. Guidelines for the diagnosis and management of *Clostridium difficile*-associated diarrhea and colitis. *Am J Gastroenterol* 1997;92:739–750.
176. Novak E, Lee JG, Seckman CE, et al. Unfavorable effect of atropine-diphenoxylate (Lomotil) therapy in lincomycin-caused diarrhea. *JAMA* 1976;235:1451–1454.
177. Wilcox MH, Howe R. Diarrhoea caused by *Clostridium difficile*: response time for treatment with metronidazole and vancomycin. *J Antimicrob Chemother* 1995;36:673–679.
178. Finegold SM, George WL. Therapy directed against *Clostridium difficile* and its toxins: complications of therapy. In: Rolfe RD, George WL, eds. Clostridium difficile: *its role in intestinal disease.* New York: Academic Press, 1988:341–357.
179. Mogg GAG, George RH, Youngs D, et al. Randomized controlled trial of colestipol in antibiotic-associated colitis. *Br J Surg* 1982;69:137–139.
180. Dudley MN, McLaughlin JC, Carrington G, et al. Oral bacitracin versus vancomycin therapy for *Clostridium difficile*-induced diarrhea: a randomized, double-blind trial. *Arch Intern Med* 1986;146:1101–1104.
181. Young GP, Ward PB, Bayley N, et al. Antibiotic-associated colitis due to *Clostridium difficile*: double-blind comparison of vancomycin with bacitracin. *Gastroenterology* 1985;89:1038–1045.
182. Wenisch C, Parschalk B, Hasenhundl M, et al. Comparison of vancomycin, teicoplanin, metronidazole, and fusidic acid for the treatment of *Clostridium difficile*-associated diarrhea. *Clin Infect Dis* 1996;22:813–818.
183. deLalla F, Nicolin R, Rinaldi E, et al. Prospective study of oral teicoplanin versus oral vancomycin for therapy of pseudomembranous colitis and *Clostridium difficile*-associated diarrhea. *Antimicrob Agents Chemother* 1992;36:2192–2196.
184. Bolton RP, Culshaw MA. Fecal metronidazole concentrations during oral and intravenous therapy for antibiotic-associated colitis due to *Clostridium difficile. Gut*1986;27:1169–1172.
185. Ings RM, McFadzean JA, Ormerod WE. The fate of metronidazole and its implications in chemotherapy. *Xenobiotica* 1975; 5:223–235.
186. Kleinfeld DI, Sharpe RJ, Donta ST. Parenteral therapy for antibiotic-associated pseudomembranous colitis. *J Infect Dis* 1988;157:389.
187. Guzman R, Kirkpatrick J, Forward K, et al. Failure of parenteral metronidazole in the treatment of pseudomembranous colitis. *J Infect Dis* 1988;158:1146.
188. Fekety R, Silva J, Kauffman C, et al. Treatment of antibiotic-associated *Clostridium difficile* colitis with oral vancomycin: comparison of two dosage regimens. *Am J Med* 1989;86:15–19.
189. Sanchez JL, Gerding DN, Olson MM, et al. Metronidazole susceptibility in *Clostridium difficile* isolates recovered from cases of *C. difficile*-associated disease treatment failures and successes. *Anaerobe* 1999;5:205–208.
190. Fekety R, Shah AB. Diagnosis and treatment of *Clostridium difficile* colitis. *JAMA* 1993;269:71–75.
191. Surawicz CM, McFarland LV, Elmer G, et al. Treatment of recurrent *Clostridium difficile* colitis with vancomycin and *Saccharomyces boulardii. Am J Gastroenterol* 1989;84:1285–1287.
192. Gorbach SL, Chang T-W, Goldin B. Successful treatment of

relapsing *Clostridium difficile* colitis with lactobacillus GG. *Lancet* 1987;2:1519.

193. Tvede M, Rask-Madsen J. Bacteriotherapy for chronic relapsing *Clostridium difficile* diarrhea in six patients. *Lancet* 1989;1: 1156–1160.
194. Seal D, Borriello SP, Barclay F, et al. Treatment of relapsing *Clostridium difficile* diarrhea by administration of a non-toxigenic strain. *Eur J Clin Microbiol* 1987;6:51–53.
195. Bassetti S, Frei R, Zimmerli W. Fungemia with *Saccharomyces cerevesiae* after treatment with *Saccharomyces boulardii. Am J Med* 1998;105:71–72.
196. Tedesco FJ, Gordon D, Fortson WC. Approach to patients with multiple relapses of antibiotic-associated pseudomembranous colitis. *Am J Gastroenterol* 1985;80:867–868.
197. Moncino MD, Falletta JM. Multiple relapses of *Clostridium difficile*-associated diarrhea in a cancer patient: successful control with long-term cholestyramine therapy. *Am J Pediatr Hematol Oncol* 1992;14:361–364.
198. Buggy BP. Fekety R, Silva J Jr. Therapy of relapsing *Clostridium difficile*-associated diarrhea and colitis with the combination of vancomycin and rifampin. *J Clin Gastroenterol* 1987;9:155–159.
199. Triadafilopoulos G, Hallstone AE. Acute abdomen as the first presentation of pseudomembranous colitis. *Gastroenterology* 1991;101:685–691.
200. Morris JB, Zollinger RM, Stellato TA. Role of surgery in antibiotic-induced pseudomembranous colitis. *Am J Surg* 1990;160: 535–539.
201. Chatila W, Manthous CA. *Clostridium difficile* causing sepsis and an acute abdomen in critically ill patients. *Crit Care Med* 1995;23:1146–1150.
202. Lowenkron SE, Waxner J, Khullar P, et al. *Clostridium difficile* infection as a cause of severe sepsis. *Intensive Care Med* 1996; 22:990.
203. Lipsett PA, Samantaray DK, Tam ML, et al. Pseudomembranous colitis: a surgical disease? *Surgery* 1994;116:491–496.
204. Grundfest-Broniatowski S, Quader M, Alexander F, et al. *Clostridium difficile* colitis in the critically ill. *Dis Colon Rectum* 1996;39:619–623.
205. Bradbury AW, Barrett S. Surgical aspects of *Clostridium difficile* colitis. *Br J Surg* 1997;84:150–159.
206. Johnson S, Gerding DN. *Clostridium difficile* infection. *Clin Infect Dis* 1998;26:1027–1036.
207. Johnson S, Gerding DN, Olson MM, et al. Prospective, controlled study of vinyl glove use to interrupt *Clostridium difficile* nosocomial transmission. *Am J Med* 1990;88:137–140.
208. Kaatz GW, Gitlin SD, Schaberg DR, et al. Acquisition of *Clostridium difficile* from the hospital environment. *Am J Epidemiol* 1988;127:1289–1294.
209. Wilcox MH, Fawley WN. Hospital disinfectants and spore formation by *Clostridium difficile. Lancet* 2000;356:1324
210. Olson MM, Shanholtzer MT, Lee JT Jr, et al. CDAD rates—reply. *Infect Control Hosp Epidemiol* 1995;16:64–65.
211. McNulty C, Logan M, Donald IP, et al. Successful control of *Clostridium difficile* infection in an elderly care unit through use of a restrictive antibiotic policy. *J Antimicrob Chemother* 1997; 40:707–711.
212. Ludlam H, Brown N, Sule O, et al. An antibiotic policy associated with reduced risk of *Clostridium difficile*-associated diarrhoea. *Age Ageing* 1999;28:578–580.
213. Freeman J, Wilcox MH. Antibiotics and *Clostridium difficile. Microbes Infection* 1999;1:377–384.
214. Starr JM, Rogers TR, Impallomeni M. Hospital-acquired *Clostridium difficile* diarrhoea and herd immunity. *Lancet* 1997;349:426–428.
215. Surawicz CM, Elmer GW, Speelman P, et al. Prevention of antibiotic-associated diarrhea by *Saccharomyces boulardii*: A prospective study. *Gastroenterology* 1989;96:981–988.
216. Siitonen S, Vapaatalo H, Salminen S, et al. Effect of *Lactobacillus* GG yogurt in prevention of antibiotic associated diarrhea. *Ann Med* 1990;22:57–59.
217. Kotz CM, Peterson LR, Moody JA, et al. Effect of yogurt on clindamycin-induced *Clostridium difficile* colitis in hamsters. *Dig Dis Sci* 1992;37:129–132.
218. Lyerly DM, Bostwick EF, Binion SB, et al. Passive immunization of hamsters against disease caused by *Clostridium difficile* by use of bovine immunoglobulin G concentrate. *Infect Immun* 1991;59:2215–2218.
219. Torres JF, Lyerly DM, Hill JE, et al. Evaluation of formalin-inactivated *Clostridium difficile* vaccines administered by parenteral and mucosal routes of immunization in hamsters. Infect Immun 1995;63:4619–4627.
220. Wilson KH, Sheagren JN. Antagonism of toxigenic *Clostridium difficile* by nontoxigenic *C. difficile. J Infect Dis* 1983;147: 733–736.
221. Borriello SP, Barclay FE. Protection of hamsters against *Clostridium difficile* ileo-caecaecitis by prior colonization with non-pathogenic strains. *J Med Microbiol* 1985;19:339–350.
222. Gerding DN. Colonization for the prevention of *Clostridium difficile* disease. *Anaerobe* 1999;5:195–199.

49

AEROMONAS, PLESIOMONAS, AND *EDWARDSIELLA*

J. MICHAEL JANDA
SHARON L. ABBOTT
DUC J. VUGIA

AEROMONAS

Description

The genus *Aeromonas* consists of oxidase-positive, gram-negative, facultatively anaerobic bacilli that ferment D-glucose as a sole source of energy (1). Although the genus originally resided within the family Vibrionaceae, with which it shares many phenotypic features, recent phylogenetic data indicate that aeromonads form a distinct lineage within the gamma subclass of the Proteobacteria (2,3). Therefore, members of this genus have been transferred to a family of their own, the Aeromonadaceae (4). The significant events in the history of *Aeromonas* as a human pathogen have been recently reviewed (5). Aeromonads are well-recognized pathogens in a number of clinical settings. These include septicemia in immunocompromised or cirrhotic patients, wound infection in traumatized persons exposed to freshwater sources, and rarely a number of other infectious processes, including peritonitis, hepatobiliary infections, ocular disease, endocarditis, and meningitis. Although controversy still surrounds the role of aeromonads as a major cause of gastroenteritis, convincing evidence indicates that at least some fecal isolates, if not many, are the cause of acute and severe cases of gastroenteritis.

Aeromonas species are routinely isolated from soil and freshwater environments and can be recovered from virtually all freshwater sources in the United States except hot springs (6). They can be recovered from estuaries and occasionally from marine life, such as shellfish (7,8). Aeromonad densities peak during the summer months, when warmer water temperatures lead to increased numbers of these microorganisms. As a result, aeromonads may be introduced into fresh produce, meat products (beef, poultry, pork), and dairy products (raw milk, ice cream) via contaminated water (9–11). The isolation of *Aeromonas* species from such a large number of foods and environmental sources, particularly during the summer, has made it difficult to link *Aeromonas*-associated gastroenteritis to specific food vehicles or ecologic niches.

The paramount association between *Aeromonas* and diseases of animals has concerned the fishing industry (12,13). Strains of *Aeromonas* that grow better at lower temperatures (25°C), termed *psychrophilic strains,* have been definitively linked to severe infections in fish, such as furunculosis and motile *Aeromonas* septicemia. This genus has caused the fishing industry, particularly salmon and catfish farms, to suffer enormous economic losses. In addition, many sporadic cases or outbreaks of infection in a variety of animals have been reported during the past several decades; these include illnesses in frogs, pigs, cattle, birds, and marine animals, such as seals and dolphins.

Microbiology

Morphologic and Cultural Characteristics

Aeromonads are typical gram-negative, facultatively anaerobic bacilli with a length of 1 to 3 μm and a width of 0.3 to 1.0 μm. Capsules, which can be detected by light microscopy of India ink-stained preparations, are produced by at least some strains, particularly those associated with two common serogroups, O:11 and O:34 (14,15). Most aeromonads grow well on selective media, such as MacConkey, Hektoen enteric (HE), and xylose–lysine–desoxycholate (XLD) agars. On nonselective media, such as blood, nutrient, and heart infusion agars, they are typically buff in appearance. Some strains elaborate a melanin-like pigment that produces a brownish discoloration to the agar surface.

J. M. Janda and **S. L. Abbott:** Microbial Diseases Laboratory, Division of Communicable Disease Control, California Department of Health Services, Berkeley, California

D. J. Vugia: Disease Investigation and Surveillance Branch, Division of Communicable Disease Control, California Department of Health Services, Berkeley, California

Such pigment-producing strains are most commonly associated with environmental species that infect fish or live in aquatic biospheres, such as *Aeromonas salmonicida* (16), certain biogroups of *Aeromonas media,* and isolates of *Aeromonas bestiarum* (17).

Structural Features

Most aeromonads are motile via a single polar flagellum. Several morphologically and antigenically distinct pili (rigid, flexible, wavy) have been isolated from the three most common species involved in human disease—namely, *Aeromonas hydrophila, Aeromonas veronii* biovar sobria, and *Aeromonas caviae.* Two classes of type IV pilins have been detected in these species. One class, the Tap pilins, have a molecular mass of approximately 17 kd and are encoded by a Tap biogenesis gene cluster (18,19). A second class of type IV pilins with a molecular mass ranging from 19 to 23 kd, the bundle-forming pilins (Bfps), are poorly characterized on a genetic basis (19,20). Recently, several different *Aeromonas* species (*A. hydrophila, A. veronii*), in addition to *A. salmonicida,* have been shown to possess a regular paracrystalline surface (S) layer that is external to the outer membrane and is composed of homogeneous protein subunits (21). These strains can be phenotypically recognized by their ability to auto-agglutinate or aggregate in broth after boiling (6). Aeromonads also display 30 to 40 distinct whole cell proteins by sodium dodecyl sulfate–polyacrylamide gel electrophoresis (SDS-PAGE); at least four to five major outer membrane proteins can be recognized in most isolates (22). The lipopolysaccharide (LPS) consists of a ladder-like construction of side chains detected by PAGE and silver staining, typical of gram-negative enteric organisms such as *Escherichia coli* and *Salmonella*; many antigenic variations in LPS composition exist (23). The LPS of some *Aeromonas* strains cross-reacts with *Vibrio cholerae* O139 biotype Bengal (24).

Biochemical Characteristics and Enzymatic Properties

One of the most interesting aspects of *Aeromonas* physiology is the vast array of substrates that the genus can utilize (25). Many isolates can ferment diverse groups of carbohydrates, such as monosaccharides, disaccharides, trisaccharides, and alcohol sugars (1). Their enzymatic machinery also is substantial; they elaborate more than 20 different extracellular enzymes, including hemolysins, proteases, DNase, RNase, gelatinase, elastase, chitinase, amylase, chondroitinase, esterase, and fibrinolysin.

Possibly one of the most difficult identifications in the clinical laboratory involves distinguishing *Aeromonas* isolates from phenotypically similar oxidase-positive members of the family Vibrionaceae (26). The problem is particularly acute in regard to the separation of *Aeromonas* from nonhalophilic *Vibrio* species because of the emergence of *V. cholerae* organisms in Southeast Asia that are resistant to the vibriostatic agent O/129 (26); the strain was recently introduced into the United States. In addition to this dilemma is the problem of phenotypically distinguishing *A. caviae* from *Vibrio fluvialis* (26). Although aeromonads by far predominate over vibriones in clinical specimens in the United States, their actual laboratory identification is often incorrect (aeromonads are misidentified as vibriones). Strains belonging to this family should be screened by a variety of biochemical techniques (salt tolerance, resistance to the vibriostatic agent O/129, string test, gas from glucose, growth on thiosulfate–citrate–bile salts–sucrose, or TCBS agar) to ensure their appropriate genus assignment (Table 49.1). For difficult strains or those possessing unusual properties, supplementary tests may be required.

TABLE 49.1. SEPARATION OF *AEROMONAS, PLESIOMONAS,* AND *VIBRIO* SPECIES WITH SCREENING TESTS

Characteristic	*Vibrio* Nonhalophilic	*Vibrio* Halophilic	*Aeromonas*	Plesiomonas
Growth on TCBS	+	+	–	–
Growth 0% NaCl	+	–	+	+
Growth 6% NaCl	+	+	–	–
O/129 (10 μg)	S[a]	V	R	S
O/129 (150 μg)	S[a]	V	R	S
String test	+	+	–	–
Ornithine decarboxylase	+	V	–[b]	+
Glucose (gas)	–	–[b]	+[b]	–

[a]An increasing number of *V. cholerae* O1 and non-O1 strains are becoming resistant.
[b]For most species.
S, susceptible (zone); V, variable (species-dependent); R, resistant; TCBS, thiosulfate–citrate–bile salts–sucrose agar.

Biochemical Identification and Species Designation

Both the number of species and the phylogenetic depth of the genus *Aeromonas* continue to increase. At present, at least 14 different species are recognized within the genus, 10 of which have been isolated from clinical specimens (Table 49.2). Only five of these 14 species have been unequivocally established as human pathogens. The identification of *Aeromonas* isolates to individual species, particularly in the clinical laboratory, is fraught with many difficulties (Table 49.3). Most commercial systems currently do not have the capability to identify most *Aeromonas* isolates to their correct genomospecies accurately. Newly described *Aeromonas* species are missing from most commercial databases at present. A further obstacle is the fact that many of the best tests for distinguishing among different *Aeromonas* species involve unusual phenotypic properties and are not included in most commercial identification systems (27, 28). However, several approaches are possible (29). At a minimum, *Aeromonas* strains should be identified to phenospecies (a group of genetically distinct species that cannot be separated biochemically) level; this approach would result in the identification of more than 90% of all aeromonads as either *A. hydrophila, A. caviae,* or *A. veronii* biovar sobria. Most commercial systems have the capacity to identify aeromonads to this level. The number of tests required for such identification is small, usually five or six. Simplified dichotomic approaches to such identifications have been published (30). In a number of circumstances, definitive genomospecies identification should be entertained, a process normally requiring the performance of more than 20 conventional biochemical tests (27). These circumstances include chronic or recurring infections involving aeromonads, recovery of stool isolates from cancer patients predisposed to systemic infection by some species, hospitalization of children for prolonged bouts of bloody diarrhea, and publication of descriptions of unusual clinical features or new presentations associated with the genus *Aeromonas.*

Isolation Methods

Aeromonads grow well on most of the selective and differential agars commonly used for fecal workups, such as MacConkey, HE, XLD, desoxycholate, and blood agars. Because the plating efficiencies of some strains (or species), such as *A. hydrophila* and *A. veronii,* are poor on one or more selective media, a nonselective agar (such as blood) should be included in fecal workups to ensure the recovery of aeromonads during the acute phase of an illness. Another problem relates to the fact that many strains of *Aeromonas* are sucrose-positive and some species (e.g., *A. caviae*) are lactose-positive (e.g., on MacConkey), so that certain media, like HE, are unsuitable for their recovery. Blood agar, with or without 20 to 30 μg of ampicillin per milliliter (to which most aeromonads are resistant), has gained favor as a common medium to isolate these bacteria from diarrheal specimens (31). Blood agar has the additional advantage that individual colonies can be screened for oxidase and indole positivity directly from the plate. One difficulty with this approach is that *Aeromonas trota* is ampicillin-susceptible and therefore cannot be isolated on ampicillin-containing media; approximately 5% of other aeromonads are also susceptible to ampicillin and are likely to be missed on ampicillin-containing media. If blood agar is not used, lactose-negative colonies can be picked and screened to Kliger iron agar (KIA) or triple sugar iron agar (TSI) and urea slants and subsequently worked up if appropriate reactions

TABLE 49.2. *AEROMONAS* SPECIES INVOLVED IN HUMAN DISEASE

Category	*Aeromonas* Species	Anatomic Specimens Isolated from
Major human pathogens	*A. hydrophila*	All major sites
	A. caviae	All major sites
	A. veronii (biovar sobria)	All major sites
Minor human pathogens	*A. veronii* (biovar veronii)	Feces, blood, wound, gallbladder, lung, sinus
	A. jandaei	Feces, blood, wound
	A. schubertii	Blood, wound
Isolated from humans; pathogenicity undetermined	*A. allosaccharophila*	Feces
	A. bestiarum	Feces
	A. media	Feces
	A. salmonicida[a]	Feces
	A. trota	Feces, appendix
Environmental species	*A. encheleia*	None at present
	A. eucrenophila	None at present
	A. popoffii	None at present
	A. sobria	None at present

[a]Some mesophilic strains of *A. salmonicida* are distinct from psychrophilic isolates that infect fish.

TABLE 49.3. MAJOR DISTINGUISHING BIOCHEMICAL FEATURES OF *AEROMONAS* SPECIES RECOVERED FROM CLINICAL SPECIMENS

Test	*A. hydrophila*	*A. caviae*	*A. veronii*[a]	*A. jandaei*	*A. schubertii*	*A. trota*[b]
Lysine decarboxylase	+	–	+	+	+	+
Ornithine decarboxylase	–	–	–	–	–	–
Arginine dihydrolase	+	+	+	+	+	+
Voges–Proskauer	+	–	+	+	+	–
Esculin hydrolysis	+	+	–	–	–	–
Acid from:						
L-Arabinose	+	+	–	–	–	–
Salicin	+	+	–	–	–	–
Sucrose	+	+	+	–	–	V
D-Mannitol	+	+	+	+	–	V
Glucose (gas)	+	–	+	+	–	V

[a]Reactions are for the predominant clinical biovar (sobria); biovar veronii is ornithine decarboxylase-positive.
[b]*A. trota* strains are susceptible to ampicillin.
+, >85% positive; –, >85% negative; V, variable, 15–85% positive.

are recorded. Cefsulodin–irgasan–novobiocin (CIN) agar, commonly used to isolate *Yersinia enterocolitica* in the laboratory, can also be used to isolate many *Aeromonas* strains (32). In our experience, this medium gives results comparable with, or better than, those of ampicillin–sheep blood agar, and its routine use in fecal examinations may be warranted if the suspected incidence of *Y. enterocolitica* and *Aeromonas* species collectively is sufficiently high to justify its inclusion.

During the acute phase of a diarrheal illness, the isolation of aeromonads in a diagnostic setting should not be a difficult task because moderate to large numbers (10^4 to 10^{10}/g of feces) of these bacteria are generally present in the fecal specimens. However, after the peak of the gastrointestinal illness or in cases of subacute or chronic diarrhea, *Aeromonas* may be overlooked if enrichment procedures are not included. Both gram-negative and Selenite-F broths, primarily used for the recovery of *Salmonella* and *Shigella* organisms, can be used to enrich for aeromonads present in the sample; alkaline peptone water (pH 8.5), used for the isolation of pathogenic *Vibrio* species, is also an excellent enrichment medium for the recovery of aeromonads (33). Such enrichment broths can then be plated onto one of a number of media used to isolate *Aeromonas* (33). It should be noted, however, that concerns have been raised about the clinical significance of *Aeromonas* strains present in such low numbers that they can be isolated only with enrichment techniques.

Epidemiology

An increasing number of medical and scientific publications indicate that at least some *Aeromonas* strains, if not all, are true enteropathogens. This evidence is based on case reports documenting the isolation of *Aeromonas* strains from the feces of persons with diarrhea in conjunction with pathologic and serologic findings that strongly link aeromonads to gastroenteritis (5). The highest attack rate appears to be in children under 5 years of age (34). These data, however, may be somewhat misleading because children are probably more likely to require medical attention for gastroenteritis than are adults. *Aeromonas* infections at any site are more likely to occur during the warmer months of the year (35), and the same seasonality has been noted in conjunction with *Aeromonas*-associated gastroenteritis (36–38).

Of the three primary settings in which *Aeromonas* gastroenteritis is seen, the most common is sporadic (episodic) diarrhea. The frequency with which *Aeromonas* has been isolated from symptomatic persons in this setting has ranged from a low of 0.7% to 0.9%, in specimens submitted to reference public health laboratories or local hospitals in the Netherlands and France, to a high of 50%, in Peruvian infants (39). The extremely high frequency with which *Aeromonas* was isolated from infants in the latter study (39) is complicated by the fact that at least one co-infecting pathogen was present in 50% or more of the fecal specimens. International studies have found high *Aeromonas* isolation rates from symptomatic persons residing in the Ivory Coast (24%), Bali (15%), Bangladesh (12%), and Japan (11%). In most of these studies, relatively high isolation rates can be attributed to the lower hygienic standards often seen in developing countries or to socioeconomic factors, such as dietary habits (6,40). Most U.S. studies have found isolation rates of 2.5% to 7.1%, depending on the study population, geographic location, and time of year in which *Aeromonas* was sought; similar frequencies (1.9% to 2.0%) have been recently reported from Scandinavian countries (41,42). Although vehicles of infection are poorly defined, one epidemiologic survey by the Centers for Disease Control and Prevention has linked the consumption of untreated well water to gastrointestinal infections with aeromonads (43); in another retrospective survey, both untreated water and prior antibiotic therapy were reported as risk factors for infection (35). A review indicates that most food-borne cases of *Aeromonas* gastroenteritis have been associated with the consumption of seafood (prawns, oysters, shrimp), fish, land snails, soups, or starchy broths (7). Molecular analysis of fecal isolates of *Aeromonas* from symptomatic persons indicate that of the 14 named species, *A. hydrophila, A. caviae,* and *A. veronii* biovar sobria account for the vast majority of isolates (6).

Aeromonas gastroenteritis is also associated with international travel. According to a recent review by Ericsson (44), the frequency of traveler's diarrhea caused by *Aeromonas* varies by geographic region; higher incidences are associated with travel to Asia (range, 1% to 57%), Africa (range, 0 to 9%), and Latin America (range, 1% to 5%). In a 1981 study by Echeverria et al. (45), *Aeromonas* species were isolated from 31% of 39 episodes of traveler's diarrhea in American Peace Corps volunteers in rural Thailand. In a subsequent 9½-year (1986 to1995) retrospective study of traveler's diarrhea in Tokyo, *Aeromonas* species were recovered from 5.5% of more than 23,000 travelers returning from trips to developing countries (46). *Aeromonas* was the fourth most common enteropathogen isolated after enterotoxigenic *E. coli, Salmonella,* and *Plesiomonas shigelloides.* Of the more than 1,200 travelers with cultures positive for *Aeromonas,* 94% were symptomatic, although 40% of these had mixed infections.

The third setting in which *Aeromonas*-associated gastroenteritis has been observed is day care. One Houston-based epidemiologic investigation of diarrheal disease in children less than 24 months of age enrolled in day care identified two outbreaks of gastroenteritis associated with *Aeromonas* (47). In the first outbreak, *Aeromonas* was the only potential enteropathogen recovered, being isolated from 6 of 25 children; 5 of the 6 children with cultures positive for *Aeromonas* had diarrhea. In a second outbreak, *Aeromonas* was isolated from 5 of 24 children with diarrhea. Genotyping of strains revealed only two isolates from the first outbreak (both *A. hydrophila*) with similar chromosomal patterns; in the second outbreak, all genotypes were distinct. A study of Ecuadorian children between the ages of 12 and 42 months identified day care as a major risk factor for the development of *Aeromonas*-associated gastroenteritis (relative risk, 10.47) in comparison with care at home (48). Risk factors identified to be associated with day care included the reuse of water to wash children's hands before meals and to wash raw vegetables (48).

In addition to the epidemiologic reports, recent case–control investigations have shown a significant association between the isolation of *Aeromonas* on primary media and the presence of gastrointestinal symptoms (6). In many of these studies, *Aeromonas* has ranked high on the list of reputed enteropathogens (41,46,49). Several studies have documented an immune response to gastrointestinal infection by *Aeromonas* in selected persons or in persons participating in cohort studies in which a variety of techniques were used, including enzyme-linked immunosorbent assay (ELISA) and immunoblotting (50–52). Kuijper et al. (50) evaluated the serum immune response in persons with presumed acute or chronic gastroenteritis caused by *Aeromonas,* in persons with diarrhea caused by other recognized enteric pathogens, and in healthy controls. Results significantly differed depending on the immunologic assay used, which included ELISA (sensitivity, 30%; specificity, 74%) and cytotoxin neutralization assays (sensitivity, 46%; specificity, 94%). Positive ELISA results correlated with immunoglobulin M (IgM) and IgG responses to the LPSs of homologous *Aeromonas* strains; tube agglutination tests were deemed unsatisfactory. Subsequent to this study, a fourfold rise in the fecal secretory IgA (sIgA) immune response (day 0 and day 5) to *Aeromonas* was detected in 11 of 12 U.S. students who became ill with diarrhea while in Mexico for summer studies (51); this immune response could be inhibited by preabsorption of the patient's fecal extract with the homologous strain. The major immune response appeared to be directed against the higher-molecular-weight bacterial LPS. Most recently, a specific IgG response to whole cell proteins of an S layer-positive strain of *A. veronii* was observed in a 24-year-old woman with ulcerative colitis (52); in addition to demonstration of the immune response, the infecting strain was isolated from feces and from the small intestine (in pure culture). An immune response to both the enterotoxin and cytolysin of an *A. veronii* strain associated with cholera-like diarrhea in a Thai woman has been previously reported (53). The effects of both microbial toxins on human embryonic fibroblasts and mouse Y1 adrenal tumor cells could be completely inhibited by the patient's acute-phase (1:40) and convalescent-phase (1:1,280) sera. Burke et al. (54) found a significantly higher rate of isolation of enterotoxigenic *Aeromonas* species (10.8%) from cases of diarrhea versus controls (0.7%) in an epidemiologic investigation of more than 900 non-aboriginal Australian children. Also reported have been a number of cases of gastroenteritis in which resolution of symptoms was accompanied by the disappearance of aeromonads from feces following therapy with agents specifically directed against this group (55).

Considerable controversy still exists regarding *Aeromonas* gastroenteritis (56,57). No clearly defined outbreaks of diarrheal illness caused by *Aeromonas* have ever been reported (even though the organism is a frequent isolate from water, food, and other environmental sources), as they have for other waterborne and food-borne pathogens. Although many epidemiologic studies have linked isolation of *Aeromonas* from stool with occurrence of disease, in some studies, the isolation rates of *Aeromonas* among asymptomatic controls have been equal to or greater than the isolation rates among case patients (58), which suggests that *Aeromonas* could simply be a nonpathogenic "fellow traveler." Immune responses after infection do not prove pathogenicity; for example, in volunteer studies with non-O1 *V. cholerae,* immune responses were seen with strains that colonized the intestine but did not cause illness (59). Finally, volunteer studies have failed to establish *Aeromonas* species as *bona fide* enteropathogens despite the fact that high doses were used for challenge (60). In summary, although most of the evidence supports a role for aeromonads in diarrheal disease, significant obstacles still remain in unequivocally establishing which *Aeromonas* strains are genuine enteric pathogens.

Pathogenesis and Immunity

It is likely that aeromonads gain entry to the digestive tract via the ingestion of contaminated food or water. Although most affected persons appear to have normal immune and physiologic mechanisms operative in the gut, George et al. (61) found evidence of reduced or absent gastric acidity in 30% of patients with *Aeromonas* infections.

Attention has recently focused on potential colonization factors produced by *Aeromonas* (6,62), particularly the type IV pilins (Bfp, Tap), and their possible relationship to intestinal disease. Bfps have been found to mediate adherence to epithelial and intestinal cell lines, freshly isolated enterocytes, and fixed human and animal intestinal tissue (63). Removal of Bfp from *Aeromonas* strains reduces *in vitro* adhesion by up to 80% (63). In contrast, experimental evidence does not support a major role for type IV Tap pilins in intestinal colonization (64). Tap mutants adhere to HEp-2 cells, Henle 407 intestinal cells, and human intestinal tissue in addition to wild-type isolates. No differences were observed in colonization rates or the incidence of diarrhea when studies were conducted in infant mice or the removable intestinal tie adult rabbit diarrheal (RITARD) model. The flexible minipilin (fxp) of Ho et al. (65) shows 91% amino acid sequence similarity to the core-encoded pilin (cep) of *V. cholerae.* This molecule is thought to play a role in intestinal colonization and is associated with the core region of the CTX genetic element (66). Expression of this flexible pilin appears to be environmentally regulated by such factors as temperature and iron availability.

Enterotoxins are the primary virulence factors identified in aeromonads and are thought to play prominent role(s) in *Aeromonas*-associated gastroenteritis (67). Two broad groups of *Aeromonas* enterotoxins (cytolytic and cytotonic) are recognized. The cytolytic enterotoxin is the more common enterotoxin. It is a β-hemolysin that is produced by many different *Aeromonas* species. This β-hemolysin is also known by a number of other names, including *aerolysin, Asao toxin,* and *cytotoxic enterotoxin* (68). The molecule is a heat-labile protein that actively induces fluid accumulation in the gut of infant mice and in rabbit ileal loops (69). At least two classes of cytolytic enterotoxins are known: one composed of 54- to 55-kd proteins belonging to the aerolysin family (70), and a second composed of 64- to 69-kd molecules that exhibit 45% to 51% amino acid sequence homology with the HlyA hemolysin of *V. cholerae* (68,71). Although immunologically and biochemically distinct versions of these molecules exist, most strains of *A. hydrophila* and *A. veronii* recovered from the feces of persons with diarrhea appear to produce a cytolytic enterotoxin (6). Some *Aeromonas* strains produce a cytotonic enterotoxin (67). The cytotonic enterotoxins are poorly characterized at present but do cause elongation of Chinese hamster ovary cells and fluid accumulation in rabbit ligated ileal loops and in suckling mice (67,72). Cytotonic enterotoxins vary in molecular mass (38 to 70 kd), physiologic properties, and cross-reactivity with cholera toxin (67). Mesophilic aeromonads are capable of invading tissue culture cells, such as HEp-2 and Caco-2 (6,73). This *in vitro* characteristic may be yet another potential enteropathogenic mechanism for aeromonads, conceivably active in cases of bloody diarrhea.

Clinical Illness

Gastrointestinal illnesses caused by members of the genus *Aeromonas* span the spectrum of symptoms and syndromes associated with other classic bacterial enteric pathogens. *Aeromonas* species have been associated with several distinctive clinical syndromes, including (a) acute, watery diarrhea; (b) dysentery; and (c) subacute or chronic diarrhea (6). The acute, secretory diarrhea syndrome is most commonly described. The fecal specimen is typically loose in consistency and watery in appearance, without red blood cells or leukocytes; mucus is occasionally observed (15% to 20%). The frequency of diarrhea in persons with this form ranges from 1 to 20 bowel movements a day (mean, ~5 to 7). In most studies of children with *Aeromonas*-associated gastroenteritis, watery diarrhea occurs at frequencies of 60% to 70%. Common symptoms associated with this type of gastroenteritis include abdominal pain (60% to 70%), fever (20% to 40%), nausea (40%), and vomiting (20% to 40%). Fever may exceed 39°C in some children (6). Approximately 10% to 15% of children with watery diarrhea from whom *Aeromonas* is isolated are co-infected with one or more other enteric pathogens. Although this infection is usually self-limited (mean duration, <7 days), between 30% and 40% of children with secretory gastroenteritis may require hospitalization for dehydration or persistent diarrhea. The most common *Aeromonas* species isolated in most of these studies is *A. caviae.* On rare occasions, profuse, cholera-like diarrhea has been reported in association with *A. veronii* infection (6). Far fewer studies of adults with *Aeromonas*-induced secretory diarrhea have been reported. The acute, secretory form in adults appears similar to that in children, causing abdominal pain (60%), fever (20%), and nausea (20%) as the prominent symptoms (27); most of these infections are community-acquired, with a mean duration of illness of 11 days.

Half of the adult patients have leukocytes in their stools, and 15% harbor multiple enteric pathogens. In approximately 15% to 25% of all cases of *Aeromonas*-associated gastroenteritis, a dysentery-like illness resembling shigellosis occurs. Cardinal features of this infection include intense abdominal pain, bloody diarrhea, and mucus with fecal polymorphonuclear leukocytes; fever, nausea, and vomiting sometimes may be present. Particularly in children, the fulminant course of this illness can require hospitalization. Many persons in whom this type of diarrheal syndrome develops are initially suspected of having ulcerative, diffuse, or segmental colitis. In some instances, colonoscopy shows superficial ulceration, erythema, and friability of the mucosa, with biopsy revealing crypt abscesses and active colitis. A third manifestation of the infection is a subacute to chronic or intermittent condition in which symptoms can persist for months to years. Although symptoms may vary, the chief complaint is a simple, nonresolving diarrhea that occurs at sporadic intervals. An example is a recent case report of a 45-year-old man in whom watery diarrhea caused by *A. caviae* developed after a trip to Turkey (74). The acute diarrhea subsequently developed into chronic enteritis of 17 months' duration. Multiple fecal isolates recovered from the patient during this interval were found to be identical by ribotyping.

Several complications can arise from *Aeromonas* gastroenteritis, particularly bloody diarrhea. Recently reported sequelae of *Aeromonas*-associated gastroenteritis include renal complications and hemolytic–uremic syndrome. At least four cases of hemolytic–uremic syndrome associated with bloody diarrhea caused by *Aeromonas* have now been reported in the literature (75–77). Three of these occurred in children, and one reported case was in a 36-year-old adult (77). An additional case of renal failure in a 6-month-old infant following an episode of bloody diarrhea was reported by Filler et al. (78). The implicated agent was a verocytotoxic strain of *Aeromonas.* However, it has also been suggested that *Aeromonas* preferentially colonizes the intestinal tract of persons with hematologic malignancies (79) and has on occasion masked the presence of more life-threatening complications, such as colonic carcinoma (80).

Aeromonas species also cause a number of extraintestinal illnesses, including wound infections and septicemia (5,62,81). Wound infections most commonly occur when freshwater sources that contain aeromonads come in contact with integument. Symptoms in such infected persons may range from a mild cellulitis to myonecrosis; those with more severe disease, especially when it is accompanied by positive blood cultures, have a much poorer prognosis. *Aeromonas* septicemia is most commonly observed in immunocompromised persons, including those with hepatobiliary disease (e.g., cirrhosis), hematologic malignancies, or solid tumors. On rare occasions, *Aeromonas* sepsis has been noted in previously healthy or non-immunocompromised persons. Fatality rates range from 30% to 50% in most surveys.

Diagnosis

The laboratory diagnosis of *Aeromonas* infections primarily depends on the isolation of aeromonads by culture. During the acute phase of a gastrointestinal illness, aeromonads should be present in moderate to large numbers (10^6 to 10^8 colony-forming units per gram of feces). If aeromonads are suspected as the causative agent of subacute or chronic diarrhea, both enrichment cultures and selective media specifically designed for the isolation of *Aeromonas* may be required because of fluctuating bacterial concentrations. In the latter situation, the simple isolation of *Aeromonas* from feces is not sufficient to identify the cause of the infection. Rather, additional tests must be performed, such as tissue biopsy (for culture and determining the presence of bacilli in histologic sections) and immunologic investigations (immunoblots for fecal sIgA or serum IgM or IgG immune responses to the infecting strain). In several recent studies, specific immune responses to *Aeromonas* have been detected in the context of intestinal infections by finding sIgA responses directed against LPS components (51) or an immune response to whole cell or outer membrane proteins of the homologous strain (50,52). Tube agglutination titers are less reliable because many healthy persons appear to have antibodies against *Aeromonas.*

In potential outbreaks in which multiple isolates of *Aeromonas* are isolated from different persons, relatedness of the isolates can be determined by a number of techniques. By far the simplest and least expensive method is to determine biochemically the genomospecies designation of each isolate (27); because aeromonads are so phenotypically diverse, such testing may also allow distinguishing between strains of the same species by biotype. If more advanced methods are required, serogrouping performed by one of several international reference centers is practical (82). All aeromonads, regardless of species designation, fall into more than 90 distinct serogroups based on the presence of unique somatic antigens; the likelihood that two given strains in the same outbreak belong to the same species and have the same biotype and serogroup is extremely remote unless they are related. Present information indicates that no single serogroup accounts for more than 10% to 20% of all clinical strains so typed. Strains may also be distinguished by a variety of molecular methods, including ribotyping, multilocus enzyme electrophoresis, and pulsed-field gel electrophoresis (83). Plasmid analysis is not a useful technique because most strains (>70%) do not carry plasmids or lose them quickly on subculture.

Antimicrobial Susceptibility

The *in vitro* antimicrobial susceptibility profile of mesophilic aeromonads is becoming an increasingly complicated subject (84). This problem is the consequence of several factors, including an expanding list of *Aeromonas* species, global recognition that these bacteria are important causes of disease, and molecular characterization of resistance determinants. The first investigation concerning the *in vitro* susceptibility of newer *Aeromonas* species to antimicrobial agents has just been published (85). Species-specific differences noted in this study include susceptibility to aminopenicillins, antipseudomonal penicillins, carbapenems, and some aminoglycosides. This study did not include less frequently encountered species that are of questionable medical significance, such as *A. bestiarum, A. media,* and *A. salmonicida.* Although a general consensus of opinion regarding the susceptibility profile of aeromonads to certain classes of therapeutic agents is still feasible (Table 49.4), such a generalization is not without certain limitations (6,85,86). For instance, aeromonads are typically resistant to first-generation cephalosporins, exhibit variable resistance to second-generation cephalosporins, and are normally susceptible to third-generation compounds. However, rare instances of the development of *in vivo* resistance to third-generation cephalosporins during a course of treatment with cefotaxime to eradicate bacteremia have been described (87). In addition, most susceptibility studies to date have been conducted in either the United States or Europe. However, one recent investigation from Taiwan (88) found much higher percentages of resistance to tetracycline, trimethoprim-sulfamethoxazole (TMP-SMX), aminoglycosides, and some extended-spectrum cephalosporins in *A. hydrophila, A. caviae,* and *A. veronii* biotype sobria isolates than was previously reported. An additional problem is that *in vitro* susceptibility data do not always correlate with *in vivo* response, partially because of the expression of inducible β-lactamases by aeromonads. Virtually all *Aeromonas* strains produce β-lactamases (85). At least three different inducible, chromosomally mediated β-lactamases can be produced by mesophilic aeromonads (68). The most interesting of these β-lactamases is a metallo-β-lactamase with activity against carbapenems (89).

Treatment

The mainstay of therapy in *Aeromonas*-associated gastroenteritis, as in any diarrheal disease, is rehydration via the oral or intravenous route. No controlled trials of antimicrobial therapy in *Aeromonas* gastroenteritis have been conducted. Illness is usually self-limited, and previously healthy persons with acute illness who are not treated with antimicrobial agents appear to do well, with rapid resolution of symptoms and clearance of the organism from stool; there is no *a priori* reason to treat such cases. At the same time, antimicrobial therapy is not contraindicated, and no evidence has been found that therapy prolongs intestinal carriage of the organism (90); additionally, some anecdotal reports suggest that antimicrobial therapy results in "prompt" resolution of symptoms (34,90,91).

Data supporting the antimicrobial therapy of chronic *Aeromonas*-associated diarrhea, although still anecdotal, are somewhat stronger. George and colleagues (61) documented clinical responses in three patients with protracted diarrhea (21 days, 28 days, and 6 months, respectively). Similarly, Holmberg et al. (90) reported five patients who took antimicrobial agents to which their *Aeromonas* isolates were suscep-

TABLE 49.4. *IN VITRO* SUSCEPTIBILITY PROFILE OF *AEROMONAS* SPECIES

	Aeromonas species	
Antimicrobial Agent	**Susceptible[a]**	**Resistant**
Aminopenicillins	*A. trota*	All other species
Aminoglycosides	All other species	*A. schubertii* (V)
Antipseudomonal penicillins	*A. trota*	*A. hydrophila, A. caviae, A. veronii* bt sobria, *A. veronii* bt veronii (V), *A. schubertii* (V)
Carbapenems	*A. hydrophila, A. caviae, A. veronii* bt *sobria, A. schubertii, A. trota*	*A. jandaei, A. veronii* bt veronii
Cephalosporins (1st generation)		All species
Cephalosporins (2nd generation; cefuroxime)	All species	
Cephalosporins (3rd generation)	All species	
Cephalosporins (4th generation)	All species	
Cephamycins (cefoxitin)	*A. veronii* bt sobria, *A. veronii* bt veronii, *A. jandaei*	*A. hydrophila, A. caviae, A. schubertii, A. trota*
Chloramphenicol	All species	
Fluoroquinolones	All species	
Monobactams	All species	
Tetracycline	All species	
Trimethoprim-sulfamethoxazole	All species	

[a]>90% of isolates susceptible based on *in vitro* testing.
(V), susceptibility or resistance is variable based on the agent tested in that class; bt, biotype.
Data from various investigations (6,83,84).

tible; within an average of 3.4 days, marked alleviation or resolution of gastrointestinal symptoms, which had lasted a mean of 47 days before treatment, was noted in all. Rautelin et al. (92) described a case of chronic diarrhea caused by *A. caviae* (17 months' duration) in a 45-year-old man. After treatment with multiple therapeutic modalities, resolution of symptoms and eradication of *Aeromonas* were achieved with a prolonged course (4 weeks) of ciprofloxacin. Based on these observations, it would appear reasonable to administer antimicrobial agents to patients who have positive stool cultures for *Aeromonas* and who have had symptoms for at least 7 to 10 days. Also, very limited data suggest that the susceptibility to septicemia is increased in patients who are immunocompromised, have malignancies or are receiving cancer chemotherapy, or have underlying hepatobiliary disease (93). In these settings, it again would appear reasonable to treat affected patients with antimicrobial agents in an effort to minimize the risk for sepsis.

Based on very limited experience, TMP-SMX may be considered the drug of choice in domestic cases of *Aeromonas* gastroenteritis (61); quinolones such as ciprofloxacin should be considered in cases acquired abroad. Although clinical efficacy data are lacking, quinolones would be a reasonable choice for empiric therapy before culture results are available. Tetracycline or doxycycline (6,61) might serve as alternatives in patients with allergies to sulfa drugs; aminoglycosides, such as gentamicin, are indicated in persons with septicemia.

PLESIOMONAS

Designated strain "C27" in 1947 by Ferguson and Henderson, *P. shigelloides* was finally and deservedly placed in its own genus in 1962 (94). Although they have resided in the family Vibrionaceae for more than 30 years, recent phylogenetic evidence based on 5S and 16S ribosomal RNA sequence data indicates that plesiomonads are more closely linked to the family Enterobacteriaceae than to vibriones (2,3,95). The next edition of *Bergey's Manual of Systematic Bacteriology* will reflect these phylogenetic relationships as the genus *Plesiomonas* is transferred to the family Enterobacteriaceae.

Plesiomonas is primarily a freshwater organism, with isolation rates increasing during warm months. Fish and shellfish, especially if associated with mud or sediment, frequently harbor plesiomonads (96). In a survey conducted by Miller and Koburger (97), plesiomonads were isolated from 58.7% of environmental samples, including water, sediment, fish, crabs, and mollusks. In a 1995 Brazilian study, plesiomonads were frequently recovered from both polluted and nonpolluted freshwater environments and from polluted salt water habitats (98). Plesiomonads can be isolated from the feces of asymptomatic cold-blooded animals and from warm-blooded animals, including cats and dogs (6,99).

Plesiomonads are straight, facultatively anaerobic, gram-negative rods, 0.8 to 1.0 μm wide to 3.0 μm long. They are motile by means of polar lophotrichous flagella (96). On non-inhibitory media, such as heart infusion or blood agar, colonies are nonhemolytic, 1 to 2 mm, opaque, and convex with entire edges. The organism grows on and can be isolated from a variety of common differential or selective agars, generally appearing as a non–lactose-fermenting colony (94). However, approximately 30% of plesiomonads ferment lactose and would be overlooked on these media. Alternatively, colonies on nutrient or blood agar can be screened for oxidase and indole production and, if the results are positive, tested further. In examinations specifically for *Plesiomonas,* inositol–brilliant green–bile salts agar is useful because few enteric bacteria other than *Plesiomonas* can utilize inositol as a carbon source; white colonies with red coloration are likely to be *Plesiomonas* (6,96). On CIN agar, plesiomonads grow as colorless colonies. Enrichment broths are effective in the isolation of *Plesiomonas* from stools; a 1988 study by Rahim and Kay (100) found enrichment with bile peptone broth or alkaline peptone broth to be superior to direct plating; 24-hour enrichment in bile peptone broth yielded 30 positive specimens versus 5 by direct plating only (n = 423). Jeppersen (101) has recently reviewed isolation, enrichment, and enumeration procedures useful in the recovery of plesiomonads from food and environmental samples.

Once isolated, *P. shigelloides* is easily identified and separated from other Vibrionaceae and Enterobacteriaceae. Key characteristics include positive oxidase, lysine and ornithine decarboxylase, and arginine dihydrolase activities; fermentation of *m*-inositol; lack of gas production from glucose; and susceptibility to O/129. As its name implies, *P. shigelloides* may antigenically cross-react with *Shigella,* most frequently with *S. sonnei* (6). The complete DNA sequence of the O antigen gene region of *P. shigelloides* O17 has been demonstrated to be identical to *S. sonnei* form I antigen (102). Patients whose strains possess cross-reacting antigens do not necessarily have longer or more severe gastrointestinal illness (103).

Despite findings of little or no *P. shigelloides* enteropathogenicity in animal and human volunteer studies and an inability to induce an sIgA immune response in colonized or infected students (51), some evidence does suggest a role for plesiomonads as enteropathogens (6,94). A pathogenic role is supported by a lessening in the severity and duration of symptoms with appropriate antibiotic therapy, an extremely low asymptomatic carriage rate (<0.1%) in humans, and outbreaks of diarrheal disease associated with contaminated water and oysters containing *Plesiomonas* (6,104). In two outbreaks reported from Japan, predominant serotypes (O17:H2, O22:H3) epidemiologically linked to each outbreak were recovered from 16 and three cases, respectively (104). A third outbreak of gastroenteritis, in Livingston County, New York, in 1996, caused by *P.*

shigelloides and *Salmonella* serotype Hartford, was recently reported by the Centers for Disease Control and Prevention (105). The implicated vehicles of infection were a contaminated water supply and potato salad. Information from case studies indicates that all age groups may be affected; symptoms usually occur 24 to 48 hours after exposure. As with most enteric pathogens, the incidence of *Plesiomonas*-associated gastroenteritis is highest when the weather is warm. *Plesiomonas* infections have been linked to travel to the Far East and Mexico (103); consumption of raw or undercooked shellfish or contaminated water also is a risk factor for gastrointestinal infection (96).

Reports of virulence-associated characteristics in *Plesiomonas* are not conclusive (6,68). Sequences of heat-labile and heat-stable toxins demonstrated in *Plesiomonas* by animal and tissue culture cell systems show no homology with genes for these toxins in *E. coli* and *V. cholerae* O1. Results of assays for invasiveness, including production of conjunctivitis in the Sereny test and internalization in HEp-2 cells, and colony blot hybridization to detect gene sequences have been negative, except for a study in which 5 (31%) of 16 freshly isolated strains of *P. shigelloides* from children with acute gastroenteritis were found to invade HeLa cells at frequencies similar to those of shigellae (106). Daskaleros et al. (107) reported the production of an iron-regulated β-hemolysin by more than 90% of all *P. shigelloides* strains (6). This hemolysin may contain enterotoxigenic activity, such as is found in *Aeromonas,* or alternatively may help release iron from erythrocytes. Colonization factors such as pilins have not been described in *Plesiomonas* to date.

Although not often encountered in the United States, *P. shigelloides* is commonly isolated in other parts of the world. One study from Bangladesh (108) listed *Plesiomonas* as the fourth leading cause of bacterial gastroenteritis (after *V. cholerae, Shigella,* and *Aeromonas*) when a single agent was involved (4% of these cases; 6.4% of cases including mixed infections); this study was limited by the lack of a control group. Features significantly associated with *Plesiomonas* enteric infection include travel to the tropics, abdominal pain, and gastrointestinal illness of 14 days' duration or longer (109). A recent Japanese study identified *P. shigelloides* as the third most common cause of traveler's diarrhea, accounting for 5.6% of all cases (46). Intestinal infections associated with *P. shigelloides* can span the entire spectrum of symptoms and sequelae associated with enteric illnesses caused by other enteropathogens. Most gastrointestinal ailments associated with *Plesiomonas* last between 2 and 14 days and often are associated with severe abdominal pain or cramping (56% to 100%). Other symptoms frequently associated with *P. shigelloides* gastroenteritis include nausea or vomiting (32% to 40%), fever (18% to 30%), and headaches (13%); approximately one-third of the persons in one study were found to be dehydrated (103). In this study, 36% of infected persons presented with frankly bloody stools, 36% described their abdominal pain as severe, and 18% had fever. Kain and Kelly (109) in a subsequent case–control investigation of 30 persons with acute gastrointestinal illnesses from which *Plesiomonas* was isolated found the chief features of infection to include abdominal pain (100%), nausea or vomiting (40%), and fever (30%). In addition to cases of secretory or colitis/proctitis-type diarrhea, subacute to chronic infections with *P. shigelloides* have been described. One case of prolonged bloody diarrhea (3 months) attributed to *P. shigelloides* was described in a 40-year-old HIV-positive man (110). Raw oysters appeared to be the source of his infection, and his illness resolved after a 2-week course of oral TMP-SMX.

Extraintestinal manifestations, such as septicemia and meningitis, are rare and have been reported mostly in immunocompromised patients, particularly neonates (110). On occasion, intestinal infections with plesiomonads have preceded subsequent bacteremic episodes in apparently healthy hosts (111); fatal outcomes of severe gastrointestinal infections without apparent dissemination caused by *Plesiomonas* also have been described (6).

In vitro susceptibility data reveal that like *Aeromonas,* most strains of *Plesiomonas* are resistant to ampicillin and susceptible to the cephalosporins, quinolones, TMP-SMX, and chloramphenicol (69,101,102). However, the susceptibility of plesiomonads to gentamicin (57% to 86%), tobramycin (36% to 97%), and amikacin (54% to 100%) has significantly varied among studies (101,102). Kain and Kelly (109) also found that, in contrast to *Aeromonas,* only 68% of the *Plesiomonas* stains tested were susceptible to tetracycline.

Observations from several studies and case reports suggest that the quinolones, cephalosporins, or TMP-SMX may be the best agents for the treatment of complicated cases of plesiomonad infection or infection in immunocompromised patients. However, whether antimicrobial treatment has any effect on diarrhea caused by *Plesiomonas* in immunocompetent persons is not yet clear. In one Canadian retrospective study (109), the treatment of *Plesiomonas* gastroenteritis with an appropriate antimicrobial agent appeared to shorten the course of diarrhea in comparison with no treatment or treatment with antibiotics to which the organism was not susceptible; on the other hand, in another retrospective study of Thai children, antibiotics did not appear to shorten the duration of *Plesiomonas* diarrhea (112). Given the potential for the organism to disseminate, even in healthy hosts, and for fatal outcomes in severe gastrointestinal infections without apparent dissemination, it would be prudent to consider antimicrobial treatment for any *Plesiomonas* infection.

EDWARDSIELLA

The genus *Edwardsiella* was first described in the early 1960s, when the species *Edwardsiella tarda* was taxonomically defined from a group of biochemically distinct strains that had been previously referred to by a number of vernacular names, including "Asakusa group" and "Bartholomew group." During the 1980s, two other species (*Edwardsiella ictaluri, Edwarsiella hoshinae*) within this genus were described. To date, *E. tarda* is the only species consistently isolated from human specimens and associated with both intestinal and extraintestinal disease. Edwardsiellae are also frequently found in the environment, and it is likely that fish, reptiles, and amphibians in aquatic ecosystems serve as the primary habitat for these organisms (113). Rarely, domestic and feral, warm-blooded animals harbor edwardsiellae (114).

The genus *Edwardsiella,* which is a member of the family Enterobacteriaceae, is composed of gram-negative, oxidase-negative rods that are facultatively anaerobic. *E. tarda,* which most closely resembles *Salmonella* biochemically, is motile by means of peritrichous flagella; fimbriae or other cell-associated structures have not been identified. Except for D-glucose and maltose, *E. tarda* fails to utilize a number of carbohydrate compounds typically oxidized as sources of energy by other gram-negative bacteria. However, this species can be easily recognized in the clinical laboratory by its chief diagnostic feature, the production of hydrogen sulfide, which is usually a red flag for colonies isolated on media such as XLD, HE, and *Salmonella–Shigella* (SS) agars. Reactions typically observed with this species include the production of indole, acid, and gas from D-glucose; the production of hydrogen sulfide on TSI slants; and lysine and ornithine decarboxylase activity. At present, two biotypes of *E. tarda* are known to exist. The most common biotype, commonly called "wild-type," is associated with all human and most animal infections. Strains of the other biogroup (biogroup 1), isolated from fresh water and snakes, are biochemically more active, producing acid from D-mannitol, L-arabinose, and sucrose. In addition, biogroup 1 strains fail to produce hydrogen sulfide on TSI slants. Recently, hydrogen sulfide-positive, D-mannitol–negative, and L-arabinose–negative strains of *E. tarda* have been described that do not belong to biogroup 1. These strains may represent a new biogroup of *E. tarda* or a new species of *Edwardsiella* (115,116). Because *E. tarda* is only infrequently encountered in the clinical laboratory, detailed studies on the best enrichment and isolation methods have not been reported; in our experience, the use of an XLD or SS plate in conjunction with Selenite produces excellent results.

Evidence supporting a definitive role for *E. tarda* as a causative agent of diarrheal illness continues to mount, although such data are hampered by the relatively infrequent isolation of this species from human specimens. A retrospective analysis of most published literature on *E. tarda* indicates isolation rates of this organism from symptomatic versus asymptomatic persons in a ratio of approximately 3:1 (117). Most asymptomatic cases from which *E. tarda* has been recovered have occurred in tropical or subtropical regions of the world, where *E. tarda* may be more common. Furthermore, the carrier rate for this organism in the general population appears to be less than 0.01% (117). In several well-described cases, serum agglutinating antibodies rose in *E. tarda*-infected persons with fulminant or prolonged bouts of diarrheal disease (118,119). Risk factors associated with such infections include the handling of ornamental fish and turtles and, rarely, other pets (119–121). Finally, recent laboratory studies have identified possible enteropathogenic mechanisms in *E. tarda* that may be operative in the gut.

Several candidate virulence factors have been associated with *E. tarda* gastrointestinal infections. Probably the best defined of these is the ability of most *E. tarda* strains to penetrate (invade) nonphagocytic cells, such as HeLa and HEp-2 cells (122–124). This process is microfilament-dependent (inhibited by cytochalasin D), and invasion may correlate with the relatively severe gastrointestinal manifestations (colitis, dysentery) often associated with enteric *Edwardsiella* infections (123). A second factor, production of a β-hemolysin, may be linked with invasive capabilities similar to those noted for *Shigella* and enteroinvasive *E. coli,* although it does not appear to be involved in cell-to-cell spread (124,125). The β-hemolysin was originally detected on modified plate or broth assays and appeared to be cell-associated, but β-hemolysin may be released extracellularly in iron-deficient media (125). This molecule could facilitate intercellular spread by releasing replicated bacterial progeny from the host cell vacuole; alternatively, it might in itself have enterotoxigenic activity.

E. tarda-associated gastroenteritis occurs as either a benign secretory diarrhea or a more invasive process resembling dysentery or enterocolitis. In a study of 10 persons with intestinal illnesses attributed to *E. tarda,* Kourany et al. (114) found the most common symptoms to be low-grade fever (38° to 38.5°C) and vomiting (70%) in addition to watery stools; only one of their patients had a more severe gastrointestinal disorder, with frankly bloody stools, fever, vomiting, and overt dehydration. Symptoms may be more severe (resembling those of pseudomembranous colitis and invasive enterocolitis), with cramping abdominal pain, nausea, tenesmus, and the passage of up to 20 bowel movements per day. Proctoscopy/sigmoidoscopy has revealed ulcerations of the mucosa, submucosal hemorrhages, and, in the case of pseudomembranous colitis, hemorrhages with a green membranous mucous layer overlying the rectal mucosa. Occasionally, disseminated *E. tarda* infections (septicemia, meningitis, hepatic abscesses) arise in patients with liver dysfunction, immunosuppression, or other underlying conditions (126,127). Cellulitis and arthritis, sequelae of systemic disease, have also been described with *E. tarda* infection (128,129).

Culture remains the diagnostic method of choice because edwardsiellae should be present in large numbers in fecal samples taken during the acute phase of an illness. When the numbers of *E. tarda* isolated are low, or the illness is in a subacute or chronic phase, acute and convalescent serum may be collected for tube agglutination assays (119). In outbreaks of gastrointestinal disease attributed to this bacterium, strains may be serotyped (somatic, flagellar) for epidemiologic purposes (130).

Only a limited number of studies on the *in vitro* susceptibility of *E. tarda* to antimicrobial agents have been performed. The results, however, indicate that virtually all strains are susceptible to a wide variety of antibiotics, including β-lactams, aminoglycosides, and quinolones (131–133). In the absence of controlled clinical trials, it is not possible to make definite recommendations regarding antimicrobial therapy. In settings of persistent diarrhea (>7 days) in which *E. tarda* is regarded as the most likely pathogen, it would appear reasonable to undertake a course of therapy. Of course, antimicrobial therapy is indicated in rare disseminated infections. Based on antimicrobial susceptibility patterns and the limited available patient data, ampicillin, TMP-SMX, or ciprofloxacin all would be a reasonable choice for antimicrobial therapy.

REFERENCES

1. Janda JM. *Vibrio, Aeromonas,* and *Plesiomonas.* In: Collier L, Balows A, Sussman, eds. *Topley & Wilson's microbiology and microbial infections,* ninth edition. London: Arnold, 1998: 1065–1089 (vol 2).
2. Martinez-Murcia AJ, Benlloch S, Collins MD. Phylogenetic interrelationships of members of the genera *Aeromonas* and *Plesiomonas* as determined by 16S ribosomal DNA sequencing: lack of congruence with results of DNA–DNA hybridizations. *Int J Syst Bacteriol* 1992;42:412–421.
3. Ruimy R, Breittmayer V, Elbaze P, et al. Phylogenetic analysis and assessment of the genera *Vibrio, Photobacterium, Aeromonas,* and *Plesiomonas* deduced from small-subunit rRNA sequences. *Int J Syst Bacteriol* 1994;44:416–426.
4. Colwell RR, MacDonell MT, De Ley J. Proposal to recognize the family Aeromonadaceae fam. nov. *Int J Syst Bacteriol* 1986; 36:473–477.
5. Janda JM, Abbott SL. Evolving concepts regarding the genus *Aeromonas*: an expanding panorama of species, disease presentations, and unanswered questions. *Clin Infect Dis* 1998;27: 332–344.
6. Janda JM, Abbott SL, Morris JG Jr. *Aeromonas, Plesiomonas,* and *Edwardsiella.* In: Blaser MJ, Smith PD, Ravdin JI, et al., eds. *Infections of the gastrointestinal tract.* New York: Raven Press, 1995:905–917.
7. Kirov SM. The public health significance of *Aeromonas* spp. in foods. *Int J Food Microbiol* 1993;20:179–198.
8. Hänninen M-L, Oivanen P, Hirvelä-Koski V. *Aeromonas* species in fish, fish eggs, shrimp, and fresh water. *Int J Food Microbiol* 1997;34:17–26.
9. Callister SM, Agger WA. Enumeration and characterization of *Aeromonas hydrophila* and *Aeromonas caviae* isolated from grocery store produce. *Appl Environ Microbiol* 1987;53:249–253.
10. Palumbo SA, Bencivengo MM, Del Corral F, et al. Characterization of the *Aeromonas hydrophila* group isolated from retail foods of animal origin. *J Clin Microbiol* 1989;27:854–859.
11. Krovacek K, Faris A, Baloda SB, et al. Prevalence and characterization of *Aeromonas* spp. isolated from foods in Uppsala, Sweden. *Food Microbiol* 1992;9:26–36.
12. Trust TJ. Pathogenesis of infectious diseases of fish. *Annu Rev Microbiol* 1986;40:479–502.
13. Joseph SW, Carnahan A. The isolation, identification, and systematics of the motile *Aeromonas* species. *Annu Rev Fish Dis* 1994;4:315–343.
14. Kuijper EJ, Steigerwalt AG, Schoenmakers BS, et al. Phenotypic characterization and DNA relatedness in human fecal isolates of *Aeromonas* spp. *J Clin Microbiol* 1989;27:132–138.
15. Martínez MJ, Simon-Pujol D, Congregado F, et al. The presence of capsular polysaccharide in mesophilic *Aeromonas hydrophila* serotypes O:11 and O:34. *FEMS Microbiol Lett* 1995; 128:69–74.
16. Pavan ME, Abbott SL, Zorzópolos J, et al. *Aeromonas salmonicida* subsp. *pectinolytica* subsp. nov., a new pectinase-positive subspecies isolated from a heavily polluted river. *Int J Syst Evol Microbiol* 2000;50:1119–1124.
17. Ali A, Carnahan AM, Altwegg M, et al. *Aeromonas bestiarum* sp. nov. (formerly genomospecies DNA group 2 *A. hydrophila*), a new species isolated from non-human sources. *Med Microbiol Lett* 1996:156–165.
18. Pepe CM, Eklund MW, Strom MS. Cloning of an *Aeromonas hydrophila* type IV pilus biogenesis gene cluster: complementation of pilus assembly functions and characterization of a type IV leader peptidase/*N*-methyltransferase required for extracellular protein secretion. *Mol Microbiol* 1996;19: 857–869.
19. Barnett TC, Kirov SM, Strom MS, et al. *Aeromonas* spp. possess at least two distinct type IV pilus families. *Microb Pathog* 1997; 23:241–247.
20. Kirov SM, Sanderson K. Characterization of a type IV bundle-forming pilus (SFP) from a gastroenteritis-associated strain of *Aeromonas veronii* biovar sobria. *Microb Pathog* 1996;21:23–34.
21. Noonan B, Trust TJ. The synthesis, secretion and role in virulence of the paracrystalline surface layers of *Aeromonas salmonicida* and *A. hydrophila. FEMS Microbiol Lett* 1997;154:1–7.
22. Aoki T, Holland BI. The outer membrane proteins of the fish pathogens *Aeromonas hydrophila, Aeromonas salmonicida,* and *Edwardsiella tarda. FEMS Microbiol Lett* 1985;27:299–305.
23. Dooley JSG, Lallier R, Shaw DH, et al. Electrophoretic and immunochemical analyses of the lipopolysaccharides from various strains of *Aeromonas hydrophila. J Bacteriol* 1985;164: 263–269.
24. Knirel YA, Senchenkova SN, Jansson P-E, et al. Structure of the O-specific polysaccharide of an *Aeromonas trota* strain cross-reactive with *Vibrio cholerae* O139 Bengal. *Eur J Biochem* 1996; 238:160–165.
25. Janda JM. Biochemical and exoenzymatic properties of *Aeromonas* species. *Diagn Microbiol Infect Dis* 1985;3:223–232.
26. Abbott SL, Seli LS, Catino Jr M, et al. Misidentification of unusual *Aeromonas* species as members of the genus *Vibrio*: a continuing problem. *J Clin Microbiol* 1998;36:1103–1104.
27. Abbott SL, Cheung WKW, Kroske-Bystrom S, et al. Identification of *Aeromonas* strains to the genospecies level in the clinical laboratory. *J Clin Microbiol* 1992;30:1262–1266.
28. Janda JM, Abbott SL, Khashe S, et al. Further studies on the biochemical characteristics and serologic properties of the genus *Aeromonas. J Clin Microbiol* 1996;34:1930–1933.
29. Millership SE. Identification. In: Austin B, Altwegg M, Gosling PJ, et al., eds. *The genus* Aeromonas. Chichester: John Wiley and Sons, 1996:85–109.
30. Carnahan AM, Behram S, Joseph SW. Aerokey II, a flexible key for identifying clinical *Aeromonas* species. *J Clin Microbiol* 1991;29:2843–2849.

31. Kelly MT, Stroh EMD, Jessop J. Comparison of blood agar, ampicillin blood agar, MacConkey–ampicillin–Tween agar, and modified cefsulodin–irgasan–novobiocin agar for isolation of *Aeromonas* spp. from stool specimens. *J Clin Microbiol* 1988; 26:1738–1740.
32. Altorfer R, Altwegg M, Zollinger J, et al. Growth of *Aeromonas* spp. on cefsulodin–irgasan–novobiocin agar selective for *Yersinia enterocolitica. J Clin Microbiol* 1985;22:478–480.
33. Moyer NP. Isolation and enumeration of aeromonads. In: Austin B, Altwegg M, Gosling PJ, et al., eds. *The genus* Aeromonas. Chichester: John Wiley and Sons, 1996:39–84.
34. Cohen MB. Etiology and mechanisms of acute infectious diarrhea in infants in the United States. *J Pediatr* 1991;118: S34–S39.
35. Moyer NP. Clinical significance of *Aeromonas* species isolated from patients with diarrhea. *J Clin Microbiol* 1987;25: 2044–2048.
36. Gracey M, Burke V, Robinson R. *Aeromonas*-associated gastroenteritis. *Lancet* 1982;2:1304–1306.
37. Janda JM, Bottone EJ, Reitano MR. *Aeromonas* species in clinical microbiology: significance, epidemiology, and speciation. *Diagn Microbiol Infect Dis* 1983;1:221–228.
38. George WL, Nakata MM, Thompson J, et al. *Aeromonas*-related diarrhea in adults. *Arch Intern Med* 1985;145:2207–2211.
39. Pazzaglia G, Sack RB, Salazar E, et al. High frequency of coinfecting enteropathogens in *Aeromonas*-associated diarrhea of hospitalized Peruvian infants. *J Clin Microbiol* 1991;29: 1151–1156.
40. Albert MJ, Faruque ASG, Faruque SM, et al. Case–control study of enteropathogens associated with childhood diarrhea in Dhaka, Bangladesh. *J Clin Microbiol* 1999;37:3458–3464.
41. Rautelin H, Sivonen A, Kuikka A, et al. Role of *Aeromonas* isolated from feces of Finnish patients. *Scand J Infect Dis* 1995;27: 207–210.
42. Svenungsson B, Lagergren A, Ekwall E, et al. Enteropathogens in adult patients with diarrhea and healthy control subjects: a 1-year prospective study in a Swedish clinic for infectious diseases. *Clin Infect Dis* 2000;30:770–778.
43. Holmberg SD, Schell WK, Fanning GR, et al. *Aeromonas* intestinal infections in the United States. *Ann Intern Med* 1986; 105:683–689.
44. Ericsson CD. Travelers' diarrhea. Epidemiology, prevention, and self-treatment. *Infect Dis Clin North Am* 1998;12:285–303.
45. Echeverria P, Blacklow NR, Sanford LB, et al. Travelers' diarrhea among American Peace Corps volunteers in rural Thailand. *J Infect Dis* 1981;143:767–771.
46. Yamada S, Matsushita S, Dejsirilert S, et al. Incidence and clinical symptoms of *Aeromonas*-associated travellers' diarrhoea in Tokyo. *Epidemiol Infect* 1997;119:121–126.
47. de la Morena ML, Van R, Singh K, et al. Diarrhea associated with *Aeromonas* species in children in day care centers. *J Infect Dis* 1993;168:215–218.
48. Sempértegui F, Estrella B, Egas J, et al. Risk of diarrheal disease in Ecuadorian day-care centers. *Pediatr Infect Dis J* 1995;14: 606–612.
49. Pazzaglia G, Sack RB, Salazar E, et al. High frequency of coinfecting enteropathogens in *Aeromonas*-associated diarrhea of hospitalized Peruvian infants. *J Clin Microbiol* 1991;29:1151–1156.
50. Kuijper EJ, van Alphen L, Peeters MF, et al. Human serum antibody response to the presence of *Aeromonas* spp. in the intestinal tract. *J Clin Microbiol* 1990;28:584–590.
51. Jiang ZD, Nelson AC, Mathewson JJ, et al. Intestinal secretory immune response to infection with *Aeromonas* species and *Plesiomonas shigelloides* among students from the United States in Mexico. *J Infect Dis* 1991;164:979–982.
52. Kokka RP, Velji AM, Clark RB, et al. Immune response to S layer-positive O:11 *Aeromonas* associated with intestinal and extraintestinal disease. *Immunol Infect Dis* 1992;2:111–114.
53. Champsaur H, Andremont A, Mathieu D, et al. Cholera-like illness due to *Aeromonas sobria. J Infect Dis* 1982;145:248–254.
54. Burke V, Gracey M, Robinson J, et al. The microbiology of childhood gastroenteritis: *Aeromonas* species and other infective agents. *J Infect Dis* 1983;148:68–74.
55. del Val A, Moles J-R, Garrigues V. Very prolonged diarrhea associated with *Aeromonas hydrophila. Am J Gastroenterol* 1990; 85:1535.
56. Golik A, Modai D, Gluskin I, et al. *Aeromonas* in adult diarrhea: an enteropathogen or an innocent bystander? *J Clin Gastroenterol* 1990;12:148–152.
57. Qadri SMH, Zafar M, Lee GC. Can isolation of *Aeromonas hydrophila* from human feces have any clinical significance? *J Clin Gastroenterol* 1991;13:537–540.
58. Kotloff KL, Wasserman SS, Steciak JY, et al. Acute diarrhea in Baltimore children attending an outpatient clinic. *Pediatr Infect Dis J* 1988;7:753–759.
59. Morris JG Jr, Takeda T, Tall BD, et al. Experimental non-O group 1 *Vibrio cholerae* gastroenteritis in humans. *J Clin Invest* 1990;85:697–705.
60. Morgan DR, Johnson PC, DuPont HL, et al. Lack of correlation between virulence properties of *Aeromonas hydrophila* and enteropathogenicity for humans. *Infect Immun* 1985;50:62–65.
61. George WL, Nakata MM, Thompson J, et al. *Aeromonas*-related diarrhea in adults. *Arch Intern Med* 1985;145:2207–2211.
62. Janda JM. Recent advances in the study of the taxonomy, pathogenicity, and infectious syndromes associated with the genus *Aeromonas. Clin Microbiol Rev* 1991;4:397–410.
63. Kirov SM, O'Donovan LA, Sanderson K. Functional characterization of type IV pili expressed on diarrhea-associated isolates of *Aeromonas* species. *Infect Immun* 1999;5447–5454.
64. Kirov SM, Barnett TC, Pepe CM, et al. Investigation of the role of type IV *Aeromonas* pilus (Tap) in the pathogenesis of *Aeromonas* gastrointestinal infection. *Infect Immun* 2000;68: 4040–4048.
65. Ho ASY, Mietzner TA, Smith AJ, et al. The pili of *Aeromonas hydrophila*: identification of an environmentally regulated "mini pilin." *J Exp Med* 1990;172:795–806.
66. Pearson GDN, Woods A, Chiang SL, et al. CTX genetic element encodes a site-specific recombination system and an intestinal colonization factor. *Proc Nat Acad Sci U S A* 1993; 90:3750–3754.
67. Chopra AK, Houston CW. Enterotoxins in *Aeromonas*-associated gastroenteritis. *Microbes Infect* 1999;1:1129–1137.
68. Janda JM. *Aeromonas* and *Plesiomonas.* In: Sussman M, ed. *Molecular medical microbiology.* London: Academic Press 2001: 1237–1270.
69. Asao T, Kinoshita Y, Kozaki S, et al. Purification and some properties of *Aeromonas hydrophila* hemolysin. *Infect Immun* 1984;46:122–127.
70. Buckley JT, Howard SP. The cytotoxic enterotoxin of *Aeromonas hydrophila* is aerolysin. *Infect Immun* 1999;67:466.
71. Wong CYF, Heuzenroeder MW, Flower RLP. Inactivation of two haemolytic toxin genes in *Aeromonas hydrophila* attenuates virulence in a suckling mouse model. *Microbiology* 1998;144: 291–298.
72. McCardell BA, Madden JM, Kothary MH, et al. Purification and characterization of a CHO cell-elongation toxin produced by *Aeromonas hydrophila. Microb Pathog* 1995;19:1–9.
73. Shaw JG, Thornley JP, Palmer I, et al. Invasion of tissue culture cells by *Aeromonas caviae. Med Microbiol Lett* 1995;4:324–331.
74. Rautelin H, Hänninen ML, Sivonen A, et al. Chronic diarrhea due to a single strain of *Aeromonas caviae. Eur J Clin Microbiol Infect Dis* 1995;14:51–53.

75. Bogdanović R, Ćobeljić M, Marković M, et al. Haemolytic–uraemic syndrome associated with *Aeromonas hydrophila* enterocolitis. *Pediatr Nephrol* 1991;5:293–295.
76. Robson WLM, Leung AKC, Trevenen CL. Haemolytic–uraemic syndrome associated with *Aeromonas hydrophila* enterocolitis [Letter]. *Pediatr Nephrol* 1992;6:221–222.
77. Fang J-S, Chen J-B, Chen W-J, et al. Haemolytic–uraemic syndrome in an adult with *Aeromonas hydrophila* enterocolitis. *Nephrol Dial Transplant* 1999;14:439–440.
78. Filler G, Ehrich JHH, Strauch E, et al. Acute renal failure in an infant associated with cytotoxic *Aeromonas sobria* isolated from patient's stool and from aquarium water as suspected source of infection [Letter]. *J Clin Microbiol* 2000;38:469–470.
79. Sherlock CH, Burdge DR, Smith JA. Does *Aeromonas hydrophila* preferentially colonize the bowels of patients with hematologic malignancies? *Diagn Microbiol Infect Dis* 1987;7:63–68.
80. Cook MA, Nedunchezian D. Colonic carcinoma manifesting as *Aeromonas* colitis. *J Clin Gastroenterol* 1994;18:242–243.
81. Ko W-C, Chuang Y-C. *Aeromonas* bacteremia: review of 59 episodes. *Clin Infect Dis* 1995;20:1298–1304.
82. Shimada T, Kosako Y. Comparison of the two O-serogrouping systems for mesophilic *Aeromonas* spp. *J Clin Microbiol* 1991; 29:197–199.
83. Hänninen M-L, Hirvelä-Koski V. Pulsed-field gel electrophoresis in the study of mesophilic and psychrophilic *Aeromonas* spp. *J Appl Bacteriol* 1997;83:493–498.
84. Jones BL, Wilcox MH. *Aeromonas* infections and their treatment. *J Antimicrob Chemother* 1995;35:453–461.
85. Overman TL, Janda JM. Antimicrobial susceptibility patterns of *Aeromonas jandaei, A. schubertii, A. trota,* and *A. veronii* biotype veronii. *J Clin Microbiol* 1999;37:706–708.
86. Morita K, Watanabe N, Kurata S, et al. β-Lactam resistance of motile *Aeromonas* isolates from clinical and environmental sources. *Antimicrob Agents Chemother* 1994;38:353–355.
87. Ko W-C, Wu H-M, Chang T-C, et al. Inducible β-lactam resistance in *Aeromonas hydrophila*: therapeutic challenge for antimicrobial therapy. *J Clin Microbiol* 1998;36:3188–3192.
88. Ko WC, Yu KW, Huang CT, et al. Increasing antibiotic resistance in clinical isolates of *Aeromonas* strains in Taiwan. *Antimicrob Agents Chemother* 1996;40:1260–1262.
89. Stunt RA, Amyes AKB, Thomson CJ, et al. The production of a novel carbapenem-hydrolysing β-lactamase in *Aeromonas veronii* biovar sobria and its association with imipenem resistance [Correspondence]. *J Antimicrob Chemother* 1998;32:835–839.
90. Holmberg SD, Schell WK, Fanning GR, et al. *Aeromonas* intestinal infections in the United States. *Ann Intern Med* 1986; 105:683–689.
91. Holmberg SD, Farmer JJ III. *Aeromonas hydrophila* and *Plesiomonas shigelloides* as causes of intestinal infections. *Rev Infect Dis* 1984;6:633–639.
92. Rautelin H, Hänninen ML, Sivonen A, et al. Chronic diarrhea due to a single strain of *Aeromonas caviae. Eur J Clin Microbiol Infect Dis* 1995;14:51–53.
93. Janda JM, Duffey PS. Mesophilic aeromonads in human disease: current taxonomy, laboratory identification, and infectious disease spectrum. *Rev Infect Dis* 1988;10:980–997.
94. Brenden RA, Miller MA, Janda JM. Clinical disease spectrum and pathogenic factors associated with *Plesiomonas shigelloides. Rev Infect Dis* 1988;10:303–316.
95. East AK, Allaway D, Collins MD. Analysis of DNA encoding 23S rRNA and 16-23S rRNA intergenic spacer regions from *Plesiomonas shigelloides. FEMS Microbiol Lett* 1992;95:57–62.
96. Janda JM, Abbott SL. Unusual food-borne pathogens: *Listeria monocytogenes, Aeromonas, Plesiomonas,* and *Edwardsiella* species. *Clin Lab Med* 1999;19:553–582.
97. Miller ML, Koburger JA. Evaluation of inositol brilliant green bile salts and *Plesiomonas* agars for recovery of *Plesiomonas shigelloides* from aquatic samples in a seasonal survey of the Suwannee river estuary. *J Food Protect* 1986;49:274–277.
98. de Mondino SSB, Nunes MP, Ricciardi ID. Occurrence of *Plesiomonas shigelloides* in water environments of Rio de Janeiro City. *Mem Inst Oswaldo Cruz* 1995;90:1–4.
99. Jagger T, Keane S, Robertson S. *Plesiomonas shigelloides*—an uncommon cause of diarrhoea in cats. *Vet Rec* 2000;146:296.
100. Rahim Z, Kay BA. Enrichment for *Plesiomonas shigelloides* from stools. *J Clin Microbiol* 1988;26:789–790.
101. Jeppersen C. Media for *Aeromonas* spp., *Plesiomonas shigelloides* and *Pseudomonas* spp. from food and environment. *Int J Food Microbiol* 1995;26:25–41.
102. Chida T, Okamura N, Ohtani K, et al. The complete DNA sequence of the O antigen gene region of *Plesiomonas shigelloides* serotype O17, which is identical to *Shigella sonnei* form I antigen. *Microbiol Immunol* 2000;44:161–172.
103. Holmberg SD, Wachsmuth K, Hickman-Brenner FW, et al. *Plesiomonas* enteric infections in the United States. *Ann Intern Med* 1986;105:690–694.
104. Tsukamoto T, Kinoshita Y, Shimada T, et al. Two epidemics of diarrhoeal disease possibly caused by *Plesiomonas shigelloides. J Hyg Camb* 1978;80:275–280.
105. Van Houten R, Farberman D, Norton J, et al. *Plesiomonas shigelloides* and *Salmonella* serotype *hartford* infections associated with a contaminated water supply—Livingston County, New York, 1996. *MMWR Morb Mortal Wkly Rep* 1998;47:394–396.
106. Binns MM, Vaughan S, Sanyal SC, et al. Invasive ability of *Plesiomonas shigelloides. Zbl Bakt Hyg* 1984;257:343–347.
107. Daskaleros PA, Stoebner JA, Payne SM. Iron uptake in *Plesiomonas shigelloides*: cloning of the genes for the heme-iron uptake system. *Infect Immun* 1991;59:2706–2711.
108. Zeaur R, Akbar A, Bradford AK. Prevalence of *Plesiomonas shigelloides* among diarrhoeal patients in Bangladesh. *Eur J Epidemiol* 1992;8:753–756.
109. Kain KC, Kelly MT. Clinical features, epidemiology, and treatment of *Plesiomonas shigelloides* diarrhea. *J Clin Microbiol* 1989; 27:998–1001.
110. Lee AC, Yuen KY, Ha SY, et al. *Plesiomonas shigelloides* septicemia: case report and literature review. *Pediatr Hematol Oncol* 1996;13:265–269.
111. Ahmad M, Aggarwal M, Ahmed A. Bloody diarrhea caused by *Plesiomonas shigelloides* proctitis in a human immunodeficiency virus-infected patient. *Clin Infect Dis* 1998;27:657.
112. Visitsunthorn N, Komolpis P. Antimicrobial therapy in *Plesiomonas shigelloides*-associated diarrhea in Thai children. *Southeast Asian J Trop Med Public Health* 1995;26:86–90.
113. Greenlees KJ, Machado J, Sundlof SF. Food-borne microbial pathogens of cultured aquatic species. *Vet Clin North Am Anim Pract* 1998;14:101–112.
114. Kourany M, Vasquez MA, Saenz R. Edwardsiellosis in man and animals in Panama: clinical and epidemiologic characteristics. *Am J Trop Med Hyg* 1977;26:1183–1190.
115. Leung MJ. *Plesiomonas shigelloides* and sucrose-positive *Edwardsiella tarda* bacteremia in a man with obstructive jaundice. *Pathology* 1996;28:68–69.
116. Walton DT, Abbott SL, Janda JM. Sucrose-positive *Edwardsiella tarda* mimicking a biogroup 1 strain isolated from a patient with cholelithiasis. *J Clin Microbiol* 1993;31:155–156.
117. Janda JM, Abbott SL. Infections associated with the genus *Edwardsiella tarda*: the role of *E. tarda* in human disease. *Clin Infect Dis* 1993;17:742–748.
118. Gilman RH, Madasamy M, Mariappan M, et al. *Edwardsiella tarda* in jungle diarrhoea and a possible association with *Entamoeba histolytica. Southeast Asian J Trop Med Public Health* 1971;2:186–189.

119. Vandepitte J, Lemmens P, De Swert L. Human edwardsiellosis traced to ornamental fish. *J Clin Microbiol* 1983;17:165–167.
120. Nagel P, Serritella A, Layden TJ. *Edwardsiella tarda* gastroenteritis associated with a pet turtle. *Gastroenterology* 1982;82: 1436–1437.
121. Fang G, Araujo V, Guerrant RL. Enteric infections associated with exposure to animals or animal products. *Infect Dis Clin North Am* 1991;5:681–701.
122. Marques LRM, Toledo MRF, Silva NP, et al. Invasion of HeLa cells by *Edwardsiella tarda. Curr Microbiol* 1984;10:129–132.
123. Janda JM, Abbott SL, Oshiro LS. Penetration and replication of *Edwardsiella* spp. in HEp-2 cells. *Infect Immun* 1991;59: 154–161.
124. Strauss EJ, Ghori N, Falkow S. An *Edwardsiella tarda* strain containing a mutation in the gene with homology to *shlB* and *hpmB* is defective for entry into epithelial cells. *Infect Immun* 1997;65:3924–3932.
125. Janda JM, Abbott SL. Expression of an iron-regulated hemolysin from *Edwardsiella tarda. FEMS Microbiol Lett* 1993;111: 275–280.
126. Wilson JP, Waterer RR, Wofford JD, et al. Serious infections with *Edwardsiella tarda*: a case report and review of the literature. *Arch Intern Med* 1989;149:208–210.
127. Zighelboim J, Williams TW Jr, Bradshaw MW, et al. Successful management of a patient with multiple hepatic abscesses due to *Edwardsiella tarda. Clin Infect Dis* 1992;14:117–120.
128. Osiri M, Tantawichien T, Deesomchock U. *Edwardsiella tarda* bacteremia and septic arthritis in a patient with diabetes mellitus. *Southeast Asian J Trop Med Pub Health* 1997;28:669–672.
129. Peyrade F, Bondiau P, Taillan B, et al. *Edwardsiella tarda* septicemia in chronic lymphoid leukemia. *Rev Med Intern* 1997; 18:233–234.
130. Tamura K, Sakazaki R, McWhorter AC, et al. *Edwardsiella tarda* serotyping scheme for international use. *J Clin Microbiol* 1988;26:2343–2346.
131. Reinhardt JF, Fowlston S, Jones J, et al. Comparative *in vitro* activities of selected antimicrobial agents against *Edwardsiella tarda. Antimicrob Agents Chemother* 1985;27:966–967.
132. Clark RB, Lister PD, Janda JM. *In vitro* susceptibilities of *Edwardsiella tarda* to 22 antibiotics and antibiotic-β-lactamase-inhibitor agents. *Diag Microbiol Infect Dis* 1991;14:173–175.
133. Reger PJ, Mockler DF, Miller MA. Comparison of antimicrobial susceptibility, β-lactamase production, plasmid analysis and serum bactericidal activity in *Edwardsiella tarda, Edwardsiella ictaluri,* and *Edwardsiella hoshinae. J Med Microbiol* 1993;39: 273–281.

50

LISTERIOSIS

PAUL MEAD
LAURENCE SLUTSKER
BRUCE G. GELLIN

Listeria monocytogenes is a facultative intracellular pathogen that causes fetal loss and serious illness among newborns, elderly, and immunocompromised persons. In addition, the organism has recently been identified as a cause of acute febrile gastroenteritis among the general population (1,2). Infection is usually acquired through ingestion of contaminated food, and although relatively uncommon, listeriosis is nevertheless a leading cause of death due to food-borne disease in the United States (3). Almost no other food-borne disease, including botulism (4), has a higher case-fatality rate.

The organism now known as *L. monocytogenes* was first identified in the mid 1920s. While investigating illness in a rabbit colony at Cambridge University, Murray et al. (5) isolated an organism they named *Bacterium monocytogenes* because of the distinctive monocytosis it caused in infected rabbits. A year after that report, Pirie (6) published an account of Tiger River disease, a fatal condition of South African rodents caused by an organism he named *Listerella hepatolytica.* The two organisms were soon shown to be the same and given the hybridized name *L. monocytogenes.* The genus name was changed to *Listeria* in 1940 when it was recognized that *Listerella* had been used previously for unrelated organisms. The genus *Listeria* contains five additional species: *grayi, innocua, ivanovii, seeligeri,* and *welshimeri*; however only *L. monocytogenes* is considered an important human pathogen.

In the decades that followed its discovery, a wealth of information accumulated on *L. monocytogenes* infections in livestock. The organism became well recognized as a cause of encephalitis, abortion, and gastrointestinal (GI) septicemia in sheep, cattle, and other livestock, and numerous studies demonstrated the role of feed, particularly contaminated silage, as a mode of infection in animals (7). In contrast, information on listeriosis in humans was slower to accrue. Although human listeriosis was recognized in the late 1920s and early 1930s, it was not until the early 1980s that food-borne transmission was firmly established as a source of human infection (8–10). In recent years, *L. monocytogenes* has drawn increasing attention as a cause of food-borne disease outbreaks and food recalls, and as a valuable model for studying the pathogenesis of intracellular parasites. Recent sequencing of the genome of *L. monocytogenes* (11) should result in a far better understanding of the molecular biology and pathogenesis of this organism over the next few years.

MICROBIOLOGY

L. monocytogenes is a gram-positive, nonspore-forming bacillus 0.5 μm wide and 1 to 2 μm long. In clinical specimens, cells are found singly or in short chains, sometimes in a *V* or "hinged" arrangement. Flagella at one pole produce characteristic tumbling motility when grown at 25°C. Biochemically, the organism is catalase positive and oxidase negative, and it produces incomplete β-hemolysis on blood agar. *L. monocytogenes* can grow under a wide variety of conditions, including substrates with high salt content (as found in many foods) and pH values ranging from 4.4 to 9.6. Growth is optimal at 30°C to 37°C; however, replication continues at temperatures as low as 1°C to 2°C. The ability to grow at low temperatures allows for selective amplification through cold enrichment and means that even low-level contamination may be problematic for refrigerated foods with a long shelf life.

L. monocytogenes is readily isolated from clinical specimens obtained from normally sterile sites such as cerebrospinal fluid (CSF), blood, and amniotic fluid, usually through direct plating on tryptic soy agar containing 5%

P. Mead: Foodborne and Diarrheal Diseases Branch, Division of Bacterial and Mycotic Diseases, Division National Center for Infectious Diseases, Centers for Disease Control and Prevention, Atlanta, Georgia.

L. Slutsker: Division of Parasitic Diseases, Centers for Disease Control and Prevention/Kenya Medical Research Institute Research Station, Kisumu, Kenya.

B. G. Gellin: Department of Preventive Medicine, Vanderbilt University School of Medicine, Nashville, Tennessee.

sheep, horse, or rabbit blood. Clinical specimens obtained from nonsterile sites, foods, and environmental specimens should be selectively enriched for *Listeria* species before being plated. Various enrichment protocols have been used; a combination of two of these enrichment protocols has been shown to be approximately 90% sensitive (12).

L. monocytogenes is ubiquitous in nature, having been isolated from soil, water, decaying vegetation, insects, and feces of wild and domestic animals (13). Consequently, the organism has many opportunities to enter food-production and -processing environments. *L. monocytogenes* has been recovered from a wide variety of foods, including meats, raw produce, seafood, and dairy products (14,15). In both natural and man-made environments, the organism can persist for months to years (13,16).

Isolates of *L. monocytogenes* can be subdivided into serotypes based on somatic (O) and flagellar (H) antigens (17). Although at least 13 different serotypes have been identified, serotypes 1/2a, 1/2b, and 4b account for most human infections. For example, among 249 clinical isolates of *L. monocytogenes* submitted to the Centers for Disease Control and Prevention (CDC) from state health departments between 1994 and 1998, 39% were serotype 4b, 31% were serotype 1/2b, and 25% were serotype 1/2a (18). Although serogroup 4b appears to have been uncommon in Europe before 1960 (19), this distribution of serotypes appears to have remained stable over the last two decades (20), with no major geographic differences in distribution of serotypes today. Other subtyping methods include phage typing and bacteriocin typing; molecular methods such as multilocus enzyme electrophoresis, chromosomal DNA restriction endonuclease analysis, ribotyping, random amplification of polymorphic DNA, repetitive element-based subtyping, and DNA macrorestriction analysis by pulsed-field gel electrophoresis (PFGE) (17). PFGE subtyping has proven extremely valuable in recent outbreak investigations (21–23), and a World Health Organization–sponsored international collaborating study has concluded that it currently provides the best balance of pattern stability and diversity (24).

PATHOGENESIS

The cellular aspects of *Listeria* pathogenesis have been studied in some detail. Nevertheless, opportunities to study the pathogenesis of listeriosis in humans are limited by the seriousness of infection, and much of the information available is derived from studies of mice, other laboratory animals, and ruminants. Differences observed among animal models suggest caution when extrapolating to human infection (25).

Human infection begins with ingestion of contaminated food. In the intestine, *L monocytogenes* is thought to induce internalization by epithelial cells. The initial stages of this process are facilitated through interaction of E-cadherin on host cells with a bacterial surface protein, internalin A (InlA); a second molecule, internalin B, may also play a role (25). Interaction with InlA is species specific and depends on the presence of proline at position 16 in the E-cadherin molecule. Although studies of mice suggest that low-level absorption through M cells may also occur (26), this mechanism may be less likely to play a role in human infection (25).

Inside the host cell, the bacterium is initially surrounded by a phagocytic vacuole. In successful infections, the vacuole membrane is disrupted through the action of a well–characterized virulence factor, listeriolysin O (LLO). LLO is a hemolysin that is encoded in the structural gene *hly* and causes the incomplete hemolysis seen on agar plates. This enzyme is most active under acidic conditions, which may explain its selective activity in disrupting the vacuole membrane. Once released from the vacuole, *L. monocytogenes* replicates within the host cell cytoplasm. This is followed by activity of another virulence factor, ActA, which induces actin polymerization at the older one pole of the bacterium. An actin "tail" forms, which pushes the organism through the cytoplasm and into neighboring cells (27). This remarkable machinery shelters the organism from the components of humoral immunity while allowing it to spread among cells of the same tissue and possibly across cell types.

After invasion of enterocytes, *L. monocytogenes* spreads to macrophages in the stroma of the intestinal villi, and from there through lymph or blood to the liver, spleen, and regional lymph nodes. Studies of animal models suggest that this occurs quickly and frequently, but that infection is rapidly controlled by a cell-mediated immune response (28). Within the liver, *L. monocytogenes* replicate within hepatocytes, spreading from cell to cell through actin polymerization. It is speculated that in persons with normal immunity, frequent exposure to listerial antigens could result in maintenance of anti-*Listeria* memory T cells. However, in debilitated and immunocompromised patients, the unrestricted proliferation of *Listeria* organisms in the liver may result in prolonged low-level bacteremia, leading to overt clinical illness through invasion of the brain, placenta, and other tissues (28). Entry into the central nervous system (CNS) probably occurs either through bacteremia with direct invasion of endothelial cells or by cell-to-cell spread from infected phagocytes to endothelial cells. In a murine model of bacteremia, nearly one-third of circulating bacteria are found in lymphocytes, primarily monocytes (29). It is also hypothesized that some forms of CNS infection may occur through alternate routes. Rhombencephalitis, the classic manifestation of listeriosis in sheep, may result from retrograde spread of *L. monocytogenes* via cranial nerves from the oral cavity (30).

Incubation Period and Infectious Dose

Information on incubation period is scant and confounded by differences in disease presentation and host characteristics. In outbreaks of invasive illness, incubation periods for patients with a single known exposure to implicated foods have been reported as anywhere from 11 to 70 days, with a median of 31 days in one outbreak (10,31). These long incubation periods are based primarily on presentations of listeriosis in pregnancy and may not be representative of infection in nonpregnant adults. Published and unpublished case reports suggest that invasive illness in nonpregnant adults can occur within 2 days of exposure (31–33) (CDC, *unpublished data*). Furthermore, Riedo et al. (31) report that in one outbreak, pregnant women who later developed culture-confirmed invasive listeriosis had symptoms of headache, myalgias and diarrhea within 4 days of the known exposure; it is conceivable that these symptoms reflected a transient bacteremia that might have presented as frank sepsis in a severely immunocompromised patient. In outbreaks of acute febrile gastroenteritis, the median incubation period has been fairly consistent at about 20 hours, with a range of 9 to 36 hours (1,2).

The infectious dose for listeriosis in humans is unknown. As with incubation period, the infectious dose may be influenced by the nature of the host, the specific syndrome, the food vehicle, and possibly the virulence of the infecting strain (34). In experiments using outbreak-associated strains, healthy primates required an oral inoculum of 10^9 organisms administered in whipped cream before becoming ill (35). In outbreaks of invasive disease in humans, implicated foods have been found to contain anywhere from less than 1 colony-forming unit (CFU) of *L. monocytogenes* per gram (CDC, *unpublished data*) to more than 1 billion CFU/g (36); however, it has been difficult to show that these levels are necessarily representative of exposure in case patients. In a recent outbreak associated with butter, careful follow-up studies showed that pathogen levels in naturally contaminated butter were relatively stable and that the patients probably consumed between 10^1 and 10^5 organisms (37). Outbreaks of acute febrile gastroenteritis have generally been associated with extremely high levels of contamination. In the 1994 outbreak linked to chocolate milk, the number of *L. monocytogenes* detected in contaminated milk was 10^9 per milliliter of milk (2).

Immunity

As with other enteric pathogens, gastric acidity provides a degree of nonspecific immunity. Use of antacids and H_2 antagonists has been reported as a risk factor for infection in at least one outbreak (9), and pretreatment with cimetidine lowers the oral infective dose in animal models (38). After invasion, cell-mediated immunity is thought to play a key role in defense against *L. monocytogenes* infections. This is consistent with the finding that conditions indicative of impaired cellular immunity (e.g., lymphoreticular malignancies and use of steroids and other immunosuppressive medications) are associated with an increased risk of listeriosis. Although virulence factors such as LLO and actin polymerization factor may illicit antibody responses, the role of humoral immunity is poorly defined. Defects in humoral immunity have not been associated with an increased risk of infection. Immunization against listeriosis has been conducted in animals but is probably impractical for humans given the relative rarity of infection (39).

CLINICAL MANIFESTATIONS

L. monocytogenes can be isolated from the stool of approximately 1% to 5% of healthy persons (40,41). Higher rates of asymptomatic carriage have been reported for laboratory workers (42) and household contacts of patients with invasive listeriosis (40,43). It is not known whether carriage among household contacts reflects a shared exposure or some degree of transmission among household members; however, the ability to recover the same strain from healthy and ill household members underscores the role of host immunity in determining susceptibility to disease. Rates of asymptomatic shedding are not markedly elevated among pregnant women (44,45) or patients with renal failure (46). Although *L. monocytogenes* has been shown to cause outbreaks of acute febrile gastroenteritis (see below), patients with diarrhea are generally no more likely to have *L. monocytogenes* in their stool than are asymptomatic persons. A study of 595 adults hospitalized with diarrhea found *L. monocytogenes* in 1% of cases, and a second study of 171 patients recovered the organism from 1.8% of patients with gastroenteritis. Asymptomatic carriage has been documented in all trimesters of pregnancy (45).

Illness caused by *L. monocytogenes* most often takes the form of either invasive disease or acute febrile gastroenteritis (Table 50.1). Invasive disease is often divided into two categories: perinatal infections, including those of pregnant woman, fetuses, and newborn children, and non-perinatal infections. Non-perinatal infections usually occur in adults with underlying medical conditions, including malignancy (particularly hematologic), immunosuppressive therapy (steroids, azathioprine, cyclosporine), organ transplants, and diabetes (18,47–51). Other disorders that may predispose to listeriosis include alcoholism, cirrhosis, collagen vascular diseases, sarcoidosis, ulcerative colitis, aplastic anemia, and conditions associated with iron overload (20,48,49,52–55). Although listeriosis is not a common opportunistic infection in persons with HIV infection, studies in the United States suggest that the risk of invasive listeriosis is 9-fold to 62-fold higher in persons with HIV infection (56,57) and 96-fold to 280-fold higher in persons with AIDS (56–58).

Invasive Disease in Nonpregnant Adults

Among nonpregnant adults, invasive listeriosis typically presents as sepsis, meningitis, or meningoencephalitis. Although historically meningitis is reported to be the most

TABLE 50.1. CLINICAL SYNDROMES ASSOCIATED WITH INFECTION WITH *LISTERIA MONOCYTOGENES*

Population	Clinical Presentation	Diagnosis	Predisposing Conditions or Circumstances
Pregnant women	Fever, ± myalgias, ± diarrhea Preterm delivery Abortion Stillbirth	Blood culture ± amniotic fluid culture	
Newborns			
<7 d old	Sepsis, pneumonia	Blood culture	Prematurity
≥7 d old	Meningitis, sepsis	Cerebrospinal fluid culture	
Nonpregnant adults	Sepsis, meningitis, focal infections	Culture of blood, cerebrospinal fluid, or other normally sterile site	Immunosuppression, advanced age
Healthy adults	Diarrhea and fever	Stool culture in selective enrichment broth	Possibly large inoculum

common presenting form, in a series of 362 U.S. cases identified through active surveillance between 1994 and 1998, 72% had bacteremia without meningitis, 11% had meningitis with concurrent bacteremia, and 13% had meningitis without documented bacteremia (18). *L. monocytogenes* accounted for 8% of all cases of bacterial meningitis in the United States in 1995, and 20% of all meningitis cases in persons older than 60 years (59).

Common presenting symptoms in nonpregnant adults with CNS listeriosis include fever, malaise, ataxia, seizures, and altered mental status. Rhombencephalitis can occur and is characterized by asymmetric cranial nerve deficits, cerebellar signs, and hemiparesis or hemisensory deficits (60–62). The CSF from patients with meningitis is usually abnormal; however, the findings are not sufficiently characteristic to differentiate listerial meningitis from other bacterial causes of meningitis. Gram stain of the CSF may show gram-positive bacilli but is often unrevealing.

Various other clinical manifestations of infection with *L. monocytogenes* have been described, including endocarditis (63,64), endophthalmitis (65), septic arthritis (66), osteomyelitis (67), pneumonia and pleural infection (68), and peritonitis (55). Cutaneous infections without bacteremia have been reported in persons handling infected animals (69) and in accidentally exposed laboratory workers (70).

Listeriosis during Pregnancy

Pregnant women with listeriosis usually present with nonspecific illness characterized by fever, headache, myalgias, and GI symptoms (71). This flulike prodrome occurs in approximately two-thirds of pregnant women with listeriosis (50,72) and is associated with the bacteremic phase of infection. Women pregnant with multiple gestations may be at increased risk for listeriosis compared with singleton pregnancies (73). Although listeriosis can occur anytime during pregnancy, it has been documented most frequently during the third trimester (72).

The major consequences of listeriosis during pregnancy are fetal loss, stillbirth, congenital infection, and neonatal disease. Fetal infection most likely results from maternal bacteremia, followed by seeding of the placenta, although some infections may occur through ascending spread from vaginal colonization (74). The frequency of fetal loss due to *L. monocytogenes* is difficult to determine because bacterial cultures are not routinely obtained from spontaneously aborted fetuses or stillborn neonates (75). In one series, *Listeria* was cultured from placental/fetal tissues in 1.6% of spontaneous abortions (76). Other adverse outcomes associated with intrauterine infection include preterm labor and amnionitis.

As with group B streptococcal infections, neonatal listeriosis can present with early or late-onset disease. Defined as illness at birth or within the first week of life, early onset neonatal listeriosis is the result of intrauterine infection. Infants with early onset disease usually present with sepsis, rather than meningitis (47). Occasionally, infants are born with granulomatosis infantiseptica, a syndrome characterized by disseminated abscesses or granulomas in multiple organs including the liver, spleen, lungs, kidney, and brain (77). Approximately 45% to 70% of neonatal listeriosis is early onset (78,79).

Late-onset neonatal disease occurs from one to several weeks after birth and is more likely to present with meningitis than early onset disease (47,80). In a review of neonatal listeriosis cases from 1967 to 1985 in Britain, 39 (93%) of 42 infants with late-onset disease had meningitis (79). Similarly, active surveillance for listeriosis in the United States in 1986 documented meningitis as the presenting syndrome in 88% of late-onset cases (47). Infants with late-onset listeriosis are usually born healthy and full term to mothers who have had uncomplicated pregnancies.

In contrast to early onset disease, the route of infection in late-onset neonatal disease is not well understood. Acquisition of infection during passage through the birth canal is likely; however, cases of late-onset disease after cesarean delivery have been reported. Clusters of late-onset neonatal listeriosis have been identified in newborn nurseries, suggesting that some nosocomial transmission also occurs (81–84). In one outbreak in Costa Rica, infection was linked to contaminated mineral oil used to bathe newborns (85).

Mortality rates for both early and late-onset neonatal infection are approximately 20% to 30% (79,86,87). Neonatal infection can be effectively prevented by antibiotic treatment during pregnancy; however, fetal or early onset neonatal infection does not invariably follow maternal listeriosis for which treatment has been delayed or not given (10,88,89). Routine microbiologic screening or antimicrobial prophylaxis for subsequent pregnancies is not generally recommended for women with a history of pregnancy-associated listeriosis (48). However, all pregnant women should be counseled on avoiding high-risk foods during pregnancy. Because of the potential adverse outcomes of maternal listeriosis and the availability of effective treatment, it is prudent to evaluate all febrile episodes during pregnancy with blood cultures.

Acute Gastroenteritis

Recent outbreak investigations provide compelling evidence that *L. monocytogenes* can cause acute gastroenteritis in persons without underlying medical conditions. Illness is characterized by fever, nonbloody diarrhea, an average incubation period less than 24 hours, and a high attack rate among exposed persons. In a 1994 outbreak in Illinois, nearly 80% of persons who consumed chocolate milk contaminated with 10^9 CFU/mL of *L. monocytogenes* developed diarrhea; 72% also reported fever (2). The median incubation period between consumption and illness was 20 hours (range, 9 to 32 hours). Diarrhea lasted a median of 42 hours, with a median of 12 stools per day at the height of symptoms. The same subtype of *L. monocytogenes* was isolated from the chocolate milk and stools of ill persons. In addition, ill persons were more likely than controls to have elevated anti-LLO titers. In a more recent outbreak in Italy, 1,566 (72%) of 2,189 persons who ate contaminated corn salad developed illness, and 292 (19%) of ill persons were hospitalized (1). Among hospitalized patients, fever and diarrhea lasted a median of 3 days. *L. monocytogenes* serotype 4b was isolated from one blood specimen, 87% of 141 stool specimens, a sample of the salad, and from environmental specimens collected from the catering plant. All isolates were identical by DNA analysis. Although the level of contamination at the time of ingestion could not be determined precisely, inoculation studies showed that the corn salad supported growth of *L. monocytogenes* when kept at 25°C for 10 hours.

Results from other outbreak investigations also support the view that *L. monocytogenes* can cause febrile gastroenteritis. In an outbreak of invasive listeriosis in the United States, case patients were significantly more likely than controls to have reported fever, vomiting, or diarrhea in the week before the case-patient's positive culture (90). In an outbreak of gastroenteritis in immunocompetent adults attending a supper party in Italy, diarrhea and fever occurred in more than 70% of the ill party-goers, and two developed bacteremia caused by *L. monocytogenes* (91). The median incubation period from the time of the supper to onset of GI symptoms was 18 hours. Although the same strain of *L. monocytogenes* that was isolated from the patients was also cultured from several foods left over from the supper, no stool specimens collected from ill persons yielded *L. monocytogenes.*

The frequency of febrile gastroenteritis caused by *L. monocytogenes* remains undetermined, as do the infectious dose and characteristics of the host that are associated with this syndrome. Clinicians and public health officials should consider culturing stools for *L. monocytogenes* in outbreaks of illness characterized by acute onset of fever and diarrhea when routine stool cultures have been negative. In such cases, the laboratory should be notified that *L. monocytogenes* is suspected so the appropriate culture media are used.

EPIDEMIOLOGY

Epidemiologic studies have established food as an important source of both sporadic and outbreak-associated listeriosis in humans. The first convincing evidence for this was obtained in 1981 when a case–control study identified coleslaw as the likely source of an outbreak involving 41 patients in Nova Scotia. The same strain of *L. monocytogenes* was recovered from patients and from unopened packages of coleslaw. It was later determined that fields where the coleslaw cabbage were grown were fertilized with raw sheep manure. Two sheep in the source flock died of listeriosis in the previous year. After harvest, the cabbage was stored in an unheated shed, possibly enhancing the growth of *L. monocytogenes* (8).

This and other early outbreaks not withstanding, most listeriosis outbreaks have involved ready-to-eat meats and dairy products (Table 50.2). This has occurred despite frequent contamination of produce items and may reflect the generally greater potential of meats and cheeses to support the growth of pathogenic organisms. Specific dairy products linked to outbreaks include 2% milk (92), various forms of soft cheese (10,93,94), and butter (95). In 1994, chocolate milk heavily contaminated with *L. monocytogenes* was identified as the source of an outbreak in which healthy persons developed acute febrile gastroenteritis but not invasive disease (2). Studies have shown that pasteurization is adequate to eliminate *L. monocytogenes* from dairy products (96), and most dairy-associated outbreaks are due to items that are unpasteurized or inadequately pasteurized or that may have been contaminated after pasteurization.

The importance of processed meats as a source of epidemic listeriosis is underscored by a series of large outbreaks.

TABLE 50.2. SELECTED OUTBREAKS OF LISTERIOSIS

Year	Location	No. of Cases (Deaths)	Implicated (or Likely) Vehicle	Perinatal Cases (%)	*Listeria Monocytogenes* Serotype	Reference
1979	Massachusetts, US	20 (5)	(Raw vegetables)	0	4b	9
1981	Nova Scotia, Canada	41 (18)	Coleslaw	83	4b	8
1983	Massachusetts, US	49 (14)	Pasteurized milk	14	4b	92
1985	California, US	142 (48)	Mexican-style cheese	66	4b	10
1983–1987	Switzerland	122 (34)	Soft cheese	53	4b	93
1988–1989	United Kingdom	NA[a]	Paté	NA[a]	4b	97
1989	Connecticut, US	10 (0)	(Shrimp)	33	4b	31
1992	France	279 (85)	Pork tongue in jelly	0	4b	121
1993	Italy	18 (0)	Rice salad	0	1/2b	91
1994	Illinois, US	48[b] (0)	Pasteurized chocolate milk	0	1/2b	2
1997	Italy	1,566 (0)	Corn and tuna salad	NA	4b	1
1998–1999	United States	101 (21)	Hot dogs	16	4b	99
1998–1999	Finland	24 (6)	Butter	0	3a	95

[a]Not available.
[b]Includes 45 cases of diarrhea and 3 cases of invasive disease.

In the United Kingdom, meat pâté from one manufacturer was identified as the source of more than 300 cases occurring between 1987 and 1989 (97). A similarly large outbreak occurred in 1992 in France when 279 cases resulted from contaminated pork tongue in jelly (98). In the United States, hot dogs were identified as the source of a 1998 outbreak involving more than 100 cases in 22 states (99).

Studies of sporadic listeriosis have confirmed the role of food as a major source of infection in the non-outbreak setting as well. In one U.S. study conducted from 1986 to 1988, patients with sporadic infection were significantly more likely than controls to have eaten non-reheated hot dogs or undercooked chicken in the month preceding their illness (100). An estimated 20% of the overall risk of listeriosis was attributable to consumption of these foods. These findings were further validated in 1989 when a single case of listeriosis was microbiologically linked to consumption of turkey franks (96). Isolates of *L. monocytogenes* serotype 1/2a with identical isoenzyme types were recovered from the blood of a patient, turkey franks from the patient's refrigerator, and from unopened packages of the turkey franks obtained from a retail store. The same strain was later isolated from equipment in the facility where the turkey franks were produced (16). In a second U.S. case–control study published in 1992, sporadic illnesses was associated with consumption of soft cheeses and eating foods from delicatessens (58). This study included a microbiologic survey of foods from the refrigerators of 123 enrolled patients (14). *L. monocytogenes* was isolated from at least one food in the refrigerators of 64% of patients, and one-third of refrigerators contained food isolates that were the same enzyme type as that isolated from the patient. Overall, 36% of beef items, 31% of poultry items, and 8% of ready-to-eat foods (processed meats, raw vegetables, leftovers, and cheeses) were contaminated.

Listeriosis was not made a nationally notifiable disease in the United States until 2000 (101), so nationwide data on incidence and demographic features of infected persons are not available. CDC and state and local health departments have conducted ongoing active surveillance for listeriosis in selected sites since 1989. Data from this system indicate that the annualized incidence of listeriosis decreased from 7.9 per million population in 1989 to 4.4 per million in 1993 (102). Results from a recently released 10-year survey demonstrate a concomitant decline in contamination of ready-to-eat meats with *L. monocytogenes* (103). These findings support the view that the decrease in human listeriosis is due in part to enforcement by regulatory agencies of a "zero-tolerance" policy for *Listeria* in ready-to-eat foods and intensified cleanup programs in meat-processing facilities (102). Published dietary recommendations for high-risk consumers may also have contributed to the decreased disease incidence (104–106).

Since 1994, overall rates of listeriosis in the United States have remained relatively constant, averaging between four and five cases per million population (18). However, the rate of infection among newborns has decreased steadily. In 1998, the rate of infection in newborns was 53 per million, representing a nearly 70% decrease since 1989 and a 39% decrease since 1994. Reasons for the decline in the rate of perinatal listeriosis are unknown; possible contributing factors may include decreased consumption of high-risk foods among pregnant women in response to education efforts and an overall decrease in the level of contamination of the food supply. Despite these changes, rates of invasive listeriosis continue to be highest in newborns and the elderly (18). Incidence rates in persons who identify themselves as Asian or African American are also higher than those in persons who identify themselves as white, although this difference was less marked in 1998 than in pervious years. Rates have generally been higher in Hispanics, and in recent years, the disparity has increased. In 1998, the rate among Hispanics was nearly fourfold higher than among non-Hispanics. This was largely due to a high rate of perinatal disease among Hispanic women (18), possibly due to frequent consumption of queso fresco and other soft cheeses in this population.

DIAGNOSIS

The isolation of *L. monocytogenes* from a normally sterile site such as blood or CSF is usually necessary for the diagnosis of invasive listeriosis. Because asymptomatic fecal carriage occurs, culture of the organism from stool in the setting of an outbreak is helpful only in the setting of an outbreak or other epidemiologic investigation. *L. monocytogenes* from sterile-site specimens usually grows well in routine media. The specimen is directly plated on tryptic soy agar containing 5% sheep, horse, or rabbit blood and is usually identified within 36 hours. Identification of *L. monocytogenes* by use of fluorescent antibody methods or approaches that use DNA probes coupled with polymerase chain reaction technology may prove useful in some specimens. Experimental serologic assays for antibody to LLO have been used in some epidemiologic investigations (2) and to support the diagnosis in culture-negative listeriosis of the CNS (107).

TREATMENT

No randomized trials have been conducted in humans to determine the optimal antibiotic or duration of therapy for listeriosis. Most *L. monocytogenes* isolates are susceptible to a wide range of antimicrobial agents *in vitro*; however, clinical efficacy may be influenced by drug uptake and compartmentalization within infected cells, the ability of specific agents to cross the blood–brain barrier, and the potential effects of subtherapeutic levels on expression of bacterial virulence factors.

Ampicillin (or amoxicillin) is currently considered the drug of choice for invasive disease based on *in vitro* activity, animal models, and available clinical experience (108). To ensure penetration of sufficient amounts into the CNS, doses of at least 6 g per day are recommended for adults (108). Furthermore, because β-lactams display only delayed killing of *Listeria in vitro,* several experts advocate the addition of gentamicin (108,109). Although likely inactive intracellularly, aminoglycosides are synergistic with penicillin *in vitro* and may be clinically beneficial by killing bacteria that are outside of host cells (108). Other drugs such as chloramphenicol and tetracycline have been associated with high treatment-failure rates (110), and reduced affinity of key penicillin-binding proteins gives most strains of *L. monocytogenes* high natural resistance to later generation cephalosporins (111). Innate resistance to penicillin derivatives has not been identified; however, relapses have been reported in immunosuppressed patients treated with 2 weeks of penicillin therapy (112). Several experts recommend that invasive illness be treated for at least 2 to 3 weeks, with longer courses for patients who are immunocompromised or who have complicated infections such as endocarditis or rhombencephalitis (108,113,114).

Patients who are allergic to penicillins should be treated with trimethoprim-sulfamethoxazole (108). Although there is less clinical experience with this drug combination, it is bactericidal, has good intracellular and CNS penetration, and has been used successfully in several settings (60). Indeed, limited evidence from the clinical literature suggests that trimethoprim-sulfamethoxazole may be more effective than ampicillin plus gentamicin. In a nonrandomized trial of 22 severely ill patients with meningoencephalitis, treatment with trimethoprim-sulfamethoxazole (±ampicillin) was associated with a 7% mortality rate, compared with a 23% mortality rate for patients treated with ampicillin plus gentamicin (115). Although vancomycin has been recommended as an alternative medication, treatment failures have occurred, and there is at least one case report of a patient developing listerial meningitis while receiving vancomycin (116). Steroids have been shown to reduce complications in some forms of bacterial meningitis; however, their use in cases of listerial meningitis is generally discouraged given their role as a risk factor of *Listeria* infection (114).

The role of antimicrobial therapy for patients with febrile gastroenteritis due to *Listeria* is unknown. Oral ampicillin or trimethoprim-sulfamethoxazole would seem reasonable choices for the reasons listed above; however, there are no studies that document the efficacy of these or other agents in reducing the duration of diarrhea or preventing progression from gastroenteritis to invasive disease. Although most patients recover spontaneously (1,2), acute gastroenteritis may be a precursor to invasive disease in a subset of high-risk patients (31).

PREVENTION

Although difficult to quantify, it is likely that some proportion of listeriosis cases can be prevented by following general consumer food safety guidelines. These include thorough cooking of raw food from animal sources; washing raw vegetables thoroughly before eating; keeping uncooked meats separate from vegetables and from cooked and ready-to-eat foods; avoiding raw (unpasteurized) milk or foods made from raw milk; and washing hands, knives, and cutting boards after handling uncooked foods (104). Pregnant women, immunocompromised persons, and others at high risk for listeriosis can take additional precautions to decrease the risk of infection. These persons should avoid foods epidemiologically linked with listeriosis including pâté and soft cheeses such as feta, Brie, Camembert, blue-veined, or Mexican-style cheese. In addition, ready-to-eat foods such as hot dogs and leftover foods should be cooked until steaming before being eaten. These persons may also reduce their risk of infection by avoiding delicatessen foods and thoroughly reheating cold cuts before eating.

Along with action on the part of the consumer, the control of listeriosis requires effort by clinicians, public health agencies, academia, and the food industry. Routine surveillance and outbreak investigations can help control listeriosis, but only if physicians and other care providers report cases promptly to public health authorities. With the advent of PulseNet, the National Molecular Subtyping Network for Foodborne Disease (117), most state public health laboratories have the ability to conduct timely molecular subtyping of *L. monocytogenes* isolates and to share subtype information electronically with other states. This system has greatly enhanced the recognition of common source outbreaks, but it relies on prompt forwarding of *L. monocytogenes* isolates to public health laboratories to be most effective.

Long-term prevention of listeriosis will require additional research to determine the infectious dose and identify virulence markers associated with human disease. The food industry should continue to develop and implement hazard analysis and critical control-point programs to control and minimize the presence of *L. monocytogenes* at important points in the processing, distribution, and marketing of processed foods (118), and regulatory agencies need to continue to enforce current regulations designed to minimize *L. monocytogenes* in ready-to-eat foods. In addition, government and academia need to continue to work with the processed meat industry to both ensure meticulous in-plant sanitation and develop practical methods for postpackaging pasteurization of processed meats. *Listeria* organisms are susceptible to irradiation (119), and this promising food safety technology (120) could be a major tool to prevent listeriosis. The recent addition of listeriosis to the list of nationally notifiable conditions should greatly enhance understanding of the epidemiology of infection in the United States and should provide a broad-based standard by which to judge the success or failure of prevention efforts.

ACKNOWLEDGMENTS

We wish to acknowledge the contributions of Anne Schuchat, MD, author of several excellent reviews on listeriosis, and to thank Ms. Colleen Crowe for her assistance with the references.

REFERENCES

1. Aureli P, Fiorucci GC, Caroli D, et al. An outbreak of febrile gastroenteritis associated with corn contaminated by *Listeria monocytogenes. N Engl J Med* 2000;342(17):1236–1241.
2. Dalton CB, Austin CC, Sobel J, et al. An outbreak of gastroenteritis and fever due to *Listeria monocytogenes* in milk. *N Engl J Med* 1997;336(2):100–105.
3. Mead PS, Slutsker L, Dietz V, et al. Food-related illness and death in the United States. *Emerging Infect Dis* 1999;5(5):607–625.
4. Shapiro RL, Hatheway C, Swerdlow DL. Botulism in the United States: a clinical and epidemiologic review. *Ann Intern Med* 1998;129(3):221–228.
5. Murray E, Webb R, Swann M. A disease of rabbits characterized by a large mononuclear leucocytosis, caused by a hitherto undescribed bacillus *Bacterium monocytogenes* (n.sp.). *J Pathol Bacteriol* 1926;29:407–439.
6. Pirie J. A new disease of veld rodents, "Tiger River disease." *Publ S Afr Inst Med Res* 1927;3:163–186.
7. Wesley I. Listeriosis in animals. In: Ryser E, Marth E, eds. Listeria, *listeriosis, and food safety,* second edition. New York: Marcel Dekker Inc, 1999:39–73.
8. Schlech WF III, Lavigne PM, Bortolussi RA, et al. Epidemic listeriosis—evidence for transmission by food. *N Engl J Med* 1983;308(4):203–206.
9. Ho JL, Shands KN, Friedland G, et al. An outbreak of type 4b *Listeria monocytogenes* infection involving patients from eight Boston hospitals. *Arch Intern Med* 1986;146(3):520–524.
10. Linnan MJ, Mascola L, Lou XD, et al. Epidemic listeriosis associated with Mexican-style cheese. *N Engl J Med* 1988;319(13): 823–828.
11. Glaser P, Frangeul L, Buchrieser C, et al. Comparative genomics of *Listeria* species. *Science* 2001;294(5543):849–852.
12. Swaminathan B, Rocourt J, Bille J. *Listeria.* In: Murray P, Baron E, Pfaller M, et al., eds. *Manual of clinical microbiology,* sixth edition. Washington, DC: American Society for Microbiology, 1995:341–348.
13. Fenlon D. *Listeria monocytogenes* in the natural environment. In: Ryser E, Marth E, eds. Listeria, *listeriosis, and food safety,* second edition. New York: Marcel Dekker Inc, 1999:21–37.
14. Pinner RW, Schuchat A, Swaminathan B, et al. Role of foods in sporadic listeriosis, II: microbiologic and epidemiologic investigation. *JAMA* 1992;267(15):2046–2050.
15. Ryser E. Foodborne listeriosis. In: Ryser E, Marth E, eds. Listeria, *listeriosis, and food safety,* second edition. New York: Marcel Dekker Inc, 1999:299–358.
16. Wenger J, Swaminathan B, Hayes P, et al. *Listeria monocytogenes* contamination of turkey franks: evaluation of a production facility. *J Food Protect* 1990;53:1015–1019.
17. Graves L, Swaminatha B, Hunter S. Subtyping *Listeria monocytogenes.* In: Ryser E, Marth E, eds. Listeria, *listeriosis, and food safety,* second edition. New York: Marcel Dekker Inc, 1999:279–299.
18. Slutsker L, Evans M, Schuchat A. Listeriosis. In: Scheld W, Craig W, Hughes J, eds. *Emerging infections.* Washington, DC: ASM Press, 2000:83–106.
19. Rocourt J. Taxonomy of the *Listeria* genus and typing of *L. monocytogenes* [in French]. *Pathol Biol (Paris)* 1996;44(9): 749–756.
20. Gellin BG, Broome CV. Listeriosis. *JAMA* 1989;261(9): 1313–1320.
21. Centers for Disease Control and Prevention. Multistate outbreak of listeriosis—United States, 1998. *MMWR Morb Mortal Wkly Rep* 1998;47(50):1085–1086.
22. Centers for Disease Control and Prevention. Multistate outbreak of listeriosis—United States, 2000. *MMWR Morb Mortal Wkly Rep* 2000;49(50):1129–1130.
23. Goulet V, Rocourt J, Rebiere I, et al. Listeriosis outbreak associated with the consumption of rillettes in France in 1993. *J Infect Dis* 1998;177(1):155–160.
24. Graves LM, Swaminathan B. PulseNet standardized protocol for subtyping *Listeria monocytogenes* by macrorestriction and

pulsed-field gel electrophoresis. *Int J Food Microbiol* 2001;65(1-2):55–62.
25. Lecuit M, Vandormael-Pournin S, Lefort J, et al. A transgenic model for listeriosis: role of internalin in crossing the intestinal barrier. *Science* 2001;292(5522):1722–1725.
26. Marco AJ, Altimira J, Prats N, et al. Penetration of *Listeria monocytogenes* in mice infected by the oral route. *Microb Pathog* 1997;23(5):255–263.
27. Cossart P, Bierne H. The use of host cell machinery in the pathogenesis of *Listeria monocytogenes. Curr Opin Immunol* 2001;13(1):96–103.
28. Vazquez-Boland JA, Kuhn M, Berche P, et al. Listeria pathogenesis and molecular virulence determinants. *Clin Microbiol Rev* 2001;14(3):584–640.
29. Drevets DA. Dissemination of *Listeria monocytogenes* by infected phagocytes. *Infect Immun* 1999;67(7):3512–3517.
30. Barlow RM, McGorum B. Ovine listerial encephalitis: analysis, hypothesis and synthesis. *Vet Rec* 1985;116(9):233–236.
31. Riedo FX, Pinner RW, Tosca ML, et al. A point-source foodborne listeriosis outbreak: documented incubation period and possible mild illness. *J Infect Dis* 1994;170(3):693–696.
32. Azadian BS, Finnerty GT, Pearson AD. Cheese-borne listeria meningitis in immunocompetent patient. *Lancet* 1989;1(8633):322–323.
33. Junttila J, Brander M. *Listeria monocytogenes* septicemia associated with consumption of salted mushrooms. *Scand J Infect Dis* 1989;21(3):339–342.
34. Pine L, Malcolm GB, Plikaytis BD. *Listeria monocytogenes* intragastric and intraperitoneal approximate 50% lethal doses for mice are comparable, but death occurs earlier by intragastric feeding. *Infect Immun* 1990;58(9):2940–2945.
35. Farber JM, Daley E, Coates F, et al. Feeding trials of *Listeria monocytogenes* with a nonhuman primate model. *J Clin Microbiol* 1991;29(11):2606–2608.
36. Farber JM, Peterkin PI. *Listeria monocytogenes,* a food-borne pathogen. *Microbiol Rev* 1991;55(3):476–511.
37. Maijala R, Lyytikainen O, Johansson T. Exposure to *Listeria monocytogenes* in an outbreak caused by butter. In: Hof H, ed. *International Symposium on Problems of Listeriosis (ISOPOL) XIV; 2001.* Mannheim, Germany: Institut fur Med Mikrobiologie und Hygiene, 2001:166.
38. Schlech WF III, Chase DP, Badley A. A model of food-borne *Listeria monocytogenes* infection in the Sprague-Dawley rat using gastric inoculation: development and effect of gastric acidity on infective dose. *Int J Food Microbiol* 1993;18(1):15–24.
39. Schlech WF. Pathogenesis and immunology of *Listeria monocytogenes. Pathol Biol (Paris)* 1996;44(9):775–782.
40. Bojsen-Moller J. Human listeriosis. Diagnostic, epidemiological and clinical studies. *Acta Pathol Microbiol Scand [B] Microbiol Immunol* 1972;229[Suppl]:1–157.
41. Muller HE. *Listeria* isolations from feces of patients with diarrhea and from healthy food handlers. *Infection* 1990;18(2):97–99.
42. Kampelmacher EH, van Noorle Jansen LM. Further studies on the isolation of *L. monocytogenes* in clinically healthy individuals [in German]. *Zentralbl Bakteriol Orig A* 1972;221(1):70–77.
43. Schuchat A, Deaver K, Hayes PS, et al. Gastrointestinal carriage of *Listeria monocytogenes* in household contacts of patients with listeriosis. *J Infect Dis* 1993;167(5):1261–1262.
44. Lamont RJ, Postlewaite R. Carriage of *Listeria monocytogenes* and related species in pregnant and non-pregnant women in Aberdeen, Scotland. *J Infect* 1986;13:187–193.
45. Gray JW, Barrett JF, Pedler SJ, et al. Faecal carriage of listeria during pregnancy. *Br J Obstet Gynaecol* 1993;100(9):873–874.
46. MacGowan AP, Marshall RJ, MacKay IM, et al. *Listeria* fecal carriage by renal transplant recipients, haemodialysis patients and patients in general practice: its relation to season, drug therapy, foreign travel, animal exposure, and diet. *Epidemiol Infect* 1991;106:157–166.
47. Gellin BG, Broome CV, Bibb WF, et al. The epidemiology of listeriosis in the United States—1986. *Am J Epidemiol* 1991;133(4):392–401.
48. Schuchat A, Swaminathan B, Broome CV. Epidemiology of human listeriosis. *Clin Microbiol Rev* 1991;4(2):169–183.
49. Nieman RE, Lorber B. Listeriosis in adults: a changing pattern. Report of eight cases and review of the literature, 1968–1978. *Rev Infect Dis* 1980;2(2):207–227.
50. McLauchlin J. Human listeriosis in Britain, 1967–85, a summary of 722 cases, II: listeriosis in non-pregnant individuals, a changing pattern of infection and seasonal incidence. *Epidemiol Infect* 1990;104(2):191–201.
51. Paul ML, Dwyer DE, Chow C, et al. Listeriosis—a review of eighty-four cases. *Med J Aust* 1994;160(8):489–493.
52. Harisdangkul V, Songcharoen S, Lin AC. Listerial infections in patients with systemic lupus erythematosus. *South Med J* 1992;85(10):957–960.
53. Kraus A, Cabral AR, Sifuentes-Osornio J, et al. Listeriosis in patients with connective tissue diseases. *J Rheumatol* 1994;21(4):635–638.
54. Mossey RT, Sondheimer J. Listeriosis in patients with long-term hemodialysis and transfusional iron overload. *Am J Med* 1985;79(3):397–400.
55. Nguyen MH, Yu VL. *Listeria monocytogenes* peritonitis in cirrhotic patients. Value of ascitic fluid gram stain and a review of literature. *Dig Dis Sci* 1994;39(1):215–218.
56. Ewert DP, Lieb L, Hayes PS, et al. *Listeria monocytogenes* infection and serotype distribution among HIV-infected persons in Los Angeles County, 1985–1992. *J Acquired Immune Defic Syndrome Hum Retrovirol* 1995;8(5):461–465.
57. Jurado RL, Farley MM, Pereira E, et al. Increased risk of meningitis and bacteremia due to *Listeria monocytogenes* in patients with human immunodeficiency virus infection. *Clin Infect Dis* 1993;17(2):224–227.
58. Schuchat A, Deaver KA, Wenger JD, et al. Role of foods in sporadic listeriosis, I: case–control study of dietary risk factors. *JAMA* 1992;267(15):2041–2045.
59. Schuchat A, Robinson K, Wenger JD, et al. Bacterial meningitis in the United States in 1995. *N Engl J Med* 1997;337(14):970–976.
60. Armstrong RW, Fung PC. Brainstem encephalitis (rhombencephalitis) due to *Listeria monocytogenes*: case report and review. *Clin Infect Dis* 1993;16(5):689–702.
61. Soo MS, Tien RD, Gray L, et al. Mesenrhombencephalitis: MR findings in nine patients. *AJR Am J Roentgenol* 1993;160(5):1089–1093.
62. Uldry PA, Kuntzer T, Bogousslavsky J, et al. Early symptoms and outcome of *Listeria monocytogenes* rhombencephalitis: 14 adult cases. *J Neurol* 1993;240(4):235–242.
63. Bassan R. Bacterial endocarditis produced by *Listeria monocytogenes*: case presentation and review of the literature. *Am J Clin Pathol* 1986;63:522–527.
64. Gallagher PG, Amedia CA, Watanakunakorn C. *Listeria monocytogenes* endocarditis in a patient on chronic hemodialysis, successfully treated with vancomycin-gentamicin. *Infection* 1986;14(3):125–128.
65. Ballen PH, Loffredo FR, Painter B. Listeria endophthalmitis. *Arch Ophthalmol* 1979;97(1):101–102.
66. Newman JH, Waycott S, Cooney LM Jr. Arthritis due to *Listeria monocytogenes. Arthritis Rheum* 1979;22(10):1139–1140.
67. Houang ET, Williams CJ, Wrigley PF. Acute *Listeria monocytogenes* osteomyelitis. *Infection* 1976;4(2):113–114.
68. Mascola L, Sorvillo F, Goulet V, et al. Fecal carriage of *Listeria*

monocytogenes—observations during a community-wide, common-source outbreak. *Clin Infect Dis* 1992;15(3):557–558.
69. Owen CR, Meis A, Jackson JW, et al. A case of primary cutaneous listeriosis. *N Engl J Med* 1960;262:1026–1028.
70. Anton W. Kritisch-experimentaller beitrag zur biologie des *Bakterium monocytogenes. Zentbl Bakteriol Mikrobiol Hyg A* 1934; 131:89–103.
71. Schuchat A. Listeriosis and pregnancy: food for thought. *Obstet Gynecol Surv* 1997;52(12):721–722.
72. Bortolussi R. Neonatal listeriosis. *Semin Perinatol* 1990;14[4 Suppl 1]:44–48.
73. Mascola L, Ewert DP, Eller A. Listeriosis: a previously unreported medical complication in women with multiple gestations. *Am J Obstet Gynecol* 1994;170[5, Pt 1]:1328–1332.
74. Mielke MEA, Held TK, Unger M. Listeriosis. In: Connor DH, Chandler FW, Schwartz DA, et al., eds. *Pathology of infectious diseases.* Stamford, CT: Appleton & Lange, 1997:621–633.
75. Anspacher R, Borchardt KA, Hannegan MW, et al. Clinical investigation of *Listeria monocytogenes* as a possible cause of human fetal wastage. *Am J Obstet Gynecol* 1966;94:386–390.
76. Giraud JR, Denis F, Gargot F, et al. Listeriosis. Occurrence in spontaneous interruptions of pregnancy [in French]. *Nouv Presse Med* 1973;2(4):215–218.
77. Gray ML, Killinger AH. *Listeria monocytogenes* and listeric infections. *Bacteriol Rev* 1966;30(2):309–382.
78. Frederiksen B, Samuelsson S. Feto-maternal listeriosis in Denmark 1981–1988. *J Infect* 1992;24(3):277–287.
79. McLauchlin J. Human listeriosis in Britain, 1967–85, a summary of 722 cases, 1: listeriosis during pregnancy and in the newborn. *Epidemiol Infect* 1990;104(2):181–189.
80. Visintine AM, Oleske JM, Nahmias AJ. Infection in infants and children. *Am J Dis Child* 1977;131(4):393–397.
81. Jean D, Croize J, Hirtz P, et al. *Listeria monocytogenes* nosocomial infection in the maternity ward [in French]. *Arch French Pediatr* 1991;48(6):419–422.
82. Larsson S, Cederberg A, Ivarsson S, et al. *Listeria monocytogenes* causing hospital-acquired enterocolitis and meningitis in newborn infants. *Br Med J* 1978;2(6135):473–474.
83. Nelson KE, Warren D, Tomasi AM, et al. Transmission of neonatal listeriosis in a delivery room. *Am J Dis Child* 1985;139 (9):903–905.
84. Simmons MD, Cockcroft PM, Okubadejo OA. Neonatal listeriosis due to cross-infection in an obstetric theatre. *J Infect* 1986;13(3):235–239.
85. Schuchat A, Lizano C, Broome CV, et al. Outbreak of neonatal listeriosis associated with mineral oil. *Pediatr Infect Dis J* 1991; 10(3):183–189.
86. Boucher M, Yonekura ML. Listeria meningitis during pregnancy. *Am J Perinatol* 1984;1(4):312–318.
87. Lorber B. Listeriosis. *Clin Infect Dis* 1997;24(1):1–9.
88. Frederiksen B. Maternal septicemia with *Listeria monocytogenes* in second trimester without infection of the fetus. *Acta Obstet Gynecol Scand* 1992;71(4):313–315.
89. Hume OS. Maternal *Listeria monocytogenes* septicemia with sparing of the fetus. *Obstet Gynecol* 1976;48[1 Suppl]:33S–34S.
90. Schwartz B, Hexter D, Broome CV, et al. Investigation of an outbreak of listeriosis: new hypotheses for the etiology of epidemic *Listeria monocytogenes* infections. *J Infect Dis* 1989;159 (4):680–685.
91. Salamina G, Dalle Donne E, Niccolini A, et al. A foodborne outbreak of gastroenteritis involving *Listeria monocytogenes. Epidemiol Infect* 1996;117(3):429–436.
92. Fleming DW, Cochi SL, MacDonald KL, et al. Pasteurized milk as a vehicle of infection in an outbreak of listeriosis. *N Engl J Med* 1985;312(7):404–407.
93. Bille J. Epidemiology of human listeriosis in Europe, with special reference to the Swiss outbreak. In: Miller A, Smith J, Somkuti G, eds. *Foodborne listeriosis.* Amsterdam: Elsevier Science, 1990:71–74.
94. Goulet V, Jacquet C, Vaillant V, et al. Listeriosis from consumption of raw-milk cheese. *Lancet* 1995;345(8964):1581–1582.
95. Lyytikainen O, Autio T, Maijala R, et al. An outbreak of *Listeria monocytogenes* serotype 3a infections from butter in Finland. *J Infect Dis* 2000;181(5):1838–1841.
96. Centers for Disease Control and Prevention. Update—listeriosis and pasteurized milk. *MMWR Morb Mortal Wkly Rep* 1988; 37:764–766.
97. McLauchlin J, Hall SM, Velani SK, et al. Human listeriosis and pate: a possible association. *BMJ* 1991;303(6805):773–775.
98. Jacquet C, Catimel B, Brosch R, et al. Investigations related to the epidemic strain involved in the French listeriosis outbreak in 1992. *Applied Environ Microbiol* 1995;61(6):2242–2246.
99. Dunne EF, Wiedmann M, Morse DL, et al. A multistate outbreak of listeriosis traced to processed meats, August 1998–February 1999. In: *37th Annual Meeting of the Infectious Disease Society of America; November 1999.* Philadelphia, PA: Infectious Disease Society of America, 1999:34.
100. Schwartz B, Ciesielski CA, Broome CV, et al. Association of sporadic listeriosis with consumption of uncooked hot dogs and undercooked chicken. *Lancet* 1988;2(8614):779–782.
101. Davis JP. Addition of listeriosis to the list of nationally notifiable diseases. In: CSTE Position Statement. Atlanta, GA: Council of State and Territorial Epidemiologists; 1999.
102. Tappero JW, Schuchat A, Deaver KA, et al. Reduction in the incidence of human listeriosis in the United States. Effectiveness of prevention efforts? The Listeriosis Study Group. *JAMA* 1995; 273(14):1118–1122.
103. Levine P, Rose B, Green S, et al. Pathogen testing of ready-to-eat meat and poultry products collected at federally inspected establishments in the United States, 1990 to 1999. *J Food Prot* 2001;64(8):1188–1193.
104. Centers for Disease Control and Prevention. *Preventing foodborne illness: listeriosis.* Atlanta, GA: Division of Bacterial and Mycotic Disease, National Center for Infectious Disease, Centers for Disease Control and Prevention, 1992.
105. Food and Drug Administration. *Eating defensively: food safety advice for persons with AIDS.* Washington, DC: Food and Drug Administration, 1992.
106. Food Safety Inspection Service. *Backgrounder: Listeria monocytogenes.* Washington, DC: US Department of Agriculture, 1992.
107. Gaillard JL, Beretti JL, Boulot-Tolle M, et al. Serological evidence for culture-negative listeriosis of central nervous system. *Lancet* 1992;340(8818):560.
108. Hof H, Nichterlein T, Kretschmar M. Management of listeriosis. *Clin Microbiol Rev* 1997;10(2):345–357.
109. Marget W, Seeliger HP. *Listeria monocytogenes* infections—therapeutic possibilities and problems. *Infection* 1988;16[Suppl 2]: S175–S177.
110. Southwick FS, Purich DL. Intracellular pathogenesis of listeriosis. *N Engl J Med* 1996;334(12):770–776.
111. Vicente MF, Perez-Daz JC, Baquero F, et al. Penicillin-binding protein 3 of *Listeria monocytogenes* as the primary lethal target for beta-lactams. *Antimicrob Agents Chemother* 1990;34(4):539–542.
112. Watson GW, Fuller TJ, Elms J, et al. Listeria cerebritis: relapse of infection in renal transplant patients. *Arch Intern Med* 1978; 138(1):83–87.
113. Schlech WF III. Foodborne listeriosis. *Clin Infect Dis* 2000;31 (3):770–775.
114. Lorber B. *Listeria monocytogenes.* In: Mandell GL, Bennett JE, Dolin R, eds. *Principles and practice of infectious diseases,* fifth edition. New York: Churchill Livingston, 2000:2208–2214.

115. Merle-Melet M, Dossou-Gbete L, Maurer P, et al. Is amoxicillin-cotrimoxazole the most appropriate antibiotic regimen for listeria meningoencephalitis? Review of 22 cases and the literature. *J Infect* 1996;33(2):79–85.
116. Baldassarre JS, Ingerman MJ, Nansteel J, et al. Development of *Listeria* meningitis during vancomycin therapy: a case report. *J Infect Dis* 1991;164(1):221–222.
117. Swaminathan B, Barrett TJ, Hunter SB, et al. PulseNet: the molecular subtyping network for foodborne bacterial disease surveillance, United States. *Emerging Infect Dis* 2001;7(3):382–389.
118. Anonymous. *Listeria monocytogenes*: recommendations by the National Advisory Committee on microbiologic criteria for foods. *Int J Food Microbiol* 1991;14:185–246.
119. Gursel B, Gurakan GC. Effects of gamma irradiation on the survival of *Listeria monocytogenes* and on its growth at refrigeration temperature in poultry and red meat. *Poultry Sci* 1997;76(12):1661–1664.
120. Tauxe RV. Food safety and irradiation: protecting the public from food-borne infections. *Emerging Infect Dis* 2001;7(3):516–521.
121. Jacquet VG, Lepoutre A, Rocourt J, et al. Epidemie de listeriose en France: bilan final et resultats de l'enquete epidemiologique. *Bull Epidemiol Hendom* 1993;4:13–14.

51

WHIPPLE'S DISEASE

DAVID N. FREDRICKS
DAVID A. RELMAN

Whipple's disease is a systemic infectious disorder, first described in 1907 (1), that affects primarily the intestinal tract and its lymphatic drainage. Despite its apparent rarity, this disease continues to capture the attention of clinicians throughout the developed countries of the world. The causative agent is an enigmatic bacterium that defied laboratory cultivation for more than 90 years and was identified by molecular methods as a previously uncharacterized actinomycete (2,3). The principal clinical features of Whipple's disease are migratory polyarthralgias, weight loss, diarrhea with evidence of malabsorption, and abdominal pain. Lymphadenopathy and skin hyperpigmentation are also prominent findings. Accompanying these features is an unusual and in some situations diagnostic pattern of tissue pathology that most often involves the proximal small intestine, the mesenteric lymphatics, and, less often, the heart and central nervous system. This clinical syndrome was described with remarkable clarity by George Whipple in his initial case report (1).

On April 12, 1907, a 36-year-old physician and medical missionary was admitted to Johns Hopkins Hospital with a 5-year history of migratory arthralgias and arthritis, cough, fever, abdominal pain, diarrhea, evidence of fat malabsorption, and weight loss. The clinical diagnosis was tuberculosis. A palpable abdominal mass prompted an exploratory laparotomy, which revealed massively enlarged mesenteric lymph nodes. At autopsy 3 days later, George Whipple found swollen small-intestinal mucosa "flecked . . .with pin-point yellowish grains," refractile "fat" deposits within mucosa and submucosa, and numerous "foamy" mononuclear cells containing vacuoles, especially within the lamina propria. Elsewhere, pleuritis, pericarditis, aortic endocarditis, and diffuse chronic lymphadenitis were noted. Whipple suspected altered fat metabolism as an etiologic factor and named this disorder "intestinal lipodystrophy"; however, he also raised the possibility of a bacterial cause (see "Microbiology").

In 1949, Black-Schaffer applied Schiff's periodic acid stain (PAS) to sections of small-intestinal and lymph node tissues from patients with intestinal lipodystrophy, with the goal of characterizing the unusual refractile tissue and cellular deposits (4). The intense "deep scarlet" staining of intracellular vacuoles indicated that the material contained carbohydrate. Having raised doubts about the etiologic importance of lipid metabolism in this disorder, Black-Schaffer argued for the use of the eponym "Whipple's disease." Alternative designations, such as *lipophagic intestinal granulomatosis* (5), fell out of favor, and the PAS stain became an important diagnostic tool. Retrospective use of this stain confirmed that macrophage vacuoles from Whipple's original case in 1907 were PAS-positive (6) and that, in addition, a case published in 1895 may have represented unrecognized Whipple's disease (7).

Two fundamental observations concerning the causation of Whipple's disease were made in the 1950s and early 1960s. Both suggested a bacterial etiology. The first was that antibiotics could cure what was otherwise a fatal disease (8). The second was that unusual-appearing monomorphic bacillary structures could be detected within affected tissues with the use of electron microscopy (9–11). George Whipple's early speculation regarding a bacterial etiology was thus supported. Studies by Silva et al. and others (12,13) showed that a portion of the bacterial cell wall reacted with the PAS stain, and that the PAS-positive macrophage vacuoles contained partially degraded remnants of this wall. Further evidence of bacterial causation followed; clinical response to antibacterial therapy was accompanied by disappearance of the bacilli, and reappearance of the bacilli heralded clinical relapse (14). Nonetheless, attempts to cultivate the microbe in the laboratory failed. Hence, it remained unidentified until the application of an approach based on amplification of bacterial riboso-

D.N. Fredricks: Department of Medicine, University of Washington; Program in Infectious Diseases, Fred Hutchinson Cancer Research Center, Seattle, Washington

D.A. Relman: Departments of Microbiology and Immunology and Medicine, Stanford University, Stanford, California; Veterans Affairs Palo Alto Health Care System, Palo Alto, California mal RNA (rRNA) gene sequences obtained directly from infected human tissues with use of the polymerase chain reaction (PCR) (15), and phylogenetic analysis of these sequences to infer evolutionary relationships between the Whipple bacillus and other known bacteria. The proposed name of the Whipple's disease bacillus is *Tropheryma whippelii* (2).

Between 1907 and 1986, approximately 700 patients with Whipple's disease were described in the medical literature (16). However, the true number of persons with clinical manifestations of infection by this organism is probably at least several times greater (17). Clinical symptoms and syndromes that are less well defined than "classic" Whipple's disease may often go unrecognized as manifestations of *T. whippelii* infection (e.g., chronic arthralgia, chronic uveitis, fever of unknown origin, and dementia with cerebellar ataxia). The ability of molecular sequence-based methods to detect this organism with great sensitivity and specificity should help define the natural ecology and the spectrum of human disease associated with this bacterium.

MICROBIOLOGY

Although Koch's postulates have not been fulfilled for Whipple's disease (18), the evidence that *T. whippelii* is the cause of Whipple's disease is compelling (19). This evidence includes the consistent observation of a uniform, sometimes dividing bacillary organism in many different affected tissues; the correlation of visible organisms and a unique rDNA sequence with clinical disease activity; their disappearance with antibacterial therapy and subsequent clinical improvement; and their return with clinical relapse (14). The localization of *T. whippelii* rRNA to affected tissues of patients with the use of *in situ* hybridization also supports a causal role for *T. whippelii* in Whipple's disease (20). No reservoir or animal host for this bacterium is known, although some animal diseases, such as *Rhodococcus equi* enteritis in foals (21), resemble Whipple's disease. In short, the natural biology of the Whipple's disease bacillus remains largely uncharacterized.

In the original description of the disease, Whipple noted "great numbers of a rod-shaped organism" that "closely resemble the tubercle bacillus" in a silver-stained lymph node (1). They were found within the foamy mononuclear cells and adjacent to them in a distribution that suggested to Whipple that they might play an etiologic role. Electron microscopy has greatly facilitated the morphologic characterization of this bacillus (9–13). Many independent investigators have described an organism of unusual but similar appearance in numerous patients with syndromes and pathologic features suggestive of Whipple's disease (Fig. 51.1). Molecular phylogenetic evidence now suggests that a single bacterial species is responsible for Whipple's disease. The Whipple bacillus is 0.15 to 0.25 μm in diameter and 1 to 2 μm in length. No evidence of flagella has been found. A 20-nm-thick cell wall lies external to the trilaminar cytoplasmic membrane (12,13). This cell wall thickness is typical of many gram-positive bacteria, and in fact the Whipple bacillus appears weakly gram-positive with the Brown and Brenn tissue stain. However, an additional thin, trilaminar membrane bilayer encompasses the cell wall. This outer membrane has symmetric phospholipid leaflets that are devoid of lipopolysaccharide, unlike the surface membranes of gram-negative bacteria. Silva et al. (13) postulated that the outer bacterial membrane might be of host origin. A bacillus with a cell wall of similar appearance was observed by Archer et al. (22) in a febrile, asplenic patient with lymphadenopathy. An inner, electron-dense, polysaccharide-containing cell wall layer is thought to account for the PAS-positive staining properties of the Whipple bacillus; accumulations of this cell wall layer within macrophage vacuoles represent remnants of partially digested intracellular bacteria and explain the PAS-positive staining properties of the vacuoles. The PAS reactivity of the Whipple bacillus is resistant to treatment with diastase, unlike that of glycogen. The Whipple bacillus is revealed by the Giemsa stain and by some silver stain procedures (e.g., Gomori), but it is not acid-fast.

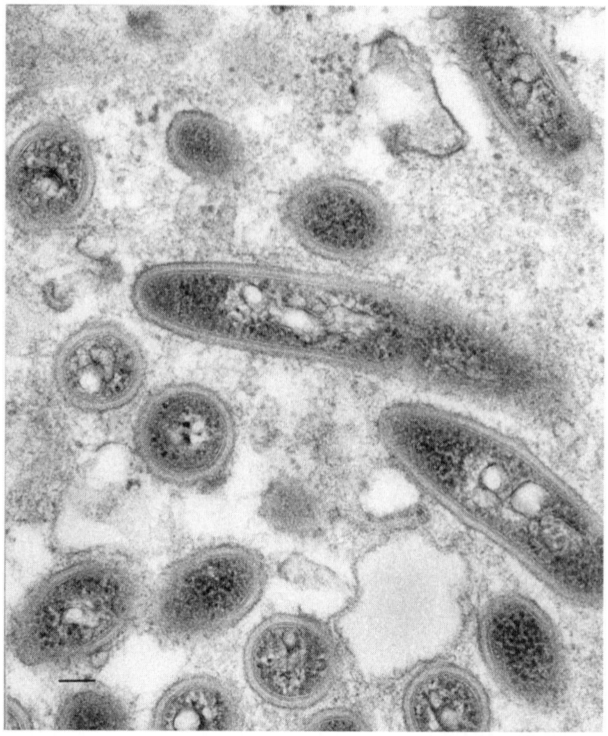

FIGURE 51.1. Electron micrograph of the Whipple's disease bacillus (*"Tropheryma whippelii"*). These extracellular bacilli are abundant within the lamina propria of patients with untreated disease. The thick cell wall has a distinctive structure, more easily appreciated at higher magnifications. Bar = 0.1 μm. (Courtesy of William O. Dobbins III.)

Whipple bacilli are most prominent in the proximal small-intestinal lamina propria, just below the epithelial basement membrane (see "Pathology"). Most intact organisms are free in the intercellular spaces, sometimes forming clusters; some are seen to undergo binary fission. On the other hand, most intracellular bacteria are found in various stages of degradation. Based on these observations, it is thought that the Whipple bacillus replicates preferentially in an extracellular environment but that it may survive for prolonged periods of time within host cells. *In situ* hybridization data also suggest that *T. whippelii* is metabolically active outside cells. An rDNA probe specific for the Whipple bacillus 16S rRNA sequence hybridizes to extracellular sites in affected tissues (20).

Numerous efforts to cultivate the Whipple bacillus in the laboratory, beginning with those of George Whipple, failed to yield any particular organism in a reproducible and consistent manner (1,23). More recently, investigators have reported the slow propagation of *T. whippelii* in the laboratory by cultivation together with human fibroblasts, and the development of a crude serologic assay (24). The estimated doubling time in culture of 18 days makes routine isolation of the Whipple bacillus unfeasible with this technique. However, the propagation of *T. whippelii* may provide opportunities for studying antibiotic susceptibility, pathogenesis, and metabolism in this unusual bacterium.

The advent of molecular phylogeny and the use of rRNA sequences to infer evolutionary relationships have paved the way for the identification of cultivation-resistant microbial pathogens (25). Broad-range PCR primers designed from known conserved bacterial 16S rDNA sequences can be used to amplify corresponding gene fragments directly from infected host tissue (26). In an initial investigation, Wilson et al. (3) studied one duodenal biopsy specimen from a patient with Whipple's disease and detected a previously uncharacterized bacterial 16S rRNA gene. Relman et al. (2) analyzed duodenal and extraintestinal tissues from five unrelated patients with the "classic" form of Whipple's disease, in addition to 14 tissues from 10 unrelated control patients without the disease. A unique 16S rRNA gene fragment was detected in all tissues obtained from patients with Whipple's disease, but not in control tissues.

Phylogenetic analysis with amplified 16S rDNA sequences indicates that the Whipple bacillus is a previously uncharacterized member of the Actinobacteria division of the domain of Bacteria (Fig. 51.2). This group was formerly classified as the "high G + C" (guanine plus cytosine) subdivision of the "gram-positive" bacterial division, based on the "high G + C" chromosomal composition of the member organisms. Most of the known bacteria that are PAS-positive after diastase digestion are members of the Actinobacteria division or of the low G + C gram-positive division (27). However, the Whipple bacillus sequence is no more than 91% similar to any known 16S rRNA sequence (2). Thus, this bacillus is not closely related to any previously characterized organism by the usual molecular phylogenetic standards. Although criteria for taxon boundaries are difficult to formulate on the basis of molecular phylogenetic analyses alone, it seems apparent that the Whipple bacillus defines a new genus and species. Each of the several more closely related bacteria belongs to a separate genus, and none of these bacteria is significantly more closely related to the Whipple bacillus than any other. The name *Tropheryma whippelii* has been proposed, from the Greek *trophe* ("nourishment") and *eryma* ("barrier") because malabsorption is a key feature of the syndrome with which it is associated, and from the name of George Whipple (2). The association between *T. whippelii* infection and Whipple's disease has been subsequently confirmed by numerous investigations (28–34).

Although current evidence suggests that one species of bacterium causes Whipple's disease, different genotypes of *T. whippelii* exist based on polymorphisms in the 16S-23S rRNA intergenic spacer DNA (35,36). Six genotypes have

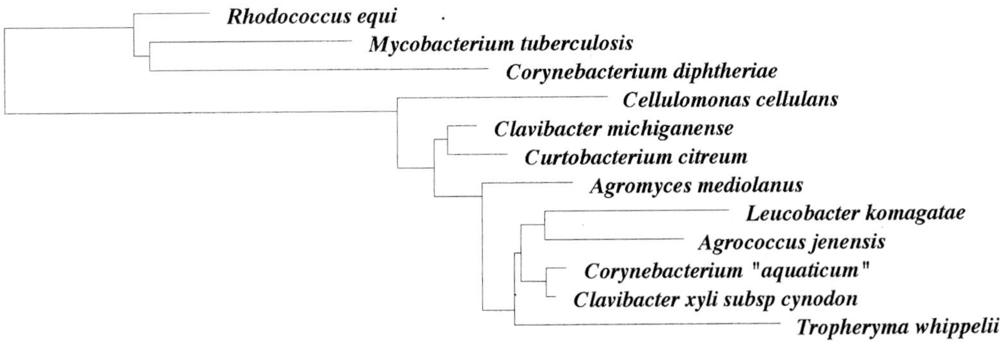

FIGURE 51.2. Evolutionary tree indicating the phylogenetic relationships of the Whipple's disease bacillus (*"Tropheryma whippelii"*). This bacterium is a novel actinomycete that is not closely related to any other characterized organism. The tree is based on comparative analysis of 16S ribosomal RNA sequences; evolutionary distance (abscissa) is proportional to the sum of the horizontal line segments connecting any two organisms (point mutations per sequence position).

been described based on this spacer sequence, but no geographic or pathologic proclivity has been attributed to any particular type.

What additional microbiological information can be inferred from the evolutionary relationships of *T. whippelii*? Many of the more closely related bacteria are common soil or water saprophytes (*Arthrobacter, Terrabacter, Streptomyces*). The actinomycetes *Mycobacterium avium* complex and *R. equi* both cause syndromes similar to Whipple's disease in HIV-seropositive persons (37–42). *Mycobacterium paratuberculosis* causes Johne's disease of cattle, with histology resembling that of Whipple's disease and Crohn's disease (43–45). *R. equi* causes a granulomatous enteritis with a PAS-positive macrophage infiltrate in foals (21). Like its close evolutionary relatives, *T. whippelii* may be a common soil or water bacterium that gains access to humans via the gastrointestinal tract. Persons in whom classic Whipple's disease develops may be particularly susceptible by virtue of a subtle immune defect. In support of this theory, Dobbins (16) previously showed that farmers are disproportionately represented among patients with Whipple's disease (see "Epidemiology").

EPIDEMIOLOGY

A number of curious and unusual features help to define the epidemiology of Whipple's disease. Although the data are limited because of the relatively low numbers of cases, the gender bias is striking, and probable predispositions have been noted based on age, race, and geography. In a review of 664 patients from the world's medical literature, Dobbins (16) found that 86.4% of patients were male. The average age at the time of diagnosis was similar for male and female patients, 49.1 and 51.0 years, respectively. Only 4.1% of all cases occurred in people 30 years of age or younger. In the same case review, whites accounted for 97.8% of patients with Whipple's disease (16). Geography may partially explain this finding. Whipple's disease is recognized primarily in the developed countries of Western Europe and North America and seems to be less common in major urban population centers. No doubt, limited disease awareness and diagnostic capabilities influence case ascertainment disproportionately in some countries. Two-thirds of all cases worldwide have been reported from the United States, Germany, and France. Few if any cases have been recognized in the Far East. In the United States, Whipple's disease has been diagnosed in persons from at least 39 states. A greater disease prevalence is suggested in portions of the northern central and mid-Atlantic states; however, the numbers are too few to conclude that regional clustering occurs. In addition, academic tertiary care facilities with a longstanding interest in Whipple's disease may draw patients from other regions and distort the geographic distribution. No reliable data are available from which to calculate disease prevalence and incidence rates accurately.

Patients' occupations, as an epidemiologic parameter, yield interesting insights into Whipple's disease. In Dobbins' compilation of reported cases (16), farmers were the most commonly represented occupational group (22.5% of all patients), and all members of the farming trades accounted for 34% of the total group. During the same period of time, the average proportion of farmers in the general workforce (e.g., United States, Britain, France, and Germany) was approximately 10%. Workers in the farming trades are more frequently and intensively exposed to soil and water than are workers in other trades. This feature of the population of patients with Whipple's disease is consistent with the natural ecology of most actinomycetes and, in particular, the Actinobacteria grouping with which *T. whippelii* seems to be most closely aligned (see "Microbiology").

The mode of transmission of Whipple's disease is still largely an area of speculation. The propensity of this disease to cause intestinal pathology and the nature of the occupations at greatest risk would suggest an oral route of entry by the causative agent. Several disease clusters have been reported during the past 40 years. Some of these clusters involved as many as seven unrelated persons living in a confined geographic area (e.g., within a 20-mile radius) or single village (46,47). In a few instances, more than one case has occurred in the same family (16,48,49).

The environmental reservoirs of *T. whippelii* are also not known, although the organisms have been detected in wastewater effluent from sewage treatment plants in Germany (50). Some investigators have detected *T. whippelii* organisms in saliva, gastric juice, and duodenal biopsy specimens from patients without Whipple's disease, which suggests that this bacterium may be a common commensal of the upper gastrointestinal tract (51–53). In contrast, other investigators have not detected *T. whippelii* in duodenal biopsy specimens from patients without Whipple's disease (54). The reasons for this discrepancy are not clear.

PATHOLOGY, IMMUNITY, AND PATHOGENESIS

Pathology

The gastrointestinal tract and its mesenteric lymphatic drainage are the most common sites of pathology in Whipple's disease (5,16,47,55) and are often involved in the absence of specific clinical manifestations related to these regions. Although the disease can lead to tissue pathology in any portion of the intestinal tract, it is most often found in the small intestine, especially within the lamina propria. Whipple commented on the "pink or red velvety swollen mucosa [of the jejunum] . . . flecked over thickly with little pin-point yellowish grains" (1). Enzinger and Helwig (56) described the small intestine as distended, with thickened and "doughy" walls, "stippled by countless yellowish white, frondlike villi." The ileum and jejunum may be more frequently abnormal by gross inspection than the duodenum. Endoscopic evaluation of the small-intestinal lining often reveals patchy areas of pale, shaggy mucosa and areas of erythematous, erosive, or friable mucosa (55); however, these grossly visible changes may not be evident in patients with subclinical gastrointestinal involvement. Whipple's disease very rarely involves the stomach or colon (16).

In "classic" Whipple's disease, the "most severe and consistent [histologic] changes are seen in the proximal small intestine" (47). On microscopic examination, the small intestine often demonstrates thickened or clubbed villi, distorted by the mononuclear cell infiltrate within the lamina propria (56). Epithelial cells usually appear normal, although they may be somewhat flattened or vacuolated. Some investigators have noted atrophy of the microvilli (9). However, the most dramatic aspects of Whipple's disease pathology are found beneath an intact basement membrane, in the lamina propria. Numerous large or plump macrophages fill this layer of the mucosa (see Color Figure 51.3). These "foamy" cells contain PAS-positive vacuoles that may sometimes appear as globules or collections of fine rod- or sickle-shaped particles (see Color Figure 51.4). Sieracki and Fine (57) suggested that this particle morphology is specific for Whipple's disease and coined the term *sickleform particle-containing cells* (57). The particles correspond to intact or partially degraded bacteria. These particles are more prominent in early untreated disease (58). Other inflammatory cells within the lamina propria include moderate numbers of lymphocytes and eosinophils, and fewer neutrophils and plasma cells. Large, neutral lipid droplets populate the lamina propria and sometimes elicit a local neutrophil response. In this circumstance, one may observe neutrophils within the epithelial layer. In addition, lymphatic channels within the lamina propria are usually dilated. These lacteals are thought to contain chylomicrons, but not the neutral lipid that accumulates in nearby sites. PAS-positive macrophages can also be detected in deeper portions of the mucosa and less often within the submucosa. In at least one patient with Whipple's disease, intestinal pathology was confined to the submucosa, although this patient had a prior history of antimicrobial therapy (59). It is also important to recognize that intestinal pathology may be patchy or mild (60). As a result, endoscopically guided biopsies may miss areas of pathology.

Several studies have confirmed and expanded on the initial electron microscopic observations of bacillary structures within the intestinal wall of patients with Whipple's disease (9–11,14,61). In untreated patients, most bacilli are extracellular, within the stroma of the lamina propria. In most cases, the density of bacilli is highest just below the epithelial basement membrane and progressively decreases from the tip of the villus toward the submucosa. Few bacteria are observed in the submucosa. Although most intracellular bacilli are found within macrophages, they were seen within intestinal epithelial cells in 11 of 13 patients in one study (12). The route and mechanism of bacterial entry into these nonprofessional phagocytes are unclear; Dobbins and Ruffin (61) proposed that the bacilli enter epithelial cells from the basolateral surface. In keeping with this hypothesis, bacilli can be observed within the epithelial intercellular space (12). Bacteria of typical appearance have also been identified within lymphatic and capillary endothelial cells, neutrophils, plasma cells, intraepithelial lymphocytes, and intestinal smooth-muscle cells. They rarely if ever localize to capillaries, lacteals, or the intestinal lumen.

Many of the pathologic features described above also characterize Whipple's disease outside the small intestine. PAS-positive, diastase-resistant macrophages are common in all anatomic sites of involvement and should raise the possibility of Whipple's disease; however, this finding alone is nonspecific. Cells of this type may accompany histoplasmosis, macroglobulinemia, and disseminated atypical mycobacterial disease (16). Morphologic or molecular evidence of the characteristic Whipple bacilli should be sought in cases with extraintestinal pathology. In addition, granulomatous responses may predominate in a number of anatomic sites, especially in lymph nodes and the liver, and were found in approximately 62 (9%) of 696 patients with Whipple's disease (16). Mesenteric lymph nodes are very frequently enlarged and matted together, with an average individual diameter of 2 to 3 cm (56). These nodes are often homogeneously cystic and spongy, and they contain an oily material of unknown composition. "Lipogranulomas" are often reported, and also interstitial fibrosis. One case of granulomatous gastritis has been attributed to Whipple's disease, but documentation of Whipple bacilli was not provided (62). PAS-positive macrophages in the stomach or rectum are likely to represent lipophages or muciphages and alone do not constitute proof of Whipple's disease (63). Conversely, PAS-negative macrophages in the context of extraintestinal granulomatous inflammation do not rule out Whipple's disease. Sarcoid-like, epithelioid, noncaseating granulomas that do not stain with PAS occur in Whipple's disease, primarily in lymph nodes, liver, spleen, and lungs, and also in the intestine (64–66) (see "Clinical Illness").

Immunity

Host immune responses in Whipple's disease appear to be relatively intact, with a few exceptions (16,67,68). The available data are derived from immunohistologic studies and the evaluation of humoral and cellular immune function in small numbers of patients. Circulating and mucosal antibody levels are usually within normal limits, and the number of plasma cells in the lamina propria, although usually decreased in untreated patients, returns to normal after treatment. On the other hand, in all patients with Whipple's disease studied so far, no circulating antibodies can be detected that are directed against the PAS-positive material in the intestinal wall (69–72). Silva et al. (13) speculated that the *T. whippelii* outer membrane is of host origin and may block the organism from eliciting a host humoral immune response.

Limited evidence suggests that subtle underlying defects in the function of cellular immune elements may be present in patients with Whipple's disease. Clearly, malnutrition contributes to cellular immune depression during clinically active phases of this disease. Poor lymphocyte mitogenic responses and cutaneous anergy (73–75) probably reflect nutritional status to a large extent. However, with antimicrobial therapy and clinical remission, mitogenic and delayed hypersensitivity responses improve only partially. Peripheral lymphocytopenia is common and persists in these patients, but the ratio of helper (CD4+) to suppressor (CD8+) T lymphocytes is normal. Of interest is an investigation of monocyte function in one patient with Whipple's disease, who was studied at five points in time during the 4 years following diagnosis (76,77). Monocyte and macrophage phagocytic and intracellular microbicidal activities did not differ significantly from those in control patients treated with antibiotics; however, the ability of these cells to degrade ingested bacteria and zymosan was impaired. The impairment persisted through a 4-year period comprising initial treatment with clinical remission, subsequent relapse, and repeated treatment with a second remission. Granulocytes from this patient behaved normally, and the patient's serum did not impair the functions of monocytes from control subjects. These results suggest a subtle defect in macrophage function in this patient (76).

The nature of this macrophage dysfunction has been suggested by some recent studies. Monocytes/macrophages from patients with Whipple's disease were noted to produce less interleukin 12 and CD11b chain of the complement 3 receptor (78,79). Peripheral blood mononuclear cells from these patients produced less interferon-γ (79). These abnormalities suggest that some patients with Whipple's disease may have a defect in macrophage activation and intracellular killing of pathogens. Such results are consistent with the widespread histologic observations of partially degraded Whipple bacilli within macrophages (see above). It is not clear to what extent these observations may represent a preexisting host defect as opposed to an acquired defect, induced by *T. whippelii* and perhaps other related bacteria (37,41,42) (see below).

Tissue-based characterizations of cellular immune responses to *T. whippelii* have not yielded substantial insight into pathogenic mechanisms or clinical manifestations. In the small-intestinal epithelium of patients with Whipple's disease, intraepithelial lymphocytes appear to be activated and have a CD8+, major histocompatibility complex (MHC) class I+ phenotype. The number of intraepithelial cells per 100 epithelial cells is probably not increased in these patients in comparison with the number in normal persons (80), but at least one study demonstrated otherwise in 15 patients at the time of diagnosis (58). In the lamina propria of patients with Whipple's disease, lymphocytes are relatively few in number, and the ratio of CD4+ to CD8+ cells is reduced. Cells that express surface immunoglobulin M (IgM) are more numerous in the lamina propria than are cells that express IgA, and the numerous plump macrophages express normal levels of MHC class II protein on their surface (58).

In the search for a genetic predisposition to Whipple's disease, most investigators have focused on human leukocyte antigen (HLA) antigen profiles. Retrospective analysis of selected cases reveals a greater representation of HLA-B27 than might be expected, even in the absence of sacroiliitis (16,81,82). However, the rarity of this disease hinders statistically meaningful population-based studies; in addition, HLA profiles may have been used for diagnostic purposes. A more recent, small study of a homogeneous population showed no association between Whipple's disease and any class I or class II HLA antigen (83). If patients with Whipple's disease do indeed bear an intrinsic immune defect, then it would seem to be subtle. These patients are not at clearly increased risk for other infections or neoplastic disorders (16). Several case reports describe an association between Whipple's disease, giardiasis, and other intestinal parasitic infections (84–86). However, the numbers of cases are too few to allow conclusions about causality, and in particular conclusions regarding the possibility of impaired intestinal mucosal immunity, to be drawn.

Pathogenesis

Microbial pathogenesis can be conceptualized as a staged process by which a microorganism establishes itself within a host and then ensures its eventual transmission to other hosts (86a). The common steps to this process include entry into a susceptible host, acquisition of a suitable niche, multiplication, avoidance or evasion of host immune defenses, and transmission to a new susceptible host. Establishment usually entails microbial multiplication, which often results in tissue damage and pathophysiology. In the case of Whipple's disease, the details of many of these steps are poorly understood.

Although definitive evidence is lacking, a reasonable hypothesis is that *T. whippelii* organisms are ingested by the oral route, cross the basal lamina by unknown mechanisms, and enter the lamina propria, where they replicate in the extracellular spaces (20). Macrophages are recruited to the lamina propria, where they engulf and destroy bacteria. However, the rate of bacterial destruction does not appear to keep pace with the rate of bacterial replication in the lamina propria, as intact extracellular bacteria can be found (13).

A number of mechanisms have been proposed to account for intestinal malabsorption in Whipple's disease. The earliest theories focused on the role of abnormal fat metabolism, leading to fat or fatty acid deposits within the intestinal mucosa (1,5); these theories soon gave way to an emphasis on lymphatic obstruction. Obstruction was presumed to result from compression of lacteals by macrophages and neutral fat deposits, and from fibrosis in the mesenteric lymphatics and lymph nodes. Observations of epithelial cell invasion and morphologic alterations suggest epithelial cell dysfunction as one possible mechanism of malabsorption (12,47). The blunting of intestinal villi and dense infiltration of the lamina propria with bacteria and inflammatory cells may also impair the absorption and transport of nutrients. In addition to all these potential mechanisms, one must consider the possible toxic effects of substances secreted by *T. whippelii* or of bacterial breakdown products.

The binary division of Whipple's disease bacilli appears to take place almost exclusively in extracellular tissue spaces. *In situ* hybridization of probe targeting *T. whippelii* rRNA shows that intact bacterial rRNA occurs mostly in the extracellular spaces, which suggests that metabolically active bacteria exist in this compartment (20). On this basis, the organism has been defined as an extracellular pathogen (12,13). However, intracellular survival may also be an important feature of the host–pathogen relationship and allow prolonged survival of the bacillus in some hosts. Two basic explanations for the rarity of this disease are the following: First, exposure to sufficient numbers of the causative agent may be uncommon. (See "Microbiology" for a discussion of possible human colonization.) For example, the bacillus may occupy an unusual environmental niche or survive only in low numbers in the external environment. Second, a putative defect in macrophage intracellular microbial killing may select rare human hosts for more severe local or systemic disease. Although classic forms of the disease are rare, it is important to remember that atypical disease or asymptomatic infection may be much more frequent.

Dissemination of the bacillus from the intestinal mucosa may occur initially by lymphatic or blood-borne routes. Detection of *T. whippelii* DNA in peripheral blood monocytes argues that blood-borne dissemination of this organism may indeed take place (87), although the frequency of this finding may be low (88). The presence of disease and visible organisms in various extraintestinal sites suggests bacterial tropism, especially for the central nervous system, heart, and reticuloendothelial system. Extraintestinal organ dysfunction probably stems largely from the mononuclear inflammatory cell response elicited by the Whipple bacillus. Later in the course of the disease, remnants of *T. whippelii* cell wall may be sufficient for continuation of the inflammatory response. Circulating immune complexes have been detected in a few patients but are of unclear significance (89,90). The similarity of Whipple's disease pathology to that of sarcoidosis in some cases argues that certain microorganisms, including *T. whippelii* and mycobacteria, may share cell wall components capable of stimulating a common host tissue response (91–93).

CLINICAL ILLNESS

Whipple's disease is a chronic, progressive, systemic disorder. Although the manifestations of Whipple's disease are most often referable to the gastrointestinal tract and its lymphatic drainage, any organ can be affected, and the manifestations can be protean. In 1963, Enzinger and Helwig (56) reviewed the literature on Whipple's disease and described three clinical stages in the untreated patient. The first is "an early and indeterminate stage, with insidious onset marked by arthralgia, weight loss, fatigue, and anemia." This is followed by a second stage with "abdominal pain and distention followed by diarrhea and steatorrhea." Finally, there comes "a short terminal stage dominated by various manifestations of malnutrition, disturbed electrolyte balance, cachexia, and often cardiac failure."

The "classic" or typical clinical presentation of Whipple's disease is characterized by weight loss in 95% of patients, diarrhea in 78%, arthralgias in 65%, and abdominal pain in 60% (47). The first two symptoms are less common in patients less than 40 years of age. Arthralgias often predate the other manifestations, usually by 3 to 24 years (94); they are migratory, usually involve large joints, and are only infrequently accompanied by evidence of joint inflammation. Among the physical signs reported, weight loss is most common (70% of patients), followed by lymphadenopathy (52%), abdominal tenderness (48%), skin hyperpigmentation (47%), and fever (38%) (47). With progressive malnutrition and subsequent hypoalbuminemia, signs of extracellular fluid accumulation, electrolyte imbalances, and anemia become more pronounced. These latter findings have become less common with early diagnosis and treatment. The results of laboratory investigations are relatively nonspecific; they most often reveal a normochromic–normocytic anemia (90% of patients), a normal or slightly elevated peripheral leukocyte count, thrombocytosis, and hypoalbuminemia.

Intestinal Disease

The known proclivity of Whipple's disease to cause pathology in the small intestines leads one to expect related clinical manifestations in nearly all patients. In fact, diarrhea is reported in approximately three-fourths of all patients, although the true proportion is probably unknown (i.e., many other persons may have no history of diarrhea and undiagnosed *T. whippelii* infection). The diarrhea may be watery or steatorrheic. In one review of Whipple's disease (47), the stool of 93% of patients exhibited an abnormally high fat content. D-Xylose absorption was deficient in 78%, although vitamin B_{12} absorption was impaired in only 13%. In a more recent study, 19 of 20 patients had a decreased serum carotene level (95). Although it is not commonly appreciated, occult gastrointestinal bleeding is common in Whipple's disease. Evidence of bleeding is found in as many as 86% of patients in some series (56); in some cases, melena or hematochezia is reported (96). Bleeding can arise in both the small and large intestine. Endoscopic examination may reveal erosions with friable mucosa or frank ulcerations. The anemia that is so common in patients with Whipple's disease may be partially a consequence of blood loss; however, the mean erythrocyte corpuscular volume in patients varies between 83 and 92 fL (47). The etiology of the mucosal erosive changes is unclear. Vascular insufficiency caused by distal capillary compression or vasculitis (97) and also nutritional factors may play a role. With respect to the latter possibility, scurvy has been a complication of Whipple's disease (98). Interestingly, weight loss may occur without any history of diarrhea or signs of malabsorption. Patients commonly experience a weight loss of 20 to 30 lb (95), usually in the later stages of the disease, but a 100-lb weight loss has been described in one patient (99). Abdominal pain in patients with Whipple's disease tends to be epigastric and intermittent.

The endoscopic appearance of the intestine may include erosions, ulcerations, raised yellow–white plaques or grains, and a shaggy pale yellow mucosa alternating with an erythematous or friable mucosa (55,100). The yellow–white lesions correspond to enlarged villi distended with PAS-positive material. Biopsy specimens should be obtained from these lesions, if apparent.

Radiographic investigations of the gastrointestinal tract frequently reveal many of the nonspecific abnormalities associated with malabsorption syndromes. The most common finding on barium studies is the presence of prominent and edematous duodenal and jejunal mucosal folds (seen in 51% to 100% of patients) (47,95). Sometimes, dilatation of the duodenum and jejunum accompanies this picture. In addition, extensive paraaortic and retroperitoneal lymphadenopathies are sometimes first discovered with the use of computerized tomography or abdominal ultrasonography (95) (see "Lymph Nodes").

Extraintestinal Disease

The clinical manifestations of Whipple's disease tend to be protean, and because this is a rare disorder, extraintestinal disease may not be recognized as such. Most of the data on the involvement of various anatomic sites in Whipple's disease are derived from small autopsy series and retrospective case reviews (5,47,56,95,101,102). Thus, these data do not give an accurate picture of the relative frequencies of involvement of the various organs. Nonetheless, some general impressions may be reliable (16). Excluding the gastrointestinal tract and its lymphatic drainage, the most commonly involved anatomic sites are the central nervous system, particularly later in the course of the disease, and the heart. Inflammation of various serosal surfaces is also common, including the pleura, pericardium, and peritoneum, and is often accompanied by a fluid exudate. Lymphadenopathy is relatively common and may be a sign of either localized or diffuse disease. In addition, numerous case reports have provided evidence of Whipple's disease in nearly all other types of tissue, organs, and anatomic compartments. Noteworthy among these relatively less frequently affected sites are the eyes and lungs.

Central Nervous System

Whipple's disease involves the central nervous system in approximately 10% of patients based on clinical manifestations, but histologic changes (PAS-positive macrophages) were found in 10 of 11 patients in an autopsy series (47). The neurologic manifestations of Whipple's disease are particularly protean, reflecting lesions at diverse locations (103). In the pre-antibiotic and early antibiotic periods, neurologic disease became evident late in the course of the clinical illness, or not until autopsy (104). In the past 20 to 30 years, a greater proportion of patients with Whipple's disease present initially with neurologic manifestations and often have no clinical signs of intestinal disease (105–107). It is hypothesized that the increasing societal use of antibiotics for unrelated diseases has partially treated or masked intestinal and other well-recognized forms of Whipple's disease, so that neurologic disease is left to emerge at a later time (108). It is clear that drugs with poor penetration of the blood–brain barrier put patients with Whipple's disease at high risk for disease relapse in the central nervous system (105,109,110) (see "Treatment and Prevention").

The three most common neurologic manifestations of Whipple's disease are dementia, ophthalmoplegia (usually external), and myoclonus (16). The dementia includes memory loss, confusion, inappropriate behavior, and apathy (105,111); it tends to progress inexorably if not treated. Personality changes, hemiparesis, and seizures also indicate cortical disease. Cognitive changes were noted in 71% of patients with Whipple's disease of the central nervous system, and 47% of patients with cognitive abnormalities also had psychiatric signs (112). Hypothalamic and endocrine symptoms feature prominently in many cases of neurologic Whipple's disease, especially disruption of sleep patterns (113), hyperphagia and polydipsia (110), and sexual dysfunction (114). Cerebellar ataxia and meningeal signs are less common. A rare but particularly important neurologic manifestation of Whipple's disease is oculomasticatory myorhythmia (OMM) or oculofacial–skeletal myorhythmia (OFSM) (115–117). OMM consists of pendular, periodic convergent–divergent oscillations of the eyes with concurrent contractions of the masticatory muscles, whereas OFSM includes the same ocular findings with myoclonus of other skeletal muscles. The frequency of these oscillations is approximately 1/s. Patients usually also have vertical gaze paralysis. The anatomic lesion is postulated to be a collection of inflammatory nodules in the rostral midbrain and brainstem. This syndrome is believed to be unique to patients with Whipple's disease and is the only pathognomonic clinical finding in this disease. Like the other neurologic forms of Whipple's disease, OMM may occur in the absence of gastrointestinal disease (117).

Histologic changes in the central nervous system include widespread inflammatory nodules, up to 2 mm in diameter, that consist of PAS-positive, sickleform particle-containing macrophages (104). They are located in the cerebral and cerebellar cortical and subcortical gray matter, hypothalamus, brainstem, and occasionally subependymal tissue (16,56). Perivascular lymphocytic infiltrates may accompany these findings. One patient who presented with signs of increased intracranial pressure was found to have multiple, ring-enhancing intracerebral mass lesions (103). Brain tissue from one lesion exhibited PAS-positive, diastase-resistant vacuolated macrophages and typical Whipple bacilli. Jejunal biopsy findings were normal. In general, it is not uncommon for extraintestinal Whipple's disease to occur in the absence of either clinical or histologic intestinal findings. This is especially true of neurologic Whipple's disease (114). In a variation on this theme, the diagnosis of Whipple's disease was made in one patient with OMM at laparotomy (118). Despite numerous negative small-intestinal biopsy findings, characteristic pathology was found in the mesenteric lymph nodes.

Cardiovascular System

The history of Whipple's disease is replete with descriptions of cardiac pathology and the resulting clinical manifestations. The autopsy on the original patient with Whipple's disease disclosed fibrinous pericarditis and aortic valve endocarditis (1). These two processes have been surprisingly common in autopsy-based studies. Plummer and colleagues (5) reviewed 34 cases of Whipple's disease and found histologic evidence of pericarditis in 71% and "verrucous" endocarditis in 50% (5). Upton (119) was the first to document typical Whipple's disease pathology in the heart. He noted eosinophils and mast cells in the pericardial exudate and a myocardial lymphocytic arteritis. Interstitial lymphocytic myocarditis was reported in a patient with Whipple's disease (120), and the notion of large-vessel arteritis is discussed by James and Bulkley (121). In a wider application of the PAS reaction, Enzinger and Helwig (56) identified PAS-positive macrophages in the pericardium of 8 of 13 autopsy cases, the myocardium of 6 of 15 cases, and the endocardium of 6 of 8 cases. In all these cardiac sites, fibrosis becomes a dominant feature in later stages of disease. The pathogenesis of cardiac lesions in Whipple's disease was later clarified by two studies in which typical Whipple's bacilli (some in the process of dividing) were revealed by electron microscopy in all three types of cardiac tissue (122,123).

Clinical evidence of cardiac disease in Whipple's disease appears to be less common than the tissue-based findings described above. However, isolated cardiac findings in the setting of nonspecific systemic signs and symptoms would probably rarely, if ever, raise the possibility of Whipple's disease in a differential diagnosis. In a series of 19 patients, 79% had gross pathologic cardiac abnormalities attributable to Whipple's disease at autopsy, but only 56% had had clinical manifestations (123). The latter included 22% with systolic murmurs, 11% with a pericardial friction rub, 6% with congestive heart failure, and 33% with electrocardiographic abnormalities. Cardiac disease may be the initial manifestation of Whipple's disease. One patient presented with aortic insufficiency; typical pathology and microorganisms were found in her native valve at surgery, but it was only at autopsy soon thereafter that evidence of intestinal involvement was discovered (124). In a separate case, mitral valve endocarditis developed in a patient with previously diagnosed intestinal Whipple's disease (125). Two years after mitral valve replacement with a Carpentier–Edwards glutaraldehyde-fixed porcine prosthesis, this patient had recurrent congestive heart failure and required a second mitral valve replacement. The removed porcine prosthesis leaflets were covered with and infiltrated by PAS-positive macrophages; extracellular and intracellular Whipple bacilli were detected by electron microscopy.

Musculoskeletal System

Musculoskeletal involvement in Whipple's disease is much more often clinically apparent than is cardiac involvement, but documentation of tissue pathology is much less available. Arthralgias are one of the most consistent complaints in these patients (see above); they usually occur in acute attacks lasting hours to days and predate the onset of intraabdominal symptomatology in more than 50% of patients (16). The mean duration of arthritis is approximately 7 years, but it may predate other manifestations by decades (56). Arthralgias tend to be migratory and involve most commonly the ankles, knees, shoulders, and wrists (47). Fluid accumulation, signs of inflammation, and radiographic or histologic evidence of joint destruction are rare (126). In these cases, however, PAS-positive macrophages and typical bacilli can be detected in the synovial membrane (127), as can *T. whippelii* rDNA (126,128,129). Whipple's disease was diagnosed in one case only following hip arthroplasty (130), and in another case Whipple's disease relapsed in a prosthetic knee (131). In addition to the syndrome of seronegative inflammatory arthropathy, Whipple's disease may also present as sacroiliitis or spondylitis (132). The latter may be more common than is clinically appreciated (133); one study detected spondylitis retrospectively in nearly 20% of those patients with Whipple's disease who underwent radiography, but ankylosing disease was found in only 10% of those with positive findings (134). In the majority of these patients, the results of tests for HLA-B27 antigen are negative.

In the setting of Whipple's disease, skeletal muscle abnormalities are relatively uncommon. Sieracki and Fine (57) first identified PAS-positive macrophages in skeletal muscle at autopsy. In one patient, a proximal myopathy developed in association with arthralgias, diarrhea, fever, and weight loss (135); type 2 fiber atrophy, variability in fiber size and shape, and PAS-positive macrophages were noted in the endomysial connective tissue, but no convincing evidence of intact bacillary structures. *T. whippelii* rDNA has been detected in muscle from a boy with juvenile dermatomyositis (136), but no other reports of this association have been published. Muscle weakness and atrophic changes are nonspecific and may also reflect malnutrition.

Eye

The ocular manifestations of Whipple's disease are diverse and reflect the potential for this disease to involve all portions of the eye and orbit. Although approximately 40 cases of ocular Whipple's disease have been reported in the literature, the clinical manifestations tend to be nonspecific; therefore, it is likely that many more cases occur and escape diagnosis. The majority of patients with ocular signs and symptoms have concurrent, clinically apparent central nervous system disease; in one review of ocular Whipple's disease, 30 of 36 cases were assigned to this category (137). In fact, many of the ocular findings in these patients (e.g., ophthalmoplegias, nystagmus, gaze palsies) are caused by central neuropathology. Most patients with ocular manifestations have had either clinical or histologic evidence of intestinal involvement (16), although exceptions are reported (138,139).

The intraocular clinical manifestations of Whipple's disease most commonly include visual loss with evidence of uveitis, vitritis, retinitis (often accompanied by retinal hemorrhage), and optic neuritis (16,137). Some patients have only anterior ocular disease, such as keratitis and corneal ulcers. The vitreous and inner retina commonly contain cellular infiltrates consisting primarily of "foamy" macrophages with vacuoles that stain intensely with PAS and are diastase-resistant (140,141). Electron microscopy reveals intact and degenerating rod-shaped bacteria within the macrophage vacuoles (141), similar to those reported in numerous studies in other affected tissues. *T. whippelii* rRNA gene sequence has been detected in the vitreous of a patient with chronic uveitis caused by Whipple's disease (138). These findings suggest that the ocular manifestations of Whipple's disease result from the local presence of *T. whippelii.*

Whipple's disease should always be suspected in patients with chronic bilateral retinitis and uveitis, especially when accompanied by a history of arthralgias, intestinal symptoms, or neurologic disease. The differential diagnosis in these settings may include rheumatoid arthritis, ulcerative colitis, sarcoidosis, Lyme disease, syphilis, tuberculosis, and reticulum cell sarcoma. Because most of the ocular manifestations of Whipple's disease are nonspecific, a definitive diagnosis usually involves vitrectomy with light and electron microscopy of the vitreous. PCR offers an alternative diagnostic method for examination of the vitreous and may be more sensitive than traditional approaches.

Respiratory Tract

Chronic cough was a clinical feature of the illness described by Whipple in 1907 (1) and continues to be reported in approximately half of patients (56). Respiratory manifestations do not usually occur without other, concurrent clinical findings and tend not to be severe. Pleuritic chest pain and mild exertional dyspnea are not uncommon (142). Pleuritis is found in approximately 72% of patients who have cough (56). In a series of 15 autopsies of patients with Whipple's disease, 14 had pleuritis and 6 had a pleural effusion (56). Winberg et al. (143) visualized Whipple bacilli in the lung parenchyma of one patient, and *T. whippelii* 16S rDNA has been detected by PCR in pleural effusion cells (87). However, the pathology of pleuropulmonary disease is variable; it includes pulmonary nodular disease on radiographs, and noncaseating granulomatous pneumonitis or pleuritis by microscopic examination (142,144).

Skin

Increased skin pigmentation was noted in many of the early descriptions of Whipple's disease. Studies have reported hyperpigmentation in 36% to 54% of patients (47,95). It tends to occur in exposed areas of skin and in scars. Despite documentation of PAS-positive macrophages in the adrenal capsule, cortex, and medulla (56,57), adrenal insufficiency does not occur. The mechanism of hyperpigmentation remains unknown. The detection of Whipple bacilli in skin nodules from a patient with Whipple's disease has been reported (145).

Lymph Nodes

Peripheral lymphadenopathy occurs in 41% to 71% of patients with Whipple's disease (5,47,56,95). Based on physical examination findings, the axillary and cervical lymphatic systems are involved most often (95). Lymph nodes may be as large as 3 to 4 cm in diameter. Nodal tenderness is unusual. Diffuse lymphadenopathy may dominate the clinical presentation of Whipple's disease (146). Computed tomography and ultrasonography may be helpful in detecting subclinical central lymphadenopathy. A few reports suggest that the high fat content of lymph nodes affected by Whipple's disease may be responsible for a distinctive pattern in which the lymph nodes appear diffusely echogenic on ultrasonography but have a low attenuation on computed tomography (147). Like the other forms of extraintestinal disease, lymph node involvement may occur in the absence of intestinal pathology (148).

Reactive hyperplasia, fibrosis, and PAS-positive macrophages are common in the enlarged peripheral lymph nodes of Whipple's disease. This picture is nonspecific, however (47). In some cases of Whipple's disease, a granulomatous inflammatory response predominates in the peripheral lymph nodes. Typical Whipple bacilli have been detected with electron microscopy in noncaseating, PAS-negative lymph node granulomas (66). This pathology can be indistinguishable from that of sarcoidosis (149).

Less Commonly Affected Extraintestinal Sites

Whipple's disease is truly a systemic disorder. Like syphilis, Lyme disease, and tuberculosis, Whipple's disease can occasionally involve any anatomic site. Among those sites less commonly affected and so far not discussed, the liver, spleen, and kidneys bear mention. Hepatomegaly and splenomegaly are detected on physical examination in fewer than 20% of patients but at autopsy are described in approximately 50% and 40% of patients, respectively (47,56). Elevated serum levels of aspartate aminotransferase were found in 38% of patients in one study (95); in this situation, one must rule out passive hepatic congestion secondary to congestive heart failure. One of the more common forms of hepatosplenic pathology is capsular fibrosis (56). In addition, granulomatous disease is relatively more frequent in the liver and spleen than in most other organs in patients with Whipple's disease. In this setting, granulomas are composed of epithelioid cells, are noncaseating, and may contain PAS-positive or PAS-negative macrophages (150). Renal complications of Whipple's disease are rarely reported, although approximately 60% of patients demonstrate abnormalities on urinalysis (95). Proteinuria and microscopic hematuria are most common. The spectrum of renal disorders associated with Whipple's disease encompasses chronic interstitial nephritis, sometimes with granulomas; glomerulonephritis; and IgA nephropathy (16,151,152). The Whipple bacillus has been visualized within the kidney parenchyma (152).

Other Systemic Syndromes Associated with Whipple's Disease

When a patient presents with arthralgias that are followed by weight loss, diarrhea, abdominal pain, lymphadenopathy, and fever, Whipple's disease is usually included in the differential diagnosis. This presentation may be considered "classic" or typical Whipple's disease. However, probably fewer than half of all persons ultimately given a diagnosis of Whipple's disease present with the classic picture. It is likely that a larger population of persons with either asymptomatic or mild, poorly defined syndromes caused by *T. whippelii* infection goes unrecognized.

Dobbins (16) summarized a group of diverse clinical syndromes that deserve to be considered within a broader definition of Whipple's disease. Intestinal signs and symptoms are not features of these nonclassic syndromes of Whipple's disease, which include (a) fever of unknown origin, sometimes accompanied by peripheral lymphadenopathy or arthralgias; (b) dementia, otherwise unexplained, sometimes accompanied by ophthalmoplegias, myoclonus, or hypothalamic symptoms; (c) chronic migratory arthropathy; (d) generalized lymphadenopathy; (e) chronic bilateral uveitis or retinitis, especially when accompanied by the neurologic manifestations listed above; (f) chronic pleuritis or pericarditis, accompanied by effusion and sometimes cough or chest pain; and (g) granulomatous hepatitis.

DIAGNOSIS

Classic Whipple's disease in its clinical presentation resembles a number of chronic systemic infectious, inflammatory, and neoplastic disorders. The original differential diagnosis for George Whipple's patient included Hodgkin's disease and gastrointestinal tuberculosis (1). Intestinal lymphoma often generates abdominal symptoms, signs, and radiographic findings similar to those of Whipple's disease (153). Other disorders that duplicate many of the clinical aspects of Whipple's disease are tropical and nontropical sprue, sarcoidosis, some collagen-vascular diseases, and disseminated *Mycobacterium avium* complex infection in HIV-infected hosts.

Extraintestinal presentations of Whipple's disease may raise questions concerning a variety of other disease entities. Central nervous system involvement is often nonspecific but may resemble multiple sclerosis and Wernicke encephalopathy. Features that distinguish these from Whipple's disease are the usual absence of supranuclear ophthalmoplegia, myoclonus, and seizures in the former (16) and a history of alcohol abuse and response to thiamine in the latter (105). OMM can be confused with palatal myoclonus, acquired pendular nystagmus, and segmental spinal myoclonus (117), and hypothalamic manifestations may suggest Kleine–Levin syndrome (110). The cerebrospinal fluid in neurologic Whipple's disease may be normal or contain small numbers of leukocytes. Some of these cells may be PAS-positive. *T. whippelii* rDNA can be detected by PCR in the cerebrospinal fluid of most patients with central nervous system Whipple's disease, and even in many patients without overt neurologic symptoms (154). The differential diagnosis of chronic uveitis and retinitis includes rheumatoid arthritis, ulcerative colitis, sarcoidosis, Lyme's disease, syphilis, tuberculosis, and reticulum cell sarcoma.

The diagnosis of Whipple's disease most often requires peroral endoscopic biopsy of the duodenal mucosa. Hematologic, chemical, and radiologic tests and procedures are nonspecific and hence not helpful. Dobbins (16) and other investigators (56,155) have emphasized the usefulness of small-intestinal mucosal biopsy in Whipple's disease. The presence of strongly PAS-reactive, diastase-resistant, acid-fast–negative macrophages in the small-intestinal lamina propria is considered sufficient for a diagnosis of Whipple's disease in the context of other typical histologic features in this tissue. (Periodic acid oxidizes glycol groups or their amino or alkylamino derivatives to dialdehydes, which then combine with Schiff reagent to form a magenta compound that is insoluble.) Electron microscopy is usually not necessary in this circumstance. Because Whipple's disease pathology can be patchy in the small-intestinal mucosa, multiple biopsies may be required (60). Another cause of false-negative histologic findings in endoscopically obtained specimens is the occurrence of Whipple's disease pathology only in the submucosa (59), as may happen after treatment with antibiotics, or only in extraintestinal tissues (see "Clinical Illness"). Amarenco et al. (118) pointed out the potential diagnostic utility of laparotomy and biopsy of intraabdominal lymph nodes in patients with extraintestinal disease, but computed tomography-guided biopsy may serve the same purpose without surgery. Granulomas in any tissue that do not stain with PAS should not exclude the diagnosis of Whipple's disease. In terms of false-positive small-intestinal histology, PAS-positive macrophages are found in several other diseases (16). *M. avium* complex and *Rhodococcus equi* infections can be ruled out with the acid-fast stain. In macroglobulinemia, the macrophages stain only weakly with PAS, and histoplasmosis can be distinguished by the typical observation of encapsulated intracellular yeast. PAS-positive macrophages in the stomach, colon, or rectum may correspond to lipophages or muciphages; thus, they are nonspecific and cannot be used as a basis for a diagnosis of Whipple's disease.

In the case of putative extraintestinal Whipple's disease, PAS-positive, diastase-resistant macrophages are again nonspecific. In lymph nodes, for example, mast cells, Russell bodies (cytoplasmic immunoglobulin globules in plasma cells), and other structures may generate a similar staining pattern. Therefore, electron microscopic detection of typical Whipple bacilli or PCR assays for *T. whippelii* are usually required to confirm a diagnosis of Whipple's disease in extraintestinal tissues. For electron microscopy, Dobbins (16) recommends fixing tissues in modified Karnovsky glutaraldehyde (2.5%) and paraformaldehyde (3%), then treatment with osmium. Accurate discrimination between *T. whippelii* and other actinomycetes (e.g., *M. avium* complex) by electron microscopy may require extensive experience.

Tissue assays based on PCR are probably more sensitive than histologic or electron microscopic tissue inspection, given that *T. whippelii* has been detected by PCR in histologically normal duodenal tissue from a patient with extraintestinal Whipple's disease (138). Fresh-frozen tissue provides more sensitive detection with PCR than does fixed tissue. Although *T. whippelii* has been detected in the peripheral blood of patients with Whipple's disease (87,156), the sensitivity of testing this fluid is not known (88). The sensitivity and specificity of PCR performed on intestinal and lymph node biopsy specimens are high (28), and this technique can be used to follow the response to antibiotic treatment (32).

In situ hybridization with a specific DNA probe targeting *T. whippelii* rRNA offers an alternative method for detecting infection in tissues (20) (see Color Figure 51.5). The sensitivity and specificity of *in situ* hybridization in comparison with those of PCR or traditional histology are not currently known. This diagnostic method may not be appropriate for patients who have been treated with antibiotics because intact bacterial rRNA is necessary. On the other hand, *in situ* hybridization may be a better method than PAS staining for following the tissue response to treatment because the degradation of PAS-positive cellular inclusions lags behind the clinical and microbiologic responses to antibiotics. PAS-positive inclusions may persist in tissues for years despite cure of Whipple's disease.

TREATMENT AND PREVENTION

Whipple's disease was uniformly fatal before the development of antibiotics. Although some partial responses have been reported following the use of corticosteroids and adrenocorticotropic hormone (ACTH) (157), these responses have been only temporary, and nearly all patients so treated ultimately succumbed to this disease (47,155). Paulley (8) in 1952 was the first to report the efficacy of antimicrobial therapy in Whipple's disease. Treatment of his patient with chloramphenicol resulted in elimination of fever and diarrhea within a week and disease remission lasting at least a year. Antibiotic therapy of Whipple's disease did not become common practice until the early 1960s, when it became clear that these drugs could dramatically alter the natural history of the illness (155,158). A variety of antibiotics besides chloramphenicol are thought to have some efficacy in the treatment of Whipple's disease (109), including penicillin, ampicillin, tetracycline, streptomycin (in combination with penicillin), trimethoprim-sulfamethoxazole, erythromycin, and, more recently, ceftriaxone (116), cefixime (159), and pefloxacin (118). Prolonged oral tetracycline was a common therapy in the 1960s. Early regimens then began to include an initial parenteral course of penicillin, sometimes accompanied by streptomycin, followed by tetracycline for approximately a year (47).

In the late 1970s and early 1980s, it became increasingly apparent that clinical relapse was a frequent problem in patients with Whipple's disease (105,110,160). Most of these relapses were manifested as neurologic disease. Keinath and co-workers (109) reviewed the response to treatment in 88 patients with at least 1 year of follow-up. Thirty-one (35%) patients suffered a relapse, at a mean of 4 years following initial diagnosis; 11 of these relapses were of a neurologic form and occurred relatively late. The most common clinical findings in patients with neurologic relapse were dementia and ataxia. Among risk factors for relapse, tetracycline therapy was the most significant; 42% of patients treated with tetracycline alone suffered relapse, and they accounted for nearly all relapses involving the central nervous system. Patients with disease relapse outside the central nervous system did well on any of a variety of antibiotic regimens, whereas those with central nervous system relapse responded poorly to repeated treatment. With encouraging reports on the use of trimethoprim-sulfamethoxazole to treat neurologic Whipple's disease, it became apparent that penetration of the blood–brain barrier is an important feature of drugs used for the initial treatment of this disorder (16,109,161,162). More recently, case reports have described the successful treatment of neurologic disease with ceftriaxone followed by doxycycline (116), with cefixime (159,163), and with pefloxacin (118).

Recommendations for the treatment of Whipple's disease are based on empiric observations and retrospective reviews of the literature. No controlled trials have been published on this subject. Although the causative agent has recently been cultivated *in vitro,* susceptibility data are currently lacking. Can the phylogenetic relationships of the Whipple bacillus, *T. whippelii,* be used to guide the selection of antibiotics in a meaningful manner? Most of the other pathogenic members of the Actinobacteria group are susceptible to penicillin, aminoglycosides, trimethoprim-sulfamethoxazole, dapsone, and the tetracyclines, many of which have been used successfully to treat Whipple's disease. Unfortunately, no known organism is closely related to *T. whippelii*; therefore, few inferences can be made regarding drug susceptibility. The current recommendation for the treatment of patients with Whipple's disease is the combination of procaine penicillin G (1.2 million U/d intramuscularly) and streptomycin (1 g/d intramuscularly) for 14 days, followed by trimethoprim-sulfamethoxazole (160 mg/800 mg orally two to three times a day) for at least a year (16,95,109). Dietary supplementation with folinic acid should be provided. Some investigators would treat patients with neurologic disease for at least 2 years, and perhaps indefinitely.

The high rate of relapse despite prolonged courses of treatment with single antibiotics raises the question of whether combinations of antibiotics should be employed. Other actinomycete pathogens, such as *Mycobacterium tuberculosis,* are usually treated with antibiotic combinations to prevent the development of antibiotic-resistant clones and produce a cure. A treatment approach employing multiple antibiotics with evidence of central nervous system penetration would seem to be a reasonable strategy, although the advantages of this approach have not been proved.

The clinical response to antibiotic therapy is more dramatic than the histologic response. Approximately 90% of treated patients experience symptomatic relief (95). Diarrhea commonly resolves within 7 days, and arthralgias improve within 1 to 3 weeks. Significant weight gain occurs within 1 month of treatment (47,158). As early as 1 week following the institution of therapy, the small-intestinal epithelium begins to revert to normal (i.e., return of epithelial cell height, loss of intraepithelial cell bacilli, and the beginning of restoration of villous architecture) (14). Extracellular bacilli in the lamina propria become degraded and are usually eliminated between 2 and 9 weeks into therapy, and the PAS staining pattern of the macrophage vacuoles becomes more homogeneous (14,16,164). Although the distribution of PAS-positive macrophages becomes sparser and patchier, these cells usually persist for at least 1 and sometimes for as many as 8 years despite clinical remission (14,95,164). Other mucosal histologic changes usually regress or resolve after approximately a year with successful treatment, although lipid deposits and some neutrophils often remain in the lamina propria (14,95).

Endoscopic examination reveals the disappearance of gross mucosal changes after 6 months of treatment (55). Correction of the small-bowel radiographic appearance occurs after a mean of 10 months (95). Bacterial DNA disappears from tissue within months of the initiation of successful antibiotic treatment (28). Neurologic disease is the most recalcitrant to treatment. Gaze palsies and confusion respond most effectively, with eventual improvement or resolution (165). Dementia and long-tract signs may stabilize but usually do not improve. Hypothalamic signs may be the least responsive to treatment. In all forms of Whipple's disease, relapse is associated with a return of previous tissue pathology and the reappearance of extracellular bacilli (14).

In the future, sensitive PCR-based assays for *T. whippelii* in natural aquatic and soil environments may lead to an appreciation of the reservoir for this organism and, subsequently, to strategies for reducing human exposure. In a general sense, further molecular characterization of this microorganism may enhance our understanding of the pathogenesis of Whipple's disease and the means by which the process may be interrupted. With the successful propagation of *T. whippelii* in the laboratory, it should now be possible to study the susceptibility of this bacterium to antibiotics and combinations of antibiotics, so that more rational treatment strategies can be pursued.

ACKNOWLEDGMENTS

We acknowledge the helpful discussions of Dr. William O. Dobbins III. D. N. F. is supported by a Physician Scientist Award from the National Institutes of Health (K11-AI01360).

REFERENCES

1. Whipple GH. A hitherto undescribed disease characterized anatomically by deposits of fat and fatty acids in the intestinal and mesenteric lymphatic tissues. *Johns Hopkins Hosp Bull* 1907;18:382–391.
2. Relman DA, Schmidt TM, MacDermott RP, et al. Identification of the uncultured bacillus of Whipple's disease. *N Engl J Med* 1992;327:293–301.
3. Wilson KH, Blitchington R, Frothingham R, et al. Phylogeny of the Whipple's disease-associated bacterium. *Lancet* 1991;338: 474–475.
4. Black-Schaffer B. The tinctorial demonstration of a glycoprotein in Whipple's disease. *Proc Soc Exp Biol Med* 1949;72: 225–227.
5. Plummer K, Russi S, Harris WHJ, et al. Lipophagic intestinal granulomatosis (Whipple's disease). Clinical and pathologic study of thirty-four cases, with special reference to clinical diagnosis and pathogenesis. *Arch Intern Med* 1950;86:280–310.
6. Yardley JH, Flemming WH. Whipple's disease: a note regarding PAS-positive granules in the original case. *Johns Hopkins Hosp Bull* 1961;109:76–79.
7. Morgan AD. The first recorded case of Whipple's disease? *Gut* 1961;2:370–372.
8. Paulley JW. A case of Whipple's disease (intestinal lipodystrophy). *Gastroenterology* 1952;22:128–133.
9. Chears WCJ, Ashworth CT. Electron microscopic study of the intestinal mucosa in Whipple's disease: demonstration of encapsulated bacilliform bodies in the lesion. *Gastroenterology* 1961; 41:129–138.
10. Cohen AS, Schimmel EM, Holt PR, et al. Ultrastructural abnormalities in Whipple's disease. *Proc Soc Exp Bio Med* 1960; 105:411–414.
11. Yardley JH, Hendrix TR. Combined electron and light microscopy in Whipple's disease: demonstration of "bacillary bodies" in the intestine. *Bull Johns Hopkins Hosp* 1961;109: 80–98.
12. Dobbins WO, Kawanishi H. Bacillary characteristics in Whipple's disease: an electron microscopic study. *Gastroenterology* 1981;80:1468–1475.
13. Silva MT, Macedo PM, Moura Nunes JF. Ultrastructure of bacilli and the bacillary origin of the macrophagic inclusions in Whipple's disease. *J Gen Microbiol* 1985;131(Pt 5):1001–1013.
14. Trier JS, Phelps PC, Eidelman S, et al. Whipple's disease: light and electron microscope correlation of jejunal mucosal histology with antibiotic treatment and clinical status. *Gastroenterology* 1965;48:684–707.
15. Relman DA, Loutit JS, Schmidt TM, et al. The agent of bacillary angiomatosis. An approach to the identification of uncultured pathogens [see Comments]. *N Engl J Med* 1990;323:1573–1580.
16. Dobbins WO. *Whipple's disease.* Springfield, IL: Charles C Thomas Publisher, 1987:242.
17. Dobbins WO. Whipple's disease: an historical perspective. *Q J Med* 1985;56:523–531.
18. Evans AS. Causation and disease: the Henle–Koch postulates revisited. *Yale J Biol Med* 1976;49:175–195.
19. Fredricks DN, Relman DA. Sequence-based identification of microbial pathogens: a reconsideration of Koch's postulates. *Clin Microbiol Rev* 1996;9:18–33.
20. Fredricks DN, Relman DA. Localization of *T. whippelii* rRNA in tissues from patients with Whipple's disease. *J Infect Dis* 2001;183:1229–1237.
21. Cimprich RE, Rooney JR. *Corynebacterium equi* enteritis in foals. *Vet Pathol* 1977;14:95–102.
22. Archer GL, Coleman PH, Cole RM, et al. Human infection from an unidentified erythrocyte-associated bacterium. *N Engl J Med* 1979;301:897–900.
23. Sherris JC, Roberts CE, Porus RL. Microbiological studies of intestinal biopsies taken during active Whipple's disease. *Gastroenterology* 1965;48:708–710.
24. Raoult D, Birg ML, La Scola B, et al. Cultivation of the bacillus of Whipple's disease. *N Engl J Med* 2000;342:620–625.
25. Woese CR. Bacterial evolution. *Microbiol Rev* 1987;51: 221–271.
26. Relman DA. The identification of uncultured microbial pathogens. *J Infect Dis* 1993;168:1–8.
27. Khavari PA, Bolognia JL, Eisen R, et al. Periodic acid–Schiff-positive organisms in primary cutaneous *Bacillus cereus* infection. Case report and an investigation of the periodic acid–Schiff staining properties of bacteria. *Arch Dermatol* 1991;127:543–546.
28. Ramzan NN, Loftus E, Burgart LJ, et al. Diagnosis and monitoring of Whipple's disease by polymerase chain reaction. *Ann Intern Med* 1997;126:520–527.
29. von Herbay A, Ditton HJ, Maiwald M. Diagnostic application of a polymerase chain reaction assay for the Whipple's disease bacterium to intestinal biopsies. *Gastroenterology* 1996;110: 1735–1743.
30. Muller C, Petermann D, Stain C, et al. Whipple's disease: comparison of histology with diagnosis based on polymerase chain reaction in four consecutive cases. *Gut* 1997;40:425–427.
31. Lynch T, Odel J, Fredricks DN, et al. Polymerase chain reaction-based detection of *Tropheryma whippelii* in central nervous system Whipple's disease. *Ann Neurol* 1997;42:120–124.
32. Petrides PE, Muller-Hocker J, Fredricks DN, et al. PCR analysis of *T. whippelii* DNA in a case of Whipple's disease: effect of antibiotics and correlation with histology. *Am J Gastroenterol* 1998;93:1579–1582.
33. Pron B, Poyart C, Abachin E, et al. Diagnosis and follow-up of Whipple's disease by amplification of the 16S rRNA gene of *Tropheryma whippelii. Eur J Clin Microbiol Infect Dis* 1999; 18:62–65.
34. Gras E, Matias-Guiu X, Garcia A, et al. PCR analysis in the pathological diagnosis of Whipple's disease: emphasis on extraintestinal involvement or atypical morphological features. *J Pathol* 1999;188:318–321.
35. Maiwald M, von Herbay A, Lepp PW, et al. Organization, structure, and variability of the rRNA operon of the Whipple's disease bacterium (*Tropheryma whippelii*). *J Bacteriol* 2000;182: 3292–3297.
36. Hinrikson HP, Dutly F, Altwegg M. Evaluation of a specific nested PCR targeting domain III of the 23S rRNA gene of "*Tropheryma whippelii*" and proposal of a classification system for its molecular variants. *J Clin Microbiol* 2000;38:595–599.
37. Gillin JS, Urmacher C, West R, et al. Disseminated *Mycobacterium avium–intracellulare* infection in acquired immunodeficiency syndrome mimicking Whipple's disease. *Gastroenterology* 1983;85:1187–1191.
38. Maliha GM, Hepps KS, Maia DM, et al. Whipple's disease can mimic chronic AIDS enteropathy. *Am J Gastroenterol* 1991; 86:79–81.
39. Roth RI, Owen RL, Keren DF. AIDS with *Mycobacterium avium–intracellulare* lesions resembling those of Whipple's disease [Letter]. *N Engl J Med* 1983;309:1324–1325.
40. Roth RI, Owen RL, Keren DF, et al. Intestinal infection with *Mycobacterium avium* in acquired immune deficiency syndrome (AIDS). Histological and clinical comparison with Whipple's disease. *Dig Dis Sci* 1985;30:497–504.
41. Strom RL, Gruninger RP. AIDS with *Mycobacterium avium–*

intracellulare lesions resembling those of Whipple's disease [Letter]. *N Engl J Med* 1983;309:1323–1324.
42. Wang HH, Tollerud D, Danar D, et al. Another Whipple-like disease in AIDS? *N Engl J Med* 1986;314:1577–1578.
43. Chiodini RJ, Van KH, Merkal RS. Ruminant paratuberculosis (Johne's disease): the current status and future prospects. *Cornell Vet* 1984;74:218–262.
44. Cornelius CE. Animal models—a neglected medical resource. *N Engl J Med* 1969;281:934–944.
45. Thoen CO, Baum KH. Current knowledge on paratuberculosis. *J Am Vet Med Assoc* 1988;192:1609–1611.
46. Capron JP, Thevenin A, Delamarre J, et al. Whipple's disease: study of 3 cases and epidemiological and radiological remarks [in French]. *Lille Med* 1975;20:842–845.
47. Maizel H, Ruffin JM, Dobbins WO. Whipple's disease: a review of 19 patients from one hospital and a review of the literature since 1950. *Medicine (Baltimore)* 1970;49:175–205.
48. Puite RH, Tesluk H. Whipple's disease. *Am J Med* 1955;19:383–400.
49. Dykman DD, Cuccherini BA, Fuss IJ, et al. Whipple's disease in a father–daughter pair. *Dig Dis Sci* 1999;44:2542–2544.
50. Maiwald M, Schuhmacher F, Ditton HJ, et al. Environmental occurrence of the Whipple's disease bacterium (*Tropheryma whippelii*). *Appl Environ Microbiol* 1998;64:760–762.
51. Ehrbar HU, Bauerfeind P, Dutly F, et al. PCR-positive tests for *Tropheryma whippelii* in patients without Whipple's disease. *Lancet* 1999;353:2214.
52. Street S, Donoghue HD, Neild GH. *Tropheryma whippelii* DNA in saliva of healthy people. *Lancet* 1999;354:1178–1179.
53. Dutly F, Hinrikson HP, Seidel T, et al. *Tropheryma whippelii* DNA in saliva of patients without Whipple's disease. *Infection* 2000;28:219–222.
54. Maiwald M, Herbay A, Persing DH, et al. *Tropheryma whippelii* DNA is rare in the intestinal mucosa of patients without other evidence of Whipple's disease. *Ann Intern Med* 2001;134:115–119.
55. Geboes K, Ectors N, Heidbuchel H, et al. Whipple's disease: endoscopic aspects before and after therapy. *Gastrointest Endosc* 1990;36:247–252.
56. Enzinger FM, Helwig EB. Whipple's disease: a review of the literature and report of fifteen patients. *Virchows Arch A Pathol Anat Histopathol* 1963;336:238–269.
57. Sieracki JC, Fine G. Whipple's disease-observations on systemic involvement. II. Gross and histologic observation. *Arch Pathol* 1959;67:81–93.
58. Ectors N, Geboes K, De Vos R, et al. Whipple's disease: a histological, immunocytochemical and electron microscopic study of the immune response in the small-intestinal mucosa. *Histopathology* 1992;21:1–12.
59. Kuhajda FP, Belitsos NJ, Keren DF, et al. A submucosal variant of Whipple's disease. *Gastroenterology* 1982;82:46–50.
60. Moorthy S, Nolley G, Hermos JA. Whipple's disease with minimal intestinal involvement. *Gut* 1977;18:152–155.
61. Dobbins WO, Ruffin JM. A light- and electron-microscopic study of bacterial invasion in Whipple's disease. *Am J Pathol* 1967;51:225–242.
62. Ectors N, Geboes K, Wynants P, et al. Granulomatous gastritis and Whipple's disease. *Am J Gastroenterol* 1992;87:509–513.
63. Gear EVJ, Dobbins WOI. Rectal biopsy: a review of its diagnostic usefulness. *Gastroenterology* 1968;55:522–544.
64. Cho C, Linscheer WG, Hirschkorn MA, et al. Sarcoidlike granulomas as an early manifestation of Whipple's disease. *Gastroenterology* 1984;87:941–947.
65. Spapen HD, Segers O, De Wit N, et al. Electron microscopic detection of Whipple's bacillus in sarcoidlike periodic acid–Schiff-negative granulomas. *Dig Dis Sci* 1989;34:640–643.
66. Wilcox GM, Tronic BS, Schecter DJ, et al. Periodic acid–Schiff-negative granulomatous lymphadenopathy in patients with Whipple's disease. Localization of the Whipple bacillus to noncaseating granulomas by electron microscopy. *Am J Med* 1987;83:165–170.
67. Keren DF. Whipple's disease: a review emphasizing immunology and microbiology. *Crit Rev Clin Lab Sci* 1981;14:75–108.
68. Dobbins WO. Is there an immune deficit in Whipple's disease? *Dig Dis Sci* 1981;26:247–252.
69. Keren DF, Weisburger WR, Yardley JH, et al. Whipple's disease: demonstration by immunofluorescence of similar bacterial antigens in macrophages from three cases. *Johns Hopkins Med J* 1976;139:51–59.
70. Groll A, Valberg LS, Simon JB, et al. Immunological defect in Whipple's disease. *Gastroenterology* 1972;63:943–950.
71. Kent TH, Layton JM, Clifton JA, et al. Whipple's disease: light and electron microscopic studies combined with clinical studies suggesting an infective nature. *Lab Invest* 1963;12:1163–1178.
72. Kirkpatrick PM, Kent SP, Mihas A, et al. Whipple's disease: case report with immunological studies. *Gastroenterology* 1978;75:297–301.
73. Feurle GE, Dorken B, Schopf E, et al. HLA-B27 and defects in the T-cell system in Whipple's disease. *Eur J Clin Invest* 1979;9:385–389.
74. Martin FF, Vilseck J, Dobbins WO, et al. Immunological alterations in patients with treated Whipple's disease. *Gastroenterology* 1972;63:6–18.
75. Veloso FT, Vaz Saleiro J, Baptista F, et al. Whipple's disease. Report of a case with clinical immunological studies. *Am J Gastroenterol* 1981;75:419–425.
76. Bjerknes R, Laerum OD, Degaard S. Impaired bacterial degradation by monocytes and macrophages from a patient with treated Whipple's disease. *Gastroenterology* 1985;89:1139–1146.
77. Bjerknes R, Odegaard S, Bjerkvig R, et al. Whipple's disease. Demonstration of a persisting monocyte and macrophage dysfunction. *Scand J Gastroenterol* 1988;23:611–619.
78. Marth T, Roux M, von Herbay A, et al. Persistent reduction of complement receptor 3 alpha-chain expressing mononuclear blood cells and transient inhibitory serum factors in Whipple's disease. *Clin Immunol Immunopathol* 1994;72:217–226.
79. Marth T, Neurath M, Cuccherini BA, et al. Defects of monocyte interleukin 12 production and humoral immunity in Whipple's disease. *Gastroenterology* 1997;113:442–448.
80. Austin LL, Dobbins WO. Intraepithelial leukocytes of the intestinal mucosa in normal man and in Whipple's disease: a light- and electron-microscopic study. *Dig Dis Sci* 1982;27:311–320.
81. Dobbins WO. HLA antigens in Whipple's disease. *Arthritis Rheum* 1987;30:102–105.
82. Feurle GE. Association of Whipple's disease with HLA-B27. *Lancet* 1985;1:1336.
83. Bai JC, Mota AH, Maurino E, et al. Class I and class II HLA antigens in a homogeneous Argentinian population with Whipple's disease: lack of association with HLA-B 27. *Am J Gastroenterol* 1991;86:992–994.
84. Oliver-Pascual E, Galan J, Oliver-Pascual A, et al. Un caso de lipodistrofia intestinal con lesions ganglionares mesentericas de granulomatosis lipofagica (Enfermedad de Whipple). *Rev Esp Enferm Apar Digest Nutr* 1947;6:213–226.
85. Meier-Willersen HJ, Maiwald M, von Herbay A. Whipple's disease associated with opportunistic infections [in German]. *Dtsch Med Wochenschr* 1993;118:854–860.
86. Bassotti G, Pelli MA, Ribacchi R, et al. *Giardia lamblia* infestation reveals underlying Whipple's disease in a patient with longstanding constipation. *Am J Gastroenterol* 1991;86:371–374.

86a. Relman DA, Falkow S. A molecular perspective of microbial pathogenicity. In: Mandell GL, Bennett JE, Dolan R, eds. *Principles and practice of infectious diseases* 4th ed. New York: Churchill Livingstone, 2000:2–13.
87. Muller C, Stain C, Burghuber O. *Tropheryma whippelii* in peripheral blood mononuclear cells and cells of pleural effusion. *Lancet* 1993;341:701.
88. Marth T, Fredericks D, Strober W, et al. Limited role for PCR-based diagnosis of Whipple's disease from peripheral blood mononuclear cells. *Lancet* 1996;348:66–67.
89. Farr M, Morris C, Hollywell CA, et al. Amyloidosis in Whipple's arthritis. *J R Soc Med* 1983;76:963–965.
90. Kwitko AO, Shearman DJ, McKenzie PE, et al. Whipple's disease: a case with circulating immune complexes. *Gastroenterology* 1980;79:1318–1323.
91. Saboor SA, Johnson NM, McFadden J. Detection of mycobacterial DNA in sarcoidosis and tuberculosis with polymerase chain reaction. *Lancet* 1992;339:1012–1015.
92. Rook GA, Stanford JL. Slow bacterial infections or autoimmunity? *Immunol Today* 1992;13:160–164.
93. Mitchell IC, Turk JL, Mitchell DN. Detection of mycobacterial rRNA in sarcoidosis with liquid-phase hybridisation. *Lancet* 1992;339:1015–1017.
94. Miksche LW, Blumcke S, Fritsche D, et al. Whipple's disease: etiopathogenesis, treatment, diagnosis, and clinical course. Case report and review of the world literature. *Acta Hepatogastroenterol (Stuttg)* 1974;21:307–326.
95. Fleming JL, Wiesner RH, Shorter RG. Whipple's disease: clinical, biochemical, and histopathologic features and assessment of treatment in 29 patients. *Mayo Clin Proc* 1988;63:539–351.
96. Feldman M, Price G. Intestinal bleeding in patients with Whipple's disease. *Gastroenterology* 1989;96:1207–1209.
97. James TN, Bulkley BH, Kent SP. Vascular lesions of the gastrointestinal system in Whipple's disease. *Am J Med Sci* 1984; 288:125–129.
98. Berger ML, Siegel DM, Lee EL. Scurvy as an initial manifestation of Whipple's disease. *Ann Intern Med* 1984;101:58–59.
99. Chears WCJ, Hargrove MD, Verner JV, et al. Whipple's disease—a review of twelve patients from one service. *Am J Med* 1961;30:226–234.
100. Volpicelli NA, Salyer WR, Milligan FD, et al. The endoscopic appearance of the duodenum in Whipple's disease. *Johns Hopkins Med J* 1976;138:19–23.
101. Feldman M. Whipple's disease. *Am J Med Sci* 1986;291:56–67.
102. Comer GM, Brandt LJ, Abissi CJ. Whipple's disease: a review. *Am J Gastroenterol* 1983;78:107–114.
103. Wroe SJ, Pires M, Harding B, et al. Whipple's disease confined to the CNS presenting with multiple intracerebral mass lesions. *J Neurol Neurosurg Psychiatry* 1991;54:989–992.
104. Sieracki JC, Fine G, Horn RCJ, et al. Central nervous system involvement in Whipple's disease. *J Neuropathol Exp Neurol* 1960;19:70–75.
105. Knox DL, Bayless TM, Pittman FE. Neurologic disease in patients with treated Whipple's disease. *Medicine (Baltimore)* 1976;55:467–476.
106. Kitamura T. Brain involvement in Whipple's disease: a case report. *Acta Neuropathol (Berl)* 1975;33:275–278.
107. Finelli PF, McEntee WJ, Lessell S, et al. Whipple's disease with predominantly neuroophthalmic manifestations. *Ann Neurol* 1977;1:247–252.
108. Riggs JE. The evolving natural history of neurologic involvement in Whipple's disease: a hypothesis. *Arch Neurol* 1988;45: 830.
109. Keinath RD, Merrell DE, Vlietstra R, et al. Antibiotic treatment and relapse in Whipple's disease. Long-term follow-up of 88 patients. *Gastroenterology* 1985;88:1867–1873.
110. Feurle GE, Volk B, Waldherr R. Cerebral Whipple's disease with negative jejunal histology. *N Engl J Med* 1979;300:907–908.
111. Manzel K, Tranel D, Cooper G. Cognitive and behavioral abnormalities in a case of central nervous system Whipple's disease. *Arch Neurol* 2000;57:399–403.
112. Louis ED, Lynch T, Kaufmann P, et al. Diagnostic guidelines in central nervous system Whipple's disease. *Ann Neurol* 1996;40: 561–568.
113. Lieb K, Maiwald M, Berger M, et al. Insomnia for 5 years. *Lancet* 1999;354:1966.
114. Mendel E, Khoo LT, Go JL, et al. Intracerebral Whipple's disease diagnosed by stereotactic biopsy: a case report and review of the literature. *Neurosurgery* 1999;44:203–209.
115. Lynch T, Fahn S, Louis ED, et al. Oculofacial–skeletal myorhythmia in Whipple's disease. *Mov Disord* 1997;12:625–626.
116. Adler CH, Galetta SL. Oculo-facial-skeletal myorhythmia in Whipple's disease: treatment with ceftriaxone. *Ann Intern Med* 1990;112:467–469.
117. Schwartz MA, Selhorst JB, Ochs AL, et al. Oculomasticatory myorhythmia: a unique movement disorder occurring in Whipple's disease. *Ann Neurol* 1986;20:677–683.
118. Amarenco P, Roullet E, Hannoun L, et al. Progressive supranuclear palsy as the sole manifestation of systemic Whipple's disease treated with pefloxacin. *J Neurol Neurosurg Psychiatry* 1991; 54:1121–1122.
119. Upton AC. Histochemical investigation of the mesenchymal lesions in Whipple's disease. *Am J Clin Pathol* 1952;22:755–764.
120. Pelech T, Fric P, Huslarova A, et al. Interstitial lymphocytic myocarditis in Whipple's disease. *Lancet* 1991;337:553–554.
121. James TN, Bulkley BH. Abnormalities of the coronary arteries in Whipple's disease. *Am Heart J* 1983;105:481–491.
122. Lie JT, Davis JS. Pancarditis in Whipple's disease: electron microscopic demonstration of intracardiac bacillary bodies. *Am J Clin Pathol* 1976;66:22–30.
123. McAllister HA, Fenoglio JJ. Cardiac involvement in Whipple's disease. *Circulation* 1975;52:152–156.
124. Bostwick DG, Bensch KG, Burke JS, et al. Whipple's disease presenting as aortic insufficiency. *N Engl J Med* 1981;305: 995–998.
125. Ratliff NB, McMahon JT, Naab TJ, et al. Whipple's disease in the porcine leaflets of a Carpentier–Edwards prosthetic mitral valve. *N Engl J Med* 1984;311:902–903.
126. Marie I, Levesque H, Levade MH, et al. Hypertrophic osteoarthropathy can indicate recurrence of Whipple's disease. *Arthritis Rheum* 1999;42:2002–2006.
127. Rubinow A, Canoso JJ, Goldenberg DL, et al. Arthritis in Whipple's disease. *Isr J Med Sci* 1981;17:445–450.
128. Delanty N, Georgescu L, Lynch T, et al. Synovial fluid polymerase chain reaction as an aid to the diagnosis of central nervous system Whipple's disease. *Ann Neurol* 1999;45:137–138.
129. O'Duffy JD, Griffing WL, Li CY, et al. Whipple's arthritis: direct detection of *Tropheryma whippelii* in synovial fluid and tissue. *Arthritis Rheum* 1999;42:812–817.
130. Farr M, Hollywell CA, Morris CJ, et al. Whipple's disease diagnosed at hip arthroplasty. *Ann Rheum Dis* 1984;43:526–529.
131. Fresard A, Guglielminotti C, Berthelot P, et al. Prosthetic joint infection caused by *Tropheryma whippelii* (Whipple's bacillus). *Clin Infect Dis* 1996;22:575–576.
132. Altwegg M, Fleisch-Marx A, Goldenberger D, et al. Spondylodiscitis caused by *Tropheryma whippelii*. *Schweiz Med Wochenschr* 1996;126:1495–1499.
133. Scheib JS, Quinet RJ. Whipple's disease with axial and peripheral joint destruction. *South Med J* 1990;83:684–687.
134. Canoso JJ, Saini M, Hermos JA. Whipple's disease and ankylosing spondylitis: simultaneous occurrence in HLA-B27 positive male. *J Rheumatol* 1978;5:79–84.

135. Swash M, Schwartz MS, Vandenburg MJ, et al. Myopathy in Whipple's disease. *Gut* 1977;18:800–804.
136. Helliwell TR, Appleton RE, Mapstone NC, et al. Dermatomyositis and Whipple's disease. *Neuromuscul Disord* 2000;10:46–51.
137. Avila MP, Jalkh AE, Feldman E, et al. Manifestations of Whipple's disease in the posterior segment of the eye. *Arch Ophthalmol* 1984;102:384–390.
138. Rickman LS, Freeman WR, Green WR, et al. Brief report: uveitis caused by *Tropheryma whippelii* (Whipple's bacillus). *N Engl J Med* 1995;332:363–366.
139. Williams JG, Edward DP, Tessler HH, et al. Ocular manifestations of Whipple's disease: an atypical presentation. *Arch Ophthalmol* 1998;116:1232–1234.
140. Durant WJ, Flood T, Goldberg MF, et al. Vitrectomy and Whipple's disease. *Arch Ophthalmol* 1984;102:848–851.
141. Font RL, Rao NA, Issarescu S, et al. Ocular involvement in Whipple's disease: light and electron microscopic observations. *Arch Ophthalmol* 1978;96:1431–1436.
142. Symmons DP, Shepherd AN, Boardman PL, et al. Pulmonary manifestations of Whipple's disease. *Q J Med* 1985;56:497–504.
143. Winberg CD, Rose ME, Rappaport H. Whipple's disease of the lung. *Am J Med* 1978;65:873–880.
144. Pequignot H, Morin Y, Grandjouan MS, et al. Sarcoidosis and Whipple's disease. Association? Relation? [in French]. *Ann Med Interne (Paris)* 1976;127:797–806.
145. Balestrieri GP, Villanacci V, Battocchio S, et al. Cutaneous involvement in Whipple's disease. *Br J Dermatol* 1996;135:666–668.
146. Aubert L, Quilichi R, Gharbi G, et al. Adenopathies in Whipple's disease [in French]. *Nouv Presse Med* 1979;8:2986.
147. Davis SJ, Patel A. Distinctive echogenic lymphadenopathy in Whipple's disease. *Clin Radiol* 1990;42:60–62.
148. Mansbach CM, Shelburne JD, Stevens RD, et al. Lymph node bacilliform bodies resembling those of Whipple's disease in a patient without intestinal involvement. *Ann Intern Med* 1978;89:64–66.
149. Rodarte JR, Garrison CO, Holley KE, et al. Whipple's disease simulating sarcoidosis. A case with unique clinical and histologic features. *Arch Intern Med* 1972;129:479–482.
150. Giradin M-FS-M, Zafrani ES, Chaumette M-T, et al. Hepatic granulomas in Whipple's disease. *Gastroenterology* 1984;86:753–756.
151. Gupta S, Pinching AJ, Onwubalili J, et al. Whipple's disease with unusual clinical, bacteriologic, and immunologic findings. *Gastroenterology* 1986;90(5 Pt 1):1286–1289.
152. Stoll T, Keusch G, Jost R, et al. IgA nephropathy and hypercalcemia in Whipple's disease. *Nephron* 1993;63:222–225.
153. Chetelat CA, Bruhlmann W, Ammann RW. Malignant-appearing retroperitoneal lymphography findings in Whipple's disease—a source of possible misdiagnosis [in German]. *Schweiz Med Wochenschr* 1985;115:364–368.
154. von Herbay A, Ditton HJ, Schuhmacher F, et al. Whipple's disease: staging and monitoring by cytology and polymerase chain reaction analysis of cerebrospinal fluid. *Gastroenterology* 1997;113:434–441.
155. Ruffin JM, Roufail WM. The diagnosis and treatment of Whipple's disease. *Am J Dig Dis* 1965;10:887–891.
156. Lowsky R, Archer GL, Fyles G, et al. Brief report: diagnosis of Whipple's disease by molecular analysis of peripheral blood. *N Engl J Med* 1994;331:1343–1346.
157. Radding J, Fiese MJ. Whipple's disease (intestinal lipodystrophy): review of the literature and report of a case successfully treated with adrenocorticotropin (ACTH) and cortisone. *Ann Intern Med* 1954;41:1066–1075.
158. Ruffin JM, Kurtz SM, Roufail WM. Intestinal lipodystrophy (Whipple's disease); the immediate and prolonged effect of antibiotic therapy. *JAMA* 1966;195:476–478.
159. Cooper GS, Blades EW, Remler BF, et al. Central nervous system Whipple's disease: relapse during therapy with trimethoprim-sulfamethoxazole and remission with cefixime. *Gastroenterology* 1994;106:782–786.
160. Feldman M, Hendler RS, Morrison EB. Acute meningoencephalitis after withdrawal of antibiotics in Whipple's disease. *Ann Intern Med* 1980;93:709–711.
161. Ryser RJ, Locksley RM, Eng SC, et al. Reversal of dementia associated with Whipple's disease by trimethoprim-sulfamethoxazole, drugs that penetrate the blood–brain barrier. *Gastroenterology* 1984;86:745–752.
162. Viteri AL, Greene JF, Chandler JB. Whipple's disease, successful response to sulfamethoxazole-trimethoprim. *Am J Gastroenterol* 1981;75:309–310.
163. Peters FP, Wouters RS, de Bruine AP, et al. Cerebral relapse of sarcoidlike Whipple's disease. *Clin Infect Dis* 1997;24:1252–1255.
164. Denholm RB, Mills PR, More IA. Electron microscopy in the long-term follow-up of Whipple's disease. Effect of antibiotics. *Am J Surg Pathol* 1981;5:507–516.
165. Pollock S, Lewis PD, Kendall B. Whipple's disease confined to the nervous system. *J Neurol Neurosurg Psychiatry* 1981;44:1104–1109.

52

MYCOBACTERIAL DISEASE OF THE GASTROINTESTINAL TRACT

C. ROBERT HORSBURGH, JR.
ANN MARIE NELSON

Mycobacteria are among the most ancient of bacteria, and mycobacterial diseases are among the most ancient of human diseases. Tuberculosis (TB) was prevalent in Egypt of the pharaohs, India of the Rig Veda, Persia of the Zoroastrians, and pre-Columbian Central America (1). The classical Greeks recognized the clinical entity of cough, fevers, and wasting, which they called *phthisis.* Hippocrates noted the grave prognosis of gastrointestinal (GI) involvement with TB; he observed that "diarrhea attacking a person with phthisis is a mortal symptom" (2).

As rates of TB in the developed countries decreased in the middle of the twentieth century, other mycobacterial diseases of the GI tract were recognized. The foremost of these is infection with organisms of the *Mycobacterium avium* complex (MAC). More recently, the severe immune suppression present in patients with AIDS has led to an increase in the occurrence of MAC infection of the alimentary canal.

GASTROINTESTINAL DISEASE CAUSED BY *M. TUBERCULOSIS* COMPLEX

Epidemiology

Human TB is acquired by either ingestion or inhalation of organisms of the *M. tuberculosis* complex. The major reservoirs for this infection are humans and cattle. Human-to-human transmission occurs when a person with active TB exhales or expectorates droplet nuclei containing organisms, which are then inhaled and cause a localized pulmonary process in the susceptible host. TB is transmitted from cattle to humans when mycobacteria from infected cattle are excreted into milk; when the organisms are ingested (as milk or milk products), they cause a localized infection of the GI tract, mostly in the terminal ileum, cecum, colon, and rectum (3,4). "Secondary" infection of the GI tract may develop when a person with active pulmonary TB swallows sputum that contains organisms, or it may be caused by hematogenous dissemination from any site (3).

In the pre-antibiotic era, secondary GI TB in persons with advanced pulmonary TB was by far the most common form of GI TB. The overwhelming number of TB cases involved the lung, and secondary TB of the GI tract eventually developed in 65% to 90% of patients with pulmonary TB (3). In an autopsy series of patients with TB reported in 1928, 184 (80%) of 230 subjects had secondary TB of the GI tract (5); isolated GI TB was rare. GI TB was more likely to develop in persons with the most severe cases of pulmonary TB; 5% to 8% of cases of "early pulmonary TB" had radiographic evidence of GI TB, versus 14% to 18% of cases of "moderately advanced TB" and 70% to 80% of cases of "far-advanced TB" (6). In the United States, the frequency of GI TB decreased as the number of TB cases overall decreased throughout the twentieth century. After the introduction of antibiotic therapy for TB, the incidence of GI TB dropped markedly. The prevalence of GI TB detected radiographically declined from 10% to 1% between 1924 and 1949 (7). During 1969 through 1973, the rate of nonperitoneal abdominal TB in a sample of the U.S. population was 0.08% of all TB cases, or 0.01 cases per 100,000 persons (8). In recent reports from India, Finland, and South Africa, fewer than 5% of persons with TB have had GI tract involvement (4,9,10).

This decrease has several probable causes. First, prompt treatment of pulmonary TB may prevent GI TB. As noted, GI involvement is uncommon in persons with

C. R. Horsburgh, Jr.: Department of Epidemiology and Biostatistics, Boston University School of Public Health; Department of Medicine, Boston University School of Medicine, Boston, Massachusetts

A. M. Nelson: AIDS Pathology Branch, Department of Infectious and Parasitic Diseases Pathology, Armed Forces Institute of Pathology, Washington, D.C.

acute TB (either primary or reactivated), but its frequency increases with the duration and severity of pulmonary disease (3,6,11). Second, because GI TB responds to antibiotic therapy for pulmonary TB, many cases of GI TB go undiagnosed and resolve with treatment of the pulmonary focus. Third, to the extent that cases of GI TB have been related to the presence of *M. tuberculosis* or *Mycobacterium bovis* organisms in unpasteurized milk, such disease has decreased with the control of TB in cattle. Recent series of patients with GI TB in developed countries have shown a predominance of isolated cases of GI TB over cases of GI TB secondary to pulmonary TB (12–16); in studies from developing countries, the majority of cases continue to be secondary (4,17).

The relationship between the two most common pathogens in the *M. tuberculosis* complex, *M. tuberculosis* and *M. bovis,* and isolated versus secondary TB of the GI tract has been the subject of much speculation. Early authors suggested that isolated infection, most likely caused by exposure to contaminated milk or milk products, would be caused most commonly by *M. bovis,* whereas secondary GI TB, resulting from the more common *M. tuberculosis* disease of the lung, would usually be caused by *M. tuberculosis* (3). However, in countries where disease of cattle is not well controlled, *M. bovis* is still rare as a cause of either isolated or secondary GI TB (4). Therefore, it appears that both species are capable of producing either isolated or secondary disease, depending on the route of exposure. Because *M. tuberculosis* is much more common than *M. bovis* worldwide, it now causes the overwhelming majority of cases of either presentation (4,18–20).

In the pre-antibiotic era, isolated GI TB was thought to be more common in children than in adults, whereas secondary GI TB was more common in adults (3). More recent studies have shown both forms to be more common in older persons; in the United States and Europe, the mean age of patients with both types appears to be 50 to 75 years, whereas in developing countries, the mean age is most often 20 to 40 years (4,21). This is most likely a reflection of the overall age distribution of cases of active TB in those areas. Despite some reports showing higher rates in women, most data indicate that the sexes are equally affected (4,22,23). The racial and ethnic distribution of cases of GI TB in the United States also mirrors that of TB cases overall, with fewer cases in whites than in nonwhites (8,24).

Persons with HIV-1 infection are uniquely susceptible to disease caused by *M. tuberculosis,* both primary acquired and reactivated disease. GI TB in patients with AIDS involves the stomach, jejunum, ileum, and rectum (25–27); both primary and secondary cases of GI TB have been reported. In patients with disseminated TB who were infected by both HIV and *M. tuberculosis,* the rate of GI tract involvement ranged from 20% in Ivory Coast to 26% in Zaire (28).

Microbiology

Mycobacteria are considered transitional forms between eubacteria and actinomycetes and so are classed in the order Actinomycetales, family Mycobacteriaceae. Mycobacteria are slender, sometimes curved, rod-shaped organisms. They are aerobic, non–spore-forming, and nonmotile, and they measure 0.2 to 0.6 μm by 1.0 to 4.0 μm. The cell walls of mycobacteria contain mycosides, which are mycolic acid-containing long-chain glycolipids or phospholipoglycans that protect these facultative intracellular parasites from lysosomal attack. Between 25% and 60% of the dry weight is lipid, in comparison with 0.5% for gram-positive and 3% for gram-negative organisms.

Mycosides retain red basic fuchsin dye after acid rinsing; this quality of acid fastness can be strong or weak. Organisms often appear beaded. Although highly specific, these stains are not very sensitive, and results are positive in sputa in only 25% to 50% of early or miliary cases of TB. Concentrations of at least 10,000 bacilli per milliliter are required for detection by this method. The auramine–rhodamine fluorescence stain is more sensitive but less specific than the carbol–fuchsin stains. The bacilli exhibit bright orange–yellow fluorescence with blue light (29–33).

The tuberculosis complex consists of four mycobacteria: *M. tuberculosis hominis, M. bovis, M. africanum,* and *M. microti. M. tuberculosis hominis* and *M. bovis* are the strains most commonly associated with human disease in the United States.

M. tuberculosis hominis

Humans are the primary reservoir of *M. tuberculosis* (more specifically known as *M. tuberculosis hominis*). It is the most common species of mycobacteria in TB of the GI tract (18,20). *In vitro,* bacilli grow at 35° to 37°C; growth is favored in 5% to 10% carbon dioxide but inhibited by a pH below 6.5 and long-chain fatty acids. Three weeks or more is required for culture because of the long doubling time (12 to 20 hours, compared with <1 hour for most bacteria). In liquid media, the organisms form cords, a phenotypic feature associated with virulence. *M. tuberculosis* is niacin-positive, reduces nitrate, is usually sensitive to isoniazid, and produces disease in guinea pigs.

M. bovis

M. bovis causes TB in cattle and is highly virulent in humans. It cannot be distinguished from *M. tuberculosis* by disease manifestations or the tuberculin (purified protein derivative, or PPD) reaction, but the two organisms have different culture characteristics. *M. bovis* is slightly smaller, grows more slowly, is niacin-negative, does not reduce nitrates, and does not produce disease in guinea pigs

(32,33). An attenuated strain of *M. bovis* was used to produce the bacille Calmette–Guérin (BCG) vaccines.

Pathogenesis and Immunity

Virulence Factors

Genetic and phenotypic differences affect the ability of mycobacteria to cause disease in humans (34). Some strains from patients in Africa and India produce attenuated disease in guinea pigs (33). Repeated passage through subcultures and exposure to ultraviolet light and air decrease the virulence of most mycobacteria. Phenotypic features, such as colony morphology and the formation of serpentine cords in either liquid or solid media, have been associated with increased virulence in guinea pigs. Cord factor (trehalose–dimycolate) inhibits polymorphonuclear leukocyte migration *in vitro* and is lethal to mice, probably by inducing microsomal enzymes and causing mitochondrial membrane dysfunction (33,35).

Pathophysiology

Although most ingested or swallowed mycobacteria are destroyed in the acid environment of the stomach, some penetrate the mucosa and are then phagocytosed by macrophages in the lamina propria. When the macrophages are unable to kill the organisms, infection spreads into Peyer patches, mucosal lymphoid follicles, or mesenteric lymph nodes. The most common sites of infection are the areas with the greatest concentration of lymphoid tissue and the slowest transit time. Thus, 50% to 90% of GI lesions are located in the ileocecal region (18,36) (Table 52.1), where multiple lesions are common. Lesions occur with decreasing frequency in the proximal portions of the small intestine; esophageal, pyloric, gastric, and anal lesions are rare and usually secondary to disseminated infection.

TABLE 52.1. LOCATION OF TUBERCULOSIS LESIONS OF THE GASTROINTESTINAL TRACT IN 184 PATIENTS

Location	Number (%)
Tongue	1 (0.6)
Stomach	1 (0.6)
Duodenum	7 (3.8)
Jejunum	39 (21.2)
Ileum	153 (83.2)
Cecum	160 (87.0)
Appendix	72 (39.1)
Colon	132 (71.7)
Sigmoid/rectum	30 (16.3)

Data from Goldberg B, Sweany NC, Brown RW. Pathological studies on tuberculous enteritis. *Am Rev Tuberc* 1928;18:744–766, with permission.

Textbooks from the pre-antibiotic era provide the best gross descriptions of tuberculous enteritis (3,37). Three anatomic forms were described: acute ulcerative, miliary, and hyperplastic. This classification has been modified slightly; a combined ulcerohypertrophic form has replaced the miliary form. The ulcerative form is the most common (60%) and is associated with the highest mortality rate, followed by the ulcerohypertrophic form (30%). Only 10% of cases are hypertrophic (36,38). In any form, healing may result in fibrosis, stricture, or stenosis (38).

Esophageal TB develops by direct extension from subcarinal lymph nodes when bacilli are swallowed. Lesions are usually located in the middle third of the esophagus; the ulcerative form is the most common and may be a rare cause of hematemesis (36,39). Healing and scar formation are associated with traction diverticula; hyperplastic lesions may cause stricture (40,41).

In gastric and duodenal TB, lesions occur as a complication of disseminated disease or, less commonly, by spread from celiac nodes. Antral and pyloric ulceration, stenosis (42), gastric outlet obstruction, upper GI bleeding, and pyloroduodenal fistulas have been reported (43). Preexisting mucosal lesions are thought to be important in the pathogenesis of both esophageal and gastric TB (44).

In the appendix, TB is often ulcerative and occurs as a local extension of ileocecal or pelvic TB. Less frequently, appendiceal TB represents an isolated extrapulmonary site of infection. Tuberculous colitis is usually segmental and associated with ileocecal disease. Colonic involvement can be ulcerative or hypertrophic; pipe stem fibrosis and aphthous ulcers of the colon have been described (45,46). The simultaneous occurrence of colonic TB and either carcinoma or ulcerative colitis has been reported (18); the mycobacteria were thought to be secondary invaders. Anorectal abscesses and fistulas were more common before antituberculous therapy (18). Such lesions, with and without fistula formation, occur infrequently today (47).

Acute Pathology (Ulcerative)

Ingested bacilli penetrate the mucosa and establish the initial lesion in the lymphoid follicles of a Peyer patch. Retrograde spread of bacilli from regional nodes and hematogenous spread in miliary TB are other sources of secondary GI infection. Subsequent follicular hyperplasia presents as a small submucosal nodule associated with edema of the overlying mucosa (38,48,49).

Caseous necrosis develops as the result of a delayed-type hypersensitivity (DTH) response to mycobacterial antigens. The center of the lesion is soft and yellow, and the necrotic center sloughs, forming a small ulcer with raised borders. As the infection spreads via the lymphatics, small satellite nodules appear that in turn ulcerate. The lesions eventually coalesce to form a large ulcer. Multiple ulcers may develop at

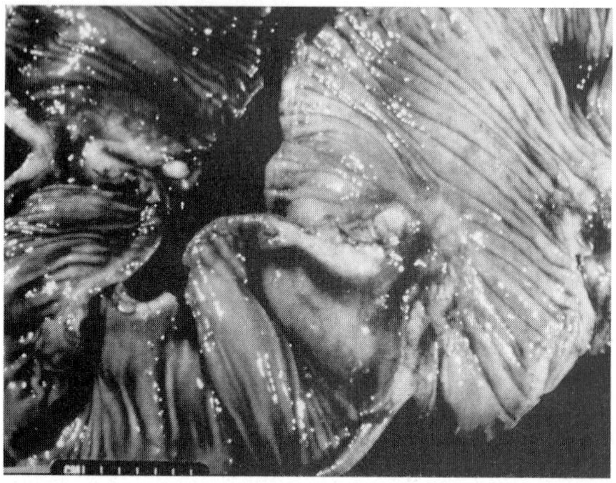

FIGURE 52.1. Photomicrograph of ulcerative tuberculous enteritis in an ileocolostomy specimen. Multiple ulcerations are present with focal thickening of the intestinal wall, especially at the ileocecal junction. (Courtesy of Mount Sinai Hospital, Miami.)

several sites, appearing radiographically as "skip lesions" (37,38,49).

The ulcers have a characteristic gross appearance with irregular, infiltrated borders and a necrotic base. They are initially round to oval, with transverse or circumferential spread. The cut surface may be white and friable (Fig. 52.1). Multiple tuberculous nodules are often present within and around the ulcer and in the adjacent serosa. Pseudopolyps may form. Adjacent lymph nodes may be involved, and focal peritonitis may occur (3,37,38).

Histologically, the early lesions show nonspecific inflammation with edema and mixed acute and chronic inflammatory cells. As the lesions progress, epithelioid macrophages accumulate, and central caseous necrosis develops. Sections of the ulcers reveal typical necrosis and granulation tissue, chronic inflammation and macrophages, and loosely formed granulomas in the surrounding tissue. Granulocytes may be found in and adjacent to areas of ulceration, and acid-fast bacilli may be found in the granuloma or ulcer bed (Fig. 52.2). Bowel involvement is often transmural.

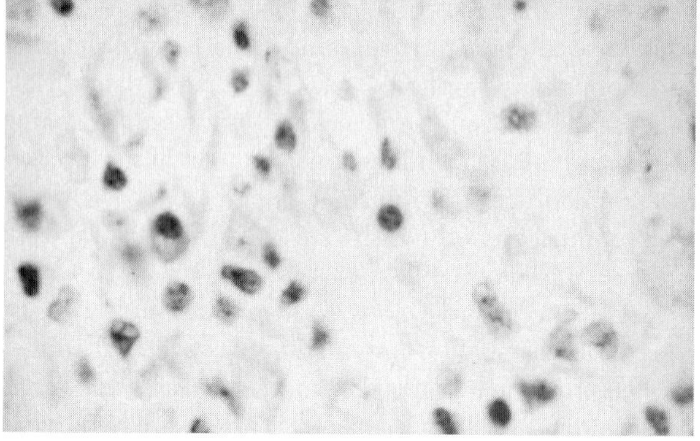

FIGURE 52.2. Histologic section of acute tuberculous enteritis. Ziehl-Neelsen–stained section of intestinal wall shows a loosely formed granuloma with numerous acid-fast bacilli. ×600. (Courtesy of Mount Sinai Hospital, Miami.)

Cellular killing and tissue destruction associated with DTH are more common in ulcerative mycobacterial disease because of the greater number of acid-fast bacilli present (see "Host Immune Response") (50). In the immunocompromised host, the ulceration may extend over a larger area of the bowel and deeper into the tissue. The disease process seems to be accelerated, usually with less fibrosis, more necrosis, and a variable inflammatory response. Cases of intestinal perforation resulting from transmural multibacillary lesions have been reported in HIV-1-associated GI TB (26,51–53).

Chronic Pathology (Hypertrophic)

Chronic infection leads to extensive granuloma formation, fibrosis, and often a palpable mass (tuberculoma) in the ileocecal or other area of the gut. This so-called chronic productive or hyperplastic form of intestinal TB is usually circumferential ("napkin ring") and is often mistaken for a neoplasm. The bowel wall may measure 1 cm or more in thickness. These strictures can be multiple and vary considerably in length. The overlying surface is often ulcerated (ulcerohypertrophic) or sclerotic (18,37,49). In cases of severe stenosis, dilatation of the proximal bowel can be significant (Figs. 52.3 and 52.4) and in rare cases can result in perforation (26).

Peritonitis occurs with or without perforation (3,18,38). Occasionally, fibrous adhesions of one or more bowel loops develop. Fistulization usually occurs in the ulcerohyper-

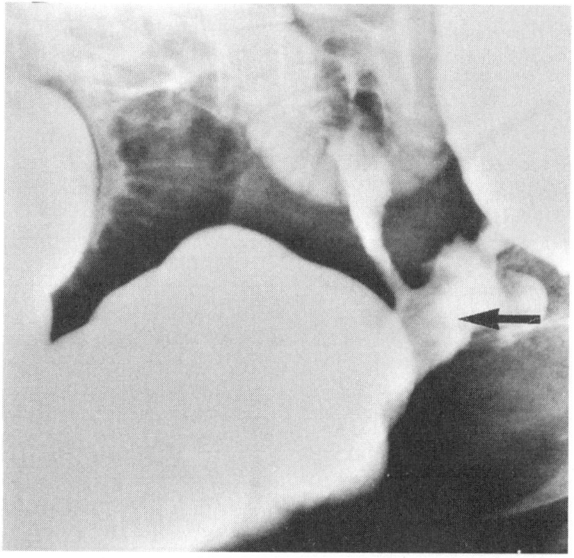

FIGURE 52.3. Radiograph of hypertrophic tuberculous enteritis with marked thickening of the intestinal wall. Note stricture and proximal dilatation of the bowel.

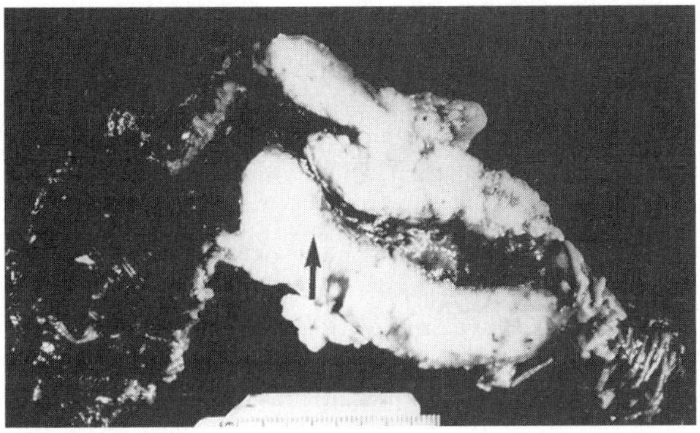

FIGURE 52.4. Photomicrograph of hypertrophic tuberculous enteritis with marked thickening of the wall. Note stricture and proximal dilatation of the bowel (*arrow*).

trophic form. It is sometimes caused by secondary bacterial invasion and can involve the adjacent bowel, the female adnexa, or the abdominal wall (18). Involvement of regional mesenteric lymph nodes is common.

Histologic examination of hypertrophic lesions shows caseating granulomas with varying degrees of fibrosis; lesions are transmural. Peyer patches and regional lymph nodes are almost invariably involved. These features may resemble Crohn's disease, but the granulomas associated with Crohn's disease are noncaseating. The presence of acid-fast bacilli in the tissue is the single most important diagnostic feature of TB (18). During active disease, acid-fast bacilli are present in areas of granulomatous changes in the bowel wall and in the affected regional lymph nodes. Caseous material can be cultured for mycobacteria. Old, healed lesions are fibrotic, sometimes calcified, with few active granulomas; acid-fast bacilli are extremely rare in these lesions (Figs. 52.4 and 52.5).

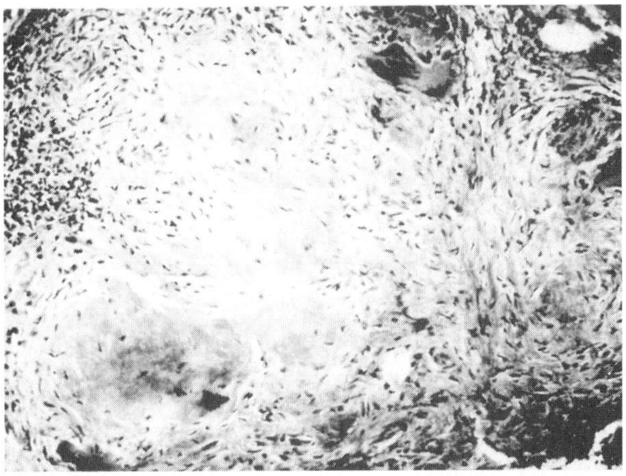

FIGURE 52.5. Histologic section of hypertrophic tuberculous enteritis showing granulomatous inflammation with abundant Langhans giant cells and fibrosis. Hematoxylin and eosin stain; ×600.

Host Immune Response

Four stages of infection and disease are described (50). Primary infection occurs in the immunologically naïve host. Inhaled or ingested mycobacteria are phagocytosed by resident pulmonary macrophages, usually in the alveoli. If the mycobacteria are able to survive and multiply, they destroy the macrophage, and the infection passes into the second or symbiotic stage. The mycobacterial antigens, along with complement component C5a and cytokines (e.g., monocyte chemotactic protein 1), induce chemotaxis, and monocytes are recruited from the peripheral blood. Bacilli undergo phagocytosis and then multiply logarithmically within these immature macrophages (50).

Approximately 4 to 8 weeks after the initial infection, the process advances to the third stage, with the onset of acquired cellular immunity. This stage is characterized by the local accumulation of large numbers of activated macrophages and lymphocytes. An indurated reaction to the intradermal injection of PPD of mycobacteria indicates the presence of cell-mediated immunity (CMI) to TB; the clonal proliferation of mycobacteria-specific T cells and the activation of macrophages leads to the intracellular killing of mycobacteria. DTH causes cell killing with formation of caseous necrosis (50). The fourth stage of mycobacterial infection pertains primarily to pulmonary TB and the formation of cavities.

The CMI-DTH interactions vary with changes in host immunity and mycobacterial concentration. CMI predominates when antigen levels are low, and DTH when large concentrations of bacilli are present or macrophage activation is impaired (50). In the immunocompromised host, bacilli that escape from the caseous centers are phagocytosed by poorly activated macrophages, which in turn are destroyed by cytotoxic lymphocytes and other DTH mechanisms. When bacillary growth is no longer controlled by effective CMI, as in persons infected with HIV-1, caseous necrosis is extended. The ratio of CMI- to DTH-mediated responses is probably an important determinant of the morphology of GI lesions.

The histologic features of TB reflect the integrity of the cellular immune response of the patient. Because little information is available regarding the effect of reduced immunity on the pathology of enteric TB, the effect of the impaired immunity associated with AIDS on pulmonary TB serves as a model. Patients with relatively intact cellular immunity have a typical granulomatous response (28,54), characterized by clustering of CD4+ T lymphocytes around epithelioid macrophages and Langhans giant cells. As the number of CD4+ T lymphocytes declines, cellular immunity decreases, and a loss of Langhans giant cells is followed by a decrease in epithelioid macrophages. This decrease in activated macrophages diminishes the intracellular killing of mycobacteria, which leads to an increase in the number of mycobacteria and a shift to DTH-mediated necrosis.

Necrosis becomes both suppurative and caseous. In the GI mucosa, these changes appear to be associated with ulcerative lesions and an increased incidence of perforation. In the final stages of AIDS, a diffuse inflammatory response ensues in which immature macrophages and polymorphonuclear leukocytes predominate; this leads to suppuration, coagulative necrosis, and an abundance of acid-fast bacilli. The large number of acid-fast bacilli within macrophages is reminiscent of proliferation in the naïve host (28).

Exaggerated local and systemic inflammatory reactions ("paradoxical reactions") develop in some patients, particularly following the initiation of highly active antiretroviral therapy (HAART), for HIV infection. This immune restoration syndrome is associated with an increase in the number of CD4+ T cells and the reconstitution of cellular immunity. The reaction is thought to be caused by increased hypersensitivity to the antigens. Such reactions have been reported during both TB and MAC disease and often involve the cervical or mesenteric lymph nodes (55,56). Fever, swelling, and, in the case of mesenteric adenopathy, abdominal pain and malabsorption may occur. Histologic features include reactive lymphoadenopathy, edema, and granulomatous reactions, often with few or no acid-fast bacilli identified. Consequently, mycobacterial cultures may be negative.

Clinical Manifestations

In the GI tract, TB may occur in single or multiple sites. Table 52.1 shows the relative distribution of lesions in a U.S. autopsy series from 1928 (5). Bhansali in India in 1977 (4) and Novis et al. in South Africa in 1973 (22) reported remarkably similar findings. The vast majority of lesions involve the small intestine, cecum, or both; disease of the esophagus and stomach is rare. Symptoms and signs manifested by patients with GI TB are nonspecific. In a series of 58 cases reported by Hoon et al. in 1950 (57), abdominal pain occurred in 88% of patients, weight loss in 77%, nausea in 52%, vomiting in 48%, anorexia in 41%, fever in 38%, diarrhea in 36%, and constipation in 24%. Disease of the esophagus may present with dysphagia or pain in the throat (39–41,58); anorectal disease may be accompanied by perianal ulcers or fistulas (47,59,60).

In the pre-antibiotic era, pulmonary TB usually accompanied enteric TB, aiding in establishing the diagnosis of TB. However, this association is no longer typical. Tuberculous peritonitis is also uncommonly associated with GI TB, presumably because tuberculous peritonitis is usually the result of hematogenous spread rather than of direct extension from an enteric focus (24). When GI TB is advanced, symptoms and signs of obstruction predominate, with nausea, vomiting, and pain; an abdominal mass may frequently be palpated (4,21), especially if the cecum is involved.

Pancreatic abscess caused by *M. tuberculosis* is a rare complication but has a high mortality rate (61–63). It occurs as an isolated lesion or can be a complication of miliary disease. Reported presentations include multicystic lesions, abscesses, tumors, and miliary foci. Late complications of GI TB include biliary obstruction, malabsorption, perforation with secondary bacterial peritonitis, and, less commonly, hemorrhage or fistula formation (4,18,24,62–64). Severe diarrhea is a rare but serious complication of GI TB; although the term *dysenteric TB* has been used, the diarrhea is secretory rather than hemorrhagic (65).

Perforation of the bowel wall is rare in GI TB but has been reported with increasing frequency in patients with HIV infection and impaired cellular immunity (26,66). It is probably caused by the large numbers of organisms and full-thickness involvement of the bowel by active, necrotizing disease. Inanition, anemia, amyloidosis, or Addison's disease may develop in patients with longstanding untreated GI TB.

Diagnosis

The diagnosis of GI TB is notoriously difficult. Confirmation of the diagnosis requires isolation of *M. tuberculosis* organisms from affected tissue or evidence of TB elsewhere with caseating granulomas in GI tissue. In 1950, Hoon et al. (57) proposed the following criteria: (a) growth of the organism from affected tissue, or (b) histologic demonstration of mycobacteria in tissue, or (c) histologic demonstration of granulomas with caseation necrosis, or (d) typical gross pathologic findings in the bowel and histologic findings of granulomas with caseation necrosis in associated lymph nodes.

Traditionally, surgical exploration was used to obtain tissue for diagnosis. Although this may be required when obstruction occurs, many cases of GI TB can now be diagnosed by endoscopic biopsy (67,68). Endoscopy may show deep ulcerative lesions, masses, or strictures, but these are not diagnostic. Biopsy specimens should be examined histologically for granulomas and acid-fast organisms and cultured for mycobacteria. Endoscopic biopsy specimens should be taken from nodular lesions and the borders of ulcers to include as much submucosal material as possible. Superficial specimens of epithelium show only nonspecific inflammation and not diagnostic granulomatous lesions or acid-fast bacilli.

Acid-fast bacilli are commonly isolated from the stool of patients with pulmonary TB and probably represent organisms from swallowed sputum rather than infection of the GI tract. Thus, feces are usually not cultured (69). When it is necessary to speciate mycobacteria, as in patients with AIDS or in cases of isolated GI infection, feces or other collected GI contents should first be examined by microscopy to detect the presence of acid-fast bacilli. In the past, cultures were recommended only if the smears were positive.

However, smears have been reported to have only a 34% sensitivity (70). The authors recommend that feces be cultured for mycobacteria whenever GI involvement is suspected (70). AIDS patients with TB often have mycobacteremia, and blood cultures may be used to detect disseminated infection.

Stool culture techniques include a decontamination procedure in which a biologic safety cabinet must be used (31). Several methods of decontamination of stool have been reported; most require a longer time than do those for decontamination of sputum (71,72). Feces should be frozen if processing cannot be performed soon after collection. A nonselective egg medium, such as Lowenstein–Jensen, is used for primary isolation; Middlebrook agar (7H10 or 7H11, with or without antibiotics) can be used for primary recovery. Species are identified by pigmentation, growth characteristics, results of biochemical tests, or nucleic acid process, as discussed in the literature (73).

Radiologic investigation can be very useful when GI TB is suspected; patients with normal findings on barium study of the upper GI tract (with small-intestinal follow-through) and lower GI tract (with ileal reflux procedure) are unlikely to have GI TB. Special attention should be paid to signs of impaired motility (e.g., accelerated transit time and hypersegmentation), as these may be the earliest defects that can be appreciated radiographically. The Stierlin sign (localized failure to retain barium), the "string sign" (persistence of a thin line of barium), discrete filling defects, or distorted GI architecture suggesting tumor all may be seen, but none is diagnostic (16–18,74,75). Newer radiographic techniques, such as computed tomography and magnetic resonance imaging, have not been shown to be of additional value for localizing affected areas or establishing a diagnosis of TB in the GI tract.

Tuberculin skin testing can be quite helpful in patients who have not received BCG vaccine and in areas, such as the United States, where tuberculous infection is uncommon. Early series showed a high rate of anergy to skin testing in patients later shown to have GI TB (3). However, this was likely a consequence of advanced TB and malnutrition, both of which may lead to failure to respond to a skin test in the face of active disease. In the current era, this clinical situation is less common, and recent reports show positive TB skin test results in 50% to 97% of patients with GI TB (4,13,20,76). When the TB skin test result is negative, control skin tests should be placed to exclude anergy, which is common in patients with TB and advanced HIV-1 infection.

Chest radiography should be performed to search for signs of TB, and abdominal films may be indicated to identify air–fluid levels in cases of suspected obstruction or free air under the diaphragm in cases of suspected perforation. Plain abdominal films may also reveal calcifications in abdominal lymph nodes in cases of reactivated TB. The differential diagnosis of GI TB includes ulcerative colitis, Crohn's disease, irritable bowel syndrome, malignancy, and other infectious processes, including bacterial abscess, diverticulitis, fungal enteritis, amebiasis, and schistosomiasis. The most common problems are differentiation of GI TB from intestinal lymphoma or Crohn's disease.

Treatment

GI TB responds well to antimycobacterial chemotherapy. Regimens for GI TB are the same as those currently recommended for pulmonary TB (Table 52.2). Patients should be started on three or preferably four agents to decrease the

TABLE 52.2. AGENTS FOR THE TREATMENT OF *M. TUBERCULOSIS* DISEASE

Agent	Adult Dose	Pediatric Dose
First-line drugs		
Isoniazid	300 mg PO qd	10–20 mg/kg/d PO
Rifampin	600 mg PO qd	10–20 mg/kg/d PO
Ethambutol	15–25 mg/kg/d PO	15–25 mg/kg/d PO[a]
Pyrazinamide	2 PO qd	15–30 mg/kg/d PO
Streptomycin	1 g IM qd	20–40 mg/kg/d IM
Amikacin	1 g IV qd	20–40 mg/kg/d IV
Alternative drugs		
Levofloxacin	400 mg PO qd	Not recommended
Paraaminosalicylic acid	3 g PO qid	150 mg/kg/d PO
Cycloserine	250–500 mg PO bid	15–20 mg/kg/d PO
Ethionamide	250–500 mg PO bid	15–20 mg/kg/d PO
Kanamycin	1 g IM qd	15–30 mg/kg/d IM
Capreomycin	1 g IM qd	15–30 mg/kg/d IM

[a]Not recommended for children less than 6 years of age.

load of organisms speedily and minimize the chances of therapeutic failure caused by drug-resistant organisms. These agents should include isoniazid, rifampin, pyrazinamide, and either ethambutol or streptomycin (77,78).

The results of *in vitro* susceptibility testing should be available by the eighth week of therapy and should be used to guide the selection of drugs for the patient. If therapy is not interrupted and the organism is not drug-resistant, a 6-month course will be adequate to effect a cure. Patients infected with HIV-1 can also be cured of TB with standard treatment regimens (77,78). All efforts should be made to ensure that therapy is not interrupted, but if interruption is necessary, the patient should not be kept on single-agent therapy because this may lead to drug resistance (79). It is critical that patients adhere to the regimen. Care providers must monitor adherence; observation of ingestion of medication by the patient ("directly observed therapy," or DOT is highly recommended). Twice- and thrice-weekly dosing schedules have been formulated to aid in adherence to DOT (78).

If the patient's TB isolate shows resistance *in vitro* to two or more of the first-line antimycobacterial agents (usually isoniazid and rifampin), it is said to be "multiply drug-resistant." Patients who have multiply drug-resistant TB can be successfully treated with alternate regimens, but therapeutic success is achieved in fewer than two-thirds of cases (80). Not only are agents other than isoniazid and rifampin less potent, they are also less well tolerated.

An important therapeutic measure for restoring immune function in the anergic TB patient is ensuring adequate nutrition. Many patients with chronic TB are visibly malnourished. When malabsorption is present, parenteral nutrition may be necessary. Surgical therapy is essential when GI TB is complicated by perforation, obstruction, or uncontrollable hemorrhage, which are associated with a poor prognosis (4,21).

GASTROINTESTINAL DISEASE CAUSED BY *M. AVIUM* COMPLEX

Epidemiology

GI MAC disease occurs most commonly in patients with AIDS (81,82). A localized MAC GI process progresses to disseminated disease within a few months (83,84), and disseminated MAC disease is largely the result of spread from a GI focus, although the GI focus may be unrecognized. Before the availability of HAART, between 15% and 24% of persons with AIDS acquired MAC disease.

The major risk factor for MAC disease is impaired immune function. Patients become at risk for MAC infection when their CD4+ T-cell count drops below $100/mm^3$. As the number of CD4+ T cells increases with HAART, the risk for MAC disease declines. The rate of MAC disease is not affected by gender, age, or the route by which HIV-1 is acquired (82,85). Also, the rate of MAC disease is similar for persons infected with HIV-1 in the United States, Europe, and Australia; in North America, MAC disease is more common in southern than in northern latitudes (86). However, MAC disease is rare in African patients, even those with advanced AIDS (87,88), possibly because of the high prevalence of TB in Africa. *M. avium* is present in animals, food, water, and soil (89), but specific risk behaviors and reservoirs for human infection have not been definitely identified; preliminary studies suggest that MAC infection may be acquired through the ingestion of contaminated water or foods (90,91).

Microbiology

The *M. avium* complex, or MAC, comprises the species *Mycobacterium avium* and *Mycobacterium intracellulare*; some authors also include *Mycobacterium scrofulaceum* in the complex, in which case the group is known as *MAIS. M. avium* causes disease similar to TB in chickens, birds, and swine. *M. intracellulare* was previously known as the *Battey bacillus*; it is usually not pathogenic in immunocompetent humans or animals, but persons with AIDS are susceptible to the organism. MAC organisms are acid-fast and stain with periodic acid–Schiff (PAS). In culture, they are thermophilic (growing at 41°C), and a pale yellow pigment develops in some strains with age (Runyon group III, nonchromogens). In addition, they are niacin-negative, do not reduce nitrates, and do not produce disease in guinea pigs. *M. scrofulaceum* is classified as a scotochromagen (Runyon group II) because it produces a yellow–orange pigment when grown in the dark. Although this mycobacterium is not thermophilic, it is similar to MAC in that it does not reduce nitrate and is negative for niacin (32,33).

The staining characteristics of MAC are the same as those of *M. tuberculosis,* and the two cannot be differentiated by microscopy. The collection and preparation of specimens and the culture conditions for MAC are the same as those for *M. tuberculosis* (see section on microbiology of *M. tuberculosis*).

Pathogenesis and Immunity

Virulence Factors

MAC organisms are ubiquitous in the environment and relatively avirulent in the normal host. Certain MAC serovars (4 and 8) are uncommon in the environment but cause most cases of disseminated disease in AIDS patients (81). Possible virulence factors include an enhanced ability to overcome the host defense, adhere to intestinal epithelium, and produce catalase, an enzyme linked to invasiveness (92,93).

Clinical isolates from patients with disseminated disease always have a smooth, transparent rather than a domed, opaque phenotype (94). Smooth, transparent colonies are more pathogenic in laboratory animals, more likely to induce monocyte production of cytokines, and usually less susceptible to antimycobacterial agents (94,95). The relationship between the two phenotypes is complicated by the ability of each isolate to transform into the other, depending on culture conditions.

Pathophysiology

The GI tract is the usual portal of entry of nontuberculous mycobacteria in the immunocompromised host. Similar to TB infection of the GI tract, GI MAC infection may be acquired through the ingestion of environmental MAC organisms, swallowing infected sputum, or hematogenous dissemination. Ingestion of environmental MAC organisms is thought to be the most common route of MAC transmission (81); colonization of the GI tract likely precedes dissemination (84,96).

After ingestion, MAC organisms invade the Peyer patches and then are transported to mesenteric lymph nodes. Most infections involve the small intestine and the macrophages of the Peyer patches, where the lamina propria becomes infected (Fig. 52.6). During severe infection, sheets of large, foamy macrophages expand the villi to such an extent that the microvilli become flattened, as in Whipple's disease (97,98). True granulomas with Langhans giant cells, epithelioid macrophages, and caseous necrosis are not typical of enteric MAC infection, probably because of the immunocompromised state of the host (99,100). The luminal surface may show mild inflammatory changes, but the enterocytes are usually intact. In tissue sections of small intestine stained with hematoxylin and eosin or with Giemsa, mycobacteria are unstained; Klatt et al. (99) and Wallace and Hannah (100) describe such organisms as "striated blue histiocytes." Acid-fast and PAS stains and silver impregnation techniques reveal masses of bacilli.

MAC disease of the colon occurs in association with disseminated disease or as a primary focus. The mucosa is usually edematous and erythematous (Figs. 52.6 and 52.7) and, during early infection, friable with multiple erosions and ulceration, features that explain the frequent association with bloody diarrhea (38). The histologic findings of colonic disease are similar to those of small-intestinal disease, described above (38,101).

Patients with MAC disease of the GI tract often exhibit marked wasting. Although diarrhea, malabsorption, and elevated circulating levels of tumor necrosis factor all have been reported in such patients, none of these findings alone can explain the marked weight loss (102). Rather, weight loss appears to be multifactorial.

Enteric MAC disease is usually associated with dissemination; the lymph nodes, liver, and spleen are the sites most commonly affected (99,100). Abdominal lymph node involvement varies from tiny foci of infection to marked lymphadenopathy with replacement of the normal architecture by sheets of foamy macrophages containing masses of mycobacteria. Because MAC disease occurs in patients with severe immunodeficiency, the normal architecture of the node is altered, and follicular atrophy is often seen. Mycobacterial spindle cell lesions, similar to those of histioid leprosy, have been reported in MAC disease (103), but pseudotumors have not been identified in the GI tract.

Host Immune Response

Enteric MAC disease occurs primarily in persons with advanced HIV-1 disease and severe immunosuppression. In most patients, macrophages and other reticuloendothelial cells are unable to kill the mycobacteria. The specific defect resulting in inability of these cells to kill MAC organisms has not been defined, but an imbalance of cytokines that inhibit intracellular MAC replication (e.g., tumor necrosis factor and migration inhibitory factor) and stimulate repli-

A

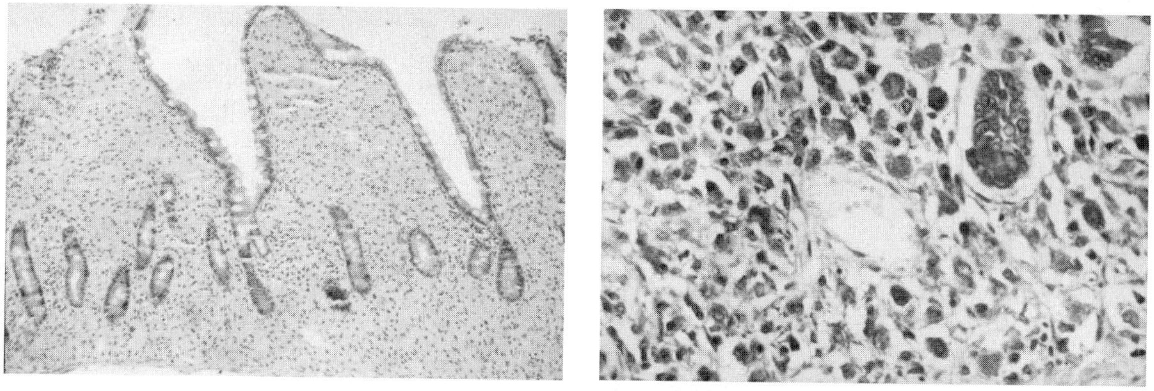

B

FIGURE 52.6. *Mycobacterium avium* complex disease. **A:** Histologic section of intestine shows marked expansion of villi and submucosa by a diffuse infiltrate of foamy histiocytes. Hematoxylin and eosin stain; ×100. (Courtesy of Dr. C. Mel Wilcox.) **B:** Ziehl-Neelsen–stained section shows histiocytes stuffed with acid-fast bacilli. ×300.

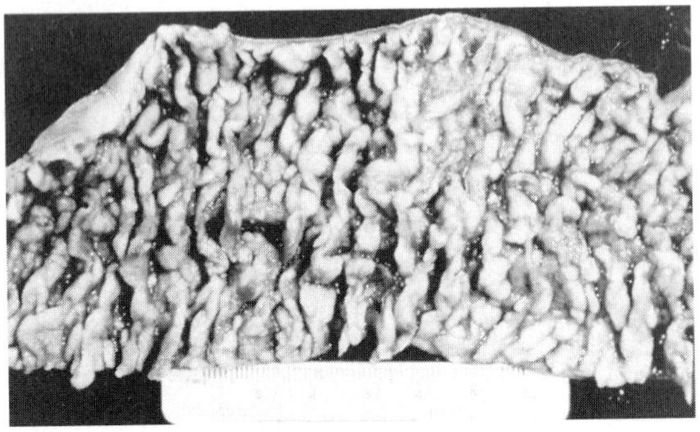

FIGURE 52.7. *Mycobacterium avium* complex disease. Gross specimen of intestine with diffuse thickening of mucosal folds. (Courtesy of Dr. C. Mel Wilcox.)

cation (e.g., interleukin 1, interleukin 6) may play a role (104). The HIV-1 envelope glycoprotein 120 has also been reported to enhance the replication of *M. avium* (105). Roles for humoral factors, such as antibodies to MAC (106–108), lactoferrin (109), and other serum factors (110), have been proposed. When HAART is initiated, the host immune response is restored, and local and systemic inflammatory reactions to MAC antigens develop (111, 112).

Clinical Manifestations

Patients with MAC disease may present with fever, night sweats, abdominal pain, diarrhea, and weight loss. Physical findings include hepatomegaly and splenomegaly; abdominal lymphadenopathy is rarely palpable, and enlarged peripheral lymph nodes are uncommon. Laboratory studies may show anemia and elevated serum levels of alkaline phosphatase, usually without a corresponding elevation in other hepatic enzymes (113,114). Severe anemia is a hallmark of this disease and should prompt a search for MAC (114–116). The frequency of signs, symptoms, and laboratory abnormalities is shown in Table 52.3.

MAC disease of the GI tract is usually a manifestation of disseminated disease. In one series, 88% of patients had duodenal involvement and 64% had rectal involvement (83). The esophagus, stomach, jejunum, ileum, and colon are less commonly involved (83,88,99,100). Enteric MAC disease may resemble Whipple's disease (117,118) or Crohn's disease (119). MAC disease of the GI tract in children infected with HIV-1 is similar to that in adults infected with HIV-1 (82,120,121).

Abdominal computed tomography may show enlarged retroperitoneal lymph nodes or thickening of the bowel wall (Fig. 52.8), and it may help differentiate MAC from TB disease (122). MAC disease of the abdomen is characterized by hepatomegaly, splenomegaly, jejunal wall thickening, and abdominal lymph nodes with a homogeneous soft-tissue density. TB of the abdomen, on the other hand, is characterized by focal visceral lesions and abdominal lymph nodes with diffuse low attenuation. Routine radiographic studies are rarely helpful.

In most patients with enteric MAC disease, the endoscopic appearance of the mucosa is normal (83). However, focal or diffuse small (2- to 4-mm) white nodules are seen in about one-third of patients (83,123). Thickened folds with a yellow mucosal discoloration (83) (Fig. 52.9), resembling those seen in Whipple's disease, may also be present (38,117,118). Ulceration or masses are rarely identified. Massive adenopathy and thickening of the bowel wall can lead to obstruction or intussusception with hemorrhage (119,124,125). As infection progresses, the bowel wall, liver, spleen, and abdominal lymph nodes are infiltrated with mycobacteria. Organ tissue is replaced by mycobacteria and inflammation, and a decline in organ function leads to abdominal pain, malabsorption, and weight loss. In contrast to GI TB, MAC GI disease rarely causes obstruction,

TABLE 52.3. FREQUENCY OF OCCURRENCE OF SIGNS, SYMPTOMS AND LABORATORY ABNORMALITIES COMMONLY ASSOCIATED WITH DISSEMINATED *M. AVIUM* COMPLEX DISEASE

Sign/Symptom/Abnormality	Percentage of Patients (%)
Fever	97
Anemia (hematocrit <26%)	96
Night sweats	62
Weight loss (≥10%)	59
Abdominal pain	56
Diarrhea	54
Serum alkaline phosphatase ≥5 times normal	39
Hepatomegaly	39
Splenomegaly	29

Data from Norsburgh CR, Metchock B, Gordon SM, et al. Predictors of survival in patients with AIDS and disseminated *Mycobacterium avium* complex disease. *J Infect Dis* 1994;170:573–577, with permission.

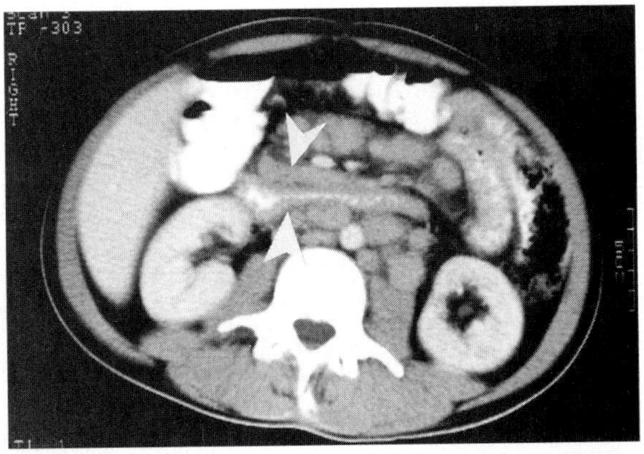

FIGURE 52.8. Abdominal computed tomogram of a patient with disseminated *Mycobacterium avium* complex disease. Note multiple enlarged abdominal lymph nodes and thickening of the duodenal wall (*arrows*).

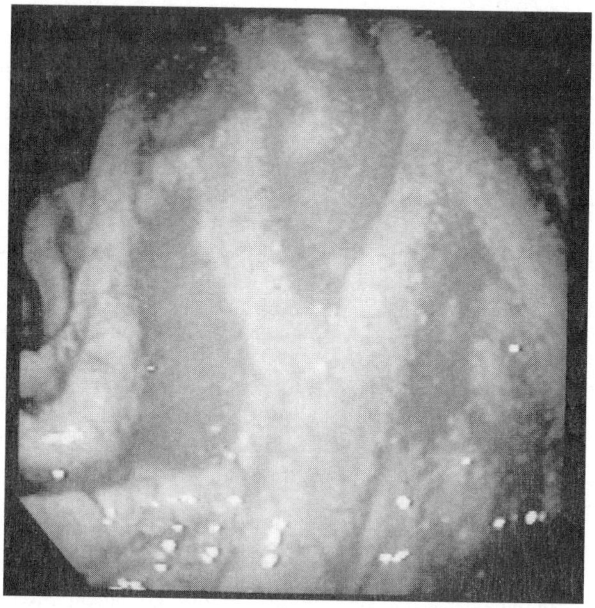

FIGURE 52.9. Endoscopic appearance of the duodenal mucosa of a patient with disseminated *Mycobacterium avium* complex disease. Intestinal folds are markedly thickened and contain multiple yellow plaques. (Courtesy of Dr. C. Mel Wilcox.)

perforation, or bleeding. Without antimycobacterial therapy, the median survival is 4 months (126); death is usually caused by superinfection or inanition (99,100).

Diagnosis

The diagnosis of GI MAC disease is based on the histologic identification of mycobacteria and confirmed by culture of the organism in tissue specimens. Endoscopic visualization and biopsy are required to obtain the tissue in most cases. Rarely, stool smear and culture may be helpful, but both are insensitive and smear is nonspecific (70,84,96). Because of the time required for MAC organisms to grow (up to 6 weeks), techniques for more rapid diagnosis are needed. The most promising of these is the detection of mycobacterial DNA by polymerase chain reaction. However, such an assay is not yet commercially available.

The diagnosis of disseminated MAC disease is usually made by blood culture. A single positive blood culture is adequate to establish the diagnosis, and negative results of two properly performed cultures can exclude disseminated MAC infection (127,128). Positive cultures in tissues from other normally sterile sites, such as bone marrow, lymph node, and liver, also indicate disseminated MAC disease. Because localized GI MAC disease may precede dissemination by several months (83,84), endoscopy is indicated when GI involvement is suspected but blood cultures are negative. Multiple biopsy specimens of all areas of the bowel should be obtained because the endoscopic appearance may be normal despite extensive mycobacterial disease. Acid-fast smears of such specimens may provide an immediate presumptive diagnosis of mycobacterial infection and accelerate the initiation of therapy, and positive cultures of biopsy specimens confirm the diagnosis.

Treatment

Therapy of MAC disease should be initiated with a minimum of two antimycobacterial agents, including one agent of the macrolide/azalide group (129–131) (Table 52.4). At least one additional agent should be administered with the macrolide to prevent the emergence of resistant organisms. Ethambutol is the preferred second agent. Amikacin is also effective, but it is more toxic and requires intravenous administration. Therapy is continued for a minimum of 12 months. After a year, therapy may be discontinued in patients with a good clinical response and a CD4+ T-cell count above 100/mm^3.

In vitro susceptibility testing of MAC isolates is not routinely performed. Only clarithromycin testing has been shown to correlate with clinical outcome. The emergence of clarithromycin-resistant MAC is uncommon in patients on multiple-drug regimens, but such resistance occurs with clarithromycin monotherapy. Clarithromycin susceptibility testing is recommended for isolates from patients with clinical relapse during clarithromycin therapy (130). Treatment without a tissue diagnosis should be avoided because many other conditions can mimic MAC disease. Patients with MAC disease rarely require hospitalization for treatment of their illness and can be treated as outpatients.

The anemia associated with MAC disease can be treated with transfusions (116) or, in some cases, erythropoietin. In general, patients with AIDS and GI MAC disease do not benefit from intravenous hyperalimentation (102). Abdominal surgery should be performed when GI MAC disease is complicated by obstruction, perforation, or bleeding (132).

Prevention

Because MAC disease is acquired from the environment, prevention by avoidance is a potential preventive strategy.

TABLE 52.4. AGENTS FOR THE TREATMENT OF *M. AVIUM* COMPLEX DISEASE

Agent	Adult Dose	Pediatric Dose
First-line drugs		
Azithromycin	600 mg PO qd	15 mg/kg/d PO
Clarithromycin	500 mg PO bid	15 mg/kg/d PO
Ethambutol	800–1200 mg PO qd	10 mg/kg/d PO
Rifabutin	300 mg PO bid	10 mg/kg/d PO
Alternative drugs		
Amikacin	25 mg/kg 3×/wk IV	25 mg/kg 3×/wk IV
Ciprofloxacin	500 mg PO bid	Not recommended
Ofloxacin	400 mg PO bid	Not recommended

However, the widespread presence of MAC organisms in the environment makes such avoidance impractical. Screening cultures to detect early disease are not useful (96). On the other hand, antimycobacterial prophylaxis has been shown to be effective (133–135). Therapy with 1,200 mg of azithromycin weekly or 500 mg of clarithromycin twice daily is associated with a 59% to 69% reduction in MAC bacteremia. Such therapy should be given to all persons with HIV infection and a CD4+ T-cell count below 50/mm^3; prophylaxis should be maintained until CD4+ T-cell counts rise above 100/mm^3 (136,137).

REFERENCES

1. Calmette A. *Tubercle bacillus infection and tuberculosis in man and animals.* Soper WB, Smith GH, translators. Baltimore: Williams & Wilkins, 1923.
2. Walsh J. Diagnosis of intestinal tuberculosis. *Trans Natl Assoc Prev Tuberc London* 1909;5:217.
3. Goldberg B. Tuberculous enterocolitis. In: Goldberg B, ed. *Clinical tuberculosis,* fifth edition. Philadelphia: FA Davis Co, 1947:H3–H33 (vol 2).
4. Bhansali SK. Abdominal tuberculosis. *Am J Gastroenterol* 1977; 67:324–337.
5. Goldberg B, Sweany HC, Brown RW. Pathological studies on tuberculous enteritis. *Am Rev Tuberc* 1928;18:744–766.
6. Blumberg A. Pathology of intestinal tuberculosis. *J Clin Lab Med* 1928;13:405.
7. Mitchell RS. The prognosis of bilateral symmetrical diffuse nodular pulmonary tuberculosis and its possible relation to intestinal tuberculosis. *Dis Chest* 1956;29:669–674.
8. Farer LS, Lowell AM, Meador MP. Extrapulmonary tuberculosis in the United States. *Am J Epidemiol* 1979;109:205–217.
9. Fraki O, Peltokallio P. Intestinal and peritoneal tuberculosis: report of two cases. *Dis Colon Rectum* 1975;18:685–693.
10. Segal I. Intestinal tuberculosis, Crohn's disease and ulcerative colitis in an urban black population. *South Afr Med J* 1984;655: 37–44.
11. Mitchell RS, Bristol LJ. Intestinal tuberculosis: an analysis of 346 cases diagnosed by routine intestinal radiography on 5,529 admissions for pulmonary tuberculosis, 1924–1949. *Am J Med Sci* 1954;227:241–251.
12. Schulze K, Warner HA, Murray D. Intestinal tuberculosis experience at a Canadian teaching institution. *Am J Med* 1977;63: 735–745.
13. Palmer KR, Patil DH, Basran GS, et al. Abdominal tuberculosis in urban Britain—a common disease. *Gut* 1985;26: 1296–1305.
14. Carrera GF, Young S, Lewicki AM. Intestinal tuberculosis. *Gastrointest Radiol* 1976;1:147–155.
15. Moshal MG, Spitaels JM. Gastrointestinal and peritoneal tuberculosis. *South Afr Med J* 1973;47:675–679.
16. Werbeloff L, Novis BH, Marks IN. The radiology of tuberculosis of the gastrointestinal tract. *Br J Radiol* 1973;46:329–336.
17. Lewis EA, Kolawole TM. Tuberculous ileocolitis in Ibadan: a clinicoradiological review. *Gut* 1972;13:646–653.
18. Paustian FF, Monto GL. Tuberculosis of the intestines. In: Bokus HL, ed. *Gastroenterology,* third edition. Philadelphia: WB Saunders, 1976:750–776 (vol 1).
19. Tandon HD, Prakash A. Pathology of intestinal tuberculosis and its distinction from Crohn's disease. *Gut* 1972;13:260–269.
20. Homan WP, Grafe WR, Dineen P. A 44-year experience with tuberculous enterocolitis. *World J Surg* 1977;1:245–250.
21. Hill GS, Tabrisky J, Peter ME. Tuberculous enteritis. *West J Med* 1976;124:440–445.
22. Novis BH, Bank S, Marks IN. Gastrointestinal and peritoneal tuberculosis. A study of cases at Groote Schuur Hospital 1962–1971. *South Afr Med J* 1973;47:365–372.
23. Freant LJ, Sawyers JL. Surgical management of tuberculous enteritis. *South J Med* 1970;63:711–714.
24. Abrams JS, Holden WD. Tuberculosis of the gastrointestinal tract. *Arch Surg* 1964;89:283–293.
25. Lax JD, Haroutiounian G, Attia A, et al. Tuberculosis of the rectum in a patient with acquired immune deficiency syndrome. *Dis Colon Rectum* 1988;31:394–397.
26. Friedenberg KA, Draguesku JO, Kiyabu M, et al. Intestinal perforation due to *Mycobacterium tuberculosis* in HIV-infected individuals: report of two cases. *Am J Gastroenterol* 1992;88: 604–607.
27. Brody JM, Miller DK, Zeman RK, et al. Gastric tuberculosis: a manifestation of acquired immunodeficiency syndrome. *Radiology* 1986;159:347–348.
28. Lucas S, Nelson AM. Pathogenesis of tuberculosis in human immunodeficiency virus-infected people. In: Bloom BR, ed. *Tuberculosis: pathogenesis, protection and control.* Washington, DC: American Society of Microbiology Press, 1994:503–513.
29. Small PM, Selcer UM. Mycobacterial infections: tuberculosis. In: Strickland GT, ed. *Hunter's tropical medicine and emerging infectious diseases,* eighth edition. Philadelphia: WB Saunders, 2000:491–513.
30. von Lichtenberg F. Mycobacterial diseases. In: *Pathology of infectious diseases.* New York: Raven Press, 1991:173–187.
31. Musial CE, Roberts GD. Tuberculosis and other mycobacteriosis. In: Wentworth BB, et al., eds. *Diagnostic procedures for bacterial infections,* seventh edition. Washington, DC: American Public Health Association, 1987:539–580.
32. Wayne LG, Willet HP. Mycobacteria. In: Sneath PHA, et al., eds. *Bergey's manual of systemic bacteriology,* vol 2. Baltimore: Williams & Wilkins, 1986:1435–1457.
33. Willet HP. Mycobacteria. In: Joklik WK, Willett HP, Amos DB, et al., eds. *Zinsser microbiology,* twentieth edition. Norwalk, CT: Appleton & Lange, 1992:497–525.
34. Dannenberg AM Jr, Rook GAW. Pathogenesis of pulmonary tuberculosis: an interplay of tissue-damaging and macrophage-activating immune responses. In: Bloom BR, ed. *Tuberculosis: pathogenesis, protection, and control.* Washington DC: American Society of Microbiology Press, 1994:459–483.
35. Edwards D, Kirkpatrick CH. The immunology of mycobacterial diseases. *Am Rev Respir Dis* 1986;134:1062–1071.
36. Marshall JB. Tuberculosis of the gastrointestinal tract and peritoneum. *Am J Gastroenterol* 1993;88:989–999.
37. Adami JG, Nicholls AG. *Principles of pathology,* vol 2. Philadelphia: Lea & Febiger, 1909:439–442.
38. Fenoglio-Preiser CM, Lantz PE, Listrom MB, et al. *Gastrointestinal pathology: an atlas and text.* New York: Raven Press, 1989:58,144,299–300,663–667,803.
39. Newman RM, Fleshner PR, Lajam F, et al. Esophageal tuberculosis: a rare presentation with hematemesis. *Am J Gastroenterol* 1991;86:751–755.
40. Gordon AH, Marshall JB. Esophageal tuberculosis: definitive diagnosis by endoscopy (case report). *Am J Gastroenterol* 1990; 85:174–177.
41. Damtew B, Frengley D, Wolinski, et al. Esophageal tuberculosis: mimicry of gastrointestinal malignancy. *Rev Infect Dis* 1987; 9:140–146.
42. Tromba JL, Inglese R, Rieders B, et al. Primary gastric tubercu-

losis presenting as pyloric outlet obstruction. *Am J Gastroenterol* 1991;86:1820–1822.
43. Nair KV, Pai CG, Rajagopal KP, et al. Unusual presentations of duodenal tuberculosis. *Am J Gastroenterol* 1991;86:756–760.
44. Palmer E. Tuberculosis of the stomach and the stomach in tuberculosis. *Am Rev Tuberc* 1950;61:116–118.
45. Kolawole TM, Lewis EA. A radiologic study of tuberculosis of the abdomen (gastrointestinal tract). *Am J Roentgenol* 1975;123: 348–358.
46. Downey DB, Nakielny RA. Aphthoid ulcers in colonic tuberculosis. *Br J Radiol* 1985;58:561–562.
47. Harland RW, Varkey B. Anal tuberculosis: report of two cases and literature review. *Am J Gastroenterol* 1992;87:1488–1491.
48. Nelson AM, Kalengayi MMR. The pathology of AIDS in Africa. In: Essex ME, et al, eds. *AIDS in Africa.* New York: Raven Press, 1994:283–323.
49. Morson BC, Dawson IMP. *Gastrointestinal pathology.* Oxford: Blackwell Science, 1972:246–250,449–450,613.
50. Dannenberg AM. Delayed-type hypersensitivity and cell-mediated immunity in the pathogenesis of tuberculosis. *Immunol Today* 1991;12:228–232.
51. Acea Nebril B, Rosales Juega D, Prada Puentes C, et al. Perforated jejunal tuberculosis in a patient with HIV infection [in Spanish]. *Rev Esp Enferm Dig* 1998;90:369–371.
52. Deb T, Singh TY, Singh NB, et al. Multiple tubercular ulcer perforations of the ileum in an AIDS patient: case report. *J Commun Dis* 1998;30:175–178.
53. Pintor E, Piret MV, Velasco M, et al. Colonic tuberculosis as a cause of rectal bleeding in 2 patients with HIV infection [in Spanish]. *Enferm Infecc Microbiol Clin* 1996;14:538–540.
54. Nambuya A, Sewankambo N, Mugerwa J, et al. Tuberculous lymphadenitis associated with human immunodeficiency virus (HIV) in Uganda. *J Clin Pathol* 1988;41:93–96.
55. Narita M, Ashkin D, Hollender ES, et al. Paradoxical worsening of tuberculosis following antiretroviral therapy in AIDS patients. *Am J Resp Crit Care Med* 1998;158:157–161.
56. Furrer H, Malinverni R. Systemic inflammatory reaction after starting highly active antiretroviral therapy in AIDS patients treated for extrapulmonary tuberculosis. *Am J Med* 1999;106: 371–372.
57. Hoon JR, Dockerty MB, Pemberton J de J, et al. Ileocecal tuberculosis including comparison of this disease with nonspecific regional enterocolitis and noncaseous tuberculated enterocolitis. *Int Abstr Surg* 1950;91:417–440.
58. Rubinstein BM, Pastrana T, Jacobson HG. Tuberculosis of the esophagus. *Radiology* 1958;70:401–403.
59. Logan VD. Anorectal tuberculosis. *Proc R Soc Med* 1969;62: 1227–1230.
60. Martin CL. Anorectal tuberculosis. In: Goldberg B, ed. *Clinical tuberculosis,* fifth edition. Philadelphia: FA Davis Co, 1947.
61. Cappell MS, Javeed M. Pancreatic abscess due to mycobacterial infection associated with the acquired immunodeficiency syndrome. *J Clin Gastroenterol* 1990;12:423–429.
62. Koduri VG, Janardhanan R, Hagan P, et al. Pancreatic TB: diagnosis by needle aspiration. *Am J Gastroenterol* 1992;87: 1206–1208.
63. Desai DC, Santhi S, Mohandas KM, et al. Tuberculosis of the pancreas: report of three cases. *Am J Gastroenterol* 1991;86: 761–763.
64. Prout WG. Multiple tuberculous perforations of ileum. *Gut* 1968;9:381–382.
65. Davis G, Corbett DB, Krejs GJ. Ileal chloride secretion as a cause of secretory diarrhea in a patient with primary intestinal tuberculosis. *Gastroenterology* 1976;76:829–835.
66. Senise JF, Hamrick PA, Guidugli RB, et al. Ileal loop perforation caused by tuberculosis in patients with the acquired immunodeficiency syndrome. *Rev Paul Med* 1991;109:61–64.
67. Moshal MG, Baker LW, Lautre G, et al. Colonoscopy: 100 examinations. *South Afr J Surg* 1973;11:73–78.
68. Bhargava DK, Tandon HD. Ileocaecal tuberculosis diagnosed by colonoscopy and biopsy. *Aust N Z J Surg* 1980;50:583–585.
69. Barnes PF, Block AB, Davidson PT, et al. Tuberculosis in patients with human immunodeficiency virus infection. *N Engl J Med* 1991;23:1644–1650.
70. Morris A, Reller LB, Salfinger M, et al. Mycobacteria in stool specimens: the nonvalue of smears for predicting culture results. *J Clin Microbiol* 1993;31:1385–1387.
71. Damsker B, Bottone EJ. *Myobacterium avium–Mycobacterium intracellulare* from the intestinal tracts of patients with the acquired immunodeficiency syndrome: concepts regarding acquisition and pathogenesis. *J Infect Dis* 1985;151:179–181.
72. Yajko DM, Nassos PS, Sanders CA, et al. Comparison of four decontamination methods for recovery of *Mycobacterium avium* complex from stools. *J Clin Microbiol* 1993;31:302–306.
73. Heifets LB, Good RC. Current laboratory methods for the diagnosis of tuberculosis. In: Bloom BR, ed. *Tuberculosis: pathogenesis, protection and control.* Washington, DC: American Society of Microbiology Press, 1994:85–110.
74. Thoeni RF, Margulis AR. Gastrointestinal tuberculosis. *Semin Roentgenol* 1979;14:283–294.
75. Tabrisky J, Lindstrom RR, Peters R, et al. Tuberculous enteritis. Review of a protean disease. *Am J Gastroenterol* 1975;63:49–57.
76. Gilinsky NH, Marks IN, Kottler RE, et al. Abdominal tuberculosis, a ten-year review. *South Afr Med J* 1983;64:849–857.
77. CDC. Initial therapy for tuberculosis in the era of multidrug resistance. *MMWR Morb Mortal Wkly Rep* 1993;42(RR-7):1–8.
78. Bass JB, Farer S, Hopewell PC, et al. Treatment of tuberculosis and tuberculosis infection in adults and children. *Am J Respir Crit Care Med* 1994;149:1359–1374.
79. Mahmoudi A, Iseman MD. Pitfalls in the care of patients with tuberculosis. *JAMA* 1993;270:65–68.
80. Goble M, Iseman MD, Madsen LA, et al. Treatment of 171 patients with pulmonary tuberculosis resistant to isoniazid and rifampin. *N Engl J Med* 1993;328:527–532.
81. Horsburgh CR. *Mycobacterium avium* complex infection in the acquired immunodeficiency syndrome. *N Engl J Med* 1991; 324:1332–1338.
82. Horsburgh CR, Selik RM. The epidemiology of disseminated nontuberculous mycobacterial infection in the acquired immunodeficiency syndrome (AIDS). *Am Rev Resp Dis* 1989;139:4–7.
83. Gray JR, Rabeneck L. Atypical mycobacterial infection of the gastrointestinal tract in AIDS patients. *Am J Gastroenterol* 1989; 12:1521–1524.
84. Horsburgh CR, Chin DP, Yajko DM, et al. Environmental risk factors for aquisition of *Mycobacterium avium* complex in persons with human immunodeficiency virus infection. *J Infect Dis* 1994;170:362–367.
85. Horsburgh CR, Caldwell MB, Simonds RJ. Epidemiology of disseminated nontuberculous mycobacterial disease in children with acquired immunodeficiency syndrome. *Pediatr Infect Dis* 1993;12:219–222.
86. Horsburgh CR, Schoenfelder JR, Gordin FM, et al. Geographic variation in risk for *M. avium* bacteremia among patients with AIDS. *Am J Med Sci* 1997;313:341–345.
87. Okello DO, Sewankambo N, Goodgame R, et al. Absence of bacteremia with *Mycobacterium avium–intracellulare* in Ugandan patients with AIDS. *J Infect Dis* 1990;162:208–210.
88. Lucas SB, Hounnou A, Peacock C, et al. The mortality and pathology of HIV infection in a West African City. *AIDS* 1993; 7:1569–1579.

89. Horsburgh CR. Epidemiology of *Mycobacterium avium* complex disease. In: Korvick JA, Benson CA, eds. Mycobacterium avium *complex infection: progress in research and treatment.* New York: Marcel Dekker Inc, 1995:1–22.
90. von Reyn CF, Maslow JN, Barber TW, et al. Persistent colonisation of potable water as a source of *Mycobacterium avium* infection in AIDS. *Lancet* 1994;343:1110–1111.
91. Horsburgh CR, Chin DP, Yajko DM, et al. Environmental risk factors for acquisition of *Mycobacterium avium* complex in persons with human immunodeficiency virus infection. *J Infect Dis* 1994;170:362–367.
92. Mapother ME, Songer JG. *In vitro* interaction of *Mycobacterium avium* with intestinal epithelial cells. *Infect Immun* 1984;45:67–73.
93. Pethel ML, Falkinham JO III. Plasmid-influenced changes in *Mycobacterium avium* catalase activity. *Infect Immun* 1989;57: 1714–1718.
94. Schafer WB, Davis CL, Cohn ML. Pathogenicity of transparent, opaque, and rough variants of *M. avium* in chicken and mice. *Am Rev Respir Dis* 1970;102:499–501.
95. Shiratsuchi H, Toosi Z, Mettler MA, et al. Colonial morphotype as a determinate of cytokine expression by human monocytes infected with *M. avium. J Immunol* 1993;150:2945–2954.
96. Havlik JA, Metchock B, Thompson SE, et al. A prospective evaluation of *Mycobacterium avium* complex colonization of the respiratory and gastrointestinal tracts of persons with HIV infection. *J Infect Dis* 1993;168:1045–1048.
97. Strom RL, Gruninger RP. AIDS with *Mycobacterium avium–intracellulare* lesions resembling those of Whipple's disease. *N Engl J Med* 1983;309:1323–1324.
98. Sohn CC, Schroff RW, Kliewer KE, et al. Disseminated *Mycobacterium avium–intracellulare* infection in homosexual men with acquired cell-mediated immunodeficiency: a histologic and immunologic study of two cases. *Am J Clin Pathol* 1983;79: 247–252.
99. Klatt EC, Jensen DF, Meyer PR. Pathology of *Mycobacterium avium–intracellulare* infection in acquired immunodeficiency syndrome. *Hum Pathol* 1987;18:709–714.
100. Wallace JM, Hannah JB. *Mycobacterium avium* complex infection in patients with the acquired immunodeficiency syndrome. *Chest* 1988;93:926–932.
101. Waisman J, Rotterdam H, Niedt GN, et al. AIDS: an overview of the pathology. *Pathol Res Pract* 1987;182:729–754.
102. Grunfeld C, Kotler DP. The wasting syndrome and nutritional support in AIDS. *Semin Gastrointest Dis* 1991;2:25–36.
103. Wood C, Nickeloff BJ, Todes-Taylor NR. Pseudo-tumor resulting from atypical mycobacterial infection: a "histoid" variety of *Mycobacterium avium–intracellulare* complex infection. *Am J Clin Pathol* 1985;83:524–527.
104. Shiratsuchi H, Johnson JL, Ellner JJ. Bidirectional effects of cytokines on growth of *M. avium* in human monocytes. *J Immunol* 1991;146:3165–3170.
105. Shiratsuchi H, Johnson JJ, Ellner JJ. Modulation of the effector function of human monocytes for *Mycobacterium avium* by human immunodeficiency virus-1 envelope protein gp120. *J Clin Invest* 1994;93:885–891.
106. Wayne WG, Young LS, Bertram M. Absence of mycobacterial antibody in patients with acquired immune deficiency syndrome. *Eur J Clin Microbiol* 1991;5:363–365.
107. Winter SM, Bernard EM, Gold JWM, et al. Humoral response to disseminated infection with *Mycobacterium avium–Mycobacterium intracellulare* in acquired immunodeficiency syndrome and hairy cell leukemia. *J Infect Dis* 1985;151:523–527.
108. Schnittman S, Lane HC, Witebsky FG, et al. Host defense against *Mycobacterium avium* complex. *J Clin Immunol* 1988; 8:234–243.
109. Douvas GS, May MH, Crowle AJ. Transferrin, iron, and serum lipids enhance or inhibit *Mycobacterium avium* replication in human macrophages. *J Infect Dis* 1993;167:857–864.
110. Crowle AJ, Cohn D, Poche P. Defects in sera from acquired immunodeficiency syndrome (AIDS) patients and from non-AIDS patients with *Mycobacterium avium* infection which decrease macrophage resistance of *M. avium. Infect Immun* 1989;57:1445–1451.
111. Race EM, Adelson-Mitty J, Kriegal GR, et al. Focal mycobacterial lymphadenitis following initiation of protease-inhibitor therapy in patients with advanced HIV-1 disease. *Lancet* 1998; 351:252–255.
112. Fonquernie L, Meynard JL, Kirstetter M, et al. Pseudotumoral abdominal granuloma concomitant with immune reconstitution after antiretroviral therapy [in French]. *Presse Med* 2000; 29:186–187.
113. Horsburgh CR, Mason UG, Farhi DC, et al. Disseminated infection with *Mycobacterium avium–intracellulare. Medicine* 1985;64:36–48.
114. Horsburgh CR, Metchock B, Gordon SM, et al. Predictors of survival in patients with AIDS and disseminated *Mycobacterium avium* complex disease. *J Infect Dis* 1994;170:573–577.
115. Sathe SS, Gascone P, Lo W, et al. Severe anemia is an important negative predictor for survival with disseminated *Mycobacterium avium–intracellulare* in acquired immunodeficiency syndrome. *Am Rev Resp Dis* 1990;142:1306–1312.
116. Jacobson MA, Peiperi L, Volberding PA, et al. Red cell transfusion therapy for anemia in patients with AIDS and ARC: incidence, associated factors, and outcome. *Transfusion* 1990;30: 133–137.
117. Roth RI, Owen RL, Keren DF, et al. Intestinal infection with *Mycobacterium avium* in acquired immune deficiency syndrome (AIDS). Histological and clinical comparison with Whipple's disease. *Dig Dis Sci* 1985;30:497–504.
118. Gillin JS, Urmacher C, West R, et al. Disseminated *Mycobacterium avium–intracellulare* infection in acquired immunodeficiency syndrome mimicking Whipple's disease. *Gastroenterology* 1983;85:1187–1191.
119. Schneebaum CW, Novick DM, Chabon AB, et al. Terminal ileitis associated with *Mycobacterium avium–intracellulare* infection in a homosexual man with acquired immune deficiency syndrome. *Gastroenterology* 1987;92:1127–1132.
120. Hoyt L, Connor E, Oleske J. Non-tuberculosis mycobacteria in children with acquired immunodeficiency syndrome. *Pediatr Infect Dis J* 1992;11:354–360.
121. Lewis LL, Butler KM, Husson RN, et al. Defining the population of human immunodeficiency virus-infected children at risk for *Mycobacterium avium–intracellulare* infection. *J Pediatr* 1992;121:677–683.
122. Radin DR. Intraabdominal *Mycobacterium tuberculosis* vs *Mycobacterium avium–intracellulare* infections in patients with AIDS: distinction based on CT findings. *AJR Am J Roentgenol* 1991;156:487–491.
123. Monsour HP Jr, Quigley EMM, Markin RS, et al. Endoscopy in the diagnosis of gastrointestinal *Mycobacterium avium–intracellulare* infection. *J Clin Gastroenterol* 1991;13:20–24.
124. Cappell MS, Hassan R, Rosenthal S, et al. Gastrointestinal obstruction due to *Mycobacterium avium–intracellulare* associated with the acquired immunodeficiency syndrome. *Am J Gastroenterol* 1992;12:1823–1827.
125. Cappell MS, Gupta A. Gastrointestinal hemorrhage due to gastrointestinal *Mycobacterium avium–intracellulare* or esophageal candidiasis in patients with the acquired immunodeficiency syndrome. *Am J Gastroenterol* 1991;87:224–229.
126. Horsburgh CR, Havlik JA, Ellis DA, et al. Survival of AIDS patients with disseminated *Mycobacterium avium* complex

infection with and without antimycobacterial chemotherapy. *Am Rev Respir Dis* 1991;144:557–559.

127. Yagupsky P, Menegus MA. Cumulative positivity rates of multiple blood cultures for *Mycobacterium avium–intracellulare* and *Cryptococcus neoformans* in patients with the acquired immunodeficiency syndrome. *Arch Pathol Lab Med* 1990;114: 923–925.
128. Barnes PF, Arevalo C. Blood culture positivity patterns in bacteremia due to *Mycobacterium avium–intracellulare. South Med J* 1988;81:1059–1060.
129. Shafran SD, Singer J, Zarowny DP, et al. A comparison of two regimens for the treatment of *Mycobacterium avium* complex bacteremia in AIDS: rifabutin, ethambutol, and clarithromycin versus rifampin, ethambutol, clofazimine, and ciprofloxacin. *N Engl J Med* 1996;335:377–383.
130. Centers for Disease Control and Prevention. 1999 USPHS/IDSA guidelines for the prevention of opportunistic infections in persons infected with human immunodeficiency virus: U.S. Public Health Service (USPHS) and Infectious Diseases Society of America (IDSA). *MMWR Morb Mortal Wkly Rep* 1999;48(RR-10):1–66.
131. Chaisson RE, Benson CA, Dube MP, et al. Clarithromycin therapy for bacteremic *Mycobacterium avium* complex disease. A randomized, double-blind, dose-ranging study in patients with AIDS. *Ann Intern Med* 1994;121:905–911.
132. Deziel DJ, Hyser MJ, Doolas A, et al. Major abdominal operations in acquired immunodeficiency syndrome. *Am Surg* 1990; 56:445–450.
133. Pierce M, Crampton S, Henry D, et al. A randomized trial of clarithromycin as prophylaxis against disseminated *Mycobacterium avium* complex infection in patients with advanced acquired immunodeficiency syndrome. *N Engl J Med* 1996;335:384–391.
134. Havlir DV, Dube MP, Sattler FR, et al. Prophylaxis against disseminated *Mycobacterium avium* complex with weekly azithromycin, daily rifabutin, or both. *N Engl J Med* 1996;335: 392–398.
135. Horsburgh CR. Advances in the prevention and treatment of *Mycobacterium avium* disease. *N Engl J Med* 1996;335:428–430.
136. El-Sadr WM, Burman WJ, Grant LB, et al. Discontinuation of prophylaxis for disseminated *Mycobacterium avium* complex disease in HIV-infected patients who have a response to antiretroviral therapy. *N Engl J Med* 2000;342:1085–1092.
137. Currier JS, Williams PL, Koletar SL, et al. Discontinuation of *Mycobacterium avium* complex prophylaxis in patients with antiretroviral therapy-induced increases in CD4+ cell count. *Ann Intern Med* 2000 133;7:493–503.

53

FUNGAL INFECTIONS OF THE GASTROINTESTINAL TRACT

DUANE R. HOSPENTHAL
JOHN E. BENNETT

The fungi are a diverse group of eucaryotic organisms that have rigid cell walls and contain the typical organelles found in higher organisms such as plants and animals. Fungi typically exist in the environment as yeasts or molds. *Yeasts* are rounded single-celled structures that reproduce by budding and appear macroscopically as creamy or mucoid colonies. *Molds* produce the typical fuzzy growth seen in culture and on organic material such as bread. Microscopically, molds produce tubular, multinucleated structures (hyphae), which may or may not have regular cross walls (septa). Those with regularly occurring septa are termed *septate hyphae,* whereas those with only rare septa are called *aseptate hyphae.* Another common fungal structure found on smear and biopsy is *pseudohyphae.* These are chains of elongated yeast, which look like hyphae, but which have constrictions where septa would normally exist. This form is seen with all *Candida* species except *C. glabrata.* Finally, many of the pathogenic fungi are described as *dimorphic.* Dimorphic fungi typically exist as molds when growing at room temperature and in the environment, and become yeasts at 37°C in culture and when causing disease.

Fungal structures may be difficult to identify on smears or tissue stained with the standard Gram stain or histopathology stain, hematoxylin and eosin (H&E). Smears of scrapings or lesional discharge are best examined with either potassium hydroxide (KOH) or calcofluor white preparations. Tissue specimens are commonly stained with Gomori methenamine silver (GMS) or periodic acid-Schiff (PAS) to better identify fungal elements. Fungi stained with GMS appear dark brown to black. Staining with PAS contrasts pink to red staining fungi against a background of yellow.

With the notable exception of *Candida* species, fungi are unusual pathogens of the gastrointestinal (GI) tract. *Candida albicans* is both the most common fungal pathogen of humans and a member of the normal GI tract flora. Finding *Candida* in the GI tract cannot be automatically interpreted as an indication of infection or pathology. Recovery of most other fungi from the GI tract should raise suspicion for infection, and usually disseminated infection. *Candida* causes disease of the GI tract through direct penetration of the mucosa, usually in the setting of immunosuppression. Local inoculation has been described with many of the other fungi, but most infections involving the other fungi follow hematogenously spread to the GI tract after inhalational respiratory infection.

Current therapy of these infections usually involves use of intravenous amphotericin B or one of the azole antifungals. Amphotericin B is the most broad spectrum of the antifungal agents and is considered the drug of choice for most life-threatening infections. This drug is associated with a range of adverse effects including fevers, chills, nausea, vomiting, and headaches during infusion, and renal and bone marrow toxicity with continued use. Care must be taken to monitor renal function, potassium, magnesium, and hematocrit with its use. Three lipid formulations of amphotericin B are now available in the United States. Whereas these formulations have been shown to have decreased renal toxicity, their higher costs and lack of efficacy data in GI infections limit use in these infections. The systemically absorbed azole agents include the triazole antifungals, fluconazole and itraconazole, and the imidazole antifungal, ketoconazole. Adverse effects with these agents are much less than amphotericin B, and all are available in oral formulations. The most important potential for adverse effects in these drugs are those due to drug-drug interactions. Ketoconazole, which has a spectrum of action similar

D. R. Hospenthal: Brooke Army Medical Center, Fort Sam Houston, Texas, F. Edward Infectious Disease Service, Department of Medicine, Hébert School of Medicine, Uniformed Services University of the Health Sciences, Bethesda, Maryland; Department of Medicine, The University of Texas Health Science Center at San Antonio, San Antonio, Texas

J. E. Bennett: Clinical Mycology Section, Laboratory of Clinical Investigation, National Institute of Allergy and Infectious Diseases, National Institutes of Health, Bethesda, Maryland to the newer itraconazole, also may interfere with steroidal hormones, and has been largely replaced by itraconazole. A wide variety of topical agents are also available for the treatment of superficial candidal infections. The fungal infections discussed in this chapter are those most commonly described. Even though other fungi have been reported to cause infection involving the GI tract, most of these are case reports with GI involvement as a manifestation of disseminated disease. Practically any fungus can cause opportunistic disease in a severely immunosuppressed host, and thus consideration of possible disease should be given to all cultures that grow fungi, even those considered common laboratory contaminants. The remainder of this chapter discusses the following mycoses: *Candida* and candidiasis—yeasts commonly recovered from culture which account for most GI fungal infections; the fungi that are found as hyphae in tissue—*Aspergillus*, the agents of mucormycosis, and *Basidiobolus ranarum;* and those fungi which are found in the human host as yeast or yeast-like organisms. Discussion of blastomycosis, cryptococcosis, histoplasmosis (including the African variant), paracoccidioidomycosis, penicilliosis, and pneumocystosis are included in this last group.

CANDIDIASIS

Mycology

Candidiasis is most commonly a mucosal infection caused by the yeast *C. albicans. C. albicans* is the most common fungal commensal of the human GI tract as well as the most common human fungal pathogen. Disease can range from superficial infection of the mucosa to life-threatening disseminated infection. Other common disease-producing *Candida* species include *C. guilliermondi, C. krusei, C. parapsilosis, C. tropicalis, C. pseudotropicalis, C. lusitaniae, C. dubliniensis*, and *C. (Torulopsis) glabrata*. These are small (4 to 6 μm) ovoid yeasts, which reproduce by budding and, with the exception of *C. glabrata*, can also exist as septate hyphae and pseudohyphae.

Epidemiology and Predisposing Factors

Candida species are common flora of the skin, vagina, and GI tract of people and other warm-blooded animals. Although person-to-person transmission can occur, most infections are secondary to overgrowth of commensal flora. Factors that predispose to overgrowth of these yeasts and potential infection include immunosuppression, hyperglycemia, broad-spectrum antibiotic exposure, and topical corticosteroid use. Common forms of immunosuppression associated with candidiasis include HIV infection and those that result from the treatment of malignancies and use of corticosteroids.

Pathogenesis and Pathology

Innate immune defenses of intact skin and mucous membranes limit invasion by these yeasts. Polymorphonuclear leukocytes and monocytes have also been shown to be important in the defense against *Candida.* Persons with decreased numbers or dysfunction of these cells, such as those receiving chemotherapy, are at the highest risk for disseminated infection. It is accepted theory that candidemia and disseminated candidiasis in persons receiving chemotherapy most likely arises from GI colonization with these yeasts. A role for cell-mediated defense in controlling the yeast flora is seen in the increased incidence of mucosal disease in persons with HIV infection and chronic mucocutaneous candidiasis. Factors produced by these yeasts to allow adherence to oral epithelium and other human structures clearly aids in colonization and pathogenicity.

Clinical Manifestations

The most common presentation of candidiasis involving the GI tract is thrush, followed by esophagitis, and then involvement of the stomach and small bowel. Oropharyngeal candidiasis (thrush) usually presents as white plaques on the oral mucosa. The plaques are white to cream colored and can be dislodged to reveal an erythematous base, which may bleed. These lesions may become confluent and appear as pseudomembranes, which make swallowing uncomfortable. Esophagitis is frequently associated with oropharyngeal disease and presents with odynophagia or dysphagia. These superficial syndromes are also described in Chapters 29, 30, 31, and 32.

Involvement of the stomach and bowel has not been associated with any specific syndrome, frequently being diagnosed after white plaques or pseudomembranes similar to oral thrush are noted on endoscopy. In addition to these typical plaques and pseudomembranes, ulcers of the stomach and bowel are also described. Care again is required in diagnosing infection in this setting because yeast recovered from stomach ulcers may represent colonization and not disease (1). Involvement of the stomach and distal GI tract has been most commonly described in autopsy series of persons treated for hematologic and other malignancies (2).

Focal pancreatitis and pancreatic abscesses due to *Candida* have also been reported (3,4). This form of candidal disease appears to occur in patients with chronic pancreatitis or another primary cause of preexisting pancreatic inflammation.

Diagnosis

Diagnosis is commonly made by observation of yeast, pseudohyphae, or hyphae on smears of plaques. These may be observed with KOH, Gram stain, or calcofluor preparations. The appearance of typical oral lesions (white plaques easily dislodged from red bases) may be specific enough to treat in the proper setting. Endoscopic lesions, which also appear pathognomonic, should be sampled, especially if ulceration is present, to rule out other coexistent infection or pathology. Culture is indicated in infection that is resistant to initial therapy or when presence of a resistant yeast is suspected. In the neutropenic patients, blood cultures may aid in diagnosis of disseminated infections. Examination of the fundi of the eyes should be included in the evaluation of any patient with deep infection or positive blood cultures to rule out endophthalmitis.

Treatment

Thrush may be treated with topical antifungals such as clotrimazole troches, 10 mg five times daily, or nystatin suspension, 4 to 6 million units five times daily for 7 to 14 days. Each troche should be held in the buccal pouch until dissolved. Nystatin suspension should be swished around the mouth and swallowed. Esophageal infection and more resistant thrush can be treated with fluconazole (100 mg daily for 7 to 14 days for thrush, 100 to 200 mg daily for 14 to 21 days for esophagitis) or itraconazole capsules (200 mg daily for 7 to 14 days for thrush, 14 to 21 days for esophagitis). In the patient whose esophageal symptoms are not controlled with fluconazole, intravenous amphotericin B 0.3 to 0.5 mg/kg or caspofungin acetate 50 mg intravenously (IV) daily is effective. Itraconazole suspension 200 mg twice a day improves symptoms in perhaps half of the patients with fluconazole-unresponsive esophageal candidiasis but the response is often temporary and partial. Neutropenic patients with esophageal candidiasis and fever are usually treated with intravenous amphotericin B using doses that would be recommended for disseminated candidiasis, that is, 0.5 to 1.0 mg/kg daily.

ASPERGILLOSIS

Mycology

Invasive aspergillosis is most commonly caused by *Aspergillus fumigatus*. Of the other species in the genus, *A. flavus, A. niger, A. terreus,* and *A. nidulans* are most commonly reported as pathogens. These fungi are molds that produce 2- to 3-μm diameter septate hyphae with consistently parallel cell walls in tissue. In culture and in nature, these molds produce large quantities of airborne conidia (asexual spores).

Epidemiology and Predisposing Factors

Aspergillus is ubiquitous in nature, growing in most organic materials and soils. Infection occurs in those patients with severe defects in neutrophil numbers or function. Aspergillosis most commonly occurs in persons with prolonged neutropenia, but persons receiving protracted courses and high doses of corticosteroids are also at increased risk.

Pathogenesis and Pathology

GI infection with *Aspergillus* species almost always occurs as part of disseminated disease in an immunosuppressed host. Phagocytic cells, including neutrophils and monocytic cells, protect against disease in the immunocompetent host. Disease begins with inhalation of conidia, as sinus or pulmonary infection. Spread may be local or hematogenous with a predilection for blood vessels. Thrombosis of blood vessels may lead to necrosis. Disease in the GI tract is usually described as submucosal ulcerations, necrotic mass lesions, or perforations.

Clinical Manifestations

Necropsy reports of immunosuppressed patients, mostly with malignancy or following liver transplantation, has found involvement of esophagus, stomach, bowel, liver, pancreas, and spleen (5–7). GI involvement can be associated with GI bleeding, found in eight of nine patients in one study (6). Disseminated disease has rarely been identified before death following GI bleeding (8). Bleeding from esophagus, stomach, duodenum, and colon has been reported in fatal cases of disseminated disease (6,8). Bowel infarction has also been described as a presentation of fatal disseminated disease (9). Even though mortality rate is high in cases of disseminated aspergillosis with GI involvement, survival of one patient with acute leukemia and *Aspergillus* peritonitis associated with colonic perforation has been reported (10).

Diagnosis

Biopsy of involved tissue reveals branching septate hyphae usually 2 to 3-μm in diameter with grossly parallel cell walls. Identification of fungal elements in tissue is best achieved with use of specific fungal stains, such as GMS. Diagnosis should be confirmed with fungal culture of biopsy material because other opportunistic mold infections (i.e., *Fusarium, Pseudallescheria, Acremonium*) also appear as branching septate hyphae in tissue. The literature abounds with reports of "aspergillosis" identified by biopsy alone. Evaluation for coexisting pulmonary infection with chest radiography or high-resolution computed tomography (CT) is also suggested.

Treatment

High-dose intravenous amphotericin B, using daily doses of 1.0 to 1.5 mg/kg, is the treatment of choice in these infections. In patients with impaired renal function or intolerance to standard amphotericin, lipid-based amphotericin B preparations can be substituted at approved doses. Itraconazole is an alternative therapy for aspergillosis, although use of this agent is usually limited to controlled or not immediately life-threatening infections. An intravenous formulation of itraconazole in cyclodextrin is available for use for up to 2 weeks. With both oral and intravenous itraconazole, a loading dose is usually given. Extended courses of oral itraconazole, at 200 mg twice daily, are usually used. Drug absorption should be documented by obtaining a drug level in persons on itraconazole long term. With normal absorption, the combined itraconazole and hydroxyitraconazole concentrations usually exceed 2 μg/mL. Treatment of peritonitis in the presence of an indwelling peritoneal catheter should include catheter removal.

MUCORMYCOSIS

Mycology

Mucormycosis is caused by the fungi of the order Mucorales in the class Zygomycetes. Zygomycosis is also used to describe disease caused by this group of fungi, but that nomenclature also includes dissimilar disease caused by fungi of other orders, such as that described in the next section on basidiobolomycosis. The most common organisms that cause this disease are the *Rhizopus* species, and species of the genera *Rhizomucor*, *Cunninghamella*, *Saksenaea*, *Mucor*, *Apophysomyces*, *Cokeromyces*, and *Absidia*. These molds grow as large-diameter (4 to 15 μm) aseptate hyphae in the environment, in culture, and in infection. These molds are common in the environment, producing cottony growth on bread, other foodstuffs, and organic matter. These organisms produce large quantities of asexual spores in nature. These spores are likely the infectious particles of mucormycosis, typically via airborne inhalation, but perhaps through ingestion in some patients with GI disease.

Epidemiology and Predisposing Factors

Disease is typically restricted to debilitated hosts, typically those with prolonged neutropenia, prolonged high-dose corticosteroid use, or uncontrolled diabetes mellitus. Other described risk factors include chronic renal insufficiency, burns, deferoxamine therapy, and aplastic anemia. GI disease is usually a manifestation of disseminated infection. Infection confined to the GI tract is only rarely (7% in one report) reported (11). Disease confined to the GI tract has been reported most commonly from South Africa and tropical countries (11,12). GI infection has been reported most commonly in malnourished children and immunosuppressed adults. Disease has also been associated with amebic colitis, typhoid, pellagra, kwashiorkor, and hepatic failure (12–14). Prematurity appears to be a risk factor for a form of mucormycosis that resembles necrotizing enterocolitis described in neonates (15).

Pathogenesis and Pathology

Polymorphonuclear leukocytes and other phagocytic cells are capable of damaging the spores and hyphae of these organisms. Lack of neutrophils or their dysfunction has been associated with infection with the agents of mucormycosis.

Clinical Manifestations

Infection of all parts of the GI tract has been described. The most common sites of GI mucormycosis are the stomach and the large intestine (11,13,16). The agents of mucormycosis may colonize or invade gastric ulcers (17,18). Vascular invasion is the hallmark of invasive disease, usually producing hard, black lesions, with hyperemic borders (17). Gastric disease commonly manifests with perforation and, as a consequence, death. Gastric mucormycosis has been associated with rapidly fatal outcomes (39 of 43 patients [91%]) in two recent reviews of the literature (19,20). Infection of the large and small bowel is the next most common form of GI mucormycosis. Disease may present as ulcerations or as inflammatory masses mimicking malignancy. This infection can present with abdominal pain and distention, and commonly fever and leukocytosis (11).

Mucormycosis confined to the GI tract occurs more frequently in children. In this group, as in adults, the stomach is most commonly involved followed by the colon, small intestine, and esophagus (21,22). An unusual form of GI mucormycosis, presenting similarly to necrotizing enterocolitis has been described in neonates (15). This form is most commonly seen in prematurely born neonates. All presentations in this group have included abdominal distention. Pneumoperitoneum was seen in 50% of these babies, hematochezia in 42% (15).

Diagnosis

Diagnosis is based on observation of the typical structures on histopathology. Fungi of this class are seen on GMS or PAS staining as ribbon-like hyphae with varying cell wall diameters. Their cell walls are thin and septations are only rarely seen. Culture of lesions may be helpful in confirming the diagnosis. No serologic testing is available to aid in diagnosis.

Treatment

Intravenous amphotericin B at high doses, 1.0 to 1.5 mg/kg daily should be used in therapy of these infections. Surgical resection of isolated lesions appears prudent. Reversing predisposing factors such as neutropenia or hyperglycemia is highly associated with therapeutic success.

BASIDIOBOLOMYCOSIS

Mycology

Basidiobolomycosis is a fungal infection caused by the mold *Basidiobolus ranarum*. Disease caused by this organism and the other members of the order Entomophthorales is sometimes grouped with that caused by members of the order Mucorales as the zygomycoses, after their shared class, Zygomycetes. Most authorities divide these two groups of dissimilar infections by order into the entomophthoramycoses and mucormycoses.

Epidemiology and Predisposing Factors

B. ranarum most commonly causes a skin or subcutaneous infection (subcutaneous zygomycosis) of children in tropical and subtropical regions of the world. Disease of the GI tract has been increasingly reported over the past decade, suggesting that this form is more common than previously believed. Most cases of GI disease have been diagnosed in the United States, chiefly from Arizona (23). The organism is found in the soil, other organic material, and in the GI tracts of amphibians, bats, fish, and reptiles.

Pathogenesis and Pathology

Subcutaneous disease is thought to occur from direct inoculation. Disease of the GI tract most likely occurs from ingestion of the fungus. Little is known of the pathogenesis of this infection or the virulence factors of the organism.

Clinical Manifestations

The most common GI presentation of this disease is that mimicking Crohn's disease, with abdominal pain, fever, and diarrhea with mucus or blood (24). Occasionally, a mass is palpated or, more commonly, noted on CT scan. These may be resected to rule out malignancy. The stomach and colon appear to be the most common sites of infection (23). On resection, tissue from these sites shows diffuse mural thickening and yellow nodules up to 3 cm in diameter (23). Luminal narrowing, cobblestone appearance, ulcers, and focal hemorrhage have been described (23).

Diagnosis

Histologically, *B. ranarum* appears as thin-walled, variably sized (8 to 40 μm), broad hyphae with few septa, often within granulomas. When stained with H&E, the hyphae are surrounded by an eosinophilic material in what is often called the *Splendore-Hoeppli phenomenon* (24). KOH examination of lesional material may aid in diagnosis. Diagnosis is confirmed by culture of the organism from biopsy material. In one case, the organism was also recovered from the urine of a subject with GI infection (25). In culture, the mold grows well both at room temperature and at 37°C. The unique formation of ballistic conidiophores (which propel conidia onto the lid of culture plates) greatly aid in the diagnosis of *B. ranarum* infection. Peripheral blood eosinophilia has been associated with some cases. An immunodiffusion test has been used to make or support this diagnosis (26).

Treatment

Cutaneous disease may remit spontaneously or resolve with surgery. GI infection has also responded to prolonged therapy with potassium iodide or trimethoprim-sulfamethoxazole. *B. ranarum* is susceptible to itraconazole and amphotericin B *in vitro*. GI disease has been treated with surgical resection followed by oral itraconazole for 2 to 12 months (23). The role of itraconazole remains uncertain.

BLASTOMYCOSIS

Mycology

Infection with the dimorphic fungus, *Blastomyces dermatitidis*, may cause localized or disseminated infection. The organism grows as a cottony mold at room temperature and as a yeast at 37°C. The yeast form of *B. dermatitidis* is unique in its large size (6 to 15 μm) and presence of broad-based budding. The walls of this organism often appear double as a result of their thickness.

Epidemiology and Predisposing Factors

Blastomycosis is most commonly seen in central and southeast United States in areas near rivers or streams. It occurs in persons without evidence of immunosuppression, occasionally in small case clusters.

Pathogenesis and Pathology

GI disease is believed to occur secondary to dissemination of organisms following pulmonary infection. Most GI disease is associated with widespread dissemination, but focal disease has been described. Histologically, pseudoepitheliomatous hyperplasia is seen in the epidermis and squamous mucosa of the mouth and esophagus in areas of the lesions. In deep tissue, pyogranulomas are seen. (27).

Clinical Manifestations

This disease is usually confined to the lungs, skin, bone, or genitourinary tract. Central nervous system (CNS) infection and GI infection is much less common. The most common GI presentation of this infection is that of oral lesions (27). These lesions are usually ulcerative, but may be verruciform or appear as granulomatous patches. Lesions are typically asymptomatic and arise from hematogenous dissemination to the submucosa or underlying bone.

Manifestations in addition to oral lesions include esophagitis, cholangitis, peritonitis, and infection of the stomach, duodenum, rectum, anus, liver and spleen (28–32). Most cases have been reported from persons with disseminated disease in other sites as well. Focal esophagitis presenting with dysphagia has been reported in four cases of infection (30). Esophageal disease has manifested in the form of strictures, and, in one case, friable, erythematous linear ulcers (33).

Diagnosis

Biopsy material reveals large (6 to 15 μm), thick-walled yeast on smear or stain. These large yeasts may be seen with H&E, but are more easily appreciated with GMS or PAS stains. On H&E staining, tissue containing *B. dermatitidis* is usually associated with a granulomatous cellular reaction. Culture is required to confirm the diagnosis. This temperature-dependent dimorphic fungus grows as a mold in culture at room temperature. When grown at 37°C, the fungus converts to a large yeast similar to that seen in biopsy material. Serology is also available for diagnostic testing but is seldom helpful. The most commonly available test, that using an immunodiffusion technique, can document prior infection, but cannot determine chronicity. Skin testing for delayed hypersensitivity to blastomycin has not been helpful in diagnosis.

Treatment

Treatment of disseminated blastomycosis is based on severity and organs involved. Serious infection and that involving the CNS is treated with intravenous amphotericin B, 0.7 to 1.0 mg/kg per day for CNS, 0.3 to 0.6 mg/kg per day for non-CNS. Stabilized, non-CNS disease of mild to moderate severity may be treated with itraconazole, 200 to 400 mg/day. Oral ketoconazole, 400 to 800 mg/day has been successful. Fluconazole, if used, should be given at a dose of 800 mg/day.

CRYPTOCOCCOSIS

Mycology

Cryptococcosis is a fungal disease caused by the encapsulated yeast *Cryptococcus neoformans. C. neoformans* is a 4- to 6-μm round yeast that displays narrow-based budding. In disease it produces a thick polysaccharide capsule. In nature this capsule is usually greatly diminished, decreasing the size of the inhaled particle and thus enhancing infectivity. Infection is initiated in the lungs and has a predilection for the CNS.

Epidemiology and Predisposing Factors

The organism is found worldwide, existing in two varieties and four mating serotypes. *C. neoformans* var. *neoformans* (serotypes A and D) is found in association with bird guano, especially that of pigeons, whereas *C. neoformans* var. *gattii* (serotypes B and C) is found in association with eucalyptus trees. Disease can affect apparently immunocompetent hosts, but is more common in those with impaired cell-mediated immunity. The incidence of this disease has increased greatly with the advent of the AIDS epidemic. Other patients at increased risk include those who have undergone solid organ transplantation, those who are taking prolonged courses of high-dose corticosteroid, and those with lymphoma or sarcoidosis.

Pathogenesis and Pathology

Cryptococcal disease of the GI tract most likely occurs via hematogenous spread from pulmonary disease, although translocation of the organism following GI tract overgrowth has been suggested in some cases of peritonitis (34). *C. neoformans* is the only fungal pathogen that produces a large polysaccharide capsule. The capsular polysaccharide is a major virulence factor of this organism. It impedes cell-mediated immunity by a variety of mechanisms including suppressing leukocyte migration and increasing resistance to phagocytosis. Melanin production is also thought to contribute to virulence. Microscopically, a granulomatous inflammatory may be seen. In AIDS patients or in CNS lesions, collections of cryptococci with little surrounding inflammation are typically seen.

Clinical Manifestations

The most common disease caused by this yeast is a chronic meningitis, most frequently in persons with AIDS. Localized pulmonary disease and focal extrapulmonary disease of the skin, bone, prostate, and kidney may also occur. Cryptococcosis can involve the entire GI tract and associated organs. Disease the esophagus, biliary tract, liver, pancreas, bowel, rectum, peritoneal cavity and omentum have been reported (35). Disease can present as ulcers, nodules, or masses. Mass lesions are often excised to rule out malignancies. Disease presenting as a large omental mass and isolated cholangitis has been reported in patients without apparent immunosuppression (36,37). Isolated esophageal disease and disease resembling Crohn's disease has been reported in two patients with hyperimmunoglobulinemia E–recurrent infection (Job) syndrome (38,39). Both of these cases, one with upper GI bleeding and an esophageal mass, and the other presenting with Crohn's-like symptoms and a constricting lesion of the colon, had documented sterile cultures of the blood, urine, and cerebrospinal fluid (CSF) and negative cryptococcal antigen testing of the serum and CSF.

In HIV-infected individuals with disseminated cryptococcosis, disease of the mouth, esophagus, stomach, biliary tract, liver, pancreas, small intestine, colon, and rectum has been described (40,41). Oral lesions include persistent ulcers of the palate, tongue, and gum line (42–44). Oral ulcerations, anal lesions, and gastric cryptococcosis has been reported as an initial presentation of AIDS (41–45).

Cryptococcal peritonitis has been described in two settings: (1) associated with continuous ambulatory peritoneal dialysis (CAPD) or ventriculoperitoneal shunting, or (2) associated with chronic liver disease. In the first group, survival rate was 90% whereas survival rate in the second group was only 12.5% (46,47). Cryptococcal peritonitis is not commonly associated with abdominal discomfort or other specific symptoms (34). Delay in diagnosis and thus treatment has been postulated to be a contributing factor in this high mortality rate. An association of recent oral or upper GI bleeding was noted in one recent review of cryptococcal peritonitis (46).

Diagnosis

Biopsy should reveal a thin-walled yeast, often within a clearing of tissue representing the unseen capsule. The capsule of the organism stains reddish pink with mucicarmine stain, making this an excellent stain for diagnosis, especially if culture confirmation is impossible. In addition to biopsy, blood, urine, and CSF culture should be obtained. Blood and urine cultures can help confirm infection with *C. neoformans* and CSF culture can help rule out concomitant CNS infection. When *C. neoformans* is discovered causing disease, CNS infection must be ruled out. Cryptococcal antigen testing can be used in both serum and CSF samples to make the diagnosis and monitor therapy. Diagnosis of cryptococcal peritonitis requires careful examination and culture of peritoneal fluid. This infection may not raise the peritoneal white blood cell count more than 500 cells/μL. Specific stains, such as India ink, are often positive in peritonitis, but Gram stain is less likely to reveal this yeast. Use of blood culture bottles to culture peritoneal fluid is likely to increase yield.

Treatment

Intravenous amphotericin B is the drug of choice in life-threatening cryptococcal infection. In chronic meningitis, amphotericin B, 0.7 to 1.0 mg/day plus flucytosine, 100 mg/kg per day is used for 6 to 10 weeks. Fluconazole, 400 mg/day has been used to complete the course of therapy in CNS infection after completion of 2 weeks of amphotericin B and flucytosine. Symptomatic pulmonary disease and other non-CNS, non–life-threatening infections can be treated with fluconazole, 200 to 400 mg/day for 6 to 12 months. Itraconazole, 200 to 400 mg/kg, can be used in non-CNS disease as an alternate drug. Removal of the peritoneal catheter and a short course of antifungal therapy, usually 6 weeks of intravenous amphotericin B, has been used successfully to treat CAPD-associated cryptococcal peritonitis (47).

HISTOPLASMOSIS

Mycology

Histoplasma capsulatum is a dimorphic fungus that may cause a wide range of disease, ranging from asymptomatic to life-threatening. *H. capsulatum* grows as a mold at lower temperatures, producing microconidia and macroconidia. In disease, the organism usually exists as a small (2 to 3 μm diameter), ovoid, intracellular yeast that displays narrow-based budding. This form is also seen when cultures are grown at 37°C.

Epidemiology and Predisposing Factors

Infection is found worldwide but is concentrated in a large endemic area in the Ohio and Mississippi River valleys of the United States. The organism is found in soil and debris enriched with bat and bird guano, including that of starlings and chickens. Disease severity is dependent on patient immunity and intensity of exposure. Life-threatening acute disseminated infection occurs most frequently in persons with advanced AIDS.

Pathogenesis and Pathology

Infection begins with inhalation of conidia and can spread hematogenously or contiguously in the chest. *H. capsulatum* parasitizes the macrophages of the lung, and these cells of the innate immune system likely aid in the dissemination of this intracellular pathogen. Infection is controlled by the cell-mediated immune system through activation of macrophages. In immunocompetent patients, a typical granulomatous reaction is seen. This reaction may be extensive in chronic disseminated disease and absent in those most immunosuppressed.

Clinical Manifestations

Symptomatic and asymptomatic infections isolated to the lung are the common presentation of this disease. Disseminated infection and focal extrapulmonary disease occur at much lower rates. Infection due to *H. capsulatum* can affect any portion of the GI tract. GI symptoms and involvement are common in the presentation of disseminated histoplasmosis (48,49). Although histoplasmosis is commonly thought of as a pulmonary disease, disseminated histoplasmosis often manifests with GI symptoms. A recent study reported 43% of 52 cases presenting with predominantly GI symptoms, with another 31% presenting with a mixture of

GI and pulmonary symptoms (50). In their review of 77 patients with GI histoplasmosis, Cappell and colleagues (51) reported diarrhea, weight loss, fever, abdominal pain, lymphadenopathy, and hepatomegaly or splenomegaly as the most common symptoms and presenting findings (51). None of these were seen in greater than one-third of all patients. Malabsorption has also been associated with disseminated infection (52). Spivak and co-workers grouped the clinical presentations of *H. capsulatum* in the GI tract into four groups. These include patients with (1) asymptomatic disease, without gross abnormalities but with yeasts in the macrophages of the lamina propria, (2) plaques or polyps, (3) ulcerative lesions and tissue necrosis presenting with abdominal pain, diarrhea, melena, or perforation, and (4) localized inflamed, thickened bowel and symptoms resembling tumor or Crohn's disease (48,53,54). In the previously mentioned study by Lamps and associates (50), gross findings included ulcers (49%), normal mucosa (23%), nodules (21%), hemorrhage (13%), and obstructive masses (6%) in their patients with disseminated disease (50). Microscopically, GI lesions in this study revealed diffuse lymphohistiocytic infiltration, ulceration, lymphohistiocytic nodules, minimal inflammatory reaction, and, rarely, granulomas. Terminal ileum and cecum, followed by isolated esophageal disease, were the most common locations of disease. Oral lesions are present in 30% to 50% of persons presenting with disseminated disease (48,55). It has been suggested that the frequency of oral lesions is lower in HIV-positive individuals with disseminated disease (55). A large study of disseminated histoplasmosis in HIV-infected individuals found 3% (8 of 280) with oral lesions (56). An isolated oral lesion also led to diagnosis of AIDS in one individual (57). Possible person-to-person spread has been suggested as a mode of transmission in one isolated case of oral histoplasmosis that presented with an oral lesion (58). Most oral lesions are painful periodontal or gingival ulcers. The periodontal lesions may lead to tooth extraction secondary to loosening. Lesions may also occur on the lips, tongue, palate, or buccal mucosa.

Diagnosis

H. capsulatum is a small budding yeast (2 to 4 μm), often found inside macrophages. Because of its size, it is difficult to identify in lesional smears and with standard stains. The organism is best seen with GMS or PAS stains. Diagnosis is best made by culture. In disseminated disease, lysis centrifugation blood cultures and bone marrow aspirate cultures may yield this yeast. Colon morphology and conversion of the mold form of *H. capsulatum* to a yeast with incubation at 37°C can be used to identify this organism, although nucleic acid hybridization is more reliable and rapid. Antigen testing of the serum and urine is useful in diagnosis of disseminated disease, though false-positive results can occur, and may also be used in monitoring response to therapy (59).

Treatment

GI histoplasmosis should be treated as any disseminated form of the infection. Severe disease is treated with intravenous amphotericin B, 0.7 mg/kg per day, until clinical improvement is noted. Itraconazole, 200 mg twice daily, can then be given for an additional 6 to 18 months. This same course of itraconazole may be used without the initial amphotericin B in patients with mild to moderate disease. Itraconazole should be continued lifelong in AIDS. It is as yet unknown whether patients responding to highly active antiretroviral therapy can have itraconazole discontinued. Ketoconazole 400 to 800 mg daily is also effective, though with increased risk of hepatotoxicity and hormonal suppression. Fluconazole is not effective at 400 mg daily but might be useful at higher doses.

AFRICAN HISTOPLASMOSIS

Mycology

African histoplasmosis caused by *H. capsulatum* var. *duboisii*, may produce GI lesions as part of disseminated or localized disease. This dimorphic fungus grows as a mold similar to *H. capsulatum* var. *capsulatum* at room temperature and in nature. In infection and at 37°C, it grows as a large (8 to 15 μm) yeast resembling *B. dermatitidis* and not as the small yeast seen in the *capsulatum* variety.

Epidemiology and Predisposing Factors

This disease is limited to Africa, specifically to tropical sub-Saharan Africa. The majority of cases have been reported from Nigeria, Zaire, Uganda, and Senegal.

Pathogenesis and Pathology

GI disease, while uncommon, usually appears as GI tract ulcers or masses. A granulomatous inflammatory reaction is commonly reported.

Clinical Manifestations

African histoplasmosis has been reported to manifest as a focal gastric lesion mimicking gastric cancer and constricting annular lesion mimicking colon cancer (60,61). Small bowel involvement and perforation has been reported, but spleen and liver are reported as the most common sites of GI involvement (60).

Diagnosis

Biopsy reveals large yeasts (8 to 15 μm), which may be seen in short chains on fungal stains. Diagnosis should be confirmed by culture.

Treatment

Many patients who have presented with GI manifestations of this infection have undergone surgical resection to remove possible malignancies. Following surgery, oral ketoconazole or intravenous amphotericin B have been given. Treatment similar to that given for *H. capsulatum* var. *capsulatum* should be effective in this disease. Amphotericin B for at least 3 months at a dose of 0.5 to 0.7 mg/kg per day have been suggested for disseminated disease (61).

PARACOCCIDIOIDOMYCOSIS

Mycology

Paracoccidioides brasiliensis is a dimorphic fungus of South America that commonly causes pulmonary disease with orofacial lesions. This fungus grows as a mold similar to *B. dermatitidis* in nature and at room temperature and as a yeast in culture at 37°C or in infection. The yeasts are round and large (2 to 30 μm) with multiple buds (daughter cells) originating from the mother cell. These are often remarked to appear as a "pilot's wheel" because of this unique morphology.

Epidemiology and Predisposing Factors

Paracoccidioidomycosis (South American blastomycosis) is a potentially fatal progressive fungal disease limited to Latin America. Disease is most frequently reported from Brazil, followed by Colombia and Venezuela, and less so from Argentina, Peru, Ecuador, Uruguay, Paraguay, Central America and southern Mexico (62). This infection has been diagnosed in individuals with past residency in this area of the world, often years after their exposure. The disease generally affects rural male farm workers, occurring more frequently in those who smoke tobacco (63,64). Oral lesions have been reported most commonly in adult white men (62). The predominance of male infection among adults but not children has led to speculation, supported by evidence of *in vitro* inhibition of *P. brasiliensis* by estrogen, that women have resistance to this infection.

Pathogenesis and Pathology

Initial infection probably begins in the lung, although this site is initially subclinical and extends from the lung to the GI tract and other sites. Histologic reaction includes pyogranulomatous inflammation with pseudoepitheliomatous hyperplasia.

Clinical Manifestations

Oral lesions have been reported as the presenting manifestation in a large number of cases of paracoccidioidomycosis. These lesions have been described as chronic, proliferative ulcerations with a mulberry appearance found on the gingiva, alveolar process, palate, or lip (62). These lesions are painful and commonly associated with pulmonary disease and tobacco use. Cervical lymph node enlargement and spontaneous drainage may occur in conjunction with oral lesions (65). Ulcerative lesions have also been reported from the small and large bowel (63,66). Chest radiograph often shows scattered infiltrates, even in patients with no pulmonary symptoms.

Diagnosis

KOH examination of lesional scrapings or discharge may lead to presumptive diagnosis based on the typical appearance of the yeasts of *P. brasiliensis*. GMS or PAS staining of biopsy material can enhance the diagnosis of this disease. Culture is essential for confirmation of the diagnosis, although growth of the mold may be slow and conversion to the yeast phase difficult to achieve. Serologic testing is available in South America and can assist in making the diagnosis of paracoccidioidomycosis.

Treatment

Paracoccidioidomycosis was treated with sulfonamides in the past but response was slow and incomplete, often followed by relapse. Itraconazole 200 mg daily is now the drug of choice, with ketoconazole being an alternative. Experience with fluconazole is encouraging but much less extensive (67). Azole therapy should be continued for at least 6 to 12 months. Intravenous amphotericin B is used in severe or unresponsive infections, followed by azole therapy long-term.

PENICILLIOSIS

Mycology

Penicillium marneffei is a dimorphic fungus that causes infection limited to Southeast Asia. This fungus grows as a mold with a red pigment diffusing into the agar at room temperature. At 37°C, the organism grows as small (2 to 6 μm diameter) yeast. In infection, the organism appears as a small intracellular yeast and as ovoid "sausage forms" extracellularly. Because the organism divides by fission, not budding, seeing a septum in the middle of a dividing yeast cell can aid identification in tissue.

Epidemiology and Predisposing Factors

Penicilliosis is typically a disseminated infection seen in severely immunosuppressed persons residing in Southeast Asia. Previously normal children also have been infected.

Disease has been associated with occupational or other exposures to soil. Most commonly seen in persons with AIDS, this disease is the third most common opportunistic infection seen in AIDS patients in Thailand (68). *P. marneffei* has been isolated from healthy bamboo rats and the soil around their burrows, although exposure to rats seems unrelated to infection.

Pathogenesis and Pathology

Infection is likely initiated via inhalation of the conidia of the mold. The high incidence in persons with AIDS indicates that the cell-mediated immune system is important in preventing or controlling infection. Granulomatous, suppurative, and necrotizing inflammation have all been described with this infection.

Clinical Manifestations

P. marneffei is commonly recovered from the liver on autopsy. Ulceration of the mouth and tonsils have been reported with disseminated disease in persons both with and without HIV infection (69). At least eight cases of intestinal penicilliosis have been reported (70,71). In these cases, shallow ulceration of the stomach, small, and large intestines were observed. Fever and diarrhea were associated with most of these cases, although these symptoms are common in AIDS patients with disseminated *P. marneffei* without documented GI invasion (69,72). Mesenteric lymphadenitis has also been described in HIV-infected children as a presentation of disseminated penicilliosis (73).

Diagnosis

Biopsy or smears of lesions may reveal the typical forms of the fungus, including the "sausage forms" with one to two septations. Blood, bone marrow, and lesional culture can be done to document infection. Positive stool cultures have been reported in a few cases (70). The organism grows as a typical *Penicillium* at room temperature and thus may be discarded as a contaminant. The red diffusable pigment and travel history should prompt further workup including diagnostic conversion of the organism to a yeast with culture at 37°C.

Treatment

Intravenous amphotericin B, 0.5–0.7 mg/kg daily should be used in serious infection. Itraconazole has been shown to be effective in the treatment of this disease and prevention of relapses. Excellent response has been shown with a regimen of 2 weeks of amphotericin B followed by oral itraconazole, 200 mg twice daily for 10 weeks in HIV-infected patients with this disease. This group should be given lifelong secondary prophylaxis with itraconazole, 200 mg daily following initial therapy.

PNEUMOCYSTOSIS

Mycology

Pneumocystis carinii has recently been included into the fungal kingdom based on genetic study. This organism has not been grown in culture or been recovered from the environment, thus most data concerning it are from human disease and animal models. In humans, the organism is seen as 1- to 4-μm trophozoites or trophic forms, often found in clumps and larger 5- to 8-μm thick-walled cysts or spore cases.

Epidemiology and Predisposing Factors

P. carinii infection is most commonly seen as a pneumonic process in persons with AIDS. Prophylaxis has been shown to greatly reduce the incidence of infection in AIDS. Use of aerosolized pentamidine as an alternative to trimethoprim/sulfamethoxazole or dapsone has been associated with disease outside the lung (74). Extrapulmonary disease is uncommon, but may affect the GI tract (74).

Pathogenesis and Pathology

In the lung, *P. carinii* initiates infection with attachment to alveolar cells. Infection is controlled by activated macrophages, requiring an intact cell-mediated immune system. Even though defects in the cell-mediated immune system as seen in AIDS have chiefly accounted for most cases of this infection, persons with humoral immunity defects also have trouble controlling this infection.

Clinical Manifestations

Although *P. carinii* is commonly an infection of the lungs, reports of disease have included virtually the entire GI tract, usually as part of a multiorgan dissemination. Isolated extrapulmonary foci of infection have included the small intestine and rectal ulcerative lesions (74,75).

Diagnosis

Diagnosis is made by observation of typical organisms in smears or biopsy sections. Calcofluor, Papanicolaou, and Wright-Giemsa stains have been used successfully to identify the organism in sputum and lesional smears. Histopathologic specimens are usually stained with GMS for best results.

Treatment

Trimethoprim-sulfamethoxazole is the preferred treatment for pneumocystosis.

DISCLAIMER

The views expressed in this manuscript are those of the authors and do not reflect the official policy or position of the Department of the Army, Department of Defense, or the U.S. Government.

REFERENCES

1. Minoli G, Terruzzi V, Rossini A. Gastroduodenal candidiasis occurring without underlying diseases (primary gastroduodenal candidiasis). *Endoscopy* 1979;1:18–22.
2. Eras P, Goldstein MJ, Sherlock P. *Candida* infection of the gastrointestinal tract. *Medicine* 1972;51:367–379.
3. Chung RT, Schapiro RH, Warshaw AL. Intraluminal pancreatic candidiasis presenting as recurrent pancreatitis. *Gastroenterology* 1993;104:1532–1534.
4. Keiser P, Keay S. Candidal pancreatic abscesses: report of two cases and review. *Clin Infect Dis* 1992;14:884–888.
5. Boon AP, O'Brien D, Adams DH. 10 Year review of invasive aspergillosis detected at necropsy. *Journal Clin Pathol* 1991;44: 452–454.
6. Meyer RD, Young LS, Armstrong D, Yu B. Aspergillosis complicating neoplastic disease. *Am J Med* 1973;54:6–15.
7. Nakamura S, Vawter G, Sallan S, et al. Fatal esophageal aspergilloma in a leukemic adolescent. *Pediatr Infect Dis J* 1992; 11:245–247.
8. Foy TM, Hawkins EP, Peters KR, et al. Colonic ulcers and lower GI bleeding due to disseminated aspergillosis. *J Pediatr Gastroenterol Nutr* 1994;18:399–403.
9. Cohen R, Heffner JE. Bowel infarction as the initial manifestation of disseminated aspergillosis. *Chest* 1992;101:877–879.
10. Weingrad DN, Knapper WH, Gold J, et al. Aspergillus peritonitis complicating perforated appendicitis in adult acute leukemia. *J Surg Oncol* 1982;19:5–8.
11. Lyon DT, Schubert TT, Mantia AG, et al. Phycomycosis of the gastrointestinal tract. *Am J Gastroenterol* 1979;72:379–394.
12. Straatsma BR, Zimmerman LE, Gass JDM. Phycomycosis. A clinicopathologic study of fifty-one cases. *Lab Invest* 1962;11: 963–985.
13. Lehrer RI, Howard DH, Sypherd PS, et al. Mucormycosis. *Ann Intern Med* 1980;93:93–108.
14. Parfrey NA. Improved diagnosis and prognosis of mucormycosis. A clinicopathologic study of 33 cases. *Medicine* 1986;65: 113–123.
15. Nissen MD, Jana AK, Cole MJ, et al. Neonatal gastrointestinal mucormycosis mimicking necrotizing enterocolitis. *Acta Paediatr* 1999;88:1290–1293.
16. Neame P, Rayner D. Mucormycosis. A report on twenty-two cases. *Arch Pathol* 1960;70:261–268.
17. Lawson HH, Schmaman A. Gastric phycomycosis. *Br J Surg* 1974;61:743–746.
18. Thomson SR, Bade PG, Taams M, et al. Gastrointestinal mucormycosis. *Br J Surg* 1991;78:952–954.
19. Cherney CL, Chutuape A, Fikrig MK. Fatal invasive gastric mucormycosis occurring with emphysematous gastritis: case report and literature review. *Am J Gastroenterol* 1999;94:-252–256.
20. Knoop C, Antoine M, Vachiéry JL, et al. Gastric perforation due to mucormycosis after heart-lung and heart transplantation. *Transplantation* 1998;66:932–935.
21. Michalak DM, Cooney DR, Rhodes KH, et al. Gastrointestinal mucormycosis in infants and children: a cause of gangrenous intestinal cellulitis and perforation. *J Pediatr Surg* 1980;15:-320–324.
22. Mooney JE, Wanger A. Mucormycosis of the gastrointestinal tract in children: report of a case and review of the literature. *Pediatr Infect Dis J* 1993;12:872–876.
23. Yousef OM, Smilack JD, Kerr DM, et al. Gastrointestinal basidiobolomycosis. Morphologic findings in a cluster of six cases. *American Journal of Clinical Pathology* 199;112:610-616.
24. Gugnani HC. A review of zygomycosis due to *Basidiobolus ranarum*. *European Journal of Epidemiology* 1999;15:923-929.
25. Zavasky D, Samowitz W, Loftus T, et al. Gastrointestinal zygomycotic infection caused by *Basidiobolus ranarum*: case report and review. *Clin Infect Dis* 1999;28:1244–1248.
26. Kaufman L, Mendoza L, Standard PG. Immunodiffusion test for serodiagnosing subcutaneous zygomycosis. *J Clin Microbiol* 1990;28:1887–1890.
27. Bell WA, Gamble J, Garrington GE. North American blastomycosis with oral lesions. *Oral Surg Oral Med Oral Pathol* 1969;-28:914–923.
28. Cherniss EI, Waisbren BA. North American blastomycosis: a clinical study of 40 cases. *Ann Intern Med* 1956;44:105–123.
29. Martin DS, Smith DT. Blastomycosis. I. A review of the literature. *Am Rev Tuberculosis* 1939;39:275–304.
30. Perez-Lasala G, Nolan RL, Chapman SW, et al. Peritoneal blastomycosis. *Am J Gastroenterol* 1991;86:357–359.
31. Ryan ME, Kirchner JP, Sell T, et al. Cholangitis due to *Blastomyces dermatitidis*. *Gastroenterology* 1989;96:1346–1349.
32. Witorsch P, Utz JP. North American blastomycosis: a study of 40 patients. *Medicine* 1968;47:169–200.
33. McKenzie R, Khakoo R. Blastomycosis of the esophagus presenting with gastrointestinal bleeding. *Gastroenterology* 1985;88:-1271–1273.
34. Mabee CL, Mabee SW, Kirkpatrick RB, et al. Cirrhosis: a risk factor for cryptococcal peritonitis. *Am J Gastroenterol* 1995;90:-2042–2045.
35. Daly JS, Porter KA, Chong FK, et al. Disseminated, nonmeningeal gastrointestinal cryptococcal infection in an HIV-negative patient. *Am J Gastroenterol* 1990;85:1421–1424.
36. Bucuvalas JC, Bove KE, Kaufman RA, et al. Cholangitis associated with *Cryptococcus neoformans*. *Gastroenterology* 1985;88:-1055–1059.
37. Chong PY, Panabokke RG, Chew KH. Omental cryptococcoma. An unusual presentation of cryptococcosis. *Arch Pathol Lab Med* 1986;110:239–241.
38. Hutto JO, Bryan CS, Greene FL, et al. Cryptococcosis of the colon resembling Crohn's disease in a patient with the hyperimmunoglobulinemia E-recurrent infection (Job's) syndrome. *Gastroenterology* 1988;94:808–812.
39. Jacobs DH, Macher AM, Handler R, et al. Esophageal cryptococcosis in a patient with the hyperimmunoglobulin E-recurrent infection (Job's) syndrome. *Gastroenterology* 1984;87:201–203.
40. Bonacini M, Nussbaum J, Ahluwalia C. Gastrointestinal, hepatic, and pancreatic involvement with *Cryptococcus neoformans* in AIDS. *J Clin Gastroenterol* 1990;12:295–297.
41. Washington K, Gottfried MR, Wilson ML. Gastrointestinal cryptpococcosis. *Mod Pathol* 1991;4:707–711.
42. Dodson TB, Perrott DH, Leonard MS. Nonhealing ulceration of oral mucosa. *J Oral Maxillofac Surg* 1989;47:849–852.
43. Glick M, Cohen SG, Cheney RT, et al. Oral manifestations of disseminated *Cryptococcus neoformans* in a patient with acquired immunodeficiency syndrome. *Oral Surg Oral Med Oral Pathol* 1987;64:454–459.
44. Lynch DP, Naftolin LZ. Oral *Cryptococcus neoformans* infection in AIDS. *Oral Surg Oral Med Oral Pathol* 1987;64:449–453.

45. Van Calck M, Motte S, Rickaert F, et al. Cryptococcal anal ulceration in a patient with AIDS. *Am J Gastroenterol* 1988;83:-1306–1308.
46. Stiefel P, Pamies E, Miranda ML, et al. Cryptococcal peritonitis: report of a case and review of the literature. *Hepatogastroenterology* 1999;46:1618–1622.
47. Yinnon AM, Solages A, Treanor JJ. Cryptococcal peritonitis: report of a case developing during continuous ambulatory peritoneal dialysis and review of the literature. *Clin Infect Dis* 1993;-17:736–741.
48. Goodwin RA, Shapiro JL, Thurman GH, et al. Disseminated histoplasmosis: clinical and pathologic correlations. *Medicine* 1980;59:1–33.
49. Heneghan SJ, Li J, Petrossian E, et al. Intestinal perforation from gastrointestinal histoplasmosis in acquired immunodeficiency syndrome. Case report and review of the literature. *Arch Surg* 1993;128:464–466.
50. Lamps LW, Molina CP, West AB, et al. The pathologic spectrum of gastrointestinal and hepatic histoplasmosis. *Am J Clin Pathol* 2000;113:64–72.
51. Cappell MS, Mandell W, Grimes MM, et al. Gastrointestinal histoplasmosis. *Dig Dis Sci* 1988;33:353–360.
52. Orchard JL, Luparello F, Brunskill D. Malabsorption syndrome occurring in the course of disseminated histoplasmosis. Case report and review of gastrointestinal histoplasmosis. *Am J Med* 1979;66:331–336.
53. Lee SH, Barnes WG, Hodges GR, et al. Perforated granulomatous colitis caused by *Histoplasma capsulatum. Dis Colon Rectum* 1985;28:171–176.
54. Spivak H, Schlasinger MH, Tabanda-Lichauco R, et al. Small bowel obstruction from gastrointestinal histoplasmosis in acquired immune deficiency syndrome. *Am Surg* 1996;62:-369–372.
55. Swindells S, Durham T, Johansson SL, et al. Oral histoplasmosis in a patient infected with HIV. *Oral Surg Oral Med Oral Pathol* 1994;77:126–130.
56. Cohen PR,Grossman ME, Silvers DN. Disseminated histoplasmosis and human immunodeficiency virus infection. *Int J Dermatol* 1991;30:614–622.
57. Oda D, McDougal L, Fritsche T, et al. Oral histoplasmosis as a presenting disease in acquired immunodeficiency syndrome. *Oral Surg Oral Med Oral Pathol* 1990;70:631–636.
58. Cohen PR, Held JL, Grossman ME, et al. Disseminated histoplasmosis presenting as an ulcerated verrucous plaque in a human immunodeficiency virus-infected man. Report of a case possibly involving human-to-human transmission of histoplasmosis. *Int J Dermatol* 1991;30:104–108.
59. Wheat LJ, Kohler RB, Tewari RP. Diagnosis of disseminated histoplasmosis by detection of *Histoplasma capsulatum* antigen in serum and urine specimens. *N Engl J Med* 1986;314:83–88.
60. Khalil M, Iwatt AR, Gugnani HC. African histoplasmosis masquerading as carcinoma of the colon. Report of a case and review of literature. *Dis Colon Rectum* 1989;32:518–520.
61. Sanguino JC, Rodrigues B Baptista A, et al. Focal lesion of African histoplasmosis presenting as a malignant gastric ulcer. *Hepatogastroenterology* 1996;43:771–775.
62. Sposto MR, Scully C, de Almeida OP, et al. Oral paracoccidioidomycosis. A study of 36 South American patients. *Oral Surg Oral Med Oral Pathol* 1993;75:461–465.
63. Peña CE. Deep mycotic infections in Colombia. A clinicopathologic study of 162 cases. *Am J Clin Pathol* 1967;47:505–520.
64. Restrepo A, Robledo M, Gutiérrez F, et al. Paracoccidioidomycosis (South American blastomycosis). A study of 39 cases observed in Medellín, Colombia. *Am J Trop Med Hyg* 1970;19:68–76.
65. de Almeida OP, Jorge J, Scully C, et al. Oral manifestations of paracoccidioidomycosis (South American blastomycosis). *Oral Surg Oral Med Oral Pathol* 1991;72:430–435.
66. Murray HW, Littman ML, Roberts RB. Disseminated paracoccidioidomycosis (South American blastomycosis) in the United States. *Am J Med* 1974;56:209–220.
67. Diaz M, Negroni R, Montero-Gei F, et al. A Pan-American 5-year study of fluconazole therapy for deep mycoses in the immunocompetent host. *Clin Infect Dis* 1992;14[Suppl 1]:-S68–S76.
68. Supparatpinyo K, Khamwan C, Baosoung V, et al. Disseminated *Penicillium marneffei* infection in Southeast Asia. *Lancet* 1994;-344:110–113.
69. Drouhet E. Penicilliosis due to *Penicillium marneffei*: a new emerging systemic mycosis in AIDS patients travelling or living in Southeast Asia. Review of 44 cases reported in HIV infected patients during the last 5 years compared to 44 cases of non AIDS patients reported over 20 years. *J Mycology Medical* 1993;-4:195–224.
70. Ko C, Hung C, Chen M, et al. Endoscopic diagnosis of intestinal penicilliosis marneffei: Report of three cases and review of the literature. *Gastrointest Endosc* 1999;50:111–114.
71. Leung R, Sung JY, Chow J, et al. Unusual cause of fever and diarrhea in a patient with AIDS. *Penicillium marneffei* infection. *Dig Dis Sci* 1996;41:1212–1215.
72. Duong TA. Infection due to *Penicillium marneffei*, an emerging pathogen: review of 155 reported cases. *Clin Infect Dis* 1996;23:-125–130.
73. Ukarapol N, Sirisanthana V, Wongsawasdi L. *Penicillium marneffei* mesenteric lymphadenitis in human immunodeficiency virus-infected children. *J Med Assoc Thai* 1998;81:637–640.
74. Dieterich DT, Lew EA, Bacon DJ, et al. Gastrointestinal pneumocystosis in HIV-infected patients on aerosolized pentamidine: report of five cases and literature review. *Am J Gastroenterol* 1992;87:1763–1770.
75. Yoshida EM, Filipenko D, Phillips P, et al. AIDS-related extrapulmonary *Pneumocystis carinii* infection presenting as a solitary rectal ulcer. *Can J Gastroenterol* 1996;10:401–404.

54

GROUP A ROTAVIRUSES

DORSEY M. BASS
HARRY B. GREENBERG

DESCRIPTION

Introduction and Historical Perspective

Since its discovery as a human pathogen almost 30 years ago, rotavirus has been recognized as an important agent of gastroenteritis in infants. In many studies throughout the world, rotavirus is the single most important cause of dehydrating diarrhea in young children. In the United States alone, rotavirus is estimated to account for $352 million in hospitalization cost (1) and as many as 20 to 40 pediatric deaths per year (2). In the developing world, rotavirus accounts for hundreds of thousands of childhood deaths each year as well as enormous morbidity (3).

Although it had long been known that a filterable agent was responsible for most childhood diarrhea, attempts to isolate such a virus via tissue culture in the 1950s and 1960s were unsuccessful. Rotaviruses had previously been identified by electron microscopy only in mice with diarrhea (4). In 1971, Mebus and co-workers (5) succeeded in isolating and propagating in tissue culture a bovine rotavirus from calves with scours (diarrhea). Bishop and co-workers (6) first described a similar agent in thin sections of duodenal mucosa from a child with acute gastroenteritis in 1973. Although several other animal rotaviruses were tissue culture adapted, it was not until 1980 that the first human strain was successfully passaged in tissue culture (7). Eventually, it was recognized that appropriate quantities of trypsin and the use of serum-free media allowed the tissue culture adaptation of large numbers of rotaviruses.

During the 1980s and 1990s monoclonal antibody (MAB) and recombinant DNA technologies were applied to the study of rotavirus with a rapid increase of our understanding about the virus, its replication cycle, epidemiology, pathogenesis, and the nature of host resistance to rotavirus disease. The later 1990s witnessed increasingly intense interest in rotavirus and particularly in vaccine development. In 1999, the first rotavirus vaccine for human infants was approved in the United States. However, an association with intussusception led to its withdrawal shortly thereafter (8,9). The rapid increase in knowledge about rotaviruses is illustrated by a review, which listed more than 990 references (10). A Medline search for rotavirus citations since the last edition of this text in 1995 found more than 1,000 additional references

Virus Structure and Physicochemical Properties

Rotaviruses are members of the Reoviridae family and consist of a three-layered protein capsid encasing a segmented double-stranded RNA (dsRNA) genome. The complete virion observed with standard negative staining by electron microscopy has a distinct appearance, resembling a short-spoked wheel. The name rotavirus (*rota,* Latin for wheel) is derived from this appearance (11). The particle size is measured as approximately 70 nM by negative stained electron microscopy and 100 nM by cryoelectron microscopy. The outer capsid has icosahedral symmetry with T = 13 (12). The outer shell of the capsid consists of two viral proteins, VP7 and VP4, which form 132 capsomeres. The inner shell consists of trimerized VP6. A core shell of rotavirus consists largely of viral proteins VP2, VP1, and VP3.

Current understanding of the three-dimensional structure of the rotavirus particle has been greatly enhanced by the technique of cryoelectron microscopy with computer-assisted image enhancement (13–16). These studies have shown that the surface of rotavirus particles has 60 spike-like projections 10 nm in length, consisting of the VP4 protein, whereas the smooth outer capsid surface is made up of VP7. This smooth surface is perforated by 132 aqueous channels (Fig. 54.1), which penetrate the virion to reach the viral core through which nascent RNA chains have been observed to protrude (17).

D. M. Bass: Department of Pediatrics, Stanford University, Stanford, California

H. B. Greenberg: Departments of Medicine and Microbiology and Immunology, Stanford University School of Medicine, Stanford, California; VA Palo Alto, Health Care System, Palo Alto, California

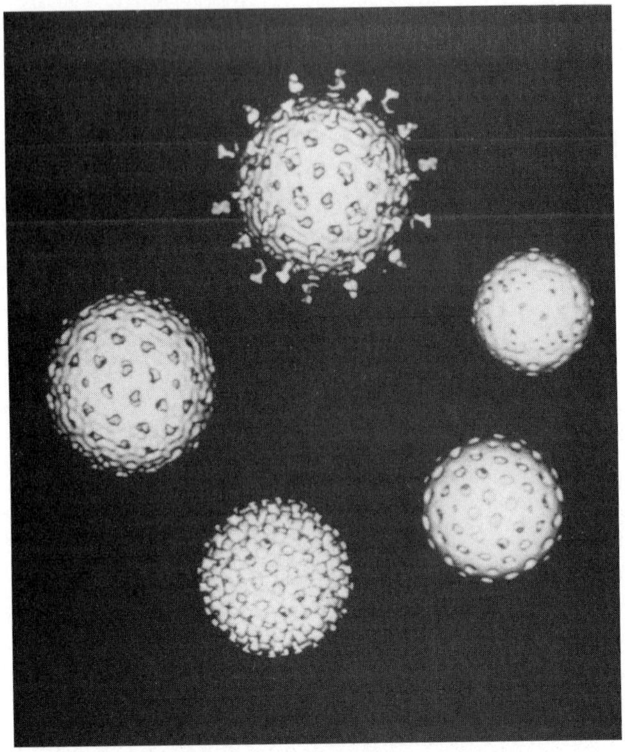

FIGURE 54.1. Three-dimensional structure of rhesus monkey rotavirus by cryoelectron microscopy. The structures are as follows: counterclockwise from the top: (a) complete double-shelled, infectious particle with 60 surface spikes consisting of VP4; (b) the smooth outer surface, attributed to VP7, with the perforating aqueous channels; (c) the inner capsid consisting of VP6 trimers; (d) the VP6 trimers merge with a smooth inner capsid shell that is perforated by channels in register with those in the outer capsid; (e) a third protein shell, the core, made up of VP1, VP2, and VP3, which contains the double-stranded, segmented RNA genome. (Courtesy of Dr. M. Yeager.)

The three forms of rotavirus particle (triple-shelled, double-shelled, and cores) can be observed readily in stool samples and tissue culture supernatants. Of the three, only triple-shelled particles are infectious under normal conditions (18). The outer capsid of triple-shelled particles may be released from the particle by calcium chelation with ethylenediamine-tetraacetic acid (EDTA) or ethyleneglycol-tetraacetic acid (EGTA) (19,20). The resultant double-shelled particles, which are transcriptionally active, may be converted to core particles by treatment with chaotropic agents. Double-shelled particles can be reconstituted to triple-shelled particles in the presence of VP7, VP4, and appropriate free calcium ion (21).

Infectious rotavirus particles (triple-shelled) have a density of 1.36 g/cm^3 in cesium chloride gradients and sediment at 520 to 530 S in sucrose. Double-shelled (noninfectious) particles have a density of 1.38 g/cm^3 and sediment at approximately 390 S. Core particles have a density of 1.44 g/cm^3 and sediment at 280 S.

Infectious triple-shelled rotavirus particles are relatively stable under a variety of environmental conditions. They are resistant to fluorocarbons, ether, chloroform, and nonionic detergents, reflecting the lack of a lipid membrane on the virion (20). Infectivity is maintained in the pH range of 4 to 9. At high pH, VP4 is selectively lost from the virion (22), whereas very low pH results in disassociation of the entire particle (23,24). Rotaviruses remain infectious for months at room temperature but repeated freezing and thawing does decrease titers. Sodium dodecyl sulfate destroys infectivity, presumably by disrupting the capsid structure. Other disinfectants that are effective against rotavirus include 95% ethanol, phenols, chlorine, and formalin (25–29).

MICROBIOLOGY

Rotavirus Classification

Rotaviruses are classified by group, subgroup, and serotype. Viruses are identified as rotaviruses by their characteristic size and morphology and by the presence of 11 double strands of RNA in their genome. The distinct groups of rotaviruses designated A, B, and C bear little or no immunologic relationship with each other and on a genomic basis share only limited homology. The group antigen is VP6, the major inner capsid protein. Most of the commercial rotavirus stool immunoassays are based on this antigen and therefore detect only group A rotaviruses. This chapter discusses only group A rotaviruses, which are the most common cause of severe watery diarrhea in infancy and early childhood. Group B and C rotaviruses are discussed in Chapter 55.

Subgroup specificity of group A rotaviruses is based on antigenic characteristics of the inner capsid protein VP6 (30). MABs can be used in an enzyme-linked immunoadsorbent assay (ELISA) to distinguish samples as either subgroup I or II (31). A small percentage of samples are not typeable or contain both subgroup I and II reactivities. With few exceptions, all human subgroup I rotaviruses belong to G serotype 2, whereas most subgroup II strains may belong to G serotypes 1, 3, 4, or 9 (32).

Rotavirus serotypes were first identified based on classic cross-neutralization studies using sera from animals hyperimmunized with purified rotaviruses. More than 12 rotavirus serotypes have been identified. Of these, only serotypes 1 through 4 and 9 are thought to be epidemiologically important human pathogens in most areas of the world. Genetic studies have identified the viral gene encoding VP7 as the primary determinant of serotype (25). The development of anti-VP7 MABs with serotype specificity allowed workers to determine the serotypes of large numbers of rotaviruses in prospective and retrospective studies (33–38). Rotavirus serotypes can also be identified on the basis of nucleic acid sequence as determined by polymerase chain reaction (PCR) based techniques. Because of the increased sensitivity of such techniques, these methods have become widely used (39–44).

A newer approach to classifying rotavirus serotypes is currently used. The previously described VP7-based serotypes are currently referred to as G types (for glycoprotein as in VP7). Because it is known that the other major outer capsid protein, VP4, also contains neutralizing epitopes, it has been proposed that rotaviruses also be categorized according to VP4 amino acid similarity into P types (45–48). The P represents the "protease" sensitivity of VP4. To date, four major P types for human viruses have been described but only two are frequently encountered. As noted, most of the P typing has been based on deduced amino acid sequence rather than serologic analysis. It is unclear whether immune responses to these different P or G types are significant predictors of protection from disease.

Genome Structure, Protein Coding Assignments, and Rotavirus Protein Function

Genome Structure

The rotavirus genome consists of 11 segments of dsRNA, which range in molecular weight from 2×10^5 to 2.2×10^6 d (49). With one exception (gene 11) (50), the segments encode one polypeptide each. The segmented genome is significant in two regards. First, the genomic RNA segments can be resolved on polyacrylamide gels relatively easily. The pattern of the segments (known as the *electropherotype*) is variable among rotaviruses and has been used as a marker for rotavirus strain variation in epidemiologic studies. The second important feature of the segmented genome is that it facilitates the development of reassortant viruses when cells are co-infected with different rotavirus strains. Because the source of individual RNA segments in progeny viruses from such "matings" can be identified either by migration on polyacrylamide gel electrophoresis (PAGE) or by hybridization, reassortant viruses have proved to be a powerful genetic tool for assigning phenotypic characteristics such as virulence, growth in tissue culture, or hemagglutination to specific rotavirus genes. Reassortant rotaviruses have also played an important role in rotavirus vaccine strategy. Reassortment occurs in nature as well and plays a role in rotavirus strain variations.

The nucleotide sequences of all 11 of the rotavirus RNA segments have been determined. Each RNA segment begins at the 5′ end with a guanidine followed by conserved noncoding sequences (51,52). The noncoding sequences are followed by the sequences encoding the protein, which terminate with a stop codon. The 3′ end consists of another set of noncoding sequences without polyadenylation. These noncoding regions on the 5′ and 3′ ends of the RNA segments contain cis-acting replication signals that are conserved on all 11 gene segments (53). The dsRNA segments are completely base paired and the 5" end of the positive strand contains a cap structure similar to that found in other members of the Reoviridae family.

Rotavirus Protein Coding Assignments and Protein Function

The coding assignments and properties of rotavirus proteins have been determined by *in vitro* translation of viral RNA, immunologic analyses with MABs, expression of rotaviral proteins via recombinant DNA, and the study of reassortant viruses (30,54–58). Table 54.1 lists the genome segments and protein products for simian SA11 virus. Both the gene segments and structural proteins are numbered from the slowest migrating on PAGE to the fastest. RNA segments 7, 8, and 9 are usually closely grouped on PAGE and the proteins encoded by these three segments may vary by rotavirus strain. Cognate RNA segments may be identified by hybridization or direct sequence analysis. In papers published before 1988, when the core protein VP3 was identified, the viral hemagglutinin (now known as VP4) was referred to as VP3.

The rotavirus inner core proteins (VP1, VP2, VP3) are the products of gene segments 1, 2, and 3, respectively. Collectively, the three proteins function as the transcriptional machinery of the virus. VP2 expressed in a baculovirus system spontaneously forms core-like particles (59). VP2 has also been shown to be an RNA-binding protein (60). VP1 has been shown to have RNA polymerase activity (61) and VP3 to have guanylyltransferase activity necessary for RNA replicase activity (62). VP6 forms the inner capsid of the virus and accounts for approximately 50% of the total virion protein. The VP6 protein is hydrophobic and spontaneously forms trimers and higher order multimers (63,64). When VP6 is coexpressed with VP2 in a baculovirus system, particles similar to native rotavirus single-shelled particles spontaneously assemble (59). VP6 is the group and subgroup antigen as noted earlier and the protein is highly immunogenic. Antibodies directed against VP6 do not have neutralization activity *in vitro* although they have been shown to protect *in vivo* in some animal models (65–67).

VP4 is one of the two outer capsid proteins of rotavirus and constitutes the spike-like projections noted in cryoelectron microscopic photographs. Genetic and biochemical studies have shown that it functions as the viral hemagglutinin (68,69), mediates permissivity for tissue culture growth and protease-enhanced plaque formation (30), and is a determinant of virulence of rotaviruses in mice (70). Both its structural role in the rotavirus particle (71) and studies employing MABs (72) have suggested that VP4 may function as the rotavirus viral attachment protein, mediating binding to target cells. Cleavage of VP4 by trypsin results in enhanced infectivity of rotaviruses, probably by facilitating membrane penetration (73). The cleavage products known as VP5* (approximately 60 kd) and VP8*

TABLE 54.1. ROTAVIRUS PROTEINS

Genome Segment	Protein	Molecular Weight	Modification	Location in Virion	Function	Percent Capsid Protein	Function
1	VP1	125,000			Core	2	RNA polymerase
2	VP2	94,000			Core	15	RNA binding
3	VP3	88,000			Core	0.5	Guanyl transferase
4	VP4	88,000	Extracellular trypsin cleavage to VP5* and VP8*		Outer capsid	1.5	Hemagglutinin, membrane penetration, cell attachment protein
5	NSVP1 [NS53]	58,700				Nonstructural	Zinc finger, RNA binding
6	VP6	44,800			Inner capsid	51	Hydrophobic trimer, group and subgroup antigen
7	NSVP2 [NS34]	34,600				Nonstructural	RNA binding
8	NSVP3 [NS35]	36,700				Nonstructural	RNA binding
9	VP7	33,900	High mannose glycosylation, endoplasmic reticulum (ER) retention		Outer capsid	30	Major outer capsid structure, neutralization
10	NSVP4 [NS28]	28,000	High mannose glycosylation, ER retention			Nonstructural	"Receptor" for single-shelled particles on surface of ER membrane. Enterotoxin?
11	NSVP5 [NS26]	26,000	Phosphorylated and O-glycosylation, two open reading frames			Nonstructural	??

(approximately 28 kd) remain virion associated (74). The trypsin cleavage sites for SA11 rotavirus have been shown to be at amino acids 241 and 247 with 247 being the preferred site (75). Studies using recombinant virus-like particles have shown that only the cleavage at amino acid 247 is necessary for activation (76). These sites are conserved in all rotavirus strains although some human strains have a third upstream cleavage site (77,78). Unlike in ortho- and paramyxoviruses, the trypsin cleavage does not expose a new hydrophobic amino terminus. The cleavage may allow a conformational change to occur, exposing amino acids 384 to 401 of VP5*, which share homology with alpha virus fusion proteins (79). VP4 is immunogenic and contains strain-specific neutralization antigens in the VP8* portion and cross-reactive neutralization regions in the VP5* portion (79).

VP7 is an outer capsid glycoprotein, which constitutes the smooth portion of the outer capsid, beneath the VP4 spikes. Approximately 30% of the virion protein is VP7. VP7 is the primary determinant of rotavirus serotype as measured by cross-neutralization studies (30). The importance of VP7 as a neutralization antigen and its unique cell biology as a model glycoprotein have led to intense study of this protein and its intracellular processing. The nucleotide sequence of VP7 predicts an open reading frame of 326 amino acids with two in-frame start codons separated by 30 codons (80). The initiation codons are followed by two stretches of hydrophobic amino acids, either of which may serve as signal sequences to direct the nascent peptide into the endoplasmic reticulum (ER) (81–83). These sequences are cleaved at amino acid 51. VP7 is retained in the ER until assembled onto complete virions and is not transported to the Golgi or the cell surface. Two sets of amino-terminal amino acids have been shown to be responsible for this retention (84). The protein is apparently an integral protein in the ER membrane with a luminal orientation (85). Glycosylation is of the high mannose type and VP7 from various rotavirus strains has one to three potential glycosylation sites although no more than two are apparently used (86,87).

During rotavirus infection at least five nonstructural proteins (NSPs) are produced. Although not components of purified, fully infectious, double-shelled rotavirus particles, these proteins undoubtedly play essential roles in virion replication and morphogenesis. Perhaps the best studied is NSP4 (segment 10), which is a 28-kd transmembrane ER glycoprotein that has been proposed as a receptor for single-shelled particles as they bud through the ER membrane (88–91). NSP4 has also been implicated as a possible viral enterotoxin (see "Pathogenesis") (92). NSP1 (RNA segment 5), NSP2 (RNA segment 7), and NSP3 (RNA segment 8) bind RNA and have been associated with intermediate replicase particles (93,94). NSP3 has been shown to bind specifically to the 3" untranslated sequences in rotavirus messenger RNAs (mRNAs) (95). NSP3 inhibits host cell translation by interaction with the mammalian translation initiation factor elF4GI (96). This interaction in which NSP3 replaces the poly A binding protein also enhances the efficiency of rotavirus mRNA translation (97). In genetic studies, NSP1 has been linked to virulence in the murine model of rotavirus disease (98), whereas in other studies, NSP4 has been linked to virulence in porcine viruses (99). NSP5, the multimeric product of the eleventh gene is both phosphorylated and O-glycosylated (50). Its role in replication is unknown.

Viral Replication Cycle

Rotavirus replication has been studied extensively in tissue culture systems. Important features of the replicative cycle are that (a) replication is strictly cytoplasmic; (b) the viral particle contains enzymatic machinery to transcribe the dsRNA genome; (c) initial +RNA transcripts serve as both mRNA for peptide synthesis and as templates for negative strand synthesis; (d) newly synthesized dsRNA strands associate with viral peptides to form subviral particles, which gain their outer capsid by budding through the ER with a transient enveloped stage; and (e) progeny virions are released mainly, but not exclusively, by cell lysis.

Cell Attachment

The process of target cell binding by viruses is a critical step in viral pathogenesis and can be an important determinant of cellular and host susceptibility to infection. Viral attachment may be a primary determinant of cell and tissue tropism and host range. There are two obvious components to the virus-cell interaction: a viral structure that serves as a ligand (viral attachment protein, or VAP) and a cellular receptor. Most studies have used tissue culture conditions to examine this interaction but they may be relevant to *in vivo* conditions. Studies have shown that only triple-shelled particles attach to cells and that neither proteolytic activation by cleavage of the VP4 outer capsid protein (100,101) nor glycosylation of VP7 (102) is required for attachment. The demonstration by immunocryoelectron microscopy that the outer capsid protein VP4 forms spike-like projections on the rotavirus particle has led to speculation that VP4 is the viral attachment protein (71). Recent studies of the mechanism by which MABs neutralize rotavirus demonstrated that antibodies against the smaller trypsin fragment of rhesus rotavirus VP4 (VP8*), but not the other major surface protein, VP7, neutralize virus by inhibition of binding to target cells (72). Previous studies had shown that a 35-kd rotavirus protein bound to target cells (100,103). Although initially thought to be VP7, this cell-binding viral protein was later shown to be NSP2, which is not thought to be present in mature virus particles (104). More recently, genetic mapping studies have identified VP4 as the rotavirus cell attachment protein (105). Furthermore, studies with variant animal rotaviruses and expressed recombinant rotavirus proteins have shown that the VP5* portion of VP4 may mediate cell attachment in a carbohydrate-independent fashion (106,107). It is possible that no single protein functions as the cell attachment protein but that a structure composed of components of several outer capsid proteins serves this purpose as has been shown for poliovirus and the rhinoviruses (108).

Studies on cellular receptors for rotavirus have shown that simian SA11 rotavirus binding to MA104 cells is saturable (approximately 13,000 binding sites per cell), sodium dependent, relatively pH independent, and sensitive to neuraminidase (101). Sialic acid–containing compounds such as fetuin and mucin inhibit binding of SA11 rotavirus to tissue culture cells (101,109). However, similar studies on human viruses have shown that virus attachment to cells and subsequent infection bear no relation to sialic acid (110,111). Large-molecular-weight, highly glycosylated surface proteins isolated from suckling murine enterocytes have been shown to specifically bind rhesus rotavirus in a sialic acid–dependent fashion (112). Other studies have suggested that sialic acid–containing gangliosides (113,114) or asialogangliosides (115) may function as rotavirus receptors. In another approach, sequence similarity to integrin ligands was noted in both VP4 and VP7, and appropriate peptides were found to inhibit rotavirus infectivity (116). Another recent report describes an MAB directed against cell surface proteins of molecular weights 220, 55, 47 KD which inhibits infection of cells by a variety of rotaviruses (117). Further studies in this area are needed to determine the nature and role of receptors in rotavirus pathogenesis and tissue tropism.

Penetration

After binding to an appropriate target cell, the viral genome must then be introduced into the cytoplasm in order for viral replication to proceed. Rotavirus entry is blocked at 4 degrees as a result of either a block in endocytosis or decreased fluidity of the cellular plasma membrane. The mechanism of penetration is not well understood. Trypsin cleavage of VP4 facilitates the entry of infectious virus, possibly unmasking fusogenic domains, which allow penetration through the lipid membrane. Indeed, recombinant expressed VP5* has been shown to permeabilize artificial liposomes (118), an effect that is lost if the putative fusogenic domain has been altered (119). Similarly, recombinant VP7 has been shown to permeabilize liposomes (120), suggesting that both outer capsid protein may play a role in this process. An *in vitro* assay of rotavirus-induced "fusion from without" has been used to demonstrate that trypsin treatment and both VP7 and VP4 are necessary for disruption of cellular membranes (76,121). These findings were replicated by others using an assay employing coentry of alpha sarcin with viral particles (122).

Early ultrastructural studies suggested that rotavirus enters cells via endocytosis and that the viral particles were transported to lysosome-like structures (123). Some studies have shown clear evidence of viral entry via coated pits and vesicles, indicating that receptor-mediated endocytosis is the major route of rotavirus entry (124). Other ultrastructural studies of a human rotavirus strain suggested that treatment of rotavirus with trypsin allowed the virus to directly penetrate the plasma membrane in a fashion analogous to bacteriophage injection of nucleic acid into bacteria (125,126). Virus that had not been treated with trypsin entered cells by endocytosis. Other studies have shown that endocytosis is a nonproductive pathway for rotavirus in cultured cells (127). It is clear from a number of studies that, unlike many viruses, rotavirus does not require acidification of endosomes for productive infection (73,124,128). Kinetic studies of the rate of entry of trypsin treated (infectious) versus untreated (noninfectious) rotavirus have supported the direct entry hypothesis (73). Other studies have shown that penetration of target cell plasma membrane is the restrictive step in some tissue culture cells that are resistant to rotavirus infection (129). Virus binds these nonpermissive cells to a comparable level to permissive cells and is efficiently internalized, but the internalized virus fails to uncoat and enter the eclipse phase. If intact rotavirus particles are transfected into nonpermissive cells via cationic liposomes, full viral replication ensues.

Uncoating

After penetration of the host cell plasma membrane, the infecting rotavirus must activate its RNA polymerase to begin replicating. *In vitro* this may be accomplished by the use of chelating agents such as EDTA, which remove the outer capsid of the virus and activate polymerase activity (19). It is thought that the low calcium concentration in the intracellular cytoplasmic microenvironment induces similar events (124).

Transcription and Translation

As noted earlier, the initiation of transcription is thought to be simultaneous with uncoating. The mechanism and precise cytoplasmic location of transcriptional activation is not known. Exquisite cryoelectron microscopic /biochemical structure-function studies suggest that the outer capsid serves as a barrier to the free movement of RNA templates past an active catalytic site (15). All initial transcripts are positive sense, full-length, single-stranded RNA (ssRNA) molecules derived from the parental strands and require adenosine triphosphate (ATP) for their synthesis (130). The positive sense RNA transcripts may then serve as templates for translation, using cellular free ribosomes for most of the rotavirus proteins or function as templates for negative sense RNA synthesis (131). Newly synthesized negative RNA strands are immediately associated with complementary positive strands within nascent subviral particles, which have been termed *replicase particles* (93). The formation of these single-shelled particles occurs in cytoplasmic electron-dense bodies referred to as *viroplasm* (132). Recent evidence suggests that NSP3 interacts with eukaryotic translation initiating factor elF4G to promote efficient translation of rotavirus mRNA (97).

Even though little is known about the mechanism of rotavirus capsid assembly in mammalian cells, it is known that baculovirus-expressed VP2 spontaneously forms core-like particles (59). Baculovirus-expressed VP6 self-assembles into oligomeric structures similar to single-shelled particles (63). Coexpression of VP2, VP6, and VP7 with or without VP4 leads to the spontaneous assembly of particles similar to triple-shelled particles (133). During rotavirus infection of mammalian cells, the two viral glycoproteins, VP7 and NS28, are synthesized in ribosomes associated with the ER and are cotranslationally inserted into the ER membrane as a result of hydrophobic amino acid signal sequences (85). Here they undergo N-linked glycosylation. The single-shelled particles then bind to the ER membrane via NS28 and bud through the ER, presumably gaining the outer capsid protein VP7 in the process. By an unknown mechanism, the particles lose their transiently acquired envelope within the ER cisternae.

The infectious cycle ends with cell lysis and release of the progeny virions. *In vitro*, some virus may be actively transported via vesicles to the cell surface before cell death (134). A significant portion of released virus remains associated with cell debris, suggesting a possible role for the cellular cytoskeleton in virus assembly or transport (135). *In vivo* the virus is released into the intestinal lumen, where it may infect other villous enterocytes.

Effects on Host Cells

As noted earlier, rotavirus is a lytic virus and infection ultimately results in death of the host cell. Observed cytopathic effects include cytoplasmic vacuolization and small cytoplasmic inclusions. Biochemical studies have shown that host protein synthesis is shut down by 4 hours (136). Other studies have shown host DNA and RNA synthesis is greatly reduced (137). It is unknown whether specific rotavirus gene products are responsible for these alterations in cellular metabolism. As noted earlier, NSP3 has been shown to inhibit host translation and NSP4 expression is associated with large cytotoxic shifts in intracellular calcium levels. Early events in rotavirus infection activate a variety of cell signaling cascades, leading to secretion of chemokines such as interleukin 8 (138). The role of this secretion in pathogenesis remains to be elucidated. As early as 4 hours after infection, infected cell membranes become increasingly permeable to calcium, sodium, and potasium (139). In certain tissue culture conditions, nonlytic persistent infections have been established (140,141). These infections could be relevant to the occasional persistent infection in immunocompromised children (142–144).

EPIDEMIOLOGY

Rotaviruses are ubiquitous and infect almost all mammalian species throughout the world. Although rotavirus may infect humans or other mammals at any age, rotavirus disease occurs mainly in the very young. The burden of rotavirus diarrhea in both the developed and developing worlds is staggering. In a recent analysis it was estimated that each year more than 125 million children in developing countries contract rotavirus gastroenteritis, with 18 million severe cases resulting in an estimated 873,000 deaths (3,110). In the United States alone, 1 to 3 million cases per year are estimated to occur with an estimated hospital expenditure in excess of $300 million (1). The costs of outpatient therapy and lost parental productivity would greatly increase the cost estimate (145). Rotavirus diarrhea accounts for an estimated 20 to 40 childhood deaths per year in the United States (2). Although rotaviruses are not always found to be the most common cause of diarrhea among children, they are usually the most common cause of severe, dehydrating disease requiring inpatient therapy. In 8 years, 34.5% of infants admitted to a Washington, DC, hospital for diarrhea had rotavirus infections (146). Similarly, in Bangladesh, rotavirus was detected in less than 4% of all pediatric diarrheal episodes but was associated with 39% of all diarrhea cases with significant dehydration (147).

Age

Greater than 90% of children have antibody directed against rotavirus by 3 years of age. In most studies, the peak incidence of rotavirus diarrhea is between 6 and 24 months of age, although recent studies from the developing world suggest that rotavirus can be an important pathogen in infants younger than 6 months of age (148), a finding that has significant implications for vaccine strategy. Most rotavirus infections in older children and adults produce minimal to no symptoms, possibly because of the acquisition of immunity. Paradoxically, neonates younger than 1 month of age often exhibit minimal symptoms with rotavirus infection. This finding may be partially explained by preexisting maternal-derived immunity or the presence in some hospital nurseries of apparently attenuated rotavirus strains (149). It has been suggested that certain sequence variations in the VP4 protein of these strains may account for their attenuation (78), but other studies have cast doubt on this hypothesis.

Region and Seasons

Like any other fecal-oral transmitted pathogen, rotavirus spreads most easily under conditions of overcrowding and poor hygiene. Thus, children in developing countries and those in crowded day care centers may be exposed to the virus many times in infancy, with many of the infections being asymptomatic. In the developed world, waves of rotavirus infection occur in regular seasonal patterns with peaks of symptomatic infection occurring in the cooler winter months (146,150). In the United States, it appears that the peak incidence of rotavirus disease begins in the fall in the Southwest and spreads eastward so that by late winter and spring, infection peaks in the Northeast (151,152). This wave of infection, however, does not represent the spread of a single strain or group of rotavirus strains as observed during influenza epidemics. The seasonality of rotavirus infection is less appreciable in tropical countries.

Serotype

In many communities, a variety of human rotavirus strains are in circulation at any one time. The strains vary by both electropherotype and serotype. Often a particular strain is predominant for 1 or 2 years before a new dominant strain emerges, perhaps as a result of immune selection. It may be that the strain diversity is most pronounced in the developing world. In a study of rotavirus isolates from rural Bangladesh during 1 year, a remarkable diversity of electropherotypically distinct strains distributed throughout the four major serotypes was observed (153). Recently, a number of reports have identified serotype G9 rotaviruses in human diarrheal stools in significant frequency in a variety of locations ranging from Philadelphia to India to Japan (154–156). It is unclear whether the emergence of these previously rare serotypes is due to increasing global surveillance using more sensitive methods such as PCR-based assays (42). The finding of these typically bovine serotypes in humans suggests that animal rotaviruses are being transmitted to humans. In a study of cattle ranchers in Panama, no evidence of cross-infection between humans and cattle could be detected (157). On the other hand, widespread asymptomatic neonatal infection with a bovine-like strain has been observed in India (158,159). The basis of the host species specificity of rotavirus strain is not known. Likewise, the epidemiologic significance of reassortment events between human and animal rotaviruses, which may occur occasionally *in vivo,* is not known. With the advent of effective rotavirus vaccines, it is important to monitor the prevalence of diverse rotavirus serotypes in various geographic areas.

The precise relationship of rotavirus serotype (both P and G types) to protective immunity is a topic of some controversy. Although the total number of distinct P and G types in humans is large, the majority of isolates fall into five G types and two P types. Most children appear to undergo only one or two significant symptomatic rotavirus infections during childhood, so it is likely that some form of heterotypic immunity develops after initial infection (160).

Transmission

Most evidence suggests that rotaviruses are transmitted by the fecal-oral route. Although respiratory transmission has been suggested, no convincing evidence supports this mechanism. Under appropriate circumstances, as little as one infectious particle can initiate disease in animal models (98,161). During rotavirus infection, large numbers of viral particles are shed in the stool. The high environmental stability of rotavirus, the low infectious dose, and the large number of virions passed during infection seem to guarantee the observed infection of virtually all children as well as occurrence of large nosocomial and day care outbreaks.

PATHOGENESIS

Rotavirus is a lytic virus and probably causes diarrhea primarily by destruction of intestinal villous epithelial cells. A number of studies of experimentally infected animals have demonstrated both morphologic and biochemical changes in the rotavirus-infected small intestine.

The pathology of the small intestine in acute viral gastroenteritis has been described in a variety of species infected naturally or experimentally with a variety of viral agents (5,162–166). Human studies have been more limited but demonstrate similar features (6,166–169). Generally, the pathology of acute viral enteritis is characterized by variable shortening of the villi, a moderate round cell infiltrate in the lamina propria, and elongation of crypts (Fig. 54.2). Early in the infection, vacuolization and shedding of enterocytes from the apical portion of villi may be observed. Lesions are often patchy in nature and symptoms may occur in the absence of a lesion demonstrable by light microscopy. In a study of 40 infants with acute rotavirus gastroenteritis, only two had definitely abnormal duodenal biopsies (169); the more distal intestine is not accessible in human infants with rotavirus disease.

A critical concept in the pathogenesis of rotavirus disease is that of cell and tissue tropism. Although occasional reports have described rotavirus antigen in the upper respiratory tract (170,171) or central nervous system (172), under normal circumstances, rotavirus infects only the epithelium of the small intestine. Hepatic infection has been described in immunocompromised hosts and under certain experimental conditions in mice, but it does not appear to be clinically important in human disease (173–175). A single report described renal and hepatic rotavirus infection in several severely immunocompromised children (176). Low levels of colonic infection may occur but are not important in the pathophysiology of rotavirus disease. Within the small intestine, rotavirus selectively infects enterocytes on the upper villi, sparing the crypt cells. Chronologically, it seems that the proximal small intestine is initially infected with subsequent spread to the distal bowel. The strongest immunofluorescence of the infected apical villous enterocytes in the proximal small bowel precedes the onset of diarrhea.

In the most generally accepted view of rotavirus diarrhea pathophysiology, the lytic infection of large numbers of highly differentiated absorptive villous enterocytes and sparing of undifferentiated crypt cells results in both (a) loss of absorptive capacity for water and sodium without impairment of crypt cell secretion and (b) loss of brush border hydrolase activity (e.g., lactase). Morphologic and biochemical studies of experimentally infected animals provide evidence to support this view.

Time course studies of histopathologic changes in experimentally infected animals have shown that, in the early hours after rotavirus or coronavirus infection, villous cells in the proximal small intestine are infected and produce viral antigen, followed by infection of the distal intestine (5,163). The

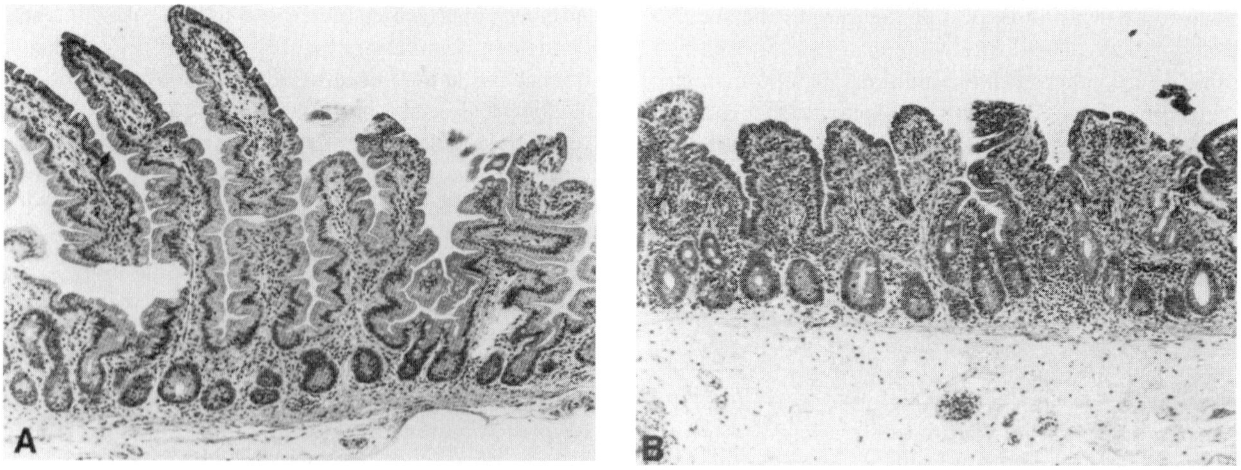

FIGURE 54.2. **A:** Normal jejunal biopsy from a volunteer before experimental infection with Norwalk virus (×100). **B:** Jejunal biopsy from the same volunteer after experimental infection with Norwalk virus, showing shortened villi and increased lymphoid cell infiltrate (×100). (From Bass DM, Baylor M, Chen C, et al. Dansylcadaverine and cytochalasin D enhance rotavirus infection of murine L cells. *Virology* 1995;212:429–437, with permission.)

infected cells become vacuolated, often containing abnormal collections of lipid-like material in their cytoplasm (177). Ultimately, the infected cells are sloughed into the intestinal lumen. It is only at this point that serious diarrhea appears. Thus, relatively little intestinal epithelial viral antigen may be demonstrable after the onset of symptoms. Some observers have noted biphasic production of infectious rotavirus, with peaks of recovered virus occurring at 2 and 4 days after inoculation of suckling mice (178). The uninfected crypt cells are stimulated by the injury to proliferate rapidly to replace the shed villous cells. These replacement cells may appear cuboidal, with poorly developed microvilli. The increased migration rate of these crypt epithelial cells is reflected in strikingly shortened cell replacement times for villi. In one study of piglets with viral enteritis, this replacement time was reduced from 11 to 2 days (179). Age-related differences in susceptibility to viral diarrhea may be related to the normally longer replacement and maturation times for villous enterocytes in young mammals than in older animals. For example, the normal life span of an enterocyte as it migrates from the crypt to a villus tip in a newborn pig is 7 to 10 days, whereas, by 3 weeks of age, the same journey requires only 3 days (180,181).

Biochemical correlates of this pattern of destruction of differentiated villus epithelium and its subsequent replacement by relatively undifferentiated cryptlike epithelium have been demonstrated (166,182–185). Levels of brush border enzymes characteristic of differentiated cells such as sucrase, alkaline phosphatase, and lactase are decreased in most studies. Sodium-coupled glucose transport and sodium-potassium ATPase are likewise reduced, whereas markers for proliferative crypt cells, such as thymidine kinase, are increased in the intestinal epithelia of animals with viral gastroenteritis. Thus, normal absorptive processes are lost and the inherent secretory capacity of the cryptlike epithelium results in excessive losses of water and salts into the gut lumen. The loss of brush border hydrolases complicates the situation as the osmotic load of undigested nutrients draws yet more fluid into the lumen (166,184). The marked reduction in glucose-coupled sodium transport might theoretically diminish the efficacy of oral rehydration solutions (ORSs) originally designed for treatment of cholera, but in actual clinical practice this does not seem to be a problem (186).

Other models for the mechanism of diarrhea associated with viral gastroenteritis have been proposed. One group of investigators has proposed that initial viral infection of a small number of enterocytes leads to release of an unidentified vasoactive agent that induces local intestinal ischemia resulting in damage to villous enterocytes (163). In subsequent studies, these investigators have observed alternating ischemic and hyperemic phases of villous circulation during rotavirus gastroenteritis, which they hypothesize are important in the imbalance between water absorption and secretion during rotaviral diarrhea in the mouse (187–189). They have also hypothesized that rapidly proliferating crypt cells may have pleomorphic junctional complexes, with resultant abnormal paracellular fluxes of salt and water (183). When mice are infected with very high doses of certain rotavirus strains from other species, diarrhea may occur with minimal evidence for productive viral replication (190,191). To date, there has been no evidence for any traditional toxin-like activity in viral gastroenteritis. Levels of adenylate and guanylate cyclases have been normal in experimental viral gastroenteritis (183–185).

Recently, the notion that the rotavirus NSP4 may function as a novel enterotoxin has been proposed (192,193). Recombinant expressed NSP4 (or a peptide derived from it) was reported to cause age-dependent diarrhea when injected into suckling mice. Physiologic *in vitro* studies show that exogenous NSP4 can mobilize intracellular calcium via a phospholipase C–inositol pathway (194). Some studies have correlated changes in deduced amino acid sequences of NSP4 with virulence in some rotaviruses (195), but in other analyses, such changes did not correlate with virulence *in vivo* (196). To date, *in vivo* intestinal secretion in response to NSP4 has been demonstrated only in mice, and some investigators have not been able to duplicate results found with the NSP4-derived peptide (196). The significance of this potential pathogenic mechanism requires further studies. NSP4 is cytotoxic to cells when expressed in the absence of other rotavirus proteins and may thus be very important in mediating intestinal cell death during the viral infection (197,198). Other recent studies have implicated activation of nerves in the gut in pathogenesis of fluid secretion during rotavirus diarrhea (199).

Some endogenous cytokines such as tumor necrosis factor and interleukin-6 have been found to be normal in rotavirus-infected intestine (200). Systemic interferon levels in children hospitalized with rotavirus gastroenteritis have been noted to be elevated during the first few days of illness (201,202). Curiously, although both types I and II interferons inhibit rotavirus infection in tissue culture (203), neither is effective in treating or preventing disease in suckling mice (204).

A number of studies have demonstrated increased small intestinal permeability to macromolecules during rotavirus gastroenteritis (205–209). It has been proposed that this decrease in mucosal barrier function may lead to abnormal host immune responses to luminal antigens such as the development of food allergy (210,211).

IMMUNITY AND HOST RESISTANCE

Many studies have investigated the immune response to rotavirus in experimental animals and in humans. Several studies have used viral reassortants and MABs to show that antibodies directed against VP4 and VP7 can neutralize rotaviruses in *in vitro* assays and protect animals from disease (reviewed in reference 212). Neutralizing antibodies against VP7 are generally serotype specific, whereas those directed against the VP5* portion of VP4 are able to neutralize a broad range of rotaviruses. Several studies have suggested that mucosal antibody protection is much more efficacious than serum antibody in preventing symptomatic disease (213–215). Measurements of both serum and intestinal antibody levels have been only fair predictors of susceptibility to rotavirus disease (216,217). Rotavirus does elicit a cytotoxic T-cell response (218–223), and passive transfer of these cells can prevent or clear rotavirus infection in both normal mice and severe combined immunodeficient (SCID) mice (224–226). It is also known that nude mice clear rotavirus infection normally (227) or after a short delay (228). Passive immunity from both transplacentally acquired immunoglobulin and breast milk immunoglobulin may provide some degree of protection. In the developed world, infants younger than 3 months of age are infrequently symptomatically infected. Although some targets of cellular and humoral immunity have been identified in model systems, it is not known which type of immune response is the best predictor of protection from disease in the field. Likewise, it is not clear which viral antigens best stimulate protective immunity in the context of vaccine development.

Host factors that may protect against rotavirus disease include diet and nutritional status, gastric secretions, mucus, intestinal flora, and age. Although colostrum feeding is a significant immunologic resistance factor in many animals (229–231), in humans the protective effect of breast-feeding on rotavirus disease is not consistently strong (232-237). Nonimmunologic protective factors in breast milk such as protease inhibitors have been proposed, but one study failed to confirm their role in ameliorating rotavirus disease (233). Mucin-like glycoproteins in human breast milk have been described, which inhibit rotavirus infection (238,239). Malnutrition, including specific micronutrient deficiencies, predisposes animals and probably humans to severe illness (206,240–247). Pepsin and acid secreted by the stomach are effective in neutralizing rotaviruses (23,24) and studies have shown that the "take" rate of orally administered live rotavirus vaccine candidates is greatly improved if the stomach contents are buffered (248,249). Intestinal mucins are inhibitors of rotavirus infection *in vitro,* although the strongest activity is directed against nonhuman sialic acid–dependent rotaviruses such as those used in most current candidate vaccine strains (250). As noted earlier, intestinal proteases such as trypsin greatly enhance rotavirus replication efficiency both *in vitro* and *in vivo* by cleaving VP4.

Human breast-fed infants with a predominance of bifidobacteria were resistant to severe rotavirus disease, suggesting a role of intestinal flora in susceptibility to rotavirus diarrhea (251). Experimental rotavirus infection caused greater growth failure in previously germ-free mice than in conventional mice (205). In animal models, dual infections with enterotoxigenic *Escherichia coli* and rotavirus appear to act synergistically to produce severe diarrhea (252,253).

CLINICAL ILLNESS

Many, if not most, rotavirus infections are asymptomatic (254–261). Such infections occur in neonates, older children, and adults and provide a reservoir that helps facilitate the transmission of rotavirus to susceptible hosts, infants, and toddlers. Symptomatic rotavirus infection follows an incubation period of 1 to 3 days, followed by the onset of fever, vomiting, and watery diarrhea. Fever and vomiting usually remit within the first 2 to 3 days of illness whereas diarrhea frequently persists for 5 to 8 days. Laboratory tests typically show mild to moderate elevation of the blood urea nitrogen level and mild metabolic acidosis (262). Minimal elevations of liver function tests during rotavirus enteritis have been noted, although their significance is uncertain (174). In a study comparing rotavirus diarrhea with other diarrheal illness, vomiting and dehydration were significantly more common in rotavirus diarrhea (262). Stools in rotavirus gastroenteritis are watery and do not contain blood or white blood cells. Although the majority of cases of rotavirus disease results in only mild to moderate dehydration, fulminant cases occur. Over a 5-year period in Toronto, the deaths of 21 children were attributed to rotavirus disease (263). More than 80% of these children were seen by a physician during the early phase of the illness, yet all the deaths occurred within the first 3 days of symptoms.

Although a variety of clinical conditions have been associated with rotavirus infection, the frequency of rotavirus infection makes it likely that many of these are coincidental associations (264). There is some evidence that rotavirus may cause some outbreaks of necrotizing enterocolitis in intensive care nurseries (265–267). Rotavirus infections in immunocompromised infections can be atypically long (months) and severe. Rotaviruses recovered from such patients often have bizarre electropherotypes resulting from gene segment rearrangements (142). There have been reports of rotavirus replication in the liver and kidney of severely immunocompromised hosts (176).

DIAGNOSIS

As noted earlier, the clinical syndrome associated with rotavirus is relatively nonspecific. Although the average clinician facing a child with acute gastroenteritis has little need for diagnostic testing, confirmation of rotavirus infection is vital for epidemiologic and vaccine studies and for the control of outbreaks of enteric illness. Therefore, a variety of diagnostic methods have been developed, including electron microscopy, solid phase immunoassays, RNA electrophoresis, nucleic acid hybridization (with and without PCR amplification), and direct cultivation of rotavirus from clinical samples in cell lines. Historically, the first diagnostic test used was electron microscopy (6). The abundance of rotavirus particles shed in the stool and their distinctive morphology result in high sensitivity and specificity with this technique. Another advantage of electron microscopy in the diagnosis of diarrheal disease is that other enteric viruses or atypical rotaviruses (non–group A rotaviruses) may be identified. The obvious disadvantage is the need for both equipment and expertise. A variety of immunoassays have been developed with several commercial kits available for detecting group A rotavirus antigen in stools (268–273). Most immunoassays have sensitivities and specificities in the 90% range. It is also possible to determine subgroup and G serotype with immunoassays employing MABs (31,35). Comparable sensitivity to electron microscopy and immunoassays can be obtained by simple protocols for isolating genomic RNA directly from stool, resolving it on polyacrylamide gels, and staining with silver to visualize the characteristic 11 segments of dsRNA (274–276). Nucleic acid hybridization tests have also been developed to not only detect rotaviruses but to serotype them as well (277–279). Some investigators have reported successful cultivation of human rotaviruses from greater than 90% of antigen-positive stools using primary African green monkey kidney cells (153). Use of human intestinal cell lines such as the Caco-2 epithelial line has been reported to be a sensitive means of isolating and amplifying human virus from clinical specimens (280). Reverse transcriptase PCR is being used increasingly for detection of rotavirus RNA in clinical material and allows for simultaneous genotyping during epidemiologic surveillance (281,282).

TREATMENT

Treatment of rotavirus diarrhea is supportive. The primary objective of therapy is to treat and prevent dehydration, which is the major cause of morbidity and mortality in infants with rotavirus disease. A worthy secondary objective is treatment and prevention of malnutrition, which is both a contributing factor in disease severity and a frequent result of moderate to severe disease.

Two major technologic advances of the twentieth century greatly decreased rotavirus mortality in the developed world. In the 1930s, the use of intravenous fluid for rehydration of infants dramatically reduced the mortality rate of infantile diarrhea. In the developing world, where facilities, equipment, and expertise in this form of therapy are lacking, great efforts have gone into developing low-cost electrolyte solutions for oral rehydration (186,283–285). Knowledge of sodium/glucose co-transporters in the intestine led eventually to solutions that had equal molar ratios of these solutes as well as potassium and bicarbonate salts for repletion of stool losses. ORS has been used successfully throughout the world in infants and children of all ages with a variety of dehydrating diarrheal illnesses and electrolyte abnormalities. Treatment failures occur only in the face of severe vomiting and frank shock. Protocols for oral rehydration differ from those for intravenous rehydration in that deficits are corrected rapidly with the oral solutions (4 to 6 hours) compared with intravenous rehydration (24 to 48 hours). Although a variety of additions to ORS have been tested, none has produced dramatically improved results in rotavirus diarrhea.

Traditional dietary management of diarrheal illness has consisted mainly of withholding food. Although this may reduce the number of stools passed, the ensuing acute malnutrition prolongs recovery from gastroenteritis (286, 287). Current recommendations are to begin refeeding with a complete diet as soon as oral rehydration is complete. Breast-feeding should continue through the rehydration process. Although secondary biochemical lactase deficiency is common in rotavirus infection, many children can be fed unrestricted diets without apparent ill effect (286–289). Likewise, the use of starchy diets low in fat and protein (BRAT or ABC diets) is without any known benefit.

Passive immunotherapy has been used in several situations. Attempts have been made to use milk antibody concentrates from rotavirus-immunized cows to treat infants with acute rotavirus infection (290,291). Although the duration of viral shedding was reduced, little effect was noted on the clinical illness. Oral immunoglobulins and colostrum have been given to immunocompromised children with chronic symptomatic rotavirus disease with resolution of their symptoms (292). More recent studies have reported somewhat more success with passive immunotherapy (reviewed in reference 293). Several studies have also reported that administration of probiotics such as *Lactobacillus* species may reduce the duration of rotavirus gastroenteritis (294,295).

Drug therapy in rotavirus gastroenteritis is generally ill advised. Antibiotics are ineffective and may lead to untoward side effects. Opiates and loperamide may reduce visible stool output but carry the risk of causing ileus or vomiting, which may preclude the use of ORS. Severe complications of such medications given to young children have been reported both in the developing and developed world (296–298) and have been observed in our own practices. Clinical trials of loperamide at the recommended doses have shown little or no benefit in children with gastroenteritis (299,300). The World Health Organization recommendation for treatment of diarrhea in children is that "antidiarrheal drugs should never be used. None has any proven practical value and some are dangerous" (301). New types of drugs for secretory diarrhea without primary effects on motility are reported to be promising for treatment of pediatric disease (302).

Specific antiviral therapy for rotavirus disease has also been studied. A variety of nucleoside analogues have been reported to inhibit rotavirus infection *in vitro* (303–306). Others have proposed the use of protease inhibitors to prevent intestinal trypsin from cleaving VP4 (307,308). Glycoproteins such as mucins, which can function as pseudoreceptors if given orally, have also been suggested as candidate therapies for rotavirus disease (109,115,238). Given the fact that much of the intestinal damage in rotavirus infection occurs before symptoms, antivirals will probably not have a large impact on rotavirus disease.

PREVENTION

The substantial morbidity and mortality associated with group A rotavirus disease clearly suggests the need for a vaccine. A quadrivalent rotavirus vaccine based on reassortant viruses derived from human strains and a simian strain, Rotashield, was licensed in the United States but withdrawn from the market due to concerns about a possible association with intussusception (8,9). The status of current vaccine development is described in a subsequent chapter.

REFERENCES

1. Matson DO, Estes MK. Impact of rotavirus infection at a large pediatric hospital. *J Infect Dis*1990;162:598–604.
2. Glass RI, Kilgore PE, Holman RC, et al. The epidemiology of rotavirus diarrhea in the United States: surveillance and estimates of disease burden. *J Infect Dis* 1996;174[Suppl 1]: S5–S11.
3. Medicine Io. The prospects for immunizing against rotavirus disease. In: *New vaccine development. Establishing priorities. Diseases of importance in developing countries.* Washington, DC: National Academy Press, 1986:308—318:
4. Adams WR, Kraft LM. Electron microscopic study of the intestinal epithelium of mice infected with the agent of epizootic diarrhea of infant mice (EDIM virus). *Am J Pathol* 1967;39–47.
5. Mebus CA, Stair EL, Underdahl NR, et al. Pathology of neonatal calf diarrhea induced by a reo-like virus. *Vet Pathol* 1973;10; 45–64.
6. Bishop RF, Davidson GP, Holmes IH, et al. Virus particles in epithelial cells of duodenal mucosa from children with viral gastroenteritis. *Lancet* 1973;2:1281–1283.
7. Wyatt RG, James WD, Bohl EH. Human rotavirus type 2: cultivation *in vitro*. *Science*1980;207:189–191.
8. Centers for Disease Control and Prevention. Withdrawal of rotavirus vaccine recommendation. *JAMA* 1999;282: 2113–2114.
9. Abramson JS, Baker CJ, Fisher MC, et al: Possible association of intussusception with rotavirus vaccination. American Academy of Pediatrics. Committee on Infectious Diseases. *Pediatrics* 1999;104:575.
10. Kapikian AZ, Chanock RM. Rotaviruses. In: Fields BN, Knipe DM, Howley PM, eds. *Field's virology.* Philadelphia: Lippincott-Raven, 1996:1657–1693.
11. Flewett TH, Bryden AS, Davies H, et al. Relation between viruses from acute gastroenteritis of children and newborn calves. *Lancet* 1974;2:61–63.
12. Ludert JE, Gil F, Liprandi F, et al. The structure of the rotavirus inner capsid studied by electron microscopy of chemically disrupted particles. *J Gen Virol* 1986;67:1721–1725.
13. Prasad BV, Chiu W. Structure of rotavirus. *Curr Top Microbiol Immunol* 1994;185:9–29.
14. Yeager M, Berriman JA, Baker TS, et al. Three-dimensional structure of the rotavirus haemagglutinin VP4 by cryo-electron microscopy and difference map analysis. *EMBO J* 1994;13: 1011–1018.
15. Lawton JA, Estes MK, Prasad BV. Comparative structural analysis of transcriptionally competent and incompetent rotavirus-antibody complexes. *Proc Natl Acad Sci U S A* 1999;96:5428–5433.
16. Lawton JA, Zeng CQ, Mukherjee SK, et al. Three-dimensional structural analysis of recombinant rotavirus-like particles with intact and amino-terminal-deleted VP2: implications for the architecture of the VP2 capsid layer. *J Virol* 1997;71:7353–7360.
17. Lawton JA, Estes MK, and Prasad BV: Three-dimensional visualization of mRNA release from actively transcribing rotavirus particles [letter]. *Nat Struct Biol* 1997;4:118–121.
18. Bridger JC, Woode GN. Charaterization of two particle types of calf rotavirus. *J Gen Virol* 1976;31:245–250.
19. Cohen J, Laporte J, Charpilienne A, et al. Activation of rotavirus RNA polymerase by calcium chelation. *Arch Virol* 1979;60:177–182.
20. Estes MK, Graham DY, Smith EM, et al. Rotavirus stability and inactivation. *J Gen Virol* 1979;43:403–408.
21. Chen D, Ramig RF. Rescue of infectivity by *in vitro* transcapsidation of rotavirus single-shelled particles. *Virology* 1993;192: 422–429.
22. Anthony ID, Bullivant S, Dayal S, et al. Rotavirus spike structure and polypeptide composition. *J Virol* 1991;65:4334–4340.
23. Bass DM, Baylor M, Broome R, et al. Molecular basis of age-dependent gastric inactivation of rhesus rotavirus in the mouse. *J Clin Invest* 1992;89:1741–1745.
24. Weiss C, Clark HF. Rapid inactivation of rotaviruses by exposure to acid buffer or acidic gastric juice. *J Gen Virol* 1985;66:2725–2730.
25. Chen YS, Vaughn JM. Inactivation of human and simian rotaviruses by chlorine dioxide. *Appl Environ Microbiol* 1990; 56:1363–1366.
26. Rodgers FG, Hufton P, Kurzawska E, et al. Morphological response of human rotavirus to ultra-violet radiation, heat and disinfectants. *J Med Microbiol*1985;20:123–130.
27. Narang HK, Codd AA. Action of commonly used disinfectants against enteroviruses. *J Hosp Infect* 1983;4:209–212.
28. Tan JA, Schnagl RD. Rotavirus inactivated by a hypochlorite-based disinfectant: a reappraisal [letter]. *Med J Aust* 1983;1:550.
29. Sattar SA, Springthorpe VS, Karim Y, et al. Chemical disinfection of non-porous inanimate surfaces experimentally contaminated with four human pathogenic viruses. *Epidemiol Infect* 1989;102:493–505.
30. Greenberg HB, Flores J, Kalica AR, et al. Gene coding assignments for growth restriction, neutralization and subgroup specificities of the W and DS-1 strains of human rotavirus. *J Gen Virol* 1983;64:313–320.
31. Greenberg H, McAuliffe V, Valdesuso J, et al. Serological analysis of the subgroup protein of rotavirus, using monoclonal antibodies. *Infect Immun* 1983;39:91–99.
32. Griffin DD, Kirkwood CD, Parashar UD, et al. Surveillance of rotavirus strains in the United States: identification of unusual strains. The National Rotavirus Strain Surveillance System Collaborating Laboratories. *J Clin Microbiol* 2000;38:2784–2787.
33. Ahmed MU, Taniguchi K, Kobayashi N, et al. Characterization by enzyme-linked immunosorbent assay using subgroup- and serotype-specific monoclonal antibodies of human rotavirus obtained from diarrheic patients in Bangladesh. *J Clin Microbiol* 1989;27:1678–1681.
34. Birch CJ, Heath RL, Gust ID. Use of serotype-specific monoclonal antibodies to study the epidemiology of rotavirus infection. *J Med Virol* 1988;24:45–53.
35. Taniguchi K, Urasawa T, Morita Y, et al. Direct serotyping of human rotavirus in stools by an enzyme-linked immunosorbent assay using serotype 1-, 2-, 3-, and 4-specific monoclonal antibodies to VP7. *J Infect Dis* 1987;155:1159–1166.

36. Beards GM. Serotyping of rotavirus by NADP-enhanced enzyme-immunoassay. *J Virol Methods* 1987;18:77–85.
37. Coulson BS, Unicomb LE, Pitson GA, et al. Simple and specific enzyme immunoassay using monoclonal antibodies for serotyping human rotaviruses. *J Clin Microbiol* 1987;25:509–515.
38. Flores J, Taniguchi K, Green K, et al. Relative frequencies of rotavirus serotypes 1, 2, 3, and 4 in Venezuelan infants with gastroenteritis. *J Clin Microbiol* 1988;26:2092–2095.
39. Gouvea V, Glass RI, Woods P, et al. Polymerase chain reaction amplification and typing of rotavirus nucleic acid from stool specimens. *J Clin Microbiol* 1990;28:276–282.
40. Gouvea V, de Castro L, Timenetsky M do C, et al. Rotavirus serotype G5 associated with diarrhea in Brazilian children. *J Clin Microbiol* 1994;32:1408–1409.
41. Munoz M, Parwani AV, Lucchelli A, et al. Detection of serotype G6 rotavirus in bovine field samples using a nonradioactive PCR-derived cDNA probe. *J Vet Diagn Invest* 1995;7:546–548.
42. Coulson BS, Gentsch JR, Das BK, et al. Comparison of enzyme immunoassay and reverse transcriptase PCR for identification of serotype G9 rotaviruses. *J Clin Microbiol* 1999;37: 3187–3193.
43. Zhou Y, Nakayama M, Hasegawa A, et al. Serotypes of human rotaviruses in 7 regions of Japan from 1984 to 1997. *Kansenshogaku Zasshi* 1999;73:35–42.
44. Wu H, Taniguchi K, Urasawa T, et al. Serological and genomic characterization of human rotaviruses detected in China. *J Med Virol* 1998;55:168–176.
45. Larralde G, Li BG, Kapikian AZ, et al. Serotype-specific epitope(s) present on the VP8 subunit of rotavirus VP4 protein. *J Virol* 1991;65:3213–3218.
46. Larralde G, Gorziglia M. Distribution of conserved and specific epitopes on the VP8 subunit of rotavirus VP4. *J Virol* 1992;66: 7438–7443.
47. Li B, Larralde G, Gorziglia M. Human rotavirus K8 strain represents a new VP4 serotype. *J Virol* 1993;67:617–620.
48. Gorziglia M, Larralde G, Kapikian AZ, et al. Antigenic relationships among human rotaviruses as determined by outer capsid protein VP4. *Proc Natl Acad Sci U S A* 1990;87:7155–7159.
49. Estes MK, Cohen J. Rotavirus gene structure and function. *Microbiol Rev* 1989;53:410–449.
50. Welch SK, Crawford SE, Estes MK. Rotavirus SA11 genome segment 11 protein is a nonstructural phosphoprotein. *J Virol* 1989;63:3974–3982.
51. Imai M, Akatani K, Ikegami N, et al. Capped and conserved terminal structures in human rotavirus genome double-stranded RNA segments. *J Virol* 1983;47:125–136.
52. McCrae MA, McCorquodale JG. Molecular biology of rotaviruses. V. Terminal structure of viral RNA species. *Virology* 1983;126:204–212.
53. Patton JT, Wentz M, Xiaobo J, et al. cis-Acting signals that promote genome replication in rotavirus mRNA. *J Virol* 1996; 70:3961–3971.
54. McCrae MA, McCorquodale JG. Genetic heterogeneity within individual bovine rotavirus isolates. *J Virol* 1982;44:813–822.
55. Mason BB, Graham DY, Estes MK. Biochemical mapping of the simian rotavirus SA11 genome. *J Virol* 1983;46:413–423.
56. Both GW, Siegman LJ, Bellamy AR, et al. Coding assignment and nucleotide sequence of simian rotavirus SA11 gene segment 10: location of glycosylation sites suggests that the signal peptide is not cleaved. *J Virol* 1983;48:335–339.
57. Kantharidis P, Dyall SM, Holmes IH. Completion of the gene coding assignments of SA11 rotavirus: gene products of segments 7, 8, and 9. *J Virol* 1983;48:330–334.
58. Both GW, Mattick JS, Bellamy AR. Serotype-specific glycoprotein of simian 11 rotavirus: coding assignment and gene sequence. *Proc Natl Acad Sci U S A* 1983;80:3091–3095.
59. Labbe M, Charpilienne A, Crawford SE, et al. Expression of rotavirus VP2 produces empty corelike particles. *J Virol* 1991; 65:2946–2952.
60. Boyle JF, Holmes KV. RNA-binding proteins of bovine rotavirus. *J Virol* 1986;58:561–568.
61. Valenzuela S, Pizarro J, Sandino AM, et al. Photoaffinity labeling of rotavirus VP1 with 8-azido-ATP: identification of the viral RNA polymerase. *J Virol* 1991;65:3964–3967.
62. Vasquez M, Sandino AM, Pizzaro JM, et al. Function of rotavirus VP3 polypeptide in viral morphogenesis. *J Gen Virol* 1993;74:937–941.
63. Estes MK, Crawford SE, Penaranda ME, et al.: Synthesis and immunogenicity of the rotavirus major capsid antigen using a baculovirus expression system. *J Virol* 1987;61:1488–1494.
64. Gorziglia M, Larrea C, Liprandi F, et al. Biochemical evidence for the oligomeric (possibly trimeric) structure of the major inner capsid polypeptide (45K) of rotaviruses. *J Gen Virol* 1985;66:1889–1900.
65. Ciarlet M, Crawford SE, Barone C, et al. Subunit rotavirus vaccine administered parenterally to rabbits induces active protective immunity. *J Virol* 1998;72:9233–9246.
66. Burns JW, Siadat-Pajouh M, Krishnaney AA, et al. Protective effect of rotavirus VP6-specific IgA monoclonal antibodies that lack neutralizing activity [see comments]. *Science* 1996;272: 104–107.
67. O'Neal CM, Clements JD, Estes MK, et al. Rotavirus 2/6 viruslike particles administered intranasally with cholera toxin, *Escherichia coli* heat-labile toxin (LT), and LT-R192G induce protection from rotavirus challenge. *J Virol* 1998;72: 3390–3393.
68. Kalica AR, Flores J, Greenberg HB. Identification of the rotaviral gene that codes for hemagglutination and protease-enhanced plaque formation. *Virology* 1983;125:194–205.
69. Mackow ER, Barnett JW, Chan H, et al. The rhesus rotavirus outer capsid protein VP4 functions as a hemagglutinin and is antigenically conserved when expressed by a baculovirus recombinant. *J Virol* 1989;63:1661–1668.
70. Offit PA, Blavat G, Greenberg HB, et al. Molecular basis of rotavirus virulence: role of gene segment 4. *J Virol* 1986;57:46–49.
71. Prasad BV, Burns JW, Marietta E, et al. Localization of VP4 neutralization sites in rotavirus by three-dimensional cryo-electron microscopy. *Nature* 1990;343:476–479.
72. Ruggeri FM, Greenberg HA. Antibodies to the trypsin cleavage peptide VP8* neutralize rotavirus by inhibiting binding of virions to target cells in culture. *J Virol* 1991;65:2211–2219.
73. Kaljot KT, Shaw RD, Rubin DH, et al. Infectious rotavirus enters cells by direct cell membrane penetration, not by endocytosis. *J Virol* 1988;62:1136–1144.
74. Estes MK, Graham DY, Mason BB. Proteolytic enhancement of rotavirus infectivity: molecular mechanisms. *J Virol* 1981;39: 879–888.
75. Lopez S, Arias CF, Bell JR, et al. Primary structure of the cleavage site associated with trypsin enhancement of rotavirus SA11 infectivity. *Virology* 1985;144:11–19.
76. Gilbert JM, Greenberg HB. Virus-like particle-induced fusion from without in tissue culture cells: role of outer-layer proteins VP4 and VP7. *J Virol* 1997;71:4555–4563.
77. Lopez S, Arias CF, Mendez E, et al. Conservation in rotaviruses of the protein region containing the two sites associated with trypsin enhancement of infectivity. *Virology* 1986;154:224–227.
78. Gorziglia M, Hoshino Y, Buckler WA, et al. Conservation of amino acid sequence of VP8 and cleavage region of 84-kDa outer capsid protein among rotaviruses recovered from asymptomatic neonatal infection [published erratum appears in *Proc Natl acad Sci U S A* 1987;84:2062]. *Proc Natl Acad Sci U S A*1986;83:7039–7043.

79. Mackow ER, Shaw RD, Matsui SM, et al. The rhesus rotavirus gene encoding protein VP3: location of amino acids involved in homologous and heterologous rotavirus neutralization and identification of a putative fusion region. *Proc Natl Acad Sci U S A* 1988;85:645–649.
80. Chan WK, Penaranda ME, Crawford SE, et al. Two glycoproteins are produced from the rotavirus neutralization gene. *Virology* 1986;151:243–252.
81. Stirzaker SC, Whitfeld PL, Christie DL, et al. Processing of rotavirus glycoprotein VP7: implications for the retention of the protein in the endoplasmic reticulum. *J Cell Biol* 1987; 105:2897–2903.
82. Stirzaker SC, Both GW. The signal peptide of the rotavirus glycoprotein VP7 is essential for its retention in the ER as an integral membrane protein. *Cell* 1989;56:741–747.
83. Stirzaker SC, Poncet D, Both GW. Sequences in rotavirus glycoprotein VP7 that mediate delayed translocation and retention of the protein in the endoplasmic reticulum. *J Cell Biol* 1990; 111:1343–1350.
84. Poruchynsky MS, Atkinson PH. Primary sequence domains required for the retention of rotavirus VP7 in the endoplasmic reticulum. *J Cell Biol* 1988;107:1697–1706.
85. Kabcenell AK, Atkinson PH. Processing of the rough endoplasmic reticulum membrane glycoproteins of rotavirus SA11. *J Cell Biol* 1985;101:1270–1280.
86. Kouvelos K, Petric M, Middleton PJ. Comparison of bovine, simian and human rotavirus structural glycoproteins. *J Gen Virol* 1984;65:1211–1214.
87. Kouvelos K, Petric M, Middleton PJ. Oligosaccharide composition of calf rotavirus. *J Gen Virol* 1984;65:1159–1164.
88. Au KS, Chan WK, Burns JW, et al. Receptor activity of rotavirus nonstructural glycoprotein NS28. *J Virol* 1989; 63:4553–4562.
89. Maass DR, Atkinson PH. Rotavirus proteins VP7, NS28, and VP4 form oligomeric structures. *J Virol* 1990;64:2632–2641.
90. Taylor JA, Meyer JC, Legge MA, et al. Transient expression and mutational analysis of the rotavirus intracellular receptor: the C-terminal methionine residue is essential for ligand binding. *J Virol* 1992;66:3566–3572.
91. Chan WK, Au KS, Estes MK. Topography of the simian rotavirus nonstructural glycoprotein (NS28) in the endoplasmic reticulum membrane. *Virology* 1988;164:435–442.
92. Estes MK, Morris AP. A viral enterotoxin. A new mechanism of virus-induced pathogenesis. *Adv Exp Med Biol* 1999;473: 73–382.
93. Patton JT, Gallegos CO. Structure and protein composition of the rotavirus replicase particle. *Virology* 1988;166:358–365.
94. Gallegos CO, Patton JT. Characterization of rotavirus replication intermediates: a model for the assembly of single-shelled particles. *Virology* 1989;172:616–627.
95. Poncet D, Aponte C, Cohen J. Rotavirus protein NSP3 (NS34) is bound to the 3′ end consensus sequence of viral mRNAs in infected cells. *J Virol* 1993;67:3159–3165.
96. Piron M, Vende P, Cohen J, et al. Rotavirus RNA-binding protein NSP3 interacts with eIF4GI and evicts the poly(A) binding protein from eIF4F. *EMBO J* 1998;17:5811–5821.
97. Vende P, Piron M, Castagné N, et al. Efficient translation of rotavirus mRNA requires simultaneous interaction of NSP3 with the eukaryotic translation initiation factor eIF4G and the mRNA 3′ end. *J Virol* 2000;74:7064–7071.
98. Broome RL, Vo PT, Ward RL, et al. Murine rotavirus genes encoding outer capsid proteins VP4 and VP7 are not major determinants of host range restriction and virulence. *J Virol* 1993;67:2448–2455.
99. Hoshino Y, Saif LJ, Kang SY, et al. Identification of group A rotavirus genes associated with virulence of a porcine rotavirus and host range restriction of a human rotavirus in the gnotobiotic piglet model. *Virology* 1995;209:274–280.
100. Fukuhara N, Yoshie O, Kitaoka S, et al. Role of VP3 in human rotavirus internalization after target cell attachment via VP7. *J Virol* 1988;62:2209–2218.
101. Keljo DJ, Smith AK. Characterization of binding of simian rotavirus SA-11 to cultured epithelial cells. *J Pediatr Gastroenterol Nutr* 1988;7:249–256.
102. Petrie BL, Estes MK, Graham DY. Effects of tunicamycin on rotavirus morphogenesis and infectivity. *J Virol* 1983;46: 270–274.
103. Sabara M, Babiuk LA. Identification of a bovine rotavirus gene and gene product influencing cellular attachment. *J Virol* 1984; 51:489–496.
104. Bass DM, Mackow ER, Greenberg HB. NS35 and not vp7 is the soluble rotavirus protein which binds to target cells. *J Virol* 1990;64:322–330.
105. Ludert JE, Feng N, Yu JH, et al. Genetic mapping indicates that VP4 is the rotavirus cell attachment protein *in vitro* and *in vivo*. *J Virol* 1996;70:487–493.
106. Méndez E, Arias CF, López S. Binding to sialic acids is not an essential step for the entry of animal rotaviruses to epithelial cells in culture. *J Virol* 1993;67:5253–5259.
107. Zarate S, Espinosa R, Romero P, et al. The VP5 domain of VP4 can mediate attachment of rotaviruses to cells. *J Virol* 2000;74: 593–599.
108. Colonno RJ, Condra JH, Mizutani S, et al. Evidence for the direct involvement of the rhinovirus canyon in receptor binding. *Proc Natl Acad Sci U S A* 1988;85:5449–5453.
109. Yolken RH, Willoughby R, Wee SB, et al. Sialic acid glycoproteins inhibit *in vitro* and *in vivo* replication of rotaviruses. *J Clin Invest* 1987;79:148–154.
110. Chen C, Baylor M, Bass DM. Murine intestinal mucins inhibit rotavirus replication. 1992;102:A919.
111. Fukudome K, Yoshie O, Konno T. Comparison of human, simian, and bovine rotaviruses for requirement of sialic acid in hemagglutination and cell absorption. *Virology* 1989;172: 196–205.
112. Bass DM, Mackow ER, Greenberg HB. Identification and partial characterization of a rhesus rotavirus binding glycoprotein on murine enterocytes. *Virology* 1991;183:602–610.
113. Superti F, Donelli G. Gangliosides as binding sites in SA-11 rotavirus infection of LLC-MK2 cells. *J Gen Virol* 1991;72: 2467–2474.
114. Kuhlenschmidt MS, Rolsma MD, Kuhlenschmidt TB, et al. Characterization of a porcine enterocyte receptor for group A rotavirus. *Adv Exp Med Biol* 1997;412:135–143.
115. Willoughby RE, Yolken RH, Schnaar RL. Rotaviruses specifically bind to the neutral glycosphingolipid asialo-GM1. *J Virol* 1990;64:4830–4835.
116. Coulson BS, Londrigan SL, Lee DJ. Rotavirus contains integrin ligand sequences and a disintegrin-like domain that are implicated in virus entry into cells. *Proc Natl Acad Sci U S A* 1997;94:5389–5394.
117. Lopez S, Espinosa R, Isa P, et al. Characterization of a monoclonal antibody directed to the surface of MA104 cells that blocks the infectivity of rotaviruses. *Virology* 2000;273: 160–168.
118. Denisova E, Dowling W, LaMonica R, et al. Rotavirus capsid protein VP5* permeabilizes membranes. *J Virol* 1999;73:3147–3153.
119. Dowling W, Denisova E, LaMonica R, et al. Selective membrane permeabilization by the rotavirus VP5* protein is abrogated by mutations in an internal hydrophobic domain. *J Virol* 2000;74:6368–6376.
120. Charpilienne A, Abad MJ, Michelangeli F, et al. Solubilized and cleaved VP7, the outer glycoprotein of rotavirus, induces perme-

abilization of cell membrane vesicles. *J Gen Virol* 1997;78: 1367–1371.

121. Falconer MM, Gilbert JM, Roper AM, et al. Rotavirus-induced fusion from without in tissue culture cells. *J Virol* 1995;69: 5582–5591.
122. Liprandi F, Moros Z, Gerder M, et al. Productive penetration of rotavirus in cultured cells induces coentry of the translation inhibitor alpha-sarcin. *Virology* 1997;237:430–438.
123. Quan CM, Doane FW. Ultrastructural evidence for the cellular uptake of rotavirus by endocytosis. *Intervirology* 1983;20: 223–231.
124. Ludert JE, Michelangeli F, Gil F, et al. Penetration and uncoating of rotaviruses in cultured cells. *Intervirology* 1987;27: 95–101.
125. Suzuki H, Kitaoka S, Konno T, et al. Two modes of human rotavirus entry into MA 104 cells. *Arch Virol* 1985;85:25–34.
126. Suzuki H, Kitaoka S, Sato T, et al. Further investigation on the mode of entry of human rotavirus into cells. *Arch Virol* 1986; 91:135–144.
127. Bass DM, Baylor M, Chen C, et al. Dansylcadaverine and cytochalasin D enhance rotavirus infection of murine L cells. *Virology* 1995;212:429–437.
128. Keljo DJ, Kuhn M, Smith A. Acidification of endosomes is not important for the entry of rotavirus into the cell. *J Pediatr Gastroenterol Nutr* 1988;7:257–263.
129. Bass DM, Baylor MR, Chen C, et al. Liposome-mediated transfection of intact viral particles reveals that plasma membrane penetration determines permissivity of tissue culture cells to rotavirus. *J Clin Invest* 1992;90:2313–2320.
130. Spencer E, Arias ML. *In vitro* transcription catalyzed by heat treated human rotavirus. *J Virol* 1981;40:1–10.
131. Patton JT, Chnaiderman J, Spencer E. Open reading frame in rotavirus mRNA specifically promotes synthesis of double-stranded RNA: template size also affects replication efficiency. *Virology* 1999;264:167–180.
132. Petrie BL, Greenberg HB, Graham DY, et al. Ultrastructural localization of rotavirus antigens using colloidal gold. *Virus Res* 1984;1:133–152.
133. Sabara M, Parker M, Aha P, et al. Assembly of double-shelled rotaviruslike particles by simultaneous expression of recombinant VP6 and VP7 proteins. *J Virol* 1991;65:6994–6997.
134. Jourdan N, Maurice M, Delautier D, et al. Rotavirus is released from the apical surface of cultured human intestinal cells through nonconventional vesicular transport that bypasses the Golgi apparatus. *J Virol* 1997;71:8268–8278.
135. Musalem C, Espejo RT. Release of progeny virus from cells infected with simian rotavirus SA11. *J Gen Virol* 1985;66: 2715–2724.
136. McCrae MA, Faulkner-Valle GP: Molecular biology of rotaviruses: I. Characterization of basic growth parameters and pattern of macromolecular synthesis. *J Virol* 1981;39: 490–496.
137. Carpio MM, Babiuk LA, Misra V, et al. Bovine rotavirus-cell interactions: effect of rotavirus infection on cellular integrity and macromolecular synthesis. *Virology* 1981;114:86–93.
138. Rollo EE, Kumar KP, Reich NC, et al. The epithelial cell response to rotavirus infection. *J Immunol* 1999;163:4442–4452.
139. Michelangeli F, Ruiz MC, del CJ, et al. Effect of rotavirus infection on intracellular calcium homeostasis in cultured cells. *Virology* 1991;181:520–527.
140. Chiarini A, Arista S, Giammanco A, et al. Rotavirus persistence in cell cultures: selection of resistant cells in the presence of foetal calf serum. *J Gen Virol* 1983;64:1101–1110.
141. Mrukowicz JZ, Wetzel JD, Goral MI, et al. Viruses and cells with mutations affecting viral entry are selected during persistent rotavirus infections of MA104 cells. *J Virol* 1998;72: 3088–3097.
142. Eiden J, Losonsky GA, Johnson J, et al. Rotavirus RNA variation during chronic infection of immunocompromised children. *Pediatr Infect Dis* 1985;4:632–637.
143. Pedley S, Hundley F, Chrystie I, et al. The genomes of rotaviruses isolated from chronically infected immunodeficient children. *J Gen Virol* 1984;65:1141–1150.
144. Wood DJ, David TJ, Chrystie IL, et al. Chronic enteric virus infection in two T-cell immunodeficient children. *J Med Virol* 1988;24:435–444.
145. Tucker AW, Haddix AC, Bresee JS, et al. Cost-effectiveness analysis of a rotavirus immunization program for the United States. *JAMA* 1998;279:1371–1376.
146. Brandt CD, Kim HW, Rodriguez WJ, et al. Pediatric viral gastroenteritis during eight years of study. *J Clin Microbiol* 1983; 18:71–78.
147. Black RE, Greenberg HB, Kapikian AZ, et al. Acquisition of serum antibody to Norwalk virus and rotavirus in relation to diarrhea in a longitudinal study of young children in rural Bangladesh. *J Infect Dis* 1982;145:483–489.
148. Huilan S, Zhen LG, Mathan MM, et al. Etiology of acute diarrhoea among children in developing countries: a multicentre study in five countries. *Bull WHO* 1991;69:549–555.
149. Haffejee IE. Neonatal rotavirus infections. *Rev Infect Dis* 1991; 13:957–962.
150. Konno T, Suzuki H, Katsushima N, et al. Influence of temperature and relative humidity on human rotavirus infection in Japan. *J Infect Dis* 1983;147:125–128.
151. Ho MS, Glass RI, Pinsky PF, et al. Rotavirus as a cause of diarrheal morbidity and mortality in the United States. *J Infect Dis* 1988;158:1112–1116.
152. Torok TJ, Kilgore PE, Clarke MJ, et al. Visualizing geographic and temporal trends in rotavirus activity in the United States, 1991 to 1996. National Respiratory and Enteric Virus Surveillance System Collaborating Laboratories. *Pediatr Infect Dis J* 1997;16:941–946.
153. Ward RL, Clemens JD, Sack DA, et al. Culture adaptation and characterization of group A rotaviruses causing diarrheal illnesses in Bangladesh from 1985 to 1986. *J Clin Microbiol* 1991; 29:1915–1923.
154. Gentsch JR, Woods PA, Ramachandran M, et al. Review of G and P typing results from a global collection of rotavirus strains: implications for vaccine development. *J Infect Dis* 1996;174 [Suppl 1]:S30–S36.
155. Ramachandran M, Vij A, Kumar R, et al. Lack of maternal antibodies to P serotypes may predispose neonates to infections with unusual rotavirus strains. *Clin Diagn Lab Immunol* 1998; 5:527–530.
156. Ramachandran M, Das BK, Vij A, et al. Unusual diversity of human rotavirus G and P genotypes in India. *J Clin Microbiol* 1996;34:436–439.
157. Ryder RW, Yolken RH, Reeves WC, et al. Enzootic bovine rotavirus is not a source of infection in Panamanian cattle ranchers and their families. *J Infect Dis* 1986;153:1139–1144.
158. Dunn SJ, Greenberg HB, Ward RL, et al. Serotypic and genotypic characterization of human serotype 10 rotaviruses from asymptomatic neonates. *J Clin Microbiol* 1993;31:165–169.
159. Das M, Dunn SJ, Woode GN, et al. Both surface proteins (VP4 and VP7) of an asymptomatic neonatal rotavirus strain (I321) have high levels of sequence identity with the homologous proteins of a serotype 10 bovine rotavirus. *Virology* 1993;194: 374–379.
160. Velázquez FR, Matson DO, Calva JJ, et al. Rotavirus infections in infants as protection against subsequent infections. *N Engl J Med* 1996;335:1022–1028.

161. Graham DY, Dufour GR, Estes MK. Minimal infective dose of rotavirus. *Arch Virol* 1987;92:261–271.
162. Snodgrass DR, Angus KW, Gray EW. Rotavirus in lambs: pathogenesis and pathology. *Arch Virol* 1977;55:263–271.
163. Osborne MP, Haddon SJ, Spencer AJ, et al. An electron microscopic investigation of time-related changes in the intestine of neonatal mice infected with murine rotavirus. *J Pediatr Gastroenterol Nutr* 1988;7:236–248.
164. Mebus CA, Wyatt RG, Kapikian AZ. Pathology of diarrhea in gnotobiotic calves induced by the human reovirus-like agent infantile gastroenteritis. *Vet Pathol* 1977;14:273–282.
165. Hall GA. Comparative pathology of infection by novel diarrhoea viruses. *Ciba Found Symp* 1987;128:192–217.
166. Davidson GP, Barnes GL. Structural and functional abnormalities of the small intestine in infants and children with rotavirus enteritis. *Acta Pediatr Scand* 1979;68:181–188.
167. Agus SG, Dolin R, Wyatt RG, et al. Acute infectious nonbacterial gastroenteritis: intestinal histopathology. Histologic and enzymatic alterations during illness produced by the Norwalk agent in man. *Ann Intern Med* 1973;79:18–25.
168. Schreiber DS, Blacklow NR, Trier JS. The small intestinal lesion induced by the Hawaii agent in infectious nonbacterial gastroenteritis. *J Infect Dis* 1974;129:705–708.
169. Kohler T, Erben U, Wiedersberg H, et al. [Histological findings of the small intestinal mucosa in rotavirus infections in infants and young children]. Histologische Befunde der Dunndarmschleimhaut bei Rotavirusinfektionen im Sauglings- und Kleinkindalter. *Kinderarztl Prax* 1990;58:323–327.
170. Fragoso M, Kumar A, Murray DL. Rotavirus in nasopharyngeal secretions of children with upper respiratory tract infections. *Diagn Microbiol Infect Dis* 1986;4:87–88.
171. Novikova NA, Al'tova EE, Noskova NV, et al. [The detection of rotavirus RNA in nasopharyngeal smears by molecular hybridization]. *Zh Mikrobiol Epidemiol Immunobiol* 1991;(4): 23–25.
172. Hongou K, Konishi T, Yagi S, et al. Rotavirus encephalitis mimicking afebrile benign convulsions in infants. *Pediatr Neurol* 1998;18:354–357.
173. Grunow JE, Dunton SF, Waner JL. Human rotavirus-like particles in a hepatic abscess. *J Pediatr* 1985;106:73–76.
174. St. Geme JW, Hyman D. Hepatic injury during rotavirus infections [letter]. *J Pediatr* 1988;113:952–953.
175. Uhnoo I, Riepenhoff TM, Dharakul T, et al. Extramucosal spread and development of hepatitis in immunodeficient and normal mice infected with rhesus rotavirus. *J Virol* 1990;64: 361–368.
176. Gilger MA, Matson DO, Conner ME, et al. Extraintestinal rotavirus infections in children with immunodeficiency. *J Pediatr* 1992;120:912–917.
177. Wolf JL, Cukor G, Blacklow NR, et al. Susceptibility of mice to rotavirus infection: effects of age and corticosteroid administration. *Infect Immun* 1981;33:565–574.
178. Riepenhoff TM, Dharakul T, Kowalski E, et al. Rotavirus infection in mice: pathogenesis and immunity. *Adv Exp Med Biol* 1987;216:1015.
179. Thake DC, Moon HW, Lambert G. Epithelial cell dynamics in transmissible gastroenteritis of neonatal pigs. *Vet Pathol* 1973; 10:330–341.
180. Moon HW. Epithelial cell migration in the alimentary mucosa of the suckling pig. *Proc Soc Exp Biol Med* 1971;137:151–159.
181. Moon HW, Joel DD. Epithelial cell migration in the small intestine of sheep and calves. *Am J Vet Res* 1975;36:187–194.
182. Davidson GP, Gall DG, Petric M, et al. Human rotavirus enteritis induced in conventional piglets: intestinal structure and transport. *J Clin Invest* 1977;60:1402-1409.
183. Collins J, Starkey WG, Wallis TS, et al. Intestinal enzyme profiles in normal and rotavirus-infected mice. *J Pediatr Gastroenterol Nutr* 1988;7:264–272.
184. Graham DY, Sackman JW, Estes MK. Pathogenesis of rotavirus-induced diarrhea. Preliminary studies in miniature swine piglet. *Dig Dis Sci* 1984;29:1028–1035.
185. Hamilton JR, Gall DG, Butler DG, et al. Viral gastroenteritis: recent progress, remaining problems. In: Elliot K, Knight J, eds. *Acute diarrhea in childhood.* p. 209-219. Amsterdam: Elsevier/Excerpta Medica/North-Holland, 1976:209–219.
186. Sack DA, Chodhury AMAK, Eusof A, et al. Oral rehydration in rotavirus diarrhea: a double blind comparison of sucrose with glucose electrolyte solution. *Lancet* 1978;2:280–283.
187. Osborne MP, Haddon SJ, Worton KJ, et al. Rotavirus-induced changes in the microcirculation of intestinal villi of neonatal mice in relation to the induction and persistence of diarrhea [see comments]. *J Pediatr Gastroenterol Nutr* 1991;12:111–120.
188. Starkey WG, Collins J, Candy DC, et al. Transport of water and electrolytes by rotavirus-infected mouse intestine: a time course study. *J Pediatr Gastroenterol Nutr* 1990;11:254–260.
189. Starkey WG, Candy DC, Thornber D, et al. An *in vitro* model to study aspects of the pathophysiology of murine rotavirus-induced diarrhoea. *J Pediatr Gastroenterol Nutr* 1990;10:361–370.
190. Offit PA, Clark HF, Kornstein MJ, et al. A murine model for oral infection with a primate rotavirus (simian SA11). *J Virol* 1984;51:233–236.
191. Ramig RF. The effects of host age, virus dose, and virus strain on heterologous rotavirus infection of suckling mice. *Microb Pathog* 1988;4:189–202.
192. Ball JM, Tian P, Zeng CQ, et al. Age-dependent diarrhea induced by a rotaviral nonstructural glycoprotein [see comments]. *Science* 1996;272:101–104.
193. Horie Y, Nakagomi O, Koshimura Y, et al. Diarrhea induction by rotavirus NSP4 in the homologous mouse model system. *Virology* 1999;262:398–407.
194. Dong Y, Zeng CQ, Ball JM, et al. The rotavirus enterotoxin NSP4 mobilizes intracellular calcium in human intestinal cells by stimulating phospholipase C-mediated inositol 1,4,5-trisphosphate production. *Proc Natl Acad Sci U S A* 1997;94:3960–3965.
195. Zhang M, Zeng CQ, Dong Y, et al. Mutations in rotavirus nonstructural glycoprotein NSP4 are associated with altered virus virulence. *J Virol* 1998;72:3666–3672.
196. Angel J, Tang B, Feng N, et al. Studies of the role for NSP4 in the pathogenesis of homologous murine rotavirus diarrhea. *J Infect Dis* 1998;177:455–458.
197. Tian P, Hu Y, Schilling WP, et al. The nonstructural glycoprotein of rotavirus affects intracellular calcium levels. *J Virol* 1994; 68:251–257.
198. Newton K, Meyer JC, Bellamy AR, et al. Rotavirus nonstructural glycoprotein NSP4 alters plasma membrane permeability in mammalian cells. *J Virol* 1997;71:9458–9465.
199. Lundgren O, Peregrin AT, Persson K, et al. Role of the enteric nervous system in the fluid and electrolyte secretion of rotavirus diarrhea [see comments]. *Science* 2000;287:491–495.
200. de Silva DG, Mendis LN, Sheron N, et al. Concentrations of interleukin 6 and tumour necrosis factor in serum and stools of children with Shigella dysenteriae 1 infection [see comments]. *Gut* 1993;34:194–198.
201. De Boissieu D, Lebon P, Badoual J, et al. Rotavirus induces alpha-interferon release in children with gastroenteritis. *J Pediatr Gastroenterol Nutr* 1993;16:29–32.
202. Mangiarotti P, Moulin F, Palmer P, et al. Interferon-alpha in viral and bacterial gastroenteritis: a comparison with C-reactive protein and interleukin-6. *Acta Paediatr* 1999;88:592–594.
203. Bass DM. Interferon gamma and interleukin 1, but not interferon alfa, inhibit rotavirus entry into human intestinal cell lines. *Gastroenterology* 1997;113:81–89.

204. Angel J, Franco MA, Greenberg HB, et al. Lack of a role for type I and type II interferons in the resolution of rotavirus-induced diarrhea and infection in mice. *J Interferon Cytokine Res* 1999;19:655–659.
205. Heyman M, Corthier G, Petit A, et al. Intestinal absorption of macromolecules during viral enteritis: an experimental study on rotavirus-infected conventional and germ-free mice. *Pediatr Res* 1987;22:72–78.
206. Uhnoo IS, Freihorst J, Riepenhoff TM, et al. Effect of rotavirus infection and malnutrition on uptake of a dietary antigen in the intestine. *Pediatr Res* 1990;27:153–160.
207. Jalonen T, Isolauri E, Heyman M, et al. Increased beta-lactoglobulin absorption during rotavirus enteritis in infants: relationship to sugar permeability. *Pediatr Res* 1991;30:290–293.
208. Isolauri E, Juntunen M, Wiren S, et al. Intestinal permeability changes in acute gastroenteritis: effects of clinical factors and nutritional management. *J Pediatr Gastroenterol Nutr* 1989;8:466–473.
209. Johansen K, Stintzing G, Magnusson KE, et al. Intestinal permeability assessed with polyethylene glycols in children with diarrhea due to rotavirus and common bacterial pathogens in a developing community. *J Pediatr Gastroenterol Nutr* 1989;9:307–313.
210. Firer MA, Hosking CS, Hill DJ. Possible role for rotavirus in the development of cows' milk enteropathy in infants. *Clin Allergy* 1988;18:53–61.
211. Ogra PL, Welliver RC, Riepenhoff TM, et al. Interaction of mucosal immune system and infections in infancy: implications in allergy. *Ann Allergy* 1984;53:523–534.
212. Matsui SM, Mackow ER, Greenberg HB. Molecular determinant of rotavirus neutralization and protection. *Adv Virus Res* 1989;36:181–214.
213. Ward RL, Bernstein DI, Shukla R, et al. Effects of antibody to rotavirus on protection of adults challenged with a human rotavirus. *J Infect Dis* 1989;159:79–88.
214. Offit PA, Clark HF. Protection against rotavirus-induced gastroenteritis in a murine model by passively acquired gastrointestinal but not circulating antibodies. *J Virol* 1985;54:58–64.
215. Offit PA, Shaw RD, Greenberg HB. Passive protection against rotavirus-induced diarrhea by monoclonal antibodies to surface proteins VP3 and VP7. *J Virol* 1986;58:700–703.
216. Ward RL, Bernstein DI, Shukla R, et al. Protection of adults rechallenged with a human rotavirus. *J Infect Dis* 1990;161:440–445.
217. Ward RL, McNeal MM, Sheridan JF. Evidence that active protection following oral immunization of mice with live rotavirus is not dependent on neutralizing antibody. *Virology* 1992;188:57–66.
218. Offit PA, Dudzik KI. Rotavirus-specific cytotoxic T lymphocytes cross-react with target cells infected with different rotavirus serotypes. *J Virol* 1988;62:127–131.
219. Offit PA, Dudzik KI. Noninfectious rotavirus (strain RRV) induces an immune response in mice which protects against rotavirus challenge. *J Clin Microbiol* 1989;27:885–888.
220. Offit PA, Svoboda YM. Rotavirus-specific cytotoxic T lymphocyte response of mice after oral inoculation with candidate rotavirus vaccine strains RRV or WC3. *J Infect Dis* 1989;160:783–788.
221. Offit PA, Dudzik KI. Rotavirus-specific cytotoxic T lymphocytes appear at the intestinal mucosal surface after rotavirus infection. *J Virol* 1989;63:3507–3512.
222. Offit PA, Hoffenberg EJ, Pia ES, et al. Rotavirus-specific helper T cell responses in newborns, infants, children, and adults. *J Infect Dis* 1992;165:1107–1111.
223. Offit PA, Cunningham SL, Dudzik KI. Memory and distribution of virus-specific cytotoxic T lymphocytes (CTLs) and CTL precursors after rotavirus infection. *J Virol* 1991;65:1318–1324.
224. Dharakul T, Rott L, Greenberg HB. Recovery from chronic rotavirus infection in mice with severe combined immunodeficiency: virus clearance mediated by adoptive transfer of immune CD8+ T lymphocytes. *J Virol* 1990;64:4375–4382.
225. Offit PA, Dudzik KI. Rotavirus-specific cytotoxic T lymphocytes passively protect against gastroenteritis in suckling mice. *J Virol* 1990;64:6325–6328.
226. Dharakul T, Labbe M, Cohen J, et al. Immunization with baculovirus-expressed recombinant rotavirus proteins VP1, VP4, VP6, and VP7 induces CD8+ T lymphocytes that mediate clearance of chronic rotavirus infection in SCID mice. *J Virol* 1991;65:5928–5932.
227. Eiden J, Lederman HM, Vonderfecht S, et al. T-cell-deficient mice display normal recovery from experimental rotavirus infection. *J Virol* 1986;57:706–708.
228. Franco MA, Greenberg HB. Immunity to rotavirus in T cell deficient mice. *Virology* 1997;238:169–179.
229. Leece JG, King MW, Dorsey WE. Rearing regimen producing piglet diarrhea (rotavirus) and its relevance to acute infantile diarrhea. *Science* 1978;199:776–778.
230. Snodgrass DR, Fahey KJ, Well PW, et al. Passive immunity in calf rotavirus infections: maternal vaccination increases and prolongs immunoglobulin G antibody secretion. *Infect Immun* 1980;28:344–349.
231. Snodgrass DR, Nagy LK, Sherwood D, et al. Passive immunity in calf diarrhea: vaccination with K99 antigen of enterotoxigenic *Escherichia coli* and rotavirus. *Infect Immun* 1982;37:586–591.
232. Totterdell BM, Chrystie IL, Banatvala JE. Cord blood and breast milk antibodies in neonatal rotavirus infection. *BMJ* 1980;280:828–830.
233. Totterdell BM, Nicholson KG, MacLeod J, et al. Neonatal rotavirus infection: role of lacteal neutralising alpha1-antitrypsin and nonimmunoglobulin antiviral activity in protection. *J Med Virol* 1982;10:37–44.
234. Totterdell BM, Banatvala JE, Chrystie IL. Studies on human lacteal rotavirus antibodies by immune electron microscopy. *J Med Virol* 1983;11:167–175.
235. Gurwith M, Wenman W, Gurwith D, et al. Diarrhea among infants and young children in Canada: a longitudinal study in three northern communities. *J Infect Dis* 1983;147:685–692.
236. Glass RI, Stoll BJ, Wyatt RG, et al. Observations questioning a protective role for breast-feeding in severe rotavirus diarrhea. *Acta Paediatr Scand* 1986;75:713–718.
237. Glass RI, Stoll BJ. The protective effect of human milk against diarrhea. A review of studies from Bangladesh. *Acta Paediatr Scand Suppl* 1989;351:131–136.
238. Yolken RH, Peterson JA, Vonderfecht SL, et al. Human milk mucin inhibits rotavirus replication and prevents experimental gastroenteritis. *J Clin Invest* 1992;90:1984–1991.
239. Newburg DS, Peterson JA, Ruiz-Palacios GM, et al. Role of human-milk lactadherin in protection against symptomatic rotavirus infection [see comments]. *Lancet* 1998;351:1160–1164.
240. Morrey JD, Sidwell RW, Noble RL, et al. Effects of folic acid malnutrition on rotaviral infection in mice. *Proc Soc Exp Biol Med* 1984;176:77–83.
241. Noble RL, Sidwell RW, Mahoney AW, et al. Influence of malnutrition and alterations in dietary protein on murine rotaviral disease. *Proc Soc Exp Biol Med* 1983;173:417–426.
242. Black RE, Merson MH, Eusof A, et al. Nutritional status, body size and severity of diarrhoea associated with rotavirus or enterotoxigenic *Escherichia coli*. *J Trop Med Hyg* 1984;87:83–89.
243. Offor E, Riepenhoff TM, Ogra PL. Effect of malnutrition on rotavirus infection in suckling mice: kinetics of early infection. *Proc Soc Exp Biol Med* 1985;178:85–90.

244. Riepenhoff TM, Offor E, Klossner K, et al. Effect of age and malnutrition on rotavirus infection in mice. *Pediatr Res* 1985; 19:1250–1253.
245. Riepenhoff TM, Uhnoo I, Chegas P, et al. Effect of nutritional deprivation on mucosal viral infections. *Immunol Invest* 1989; 18:127–139.
246. Ahmed F, Jones DB, Jackson AA. The interaction of vitamin A deficiency and rotavirus infection in the mouse. *Br J Nutr* 1990;63:363–373.
247. Ahmed F, Jones DB, Jackson AA. Effect of vitamin A deficiency on the immune response to epizootic diarrhoea of infant mice (EDIM) rotavirus infection in mice. *Br J Nutr* 1991;65: 475–485.
248. Pichichero ME, Losonsky GA, Rennels MB, et al. Effect of dose and a comparison of measures of vaccine take for oral rhesus rotavirus vaccine. The Maryland Clinical Studies Group. *Pediatr Infect Dis J* 1990;9:339–344.
249. Ing DJ, Glass RI, Woods PA, et al. Immunogenicity of tetravalent rhesus rotavirus vaccine administered with buffer and oral polio vaccine. *Am J Dis Child* 1991;145:892–897.
250. Chen CC, Baylor M, Bass DM. Murine intestinal mucins inhibit rotavirus infection. *Gastroenterology* 1993;105:84–92.
251. Duffy LC, Riepenhoff TM, Byers TE, et al. Modulation of rotavirus enteritis during breast-feeding. Implications on alterations in the intestinal bacterial flora. *Am J Dis Child* 1986; 140:1164–1168.
252. Stiglmair HM, Pospischil A, Hess RG, et al. Enzyme histochemistry of the small intestinal mucosa in experimental infections of calves with rotavirus and enterotoxigenic *Escherichia coli*. *Vet Pathol* 1986;23:125–131.
253. Tzipori S, Chandler D, Smith M. The clinical manifestation and pathogenesis of enteritis associated with rotavirus and enterotoxigenic *Escherichia coli* infections in domestic animals. *Prog Food Nutr Sci* 1983;7:193–205.
254. Pickering LK O'Ryan M. Serotypes of rotavirus that infect infants symptomatically and asymptomatically. *Adv Exp Med Biol* 1991;310:241–247.
255. Abiodun PO, Ihongbe JC, Ogbimi A. Asymptomatic rotavirus infection in Nigerian day-care centres. *Ann Trop Paediatr* 1985; 5:163–165.
256. Araya M, Figueroa G, Espinoza J, et al. Acute diarrhoea and asymptomatic infection in Chilean preschoolers of low and high socio-economic strata. *Acta Paediatr Scand* 1986;75:645–651.
257. Barron RB, Barreda GJ, Doval UR, et al. Asymptomatic rotavirus infections in day care centers. *J Clin Microbiol* 1985; 22:116–118.
258. Champsaur H, Henry AM, Goldszmidt D, et al. Rotavirus carriage, asymptomatic infection, and disease in the first two years of life. II. Serological response. *J Infect Dis* 1984;149:675–682.
259. Eiden JJ, Verleur DG, Vonderfecht SL, et al. Duration and pattern of asymptomatic rotavirus shedding by hospitalized children. *Pediatr Infect Dis J* 1988;7:564–569.
260. Losonsky GA, Reymann M. The immune response in primary asymptomatic and symptomatic rotavirus infection in newborn infants. *J Infect Dis* 1990;161:330–332.
261. Walther FJ, Bruggeman C, Daniels BM, et al. Symptomatic and asymptomatic rotavirus infections in hospitalized children. *Acta Paediatr Scand* 1983;72:659–663.
262. Rodriguez WJ, Kim HW, Brandt CD, et al. Fecal adenoviruses from a longitudinal study of families in metropolitan Washington, D.C.: laboratory, clinical, and epidemiologic observations. *J Pediatr* 1985;107:514–520.
263. Carlson JAK, Middleton PJ, Shaw RD, et al. Fatal rotavirus gastroenteritis. An analysis of 22 cases. *Am J Dis Child* 1978;132: 477–479.
264. Schumacher RF, Forster J. The CNS symptoms of rotavirus infections under the age of two. *Klinische Padiatrie* 1999;211: 61–64.
265. Rotbart HA, Levin MJ, Yolken RH, et al. An outbreak of rotavirus-associated neonatal necrotizing enterocolitis. *J Pediatr* 1983;103:454–459.
266. Rotbart HA, Nelson WL, Glode MP, et al. Neonatal rotavirus-associated necrotizing enterocolitis: case control study and prospective surveillance during an outbreak. *J Pediatr* 1988; 112:87–93.
267. Keller KM, Schmidt H, Wirth S, et al. Differences in the clinical and radiologic patterns of rotavirus and non-rotavirus necrotizing enterocolitis. *Pediatr Infect Dis J* 1991;10:734–738.
268. Yolken RH, Leggiadro RJ. Immunoassays for the diagnosis of viral enteric pathogens. *Diagn Microbiol Infect Dis* 1986;4: 61S–69S.
269. Christy C, Vosefski D, Madore HP. Comparison of three enzyme immunoassays to tissue culture for the diagnosis of rotavirus gastroenteritis in infants and young children. *J Clin Microbiol* 1990;28:1428–1430.
270. Honma H, Ushijimma H, Takagi M, et al. Evaluation of a new enzyme immunoassay (TESTPACK ROTAVIRUS) for diagnosis of viral gastroenteritis. *Kansenshogaku Zasshi* 1990;64: 174–178.
271. Chernesky M, Castriciano S, Mahony J, et al. Examination of the Rotazyme II enzyme immunoassay for the diagnosis of rotavirus gastroenteritis. *J Clin Microbiol* 1985;22:462–464.
272. Steele AD, Williams MM, Bos P, et al. Comparison of two rapid enzyme immunoassays with standard enzyme immunoassay and latex agglutination for the detection of human rotavirus in stools. *J Diarrhoeal Dis Res* 1994;12:117–120.
273. Rabenau H, Knoll B, Allwinn R, et al. Improvement of the specificity of enzyme immunoassays for the detection of rotavirus and adenovirus in fecal specimens. *Intervirology* 1998;41: 55–62.
274. Herring AJ, Inglis NF, Ojeh CK, et al. Rapid diagnosis of rotavirus infection by direct detection of viral nucleic acid in silver-stained polyacrylamide gels. *J Clin Microbiol* 1982;16: 473–477.
275. Avendano LF, Dubinovsky S, James HJ. Comparison of viral RNA electrophoresis and indirect ELISA methods in the diagnosis of human rotavirus infection. *Bull Pan Am Health Org* 1984;18:245–249.
276. Chudzio T, Kasatiya S, Irvine N, et al. Rapid screening test for the diagnosis of rotavirus infection. *J Clin Microbiol* 1989;27: 2394–2396.
277. Flores J, Green KY, Garcia D, et al. Dot hybridization assay for distinction of rotavirus serotypes. *J Clin Microbiol* 1989;27: 29–34.
278. Flores J, Sears J, Schael IP, et al. Identification of human rotavirus serotype by hybridization to polymerase chain reaction-generated probes derived from a hyperdivergent region of the gene encoding outer capsid protein VP7. *J Virol* 1990;64: 4021–4024.
279. Fernandez J, Sandino A, Yudelevich A, et al. Rotavirus detection by dot blot hybridization assay using a non-radioactive synthetic oligodeoxynucleotide probe. *Epidemiol Infect* 1992;108: 175–184.
280. Cumino AC, Giordano MO, Martínez LC, et al. Culture amplification in human colon adenocarcinoma cell line (CaCo-2) combined with an ELISA as a supplementary assay for accurate diagnosis of rotavirus. *J Virol Methods* 1998;76:81–85.
281. Husain M, Seth P, Broor S. Detection of group A rotavirus by reverse transcriptase and polymerase chain reaction in feces from children with acute gastroenteritis. *Arch Virol* 1995;140: 1225–1233.
282. Arguelles MH, Villegas GA, Castello A, et al. VP7 and VP4

genotyping of human group A rotavirus in Buenos Aires, Argentina. *J Clin Microbiol* 2000;38:252–259.
283. Marin L, Gunoz H, Sokucu S, et al. Oral rehydration therapy in malnourished infants with infectious diarrhoea. *Acta Paediatr Scand* 1986;75:477–482.
284. Sokucu S, Marin L, Gunoz H, et al. Oral rehydration therapy in infectious diarrhoea. Comparison of rehydration solutions with 60 and 90 mmol sodium per litre. *Acta Paediatr Scand* 1985;74:489–494.
285. Farthing MJ. History and rationale of oral rehydration and recent developments in formulating an optimal solution. *Drugs* 1988;38:80–90.
286. Hjelt K, Paerregaard A, Petersen W, et al. Rapid versus gradual refeeding in acute gastroenteritis in childhood: energy intake and weight gain. *J Pediatr Gastroenterol Nutr* 1989;8:75–80.
287. Armitstead J, Kelly D, Walker-Smith J. Evaluation of infant feeding in acute gastroenteritis. *J Pediatr Gastroenterol Nutr* 1989;8:240–244.
288. Quak SH, Low PS, Quah TC, et al. Oral refeeding following acute gastro-enteritis: a clinical trial using four refeeding regimes. *Ann Trop Paediatr* 1989;9:152–155.
289. Haffejee IE. Cow's milk-based formula, human milk, and soya feeds in acute infantile diarrhea: a therapeutic trial. *J Pediatr Gastroenterol Nutr* 1990;10:193–198.
290. Brussow H, Hilpert H, Walther I, et al. Bovine milk immunoglobulins for passive immunity to infantile rotavirus gastroenteritis. *J Clin Microbiol* 1987;25:982–986.
291. Hilpert H, Brussow H, Mietens C, et al. Use of bovine milk concentrate containing antibody to rotavirus to treat rotavirus gastroenteritis in infants. *J Infect Dis* 1987;156:158–166.
292. Guarino A, Guandalini S, Albano F, et al. Enteral immunoglobulins for treatment of protracted rotaviral diarrhea. *Pediatr Infect Dis J* 1991;10:612–614.
293. Hammarstrom L. Passive immunity against rotavirus in infants. *Acta Paediatr Suppl* 1999;88:127–132.
294. Guarino A, Canani RB, Spagnuolo MI, et al. Oral bacterial therapy reduces the duration of symptoms and of viral excretion in children with mild diarrhea. *J Pediatr Gastroenterol Nutr* 1997;25:516–519.
295. Guandalini S, Pensabene L, Zikri MA, et al. Lactobacillus GG administered in oral rehydration solution to children with acute diarrhea: a multicenter European trial. *J Pediatr Gastroenterol Nutr* 2000;30:54–60.
296. Bhutta TI, Tahir KI. Loperamide poisoning in children [letter] [see comments]. *Lancet* 1990;335:363.
297. Minton NA, Henry JA. Loperamide poisoning in children [letter; comment]. *Lancet* 1990;335:788.
298. Schwartz RH, Rodriquez WJ. Toxic delirium possibly caused by loperamide [letter; comment]. *J Pediatr* 1991;118: 656–657.
299. Kassaem AS, Madkour AB, Massoub BS, et al. Loperamide in acute childhood diarrhea. *J Diarrhoeal Dis Res* 1983;1:10–16.
300. Owens JR, Broadhead R, Hendrickse RG, et al. Loperamide in the treatment of acute gastroenteritis in children: report on a two centre double-blind controlled clinical trial. *Ann Trop Pediatr* 1981;1:135–141.
301. World Health Organization. *WHO, The rational use of drugs in the management of acute diarrhea in children.* Geneva: World Health Organization, 1990.
302. Salazar-Lindo E, Santisteban-Ponce J, Chea-Woo E, et al. Racecadotril in the treatment of acute watery diarrhea in children. *N Engl J Med* 2000;343:463–467.
303. De CE, Bergstrom DE, Holy A, et al. Broad-spectrum antiviral activity of adenosine analogues. *Antiviral Res* 1984;4:119–133.
304. De CE, Cools M, Balzarini J, et al. Broad-spectrum antiviral activities of neplanocin A, 3-deazaneplanocin A, and their 5′-nor derivatives. *Antimicrob Agents Chemother* 1989;33:1291–1297.
305. Kitaoka S, Konno T, De CE. Comparative efficacy of broad-spectrum antiviral agents as inhibitors of rotavirus replication *in vitro*. *Antiviral Res* 1986;6:57–65.
306. Linhares RE, Wigg MD, Lagrota MH, et al. The *in vitro* antiviral activity of isoprinosine on simian rotavirus (SA-11). *Braz J Med Biol Res* 1989;22:1095–1103.
307. Ebina T, Tsukada K. Protease inhibitors prevent the development of human rotavirus-induced diarrhea in suckling mice. *Microbiol Immunol* 1991;35:583–588.
308. Vonderfecht SL, Miskuff RL, Wee SB, et al. Protease inhibitors suppress the *in vitro* and *in vivo* replication of rotavirus. *J Clin Invest* 1988;82:2011–2016.

55

HUMAN GROUP B AND C ROTAVIRUSES

ERICH R. MACKOW

Group A rotaviruses are the most common cause of diarrheal disease in infants and young children. However, the identification of genetically and antigenically distinct human group B and C rotaviruses has stimulated interest in their contribution to diarrheal disease in various populations. Group C rotaviruses, like group A strains, cause diarrhea in young children age 4 months to 4 years, although some reports implicate group C rotaviruses as the cause of clinical disease primarily in children older than 4 years and in some adults (1). Group C rotaviruses have been identified as the causative agents of food-borne institutional diarrheal outbreaks in Japanese and English elementary schools and have also been identified in children in the United States (2–8).

In contrast to other human rotaviruses, group B rotaviruses are responsible for predominantly adult diarrheal disease (9,10). Group B rotaviruses were first identified as the cause of human disease in 1983 (9). At that time, a group B rotavirus named ADRV—*a*dult *d*iarrheal *r*ota*v*irus—was identified as the causative agent of severe "cholera-like" diarrheal outbreaks in large portions (5% to 45 %) of the rural Chinese population (9–14). Contamination of water supplies during the outbreaks suggest that ADRV was introduced via drinking water. Outbreaks of ADRV-induced diarrhea have continued to appear in China. Although Group B rotavirus outbreaks have not been widely encountered elsewhere, there are reports from outside of China where Group B rotaviruses have been identified as the etiologic agent of diarrheal disease. There is only one report of a group B rotavirus outbreak in the United States (15). However, recent epidemiologic studies suggest that approximately 5% of the U. S. population are seropositive for ADRV and all of those identified are adult. The presence of human group B rotavirus antibodies has also been documented in other parts of the world including Bangladesh, India, Japan, Thailand, Mexico, Australia, and the United Kingdom, suggesting that ADRV may be a more widespread cause of adult diarrhea than previously estimated (12,13,16–20).

One caveat to the infrequent detection of both group B and C rotaviruses is that standardized diagnostic assays for these viruses are not widely available. The Rotazyme assay is the only available clinical diagnostic assay for rotavirus and this assay detects exclusively group A rotaviruses. Another consideration for the infrequent detection of these viruses is that adults rarely report their clinical disease. Recent progress on the study of group B and C rotavirus strains promises the development of clinical diagnostic tests for these viruses in the near future.

Rotaviruses from groups A, B, and C cause disease in both human and animal populations (9,11,15,21–27). In animals, rotavirus infections are endemic and provide a reservoir of virus for potential human infections. Further suggesting the potential for zoonotic infections in humans is the fact that U.S. pigs are 70% to 99% seropositive for groups A, B, and C rotaviruses (16). Additionally, rotaviruses contain a segmented RNA genome and individual gene segments can be reassorted upon mixed infection (28). Segmented viruses, such as influenza and rotavirus, permit for rapid genetic shifts and, as a result, the rapid development of new viral strains with altered host range restrictions and virulence characteristics. One possibility for the outbreaks of human group B rotavirus disease in China is the reassortment of normally benign human viruses to new more virulent strains. Alternatively, the reassortment or genetic drift of zoonotic group B rotaviruses may have altered viral host ranges to include humans.

Studies of group B and C rotaviruses in human populations are only beginning to shed light on their contributions to diarrheal disease. The roles of group B and C rotavirus strains in worldwide human disease are poised to unfold with the implementation of newly developing diagnostic tests, the recent cultivation of group C strains, and the increasing use of recombinant DNA techniques to study these viruses.

E. R. Mackow: Departments of Medicine and Molecular Genetics and Microbiology, Stony Brook University, Stony Brook, New York; Northport VA Medical Center, Northport, New York

HISTORY

Atypical Rotaviruses

Historically rotaviruses were identified by their electron microscopic morphology and by their genetic content of 11 double-stranded RNA segments (29,30). Rotaviruses that were antigenically distinct or contained a unique electrophoretic pattern of dsRNA segments were referred to as atypical rotavirus strains, pararotaviruses, novel rotaviruses, or rotavirus-like viruses, because they differed from group A rotavirus strains (9,22,24,26,27,31–41A). In 1983, Pedley and colleagues (36) proposed the classification of rotaviruses into serologically related groups A, B, and C. In 1984, avian serogroup D was defined and, in 1986, serogroup E rotaviruses were identified (37). With more specific serogroup definitions, still more rotavirus groups were identified by their antigenic similarity to other rotavirus strains. Antigenically distinct rotavirus groups A to G have been defined for rotavirus strains (41,42). Each group is also genetically distinct and gene reassortment that occurs between some rotavirus strains of the same group has not been observed to occur between strains of different groups (43).

Among rotavirus groups, only group A, B, and C strains have been identified as clinical pathogens in humans (9,19,29,30,32,44). However, there are reports of human rotavirus isolates that are not from serogroups A, B, C, or D and that have unique electrophoretic patterns (42,45). These viruses may define new serogroups that cause human disease.

ADRV

Group B rotaviruses were first identified as human pathogens in 1983 following epidemic outbreaks of severe dehydrating diarrhea in the Chinese population (9–11). Interestingly, these outbreaks primarily occurred in individuals age 15 years and older with the highest infection rate occurring in individuals older than age 30 years (1.6% to 2.3 %) (12–14). Initially, the causative agent was referred to as rotavirus-like or novel because its morphology resembled other rotavirus strains, it lacked serologic cross-reactivity with group A and C rotavirus strains, and it contained a unique dsRNA electrophoretic pattern (9). It was later confirmed to be antigenically related to group B rotavirus strains (11). Of those infected, 85% were older than 15 years of age and only 2.8% were 0 to 4 years of age (12). As a result, the rotavirus agent was named the adult diarrheal rotavirus, or ADRV.

IDIR

In 1984, a group B rotavirus was detected as the cause of infectious diarrhea of infant rats, or IDIR (27). This virus caused the formation of syncytia in the villous epithelium of the infected animals, which contained 80 nm rotavirus-like particles (27). The viral dsRNAs were distinct from group A strains and were later demonstrated to be antigenically related to group B rotaviruses (27,46). The RNA electrophoretic pattern of IDIR is not identical to that of ADRV but the patterns are similar. The two viruses have since been found to be related both antigenically and genetically (46). IDIR and ADRV are also able to fuse cells forming multinucleate syncytia in the infected cell monolayer (27). Syncytia are hallmarks of group B rotavirus strains and are absent from all other rotaviruses (23,24,27,31,41A,47).

There is one report of a rat group B rotavirus infecting humans (15). In 1985, IDIR infections were reported during an analysis of non–group A rotavirus infections of children and adults in Baltimore, MD. Six fecal specimens from three children and three adults were able to confer IDIR infections to rats (15). The three adults were physicians at the same hospital and one physician worked with IDIR-infected rats, so there is some question as to whether the virus was inadvertently introduced into others by contact or whether the children were the source of the virus. Of the three children infected, one was a child of one of the physicians, one was admitted with diarrhea, and diarrhea developed in the third after admission (15). Regardless of the source of the inoculum, this study indicates that IDIR can infect humans and that it is a potential source of human disease.

Group C Rotavirus

Group C rotaviruses were originally referred to as *pararotaviruses* for their similarity to typical group A rotaviruses (35,48). The first report of human pararotavirus appeared in 1982 in the infection of an infant in Australia (49). Two additional reports of human group C rotaviruses in Brazil and France also appeared in 1983 (35,38). In each case, a single infant was infected with a group C rotavirus. Since then, many clinical diarrheal cases in infants and adults have been attributed to group C rotavirus infections (1,3, 5,6,32,34,44,50–60). One report associates group C rotaviruses with infections of infants with extrahepatic biliary atresia, although there is no further reports on this association (61). In contrast to other rotaviruses, group C rotavirus infections have only been reported in humans and pigs. A high percentage of pigs are seropositive in both North America and the United Kingdom (17,25).

Human group C rotavirus infections have been reported in Argentina, Australia, Brazil, Bulgaria, Chile, China, Ecuador, England, Finland, France, Germany, India, Italy, Japan, Malaysia, Mexico, Nepal, South Africa, Thailand, and the United States (1,3,4,5,8,32,34,35,38,44,49,50–60, 62–67). Recent epidemic outbreaks of group C rotavirus infections were reported in England, Brazil, and Japan in 1989 (2,7,8,57,59,68,69). In each case, large numbers of school children became ill, with vomiting being the primary symptom of the infection. In the Japanese outbreak, both children and adults were infected (ages 7 to 54 years) and the outbreak included 22% (675) of the elementary school students (59,70). In one British outbreak, 28 of 130 school children, age 4 to 10 years became ill (2). In both of these outbreaks, a school lunch was a common factor. The Japanese outbreak involved seven separate schools that were served by a common regional food preparation service, although the cause of the outbreak was not linked to a common food source. Others have also indicated that group C rotavirus infections occur in adults and children and that group C infections are the most common cause of gastroenteritis in children between 4 and 7 years of age (1,4,70,71).

CLASSIFICATION AND VIRAL STRUCTURE

Rotaviruses are members of the family Reoviridae by virtue of their icosahedral triple-layered protein capsid structure and the presence of a segmented dsRNA genome. Complete group B and C rotavirus particles are approximately 70 nm in diameter and indistinguishable from group A rotaviruses by electron microscopy (EM) (41). Rotaviruses are not enveloped and, as a result, they are resistant to lipid solvents. The IDIR group B rotavirus is reported to be labile at pH 3 but stable to ether or pH 5 (27). ADRV viral particles are reported to be 70 nm in diameter (9,12), but more often than not, ADRV virions are found as degraded 45- to 52-nm viral corelike particles (12). ADRV is also reported to be more stable at 40°C than at −20°C (12).

Treatment of viral particles with calcium chelators, EGTA or EDTA, results in the production of single-shelled particles approximately 55 nm in diameter and activates the viral transcriptase (72). Predominant corelike particles in ADRV preparations may be attributable to preparation of the virus for EM. Group C rotaviruses are reported to be insensitive to 1.5 M $CaCl_2$ treatments, which disrupt double-shelled group A rotavirus particles (73).

All Reoviridae are transcriptionally active and contain a dsRNA-dependent RNA polymerase within their viral cores (41). The RNA polymerase complex synthesizes capped but not polyadenylated mRNAs, which exit pores in the double-shelled virus particle into the cell cytoplasm. Virus replication is fully cytoplasmic and genomic dsRNAs are synthesized within replicase particles, which include the viral proteins VP1, VP2, and VP3 and 11 single-stranded template RNAs (41).

SEROGROUPS

Rotaviruses are distinguished serologically into groups A through G (42). Viruses from a single rotavirus group are antigenically unique and are not recognized by infection serum from other rotavirus groups. Cross-reactive epitopes present on the major inner capsid protein VP6 are primarily involved in differentiating rotavirus groups, because this highly antigenic protein comprises approximately 50% of viral protein content (41,74). The VP6 protein is also the target of most diagnostic virus and serum antibody detection assays. Although tests for the group specificity of rotaviruses have been used for many years in research laboratories, the wide availability of standardized tests for group B and C rotaviruses is just beginning. Group B and C diagnostic assays have been reported using recombinant VP6 proteins and monoclonal antibodies to the VP6 antigen (70,75–80). These polymerase chain reaction (PCR) and neutralization-based detection assays should offer the same rapid diagnostic testing currently available for group A rotaviruses in the Rotazyme clinical diagnostic assay (67,71,77,81–86).

GROUP B AND C ROTAVIRUS SEROTYPES

Two proteins of the rotavirus outer capsid have been shown to be involved in neutralization specificity. The VP4 and VP7 proteins of the outer capsid are recognized by antibodies that neutralize rotaviruses (41,87–89). Within each rotavirus group are a variety of different VP4 and VP7 neutralization antigens, which form the basis of rotavirus serotypes (42). Infection sera from viruses of the same serotype can prevent or neutralize the infectivity of each other. Within group A rotaviruses, serotyping nomenclature has been developed based on these two proteins. The VP4 protein, which is proteolytically cleaved, defines the P serotype of the virus, and the VP7 glycoprotein defines the G serotype (87,88,90).

Serotypes have not been defined for group B rotavirus strains, largely because of the inability to cultivate these viruses and, as a result, develop neutralization tests. However, the cultivation of group B rotaviruses has recently been reported, suggesting that a complete understanding of group B rotavirus neutralization determinants is open to investigation (91). The ability of antibodies to the ADRV VP4 protein to neutralize ADRV has been presented, indicating that the VP4 protein plays a role in viral neutralization and that at least one P type exists for group B strains. However, multiple group B rotavirus P types are likely to exist because of the low level of identical amino acids between the VP4 proteins of ADRV and IDIR (58%) (92,93) and because of the low level of antibody cross-reactivity between the VP4 proteins of ADRV, IDIR, and a porcine strain, SRV-1 (92,94).

More than one ADRV isolate has been derived from the outbreaks in China (9,12,95–97). The serotypic diversity of the VP7 protein of group B strains has not been investigated, but there are likely to be multiple serotypes similar to that of group A rotaviruses (98). The low level of homology between the IDIR and ADRV VP7 proteins (52% identical amino acids) (98–100) is much less than the 85% homology of group A VP7 proteins that define different serotypes. The genes encoding the VP4 and VP7 proteins of ADRV and IDIR strains have been cloned and expressed, and, with information from the recent identification of an Indian ADRV strain, CAL, should permit studies of group B rotavirus serotypic diversity (86,92,93,99,100).

GROUP C SEROTYPES

In the past, the serotypic evaluation of group C rotaviruses has been hampered by the inability to cultivate group C strains. However, this obstacle has reportedly been overcome and there are several reports of group C rotaviruses that have been adapted to growth in tissue culture (101–104). In addition, the cloning of human group C rotavirus genes encoding the VP6, VP7, and NSP5 proteins have been reported, and the VP4 protein has been cloned from animal strains (105–114). With these developments, the tools for evaluating the serotypic diversity of human and animal group C rotavirus strains are available. Initial studies with hyperimmune sera to human (Ehime 86-542) (59), porcine (Cowden) (101), and bovine (Shintoku) (103) strains of group C rotavirus have indicated that at least two different serotypes exist (115). Hyperimmune or convalescent sera to the Ehime strain and two porcine strains can neutralize the Cowden group C rotavirus, but they have no effect on the bovine, Shintoku, or porcine, HF, rotavirus strains (202). The human Bristol strain was not tested in this study (3).

Although these studies were not able to consider the two different neutralization antigens on the virus, it is likely that many G or P group C serotypes will be identified because there are many diverse group C isolates and hosts (human, porcine, and bovine) (115). Defining human and animal group C serotypes should help resolve the source of human infections.

ELECTROPHEROTYPES

Group B and C rotaviruses each have unique electrophoretic RNA profiles from group A rotavirus strains (Fig. 55.1). Each virus contains 11 dsRNA segments in its

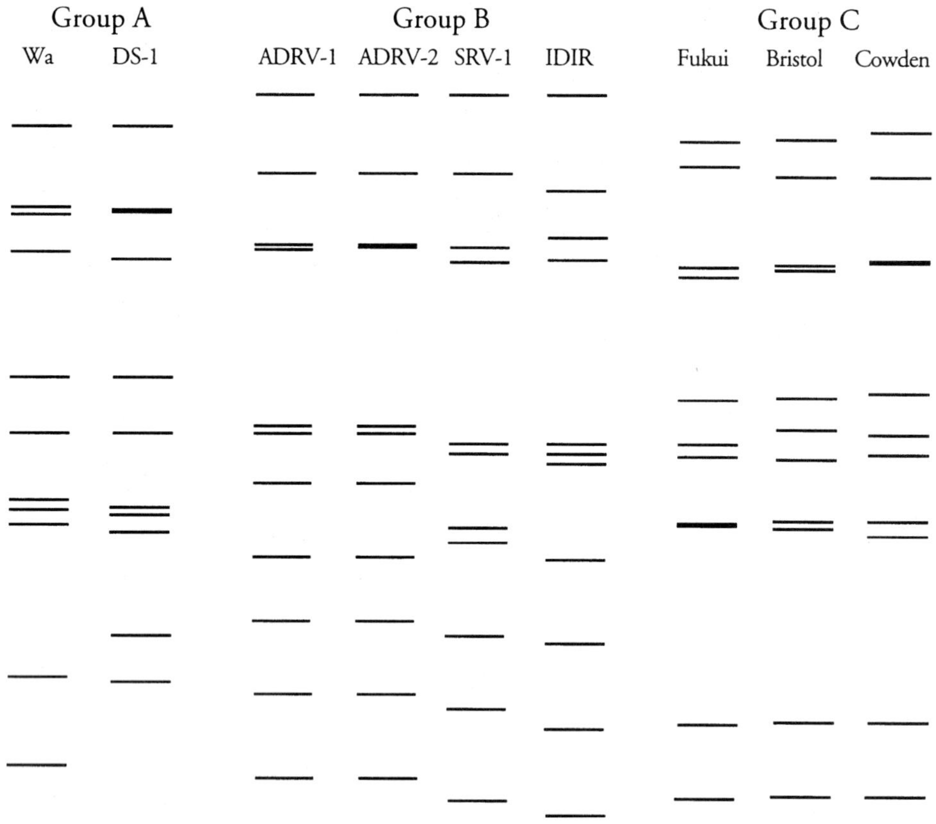

FIGURE 55.1. Electropherotypes of group A, B, and C rotaviruses. Genomic double-stranded RNA is extracted from rotavirus isolates and separated by 7.5% to 12% polyacrylamide gel electrophoresis (PAGE) under neutral conditions. Gels are fixed and silver stained in order to visualize dsRNA segments. This diagram represents the position of dsRNA segments separated from human group A, B, and C rotaviruses by PAGE. All strains listed are human rotaviruses except for the IDIR rat group B rotavirus strain and the Cowden porcine group C rotavirus. DsRNA patterns are referred to as *electropherotypes* because patterns are fingerprints of individual viruses and often can be used to designate their group specificity.

genome; however, the length of the gene segments and their migration by neutral polyacrylamide gel electrophoresis (PAGE) vary between groups. The electrophoretic migration of rotavirus gene segments is characteristic of the virus and is similar within each rotavirus group. Because of this, the electrophoretic profile of dsRNAs (or their "electropherotype") has been used to characterize strains and to preliminarily specify their rotavirus group (116). However, as described later, substantial nucleic acid sequence differences between viruses of the same group may not result in changes in gene migration patterns and, therefore, electropherotyping patterns of viruses are not definitive determinants of viral groups.

Group A strains fall into four size classes in a 4-2-3-2 pattern from top to bottom of the gel. Group B and C rotaviruses also contain several patterns of gene segments with common elements. ADRV has a 4-2-1-1-1-1-1 pattern, IDIR a 4-3-1-1-1-1, whereas bovine and porcine group B rotaviruses have a pattern of 4-2-2-3. Common elements are the four large RNA segments and the equal distribution of the smallest three gene segments with variation occurring in gene segments 5 through 8. Group C rotaviruses have a 4-3-2-2 pattern (17,25). Although these represent typical patterns of rotavirus RNA segments, variations of these patterns, usually involve the decreased migration (increased size) of a small RNA segment, designated as "short" RNA patterns. Bovine strains of group B rotavirus have been identified in dairy cattle that display short genome electropherotypes (117,118).

The gross electropherotyping patterns of rotaviruses contain additional differences between rotavirus groups. The four largest gene segments of groups A, B, and C rotaviruses have unique electrophoretic patterns. In group A strains, gene segments 2 and 3 are usually close together, whereas, in group B strains, gene segments 3 and 4 comigrate, and, in group C, rotaviruses tend to have the four large gene segments more equally distributed. Group B strains also have the largest gene segment 2. Gene segments 5 and 6 of group B strains migrate close together or comigrate, in contrast to A or C strains, in which these genes are discrete. In addition, the size of dsRNA gene segment pairs and triplets are specific to each rotavirus group. Most rotaviruses can be tentatively classified by their electropherotype, although final serogrouping is dependent on serologic testing.

Variations in the electropherotype of rotaviruses often reflect minor changes in the RNA, which affect their migration on the gel. These changes may not reflect antigenic differences between viruses or differences in the size of the RNA segments. An example of this is the variable migration of group A gene segments 7 to 9. Nearly all of these gene segments are the same length and the apparent differences in their electrophoretic mobility are only the result of sequence-induced differences, which change the migration of their RNA segments on PAGE. Another example of this migrational anomaly is the apparent size of gene segments 5 and 6 of ADRV. Sequencing full-length clones of these segments has revealed that gene 6 is actually 7 bases longer than gene 5, even though gene 6 appears smaller and migrates below gene 5 on electropherotyping gels (119). Numbering of electrophoretically separated RNAs rather than their sequence length is the convention for naming Reoviridae RNA segments.

During ADRV outbreaks in different parts of China, a variety of group B isolates were compared electrophoretically (12,13). These isolates were mostly identical by electropherotype but slight variations in genome profiles were detected (Fig. 55.1). In the two most distant outbreaks in Lanzhou and Jinzhou, China, 1,100 miles apart, electrophoretic RNA profiles were very similar but oligonucleotide mapping of the RNA segments suggested substantial differences in these viruses (12,13).

HYBRIDIZATION

Hybridization of nucleic acids between rotavirus strains has also been used to define group specificity (46,110,111, 120–125). In general, RNA from rotaviruses of one group hybridize only to viruses within the group and do not cross-hybridize with those from other rotavirus groups (110,111,122,123,125). This distinction can be used as a way of grouping rotaviruses and has also been used to detect group B strains in a dot blot hybridization format (46,110,122). Group B rotavirus ADRV cross-hybridizes with both porcine and rat group B strains and does not hybridize with the group A or C strains tested (17,111,122, 126). It has also been reported that gene segment 1 of groups A and B or A and C rotaviruses hybridizes but that probes to group B or C do not cross-hybridize with each other (25).

Recombinant approaches to the study of group A, B, and C rotaviruses have led to the development of gene-specific probes for these viruses. Clones for each RNA segment of the group B rotavirus ADRV were reported in 1990 as indicated in Figure 55.2 (72). Probes for the IDIR and porcine strains have also been developed. Virtually all group C rotavirus genes have also been cloned and probes have been made for their detection. Porcine and human group C rotavirus RNA segments are highly conserved by hybridization analysis. Gene segment 7 shares the least homology with group C rotaviruses. Known sequences and PCR have provided new means for rotavirus detection (82,83,85,86). PCR has dramatically improved our ability to identify and type rotaviruses from minute quantities of sample and has recently been used to diagnose rotavirus infection in new human populations (4,67,75,77,81,82,86,98,117,127–129). Sensitive PCR diagnostics using conserved group-specific nucleic acid sequences should enhance progress in identifying group B and C rotavirus-induced disease (81,86).

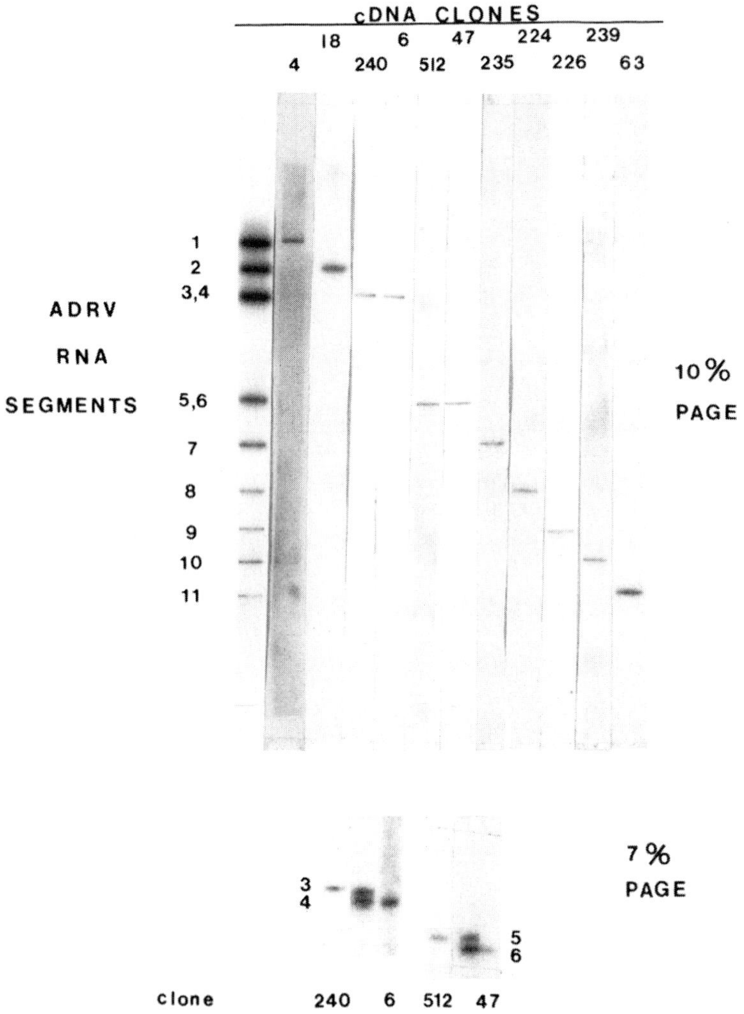

FIGURE 55.2. Hybridization of group B rotavirus clones to ADRV viral dsRNAs. ADRV virion dsRNAs were separated by polyacrylamide gel (PAGE) electrophoresis and blotted onto nitrocellulose. cDNA clones of ADRV gene segments were used to probe strips of the nitrocellulose blot in order to determine their genetic specificity. RNA segments 3,4 and 5,6, which comigrate on 10% gels, were resolved by 7% PAGE as shown. Each clone hybridizes to a single dsRNA segment and is compared with a control hybridization (Lane 1) to all 11 segments. Representative clones from each ADRV RNA segment have been identified.

VIRAL STABILITY

Group C rotaviruses are purified by techniques used for group A rotaviruses (25). However, ADRV is purified by ammonium sulfate (18%) fractionating the virus from specimens (36). After resuspending the viral concentrate, ADRV is pelleted through a 20% to 40% sucrose gradient for 2 hours onto a 1.5 g/mL CsCl cushion. Virus at the interface is applied directly to 1.37 g/mL CsCl gradients and banded by isopycnic centrifugation (72). A visible virus band is present at 1.385 g/mL CsCl and harvested by pelleting (27,72).

Some parameters affecting the viability of infectious ADRV have been analyzed using the ability of the virus to transiently infect Ma104 cells in tissue culture. Interestingly, group A and C rotaviruses are completely resistant to many agents that inactivate ADRV (25). ADRV infectivity is inactivated by many of the manipulations used for purification, such as hydrocarbon (tri-chloro-trifluoroethane, Genetron, chloroform, ether) or detergent (deoxycholate, SDS, Triton X-100, Tween 20) extraction and titers are reduced by even brief sonication. Trypsin, chymotrypsin, and pancreatin at a variety of concentrations also appear to completely inactivate ADRV for infecting MA104 cells. Calcium chelators EDTA and EGTA, reducing agents, pH less than 6, heat (42° or 50°C), and freezing and thawing all inactivate ADRV as assayed by transient infection of tissue culture cells.

GENE STRUCTURE

All rotaviruses contain a genome of 11 double-stranded (ds) RNA segments at the core of the virus (29,41). Genomic RNA serves as a template for mRNA synthesis by the endogenous dsRNA-dependent RNA polymerase present within the core particle (41,130,131). In addition, replication of genomic dsRNA from cytoplasmic mRNAs occurs within replicase particles, which self-assemble in the cytoplasm during infection (132,133,134,135).

Rotavirus dsRNAs have short conserved sequences at their 5′ and 3′ termini (41). Group A, B, and C rotaviruses differ in the sequence of their genomic end-terminal sequences and these differences may be prime factors that prevent gene reassortment between different rotavirus groups (43). The sequence at the ends of 9 of 11 ADRV gene segments have been determined and provide consensus sequences for human group B rotavirus strains (Fig. 55.3). Substantial end-terminal RNA sequence differences between ADRV and IDIR gene segments further demonstrate the divergence of these two group B rotavirus strains (136).

The 5′ consensus sequence is extremely short [GG(C/U)A] and precedes six A or U residues at the beginning of each gene segment. A longer region of nine nucleotides are conserved at the 3′ end of ADRV gene segments. Only gene segment 10 contains mismatches with the consensus sequence in the first seven nucleotide residues at the 3′ end. The eighth and ninth residues from the 3′ end are AU, respectively, in 7/9 of the ADRV genes. The 3′ terminal conservation identified in these genes could represent a mechanism by which viral messenger RNAs are recognized and assembled into replicase particles prior to negative strand RNA synthesis or they could be required for polymerase initiation during viral replication. Hairpin structures at the 3′ end of RNA segments may also be required to stabilize and prevent the degradation of plus-stranded RNAs or as gene-specific viral replication signals that allow the virus to select 11 different RNA segments for replication within viral particles. The 5′ end of each gene segment also contains large hairpin structures that extend well into the coding sequences of the viral genes and thus could be used as gene-specific recognition sequences for viral RNA packaging. In addition, the 5′ and 3′ end-terminal structures can base pair to each other and thus provide gene-specific panhandle structures that could be used for RNA packaging and for initiation of transcription within replicase particles (72).

Group C rotaviruses contain even less conservation at their RNA termini than group B rotaviruses. The 5′ sequence 5′-G(GCU)(AC)AU occurs in each gene segment sequenced. As in group B rotaviruses, the 3′ end is more highly conserved, having a unique UGUGGCU-3′ sequence. The only discrepancy with this is derived from a few sequences that reportedly lack the terminal CU or U residues, although these findings may also result from incomplete end-terminal sequences for these segments. Consensus sequences may change as larger numbers of terminal sequences are determined for group C rotavirus genes. To date, group C strains are the only rotaviruses reported to lack CC at their 3′ termini.

Transcription

Virus purification has been used as a means of generating large amounts of viral mRNA *in vitro*. Rotaviruses contain an endogenous transcriptase that permits transcription of capped mRNAs either *in vivo* or *in vitro* (130,131,137,138). Purified triple-layered particles are transcriptionally activated by chelating calcium or by brief heat treatment of the virus, which removes the outer capsid (119,131,139,138). Transcriptionally active double-shelled particles are permeable, permitting nucleoside entry and the extrusion of mRNAs synthesized within the particle (131,138).

Group B and C rotaviruses are activated in roughly the same way as group A strains, although each may have slightly different pH or nucleotide concentration optima. Both group B and C rotaviruses have been used to generate mRNAs in order to amplify viral-specific nucleic acids. Opti-

Gene	5′	3′
2	GGCAAUUGUCGUGAUGG	GACAUGAUAUUUUAAAAACCC
4	GGCAAUAUAUUUGCUAUGU	UGCAAAUACAUAUAAAAACCC
5	GGUUUAAAUAGCCCAACCGGUGAUUCAAGCAUGG	AAAAAAUAAGCAAUAAAACCC
6	GGUAUAAUUAGAUUGUCAGUAUCCAGGUUUGGGAAACCUAUGG	UACAUAUCUAAAUAAAAACCC
7	GGUAUAAUUACGUUUGAUUCAGAUAGUACUUCGGGUUACUGAGAAACAAACGUAAUGG	CAACCAAAGUAAUAAAAACCC
8	GGUAGAAAUUAAUCUAUUCAGUGUGUCGUGAGAGGGCUCCAUCACCCUGGUCACCAUGA	UAACGGCUAUUUUUAAAACCC
9	GGCAAUAAAAUGG	UAGCCGAAGCUGUAAAAACCC
10	GGCAAUUAAAAGUCCAGUUAUGG	UGAUCAAACUGAUAAGGACCC
11	GGUAUAUAAAAGUCAGUAGACGGCUGGAAACGUUGCACGUACUACUCACUACCCAGAGAUGG	UGAGUUAUAUUUAAAAAACCC

Consensus

	U AAAAAA	AAA
5′	GGCAUUUUUU	UUUAAAACCC 3′

FIGURE 55.3. End-terminal RNA sequences of ADRV cDNA clones and viral mRNAs were sequenced and the end-terminal sequences of known gene segments are presented. Each 5′- and 3′-terminal RNA sequence maintains a small consensus sequence, which is common to each RNA segment. 5′-Terminal sequences differ widely in the position of their methionine initiation codons, AUG. Gene segment 9 initiates at base 10 from the 5′-end and contains the shortest non-coding 5′-terminal sequence.

mized transcription from the ADRV RNA polymerase includes viral activation by a combination of heating at 55°C for 1 minute and the presence of 5 mM EGTA (119). RNA transcription is maximal at pH 8.5 with a temperature optimum of 42°C (92,119). Transcription is inhibited by magnesium ion concentrations that deviate from 2 mM and is optimized in 8 mM rXTPs. *In vitro*, synthesized mRNAs can be used to express ADRV proteins *in vitro* for the purpose of determining gene coding assignments and for obtaining full-length clones of gene segments (92,119,140,141).

Table 55.1 shows the DRV gene coding assignments.

Cloning and Expression of ADRV Genes and Proteins

Molecular Analysis of Group B Strains

Group B rotaviruses have been isolated from humans and from a variety of animals (9–11,21–24,26,27,31,33,47,101, 142,143). The genes from humans, ADRV, and from rats, IDIR, group B rotavirus strains have been cloned, sequenced, and expressed (72,92,94,99,100,119,141,144–147). ADRV gene segments 2, 4, 5, and 9 encoding structural proteins VP2, VP4, VP6, and VP7 have been expressed via baculovirus recombinants (92,94,141,147,148).

The nucleic acid sequences and encoded polypeptides of group B rotaviruses, IDIR and ADRV, are dramatically different from group A and C rotavirus strains (72,92,94,99, 100,119,141,144–147). Each ADRV protein contains low-level amino acid identity (18% to 28%) with corresponding group A rotavirus structural proteins. Although group A equivalent proteins are likely to be involved in analogous ADRV functions, little information has been presented to directly verify the function of group B rotavirus proteins.

Structural Proteins

ADRV gene segments 2, 4, 5, and 9 encode the major structural proteins of the viral capsid. Gene segment 5 of ADRV encodes the major inner capsid protein, VP6 (119). The *in vitro* expressed gene 5 polypeptide comigrates with the 44-kd protein present on EDTA-treated iodinated ADRV virions. The baculovirus-expressed VP6 protein is oligomeric and multimerizes to apparent trimer, hexamer, and greater molecular mass products as assayed by SDS PAGE (148). Antibodies made to the expressed protein, recognize ADRV virions (148) and could prove useful as diagnostic reagents.

The ADRV VP6 equivalent protein contains 25% and 20% identical amino acids to the group C and group A rotavirus VP6 proteins (119). The similarity of these proteins suggests an evolutionary relationship among the three, which distantly relates ADRV to both group A and C rotaviruses and suggests that group B rotaviruses are more closely related to group C rotaviruses (119).

The VP6 proteins of ADRV (gene 5) and IDIR (gene 6) are highly related (119,144). IDIR and ADRV genes are

TABLE 55.1. ADRV GENE CODING ASSIGNMENTS[a]

ADRV Gene		ADRV Protein	Group A Rotavirus				
Segment	Length (Bases)	# Amino Acids (kd)	Capsid Location If Determined	Protein Equivalent (kd)	Group A Gene	ADRV Equivalency Determined By	ADRV Protein Attributes
1	Incomplete	(?) Inc.		VP1 (125)	1	AA alignment	
2	2,844	933 (105)	Inner	VP2 (103)	2	AA alignment Viral comp/IgG	GTP binding domain
3	Incomplete	(?) Inc.		VP3 (88?)	3	AA alignment	
4	2,303	749 (84)	Outer	VP4 (86.5)	4	AA alignment Viral comp/IgG	Neutralization, spike Trypsin cleavage sites
5	1,269	391 (44)	Inner	VP6 (45)	6	AA alignment Viral comp/IgG	Trimer, hexamer formation
6	1,276	107 AAs. (11.7) ORF 40-360		None			Fusion, myristoylated AD6F1 frame 1
		321 (37) ORF 257-1219		NSP1 (58.5)	5	NBRF FastA	Zinc finger AD6F2 frame 2
7	1,179	324 (37.5)		NSP3 (36)	7	AA alignment	Acidic
8	1,006	279 (32)		NSP2 (36.5)	8	AA alignment	Basic
9	814	249 (28.5)	Outer	VP7 (34)	9	AA alignment Viral comp/IgG	Glycosylated to 36 kd Neutralization?
10	751	219 (25.4)		NSP4 (28)	10	Hydrophilicity and AA comp	Glycosylated
11	631	170 (20)		NSP5 (22)	11	AA alignment	

[a]ADRV gene segments have been cloned and sequenced and are available from Genbank at the following accession numbers M91433, M91434, M55982, M91435, M91436, M91437, X56143, M33872, M33873.
AA, amino acid; NBRF, Natural Biomedicaal Research Foundation; ORF, open reading frame.

73% identical at the nucleic acid level. Cloned IDIR and porcine group B genes encoding the VP6 protein have permitted amino acid comparisons of three group B rotavirus VP6 proteins (119,144). Sequence comparisons indicate that group B VP6 proteins share approximately 80% to 84% identical and 92% to 95% similar VP6 amino acids. The similarity between group B VP6 proteins serves as a counterpoint to the divergence of outer capsid proteins VP4 and VP7, discussed later.

The ADRV VP6 equivalent protein is recognized by hyperimmune serum to ADRV or the porcine group B rotavirus, by human ADRV convalescent serum from Chinese or U. S. adults, by group B–specific monoclonal antibodies, and by some but not all IDIR-specific antibodies (12,119,147–149). The group B VP6 protein is not recognized by group A hyperimmune sera.

Gene segment 2 of ADRV and IDIR encodes a single 105- to 106-kd protein, which is similar to the group A rotavirus VP2 protein, present in the viral core (141,150). The gene 2 protein has been expressed *in vitro* and via baculovirus, and the expressed protein has the same molecular mass as a 105-kd protein present on single-shelled ADRV virions. The protein is recognized by anti-ADRV hyperimmune and convalescent serum and does not cross-react with group A rotavirus sera (141).

Viral Glycoprotein

ADRV gene segment 9 encodes a protein with low-level amino acid homology to the group A rotavirus outer capsid protein VP7 (48% similarity, 28% identity) (99,151–153). The likely VP7-equivalent protein contains three potential N-linked glycosylation sites and an amino-terminal signal sequence that could be used to translocate the protein into the lumen of the endoplasmic reticulum (ER) or associate it with plasma membranes (99). Interestingly, early observations of intracellular group B rotaviruses suggest that they are associated with smooth ER membranes in contrast to the rough ER association of group A rotavirus particles (47). It is unknown whether translocation of the VP7 protein, viral budding at the ER, or both direct group B rotaviruses to smooth ER membranes; however, this could represent a fundamental difference in group B rotavirus assembly.

The gene 9–encoded protein also contains a conserved cleavage site, which is used in group A rotavirus strains to cleave the amino-terminal signal sequence from the VP7 protein (99,87). The *in vitro* translated gene 9 protein is glycosylated and increases in size from 29 to 37 kd in the presence of canine microsomes. The protein comigrates with a protein present on iodinated ADRV virions, further suggesting its VP7-equivalency on ADRV (119). It is anticipated that antibodies to the VP7 protein will neutralize the virus and protect animals from disease just as VP7 does in group A strains.

The VP7 protein from the IDIR group B strain contains only 52% identical residues with the ADRV VP7 (99,100). Three bovine strains had more than 90% nucleotide and deduced amino acid homologies among themselves, but they had only 48% to 61% homology with genes from IDIR and ADRV group B rotaviruses (75). In group A strains, different serotypes are defined by VP7 proteins with approximately 85% identical amino acids. The low level of identity between these proteins suggests that ADRV and IDIR are completely discrete group B rotavirus glycoprotein serotypes.

VP4 Protein Conservation

Group A, B, and C strains share limited amino acid identity among their VP4 polypeptides (20% identical, 42% similar residues) (92–94,106,154). Expression and sequencing studies determined that gene segment 4 encodes an 84-kd protein and that the encoded protein comigrates with a protein present on the ADRV outer capsid (92). In group A strains, the VP4 protein is the viral spike protein (86.5 kd), which is proteolytically cleaved to activate virus for infection (87,155). The group A VP4 protein is also the viral hemagglutinin, a determinant of viral neutralization, and confers its P serotype designation (87,88,156–160). Although there is one report of a group B rotavirus isolated from a Chinese infant that hemagglutinates rhesus monkey erythrocytes (161), no further reports of group B rotavirus hemagglutination have been presented. This includes studies on ADRV, IDIR, and other group B rotaviruses, as well as recombinant baculovirus-expressed ADRV VP4 preparations.

There are several potential proteolytic cleavage sites on the VP4 protein at approximately the same positions as the group A VP4 protein (92). However, the importance of proteolytic processing of group B rotavirus VP4 proteins has not been demonstrated. Like for group A rotavirus VP4 proteins, antibodies to the baculovirus-expressed ADRV VP4 protein are anticipated to neutralize the virus (92).

The ADRV and IDIR VP4 proteins are only 58% identical at the amino acid level (92,94). In group A rotaviruses, amino acid differences of only 8% define different serotypes. Substantial differences between the rat and human VP4 proteins suggest that they are distantly related and likely to define unique group B rotavirus P types.

Potential Fusion Protein

Gene 6 of ADRV encodes two proteins in two different overlapping open reading frames (ORFs). The encoded proteins have been termed AD6F1 and AD6F2 for their origin in ADRV gene segment 6 and the open reading frame from which they are derived. The second ORF in gene 6, AD6F2, tentatively encodes a protein similar to the NSP1 protein of group A rotavirus strains. The first ORF, called AD6F1, is a 107–amino acid protein. AD6F1 does not share amino acid similarity with any group A rotavirus protein. However, AD6F1 shares significant amino acid similarity with the respiratory syncytial virus (RSV) and Newcastle disease virus (NDV) fusion (F) proteins. This finding is interesting because both RSV and NDV fuse cells and form syncytia via the F protein (162,163). An NBRF database search for proteins with similarities to AD6F1 revealed that the NDV F protein contains 24% identical and 43% similar amino acids, whereas the RSV F protein is 22% identical and 53% similar to AD6F1 (more than 91 amino acids). The region of similarity comprises nearly the entire length of the 107–amino acid long AD6F1 protein (Fig. 55.4).

The AD6F1 protein contains a potential N-terminal myristoylation site and several potential proteolytic cleavage sites (Fig. 55.4). AD6F1 also contains one long, potentially membrane-spanning, hydrophobic domain. Within this domain are α-helical heptad repeats, which form a hydrophobic face on the protein and a leucine zipper. Each of these transmembrane elements can be involved in protein oligomerization and membrane integration. Interestingly, the NDV fusion protein is acylated, containing a fatty acid moiety at its carboxyl terminus (164,165). Although the role of acylation has not been defined in NDV cell fusion, it could serve to associate the protein with cell membranes similar to a myristoyl group on the group B rotavirus AD6F1 protein. This interesting finding may suggest a role for myristoylation in icosahedral virus-induced cell fusion.

AD6F1 contains two N/G cleavage sites, which are associated with the proteolytic cleavage of myristoylated poliovirus and HIV polyproteins and the reovirus μ1 protein to produce mature myristoylated structural proteins (166–171). Proteolytic processing of AD6F1 at the N/G cleavage site or several adjacent trypsin or chymotrypsin sites would yield a mature amino-terminal polypeptide of 7 kd. These potential cleavages of AD6F1 would contain both the N-terminal myristoyl group and a carboxyl terminal transmembrane domain that

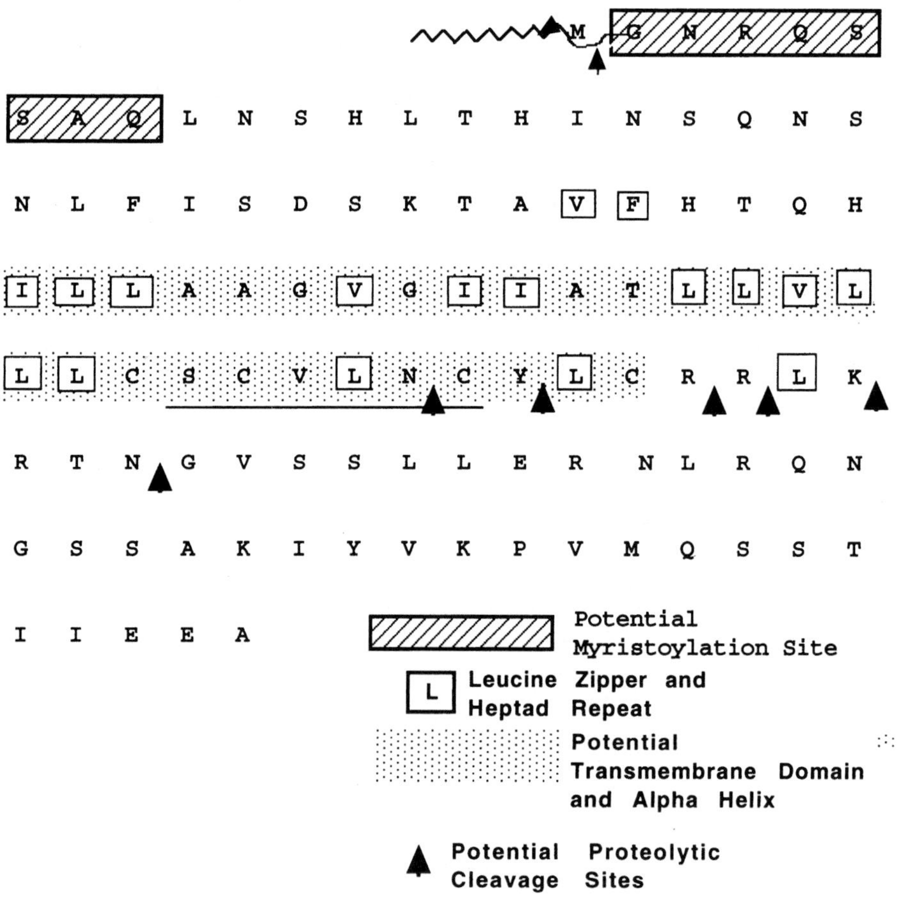

FIGURE 55.4. AD6F1 protein attributes. The AD6F1 protein contains a consensus sequence for N-terminal myristoylation and one long hydrophobic, potentially membrane-spanning, domain downstream. Each of these attributes can associate proteins with membranes. Within the hydrophobic domain is an α-helical heptad repeat with a leucine zipper-like sequence, which is often associated with protein oligomerization and with integral membrane proteins. Several potential proteolytic cleavage sites are present just downstream of the hydrophobic domain, including trypsin and chymotrypsin sites as well as two sites similar to those used to cleave myristoylated polio virus, reovirus, and HIV polyproteins.

could associate the protein with one or more cell membranes and thereby contribute to cell fusion.

Other Group B Rotavirus Genes

Gene 11 of ADRV is 631 bases long and encodes a 20-kd protein (72). The gene 11 protein from group A rotavirus (NSP5) shares 40% similar amino acids (25% identical) with the ADRV gene 11 product. A comparison of IDIR and ADRV gene 11 sequences indicates that they are 72% and 67% identical at the nucleic acid and amino acid levels, respectively (72,100).

Gene segments 7, 8, and 10 are likely to encode nonstructural proteins NSP2, NSP3, and NSP4 based on amino acid similarities with group A strains. Gene segment 7 of ADRV and gene 5 of IDIR encode homologous NSP3 protein equivalents to group A rotaviruses (144,172). It has been reported that the IDIR gene segment 8 encoded protein is immunoprecipitated by three human (IDIR-specific) sera but not by ADRV-specific sera, suggesting variation in this gene product between group B rotavirus strains (140). It has not been demonstrated that any nonstructural ADRV protein is functionally equivalent to group A rotavirus proteins.

Genes encoding VP1 protein equivalent in IDIR have been cloned and sequenced, and appear to contain a polypeptide correlating to the group A rotavirus VP1 protein present in transcriptionally active viral cores (145).The gene segment 1–encoded protein is 28% identical and 50% similar to the group A rotavirus VP1 protein and contains RNA polymerase-specific domains, including a GDD amino acid sequence (145).

Group C Gene Coding Assignments

Group C rotavirus gene segments from porcine or bovine strains have been cloned and sequenced (105,106, 109–114,173–178). Group C rotaviruses, are highly related to group A rotavirus strains. An example of this is the cross-hybridization of gene segment 1 from group C and group A rotaviruses (25,46). Antigenic cross-reactivity between group C and A rotavirus VP6 proteins has also been noted (179). Along with hybridization, amino acid alignments have been used to define protein homologies between group C and A rotaviruses as described earlier for group B rotavirus proteins. A summary of group C rotavirus gene coding assignments is presented in Table 55.2, and a detailed description of animal rotaviruses has been presented by Linda Saif and Janis Bridger (16, 17,25,32).

Structural Proteins

Several reports describe the structural proteins of group C rotaviruses (180,181). Sequences of six structural proteins of the group C rotavirus virion were recently completed (176,177). In one study, 52,000- and 39,000-kd virion proteins of the outer shell were lost by EDTA treatment of the virus (180). The 39,000-kd protein was reported to be glycosylated because it is sensitive to endoglycosidase F and likely represents the viral VP7 protein. It has been further suggested that 44-kd and 93-kd proteins are likely to be the group C rotavirus VP6 and VP2 proteins of the inner capsid (180). Another report described the four inner shell structural proteins of 125-, 93-, 74-, and 41-kd, two nonstructural proteins of 39 and 35 kd, and a 37- and 33-kd outer shell proteins (181). The 37-kd protein is glycoslyated and there is some question about the association of a 25-kd protein with the virion and whether this protein is also glycosylated (181). Human group C rotavirus genome segment 3 contains 2,283 bp and encodes the VP4 gene with an open reading frame of 744 amino acids (176,182). The large number of amino acid differences between the human and

TABLE 55.2. GROUP C GENE CODING ASSIGNMENTS[a]

Group C Gene		Protein		Group A Rotavirus					
Segment	Length (Bases)	# Amino Acids (kd)	Capsid Location If Determined	Protein Equivalent (kd)	% Amino Acid Identity	Equivalency Group A Gene	Determined By	Source	Protein Attributes
1	3,313	1082 (125)		VP1 (125)	48.2	1	Hybridization/AA	Porcine	Polymerase
2	2,655	873 (101)	Core	VP2 (103)	43.6	2	Hybridization/AA	Porcine	GTP binding domain
3	2,646	736 (83)	Outer	VP4	33.2	4	Hybridization/AA	Porcine	Neutralization, spike
4	2,145	692 (81)		VP3	34.5	3	Hybridization/AA	Hu/Por	Nuc. binding motif
5	1,352	395 (44.5)	Inner	VP6	41.3	6	Alignment	Hum/Por/Bov	Major viral antigen
6	1,348	402 (39)		NSP3	23	7	Alignment	Por/Bov	
7	1,235	393 (46.4)		NSP1	15	5	Alignment	Porcine	Zinc finger
8	1,063	332 (37.3)	Outer	VP7	<30	9	Alignment	Hu/Por	Glycosylation
9	995	312 (35.8)		NSP2	37	8	Alignment	Porcine	Basic
10	693	210–212 (923.4)		NSP5	16	11	Alignment	Hu/Por/Bov	
11	613	150 (17.7)		NSP4	Not sig	10	Hydropathy	Hu/Por	Glycosylation—4 sites

[a]Gene segments have been cloned and sequenced and are available from Genbank at the following: L12390, L12391, M29287, M81488, M74216, M74217, M74218, M74219, M88768, M61100, M61101, X60546, X65938, and X65939.

porcine VP4s suggests that the porcine C/Cowden isolate may belong to a different group C rotavirus P type (182).

Within group C rotaviruses, nucleic acid and amino acid comparisons have been performed between individual genes and proteins. The VP6 proteins from the bovine (Shintoku), porcine (Cowden), and three human strains (Bristol, Belem, and Preston) of group C rotavirus have been compared (105,107,108,183). The bovine, porcine and Bristol VP6 proteins share 88% to 92% identical amino acids. Differences between group C rotavirus VP6 proteins are greater than any two subgroups of group A rotaviruses, suggesting that these viruses are likely to define clearly distinguishable subgroup antigenic determinants.

Within human group C rotavirus strains, the VP6 genes are 97.9% to 99.6% identical, with 100% identical amino acid sequence (107,183). Even Brazilian and U. K. isolates share 100% identical amino acid sequences, suggesting similar origins and the recent divergence of human group C rotavirus strains (183). A table of human group C rotavirus nucleic acid and amino acid homologies with the porcine Cowden strain illustrates the relationship of group C rotavirus strains (Table 55.3).

Porcine and human group C rotavirus VP7 proteins contain 83% nucleic acid identity and 88% amino acid identity (113,184,185), suggesting that human and porcine group C strains may comprise their own glycoprotein-specific serotypes. In contrast, the Cowden and a second human group C rotavirus strain, Ehime 86-542, are probably within the same group C serotype because antibodies to Cowden neutralizes Ehime (115). Like for group B homologies, the group C rotavirus VP7 protein shares less than 30% amino acid identity with group A rotavirus VP7 protein.

Nonstructural Proteins

Nonstructural proteins of group C strains have been aligned and compared. Porcine and bovine NSP3 proteins share only 81% identical amino acids, whereas NSP5 proteins from bovine and human group C strains share 68% identical amino acids, while both have a relatively constant (78%) nucleic acid homology (109,114,186). As in group A strains, viral nonstructural proteins are more divergent than their structural protein counterparts.

Identical amino acids shared between group C and group A rotavirus strains are listed in Table 55.3. Identical amino acids shared between group A and C rotaviruses are approximately 15% to 20% greater for most proteins (except for VP7) than comparable group B to group A protein homologies. This indicates that group C and A strains are more closely related and that group B strains are distant relatives to other rotavirus groups. However the NSP5, NSP1, and NSP3 proteins share only 15% to 23% amino acid identity and are almost completely different between group A, B, and C rotaviruses.

NSP3

The porcine group C rotavirus NSP3 protein shares homology with a known double-stranded RNA-dependent protein kinase PKR (187). The full-length protein and an 8-kd C-terminal product, both of which contain the motif present in double-stranded RNA-binding proteins and bound specifically to double-stranded RNA (187). NSP3 products expressed in HeLa cells were capable of rescuing the replication of an interferon-sensitive deletion mutant of vaccinia virus, suggesting that this protein may inhibit cellular blockades to viral protein synthesis (187). Interestingly, corresponding motifs were not identified in any group A rotavirus proteins, suggesting either that this is a function unique to group C rotaviruses or that group A rotaviruses use other means for altering host cell protein synthesis blockades during viral infection.

NSP4

The complete nucleotide sequence of genome segment 11 from the noncultivable human group C rotavirus (Bristol strain) is 613 bp long and encodes a single open reading frame of 150 amino acids (188). The predicted translation product is 17.7 kd and contains four potential N-linked glycosylation sites but lacks significant homologies to other rotaviral proteins (188). However, hydropathy and structural features are analogous to the integral membrane glycoprotein NSP4 encoded by group A rotavirus gene 10 (188,189).

The NSP4 protein has been reported as the viral enterotoxin in group A rotaviruses, suggesting that it has potential importance for other rotaviruses (190). One report docu-

TABLE 55.3. GROUP C ROTAVIRUS VP6 GENE AND PROTEIN HOMOLOGY

	Cowden NA AA	Bristol NA AA	Belem NA AA	Preston NA AA
Cowden (porcine)	——	84% 92%	83% 92%	84% 92%
Bristol (human)		——	98% 100%	99.6% 100%
Belem (human)			——	98% 100%
Preston (human)				——

NA, percentage of identical nucleic acids between group C rotavirus VP6 proteins; AA, percentage of identical amino acids between group C rotavirus VP6 proteins.

ments amino acid differences between pathogenic and non-pathogenic group C rotavirus NSP4 proteins (128). However, the lack of amino acid homology between group C and group A NSP4 proteins provides little indication that these proteins impart equivalent functions (188). There is also no indication whether the amino acid differences identified between group C NSP4 proteins and group A NSP4 proteins are related to the pathogenicity of these viruses. Because changes in other viral proteins were not evaluated and single gene reassortants were not used to establish a correlation of the changes with pathogenesis, it is just as likely that pathogenic differences between these viruses stem from differences between other viral proteins or are multifactorial.

Protein Functions

As with group B strains, very little has been done to define functional properties of group C rotavirus proteins. The proteins involved in group C rotavirus neutralization and serotype specificity have not been defined but are presumed to be the VP7 and VP4 equivalent proteins of group C strains.

Hemagglutination

Group C rotaviruses have been determined to agglutinate human and sheep erythrocytes (191). In group A rotaviruses, this function has been attributed to the VP8 proteolytic cleavage fragment of the outer capsid spike protein VP4 (156). It is likely that the VP4 protein of group C strains is also the viral hemagglutinin in group C rotaviruses.

Coexpression Studies

In group A strains, coexpression of VP2 and VP6 proteins results in the assembly of single-shelled–like particles (192). When the VP6 protein of group C rotavirus was coexpressed with the group A rotavirus VP2 protein, similar single-shelled–like particles were obtained (193). This result demonstrates the functional similarity of these viral proteins and suggests conservation of VP2-binding domains within VP6 proteins. Differences between the group A and C rotavirus VP6 proteins were also demonstrated by coexpression because mixed trimers or hexamers were not formed by these proteins. This finding suggests that there are group-specific determinants of VP6 oligomerization.

HOST RANGE: ANIMAL AND HUMAN INFECTION

There are a variety of hosts for both group B and C rotavirus infections (1,3,5,9,10,17,18,21,22,24–27,32,34,40,41A,47,50,51,55–60,98,117,143,194–199). Thus far, group B rotavirus infections have been identified in humans, rats, swine, calves, and sheep. Interestingly, the only rotavirus group to infect rats is the group B rotavirus IDIR (27). Pigs in particular are reported to be seropositive for group A, B, and C rotaviruses at 99%, 86%, and 77% levels in the United States, suggesting the possibility of zoonotic infections of humans from endemic porcine strains (16,18,19,73,143,196). Serologic evidence of animal and human group B rotavirus infections in the United States, United Kingdom, and China and the recent identification of human group B rotaviruses in India suggest that these viruses are not geographically limited (86). Group C rotaviruses have been identified predominantly in humans (Bristol), swine (Cowden), and calves (Shintoku), and evidence of group C rotavirus infections has been documented throughout the world in animal and human populations (1,3,5,32,50,51,55–60,194,196,199).

ANIMAL MODELS

Attempts have been made to infect rats and pigs with the human group B rotavirus strain but none of these trials has resulted in infection or viral shedding. With the large differences reported in the outer capsid proteins of group B rotaviruses, it is not necessarily surprising that viral isolates are host restricted and fail to infect other mammalian species.

Studies on the human group B rotavirus ADRV have been severely limited by the inability to study the virus in tissue culture or animal models. However, a report describing the cultivation of porcine group B rotavirus cultivation has been presented and should foster basic studies of these viruses (91). Rat (IDIR), porcine (Ohio and SRV-1), and bovine (Ohio strain) strains have been studied in animals, providing viable animal models for the study of group B rotavirus infections (23,25–27,143).

Rats and pigs infected with group B rotavirus shed small amounts of virus by group A rotavirus standards (26,27). In the rat model, the infected animal must also be sacrificed in order to harvest high titer virus from washes of the small intestine (27). Very little virus is shed in the stool, and virus that is obtained from stool is less infectious than virus from gut washes. Porcine rotavirus infection also produces only a small amount of virus, even though it induces acute transient diarrhea in the animal (26,143). Small amounts of high titer virus have been obtained from porcine, rat, and human group B rotavirus infections. These preparations have been used in most of the molecular biology studies of group B rotavirus strains.

Group C rotaviruses can be passed serially to new animals for the purposes of generating more virus and for studying viral pathogenesis. Representative strains exist for each species infected by group C rotaviruses, although the Cowden porcine strain has been cultivated and is the most extensively studied (101–104). A complete discussion of animal group C rotavirus strains is presented in reference 25.

TISSUE CULTURE PROPAGATION OF GROUP B AND C ROTAVIRUSES

In an attempt to infect tissue culture cell lines, porcine group B rotavirus strains were originally added to cells in tissue culture monolayers. The presence of infected cells was detected by immunofluorescence and by the formation of syncytia in the monolayer (143). The formation of syncytia is characteristic of group B rotavirus strains and syncytia were used to screen for new group B rotavirus isolates. Rat, bovine, and ovine rotaviruses were all identified as group B rotavirus strains by their ability to form syncytia in infected cell monolayers and by their reactivity with antisera by immunofluorescence or immunostaining (23,24,27,33, 41A,47,143). However, early attempts to cultivate group B rotaviruses did not lead to the productive infection of tissue culture cells.

In 1996, porcine group B rotaviruses were reportedly cultivated (91). The virus was grown in swine kidney cells, and pancreatin was determined to be essential for the propagation of group B rotaviruses (91). However, no further studies of group B rotavirus propagation have been published with the porcine or other group B rotaviruses.

Several reports have described the cultivation of group C rotavirus strains. Porcine and human group C rotaviruses have been adapted to growth in tissue culture on primary AGMK cell lines, CaCo2 cells, Ma104 cells, or ST cells (101–104,200). Essential to the growth process was the use of roller tubes and high concentrations of proteolytic enzyme trypsin or pancreatin in the maintenance medium (101–104). Infection of monolayers was monitored by immunofluorescence of infected cells, and virus was passed 16 times until 107 focus-forming units were obtained. The origin of the virus was confirmed by immune electron microscopy and electropherotyping, demonstrating that the input viral dsRNA was the same as that of the isolated progeny virus.

PATHOGENESIS

Rotaviruses of all groups infect the epithelium of the small intestine. Differences in the location of infection have been reported, indicating that group B rotavirus infections occur primarily in the distal small intestine, whereas group A and C rotaviruses infect primarily the proximal small intestinal epithelium (47). The mechanism by which group B and C rotaviruses induce watery diarrhea is still unclear and may be multifactorial in cause. Tissue injury, toxin-like effects, increased luminal solutes, failure to absorb water from the lumen, and cellular responses to rotavirus infection all may contribute to disease. Group B rotaviruses have an additional effect on the epithelial cells in that infection fuses intestinal epithelial cells into syncytia, further compromising epithelial barrier functions (21,23,24,26,27,31,41A,47,143).

SYNCYTIUM FORMATION

There are few icosahedral viruses that have been demonstrated to fuse infected cells. However, group B rotaviruses, avian reoviruses, and Nelson Bay virus are all icosahedral viruses of the Reoviridae family, which fuse cells and form syncytia during infection (22–24,26,47,201–204). Syncytia formation during animal group B rotavirus infections has been demonstrated for some time (21,23,24,26,27,41A, 47,143), and the human group B rotavirus, ADRV, was shown to form syncytia in infected Ma104 cells (Fig. 55.5). Syncytium formation is a hallmark of group B rotavirus infections and has not been demonstrated in other rotavirus groups.

Neutralization of ADRV

The transient infection of MA104 cells has recently been used as the basis of focus reduction neutralization (FRN) assays. ADRV-1 and ADRV-2 have been treated with hyperimmune serum to ADRV virus (1/1,600) or anti-VP4 hyperimmune serum (1/400) before infecting tissue culture monolayers. In each case, virus is neutralized by anti–ADRV-specific sera, but VP6-specific and group A–specific hyperimmune sera have no effect. Because high concentrations of anti-VP4 sera are required for neutralization, it is possible that other neutralization antigens besides VP4 are present on the virion or that most of the VP4 in the sample is dissociated from virion. The fusion protein and VP7 protein of ADRV are other likely neutralization targets.

EPIDEMIOLOGY

ADRV

The human group B rotavirus, ADRV, was initially isolated in 1982 and 1983 from epidemic gastroenteritis outbreaks in Chinese adults (9–12). The outbreaks were unique in their host range in that infection was limited primarily to adults. ADRV predominantly infects individuals older than age 15 years and results in a low mortality rate (0.1%) in elderly or infirm individuals (9,13). Interestingly, the incidence of ADRV disease in individuals age 20 to 29 years old was 10 times that of infants and young children (0 to 4 years of age) (9,13). In, fact 85% of those infected were older than 15 years of age. Even among families where the virus spread from familial contacts, infants and young children were often spared from the disease (9,13). However, infection of infants and young children has been documented by studies of hospitalized individuals during the Chinese ADRV outbreaks (161).

In 1982 and 1983, the People's Republic of China experienced nationwide outbreaks of severe adult diarrheal disease caused by ADRV. Outbreaks originated in the northeast of China in the Heilongjiang province in the spring of

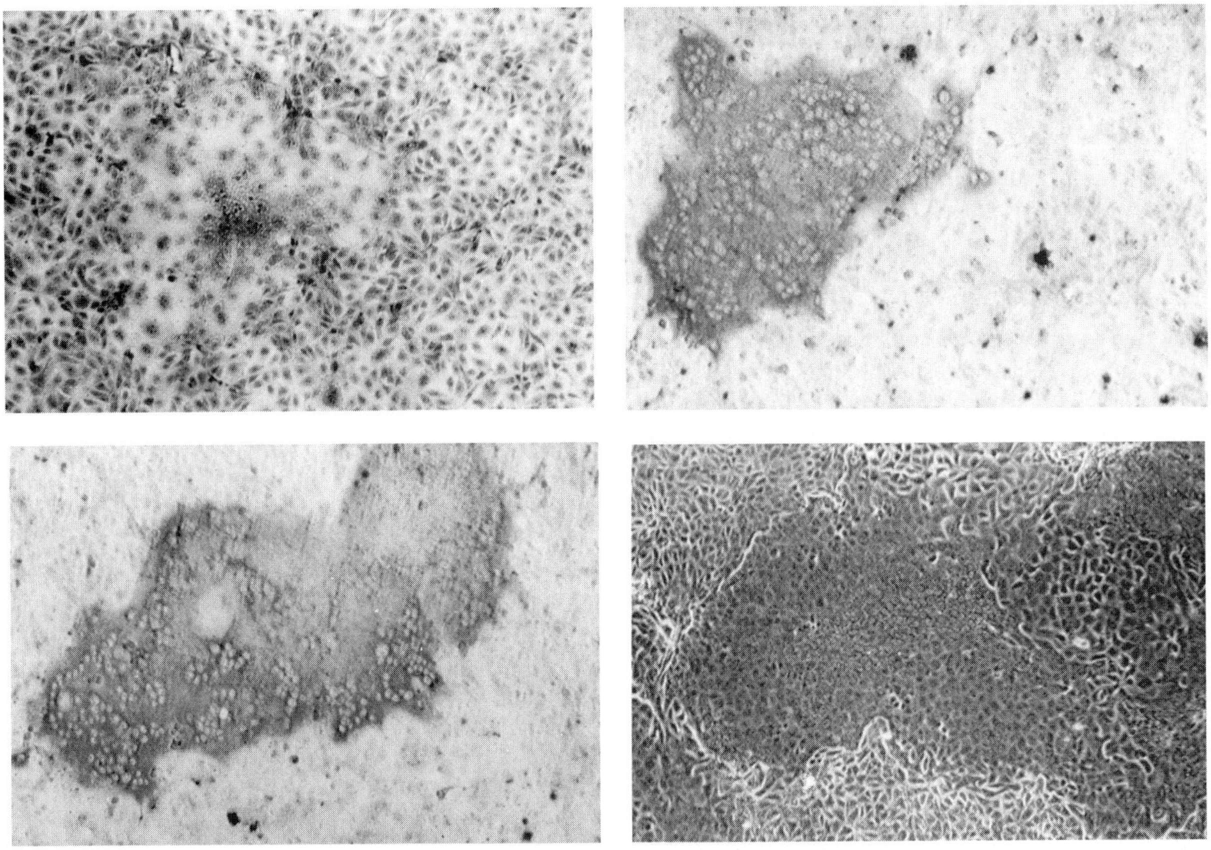

FIGURE 55.5. ADRV-Induced syncytia cells transiently infected with ADRV virus cause the formation of syncytia by fusing adjacent cells. Shown are syncytia formed from the infection of AGMK cells.

1982 (12,13). In the initial outbreak, one-fourth of all counties were affected with a very low mortality rate associated with elderly and infirm individuals. The incidence of ADRV-induced disease continued into 1983 and included approximately one-half of the counties and more than 1 million people (12).

In the fall of 1982 and spring of 1983, a separate outbreak of adult diarrheal disease of epidemic proportions was reported in the distant northwest of China in the Gansu province (12,13). This outbreak began in a coal mining area near Lanzhou City and spread rapidly to the city. The prevalence of ADRV in Lanzhou included as many as 3.45% of the city population (12).

In each of these initial outbreaks, it was demonstrated that the water was either fecally contaminated or the water system was not chlorinated for several days before the outbreak and that the causative agent, ADRV, was probably transmitted as a waterborne pathogen (12). Subsequent to primary infections from drinking water, ADRV spread via close personal contacts. Epidemics quickly subsided following chlorination of the water supply.

The incidence of disease during the Chinese ADRV outbreaks were of epidemic proportions and ranged from 5% to 44% of the local population (12). ADRV-induced diarrhea is severe and has been described as "cholera-like" in its ability to induce voluminous diarrhea (9,10,12). The average incubation period for ADRV infection is 56 hours, followed by the sudden onset of severe and frequent cramping diarrhea (100%). Vomiting is associated with 80% of cases reported and nearly one-half of cases studied demonstrated signs of dehydration (9,10,12). Fever is not normally associated with ADRV infections, and only 1% of affected persons had low-grade fevers. Symptoms lasted 1 to 14 days and averaged 6 days in duration. There is a very low mortality rate associated with the infection, which may be the result of secondary complications in elderly or infirm individuals.

High titer virus is shed in human stools approximately 24 hours following ADRV infection at a time when diarrhea is minimal (9,10,12). By the time large quantities of watery diarrhea are observed (approximately 48 hours), shedding is diminished. Stools from outbreaks of ADRV-induced diarrhea in China are the primary source of high titer ADRV virus in the world.

In contrast to disease caused by other rotavirus groups, ADRV disease does not appear to have a seasonal distribution. Chinese outbreaks occurred in the winter in the northwest and northeast of China and in the early summer in southern provinces (12–14). Outbreaks are not likely to represent the first human infections by group B rotaviruses because gamma globulin pools, which preceded the outbreak, contain antibodies to ADRV (205). Epidemic outbreaks have continued to be reported periodically in China. In April 1997, an outbreak of adult diarrhea caused more than 1,000 hospitalized cases (47%) among graduates in a university in Shi Jiazhuang City (Hebei province) (97). Rotavirus was confirmed to be the cause by PAGE, with 14 samples having the same nucleic acid electrophoresis pattern of 4-2-1-1-1-1-1. The viral nucleic acid was not amplified by ADRV-specific primers, suggesting that the virus differs from ADRV, although it was not tested whether samples contained group B–specific VP6 antigen. A recent outbreak of group B rotavirus diarrhea in India further demonstrates that group B disease is not limited to China (86).

Antibodies to group B rotaviruses are common in China and have been detected in 5% to 15% of human serum samples from India, Australia, the United States (12,13), and England (19). In a separate study, antibody to group B rotavirus was detected much less frequently in serum from individuals from the United States (1 in 155), Kenya (1 in 10), Thailand (1 in 20), and Canada (1 in 15) (206). Recent studies using recombinant ADRV antigens are just beginning to define the prevalence of group B rotavirus disease in human populations; however, these studies demonstrate that approximately 1% to 8% of the worldwide human population has been exposed to some form of group B rotavirus and that the exposure rates are highest in adults (76).

GROUP C

Human and animal group C rotavirus infections have been documented in Africa, Argentina, Australia, Europe, North and South America, Japan, and Thailand (2,3,5,32,35,39, 44,50,51,58,59,60,65,66,116,127,207). It is, therefore, likely that group C rotaviruses are endemic in human populations throughout the world because they are for porcine and bovine populations. However, pre-1984 pooled immunoglobulins from the United Kingdom, Belgium, the United States, Canada, and Japan indicate no signs of group C rotaviruses in human populations (32). Sera since 1984 have demonstrated an 8% prevalence rate for group C rotavirus in the United Kingdom and a worldwide prevalence of 6% to 29% (16). One report using an immunofluorescence assay for group C indicated that 30% of women of childbearing age were seropositive for group C rotavirus (208). A separate study in the United Kingdom indicated that seroprevalence increases with age with an average prevalence of 43% and a 66% seroprevalence rate in individuals 71 to 75 years of age (77,78). Data from Sweden similarly suggest that symptomatic group C rotavirus infections occur more frequently in adults than was previously recognized (71). There is one report that co-infection of group C and A rotaviruses in gnotobiotic pigs influences the pathogenesis of group C rotaviruses (129).

Human group C rotavirus outbreaks of gastroenteritis have been documented in several institutional settings. Group C rotavirus infections are the most frequent among children age 4 to 7 years, but the virus has also been documented in infants and adults (2,5,209,210). However the frequency of group C rotavirus disease is much lower than that for group A strains. The most dramatic outbreak of group C rotavirus occurred in Japan, where 675 of 3,102 (21.8%) school children were infected (5). A food-borne origin is suspected in this outbreak because all affected children had lunch from a single food preparation center. The outbreak encompassed seven different elementary schools, although a common food source for the infection was not determined. Virus was determined to be group C specific by immunoelectron microscopy and did not react with group A- or B-specific reference sera (5).

Of the children infected, 46% presented with abdominal pain, 44.6% with acute vomiting, 41.3% with nausea, 41.1% with temperature greater than 37°C, and only 27.6% with diarrhea (5). Thus, vomiting and fevers are the main clinical symptoms for group C rotavirus infections, and diarrhea was less associated with group C rotavirus infections than with group A or B rotaviruses.

IMMUNITY, DIAGNOSIS, AND PREVENTION

The determinants of group B and C rotavirus immunity and protection are currently based on presumptions made from experiences with group A rotaviruses. From group A rotavirus studies, the outer capsid VP4 and VP7 proteins of group B and C rotavirus strains are likely to be involved in viral neutralization and host immunity to rotavirus disease. In the case of group B rotaviruses, antibodies to the recombinant VP4 protein reportedly neutralize the virus, suggesting that these presumptions are likely to be true. In group C rotavirus, recent progress has also defined at least two serotypes based on one-way neutralization assays of cultivable strains (115). The basis for host-attenuated vaccines for the prevention of group C rotavirus disease may already reside within the serotypically similar porcine and human strains available.

Diagnostic Assays

The cause of approximately 50% of all clinical diarrhea cases remain unresolved. Group B and C rotavirus infections are among the causes of undiagnosed human diarrheal disease (211,212). Except for the general detection of rotavirus particles by electron microscopy, clinical diagnostic assays for group B and C rotaviruses have not been established. Outside research laboratories, there is no current means of diagnosing infections caused by these agents or determining the seroprevalence of group B and C rotavirus infections. Detection of group B and C rotaviruses has traditionally been approached by electropherotyping assays in which atypical patterns of nucleic acids are detected on polyacrylamide gels (25,29,30,42). Another assay that is used to differentiate group A, B, and C rotavirus infections is immune electron microscopy (IEM). This technique uses hyperimmune sera to aggregate viruses from specific viral groups and aggregates are detected visually by EM.

Initial ELISAs to detect group-specific antibodies in serum have also been performed, but these assays have suffered from the poor sensitivity and high background problems associated with the use of stool-derived virus as the antigen coat on ELISA plates. One assay reports the detection of rat, porcine, and bovine group B rotavirus in fecal specimens by solid-phase enzyme immunoassay, suggesting the utility and success of more recently generated reagents (213). Assays using monoclonal antibodies to detect group B–specific viral antigens in stools have also been developed and presented (12,206,214,215). ELISA and MAb diagnostic assays for ADRV have also been reported and, in one study, three MAbs to ADRV were prepared to outer capsid proteins (214,83,12,13,14,215,216). One of these MAbs has since been reported to immunoprecipitate the ADRV VP4 protein expressed from baculovirus recombinants (92,214). There are also two reports of MAbs made to the group B rotavirus VP6 protein, which have been used in ELISA and immunofluorescence assays (12,215).

Recently, the Calcutta strain (CAL) of group B rotavirus was identified in India (86). Primers made to ADRV sequences were also found to amplify gene segments 4, 5, 6, 7, and 9 from the different CAL isolates (86). This establishes a functional set of primers suitable for the detection of various genes of human group B rotaviruses using a rapid reverse transcriptase PCR assay and suggests the utility of PCR diagnostics in detecting group B rotavirus infections (86).

Antibodies to the recombinant ADRV VP6 protein have also been used in an ADRV antigen detection assay using a rabbit anti-ADRV capture serum and detected with an ADRV VP6-specific mAb (148). The development of monoclonal antibody reagents to group B and C rotaviruses is important for detecting clinical rotavirus disease. The use of recombinant group B and C viral antigens should translate into the development of sensitive ELISA diagnostic assays for these viruses.

There is one report of a counter immunoelectrophoresis (CIE) assay for group B rotavirus detection. In this study, 47% of rats, 36% of pigs, less than 1% of chickens, and 0% of horses were seropositive for group B rotaviruses in China (12). CIE was also used to assess the prevalence of group B rotavirus disease in some human populations (12). In China, 12% to 41% of persons surveyed were seropositive for group B rotavirus. However, only 15% of Australians, 9.5% of Americans and 12.5% of Canadians surveyed were group B rotavirus positive by this assay. There is also one report of a latex agglutination assay for the rapid detection of ADRV using monoclonal antibodies bound to latex beads, although no further reports of this assay have been presented (12).

In two studies, the seroprevalence of group B rotavirus infections was investigated using IDIR as the target antigen in human serum ELISAs (15,76). These studies analyzed human serum antibodies to IDIR and determined that 43.4% of U. S. children younger than 1 year of age were seropositive for IDIR. Children younger than 2 years of age had an IDIR seroprevalence rate of 51.4%, and 87.9 % of individuals older than 20 years were determined to have serum antibodies to IDIR (15). These percentages represent the highest seroprevalence rates reported for group B rotavirus disease in any human cohort and may represent false-positive results from the assay used. In the second study, individuals (1%) exhibited serum antibodies directed against the recombinant VP6 (ages, 54 to 95 years; mean age, 77 years) (76).

GROUP C ROTAVIRUS DIAGNOSTICS

Several reports of group C rotavirus monoclonal antibodies and ELISAs have recently appeared. In one report, three mAbs to the porcine group C rotavirus were generated which immunoprecipitate the VP6 protein of group C strains and do not cross-react with group A or B strains (217). In another report, five mAbs were generated that cross-react with both group A and C rotaviruses in cell culture immunofluorescence tests (179). These mAbs recognized the VP6 protein of each strain by Western blot. This report suggested that three overlapping epitopes within a single antigenic domain are shared by the mAbs (179). There are no further reports of cross-reactive epitopes between the VP6 proteins of group A and C rotavirus strains.

Several other group C rotavirus studies have made use of monoclonal antibodies in diagnostic assays for group C rotaviruses (54,73,79,179,217–219). A majority of these diagnostics have relied on sandwich ELISA assays in which monoclonal antibodies are used to capture group C rotavirus antigens and the antigen is subsequently detected with a polyclonal serum. These tests are 63% to 100% accurate for the detection of group C rotaviruses (54,73,79,179,217–219). However, tests that report 100% accuracy have not been tested on a diverse set of group C rotavirus isolates used in other assays.

There are reports of rapid diagnostic assays for group C rotaviruses using a reverse passive hemagglutination assay (RHPA) and a latex agglutination test, and a separate report using this as a neutralization assay (54,84,79). In these tests, sheep erythrocytes or latex beads are coated with group C–specific MAbs and used to assay samples containing group C rotaviruses. In the presence of group C–specific antigen, the erythrocytes or latex beads agglutinate and precipitate from the diagnostic solution (79). These tests are reported to be 96% to 100% accurate at detecting group C rotavirus antigens and the latex agglutination test is complete in 2 minutes (79). With a number of MAbs and other reagents for group C strains already developed, clinical diagnostic assays for these viruses should soon be widely available.

Nucleic acid–based assays have also been used to detect viral groups by hybridization (27,127,167). Group C rotavirus hybridization studies have been used to categorize similar group C rotavirus strains. The similarities identified by hybridization have subsequently been shown to be significant by cross-neutralization studies performed on hybridization-related viruses. The PCR has more effectively been used to detect group B and C viruses and promises the best sensitivity of any assay to date (67,75,81,85,86,98,127–129,220). However, the oligonucleotide primers chosen to detect virus by PCR are extremely important and must be complementary to highly conserved nucleic acid sequences in order for this strategy to be used successfully. Although group-specific PCR assays have been proposed, the ability of these assays to detect all viruses of a group have not been adequately tested. With the sequencing of more group B and C rotavirus genes, comparative sequence analysis may be used in reliable group-specific viral screens (67,75,81,86,98,127–129).

ELISAs for serum antibodies to group B or C viruses or for viral antigens still represent the best diagnostic choice for the specific, sensitive, and timely detection of rotaviruses. With the development of cultivable viruses that can be purified and of recombinant expressed proteins, assays for group B and C rotaviruses can be developed and used coordinately with group A–specific Rotazyme assays for detecting human rotavirus infections. However, the lack of widespread human group B and C rotavirus disease has limited the rationale for reagent development and widespread testing for these viruses.

CONCLUSION

Group B and C rotaviruses are potentially important human pathogens with a broad animal host reservoir. The development of MAbs, cultivated viral strains, and recombinant diagnostic reagents should permit further study and detection of these viruses, although a rationale for widespread diagnosis of group B and C rotaviruses is not apparent in most clinical settings. Diagnostic assays for group B and C rotaviruses should permit more accurate assessments of their contribution to human disease and help to define the cause of some of the 25% to 50% of diarrheal cases that remain undiagnosed each year (211,212). The functions of group B and C rotavirus proteins are only beginning to be discovered. Defining the means in which similar viral functions can be performed from dissimilar proteins among group A, B, and C rotaviruses will provide a basic understanding of required rotavirus functions and may present common means for disease intervention. Unique group B and C rotavirus proteins will also allow definition of new elements that contribute to rotavirus pathogenesis. Group B rotavirus–induced cell fusion and the enhanced pathogenesis accompanying epithelial syncytia is particularly interesting in that the means by which nonenveloped viruses interact with lipid bilayers is poorly understood. The ability to antigenically discriminate group B and C isolates will permit the definition of rotavirus subgroups and serotypes. Establishing antigenic differences of circulating group B and C rotaviruses will permit a rational approach to questions concerning the necessity and feasibility of preventive measures or diagnostic testing for human group B and C rotaviruses.

REFERENCES

1. Ishimaru Y, Nakano H, Oseto M, et al. Group C rotavirus infection and infiltration. *Acta Paediatr Jpn* [Overseas Edition] 1990;32:523–529.
2. Brown DW, Campbell L, Tomkins DS, et al. School outbreak of gastroenteritis due to atypical rotavirus [Letter]. *Lancet* 1989;2:737–738.
3. Caul EO, Ashley CR, Darville JM, et al. Group C rotavirus associated with fatal enteritis in a family outbreak. *J Med Virol* 1990;30:201–205.
4. Jiang B, Dennehy PH, Spangenberger S, et al. First detection of group C rotavirus in fecal specimens of children with diarrhea in the United States. *J Infect Dis* 1995;172:45–50.
5. Matsumoto K, Hatano M, Kobayashi K, et al. An outbreak of gastroenteritis associated with acute rotaviral infection in schoolchildren. *J Infect Dis* 1989;160:611–615.
6. Oishi I, Yamazaki K, Minekawa Y. An occurrence of diarrheal cases associated with group C rotavirus in adults. *Microbiol Immunol* 1993;37:505–509.
7. Otsu R. A mass outbreak of gastroenteritis associated with group C rotaviral infection in schoolchildren. *Comp Immunol Microbiol Infect Dis* 1998;21:75–80.
8. Sekine S, Hayashi Y, Ando T, et al. [An outbreak of gastroenteritis due to group C rotavirus in Tokyo]. *Kansenshogaku Zasshi* 1993;67:110–115.
9. Hung T, Chen GM, Wang CG, et al. Rotavirus-like agent in adult non-bacterial diarrhoea in China [Letter]. *Lancet* 1983;2:1078–1079.
10. Hung T, Chen GM, Wang CG, et al. Waterborne outbreak of rotavirus diarrhoea in adults in China caused by a novel rotavirus. *Lancet* 1984;1:1139–1142.
11. Chen,CM., Hung T, Bridger JC, et al. Chinese adult rotavirus is a group B rotavirus [Letter]. *Lancet* 1985;2:1123–1124.
12. Hung T. Rotavirus and adult diarrhea. *Adv Virus Res* 1988;35:193–218.
13. Hung T, Chen GM, Wang CG, et al. Seroepidemiology and molecular epidemiology of the Chinese rotavirus. *Ciba Found Symp* 1987;128:49–62.
14. Hung T, Fan RL, Wang CA, et al. Seroepidemiology of adult rotavirus [Letter]. *Lancet* 1985;2:325–326.
15. Eiden J, Vonderfecht S, Yolken RH. Evidence that a novel rotavirus-like agent of rats can cause gastroenteritis in man. *Lancet* 1985;2:8–11.
16. Bridger JC. New and emerging gut viruses: structure, pathophys-

iology and clinical manifestations. Non-group-A rotaviruses. In *Viruses and the Gut*. Windsor, Berkshire, England: Smith Kline and French Laboratories, 1988:79–82.

17. Bridger JC. Novel rotaviruses in animals and man. In Symposium CF, ed. *Novel Diarrheal Viruses*, vol. 128. Chichester, England: Wiley, 1987:5–23.
18. Bridger JC, Brown JF. Prevalence of antibody to typical and atypical rotaviruses in pigs. *Vet Rec* 1985;116:50.
19. Brown DW, Beards GM, Chen GM, et al. Prevalence of antibody to group B (atypical) rotavirus in humans and animals. *J Clin Microbiol* 1987;25:316–319.
20. Ushijima H, Shinozaki T, Fang ZY, et al. Group B rotavirus antibody in Japanese children [Letter]. *J Diarrhoeal Dis Res* 1992;10:41.
21. Chasey D, Banks J. The commonest rotaviruses from neonatal lamb diarrhoea in England and Wales have atypical electropherotypes. *Vet Rec* 1984;115:326–327.
22. Chasey D, Davies P. Atypical rotaviruses in pigs and cattle. *Vet Rec* 1984;114:16–17.
23. Chasey D, Higgins RJ, Jeffrey M, et al. Atypical rotavirus and villous epithelial cell syncytia in piglets. *J Comp Pathol* 1989; 100:217–222.
24. Mebus CA, Rhodes MB, Underdahl NR. Neonatal calf diarrhea caused by a virus that induces villous epithelial cell syncytia. *Am J Vet Res* 1978;39:1223–1228.
25. Saif LJ. Non group A rotaviruses. In: Saif LJ, Theil, KW, eds. *Viral diarrheas of man and animals*. Boca Raton, FL: CRC Press, 1990:73–95.
26. Theil KW, Saif LJ, Moorhead PD, et al. Porcine rotavirus-like virus (group B rotavirus): characterization and pathogenicity for gnotobiotic pigs. *J Clin Microbiol* 1985;21:340–345.
27. Vonderfecht SL, Huber AC, Eiden J, et al. Infectious diarrhea of infant rats produced by a rotavirus-like agent. *J Virol* 1984; 52:94–98.
28. Greenberg HB, Kalica AR, Wyatt RG, et al. Rescue of noncultivatable human rotavirus by gene reassortment during mixed infection with ts mutants of a cultivatable bovine rotavirus. *Proc Natl Acad Sci U S A* 1981;78:420–424.
29. Estes MK, Palmer EL, Obijeski JF. Rotaviruses: a review. *Curr Top Microbiol Immunol* 1983;105:123–184.
30. Holmes I. Rotaviruses. In: Joklik WK, ed. *Reoviridae*. New York: Plenum Press, 1983:359–423.
31. Askaa J, Bloch B. Infection in piglets with a porcine rotavirus-like virus. Experimental inoculation and ultrastructural examination. *Arch Virol* 1984;80:291–303.
32. Bridger JC, Pedley S, McCrae MA. Group C rotaviruses in humans. *J Clin Microbiol* 1986;23:760–763.
33. Chasey D, Bridger JC, McCrae MA. A new type of atypical rotavirus in pigs. *Arch Virol* 1986;89:235–243.
34. Espejo RT, Puerto F, Soler C, et al. Characterization of a human pararotavirus. *Infect Immun* 1984;44:112–116.
35. Nicolas JC, Cohen J, Fortier B, et al. Isolation of a human pararotavirus. *Virology* 1983;124:181–184.
36. Pedley S, Bridger JC, Brown JF, et al. Molecular characterization of rotaviruses with distinct group antigens. *J Gen Virol* 1983;64:2093.
37. Pedley S, Bridger JC, Chasey D, et al. Definition of two new groups of atypical rotaviruses. *J Gen Virol* 1986;67:131.
38. Pereira HG, Leite JP, Azeredo RS, et al. An atypical rotavirus detected in a child with gastroenteritis in Rio de Janeiro, Brazil. *Memorias Do Instituto Oswaldo Cruz* 1983;78:245–250.
39. Snodgrass DR, Herring AJ, Campbell I, et al. Comparison of atypical rotaviruses from calves, piglets, lambs and man. *J Gen Virol* 1984;65:909.
40. Thouless ME, DiGiacomo RF, Neuman DS. A new type of atypical rotavirus in pigs. *Arch Virol* 1986;89:235–243.
41. Estes MK. Rotaviruses and their replication. In: Fields BN, Knipe DM, eds. *Virology*. New York: Raven Press, 1990:1329–1352.

41A. Vonderfecht SL, Eiden JJ, Torres A, et al. Identification of a bovine enteric syncytial virus as a nongroup A rotavirus. *Am J Vet Res* 1986;47:1913–1918.

42. Kapikian AZ, Chanock RM. Rotaviruses. In: Fields BN, Knipe DM, Chanock RM, et al., eds. *Virology*, vol. 2, second edition. New York: Raven Press, 1990:1353–1404.
43. Yolken R, Arango JS, Eiden J, et al. Lack of genomic reassortment following infection of infant rats with group A and group B rotaviruses. *J Infect Dis* 1988;158:1120–1123.
44. Beards GM, Desselberger U, Flewett TH. Temporal and geographical distributions of human rotavirus serotypes, 1983 to 1988. *J Clin Microbiol* 1989;27:2827–2833.
45. Steele JC Jr. Rotavirus. *Clin Lab Med* 1999;19:691–703.
46. Eiden J, Vonderfecht S, Theil K, et al. Genetic and antigenic relatedness of human and animal strains of antigenically distinct rotaviruses. *J Infect Dis* 1986;154:972–982.
47. Chasey D, Banks J. Replication of atypical ovine rotavirus in small intestine and cell culture. *J Gen Virol* 1986;67:567–576.
48. Bohl EH, Saif LJ, Theil KW, et al. Porcine pararotavirus: detection, differentiation from rotavirus, and pathogenesis in gnotobiotic pigs. *J Clin Microbiol* 1982;15:312–319.
49. Rodger SM, Bishop RF, Holmes IH. Detection of a rotavirus-like agent associated with diarrhea in an infant. *J Clin Microbiol* 1982;16:724–726.
50. Bothig B, Schulze P, Schreier E, et al. Atypical human rotaviruses in the G.D.R. *Acta Virol* 1989;33:320–326.
51. Brown DW, Mathan MM, Mathew M, et al. Rotavirus epidemiology in Vellore, south India: group, subgroup, serotype, and electrophoretype. *J Clin Microbiol* 1988;26:2410–2414.
52. Dimitrov DH, Estes MK, Rangelova SM, et al. Detection of antigenically distinct rotaviruses from infants. *Infect Immun* 1983;41:523–526.
53. Dimitrov DH, Graham DY, Lopez J, et al. RNA electropherotypes of human rotaviruses from North and South America. *Bull WHO* 1984;62:321–329.
54. Fujii R, Kuzuya M, Hamano M, et al. Detection of human group C rotaviruses by an enzyme-linked immunosorbent assay using monoclonal antibodies. *J Clin Microbiol* 1992;30:1307–1311.
55. Gabbay YB, Mascarenhas JD, Linhares AC, et al. Atypical rotavirus among diarrhoeic children living in Belem, Brazil. *Memorias Do Instituto Oswaldo Cruz* 1990;84:5–8.
56. Ishimaru Y, Nakano S, Nakano H, et al. Epidemiology of group C rotavirus gastroenteritis in Matsuyama, Japan. *Acta Paediatr Jpn* [Overseas Edition] 1991;33:50–56.
57. Maunula L, Svensson L, von Bonsdorff BC. A family outbreak of gastroenteritis caused by group C rotavirus. *Arch Virol* 1992; 124:269–278.
58. Penaranda ME, Cubitt WD, Sinarachatanant P, et al. Group C rotavirus infections in patients with diarrhea in Thailand, Nepal, and England. *J Infect Dis* 1989;160:392–397.
59. Ushijima H, Honma H, Mukoyama A, et al. Detection of group C rotaviruses in Tokyo. *J Med Virol* 1989;27:299–303.
60. Von Bonsdorf C-H, Svensson L. Human serogroup C rotavirus in Finland. *Scand J Infect Dis* 1988;20:475–478.
61. Riepenhoff-Talty M, Gouvea V, Evans MJ, et al. Detection of group C rotavirus in infants with extrahepatic biliary atresia. *J Infect Dis* 1996;174:8–15.
62. Cox MJ, James VL, Azevedo RS, et al. Infection with group C rotavirus in a suburban community in Brazil. *Trop Med Int Health* 1998;3:891–895.
63. Dimitrov DH, Shindarov LM, Rangelova S. Occurrence of antigenically distinct rotaviruses in infants in Bulgaria. *Eur J Clin Microbiol* 1986;5:471–473.
64. Rasool NB, Hamzah M, Jegathesan M, et al. Identification of a

human group C rotavirus in Malaysia. *J Med Virol* 1994;43: 209–211.
65. Sorrentino A, Scodeller EA, Bellinzoni R, et al. Detection of an atypical rotavirus associated with diarrhoea in Chaco, Argentina. *Trans R Soc Trop Med Hyg* 1986;80:120–122.
66. Suzuki H, Sato T, Kitaoka S, et al. Epidemiology of rotavirus in Guayaquil, Ecuador. *Am J Trop Med Hyg* 1986;35:372–375.
67. Teixeira JM, Camara GN, Pimentel PF, et al. Human group C rotavirus in children with diarrhea in the Federal District, Brazil. *Braz J Med Biol Res* 1998;31:1397–1403.
68. Hamano M, Kuzuya M, Fujii R, et al. Outbreak of acute gastroenteritis caused by human group C rotavirus in a primary school. Jpn *J Infect Dis* 1999;52:170–171.
69. Souza DF, Kisielius JJ, Ueda M, et al. An outbreak of group C rotavirus gastroenteritis among adults living in Valentim Gentil, Sao Paulo State, Brazil. *J Diarrhoeal Dis Res* 1998;16:59–65.
70. Kuzuya M, Fujii R, Hamano M, et al. Survey of human group C rotaviruses in Japan during the winter of 1992 to 1993. *J Clin Microbiol* 1998;36:6–10.
71. Nilsson M, Svenungsson B, Hedlund KO, et al. Incidence and genetic diversity of group C rotavirus among adults. *J Infect Dis* 2000;182:678–684.
72. Chen GM, Hung T, Mackow ER. cDNA cloning of each genomic segment of the group B rotavirus ADRV: molecular characterization of the 11th RNA segment. *Virology* 1990;175: 605–609.
73. Terrett LA, Saif LJ, Theil KW, et al. Physicochemical characterization of porcine pararotavirus and detection of virus and viral antibodies using cell culture immunofluorescence. *J Clin Microbiol* 1987;25:268–272.
74. Estes MK, Crawford SE, Penaranda ME, et al. Synthesis and immunogenicity of the rotavirus major capsid antigen using a baculovirus expression system. *J Virol* 1987;61:1488–1494.
75. Chang KO, Parwani AV, Smith D, et al. Detection of group B rotaviruses in fecal samples from diarrheic calves and adult cows and characterization of their VP7 genes. *J Clin Microbiol* 1997;35:2107–2110.
76. Eiden JJ, Mouzinho A, Lindsay DA, et al. Serum antibody response to recombinant major inner capsid protein following human infection with group B rotavirus. *J Clin Microbiol* 1994; 32:1599–603.
77. James VL, Lambden PR, Caul EO, et al. Enzyme-linked immunosorbent assay based on recombinant human group C rotavirus inner capsid protein (VP6) to detect human group C rotaviruses in fecal samples. *J Clin Microbiol* 1998;36: 3178–3181.
78. James VL, Lambden PR, Caul EO, et al. Seroepidemiology of human group C rotavirus in the UK. *J Med Virol* 1997;52:86–91.
79. Kuzuya M, Fujii R, Hamano M, et al. rapid detection of human group c rotaviruses by reverse passive hemagglutination and latex agglutination tests using monoclonal antibodies. *J Clin Microbiol* 1993;31:1308–1311.
80. Mackow ER, FayME, Werner-Eckert R, et al. Baculovirus expression of the ADRV gene 5 encoded protein produces an oligomerized, antigenic, and immunogenic VP6 protein. *Virology* 1993;193:537–542.
81. Alfieri AA, Leite JP, Alfieri AF, et al. Detection of field isolates of human and animal group C rotavirus by reverse transcription-polymerase chain reaction and digoxigenin-labeled oligonucleotide probes. *J Virol Methods* 1999;83:35–43.
82. Chinsangaram J, Akita GY, Osburn BI. Detection of bovine group B rotaviruses in feces by polymerase chain reaction. *J Vet Diagn Invest* 1994;6:302–307.
83. Eiden JJ, Wilde J, Firoozmand F, et al. Detection of animal and human group B rotaviruses in fecal specimens by polymerase chain reaction. *J Clin Microbiol* 1991;29:539–543.
84. Fujii R, Kuzuya M, Hamano M, et al. Neutralization assay for human group C rotaviruses using a reverse passive hemagglutination test for endpoint determination. *J Clin Microbiol* 1000; 38:50–54.
85. Gouvea V, Allen JR, Glass RI, et al. Detection of group B and C rotaviruses by polymerase chain reaction. *J Clin Microbiol* 1991;29:519–523.
86. Sen A, Kobayashi N, Das S, et al. Amplification of various genes of human group B rotavirus from stool specimens by RT-PCR. *J Clin Virol* 2000;17:177–181.
87. Estes MK, Cohen J. Rotavirus gene structure and function. *Microbiol Rev* 1989;53:410–449.
88. Estes MK, Conner ME, Gilger MA, et al. Molecular biology and immunology of rotavirus infections. *Immunol Invest* 1989; 18:571–581.
89. Matsui SM, Mackow ER, Greenberg HB. Molecular determinant of rotavirus neutralization and protection. *Adv Virus Res* 1989;36:181–214.
90. Snodgrass DR, Hoshino Y, Fitzgerald TA, et al. Identification of four VP4 serological types (P serotypes) of bovine rotavirus using viral reassortants. *J Gen Virol* 1992;73:2319–2325.
91. Sanekata T, Kuwamoto Y, Akamatsu S, et al. Isolation of group B porcine rotavirus in cell culture. *J Clin Microbiol* 1996;34: 759–761.
92. Mackow ER, Werner-Eckert R, Fay ME, et al. Identification and baculovirus expression of the VP4 protein of the human group B rotavirus ADRV. *J Virol* 1993;67:2730–2738.
93. Sato S, Yolken RH, Eiden JJ. The complete nucleic acid sequence of gene segment 3 of the IDIR strain of group B rotavirus. *Nucleic Acids Res* 1989;17:10113.
94. Lindsay DA, Vonderfecht SS, Willoughby R, et al. Identification and expression of the outer capsid protein (VP4) of the IDIR strain of group B rotavirus. *Virology* 1993;194:724–733.
95. Hong T. Human group B rotavirus: adult diarrhea rotavirus. *Chin Med J (Engl)* 1996;109:11–12.
96. Li YY, Li X, Zheng CX. [Adult diarrhea rotavirus in Jilin, China]. *Uirusu* 1990;40:9–12.
97. Yang H, Chen S, et al. [A novel rotavirus causing large scale of adult diarrhea in Shi Jiazhuang]. *Chung Hua Liu Hsing Ping Hsueh Tsa Chih* 1998;19:336–338.
98. Tsunemitsu H, Morita D, Takaku H, et al. First detection of bovine group B rotavirus in Japan and sequence of its VP7 gene. *Arch Virol* 1999;144:805–815.
99. Chen GM, Hung T, Mackow ER. Identification of the gene encoding the group B rotavirus VP7 equivalent: primary characterization of the ADRV segment 9 RNA. *Virology* 1990;178: 311–315.
100. Petric M, Mayur K, Vonderfecht S, et al. Comparison of group B rotavirus genes 9 and 11. *J Gen Virol* 1991;72:2801–2804.
101. Saif LJ, Terrett LA, Miller KL, et al. Serial propagation of porcine group C rotavirus (pararotavirus) in a continuous cell line and characterization of the passaged virus. *J Clin Microbiol* 1988;26:1277–1282.
102. Terrett LA, Saif LJ. Serial propagation of porcine group C rotavirus (pararotavirus) in primary porcine kidney cell cultures. *J Clin Microbiol* 1987;25:1316–1319.
103. Tsunemitsu H, Saif LJ, Jiang BM, et al. Isolation, characterization, and serial propagation of a bovine group C rotavirus in a monkey kidney cell line (MA104). *J Clin Microbiol* 1994;29:2609–2613.
104. Welter MW, Welter CJ, Chambers DM, et al. Adaptation and serial passage of porcine group C rotavirus in ST-cells, an established diploid swine testicular cell line. *Arch Virol* 1991;120: 297–304.
105. Bremont M, Chabanne VD, Vannier P, et al. Sequence analysis of the gene (6) encoding the major capsid protein (VP6) of

group C rotavirus: higher than expected homology to the corresponding protein from group A virus. *Virology* 1990;178: 579–583.
106. Bremont M, Juste LP, Chabanne VD, et al. Sequences of the four larger proteins of a porcine group C rotavirus and comparison with the equivalent group A rotavirus proteins. *Virology* 1992;186:684–692.
107. Cooke SJ, Lambden PR, Caul EO, et al. Molecular cloning, sequence analysis and coding assignment of the major inner capsid protein gene of human group C rotavirus. *Virology* 1991;184:781–785.
108. Jiang B, Tsunemitsu H, Gentsch JR, et al. Nucleotide sequence of gene 5 encoding the inner capsid protein (VP6) of bovine group C rotavirus: comparison with corresponding genes of group C, A and B rotaviruses. *Virology* 1992;190:542–547.
109. Jiang B, Tsunemitsu H, Gentsch JR, et al. Nucleotide sequences of genes 6 and 10 of a bovine group C rotavirus. *Nucleic Acids Res* 1993;21:2250.
110. Jiang BM, Qian Y, Tsunemitsu H, et al. Analysis of the gene encoding the outer capsid glycoprotein (VP7) of group C rotaviruses by northern and dot blot hybridization. *Virology* 1991;184:433–436.
111. Jiang BM, Tsunemitsu H, Qian Y, et al. Analysis of the genetic diversity of genes 5 and 6 among group C rotaviruses using cDNA probes. *Arch Virol* 1992;126:45–56.
112. Lambden PR, Cooke SJ, Caul EO, et al. Cloning of noncultivatable human rotavirus by single primer amplification. *J Virol* 1992;66:1817–1822.
113. Qian YA, Jiang BM, Saif LJ, et al. Sequence conservation of gene 8 between human and porcine group C rotaviruses and its relationship to the VP7 gene of group A rotaviruses. *Virology* 1991;182:562–569.
114. Qian YA, Jiang BM, Saif LJ, et al. Molecular analysis of the gene 6 from a porcine group C rotavirus that encodes the NS34 equivalent of group A rotaviruses. *Virology* 1991;184:752–757.
115. Tsunemitsu H, Jiang B, Yamashita Y, et al. Evidence of serologic diversity within group C rotaviruses. *J Clin Microbiol* 1992;30: 3009–3012.
116. Arista S, Giovannelli L, Pistoia D, et al. Electropherotypes, subgroups and serotypes of human rotavirus strains causing gastroenteritis in infants and young children in Palermo, Italy, from 1985 to 1989. AD - Institute of Microbiology, University of Palermo, Italy. *Res Virol* 1990;141:435–448.
117. Chinsangaram J, Schore CE, Guterbock W, et al. Prevalence of group A and group B rotaviruses in the feces of neonatal dairy calves from California. *Comp Immunol Microbiol Infect Dis* 1995;18:93–103.
118. Parwani AV, Lucchelli A, Saif LJ. Identification of group B rotaviruses with short genome electropherotypes from adult cows with diarrhea. *J Clin Microbiol* 1996;34:1303–1305.
119. Chen GM, Werner ER, Tao H, et al. Expression of the major inner capsid protein of the group B rotavirus ADRV: primary characterization of genome segment 5. *Virology* 1991;182: 820–829.
120. Dimitrov DH, Graham DY, Estes MK. Detection of rotaviruses by nucleic acid hybridization with cloned DNA of simian rotavirus SA11 genes. *J Infect Dis* 1985;152:293–300.
121. Eiden J, Sato S, Yolken R. Specificity of dot hybridization assay in the presence of rRNA for detection of rotaviruses in clinical specimens. *J Clin Microbiol* 1987;25:1809–1811.
122. Eiden JJ, Firoozmand F, Sato S, et al. Detection of group B rotavirus in fecal specimens by dot hybridization with a cloned cDNA probe. *J Clin Microbiol* 1989;27:422–426.
123. Lin M, Imai M, Ikegami N, et al. cDNA probes of individual genes of human rotavirus distinguish viral subgroups and serotypes. *J Virol Methods* 1987;15:285–289.
124. Mason BB, Graham DY, Estes MK. Biochemical mapping of the simian rotavirus SA11 genome. *J Virol* 1983;46:413–423.
125. Rosen BI, Saif LJ, Jackwood DJ, et al. Serotypic differentiation of group A rotaviruses with porcine rotavirus gene 9 probes. *J Clin Microbiol* 1990;28:2526–2533.
126. McCrae MA. Nucleic acid-based analyses of non-group A rotaviruses. *Ciba Found Symp* 1987;128:24–48.
127. Castello AA, Arguelles MH, Villegas GA, et al. Characterization of human group C rotavirus in argentina. *J Med Virol* 2000; 62:199–207.
128. Chang KO, Kim YJ, Saif LJ. Comparisons of nucleotide and deduced amino acid sequences of NSP4 genes of virulent and attenuated pairs of group A and C rotaviruses. *Virus Genes* 1999;18:229–233.
129. Chang KO, Nielsen PR, Ward LA, et al. Dual infection of gnotobiotic calves with bovine strains of group A and porcine-like group C rotaviruses influences pathogenesis of the group C rotavirus. *J Virol* 1999;73:9284–9293.
130. Flores J, Myslinski J, Kalica AR, et al. *In vitro* transcription of two human rotaviruses. *J Virol* 1982;43:1032–1037.
131. Spencer E, Arias ML. *In vitro* transcription catalyzed by heat-treated human rotavirus. *J Virol* 1981;40:1–10.
132. Gallegos CO, Patton JT. Characterization of rotavirus replication intermediates: a model for the assembly of single-shelled particles. *Virology* 1989;172:616–627.
133. Mansell EA, Patton JT. Rotavirus RNA replication: VP2, but not VP6, is necessary for viral replicase activity. *J Virol* 1990;64: 4988–4996.
134. Patton JT, Gallegos CO. Rotavirus RNA replication: single-stranded RNA extends from the replicase particle. *J Gen Virol* 1990;71:1087–1094.
135. Patton JT, Gallegos CO. Structure and protein composition of the rotavirus replicase particle. *Virology* 1988;166:358–365.
136. Eiden JJ, Vonderfecht S, Petric M. Terminal sequence conservation among the genomic segments of a group B rotavirus (IDIR strain). *Virology* 1992;191:495–497.
137. Sandino AM, Jashes M, Faundez G, et al. Role of the inner protein capsid on *in vitro* human rotavirus transcription. *J Virol* 1986;60:797–802.
138. Spencer E, Garcia BI. Effect of S-adenosylmethionine on human rotavirus RNA synthesis. *J Virol* 1984;52:188–197.
139. Jiang BM, Saif LJ. *In vitro* transcription and translation of genomic RNA from a porcine group C rotavirus. *Arch. Virol* 1992;124:181–185.
140. Eiden JJ, Wee SB, Vonderfecht SL. *In vitro* transcription and translation of group B rotavirus strain IDIR gene 8 and immunoprecipitation by human sera. *J Clin Microbiol* 1992;30: 440–443.
141. Mackow ER, Fay ME, Hung T, et al. Cloning, sequencing and expression of the gene encoding the VP2 protein of the human group B rotavirus, ADRV. *Virology* 1994;201:162.
142. Theil KW, McCloskey CM. Rabbit syncytium virus is a Kemerovo serogroup orbivirus. *J Clin Microbiol* 1991;29:2059–2062.
143. Theil KW, Saif LJ. *In vitro* detection of porcine rotavirus-like virus (group B rotavirus) and its antibody. *J Clin Microbiol* 1985;21:844–846.
144. Eiden JJ. Gene 5 of the IDIR agent (group B rotavirus) encodes a protein equivalent to NS34 of group A rotavirus. *Virology* 1993;196:298–302.
145. Eiden JJ, Hirshon C. Sequence analysis of Group B Rotavirus Gene 1 and definition of a rotavirus-specific sequence motif within the RNA polymerase. *Virology* 1993;192:154–160.
146. Eiden JJ, Nataro J, Vonderfecht S, et al. Molecular cloning, sequence analysis, *in vitro* expression, and immunoprecipitation of the major inner capsid protein of the IDIR strain of group B rotavirus (GBR). *Virology* 1992;188:580–589.

147. Lindsay DA, Vonderfecht SL, Betenbaugh MJ, et al. Baculovirus expression of gene 6 of the IDIR strain of group B rotavirus (GBR): coding assignment of the major inner capsid protein. *Virology* 1993;193:367–375.
148. Mackow ER, FayME, Werner-Eckert R, et al. Baculovirus expression of the ADRV gene 5 encoded protein produces an oligomerized, antigenic, and immunogenic VP6 protein. *Virology* 1993;193:537–542.
149. Vonderfecht SL, Schemmer JK. Purification of the IDIR strain of group B rotavirus and identification of viral structural proteins. Virology 1993;194:277–283.
150. Lindsay DA, Vonderfecht SL, Eiden JJ. Group B rotavirus VP2: sequence analysis, expression, and gene coding assignment. *Virology* 1994;199:141–150.
151. Both GW, Mattick JS, Bellamy AR. Serotype-specific glycoprotein of simian 11 rotavirus: coding assignment and gene sequence. *Proc Natl Acad Sci U S A* 1983;80:3091–3095.
152. Estes MK, Mason BB, Crawford S, et al. Cloning and nucleotide sequence of the simian rotavirus gene 6 that codes for the major inner capsid protein. *Nucleic Acids Res* 1984;12: 1875–1887.
153. Mackow ER, Shaw RD, Matsui SM, et al. Characterization of homotypic and heterotypic VP7 neutralization sites of rhesus rotavirus. *Virology* 1988;165:511–517.
154. Mackow ER, Shaw RD, Matsui SM, et al. the rhesus rotavirus gene encoding protein vp3: location of amino acids involved in homologous and heterologous rotavirus neutralization and identification of a putative fusion region. *Proc Natl Acad Sci U S A* 1988;85:645–649.
155. Prasad BV, Burns JW, Marietta E, et al. Localization of VP4 neutralization sites in rotavirus by three-dimensional cryo-electron microscopy. *Nature* 1990;343:476–479.
156. Fiore L, Greenberg HB, Mackow ER. The VP8 fragment of VP4 is the rhesus rotavirus hemagglutinin. *Virology* 1991;181: 553–563.
157. Kalica AR, Flores J, Greenberg HB. Identification of the rotaviral gene that codes for hemagglutination and protease-enhanced plaque formation. *Virology* 1983125:194–205.
158. Mackow ER, Barnett JW, Chan H, et al. The rhesus rotavirus outer capsid protein VP4 functions as a hemagglutinin and is antigenically conserved when expressed by a baculovirus recombinant. *J Virol* 1989;63:1661–1668.
159. Offit PA, Blavat G. Identification of the two rotavirus genes virus genes determining neutralization specificities. *J Virol* 1986;57:376–378.
160. Offit PA, Blavat G, Greenberg HB, et al. Molecular basis of rotavirus virulence: role of gene segment 4. *J Virol* 1986;57: 46–49.
161. Dai GZ, Sun MS, Liu SQ, et al. First report of an epidemic of diarrhoea in human neonates involving the new rotavirus and biological characteristics of the epidemic virus strain (KMB/R85). *J Med Virol* 1987;22:365–373.
162. Spear PG. Virus-induced cell fusion. In: Sowers AE, ed. *Cell fusion*. New York: Plenum, 1987:3–31.
163. White J. Membrane fusion. *Science* 1992;258:917–924.
164. Schmidt MFG. Acylation of viral spike glycoproteins: a feature of enveloped RNA viruses. *Virology* 1982;116:327–338.
165. Towler DA, Gordon JI, Adams SP, et al. The biology and enzymology of eukaryotic protein acylation. *Annu Rev Biochem* 1988;57:69–99.
166. Bryant M, Ratner L, Duronio R, et al. Incorporation of 12-methoxydodecanoate into the HIV 1 gag polyprotein precursor inhibits its proteolytic processing and virus production in a chronically infected human lymphoid cell line. *Proc Natl Acad Sci U S A* 1991;88:2055–2059.
167. Krausslich HG, Holscher C, Reuer Q, et al. Myristoylation of the poliovirus polyprotein is required for proteolytic processing of the capsid and for viral infectivity. *J Virol* 1990;64:2433–2436.
168. Moscufo N, Chow M. Myristate-protein interactions in poliovirus: interactions of VP4 threonine 28 contribute to the structural conformation of assembly intermediates and the stability of assembled virions. *J Virol* 1992;66:6849–6857.
169. Nibert M, Fields BN. A carboxy-terminal fragment of protein 1/mu 1C is present in infectious subvirion particles of mammalian reoviruses and is proposed to have a role in penetration. *J Virol* 1992;66:6408–6418.
170. Nibert ML, Schiff LA, Fields BN. Mammalian reoviruses contain a myristoylated structural protein. *J Virol* 1991;65:1960–1967.
171. Wang C, Barklis E. Assembly, processing, and infectivity of HIV type 1 Gag mutants. *J Virol* 1993;67:4264–4273.
172. Eiden JJ. Expression and sequence analysis of gene 7 of the IDIR agent (group B rotavirus): similarity with NS53 of group A rotavirus. *Virology* 1994;199:212–218.
173. Bremont M, Chabanne-Vautherot D, Cohen J. Sequence analysis of three non structural proteins of a porcine group C (Cowden strain) rotavirus. *Arch Virol* 1993;130:85–92.
174. Bremont M, Juste LP, Chabanne VD, et al. Erratum: sequences of the four larger proteins of a porcine group C rotavirus and comparison with the equivalent group A rotavirus proteins. *Virology* 1992;189:402.
175. Grice AS, Lambden PR, Caul EO, et al. Sequence conservation of the major outer capsid glycoprotein of human group C rotaviruses. *J Med Virol* 1994;44:166–171.
176. Jiang B, Gentsch JR, Tsunemitsu H, et al. Sequence analysis of the gene encoding VP4 of a bovine group C rotavirus: molecular evidence for a new P genotype. *Virus Genes* 1999;19:85–88.
177. Jiang B, Saif LJ, Gentsch JR, et al. Completion of the four large gene sequences of porcine group C Cowden rotavirus. *Virus Genes* 2000;20:193–194.
178. Samarbaf-Zadeh AR, Lambden PR, Green SM, et al. The VP3 gene of human group C rotavirus. *Virus Genes* 1996;13: 169–173.
179. Tsunemitsu H, Ojeh CK, Jiang B, et al. Production and characterization of monoclonal antibodies to porcine group C rotaviruses cross-reactive with group A rotaviruses. *Virology* 1992;191:272–281.
180. Bremont M, Cohen J, and McCrae MA. Analysis of the structural polypeptides of a porcine group C rotavirus. *J Virol* 1988; 62:2183–2185.
181. Jiang BM, Saif LJ, Kang SY, et al. Biochemical characterization of the structural and nonstructural polypeptides of a porcine group C rotavirus. *J Virol* 1990;64:3171–3178.
182. Fielding PA, Lambden PR, Caul EO, et al. Molecular characterization of the outer capsid spike protein (VP4) gene from human group C rotavirus. *Virology* 1994;204:442–446.
183. Cooke SJ, Clarke IN, Freitas RB, et al. The correct sequence of the porcine group C/Cowden rotavirus major inner capsid protein shows close homology with human isolates from Brazil and the U.K. *Virology* 1992;190:531–537.
184. Jiang B, Tsunemitsu H, Dennehy PH, et al. Sequence conservation and expression of the gene encoding the outer capsid glycoprotein among human group C rotaviruses of global distribution. *Arch Virol* 1996;141:381–390.
185. Tsunemitsu H, Jiang B, Saif LJ. Sequence comparison of the VP7 gene encoding the outer capsid glycoprotein among animal and human group C rotaviruses. *Arch Virol* 1996;141: 705–713.
186. James VL, Lambden PR, Deng Y, et al. Molecular characterization of human group C rotavirus genes 6, 7 and 9. *J Gen Virol* 1999;80:3181–3187.
187. Langland JO, Pettiford S, Jiang B, et al. Products of the porcine group C rotavirus NSP3 gene bind specifically to double-

stranded RNA and inhibit activation of the interferon-induced protein kinase PKR. *J Virol* 1994;68:3821–3829.
188. Deng Y, Fielding PA, Lambden PR, et al. Molecular characterization of the 11th RNA segment from human group C rotavirus. *Virus Genes* 1995;10:239–243.
189. Horie Y, Nakagomi T, Oseto M, et al. Conserved structural features of nonstructural glycoprotein NSP4 between group A and group C rotaviruses. *Arch Virol* 1997;142:1865–1872.
190. Ball JM., Tian P, Zeng CQ, et al. Age-dependent diarrhea induced by a rotaviral nonstructural glycoprotein [see comments]. *Science* 1996;272:101–104.
191. Svensson L. Group C rotavirus requires sialic acid for erythrocyte and cell receptor binding. *J Virol* 1992;66:5582–5585.
192. Labbe M, Charpilienne A, Crawford SE, et al. Expression of rotavirus VP2 produces empty corelike particles. *J Virol* 1991; 65:2946–2952.
193. Tosser G, Labbe M, Bremont M, et al. Expression of the major capsid protein of Group C rotavirus and synthesis of chimeric single-shelled particles by using recombinant Baculoviruses. *J Virol* 1992;66:5825–5831.
194. Alpers D, Sanders RC, Hampson DJ. Rotavirus excretion by village pigs in Papua New Guinea. *Aust Vet J* 1991;68:65–67.
195. Clark KJ, Tamborello TJ, Xu Z, et al. An unusual group-A rotavirus associated with an epidemic of diarrhea among three-month-old calves. *J Am Vet Med Assoc* 1996;208:552–554.
196. Geyer A, Sebata T, Peenze I, et al. Group B and C porcine rotaviruses identified for the first time in South Africa. *J S Afr Vet Assoc* 1996;67:115–116.
197. Gueguen C, Maga A, McCrae MA, et al. Caprine and bovine B rotaviruses in western France: group identification by Northern hybridization. *Vet Res* 1996;27:171–176.
198. Legrottaglie R, Rizzi V, Agrimi P. Molecular epidemiology of bovine rotaviruses. Characterization of rotaviruses isolated from diarrhoeic calves by genome profile analysis. *New Microbiol* 1995;18:193–200.
199. Noel JS, Beards GM, Cubitt WD. Epidemiological survey of human rotavirus serotypes and electropherotypes in young children admitted to two children's hospitals in northeast London from 1984 to 1990. *J Clin Microbiol* 1994;29:2213–2219.
200. Shinozaki K, Yamanaka T, Tokieda M, et al. Isolation and serial propagation of human group C rotaviruses in a cell line (CaCo-2). *J Med Virol* 1996;48:48–52.
201. Kawamura H, Shimizu F, Maeda M, et al. Avian reovirus: its properties and serological classification. *Ntl Inst Anim Health Q (Tokyo)* 1965;5:115–124.
202. Ni Y, Ramig RF. Characterization of avian reovirus-induced cell fusion: the role of structural proteins. *Virology* 1993;194: 705–714.
203. Wilcox GE, Compans RW. Cell fusion induced by Nelson Bay virus. *Virology* 1982;123:312–322.
204. Wilcox GE, Compans RW. Characterization of Nelson Bay virus and virus-induced cell fusion. In: Compans RW and Bishop DHL, ed. *Double-stranded RNA viruses*. Elsevier, 1983: 391–403.
205. Penaranda ME, Ho MS, Fang ZY, et al. Seroepidemiology of adult diarrhea rotavirus in China, 1977 to 1987. *J Clin Microbiol* 1989;27:2180–2183.
206. Nakata S, Estes MK, Graham DY, et al. Detection of antibody to group B adult diarrhea rotaviruses in humans. *J Clin Microbiol* 1987;25:812–818.
207. Besselaar TG, Rosenblatt A, Kidd AH. Atypical rotavirus from South African neonates. Brief report. *Arch Virol* 1986;87: 327–330.
208. Riepenhoff-Talty M, Morse K, Wang CH, et al. Epidemiology of group C rotavirus infection in Western New York women of childbearing age. *J Clin Microbiol* 1997;35:486–488.
209. Fujita Y, Yamada H, Araki K, et al. [Detection of group C rotavirus in the day care center]. *Kansenshogaku Zasshi* 1994; 68:723–727.
210. Qian Y, Saif LJ, Kapikian AZ, et al. Comparison of human and porcine group C rotaviruses by northern blot hybridization analysis. *Arch Virol* 1991;118:269–277.
211. Flewett TH, Beards GM, Brown DW, et al. The diagnostic gap in diarrhoeal aetiology. *Ciba Found Symp* 1987;128:238–249.
212. Lebaron CW, Furutan NP, Lew JF, et al. Viral agents of gastroenteritis. *MMWR Morbid Mortal Wkly Rep* 1990;39:1–24.
213. Vonderfecht SL, Lindsay DA, Eiden JJ. Detection of rat, porcine, and bovine group B rotavirus in fecal specimens by solid-phase enzyme immunoassay. *J Clin Microbiol* 1994;32:1107–1108.
214. Burns JW, Welch SK, Nakata S, et al. Characterization of monoclonal antibodies to human group B rotavirus and their use in an antigen detection enzyme-linked immunosorbent assay. *J Clin Microbiol* 1989;27:245–250.
215. Yolken R, Wee SB, Eiden J, et al. Identification of a group-reactive epitope of group B rotaviruses recognized by monoclonal antibody and application to the development of a sensitive immunoassay for viral characterization. *J Clin Microbiol* 1988; 26:1853–1858.
216. Nakata S, Estes MK, Graham DY, et al. Antigenic characterization and ELISA detection of adult diarrhea rotaviruses [published erratum appears in *J Infect Dis* 1987;155:162]. *J Infect Dis* 1986;154:448–455.
217. Ojeh CK, Jiang BM, Tsunemitsu H, et al. Reactivity of monoclonal antibodies to the 41- kilodalton protein of porcine group C rotavirus with homologous and heterologous rotavirus serogroups in immunofluorescence tests. *J Clin Microbiol* 1991; 29:2051–2055.
218. Ojeh CK, Tsunemitsu H, Simkins RA, et al. Development of a biotin-streptavidin-enhanced enzyme-linked immunosorbent assay which uses monoclonal antibodies for detection of group C rotaviruses. *J Clin Microbiol* 1992;30:1667–1673.
219. Tsunemitsu H, Jiang B, Saif LJ. Detection of group C rotavirus antigens and antibodies in animals and humans by enzyme-linked immunosorbent assays. *J Clin Microbiol* 1992;30: 2129–2134.
220. Wu H, Taniguchi K, Urasawa T, et al. Serological and genomic characterization of human rotaviruses detected in China. *J Med Virol* 1998;55:168–176.

56

NORWALK VIRUS AND THE HUMAN ENTERIC CALICIVIRUSES

MICHELE E. HARDY
MARY K. ESTES

The first virus identified as a cause of gastroenteritis was the Norwalk virus (NV). This virus originated from an outbreak of epidemic gastroenteritis in an elementary school in Norwalk, Ohio, in 1968. During this outbreak, 50% of the students and teachers became ill and secondary spread to 32% of family contacts was documented (1). Ultimately, NV was visualized by immune electron microscopy (IEM) and was described as a filterable agent 27 nm × 32 nm (2). This report provided definitive proof that viruses can cause diarrhea, a hypothesis based on studies performed during the 1940s and 1950s in which filterable infectious agents could be passaged serially in volunteers, yet no virus was successfully cultivated using available tissue culture techniques. Administration of a bacteria-free fecal filtrate of NV to volunteers resulted in the first clear description of the basic virologic, clinical, and immunologic responses to nonbacterial infections (3). Thus, visualization of NV opened a new era in characterization of viral agents associated with diarrheal disease. In a seemingly short time, the large rotaviruses, enteric adenoviruses, coronaviruses, and toroviruses, and the smaller caliciviruses and astroviruses were identified. Rotaviruses were quickly recognized to be the major viral agents responsible for life-threatening diarrheal illness in young children and neonatal animals (see Chapters 54 and 55).

The last decade has ushered in significant advances in our understanding of NV and Norwalk-like viruses (NLVs), despite the lack of a cell culture system to propagate virus in the laboratory. These human enteric caliciviruses (HuCV) currently are recognized as the most important viral cause of food-borne outbreaks of acute, nonbacterial gastroenteritis and are implicated in outbreaks stemming from contaminated water supplies (4). Molecular epidemiologic studies are defining the extensive genetic diversity of this group of viruses (5–12). Recombinant virus-like particles (rVLPs) representative of different antigenic types are being used to characterize antigenic relationships and to develop assays that evaluate antibody responses in infected people (7,13–15). The atomic resolution structure of the NV capsid was solved and provides a detailed map of regions of the capsid that may be important in virus assembly and presentation of virus-neutralizing epitopes (16). The molecular details of the replication strategy are starting to be unraveled, as researchers take advantage of full-length complementary DNA (cDNA) clones and *in vitro* expression systems (17–19). Finally, genome sequences of two animal viruses—the porcine enteric calicivirus (PEC) and bovine enteric calicivirus—were determined and found to be closely related genetically to HuCVs (20–22). In this chapter, we review the most recent data available and include historical perspectives where appropriate. The reader is referred to excellent resources for a full description of the history of isolation and characterization of the HuCV (23,24).

MORPHOLOGY AND CLASSIFICATION

HuCVs are difficult to study. These viruses are refractory to cultivation and there are no animal models to produce infectious virus particles. In the past, these complications limited study of HuCV to a few research laboratories or to public health or hospital laboratories that were able to identify viruses by methods such as IEM. Very low concentrations of virus are present in stool samples, making detection and purification difficult. Despite these limitations, once NV was recognized in stools by IEM, an explosion of studies rapidly reported many morphologically similar agents, including the Hawaii agent (25), Snow Mountain agent

M. E. Hardy: Veterinary Molecular Biology Laboratory, Montana State University, Bozeman, Montana

M. K. Estes: Department of Molecular Virology and Microbiology, Baylor College of Medicine, Houston, Texas

(26), Montgomery County agent (27), Taunton agent (28), and Otofuke, Sapporo, and Osaka agents (29–31).

Historically, NV and related viruses were classified based on morphology. Geographic names that denoted the location of the outbreak were used as a way to describe these morphologically ill-defined particles. In an interim classification system, viruses were first characterized according to whether they had visible structural features, and NV was classified as a small round structured virus (SRSV) (32,33). Table 56.1 illustrates morphologic and biophysical properties of fecal viruses on which the interim classification system was based. The classification system for fecal viruses helped researchers to compare agents but suffered from being simply morphologic, with success dependent on the timing and quality of samples collected and on the skill and interpretation of individual electron microscopists. These inherent difficulties were compounded for stool samples, which are not clear or easy samples to study, and which may contain fecal immunoglobulins or other factors (e.g., proteolytic enzymes and mucins) that obscure or degrade the surface structure of viruses. The interim classification system served a valuable need with the recognized caveat that conclusions based on electron microscopy (EM) classification alone must be regarded as tentative. Recent studies in which new methods applied to samples previously characterized by EM alone highlight this point, because some agents previously classified solely by morphology were incorrectly identified (34). Similarly, molecular methods have shown that particles previously characterized as other agents (e.g., minireoviruses) are actually NLV, and viruses with or without typical calicivirus morphology also may be NLV.

Biochemical studies on the viral proteins isolated from stools of infected volunteers predicted NV to be a calicivirus based on the presence of a single virion-associated protein with an apparent molecular weight of approximately 59,000 (35). This characteristic was consistent with the prototypical caliciviruses that have a single structural protein with molecular weights ranging from 60,000 to 70,000 Kd (36–38). Molecular cloning and characterization of the NV and Southampton virus (SV) genomes allowed these viruses to be unequivocally classified as members of the family *Caliciviridae* (39,40). The name calicivirus is derived from the Latin word *calyx,* meaning *cup* or *goblet* referring to cup-shaped depressions observed by EM. The International

TABLE 56.1. CHARACTERISTICS OF SMALL ROUND FECAL VIRUSES ACCORDING TO MORPHOLOGY BY ELECTRON MICROSCOPY

Morphology	Type of Virus	Morphologic/Biophysical Properties/Genome	Examples	Comment
Featureless (no surface structure; smooth outer edge)	Picornavirus	BD 1.34 g/cm^3 Size ~23–30 nm RNA genome	Poliovirus, coxsackievirus, hepatitis A virus	
	Parvovirus	BD 1.38–1.46 g/cm^3 Size ~18–26 nm ssDNA	Mink enteritis virus, feline/canine/bovine parvoviruses	
	Small round viruses	BD 1.38–1.40 g/cm^3 Size ~22–26 nm DNA?	Wollan, Parramatta, Ditchling, cockle agents	May be parvoviruses or bacteriophage heads carried in feces and unrelated to gastroenteritis. Ditchling virus originally classified here later shown to be an astrovirus.
Structured (surface structure and/or ragged edge)	Astrovirus	5–6 pointed surface star BD 1.36–1.38 g/cm^3 Size ~28–30 nm RNA	Lamb, human astroviruses (five serotypes)	
	Calicivirus	Surface hollows, ragged outline, "Star of David" configuration BD 1.36–1.39 g/cm^3 Size ~30–38 nm RNA	Human (UK1–4 and Sapporo), Newbury bovine, porcine	
	SRSV	Amorphous surface, ragged outline BD 1.36–1.41 g/cm^3 Size ~30–35 nm RNA	Norwalk, Hawaii, Snow Mountain, Montgomery County, Taunton, Otofuke, Sapporo, Osaka, minireoviruses	Norwalk, Hawaii, Snow Mountain, and most SRSVs now shown to be human caliciviruses based on sequence analysis: others still not tested now called NLVs (see text)

BD, bouyant density; SRSV, small round structured virus.
From Cubitt WD, Green KY, Payment P. Prevalence of antibodies to the Hawaii strain of human calicivirus as measured by recombinant protein based immunoassay. *J Med Virol* 1998;54:135–139, with permission.

Committee on Taxonomy of Viruses has recently accepted an updated classification scheme for the Caliciviridae based on new molecular data that divide the family into four genera, with a type species for each (41). The HuCVs belong to two genera, the NLVs and the "Sapporo-like viruses" (SLVs), with NV and the Sapporo virus as type species, respectively. This division is based primarily on genome organization and phylogenetic analyses. Viruses in both genera cause similar clinical illness, yet there are differences between the strains that segregate into each genus. Viruses in the NLV genus usually are associated with epidemic gastroenteritis outbreaks in school-age children and adults and lack prominent cupshaped depressions when observed by EM. The SLVs are typically found in sporadic cases of pediatric gastroenteritis, and classic calicivirus morphology is readily apparent by EM. These segregations are useful to make generalities about the HuCV but are tenuous at best, given that some virus strains with typical morphology are more related genetically to the NLV and some animal viruses are related genetically to the NLV and SLV. Thus, until well-characterized serologic reagents are widely available, division of the HuCV into NLV and SLV genera is based on sequence analysis and phylogenetic grouping. The remaining two genera in the family *Caliciviridae* include the genus Lagovirus with rabbit hemorrhagic disease virus (RHDV) as the type species, and the genus Vesivirus, represented by vesicular exanthema of swine virus (VESV) as the type species.

A comparison of the properties of HuCV with animal caliciviruses identifies three key features (Table 56.2): (a) The only cultivable caliciviruses are animal strains, (b) animal caliciviruses cause a spectrum of diseases, in addition to diarrheal disease, and (c) some caliciviruses have a broad host range and infect more than one species. HuCVs remain relatively poorly studied compared with some of the animal caliciviruses. It is possible that additional human illnesses and cross-species transmission will be discovered as HuCVs become well characterized. This idea is fortified by the rapid changes observed in the epidemiology of HuCV infections now that new methods of virus detection are available.

VIRUS STRUCTURE

NV was classically described as a 27-nm particle based on analysis of particles obtained from stools that were aggregated with antibody (2). One limitation to the EM analysis of particles from stool has been the necessity to perform IEM due to the low numbers of particles present in most stool preparations. However, based on these micrographs, it was rare to see particles with typical calicivirus structure, having distinct cuplike indentations in the surface of particles (Fig. 56.1A and B). Instead, the NV appeared to have a feathery outer edge that lacked a definitive surface sub-

TABLE 56.2. COMPARISON OF HUMAN CALICIVIRUS (NORWALK) WITH ANIMAL CALICIVIRUSES

Virus Strain	Host Range Origin (Secondary Hosts)	Designation	Disease	Typical Calicivirus Structure	Cultivated	Other Comments
Norwalk virus	Humans	HuCV/NV/8FIIa/68/US	Diarrhea	No	No	Prototype human calicivirus; several genotypes
Porcine enteric calicivirus	Pigs	PEC	Diarrhea	Yes	Yes	Cultivation requires adding large intestinal content fluids
Bovine enteric calicivirus	Calves	Newbury agents 1 and 2	Diarrhea	Yes	No	
Feline calicivirus	Cats, dogs (humans?)	FCV	Respiratory illness, arthritis	Yes	Yes	One serotype with many variants, persistent infections
Rabbit hemorrhagic disease virus	Rabbits	RHDV	Hemorrhagic diarrheal disease—often lethal; liver infected	Yes	No	Recently isolated in United States; found in Europe, China, Mexico
San Miguel sea lion virus	Sea lions (humans)	SMSV	Abortions, vesicular lesions	Yes	Yes	Possibly the same virus as VESV
Vesicular exanthema of swine virus	Pigs (fish; sea lions?)	VESV	Skin lesions, glossitis, diarrhea	Yes	Yes	Possibly the same virus as SMSV
Primate calicivirus	Pigmy chimpanzees	PrCV-Pan 1/82	None	Yes	Yes	Persistent infections
Chicken enteric calicivirus	Chickens	ChCV	Diarrhea	Yes	No	

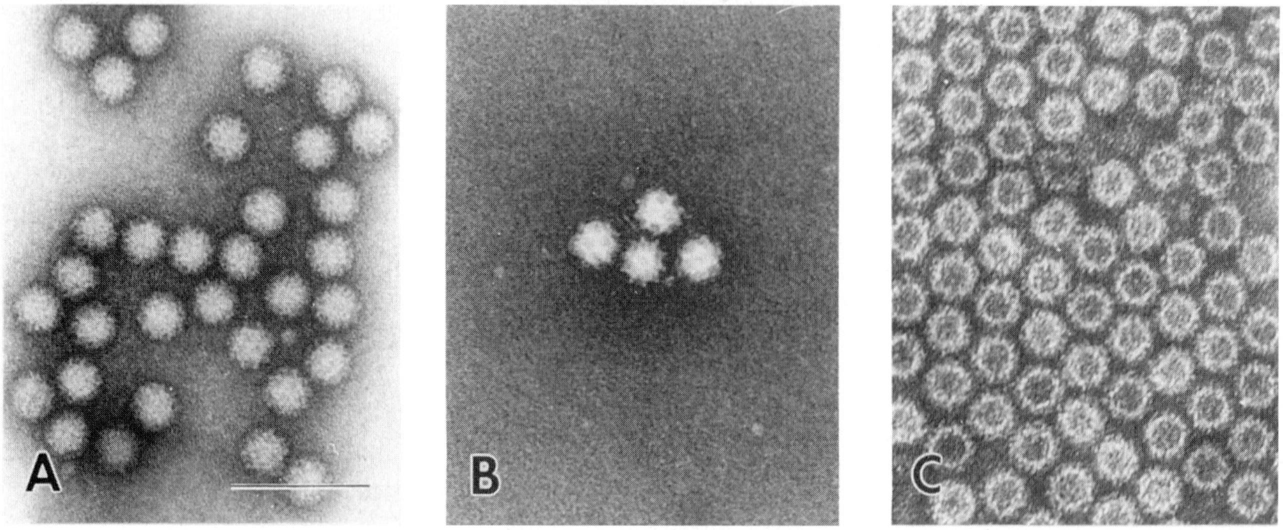

FIGURE 56.1. Electron micrographs of caliciviruses. Negative-stain electron micrographs of **(A)** Norwalk virus from the stool of a volunteer given human calicivirus (HuCV)/Norwalk virus (NV)/8FIIa; **(B)** a HuCV with typical structure including distinct cuplike indentations in the surface of particles, taken from the stool of a child containing HuCV/Sapporo; and **(C)** recombinant NV particles produced and purified from insect cells infected with a baculovirus recombinant that expresses the NV VP1. (Bar, 50 nm.)

structure (Fig. 56.1A); in certain orientations, NV appeared to have minor surface indentations.

A precise description of the structure of NV is now available based on analyses of recombinant NV (rNV) particles produced in insect cells infected with a baculovirus recombinant expressing the cDNA that encodes the capsid protein (42). The NV capsid is unique among animal viruses in that it is composed of 180 molecules of a single, major capsid protein encoded in open reading frame 2 (ORF2) called viral protein 1 (VP1). A few molecules (less than five) of a second protein (ORF3 or VP2) are also present in virions, possibly associated with the viral genome (43). Although a single capsid protein is common among plant viruses, it is unusual among animal viruses and the only other known animal viruses to share this feature, apart from caliciviruses, are the nodaviruses (44). By negative-stain EM, rNV particles have a similar morphology to the native NV (Fig. 56.1A and C). Analysis of these rNV particles by electron cryomicroscopy and computer image processing has shown the rNV particles have a distinct architecture and exhibit T = 3 icosahedral symmetry (Fig. 56.2A) (45). The capsid is made of 90 dimers of the capsid protein that form a shell (S) domain from which archlike capsomers protrude to form a protruding domain (P) (Fig. 56.2B–C). These arches are arranged in such a way that there are large hollows at the icosahedral fivefold and threefold positions (see Fig. 56.2B). These hollows are what appear as the cuplike structures in typical caliciviruses. The three-dimensional structure of a typical calicivirus (the primate PrCV Pan-1) also has been determined (46); this typical calicivirus structure differs from that of NV primarily in the length and shape of the protruding archlike domains. That is, the P domain in the typical calicivirus is longer than that for NV and the shape of the top of the arch also differs in such a way that the NV would show a feathery appearance by negative-stain EM.

These three-dimensional structures are valuable because they provide independent evidence of the similarities of these two distinct types of caliciviruses. An atomic resolution structure of the rNV VLPs is now available (16), and the structure exhibits both classic and novel features (Fig. 56.2C). The N-terminal 225 residues constitute the S domain and fold into a classic eight-stranded β-sandwich. The rest of the protein constitutes the P domain that has a fold unlike any other viral protein. The P domain consists of two subdomains: P2 and P1 (Fig. 56.2B and C). The P2 subdomain is located at the exterior of the capsid and exhibits the largest sequence variation among NLV, unlike the S and P1 domains that are better conserved. The variable P2 domain is likely to contain the determinants of strain specificity and cell binding, and it may serve as a replaceable module to alter strain specificity.

Regions of sequence conservation and variability are easily identified by analysis of the predicted amino acid sequences of the capsid proteins of different NLV strains. These regions of sequence variability are of interest because they often represent regions where neutralization epitopes are present on viral capsid proteins. The NV capsid protein can be divided into three domains based on sequence comparisons (47) (Fig. 56.3). Region 1 (aa 1 to 280) is relatively conserved and contains the region that forms the S domain of the capsid (45). This region corresponds to the B domain

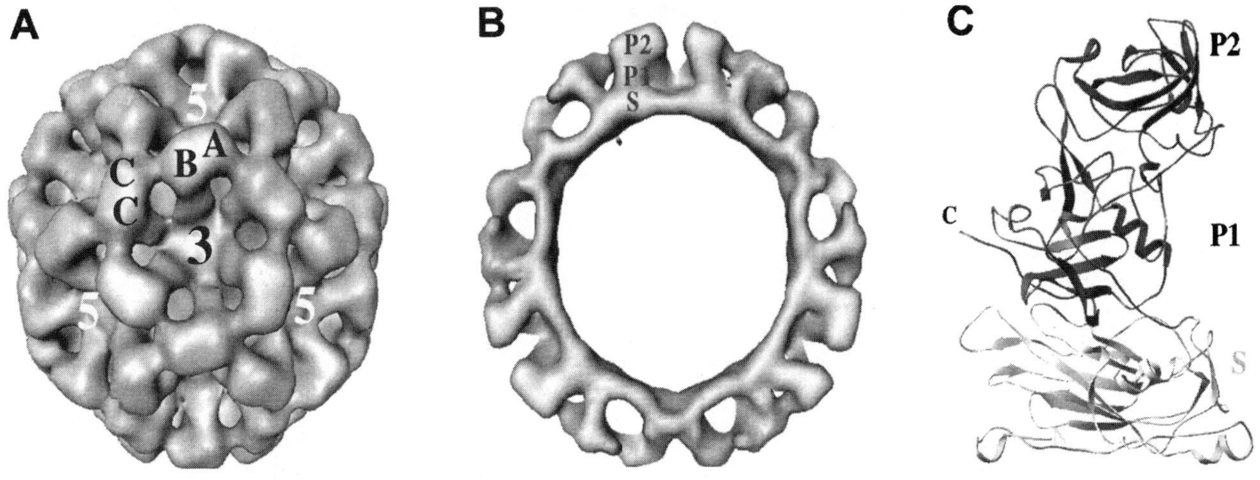

FIGURE 56.2. The structure of Norwalk virus (NV) particles. **A:** The three-dimensional structure of recombinant NV (rNV) particles viewed along the icosahedral threefold axis. This structure was determined by image processing of the rNV particles. The rNV particles have a distinct architecture and they exhibit T = 3 icosahedral symmetry; the threefold and fivefold axes of symmetry are shown and the cuplike depressions are evident at the threefold and fivefold axes. The capsid structure is made up of 90 dimers of a single protein that form a shell domain from which archlike capsomers protrude (Fig. 55.1B and C). (*A, B,* and *C* on the particle image denote subunit contacts.) **B:** A central section of the particle perpendicular to the icosahedral threefold axis. The arch is composed of two domains: the protruding (P) domain that is divided into two subdomains (P1 and P2) and the shell (S) domain. **C:** Ribbon representation of a single subunit from the rNV crystal structure. (From Prasad BV, Hardy ME, Dokland T, et al. X-ray crystallographic structure of the Norwalk virus capsid. *Science* 1999;286:287–290, and Prasad BV, Rothnagel R, Jiang X, et al. Three-dimensional structure of baculovirus-expressed Norwalk virus capsids. *J Virol* 1994;68: 5117–5125, with permission.)

described for animal caliciviruses (48). Region 2 (aa 281 to 404 for NV) shows high sequence variability and corresponds to variable domains C to E described for animal caliciviruses by Neill (48). The third region (aa 405 to the carboxyl terminus [C-terminus] for NV) is more conserved but still displays some variability. Regions 2 and 3 form the protruding archlike capsomeres.

GENOME ORGANIZATION AND REPLICATION STRATEGIES

Complete genome sequences for several calicivirus strains are known (Fig. 56.4) (21,22,39,40,49–53). The calicivirus genome is a positive sense, single-stranded RNA molecule 7 to 8 kilobases (kb) in length. The genome is polyadenylated at the 3′ end and has a small protein (VPg) covalently linked to the 5′ end in place of a 7-methylguanosine cap structure typically associated with eukaryotic messenger RNAs (mRNAs). The presence of VPg has been shown experimentally only for the animal viruses (54–56) but is assumed to be present on the HuCV RNA. All calicivirus genomes encode a large polyprotein, the major capsid protein, and a small minor structural protein in either two or three ORFs. The HuCVs display the two main genome organizations. In viruses with only two ORFs, the capsid protein is part of the polyprotein and is released by proteolytic cleavage. The NLV genome encodes three ORFs. ORF1 encodes the polyprotein precursor to viral nonstructural proteins. The second ORF encodes the major capsid protein and ORF3 encodes a minor structural protein. Viruses in the SLV have the major capsid protein coding sequences fused to the nonstructural protein coding sequences and thus have only two ORFs, with the second encoding the minor structural protein. It recently has been proposed that the major capsid protein be referred to as VP-1 and the minor 3′ terminal protein as VP2, to facilitate comparisons between caliciviruses with two and three ORFs (57).

There are additional differences among the calicivirus genomes. The NLV Southampton strain has a predicted fourth ORF; this has not been seen in other NLV and its significance remains unclear. The sizes of VP1 are different, with VP1 of feline calicivirus (FCV) (53), RHDV (52), and San Miguel sea lion virus serotypes 1 and 4 (SMSV, not shown) (48) being longer than that of the NV VP1. This larger size of the predicted VP1 is due to the presence of additional amino acids at the N-terminus of these other viruses; in some cases, these sequences are removed by cleavage of a precursor, so the mature VP1 is smaller. However, the mature capsid proteins of these viruses also are larger than the capsid protein of NV. Finally, the relative

```
           1                                                                                                                          120
NV-8fIIa   MMMASKDATS SVDGASGAGQ LVPEVNASDP LAMDPVAGSS TAVATAGQVN PIDPWIINNF VQAPQGEFTI SPNNTPGDVL FDLSLGPHLN PFLLHLSQMY NGWVGNMRVR IMLAGNAFTA
KY-89      MMMASKDATS SVDGASASVQ LVPEVNASDP LAMDPVAGSS TAVATAGQVN PIDPWIINNF VQAPQGEFTI SPNNTPGDVL FDLSLGPHLN PFLLHLSQMY NGWVGNMRVR IMLAGNAFTA
SHV        MMMASKDAPQ SADGASGAGQ LVPEVNTADP LPMEPVAGPT TAVATAGQVN MIDPWIVNNF VQSPQGEFTI SPNNTPGDIL FDLQLGPHLN PFLSHLSQMY NGWVGNMRVR ILLAGNAFSA
DSV        MMMASKDAPT NMDGTSGAGQ LVPEANTAEP ISMEPVAGAA TAAATAGQVN MIDPWIMSNY VQAPQGEFTI SPNNTPGDIL FDLQLGPHLN PFLSHLAQMY NGWVGNMRVK VLLAGNAFTA
OTH-25     MKMASNDAAP SNDGAAG... LVPEIN.NEA MALDPVAGAA IAAPLTGQQN IIDPWIMNNF VQAPGGEFTV SPRNSPGEVL LNLELGPEIN PYLAHLARMY NGYAGGFEVQ VVLAGNAFTA
TV         MKMASNDAAP SNDGAAC... LVPEIN.NEA MALEPVAGSA IAAPLTGQQN IIDPWIMNNF VQAPGGEFTV SPRNSPGEVL LNLELGPEIN PYLAHLARMY NGYAGGFEVQ VVLAGNAFTA
HV         MKMASNDAAP SNDGAAG... LVPEVN.NET MALEPVAGAS IAAPLTGQNN VIDPWIRMNF VQAPNGEFTV SPRNSPGEIL LNLELGPELN PFLAHLSRMY NGYAGGVEVQ VLLAGNAFTA
BV         MKMASNDANP SDGSAAN... LVPEVN.NEV MALEPVVGAA IAAPVAGQQN VIDPWIRNNF VQAPGGEFTV SPRNAPGEIL WSAPLGPDLN PYLSHLSRMY NGYAGGFEVQ VILAGNAFTA
Consensus  M-MAS-DA-- ---------- LVPE-N---- ----PV-G-- -A----GQ-N -IDPWI--N- VQ-P-GEFT- SP-N-PG--L ----LGP--N P-L-HL--MY NG--G---V- --LAGNAF-A
           ---------- ---------- ---------- ---------- ---------- ---------- ---------- ------G--L ------P--N P--------Y ----G----- ----G-----

                                                                      Region 1
           121                                                                                                                        238
NV-8fIIa   GKIIVSCIPP GFGSHNLTIA QATLFPHVIA DVRTLDPIEV PLEDVRNVLF HNNDRNQQTM RLVCMLYTPL RTGGGTG..D SFVVAGRVMT CPSPDFNFLF LVPPTVEQKT RPFTLPNLPL
KY-89      GKIIVSCIPP GFGSQQLTIA QATLFPHVIA DVRTLDPIEV PLEDVRNVLF HNNDRNQQTM RLVCMLYTPL STGGGTG..D SFVVAGRVMT CPSPDFNFLF LVPPTVEQKT RPFTLPNLPL
SHV        GKIIVCCVPP GFTSSSLTIA QATLFPHVIA DVRTLEPIEM PLEDVRNVLY HTND.NQPTM RLVCMLYTPL RTGGGSGNSD SFVVAGRVLT APSSDFSFLF LVPPTIEQKT RAFTVPNIPL
DSV        GKIIISCIPP GFAAQNISIA QATMFPHVIA DVRVLEPIEV PLEDVRNVLF HNNDSS.PTM RLVCMLYTPL RASGSSSGTD PFVIAGRVLT CPSPDFSFLF LVPPNVEQKT KPFSVPNLPL
OTH-25     AKVIFAAIPP NFPIDNLSAA QITMCPHVIV DVRQLEPINL PMPDVRNNFF HYNQGSDSRL RLIAMLYTPL RANNSGD..D VFTVSCRVLT RPSPDFSFNF LVPSTMESKT KPFTLPILTI
TV         GKIIFAAIPP NFPIDNLSAA QITMCPHVIV DVRQLEPINL PMPDVRNNFF HYNQGSDSRL RLIAMLYTPL RANNSGD..D VFTVSCRVLT RPSPDFSFNF LVPPTVESKT KPFTLPILTI
HV         GKLVFAAIPP HFPLENLSPG QITMFPHVII DVRTLEPVLL PLPDVRNNFF HYNQQPEPRM RLVAMLYTPL RSNGSGD..D VFTVSCRVLT RPSPDFDFNY LVPPTVESKT KPFTLPILTI
BV         GKVIFAAVPP NFPTEGLSPS QVTMFPHIIV DVRQLEPVLI PLPDVRNNFY HYNQANDSTL KLIAMLYTPL RANNAGD..D VFTVSCRVLT RPSPDFDFIF LVPPTVESRT KPFTVPVLTV
Consensus  -K------PP -F-------- Q-T--PH-I- DVR-L-P--- P--DVRN--- H-N------- -L--MLYTPL ---------D -F----RV-T -PS-DF-F-- LVP---E--T --F--P----
           --------PP ---------- -----PH--- D-R---P--- ---D-R---- H--------- -L-------- ---------- -------V-T -P--DF-F-- ---------- ----------

           239                                                                                                                        337
NV-8fIIa   SSLSNSRAPL PISSIGISPD NVQSVQFQNG RCTLDGRLVG TTPVSLSHVA KIRGT..... .....SNGTV .......... INLTELDGTP FHPFEG.PAP IGFPDLGGCD WHINMTQFGH
KY-89      SSLSNSRAPL PISGMGISPD NVQSVQFQNG RCTLDGRLVG TTPVSLSHVA KIRGT..... ...SN..GTV .......... INLTELDGTP FHPFEG.PAP IGFPDLGGCD WHINMTQFGH
SHV        QTLSNSRFPS LIQGMILSPD ASQVVQFQNG RCLIDGQLLG TTPATSGQLF RVRGK..... ...INQGART .......... LNLTEVDGKP FMAFDS.PAP VGFPDFGKCD WHMRISKTPN
DSV        NTLSNSRVPS LINAMMISRD HGQMVQFQNG RVTLDGQLQG TTPTSLSQLC KIRGKVFHAS GGNG...... .......... LNLTELDGSA YHAFES.PAP IGFPDIGDCD WHMSATATNN
OTH-25     SEMSNSRFPV PIDSLHTSPT ESIVVQCQNG RVTLDGELMG TTQLLPNQIC AFRGTLTRST NRASDQADTA TPRLFNHHWH IQLDNLNGTP YDPAEDIPAP LGTPDFRGKV FGVA...GQR
TV         SEMSNSRFPV PIDSLHTSPT ENIVVQCQNG RVTLDGELMG TTQLLPSQIC AFRGTLTRST SRASDQADTP TPRLFNYYWH IQLDNLNGTP YDPAEDIPAP LGTPDFRGKV FGVA...SQR
HV         GELSNSRFPV PIDELYTSPN EGVIVQPQNG RSTLDGELLG TTQLVPSNIC ALRG...RIN AQVPDD.... .....HHQWN LQVTNTNGTP FDPTEDVPAP LGTPDFLANI YGVT...SQR
BV         EEMSNSRFPI PLEKLYTGPS SAFVVQPQNG RCTTDGVLLG TTQLSAVNIC NFRGDVTHIA G......... .....SHDYT MNLASQNWSN YDPTEEIPAP LGTPDFVGKI QGLLTQTTR.
Consensus  ---SNSR-P- ---------- ----VQ-QNG R---DG-L-G TT-------- --RG------ ---------- ---------- ---------- -------PAP -G-PD----- ----------
           ---------- ---------- ---------- R--------- T--------- ---------- ---------- ---------- ---------- ---------- ---------- ----------

                                                                      Region 2
           338                                                                                                                        440
NV-8fIIa   SSQTQ..... YDVDTTPDTF VPHLGSIQA. ....NGI... GSGNYVGVLS WISPPSHPSG SQVDLWKIPN YGSSITEATH LAPSVYPPGF GEVLVFFMSK MPGP....GA YNLPCLLPQE
KY-89      SSQTQ..... YDVDTTPDTS VPHLGSIQA. ....NGI... GSGNYIGVLS WVSPPSHPSG SQVDLWKIPN YGSSITEATH LAPSVYSPGF GEVLVFFMSK IPGP....GG DSLPCLLPQG
SHV        NTGSGDPMRS VSVQTNVQGF VPHLGSIQF. ....DEVFNH PTGDYIGTIE WISQPSTPPG TDINLWEIPD YGSSLSQAAN LAPPVFPPGF GEALVYFVSA FPGPNNRSAP NDVPCLLPQE
DSV        FTGSSNEYQI LIKQES..AF APHLGHVQA. ....DNLSAG ANTDLIVSLS WISPVSDQHR HDVDPWVIPR YGSSLTEAAQ LAPPIYPPGF GEAIVFFMSD FPVVSGVNGM .RIPCTLPQE
OTH-25     NPDSTTRAHE AKVDTTSGRF TPKLGSLEIT T.ESDDFDPN QSTKFTPVG. ..I..GVDNE ADFQQWSLPD YSGQFTHNMN LAPAVAPNFP GEQLLFFRSQ LPSSGGRSNG I.LDCLVPQE
TV         NPDSTTRAHE AKVDTTSGRF TPKLGSLEIT T.ESDDFDPN QPTKFTPVG. ..V..GVDNE AEFQQWSLPN YSGQFTHNMN LAPAVAPNFP GEQLLFFRSQ LPSSGGRSNG V.LDCLVPQE
HV         NPNNTCRAHD GVLATWSPKF TPKLGSVILG TWEESDLDLN QPTRFTPVG. .LF..NTDH. ..FDQWALPS YSGRLTLNMN LAPSVSPLFP LEQLLFFRSH IPLKGGTSDG A.IDCLLPQE
BV         .ADGSTRAHK ATVSTGSVHF TPKLGSVQFT TDTNNDFQAG QNTKFTPVG. .VIQDGDHHQ NEPQQWLLPN YSGRTGHNVH LAPAVAPTFP GEQLLFFRST MPGCSGYPN. MNLDCLLPQE
Consensus  ---------- ---------- -P-LG----- ---------- ---------- ---------- -----W--P- Y--------- LAP------- -E----F-S- -P-------- ----C--PQ-
           ---------- ---------- ---------- ---------- ---------- ---------- ---------- ---------- ---------- ---------- -P-------- ----------

                                                                      Region 3
           441                                                                                530
NV-8fIIa   YISHLASEQA PTVGEAALLH YVDPDTGRNL GEFKAYPDGF LTCVPNGASS GPQQLPINGV FVFVSWVSRF YQLKPVGTAS SARGRLGLRR
KY-89      YISHLASEQA PTVGEGPLLH YVDPDTDRNL GEFKAYPDGF LTCVPNGASS GPQQLPINGV FVFVSWVSRF YQLKPVGTAS TARGRLGLRR   530
SHV        YITHFVSEQA PTMGDAALLH YVDPDTNRNL GEFKLYPGGY LTCVPNGVGA GPQQLPLNGV FLFVSWVSRF YQLKPVGTAS TARGRLGVRR I 546
DSV        YVAHFVNEQA PTRGEAALLH YVDPDTHRNL GEFKMYPEGF MTCVPNSSGS GPQTLPINGV FTFVSWVSRF YQLKPVGTAG PAR.RLGIRR S 545
OTH-25     WVQHFYQESA PAQTQVALVR YVNPDTGRVL FEAKLHKLGF MTIAKNGDS. .PITVPPNGY FRFESWVNPF YTLAPMGTGN .GRRRIQ...   548
TV         WVQHFYQESA PAQTQVALVR YVNPDTGRVL FEAKLHKLGF MTIAKNGDS. .PITVPPNGY FRFESWVNPF YTLAPMGTGN .GRRRIQ ..   549
HV         WIQHFYQESA PAATDVALIR YTNPDTGRVL FEAKLHRQGF ITVANSGSR. .PIVVPPNGY FRFDSWVNQF YSLAPMGTGN .GRRRVQ ..   536
BV         WVLHFYQEAA PAQSDVALLR FVNPDTGRVL FECKLHKSGY ITVAHTGP.. YDLVLPPNGY FRFDSWVNQF YTLAPMGNGT GRRRAL ...   540
Consensus  ---H---E-A P------L-- ---PDT-R-L -E-K----G- -T-------- -----P-NG- F-F-SWV--F Y-L-P-G--- --R------- --
           ---------- ---------- ---------- ---------- ---------- ---------- ---------- ---------- ---------- --
```

sizes of VP1 and the VP2 are distinctly different among these different caliciviruses.

The first characterization of the calicivirus genome included identification of sequence motifs in ORF1 with similarity to those in the nonstructural protein-coding region of the picornaviruses (58). These conserved motifs include an nucleoside 5′-triphosphate (NTP)-binding motif (putative 2C-like helicase), 3C-like protease, and 3D-like RNA-dependent RNA polymerase (RdRp). Enzymatic activity has been shown experimentally for the HuCV protease (18) and nucleoside triphosphatase (NTPase) (59), and RdRp activity was reported for RHDV and FCV (60,61). Interestingly, the most efficient RdRp activity of the FCV was exhibited by a large precursor protein that contained both protease and polymerase domains (61).

ORF1 encodes additional proteins, some with as yet unknown function. The actual number of fully processed nonstructural proteins encoded by ORF1 remains unclear, and at least for the HuCV, awaits a cell culture system. Translation of *in vitro* transcribed SV RNA in rabbit reticulocyte lysates resulted in ORF1 being processed into three major proteins with apparent molecular weights of 113,000, 48,000, and 41,000 (18). Site-directed mutagenesis and immunoprecipitation showed the 113-K protein (p113) contained protease and polymerase domains, p41 was the NTPase, and p48 represented the N-terminal 398 amino acids. VPg has been mapped in the FCV (57), RHDV (62), and the primate calicivirus Pan-1 genomes (63), and amino acid sequence comparisons suggest a similar location in HuCV (aa 963 to 1,100). Additional processing sites that represented release of the protease domain were subsequently found when portions of ORF-1 were expressed in bacteria. Expression of ORF-1 of the Camberwell virus (CV) in COS cells confirmed these additional processing sites (17).

The protease is the best characterized of the calicivirus nonstructural proteins. The composition and spacing of the catalytic residues and cleavage site specificities show that the calicivirus protease is similar to the picornavirus 3C protease ($3C^{pro}$). Enzymatic activity and cleavage site specificities of the calicivirus 3C-like protease ($3CL^{pro}$) of HuCV and animal caliciviruses RHDV and FCV have been reported (18,64–66). Analysis of data from these studies suggests that like the picornaviruses, the calicivirus $3CL^{pro}$ and its substrate recognition preferences differ somewhat between viruses belonging to different genera. The kinetics of proteolytic processing by the calicivirus protease and potential hierarchal regulation of proteolysis are important to understand, because viral proteases present a clear target for development of antiviral compounds. A map of the RHDV polyprotein discerned by transient expression of cDNA constructs has been proposed and closely resembles that of the P2/P3 region of the poliovirus polyprotein (62,67). This and other polyprotein maps await confirmation in an infectious system, because it is difficult to extrapolate the complex regulatory controls likely to occur in the context of an authentic virus infection.

A description of the replication strategy remains speculative for HuCV because of the lack of a cell culture model to study basic steps in virus entry and uncoating protein synthesis, RNA replication and packaging, and virus maturation and egress. A few predictions can be made based on genome homology with other RNA viruses and animal caliciviruses for which mechanisms of replication have been described. These predictions and the supporting data, though limited, are summarized in the following paragraphs.

The organization of the ORF1 polyprotein and the presence of a protease that cleaves co-translationally to generate nonstructural proteins are similar to the genome expression strategy exhibited by other positive strand RNA viruses. Proteolytic processing affords these viruses a mechanism to regulate gene expression where transcriptional control is not possible or is limited to synthesis of subgenomic mRNA. It has been shown experimentally that animal calicivirus strains make at least one major species of subgenomic RNA during virus replication (68). Thus, the strategy of calicivirus genome expression resembles that of the alphaviruses that employ both proteolytic processing of large

FIGURE 56.3. Alignment comparing the deduced amino acid sequences of the capsid protein of Norwalk virus (NV) and other human caliciviruses. This alignment compares the capsid sequence of NV, OTH-25, a virus similar to Snow Mountain agent (87), Toronto virus, Hawaii virus, Bristol virus, Southampton virus, and Desert Shield virus. Alignment of these sequences was obtained using the GAP and PILEUP programs of GCG. The two bottom lines show consensus sequences; *dots* correspond to a deletion or insertion; *dashes* indicate the absence of consensus. The first line of the consensus sequence represents consensus amino acids among human caliciviruses. The second line of the consensus shows consensus amino acids among these human caliciviruses and animal caliciviruses including feline calicivirus, rabbit hemorrhagic disease virus, and San Miguel sea lion virus type 1 and type 4. The numbers shown correspond to the amino acid sequence number of the NV capsid protein, which is shown first because it is the prototype virus. The highly conserved region of animal caliciviruses would span aa 1 to 280 (region 1). Regions C to E, which were characterized as variable, would correspond to aa 281 to 404 (region 2), and the conserved C-terminal domains would correspond to aa 405 to 530 (region 3). The conserved PPG similar to that in viral protein 3 of picornaviruses is highlighted by a *bar,* the cleavage site detected for NV in insect cells is shown by an *arrow,* and one conserved cysteine is highlighted by an *asterisk.*

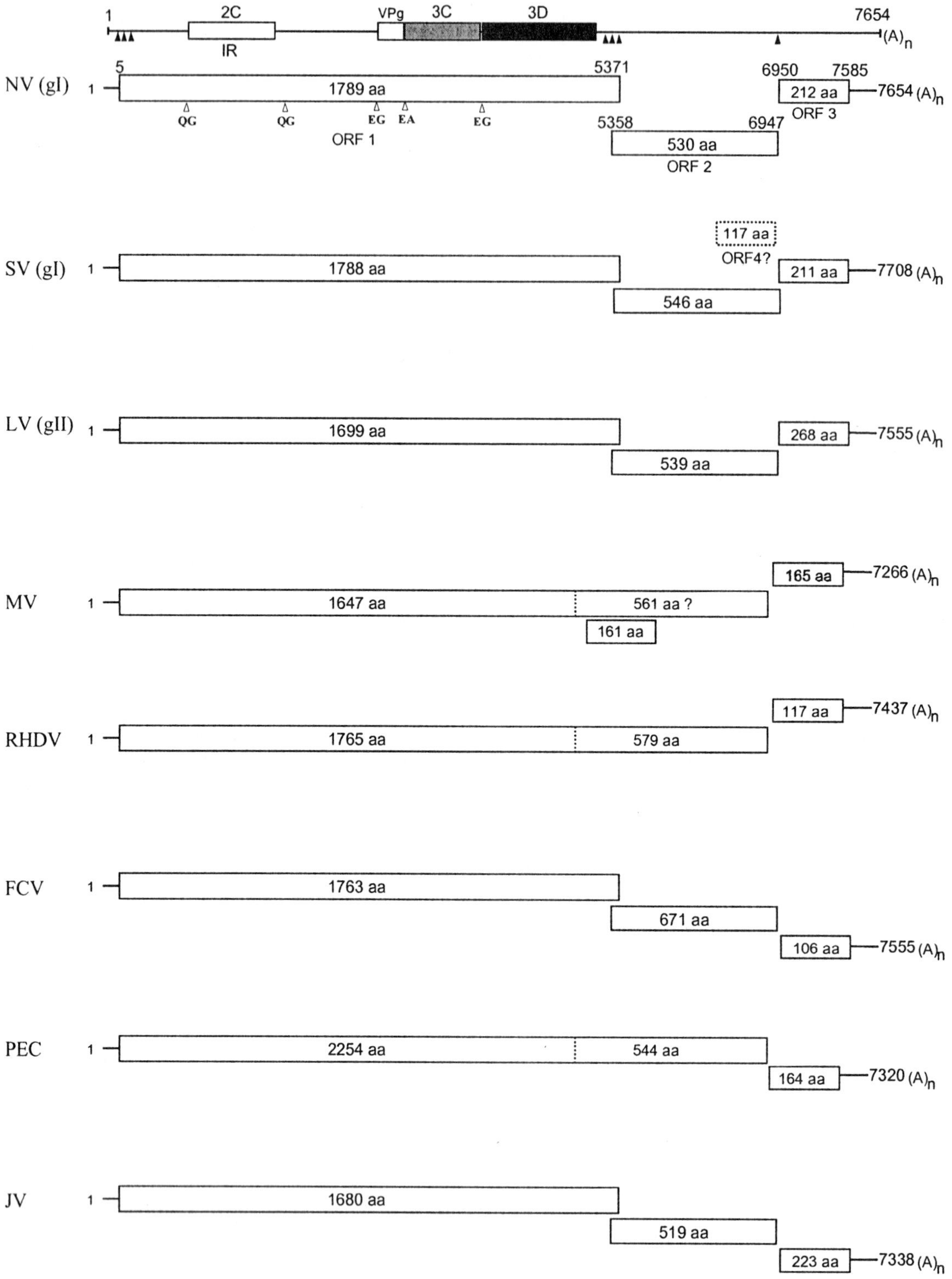

FIGURE 56.4. Genomic organization of Norwalk virus and other caliciviruses. Predicted open reading frames (ORFs) include ORF1, a polyprotein that contains the nucleoside triphosphatase, 3C-like protease, and the 3D RNA-dependent RNA polymerase. ORF2 encodes viral protein 1 (VP1) of the Norwalk-like virus (NLV), bovine NLV-like Jena virus (JV), and feline calicivirus (FCV); and ORF3 that codes for VP2 in the NLV, JV, and FCV. In the Sapporo-like viruses, porcine enteric calicivirus, and rabbit hemorrhagic disease virus, VP1 is contiguous with the polyprotein in ORF-1 and VP2 is encoded in the 3′ terminal ORF2. A fourth ORF is predicted for Southampton virus and Manchester virus. Locations of the AUG *(arrowheads)* initiation codons, and *IR* denotes an immunoreactive region in ORF1 of NV reported by Matsui et al. (187).

polyprotein and synthesis of a subgenomic RNA. Molecular details of HuCV RNA replication and packaging await the establishment of a cell culture system or an *in vitro* replication model.

The exact site of NLV replication in the intestine is not known. Early studies suggested that NV replicated in the mature enterocytes in the villus tips of the proximal small intestine (69–71). Jejunal biopsies from infected volunteers showed that symptomatic illness correlated with broadening and blunting of the villi and crypt cell hyperplasia. These observations provided strong suggestive evidence that NLVs have an enteric tropism that may be restricted to the proximal small intestine. To date, cultured cell lines, even those human in origin, have not supported NLV replication in the laboratory. The reasons for the failure to establish suitable *in vitro* culture media for NLV are not clear, but it is most likely that conditions that mimic the complex natural intestinal environment are important for a productive replication cycle, and these conditions have not been successfully reproduced in culture. Although there currently is no cell line that supports a complete NLV replication cycle, early events such as binding and internalization have been explored using available intestinal cell lines and baculovirus expressed VLPs. Binding of rNV capsids to cells in culture has been used to study virus–receptor interactions (72). rNV particles purified from insect cell cultures bind to a number of cell lines from various tissues of human and animal origin. The particles bind specifically to a saturable number of molecules on the surfaces of all cell lines tested. The highest binding percentage (about 20%) occurs with the human colon carcinoma cell line Caco-2, whereas cell lines from other species and tissue sources show binding percentages of 5% or less. Three human intestinal cell lines also bind rNV inefficiently, at less than 5%. Although 20% binding efficiency is low, the binding affinities of 10^8 to 10^9 M^{-1} are within the range for virus–receptor interactions (73). It is not known if 20% binding is all that is necessary for a productive infection or if the cell types examined do not express the appropriate receptor. A second study on VLP binding to cells in culture reported identification of a 105-kd cellular protein present in membrane fractions of six mammalian cell lines including Caco-2s that bound serologically distinct VLPs (74). The significance of these data is not clear in light of the fact that there is no way to test the functionality of this putative attachment molecule.

The ability of several sources of antibodies to block binding also was investigated for rNV particles (72). One monoclonal antibody (MAB) (75) of 10 tested blocks binding of rNV to Caco-2 cells. The precise domain of the capsid recognized by this MAB is not known, but peptides synthesized to the predicted regions of the capsid were unable to compete with rNV for binding. Reactivity with deletion mutants of the capsid protein mapped the putative virus attachment site to a conformational epitope between amino acids 300 and 384. Several polyclonal sera also were tested in the binding assays. Interestingly, serum from rabbits, guinea pigs, and mice that were hyperimmunized with rNV, as well as convalescent human serum from infected volunteers, was unable to block binding, suggesting that perhaps the most immunodominant epitopes of the NV capsid are nonneutralizing.

The PEC is currently the only enteric calicivirus that can be grown in cell culture (76). Propagation of the PEC requires addition of intestinal contents from uninfected gnotobiotic piglets, and this requirement is not alleviated on continued passage of the virus. The biologic basis of the necessity for intestinal contents is not known, but it is tempting to speculate that some factor in the intestinal contents (e.g., cytokine and growth factor) results in a physiologic alteration in the cells that renders them permissive for infection. The genome of PEC has been cloned and sequenced and is most closely related based on phylogenetic grouping to the SLV (22). Comparison of the sequence of the wild-type PEC (Cowden strain) with that of the tissue culture-adapted strain showed a total of eight nucleotide differences. Three of the nucleotide changes were silent. Two amino acid changes were located in the RdRp and three amino acids changes in VP1. These amino acid changes are located in the hypervariable region of VP1 and lead to a higher predicted localized hydrophilicity. Intriguingly, this region corresponds to a similar region of the NV VP1 shown to be important in cell binding, as described above. It will be interesting to analyze the cell binding characteristics of recombinant capsids bearing these substitutions and to investigate the effects of these substitutions on infectivity, once infectious clones for PEC are available.

Three double-stem RNA loops are predicted in the 5′ and of the genomic RNA (nucleotide [nt] 32 to 110) and upstream of ORF2 (nt 5,280 to 5,356) and ORF3 (nt 6,848 to 6,941) in the NV genome (39). These structures may be important not only for synthesis of viral genomic but also for subgenomic RNA replication. A consensus sequence also is located at the 5′ end of the viral genome and upstream of ORF2 (nt 5,300 to 5,369), and may be a packaging signal for genomic and subgenomic RNA (49). A recent study analyzed binding of cellular proteins to the 5′ about 200 nucleotides that included the double-stem RNA loop structure and showed specific binding of La, PCBP-2, PTB, and hnRNP L (77). These cellular proteins are known to be important in directing internal ribosome entry site (IRES)-mediated translation of poliovirus RNA. Although still lacking functional analyses, these RNA binding data have implications in predicting how the NLV genome may be translated. The first in-context initiation codon begins at nucleotide 11. Studies on translation initiation on eukaryotic mRNA suggest that shorter 5′ noncoding regions translate inefficiently, and AUG codons so near the 5′ terminus may be ignored by the ribosome (78). The next in-frame in-context AUG codon of NV is at nucleotide 158. An IRES this short has not been described, so it is possible that the caliciviruses utilize a novel mechanism of translation initiation. Competition with the cap analogue 7-methyl-guonosine triphosphate had no effect on translation of FCV RNA *in vitro,* suggesting a cap-independent mechanism of initiation (79). Furthermore, treatment of FCV RNA isolated from infected cells with proteinase K abolished the ability of the RNA to program translation *in vitro.* These data suggest that VPg plays a role in translation of calicivirus RNA, perhaps as a cap analogue that binds translation initiation factors. The functional interactions of VPg with the cellular translational apparatus remain to be experimentally demonstrated.

The small 3′ terminal protein VP2 is the most variable in sequence in the calicivirus genome (80,81). VP2 ranges from 208 to 268 amino acids in length in the HuCV, with calculated molecular weights ranging from 23 to 29 K. VP2 of FCV and RHDV are smaller at approximately 10 and 12 K, respectively. VP2 is a basic protein recently identified as a minor structural protein in rNV particles, RHDV and FCV virions (43,57,62). The function of VP2 as a structural protein is unclear. VLPs assemble in the absence of VP2, so this protein is not necessary for assembly of empty capsids. As noted earlier, the NLV capsid is composed predominately of 180 copies of VP1, an unusual property among animal viruses, but common among plant viruses. A distinguishing difference however is the presence of an N-terminal basic domain in the plant virus capsid proteins that is thought to bind RNA. The NLV VP1 lacks this domain. Thus, it has been proposed that perhaps VP2 binds viral RNA and plays a role in genome encapsidation. RNA binding studies with VP2 have not been reported for the caliciviruses. Preliminary studies using mutants of the FCV infectious cDNA clone have suggested that VP2 is necessary for virus replication but the precise role of VP2 in the replication cycle has not been elucidated (57).

GENETIC AND ANTIGENIC VARIABILITY OF THE NLV

The availability of the NV sequence opened a new era in the characterization of NLVs, including many agents previously characterized as SRSVs. The initial sequencing of the NV and SV genomes allowed primers to be selected that would amplify similar and more genetically diverse agents. New methods were developed to reduce the presence of PCR inhibitors in stool, allowing detection and characterization of the small amounts of nucleic acid that are typical in HuCV samples. These advances resulted in sequence analysis of numerous HuCV during the past decade (40,47,82–93). Most studies characterized a portion of the viral genome in the RNA polymerase region because this region of the genome was the first published and was expected to be conserved; consistent with this idea, many viruses could be amplified with primers designed based on the NV polymerase sequence. Because the original description of primers that successfully amplified NLV, many primers to regions of the genome, including capsid sequences and NTPase sequences, have been used to detect genetically diverse viruses. Previously well-characterized NLVs (Snow Mountain agent [SMA] [26,94] and Hawaii agent [HV] [27]) were amplified and sequenced and their relatedness to NV was determined (83,87). These studies were important because they provided a foundation for genetic comparisons based on previous antigenic relationships defined either by human volunteer cross-challenge studies or IEM, using well-characterized sera from human volunteer studies. HV had previously been shown to be distinct from NV based on the findings that human volunteers initially challenged with NV were not protected from subsequent challenge with HV. These distinct serologic differences were confirmed by IEM studies (27). In addition, SMA was characterized as antigenically distinct from NV and HV based on IEM. Comparisons of the sequences of these viruses showed initially that NV and SMA represented the two genogroups I and II. Analysis of HV showed this virus was also genogroup II; this result was unexpected because it had been assumed that SMA and HV were distinct viruses based on previous IEM data. These observations highlight the difficulties in correlating genetic and antigenic relationships.

A number of important questions related to the classification, genetic relatedness, detection ability, molecular epidemiology, and evolution of the NLVs have been addressed by such molecular assays and subsequent sequence and phylogenetic analyses (10–12,95). The most recent studies describe the diversity of the HuCV (7,96). Previous analysis suggested that within a genogroup, the aa similarity between two different strains ranged from 80% to 96% for the polymerase region and from 77% to 98% for the capsid region. A recent comprehensive analysis of genetic diversity in all three ORFs of NLV shows that extensive genetic variation exists even within genogroups, and phylogenetic grouping is the same whether nucleotide or amino acid sequences are used in the comparisons (96). Genetic relationships within ORF-2 are most robust and show good correlation with eight antigenic types defined by solid phase (SPIEM). A good correlation between clustering of NLV strains based on sequence analysis of the 5′ end of ORF-2 and patient immune responses also is found if distinct NLV capsid types are defined by more than 80% nucleotide sequence identity (7). Likewise, Green et al. (7) suggested more than 20% amino acid divergence in the complete capsid protein may represent antigenically distinct capsid types. These types of studies are important in classifying the NLV because it currently is not possible to perform virus neutralization assays that serve as the gold standard for defining antigenic relationships among virus isolates.

Sequence analysis of NV and other morphologically typical human and animal caliciviruses is beginning to unravel the genetic relationships between these viruses. Sequence analysis of the polymerase region initially was done on a limited number (three) of morphologically typical HuCVs all previously characterized by EM and obtained from infants and young children; the sequences of these viruses were found to be closely related to SMA and clustered in genogroup II (88). Thus, at least some morphologically typical HuCVs are genetically related to SMA. It was a great surprise when a previously uncharacterized agent, called minireovirus or Toronto virus (TV) found in stool samples from children hospitalized in Toronto, was studied and also shown to be an HuCV with a polymerase sequence similar to that of SMA (47). If these HuCVs also prove to be antigenically similar to SMA, then physical or chemical factors must be the reason for the morphologic differences between viruses previously called HuCVs and SRSVs. This would not be surprising because it is known that other caliciviruses—that is, VESV (97), and amyelosis chronic stunt virus (98)—are degraded by adverse physical conditions and/or proteolytic enzymes.

Different results have recently been obtained from the study of other morphologically typical HuCVs. Analysis of the predicted sequence of the polymerase region of the HuCV prototype Sapporo virus and of other antigenically uncharacterized viruses with typical calicivirus morphology has indicated that these viruses are more closely related to feline caliciviruses (89,90). The significance of this finding remains unknown, and it may simply indicate that some HuCVs have evolved from animal caliciviruses. The sequence similarity observed in the short regions of genome studied is not extremely high (less than 40%) when compared to the limited number of FCV sequences currently available. Therefore, it is not possible with our current knowledge to know whether direct transmission of virus from cats to humans occurred sometime in the past, followed by virus mutation as it became adapted to growth in humans. It is of interest that transmission of animal caliciviruses to humans has been suggested previously (99,100), and transmission of caliciviruses likely occurs among animals (101,102). Transmission of viruses among animals is supported by recent sequence analyses that have shown that several SMSV serotypes, VESV, and a newly isolated skunk calicivirus appear to be closely related (101). These results raise interesting epidemiologic and evolutionary questions that will need to be answered in future studies.

Some of the new sequence studies included a preliminary analysis of whether these RNA viruses undergo rapid mutation, resulting in continual appearance of new serotypes. This question was addressed by determining whether currently circulating viruses are very similar to the prototype NV, SMA, and HV. Comparisons of the sequences of viruses found to have similar antigenic reactivity, but isolated at different times and geographic locations, indicate that the amino acid sequences are not rapidly changing. Recombination between calicivirus strains has recently been reported and may contribute to the overall genetic diversity of the HuCV (96,103,104). So far, the evidence for recombination is only for that between HuCV. It will be of interest to determine if recombination between cultivable animal caliciviruses and the HuCV is possible, and if such a system can be exploited to study the replication cycle of the HuCV.

Viruses with very similar sequences to prototype NV have been found. Thus, a virus (HuCV/KY-89/89/J) was found to be antigenically similar to prototype NV based on its reactivity in an enzyme-linked immunosorbent assay (ELISA) that uses polyclonal antibody to the baculovirus-expressed rNV, but this virus was isolated 21 years later in Japan (105). Sequence analysis of KY-89 and comparison with NV showed 87.2% nt similarity over 2,516 continuous nucleotides amounting to 96% to 98% amino acid similarity in two ORFs (87). Distinct strains related to SMA but isolated 13 to 16 years later in Japan or the United Kingdom also have shown 80% nucleotide and 88% to 92% amino acid similarity to the prototype strain. Thus, viruses antigenically similar to the prototype viruses are still circulating, and these have been found to show relatively good conservation of amino acid sequences over long periods of time. Although variable regions in the capsid protein have been identified, it is noteworthy that these did not change more dramatically within a specific antigenic virus type than did other regions of the genome. A larger sequence database over larger regions of the genome is needed to permit extensive analysis of the evolutionary relationships of these viruses.

A number of the viruses whose sequences have been characterized were initially identified as NV based on the NV ELISA with convalescent serum from volunteers. A subset also has been tested by the new NV ELISA that uses hyperimmune antiserum made to the baculovirus-expressed rNV particles. Unexpectedly, only some of the viruses positive by the human reagent ELISA also were positive by the rNV antigen ELISA. Sequence analysis of the strains showing different reactivities in each test was performed to determine the basis for this different reactivity. The results showed that viruses that were positive in both the human and the rNV antigen ELISA were genetically very similar to the prototype NV within the polymerase region, with similarities ranging from between 80% to 87% nt and 89% to 99% amino acid, respectively. In contrast, viruses that were positive in the human ELISA but negative in the rNV antigen test showed polymerase similarities with prototype NV of 71% to 75% nucleotide and 82% to 87% amino acid, respectively (summarized in reference 106). Because the rNV ELISA only detects the capsid protein, these results indicate either (a) there are other proteins in stool samples that are cross-reactive with human convalescent serum or (b) human convalescent serum contains antibodies that detect a different form of the capsid protein that contains more cross-reactive epitopes, whereas the hyperimmune antiserum made to rNV particles is highly specific for conformationally specific epitopes on virus particles. Production of MABs to the distinct regions of the capsid protein may help distinguish between these possibilities.

DIAGNOSTIC ASSAYS

It is not possible to make a specific diagnosis of infection with the NLV group on the sole basis of clinical findings. However, a provisional diagnosis of infection during outbreaks of gastroenteritis is possible if the following criteria are met: (a) absence of bacterial or parasitic pathogens, (b) vomiting in more than 50% of cases, (c) duration of illness (mean or median ranges) from 12 to 60 hours, and (d) an incubation period of 24 to 48 hours. These criteria were met in 81% to 100% of ill individuals in 38 NLV outbreaks (107) and have been used successfully in several epidemiologic studies. A definitive diagnosis desirable for both clinical and epidemiologic studies requires the availability of detection methods for viral nucleic acid, viral antigen, or antibody responses. Previous and current epidemiologic studies rely on detection of infection based on available diagnostic assays, and first-generation and current diagnostic assays have recently been reviewed (108). Below is a synopsis of the methods currently in use to detect NLVs (Fig. 56.5).

The inability to grow the NLVs in cell culture, the expectedly high sequence variability of the genome, and the low numbers of particles in stools from infected individuals continue to present challenges for detecting virus. However, cloning, sequencing, and expression of the NV capsid protein permitted a number of new assays to be developed that

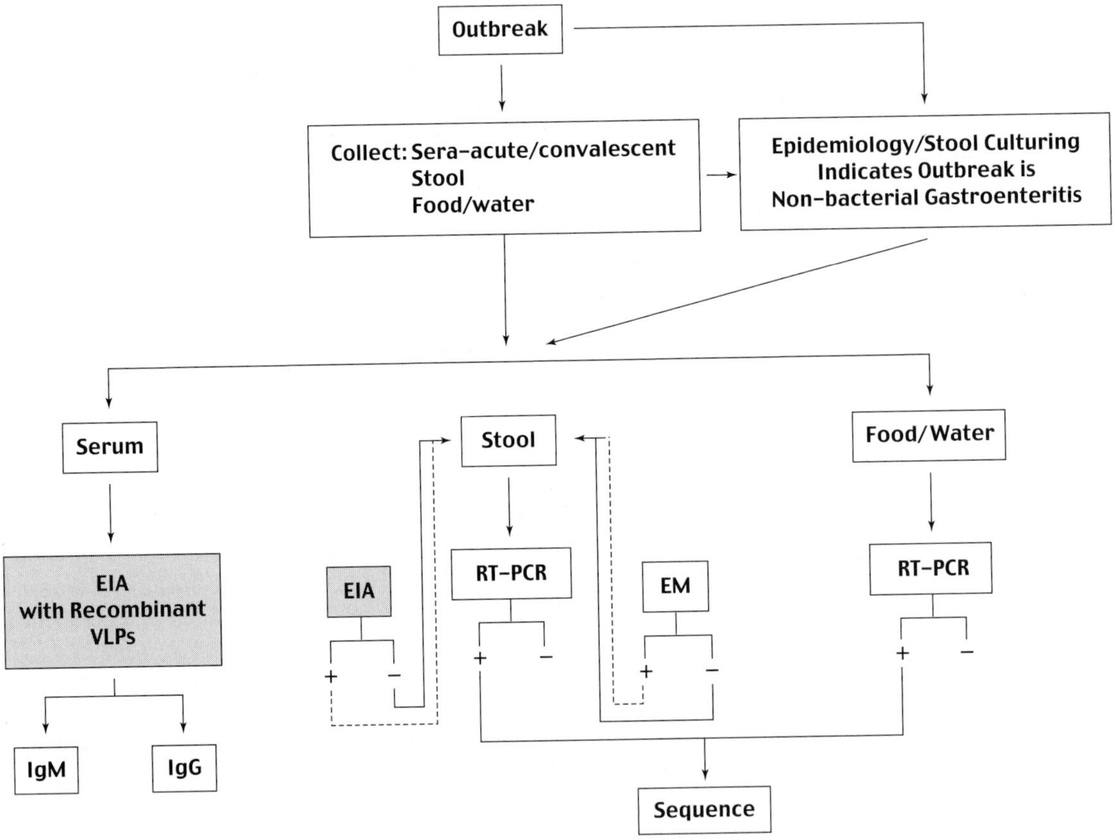

FIGURE 56.5. Schematic of approaches to determine if an outbreak of gastroenteritis is caused by a human calicivirus. After an outbreak, clinical samples (serum and stool) and possible vehicles of transmission (food/water) are collected for analysis. These can be tested directly for bacterial pathogens, and if the results are negative, then they are tested for viruses or they can be tested for viruses directly if the epidemiologic and/or clinical data suggest nonbacterial gastroenteritis. Stool samples can be evaluated by electron microscopy and reverse transcriptase polymerase chain reaction (RT-PCR) for virus, and enzyme immunoassays for human calicivirus detection can currently be performed in selected research laboratories. RT-PCR can be performed on the potential vehicles of transmission and if amplicons are found, sequence analysis can be used to compare with sequence obtained from stools. Antibody responses can also be used in selected research laboratories to confirm infection; immunoglobulin G responses require paired sera while immunoglobulin M are performed on single serum sample. (Modified from Atmar RL, Estes MK. Diagnosis of noncultivatable gastroenteritis viruses, the human caliciviruses. *Clin Microbiol Rev* 2001;14:15–37, with permission. Details for collecting specimens are given in Parashar et al. [114].)

quickly replaced the first-generation assays that used reagents from volunteers (108). The new assays for virus detection include reverse transcriptase polymerase chain reaction (RT-PCR) to detect the viral genome and new ELISAs to detect both antibody responses and viral antigen. The usefulness of each of these assays to detect infections with specific viruses is summarized briefly here (Fig. 56.5).

The most used molecular assays developed to detect NLVs are based on detection of the viral genome. Nucleic acid hybridization assays and RT-PCR assays to amplify the small amount of nucleic acid found in many stools are about as sensitive as previous radioimmune assays (RIAs) to detect virus in stools of volunteers and in oysters seeded with NV (85,106,109–112). Two key points must be considered for the success of using RT-PCR as a routine diagnostic method. First, the availability of universal primers to detect all HuCVs facilitates their use in diagnostic settings. Second, the exquisite sensitivity of these assays is both an asset and a problem because extreme caution must be taken to ensure that any results obtained are not false positives caused by contamination within a laboratory. The use of primers initially developed to detect the polymerase region of the NV genome proved useful for obtaining amplification and subsequent sequence information of a broad range of HuCVs (106). These results and the sequence data obtained from a relatively large number of studies indicate that it is not possible to select a single set of primer pairs that will detect a broad range of viruses. Instead, investigators use either (a) several sets of primer pairs that detect the polymerase region, as well as the capsid region, of viruses in the distinct genogroups, or (b) degenerate primers to detect most enteric caliciviruses. Use of several primer sets now detects about 80% of viruses in samples from outbreaks (96,106,113). Guidelines for data and sample collection for outbreak analysis have been published (108,114).

ELISAs to detect virus antigen and antibody responses also have been developed to detect NV. These assays were developed after the successful expression and self-assembly of the NV capsid protein into stable VLPs. The rNV particles were first used to develop an ELISA to detect antibody responses, and in this assay, rNV particles are used to coat the wells of microtiter plates (42). Initially, this assay was developed and validated using samples from human volunteers and well-characterized samples tested with previous assays (15,115,116). These studies showed that the rNV ELISA to detect antibody is as specific, sensitive, and efficient as previously described methods for detecting NV infection, and often more sensitive. The increased test sensitivity can be attributed to the very low assay background, which enables serum lacking antibody or containing very low levels of antibody to be detected, and these test results can easily be documented by use of the readily available rNV antigen for antibody absorption (115). In addition, higher antibody titers are obtained using the rNV antibody ELISA (15). The rNV antibody assay also has been shown to be broadly reactive in that it is able to detect seroresponses in volunteers given NV, HV, or SMA, although the highest increases in antibody titer are in NV-infected individuals (116). This assay has already been used in several small and large-scale epidemiologic studies (15,117–119).

The rNV particles also were used to produce the first hyperimmune antiserum to NV, and antiserum produced in guinea pigs, mice, and rabbits contains high titer antibodies to the immunogen and native NV in stool (42, 15,115). These results show that the previous lack of success of producing high titer antiserum was not due to any inherent poor antigenicity of NV, but to the paucity of pure antigen. The hyperimmune antiserum was subsequently used to develop an antigen ELISA, which has been shown to be a highly sensitive and specific assay for NV antigen and closely related virus strains (106,115). The test sensitivity of the standard antigen ELISA was determined to be 1.4×10^6 virions without using any enhanced methods of signal amplification, and antigen was detected in the stools of volunteers diluted as much as 1 : 10,000. Comparison of the sensitivity of the ELISA, RT-PCR, dot-blot hybridization, and RIA (using human volunteer reagents) to detect NV in stool showed that the sensitivity of the ELISA was similar to that of RT-PCR, and the ELISA was more sensitive than dot-blot hybridization and RIA. The rNV antigen ELISA can detect both virus particles and soluble protein, and the presence and detection of such large amounts of soluble protein in stools likely explain the comparable sensitivities of the ELISA and RT-PCR.

The relative simplicity of performing an ELISA theoretically makes it the assay of choice for virus detection. This asset currently is offset by the finding that the NV antigen ELISA is specific for NV and closely related NLVs, and many of the HuCVs do not react in this simple, sensitive, and specific assay. Similar results have been obtained for ELISAs made to other NLVs (reviewed in reference 108). Current efforts are seeking antibodies that detect common, cross-reactive epitopes on the capsids of NLVs and other HuCvs. An MAB-based ELISA that recognizes a common epitope on genogroup I NLVs has been developed (120). New MABs that recognize common epitopes on genogroup II NLVs, as well as cross-reactive epitopes on both genogroup I and genogroup II NLVs, and SLVs are now characterized (121). These new reagents offer promise that sensitive and broadly cross-reactive ELISAs will become available for the diagnosis, basic research, epidemiology, and environmental monitoring of all HuCVs.

ANTIBODY PREVALENCE AND INCIDENCE

Our knowledge of the epidemiology of NV and HuCV infections is changing rapidly. This is because the cloning and expression of the NLV genomes have permitted large-scale epidemiologic studies to be performed, and results from such studies are indicating that infection with NLVs is much more widespread than previously recognized. Here, we briefly review the previous understanding of NLV epidemiology, which has been reviewed extensively elsewhere (24,122), and summarize how some of this previous dogma is changing with results from new studies based on widespread use of more sensitive molecular assays.

NV antibody prevalence initially was studied using an RIA or immune adherence hemagglutination assay in relatively large studies (123–125). One classic study examined acquisition of antibody in the United States to NV or rotavirus, the virus known to cause severe life-threatening disease in young children (123). In this study, NV antibody was acquired gradually, beginning slowly in childhood and accelerating in adult years, so that 50% of adults possessed antibody by age 50 years. Similar observations have been made in the United Kingdom and Japan using rNV capsid antibody (118,126,127). This pattern of antibody acquisition was similar to that observed for hepatitis A in similar populations, and it contrasted with antibody acquisition to rotavirus, which occurs more rapidly, with 90% of children possessing rotavirus antibody by age 3 years (123). Other studies showed the rate of antibody acquisition varied between locations, with antibody acquisition occurring earlier in less developed countries (125). Thus, it was found that in countries such as Bangladesh and Ecuador, most people had antibody to NV by the age of 5 years, whereas in the United States and the former Yugoslavia, antibody acquisition occurs gradually over the first two decades of life (124,125,128–130). A recent study on the seroprevalence of NV antibody in isolated communities in the Amazon region using the new rNV antibody assay showed a range of antibody prevalence from 38% to 100% for different communities (131). In addition, children age 6 to 10 years had NV antibody levels similar to those of adults. Taken together, these data suggest that transmission occurs largely by the fecal-oral route and exposure risks decrease as sanitary conditions improve. However, this may not be the only route of NV transmission because some evidence suggests that certain hospital outbreaks may be due to airborne or fomite transmission (132,133).

The lack of detection of antibodies to NV in infants and young children in the United States and other developed countries (using the original antibody assays with reagents from human volunteers) suggested that this virus was not an important cause of severe infantile diarrhea. However, this role of NV and other related agents in diarrheal illness in infants or young children is being reevaluated. In a recent longitudinal study, infection with the NV detected by ELISA using the rNV antigen was observed in 49% of 154 infants and young children in Finland over almost 2 years (15,117). There are several explanations for the lack of detection of antibody in the earlier studies. First, the new rNV assay is more sensitive than the previous human reagent assays (15,115,116,134). In addition, the sensitivity of detecting low-avidity antibody after primary infections in young children remains unknown and it is not yet clear how well the rNV antibody assay will detect seroresponses in young children infected with antigenically distinct NLVs. Thus, similar assays based on the expression of antigens from viruses in the other genogroups need to be developed and compared for their respective abilities to detect responses in children infected with different NLVs or SLVs. It is known that the rNV assay is broadly reactive and it does detect antibody responses in adults who were infected with SMA or HV, but the magnitude of responses in individuals with heterologous infections generally was not as great as the responses seen in volunteers given NV (116). Responses to rNV antigen in children with heterologous NLV infections may be even weaker.

The discovery that the minireovirus (i.e., TV) is an HuCV most closely related to the SMA is one example that highlights the possible importance of HuCVs in causing more than mild diarrhea in young children (47). Minireoviruses originally were detected by EM and described as second to rotavirus in causing young children to be hospitalized for diarrheal illness in Toronto (135,136). TV originally was only able to be detected using EM and more recently by other molecular techniques such as RT-PCR. TV does not react in the new antigen ELISA that uses hyperimmune antiserum made to the rNV that detects NV and closely related viruses (47,106,115). This result illustrates that the hyperimmune antiserum made to the rNV is very specific, and detection of other virus types will require the development of similar antigen ELISAs using particles expressed from the other virus types, or the development of other assays that can detect more broadly reactive antigenic epitopes. The type specificity of the rNV antigen assay and the broader reactivity of the rNV antibody assay is reminiscent of the results obtained in the early studies using the first HuCV ELISA developed to detect the HuCV Sapporo strain (137,138).

Given the current new information concerning the relatedness between different HuCVs, it is clear that our understanding of the epidemiology of these infections is just beginning. Antibody prevalence data available to date based on previous and possibly even new assays appear to measure primarily group-reactive antibodies; therefore, we really have little idea of the relative importance of any given strain or serotype in different geographic locations. Because of the apparent broader reactivity of the rNV antibody assay, data with these new assays also may not provide serotype-specific information. However, further clarification of these issues is likely to come as the domains containing common and serotype-specific antigenic epitopes are characterized and as new tests are developed and used based on this more precise information.

IMPORTANCE OF THE ENTERIC CALICIVIRUSES IN CAUSING DISEASE

Norwalk and related viruses have been well documented as the major causes of epidemic gastroenteritis in both developed and developing countries. These viruses have been documented on all continents where they have been sought, and it is expected that they will be found worldwide, as have rotaviruses, once diagnostic assays are readily available. Because of the limited availability of diagnostic assays, our current understanding of the importance of NV disease comes primarily from studies from a few laboratories that have had access to these diagnostic reagents.

The application of the newer diagnostic tests has changed our understanding of the epidemiology of infections caused by the HuCVs, particularly the NLVs. NLVs are now recognized to be the principal cause of outbreaks of nonbacterial gastroenteritis, and new estimates suggest they are the most common cause of all food-borne illnesses (4,8,11). Before the development of new assays, NLVs were not thought to be a common cause of gastroenteritis in young children, but several recent studies have found NLVs to be second only to rotaviruses as a cause of viral gastroenteritis in young children, and seroprevalence studies suggest that infection in young children in developed countries is common (117,118,139,140). Although multiple strains may circulate within a community at one time, a single strain or strains within an antigenic cluster may predominate (12,120,141). In addition, the duration of virus shedding has been found to be longer than previously recognized (115), providing a potential explanation for the occurrence of food-borne outbreaks traced to postsymptomatic individuals (142,143). In many outbreaks, oysters are the vehicle of transmission. In fact, the largest outbreak of food-borne illness affecting more than 2,000 persons resulted from consumption of shellfish in Australia (144). Outbreaks have occurred in recreational camps, cruise ships, communities, hospitals, schools (elementary or college), nursing homes, and families, and they have been associated with contaminated drinking water, swimming water, consumption of uncooked or poorly cooked shellfish, ice, and bakery products (frosting), various types of salads (potato, fruit, tossed), and cold foods (celery, melon, vermicelli consommé, sandwiches, and cold cooked ham). Outbreaks have occurred year-round and have affected primarily young children (age 4 years and older) and adults.

The spectrum of infections is widened when one includes the outbreaks associated with SLVs. Infections with these viruses have been documented almost exclusively by EM and with a worldwide distribution in Europe, North America, Africa, Asia, and Australia (reviewed in reference 145). Infections with SLVs were first detected among infants with gastroenteritis (146), and such infections among infants and young children have been confirmed and extended to adults and the elderly; they have been associated with outbreaks in orphanages, day care centers, schools, and hospital wards. New studies in Finland and Japan have reported NLVs and SLVs to be common causes of viral gastroenteritis in children younger than 2 years and they were as prevalent as, or more prevalent than, group A rotaviruses; the NLVs caused more severe disease than SLVs (140,147).

Nosocomial infection with HuCV has been documented (135) and may be quite common, and asymptomatic infections can occur (148). The high rate of nosocomial infection in children in Toronto often was associated with immunocompromised children (135,136). Although NV has been found in the stools of HIV-positive patients, its role in the cause of gastroenteritis or infection in this group has not been reported to be greater than that in non-HIV-infected controls (149,150). Because of the discovery that the minireovirus in many immunocompromised children is an NLV, it may be worthwhile to reevaluate the role of these infections in other immunocompromised populations using the new assays.

The types of clinical manifestations caused by enteric animal caliciviruses are important to consider, because historically, comparative virology has shown that human viral infections ultimately are found to mimic previously described animal virus infections. The best studied animal calicivirus is FCV, which causes respiratory infections, conjunctivitis, pneumonia, vesicles, diarrhea, and possibly an arthritic-like limping disease in infected kittens (reviewed in reference 151). Infected cats may become persistently infected with virus remaining in the tonsils (152). These viruses are interesting because they appear to fall into one serotype with many variants that give one-way reactions in cross-neutralization assays (151,153). In spite of this, a vaccine composed of one serotype appears to provide broad protection. The marine caliciviruses (i.e., SMSVs) are of interest because they have a broader host range, and feeding of uncooked fish or pinniped containing caliciviruses to piglets resulted in epidemic outbreaks of VESV in pigs (reviewed in references 154 and 155). The clinical manifestations were indistinguishable from foot-and-mouth disease, including vesicles in the mouth, on the tongue, lips, and snout, and between the toes. In addition, VESV may cause encephalitis, myocarditis, fever, diarrhea, failure of infected animals to survive, and pregnant sows and sea lions to abort.

PECs cause diarrhea in pigs. This is one of the few enteric viruses successfully cultivated and is closely related genetically to SLV (156,157). Sugieda et al. (158) recently reported detection of NLV sequences in the cecum contents of healthy slaughtered pigs in Japan, but the role of these viruses as disease-causing agents is not known. The genomes of two bovine enteric caliciviruses, the Jena virus and Newbury agent, have been cloned and are closely related genetically to the NLV (20–22). A survey for the presence of calicivirus sequences in food animals showed a relatively high prevalence (33% of veal calf farms tested) of NLV sequences (159). That both genogroup I and genogroup II NLV sequences are present provides a sound basis for the development of hypotheses that describe emergence of epidemics, as well as the existence of nonhuman reservoirs for the HuCV.

A devastating but relatively recently recognized disease in rabbits, RHDV, is noteworthy because it causes a hemorrhagic diarrheal disease, with hemorrhagic septicemia, infectious necrosis of the liver in rabbits, and high mortality in adult animals (160,161). Although this virus cannot be cultivated in tissue culture, it has been cloned, and recombinant RHDV capsids expressed using baculovirus recombinants in a manner similar to NV have been shown to be an effective vaccine (162). A chicken calicivirus also causes diarrhea in infected animals (163), whereas other caliciviruses, such as the primate calicivirus, cause no detectable illness but do cause persistent infections (164).

CLINICAL FEATURES OF INFECTION, PATHOGENESIS, AND TREATMENT

The clinical manifestations of NV infections have been reported both from natural outbreaks and from volunteer studies. The illness is generally mild and self-limited, with symptoms lasting 12 to 24 hours, with a mean incubation time of 48 hours. The main clinical features include the sudden onset of vomiting and/or diarrhea, and a wide spectrum of disease may be seen in individual volunteers. For example, in one study, within 24 hours, one volunteer vomited 20 times and required parenteral fluid therapy, whereas other volunteers had no vomiting but had diarrhea with up to eight stools (3). The diarrheal stools are often liquid, without mucus, blood, or leukocytes (165). It has been estimated that about 50% of people exposed to NV become ill and secondary cases often occur. Hospitalization or rehydration is rarely required for adults and the major impact of this disease has been morbidity and loss of time from work and school.

An analysis of the clinical, virologic, and immunologic responses in a volunteer study using the newly developed diagnostic assays confirmed and extended conclusions about NV infection of adults (Table 56.3) (115). Specifically, this study showed a higher infection rate, more subclinical infections, and longer virus excretion after NV inoculation than previously recognized. Of 50 volunteers administered NV, 41 (82%) became infected; of these infections, 68% were symptomatic and 32% were asymptomatic. The peak of virus shedding was between 25 and 72 hours and virus first appeared in stool 15 hours after virus administration. Surprisingly, stool specimens collected 7 days after inoculation remained ELISA positive for both individuals with symptomatic and individuals with asymptomatic infection. These new data add to our understanding of the clinical manifestations of NV-induced acute gastroenteritis and have implications for the diagnosis of NV infections and the natural history and epidemiology of NV. For example, the findings of prolonged virus shedding and a higher rate of subclinical infections are important for understanding virus transmissions and for planning intervention measures to control disease spread. Previously, it had been thought that virus shedding began with the onset of clinical illness and usually did not last more than 72 hours (3,166). These new results indicate that although virus excretion peaks at 3 days, virus antigen is still being shed in the latest samples available for testing (7 days postinoculation). The high rate of asymptomatic infection, with one individual still shedding virus at day 6, also may facilitate virus transmission; this could help explain those food-borne epidemics in which food handlers report no previous illness (167). It will be important to determine the maximal time of virus shedding, and whether the viral antigen excreted at late times is infectious (and not simply solu-

TABLE 56.3. CLINICAL STATUS IN RELATION TO MAGNITUDE OF SERORESPONSE TO NORWALK VIRUS

			No. (%) of Subjects with Symptoms						
Antibody Response (-fold)	No. of Cases	No. Antigen Positive	Diarrhea (38 [15–55])	Vomiting[a] (24 [23–31])	Nausea[b] (25 [15–51])	Cramps (28 [7–55])	Headache/ Body Ache[c] (29 [3–55])	Chills (27 [19–55])	Fever >37.8°C[d] (33 [15–55])
0	10[e]	1[e] (10)	1[e] (10)	0	1 (10)	0	4 (40)	0	0
4	3	0	0	0	0	1 (33)	0	0	0
16	15	13 (87)	9 (60)	4 (27)	10 (67)	10 (67)	11 (73)	4 (27)	3 (20)
64	17	17 (100)	11 (65)	9 (53)	13 (76)	12 (71)	12 (71)	5 (29)	3 (18)
256	5	5 (100)	3 (60)	3 (60)	4 (80)	4 (80)	4 (80)	1 (20)	3 (60)
Total	50[f]	36 (88)	24 (59)	16 (39)	27 (66)	27 (66)	27 (66)	10 (24)	9 (22)

Symptom headings show (median hours of incubation [range]).
[a] $P = .02$, χ^2 for trend = 5.4.
[b] $P \leq .02$, χ^2 for trend = 5.9.
[c] $P = .04$, χ^2 for trend = 4.2.
[d] $P = .08$, χ^2 for trend = 3.2.
[e] Includes one infected subject with no antibody response but who had watery diarrhea and excreted virus and had antibody titers of 1:2,560.
[f] Norwalk infection was confirmed in 41 subjects by either antigen excretion or seroconversion; percentages were calculated on 41 as total.
From Graham DY, Jiang X, Tanaka T, et al. Norwalk virus infection of volunteers: new insights based on improved assays. *J Infect Dis* 1994;170:34–43, with permission.)

ble antigen); if infectious virus is routinely shed for long times, this information will need to be considered in planning outbreak control efforts in hospitals, nursing homes, and the food industry.

Illnesses induced in volunteers with the Hawaii agent, the Montgomery County agent, SMA, and one strain of morphologically typical HuCV, as well as naturally occurring illnesses with the morphologically typical HuCV (SLVs) in infants, older children, and adults, appear clinically indistinguishable from those observed with the NV (reviewed in reference 145). Abdominal pain has been noted as a symptom that accompanies the vomiting and diarrhea in older children and adults, and in some outbreaks, symptoms have been described as "flulike," with aching limbs, headache, malaise, and fever being noted. With the new tests available for diagnosis, it will be of interest to monitor flulike illnesses not attributable to influenza and determine whether a significant percentage of these illnesses are actually due to HuCV infections.

The pathogenesis of NV and HV illness has been examined in volunteer studies in which proximal intestinal biopsies were taken (69,70,168). Histologic changes were seen in jejunal biopsies from ill volunteers. Symptomatic illness was correlated with a broadening and blunting of the intestinal villi, crypt cell hyperplasia, cytoplasmic vacuolization, and infiltration of polymorphonuclear and mononuclear cells into the lamina propria, but the mucosa itself remained intact. Histologic changes were not seen in the gastric fundus, antrum, or colonic mucosa or in convalescent phase biopsies. The extent of small intestinal involvement remains unknown because studies have only examined the proximal small intestine, and the site of virus replication has not been identified. Clinical studies also showed that small intestinal brush border enzymatic activities (alkaline phosphatase, sucrase, and trehalase) were decreased, resulting in mild steatorrhea and transient carbohydrate malabsorption. Jejunal adenylate cyclase activity was not elevated (169), gastric secretion of HCl, pepsin, and intrinsic factor was associated with these histologic changes, and gastric emptying was delayed (170). It has been suggested that reduced gastric motility may be responsible for the nausea and vomiting associated with this gastroenteritis. Attempts to detect interferon in serum, jejunal aspirates, or jejunal biopsy specimens from volunteers inoculated with NV or HV were not successful; however, it is unclear whether these viruses do not induce interferon production in the gut or whether there are alternative physiologic explanations for lack of detection (171).

It is of interest to consider data on the pathogenesis of PEC infections in piglets, and infection of calves with Newbury agent (a bovine enteric calicivirus), because the consequences of calicivirus infection in the gut by these viruses appear similar to what is known about HuCV (156,172–174). Oral inoculation in piglets and/or calves results in diarrhea and anorexia 2 to 4 days postinoculation and loss of digestive and absorptive function. Mature enterocytes are infected, villi are stunted, and lesions are restricted to the anterior portion of the small intestine. In calves, histologic changes in the stomach, large intestine, liver, or lungs are not observed. It may be that calicivirus infection in these animals is similar enough to HuCV infections that supportive evidence for the mechanisms of calicivirus pathogenesis in humans can be provided by these models.

As discussed earlier, the illnesses caused by these enteric caliciviruses are generally mild and self-limited, and resolution occurs without sequelae. Treatment involves symptomatic therapy, with oral rehydration generally being sufficient. In rare cases, parenteral administration of intravenous fluids is required. Deaths in the elderly infected with NV and in immunocompromised children infected with HuCV have been reported, but these have generally been attributed to other primary causes.

IMMUNITY, PREVENTION, AND CONTROL

Studies of viral immunity have been relatively limited and have monitored the clinical resistance to infection or illness as correlated with preinfection antibody status of volunteers administered NV, SMA, or HV and of individuals involved in outbreaks (27,175,176). The development of immunity also has been monitored in similar settings by characterizing the seroresponses of individuals exposed to virus and with various clinical or infection outcomes. The assays used for most analyses of immunity have been the first-generation tests such as IEM, RIAs, and ELISAs that used human reagents. The inability to cultivate NV and other enteric HuCVs has hampered studies of viral immunity because *in vitro* neutralization assays are not available. Thus, the analyses of immunity in volunteers are complicated by several factors, including the following: (a) the preinfection exposure status to any of the HuCV agents of any adult volunteer is not known, so interpretation of results is never completely clear; and (b) neutralization assays with well-characterized cultivated viruses are not available, so the results of available assays may reflect responses to common or shared nonneutralizing epitopes.

Few studies have examined immunity to typical calicivirus infections in young children. However, one study that measured immunity to the HuCV Sapporo strain using an RIA with hyperimmune antiserum and apparently measured type-specific antibodies found that the presence of serum antibody was correlated with resistance to illness, but not infection (177). These results are of interest with the knowledge that this virus strain is in a separate genus from the NLV, and that children become infected with other virus serotypes (178).

Studies of clinical immunity in volunteers to NLVs have resulted in a more complex picture. Initial studies indicated that at least 50% of adult volunteers are susceptible to illness after administration of NV, HV, SMA, or a strain of HuCV. Early volunteer studies also showed that short-term homologous immunity develops, because volunteers who became ill after an initial NV challenge failed to become ill on rechallenge 6 to 14 weeks later with the same agent (176). It would be interesting to determine whether any of these individuals actually had asymptomatic infections using the new more sensitive assays. Several volunteer studies were unable to correlate elevated preexisting levels of serum or intestinal antibody to NV with long-term resistance to illness but showed an unexpected reciprocal relationship between prechallenge NV antibody levels and susceptibility to illness (176,179). In other volunteer studies, short-term resistance to infection was induced by prior homologous infection and was correlated with high antibody levels (27,179). Other epidemiologic studies found the level of antibody does not correlate with protection (180,181), so a clear correlate of protection remains to be identified.

The recent analysis of volunteers given NV using the new molecular assays has confirmed that 50% of volunteers are susceptible to illness, but a larger number (80%) of volunteers may be infected, with many of these infections being asymptomatic (115). Analysis of the preinfection serum antibody levels confirmed and extended the conclusions summarized earlier about clinical immunity. In this study, the volunteers were divided into five groups based on infection status and clinical outcome and severity of the infection (Fig. 56.6). Uninfected individuals were more likely to have lower preexisting antibody titers compared with any of the infected groups ($p < 0.001$). In addition, individuals who got watery diarrhea but no vomiting had significantly higher preexisting antibody titers when compared to uninfected individuals. For all the infected groups, there were significant increases in the geometric mean titers after infection, and among the groups of infected volunteers, the rises in antibody titers in the convalescent sera were significantly higher in volunteers who vomited (groups 3 and 5 versus groups 2 and 4) and in volunteers who vomited and had diarrhea (group 5 versus groups 2, 3, and 5). This result suggests that volunteers who vomit have high titer antibody responses and these could be prolonged responses. If true, this could explain the association of diarrheal disease with vomiting with seroresponses to NV in epidemiology studies.

An analysis of the infection outcome of volunteers relative to their preexisting antibody status also showed that individuals lacking antibody were not resistant to infection or illness (Table 56.4). Instead, there was a 60% seroconversion in volunteers lacking preexisting serum antibody (titers less than 10), so the lack of detectable serum antibody did not fully correlate with protection from infection. Although some volunteers with preexisting serum antibody titers of less than 1 : 50 (determined by the human reagent RIA) previously had been reported to become ill (124), it was not clear whether these individuals really lacked antibody or whether they simply possessed low titers. The lack of antibody in these volunteers was confirmed by adsorption of the prechallenge serum with rNV particles. How-

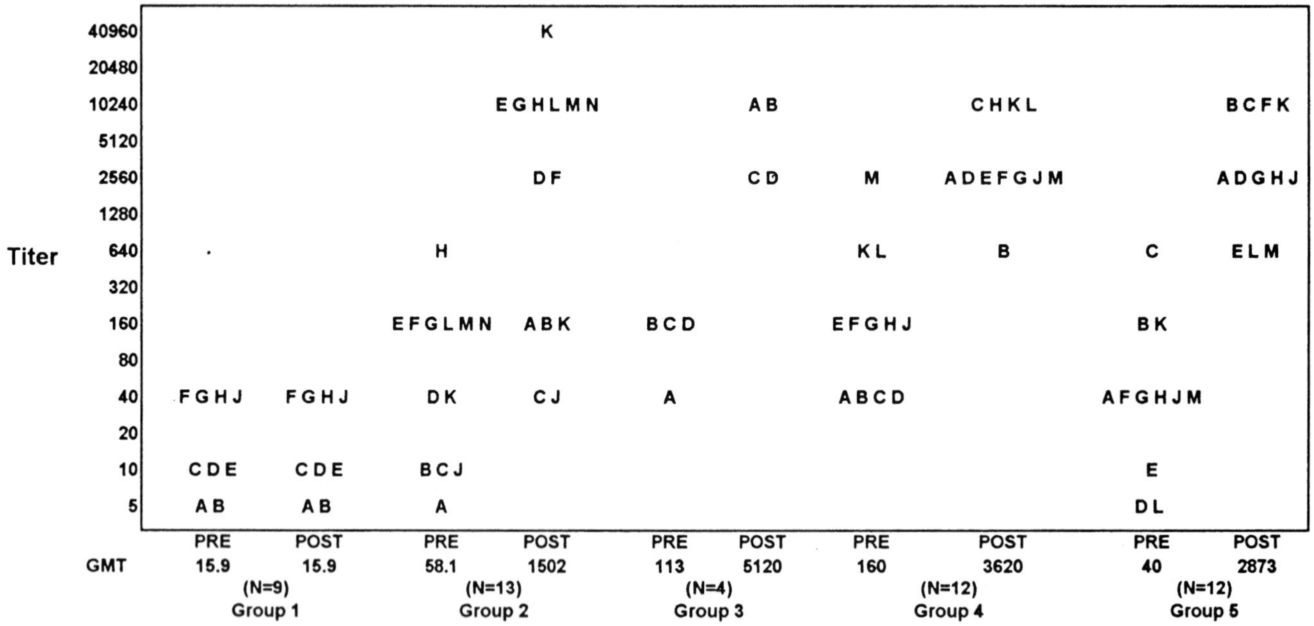

FIGURE 56.6. Serologic status of volunteers inoculated with Norwalk virus relative to clinical illness. Group 1, uninfected (no seroconversion and no antigen shedding); group 2, asymptomatic or mild symptomatic infection (no vomiting and no diarrhea); group 3, symptomatic infection (vomiting, no diarrhea); group 4, symptomatic infection (no vomiting but watery diarrhea); group 5, symptomatic infection (vomiting and watery diarrhea). Preinoculation and postinoculation titers for each subject are shown (individual letters); geometric means *(GMT)* are at bottom. Cutoff was A_{414nm} of 0.1. (From Graham DY, Jiang X, Tanaka T, et al. Norwalk virus infection of volunteers: new insights based on improved assays. *J Infect Dis* 1994;170:34–43, with permission.)

TABLE 56.4. INFECTION OUTCOME RELATIVE TO PREEXISTING NORWALK VIRUS ANTIBODY STATUS

Serum Titers	Number of Cases	Number of Volunteers (%) Who Had								
		Seroconversion[a]	Virus Shedding[b]	Diarrhea	Vomiting	Nausea[a]	Cramps	Headache	Chills	Fever
<10[c]	5	3 (60)	2 (40)	2 (40)	2 (40)	2 (40)	2 (40)	4 (80)	1 (20)	1 (20)
10	7	4 (57)	2 (29)	1 (14)	1 (14)	1 (14)	1 (14)	3 (42)	0 (0)	0 (0)
40	17	13 (76)	12 (70)	10 (59)	7 (41)	11 (65)	12 (70)	12 (70)	5 (29)	4 (23)
160	16	16 (100)	16 (100)	7 (44)	5 (31)	10 (62)	10 (62)	9 (56)	3 (19)	3 (19)
640	4	4 (100)	3 (75)	3 (75)	1 (25)	4 (100)	2 (50)	3 (75)	1 (25)	1 (25)
2,560	1	0 (0)	1 (100)	1 (100)	0 (0)	0 (0)	0 (0)	0 (0)	0 (0)	0 (0)

[a] $P = .065$, χ^2 for trend = 3.4.
[b] $P = .0012$, χ^2 for trend = 10.5.
[c] Subjects did not have preexisting antibody; blocking also was consistent with lacking antibody.
From Graham DY, Jiang X, Tanaka T, et al. Norwalk virus infection of volunteers: new insights based on improved assays. *J Infect Dis* 1994;170:34–43, with permission.)

ever, individuals who excreted virus had significantly higher preexisting antibody titers, and there was a trend for higher preexisting antibody titers in those who seroconverted.

Taken together, these results suggest that our knowledge about immunity to HuCV infections remains incomplete and the conflicting data may be clarified once assays that measure neutralizing epitopes become available (182). Currently, it appears that short-term resistance to illness can be induced by infection, and this immunity appears to correlate with the level of serum antibody. On the other hand, long-term resistance to illness appears to be more complicated and may be influenced by other factors; for example, there may be a genetic susceptibility to infection determined by the presence or absence of a specific virus receptor. It has been suggested that there is a subset of individuals who are relatively resistant to NV infection, and these individuals tend to have lower levels of antibody to NV, probably because they are less frequently infected (176). Whether these individuals would be resistant to infections with all HuCVs or only to a subset of such agents remains to be determined. Again, cultivation of these agents will facilitate answering these questions and likely will lead to resolution of whether individual serotypes of these viruses use distinct receptors to infect the gastrointestinal tract.

Because of our incomplete understanding of protective immunity to NV and other HuCVs, it is unclear whether vaccination strategies will be able to prevent such illnesses. Vaccines might prove effective, if the evidence for widespread and broad immunity to the morphologically typical caliciviruses is correct and if the results in less-developed countries reflect the ability to induce protection, possibly with repeated exposure. Some of these data are reminiscent of early reports for poliovirus exposure and resistance. It clearly is important to determine the number of serotypes of HuCVs and the relationship of serotypes to specific syndromes. It is possible that repeated immunization will be required to induce long-lasting immunity, and the availability of large amounts of stable recombinant particles makes it feasible if these induce protective immunity. Co-administration of rNV particles to mice with mucosal adjuvants can induce good mucosal responses (183,184). The rNV particles are safe and immunogenic when given to volunteers in water or as an edible vaccine (182,185,186), and it is likely that evaluation of the immune response to these particles will help us understand immunity to these enteric infections.

SUMMARY

Significant advances in our knowledge about NV and related viruses have come from the cloning, sequencing and expression of cDNAs of the genomes of these viruses. The availability of new diagnostic assays based on unlimited recombinant antigen and molecular assays based on knowledge of the genome sequences are allowing large-scale epidemiologic studies and characterization of the similarity and diversity of virus strains to proceed. The new information already obtained indicates that infections with these viruses occur much more frequently than previously recognized, and our understanding of the epidemiology of these infections can be expected to continue to change. There is little doubt that further studies of the molecular biology and epidemiology of these viruses will reveal unexpected and exciting new information about the interactions of these viruses with a diversity of cells of the gastrointestinal tract and possibly extraintestinally, as have similar studies with the rotaviruses over the past 20 years. We predict that as the HuCVs are studied, they may be found to play roles in both acute and chronic human illness whose etiologies currently are unknown.

ACKNOWLEDGMENTS

We gratefully acknowledge support for our research on NV and HuCVs provided by the National Institutes of Health, the Food and Drug Administration, Thrasher Research Fund, NOAA, and the Montana AES.

REFERENCES

1. Adler I, Zickl R. Winter vomiting disease. *J Infect Dis* 1969; 119:668–673.
2. Kapikian AZ, Wyatt RG, Dolin R, et al. Visualization by immune electron microscopy of a 27-nm particle associated with acute infectious nonbacterial gastroenteritis. *J Virol* 1972; 10:1075–1081.
3. Dolin R, Blacklow NR, DuPont H, et al. Transmission of acute infectious nonbacterial gastroenteritis to volunteers by oral administration of stool filtrates. *J Infect Dis* 1971;123:307–312.
4. Mead PS, Slutsker L, Dietz V, et al. Food-related illness and death in the United States. *Emerg Infect Dis* 1999;5:607–625.
5. Koopmans M, Vinje J, de Wit M, et al. Molecular epidemiology of human enteric caliciviruses in the Netherlands. *J Infect Dis* 2000;181[Suppl 2]:S262–S269.
6. Glass RI, Noel J, Ando T, et al. The epidemiology of enteric caliciviruses from humans: a reassessment using new diagnostics. *J Infect Dis* 2000;181[Suppl 2]:S254–S261.
7. Noel JS, Ando T, Leite JP, et al. Correlation of patient immune responses with genetically characterized small round-structured viruses involved in outbreaks of nonbacterial acute gastroenteritis in the United States, 1990 to 1995. *J Med Virol* 1997;53: 372–383.
8. Vinje J, Koopmans MP. Molecular detection and epidemiology of small round-structured viruses in outbreaks of gastroenteritis in the Netherlands. *J Infect Dis* 1996;174:610–615.
9. Vinje J, Deijl H, van der HR, et al. Molecular detection and epidemiology of Sapporo-like viruses. *J Clin Microbiol* 2000;38: 530–536.
10. Ando T, Jin Q, Gentsch JR, et al. Epidemiologic applications of novel molecular methods to detect and differentiate small round structured viruses (Norwalk-like viruses). *J Med Virol* 1995;47:145–152.
11. Fankhauser RL, Noel JS, Monroe SS, et al. Molecular epidemiology of "Norwalk-like viruses" in outbreaks of gastroenteritis in the United States. *J Infect Dis* 1998;178:1571–1578.
12. Noel JS, Fankhauser RL, Ando T, et al. Identification of a distinct common strain of "Norwalk-like viruses" having a global distribution. *J Infect Dis* 1999;179:1334–1344.
13. Cubitt WD, Green KY, Payment P. Prevalence of antibodies to the Hawaii strain of human calicivirus as measured by a recombinant protein based immunoassay. *J Med Virol* 1998; 54:135–139.
14. Cubitt WD, Jiang X. Study on occurrence of human calicivirus (Mexico strain) as cause of sporadic cases and outbreaks of calicivirus-associated diarrhea in the United Kingdom, 1983–1995. *J Med Virol* 1996;48:273–277.
15. Green KY, Lew JF, Jiang X, et al. Comparison of the reactivities of baculovirus-expressed recombinant Norwalk virus capsid antigen with those of the native Norwalk virus antigen in serologic assays and some epidemiologic observations. *J Clin Microbiol* 1993;31:2185–2191.
16. Prasad BV, Hardy ME, Dokland T, et al. X-ray crystallographic structure of the Norwalk virus capsid. *Science* 1999;286:287–290.
17. Seah EL, Marshall JA, Wright PJ. Open reading frame 1 of the Norwalk-like virus Camberwell: completion of sequence and expression in mammalian cells. *J Virol* 1999;73:10531–10535.
18. Liu B, Clarke IN, Lambden PR. Polyprotein processing in Southampton virus: identification of 3C-like protease cleavage sites by in vitro mutagenesis. *J Virol* 1996;70:2605–2610.
19. Liu BL, Viljoen GJ, Clarke IN, et al. Identification of further proteolytic cleavage sites in the Southampton calicivirus polyprotein by expression of the viral protease in *E. coli*. *J Gen Virol* 1999;80[Pt 2]:291–296.
20. Dastjerdi AM, Green J, Gallimore CI, et al. The bovine Newbury agent-2 is genetically more closely related to human SRSVs than to animal caliciviruses. *Virology* 1999;254:1–5.
21. Liu BL, Lambden PR, Gunther H, et al. Molecular characterization of a bovine enteric calicivirus: relationship to the Norwalk-like viruses. *J Virol* 1999;73:819–825.
22. Guo M, Chang KO, Hardy ME, et al. Molecular characterization of a porcine enteric calicivirus genetically related to Sapporo-like human caliciviruses. *J Virol* 1999;73:9625–9631.
23. Kapikian AZ. The discovery of the 27-nm Norwalk virus: an historic perspective. *J Infect Dis* 2000;181[Suppl 2]:S295–S302.
24. Green KY, Ando T, Balayan MS. Taxonomy of the Caliciviruses. *J Infect Dis* 2000;181:5322–5330.
25. Thornhill TS, Wyatt RG, Kalica AR, et al. Detection by immune electron microscopy of 26- to 27-nm viruslike particles associated with two family outbreaks of gastroenteritis. *J Infect Dis* 1977;135:20–27.
26. Morens DM, Zweighaft RM, Vernon TM, et al. A waterborne outbreak of gastroenteritis with secondary person-to-person spread. Association with a viral agent. *Lancet* 1979;1:964–966.
27. Wyatt RG, Dolin R, Blacklow NR, et al. Comparison of three agents of acute infectious nonbacterial gastroenteritis by cross-challenge in volunteers. *J Infect Dis* 1974;129:709–714.
28. Agus SG, Falchuk ZM, Sessoms CS, et al. Increased jejunal IgA synthesis *in vitro* during acute infectious nonbacterial gastroenteritis. *Am J Dig Dis* 1974;19:127–131.
29. Taniguchi K, Urasawa S, Urasawa T. Virus-like particle, 35 to 40 nm, associated with an institutional outbreak of acute gastroenteritis in adults. *J Clin Microbiol* 1979;10:730–736.
30. Kogasaka R, Nakamura S, Chiba S, et al. The 33- to 39-nm virus-like particles, tentatively designed as Sapporo agent, associated with an outbreak of acute gastroenteritis. *J Med Virol* 1981;8:187–193.
31. Oishi I, Yamazaki K, Minekawa Y, et al. Three-year survey of the epidemiology of rotavirus, enteric adenovirus, and some small spherical viruses including "Osaka-agent" associated with infantile diarrhea. *Biken J* 1985;28:9–19.
32. Caul EO, Appleton H. The electron microscopical and physical characteristics of small round human fecal viruses: an interim scheme for classification. *J Med Virol* 1982;9:257–265.
33. Appleton H. Small round viruses: classification and role in food-borne infections. *Ciba Found Symp* 1987;128:108–125.
34. Herrmann JE, Hudson RW, Blacklow NR. Marin County agent, an astrovirus. *Lancet* 1987;2:743.
35. Greenberg HB, Valdesuso JR, Kalica AR, et al. Proteins of Norwalk virus. *J Virol* 1981;37:994–999.
36. Burroughs JN, Brown F. Physico-chemical evidence for the reclassification of the caliciviruses. *J Gen Virol* 1974;22: 281–286.
37. Schaffer FL, Soergel ME. Single major polypeptide of a calicivirus: characterization by polyacrylamide gel electrophoresis and stabilization of virions by cross-linking with dimethyl suberimidate. *J Virol* 1976;19:925–931.
38. Bachrach HL, Hess WR. Animal picornaviruses with a single major species of capsid protein. *Biochem Biophys Res Commun* 1973;55:141–149.
39. Jiang X, Wang M, Wang K, et al. Sequence and genomic organization of Norwalk virus. *Virology* 1993;195:51–61.
40. Lambden PR, Caul EO, Ashley CR, et al. Sequence and genome organization of a human small round-structured (Norwalk-like) virus. *Science* 1993;259:516–519.
41. Green KY, Ando T, Balayan MS, et al. Taxonomy of the caliciviruses. *J Infect Dis* 2000;181[Suppl 2]:S322–S330.
42. Jiang X, Wang M, Graham DY, et al. Expression, self-assembly, and antigenicity of the Norwalk virus capsid protein. *J Virol* 1992;66:6527–6532.

43. Glass PJ, White LJ, Ball JM, et al. Norwalk virus open reading frame 3 encodes a minor structural protein. *J Virol* 2000;74: 6581–6591.
44. Hendry DA. Nodaviridae in invertebrates. In: Kurstak E, ed. Viruses of invertebrates. New York: Marcel Deker, 1991:227–276.
45. Prasad BV, Rothnagel R, Jiang X, et al. Three-dimensional structure of baculovirus-expressed Norwalk virus capsids. *J Virol* 1994;68:5117–5125.
46. Prasad BV, Matson DO, Smith AW. Three-dimensional structure of calicivirus. *J Mol Biol* 1994;240:256–264.
47. Lew JF, Petric M, Kapikian AZ, et al. Identification of minireovirus as a Norwalk-like virus in pediatric patients with gastroenteritis. *J Virol* 1994;68:3391–3396.
48. Neill JD. Nucleotide sequence of the capsid protein gene of two serotypes of San Miguel sea lion virus: identification of conserved and non-conserved amino acid sequences among calicivirus capsid proteins. *Virus Res* 1992;24:211–222.
49. Hardy ME, Estes MK. Completion of the Norwalk virus genome sequence. *Virus Genes* 1996;12:287–290.
50. Dingle KE, Lambden PR, Caul EO, et al. Human enteric Caliciviridae: the complete genome sequence and expression of virus-like particles from a genetic group II small round structured virus. *J Gen Virol* 1995;76[Pt 9]:2349–2355.
51. Liu BL, Clarke IN, Caul EO, et al. Human enteric caliciviruses have a unique genome structure and are distinct from the Norwalk-like viruses. *Arch Virol* 1995;140:1345–1356.
52. Meyers G, Wirblich C, Thiel HJ. Rabbit hemorrhagic disease virus—molecular cloning and nucleotide sequencing of a calicivirus genome. *Virology* 1991;184:664–676.
53. Carter MJ, Milton ID, Meanger J, et al. The complete nucleotide sequence of a feline calicivirus. *Virology* 1992;190:443–448.
54. Burroughs JN, Brown F. Presence of a covalently linked protein on calicivirus RNA. *J Gen Virol* 1978;41:443–446.
55. Schaffer FL, Ehresmann DW, Fretz MK, et al. A protein, VPg, covalently linked to 36S calicivirus RNA. *J Gen Virol* 1980;47: 215–220.
56. Meyers G, Wirblich C, Thiel HJ. Genomic and subgenomic RNAs of rabbit hemorrhagic disease virus are both protein-linked and packaged into particles. *Virology* 1991;184:677–686.
57. Sosnovtsev SV, Green KY. Identification and genomic mapping of the ORF3 and VPg proteins in feline calicivirus virions. *Virology* 2000;277:193–203.
58. Neill JD. Nucleotide sequence of a region of the feline calicivirus genome which encodes picornavirus-like RNA-dependent RNA polymerase, cysteine protease and 2C polypeptides. *Virus Res* 1990;17:145–160.
59. Pfister T, Wimmer E. Polypeptide p41 of a Norwalk-like virus is a nucleic acid-independent nucleoside triphosphatase. *J Virol* 2001;75:1611–1619.
60. Vazquez AL, Martin Alonso JM, Casais R, et al. Expression of enzymatically active rabbit hemorrhagic disease virus RNA-dependent RNA polymerase in Escherichia coli. *J Virol* 1998; 72:2999–3004.
61. Wei L, Huhn JS, Mory A, et al. Proteinase-polymerase precursor as the active form of feline calicivirus RNA-dependent RNA polymerase. *J Virol* 2001;75:1211–1219.
62. Wirblich C, Thiel HJ, Meyers G. Genetic map of the calicivirus rabbit hemorrhagic disease virus as deduced from in vitro translation studies. *J Virol* 1996;70:7974–7983.
63. Dunham DM, Jiang X, Berke T, et al. Genomic mapping of a calicivirus VPg. *Arch Virol* 1998;143:2421–2430.
64. Boniotti B, Wirblich C, Sibilia M, et al. Identification and characterization of a 3C-like protease from rabbit hemorrhagic disease virus, a calicivirus. *J Virol* 1994;68:6487–6495.
65. Wirblich C, Sibilia M, Boniotti MB, et al. 3C-like protease of rabbit hemorrhagic disease virus: identification of cleavage sites in the ORF-1 polyprotein and analysis of cleavage specificity. *J Virol* 1995;69:7159–7168.
66. Sosnovtseva SA, Sosnovtsev SV, Green KY. Mapping of the feline calicivirus proteinase responsible for autocatalytic processing of the nonstructural polyprotein and identification of a stable proteinase-polymerase precursor protein. *J Virol* 1999;73:6626–6633.
67. Meyers G, Wirblich C, Thiel HJ, et al. Rabbit hemorrhagic disease virus: genome organization and polyprotein processing of a calicivirus studied after transient expression of cDNA constructs [In Process Citation]. *Virology* 2000;276:349–363.
68. Meanger J, Carter MJ, Milton ID, et al. Scheme of RNA transcription in calicivirus-infected cells. *Biochem Soc Trans* 1993; 21:67S.
69. Agus SG, Dolin R, Wyatt RG, et al. Acute infectious nonbacterial gastroenteritis: intestinal histopathology. Histologic and enzymatic alterations during illness produced by the Norwalk agent in man. *Ann Intern Med* 1973;79:18–25.
70. Schreiber DS, Blacklow NR, Trier JS. The small intestinal lesion induced by Hawaii agent acute infectious nonbacterial gastroenteritis. *J Infect Dis* 1974;129:705–708.
71. Favorov MO, Khudyakov YE, Mast EE, et al. IgM and IgG antibodies to hepatitis E virus (HEV) detected by an enzyme immunoassay based on an HEV-specific artificial recombinant mosaic protein. *J Med Virol* 1996;50:50–58.
72. White LJ, Ball JM, Hardy ME, et al. Attachment and entry of recombinant Norwalk virus capsids to cultured human and animal cell lines. *J Virol* 1996;70:6589–6597.
73. Wickham TJ, Granados RR, Wood HA, et al. General analysis of receptor-mediated viral attachment to cell surfaces. *Biophys J* 1990;58:1501–1516.
74. Tamura M, Natori K, Kobayashi M, et al. Interaction of recombinant Norwalk virus particles with the 105-kilodalton cellular binding protein, a candidate receptor molecule for virus attachment. *J Virol* 2000;74:11589–11597.
75. Hardy ME, Tanaka TN, Kitamoto N, et al. Antigenic mapping of the recombinant Norwalk virus capsid protein using monoclonal antibodies. *Virology* 1996;217:252–261.
76. Flynn WT, Saif LJ. Serial propagation of porcine enteric calicivirus-like virus in primary porcine kidney cell cultures. *J Clin Microbiol* 1988;26:206–212.
77. Gutierrez-Escolano AL, Brito ZU, del Angel RM, et al. Interaction of cellular proteins with the 5′ end of Norwalk virus genomic RNA. *J Virol* 2000;74:8558–8562.
78. Kozak M. Effects of long 5′ leader sequences on initiation by eukaryotic ribosomes in vitro. *Gene Expr* 1991;1:117–125.
79. Herbert TP, Brierley I, Brown TD. Identification of a protein linked to the genomic and subgenomic mRNAs of feline calicivirus and its role in translation. *J Gen Virol* 1997;78[Pt 5]: 1033–1040.
80. Cauchi MR, Doultree JC, Marshall JA, et al. Molecular characterization of Camberwell virus and sequence variation in ORF3 of small round-structured (Norwalk-like) viruses. *J Med Virol* 1996;49:70–76.
81. Seah EL, Gunesekere IC, Marshall JA, et al. Variation in ORF3 of genogroup 2 Norwalk-like viruses. *Arch Virol* 1999;144: 1007–1014.
82. Lew JF, Kapikian AZ, Jiang X, et al. Molecular characterization and expression of the capsid protein of a Norwalk-like virus recovered from a Desert Shield troop with gastroenteritis. *Virology* 1994;200:319–325.
83. Lew JF, Kapikian AZ, Valdesuso J, et al. Molecular characterization of Hawaii virus and other Norwalk-like viruses: evidence for genetic polymorphism among human caliciviruses. *J Infect Dis* 1994;170:535–542.
84. Ando T, Mulders MN, Lewis DC, et al. Comparison of the polymerase region of small round structured virus strains previ-

ously classified in three antigenic types by solid-phase immune electron microscopy. *Arch Virol* 1994;135:217–226.
85. Green J, Norcott JP, Lewis D, et al. Norwalk-like viruses: demonstration of genomic diversity by polymerase chain reaction. *J Clin Microbiol* 1993;31:3007–3012.
86. Norcott JP, Green J, Lewis D, et al. Genomic diversity of small round structured viruses in the United Kingdom. *J Med Virol* 1994;44:280–286.
87. Wang J, Jiang X, Madore HP, et al. Sequence diversity of small, round-structured viruses in the Norwalk virus group. *J Virol* 1994;68:5982–5990.
88. Cubitt WD, Jiang XJ, Wang J, et al. Sequence similarity of human caliciviruses and small round structured viruses. *J Med Virol* 1994;43:252–258.
89. Matson DO, Zhong WM, Nakata S, et al. Molecular characterization of a human calicivirus with sequence relationships closer to animal caliciviruses than other known human caliciviruses. *J Med Virol* 1995;45:215–222.
90. Lambden PR, Caul EO, Ashley CR, et al. Human enteric caliciviruses are genetically distinct from small round structured viruses [Letter]. *Lancet* 1994;343:666–667.
91. Moe CL, Gentsch J, Ando T, et al. Application of PCR to detect Norwalk virus in fecal specimens from outbreaks of gastroenteritis. *J Clin Microbiol* 1994;32:642–648.
92. Green SM, Dingle KE, Lambden PR, et al. Human enteric Caliciviridae: a new prevalent small round-structured virus group defined by RNA-dependent RNA polymerase and capsid diversity. *J Gen Virol* 1994;75[Pt 8]:1883–1888.
93. Moussa A, Chasey D, Lavazza A, et al. Haemorrhagic disease of lagomorphs: evidence for a calicivirus. *Vet Microbiol* 1992;33: 375–381.
94. Dolin R, Reichman RC, Roessner KD, et al. Detection by immune electron microscopy of the Snow Mountain agent of acute viral gastroenteritis. *J Infect Dis* 1982;146:184–189.
95. Ando T, Noel JS, Fankhauser RL. Genetic classification of "Norwalk-like viruses." *J Infect Dis* 2000;181[Suppl 2]:S336–S348.
96. Vinje J, Green J, Lewis DC, et al. Genetic polymorphism across regions of the three open reading frames of "Norwalk-like viruses." *Arch Virol* 2000;145:223–241.
97. Oglesby AS, Schaffer FL, Madin SH. Biochemical and biophysical properties of vesicular exanthema of swine virus. *Virology* 1971;44:329–341.
98. Hillman B, Morris TJ, Kellen WR, et al. An invertebrate calici-like virus. Evidence for partial virion disintegration in host excreta. *J Gen Virol* 1982;60:115–123.
99. Smith AW, Prato C, Skilling DE. Caliciviruses infecting monkeys and possibly man. *Am J Vet Res* 1978;39:287–289.
100. Humphrey TJ, Cruickshank JG, Cubitt WD. An outbreak of calicivirus associated gastroenteritis in an elderly persons home. A possible zoonosis? *J Hyg (Lond)* 1984;93:293–299.
101. Neill JD, Meyer RF, Seal BS. Genetic relatedness of the caliciviruses: San Miguel sea lion and vesicular exanthema of swine viruses constitute a single genotype within the Caliciviridae. *J Virol* 1995;69:4484–4488.
102. Barlough JE, Berry ES, Skilling DE, et al. Antibodies to marine caliciviruses in the Pacific walrus (Odobenus rosmarus divergens Illiger). *J Wildl Dis* 1986;22:165–168.
103. Hardy ME, Kramer SF, Treanor JJ, et al. Human calicivirus genogroup II capsid sequence diversity revealed by analyses of the prototype Snow Mountain agent. *Arch Virol* 1997;142: 1469–1479.
104. Jiang X, Espul C, Zhong WM, et al. Characterization of a novel human calicivirus that may be a naturally occurring recombinant. *Arch Virol* 1999;144:2377–2387.
105. Oishi I, Yamazaki K, Kimoto T, et al. Demonstration of low molecular weight polypeptides associated with small, round-structured viruses by western immunoblot analysis. *Microbiol Immunol* 1992;36:1105–1112.
106. Jiang X, Wang J, Estes MK. Characterization of SRSVs using RT-PCR and a new antigen ELISA. *Arch Virol* 1995;140: 363–374.
107. Kaplan JE, Feldman R, Campbell DS, et al. The frequency of a Norwalk-like pattern of illness in outbreaks of acute gastroenteritis. *Am J Public Health* 1982;72:1329–1332.
108. Atmar RL, Estes MK. Diagnosis of noncultivatable gastroenteritis viruses, the human caliciviruses. *Clin Microbiol Rev* 2001; 14:15–37.
109. Jiang X, Wang J, Graham DY, et al. Detection of Norwalk virus in stool by polymerase chain reaction. *J Clin Microbiol* 1992; 30:2529–2534.
110. Atmar RL, Metcalf TG, Neill FH, et al. Detection of enteric viruses in oysters by using the polymerase chain reaction. *Appl Environ Microbiol* 1993;59:631–635.
111. De Leon R, Matsui SM, Baric RS, et al. Detection of Norwalk virus in stool specimens by reverse transcriptase-polymerase chain reaction and nonradioactive oligoprobes. *J Clin Microbiol* 1992;30:3151–3157.
112. Willcocks MM, Silcock JG, Carter MJ. Detection of Norwalk virus in the UK by the polymerase chain reaction. *FEMS Microbiol Lett* 1993;112:7–12.
113. Ando T, Monroe SS, Gentsch JR, et al. Detection and differentiation of antigenically distinct small round-structured viruses (Norwalk-like viruses) by reverse transcription-PCR and southern hybridization. *J Clin Microbiol* 1995;33:64–71.
114. Parashar UD, Quiroz ES, Mounts AW, et al. "Norwalk-like viruses" Public health consequences and outbreak management. 2001;50(RR-9):1–17.
115. Graham DY, Jiang X, Tanaka T, et al. Norwalk virus infection of volunteers: new insights based on improved assays. *J Infect Dis* 1994;170:34–43.
116. Treanor JJ, Jiang X, Madore HP, et al. Subclass-specific serum antibody responses to recombinant Norwalk virus capsid antigen (rNV) in adults infected with Norwalk, Snow Mountain, or Hawaii virus. *J Clin Microbiol* 1993;31:1630–1634.
117. Lew JF, Valdesuso J, Vesikari T, et al. Detection of Norwalk virus or Norwalk-like virus infections in Finnish infants and young children. *J Infect Dis* 1994;169:1364–1367.
118. Gray JJ, Jiang X, Morgan-Capner P, et al. Prevalence of antibodies to Norwalk virus in England: detection by enzyme-linked immunosorbent assay using baculovirus-expressed Norwalk virus capsid antigen. *J Clin Microbiol* 1993;31: 1022–1025.
119. Khan AS, Moe CL, Glass RI, et al. Norwalk virus-associated gastroenteritis traced to ice consumption aboard a cruise ship in Hawaii: comparison and application of molecular method-based assays. *J Clin Microbiol* 1994;32:318–322.
120. Hale AD, Tanaka TN, Kitamoto N, et al. Identification of an epitope common to genogroup 1 "Norwalk-like viruses." *J Clin Microbiol* 2000;38:1656–1660.
121. Kitamoto N, Tanaka TN, Natori K, et al. Cross-reactivity among several recombinant calicivirus virus-like (VLPs) with monoclonal antibodies obtained from mice immunized orally with one type of VLP. 2001 *(in press)*.
122. Blacklow NR, Greenberg HB. Viral gastroenteritis. *N Engl J Med* 1991;325:252–264.
123. Kapikian AZ, Greenberg HB, Cline WL, et al. Prevalence of antibody to the Norwalk agent by a newly developed immune adherence hemagglutination assay. *J Med Virol* 1978;2:281–294.
124. Blacklow NR, Cukor G, Bedigian MK, et al. Immune response and prevalence of antibody to Norwalk enteritis virus as determined by radioimmunoassay. *J Clin Microbiol* 1979;10: 903–909.

125. Greenberg HB, Valdesuso J, Kapikian AZ, et al. Prevalence of antibody to the Norwalk virus in various countries. *Infect Immun* 1979;26:270–273.
126. Parker SP, Cubitt WD, Jiang XJ, et al. Seroprevalence studies using a recombinant Norwalk virus protein enzyme immunoassay. *J Med Virol* 1994;42:146–150.
127. Numata K, Nakata S, Jiang X, et al. Epidemiological study of Norwalk virus infections in Japan and Southeast Asia by enzyme-linked immunosorbent assays with Norwalk virus capsid protein produced by the baculovirus expression system. *J Clin Microbiol* 1994;32:121–126.
128. Cukor G, Blacklow NR, Echeverria P, et al. Comparative study of the acquisition of antibody to Norwalk virus in pediatric populations. *Infect Immun* 1980;29:822–823.
129. Echeverria P, Burke DS, Blacklow NR, et al. Age-specific prevalence of antibody to rotavirus, Escherichia coli heat-labile enterotoxin, Norwalk virus, and hepatitis A virus in a rural community in Thailand. *J Clin Microbiol* 1983;17:923–925.
130. Black RE, Greenberg HB, Kapikian AZ, et al. Acquisition of serum antibody to Norwalk Virus and rotavirus and relation to diarrhea in a longitudinal study of young children in rural Bangladesh. *J Infect Dis* 1982;145:483–489.
131. Gabbay YB, Glass RI, Monroe SS, et al. Prevalence of antibodies to Norwalk virus among Amerindians in isolated Amazonian communities. *Am J Epidemiol* 1994;139:728–733.
132. Sawyer LA, Murphy JJ, Kaplan JE, et al. 25- to 30-nm virus particle associated with a hospital outbreak of acute gastroenteritis with evidence for airborne transmission. *Am J Epidemiol* 1988;127:1261–1271.
133. Ho MS, Glass RI, Monroe SS, et al. Viral gastroenteritis aboard a cruise ship. *Lancet* 1989;2:961–965.
134. Monroe SS, Stine SE, Jiang X, et al. Detection of antibody to recombinant Norwalk virus antigen in specimens from outbreaks of gastroenteritis. *J Clin Microbiol* 1993;31:2866–2872.
135. Spratt HC, Marks MI, Gomersall M, et al. Nosocomial infantile gastroenteritis associated with minirotavirus and calicivirus. *J Pediatr* 1978;93:922–926.
136. Middleton PJ, Szymanski MT, Petric M. Viruses associated with acute gastroenteritis in young children. *Am J Dis Child* 1977;131:733–737.
137. Nakata S, Estes MK, Chiba S. Detection of human calicivirus antigen and antibody by enzyme-linked immunosorbent assays. *J Clin Microbiol* 1988;26:2001–2005.
138. Cubitt WD, Blacklow NR, Herrmann JE, et al. Antigenic relationships between human caliciviruses and Norwalk virus. *J Infect Dis* 1987;156:806–814.
139. Bon F, Fascia P, Dauvergne M, et al. Prevalence of group A rotavirus, human calicivirus, astrovirus, and adenovirus type 40 and 41 infections among children with acute gastroenteritis in Dijon, France. *J Clin Microbiol* 1999;37:3055–3058.
140. Pang XL, Honma S, Nakata S, et al. Human caliciviruses in acute gastroenteritis of young children in the community. *J Infect Dis* 2000;181[Suppl 2]:S288–S294.
141. Maguire AJ, Green J, Brown DW, et al. Molecular epidemiology of outbreaks of gastroenteritis associated with small round-structured viruses in East Anglia, United Kingdom, during the 1996–1997 season. *J Clin Microbiol* 1999;37:81–89.
142. Patterson T, Hutchings P, Palmer S. Outbreak of SRSV gastroenteritis at an international conference traced to food handled by a post-symptomatic caterer. *Epidemiol Infect* 1993;111:157–162.
143. White KE, Osterholm MT, Mariotti JA, et al. A foodborne outbreak of Norwalk virus gastroenteritis. Evidence for post-recovery transmission. *Am J Epidemiol* 1986;124:120–126.
144. Murphy AM, Grohmann GS, Christopher PJ, et al. An Australia-wide outbreak of gastroenteritis from oysters caused by Norwalk virus. *Med J Aust* 1979;2:329–333.
145. Cubitt WD. Diagnosis, occurrence and clinical significance of the human 'candidate' caliciviruses. *Prog Med Virol* 1989;36: 103–119.
146. Madeley CR, Cosgrove BP. Caliciviruses in man [Letter]. *Lancet* 1976;1:199–200.
147. Nakata S, Honma S, Numata KK, et al. Members of the family Caliciviridae (Norwalk virus and Sapporo virus) are the most prevalent cause of gastroenteritis outbreaks among infants in Japan. *J Infect Dis* 2000;181:2029–2032.
148. Matson DO, Estes MK, Tanaka T, et al. Asymptomatic human calicivirus infection in a day care center. *Pediatr Infect Dis J* 1990;9:190–196.
149. Kaljot KT, Ling JP, Gold JW, et al. Prevalence of acute enteric viral pathogens in acquired immunodeficiency syndrome patients with diarrhea. *Gastroenterology* 1989;97:1031–1032.
150. Cunningham AL, Grohman GS, Harkness J, et al. Gastrointestinal viral infections in homosexual men who were symptomatic and seropositive for human immunodeficiency virus. *J Infect Dis* 1988;158:386–391.
151. Studdert MJ. Caliciviruses. Brief review. *Arch Virol* 1978;58: 157–191.
152. Dick CP, Johnson RP, Yamashiro S. Sites of persistence of feline calicivirus. *Res Vet Sci* 1989;47:367–373.
153. Kalunda M, Lee KM, Holmes DF, et al. Serologic classification of feline caliciviruses by plaque-reduction neutralization and immunodiffusion. *Am J Vet Res* 1975;36:353–356.
154. Barlough JE, Berry ES, Skilling DE, et al. The marine calicivirus story—part I. *Comp Contin Ed Pract Vet* 1986;8:F5–F14.
155. Barlough JE, Berry ES, Skilling DE, et al. The marine calicivirus story—part II. *Comp Contin Ed Pract Vet* 1986;8: F75–F82.
156. Saif LJ, Bohl EH, Theil KW, et al. Rotavirus-like, calicivirus-like, and 23-nm virus-like particles associated with diarrhea in young pigs. *J Clin Microbiol* 1980;12:105–111.
157. Parwani AV, Flynn WT, Gadfield KL, et al. Serial propagation of porcine enteric calicivirus in a continuous cell line. Effect of medium supplementation with intestinal contents or enzymes. *Arch Virol* 1991;120:115–122.
158. Sugieda M, Nagaoka H, Kakishima Y, et al. Detection of Norwalk-like virus genes in the caecum contents of pigs. *Arch Virol* 1998;143:1215–1221.
159. Der Poel WH, Vinje J, van der HR, et al. Norwalk-like calicivirus genes in farm animals. *Emerg Infect Dis* 2000;6:36–41.
160. Parra F, Prieto M. Purification and characterization of a calicivirus as the causative agent of a lethal hemorrhagic disease in rabbits. *J Virol* 1990;64:4013–4015.
161. Ohlinger VF, Haas B, Thiel HJ. Rabbit hemorrhagic disease (RHD): characterization of the causative calicivirus. *Vet Res* 1993;24:103–116.
162. Laurent S, Vautherot JF, Madelaine MF, et al. Recombinant rabbit hemorrhagic disease virus capsid protein expressed in baculovirus self-assembles into viruslike particles and induces protection. *J Virol* 1994;68:6794–6798.
163. Cubitt WD, Barrett AD. Propagation and preliminary characterization of a chicken candidate calicivirus. *J Gen Virol* 1985; 66[Pt 7]:1431–1438.
164. Smith AW, Skilling DE, Ensley PK, et al. Calicivirus isolation and persistence in a pygmy chimpanzee (Pan paniscus). *Science* 1983;221:79–81.
165. Dolin R, Reichman RC, Fauci AS. Lymphocyte populations in acute viral gastroenteritis. *Infect Immun* 1976;14:422–428.
166. Thornhill TS, Kalica AR, Wyatt RG, et al. Pattern of shedding of the Norwalk particle in stools during experimentally induced gastroenteritis in volunteers as determined by immune electron microscopy. *J Infect Dis* 1975;132:28–34.
167. Hedberg CW, Osterholm MT. Outbreaks of food-borne and

waterborne viral gastroenteritis. *Clin Microbiol Rev* 1993;6: 199–210.
168. Widerlite L, Trier JS, Blacklow NR, et al. Structure of the gastric mucosa in acute infectious bacterial gastroenteritis. *Gastroenterology* 1975;68:425–430.
169. Levy AG, Widerlite L, Schwartz CJ, et al. Jejunal adenylate cyclase activity in human subjects during viral gastroenteritis. *Gastroenterology* 1976;70:321–325.
170. Meeroff JC, Schreiber DS, Trier JS, et al. Abnormal gastric motor function in viral gastroenteritis. *Ann Intern Med* 1980; 92:370–373.
171. Dolin R, Baron S. Absence of detectable interferon in jejunal biopsies, jejunal aspirates, and sera in experimentally induced viral gastroenteritis in man. *Proc Soc Exp Biol Med* 1975;150: 337–339.
172. Bridger JC. Detection by electron microscopy of caliciviruses, astroviruses and rotavirus-like particles in the faeces of piglets with diarrhea. *Vet Rec* 1980;107:532–533.
173. Flynn WT, Saif LJ, Moorhead PD. Pathogenesis of porcine enteric calicivirus-like virus in four-day-old gnotobiotic pigs. *Am J Vet Res* 1988;49:819–825.
174. Woode GN, Bridger JC. Isolation of small viruses resembling astroviruses and caliciviruses from acute enteritis of calves. *J Med Microbiol* 1978;11:441–452.
175. Dolin R, Blacklow NR, DuPont H, et al. Biological properties of Norwalk agent of acute infectious nonbacterial gastroenteritis. *Proc Soc Exp Biol Med* 1972;140:578–583.
176. Parrino TA, Schreiber DS, Trier JS, et al. Clinical immunity in acute gastroenteritis caused by Norwalk agent. *N Engl J Med* 1977;297:86–89.
177. Nakata S, Chiba S, Terashima H, et al. Humoral immunity in infants with gastroenteritis caused by human calicivirus. *J Infect Dis* 1985;152:274–279.
178. Cubitt WD, McSwiggan DA. Seroepidemiological survey of the prevalence of antibodies to a strain of human calicivirus. *J Med Virol* 1987;21:361–368.
179. Johnson PC, Mathewson JJ, DuPont HL, et al. Multiple-challenge study of host susceptibility to Norwalk gastroenteritis in US adults. *J Infect Dis* 1990;161:18–21.
180. Baron RC, Greenberg HB, Cukor G, et al. Serological responses among teenagers after natural exposure to Norwalk virus. *J Infect Dis* 1984;150:531–534.
181. Ryder RW, Singh N, Reeves WC, et al. Evidence of immunity induced by naturally acquired rotavirus and Norwalk virus infection on two remote Panamanian islands. *J Infect Dis* 1985; 151:99–105.
182. Estes MK, Ball JM, Guerrero RA, et al. Norwalk virus vaccines: challenges and progress. *J Infect Dis* 2000;181[Suppl 2]: S367–S373.
183. Ball JM, Hardy ME, Atmar RL, et al. Oral immunization with recombinant Norwalk virus-like particles induces a systemic and mucosal immune response in mice. *J Virol* 1998;72:1345–1353.
184. Guerrero RA, Ball JM, Krater SS, et al. Recombinant Norwalk virus-like particles administered intranasally to mice induce systemic and mucosal (fecal and vaginal) immune responses. *J Virol* 2001;75:9713–9722.
185. Mason HS, Ball JM, Shi JJ, et al. Expression of Norwalk virus capsid protein in transgenic tobacco and potato and its oral immunogenicity in mice. *Proc Natl Acad Sci U S A* 1996;93: 5335–5340.
186. Tacket CO, Mason HS, Losonsky G, et al. Human immune responses to a novel Norwalk virus vaccine delivered in transgenic potatoes. *J Infect Dis* 2000;182:302–305.
187. Matsui SM, Kim JP, Greenberg HB, et al. The isolation and characterization of a Norwalk virus-specific cDNA. *J Clin Invest* 1991;87:1456–1461.

57

ASTROVIRUSES

SUZANNE M. MATSUI
DAVID KIANG

Astrovirus was first described in association with gastroenteritis in 1975 (1,2). Appleton and Higgins (1) examined fecal samples from 14 newborn infants with diarrhea and vomiting and visualized by electron microscopy (EM) 29- to 30-nm-diameter viral particles in the specimens from 8 babies. These particles differed morphologically from rotavirus and Norwalk virus and were subsequently confirmed to be astrovirus (3). In the same year, Madeley and Cosgrove (2) reported finding a 28-nm-diameter, small round virus with a distinctive surface structure in the stools of infants with diarrhea. This virus was named astrovirus for the characteristic five- or six-pointed star configuration that was evident on the surface of approximately 10% of the viral particles examined (4). A major breakthrough in the study of these viruses occurred in 1981 when Lee and Kurtz (5) demonstrated serial passage of astrovirus in cell culture with the use of trypsin. This enabled more detailed characterization of the virus, in terms of its epidemiology, pathogenesis, and its molecular biology. Astrovirus has emerged as a medically important pathogen with notable features (described later) and as such has now been assigned its own viral family, Astroviridae.

Eight serotypes of human astrovirus (HAstV-1 to HAstV-8) have been described (6–10). In addition, morphologically indistinguishable, but serologically distinct, astroviruses have been found by EM in the feces of cats (11), calves (12), deer (13), dogs (14), mice (15), pigs (16,17), lambs (18), turkeys (19–21), ducks (22), and chickens (23). Infection with astroviruses appears to be species specific (24), and as a consequence, no animal model for human infection currently exists. In general, astrovirus infection results in diarrhea, but fatal hepatitis in 3- to 6-week-old ducklings (22), nephritis in chicks (23), and enteritis associated with immunosuppression in turkey poults (19) have been reported.

S. M. Matsui: Department of Medicine, Stanford University School of Medicine, Stanford, California; Department of Gastroenterology, VA Palo Alto Health Care System, Palo Alto, California

D. Kiang: Genemed Biotechnologies, Inc., South San Francisco, California

ASTROVIRUS PHYSICAL FEATURES

To facilitate classification of small, round viruses found in feces, Caul and Appleton (3) proposed a scheme based on the physical and EM features of these viruses (Table 57.1). In this scheme, astroviruses comprise a unique subgroup of small, round viruses with surface structure, separate from other viruses such as the classic human caliciviruses and Norwalk virus (Fig. 57.1). Astroviruses visualized by EM display a smooth circular border, triangular surface hollows, and a characteristic five- or six-pointed surface star with a stain-displacing center that appears white on negatively stained preparations (4,25). Although the stellate surface configuration is its most distinct feature, it is not present on all particles (3,4) and may be obscured by antibody coating of viral aggregates in stool (24,26) or in preparations for immune EM (IEM) (27). "Bridging structures" between astrovirus particles are observed occasionally and may represent surface extensions of the virus (4,18). An array of surface spikes has been observed by EM and electron cryomicroscopy of purified preparations of cell culture-adapted

TABLE 57.1. PHYSICAL FEATURES

27–34-nm diameter, spherical, nonenveloped particles
Characteristic starlike surface appearance by direct electron microscopy
Smooth capsid with short spikes emanating from surface
Particles may be sensitive to cesium chloride, repeated freezing/thawing
Buoyant density: 1.35–1.38 g/mL (cesium chloride), 1.32 g/mL (potassium tartrate)
Single-stranded, plus-sense, poly(A)+, 6.8-kb RNA genome
2.4-kb, poly(A)+, subgenomic RNA produced during infection
M_r 87K structural protein produced in infected cells
Encoded by subgenomic RNA
Cleavage at R70 yields an M_r 79K capsid protein intracellularly
At least three smaller capsid proteins derived by trypsin cleavage
Eight serotypes by immune electron microscopy and enzyme immunoassay

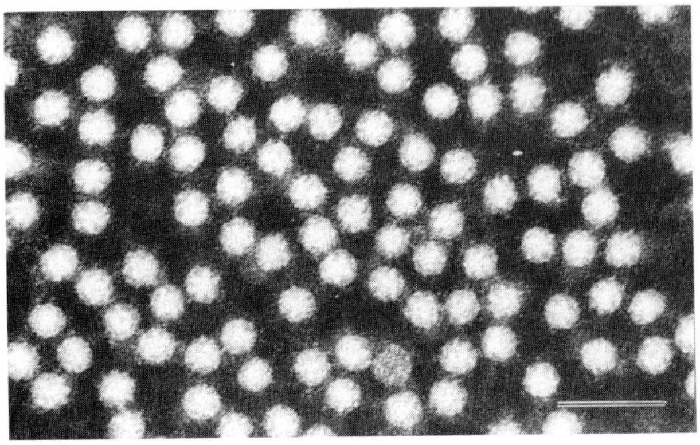

FIGURE 57.1. Astroviruses. Electron micrograph of astrovirus particles in a human fecal specimen. Bar marker represents 100 nm. (Courtesy of Dr. Charles D. Humphrey.)

human astroviruses, serotypes 2 and 1, respectively (28,29). The three-dimensional map generated by electron cryomicroscopy indicates viral particles consist of a solid capsid shell (330 Å in diameter) with 30 dimeric spikes (50 Å) protruding from the surface (29).

Astrovirus particles are stable at a pH of 3 and are chloroform resistant. Human astrovirus remains active after 5 minutes at 60°C but is inactivated after 10 minutes at that temperature (24). Characteristic astrovirus morphology is retained in infected fecal specimens that were stored at ultralow temperatures of −70°C to −85°C for 6 to 10 years (30). Repeated freezing and thawing, however, may disrupt the integrity of astrovirus particles.

The diameter of astrovirus particles varies depending on the species of origin and method of fixation. Average diameters in the range of 27 to 34 nm are reported. Madeley (25) systematically measured more than 1,000 negatively stained (3% potassium phosphotungstate) astroviruses from stool specimens of infected infants and found a mean viral diameter of 28 ± 1.6 nm. At the other end of the spectrum, bovine astrovirus 2, shed by experimentally infected gnotobiotic calves and prepared for EM with glutaraldehyde and 1% osmium tetroxide, ranged in diameter from 30 to 37 nm and averaged 34 nm (31).

Human astroviruses typically band at a buoyant density of 1.35 to 1.37 g/mL in cesium chloride (CsCl) (3,24,32). In outbreaks of astrovirus gastroenteritis at a school in Japan (33) and a convalescent home in the United States (34), the buoyant density of the astrovirus particles was slightly higher, 1.39 to 1.40 g/mL. In animal infections, buoyant densities of astrovirus have ranged from 1.34 g/mL in beagle pups (14) to 1.38 to 1.40 g/mL in lambs (35). Astrovirus morphology may be disrupted after viral particles are pelleted from a CsCl density gradient (36). Improved recovery of intact astrovirus particles from fecal extracts was reported using separation on a potassium tartrate glycerol density gradient, then concentration by pelleting. The buoyant density for human astrovirus in this medium was 1.32 g/mL (36).

In a description of human astrovirus adapted to growth in Caco-2 cells (see later discussion), Willcocks et al. (37) found astrovirus particles at two densities in a CsCl gradient. They speculated that the fraction with a density of 1.35 g/mL likely represented complete viral particles, whereas the fraction with a density of 1.32 g/mL possibly represented empty particles. The particles had identical polypeptide profiles, but no attempt was made to determine the nature of the nucleic acid contained within these particles. A similar observation was made by Matsui et al. (32) for astrovirus serotype 1 grown in LLCMK2 cells. Enzyme immunoassay (EIA) (38,39) performed on CsCl gradient fractions identified two peaks of astrovirus antigen activity, one at a density of 1.37 g/mL (major peak) and the other at 1.33 g/mL (minor peak). RNA extracted from the major peak fraction hybridized with probes from two different regions of the viral genome, whereas that extracted from the minor peak did not hybridize to either probe. This suggests that the lower density particles do not contain viral nucleic acid. These limited experiments do not suggest a subpopulation of viral particles containing subgenomic RNA only forms during infection, as is the case for the calicivirus, rabbit hemorrhagic disease virus (40).

MICROBIOLOGY

Growth In Cell Culture

The progress made in adapting human astroviruses to growth in cell culture parallels, to a large degree, the strides made in cultivating rotaviruses during the late 1970s (41,42). Both viruses are now cultivatable in continuous lines of monkey kidney epithelial cells, in the presence of trypsin. In rotaviruses, trypsin facilitates viral uncoating by cleaving the outer capsid protein VP-4. Although trypsin is definitely required for astrovirus infection to occur in cell culture, the mechanism by which trypsin influences viral infectivity is not fully understood at this time. A recent report by Bass and Qiu (43) suggests that the ability of trypsin to enhance viral infectivity is not due to an increase in cell binding.

Two years after the identification of astroviruses in human fecal specimens, Lee and Kurtz (44) described the detection of astrovirus antigen in primary cells by immunofluorescence. For these studies, primary human embryonic kidney (HEK) cells were incubated for 24 hours with 10% fecal extracts then were washed and fixed. The fixed cells were subsequently incubated with convalescent serum from an astrovirus-infected individual, followed by a sheep anti-human immunoglobulin conjugate. Specific fluorescence was detectable with the convalescent serum, but not with acute serum from the same person or convalescent serum that had been adsorbed with astrovirus-containing fecal extracts. Furthermore, convalescent serum from other individuals who had been ill with astrovirus gastroenteritis reacted specifically with infected HEK cells, as demonstrated by IEM and immunofluorescence.

In 1981, these investigators reported the successful serial passage of astrovirus in tissue culture with trypsin in the growth medium (5). Trypsin at a concentration of 10 μg/mL was reported to be the optimal concentration required for productive infection. Increasing the trypsin concentration to 50 μg/mL did not enhance viral growth. Lower trypsin concentrations, such as the 0.5-μg/mL concentration used for rotavirus propagation, were not sufficient for astrovirus. The greatest number of viral particles were detected in the cell-free supernatant of primary HEK cell monolayers after 48 hours of growth in trypsin-containing medium. Viral titers of 10^5 to 10^7/mL were observed. Primary baboon kidney (PBK) cells and a continuous line of LLCMK2 cells were infectible with astrovirus (originally from feces) after six passages in HEK cells, but direct inoculation of either PBK or LLCMK2 cells with fecal extracts was not successful. Viral yield was significantly reduced by diminishing the concentration of trypsin in the medium of LLCMK2 cells in which serial passage had been established. All five serotypes of astrovirus described by Kurtz and Lee (6,7) have been adapted to growth in LLCMK2 cells. Although cytopathic effect is not demonstrated easily in LLCMK2 cells, assays to quantify astrovirus infectivity and study viral neutralization have been developed for at least three serotypes (types 1, 2, and 5) (45).

A continuous line of human colon carcinoma (Caco-2) cells was used for direct infection with an astrovirus-containing fecal extract, isolate A88/2 (Newcastle), from a 1988 outbreak of gastroenteritis in the United Kingdom (37). Trypsin at a concentration of 5 μg/mL was required for growth of the virus. Cytopathic effect was apparent at 2 days postinfection and progressed substantially over the next 2 days. After five passages in Caco-2 cells, astrovirus particles were indistinguishable from astroviruses derived from feces. This provides an expedient way to adapt wild-type astroviruses to cell culture without first having to pass the virus in primary HEK cells. Cell culture-adapted reference strains, as well as human astrovirus, from fecal samples can also be propagated in a hepatoma cell line (PLC/PRF/5) (46). In addition, human astrovirus from clinical samples can be isolated in human intestinal cell line T84 (47). This study also found HAstV-1 to HAstV-7 could be propagated in Caco-2, T84, HT-29 (human intestinal cell line), and MA-104 (African green monkey kidney epithelial cells) cells, and nonprimate baby hamster kidney (BHK) cells supported passage of HAstV-2 (47). In a separate study (48), BHK cells supported astrovirus infection after transfection of genome-length HAstV-1 RNA transcripts.

Astrovirus Serotypes

Eight serotypes of human astrovirus have been identified by immunofluorescence and IEM (6–10). Each of the prototype (Oxford) strains was isolated from natural infections and adapted to growth in cell culture by Kurtz and Lee (5). In the Oxford region of the United Kingdom, where community-acquired strains of astrovirus were monitored between 1975 and 1987, serotype 1 emerged as the most common serotype found and accounted for 72%. Each of the other serotypes was responsible for 6% to 8% of the community-acquired astrovirus strains in this region. Similar results were obtained by other investigators (7,8,24, 49–59,123), although the predominant serotype may also be dependent on location (60).

Hyperimmune serum produced to each of the reference strains of human astrovirus appear to be largely serotype specific when used in immunofluorescence tests and IEM (24, 38). A monoclonal antibody (MAb) developed by Herrmann et al. (39) reacts with all eight serotypes of human astrovirus (8,). This nonneutralizing MAb is used in EIAs to detect astrovirus antigen (see later discussion and reference 39). The antibody is directed to a viral structural protein (61), most probably to an epitope located in the amine-terminus (N-terminus) half of the open reading frame 2 (ORF2) product (Geigenmüller and Matsui, *unpublished data*).

Molecular Biology And Genome Organization

The astrovirus genome consists of single-stranded, positive-sense RNA that is approximately 6,800 nucleotides long, excluding the poly(A) tail at the 3′ end. Of the eight astrovirus serotypes described (6–10), the complete nucleotide sequences of four serotypes (human astrovirus serotype 1, 2, 3, and 8) are now available (GenBank accession L23513, Z25771, L13745, AF141381, and AF260508). Two serotype 1 strains, the prototype Oxford strain adapted to growth in LLCMK2 cells and the Newcastle strain isolated and adapted to growth in Caco-2 cells, have been cloned and sequenced (62–64). A full-length complementary DNA (cDNA) clone of HAstV-1 from which infectious viral RNA can be transcribed has been described (48). The complete sequences of the reference Oxford serotype 2 astrovirus (65), a serotype 3 isolate (AF141381) and a Mexican serotype 8 strain (66) also have been reported. Complete capsid-encoding sequences of serotypes 4 to 7 (described later) are available as well (GenBank accession numbers AB025812, AB037274, Z46658, and Y08632). For other animal astroviruses, full genomic sequences of turkey and sheep astrovirus and avian nephritis virus are available (GenBank accession Y15937, AF206663, and AB033998).

During infection of susceptible cells, two populations of positive-sense astrovirus RNA that are co-terminal at the 3′ end are produced: (a) full-length, 6.8-kilobase (kb) genomic RNA and (b) a 2.4-kb subgenomic RNA (Fig. 57.2) (32,67). The astrovirus genome consists of three long ORFs. The 5′-most ORF, designated ORF1a by the International Committee on the Taxonomy of Viruses (ICTV) (68), is preceded in

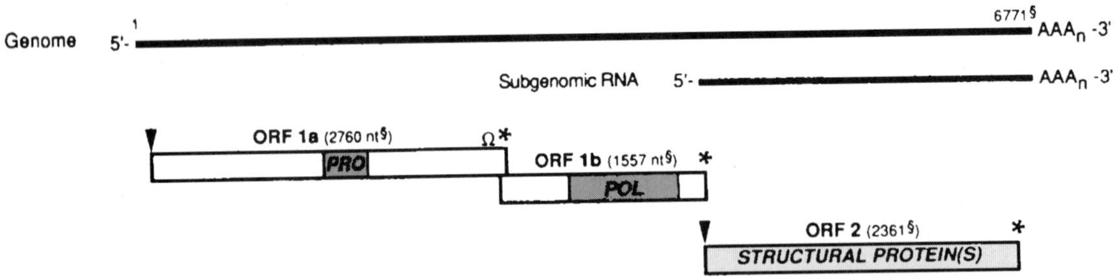

FIGURE 57.2. Genome organization for astrovirus serotype 1 (Oxford reference strain) is shown. Genome and open reading frame (ORF) lengths (shown in nucleotides *[nt]*) vary slightly, depending on the strain of astrovirus examined (§). For example, in another strain of serotype 1 astrovirus (Caco-2 cells adapted) (37), the genome is 6,813 nt, ORF1a is 2,808 nt, ORF1b is the same as shown, and ORF2 is 2,361 nt. For serotype 2 (Oxford reference strain), the genome is 6,797 nt, ORF1a and ORF1b are the same as shown, and ORF2 is 2391 nt (63). Shown are an *(arrowhead)* initiation codon and a *(asterisk)* termination codon. The ribosomal frameshift region is found toward the 3′ end of ORF1a (Ω). The locations of the protease (*PRO*) and RNA-dependent RNA polymerase (*POL*) motifs are shaded (▭).

human astrovirus by a 5′-untranslated region of 80 (serotype 8) to 85 (serotypes 1 and 3) nucleotides (nt). ORF1a ranges in length from 2,763 to 2,808 nt and overlaps the second ORF, designated ORF1b by 61 (serotype 3) to 73 nt (serotypes 1, 2, and 8). ORF1b is 1,548 nt (serotype 3) to 1,560 nt (serotypes 1, 2, and 8) in length (62,64,65) and overlaps the third 3′-most ORF, designated ORF2 by 8 nt. ORF2 is encoded in both genomic and subgenomic RNAs. Its length differs for each of the eight strains sequenced thus far, ranging from 2,316 (serotype 4) to 2,391 (Oxford serotype 2) (65) nt in length. The 3′-untranslated region consists of 80 (serotype 1) to 85 nt (serotype 5 and 8) that precede the poly(adenylic acid) (poly[A]) tail. General features of the 3′-untranslated region, such as distance to the poly(A) tail and predicted secondary structure, suggest similarities between astrovirus and picornaviruses (64). Conservation of the terminal 19 nt of ORF2 and the 3′-untranslated region was observed for all eight human astrovirus serotypes (69). Jonassen et al. (70) found that the 3′-noncoding region of infectious bronchitis virus and equine rhinovirus serotype 2 contained a motif similar both in sequence and folding to the second RNA stem loop in the 3′ end of human astrovirus genome. The presence of the same motif in astroviruses of sheep, pig, and turkey suggests that RNA recombination events have occurred (70).

Sequence analysis of the polypeptides encoded by the ORFs indicates that viral nonstructural proteins are encoded by ORFs 1a and 1b. ORF1a encodes a polypeptide of 920 (62,65) to 935 (64) aa that contains a viral serine protease motif, whereas ORF1b encodes a polypeptide of 515 (serotype 3) to 519 aa (serotype 1 [Oxford and Newcastle] and 2) that contains an RNA-dependent RNA polymerase motif. Sequences suggesting a nuclear localization signal and potential transmembrane helices have been found in ORF1a (65,71). The significance of these observations remains largely speculative, although recent studies have indicated that the nuclear localization signal is functional (72). A clear VPg domain has not been identified. The region between the putative transmembrane domain and the protease motif contains one serine at position 420 that may link the hypothetical astrovirus VPg to its genomic RNA (65).

Comparison of the complete nucleotide sequence of serotype 1 (Oxford strain) and the other serotypes sequenced to date indicates a homology of 81% (serotype 3) to 97% (serotype 1 Newcastle strain). The slight differences found between the two serotype 1 strains may be influenced by passage number and viral adaptation to different host cells. In astroviruses isolated in primary HEK cells, a 45-nt deletion in ORF1a was consistently observed, relative to fecal viruses or isolates from Caco-2 cells (73). The human astrovirus 3C-like serine protease and polymerase motifs are highly conserved among all serotypes for which sequence is available. Phylogenetic analysis (GrowTree, Genetics Computer Group, University of Wisconsin) of the known astrovirus protease motifs encoded by ORF1a groups the human motifs apart from the animal astrovirus motifs with the lowest level of relatedness between human and avian astroviruses (Fig. 57.3A). The phylogram of the astrovirus polymerase motifs also exhibits similar relationships (Fig. 57.3B). Analysis of the deduced amino acid sequences of the human astrovirus ORF1a product, of serotypes 1 to 8, by Belliot et al. (10) suggest the existence of two genogroups: A (types 1 to 5 and 8) and B (types 6 and 7). ORF1b and ORF2 sequences showed large and equal pair-wise distances between all eight serotypes (10).

The mechanism by which ORF1b is translated is not immediately evident from routine sequence analysis, because the first AUG codon occurs at nt 454 to 456 of ORF1b and is in a suboptimal context for initiation according to Kozak's rules (74). With more detailed analysis, however, it has been possible to identify highly conserved sequences (in three available astrovirus serotypes that were examined) that strongly suggest a (−1) ribosomal frameshifting mechanism

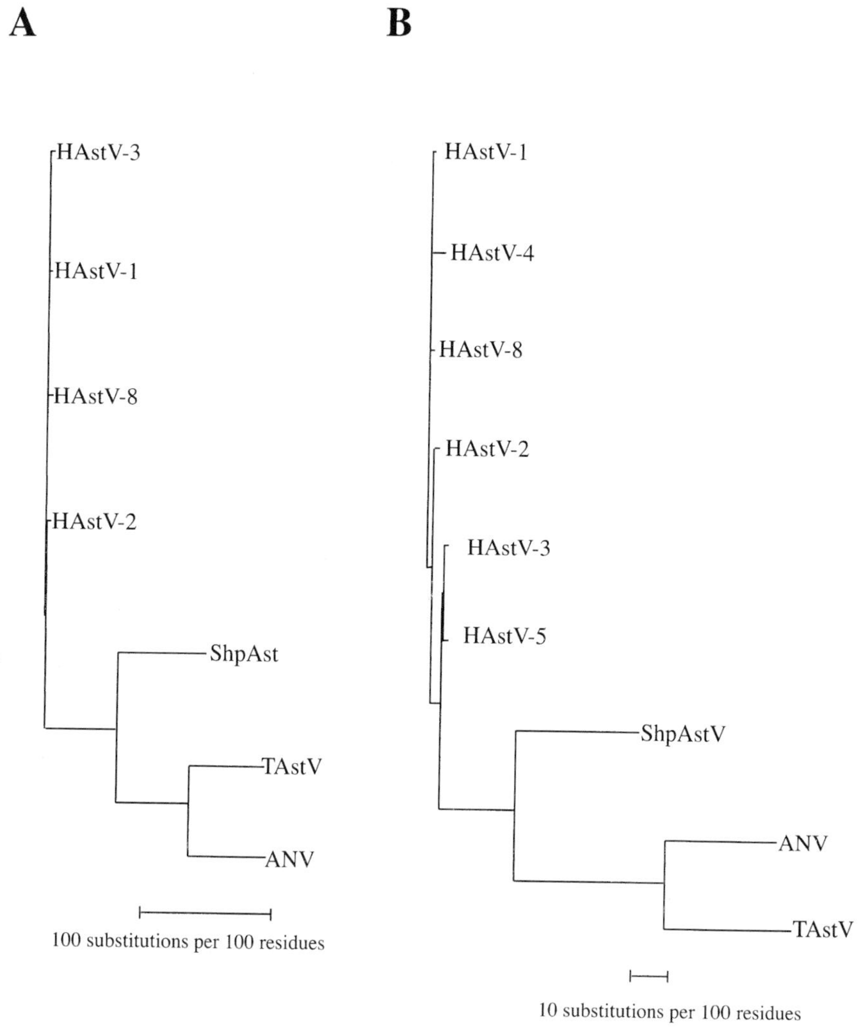

FIGURE 57.3. Phylogenetic analysis of deduced amino acid sequences of the 3C-like serine protease **(A)** and RNA-dependent RNA polymerase **(B)** motifs of various astroviruses (human astroviruses [*HAst-V-1 to 5, and 8*]), avian nephritis virus (*ANV*), turkey astrovirus (*TAstV*), and sheep astrovirus (*ShpAstV*) using the GrowTree program of the GCG software package (SeqWeb version 1.2, Wisconsin Package version 10.1).

for translation of ORF1b (62,64,65). These sequences include a heptameric shift sequence (A AAA AAC) and downstream stem-loop structure that resembles the required elements for the translation of retrovirus protease and polymerase (75–78) and coronavirus polymerase (79).

Currently, the processing of the astrovirus nonstructural proteins is not well understood. Gibson et al. (80) observed a lack of processing of the full-length ORF1a and ORF1a/1b products expressed using an *in vitro* system (80). Willcocks et al. (72) identified products with relative molecular masses (M_r) of 160, 75, 34, 20, 6.5, and 5.5K in infected Caco-2 cells by Western analysis using antibodies directed toward the end of the ORF1a protein product (aa 643 to 940) (72). Antibodies to an ORF1b protein detected products with an M_r of 160 and 59K, suggesting possible processing at the boundary of the ORF1a/1b polyprotein. A separate report that examines processing of the ORF1a product in an *in vitro* system with immunoprecipitation by N-terminus and carboxyl terminus (C-terminus)-specific antibodies identified the full-length M_r 101K product (p101) and the N-terminus and C-terminus cleavage products, p64 and p38, respectively. Mutations of the catalytic triad (Ser-551, Asp-489, and His-461) and deletion analysis suggest that processing is mediated by the 3C-like serine protease encoded by ORF1a (81). Expression of ORF1a in a vaccinia virus infection–transfection system suggests that p64 is being further processed in cells (82).

Because ORF2 is encoded by both the genomic and subgenomic RNA, it was hypothesized that ORF2 encodes a structural protein (83). Other viruses, such as the enveloped alphaviruses, use their subgenomic RNA to produce large quantities of the structural proteins that are required for assembly of intact progeny viruses (84). The role of the astrovirus subgenomic RNA was proved by immunoprecipitation of the M_r 87K ORF2 product (Oxford serotype 1) with antibodies produced to purified astrovirus particles (62). This protein is likely the precursor of the three to five M_r 20 to 40K structural proteins that were identified in earlier analyses of human and animal astroviruses (see later discussion and references 62 and 67).

The astrovirus genome is thus organized with nonstructural proteins encoded by the 5′-end ORFs 1a and 1b and a structural protein by ORF2 at the 3′ end. Although this general genome organization is similar to that found in caliciviruses (85), some of the key features that distinguish astroviruses from caliciviruses include the size and number of structural proteins and the strategies used to translate the viral RNA-dependent RNA polymerase as well as the M_r 87K structural protein. Based on these distinctive characteristics, astroviruses have been classified in a new, separate viral family, the Astroviridae (68,83).

Structural Proteins

The size and number of astrovirus structural proteins described have varied from study to study. To date, the polypeptide profiles of ovine, porcine, and several serotypes of human astrovirus have been examined. Ovine astrovirus was studied first. Herring et al. (35) purified astrovirus particles shed by experimentally infected lambs and found two polypeptides that migrated at an M_r of about 33K. Five proteins have been described for porcine astrovirus. They range in mass from 13 to 39K (17). The studies of human astrovirus have been done on tissue culture-adapted strains of the virus. Kurtz and Lee (24) described four proteins with M_r of 36.5, 34, 33, and 32K for astrovirus serotype 4 that was grown in cell culture in the presence of trypsin. They postulated that the faint M_r 36.5K band might be a precursor protein that is processed to one of the smaller proteins, in a manner analogous to the enterovirus VP0 protein (86). In a later report, Kurtz (87) identified two additional proteins (M_r = 24 and 5.2K) in astrovirus serotype 1-infected cells. Willcocks et al. (37) studied the astrovirus-specific polypeptides in Caco-2 cells infected with purified astrovirus (serotype 1). Three proteins with M_r of 33.5, 31.5, and 24K were consistently detected in purified astrovirus particles by astrovirus serotype 1-specific antiserum. The M_r 24K polypeptide was sensitive to treatment with sodium dodecyl sulfate and was hypothesized to be a protein that is not securely attached to the viral particle. An additional M_r 27K polypeptide was seen in some preparations, and it was suggested that this may be a proteolytic digestion product of one of the larger proteins. In studies of astrovirus serotype 5 (Marin County strain [34]) proteins, a single structural protein with an M_r of 30K was immunoprecipitated.

Monroe et al. (67) used a different approach to examine the protein composition of astrovirus particles. Protein synthesis in astrovirus-infected LLCMK2 cells was examined in the absence of trypsin. With this strategy, a single protein with an M_r of about 90K was immunoprecipitated from infected cell lysates. If the infected cell lysates were pretreated with trypsin, a predominant M_r 29K protein and two other proteins (M_r 31 and 20K) were immunoprecipitated. This suggested that the protein with an M_r of about 90K might be a precursor protein that is proteolytically cleaved to yield the smaller proteins described in previous studies. In cells infected with HAstV-1 in a virtually trypsin-free environment, Bass and Qiu (88) detected an M_r 87K capsid protein that was rapidly converted to an M_r 79K product that was incorporated into viral particles. The addition of trypsin resulted in viral capsid proteins of M_r 34, 29, and 26K and enhanced infectivity of the virus (88). In LLCMK2 cells infected with human astrovirus (serotype 2) grown in media containing trypsin, Sanchez-Fauquier et al. (89) detected a major M_r 26K (VP26) and a minor M_r 29K (VP29) capsid protein using a neutralizing MAb (PL-2). In addition, several intermediate-sided proteins (p74-p35) were also identified (89). These proteins were believed to be derived from an M_r 86K precursor.

Belliot et al. (61) analyzed partially purified reference strains of human astrovirus (serotypes 1 to 7). Based on immunoprecipitation with homologous rabbit serum, three proteins, P1, P2, and P3 (Mr 25-33K), were identified in serotypes 1 to 4 and only P2 and P3 in serotypes 5 to 7 (61).

EPIDEMIOLOGY

Role In Disease

Astrovirus infections occur worldwide, as evidenced by reports from far-reaching parts of the globe (1,2,33,36,37, 49,50,52,55,57,60,90–128). These infections may be community acquired (97,98,124,128,129) or nosocomial (1,2, 36,94,95,98,99,119,120,127–130) (Table 57.2). Although astrovirus, like rotavirus, primarily causes disease in young children, it is also a cause of outbreaks of gastroenteritis among elderly patients (103,131–133), immunocompromised adults (92,96,134,135), and military recruits (125). Peak incidence is in the winter months in temperate regions (91,101,106,136) and in the rainy season in tropical areas (93), similar to human rotavirus infections. Viral transmission occurs through the fecal-oral route with spread via person-to-person contacts, contaminated food or water, and possibly fomites (24,137–144). The virus has also been found in sludge biosolids (140).

TABLE 57.2. EPIDEMIOLOGIC FEATURES

Worldwide distribution
Primarily a pediatric pathogen
Outbreaks in elderly and immunocompromised patients also
Antibody acquisition in childhood
Antibody prevalence 75% by age 10 y
Antibody to serotypes 1–5 in U.S. gamma globulin pools
Serotype 1 is generally most common
Fecal-oral transmission (person-to-person, contaminated food/water, ?fomites)
Peak incidence in winter in northern temperate regions

The true incidence of astrovirus gastroenteritis and its role in disease have been difficult to assess for various reasons. Astrovirus gastroenteritis is generally a mild, self-limiting illness that does not routinely lead to hospitalization, extensive outpatient evaluation, or clinic visits. The virus may be difficult to detect by EM because only about 10% of the viral particles exhibit the characteristic starlike ultrastructure. Newer detection methods have been devised (38,39,105,145) but have only recently been implemented.

Herrmann et al. (38,39) developed an EIA for detecting astrovirus antigen in fecal specimens. The EIA uses an MAb as a capture antibody that recognizes all eight serotypes of astrovirus and rabbit polyclonal antiserum as the detector antibody (39). With this EIA, they performed controlled studies in Thailand (97) to determine the incidence of astrovirus gastroenteritis in a pediatric outpatient setting and its importance as a pathogen, relative to rotavirus and enteric adenovirus. Rotavirus, as expected, was the most frequently detected viral pathogen and was found in 19% of patients with gastroenteritis. Astrovirus was the second most frequently detected virus, found in 8.6% of patients with diarrhea. Enteric adenovirus was found in only 2.6% of these patients with diarrhea. In a similar study of rural Guatemalan children, astrovirus was found in 7.3% of those with diarrhea (93). A study in Australia showed that astrovirus is the second leading cause of gastroenteritis in children (55). In addition, during a prospective study of oral poliovirus immunogenicity in Mayan infants, astrovirus was identified as the most common enteric pathogen in diarrheic stool samples (50). These findings are in contrast to hospital-based EM studies that indicate enteric adenovirus is the second most common cause of viral diarrhea in young children and typically quote the incidence of astrovirus diarrhea to be in the 1% to 4% range (58, 91, 101).

Adult volunteer studies have helped to evaluate astrovirus pathogenicity. The first study (146), conducted in the United Kingdom, administered fecal extracts containing astrovirus from a child to eight adults who had little or no astrovirus-specific antibody at entry. Only one volunteer developed overt illness. Fecal filtrates containing large numbers of astrovirus from this individual were administered to nine other volunteers. Five of the nine developed mild symptoms, but no vomiting or diarrhea. Of the 17 volunteers in the two phases of the study, viral shedding was documented in four, with the largest number of viral particles shed by the most symptomatic volunteer. In 16 of the volunteers, seroconversion was demonstrated in 13 by immunofluorescence and in 10 by IEM.

A second study (34) by investigators in the United States administered serotype 5 astrovirus (from an outbreak at a northern California elderly care facility) to 19 adult volunteers. One of the volunteers became ill on days 5 to 6 and had a serologic response, whereas seven others developed a serologic response only. These studies demonstrate that astrovirus, unlike Norwalk virus, is of relatively low pathogenicity in adults.

Antibody Prevalence

Antibody to human astrovirus has been found in γ-globulin pools from the United States (136), Japan (33), and other regions of the world (59,147), indicating that astrovirus infection is common. Detecting these astrovirus infections, however, is a more difficult task (see earlier discussion).

Antibody acquisition occurs in early childhood in most cases (148). In a survey of 87 children younger than 10 years in Oxford, United Kingdom, Kurtz and Lee (149) found that antibody prevalence increases from 7% in 6- to 12-month-old infants to 70% by the time children enter school. Seventy-five percent of children age 10 years had such antibodies, a level comparable to that found in nursing students (77%) who were concurrently tested. Other surveys of seroprevalence according to serotype found rates of (a) 86% (serotype 1), 1% (type 2), 8% (type 3), and 6% (type 4) in the United Kingdom (53); (b) 91% (type 1 neutralizing antibodies), 31% (type 2), 69% (type 3), 56% (type 4), 36% (type 5), 16% (type 6), and 10% (type 7) in the Netherlands (123); and (c) 94% (type 1) and 42% (type 3) in the United States (117).

The characteristics of immunity to astrovirus are not well understood. Symptomatic astrovirus infection involves primarily two age-groups, young children and elderly patients, suggesting that antibody acquired in childhood may afford protection from illness during early adulthood. In one volunteer study (146), those with detectable anti-astrovirus antibody in serum did not develop diarrhea after ingesting the inoculum. Studies by Wilson and Cubitt (59) demonstrated both immunoglobulin M (IgM) and immunoglobulin G (IgG) responses to serotype 1 astrovirus in a volunteer infected with the Marin County agent, a serotype 5 astrovirus. They speculated that the anamnestic response observed in this individual was due to prior infection with astrovirus serotype 1 and the antigenic relatedness of these two serotypes.

Importance of the mucosal defense against recurrent astrovirus infections was demonstrated when normal small intestinal biopsy specimens were challenged in an organ culture system with inactivated human astrovirus. Upon viral challenge, human astrovirus-specific CD4+ T cells, which produced Th1-type cytokines were isolated. This suggests that these cells may be dispersed throughout the lamina propria, conferring protective immunity to recurrent astrovirus infections (150). The importance of CD4+ T cells is also suggested by reports of patients developing astrovirus infection after treatment with fludarabine monophosphate, which significantly decreases the CD4+ T cell count (134,151). In another report, the production of CD16+ and CD8+ T cells in a patient with prolonged viral shedding correlated with decreased levels of viral shedding, suggesting that several types of T cells participate in controlling infection (152). The specifics of immunity to astrovirus infection and the determinants of astrovirus infectivity require further investigation.

VIRAL PATHOGENESIS

Astrovirus pathogenesis in humans is not well studied. In the only study reported to date, astrovirus shedding in diarrheal feces was correlated with the visualization of astrovirus particles in intestinal epithelial cells by EM (153). This suggests that the intestine is the site of viral replication in humans. Small intestinal biopsy from one of the patients demonstrated astrovirus in epithelial cells located in the lower part of the villus. In the other patient, astrovirus was found in "exposed" surface epithelial cells. Both children described in this report had a history of gastrointestinal problems including chronic diarrhea, sucrase-isomaltase deficiency or cow's milk sensitive enteropathy, and prior shedding of *Escherichia coli* O86 or rotavirus in the stool. Neither of the human volunteer studies (described earlier) (34,146) were designed to examine histologic effects of the infection.

Viral pathogenesis has been studied more extensively in lambs and calves. Gnotobiotic lambs infected with an outbreak strain of ovine astrovirus developed illness on day 4 and shed astrovirus in feces from day 3 to day 9 postinoculation (18,154,155). Histologic examination of the intestines indicated that only mature enterocytes and subepithelial macrophages in the small intestine were infected and resulted in transient villus atrophy and crypt hypertrophy. Some enterocytes contained aggregates of virus particles along the microvilli and in lysosomes and autophagic vacuoles. Other enterocytes demonstrated only indirect evidence of infection such as intracytoplasmic inclusions, vacuoles, and degenerate nuclei.

Bovine astroviruses are antigenically distinct from ovine astroviruses (156). Although bovine astroviruses may be one of several groups of small, round viruses isolated from feces of calves with diarrhea, they are generally considered nonpathogenic because inoculation with bovine astrovirus alone does not result in diarrhea in gnotobiotic calves (12,157). Bovine astroviruses, in contrast to ovine astroviruses, preferentially infect M cells and absorptive enterocytes overlying the dome villi of small intestinal Peyer patches (12,158). When bovine astrovirus infection accompanies infection with bovine rotavirus or Breda virus 2, more severe diarrhea (than with either virus alone), more extensive infection of the dome epithelial cells, and an active inflammatory reaction are noted (12).

Viral Infection in Cell Culture Systems

Given the above observations, it seems reasonable to expect that astroviruses enter cells through the apical surface. However, in polarized Caco-2 cells, wild-type human astroviruses appear to enter through the basolateral surface (37). Willcocks et al. (71) have suggested that this may be an artifact of the cell culture system and that differentiated intestinal epithelial cells may well have receptors for astrovirus infection on the apical surface.

Entry of astrovirus has also been studied in Graham 293 cells, a transformed line of primary human embryonal kidney cells (159). Graham 293 cell monolayers were infected with astrovirus serotype 1 and treated with lysosomotropic agents (ammonium chloride, methylamine, dansylcadaverine) or the ionophore monensin. These agents inhibited the early stages of infection, distal to viral attachment to the cell membrane, and did not appear to have a direct virucidal effect. In these experiments, all the chemicals at nontoxic levels inhibited viral infection, suggesting that the endocytic pathway may be critical to delivery of the astrovirus genome into the cytoplasm. Ultrastructural analysis corroborated these biochemical results. Viral particles were found attached at various sites on the cell membrane, and after about 10 minutes, they were internalized by membrane invagination at coated pits. After about 30 minutes, larger smooth vacuoles containing multiple viral particles were observed. In other studies, flavonoids that inhibit early steps in picornavirus replication have been shown to inhibit astrovirus antigen synthesis in LLCMK2 cells in a dose-dependent fashion (160). The precise mechanism by which these chemicals act in astrovirus infection is not known.

A cell culture model of bovine astrovirus infection also has been achieved. In this system, bovine astrovirus serotype 2 (US2) was adapted to growth in primary neonatal bovine kidney (NBK) cells in the presence of 50 μg/mL of trypsin (31). By using immunofluorescent probes to track the expression of viral antigens, the following was observed. The first indication of viral infection and production of viral antigens was at 7 hours postinfection when viral antigen was observed in the cytoplasm. Soon thereafter, two or three brilliant immunofluorescent granules were seen in the nucleus, in a pattern that suggested nucleolar involvement. Subsequently, dense immunofluorescent granules were seen in the perinuclear region of the cytoplasm, followed by diffuse cytoplasmic staining. Typically about 2%, and occasionally 10% to 20%, of the cells were infected when administered an inoculum with a multiplicity of infection (MOI) level of more than 1. The role of the nucleus and nucleoli in astrovirus replication is not known. Because astrovirus infection was not inhibited by the addition of the DNA transcription inhibitor, these investigators concluded that either the nucleoli are not affected by actinomycin D or they are not essential for viral replication.

CLINICAL ILLNESS

Astrovirus gastroenteritis is primarily a disease that affects pediatric populations throughout the world (Table 57.3).

Its medical importance was established when it was shown to be the second most common viral agent in young children with diarrhea who were evaluated in an outpatient setting (97). Although serotype 1 appears to be the most common human astrovirus (24,59), severe infections with astrovirus serotype 4 have been noted in young adults (9). Acquisition of serotype 5 antibodies may occur later in life than antibodies for serotypes 1 to 4 (123).

The incubation period determined by adult human volunteer studies is 3 to 4 days (34,146). A shorter incubation period of 24 to 36 hours was extrapolated from the secondary spread characteristics during an outbreak of gastroenteritis in a kindergarten (33). In general, the illness caused by human astrovirus consists of a mild, watery diarrhea, 2 to 3 days in duration, with vomiting, fever, anorexia, abdominal pain, and various constitutional symptoms that last about 4 days (24,26,136,161,162). Diarrhea lasting 7 to 14 days and prolonged viral shedding occur in some individuals (24). In children, the diarrhea due to astrovirus may be indistinguishable from that due to rotavirus (24,93), but it is frequently milder (99,128). Astrovirus diarrhea typically does not cause significant dehydration and may result in fewer hospitalizations (97). Certain patients may develop prolonged lactose intolerance (94,99, 128). Deaths associated with astrovirus infection are rare but have been reported (163).

The significance of astrovirus infection in immunocompromised patients remains controversial. In a case–control study of HIV-infected individuals with diarrhea (96), astrovirus was found in 13 (12%) of 109 fecal specimens from 65 patients with diarrhea and 2 (2%) of 113 fecal specimens from 65 controls without diarrhea. Seven different types of viruses were identified in 35% of patients with diarrhea; single agents were detected in most cases, and bacteria and parasite detections were far less common. In a similar study of bone marrow transplant recipients with diarrhea (92), an enteric pathogen was found in 13% of cases. Among the enteric pathogens, astrovirus was identified most frequently and accounted for 7 (4.7%) of 150 episodes of diarrhea. In these patients, diarrhea developed in the hospital between days 21 and 65 and lasted 2 to 31 days. In a separate case (24), a child with combined immunodeficiency developed chronic astrovirus diarrhea with viral shedding for more than 4 months after undergoing bone marrow transplantation. This illness persisted until the child's death. In contrast, astrovirus was not correlated with diarrhea in studies of HIV-infected patients in Venezuela (164) and Argentina (165) or in those with AIDS in Venezuela (121).

TABLE 57.3. CLINICAL FEATURES

Incubation period: 3–4 d
Duration of illness: 1–4 d
Self-limiting disease in otherwise healthy individuals
  May be prolonged in immunocompromised patients
Signs and symptoms: watery diarrhea, anorexia, fever, vomiting
Symptomatic infection in young children, elderly patients, and immunocompromised individuals

DIAGNOSIS

Traditionally, direct EM has been the cornerstone of astrovirus detection in fecal specimens. Patients with acute astrovirus diarrhea have been noted to shed as many as 10^{10} virus particles per milliliter (or 10^8 viable particles) (24). IEM has also been described for the detection of astrovirus and the evaluation of immune responses (33,166,167). This technique may be useful in evaluating specimens that contain fewer viral particles or may help to establish etiology if paired acute and convalescent sera are available.

Although the virus has distinctive surface features (described earlier), only about 10% of the particles display these features, and identification may require an experienced microscopist (168). A retrospective study of fecal viruses, previously identified as small, round featureless viruses (SRVs) by EM alone, revealed that many of the viruses had been misclassified (169). By using complementary techniques, these investigators found that astroviruses, in particular, were prone to misclassification. Fourteen (26%) of 53 SRV samples were shown to be astrovirus by careful reexamination of the morphologic features and IEM with convalescent human serum, as well as astrovirus serotype 1-specific rabbit antiserum. Two caliciviruses and one Norwalk-like virus were also found to be misclassified. Another example of misclassification is the Marin County virus, which was isolated from a nursing home outbreak in 1981 and initially identified as a "Norwalk-like" virus (132). It was later proved to be an astrovirus (170,171) and is now considered to be an astrovirus serotype 5 prototype strain.

An EIA that uses a group reactive MAB (8E7) to capture viral antigen and polyclonal antiserum as the detector antibody has been developed by Herrmann et al. (38,39). A biotinylated detector antibody has been incorporated into the modified EIA described by Moe et al. (105). Both EIAs have comparable sensitivity (91%) and specificity (98%) when compared with IEM. Several studies have relied on these tests for rapid identification of astrovirus infection (93,97,102,105). A commercial EIA based on MAb 8E7 was found to have a sensitivity of 100% and a specificity of 98.6% when tested in Australia (172).

Detection strategies using molecular probes and reverse transcriptase polymerase chain reaction (RT-PCR) have also been described (105,112,145,173–175). Complete sequence information of five astrovirus strains, representing four serotypes, is available (see earlier discussion). Primers derived from the 3′ end of the genome reportedly have been successful in amplifying astrovirus-specific products from five reference serotypes (83). Other primers derived from the RNA-dependent RNA polymerase motif are also suitable candidates for RT-PCR amplification of different human astrovirus serotypes (62). Good correlation has been observed when RT-PCR was used to confirm EIA diagnosis of astrovirus (50,92,96,104).

Regions encoding immunoreactive viral epitopes may be important in the future development of recombinant antigens and more specifically targeted antibodies that can be produced in large quantities. Although tests to detect astrovirus antibody may be useful in epidemiologic investigations, tests that rapidly and accurately identify astrovirus antigen are likely to be preferable in the clinical setting.

TREATMENT AND PREVENTION

Astrovirus gastroenteritis is generally a mild, self-limiting illness that may disrupt one's normal activities for a few days but does not require specific therapy. Dehydration, requiring fluid resuscitation, may develop in those patients with underlying gastrointestinal disease, poor nutritional status, severe mixed infection, or prolonged illness (24,93).

To prevent astrovirus infection, its transmission must be interrupted. This is particularly important in hospitals and other institutions, day care centers, and families in which person-to-person transmission is likely to occur. Strict implementation of universal hygienic procedures is essential. The virus is relatively resistant to alcohols, including isopropanol, ethanol, and methanol (176). Of these alcohols, methanol was shown to be the most effective in reducing astrovirus infectivity. Seventy percent methanol reduced astrovirus infectivity by 3 log_{10}, whereas 90% methanol reduced viral titers to less than 10 infective units per milliliter.

For food handlers, it is important to keep in mind that viral shedding in feces may begin a day before symptoms and continue for several days after diarrhea resolves. A rapid diagnostic test that detects astrovirus in stool may be useful in this setting. Careful selection and preparation of foods that have been implicated in outbreaks of astrovirus gastroenteritis, such as shellfish, are advisable.

The feasibility of developing a vaccine to prevent astrovirus illness has not been fully evaluated. Recent epidemiologic studies have demonstrated the medical importance of astrovirus. More work is required to understand the fundamentals of immunity to astrovirus (147).

SUMMARY

Astrovirus gastroenteritis is largely a disease of childhood but is also found among immunocompromised individuals and elderly institutionalized patients. Human astrovirus, a member of the viral family Astroviridae, has many unique characteristics that range from its ultrastructural appearance to its strategies for viral protein expression. As our ability to detect this virus has improved, it has been possible to establish its medical importance, identify outbreaks due to this agent, and study its cellular localization. Important information regarding viral replication and morphogenesis, as well as mechanisms of immunity, remain to be elucidated.

REFERENCES

1. Appleton H, Higgins PG. Viruses and gastroenteritis in infants. *Lancet* 1975;1:1297.
2. Madeley CR, Cosgrove BP. Viruses in infantile gastroenteritis. *Lancet* 1975;2:124.
3. Caul EO, Appleton H. The electron microscopical and physical characteristics of small round human fecal viruses: an interim scheme for classification. *J Med Virol* 1982;9:257–265.
4. Madeley CR, Cosgrove BP. 28 nm particles in faeces in infantile gastroenteritis. *Lancet* 1975;2:451–452.
5. Lee TW, Kurtz JB. Serial propagation of astrovirus in tissue culture with the aid of trypsin. *J Gen Virol* 1981;57:421–424.
6. Lee TW, Kurtz JB. Human astrovirus serotypes. *J Hyg (Camb)* 1982;89:539–540.
7. Kurtz JB, Lee TW. Human astrovirus serotypes. *Lancet* 1984;2:1405.
8. Lee TW, Kurtz JB. Prevalence of human astrovirus serotypes in the Oxford region 1976–92, with evidence for two new serotypes. *Epidemiol Infect* 1994;112:187–193.
9. Cubitt WD. Human, small round structured viruses, caliciviruses and astroviruses. *Baillieres Clin Gastroenterol* 1990;4:643–656.
10. Belliot G, Lee T, Kurtz JL, et al. Protein and genetic characterization of an astrovirus type 8. In: *Abstracts of the American Society for Virology Meeting.* Amherst, MA: American Society for Virology, 1999:176.
11. Hoshino Y, Zimmer JF, Moise NS, et al. Detection of astroviruses in faeces of a cat with diarrhea. *Arch Virol* 1981;70:373–376.
12. Woode GN, Bridger JC. Isolation of small viruses resembling astroviruses and caliciviruses from acute enteritis of calves. *J Med Microbiol* 1978;11:441–452.
13. Tzipori S, Menzies JD, Gray EW. Detection of astroviruses in the faeces of red deer. *Vet Rec* 1981;108:286.
14. Williams FP. Astrovirus-like, coronavirus-like, and parvovirus-like particles detected in the diarrheal stools of beagle pups. *Arch Virol* 1980;66:216–226.
15. Kjeldsberg E, Hem A. Detection of astroviruses in gut contents of nude and normal mice. *Arch Virol* 1985;84:135–140.
16. Bridger JC. Detection by electron microscope of caliciviruses, astroviruses and rotavirus-like particles in the faeces of piglets with diarrhea. *Vet Rec* 1980;107:532–533.
17. Shimizu M, Shirai J, Narita M, et al. Cytopathic astrovirus isolated from porcine acute gastroenteritis in an established cell line derived from porcine embryonic kidney. *J Clin Microbiol* 1990;28:201–206.
18. Snodgrass DR, Gray EW. Detection and transmission of 30 nm virus particles (astroviruses) in faeces of lambs with diarrhea. *Arch Virol* 1977;55:287–291.
19. Reynolds DL, Saif YM. Astrovirus: a cause of an enteric disease in turkey poults. *Avian Dis* 1986;30:728–735.
20. McNulty MS, Curran WL, McFerran JB. Detection of astroviruses in turkey faeces by direct electron microscopy. *Vet Rec* 1980;106:561.
21. Koci MD, Seal BS, Schultz-Cherry S. Molecular characterization of an avian astrovirus. *J Virol* 2000;74:6173–6177.
22. Gough RE, Collins MS, Borland E, et al. Astrovirus-like particles associated with hepatitis in ducklings. *Vet Rec* 1984;114:279.

23. Imada T, Yamaguchi S, Mase M, et al. Avian nephritis virus (ANV) as a new member of the family Astroviridae and construction of infectious ANV cDNA. *J Virol* 2000;74:8487–8493.
24. Kurtz JB, Lee TW. Astroviruses: human and animal. In: Bock G, Whelan J, eds. *Novel diarrhea viruses.* Ciba Foundation Symposium 128. Chichester: Wiley, 1987:92–107.
25. Madeley C. Comparison of the features of astroviruses and caliciviruses seen in samples of feces by electron microscopy. *J Infect Dis* 1979;139:519–523.
26. Kurtz J, Cubitt WD. Astroviruses and caliciviruses. In: Farthing MJG, Keusch GT, eds. *Enteric infection: mechanisms, manifestations, and management.* New York: Raven Press, 1989:205–215.
27. Ashley CR, Caul EO, Paver WK. Astrovirus-associated gastroenteritis in children. *J Clin Pathol* 1978;31:939–943.
28. Risco C, Carrascosa JL, Pedregosa AM, et al. Ultrastructure of human astrovirus serotype 2. *J Gen Virol* 1995;76:2075–2080.
29. Yeager M, Tihova M, Nowotny N, et al. Icosahedral design of human astrovirus. 2001 *(submitted).*
30. Williams FP Jr. Electron microscopy of stool-shed viruses: retention of characteristic morphologies after long-term storage at ultralow temperatures. *J Med Virol* 1989;29:192–195.
31. Aroonprasert D, Fagerland JA, Kelso NE, et al. Cultivation and partial characterization of bovine astrovirus. *Vet Microbiol* 1989; 19:113–125.
32. Matsui SM, et al. Cloning and characterization of human astrovirus immunoreactive epitopes. *J Virol* 1993;67:1712–1715.
33. Konno T, Suzuki H, Ishida N, et al. Astrovirus-associated epidemic gastroenteritis in Japan. *J Med Virol* 1982;9:11–17.
34. Midthun K, Greenberg HB, Kurtz JB, et al. Characterization and seroepidemiology of a type 5 astrovirus associated with an outbreak of gastroenteritis in Marin County, California. *J Clin Microbiol* 1993;31:955–962.
35. Herring AJ, Gray EW, Snodgrass DR. Purification and characterization of ovine astrovirus. *J Gen Virol* 1981;53:47–55.
36. Ashley CR, Caul EO. Potassium tartrate-glycerol as a density gradient substrate for separation of small, round viruses from human feces. *J Clin Microbiol* 1982;16:377–381.
37. Willcocks MM, Carter MJ, Laidler FR, et al. Growth and characterisation of human faecal astrovirus in a continuous cell line. *Arch Virol* 1990;113:73–81.
38. Herrmann JE, Hudson RW, Perron-Henry DM, et al. Antigenic characterization of cell-cultivated astrovirus serotypes and development of astrovirus-specific monoclonal antibodies. *J Infect Dis* 1988;158:182–185.
39. Herrmann JE, Nowak NA, Perron-Henry DM, et al. Diagnosis of astrovirus gastroenteritis by antigen detection with monoclonal antibodies. *J Infect Dis* 1990;161:226–229.
40. Meyers G, Wirblich C, Thiel H-J. Genomic and subgenomic RNAs of rabbit hemorrhagic disease virus are both protein-linked and packaged into particles. *Virology* 1991;184:677–686.
41. Banatvala JE, Totterdell BM, Chrystie IL, et al. *In vitro* detection of human rotaviruses. *Lancet* 1975;2:821.
42. Graham DY, Estes MK. Proteolytic enhancement of rotavirus infectivity: biologic mechanisms. *Virology* 1980;101:432–439.
43. Bass DM, Qiu SQ. Trypsin activation of astrovirus does not enhance target cell binding. In: *Abstracts of the American Society for Virology Meeting.* Fort Collins, CO: American Society for Virology, 2000:81.
44. Lee TW, Kurtz JB. Astroviruses detected by immunofluorescence [Letter]. *Lancet* 1977;2:406.
45. Hudson RW, Herrmann JE, Blacklow NR. Plaque quantitation and virus neutralization assays for human astroviruses. *Arch Virol* 1989;108:33–38.
46. Taylor MB, Grabow WO, Cubitt WD. Propagation of human astrovirus in the PLC/PRF/5 hepatoma cell line. *J Virol Methods* 1997;67:13–18.
47. Brinker JP, Blacklow NR, Herrmann JE. Human astrovirus isolation and propagation in multiple cell lines. *Arch Virol* 2000; 145:1847–1856.
48. Geigenmüller U, Ginzton NH, Matsui SM. Construction of a genome-length cDNA clone for human astrovirus serotype 1 and synthesis of infectious RNA transcripts. *J Virol* 1997;71: 1713–1717.
49. Gaggero A, et al. Prevalence of astrovirus infection among Chilean children with acute gastroenteritis. *J Clin Microbiol* 1998;36:3691–3693.
50. Maldonado Y, et al. Population-based prevalence of symptomatic and asymptomatic astrovirus infection in rural Mayan infants. *J Infect Dis* 1998;178:334–339.
51. Jonassen TO, Monceyron C, Lee TW, et al. Detection of all serotypes of human astrovirus by the polymerase chain reaction. *J Virol Methods* 1995;52:327–334.
52. Mustafa H, Palombo EA, Bishop RF. Epidemiology of astrovirus infection in young children hospitalized with acute gastroenteritis in Melbourne, Australia, over a period of four consecutive years, 1995 to 1998. *J Clin Microbiol* 2000;38:1058–1062.
53. Noel J, Cubitt D. Identification of astrovirus serotypes from children treated at the Hospitals for Sick Children, London 1981–93. *Epidemiol Infect* 1994;113:153–159.
54. Noel JS, Lee TW, Kurtz JB, et al. Typing of human astroviruses from clinical isolates by enzyme immunoassay and nucleotide sequencing. *J Clin Microbiol* 1995;33:797–801.
55. Palombo EA, Bishop RF. Annual incidence, serotype distribution, and genetic diversity of human astrovirus isolates from hospitalized children in Melbourne, Australia. *J Clin Microbiol* 1996;34:1750–1753.
56. Saito K, et al. Detection of astroviruses from stool samples in Japan using reverse transcription and polymerase chain reaction amplification. *Microbiol Immunol* 1995;39:825–828.
57. Naficy AB, et al. Astrovirus diarrhea in Egyptian children. *J Infect Dis* 2000;182:685–690.
58. Kapikian A. Viral gastroenteritis. *JAMA* 1993;269:627–630.
59. Wilson SA, Cubitt WD. The development and evaluation of radioimmune assays for the detection of immune globulins M and G against astrovirus. *J Virol Methods* 1988;19:151–159.
60. Guerrero ML, et al. A prospective study of astrovirus diarrhea of infancy in Mexico City. *Pediatr Infect Dis J* 1998;17:723–727.
61. Belliot G, Laveran H, Monroe SS. Capsid protein composition of reference strains and wild isolates of human astroviruses. *Virus Res* 1997;49:49–57.
62. Lewis TL, Greenberg HB, Herrmann JE, et al. Analysis of astrovirus serotype 1 RNA, identification of the viral RNA-dependent RNA polymerase motif, and expression of a viral structural protein. *J Virol* 1994;68:77–83.
63. Willcocks MM, Carter MJ. Identification and sequence determination of the capsid protein gene of human astrovirus serotype 1. *FEMS Microbiol Lett* 1993;114:1–7.
64. Willcocks MM, Brown TD, Madeley CR, et al. The complete sequence of a human astrovirus. *J Gen Virol* 1994;75:1785–1788.
65. Jiang B, Monroe SS, Koonin EV, et al. RNA sequence of astrovirus: distinctive genomic organization and a putative retrovirus-like ribosomal frameshifting signal that directs the viral replicase synthesis. *Proc Natl Acad Sci U S A* 1993;90:10539–10543.
66. Mendez-Toss M, Romero-Guido P, Munguia ME, et al. Molecular analysis of a serotype 8 human astrovirus genome [In Process Citation]. *J Gen Virol* 2000;81[Pt 12]:2891–2897.
67. Monroe SS, Stine SE, Gorelkin L, et al. Temporal synthesis of proteins and RNAs during human astrovirus infection of cultured cells. *J Virol* 1991;65:641–648.
68. Monroe SS, Carter MJ, Herrmann JE, et al. Family Astroviridae. In: Murphy FA, et al., eds. *Classification and nomenclature of viruses. Sixth Report of the International Committee on Tax-*

onomy of Viruses. New York, NY: Springer-Verlag, 1995: 364–367.
69. Monceyron C, Grinde B, Jonassen TO. Molecular characterisation of the 3′-end of the astrovirus genome. *Arch Virol* 1997;142:699–706.
70. Jonassen CM, Jonassen TO, Grinde B. A common RNA motif in the 3′ end of the genomes of astroviruses, avian infectious bronchitis virus and an equine rhinovirus. *J Gen Virol* 1998;79: 715–718.
71. Willcocks MM, Carter MJ, Madeley CR. Astroviruses. *Rev Med Virol* 1992;1992:97–106.
72. Willcocks MM, Boxall AS, Carter MJ. Processing and intracellular location of human astrovirus non-structural proteins. *J Gen Virol* 1999;80:2607–2611.
73. Willcocks MM, Ashton N, Kurtz JB, et al. Cell culture adaptation of astrovirus involves a deletion. *J Virol* 1994;68:6057–6058.
74. Kozak M. An analysis of 5′-noncoding sequences from 699 vertebrate messenger RNAs. *Nucleic Acid Res* 1987;15:8125–8148.
75. Chamorro M, Parkin N, Varmus HE. An RNA pseudoknot and an optimal heptameric shift site are required for highly efficient ribosomal frameshifting on a retroviral messenger RNA. *Proc Natl Acad Sci U S A* 1992;89:713–717.
76. Jacks T, Madhani HD, Masiarz FR, et al. Signals for ribosomal frameshifting in the Rous sarcoma virus. *Cell* 1988;55:447–458.
77. Jacks T, Power M, Masiarz F, et al. Characterization of ribosomal frameshifting in HIV-1 gag-pol expression. *Nature* 1988; 331:280–283.
78. Wilson W, Braddock M, Adams SE, et al. HIV expression strategies: ribosomal frameshifting is directed by a short sequence in both mammalian and yeast systems. *Cell* 1988;55:1159–1169.
79. Brierley I, Digard P, Inglis SC. Characterization of an efficient coronavirus ribosomal frameshifting signal: requirement for an RNA pseudoknot. *Cell* 1989;57:537–547.
80. Gibson CA, Chen J, Monroe SA, et al. Expression and processing of nonstructural proteins of the human astroviruses. *Adv Exp Med Biol* 1998;440:387–391.
81. Kiang D, Matsui S. Proteolytic processing of a human astrovirus nonstructural protein. *J Gen Virol* 2002;83 (*in press*).
82. Kiang D, Chew T, Matsui S. Processing of the astrovirus ORF1a encoded polyprotein. In: *Abstracts of the American Society for Virology Meeting.* Fort Collins, CO: American Society for Virology, 2000:120.
83. Monroe SS, Jiang B, Stine SE, et al. Subgenomic RNA sequence of human astrovirus supports classification of Astroviridae as a new family of RNA viruses. *J Virol* 1993;67:3611–3614.
84. Strauss JH, Strauss EG. Replication of the RNAs of alphaviruses and flaviviruses. In: Domingo E, Holland JJ, Ahlquist P, eds. *RNA genetics. Volume 1: RNA-directed virus replication.* Boca Raton: CRC Press, 1988:71–90.
85. Studdert MJ. Caliciviruses. *Arch Virol* 1978;58:157–191.
86. Semler BL, Kuhn RJ, Wimmer E. Replication of the poliovirus genome. In: Domingo E, Holland JJ, Ahlquist P, eds. *RNA genetics. Volume 1: RNA-directed virus replication.* Boca Raton: CRC Press, 1988.
87. Kurtz J. Astroviruses. In: Farthing MJG, ed. *Viruses and the gut; Proceedings of the Ninth British Society of Gastroenterology.* Welwyn Garden City, UK: Smith Kline & French Laboratories, LTD, 1988:84–87.
88. Bass DM, Qiu S. Proteolytic processing of the astrovirus capsid. *J Virol* 2000;74:1810–1814.
89. Sanchez-Fauquier A, et al. Characterization of a human astrovirus serotype 2 structural protein (VP26) that contains an epitope involved in virus neutralization. *Virology* 1994;201: 312–320.
90. Avery RM, Shelton AP, Beards GM, et al. Viral agents associated with infantile gastroenteritis in Nigeria: relative prevalence of adenovirus serotypes 40 and 41, astrovirus, and rotavirus serotypes 1 to 4. *J Diarrhoeal Dis Res* 1992;10:105–108.
91. Bates PR, Bailey AS, Wood DJ, et al. Comparative epidemiology of rotavirus, subgenus F (types 40 and 41) adenovirus and astrovirus gastroenteritis in children. *J Med Virol* 1993;39:224–228.
92. Cox GJ, et al. Etiology and outcome of diarrhea after marrow transplantation: a prospective study. *Gastroenterology* 1994;107: 1398–1407.
93. Cruz JR, Bartlett AV, Herrmann JE, et al. Astrovirus-associated diarrhea among Guatemalan ambulatory rural children. *J Clin Microbiol* 1992;30:1140–1144.
94. Esahli H, Breback K, Bennet R, et al. Astroviruses as a cause of nosocomial outbreaks of infant diarrhea. *Pediatr Infect Dis J* 1991;10:511–515.
95. Ford-Jones EL, Mindorff CM, Gold R, et al. The incidence of viral-associated diarrhea after admission to a pediatric hospital. *Am J Epidemiol* 1990;131:711–718.
96. Grohmann GS, et al. Enteric viruses and diarrhea in HIV-infected patients. Enteric Opportunistic Infections Working Group. *N Engl J Med* 1993;329:14–20.
97. Herrmann JE, Taylor DN, Echeverria P, et al. Astroviruses as a cause of gastroenteritis in children. *N Engl J Med* 1991;324: 1757–1760.
98. Kotloff KL, et al. The frequency of astrovirus as a cause of diarrhea in Baltimore children. *Pediatr Infect Dis J* 1992;11:587–589.
99. Kurtz JB, Lee TW, Pickering D. Astrovirus associated gastroenteritis in a children's ward. *J Clin Pathol* 1977;30:948–952.
100. Leite JP, Barth OM, Schatzmayr HG. Astrovirus in faeces of children with acute gastroenteritis in Rio de Janeiro, Brazil. *Memorias Instit Oswaldo Cruz* 1991;86:489–490.
101. Lew JF, et al. Six-year retrospective surveillance of gastroenteritis viruses identified at ten electron microscopy centers in the United States and Canada. *Pediatr Infect Dis J* 1990;9:709–714.
102. Lew JF, et al. Astrovirus and adenovirus associated with diarrhea in children in day care settings. *J Infect Dis* 1991;164:673–678.
103. Lewis DC, Lightfoot NF, Cubitt WD, et al. Outbreaks of astrovirus type 1 and rotavirus gastroenteritis in a geriatric in-patient population. *J Hosp Infect* 1989;14:9–14.
104. Mitchell DK, Van R, Morrow AL, et al. Outbreaks of astrovirus gastroenteritis in day care centers. *J Pediatr* 1993;123:725–732.
105. Moe CL, et al. Detection of astrovirus in pediatric stool samples by immunoassay and RNA probe. *J Clin Microbiol* 1991;29: 2390–2395.
106. Monroe SS, et al. Electron microscopic reporting of gastrointestinal viruses in the United Kingdom, 1985–1987. *J Med Virol* 1991;33:193–198.
107. Pavone R, Schinaia N, Hart CA, et al. Viral gastro-enteritis in children in Malawi. *Ann Trop Paediatr* 1990;10:15–20.
108. Stewien KE, et al. Viral, bacterial and parasitic pathogens associated with severe diarrhoea in the city of Sao Paulo, Brazil. *J Diarrhoeal Dis Res* 1993;11:148–152.
109. Medina SM, Gutierrez MF, Liprandi F, et al. Identification and type distribution of astroviruses among children with gastroenteritis in Colombia and Venezuela. *J Clin Microbiol* 2000;38: 3481–3483.
110. Schulz K, Wegner U, Gurtler L, et al. Analysis of genotypes of human astrovirus isolates from hospitalized children in north-eastern Germany. *Eur J Clin Microbiol Infect Dis* 2000;19: 563–565.
111. Lopez L, et al. Astrovirus infection among children with gastroenteritis in the city of Zaragoza, Spain. *Eur J Clin Microbiol Infect Dis* 2000;19:545–547.
112. Sakamoto T, et al. Molecular epidemiology of astroviruses in Japan from 1995 to 1998 by reverse transcription-polymerase chain reaction with serotype-specific primers (1 to 8). *J Med Virol* 2000;61:326–331.

113. Foley B, O'Mahony J, Morgan SM, et al. Detection of sporadic cases of Norwalk-like virus (NLV) and astrovirus infection in a single Irish hospital from 1996 to 1998. *J Clin Virol* 2000;17: 109–117.
114. Putzker M, Sauer H, Kirchner G, et al. Community acquired diarrhea—the incidence of astrovirus infections in Germany. *Clin Lab* 2000;46:269–273.
115. Hachiya M, Matsui M, Sanogo M, et al. Genetic variation in the capsid region of human astrovirus serotype 4 isolated in Japan. *Microbiol Immunol* 1999;43:1067–1070.
116. Oseto M, et al. Serotypes of astrovirus isolated from children in sporadic gastroenteritis cases in Ehime Prefecture 1981–1997. *Jpn J Infect Dis* 1999;52:134–135.
117. Mitchell DK, et al. Prevalence of antibodies to astrovirus types 1 and 3 in children and adolescents in Norfolk, Virginia. *Pediatr Infect Dis J* 1999;18:249–254.
118. Steele AD, Basetse HR, Blacklow NR, et al. Astrovirus infection in South Africa: a pilot study. *Ann Trop Paediatr* 1998;18: 315–319.
119. Shastri S, Doane AM, Gonzales J, et al. Prevalence of astroviruses in a children's hospital. *J Clin Microbiol* 1998;36:2571–2574.
120. Unicomb LE, et al. Astrovirus infection in association with acute, persistent and nosocomial diarrhea in Bangladesh. *Pediatr Infect Dis J* 1998;17:611–614.
121. Gonzalez GG, Pujol FH, Liprandi F, et al. Prevalence of enteric viruses in human immunodeficiency virus seropositive patients in Venezuela. *J Med Virol* 1998;55:288–292.
122. Araki K, Kobayashi S, Utagawa E, et al. Prevalence of human astrovirus serotypes in Shizuoka 1991–96 [in Japanese]. *Kansenshogaku Zasshi* 1998;72:12–16.
123. Koopmans MP, Bijen MH, Monroe SS, et al. Age-stratified seroprevalence of neutralizing antibodies to astrovirus types 1 to 7 in humans in The Netherlands. *Clin Diagn Lab Immunol* 1998;5:33–37.
124. Taylor MB, Marx FE, Grabow WO. Rotavirus, astrovirus and adenovirus associated with an outbreak of gastroenteritis in a South African child care centre. *Epidemiol Infect* 1997;119: 227–230.
125. Belliot G, Laveran H, Monroe SS. Outbreak of gastroenteritis in military recruits associated with serotype 3 astrovirus infection. *J Med Virol* 1997;51:101–106.
126. Kriston S, Willcocks MM, Carter MJ, et al. Seroprevalence of astrovirus types 1 and 6 in London, determined using recombinant virus antigen. *Epidemiol Infect* 1996;117:159–164.
127. Bon F, et al. Prevalence of group A rotavirus, human calicivirus, astrovirus, and adenovirus type 40 and 41 infections among children with acute gastroenteritis in Dijon, France. *J Clin Microbiol* 1999;37:3055–3058.
128. Nazer H, Rice S, Walker-Smith JA. Clinical associations of stool astrovirus in childhood. *J Pediatr Gastroenterol Nutr* 1982;1: 555–558.
129. Madeley CR, Cosgrove BP, Bell EJ, et al. Stool viruses in babies in Glasgow. I. Hospital admissions with diarrhoea. *J Hyg* 1977; 78:261–273.
130. Riepenhoff-Talty M, Saif LJ, Barrett HJ, et al. Potential spectrum of etiological agents of viral enteritis in hospitalized infants. *J Clin Microbiol* 1983;17:352–356.
131. Gray JJ, Wreghitt TG, Cubitt WD, et al. An outbreak of gastroenteritis in a home for the elderly associated with astrovirus type 1 and human calicivirus. *J Med Virol* 1987;23:377–381.
132. Oshiro LS, et al. A 27-nm virus isolated during an outbreak of acute infectious nonbacterial gastroenteritis in a convalescent hospital: a possible new serotype. *J Infect Dis* 1981;143:791–795.
133. Matsui SM, et al. An outbreak of astrovirus gastroenteritis in a nursing home and molecular characterization of the virus. *Gastroenterology* 1994;106:A730.
134. Coppo P, Scieux C, Ferchal F, et al. Astrovirus enteritis in a chronic lymphocytic leukemia patient treated with fludarabine monophosphate. *Ann Hematol* 2000;79:43–45.
135. Bjorkholm M, Celsing F, Runarsson G, et al. Successful intravenous immunoglobulin therapy for severe and persistent astrovirus gastroenteritis after fludarabine treatment in a patient with Waldenstrom's macroglobulinemia. *Int J Hematol* 1995;62: 117–120.
136. LeBaron CW, et al. Viral agents of gastroenteritis. Public health importance and outbreak management. *MMWR Morb Mortal Wkly Rep* 1990;39:1–24.
137. Appleton H. Small round viruses: classification and role in food-borne infections. In: Bock G, Whelans J, eds. *Novel diarrhoea viruses.* Ciba Foundation Symposium 128. Chichester: Wiley, 1987:108–125.
138. Pinto RM, Abad FX, Gajardo R, et al. Detection of infectious astroviruses in water. *Appl Environ Microbiol* 1996;62: 1811–1813.
139. Myint S, Manley R, Cubitt D. Viruses in bathing waters [Letter; Comment] [published erratum appears in *Lancet* Dec. 23–30, 1995;346(8991-8892):1716]. *Lancet* 1994;343:1640–1641.
140. Chapron CD, Ballester NA, Margolin AB. The detection of astrovirus in sludge biosolids using an integrated cell culture nested PCR technique. *J Appl Microbiol* 2000;89:11–15.
141. LeGuyader F, Haugarreau L, Miossec L, et al. Three year study to assess human enteric viruses in shellfish. *Appl Environ Microbiol* 2000;66:3241–3248.
142. Chapron CD, Ballester NA, Fontaine JH, et al. Detection of astroviruses, enteroviruses, and adenovirus types 40 and 41 in surface waters collected and evaluated by the information collection rule and an integrated cell culture-nested PCR procedure. *Appl Environ Microbiol* 2000;66:2520–2525.
143. Abad FX, Pinto RM, Villena C, et al. Astrovirus survival in drinking water. *Appl Environ Microbiol* 1997;63:3119–3122.
144. Abad FX, Pinto RM, Diez JM, et al. Disinfection of human enteric viruses in water by copper and silver in combination with low levels of chlorine. *Appl Environ Microbiol* 1994;60: 2377–2383.
145. Jonassen TO, Kjeldsberg E, Grinde B. Detection of human astrovirus serotype 1 by the polymerase chain reaction. *J Virol Methods* 1993;44:83–88.
146. Kurtz JB, Lee TW, Craig JW, et al. Astrovirus infection in volunteers. *J Med Virol* 1979;3:221–230.
147. Glass RI, et al. The changing epidemiology of astrovirus-associated gastroenteritis: a review. *Arch Virol* 1996;12[Suppl]: 287–300.
148. Walter JE, Mitchell DK. Role of astroviruses in childhood diarrhea. *Curr Opin Pediatr* 2000;12:275–279.
149. Kurtz J, Lee T. Astrovirus gastroenteritis age distribution of antibody. *Med Microbiol Immunol* 1978;166:227–230.
150. Molberg O, et al. CD4+ T cells with specific reactivity against astrovirus isolated from normal human small intestine [see Comments]. *Gastroenterology* 1998;114:115–122.
151. Bergmann L, Fenchel K, Jahn B, et al. Immunosuppressive effects and clinical response of fludarabine in refractory chronic lymphocytic leukemia. *Ann Oncol* 1993;4:371–375.
152. Cubitt WD, Mitchell DK, Carter MJ, et al. Application of electronmicroscopy, enzyme immunoassay, and RT-PCR to monitor an outbreak of astrovirus type 1 in a paediatric bone marrow transplant unit. *J Med Virol* 1999;57:313–321.
153. Philips AD, Rice SJ, Walker-Smith JA. Astrovirus within human small intestinal mucosa. *Gut* 1982;23:A923–A924.
154. Snodgrass DR, Angus KW, Gray EW, et al. Pathogenesis of diarrhoea caused by astrovirus infections in lambs. *Arch Virol* 1979;60:217–226.
155. Gray EW, Angus KW, Snodgrass DR. Ultrastructure of the

small intestine in astrovirus-infected lambs. *J Gen Virol* 1980; 49:71–82.
156. Woode GN, Pohlenz JF, Gourley NE, et al. Astrovirus and Breda virus infections of dome cell epithelium of bovine ileum. *J Clin Microbiol* 1984;19:623–630.
157. Bridger JC, Hall GA, Brown JF. Characterization of a calici-like virus (Newbury agent) found in association with astrovirus in bovine diarrhea. *Infect Immun* 1984;43:133–138.
158. Hall GA. Comparative pathology of infection by novel diarrhoea viruses. In: Bock G, Whelan J, eds. *Novel diarrhoea viruses.* Ciba Foundation Symposium 128. Chichester: Wiley, 1987:192–217.
159. Donelli G, Superti F, Tinari A, et al. Mechanism of astrovirus entry into Graham 293 cells. *J Med Virol* 1992;38:271–277.
160. Superti F, et al. *In vitro* effect of synthetic flavonoids on astrovirus infection. *Antiviral Res* 1990;13:201–208.
161. Greenberg HB, Matsui SM. Astroviruses and caliciviruses: emerging enteric pathogens. *Infect Agents Dis* 1992;1:71–91.
162. Blacklow NR, Greenberg HB. Viral gastroenteritis. *N Engl J Med* 1991;325:252–264.
163. Singh PB, Sreenivasan MA, Pavri KM. Viruses in acute gastroenteritis in children in Pune, India. *Epidemiol Infect* 1989; 102:345–353.
164. Liste MB, Natera I, Suarez JA, et al. Enteric virus infections and diarrhea in healthy and human immunodeficiency virus-infected children. *J Clin Microbiol* 2000;38:2873–2877.
165. Giordano MO, et al. Diarrhea and enteric emerging viruses in HIV-infected patients. *AIDS Res Hum Retroviruses* 1999;15: 1427–1432.
166. Kjeldsberg E. Small spherical viruses in faeces from gastroenteritis patients. *Acta Pathol Microbiol Scand Section B Microbiol* 1977;85B:351–354.
167. Berthiaume L, Alain R, McLaughlin B, et al. Rapid detection of human viruses in faeces by a simple and routine immune electron microscopy technique. *J Gen Virol* 1981;55:223–227.
168. Madeley D. Viruses and diarrhoea—where are we now? *APMIS* 1993;101:497–504.
169. Oliver AR, Phillips AD. An electron microscopical investigation of faecal small round viruses. *J Med Virol* 1988;24:211–218.
170. Herrmann JE, Cubitt WD, Hudson RW, et al. Immunological characterization of the Marin County strain of astrovirus. *Arch Virol* 1990;110:213–220.
171. Herrmann JE, Hudson RW, Blacklow NR. Marin County agent, an astrovirus [Letter]. *Lancet* 1987;2:743.
172. McIver CJ, Palombo EA, Doultree JC, et al. Detection of astrovirus gastroenteritis in children. *J Virol Methods* 2000;84:99–105.
173. Willcocks MM, Carter MJ, Silcock JG, et al. A dot-blot hybridization procedure for the detection of astrovirus in stool samples. *Epidemiol Infect* 1991;107:405–410.
174. Willcocks MM, Silcock JG, Carter MJ. Detection of Norwalk virus in the UK by the polymerase chain reaction. *FEMS Microbiol Lett* 1993;112:7–12.
175. Sakon N, Yamazaki K, Utagawa E, et al. Genomic characterization of human astrovirus type 6 Katano virus and the establishment of a rapid and effective reverse transcription-polymerase chain reaction to detect all serotypes of human astrovirus. *J Med Virol* 2000;61:125–131.
176. Kurtz JB, Lee TW, Parsons AJ. The action of alcohols on rotavirus, astrovirus and enterovirus *J Hosp Infect* 1980;1: 321–325.

58

ENTERIC ADENOVIRUSES

JOHN E. HERRMANN
NEIL R. BLACKLOW

Two distinct serotypes of adenovirus, types 40 and 41, now categorized as subgroup F adenoviruses, have been commonly identified in the stools of infants and young children with gastroenteritis in temperate countries (1–12). These viruses have been isolated from cases of diarrhea in Asia, Africa, and South America as well (13–18). The percentage of cases of pediatric gastroenteritis found to be due to enteric adenoviruses has been quite variable, ranging from approximately 1% to 16%.

Other types of adenoviruses have also been isolated from stools, and some have been associated with gastroenteritis (19–21), but only types 40 and 41 have been consistently associated with gastroenteritis. These enteric types also appear in higher concentrations in stools than other adenovirus types as determined by electron microscopy (EM) studies (22). The number of particles shed, like rotavirus, may exceed 10^{11} particles per gram of feces in children with diarrhea (23).

Enteric adenoviruses were originally described as being noncultivatable or fastidious viruses, because they could be seen in large numbers by EM in stools (6,7,24) but could not be cultivated in cell lines generally used to isolate other adenovirus types. In 1981, Takiff et al. (25) showed that these viruses could be cultivated in Graham 293 cells, a line of human embryonic kidney (HEK) cells transformed with sheared adenovirus type 5 DNA. Subsequently, it has been found that some subgroup F adenoviruses can be isolated in HEp-2 cells, Chang conjunctiva cells, Caco-2 cells (26–29), or PLC/PRF/5 cells (30), as well as Graham 293 cells and can be propagated in HeLa, H1407 cells (31) KB, A549 cells, or Caco-2 cells (29).

J. E. Herrmann: Division of Infectious Diseases and Immunology, University of Massachusetts Medical School, Worcester, Massachusetts

N. R. Blacklow: Division of Infectious Diseases, University of Massachusetts Medical School and University of Massachusetts Memorial Medical Center, Worcester, Massachusetts

DESCRIPTION OF THE VIRUSES

Morphology and Physical Properties

Like other adenoviruses, enteric adenoviruses are nonenveloped, icosahedral, double-stranded DNA viruses of 80-nm diameter. They have 252 capsomeres, which consist of 20 equilateral triangular sides and 12 vertices, and no morphologic differences are seen by EM between the enteric and nonenteric types (Fig. 58.1). Complete enteric adenovirus particles form a band at a density of 1.34 g/mL and incomplete particles form a band at a density of 1.30 g/mL in cesium chloride. The enteric serotypes, 40 and 41, share the adenovirus group antigen and are distinguished from each other and from the nonenteric serotypes serologically and by their genome profiles after cleavage with restriction endonucleases followed by gel electrophoresis. The two serotypes collectively have been designated as subgroup F adenoviruses, but each of the two enteric serotypes gives an electrophoretic pattern distinct from any of the other adenovirus serotypes (23).

Enteric adenoviruses have been shown to survive on environmental surfaces but are less resistant to inactivation than rotavirus or hepatitis A virus (32). Adenovirus 41 was able to be detected by enzyme-linked immunosorbent assay (ELISA) in virus-seeded sewage samples, suggesting that the virus is stable in this environment (33). It can be assumed, based on their biophysical and biochemical properties, that other stability characteristics are similar to those of the nonenteric adenoviruses.

Propagation in Cell Cultures

The subgroup F adenoviruses, unlike other adenoviruses, cannot be serially cultivated on primary HEK cells. Takiff et al. (25) found that these viruses could be cultivated in cell line of HEK cells transformed by adenovirus type 5, Graham 293 cells. Because of this, they postulated that the adenovirus 41 strain that they examined in detail was similar in action to an adenovirus host-range mutant deficient in early gene functions (34). It was further suggested by Van Loon

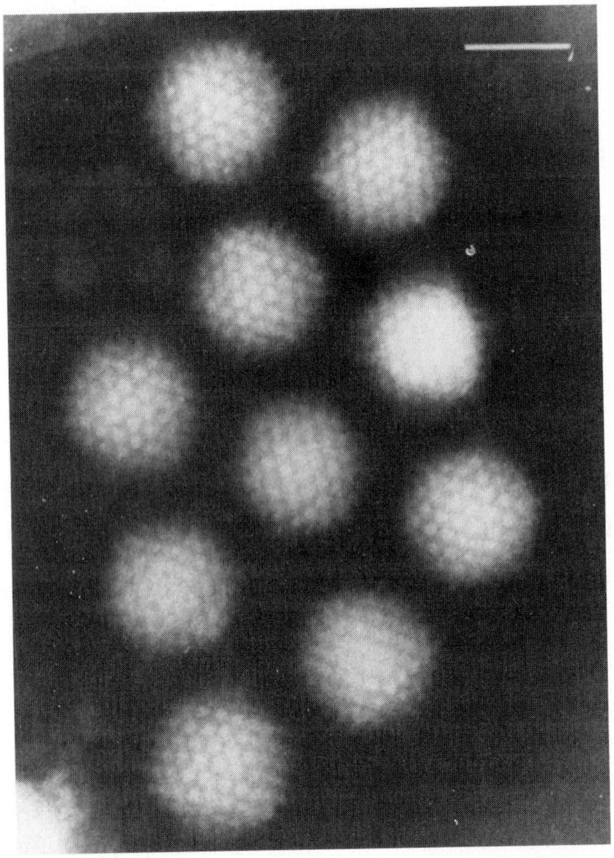

FIGURE 58.1. Electron micrograph of enteric adenovirus type 40, isolated from a stool specimen in Graham 393 cells. Negatively stained with phosphotungstic acid. Size bar = 50 nm. (Courtesy of W. D. Cubitt.)

et al. (35) that the inability of adenovirus types 40 and 41 to be cultivated on cell lines normally supportive for other adenovirus types was due to the relative inability of the adenovirus 41 E1A gene to transactivate other adenovirus 41 early genes. Thus, these reports indicated that the enteric adenoviruses required early gene products from other adenovirus types for efficient growth.

Studies by Pieniazek et al. (31) questioned the conclusions of Van Loon et al. (35). In their study (31), the prototype strain of adenovirus, strain TAK, lost more than 90% of its infectivity on the first passage in Graham 293 cells and lost 100% by the second passage. In contrast to these results, adenovirus 41 strain TAK was able to be serially cultivated to high titers in HeLa, H1407, or HEp-2 cells. The basis for the loss of infectivity of this virus strain in Graham 293 cells was found to due to a defect in assembly of the virion. In Graham 293 cells, only traces of adenovirus protein V could be found by Western blot analysis, whereas in adenovirus 41 strain TAK virions obtained from HEp-2-infected cells, a strong band in the position of protein V was found.

Grabow et al. (30) have also reported a cell line that showed greater efficiency for propagating laboratory strains of adenovirus types 40 and 41 than Graham 293 cells or Chang conjunctiva cells. The cell line used was PLC/PRF/5, a cell line derived from a human hepatocellular carcinoma. The reason for the high susceptibility of the cell line was not determined. Efficient replication of adenovirus types 40 and 41 in Caco-2 cells has also been reported (29).

Immunotypes

Currently, 49 serotypes of human adenoviruses are recognized (36), subdivided into six subgenera (or subgroups) A through F. Two additional serotypes, 50 and 51, have been proposed (37). All of these serotypes share a cross-reacting common antigen. Several antigens are associated with the major structural proteins, proteins that have been resolved by polyacrylamide gel electrophoresis. The most abundant, the hexon (polypeptide II) contains the common genus, species-specific, and subgenus-specific antigens. The penton base (polypeptide III) and the fiber antigens (polypeptide IV) have genus and species reactivities, respectively, as well as subgenus specificity. There are also core proteins (polypeptides V and VII) and other virion polypeptides IIIa and IX (38). The molecular weights of the internal polypeptides of adenovirus 40 and 41 were sufficiently different from those of subgroups A through E to establish them as group F and G (23), now collectively classified as subgenus F adenoviruses.

A comparison of the predicted amino acid sequence of the adenovirus 40 hexon with that of adenovirus 41 revealed an overall identity of 88% (39). The regions in the hexon protein that varied between adenovirus 40 and adenovirus 41 were the same regions that varied between adenovirus 2 and adenovirus 5 (subgroup C), suggesting that these are the areas of the protein that represent type-specific determinants.

Cross-reactions between adenoviruses 40 and adenoviruses 41 are seen with antiserum raised to either type, and a one-way cross-reaction has been noted between antiserum to type 4 and type 40 (40). One epitope on protein VI of subgenus F adenoviruses is shared by members of subgenus A. Monoclonal antibodies (MABs) have been prepared, which are specific for each type (41–46), antibodies that may or may not neutralize virus infectivity. Various DNA variants of adenovirus 41 have been described, which may not be neutralized by some MABs that neutralize prototype stains (41). Variants of adenovirus 40 have also been detected but have not been found to differ in their ability to be neutralized by adenovirus 40 MABs (41).

Genome Profiles

Adenoviruses contain double-stranded DNA of approximately 2.3×10^7 Da. DNA restriction patterns for adenoviruses in subgenera A to F have been published for restriction endonucleases *Bam*HI, *Bg*III, *Bst*E11, *Hind*III, and

*Sma*I (47). Both adenovirus 40 and adenovirus 41 give genome profiles distinct from the other known adenovirus serotypes. Genome variants have also been described for adenovirus 40 and adenovirus 41 (48–51). An extensive study of variants among 48 strains of adenovirus 40 and 128 strains of adenovirus 4l, using 9 and 10 different restriction endonucleases, respectively, has been reported by van der Avoort et al. (52). Variants among both adenovirus 40 and adenovirus 41 were found, but variants that resulted in antigenic changes detectable by neutralization studies with MABs or later by MAB-based ELISA (41,52) seemed to be among adenovirus 41 strains only. In some studies, strains of adenovirus 40 or adenovirus 41 did not show variation after treatment with *Sma*I (49), but in other studies, variants have been detected with this enzyme as well (52). Studies in South Africa suggest that emergence of adenovirus 41 variants is an ongoing process (53).

EPIDEMIOLOGY

Studies on the incidence of infection with the enteric types of adenoviruses, as determined by detection of viruses in stool samples and by seroepidemiologic studies, indicate that these viruses cause infections worldwide. Unlike rotavirus infection, most studies do not indicate seasonal variation, although an increased number of cases during the summer in Sweden (54) and in a rural area of South Africa (18) have been noted. A slight peak of incidence was also observed in the cool, dry months in a study in Bangladesh (17). Most infections (approximately 95%) occur in infants younger than 2 years. When the incidence of the two serotypes has been compared, adenovirus 41 is from two to six times more common than adenovirus 40 (5–57).

Where extensive studies have been done, it appears that enteric adenoviruses may be proportionately more important as causes of diarrhea in developed countries than in developing countries. The incidence of infection reported for children with acute gastroenteritis in developed countries has usually been between 4% and 10%, and these viruses were considered to be second in importance only to rotaviruses. Other gastroenteritis viruses, such as astroviruses and Norwalk-like viruses, are now being more commonly found than enteric adenoviruses (58). The incidence from year to year in the same geographic area, however, may be highly variable. For example, in an EM study of stools from children in the Washington, DC, area, Brandt et al. (59) detected adenovirus (all serotypes) from a low of 1.4% to a high of 10.7% during eight successive years of study.

In developing countries, the incidence of enteric adenovirus gastroenteritis has generally been low, 2% to 3%. In a study of Thai children, 2% (22 of 1,114) with gastroenteritis were found to have enteric adenoviruses. In a study in rural Bangladesh, the incidence was 2.8% (125 of 4,409) of children younger than 5 years with diarrhea (16). In India, there was no significant difference in the infection rate with enteric adenoviruses for children with and without gastroenteritis in a 1-year survey (60). In Australian aboriginal children, a 1-year survey on stools from children with gastroenteritis showed that only 1.3% (18 of 1,343) harbored enteric adenoviruses, compared with 6.8% (91 of 1,343) who were positive for group A rotaviruses and 5.5% (74 of 1,343) who were positive for astroviruses (61). However, the incidence in a study in Melbourne, Australia, was also low (3.1%) (57).

Higher rates have been reported in some developing countries. In a 1-year survey of children in rural Guatemala (13), children had a greater incidence of enteric adenoviruses associated with diarrheal episodes (14.0%; 54 of 385) than rotaviruses (4.7%; 18 of 385). A 1-year survey in a rural African area (18) found that 13.2% (41 of 432) were positive for enteric adenoviruses by a dot-blot hybridization test, although only 3 of these 41 were positive by EM or isolation in cell culture, and 9 of 432 (2.1%) were positive by ELISA. In South Africa, Steele et al. (62) found a rate of 3.0% but suggested in a later study that the incidence of enteric adenovirus infection in South Africa may be underestimated (53).

Seroepidemiologic studies also indicate that infection with enteric adenoviruses is widespread and occurs in both developed and developing countries. In a serologic survey (63), more than one-third of the serum samples from the United Kingdom, New Zealand, Hong Kong, and Gambia were positive for neutralizing antibodies against a strain of enteric adenovirus that could be neutralized by antiserum to both serotypes 40 and 41. None of the 16 serum samples from Guatemala were positive and 15% of Kuwaiti serum samples were positive. It was noted that the proportion of positive serum increased with age, generally being more than double in children 2 to 4 years of age, than in children 2 years or younger.

PATHOGENESIS

Adenovirus particles have been seen within the nucleus of small intestinal mucosal cells in a fatal case of adenovirus gastroenteritis and enteric adenoviruses have been recovered from fluids in the small intestine (64). The high number of enteric particles shed (up to 10^{11} particles per gram) in stools also indicates that these viruses actively multiply in the intestinal tract. Detailed studies regarding mechanisms of enteric adenovirus gastroenteritis have not been reported.

Enteric adenoviruses and other adenoviruses have also been frequently isolated from patients with AIDS and immunocompromised patients (65–72). However, there does not seem to be a major involvement of the enteric types or of any other particular serotype. In a study of 67 adenovirus isolates from 48 patients with AIDS, there were isolates from subgenera A, B, C, and D, including five new serotypes

(types 43 to 47) of subgenus D (72). Because of the variety of serotypes obtained from liver, lung, blood, urine, and stool samples, we could not assign any epidemiologic significance to a particular serotype. Chronic diarrhea is also common in patients with AIDS. Adenoviruses have been associated with this chronic diarrhea in some studies (66,68), but diarrhea has not been specifically associated with the enteric types, 40 and 41 (66,68). Whether further studies on adenovirus-induced diarrhea in patients with AIDS will implicate specific serotypes remains to be determined.

Transmission of these viruses appears to be by person-to-person spread, as with rotaviruses, and no waterborne or food-borne outbreaks have been reported. It has also been suggested that nosocomial infections occur (73). Spread to adults is uncommon. Asymptomatic infections may occur in approximately 2% of those studied in one report (54) and up to 8% (74) and 17% (75) in studies done in day care centers.

CLINICAL ILLNESS

The clinical course of gastroenteritis caused by enteric adenoviruses is similar to that caused by rotavirus, with diarrhea being the most frequent symptom. Vomiting is also a common finding. Fever and respiratory symptoms may also be present. The age-groups mainly affected are infants and young children. The illness is usually mild and asymptomatic infections are known to occur, but the disease can be severe and fatal cases have been reported (64). The incubation period is approximately 7 days and virus excretion in stools lasts 10 to 14 days (76). However, persistent diarrhea (≥14 days) has been documented (77).

Detailed studies on the symptoms of enteric adenovirus gastroenteritis have been reported by Uhnoo et al. (76). The characteristics of patients with gastroenteritis caused by enteric adenoviruses and rotaviruses are shown in Table 58.1. These data were obtained in a prospective 1-year study, comprising children with acute gastroenteritis admitted to a hospital or treated as outpatients. Significant differences between group A rotavirus and enteric adenovirus gastroenteritis were found for a temperature higher than 39°C, where 42% of the rotavirus patients showed a temperature higher than 39°C compared with 3% of the enteric adenovirus patients, and for duration of diarrhea. Those infected with enteric adenoviruses had diarrhea for a mean duration of 10.8 days, compared with 5.9 days for the rotavirus patients.

In an earlier study by Uhnoo et al. (54), a follow-up study of three children who recovered from enteric adenovirus gastroenteritis showed that they had lactose intolerance for up to 5 to 7 months after recovery. Evidence of malabsorption using the D-xylose absorption test during acute enteric adenovirus disease was shown by Mavromichalis et al. (78). A possible role for adenoviruses in celiac disease, characterized by small intestinal mucosal injury and malabsorption, has also been suggested (79).

The clinical picture for infants in developing countries is similar to that seen in developed countries. In a study of infants younger than 5 years in Bangladesh who had enteric adenovirus gastroenteritis, the symptoms experienced by 80 children examined were similar to symptoms in infants infected with group A rotaviruses (17). The most common clinical features were watery diarrhea (88%; 69% more than eight times per day), vomiting (80%), abdominal pain

TABLE 58.1. COMPARISON OF CLINICAL FEATURES OF CHILDREN INFECTED WITH ENTERIC ADENOVIRUSES OR ROTAVIRUSES

	No. Infected (% Infected) Virus Infection	
Clinical Feature	Enteric Adenovirus (n = 32)	Rotavirus (n = 168)
Diarrhea	31 (97)	164 (98)
Diarrhea >10 times daily	7 (22)	36 (21)
Vomiting	25 (78)	146 (87)
Fever	14 (44)	141 (84)
Fever >39°C	1 (3)	71 (42)
Abdominal pain	8 (25)	31 (18)
Blood in stools	1 (3)	2 (1)
Mucus in stools	6 (19)	28 (17)
Respiratory symptoms	6 (19)	56 (33)
Admission to hospital	9 (28)	65 (39)
Duration (mean days)		
Hospital stay	3.6	2.4
Diarrhea	10.8	5.9
Vomiting	3.2	2.5

Adapted from data presented by Uhnoo I, Olding-Stenkvist E, Kreuger A. Clinical features of acute gastroenteritis associated with rotavirus enteric adenoviruses, and bacteria. *Arch Dis Child* 1986;61:732–738, with permission.

(76%), and low-grade fever (95%). Mild to moderate dehydration was also commonly found. There was no significant difference in the degree of dehydration seen in patients with enteric adenovirus gastroenteritis and those with gastroenteritis caused by group A rotaviruses.

DIAGNOSIS

Electron Microscopy

The enteric adenoviruses were first associated with diarrheal disease based on EM studies, and the viral particles are generally seen in high numbers, up to 10^{11}/g of feces. Because they occur in higher numbers other than nonenteric types, Brandt et al. (21) has reported that the likelihood of detecting the enteric types by EM alone was increased when one or more particles were detected per minute of viewing. For definitive identification however, immune EM using type-specific antiserum is required (80,81).

Enzyme-linked Immunosorbent Assay

In earlier studies, ELISAs specific for each of the enteric types (40 and 41) were developed with polyclonal serum that had been absorbed with adenovirus antigens from other subgenera (82,83). Since then, ELISA tests have been described, using MAB specific for type 40 and 41 (41–46). For direct detection in stool samples, we developed an indirect ELISA that uses a polyclonal capture antibody directed against adenovirus group antigen and murine MAB to each of the two enteric types as detector antibodies (44). MAB-based ELISA tests for group F adenoviruses are now commercially available as well and have been evaluated in epidemiologic and other studies (13,75,84). Because of the ease of performance, commercial availability, and the high sensitivity and specificity obtained, MAB-based ELISA is the method of choice for routine diagnosis of enteric adenovirus infections.

Detection Of Viral DNA

Detection of viral DNA has been applied to adenovirus type 40 and type 41. In earlier studies, cloned DNA fragments used by Takiff et al. (85) in a dot-blot hybridization system were found to detect less than 20 pg of enteric adenovirus DNA. A hybridization test was also described that had a similar sensitivity to a radioimmunoassay for enteric adenovirus (86). Later studies have concentrated on polymerase chain reaction (PCR) techniques (87). By use of primers from genes encoding early regions E1A and E1B of subgroup F adenoviruses, PCR was found effective for detecting enteric adenoviruses at a level of 103 virus particles (380 fg). Although this PCR was not tested extensively on stool samples known to contain enteric adenoviruses, preliminary studies (87) and later studies (88,89) suggested that PCR was potentially an effective means for diagnosing enteric adenovirus infection. No commercial PCR assays are available yet. PCR has been used for typing enteric adenoviruses as well (90).

Another method for detection of enteric adenoviruses is the use of synthetic oligonucleotide probes (73). When tested on clinical stool samples, hybridization with the probes was found to have a sensitivity approximately equal to that obtained with a commercial MAB-based ELISA but was less specific than the ELISA.

Isolation In Cell Culture

For isolation of enteric adenoviruses, stool samples are prepared by dilution in phosphate-buffered saline (PBS) and clarification by centrifugation. The clarified stool suspensions are inoculated onto monolayers of Graham 293 cells, maintenance medium is added (Eagle minimum essential medium plus 2% fetal calf serum and antibiotics) and the cells held for 7 to 10 days at 37°C. Cultures should be passaged at least once if no cytopathic effect is evident on the first passage. Use of a shell vial culture technique was less sensitive than conventional culture for detection of adenovirus 41 (93). Modification of conventional culture by centrifugation of specimens onto cells of 24-well culture plates resulted in improved sensitivity for detecting both adenovirus 40 and adenovirus 41 and reduced the culture time required to 48 hours of incubation (94).

Adenoviruses can be identified as enteric types by ELISA with MABs as discussed above or by examination of the DNA patterns obtained on agarose gels after the DNA is treated with restriction endonucleases (23,92). Several enzymes have been used to classify adenoviruses, but *Sma*I has been favored for identification of the enteric types. The procedure for preparation and treatment of the virus samples has been described (92).

Electrophoresis can be done in polyacrylamide gels (92) or in agarose minigels (95). The bands are visualized with an ultraviolet illuminator, or a silver stain can be used (92). The bands are compared with those obtained with known prototype strains of type 40 and 41 viruses. Additional unclassified types may also be found in adenovirus-associated gastroenteritis (19), but their significance remains to be established.

Other Methods

Other methods for the direct detection of enteric adenoviruses in stools have been described, most of which have now been replaced by MAB-based ELISAs. Extraction of DNA directly from stools, followed by treatment with restriction endonucleases and electrophoresis in agarose (95) or polyacrylamide gels (96), has been reported. A latex agglutination test has also been applied to detection of enteric adenoviruses in stools. However, this test detects adenoviral group antigen and is not specific for the enteric types (97).

TREATMENT AND PREVENTION

There is presently no specific antiviral therapy for treatment of enteric adenovirus infection. As with diarrheal diseases caused by rotaviruses and other viral agents, treatment is directed at prevention of severe dehydration and electrolyte imbalance. Use of oral rehydration salt solutions containing glucose or sucrose has recently been shown to be as effective as intravenous fluid therapy for mild to moderately severe dehydrating rotavirus gastroenteritis, and presumably this would apply to dehydrating enteric adenovirus gastroenteritis as well. The standard World Health Organization formula consists of per liter of water, glucose 20 g, sodium chloride 3.5 g, sodium bicarbonate 2.5 g, and potassium chloride 1.5 g. Oral rehydration solutions are also commercially available. Intravenous therapy must be administered if oral rehydration is not successful in replacing fluids and electrolytes or if the patient is in shock or is severely dehydrated.

Little is known about immune responses to enteric adenoviruses, immunity, or duration of immunity should it occur. It has been reported that in eight children, previous infection with enteric adenoviruses did not protect against subsequent symptomatic infection (98). Persistence of neutralizing antibodies as seen in seroepidemiologic studies and the successful development of vaccines against adenoviral acute respiratory disease suggest the possibility for the development of vaccines against enteric adenovirus infection. However, because enteric adenoviruses do not appear to be of high importance in developing countries, where diarrheal diseases are major causes of morbidity and mortality, development of a vaccine would not appear to be of high priority. Whether further epidemiologic studies will demonstrate a greater need for vaccine development remains to be determined.

REFERENCES

1. Brandt CD, Kim HW, Rodriguez WJ, et al. Adenoviruses and pediatric gastroenteritis. *J Infect Dis* 1985;151:437–443.
2. Albert MJ, Enteric adenoviruses. *Arch Virol* 1986;88:1–17.
3. Yolken RH, Lawrence F, Leister F, et al. Gastroenteritis associated with enteric type adenovirus in hospitalized infants. *J Pediatr* 1982;101:21–26.
4. Wood DJ. Adenovirus gastroenteritis. *Br Med J* 1988;296: 229–230.
5. Wood DJ, Longhurst D, Killough RI, et al. One-year prospective cross-sectional study to assess the importance of group F adenovirus infections in children under 2 years admitted to hospital. *J Med Virol* 1988;26:429–435.
6. Brandt CD, Kim HW, Yolken RH, et al. Comparative epidemiology of two rotavirus serotypes and other viral agents associated with pediatric gastroenteritis. *Am J Epidemiol* 1979;110:243–254.
7. Gary GW Jr., Hierholzer JC, Black RE. Characteristic of non-cultivable adenoviruses associated with diarrhea in infants: a new subgroup of human adenoviruses. *J Clin Microbiol* 1979;10: 96–103.
8. Uhnoo I, Wadell G., Svensson L, et al. Two new serotypes of enteric adenovirus causing infantile diarrhea. *Develop Biol Standard* 1983;53:311–318.
9. Madeley CR. The emerging role of adenoviruses as inducers of gastroenteritis. *Pediatr Infect Dis* 1986;5:S63–S74.
10. Schoenemann W. The importance of infections with adenoviruses in infancy. *Monatsschrift Kinderheilkunde* 1988;136:680–685.
11. Cevenini R, Mazzaracchio R, Rumpianesi F, et al. Prevalence of enteric adenovirus from acute gastroenteritis: a five year study. *Eur J Epidemiol* 1987;3:147–150.
12. Richmond SJ, Dunn SM, Caul EO, et al. An outbreak of gastroenteritis in young children caused by adenoviruses. *Lancet* 1979;1:1178.
13. Cruz JR, Caceres P, Cano F, et al. Adenovirus types 40 and 41 and rotaviruses associated with diarrhea in children from Guatemala. *J Clin Microbiol* 1990;28:1780–1784.
14. Oishi I, Yamazaki K, Minekawa Y, et al. Three-year survey of the epidemiology of rotavirus, enteric adenovirus, and some small spherical viruses including "Osaka agent" associated with infantile diarrhea. *Biken J* 1985;28:9–19.
15. Shinozaki, Arakf K, Fujita Y, et al. Epidemiology of enteric adenoviruses 40 and 41 in acute gastroenteritis in infants and young children in the Tokyo area. *Scand J Infect Dis* 1991;23:543–547.
16. Herrmann JE, Blacklow NR, Perron-Henry DM, et al. Incidence of enteric adenoviruses among children in Thailand and the significance of these viruses in gastroenteritis. *J Clin Microbiol* 1988;26:1783–1786.
17. Jarecki-Khan K, Tzipori SR, Unicomb LE. Enteric adenovirus infection among infants with diarrhea in rural Bangladesh. *J Clin Microbiol* 1993;31:484–489.
18. Tiemessen CT, Wegerhoff MJ, Erasmus MJ, et al. Infection by enteric adenoviruses, rotaviruses, and other agents in a rural African environment. *J Med Virol* 1989;28:176–182.
19. Bishai FR, Yolken RH, Chernesky MA, et al. Studies on fastidious adenoviruses in Ontario: a distinct strain associated with gastroenteritis. *J Clin Microbiol* 1986;23:398–400.
20. Brown M. Laboratory identification of adenoviruses associated with gastroenteritis in Canada from 1983 to 1986. *J Clin Microbiol* 1986;28:1525–1529.
21. Sakata H, Taketazu G, Nagaya K, et al. Outbreak of severe infection due to adenovirus type 7 in a paediatric ward in Japan. *J Hosp Infect* 1998;39:207–211.
22. Brandt CD, Rodriguez WJ, Kim HW, et al. Rapid presumptive recognition of diarrhea-associated adenoviruses. *J Clin Microbiol* 1984;20:1008–1009.
23. Wadell G. Molecular epidemiology of human adenoviruses. current topics. *Microbiol Immunol* 1984;110:191–220.
24. Madeley CR, Cosgrove BP, Bell EJ, et al. Stool viruses in babies in Glasgow. 1. Hospital admissions with diarrhea. *J Hyg (London)* 1977;261–273.
25. Takiff HE, Straus SE, Garon CF. Propagation and *in vitro* studies of previously non-cultivable enteral adenoviruses in 293 cells. *Lancet* 1981;2:832.
26. Kidd AH, Madeley CA. *In vitro* growth of some fastidious adenoviruses from stool specimens. *J Clin Pathol* 1981;34:213–316.
27. de Jong JC, Wigand R, Kidd AH, et al. Candidate adenoviruses 40 and 41: fastidious adenoviruses from human infant stool. *J Med Virol* 1983;11:215–231.
28. Perron-Henry DM, Herrmann JE, Blacklow NR. Isolation and propagation of enteric adenoviruses in HEp-2 cells. *J Clin Microbiol* 1988;26:1445–1447.
29. Pinto RM, Diez JM, Bosch A. Use of the colonic carcinoma cell line CaCo-2 for *in vivo* amplification and detection of enteric viruses. *J Med Virol* 1994;44:310–315.

30. Grabow WOK, Puttergill DL, Bosch A. Propagation of adenovirus types 40 and 41 in the PLC/PRF/5 primary liver carcinoma cell line. *J Virol Methods* 1992;37:201–208.
31. Pieniazek D, Pieniazek N, Macejak D, et al. Differential growth of human enteric adenovirus 41 (TAK) in continuous cell lines. *Virology* 1990;174:239–249.
32. Abad FX, Pinto RM, Bosch A. Survival of enteric viruses on environmental fomites. *Applications Environ Microbiol* 1994;50: 3704–3710.
33. Dahling DR, Wright BA, Williams FP Jr. Detection of viruses in environmental samples: suitability of commercial rotavirus and adenovirus test kits. *J Virol Methods* 1993;45:137–147.
34. Takiff HE, Straus SE. Early replicative block prevents the efficient growth of fastidious diarrhea-associated adenovirus in cell culture. *J Med Virol* 1982;9:93–100.
35. Van Loon AE, Maas R, Vaessen RTMJ, et al. Cell transformation by the left terminal regions of the adenovirus 40 and 41 genomes. *Virology* 1985;147:227–230.
36. Brown M, Grydsuk JD, Fortsas E, et al. Structural features unique to enteric adenoviruses. *Arch Virol* 1996;12[Suppl]:301–307.
37. DeJong JC, Wermenbol AC, Verweij-Uijterwaal MW, et al. Adenoviruses from human immunodeficiency virus-infected individuals, including two strains that represent new candidate serotypes Ad50 and Ad51 of species B1 and D, respectively. *J Clin Microbiol* 1999;37:3940–3945.
38. Philipson L. Structure and assembly of adenoviruses. *Curr Topics Microbiol Immunol* 1983;109:1–52.
39. Toogood CIA, Murali R, Burnett RM, et al. The adenovirus type 40 hexon: sequence, predicted structure and relationship to other adenovirus hexons. *J Gen Virol* 1989;70:3203–3214.
40. Svensson L, Wadell G, Uhnoo I, et al. Cross-reactivity between enteric adenoviruses and adenovirus type 4: analysis of epitopes by solid-phase immune electron microscopy. *J Gen Virol* 1983; 64:2517–2520.
41. de Jong JC, Bijlsma K, Wermenbol AG, et al. Detection, typing and subtyping of enteric adenoviruses 40 and 41 from fecal samples and observation of changing incidence of infections with these types and subtypes. *J Clin Microbiol* 1993;31:1562–1569.
42. Wood DJ, deJong JC, Bijlsma K, et al. Development and evaluation of monoclonal antibody-based immune electron microscopy for diagnosis of adenovirus types 40 and 41. *J Virol Methods* 1989; 25:241–250.
43. Herrmann JE, Perron-Henry DM, Stobbs-Walro D, et al. Preparation and characterization of monoclonal antibodies to enteric adenovirus types 40 and 41. *Arch Virol* 1987;94:259—265.
44. Herrmann JE, Perron-Henry DM, Blacklow NR. Antigen detection with monoclonal antibodies for the diagnosis of adenovirus gastroenteritis. *J Infect Dis* 1987;155:1167–1171.
45. Singh-Naz N, Naz RK. Development and application of monoclonal antibodies for specific detection of human enteric adenoviruses. *J Clin Microbiol* 1986;23:840–842.
46. Singh-Naz N, Rodriguez WJ, Kidd AH, et al. Monoclonal antibody enzyme-linked immunosorbent assay for specific identification and typing of subgroup F adenoviruses. *J Clin Microbiol* 1988;26:297–300.
47. Adrian T, Wadell G, Hierholzer JC, et al. DNA restriction analysis of adenovirus prototypes 1 to 41. *Arch Virol* 1986;91:277–290.
48. Willcocks MM, Carter MJ, Laidler FR, et al. Restriction enzyme analysis of faecal adenoviruses in Newcastle upon Tyne. *Epidemiol Infect* 1988;101:445–458.
49. Kidd AH. Genome variants of adenovirus 41 (subgroup G) from children with diarrhoea in South Africa. *J Med Virol* 1984;14: 49–59.
50. Shinozaki T, Araki K, Kobayashi M, et al. Genome variants of human adenovirus types 40 and 41(subgroup F) in Japan. *J Clin Microbiol* 1988;26:2567–2571.
51. Kidd AH, Berkowitz FE, Blaskovic PJ, et al. Genome variants of human adenovirus 40 (subgroup F). *J Med Virol* 1984;14:235–246.
52. van der Avoort HGAM, Wermenbol AG, Zomerdijk TPL, et al. Characterization of fastidious adenovirus types 40 and 41 by DNA restriction enzyme analysis and by neutralizing monoclonal antibodies. *Virus Res* 1989;12:139–158.
53. Moore PL, Steele AD, Alexander JJ. Relevance of commercial diagnostic tests to detection of enteric adenovirus infections in South Africa. *J Clin Microbiol* 2000;38:1661–1663.
54. Uhnoo I, Wadell G, Svensson L, et al. Importance of enteric adenoviruses 40 and 41 in acute gastroenteritis in infants and young children. *J Clin Microbiol* 1984;20:365–372.
55. Bryden AS, Curry A, Cotterill H, et al. Adenovirus-associated gastro-enteritis in the northwest of England: 1991–1994. *Br J Biomed Sci* 1997;54:273–277
56. Noel J, Mansoor A, Thaker U, et al. Identification of adenoviruses in faeces from patients with diarrhoea at the Hospitals for Sick Children, London, 1989–1992. *J Med Virol* 1994;43:84–90.
57. Grimwood K, Carzino R, Barnes GL, et al. Patients with enteric adenovirus gastroenteritis admitted to an Australian pediatric teaching hospital from 1981 to 1992. *J Clin Microbiol* 1995;33: 131–136.
58. Pang XL, Honma S, Nakata S, et al. Human caliciviruses in acute gastroenteritis of young children in the community. *J Infect Dis* 2000;181[Suppl 2]:S288–S294.
59. Brandt CD, Kim HW, Rodgriguez WJ, et al. Pediatric viral gastroenteritis during eight years of study. *J Clin Microbiol* 1983; 18:71–78.
60. Bhan MK, Raj P, Bhandari N, et al. Role of enteric adenoviruses and rotaviruses in mild and severe acute enteritis. *Pediatr Infect Dis J* 1988;7:320–323.
61. Herrmann JE, Henry DM, Albert MJ, et al. Incidence of astroviruses in Australian aboriginal children and comparison with other gastroenteritis viruses [Abstract]. *Int Congress Virol* 1993;P7-6:138.
62. Steele AD, Basetse HR, Blacklow NR, et al. Astrovirus infection in South Africa: a pilot study. *Ann Trop Pediatr* 1998;18:315–319.
63. Kidd AH, Banatvala JE, De Jong JC. Antibodies to fastidious faecal adenoviruses (species 40 and 41) in sera from children. *J Med Virol* 1983;11:333–341.
64. Whitelaw A, Davies H, Parry J. Electron microscopy of fatal adenovirus gastroenteritis. *Lancet* 1977;1:361.
65. Grohmann GS, Glass RI, Pereira HG, et al. Enteric viruses and diarrhea in HIV-infected patients. *N Engl J Med* 1993;329:14–20.
66. Smith PD, Quinn TC, Strober W, et al. Gastrointestinal infection in AIDS. *Ann Intern Med* 1992;116:63–67.
67. Smith PD, Saini SS, Orenstein JM. Infections of the large intestine in the immunocompromised host. In: Philips SF, Pemberton JH, Shorter RG, eds. *The large intestine: physiology, pathophysiology, and disease.* Philadelphia: Raven Press, 1991:437.
68. Janoff EN, Orenstein JM, Manischewitz JF, et al. Adenovirus colitis in the acquired immunodeficiency syndrome. *Gastroenterology* 1991;100:976–979.
69. Giordano MO, Martinez LC, Rinaldi D, et al. Diarrhea and enteric emerging viruses in HIV-infected patients. *AIDS Res Hum Retroviruses* 1999;15:1427–1432.
70. Schofield KP, Morris DJ, Bailey AS, et al. Gastroenteritis due to adenovirus type 41 in an adult with chronic lymphocytic leukemia. *Clin Infect Dis* 1994;19:311–312.
71. Gonzalez GG, Pujol FH, Liprandi F, et al. Prevalence of enteric viruses in human immunodeficiency virus seropositive patients in Venezuela. *J Med Virol* 1998;55:288–292.
72. Hierholzer JC, Wigand R, Anderson LJ, et al. Adenoviruses from patients with AIDS: a plethora of serotypes and a description of five new serotypes of subgenus D (types 43–47). *J Infect Dis* 1988;158:804–813.
73. Kotloff KL, Losonsky GA, Morris JG Jr, et al. Enteric adenovirus

infection and childhood diarrhea: an epidemiologic study in three clinical settings. *Pediatrics* 1989;84:219–225.
74. Lew JF, Moe CL, Monroe SS, et al. Astrovirus and adenovirus associated with diarrhea in children in day care settings. *J Infect Dis* 1991;164:673–678.
75. Van R, Wun C-C, O'Ryan ML, et al. outbreaks of human enteric adenovirus types 40 and 41 in Houston day care centers. *J Pediatr* 1992;120:516–521.
76. Uhnoo I, Olding-Stenkvist E, Kreuger A. Clinical features of acute gastroenteritis associated with rotavirus enteric adenoviruses, and bacteria. *Arch Dis Child* 1986;61:732–738.
77. Lima AA, Moore SR, Barboza MS Jr, et al. Persistent diarrhea signals a critical period of increased diarrhea burdens and nutritional shortfalls: a prospective cohort study among children in Northeastern Brazil. *J Infect Dis* 2000;181:1643–1651.
78. Mavromichalis J, Evans N, McNeish AS, et al. Intestinal damage in rotavirus and adenovirus gastroenteritis assessed by D-xylose malabsorption. *Arch Dis Child* 1977;52:589–591.
79. Kagnoff MF, Austin RK, Hubert JJ, et al. Possible role for a human adenovirus in the pathogenesis of celiac disease. *J Exp Med* 1984;160:1544–1557.
80. Leite JPG, Pereira HG, Azeredo RS, et al. Adenoviruses in faeces of children with acute gastroenteritis in Rio De Janeiro, Brazil. *J Med Virol* 1985;15:203–209.
81. Wood DJ, Bailey AS. Detection of adenovirus types 40 and 41 in stool specimens by immune electron microscopy. *J Med Virol* 1987;21:191–199.
82. Johansson ME, Uhnoo I, Svensson L, et al. Enzyme-linked immunosorbent assay for detection of enteric adenovirus 41. *J Med Virol* 1985;17:19–27.
83. Johansson RE, Uhnoo I, Kidd AH, et al. Direct identification of enteric adenovirus, a candidate new serotype, associated with infantile gastroenteritis. *J Clin Microbiol* 1980;12:95–100.
84. Wood DJ, Bijlsma K, DeJong JC, et al. Evaluation of a commercial monoclonal antibody-based enzyme immunoassay for detection of adenovirus types 40 and 41 in stool specimens. *J Clin Microbiol* 1989;27:1155–1158.
85. Takiff HE, Seidlin M, Krause P, et al. Detection of enteric adenoviruses by dot-blot hybridization using a molecularly cloned viral DNA probe. *J Med Virol* 1985;16:107–118.
86. Stalhandske P, Hyypia T, Allard A, et al. Detection of adenoviruses in stool specimens by nucleic acid spot hybridization. *J Med Virol* 1985;16:213–218.
87. Allard A, Girones R, Juto P, et al. Polymerase chain reaction for detection of adenoviruses in stool samples. *Clin Microbiol* 1990; 28:2659–2667.
88. Allard A, Albinsson B, Wadell G. Detection of adenoviruses in stools from healthy persons and patients with diarrhea by two-step polymerase chain reaction. *J Med Virol* 1992;37:149–157.
89. Rousell J, Zajdel ME, Howdle PD, et al. Rapid Detection of enteric adenoviruses by means of the polymerase chain reaction. *J Infect* 1993;27:271–275.
90. Allard A, Kajon A, Wadell G. Simple procedure for discrimination and typing of enteric adenoviruses after detection by polymerase chain reaction. *J Med Virol* 1994;44:250–257.
91. Scott-Taylor TH, Ahluwalia G, Dawood M, et al. Detection of enteric adenoviruses with synthetic oligonucleotide probes. *J Med Virol* 1993;41:328–337.
92. Brown M, Petric M, Middleton PJ. Silver staining of DNA restriction fragments for the rapid identification of adenovirus isolates: application during nosocomial outbreaks. *J Virol Methods* 1985;10:39–44.
93. VanDoornum GJ, DeJong JC. Rapid shell vial culture technique for detection of enteroviruses and adenoviruses in fecal specimens: comparison with conventional virus isolation methods. *J Clin Microbiol* 1998;36: 2865–2869.
94. Durepaire N, Ranger-Rogez S, Denis F. Evaluation of rapid culture centrifugation method for adenovirus detection in stools. *Diagn Microbiol Infect Dis* 1996;24:25–29.
95. Buitenwerf J, Louwerens JJ, de Jong JC. A simple and rapid method for typing adenoviruses 40 and 41 without cultivation. *J Virol Methods* 1985;10:39–44.
96. Moosai RB, Carter MJ, Madeley CR. Rapid detection of enteric adenovirus and rotavirus: a simple method using polyacrylamide gel electrophoresis. *J Clin Pathol*1984;37:1404–1408.
97. Grandien M, Pettersson CA, Svensson L, et al. Latex agglutination test for adenovirus diagnosis in diarrheal disease. *J Med Virol* 1987;23:311–316.
98. Unicomb LE, Jarecki-Khan K, Hall A, et al. Previous enteric adenovirus infection does not protect against subsequent symptomatic infection: longitudinal follow-up of eight infants. *Microbiol Immunol* 1996;161–168.

59

OTHER VIRAL AGENTS OF GASTROENTERITIS

ROGER I. GLASS

More than 15 different groups of viruses encompassing more than 100 serotypes can be found in the gut. The continual turnover of this massive epithelial cell pool provides a constant supply of new tissue to support the propagation or passage of a wide variety of viruses. However, although many viruses are present in the gut, relatively few are causative agents of diarrhea. Some either are not pathogenic to the intestinal epithelium or cause other unrelated illnesses; these include hepatitis A virus, reoviruses, nonenteric adenoviruses, poliovirus, coxsackieviruses A and B, echovirus, and most if not all of the other human enteroviruses (1). Others, such as cytomegalovirus, varicella zoster, measles, mumps, parainfluenza, papillomavirus, herpes simplex virus, and perhaps HIV, commonly infect other parts of the body but can occasionally cause opportunistic infections in the gut. When these viruses opportunistically infect epithelial cells at different sites in the gastrointestinal (GI) tract from the mouth to the rectum, they cause illnesses such as malabsorption, esophagitis, proctitis, and colitis, which may have GI signs and symptoms, but for which diarrhea is usually only a secondary problem (see Chapter 54).

A relatively small group of viruses has been incriminated to cause acute gastroenteritis in humans, and fewer have proved true etiologic agents. Before the 1970s, viruses were suspected to be the cause of a majority of diarrheal episodes because the recognized bacterial and parasitic agents could be found in only a small fraction of diarrheal specimens (2,3). Volunteer studies in the 1940s and 1950s supported this hypothesis because bacteria-free stool filtrates from patients with gastroenteritis were found to cause diarrhea in volunteers and could be passaged serially in volunteers, suggesting that viruses, not toxins, were the causative agents (4,5).

The identification of specific viruses and their association with gastroenteritis were boosted with each major advance in diagnostic virology (Table 59.1). In the 1950s and 1960s, the development of tissue culture techniques led to the cultivation and identification of echoviruses, adenoviruses, coxsackieviruses A and B, and reovirus from stool and led to their identification as putative diarrheal pathogens. The development of electron microscopic (EM) methods in the 1970s and their application to screening fecal specimens led to breakthroughs in the identification of new enteric viruses that were difficult to culture, including the Norwalk agent (6), rotavirus (7), caliciviruses, astroviruses (8,9), adenovirus (10,11), coronavirus (12,13), parvovirus (14,15), torovirus (16,17), the Aichi virus (18,19), and other small round structured viruses (SRSVs) that looked like the Norwalk agent but were antigenically distinct by immune EM (IEM). Although many viruses could be identified in fecal specimens from patients with diarrhea, not all these agents were necessarily causative agents of gastroenteritis.

This chapter begins with a review of the types of evidence required to establish that a virus is a causative agent of gastroenteritis and then describes a collection of viruses not discussed elsewhere in this book that have been implicated as causative agents, but for which a causal relationship is still unproved (Table 59.1). Much research is ongoing to establish whether these agents actually cause gastroenteritis.

WHEN IS A NOVEL VIRUS AN ENTERIC PATHOGEN?

Evidence To Establish A Causal Relationship

The observation of a virus in a fecal specimen from a patient with diarrhea raises two questions: (a) What is the true identity of the virus seen by EM or grown in culture, and (b) can the virus be implicated as the causative agent of the patient's diarrhea? The first question relates to virus detection and characterization (Table 59.2). Some viruses, such as the coronaviruses or toroviruses, have a pleomor-

R. I. Glass: Viral Gastroenteritis Section, National Centers for Infectious Diseases, Centers for Disease Control and Prevention, Atlanta, Georgia

TABLE 59.1. HISTORY OF THE IDENTIFICATION OF VIRAL AGENTS ASSOCIATED WITH DIARRHEA

Time	Recognized Agents	Putative Pathogens
Cultivation period		
1940–1950s		Transmissible agents
1958		Echovirus 14, 18, 19 and others
1960		Adenovirus (1, 2, 3, 4, 5, 7) and others
1970		Coxsackievirus A and B
EM period		
1972	Norwalk	Parvovirus
1973	Rotavirus group A	
1975	Enteric adenoviruses 40, 41, 31	Coronavirus
	Astrovirus	
	Calicivirus	
1980s	Rotavirus groups B and C	
1974 to present	Small round structured viruses, Norwalk, Snow Mountain, Hawaii, Taunton, Paramatta	
1984		Toroviruses (Berne/Breda)
1988		Picobirnavirus
1991	Aichi virus	

phic structure as seen by EM that can often be confused with other membranous material from the patient's gut that is seen in fecal specimens. Similarly, viruses that produce a cytopathic effect (CPE) in cell culture, such as enteroviruses and adenoviruses, may be enteric agents that are easy to cultivate but not necessarily the cause of disease. With the exception of the enteroviruses and reoviruses, the enteric viral pathogens described in this chapter either are noncultivatable or grow poorly in cell culture and have only a single principal method for identification, usually EM.

When possible, one way to avoid problems in virus identification is to establish more than one detection method. The development or availability of alternative assay systems to EM and IEM, such as immunoassays, molecular-based detection techniques, or cultivation methods, can help confirm the identity of a viral agent seen initially by EM. For example, work to establish the pathogenic role of coronaviruses as agents of gastroenteritis has been inhibited by the lack of alternative, confirmatory assays that are needed to distinguish particles that appear to be coronaviruses from cellular debris with comparable morphologic features. Consequently, the observation of a fringed agent with a crown-like appearance and size in a stool specimen is often termed a "coronavirus-like particle" (CVLP) because no method is available to confirm this observation.

TABLE 59.2. REQUIREMENTS FOR A NOVEL VIRUS TO BE CONSIDERED AN ETIOLOGIC AGENT

1. Strength/consistency of the association: more common in cases with diseases than in controls.
2. Documented immune response to the agent.
3. Consistency/temporality:
   Onset of disease corresponds to onset of infection; termination of disease corresponds to termination of infection.
4. Biologically *plausible analogy* (e.g., evidence from animal models).
5. Specificity.
6. Biologic gradient–dose response (21).
7. Volunteer studies (Koch postulates).

Once an agent has been found in a fecal specimen from a patient with diarrhea, the establishment of its role as the etiologic agent can be difficult. For an individual patient, one first would have to rule out the presence of more than two dozen other etiologic agents and toxins that are known to cause gastroenteritis, a very difficult task. The issue is less problematic in an epidemic, because one assumes that all patients were infected with the same agent, and so the finding of an etiologic agent in most of these patients and the failure to identify the same agent among controls without illness provides strong epidemiologic evidence of causality. To establish that the agent is not only present in the intestine but that it is actually replicating and causing disease, one would like to document an immune response, which can be measured by a difference in antibody titers between acute and convalescent-phase sera. For example, the pathogenicity of parvoviruses was questioned early by difficulty in documenting an immune response to this agent, whereas the immune response to the Norwalk agent could be clearly demonstrated.

Most of the novel viral agents found in diarrheal specimens from humans are known to be agents of gastroenteritis in different animal species. Toroviruses and coronaviruses were established pathogens in animals, and picobirnaviruses were originally associated with diarrhea in pigs and passaged in the same species. The fact that a virus can cause diarrhea in another animal model provides a measure of biologic plausibility and affirms that the virus can home to gut cells in the animal, replicate in a mammalian host, and is not a pathogen of another microorganism in the gut (e.g., parasite, helminth, or bacteria). Consequently, although phages can be seen in many fecal specimens, they have never been associated with diarrhea in animals or humans, cause no immune response in the host, and are recognized pathogens of bacteria rather than the human host.

In establishing causality, several other lines of evidence are helpful, though often difficult, to establish (20,21). In general, one would expect the onset of disease to correspond with the onset of infection and the termination of disease to correspond with the termination of infection. At the period of most intense diarrhea, the virus is often shed in its highest concentration. For all viral pathogens that have been intensively studied, asymptomatic infections can occur, although virus is often present in substantially lower titers than in patients with acute diarrhea. New diagnostic tests such as polymerase chain reaction (PCR) and cultivation may detect very low titers of virus that may be normally present in the gut but not be pathogenic. As more sensitive assays are employed, we will learn more about the normal viral flora of the gut and what level of virus might be associated with illness. Finally, many different microorganisms, as well as toxins, drugs, allergies, and other conditions, have been associated with gastroenteritis. In establishing the pathogenicity of a new viral agent, one would like to make certain that these other etiologic agents or conditions are not present simultaneously. These requirements for a novel agent to be considered an etiologic agent are similar to those postulates outlined by Robert Koch for infectious agents and Hill (21) for use with epidemiologic data.

REVIEW OF AGENTS

Table 59.3 provides a listing of viruses that may cause gastroenteritis in humans and includes details on their sizes and morphology. Illustrations are shown in Figure 59.1.

Picobirnavirus

Picobirnaviruses are small (pico), bi-segmented (bi), double-stranded RNA (dsRNA) viruses that were first identified by Pereira et al. in 1988 (22). The virus was first found by polyacrylamide gel electrophoresis (PAGE) analysis of RNA extracted from the intestinal contents of a rat. The bands were determined to be dsRNA with lengths of approximately 2.6 and 1.5 kb. The virus has a density of 1.38 to 1.40 g/mL and appears as a 35-nm discrete small round virus (SRV) without distinctive surface structure. Because of the original description of the virus, picobirnaviruses have been detected in fecal specimens of a variety of animal species, including guinea pigs (23), pigs (24,25), calves (26), rabbits (27), birds (28), and humans (29), and have varied, with some strains having two segmented dsRNA bands and others with three distinct dsRNA bands (trirnaviruses) (30). Gatti et al. (24) observed that the virus was more common in pigs with diarrhea than in control animals, thereby linking the presence of the picobirnaviruses with diarrhea. Picobirnaviruses have been propagated in mammalian cell cultures as well (31).

TABLE 59.3. VIRUSES THAT MAY CAUSE GASTROENTERITIS IN HUMANS

		Virus Description			Enteric Disease in	
Virus	Family	Size (nm)	Nucleic Acid	Morphology—Electron Microscopy	Animals	Humans
Coronavirus	Coronaviridae	60–2,200	+ ssRNA	Enveloped, pleomorphic, fringed	Diarrhea in cows and other animals	?diarrhea, ?NEC, ?tropical sprue
Torovirus	Coronaviridae genus *Torovirus*	100–150	+ ssRNA	Enveloped, pleomorphic, fringed	Diarrhea in cows (Breda)	?Diarrhea in children
Picobirnavirus	Not classified	35	dsRNA, two segments	SRV	Diarrhea in pigs; infections in pigs, hamsters, rabbits, and birds	?Diarrhea in HIV-infected humans
Reovirus	Reoviridae	70–75	dsRNA, ten segments	Spoked wheel-shape, double capsid		?Diarrhea, no confirmed disease, ?biliary atresia
Enterovirus	Picornaviridae	26–28	ssRNA	SRV		?Outbreaks of diarrhea due to select types
Parvovirus	Parvoviridae	20–30	ssDNA	SRV	Diarrhea in cows, cats, mink, and dogs	?Diarrhea

SRV, small round virus.

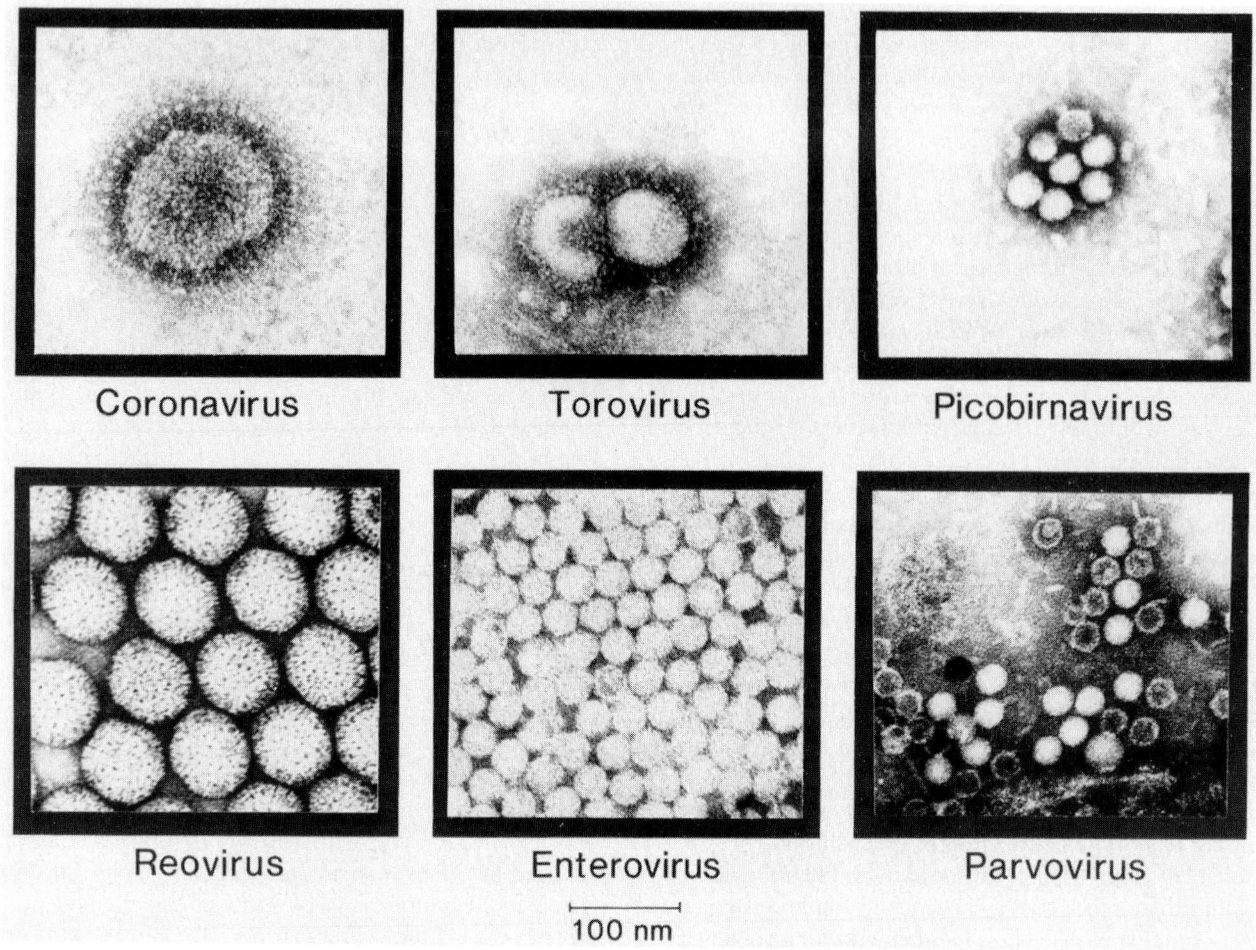

FIGURE 59.1. Viruses that may cause gastroenteritis in humans.

In humans, picobirnaviruses have been identified in fecal specimens collected in various settings. After the original identification from fecal specimens in Brazil, these viruses were identified in fecal specimens from children or adults with gastroenteritis in Venezuela (30,32), England (27), Argentina (33,34), and the United States (35), and in people without diarrhea in England (27). In both the American and Argentine studies, picobirnavirus was significantly linked with diarrhea in HIV-infected patients (35). In the U.S. study, 6 of 65 HIV-infected patients with diarrhea excreted picobirnavirus, compared with 1 of 65 HIV-infected patients without diarrhea ($p = .11$) (35). Nonetheless, these patients had 10 distinct episodes of diarrhea from which picobirnavirus was detected, compared with only 2 episodes in a control group without diarrhea ($p = .02$). Infected patients tended to excrete the virus for prolonged periods and one patient excreted the virus for 8 months. No immune response could be detected in the serum of these patients by IEM, an observation that was difficult to assess given the severe stage of disease of these immunocompromised patients. In Argentina, picobirnaviruses were detected in 15% of 82 HIV-infected patients with diarrhea, but in none of the HIV-infected patients without diarrhea (33,34). Similar rates of detection have been found among HIV-infected persons in Australia (G. S. Grohmann, *personal communication*) and Venezuela (30,32).

Although no immune response could be documented in these HIV-infected patients, an immune response could be documented by solid-phase IEM in rabbits experimentally infected with picobirnavirus. The demonstration of an immune response that was associated in time with the period of virus excretion and the ability to culture an animal strain in a mammalian cell line both suggest that picobirnavirus is a virus of vertebrates.

Diagnosis of picobirnavirus rests with the identification of two segments by PAGE examination of RNA extracted from fecal specimens. New evidence suggests that the sensitivity of detection can be increased at least fourfold if the RNA is first concentrated (35). Recent cloning and sequencing of the segmented genome has provided new approaches for diagnosis by reverse transcriptase polymerase chain reaction (RT-PCR) (36). The role of the virus as a pathogen in humans remains in question, and improvements in diagnostic assays are needed to examine the epidemiology and association of this novel agent with diarrhea (27,36).

Toroviruses

Toroviruses are enveloped, positive-strand RNA viruses that cause enteric infections and diarrhea in animals and, perhaps, humans (37). The virus was first identified in Berne, Switzerland, from the rectal swab of a horse with pseudomembranous enteritis attributed to *Salmonella,* as well as the prototype strain Berne virus (BEV) (38). The enteropathogenic role of toroviruses was supported by studies of Woode et al. (39) in Breda, Iowa, who found a bovine torovirus (the Breda agent [BRV]) to be present in stool specimens obtained from calves with severe diarrhea during an outbreak in a dairy herd. The discovery and description of toroviruses as enteric pathogens in cows and their finding in a broad group of higher vertebrates (e.g., pigs, cats, and mice) led to an intense search to ascertain whether torovirus was also a cause of diarrhea in humans.

Studies of animals led to a broader understanding of the pathogenicity, clinical features, and epidemiology of toroviruses that has helped guide the search for human disease. Although the importance of BEV as an etiologic agent of diarrhea in horses is unclear, BRV strains cause watery diarrhea in gnotobiotic calves 24 to 48 hours after experimental infection (40). This diarrhea is accompanied by dehydration, weakness, and malabsorption measured as a reduction in xylose resorption. Infection occurs primarily in the crypt cells of the intestinal villi, particularly in the large intestine. Koopmans et al. (37,41) described a high attack rate of torovirus-associated diarrhea under field conditions in the Netherlands when colostrum-fed calves were monitored prospectively. Diarrhea occurred in 9 of 10 calves, lasted 2 to 13 days, and caused dehydration in 4 animals. Symptoms were similar to those of calf rotavirus and coronavirus. Toroviruses appeared to cause respiratory tract or generalized infections as well and have been identified in respiratory secretions and the respiratory tract on postmortem examination. The intestines of experimentally infected cows examined on postmortem show involvement from the midjejunum to the lower small intestine, with thinning of the wall, villus fusion, atrophy, and epithelial disorientation.

Virologic studies of animal toroviruses have provided diagnostic tools that have helped in the search for toroviruses in humans. The virus, which belongs to the genus *Torovirus* and the family Coronaviridae, has an unusual, pleomorphic structure by EM (42). The viruses often appear like a misshaped donut (torus) that can be deformed to biconcave disks, or membranous particles with various intermediate forms that make them difficult to identify except to the alert and motivated electron microscopist (43). They are 100 to 150 nm in length and have 20-nm peplomers that project from the surface like clubs or fringe. BEV is the only strain successfully adapted to grow in tissue culture.

Torovirus contains a single positive strand of RNA 25 to 30 kb long that is polyadenylated and has six open reading frames, which encode for various proteins that have not been fully characterized. Several of these proteins are antigenic and lead to an immune response in experimentally infected calves (44). An immunoglobulin M response can be measured early after infection, and seroconversion by immunoglobulin G (IgG) occurs subsequently. Serosurveys of herds of cows indicate that most adult cows from various countries surveyed have IgG antibodies; maternal antibody is present in most newborn calves, disappears after 3 to 4 months, and is replaced by age 2 years with antibody acquired through natural infection (45). In serosurveys, most adult horses also have antibodies to toroviruses (BEV) (46). The observation that antibodies to BEV and BRV are partially cross-reactive is based on experiments in which assays for these viruses detected antibodies in other species (e.g., goats, sheep, pigs, rabbits, and mice), suggesting that these assays might be used for serosurveys in humans (47). However, serosurveys of veterinarians and farm workers in Great Britain (47) and Switzerland and in Indians with tropical sprue (48) were negative for antibodies to BRV, indicating either that humans have little exposure to the virus or that the human strain does not cross-react with the animal strains (47,48).

Work with animal torovirus has also led to the development of assays to detect torovirus antigen in fecal specimens. Besides EM and IEM, an enzyme-linked immunoadsorbent assay (ELISA) has been developed using bovine reagents (47), as well as complementary DNA (cDNA) probes for hybridization made from the BEV strain (49). Finally, RT-PCR has been used to detect RNA from the conserved 3N ends of the virus, and this method can detect both equine (BEV) and bovine (BRV) strains (50). These assays have not been used extensively to search for toroviruses in human fecal specimens.

The role of toroviruses as a cause of diarrhea in humans remains unanswered. Torovirus-like particles (TVLPs) have been seen by EM in fecal specimens from children and adults with diarrhea in Great Britain, France (16), and the Netherlands. However, no other assays were applied to confirm the identity of the particle or assess its etiologic role as the cause of diarrhea. Koopmans et al. (49) identified toroviral RNA by using a hybridization assay with a cDNA probe prepared from BEV, but the results were not unequivocal due to high background levels and rapid degradation of RNA in stool specimens. In Toronto, a recent survey of patients with diarrhea whose fecal specimens were screened by EM identified TVLPs in 224 (8%) of 2,800 specimens screened, suggesting that TVLPs may be more common in human fecal specimens than was previously determined (50). Koopmans et al. (49) tested a subset of these specimens with various additional diagnostic tests to determine the true identity of these particles. Although molecular assays used previously gave inconclusive results, an ELISA using bovine torovirus reference reagents distinguished between those stools found to be positive for TVLPs by EM and those that were negative. This finding suggested that a two-way antigenic cross-reactivity existed between human TVLPs and bovine TVLPs and led to the use of human reagents from which human TVLP-specific antiserum was raised, and this antiserum was found to be more specific than antiserum to the bovine strain. These assays and reagents need to be applied further to other surveys to detect TVLPs.

Recently, the Toronto group has identified toroviruses in 72 (35%) of 206 children with gastroenteritis, and in 30 (14%) of 206 controls (51). Compared with patients with rotavirus or astrovirus, patients infected with torovirus were more often immunocompromised and nosocomially infected and had less vomiting, but more bloody diarrhea. Toroviruses have been identified in Indian children as well, but EM observations were not followed up with confirmatory diagnostic assays (52).

In summary, toroviruses have been found in human stools by EM and their presence has been confirmed by immunoassay based on reagents to bovine toroviruses. Their role as etiologic agents of diarrhea in the human population remains to be determined and will rest, in part, upon finding an immune response, which is a *sine qua non* of infection (47). Improved diagnostics, particularly molecular assays based on sequence information of human TVLPs, will assist in confirming those specimens that appear to be positive by EM. This should be aided by improved molecular characterization of the virus (17). The availability of new assays for TVLPs should lead rapidly to more information about their etiologic role in humans.

Coronavirus

Coronaviruses are large, enveloped, positive-strand RNA viruses belonging to the family Coronaviridae that cause gastroenteritis in many animal species but are most commonly associated with respiratory infections in humans (53). They were first reported to cause explosive diarrhea in adults (12) and were later found to be associated with tropical sprue in Indian children and adults (13). The regular finding of coronaviruses in the feces of patients with nonbacterial gastroenteritis and the recognition that coronaviruses are a common cause of diarrhea in other animal species has led many investigators to seek an etiologic role for the human enteric coronaviruses as an agent of gastroenteritis in humans (54,55). Despite two decades of research to test this association, the findings have been inconclusive, leaving this question unanswered.

The virus can be detected in human feces by direct EM with negative stain and appears as a pleomorphic particle 60 to 2,200 nm in diameter, covered with a distinct, crownlike (corona) fringe made up of regularly spaced, club-shaped projections approximately 20 nm long (56). This fringe is often disrupted, leaving a particle that could easily be confused with cellular debris in the stool (57). In the absence of any confirmatory assay, all particles found in fecal specimens are referred to as CVLPs. These are distinct from the coronaviruses present in the human respiratory tract that are a recognized cause of acute infections and for which confirmatory diagnostic assays are available. Human respiratory coronaviruses cross-react with enteric coronaviruses by IEM (58,59), but not by ELISA or immunoblot assays (60,61).

Because EM is the only method routinely used to search for coronaviruses in fecal specimens, and because the particles are pleomorphic, variations in the prevalence of infection observed in epidemiologic studies may reflect more the ability of and the criteria used by the electron microscopist than the true prevalence of infection. The prevalence of CVLPs observed in a recent 3-year survey of more than 50,000 stool examinations conducted by electron microscopists in England indicated that about 0.7 CVLPs were detected for every 100 rotaviruses, and this rate varied from 0% to 2.3% (62). A similar 6-year survey of electron microscopists at 10 centers in the United States indicated that from more than 50,000 EM examinations, CVLPs were detected in about 6% of specimens and detection rates ranged from 0% at three centers to 13% at one center, where rates have always been reported high (63–65). CVLPs had no distinct seasonality and were found in both children and adults. Given the variable range and prevalence within a single country, the results obtained from surveys in many other countries are difficult to interpret. What is clear is that CVLPs appear to have a global distribution (66–70), are more commonly found in the stools of infants and children than in adults, and do not appear to have a distinct seasonality in their distribution or known mode of transmission. Fewer studies have compared the rates of CVLPs among patients with diarrhea and among controls or have monitored the duration of viral shedding. Some investigators have found more CVLPs in patients with diarrhea than in controls (58,71). Others have found CVLPs to be as common in patients with diarrhea as in controls without diarrhea (56,68,72), raising doubts about their etiologic role. Because asymptomatic shedding is common, and because CVLPs can be excreted for long periods in healthy people, it may be difficult to prove pathogenicity merely by comparing prevalence in patients with and without diarrhea.

Several investigators have identified CVLPs in stools of infants with necrotizing enterocolitis (NEC) and tried to implicate this virus as the causative agent (73,74). In 1985, Resta et al. (60) reported the first successful propagation of one such CVLP and the development of confirmatory assays for this infection. In the subsequent decade, efforts to reproduce these results have been unsuccessful, raising doubts about their initial validity. Others have found CVLPs in intestinal lesions of patients with NEC, but in the absence of confirmatory assays, the virus could not be distinguished from other cellular material with similar morphologic features (75). In 1975, Mathan et al. (13) found CVLPs to be more common in fecal specimens from patients with tropical sprue. They later described virus-like particles in the cisternae of the smooth endoplasmic reticulum of damaged crypt cells (76). Despite these observations, the etiology of tropical sprue remains unknown and the association with coronavirus has not been confirmed.

In summary, CVLPs are found in fecal specimens from humans and are most frequently detected in specimens from infants and young children by EM. It is often difficult to distinguish CVLPs from other cellular debris present in stool, and no independent culture method or antigenic or molecular-based assays are currently available to confirm the identity of the virus. Hence, any attempt to prove the association of CVLPs with human disease must await the development of diagnostic reagents prepared from fecal specimens or cultures of virus of human origin.

Enteroviruses

The enteroviruses were among the first viral agents suggested to be causative agents of nonbacterial gastroenteritis in humans (77). These viruses were among the first to be successfully cultivated from stools, and their considerable antigenic diversity with multiple serotypes perhaps ensured that at least some might be implicated as an agent of gastroenteritis in humans. Some of these viruses appeared to cause respiratory tract infections or viral syndrome in which gastroenteritis might be an associated symptom rather than the prime presentation of infection. In many early studies, individual serotypes of enteroviruses (echoviruses 4, 11, 14, 18, and 19) were tentatively associated with gastroenteritis, even though full evidence for causality was lacking (1,78). Over time, these associations have been put aside, and today, enteroviruses are not generally considered to be causative agents of gastroenteritis in humans, even though several serotypes may well be diarrheal pathogens.

The enteroviruses are positive-strand RNA viruses that combine the polioviruses, coxsackieviruses, and echoviruses, all of which are found in the human intestine. Enteroviruses are small (20 to 30 nm), nonenveloped viruses that appear as SRVs or small round featureless viruses by EM, because they have none of the distinct morphologic features of the SRSVs, which include both the caliciviruses and astroviruses (79). More than 70 serotypes of enteroviruses have been identified, and in humans these are associated with a variety of clinical illnesses, ranging from acute respiratory tract infections, hemorrhagic conjunctivitis, aseptic meningitis, and encephalitis to carditis. Because of the great antigenic diversity of this group, neutralization tests are required to characterize the agent and to detect a type-specific immune response in infected patients. Detection is by cultivation of stool specimens, EM detection of SRVs, or hybridization using oligonucleotide probes common to all enteroviruses, and subsequent typing by neutralization (80).

Epidemiologic studies to examine whether enteroviruses cause diarrhea have rested either on the investigation of specimens collected from longitudinal studies, on case–control studies of diarrhea in children, or on the examination of fecal specimens collected in outbreaks of nonbacterial gastroenteritis. In outbreaks, one assumes that a single serotype would be involved and that this serotype would be detected more frequently among cases with diarrhea than controls who were well. Eichenwald et al. (81) identified echovirus 18 among premature infants with diarrhea in a nursery and in sick infants younger than 5 months on a hospital ward. Investigations of other outbreaks have implicated serotypes 1, 2, 6, 7, 11, 14, 19, 20, and 22 to be associated with diarrhea (78,82–89). Here, the finding of the same organism in more than one child with symptoms supported an etiologic role but did not confirm it. Moreover, the virus was often identified in other children who did not have diarrhea. At the time of these studies, many other diarrheal pathogens that are currently recognized had not yet been discovered and could, therefore, not be ruled out.

Case–control and longitudinal studies have compared detection rates and serotypes of enteroviruses in children with diarrhea and in those without diarrhea. Ramos-Alvarez and Sabin (89) implicated enterovirus types 2, 6, 7, 8, 10, 11, 12, 14, 18, and 19 as the agents of summer diarrhea in 42% of young children with diarrhea compared with 13% of those without diarrhea. Sommerville (90) isolated echovirus strains 6, 7, 9, 11, and 13 from 8.5% of 338 children with diarrhea but only 2.5% of 115 children the same age with respiratory tract infections. Other investigators have failed to support these findings. Yow et al. (91), for example, isolated enteroviruses in 5.6% of 390 infants with diarrhea compared with 4.4% of 380 controls, giving numbers too small to establish an etiologic role for all enteroviruses or for any individual serotype. Because many of these serotypes are common respiratory tract pathogens in children, it is difficult to determine whether these were primary enteric infections or whether the diarrheal illness was secondary to a respiratory tract infection, possibly mediated by use of medications or altered diet.

Despite the wealth of early studies implicating enteroviruses as potential causes of diarrhea, the large number of types and the low frequency of any single type have made it difficult to unequivocally implicate individual strains as a cause of diarrhea (82). In outbreaks, a number of enteroviruses have been identified from patients with gastroenteritis, suggesting that they may have an etiologic role in some settings. Nonetheless, given the large number of serotypes and a relatively small contribution of any individual serotype, very large longitudinal studies or more outbreak investigations are required to arrive at a conclusion concerning causality. Even then, it may be difficult to separate infections for which diarrhea is the prime illness from those in which GI symptoms were secondary to other infections.

Reoviruses

The first reoviruses were identified in the early 1950s from fecal specimens of persons who clinically did not have a GI illness (92). Although these viruses were initially thought to be in the enterovirus group, they were later distinguished by their larger size (75 nm), cytoplasmic inclusions produced in monkey kidney tissue cells, patterns of hemagglutination of human type O erythrocytes, and pathogenicity for newborn mice. Sabin proposed the name reovirus to emphasize that they were respiratory tract and enteric isolates that were not associated with disease (orphan). Later, the virus was found to contain 10 segments of dsRNA that was specific for this virus group, and these viruses were reclassified in a new family, Reoviridae.

Members of the Reoviridae family are found in a wide host of animals, from insects and crustaceans to vertebrates, including mammals. In mammals other than humans, they produce a range of upper respiratory tract and enteric symptoms, with diarrhea occurring as one of the many presentations in mice, infant and adult cows, sheep, pigs, and dogs. Although reoviruses have been periodically implicated as etiologic agents of diarrhea in humans (87,89,93,94), study results so far have been inconclusive, and they are currently not considered causative agents of diarrhea. Reoviruses have also been implicated in biliary atresia (95–98), but this association has never been confirmed. Despite the availability of good diagnostic assays for detecting these agents in humans, the reoviruses are only occasionally identified in a human fecal specimen and are probably unrelated to diarrhea.

Parvovirus

Parvoviruses are small (20 to 30 nm), round, featureless, single-stranded DNA viruses that can be distinguished from the enteroviruses by their different buoyant density in cesium chloride, from the Norwalk viruses by their featureless surface and slightly smaller size, and from both of these RNA viruses by their nucleic acids (99). Several animal parvoviruses, including strains from cows, cats, mink, and dogs, have been well characterized and appear to cause gastroenteritis in these species (100). In humans, the search for a comparable pathogenic strain has been elusive.

Several outbreaks of gastroenteritis have been identified in which an SRV was seen by EM that could not be cultivated but resembled parvovirus in morphology, size, or buoyant density (14,15,101). These SRVs were often found with other established pathogens (e.g., astroviruses, caliciviruses, or SRSVs). In the absence of alternative immune or nucleic acid-based assays to characterize the strain, no final identification was made. No distinct seroconversion could be observed in paired sera collected from patients involved in these outbreaks, raising questions about their true infectious potential. Parvovirus B19, the only recognized parvovirus in humans, causes aplastic anemia, erythema infectiosum (fifth disease), and possible birth defects but is not associated with gastroenteritis. Parvovirus B19 is distinct from the enteric candidate parvoviruses based on the lack of antigenic cross-reactivity and failure to cross-hybridize using nucleic acid probes. Both the identity of the fecal parvoviruses and their role in gastroenteritis remain in question.

Aichi Virus

The Aichi virus was first identified in fecal specimens from 12 of 15 subjects in Aichi Prefecture, Japan, who developed gastroenteritis after consumption of oysters (18,102). The virus caused apparent CPEs on BS-C-1 cells and Aichi antigen was detected by ELISA in 13 (28%) of 47 fecal specimens from patients involved in five different outbreaks of oyster-associated gastroenteritis (103). Nearly half of affected patients demonstrated a fourfold or greater risk in neutralizing antibodies to the infecting strain. The virus was also identified in 5 (2.3%) of 222 Pakistani children with gastroenteritis and 5 (0.7%) of 722 Japanese tourists returning home from travel in Southeast Asia (104).

The virus was recently sequenced, and it has distinct gene coding arrangements that have distinguished it from other genera of the Picornaviridae family and that have led the investigators to propose that it be regarded as a new genus (105). The availability of molecular and immune diagnostics and the ability to cultivate this virus clear the way for other groups to investigate the prevalence of the Aichi virus in other clinical and epidemic settings (106).

SUMMARY

Although many viruses inhabit the gut, relatively few directly cause diarrhea. Some agents, such as the reoviruses and enteroviruses, survive well in the human intestine, can easily be identified and characterized by culture, and probably cause little, if any, diarrhea. Others that grow poorly, like toroviruses, picobirnaviruses, and coronaviruses, cause diarrhea in animals and may well cause diarrhea in humans, although this may not be common. Finally, a third group of viruses are generally found elsewhere in the body but can be opportunists in the gut and are infrequently, if ever, even secondarily associated with gastroenteritis. When a virus is identified in the stool of a patient with gastroenteritis, its identity must be confirmed, other common agents of gastroenteritis must be ruled out, and an immune response must be documented before any thought can be given to its role as the causative agent.

REFERENCES

1. Madeley CR. Epidemiology of gut viruses. In: Farthing MJG, ed. *Viruses and the gut.* London: Smith Kline and French Laboratories Ltd, 1989:5–15.
2. Kapikian AZ, Estes MK, Chanock RM. Norwalk group of viruses. In: Fields BN, Knipe DM, Howley PM, et al., eds. *Fields virology,* third edition, volume 1. Philadelphia: Lippincott–Raven Publishers, 1996:783–810.

3. Yow MD, Melnick JL, Blattner RJ, et al. The association of viruses and bacteria with infantile diarrhea. *Am J Epidemiol* 1970;92:33–39.
4. Reiman HA, Price AH, Hodges JH. The cause of epidemic diarrhea, nausea and vomiting (viral dysentery?). *Proc Soc Exp Biol Med* 1945;59:8–9.
5. Gordon I, Ingraham HS, Korns RF. Transmission of epidemic gastroenteritis to human volunteers by oral administration of fecal filtrates. *J Exp Med* 1947;86:409–422.
6. Kapikian AZ, Wyatt RG, Dolin R, et al. Visualization by immune electron microscopy of a 27 nm particle associated with acute infectious nonbacterial gastroenteritis. *J Virol* 1972; 10:1075–1081.
7. Bishop RF, Davidson GP, Holmes IH, et al. Virus particles in epithelial cells of duodenal mucosa from children with viral gastroenteritis. *Lancet* 1973;1:1281–1283.
8. Madeley CR, Cosgrove BP. 28 nm particles in faeces in infantile gastroenteritis. *Lancet* 1975;2:451–452.
9. Madeley CR, Cosgrove BP. Viruses in infantile gastroenteritis [Letter]. *Lancet* 1975;2:124.
10. Johansson ME, Uhnoo I, Kidd AH, et al. Direct identification of enteric adenovirus, a candidate new serotype, associated with infantile gastroenteritis. *J Clin Microbiol* 1980;12:95–100.
11. DeJong JC, Wigand R, Kidd AH, et al. Candidate adenoviruses 40 and 41: fastidious adenoviruses from human infant stool. *J Med Virol* 1983;11:215–231.
12. Caul EO, Paver WK, Clarke SK. Coronavirus particles in faeces from patients with gastroenteritis [Letter]. *Lancet* 1975;1:1192.
13. Mathan M, Mathan VI, Swaminathan SP, et al. Pleomorphic virus-like particles in human faeces. *Lancet* 1975;1:1068–1069.
14. Appleton H, Higgins PG. Viruses and gastroenteritis in infants [Letter]. *Lancet* 1975;1:1297.
15. Clarke SKR, Cook GT, Egglestone SI, et al. A virus from epidemic vomiting disease. *Br Med J* 1972;3:86–89.
16. Beards GM, Green J, Hall C, et al. An enveloped virus in stools of children and adults with gastroenteritis that resembles the Breda virus of calves. *Lancet* 1984;1:1050–1052.
17. Duckmanton L, Luan B, Devenish J, et al. Characterization of torovirus from human fecal specimens. *Virology* 1997;239: 158–168.
18. Yamashita T, Kobayashi S, Sakae K, et al. Isolation of cytopathic small round viruses with BS-C-1 cells from patients with gastroenteritis. *J Infect Dis* 1991;164:954–957.
19. Yamashita T, Sakae K, Tsuzuki H, et al. Complete nucleotide sequence and genetic organization of Aichi virus, a distinct member of the Picornaviridae associated with acute gastroenteritis in humans. *J Virol* 1998;72:8408–8412.
20. Huebner RJ. Criteria for etiologic association of prevalent viruses with prevalent diseases. *Ann N Y Acad Sci* 1957;67: 430–438.
21. Hill AB. The environment and disease: association or causation. *Proc Royal Soc Med* 1965;58:295–300.
22. Pereira HG, Flewett TH, Candeias JN, et al. A virus with bisegmented double-stranded RNA genome in rat (*Oryzomys-nigripes*) intestines. *J Gen Virol* 1988;69:2749–2754.
23. Pereira HG, de Araujo HP, Fialho AM, et al. A virus with bisegmented double-stranded RNA genome in guinea pig intestines. *Mem Inst Oswaldo Cruz* 1989;84:137–140.
24. Gatti MSV, Pestana de Castro AF, Ferraz MMG, et al. Viruses with bisegmented double-stranded RNA in pig faeces. *Res Vet Sci* 1989;47:397–398.
25. Chasey D. Porcine picobirnavirus in UK? *Vet Rec* 1990;126:465.
26. Vanopdenbosch E, Wellemans G. Bovine birna type virus: a new etiological agent of neonatal calf diarrhoea? *Vlaams Diergeneeskd Tijdschr* 1990;59:1–4.
27. Gallimore C, Lewis D, Brown D. Detection and characterization of a novel bisegmented double-stranded RNA virus (picobirnavirus) from rabbit faeces. *Arch Virol* 1993;133:63–73.
28. Leite JPG, Monteiro SP, Fialho AM, et al. A novel avian virus with trisegmented double-stranded RNA and further observations on previously described similar viruses with bisegmented genome. *Virus Res* 1990;16:119–126.
29. Pereira HG, Fialho AM, Flewett TH, et al. Novel viruses in human feces. *Lancet* 1988;2:103–104.
30. Ludert JE, Liprandi F. Identification of viruses with bi- and trisegmented double-stranded RNA genome in faeces of children with gastroenteritis. *Institut PasteurElsevier* 1993;144:219–224.
31. Pereira HG. Double-stranded RNA viruses. *Semin Virol* 1991; 2:39–53.
32. Ludert JE, Abdul-Latiff L, Liprandi A, et al. Identification of picobirnavirus, viruses with bisegmented double stranded RNA, in rabbit faeces. *Res Vet Sci* 1995;59(3):222–225.
33. Giordano MO, Martinez LC, Espul C, et al. Diarrhea and enteric emerging viruses in HIV-infected patients. *AIDS Res Hum Retroviruses* 1999;15:1427–1432.
34. Giordano MO, Martinez LC, Rinaldi D, et al. Detection of picobirnavirus in HIV-infected patients with diarrhea in Argentina. *J Acquired Immune Defic Syn Hum Retrovirol* 1998; 18:380–383.
35. Grohmann GS, Glass RI, Pereira HG, et al. Enteric viruses and diarrhea in HIV-infected patients. *N Engl J Med* 1993;329: 14–20.
36. Rosen BI, Fang Z-Y, Glass RI, et al. Cloning of human picobirnavirus gene segments and development of an RT-PCR detection assay. *Virology* 2000;277:316–329.
37. Koopmans M, Horzinek M. Toroviruses of animals and humans (a review). *Adv Virus Res* 1994;43:233–273.
38. Weiss M, Steck F, Horzinek MC. Purification and partial characterization of a new enveloped RNA virus (Berne virus). *J Gen Virol* 1983;64:1849.
39. Woode GN, Reed DE, Runnels PL, et al. Studies with an unclassified virus isolated from diarrheic calves. *Vet Microbiol* 1982;7:221–240.
40. Pohlenz JFL, Cheville NF, Woode GN, et al. Cellular lesions in intestinal mucosa of gnotobiotic calves experimentally infected with a new unclassified bovine virus (Breda virus). *Vet Pathol* 1984;21:407.
41. Koopmans M, van Wuijckhuise-Sjouke L, Schukken YH, et al. Association of diarrhea in cattle with torovirus infections on farms. *Am J Vet Res* 1991;52:1769–1773.
42. Weiss M, Horzinek M. The proposed family Toroviridae: agents of enteric infections. *Arch Virol* 1987;92:1–15.
43. Fagerland JA, Pohlenz JFL, Woode GN. A morphologic study of the replication of Breda virus (proposed family Toroviridae) in bovine intestinal cells. *J Gen Virol* 1986;67:1293–1304.
44. Koopmans M, van den Boom U, Woode G, et al. Seroepidemiology of Breda virus in cattle using ELISA. *Vet Microbiol* 1989; 19:223–243.
45. Koopmans M, Cremers H, Woode G, et al. Breda virus (Toroviridae) infection and systemic antibody response in sentinel calves. *Am J Vet Res* 1990;51:1443–1448.
46. Weiss M, Steck F, Kaderli R, et al. Antibodies to Berne virus in horses and other animals. *Vet Microbiol* 1984;9:523–531.
47. Brown DWG, Beards GM, Flewett TH. Detection of Breda virus antigen and antibody in humans and animals by enzyme immunoassay. *J Clin Microbiol* 1987;24:637–640.
48. Brown DWG, Selvakumar R, Daniel DJ, Et al. Prevalence of neutralizing antibodies to Berne virus in animals and humans in Vellore, South India. *Arch Virol* 1988;98:267–269.
49. Koopmans M, Snijder EJ, Horzinek MC. cDNA probes for the detection of bovine torovirus (Breda virus) infections. *J Clin Microbiol* 1991;29:493–497.

50. Koopmans M, Petric M, Glass RI, et al. Enzyme-linked immunosorbent assay reactivity of torovirus-like particles in fecal specimens from humans with diarrhea. *J Clin Microbiol* 1993;31:2738–2744.
51. Jamieson FB, Wang EEL, Bain C, et al. Human torovirus: a new nosocomial gastrointestinal pathogen. *J Infect Dis* 1998; 178:1263–1269.
52. Krishnam T, Naik TN. Electron microscopic evidence of torovirus like particles in children with diarrhoea. *Indian J Med Res* 1997;105:108–110.
53. McIntosh K. Coronaviruses. In: Fields BN, Knipe DM, Chanock RM, et al., eds. *Virology,* second edition, volume 1. New York: Raven Press, 1990:857–864.
54. Macnaughton MR, Davies HA. Human enteric coronaviruses. *Arch Virol* 1981;70(4):301–313.
55. Clarke SK, Caul EO, Egglestone SI. The human enteric coronaviruses. *Postgrad Med J* 1979;55:135–142.
56. Saif LJ, Heckert RA. Enteric coronaviruses. In: Saif LJ, Theil KW, eds. *Viral diarrheas of man and animals.* Boca Raton: CRC Press, 1990:185–252.
57. Dourmashkin RR, Davies HA, Smith H, et al. Are coronavirus-like particles seen in diarrhoea stools really viruses? *Lancet* 1980; 2:971.
58. Gerna G, Passarani N, Battaglia M, et al. Coronaviruses and gastroenteritis: evidence of antigenic relatedness between human enteric coronavirus strains and human coronavirus OC43. *Microbiol Rev* 1984;7:315.
59. Gerna G, Passerani N, Cereda PM, et al. Antigenic relatedness of human enteric coronavirus strains to human coronavirus OC43: a preliminary report. *J Infect Dis* 1984;150:618.
60. Resta S, Luby JP, Rosenfeld CR, et al. Isolation and propagation of a human enteric coronavirus. *Science* 1985;229:978–981.
61. Battaglia M, Passarani N, Di Matteo A, et al. Human enteric coronaviruses: further characterizations and immunoblotting of viral proteins. *J Infect Dis* 1987;155:140–143.
62. Monroe SS, Glass RI, Noah N, et al. Electron microscopic reporting of gastrointestinal viruses in the United Kingdom, 1985–87. *J Med Virol* 1991;33:193–198.
63. Lew JF, Glass RI, Petric M, et al. Six year retrospective surveillance of gastroenteritis viruses identified at ten electron microscopy centers in the United States and Canada. *Pediatr Infect Dis J* 1990;9:709–714.
64. Payne CM, Ray CG, Bourdin V, et al. An eight-year study of the viral agents of acute gastroenteritis in humans: ultrastructural observations and seasonal distribution with a major emphasis on coronavirus-like particles. *Diagn Microbiol Infect Dis* 1986;5:39–54.
65. Mortensen ML, Ray CG, Payne CM, et al. Coronavirus-like particles in human gastrointestinal disease. *Am J Dis Child* 1985;139:928.
66. Schnagl RD, Morey R, Homes IH. Rotavirus and coronavirus-like particles in aboriginal and non-aboriginal neonates in Kalgoorlie and Alice Springs. *Med J Aust* 1979;2:178.
67. Yongnian H, Wang NL, Lo HN, et al. A finding of coronavirus particles in feces of patients with diarrhea. *Chin J Epidemiol* 1987;8:25.
68. Bennett PH, Gust ID. Coronavirus-like particles and other agents in the faeces of children in Efate, Vanuatu. *J Trop Med Hyg* 1982;85:213.
69. Simhon A, Mata L. Fecal rotaviruses, adenoviruses, coronavirus-like particles, and small round viruses in a cohort of rural Costa Rican children. *Am J Trop Med Hyg* 1985;34:931–936.
70. Sitbon M. Human-enteric-coronavirus-like particles (CVLP) with different epidemiological characteristics. *J Med Virol* 1985; 16:67.
71. Vaucher YE, Ray CG, Minnich LL, et al. Pleomorphic, enveloped, virus-like particles associated with gastrointestinal illness in neonates. *J Infect Dis* 1982;145:27.
72. Maass G, Baumeister HG. Coronavirus-like particles as aetiological agents of acute non-bacterial gastroenteritis in humans. In: Karger S, Basel, eds. Develop. Biol. Standards International Symposium of enteric infection in man and animals: standards of immunology, Proceedings edition, volume 5. Dublin:, 1982:319.
73. Siegel JD, Luby JP, Laptook AR, et al. Identification of coronavirus (CRNV) in a premature nursery during an outbreak of necrotizing enterocolitis (NEC) and diarrhea (D). *Pediatr Res* 1983;17:181A.
74. Chany C, Moscovici O, Lebon P, et al. Association of coronavirus-like infection with neonatal necrotizing enterocolitis. *Pediatrics* 1982;69:209.
75. Moscovici O, Chany C, Lebon P, et al. Association d'infection a coronavirus avec l'enterocolite hemorragique du nouveau-ne. *CR Acad Sci Paris* 1980;290:869–872.
76. Baker SJ, Mathan M, Mathan VI, et al. Chronic enterocyte infection with coronavirus: one possible cause of the syndrome of tropical sprue? *Dig Dis Sci* 1982;27:1039–1043.
77. Melnick JL. Enteroviruses: polioviruses, coxsackieviruses, echoviruses, and newer enteroviruses. In: Fields BN, Knipe DN, Chanock RN, eds. *Virology,* second edition, volume 1. New York: Raven Press, 1990:549–605.
78. Kibrick S. Current status of Coxsackie and ECHO viruses in human disease. *Prog Med Virol* 1964;6:27–70.
79. Caul EO, Appleton H. The electron microscopical and physical characteristics of small round human fecal viruses: an interim scheme for classification. *J Med Virol* 1982;9:257–265.
80. Morens DM, Pallansch MA, Moore M. Polioviruses and other enteroviruses. In: Belshe RB, ed. *Textbook of human virology,* second edition. St. Louis, MO: Mosby–Year Book, 1991:484–494.
81. Eichenwald HF, Ababio A, Arky AM, et al. Epidemic diarrhea in premature and older infants caused by ECHO virus type 18. *JAMA* 1958;166:1563–1566.
82. Melnick JL. Enteroviruses. In: Evans AS, ed. *Viral infections of humans, epidemiology and control.* New York: Plenum Publishing, 1978.
83. (deleted by author)
84. McAllister RM. Echovirus infections. *Pediatr Clin North Am* 1960;7:927–945.
85. Parrott RH. The clinical importance of group A coxsackieviruses. *Annotated N Y Acad Sci* 1957;67:230–240.
86. Sanford JP, Sulkin SE. The clinical spectrum of echovirus infection. *N Engl J Med* 1959;261:1113–1122.
87. Ramos-Alvarez M. Cytopathogenic enteric viruses associated with undifferentiated diarrheal syndromes in early childhood. *Ann N Y Acad Sci* 1957;67:326–331.
88. Klein JO, Lerner AM, Finland M. Acute gastroenteritis associated with ECHO virus, type 11. *Am J Med Sci* 1960;240:749–753.
89. Ramos-Alvarez M, Sabin AB. Enteropathogenic viruses and bacteria. Role in summer diarrheal diseases of infancy and early childhood. *JAMA* 1958;167:147–156.
90. Sommerville RG. Enteroviruses and diarrhoea in young persons. *Lancet* 1958;2:1347–1349.
91. Yow MD, Melnick JL, Blattner RJ, et al. Enteroviruses in infantile diarrhea. *Am J Hyg* 1963;77:283–292.
92. Tyler KL, Fields BN. Reoviruses. In: Fields BN, Knipe DM, Chanock RM, eds. *Virology,* second edition, volume 2. New York: Raven Press, 1990:1307–1328.
93. Ramos-Alvarez M, Sabin AB. Characteristics of poliomyelitis and other enteric viruses recovered in tissue culture from healthy American children. *Proc Soc Exp Biol Med* 1954;87: 655–661.

94. Rosen L, Hovis JF, Mastrota FM, et al. An outbreak of infection with a type 1 reovirus among children in an institution. *Am J Hyg* 1960;71:266–274.
95. Bangaru B, Morecki R, Glaser JH, et al. Comparative studies of biliary atresia in human newborn and reovirus-induced cholangitis in weanling mice. *Lab Invest* 1980:456–462.
96. Glaser JH, Balistreri WF, Morecki R. Role of reovirus type 3 in persistent infantile cholestasis. *Pediatrics* 1984;105:912–915.
97. Glaser JH, Morecki R. Reovirus type 3 and neonatal cholestasis. *Semin Liver Dis* 1987;7:100–107.
98. Morecki R, Glaser JH, Cho S, et al. Biliary atresia and reovirus type 3 infection. *N Engl J Med* 1982;307:481–484.
99. Pattison JR. Parvoviruses: medical and biological aspects. In: Fields BN, Knipe DM, eds. *Virology,* second edition, volume 2. New York: Raven Press, 1990:1766–1784.
100. Bridger JC. Small viruses associated with gastroenteritis in animals. In: Saif LJ, Thiel KW, eds. *Viral diarrheas of man and animals.* Boca Raton: CRC Press, 1989:161–182.
101. Appleton H. Small round viruses: classification and role in food-borne infections. In: Ciba Foundation Symposium 128, editor. *Novel diarrhoea viruses.* New York: John Wiley and Sons, 1987:108–125.
102. Yamashita T. Biological and epidemiological characteristics of Aichi virus, as a new member of Picornaviridae [Review]. *Virus* 1999;49:183–191.
103. Yamashita T, Sakae K, Ishihara Y, et al. Prevalence of newly isolated, cytopathic small round virus (Aichi strain) in Japan. *J Clin Microbiol* 1993;31(11):2938–2943.
104. Yamashita T, Sakae K, Kobayashi S, et al. Isolation of cytopathic small round virus (Aichi Virus) from Pakistani children and Japanese travelers from Southeast Asia. *Microbiol Immunol* 1995;39:433–435.
105. Su-Arehawaratana P, Singharaj P, Taylor DN, et al. Safety and immunogenicity of different immunization regimens of CVD 103-HgR live oral cholera vaccine in soldiers and civilians in Thailand. *J Infect Dis* 1992;165:1042–1048.
106. Yamashita T, Tsuzuki H, Kobayashi S, Sakae K, Suzuki Y. Application of RT-PCR to detect Aichi virus as a new member of Picornaviridae isolated from patients with gastroenteritis. *Clin Virol (Jpn)* 1999;27:127–132.

60

AMEBIASIS

SHARON L. REED
JONATHAN I. RAVDIN

Invasive amebiasis due to infection by *Entamoeba histolytica* is one of the most important parasitic diseases of humans. This enteric protozoan is the third leading parasitic cause of death worldwide (1); there is no vaccine or form of chemoprophylaxis available. The organism spreads by direct fecal-oral contact or contamination of food and water due to poor sanitary facilities and practices; therefore, the disease burden is concentrated in the poorest, least developed regions. Continually expanding knowledge of the parasite's pathogenic mechanisms and the host's immune response provides promise for future vaccine development.

BIOLOGY

The life cycle of *E. histolytica* is relatively straightforward, in comparison to the nematodes and cestodes that parasitize the gut (Fig. 60.1). The cyst is the infective form because of its chitinous cell wall (a polymer of *N*-acetyl-D-glucosamine) (2). Cysts can survive for weeks at an appropriate temperature and humidity. Following ingestion of the cyst, stimulation by stomach acid apparently induces excystation in the small bowel. Trophozoites go on to colonize the large bowel, feed on bacteria, and multiply or encyst depending on local conditions. The infective dose can be as little as a single cyst; the incubation period appears to diminish with the size of the infective dose (from weeks to a few days) (3). Trophozoites are not transmissible because of their rapid disintegration outside the body and susceptibility to the low pH environment of the stomach.

Entamoeba histolytica belongs to the pseudopod-forming protozoan superclass Rhizopoda within the subphylum Sarcodina (4). There is definitive evidence for the existence of morphologically identical but distinct pathogenic and nonpathogenic species of *Entamoeba, E. histolytica,* and *E. dispar,* respectively (5). Studies of zymodeme analysis, the pattern of electrophoretic mobility of certain parasite isoenzymes, first revealed an association of distinct zymodemes with symptomatic invasive amebic disease (6). Studies with RNA and DNA probes demonstrated genetic differences between *E. histolytica* and *E. dispar* (7–9). Ribosomal RNA probes have also indicated species specificity (10). The existence and (**names**) of these two distinct species were first proposed in 1925 (11); it is essential to differentiate *E. histolytica* from *E. dispar* for any study of the epidemiology and clinical management of amebiasis.

Entamoeba histolytica has numerous antigenic differences from *E. dispar.* Distinct epitopes of the 170-kd heavy subunit of the galactose-inhibitable adherence protein exist in *E. histolytica* (12). Murine monoclonal antibodies distinguish between *E. histolytica* and *E. dispar* isolates (13–15). For example, antibodies to a recombinant form of the 29-kd amebic surface antigen differentiated *E. histolytica* from

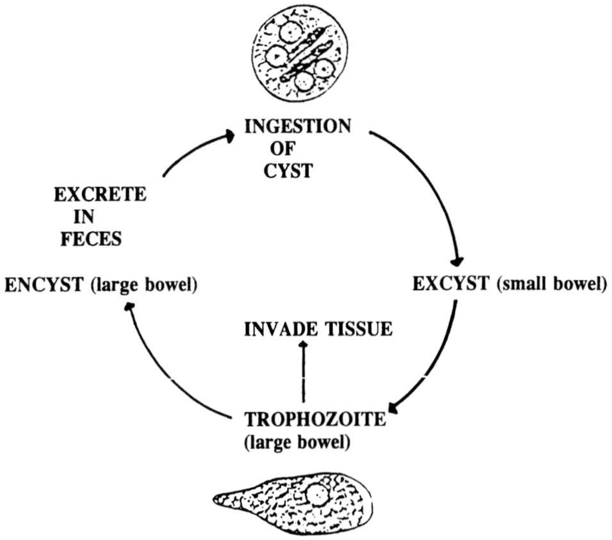

FIGURE 60.1. Life cycle of *Entamoeba histolytica*.

S. L. Reed: Department of Pathology and Medicine, University of California San Diego Medical Center, San Diego, California
J. I. Ravdin: Department of Medicine, University of Minnesota, Minneapolis, Minnesota

E. dispar (16), even though the gene encoding the protein was present in all isolates. The first demonstration of genomic DNA differences was made by screening a complementary DNA (cDNA) library with pooled human immune sera to identify a cDNA clone unique to *E. histolytica* (17). Southern blotting of the cDNA probe and hybridization with an actin cDNA probe revealed significant genomic DNA differences between species (15). The restriction fragment patterns of specific polymerase chain reaction (PCR) amplified genomic DNA fragments were also able to differentiate *E. histolytica* and *E. dispar* isolates; additional strain-specific cDNA clones have been produced (18,19). Now a number of PCR methods have been developed based on DNA sequence differences between *E. histolytica* and *E. dispar* (20,21) (E. Tannich, personal communication).

The *E. dispar* and *E. histolytica* trophozoites range in size from 10 to 60 µm with a single 3- to 5-µm nucleus containing fine peripheral chromatin and a central nucleolus. The *E. histolytica* trophozoites may contain ingested erythrocytes. The amebic cytoplasm consists of a clear ectoplasm with a granular endoplasm and numerous vacuoles. Cysts of *E. dispar* and *E. histolytica* average 12 µm in diameter (range, 5 to 20 µm) and contain one to four nuclei dependent on maturity; nuclei are morphologically identical to those in trophozoites. Young cysts contain chromatoid bodies with smooth, rounded edges; these are composed of ribosome particles in crystalline arrays (22). Immature cysts often contain clumps of glycogen that stain with iodine.

To recognize patients with amebiasis, clinicians should have an in-depth knowledge of the epidemiology of the organism (Table 60.1). Epidemiologic surveys are difficult to interpret because of the insensitivity of a single stool examination (23,24), the frequent laboratory errors made in identification of *E. dispar* (25), and the variability in detection of serum antiamebic antibodies. *E. dispar* does not elicit a humoral immune response to the *E. histolytica* antigens used in serologic assays (26,27). It is estimated that 10% of the world's population is infected with *E. dispar* or *E. histolytica* (1). Excluding the People's Republic of China, each year, worldwide, approximately 50 million cases of invasive disease occur, resulting in up to 100,000 deaths (1). The prevalence of infection may be as high as 50% in certain underdeveloped areas (28,29). Serologic studies in Mexico City indicate that up to 9% of the population were infected with *E. histolytica* in the last 5 to 10 years (8,26). The prevalence of amebic infection depends on cultural habits, age (increased in school-age children), level of sanitation, crowding, and socioeconomic status (28,30). For example, there was a recent outbreak of amebic liver abscesses associated with a contaminated water supply in Tbillisi, Republic of Georgia (31).

TABLE 60.1. EPIDEMIOLOGIC RISK FACTORS THAT APPARENTLY PREDISPOSE TO *E. HISTOLYTICA* INFECTION AND INCREASED SEVERITY OF DISEASE

Prevalence	Increased Severity
Lower socioeconomic status in an endemic area, including crowding and lack of indoor plumbing	Children, especially neonates
Immigrants from endemic area	Pregnancy and postpartum states
Institutionalized population, especially mentally retarded	Corticosteroid use
Communal living	Malignancy
Promiscuous male homosexuals	Malnutrition

From Sullam PM, Slutkin G, Gottlieb AB, et al. Paromycin therapy of endemic amebiasis in homosexual men. *Sex Transm Dis* 1986;13: 151–155.

Intestinal infection with *E. histolytica* is usually asymptomatic (23,24,32–34); the parasite is eliminated from the gut within 12 months, possibly because of competition with the host's intestinal flora or as yet undefined mucosal immune mechanisms (35). In Durban, South Africa, a 10% combined prevalence of *E. dispar* and *E. histolytica* infection resulted in 0.1% of the population suffering invasive amebiasis annually (36,37). In another study, there was a 10% risk per year for development of symptomatic invasive amebiasis following acquisition of *E. histolytica* (37). The percentage of asymptomatic *E. histolytica* intestinal infections range from 10% in Durban, South Africa, to 96% in southeastern Mexico (38). In the latter study, PCR methods revealed a high prevalence of mixed infection with *E. dispar* and *E. histolytica* (56%). The occurrence of asymptomatic *E. histolytica* infection in endemic areas accounts for the high prevalence of serum antiamebic antibodies observed.

In the United States, the combined prevalence of *E. dispar* and *E. histolytica* infection is approximately 4%; however, certain high-risk groups have a high incidence of infection and disease. Institutionalized populations, especially the mentally retarded, have a very high rate of infection concomitant with invasive amebiasis and significant mortality (39–41). Mass therapy or isolation of stool carriers has been unsuccessful in the long-term prevention of amebiasis within institutions (39,42). Improved housing conditions and staffing of health care personnel appear to make a substantial impact (43). In the late 1970s, there was a markedly increased prevalence of amebic infection among sexually promiscuous male homosexuals. The prevalence of *Entamoeba* infection in the gay male population of New York City, San Francisco, and London approached 40% to 50%; however, this only resulted in occasional cases of amebic colitis, because most of the men were infected with *E. dispar* (44–48). The prevalence of *E. histolytica* infection in this population has now declined as a result of the changes in sexual practices in response to the fear of acquisition of HIV (49). In HIV-infected subjects followed up from 1990 to 1998, only 111 of 34,063 patients were confirmed to be infected with *E. histolytica* or *E. dispar* (50). Of those with *Entamoeba* species infection, 92% were in men who had sex with men; high risk was also associated with being born in Latin America (compared with nonendemic sites) and decreasing CD4⁺ cell counts. Nevertheless, amebiasis is one of the causes of diarrhea in individuals with AIDS (49). Axenic *E. histolytica* trophozoites take up the HIV *in vitro* but do not transfer it to uninfected human cells (51). Some risk factors for amebic infection are unanticipated; for example, at a chiropractic clinic in Colorado, infection was spread by colonic irrigation without proper sterilization of equipment (52). New immigrants or migrant workers from endemic areas such as Mexico are an important foci of disease in the United States. Most cases of invasive amebiasis reported from academic institutions in the southwestern United States occurred in Mexican-Americans (53–58). Foreign travel to any endemic area in the world is associated with increased risk of amebiasis, especially when precautions to avoid enteric infection are not taken (59). The acquisition of *E. dispar* and *E. histolytica* is associated with long-term (greater than 1 month) residence in endemic areas and is usually detected only when symptomatic disease results (60,61).

PATHOGENESIS AND HOST IMMUNITY

Entamoeba histolytica is named for its lytic effect on tissue. Trophozoites appear to invade the colonic epithelium directly with diffuse mucosal damage before amebic invasion (62–64). An amorphous, granular, eosinophilic material surrounds trophozoites in tissue, whether in colon, liver, or lung (62,64,65). Inflammatory cells are found only at the periphery of established amebic lesions (62,64) because of the contact-dependent amebic lysis of neutrophils (66,67). This results in the release of toxic nonoxidative neutrophil products that contribute to the destruction of host tissues (68,69).

Colonic amebic lesions may manifest as nonspecific thickening of the mucosa or as the classic flask-shaped ulcer (3,64) (Fig. 60.2). *E. histolytica* trophozoites in tissue can be recognized by a surrounding clear halo caused by fixation artifact, the presence of characteristic nuclear morphology, ingested erythrocytes, and intense staining with periodic acid-Schiff stain or detection of ingested erythrocytes by Gridley stain (70). The amebic liver "abscess" contains acellular, proteinaceous debris rather than white cells, with trophozoites invading tissue in the surrounding rim (62,65). Amebae establish hepatic infection by ascending the portal venous system; triangular areas of hepatic necrosis may occur, apparently due to ischemia from amebic obstruction of portal vessels (62,71,72). Liver enzyme abnormalities, frequently present with intestinal amebiasis, are associated with periportal inflammation without demonstrable trophozoites (65,73). Periportal fibrosis has

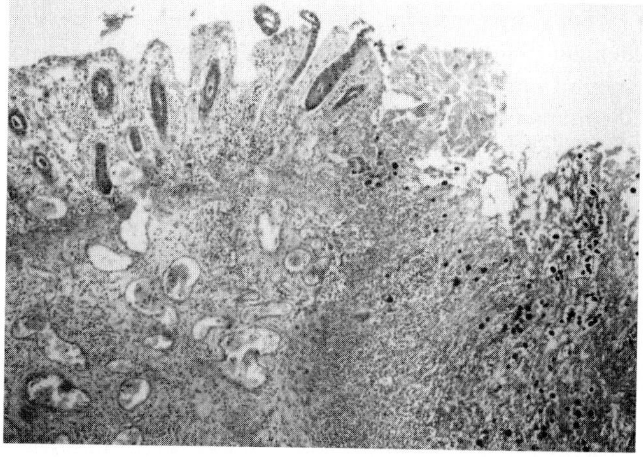

FIGURE 60.2. Pathology of amebic colitis. Undermined colonic ulcer with trophozoites on periphery of lesion (*arrow*). Hematoxylin and eosin stain, ×100. (From McAuley JB, Herwaldt BL, Stokes SL, et al. Diloxanide furoate for treating asymptomatic *Entamoeba histolytica* cyst passers: 14 years' experience in the United States. *Clin Infect Dis* 1992;15:464–468, with permission.)

been reported and may reflect past trophozoite invasion or host reaction to amebic antigens and toxins.

The development of an axenic culture medium for *E. histolytica* stimulated a rapid expansion of research into the pathogenic mechanisms of the parasite. The pathogenesis of invasive amebiasis commences with the adherence of trophozoites to the mucins lining the luminal surface of the large bowel, followed by proteolytic degradation of the basement membrane of the mucosa, direct amebic cytolytic and proteolytic effects on tissue, and, lastly, the resistance of the parasite to host luminal and cellular defense mechanisms (74). Adherence of *E. histolytica* trophozoites to Chinese hamster ovary (CHO) cells and human colonic mucins *in vitro* is mediated by the parasite's galactose inhibitable adherence lectin (75–78). The lectin participates in adherence of *E. histolytica* trophozoites to human leukocytes (67,79), rat and human colonic mucosa and submucosa (78), human erythrocytes (75,80), opsonized bacteria or bacteria with galactose-containing lipopolysaccharide, and rat colonic epithelial cells (77). The adherence lectin is a 260-kd surface protein, consisting of 170- and 35-kd subunits (76). The heavy subunit has been found to mediate attachment, as evidenced by its recognition by adherence-inhibitory monoclonal antibodies (81,82) and the direct galactose-binding *in vitro* activity of recombinant heavy subunit produced by expression-PCR methodology (83). A multigene family encodes the heavy and light subunits of the lectin (84,85). The heavy subunit has a short cytoplasmic domain, a transmembrane domain, and a large extracellular portion with a highly antigenic distinct cysteine-rich area. The light subunit, in contrast, attaches to the membrane via a glycosyl-phosphatidylinositol anchor (85). There are at least seven discrete epitopes in the heavy subunit as found by monoclonal immunoglobulin G (IgG) antibody mapping (82); all are located in the cysteine-rich domain. Binding by monoclonal antibodies to the 170-kd subunit can abrogate amebic resistance to the lytic effect of the human complement, apparently by blocking the interference of the lectin with the C5b-9 membrane attack complex at the steps of C8 and C9 assembly. The lectin has sequence and antigenic similarities to the human CD59 inhibitor of C8 and C9 (86).

Axenic *E. histolytica* trophozoites kill target cells only upon direct contact in a calcium-dependent manner (77,87, 88). Adherence mediated by the galactose-inhibitable lectin is absolutely required for the *in vitro* lysis of target cells. Target cell death occurs up to 20 minutes after attachment by trophozoites; a lethal hit can be delivered within seconds (87,88). Amebic cytolytic activity is dependent on parasite microfilament function (75,87), calcium (89,90), Ca^{2+}-dependent parasite phospholipase A (PLA) enzyme activity (89,90), and maintenance of an acid pH in amebic endocytic vesicles (91). Attachment by *E. histolytica* trophozoites results in a sustained elevation of target cell–free intracellular calcium concentration ($[Ca^{2+}]_i$) in the target cell, which contributes to, but may not be totally sufficient for, target cell death (88). Phorbol esters and protein kinase C activators specifically augment parasite cytolytic activity (92). The relevance of calcium as a second messenger mechanism in amebic cytolytic activity is supported by identification of Ca^+ binding parasite proteins and kinases (93); a Rho-dependent signal transduction mechanism also appears to have a role in amebic cytolysis (94). *E. histolytica* contains an ionophore-like protein of 77 amino acids, with sequence homology to the saponins and to surfactant-associated protein B, which induces lipid bilayers or vesicles to leak Na^+, K^+, and, to a lesser degree, Ca^{2+} (95–97). This ionophore is packaged in dense intracellular aggregates; purified preparations can depolarize erythrocytes (98). There are three protein isoforms, all well characterized by their protein and cDNA sequences (99). Monomers of the protein oligomerize after insertion into the membrane, forming an ion channel (100). Amebapore has potent antibacterial defensin activity and is also present in the nonpathogenic *E. dispar* species. It is unclear whether amebapore has a direct role in amebic cytolysis of target cells, which appears to occur by necrosis rather than apoptosis (99). *E. histolytica* contains numerous proteolytic enzymes, including a cathepsin B proteinase, an acidic proteinase (101), a collagenase (102), and a well-characterized major neutral proteinase (103). Cysteine proteinases undoubtedly are involved in dissolution of the extracellular matrix anchoring cells and tissue structure by invading trophozoites (104).

Parasite cysteine proteinases degrade human secretory IgA (105) and IgG molecules (106), a possible means of immune evasion. The 56-kd cysteine proteinase activates complement by cleavage of C3 (107); pathogenic organisms were found to release greater amounts of the enzyme (108). Reed and co-workers (109) succeeded in cloning the amebic cysteine proteinase genes; there are now known to be three genes in total encoding the cysteine proteinase (110). *E. histolytica* trophozoites have larger amounts of proteinase mRNA and secrete more enzyme than *E. dispar* (104). *E. histolytica* cysteine proteinases may also have a role in initiating gut inflammation by stimulating release of proinflammatory cytokines from intestinal epithelium (111). Amebic glycosidases, such as β-glucosaminidase (112) and a surface membrane–associated neuraminidase (113), may be involved in the degradation of colonic mucins or alteration of target cell surface membrane glycoproteins.

Host polymorphonuclear leukocytes constitute the initial host response to *E. histolytica* (68,69). Neutrophils chemotax to trophozoites (114); however, their lysis by the ameba enhances the destruction of host tissues. A further understanding of the biochemical and molecular basis for pathogenicity of *E. histolytica* is necessary for development of an amebiasis vaccine or other intervention strategy.

Cure of amebic colitis or liver abscess apparently results in some immunity to a recurrence of invasive amebiasis. In a 5-year follow-up study of 1,021 subjects in Mexico City with amebic liver abscess, only five recurrences developed (115). In a study of 982 subjects in a highly endemic area of India, the presence of serum antiamebic antibodies was associated with a lower rate of intestinal infection (29). As discussed, asymptomatic infection with *E. dispar* or *E. histolytica* spontaneously clears within 8 to 12 months (35). The human immune response to *E. histolytica* has been well characterized, mainly following treatment of amebic liver abscess.

In patients with amebic liver abscess, high titers of serum antiamebic antibodies (55) develop by the seventh day of illness, which persist for up to 10 years. However, amebic liver abscess is a progressive, unremitting disease despite the presence of serum antibodies that are capable of inhibiting amebic adherence *in vitro* (116). By immunoblotting human sera to total parasite protein, a set of highly conserved *E. histolytica* antigens of approximately 37, 43, 59, 90, 110, and 170 kd was defined (117). The 170-kd antigen is the heavy subunit of the galactose-inhibitable lectin, which is recognized by antibodies in more than 95% of sera from hundreds of subjects with invasive amebiasis (27,116). Serum antibodies from subjects residing in India, Mexico, Zaire, Egypt, South Africa, and the United States all recognize the native lectin heavy subunit, which was purified from a single clone of an axenic strain originally isolated in Mexico City (strain HMI:IMSS), indicating a high degree of conserved antigenicity (27,116,118). Sera from healthy control subjects or infected patients (with high antibody titers to *E. histolytica*) have amebicidal activity through activation of the alternate and classic complement pathways (119,120). However, trophozoites isolated from amebic liver abscesses or colonic lesions are resistant to complement-mediated lysis (120). In addition, complement-resistant amebae can be selected *in vitro* by culture in normal human serum (121). Complement activation occurs at least in part via cleavage of C3 by the 56-kd neutral cysteine proteinase of the parasite (107). As mentioned, the lectin 170-kd subunit inhibits assembly of C8 and C9 into the membrane attack complex, contributing to the resistance of the parasite to complement-mediated lysis (86).

Recently, investigations of the mucosal immune response to *E. histolytica* revealed an antiamebic sIgA response during infection (122,123). Colostral antiamebic sIgA antibodies are found during asymptomatic intestinal infection, without serum antiamebic IgA or IgG antibodies being present. Study of salivary IgA responses to *E. histolytica* infection yielded conflicting results (124–126). Initially, an infrequent association was found between salivary antiamebic IgA and intestinal infection (124), with none to only 36% being positive. In contrast, a strikingly positive correlation was reported between anti-*E. histolytica* IgA in whole clarified saliva and amebic infection in asymptomatic school children in Mexico (125).

It is highly unlikely that all these asymptomatic children had *E. histolytica* infections, zymodeme analysis and serum antibody studies were not performed. In contrast, a follow-up study of subjects with seropositive invasive amebiasis, asymptomatic intestinal infection, and uninfected control subjects demonstrated that salivary antiamebic IgA was found exclusively during invasive amebiasis (126). In Durban, South Africa, fecal anti-lectin IgA responses were found in all subjects following amebic liver abscess and persisted for 12 to 18 months (J. Ravdin, unpublished observation). *E. dispar* infection is associated with a mucosal anti-lectin IgA response in a minority of subjects; up to 20% of uninfected subjects in endemic areas may at any time have anti-lectin IgA in feces.

Cell-mediated immune defense mechanisms clearly have an important role in limiting invasive disease and resisting a recurrence after appropriate therapy. The cell-mediated response consists of antigen-specific lymphocyte blastogenesis with production of lymphokines (including gamma-interferon) capable of activating monocyte-derived macrophages to kill *E. histolytica* trophozoites *in vitro* (79,127). In addition, incubation of immune T cells with *E. histolytica* antigen *in vitro* elicits cytotoxic T-lymphocyte activity against trophozoites (128). Purified 260-kd galactose-inhibitable lectin is a highly conserved T- as well as B-cell antigen, eliciting lymphocyte responses in seropositive subjects (129). However, in acute disease, the T-lymphocyte responses to *E. histolytica* appear to be specifically suppressed by a parasite-induced serum factor (130). The lack of an increased incidence of severe invasive or extraintestinal amebiasis in AIDS patients (48) suggests that host resistance to the initial amebic invasion of the colonic mucosa does not involve cell-mediated mechanisms. Clinical correlation of the severity of established invasive disease with cell-mediated immune function include the depression of T-cell numbers and delayed hypersensitivity in patients with an amebic liver abscess (114,131), the severe exacerbation of intestinal amebiasis with the occurrence of toxic megacolon during corticosteroid therapy (132,133), and the fulminant amebic disease found in young infants and pregnant women (134–136). Studies in an SCID mouse model of amebic liver abscess indicate that gamma-interferon and macrophage nitric oxide are important host defenses that limit abscess size (137).

Nonimmune host defenses are crucial for resistance to symptomatic invasive amebiasis. In animal models, mucous trapping of *E. histolytica* trophozoites occurs (138), and depletion of the colonic mucous blanket is seen before parasites invade (139). Chadee and co-workers (77,140) demonstrated that purified rat and human colonic mucins, rich in terminal galactose residues, act as high-affinity receptors for the *E. histolytica* galactose-inhibitable lectin. Colonic mucins inhibit amebic adherence to colonic epithelial cells and their lysis by trophozoites *in vitro* (77). *E. histolytica* trophozoites also release a potent mucous secretagogue (141). Therefore, colonic mucin glycoproteins act as an important host defense by binding to the parasite's adherence lectin; this interaction apparently prevents invasion and facilitates intestinal colonization and thus parasitism by *E. histolytica.*

Interruption of transmission of *E. histolytica* cysts depends on socioeconomic problems and sanitation. Vaccine development would be the most efficient and cost-effective means of disease prevention. Native galactose lectin protein is highly effective as a vaccine in the experimental gerbil model of amebic liver abscess (142). The recombinant subunit LC3 vaccine was also efficacious in the gerbil model of amebic liver abscess via systemic immunization (143). The use of attenuated *Salmonella* bacteria expressing fragments of the lectin 170-kd subunit also provides partial protection (144). Protective immunity in gerbils immunized with recombinant portions of the lectin 170-kd subunit correlates with the induction of antibodies to a 25-amino acid region of the molecule (145). Gerbils were provided partial protection by immunization with the synthetic 25-mer peptide linked to keyhole limpet hemocyanin, less so when linked to the β-subunit of cholera toxin (146). The native amebic lectin has mitogenic activity, inducing production of interleukin-12 in human macrophages (147). Immunization with polyclonal antibodies to a recombinant serine-rich protein or with monoclonal antibody to a lipophosphoglycan antigen also provides protection against amebic liver abscess in the SCID mouse model of amebic liver abscess (148,149). Numerous research groups are working on the development of different recombinant vaccines to induce amebicidal cell-mediated immunity, adherence-inhibitory secretory IgA responses, or humoral immunity that contributes to protection against invasive amebiasis.

Clinical Syndromes of Amebiasis

Intestinal Amebiasis

Intestinal infection with *E. histolytica* causes a wide spectrum of disease. The major clinical syndromes fall into four groups: asymptomatic cyst passers, acute colitis, fulminant colitis, and ameboma (reviewed in references 149 and 150).

Asymptomatic Cyst Passers

Because an estimated 90% of patients infected with *E. histolytica* are asymptomatic (1), cyst passers are the most common presentation physicians encounter worldwide, particularly in developed countries. Interpretation of most of the early clinical studies is difficult because they predated techniques allowing specific identification of *E. histolytica,* including isoenzyme techniques (6), PCR (21), and antigen detection (21,151), and thus probably involved mixed populations of carriers of *E. histolytica* and *E. dispar.* In a recent study of the prevalence of infection by *E. histolytica* and *E. dispar* in 2000 children in Bangladesh, 8% of asymptomatic children where found to be colonized with *E. histolytica-E. dispar* cysts, but only 1% had *E. histolytica,* as determined by isoenzymes or specific antigen detection (151). In symptomatic children with diarrhea, 10.7% had *E. histolytica-E. dispar* cysts or trophozoites, but only 4.2% harbored *E. histolytica.* Thus, the majority of patients infected with *Entamoeba* harbor *E. dispar,* even in developing countries.

In developed countries, a physician is most likely to encounter *E. histolytica-E. dispar* cysts in homosexual men, with colonization rates on routine stool examinations being as high as 30% (152). A recent large survey of HIV-infected patients in the U.S. found a signficant decrease in prevalence of *E. histolytica-E. dispar* infection to 3.3% (152a). Unfortunately, the study was retrospective so additional tests to differentiate *E. histolytica* from *E. dispar* infection were not possible (153). Several large studies from London have characterized the prevalence and clinical impact of infection in homosexual patients (45). All 100 patients who were culture positive were carriers of *E. dispar,* had negative amebic serology, and had no histologic evidence of invasive amebiasis (49). Because T-cell–mediated immunity is an important defense against amebiasis (128–130), one might anticipate that colonization, even with *E. dispar,* might cause significant disease in these patients. Instead, a benign clinical course was found in follow-up of 19 AIDS patients (153). All were colonized with *E. dispar,* none had positive amebic serology, and all untreated patients became culture-negative in an average of 11 weeks. A majority of the symptomatic patients (64%) had other potential pathogens isolated at the same time, suggesting that a search for other causes is always appropriate in a symptomatic AIDS patient with diarrhea and *E. histolytica-E. dispar* cysts.

A variable percentage of asymptomatic patients will be carriers of *E. histolytica,* however. In South Africa, Gathiram and Jackson (37) identified 20 asymptomatic carriers with *E. histolytica* (10% of all infections, incidence of 1%). Within 1 year, amebic colitis had developed in 10% and the rest remained asymptomatic with spontaneous cure. Studies in Mexico and other regions have found that a higher percentage of asymptomatic infections may be due to pathogenic organisms (38). These patients would be particularly important to identify and treat because they are a potential source of disease transmission.

Acute Colitis

Patients with acute amebic colitis usually present with the gradual onset of abdominal pain and frequent, loose, watery stools containing blood and mucus. Associated symptoms may include back pain, tenesmus, or flatulence (Table 60.2). Most patients have symptoms for 1 to 2 weeks before presentation, but the occasional patient may have profuse diarrhea leading to rapid dehydration. A minority of patients are febrile, in contrast to patients with bacterial dysentery. Most patients have abdominal tenderness on examination, often localized to the lower abdomen. The characteristic appearance of the punctuate, hemorrhagic ulcers with relatively normal intervening mucosa on rectal or sigmoidoscopic examination may be helpful in the diagnosis (see Color Figure 60.3).

Fulminant Colitis

Fulminant colitis is an unusual complication of amebic dysentery, which carries a grave prognosis with survival

TABLE 60.2. PRESENTING SYMPTOMS AND SIGNS OF PATIENTS WITH AMEBIC COLITIS

Presentation	Percentage
Symptoms	
Diarrhea	100
Dysentery	99
Abdominal pain	85
Low back pain	66
Signs	
Fever	38
Abdominal tenderness	83
Localized	42
Generalized	41
Dehydration	5
Length of symptoms	
0–1 week	48
2–4 weeks	37
>4 weeks	15

Adapted from Adams EB, MacLeod IN. Invasive amebiasis. I. Amebic dysentery and its complications. *Medicine (Baltimore)* 1977;56: 315–323.

TABLE 60.3. FINDINGS AT LAPAROTOMY IN PATIENTS WITH FULMINANT AMEBIC COLITIS

Finding	Percentage
Multiple perforations	60
Colonic gangrene	16
Single perforation	10
Perforated ameboma	2
Microscopic perforation	12

Adapted from Aristizabal H, Acevedo J, Botero M. Fulminant amebic colitis. *World J Surg* 1991;15:216–221.

rates rarely greater than 40% (154). Clinically, patients present with more severe bloody diarrhea and fever, followed by rapid progression to diffuse abdominal tenderness. The progression may be so rapid, however, that only 25% of adults who ultimately had perforations detected at surgery presented with a rigid abdomen (154) (Table 60.3). Young children appear to be at increased risk for fulminant colitis (155). The clinical development of fulminant colitis is associated with the pathologic progression from superficial ulceration of the bowel to transmural necrosis (Table 60.3).

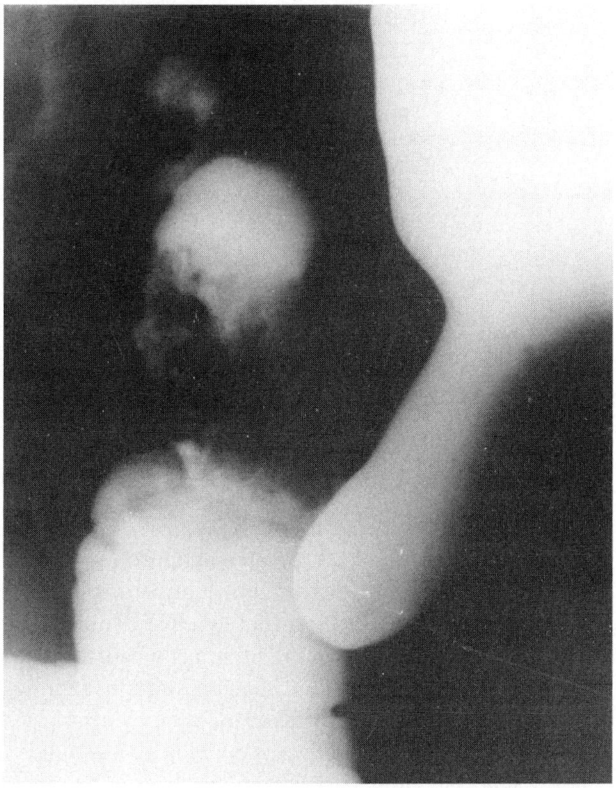

FIGURE 60.4. Barium enema examination on 26-year-old Filipino man with asymptomatic left lower quadrant mass. (Courtesy of Department of Radiology, UCSD Medical Center.)

Ameboma

Ameboma is an unusual presentation of amebic intestinal infection, occurring in less than 1% of patients with invasive intestinal disease (156). The majority of patients present with an abdominal mass, which may be tender, but are otherwise asymptomatic. The appearance on radiographic studies mimics a carcinoma presenting as an "apple core-like" lesion (157) (Fig. 60.4). A positive amebic serology or biopsy by colonoscopy can prevent an unnecessary surgical procedure, although an ameboma and carcinoma may coexist (158).

Other Syndromes

The clinical significance of persistent diarrhea following adequate therapy of intestinal amebic infection, called *chronic nondysenteric colitis* (156) or *ulcerative postdysenteric* colitis (158), is unclear. Recurrent amebic infection cannot be identified, and these patients do not respond to additional antiparasitic therapy.

Complications

The most common complication of acute amebic colitis is peritonitis. Usually, slow leakage develops with a delay in clinical signs of peritonitis, but fulminant colitis and acute perforation may also occur (156). Less frequent complications include sudden hemorrhage requiring transfusion and amebic strictures of the anus, rectum, or sigmoid colon (156). Cutaneous amebiasis results from direct spread of intestinal infection. These lesions are usually painful ulcers, which are easily confused with squamous cell carcinoma (159). Amebic trophozoites are usually apparent on biopsy, and patients respond well to medical therapy alone. Cutaneous amebiasis and carcinomas may coexist, so a follow-up biopsy of any nonresolving lesion is important (159).

Differential Diagnosis

Acute amebic colitis must be distinguished from bacterial causes of dysentery, including *Shigella, Campylobacter, Salmonella, Vibrio, Salmonella,* and enteroinvasive *Escherichia coli.* One clinical clue to amebiasis is the relative lack of fever or possible absence of fecal leukocytes; however, examination of stool for parasites, cultures, and amebic serology is usually required to make the definitive diagnosis. It is particularly important to exclude amebic colitis before treating any patient with presumptive inflammatory bowel disease with steroids (160) because potentially fatal toxic megacolon may develop.

Amebic Liver Abscess

Amebic liver abscess is the most common complication of invasive amebiasis (reviewed in references 149 and 150).

TABLE 60.4. SIGNS AND SYMPTOMS OF AMEBIC LIVER ABSCESS

Presentation	Adams and MacLeod (161) (N = 2,074)	Katzenstein et al. (55) (N = 67)	
		Acute	Chronic
Symptom			
Abdominal pain	94	85	38
Fever	75	85	32
Diarrhea	14	30	30
Weight loss	NR	20	60
Cough	11	5	7
Sign			
Tender liver	80	90	90
Hepatomegaly	80	25	60
Rales/rhonchi	47	27	60

NR, not reported.

Diagnosis is hindered by the nonspecific nature of the symptoms and the potential for presentation months after leaving an endemic area. The majority of patients present acutely with less than 10 days of fever and abdominal pain (Table 60.4) (55,161). Dull, right upper quadrant pain, which may radiate to the shoulder, is the most common symptom, but diffuse epigastric or pleuritic pain may also occur. An enlarged, painful liver is the most useful sign but is not diagnostic. Most patients are febrile (>80%), and a minority of patients (10%) may actually present with a fever of unknown origin (161). Although all patients have had intestinal infection preceding development of a liver abscess, less than 30% have active diarrhea at any time before presentation. A subset of patients have a more chronic course with subacute symptoms for more than 2 weeks (161). These cases are more likely to manifest as a wasting disease with hepatomegaly, weight loss, and anemia. Atypical presentations may include shortness of breath and cough secondary to pleural effusions or rupture into the pleural space.

Complications of Amebic Liver Abscess

Mortality rate from uncomplicated amebic liver abscess is less than 1%, but mortality rate increases at least 10-fold with rupture (161,162) (Table 60.5).

Pleuropulmonary Complications

Pleuropulmonary complications of amebic abscess, including localized rupture, empyema, and hepatobronchial fistulas, are most common, occurring in approximately 10% of patients. Up to half of patients may have a small to moderate, serous pleural effusion, which may be the first radiographic clue to underlying liver disease. Localized rupture by contiguous spread into the pleural cavity is usually benign and responds to medical therapy alone (Fig. 60.5). Formation of an empyema is much more serious and is usually heralded by sudden pleuritic pain and shortness of breath, necessitating aggressive drainage and medical therapy. The development of an hepatobronchial fistula is potentially the most dramatic complication of an amebic abscess with the patient coughing up large amounts of necrotic debris, which may contain trophozoites. This complication usually responds well to medical therapy unless aspiration of the abscess contents into the lungs occurs.

Peritoneal Rupture

Rupture of amebic liver abscesses into the peritoneum occurs in 2% to 5% of patients (161). Because the contents are sterile, the prognosis is much better than with rupture of infected bowel. Mortality rate from this complication has decreased dramatically following the advent of percutaneous catheter drainage (163).

TABLE 60.5. COMPLICATIONS OF AMEBIC LIVER ABSCESSES

Complications	Cases	Percentage	Mortality (%)
Pulmonary	146	7.8	6.2
Pleural effusion and empyema		29	
Hepatobronchial fistula		47	
Lung abscess		14	
Consolidation		10	
Abdominal rupture	38	2.0	18.4
Pericardial rupture	27	1.4	29.6

Adapted from Adams EB, MacLeod IN. Invasive amebiasis. II. Amebic liver abscess and its complications. *Medicine (Baltimore)* 1977;56:325–334.

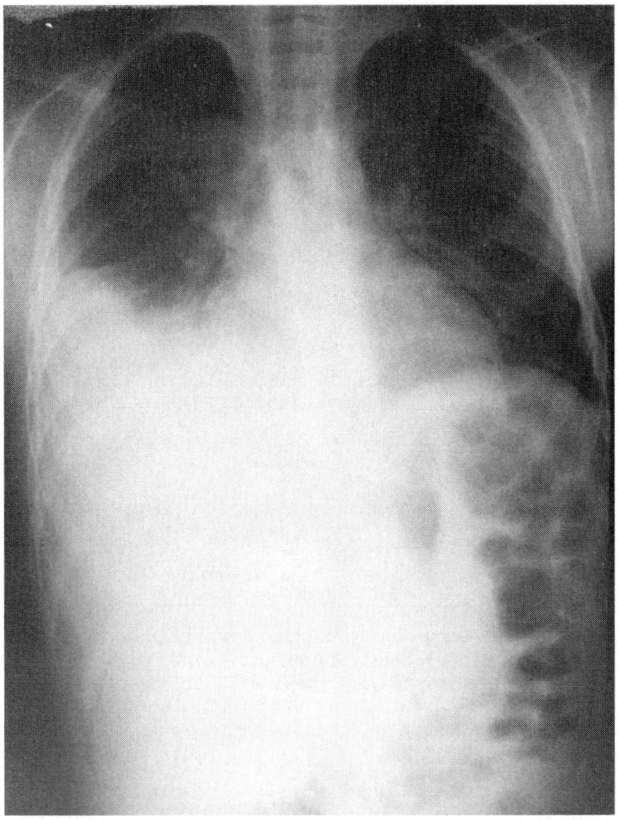

FIGURE 60.5. Chest radiograph of 8-year-old girl with local rupture of amebic liver abscess. (Courtesy of Department of Radiology, UCSD Medical Center.)

Pericardial Rupture

Rupture of an amebic liver abscess into the pericardium is the most serious complication, with a mortality rate of more than 70% if not recognized early (164). Rupture into the pericardium may occur even when the patient is on adequate medical therapy and is usually preceded by the development of a serous effusion (161). Rapid clinical deterioration from cardiac tamponade is usually the rule (161), although aggressive drainage and medical therapy may be curative. Early drainage of left lobe abscesses of the liver is recommended to prevent this potentially fatal complication (165).

Differential Diagnosis of Amebic Liver Abscess

The diagnosis of an amebic liver abscess should be considered in any patient from an endemic area with fever and right upper quadrant abdominal tenderness. Although infection of the biliary tract may be suspected initially, with the advent of modern imaging techniques, the differential diagnosis is usually limited to a pyogenic abscess or necrotic tumor. Patients with pyogenic liver abscesses are more likely to be older and have underlying gallbladder or bowel disease (166). A positive amebic serology result confirms the diagnosis, but in an ill patient with multiple abscesses, percutaneous aspiration for bacterial cultures, pathologic examination, and treatment may be indicated.

Diagnosis of Amebic Infection

Laboratory Tests

Routine hematology or chemistry tests are rarely helpful in the diagnosis of invasive amebiasis. Sixty percent of patients with an amebic liver abscess have a white blood cell count greater than 15,000. Invasion with *E. histolytica* does not cause eosinophilia. An elevated alkaline phosphatase was the most consistent biochemical indicator of an amebic liver abscess, increased in 84% of patients (55). Transaminases were only elevated in 50% of patients, and abnormal values were more frequent in patients with acute infection and complications such as rupture (55).

Microscopic Diagnosis

Early diagnosis is critical for successful treatment of invasive amebiasis. Intestinal infection is diagnosed by the presence of the hematophagous trophozoites of *E. histolytica* on wet mount or trichrome stain of stool concentrates (Fig. 4, Chapter 72). Unfortunately, the cysts of *E. histolytica* and *E. dispar* cannot be distinguished by microscopic examination. Shedding of cysts may be intermittent, so examination of at least three stools is recommended. Although patients with frank colitis usually have a large number of motile trophozoites in their stool, specimens must be examined immediately because the trophozoites are rapidly killed by drying, water, urine, barium, or a number of antibiotics. Biopsy or scrapings from the edge of bowel ulcers may increase the diagnostic yield but should be avoided in patients with fulminant colitis. Of all children in a study from Bangladesh diagnosed with amebiasis by microscopy, only 40% were proven to harbor *E. histolytica* when tested by the more specific methods of antigen detection, culture and isoenzyme analysis, or PCR (151).

Less than 30% of patients with amebic liver abscess have symptomatic intestinal infection, but recent studies in which daily stool cultures were obtained from patients with amebic liver abscesses suggest that more than 70% may have asymptomatic colonization (167). Trophozoites are rarely seen in aspirates of the necrotic debris, which forms the bulk of amebic liver abscesses.

Serologic Tests

Amebic serology is very useful in the diagnosis of invasive amebiasis. The most commonly used tests, counterimmunoelectrophoresis (CIE), agar gel diffusion (AGD), indirect hemagglutination (IHA), and enzyme-linked immunoadsorbent assay (ELISA), are positive in 85% to 95% of patients with amebic colitis or liver abscesses (168). The titer correlates with the duration of illness rather than severity of disease. Serologic tests were initially negative in 10% of patients who presented acutely with an amebic liver abscess, but all were positive within 2 weeks (55). Caution must be taken with the interpretation of IHA titers because they may remain elevated for several years following successful treatment (168). In contrast, CIE and AGD results usually revert to negative within months. In asymptomatic carriers of pathogenic *E. histolytica,* a serum antibody response develops that serves as a useful marker of both active and potential disease (26).

Antigen detection tests

The development of an antigen detection assay specific for *E. histolytica* in the stool is an important advance. The assay is based on *E. histolytica*-specific epitopes of the galactose-inhabitable lectin (14). In large field trials, the sensitivity of the assay was 85% compared to isoenzyme analysis and 93% compared to PCR (21).

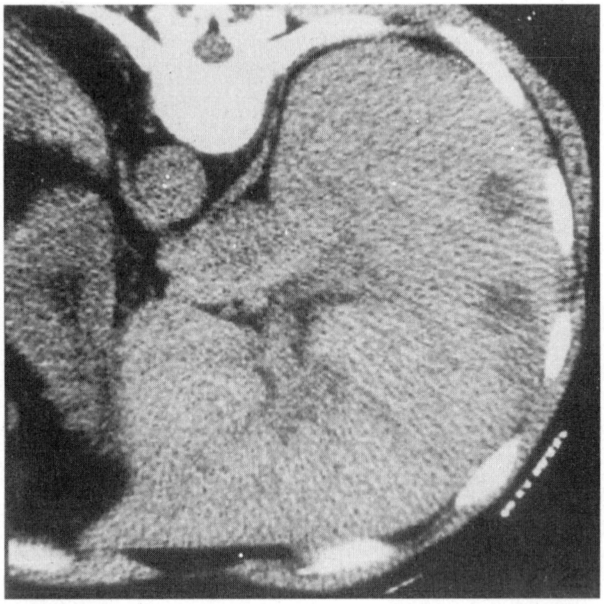

FIGURE 60.7. Computed tomography scan of patient with multiple liver abscesses. Liver aspirate grew *Entamoeba histolytica* on culture. (Courtesy of Department of Radiology, UCSD Medical Center.)

Radiographic Studies

Barium studies are relatively contraindicated in the workup of a patient with acute dysentery because of the risk of perforation. Patients with amebomas rarely have acute diarrhea, however, and the lesions are usually identified on barium studies to define an abdominal mass.

Noninvasive radiographic studies, including ultrasound, computed tomography (CT) scan, and magnetic resonance imaging (MRI), have dramatically improved the early diagnosis of amebic liver abscesses. The classic ultrasound appearance is a round or cystic mass with well-defined borders (Fig. 60.6). The majority of patients (75%) have single abscesses of the right lobe of the liver (169), but up to 50% of patients who present acutely may have multiple lesions, which may be difficult to distinguish from a pyogenic abscess (55) (Fig. 60.7). The time for complete resolution of abscesses is variable, ranging from 1½ to 23 months (170). Abscesses may actually increase in size early in the

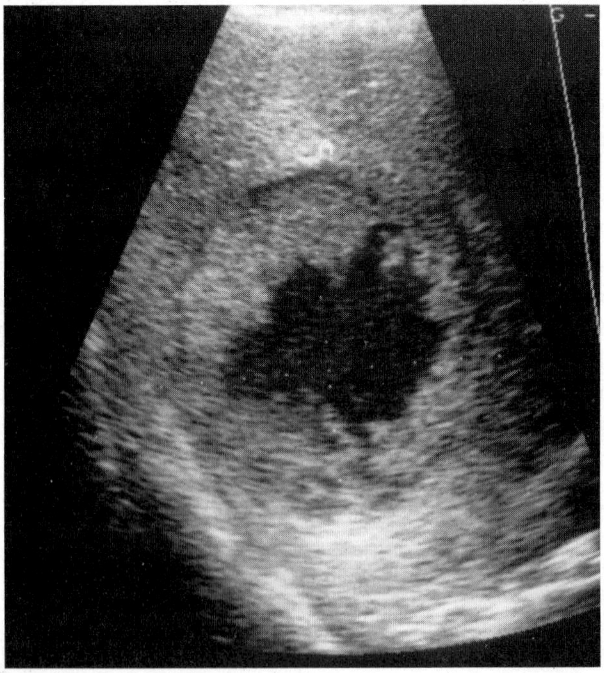

FIGURE 60.6. Liver ultrasound of same 8-year-old girl as in Fig. 60.5 showing a large cystic mass. (Courtesy of Department of Radiology, UCSD Medical Center.)

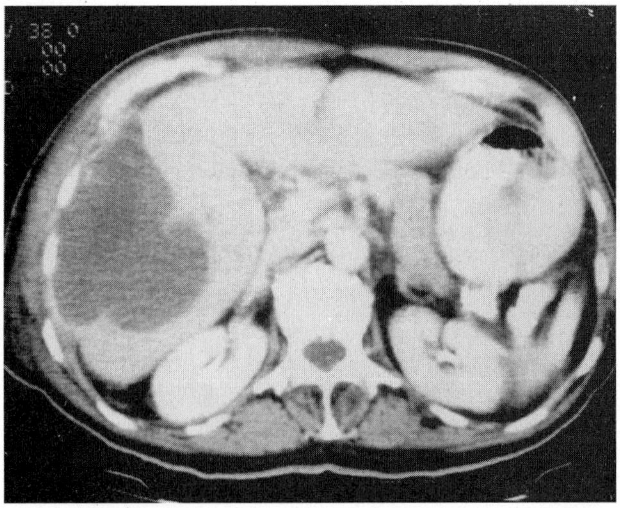

FIGURE 60.8. Patient with localized rupture of amebic liver abscess detected by computed tomography scan. (Courtesy of Department of Radiology, UCSD Medical Center.)

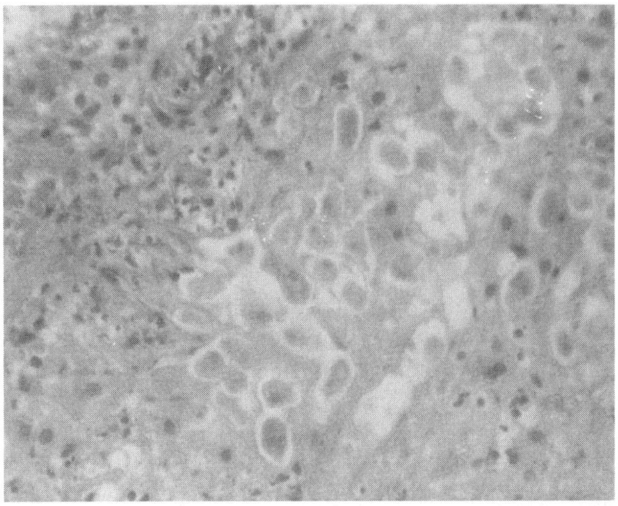

FIGURE 60.9. Pathology of amebic liver abscess. Trophozoites seen on edge of necrotic liver abscess. Hematoxylin and eosin stain, ×100.

course of successful therapy, so it is important not to obtain follow-up studies too early (35). CT scans have also enhanced the detection of early rupture (Fig. 60.8).

Pathology

Amebic trophozoites invade the colonic epithelium, forming an ulcer that progresses through the lamina propria to the muscularis mucosa and extends laterally under normal-appearing mucosa, forming a flask-shaped ulcer (62). Significant tissue necrosis is detected with a relative paucity of inflammation. Amebic trophozoites are usually seen in clusters in the periphery of necrotic areas (62) (Fig. 60.9). Although trophozoites are detectable by standard hematoxylin and eosin staining of tissues, the distinct pink color seen with periodic acid-Schiff stain helps differentiate trophozoites from phagocytic cells (reviewed in reference 70).

In an amebic liver abscess, the liver parenchyma is completely replaced with necrotic debris with a paucity of inflammatory cells or amebic trophozoites (62). The color of the fluid may range from yellow to brown and has been described as "anchovy paste" from its consistency and color when it is mixed with blood. Trophozoites are usually only found near the capsule of the abscess (Fig. 60.9).

Treatment of Amebic Infection

Treatment of Cyst Passers

Two main classes of drugs are used to treat amebiasis: (a) luminal agents that are poorly absorbed in tissues and (b) agents with good tissue penetration. Three major luminal agents are available: iodoquinol, diloxanide furoate, and paromomycin but only paromomycin is available in the U.S. (Table 60.6). All have efficacy rates of 85% to 95% for the eradication of cyst passage (177). Iodoquinol, a halogenated hydroxyquinoline, is effective but must be given for a 20-day course. Diloxanide furoate, a substituted acetanilide, has been widely used outside the United States (178). Paromomycin is a nonabsorbable aminoglycoside that is active against both trophozoites and cysts (179). The most important indication for use of a luminal agent is adjunctive therapy in all patients with invasive amebiasis; metronidazole is not effective therapy for cysts. Although all three luminal active drugs are very effective, the treatment of asymptomatic cyst passers is perhaps the biggest dilemma in the management of amebiasis. If the patient is asymptomatic and has a negative serology, and if the infecting strain can be characterized as *E. dispar*, then follow-up without

TABLE 60.6. TREATMENT OF AMEBIASIS

Syndrome	Adult Dose
Asymptomatic cyst passer, luminal agent	
Iodoquinol (650-mg tablets)[a]	650 mg tid × 20 days
Paromomycin (250-mg tablets)	500 mg tid × 7 days
Diloxanide furoate (500-mg tablets)[a]	500 mg tid × 10 days
Acute colitis	
Metronidazole (250- or 500-mg tablets)	750 mg tid × 5–10 days
+	
Luminal agent (above)	
Amebic liver abscess	
Metronidazole	750 mg tid IV or PO × 5–10 days
Tinidazole[a]	2 g PO
Ornidazole[a]	2 g PO
+	
Luminal agent (above)	

[a]Not available in the United States.

treatment is advised (45). If serologic tests or amebic cultures are not available to identify carriers of *E. histolytica*, it is most prudent to treat all patients. The treatment of pregnant patients is particularly a difficult issue because there is anecdotal evidence that invasive amebiasis is more severe and there is theoretic teratogenic risk of metronidazole. Some authors argue that an asymptomatic woman with a negative amebic serology should be carefully followed up without therapy and treatment with metronidazole should be reserved for those with invasive disease (149). Others advise that all pregnant women with "mild-to-moderate" intestinal disease should be treated with paromomycin (177).

Intestinal Amebiasis

The therapy of invasive amebiasis has dramatically improved since the introduction of imidazoles, particularly metronidazole. Metronidazole is the most effective amebicide for treatment of both colonic and extracolonic disease. Standard oral doses of 750 mg (10 mg/kg) three times a day for 5 to 10 days are indicated, followed by a luminal agent to prevent recurrence. The main side effects of metronidazole are nausea, vomiting, and a disulfiram-like effect with alcohol. Potential teratogenic effects of metronidazole have been noted *in vitro,* but long-term follow-up of several thousand women inadvertently given therapy for trichomoniasis during pregnancy failed to reveal any problems (180).

Amebic Liver Abscess

Mortality rate from uncomplicated amebic liver abscesses has decreased to less than 1% with early therapy with imidazoles. Single-dose therapies with metronidazole, tinidazole, and ornidazole have efficacies greater than 80%, but only metronidazole is available in the United States. Follow-up therapy with a luminal agent is very important even in patients without active diarrhea because asymptomatic colonization rates of up to 72% were detected in patients with amebic liver abscesses (167). Although all 50 patients in the South African study with amebic liver abscesses responded rapidly to metronidazole, cysts were not eradicated in 55% by metronidazole alone, creating potential sources for recurrence of invasive amebiasis or transmission (167).

The majority of patients respond dramatically within 72 hours of instituting metronidazole therapy (181). In patients who do not, evaluation for possible rupture should be instituted. Some authors advocate the addition of emetine 65 mg per day intramuscularly and oral chloroquine 600 mg followed by 300 mg per day (181), but we have found this unnecessary because all patients responded to percutaneous drainage (185). The primary indications for drainage include the following (165): (a) for initial diagnosis to exclude a pyogenic liver abscess, (b) for imminent rupture (usually >12 cm), (c) for failure to respond to medical therapy after 72 hours, (d) to drain a left lobe abscess and prevent pericardial rupture, and (e) to drain a ruptured abscess (163). Open surgery is relatively contraindicated except in cases of bowel perforation.

Prevention of Amebiasis

Transmission of amebiasis, like all fecally spread infections, could be completely prevented with adequate sanitation. The four critical areas to limit infection are adequate sanitation, health education, early treatment of potentially infectious cases, and surveillance and control programs (reviewed in reference 182). Effective prevention through sanitation requires both adequate disposal of human stools and sterilization of water. Asymptomatic carriers may excrete up to 15 million cysts a day, which can survive in water for several weeks and are resistant to levels of chlorination used in water purification. Although filtration and precipitation usually eliminate cysts, recontamination must be prevented. Infected food handlers are major sources of transmission, and health education emphasizing basic sanitation is required. Early treatment of patients with invasive disease and those shedding pathogenic cysts is critical. In the future, such targeted therapy will be helped significantly by more sensitive diagnostic tests. Mass chemotherapy trials for high-risk populations, such as in chronically institutionalized, mentally challenged populations, have been disappointing (183). Targeted surveillance in endemic areas, particularly using serologic testing and identification of pathogenic strains, will be important, particularly when integrated into programs for control of diarrheal diseases. For the individual traveler, no effective chemoprophylaxis for amebiasis exists. Risk of infection is best minimized by avoiding unpeeled fruits and vegetables and using bottled water. Boiling water or disinfection by iodination (tetraglycine hydroperiodide) is most effective (184).

REFERENCES

1. Walsh JA. Prevalence of *Entamoeba histolytica* infection. In: Ravdin JI, ed. *Amebiasis: human infection by* Entamoeba histolytica. New York: Churchill Livingstone, 1988:93–105.
2. Chayen A, Avron B, Nuchamowitz Y, et al. Appearance of sialoglycoproteins in encysting cells of *Entamoeba histolytica. Infect Immun* 1988;56:673–681.
3. Walker EL, Sellards AW. Experimental entamoebic dysentery. *Philippine J Sci B Trop Med* 1913;8:253–330.
4. Levine ND, Corliss JO, Cox FEG. A newly revised classification of the protozoa. *J Protozool* 1980;27:37–58.
5. Clark CG. The evolution of *Entamoeba*, a cautionary tale. *Res Microbiol* 2000;151:599–603.
6. Sargeaunt PG, Williams JE, Grene JD. The differentiation of invasive and non-invasive *Entamoeba histolytica* by isoenzyme electrophoresis. *Trans R Soc Trop Med Hyg* 1978;72:519–521.

7. Clark CG, Diamond LS. Ribosomal RNA genes of "pathogenic" *Entamoeba histolytica* are distinct. *Mol Biochem Parisitol* 1991;49:297–302.
8. Garfinkel LI, Gilandi M, Huber M, et al. DNA probes specific for *Entamoeba histolytica* possessing pathogenic and nonpathogenic zymodemes. *Infect Immun* 1989;57:926–931.
9. Tannich E, Burchard GD. Differentiation of pathogenic from nonpathogenic *Entamoeba histolytica* by restriction fragment analysis of a single gene amplified *in vitro. J Clin Microbiol* 1991;29:250–255.
10. Clark CG, Diamond LS. Intraspecific variation and phylogenetic relationships in the genus *Entamoeba* as revealed by riboprinting, *J.Eukaryot Microbiol* 1997;44:142–154.
11. Diamond LS, Clark CG. A redescription of *Entamoeba histolytica* Schaudinn, 1903 (Emended Walker, 1911) separating it from *Entamoeba dispar* Brumpt, 1925, *J Eukaryot Microbiol* 1993;40:340–344.
12. Petri WA Jr, Jackson TFHG, Gathiram V, et al. Pathogenic and nonpathogenic strains of *Entamoeba histolytica* can be differentiated by monoclonal antibodies to the galactose-specific adherence lectin. *Infect Immun* 1990;58:1802–1806.
13. Strachan WD, Spice WM, Chiodini PL, et al. Immunological differentiation of pathogenic and nonpathogenic isolates of *Entamoeba histolytica. Lancet* 1988;1:561–562.
14. Tachibana H, Kobayashi S, Nagakura K. Reactivity of monoclonal antibodies to species-specific antigens of *Entamoeba histolytica. J Protozool* 1991;38:329–334.
15. Bhattacharya A, Bhattacharya S, Sharma MP, et al. Metabolic labeling of *Entamoeba histolytica* antigens: characterization of a 28-kDa major intracellular antigen. *Exp Parasitol* 1990;70: 255–263.
16. Reed SL, Flores BM, Batzer MA, et al. Molecular and cellular characterization of the 29-kilodalton peripheral membrane protein of *Entamoeba histolytica:* differentiation between pathogenic and nonpathogenic isolates. *Infect Immun* 1992;60: 542–549.
17. Tannich E, Horstmann RD, Knobloch J, et al. Genomic DNA differences between pathogenic and nonpathogenic *Entamoeba histolytica. Proc Natl Acad Sci U S A* 1989;86:5118–5122.
18. Tachibana H, Kobayashi S, Paz KC, et al. Analysis of pathogenicity by restriction-endonuclease digestion of amplified genomic DNA of *Entamoeba histolytica* isolated in Pernambuco, Brazil. *Parasitol Res* 1992;78:433–436.
19. Burch DJ, Li E, Reed S, et al. Isolation of a strain-specific *Entamoeba histolytica* cDNA clone. *J Clin Microbiol* 1991;29: 696–701.
20. Verweij JJ, Blotkamp J, Brienen EAT, et al. Differentiation of *Entamoeba histolytica* and *Entamoeba dispar* cysts using polymerase chain reaction on DNA isolated from faeces with spin columns. *Eur J Clin Microbiol Infect Dis* 2000;19: 358–361.
21. Haque R, et al. Comparison of PCR, isoenzyme analysis, and antigen detection for diagnosis of *Entamoeba histolytica* infection. *J Clin Microbiol* 1998;36:449–452
22. Barker DC. Differentiation of *Entamoeba.* Patterns of nucleic acids and ribosomes during encystation and excystation. In: Van den Bossche H, ed. *Biochemistry of parasites and host-parasite relationships.* Amsterdam: Elsevier Biomedical, 1976:253.
23. Healy GR. Diagnostic techniques for stool samples. In: Ravdin JI, ed. *Amebiasis: human infection of* Entamoeba histolytica. New York: Churchill Livingstone, 1988:635–649.
24. Mathur TN, Kaur J. The frequency of excretion of cysts of *Entamoeba histolytica* in known cases of nondysenteric amoebic colitis based on 21 stool examinations. *Indian J Med Res* 1973; 61:330–334.
25. Krogstad DJ, Spencer HC, Healy GR, et al. Amebiasis: epidemiologic studies in the United States, 1971–1974. *Ann Intern Med* 1978;88:89–97.
26. Jackson TFHG, Gathiram V, Simjee AE. Seroepidemiological study of antibody responses to the zymodemes of *Entamoeba histolytica. Lancet* 1985;1:716–719.
27. Ravdin JI, Jackson TF, Petri WA Jr, et al. Association of serum antibodies to adherence lectin with invasive amebiasis and asymptomatic infection with *Entamoeba histolytica. J Infect Dis* 1990;162:768–772.
28. Bray RS, Harris WG. The epidemiology of infection with *Entamoeba histolytica* in The Gambia, West Africa. *Trans R Soc Trop Med Hyg* 1977;71:401–407.
29. Choudhuri G, Prakash V, Kumar A, et al. Protective immunity to *Entamoeba histolytica* infection in subjects with antiamoebic antibodies residing in a hyperendemic zone. *Scand J Infect Dis* 1991;23:771–776.
30. Caballero-Salcedo A, Viveros-Rogel M, Salvatiena B, et al. Seroepidemiology of amebiasis in Mexico. *Am J Trop Med Hyg* 1994;50:412–419.
31. Petri WA Jr, Haque R, Lyerly D, et al. Estimating the impact of amebiasis on health. *Parasitology Today* 2000;16:320–321.
32. Walsh JA. Transmission of *Entamoeba histolytica* infection. In: Ravdin JI, ed. *Amebiasis:* human infection by *Entamoeba histolytica.* New York: Churchill Livingstone, 1988:106–119.
33. Gutierez G, Ludlow A, Espinos G, et al. National serologic survey II. Search for antibodies against *Entamoeba histolytica* in Mexico. In: Sepulveda B, Diamond LS, eds. Proceedings of the International Conference on Amebiasis. *Amebiasis.* Mexico City: Instito Mexicano del Seguro Social, 1976:609–618.
34. Abdel-Hafez MM, el-Kady N, Bolbol AS, et al. Prevalence of intestinal parasitic infections in Riyadh district, Saudi Arabia. *Ann Trop Med Parasitol* 1986;80:631–634.
35. Gathiram V, Jackson TFHG. Frequency distribution of *Entamoeba histolytica* zymodemes in a rural South African population. *Lancet* 1985;1:719–721.
36. Nanda R, Baveja U, Anand BS. *Entamoeba histolytica* cyst passers: clinical features and outcome in untreated subjects. *Lancet* 1984;2:301–303.
37. Gathiram V, Jackson TFHG. A longitudinal study of asymptomatic carriers of pathogenic zymodemes of *Entamoeba histolytica. S Afr Med J* 1987;72:669–672.
38. Acuna-Soto R, Samuelson J, De Girolami P, et al. Application of the polymerase chain reaction to the epidemiology of pathogenic and nonpathogenic *Entamoeba histolytica. Am J Trop Med Hyg* 1993;48:58–70.
39. Thacker SB, Simpson S, Gordon TJ, et al. Parasitic disease control in a residential facility for the mentally retarded. *Am J Public Health* 1979;69:1279–1281.
40. Sexton DJ, Krogstad DJ, Spencer HC, et al. Amebiasis in a mental institution: serologic and epidemiologic studies. *Am J Epidemiol* 1974;100:414–423.
41. Petri WA, Ravdin JI. Amebiasis in institutionalized populations. In: Ravdin JI, ed. *Amebiasis: human infection by* Entamoeba histolytica. New York: Churchill Livingstone, 1988.
42. Thacker SB, Kimball AM, Wolfe M, et al. Parasitic disease control in a residential facility for the mentally retarded: failure of selected isolation procedures. *Am J Public Health* 1981;71:303.
43. Brooke MM. Epidemiology and control of amebiasis in institutions for the mentally retarded. *Am J Ment Defic* 1963;68:187.
44. Kean BH, William DC, Luminais SK. Epidemic of amoebiasis and giardiasis in a biased population. *Br J Vener Dis* 1979;55: 375–378.
45. Allason-Jones E, Mindel A, Sargeaunt P, et al. *Entamoeba histolytica* is a commensal intestinal parasite in homosexual men. *N Engl J Med* 1986;515:353–356.
46. Markell EK, Havens RF, Kuritsubo RA, et al. Intestinal protozoa

in homosexual men of the San Francisco Bay area: prevalence and correlates of infection. *Am J Trop Med Hyg* 1984;33:239–245.
47. Ortega HB, Borchardt KA, Hamilton R, et al. Enteric pathogenic protozoa in homosexual men from San Francisco. *Sex Transm Dis* 1983;11:59.
48. Sorvillo FJ, Strassburg MA, Seidel J, et al. Amebic infections in asymptomatic homosexual men, lack of evidence of invasive disease, *Am J Public Health* 1986;76:1137–1139.
49. Druckman DA, Quinn TC. *Entamoeba histolytica* infection in homosexual men. In: Ravdin JI, ed. *Amebiasis: human infection by* Entamoeba histolytica. New York: Churchill Livingstone, 1988:563–575.
50. Lowther SA, Dworkin MS, Hanson DL, et al. *Entamoeba histolytica Entamoeba dispar* infections in human immunodeficiency virus-infected patients in the United States. *Clin Infec Dis* 2000;30:955–959.
51. Brown M, Reed S, Levy JA, et al. Detection of HIV-1 in *Entamoeba histolytica* without evidence of transmission to human cells. *AIDS* 1991;5:93–96.
52. Istre GR, Kriess K, Hopkins RS, et al. An outbreak of amebiasis spread by colonic irrigation at a chiropractic clinic. *N Engl J Med* 1982;309:339–342.
53. Sabot JM, Patterson M. Amebic liver abscess: 1966–1976. *Dig Dis* 1978;23:110.
54. Abuabara SF, Barrett JA, Hau T, et al. Amebic liver abscess. *Arch Surg* 1982;117:239–244.
55. Katzenstein D, Rickerson V, Braude A. New concepts of amebic liver abscess derived from hepatic imaging, serodiagnosis, and hepatic enzymes in 67 consecutive cases in San Diego. *Medicine (Baltimore)* 1982;61:237–246.
56. Thompson JE Jr, Forlenza S, Verma R. Amebic liver abscess: a therapeutic approach. *Rev Infect Dis* 1985;7:171–179.
57. Barnes PF, DeCock KM, Reynolds TN, et al. A comparison of amebic and pyogenic abscess of the liver. *Medicine (Baltimore)* 1987;66:472–483.
58. Thompson JE Jr, Glasser AJ. Amebic abscess of the liver. Diagnostic features. *J Clin Gastroenterol* 1986;8:550–554.
59. Pearson RD, Hewlett EL. Amebiasis in travelers. In: Ravdin JI, ed. *Amebiasis: human infection by* Entamoeba histolytica. New York: Churchill Livingstone, 1988:556–562.
60. Pehrson PO. Amoebiasis in a non-endemic country. *Scand J Infect Dis* 1983;15:207–214.
61. Merson MH, Morris GK, Sack DA, et al. Traveler's diarrhea in Mexico: a prospective study. *N Engl J Med* 1976;294:1299.
62. Brandt H, Perez Tamayo R. Pathology of human amebiasis. *Hum Pathol* 1970;1:351–385.
63. Griffin JL, Juniper K Jr. Ultrastructure of *Entamoeba histolytica* from human amebic dysentery. *Arch Pathol* 1971;91:271–280.
64. Prahap K, Gilman R. The histopathology of acute intestinal amebiasis. *Am J Pathol* 1970;60:229–239.
65. Chatgidakis CB. The pathology of hepatic amoebiasis as seen on the Witwatersrand. *S Afr J Clin Sci* 1953;4:230.
66. Guerrant RL, Brush J, Ravdin JI, et al. Interaction between *Entamoeba histolytica* and human polymorphonuclear neutrophils. *J Infect Dis* 1981;143:83–93.
67. Ravdin JI, Murphy CF, Salata RA, et al. The *N*-acetyl-D-galactosamine-inhibitable adherence lectin of *Entamoeba histolytica.* I. Partial purification and relation to amoebic virulence *in vitro. J Infect Dis* 1985;151:804–815.
68. Tsutsumi V, Mena-Lopez R, Anaya-Velazquez F, et al. Cellular basis of experimental amebic liver abscess formation. *Am J Pathol* 1984;117:81–91.
69. Salata RA, Ravdin JI. The interaction of human neutrophils and *Entamoeba histolytica* increases cytopathogenicity for liver cell monolayers. *J Infect Dis* 1986;154:19–26.
70. Joyce MP, Ravdin JI. Pathology of human amebiasis. In: Ravdin JI, ed. *Amebiasis: human infection by* Entamoeba histolytica. New York: Churchill Livingstone, 1988:129–146.
71. Aikat BK, Bhusnurmath SR, Pal AK, et al. The pathology and pathogenesis of fatal hepatic amoebiasis: a study based on 79 autopsy cases. *Trans R Soc Trop Med Hyg* 1979;73:188–192.
72. Gulati PD, Gupta DN, Chuttani HK. Amoebic liver abscess and disturbances of portal circulation. *Am J Med* 1967;45: 852–854.
73. Tandon BN, Tandon HD, Puri BK. An electron microscopic study of liver in hepatomegaly presumably caused by amebiasis. *Exp Mol Pathol* 1975;22:118.
74. Ravdin JI. *Entamoeba histolytica:* pathogenic mechanisms, human immune response, and vaccine development. *Clin Res* 1990;38:215–225.
75. Ravdin JI, Guerrant RL. Role of adherence in cytopathogenic mechanisms of *Entamoeba histolytica. J Clin Invest* 1981;68: 1305–1313.
76. Petri WA, Smith RD, Schlesinger PH, et al. Isolation of the galactose-binding lectin which mediates the *in vitro* adherence of *Entamoeba histolytica. J Clin Invest* 1987;80:1238–1244.
77. Chadee K, Petri WA, Innes DJ, et al. Rat and human colonic mucins bind to and inhibit the adherence of lectin of *Entamoeba histolytica. J Clin Invest* 1987;80:1245–1254.
78. Ravdin JI, John JE, Johnston LI, et al. Adherence of *Entamoeba histolytica* trophozoites to rat and human colonic mucosa. *Infect Immuun* 1985;48:292–297.
79. Salata RA, Pearson RD, Ravdin JI. Interaction of human leukocytes with *Entamoeba histolytica:* killing of virulent amebae by the activated macrophage. *J Clin Invest* 1985;76:491–499.
80. Orozco ME, Rodriguez M, Murphy CF, et al. *Entamoeba histolytica:* cytopathogenicity and lectin activity of avirulent mutants. *Exp Parasitol* 1987;63:157–165.
81. Petri WA Jr, Chapman MD, Snodgrass T, et al. Subunit structure of the galactose and *N*-acetyl-D-galactosamine-inhibitable adherence lectin of *Entamoeba histolytica. J Biol Chem* 1989; 264:3007–3012.
82. Mann BJ, Chung CY, Dodson JM, et al. Neutralizing monoclonal antibody epitopes of the *Entamoeba histolytica* galactose adhesin map to the cysteine-rich extracellular domain of the 170-kilodalton heavy subunit. *Infect Immun* 1993;61:1772–1778.
83. Pillai DR, Wan WSK, Yau YCW, et al. The cysteine-rich region of the *Entamoeba histolytica* adherence lectin (170-kilodalton subunit) is sufficient for high-affinity Gal / GalNAc-specific binding in vitro. *Infect Immun* 1999;67:3836–3841.
84. Tannich E, Ebert F, Horstmann RD. Primary structure of the 170-kDa surface lectin of pathogenic *Entamoeba histolytica. Proc Natl Acad Sci U S A* 1991;88:1849–1853.
85. McCoy JJ, Mann BJ, Vedvick T, et al. Structural analysis of the light subunit of the *Entamoeba histolytica* adherence lectin. *J Biol Chem* 1993;24:223–231.
86. Braga LL, Ninomiya H, McCoy JJ, et al. Inhibition of the complement membrane attack complex by the galactose-specific adhesion of *Entamoeba histolytica. J Clin Invest* 1992;90:1131–1137.
87. Ravdin JI, Croft BY, Guerrant RL. Cytopathogenic mechanisms of *Entamoeba histolytica. J Exp Med* 1980;152:377–390.
88. Ravdin JI, Moreau F, Sullivan JA, et al. The relationship of free intracellular calcium ions to the cytolytic activity of *Entamoeba histolytica. Infect Immun* 1988;56:1505–1512.
89. Ravdin JI, Murphy CF, Guerrant RL, et al. Effect of calcium and phospholipase A antagonists on the cytopathogenicity of *Entamoeba histolytica. J Infect Dis* 1985;152:542–549.
90. Long-Krug SA, Hysmith RM, Fischer KJ, et al. The phospholipase A enzymes of *Entamoeba histolytica:* description and subcellular localization. *J Infect Dis* 1985;152:536–541.

91. Ravdin JI, Schlesinger PH, Murphy CF, et al. Acid intracellular vesicles and the cytolysis of mammalian target cells by *Entamoeba histolytica* trophozoites. *J Protozool* 1986;33:478–486.
92. Weikel CS, Murphy CF, Orozco ME, et al. Phorbol esters specifically enhance the cytolytic activity of *Entamoeba histolytica. Infect Immun* 1988;56:1485–1491.
93. Yadava N, Chandok MR, Prasad J, et al. Characterization of EhCaBP, a calcium-building protein of *Entamoeba histolytica* and its binding proteins. *Mol Biochem Parasitol.* 1997;84: 69–82.
94. Godbold GD, Mann BJ. Cell killing by the human parasite *Entamoeba histolytica* is inhibited by the Rho-inactivating C3 exoenzyme. *Mol Biochem Parasitol* 2000;108:147–151.
95. Young JE, Young TM, Lu LP, et al. Characterization of a membrane pore-forming protein from *Entamoeba histolytica. J Exp Med* 1982;156:1677–1690.
96. Lynch EC, Rosenberg IM, Gitler C. An ion-channel forming protein produced by *Entamoeba histolytica. EMBO J* 1982;1: 801–804.
97. Leippe M, Tannich E, et al. Primary and secondary structure of the pore-forming peptide of pathogenic *Entamoeba histolytica. EMBO J* 1992;11:3501–3506.
98. Young JD-E, Cohn ZA. Molecular mechanisms of cytotoxicity mediated by *Entamoeba histolytica:* characterization of a pore-forming protein (PFP). *J Cell Biochem* 1985;29:299–308.
99. Leippe M. Amoebapores. *Parasitol Today* 1997;13:178–183.
100. Leippe M, at al. Comparison of pore-forming peptides from pathogenic and nonpathogenic *Entamoeba histolytica. Mol Biol Parasitol* 1997;59:101–110.
101. Scholze H, Werries E. A weakly acidic protease has a powerful proteolytic activity in *Entamoeba histolytica. Mol Biochem Parasitol* 1984;11:293–300.
102. Munoz MDL, Calderon J, Rojkind M. The collagenase of *Entamoeba histolytica. J Exp Med* 1982;155:42–51.
103. Keene WE, Petitt MG, Allen S, et al. The major neutral proteinase of *Entamoeba histolytica. J Exp Med* 1986;163:536–549.
104. Reed SL. *Entamoeba* infections in human immunodeficiency virus-infected patients: not just a tropical problem. *Clin Infect Dis* 2000;30:959–961.
105. Kelsall BL, Ravdin JI. Proteolytic degradation of human IgA by *Entamoeba histolytica. J Infect Dis* 1993;168:1319–1322.
106. Tran VQ, Herdman DS, Torian BE, et al. The natural cysteine proteinase of *Entamoeba histolytica* degrades IgG and prevents its binding. *J Infect Dis* 1998;177:508–511.
107. Reed SL, Gigli I. Lysis of complement-sensitive *Entamoeba histolytica* by activated terminal complement components. *J Clin Invest* 1990;86:1815–1822.
108. Reed SL, Keene WE, McKerrow JH. Thiol proteinase expression and pathogenicity of *Entamoeba histolytica. J Clin Microbiol* 1989;27:2772–2777.
109. Reed S, Bouvier J, Pollack AS, et al. Cloning of a virulence factor of *Entamoeba histolytica. J Clin Invest* 1993;91:1532–1540.
110. Bruchhaus I, Jacobs T, Leippe M, et al. *Entamoeba histolytica* and *Entamoeba dispar*: differences in numbers and expression of cysteine proteinase genes. *Mol Microbiol* 1996;22:255–263.
111. Zhang Z, Yan L, Wang L, et al. *Entamoeba histolytica* cysteine proteinases with interleukin-1 beta converting enzyme (ICE) activity cause intestinal inflammation and tissue damage in amoebiasis. *Mol Microbiol* 2000;37:542–548.
112. Werries E, Nebinger P, Franz A. Degradation of biogene oligosaccharides by beta-*N*-acetylglucosaminidase secreted by *Entamoeba histolytica. Mol Biochem Parasitol* 1983;7:127–140.
113. Udezulu IA, Leitch GJ. A membrane-associated neuraminidase in *Entamoeba histolytica* trophozoites. *Infect Immun* 1981;36: 795–801.
114. Salata RA, Ahmed P, Ravdin JI. *Entamoeba histolytica* chemoattractant activity of human polymorphonuclear neutrophils. *J Parasitol* 1989;75:644–646.
115. DeLeon A. Prognostico tardio en el absceso hepatico amibiano. *Arch Invest Med (Mex)* 1970;1[Suppl 1]:205–206.
116. Petri WA, Joyce MP, Broman J, et al. Recognition of the galactose- or *N*-acetylgalactosamine-binding lectin of *Entamoeba histolytica* by human immune sera. *Infect Immun* 1987;55: 2327–2331.
117. Joyce MP, Ravdin JI. Antigens of *Entamoeba histolytica* recognized by immune sera from liver abscess patients. *Am J Trop Med Hyg* 1988;38:74–80.
118. Abd-Alla M, El-Hawey AM, Ravdin JI. Use of an enzyme-linked immunosorbent assay to detect anti-adherence protein antibodies in sera of patients with invasive amebiasis in Cairo, Egypt. *Am J Trop Med Hyg* 1992;47:800–804.
119. Ortiz-Ortiz L, Capin R, Capin NR, et al. Activation of the alternative pathway of complement by *Entamoeba histolytica. Clin Exp Immunol* 1978;34:10–18.
120. Reed SL, Sargeaunt PG, Braude AI. Resistance to lysis by human serum of pathogenic *Entamoeba histolytica. Trans R Soc Trop Med Hyg* 1983;77:248–253.
121. Calderon J, Tovar R. Loss of susceptibility to complement lysis in *Entamoeba histolytica* HM1 by treatment with human serum. *Immunology* 1986;58:467–471.
122. Grundy MS, Cartwright TL, Lundin L, et al. Antibodies against *Entamoeba histolytica* in human milk and serum in Kenya. *J Clin Microbiol* 1983;17:753–758.
123. Islam A, Stoll BJ, Ljungstrom I, et al. The prevalence of *Entamoeba histolytica* in lactating women and in their infants in Bangladesh. *Trans R Soc Trop Med Hyg* 1988;82:99–103.
124. Speelman P, Ljungstrom I. Protozoal enteric infections among expatriates in Bangladesh. *Am J Trop Med Hyg* 1986;35: 1140–1145.
125. del Muro R, Acosta E, Merino E, et al. Diagnosis of intestinal amebiasis using salivary IgA antibody detection. *J Infect Dis* 1990;162:1360–1364.
126. Aceti A, Pennica A, Celestino D, et al. Salivary IgA antibody detection in invasive amebiasis and in asymptomatic infection. *J Infect Dis* 1991;164:613–615.
127. Salta RA, Murray HW, Rubin BY, et al. The role of gamma interferon in the generation of human macrophages and T lymphocytes cytotoxic for *Entamoeba histolytica. Am J Trop Med Hyg* 1987;37:72–78.
128. Salata RA, Martinez-Palomo A, Murphy CF, et al. Patients treated for amebic liver abscess develop a cell-mediated immune response effective *in vitro* against *Entamoeba histolytica. J Immunol* 1986;136:2633–2639.
129. Schain DS, Salata RA, Ravdin JI. Human T-lymphocyte proliferation, lymphokine production, and amebicidal activity elicited by the galactose-inhibitable adherence protein of *Entamoeba histolytica. Infect Immun* 1992;60:2143–2146.
130. Salata RA, Martinez-Palomo A, Conales L, et al. Immune sera suppresses the antigen specific proliferative response in T lymphocytes from patients cured of amebic liver abscess. *Infect Immun* 190;58:3941–3946.
131. Sepulveda B, Martinez-Palomo A. Immunology of amoebiasis by *Entamoeba histolytica.* In: Cohen S, Warren VS, eds. *Immunology of parasitic infections,* vol 1, second edition. Oxford: Blackwell Scientific, 1982:70–91.
132. Kanani SR, Knight R. Relapsing amoebic colitis of 12 years' standing exacerbated by corticosteroids. *BMJ* 1969;2:613–614.
133. Balikian JP, Bitar JG, Rishani KI, et al. Fulminating necrotizing amebic colitis in children. *Am J Proctol* 1977;28:69.
134. Tucker PC, Webster PD, Kilpatrick ZM. Amebic colitis mistaken for inflammatory bowel disease. *Arch Intern Med* 1975; 135:681.

135. Lewis EA, Anitia AU. Amoebic colitis: review of 295 cases. *Trans R Soc Trop Med Hyg* 1969;63:633–638.
136. Fuchs G, Ruiz-Palacios G, Pickering LK. Amebiasis in the pediatric population. In: Ravdin JI, ed. *Amebiasis: human infection by* Entamoeba histolytica. New York: Churchill Livingstone, 1988:594–613.
137. Seydel KB, Smith SJ, Stanley SL Jr. Innate immunity to amebic liver abscess is dependent on gamma interferon and nitric oxide in a murine model of disease. *Infect Immun* 2000;68:400–402.
138. Leitch GJ, Dickey AD, Udezulu IA, et al. *Entamoeba histolytica* trophozoites in the lumen and mucus blanket of rat colons studied *in vitro*. *Infect Immun* 1985;47:68–73.
139. Chadee K, Meerovitch E. *Entamoeba histolytica:* early progressive pathology in the cecum of the gerbil (*Meriones unguiculatus*). *Am J Trop Med Hyg* 1985;34:283–291.
140. Chadee K, Petri WA, Johnson M, et al. Binding and internalization of purified rat colonic mucins by the Gal/GalNAc adherence lectin of *Entamoeba histolytica. J Infect Dis* 1988; 158:398–406.
141. Chadee K, Innes DJ, Ravdin JI. Mucin and nonmucin secretagogue activity of *Entamoeba histolytica* and cholera toxin in rat colon. *Gastroenterology* 1991;100:986–997.
142. Petri WA Jr, Ravdin JI. Protection of gerbils from amebic liver abscess by immunization with the galactose-specific adherence lectin of *Entamoeba histolytica. Infect Immun* 1991; 59:97–101.
143. Soong CJG, Kain KC, Abd-Alla M, et al. A recombinant lectin is efficacious as a subunit vaccine in the gerbil model of amebic liver abscess. *J Infect Dis* 1995;171:645–651.
144. Mann BJ, Burkholker BV, Lockhart LA. Protection in a gerbil model of amebiasis by oral immunization with *Salmonella* by expressing the galactose / N-acetyl D-galactosamine inhibitable lectin of *Entamoeba histolytica. Vaccine* 1997;15:659–663.
145. Lotter H, Zhang T, Seydel KB, et al. Identification of an epitope on the *Entamoeba histolytica* 170-kd lectin conferring antibody-medicated protection against invasive amebiasis. *J Exp Med* 1997;185:1793–1801.
146. Lotter H, Khajawa F, Stanley SL Jr, et al. Protection of gerbils from amebic liver abscess by vaccination with a 25-mer peptide derived from the cysteine-rich region of *Entamoeba histolytica* galactose-specific adherence lectin. *Infect Immun* 2000;68: 4416–4421.
147. Campbell D, Mann BJ, Chadee K. A subunit vaccine candidate region of the *Entamoeba histolytica* galactose-adherence lectin promotes interleukin-12 gene transcription and protein production in human macrophages. *Eur J Immunol* 2000;30: 423–430.
148. Marinets A, Zhang T, Guillen N, et al. Protection against invasive amebiasis by a single monoclonal antibody directed against a lipophosphoglycan antigen localized on the surface of *Entamoeba histolytica. J Exp Med* 1997;186:1557–1565.
149. Reed SL. Amebiasis: an update. *Clin Infect Dis* 1992;14: 385–393.
150. Petri WA, Singh U. Diagnosis and management of amebiasis. *Clin Infect Dis* 1999;29:1119–1125.
151. Haque R., Faruque ASG, Hahn P, et al. *Entemoeba histolytica* and *Entamoeba dispar* infection in children in Bangladesh. *J Infect Dis* 1997;175:734–736.
152. Quinn TC, Stamm WE, Goodell SE, et al. The polymicrobial origin of intestinal infections in homosexual men. *N Engl J Med* 1983;309:576–582.
152a. Lowther SA, Dworkin MS, Hanson DL. *Entamoeba histolytica/dispar* infections among HIV-infected patients in the United States. *Clin Infect Dis* 2000;30:955–959.
153. Reed SL, Wessel DW, Davis CE. *Entamoeba histolytica* infection and AIDS. *Am J Med* 1991;90:269–270.
154. Aristizabal H, Acevedo J, Botero M. Fulminant amebic colitis. *World J Surg* 1991;15:216–221.
155. Fuchs G, Ruiz-Palacios G, Pickering LK. Amebiasis in the pediatric population. In: Ravdin JI, ed. *Amebiasis: human infection by* Entamoeba histolytica. New York: Churchill Livingstone, 1988:594–613.
156. Adams EB, MacLeod IN. Invasive amebiasis. I. Amebic dysentery and its complications. *Medicine* (*Baltimore*) 1977;56: 315–323.
157. Radke RA. Ameboma of the intestine: an analysis of the disease as presented in 78 collected and 41 previously unreported cases. *Ann Intern Med* 1955;43:1048–1066.
158. Powell SJ, Wilmot AJ. Ulcerative post-dysenteric colitis. *Gut* 1966;7:438–443.
159. Mhlanga BR, Lanoie LO, Norris HJ, et al. Amebiasis complicating carcinomas: a diagnostic dilemma. *Am J Trop Med Hyg* 1992;759:764.
160. Patel AS, DeRidder PH. Amebic colitis masquerading as acute inflammatory bowel disease: the role of serology in its diagnosis. *J Clin Gastroenterol* 1989;11:407–410.
161. Adams EB, MacLeod IN. Invasive amebiasis. II. Amebic liver abscess and its complications. *Medicine* (*Baltimore*) 1977;56: 325–334.
162. Ibarra-Perez C. Thoracic complications of amebic abscess of the liver. Report of 501 cases. *Chest* 1981;79:672–677.
163. Ken JG, vanSonnenberg E, Casola G, et al. Perforated amebic liver abscesses: successful percutaneous treatment. *Radiology* 1989;170:195–197.
164. Ibarra-Perez C, Green L, Calvillo-Juarez M, et al. Diagnosis and treatment of rupture of amebic abscess of the liver into the pericardium. *J Thorac Cardiovasc Surg* 1972;64:11–17.
165. vanSonnenberg E, Mueller PR, Schiffman HR, et al. Intrahepatic amebic abscesses: indications for and results of percutaneous catheter drainage. *Radiology* 1985;156:631–635.
166. Barnes PF, DeCock KM, Reynolds TR, et al. A comparison of amebic and pyogenic abscess of the liver. *Medicine* (*Baltimore*) 1987;66:472–483.
167. Irusen EM, Jackson TFHG, Simjee AE. Asymptomatic intestinal colonization by pathogenic *Entamoeba histolytica* in amebic liver abscess: prevalence, response to therapy, and pathogenic potential. *Clin Infect Dis* 1992;14:889–893.
168. Healy GR. Immunologic tools in the diagnosis of amebiasis: epidemiology in the United States. *Rev Infect Dis* 1986;8: 239–245.
169. Ahmed L, El Rooby A, Kassem MI, et al. Ultrasonography in the diagnosis and management of 52 patients with amebic liver abscess in Cairo. *Rev Infect Dis* 1990;12:330–337.
170. Ralls PW, Quinn MF, Boswell WD, et al. Patterns of resolution in successfully treated hepatic amebic abscess: sonographic evaluation. *Radiology* 1983;149:541–543.
171. Joyce MP, Ravdin JI. Pathology of human amebiasis. In: Ravdin JI, ed. *Amebiasis: human infection by* Entamoeba histolytica. New York: Churchill Livingstone, 1988:129–146.
172. Reed SL, Flores BM, Batzer MA, et al. Molecular and cellular characterization of the 29-kDa peripheral membrane protein of *Entamoeba histolytica:* differentiation between pathogenic and nonpathogenic isolates. *Infect Immun* 1992;60:542–549.
173. Tachibana H, Kobayashi S, Kato Y, et al. Identification of a pathogenic isolate-specific 30,000-Mr antigen of *Entamoeba histolytica* by using a monoclonal antibody. *Infect Immun* 1990; 58:955–960.
174. Haque R, Neville L, Hahn P, Petri WA. Rapid diagnosis of *Entamoeba* infection by using *Entamoeba* and *Entamoeba histolytica* stool antigen detection kits. *J Clinical Microbiol* 1995; 33:2558–2561.
175. Abd-Alla M, Jackson TFHG, Gathirim V, et al. Differentiation

of pathogenic from nonpathogenic *Entamoeba histolytica* infection by detection of galactose-inhibitable adherence protein antigen in sera and feces. *J Clin Microbiol* 1993;31:2845–2850.

176. Luaces AL, Pico T, Barrett AJ. The ENZYMEBA test: detection of intestinal *Entamoeba histolytica* infection by immuno-enzymatic detection of histolysin. *Parasitology* 1992;105:203–205.
177. McAuley JB, Juranek DD. Luminal agents in the treatment of amebiasis. *Clin Infect Dis* 1992;14:1161–1162.
178. McAuley JB, Herwaldt BL, Stokes SL, et al. Diloxanide furoate for treating asymptomatic *Entamoeba histolytica* cyst passers: 14 years' experience in the United States. *Clin Infect Dis* 1992;15:464–468.
179. Sullam PM, Slutkin G, Gottlieb AB, Mills J. Paromomycin therapy of endemic amebiasis in homosexual men. *Sex Transm Dis* 1986;13:151–155.
180. Beard CM, Noller KL, O'Fallon WM, et al. Lack of evidence for cancer due to use of metronidazole. *N Engl J Med* 1979;301:519–522.
181. Thompson JE, Forlenza S, Verma R. Amebic liver abscess: a therapeutic approach. *Rev Infect Dis* 1985;7:171–179.
182. Martinez-Palomo A, Martinez-Baez M. Selective primary health care: strategies for control of disease in the developing world. X. Amebiasis. *Rev Infect Dis* 1983;5:1093–1102.
183. Sexton DJ, Krogstad DJ, Spencer HC, et al. Amebiasis in a mental institution: serologic and epidemiologic studies. *Am J Epidemiol* 1974;100:414–423.
184. Backer H. Field water disinfection. In: Auerbach PS, Geehr EC, eds. *Management of wilderness and environmental emergencies.* St Louis: CV Mosby, 1989:805–829.
185. Ravdin JI, Guerrant RL. A review of the parasite cellular mechanisms involved in the pathogenesis of amebiasis. *Rev Infect Dis* 1982;4:1185–1207.
186. Ravdin JI. Intestinal disease caused by *Entamoeba histolytica.* In: Ravdin JI, ed. *Amebiasis: human infection by* Entamoeba histolytica. New York: Churchill Livingstone, 1988:495–509.

61

GIARDIA DUODENALIS

GAÉTAN M. FAUBERT
PETER LEE
AWS ABDUL-WAHID

Giardia duodenalis is the most common intestinal protozoan enteropathogen worldwide. This flagellated protozoan inhabits the upper part of the small intestine of its host and has a direct life cycle. After the host ingests the cysts (Fig. 61.1), which are the infective stage, the trophozoites usually emerge from the cysts in the duodenum and attach to the intestinal mucosa (Fig. 61.2). They undergo mitotic division in the intestinal lumen; some will encyst to protect themselves and will be eliminated from the host in the feces. For many years, there has been a debate over whether this protozoan was a pathogen or merely a harmless commensal. There is now compelling evidence to indicate that *Giardia* is an important cause of acute and chronic diarrhea, which may be associated with intestinal malabsorption and growth retardation in infants and young children (1–3). In some cases, disease symptoms of diarrhea and malabsorption can be severe and chronic; it had been reported to last 10 years in a patient with underlying hypogammaglobulinemia (4). Giardiasis may be profoundly incapacitating to infants, children, persons with immunodeficiencies, the elderly, and individuals with protein malnutrition (5). Giardiasis has been reported as the cause of urticaria in children and adults (6–9). In one patient, the chronic urticaria was resolved with treatment of giardiasis (7). There is still no adequate explanation for the diverse clinical spectrum of symptoms associated with giardiasis, which range from asymptomatic infection to acute self-limiting diarrhea or sometimes persistent diarrhea that may fail to respond to appropriate therapy, even in immunocompetent individuals. In addition, the mechanisms by which *Giardia* infection produces diarrhea and malabsorption of nutrients by the host are poorly understood, although several theories have been put forward. Finally, despite extensive study in animal models and in humans, the key immunologic determinants required for clearance of acute infection and development of protective immunity remain ill defined.

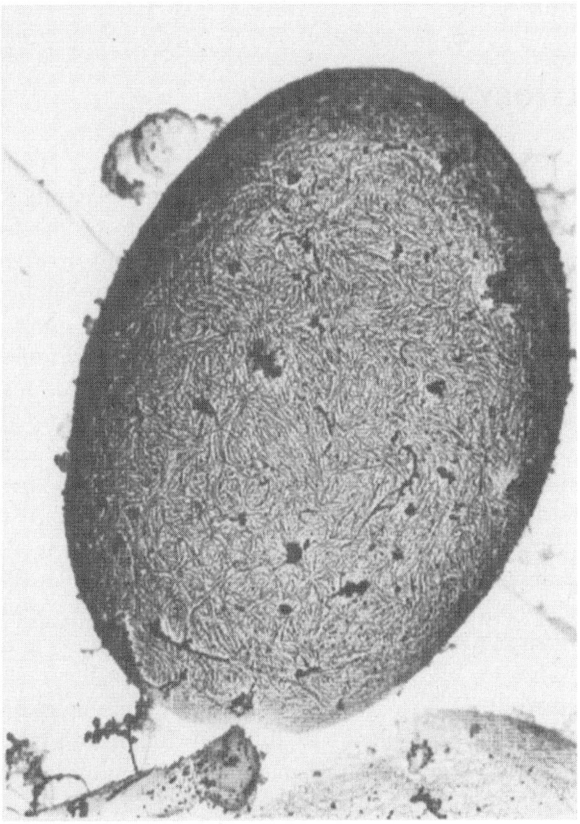

FIGURE 61.1. High-resolution, low-voltage scanning electron micrograph of a *Giardia duodenalis* (×7,700) showing the filamentous structure of the cyst wall. (From Erlandsen SL, Bemrick WJ, Pawley J. High-resolution electron microscopic evidence for the filamentous structure of the cyst wall in *Giardia muris* and *Giardia duodenalis*. *J Parasitol* 75:787–797, with permission.)

G.M. Faubert, P. Lee, and A. Abdul-Wahid: Institute of Parasitology, McGill University, Ste. Anne-de-Bellevue, Quebec, Canada

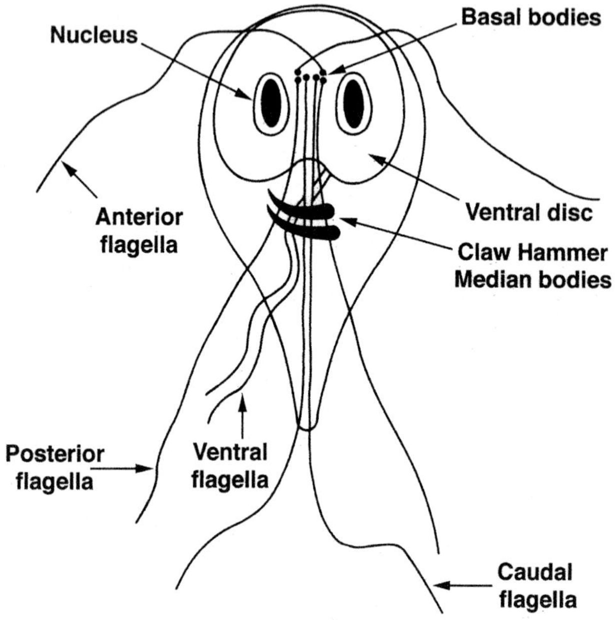

FIGURE 61.2. Trophozoite of the *Giardia duodenalis* showing the median bodies in the shape of a claw hammer that is characteristic of the *duodenalis*-type organisms.

HISTORY

Anton van Leeuwenhoek wrote a letter to Robert Hooke, secretary of the Royal Society, London, dated November 4, 1681, in which he gives what is believed to be the first account identifying *Giardia,* using his hand lenses to examine specimens of his diarrheal stools (10). Vilem Lambl in 1859 rediscovered the parasite in the diarrheic stools of children and named the organism *Cercomonas intestinalis,* again making a link between the presence of this organism and diarrhea. The name *lamblia* was first applied to the genus by Blanchard in 1888. Kunstler in 1882 discovered a similar organism in tadpoles and named it *Giardia agilis,* after his teacher and mentor Professor Alfred Giard. As far as can be ascertained, Giard had no direct involvement in the discovery of this organism or in the description of its biology. Although discovery of the cyst form of the parasite is often attributed to Grassi in 1879, cysts are present in the sketches of Vilem Lambl, which he published in 1860. Interest in the biology and pathology of this group of protozoa began in the mid-1970s when *Giardia* organisms were isolated from mammalian, avian, and amphibian hosts (11,12).

TAXONOMY

Morphologic Systematics

Giardia has traditionally been placed in the subphylum Sarcomastigophora, in the superclass Mastigophora, and in the order Diplomonadida. In addition, *Giardia* belongs to the family Hexamitidae, which contains six genera, three of which, including *Giardia,* are exclusively parasitic (13). Organisms in the genus *Giardia* possess an adhesive disc on the ventral surface, which distinguishes it from other members of the family Hexamitidae. Different *Giardia* species were initially assigned on the basis of the host from which they were derived, which produced more than 40 *Giardia* "species." Filice (14) in 1952 considered host specificity unreliable and emphasized the shape of the median body as an approach to distinguish between the three major morphologic types: *G. agilis* from amphibians, which has a long teardrop-shaped median body; *Giardia muris* from mice with two small, rounded median bodies; and *G. duodenalis* (*intestinalis* = *lamblia*) infecting humans and other mammals, birds, and reptiles, which has median bodies resembling the claw of a claw hammer. In addition to these three major morphologic subtypes, two other *Giardia* isolates have been described and have been assigned to separate species: *Giardia psittaci,* an isolate from a budgerigar (15) that has median bodies of the *G. duodenalis* type but lacks the ventrolateral flange and thus the marginal groove bordering the adhesive disk; and *Giardia ardea,* an isolate from the great blue heron (16), which has a median body similar to those of *G. muris* and *G. duodenalis* but a ventral disk and single caudal flagellum more similar to those of *G. muris.* A sixth species, *Giardia microti,* has been proposed on the basis of cyst morphology and small subunit ribosomal RNA (rRNA) sequence analysis (17). It is likely that new *Giardia* species will be described. In this chapter because Filice's classification is followed, the name *G. duodenalis* is used to describe the human type of *Giardia.*

Molecular Systematics

Isoenzyme Electrophoretic Analysis

The electrophoretic analysis of gene products has been used to study genetic variation in a wide range of organisms. Isolates with identical banding patterns after the application of specific enzyme stains are referred to as zymodemes. These studies in the genus *Giardia* have been limited to the morphologic group *G. duodenalis* (18). Essentially, electrophoretic studies have demonstrated that some isolates have identical proteins and enzymes while others differ substantially among them. Interestingly, regardless of the nature of genetic diversity among isolates of *G duodenalis,* there appears to be no simple correlation with either host or geographic origin. Twenty-seven *G. duodenalis* cyst-positive specimens (humans, animals, water) obtained from a waterborne outbreak in a community in British Columbia, Canada, were used to evaluate the sensitivity of molecular techniques to biotype these isolates from different sources (19). The polymerase chain reaction (PCR), followed by restriction fragment length polymorphism (RFLP) analysis, pulsed-field gel electrophoresis, and isoenzyme electrophoresis analysis, failed to detect different biotypes in the variety of samples obtained from the waterborne outbreak. The authors concluded that more-sensitive methods must be developed to detect and characterize *Giardia* from an original host that is eventually spread into the environment (19). Differences have been found in genetic products from isolates taken from the same host species. Moreover, differences were seen among isolates obtained from waterborne outbreaks. For example, differences in genetic products were observed between isolates taken from the contaminated water and those taken from animals and humans who drank the contaminated water (20,21). On the other hand, it has been reported that human and cat isolates were identical at 10 enzyme loci (22). Therefore, in view of these results, the analysis of *Giardia* gene products by electrophoresis appears to be an unreliable and unpredictable method for the taxonomy of *Giardia.* Isoenzyme electrophoresis studies have demonstrated the extensive genetic variation within the morphologically *G. duodenalis* group. *Giardia* trophozoites reproduce asexually and antigenic variation is a common occurrence (23); these two biologic characteristics may contribute to the variation observed in these studies.

DNA Hybridization

The advantage of DNA hybridization technology is that it offers a method for direct genetic characterization of *Giardia* isolates. For taxonomy, this technique has at least two advantages over protein electrophoresis because both expressed and nonexpressed genome sequences can be examined and second genomic DNA is less susceptible to environmental influences. Restriction endonuclease analysis, followed by hybridization to nucleic acid probes, has been used to detect genetic variation in *Giardia.* Pulsed-field gel electrophoresis separations of intact chromosomes have shown that *Giardia* possesses at least five distinct sets of chromosomes varying in size between 1×10^6 and 4×10^6 base pairs (bp) (24,25). Using this technique, variations between human isolates and animal isolates have been detected (26). *Giardia* heterogeneity between isolates can also be demonstrated by RFLP analysis and DNA fingerprinting using the bacteriophage M13 genome as a probe (27,28). However no universally accepted typing system has emerged that will reliably distinguish any particular human or animal subspecies of *G. duodenalis.* Thus, the consensus of opinion indicates that further attempts to phenotype or genotype *Giardia* isolates should not be made until they can be related to differences in subspecies biology. Because DNA analysis has shown close similarity between *G. duodenalis* isolates from humans and those from domestic and wild animals, there is extra support to the view that giardiasis is a zoonosis (29).

Using data generated by phenotypic and genetic studies, attempts have been made to classify *Giardia* isolates recovered from humans and several other mammalian species into two major genetic assemblages. These genetic assemblages have been described in Europe as Polish and Belgian, in North America as groups 1\2 and 3, and in Australia as assemblages A and B (30). However no universal consensus regarding the nomenclature of these two different groups of *Giardia* has been reached in spite of the fact that a comparative analysis has shown that these variously named groups are in fact genetically equivalent (31). These two groups could conceivably be viewed as representing the species *G. duodenalis,* whereas the host-adapted genotypes would represent other species.

BIOLOGY OF *GIARDIA* SPECIES

Giardia species exist in two forms: the motile trophozoite that is exclusively found within the intestinal tract and that produces diarrheal disease; and the cyst that survives outside the host in harsh conditions and transmits the infection.

Trophozoite

Giardia trophozoites divide by binary fission under a relatively low oxygen tension that is present in the intestinal lumen. There is no evidence that a sexual stage is involved in parasite replication. It is essentially a luminal parasite, so it is predominantly dependent on factors within the intestinal lumen for growth and multiplication. The trophozoite measures approximately 12 to 15 μm in length and 5 to 9 μm in width. It has two nuclei and four pairs of flagella originating from basal bodies at the anterior pole of the nuclei (Fig. 61.2). The basal bodies are the major microtubule organizing centers and one functionally equivalent to the centrosome of higher cells. The flagella have the usual eukaryotic pattern of nine pairs and two central single microtubules. Flagella contain axonemal proteins and an additional set of polypeptides of approximately 30 kd. The median body, which is the "frown" in the giardial "face," is found in the posterior portion of the cell and has a different form characteristic of the three morphologic types of *Giardia.* This structure, unique to *Giardia* species, is composed largely of microtubules. No specific function has been ascribed to the median body yet. It contains giardins, actin, and α-actinin, suggesting that the median body may be involved in disk synthesis during cell division or possibly acting as a reservoir or nucleating template for new disk fibers (32). Scanning electron microscopy clearly shows the convex dorsal surface of the trophozoite and the concave ventral surface containing the attachment organelle, the ventral disk. The ventral striated disk is the most distinctive structure of the trophozoite. It is a rigid structure consisting of a platform of microtubules, 50 to 60 nm apart, each of which appears to be linked to the cytoplasmic face of the ventral plasmalemma by two short arms reported to have adenosine triphosphatase activity (32). The proteins found in the striated disk have been called giardins, which range in size from 29 to 38 kd (33). The rim of the disk contains contractile proteins, actin, α-actinin, myosin, and tropomyosin, which give the outer portion of the disk its flexibility and are presumed to be involved in attachment of the trophozoite to the intestinal epithelium (32).

Giardia is generally thought to belong to the earliest lineage to diverge from the major eukaryotic line of descent and lacks several of the prominent organelles, particularly mitochondria and peroxisomes, characteristic of most eukaryotic cells. (34). However, the trophozoite has many of the endomembrane protein transport elements of higher cells, indicating that they appeared very early in the evolution of eukaryotic cells (35). There are multiple ovoid vacuoles 0.1 to 0.4 µm in diameter, usually situated immediately beneath the plasma membrane. These vacuoles appear to be lysosomal in function, because they contain various hydrolyses, including acid phosphatase, thiol-dependent and thiol-independent proteinases, DNases, and RNases (31,36). The function of these structures in the parasite's life cycle and in the pathogenesis of infection remains to be established.

Although no classic Golgi apparatus has been described in *Giardia,* a structure containing encystation-specific antigens has been detected in encysting trophozoites (37–39). Evidence has been presented that these structures are involved in protein sorting and it seems likely that they will also be present in nonencysting trophozoites. For a critical review of the existence or absence of a Golgi apparatus and endoplasmic reticulum in *Giardia,* the reader is referred to reference 35. *Giardia* species have two nuclei that are morphologically indistinguishable, replicate at approximately the same time, and are transcriptionally active with linear chromosomes; hence, the nuclei appear to have similar functions (40). In this case, *Giardia* species, as well as *Hexamita* belong to a group of binucleate organisms called diplomads.

Cysts

Cysts are ovoid or elliptical in shape and measure approximately 7 to 10 µm in length. The dormant, quadrinucleate, ovoid cysts, which are responsible for transmission of giardiasis, are somewhat resistant to the environment and may remain viable for days to months if kept wet, cold, and free of fecal materials. High-resolution scanning electron microscopic morphologic studies (Fig. 61.1) of the cyst wall of *Giardia* species have demonstrated that it is composed of membranous and filamentous layers (41). The chemical structure of the cyst wall remains controversial. Lectin-binding studies have suggested that *N*-acetylglucosamine was the major cyst wall sugar (42), and the finding that encysting trophozoites contained chitin synthetase activity suggested that chitin was a major component of the cyst wall (42,43). Subsequent studies have suggested that galactosamine is the major cyst wall sugar accompanied by glucose, probably in the form of glycogen (44). *N*-acetylgalactosamine (GalNAc) is not detected in trophozoites, but a biosynthetic pathway operates during encystation. Uridine diphosphate *N*-acetylglucosamine (UDP-GlcNAc) 4-epimerase is detectable during the encystation process and is involved in the synthesis of GalNAc from glucose. Cyst wall proteins (CWPs) with a molecular weight ranging from 29 to 102 kd have been detected by immunostaining (45), but their final structure remains to be determined.

Endosymbionts

Infection of protozoan parasites of the genus *Giardia* with various microorganisms including bacteria, mycoplasma, and virus have been well documented (46). Among the most well characterized of these microinvaders are the viruses. These *Giardia*-specific viruses share several common features: They are double-stranded RNA (dsRNA) viruses with nonsegmented genomes ranging between 5 and 7 kilobases (kb); and they are spherical or icosahedral with an average diameter of 30 to 40 nm (46). Spherical virus consists of a linear open-ended 7-kb dsRNA molecule encapsulated by a 100-kd capsid protein at an RNA-to-protein molecular ratio of 1 : 420. The virus is present in the nuclei of infected trophozoites and is eventually released into the culture medium (46). It has been reported that a single trophozoite can contain approximately 5×10^5 viral particles. This number would represent the threshold intracellular density of viral particles that arrest the growth of *G. duodenalis* (47). There were dsRNA viruses isolated in the trophozoites of *G. duodenalis* Portland I strain. The viral dsRNA has been found in 28 of the 76 isolates examined (47). Trophozoites that were virus free were susceptible to infection with the virus. On the other hand, the *Giardia* dsRNA virus failed to infect other parasitic protozoa, thereby confirming the genus specificity of the virus (46).

Nucleus And Chromosomes Transcription

Each nucleus contains approximately equal numbers of rRNA genes (48). There is a possibility that the two nuclei contain different complements of DNA; however, it has yet to be determined (35). In each cell cycle, both nuclei divide, giving rise to a total of four daughter nuclei. On the basis of static microscopy, it has been proposed that the two daughters of a single nucleus segregate to different trophozoites (equational segregation) (14,48–51), although this has yet to be proven.

Giardia has five different major chromosomes, varying in size between 1×10^6 and 4×10^6 bp, which have been faithfully maintained in each of the nuclei in parasites grown after many generations *in vitro* (24,52). Moreover, *Giardia* has at least four, perhaps eight or more, copies of each of the five chromosomes and has an estimated genome complexity of 1.2×10^7 bp of DNA and a guanylate cyclase content of 46%. There are also a number of variable minor chromosomes (in representation) that are partial duplications of major chromosomes (53–56) with loss of substantial subtelomeric regions from different chromosome terminals. The appearance of such minor chromosomes has been identified in several drug-resistant lines and has led to the idea that *Giardia* chromosomes could rearrange and segments could be lost.

Giardia has been classified as diploid on a morphologic basis; however, on a physiologic basis, it is not clear if they are diploid or aneuploid. Other than its two nuclei and partial duplications, many chromosomes are present in greater copy number than others, and chromosome representation varies from isolate to isolate (55). The extensive duplication and rearrangement undergone of the *Giardia* genome include whole and partial chromosome duplications, subtelomeric loss followed by duplication or partial duplication under stress, and extensive internal duplications among different chromosomes when different isolates are compared (35). Instead, *Giardia* is sometimes considered as polyploid (more than two haploid sets of chromosomes) and sometimes aneuploid (having an inexact multiple of the typical haploid set of chromosomes by gaining or losing individual chromosomes). The plasticity and aneuploidy are presumably allowed by the lack of a requirement for meiotic pairing, because *Giardia* is asexual; yet, it has successfully survived as an asexual organism perhaps with the aid of mobile and transposable elements (i.e., *Giardia* plasmid). It has been suggested that polyploidy may also be the asexual means to replace and repair defective genes and mutations in three-way genetic crosses (35). It has been speculated that three copies of any given gene allow for a versatile mechanism that is capable of self-repair (57).

None of the reported *G. duodenalis* sequences appear to have introns, a feature that seems to be characteristic of many protozoan parasites that branched off from the main eukaryotic cell lineage. Therefore, if its genome contains introns, they are found in a relatively small number of genes. The first *G. duodenalis* messenger RNA (mRNA) transcript to be analyzed was the β-tubulin gene, which revealed a short six-nucleotide 5′ untranslated region (UTR) (58). Analyses of other mRNA transcripts also suggest that the gene transcription start sites lie very near the ATG initiation codon, giving rise to unusual 5′ UTRs ranging from 0 to 14 nucleotides in length (35). A comparison of the upstream sequences from seven genes encoding cytoskeletal proteins revealed a conserved sequence at the transcription start site, as well as a conserved region at −30 bp and another at approximately −40 to −70 bp (59).

LIFE CYCLE

Giardia species have two life cycle stages that are remarkably adapted to survival in harsh environments. Infection is initiated by ingestion of *Giardia* cysts generally through contaminated water or food, although direct person-to-person transfer does occur. Infection can be initiated with as few as 10 to 100 cysts (60). Exposure of cysts to gastric acid during their passage through the stomach triggers excystation and the trophozoites emerge. Excystation occurs in the proximal small intestine where the new trophozoites emerge, quickly divide by binary fission, attach, and colonize the small intestine of its host. To attach to the intestinal epithelial cells via the unique adhesive disk, they penetrate the mucous layer. As trophozoites pass distally along the small intestine, they are bathed in changing mixtures of hydrogen gas, bile, proteases, digestive enzymes, and ingested food; these gradual changes in the trophozoite microenvironment are thought to be important for triggering encystation. In humans, 150 to 20,000 cysts per gram of feces are excreted daily (61). Cyst excretion seems to have a cyclic pattern, because on some days, cyst counts may be below the detection limit of light microscopy. The *Giardia* life cycle is completed when cysts are ingested by another human or animal host. Although the infection can occur after person-to-person contact, water is usually the main source of contamination. Giardiasis can be transmitted via a domestic or a sylvatic cycle (Fig. 61.3). In the domestic cycle, humans, pets, and farm animals are the major source of contamination of surface water and wildlife becomes the victim. In the sylvatic cycle, wildlife is the major contamination of surface water and humans, pets, and farm animals are the victims.

ENCYSTATION

The Cellular Basis Of Encystment

The process of encystation involves the transformation of the trophozoite stage to a cyst, a key step in the life cycle of *Giardia* that allows the parasite to survive between hosts during person-to-person, waterborne, or food-borne transmission. Exposure of trophozoites to bile salts has been proposed to be the trigger causing cells to encyst (43). Cholesterol deprivation caused by bile has also been advanced as a likely inducer of encystment rather than some components of bile itself (62). A modification of the TY1-S-33 culture medium, originally developed to grow the *Giardia* trophozoites, allows the trophozoite to encyst *in vitro* (43). In the modified medium, the pH level is adjusted to 7.8 and the trophozoites are exposed to a higher concentration of conjugated bile salts and myristic acids (63,64). Recently, several studies have appeared in the literature concerning the composition, synthesis, and transport of components from the trophozoites to the nascent cyst wall. The identification of fibrous components containing polymers of galactosamine or GalNAc has significantly contributed to our understanding of the biochemical nature of the cyst wall (44). During encystment, trophozoites appear to develop a Golgi-like complex, begin to express cyst

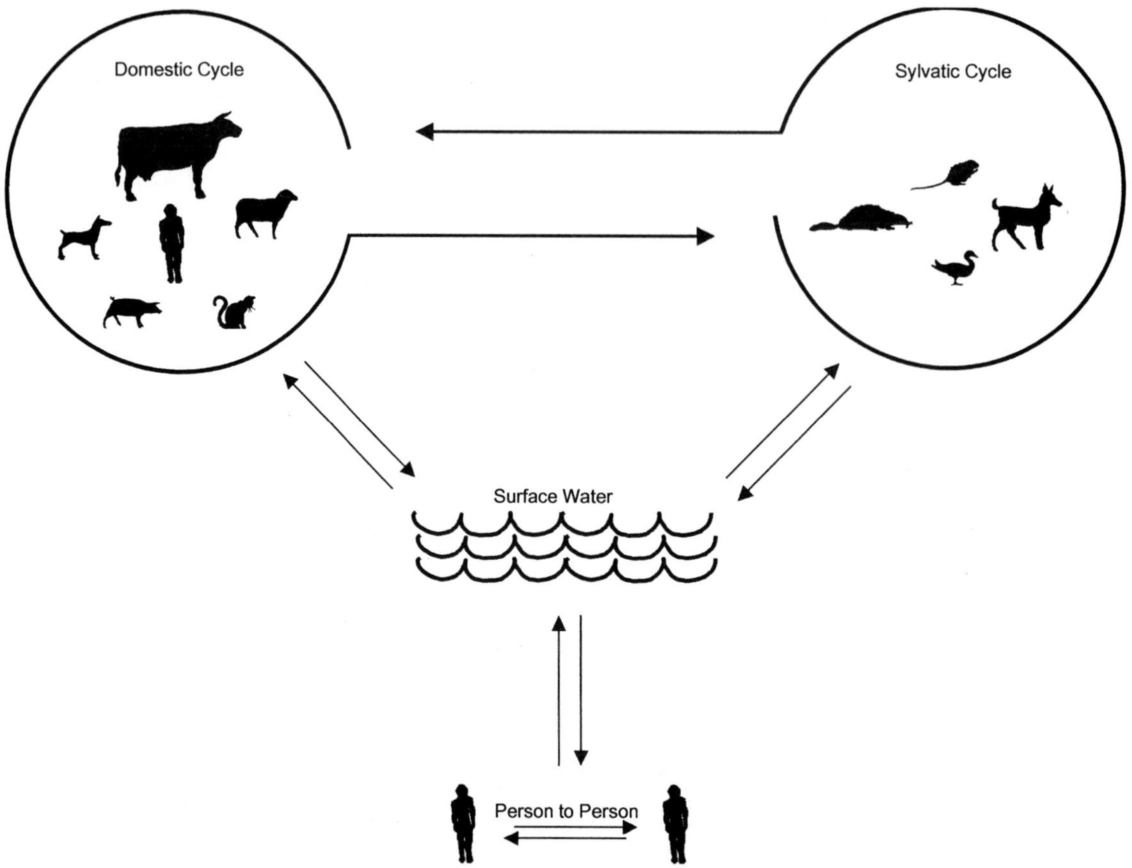

FIGURE 61.3. Life cycle of *Giradia duodenalis*-type of organisms, showing water as the major source of contamination. In the domestic cycle, humans, domestic, and farm animals play a major role in contaminating the water. However, in the sylvatic cycle, the wildlife plays a major role in contaminating the water.

antigens, and produce encystment-specific vesicles (ESVs) (65). The development of monoclonal antibodies specific to cyst antigens (66–68) has contributed to the advancement of our knowledge about encystation. These antibodies were invaluable reagents to study the chronologic events taking place during encystation (38,44). Lujan et al. (69) cloned two genes encoding for two CWPs with leucine-rich repeats: CWP-1 is a 26-kd protein and CWP-2 is a 39-kd protein. After synthesis, CWP-1 and CWP-2 combine to form a stable complex that is found mainly in the ESVs (66,69). The expression of a series of chimeric CWP-1 green fluorescent protein reporter proteins has demonstrated that a short 110-bp 5′ flanking region on the CWP1 gene harbors all necessary *cis*-DNA elements for encystation-specific expression of a reporter gene during *in vitro* encystation. The sequences at the 3′ flanking region are proposed to be involved in the modulation of steady-state mRNA levels of the CWP-1 transcript during encystation (70).

The first sign, visible by light microscopy, that a trophozoite entering encystation is the formation of ESVs that transport regulated antigens to the nascent cyst wall. Then, the trophozoite rounds up, detaches from its substratum, losses its remarkable mobility, and becomes optically refractive (71). ESVs are only present during encystation; in encysting culture medium, ESVs start to appear at 5 hours, and by 15 hours, most cells have visible excretory vesicles (37,66,71). ESVs have a very uniform density and are more electron opaque than the cytoplasm. This observation suggests that if the proteins transported by these structures associate with the fibrous portion of the cyst wall, the association may occur after exocytosis of the vesicle content into the extracellular milieu (72,73).

Physiology Of Encystation

During the process of encystation, *Giardia* undergoes fundamental changes in its metabolism. Most of the changes are related to the formation of the cyst wall and the penultimate transformation from trophozoite to cyst. A change in membrane transport activity is observed with encysting trophozoites. After 10 hours in encysting medium, trophozoites can no longer use exogenous glucose and become resistant to metronidazole (MTZ), the drug most commonly used for treating *Giardia.*

Originally, direct analysis of cyst wall filaments was impossible due to their insoluble nature. However, soluble material can now be obtained through partial hydrolysis in trifluoroacetic acid. Analysis of the soluble material has revealed that *Giardia* outer cyst wall filaments is a [D-GalNAc (β1—>3)-D-GalNAc]$_n$ homopolymer where *n* equals at least 23 (74). Weight analysis of the filaments has shown that D-GalNAc accounts for 63% of the filaments, with the remaining 37% containing protein as demonstrated by amino acid analysis. No fatty acids were detected. It is uncertain whether GalNAc occurs as a polysaccharide alone or if it is linked to protein/peptide. *Giardia* synthesizes GalNAc, rather than salvaging it (74). It has an inducible carbohydrate-synthesizing pathway and all of the GalNAc synthesizing enzymes' activities in the pathway increase significantly during encystation (Fig. 61.4) (75). Within the first 6 hours of encystment, mRNA for glucosamine-6-phosphate isomerase (GPI), the first inducible enzyme in the pathway appears, and its product appears to allosterically activate UDP-GlcNAc pyrophosphate and shift the dynamics of the equation in favor of GlcNAc and subsequently GalNAc synthesis (74). Two genes for GPI

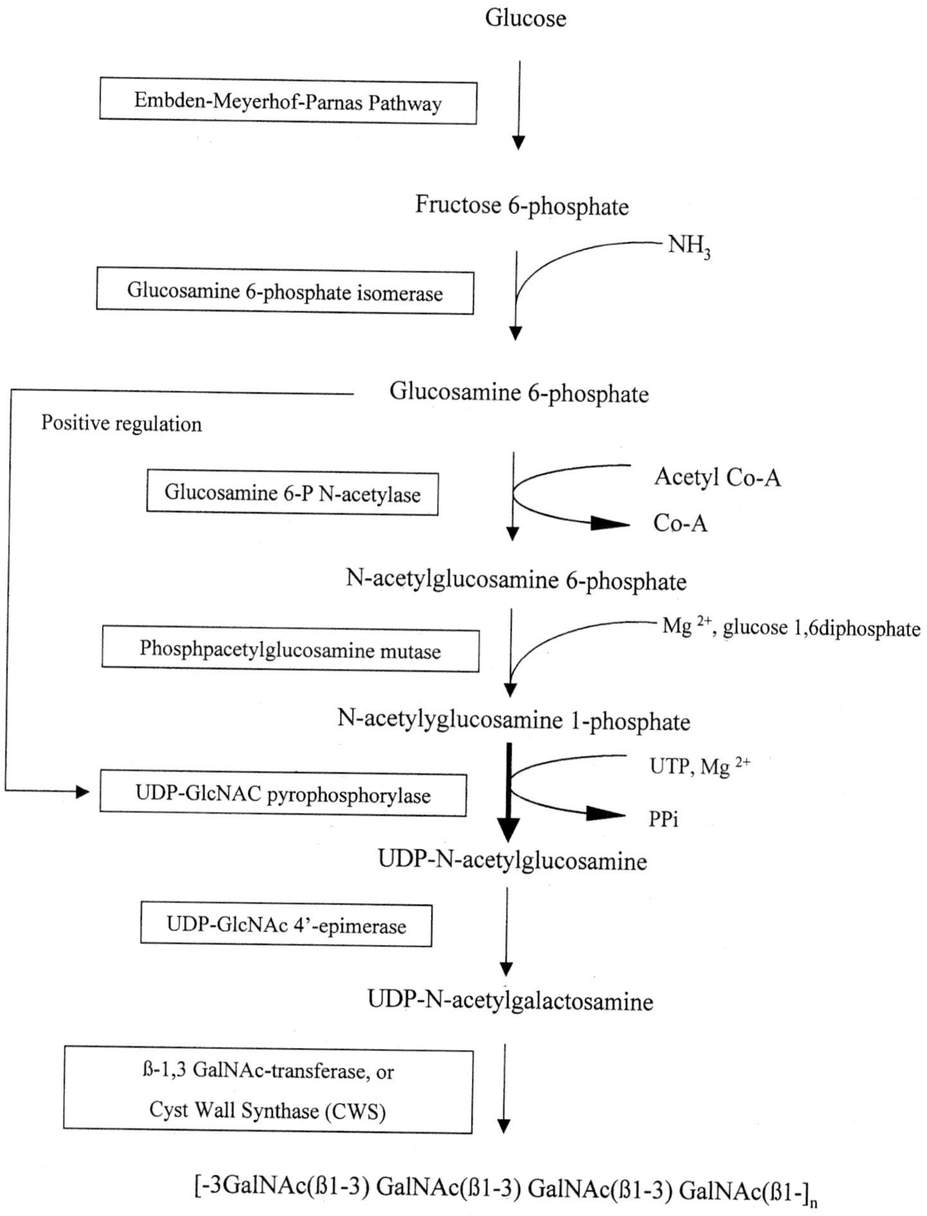

FIGURE 61.4. The pathway of uridine diphosphate *N*-acetylglucosamine synthesis that is induced when *Giardia* encysts. (From Jarroll EA, Macechko PT, Steimle PA, et al. Regulation of carbohydrate mechanism during *Giardia* encystment. *J Eukaryot Microbiol* 2001;48:22–26, with permission.)

have been cloned and sequenced, *gpi1* and *gpi2*. (74). However, *gpi1* represents the inducible GPI. Using reverse transcriptase PCR, probes specific for *gpi2* do not show mRNA present in encysting or nonencysting trophozoites; whereas, *gpi1*-specific probes demonstrate that mRNA for the isomerase is detectable within 5 to 6 hours postinduction with bile (74).

It was also observed that the amino acids associated with the D-GalNAc polysaccharide had a relatively large amount of leucine, which implicates leucine-rich CWPs encoded by CWP-1 and CWP-2 (67,69). CWP-1 and CWP-2 are the only CWP genes that have been cloned. The *cwp1* and *cwp2* genes predict acidic and leucine-rich proteins with molecular weights of 26 and 39 kd, respectively, which are targeted to the secretory pathway by amine terminus signal peptides. Additionally, both proteins contain a cysteine-rich region and five tandem copies of a leucine-rich repeat, and both co-localize within ESVs of encysting trophozoites and the cyst wall of mature cysts (73).

EXCYSTATION

Excystation *in vitro* has been achieved by exposure of cysts to drastic changes in temperature, osmolarity, pH, and proteases. For example, exposure of cysts to a pH level of 1.3, followed by transfer to neutral pH, results in a rapid transition of the parasite from a dormant, immobile form to an active one that attaches to a substratum and begins to enter into division (76). This rapid transition requires coordinated partitioning of the cytoskeleton and nuclei between the daughter cells (72). From the cyst emerges a tetranucleate organism that rapidly undergoes cytokinesis to yield two binucleate trophozoites (74). Recent work has shown that antibodies to CWP or lectin that binds to CWP inhibits excystation in a specific manner, demonstrating the role that glycoproteins may play in excystation (77). Furthermore, excystation has been blocked by specific cysteine protease inhibitors; the target protease was identified and its corresponding gene cloned (78). Calmodulin is a ubiquitous protein found in all eukaryotic cells, which is widely recognized as the common primary intracellular receptor for calcium. Among various functions, calmodulin can activate enzymes such as protein kinases. Trifluoperazine, a calmodulin antagonist, can inhibit excystation, demonstrating the role calcium plays in *Giardia* cyst excystation activity (79). In eukaryotic cells, cyclic adenosine monophosphate (cAMP)-dependent signaling pathways play a critical role in regulating cell growth, metabolism, and differentiation (80). Protein kinase A (PKA), the defining enzyme of the cAMP-dependent signaling pathway, is the simplest protein kinase known because of its dissociative mechanism of activation. PKA inhibitors lead to a reduction of giardial excystation (80). Excystation entails not only molecular responses but also detection of environmental stimuli across the tough extracellular cyst wall, leading to highly coordinated physiologic and structural responses. For example, cytoplasmic pH changes occur within the cyst wall in the earliest stage of excystation in response to conditions modeling cyst ingestion and passage into human stomach (81). These findings show that excystation of this primitive eukaryotic cell is a highly complex and active process.

ATTACHMENT

Giardia trophozoites attach intimately to the intestinal epithelium and to various inert substrates such as glass and plastic. *In vivo* attachment is considered a feature of the relationship between trophozoite and its host and an indicator of trophozoite vitality. The ventral disk is thought to be the primary organelle of attachment. It has been suggested that the attachment process is mediated by the continuous activity of the ventral flagella, which generate a hydrodynamic force between the disk and attachment surface (82). It also has been proposed that flagella activity causes a low-pressure area under the ventral disk due to fluid fluxes around the ventral and marginal grooves. However, attachment occurs in *G. psittaci* in which the ventrolateral flange is incomplete (15), thus making it unlikely that hydrodynamic forces can be the sole explanation for disk-mediated attachment. The presence of contractile proteins in the peripheral regions of the ventral disk suggests that they participate in attachment (82). Inhibitors of microfilament function such as cytochalasin B and low calcium concentration inhibit attachment (83).

Many enteropathogens possess lectin or lectin-like substances on surface structures. These sugar-binding proteins, which recognize oligosaccharide ligands on the intestinal epithelium, are now considered to have a central role in mediating attachment. Several lectins have been isolated from *G. duodenalis* trophozoites. A mannose-binding surface lectin has been described using the classic approach of mixed-cell agglutination with mammalian erythrocytes. This lectin is distributed throughout the trophozoite surface and is not specifically localized to the ventral disk (84). It is present as a prolectin, which can be activated by trypsin (85). Taglin, which is a trypsin-activated lectin, has been identified from the trophozoite (86). *Giardia* trophozoites adhere to isolated mammalian intestinal epithelial cells *in vitro* by mechanisms consistent with lectin-mediated attachment (87). They attach to Caco-2 cells, the small intestinal epithelial cell line, by mechanisms that incorporate both contractile proteins and surface lectin-mediated processes (88). The relative importance of mechanical and lectin-mediated attachment mechanisms has not been established *in vivo*. The surface lectin may operate in the initial attachment between *Giardia* and the intestinal epithelium, because unlike ventral disk-related attachment, the parasite does not need to be in a specific orientation to the mucosa. Subsequently, the parasite may reorient itself in a ventral surface-down position when mechanical forces may be more effective.

IN VITRO CULTURE

Of the three morphologic types of *Giardia* only some of the *G. duodenalis* isolates have been successfully cultivated *in vitro* (18,89). Isolates obtained from cats and dogs that had the characteristics of the *G. duodenalis* group could not be cultivated *in vitro* (Gaétan Faubert, *unpublished observations*). Axenic cultivation of isolates of *G. muris* and *G. ardea* has been reported (89). Karapetyan (90) first described methods for *in vitro* cultivation of *Giardia* using complex media with the addition of *Candida* species and chick fibroblasts. In 1970, Meyer (91) described a method for axenically culturing *Giardia* trophozoites from rabbit, chinchilla, cat, and later humans using the Hank's balanced saline solution supplemented with bovine serum, yeast extract, and cysteine. Since then, various modifications have been made to the culture medium. The most commonly used medium is TY1-S-33, which includes a casein digest (trypticase), yeast extract, iron (ferric ammonium citrate), dextrose, bovine serum, ascorbic acid, bile salts, and cysteine (92). Cultures are usually maintained in screw-capped glass tubes or flasks with very limited airspace to maintain a low oxygen concentration. Cysteine is added to the medium and serves as a reducing agent. The modification of the TY1-S-33 medium for induction of encystation (43) *in vitro* has contributed significantly to the advancement of our knowledge on the biology of this primitive eukaryotic cell (43). Because the life cycle of *G. duodenalis* can be completed in axenic cultures (64), it is now possible to study in detail the molecular process involved in the cyst wall formation.

METABOLISM

Giardia species are clearly eukaryotic organisms, because they possess the hallmark organelles, nuclei, ribosomes, lysosomal vacuoles, and multiple linear chromosomes. However, they lack a number of organelles and features typical of higher eukaryotes (35). For example, *Giardia* species lack mitochondria, peroxisomes, and nucleoli and are dependent on anaerobic metabolism (35). In addition, trophozoites lack a readily discernible Golgi apparatus, although a Golgi-like structure becomes apparent during encystation (34). *Giardia* metabolism is fermentative, and electron transport proceeds in the absence of oxidative phosphorylation found in organisms with mitochondria (93).

Carbohydrate

Giardia is an aerotolerant anaerobe and thus differs from most eukaryotes, which have a predominantly aerobic metabolism. *Giardia* lacks mitochondria and mitochondrial enzymes and respires in the presence of oxygen by a flavin–iron–sulfur protein-mediated electron transport system. The Embden–Meyerhof–Parnas and hexose monophosphate pathways catabolize glucose, and energy is produced, at least in part, by substrate level phosphorylation (94,95). Substrates are incompletely oxidized to CO_2, acetate, ethanol, and alanine. The acetate formed may not come from glucose. The predominant oxidative metabolic pathway appears to vary depending on the oxygen concentration. In a strictly anaerobic environment, alanine is produced from pyruvate and ketoglutarate, whereas in the presence of low oxygen concentrations, ethanol production increases and alanine production is reduced (96,97).

Fatty Acids

Giardia is unable to synthesize phospholipids, long chain fatty acids, and sterols *de novo.*Therefore it is reliant on exogenous sources of fatty acids and phospholipids (98,99). It is possible that the parasite has developed a special process for acquiring lipids from its host. Exogenously supplied, unsaturated, fatty acids can be taken up by *Giardia* and incorporated into various phosphoglycerides, including phosphatidylglycerol and other glycerol-based phospholipids; however, the process is poorly understood. This phosphatidylglycerol is an important phospholipid of *Giardia* because it has been shown that various synthetic phosphatidylglycerol analogues inhibit the growth of the parasite *in vitro* (98). Fatty acids are precursors to triglycerides and other lipid components that comprise integral structural components of trophozoite plasma and endomembranes. They are also involved in transducing intracellular signals for gene expression. Biliary lipids may be an extremely important source of membrane phospholipid for *Giardia,* with the uptake of phospholipid and cholesterol being facilitated by conjugated bile salts (100,101).

Nucleic Acids

Like most protozoan parasites, *Giardia* is unable to synthesize purines and pyrimidines, which distinguishes this cell from most other eukaryotes cells (102–104). *Giardia* is therefore dependent on salvage pathways for acquisition of exogenous nucleobase, the precursors for DNA and RNA synthesis. Pyrimidines appear to be taken up by active transport mechanisms. Two classes of nucleotide transporters have been described, one that is specific for uridine and cytosine while the other uses only thymidine as a substrate (105).

Oxidative Stress Management

All organisms have detoxifying mechanisms against harmful radicals, and glutathione (GSH) cycling has been regarded as the primary defense mechanism in organisms ranging from *Escherichia coli* to humans (106). *Giardia* lacks conventional pathways of oxygen stress management (e.g., superoxide dismutase, catalase, peroxidase, and GSH cycling) and energy production, which are found in most eukaryotes (107). Instead, novel prokaryotic oxidation stress management mechanisms are used to protect oxygen-labile electron transport proteins (107–110). For example, *Giardia* contains cysteine and an active bacterial thioredoxin reductase-like disulfide reductase, which serve as intracellular reductants to maintain the intracellular environment (109,110). Additionally, it contains a nicotinamide adenine dinucleotide (NADH) oxidase, which removes oxygen by reducing it to water (107,108) and a membrane-associated NADH peroxidase to degrade H_2O_2. The presence of cysteine and thioglycolate (109) scavenge superoxide and other low intracellular free radicals. Interestingly, *Giardia* trophozoites are coated with cysteine-rich variable surface proteins (VSPs), thereby using this mechanism for protection against a hostile external environment (111).

ANIMAL MODELS OF GIARDIASIS

The development of animal models for giardiasis has greatly improved the understanding of the basic parameters underlying host–parasite interactions. The *G. muris* mouse model has been extensively used as a model for human infection (112). Oral infection of mice with *G. muris* cysts results in a reproducible pattern of infection, intestinal villous atrophy, and impairment of weight gain (112,113). However, major biologic differences exist between *G. muris* and *G. duodenalis.* For instance, *G. duodenalis*-type organisms can be cultured *in vitro,* are infective to a wide variety of animals, and are genetically and morphologically distinct from *G. muris.* Therefore, the availability of an animal model that is susceptible to infection with *G. duodenalis*-type organisms remains essential to investigate the mechanisms of pathogenesis of human giardiasis.

Adult rats were first used by Hegner (114), and subsequently by Armaghan (115) to determine their susceptibility to infection with *Giardia* isolated from humans. They found that a low percentage of animals established the infection, and the duration of infection was short with no cysts being shed in the feces of the rats. On the other hand, weanling rats were found to be susceptible to infection with *G. duodenalis,* and their susceptibility was enhanced by serial passage in rats. A recent study has demonstrated that infection of 8-day-old neonatal rats with virulent *G. duodenalis* isolates results in abnormal intestinal absorption, without significant alterations in the architecture of the small intestinal mucosa (116). Similarly, weanling mice exhibit a higher susceptibility to infection with *G. duodenalis* than adult animals (117). However, as the animals aged, susceptibility to infection significantly decreased. Weanling mice have been used to study antigenic variation (118,119). Dogs, cats, rabbits, and small ruminants have been used to study giardiasis with different degrees of success.

Belosovic et al. (113) were first to propose the Mongolian gerbil (*Meriones unguiculatus*) as an animal model to study human giardiasis. Not only were adult gerbils found to be highly susceptible to infection with *G. duodenalis*-type organisms, but the pattern and duration of cyst shedding was comparable to that seen in human infection. In addition, the pathophysiologic changes associated with gerbil infection are similar to those observed in human infection (113). Mongolian gerbils have been extensively used to investigate several aspects of giardiasis, including antigenic variation (120), virulence of *Giardia* isolates (121), pathophysiology of giardiasis (122–124), and epidemiology (117).

THE IMMUNE RESPONSE TO *GIARDIA* IN HUMANS

It is known that the immune system is playing a determining role in the control of the infection with respect to eradicating acute infection and in the development of protective immunity. This knowledge comes mainly from four sources: (a) *in vitro* studies involving the growth of *G. duodenalis* trophozoites together with immune cells from various hosts; (b) studies of mice infected with their natural parasite *G. muris;* (c) animal models involving *G. duodenalis*-infected adult gerbils or weanling mice; and (d) studies of humans naturally infected with *Giardia* or those who have volunteered to be infected with *Giardia* (125). Both humoral and cell-mediated immune responses occur in human giardiasis.

Epidemiologic evidence indicates that age-specific prevalence of giardiasis rises during childhood, and the observation that it only begins to decline during early adolescence is indicative of the requirement of a protective immunity to control the infection (126). Further evidence for the development of protective immunity during giardiasis comes from studies of the prevalence of symptomatic giardiasis reported after waterborne epidemics. Furthermore, prevalence is lower in the indigenous population compared with individuals who had recently arrived in an endemic area. Individuals with recurrent or chronic exposure to the parasite appear more likely to develop asymptomatic infections in comparison to individuals exposed to the parasite for the first time or at infrequent intervals who invariably develop disease pathology (127). This observation probably accounts for the relative infrequency of symptomatic infections in homosexual men, those living in developing countries, and residents of high prevalence areas in the industrialized world such as the American and Canadian Rockies regions. All these studies suggest that exposure to the parasite does produce immune protection in humans that is able to control not only the parasite load but also the symptoms of the disease.

Innate Immunity

In some patients, giardiasis may resolve within a few days, whereas in others symptoms can last for years, even in the presence of circulating antibodies in serum, secretory antibodies at mucosal sites, and cell-mediated immunity. Because of the biologic characteristics of *Giardia,* it is likely that non-immune factors play a role in susceptibility to infection or duration and severity of the disease. For example, normal human milk kills *G. duodenalis* trophozoites independently of specific secretory immunoglobulin A (sIgA) antibodies (128). A number of laboratories have demonstrated *Giardia* cidal factors present in the milk, such as conjugated bile salts (129), unsaturated fatty acids (130), or free fatty acids (131). *G. duodenalis* trophozoites are killed by products of lipolysis present in human duodenal and upper jejunal fluid (132). Aley et al. (133) have reported that human neutrophil defensins and indolicidin have antitrophozoite activities when they are added to the culture medium. These results demonstrate the importance of non-immune mechanisms to the control of parasite population in the intestine. On the other hand, innate immunity mechanisms may protect the parasite from destruction. For example, mucus has been reported to protect the trophozoites from killing by lipolytic products in the intestinal fluid (134). These results were confirmed since *G. duodenalis* trophozoites grown *in vitro* were protected from the *Giardia* cidal effect of human milk by addition of intestinal mucus to culture medium (135). The effect of nitric oxide (NO) produced by HT-29 and HCT-8 human intestinal epithelial cells on *G. duodenalis* trophozoites has been studied (136) and was found that NO inhibits growth, encystation, and excystation of *Giardia* cells but has no effect on parasite viability; suggesting that for *G. duodenalis,* NO is cytostatic rather than cytotoxic. Again these results emphasize the involvement of defense mechanisms in the control of this intestinal innate infectious agent.

Acquired Immunity

Cell-mediated Immunity

Due to the invasive techniques required for harvesting trophozoites at the mucosal sites, studies of cell-mediated immunity in human giardiasis are limited. Most of our knowledge is derived from experiments done with *G. duodenalis* trophozoites grown *in vitro.* T cells play a major role in the control of the infection, because *Giardia* antigens are T-cell-dependent antigens (125). There is only one study reported in the literature on the production of cytokines by human lymphocytes stimulated by live *Giardia* trophozoites. The addition of *in vitro*-derived trophozoites to intraepithelial, lamina propria, or peripheral blood lymphocytes resulted in the production of interferon-γ (IFN-γ) by these lymphocytes (137). It was concluded that live *Giardia* induces the production of equal amounts of IFN-γ in CD4+ lymphocytes isolated from peripheral blood lymphocytes or from the intestines (137). An inflammatory cell infiltrate in the small intestinal mucosa often accompanies human infection with *Giardia* (138,139). The number of plasma cells present in the gut lymphoid tissues is also increasing. Both the immunoglobulin M (IgM) and IgA bearing cells are the prominent subtype (139). As expected, secretory IgM (sIgM) cells are prominent early in the infection, whereas the IgA cells are prominent during the acute phase (139). The intraepithelial lymphocyte numbers decrease with resolution of the infection, confirming their role in acquired immunity.

It is well known that tissue macrophages and related cells such as dendritic cells play a critical role in the mucosal immune response as antigen-presenting cells. Unfortunately, the role they play in human giardiasis is unknown. However, several studies using the *G. muris* mouse model of infection have demonstrated that macrophages act as effector cells in the resolution of the infection (125). For example, macrophages beneath the basal lamina extend pseudopodia into the epithelium, trapping invading *G. muris* trophozoites and enclosing them in phagolysosomes (140). Mouse peritoneal macrophages will also kill *G. muris* trophozoites *in vitro;* this effect is enhanced by the addition of immune serum (141) or milk containing anti-*Giardia* IgG and IgA antibodies (125,139). The role of mast cells in human giardiasis has not been addressed. It is likely that these cells, which represent a prominent population of the mucosal epithelial tissue, play a role, because degranulation of mast cells releases mediators that are toxic to the parasite or can improve access to other effector cells into the mucosa. There are other polymorphonuclear leukocytes such as antibody-dependent cell-mediated cytotoxicity cells that have been reported to play an effector role in human giardiasis. Unfortunately, it is not known whether similar effector mechanisms exist in human giardiasis; these experiments were done *in vitro* and the trophozoites were kept under conditions suitable for the leukocytes, but not for the parasite, making the latter vulnerable to immunologic attack (142). Because of this, the interpretation of many *in vitro* studies on the effector mechanisms implicated in the immune response to *G. duodenalis* trophozoites is problematic.

Humoral Antibody Response

The presence of serum antibody specific for *Giardia* was first demonstrated in patients with giardiasis in 1946 (143). The lethal effect of human serum for *G. duodenalis* trophozoites appears to be dependent on the presence of an intact classic pathway of complement activation. When human serum containing anti-*G. duodenalis* antibodies was added to culture medium, more than 98% of the trophozoites were killed (144). The killing effect of human serum was abrogated when the serum was chelated with ethylenediaminetetraacetic acid or was heat inactivated at 56°C for 30 minutes, conditions known to inactivate complement. Although these results were obtained from experiments done *in vitro,* they nevertheless demonstrate the potential role of antibodies and complement in the control of the infection. Anti-*Giardia* IgG antibodies can be detected in more than 80% of patients with symptomatic infection and antibody titers may remain elevated for months or even years after primary infection (145). IgG titers are often raised in non-infected individuals in endemic areas, indicating previous exposure to the parasite (146,147). The relationship between the presence of anti-*Giardia* IgG and protective immunity has not been established. Anti-*Giardia* IgM titers increase early in infection and then decline within 3 weeks (147,149). Specific IgM antibodies have been detected in naturally infected individuals in India, The Gambia, and the United Kingdom (147,149) and during experimental human infection (148). Several studies have reported the presence of anti-*Giardia* IgA in serum from patients with giardiasis, although studies in India and The Gambia suggest that only about 30% of patients with active infection have detectable IgA antibody levels (150). Occasionally, giardiasis has been associated with an increase in total serum immunoglobulin E (IgE). The authors concluded that infection had increased intestinal permeability, allowing entry of food antigens, which then became the target of the IgE response (151). It is difficult to determine the significance of antibodies present in the serum of infected patients, because *G. duodenalis* is a non-tissue-invading intestinal protozoan that is recognized to stimulate mainly the local immune response. Therefore, the presence of antibodies in the serum appears to be an accidental event that could be due to a leakage of antigens through the intestinal mucosa occurring when a patient has been infected with a large number of cysts or when the infection becomes chronic.

There is relatively little information on the role of secretory immunoglobulin in human giardiasis, although there is evidence to suggest that individuals with sIgA deficiency are more susceptible to infection (152). sIgA has been demonstrated on the surface of *G. duodenalis* trophozoites in human jejunal biopsies (153), and specific anti-*Giardia* sIgA antibodies have been shown to be present in human duodenal fluid by enzyme-linked immunosorbent assay (ELISA). Total sIgA concentration in duodenal fluid from infected patients has been found to be within the normal range (154). Specific anti-*Giardia* sIgA antibodies have been detected in human milk and saliva. Epidemiologic studies suggest that these antibodies may protect breast-fed infants from giardiasis (126,155,156). Considering the biologic activities of *Giardia* trophozoites in its intestinal niche, it is not surprising to see the efficacy of sIgA as the mediator of the infection. sIgA present at mucosal surfaces mediates protection by inhibiting adherence of pathogenic microorganisms to the mucosal wall; agglutinating microbes; interfering with microorganisms motility by interacting with their flagella; or neutralizing the action of microorganisms products such as enzymes and toxins (157).

ANTIGENS OF *GIARDIA*

Polypeptides

The identification of *G. duodenalis* antigens that play a role in acquired immunity has been difficult for various reasons: (a) Usually the trophozoites do not invade the tissues; if there is a stimulation of the immune system, it remains localized; (b) occurrence of antigenic variation; and (c) investigators have used different isolates of *G. duodenalis,* different antibody reagents, and various assays in studies on the immune response to *Giardia.* Therefore, it is difficult to compare the results obtained by different laboratories. Crude antigenic extracts prepared from *G. duodenalis* trophozoites cultured *in vitro* have revealed different antigenic polypeptides depending on the characterization techniques. For example, a minimum of 20 possible antigenic polypeptides were detected by Western blotting, ranging in molecular weight from 14 to 125 kd (158). Western blot has been useful in demonstrating similarities in the antigens profile of *G. duodenalis* isolates from different geographic areas. For example, similarities in the proteins were reported for isolates from Afghanistan, Puerto Rico, Ecuador, and Oregon. The molecular mass of common molecules ranged from 12 to 140 kd (159–160). However, isoenzymes and isoelectric focusing techniques show differences between isolates from the same geographic region or even the same localities (20,21).

Nash and Keister (161) were able to classify 19 isolates of *G. duodenalis* into three groups on the basis of reactivity with antibodies raised against excretory–secretory (ES) products released by each isolate into culture medium. Five isolates showed major antibody cross-reactivity among them, and 11 had moderate antibody cross-reactivity. Three isolates released identical ES products. Similarities were also observed in the antigens present on the surface of the trophozoites of the 19 isolates even if patients had been infected in different geographic areas (161). None of these antigenic profile studies in geographic areas were able to identify a single common dominant protein among the isolates.

The identification of a major surface antigen on *G. duodenalis* trophozoite isolates will be an asset to the development of immunodiagnostic tests, characterization of isolates, or design of a vaccine. The existence of an 82-kd dominant surface antigen on the trophozoite of *G. duodenalis* grown in culture medium was first reported by Einfeld and Stibbs (162). The characterization of this surface antigen revealed that it was pronase and periodate, modifiable and heat labile (162), suggesting it was a glycoprotein. Using surface iodination techniques, Edson et al. (163) identified an 88-kd major trophozoite surface antigen proposed to be similar to the 82-kd polypeptide reported by Einfeld and Stibbs (162). Although antibodies against the 88-kd polypeptide were detected in serum of infected patients, no clear correlation was established between the appearance of specific serum antibodies to a major *G. duodenalis* antigen and protective immunity. Crossley and Holberton (164) introduced methods to study *Giardia* molecules from Percoll gradient purified plasma membranes. Membrane preparations revealed a major 75-kd band, which these investigators concluded corresponded to the iodinatable and antibody-precipitated 82/88-kd antigen reported earlier (162).

Heat Shock Proteins

Heat shock proteins (Hsps) are synthesized by mammal, bacterium, protozoan, helminth, and plant cells in response to abrupt rises in temperature, pH, or other stressful treatments. *Giardia* trophozoites live in the small intestines, a habitat characterized by harsh stressful conditions caused by the host's local immune response, as well as ever-changing luminal factors (e.g., bacteria, digestive enzymes, or ingested food). The presence of Hsp has been identified on *G. duodenalis* surface membrane of trophozoite isolates obtained from symptomatic and asymptomatic patients. Using Western blots 65- and 70-kd antigens were identified in the feces of gerbils infected with strains obtained from symptomatic and nonsymptomatic patients, respectively (165,166). The synthesis of [^{35}S]methionine-labeled proteins of 30, 70, 83, and 100 kd increased when trophozoites were heat stressed by incubating cultures at 43°C (165). During *in vitro* encystation, several stage-specific proteins were recognized in Western blot using antiserum raised against antigens of the Hsp60 family from *Mycobacterium bovis* and Hsp70 from *Plasmodium falciparum* (166).

Lectins

Lectins are glycoproteins that bind to specific sugars and oligosaccharides and are linked to glycoproteins or glycolipids present on the cell surface of eukaryotes. Trophozoites of *G. duodenalis* have lectins on their surface membrane with specificity for D-glucosyl and D-mannose residues (84). Taglin, a mannose 6-phosphate-binding, trypsin-activated lectin was isolated from the trophozoite plasma membrane (85,86). Activation of *G. duodenalis* lectin by proteases from the human duodenum has been reported (85). After activation, the lectin agglutinated intestinal cells to which the parasite adheres *in vitro.* A systematic analysis of *G. duodenalis* trophozoite surface carbohydrate residues using lectins and glycosidases revealed that GlcNAc was the only detectable specific saccharide on the plasma membrane (68). The exact biologic functions of lectins are unknown, but it appears that they play a role in the attachment of trophozoites to the site of colonization (84). Whether lectins play a role in the immune response to *Giardia* is unknown.

Giardins

The giardins are defined as a family of about 30-kd structural proteins found in microribbons attached to microtubules in the disk cytoskeleton of *Giardia* trophozoites (164). Giardins are unique proteins of *Giardia* cells (167); similar cytoskeleton proteins have not been reported for eukaryotic cells. These *Giardia* proteins were found at the edges of disk microribbons of the trophozoite and are named α_1-giardin, α_2-giardin, and γ-giardin (33,168). The interest in giardins as primary antigens in the immune response to *Giardia* stems from the fact that these proteins are unique to this parasite, are surface antigens, and probably comprise the first set of antigens the local immune system detects after attachment to the mucosal surfaces.

ANTIGENIC VARIATION AND ITS BIOLOGIC SIGNIFICANCE IN GIARDIASIS

Antigenic variation represents a mechanism whereby viruses, bacteria, and parasites evade the host immune response by varying the structure of surface exposed antigens. By the time the host has developed a protective immune response against the antigens originally present, the pathogen has been successful in replacing these molecules with new antigens. Nash's laboratory was the first to report the phenomenon of antigenic variation in giardiasis (23). These antigens are a family of cysteine-rich proteins encoded by a complex of 20 to 184 genes (23). In contrast to African trypanosomiasis, in which genes encoding variant surface antigens are expressed from telomere-associated sites, the VSP genes for the *Giardia* surface proteins have no telomere association. The unique characteristics of antigenic variation in giardiasis are as follows: (a) Certain epitopes are reexpressed in clones, suggesting the presence of a favored set in the repertoire of epitopes; (b) the repertoires of VSPs may differ among isolates; and (c) the same epitope detected on the surfaces of independent isolates is present in molecules of varying molecular mass (23). Contrary to other parasitic systems in which it has been reported, antigenic variation in giardiasis was first observed as a phenomenon occurring *in vitro* (169). The finding of antigenic variation of a cysteine-rich protein in *Giardia* trophozoites (170,171) was expected, because this protozoan has a high nutritional requirement for cysteine (172).

The importance of antigenic variation as a parameter in the immune response to *Giardia* was realized when the phenomenon was documented *in vivo* in humans, mice, and gerbils (173,174). Gerbils were inoculated orally with live trophozoites of *G. duodenalis;* clone WB C1-6E7, which expresses a major 179-kd surface membrane protein, was found to lose this surface antigen 7 days postinfection and replaced this protein by a series of new antigens, including a major protein at 92 kd (174). It is hypothesized that B-cell-dependent mechanisms are most likely responsible for the surface antigen switch (173).

SUMMARY OF THE IMMUNE RESPONSE IN GIARDIASIS

Parasite Clearance

Current evidence suggests that both antibody- and cell-mediated mechanisms are involved in parasite eradication. The appearance of increasing concentrations of sIgA in intestinal fluid and its association with clearance of *Giardia* in the mouse model strongly supports the role of sIgA in parasite clearance. Anti-*Giardia* sIgA antibodies agglutinate trophozoites *in vitro* and thus may interfere with motility and cell division. Antibody-dependent cell cytotoxicity (ADCC), neutrophils, and macrophages may also be important within the intestinal lumen.

Control Of Mucosal Invasion

Although mucosal invasion is a rare event, potential pathways for preventing this include cytotoxic intraepithelial lymphocytes and ADCC by lamina propria lymphocytes (175). Activation of the classic complement pathway and a unique pathway involving calcium and complement components C1 and factor B will also effect trophozoite lysis within the mucosa (175,176).

Protective Immunity

Immune milk appears to passively prevent giardiasis in humans (128). Active immunity does appear to be acquired, although this may not be complete or long-lasting. Continued exposure to the parasite may be required to maintain effective protective immunity. It is unclear as to exactly which pathways are involved in immune protection, although secretion of *Giardia*-specific sIgA antibody would seem to be the first line of defense. The antigens involved in the production of protective immunity have not been defined yet.

EPIDEMIOLOGY

There is wide variation in the prevalence of *Giardia* infection between countries and within regions of the same country. It occurs throughout temperate and tropical locations, with prevalence rates varying between 2% and 5% in the industrialized world and up to 20% to 30% in the developing world (177). Social, environmental, and climatic factors may influence the prevalence of infections. The infection is transmitted by the fecal-oral route. Waterborne outbreaks of giardiasis do occur after contamination of water by fecal material containing cysts that are resistant to disinfection procedures such as chlorination. Food-borne outbreaks can occur after fresh food has been washed with contaminated water or handled by infected people having poor hygiene. Direct person-to-person spread by fecal-oral transmission is another major mechanism by which the disease is transmitted. One of the earliest systematic surveys of prevalence was performed by Dobell in 1921 (178). Giardiasis was found to be endemic in Great Britain in the early 1920s, with prevalence rates from 3.8% to 9.3%. He also made the highly relevant observation that infection was two to three times more common in children. Nevertheless, he remained unconvinced of the importance of *Giardia* as a cause of diarrheal disease at this time. It is now well recognized that giardiasis is common in children in the developing and industrialized world. In rural Guatemala, 45 children were followed from birth through the first 3 years of life, and all were found to have had giardiasis during this period, many having had recurrent infections (126). Prevalence in Peruvian children reached 40% by the age of 6 months, whereas stool examination confirmed prevalence rates of about 20% in children in Zimbabwe and Bangladesh (179). Age-specific prevalence of giardiasis continues to rise through infancy and childhood and only begins to decline after adolescence (180).

High-risk Groups

Infants and young children have increased susceptibility to giardiasis, although infection is rare during the first 6 months of life when breast-feeding is common (126,177). In the United States, Canada, and other industrialized countries, the number of day care facilities has grown over the past 15 years. These centers are of increasing importance in the spread of communicable diseases among a population not previously at risk. Outbreaks of giardiasis at day care nurseries have been reported on several occasions (181–183). For instance, the prevalence of *G. duodenalis* in children attending day care at ages 1 to 3 years was significantly higher than the 2% prevalence in age-matched children not in day care centers (181). Moreover, infected children returning home may become a source of contamination for other members of the family (183). Canadian children were more likely to be infected and symptomatic than immigrant children attending nurseries (183). Nutritional insufficiency in children may be an additional risk factor, possibly contributing to chronicity of disease and a downward spiral in the infection–undernutrition cycle. A recent study of 31 Gambian children with chronic diarrhea and malnutrition showed that 45% had giardiasis, compared with only 12% of healthy age- and sex-matched control children (184). The study indicates that *Giardia* is highly prevalent in children with chronic diarrhea and malnutrition and supports the view that chronic infection is strongly associated with persistent diarrhea and undernutrition.

Because of the paucity of epidemiologic studies with regard to pregnancy and giardiasis, it is difficult to determine whether pregnant women are at risk of getting the infection or losing immunologic control over a preexisting infection. A study in Bangladesh has shown that pregnant women at 6-months of gestation who were infected with *Giardia* excreted a significantly higher number of cysts compared with nonpregnant infected women (185). A similar observation has been reported in the mouse animal model of the disease (186). The sudden increase in the shedding of cysts in fecal material is not unique to *Giardia.* It has been reported with other intestinal protozoan infections (187).

Giardiasis has long been recognized to be a disease of travelers (177). British soldiers returning from northern France and the eastern Mediterranean during World War I were among the first well-documented cases (188). Subsequently, attention focused on European and North American tourists traveling to the European continents or locations within the developing world (189,190). Overall, the risk to the travelers of acquiring giardiasis is relatively low, usually accounting for fewer than 5% of cases of traveler's diarrhea. However, 30% of travelers to the Soviet Union acquired *Giardia* infection and more than 40% of Scandinavian visitors to St. Petersburg acquired the infection (177). However, it is not essential to move from the industrialized to the developing world to become infected with *Giardia.* For example, American or Canadian tourists visiting their respective countries can acquire the infection (191,192).

Immunocompromised Hosts

Because *Giardia* is an opportunistic organism, the following groups of peoples are at risk: infants whose immune system is not fully developed; individuals born with an immunologic defect; individuals having co-infections (e.g., *Plasmodium* and *Giardia*); individuals using immunosuppressive drugs; individuals on cancer therapy; and aging people whose immune system is going to senescence. Ament and Rubin (193) found that approximately 90% of the hypogammaglobulinemic patients passing *Giardia* cysts were symptomatic (chronic diarrhea). Symptomatic giardiasis has been observed in X-linked infantile congenital hypogammaglobulinemia (Bruton's syndrome) and in the common variably (late-onset) acquired hypogammaglobulinemia (194). In the former case of congenital defect, the syndrome represents a pure B-cell deficiency characterized by low levels of all immunoglobulins and normal T-cell function, whereas in the case of acquired hypogammaglobulinemia, only the IgG and IgA levels are decreased, but a T-cell dysfunction may also occur. Some of these hypogammaglobulinemic patients also have severe deficiency of IgM (195). These observations in immunocompromised patients confirm that the development of symptomatic giardiasis cannot be associated with a particular arm of the immune system. Hypogammaglobulinemic patients with giardiasis have a decrease in sIgA anti-*Giardia*-specific antibodies and the infection is mild (196). Serum antibody response in malnourished patients is often normal, but sIgA antibody level is reduced on mucosal surfaces (197). Children with a severe T-cell deficiency due to thymic aplasia (DiGeorge's syndrome) or purine-nucleoside phosphorylase deficiency are not more susceptible to giardiasis, and the morbidity rate is comparable to that of immunocompetent children (195). AIDS patients with a low CD4+ T-cell count do not have persistent or severe diarrheal episodes (198). These results are surprising, because in the mouse model of the disease, the CD4+ T cells and other T-cell subsets have been reported to play a role in the elimination of the parasite from the small intestine (199).

Usually, clinical studies are required to establish whether recrudescence of preexisting opportunistic infections is an important cause of morbidity when immunosuppressive therapy is given to patients in areas where the infection is endemic. There are no reports in the literature on the effects of drugs such as corticosteroids, cyclosporin A, or other immunosuppressive agents of cell-mediated immunity on the outcome of preexisting *Giardia* infections in humans.

Reservoirs

Giardia is a ubiquitous organism with poor host specificity. It is the most common parasite of domestic dogs (30) and cattle (200). It has also been reported in wildlife (192). In this case, various mammalian hosts infected with the *duodenalis* type can serve as a reservoir of the infection for humans. There is evidence in the literature supporting World Health Organization (WHO) classification of giardiasis as a zoonosis (201–203). Zoonotic organisms are characterized by their ability to infect both humans and animals and by the requirement that the infection can be transmitted between them. This is difficult to establish in infections, such as giardiasis, which are transmitted by the fecal-oral route, so the WHO classification is not widely accepted (203). The ongoing confusion regarding the taxonomy of *Giardia* has also contributed to the nonacceptance. However, giardiasis has been constantly reported in various farm animals including cattle, pigs, and sheep, and they may serve as an environmental reservoir of the infection (204). Manure from farm animals is usually spread onto the field as organic fertilizer. In a recent study, we have reported a range of 700 to 1,000 *Giardia* cysts per gram of manure (200). Because giardiasis can develop into a chronic infection in calves (205), it is not surprising to see that a significantly higher number of *Giardia* cysts have been reported from farm effluents by comparison to effluents from municipalities (206,207).

DIAGNOSIS

Clinical Diagnosis

Clinical diagnosis of giardiasis is often suggested by a typical history, particularly if one recently traveled to a foreign country, visited a farm, went on a backpacking excursion, or drank unfiltered water or if children attend day care centers. For the traveler, diarrhea usually begins toward the end of the holiday and persists on return, unlike most other forms of traveler's diarrhea that occur early and resolve rapidly. Many clinicians will treat empirically at this stage even without knowing the results of fecal examinations.

Microscopy

Light microscopic detection of *Giardia* forms (cysts and less frequently trophozoites) continues to be the mainstay of diagnosis and is considered the gold standard method. Stool specimens are examined either fresh for the presence of trophozoites or fixed with formalin ethyl acetate or 10% formaldehyde for eventual examination of cysts and trophozoites after using staining methods. Cyst detection can be improved by using flotation concentration methods. Cyst detection in fecal specimens can be assisted by use of an immunofluorescent antibody to cyst protein. Examination of a single stool specimen may detect up to 70% of cases of giardiasis, rising to 85% after examination of three separate specimens (208). The sensitivity of this method is rather low because cysts are excreted intermittently or in some cases released in numbers too small to be detected (125). Trophozoites are usually only found in watery diarrhea and stools should be examined as a saline wet mount immediately after they have been passed. Trophozoites may also be detected in duodenal fluid, and although some studies have suggested that this is a more reliable approach to diagnosis than fecal examination, only 44% of 74 South Indian patients with giardiasis had a positive duodenal aspirate (208). Stool positivity in these subjects was only 85%, indicating that the two diagnostic approaches are complementary.

Immunodiagnosis

The immunodiagnosis of giardiasis has received much attention. Knowledge about *Giardia* antigens and the need for improved diagnostic tests are two factors that have contributed to the increased number of publications in this area (125). In spite of the identification of novel antigens and the use of various assays, unfortunately, this has not resulted in a very highly rewarding exercise.

Serologic Assays

Anti-*Giardia* antibodies are found in infected and noninfected individuals in endemic areas, presumably because of continued exposure to the parasite. It is likely that most of the population may have anti-*Giardia* circulating antibodies in their fluids. This represents a major problem in diagnosis because serology becomes unhelpful in distinguishing past from current infection. Moreover, because of the sensitivity of the serologic assays, a negative result clearly does not exclude infection.

When crude extracts of trophozoites are processed for antigen usage in an ELISA, the sensitivity varies with the immunoglobulin isotype used as a second antibody. For example, when the IgM isotype was used as the second antibody, 59% (75/128) of the serum from persons with proven cases tested positive, compared with only 35% (15/43) when the whole immunoglobulin was used (125). It appears that anti-*Giardia* IgM titers are usually only elevated in individuals with current infection, with antibody concentrations falling rapidly once the infection has been cleared. Anti-*Giardia* IgM antibodies are useful in identifying individuals with acute giardiasis, even in endemic areas such as India and The Gambia (147,149). The ELISA has a comparable sensitivity when IgA or IgG is used as the second antibody (125). Like anti-*Giardia* IgM antibodies, antibodies of the IgA isotype are short-lived and thus may be of value in the diagnosis of ongoing infection in patients with raised IgA titers (150). It has been reported that the use of intact trophozoites instead of a crude extract increases the sensitivity of the ELISA assay (125). The sensitivity of the immunofluorescent assay (IFA) in the detection of anti-*Giardia* antibodies in the serum of persons with proven infection is comparable to that of the ELISA. The sensitivity of the IFA increases when cysts are used as antigen instead of trophozoites.

The variation in the results obtained in the serologic survey done in the field (156) or experimental infection of healthy individuals (148) demonstrates the poor sensitivity of serologic assays presently available for the diagnosis of giardiasis. Except for the different levels of antibodies detected, serodiagnostic assays failed to show differences in serum antibody responses between symptomatic and asymptomatic patients. Since *Giardia* trophozoites rarely invade the tissues, the systemic immune response is practically never stimulated, and searching for antibodies to *Giardia* in the serum remains an unreliable exercise. Although many commercial kits are available for detecting anti-*Giardia* antibodies in infected patients, it is unfortunate that no investigators have reported their efficacy in the literature.

Detection Of Antigens In Feces

The availability of an immunodiagnostic assay that can detect small amounts of antigens in feces would have the potential to improve the microscopic diagnosis and serology in many ways. For example, it would be more indicative of an active giardial infection and would, therefore, represent a more meaningful clinical finding than the detection of antibodies in the serum. Various assays have been commercialized (125). Contrary to the commercial kits available for the detection of antibodies in the serum, the sensitivity of the ELISA for the detection of antigens in the stools has been evaluated by several laboratories. The ELISA-GSA 65 assay detects a *G. duodenalis*-specific antigen that is excreted in the stool (209). The ELISA-GSA 65 is available commercially as a kit and its sensitivity and specificity are comparable to those of microscopic examination for cysts in the stool. This kit can detect *Giardia* infection in at least 30% more cases than the microscopic examination (210). In an epidemiologic study on the prevalence of *G. duodenalis* infection in 328 patients admitted to the University Hospital of the West Indies for various illnesses, the commercial rapid enzyme assay for detecting antigens in a single stool specimen was compared with the formalin ether concentration method for the detection of cysts in stool (211,212). The formalin ether concentration method detected 6 cases of giardiasis, whereas the assay for detecting antigens in stool detected these 6 cases plus an additional 11 cases.

PATHOLOGY

Etiology Of Diarrhea

The mechanisms by which *Giardia* causes diarrhea and intestinal malabsorption of nutrients remain a controversial subject. Early hypotheses proposed to explain the disease pathogenesis suggested that *Giardia* trophozoites act as a mechanical barrier to absorption or competed for host nutrients. Although *Giardia* is known to physically attach to the surface of the intestinal epithelium, the size and number of trophozoites lining the intestinal mucosa during peak infection are insufficient to create a mechanical barrier capable of significantly interfering with the absorption of nutrients across the intestinal wall. A recent study performed in gerbils infected with various human isolates of *G. duodenalis* suggests that trophozoites do not have a uniform distribution with the host gut but demonstrate the existence of colonization niches (121), thus contradicting earlier hypotheses. Evidence exists that *Giardia* can directly produce varying degrees of mucosal injury while influencing conditions in the intestinal lumen, which could impair nutrient digestion and absorption (213). The precise mechanism by which diarrhea is produced in giardiasis remains unknown. However, several experimental systems employing parasite extracts or metabolites have repeatedly demonstrated the production of intestinal abnormalities such as disaccharidase deficiencies and villous atrophy (122,214, 215).

Alterations Of Intestinal Function And Morphology

Various structural and functional abnormalities of the small intestinal mucosa occur during human infection and in giardiasis animal models. Abnormalities include villous atrophy (216–218) and a shortening of the villus, which is associated with an increase in crypt depth (Fig. 61.5). Changes in crypt morphology occur in the absence of major inflammatory infiltrate in the lamina propria and without an increase in the number of intraepithelial lymphocytes. Ultrastructural changes such as shortening and disruption of microvilli have been reported in human giardiasis even when villous architecture appears normal by light microscopy (219–221). A nonuniform reduction in microvillous membrane surface area in both the jejunum and the ileum has also been reported in the gerbil model (217), although these abnormalities were extremely transient and their importance in the production of diarrhea has been questioned.

Alterations in the microvillous membrane do not correlate with trophozoite attachment. Furthermore, recent studies have shown that loss of the brush border surface area may be mediated in part by thymus-derived T lymphocytes (222), and that morphologic changes in the jejunal mucosa are accompanied by mast cell hyperplasia (124). In human infection, evidence suggests that the extent of mucosal abnormality relates to the severity of diarrhea (223,224).

In gerbils, basal transport of sodium and chloride ions was similar to that in non-infected controls, but glucose-

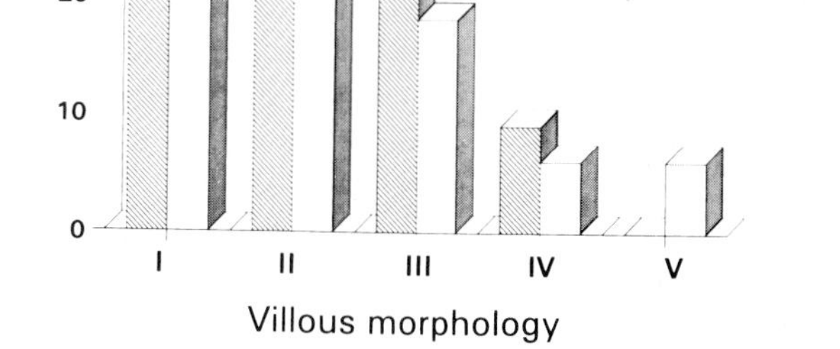

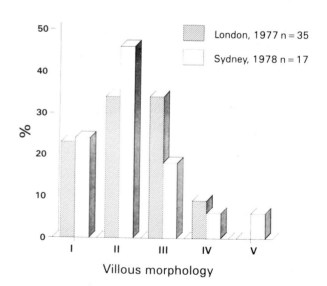

FIGURE 61.5. Percentage of subjects with villous architectural abnormalities (I, normal; II, mild partial villous atrophy; III, moderate partial villous atrophy; IV, severe partial villous atrophy; V, subtotal villous atrophy). (Data from Wright SG, Tomkins AM, Ridley DS. Giardiasis: clinical and therapeutic aspects. *Gut* 1977;18:343–350; and from Ducombe VM, Bolin TD, Davis AE, et al. Histopathology in giardiasis: a correlation with diarrhoea. *Aust N Z J Med* 1978;8:392–396, with permission.)

stimulated sodium absorption was significantly reduced in stripped jejunal mucosal segments mounted in Ussing chambers (217). *In vivo* perfusion studies in animals have also shown impaired water, sodium, and chloride absorption in response to glucose, although basal transport was similar to that of controls (217).

Disaccharidase Activity

Human and experimental models of giardiasis have been associated with reductions in lactase, sucrase, trehalase, and maltase activities in the microvillous membrane (216,224, 242). The reduction in disaccharidase activities is maximal when diarrhea and villous morphologic abnormalities are most profound (29). From the available evidence, it appears that disaccharidase deficiencies associated with primary infections represent direct parasite-mediated damage to the intestinal mucosa. Alternatively, deficiencies observed during secondary exposures may be the result of the host's local immune response to giardial antigens (122,215).

Mechanisms Of Parasite-mediated Mucosal Damage And Pathology

The mechanisms by which these abnormalities occur are poorly defined. Although there have been a few reports of epithelial invasion (225,226), *Giardia* is predominantly a luminal parasite, so invasive episodes must be regarded as exceptional and cannot be evoked as a major mechanism for disrupting mucosal structure and function. *Giardia* trophozoites, however, do attach to the epithelium and have been shown by electron microscopy to disrupt and distort microvilli at the site where the ventral adhesive disk interfaces with the microvillous membrane (227). In the mouse model of giardiasis, ventral disk imprints are particularly marked; similar but less-impressive attachment imprints have been reported in infected human small intestines. It seems unlikely, however, that the localized attachment sites can account for the widespread changes in microvillous membrane surface area observed in the small intestine (217).

In vitro models using live *G. duodenalis* trophozoites, trophozoite extracts, or secreted *Giardia* metabolites on human colonic or duodenal cell monolayers have been developed to study the mechanisms for causing brush border injury and malabsorption associated with giardiasis (214). These models effects on enterocytes were associated with a rearrangement of the cytoskeletal proteins filamentous actin and α-actinin (214).

Bacterial Overgrowth

It has been reported that some patients with symptomatic giardiasis have secondary bacterial overgrowth in the proximal small intestines (228). Although individual species of bacteria have not been identified, the importance of bacterial overgrowth in giardiasis relates to the deconjugation of bile salts by bacteria. The removal of the glycine or taurine conjugates from bile salts reduces bile salt solubility in aqueous solution and thus reduces their efficacy for micelle formation within the intestinal lumen. In addition, free bile salts are membranotoxic and can cause intestinal secretion, thereby contributing to the production of diarrhea (29). In one study, evidence of bile salt deconjugation was found in all patients with bacterial overgrowth and in 40% of giardiasis controls without malabsorption (228). Moreover, increases in aerobic bacterial counts were repeatedly observed in patients with symptomatic giardiasis having signs of steatorrhea (228,229). However, this is not a universal finding (other studies have failed to confirm it) and may reflect the nature of the intestinal microbiota of the studied subjects (3,100,121).

Inhibition Of Hydrolytic Enzymes

Duodenal concentrations of trypsin, chymotrypsin, amylase, and lipase were shown to be lower during an infection with *Giardia* (230–232). However, there is no evidence that the variation is due to a failure of pancreatic exocrine secretion but would be the result of the presence of live parasites in the intestines or release of antigens. Live *Giardia* trophozoites or a trophozoite sonicate inhibits trypsin activity and lipolysis *in vitro* (233–235). Children suffering from giardiasis have a significant reduction in pancreatic lipase activity. The finding was correlated with the presence of steatorrhea (230). The mechanism by which the parasite or their antigens inhibit these enzyme activities has not been established but could be related to the direct interaction between a parasite product, such as its own proteinases, and the host enzymes. A number of giardial proteases have been discovered, most of which are cysteine proteases (95). Interestingly, some ES products from the trophozoites have proteolytic activities (236). The role these proteases play in the pathogenesis of giardiasis merits further investigations because proteases are known to play a key role in the pathogenesis of other enteric protozoan parasites such as *Entamoeba histolytica* (237).

CLINICAL PRESENTATION OF GIARDIASIS

Few symptoms, if any, are associated with asymptomatic infections and patients usually resolve the diarrhea in 3 to 4 days (238); without any intestinal pathology, the enteropathy and intestinal dysfunction are subclinical (29). The clinical syndrome of acute giardiasis has been well characterized in travelers moving to an area of high endemicity (239,240) (Table 61.1). Acute giardiasis is mainly characterized by diarrhea, which is usually initially watery but can be accompanied by steatorrhea, nausea, abdominal discomfort, bloating, and often weight loss (Table 61.1). Patients

TABLE 61.1. SYMPTOMS OF ACUTE GIARDIASIS IN TRAVELERS

Clinical Features	Aspen, Colorado (Reference 193) (n = 324) (%)	Soviet Union (Reference 243) (n = 56) (%)
Diarrhea	96	93
Weakness	72	80
Weight loss	62	73
Abdominal pain	61	77
Nausea	60	59
Steatorrhea	57	55
Flatulence	35	—
Vomiting	29	—
Fever	17	—

with the acute form of the disease suffer from disaccharidases deficiencies, reversible ultrastructural damage of the intestines, and inflammation (Fig. 61.5) Although most patients resolve the acute infection, some develop chronic diarrhea, steatorrhea, and malabsorption of nutrients that results in severe weight loss. These symptoms usually begin within 3 to 20 days of arrival in the high-risk area, and for most patients, the symptoms disappear within 2 to 4 weeks. However, in some travelers, symptoms may persist for 7 or more weeks. A possible link between the genotypes of different *Giardia* isolates and clinical symptomology has been recently reported (241). A 100% correlation between the severity of diarrheal complaints and genotypes was established. Isolates belonging to assemblage A were solely detected in patients with intermittent diarrheal complaints, whereas isolates belonging to assemblage B were present in patients with persistent diarrheal complaints (241).

Intestinal malabsorption occurs in patients with chronic giardiasis, with malabsorption of fat and other nutrients such as vitamins A and B_{12} (242) (Table 61.2). Indirect evidence of carbohydrate malabsorption is suggested by reduced D-xylose absorption (243,244). Secondary lactase deficiency with lactose malabsorption is, however, well recognized to occur in giardiasis and may take several weeks to recover, even after clearance of the parasite.

Growth Impairment

Earlier studies have elucidated an existing association between giardiasis and growth retardation in infants and young children in underdeveloped and developing countries (3,242). However, observations of well-nourished children attending day care centers did not document any evidence of growth failure in this population (245,246). Lunn et al. (247) found significant physiologic alterations in the gross intestinal function of infants between the ages of 2 and 8 months, which positively correlated with the appearance of parasite-specific antibodies. The authors concluded that infant growth over the whole 6-month study period was unrelated to *Giardia*-specific antibody titers or to the time of infection.

Allergic And Inflammatory Phenomena

Although immediate-type hypersensitivity is a relatively common association with helminthic infections, it is rare in protozoan infections. However, urticaria, arthralgia, and other allergic occurrences have been reported in patients with giardiasis. Acute urticaria in one case was associated with increased serum IgE concentrations, although there was no increase in anti-*Giardia* IgE (151). Lymphoid nodular hyperplasia has been associated with both chronic giardiasis and immune deficiency (248–250). In one study from Venezuela, 125 children were classified into three groups: those parasitized by *Giardia* and other gastrointestinal parasites, those parasitized with other gastrointestinal parasites, or those unparasitized. Total serum IgE was measured in the studied groups, and the levels of giardial-specific and food-protein-specific serum IgE were consistently higher in the *Giardia*-parasitized group of children. In addition, allergic manifestations were significantly higher in *Giardia*-parasitized children (251). The mechanisms behind the occurrence of allergic phenomena in patients suffering from giardiasis are unknown. A recent study has demonstrated that food antigen uptake was significantly higher in Mongolian gerbils infected with a virulent strain of *G. duodenalis* compared with sham-treated animals (124). The mucosal mast cell count was at a normal level in all animals at 6 days postinfection but

TABLE 61.2. INTESTINAL MALABSORPTION IN GIARDIASIS

	Malabsorbed Elements				
	D-Xylose	Lactose	Fat	Vitamin A	Vitamin B_{12}
Number of surveyed subjects	224	61	335	19	191
Number of positive subjects	105	30	184	19	117
Percentage of positive cases	47	49	55	100	61

Source: From Farthing MJG. *Giardia lamblia.* In: Blaser J, Smith PD, Ravdin JI, et al. *Infections of the gastrointestinal tract.* New York, NY: Raven Press, 1995:1081–1105, with permission.

was significantly elevated at 21 days postinfection in *Giardia*-infected gerbils (124). The authors concluded that the increased number of mast cells during the acute phase was due to an increase in antigen uptake in the jejunum, leading to the development of allergies (124). Alternatively, it is also possible that the development of allergies is the result of the interaction between *Giardia*-specific sIgA and its antigen epitopes, because sIgA antibodies have been reported to play a role in inflammatory reactions occurring at the gut level (157).

Ocular Complications

The first description of ocular complications in patients with giardiasis was reported in the late 1930s (252). Cases of iridocyclitis, choroiditis, retinal hemorrhages, anterior and posterior uveitis, retinal vasculitis, and a "salt and pepper" form of degeneration of the retinal pigmented epithelium were later associated with giardiasis (253,254). A recent study investigating the ocular changes associated with giardiasis in 141 children has demonstrated that asymptomatic, nonprogressive retinal lesions were common in approximately 20% of cases (255). In all of the studied cohorts, retinal changes were consistently observed in younger children (mean age, 3.5 years).

TREATMENT OF GIARDIASIS

The four major classes of drugs used to treat giardiasis are as follows: (a) the nitroimidazole derivatives such as MTZ, tinidazole, and ornidazole; (b) the acridine dyes such as quinacrine (mepacrine); (c) aminoglycosides such as paromomycin; and (d) the nitrofurans such as furazolidone (2,256,259). The recommended doses and efficacy of these drugs are summarized in Table 61.3. Nitroimidazole derivatives such as MTZ, tinidazole, and ornidazole are probably the drugs of choice because the treatment period is brief and compliance is generally good (256) (Table 61.3). Although the Food and Drug Administration has not approved the use of MTZ for the treatment of giardiasis, the drug is still prescribed in the United States for this purpose. In addition, tinidazole and ornidazole are not available in the United States.

The mode of action of nitroimidazoles in *Giardia* has not been examined in detail. MTZ is also the drug commonly used to treat infections caused by anaerobic protozoan parasites such as *Trichomonas vaginalis, G. duodenalis,* and *E. histolytica* (40). It has been proposed that toxic radicals binding to DNA or cumulative DNA strand breaks are the mechanisms of cell death (40,257).

Quinacrine, an antimalarial, is also effective against *Giardia;* unfortunately, it is no longer commercially available in the United States (257). Quinacrine acts by interfering with flavin enzymes, causing depression in oxygen consumption. Quinacrine also incorporates into DNA by intercalating between nucleobase pairs, thus causing genetic damage to the parasite (258).

Furazolidone appears to be a less effective drug in giardiasis but is widely used for the treatment of giardiasis in the United States, particularly in pediatric populations because the drug is available as a suspension in a syrup form (259,260). The drug is metabolically reduced to cytotoxic products in a similar manner to MTZ, but not via ferredoxin (40). NADH oxidase activates furazolidone, forming superoxides and other toxic radicals (261). None of the aforementioned drugs are regarded safe for use during pregnancy because they have unpleasant adverse effects and potential teratogenicity (Table 61.4). Although paromomycin is not a highly effective anti-giardial agent, it is currently the only chemotherapeutic agent suggested for use in pregnant patients because the drug is poorly absorbed. Paromomycin exerts its anti-giardial effects by interfering with the *Giardia* 50S and 30S ribosomal subunits, causing misreading of mRNA codons and inhibiting protein synthesis (40). Table 61.4 lists adverse effects associated with the common anti-*Giardia* therapeutic agents.

TABLE 61.3. DOSING AND EFFICACY OF STANDARD DRUG TREATMENTS OF GIARDIASIS

Drug	Adult Dose	Pediatric Dose	Efficacy
Metronidazole	250 mg tid for 5–7 days PO	5 mg/kg tid PO for 5–7 days	>90%
Tinidazole	2-g single dose PO	50 mg/kg single PO dose[a]	>90%
Ornidazole	2-g single dose PO	40–50 mg/kg single PO dose[a]	>90%
Quinacrine	100 mg tid for 5–7 days PO	2 mg/kg tid PO for 7 days	>90%
Furazolidone	100 mg qid for 7–10 days PO	2 mg/kg qid PO for 10 days	80–96%
Paromomycin	500 mg tid for 5–10 days PO	30 mg/kg tid PO for 5–10 days	55–88%

[a]Administered to a maximum dose of 2 g.
tid, three times a day; PO, orally; qid, four times a day.
Source: From Farthing MJG. *Giardia lamblia.* In: Blaser J, Smith PD, Ravdin JI, et al. *Infections of the gastrointestinal tract.* New York, NY: Raven Press, 1995:1081–1105.

TABLE 61.4. ADVERSE EFFECTS OF ANTIGIARDIAL DRUGS

Drug	Side Effects	
	Common	Rare
Nitroimidazoles (including metronidazole, tinidazole and ornidazole)	Nausea, vomiting metallic taste, gastrointestinal unrest, rashes, vertigo, urticaria, disulfuram-like reaction with consumption of alcohol	Pancreatitis, central nervous system toxicity, reversible neutropenia, peripheral neuropathy, T-wave flattening with prolonged use, carcinogenesis/mutagenesis?
Mepacrine	Gastrointestinal unrest, dizziness, headache, nausea, vomiting, yellow-orange discoloration of the skin and mucous membranes	Toxic psychosis, chronic dermatoses, hepatitis, aplastic anemia
Furazolidone	Nausea, vomiting, hemolysis in glucose-6-phosphate dehydrogenase-deficient patients, diarrhea, brown discoloration of urine	disulfuram-like reaction with alcohol consumption, furazolidone-induced mania
Paromomycin	Ototoxicity and nephrotoxicity with systemic administrations	Remains to be reported

Source: From Farthing MJG. *Giardia lamblia.* In: Blaser J, Smith PD, Ravdin JI, et al. *Infections of the gastrointestinal tract.* New York, NY: Raven Press, 1995:1081–1105.

New Anti-giardial Agents

Recent studies suggest that benzimidazoles, albendazole and mebendazole, which are well recognized for their broad-spectrum antihelminthic activity, are effective in the treatment of giardiasis (257,262). The anti-*Giardia* activity relates to the interaction with the cytoskeletal protein β-tubulin, which inhibits cytoskeleton polymerization and impairs glucose uptake (257). Incubation of *Giardia* trophozoites with benzimidazoles inhibits the attachment of trophozoites to mammalian cell monolayers (263). Albendazole has been proven to be an effective anti-giardial agent both in *in vitro* and in clinical trials (262). This drug may be particularly useful in children in the developing world because it can serve a dual purpose of treating against intestinal helminths and *Giardia.* Mebendazole has also been reported to be effective in treating giardiasis in children (264).

Other drugs reported to have anti-*Giardia* activity including the antimalarial mefloquine, the antibiotic bacitracin zinc (257), and nitazoxanide. The latter drug has been used with great success in a patient with AIDS chronically infected with MTZ- and albendazole-resistant *Giardia* (265). Drug combinations may be more effective than single-agent therapies for treating giardiasis. In a recent study, patients with refractory giardiasis, including immunodepressed individuals, treated with a combination of quinacrine and MTZ exhibited a cure rate of 83% (266). Alternatively, an albendazole–MTZ combination was shown to be 100% effective in 20 patients afflicted by MTZ-resistant giardiasis that had failed to respond to three to five courses of standard oral MTZ therapy alone (267).

Drug Sensitivity Testing

Various approaches have been developed to measure drug sensitivity profiles of *Giardia* isolates in axenic culture (268–273). Previously published methods for assessing anti-giardial activity *in vitro* rely on the viability of *G. duodenalis* trophozoites *in vitro.* But these studies have been hampered by the lack of good standardized methods. Hence, a reliable viability assay is needed for *in vitro* susceptibility studies and to screen drugs for anti-giardial activity.

VACCINES

The question remains as to whether giardiasis can be prevented by the administration of an appropriate vaccine. Experimental infection in human volunteers (60) and epidemiologic studies (274) suggest that protective immunity is acquired after exposure to *Giardia.* It seems likely that protective immunity does not necessarily develop after a single infection, because in rural Guatemala, many infants and children experienced multiple infections during the first 3 years of life (275), and age-specific prevalence of the disease is known to rise throughout childhood and only begins to abate to adult levels during adolescence (272). Although, the question as to why the development of protective immunity during natural infection appears to be a lengthy process is intriguing, it is possible that the presence of many immunologic subtypes, together with the antigenic complexity of different parasite isolates (159,276), may account for these phenomena. As indicated above, even within a single isolate antigen, expression can vary (23).

Veterinary vaccines for *Giardia* are highly desirable because of the high prevalence of infection in domestic animals, which poses a serious concern for zoonotic transmission (277). In experimentally infected animals and humans, elevated levels of serum and mucosal antibodies are found during the elimination phase of the infection. Moreover, the host produces specific serum and mucosal antibodies directed against both surface and cytosolic antigens (278–279). There are few studies in the literature on the induction of active immunity against *G. duodenalis.* Subcutaneous immunization of 3-week-old mice with a 56-kd protein, followed by an oral immunization boost, resulted in a lower load of trophozoites within the small intestine when animals were challenged with 10^7 trophozoites 7 days after the last immunization (277).

The immunization stimulated an increase in the number of CD4+ T cells, which dropped to normal levels by day 30 postimmunization. Moreover, a significant elevation in the IgA- and IgG-secreting plasma cells was observed in the lamina propria and jejunum of immunized mice (277). The vaccination of 6-week-old kittens with a crude extract of *G. duodenalis* trophozoites resulted in a smaller number of cysts excreted in the feces when animals were challenged intraduodenally with 10^6 trophozoites 14 days after the last immunization (277). Vaccination of kittens was also observed to increase serum anti-*Giardia* IgG and IgA antibodies, as well as the mucosal anti-*Giardia* IgA antibody titer. Similar results were also observed with 6-week-old puppies (277).

ACKNOWLEDGMENTS

We gratefully acknowledge Drs. J-D MacLean and A. Jardim for their critical review of the manuscript. Gaétan Faubert is supported by a grant from the National Sciences and Engineering Research Council of Canada. Peter Lee is the grateful recipient of a Fonds pour la Formation des Chercheurs et l'aide à la Recherche (FCAR) scholarship. Research at the Institute of Parasitology is supported by FCAR.

REFERENCES

1. Farthing MJG. Host–parasite interactions in human giardiasis. *J Med* 1989;70:191–204.
2. Adam RD. The biology of *Giardia* spp. *Microbiol Rev* 1991;55: 706–732
3. Farthing MJG. Giardiasis as a disease. In: Reynoldson JA, Thompson RCA, Lymbery AJ, eds. Giardia*: from molecules to disease and beyond.* Oxford: CAB International, 1993:1537.
4. Ament ME, Rubin CE. Relation of giardiasis to abnormal intestinal structure and function in immunodeficiency syndromes. *Gastroenterology* 1972;62:216–226.
5. Smith PD. Pathophysiology and immunology of giardiasis. *Ann Rev Med* 1985;36:295–307.
6. Wolfe MS. Giardiasis. *JAMA* 1975;233:1362–1365.
7. Harris RH, Mitchell JH. Chronic urticaria due to *Giardia lamblia. Arch Dermatol* 1949;59:587–589.
8. Webster BH. Human infection with *Giardia lamblia. Dig Dis Sci* 1958;3:64–71.
9. Hamrick HJ, Moore WJ. Giardiasis causing urticaria in a child. *Am J Dis Child* 1983;137:761–763.
10. Dobell CA. The discovery of intestinal protozoa in man. *Proc R Soc Med* 1920;13:1–15.
11. Meyer EA, Jarrol EL. *Giardia* and giardiasis. *Am J Epidemiol* 1980;111:1–12.
12. Kulda J, Nohynkova E. Flagellates of the human intestine and of intestines of other species. In: JP Kreir, ed. *Protozoa of veterinary and medical interest.* New York, NY: Academic Press, 1978: 69.
13. Meyer EA. Taxonomy and nomenclature. In: Meyer EA, ed. *Giardiasis.* Amsterdam: Elsevier Science, 1990:51–60.
14. Filice PP. Studies on the cytology and life history of *Giardia* from the laboratory rat. *Calif Publ Zool* 1952;57:53–143.
15. Erlandsen SL, Bemrick WJ. SEM evidence for a new species. *Giardia psittaci. J Parasitol* 1987;73:623–629.
16. Erlandsen SL. Axenic culture and characterization of *Giardia ardea* from the great blue heron (*Ardea herodias*) *J Parasitol* 1990;76:717–724.
17. Van Keulen H, Feely D, Macechko E, et al. The sequence of *Giardia* small sub-unit rRNA shows that voles and muskrats are parasitized by a unique species *Giardia microti. J Parasitol* 1998; 84:294–300.
18. Thompson RCA, Lymbery AJ, Meloni BP. Genetic variation in *Giardia* Kunstler, 1882: taxonomic and epidemiological significance. CAB International, 1990;14:1–28.
19. McIntyre L, Hoang L, Ong CSL, et al. Evaluation of molecular techniques to biotype *Giardia duodenalis* collected during an outbreak. *J Parasitol* 2000;86:172–177.
20. Isaac-Renton JL, Byrne SK, Prameya R. Isoelectric focusing of 10 strains of *Giardia duodenalis. J Parasitol* 1988;74: 1054–1056.
21. Meloni BP, Lymbery AJ, Thompson RCA. Isoenzyme electrophoresis of 30 isolates of *Giardia* from humans and felines. *Am J Trop Med Hyg* 1988;38:65–73.
22. Meloni BP, Lymbery AJ, Thompson RCA. Genetic characterization of isolates of *Giardia duodenalis* by enzyme electrophoresis: implications for reproductive biology, population structure, taxonomy, and epidemiology. *J Parasitol* 1995;81:368–383.
23. Nash T. Surface antigen variability and variation in *Giardia lamblia. Parasitol Today* 1992;8:229–243
24. Upcroft JA, Boreham PFL, Upcroft P. Geographic variation in *Giardia* karyotypes. *Int J Parasitol* 1989;19:519–527.
25. Korman SH, LeBlancq SM, Deckelbaum RI, et al. Investigation of human giardiasis by karyotype analysis. *J Clin Invest* 1992; 89:1725–1733.
26. Nash TE, McCutchan T, Keister D, et al. Restriction endonuclease analysis of DNA from 15 *Giardia* isolates from humans and animals. *J Infect Dis* 1985;152:64–73.
27. Upcroft P, Mitchell R, Boreham FP. DNA fingerprinting of the intestinal parasite *Giardia duodenalis* with the M13 phage genome. *Int J Parasitol* 1990;20:319–323.
28. Butcher PD, Cevallos AM, Camaby S, et al. Phenotypic and genotypic variation in *Giardia lamblia* isolates during chronic infection. *Gut* 1993;34:51–54.
29. Farthing MJG. The molecular pathogenesis of giardiasis. *J Pediatr Gastroenterol Nutr* 1997;24:79–88.
30. Thompson RCA, Hopkins RM, Homan WL. Nomenclature and genetic groupings of *Giardia* infecting mammals. *Parasitol Today* 2000;16:210–217.
31. Lindmark DG. *Giardia lamblia:* localization of hydrolase activities in lysosome-like organelles of trophozoites. *Exp Parasitol* 1988;65:141–147.
32. Holberton DV. Arrangements of subunits in microribbons from *Giardia. J Cell Sci* 1981;47:167–185.
33. Peattie DA, Alonso RA, Hem A, et al. Ultrastructural localization of giardins to the edges of disk microribbons of *Giardia*

lamblia and the nucleotide and deduced protein sequence of alpha-giardin. *J Cell Biol* 1989;109:2323–2335.

34. Reiner DS, McCaffery M, Gillin FD. Sorting of cyst wall proteins to a regulated secretory pathway during differentiation of the primitive eukaryote, *Giardia lamblia. Eur J Cell Biol* 1990; 53:142–153.
35. Adam RD. The *Giardia lamblia* genome. *Int J Parasitol* 2000; 30:475–484.
36. Feely DE, Dyer JK. Localization of acid phosphatase activity in *Giardia lamblia* and *Giardia muris* trophozoites. *J Protozool* 1987;34:80–83.
37. McCaffery JM, Faubert GM, Gillin FD. *Giardia lamblia:* traffic of a trophozoite variant surface protein and a major cyst wall epitope during growth, encystation, and antigenic switching. *Exp Parasitol* 1994;79:236–249.
38. McCaffery JM, Gillin FD. *Giardia lamblia:* ultrastructural basis of protein transport during growth and encystation. *Exp Parasitol* 1994;79:220–235.
39. McCaffery JM, Gillin FD. Sorting of cyst wall proteins to a regulated secretory pathway during differentiation of the primitive eukaryote, *Giardia lamblia. Eur J Cell Biol* 1990;53:142–153.
40. Upcroft J, Upcroft P. My favorite cell: *Giardia. BioEssays* 1998; 20:256–263.
41. Erlandsen SL, Macechko PT, van Keulen H, et al. Formation of the *Giardia* cyst wall: studies on extracellular assembly using immunogold labeling and high resolution field emission SEM. *J Eukaryot Microbiol* 1996;43:416–429.
42. Ward HD, Alroy J, Lev BI, et al. Identification of chitin as a structural component of *Giardia* cysts. *Infect Immun* 1985;49: 629–634.
43. Gillin FD, Reiner DS, Gault MJ, et al. Encystation and expression of cyst antigens by *Giardia lamblia in vitro. Science* 1987; 235:1040–1043.
44. Jarroll EL, Manning P, Lindmark DG, et al. *Giardia* cyst wall-specific carbohydrate: evidence for the presence of galactosamine. *Mol Biochem Parasitol* 1989;32:121–132.
45. Erlandsen SL, Bemrick WJ, Schupp DE, et al. High resolution immunogold localization of *Giardia* cyst wall antigens using field emission SEM with secondary and backscatter electron imaging. *J Histochem Cytochem* 1990;38:625–632.
46. Wang AL, Wang CC. Discovery of a specific double-stranded RNA virus in *Giardia lamblia. Mol Biochem Parasitol* 1986;21: 269–276.
47. Wang AL, Wang CC. Viruses of parasitic protozoa. *Parasitol Today* 1991;7:76–80.
48. Kabnick KS, Peattie DA. *In situ* analyses reveal that the two nuclei of *Giardia lamblia* are equivalent. *J Cell Sci* 1990;95: 353–360.
49. Kofoid CA, Christensen EB. On binary and multiple fission in *Giardia. Univ Calif Publ Zool* 1915;16:30–54.
50. Boeck W. Mitosis in *Giardia microtus. Univ Calif Publ Zool* 1917;18:1–26.
51. Boeck W. Studies on *Giardia microtus. Univ Calif Publ Zool* 1919;19:1–26.
52. Adam RD, Nash TE, Wellems TE. The *Giardia lamblia* trophozoite contains a set of closely related chromosomes. *Nucleic Acids Res* 1988;16:4555–4567.
53. Upcroft JA, Healey A, Upcroft P. Chromosomal duplication in *Giardia duodenalis. Int J Parasitol* 1993;23:609–616.
54. Chen N, Upcroft JA, Upcroft P. Physical map of 2Mb chromosome of the intestinal protozoan parasite *Giardia duodenalis* karyotypes. *Chromosome Res* 1994;2:307–313.
55. Upcroft JA, Chen N, Upcroft P. Mapping variation in chromosome homologues of different *Giardia* strains. *Mol Biochem Parasitol* 1996;76:135–143.
56. Adam RD. Chromosome-sized variation in *Giardia lamblia:* the role of rDNA repeats. *Nucleic Acids Res* 1992;20:3057–3061.
57. Bell G. Sex and death in protozoa. The history of an obsession. Cambridge: Cambridge University Press, 1989.
58. Kirk-Mason KE, Turner MJ, Chakraborty PR. Evidence for unusually short tubulin mRNA leaders and characterization of tubulin genes in *Giardia lamblia. Mol Biochem Parasitol* 1989; 36:87–99.
59. Holberton DV, Marshall J. Analysis of consensus sequence patterns in *Giardia* cytoskeleton gene promoters. *Nucleic Acids Res* 1995;23:2945–53.
60. Rendtorff RC. The experimental transmission of human intestinal protozoan parasites: II *Giardia lambliacysts* given in capsules. *Am J Hyg* 1954;59:209–220.
61. Porter A. An enumerative study of the cysts of *Giardia (lamblia) intestinalis* in human dysenteric faeces. *Lancet* 1916;1: 1166–1169.
62. Lujan H, Mowatt M, Byrd L, et al. Cholesterol starvation induces differentiation of the intestinal parasite *Giardia lamblia. Proc Natl Acad Sci U S A* 1996;93:7628–7633.
63. Gillin FD, Reiner DS, Boucher SE. Small intestinal factors promote encystation of *Giardia lamblia in vitro. Infect Immun* 1988;56:705–707.
64. Boucher SEM, Gillin FD. Excystation of *in vitro*-derived *Giardia lamblia* cysts. *Infect Immun* 1990;58:3516-3522.
65. Reiner D, Douglas H, Gillin F. Identification and localization of cyst-specific antigens of *Giardia lamblia. Infect Immun* 1989; 57:963–968.
66. Campbell JD, Faubert GM. Recognition of *Giardia lamblia* cyst-specific antigens by monoclonal antibodies. *Parasite Immunol* 1994;16:211–219.
67. Mowatt MR, Lujan HD, Cotten DB, et al. Developmentally regulated expression of a *Giardia lamblia* cyst wall protein gene. *Mol Microbiol* 1995;15:955–963.
68. Ward HD, Kane AV, Ortega-Barria E, et al. Identification of developmentally regulated *Giardia lamblia* cyst antigens using GCSA-1, a cyst-specific monoclonal antibody. *Mol Microbiol* 1990;4:2095–2102.
69. Lujan HD, Mowatt MR, Conrad JT, et al. Identification of a novel *Giardia lamblia* cyst wall protein with leucine-rich repeats. *J Biol Chem* 1995;270:29307–29313.
70. Hehl AB, Marti M, Köhler P. Stage-specific expression and targeting of cyst wall protein-green fluorescent protein chimeras in *Giardia. Mol Biol Cell* 2000;11:1789–1800.
71. Faubert G, Reiner DS, Gillin FD. *Giardia lamblia:* regulation of secretory vesicle formation and loss of ability to reattach during encystation *in vitro. Exp Parasitol* 1991;72:345–354.
72. Gillin FD, Reiner DS, McCaffery JM. Cell biology of the primitive eukaryote *Giardia lamblia. Annu Rev Microbiol* 1996;50: 679–705.
73. Lujan HD, Mowatt MR, Nash TE. Mechanisms of *Giardia lamblia* differentiation into cysts. *Microbiol Mol Biol Rev* 1997; 61:294–304.
74. Jarroll EA, Macechko PT, Steimle PA, et al. Regulation of carbohydrate mechanism during *Giardia* encystment. *J Eukaryot Microbiol* 2001;48:22–26.
75. Macechko PT, Steimle P, Lindmark D, et al. Galactosamine synthesizing enzymes are induced when *Giardia* encyst. *Mol Biochem Parasitol* 1992;56:301–310.
76. Bingham AK, Meyer EA. *Giardia* excystation can be induced *in vitro* in acidic solutions. *Nature* 1979;277:301–302.
77. Meng TC, Hetsko ML, Gillin FD. Inhibition of *Giardia lamblia* excystation by antibodies against cyst walls proteins and by wheat germ agglutinin. *Infect Immun* 1996;64:2144–2150.
78. Ward W, Alvaredo L, Rawlings ND, et al. A primitive enzyme

for a primitive cell: the protease required for excystation of *Giardia. Cell* 1997;89:437–444.
79. Bernal RM, Tovar R, Santos JI, et al. Possible role of calmodulin in excystation of *Giardia lamblia. Parasitol Res* 1998;84: 687–693.
80. Abel ES, Davids BJ, Robles LD, et al. Possible roles of protein kinase A in cell motility and excystation of the early diverging eukaryote *Giardia lamblia. J Biol Chem* 2001;276:10320–10329.
81. Hetsko ML, McCaffery JM, Svard SG, et al. Cellular and transcriptional changes during excystation of *Giardia lamblia in vitro. Exp Parasitol* 1998;88:172–183.
82. Holberton DV. Attachment of *Giardia* hydrodynamic model based on flagellar activity. *J Exp Biol* 1974;60:207–221.
83. Erlandsen SL, Feely DE. Trophozoite motility and the mechanism of attachment. In: Meyer EA, Erlandsen SL, eds. Giardia *and giardiasis.* New York, NY: Plenum Publishing, 1984:33–60.
84. Farthing MJG, Pereira MEA, Keusch GT. Description and characterization of a surface lectin from *Giardia lamblia. Infect Immun* 1986;51:661–667.
85. Lev B, Ward H, Keusch GT, et al. Lectin activation of *Giardia lamblia* by host protease: a novel host-parasite interaction. *Science* 1986;232:71–73.
86. Ward HD, Lev BI, Kane AU, et al. Identification and characterization of taglin, a mannose-6-phosphate binding, trypsin-activated lectin from *Giardia lamblia. Biochemistry* 1987;26: 8669–8675.
87. Inge PMG, Edson CM, Farthing MJG. Attachment of *Giardia lamblia* to mammalian intestinal cells. *Gut* 1988;29: 795–801.
88. Katelaris PH, Naeem A, Farthing MJG. An *in vitro* model of attachment of *Giardia lamblia* to an intestinal cell line and potential use as an assay of drug sensitivity. *Gut* 1992;33 [Suppl]:S45.
89. Thompson RCA, Reynoldson JA. *Giardia* and giardiasis. *Adv Parasitol* 1993;32:71–160.
90. Karapetyan A. *In vitro* cultivation of *Giardia duodenalis. J Parasitol* 1962;46:337–340.
91. Meyer EA. *Giardia lamblia*: isolation and axenic cultivation. *Exp Parasitol* 1976;39:101–105.
92. Keister DB. Axenic culture of *Giardia lamblia* in TYI-S-33 medium supplemented with bile. *Trans Royal Soc Trop Med Hyg* 1983;77:487–488.
93. Müller M. Energy metabolism of protozoa without mitochondria. *Annu Rev Microbiol* 1988;42:465–488.
94. Lindmark DG. Energy metabolism for the anaerobic protozoan *Giardia lamblia. Mol Biochem Parasitol* 1980;1:1–12.
95. Jarroll EL, Muller PJ, Meyer EA, et al. Lipid and carbohydrate metabolism of *Giardia lamblia. Mol Biochem Parasitol* 1981;2: 187–196.
96. Paget TA, Raynor MH, Shipp DWE, et al. *Giardia lamblia* produces alanine anaerobically but not in the presence of oxygen. *Mol Biochem Parasitol* 1990;42:63–68.
97. Paget TA, Kelly ML, Jarroll EL, et al. The effects of oxygen on fermentation in the intestinal protozoal parasite *Giardia lamblia. Mol Biochem Parasitol* 1993;57:65–72.
98. Gibson GR, Ramirez D, Maier J, et al. *Giardia lamblia:* incorporation of free and conjugated fatty acids into glycerol-based phospholipids. *Exp Parasitol* 1999;92:1–11.
99. Stevens TL, Gibson GR, Adam R, et al. Uptake and cellular localization of exogenous lipids by *Giardia lamblia,* a primitive eukaryote. *Exp Parasitol* 1997;86:133–143.
100. Halliday CEW, Inge PMG, Farthing MJG. *Giardia* bile salt interactions *in vitro* and *in vivo. Trans Royal Soc Trop Med Hyg* 1988;82:428–432.
101. Farthing MJG, Keusch GT, Carey MC. Effects of bile and bile salts on growth and membrane lipid uptake by *Giardia lamblia:* possible implications for pathogenesis of intestinal disease. *J Clin Invest* 1985;76:1727–1732.
102. Gillin FD, Reiner DS, Boucher SE. Small intestinal factors promote encystation of *Giardia lamblia in vitro. Infect Immun* 1988;56:705–707.
103. Lindmark DG, Jarroll EL. Pyrimidine metabolism in *Giardia lamblia* trophozoites. *Mol Biochem Parasitol* 1982;5:291–296.
104. Wang CC, Aldritt S. Purine salvage networks in *Giardia lamblia. J Exp Med* 1983;158:1703–1712.
105. Jarroll EL, Hammond MM, Lindmark DG. *Giardia lamblia:* uptake of pyrimidine nucleosides. *Exp Parasitol* 1987;63: 152–156.
106. Fahey RC, Sundquist AR. Evolution of glutathione metabolism. *Adv Enzymol* 1991;64:1–53.
107. Brown DM, Upcroft JA, Upcroft P. Free radical detoxification in *Giardia duodenalis. Mol Biochem Parasitol* 1995;72: 47–56.
108. Brown DM, Upcroft JA, Upcroft P. A H2O-producing NADH oxidase from the protozoan parasite *Giardia duodenalis. Eur J Biochem* 1996;241:155–161.
109. Brown DM, Upcroft JA, Upcroft P. Cysteine is the major low molecular weight thiol in *Giardia duodenalis. Mol Biochem Parasitol* 1993;61:155–158.
110. Brown DM, Upcroft JA, Upcroft P. Thiol redox management by disulfide reductase in the protozoan parasite *Giardia duodenalis. Mol Biochem Parasitol* 1996;83:211–220.
111. Gillin FD, Hagblom P, Harwood J, et al. Isolation and expression of the gene for a major surface protein of *Giardia lamblia. Proc Natl Acad Sci U S A* 1990;87:4463–4467.
112. Roberts-Thompson IC, Stevens DP, Mahmoud AAF, et al. Giardiasis in the mouse: an animal model. *Gasteroenterology* 1976;71:57–61.
113. Belosovic M, Faubert GM, MacLean JD, et al. *Giardia lamblia* infections in Mongolian gerbils: an animal model. *J Infect Dis* 1983;147:222–226.
114. Hegner RW. Excystation and infection in the rat with *Giardia lamblia* from man. *Am J Hyg* 1927;7:782–785.
115. Armaghan V. Biological studies on the *Giardia* of rats. *Am J Hyg* 1937;26:236–258.
116. Cevallos AM, James M, Farthing MJG. Small intestinal injury in a neonatal rat model is strain dependent. *Gasteroenterology* 1995;109:766–773.
117. Faubert GM, Belosovic M. Animal models for *Giardia duodenalis* type organisms. In: Meyer EA, ed. *Giardiasis.* New York: Elsevier Science, 1990:77–90.
118. Byrd LA, Conrad JT, Nash TE. *Giardia lamblia* infections in adult mice. *Infect Immun* 1994;62:3583–3585.
119. Muller N, Gottestein B. Antigenic variation and the murine immune response to *Giardia lamblia. Int J Parasitol* 1998;28: 1829–1839.
120. Aggarwal A, Nash TE. Antigenic variation of *Giardia lamblia in vivo. Infect Immun* 1988;56:1420–1423.
121. Astiazaran-Garcia H, Espinosa-Cantenellano M, Castanon G, et al. *Giardia lamblia:* effect of infection with symptomatic and asymptomatic isolates on the growth of gerbils (*Meriones unguiculatus*). *Exp Parasitol* 2000;95:128–135.
122. Belosovic M, Faubert GM, MacLean JD. Disaccharidase activity in the small intestines of gerbils (*Meriones unguiculatus*) during primary and challenge infections with *Giardia lamblia. Gut* 1989;30:1213–1219.
123. Mohammed SR, Faubert GM. Disaccharidase deficiencies in Mongolian gerbils (*Meriones unguiculatus*) protected against *Giardia lamblia. Parasitol Res* 1995;81:582–590.
124. Hardin JA, Buret AG, Olson ME, et al. Mast cell hyperplasia and increased macromolecular uptake in an animal model of giardiasis. *J Parasitol* 1997;83:908–912.

125. Faubert G. Immune response to *Giardia duodenalis. Clin Microbiol Rev* 2000;13:35–54.
126. Farthing MJG, Mata L, Urrutia JJ, et al. Natural history of *Giardia* infection of infants and children in rural Guatemala and its impact on physical growth. *Am J Clin Nutr* 1986;43:393–403.
127. Istre GR, Dunlop TS, Gaspard B, et al. Waterborne giardiasis at a mountain resort: evidence for acquired immunity. *Am J Public Health* 1984;74:602–604.
128. Gillin FD, Reiner D, Wang CS. Human milk kills parasitic intestinal protozoa. *Science* 1983;221:1290–1292.
129. Gillin FD. *Giardia lamblia* the role of conjugated and unconjugated bile salts in killing by human milk. *Exp Parasitol* 1987;63: 74–83.
130. Rohrer L, Winterhalter KH, Eckert J, et al. Killing of *Giardia lamblia* by human milk is mediated by unsaturated fatty acids. *Antimicrob Agents Chemother* 1986;30:254–257.
131. Reiner DS, Wang CS, Gillin FD. Human milk kills *Giardia lamblia* by generating toxic lipolytic products. *J Infect Dis* 1986; 154:825–832.
132. Das S, Reiner DS, Zenian J, et al. Killing of *Giardia lamblia* trophozoites by human intestinal fluid *in vitro. J Infect Dis* 1988;157:1257–1260.
133. Aley S, Zimmerman M, Hetsko M, et al. Killing of *Giardia lamblia* by cryptidins and cationic neutrophil peptides. *Infect Immun* 1994;62:5397–5403.
134. Zinneman HH, Kaplan AP. The association of giardiasis with reduced intestinal secretory immunoglobulin A. *Am J Dig Dis* 1972;17:793–799.
135. Zenian AJ, Gillin FD. Intestinal mucus protects *Giardia lamblia* from killing by human milk. *J Protozool* 1987;34:22–26.
136. Eckmann L, Fabrice L, Langford DT, et al. Nitric oxide production by human intestinal epithelial cells and competition for arginine as potential determinants of host defense against the lumen-dwelling pathogen *Giardia lamblia. J Immunol* 2000; 164:1478–1487.
137. Ebert EC. *Giardia* induces proliferation and interferon γ production by intestinal lymphocytes. *Gut* 1999;44:342–346.
138. Rosekrans PCM, Lindeman J, Meijer CJLM. Quantitative histological and immunohistochemical findings in jejunal biopsy specimens in giardiasis. *Virch Arch Pathol Anat Histopathol* 1981;393:145–151.
139. Den Hollander N, Riley D, Befus D. Immunology of giardiasis. *Parasitol Today* 1988;4:124–131.
140. Owen RL, Allen CL, Stevens DP. Phagocytosis of *Giardia muris* by macrophages in Peyer's patch epithelium in mice. *Infect Immun* 1981;32:591–601.
141. Belosevic M, Faubert GM. Killing of *Giardia muris* trophozoites *in vitro* by spleen, mesenteric lymph node and peritoneal cells from susceptible and resistant mice. *Immunology* 1986;59: 267–275.
142. Guy RA, Bertrand S, Faubert GM. Modification of RPMI 1640 for use in *in vitro* immunological studies of host-parasite interactions in giardiasis. *J Clin Microbiol* 1991;29:627–629.
143. Halita M, Isaicu U. Reactia de fixare a complementului, in lambliaza intestinula. *Ardealul Med* 1946;6:154.
144. Hill DR, Burge JJ, Pearson RD. Susceptibility of *Giardia lamblia* trophozoites to the lethal effect of human serum. *J Immunol* 1984;132:2046–2052.
145. Farthing MJG, Goka AKJ, Butcher PD, et al. Serodiagnosis of giardiasis. *Serodiagn Immunother* 1987;1:233–238.
146. Gilman RH, Brown KH, Visvesvara GS, et al. Epidemiology and serology of *Giardia lamblia* in a developing country: Bangladesh. *Trans Royal Soc Trop Med Hyg* 1985;79:469–473.
147. Goka AKJ, Rolston DDK, Mathan VI, et al. Diagnosis of giardiasis by specific IgM antibody enzyme-linked immunosorbent assay. *Lancet* 1986;2:184–186.
148. Nash TE, Herrington DA, Losonsky GA, et al. Experimental human infections with *Giardia lamblia. J Infect Dis* 1987;156: 974–984.
149. Sullivan PB, Neale G, Cevallos AM, et al. Evaluation of specific serum anti-*Giardia* IgM antibody response in diagnosis of giardiasis. *Trans Royal Soc Trop Med Hyg* 1991;85:748–749.
150. Goka AKJ, Rolston DDK, Mathan VI, et al. Serum IgA response in human *Giardia lamblia* infection. *Serodiagn Immunother* 1989;3:273–277.
151. Farthing MJG, Chong S, Walker-Smith IA. Acute allergic phenomena in giardiasis. *Lancet* 1984;2:1428.
152. Popovic O, Pendic B, Paljm A, et al. Giardiasis: local immune defense and responses. *Eur Soc Clin Invest* 1974;4:380.
153. Briaud M, Morichau-Beauchant M, Matuchansky C, et al. Intestinal immune response in giardiasis. *Lancet* 1981;2:358.
154. Naik SR, Kumar U, Sehgal S, et al. Immunological studies in giardiasis. *Ann Trop Med Parasitol* 1979;73:291.
155. Speelman P, Ljungstrom I. Protozoal enteric infections among expatriates in Bangladesh. *Am J Trop Med* 1986;35:1140–1145.
156. Miotti PG, Gilmore RH, Pickering UK, et al. Prevalence of serum and milk antibodies to *Giardia lamblia* in different populations of lactating women. *J Infect Dis* 1985;152:1025–1031.
157. Van Egmond M, Damen CA, van Spriel AB, et al. IgA and the IgA Fc receptor. *Trends Immunol* 2001;22:205–211.
158. Moore GW, Sogandares-Bernal F, Dennis MV, et al. Characterization of *Giardia lamblia* trophozoite antigens using polyacrylamide gel electrophoresis, high-performance liquid chromatography, and enzyme-labeled immunosorbent assay. *Vet Parasitol* 1982;10:229–237.
159. Smith PD, Gillin FD, Kaushal NA, et al. Antigenic analysis of *Giardia lamblia* from Afghanistan, Puerto Rico, Ecuador and Oregon. *Infect Immun* 1982;36:714–719.
160. Wenman WM, Meuser RU, Wallis PM. Antigenic analysis of *Giardia duodenalis* strains isolated in Alberta. *Can J Microbiol* 1986;32:926–929.
161. Nash TE, Keister DB. Differences in excretory-secretory products and surface antigens among 19 isolates of *Giardia. J Infect Dis* 1985;152:1166–1171.
162. Einfeld DA, Stibbs HH. Identification and characterization of a major surface antigen of *Giardia lamblia. Infect Immun* 1984; 46:377–383.
163. Edson CM, Farthing MJG, Thorley-Lawson DA, et al. An 88,000-Mr *Giardia lamblia* surface protein which is immunogenic in humans. *Infect Immun* 1986;54:62l–625.
164. Crossley R, Holberton D. Assembly of 2.5nm filaments from giardin, a protein associated with cytoskeletal microtubules in *Giardia. J Cell Sci* 1985;78:205–231.
165. Lindley TA, Chakraborty PR, Edlind TD. Heat shock and stress response in *Giardia lamblia. Mol Biochem Parasitol* 1988;28: 135–144.
166. Reiner DS, Shinnick TM, Ardeshir F, et al. Encystation of *Giardia lamblia* leads to expression of antigens recognized by antibodies against conserved heat shock protein. *Infect Immun* 1992;60:5312–5315.
167. Crossley R, Holberton DV. Characterization of proteins from the cytoskeleton of *Giardia lamblia. J Cell Sci* 1983;59:81–103.
168. Nohria A, Alfonso RA, Peattie DA. Identification and characterization of γ-giardin and the γ-giardin gene from *Giardia lamblia. Mol Biochem Parasitol* 1992;56:27–38.
169. Nash TE, Aggarwal A, Adam RD, et al. Antigenic variation in *Giardia lamblia. J Immunol* 1988;141:636–641.
170. Adam RD, Aggarwal A, Lal AA, et al. Antigenic variation of a cysteine-rich protein in *Giardia lamblia. J Exp Med* 1988;167: 109–118.
171. Nash TE, Banks SM, Alling DW, et al. Frequency of variant antigens in *Giardia lamblia. Exp Parasitol* 1990;71:415–421.

172. Gillin FD, Diamond LS. *Entamoeba histolytica* and *Giardia lamblia:* effects of cysteine and oxygen tension on trophozoite attachment to glass and survival in culture media. *Exp Parasitol* 1981;52:9–17.
173. Gottstein B, Nash TE. Antigenic variation in *Giardia lamblia*: infection of congenitically athymic nude and SCID mice. *Parasite Immunol* 1991;13:649–659.
174. Aggarwal A, Nash TE. Antigenic variation of *Giardia lamblia in vivo. Infect Immun* 1988;56:1420–1423.
175. Kanwar SS, Ganguly NK, Walia BNS, et al. Direct and antibody dependent cell mediated cytotoxicity against *Giardia lamblia* by splenic and intestinal lymphoid cells in mice. *Gut* 1986; 27:73–77.
176. Deguchi M, Gillin FD, Gigli I. Mechanism of killing of *Giardia lamblia* trophozoites by complement. *J Clin Invest* 1987;79:1296–1302
177. Islam A. Giardiasis in developing countries. In: Meyer ED, ed. *Giardiasis.* Amsterdam, NY: Elsevier Science, 1990:236–266.
178. Dobell C. *A report on the occurrence of intestinal protozoa in the inhabitants of Britain.* Medical Research Council Special Report; 1921. Series No. 59.
179. Mason PR, Patterson BA. Epidemiology of *Giardia lamblia* infection in children: cross-sectional and longitudinal studies in urban and rural communities in Zimbabwe. *Am J Trop Med Hyg* 1987;37:277–282.
180. Oyerinde JPO, Ogunbi O, Alonge AA. Age and sex distribution of infections with *Entamoeba histolytica* and *Giardia intestinalis* in the Lagos population. *Int J Epidemiol* 1977;6:231–234.
181. Black RE, Dykes CA, Sinclair SP, et al. Giardiasis in day-care centers: evidence of person-to-person transmission. *Pediatrics* 1977;60:486–491.
182. White KE, Hedberg CW, Edmonson LM, et al. An outbreak of giardiasis in a nursing home with evidence for multiple modes of transmission. *J Infect Dis* 1989;160:298–304.
183. Keystone JS, Krajden S, Warren MR. Person-to-person transmission of *Giardia lamblia* in day-care nurseries. *Can Med Assoc J* 1978;119:241–248.
184. Sullivan PB, Marsh MN, Phillips MB, et al. Prevalence and treatment of giardiasis in chronic diarrhoea and malnutrition. *Arch Dis Child* 1991;66:304–306.
185. Ljungstrom I, Stoll B, Islam A. *Giardia* infection during pregnancy and lactation. *Trans Royal Soc Trop Med Hyg* 1987;81:161.
186. Stevens DP, Frank DM, Mahmoud AAF. Thymus dependency of host resistance to *Giardia muris* infection: studies in nude mice. *J Immunol* 1978;120:680–682.
187. Faubert GM, Litvinsky Y. Natural transmission of *Cryptosporidium parvum* between dams and calves on a dairy farm. *J Parasitol* 2000;86:495–500.
188. Fantham HB. Remarks on the nature and distribution of the parasites observed in the stools of 1,305 dysenteric patients. *Lancet* 1916;190:1165–1166.
189. Brandborg LL. Giardiasis and traveler's diarrhea. *Gastroenterology* 1980;78:1602–1614.
190. Speelman P, Ljungstrom I. Protozoal enteric infections among expatriates in Bangladesh. *Am J Trop Med* 1986;35:1140–1145
191. Moore GT, Cross WM, McGuire D, et al. Epidemic giardiasis at a ski resort. *N Engl J Med* 1969;281:402–407.
192. Isaac-Renton J, Moorehead W, Ross A. Longitudinal studies on *Giardia* contamination in two community drinking water supplies: cyst levels, parasite viability, and health impact. *Appl Environ Microbiol* 1996;62:47–54.
193. Ament ME, Rubin CE. Relation of giardiasis to abnormal intestinal structure and function in gastrointestinal syndrome. *Gastroenterology* 1972;62:216–226.
194. Boyd WP, Bachman BA. Gastrointestinal infections in the compromised host. *Med Clin North Am* 1982;66:743–753.
195. Webster ADB. Giardiasis and immunodeficiency diseases. *Trans Royal Soc Trop Med Hyg* 1980;74:440–443.
196. Zinneman HH, Kaplan AP. The association of giardiasis with reduced intestinal secretory immunoglobulin A. *Am J Dig Dis* 1972;17:793–799.
197. Chandra RK. Parasitic infection, nutrition, and immune response. *Fed Proc* 1984;43:251–255.
198. Janoff EN, Smith PD, Blaser MJ. Acute antibody responses to *Giardia lamblia* are depressed in patients with AIDS. *J Infect Dis* 1988;157:798–804.
199. Vinayak VK, Khanna R, Kum K. 1991. Kinetics of intraepithelium and lamina propria lymphocyte responses during *Giardia lamblia* infection in mice. *Microb Pathol* 1991;10:343–350.
200. Ruest N, Faubert GM, Couture Y. Prevalence and geographical distribution of *Giardia* spp. and *Cryptosporidium* spp. in dairy farms in Quebec. *Can Vet J* 1998;39:697–700.
201. Faubert GM. Is giardiasis a true zoonosis? *Parasitol Today* 1988; 4:66–71.
202. Buret A, denHollander N, Wallis PM, et al. Zoonotic potential of giardiasis in domestic ruminants. *J Infect Diseases* 1990;162: 231–237.
203. World Health Organization. *Parasitic zoonosis.* World Health Organization; 1979. Technical Report Series, No. 637.
204. Atwill EA, Sweitzer RA, Pereira M, et al. Prevalence of an associated risk factor for shedding *Cryptosporidium parvum* oocysts and *Giardia* cysts within feral pig population in California. *Appl Environ Microbiol* 1997;63:3946–3949.
205. O'Handley RM, Cockwill C, McAllister TA, et al. Duration of naturally acquired giardiasis and cryptosporidiosis in dairy calves and their association with diarrhea. *JAVMA* 1999;214: 391–396.
206. Wallis PM, Erlandsen SL, Isaac-Renton J, et al. Prevalence of *Giardia* cysts and *Cryptosporidium* oocysts and characterization of *Giardia* spp. isolated from drinking water in Canada. *Appl Environ Microbiol* 1996;62:2789–2797.
207. Cifuentes E, Gomez M, Blumenthal U, et al. Risk factors for *Giardia intestinalis* infection in agricultural villages practicing wastewater irrigation in Mexico. *Am J Trop Med Hyg* 2000;62: 388–392.
208. Goka AKI, Rolston DDK, Mathan VI, et al. The relative merits of faecal and duodenal juice microscopy in the diagnosis of giardiasis. *Trans Royal Soc Trop Med Hyg* 1990;84:66–67.
209. Rosoff ID, Stibbs HH. Isolation and identification of a *Giardia lamblia*-specific stool antigen (GSA 65) useful in coprodiagnosis of giardiasis. *J Clin Microbiol* 1986;23:905–910.
210. Rosoff ID, Sanders CA, Sanders SS, et al. Stool diagnosis of giardiasis using a commercially available enzyme immunoassay to detect *Giardia*-specific antigen 65 (GSA 65). *J Clin Microbiol* 1989;27:1997–2002.
211. Lindo JF, Levy VA, Baum MK, et al. Epidemiology of giardiasis and cryptosporidiosis in Jamaica. *Am J Trop Med Hyg* 1998; 59:717–721.
212. Behr MA, Kokoskin E, Gyorkos TW, et al. Laboratory diagnosis for *Giardia lamblia* infection: a comparison of microscopy, coprodiagnosis and serology. *Can J Infect Dis* 1997;8:33–38.
213. Katelaris PH, Farthing MJG. Diarrhoea and malabsorption in giardiasis: a multifactorial process. *Gut* 1992;33:295–297.
214. Desiree AT, Dorota K, Pang G, et al. *Giardia lamblia* rearranges F-actin and ?-actinin in human colonic and duodenal monolayers and reduces transepithelial electrical resistance. *J Parasitol* 2000;86:800–806.
215. Mohammed SR, Faubert GM. Purification of a fraction of *Giardia lamblia* trophozoite extract associated with disaccharidase deficiencies in immune gerbils (*Meriones unguiculatus*). *Parasite* 1995;2:31–39.
216. Buret A, Gall DG, Olson ME. Growth, activities of enzymes in

the small intestine and ultrastructure of the microvillus border in gerbils infected with *Giardia duodenalis. Parasitol Res* 1991; 77:109–114.
217. Buret A, Hardin JA, Olson ME, et al. Pathophysiology of small intestinal malabsorption in gerbils infected with *Giardia lamblia. Gastroenterology* 1992;103:506–513.
218. Oberhuber G, Kastner N, Stolte M. Giardiasis: a histologic analysis of 567 cases. *Scand J Gastroenterol* 1997;32:48–51.
219. Hoskins LC, Winawer SY, Broitman SA, et al. Clinical giardiasis and intestinal malabsorption. *Gastroenterology* 1967;53: 265–279.
220. Takano J, Yardley JH. Jejunal lesions in patients with giardiasis and malabsorption. An electron microscopic study. *Bull Johns Hopkins Hosp* 1965;116:413–429.
221. Morecki R, Parker JG. Ultrastructural studies of the human *Giardia lamblia* and subjacent jejunal mucosa in a subject with steatorrhea. *Gastroenterology* 1967;52:151–164.
222. Scott KGE, Logan MR, Klammer GM, et al. Jejunal brush border microvillus alterations in *Giardia muris*-infected mice: role of T lymphocytes and interleukin-6. *Infect Immun* 2000;68: 3412– 3418.
223. Wright SG, Tomkins AM, Ridley DS. Giardiasis: clinical and therapeutic aspects. *Gut* 1977;18:343–350.
224. Ducombe VM, Bolin TD, Davis AE, et al. Histopathology in giardiasis: a correlation with diarrhoea. *Aust N Z J Med* 1978;8: 392–396.
225. Brandborg LL, Tankersley CB, Gottlieb S, et al. Histological demonstration of mucosal invasion of *Giardia lamblia* in man. *Gastroenterol* 1967;52:143–150.
226. Saha TK, Ghosh TK. Invasion of small intestinal mucosa by *Giardia lamblia. Gastroenterology* 1977;72:402–405.
227. Erlandsen SL, Chase DG. Morphological alterations in the microvillus border of villous epithelial cells produced by intestinal micro-organisms. *Am J Clin Nutr* 1974;27:1277–1286.
228. Tandon BN, Tandon RK, Satpathy BK, et al. Mechanism of malabsorption in giardiasis: a study of bacterial flora and bile salt deconjugation in upper jejunum. *Gut* 1977;18:176–181.
229. Tomkins AM, Drasar BS, Bradley AK, et al. Bacterial colonization of jejunal mucosa in giardiasis. *Trans Royal Soc Trop Med Hyg* 1978;72:33–36.
230. Gupta RK, Mehta S. Giardiasis in children: a study of pancreatic functions. *Indian J Med Res* 1973;61:743–748.
231. Chawla LS, Sehgal AK, Broor SL, et al. Tryptic activity in the duodenal aspirate following a standard test meal in giardiasis. *Scand J Gastroenterol* 1975;10:445–447.
232. Okada M, Fuchigami T, Ri S, et al. The BTPABA pancreatic function test in giardiasis. *Postgrad Med J* 1983;59:79–82.
233. Smith PD, Horsburgh CR, Brown WR. *In vitro* studies on bile acid deconjugation and lipolysis inhibition by *Giardia lamblia. Dig Dis Sci* 1981;26:700–704.
234. Katelaris PH, Seow F, Ngu MC. The effect of *Giardia lamblia* trophozoites on lipolysis *in vitro. Parasitology* 1991;103:35–39.
235. Seow F, Katelaris PH, Ngu M. The effect of *Giardia lamblia* trophozoites on trypsin, chymotrypsin and amylase *in vitro. Parasitology* 1993;106:233–238.
236. Jimenez JC, Uzcanga G, Zambrano A, et al. identification and partial characterization of excretory/secretory products with proteolytic activity in *Giardia intestinalis. J Parasitol* 2000;86:859–862.
237. Que X, Reed SL. Cysteine proteinases and the pathogenesis of amebiasis. *Clin Microbiol Rev* 2000;3:196–206.
238. Backer HD. Giardiasis: an elusive case of gastrointestinal distress. *Phys Sportsmed* 2000;28:46–57.
239. Brodsky RE, Spencer HC, Schultz MG. Giardiasis in American travelers to the Soviet Union. *J Infect Dis* 1974;130:319–323.
240. Moore GT, Cross WM, McGuire D, et al. Epidemic giardiasis at a ski resort. *N Engl J Med* 1969;281:402–407.
241. Homan WL, Mank TG. Human giardiasis: genotype linked differences in clinical symptomology. *Int J Parasitol* 2001;31: 822–826.
242. Farthing MJG. *Giardia lamblia.* In: Blaser J, Smith PD, Ravdin JI, et al. *Infections of the gastrointestinal tract.* New York, NY: Raven Press, 1995:1081–1105.
243. Tolboom JJM. Milk intolerance due to lactose and giardiasis. *Am J Clin Nutr* 1988;48:178–179.
244. Mantovani MP, Guandalini S, Ecuba P, et al. Lactose malabsorption in children with symptomatic *Giardia lamblia* infection: feasibility of yogurt supplementation. *J Pediatr Gastroenterol Nutr* 1989;9:295–300.
245. Pickering LK, Woodward WE, Du Pont HL, et al. Occurrence of *Giardia lamblia* in children in day care centers. *J Pediatr* 1984;104:522–536.
246. Ish-Horowicz M, Korman SH, Shapiro M, et al. Asymptomatic giardiasis in children. *Pediatr Infect Dis J* 1989;8:773–779.
247. Lunn PG, Erinoso HO, Northrop-Clewes CA, et al. Giardia intestinalis is unlikely to be a major cause of the poor growth of rural Gambian infants. *J Nutr* 1998;129:872–877.
248. Webster ADB, Kenwright S, Ballard J, et al. Nodular lymphoid hyperplasia of the bowel in primary hypogammaglobulinaemia. *Gut* 1977;18:364–372.
249. Ajdukiewicz AB, Youngs GR, Bouchier IAD. Nodular lymphoid hyperplasia and hypogammaglobulinaemia. *Gut* 1972; 13:589–595.
250. Nagura H, Kohler PF, Brown WR. Immunocytochemical characterisation of lymphocytes in nodular lymphoid hyperplasia of the bowel. *Lab Invest* 1979;40:66.
251. Di Prisco MC, Hagel I, Lynch NR, et al. Association between giardiasis and allergy. *Ann Allergy Asthma Immunol* 1998;81: 261– 265.
252. Barraquer I. Sur la coincidence de la lambliase et de certains lesions du fond de l'oeil. *Bull Soc Pathol Exot (Paris)* 1938;31: 55–58.
253. Knox DL, King J. Retinal arteritis, iridocyclitis and giardiasis. *Ophthalmology* 1982;89:133–139.
254. Pettoello-Mantovani M, Giardino I, Magli A, et al. Intestinal giardiasis associated with ophthalmologic changes. *J Pediatr Gastroenterol Nutr* 1990;11:196–200.
255. Corsi A, Nucci C, Knafelz D, et al. Ocular changes associated with *Giardia lamblia* infection in children. *Br J Ophthal* 1998; 82:59–62.
256. Davidson RA. Issues in clinical parasitology: the treatment of giardiasis. *Am J Gastroenterol* 1984;79:256–261.
257. Gardner TB, Hill DR. Treatment of giardiasis. *Clin Microbiol Rev* 2001;14:114–128.
258. Paget TA, Jarroll EL, Manning P, et al. Respiration in the cysts and trophozoites of *Giardia muris. J Gen Microbiol* 1989;135: 145–154.
259. Mendelson R. The treatment of giardiasis. *Trans Royal Soc Trop Med* 1980;74:438–439.
260. Schofield PJ, Edwards MR, Kranz P. Glucose metabolism in *Giardia lamblia. Mol Biochem Parasitol* 1991;45:39–48.
261. Crouch AA, Seow WK, Thong YH. Effect of twenty-three chemotherapeutic agents on the adherence and growth of *Giardia lamblia in vitro. Trans Royal Soc Trop Med Hyg* 1986;80: 893–896.
262. Gascon J, Abos R, Valls ME, et al. Mebendazole and metronidazole in giardial infections. *Trans Royal Soc Trop Med Hyg* 1990;84:694.
263. Meloni BP, Thompson RCA, Reynoldson JA, et al. Albendazole: a more effective anti-giardial agent *in vitro* than metronidazole or tinidazole. *Trans Royal Soc Trop Med Hyg* 1990;84: 375–379.
264. Al Waili NSD, Hasan NU. Mebendazole in giardial infections:

a comparative study with metronidazole. *J Infect Dis* 1992;165: 1170–1171.
265. Abboud P, Lemee V, Gargala G, et al. Successful treatment of metronidazole- and albendazole-resistant giardiasis with nitazoxanide in a patient with acquired immunodeficiency syndrome. *Clin Infect Dis* 2001;32:1792– 1794.
266. Nash TE, Ohl CA, Thomas E, et al. Treatment of patients with refractory giardiasis. *Clin Infect Dis* 2001;33:22–28.
267. Cacopardo BI, Patamia V, Bonaccorso O, et al. Efficacia sinergica dell'associazione albendazole-metronidazolo nella giardiasi refrattaria a monoterapia con metronidazolo. *Clin Ter* 1995; 146:761–767.
268. Gillin FD, Diamond LS. Inhibition of clonal growth of *Giardia lamblia* and *Entamoeba histolytica* by metronidazole, quinacrine and other antimicrobial agents. *J Antimicrob Chemother* 1981;8: 305–316.
269. Boreham PF, Phillips RE, Shepherd RW. The sensitivity of *Giardia intestinalis* to drugs *in vitro. J Antimicrob Chemother* 1984;14:449–461.
270. Gordts B, Hemelhof W, Asselman C, et al. *In vitro* susceptibility of 25 *Giardia lamblia* isolates of human origin to six commonly used anti-protozoal agents. *Antimicrob Agents Chemother* 1985;28:378–380.
271. Hoyne GF, Boreham PFL, Parsons PG, et al. The effect of drugs on the cell cycle of *Giardia intestinalis. Parasitology* 1989;99: 333–339.
272. Inge PMG, Farthing MJG. A radiometric assay for anti-giardial drugs. *Trans Royal Soc Trop Med Hyg* 1987;81:345–347.
273. Sousa MC, Poiares-da-Silva J. A new method for assessing metronidazole susceptibility of Giardia lamblia trophozoites. *Antimicrob Agents Chemother* 1999;43:2939–2942.
274. Farthing MJG. Immunopathology of giardiasis. *Springer Semin Immunopathol* 1990;12:269–282.
275. Farthing MJG, Mata L, Urrutia JJ, et al. Natural history of *Giardia* infection of infants and children in rural Guatemala and its impact on physical growth. *Am J Clin Nutr* 1986;43: 393–403.
276. Udezulu IA, Visvesvara GS, Moss DM, et al. Isolation of two *Giardia lamblia* (WB strain) clones with distinct surface protein and antigenic profiles and differing infectivity and virulence. *Infect Immun* 1992;60:2274–2280.
277. Olson ME, Ceri H, Morck DW. *Giardia* vaccination. *Parasitol Today* 2000;16:213–217.
278. Faubert GM. The immune response to *Giardia. Parasitol Today* 1996;12:140–145.
279. Yanke SJ, Ceri H, McAllister TA, et al. Serum immune response to *Giardia duodenalis* in experimentally infected lambs. *Vet Parasitol* 1998;75:9–19.

62

CRYPTOSPORIDIUM

CHARLES R. STERLING
RICHARD L. GUERRANT

Cryptosporidium parvum is a small intracellular protozoan parasite that has become the focus of increased attention. Recognized as a veterinary pathogen since the early 1970s, widespread interest in this organism as a human pathogen was fueled by patients with AIDS and other immunosuppressed patients, in whom it causes a debilitating chronic diarrhea. We now know, however, that it is also an important cause of diarrheal illness in immunocompetent people, and it is increasingly recognized as a cause of diarrhea in children in developing areas worldwide and as a troublesome waterborne pathogen.

HISTORICAL ASPECTS

In 1907, Tyzzer (1) described a new protozoan genus that he identified in the gastric epithelium of laboratory mice and named *Cryptosporidium.* The name *Cryptosporidium,* meaning "hidden spore" in Greek, reflects the unusual absence of sporocysts surrounding the sporozoites. In 1912, he identified and named *C. parvum* (2). Until recently, *Cryptosporidium* species were mainly of interest to the veterinary profession as etiologic agents of avian and bovine diarrheal disease. However, in 1976, infections in humans were first reported in an immunocompetent child with enterocolitis in whom it was diagnosed by rectal biopsy (3) and in an adult with bullous pemphigoid treated with cyclophosphamide and prednisolone (4). With an additional six case reports over the ensuing 5 years, including five patients with immune compromise (one with congenital hypogammaglobulinemia and one with immunoglobulin A [IgA] deficiency), only eight human cases (six immunocompromised) were reported before 1982 (5–10). Nevertheless, it was not until the advent of AIDS that the medical profession really took notice of this organism (11) and later considered it an AIDS-defining illness (12). Most of our knowledge of the clinical significance and presentation, pathogenesis, epidemiology, and treatment of cryptosporidial infection has been accumulated in the last two decades.

C. R. Sterling: Department of Veterinary Science and Microbiology, University of Arizona, Tucson, Arizona

R. L. Guerrant: Department of Medicine, University of Virginia School of Medicine; Division of Geographic Medicine, University of Virginia Hospital, Charlottesville, Virginia

MICROBIOLOGY

Taxonomy

The early belief that *Cryptosporidium* was host specific led to the naming of numerous species according to the host from which they were described. At least 23 species have been reported (13,14). Studies involving cross-transmission and more careful morphometric analysis, however, have either invalidated species distinctions or placed the validity of many in doubt. The *Cryptosporidium* species currently recognized as valid by many researchers include *Cryptosporidium muris* from mice and cattle, *C. parvum* from a wide variety of mammalian species including humans, *Cryptosporidium wrairi* from guinea pigs, *Cryptosporidium felis* from cats, *Cryptosporidium baileyi* from chickens, *Cryptosporidium meleagridis* from turkeys, *Cryptosporidium serpentis* from snakes, and *Cryptosporidium nasorum* from a fish (13–15). Recent genetic studies, based on analysis of small subunit ribosomal RNA sequences confirms at least four *Cryptosporidium* species: *C. muris, C. serpentis, C. baileyi,* and *C. parvum* (16–18) (Fig. 62.1). The other four listed above are considered species by biologic characteristics, clustered together or within different *C. parvum* isolates. This work suggests that a revision in the taxonomy of *Cryptosporidium* species may be warranted. Within the taxon *C. parvum,* it has become clear that two distinct genotypes exist (16–28). One genotype, type 1, is confined to human infections, whereas the other genotype, type 2, is found mostly in domestic and farm animals but also has been associated with human infections (29,30).

C. parvum is the primary species responsible for producing infection and disease in humans. There is one report of

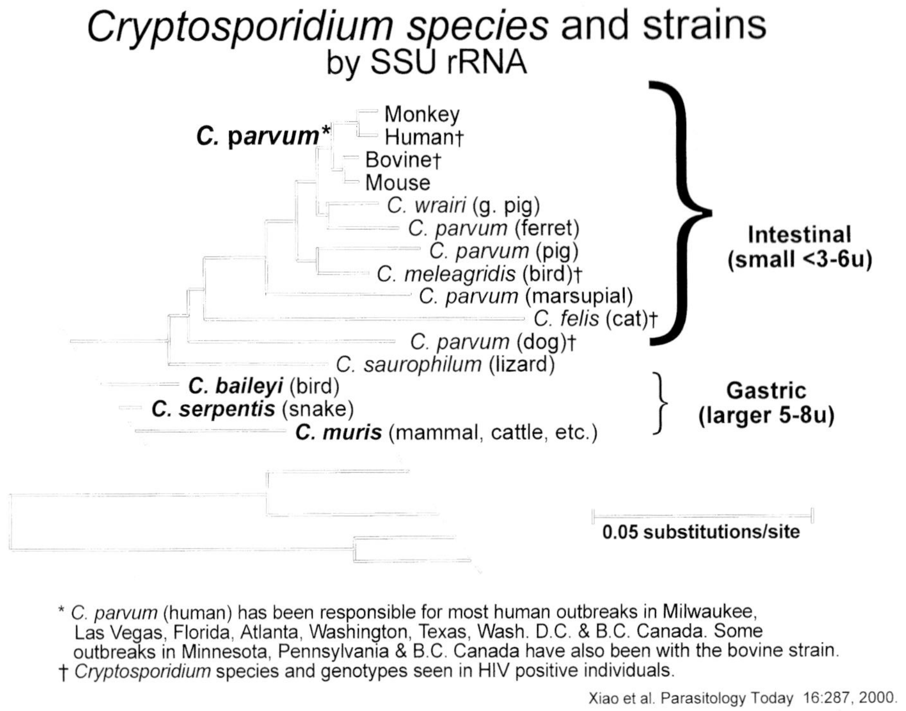

FIGURE 62.1. Recent genetic studies, based on analysis of small subunit rRNA sequences confirms at least 4 Cryptosporidium species: *C. muris, C. serpentis, C. baileyi,* and *C. parvum* (16–18). **C. parvum* (human) has been responsible for most human outbreaks in Milwaukee, Las Vegas, Florida, Atlanta, Washington, Texas, Wash. D.C., and B.C. Canada. Some outbreaks in Minnesota, Pennsylvania, and B.C. Canada have also been with the bovine strain. *Cryptosporidium* species and genotypes seen in HIV positive individuals. From Xiao et al. Cryptosporidium systematics and implications for public health. *Parasitol Today* 2000;16:287–292.

C. baileyi infecting an immunodeficient individual (31), but the parasite's identity was subsequently questioned after base sequence and polymerase chain reaction (PCR) analysis showed it to be *C. parvum* (32). Recent molecular characterization of *Cryptosporidium* isolated from patients with AIDS in the United States, Kenya, and Switzerland and from children in Peru have demonstrated the presence of non-*C. parvum* cryptosporidial parasites (*C. felis, C. meleagridis,* and a *Cryptosporidium* genotype from dogs), underscoring zoonotic transmission (33–35). Both *C. felis* and *C. meleagridis* have recently been shown to be genetically related to *C. parvum,* thereby raising questions about the taxonomic designation of these species (18). The advances being made by PCR and sequencing techniques will help define the significance of the genetic diversity within *C. parvum* and determine whether non-*parvum Cryptosporidium* species and other genotypes of *C. parvum* are infectious to humans.

Life Cycle And Morphology

The oocyst is the final development stage in the life cycle of *Cryptosporidium* and can be found in the feces of an infected host. It must be ingested or inhaled to initiate infection of a new susceptible host (Fig. 62.2). Oocysts of *C. parvum* measure 4 to 6 μm in diameter and are fully sporulated (contain four free, fully developed, and infectious sporozoites) when they leave their host.

Approximately 80% of the oocysts formed within an infected host are thick walled. This oocyst population constitutes the environmentally resistant infectious forms that must find their way into a new host to initiate infection. The remaining 20% are referred to as thin-walled oocysts and are only rarely encountered within the feces of an infected host. These forms, which are enveloped by a single limiting membrane and can excyst spontaneously within the intestine or at extraintestinal sites, presumably account for the persistent infections frequently encountered in immunocompromised hosts (36).

Upon ingestion, oocysts must undergo a process of excystation (release of infective sporozoites) for the life cycle to continue. This necessary step usually occurs in the environment of the small intestine of a susceptible host (37). Exposure to reducing conditions, enzymes, and bile salts are all important contributors to this process within the host. The process of excystation results from the dissolution of a suture at one end of the oocyst wall. Sporozoites then escape through the opening created by the breakdown of this suture (38).

Newly excysted sporozoites must attach to and invade appropriate susceptible host cells to initiate the ensuing asexual merogonic cycle. Enterocytes of the terminal ileum appear to be preferentially invaded by *C. parvum* sporozoites in many mammalian hosts. In addition, parasite development has been reported at such extraintestinal sites as the conjunctiva of the eye and within cells of the respiratory and biliary tree of immune compromised human hosts. *Cryptosporidium* sporozoites are unique among the Coccidia because they invade cells only to the level of the extracytoplasmic compartment beneath the infected cell's outer limiting membrane.

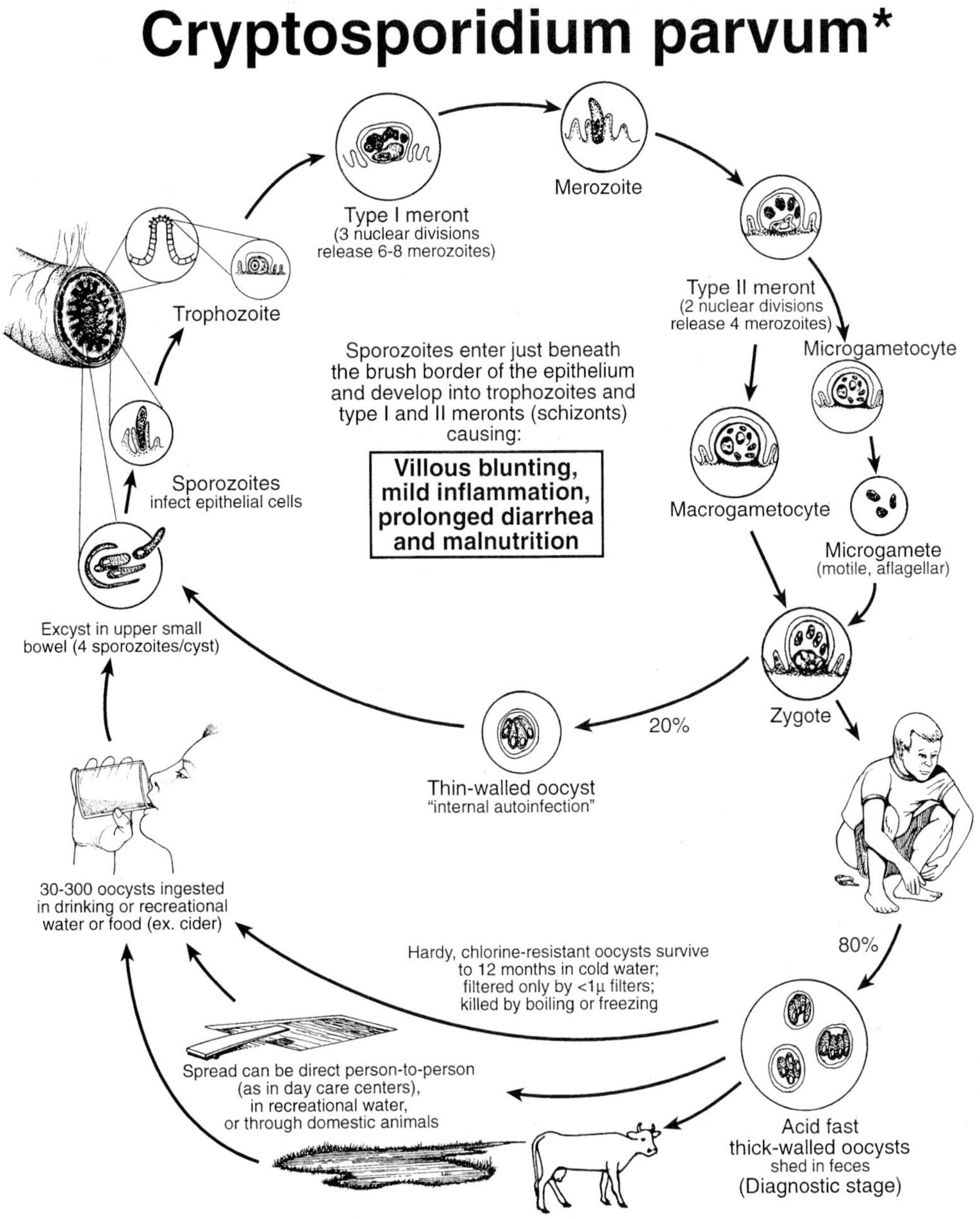

FIGURE 62.2. Reservoirs and routes of spread of *Cryptosporidium.* *Although less is known about the life cycles of *Cyclospora* and *Isospora*, both penetrate into epithelial cytoplasm and both *Cyclospora* and *Isospora* (which are larger), unlike *Cryptosporidium*, require development outside the host, and thus lack the same risk for secondary person-to-person spread. All three are acid fast. From Steinar TS Pape JW, Guerrant RL. Interstitial coccidial infections. In: Guerrant RL, Walter DH, and Weller IVD, eds. *Tropical infectious diseases: principles, pathogens & practice.* Churchill Livingston, 1999:721–735.

Sporozoite attachment and subsequent internalization have been described in detail (39). The process is very much like that described for cell invasion by malaria and other Apicomplexa parasites. Sporozoite probing and the release of contents from apical end organelles (rhoptries and micronemes) presumably cause an indentation and folding of the host cell limiting membrane, which ultimately encompasses the parasite within a parasitophorous vacuole of host cell origin. Membrane junctions form at the vacuole base nearest the sporozoite apical end and this region ultimately differentiates into a complex "feeder organelle." The membranous folds of this organelle tremendously increase the available surface area between host cell and parasite, possibly to facilitate the exchange of materials. Recently, a parasite-encoded transport protein has been localized at this interface (40).

Each sporozoite that has successfully invaded a cell dedifferentiates and rounds up within the parasitophorous vacuole to become a uninucleate trophozoite. Trophozoites undergo a complex cycle of growth and differentiation (merogony) to become type I meronts with six to eight merozoites. Studies in mice indicate that this process occurs between 8 and 16 hours after infection (41). Type I meronts persist throughout an infection and likely contribute to the severity of disease manifested in patients with AIDS.

Type I meronts rupture, releasing six to eight merozoites to invade adjacent susceptible host cells. Parasites developing from these merozoites can become type I meronts again or type II meronts. The latter have been described from animals 24 hours after the infection. The persistence of type II meronts seen in infections is presumably the result of a cycle involving the continued production of auto-infective thin-walled oocysts and type I meronts. Four merozoites are produced in type II meronts and presumably are destined only to become gamonts. Merozoites of type I and type II meronts are morphologically similar and measure approximately 5.0 × 1.0 μm.

Merozoites from type II meronts invade host cells to become microgamonts (male) or macrogamonts (female); most differentiate into the latter. Gamonts have been seen at 36 (microgamont) and 48 (macrogamont) hours after the infection of animals.

Microgamonts show a more extensive nuclear division than that observed in meronts, and as many as 16 nuclei have been observed. These migrate to the periphery of the microgamont cytoplasm and bud to form the bullet-shaped microgametes, which measure about 1.4 × 0.4 μm. Fertilization with ensuing zygote formation occurs when microgametes attach to and fuse with mature macrogametes.

Zygotes develop into either thick-walled or thin-walled oocysts having four naked sporozoites. The process of sporogony is similar to that of merogony, except that the first nuclear division is meiotic, restoring the haploid genomic complement of sporozoites. Sporulated oocysts can be observed in infected animals at 72 hours and subsequently during the course of an infection (41). Factors that influence the development of the two discrete oocyst forms are unknown. Sporozoites are structurally similar to merozoites, except they possess a more tapered anterior end, centrally located amylopectin granules, and a posteriorly situated nucleus.

Cultivation

The complete growth and development of *C. parvum* apart from animals of its normal host range have been accomplished using *in ovo* and *in vitro* cultivation systems. In the former, inoculation of purified sporozoites from calf and human isolates of *C. parvum* into the chorioallantoic membrane (CAM) of chicken embryos results in parasite multiplication in endoderm cells with the eventual release of oocysts into the chorioallantoic fluid (42).

Parasite development in eggs appears similar to what has been reported in the ileum of experimentally infected neonatal mice. Drawbacks to the use of eggs are that not all eggs from different types or even the same type of chicken are equally susceptible to infection, and that oocysts are not easily released from the CAM into the chorioallantoic fluid, making large-scale recovery difficult.

The *in vitro* development of *C. parvum* has been accomplished within various epithelial-like cell lines. The most successful host cell lines include human Caco-2, RL95-2, HT-29.74, HCT-8, and canine MDCK (43). In comparative studies, parasite yields were best in HCT-8 and MDCK cell lines (44,45). Improvements to medium formulation have been made such that up to 10-fold enhancement of growth *in vitro* can be accomplished (46). Claims of complete development from sporozoite to infectious oocyst *in vitro* have been made but have been difficult to reproduce. It has been hypothesized that a major reason for this lies in the inability of the parasite to produce thin-walled auto-infective oocysts *in vitro* (47).

EPIDEMIOLOGY

Transmission Routes

Cryptosporidium species are ubiquitous and infect a wide variety of hosts, from fish, reptiles, and birds to rodents, primates, and other mammals (37,48). Human infections are primarily due to *C. parvum,* a species that is infectious for most mammals and that is particularly prevalent in ruminants. Calves are a source of human infection (49–56) and contact with farm animals is frequently reported in sporadic cases (57–60). Other animal species also believed to be important as potential reservoirs include rodents, sheep (59,61,62), and house pets such as cats and dogs, particularly kittens and puppies (63–69). Many infections are therefore the result of zoonotic transmission. Person-to-person transmission from fecal-oral spread is an important means of transmission in urban settings (70), day care centers, nosocomial outbreaks, and between family members, and there is evidence for transmission during male homosexual intercourse (71,72). *Cryptosporidium* infection is becoming more prominent in the differential diagnosis of traveler's diarrhea. Additional transmission routes of this parasite to humans have been suggested through studies of the ability of marine and freshwater bivalves and house flies to concentrate and serve as transport hosts for viable oocysts (73–77).

The 1993 waterborne outbreak of diarrheal illness in Wisconsin, with an estimated 403,000 cases of diarrhea over the span of 2 months (78,79), of which more than 600 were confirmed cases of cryptosporidiosis, provides another unfortunate reminder that routine chlorination of drinking water is relatively ineffective at killing the *Cryptosporidium* oocysts. They are several-fold more resistant to disinfectants than *Giardia lamblia* cysts, and because of their small size, they may not be completely filtered by routine filtering devices (80) or totally removed by activated sludge treatment of sewage (81,82). Outbreaks of swimming pool-associated cryptosporidiosis are further evidence of the highly infective nature of the organism and its resistance to disinfection and filtering (83–85). Waterborne outbreaks are being documented with increasing frequency (86–96). Many of these have been attributed to errors in the handling of filtering systems of water purification plants or to raw sewage and agricultural runoff contaminating surface waters not being filtered. The detection of *Cryptosporidium* oocysts in water samples is obviously an important issue. It is far more difficult than detection in stool, but as more sensitive techniques are developed, the prevalence of *Cryptosporidium* oocysts in drinking water and the environment is becoming increasingly recognized (80,81,97–103). Immunomagnetic separation has replaced differential centrifugation techniques as a means to enhance oocyst concentration from water samples and combined PCR–restriction fragment length polymorphism techniques have permitted the development of species- and strain-specific tools that might be used to identify *Cryptosporidium* from these samples (16,104–108).

The interplay of environmental reservoirs and hosts of *Cryptosporidium* is complex and the interactions and transmission patterns are only beginning to be understood. Interestingly, type I *C. parvum* infections from humans do not appear to be transmissible to most other mammalian hosts (23).

Demographics

Cryptosporidium is associated with diarrheal illness in most areas of the world. Numerous studies have documented its presence in more than 40 countries spanning all six continents. Prevalence rates in patients with diarrhea have varied from as low as 1% in Europe and North America to up to 30% on other continents. If one pools data from multiple studies, an average of 6.1% of diarrheal illnesses in developing countries are due to *Cryptosporidium,* compared with 2.1% in developed countries (Table 62.1) (109). The prevalence in control patients averages 1.5% and 0.2% in developing countries and developed countries, respectively, suggesting that asymptomatic infections occur. Serologic studies confirm these results, with a higher seroprevalence in developing countries than in developed countries (110). An asymptomatic carrier state has now been clearly demonstrated in numerous patients. One study from the United States reports a prevalence of 12.7% in immunocompetent patients undergoing routine upper endoscopy (111). In Peru, where infections are commonly encountered in children in the 1- to 5-year-old age-group, as many as 63% were found to be asymptomatic in one study (112).

Developing Countries

In poorly developed regions where standards of sanitation and water treatment technology are low and crowded living conditions predominate, the prevalence of cryptosporidiosis is much higher. Although less than 20% of persons acquire serologic evidence of cryptosporidiosis by young adulthood in developed areas, less-developed areas have seroprevalence rates that exceed 60% by 10 years of life in China and 95% by 2 years of life in northeastern Brazil (113). There is often a seasonal pattern of increased infections during warmer and rainy seasons (67,114–123), although other studies have found an increased prevalence during the dry and warm season (48,124–126). Other risk factors include weaning, crowding, lower birth weight, and younger age (<2 years); and breast-feeding seems to have a protective effect, with significantly lower rates of cryptosporidiosis in breast-fed infants (115,117,118,120, 127–136). Despite earlier speculations, the transfer of passive immunity via milk to the infant is apparently not the mechanism responsible for the lower incidence rate (137). Decreased exposure to the parasite in breast-fed infants may be a potential explanation. In a Peruvian study, both symptomatic and asymptomatic infections with cryptosporidia were shown to have an adverse effect on weight gain during the first month of infection; the effect being less severe for the asymptomatic individuals. Anthropometric data from these children established that a growth faltering occurred several months after infection, followed by a period of catch-up growth. Younger children took longer to catch up than older children, whereas those infected between age 0

TABLE 62.1. FREQUENCIES OF *CRYPTOSPORIDIUM* INFECTION IN PRESUMABLY IMMUNOCOMPETENT PATIENTS WITH SPORADIC DIARRHEAL ILLNESS AND CONTROLS FROM 43 STUDIES IN DEVELOPING COUNTRIES (ASIA, AFRICA, AND LATIN AMERICA) AND 35 STUDIES IN DEVELOPED COUNTRIES (EUROPE, NORTH AMERICA, AND AUSTRALIA)

Area	*Cryptosporidium* Cases/ Total Diarrhea Patients Screened (% Positive)	Positive Controls/ Total Control Patients Screened (% Positive)
Developing countries	1,486/24,269 (6.1%)	61/4,146 (1.5%)
Developed countries	2,232/107,329 (2.1%)	3/1,941 (0.15%)

TABLE 62.2. FREQUENCIES OF *CRYPTOSPORIDIUM* INFECTION IN HIV-POSITIVE PATIENTS WITH DIARRHEA AND HIV-POSITIVE CONTROLS WITHOUT DIARRHEA FROM 9 STUDIES IN DEVELOPING COUNTRIES (AFRICA AND LATIN AMERICA) AND 13 STUDIES IN DEVELOPED COUNTRIES (EUROPE, NORTH AMERICA, AND AUSTRALIA)

Area	*Cryptosporidium* Cases/ Total Diarrhea Patients Screened (% Positive)	Positive Controls/ Total Control Patients Screened (% Positive)
Developing countries	120/503 (24%)	5/101 (5%)
Developed countries	148/1,074 (13.8%)	0/35

and 5 months, or already stunted, did not catch up at 1-year postinfection. This study suggests that *Cryptosporidium* infection at an early age may have a lasting affect on linear growth (138). Furthermore, studies in northeast Brazil show that cryptosporidiosis in young children predisposes to protracted periods of increased diarrheal illnesses and growth shortfalls (139), as well as to long-term deficits in physical fitness and cognitive function (140). There is a significant association of cryptosporidiosis with malnutrition and a higher mortality rate.

Patients in developing countries who have AIDS have a higher incidence of chronic diarrhea than patients with AIDS in developed countries and seem to have a higher rate (up to 48%) of *Cryptosporidium* infection as the etiology of their diarrhea (Table 62.2) (109).

Developed Countries

In the immunocompetent host in developed countries, disease outbreaks have been reported in day care centers (141–154), veterinary students and animal caretakers (49,50,155–158), and health care workers. Rates of infection during outbreaks in day care centers may reach as high as 43%, with significant secondary spread in family contacts (144,151). Asymptomatic cryptosporidiosis in day care centers has also been reported (159–161). A report of a nosocomial outbreak described serologic evidence for the transmission of *Cryptosporidium* to 31% of hospital personnel who came in contact with an infected patient with diarrhea (162). Other nosocomial outbreaks have been documented, some in immunocompromised patients and patients with AIDS (162–168). *Cryptosporidium* is becoming an increasingly recognized cause of traveler's diarrhea in people traveling to areas with an increased prevalence of cryptosporidiosis (169–182). It is also the etiologic organism in sporadic cases in patients with gastroenteritis (145), and children are again most vulnerable (183,184), with transmission to other family members (141,151,170,185).

In the immunocompromised host, most cases of cryptosporidiosis are being reported in patients with AIDS, in whom it is being recognized as a leading cause of chronic diarrhea (186–193). Data derived before the introduction of highly active antiretroviral therapy (HAART) in HIV-infected individuals suggested that up to 15% of patients with AIDS in the United States were infected with *Cryptosporidium* (187–189), with homosexual men having higher rates of infection than heterosexual patients (71). Since HAART, morbidity and mortality rates due to opportunistic infections and *Cryptosporidium* specifically have declined significantly (194–196). Other patient populations, however, are also at increased risk, such as patients with various forms of hypogammaglobulinemia including selective IgA deficiency (8,9,197–202), patients taking corticosteroids and other immunosuppressive agents (4,203), patients with malignancies or undergoing chemotherapy (64,204–212), organ transplant recipients (10,312–215), and bone marrow transplant recipients (166,167,207,209, 216–219).

PATHOLOGY AND PATHOGENESIS

Pathologic manifestations of cryptosporidiosis appear to be similar in all infected animal species and are largely a function of where infection occurs. In immunocompetent hosts, parasite replication is principally confined to the apical border of enterocytes in the lower jejunum and ileum. The entire gastrointestinal (GI) tract, as well as ancillary extraintestinal sites including biliary and pancreatic ducts and portions of the respiratory tract, may become infected in immunocompromised hosts. Mild to severe intestinal villous atrophy is observed. Villous stunting, broadening, and fusion may occur (7,10). Inflammation, accompanied by plasma cell, neutrophil, macrophage, and lymphocyte infiltration into the subepithelial lamina propria, has been noted (4,7). Crypts may appear enlarged and hyperplastic and Peyer patches appear reactive (220,221). At the ultrastructural level, infected cells lack microvilli at the site of parasite attachment and the cytoplasm may appear excessively vacuolated. Mitochondria may also appear swollen and vacuolated (4,222). Similar changes are seen in epithelial cells of the respiratory tree and may be accompanied by hypertrophy, loss of cilia, and excess mucus production.

Pathogenic mechanisms operative during cryptosporidiosis still remain poorly defined. Much of what has been learned has come from animal models. Malabsorption in both the small and large intestine and impaired digestion in the small intestine underlie diarrhea in germ-free calves infected with *C.*

parvum (223). Similar malabsorption, involving impairment to glucose-stimulated sodium and water absorption and/or increased chloride secretion, has been reported in neonatal pig models of infection (224,225). D-Xylose and vitamin B_{12} malabsorption has been described in infected patients with AIDS (226). In addition, permeability defects and decreased resistance across *C. parvum*-infected cell lines indicate that alterations to barrier properties and intercellular junctional complexes may contribute to the observed diarrhea (227,228). The end result may include bacterial overgrowth, osmotic pressure changes across the gut wall, and an excessive release of fluid into the intestinal lumen (229). The often described cholera-like diarrhea also suggests enterotoxin-like activity. Such activity, which has been reported in cell-free extracts from *C. parvum*-infected tissue (230), has not been confirmed by others (231). Additional studies demonstrate enterotoxic activity on human jejunum by stool filtrates from infected calves (232). Whether this effect is of host or parasite origin remains unclear (233).

Alterations in cellular enzyme activities also have been noted in association with *C. parvum* infections. Marked reductions in the brush border enzymes lactase and alkaline phosphatase have been reported from infected athymic rats (234). Decreases in these enzyme levels, along with sucrase, have been observed in neonatal pig models of infection (231). Lactase deficiency, along with xylose malabsorption, has been reported from infected calves (235). Epithelial barrier dysfunction, which is the site of parasite replication, is documented but may involve transcellular and paracellular pathways (233,236).

IMMUNITY

Overview Of Animal Models

On the basis of clinical data from humans and experimental data from animals, a role for both humoral and cellular responses in resolving *C. parvum* infections has been accepted (113). Several reports note that either hypogammaglobulinemic or anergic patients have presented with severe protracted diarrhea with *Cryptosporidium* infection (4,8,197,198). Animal models, particularly those using mice of different strains and genetic backgrounds, have focused largely on the role of cell-mediated responses. The use of athymic (237), CD4 (helper T cell), and interferon-γ (IFNγ)-depleted (238,239), severe combined immunodeficient (SCID) (240–242), and murine retrovirus-infected (243) mouse models and the use of an athymic rat model (234) demonstrate that a loss of T-cell function leads to a variable, but persistent, cryptosporidiosis similar to what might be seen in patients with AIDS. Resolution of an established infection in reconstituted SCID mice was shown to be dependent on CD4 cells and IFN-γ. It has been argued, however, that because patients with AIDS show increasing levels of IFN-γ as their disease progresses, the models rendering mice deficient in CD4 and IFN-γ may not resemble what is seen in patients with AIDS and cryptosporidiosis (244). Cytotoxic CD8 cells appear to have little or no role in recovery from infection (239,242). A role for natural killer cells in resolving cryptosporidiosis has been suggested but also appears to be minimal (245, 246).

Although it is clear that different animal species can mount antibody responses of all subclasses to a variety of cryptosporidial antigens, their role in conferring protection is unclear. Neonatal BALB/c mice exhibit antibody responses that do not correlate with either the severity or the duration of infection (247). Furthermore, if these mice were depleted of B cells, they did not differ from controls in the onset, peak, or duration of infection. Also, adult B-cell-depleted mice were impossible to infect regardless of the infectious dose given, further suggesting that the development of antiparasite antibody plays a less important role than CD4 cells in resolving this murine infection. Specific antiparasite antibody, however, might prove valuable in therapeutic regimens for controlling cryptosporidiosis.

Although animal models have been useful in studying immune parameters involved in cryptosporidiosis, it must be kept in mind that they do not show all the clinical and immunologic abnormalities associated with cryptosporidiosis in the AIDS population. Exceptions to this have recently been encountered in IFN-γ knockout mice, which exhibit weight loss, wasting, and death after infection with relatively few oocysts (248,249). Because of this, we constantly have to evaluate and question the meaning of results coming from such models. In this context, it is perhaps relevant to exploit models such as monkeys infected with HIV or the simian immunodeficiency virus.

Humoral Immunity

Much of our knowledge concerning immune responses to cryptosporidial infection in humans derives from serologic surveys and clinical case reports of immunocompetent and immunocompromised populations. The notion that humoral responses play a role in *C. parvum* infections comes from observations of persistent infections in congenitally immunodeficient patients with hypogammaglobulinemias or agammaglobulinemias (8,49,250).

Immunofluorescent assays have been used to demonstrate seroconversion in immunocompetent patients, a lack of responsiveness in hypogammaglobulinemic patients, low-level responses in patients with AIDS (250), and isotype-specific seroconversion responses in immunocompetent patients (251).

Enzyme-linked immunoadsorbent assays (ELISAs) also have been used to detect humoral responses to cryptosporidial infections. Elevated and persistent (up to 10 months) immunoglobulin G (IgG) responses have been detected in immunocompetent and immunocompromised patients. Immunoglobulin M (IgM) responses in the same patients usually were detectable for only 4 months after infection (252). Subsequent studies centered on populations living in areas endemic for cryptosporidiosis have demonstrated persistently elevated titers for IgG, and in some cases, IgM and IgA (110,175,253,254). It could be argued that antibody persistence in these instances may be indicative of constant or recurrent parasite exposure. Immunocompetent individuals involved in human infectivity studies showed noticeable IgM serum responses after primary exposure to infection and predominantly IgG and IgA serum responses after rechallenge 1 year later (255). In this study, there was no correlation between the appearance of these antibodies after primary challenge and subsequent protection as measured by symptoms, diarrhea, and the presence of oocysts. *C. parvum*-specific antibody responses have also been detected at mucosal sites in immunocompetent and immunocompromised patients. Most of these studies have focused on IgA responses but were unable to correlate antibody titers or specificity with alterations in fecal volume or oocyst output (256–258). In a recent study, however, fecal IgA reactivity was reported to be greatest in healthy volunteers who received the highest challenge doses and who were shedding oocysts and experiencing diarrheal illness (259). Recent improvements to the sensitivity and specificity of the ELISA procedure have been reported, which should prove useful in future epidemiologic studies.

The serum of infected patients also has been used in immunoblotting techniques to study antigen-specific immunoglobulin responses to *C. parvum.* A large number of antigens ranging from 3 to more than 200 kd react with human serum (260,261). Prominent among them is reactivity to antigens of 15 and 23 kd, which are localized on the surface of sporozoites. These antigens have also been shown to possess neutralization sensitive epitopes (262). Immunoblot studies employing animal serum also have identified a number of other immunodominant antigens (263–268). The extent to which any demonstrable antibodies play a real role in protective immunity remains unclear.

Cellular Immunity

Even fewer studies have been performed in humans to assess the role of cellular immunity in relation to *Cryptosporidium* infection. The association of *C. parvum* infection and disease in the HIV-infected population, however, underscores the role of cellular responses in controlling this infection. Patients with underlying lymphocyte malignancies have also proved highly susceptible to persistent cryptosporidiosis (205,207,209–211).

The results of two studies in HIV-infected patients clearly demonstrate that the severity of disease associated with cryptosporidiosis is a function of CD4 lymphocyte counts (269–270). Transient disease conditions were noted in patients with a wide range of lymphocyte counts and infections usually resolved when CD4 counts were greater than 180 cells/mm^3. Fulminating disease, resulting in death, was usually seen in patients with CD4 counts of less than 50 cells/mm^3. Protracted cryptosporidiosis has been observed in a non-HIV pediatric patient with IFN-γ deficiency, underscoring the potential importance of the regulatory cytokines in controlling infection through cellular responses (271).

Further studies to define the role of cellular immunity in humans, such as *in vitro* antigen-induced lymphocyte proliferative assays, are just now receiving attention. Along with appropriately designed animal studies, a clearer understanding of the role of accessory cells and products (cytokines) in controlling cryptosporidial infection may emerge. C-X-C chemokines, tumor necrosis factor-α, interleukin 8, and transforming growth factor-β have all been detected from infected human tissue (272–274). Their ultimate role in controlling infections and promoting intestinal healing has not been fully defined, however.

CLINICAL ILLNESS

The clinical manifestations of *Cryptosporidium* infection are influenced by the immune status of the host. After an incubation period of approximately 1 week (179,275), the disease becomes manifest by a watery, noninflammatory, foul-smelling diarrhea. However, the severity and duration of the disease will vary greatly depending on the status of the host's immune system. Patients at either end of the age spectrum or patients with nutritional deficiencies may behave similar to immunocompromised patients (121,276). There is an important interplay between cryptosporidial infection and malnutrition, and it is becoming apparent that malnutrition predisposes to a more prolonged and severe diarrheal illness, whereas failure to thrive, increased diarrhea burdens, and long-term deficits in growth, fitness, and schooling can be significant manifestations of *Cryptosporidium* infections in younger patients (112,121,126,133,136,138–140,253,277–279).

Immunocompetent Host

In immunocompetent patients, *C. parvum* causes a self-limited diarrheal illness that typically lasts 10 to 14 days but may last anywhere from 3 days to longer than 1 month. The diarrhea is characteristically profuse and watery, sometimes containing mucus. Patients often complain of crampy abdominal pain, flatulence, nausea, and vomiting and may have constitutional symptoms (anorexia, malaise, weakness, myalgias, and headaches). The diarrhea and abdominal pain are often exacerbated by eating. Fever is rarely significant. The disease can rarely be protracted, severe, and associated with significant weight loss (66,182,185,280). Mortality is rare, usually only occurring in severely malnourished children (133). Spontaneous complete recovery is the rule. A low median infectious dose level (ID_{50} = 132 oocysts) was established in healthy volunteers who had no evidence of prior exposure to the parasite (281). Symptoms associated with infection in this study tended to be mild and prompted further studies in which the same volunteers were rechallenged, other volunteers who had a prior history of exposure as determined by the presence of serum antibodies were challenged, or new volunteers with no history of prior exposure were challenged with different strains of the parasite (255,282,283). In the volunteer group rechallanged 1 year after initial infection, the illness attack rate was equal to that of the primary challenge group, fostering the notion that it might take multiple exposures to the parasite to develop protection. Interestingly, in the seropositive and challenged group, the data strongly suggested that prior exposure to *C. parvum* at least provides protection from infection and illness at low oocyst dose exposure levels. Lastly, there was a variance in the ID_{50} and clinical illness observed in volunteers challenged with different isolates of *Cryptosporidium,* with a Texas isolate (i.e., TAMU) being the most infectious.

Respiratory symptoms are significantly more frequent in children with cryptosporidial diarrhea than in patients with diarrhea of a different etiology (116,124,128,280,284), raising the issue that *Cryptosporidium* may indeed be a pulmonary pathogen as well. *Cryptosporidium* infection was documented by the demonstration of organisms in a tracheal aspirate of an immunocompetent child with laryngotracheitis and cryptosporidial diarrhea (286) and, as discussed later, is now recognized as a cause of pneumonia in the immunocompromised host. *Cryptosporidium* was the cause of acute pancreatitis in a 14-year-old farmer's daughter who drank unpasteurized milk (287) and caused symptoms mimicking those of acute appendicitis in one case (288). It was associated with recurrent urticaria and angioedema in one patient (289) and reactive arthritis in several others (290–292).

Immunocompromised Host

In contrast to the presentation and course in the immunocompetent patient, *Cryptosporidium* infection in the immunocompromised patient usually presents as a more severe, prolonged, cholera-like illness that can be life threatening, with as many as 71 stools per day and up to 17 L per day reported (11,293). From 2 to 3 L of diarrheic stool is common, and malabsorption can become a serious problem in these patients, with significant resulting dehydration and malnutrition and profound weight loss (up to 20 kg reported in one patient [294]). Patients may complain of crampy upper abdominal pain. Uncontrolled disease may contribute or lead to the death of patients (164,198,204, 207,226,295–297). Spontaneous clinical recovery occurs, with or without clearing of oocyst shedding (164,210, 295,298–300) and correlates with higher CD4 counts in patients with AIDS (164,269,301). Some patients have mild disease or are asymptomatic (209,215,302–305). Most often the disease is chronic in nature, with symptoms waxing and waning depending on a multiplicity of factors, including therapy, nutritional status, and variations in the immunologic status of the patient. Four clinical patterns of disease have been described in HIV-positive patients (270): transient in 29%, chronic in 60%, fulminant (more than 2 L of stool per day) in 8%, and asymptomatic in 4%. Fulminant disease only occurred in patients with a CD4 count less than 50 cells/mm^3, who survived only 5 weeks on average, compared with 20 weeks for those with chronic diarrhea and 36 weeks for those with transient infection.

All segments of the GI tract have been reported to be involved, including the pharynx, esophagus, stomach, duodenum, jejunum, ileum, appendix, colon, and rectum (9,306–310). Pancreatic duct involvement has been reported, with or without resultant pancreatitis (311,312), and cryptosporidial enteritis was associated with an enterovesical fistula in one patient (313). *Cryptosporidium* infection of the gallbladder and biliary tract is not uncommon (10% to 26% of patients with cryptosporidiosis in various studies [301,314]), resulting in acalculous cholecystitis, extrahepatic bile duct stenosis, and sclerosing cholangitis (201,270,301,315–326). Biliary duct involvement appears to predict a worse prognosis (295). The gallbladder may play a role as a reservoir of organisms, leading to persistent diarrhea, and in one patient cholecystectomy resulted in resolution of the diarrhea (327).

Although the literature debates whether respiratory tree involvement reflects true infection versus colonization or contamination, respiratory tract infection is well documented (sometimes at autopsy), often presenting as pneumonia (197,208,209,211,216,270,328–340). In one patient, *Cryptosporidium* was the only pathogen found during the workup of sinusitis (338). Infection at these extraintestinal sites is felt to occur via mucosal luminal spread, rather than systemic dissemination or direct tissue invasion.

DIAGNOSIS

Serologic testing (56,110,162,175,250–254,341) is mainly used for epidemiologic purposes and has little diagnostic application. As already noted, antibodies to *Cryptosporidium* can be detected by indirect immunofluorescent assay, ELISA, and other methods. Elevated serum IgM or IgG titers can be detected within 2 weeks of onset of symptoms in most patients. IgG and even IgM titers persist for long periods in most patients, the latter suggesting possible reexposure in highly endemic areas. Fecal IgA responses are significant in individuals with evidence of recent *Cryptosporidium* infection, suggesting that detection of these antibodies may be useful in detecting recent infections (259).

Sonographic or computed tomographic examination may be helpful for the diagnosis of cryptosporidial cholangitis (342–344), and endoscopic retrograde cholangiography is often necessary for diagnosis and therapeutic intervention (311,321,345). Infection at extraintestinal sites usually requires biopsy for diagnosis, although it may be achievable by staining of bile, sputum, or bronchial washings.

The mainstay of diagnosis is the identification of the oocysts in stool specimens. Three or more specimens are sometimes needed for the diagnosis, because oocyst excretion varies throughout the day and from day to day (346). Aspiration of duodenal fluid (347) or small intestinal brushing (348) can be used for diagnosis when upper GI endoscopy is performed, particularly if biopsies are contraindicated. There is little need for performing intestinal biopsies or electron microscopy for the diagnosis of cryptosporidiosis (349). Concentration of stool specimens is mainly necessary in epidemiologic studies and in the evaluation of contacts of infected patients in whom the number of parasites may be small, but it is usually unnecessary for the evaluation of the patient with diarrhea. Various methods (most commonly the formalin ethyl acetate method) are used, including the use of a disposable parasite concentrator (350), and various fecal concentration devices (351). Newer concentration techniques are more sensitive, lowering the threshold of detection of oocysts in formed stool specimens to 5,000 oocysts per gram of stool (352).

The most convenient, and widely used methods for identifying oocysts in stool samples are acid-fast or immunofluorescent stains (see Color Figure 62.3) (353–369). Care in measuring oocysts after staining must be exercised, however, because they can readily be confused with the larger (8 to 10 μm) oocysts of *Cyclospora* (370).

Several differently formulated immunoassays have recently become available to enhance *Cryptosporidium* detection. Commercially available immunofluorescent antibody kits are highly sensitive and specific for detecting *Cryptosporidium* in clinical laboratory samples but show varying degrees of cross-reactivity with other *Cryptosporidium* species and, therefore, could detect nonhuman cryptosporidia in environmental samples (371,372). Enzyme immunoassays with nearly the same sensitivity and specificity have also become available commercially. The latter have great utility where sample batching can be done, such as in epidemiologic studies (371,372).

PCR-based detection methods have also been applied to clinical and environmental samples (373–375). The advantages of this technology are that the limits of detection may extend to a single oocyst and that genotyping can also be performed. This technology, which has already enhanced our knowledge of the epidemiology of this parasite, when perfected has the ability to enhance it to an even greater degree. The current greatest challenge to the technique is in removing substances found in stool and environmental samples that can inhibit the PCR reaction.

Often overlooked is the fact that infection with *Cryptosporidium* is likely underdiagnosed either because clinicians do not consider this diagnosis in immunocompetent individuals or because this is not tested for in routine stool analysis. In addition, other causes of noninflammatory diarrhea must obviously be considered during the workup. It is also important to realize that *Cryptosporidium* will sometimes be one of two or more organisms found during a workup for diarrhea, likely secondary to similar environmental transmission profiles. Careful epidemiologic questioning may help guide the clinician to the most likely pathogen. In the healthy host, other parasitic causes of persistent diarrhea include *Giardia lamblia, Cyclospora* and *Isospora.* In addition, enterotoxigenic *Escherichia coli,* viral infections (rotavirus and Norwalk virus) should be considered. In immunocompromised patients, one also has to consider the microsporidians, *Campylobacter, Salmonella, Clostridium difficile,* adenovirus, cytomegalovirus, and *Mycobacterium avium–intracellulare* as potential etiologies.

TREATMENT

Treating cryptosporidiosis using conventional chemotherapeutic approaches has proven very frustrating. Over the last two decades, more than 100 compounds have been screened *in vitro* and *in vivo* for anticryptosporidial activity or tried empirically, mostly with negative results (376). These have included sulfonamides, clindamycin, metronidazole, and other antiprotozoal agents. This failure, in part, has been ascribed to the parasite's unique intracellular but extracytoplasmic location (377,378). Recently, a parasite-encoded transport protein has been localized at the parasite–host cell interface, which may represent a potential target for drug intervention (40).

Treatment of patients with AIDS with HAART is key to improvement of the diarrhea and clearing of the oocysts from the stool. A resolution of diarrhea in patients with AIDS was seen concomitant with a rise in CD4 counts with this type of antiretroviral therapy (379–381). Unfortunately, such therapy is not available to everyone, particularly to those with AIDS in developing countries. In patients with exogenous immune suppression, immunosuppressive therapy should ideally be discontinued or tapered (4,64, 207). In gallbladder disease, papillotomy may be helpful when there is evidence of obstruction due to papillary stenosis (318,345).

Some patients will present with significant volume loss and will need hospitalization for intravenous fluid repletion. Oral rehydration also needs to be encouraged. Careful attention to electrolytes is necessary. In immunocompromised patients, malabsorption may be significant and may contribute to severe malnutrition and weight loss. Nutritional supplementation intravenously may be needed, and total parenteral nutrition is occasionally used (176,201). Drugs that affect gut motility (e.g., loperamide, diphenoxylate, and opiates) should be used in an attempt to slow the increased peristalsis of the intestinal tract and the resulting volume loss and decreased transit time of nutrients (382).

In spite of the numerous chemotherapeutic failures attendant with treating cryptosporidiosis in patients with AIDS, encouraging results recently have been obtained using a few drugs. These have been reported with paromomycin, a combination of paromomycin plus azithromycin, and with nitazoxanide (NTZ). Paromomycin, an aminoglycoside, may reach the parasite by being absorbed in limited quantities across the apical membrane of infected cells and has displayed at least partial activity in clinical trials (383). Its activity was reportedly enhanced when given concomitantly with the macrolide antibiotic azithromycin, but there were inconsistencies noted in stool volumes versus reductions in parasite excretion and stool frequency (384). In both cases, biliary disease, when present, remained a problem. The most promising treatment results have been reported after treatment with NTZ, a nitrothiazole benzamide with reported wide-spectrum antimicrobial and antiparasite activity. In a placebo-controlled trial in Mexico, 22 (about 65%) of 34 patients receiving differing doses of NTZ were parasitologically cured, and of the cured, 19 (86%) had complete resolution of their diarrhea (385). Interestingly and unexplainably, parasitologic and clinical resolution rates of 25% and 50%, respectively, were reported in the placebo group. A somewhat similar large-scale clinical trial in the United States produced less-encouraging results, yet clinical responses were still favorable in many who had not responded to other therapies (386). In 1998 the clinical trials were shut down because of the impact of HAART, with the attendant enrollment decline in those presenting with cryptosporidiosis. In May 1998, the Food and Drug Administration (FDA), under committee advisement, declined to recommend accelerated approval of NTZ, citing problems with study design (open label), baseline data, and efficacy endpoints (387). This drug is still available for compassionate use (FDA-253B) and has *de facto* become the drug of treatment choice because of availability through various AIDS networks.

A novel approach to treating cryptosporidiosis in patients with AIDS has involved the use of polyclonal antibody-based immunotherapies. The most widely tested has involved administration of hyperimmune bovine colostrum. Early studies showed promise for this type of therapy with limited patient numbers (325,388). As with so many other experiences in treating this infection, however, follow-up clinical studies involving this product or a hyperimmune egg yolk preparation showed highly variable clinical benefits attendant with this therapy (389; R. Soave, *personal communication*). In these cases, failure may be due to the means of delivery, because the antibodies must survive passage through the stomach to be effective when needed.

There is the persistent concern that the impact of HAART on the number of cases of cryptosporidiosis will cause drug companies to lose interest in developing an effective therapy against this disease. Still, it must be kept in mind that most of the worldwide patients with AIDS affected by this parasite do not have access to HAART and that children of developing countries and individuals exposed to waterborne outbreaks or to animals with this disease might benefit significantly from effective therapy. Furthermore, cryptosporidiosis may impair absorption of antiretroviral drugs. Because of these concerns, all rational manners of drug development and testing should be encouraged.

PREVENTION

Environmental Eradication

Cryptosporidium oocysts are very resistant to a wide variety of environmental conditions and disinfection methods. They can survive for months when kept cold and moist. They are killed by exposure to temperatures higher than 60°C or lower than −20°C for longer than 30 minutes (48). One study subjected the oocysts to conditions similar to milk pasteurization specifications and found effective neutralization of their infectivity (390). Most common disinfectants used routinely in hospitals and clinical laboratories do not kill *Cryptosporidium* oocysts when used at the usual recommended dilutions. Exposure to 5% ammonia or 10% formol saline for 18 hours is needed to kill the cysts (58). Routine chlorination and various water treatment processes used for water purification are not very effective at killing *Cryptosporidium* oocysts (391), particularly when there is a sudden discharge of oocysts into the water, such as after a heavy rainfall. Recent studies indicate that ozone, chlorine dioxide, and sand filtration are more effective means of eradicating the oocysts from drinking water (392–394), giving some hope that a practical solution may be within reach. Ultraviolet light is receiving increased attention as a means of disinfecting water contaminated with *Cryptosporidium* and has been shown to inactivate oocysts at low- and medium-dose levels, including in water with turbidity of more than 1 NTU (395). Both technical and financial problems for the commercial application of effective systems in the developing world remain a formidable challenge.

An important issue is the decontamination of the instruments used for GI and pulmonary endoscopies. As mentioned earlier, one study found a high prevalence of *Cryptosporidium* oocysts in patients undergoing upper endoscopy for presumably unrelated diagnoses (111), raising a valid concern about the potential for patient-to-patient transmission by means of contaminated endoscopes. The need for and difficulty of disinfection have been addressed in some publications, and the reader is referred to them for further information (396,397).

Enteric Precautions

Careful hand washing is of utmost importance in preventing spread in hospitals and day care centers, and the use of gowns and gloves and appropriate disposal of contaminated feces are necessary for caretakers of hospitalized patients. These patients should ideally be in private rooms. Contaminated equipment should be autoclaved, and contaminated surfaces should be washed with commercial bleach that ideally is left on to soak for at least 15 minutes. Shedding of oocysts usually stops 1 to 2 weeks after the onset of symptoms in immunocompetent patients (398), but a small number of oocysts may remain present in feces for 2 weeks or longer after the resolution of diarrhea (65,114,127,134, 142,147,150,154,159,213,275,399,400). These persons and asymptomatic carriers are likely to be important reservoirs of infection.

Travelers should follow routine recommendations of avoiding unboiled or uncooked drinks and foods when traveling to endemic areas. Immunocompromised patients who go camping or take trips to endemic areas should be particularly careful in avoiding any potentially contaminated water or foods.

Education

Health care professionals need to educate the medical community about the importance of including cryptosporidiosis in the differential diagnosis of diarrheal diseases, even in immunocompetent hosts and in developed countries and urban settings. The public needs to be educated about diarrheal diseases in general and routine precautions that need to be followed when a family member has a diarrheal illness. Immunocompromised patients should be advised to avoid, when possible, contact with animals with diarrhea.

ACKNOWLEDGMENT

We thank Dr. Karim Adal who prepared much of the original edition on which this chapter is based.

REFERENCES

1. Tyzzer EE. A sporozoan found in the peptic glands of the common mouse. *Proc Soc Exp Biol Med* 1907;5:12–13.
2. Tyzzer EE. *Cryptosporidium parvum* (sp. nov.), a coccidium found in the small intestine of the common mouse. *Arch Protistenkd* 1912;26:394–412.
3. Nime FA, Burek JD, Page DL, et al. Acute enterocolitis in a human being infected with the protozoan *Cryptosporidium. Gastroenterology* 1976;70:592–598.
4. Meisel JL, Perera DR, Meligro C, et al. Overwhelming watery diarrhea associated with a *Cryptosporidium* in an immunosuppressed patient. *Gastroenterology* 1976;70:1156–1160.
5. Weinstein L, Edelstein SM, Madara JL, et al. Intestinal cryptosporidiosis complicated by disseminated cytomegalovirus infection. *Gastroenterology* 1981;81:584–591.
6. Tzipori S, Angus KW, Campbell I, et al. Vomiting and diarrhea associated with cryptosporidial infection. *N Engl J Med* 1980; 303:818.
7. Stemmermann GN, Hayashi T, Glober GA, et al. Cryptosporidiosis: report of a fatal case complicated by disseminated toxoplasmosis. *Am J Med* 1980;69:637–642.
8. Lasser KH, Lewin KJ, Ryning FW. Cryptosporidial enteritis in a patient with congenital hypogammaglobulinemia. *Hum Pathol* 1979;10:234–240.
9. Booth CC, Slavin G, Dourmashkin RR, et al. Immunodeficiency and cryptosporidiosis. Demonstration at the Royal College of Physicians of London. *Br Med J* 1980;281:1123–1127.
10. Weisburger WR, Hutcheon DF, Yardley JH, et al. Cryptosporidiosis in an immunosuppressed renal-transplant recipient with IgA deficiency. *Am J Clin Pathol* 1979;72:473–478.
11. Centers for Disease Control and Prevention. Cryptosporidiosis: an assessment of chemotherapy of males with acquired immune deficiency syndrome (AIDS). *MMWR Morb Mortal Wkly Rep* 1982;31:589–592.
12. Centers for Disease Control and Prevention. 1993 Revised classification for HIV infection and expanded surveillance case definition for AIDS among adolescents and adults. *MMWR Morb Mortal Wkly Rep* 1993;41:1–19.
13. O'Donoghue PJ. *Cryptosporidium* and cryptosporidiosis in man and animals. *Int J Parasitol* 1995;25:139–195.
14. Fayer R, Speer CA, Dubey JP. The general biology of *Cryptosporidium.* In: Fayer R, ed. Cryptosporidium and *cryptosporidiosis.* Boca Raton, FL: CRC Press, 1997;1–41.
15. Morgan UM, Xiao L, Fayer R, et al. Variation in *Cryptosporidium:* towards a taxonomic revision of the genus. *Int J Parasitol* 1999;29:1733–1751.
16. Xiao L, Escalante L, Yang C, et al. Phylogenetic analysis of *Cryptosporidium* parasites based on the small-subunit rRNA gene locus. *Appl Environ Microbiol* 1999;65:1578–1583.
17. Xiao L, Morgan UM, Limor J, et al. Genetic diversity within *Cryptosporidium parvum* and related *Cryptosporidium* species. *Appl Environ Microbiol* 1999;65:3386–3391.
18. Xiao L, Morgan UM, Fayer R, et al. *Cryptosporidium* systematics and implications for public health. *Parasitol Today* 2000;16: 287–292.
19. Bonnin A, Fourmaux MN, Dubremetz JF, et al. Genotyping human and bovine isolates of *Cryptosporidium parvum* by polymerase chain reaction–restriction fragment length polymorphism analysis of a repetitive DNA sequence. *FEMS Microbiol Lett* 1996;137:207–211.
20. Carraway MS, Tzipori S, Widmer G. Identification of genetic heterogeneity in the *Cryptosporidium parvum* ribosomal repeat. *Appl Environ Microbiol* 1996;62:712–716.
21. Carraway MS, Tzipori S, Widmer G. A new restriction fragment length polymorphism from *Cryptosporidium parvum* identifies genetically heterogeneous parasite populations and genotypic changes following transmission from bovine to human hosts. *Infect Immun* 1997;65:3958–3960.
22. Morgan UM, Clare C, Constantine CC, et al. Differentiation between human and animal isolates of *Cryptosporidium parvum* using rDNA sequencing and direct PCR analysis. *J Parasitol* 1997;83:825–830.
23. Peng MM, Xiao L, Freeman AR, et al. Genetic polymorphism

among *Cryptosporidium parvum* isolates: evidence of two distinct human transmission cycles. *Emerging Infect Dis* 1997;3: 567–573.

24. Spano F, Putignani L, Mclauchlin J, et al. PCR-RFLP analysis of the *Cryptosporidium* oocyst wall protein (COWP) discriminates between *C. wrairi* and *C. parvum,* and between *C. parvum* isolates of human and animal origin. *FEMS Microbiol Lett* 1997;150:209–217.
25. Awad-El-Kariem FM, Robinson HA, Petry F, et al. Differentiation between human and animal isolates of *Cryptosporidium parvum* using molecular and biologic markers. *Parasitol Res* 1998;84:297–301.
26. Morgan UM, Sargent KD, Depazes P, et al. Molecular characterization of *Cryptosporidium* from various hosts. *Parasitology* 1998;117:31–37.
27. Spano F, Putignani L, Guida S, et al. *Cryptosporidium parvum:* PCR-RFLP analysis of the TRAP-C1 (thrombospondin-related adhesive protein of *Cryptosporidium*-1) gene discriminates between two alleles differentially associates with parasite isolates of animal and human origin. *Exp Parasitol* 1998;90:195–198.
28. Sulaiman IM, Xiao L, Yang C, et al. Differentiating human from animal isolates of *Cryptosporidium parvum. Emerging Infect Dis* 1998;4:681–685.
29. Xiao L, Sulaiman IM, Fayer R, et al. Species and strain-specific typing of *Cryptosporidium* parasites in clinical and environmental samples. *Mem Inst Oswaldo Cruz* 1998;93:687–692.
30. Sulaiman IM, Xiao L, Lal AA. Evaluation of *Cryptosporidium parvum* genotyping techniques. *Appl Environ Microbiol* 1999; 65:4431–4435.
31. Ditrich O, Palkovic L, Sterba J, et al. The first finding of *Cryptosporidium baileyi* in man. *Parasitol Res* 1991;77:44–47.
32. Slemenda S. Paper presented at: the Microsporidiosis and Cryptosporidiosis in Immunodeficient Patients Conference; 1993; Ceské Budejovice, Czech Republic.
33. Pieniazek NJ, Bornay-Llinares FJ, Slemenda SB, et al. New *Cryptosporidium* genotypes in HIV-infected persons. *Emerging Infect Dis* 1999;5:444–449.
34. Morgan UM, Weber R, Xiao L, et al. Molecular characterization of *Cryptosporidium* isolates obtained from human immunodeficiency virus-infected individuals living in Switzerland, Kenya, and the United States. *J Clin Microbiol* 2000;38:1180–1183.
35. Xiao L, Bern C, Limor J, et al. Non-*C. parvum Cryptosporidium* parasites as an emerging cause of human infection. In: Programs and abstract of the International Conference of Emerging Infectious Disease; 2000; Atlanta, GA. Abstract 8/125.
36. Crawford FG, Vermund SH. Human cryptosporidiosis. *CRC Crit Rev Microbiol* 1988;16:113–159.
37. Fayer R, Ungar BLP. *Cryptosporidium* spp. and cryptosporidiosis. *Microbiol Rev* 1986;50:458–483.
38. Reduker DW, Speer CA, Blixt JA. Ultrastructure of *Cryptosporidium parvum* oocysts and excysting sporozoites as revealed by high resolution scanning electron microscopy. *J Protozool* 1985;32:708–711.
39. Lumb R, Smith K, O'Donoghue PJ, et al. Ultrastructure of the attachment of *Cryptosporidium* sporozoites to tissue culture cells. *Parasitol Res* 1988;74:531–536.
40. Perkins ME, Riojas YA, Wu TW, et al. CpABC, a *Cryptosporidium parvum* ATP-binding cassette protein at the host–parasite boundary in intracellular stages. *Proc Natl Acad Sci U S A* 1999; 96:5734–5739.
41. Current WL, Reese NC. A comparison of endogenous development of three isolates of *Cryptosporidium* in suckling mice. *J Protozool* 1986;33:98–108.
42. Current WL, Long PL. Development of human and calf *Cryptosporidium* in chicken embryos. *J Infect Dis* 1983;148: 1108–1113.
43. Upton SJ. *In vitro* cultivation. In: Fayer R, ed. Cryptosporidium *and cryptosporidiosis.* Boca Raton, FL: CRC Press, 1997: 181–207.
44. Upton SJ, Tilley M, Brillhart DB. Comparative development of *Cryptosporidium parvum* (Apicomplexa) in 11 continuous host cell lines. *FEMS Microbiol Lett* 1994;118:233–236.
45. Gut J, Petersen C, Nelson RG, et al. *Cryptosporidium parvum: in vitro* cultivation in Madin-Darby canine kidney cells. *J Protozool* 1991;38:72S–73S.
46. Upton SJ, Tilley M, Brillhart DB. Effects of select medium supplements on *in vitro* development of *Cryptosporidium parvum* in JCT-8 cells. *J Clin Microbiol* 1995;33:371–375.
47. Current WL, Haynes TB. Complete development of *Cryptosporidium* in cell culture. *Science* 1984;224:603–605.
48. Tzipori S. Cryptosporidiosis in animals and humans. *Microbiol Rev* 1983;47:84–96.
49. Current WL, Reese NC, Ernst JV, et al. Human cryptosporidiosis in immunocompetent and immunodeficient persons: studies of an outbreak and experimental transmission. *N Engl J Med* 1983;308:1252–1257.
50. Anderson BC, Donndelinger T, Wilkins RM, et al. Cryptosporidiosis in a veterinary student. *J Am Vet Med Assoc* 1982; 180:408–409.
51. Holten-Andersen W, Gerstoft J, Henriksen SA. Human cryptosporidiosis. *N Engl J Med* 1983;309:1325–1326.
52. Nouri M, Toroghi R. Asymptomatic cryptosporidiosis in cattle and humans in Iran. *Vet Rec* 1991;128:358–359.
53. Pohjola S, Jokipii AMM, Jokipii L. Sporadic cryptosporidiosis in a rural population is asymptomatic and associated with contact to cattle. *Acta Vet Scand* 1986;27:91–102.
54. Miron D, Kenes J, Dagan R. Calves as a source of an outbreak of cryptosporidiosis among young children in an agricultural closed community. *Pediatr Infect Dis J* 1991;10:438–441.
55. Rahman ASMH, Sanyal SC, Al-Mahmud KA, et al. Cryptosporidiosis in calves and their handlers in Bangladesh. *Lancet* 1984;2:221.
56. Lengerich EJ, Addiss DG, Marx JJ, et al. Increased exposure to cryptosporidia among dairy farmers in Wisconsin. *J Infect Dis* 1993;167:1252–1255.
57. Shield J, Baumer JH, Dawson JA, et al. Cryptosporidiosis—an educational experience. *J Infect* 1990;21:297–301.
58. Campbell I, Tzipori S, Hutchison G, et al. Effect of disinfectants on survival of *Cryptosporidium* oocysts. *Vet Rec* 1982;111: 414–415.
59. Casemore DP. Sheep as a source of human cryptosporidiosis. *J Infect* 1989;19:101–104.
60. Public Health Laboratory Service Study Group. Cryptosporidiosis in England and Wales: prevalence and clinical and epidemiological features. *BMJ*1990;300:774–777.
61. Nouri M, Karami M. Asymptomatic cryptosporidiosis in nomadic shepherds and their sheep. *J Infect* 1991;23:331–333.
62. Nouri M, Mahdavi Rad S. Effect of nomadic shepherds and their sheep on the incidence of cryptosporidiosis in an adjacent town. *J Infect* 1993;26:105–106.
63. Egger M, Mai Nguyen X, Schaad UB, et al. Intestinal cryptosporidiosis acquired from a cat. *Infection* 1990;18:177–178.
64. Lewis IJ, Hart CA, Baxby D. Diarrhoea due to *Cryptosporidium* in acute lymphoblastic leukaemia. *Arch Dis Child* 1985;60: 60–62.
65. Hart CA, Baxby D, Blundell N. Gastro-enteritis due to *Cryptosporidium:* a prospective survey in a children's hospital. *J Infect* 1984;9:264–270.
66. Edelman MJ, Oldfield EC. Severe cryptosporidiosis in an immunocompetent host. *Arch Intern Med* 1988;148: 1873–1874.
67. Newman RD, Wuhib T, Lima AAM, et al. Environmental

sources of *Cryptosporidium* in an urban slum in northeastern Brazil. *Am J Trop Med Hyg*1993;49:270–275.
68. Mtambo MMA, Nash AS, Blewett DA, et al. *Cryptosporidium* infection in cats: prevalence of infection in domestic and feral cats in the Glasgow area. *Vet Rec* 1991;129:502–504.
69. Koch KL, Shankey TV, Weinstein GS, et al. Cryptosporidiosis in a patient with hemophilia, common variable hypogammaglobulinemia and the acquired immunodeficiency syndrome. *Ann Intern Med* 1983;99:337–340.
70. Brown EAE, Casemore DP, Gerken A, et al. Cryptosporidiosis in Great Yarmouth—the investigation of an outbreak. *Public Health* 1989;103:3–9.
71. Navin TR, Hardy AM. Cryptosporidiosis in patients with AIDS. *J Infect Dis* 1987;155:150.
72. Weber J, Philip S. Human cryptosporidiosis. *N Engl J Med* 1983;309:1326.
73. Fayer R, Graczyk TK, Lewis EJ, et al. Survival of infectious *Cryptosporidium parvum* oocysts in seawater and eastern oysters (*Crassostrea virginica*) in the Chesapeake Bay. *Appl Environ Microbiol* 1998;64:1070–1074.
74. Graczyk TK, Fayer R, Cranfield MR, et al. Recovery of waterborne *Cryptosporidium parvum* oocysts by freshwater benthic clams (Corbicula fluminea). *Appl Environ Microbiol* 1998;64: 427–430.
75. *Graczyk TK, Fayer R, Lewis EJ, et al.* Cryptosporidium oocysts in Bent mussels (*Ischadium recurvum*) in the Chesapeake Bay. *Parasitol Res* 1999;85:30–34.
76. Fayer R, Lewis EJ, Trout JM, et al. *Cryptosporidium parvum* in oysters from commercial harvesting sites in the Chesapeake Bay. *Emerging Infect Dis* 1999;5:706–710.
77. Graczyk TK, Cranfield MR, Fayer R, et al. House flies (*Musca domestica*) as transport hosts of *Cryptosporidium parvum. Am J Trop Med Hyg* 1999;61:500–504.
78. Edwards DD. Troubled waters in Milwaukee. *ASM News* 1993; 59:342–345.
79. MacKenzie WR. A massive outbreak in Milwaukee of *Cryptosporidium* infection transmitted through the public water supply. *N Engl J Med* 1994;331:161–167.
80. LeChevallier MW, Norton WD, Lee RG. *Giardia* and *Cryptosporidium* spp. in filtered drinking water supplies. *Appl Environ Microbiol* 1991;57:2617–2621.
81. Madore MS, Rose JB, Gerba CP, et al. Occurrence of *Cryptosporidium* oocysts in sewage effluents and selected surface waters. *J Parasitol* 1987;73:702–705.
82. Villacorta-Martinez de Maturana I, Ares-Mazas ME, Duran-Oreiro D, et al. Efficacy of activated sludge in removing *Cryptosporidium parvum* oocysts from sewage. *Appl Environ Microbiol* 1992;58:3514–3516.
83. Sorvillo FJ, Fujioka K, Nahlen B, et al. Swimming-associated cryptosporidiosis. *Am J Public Health* 1992;82:742–744.
84. Joce RE, Bruce J, Kiely D, et al. An outbreak of cryptosporidiosis associated with a swimming pool. *Epidemiol Infect* 1991;107:497–508.
85. Centers for Disease Control and Prevention. Swimming-associated cryptosporidiosis—Los Angeles County. *MMWR Morb Mortal Wkly Rep* 1990;39:343–345.
86. Richardson AJ, Frankenberg RA, Buck AC, et al. An outbreak of waterborne cryptosporidiosis in Swindon and Oxfordshire. *Epidemiol Infect* 1991;107:485–495.
87. Rush BA, Chapman PA, Ineson RW. *Cryptosporidium* and drinking water. *Lancet* 1987;2:632–633.
88. Rush BA, Chapman PA, Ineson RW. A probable waterborne outbreak of cryptosporidiosis in the Sheffield area. *J Med Microbiol* 1990;32:239–242.
89. Smith HV, Girwood RWA, Patterson WJ, et al. Waterborne outbreak of cryptosporidiosis. *Lancet* 1988;2:1484.
90. Smith HV, Patterson WJ, Hardie R, et al. An outbreak of waterborne cryptosporidiosis caused by post-treatment contamination. *Epidemiol Infect* 1989;103:703–715.
91. D'Antonio RG, Winn RE, Taylor JP, et al. A waterborne outbreak of cryptosporidiosis in normal hosts. *Ann Intern Med* 1986;103:886–888.
92. Joseph C, Hamilton G, O'Connor M, et al. Cryptosporidiosis in the Isle of Thanet; an outbreak associated with local drinking water. *Epidemiol Infect* 1991;107:509–519.
93. Gallaher MM, Herndon JL, Nims LJ, et al. Cryptosporidiosis and surface water. *Am J Public Health* 1989;79:39–42.
94. Hayes EB, Matte TD, O'Brien TR, et al. Large community outbreak of cryptosporidiosis due to contamination of a filtered public water supply. *N Engl J Med* 1989;320:1372–1376.
95. Weinstein P, Macaitis M, Walker C, et al. Cryptosporidial diarrhoea in South Australia: an exploratory case–control study of risk factors for transmission. *Med J Aust* 1993;158: 117–119.
96. McNaulty JM, Keene WE, Fleming DW. A water system in one town causing an outbreak of cryptosporidiosis in another town. *Program and abstracts of the 33rd Interscience Conference on Antimicrobial Agents and Chemotherapy.* New Orleans, LA: American Society for Microbiology; 1993:387. Abstract 1463.
97. Hansen JS, Ongerth JE. Effects of time and watershed characteristics on the concentration of *Cryptosporidium* oocysts in river water. *Appl Environ Microbiol* 1991;57:2790–2795.
98. Musial CE, Arrowood MJ, Sterling CR, et al. Detection of *Cryptosporidium* in water by using polypropylene cartridge filters. *Appl Environ Microbiol* 1987;53:687–692.
99. Ongerth JE, Stibbs HH. Identification of *Cryptosporidium* oocysts in river water. *Appl Environ Microbiol* 1987;53: 672–676.
100. Rose JB. Occurrence and significance of *Cryptosporidium* in water. *J Am Water Works Assoc* 1988;80:53–58.
101. LeChevallier MW, Norton WD, Lee RG. Occurrence of *Giardia* and *Cryptosporidium* spp. in surface water supplies. *Appl Environ Microbiol* 1991;57:2610–2616.
102. Isaac-Renton JL, Fogel D, Stibbs HH, et al. *Giardia* and *Cryptosporidium* in drinking water. *Lancet* 1987;1:973–974.
103. Stetzenbach LD, Arrowood MJ, Marshall MM, et al. Monoclonal antibody based immunofluorescent assay for *Giardia* and *Cryptosporidium* detection in water samples. *Water Sci Technol* 1988;20:193–198.
104. Bukhari Z, McCuin RM, Fricker CR, et al. Immunomagnetic separation of *Cryptosporidium parvum* from source water samples of various turbidities. *Appl Environ Microbiol* 1998;64: 4495–4499.
105. Clancy JL, Bukhari Z, McCuin RM, et al. USEPA method 1622. *J Am Water Works Assoc* 1999;91:58–68.
106. Rochelle PA, DeLeon R, Johnson A, et al. Evaluation of immunomagnetic separation for recovery of infectious *Cryptosporidium parvum* oocysts from environmental samples. *Appl Environ Microbiol* 1999;65:841–845.
107. Rochelle RA, Jutras EM, Atwill ER, et al. Polymorphisms in the β-tubulin gene of *Cryptosporidium parvum* differentiate between isolates based on animal host but not geographic origin. *J Parasitol* 1999;85:986–988.
108. Widmer G, Tzipori S, Fichtenbaum CJ, et al. Genotypic and phenotypic characterization of *Cryptosporidium parvum* isolates from people with AIDS. *J Infect Dis* 1998;178:834–840.
109. Guerrant RL. Cryptosporidiosis: an emerging, highly infectious threat. *Emerging Infect Dis* 1997;3:51–57.
110. Ungar BLP, Gilman RH, Lanata CF, et al. Seroepidemiology of *Cryptosporidium* infection in two Latin American populations. *J Infect Dis* 1988;157:551–556.
111. Roberts WG, Green PHR, Ma J, et al. Prevalence of cryp-

tosporidiosis in patients undergoing endoscopy: evidence for an asymptomatic carrier state. *Am J Med* 1989;87:537–539.
112. Checkley W, Gilman RH, Epstein LD, et al. Asymptomatic and symptomatic cryptosporidiosis: their acute effect on weight gain in Peruvian children. *Am J Epidemiol* 1997;145:156–163.
113. Zu S-X, Li J-F, Barrett LJ, et al. Seroepidemiologic study of *Cryptosporidium* infection in children from rural communities of Anhui, China, and Fortaleza, Brazil. *Am J Trop Med Hyg* 1994;51:1–10.
114. Hojlyng N, Molbak K, Jepsen S, et al. Cryptosporidiosis in Liberian children. *Lancet* 1984;1:734.
115. Pal S, Bhattacharya SK, Das P, et al. Occurrence and significance of *Cryptosporidium* infection in Calcutta. *Trans royal Soc Trop Med Hyg* 1989;83:520–521.
116. Shahid NS, Rahman ASMH, Anderson BC, et al. Cryptosporidiosis in Bangladesh. *Br Med J* 1985;290:114–115.
117. Shahid NS, Rahman ASMH, Sanyal SC. *Cryptosporidium* as a pathogen for diarrhoea in Bangladesh. *Trop Geogr Med* 1987; 39:265–270.
118. Mata L, Bolaños H, Pizarro D, et al. Cryptosporidiosis in children from some highland Costa Rican rural and urban areas. *Am J Trop Med Hyg* 1984;33:24–29.
119. Moodley D, Jackson TFHG, Gathiram V, et al. *Cryptosporidium* infections in children in Durban: seasonal variation, age distribution and disease status. *S Afr Med J* 1991;79:295–297.
120. Molbak K, Hojlyng N, Ingholt L, et al. An epidemic outbreak of cryptosporidiosis: a prospective community study from Guinea Bissau. *Pediatr Infect Dis J* 1990;9:566–570.
121. Bogaerts J, Lepage P, Rouvroy D, et al. *Cryptosporidium* spp., a frequent cause of diarrhea in Central Africa. *J Clin Microbiol* 1984;20:874–876.
122. Rahman M, Shahid NS, Rahman H, et al. Cryptosporidiosis: a cause of diarrhea in Bangladesh. *Am J Trop Med Hyg* 1990;42: 127–130.
123. Steele AD, Gove E, Meewes PJ. Cryptosporidiosis in white patients in South Africa. *J Infect* 1989;19:281–285.
124. Sallon S, El Showwa R, El-Masri M, et al. Cryptosporidiosis in children in Gaza. *Ann Trop Paediatr* 1990;11:277–281.
125. Dagan R, Bar-David Y, Kassis I, et al. *Cryptosporidium* in Bedouin and Jewish infants and children in southern Israel. *Isr J Med Sci* 1991;27:380–385.
126. Cruz JR, Cano F, Caceres P, et al. Infection and diarrhea caused by *Cryptosporidium* sp. among Guatemalan infants. *J Clin Microbiol* 1988;26:88–91.
127. Addy PA-K, Aikins-Bekoe P. Cryptosporidiosis in diarrhoeal children in Kumasi, Ghana. *Lancet* 1986;1:735.
128. Weikel CS, Johnston LI, De Sousa MA, et al. Cryptosporidiosis in northeastern Brazil: association with sporadic diarrhea. *J Infect Dis* 1985;151:963–965.
129. Guessous-Idrissi N, Essadki O, Bennis M, et al. Prévalence des cryptosporidies dans les diarrhées infantiles à Casablanca. *Presse Med* 1990;19:379.
130. Das P, Sengupta K, Dutta P, et al. Significance of *Cryptosporidium* as an aetiologic agent of acute diarrhoea in Calcutta: a hospital based study. *J Trop Med Hyg* 1993;96:124–127.
131. Carstensen H, Hansen HL, Kristiansen HO, et al. The epidemiology of cryptosporidiosis and other intestinal parasitoses in children in southern Guinea-Bissau. *Trans Royal Soc Trop Med Hyg* 1987;81:860–864.
132. Smith G, Van den Ende J. Cryptosporidiosis among black children in hospital in South Africa. *J Infect* 1986;13:25–30.
133. MacFarlane DE, Horner-Bryce J. Cryptosporidiosis in well-nourished and malnourished children. *Acta Paediatr* 1987;76: 474–477.
134. Pape JW, Levine E, Beaulieu ME, et al. Cryptosporidiosis in Haitian children. *Am J Trop Med Hyg* 1987;36:333–337.
135. Newman RD, Sears SL, Moore SR, et al. Longitudinal study of *Cryptosporidium* infection in children of northeastern Brazil. *J Infect Dis* 1999;180:167–175.
136. Lima AAM, Moore SR, Barboza MS Jr, et al. Persistent diarrhea signals a critical period of increased diarrhea burdens and nutritional shortfalls: a prospective cohort study among children in northeastern Brazil. *J Infect Dis* 2000;181:1643–1651.
137. Sterling CR, Gilman RH, Sinclair NA, et al. The role of breast milk in protecting urban Peruvian children against cryptosporidiosis. *J Protozool* 1991;38:23S–25S.
138. Checkley W, Epstein LD, Gilman RH, et al. Effects of *Cryptosporidium parvum* infection in Peruvian children: growth faltering and subsequent catch-up growth. *Am J Epidemiol* 1998; 148:497–506.
139. Agnew DG, Lima AAM, Newman RD, et al. Cryptosporidiosis in northeastern Brazilian children: association with increased diarrheal morbidity. *J Infect Dis* 1998;111:754–760.
140. Guerrant DI, Moore SR, Lima AAM, et al. Association of early childhood diarrhea and cryptosporidiosis with impaired physical fitness and cognitive function four-seven years later in a poor urban community in northeastern Brazil. *Am J Trop Med Hyg* 1999;61:707–713.
141. Cruickshank R, Ashdown L, Croese J. Human cryptosporidiosis in north Queenland. *Aust N Z J Med* 1988;18:582–586.
142. Stehr-Green JK, McCaig L, Remsen HM, et al. Shedding of oocysts in immunocompetent individuals infected with *Cryptosporidium. Am J Trop Med Hyg* 1987;36:338–342.
143. Ferson MJ, Young LC. *Cryptosporidium* and coxsackievirus B5 causing epidemic diarrhoea in a child-care centre. *Med J Aust* 1992;156:813.
144. Alpert G, Bell LM, Kirkpatrick CE, et al. Outbreak of cryptosporidiosis in a day-care center. *Pediatrics* 1986;77:152–157.
145. Wolfson JS, Richter JM, Waldron MA, et al. Cryptosporidiosis in immunocompetent patients. *N Engl J Med* 1985;312:1278–1282.
146. McNabb SJN, Hensel DM, Welch DF, et al. Comparison of sedimentation and flotation techniques for identification of *Cryptosporidium* sp. oocysts in a large outbreak of human diarrhea. *J Clin Microbiol* 1985;22:587–589.
147. Melo Christino JAG, Carvalho MIP, Salgado MJ. An outbreak of cryptosporidiosis in a hospital day-care centre. *Epidemiol Infect* 1988;101:355–359.
148. Skeels MR, Sokolow R, Hubbard CV, et al. *Cryptosporidium* infection in Oregon public health clinic patients 1985–88: the value of statewide laboratory surveillance. *Am J Public Health* 1990;80:305–308.
149. Centers for Disease Control and Prevention. Cryptosporidiosis among children attending day care centers—Georgia, Pennsylvania, Michigan, California, New Mexico. *MMWR Morb Mortal Wkly Rep* 1984;33:599–601.
150. Combee CL, Collinge ML, Britt EM. Cryptosporidiosis in a hospital-associated day care center. *Pediatr Infect Dis* 1986;5: 528–532.
151. Heijbel H, Slaine K, Seigel B, et al. Outbreak of diarrhea in a day care center with spread to household members: the role of *Cryptosporidium. Pediatr Infect Dis J* 1987;6:532–535.
152. Nwanyanwu OC, Baird JN, Reeve GR. Cryptosporidiosis in a day-care center. *Tex Med* 1989;85:40–43.
153. Taylor JP, Perdue JN, Dingley D, et al. Cryptosporidiosis outbreak in a day-care center. *Am J Dis Child* 1985;139: 1023–1025.
154. Walters IN, Miller NM, Van den Ende J, et al. Outbreak of cryptosporidiosis among young children attending a day-care centre in Durban. *S Afr Med J* 1988;74:496–499.
155. Reif JS, Wimmer L, Smith JA, et al. Human cryptosporidiosis associated with an epizootic in calves. *Am J Public Health* 1989; 79:1528–1530.

156. Pohjola S, Oksanen H, Jokipii L, et al. Outbreak of cryptosporidiosis among veterinary students. *Scand J Infect Dis* 1986;18:173–178.
157. Levine JF, Levy MG, Walker RL, et al. Cryptosporidiosis in veterinary students. *J Am Vet Med Assoc* 1988;193:1413–1414.
158. Hojlyng N, Holten-Andersen W, et al. Cryptosporidiosis: a case of airborne transmission. *Lancet* 1987;2:271–272.
159. Tangermann RH, Gordon S, Wiesner P, et al. An outbreak of cryptosporidiosis in a day-care center in Georgia. *Am J Epidemiol* 1991;133:471–476.
160. Crawford FG, Vermund SH, Ma JY, et al. Asymptomatic cryptosporidiosis in a New York City day care center. *Pediatr Infect Dis J* 1988;7:806–807.
161. Diers J, McCallister GL. Occurrence of *Cryptosporidium* in home daycare centers in West-Central Colorado. *J Parasitol* 1989;75:637–638.
162. Koch KL, Phillips DJ, Aber RC, et al. Cryptosporidiosis in hospital personnel: evidence for person-to-person transmission. *Ann Intern Med* 1985;102:593–596.
163. Heald AE, Bartlett JA. *Cryptosporidium* spread in a group residential home. *Ann Intern Med* 1994;121:647–648.
164. Ravn P, Lundgren JD, Kjaeldgaard P, et al. Nosocomial outbreak of cryptosporidiosis in AIDS patients. *BMJ*1991; 302:277–280.
165. Navarrete S, Stetler HC, Avila C, et al. An outbreak of *Cryptosporidium* diarrhea in a pediatric hospital. *Pediatr Infect Dis J* 1991;10:248–250.
166. Martino P, Gentile G, Captrioli A, et al. Hospital-acquired cryptosporidiosis in a bone marrow transplantation unit. *J Infect Dis* 1988;158:647–648.
167. Collier AC, Miller RA, Meyers JD. Cryptosporidiosis after marrow transplantation: person-to-person transmission and treatment with spiramycin. *Ann Intern Med* 1984;101:205–206.
168. Baxby D, Hart CA, Taylor C. Human cryptosporidiosis: a possible case of hospital cross infection. *Br Med J* 1983;287: 1760–1761.
169. Atterholm I, Castor B, Norlin K. Cryptosporidiosis in southern Sweden. *Scand J Infect Dis* 1987;19:231–234.
170. Biggs B-A, Megna R, Wickremesinghe S, et al. Human infection with *Cryptosporidium* spp.: results of a 24 month survey. *Med J Aust* 1987;147:175–177.
171. Ma P, Kaufman DL, Helmick CG, D'Souza AJ, Navin TR. Cryptosporidiosis in tourists returning from the Caribbean. *N Engl J Med* 1985;312:647–648.
172. Soave R, Ma P. Cryptosporidiosis: traveler's diarrhea in two families. *Arch Intern Med* 1985;145:70–72.
173. Sterling CR, Seegar K, Sinclair NA. *Cryptosporidium* as a causative agent of traveler's diarrhea. *J Infect Dis* 1986;153: 380–381.
174. Taylor DN, Houston R, Shlim DR, et al. Etiology of diarrhea among travelers and foreign residents in Nepal. *JAMA* 1988; 260:1245–1248.
175. Ungar BLP, Mulligan M, Nutman TR. Serologic evidence of *Cryptosporidium* infection in US volunteers before and during Peace Corps service in Africa. *Arch Intern Med* 1989;149: 894–897.
176. Flegg PJ. *Cryptosporidium* in travelers from Pakistan. *Trans Royal Soc Trop Med Hyg*1987;81:171.
177. Jokipii L, Pohjola S, Jokipii AMM. *Cryptosporidium:* a frequent finding in patients with gastrointestinal symptoms. *Lancet* 1983;2:358–361.
178. Jokipii L, Pohjola S, Jokipii AMM. Cryptosporidiosis associated with traveling and giardiasis. *Gastroenterology* 1985;89:838–842.
179. Jokipii AMM, Hemilä M, Jokipii L. Prospective study of acquisition of *Cryptosporidium, Giardia lamblia,* and gastrointestinal illness. *Lancet* 1985;2:487–489.
180. Gatti S, Cevini C, Bruno A, et al. Cryptosporidiosis in tourists returning from Egypt and the island of Mauritius. *Clin Infect Dis* 1993;16:344–345.
181. Elsser KA, Moricz M, Proctor EM. *Cryptosporidium* infections: a laboratory survey. *Can Med Assoc J* 1986;135:211–213.
182. Fafard J, Lalonde R. Long-standing symptomatic cryptosporidiosis in a normal man: clinical response to spiramycin. *J Clin Gastroenterol* 1990;12:190–191.
183. Hunt DA, Shannon R, Palmer SR, et al. Cryptosporidiosis in an urban community. *Br Med J* 1984;289:814–816.
184. Baxby D, Hart CA. The incidence of cryptosporidiosis: a two-year prospective study in a children's hospital. *J Hyg* 1986; 96:107–111.
185. Issacs D, Hunt GH, Phillips AD, et al. Cryptosporidiosis in immunocompetent children. *J Clin Pathol* 1985;38:76–81.
186. Dryden MS, Shanson DC. The microbial causes of diarrhoea in patients infected with the human immunodeficiency virus. *J Infect* 1988;17:107–114.
187. Antony MA, Brandt LJ, Klein RS, et al. Infectious diarrhea in patients with AIDS. *Dig Dis Sci* 1988;33:1141–1146.
188. Laughon BE, Druckman DA, Vernon A, et al. Prevalence of enteric pathogens in homosexual men with and without acquired immunodeficiency syndrome. *Gastroenterology* 1988; 94:984–993.
189. Smith PD, Lane HC, Gill VJ, et al. Intestinal infections in patients with the acquired immunodeficiency syndrome (AIDS): etiology and response to therapy. *Ann Intern Med* 1988;108:328–333.
190. Connolly GM, Dryden MS, Shanson DC, et al. Cryptosporidial diarrhoea in AIDS and its treatment. *Gut* 1988;29: 593–597.
191. Connolly GM, Forbes A, Gazzard BG. Investigation of seemingly pathogen-negative diarrhoea in patients infected with HIV1. *Gut* 1990;31:886–889.
192. René E, Marche C, Regnier B, et al. Intestinal infections in patients with acquired immunodeficiency syndrome: a prospective study in 132 patients. *Dig Dis Sci* 1989;34:773–780.
193. Kotler DP, Francisco A, Clayton F, et al. Small intestinal injury and parasitic diseases in AIDS. *Ann Intern Med* 1990;113: 444–449.
194. Kim LS, Hadley WK, Stansell J, et al. Declining prevalence of cryptosporidiosis in San Francisco. *Clin Infect Dis* 1998;27: 655–656.
195. Lemoing V, Bissuel F, Costagliola D, et al. Decreased prevalence of intestinal cryptosporidiosis in HIV-infected patients concomitant to the widespread use of protease inhibitors. *AIDS* 1998;12:1395–1397.
196. Miller JR. Decreasing cryptosporidiosis among HIV-infected persons in New York City, 1995–1997. *J Urban Health* 1998; 75:601–602.
197. Kocoshis SA, Cibull ML, Davis TE, et al. Intestinal and pulmonary cryptosporidiosis in an infant with severe combined immune deficiency. *J Pediatr Gastroenterol Nutr* 1984;3: 149–157.
198. Sloper KS, Dourmashkin RR, Bird RB, et al. Chronic malabsorption due to cryptosporidiosis in a child with immunoglobulin deficiency. *Gut* 1982;23:80–82.
199. Jacyna MR, Parkin J, Goldin R, et al. Protracted enteric cryptosporidial infection in selective immunoglobulin A and saccharomyces opsonin deficiencies. *Gut* 1990;31:714–716.
200. Heaton P. Cryptosporidiosis and acute leukaemia. *Arch Dis Child* 1990;65:813–814.
201. Davis JJ, Heyman MB, Ferrell L, et al. Sclerosing cholangitis associated with chronic cryptosporidiosis in a child with a congenital immunodeficiency disorder. *Am J Gastroenterol* 1987; 82:1196–1202.

202. Chng HH, Shaw D, Klesius P, et al. Inability of oral bovine transfer factor to eradicate cryptosporidial infection in a patient with congenital dysgammaglobulinemia. *Clin Immunol Immunopathol* 1989;50:402–406.
203. Holley HP, Thiers BH. Cryptosporidiosis in a patient receiving immunosuppressive therapy: possible activation of latent infection. *Dig Dis Sci* 1986;31:1004–1007.
204. Mead GM, Sweetenham JW, Ewins DL, et al. Intestinal cryptosporidiosis: a complication of cancer treatment. *Cancer Treat Rep* 1986;70:769–770.
205. Miller RA, Holmberg RE Jr, Clausen CR. Life-threatening diarrhea caused by *Cryptosporidium* in a child undergoing therapy for acute lymphocytic leukemia. *J Pediatr* 1983;103:256–259.
206. Oh SH, Jaffe N, Fainstein V, et al. Cryptosporidiosis and anticancer chemotherapy. *J Pediatr* 1984;104:963–964.
207. Foot ABM, Oakhill A, Mott MG. Cryptosporidiosis and acute leukaemia. *Arch Dis Child* 1990;65:236–237.
208. Gentile G, Baldassarri L, Caprioli A, et al. Colonic vascular invasion as a possible route of extraintestinal cryptosporidiosis. *Am J Med* 1987;82:574–575.
209. Gentile G, Venditti M, Micozzi A, et al. Cryptosporidiosis in patients with hematologic malignancies. *Rev Infect Dis* 1991;13: 842–846.
210. Stine KC, Harris J-AS, Lindsey NJ, et al. Spontaneous remission of cryptosporidiosis in a child with acute lymphocytic leukemia. *Clin Pediatr* 1985;24:722–724.
211. Travis WD, Schmidt K, MacLowry JD, et al. Respiratory cryptosporidiosis in a patient with malignant lymphoma. *Arch Pathol Lab Med* 1990;114:519–522.
212. Borowitz SM, Saulsbury FT. Treatment of chronic cryptosporidial infection with orally administered human serum immune globulin. *J Pediatr* 1991;119:593–595.
213. Roncoroni AJ, Gomez MA, Mera J, et al. *Cryptosporidium* infection in renal transplant patients. *J Infect Dis* 1989;160:559.
214. Ona ET. Early pitfalls in renal transplantation. *Transplant Proc* 1992;24:1280–1282.
215. Vajro P, di Martino L, Scotti S, et al. Intestinal *Cryptosporidium* carriage in two liver-transplanted children. *J Pediatr Gastroenterol Nutr* 1991;12:139.
216. Kibbler CC, Smith A, Hamilton-Dutoit SJ, et al. Pulmonary cryptosporidiosis occurring in a bone marrow transplant patient. *Scand J Infect Dis* 1987;19:581–584.
217. Manivel C, Filipovich A, Snover DC. Cryptosporidiosis as a cause of diarrhea following bone marrow transplantation. *Dis Colon Rectum* 1985;28:741–742.
218. Portnoy D, Whiteside ME, Buckley E III, et al. Treatment of intestinal cryptosporidiosis with spiramycin. *Ann Intern Med* 1984;101:202–204.
219. Blakey JL, Barnes GL, Bishop RJ, et al. Infectious diarrhea in children undergoing bone-marrow transplantation. *Aust N Z J Med* 1989;19:31–36.
220. Fletcher A, Sims TA, Talbot IC. Cryptosporidial enteritis without general or selective immune deficiency. *Br Med J* 1982; 285:22–23.
221. Petras RE, Carey WD, Alanis A. Cryptosporidial enteritis in a homosexual male with acquired immunodeficiency syndrome. *Cleve Clin Q* 1983;50:41–45.
222. Bird RG, Smith MD. Cryptosporidiosis in man: parasite life cycle and fine structural pathology. *J Pathol* 1980;132:217–233.
223. Heine J, Pohlenz JFL, Moon HW, et al. Enteric lesions and diarrhea in gnotobiotic calves monoinfected with *Cryptosporidium* species. *J Infect Dis* 1984;150:768–775.
224. Argenzio RA, Liacos JA, Levy ML, et al. Villous atrophy, crypt hyperplasia, cellular infiltration, and impaired glucose-Na absorption in enteric cryptosporidiosis of pigs. *Gastroenterology* 1990;98:1129–1140.
225. Moore R, Tzipori S, Griffiths JK, et al. Temporal changes in permeability and structure of piglet ileum after site-specific infection by *Cryptosporidium parvum. Gastroenterology* 1995; 108:1030–1039.
226. Modigliani R, Bories C, Le Charpentier Y, et al. Diarrhoea and malabsorption in acquired immune deficiency syndrome: a study of four cases with special emphasis on opportunistic protozoan infestations. *Gut* 1985;26:179–187.
227. Adams RB, Guerrant RL, Zu S, et al. *Cryptosporidium parvum* infection of intestinal epithelium: Morphologic and functional studies in an in vitro model. *J Infect Dis* 1994;169:170–177.
228. Griffiths JK, Moore R, Dooley S, et al. *Cryptosporidium parvum* infection of Caco-2 cell monolayers induces an apical monolayer defect, selectively increases transmonolayer permeability, and causes epithelial cell death. *Infect Immun* 1994;62: 4506–4514.
229. Current WL, Garcia LS. Cryptosporidiosis. *Clin Microbiol Rev* 1991;4:325–358.
230. Garza DH, Fedorak RN, Soave R. Enterotoxin-like activity in cultured cryptosporidia: role in diarrhea. *Gastroenterology* 1986; 90:1424.
231. Guerrant RL, Petri WA, Weikel CS. Parasitic causes of diarrhea. In: Lebenthal E, Duffey M, eds. *Textbook of secretory diarrhea.* New York: Raven Press, 1990:273–280.
232. Guarino A, Canani RB, Pozio E, et al. Enterotoxic effect of stool supernatant of *Cryptosporidium*-infected calves on human jejunum. *Gastroenterology* 1994;106:28–34.
233. Sears CL, Guerrant RL. Cryptosporidiosis: the complexity of intestinal pathophysiology. *Gastroenterology* 1994;106: 252–254.
234. Gardner AL, Roche JK, Weikel CS, et al. Intestinal cryptosporidiosis: pathophysiologic alterations and specific cellular and humoral immune responses in rnu/+ and rnu/rnu (athymic) rats. *Am J Trop Med Hyg* 1991;44:49–62.
235. Moon HW, Pohlenz JFL, Woodmansee DB, et al. Intestinal cryptosporidiosis: pathogenesis and immunity. *Microecol Ther* 1985;15:103–120.
236. Adams RB, Guerrant RL, Zu S, et al. *Cryptosporidium parvum* infection of intestinal epithelium: morphologic and functional studies in an in vitro model. *J Infect Dis* 1994;169:170–177.
237. Heine J, Moon HW, Woodmansee DB. Persistent *Cryptosporidium* infection in congenitally athymic (nude) mice. *Infect Immun* 1984;43:856–859.
238. Ungar BLP, Burris JA, Quinn CA, et al. New mouse models for chronic *Cryptosporidium* infection in immunodeficient hosts. *Infect Immun* 1990;58:961–969.
239. Ungar BLP, Kao T-C, Burris JA, et al. *Cryptosporidium* infection in an adult mouse model. Independent roles for IFN-gamma and CD4+ T lymphocytes in protective immunity. *J Immunol* 1991;147:1014–1022.
240. Mead JR, Arrowood MJ, Healey MC, et al. Cryptosporidial infections in SCID mice reconstituted with human or murine lymphocytes. *J Protozool* 1991;38:59S–61S.
241. Mead JR, Arrowood MJ, Sidwell RW, et al. Chronic *Cryptosporidium parvum* infections in congenitally immunodeficient SCID and nude mice. *J Infect Dis* 1991;163:1297–1304.
242. Chen W, Harp JA, Harmsen AG. Requirements for CD4+ cells and gamma interferon in resolution of established *Cryptosporidium parvum* infection in mice. *Infect Immun* 1993;61: 3928–3932.
243. Darban H, Enriquez J, Sterling CR, et al. Cryptosporidiosis facilitated by murine retroviral infection with LP-BM5. *J Infect Dis* 1991;164:741–745.
244. Petersen C. Cryptosporidiosis in patients infected with the human immunodeficiency virus. *Clin Infect Dis* 1992;15: 903–909.

245. Enriquez FJ, Sterling CR. *Cryptosporidium* infections in inbred strains of mice. *J Protozool* 1991;38:100S–102S.
246. Harp JA, Moon HW. Susceptibility of mast cell-deficient W/W^v mice to *Cryptosporidium parvum. Infect Immun* 1991;59: 718–720.
247. Taghi-Kilani R, Sekla L, Hayglass KT. The role of humoral immunity in *Cryptosporidium* spp. infection. Studies with B cell-depleted mice. *J Immunol* 1990;145:1571–1576.
248. Griffiths JK, Theodos C, Paris M, et al. The gamma interferon gene knockout mouse: a highly sensitive model for evaluation of therapeutic agents against *Cryptosporidium parvum. J Clin Microbiol* 1998;36:2503–2508.
249. Mead JR, You XD. Susceptibility differences to *Cryptosporidium parvum* infection in two strains of gamma interferon knockout mice. *J Parasitol* 1998;84:1045–1048.
250. Campbell PN, Current WL. Demonstration of serum antibodies to *Cryptosporidium* sp. in normal and immunodeficient humans with confirmed infections. *J Clin Microbiol* 1983;18: 165–169.
251. Casemore DP. The antibody response to *Cryptosporidium:* development of a serological test and its use in a study of immunologically normal persons. *J Infect* 1987;14:125–134.
252. Ungar BLP, Soave R, Fayer R, et al. Enzyme immunoassay detection of immunoglobulin M and G antibodies to *Cryptosporidium* in immunocompetent and immunocompromised persons. *J Infect Dis* 1986;153:570–578.
253. Janoff EN, Mead PS, Mead JR, et al. Endemic *Cryptosporidium* and *Giardia lamblia* infections in a Thai orphanage. *Am J Trop Med Hyg* 1990;43:248–256.
254. Laxer MA, Alcantara AK, Javato-Laxer M, et al. Immune response to cryptosporidiosis in Philippine children. *Am J Trop Med Hyg* 1990;42:131–139.
255. Okhuysen PC, Chappell CL, Sterling CR, et al. Susceptibility and serologic response of healthy adults to reinfection with *Cryptosporidium parvum. Infect Immun* 1998;66:441–443.
256. Kapel N, Meillet D, Buraud M, et al. Determination of anti-*Cryptosporidium* coproantibodies by time-resolved immunofluorometric assay. *Trans Royal Soc Trop Med Hyg* 1993;87: 330–332.
257. Flanigan TP. Human immunodeficiency virus infection and cryptosporidiosis: protective immune responses. *Am J Trop Med Hyg* 1994;50:29–35.
258. Benhamou Y, Kapel N, Hoang C, et al. Inefficacy of intestinal secretory immune response to *Cryptosporidium* in acquired immunodeficiency syndrome. *Gastroenterology* 1995;108: 627–635.
259. Dann SM, Okhuysen PC, Salameh BM, et al. Fecal antibodies to *Cryptosporidium parvum* in healthy volunteers. *Infect Immun* 2000;68:5068–5074.
260. Ungar BLP, Nash TE. Quantification of specific antibody response to *Cryptosporidium* antigens by laser densitometry. *Infect Immun* 1986;53:124–128.
261. Mead JR, Arrowood MJ, Sterling CR. Antigens of *Cryptosporidium* sporozoites recognized by immune sera of infected animals and humans. *J Parasitol* 1988;74:135–143.
262. Riggs MW. Immunology: host response and development of passive immunotherapy and vaccines. In: Fayer R, ed. Cryptosporidium*and cryptosporidiosis.* Boca Raton, FL: CRC Press, 1997:129–162.
263. Tilley M, Upton SJ, Fayer R, et al. Identification of a 15-kilodalton surface glycoprotein on sporozoites of *Cryptosporidium parvum. Infect Immun* 1991;59:1002–1007.
264. Reperant J-M, Naciri M, Chardes T, et al. Immunological characterization of a 17-kDa antigen from *Cryptosporidium parvum* recognized early by mucosal IgA antibodies. *FEMS Microbiol Lett* 1992;99:7–14.
265. Whitmire WM, Harp JA. Characterization of bovine cellular and serum antibody responses during infection by *Cryptosporidium parvum. Infect Immun* 1991;59:990–995.
266. Lumb R, Lanser JA, O'Donoghue PJ. Electrophoretic and immunoblot analysis of *Cryptosporidium* oocysts. *Immunol Cell Biol* 1988;66:369–376.
267. Hill BD, Blewett DA, Dawson AM, et al. Analysis of the kinetics, isotype and specificity of serum and coproantibody in lambs infected with *Cryptosporidium parvum. Res Vet Sci* 1990;48:76–81.
268. Tilley M, Upton SJ. Electrophoretic characterization of *Cryptosporidium parvum* (KSU-1 isolate) (Apicomplexa: Cryptosporiidae). *Can J Zool* 1990;68:1513–1519.
269. Flanigan T, Whalen C, Turner J, et al. *Cryptosporidium* infection and CD4 counts. *Ann Intern Med* 1992;116:840–842.
270. Blanshard C, Jackson AM, Shanson DC, et al. Cryptosporidiosis in HIV-seropositive patients. *Q J Med* 1992;85:813–823.
271. Gomez Moralez MA, Ausiello CM, Guarino A, et al. Severe, protracted intestinal cryptosporidiosis associated with interferon γ deficiency: pediatric case report. *Clin Infect Dis* 1996; 22:848–850.
272. Laurent F, Eckmann L, Savidge T, et al. *Cryptosporidium parvum* infection of human intestinal epithelial cells induces the polarized secretion of C-X-C chemokines. *Infect Immun* 1997; 65:5067–5073.
273. Seydel KB, Zhang T, Champion GA, et al. *Cryptosporidium parvum* infection of human intestinal xenografts in SCID mice induces production of tumor necrosis factor alpha and interleukin-8. *Infect Immun* 1998;66:2379–2382.
274. Robinson P, Okhuysen PC, Chappell CL, et al. Transforming growth factor β1 is expressed in the jejunum after experimental *Cryptosporidium parvum* infection in humans. *Infect Immun* 2000;68:5405–5407.
275. Jokipii L, Jokipii AMM. Timing of symptoms and oocyst excretion in human cryptosporidiosis. *N Engl J Med* 1986;315: 1643–1647.
276. Bannister P, Mountford RA. *Cryptosporidium* in the elderly: a cause of life-threatening diarrhea. *Am J Med* 1989;86:507–508.
277. Sallon S, Deckelbaum RJ, Schmid II, et al. *Cryptosporidium,* malnutrition, and chronic diarrhea in children. *Am J Dis Child* 1988;142:312–315.
278. Sarabia-Arce S, Salazar-Lindo E, Gilman RH, et al. Case–control study of *Cryptosporidium parvum* infection in Peruvian children hospitalized for diarrhea: possible association with malnutrition and nosocomial infection. *Pediatr Infect Dis J* 1990;9: 627–631.
279. Lima AAM, Fang G, Schorling JB, et al. Persistent diarrhea in northeast Brazil: etiologies and interactions with malnutrition. *Acta Paediatr* 1992;81[Suppl 381]:39–44.
280. Keren G, Barzilai A, Barzilay Z, et al. Life-threatening cryptosporidiosis in immunocompetent infants. *Eur J Pediatr* 1987; 146:187–189.
281. DuPont HL, Chappell CL, Sterling CR, et al. The infectivity of *Cryptosporidium parvum* in healthy volunteers. *N Engl J Med* 1995;332:855–859.
282. Chappell CL, Okhuysen PC, Sterling CR, et al. Infectivity of *Cryptosporidium parvum* in healthy adults with pre-existing anti-*C. parvum* serum immunoglobulin G. *Am J Trop Med Hyg* 1999;60:157–164.
283. Okhuysen PC, Chappell CL, Crabb JH, et al. Virulence of three distinct *Cryptosporidium parvum* isolates for healthy adults. *J Infect Dis* 1999;180:1275–1281.
284. Egger M, Mausezahl D, Odermatt P, et al. Symptoms and transmission of intestinal cryptosporidiosis. *Arch Dis Child* 1990; 65:445–447.
285. Thomson MA, Benson JWT, Wright PA. Two year study of *Cryptosporidium* infection. *Arch Dis Child* 1987;62:559–563.

286. Harari MD, West B, Dwyer B. *Cryptosporidium* as a cause of laryngotracheitis in an infant. *Lancet* 1986;1:1207.
287. Hawkins SP, Thomas RP, Teasdale C. Acute pancreatitis: a new finding in *Cryptosporidium* enteritis. *Br Med J* 1987;294: 483–484.
288. Ramsden K, Freeth M. Cryptosporidial infection presenting as an acute appendicitis. *Histopathology* 1989;14:209–211.
289. Merino FJ, Lopez-Serrano MC, Velasco AC. Diarrhea por *Cryptosporidium*asociada a urticaria y angiodema. *Enferm Infect Microbiol Clin* 1989;7:78.
290. Hay EM, Winfield J, McKendrick MW. Reactive arthritis associated with *Cryptosporidium* enteritis. *Br Med J* 1987;295:248.
291. Shepherd RC, Sinha GP, Reed CL, et al. Cryptosporidiosis in the West of Scotland. *Scott Med J* 1988;33:365–368.
292. Shepherd RC, Smail PJ, Sinha GP. Reactive arthritis complicating cryptosporidial infection. *Arch Dis Child* 1989;64:743–744.
293. Andreani T, Modigliani R, le Charpentier Y, et al. Acquired immunodeficiency with intestinal cryptosporidiosis: possible transmission by Haitian whole blood. *Lancet* 1983;1: 1187–1191.
294. Cooper DA, Wodak A, Marriot DJE, et al. Cryptosporidiosis in the acquired immune deficiency syndrome. *Pathology* 1984;16: 455–457.
295. Gerard L, Daleine G, Longuet P, et al. Intestinal cryptosporidiosis in 37 HIV infected patients: prognostic significance of biliary tract involvement. In: Programs and abstracts of the IXth International Conference on AIDS; 1993; Berlin, Germany. Abstract WS-B13-4.
296. Pitlik SD, Fainstein V, Garza D, et al. Human cryptosporidiosis: spectrum of disease. *Arch Intern Med* 1983;143:2269–2275.
297. Soave R, Danner RL, Honig CL, et al. Cryptosporidiosis in homosexual men. *Ann Intern Med* 1984;100:504–511.
298. Saltzberg DM, Kotloff KL, Newman JL, et al. *Cryptosporidium* infection in acquired immunodeficiency syndrome: not always a poor prognosis. *J Clin Gastroenterol* 1991;13:94–97.
299. Berkowitz CD, Seidel JS. Spontaneous resolution of cryptosporidiosis in a child with acquired immunodeficiency syndrome. *Am J Dis Child* 1985;139:967.
300. Lerner CW, Tapper ML. Opportunistic infection complicating acquired immune deficiency syndrome: clinical features of 25 cases. *Medicine (Baltimore)* 1984;63:155–164.
301. Mc Gowan I, Hawkins AS, Weller IVD. The natural history of cryptosporidial diarrhoea in HIV-infected patients. *AIDS* 1993; 7:349–354.
302. Scaglia M, Senaldi G, Di Perri G, et al. Unusual low-grade cryptosporidial enteritis in AIDS: a case report. *Infection* 1986;14: 87–88.
303. Janoff EN, Limas C, Gebhard RL, et al. Cryptosporidial carriage without symptoms in the acquired immunodeficiency syndrome (AIDS). *Ann Intern Med* 1990;112:75–76.
304. Gentile G, Caprioli A, Donelli G, et al. Asymptomatic carriage of *Cryptosporidium* in two patients with leukemia. *Am J Infect Control* 1990;18:127–128.
305. Zar F, Geiseler PJ, Brown VA. Asymptomatic carriage of *Cryptosporidium* in the stool of a patient with acquired immunodeficiency syndrome. *J Infect Dis* 1985;151:195.
306. Godwin TA. Cryptosporidiosis in the acquired immunodeficiency syndrome: a study of 15 autopsy cases. *Hum Pathol* 1991;22:1215–1223.
307. Berk RN, Wall SD, McArdle CB, et al. Cryptosporidiosis of the stomach and small intestine in patients with AIDS. *AJR Am J Roentgenol* 1984;143:549–554.
308. Kazlow PG, Shah K, Benkov KJ, et al. Esophageal cryptosporidiosis in a child with acquired immune deficiency syndrome. *Gastroenterology* 1986;91:1301–1303.
309. Oberhuber G, Lauer E, Stolte M, et al. Cryptosporidiosis of the appendix vermiformis: a case report. *Z Gastroenterol* 1991;29: 606–608.
310. Zambrano Nunez MR, Sakai P, Ishioka S, et al. Erosive gastroduodenitis with cryptosporidiosis in a patient with acquired immunodeficiency syndrome. *Rev Hosp Clin Fac Med Sao Paulo* 1990;45:188–189.
311. Gross TL, Wheat J, Bartlett M, O'Connor KW. AIDS and multiple system involvement with *Cryptosporidium. Am J Gastroenterol* 1986;81:456–458.
312. Orenstein J, Steinberg W, Simon G. *Cryptosporidiosis of the pancreas [Abstract 1224]. In: Program and abstracts of the 33rd Interscience Conference on Antimicrobial Agents and Chemotherapy.* New Orleans, LA: American Society for Microbiology, 1993;344.
313. Meyers SA, Kuhlman JE, Fishman EK. Enterovesical fistula in a patient with cryptosporidiosis and AIDS: CT demonstration. *Clin Imaging* 1990;14:143–145.
314. Soave R, Johnson WD Jr. *Cryptosporidium* and *Isospora belli* infections. *J Infect Dis* 1988;157:225–229.
315. Lee JG, Grech P, Edwards P, et al. AIDS cholangiopathy as the first sign of HIV infection. *N C Med J* 1993;54:16–17.
316. Kahn DG, Garfinkle JM, Klonoff DC, et al. Cryptosporidial and cytomegaloviral hepatitis and cholecystitis. *Arch Pathol Lab Med* 1987;111:879–881.
317. Pitlik SD, Fainstein V, Rios A, et al. Cryptosporidial cholecystitis. *N Engl J Med* 1983;308:967.
318. Dowsett JF, Miller R, Davidson R, et al. Sclerosing cholangitis in acquired immunodeficiency syndrome: case reports and review of the literature. *Scand J Gastroenterol* 1988;23:1267–1274.
319. Hasan FA, Jeffers LJ, Dickinson G, et al. Hepatobiliary cryptosporidiosis and cytomegalovirus infection mimicking metastatic cancer to the liver. *Gastroenterology* 1991;100:1743–1748.
320. Hinnant K, Schwartz A, Rotterdam H, et al. Cytomegaloviral and cryptosporidial cholecystitis in two patients with AIDS. *Am J Surg Pathol* 1989;13:57–60.
321. Forbes A, Blanshard C, Gazzard B. Natural history of AIDS related sclerosing cholangitis: a study of 20 cases. *Gut* 1993;34: 116–121.
322. Blumberg RS, Kelsey P, Perrone T, et a;. Cytomegalovirus- and *Cryptosporidium*-associated acalculous gangrenous cholecystitis. *Am J Med* 1984;76:1118–1123.
323. Cello JP. Acquired immunodeficiency syndrome cholangiopathy: spectrum of disease. *Am J Med* 1989;86:539–546.
324. Tzipori S, Roberton D, Chapman C. Remission of diarrhoea due to cryptosporidiosis in an immunodeficient child treated with hyperimmune bovine colostrum. *Br Med J* 1986;293: 1276–1277.
325. Tzipori S, Roberton D, Cooper DA, et al. Chronic cryptosporidial diarrhoea and hyperimmune cow colostrum. *Lancet* 1987;2:344–345.
326. Margulis SJ, Honig CL, Soave R, et al. Biliary tract obstruction in the acquired immunodeficiency syndrome. *Ann Intern Med* 1986;105:207–210.
327. Amiel C, May T, Mansuy L, et al. *Cryptosporidium* cholangitis treated by celioscopic cholecystectomy and sphincterotomy. In: Program and abstracts of the IXth International Conference on AIDS; 1993; Berlin, Germany. Abstract PO-B10-1460.
328. Ma P, Villanueva TG, Kaufman D, et al. Respiratory cryptosporidiosis in the acquired immune deficiency syndrome: use of modified Kinyoun and Hemacolor stains for rapid diagnoses. *JAMA* 1984;252:1298–1301.
329. Miller RA, Wasserheit JN, Kirihara J, et al. Detection of *Cryptosporidium* oocysts in sputum during screening for mycobacteria. *J Clin Microbiol* 1984;20:1192–1193.
330. Moore JA, Frenkel JK. Respiratory and enteric cryptosporidiosis in humans. *Arch Pathol Lab Med* 1991;115:1160–1162.

331. Forgacs P, Tarshis A, Ma P, et al. Intestinal and bronchial cryptosporidiosis in an immunodeficient homosexual man. *Ann Intern Med* 1983;99:793–794.
332. Fripp PJ, Bothma MT, Crewe-Brown HH. Four years of cryptosporidiosis at GaRankuwa Hospital. *J Infect* 1991;23:93–100.
333. Hojlyng N, Jensen BN. Respiratory cryptosporidiosis in HIV-positive patients. *Lancet* 1988;1:590–591.
334. Goodstein RS, Colombo CS, Illfelder MA, et al. Bronchial and gastrointestinal cryptosporidiosis in AIDS. *J Am Osteopath Assoc* 1989;89:195–197.
335. Jensen BN, Gerstoft J, Hojlyng N, et al. Pulmonary pathogens in HIV-infected patients. *Scand J Infect Dis* 1990;22:413–420.
336. Jensen BN, Gerstoft J, Skinhoj P. The prognosis in HIV-infected patients with pneumonia. Relation to microbiological diagnoses. *Dan Med Bull* 1991;38:468–470.
337. Brady EM, Margolis ML, Korzeniowski OM. Pulmonary cryptosporidiosis in acquired immune deficiency syndrome. *JAMA* 1984;252:89–90.
338. Davis JJ, Heyman MB. Cryptosporidiosis and sinusitis in an immunodeficient adolescent. *J Infect Dis* 1988;158:649.
339. Martin Sanchez AM, Rodriguez Hernandez J, Fuertes Martin A, et al. Cryptosporidiasis respiratoria: a proposito de un nuevo caso. *Rev Clin Esp* 1991;189:300–301.
340. Rodriguez Perez R, Fernandez Perez B, Dominguez Alvarez LM, et al. Criptosporidiasis respiratoria en pacientes VIH. Descripcion de dos casos. *Rev Clin Esp* 1992;190:210–211.
341. Gomez Morales MA, Pozio E, Croppo GP. Serodiagnosis of cryptosporidiosis in Italian HIV-positive patients by means of an oocyst soluble antigen in an ELISA. *J Infect* 1992;25:229–236.
342. McCarty M, Choudhri AH, Helbert M, et al. Radiological features of AIDS related cholangitis. *Clin Radiol* 1989;40: 582–585.
343. Bonato C, Vigano MG, Nicoletti R, et al. Sonographic diagnosis of cholangitis in AIDS patients. In: Programs and abstracts of the IXth International Conference on AIDS; 1993; Berlin, Germany. Abstract PO-B10-1437.
344. Teixidor HS, Godwin TA, Ramirez EA. Cryptosporidiosis of the biliary tract in AIDS. *Radiology* 1991;180:51–56.
345. Schneiderman DJ, Cello JP, Laing FC. Papillary stenosis and sclerosing cholangitis in the acquired immunodeficiency syndrome. *Ann Intern Med* 1987;106:546–549.
346. Goodgame RW, Genta RM, Clinton White A, et al. Intensity of infection in AIDS-associated cryptosporidiosis. *J Infect Dis* 1993;167:704–709.
347. Floch JJ, Laroche R, Kadende P, et al. Les parasites, agents etiologiques des diarrhées du SIDA: intérêt de l'examen du liquide d'aspiration duodénale. *Bull Soc Pathol Exot Filiales* 1989;82: 316–320.
348. Silverman JF, Levine J, Finley JL, et al. Small-intestinal brushing cytology in the diagnosis of cryptosporidiosis in AIDS. *Diagn Cytopathol* 1990;6:193–196.
349. Connolly GMM, Ellis DS, Williams JE, et al. Use of electron microscopy in examination of faeces and rectal and jejunal biopsy specimens. *J Clin Pathol* 1991;44:313–316.
350. Zierdt WS. Concentration and identification of *Cryptosporidium* sp. by use of a parasite concentrator. *J Clin Microbiol* 1984; 20:860–861.
351. Perry JL, Matthews JS, Miller GR. Parasite detection efficiencies of five stool concentration systems. *J Clin Microbiol* 1990; 28:1094–1097.
352. Weber R, Bryan RT, Juranek DD. Improved stool concentration procedure for detection of *Cryptosporidium* oocysts in fecal specimens. *J Clin Microbiol* 1992;30:2869–2873.
353. Smith HV, McDiarmid A, Smith AL, et al. An analysis of staining methods for the detection of *Cryptosporidium* spp. oocysts in water-related samples. *Parasitology* 1989;99:323–327.
354. Garcia LS, Bruckner DA, Brewer TC, et al. Techniques for the recovery and identification of *Cryptosporidium* oocysts from stool specimens. *J Clin Microbiol* 1983;18:185–190.
355. Garza D, Hopfer RL, Eichelberger C, et al. Fecal staining methods for screening *Cryptosporidium* oocysts. *J Med Technol* 1984; 1:560–563.
356. Ma P, Soave R. Three-step stool examination for cryptosporidiosis in 10 homosexual men with protracted watery diarrhea. *J Infect Dis* 1983;147:824–828.
357. Garcia LS, Current WL. Cryptosporidiosis: clinical features and diagnosis. *Crit Rev Clin Lab Sci* 1989;27:439–460.
358. Casemore DP. ACP Broadsheet 128: June 1991, laboratory methods for diagnosing cryptosporidiosis. *J Clin Pathol* 1991; 44:445–451.
359. Chichino G, Bruno A, Cevini C, et al. New rapid staining methods of *Cryptosporidium* oocysts in stool. *J Protozool* 1991; 38:212S–214S.
360. MacPherson DW, McQueen R. Cryptosporidiosis: multiattribute evaluation of six diagnostic methods. *J Clin Microbiol* 1993;31:198–202.
361. Casemore DP, Sands RL, Curry A. *Cryptosporidium* species: a "new" human pathogen. *J Clin Pathol* 1985;38:1321–1336.
362. Casemore DP, Armstrong M, Sands RL. Laboratory diagnosis of cryptosporidiosis. *J Clin Pathol* 1985;38:1337–1341.
363. Payne P, Lancaster LA, Heinzman M, et al. Identification of *Cryptosporidium* in patients with the acquired immunodeficiency syndrome. *N Engl J Med* 1983;309:613–614.
364. Ungureanu EM, Dontu GE. A new staining technique for the identification of *Cryptosporidium* oocysts in faecal smears. *Trans royal Soc Trop Med Hyg* 1992;86:638.
365. Garcia LS, Brewer TC, Bruckner DA. Fluorescence detection of *Cryptosporidium* oocysts in human fecal specimens by using monoclonal antibodies. *J Clin Microbiol* 1987;25:119–121.
366. Garcia LS, Brewer TC, Bruckner DA. Incidence of *Cryptosporidium* in all patients submitting stool specimens for ova and parasite examination: monoclonal antibody IFA method. *Diagn Microbiol Infect Dis* 1989;11:25–27.
367. Garcia LS, Shum AC, Bruckner DA. Evaluation of a new monoclonal antibody combination reagent for direct fluorescence detection of *Giardia* cysts and *Cryptosporidium* oocysts in human fecal specimens. *J Clin Microbiol* 1992;30: 3255–3257.
368. Arrowood MJ, Sterling CR. Comparison of conventional staining methods and monoclonal antibody-based methods for *Cryptosporidium* oocyst detection. *J Clin Microbiol* 1989;27: 1490–1495.
369. Rusnak J, Hadfield TL, Rhodes MM, et al. Detection of *Cryptosporidium* oocysts in human fecal specimens by an indirect immunofluorescence assay with monoclonal antibodies. *J Clin Microbiol* 1989;27:1135–1136.
370. Ortega YR, Sterling CR, Gilman RH, et al. *Cyclospora* species—a new protozoan pathogen of humans. *N Engl J Med* 1993; 328:1308–1312.
371. Graczyk TK, Cranfield MR, Fayer R. Evaluation of commercial enzyme immunoassay (EIA) and immunofluorescent antibody (IFA) test kits for detection of *Cryptosporidium* oocysts of species other than *Cryptosporidium*. *Am J Trop Med Hyg* 1996; 54:274–279.
372. Garcia LS, Shimizu RY. Evaluation of nine immunoassay kits (enzyme immunoassay and direct fluorescence) for detection of *Giardia lamblia* and *Cryptosporidium parvum* in human fecal specimens. *J Clin Microbiol* 1997;35:1526–1529.
373. Fricker CR, Crabb JH. Water-borne cryptosporidiosis: detection methods and treatment options. *Adv Parasitol* 1998;40: 241–278.
374. Morgan UM, Thompson RCA. PCR detection of *Cryptosporid-*

ium parvum: the way forward? *Parasitol Today* 1998;14: 241–246.
375. Widmer G. Genetic heterogeneity and PCR detection of *Cryptosporidium parvum. Adv Parasitol* 1998;40:223–240.
376. Blagburn BL, Soave R. Prophylaxis and chemotherapy: human and animal. In: Fayer R, ed. Cryptosporidium*and cryptosporidiosis.* Boca Raton, FL: CRC Press, 1997:111–128.
377. Griffiths JK. Human cryptosporidiosis: epidemiology, transmission, clinical disease, treatment, and diagnosis. In: Baker JR, Muller R, Rollinson D, eds. *Opportunistic protozoa in humans. Advances in parasitology,* vol 40. San Diego, CA: Academic Press, 1998:37–85.
378. Griffiths JK, Balakrishnan R, Widmer G, et al. Paromomycin and geneticin inhibit intracellular *Cryptosporidium parvum* without trafficking through the host cell cytoplasm: implications for drug delivery. *Infect Immun* 1998;66:3874–3883.
379. Bodin S, Bouhour D, Durupt S, et al. Value of protease inhibitors in the treatment of infections due to microsporidium and/or *Cryptosporidium* in patients with HIV. *Pathol Biol* 1998;46:418–419.
380. Carr A, Marriott D, Field A, et al. Treatment of HIV-1 associated microsporidiosis and cryptosporidiosis with combination antiretroviral therapy. *Lancet* 1998;351:256–261.
381. Foudraine NA, Weverling GJ, van Gool T, et al. Improvement of chronic diarrhoea in patients with advanced HIV-1 infection during potent antiretroviral therapy. *AIDS* 1998;12:35–41.
382. Clark DP. New insights into human cryptosporidiosis. *Clin Microbiol Rev* 1999;12:554–563.
383. White AC, Chappell CL, Hayat CS, et al. Paromomycin for cryptosporidiosis in AIDS: a prospective, double-blind trial. *J Infect Dis* 1994;170:419–424.
384. Smith NH, Cron S, Valdez LM, et al. Combination drug therapy for cryptosporidiosis in AIDS. *J Infect Dis* 1998;178: 900–903.
385. Rossignol J-F, Hidalgo H, Feregrino M, et al. A double-blind placebo-controlled study of nitazoxanide in the treatment of cryptosporidial diarrhoea in AIDS patients in Mexico. *Trans royal Soc Trop Med Hyg* 1998;92:663–666.
386. Davis LJ, Soave RE, Dudley RE, et al. *Nitazoxanide (NTZ for AIDS-related cryptosporidial diarrhea (CD): an open-label safety, efficacy and pharmacologic study. In: Program and abstracts of the 36th Interscience Conference on Antimicrobial Agents and Chemotherapy.* Washington, DC: American Society for Microbiology; 1996:289.
387. Roehr B. Another failed promise? Nitazoxanide gets the NIX. *J Int Assoc Phys AIDS Care* August 1998.
388. Ungar BLP, Ward DJ, Fayer R, et al. Cessation of *Cryptosporidium*-associated diarrhea in an acquired immunodeficiency syndrome patient after treatment with hyperimmune bovine colostrum. *Gastroenterology* 1990;98:486–489.
389. Crabb JH. Antibody-based immunotherapy of cryptosporidiosis. In: Baker JR, Muller R, Rollinson D, eds. *Opportunistic protozoa in humans. Advances in parasitology,* vol 40. San Diego, CA: Academic Press, 1998:121–149.
390. Anderson BC. Moist heat inactivation of *Cryptosporidium* sp. *Am J Public Health* 1985;75:1433–1434.
391. Robertson LJ, Campbell AT, Smith HV. Survival of *Cryptosporidium parvum* oocysts under various environmental pressures. *Appl Environ Microbiol* 1992;58:3494–3500.
392. Peeters JE, Mazas EA, Masschelein WJ, et al. Effect of disinfection of drinking water with ozone or chlorine dioxide on survival of *Cryptosporidium parvum* oocysts. *Appl Environ Microbiol* 1989;55:1519–1522.
393. Chapman PA, Rush BA. Efficiency of sand filtration for removing *Cryptosporidium* oocysts from water. *J Med Microbiol* 1990; 32:243–245.
394. Korich DG, Mead JR, Madore MS, et al. Effects of ozone, chlorine dioxide, chlorine, and monochloramine on *Cryptosporidium parvum* oocyst viability. *Appl Environ Microbiol* 1990;56: 1423–1428.
395. Clancy JL, Bukhari Z, Hargy TM, et al. Using UV to inactivate *Cryptosporidium. J Am Water Works Assoc* 2000;92:97–104.
396. Weller IVD, Williams CB, Jeffries DJ, et al. Cleaning and disinfection of equipment for gastrointestinal flexible endoscopy: interim recommendations of a Working Party of the British Society of Gastroenterology. *Gut* 1988;29:1134–1151.
397. Casemore DP, Blewett DA, Wright SE. Cleaning and disinfection of equipment for gastrointestinal flexible endoscopy: interim recommendations of a Working Party of the British Society of Gastroenterology. *Gut* 1989;30:1156–1157.
398. Shepherd RC, Reed CL, Sinha GP. Shedding of oocysts of *Cryptosporidium* in immunocompetent patients. *J Clin Pathol* 1988; 41:1104–1106.
399. Ratnam S, Paddock J, McDonald E, et al. Occurrence of *Cryptosporidium* oocysts in fecal samples submitted for routine microbiological examination. *J Clin Microbiol* 1985;22:402–404.
400. Baxby D, Hart CA. Cryptosporidiosis. *Br Med J* 1984;289: 1148.

63

CYCLOSPORA

BRADLEY A. CONNOR
BARBARA HERWALDT

Cyclospora cayetanensis is a protozoan parasite, 8 to 10 µm in diameter (i.e., about twice as large as *Cryptosporidium parvum*), that causes a syndrome characterized by prolonged diarrhea, anorexia, weight loss, and fatigue. In the two decades since this organism was first described, much has been learned about its microbiologic characteristics and taxonomic position and about the clinical illness it causes; furthermore, methods for detecting the organism in stool specimens and environmental samples have improved, effective therapy [i.e., treatment with trimethoprim-sulfamethoxazole (TMP-SMX)] has been identified, and multiple outbreaks of illness caused by this parasite, including the large, multistate, food-borne outbreaks in North America associated with various types of produce, have been investigated. However, many questions remain, such as how implicated food items become contaminated, what accounts for the striking seasonality of infection, and how the organism responds to various environmental conditions. In addition, alternative therapies are needed for persons who cannot tolerate treatment with TMP-SMX.

HISTORICAL ASPECTS

The organism now called *C. cayetanensis* first came to worldwide attention in 1990 and 1991 after the publication of four reports (1–4). One of these, the report by Shlim and colleagues (2) of the Canadian International Water and Energy Consultants Clinic in Kathmandu, Nepal, provided the first detailed clinical description of the illness associated with this organism, based on the largest series of cases up to that time ($n = 55$). The novel organism was found in association with a syndrome of prolonged diarrhea, anorexia, weight loss, and fatigue. The illness was not cured by various antimicrobial agents that were tried (therapy was directed at other agents of gastroenteritis because it was unclear whether this organism was a pathogen), but disappearance of the organism from stool usually was associated with remission of symptoms.

About the same time that the report of Shlim et al. (2) was published, Long and colleagues (1,4) published two reports about an identical-appearing organism detected in stool specimens from travelers, case patients in outbreaks, and patients with AIDS, and they speculated about the nature of the organism. On the one hand, they thought it had a prokaryotic appearance; by electron microscopy, its internal organelles resembled the photosynthesizing organelles of blue–green algae. On the other hand, they also noted that it had sporocysts and thus resembled a coccidian oocyst. In their 1991 publication (4), they referred to this enigmatic organism as a "cyanobacterium-like or coccidian-like body."

It turned out that what apparently was a newly described organism actually had been identified earlier. In 1986 in New York, Soave et al. (5) had described it in the stool of immunocompetent travelers to Mexico and Haiti in whom gastrointestinal symptoms had developed. They thought the structure resembled an unsporulated coccidian parasite but could not exclude the possibility that it was a fungal spore. According to a report published in 1994 (6), researchers in Haiti treating patients with AIDS had noted the organism in stool specimens as early as 1983. In an abstract in 1989 (7), researchers working in Peru described having seen "*Cryptosporidium muris*-like objects" that might represent "cysts of an unidentified flagellate" in stool specimens from three patients between 1985 and 1987 and from persons in cohort studies begun in 1988 that were focused on *C. parvum.*

However, even the descriptions of the organism in the 1980s were not the earliest. In 1979, Ashford (8) had reported his discovery in 1977 and 1978 of an "undescribed coccidian" in stool from three persons in Papua New Guinea, two of whom were symptomatic. Although he had correctly deduced that the structure was a coccidian para-

B. A. Connor: Department of Medicine, Weill Medical College of Cornell University and New York Presbyterian Hospital, New York, New York

B. Herwaldt: Division of Parasitic Diseases, Centers for Disease Control and Prevention, Atlanta, Georgia site, he was uncertain how to classify it by genus because he had been unable to characterize the morphologic features of fully developed oocysts (i.e., the number of sporozoites in each of the two sporocysts in a fully sporulated oocyst). Unfortunately, his report went virtually unnoticed until it was rediscovered in 1993.

The uncertainty surrounding this organism—whether it was a parasite or some other type of microbe or structure—was finally resolved with the 1993 report of Ortega and colleagues (9), who had succeeded in getting the organism to sporulate fully and had demonstrated that each of the two sporocysts in a fully sporulated oocyst contained two sporozoites. Based on these morphologic characteristics, the researchers concluded that the organism was a coccidian parasite of the genus *Cyclospora.* They proposed the name *C. cayetanensis* after the university in Lima (Universidad Peruana Cayetano Heredia) where their principal studies had been conducted (10).

Although *C. cayetanensis* was the first *Cyclospora* species found to infect humans, cyclosporan organisms were probably first identified by Eimer in 1870 in the intestine of the mole (10). In 1881, Schneider, who described a *Cyclospora* species (*C. glomerica*) in a myriapod, created the genus *Cyclospora.* In 1902, Schaudinn described tissue stages of *C. caryolytica,* the species that infects moles, in intestinal epithelium. Subsequently, other *Cyclospora* species that affect animals were described (10).

At least three factors contributed to the apparent emergence of *Cyclospora* as a human pathogen. First, the popularization of the acid-fast stain in the early 1980s for detecting *Cryptosporidium* species in stool specimens set the stage for the recognition of *Cyclospora* oocysts, which also are acid-fast. A second factor may have been the change in the empiric treatment of traveler's diarrhea from TMP-SMX, which eradicates the organism, to quinolone antibiotics, which apparently have limited effects on the parasite; this change may have facilitated the detection of *Cyclospora* infection among travelers and expatriates in Nepal. Third, the emergence of travel medicine as a specialty and the recognition of a "new" traveler's disease helped to generate interest in tropical diseases in general and diseases in travelers in particular and to motivate research in these areas.

TAXONOMY, MORPHOLOGY AND LIFE CYCLE

Taxonomy

Confusion about the precise taxonomy of the organism now called *C. cayetanensis* was manifested early on, with the organism being described variably as an oocyst-like body (8), cyanobacterium-like body (4), coccidian-like body (4), fungal spore, and large *Cryptosporidium* (5,11,12). Demonstration that the organism sporulated and identification of the morphologic characteristics of sporulated oocysts supported its reclassification as a member of the genus *Cyclospora* in the coccidian family Eimeriidae (9,10).

Historically, the taxonomy of coccidia in general has been based on such features as oocyst morphology, staining properties, life cycle, and sporulation characteristics. However, based on phylogenetic analyses of the small-subunit (18S) ribosomal RNA (rRNA) gene, human-associated *Cyclospora* has been found to be closely related to members of the *Eimeria* genus (13). Because *Cyclospora* organisms appear to be as closely related to some *Eimeria* species as they are to each other, the possibility of reclassifying *C. cayetanensis* as a member of the genus *Eimeria* has been raised (14).

Morphology

By light microscopy, *C. cayetanensis* oocysts appear as nonrefractile, double-walled spheres, 8 to 10 μm in diameter, with a bilayered wall approximately 113 nm thick (10). The outer layer is rough and about 63 nm thick, and the inner layer is smooth and about 50 nm thick (10). Each oocyst contains two ovoidal sporocysts (~4.0 × ~6.3 μm), and each sporocyst contains two crescent-shaped sporozoites (~1.2 × ~9.0 μm) (10). The sporozoites have an apical complex, rhoptries, micronemes, and a membrane-bound nucleus, features characteristic of coccidian parasites of the phylum Apicomplexa, family Eimeriidae.

Life Cycle

Except for the fact that *C. cayetanensis* oocysts sporulate outside the host, in the environment, *Cyclospora* completes its asexual and sexual life cycles within the same host. Both asexual and sexual stages have been detected in human intestinal epithelial cells, specifically in membrane-bound, parasitophorous vacuoles concentrated at the luminal end of enterocytes (15–17). The host becomes infected by ingesting sporulated oocysts, which excyst in the proximal small bowel and release sporozoites, which are the infective units. The sporozoites then invade intestinal epithelial cells, where they develop into trophozoites and undergo schizogony to form merozoite-containing schizonts. After the merozoites are released, they can invade other epithelial cells, undergo further asexual cycles, and thus propagate the infection, or they can develop into microgametes or macrogametes. When a microgamete fertilizes a macrogamete, an oocyst results, which subsequently is passed in the stool.

Unlike *Cryptosporidium* oocysts, which are fully sporulated and infective when shed in stool, *Cyclospora* oocysts must sporulate outside the host before they become infectious for the next host. Although the amount of time required for sporulation in nature is unknown, in the laboratory setting, sporulation usually takes at least 1 week. Organisms were noted to sporulate within 7 to 13 days in

2.5% potassium dichromate at temperatures of 25°C or 32°C (9).

PATHOLOGY, PATHOGENESIS, AND HISTOPATHOLOGY

Early descriptions of the clinical illness associated with *Cyclospora* infection, including evidence of D-xylose malabsorption, suggested that small-bowel pathology might be a factor in the pathogenesis of the disease cyclosporiasis. Endoscopic examination of the upper gastrointestinal tract and light and electron microscopic examination of distal duodenal and jejunal biopsy specimens have provided evidence that human-associated *Cyclospora* organisms parasitize the enterocytes of the upper small bowel.

In a study of infected travelers and expatriates in Nepal, upper gastrointestinal endoscopy showed moderate to marked erythema of the distal duodenum in five of nine patients (18). The parasite was detected in duodenal aspirates from two patients. Histopathologic examination of small-bowel biopsy specimens showed epithelial disarray, with acute and chronic inflammation, partial villous atrophy, and crypt hyperplasia. The villus-to-crypt ratio ranged from 0.6:1 to 1.5:1, whereas the normal range is 3.1 to 4:1 (18). Biopsy specimens from the gastric antrum and colon (one patient each) did not show histopathologic changes or organisms. Similar histopathologic changes in jejunal biopsy specimens were noted in other studies (15,17). Some inflammatory changes appear to persist beyond parasite eradication; a dense, myelin-like material can be seen in association with enterocytes, particularly in patients with prolonged disease (19). Electron microscopic examination of intestinal biopsy specimens from infected patients has demonstrated both asexual stages (comprised of trophozoites, schizonts, and merozoites) and sexual stages (microgametes and macrogametes) (15–17).

IMMUNITY

One way to assess indirectly whether immunity to *Cyclospora* can develop in infected persons is to investigate whether the rates of infection and disease in areas where *Cyclospora* is endemic decrease as age increases. In a 2-year, community-based, cross-sectional study that included stool specimens from 5,836 persons younger than 18 years in a Peruvian shantytown, the infection rate was highest among children ages 2 to less than 4 years (the rate was about 2% for the study period as a whole and was higher during the transmission season), and no cases of infection were detected in persons older than 11 years (20). Overall, 20 (32%) of the 63 infected children were symptomatic sometime during the period of oocyst excretion. These age-specific data suggest that immunity develops with time in persons living in areas where *Cyclospora* is endemic, probably because of repeated exposure. Similarly, the infection rate was highest among children ages 1.5 to 9 years during 1 year of surveillance in outpatient health care facilities in Guatemala (21).

In a case–control study comparing infected and uninfected foreigners in Nepal, a longer duration of stay appeared to be associated with a protective effect; the infected residents in the study had lived in Nepal for a median of 11 months (interquartile range, 4 to 21 months), whereas the uninfected residents had lived there for a median of 24 months (interquartile range, 9 to 72 months) ($p < .001$) (22). On the other hand, symptomatic reinfection during successive transmission seasons has been documented (18,19,22), but it appears to become less common after repeated exposure. In a study of the incidence of diarrhea during long-term residence in Nepal, one infected person apparently became reinfected during the same year, with a symptom-free period between the two episodes of longer than 3 months (23). However, no information was provided in the report about whether negative stools had been documented during the symptom-free interval.

The components of the immune system relevant to the clearance of *Cyclospora* infection and protection from relapses and symptomatic reinfections are unknown, as are the effectiveness and duration of the immune response. Conflicting reports have been published about whether increases in anti-*Cyclospora* antibody titers can be detected during convalescence from infection (4,24). The importance of having an intact immune system is evidenced by data showing a high incidence of recurrent cyclosporiasis among patients with AIDS (6).

CLINICAL ILLNESS

The clinical illness associated with *Cyclospora* infection has been well described in travelers and expatriates in developing countries, native immunocompetent and immunocompromised persons in the developing world, and nonimmune adults in the developed world (2,3,6,12,19,21, 22,25–42). Illness typically is the most severe and lasts the longest in infected non-immune adults (e.g., foreigners in Nepal, upper and middle class adults in Peru, and case patients in outbreaks in North America) (2,17,20,27,34). The first detailed clinical description of cyclosporiasis was from a clinic-based study of 55 symptomatic foreigners in Nepal, most of whom were adults and quite sick (2).

Symptomatic, non-immune patients typically report the acute onset of gastroenteritis, characterized by frequent bouts of diarrhea. The stool, described variably as watery, soft, or semiformed, usually does not contain blood or inflammatory cells, and the diarrhea occurs in a cyclic pattern, sometimes alternating with constipation. Abdominal cramps, nausea, and upper intestinal gas and bloating are frequently noted. Some patients have low-grade fever and vomiting. Progressive fatigue, anorexia, and weight loss often predominate and may overshadow the diarrhea. Weight loss is common, with a mean loss of 3.6 kg (range, 0 to 15 kg) among 48 foreigners in Nepal (2) and 3.6 kg (range, 0.9 to 18.2 kg) among 384 persons in the multistate outbreak in North America in 1996 (27). Fatigue as a hallmark symptom is nearly universal and often is severe. Half of 66 patients identified at one hospital reported absence from work because of extreme fatigue (43).

The acute phase of the illness typically subsides after a few days, and a characteristic pattern of unusually severe fatigue, along with anorexia, diarrhea, and nausea ensues. The symptoms can be described as consistent from day to day or as intermittent, with remissions and exacerbations occurring every few days. Complications of infection can include dehydration, malabsorption, and possibly Guillain-Barré syndrome (44) and Reiter syndrome (45).

Investigations of multiple outbreaks in North America have shown that diarrhea, anorexia, weight loss, and fatigue are the four most common symptoms in symptomatic, non-immune adults (27,32,41). In the multistate outbreak in 1996, each of these symptoms occurred in more than 90% of 760 patients with laboratory-confirmed cases (data about these four symptoms were available for from 507 to 759 patients) (27). The same four symptoms were those most commonly reported in a wedding-associated cluster of cases in Boston that was part of the multistate outbreak (41). Most (51 of 57, or 89%) of the case patients had recurring symptoms, characterized by a waxing and waning course, and most (35 of 57, or 61%) reported being ill for more than 3 weeks. No illness was noted among household contacts who had not attended the event, consistent with the presumed non-infectivity of excreted, unsporulated oocysts.

Similarly, in a cluster of cases in New York City that was part of the same multistate outbreak, the same four symptoms predominated (B. Connor, *unpublished data*). A flu-like prodrome, with accompanying myalgia and arthralgia, often preceded the onset of the other symptoms. The median number of stools in a 24-hour period at the onset of illness was 6 (range, 1 to 80). Some of the infected persons did not have diarrhea but noted a change in bowel habits associated with bloating, abdominal gas, and, in some patients, constipation.

The incubation period from ingestion of oocysts to onset of clinical symptoms averages 1 week. Data from the social event-associated clusters of cases in the North American outbreaks of cyclosporiasis consistently show that the median incubation period is about 7 days (27–29,41,43). However, individual cases with shorter and longer incubation periods have been reported (2,27,28). Whether the size of the inoculum affects the incubation period is unknown.

Illness in untreated, non-immune adults can persist for weeks, sometimes months (2,12,22,27,32,46,47). The mean duration of symptoms in the initial report from Nepal was 43 days (range, 4 to 107 days) (2). In a subsequent study among foreigners in Nepal, the median duration of illness was 7 weeks (interquartile range, 4 to 9 weeks) for patients infected with *Cyclospora,* in comparison with 9 days (range, 4 to 19 days) for patients who had diarrhea but were not infected with *Cyclospora* (22). In some outbreaks in North America, the median durations of diarrheal disease were 10 days (range, 1 to 60 days) (27), 10.5 days (range, 1 to 42 days), 11.4 days (range, 1 to 18 days) (32), 21 days (range, 1 to 47 days) (12), and 24 days (range, 1 to 27 days) (32); these data are underestimates because it is possible that some case patients had already been treated or were still sick when interviewed.

Shedding of oocysts by untreated persons has been reported to last up to 12.5 weeks (2), up to 8 weeks (26), and 8 weeks (in an asymptomatic patient with antibodies to both HIV and human T-lymphotropic virus type 1) (48). Although symptoms usually resolve at about the same time that stool examinations become negative, excretion of oocysts can persist for more than 1 month after symptoms resolve (2,26), and symptoms can persist for several weeks longer than oocyst excretion is documented (22). An infected person identified in a community-based study in Haiti was found to be excreting oocysts in January, March, and July (49); the exact duration of excretion and whether reinfection had occurred were not known. In two cohort studies in Peruvian shanty towns, in which the prevalence rates for infection at presentation in children ages 1 month to 2.5 years were 18% (26 of 147) and 6% (15 of 230), infected children shed organisms for a mean of 22 to 23 days (range, 7 to 70 days) (9); only small proportions of the infected children (28% in one study and 11% in the other) had diarrhea when evaluated. Excretion of oocysts usually stops during therapy or by several days to 1 week after therapy (20,38,50,51).

Cyclospora infection has been detected in immunocompromised hosts; most of the data are for HIV-infected persons (6,36). Research in Haiti has shown that clinical illness in these patients is often prolonged and recurrent (6). Indirect evidence for biliary tract infection in two patients with AIDS has been reported (52).

DIAGNOSIS

Now that *Cyclospora* has been added to the list of pathogens that cause gastroenteritis, infection with this organism should be considered when patients with appropriate clinical manifestations are evaluated. Physicians should be aware that most laboratories do not test for *Cyclospora* unless such testing is specifically requested. Confirming the diagnosis is important because therapy for *Cyclospora* infection is highly effective and differs from that for most of the other parasitic gastroenteritides. Certain clinical characteristics, besides diarrhea, should prompt a consideration of *Cyclospora* as a possible etiologic agent, with the fact that cases can differ with respect to symptomatology and severity of illness kept in mind. Extreme fatigue out of proportion to other symptoms and a waxing and waning course, with intermittent diarrhea and anorexia, are hallmarks of the disease in nonimmune adults. The season in which the symptoms occur can also provide a helpful clue. However, as discussed below, the seasonality varies around the world, and cases in North America that are linked to the ingestion of imported produce can be noted at various times of the year, depending on the source of the food.

As discussed above, *Cyclospora* oocysts by light microscopy appear as nonrefractile, double-walled spheres, 8 to 10 μm in diameter (4,9,12,53,54) (see Color Figure 63.1). Microscopists familiar with the organism can easily identify it on direct wet mounts or on wet mounts after Sheather sucrose flotation. With modified acid-fast staining, *Cyclospora* oocysts appear variably red; some oocysts resist the stain and appear as "ghosts" (12,54).

In one study in which multiple stool specimens per infected patient were examined by direct microscopy and after modified acid-fast staining, *Cyclospora* oocysts were almost always present in the stool (i.e., negative stools were uncommonly found between two positive stools); the organism was identified in 88 (96%) of 92 stool examinations (2). However, the results of this study of patients with multiple positive stool examinations may not be applicable to all infected patients. Experience in outbreak investigations in North America has shown that detecting the organism in stool can be difficult, even if the patient is symptomatic and the microscopist is experienced, because oocysts often are excreted in relatively low to modest numbers.

To facilitate the detection of oocysts, stool specimens may first have to be processed by a method, such as formalin–ethyl acetate concentration, that concentrates parasites (54). Specimens preserved in formalin for prolonged periods may become more resistant to staining. An alternative to the modified acid-fast stain, which results in variable degrees of staining of oocysts, is a safranin-based stain that uniformly stains oocysts a brilliant reddish orange if fecal smears are heated during staining (55). Ultraviolet fluorescence microscopy is a useful technique for initial screening of wet mounts of stool for *Cyclospora* oocysts, which autofluoresce and thus are easily detectable (12,54). Either the narrow-band filter sets (360 to 370 nm, with the peak at 365 nm) or the wide-band filter sets (range, 330 to 385 nm) can be used. If characteristic autofluorescent structures are seen, their morphologic features should be confirmed by bright field, phase contrast, or differential interference contrast microscopy. Studies have shown that the use of fluorescence microscopy as a screening technique increases the diagnostic yield (56,57); in a study of 143 positive specimens, the estimated sensitivity of modified acid-fast staining versus fluorescence microscopy was 78% (56).

The diagnosis of *Cyclospora* infection can also be confirmed by demonstrating sporulation of oocysts (9,12). However, this is not a practical means of diagnosis for clinical microbiology laboratories, in part because of the prolonged time required for sporulation. Molecular biologic techniques, such as polymerase chain reaction-based methods to detect *Cyclospora* in fecal and environmental samples, are being developed and may enhance diagnostic capabilities (13,58). Detection of the parasite in intestinal tissue by light microscopy can be difficult, and electron microscopy is often required for confirmation. A hematoxylin-enhancement histologic technique was recently described that may obviate the need for electron microscopy (59).

TREATMENT

The current treatment of choice for persons infected with *Cyclospora* is a 7- to 10-day course of therapy with TMP-SMX [adult dose, one double-strength tablet (160 mg of TMP and 800 mg of SMX) twice daily] (50). The effectiveness of TMP-SMX was first suggested in 1993 by a report that TMP-SMX therapy had attenuated symptoms in an infected patient with AIDS (36). Later in 1993, researchers reported that five infected Peruvian patients (one adult and four children) were successfully treated, with resolution of symptoms and clearance of the organism from stool specimens (60). In 1994, researchers reported their experience with TMP-SMX (one double-strength tablet four times daily for 10 days) in an open trial in 43 HIV-infected Haitian patients (6). Diarrhea and abdominal cramps resolved by a mean of 2.5 days (range, 1 to 5 days). All the stools reexamined on days 5 (n = 23) and 10 (n = 43) were negative for *Cyclospora.* Almost half (12 of 28, or 43%) of the patients had symptomatic, stool-positive relapses, which also responded to TMP-SMX therapy. During a mean monitoring period of 7 months, TMP-SMX prophylaxis (one double-strength tablet thrice weekly) was effective in preventing relapses in most (11 of 12) patients. In settings in which TMP-SMX was used as prophylaxis against toxoplasmosis and *Pneumocystis carinii* pneumonia in patients with AIDS, TMP-SMX may have decreased the incidence rate of *Cyclospora* infection (6). In 1995, the results of a trial comparing TMP-SMX (one double-strength tablet twice daily for 7 days) and placebo for the treatment of infection in 40 immunocompetent foreigners in Nepal were published (50). Twenty-one patients were treated with TMP-SMX and 19 with placebo. After 3 days, *Cyclospora* was still detectable in stool from 12 (71%) of 17 in the treatment group and 19 (100%) of 19 in the placebo group (p = .016). However, on day 7, *Cyclospora* was still detectable in stool from only 1 (6%) of 16 in the treatment group, compared with 15 (88%) of 17 in the placebo group (p <.001). The patient treated with TMP-SMX who still had a positive stool at 7 days responded to an additional 7-day course of therapy. Two other patients received an additional week of therapy because they had experienced only moderate relief of their symptoms after the first week of therapy. Similarly, experience during the subsequent outbreaks of cyclosporiasis in North America has suggested that a longer course of therapy (perhaps 10 to 14 days) may be indicated for patients who have persistent symptoms.

No alternatives to TMP-SMX for the treatment of *Cyclospora* infection have been identified yet. In the study in 1989 in Nepal, 34 patients received 78 courses of antimicrobial therapy (2); the most commonly used agents were norfloxacin, tinidazole, quinacrine, nalidixic acid, and diloxanide furoate. No difference was noted in duration of illness between untreated and treated patients. An open-label trial of azithromycin therapy (500 mg once daily for 7 days) in 14 patients in Nepal also showed no benefit (61). Limited data suggest that therapy with albendazole (B. Connor, *unpublished data*), TMP alone (62), and tetracycline (2) also is ineffective. The treatment of patients who reportedly are allergic to sulfa drugs is problematic. Approaches that can be considered include observation, symptomatic treatment, or the use of an antimicrobial agent of unknown effectiveness against *Cyclospora.* Although a recent report from a clinical trial among HIV-infected Haitians suggested that ciprofloxacin is moderately effective in the treatment of *Cyclospora* infection (51), substantial clinical experience in treating immunocompetent patients in Nepal and North America has suggested that ciprofloxacin therapy is ineffective.

EPIDEMIOLOGY

Geographic Distribution and Seasonality of Infection

Cyclospora infection appears to be most prevalent in tropical and subtropical areas of the world. Although unexplained cases of cyclosporiasis occasionally are reported in developed countries, infection typically has been associated with overseas travel or the ingestion of imported produce. The proportion of stool specimens positive for *Cyclospora* has been less than 0.5% in laboratory surveys conducted during non-outbreak periods in North America and the United Kingdom (35,36,63–65).

The studies conducted to date among native populations and foreigners in developing countries have shown that the prevalence of *Cyclospora* infection and the likelihood that infected persons are symptomatic are highly variable. Some of the factors that contribute to the variability include characteristics of the study (e.g., clinic- vs. community-based), area of the world, time of year, sanitary conditions, and attributes of the persons being studied, such as age, immune competence, socioeconomic status, duration of stay in the area, and likelihood of previous *Cyclospora* infection (2,9,12,20–22,25,34,66).

The specifics of the seasonality of *Cyclospora* infection vary around the world. In Kathmandu, Nepal, cases of infection usually cluster from May through August and peak in June and July (2,18,22,66); infection rates are highest just before and during the warm monsoon months and decrease markedly before the rains end. The months during which cases occur and peak are similar for Guatemala and Nepal (21). In Indonesia, preliminary data indicate that cases are most common during the cooler wet season of October through May (34). In a coastal area of Haiti, cases peak during the first quarter of the year, which includes the relatively drier and cooler months (49). In contrast, in a dry, coastal area near Lima, Peru, the season for infection (i.e., from December or January through May and sometimes June and July) includes the relatively warmer months for this area, which are cooler than the peak infection months in Haiti (9,10,20). The ways in which *Cyclospora* is "carried" from one season to the next are poorly understood, as are the environmental or other triggers that initiate the onset of a new season (12).

General Points about Modes of Transmission

Infected persons excrete *C. cayetanensis* oocysts in their feces. Whether animals can become infected with this (vs. only with other) *Cyclospora* species and serve as sources of infection for humans is not yet known (12). Direct person-to-person transmission by fecal exposure is unlikely because excreted oocysts must sporulate in the environment to become infectious. However, indirect transmission can occur if an infected person contaminates the environment and the excreted oocysts remain viable during the time required to become infectious and be ingested by the next host. For example, as discussed below, *Cyclospora* can be transmitted by the ingestion of food or water contaminated with oocysts. The oocysts must already have sporulated before the food or water becomes contaminated, or, if they are unsporulated at the time of contamination, they must have time thereafter to sporulate before consumption. Thus, food or water contaminated with unsporulated oocysts shortly before consumption (e.g., by a chef) should not cause infection.

Limited information is available about the conditions required to kill oocysts during routine commercial handling or processing of food and water, in part because no methods are available yet to assess the viability of *Cyclospora* oocysts, beyond determining whether sporulation and excystation have occurred. However, no documented outbreaks have been associated with cooked or commercially frozen food. Because *C. cayetanensis* oocysts are about twice as big as *C. parvum* oocysts, *Cyclospora* oocysts are more easily removed by conventional water filtration.

Food-borne Outbreaks in North America

Definite or probable food-borne outbreaks of cyclosporiasis were documented in North America (in the United States and sometimes also in Canada) each year from 1995 to 2000 (12). Overall, at least 12 distinct food-borne outbreaks were documented during that period (12), and the number of cases reported for the series of outbreaks as a whole was at least about 3,700. Two of the outbreaks, each of which comprised more than 1,000 reported cases, accounted for a large proportion of the reported cases for the series of outbreaks as a whole (27,28); the other outbreaks were smaller, with up to several hundred reported cases per outbreak (12). The magnitudes of some of the outbreaks probably were underestimated because of under-recognition and under-reporting of cases (12). Similarly, other outbreaks may have occurred but not been recognized.

All the outbreaks that were recognized and investigated were associated with the consumption of produce (12). A foreign country was always found to be one of the possible sources of the produce in those outbreaks for which traceback investigations were conducted. The seasonality of the outbreaks largely reflected the seasonality of *Cyclospora* infection in the countries in which the various types of implicated produce were grown.

The outbreaks that brought *Cyclospora* to prominence were the two widespread, multistate outbreaks that occurred in the United States and Canada in 1996 and 1997 (27,28). These outbreaks were strikingly similar; both occurred in the spring, both were associated with more than 1,000 reported cases (1,465 and 1,012 cases, respectively), and both were linked to fresh raspberries imported from Guatemala (27,28). The fact that outbreaks associated with Guatemalan raspberries were first recognized in the mid-1990s may be attributable at least in part to the marked increase at that time in the volume of raspberries exported to the United States from Guatemala (67).

Unfortunately, the specific means by which the raspberries became contaminated was not determined. However, the leading hypothesis is that contamination resulted from exposure to contaminated water, specifically when raspberries were sprayed with insecticides, fungicides, and fertilizers that had been mixed with water (12,27). In this scenario, infected humans (or animals, if they can serve as reservoir hosts of infection, which is uncertain) contaminated the water, either directly or indirectly (e.g., by contaminating the environment, so that the water supplies were then contaminated), and the water in turn contaminated the raspberries.

After the outbreak in 1996, during preparations for the 1997 spring export season, the Guatemalan Berry Commission instituted control measures on raspberry farms (12,27,28). The measures focused on improving the quality of water used in agriculture and on raising the standards for employee hygiene and sanitation. In addition, the Commission specified that only farms classified as low-risk in such regards could export fresh raspberries to the United States in the spring of 1997. The fact that another large outbreak linked to fresh raspberries then occurred suggests that some farms did not fully implement the control measures or instituted them too late, that the measures were ineffective, or that the measures were not directed against the true mode of contamination (12,28). The outbreak ended shortly after the exportation of fresh Guatemalan raspberries stopped at the end of May 1997 (28).

In the spring of 1998, importation of fresh Guatemalan raspberries into the United States was not permitted by the U.S. Food and Drug Administration, but importation into Canada continued. The outcome of this inadvertent intervention trial was that an outbreak linked to fresh Guatemalan raspberries was documented in Canada that spring (12,31). In the spring of 1999 and the spring of 2000, the United States imported Guatemalan raspberries from some farms that met stricter standards. Although no outbreaks associated with Guatemalan raspberries were documented in 1999, two U.S. clusters of cases that might have been related to each other and associated with Guatemalan raspberries were documented in 2000 (12).

In addition, in 1997, 1998, and 1999, several outbreaks of cyclosporiasis that were associated with the consumption of fresh fruit but not of Guatemalan raspberries were documented in North America (12). The specific vehicles were unclear because mixed-fruit items had been served at the events associated with the outbreaks. The possibility that Guatemalan blackberries caused illness was raised for some of these outbreaks, and also for some of the cases in the outbreaks of 1996 through 1998 that were largely attributable to raspberries. Overall, for the outbreak investigations in the 1990s, the evidence linking Guatemalan blackberries to outbreaks of cyclosporiasis was suggestive but not as strong as the evidence for raspberries, even though the two types of berries often are grown on the same farms and Guatemala exports more blackberries than raspberries (12). Whether the structure of the produce influences the risk for contamination with *Cyclospora* or for its adherence to produce is unknown (12).

Other U.S. outbreaks of cyclosporiasis have been linked to other types of fresh produce—specifically, mesclun lettuce (i.e., a mixture of young lettuce leaves of various types, also known as spring mix, field greens, baby greens, and gourmet salad mix) and basil (12,30,32). Outbreaks associated with mesclun lettuce occurred in Florida in 1997. These included at least one outbreak that began in March and another that occurred in December. For the March outbreak, the vehicle definitely was mesclun lettuce, but more than one possible source of the lettuce was identified (i.e., Peru and the United States). For the December outbreak, a salad with multiple ingredients, including mesclun lettuce, was the vehicle, and the only possible source of the lettuce was Peru. If the evidence from both outbreaks is combined, then mesclun lettuce was the probable vehicle for both outbreaks and Peru was the probable source of the lettuce (12). Two outbreaks linked to fresh basil have been documented, including one in June and July of 1997 in the northern Virginia–Washington–Baltimore metropolitan area and another in July 1999 in Missouri (30,32). The two possible sources of the basil in the 1999 outbreak included a Mexican farm and a U.S. farm. Different Mexican farms were among the multiple possible sources of the basil in the 1997 outbreak.

Waterborne Transmission

In June 1994, a waterborne outbreak of cyclosporiasis occurred in a military detachment in Pokhara, Nepal, in association with a chlorinated mixture of river and municipal water (68). Also in Nepal, consumption of untreated water was identified as a risk factor for *Cyclospora* infection in 1992 in a case–control study of travelers and expatriates (22).

In the United States, one outbreak of cyclosporiasis and several sporadic cases of infection might have been caused by waterborne transmission, but the evidence was not definitive (12). The outbreak occurred in a physicians' dormitory in Chicago in the early summer of 1990 and was the first outbreak of cyclosporiasis documented in the United States (26). The water for the dormitory was stored in the penthouse area in two tanks; these had recently been refilled after repair of a broken water pump. However, how the water in the tanks could have become contaminated with *Cyclospora* is unclear, and the possibility that the outbreak might have been food-borne rather than waterborne has been raised (12,26).

No community-wide waterborne outbreaks of cyclosporiasis have been documented in the United States. Contamination of U.S. water supplies with *Cyclospora* probably is uncommon (12). Although waterborne transmission of *Cyclospora* has been documented less often than food-borne transmission, the implicated produce in at least some of the food-borne outbreaks discussed above may have become contaminated through exposure to water (12). Water likely serves as a milieu that facilitates the survival of *Cyclospora* for relatively long periods in the environment.

REFERENCES

1. Long EG, Ebrahimzadeh A, White EH, et al. Alga associated with diarrhea in patients with acquired immunodeficiency syndrome and in travelers. *J Clin Microbiol* 1990;28:1101–1104.
2. Shlim DR, Cohen MT, Eaton M, et al. An alga-like organism associated with an outbreak of prolonged diarrhea among foreigners in Nepal. *Am J Trop Med Hyg* 1991;45:383–389.
3. Centers for Disease Control and Prevention. Outbreaks of diarrheal illness associated with cyanobacteria (blue–green algae)-like bodies: Chicago and Nepal, 1989 and 1990. *MMWR Morb Mortal Wkly Rep* 1991;40:325–327.
4. Long EG, White EH, Carmichael WW, et al. Morphologic and staining characteristics of a cyanobacterium-like organism associated with diarrhea. *J Infect Dis* 1991;164:199–202.
5. Soave R, Dubey JP, Ramos LJ, et al. A new intestinal pathogen? *Clin Res* 1986;34:533A(abst).
6. Pape JW, Verdier R-I, Boncy M, et al. *Cyclospora* infection in adults infected with HIV: clinical manifestations, treatment, and prophylaxis. *Ann Intern Med* 1994;121:654–657.
7. Naranjo [*sic*] J, Sterling C, Gilman R, et al. *Cryptosporidium muris*-like objects from fecal samples of Peruvians. In: *Program and abstracts of the 38th annual meeting of the American Society of Tropical Medicine and Hygiene,* Honolulu, 10–14 December, 1989:243(abst 324).
8. Ashford RW. Occurrence of an undescribed coccidian in man in Papua New Guinea. *Ann Trop Med Parasitol* 1979;73:497–500.
9. Ortega YR, Sterling CR, Gilman RH, et al. *Cyclospora* species: a new protozoan pathogen of humans. *N Engl J Med* 1993;328: 1308–1312.
10. Ortega YR, Gilman RH, Sterling CR. A new coccidian parasite (Apicomplexa: Eimeriidae) from humans. *J Parasitol* 1994;80: 625–629.
11. Soave R. *Cyclospora*: an overview. *Clin Infect Dis* 1996;23: 429–437.
12. Herwaldt BL. *Cyclospora cayetanensis*: a review, focusing on the outbreaks of cyclosporiasis in the 1990s. *Clin Infect Dis* 2000;31: 1040–1057.
13. Relman DA, Schmidt TM, Gajadhar A, et al. Molecular phylogenetic analysis of *Cyclospora,* the human intestinal pathogen, suggests that it is closely related to *Eimeria* species. *J Infect Dis* 1996;173:440–445.
14. Pieniazek NJ, Herwaldt BL. Reevaluating the molecular taxonomy: is human-associated *Cyclospora* a mammalian *Eimeria* species? *Emerging Infect Dis* 1997;3:381–383.
15. Bendall RP, Lucas S, Moody A, et al. Diarrhoea associated with cyanobacterium-like bodies: a new coccidian enteritis of man. *Lancet* 1993;341:590–592.
16. Sun T, Ilardi CF, Asnis D, et al. Light and electron microscopic identification of *Cyclospora* species in the small intestine: evidence of the presence of asexual life cycle in human host. *Am J Clin Pathol* 1996;105:216–220.
17. Ortega YR, Nagle R, Gilman RH, et al. Pathologic and clinical findings in patients with cyclosporiasis and a description of intracellular parasite life-cycle stages. *J Infect Dis* 1997;176: 1584–1589.
18. Connor BA, Shlim DR, Scholes JV, et al. Pathologic changes in the small bowel in nine patients with diarrhea associated with a coccidian-like body. *Ann Intern Med* 1993;119:377–382.
19. Connor BA, Reidy J, Soave R. Cyclosporiasis: clinical and histopathologic correlates. *Clin Infect Dis* 1999;28:1216–1222.
20. Madico G, McDonald J, Gilman RH, et al. Epidemiology and treatment of *Cyclospora cayetanensis* infection in Peruvian children. *Clin Infect Dis* 1997;24:977–981.
21. Bern C, Hernandez B, Lopez MB, et al. Epidemiologic studies of *Cyclospora cayetanensis* in Guatemala. *Emerging Infect Dis* 1999;5: 766–774.
22. Hoge CW, Shlim DR, Rajah R, et al. Epidemiology of diarrhoeal illness associated with coccidian-like organism among travellers and foreign residents in Nepal. *Lancet* 1993;341:1175–1179.
23. Shlim DR, Hoge CW, Rajah R, et al. Persistent high risk of diarrhea among foreigners in Nepal during the first 2 years of residence. *Clin Infect Dis* 1999;29:613–616.
24. Clarke SC, McIntyre M. An attempt to demonstrate a serological immune response in patients infected with *Cyclospora cayetanensis* [Letter]. *Br J Biomed Sci* 1997;54:73–74.
25. Hoge CW, Echeverria P, Rajah R, et al. Prevalence of *Cyclospora* species and other enteric pathogens among children less than 5 years of age in Nepal. *J Clin Microbiol* 1995;33:3058–3060.
26. Huang P, Weber JT, Sosin DM, et al. The first reported outbreak of diarrheal illness associated with *Cyclospora* in the United States. *Ann Intern Med* 1995;123:409–414.
27. Herwaldt BL, Ackers M-L, Cyclospora Working Group. An out-

break in 1996 of cyclosporiasis associated with imported raspberries. *N Engl J Med* 1997;336:1548–1556.
28. Herwaldt BL, Beach MJ, Cyclospora Working Group. The return of *Cyclospora* in 1997: another outbreak of cyclosporiasis in North America associated with imported raspberries. *Ann Intern Med* 1999;130:210–220.
29. Koumans EHA, Katz DJ, Malecki JM, et al. An outbreak of cyclosporiasis in Florida in 1995: a harbinger of multistate outbreaks in 1996 and 1997. *Am J Trop Med Hyg* 1998;59:235–242.
30. Centers for Disease Control and Prevention. Outbreak of cyclosporiasis: Northern Virginia–Washington, DC–Baltimore, Maryland, metropolitan area, 1997. *MMWR Morb Mortal Wkly Rep* 1997;46:689–691.
31. Centers for Disease Control and Prevention. Outbreak of cyclosporiasis: Ontario, Canada, May 1998. *MMWR Morb Mortal Wkly Rep* 1998;47:806–809.
32. Lopez AS, Dodson DR, Arrowood MJ, et al. Outbreak of cyclosporiasis associated with basil in Missouri in 1999. *Clin Infect Dis* 2001;32:1010–1017.
33. Zerpa R, Uchima N, Huicho L. *Cyclospora cayetanensis* associated with watery diarrhoea in Peruvian patients. *J Trop Med Hyg* 1995; 98:325–329.
34. Fryauff DJ, Krippner R, Prodjodipuro P, et al. *Cyclospora cayetanensis* among expatriate and indigenous populations of West Java, Indonesia. *Emerging Infect Dis* 1999;5:585–588.
35. Ooi WW, Zimmerman SK, Needham CA. *Cyclospora* species as a gastrointestinal pathogen in immunocompetent hosts. *J Clin Microbiol* 1995;33:1267–1269.
36. Wurtz RM, Kocka FE, Peters CS, et al. Clinical characteristics of seven cases of diarrhea associated with a novel acid-fast organism in the stool. *Clin Infect Dis* 1993;16:136–138.
37. Jelinek T, Lotze M, Eichenlaub S, et al. Prevalence of infection with *Cryptosporidium parvum* and *Cyclospora cayetanensis* among international travellers. *Gut* 1997;41:801–804.
38. Fryauff DJ, Krippner R, Purnomo, et al. Short report: case report of *Cyclospora* infection acquired in Indonesia and treated with cotrimoxazole. *Am J Trop Med Hyg* 1996;55:584–585.
39. Wurtz R. *Cyclospora*: a newly identified intestinal pathogen of humans. *Clin Infect Dis* 1994;18:620–623.
40. Hale D, Aldeen W, Carroll K. Diarrhea associated with cyanobacteria-like bodies in an immunocompetent host. *JAMA* 1994;271:144–145.
41. Fleming CA, Caron D, Gunn JE, et al. A food-borne outbreak of *Cyclospora cayetanensis* at a wedding. *Arch Intern Med* 1998;158: 1121–1125.
42. Manuel DG, Shahin R, Lee W, et al. The first reported cluster of food-borne cyclosporiasis in Canada. *Can J Public Health* 1999; 90:399–402.
43. Connor BA, Soave R. *Cyclospora*: clinical manifestations. Food and Drug Administration (FDA)/Center for Food Safety and Applied Nutrition, Food Advisory Committee Meeting. *Federal Register* July 1997.
44. Richardson RF, Remler BF, Katirji B, et al. Guillain-Barré syndrome after *Cyclospora* infection. *Muscle Nerve* 1998;21: 669–671.
45. Connor BA, Johnson E, Soave R. Reiter's syndrome following protracted symptoms of *Cyclospora* infection. *Emerging Infect Dis* 2001;7:453–454.
46. Berlin OGW, Novak SM, Porschen RK, et al. Recovery of *Cyclospora* organisms from patients with prolonged diarrhea. *Clin Infect Dis* 1994;18:606–609.
47. Pollok RCG, Bendall RP, Moody A, et al. Traveller's diarrhoea associated with cyanobacterium-like bodies. *Lancet* 1992;340: 556–557.
48. Schubach TM, Neves ES, Leite AC, et al. *Cyclospora cayetanensis* in an asymptomatic patient infected with HIV and HTLV-1. *Trans R Soc Trop Med Hyg* 1997;91:175.
49. Eberhard ML, Nace EK, Freeman AR, et al. *Cyclospora cayetanensis* infections in Haiti: a common occurrence in the absence of watery diarrhea. *Am J Trop Med Hyg* 1999;60:584–586.
50. Hoge CW, Shlim DR, Ghimire M, et al. Placebo-controlled trial of co-trimoxazole for *Cyclospora* infections among travellers and foreign residents in Nepal. *Lancet* 1995;345:691–693.
51. Verdier R-I, Fitzgerald DW, Johnson WD, et al. Trimethoprim-sulfamethoxazole compared with ciprofloxacin for treatment and prophylaxis of *Isospora belli* and *Cyclospora cayetanensis* infection in HIV-infected patients. *Ann Intern Med* 2000;132:885–888.
52. Sifuentes-Osornio J, Porras-Cortés G, Bendall RP, et al. *Cyclospora cayetanensis* infection in patients with and without AIDS: biliary disease as another clinical manifestation. *Clin Infect Dis* 1995;21:1092–1097.
53. Ortega YR, Sterling CR, Gilman RH. *Cyclospora cayetanensis. Adv Parasitol* 1998;40:399–418.
54. Eberhard ML, Pieniazek NJ, Arrowood MJ. Laboratory diagnosis of *Cyclospora* infections. *Arch Pathol Lab Med* 1997;121: 792–797.
55. Visvesvara GS, Moura H, Kovacs-Nace E, et al. Uniform staining of *Cyclospora* oocysts in fecal smears by a modified safranin technique with microwave heating. *J Clin Microbiol* 1997;35: 730–733.
56. Lopez B, de Merida AM, Arrowood MJ, et al. Comparison of two microscopic diagnostic methods for *Cyclospora cayetanensis*. In: *Program and abstracts of the International Conference on Emerging Infectious Diseases,* Atlanta, March 8–11, 1998:80(abst P-2.3).
57. Berlin OGW, Peter JB, Gagne C, et al. Autofluorescence and the detection of *Cyclospora* oocysts [Letter]. *Emerging Infect Dis* 1998;4:127–128.
58. Orlandi PA, Lampel KA. Extraction-free, filter-based template preparation for the rapid and sensitive PCR detection of pathogenic parasitic protozoa. *J Clin Microbiol* 2000;38:2271–2277.
59. Van Nhieu JT, Nin F, Fleury-Feith J, et al. Identification of intracellular stages of *Cyclospora* species by light microscopy of thick sections using hematoxylin. *Hum Pathol* 1996;27:1107–1109.
60. Madico G, Gilman RH, Miranda E, et al. Treatment of *Cyclospora* infections with co-trimoxazole. *Lancet* 1993;342: 122–123.
61. Shear M, Connor BA, Shlim DR, et al. Azithromycin treatment of *Cyclospora* infections. *Gastroenterology* 1994;106[Suppl 4]: 772A(abst).
62. Shlim DR, Pandey P, Rabold JG, et al. An open trial of trimethoprim alone against *Cyclospora* infections. *J Travel Med* 1997;4: 44–45.
63. Ebrahimzadeh A, Rogers L. Diarrhea caused by a cyanobacterium-like organism. *Eur J Epidemiol* 1995;11:661–664.
64. Clarke SC, McIntyre M. The incidence of *Cyclospora cayetanensis* in stool samples submitted to a district general hospital. *Epidemiol Infect* 1996;117:189–193.
65. Brennan MK, MacPherson DW, Palmer J, et al. Cyclosporiasis: a new cause of diarrhea. *Can Med Assoc J* 1996;155:1293–1296.
66. Sherchand JB, Cross JH, Jimba M, et al. Study of *Cyclospora cayetanensis* in health care facilities, sewage water and green leafy vegetables in Nepal. *Southeast Asian J Trop Med Public Health* 1999;30:58–63.
67. Katz D, Kumar S, Malecki J, et al. Cyclosporiasis associated with imported raspberries, Florida, 1996. *Public Health Rep* 1999;114: 427–438.
68. Rabold JG, Hoge CW, Shlim DR, et al. *Cyclospora* outbreak associated with chlorinated drinking water [Letter]. *Lancet* 1994;344: 1360–1361.

64

MICROSPORIDIA

DONALD P. KOTLER
JAN M. ORENSTEIN

DESCRIPTION

Microsporidians are protozoans that exist as obligate intracellular parasites. They are ubiquitous in nature, infecting species in all five classes of vertebrates, in addition to invertebrates including arthropods and fish. The phylum Microspora is large, containing approximately 100 genera and 1,000 species. As primitive eukaryotes, microsporidians have nuclear membranes but lack mitochondria, peroxisomes, and Golgi apparatus, which are characteristic of most eukaryotes. Microsporidians are thought to have diverged from prototype eukaryotes, based on molecular taxonomic studies of ribosomal RNA (1).

Microsporidians have a unique mode of transmission (2). Microsporidial spores contain an extrusion apparatus consisting of a coiled polar filament and an anchoring disk. Cellular infection is believed to occur through extrusion of the polar filament, followed by ejection of the sporoplasm through the hollow tube. The process of filament extrusion appears to involve an influx of calcium and water into the spore, causing a rise in internal pressure. If the plasma membrane of the target cell is breached during this process, the sporoplasm is passed into the cell cytoplasm to continue the parasite's life cycle.

Microsporidians were first described in tissue sections about 70 years ago (3) and recognized as a cause of tissue injury and disease about 30 years ago (4,5). Microsporidians have been identified as a cause of disease in several species of mammals. Most infections occur in young animals or in association with immune deficiencies. Six genera have been identified as pathogens in humans, three related to species causing disease in animals.

The clinical syndromes associated with microsporidiosis in patients with AIDS, include diarrhea, keratoconjunctivitis, nephritis, hepatitis, and myositis; diarrhea and its attendant malabsorption are the most common. The detection of microsporidians in clinical specimens increased until 1996, then fell as a result of highly active antiretroviral therapy (HAART). The aim of this chapter is to describe the clinical features, diagnostic modalities, and treatment of intestinal disease by *Enterocytozoon bieneusi* and *Encephalitozoon intestinalis,* the two most clinically relevant species of Microsporidia known to infect patients with AIDS.

E. BIENEUSI

Intestinal microsporidiosis in patients with AIDS was recognized almost simultaneously in different areas of the world. *E. bieneusi* organisms were first observed in 1982 in small intestinal biopsies from patients with AIDS in Texas and Washington, D.C. (6). The first case reports from the United States (7) and France (8), the latter involving a Haitian patient (7–8), were followed by additional reports confirming the syndrome (9–14). More than 500 cases had been recognized by mid 1993. Cases of *E. bieneusi* have been reported from all continents with prevalence rates comparable to other AIDS-associated opportunistic enteric infections, such as *Cryptosporidium* (15). Recent reports identified *E. bieneusi* in patients with other immune deficiencies, including iatrogenic immune suppression (16–20), as well as persons without evident immune deficiencies (21–28), indicating that microsporidiosis is more widespread than previously suspected.

Microbiology

Taxonomy

The characteristic features of *E. bieneusi* are its development as a multinucleate plasmodium in intimate contact with the cell cytoplasm, cleftlike structures called electron-lucent inclusions, and electron-dense disks that fuse to form the polar tubule. Other distinctive features include precocious development of the injection apparatus within the intact

D. P. Kotler: Department of Medicine, College of Physicians and Surgeons, Columbia University; Gastrointestinal Division, Department of Medicine, St. Luke's–Roosevelt Hospital Center, New York, New York

J. M. Orenstein: Department of Pathology, George Washington University, Washington, D.C.

plasmodium, six turns of the polar tubule arranged in two layers, and mononuclear spores (1 × 1.5 μm), which are the smallest of all known microsporidians.

Recent reports describe *Enterocytozoon* species in other mammals, including monkeys, domestic dogs and cats, and pigs and cattle (29–35). The organisms that infect monkeys appear identical to those that infect humans. In monkeys, the parasite appears to localize in the hepatobiliary tree, rather than the small intestinal mucosa (34). Persistent infection with *E. bieneusi* has been established in a simian immunodeficiency virus-infected monkey with spores isolated from a patient with AIDS (35).

Life Cycle

The different stages in the life cycle of *E. bieneusi* have been characterized by transmission electron microscopy (TEM) in several laboratories (6,36). Because no experimental system for *in vitro* culture of *E. bieneusi* is available, the various developmental stages have been characterized in clinical specimens and their sequence inferred from studies of other microsporidians. A single infected enterocyte may contain microsporidial forms in different stages of development. Whether this occurs as a result of multiple infections in the same cell, binary or multiple fission of plasmodial forms, or variable rates of maturation of infectious sporoplasm is unclear.

The earliest stage identified in clinical material is the proliferating plasmodium or meront (Fig. 64.1A). These are small (1 μm in diameter), oval, membrane-bound inclusions, usually seen in the apical cytoplasm and usually associated with cellular mitochondria. The meront is more electron lucent than the surrounding cytoplasm and contains free ribosomes but no other recognizable structures. A nucleus is the next structure identified during the maturation process; subsequent development is indicated by nuclear division, emergence of rough endoplasmic reticulum, and the appearance of electron-lucent inclusions (Fig. 64.1B). These inclusions are lined by electron-dense material (best demonstrated by ferric–osmium staining) that is destined to form the polar tubule. Later in this stage, electron-dense disklike structures begin to develop from the clefts (Fig. 64.1C) as the parasite enters sporogony. Future spores are defined by progressive development and association of the polar tube with its anchoring plate, polaroplast membrane, nucleus, and posterior vacuole. Through a complicated process of membrane invaginations, the sporogonial plasmodium divides into multiple sporonts. With development of the endospore and ectospore, first the sporoblast and then the mature electron-dense egg-shaped spore is formed.

The electron-dense disks, whose appearance indicates the beginning of sporogony, increase in number and size and form flat stacks within the plasmodia (Fig. 64.1C). In some sections, the disks appear ringlike. Interconnections develop, both end to end and in a syncytial-like pattern, leading to the coiled tubule. The coiled tube contains six turns in *E. bieneusi* and appears organized into two tiers of three turns each; the two tiers are consistently out of register by about 45 degrees.

Mature spores have been identified during eruption through the lysing enterocyte membrane and in sloughed, usually dying epithelial cells (Fig. 64.1D). However, some cells retain viability for a period after sloughing. For this reason, it is possible that spore maturation could proceed after the enterocyte has been extruded into the intestinal lumen.

Epidemiology

Although *E. bieneusi* was initially thought to be an uncommon pathogen, it is recognized now as a common enteric infection in patients with AIDS. Prevalence rates among patients with AIDS have varied between 2% and 50% (37–46), depending on the study group and methods of diagnosis. Several studies have shown that the prevalence of microsporidiosis is higher in AIDS patients with diarrhea than in those without diarrhea, and more common in patients with chronic than acute diarrhea (45,46). A single study showed equivalent prevalence rates of *E. bieneusi* in AIDS patients with and without diarrhea, irrespective of the number of CD4+ lymphocytes, the presence of co-infections, or other clinical parameters (42). However, many studies have shown that clinical and parasitologic remission occurs commonly in patients receiving HAART (see below).

The mode of transmission of *E. bieneusi* has not been completely defined. An outbreak of microsporidiosis that was traced to a water distribution system caused at least 338 infections among HIV-infected patients, other immunosuppressed patients, and immunocompetent subjects (47). The parasite likely is acquired by ingestion of contaminated food or water or by direct human-to-human contact (48, 49). Seasonal variation in the incidence of infection is controversial (50,51).

Several studies have suggested an inverse relationship between the development of symptomatic microsporidiosis and immune function (43–45,52). Microsporidiosis is typically diagnosed in patients with severe depletion of CD4+ lymphocytes (18 to 30 cells/mm^3).

Pathogenesis Of Diarrhea

Current understanding of disease pathogenesis related to *E. bieneusi* infection is based on clinicopathologic correlations and the pattern of intestinal injury. After passage of ingested spores into the intestinal lumen, the polar filament is extruded, possibly in response to the higher pH level in the small intestinal lumen and other local factors (2). The polar filament likely facilitates infection of epithelial cells, which

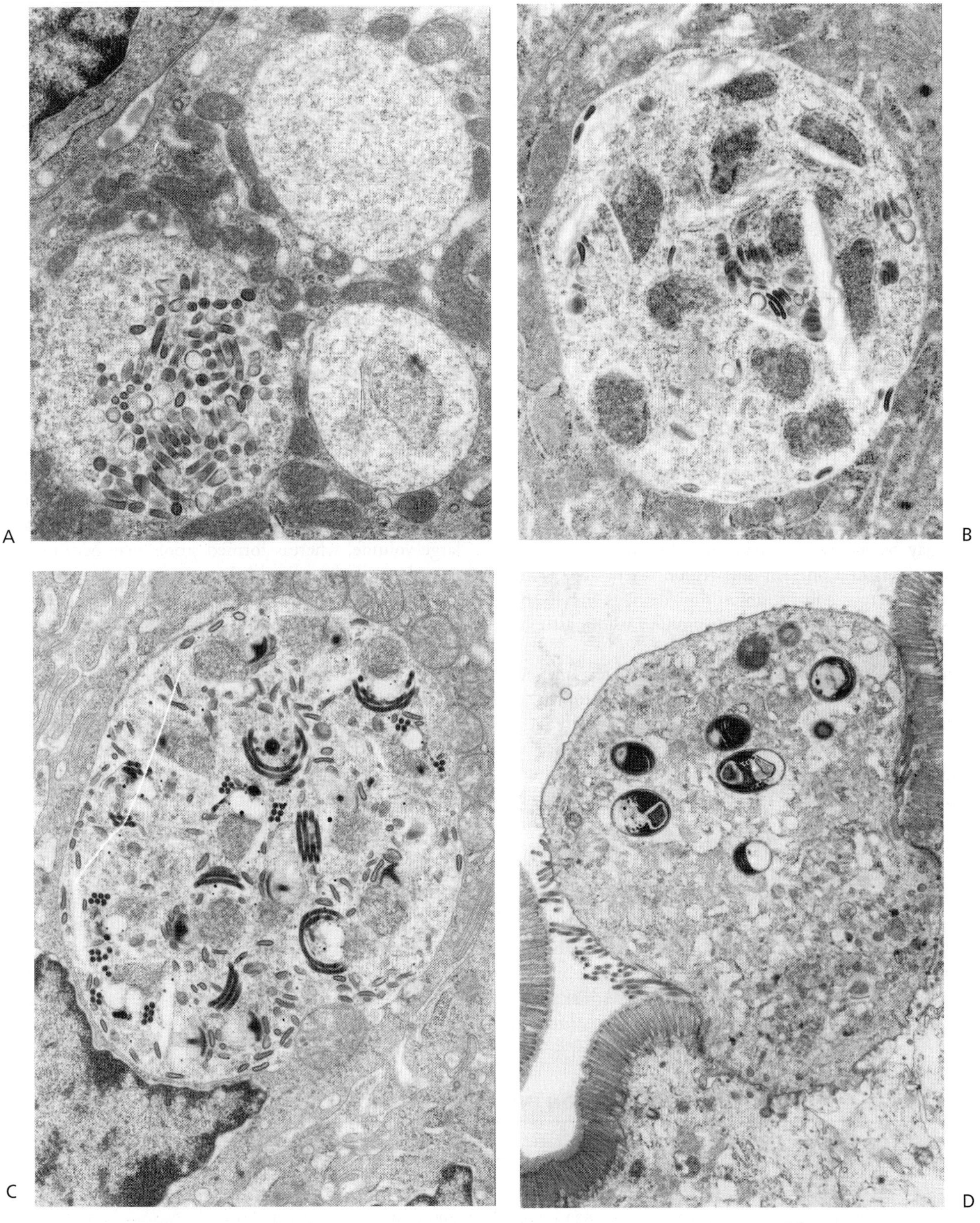

FIGURE 64.1. Transmission electron microscopy of *Enterocytozoon bieneusi*. **A:** Two proliferative plasmodia, a very early one without a nucleus (**upper right**) and one with a single nucleus (**lower right**), and a sporogonial plasmodium (**lower left**) containing electron-dense disk and rod-shaped precursors of polar tubes. Note the intimate association of the cell's electron-dense mitochondria with the plasmodia. Stain; ×16,500. **B:** An early sporogonial plasmodium with several electron-dense nuclei and disks and prominent electron-lucent clefts. Stain; ×15,500. **C:** A single late sporogonial plasmodium molding the apical nuclear pole. Future spores are identified by the polar tubes coiling around nuclei and polar vacuoles. When cut on end, the double layer of three turns is visible. Stain; ×14,600. **D:** A shedding cell, with few microvilli, contains several spores with polar vacuoles. Stain; ×8,000.

are eventually destroyed. The sloughed cells release mature spores into the lumen, and the infection continues via autoinfection. Spores may travel from cell to cell beneath the mucous layer, infecting contiguous cells, or may enter the luminal fluid and potentially infect a noncontiguous cell. It is unclear which mechanism is more important or if alternative mechanisms of cell-to-cell transmission occur.

The development of clinical disease is likely due to the excessive loss of epithelial cells. Differences in the intensity of infection may correlate with variability in clinical severity of disease (43,53). Although the etiologies differ, intestinal dysfunction in *E. bieneusi* infection resembles that of patients with tropical sprue and celiac disease, two diseases characterized by excessive loss of villous enterocytes (54). The rates of cell proliferation and loss are affected by many physiologic and pathologic stimuli. Under conditions of increased cell loss, such as during enteric infections, compensatory crypt hyperplasia returns villous architecture toward normal. The migration rate of newly formed enterocytes may be increased, leaving insufficient time for full functional maturation. For this reason, there are greater deficits in lactose and fat absorption than in starch and sucrose absorption in diseases that produce villous atrophy and crypt hyperplasia.

The relationship between *E. bieneusi* infection and intestinal structure and function has been examined in patients with AIDS (55). Partial villous atrophy and crypt hyperplasia were present in AIDS patients with microsporidiosis and cryptosporidiosis, but not in those without enteric pathogens (Table 64.1). Similarly, decreased levels of sucrase, lactase, and maltase were found in biopsies from AIDS patients with cryptosporidiosis and microsporidiosis, whereas normal levels were present in those without enteric pathogens. The ratios of sucrase to lactase and maltase to lactase were higher in the patients with parasitoses, implying a disproportionate loss of lactase. D-Xylose malabsorption also was prevalent in patients with parasitoses, but not in those without infections. Finally, small intestinal structure and function was fully preserved at the ultrastructural level in many patients without enteric pathogens identified by TEM. Other studies have confirmed a decrease in mucosal surface area and decreased lactase-specific activity in the jejunum of patients with microsporidiosis (56). Malabsorption may be exacerbated by alterations in intestinal transit in some patients (57).

Information regarding immunity to *E. bieneusi* infection has been limited by the inability to grow the organism *in vitro* or propagate the infection experimentally.

Clinical Illness

The clinical features of *E. bieneusi* enteritis are characteristic but vary in intensity (58). Typically, 3 to 10 nonbloody bowel movements of variable volume and consistency occur at irregular intervals. The bowel movements tend to be clustered during one portion of the day, usually late evening or early morning. Nocturnal diarrhea is uncommon. Some of the bowel movements are watery and of large volume, whereas formed stools may occasionally be passed. Although diarrhea may not be present in every patient with *E. bieneusi* infection, evidence of enteropathy has been found in all patients studied. Excessive flatus and an alteration in the odor of feces and flatus are often present. The infection is not accompanied by fever. Patients with mild disease may describe intolerance to lactose and fat, whereas those with more severe disease are intolerant to almost all foods. When severe, the diarrhea is associated with dehydration and electrolyte abnormalities, predominantly hypokalemia and hypomagnesemia. Serum bicarbonate concentrations may be subnormal, reflecting fecal losses.

The pathogenesis of weight loss is complex. Nutrient malabsorption and excess fecal energy losses have been reported (59,60). Resting energy expenditure is reduced in patients with microsporidiosis and other protozoal diarrhea (61,62). However, weight loss is related more to decreased caloric intake than to the severity of measured malabsorption or the reduction in energy expenditure. Patients may

TABLE 64.1. EFFECT OF MICROSPORIDIOSIS ON INTESTINAL STRUCTURE AND FUNCTION

	Villus Height*	Crypt Depth**	Sucrase*	Lactase***	Maltase	D-Xylose Absorption***
Micro	50 ± 3	92 ± 11	140 ± 30	40 ± 10	1,300 ± 430	16.1 ± 1.3
AIDS	86 ± 15	71 ± 8	500 ± 100	210 ± 30	2,050 ± 310	31.2 ± 3.8
Controls	85 ± 8	52 ± 5	530 ± 130	190 ± 10	2,040 ± 310	20–50

Data are presented as mean ± standard error; villus height and crypt depth in micrometers; sucrase, lactase, maltase levels in units per milligram of protein; D-xylose as 1-h serum value after 25-g oral dose.

*$p < .01$; **$p < .005$; ***$p < .001$ for overall analysis of variance.

Micro, patients with microsporidiosis; AIDS, patients with AIDS with no pathogens detected by transmission electron microscopy of jejunal biopsies.

Source: Adapted from Kotler DP. Gastrointestinal complications of the acquired immunodeficiency syndrome. In: Yamada T, ed. *Textbook of gastroenterology.* Philadelphia, PA: Lippincott, 1991:86–103, with permission.

note that appetite is intermittently normal, but formal calorie counts often reveal inadequate food intake, similar to that seen in other clinical and experimental malabsorption syndromes (63), and is related to the presence of unabsorbed nutrients in the lower intestine. Changes in gastric and pancreatic secretion and disturbances in gastric emptying and small intestinal transit are associated with microsporidiosis (64–66).

Weight loss occurs slowly, and the rate of weight loss may diminish over time (67). Rapid changes in weight usually are related to alterations in fluid balance associated with a change in the intensity of diarrhea. Studies of hydration status have shown that patients with microsporidiosis are chronically dehydrated compared with healthy subjects and AIDS patients without malabsorption (68).

Microsporidiosis is associated with biliary tract disease (69–71) and is a potential cause of AIDS-associated cholangiopathy (72). Microsporidia-associated biliary tract disease may resemble primary sclerosing cholangitis (73), similar to the cholangiopathy associated with cryptosporidiosis and cytomegalovirus infection. Sclerosing cholangitis may be the final result of bile duct epithelial injury. The biliary tract syndrome associated with microsporidiosis is characterized biochemically by progressive elevations in serum activities of alkaline phosphatase and γ-glutamyl transpeptidase. Transaminase levels are only mildly elevated, and bilirubin concentrations usually are within the normal reference range. Some patients complain of epigastric or right upper quadrant discomfort or pruritus; others are asymptomatic. Abdominal pain appears to be related to papillitis and papillary stenosis. AIDS cholangiopathy has been associated with progressive liver disease and liver failure in a few patients (D. P. Kotler, *unpublished observations*). We have seen subacute pancreatitis associated with chronic pain in a pediatric patient with *E. bieneusi* infection, although histologic examination of the pancreas and pancreatic ducts was not performed.

Diagnosis

Initially, the diagnosis of *E. bieneusi* infection was based exclusively on TEM. Recognition that the parasite can be identified in tissue sections by light microscopy (74–76), coupled with confirmatory special stains (77,78), coincided with a marked increase in the number of infections that were diagnosed. More recently, techniques for the diagnosis of microsporidiosis have been applied to fecal specimens, broadening the pool of patients in whom a search for microsporidiosis is possible. Studies to correlate the sensitivities, specificities, and predictive values for the various diagnostic modalities will allow standardization of these techniques. Development of molecular techniques for the identification of *E. bieneusi* carries the promise of increased diagnostic sensitivity.

Electron Microscopy

The diagnosis of *E. bieneusi* infection by TEM is based on detection of the developing forms within enterocytes (see above). Ultrastructural studies can be performed without regard to tissue orientation. All forms are readily detected, except the early meronts, which may resemble tangential sections of intraepithelial lymphocytes; meronts are intracellular whereas intraepithelial lymphocytes are intercellular in location. Enterocyte injury occurs, but it is nonspecific.

Light Microscopy

The endoscopist is advised to take multiple biopsies from the most distal site possible, because the distal duodenum and proximal jejunum have higher parasite burdens than the proximal duodenum (79). Some biopsies may be denuded of enterocytes, which hinders interpretation. Although a well-oriented specimen is not a requirement for proper identification, it greatly assists the observer in diagnosis. Biopsies containing long, slender villi and short crypts usually do not harbor *E. bieneusi.*

E. bieneusi infection is associated with partial villous atrophy and crypt hyperplasia (Fig. 64.2A). In some infections, villus height is nearly normal and marked crypt hyperplasia is present, whereas other infections demonstrate significant villous atrophy with little crypt hyperplasia, possibly reflecting differences in parasite burden or other factors such as nutritional status. The degree of injury usually is similar in different biopsies obtained from the same area. Typically, the number of intraepithelial lymphocytes, but not neutrophils or eosinophils, is increased. Microsporidial infection of colonic epithelium has been reported (80) but appears to be rare.

Cell injury is most prominent in the upper one-third of the villus. The villous tips show piling up of cells, many of which are infected and in the process of being sloughed from the surface (Fig. 64.2B). Individually sloughed cells appear as teardrop-shaped cells containing refractile spores (Fig. 64.2C). This is a characteristic feature of microsporidiosis and the most readily recognized diagnostic feature. Nuclear alterations include pleomorphism, hyperchromicity, and loss of basal orientation. Cytoplasmic alterations include increased numbers of lysosomes, vesiculation, vacuolization, and accumulation. The lamina propria may contain increased numbers of plasma cells and macrophages, but not neutrophils.

Light microscopic examination of one micron, plastic-embedded sections stained with either toluidine blue or trichrome (methylene blue, basic fuchsin, azure II) increase the diagnostic sensitivity to that of TEM. The organisms frequently affect nuclear shape, with a flattening or cupping of the apical pole (Fig. 64.2D). Electron-lucent clefts also may be visible, particularly when flanked by material that picks up

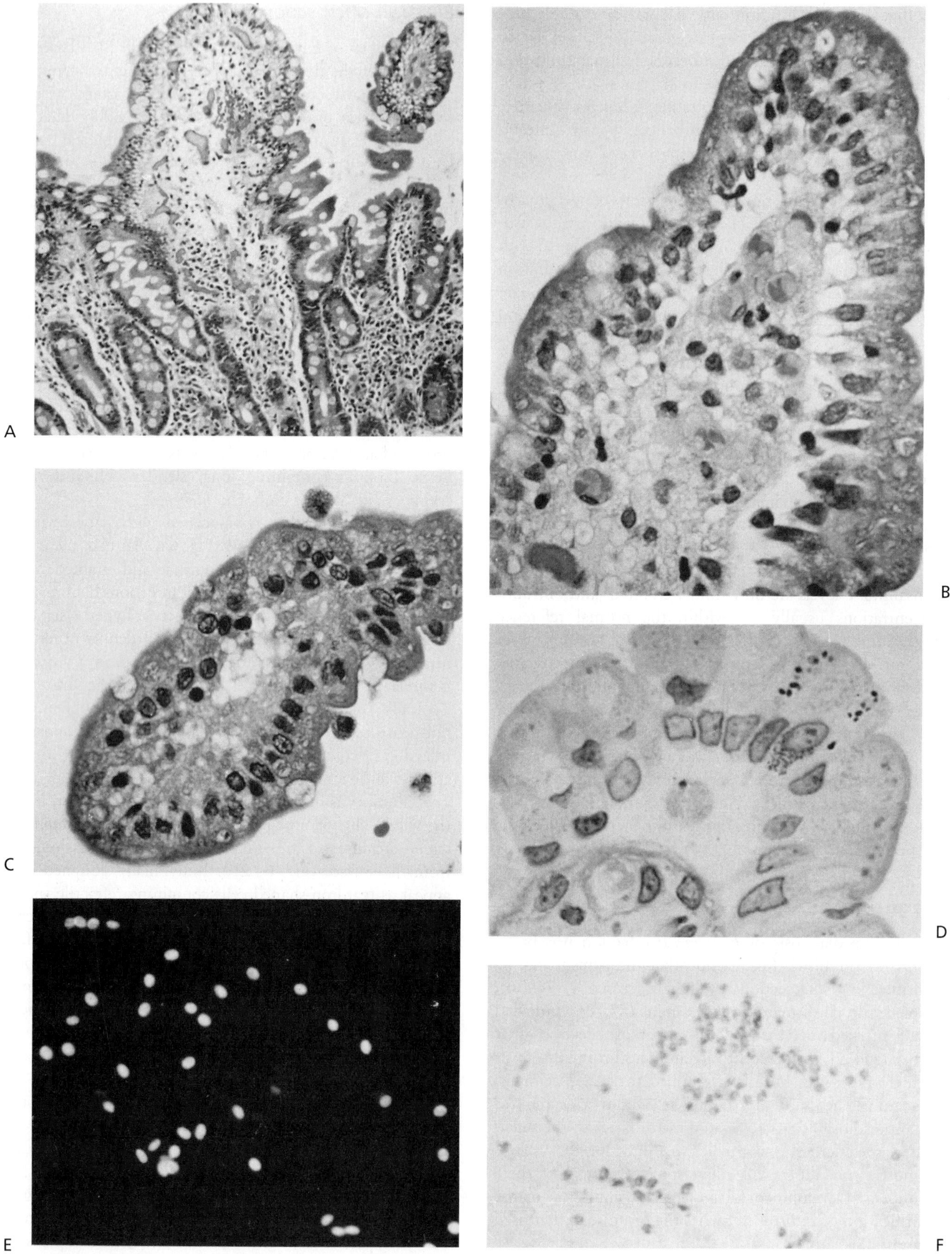
A
B
C
D
E
F

the hematoxylin stain, resulting in a cat's eye appearance. Rarely, spores are detected as clusters of negatively staining or refractile granular material in the cytoplasm of individual cells, particularly sloughed cells (Fig. 64.2C).

Special Preparations And Procedures

Special stains and preparations can facilitate the diagnosis of microsporidiosis by light microscopy. These stains include Gram, Giemsa, acid-fast, Warthin–Starry, and a modified tissue trichrome–chromotrope 2R stain, as described for examination of fecal specimens (81). Examination under polarized light is useful for detecting *E. bieneusi,* because the spores are birefringent, particularly in Gram-stained sections. In addition, Giemsa-stained touch preparations of fresh mucosal biopsies may be helpful (82–83). The sensitivities and negative predictive values of these techniques ranged between 57% and 88%, whereas the specificities and positive predictive values ranged between 94% and 100% (Table 64.2) (83). A false-negative diagnosis was related to a low parasite burden. A surprising finding was the excellent sensitivity of hematoxylin and eosin-stained sections for the diagnosis, albeit by observers with large clinical experience. The ability to correctly diagnose microsporidiosis by hematoxylin and eosin-stained sections has been noted by several investigators (74–76,80,82,83).

Intestinal fluid obtained by aspiration or lavage, or mucosal cytobrush preparations also may be helpful for the detection of microsporidians (84). Spores are readily identified in duodenal brush specimens with Giemsa, Gram, Diff-Quik, and modified trichrome stains. The chromotrope 2R stain allows differentiation between microsporidial spores and bacteria, because bacteria (light-green counterstain) do not take up the chromotrope stain.

Stool Examination

The use of special stains and light microscopy has increased the ability to diagnose *E. bieneusi* infection, but these are of limited value because endoscopy with biopsy, passage of a small intestinal tube for fluid aspiration, or passage of a capsule biopsy is required. The use of fecal specimens for diagnosis would greatly simplify diagnosis. Several techniques have been applied successfully. Giemsa staining of a fecal preparation that was homogenized, sieved, centrifuged, and extensively washed revealed *E. bieneusi* spores (85). The chromotrope 2R modified trichrome stain also can facilitate visualization of spores in stool; *E. bieneusi* spores become pink and most other material green (86) (Fig. 64.2F). Occasional yeast forms or bacteria take up the chromotrope stain, but they differ from *E. bieneusi* in size and shape. The advantage of this stain is that specimens without special preparation or formalin-fixed stool may be used. However, attention to the staining conditions, particularly decolorization, is required. A further modification of this method, staining at 56°C, decreases the time required for the parasite to take up the stain (87). An alternative method for studying fecal specimens is based on binding of the fluorochrome, uvitex 2B of calcofluor, to chitin, which is a component of the microsporidial cell wall (88). This technique is quite sensitive and works well with fresh or concentrated preparations (Fig. 64.2E). Although prior formalin fixation reduces the staining, it is still within acceptable diagnostic levels.

Several laboratories have successfully identified microsporidians in stool and clinical specimens using various techniques, such as *in situ* hybridization and polymerase chain reaction (89–100). Separate primers are available to distinguish among the different species of microsporidians. The availability of these techniques may facilitate the diagnosis of microsporidiosis and the epidemiologic studies of both prevalence and nonhuman reservoirs.

Treatment

Drug Therapy

Spontaneous remission of symptoms in patients with *E. bieneusi* infection was an early finding in patients receiving HAART (101–106), as a result of immune reconstitution due to HIV-1 suppression. In some patients, symptoms returned when therapy failed, suggesting that infection was

FIGURE 64.2. Light microscopy of *Enterocytozoon bieneusi.* **A:** A distorted villus and elongated crypts typical of microsporidia infection. Several shed enterocytes are visible. Hematoxylin and eosin stain; ×160. **B:** Clear clefts are visible in some of the many bluish supranuclear plasmodia at the tip of a villus. Note the characteristic vacuolization and separation of enterocytes at the basement membrane. ×640. H&E. **C:** The spores in one (upper) of the 2 shedding enterocytes are slightly refractile. Many bluish supranuclear plasmodia are visible. Hematoxylin and eosin stain; ×640. **D:** The spores stain dark blue, whereas the plasmodia stain lighter than the cytoplasm in semithin plastic sections. The darker "dots" within the plasmodia are nuclei. A spore is present in a shed cell within the space created by the sloughing enterocytes. Methylene blue–basic fuchsin–azure II stain; ×1,000. **E:** The spores fluoresce white to pink using the calcofluor whitening agent. (Courtesy of Dr. Elizabeth Didier.) Duodenal fluid stain; ×1,600. **F:** The spores stain pink and the background light blue in the modified trichrome, chromotrope 2R stain (Giang T, Kotler DP, Garro ML, et al. Tissue diagnosis of intestinal microsporidiosis using the chromotrope-2R trichrome stain. *J Clin Pathol* 1993;117:1249–1253.). The polar vacuole and a central band can be seen in several of the spores. Stain; ×1,500.

TABLE 64.2. DIAGNOSIS OF MICROSPORIDIOSIS BY LIGHT MICROSCOPY

	Hematoxylin and Eosin	Gram	Giemsa	Chromotrope	Touch
Sensitivity	83	77	57	83	83
Specificity	95	100	100	100	100
Positive predictive value	94	100	100	100	100
Negative predictive value	88	88	75	88	88

Gram, Brown–Hopp's tissue Gram-stain; chromotrope, chromotrope 2R-modified trichrome stain; touch, Giemsa stain of mucosal touch preparations.
Source: Adapted from Weber R, Bryan RT, Owen RL, et al. Improved light-microscopical detection of microsporidia spores in stool and duodenal aspirates. *N Engl J Med* 1992;326:161–166, with permission.

suppressed but not eradicated. Unfortunately, an effective antiparasitic agent for *E. bieneusi* infection has not been identified. Decreased diarrhea and weight stabilization have been noted with several agents, including metronidazole and albendazole, but histologic evidence of infection persists and the disease recurs once therapy is discontinued (117–113). Fumagillin was identified as a potentially effective agent against *E. bieneusi,* a finding confirmed in a randomized clinical trial, although the agent may cause significant toxicities, including thrombocytopenia (114,115).

Fluid, Electrolyte, And Nutritional Therapies

Patients with *E. bieneusi* infection are often chronically dehydrated (68) and may be depleted of both macronutrients and micronutrients. Electrolyte and mineral deficits, particularly K^{2+}, Ca^{2+}, and Mg^{2+}, may be severe and necessitate replacement therapy. Diet modification may be helpful in patients with mild to moderate disease. A lactose-free, low-fat diet with calorie-rich fluid supplements containing extra protein may be well tolerated. Symptoms may improve and weight may increase during the administration of nutritional formulas, including semi-elemental diets and those containing medium-chain triglycerides (116,117). Parenteral nutritional therapy results in nutritional repletion in some patients (117,118). Hydrophilic bulking agents are variably effective, depending on the level of malabsorption. Opiates such as diphenoxylate, paregoric, or tincture of opium may be effective, although the dose required sometimes causes excessive sedation.

Prevention

Recommendations for prevention of microsporidiosis are not available, since the reservoirs and routes of transmission of *E. bieneusi* have not been elucidated.

E. INTESTINALIS

In 1988, we identified a microsporidian by TEM that differed ultrastructurally from *E. bieneusi* (119). Two years later, three additional cases were identified. Since then, the second microsporidian, named *E. intestinalis* (120), which has a prevalence about one-tenth that of *E. bieneusi,* has been identified in the United States, Europe, and Australia.

Microbiology

Taxonomic analysis permitted the classification of *E. intestinalis* as a new species (120). Although originally thought to be a new genus, collection of sufficient material to allow DNA sequencing showed that the parasite had a high level of DNA homology to *Encephalitozoon* species. Distinctive morphologic features include a unique development of individual cells within separate chambers of a parasitophorous vacuole (Fig. 64.3A) and separation of developing organisms by septa of parasite origin. Other unique features are the completion of merogony before the development of the polar tubule, the lack of electron-lucent inclusions and electron-dense disks, presence of the polar tubule with a single tier of five to six turns, and spores of 2.2×1.2 μm in diameter (Fig. 64.3B).

Epidemiology, Pathogenesis, and Immunity

The epidemiology, pathogenesis, and immunity of *E. intestinalis* have not been studied but are presumed to be the same as those for *E. bieneusi.* Transmission likely is to occur through the oral route. The organism affects immune-competent and immune-deficient subjects (121). Species other than humans may be infected (122). In contrast to infection with *E. bieneusi,* in which the infection is limited to epithelial cells, *E. intestinalis* organisms infect epithelial cells and lamina propria macrophages. Renal involvement has been confirmed by the identification of spores, both free and within cells, in urinary sediment (Fig. 64.3B). Ultrastructural analysis of cell preparations revealed infection of both tubule cells (microvilli) and transitional cells (elongated cells with prominent cytokeratin). Granulomatous interstitial nephritis with *E. intestinalis* in the proximal and distal convoluted tubule has been confirmed in autopsy material. Parasites have also been identified in

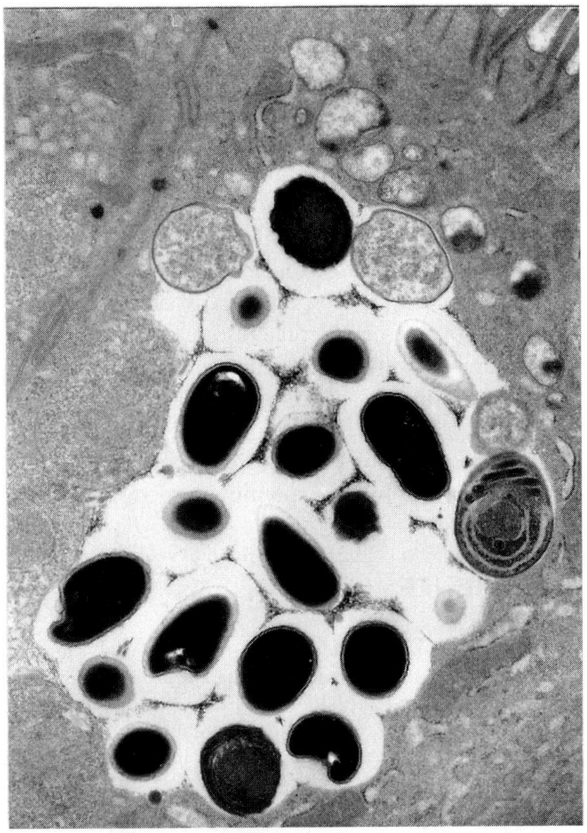

A

FIGURE 64.3. Transmission electron microscopy of *Encephalitozoon intestinalis.* **A:** Electron-dense fibrillar material divides the parasitophorous vacuole into chambers containing irregular light-staining meronts (on the vacuole edge) and oval sporoblasts/sporonts (coils visible in one), and more central electron-dense spores. Stain; ×11,000. **B:** Spores of *E. intestinalis* detected in urine have a single row of five to seven coils. Note the prominent polar vacuole. Stain; ×60,000. **C:** Spores of *Enterocytozoon bieneusi* detected in stool have a double row of three turns each. Note the single nucleus and the ectospore and endospore layers. Stain; ×77,000.

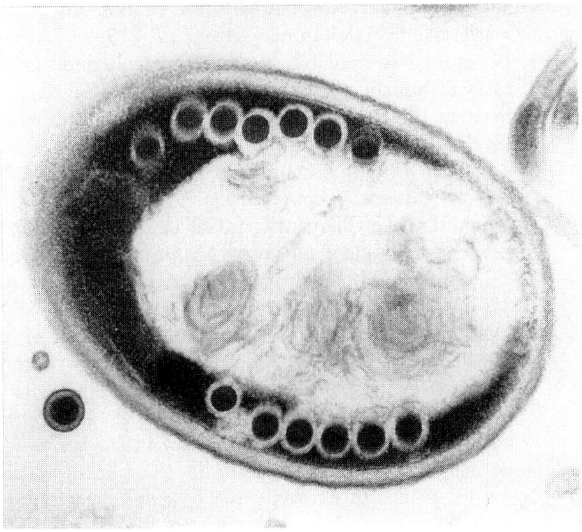

B

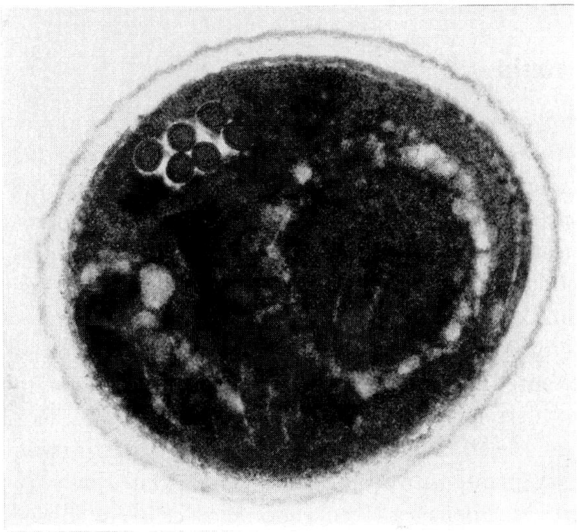

C

the liver both free and within cells of the portal vein, and endothelial and Kupffer cells, as well as in the gall bladder and biliary epithelium (123). Recently, *E. intestinalis* also was identified in the upper respiratory tract (124). Thus, in contrast to *E. bieneusi, E. intestinalis* disseminates widely to extraintestinal sites.

E. intestinalis probably enters host enterocytes by diacytosis (i.e., the injection of microsporidian sporoplasm through the polar tubule into the host cell). A recent *in vitro* study suggested that entry was mediated by directed phagocytosis, based on inhibition by cytochalasin D, colocalization of *E. intestinalis* and filamentous actin, and engulfment of *E. intestinalis* into Caco-2 cell protrusions (125).

More information is available about the immune response to *E. intestinalis* than *E. bieneusi* infection, because *E. intestinalis* can be grown *in vitro,* allowing production of parasite antigen. Seropositivity to *Encephalitozoon* infection is common, occurring in 5% to 10% of healthy, immune-competent individuals in one study (126–128). Cell-mediated immunity is an important defense against *Encephalitozoon* species, with interferon-γ (IFN-γ) an important mediator of protection from this parasite (129,130). Systemic dissemination of infection occurs in IFN-γ gene-deficient mice (131). In addition, animals lacking CD4+, but not CD8+, T lymphocytes are able to resist infection, implying that a CD8+ T-cell response involving IFN-γ secretion is important (132,133).

Clinical Illness

Clinically, *E. intestinalis* may produce a diarrheal syndrome with weight loss and malabsorption, similar to that associated with *E. bieneusi* infection. AIDS cholangiopathy also has been associated with *E. intestinalis* infection (123). Although patients with spores in their urine sediment may be asymptomatic, flank pain and symptoms of urethritis occur in some patients. Parasites have been associated with a rectal ulcer and chronic sinusitis. Whether *E. intestinalis* infects the central nervous system and causes neurologic syndromes in patients with AIDS is not known. Interestingly, the first patient reported died from sudden multiorgan system failure, including encephalopathy (119), and intestinal perforation was documented in another patient (134).

Diagnosis

E. intestinalis infection is diagnosed by the same techniques as *E. bieneusi.* The organism is usually easier to detect, due to its larger size, greater refractivity, birefringence, staining qualities, and larger parasite burden. The electron microscopic features are noted above. As with *E. bieneusi,* the parasite and its associated pathology localize to the distal villus. Individual cell shedding is less frequent than sloughing of whole groups of attached enterocytes. Epithelial disarray is also present. The spores are brightly birefringent and stain to a much greater degree than *E. bieneusi* spores (see Color Figure 64.4A–D). Typical of microsporidians, *E. intestinalis* spores are gram-positive (not easily demonstrated with *E. bieneusi*). Macrophages (even endothelial cells and fibroblasts) containing spores can be seen in the lamina propria. As noted above, free spores and cells containing spores can be found in urinary sediment, and spores can be detected in stool.

Treatment

E. intestinalis differs from *E. bieneusi* in its uniformly good response to albendazole therapy (134–136). Although relatively few cases have been studied, all have responded clinically with a decrease or disappearance of diarrhea and clearing of spores from the urine and stool. Follow-up biopsies have shown disappearance of spores and only ghosts of spores within macrophage lysosomes. Improvement in D-xylose absorption has been noted (124). Whether or not viable sporoplasm and spores are being sequestered in some location is unknown. Studies of antiparasitic agents performed *in vitro* have documented efficacy of some agents against *Encephalitozoon* species *in vitro* (137–139). Management of fluid and electrolyte status and nutritional therapy are similar to those for *E. bieneusi.*

In summary, microsporidiosis is now recognized as an important cause of intestinal disease in patients with HIV-1 infection and other immunodeficiency diseases and rarely immunocompetent persons. Further study should fill the major gaps in our understanding of the transmission, life cycle, and immunobiology of microsporidians, and hopefully facilitate development of specific antimicrosporidial therapies.

REFERENCES

1. Vossbrinck CR, Maddox JV, Friedman S, et al. Ribosomal RNA sequence suggests microsporidia are extremely ancient eukaryotes. *Nature* 1987;326:411–414.
2. Canning EU, Hollister WS. Microsporidia of mammals—widespread pathogens or opportunistic curiosities? *Parasitol Today* 1987;3:267–73.
3. Levaditi C, Nicolau S, Schoen R. L'etiologie de l'encephalite. *Comptes Rendus Acad Sci* 1923;177:985–988.
4. Matsubayashi H, Koike T, Mikata I, et al. A case of *Encephalitozoon*-like infection in man. *Arch Pathol* 1959;67:181–187.
5. Bergquist NR, Waller T, Mravak S, et al. Report of two recent cases of human microsporidiosis. Paper presented at: Annual meeting of the American Society of Tropical Medicine and Hygiene; 1983; San Antonio, Texas. Abstract.
6. Orenstein JM. Microsporidiosis in the acquired immunodeficiency syndrome. *J Parasitol* 1991;77:843–864.
7. Desportes I, Le Charpentier Y, Galian A, et al. Occurrence of a new microsporidan: *Enterocytozoon bieneusi* n.g., n.sp., in the enterocytes of a human patient with AIDS. *J Protozool* 1985;32: 250–254.
8. Dobbins W, Weinstein WM. Electron microscopy of the intestine and rectum in acquired immunodeficiency syndrome. *Gastroenterology* 1985;88:738–749.
9. Curry A, McWilliam LJ, Haboubi NY, et al Microsporidiosis in a British patient with AIDS. *Br Med J* 1988;41:477–478.
10. Bernard E, Michiels JF, Durant J, et al. Intestinal microsporidiosis due to *Enterocytozoon bieneusi:* a new case report in an AIDS patient. *AIDS* 1991;5:606–607.
11. Michiels JF, Hofman P, Saint Paul MC, et al. Microsporidiose intestinale: 3 cas chez des sujets seropositifs pour le VIH. *Ann Pathol* 1991;11:169–175.
12. Ullrich R, Zeitz M, Bergs C, et al. Intestinal microsporidiosis in a German patient with AIDS. *Klin Wochenschr* 1991;69: 443–445.
13. Modigliani R, Bories C, Le Charpentier Y, et al. Diarrhoea and malabsorption in acquired immune deficiency syndrome: a study of four cases with special emphasis on opportunistic protozoan infestations. *Gut* 1985;26:179–187.
14. Orenstein JM, Chiang J, Steinberg W, et al Intestinal microsporidiosis as a cause of diarrhea in human immunodeficiency virus-infected patients: a report of 20 cases. *Hum Pathol* 1990;21:475–1481.

15. Kotler DP, Francisco A, Clayton F, et al. Small intestinal injury and parasitic disease in AIDS. *Ann Intern Med* 1990;113:444–449.
16. Sax PE, Rich JD, Pieciak WS, et al. Intestinal microsporidiosis occurring in a liver transplant recipient. *Transplantation* 1995;60:617–618.
17. Guerard A, Rabodonirina M, Cotte L, et al. Intestinal microsporidiosis occurring in two renal transplant recipients treated with mycophenolate mofetil. *Transplantation* 1999;68:699–707.
18. Gumbo T, Hobbs RE, Carlyn C, et al. Microsporidia infection in transplant patients. *Transplantation* 1999;67:482–484.
19. Metge S, Van Nhieu JT, Dahmane D, et al. A case of *Enterocytozoon bieneusi* infection in an HIV-negative renal transplant recipient. *Eur J Clin Microbiol Infect Dis* 2000;19:221–223.
20. Goetz M, Eichenlaub S, Pape GR, et al. Chronic diarrhea as a result of intestinal microsporidiosis in a liver transplant recipient. *Transplantation* 2001;71:334–337.
21. Hautvast JL, Tolboom JJ, Derks TJ, et al. Asymptomatic intestinal microsporidiosis in a human immunodeficiency virus-seronegative, immunocompetent Zambian child. *Pediatr Infect Dis J* 1997;16:415–416.
22. Desportes-Livage I, Doumbo O, Pichard E, et al. Microsporidiosis in HIV-seronegative patients in Mali. *Trans Royal Soc Trop Med Hyg* 1998;92:423–424.
23. Fournier S, Liguory O, Garrait V, et al. Microsporidiosis due to *Enterocytozoon bieneusi* infection as a possible cause of traveller's diarrhea. *Eur J Clin Microbiol Infect Dis* 1998;17:743–744.
24. Gainzarain JC, Canut A, Lozano M, et al. Detection of *Enterocytozoon bieneusi* in two human immunodeficiency virus-negative patients with chronic diarrhea by polymerase chain reaction in duodenal biopsy specimens and review. *Clin Infect Dis* 1998;27:394–398.
25. Svenungsson B, Capraru T, Evengard B, et al. Intestinal microsporidiosis in a HIV-seronegative patient. *Scand J Infect Dis* 1998;30:314–316.
26. Lopez-Velez R, Turrientes MC, Garron C, et al. Microsporidiosis in travelers with diarrhea from the tropics. *J Travel Med* 1999;6:223–227.
27. Gumbo T, Gangaidzo IT, Sarbah S, et al. *Enterocytozoon bieneusi* infection in patients without evidence of immunosuppression: two cases from Zimbabwe found to have positive stools by PCR. *Ann Trop Med Parasitol* 2000;94:699–702.
28. Muller A, Bialek R, Kamper A, et al. Detection of microsporidia in travelers with diarrhea. *J Clin Microbiol* 2001;39:1630–1632.
29. Mansfield KG, Carville A, Shvetz D, et al. Identification of an *Enterocytozoon bieneusi*-like microsporidian parasite in simian-immunodeficiency-virus-inoculated macaques with hepatobiliary disease. *Am J Pathol* 1997;150:1395–1405.
30. Breitenmoser AC, Mathis A, Burgi E, et al. High prevalence of *Enterocytozoon bieneusi* in swine with four genotypes that differ from those identified in humans. *Parasitology* 1999;118:447–453.
31. Mathis A, Breitenmoser AC, Deplazes P. Detection of new *Enterocytozoon* genotypes in faecal samples of farm dogs and a cat. *Parasite* 1999;6:189–193.
32. Rinder H, Thomschke A, Dengjel B, et al. Close genotypic relationship between *Enterocytozoon bieneusi* from humans and pigs and first detection in cattle. *J Parasitol* 2000;86:185–188.
33. Chalifoux LV, Carville A, Pauley D, et al. *Enterocytozoon bieneusi* as a cause of proliferative serositis in simian immunodeficiency virus-infected immunodeficient macaques (*Macaca mulatta*). *Arch Pathol Lab Med* 2000;124:1480–1484.
34. Mansfield KG, Carville A, Hebert D, et al. Localization of persistent *Enterocytozoon bieneusi* infection in normal rhesus macaques (*Macaca mulatta*) to the hepatobiliary tree. *J Clin Microbiol* 1998;36:2336–2338.
35. Tzipori S, Carville A, Widner G, et al. Transmission and establishment of a persistent infection of *Enterocytozoon bieneusi* derived from a human with AIDS in SIV-infected rhesus monkeys. *J Infect Dis* 1997;175:1016–1020.
36. Cali A, Owen RI. Intracellular development of *Enterocytozoon*, a unique microsporidian found in the intestine of AIDS patients. *J Protozool* 1990;37:145–155.
37. Canning EU, Hollister WS. *Enterocytozoon bieneusi* (Microspora): prevalence and pathogenicity in AIDS patients. *Trans Royal Soc Trop Med* 1990;84:181–186.
38. Greenson J, Belitsos P, Yardley J, et al. AIDS enteropathy: occult enteric infections and duodenal mucosal alterations in chronic diarrhea. *Ann Intern Med* 1991;114:366–372.
39. Swenson J, MacLean JD, Kokoskin-Nelson E, et al. Microsporidiosis in AIDS patients. *Can Commun Dis Rep* 1993;19:13–15.
40. Cotte L, Rabodonirina M, Piens A, et al.. Prevalence of intestinal protozoons in french patients infected with HIV. *J Acquired Immunodefic Syndrome* 1993;6:1024–1029.
41. Simon D, Weiss L, Wittner M, et al. Prevalence of microsporidia in AIDS patients with refractory diarrhea. *Am J Gastroenterol* 1991;86:1348(abst).
42. Rabeneck L, Gyorkey F, Genta R, et al. The role of microsporidia in the pathogenesis of HIV-related chronic diarrhea. *Ann Intern Med* 1993;119:895–899.
43. Kotler DP, Orenstein JM. Prevalence of intestinal microsporidiosis in HIV-infected individuals for gastroenterological evaluation. *Am J Gastroenterol* 1994;89:1998–2002.
44. Molina JM, Sarfati C, Beauvais B, et al. Intestinal microsporidiosis in human immunodeficiency virus-infected patients with chronic unexplained diarrhea: prevalence and clinical and biologic features. *J Infect Dis* 1993;167:217–221.
45. Coyle CM, Orenstein JM, Wittner M, et al. Prevalence of microsporidiosis in AIDS related diarrhea as determined by polymerase chain reaction to microsporidian ribosomal RNA. *Clin Infect Dis* 1996;23:1002–1006.
46. Sobottka I, Schwartz DA, Schottelius J, et al. Prevalence and clinical significance of intestinal microsporidiosis in human immunodeficiency virus-infected patients with and without diarrhea in Germany: a prospective coprodiagnostic study. *Clin Infect Dis* 1998;26:475–480.
47. Cotte L, Rabodonirina M, Chapuis F, et al. Waterborne outbreak of intestinal microsporidiosis in persons with and without human immunodeficiency virus infection. *J Infect Dis* 1999;-180:2003–2008.
48. Hutin YJ, Sombardier MN, Liguory O, et al. Risk factors for intestinal microsporidiosis in patients with human immunodeficiency virus infection: a case–control study. *J Infect Dis* 1998;178:904–907.
49. Mota P, Rauch CA, Edberg SC. Microsporidia and Cyclospora: epidemiology and assessment of risk from the environment. *Crit Rev Microbiol* 2000;26:69–90.
50. Conteas CN, Berlin OG, Lariviere MJ, et al. Examination of the prevalence and seasonal variation of intestinal microsporidiosis in the stools of persons with chronic diarrhea and human immunodeficiency virus infection. *Am J Trop Med Hyg* 1998;58:559–561.
51. Kopicko JJ, Frazer T, Dascomb K, et al. Influence of seasonal variation with enteric microsporidiosis among HIV-infected individuals. *J Acquired Immunodefic Syndrome* 1999;22:408–409.
52. Eeftinck Schattenkerk JKM, van Gool T, van Ketel RJ, et al. Clinical significance of small-intestinal microsporidiosis in HIV-1infected individuals. *Lancet* 1991;337:895–898.
53. Goodgame R, Stager C, Marcantel B, et al. Intensity of infection in AIDS-related intestinal microsporidiosis. *J Infect Dis* 1999;180:929–932.

54. Brunner O, Edelman S, Klipstein FA. Intestinal morphology of rural Haitians: a comparison between overt tropical sprue and asymptomatic subjects. *Gastroenterology* 1970;58:655–672.
55. Kotler DP, Reka S, Chow K, et al. Effects of enteric parasitoses and HIV infection upon small intestinal structure and function in patients with AIDS. *J Clin Gastroenterol* 1993;16:10–15.
56. Schmidt W, Schneider T, Heise W, et al. Mucosal abnormalities in microsporidiosis. *AIDS* 1997;11:1589–1594.
57. Sharpstone D, Neild P, Crane R, et al. Small intestinal transit, absorption, and permeability in patients with AIDS with and without diarrhoea. *Gut* 1999;45:70–76.
58. Kotler DP. Gastrointestinal complications of the acquired immunodeficiency syndrome. In: Yamada T, ed. *Textbook of gastroenterology.* Philadelphia, PA: Lippincott, 1991:86–103.
59. Carbonnel F, Beaugerie L, Abou Rached A, et al. Macronutrient intake and malabsorption in HIV infection: a comparison with other malabsorptive states. *Gut* 1997;41:805–810.
60. Beaugerie L, Carbonnel F, Carrat F, et al. Factors of weight loss in patients with HIV and chronic diarrhea. *J Acquired Immunodefic Syndrome Hum Retrovirol* 1998;19:34–39.
61. Kotler DP, Tierney AR, Brenner SK, et al. Preservation of short-term energy balance in clinically stable patients with AIDS. *Am J Clin Nutr* 1990;57:7–13.
62. Sharpstone DR, Ross HM, Gazzard BG. The metabolic response to opportunistic infections in AIDS. *AIDS* 1996;10: 1529–1533.
63. Sclafani A, Koopmans HS, Vasselli J, et al. Effects of intestinal bypass surgery on appetite, food intake, and body weight in obese and lean rate. *Am J Physiol* 1978;234:E389–E398.
64. Spiller RC, Trotman IF, Higgins BE, et al. The ileal brake—inhibition of jejunal motility after ileal fat perfusion in man. *Gut* 1984;25:365–374.
65. Owyang C, Green L, Rader D. Colonic inhibition of pancreatic and biliary secretion. *Gastroenterology* 1983;84:470–475.
66. Burn-Murdoch RA, Fischer M, Hunt JN. The slowing of gastric emptying by proteins in test meals. *J Physiol* 1978;274: 477–485.
67. Macallan DC, Noble C, Baldwin C, et al. Prospective analysis of patterns of weight change in stage IV human immunodeficiency virus infection. *Am J Clin Nutr* 1993;58:417–424.
68. Babameto G, Kotler DP, Burastero S, et al. Alterations in hydration in HIV-infected individuals. *Clin Res* 1994;42:279(abst).
69. McWhinney PHM, Nathwani D, Green ST, et al. Microsporidiosis detected in association with AIDS-related sclerosing cholangitis. *AIDS* 1991;5:1394–1395.
70. Beaugerie L, Teilhac M-F, Deluol A-M, et al. Cholangiopathy associated with microsporidia infection of the common bile duct mucosa in a patient with HIV infection. *Ann Intern Med* 1992;117:401–402.
71. Pol S, Romana CA, Richard S, et al. Microsporidia infection in patients with the human immunodeficiency virus and unexplained cholangitis. *N Engl J Med* 1993;328:95–99.
72. Cello J. Acquired immunodeficiency syndrome cholangiopathy: spectrum of disease. *Am J Med* 1989;86:539–546.
73. Chen LY, Goldberg H. Sclerosing cholangitis. Broad spectrum of radiographic features. *Gastrointest Radiol* 1984;9:39–46.
74. Peacock CS, Blanshard C, Tovey DG, et al. Histological diagnosis of intestinal microsporidiosis in patients with AIDS. *J Clin Pathol* 1991;44:558–563.
75. Lucas SB, Papadaki L, Conlon C, et al. Diagnosis of intestinal microsporidiosis in patients with AIDS. *J Clin Pathol* 1989;42: 885–887.
76. Simon D, Weiss L, Tanowitz H, et al. Light microscope diagnosis of human microsporidiosis and variable response to octreotide. *Gastroenterology* 1991;100:271–273.
77. Giang T, Kotler DP, Garro ML, et al. Tissue diagnosis of intestinal microsporidiosis using the chromotrope-2R trichrome stain. *J Clin Pathol* 1993;117:1249–1253.
78. Bryan RT, Weber R. Microsporidia. Emerging pathogens in immunodeficient persons [Editorial]. *Arch Pathol Lab Med* 1993;117:1243–1245.
79. Orenstein JM, Tenner M, Kotler DP. Localization of infection by the microsporidian *Enterocytozoon bieneusi* in the gastrointestinal tract of AIDS patients with diarrhea. *AIDS* 1992;6: 195–197.
80. Weber R, Muller A, Spycher MA, et al. Intestinal *Enterocytozoon bieneusi* microsporidiosis in an HIV-infected patient: diagnosis by ileo-colonoscopic biopsies and long-term follow up. *Clin Invest* 1992;70:1019–1023.
81. Verre J, Marriott D, Hing M, et al. Evaluation of light microscopic detection of microsporidial spores in faeces from HIV infected patients. In: Program and abstracts of the Workshop on Intestinal Microsporidia in HIV Infection; December 15–16, 1992; Paris, France. Abstract.
82. Rijpstra AC, Canning EU, Van Ketel RJ, et al. Use of light microscopy to diagnose small-intestinal microsporidiosis in patients with AIDS. *J Infect Dis* 1988;157:827–831.
83. Kotler DP, Giang TT, Garro ML, et al. Light microscopic diagnosis of microsporidiosis in patients with AIDS. *Am J Gastroenterol* 1994;89:540–544.
84. Orenstein JM, Zierdt W, Zierdt C, et al. Identification of spores of the Microspora, *Enterocytozoon bieneusi* in stool and duodenal fluid from AIDS patients with diarrhea. *Lancet* 1991;336: 1127–1128.
85. van Gool T, Hollister WS, Schattenkerk JE, et al. Diagnosis of *Enterocytozoon bieneusi* microsporidiosis in AIDS patients by recovery of spores from faeces. *Lancet* 1990;2:697–698.
86. Weber R, Bryan RT, Owen RL, et al. Improved light-microscopical detection of microsporidia spores in stool and duodenal aspirates. *N Engl J Med* 1992;326:161–166.
87. Bryan RT, Weber R, Stewart JM, et al. New manifestations and simplified diagnosis of human microsporidiosis. *Am J Trop Med Hyg* 1991;45:133–134.
88. van Gool T, Snijders F, Reiss P, et al. Diagnosis of intestinal and disseminated microsporidial infections in patients with HIV by a new rapid fluorescence technique. *J Clin Pathol* 1993;46: 694–699.
89. Zhu X, Wittner M, Tanowitz H, et al. Small subunit rRNA sequence of *Enterocytozoon bieneusi* and its potential diagnostic role with use of the polymerase chain reaction. *J Infect Dis* 1993;168:1570–1575.
90. Zhu X, Wittner M, Tanowitz HB, et al. Nucleotide sequence of the small subunit rRNA of *Encephalitozoon intestinalis. Nucleic Acids Res* 1993;20:4846.
91. Weiss LM, Zhu X, Cali A, et al. Utility of microsporidian rRNA in diagnosis and phylogeny: a review. *Folia Parasitol* 1994;41: 81–90.
92. Franzen C, Muller A, Hegener P, et al. Detection of microsporidia (*Enterocytozoon bieneusi*) in intestinal biopsy specimens from human immunodeficiency virus-infected patients by PCR. *J Clin Microbiol* 1995;33:2294–2296.
93. David F, Molina JM, Derouin F, et al. Detection and species identification of intestinal microsporidia by polymerase chain reaction in duodenal biopsies from human immunodeficiency virus-infected patients. *J Infect Dis* 1996;174:874–877.
94. Velasquez JN, Rodriguez MI, Cabrera MG, et al. Detection of the microsporidian parasite *Enterocytozoon bieneusi* in specimens from patients with AIDS by PCR. *J Clin Microbiol* 1996; 34:3230–3232.
95. Ombrouck C, Desportes-Livage I, Danis M, et al. Specific PCR assay for direct detection of intestinal microsporidia *Enterocytozoon bieneusi* and *Encephalitozoon intestinalis* in fecal specimens

from human immunodeficiency virus-infected patients. *J Clin Microbiol* 1997;35:652–655.

96. Liguory O, Molina JM, Modai J, et al. Diagnosis of infections caused by *Enterocytozoon bieneusi* and *Encephalitozoon intestinalis* using polymerase chain reaction in stool specimens. *AIDS* 1997;11:723–726.
97. Kock NP, Schottelius J, Albrecht H, et al. Species-specific identification of microsporidia in stool and intestinal biopsy specimens by the polymerase chain reaction. *Eur J Clin Microbiol Infect Dis* 1997;16:369–376.
98. Talal AH, Kotler DP, Weiss LW. Detection of *Enterocytozoon bieneusi* by PCR using primers to the small-subunit rRNA. *Clin Infect Dis* 1998;26:673–675.
99. da Silva AJ, Bornay-Llinares FJ, del Aguila de la Puente CD, et al. Diagnosis of *Enterocytozoon bieneusi* (microsporidia) infections by polymerase chain reaction in stool samples using primers based on the region coding for small-subunit ribosomal RNA. *Arch Pathol Lab Med* 1997;121:874–879.
100. Carnevale S, Velasquez JN, Labbe JH, et al. Diagnosis of *Enterocytozoon bieneusi* by PCR in stool samples eluted from filter paper disks. *Clin Diagn Lab Immunol* 2000;7:504–506.
101. Goguel J, Katlama C, Sarfati C, et al. Remission of AIDS-associated intestinal microsporidiosis with highly active antiretroviral therapy. *AIDS* 1997;11:1658–1659.
102. Conteas CN, Berlin OG, Speck CE, et al. Modification of the clinical course of intestinal microsporidiosis in acquired immunodeficiency syndrome patients by immune status and anti-human immunodeficiency virus therapy. *Am J Trop Med Hyg* 1998;58:555–558.
103. Carr A, Marriott D, Field A, et al. Treatment of HIV-1-associated microsporidiosis and cryptosporidiosis with combination antiretroviral therapy. *Lancet* 1998;351:256–261.
104. Maggi P, Larocca AM, Quarto M, et al. Effect of antiretroviral therapy on cryptosporidiosis and microsporidiosis in patients infected with human immunodeficiency virus type 1. *Eur J Clin Microbiol Infect Dis* 2000;19:213–217.
105. Foudraine NA, Weverling GJ, van Gool T, et al. Improvement of chronic diarrhoea in patients with advanced HIV-1 infection during potent antiretroviral therapy. *AIDS* 1998;12:35–41.
106. Miao YM, Awad-El-Kariem FM, Franzen C, et al. Eradication of cryptosporidia and microsporidia following successful antiretroviral therapy. *J Acquired Immunodefic Syndrome* 2000;25:124–129.
107. Field HM, Harkness A, Marriott D. Enteric microsporidiosis: incidence and response to albendazole or metronidazole. In: Program and abstracts of the VII International Conference on AIDS; 1992; Amsterdam. Abstract PoB 3344.
108. Blanshard C, Ellis DS, Tovey DG, et al. Treatment of intestinal microsporidiosis with albendazole in patients with AIDS. *AIDS* 1992;6:311–313.
109. Dieterich DT, Lew E, Kotler DP, et al. Treatment with albendazole for intestinal disease due to *Enterocytozoon bieneusi* in patients with AIDS. *J Infect Dis* 1994;169:173–183.
110. Dieterich DT, Lew E, Kotler DP, et al. Divergence between clinical and histologic responses during treatment of *Enterocytozoon bieneusi* infection with albendazole: prospective study and review of the literature. *AIDS* 1993;7[Suppl 3]:S43–S44.
111. Dionisio D, Manneschi LI, Di Lollo S, et al. *Enterocytozoon bieneusi* in AIDS: symptomatic relief and parasite changes after furazolidone. *J Clin Pathol* 1997;50:472–476.
112. Dionisio D, Manneschi LI, Di Lollo S, et al. Persistent damage to *Enterocytozoon bieneusi,* with persistent symptomatic relief, after combined furazolidone and albendazole in AIDS patients. *J Clin Pathol* 1998;51:731–736.
113. Bicart-See A, Massip P, Linas MD, et al. Successful treatment with nitazoxanide of *Enterocytozoon bieneusi* microsporidiosis in a patient with AIDS. *Antimicrob Agents Chemother* 2000;44:167–168.
114. Molina JM, Goguel J, Sarfati C, et al. Potential efficacy of fumagillin in intestinal microsporidiosis due to *Enterocytozoon bieneusi* in patients with HIV infection: results of a drug screening study. The French Microsporidiosis Study Group. *AIDS* 1997;11:1603–1610.
115. Molina JM, Goguel J, Sarfati C, et al. Trial of oral fumagillin for the treatment of intestinal microsporidiosis in patients with HIV infection. ANRS 054 Study Group. Agence Nationale de Recherche sur le SIDA. *AIDS* 2000;14:1341–1348.
116. Wanke CA, Pleskow D, Degirolami PC, et al. A medium chain triglyceride-based diet in patients with HIV and chronic diarrhea reduces diarrhea and malabsorption: a prospective, controlled trial. *Nutrition* 1996;12:766–771.
117. Kotler DP, Fogleman L, Tierney AR. Comparison of total parenteral nutrition and an oral, semielemental diet on body composition, physical function, and nutrition-related costs in patients with malabsorption due to acquired immunodeficiency syndrome. *J Parenter Enteral Nutr* 1998;22:120–126.
118. Kotler DP, Tierney AR, Wang J, et al. Effect of home total parenteral nutrition upon body composition in AIDS. *J Parenter Enteral Nutr* 1990;14:454–458 .
119. Orenstein JM, Tenner M, Cali A, et al. A microsporidian previously undescribed in humans, infecting enterocytes and macrophages and associated with diarrhea in an AIDS patient. *Hum Pathol* 1992;23:722–728.
120. Cali A, Kotler DP, Orenstein JM. *Encephalitozoon intestinalis,* N.G., N.Sp., an intestinal microsporidian associated with chronic diarrhea and dissemination in AIDS patients. *J Euk Microbiol* 1993;40:101–112.
121. Raynaud L, Delbac F, Broussolle V, et al. Identification of *Encephalitozoon intestinalis* in travelers with chronic diarrhea by specific PCR amplification. *J Clin Microbiol* 1998;36:37–40.
122. Bornay-Llinares FJ, da Silva AJ, Moura H, et al. Immunologic, microscopic, and molecular evidence of *Encephalitozoon intestinalis* (*Septata intestinalis*) infection in mammals other than humans. *J Infect Dis* 1998;178:820–826.
123. Orenstein JM, Dieterich DT, Kotler DP. Systemic dissemination by a newly recognized microsporidia species in AIDS. *AIDS* 1992;6:1143–1150.
124. Orenstein JM, Dieterich DT, Lew EA, Kotler DP. Albendazole as a treatment for disseminated microsporidiosis due to *Encephalitozoon intestinalis* in AIDS patients. *AIDS* 1993;7[Suppl 3]:S40–S42.
125. Foucault C, Drancourt M. Actin mediates *Encephalitozoon intestinalis* entry into the human enterocyte-like cell line, Caco-2. *Microb Pathol* 2000;28:51–58.
126. Didier ES, Kotler DP, Dieterich DT, et al. Serologic studies in human microsporidiosis. *AIDS* 1993;7[Suppl 3]:S8–S11.
127. Weiss LM, Cali A, Levee E, et al. Diagnosis of *Encephalitozoon cuniculi* infection by Western blot and the use of cross-reactive antigens for the possible detection of microsporidiosis in humans. *Am J Trop Med Hyg* 1992;47:456–462.
128. van Gool T, Vetter JC, Weinmayr B, et al. High seroprevalence of Encephalitozoon species in immunocompetent subjects. *J Infect Dis* 1997;175:1020–1024.
129. Braunfuchsova P, Kopecky J, Ditrich O, et al. Cytokine response to infection with the microsporidian, Encephalitozoon cuniculi. *Folia Parasitol (Praha)* 1999;46:91–95.
130. Khan IA, Moretto M. Role of gamma interferon in cellular immune response against murine *Encephalitozoon cuniculi* infection. *Infect Immun* 1999;67:1887–1893.
131. El Fakhry Y, Achbarou A, Franetich JF, et al. Dissemination of *Encephalitozoon intestinalis,* a causative agent of human

microsporidiosis, in IFN-gamma receptor knockout mice. *Parasite Immunol* 2001;23:19–25.

132. Moretto M, Casciotti L, Durell B, et al. Lack of CD4(+) T cells does not affect induction of CD8(+) T-cell immunity against *Encephalitozoon cuniculi* infection. *Infect Immun* 2000;68: 6223–6232.
133. Khan IA, Schwartzman JD, Kasper LH, et al. CD8+ CTLs are essential for protective immunity against *Encephalitozoon cuniculi* infection. *J Immunol* 1999;162:6086–6091.
134. Soule JB, Halverson AL, Becker RB, et al. A patient with acquired immunodeficiency syndrome and untreated *Encephalitozoon (Septata) intestinalis* microsporidiosis leading to small bowel perforation. Response to albendazole. *Arch Pathol Lab Med* 1997;121:880–887.
135. Case records of the Massachusetts General Hospital. *N Engl J Med* 1993;329:1946–1954.
136. Molina JM, Chastang C, Goguel J, et al. Albendazole for treatment and prophylaxis of microsporidiosis due to *Encephalitozoon intestinalis* in patients with AIDS: a randomized double-blind controlled trial. *J Infect Dis* 1998;177:1373–1377.
137. Coyle C, Kent M, Tanowitz HB, et al. TNP-470 is an effective antimicrosporidial agent. *J Infect Dis* 1998;177:515–518.
138. Didier ES. Effects of albendazole, fumagillin, and TNP-470 on microsporidial replication in vitro. *Antimicrob Agents Chemother* 1997;41:1541–1546.
139. Ridoux O, Drancourt M. Lack of *in vitro* antimicrosporidian activity of thalidomide. *Antimicrob Agents Chemother* 1999;43: 2305–2306.

65

INTESTINAL INFECTION WITH OTHER PROTOZOA, INCLUDING *ISOSPORA BELLI*, *BLASTOCYSTIS HOMINIS*, AND *DIENTAMOEBA FRAGILIS*

KEVIN C. KAIN
JAY S. KEYSTONE

This chapter focuses on other intestinal protozoa that are either proven or probable human pathogens, and on the nonpathogenic protozoa from which they must be differentiated (Table 65.1; Figs. 65.1 and 65.2). Most of these protozoa exist in two forms: a motile trophozoite that replicates in the bowel lumen and a nonreplicating infective cyst that resists the external environment.

For an optimal laboratory diagnosis of intestinal protozoal infection, the examination of at least three stool specimens collected over several days is generally required. However, recent studies suggest that the examination of one or two stool samples will detect up to 90% of the protozoa present (1). Any examination for parasites in fecal samples must include the use of a permanent stained smear and a micrometer. The identification of intestinal protozoa is based on unique characteristics of the trophozoite and cyst stages, including size and shape, number and structure of nuclei, nuclear characteristics, motility (trophozoites), inclusions, and chromatoidal bodies (2). These features are most readily demonstrated by using permanently stained fecal smears (trichrome or iron hematoxylin for amebae; modified acid-fast stain for coccidia), together with wet mounts and iodine-stained smears of direct and concentrated stool samples.

ISOSPORIASIS

Isosporiasis is caused by the intestinal sporozoan *Isospora belli,* which is related to *Cryptosporidium* and *Sarcocystis. I. belli* was first described by Virchow in 1860 but was named in 1923 (3). Isosporiasis is an important cause of protracted diarrhea in immunocompromised hosts, particularly in patients with AIDS, and is occasionally a cause of traveler's diarrhea (4,5).

TABLE 65.1. COMMONLY IDENTIFIED INTESTINAL PROTOZOA OF HUMANS

Organism	Potentially Pathogenic
Coccidia	
Cryptosporidium species	+
Isospora belli	+
Cyclospora[a] species	+
Sarcocystis species	+
Amebae	
Entamoeba histolytica	+
E. polecki	?
E. hartmanni	–
E. coli	–
Iodamoeba bütschlii	–
Endolimax nana	–
Flagellates	
Giardia duodenalis[b]	+
Dientamoeba fragilis[c]	+
Chilomastix mesnili	–
Pentatrichomonas hominis	–
Retortamonas intestinalis	–
Enteromonas hominis	–
Ciliates	
Balantidium coli	+
Other	
Blastocystis hominis	?

[a]A coccidium-like protozoan; proposed name is *Cyclospora cayetanensis.*
[b]Formerly *Giardia lamblia.*
[c]An ameba-like flagellate.

K.C. Kain and **J.S. Keystone:** Tropical Disease Unit, Department of Medicine, The Toronto Hospital, and the University of Toronto, Toronto, Ontario, Canada.

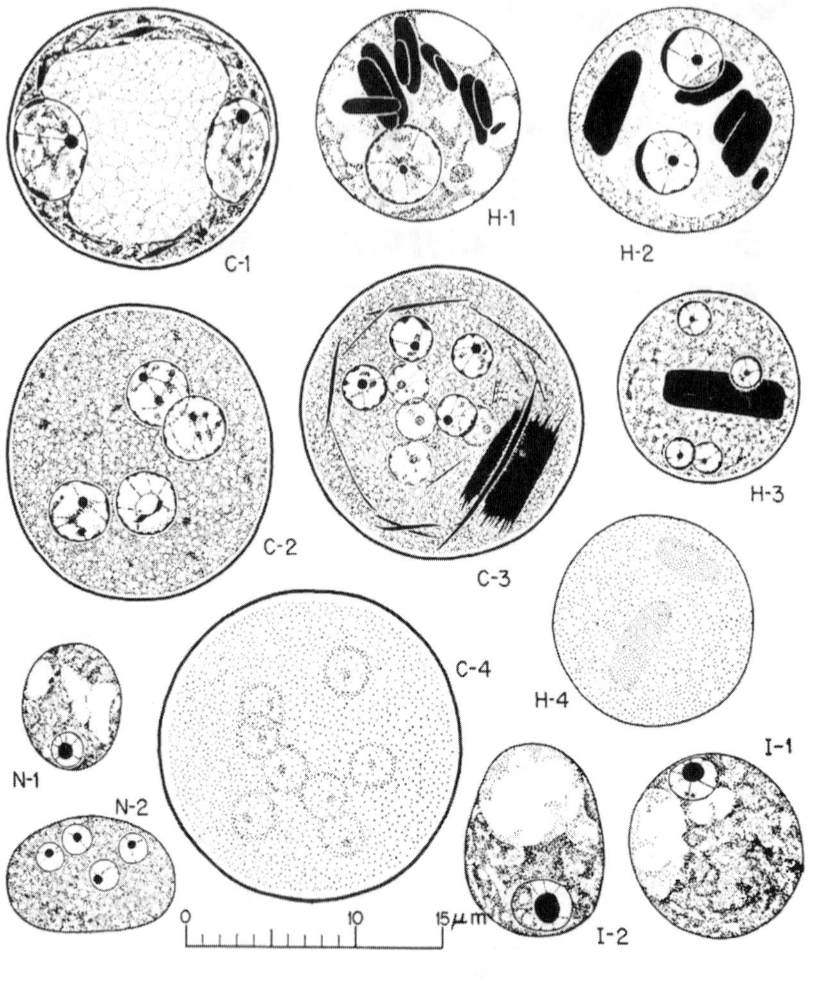

FIGURE 65.1. Cysts of intestinal amebae. *C-1–C-3*: Cysts of *Entamoeba coli.* Iron hematoxylin stain. *C-4*: Mature cyst of *E. coli.* Unstained. *H-2, H-3*: Cysts of *Entamoeba histolytica.* Iron hematoxylin stain. *H-4*: Unstained cyst of *E. histolytica* showing chromatoidal bars. *N-1, N-2*: Cysts of *Endolimax nana.* Iron hematoxylin stain. *I-1, I-2*: Cysts of *Iodamoeba bütschlii.* Iron hematoxylin stain. (From Strickland GI, ed. *Hunter's tropical medicine,* seventh edition. Philadelphia: WB Saunders, 1991, with permission.)

Microbiology

I. belli is an obligate, intracellular, coccidian protozoon of the phylum Apicomplexa (class Sporozoea). The life cycle of *I. belli* is similar to that of cryptosporidia and other coccidia, consisting of alternating asexual (schizogony) and sexual (sporogony) cycles in the enterocytes of the proximal small bowel (6–8). Human infection follows the ingestion of mature sporulated oocysts containing two sporocysts, each of which has four sporozoites (Figs. 65.3 and 65.4). The sporulated oocyst is the infective stage that excysts in the small bowel and releases sporozoites. Liberated sporozoites invade the small-bowel enterocytes and initiate asexual reproduction. In the sexual cycle, which follows soon after, oocysts are produced that are not infectious; they pass unsporulated in the feces approximately 9 to 15 days after ingestion. For sporulation to occur, a period of 24 to 48 hours outside the host is required, depending on environmental conditions. For this reason, exogenous autoinfection with *I. belli* is less likely to occur than with cryptosporidia.

Epidemiology

Isosporiasis has a worldwide distribution but is most prevalent in the tropics and subtropics (9,10). Humans are the only recognized source of infection (11,12). The true prevalence in humans is unknown. As an opportunistic pathogen in HIV-1–infected persons in the United States, *I. belli* remains an unusual cause of chronic diarrhea; it is identified in approximately 0.2% of patients. However, prevalence rates are much higher in the tropics. In some studies, more than 15% of AIDS patients in Africa and Haiti were infected with *I. belli* (10,12,13).

The mode of transmission is by ingestion of food or water contaminated with mature sporulated oocysts. Direct person-to-person transmission is also possible but probably less common (14). The incubation period is approximately 7 days. Like those of other coccidia, *I. belli* oocysts are highly resistant to common disinfectants and changes in environmental conditions; oocysts may remain viable for months if kept moist and cool (12). Sporadic outbreaks have occurred in institutions and day care centers in the United States (15,16).

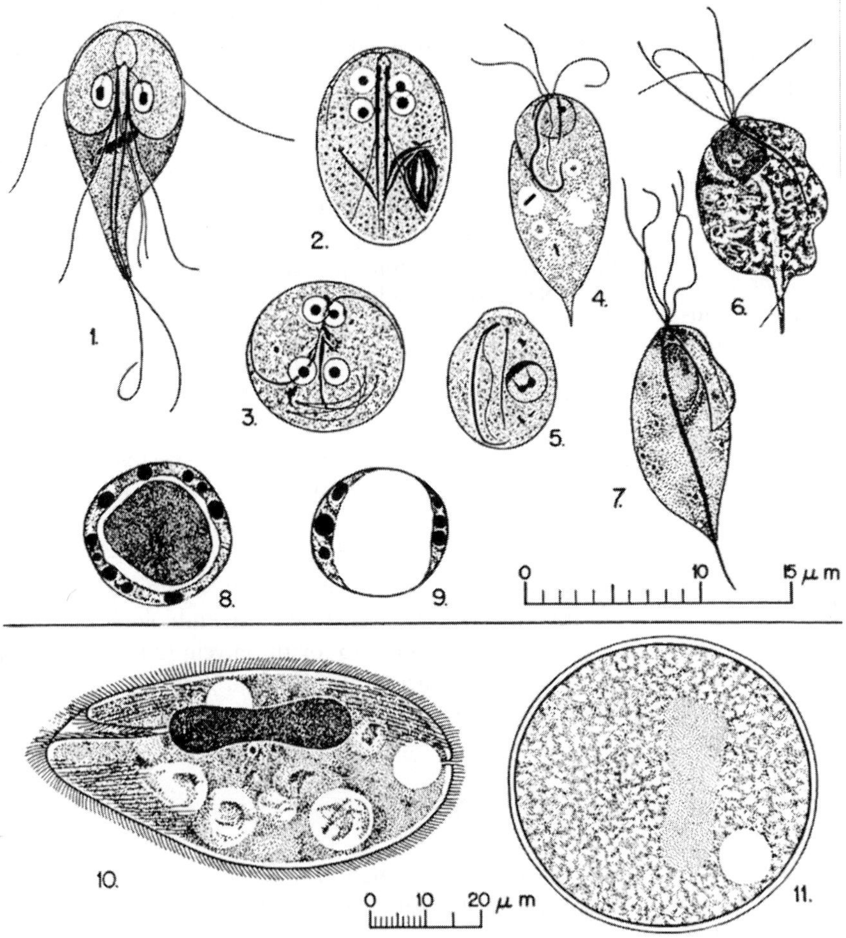

FIGURE 65.2. Intestinal flagellates and ciliates. *1*: Trophozoite of *Giardia duodenalis.* Iron hematoxylin stain. *2, 3*: Cysts of *G. duodenalis.* Iron hematoxylin stain. *4*: Trophozoite of *Chilomastix mesnili.* Iron hematoxylin stain. *5*: Cysts of *C. mesnili.* Iron hematoxylin stain. *6*: Trophozoite of *Pentatrichomonas hominis.* Iron hematoxylin stain. *7*: Trophozoite of *Trichomonas vaginalis.* Iron hematoxylin stain. *8*: *Blastocystis hominis.* Iron hematoxylin stain. *9*: *Blastocystis hominis.* Unstained. *10*: Trophozoite of *Balantidium coli.* *11*: Cyst of *B. coli.* Unstained. (From Strickland GI, ed. *Hunter's tropical medicine*, seventh edition. Philadelphia: WB Saunders, 1991, with permission.)

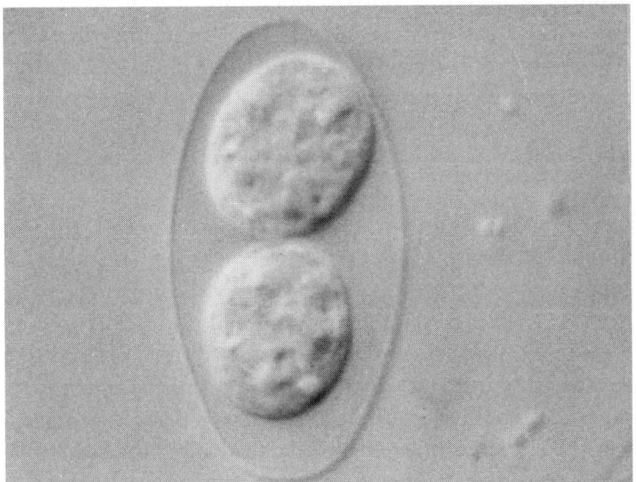

FIGURE 65.3. Oocyst of *Isospora belli.* A mature sporulated oocyst containing two sporocysts is revealed with the use of Nomarski optics. ×1,250. (Courtesy of Dr. Murray Wittner.)

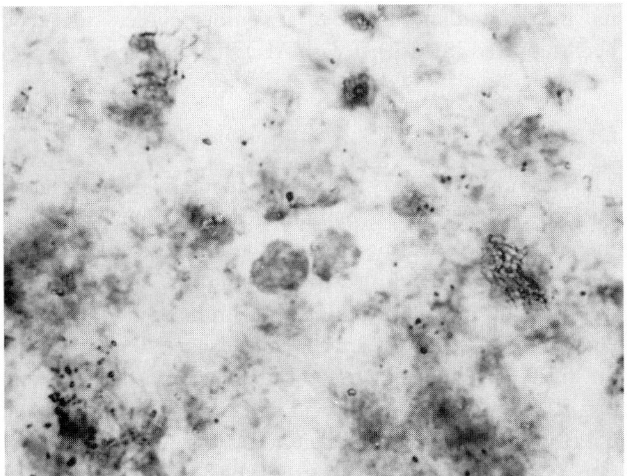

FIGURE 65.4. Direct smear of stool sample from a patient with isosporiasis. Modified acid-fast stain; ×600. (Courtesy of Dr. Jim Yang.)

Pathogenesis and Immunity

Little is known about the pathogenesis of isosporiasis. Infection is associated with villous atrophy and increased numbers of inflammatory cells in the lamina propria of the proximal small bowel (6). Developmental stages of *I. belli* may be found within the epithelial cells and occasionally in the lamina propria. Lymph node involvement has been reported in AIDS patients.

The mechanisms of host immunity to *I. belli* are unknown. However, persons with depressed cellular immunity are at greatest risk for the development of persistent diarrhea. Isosporiasis that is associated with persistent diarrhea (lasting more than 1 month) is an AIDS-indicator condition in HIV-1–infected persons. Some evidence suggests that *I. belli* oocysts may occasionally sporulate within the intestine, excyst, and reinitiate the endogenous cycle (autoinfection). Autoinfection and recycling of schizonts may, at least in part, be responsible for the prolonged diarrhea observed in immune-deficient hosts.

Clinical Presentation

The clinical presentation of isosporiasis often resembles that of cryptosporidiosis or giardiasis. In immunocompetent hosts, isosporiasis is characterized by the acute onset of watery diarrhea, colicky abdominal pain, and low-grade fever. In almost all immunologically intact hosts, it is a self-limited infection, lasting less than 1 month. In immunodeficient hosts, particularly in patients with AIDS, infection is associated with protracted watery diarrhea, abdominal pain, nausea, weight loss, and malabsorption. If left untreated, infection may persist for years. Two reports of extraintestinal isosporiasis and a case of acalculous cholecystitis have been reported in patients with AIDS (17–19).

Diagnosis

The diagnosis of isosporiasis can be made by demonstrating oocysts in stool samples or finding developmental stages of the parasite in small-bowel biopsy specimens. Oocysts are most commonly identified in fecal samples with the use of wet preparations and auramine–rhodamine or modified acid-fast stains (12,20). They are elliptic in shape (20 to 30 μm by 10 to 20 μm) and, like the oocysts of cryptosporidia, stain bright red with modified acid-fast stains (Figs. 65.3 and 65.4). Oocysts may not be detected in the feces at presentation but may be shed for up to 120 days following recovery. Unlike the oocysts of cryptosporidia, *I. belli* oocysts may be shed intermittently in small numbers and can easily be overlooked in standard ova and parasite examinations. The identification of isosporiasis may be facilitated by the examination of several stool samples (at least four) collected during several days (13) and the use of a concentration technique, such as the Sheather sugar flotation method (12), and a wet preparation. Occasionally, small-bowel biopsy specimens yield a positive result when stool samples are negative.

Treatment

Unlike cryptosporidiosis, isosporiasis responds promptly to appropriate antimicrobial therapy. The treatment of choice is trimethoprim (160 mg) and sulfamethoxazole (800 mg) (TMP-SMX) four times per day for 10 days, followed by TMP-SMX twice daily for 21 days (13,21). In approximately 50% of immunosuppressed patients, symptomatic isosporiasis recurs unless they receive maintenance therapy. Pyrimethamine (25 mg daily) and folinic acid (5 to 10 mg daily), TMP-SMX three times per week, or sulfadoxine and pyrimethamine (500 mg and 25 mg, respectively, weekly) have all been used successfully to prevent relapses. In persons who cannot tolerate sulfa drugs, pyrimethamine (75 mg daily) and folinic acid (10 mg daily) for 14 days followed by maintenance doses of pyrimethamine have been effective (22). Ciprofloxacin has a microbiologic cure rate of 75% (23). Responses to roxithromycin (24), metronidazole, quinacrine, diclazuril (25), furazolidone, and nitazoxanide (26) have been reported anecdotally.

SARCOCYSTOSIS

Sarcocystosis is a rare zoonotic infection of humans that was first described by Kartoulis in 1893 (27). *Sarcocystis* species are unique among coccidian infectious agents in that humans can act as both the intermediate and the definitive host. This section focuses on the sexual stage of infection (human as definitive host) because this stage is associated with gastrointestinal infection and may result in intestinal symptoms. For a review of extraintestinal disease caused by sarcocystosis, the reader is referred to Beaver et al. (28).

Microbiology

Sarcocystis species are intracellular coccidian protozoa of the phylum Apicomplexa. The life cycle requires two hosts, a predator and a prey; these are generally a carnivore and a herbivore, respectively. The sexual stages develop in the intestinal tract of the definitive host (the predator) and the asexual stages in the tissues of the intermediate host (the prey). Humans become definitive hosts of *Sarcocystis* organisms by ingesting inadequately cooked meat that contains tissue cysts (sarcocysts) of either of two species, *S. bovihominis* (beef) or *S. suihominis* (pork). Zoites (also called *bradyzoites* or *cystozoites*) contained in the sarcocysts are released by digestive enzymes and penetrate the enterocytes of the small bowel. Zoites invade the lamina propria and differentiate into microgametocytes (male) and macrogametocytes (female). Fertilization of macrogametocytes by microgametocytes occurs in approximately 24 hours, and

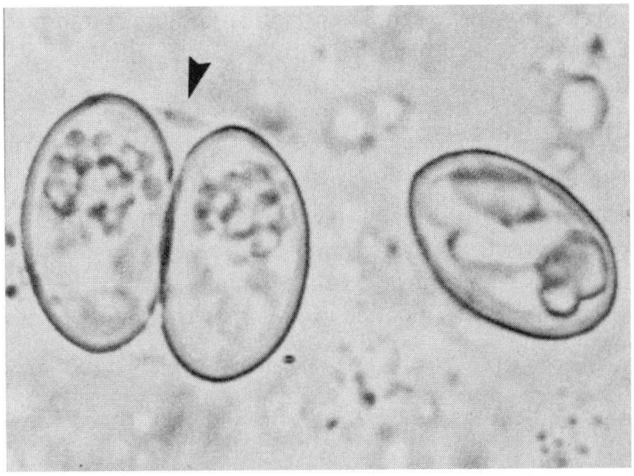

FIGURE 65.5. Oocyst and free sporocyst of *Sarcocystis* species. The thin-walled oocyst (*arrow*) usually ruptures, so that individual sporocysts are more commonly seen. In the oocyst, residual bodies in each sporocyst overlie the individual sporozoites. Formalin-fixed wet preparation; ×800. (From Ash LR, Orihel TC. *Atlas of human parasitology,* third edition. Chicago: American Society of Clinical Pathologists, 1990, with permission.)

the resulting zygotes undergo oocyst wall formation and sporulation. Sporulated oocysts consist of a thin wall containing two sporocysts, each of which contains four sporozoites (Fig. 65.5). Oocyst walls are thin and easily ruptured, so that free sporocysts are the form most commonly seen in the feces, approximately 2 to 3 weeks after ingestion of infected meat.

Tissue cysts develop in intermediate hosts, including humans, who become infected by ingesting oocysts or free sporocysts. Sporozoites excyst from the sporocysts and enter vascular endothelium, where they develop into schizonts that produce merozoites. These in turn enter striated muscle cells and produce sarcocysts. Tissue sarcocystosis is more common than was previously recognized, particularly in Southeast Asia, where up to 21% of persons were infected in some series (30,31). However, sarcocysts rarely cause symptoms (28,32,33).

Epidemiology (Human As Definitive Host)

Sarcocystosis is found worldwide, but its prevalence and incidence are unknown. It is speculated that many infections go unrecognized (34). In three surveys, 10% of Laotians (35), 22% of Tibetans (36), and 1% to 5.3% of Bolivian children (37) were found to be excreting oocysts; most were asymptomatic. A higher prevalence of infection may be found in agricultural societies or where inadequately cooked beef, pork, and occasionally caribou are consumed (38). Nonhuman primates may also serve as definitive hosts, but their importance as reservoirs for human infection is unknown (39).

Pathology

The histology of intestinal sarcocystosis ranges from segmental eosinophilic enteritis to necrotizing enteritis (34). In contrast to cryptosporidiosis and isosporiasis, intestinal sarcocystosis is not associated with villous blunting. Developmental stages of *Sarcocystis* species are occasionally identified in the lamina propria and submucosa in small-bowel biopsy specimens.

Clinical (Intestinal) Presentation

Sarcocystis species are generally not pathogenic to carnivores; however, severe intestinal symptoms may develop in humans. The spectrum of disease ranges from asymptomatic to necrotizing enteritis with intestinal obstruction. Abdominal pain, nausea, and diarrhea that lasted approximately 48 hours and appeared to coincide with zoite invasion of enterocytes of the small bowel developed in volunteers 3 to 6 hours after they ingested beef and pork infected with *Sarcocystis* organisms (40). Milder pain and diarrhea were associated with the appearance of sporocysts in the stool approximately 2 to 3 weeks after the consumption of infected meat. Severe disease is occasionally reported; severe abdominal pain, fever, and intestinal obstruction developed in six patients in Thailand who consumed *Sarcocystis*-infected raw beef (35). The condition of all six was improved by resection of the small bowel, which demonstrated multiple organisms. This report also noted that local market beef was infected with sarcocysts and speculated that many milder cases go unrecognized.

Diagnosis

The diagnosis of intestinal sarcocystosis is confirmed by the demonstration of oocysts or, more likely, free sporocysts (approximately 16 × 10 μm) in fresh stool samples, or by the finding of developmental sexual stages of the parasite in biopsy specimens or resected tissue (Fig. 65.5). Oocysts and sporocysts are shed sporadically, and an optimal diagnosis requires the use of a concentration technique, such as the Sheather sugar flotation method, and the examination of multiple stool samples collected during several days (12). Diagnostic stages in the stool may take 2 to 3 weeks to appear after the gastrointestinal symptoms first develop. Oocysts and sporocysts may be identified in wet preparations or by modified acid-fast or auramine staining. Oocysts stain bright red with modified acid-fast stains, like the oocysts of cryptosporidia and *I. belli.*

Treatment

The optimal therapy for intestinal sarcocystosis is unknown. Many mild infections appear to be self-limited. However, severe infections may require bowel resection.

E. POLECKI INFECTION

Entamoeba polecki is a frequent intestinal protozoan of monkeys and pigs that in rare instances causes human infections. The pathogenic potential of *E. polecki* in humans is at present unresolved.

Microbiology

Both the trophozoite and cyst stages of *E. polecki* have been identified in human stool samples, but the cyst is the form most frequently recognized. *E. polecki,* particularly the trophozoite stage, morphologically resembles both *Entamoeba histolytica* and *Entamoeba coli* and may frequently be misdiagnosed unless permanently stained fecal smears are carefully examined. The cyst stage is most helpful in differentiating *E. polecki* from other amebae; it is characterized by the presence of a single nucleus with a prominent karyosome and large numbers of chromatoid bodies of varied morphology (Fig. 65.6). The isoenzyme patterns of *E. polecki* are almost identical to those of *Entamoeba dispar,* so that the validity of this species (41) and its pathogenicity for humans are somewhat doubtful.

Epidemiology

E. polecki has a worldwide distribution, but most human infections have been reported from Papua New Guinea, where up to 19% of children were infected in one study (42). The most common mode of transmission appears to be the ingestion of cysts in food or water contaminated by infected monkey or pig feces. Human-to-human transmission has also been reported.

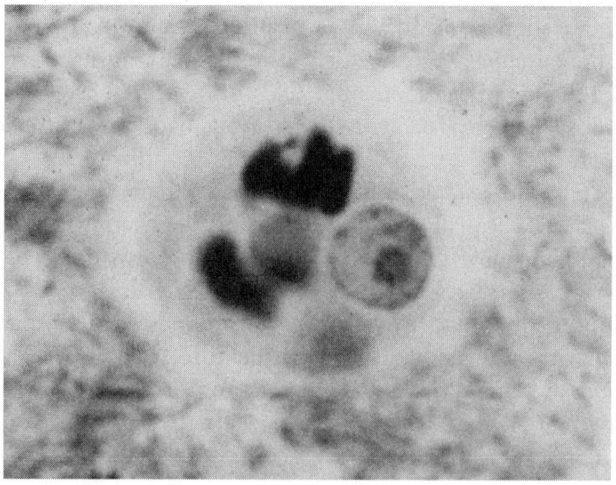

FIGURE 65.6. Cyst of *Entamoeba polecki.* This photograph illustrates some of the morphologic features that distinguish *E. polecki* from other intestinal amebae. Uninucleate cysts with large numbers of chromatoid bodies of varied morphology strongly suggest *E. polecki* infection. Iron hematoxylin stain. (From Ash LR, Orihel TC. *Atlas of human parasitology,* third edition. Chicago: American Society of Clinical Pathologists, 1990, with permission.)

Clinical Presentation

The vast majority of infected persons are asymptomatic, which is not surprising in view of the nonpathogenic isoenzyme patterns of this parasite. However, gastrointestinal symptoms, including diarrhea, cramps, anorexia, and malaise, have been reported in patients with heavy *E. polecki* infections.

Diagnosis

Many *E. polecki* infections may go unrecognized because of the difficulty of identifying this protozoan. Differentiating *E. polecki* cysts and trophozoites from those of *E. histolytica* and *E. coli* requires careful examination of permanently stained fecal smears (Fig. 65.6). The presence of uninucleate cysts with many chromatoid bodies should strongly suggest *E. polecki* infection.

Treatment

To date, no convincing evidence has been found that *E. polecki* is pathogenic for humans; hence, routine treatment is not warranted. In a limited number of anecdotal reports in which *E. polecki* was implicated in human disease, patients responded to treatment with 750 mg of metronidazole three times daily for 5 to 10 days. Diloxanide furoate (Furamide; 500 mg three times daily for 10 days) combined with metronidazole has also been used successfully to eradicate *E. polecki* infection.

D. FRAGILIS INFECTION

Dientamoeba fragilis, a protozoan parasite of the large intestine, was first discovered by Wenyon in 1909; however, it was not until 1918 that Jepps and Dobell (43) described the parasite as a new species. An excellent comprehensive review of the parasite by Windsor and Johnson was recently published (44).

Microbiology

D. fragilis was initially classified with the Sarcodina, but more recent electron microscopy, nucleic acid sequencing, and immunofluorescence studies suggest that it is a flagellate (without a flagellum) of the genera *Histomonas* and *Trichomonas* (45–47). The trophozoite may contain from one to four nuclei but is normally seen in the typical binucleate form (Fig. 65.7). It usually measures 5 to 12 μm in diameter but shows considerable variation in size. The nuclei contain four to six large granules clumped in the center, and the

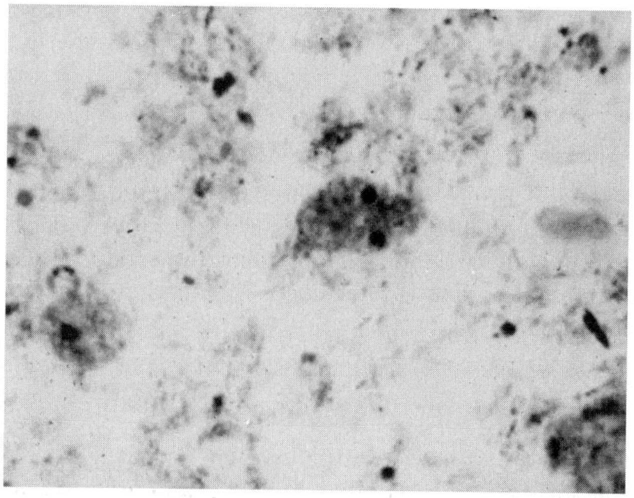

FIGURE 65.7. Trophozoites of *Dientamoeba fragilis.* Uninucleate and more typical binucleate trophozoites of *D. fragilis.* A typical nucleus with a karyosome in the form of a tetrad is observed in the binucleate organism. Iron hematoxylin stain; ×600.

cytoplasm may contain numerous food vacuoles. No cyst form has been described. The organism is usually found in the cecum and proximal large intestine. Its life span is unknown, but infection appears to persist for years.

Epidemiology

Dientamoebiasis is found worldwide, with prevalence rates of 1.4% to 19% in population-based surveys (48–52). However, the actual prevalence may be higher because in many early studies stools were not preserved or examined with permanently stained smears (53,54). The highest prevalence of infection (8% to 69%) has been found in children, institutionalized persons, native Americans, children in day care centers, and persons with poor personal hygiene (55–60). In a relatively recent study, *D. fragilis* antibodies were detected in 91% of 189 healthy children (61). It is interesting to note that the parasite is not seen with greater frequency in sexually active male homosexuals (62–64). Although the mode of transmission has not been determined, several observations suggest that transmission is likely by the direct fecal–oral transmission of pinworm eggs, which contain the organism. This mode of transmission is analogous to that of *Histomonas meleagridis,* the poultry pathogen transmitted by ova of the nematode *Heterakis gallinae.* Several studies have shown an 8- to 20-fold higher association of pinworm and *D. fragilis* infections than expected (65–67) and no association with other helminth infections. Two investigators who accidentally or deliberately infected themselves with one parasite subsequently noted a co-infection with the other (65,68). However, attempts to infect a human volunteer with *D. fragilis* alone failed (69,70). The parasite does not survive in water or simulated gastric juice (67,69). Finally, Burrows and Swendlow (65) did find structures resembling *D. fragilis* in the eggs of pinworms, but this study has not been confirmed by means of electron microscopy.

Pathogenesis and Immunity

Little is known about the pathogenesis of dientamoebiasis. To date, no studies have documented tissue invasion by this parasite, although the authors of two case reports proposed, without proof, that their patients' cases of colitis were caused by *D. fragilis* (71,72). Clinical experience with dientamoebiasis suggests that immunity to infection is incomplete because patients may be reinfected and become symptomatic with subsequent infections.

Clinical Presentation

For many years, *D. fragilis* was felt to be a harmless commensal, although the literature contained many reports of illness associated with infection (73–75). In 1966, Kean and Malloch (76) published for the first time a large case series of 100 patients with symptomatic infections. Spencer and co-workers (77,78) brought the infection to the attention of physicians once again with two retrospective case series in 1979 and 1982, in which they reviewed the clinical picture and response to therapy of children and adults infected with *D. fragilis* alone. The most convincing evidence that *D. fragilis* is a human pathogen comes from a randomized, placebo-controlled treatment trial of patients infected with *D. fragilis* alone (79); eradication of the parasite resulted in significantly greater relief of gastrointestinal symptoms in infected children than did placebo therapy.

Most symptomatic patients have abdominal pain (45% to 78%), diarrhea (46% to 68%), nausea (42%), or anorexia (20% to 31%). Less frequently, vomiting (17% to 22%), bloating/flatulence (16%), weight loss (22% to 26%), fatigue (6% to 13%), headache (24%), fever (12% to 26%), and irritability (12% to 20%) are described. Diarrhea occurs most often during the first week or two of illness, and abdominal pain appears to predominate after 1 or 2 months. The incidence of symptomatic infection is unclear because most retrospective studies suffer from referral bias in that they are more likely to review symptomatic persons. In a prospective study of children in 22 Canadian day care nurseries, only 10% of 72 infected children were symptomatic (58). This compares with rates of 42% to 58% reported in retrospective studies (53). Urticaria and pruritus were described in 6.7% and 12% of patients in two studies (67,78).

Diagnosis

The index of suspicion for dientamoebiasis should be high when someone with symptomatic enterobiasis (pruritus ani) presents with abdominal pain or diarrhea, two symptoms that do not usually accompany the latter infection. The corollary, pruritus ani in a patient with dientamoebiasis, should suggest the likelihood of co-infection with pinworm.

Dientamoebiasis has been associated with peripheral eosinophilia in up to 50% of infected persons (73,77,78). However, these reports require confirmation because absolute counts were not assessed and enterobiasis was not excluded. Absolute eosinophilia was detected in only 2 of 29 patients with dientamoebiasis in whom enterobiasis had been ruled out (79).

The diagnosis depends largely on proper stool collection and processing techniques. Several stool samples taken at intervals of 1 day or more should be examined because excretion in stool is variable (67,80). Samples must be examined soon after defecation or preserved in a suitable fixative immediately after passage (53). Appropriate fixatives include polyvinyl alcohol (81), modified Schaudinn fixative (82), and sodium acetate–acetic acid–formalin (83). A permanent stain of fecal films from fresh or preserved material is essential because concentration procedures alone are not reliable diagnostic techniques for this infection (53). Permanent staining with hematoxylin (53), trichrome (84), or celestine blue B (85) may be used. Commercial fixatives and stains appear to be superior to traditional ones (86). Although culture techniques are by far the most sensitive method of detecting *D. fragilis,* they are beyond the scope of most laboratories (87).

Treatment

In view of the high prevalence of dientamoebiasis in the community and the apparently low incidence of symptomatic infections, treatment is recommended only for symptomatic persons. Iodoquinol, metronidazole, tetracycline, and paromomycin clear infection in a majority of cases, but efficacy data are lacking. When patients with dientamoebiasis have pruritus ani, a search for or presumptive treatment of enterobiasis is indicated. Because in theory *D. fragilis* is transmitted in pinworm eggs, concomitant treatment of enterobiasis is recommended to prevent recurrence, regardless of whether symptoms of pinworm infection are present.

Screening and the treatment of all infected persons in institutions or day care centers are likely to reduce the prevalence of infection only temporarily (88).

BALANTIDIASIS

Balantidiasis is caused by the protozoan *Balantidium coli.* It is the only ciliate known to parasitize humans. In rare instances, *B. coli* invades the large-bowel mucosa and causes intestinal symptoms.

Microbiology

B. coli is the largest protozoan that infects humans. The rapid, rotary motion of the large (50 to 200 μm), oval trophozoite is accomplished by synchronized beating of its cilia. Its pointed anterior end contains a cytostome. The cyst stage is spherical to oval in shape and measures 50 to 70 μm. Both the trophozoite and cyst stages have a characteristic, easily identifiable macronucleus and a smaller micronucleus that is difficult to discern, even in stained organisms.

Epidemiology

B. coli has a worldwide distribution and frequently inhabits the intestinal tract of insects, fish, and mammals, particularly primates and swine; however, balantidiasis in humans is infrequently reported. Pigs appear to be the major reservoir of human infection in both tropical and temperate regions. Most cases of *B. coli* infection are described in Central America, Papua New Guinea, and Asia, particularly in areas of poor hygiene where swine and humans are in close contact. Incidence rates in swine farmers or slaughterhouse employees may approach 30%. Contact with pigs has been reported in approximately 50% of cases in Papua New Guinea. Human infection is rarer in temperate areas, but epidemics have been described in overcrowded institutions where personal hygiene was poor (89). Transmission occurs by ingestion of the infective cyst stage, which may remain viable for weeks in moist feces or soil. On ingestion, cysts excyst and release trophozoites, which reside in the lumen of the large bowel or invade the colonic mucosa.

Pathogenesis

B. coli trophozoites may invade the colonic mucosa; invasion is in part facilitated by parasite-derived hyaluronidase. They multiply in the submucosa, causing necrosis and ulceration, as in *E. histolytica* infection. Typically, the resulting ulcers are flask-shaped with undermined edges, and they may involve the entire thickness of the colon. Secondary bacterial infection may follow mucosal invasion by the parasite, so that the inflammatory response is increased. Rarely, balantidiasis is complicated by colonic perforation and metastatic spread to the liver, bladder, or vagina.

Clinical Presentation

Balantidiasis represents a spectrum of disease that ranges from the silent carrier state to fulminant dysentery, but most infections are asymptomatic. Symptomatic infection may resemble amebiasis, with symptoms that vary from chronic intermittent diarrhea, abdominal pain, and weight loss to fulminant dysentery with discharge of blood and mucus per rectum, colonic tenderness, and fever. The dysenteric presentation is occasionally complicated by colonic hemorrhage and perforation. Rarely, extraintestinal spread to liver, lungs, lymph nodes, and appendix has been reported (90,91). Eosinophilia is not a feature of infection.

Diagnosis

Unlike the diagnosis of other intestinal protozoan infections, that of balantidiasis depends on the identification of trophozoites (50 to 200 μm by 40 to 70 μm) in stool samples, biopsy specimens, or resected material. Cysts, which measure from 50 to 70 μm, are rarely identified in feces. In direct wet preparations, viable trophozoites show a rapid rotary motion. The large size of this parasite makes identification possible by low-power microscopy. Both unstained and stained fecal preparations frequently demonstrate the characteristic kidney bean-shaped macronucleus and prominent cytostome of the trophozoite (Figs. 65.8 and 65.9).

Treatment

Tetracycline (500 mg four times daily for 10 days) is the treatment of choice for balantidiasis. Alternatives include iodoquinol (650 mg three times daily for 20 days), metronidazole (750 mg three times daily for 5 days), or paromomycin (30 mg/kg per day for 7 days).

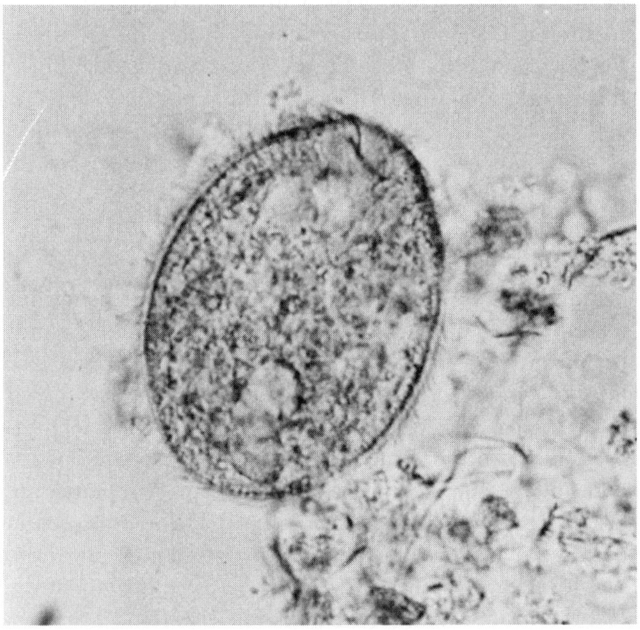

FIGURE 65.8. *Balantidium coli* trophozoite in stool. These organisms can be recognized by their large size, ciliated surface, prominent cytosome, and large, kidney bean-shaped macronucleus. Formalin-preserved wet mount. (From Ash LR, Orihel TC. *Atlas of human parasitology,* third edition. Chicago: American Society of Clinical Pathologists, 1990, with permission.)

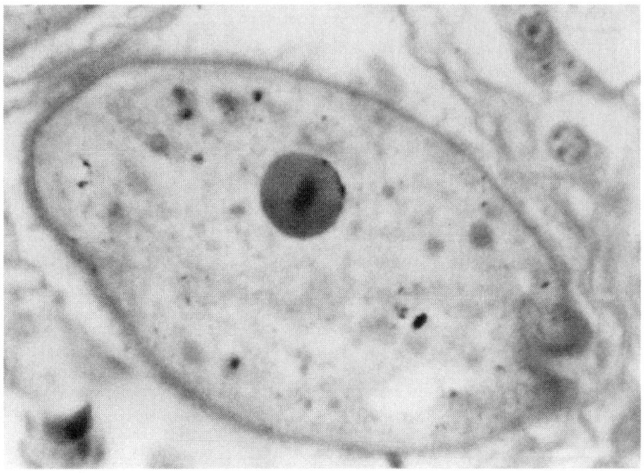

FIGURE 65.9. Colonic biopsy specimen with trophozoite of *Balantidium coli.* Trichrome stain shows the prominent cytosome and usual kidney bean-shaped macronucleus, which has been bisected in this tissue section. (Courtesy of Dr. Jim Yang.)

B. HOMINIS INFECTION

Blastocystis hominis, initially described by Alexieff in 1911, is a common inhabitant of the human gastrointestinal tract. It was named in 1912 by Brumpt (92), who considered it to be a yeast. At present, *B. hominis* is an organism of uncertain taxonomic classification. Zierdt (93) recently classified *B. hominis* as a protozoan and placed it in the suborder Blastocystina, order Amoebida, pending confirmation at a molecular level (93,94). The role of *B. hominis* as a human pathogen is controversial and at present unresolved (95).

Microbiology

B. hominis is a strict anaerobic protozoan of variable size (5 to 40 μm) that resides primarily in the cecum and large bowel. It lacks a cell wall, divides by binary fission, and has three morphologic forms: vacuolated, ameba-like, and granular (94). The vacuolated form, characterized by a large membrane-bound central body, is most commonly identified in human fecal samples (Fig. 65.10). The cyst stage has now been shown in an animal model to represent the infective stage of the parasite. (96–98). Restriction site analysis of ribosomal DNA amplified by polymerase chain reaction (PCR) and isoenzyme analysis studies show that *B. hominis* is highly polymorphic, and that no correlation exists between isoenzyme patterns, DNA subgroups, and disease in infected humans (99).

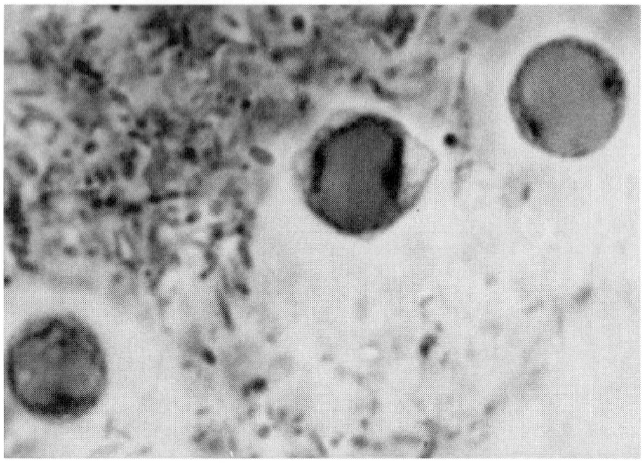

FIGURE 65.10. *Blastocystis hominis.* Direct smear of stool sample from patient infected with *B. hominis* showing the typical vacuolated form of this parasite. Iron hematoxylin stain; ×750.

Epidemiology

B. hominis has a worldwide distribution, but some evidence suggests that it may be more common in the tropics and subtropics. Prevalence rates range from 3% to 20% in samples submitted to microbiology laboratories to 52% in male homosexuals. Recent studies have not demonstrated a significant difference in the prevalence of infection between symptomatic and asymptomatic persons, even when they are infected with HIV (101–104). The mode of transmission of *B. hominis* has not been determined but is presumed to be fecal–oral because of the association of infection with the consumption of untreated water and travel to the tropics (105–107). Rare outbreaks of blastocystosis have been reported (108,109). Also, infection appears to be widely distributed in the animal kingdom and has been reported in pigs, monkeys, reptiles, poultry, and rodents (93). However, it is not known whether animals are significant reservoirs of human infection.

Pathogenesis

Pathogenic mechanisms for *B. hominis* have not been identified. Attempts to infect gnotobiotic guinea pigs did not provide convincing evidence of pathogenicity unless large numbers of organisms were inoculated together with enteric flora. Symptomatic infection and superficial invasion of the cecal mucosa developed in 22% of these germ-free guinea pigs (110). Isolates of *B. hominis* from both asymptomatic and symptomatic patients caused significant and cytopathic effects on monolayers of Chinese hamster ovary cells (111). Properly controlled prospective studies of the pathogenicity of *B. hominis* in humans have not been performed.

Clinical Presentation

Infections with *B. hominis* were increasingly reported in the 1980s and 1990s in both immunocompromised and immunologically intact hosts. In the absence of other identified microorganisms, several authors consider *B. hominis* to be a possible pathogen (93,94,112,113). Symptoms attributed to infection include diarrhea, abdominal pain, flatus, nausea, vomiting, anorexia, and malaise. However, virtually all the studies that have evaluated the clinical significance of blastocystosis have been retrospective case series from which a definitive answer is not forthcoming. Two prospective case–control studies assessing the role of *B. hominis* as a possible intestinal pathogen in travelers gave opposite results (114,115). Earlier reports of a correlation between gastrointestinal symptoms and the number of *B. hominis* organisms identified in stool samples have not been confirmed by more recent studies (101,102,106). Peripheral eosinophilia has been reported in some cases; however, alternative causes of eosinophilia were often not excluded. Fecal leukocytes are rarely observed with *B. hominis* infection. The results of endoscopic, histopathologic, and radiologic studies of infected patients are usually normal (106,109).

Diagnosis

The diagnosis of blastocystosis is made by demonstrating the organism in unstained or permanently stained stool smears (Fig. 65.10). The vacuolated form is most often identified and stains well with iron hematoxylin or trichrome. Concentration techniques may result in lysis of the organism. Heavy infections may obscure the identification of other intestinal protozoa in stool (116).

Treatment

Controlled prospective treatment trials for *B. hominis* have not been performed. No antimicrobial agents have been demonstrated to eradicate *B. hominis* infection reliably, but metronidazole is frequently prescribed. However, it has not been convincingly shown to alter the natural history of infection. Limited *in vitro* susceptibility testing has shown activity against *B. hominis* by emetine, metronidazole, furazolidone, co-trimoxazole, quinacrine, and pentamidine (in order of efficacy) (117). Ketoconazole and iodoquinol are less active *in vitro* than metronidazole (118). Some reports indicate that iodoquinol and co-trimoxazole may have activity (105,119,120). *In vitro* studies have shown that the cyst form is resistant to metronidazole (122).

In summary, *B. hominis* is a frequently recognized colonic protozoan of uncertain pathogenic potential. Clarification of its role in human disease will require properly controlled prospective studies of pathogenicity and specific therapy. At present, little evidence is available to support the routine use of antimicrobial therapy for blastocystosis.

NONPATHOGENIC INTESTINAL PROTOZOA

Nonpathogenic amebae and flagellates are frequently found on stool examination (Figs. 65.1 and 65.2) and must be differentiated from potentially pathogenic protozoa. They are usually distinguished from known pathogens, such as *E. histolytica,* on the basis of (a) the number of nuclei and nuclear detail (best seen with permanent stains, such as iron hematoxylin); (b) the size and shape of cysts and trophozoites; (c) the presence of characteristic chromatoidal or inclusion bodies; and (d) the lack of rapid directional motility and erythrocyte ingestion by trophozoites.

The presence of these organisms may imply host consumption of fecally contaminated water or food. However, there is no evidence to suggest that any of these protozoa have pathogenic potential, even in immunocompromised hosts, so that therapy directed at eradicating carriage is not indicated. A recent study showed that costs could be reduced considerably if nonpathogenic protozoa were not reported by clinical laboratories or were reported with a qualifier, such as "not medically significant" (125). When nonpathogenic amebae are identified in symptomatic persons, further investigation should be undertaken to search for recognized pathogens.

Amebae

Entamoeba hartmanni

E. hartmanni is found worldwide and was once considered to be a small race of *E. histolytica.* However, *E. hartmanni* has a unique isoenzyme pattern and is now considered to be a separate species (126). *E. hartmanni* is morphologically similar to *E. histolytica,* but the cysts (<10 μm on wet preparation, <9 μm on permanent stained smear) and trophozoites (<12 μm on wet preparation, <11 μm on permanent stained smear) of *E. hartmanni* are smaller.

Entamoeba coli

E. coli is a common gut protozoan that is also widely distributed. *E. coli* trophozoites and cysts are usually distinguished from those of *E. histolytica* on the basis of nuclear morphology. The *E. coli* nucleus generally has a larger and often eccentric karyosome. In addition, most mature cysts have more than five nuclei and are 15 μm or larger in diameter; in comparison, *E. histolytica* cysts have four or fewer nuclei and are 10 to 15 μm in diameter.

Endolimax nana

E. nana is a small, nonpathogenic ameba that is at least as prevalent as *E. coli.* The cysts and trophozoites of *E. nana* are smaller than those of *E. histolytica* and have a nuclear structure characterized by a lack of peripheral chromatin on the nuclear membrane and the presence of a large central or eccentric karyosome.

Iodamoeba bütschlii

This nonpathogenic ameba is less commonly encountered than *E. coli* or *E. nana.* The cysts of *I. bütschlii* are characterized by a large glycogen vacuole that stains with iodine on a wet preparation. The trophozoites have vacuolated cytoplasm.

Flagellates

Chilomastix mesnili is the most common nonpathogenic flagellate observed in fecal specimens. It is differentiated from *Giardia duodenalis* by its lemon-shaped cysts and the presence of a single nucleus. Other nonpathogenic flagellates, such as *Enteromonas hominis, Retortamonas intestinalis,* and *Pentatrichomonas hominis,* are rarely encountered.

REFERENCES

1. Senay H, MacPherson D. Parasitology: diagnostic yield of stool examination. *Can Med Assoc J* 1989;140:1329–1331.
2. Strickland GI, ed. *Hunter's tropical medicine,* seventh edition. Philadelphia: WB Saunders, 1991.
3. Wenyon CM. Coccidiosis of cats and dogs and the status of the *Isospora* of man. *Ann Trop Med Parasitol* 1923;17:231–239.
4. Godiwala T, Yaeger R. *Isospora* and traveler's diarrhea. *Ann Intern Med* 1987;106:909–910.
5. Shaffer N, Moore L. Chronic traveler's diarrhea in a normal host due to *Isospora belli. J Infect Dis* 1989;159:596–597.
6. Brandborg LL, Goldberg SB, Breidenbach WC. Human coccidiosis—a possible cause of malabsorption. *N Engl J Med* 1970;283:1306–1313.
7. Trier JS, Moxey PC, Schimmel EM, et al. Chronic intestinal coccidiosis in men: intestinal morphology and response to treatment. *Gastroenterology* 1974;66:923–935.
8. Lindsay DS, Dubey JP, Blagburn BL. Biology of *Isospora* spp. from humans, nonhuman primates, and domestic animals. *Clin Microbiol Rev* 1997;10:19–34.
9. Faust EC, Giraldo LE, Caicedo G, et al. Human isosporiasis in the Western Hemisphere. *Am J Trop Med Hyg* 1961;10:343–349.
10. Soave R, Johnson WD Jr. *Cryptosporidium* and *Isospora belli* infections. *J Infect Dis* 1988;157:225–229.
11. Kirkpatrick CE. Animal reservoirs of *Cryptosporidium* spp. and *Isospora belli. J Infect Dis* 1988;158:909–910.
12. Current WL. Human enteric coccidia. II. *Isospora belli* and *Sarcocystis* spp. *Clin Microbiol Newslett* 1985;7:175–182.
13. DeHovitz JA, Pape JW, Boncy M, et al. Clinical manifestations and therapy of *Isospora belli* infection in patients with the

acquired immunodeficiency syndrome. *N Engl J Med* 1986; 315:87–90.

14. Forthal DN, Guest SS. *Isospora belli* enteritis in three homosexual men. *Am J Trop Med Hyg* 1984;33:1060–1064.
15. Jeffery GM. Epidemiologic considerations of isosporiasis in a school for mental defectives. *Am J Hyg* 1958;67:251–255.
16. Current WL, Reese NC, Ernst JV, et al. Human cryptosporidiosis in immunocompetent and immunodeficient persons: studies of an outbreak and experimental transmission. *N Engl J Med* 1983;308:1252–1257.
17. Restrepo C, Macher AM, Radany EH. Disseminated extraintestinal isosporiasis in a patient with acquired immune deficiency syndrome. *Am J Clin Pathol* 1987;87:536–542.
18. Michels JF, Hafman P, Bernard E, et al. Intestinal and extraintestinal *Isospora belli* infection in an AIDS patient. A second case report. *Pathol Res Pract* 1994;190:1089–1093.
19. Benator DA, French AL, Beaudet LM, et al. *Isospora belli* infection associated with acalculous cholecystitis in a patient with AIDS. *Ann Intern Med* 1994;121:663–664.
20. Ng E, Markell EK, Fleming RI, et al. Demonstration of *Isospora belli* by acid-fast stain in a patient with acquired immune deficiency syndrome. *J Clin Microbiol* 1984;20:384–386.
21. Pape JW, Verdier RI, Johnson WD Jr. Treatment and prophylaxis of *Isospora belli* infection in patients with the acquired immunodeficiency syndrome. *N Engl J Med* 1989;320: 1044–1047.
22. Weiss LM, Perlman DC, Sherman J, et al. *Isospora belli* infection: treatment with pyrimethamine. *Ann Intern Med* 1988; 109:474–475.
23. Verdier R-I, Fitzgerald DW, Johnson JW Jr, et al. Trimethoprim-sulfamethoxazole compared with ciprofloxacin for treatment and prophylaxis of *Isospora belli* and *Cyclospora cayetanensis* infection in HIV-infected patients. A randomized, controlled trial. *Ann Intern Med* 2000;132:885–888.
24. Musey KL, Chidiac C, Beaucaire G, et al. Effectiveness of roxithromycin for treating *Isospora belli* infection. *J Infect Dis* 1988; 158:646.
25. Kayembe K, Desmet P, Henry MC, et al. Diclazuril for *Isospora belli* infection in AIDS. *Lancet* 1989;1:1397–1398.
26. Cabello RR, Guerrero LR, Garcia MDRM, et al. Nitazoxanide for the treatment of intestinal protozoan and helminth infections in Mexico. *Trans R Soc Trop Med Hyg* 1997;91:701–703.
27. Kartulis S. Ueber pathogene protozoen bei dem Menschen. I. Gregarinose der Leber und der Bauchmuskeln. II. Amoben bei Knochennekrose (Osteomyelitis) der Unterkiefers. *Z Hyg Infectionskr* 1893;13:1–14.
28. Beaver PC, Gadgill K, Morera P. *Sarcocystis* in man: a review and report of five cases. *Am J Trop Med Hyg* 1979;28:819–844.
29. Ash LR, Orihel TC. *Atlas of human parasitology,* third edition. Chicago: American Society of Clinical Pathologists, 1990.
30. Wong KT, Pathmanathan R. High prevalence of human skeletal muscle sarcocystosis in Southeast Asia. *Trans R Soc Trop Med Hyg* 1992;86:631–632.
31. Kan SP, Pathmanathan R. Review of sarcocystosis in Malaysia. *Southeast Asian J Trop Med Public Health* 1991;22[Suppl]: 129–134.
32. Kimmig P, Piekarski G, Heydorn AO. Sarcosporidiosis (*Sarcocystis suihominis*) in man. *Immunol Infect* 1979;7:170–177.
33. Piekarski G, Heydorn AO, Aryeetey ME, et al. Clinical, parasitological and serological investigations in sarcosporidiosis (*Sarcocystis suihominis*) of man. *Immunol Infect* 1978;6:153–159.
34. Bunyaratvej S, Bunyawongwiroj P, Nitiyanant P. Human intestinal sarcosporidiosis: report of six cases. *Am J Trop Med Hyg* 1982;31:36–41.
35. Giboda M, Ditrich O, Scholz T, et al. Current status of food-borne parasitic zoonoses in Laos. *Southeast Asian J Trop Med Public Health* 1991;22[Suppl]:56–61.
36. Yu S. Field survey of *Sarcocystis* infection in the Tibet autonomous region. *Chung Kuo I Hsueh Ko Hsueh Yuan Hsueh Pao* 1991;13:29–32.
37. Esteban JG, Aguirre C, Angles R, et al. Balantidiasis in Aymara children in the northern Bolivian Altiplano. *Am J Trop Med Hyg* 1998;59:922–927.
38. Khan RA, Fong D. *Sarcocystis* in caribou (*Rangifer tarandus terraenorae*) in Newfoundland. *Southeast Asian J Trop Med Public Health* 1991;22[Suppl]:142–143.
39. Fayer R, Heydorn AO, Johnson AJ. Transmission of *Sarcocystis suihominis* from humans to swine to nonhuman primates. *Z Parasitenkd* 1979;59:15–20.
40. Dubey JP, Fayer R. Sarcocystosis. *Br Vet J* 1983;139:371–377.
41. Sargeaunt PG, Williams JE, Neal RA. A comparative study of *Entamoeba histolytica,* "*E. histolytica*-like" and other morphologically identical amoebae using isoenzyme electrophoresis. *Trans R Soc Trop Med Hyg* 1980;74:469–474.
42. Desowitz RS, Barnish G. *Entamoeba polecki* and other intestinal protozoa in Papua New Guinea highland children. *Ann Trop Med Parasitol* 1986;80:399–402.
43. Jepps MW, Dobell C. *Dientamoeba fragilis,* n.g., n.sp., a new intestinal amoeba from man. *Parasitology* 1918;10:352–367.
44. Windsor JJ, Johnson EH. *Dientamoeba fragilis*: the unflagellated human flagellate. *Br J Biomed Sci* 1999;56:295–306.
45. Dwyer DM. Analysis of the antigenic relationships among *Trichomonas, Histomonas, Dientamoeba* and *Entamoeba.* III. Immunoelectrophoresis techniques. *J Protozool* 1974;21: 139–145.
46. Camp RR, Mattera CFT, Honigberg BM. Study of *Dientamoeba fragilis.* Jepps and Dobell. I. Electron microscopic observations of the binucleate stages. II. Taxonomic position and revision of the genus. *J Protozool* 1974;21:69–82.
47. Silverman JD, Clark CG, Sogin ML. *Dientamoeba fragilis* shares a recent common evolutionary history with trichomonads. *Mol Biochem Parasitol* 1996;76:311–314.
48. Svensson RM. A survey of human intestinal protozoa in Sweden and Finland. *Parasitology* 1928;20:237–249.
49. Wenrich DH, Stabler RM, Arnelt JH. *Entamoeba histolytica* and other intestinal protozoa in 1,060 college freshmen. *Am J Trop Med* 1935;15:331–345.
50. Miller MJ. The intestinal protozoa of man in midwestern Canada. *J Parasitol* 1939;25:355–357.
51. Boe J. The occurrence of human intestinal protozoa in Norway. *Acta Med Scand* 1943;113:321–328.
52. Mackie TT, Larsh JE Jr, Mackie JW. A survey of intestinal parasitic infections in the Dominican Republic. *Am J Trop Med* 1951;31:825–832.
53. Scholten TH, Yang J. Evaluation of unpreserved and preserved stools for the detection and identification of intestinal parasites. *Am J Clin Pathol* 1974;62:563–567.
54. Garcia LS, Brewer TC, Bruckner DA. A comparison of the formalin-ether concentration and trichrome-stained smear methods for the recovery and identification of intestinal protozoa. *Am J Med Technol* 1979;45:932–935.
55. Weiner D, Brooke MM, Witkow A. Investigation of parasitic infections in the central area of Philadelphia. *Am J Trop Med Hyg* 1959;8:625–629.
56. Melvin DM, Brooke MM. Parasitologic surveys on Indian reservations in Montana, South Dakota, New Mexico, Arizona and Wisconsin. *Am J Trop Med Hyg* 1962;11:765–772.
57. Millet VE, Spencer MJ, Chapin MR, et al. Intestinal protozoan infection in a semicommunal group. *Am J Trop Med Hyg* 1983; 32:54–60.
58. Keystone JS, Yang J, Grisdale D, et al. Intestinal parasites in

metropolitan Toronto day-care centres. *Can Med Assoc J* 1984; 131:733–735.
59. Spencer MJ, Millet VE, Garcia LS, et al. Parasitic infections in a pediatric population. *Pediatr Infect Dis* 1983;2:110–113.
60. Naiman HK, Sckla L, Albritton WL. Giardiasis and other intestinal parasitic infections in a Manitoba residential school for the mentally retarded. *Can Med Assoc J* 1980;122:185–188.
61. Chan F, Stewart N, Guan M, et al. Prevalence of Dientamoeba fragilis antibodies in children and recognition of a 39 kDa immunodominant protein antigen of the organism. *Eur J Clin Microbiol Infect Dis* 1996;15:950–954.
62. Keystone JS, Keystone DL, Proctor EM. Intestinal parasitic infections in homosexual men: prevalence, symptoms and factors in transmission. *Can Med Assoc J* 1980;123:512–514.
63. Peters CS, Sable R, Janda WM, et al. Prevalence of enteric parasites in homosexual patients attending an out-patient clinic. *J Clin Microbiol* 1986;24:684–685.
64. Ortega HB, Borchardt KA, Hamilton R, et al. Enteric pathogenic protozoa in homosexual men from San Francisco. *Sex Transm Dis* 1984;11:59–63.
65. Burrows RB, Swerdlow MA. *Enterobius vermicularis* as a probable vector of *Dientamoeba fragilis. Am J Trop Med Hyg* 1956;5: 258–265.
66. Chang SL. Parasitization of the parasite. *JAMA* 1973;223:1510.
67. Yang J, Scholten TH. *Dientamoeba fragilis*: a review with notes on the epidemiology, pathogenicity, mode of transmission and diagnosis. *Am J Trop Med Hyg* 1977;26:16–22.
68. Ockert G. Zur Epidemiologic von *Dientamoeba fragilis* II Mitteilung: Versuch der Ubertragungdee der Art mit Enterobius. *Eur J Hyg Epidemiol Microbiol Immunol* 1972;16:222–225.
69. Wenrich DH. Studies on *Dientamoeba fragilis* (protozoa). IV. Further observations, with an outline of present day knowledge of this species. *J Parasitol* 1944;30:322–338.
70. Knoll EW, Howel KM. Studies on *Dientamoeba fragilis*: its incidence and possible pathogenicity. *Am J Clin Pathol* 1945;15: 178–183.
71. Skein R, Gelb A. Colitis due to *Dientamoeba fragilis. Am J Gastroenterol* 1983;78:634–636.
72. Cuffari C, Oligny L, Seidman EG, et al. *Dientamoeba fragilis* masquerading as allergic colitis. *J Pediatr Gastroenterol Nutr* 1998;26:16–20.
73. Hood M. Diarrhea caused by *Dientamoeba fragilis. J Lab Clin Med* 1940;25:914–918.
74. Hakansoon EG. *Dientamoeba fragilis,* a cause of illness. *Am J Trop Med Hyg* 1936;16:175–183.
75. Yoeli M. A report of intestinal disorders accompanied by large numbers of *Dientamoeba fragilis. J Trop Med Hyg* 1955;58:38–41.
76. Kean BH, Malloch CL. The neglected amoeba: *Dientamoeba fragilis*: a report of 100 "pure" infections. *Am J Dig Dis Nutr Sci* 1966;11:735–746.
77. Spencer MJ, Garcia LS, Chapin MR. *Dientamoeba fragilis*: an intestinal pathogen in children. *Am J Dis Child* 1979;133: 390–393.
78. Spencer MJ, Chapin MR, Garcia LS. *Dientamoeba fragilis*: a gastrointestinal protozoan infection in adults 1982. *Am J Gastroenterol* 1982;77:565–569.
79. Keystone JS, MacPherson D, Navas L. The clinical significance of dientamoebiasis. Presented at the 41st annual meeting of the American Society of Tropical Medicine, Seattle, November 15–19, 1992(abst).
80. Hiatt RA, Markell EK, Ng E. How many stool examinations are necessary to detect pathogenic intestinal protozoa? *Am J Trop Med Hyg* 1995;53:36–39.
81. Goldman M, Brooke MM. Protozoans in stools unpreserved and preserved in PVA fixative. *Public Health Rep* 1953;68: 703–706.
82. Scholten T. An improved technique for the recovery of intestinal protozoa. *J Parasitol* 1972;58:633–634.
83. Yang J, Scholten T. An alternative to Schaudinn's fixative for the recovery and identification of intestinal parasites. *Can J Public Health* 1976;67:138.
84. Alger N. A simple, rapid, precise stain for intestinal protozoa. *Am J Clin Pathol* 1966;45:361–362.
85. Yang J, Scholten T. Celestin blue B stain for intestinal protozoa. *Am J Clin Pathol* 1976;65:715–718.
86. Garcia LS, Shimizu RY. Evaluation of intestinal protozoan morphology in human faecal specimens preserved in EcoFix: comparison of Wheatley's trichrome stain and EcoStain. *J Clin Microbiol* 1998;36:174–176.
87. Robinson GL. The laboratory diagnosis of human parasitic amoeba. *Trans R Soc Trop Med Hyg* 1968;62:285–294.
88. Thacker SB, Kimball AM, Wolfe M, et al. Parasitic control in a residential facility for the mentally retarded: failure of selected isolation procedure. *Am J Public Health* 1981;71:303–305.
89. Walzer PD, Judson FN, Murphy KB, et al. Balantidiasis outbreak in Truk. *Am J Trop Med Hyg* 1973;22:33.
90. Dodd LG. *Balantidium coli* infestation as a cause of acute appendicitis. *J Infect Dis* 1991;163:1392.
91. Dorfman S, Rangel O, Bravo LG. Balantidiasis: report of a fatal case with appendicular and pulmonary involvement. *Trans R Soc Trop Med Hyg* 1984;78:833–834.
92. Brumpt E. *Blastocystis hominis* n. sp. et formes voisines. *Bull Soc Pathol Exot Filiales* 1912;5:725–730.
93. Zierdt CH. *Blastocystis hominis,* a long misunderstood intestinal pathogen. *Parasitol Today* 1988;4:15–17.
94. Zierdt CH. *Blastocystis hominis*—past and future. *Clin Microbiol Rev* 1991;4:61–79.
95. Stenzel DJ, Boreham PFL. *Blastocystis hominis* revisited. *Clin Microbiol Rev* 1996;9:563–584.
96. Stenzel DJ, Boreham PF. A cyst-like stage of *Blastocystis hominis. Int J Parasitol* 1991;21:613–615.
97. Stenzel DJ, Boreham PF, McDougall R. Ultrastructure of *Blastocystis hominis* in human stool samples. *Int J Parasitol* 1991; 21:807–812.
98. Moe KT, Singh M, Howe J, et al. Experimental *Blastocystis hominis* infection in laboratory mice. *Parasitol Res* 1997;83: 319–325.
99. Gericke AS, Buchard GD, Knoblock J, et al. Isoenzyme patterns of Blastocystis hominis patient isolates derived from symptomatic and healthy carriers. *Trop Med Int Health* 1997;2: 245–253.
100. Boreham PF, Upcroft JA, Dunn LA. Protein and DNA evidence for two demes of *Blastocystis hominis* from humans. *Int J Parasitol* 1992;22:49–53.
101. Senay H, MacPherson D. *Blastocystis hominis*: epidemiology and natural history. *J Infect Dis* 1990;162:987–990.
102. Udkow MP, Markell EK. *Blastocystis hominis*: prevalence in asymptomatic versus symptomatic hosts. *J Infect Dis* 1993;168: 242–244.
103. Albrecht H, Stellbrink H-J, Koperski K, et al. *Blastocystis hominis* in human immunodeficiency virus-related diarrhea. *Scand J Gastroenterol* 1995;30:309–314.
104. Storgaard M, Lauren AL, Andersen PL. The occurrence of *Blastocystis hominis* in HIV-infected patients. *AIDS* 1996;10:44–45.
105. Taylor DN, Echeverria P, Blaser MJ, et al. Polymicrobial aetiology of traveller's diarrhoea. *Lancet* 1985;1:381.
106. Kain KC, Noble MA, Freeman HJ, et al. Epidemiology and clinical features associated with *Blastocystis hominis* infection. *Diagn Microbiol Infect Dis* 1987;8:235–244.
107. O'Gorman MA, Orenstein SR, Proujansky R, et al. Prevalence and characteristics of *Blastocystis hominis* infection in children. *Clin Pediatr (Phila)* 1993;32:91–96.

108. Gugliemetti P, Cellesi C, Figura N, et al. Family outbreak of *Blastocystis hominis* associated with gastroenteritis. *Lancet* 1989; 3:1394.
109. *Blastocystis hominis*: a commensal or pathogen? [Editorial]. *Lancet* 1991;337:521–522.
110. Phillips BP, Zierdt CH. *Blastocystis hominis*: pathogenic potential in human patients and gnotobiotes. *Exp Parasitol* 1976;39: 358–364.
111. Walderich B, Bernaver S, Renner M, et al. Cytopathic effects of *Blastocystis hominis* or Chinese hampster ovary (CHO) on adenocarcinoma HT29 cell cultures. *Trop Med Int Health* 1998;3: 385–390.
112. Sheehan DJ, Raucher BC, McKitrick JC. Association of *Blastocystis hominis* with signs and symptoms of human disease. *J Clin Microbiol* 1986;24:548.
113. Giacometti A, Cirioni O, Fiorentini A, et al. Irritable bowel syndrome in patients with *Blastocystis hominis* infection. *Eur J Clin Microbial Infect Dis* 1999;18:436–439.
114. Shlim DR, Hoge CW, Rajah R, et al. Is *Blastocystis hominis* a cause of diarrhea in travelers? A prospective controlled study in Nepal. *Clin Infect Dis* 1995;21:97–101.
115. Jelinek T, Peyerl G, Loscher T, et al. The role of *Blastocystis hominis* as a possible intestinal pathogen in travellers. *J Infect* 1997;35:63–66.
116. Markell EK, Udkow MP. *Blastocystis hominis*: pathogen or fellow traveler? *Am J Trop Med Hyg* 1986;35:1023–1026.
117. Zierdt CH. *In vitro* response of *Blastocystis hominis* to antiprotozoal drugs. *J Protozool* 1983;30:332–334.
118. Dunn LA, Boreham PF. The *in vitro* activity of drugs against *Blastocystis hominis. J Antimicrob Chemother* 1991;27:507–516.
119. Grossman I, Weiss LM, Simon D, et al. *Blastocystis hominis* in hospital employees. *Am J Gastroenterol* 1992;87:729–732.
120. Schwartz E, Houston R. Effect of co-trimoxazole on stool recovery of *Blastocystis hominis. Lancet* 1992;339:428.
121. Ulgen Z, Girginkardesler N, Balcioglu C, et al. Effect of trimethoprim-sulfamethoxazole in *Blastocystis hominis* infection. *Am J Gastroenterol* 1999;94:3245–3247.
122. Zaman V, Zaki M. Resistance of *Blastocystis hominis* cysts to metronidazole. *Trop Med Int Health* 1996;1:677–678.
123. Lee MB, Kain KC, Keystone JS. Cost implications of reporting nonpathogenic protozoa. *Clin Infect Dis* 2000;30:401–402.
124. Sargeaunt PG, Williams JE. Electrophoretic isoenzyme patterns of pathogenic and nonpathogenic intestinal amoebae of man. *Trans R Soc Trop Med Hyg* 1979;73:225–227.

66

CESTODES

MICHAEL CAPPELLO
MICHELE BARRY

Cestodes (class Cestoidea in the phylum Platyhelminthes), parasitic tapeworms of the gastrointestinal tract, have been known to cause disease in humans since the time of Aristotle (1). Tapeworms of mammals have a flat, segmented body consisting of a head or scolex and a series of segments (proglottids); they do not possess a true body cavity (2–5). The adult tapeworm grows in an anterior to posterior direction by a process called *strobilation,* or formation of new proglottids, in which the most posterior proglottids become mature and then gravid. Tapeworms can range in length from 25 to 35 mm (*Hymenolepis nana*) to 25 to 30 m (*Taenia saginata*) and are primarily parasites of vertebrates. Cestodes lack a true digestive tract and absorb all nutrient molecules from the host through a surface membrane, a syncytial surface layer with minute projections that usually abuts the host's intestinal villi. Tapeworms are hermaphroditic, with proglottids that contain both an ovary and testes. All but one human cestode (*H. nana*) must pass through one or more intermediate hosts before it can develop in the definitive host.

Of the four main groups of cestodes, only two are important parasites of humans: the order Pseudophyllidea, in which the parasites have a scolex containing two sucking grooves (e.g., *Diphyllobothrium latum*), and the order Cyclophyllidea, in which the parasites have a scolex with four suckers (e.g., *T. saginata, Taenia solium, Echinococcus* species, H. nana, Hymenolepis diminuta, Mesocestoides species, and *Dipylidium caninum*) (2–5). Humans are the only definitive host for two cestode species (*T. saginata* and *T. solium*) but are accidentally involved in the life cycles of others. Clinical manifestations of cestode infection are attributable to the adult or larval stages, although only the adult stage of some parasite species is found in humans. This chapter describes adult cestode infections of the human gastrointestinal tract, excluding those caused by *Echinococcus* species.

M. Cappello: Division of Infectious Diseases, Departments of Pediatrics and Epidemiology and Public Health, Yale University School of Medicine, New Haven, Connecticut

M. Barry: Department of Medicine and Public Health, Yale University School of Medicine; and Department of International Heath, Yale–New Haven Hospital, New Haven, Connecticut

T. SAGINATA

Epidemiology

T. saginata, the beef tapeworm, is highly endemic in Latin America and Africa; its prevalence is moderate in Europe, South Asia, and Japan and low in Australia, Canada, and the United States (2,3). In areas where infection is highly endemic (e.g., among certain indigenous populations of sub-Saharan Africa), the prevalence may exceed 90% (6). Populations at greatest epidemiologic risk for infection include those that rely on raising cattle in areas where exposure to human excreta occurs commonly.

Life Cycle

Humans are definitive hosts for the adult *T. saginata* tapeworm, which may survive within the intestine for up to 25 years. Infection is acquired by eating undercooked beef ("measly beef") that contains living larval forms of *T. saginata* within cysts (cysticerci) (Fig. 66.1). Once in the small intestine, the larva is released from its cyst and attaches to the surface with the aid of four suckers located on the anterior scolex. The parasite then grows distally by segment differentiation (proglottid formation), ultimately reaching lengths of 10 to 25 m (Fig. 66.2). On reaching adulthood, the worm sheds 6 to 10 distal proglottids daily, each containing up to 80,000 eggs. These segments can actively migrate through the large intestine and rectum and pass out through the anus. Rarely, some of the eggs may burst from the segments, but typically *T. saginata* proglottids are passed intact in the feces or migrate via independent muscular activity. After eggs or proglottids are ingested by the intermediate host (cattle), the hexacanth embryos emerge from the eggs, invade the intestinal mucosa, and disseminate via

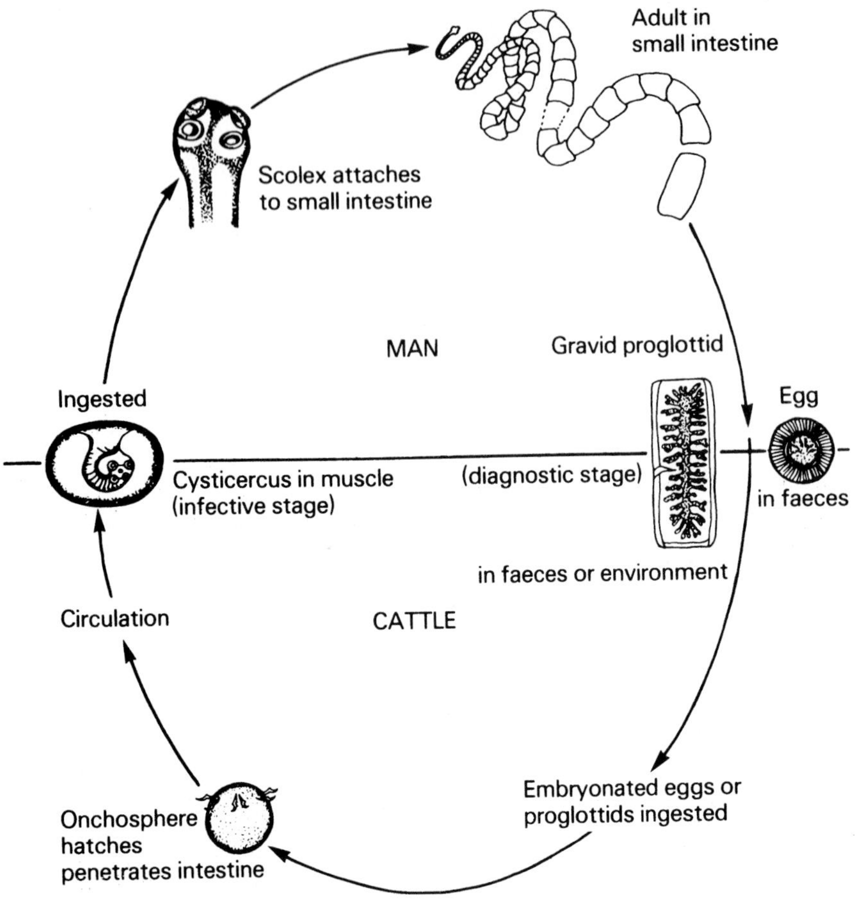

FIGURE 66.1. Life cycle of *Taenia saginata.* (From Zaman V. *Atlas of Medical parasitology,* second edition. Australia: ADIS Health Science Press, 1984, with permission.)

the bloodstream or lymphatics to subcutaneous tissues, where they form viable cysticerci. The life cycle resumes when a definitive host (human) eats undercooked beef containing larval cysts. Importantly, *T. saginata* eggs do not develop into cysticerci in humans, nor do they disseminate. It is primarily by eating contaminated beef infected with cysticerci that humans acquire the adult *T. saginata* tapeworm.

Clinical Manifestations

The incubation period from the time of infection to the passage of segments is 10 to 12 weeks. The majority of patients infected with *T. saginata* are usually infected with a single tapeworm (Fig. 66.2). Most are asymptomatic unless they become aware of tapeworm segments passing in feces (6–8). However, mild intermittent gastrointestinal symptoms, such as nausea, postprandial fullness, and vague epigastric pain, have been associated with *T. saginata* infection. Vomiting, diarrhea, and intestinal obstruction have also been described. Occasionally, proglottids emerge from the anus and migrate actively down the thigh, resulting in pruritus. However, in a survey in Kenya, Hall et al. (6) noted that unless proglottids are actively crawling out of the anal sphincter, most tapeworm proglottids are excreted asymptomatically. Kaminsky (8), in a study of rural populations in Honduras, noted that more than half of all infections are asymptomatic. Rarely, proglottid segments can be vomited or migrate aberrantly, ultimately leading to appendicitis, cholecystitis, or even colonic perforation (9,10) (Fig. 66.3). Usually, no malabsorption or weight loss is associated with *T. saginata* infection. Moderate eosinophilia may be present.

Diagnostic Tests

Definitive diagnosis depends on the identification of proglottids from an infected person. Specimens should be collected in water or saline solution (6,11,12) (Fig. 66.4). To distinguish *T. saginata* from *T. solium,* proglottids can be pressed gently between two microscope slides and then injected with India ink through the lateral pore to count uterine branches. *T. saginata* has 15 or more primary uterine branches on each side of the central core, whereas *T. solium* usually has fewer than 13 uterine branches per side (3). Gravid proglottids can also be fixed in 10% formalin for permanent carmine staining. Staining with hematoxylin and eosin has also been reported to be effective for speciation (13,14). Eggs from both species are indistinguishable by light microscopy and are only intermittently detected by

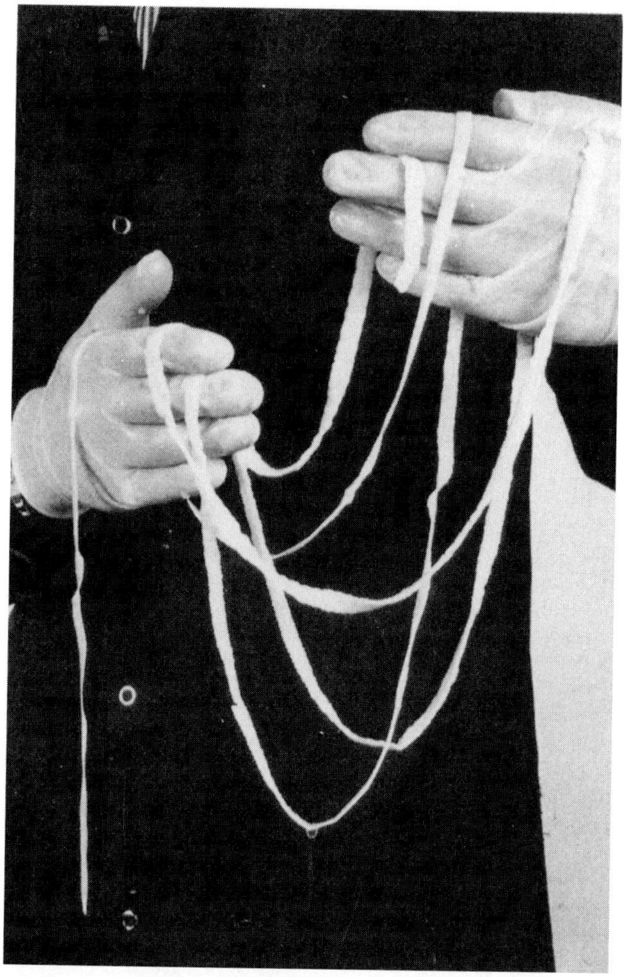

FIGURE 66.2. Adult *Taenia saginata* tapeworm. (From Manson-Bahr PEC, Bell DR. Tapeworms (cestoids). In: *Manson's tropical diseases.* London: Bailliere Tindall, 1987:521–557, with permission.)

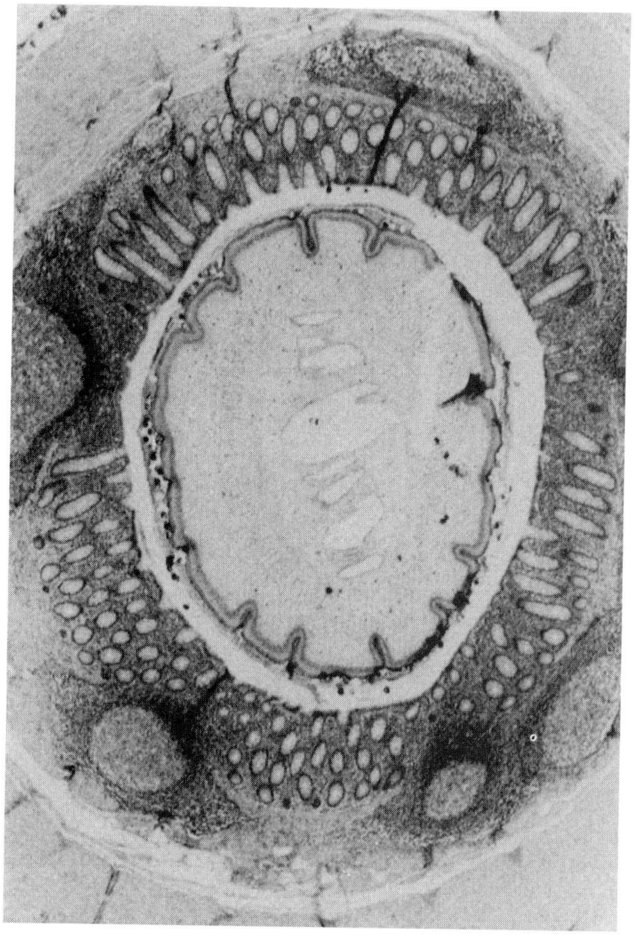

FIGURE 66.3. Low-power view of appendix with a cross-section of *Taenia saginata* proglottid filling the lumen. (From Gutierrez Y. Introduction to cestodes. In: *Diagnostic pathology of parasitic infections with clinical correlations.* Philadelphia: Lea & Febiger, 1990, with permission.)

routine fecal examination (Fig. 66.5). Microscopic examination of adhesive tape applied to perianal skin, as is recommended for the diagnosis of *Enterobius vermicularis* (pinworm) infection, may also be useful.

Coproantigen detection of *Taenia*-specific antigens by enzyme-linked immunosorbent assay (ELISA) is a sensitive diagnostic tool, although cross-reactivity with other *Taenia* species, including *T. solium,* can occur (15,16). At least two molecular techniques that utilize polymerase chain reaction with restriction enzyme analysis have been developed for differentiating between *T. saginata* and *T. solium* (13,17). Whether either of these will ultimately be of use in areas where infection is highly endemic remains to be determined.

Treatment

Anthelmintic drug therapy is extremely effective at eradicating tapeworm infections in adults and children. Praziquantel administered orally in a single dose (5 to 10 mg/kg) is the drug of choice for *T. saginata* infections (18,19). Niclosamide, which until recently has been commonly prescribed for the treatment of tapeworm infections, is no longer available in the United States. Paromomycin produces reasonable cure rates, but common side effects such as diarrhea make it a less attractive option (20,21). Paromomycin does have the advantage of not being absorbed and therefore may be safer in pregnancy. Albendazole, although effective for treating larval cysticercosis caused by *T. solium,* has variable activity against the adult intestinal stage of the tapeworm parasite and is therefore not routinely recommended (8,22).

The passage of intact or disintegrating segments containing eggs may continue for days after treatment. A second stool examination for proglottids or eggs should be performed 3 months following anthelmintic therapy (regeneration period for the scolex) to ensure that cure has been accomplished. Reinfection is common in areas where

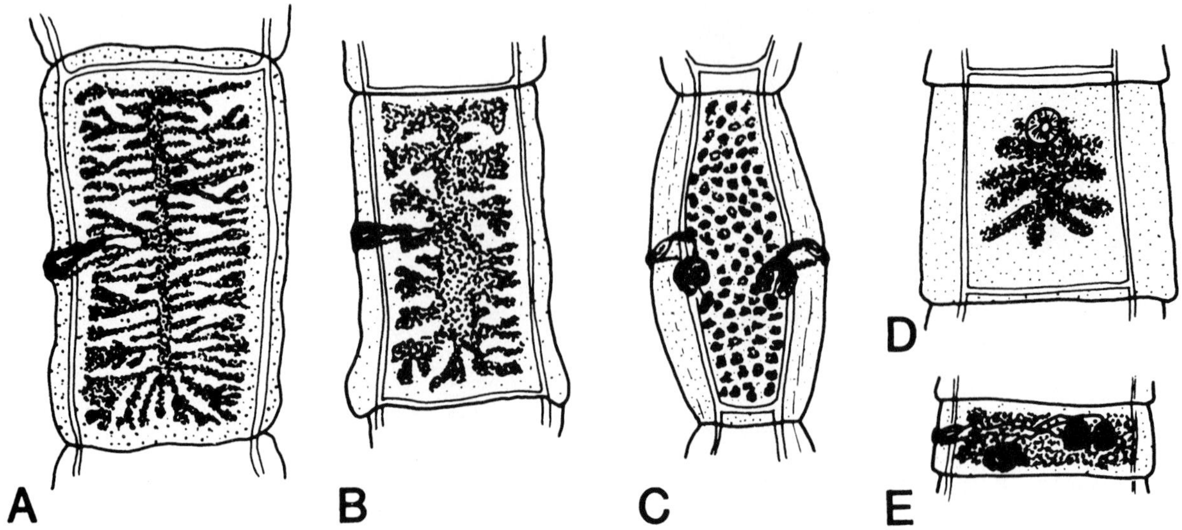

FIGURE 66.4. Schematic representation (not at scale) of gravid proglottids of some common intestinal tapeworms of humans. **A:** *Taenia saginata* (12 or more uterine branches). **B:** *Taenia solium* (10 or fewer uterine branches). **C:** *Dipylidium caninum.* **D:** *Diphyllobothrium.* **E:** *Hymenolepis.* (From Smith JW, Gutierrez Y. Medical parasitology. In: Henry JB, ed. *Todd, Sanford, and Davidsohn's clinical diagnosis and management by laboratory methods,* seventeenth edition. Philadelphia: WB Saunders, 1984, with permission.)

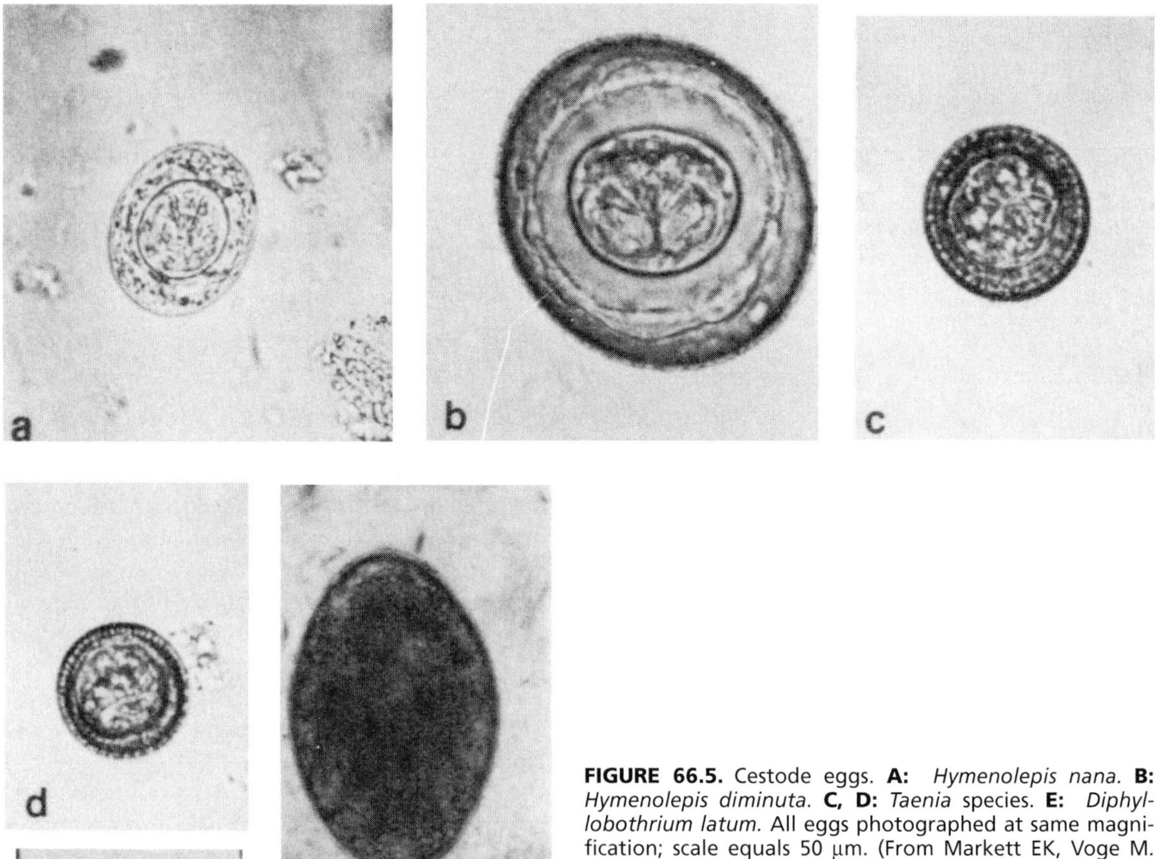

FIGURE 66.5. Cestode eggs. **A:** *Hymenolepis nana.* **B:** *Hymenolepis diminuta.* **C, D:** *Taenia* species. **E:** *Diphyllobothrium latum.* All eggs photographed at same magnification; scale equals 50 μm. (From Markett EK, Voge M. *Medical parasitology,* fifth edition. Philadelphia: WB Saunders, 1981, with permission.)

the disease is highly endemic, so that repeated courses of therapy may be necessary for long-term control.

Prevention and Control

Thorough cooking of meat is a key individual measure for the prevention of infection with *T. saginata.* However, because sociocultural factors, such as the consumption of raw meat in local ceremonial practices or as a traditional treatment for anemia, play a role in *T. saginata* infection, culturally sensitive educational control programs are important. Public health measures such as sanitary disposal of human feces and restriction of cattle from land contaminated by human feces may also prevent transmission. Although freezing beef at −20°C for 5 days kills cysticerci, this is often not practical in areas of endemicity.

T. SOLIUM

Epidemiology

T. solium, the pork tapeworm, is a major cause of morbidity in developing countries. Unlike *T. saginata,* T. solium is capable of causing disease in humans in both its adult and larval stages. Intestinal adult tapeworm infection (taeniasis) is acquired by eating undercooked pork containing cysticerci, whereas ingestion of *T. solium* eggs leads to tissue dissemination of larvae and cyst formation (cysticercosis). Neurocysticercosis, or infection of the central nervous system with *T. solium,* is the leading cause of seizures in areas of endemicity, particularly Latin America and India (23). Importantly, adult tapeworm carriers are the primary source of transmission of the larval stages in humans (23,24).

T. solium has a worldwide geographic distribution, occurring most frequently in rural communities where raising pigs is a common practice. Areas where infection is highly endemic include Central and South America, Mexico, Southeast Asia, the Philippines, Micronesia, Africa, India, and eastern Europe. Transmission of *T. solium* has been described in the United States, although the majority of these locally acquired cases involve infection with the larval stages (cysticercosis), not intestinal taeniasis (25).

Life Cycle

Intestinal infection with *T. solium,* like that with *T. saginata,* follows the ingestion of undercooked pork containing cysticerci (Fig. 66.6). After degradation of the cyst wall, the scolex attaches to the duodenal mucosa and develops into an

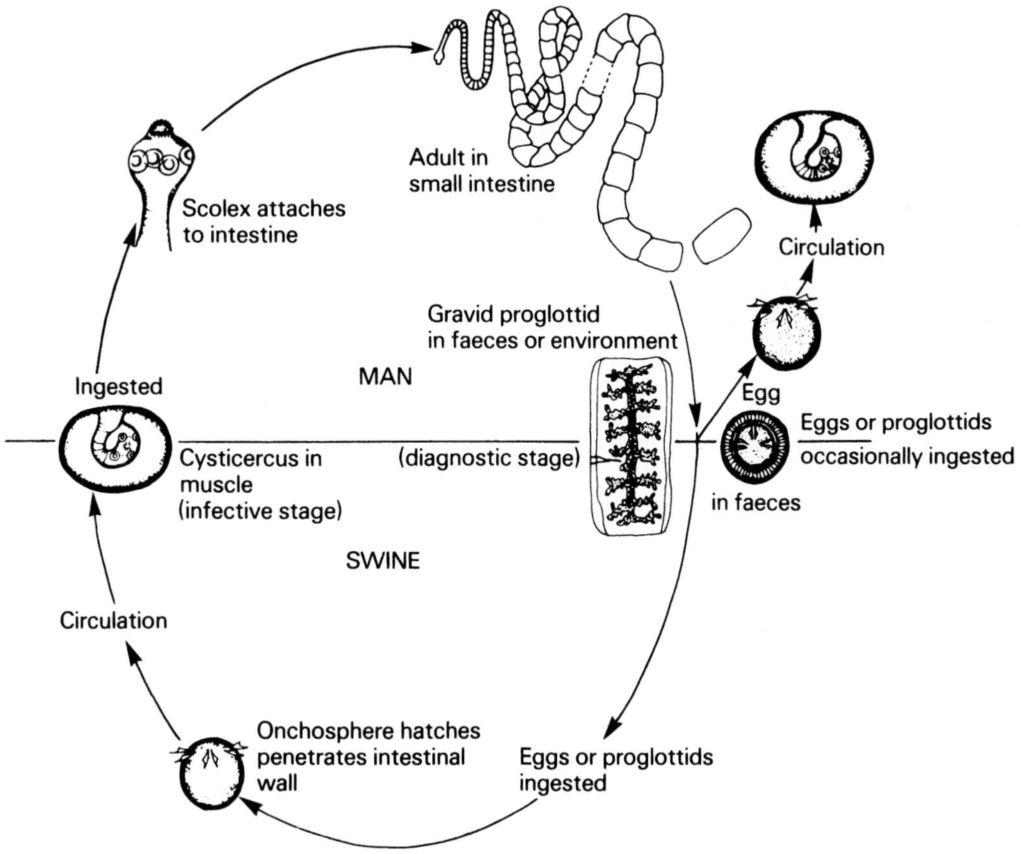

FIGURE 66.6. Life cycle of *Taenia solium.* (From Zaman V. *Atlas of medical parasitology,* second edition. Australia: ADIS Health Science Press, 1984, with permission.)

adult worm in 6 to 8 weeks. The adult tapeworm sheds fewer than 10 proglottids per day, each containing 50,000 to 100,000 eggs. Unlike those of *T. saginata,* these proglottids are rarely motile and therefore are found mostly in feces. Pigs, the coprophagic intermediate hosts, ingest the eggs contained in human waste. The eggs hatch in the stomach, releasing hexacanth embryos that ultimately penetrate the intestinal wall of the pig. Ultimately, the larval stages migrate via the bloodstream and lymphatics to muscle, subcutaneous tissues, or viscera. Humans complete the *T. solium* life cycle by eating pork containing viable cysticerci.

Cysticercosis, caused by the dissemination of *T. solium* larvae, occurs following the ingestion of tapeworm eggs excreted in human feces. Although transmission via fecal contamination of food or water is the most common means of acquiring cysticercosis, autoinfection within a single tapeworm carrier caused by direct ingestion of excreted eggs is also a potential route. A recent outbreak of neurocysticercosis in an orthodox Jewish community underscores the point that the consumption of pork is not necessary for larval infection with *T. solium* (26). In this outbreak, tapeworm carriers working in the homes of this community were the source of tapeworm dissemination; several cases of neurocysticercosis were documented.

Clinical Manifestations

Intestinal Taeniasis

Persons infected with *T. solium* are frequently asymptomatic, becoming aware of tapeworm infection only after the fecal passage of proglottids. The *T. solium* proglottid segments are less motile than those of *T. saginata,* so that migration onto the perianal skin is less commonly noted. Anal pruritus and urticaria have been described with heavy infections, and eosinophilia may be present in early infection. Intestinal symptoms noted in patients with *T. solium* infection include vague abdominal pain, nausea, anorexia or increased appetite, and diarrhea (2,3). However, the degree to which these symptoms are attributable to tapeworm infection is controversial, as many patients are also infected with other intestinal parasites.

Cysticercosis

In humans, the ingestion of *T. solium* eggs leads to tissue dissemination and the formation of larval cysts. *T. solium* cysticerci can develop in a number of somatic tissues, including skeletal muscle, skin, eye, heart, and, most importantly, the central nervous system. The most common presenting clinical feature of cysticercosis in areas of endemicity is localized seizures, which often result from inflammation in the brain directed at degenerating parenchymal cysts. However, other neurologic sequelae have also been described, including meningitis, encephalopathy, hydrocephalus, and spinal cord involvement (23).

Diagnostic Tests

Adult *T. solium* and *T. saginata* parasites are similar, although certain useful morphologic features allow for differentiation of the two species. Because patients infected with adult *T. solium* are at additional risk for cysticercosis secondary to autoinfection, attempts should be made to discriminate between *T. saginata* and *T. solium* infection. Microscopic examination of proglottid segments is the most reliable means of differentiating between the two species of adult tapeworm (Fig. 66.4). A gravid proglottid of *T. solium* should have fewer than 13 lateral branches on each side of the uterine stem. Unlike the scolex of *T. saginata,* that of *T. solium* possesses two rows of rostellar hooks, which it uses along with four suckers to attach to the mucosa of the small intestine (Fig. 66.7). However, because the scolex is rarely present in fecal samples, the diagnosis of *T. solium* infection is usually made by identifying proglottids or eggs passed in feces. Egg excretion is sporadic because proglottids are usually passed intact. However, eggs can be identified in fecal smears or stool concentrates or by perianal swabs. Because infection with multiple tapeworm species has been noted, thorough analysis of positive stool samples is necessary. It is important to recognize that the eggs of *T. solium* and *T. saginata* cannot be differentiated by microscopic examination.

Coproantigen testing with a capture-type ELISA for *Taenia*-specific fecal antigen is highly sensitive and may be particularly effective in identifying more lightly infected tapeworm carriers than are routine stool examinations (15,27). However, this test may not be useful in distinguishing between *T. solium* and *T. saginata* infection. A recently developed monoclonal antibody has been shown to be highly sensitive and extremely specific for detecting *T. solium* eggs in the feces of infected persons (28). To date, serodiagnostic testing for intestinal taeniasis has not been helpful, although immunologic testing with indirect hemagglutination antibody, ELISA, and specific serologic markers in immunoblot assays has been utilized for the diagnosis of cysticercosis, particularly when it involves the central nervous system (23,29).

Treatment

The treatment of intestinal taeniasis caused by *T. solium* is similar to that recommended for *T. saginata* infection. Praziquantel is the drug of choice, given as a single oral dose of 5 to 10 mg/kg (18). Larger doses of praziquantel may trigger the destruction of occult central nervous system cysts, particularly those in the brain parenchyma, and so lead to seizures (30). In fact, doses as low as 2.5 mg/kg may be effective in treating intestinal tapeworm infections (31). Following treatment, which results in disintegration of the scolex and the destruction of proglottids, anterograde regurgitation of eggs into the stomach, exposing the patient to larval invasion and subsequent cysticercosis, is theoretically possible. For this reason, agents that might induce vomiting should be avoided.

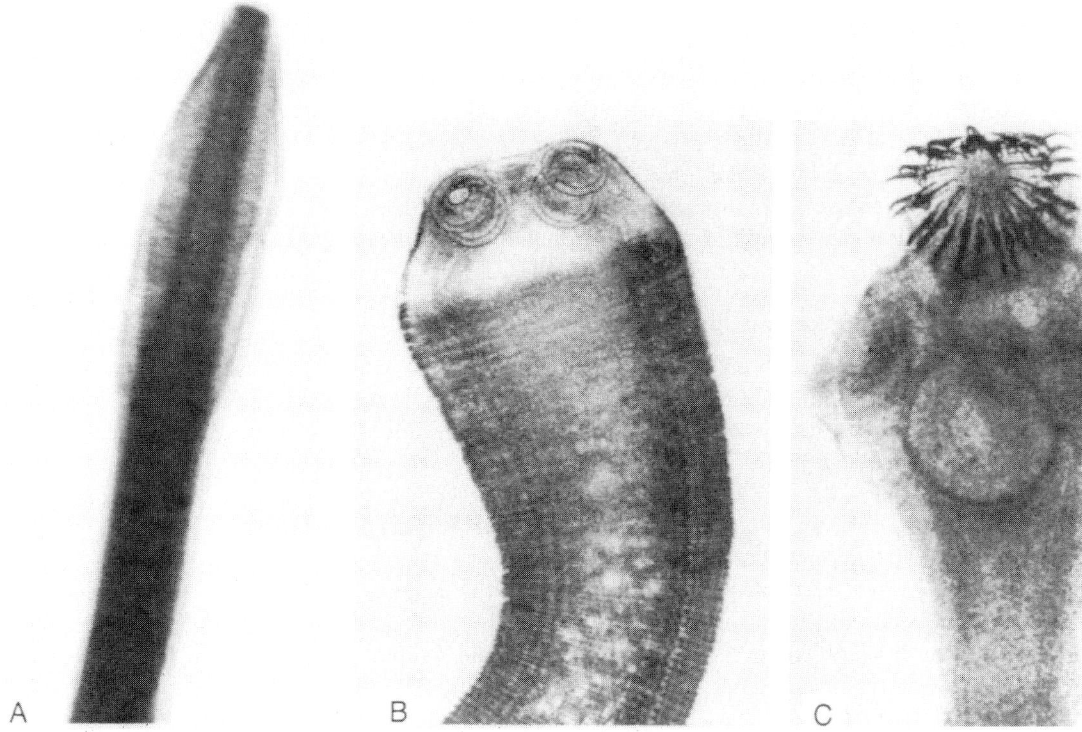

FIGURE 66.7. Scolices of various tapeworms. **A:** *Diphyllobothrium latum.* **B:** *Taenia saginata.* **C:** *Taenia solium.* (From Markett EK, Voge M. *Medical parasitology,* fifth edition. Philadelphia: WB Saunders, 1981, with permission.)

The use of purgatives is of no proven benefit, although it has been suggested that they may reduce the theoretic possibility of autoinfection following proglottid disintegration (32). We do not recommend the use of purgatives. However, it is recommended that a follow-up stool evaluation be performed 3 months after treatment to ensure eradication.

Prevention and Control

T. solium intestinal infection can be totally prevented by protecting pig feed from contamination with human feces. Effective measures to prevent infection include thorough cooking of pork or freezing at −20°C for 12 to 24 hours. Mass chemotherapy programs targeting communities where taeniasis is highly prevalent may reduce transmission from humans to pigs, thereby interrupting the natural life cycle of *T. solium.* In one intervention study, the prevalence of human taeniasis was reduced from 3.5% to 1% within 10 months following niclosamide treatment, and the seroprevalence of *T. solium* infection in pigs was concomitantly reduced from 55% to 7% (33). Such strategies will likely be of long-term benefit only if education succeeds in reducing the behaviors that encourage the proliferation and transmission of the parasite within high-risk communities.

D. LATUM

Epidemiology

Diphyllobothriasis is caused by infection with adult fish tapeworms of the genus *Diphyllobothrium.* The majority of cases are caused by *D. latum,* but other species are capable of infecting humans, including *D. dendriticum, D. pacificum, D. alascence, D. nihonkaiense,* and *D. ursi* (34,35). The disease is most common in northern Europe, including Scandinavia, and Asia, although cases have been reported from most areas of the world (36–42). In North America, diphyllobothriasis has frequently been reported in the Great Lakes region, probably having been introduced to that area by Scandinavian settlers. Native American populations in northern Canada and Alaska also carry these species of tapeworm (40).

The practice of eating raw fish is perhaps the greatest risk factor for acquiring this infection (43,44). As such, the prevalence of diphyllobothriasis tends to be increased in cultures that rely heavily on this tradition. Frequent cases have been reported in women who prepare gefilte fish, a popular Jewish delicacy that is often sampled before cooking to test for proper flavoring. Also, the rising popularity of sushi has increased the risk for *D. latum* infection in the

United States during the past two decades, with reports documenting a potential risk from eating raw, inadequately frozen salmon (41,42). Infection with *D. pacificum* has been reported in Japan following the ingestion of contaminated sushi, whereas a common source of this parasite in Peru is ceviche, a popular dish containing marinated raw fish (3). Overall, however, the incidence of diphyllobothriasis worldwide, even in areas where infection is traditionally highly endemic, has fallen dramatically in recent years.

Life Cycle

D. latum requires at least two intermediate hosts before completing its life cycle in humans (Fig. 66.8). When eggs passed in feces are deposited in freshwater streams or ponds, they must hatch and be eaten by suitable species of copepods. These freshwater crustaceans allow the eggs to develop from ciliated coracidia into procercoid larvae. When a small fish feeds on an infected copepod, the procercoids invade the stomach wall and penetrate the secondary host's musculature. Here, the procercoid matures into a plerocercoid, growing from 500 μm to 5 mm in length within a 4-week period. Humans become infected by eating a fish that harbors a viable plerocercoid larva, which then matures into an adult tapeworm and attaches by its scolex to the wall of the small intestine. Species of fish known to carry *D. latum* include pike, turbot, perch, and salmon. Eggs appear in the stool approximately 3 weeks after infection. The adult *D. latum* parasite can grow at a rate of 5 cm/d and reach a length of more than 20 m. The scolex is rounded, with dorsal and ventral sucking grooves (Fig. 66.6). Each tapeworm can release up to 1 million eggs per day, which must be deposited in suitable fresh water (high oxygen content and a temperature below 22°C) to remain viable. A single parasite can survive many years within its human host. Other mammals, including bears, wolves, foxes, and cats, are capable of serving as definitive hosts to many species of *Diphyllobothrium,* including *D. latum.*

Clinical Manifestations

Despite the large size of this tapeworm, the majority of *D. latum* infections are asymptomatic. In a controlled trial, however, certain symptoms were found to be more common in

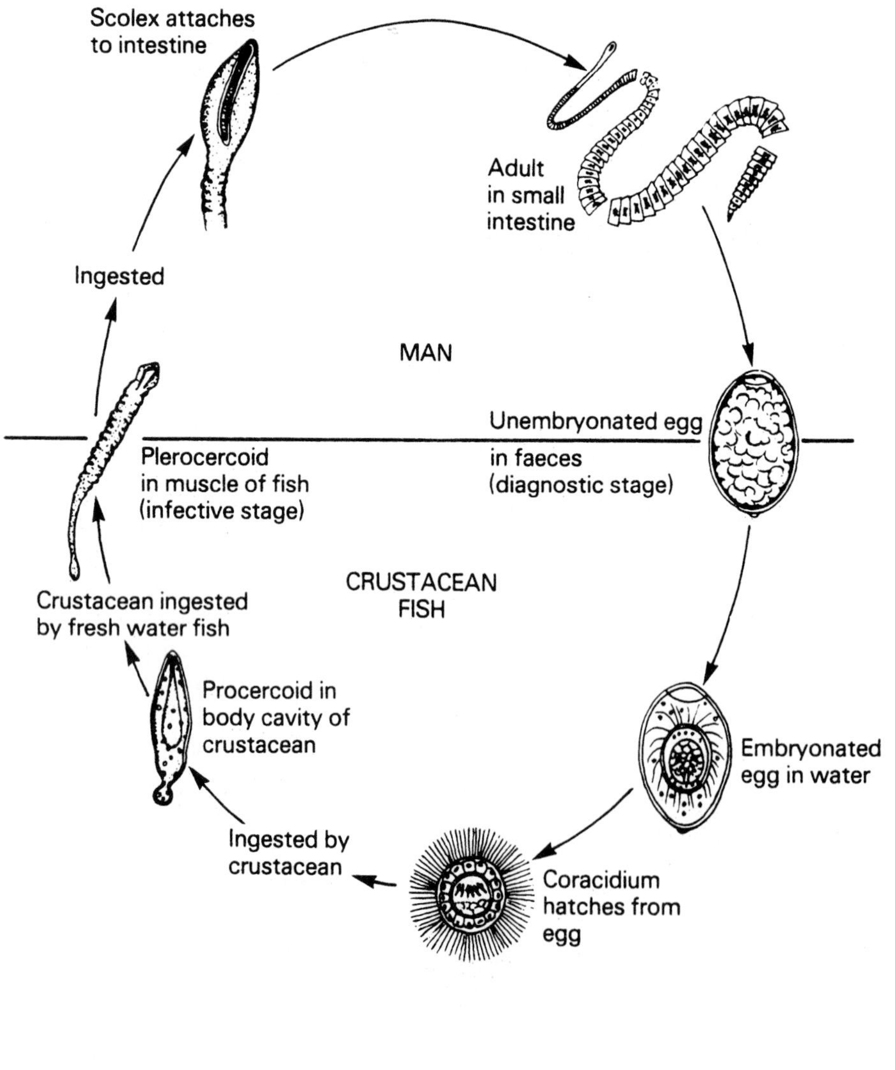

FIGURE 66.8. Life cycle of *Diphyllobothrium latum.* (From Zaman V. *Atlas of medical parasitology,* second edition. Australia: ADIS Health Science Press, 1984, with permission.)

otherwise healthy tapeworm carriers than in uninfected controls, including diarrhea, fatigue, dizziness, distal paresthesias, and a sensation of hunger (45). Abdominal pain, although not a common feature of diphyllobothriasis, can occur in persons with large tapeworm burdens or multiple infections (46). A rare but striking clinical sequela of *D. latum* infection is tapeworm-associated pernicious anemia. This entity is virtually indistinguishable from the idiopathic form, with decreased serum levels of vitamin B_{12}, megaloblastosis, glossitis, and peripheral neuropathy. Although anemia develops in only 2% of persons, subclinical vitamin B_{12} deficiency can be detected in a much higher percentage of non-anemic persons with diphyllobothriasis than in uninfected controls (47–48). It has been demonstrated that the tapeworm actively absorbs free B_{12} from the small intestine, and it also appears capable of dissociating the host intrinsic factor–vitamin B_{12} complex (48).

Diagnostic Tests

The diagnosis of diphyllobothriasis relies on the identification of ova in the stool of an infected person. The eggs measure approximately 60×40 μm and have a characteristic operculum at one pole (Fig. 66.5). The proglottids, which may be passed in the stool or occasionally vomited, can also be used for identification. These segments are wider than long and contain both male and female reproductive organs (Fig. 66.4). An egg-filled uterus leads to a midventral genital pore, through which the ova are expelled into the small intestine. It may be necessary to collect multiple stool samples to detect sporadic egg output. Serum B_{12} levels may be diminished even in the absence of megaloblastic anemia. To date, no serologic test is available to detect infection with *D. latum*. Persons infected with *D. latum* may have a mild leukocytosis and moderate peripheral blood eosinophilia (5% to 10%).

Patients with pernicious anemia or vitamin B_{12} deficiency who have a history of eating raw fish should be examined for fecal excretion of *Diphyllobothrium* eggs. In addition, those who have lived in areas where the infection is highly endemic, particularly Scandinavia or the Great Lakes region of North America, may be at increased risk for the development of this infrequent but treatable complication of diphyllobothriasis.

Treatment

Praziquantel (5 to 10 mg/kg in a single dose) is an effective treatment for diphyllobothriasis (18). Although niclosamide is also effective, this agent is no longer available in the United States. Most of the strobila is usually evacuated quickly, although the scolex itself may not be recovered. A posttreatment purge is not required. Follow-up stool examinations are recommended 6 to 8 weeks following therapy. Tapeworm-associated pernicious anemia generally resolves with eradication of the parasite. However, supplemental vitamin B_{12} therapy is warranted in cases of symptomatic deficiency associated with tapeworm infection.

Prevention and Control

The most reliable means of preventing diphyllobothriasis is to prepare all types of seafood adequately before it is consumed. Fish and hard roe should be thoroughly cooked to ensure that all viable procercoids are killed. Raw fish can be safely eaten only if it has been frozen at −18°C for at least 24 hours, or at −10° degrees for 72 hours (42). As stated, numerous mammalian species appear to be suitable hosts for the development of *D. latum*. Therefore, it is unlikely that preventive measures will succeed in eradicating diphyllobothriasis. However, proper disposal and treatment of sewage should help to reduce the transmission of this tapeworm significantly in areas where infection is endemic.

H. NANA

Epidemiology

H. nana, the dwarf tapeworm, is the cestode that most commonly infects humans, with up to 50 million cases estimated worldwide (2,3). The geographic distribution of *H. nana* is extensive and includes Europe, Africa, Asia, and the Americas. Transmission occurs most commonly via the fecal–oral route, so that high rates of disease spread are generally found in children living in places where sanitary conditions are poor (49–51). In the United States and elsewhere, outbreaks of hymenolepiasis have been reported most frequently in long-term care facilities, where poor hygiene and crowded living conditions likely facilitate transmission of the parasite (52,53).

Life Cycle

H. nana is the only human tapeworm with a life cycle that does not require an intermediate host (Fig. 66.9). When infective eggs are ingested, they hatch in the duodenum, releasing a double-membraned oncosphere. After penetrating the intestinal mucosa, the oncosphere develops into a cysticercoid larva within the lymphatics of the intestinal villi. In 4 to 7 days, the cysticercoid migrates back into the lumen of the small bowel, attaches by its scolex to the intestinal wall, and eventually matures into a gravid adult. Importantly, this life cycle can be repeated within the same host, a phenomenon referred to as *internal autoinfection*. It takes approximately 3 to 4 weeks from the time of infection for eggs to appear in the stool. The adult tapeworm measures approximately 20 to 40 mm in length and up to 1 mm in width. Four suckers are located on its scolex, along with a retractable rostellum that contain approximately 25 hooks. The proglottids are wider than they are long, with

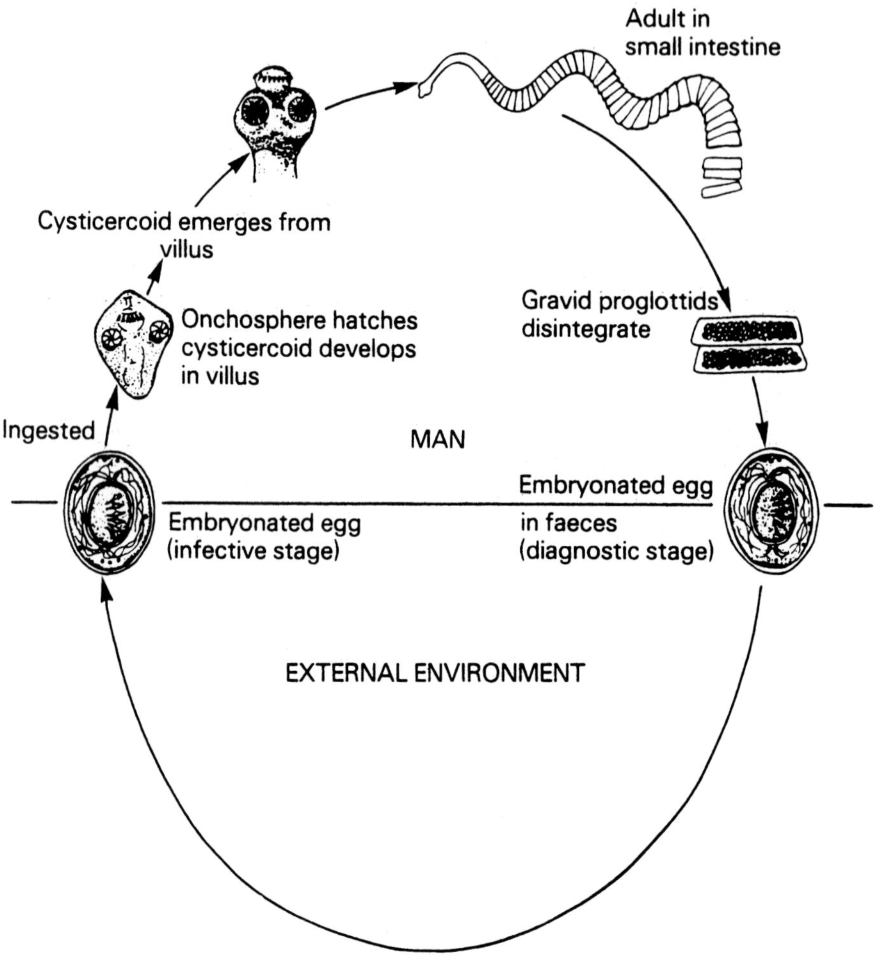

FIGURE 66.9. Life cycle of *Hymenolepis nana.* (From Zaman V. *Atlas of medical parasitology,* second edition. Australia: ADIS Health Science Press, 1984, with permission.)

three testes and one ovary (Fig. 66.4). When gravid, each proglottid may contain up to 200 eggs.

Clinical Manifestations

Although most infections are asymptomatic, heavy infestation with *H. nana* can cause significant intestinal inflammation, particularly in children. Diarrhea, abdominal cramping, pruritus ani, and anorexia are the most frequent gastrointestinal symptoms noted. Systemic illness, characterized by dizziness, irritability, and even generalized seizures, has been associated with hymenolepiasis, although the etiology of these central nervous system sequelae remains unknown. In addition, an association has been noted between intestinal *H. nana* infection and phlyctenular keratoconjunctivitis, an allergic inflammatory condition of the eye, perhaps mediated by a parasite-released toxin (54). Also, in patients with immune suppression caused by an underlying illness or systemic chemotherapy, an overwhelming intestinal worm burden may develop as a result of increased rates of *H. nana* autoinfection in certain compromised hosts. Lastly, disseminated hymenolepiasis, characterized by systemic tissue invasion by larvae, is an infrequent complication of *H. nana* infection (55).

Diagnostic Tests

The diagnosis of *H. nana* infection is made by identifying the characteristic double-membraned eggs in the stool of an infected person (Fig. 66.5). These ova are small, measuring approximately 40 μm in diameter, and samples should be handled carefully during processing to preserve their morphology. Multiple stool examinations with the use of concentrating techniques may be necessary to detect light infections because egg output can be irregular. ELISA has been used to detect antibodies to *H. nana* in the serum of infected patients (56,57). However, the specificity of this test is poor because false-positive results are frequently obtained in persons with cysticercosis or hydatid disease. Therefore, it is not recommended for routine clinical use in the diagnosis of hymenolepiasis. Moderate peripheral blood eosinophilia (5% to 10%) may be the only laboratory abnormality in *H. nana* infection.

Treatment

The drug of choice for *H. nana* infection is praziquantel, given in a single oral dose of 25 mg/kg (18). Cure rates above 98% have been reported with this dose (58,59). Niclosamide, which is no longer available in the United States, is active only against the adult stage of the worm and therefore does not affect larvae encysted in the intestinal villi. A posttreatment purge is not necessary, although stool examinations should be repeated 8 to 12 weeks after therapy to confirm successful elimination of the parasite.

Prevention and Control

Efforts aimed at interrupting the spread of *H. nana* should be directed at preventing fecal–oral contamination in populations at risk for infection, particularly young children. In addition, proper hygienic conditions must be rigidly maintained in long-term care facilities found to harbor this tapeworm.

H. DIMINUTA

Epidemiology

H. diminuta, a tapeworm of rodents, can also cause disease in humans (60–63). The majority of infections occur in children, often in urban settings, and are associated with impoverished living conditions and rodent infestation.

Life Cycle

The life cycle of *H. diminuta* begins with the ingestion of eggs by any one of a number of arthropod species, including fleas, cockroaches, and beetles (Fig. 66.10). The eggs develop into cysticercoid larvae within the intestine of the intermediate host. Most infections in humans develop when an insect harboring *H. diminuta* is inadvertently ingested, usually after having contaminated a source of cereal or grain. The larvae then attach to the mucosa of the small intestine, where they mature into adults. The adult scolex bears four suckers but lacks an armed rostellum. The mature proglottids are similar in appearance to those of *H.*

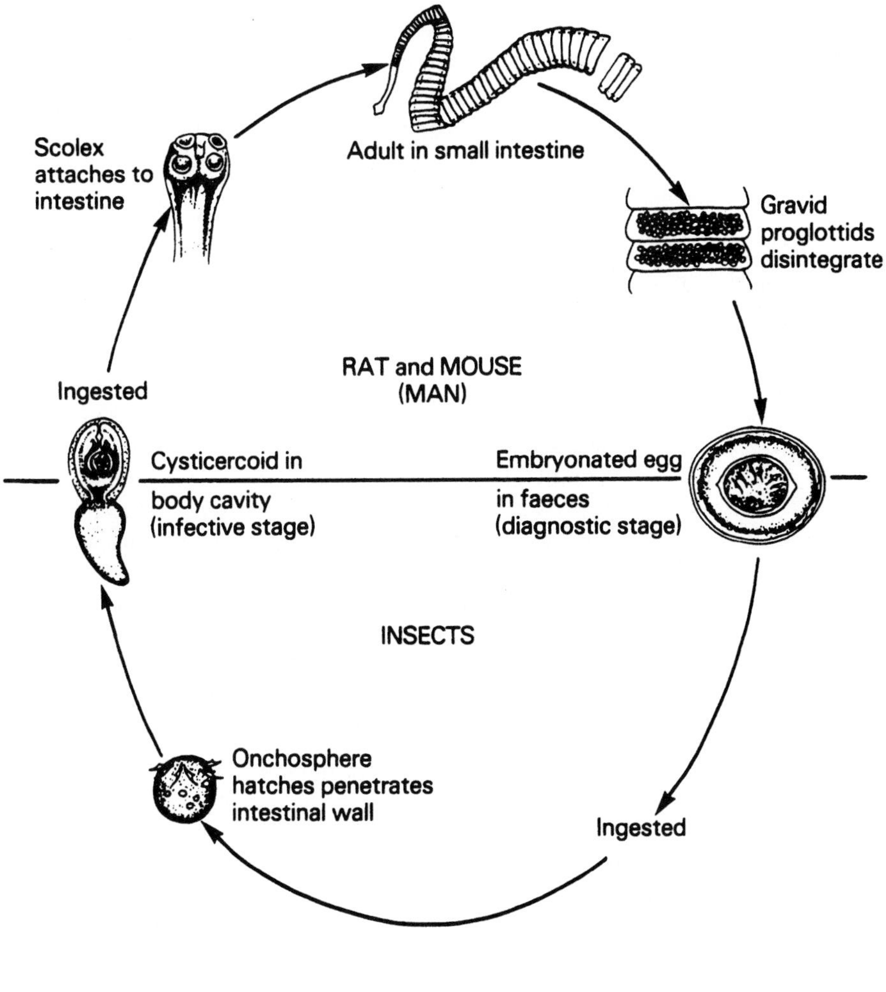

FIGURE 66.10. Life cycle of *Hymenolepis diminuta.* (From Zaman V. *Atlas of medical parasitology,* second edition. Australia: ADIS Health Science Press, 1984, with permission.)

nana. Adult worms can grow to 90 cm in length and up to 4 mm in width. Eggs are deposited in the stool when gravid proglottids are released into the bowel lumen and can generally be detected 2 to 3 weeks after infection.

Clinical Manifestations

The symptoms of *H. diminuta* infection are similar to those associated with *H. nana* infection and include diarrhea, abdominal pain, and anorexia. Most infections, however, appear to be asymptomatic.

Diagnostic Tests

Identification of *H. diminuta* eggs in stool confirms the diagnosis of infection. The characteristic ova measure approximately 60 μm in diameter (nearly twice the size of the ova of *H. nana*) and have a thick outer membrane (Fig. 66.5).

Treatment

Single-dose therapy with praziquantel (10 mg/kg) is recommended for persons with *H. diminuta* infection (18). However, at least one report has suggested that higher doses or multiple courses of treatment may be necessary (63). Of note, tapeworm segments may continue to be passed in the stool for several days following successful treatment. Purgative therapy is not necessary.

Prevention and Control

Prevention of *H. diminuta* infection requires careful storage of dried food products, particularly grains and cereals, to avoid contamination by rodents and insects.

UNCOMMON INTESTINAL CESTODES

D. caninum

D. caninum is a rare zoonotic cause of intestinal disease in humans (64–66). The most common tapeworm of domestic dogs and cats, *D. caninum* has a worldwide geographic distribution. Infection usually occurs in young children and infants (67–74). Infection follows the ingestion of an intermediate host, usually a dog or cat flea (*Ctenocephalides canis* and *Ctenocephalides felis*) containing the larvae (cysticercoids) of *D. caninum.* In rare cases, the human flea (*Pulex irritans*) or dog louse (*Trichodectis canis*) may serve as an intermediate host. Attached to the intestinal mucosa, the adult tapeworm ultimately grows to 15 to 70 cm in length. Although most infections are asymptomatic, actively mobile gravid proglottids with the size and shape of cucumber seeds can migrate out through the anus or be passed in feces (Fig. 66.4). Parents may also report seeing proglottids on diapers or in a child's feces. In clinically documented infections, symptoms include transient diarrhea, abdominal pain, anal pruritus, and irritability. Urticaria and eosinophilia have been reported (74). Praziquantel in a single oral dose of 5 to 10 mg/kg is the drug of choice for adults and children. (18,71). Infection can also be effectively treated with a single dose of niclosamide, although this agent is no longer available in the United States. The most effective means of prevention is to control the flea infestation of pet dogs and cats. Frequent deworming of pets may also help to interrupt the natural life cycle of *D. caninum.*

Bertiella Species

Tapeworms of the genus *Bertiella* primarily infect nonhuman primates. To date, however, at least 55 cases of human bertiellosis have been reported involving three related species: *B. studeri, B. satyri,* and *B. mucronata* (75). Both adults and children are at risk, and cases have been reported from most parts of the world, including the United States (76–86). Infection develops following the ingestion of oribatid mites that contain the cysticercoid stage of the parasite. These mites typically infect nonhuman primates, so most patients with bertiellosis have a history of close contact with monkeys, either in the wild or in captivity. Diarrhea, abdominal pain, weight loss, and anorexia have all been associated with bertiellosis. The diagnosis is made by identifying the characteristic eggs or proglottids in feces (78). Praziquantel in a single oral dose of 10 mg/kg is the treatment of choice for *Bertiella* infections (18,75,86).

Mesocestoides

Mesocestoides is a tapeworm primarily of small mammals that requires multiple intermediate hosts to complete its life cycle. When an infected arthropod vector (first intermediate host) is ingested by a bird or reptile (second intermediate host), the cysticercoid larvae migrate to the liver and peritoneum. There, the larvae develop to the tetrathyridial stage, which is infectious for humans and other mammals (definitive host), including foxes, raccoons, dogs, cats, and skunks. The adult tapeworm develops within the intestine of the definitive host, releasing proglottids into the feces. Most human cases of *Mesocestoides* infection occur following ingestion of the liver or blood of second intermediate hosts, including birds, lizards, and turtles (3,87–89). A recent case report describing infection in a 22-month-old child in a day care setting could not document the route of transmission, although a variety of reptiles and amphibians were housed as pets in the center (87). To date, 22 cases of human infection have been reported worldwide, including six in children from the United States (87–89). The diagnosis is made following the identification of proglottid segments in the feces of an infected person. Egg excretion is variable. Although no longer available in the United States, niclosamide has been reported to be effective in eradicating *Mesocestoides* infections in adults and children. Few data are available on the efficacy of praziquantel in the treatment of this infection.

REFERENCES

1. Grove DI. *A history of human helminthology.* Wallingford, UK: CAB, International, 1990.
2. Schantz PM. Tapeworms. *Gastroenterol Clin North Am* 1996;25: 637–653.
3. Wittner M, Tanowitz HB. Cestode infections. In: Guerrant RL, Walker DH, Weller PF, eds. *Tropical infectious diseases.* New York: Churchill Livingstone, 1999.
4. Manson-Bahr PEC, Bell DR. Tapeworms (cestoids). In: *Manson's tropical diseases.* London: Bailliere Tindall, 1987:521–557.
5. Gutierrez Y. Introduction to cestodes. In: *Diagnostic pathology of parasitic infections with clinical correlations.* Philadelphia: Lea & Febiger, 1990:423–431.
6. Hall A, Latham MC, Crompton DWT, et al. *Taenia saginata* (Cestoda) in western Kenya: reliability of faecal examination in diagnosis. *Parasitology* 1981;83:91–101.
7. Zaman V. *Atlas of medical parasitology,* second edition. Australia: ADIS Health Science Press, 1984.
8. Kaminsky RG. Albendazole treatment in human taeniasis. *Trans R Soc Trop Med Hyg* 1991;85:648–650.
9. Demiriz M, Gunhan O, Celasun B, et al. Colonic perforation caused by taeniasis. *Trop Geogr Med* 1995;47:180–182.
10. Ozbek A, Guzel C, Babacan M, et al. An infestation due to a *Taenia saginata* with an atypical location. *Am J Gastroenterol* 1999;94:1712–1713.
11. Smith JW, Gutierrez Y. Medical parasitology. In: Henry JB, ed. *Todd, Sanford, and Davidsohn's clinical diagnosis and management by laboratory methods,* seventeenth edition. Philadelphia: WB Saunders, 1984.
12. Tanowitz HB, Weiss LM, Wittner M. Diagnosis and treatment of intestinal helminths I. Common intestinal cestodes. *Gastroenterologist* 1993;1:265–273.
13. Mayta H, Talley A, Gilman RH, et al. Differentiating *Taenia solium* and *Taenia saginata* infections by simple hematoxylin-eosin staining and PCR-restriction enzyme analysis. *J Clin Microbiol* 2000;38:133–137.
14. Markell EK, Voge M. *Medical parasitology,* fifth edition. Philadelphia: WB Saunders, 1981:177–205.
15. Allan JC, Noval JC, Flisser A, et al. Immunodiagnosis of taeniasis by coproantigen detection. *Parasitology* 1990;101:473–477.
16. Deplazes P, Ecker J, Pawlowski ZS, et al. An enzyme-linked immunosorbent assay for diagnostic detection of *Taenia saginata* copro-antigens in humans. *Trans R Soc Trop Med Hyg* 1991; 85:391–396.
17. Gonzalez LM, Montero E, Harrson LJ, et al. Differential diagnosis of *Taenia saginata* and *Taenia solium* infection by PCR. *J Clin Microbiol* 2000;38:737–744.
18. Drugs for parasitic infections. *Med Lett Drugs Ther* 1998;40: 1–12 (updated electronic version available at *http:www.medletter.comhtml_filespublicreading.htm#Parasitic*).
19. Ruiz Perez A, Santana Ane M, Villaverde Ane B, et al. The minimum dosage of praziquantel in the treatment of *Taenia saginata,* 1986–1993. *Rev Cubana Med Trop* 1995;47:219–220.
20. Vermund SH, MacLeod S, Goldstein RE. Taeniasis unresponsive to a single dose of niclosamide: case report of persistent infection with *Taenia saginata* and a review of therapy. *Rev Infect Dis* 1986; 8:423–426.
21. Botero D. Paromomycin as effective treatment of *Taenia* infections. *Am J Trop Med Hyg* 1970;19:234–237.
22. Chung WC, Fan PC, Lin CY, et al. Poor efficacy of albendazole for the treatment of human taeniasis. *Int J Parasitol* 1991;21: 269–270.
23. White AC Jr. Neurocysticercosis: updates on epidemiology, pathogenesis, diagnosis, and management. *Annu Rev Med* 2000; 51:187–206.
24. Rodriguez-Canul R, Fraser A, Allan JC, et al. Epidemiological study of *Taenia solium* taeniasis cysticercosis in a rural village in Yucatan state, Mexico. *Ann Trop Med Parasitol* 1999;93:57–67.
25. Centers for Disease Control and Prevention. Locally acquired neurocysticercosis—North Carolina, Massachusetts, and South Carolina, 1989–1991. *MMWR Morb Mortal Wkly Rep* 1992;41: 1–4.
26. Schantz PM, Moore AC, Muñoz JL, et al. Neurocysticercosis in an orthodox Jewish community in New York City. *N Engl J Med* 1992;327:692–695.
27. Allen JC, Velasquez-Tohom M, Torres-Alvarez R, et al. Field trial of coproantigen-based diagnosis of *Taenia solium* taeniasis by enzyme-linked immunosorbent assay. *Am J Trop Med Hyg* 1996;54:352–356.
28. Montenegro TC, Miranda EA, Gilman R. Production of monoclonal antibodies for the identification of the eggs of *Taenia solium. Ann Trop Med Parasitol* 1996;90:145–155.
29. Del Brutto OH, Wadia NH, Dumas M, et al: Proposal of diagnostic criteria for human cysticercosis and neurocysticercosis. *J Neurol Sci* 1996;142:1–6.
30. Flisser A, Madrazo I, Plancarte A, et al. Neurological symptoms in occult neurocysticercosis after a single taeniacidal dose of praziquantel. *Lancet* 1993;342:748.
31. Pawlowski ZS. Efficacy of low doses of praziquantel in taeniasis. *Acta Trop* 1991;48:83–88.
32. Richards F, Schantz P. Dogma disputed. Treatment of *Taenia solium* infection. *Lancet* 1985;1:1264–1265.
33. Allan JC, Velasquez-Tohom M, Fletes C, et al. Mass chemotherapy for intestinal *Taenia solium* infection: effect on prevalence in humans and pigs. *Trans R Soc Trop Med Hyg* 1997;91:595–598.
34. Von Bonsdorf B. *Diphyllobothriasis in man.* London: Academic Press, 1977.
35. Ohnishi K, Murata M. Single-dose treatment with praziquantel for human *Diphyllobothrium nihonkaiense* infections. *Trans R Soc Trop Med Hyg* 1993;84:482–483.
36. Mercado R, Arias B. *Taenia* sp and other intestinal cestode infections in individuals from public outpatient clinics and hospitals from the northern section of Santiago, Chile (1985–1994). *Bol Chil Parasitol.* 1995;50:80–83.
37. Kyronseppa H. The occurrence of human intestinal parasites in Finland. *Scand J Infect Dis* 1993;25:671–673.
38. Nozaki T, Nagakura K, Fusegawa H, et al. Brief survey of common intestinal parasites in the Tokyo metropolitan area. *Kansenshogaku Zasshi* 1998;72:865–869.
39. Chung PR, Sohn WM, Jung Y, et al. Five human cases of *Diphyllobothrium latum* infection through eating raw flesh of redlip mullet, *Liza haematocheila. Korean J Parasitol* 1997;35:283–289.
40. Rausch RL, Scott EM, Rausch VR. Helminths in Eskimos in western Alaska, with particular reference to *Diphyllobothrium* infection and anaemia. *Trans R Soc Trop Med Hyg* 1967;61: 351–357.
41. Hutchinson JW, Bass JW, Demers DM, et al. Diphyllobothriasis after eating raw salmon. *Hawaii Med J* 1997;56:176–177
42. Centers for Disease Control and Prevention. Diphyllobothriasis associated with salmon—United States. *MMWR Morb Mortal Wkly Rep* 1981;30:331–332, 337–338.
43. Bruckner DA. Helminthic food-borne infections. *Clin Lab Med* 1999;19:639–660.

44. Adams AM, Murrell KD, Cross JH. Parasites of fish and risks to public health. *Rev Sci Tech* 1997;16:652–660.
45. Saarni M, Nyberg W, Grasbeck R, et al. Symptoms in carriers of *Diphyllobothrium latum* and in non-infected controls. *Acta Med Scand* 1963;173:147–154.
46. Waki K, Oi H, Takahashi S, et al. Successful treatment of *Diphyllobothrium latum* and *Taenia saginata* infection by intraduodenal "Gastrografin" injection. *Lancet* 1986;2:1124–1126.
47. Nyberg W, Grasbeck R, Saarni M, et al. Serum vitamin B_{12} levels and incidence of tapeworm-associated anemia in a population heavily infected with *Diphyllobothrium latum. Am J Clin Nutr* 1961;9:606–612.
48. von Bonsdorff B, Gordin R. Castle's test (with vitamin B_{12} and normal gastric juice) in the ileum in patients with genuine and patients with tapeworm pernicious anaemia. *Acta Med Scand* 1980;208:193–197.
49. Weisse ME, Raszka WV. Cestode infection in children. *Adv Pediatr Infect Dis* 1996;12:109–153.
50. Ludwig KM, Frei F, Alvares Filho F, et al. Correlation between sanitation conditions and intestinal parasitosis in the population of Assis, State of Sao Paulo. *Rev Soc Bras Med Trop* 1999;32: 547–555.
51. Rai SK, Uga S, Ono K, et al. Contamination of soil with helminth parasite eggs in Nepal. *Southeast Asian J Trop Med Public Health* 2000;31:388–393.
52. Yoeli M, Most H, Hammond J, et al. Parasitic infections in a closed community: results of a 10-year survey in Willowbrook State School. *Trans R Soc Trop Med Hyg* 1972;66:764–776.
53. Sirivichayakul C, Radomyos P, Praevanit R, et al. *Hymenolepis nana* infection in Thai children. *J Med Assoc Thai* 2000;83: 1035–1038.
54. Al-Hussaini MK, Khalifa R, Al-Ansary ATA, et al. Phlyctenular eye disease in association with *Hymenolepis nana* in Egypt. *Br J Ophthalmol* 1979;63:627–631.
55. Gamal-Eddin FM, Aboul-Atta AM, Hassounah OA. Extraintestinal nana cysticercoidiasis in asthmatic and filarised Egyptian patients. *J Egypt Soc Parasitol* 1986;16:517–520.
56. Gomez-Priego A, Godinez-Hana AL, Gutierrez-Quiroz M. Detection of serum antibodies in human *Hymenolepis* infection by enzyme immunoassay. *Trans R Soc Trop Med Hyg* 1991;85: 645–647.
57. Castillo RM, Grados P, Carcamo CC, et al. Effect of treatment on serum antibody to *Hymenolepis nana* detected by enzyme-linked immunosorbent assay. *J Clin Microbiol* 1991;29:413–414.
58. Schenone H. Praziquantel in the treatment of *Hymenolepis nana* infections in children. *Am J Trop Med Hyg* 1980;29:320–321.
59. Groll E. Praziquantel for cestode infections in man. *Acta Trop* 1980;37:293–296.
60. Hamrick HJ, Bowdre JH, Church SM. Rat tapeworm (*Hymenolepis diminuta*) infection in a child. *Pediatr Infect Dis J* 1990;9:216–219.
61. Edelman MH, Spingarn CL, Nauenberg WG, et al. *Hymenolepis diminuta* (rat tapeworm) infection in man. *Am J Med* 1965;38: 951–953.
62. Verghese SL, Sudha P, Padmaja P, et al. *Hymenolepis diminuta* infestation in a child. *J Commun Dis* 1998;30:201–203.
63. Tena D, Perez Simon M, Gimeno C, et al. Human infection with *Hymenolepis diminuta*: case report from Spain. *J Clin Microbiol* 1998;36:2375–2376.
64. Marx M. Parasites, pets and people. *Prim Care* 1991;18: 153–165.
65. Brandstetter W, Auer H. *Dipylidium caninum,* a rare parasite in man. *Wien Klin Wochenschr* 1994;106:115–116.
66. Neafie RC, Marty AM. Unusual infections in humans. *Clin Microbiol Rev* 1993;6:34–356.
67. Gadre DV, Kumar A, Mathur M. Infection by *Dipylidium caninum* through pet cats. *Indian J Pediatr* 1993;60:151–152.
68. Ferraris S, Reverso E, Parravicini LP, et al. *Dipylidium caninum* in an infant. *Eur J Pediatr* 1993;152:702.
69. Reid CJ, Perry FM, Evans N. *Dipylidium caninum* in an infant. *Eur J Pediatr* 1992;151:502–503.
70. Chappell CL, Enos JP, Penn HM. *Dipylidium caninum,* an underrecognized infection in infants and children. *Pediatr Infect Dis J* 1990;9:745–747.
71. Wijesundera M. The use of praziquantel in human infection with *Dipylidium. Trans R Soc Trop Med Hyg* 1989;83:383.
72. Raitiere C. Dog tapeworm (*Dipylidium caninum*) infestation in a 6-month-old infant. *J Fam Pract* 1992;34:101–102.
73. Turner JA. Human *Dipylidium* in the United States. *J Pediatr* 1962;61:763–768.
74. Neafie R, Marty A. Unusual infections in humans. *Clin Microbiol Rev* 1993;6:37–39.
75. Denegri GM, Perez-Serrano J. Bertiellosis in man: a review of cases. *Rev Inst Med Trop Sao Paulo* 1997;39:123–127.
76. Stunkard H, Koivastik T, Healy G. Infection of a child in Minnesota by *Bertiella studeri* (Cestoda-Anoplocephalidae). *Am J Trop Med Hyg* 1964;13:402–409.
77. Galan-Puchades MT, Fuentes MV, Simarro PP, et al. Human *Bertiella studeri* in equatorial Guinea. *Trans R Soc Trop Med Hyg* 1997;91:680.
78. Galan-Puchades MT, Fuentes MV, Mas-Coma S. Human *Bertiella studeri* in Spain, probably of African origin. *Am J Trop Med Hyg* 1997;56:610–612.
79. Ando K, Ito T, Miura K, et al. Infection of an adult in Mie Prefecture, Japan, by *Bertiella studeri. Southeast Asian J Trop Med Public Health* 1996;27:200–201.
80. Panda DN, Panda MR. Record of *Bertiella studeri* (Blanchard, 1891), an anaplocephalid tapeworm, from a child. *Ann Trop Med Parasitol* 1994;88:451–452.
81. Richard-Lenoble D, Kombila M, Maganga ML, et al. *Bertiella* infection in a Gabon-born girl. *Am J Trop Med Hyg* 1986;35:134.
82. Bolbol AS. *Bertiella* sp. infection in man in Saudi Arabia. *Ann Trop Med Parasitol* 1985;79:643–644.
83. Bhaibulaya M. Human infection with *Bertiella studeri* in Thailand. *Southeast Asian J Trop Med Public Health* 1985;16:505–507.
84. Subbannayya K, Achyutha Rao KN, Shivananda PG, et al. *Bertiella* infection in an adult male in Karnataka. A case report. *Indian J Pathol Microbiol* 1984;27:269–271.
85. Banyopadhyah AK, Manna B. The pathogenic and zoonotic potential of *Bertiella studeri. Ann Trop Med Parasitol* 1987;81: 465–466.
86. Conder GA, Roehm PA, Duprey DA, et al. Treatment of bertiellosis in *Macaca fascicularis* with praziquantel. *J Helminthol Soc Wash* 1991;58:128.
87. Schultz L, Hummet B, Lubell I. *Mesocestoides* (Cestoda) infection in a California child. *Pediatr Infect Dis J* 1992;11:332–333.
88. Gutierrez NN, Buchino JJ, Schubert WK. *Mesocestoides* (Cestoda) infection in children in the United States. *J Pediatr* 1978; 93:245–247.
89. Eom KS, Kim SH, Rim HJ Second case of human infection with *Mesocestoides lineatus* in Korea. *Kisaengchunghak Chapchi* 1992; 30:147–150.

67

ASCARIASIS, TRICHURIASIS, AND ENTEROBIASIS

KATHRYN N. SUH
JAY S. KEYSTONE

Helminths are among the most prevalent human parasites and are a major cause of morbidity and mortality, particularly in developing countries. Current estimates suggest that 1.4 billion people worldwide are infected with *Ascaris,* 1.2 billion with hookworm (*Ancylostoma duodenale* and *Necator americanus*), and 1 billion with *Trichuris trichiura* (1). Ascariasis is the most common soil-transmitted helminthic (geohelminthic) infection globally, but hookworm infection is the most common in North America (2). Many persons are infected with multiple species of helminths, and for prolonged periods. The prevalence and intensity of geohelminthic infections are related to socioeconomic factors (e.g., poverty, population density, poor sanitation, low educational standards, lack of safe drinking water) to a greater extent than to ecologic factors.

ASCARIASIS

Ascaris, the largest and one of the most prevalent human helminths, is also among the earliest recorded, with references dating to ancient Greece, Rome, and China (2). Human infections are caused by *Ascaris lumbricoides,* which although specific for humans has been found accidentally in other mammalian species. The closely related *Ascaris suum,* endemic to pigs, has caused disease in humans following accidental ingestion of large quantities of ova, but maturation to adult worms has not occurred in such cases (3). Little evidence exists to suggest that natural cross-infection between pigs and humans is a significant problem.

K. N. Suh: Division of Infectious Diseases, Department of Medicine, Queen's University; Department of Medicine, Kingston General Hospital, Kingston, Ontario, Canada

J. S. Keystone: Department of Medicine, University of Toronto; Centre for Travel and Tropical Medicine, Division of Infectious Diseases, Toronto General Hospital, Toronto, Ontario, Canada

Epidemiology

Ascaris is widely distributed throughout the world, found in at least two-thirds of the world's nations as of 1989 (4). Its distribution is closely related to that of *T. trichiura,* and the prevalence of co-infection is high. Ascariasis is most prevalent in Asia; an estimated 73% of the global pool is found there (especially in China, India, and Southeast Asia), followed by 12% in Africa and 8% in Latin America (5). However, prevalence estimates can vary markedly within a given country; for example, in different Nigerian communities, the prevalence ranges from 0.9% to 98.2% (6). In tropical climates, soil conditions are optimal for year-round transmission of infective eggs, whereas in temperate climates, fluctuations in temperature and humidity result in a seasonal pattern of infection. In North America, ascariasis is the third most commonly diagnosed geohelminthic infection (after hookworm infection and trichuriasis); most cases are attributable to immigrants from areas where infection is endemic.

The prevalence of ascariasis is highest in children, reaching a peak between the ages of 4 and 14 years in areas of endemicity (2). The worm burden is generally higher in children than in adults, but it is unclear whether this age-dependent intensity is a consequence of decreased exposure or increased immunity in adults. In most infected persons, the worm burden is low; the majority of adult worms (80%) are harbored by a small proportion of potential hosts (20%) (2). In addition, both the predisposition to acquiring infection and the intensity of infection appear to vary among individuals in relation to a variety of host factors (7,8).

The morbidity and mortality associated with ascariasis are extremely difficult to estimate, given the often inadequate records and surveillance methods employed in areas of endemicity. Morbidity usually depends on the worm burden and is therefore higher in children. In regions of endemicity, ascariasis during childhood is associated with malnutrition and impaired growth, reduced vitamin A absorption, and possibly impaired cognitive function, although the latter association has not been definitively proved (9). Gastrointestinal and biliary tract complications account for most of the clinical illness and deaths caused by ascariasis. Estimates of attributable deaths range from 20,000 to more than 100,000 annually (10,11).

Morphology

Adult *Ascaris* organisms are flesh-colored, cylindric, unsegmented, and tapered at both ends. Sexual dimorphism is well expressed, with females being larger than males. On average, females are 20 to 49 cm long and 3 to 6 mm in diameter, whereas males are 15 to 30 cm in length and 2 to 4 mm in diameter (Fig. 67.1). The head or anterior end consists of three toothed lips. All viscera are contained in the body cavity or pseudocoelom; the worms have no circulatory system. The excretory system consists of two lateral excretory canals that run along the length of the worm. The female has a ventral vulvar opening located at the junction of the anterior and middle thirds of the body; the male has two copulatory spicules and numerous papillae on its curved posterior end.

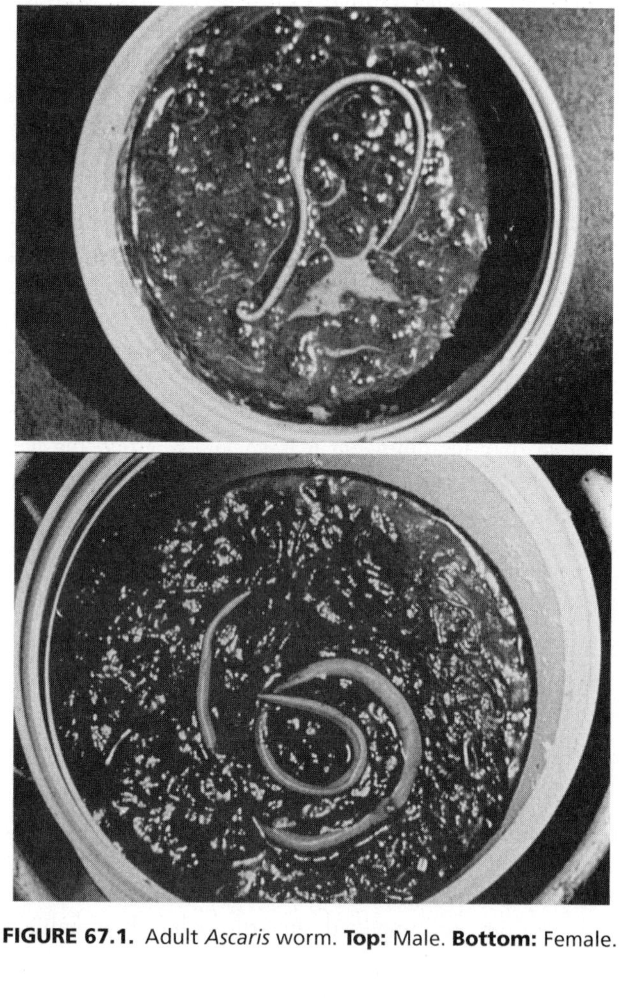

FIGURE 67.1. Adult *Ascaris* worm. **Top:** Male. **Bottom:** Female.

Characteristic fertilized eggs are ovoid and brown; they have a thick, multilayered outer shell and measure 45 to 70 μm by 30 to 50 μm. Unfertilized eggs may be more difficult to identify and can be confused with ova from other nematodes. They are more irregular in shape, longer, and narrower, and their shell is thinner than that of the fertilized eggs.

Life Cycle and Transmission

The life cycle of *Ascaris* is shown in Fig. 67.2. Soil is necessary for the development of *Ascaris* eggs and acts as a reservoir. Eggs produced by mature female worms in the small intestine are fertilized, and excreted in stool. Optimal soil conditions for maturation include a temperature of 28°C to 32°C and high levels of moisture; eggs are sensitive to high temperatures and desiccation but can otherwise survive in soil for up to 6 years in temperate climates. The eggs embryonate following weeks to months of development in soil, depending on environmental conditions. One to two days after the embryonated eggs are ingested, larvae hatch in the small bowel and penetrate the intestinal wall, entering the portal circulation. Within 2 weeks, larvae reach the pulmonary circulation and enter the alveoli, occasionally producing clinical pulmonary disease. They then ascend the tracheobronchial tree, are swallowed, and reach the small intestine, where they develop into mature adults and live for 10 to 18 months. Most adult worms reside in the jejunum. Sexual maturation and egg production begin 3 to 4 months after initial ingestion. Females have a prodigious reproductive potential and can each produce more than 200,000 eggs per day, which accounts for the high infection rate in areas of endemicity. Person-to-person transmission does not occur because fertilized eggs must incubate in soil to become infective.

Pathology

The host response to infection and the clinical picture vary according to the stage of infection. The initial passage of larvae in the lungs usually causes no symptoms or pathologic changes. However, subsequent larval migration during reinfection is characterized by an immunologic and inflammatory reaction with eosinophilia. Masses of acidophilic material are concentrated around the larvae (the Splendore–Hoeppli phenomenon), consistent with a hypersensitivity reaction. The hypersensitivity reaction that occurs in the lungs is responsible for the clinical manifestations of Loeffler syndrome. The intensity of the host response, which is proportional to the number of larvae destroyed during migration, varies greatly and appears to be maximal in populations sensitized by repeated exposure (12).

In contrast, the intestinal phase of infection is usually asymptomatic. Adult worms brace themselves against the intestinal wall and can migrate within the intestinal lumen. Pathologic findings represent complications resulting from

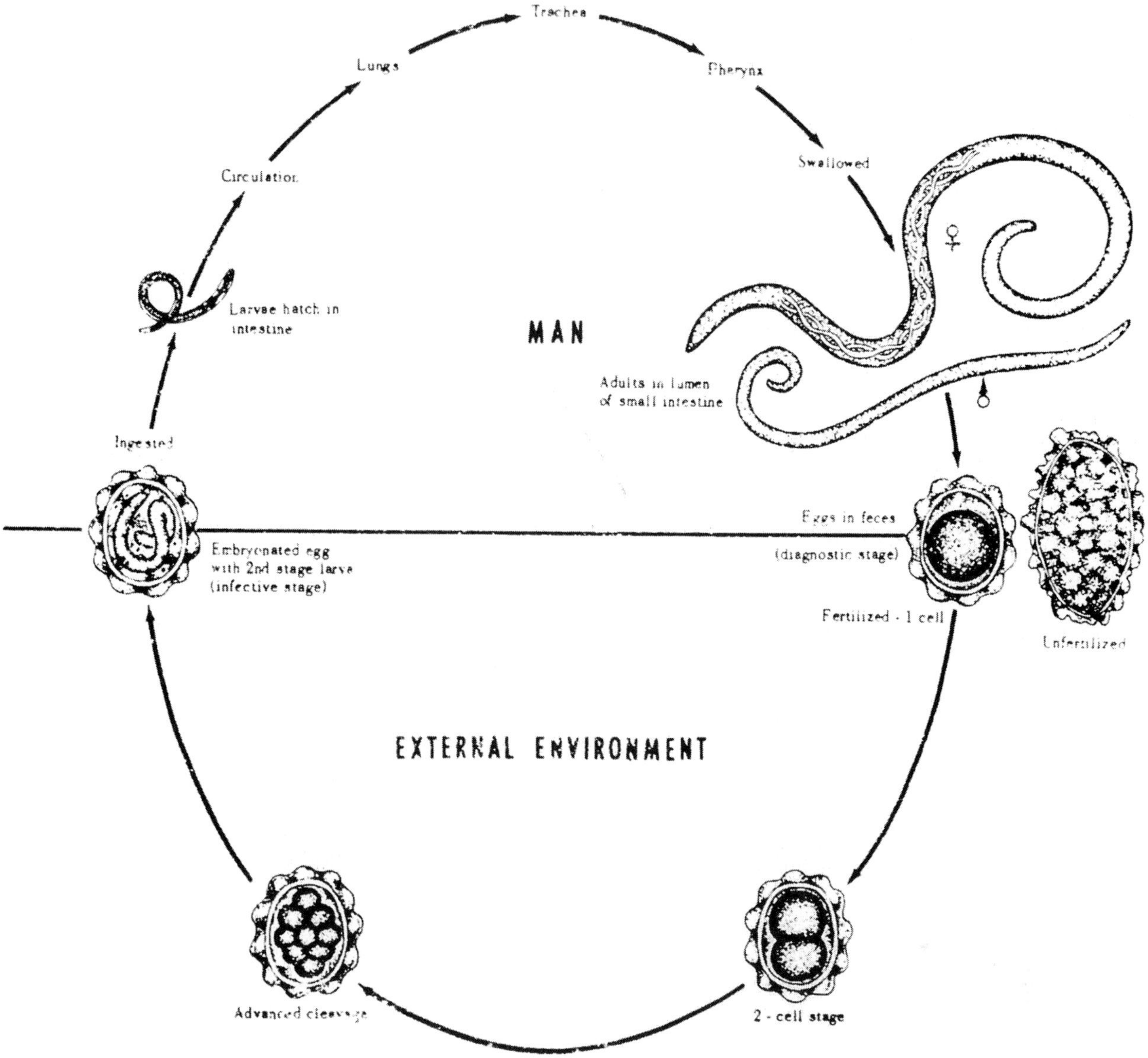

FIGURE 67.2. Life cycle of *Ascaris lumbricoides.*

either an excessive worm burden or extraintestinal worm migration (e.g., into the biliary tract). Migrating worms may release eggs in ectopic sites (e.g., liver, lung), sometimes causing granulomatous inflammation and necrosis with subsequent tissue scarring. Certain medications or fever may cause worms to migrate from the intestine (13).

Immunology and Immunity

Infection with *Ascaris* stimulates the production of a variety of antibodies, including immunoglobulin M (IgM) and both parasite-specific and nonspecific IgE. The major *Ascaris* antigen, a 25-kd molecule known as ABA-1 (*Ascaris* body fluid allergen), is a potent allergen and accounts for most of the allergenic activity of adult ascarids (14). Individual immune responses vary markedly, but high worm burdens in general result in higher antibody levels (15). High antibody titers are found in persons with repeated and more intense contact with *Ascaris* organisms and presumably confer some immunity, evidenced by low egg counts and few adult worms in such people (16).

A thorough understanding of the role of IgE in protection against *Ascaris* and other helminths is lacking. The participation of IgE in immediate hypersensitivity reactions, although occasionally severe or fatal, appears to have evolved as a specific immune defense against helminths. *Schistosoma hematobium*-specific IgE has been clearly associated with resistance to reinfection (17), and a similar role has been suggested for *Ascaris*-specific IgE. In one study of Venezuelan children, reinfection with *Ascaris,* although associated with an increase in total IgE levels, occurred in those children who were unable to maintain high levels of *Ascaris*-specific IgE (18). High levels of nonspecific IgE may benefit the parasite by limiting the opportunity for parasite-specific IgE to elicit an antibody-dependent cellular cytotoxicity response from the host (19). Alternatively, nonspecific IgE may protect the host against overwhelming hypersensitivity reactions and anaphylaxis (20). Clearly, much work remains to be done in this area.

Clinical Features

Most infections with *Ascaris* are asymptomatic. Pulmonary ascariasis, a result of larval migration through the alveoli, occurs 5 to 26 days after initial infection. It is among the most common causes of Loeffler syndrome but overall is rare, even in areas of endemicity (21). Symptoms are more common in children and persons with reinfection and may be seasonal (2,12); they include low-grade fever, chills, dyspnea, wheezing, and dry cough. Marked peripheral eosinophilia is the rule. Chest radiographs show bilateral patchy infiltrates. Symptoms resolve within 2 weeks, although eosinophilia can persist for much longer.

Gastrointestinal ascariasis caused by worm masses or worm migration accounts for most cases of clinically apparent infection; however, adult worms generally cause no symptoms. Vague abdominal pain, nausea, anorexia, and diarrhea may be present. Eosinophilia is not generally associated with adult worm infections, or is mild. Intestinal obstruction is the most common complication caused by adult worms (Fig. 67.3). In one series of 4,793 complicated cases of ascariasis, 62.4% were caused by obstruction (9). In areas of endemicity, up to 35% of all cases of intestinal obstruction are caused by *Ascaris,* with a case fatality rate of up to 8.6%. Obstruction is 30 times more likely to develop in children than in adults. Symptoms are indistinguishable from those of obstruction with other causes. Intussusception, volvulus, bowel infarction, or perforation may also occur.

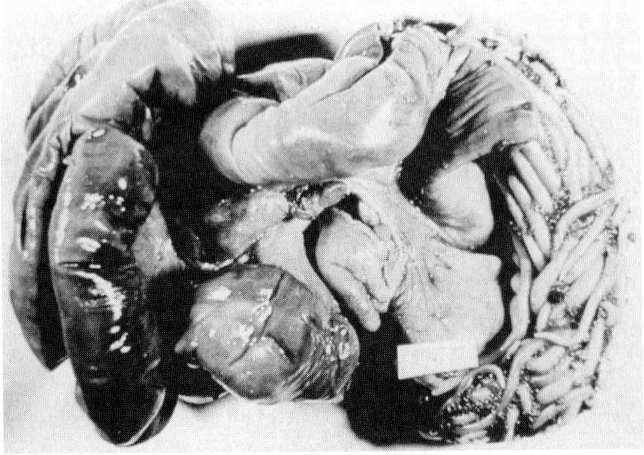

FIGURE 67.3. Resected bowel obstructed by *Ascaris lumbricoides.*

Extraintestinal ascariasis results from worm migration. The hepatobiliary tract and pancreas are the most commonly involved extraintestinal sites. Presentations in one series of 507 patients in India included biliary colic (55.2%), acute cholangitis (23.9%), acalculous cholecystitis (12.6%), acute pancreatitis (7.5%), and liver abscess (0.7%) (22). *Ascaris* biliary disease shows a marked female preponderance and tends to occur in persons who have previously had biliary tract disease or undergone manipulation of the biliary tract (23). *Ascaris* has also been associated with recurrent pyogenic cholangitis in areas of endemicity (24).

Live worms may be coughed up, vomited, or extruded through the nose. Occasionally, worms can migrate to the upper airway and cause asphyxia. Complications caused by adult worms in other organs are exceedingly rare.

Diagnosis

The diagnosis of ascariasis relies on the demonstration of *Ascaris* larvae, ova, or worms. In pulmonary disease, eosinophils and Charcot–Leyden crystals can be found in sputum, and larvae may be recovered from sputum and gastric aspirates. Because lung involvement precedes egg production by 8 to 10 weeks, the result of stool examination for ova is usually negative. Intestinal ascariasis is most reliably diagnosed by the identification of ova in fresh or fixed stool specimens. The Kato–Miura thick smear is commonly used to detect eggs in feces, but most standard concentration tests, usually based on centrifugation, are effective.

Adult worms can be readily identified when expelled in feces or from other sites. They can also be visualized radiographically; worms are usually outlined by barium during contrast studies, but they also ingest barium and can be identified by visualizing barium within the gut of the worm (Fig. 67.4). Infections with adult worms can also be diagnosed with ultrasonography or endoscopy and at surgery.

Indirect methods of diagnosis include demonstration of IgM antibodies by agar gel diffusion or immunoelectrophoresis. Solid-phase radioimmunoassay, indirect immunofluorescence, and hemagglutination methods are of limited use because of cross-reactivity with blood group and other parasite antibodies. In general, the use of serodiagnostic methods is limited to the diagnosis of early *Ascaris* infections (before egg production begins) and to epidemiologic studies.

Treatment

Ascaris pneumonia is self-limited. Bronchodilators, antitussives, and, in extreme cases, steroids may be required to control symptoms. Anthelmintic therapy is ineffective against larvae and is of no benefit in pulmonary disease.

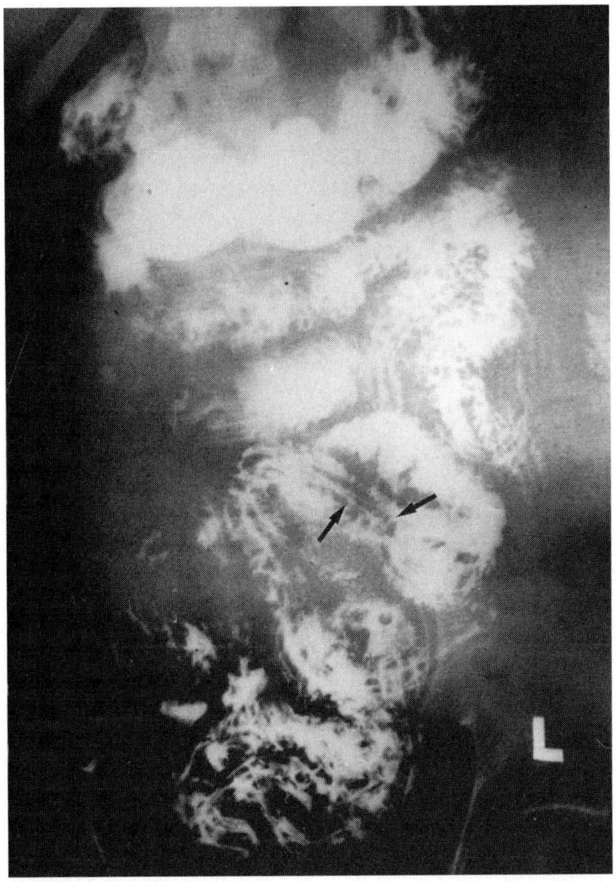

FIGURE 67.4. Small-bowel follow-through outlining an adult *Ascaris* worm. Barium is seen within the gut of the worm (*arrow, left*) and outlining the worm (*arrow, right*).

Intestinal ascariasis should always be treated. Drugs of choice include pyrantel pamoate, mebendazole, and albendazole. Pyrantel pamoate is a cyclic amidine compound that causes spastic paralysis of the worm. A single dose of 11 mg/kg (maximum of 1 g) is more than 90% effective in *Ascaris* infections. Its action is slow, however, and it may take several days before the worms are killed and cleared. Pyrantel pamoate is contraindicated in persons with liver disease and should be used with caution in pregnancy. Gastrointestinal side effects are common but mild.

Mebendazole and albendazole are benzimidazole compounds that block helminthic glucose uptake, inhibit microtubule formation, and lead to parasite death. Mebendazole (100 mg twice daily for 3 days or 500 mg once) and albendazole (400 mg as a single dose) are equally effective (all doses are regardless of age), with median cure rates of 95% to 97% (25). Resistance to these drugs has not yet been demonstrated. Both are contraindicated during pregnancy.

Piperazine temporarily paralyzes *Ascaris* organisms by inhibiting cholinergic activity; worms are evacuated by natural peristalsis. A dose of 75 mg/kg per day for 2 days (maximum daily dose of 4 g in children older than 12 years and adults, and 2.5 g in children ages 2 to 12 years) is more than 90% effective but can cause neurotoxicity and hypersensitivity reactions. With the availability of more effective and less toxic agents, piperazine has fallen out of favor in industrialized nations, but because of its low cost it is still an attractive alternative in the developing world. Other effective agents include ivermectin and levamisole. Endoscopic and surgical intervention may be indicated for biliary tract disease or intestinal obstruction, especially if conservative measures fail.

Prevention and Control

Strategies for the prevention and control of ascariasis include individual and community measures and mass chemotherapy programs. Individual interventions include hand washing, attention to hygienic preparation of food, water purification by boiling, and close supervision of children. At the community level, significant changes may be required to improve health education and levels of sanitation. Mass chemotherapy has emerged as a safe, rapidly effective alternative for reducing the transmission of helminthic infections in areas of endemicity. Chemotherapy can be universal (treat everyone), targeted (treat only specific groups; e.g., children), or selective (treat based on current infection status; e.g., screen for infection and treat only heavily infected persons). Universal chemotherapy may be more likely than the other approaches to reduce worm burden and egg output and thereby reduce morbidity (26,27). However, no chemotherapy program can provide effective long-term prevention without concomitant improvements in sanitation and health education.

TRICHURIASIS

T. trichiura, commonly known as *whipworm* because of the morphology of the adult worms, causes varying degrees of intestinal symptomatology. It differs from the other geohelminths in two respects: its life cycle lacks a pulmonary phase, and adult worms reside in the large (not small) bowel.

Epidemiology

Trichuriasis is one of the most prevalent parasitic infections, affecting an estimated 1 billion persons. Although concentrated in the tropics, *Trichuris* is distributed worldwide and is common even in temperate climates. In the United States, *T. trichiura* is identified in 1.2% of stool specimens submitted for parasitology studies (28). Humans are the primary hosts for *T trichiura*; rarely, human infection may be caused by *Trichiura suis* (pig whipworm) or *Trichiura vulpis* (dog whipworm). Co-infection with *Ascaris* is common.

The age distribution of trichuriasis parallels that of ascariasis, with a higher prevalence of both infections during childhood. Infection often occurs by 2 years of age and is most prevalent in 5- to 10-year-olds. Generally, the worm burden is significantly reduced in adults; this may be a consequence of decreased exposure or related to a person's intrinsic susceptibility to reinfection. The intensity of infection, even within a given community, varies greatly; most people harbor few worms, and 70% of the worm population is found in fewer than 15% of infected persons. The worm burden is also highly aggregated, with familial clustering (29).

Until recently, trichuriasis was considered to be benign, but it is now well recognized that gastrointestinal symptoms can result from infection. Trichuriasis has been suggested as one contributing factor to chronic diarrheal disease in the tropics, but the overall morbidity attributable to this parasite is unclear.

Morphology

The adult worm is characterized by its whiplike anterior end, which comprises three-fifths of its length. The posterior two-fifths are thicker and contain the intestines and reproductive organs. The female measures 30 to 50 mm in length and has an uncoiled posterior end, whereas the male may be slightly smaller (30 to 45 mm long) and has a coiled posterior with a copulatory spicule (Fig. 67.5). *Trichuris* eggs measure approximately 50 by 20 μm and are typically barrel-shaped, with thick shells and hyaline plug-like prominences at either pole.

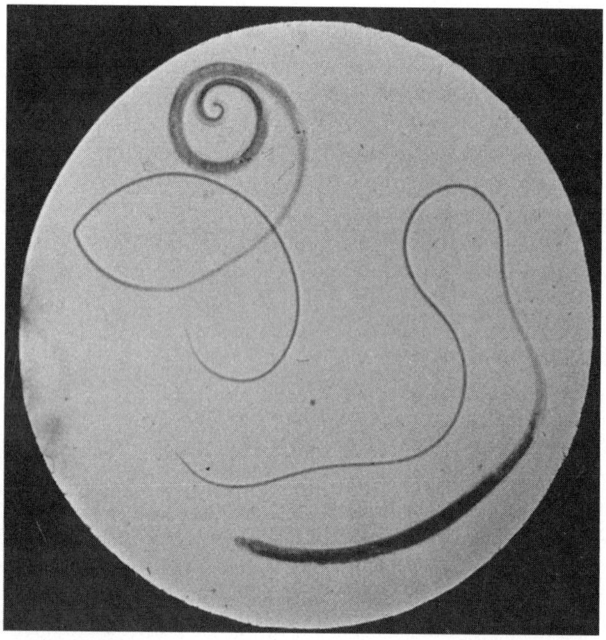

FIGURE 67.5. Adult *Trichuris* worm. **Top:** Male. **Bottom:** Female.

Life Cycle and Transmission

Person-to-person transmission of *Trichuris* does not occur because eggs require incubation in soil before becoming infective. Eggs passed in stool require 2 to 4 weeks to embryonate in warm, moist soil. The eggs are less hardy than those of *Ascaris* and are more sensitive to cold and desiccation. However, in ideal conditions, they can survive in soil for up to 1 year. After infective eggs are ingested, larvae hatch in the cecum and penetrate the intestinal crypts, where they mature during several days (Fig. 67.6). No tissue migration occurs during the larval phase of *Trichuris* infection. Adult worms emerge in the cecum, attaching themselves to the intestinal mucosa by their anterior ends, and they remain this way throughout their lives. Egg production begins 2 to 3 months after initial infection; females can each produce between 3,000 and 20,000 eggs per day. The life span of the adult worm ranges from 1 to 8 years.

Pathology

Adult worms generally inhabit the cecum, but in cases of more intense infection they may be found in the entire colon (Fig. 67.7) and also in the terminal ileum. The mucosa may not be markedly abnormal in appearance or may be edematous with increased vascularity. Mucosal findings at the site of attachment of the worm include petechial or subepithelial hemorrhages, mucosal cell destruction, and a superficial infiltrate of eosinophils, lymphocytes, and plasma cells. In heavy infections, the mucosa may be friable and ulcerated, with a tendency to bleed easily. Anemia, when it occurs, is caused by chronic occult blood loss from the inflamed intestine; adult worms do not actively ingest blood (30).

Immunology and Immunity

In murine trichuriasis, antibody and lymphoid cell immune responses result in worm expulsion. Mice resistant to *T. muris* infection exhibit a helper T-cell type 2 (Th2) response, with production of interleukins 5 and 9, whereas a Th1 response and interferon-α production predominate in susceptible mice (31). In contrast, worms are not expelled in humans, and reinfection is the rule. *Trichuris* infection elicits a local immediate hypersensitivity reaction in the colonic mucosa (32). Despite a strong humoral immune response with production of IgG, IgE, and IgA in humans (33) and a correlation between IgA antibodies and lower worm burdens (34), significant immunity to *Trichuris* does not develop. The humoral response is age-dependent; a rapid increase in antibody levels is observed during the initial infection in childhood, followed in adulthood by decreases in both intensity of infection and antibody levels (34).

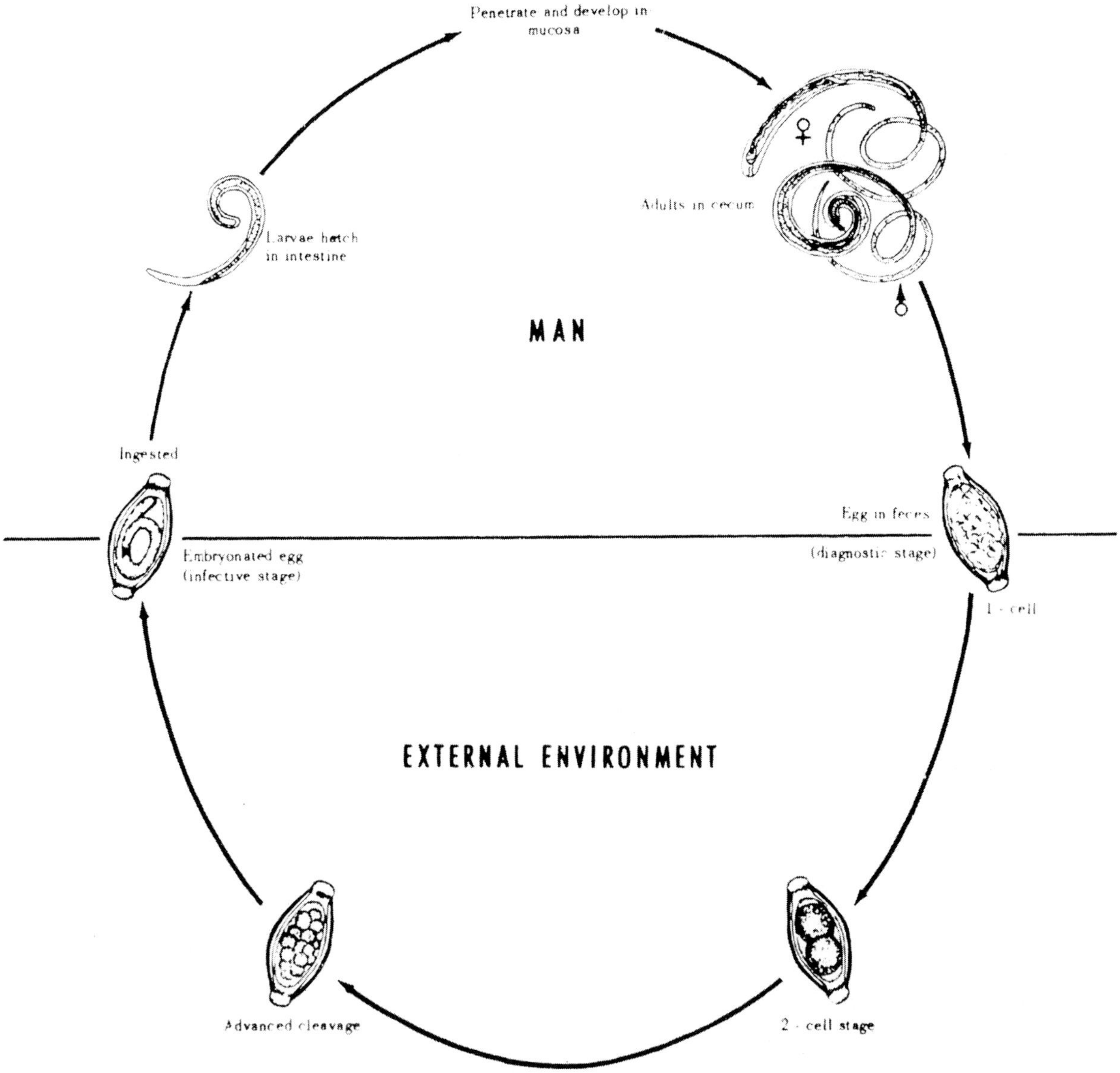

FIGURE 67.6. Life cycle of *Trichuris trichiura.*

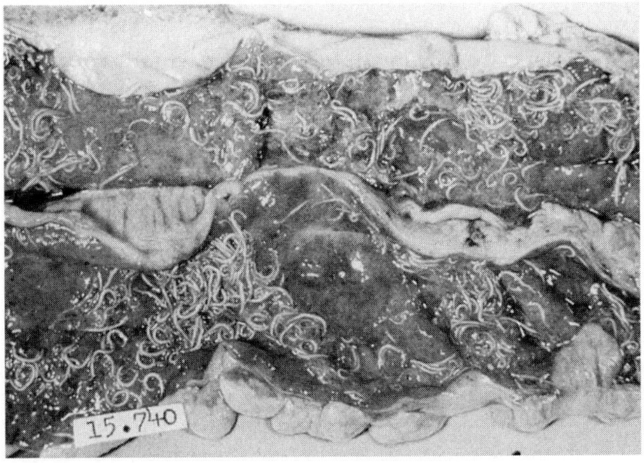

FIGURE 67.7. *Trichuris trichiura* in resected colon.

Clinical Features

Most infected persons are asymptomatic. Moderate worm burdens (50 to 150 worms) may cause lower abdominal pain, diarrhea, distention, anorexia, and weight loss. Intense infection typically occurs in children and may lead to *Trichuris* dysentery syndrome; this is characterized by chronic diarrhea, which may be profuse and bloody, growth retardation, and anemia. Abdominal cramps, fecal urgency, tenesmus, and rectal prolapse—a hallmark of trichuriasis in areas of endemicity—may also occur, and pica is not uncommon. Growth retardation can also occur with milder infections and is reversible with anthelmintic therapy (35). Anemia secondary to chronic blood loss from the gastrointestinal tract can be severe. Clubbing of the fingers and toes may also be observed in severe infection. Some evidence suggests that cognitive function may be reversibly impaired in children with chronic infection (36).

Diagnosis

The diagnosis of trichuriasis is usually made by finding the characteristic eggs in stool specimens. Adult worms and Charcot–Leyden crystals may also be seen. Air–contrast barium enemas may demonstrate worms as linear or coiled translucencies. Proctoscopy or colonoscopy may reveal mucosal inflammation, and adult worms may be noted hanging into the intestinal lumen. Microcytic anemia resulting from iron deficiency may be present in heavy infection. Peripheral eosinophilia, if present, is usually mild and is not correlated with worm burden or symptoms.

Treatment

T. trichiura is generally more resistant to therapy than are other geohelminths. Current drugs of choice are mebendazole and albendazole. Single-dose therapy with 500 mg of mebendazole is slightly more effective than one 400-mg dose of albendazole (37,38); however, the median cure rate in several studies in which either regimen was used was still less than 40% (25). Despite these low cure rates, single-dose therapy can significantly reduce fecal egg counts, which may be important at least in controlling symptoms and morbidity (37). Three-day regimens with either mebendazole (100 mg twice daily) or albendazole (400 mg once daily) are considered curative, even in heavy infections (30). Benzimidazole therapy of *T. trichiura* is also highly effective against *A. lumbricoides.*

Prevention and Control

The approach to the prevention and control of trichuriasis is similar to that for ascariasis. Control of trichuriasis may be more challenging, however, because the prevalence of infection falls slowly despite control of transmission, and *T. trichiura* is inherently less susceptible to chemotherapy.

ENTEROBIASIS

Enterobiasis is caused by *Enterobius vermicularis,* otherwise known as *pinworm* or *threadworm.* It is the most common helminthic infection of humans in North America and probably throughout the world. Humans are the only hosts for *E. vermicularis*; related species can infect other animals.

Epidemiology

E. vermicularis is distributed worldwide in both rural and urban settings. It is somewhat more common in temperate climates, where transmission may be enhanced by closer contact between persons in these regions. Prevalence rates of 100% have been reported in areas of the United States and northwestern Europe (39), although the incidence and prevalence in the United States have declined in recent years (40).

Enterobiasis is most common in children of both sexes between the ages of 5 and 10 years and is relatively rare in children younger than 2 years (41). *Enterobius* does not respect socioeconomic boundaries; however, close contact with infected persons, overcrowding, and poor personal hygiene facilitate transmission. Infection may therefore be difficult to cure within families and institutions, as reinfection can occur easily in these settings. High rates of infection have also been documented in homosexual men (42). As with ascariasis and trichuriasis, a relatively few infected persons harbor most of the worm population.

When it is symptomatic, enterobiasis is generally a nuisance disease, but nocturnal symptoms and insomnia can be problematic. Thus, morbidity can be significant despite the lack of serious complications of this infection.

Morphology

Sexual dimorphism is well expressed in *E. vermicularis.* Adult females are 8 to 13 mm long and 0.5 mm wide and have an attenuated, pointed tail. The anterior end of the female contains the digestive and reproductive systems, the latter opening onto the ventral surface at the junction of the anterior and middle thirds of the body. The adult male is much smaller, measuring only 2 to 5 mm in length and 0.2 mm in width, and has a curved posterior end with a single copulatory spicule. *Enterobius* eggs are ovoid in shape, measuring 50 to 60 by 20 to 30 μm, have a thick shell, and are distinctively flattened on one side.

Life Cycle and Transmission

The life cycle of *E. vermicularis* takes place entirely within the human gastrointestinal tract (Fig. 67.8); a soil phase is not required. Non-infective eggs are laid in the perianal region or released when the adult female dies or the worm is mechanically disrupted (e.g., by scratching). At body temperature, the eggs require a maximum of 6 hours (less with exposure to oxygen) to become infective. They lose their infectivity quickly, within 1 to 2 days, and are viable for less than 2 weeks. Survival is optimal at lower temperatures and high humidity. After the eggs are ingested, larvae hatch in the stomach and duodenum and molt twice before they mature into adults. Adult worms mate in the distal small intestine and subsequently settle in the appendix, cecum, and colon. Egg production begins 5 weeks after initial infection. Adult females live for 12 weeks, and adult males for 7 weeks.

Transmission can occur in several ways (43): direct fecal–oral transmission, including autoinfection; exposure

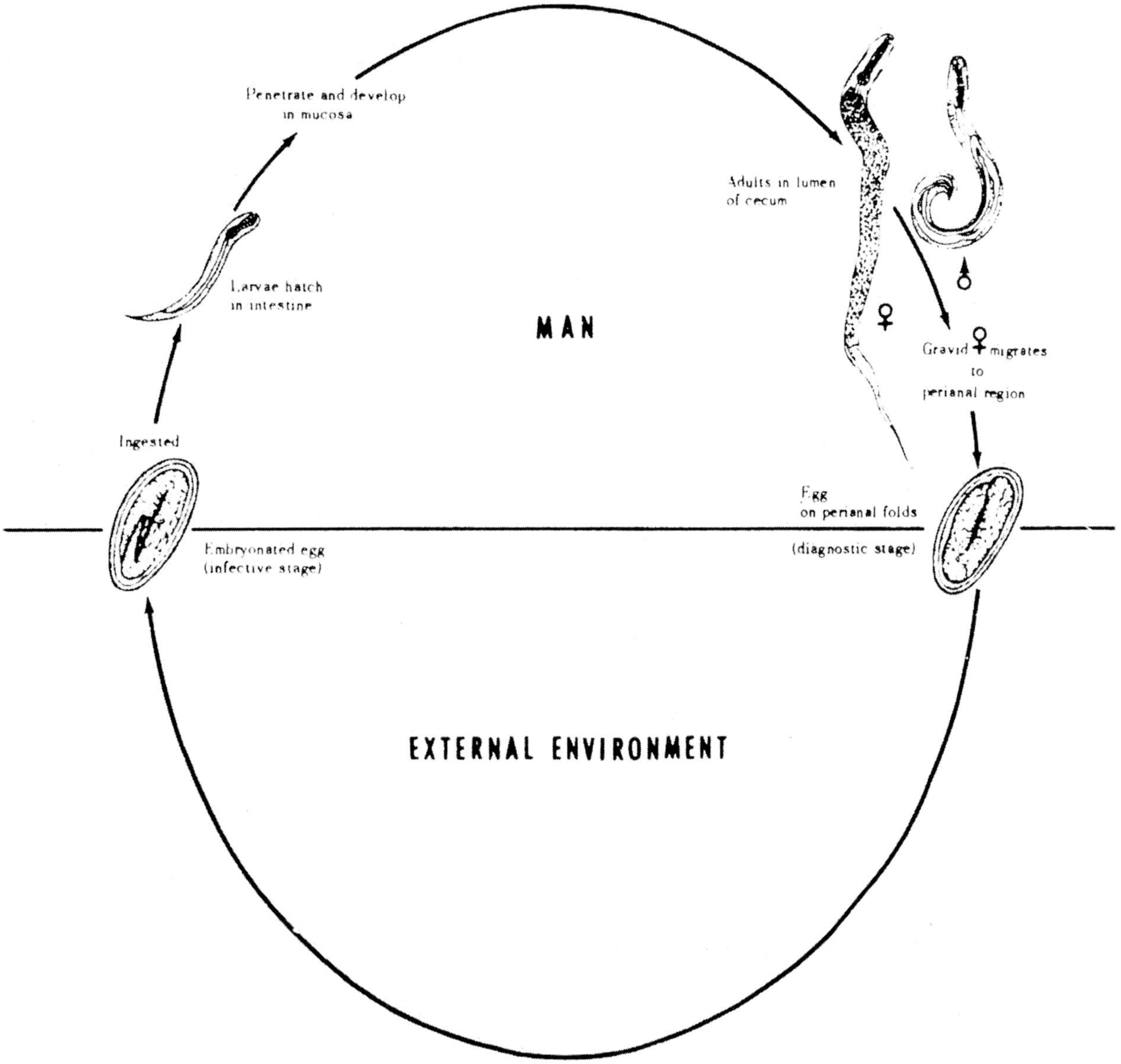

FIGURE 67.8. Life cycle of *Enterobius vermicularis.*

to viable eggs on fomites; ingestion of eggs in contaminated dust; and retroinfection, in which larvae migrate back into the large bowel after hatching in the perianal mucosa.

Pathology

On pathologic examination, the most common site of infection in enterobiasis is the appendix; 86.5% of 259 infections were localized to the appendix in one series (44). However, no evidence supports the notion that *Enterobius* causes acute appendicitis. Within the bowel, worms do not cause an inflammatory reaction, although eosinophilic colitis has been described (45). Ulceration and hemorrhage may be noted at the site of worm attachment to the mucosa, sometimes with secondary abscess formation (43). Ectopic worms are most commonly found in the peritoneal cavity and female genital tract, where they may elicit a granulomatous reaction with lymphocytes, eosinophils, Charcot–Leyden crystals, and occasionally calcification. Lesions appear grossly as white or yellow nodules. Eggs laid by ectopic worms may also be encased by granulomas and Splendore–Hoeppli substance.

Immunology and Immunity

Little literature is available regarding human immune responses in enterobiasis. No local IgE-mediated allergic response is caused by *E. vermicularis.* Some evidence indicates that immune responses mediated by T cells may play a role in intestinal inflammation in rodent models of infection (41). Seroepidemiologic studies in enterobiasis are lacking.

Clinical Features

The majority of infections are asymptomatic. The most common symptom, which occurs in one-third of infected patients, is perianal pruritus caused by the female worm or her eggs. Insomnia, irritability, and restlessness may be attributed to sleep disturbed by nocturnal itching. Complications of pruritus ani include eczematous perianal skin lesions, which may become secondarily infected. Abdominal pain appears to be uncommon, but the exact incidence is unclear because most studies have not controlled for duration or intensity of infection or for coexisting conditions. Children occasionally demonstrate anorexia and weight loss. In female patients, worms may migrate through the vagina and uterus, causing vulvovaginitis with vaginal discharge, endometritis, or salpingitis. Enuresis and recurrent urinary tract infections have been reported with enterobiasis. Worms have also been identified in remote sites (e.g., lung, eye), but these cases are extremely unusual. No evidence supports an association between enterobiasis and conditions such as tooth grinding, thumb sucking, or nail biting in children. Eosinophilia is not a feature of enterobiasis.

Diagnosis

Examination of stool for ova or adult worms is an insensitive method for diagnosing enterobiasis; results are positive in fewer than 15% of examinations. Adult worms or eggs can sometimes be seen on inspection of the perianal region, particularly at night. The most reliable test is the cellulose acetate ("Scotch tape") test, performed by affixing adhesive tape to both sides of a tongue depressor (adhesive side out), spreading the buttocks, and applying the tape firmly against the perianal skin. The test is best performed on awakening in the morning. The tape is then placed on a microscope slide, adhesive side down, and examined for eggs (and worms) (Fig. 67.9). One test is 50% sensitive, and sensitivity increases with multiple applications on consecutive days: 90% with three, 99% with five, and 100% with seven tests (46). However, enterobiasis can be excluded only after the results of six consecutive tests (on separate days) are negative (43). Commercially manufactured applicators for this purpose are also available. Eggs can also be detected in perianal scrapings or swabs and underneath the fingernails. Proctoscopy or colonoscopy should not be required to establish the diagnosis, but adult worms may be visualized during these procedures.

Co-infection with *Dientamoeba fragilis* is present in up to 50% of persons with enterobiasis (47). Identification of one parasite should therefore suggest the presence of the other.

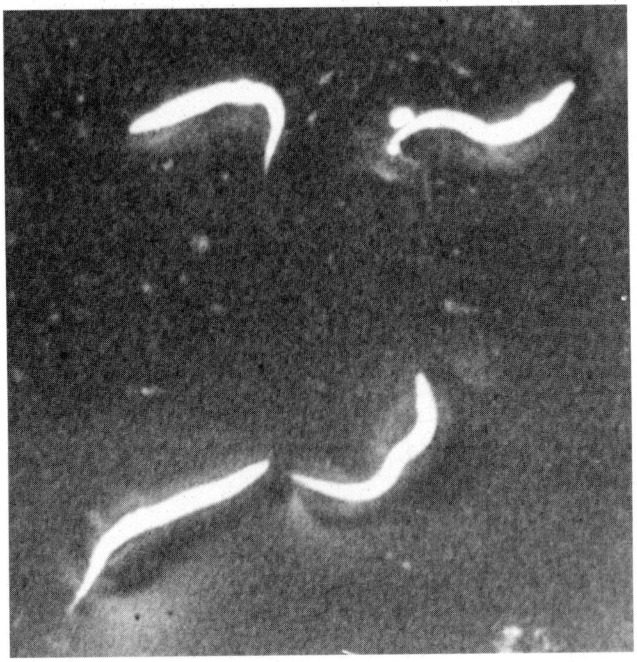

FIGURE 67.9. Adult *Enterobius vermicularis* worm on cellulose acetate.

Treatment

Personal hygiene measures can reduce reinfection and transmission rates. Attention must be paid to scrupulous hand washing, trimming of fingernails, and adequate hygiene. Although gloves can be worn by children during sleep as a preventative measure, this is not usually necessary if they wear underwear and pajamas. Frequent changes of underwear (daily) and linens (weekly) are ideal; regular laundering is adequate for disinfection. Regular vacuuming of areas likely to be contaminated may also contribute to breaking the transmission cycle.

Primary infections with *E. vermicularis* usually clear spontaneously in 30 to 45 days. However, anthelmintic therapy is always recommended, regardless of symptoms, because of the risk for reinfection and transmission to others. All members of an infected household should be treated concurrently with the index case. *E. vermicularis* infection is amenable to therapy with several anthelmintic agents. Albendazole is the most effective (43), with 100% cure rates reported in several studies. Mebendazole, pyrantel pamoate, and piperazine are also highly effective, with cure rates of better than 90%. Doses and duration of therapy are listed in Table 67.1. Regardless of the agent used, a second course of treatment should be administered 2 to 4 weeks after the first because therapy is more effective against adult worms than against newly ingested eggs and developing larvae. Recurrent infections may require several (four or more) courses of therapy. Treatment may be withheld during pregnancy; benzimidazole agents should be avoided.

TABLE 67.1. RECOMMENDED THERAPY FOR ENTEROBIUS VERMICULARIS INFECTION

Drug	Dose[a]
Albendazole	Adults and children >2 years: 400 mg once Children <2 years: 100 mg once
Mebendazole	100 mg once
Pyrantel pamoate	11 mg/kg once (maximum, 1 g)
Piperazine	50 mg/kg daily (maximum, 2 g) for 7 days

[a]Dose regardless of age, except as noted. A second course of therapy must be repeated 2 to 4 weeks after the first, regardless of the agent used.

Prevention and Control

Personal hygiene measures and cleanliness of accommodations must be emphasized to control transmission. A social stigma is often attached to pinworm infection, but this is a very common infection that occurs in all social strata. In addition to individual/household therapy, "prophylactic" chemotherapy (e.g., every 2 to 4 months) for persons continually exposed to *E. vermicularis* may be used (43). Mass chemotherapy is also effective in selected settings.

REFERENCES

1. Crompton DWT. How much human helminthiasis is there in the world? *J Parasitol* 1999;85:397–403.
2. Khuroo MS. Ascariasis. *Gastroenterol Clin North Am* 1996;25: 553–577.
3. Phills JA, Harrold AJ, Whiteman GV, et al. Pulmonary infiltrates, asthma, and eosinophilia due to *Ascaris suum* infestation in man. *N Engl J Med* 1972;286:965–970.
4. Crompton DWT. Prevalence of ascariasis. In: Crompton DWT, Nesheim MC, Pawlowski ZS, eds. *Ascariasis and its prevention and control.* London: Taylor and Francis, 1989:45–69.
5. Peters W. Medical aspects—comments and discussion II. *Symp Br Soc Parasitol* 1978;16:25–40.
6. Crompton DWT, Tulley JJ. How much ascariasis is there in Africa? *Parasitol Today* 1987;3:123–127.
7. World Health Organization. *Prevention and control of intestinal parasitic infections.* WHO Technical Report Series No. 749. Geneva: World Health Organization, 1987.
8. Croll NA, Ghadarian F. Wormy persons: contribution to the nature and patterns of overdispersion with *Ascaris lumbricoides, Ancyclostoma duodenale, Necator americanus,* and *Trichuris trichiura. Trop Geogr Med* 1981;33:241–248.
9. Crompton DWT. *Ascaris* and ascariasis. *Adv Parasitol* 2001; 48:285–375.
10. Walsh JA, Warren KS. Selective primary health care: an interim strategy for disease control in developing countries. *N Engl J Med* 1979;301:967–974.
11. Pawlowski ZS, Davis A. Morbidity and mortality in ascariasis. In: Crompton DWT, Nesheim MC, Pawlowski ZS, eds. *Ascariasis and its prevention and control.* London: Taylor and Francis, 1989: 71–86.
12. Gelpi AP, Mustafa A. Seasonal pneumonia with eosinophilia. A study of larval ascariasis in Saudi Arabia. *Am J Trop Med Hyg* 1967;16:646–657.
13. Ochoa B. Surgical complications of ascariasis. *World J Surg* 1991;15:222–229.
14. McGibbon AM, Christie JF, Kennedy MW, et al. Identification of the major *Ascaris* allergen and its purification to homogeneity by high-performance liquid chromatography. *Mol Biochem Parasitol* 1990;39:163–172.
15. Haswell-Elkins MR, Kennedy MW, Maizels RM, et al. The antibody recognition profiles of humans naturally infected with *Ascaris lumbricoides. Parasite Immunol* 1989;11:615–627.
16. Jones HI. Haemagglutination tests in the study of *Ascaris* epidemiology. *Ann Trop Med Parasitol* 1977;71:219–226.
17. Hagan P, Blumenthal UJ, Dunn D, et al. Human IgE, IgG4 and resistance to infection with *Schistosoma haematobium. Nature* 1991;349:243–245.
18. Hagel I, Lynch NR, Di Priscio MC, et al. *Ascaris* reinfection of slum children: relation with the IgE response. *Clin Exp Immunol* 1993;94:80–83.
19. Pritchard DI. Immunity to helminths: is too much IgE parasite-rather than host-protective? *Parasite Immunol* 1993;15:5–9.
20. Hagan P. IgE and protective immunity to helminth infections. *Parasite Immunol* 1993;15:1–4.
21. Spillman RK. Pulmonary ascariasis in tropical communities. *Am J Trop Med Hyg* 1995;24:791–800.
22. Khuroo MS, Zargar SA, Mahajan R. Hepatobiliary and pancreatic ascariasis in India. *Lancet* 1990;335:1503–1506.
23. Sandouk F, Haffar S, Zada MM, et al. Pancreatic–biliary ascariasis: experience of 300 cases. *Am J Gastroenterol* 1997;92: 2264–2267.
24. Shulman A. Intrahepatic biliary stones: imaging features and a possible relationship with *Ascaris lumbricoides. Clin Radiol* 1993; 47:325–332.
25. Bennett A, Guyatt H. Reducing intestinal nematode infection: efficacy of albendazole and mebendazole. *Parasitol Today* 2000; 16:71–74.
26. Asaolu SO, Holland CV, Crompton DWT. Community control of *Ascaris lumbricoides* in rural Oyo State, Nigeria: mass, targeted, and selected treatment with levamisole. *Parasitology* 1991;103(Pt 2):291–298.
27. Hall A, Anwar KS, Tomkins AM. Intensity of reinfection with *Ascaris lumbricoides* and its implications for parasite control. *Lancet* 1992;339:1253–1257.
28. Kappus KD, Lundgren RG, Juranek DD, et al. Intestinal parasitism in the United States: update on a continuing problem. *Am J Trop Med Hyg* 1994;50:705–713.
29. Bundy DA, Cooper ES, Thompson DE, et al. Age-related prevalence and intensity of *Trichuris trichiura* infection in a St. Lucian community. *Trans R Soc Trop Med Hyg* 1987;81:85–94.
30. Bundy DAP, Cooper E. Trichuriasis. In: Strickland GT, ed. *Hunter's tropical medicine and emerging infectious diseases,* eighth edition. Philadelphia: WB Saunders, 2000:722–724.
31. Else KJ, Hultner L, Grencis RK. Modulation of cytokine production and response phenotypes in murine trichuriasis. *Parasite Immunol* 1992;14:441–449.
32. Cooper ES, Spencer J, Whyte-Alleng CAM, et al. Immediate hypersensitivity in colon of children with chronic *Trichuris trichiura. Lancet* 1991;338:1104–1107.
33. Lillywhite JE, Bundy DA, Didier JM, et al. Humoral immune responses in human infection with the whipworm *Trichuris trichiura. Parasite Immunol* 1991;13:491–507.
34. Bundy DA, Lillywhite JE, Didier JM, et al. Age dependency of infection status and serum antibody levels in human whipworm (*Trichuris trichiura*) infection. *Parasite Immunol* 1991;13: 629–638.
35. Cooper ES, Bundy DA, MacDonald TT, et al. Growth suppression in the *Trichuris* dysentery syndrome. *Eur J Clin Nutr* 1990; 44:285–291.

36. Nokes C, Grantham-McGregor SM, Sawyer AW, et al. Moderate to heavy infections of *Trichuris trichiura* affect cognitive function in Jamaican schoolchildren. *Parasitology* 1992;104:539–547.
37. Albonico M, Smith PG, Hall A, et al. A randomized controlled trial comparing mebendazole and albendazole against *Ascaris, Trichuris,* and hookworm infections. *Trans R Soc Trop Med Hyg* 1994;88:585–589.
38. Jackson TF, Epstein SR, Gouws E, et al. A comparison of mebendazole and albendazole in treating children with *Trichuris trichiura* infection in Durban, South Africa. *S Afr Med J* 1998;88: 880–883.
39. Cook GC. In: *Parasitic diseases in clinical practice.* London: Springer-Verlag, 1990:114–116.
40. Vermund SH, Macleod S. Is pinworm a vanishing infection? Laboratory surveillance in a New York City medical center from 1971 to 1986. *Am J Dis Child* 1988;142:566–568.
41. Grencis RK, Cooper ES. *Enterobius, Trichuris, Capillaria,* and hookworm including *Ancylostoma caninum. Gastroenterol Clin North Am* 1996;25:579–597.
42. Weller IVD. The gay bowel. *Gut* 1985;26:869–875.
43. Cook GC. *Enterobius vermicularis* infection. *Gut* 1994;35: 1159–1162.
44. Sinniah B, Leopairut J, Neafie RC, et al. Enterobiasis: a histopathological study of 259 patients. *Ann Trop Med Parasitol* 1991;85:625–635.
45. Liu LX, Chi J, Upton MP. Eosinophilic colitis associated with larvae of the pinworm *Enterobius vermicularis. Lancet* 1995;346: 410–412.
46. Keystone JS. Enterobiasis. In: Goldsmith R, Heyneman D, eds. *Tropical medicine and parasitology.* Norwalk, CT: Appleton & Lange, 1989:357–361.
47. Yang J, Scholten T. *Dientamoeba fragilis*: a review with notes on its epidemiology, pathogenicity, mode of transmission, and diagnosis. *Am J Trop Med Hyg* 1977:26:16–22.

68

TRICHINELLA SPIRALIS

DICKSON D. DESPOMMIER

The genus *Trichinella* has undergone extensive revision during the last few years, largely because of the advent of reliable DNA probes that can be used in the polymerase chain reaction (PCR). Nine distinct genotypes and seven species (two are provisional) are now recognized (1). Because members of the genus *Trichinella* infect a broad spectrum of mammalian hosts, these nematodes have become one of the world's most widely distributed parasite groups. They are distantly related to *Trichuris trichiura* and *Capillaria* species; all belong to the order Trichurida. These roundworms constitute an unusual group of organisms in the phylum Nematoda in that all of them live as intracellular parasites.

The diseases that *Trichinella* species cause are collectively referred to as *trichinellosis.* Currently, the prevalence of trichinellosis is low within the United States; it occurs mostly as scattered outbreaks (2). The majority of human cases are caused by *Trichinella spiralis,* and the information that follows is largely about this species. The domestic pig is the main reservoir host for *T. spiralis.* The prevalence of *T. spiralis* infection is significantly higher in parts of Europe, Asia, and Southeast Asia than in the United States, and is *T. spiralis* is now considered endemic in Japan and China. A large outbreak of trichinellosis occurred in Lebanon in 1997, in which more than 200 people were infected (3). *T. spiralis* infection in humans has been reported from Korea for the first time (4). In contrast, *Trichinella* infections in wildlife within the United States are now thought to be caused largely by the T5 strain, tentatively designated *Trichinella murrelli* (5).

An outbreak of *Trichinella pseudospiralis* infection in Thailand has been reported (6). This species can also infect birds of prey. *Trichinella paupae* (provisional), apparently similar in biology to *T. pseudospiralis,* has been described in wild and domestic pigs in Papua New Guinea (7).

Human infections are also caused by *Trichinella nativa* and *Trichinella britovi* (8,9). Reservoir hosts for *T. nativa* include sled dogs, walruses, and polar bears. *T. britovi* causes the sylvatic form of trichinellosis throughout most of Asia and Europe. Numerous reports have appeared in the literature of infections with this parasite in foxes, raccoon dogs, opossums, domestic and wild dogs, and cats.

Trichinella nelsoni is restricted to mammals in equatorial Africa, such as hyenas and the large predatory cats (10). Occasionally, people become infected with *T. nelsoni.* Most animals in the wild, regardless of their geographic location, acquire *Trichinella* infection by scavenging. As of this writing, Puerto Rico and mainland Australia remain free of *Trichinella.*

BIOLOGY AND LIFE CYCLE

The life cycle is depicted in Fig. 68.1. Infection is initiated when raw or undercooked meats harboring the Nurse cell–larva complex are ingested (Fig. 68.2). Infective larvae (Fig. 68.3) are released from muscle tissue by digestive enzymes in the stomach and migrate to the upper two-thirds of the small intestine (Fig. 68.4). Partial digestion of the outermost cuticular layer (epicuticle) by alkaline conditions and pancreatic enzymes (11,12) allows the parasites to receive environmental cues (13). The worms are then able to select sites within the host. The immature parasites penetrate the columnar epithelium at the base of the villus. They live within a row of these cells and are considered intra-multicellular organisms (14,15).

Larvae molt four times in rapid succession during a 30-hour period, developing into adults (16) (Fig. 68.5). The female is 3 mm in length and 36 μm in diameter; the male is 1.5 mm in length and 36 μm in diameter.

Patency occurs within 5 days after mating. Adult females produce live offspring, the newborn larvae (Fig. 68.6), which are 0.08 mm in length and 7 μm in diameter. The female produces offspring as long as host immunity does not develop. Eventually, acquired protective responses interfere with the overall process of embryogenesis and create conditions in the local area of infection that force the adult parasites to evacuate and relocate in a more distal portion of the intestinal tract. Expulsion of worms from the host is the

D. D. Despommier: Department of Environmental Health Sciences and Microbiology, Columbia University, New York, New York

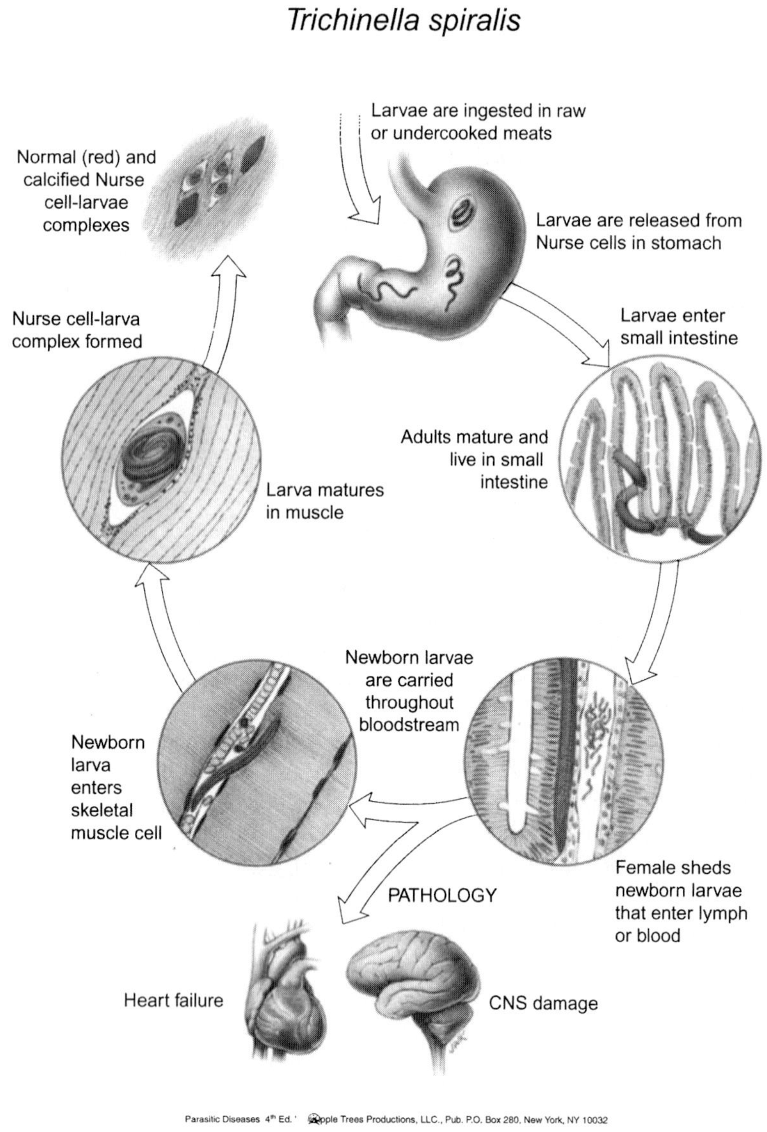
Trichinella spiralis
Larvae are ingested in raw or undercooked meats
Normal (red) and calcified Nurse cell-larvae complexes
Larvae are released from Nurse cells in stomach
Nurse cell-larva complex formed
Larvae enter small intestine
Adults mature and live in small intestine
Larva matures in muscle
Newborn larvae are carried throughout bloodstream
Newborn larva enters skeletal muscle cell
PATHOLOGY
Female sheds newborn larvae that enter lymph or blood
Heart failure
CNS damage
Parasitic Diseases 4th Ed. Apple Trees Productions, LLC., Pub. P.O. Box 280, New York, NY 10032

FIGURE 68.1. Life cycle of *Trichinella spiralis*. (Adapted from Despommier DD, Karapelou JW. *Parasite life cycles*. New York: Springer-Verlag, 1987.)

final expression of immunity and may take several weeks to reach effective levels (17).

The newborn larva is the only stage at which the parasite possesses a swordlike stylet, located in its oral cavity. The stylet is used to create an entry hole in potential host cells. Larvae enter the lamina propria in this fashion and penetrate either the mesenteric lymphatics or the bloodstream. Most newborn larvae enter the general circulation and are distributed throughout the body (16).

Migrating newborns leave capillaries and enter cells (Fig. 68.7). No tropism for any particular cell type is apparent. Once inside, the parasites either remain or leave, depending on the environmental cues (yet to be determined) they receive. Most cell types die as a result of invasion. Skeletal muscle cells are the only exception. Not only do the parasites remain inside them after invasion, they induce a remarkable series of changes, causing a fully differentiated muscle cell to transform into one that supports the growth and development of the larva. This process is termed *Nurse cell formation* (18) (Fig. 68.8). Parasite and host cell develop in a coordinated fashion (19). *T. spiralis* is infective by day 14 of infection, but the worm continues to grow through day 20 (20). The significance of this precocious behavior has yet to be appreciated.

Parasites inside cells other than striated muscle cells fail to induce Nurse cells; they either reenter the general circulation or die.

A fascinating aspect of the parenteral phase is the formation of the Nurse cell–parasite complex, which results in an intimate and permanent association between the worm and its intracellular niche (19). Some of the cellular and molecular events leading up to Nurse cell formation have been investigated in synchronously infected animals.

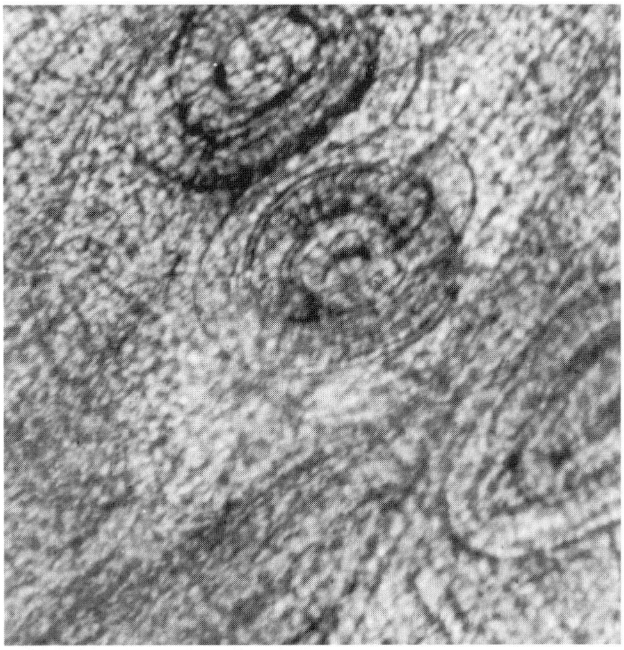

FIGURE 68.2. Unstained muscle biopsy specimen with three larvae of *Trichinella spiralis.* ×235.

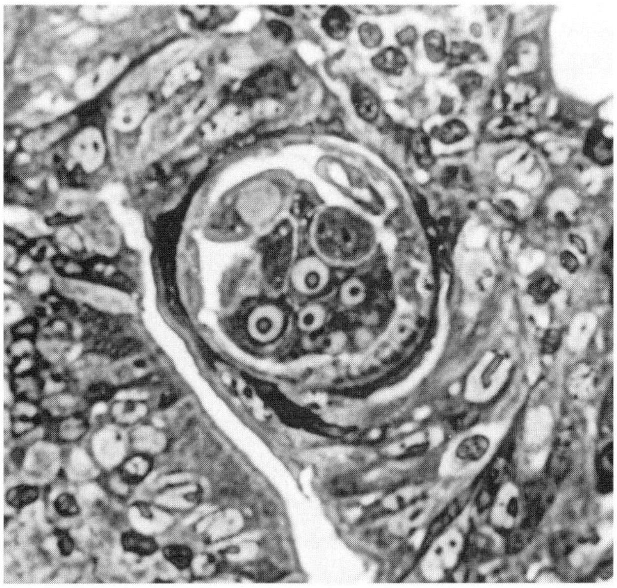

FIGURE 68.4. Adult *Trichinella spiralis in situ.* ×715.

At the cellular level, myofilaments and other related muscle cell components are replaced during a 14- to 16-day period by whorls of smooth membranes and clusters of dysfunctional mitochondria (21) (Fig. 68.9). The net result is that the host cell switches from an aerobic to an anaerobic metabolism. Nuclei enlarge and divide (22), amplifying the host's genome within the Nurse cell cytoplasm (23).

Similar dramatic changes in the host cell can be discerned at the molecular level. Overexpression of collagen types IV and VI messenger RNA, initiated on days 10 through 12, results in the laying down of a thick, acellular capsule along the entire outer surface of the Nurse cell (24). Collagen deposits are thickest at the poles of the Nurse cell. Reticular fibers and other fibrous macromolecules also accumulate in this region, facilitating the attachment of the Nurse cell to adjacent normal portions of the same muscle cell. In this way, even heavily infected animals (e.g., nude mice) seem to behave normally.

Angiogenesis is facilitated by the induction of vascular endothelial growth factor (VEGF) synthesis within the developing Nurse cell beginning on day 7 (25). VEGF synthesis continues throughout the infection and results in the development, some 10 days later, of the circulatory rete

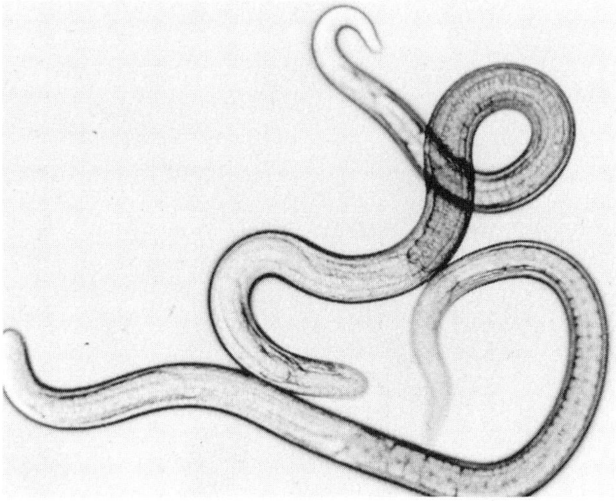

FIGURE 68.3. Infective L1 larvae of *Trichinella spiralis* isolated from an infected animal by digestion of muscle tissue for 1 hour at 37°C in pepsin hydrochloride. ×180.

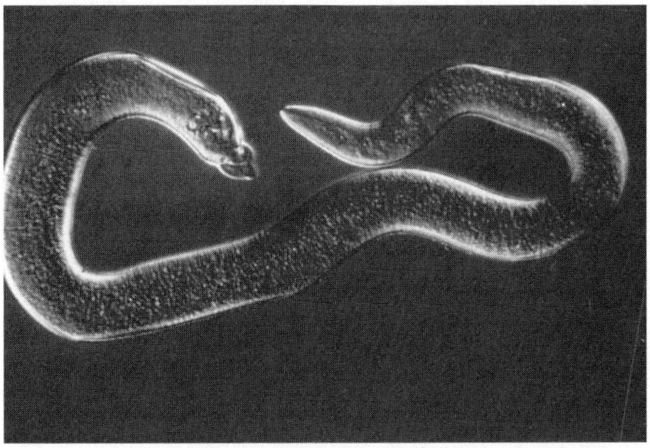

FIGURE 68.5. Adult male *Trichinella spiralis* organism, 1.5 mm × 36 μm. Normarski-phase interference photomicrograph. ×300. (Courtesy of Eric Grave.)

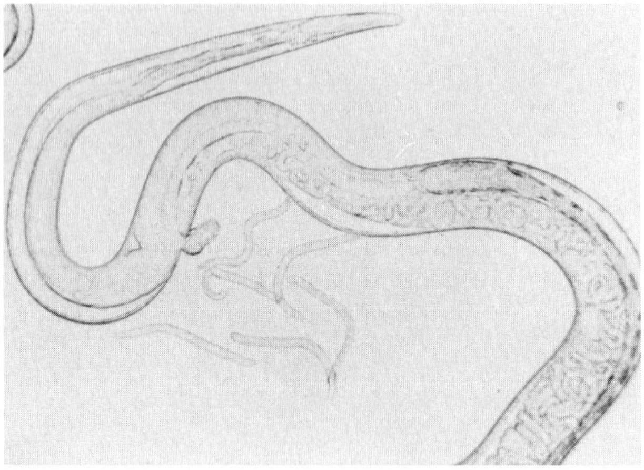

FIGURE 68.6. Newborn larvae (80 μm × 7 μm) *in utero* and expressed from a female adult *Trichinella spiralis* organism. ×250.

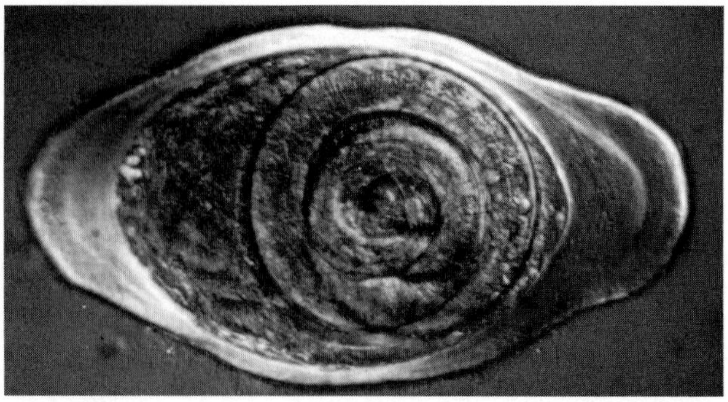

FIGURE 68.8. Nurse cell–parasite complex. Normarski-phase photomicrograph. ×200. (Courtesy of Eric Grave.)

(26). The rete consists of a complex network of vessels, similar in diameter to sinusoids (30 to 40 μm). Many vessels in the rete end blindly (27). Sinusoids would facilitate the rapid exchange of nutrients and wastes. When one considers the high metabolic demand for glucose that the Nurse cell–parasite complex, in its anaerobic environment, places on the host, the evolution of sinusoidal vessels may be an absolute requirement for the long-term maintenance (months and years in some cases) of this intimate relationship.

Nurse cells are generally believed to result from a series of exposures to the proteins secreted by the developing larva (28–30). They consist of some hundred or so novel peptides (31) and emanate from the stichosome of the parasite while it grows and develops within its intracellular niche. The stichosome consists of a row of discoid cells, each of which contains secretory granules of a single morphologic type. At least five unique stichocyte types are known.

A few secreted proteins enter host cell nuclei and remain there throughout the infection (28). Speculation favors a transcriptional role for these tyvelosylated, secreted parasite products (30,31). Their presence in hypertrophic nuclei within the Nurse cell can be reversed by the administration of low doses (i.e., noncurative) of mebendazole (32). However, none of these secreted proteins has yet been characterized in terms of its potential role(s) in Nurse cell formation.

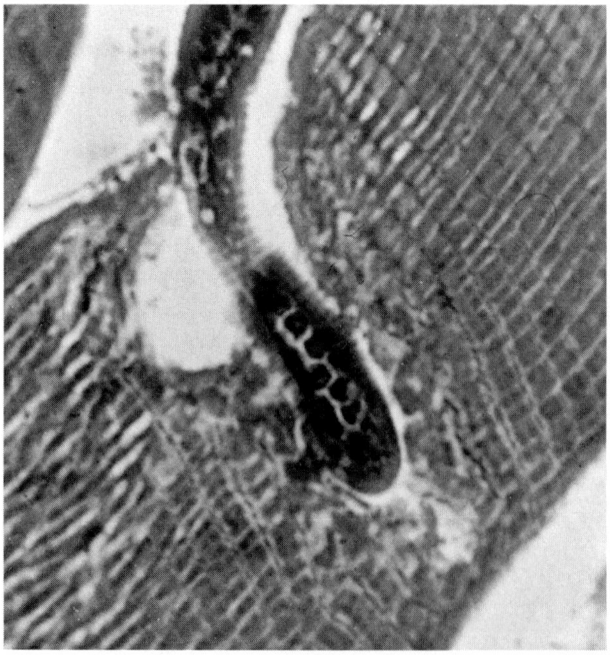

FIGURE 68.7. Newborn larva in *Trichinella spiralis* organism penetrating a muscle fiber. ×1,760.

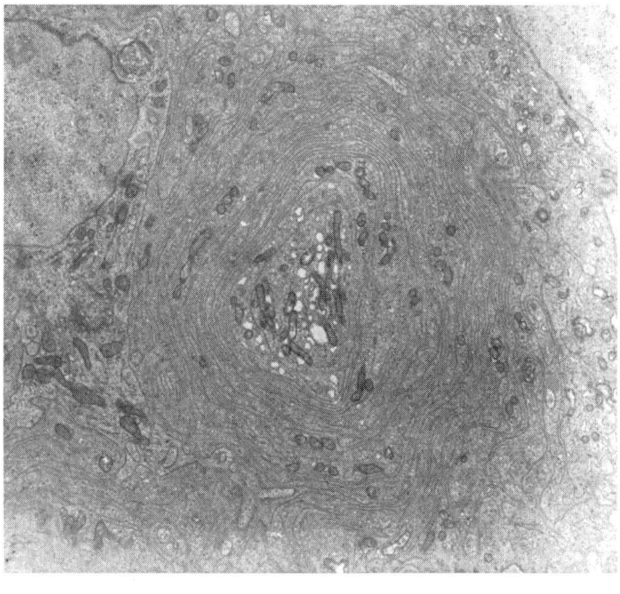

FIGURE 68.9. The cytoplasm of the mature Nurse cell–parasite complex consists of whorls of smooth membranes and collections of dysfunctional mitochondria. Electron micrograph. ×4,800.

EPIDEMIOLOGY

Within the last 10 years, outbreaks of trichinellosis in the United States have been rare and sporadic in nature (2). Most have been associated with the ingestion of raw or undercooked meats obtained from commercial sources. Pigs raised on individual farms, rather than on commercial factory farms, such as the ones in North Carolina, are more likely to be fed uncooked garbage and so acquire the infection. Feeding unprocessed garbage containing meat scraps is against federally mandated regulations, but the enforcement of laws governing the running of large production facilities is a full-time activity, and thousands of small farms throughout the country often escape the constant oversight of the U.S. Department of Agriculture inspectors.

In addition, hunters and those sharing their kills of carnivorous mammals—bear, fox, cougar, and the like—sometimes become infected by eating such meats undercooked or raw. Herbivores can harbor the infection (33–35) because most plant eaters occasionally ingest meat when the opportunity arises. Epidemics after the ingestion of raw horse meat have been reported in France and Italy (36,37).

In the United States, meat from slaughtered animals is not inspected for *Trichinella* larvae (Fig. 68.10). In Europe, the countries participating in the common market employ several strategies to examine meat for muscle larvae (38,39). Most serve to identify herds of infected animals from a given region. If pooled samples from any country are consistently negative after several years of inspection, then a *Trichinella*-free designation is applied to meat from that zone. Nonetheless, rare outbreaks occur even within these zones despite the system of inspection, primarily because of the existence of sylvatic cycles.

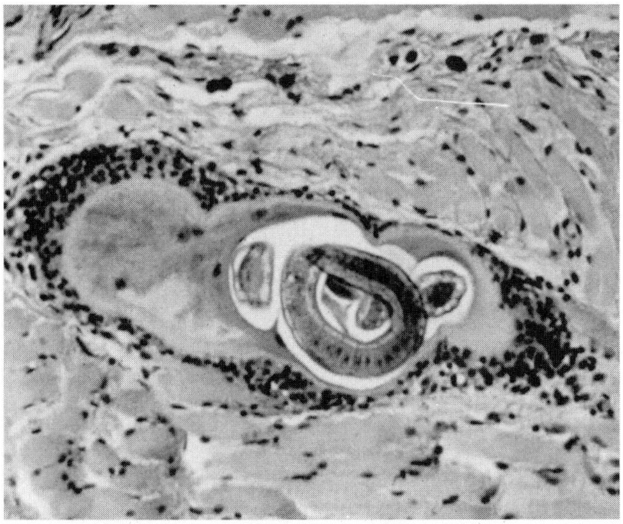

FIGURE 68.10. The Nurse cell–parasite complex elicits an intense mixed cellular inflammatory response during the first 40 to 50 days after the parasite enters the host cell. ×200.

PATHOGENESIS AND IMMUNITY

The enteral (intestinal) phase includes larval stages 1 through 4 and the immature and reproductive adult stages. In humans, this phase can last up to 3 weeks or more. Developing worms damage columnar epithelium, depositing shed cuticula there. Later in the infection, at the onset of the production of newborns, local inflammation, consisting of infiltration by eosinophils, neutrophils, and lymphocytes, intensifies in the local area (40) (Fig. 68.11). Villi flatten and become somewhat less absorbent, but not sufficiently for a malabsorption syndrome to develop.

When larvae penetrate the lymphatic circulation or bloodstream, a bacteremia caused by enteric flora may result. Circulating eosinophils are not elevated in this case. Severe infection can lead to death from sepsis (41). Wheat germ agglutinin receptors are lost along the entire small intestine (40). The myenteric electric potential is interrupted during the enteral phase, and as the result, gut motility slows down (40).

The parenteral phase of infection induces most of the pathologic consequences. It is dose-dependent (42,43) and directly attributable to the random penetration of cells (e.g., brain, liver, kidney, heart) by migrating newborn larvae as

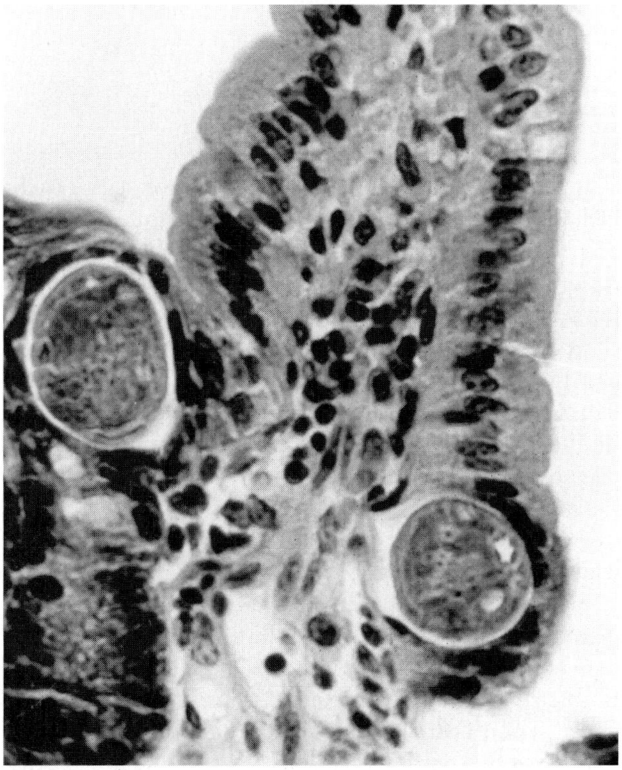

FIGURE 68.11. The enteral phase of the infection elicits an intense mixed cellular inflammatory response that is thought to be the dominant immune mechanism for expelling the worms from the host. This reaction is thought to be elicited by the adult worms during a primary infection. ×565.

they search for striated skeletal muscle cells. Cell death is the usual result of these events. The greater the number of penetration events that occur, the more severe the ensuing pathology (41). As a result, during heavy infection, a generalized edema develops (43). Proteinuria may follow. Cardiomyopathies and central nervous system abnormalities are also common in persons experiencing moderate to heavy infection (41).

Experimental infections in immunologically defined strains of rodents have shown that the total number of muscle larvae produced depends on numerous factors related to the immune capabilities of a given strain (16,44,45). The induction of interleukin-4 (IL-4) (46,47) and IL-9 (48), and the production of eosinophils and immunoglobulin E antibodies (IL-5 and IL-6) (46), appear to be essential for limiting the production of newborn larvae and expelling adult worms.

However, the induction of nitric oxide (NO) by tumor necrosis factor is not one of the effector mechanisms (49); knockout mice unable to produce NO expelled their parasites in normal fashion in the absence of local gut damage. In NO+ mice, the expulsion of adults was accompanied by cellular pathology surrounding the worms. Hence, the local production of NO during inflammation may have been a contributing factor in the development of intestinal pathology in infection with *T. spiralis.* Whether or not these mechanisms are invoked during human infection is not known.

CLINICAL DISEASE

The clinical features of mild, moderate, and severe trichinellosis have been reviewed (42,43). The nature of the disease state varies with time; as a result, trichinellosis can resemble a wide variety of clinical conditions. It is often misdiagnosed for this reason. As mentioned, the severity of clinical trichinellosis is dose-dependent, so that a diagnosis based solely on symptoms is difficult at best. However, certain clues, even in the early stages of the disease, should alert the physician to include trichinellosis in the differential diagnosis.

The first few days of infection are characterized by gastroenteritis associated with diarrhea, abdominal pain, and vomiting. Enteritis ensues that is secretory in nature (40). This phase is transitory and abates within 10 days after the ingestion of infected tissue. A history of eating raw or undercooked meats suggests the diagnosis of trichinellosis. If others who ate the same meats have similar symptoms, the suspicion of trichinellosis is reinforced. Unfortunately, most clinicians opt for a scenario of food poisoning at this point in the course of the infection.

The parenteral phase begins approximately 1 week after infection and may last several weeks. Typically, the patient has fever and myalgia, bilateral periorbital edema, and petechial hemorrhages, which are seen most clearly in the subungual skin but are also observed in the conjunctivae and mucous membranes. Muscle tenderness can be readily detected. Laboratory studies reveal a moderately elevated white blood cell count (12,000 to 15,000/mm^3) and a circulating eosinophilia ranging from 5% to 50% (41,50).

The penetration of tissues other than muscle by larvae gives rise to more serious sequelae (41). In many cases of moderate to severe infection, cardiovascular involvement leads to myocarditis. Electrocardiographic changes are frequently noted during this phase. Parasite invasion of the diaphragm and accessory muscles of respiration results in dyspnea. Neurotrichinellosis occurs in association with central nervous system invasion.

A convalescent phase follows the acute phase. Many Nurse cell–parasite complexes are destroyed by calcification following recovery. However, a few remain alive, even after some 30 years of exposure in one case (51).

Two clinical presentations have been described for *T. nativa* infections resulting from the ingestion of infected polar bear or walrus meat: a classic myopathic form and a second form that presents as a persistent diarrheal illness (52). The second form is thought to represent a secondary infection in previously sensitized persons.

DIAGNOSIS

The definitive diagnosis depends on the finding of Nurse cell–parasite complexes in muscle biopsy specimens by microscopic examination (Fig. 68.12) or the detection of *Trichinella*-specific DNA by PCR (53). PCR is very sensitive and specific for detecting small numbers of larvae in muscle tissue, but because it is infrequently requested and because it is expensive to maintain such a capability, PCR is not available in most hospital laboratories. This situation will undoubtedly change in the near future as more and more parasitic infections are diagnosed routinely by PCR-based methods.

Even in the heaviest of infections, sampling errors can cause a negative muscle biopsy result. In addition, the larvae may be at an early stage of development, so that they are inconspicuous even to the best-trained pathologist. A rising, plateauing, and falling level of circulating eosinophils throughout the infection period is not direct proof of infection, but with such information in hand, the clinician can treat as if the diagnosis of trichinellosis had been made. Bilateral periorbital edema, subungual petechiae, and high fever, coupled with a history of eating raw or undercooked meats, are further indirect evidence of this infection.

Muscle enzymes, such as creatine phosphokinase and lactate dehydrogenase, are released into the circulation, so that serum levels increase. The results of serologic tests become positive within 2 weeks. Enzyme-linked immunosorbent assay (ELISA) can detect antibodies in some patients as early as 12 days after infection (54).

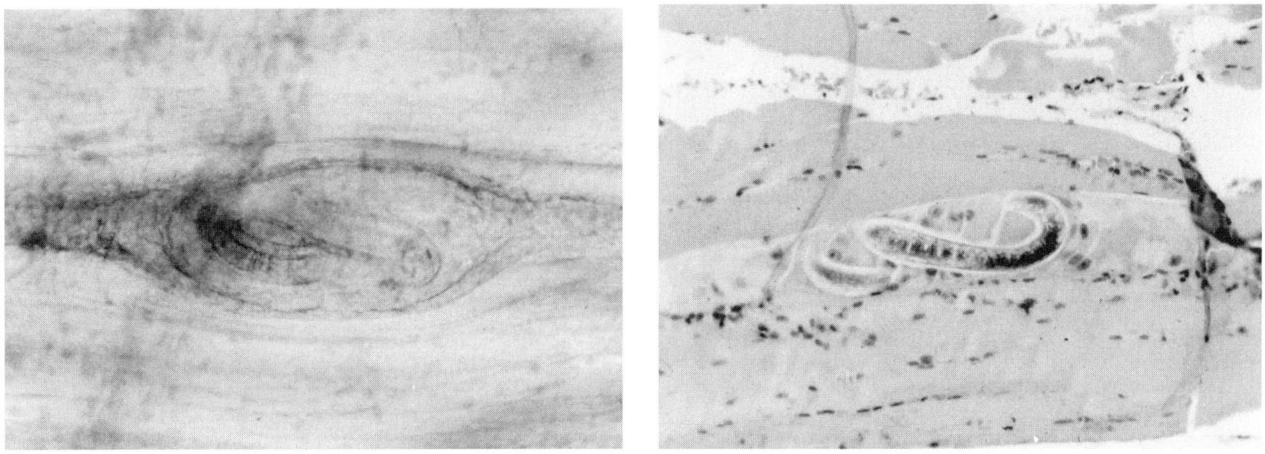

A B

FIGURE 68.12. Muscle biopsy specimen from two infected patients with clinical trichinellosis. **A:** The fact that the larva is mature indicates that the biopsy specimen was obtained 25 days or more after the patient ingested infected larvae. ×170. **B:** The larva has yet to achieve its full length, which suggests that the patient was recently infected (i.e., 15 to 20 days before the biopsy). ×175.

TREATMENT

No anthelmintic therapy is specific, even after a definitive diagnosis has been made. Mebendazole, if given early during the infection, may help reduce the number of larvae and so prevent further clinical complications, but the likelihood of obtaining a diagnosis in time to do so is remote (55). The dosage for both adults and children is 200 to 400 mg three times daily for 3 days, then 400 to 500 mg three times daily for 10 days, as recommended in the March 2000 issue of the *Medical Letter on Drugs and Therapeutics* (1000 Main Street, New Rochelle, New York 10801). Antiinflammatory corticosteroids, particularly prednisolone, are recommended if the diagnosis is secure. Rapidly destroying larvae with anthelmintics without the use of steroids may actually exacerbate host inflammatory responses and worsen disease (e.g., Jarisch–Herxheimer reaction). The myopathic phase is treated with antipyretics and analgesics (aspirin, acetaminophen), and these should be continued until the fever and allergic signs recede. Because of their immunosuppressive potential, steroids should be administered with caution.

PREVENTION

Trichinellosis caused by *T. spiralis* can be prevented either by cooking meat thoroughly at 58.5°C for 10 minutes or by freezing it at −20°C for 3 days. The U.S. Department of Agriculture issued the following statement on its Web site regarding the control and prevention of *T. spiralis* infection:

> "Trichinosis is unique among the parasites encountered in meat inspection in that it cannot be diagnosed by gross examination of the carcass and, as yet, there is no test that will guarantee absolute freedom from the presence of the parasite in pork. We must therefore assume that all swine are infested and must be sufficiently treated to destroy trichinae by heating, freezing, curing, or use of irradiation. The consumer is expected to thoroughly cook those fresh pork cuts that have not been processed to destroy trichinae."

Nevertheless, no coordinated educational program from the U.S. Department of Agriculture conveys this important message to the consumer. Nor is it required that the warning and advice appear on labels on all fresh cuts of pork.

A different strategy is required to prevent infection with other species of *Trichinella* because they are found mostly in wild animals. For example, substances in the muscles of bears and raccoons that prevent the formation of ice crystals during hibernation inadvertently permit the larvae to survive at temperatures below freezing. Hence, the only way to render those meats edible is to cook them thoroughly.

In the United States, most (90% to 95%) infections with *T. spiralis* can be traced back to a single episode of eating undercooked or raw pork purchased from commercial sources (e.g., sausage) (2). In addition, some outbreaks have been traced to ground beef adulterated with pork scraps.

In the United States, tracing a sample of contaminated pork that has been sold commercially back to its farm source is often futile because the origin of individual pigs cannot be identified after the animals are sold at auction. As pointed out, small farms that raise pigs for local consumption are not usually subjected to the same enforcement of U.S. Department of Agriculture regulations as are large-scale factory hog operations (so-called factory farms). Hence, meat scraps and wild rodents often enter the digestive tract of solitary animals raised more as an afterthought than for food. For this reason alone, trichinellosis will always present as sporadic epidemics.

REFERENCES

1. Zarlenga DS, Chute MB, Martin A, et al. A multiplex PCR for unequivocal differentiation of all encapsulated and non-encapsulated genotypes of *Trichinella. Int J Parasitol* 1999;29: 1859–1867.
2. Moorehead A, Grunenwald PE, Deitz VJ, et al. Trichinellosis in the United States, 1991–1996: declining but not gone. *Am J Trop Med Hyg* 1999;60:66–69.
3. Haim M, Efrat M, Wilson M, et al. An outbreak of *Trichinella spiralis* infection in southern Lebanon. *Epidemiol Infect* 1997; 119:357–362.
4. Sohn WM, Kim HM, Chung DI, et al. The first human case of *Trichinella spiralis* infection in Korea. *Korean J Parasitol* 2000; 38:111–115.
5. Pozio E, La Rosa G. *Trichinella murrelli* n. sp: etiological agent of sylvatic trichinellosis in temperate areas of North America. *J Parasitol* 2000;86:134–139.
6. Jongwutiwes S, Chantachum N, Kravichina P, et al. First outbreak of human trichinellosis caused by *Trichinella pseudospiralis. Clin Infect Dis* 1998;26:111–115.
7. Pozio E, Owen IL, LaRosa G, et al. *Trichinella paupae* n. sp. (Nematoda), a new non-encapsulated species from domestic and sylvatic swine. *Int J Parasitol* 1999;29:1825–1839.
8. Pozio E, Kapel CM. *Trichinella nativa* in sylvatic wild boars. *J Helminthol* 1999;73:87–89.
9. Pozio E, Miller I, Jarvis T, et al. Distribution of sylvatic species of *Trichinella* in Estonia according to climate zones. *J Parasitol* 1998;84:193–195.
10. La Rosa G, Pozio E. Molecular investigation of African isolates of *Trichinella* reveals genetic polymorphism in *Trichinella nelsoni. Int J Parasitol* 2000;30:663–667.
11. Stewart GL, Despommier DD, Burnham J, et al. *Trichinella spiralis*: behavioral, structural, and biochemical studies on larvae following exposure to components of the host enteric environment. *Exp Parasitol* 1987;63:195–204.
12. Modha J, Roberts MC, Robertson WM, et al. The surface coat of infective larvae of *Trichinella spiralis. Parasitology* 1999;118: 509–522.
13. Despommier D. Behavioral cues in migration and location of parasitic nematodes, with special emphasis on *Trichinella spiralis.* In: Bailey WS, ed. *Cues that influence behavior of internal parasites.* Auburn, AL: Agricultural Research Service Workshop, May, 1982:110–126.
14. Wright K. *Trichinella spiralis*: an intracellular parasite in the intestinal phase. *J Parasitol* 1979;65:441–445.
15. Despommier DD. *Trichinella spiralis* and the concept of niche. *J Parasitol* 1993;79:472–482.
16. Despommier DD. Biology. In: Campbell WC, ed. *Trichinella and trichinellosis.* New York: Plenum Publishing, 1983:75–152.
17. Bell RG. The generation and expression of immunity to *Trichinella spiralis* in laboratory rodents. *Adv Parasitol* 1998; 41:149–217.
18. Despommier DD. How does *Trichinella* make itself a home? *Parasitol Today* 1998;14:318–323.
19. Despommier DD. The worm that would be virus. *Parasitol Today* 1990;6:193–196.
20. Despommier DD, Aron L, Turgeon L. *Trichinella spiralis*: growth of the intracellular (muscle) larva. *Exp Parasitol* 1975;37:108–116.
21. Despommier DD. Adaptive changes in muscle fibers infected with *Trichinella spiralis. Am J Pathol* 1975;78:477–484.
22. Despommier DD, Symmans WF, Dell R. Changes in Nurse cell nuclei during synchronous infection with *Trichinella spiralis. J Parasitol* 1991;77:290–295.
23. Jasmer DP. *Trichinella spiralis*-infected skeletal muscle cells arrest in G2/M and cease muscle gene expression. *J Cell Biol* 1993;121: 785–793.
24. Polvere RI, Kabash C, Kadan I, et al. *Trichinella spiralis*: collagen type IV and type VI synthesis. *Exp Parasitol* 1997;86:191–199.
25. Capo V, Despommier DD, Polvere RI. *Trichinella spiralis*: vascular endothelial growth factor is up-regulated within the Nurse cell during the early phase of its formation. *J Parasitol* 1998;84: 209–214.
26. Pagenstecher HA. *Die Trichinen.* Leipzig: Engelsmanns, 1865. 116 pp.
27. Baruch AM, Despommier DD. Blood vessels in *Trichinella spiralis* infections: a study using vascular casts. *J Parasitol* 1991;77: 290–295.
28. Despommier DD, Gold AM, Buck SW, et al. *Trichinella spiralis*: a secreted antigen of the infective Ll larva localizes to the cytoplasm and nucleoplasm of infected host cells. *Exp Parasitol* 1990; 72:27–38.
29. Li CK, Chung YY, Ko RC. The distribution of excretory/secretory antigens during the muscle phase of *Trichinella spiralis* and *T. pseudospiralis* infections. *Parasitol Res* 1999;85:993–998.
30. Yao C, Jasmer DP. Nuclear antigens in *Trichinella spiralis*-infected muscle cells: nuclear extraction, compartmentalization and complex formation. *Mol Biochem Parasitol* 1998;92:207–218.
31. Wu Z, Nagano I, Takahashi Y. A panel of antigens of muscle larvae of *Trichinella spiralis* and *T. pseudospiralis* as revealed by two-dimensional Western blot and immunoelectron microscopy. *Parasitology* 1999;118:615–622.
32. Yao C, Bohnet S, Jasmer DP. Host nuclear abnormalities and depletion of nuclear antigens induced in *Trichinella spiralis*-infected muscle cells by the anthelmintic mebendazole. *Mol Biochem Parasitol* 1998;96:1–13.
33. Dworkin MS, Gamble HR, Zarlenga DS, et al. Outbreak of trichinellosis associated with eating cougar jerky. *J Infect Dis* 1996;174:663–666.
34. Malczewska M, Malczewski A, Rocki B, et al. The red fox (*Vulpes vulpes*) as reservoir of *Trichinella* sp in Poland. *Wiad Parazytol* 1997;43:303–306.
35. Nutter FB, Levine JF, Stoskopf MK, et al. Seroprevalence of *Toxoplasma gondii*and *Trichinella spiralis* in North Carolina black bears (*Ursus americanus*). *J Parasitol* 1998;84:1048–1050.
36. Arriaga C, Yepez-Mulia L, Viveros N, et al. Detection of *Trichinella spiralis* muscle larvae in naturally infected horses. *J Parasitol* 1995;81:781–783.
37. Dupouy-Camet J, Soule C, Ancelle T. Recent news on trichinellosis: another outbreak due to horse meat consumption in France in 1993. *Parasite* 1994;1:99–103.
38. Nockler K, Voigt WP, Protz D, et al. Intravitale Diagnostik der Trichinellose beim Schwein mit dem indirekten ELISA. *Berl Munch TerarztWochenschr* 1995;108:167–174.
39. Gamble HR. Factors affecting the efficiency of pooled sample digestion for the recovery of *Trichinella spiralis* from muscle tissue. *Int J Food Microbiol* 1999;48:73–78.
40. Castro GA, Bullock GR. Pathophysiology of the gastrointestinal phase. In: Campbell WC, ed. *Trichinella and trichinellosis.* New York: Plenum Publishing,1983:209–241.
41. Kociecka W. Early clinical syndromes of severe trichinellosis. In: Campbell WC, Pozio E, Bruschi F, eds. *Trichinellosis. Proceedings of the Eighth International Conference on Trichinellosis,* Orvieto, Italy, 1993:475–480.
42. Murrell D, Bruschi F. Clinical trichinellosis. In: Sun T, ed. *Progress in clinical parasitology.* Boca Raton, FL: CRC Press, 1994: 117–150.
43. Capo V, Despommier DD. Clinical aspects of infection with *Trichinella* spp. *Clin Microbiol Rev* 1996;9:47–54.
44. Finkleman FD, Shea-Donahue T, Goldhill J, et al. Cytokine regulation of host defense against parasitic gastrointestinal nema-

todes: lessons from studies with rodent models. *Annu Rev Immunol* 1997;15:505–533.
45. Stear MJ, Wakelin D. Genetic resistance to parasitic infection. *Rev Sci Tech* 1998;17:143–153.
46. Hermanek J, Goyal PK, Wakelin D. Lymphocyte, antibody and cytokine responses during concurrent infections between helminths that selectively promote T-helper-1 or T-helper-2 activity. *Parasite Immunol* 1994;16:111–117.
47. Lawrence CE, Paterson JC, Higgins LM, et al. IL-4–regulated enteropathy in an intestinal nematode infection. *Eur J Immunol* 1998;28:2672–2684.
48. Wakelin D. Immune responses to intestinal parasites: protection, pathology and prophylaxis. *Parassitologia* 1997;39:269–274.
49. Lawrence CE, Paterson JC, Wei XQ, et al. Nitric oxide mediates intestinal pathology but not immune expulsion during *Trichinella spiralis* infection in mice. *J Immunol* 2000;164:4229–4234.
50. Kociecka W, Mrozewicz B, Gustowska L. Clinical aspects of late sequelae of trichinellosis. *Wiad Parazytol* 1997;43:309–311.
51. Froscher W, Gullotta M, Saatoff M, et al. Chronic trichinosis. Clinical, bioptic, serologic, and electromyographic observations. *Eur Neurol* 1989;28:221–226.
52. MacClean JD, Poirier L, Gyorkos TW, et al. Epidemiologic and serologic definition of primary and secondary trichinosis in the arctic. *J Infect Dis* 1992;165:908–912.
53. Wu Z, Nagano I, Pozio E, et al. Polymerase chain reaction-restriction fragment length polymorphism (PCR-RLFP) for the identification of *Trichinella* isolates. *Parasitology* 1999;118: 211–218.
54. Despommier DD. Trichinellosis. In: Schantz PM, Walls KW, eds. *Helminth diseases.* Orlando, FL: Academic Press, 1987: 43–60 (*Immunodiagnosis of parasitic diseases,* vol 1).
55. Drugs for parasitic infections. *Med Lett Drugs Ther* 2000.

69

HOOKWORM INFECTIONS

PETER J. HOTEZ

Approximately 1 billion persons are thought to harbor one or more species of hookworms, which cause intestinal blood loss that leads to iron deficiency and anemia (1). Certain human populations are particularly susceptible to the effects of chronic hookworm anemia. Deficits in physical, intellectual, psychomotor, and cognitive development are frequently seen in children with moderate or heavy hookworm infection (2); therefore, hookworm infection affects both the health and education of school-age children. Hookworm also affects an estimated 44 million pregnant women, of whom 3 to 5 million have worm burdens sufficiently heavy to affect the fetus (3). Because it occurs insidiously, hookworm infection is frequently overlooked as a major cause of global morbidity.

Hookworms were not recognized as etiologic agents of disease until the middle of the nineteenth century and did not receive widespread attention until they were implicated as the cause of "miner's anemia" among Italian laborers constructing the Saint Gotthard railway tunnel in the Swiss Alps (4). The life cycle of *Ancylostoma duodenale* was elucidated by Looss (5), a German scientist working in Egypt, and the life cycle of *Necator americanus* was elucidated by Stiles (6), a U.S. government scientist. At one time, hookworm infection was common throughout the southeastern United States. In the early part of the twentieth century, the South was the target of a vigorous hookworm control campaign carried out by the Rockefeller Sanitary Commission (7).

MICROBIOLOGY AND LIFE CYCLE

Hookworms are bursate nematodes (order Strongyloidea) of the family Ancylostomidae, which are distinguished by their highly cuticularized buccal capsules provided with teeth or cutting plates (8). *Ancylostoma* and *Necator* are the only medically important genera (Fig. 69.1).

Necator

N. americanus is the only human pathogen of this genus. It is known as the "New World" hookworm because of its widespread distribution in the Caribbean and the Americas. Small foci still remain in North America, particularly in Mexico and possibly even the southeastern United States. Despite its "New World" designation, *N. ameri-*

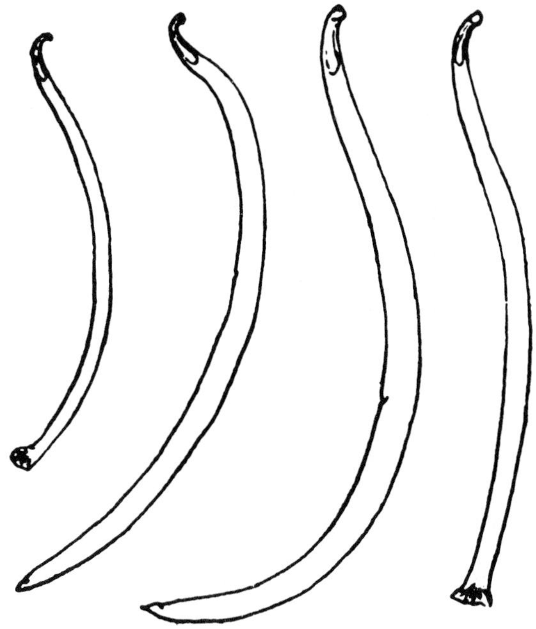

FIGURE 69.1. Outline drawings showing relative length and shape of *Necator americanus* and *Ancylostoma duodenale*. **Left to right:** *N. americanus* male, *N. americanus* female, *A. duodenale* female, *A. duodenale* male. ×10. (From Chandler AC. *Hookworm disease: its distribution, biology, epidemiology, pathology, diagnosis, treatment, and control*. New York: Macmillan, 1929.)

P. J. Hotez: Department of Microbiology and Tropical Medicine, George Washington University Medical Center, Washington D.C.

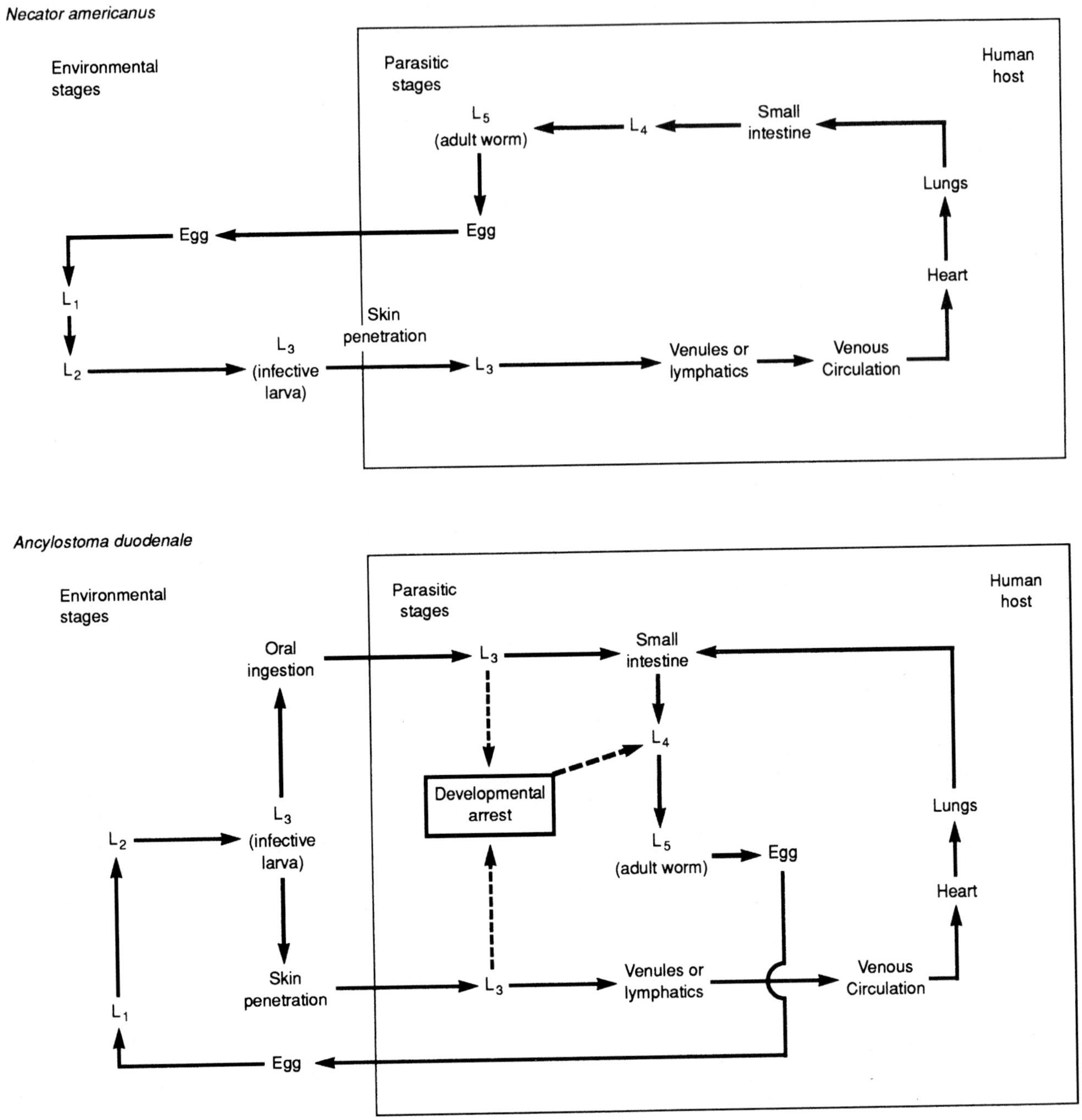

FIGURE 69.2. Life cycles of *Necator americanus* and *Ancylostoma duodenale*, showing environmental and parasitic stages.

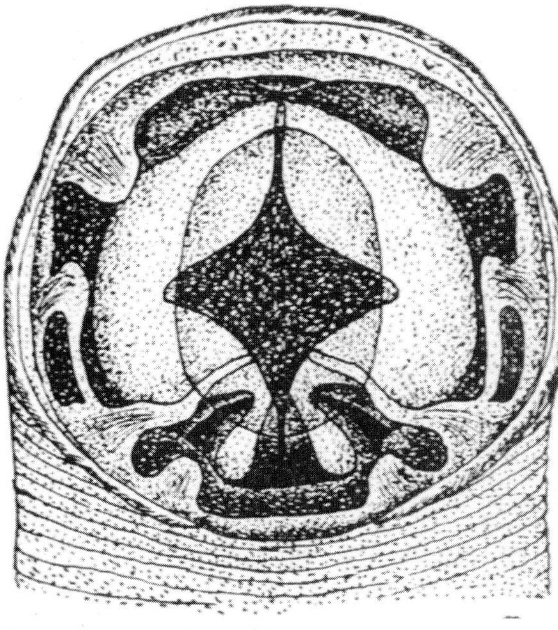

FIGURE 69.3. Mouth capsule of *Necator americanus.* (From Chandler AC. *Hookworm disease: its distribution, biology, epidemiology, pathology, diagnosis, treatment, and control.* New York: Macmillan, 1929.)

canus is also a major pathogen in sub-Saharan Africa, Southeast Asia, and the Pacific Islands. It is presumed to have been introduced to the Americas by slaves and colonists from Africa (8). In terms of distribution, *N. americanus* is the predominant hookworm affecting humans. *N. americanus* has only a single route of infection, which is the percutaneous entry of third-stage infective larvae (Fig. 69.2). On entering the host, the larvae are swept from the skin in lymphatics and venules to the right side of the heart and then to pulmonary capillaries. The larvae enter the lung parenchyma, ascending the alveoli, bronchioles, bronchi, and trachea before being coughed and swallowed. The larvae molt twice and sexually differentiate into male (7 to 9 mm in length) and female (9 to 11 mm in length) adults, which live for 5 to 6 years (9). *N. americanus* has a relatively small buccal capsule, which is armed with cutting plates that facilitate attachment to the intestinal mucosa (Fig. 69.3). A single female *N. americanus* organism produces 6,000 to 11,000 eggs a day (after a prepatent period of 45 to 60 days); these develop optimally at temperatures of 25°C to 28°C when deposited in feces onto moist soil (8). The resulting first-stage larva undergoes two successive molts to become an infective filariform larva (Fig. 69.4). The third larval stage is nonfeeding and capable of considerable vertical movement, migrating to the soil surface or low vegetation to facilitate human contact and renew the life cycle (10).

Ancylostoma

Three members of the genus *Ancylostoma* have been found to be parasites of humans (Fig. 69.5). Of these, *A. duodenale* is by far the most important human pathogen, whereas infection with *A. ceylanicum* or the dog hookworm *A. caninum* has been described in humans within restricted geographic areas.

A. duodenale is known as the "Old World" hookworm, a term that refers to its distribution in the Mediterranean regions of Africa and Europe and in India and China. However, even in India and China, *N. americanus* is still the predominant hookworm, with *A. duodenale* restricted primarily to somewhat more northerly latitudes. Focal pockets of distribution also exist in Latin America (11). A number of features of *A. duodenale* distinguish it from *N. americanus,* including its larger size (8 to 11 mm for an adult male, 10 to 13 mm for an adult female), greater fecundity (10,000 to 30,000 eggs per day), greater virulence (adult worms cause greater blood loss), and shortened life span. These features led Hoagland and Schad (12) to postulate that *A. duodenale* is the more "opportunistic species." Like the larvae of *N. americanus, A. duodenale* larvae can infect humans percutaneously. However, *A. duodenale* larvae are also infective via the oral route. In some geographic areas, oral ingestion may be the predominant route of transmission. Another unusual feature of *A. duodenale* larvae is their capacity for arrested development in the tissues after host entry (13). It has been suggested that the phenomenon of arrested development explains the seasonal variation in the egg output of humans with *A. duodenale* infection (13). It has been further hypothesized that the arrested larvae can mobilize from the tissues to the colostrum and breast milk, so that vertical transmission of ancylostomiasis to infants occurs (2,14). The mechanisms by which hookworm larvae remain in an arrested state is not known, although a phenotypic similarity between arrested hookworm larvae and the "dauer" larval stage of the free-living nematode *Caenorhabditis elegans* has been noted (15). Conceivably, similar environmental cues and signal transduction molecules have a role in *A. duodenale.*

A. ceylanicum is primarily a hookworm of dogs and cats. However, it is also a minor parasite of humans in India and Southeast Asia. Unlike *A. duodenale, A. ceylanicum* does not cause significant blood loss (16). The classic cause of canine hookworm infection, *A. caninum,* may under some circumstances be transmitted as a zoonotic agent to humans. A single acquired adult *A. caninum* worm in the gastrointestinal tract causes an eosinophilic enteritis syndrome (see later discussion). Eosinophilic enteritis associated with *A. caninum* infection has been reported only from northern Queensland, Australia (17), although some evidence indicates that it may occur in other parts of the world. The dog and cat hookworm, *A. braziliense,* cannot complete its life cycle in

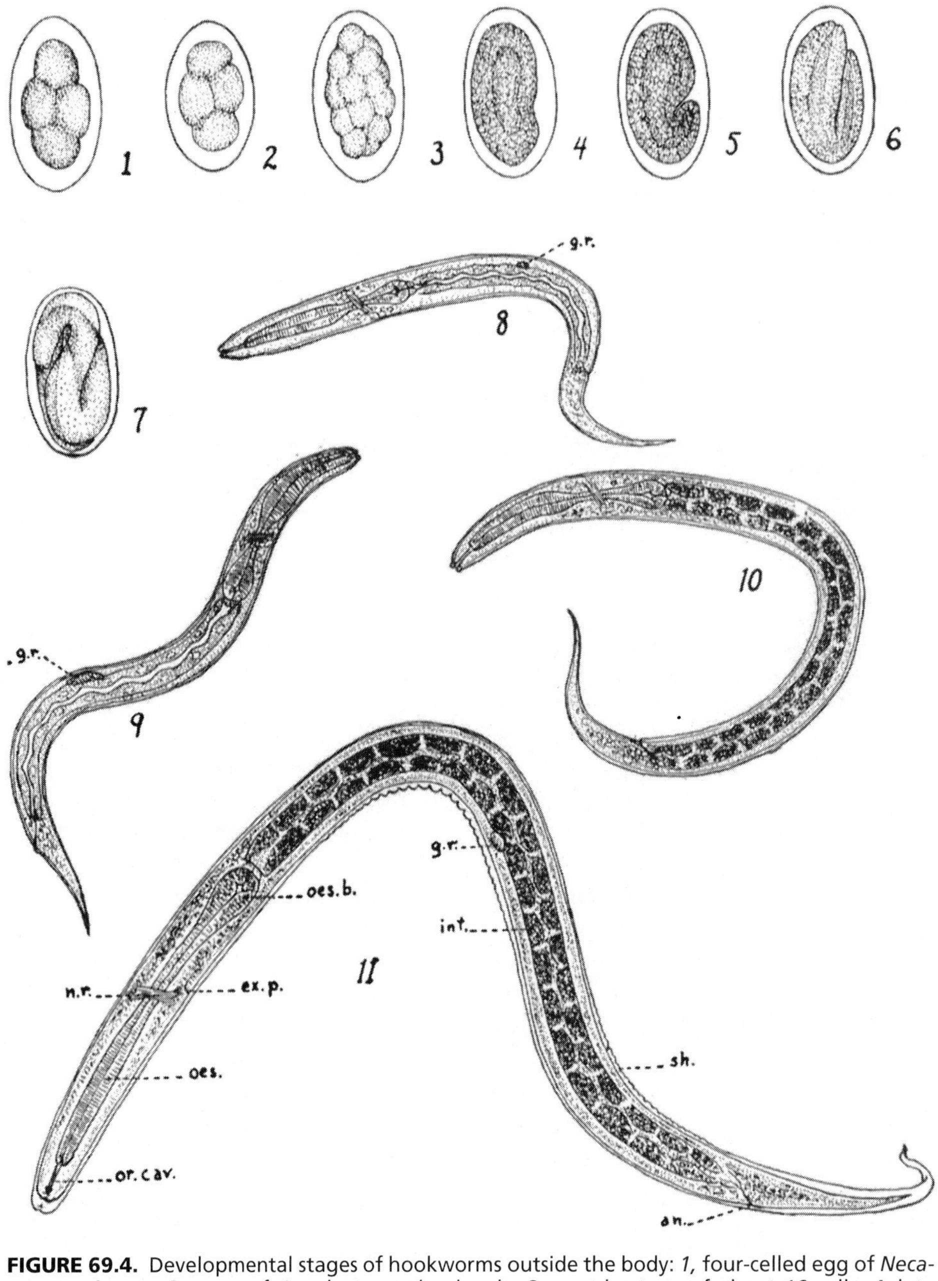

FIGURE 69.4. Developmental stages of hookworms outside the body: *1,* four-celled egg of *Necator americanus*; *2,* same of *Ancylostoma duodenale*; *3,* morula stage of about 16 cells; *4,* late morula stage; *5,* early tadpole stage; *6,* late tadpole stage; *7,* developed embryo in egg; *8,* newly hatched embryo; *9,* newly hatched *Strongyloides* embryo for comparison; *10,* larva after first molt; *11,* infective larva. ×500. (From Chandler AC. *Hookworm disease: its distribution, biology, epidemiology, pathology, diagnosis, treatment, and control*. New York: Macmillan, 1929.)

humans; rather, it migrates aberrantly in the skin to cause cutaneous larva migrans (18).

EPIDEMIOLOGY

Because appropriate soil conditions are needed to facilitate egg development and permit survival of the larval stages, the epidemiology of hookworm infection is intimately connected to the soil and human agricultural pursuits. In general, favorable transmission requires moist soil (either through rainfall or irrigation), humidity, warm temperatures, and shade. These conditions can also frequently be met in mines and tunnels. In contrast, unshaded open areas, salinity, and compacted and water-logged soils are unfavorable for transmission (10).

With the appropriate climactic and soil conditions, high-intensity hookworm infection will develop in a

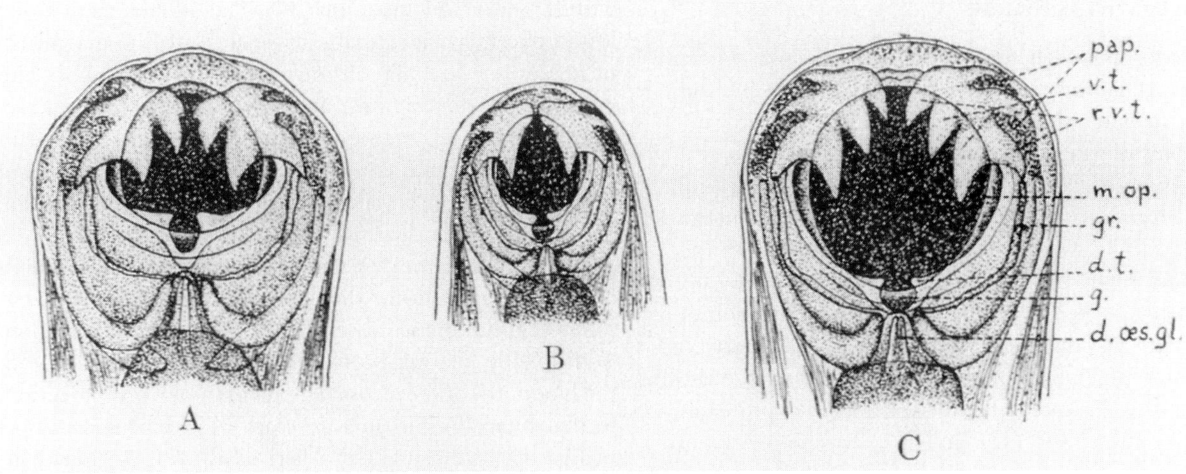

FIGURE 69.5. Buccal capsules of three species of *Ancylostoma*: *A. duodenale* **(A)**, *A. braziliense* **(B)**, and *A. caninum* **(C)**. (From Chandler AC. *Hookworm disease: its distribution, biology, epidemiology, pathology, diagnosis, treatment, and control*. New York: Macmillan, 1929.)

community provided its members are likely to come into contact with human feces (11). This generally occurs in one of three settings (10): (a) areas lacking appropriate sanitation or where indiscriminate defecation occurs; (b) areas where inadequately composted human excreta are used as fertilizer; or (c) highly focal areas of human defecation, such as in mines and tunnels and on plantations. Certain agricultural pursuits, such as the cultivation of coffee beans, tea, mulberry leaves, and sugar cane, are notorious for facilitating high rates of hookworm transmission.

In any given area of endemicity, the distribution of infection in a community often varies widely (10). Most persons usually harbor a light infection, whereas only a few harbor a heavy infection. Curiously, the subset of people who harbor large numbers of worms will, if treated, reacquire heavy worm burdens if left to live in the same area of endemicity (19). This predisposition to infection has been noted with other human helminth infections; its basis is unknown.

Endemic hookworm infection frequently shows an age-associated prevalence and intensity that differ from those of infections with other so-called geohelminths (e.g., *Ascaris* and *Trichuris*). For instance, in *Ascaris* and *Trichuris* infections, the prevalence and intensity classically are highest among school-age children. However, the age-associated pattern of hookworm infection in areas of endemicity is frequently not straightforward. Although heavy infections are noted among children in some regions, it is also common to find a rise in the prevalence and intensity of hookworm infection as a function of age. This appears to be particularly true of *N. americanus* infections, the most severe cases of which can sometimes be identified among elderly populations.

PATHOGENESIS AND IMMUNITY

Migratory Phase

Infective hookworm larvae elicit two types of histopathology, depending on their mode of host entry.

Third-stage larvae that infect percutaneously cause mechanical, chemical, and inflammatory damage to all layers of the skin. In the epidermis, the larvae separate epidermal keratinocytes, a process facilitated by the release of a parasite hyaluronidase that breaks the hyaluronan bridges connecting these cells (20). Epidermal entry is usually followed by penetration through the basement membrane into the dermis. A zinc metalloprotease released by invading larvae (21,22) may help to dissolve the major connective tissue macromolecular barriers chemically. Hookworm larvae also release a family of cysteine-rich secretory proteins during host entry. Known as *Ancylostoma*-secreted proteins (ASPs), these polypeptides have partial homology to the venom proteins of stinging insects (23–25). The function of the ASPs is not known.

When hookworm larvae invade the skin, the host responds by mounting an intense inflammatory response ("ground itch"). The features of ground itch resemble those of both immediate and delayed-type hypersensitivity reactions; the condition probably results from the elaboration of cytokines by keratinocytes and the infiltration of immunocompetent cells into the skin. Eicosanoids released by hookworm larvae may also contribute to cutaneous inflammation (26).

As noted earlier, hookworm larvae of the species *A. duodenale* may also enter the gastrointestinal tract directly by oral ingestion. When large numbers of larvae enter at once, a second type of hookworm-associated hypersensitivity syndrome, known as *Wakana disease,* may occur (27).

Gastrointestinal Phase

Adult hookworms attach to the intestinal mucosa, where they cause mechanical and chemical damage. Mechanical damage occurs when the buccal capsule of the parasite surrounds a bolus of intestinal mucosa and holds onto it by a combination of specialized teeth (*A. duodenale*) or cutting plates (*N. americanus*). As the esophageal muscles of the parasite contract, a small vacuum is created that fixes the bolus of mucosa in the buccal capsule (28) (Fig. 69.6). Chemical damage to the intestinal mucosal bolus subsequently occurs via the action of several parasite-derived hydrolytic enzymes, which presumably are released into the buccal capsule. Released hydrolases include proteases (29–31), a hyaluronidase (32), and an acetylcholinesterase (33). Ultimately, the ingested mucosal bolus is degraded (28).

One consequence of hookworm attachment is the ultimate rupture and destruction of capillaries contained within the lamina propria, resulting in blood extravasation (28). Some blood leaks at the site of attachment, although much of it is ingested by the worm. A continuous flow of blood is guaranteed by the release of parasite-derived anticoagulants, including a small polypeptide that inhibits factor Xa (34), an antiinflammatory polypeptide (35), and a platelet anti-aggregating factor (36). The degree of hookworm-associated blood loss is species-dependent; the greatest loss occurs with *A. duodenale* infection, approximately 10-fold less with *N. americanus* infection, and almost none with *A. ceylanicum* infection (37). The differences in blood loss between species usually correlate with the magnitude of hookworm anemia, although the onset of anemia also depends on dietary iron intake and host iron reserves (38,39). However, even iron deficiency that does not result in clinical anemia can severely impair the host. For instance, iron is essential for the development and function of dopaminergic neurons and as a prosthetic group in biosynthetic enzymes for neurotransmitters (40); iron deficiency may account for the deficits in intellectual and cognitive development observed in hookworm infection. Additionally, plasma proteins are lost in association with the blood loss and mucosal edema of hookworm infection, so that hypoalbuminemia develops (41). Changes in normal gastric acidity (41) and peristalsis (42) also may contribute to the gastrointestinal pathology of hookworm infection.

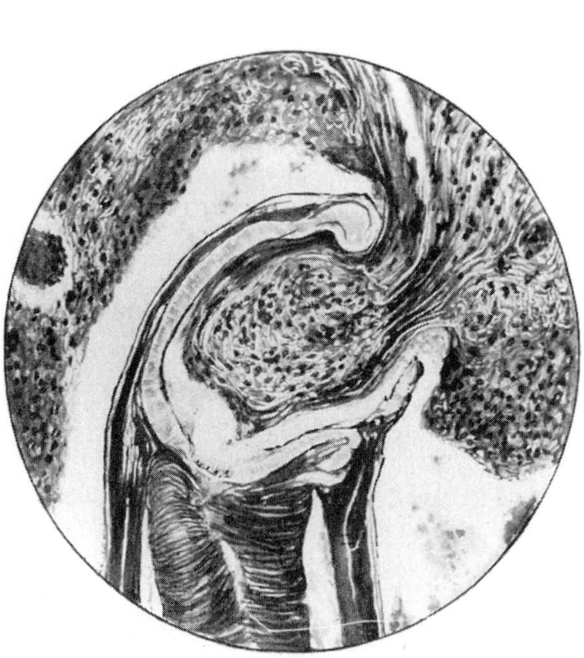

FIGURE 69.6. Photomicrograph of *Necator americanus* attached to intestinal mucosa. (From Dock G and Bass CC. *Hookworm disease, etiology, pathology, diagnosis, disease, prognosis, and treatment.* St. Louis: Mosby, 1910.)

Immunity

No compelling evidence indicates that humans mount an effective immune response to naturally acquired hookworm infection. In contrast, age-acquired resistance can be demonstrated during infection with other geohelminths (43). Hookworm-infected persons have circulating antibodies to hookworm antigens, but they do not correlate with resistance (44). The absence of clear-cut immunity has led a number of investigators to postulate the existence of different means of immune evasion and escape.

CLINICAL DISEASE

Migratory Phase

Ground itch is an intensely pruritic papular dermatitis, usually on the hands and feet. A distinct cutaneous manifestation, known as *cutaneous larva migrans* ("creeping eruption") develops when canine or feline hookworm larvae (especially *A. braziliense*) enter the epidermis and migrate laterally to elicit long, serpiginous tracks that become raised and crusted (18). Both of these cutaneous manifestations are frequently accompanied by secondary bacterial invasion.

Lung involvement secondary to the pulmonary migration of hookworm larvae is usually not severe but may result in a pneumonitis with dyspnea, cough, and wheezing. Wakana disease is a gastrointestinal syndrome associated with the ingestion of large numbers of *A. duodenale* infective larvae; it is characterized by nausea, vomiting, cough, dyspnea, and eosinophilia (26).

Gastrointestinal Phase

The hallmark of the gastrointestinal phase of hookworm infection is iron deficiency and iron deficiency anemia resulting from intestinal blood loss. This phase usually begins 10 to 20 weeks after the initial exposure to infective hookworm larvae. However, with strains of *A. duodenale* larvae that are prone to undergo arrest, the gastrointestinal phase may not occur for several months (45).

A variety of gastrointestinal symptoms have been described in naturally infected patients and human volunteers, including postprandial epigastric pain, nausea, and mild diarrhea (46,47). Patients with gastrointestinal symptoms of hookworm infection often report some relief after eating clay or other bulky substances.

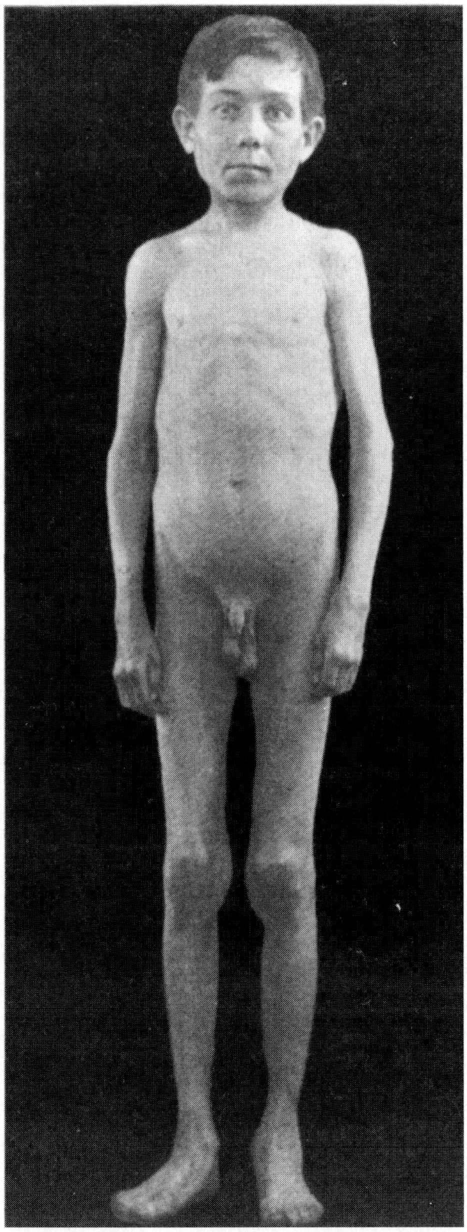

FIGURE 69.7. Hookworm subject, 22 years old. Three hundred hookworms were expelled from this patient, but he became reinfected. (From Dock G and Bass CC. *Hookworm disease, etiology, pathology, diagnosis, disease, prognosis, and treatment*. St. Louis: Mosby, 1910.)

Hookworm anemia can be severe enough to cause exertional dyspnea, lassitude, palpitations, and even high-output heart failure. The physical signs of hookworm anemia include pale sclerae, koilonychia, and cardiac flow murmurs. An extreme form of hookworm anemia associated with a high mortality rate has been described in infants with ancylostomiasis in whom melena, extreme paleness, diarrhea, and anorexia develop (14).

More commonly, however, heavily infected persons have chronic hookworm anemia, which is often exacerbated by underlying malnutrition (Fig. 69.7). Children especially can manifest signs and symptoms of moderate kwashiorkor (2). Curiously, the skin of these patients often acquires a yellow–green pallor, known as *chlorosis* (48); in dark-skinned patients, areas of depigmentation may develop. Probably the most devastating effect of chronic hookworm anemia in childhood is the long-term impairment of intellectual and physical growth. Although growth retardation is most apparent at the time of puberty (49), it is probably a continuous process throughout childhood; however, it can be partly reversed by interventions with either specific anthelmintic chemotherapy (50,51) or oral iron supplementation (52). Delays in intellectual, cognitive, and psychomotor development also occur in association with chronic hookworm anemia (53–55), probably as a direct consequence of long-standing iron deficiency (1,52). Unlike growth retardation, which can be reversed with "catch-up" growth, these delays in mental development may be permanent when they occur in infancy and early childhood.

Eosinophilic Enteritis

Eosinophilic enteritis was described recently in a series of patients from northern Queensland, Australia, who harbored the adult dog hookworm, *A. caninum* (17). The patients presented with severe abdominal pain, weight loss, and melena in association with elevated serum immunoglobulin E (IgE) and eosinophilia. This syndrome often occurs in the setting of infection with a single adult *A. caninum* hookworm attached to an ectopic site in the gastrointestinal tract (e.g., stomach, large intestine).

DIAGNOSIS

Hookworm infection is diagnosed by identifying the characteristic eggs in the stools. Because only heavy hookworm infection is associated with anemia, it has been argued that it is pointless to carry out concentration techniques to identify persons with very light infection. A number of quantitative egg-counting techniques are available that allow for indirect estimates of the worm burden, including the

Kato–Katz technique, Beaver's direct egg-count technique, Stoll's dilution egg-count technique, and the McMaster technique (10). All these techniques assume that the fecundity of the female hookworm population is constant, whereas in reality fecundity is strongly affected by worm crowding and host resistance (54,55). In addition, because of arrested development, marked seasonal fluctuations in the egg counts for *A. duodenale* can occur (13).

Because the eggs of *N. americanus* and *A. duodenale* are highly similar in respect to morphology, it is usually necessary to differentiate the two species on the basis of differences between third-stage larvae (10). Currently, no reliable means of immunodiagnosis for differentiating these two species is available.

A specific diagnosis of eosinophilic enteritis has been made by recovering *A. caninum* at colonoscopy from the terminal ileum of a patient (17).

TREATMENT

A large number of anthelmintic agents are available that can remove adult hookworms from the small intestine (56). The benzimidazole anthelmintics mebendazole (100 mg twice daily for 3 consecutive days) and albendazole (400 mg as a single dose or for 3 days consecutively to ensure complete removal) are the drugs of choice. The benzimidazoles have both theoretic and actual toxicities, including embryotoxicity and teratogenicity in laboratory animals, and are contraindicated in patients with blood dyscrasias, leukopenia, and liver disease. Because of the former, and the fact that the safety of the benzimidazoles has not been established in infants, pyrantel pamoate in suspension (11 mg/kg per day, not to exceed 1 g) has been suggested as an alternative for young children. However, many thousands of children from Papua New Guinea were recently reported to have received mebendazole and albendazole with no side effects (57). Similarly, the World Health Organization now recommends albendazole for the treatment of pregnant women beyond the first trimester (58). Many anthelmintics are poorly absorbed, and no evidence has been found that they eradicate populations of arrested *A. duodenale* larvae in the tissue.

In addition to specific anthelmintic therapy, dietary supplementation with iron in the form of ferrous sulfate can relieve many of the short- and long-term effects of hookworm anemia (9,52).

PREVENTION

General improvements in living standards, sanitation, and water supplies have been the most effective means of controlling human hookworm infection (10). More than anything else, such improvements account for the widespread eradication of hookworm infection in the United States. However, it is not always possible to improve living standards, and combination programs consisting of sanitation with appropriate disposal of feces, health education, oral iron supplementation, and mass or targeted chemotherapy have been effective in the control of human hookworm infection. Unfortunately, these efforts can be expensive and require large investments of human energy. In many parts of the developing world, it has been extremely difficult to implement them, particularly in regions of endemicity where reinfection can occur just a few months after specific anthelminthic chemotherapy (59). A better understanding of the biochemistry and molecular biology of human hookworm infection may ultimately provide the basis for rational vaccine development (60).

REFERENCES

1. Hotez PJ, Pritchard DI. Hookworm infection. *Sci Am* 1995;272: 68–74.
2. Hotez PJ. Hookworm disease in children. *Pediatr Infect Dis J* 1989;8:516–520.
3. Bundy DAP, Chan MS, Savioli L. Hookworm infection in pregnancy. *Trans R Soc Trop Med Hyg* 1995;89:520–521.
4. Peduzzi R, Piffaretti JC. *Ancylostoma duodenale* and the Saint Gotthard anemia. *Lancet* 1983;287:1942–1945.
5. Looss A. On the penetration of *Ancylostoma* larvae into the human skin. *Zentralbl Bakteriol Parasitenkd* 1901;29:733–739.
6. Stiles CW. A new species of hookworm (*Uncinaria americana*) parasitic in man. *Am Med* 1902;3:777–778.
7. Ettling J. *The germ of laziness, Rockefeller philanthropy and public health in the New South.* Cambridge, MA: Harvard University Press, 1981.
8. Anderson RC. *Nematode parasites of vertebrates, their development and transmission.* Wallingford, UK: CAB International, 1992.
9. Kendrick JF. The length of life and rate of loss of hookworms *Ancylostoma duodenale* and *Necator americanus*. *Am J Trop Med Hyg* 1934;14:363–379.
10. Pawlowski ZS, Schad GA, Stott GJ. *Hookworm infection and anemia, approaches to prevention and control.* Geneva: World Health Organization, 1991.
11. Soper FL. The report of a nearly pure *Ancylostoma duodenale* infestation in native South American Indians and a discussion of its ethnological significance. *Am J Hyg* 1927;7:174–184.
12. Hoagland KE, Schad GA. *Necator americanus* and *Ancylostoma duodenale*: life history parameters and epidemiological implications of two sympatric hookworms on humans. *Exp Parasitol* 1978;44:36–49.
13. Schad GA, Chowdhury AF, Dean CG, et al. Arrested development in human hookworm infections: an adaptation to a seasonally unfavorable external environment. *Science* 1973;180:502–504.
14. Sen-hai Y, Wei-xia S. Hookworm infection and disease in China. In: Schad GA, Warren KS, eds. *Hookworm disease, current status and new directions.* London: Taylor and Francis, 1990.
15. Hotez PJ, Hawdon J, Schad GA. Hookworm larval infectivity, arrest and amphiparatenesis: the *Caenorhabditis elegans* Daf-c paradigm. *Parasitol Today* 1993;9:23–26.
16. Rep BH, Van Joost KS, Vetter JCM. Pathogenicity of *Ancylostoma ceylonicum. Trop Geogr Med* 1971;23:183–192.
17. Prociv P, Croese J. Human eosinophilic enteritis caused by dog hookworm *Ancylostoma caninum. Lancet* 1990;335: 1299–1302.
18. Sulica VI, Berberian B, Kao GF. Histopathologic findings of cutaneous larva migrans. *J Cutan Pathol* 1988;15:346.

19. Schad GA, Anderson RM. Predisposition to hookworm infection. *Science* 1985;228:1537–1540.
20. Hotez PJ, Narasimhan S, Haggerty J, et al. Hyaluronidase from infective *Ancylostoma* hookworm larvae and its possible function as a virulence factor in tissue invasion and in cutaneous larva migrans. *Infect Immun* 1992;60:1018–1023.
21. Hawdon JM, Jones BF, Perregaux MA, et al. *Ancylostoma caninum*: metalloprotease release coincides with activation of infective larvae *in vitro*. *Exp Parasitol* 1995;80:205–211.
22. Kumar S, Pritchard DI. Secretion of metalloproteases by living infective larvae of *Necator americanus*. *J Parasitol* 1992;78:917–919.
23. Hawdon JM, Jones BF, Hoffman DR, et al. Cloning and characterization of *Ancylostoma*-secreted protein: a novel protein associated with the transition to parasitism by infective hookworm larvae. *J Biol Chem* 1996;271:6672–6678.
24. Hawdon JM, Narasimhan S, Hotez PJ. *Ancylostoma*-secreted protein 2: cloning and characterization of a second member of a family of nematode-secreted proteins from *Ancylostoma caninum*. *Mol Biochem Parasitol* 1999;99:149–165.
25. Zhan B, Hawdon J, Shan Q, et al. *Ancylostoma*-secreted protein 1 (ASP-1) homologues in human hookworms. *Mol Biochem Parasitol* 1999;98:143–149.
26. Salafsky B, Fusco AC, Siddiqui A. *Necator americanus*: factors influencing skin penetration by larvae. In: Schad GA, Warren KS, eds. *Hookworm disease, current status and new directions.* London: Taylor and Francis, 1990.
27. Yoshida Y, Nakanishi Y, Mitani W. Experimental studies on the infection modes of *Ancylostoma duodenale* and *Necator americanus* to the definitive host. *Jpn J Parasitol* 1958;7:102–112.
28. Kalkofen UP. Intestinal trauma resulting from feeding activities of *Ancylostoma caninum*. *Am J Trop Med Hyg* 1974;23: 1046–1053.
29. Harrop SA, Sawangjaroen N, Prociv P, et al. Characterization and localization of cathepsin B proteinases expressed by adult *Ancylostoma caninum* hookworms. *Mol Biochem Parasitol* 1995;71: 163–171.
30. Harrop SA, Prociv P, Brindley PJ. *Acasp*, a gene encoding a cathepsin D-like aspartic protease from the hookworm *Ancylostoma caninum*. *Biochem Biophys Res Commun* 1996;227:294–302.
31. Hotez PJ, Trang NL, McKerrow JH, et al. Isolation and characterization of a protease from the hookworm *Ancylostoma caninum*. *J Biol Chem* 1985;260:7343–7348.
32. Hotez P, Capello MC, Hawdon J, et al. Hyaluronidases of the gastrointestinal invasive nematodes *Ancylostoma caninum* and *Anisakis simplex*: possible functions in the pathogenesis of human zoonoses. *J Infect Dis* 1994;170:918–926.
33. Daub J, Loukas A, Pritchard DI, et al. A survey of genes expressed in adults of the human hookworm *Necator americanus*. *Parasitology* 2000;120:171–184.
34. Cappello M, Vlasuk GP, Bergum PW, et al. *Ancylostoma caninum* anticoagulant peptide (AcAP): a novel hookworm-derived inhibitor of human coagulation factor Xa. *Proc Natl Acad Sci U S A* 1995;92:6152–6156.
35. Moyle M, Foster DL, McGrath DE, et al. A hookworm glycoprotein that inhibits neutrophil function is a ligand of the integrin CD11b/CD18. *J Biol Chem* 1994;269:1008–10015.
36. Chadderdon RC, Cappello M. The hookworm platelet inhibitor: functional blockage of GPIIb-IIIa and GPIa-IIa inhibits platelet aggregation and adhesion *in vitro*. *J Infect Dis* 1999;179: 1235–1241.
37. Roche M, Layrisse M. Nature and causes of hookworm anemia. *Am J Trop Med Hyg* 1966;15:1029–1102.
38. Gilles HM. Selective primary health care: strategies for control of disease in the developing world. XVII. Hookworm infection and anemia. *Rev Infect Dis* 1985;7:111–118.
39. Stoltzfus RJ, Chwaya HM, Tielsch J, et al. Epidemiology of iron deficiency anemia in Zanzibari school children: the importance of hookworms. *Am J Clin Nutr* 1997;65:153–159.
40. Scrimshaw NS. Iron deficiency. *Sci Am* 1991;265:46–52.
41. Miller TA. Hookworm infection in man. *Adv Parasitol* 1979;17: 315–384.
42. Castro GA, Behnke JM, Weisbrodt NW. Hookworm infection and malabsorption: a critical review. In: Schad GA, Warren KS, eds. *Hookworm disease, current status and new directions.* London: Taylor and Francis, 1990.
43. Schad GA, Soulsby EJL, Chowdhury AB, et al. In: *Nuclear techniques in helminthological research.* Vienna: International Atomic Energy Agency, 1975:41–54.
44. Pritchard DI, Quinnell RJ, Slater AFG, et al. Epidemiology and immunology of *Necator americanus* infection in a community in Papua New Guinea: humoral responses to excretory–secretory and cuticular collagen antigens. *Parasitology* 1990;100:317–326.
45. Nawalinski TA, Schad GA. Arrested development in *Ancylostoma duodenale*: course of self-induced infection in man. *Am J Trop Med Hyg* 1974;23:895–898.
46. Maxwell C, Hussain R, Nutman TB, et al. Clinical and immunologic responses of normal volunteers to low-dose hookworm (*Necator americanus*) infection. *Am J Trop Med Hyg* 1987;37:126–134.
47. Carroll SM, Grove DI. Experimental infections of humans with *Ancylostoma ceylonicum*: clinical, parasitological, haematological and immunological findings. *Trop Geogr Med* 1986;38:38–45.
48. Crosby WH. What became of chlorosis? *JAMA* 1987;257: 2799–2800.
49. Smillie WG, Augustine DL. Hookworm infestation: the effect of varying intensities on the physical condition of schoolchildren. *Am J Dis Child* 1926;31:151–168.
50. Stephenson LS, Latham MC, Kurz KM, et al. Treatment with a single dose of albendazole improves growth of Kenyan schoolchildren with hookworm, *Trichuris trichiura,* and *Ascaris lumbricoides* infections. *Am J Trop Med Hyg* 1989;41:78–87.
51. Stephenson LS, Latham MC, Kinoti SN, et al. Improvements in physical fitness of Kenyan schoolboys infected with hookworm, *Trichuris trichiura,* and *Ascaris lumbricoides* following a single dose of albendazole. *Trans R Soc Trop Med Hyg* 1990;84:277–282.
52. Crompton DWT, Stephenson LS. Hookworm infection, nutritional status and productivity. In: Schad GA, Warren KS, eds. *Hookworm disease, current status and new directions.* London: Taylor and Francis, 1990.
53. Smillie WG, Spencer CR. Mental retardation in schoolchildren with hookworm. *J Educ Psychol* 1926;17:314–321.
54. Watkins WE, Pollitt E. "Stupidity or worms": do intestinal worms impair mental performance *Psychol Bull* 1997;121:171–191.
55. Albonico M, Crompton DWT, Savioli L. Control strategies for human intestinal nematode infections. *Adv Parasitol* 1999;42: 277–341.
56. Rossignol JF. Chemotherapy: present status. In: Schad GA, Warren KS, eds. *Hookworm disease, current status and new directions.* London: Taylor and Francis, 1990.
57. Biddulph J. Mebendazole and albendazole for infants. *Pediatr Infect Dis J* 1990;9:373.
58. World Health Organization. Report of the WHO informal consultation on the use of chemotherapy for the control of morbidity due to soil-transmitted nematodes in humans. Division of control of tropical diseases. Geneva: World Health Organization, 1996:WHO/CTD/SIP.96.1.
59. Albonico M, Smith PG, Ercole E, et al. Rate of reinfection with intestinal nematodes after treatment of children with mebendazole or albendazole in a highly endemic area. *Trans R Soc Trop Med Hyg* 1995;89:538–541
60. Hotez PJ, Ghosh K, Hawdon JM, et al. Experimental approaches to the development of a recombinant hookworm vaccine. *Immunol Rev* 1999;171:163–172

70

STRONGYLOIDES STERCORALIS

AFZAL A. SIDDIQUI
ROBERT M. GENTA
STEVEN L. BERK

Strongyloidiasis is an intestinal infection caused by a geohelminth, *Strongyloides stercoralis.* In some parts of the world, notably Africa and Papua New Guinea, human infections with *Strongyloides fuelleborni* have also been reported (1–4). The growing importance of strongyloidiasis is related to the unique ability of this nematode to replicate within its host. Because of this ability, cycles of autoinfection with the development of chronic disease are possible (5,6). Infection of humans with *S. stercoralis* usually results in an asymptomatic chronic disease of the gastrointestinal tract that can remain undetected for up to 40 years (7). However, in immunocompromised hosts, particularly those receiving corticosteroids (8–10), hyperinfection can occur, with the dissemination of larvae to other organs not ordinarily involved in the life cycle. Mortality rates associated with hyperinfection can be as high as 70% to 87% (11–14). Furthermore, almost all deaths caused by helminths in the United States are a consequence of *S. stercoralis* hyperinfection (15,16).

MICROBIOLOGY

Taxonomy

The family Strongylidae (class Secernentia, order Rhabditidae) comprises only one genus, *Strongyloides* Grassi, 1879. The members of this genus, also called *threadworms,* are heterogenetic, with free-living and parasitic generations, and include at least 40 named species (17). Most of these are parasites of mammals, but some can also be found in birds, reptiles, and amphibians. The only species discussed in this chapter is *S. stercoralis* Bavay, 1876 (synonyms: *Anguillula stercoralis, Strongyloides intestinalis, Strongyloides canis, Strongyloides felis*). *S. fuelleborni* von Listow, 1905 is a parasite of primates that may also infect humans (1,2). Several other species are also important because they can cause disease in livestock (*Strongyloides ransomi, Strongyloides westeri, Strongyloides papillosus*) (18) or because they can be used as models of human strongyloidiasis (*Strongyloides ratti*) (19–23).

Morphology

The parasitic female is rarely identified in the stools of infected patients but is one of the stages found in tissue sections of small intestine. It measures 1.5 to 10 mm in length and 27 to 95 μm in width. Its cuticle is finely striated, and in tissue sections, it is often wrinkled. In cross-sections, depending on the level, one may see a muscular esophagus, intestine, ovaries, and eggs. Rhabditiform larvae are identified most commonly in the stools. They measure approximately 400 μm in length and 20 to 25 μm in diameter and are characterized by a bulbar esophagus and a thinner, longer intestine. In tissue sections, they are often found in the intestinal submucosa and within small intestinal crypts, and only exceptionally in the lungs, but they cannot be specifically identified based on their morphologic characteristics. Filariform or strongyliform (third-stage) larvae are the stage most frequently identified in the extraintestinal tissues and fluids (most often the sputum) of patients with disseminated infection. They are long and slender (400 to 700 μm in length and 12 to 20 μm in width), with a cylindric esophagus that occupies half of the body length. In transverse sections, the cuticle shows four characteristic lateral alae, which can be used for species identification (24).

Life Cycle and Pathophysiology

The life cycle of *S. stercoralis* (Fig. 70.1) begins when filariform larvae penetrate the skin of a susceptible host. The larvae migrate via the lymphatic and venous circulation, pass

A. A. Siddiqui: Texas Tech University Health Sciences Center and Amarillo Veterans Affairs Healthcare System, Amarillo, Texas.
R. M. Genta: Baylor College of Medicine and Houston Veterans Affairs Medical Center, Houston, Texas.
S. L. Berk: Texas Tech University Health Sciences Center, Amarillo, Texas.

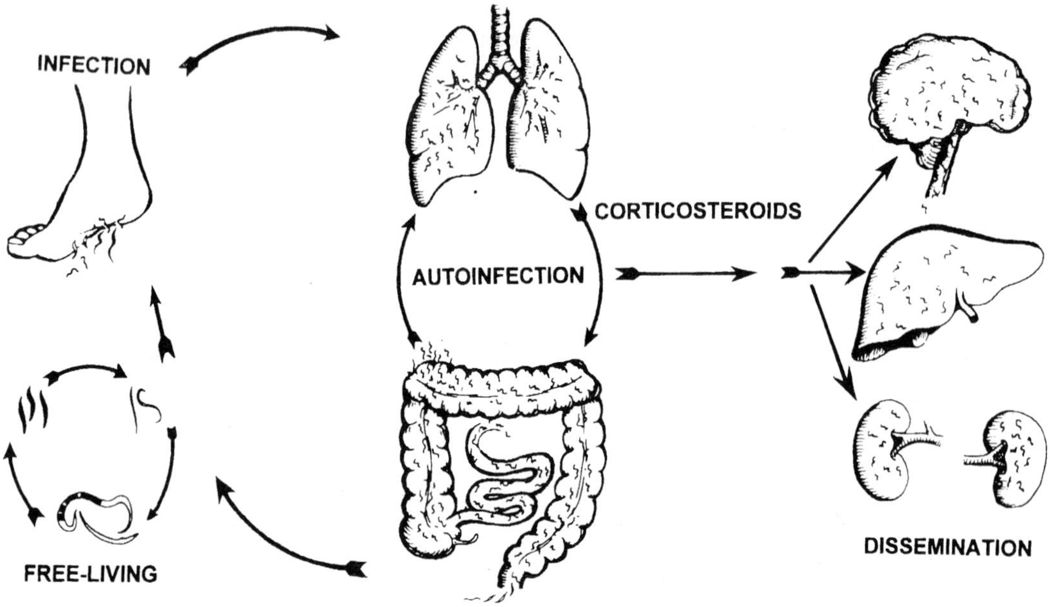

FIGURE 70.1. The life cycle of *Strongyloides stercoralis*. The administration of corticosteroids disrupts the usually well-regulated autoinfection and results in the dissemination of larvae throughout the body. Steroids may act by depressing certain host immune responses or by directly stimulating parasite ecdysis.

through the right side of the heart, settle in the capillary bed of the lungs, and then penetrate the capillary walls and enter the alveoli (11,12,25). The larvae subsequently climb the tracheobronchial tree to the larynx (11,112,24–26). They are eventually swallowed and reach the duodenum and upper part of the small intestine, where they mature into adult egg-laying females (11,12,24,27). However, Schad (24) and co-workers have argued that the pulmonary route is just one of several possible pathways by which the larvae reach the duodenum, whether they begin their journey in the subcutaneous tissue, the inguinal area, or the distal part of the ileum. Males have been identified in the stools of infected patients and dogs (24), but these findings have been largely ignored. In the duodenum and first part of the jejunum, parasitic adult females enter the lamina propria, where they deposit a small number of eggs each day. After the eggs hatch, rhabditiform larvae emerge and migrate into the intestinal lumen, eventually passing with the feces into the external environment. Here, depending on poorly understood conditions of temperature and humidity, the rhabditiform larvae either molt directly into infective parasitic filariform larvae, capable of repenetrating the skin of a suitable host (direct cycle), or pass through four ecdyses (molts) to become adult male and female worms that mate and produce offspring; these in turn develop into filariform larvae and reenter parasitic life (indirect or heterogonic cycle).

A small portion of the rhabditiform larvae that hatch from the eggs deposited in the intestine are believed to molt within the intestine into the filariform stage. These larvae penetrate the colonic wall or perianal skin, complete the internal cycle, and establish themselves as mature adult females in the small intestine. This process, known as *autoinfection,* is believed to represent the mechanism by which *S. stercoralis* can persist virtually indefinitely in infected hosts (28,29).

EPIDEMIOLOGY

Although information regarding the worldwide prevalence of strongyloidiasis is fragmentary, 3 million to 100 million persons are estimated to be infected worldwide (1,30). The unreliability of these estimates is reflected in the wide range of prevalence rates, varying between less than 1% and 85%, of populations living in adjacent regions of the same country (31–33) (Table 70.1). Some of these estimates are probably artifactually low because obtaining epidemiologic data on the prevalence of *S. stercoralis* has been difficult in the past, mainly because a diagnosis based on the direct wet mount analysis of stool has always been extremely difficult to obtain in cases of chronic, low-level *S. stercoralis* infection. It is only recently, with the advent of a sensitive agar plate method, that interest in *S. stercoralis* infection has been renewed. Provided these limitations are kept in mind, one can assume that *S. stercoralis* is present in virtually all tropical and subtropical regions of the world. Pockets of low endemicity (<1% to 3%) exist in several industrialized

TABLE 70.1. PREVALENCE OF STRONGYLOIDES STERCORALIS IN SOME OF THE DEVELOPING COUNTRIES

Country	No. Specimens Examined	Percentage Positive	Reference
Abidjan	1,001	1.4	(204)
Argentina	36	83.3	(205)
Argentina	207	2.0	(206)
Brazil	200	2.5	(207)
Brazil	900	13.0	(208)
Ethiopia	1,239	13.0	(209)
Guinea	800	6.4	(210)
Honduras	266	2.6	(175)
Israel	106	0.9	(211)
Kenya	230	4.0	(212)
Laos	669	19.0	(213)
Mexico	100	2.0	(214)
Nigeria	2,008	25.1	(215)
Romania	231	6.9	(216)
Sierra Leone	1,164	3.8	(217)
Sudan	275	3.3	(218)
Thailand	491	11.2	(219)

countries of western Europe (e.g., Italy, France, and Switzerland) (31–40), eastern Europe (e.g., Poland and many parts of the former Soviet Union) (41–43), the United States (Appalachian region and southern states) (44,45), Japan (Okinawa) (46), and Australia (aboriginal populations) (47,48). Significant prevalence rates of strongyloidiasis have been found in institutionalized patients, even in Pennsylvania and British Columbia, where the parasite is not known to be endemic in the general population (49–51). Because of the long persistence of this parasite in its host and its relatively high prevalence among some populations, physicians practicing in industrialized countries should consider the possibility of strongyloidiasis in immigrant or refugee patients born in tropical or subtropical regions and also in persons from local areas of endemicity.

Strongyloidiasis and AIDS

Because cell-mediated immunity is thought to regulate *S. stercoralis* autoinfection, it was expected that patients with AIDS would have more frequent and severe infections with *S. stercoralis.* However, in areas of the world where both *S. stercoralis* and AIDS are endemic, a higher incidence of chronic strongyloidiasis in association with AIDS has not been detected (52). For this reason, several authors speculated that strongyloidiasis is regulated by other factors and that it would remain one of the missing infections in AIDS (1,53–56). During the past few years, a very limited number of patients with AIDS and extraintestinal strongyloidiasis have been reported (57–62). As Karp and Neva (10) correctly pointed out, some conditions that co-segregate with HIV infection are known to predispose to hyperinfection syndrome, including inanition and the use of steroids. In fact, a common denominator of the immunosuppressive diseases associated with hyperinfection is treatment with corticosteroids. It is apparent that strongyloidiasis is not an important opportunistic infection associated with AIDS; however, the infection should still be sought and promptly treated in HIV-infected patients with a suggestive geographic history. On the other hand, strongyloidiasis appears to be a relevant opportunistic infection in persons with human T-cell lymphotropic virus type 1 (HTLV-1) infection (10,63).

PATHOGENESIS AND IMMUNITY

According to the cycle outlined above, chronic infection is sustained by a relatively low and stable number of adult worms that reside in harmony within their host's intestine and survive by means of well-regulated autoinfection (26). The rate of autoinfection is believed to be regulated by the host's cell-mediated immunity (27,64,65). When this regulatory function becomes impaired during immunosuppression, increasing numbers of autoinfective larvae complete the cycle, and the population of parasitic adult worms increases (hyperinfection). Eventually, the extraordinary numbers of migrating larvae deviate from the presumed route (intestine → venous bed → lungs → trachea → intestine) and disseminate to other organs, including meningeal spaces and brain, liver, kidneys, lymph nodes, and cutaneous and subcutaneous tissues. In these organs, the larvae cause hemorrhage by breaking capillaries, elicit inflammatory responses, and implant gram-negative bacteria carried from fecal material. The resulting syndrome, known as *disseminated strongyloidiasis,* is nearly always fatal (64,65).

The validity of the above model has been questioned by Schad et al. (66,67), who used an experimental canine model of disseminated strongyloidiasis to show that only a few larvae could be recovered from the lungs of dogs with massive hyperinfection. Later, in a series of experiments based on a compartmental analysis of larvae labeled with radioactive isotopes and mathematical modeling, they presented convincing evidence that the tracheobronchial route in the dog is not used by the majority of migrating larvae (68). According to their model, larvae that began their migration in the skin (primary infection) or distal ileum (autoinfection) are not more likely to pass through the lungs than through any other organ, which suggests that the migratory pathway involves random dissemination throughout the body. However, this conclusion has not been fully accepted because large numbers of larvae are frequently identified in bronchoalveolar lavage fluid from hyperinfected patients (8,69).

Determining the migratory pathway involved in autoinfection is important for understanding the biology of *S. stercoralis* and the host mechanisms that regulate internal infection. Recently, the accepted paradigm that host mechanisms regulate hyperinfection and dissemination has been challenged (26). The theory that host immunity controls infection fails to consider the role that parasites may play in such regulation. In this regard, the adverse impact of increased parasite density on egg production and growth ("crowding effect") has been demonstrated for several intestinal nematodes. Although it may be difficult to distinguish between host resistance and direct parasite-to-parasite effects, it seems clear that in a normal host–parasite relationship, the parasite may reach a particular population size or critical biomass, after which regulatory mechanisms yet unknown intervene to limit the population (70).

We have proposed that during the parallel evolution of humans and their parasites, *S. stercoralis* acquired the ability to reach an optimal population size in the human duodenum. If the initial infective dose of larvae is low, intraluminal molting occurs at a higher rate until the "optimal" size of the adult population is reached. In this model, it is assumed that *S. stercoralis* organisms, like other nematodes, transmit their molting signal by molting hormones (ecdysteroids) (71,72). When the size of the parasite population reaches a certain level, adult females decrease their production of ecdysteroids, and a lowered molting rate (i.e., just sufficient to replace the dying adults) results. During the initial phase of infection, the host mounts humoral and cellular immune responses directed at all tissue stages of the parasite. These well-characterized responses (32,36,73–83) do not eradicate all the parasites but do limit the size of the parasite population. Impaired immune responses may allow the growth of larger numbers of parasites, as reported in patients with agammaglobulinemia (84–85), but total dysregulation of the parasite population does not occur because worms, in part, regulate their own growth. Conversely, the presence of intact immune responses is not sufficient to prevent dissemination should the parasites' own regulatory mechanisms fail (86).

The levels of ecdysteroid-like substances are generally negligible in healthy subjects (71,72). The administration of exogenous or endogenous corticosteroids may result in increased amounts of ecdysteroid-like substances in the host's tissues, including in the intestinal wall, where adult females reside. These substances may act as molting signals for the eggs or rhabditiform larvae, which transform intraluminally into excessive numbers of filariform larvae. Available data are not sufficient to prove a dose-dependent effect, but it is indeed remarkable that patients in whom fulminating hyperinfection develops after only a few days of steroid administration are usually those who have received intravenous methylprednisolone (87–91). Once a population has become very large (e.g., 100,000 adult worms), it may continue to expand rapidly, even at low molting rates, and the discontinuation of steroids may not be sufficient to arrest the relentless growth process that leads to the host's death. We further postulate that like mammals, *S. stercoralis* metabolizes steroids via a receptor-mediated pathway (92). We have demonstrated the presence of a steroid receptor in *S. stercoralis* (93). The nucleotide sequence of the *S. stercoralis* steroid receptor shows appreciable identity with a number of nuclear hormone receptors, including the Daf-12 protein of *Caenorhabditis elegans* and ecdysone receptors of insects (93). Daf-12 regulates the dauer diapause and developmental age in *C. elegans,* which strengthens the basis of further research on this phenomenon in *Strongyloides.*

Pathology

The pathologic lesions associated with chronic, uncomplicated *S. stercoralis* infection have received little attention; only rarely have patients with such lesions come to autopsy. However, pathologic descriptions of the lesions in patients in whom strongyloidiasis was an incidental finding and our studies indicate that the worms reside in the intestinal mucosa without causing significant inflammatory responses or tissue damage. The classic description of the pathology of strongyloidiasis was made by De Paola et al. in 1962 (94) and later updated by Genta and Caymmi-Gomes (95). These authors proposed the subdivision of the intestinal lesions into three distinct forms.

In "catarrhal" enteritis (presumably associated with light infections), the small intestine is congested, the mucosa is covered with abundant mucoid secretions, and scattered petechial hemorrhages are present. The most remarkable histologic feature is an increased mononuclear infiltrate in the submucosa, although parasites are rare. In the more severe "edematous" enteritis, the intestinal wall is grossly thickened, the mucosal folds are flattened, and the affected intestinal segments have a rubbery consistency. Histologic findings include submucosal edema, flattening of the villi, and a scattering of parasites throughout the lamina propria. The most severe form, "ulcerative" enteritis, is almost exclusively seen in association with hyperinfection. The intestinal walls may be made rigid by the edema and fibrosis that result from long-standing inflammation, and the mucosa may exhibit atrophy, erosions, and ulcerations. An abundant inflammatory infiltrate, most often consisting of neutrophils, and all the life cycle stages of *S. stercoralis* are seen throughout the intestinal mucosa. Jejunal perforation has been reported in patients with the ulcerative enteritis form of strongyloidiasis (96). Uncommonly, the mucosal damage occurs predominantly in the large intestine, simulating ulcerative colitis and pseudopolyposis (97,98). *S. stercoralis* larvae have been found in the appendix, and eosinophilic appendicitis apparently caused by this parasite has been reported (99–101). In patients with disseminated strongyloidiasis, the intestinal lesions reflect the large number of worms dwelling within the intestinal mucosa and penetrating the walls of the small intestine (Fig. 70.2). In addition, the stomach (102) and peritoneal cavity (29,103) may be invaded by migrating parasites. However, because most of

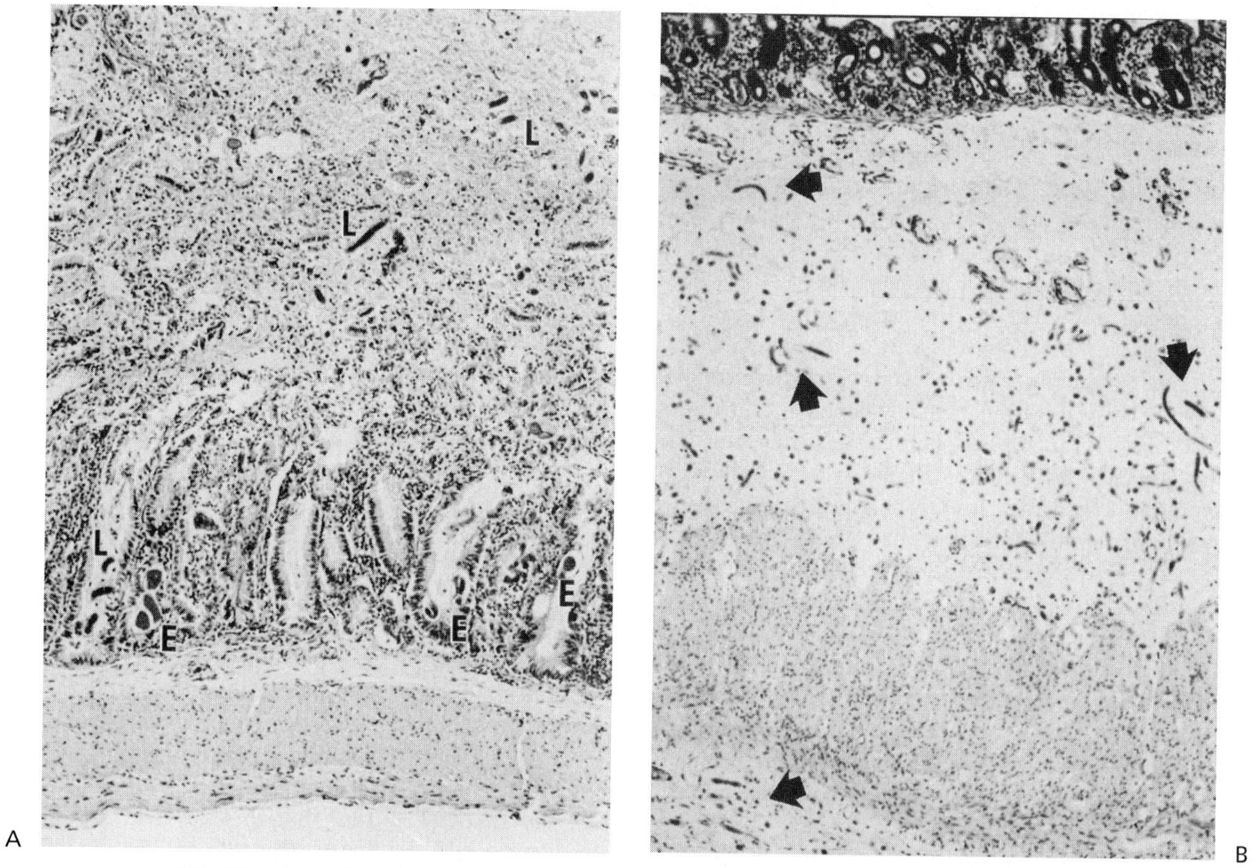

FIGURE 70.2. Sections from the intestine of a host who died of disseminated strongyloidiasis following high-dose corticosteroid therapy. The architecture of the jejunal mucosa (*left*) is completely effaced, and large numbers of larvae (*L*) and eggs (*E*) of *Strongyloides stercoralis* are visible on the surface and within the mucosa. The colonic wall (*right*) shows preservation of the mucosa and a high degree of submucosal edema. Innumerable migrating filariform larvae (*arrows*) are present within the edematous spaces.

these patients are receiving immunosuppressive doses of corticosteroids, inflammatory responses are often minimal despite extensive tissue damage. The gastrointestinal pathology is often overshadowed by the lesions found in other organs, particularly in patients who receive anthelmintic therapy before succumbing to disseminated strongyloidiasis.

Migrating parasites may cause mechanical damage in addition to inflammation. In human patients, the extraintestinal organ most commonly affected by migratory damage is the lung. In severe disseminated infection, when hundreds of thousands of adult parasites dwell in the intestine and millions of larvae migrate throughout the body, alveolar microhemorrhages may result in massive pulmonary bleeding. As larvae penetrate the large intestine, they create small breaks in the mucosa that facilitate bloodstream invasion by enteric bacteria. The larvae themselves carry bacteria on their cuticle to distant sites. Regardless of the mechanism, the widespread dissemination of larvae is frequently associated with polymicrobial sepsis, diffuse or patchy bronchopneumonia, pulmonary and cerebral abscesses, and meningitis. Filariform larvae, and occasionally rhabditiform larvae and adult worms, also may disseminate to the mesenteric lymph nodes, biliary tract, liver, pancreas, spleen, heart, endocrine glands, and ovaries (95). In these locations, the parasite frequently induces a granulomatous response (104).

CLINICAL ILLNESS

No other nematode has been associated with so broad a spectrum of manifestations or implicated as the cause of so many different clinical syndromes as *S. stercoralis.* Although some of these manifestations are dramatic, the majority of persons with chronic infection are either asymptomatic or have mild, nonspecific symptoms.

Gastrointestinal Manifestations

The gastrointestinal manifestations of chronic strongyloidiasis are usually nonspecific (32,105). Epigastric abdominal pain, postprandial fullness or bloating, and heartburn are among the symptoms most commonly reported (106,107). Brief episodes of diarrhea alternating with constipation may also occur. The diarrhea usually consists of semiformed, nonbloody stools (33). Persons who have chronic infection occasionally pass stools with occult blood (97), and even massive colonic hemorrhage has been reported (108). A severe, cholera-like diarrhea with electrolyte imbalance and cardiac arrest has been reported in two patients, but this is exceedingly uncommon (109,110).

On physical examination, chronically infected patients appear normal, or palpation reveals only mild abdominal tenderness. Less commonly, chronic strongyloidiasis resembles inflammatory bowel disease, particularly ulcerative colitis, and the endoscopic appearance may be that of pseudopolyposis (97). Rarely, patients have undergone surgery for "chronic colitis," with the correct diagnosis established by pathologic examination of the resected colon (98). Malabsorption frequently occurs in patients with strongyloidiasis (111–113). The majority of these patients, however, are from areas of the world where tropical sprue and spruelike conditions are widespread, so that a clear relationship of cause and effect between *S. stercoralis* infection and malabsorption is difficult to determine. Garcia et al. (114) convincingly argued that malnutrition was the cause rather than the effect of severe strongyloidiasis in a group of Colombian patients. Experimental work in rodents seems to support this conclusion (115).

In contrast to the asymptomatic nature of chronic strongyloidiasis, the gastrointestinal manifestations of disseminated strongyloidiasis are dramatic and often catastrophic. Hyperinfection is often heralded by profuse diarrhea, which may be watery, mucoid, and bloody. The diarrhea is a consequence of the erosions, ulcerations, and edema caused by millions of adult worms and filariform larvae in the mucosa of the small and large intestine (64,65,71). Depending on the extent, severity, and location of these lesions, malabsorption, exudation, and altered motility result. These mucosal changes predispose the patient to bacterial enterocolitis (116) and, after variable periods of diarrhea, paralytic ileus (91,117). Probably because of the large numbers of larvae migrating from the large intestine into the circulation, polymicrobial (predominantly gram-negative) sepsis may occur, with the development of local infections and abscesses in virtually any organ (64,65). Larvae have been identified in other gastrointestinal organs, including the liver, stomach, and pancreas of patients with overwhelming infection (71), but the presence of parasites in these locations does not cause characteristic symptoms.

Pulmonary Manifestations

Although the risk for strongyloidiasis may be increased in patients with chronic obstructive pulmonary disease (118), no respiratory signs or symptoms are associated with acute or chronic strongyloidiasis. In these infections, the number of larvae passing through the lungs is probably negligible. Occasionally, disseminated strongyloidiasis has developed in patients who presented with asthma and were treated with corticosteroids (119–126), but these patients are often on low-dose steroid therapy, which predisposes to strongyloidiasis (105). Chronic obstructive pulmonary disease has been associated with strongyloidiasis in some series of American patients (105,118,127). How hyperinfection can develop in patients with chronic obstructive pulmonary disease is illustrated in a conceptual model presented in Fig. 70.3.

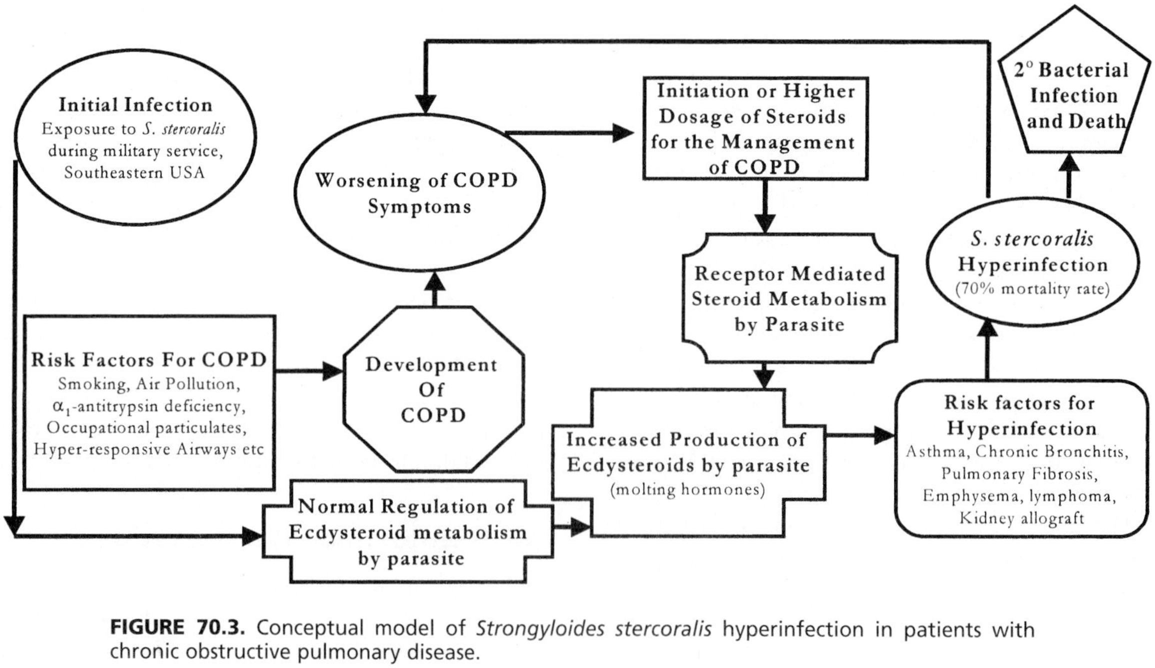

FIGURE 70.3. Conceptual model of *Strongyloides stercoralis* hyperinfection in patients with chronic obstructive pulmonary disease.

Although peculiar microcalcifications have been observed in the lungs of chronically infected dogs (128), a direct effect of parasites on the pulmonary parenchyma has not been documented in humans and appears unlikely. Among patients with disseminated strongyloidiasis, pulmonary manifestations are common, particularly diffuse bronchopneumonia (64,129–131). Pulmonary abscesses have also been reported (132). Intraalveolar hemorrhage, often sufficiently severe to cause the patient's death, is a frequent event during the course of disseminated strongyloidiasis. In some cases, fatal pulmonary hemorrhages occur a few days after apparently successful treatment of the parasite, which suggests an immunologically mediated mechanism of vascular damage (133,134).

Neurologic Manifestations

Gram-negative polymicrobial meningitis is the most frequent central nervous system manifestation of disseminated strongyloidiasis (135–141). In some cases, larvae have been identified in the cerebrospinal fluid. Rarely, larvae have been found in the absence of bacteria in patients with signs of meningeal involvement, suggesting the possibility of parasitic (aseptic) meningitis (142–144). Eosinophilic meningitis has not been described in association with strongyloidiasis, possibly because most patients with strongyloidiasis receive corticosteroids and their eosinophilic counts are generally low. In a less common form of central nervous system involvement, cerebral and cerebellar abscesses containing *S. stercoralis* larvae develop (145).

Other Systemic Manifestations

Arthritis is an unusual manifestation of strongyloidiasis and is associated with the local deposition of immune complexes containing *S. stercoralis* antigens (146–149). Cardiac arrhythmias and arrest are rare and have been attributed to direct myocardial damage by the migrating larvae (150) or to electrolyte imbalance precipitated by severe intestinal strongyloidiasis (109,110). Depression and neurosis have been associated with chronic strongyloidiasis (151), but they likely represent a reaction to the long duration of symptoms. The passage of larvae in the sperm and the development of genital lesions in association with strongyloidiasis have also been described (152).

Cutaneous Manifestations

Three types of cutaneous manifestation have been described in patients with chronic strongyloidiasis. Urticarial rashes, possibly caused by a sensitization to parasite antigens, have occurred sporadically in patients from all parts of the world (45,74,153–155). In contrast, a characteristic dermatitis caused by the subcutaneous migration of filariform larvae (larva currens) has been reported almost exclusively in white patients who acquired the infection in Southeast Asia (109,155–161). In many of these patients, larva currens was the only sign of strongyloidiasis, and permanent eradication of the dermatitis was achieved with thiabendazole therapy (161–164). Finally, generalized cutaneous purpura has been recently described in several patients with leukopenia, various degrees of thrombocytopenia, and disseminated infection (155,165–167). In two of these cases, the purpuric lesions were related to the migration of filariform larvae in the dermis (155,167).

DIAGNOSIS

The diagnosis of strongyloidiasis is suspected by clinical signs and symptoms, eosinophilia, and serologic findings (6,25,127,168). A definitive diagnosis of strongyloidiasis is usually accomplished by the detection of larvae in the stool. However, in a majority of uncomplicated cases of strongyloidiasis, the intestinal worm load is very low and larval output is minimal (168). Eosinophilia is usually the only indication of the presence of *S. stercoralis* infection but is mild (5% to 15%) and nonspecific (6,25,127,168). In more than two-thirds of cases, no more than 25 larvae are present per gram of stool (168). Single examination of a stool sample has been shown to yield a negative result in up to 70% of cases. Repeated examinations of stool specimens improve the chances of finding parasites; in some studies, diagnostic sensitivity increases to 50% with three stool examinations and can approach 100% if seven serial stool samples are examined (169).

A number of techniques have been used to discern larvae in stool samples, including direct smear of feces in saline solution/Lugol iodine stain, Baermann concentration, formalin–ethyl acetate concentration, Harada–Mori filter paper culture, and nutrient agar plate culture (170–172). Concentrating the stool with formalin–ethyl acetate increases the yield, but dead individual larvae are more difficult to visualize at low magnification. The Baermann method and the Harada–Mori filter paper culture capitalize on the ability of *S. stercoralis* to enter a free-living cycle of development. They are much more sensitive than single stool smears but are rarely standard procedures in clinical parasitology laboratories (173). In a comparative study of more than 1,300 stool samples in which four different methods of stool examination (direct fecal smear, formalin–ethyl acetate concentration, Harada–Mori filter paper culture, and agar plate culture) were used, the agar plate culture method was found to be 96% sensitive (174). In another study, the agar plate culture method was found to be 4.4 times more efficient than the direct smear procedure (175). Although the agar plate method is laborious and time-consuming (it takes about 2 to 3 days), it is more sensitive than other procedures (e.g., wet mount analysis) for the detection of larvae in feces (176). As Grove (6) points out, "the balance of opinion probably favors the agar plate culture method but this is perhaps more expensive and complex."

Although in some studies the examination of duodenal aspirate is reportedly very sensitive, this invasive method is recommended only in pediatric cases when it is necessary to achieve a rapid demonstration of parasites, as in an immunocompromised child with suspected overwhelming infection (168). Microscopic examination of a single specimen of duodenal fluid was found to be more sensitive than wet mount analysis of stools samples for the detection of larvae, identifying 76% of patients; the parasite was found exclusively in duodenal fluid (not in feces) in 67% of patients. The "string test," in which a gelatin capsule containing a string is swallowed by the patient and retrieved after a few hours, enjoyed a brief period of popularity a few years ago, but currently it is used infrequently (177). In some cases, histologic examination of duodenal or jejunal biopsy specimens may reveal *S. stercoralis* organisms embedded in the mucosa (25).

The detection of *S. stercoralis* larvae is usually easier in cases of hyperinfection because large numbers of worms are involved in disseminated infection (11,12,25,168). The larvae can be identified in wet preparations of sputum, bronchoalveolar lavage fluid, bronchial washings and brushings, or lung biopsy specimens, or by examining pleural fluid with either Gram, Papanicolaou, or acid-fast (auramine O and Kinyoun) staining procedures (8,11,12,168,173,178). Findings on chest films are usually variable; pulmonary infiltrates, when present, may be alveolar or interstitial, diffuse or focal, unilateral or bilateral (179). Lung consolidation, occasional cavitation, and even abscess formation have also been reported (11,12). Varying chest roentgenographic pictures are explained by different types of bacterial superinfection, particularly with gram-negative bacilli.

Because it is imperative to examine stool samples repeatedly to achieve a correct diagnosis, it is important to note that a negative result does not necessarily indicate unequivocally the absence of infection (6,168). Therefore, a highly specific and efficient serodiagnostic test for *S. stercoralis,* with a potential for use even in multiple helminth infections, is greatly needed. Several immunodiagnostic assays have been tested through the years with limited success, including skin testing with larval extracts, indirect immunofluorescence with fixed larvae, and radioallergosorbent testing for specific immunoglobulin E and gelatin particle agglutination (6,27,168,180,181). An enzyme-linked immunoadsorbent assay (ELISA) ("*Strongyloides* antibody") for detecting serum immunoglobulin G against a crude extract of the filariform larvae of *S. stercoralis* is available only at specialized centers (6,168,182–185). The sensitivity and specificity of this ELISA can be improved if the serum samples are preincubated with *Onchocerca* antigens before testing (182,186). The question of the specificity of this ELISA has been thoroughly reviewed. Briefly, Genta (184) claimed that the ELISA is 88% sensitive and 99% specific, and that it has positive and negative predictive values of 97% and 95%, respectively. With the use of state-of-the-art statistical models in another study, of Indochinese refugees in Canada, these figures were calculated as 95%, 29%, 30%, and 95%, respectively (187). The difficulty in calculating diagnostic efficiency parameters can be attributed to the lack of a definitive gold standard for *S. stercoralis* (188). In population-based studies, it is widely believed that stool examination generally underestimates the prevalence of *S. stercoralis* infection, whereas serology generally results in an overestimation (6). Furthermore, positive serology does not distinguish between past and current infection because antibody levels remain detectable for years following anthelmintic treatment (6,168), and it is difficult to know whether or not low-level autoinfection is present (6). The "*Strongyloides* antibody" test exhibits cross-reactivity with other helminthic infections, including filariasis, *Ascaris lumbricoides* infection, and acute schistosomiasis (183,189), but for the general population in the United States, these infections are rarely considered in the differential diagnosis of symptomatic strongyloidiasis (168). However, this does not hold true for veterans and international travelers, who may have been exposed to "cross-reactive" antigens of other helminths and have antibodies that can be detected for many years after exposure (190). On a practical basis, this serologic test is unlikely to be widely available because of the need for *S. stercoralis* filariform larval and *Onchocerca* antigens. The major value of serology is as a screening test; a positive result indicates the need for a further search for the parasite (6,168).

To improve serodiagnosis, a number of antigenic proteins on the surface of *S. stercoralis* infective larvae or in their excretory/secretory products have been identified (6), some of which are immunoreactive with sera from infected humans (74,191). Although considerable variability is noted, the most prominent antigenic proteins of *S. stercoralis* appear to be 28, 31, and 41 kd in size (192,193). However, the specificity of these antigens has yet to be tested. Two recombinant *S. stercoralis* antigens have been identified, 5a and 12a, that show no cross-reactivity with sera from patients with filarial or non-*Strongyloides* intestinal nematode infections (194). Three *S. stercoralis* antigens (P1, P4, and P5) recognized by human antibodies exhibit no immunoreactivity with sera obtained from patients infected with schistosomes, filarial parasites, hookworms, or *Onchocerca* (195). Screening of an *S. stercoralis* complementary DNA library with affinity-purified antibodies against antigens P1, P4, and P5 has led to the identification of these antigens as oxoglutarate dehydrogenase, alkaline phosphatase, and isocitrate dehydrogenase (196,197). It is expected that a test based on these three antigens will be extremely useful in detecting chronic, latent, and *de novo* infections of *S. stercoralis* and in monitoring the effectiveness of therapy.

TREATMENT

Strongyloidiasis is a difficult infection to treat because with many helminths, a treatment is considered sufficient if the worm burden is kept below the level at which clinical disease develops (6,168). With *S. stercoralis,* however, only complete eradication of the parasites removes the danger of potentially serious disease; a truly effective anthelmintic must kill the autoinfective L3 larvae, which are relatively resistant to chemical agents (6,168). Additionally, the poor sensitivity of diagnostic stool examination makes it even harder to determine the efficacy of treatment. Thiabendazole (Mintezol), has been the drug of choice for the treatment of strongyloidiasis despite gastrointestinal side effects and a high relapse rate (6,176). However, recent studies have shown ivermectin (Stromectol) to be the best drug for the treatment of uncomplicated *S. stercoralis* infection (198,199). It is well tolerated, and the cure rate is higher than with thiabendazole. Other drugs, such as mebendazole (Vermox) and albendazole, have shown variable therapeutic efficacy (168). Ivermectin has been found to be the most effective drug in treating disseminated strongyloidiasis (200) and chronic intestinal disease in both children (201) and adults (202). Recently, ivermectin has been registered as the drug of choice in the World Health Organization essential drug list for the treatment of *S. stercoralis* infection (203).

PREVENTION

The transmission of *S. stercoralis* can be prevented by implementing public health measures aimed at ensuring the proper disposal and treatment of excrement and by avoiding skin contact with contaminated soil. In patients from areas of endemicity who may harbor asymptomatic chronic strongyloidiasis, life-threatening disseminated hyperinfection can be prevented by seeking and eradicating the parasite before corticosteroid, immunosuppressive, or antineoplastic therapy is started.

REFERENCES

1. Genta RM. Global prevalence of strongyloidiasis: critical review with epidemiologic insights into the prevention of disseminated disease. *Rev Infect Dis* 1989;11:755–767.
2. Barnish G, Ashford RW. *Strongyloides fuelleborni* in Papua New Guinea: epidemiology in an isolated community, and results of an intervention study. *Ann Trop Med Parasitol* 1989;83: 499–506.
3. Hira PR, Patel BG. Human strongyloidiasis due to the primate species *Strongyloides fuelleborni. Trop Geogr Med* 1980;32: 23–29.
4. Ashford, RW, Barnish G, Viney ME. *Strongyloides fuelleborni kellyi*: infection and disease in Papua New Guinea. *Parasitol Today* 1992;8:314–318.
5. Mansfield LS, Niamatali S, Bhopale V, et al. *Strongyloides stercoralis*: maintenance of exceedingly chronic infections. *Am J Trop Med Hyg* 1996;55:617–624.
6. Grove DI. Human strongyloidiasis. *Adv Parasitol* 1996;38: 251–309.
7. Kerlin RL, Nolan TJ, Schad GA. *Strongyloides stercoralis*: histopathology of uncomplicated and hyperinfective strongyloidiasis in the Mongolian gerbil, a rodent model for human strongyloidiasis. *Int J Parasitol* 1995;25:411–420.
8. Berk SL, Verghese A. Parasitic pneumonia. *Semin Respir Infect* 1988;3:172–178.
9. Wehner JH, Kirsch CM. Pulmonary manifestations of strongyloidiasis. *Semin Respir Infect* 1997;12:122–129.
10. Karp CL, Neva FA. Tropical infectious diseases in human immunodeficiency virus-infected patients. *Clin Infect Dis* 1999; 28:947–963.
11. Woodring JH, Halfhill H 2nd, Reed JC. Pulmonary strongyloidiasis: clinical and imaging features. *AJR Am J Roentgenol* 1994;162:537–542.
12. Woodring JH, Halfhill H 2nd, Berger R, et al. Clinical and imaging features of pulmonary strongyloidiasis. *South Med J* 1996;89:10–19.
13. Link K, Orenstein R. Bacterial complications of strongyloidiasis: *Streptococcus bovis* meningitis. *South Med J* 1999;92: 728–731.
14. Ting YM. Pulmonary strongyloidiasis—case report of 2 cases. *Kao Hsiung J Med Sci* 2000;16:269–274.
15. Muenning P, Pallin D, Sell RL, et al. The cost-effectiveness of strategies for the treatment of intestinal parasites in immigrants. *N Engl J Med* 1999;340:773–779.
16. Mitre E. Treatment of intestinal parasites in immigrants. *N Engl J Med* 1999;341:377–378.
17. Anderson RC. *Nematode parasites of vertebrates: their development and transmission,* second edition. New York, CABI Publishing, 2000;61–65.
18. Little MD. Comparative morphology of six species of *Strongyloides* (Nematoda) and redefinition of the genus. *J Parasitol* 1966;48:41–47.
19. Abe T, Nawa Y, Yoshimura K. Protease-resistant interleukin-3–stimulating components in excretory and secretory products from adult worms of *Strongyloides ratti. J Helminthol* 1992;66: 155–158.
20. Grove DI, Northern C. Dissociation of the protective immune response in the mouse to *Strongyloides ratti. J Helminthol* 1989; 63:307–314.
21. Genta RM, Ottesen EA, Gam AA, et al. Immunologic responses to experimental strongyloidiasis in rats. *Z Parasitenkd* 1983;69:667–675.
22. Grove DI, Dawkins HJ. Effects of prednisolone on murine strongyloidiasis. *Parasitology* 1981;83:401–409.
23. Genta RM, Ward PA. The histopathology of experimental strongyloidiasis. *Am J Pathol* 1980;99:207–220.
24. Schad GA. Morphology and life history of *Strongyloides stercoralis.* In: Grove DI, ed. *Strongyloidiasis: a major roundworm infection of man.* London: Taylor and Francis, 1989:85–104.
25. Heyworth MF. Parasitic diseases in immunocompromised hosts. Cryptosporidiosis, isosporiasis, and strongyloidiasis. *Gastroenterol Clin North Am* 1996;25:691–707.
26. Genta RM. Dysregulation of strongyloidiasis: a new hypothesis. *Clin Microbiol Rev* 1992;5:345–355.
27. Mansfield LS, Schad GA. Ivermectin treatment of naturally acquired and experimentally induced *Strongyloides stercoralis* infections in dogs. *J Am Vet Med Assoc* 1992;201:726–730.
28. Neva FA. Biology and immunology of human strongyloidiasis. *J Infect Dis* 1986;153:397–406.
29. Lintermans JP. Fatal peritonitis, an unusual complication of

Strongyloides stercoralis infestation. *Clin Pediatr (Phila)* 1975;14: 974–975.
30. Pawlowski ZS. Epidemiology, prevention and control. In: Grove DI, ed. *Strongyloidiasis: a major roundworm infection of man.* London: Taylor and Francis, 1989:233–249.
31. Subbannayya K, Babu MH, Kumar A, et al. *Entamoeba histolytica* and other parasitic infections in south Kanara district, Karnataka. *J Commun Dis* 1989;21:207–213.
32. de Messias IT, Telles FQ, Boaretti AC, et al. Clinical, immunological and epidemiological aspects of strongyloidiasis in an endemic area of Brazil. *Allergol Immunopathol (Madr)* 1987;15: 37–41.
33. Carvalho Filho E. Strongyloidiasis. *Clin Gastroenterol* 1978;7: 179–200.
34. Poirriez J, Becquet R, Dutoit E, et al. Autochthonous strongyloidiasis in the north of France. *Bull Soc Pathol Exot* 1992;85: 292–295.
35. Doury P. Autochthonous anguilluliasis in France. *Bull Soc Pathol Exot* 1993;86:116.
36. Genta RM, Gatti S, Linke MJ, et al. Endemic strongyloidiasis in northern Italy: clinical and immunological aspects. *Q J Med* 1988;68:679–690.
37. Cadi Soussi M, Kerkeb O, Mellouki W. Autochthonous anguilluliasis. Apropos of 3 cases. *Maroc Med* 1986;8:476–480.
38. Eyckmans L, Van Landuyt H, Vermylen J, et al. Autochthonous strongyloidiasis in Belgium. *Ann Soc Belg Med Trop* 1967;47: 265–270.
39. Castelli D, Vercellino E. On strongyloidiasis endemy in Piedmont. *G Mal Infett Parassit* 1967;19:453–455.
40. Berthoud F, Berthoud S. Eighteen cases of anguilluliasis diagnosed at Geneva. *Schweiz Med Wochenschr* 1975;105: 1110–1115.
41. Shimanskaia GA. Strongyloidiasis in the population of Vladimir-Volynsk district of the Volynsk region. *Med Parazitol (Mosk)* 1973;42:612.
42. Borisenko VS. Strongyloidiasis in psychoneurological boarding houses of Dniepropetrovsk region. *Vrach Delo* 1974;7:140–143.
43. Prokhorov AF, Isupov IUI, Golovan TV, et al. Epidemiology of strongyloidiasis in the northern Caucasus. *Med Parazitol (Mosk)* 1983;52:34–38.
44. Genta RM, Weesner R, Douce RW, et al. Strongyloidiasis in US veterans of the Vietnam and other wars. *JAMA* 1987;258: 49–52.
45. Walzer PD, Milder JE, Banwell JG, et al. Epidemiologic features of *Strongyloides stercoralis* infection in an endemic area of the United States. *Am J Trop Med Hyg* 1982;31:313–319.
46. Arakaki T, Kohakura M, Asato R, et al. Epidemiological aspects of *Strongyloides stercoralis* infection in Okinawa, Japan. *J Trop Med Hyg* 1992;95:210–213.
47. Fisher D, McCarry F, Currie B. Strongyloidiasis in the Northern Territory. Under-recognised and under-treated? *Med J Aust* 1993;159:88–90.
48. Prociv P, Luke R. Observations on strongyloidiasis in Queensland aboriginal communities. *Med J Aust* 1993;158:160–163.
49. Braun TI, Fekete T, Lynch A. Strongyloidiasis in an institution for mentally retarded adults. *Arch Intern Med* 1988;148:634–636.
50. Proctor EM, Muth HA, Proudfoot DL, et al. Endemic institutional strongyloidiasis in British Columbia. *Can Med Assoc J* 1987;136:1173–1176.
51. Sargent RG. Parasitic infection among residents of an institution for mentally retarded persons. *Am J Ment Defic* 1983;87: 566–569.
52. Dias RM, Mangini AC, Torres DM, et al. Ocorrencia de *Strongyloides stercoralis* em pacientes portadores da sindrome de imunodeficiencia adquirida (AIDS). *Rev Inst Med Trop Sao Paulo* 1992;34:15–17.
53. Hunter G, Bagshawe AF, Baboo KS, et al. Intestinal parasites in Zambian patients with AIDS. *Trans R Soc Trop Med Hyg* 1992; 86:543–545.
54. Lucas SB. Missing infections in AIDS. *Trans R Soc Trop Med Hyg* 1990;84[Suppl 1]:34–38.
55. Petithory JC, Derouin F. AIDS and strongyloidiasis in Africa [Letter]. *Lancet* 1987;1:921.
56. Guerin JM, Leibinger F, Mofredj A. *Strongyloides stercoralis* infection in patients infected with human immunodeficiency virus. *Clin Infect Dis* 1997;24:95.
57. Kramer MR, Gregg PA, Goldstein M, et al. Disseminated strongyloidiasis in AIDS and non-AIDS immunocompromised hosts: diagnosis by sputum and bronchoalveolar lavage. *South Med J* 1990;83:1226–1229.
58. Maayan S, Wormser GP, Widerhorn J, et al. *Strongyloides stercoralis* hyperinfection in a patient with the acquired immune deficiency syndrome. *Am J Med* 1987;83:945–948.
59. Makris AN, Sher S, Bertoli C, et al. Pulmonary strongyloidiasis: an unusual opportunistic pneumonia in a patient with AIDS. *AJR Am J Roentgenol* 1993;161:545–547.
60. Schainberg L, Scheinberg MA. Recovery of *Strongyloides stercoralis* by bronchoalveolar lavage in a patient with acquired immunodeficiency syndrome. *Am J Med* 1989;87:486.
61. Vieyra Herrera G, Becerril Carmona G, Padua Gabriel A, et al. *Strongyloides stercoralis* hyperinfection in a patient with the acquired immune deficiency syndrome. *Acta Cytol* 1988;32: 277–278.
62. Lee BE, Robinson JL. Strongyloidiasis and infection due to human immunodeficiency virus: 25 cases at a Brazilian teaching hospital, including seven cases of hyperinfection syndrome. *Clin Infect Dis* 1999;28:154.
63. Marsh BJ. Infectious complications of human T cell leukemia/ lymphoma virus type I infection. *Clin Infect Dis* 1996;23: 138–145.
64. Igra-Siegman Y, Kapila R, Sen P, et al. Syndrome of hyperinfection with *Strongyloides stercoralis. Rev Infect Dis* 1981;3: 397–407.
65. Scowden EB, Schaffner W, Stone WJ. Overwhelming strongyloidiasis: an unappreciated opportunistic infection. *Medicine (Baltimore)* 1978;57:527–544.
66. Schad GA, Hellman ME, Muncey DW. *Strongyloides stercoralis*: hyperinfection in immunosuppressed dogs. *Exp Parasitol* 1984; 57:287–296.
67. Genta RM, Schad GA, Hellman ME. *Strongyloides stercoralis*: parasitological, immunological and pathological observations in immunosuppressed dogs. *Trans R Soc Trop Med* Hyg 1986;80: 34–41.
68. Schad GA, Aikens LM, Smith G. *Strongyloides stercoralis*: is there a canonical migratory route through the host? *J Parasitol* 1989;75:740–749.
69. Genta RM, Miles P, Fields K. Opportunistic *Strongyloides stercoralis* infection in lymphoma patients. Report of a case and review of the literature. *Cancer* 1989;63:1407–1411.
70. Schad GA, Smith G, Megyeri Z, et al. *Strongyloides stercoralis*: an initial autoinfective burst amplifies primary infection. *Am J Trop Med Hyg* 1993;48:716–725.
71. Koolman J, Moeller H. Diagnosis of major helminthic infections by RIA detection of ecdysteroids in urine and serum. *Insect Biochem* 1986;16:287–291.
72. Koolman J, Walter J, Zahner H. Ecdysteroids in helminths. In: Hoffmann J, Porchet M, eds. *Metabolism and mode of action of invertebrate hormones.* Berlin: Springer-Verlag, 1984:323–330.
73. Sato Y, Shiroma Y. Peripheral lymphocyte subsets and their responsiveness in human strongyloidiasis. *Clin Immunol Immunopathol* 1989;53:430–438.
74. Sato Y, Inoue F, Matsuyama R, et al. Immunoblot analysis of

antibodies in human strongyloidiasis. *Trans R Soc Trop Med Hyg* 1990;84:403–406.
75. Northern C, Grove DI. *Strongyloides stercoralis*: antigenic analysis of infective larvae and adult worms. *Int J Parasitol* 1990; 20:381–387.
76. Genta RM, Lillibridge JP. Prominence of IgG4 antibodies in the human responses to *Strongyloides stercoralis* infection. *J Infect Dis* 1989;160:692–699.
77. Badaro R, Carvalho EM, Santos RB, et al. Parasite-specific humoral responses in different clinical forms of strongyloidiasis. *Trans R Soc Trop Med Hyg* 1987;81:149–150.
78. Northern C, Grove DI. Western blot analysis of reactivity to larval and adult *Strongyloides ratti* antigens in mice. *Parasite Immunol* 1988;10:681–691.
79. Genta RM, Frei DF, Linke MJ. Demonstration and partial characterization of parasite-specific immunoglobulin A responses in human strongyloidiasis. *J Clin Microbiol* 1987;25: 1505–1510.
80. McRury J, de Messias IT, Walzer PD, et al. Specific IgE responses in human strongyloidiasis. *Clin Exp Immunol* 1986; 65:631–638.
81. Genta RM, Ottesen EA, Neva FA, et al. Cellular responses in human strongyloidiasis. *Am J Trop Med Hyg* 1983;32:990–994.
82. Genta RM, Ottesen EA, Poindexter R, et al. Specific allergic sensitization to *Strongyloides* antigens in human strongyloidiasis. *Lab Invest* 1983;48:633–638.
83. Genta RM, Weil GJ. Antibodies to *Strongyloides stercoralis* larval surface antigens in chronic strongyloidiasis. *Lab Invest* 1982; 47:87–90.
84. Shelhamer JH, Neva FA, Finn DR. Persistent strongyloidiasis in an immunodeficient patient. *Am J Trop Med Hyg* 1982;31: 746–751.
85. Brandt de Oliveira R, Voltarelli JC, Meneghelli UG. Severe strongyloidiasis associated with hypogammaglobulinaemia. *Parasite Immunol* 1981;3:165–169.
86. Genta RM, Douce RW, Walzer PD. Diagnostic implications of parasite-specific immune responses in immunocompromised patients with strongyloidiasis. *J Clin Microbiol* 1986;23: 1099–1103.
87. Morgan JS, Schaffner W, Stone WJ. Opportunistic strongyloidiasis in renal transplant recipients. *Transplantation* 1986;42: 518–524.
88. DeVault GA Jr, Brown ST, Montoya SF Jr, et al. Disseminated strongyloidiasis complicating acute renal allograft rejection. Prolonged thiabendazole administration and successful retransplantation. *Transplantation* 1982;34:220–221.
89. Weller IV, Copland P, Gabriel R. *Strongyloides stercoralis* infection in renal transplant recipients. *Br Med J (Clin Res Ed)* 1981;282:524.
90. Scoggin CH, Call NB. Acute respiratory failure due to disseminated strongyloidiasis in a renal transplant recipient. *Ann Intern Med* 1977;87:456–458.
91. Hakim SZ, Genta RM. Fatal disseminated strongyloidiasis in a Vietnam War veteran. *Arch Pathol Lab Med* 1986;110:809–812.
92. Krzanowski JJ. Mechanism of glucocorticoid action. *J Fla Med Assoc* 1993;80:697–700.
93. Siddiqui AA, Stanley CS, Skelly PJ, et al. A cDNA encoding a nuclear hormone receptor of the steroid/thyroid hormone-receptor superfamily from the human parasitic nematode *Strongyloides stercoralis. Parasitol Res* 2000;86:24–29.
94. De Paola D, Braga-Dias L, da Silva JR. Enteritis due to *Strongyloides stercoralis. Am J Dig Dis* 1962;7:1086–1098.
95. Genta RM, Caymmi-Gomes M. Pathology. In: Grove DI, ed. *Strongyloidiasis: a major roundworm infection of man.* London: Taylor and Francis, 1989:105–132.
96. Kennedy S, Campbell RM, Lawrence JE, et al. A case of severe *Strongyloides stercoralis* infection with jejunal perforation in an Australian ex-prisoner-of-war. *Med J Aust* 1989;150:92–93.
97. Carp NZ, Nejman JH, Kelly JJ. Strongyloidiasis. An unusual cause of colonic pseudopolyposis and gastrointestinal bleeding. *Surg Endosc* 1987;1:175–177.
98. Berry AJ, Long EG, Smith JH, et al. Chronic relapsing colitis due to *Strongyloides stercoralis. Am J Trop Med Hyg* 1983;32: 1289–1293.
99. Nadler S, Cappell MS, Bhatt B, et al. Appendiceal infection by *Entamoeba histolytica* and *Strongyloides stercoralis* presenting like acute appendicitis. *Dig Dis Sci* 1990;35:603–608.
100. Shakir AA, Youngberg G, Alvarez S. *Strongyloides* infestation as a cause of acute appendicitis. *J Tenn Med Assoc* 1986;79:543–544.
101. Noodleman JS. Eosinophilic appendicitis. Demonstration of *Strongyloides stercoralis* as a causative agent. *Arch Pathol Lab Med* 1981;105:148–149.
102. Williford ME, Foster WL Jr, Halvorsen RA, et al. Emphysematous gastritis secondary to disseminated strongyloidiasis. *Gastrointest Radiol* 1982;7:123–126.
103. Olurin EO. Strongyloidiasis causing fatal peritonitis. *West Afr Med J Niger Pract* 1970;19:102–104.
104. Poltera AA, Katsimbura N. Granulomatous hepatitis due to *Strongyloides stercoralis. J Pathol* 1974;113:241–246.
105. Davidson RA, Fletcher RH, Chapman LE. Risk factors for strongyloidiasis. A case–control study. *Arch Intern Med* 1984; 144:321–324.
106. Davidson RA. Strongyloidiasis: a presentation of 63 cases. *N C Med J* 1982;43:23–25.
107. Milder JE, Walzer PD, Kilgore G, et al. Clinical features of *Strongyloides stercoralis* infection in an endemic area of the United States. *Gastroenterology* 1981;80:1481–1488.
108. Dellacona S, Spier N, Wessely Z, et al. Massive colonic hemorrhage secondary to infection with *Strongyloides stercoralis. N Y State J Med* 1984;84:397–399.
109. Cunliffe WJ, Garcia S. Linear urticaria due to larva currens—strongyloidiasis. *Br J Dermatol* 1968;80:108–110.
110. Kane MG, Luby JP, Krejs GJ. Intestinal secretion as a cause of hypokalemia and cardiac arrest in a patient with strongyloidiasis. *Dig Dis Sci* 1984;29:768–772.
111. Milner PF, Irvine RA, Barton CJ, et al. Intestinal malabsorption in *Strongyloides stercoralis* infestation. *Gut* 1965;6:574–581.
112. Laudanna AA, Polack M, Betarello A, et al. Evidence of protein-losing enteropathy in strongyloidiasis. *Rev Inst Med Trop Sao Paulo* 1973;15:222–226.
113. Alam SZ, Purohit D. A case report. Malabsorption secondary to *S. stercoralis* infestation. *Med J Zambia* 1982;16:85.
114. Garcia FT, Sessions JT, Strum WB, et al. Intestinal function and morphology in strongyloidiasis. *Am J Trop Med Hyg* 1977;26: 859–865.
115. Weesner RE, Kolinjivadi J, Giannella RA, et al. Effect of *Strongyloides ratti* on small-bowel function in normal and immunosuppressed host rats. *Dig Dis Sci* 1988;33:1316–1321.
116. Genta RM. Diarrhea in helminthic infections. *Clin Infect Dis* 1993;16[Suppl 2]:S122–S129.
117. Cookson JB, Montgomery RD, Morgan HV, et al. Fatal paralytic ileus due to strongyloidiasis. *Br Med J* 1972;4:771–772.
118. Davidson RA. Infection due to *Strongyloides stercoralis* in patients with pulmonary disease. *South Med J* 1992;85:28–31.
119. Kaslow JE, Novey HS, Zuch RH, et al. Disseminated strongyloidiasis: an unheralded risk of corticosteroid therapy [Letter]. *J Allergy Clin Immunol* 1990;86:138.
120. Prociv P. Verminous asthma [Letter; Comment]. *Med J Aust* 1993;158:69.
121. Sadowska H, Konieczny B. Przypadek hiperinwazji *Strongyloides stercoralis* w przebiegu dychawicy oskrzelowej. *Pol Tyg Lek* 1990;45:628–629.

122. Sim TC, Alam R, Grant JA. Refractory wheezing and septicemia in a 57-year-old man with asthma [Clinical Conference]. *Ann Allergy* 1990;65:180–184.
123. Nwokolo C, Imohiosen EA. Strongyloidiasis of respiratory tract presenting as "asthma." *Br Med J* 1973;2:153–154.
124. Ujda J. Case of bronchial asthma in the course of infestation with *Strongyloides stercoralis. Wiad Lek* 1972;25:1089–1091.
125. Klein A, Kaufman H, Most H. Intestinal parasites and asthma. *N Engl J Med* 1971;285:179.
126. Quoix E, Hardy A, Kouao-Bile I, et al. Bronchial asthma associated with anguilluliasis [in French]. *Rev Pneumol Clin* 1984; 40:385–387.
127. Berk SL, Verghese A, Alvarez S, et al. Clinical and epidemiologic features of strongyloidiasis. A prospective study in rural Tennessee. *Arch Intern Med* 1987;147:1257–1261.
128. Caceres MH, Genta RM. Pulmonary microcalcifications associated with *Strongyloides stercoralis* infection. *Chest* 1988;94: 862–865.
129. Marsan C, Marais MH, Sollet JP, et al. Disseminated strongyloidiasis: a case report. *Cytopathology* 1993;4:123–126.
130. Cook GA, Rodriguez H, Silva H, et al. Adult respiratory distress secondary to strongyloidiasis. *Chest* 1987;92:1115–1116.
131. Dwork KG, Jaffe JR, Lieberman HD. Strongyloidiasis with massive hyperinfection. *N Y State J Med* 1975;75:1230–1234.
132. Ford J, Reiss-Levy E, Clark E, et al. Pulmonary strongyloidiasis and lung abscess. *Chest* 1981;79:239–240.
133. Genta RM, Harper JS, Gam AA, et al. Experimental disseminated strongyloidiasis in *Erythrocebus patas.* II. Immunology. *Am J Trop Med Hyg* 1984;33:444–450.
134. Thompson JR, Berger R. Fatal adult respiratory distress syndrome following successful treatment of pulmonary strongyloidiasis. *Chest* 1991;99:772–774.
135. Thompson AJ, Brown MM, Ridley A. *Escherichia coli* meningitis and disseminated strongyloidiasis [Letter]. *J Neurol Neurosurg Psychiatry* 1988;51:1596–1597.
136. Tabacof J, Feher O, Katz A, et al. *Strongyloides* hyperinfection in two patients with lymphoma, purulent meningitis, and sepsis. *Cancer* 1991;68:1821–1823.
137. Schindzielorz A, Edberg SC, Bia FJ. *Strongyloides stercoralis* hyperinfection and central nervous system involvement in a patient with relapsing polychondritis. *South Med J* 1991;84:1055–1057.
138. Chirgwin K. Meningitis and an unusual pathogen. *Hosp Pract* 1990;25:47–48, 51.
139. Furuya N, Shimozi K, Nakamura H, et al. A case report of meningitis and sepsis due to *Enterococcus faecium* complicated with strongyloidiasis. *Kansenshogaku Zasshi* 1989;63:1344–1349.
140. Saito A, Aragaki T, Kinjou F. *Strongyloides* infection and bacterial meningitis in immunocompromised host, especially anti-HTLV-1 antibody–positive patients. *Kansenshogaku Zasshi* 1988;62[Suppl]:71–72.
141. Vishwanath S, Baker RA, Mansheim BJ. *Strongyloides* infection and meningitis in an immunocompromised host. *Am J Trop Med Hyg* 1982;31:857–858.
142. Neefe LI, Pinilla O, Garagusi VF, et al. Disseminated strongyloidiasis with cerebral involvement. A complication of corticosteroid therapy. *Am J Med* 1973;55:832–838.
143. Meltzer RS, Singer C, Armstrong D, et al. Case report: antemortem diagnosis of central nervous system strongyloidiasis. *Am J Med Sci* 1979;277:91–98.
144. Owor R, Wamukota WM. A fatal case of strongyloidiasis with *Strongyloides* larvae in the meninges. *Trans R Soc Trop Med Hyg* 1977;70:497–499.
145. Masdeu JC, Tantulavanich S, Gorelick PP, et al. Brain abscess caused by *Strongyloides stercoralis. Arch Neurol* 1982;39:62–63.
146. Forzy G, Dhondt JL, Leloire O, et al. Reactive arthritis and *Strongyloides* [Letter]. *JAMA* 1988;259:2546–2547.
147. Akoglu T, Tuncer I, Erken E, et al. Parasitic arthritis induced by *Strongyloides stercoralis. Ann Rheum Dis* 1984;43:523–525.
148. Doury P. Parasitic rheumatism [Letter]. *Arthritis Rheum* 1981; 24:638–639.
149. Bocanegra TS, Espinoza LR, Bridgeford PH, et al. Reactive arthritis induced by parasitic infestation. *Ann Intern Med* 1981; 94:207–209.
150. Becquet R, Dutoit E, Poirriez J, et al. Cardiac form of anguillulosis [Letter]. *Presse Med* 1983;12:1366–1367.
151. Haggerty JJ Jr, Sandler R. Strongyloidiasis presenting as depression: a case report. *J Clin Psychiatry* 1982;43:340–341.
152. Agbo K, Deniau M. Anguillulospermia resistant to treatment. Apropos of a case diagnosed in Togo [in French]. *Bull Soc Pathol Exot Filiales* 1987;80:271–273.
153. Corsini AC. Strongyloidiasis and chronic urticaria. *Postgrad Med J* 1982;58:247–248.
154. Leighton PM, MacSween HM. *Strongyloides stercoralis.* The cause of an urticarial-like eruption of 65 years' duration. *Arch Intern Med* 1990;150:1747–1748.
155. von Kuster LC, Genta RM. Cutaneous manifestations of strongyloidiasis. *Arch Dermatol* 1988;124:1826–1830.
156. Flensted-Jensen J. Cutaneous strongyloidiasis. *Ugeskr Laeger* 1982;144:721–722.
157. Lapierre J. Often unrecognized cutaneous manifestations of strongyloidosis: linear dermatitis or larva currens. *Semin Hop* 1980;56:409–413.
158. Orecchia G, Pazzaglia A, Scaglia M, et al. Larva currens following systemic steroid therapy in a case of strongyloidiasis. *Dermatologica* 1985;171:366–367.
159. Pelletier LL Jr, Baker CB, Gam AA, et al. Diagnosis and evaluation of treatment of chronic strongyloidiasis in ex-prisoners of war. *J Infect Dis* 1988;157:573–576.
160. Stone OJ, Newell GB, Mullins JF. Cutaneous strongyloidiasis: larva currens. *Arch Dermatol* 1972;106:734–736.
161. Verburg GP, de Geus A. Strongyloidiasis bij voormalige krijgsgevangenen en geinterneerden die tijdens de Tweede Wereldoorlog in Zuidoost-Azie verbleven. *Ned Tijdschr Geneeskd* 1990;134:2529–2533.
162. Pelletier LL Jr. Chronic strongyloidiasis in World War II Far East ex-prisoners of war. *Am J Trop Med Hyg* 1984;33:55–61.
163. Grove DI. Strongyloidiasis in Allied ex-prisoners of war in southeast Asia. *Br Med J* 1980;280:598–601.
164. Gill GV, Bell DR. *Strongyloides stercoralis* infection in former Far East prisoners of war. *Br Med J* 1979;2:572–574.
165. Bank DE, Grossman ME, Kohn SR, et al. The thumbprint sign: rapid diagnosis of disseminated strongyloidiasis. *J Am Acad Dermatol* 1990;23:324–326.
166. Berenson CS, Dobuler KJ, Bia FJ. Fever, petechiae, and pulmonary infiltrates in an immunocompromised Peruvian man. *Yale J Biol Med* 1987;60:437–445.
167. Kalb RE, Grossman ME. Periumbilical purpura in disseminated strongyloidiasis. *JAMA* 1986;256:1170–1171.
168. Liu LX, Weller PF. Strongyloidiasis and other intestinal nematode infections. *Infect Dis Clin North Am* 1993;7: 655–682.
169. Nielsen PB, Mojon M. Improved diagnosis of *Strongyloides stercoralis* by seven consecutive stool specimens. *Zentralbl Bakteriol Mikrobiol Hyg [A]* 1987;263:616–618.
170. Garcia LS, Bruckner DA. *Diagnostic medical parasitology.* Washington, DC: American Society for Microbiology Press, 1993; 203–212.
171. Siddiqui AA, Berk SL. Diagnosis of *Strongyloides stereoralis* infection. *Clin Infect Dis* 2001;33:1040–1047.
172. Gutierrez Y. *Diagnostic pathology of parasitic infections with clinical correlations,* second edition. Oxford: Oxford University Press, 2000;283–313.

173. Kemp L, Hawley T. Clinical pathology rounds. Strongyloidiasis in a hyperinfected patient. *Lab Med* 1996;27:237–240.
174. Sato Y, Kobayashi J, Toma H, et al. Efficacy of stool examination for detection of *Strongyloides* infection. *Am J Trop Med Hyg* 1995;53:248–250.
175. de Kaminsky RG. Evaluation of three methods for laboratory diagnosis of *Strongyloides stercoralis* infection. *J Parasitol* 1993; 79:277–280.
176. Zaha O, Hirata T, Kinjo F, et al. Strongyloidiasis—progress in diagnosis and treatment. *Intern Med* 2000;39:695–700.
177. Beal CB, Viens P, Grant RG, et al. A new technique for sampling duodenal contents: demonstration of upper small-bowel pathogens. *Am J Trop Med Hyg* 1970;19:349–352.
178. Siddiqui AA, Gutierrez C, Berk SL. Diagnosis of *Strongyloides stercoralis* by acid-fast staining. *J Helminthol* 1999;73:187–188.
179. Ansari TM, Couch L, Idell S. *Strongyloides*-induced lung disease. *Emerg Med* 1997;4:127–136.
180. Sato Y, Otsuru M, Takara M, et al. Intradermal reactions in strongyloidiasis. *Int J Parasitol* 1986;16:87–91.
181. Sato Y, Toma H, Kiyuna S, et al. Gelatin particle indirect agglutination test for mass examination for strongyloidiasis. *Trans R Soc Trop Med Hyg* 1991;85:515–518.
182. Lindo JF, Conway DJ, Atkins NS, et al. Prospective evaluation of enzyme-linked immunosorbent assay and immunoblot methods for the diagnosis of endemic *Strongyloides stercoralis* infection. *Am J Trop Med Hyg* 1994;51:175–179.
183. Gam AA, Neva FA, Krotoski WA. Comparative sensitivity and specificity of ELISA and IHA for serodiagnosis of strongyloidiasis with larval antigens. *Am J Trop Med Hyg* 1987;37:157–161.
184. Genta RM. Predictive value of an enzyme-linked immunosorbent assay (ELISA) for the serodiagnosis of strongyloidiasis. *Am J Clin Pathol* 1988;89:391–394.
185. Sato Y, Kobayashi J, Shiroma Y. Serodiagnosis of strongyloidiasis. The application and significance. *Rev Inst Med Trop Sao Paulo* 1995;37:35–41.
186. Conway DJ, Atkins NS, Lillywhite JE, et al. Immunodiagnosis of *Strongyloides stercoralis* infection: a method for increasing the specificity of the indirect ELISA. *Trans R Soc Trop Med Hyg* 1993;87:173–176.
187. Gyorkos TW, Genta RM, Viens P, et al. Seroepidemiology of *Strongyloides* infection in the Southeast Asian refugee population in Canada. *Am J Epidemiol* 1990;132:257–264.
188. Joseph L, Gyorkos TW, Coupal L. Bayesian estimation of disease prevalence and the parameters of diagnostic tests in the absence of a gold standard. *Am J Epidemiol* 1995;141:263–272.
189. Lindo JF, Atkins NS, Lee MG, et al. Parasite-specific serum IgG following successful treatment of endemic strongyloidiasis using ivermectin. *Trans R Soc Trop Med Hyg* 1996;90:702–703.
190. Maizels RM, Bundy DAP, Selkirk ME, et al. Immunological modulations and evasion by helminth parasites in human populations. *Nature* 1993;365:797–805.
191. Brindley PJ, Gam AA, Pearce EJ, et al. Antigens from the surface and excretions/secretions of the filariform larva of *Strongyloides stercoralis. Mol Biochem Parasitol* 1988;28:171–180.
192. Conway DJ, Bailey JW, Lindo JF, et al. Serum IgG reactivity with 41-, 31-, and 28-kDa larval proteins of *Strongyloides stercoralis* in individuals with strongyloidiasis. *J Infect Dis* 1993; 168:784–787.
193. Conway DJ, Lindo JF, Robinson RD, et al. *Strongyloides stercoralis*: characterization of immunodiagnostic larval antigens. *Exp Parasitol* 1994;79:99–105.
194. Ramachandran S, Thompson RW, Gam AA, et al. Recombinant cDNA clones for immunodiagnosis of strongyloidiasis. *J Infect Dis* 1998;177:196–203.
195. Siddiqui AA, Koenig NM, Sinensky M, et al. *Strongyloides stercoralis*: identification of antigens in natural human infections from endemic areas of the United States. *Parasitol Res* 1997;83: 655–658.
196. Siddiqui AA, Stanley CS, Berk SL. Cloning and expression of isocitrate lyase from human round worm *Strongyloides stercoralis. Parasite* 2000;7:233–236.
197. Siddiqui AA, Stanley CS, Berk SL. A cDNA encoding the highly immunodominant antigen of *Strongyloides stercoralis*: gamma-subunit of isocitrate dehydrogenase (NAD+). *Parasitol Res* 2000;86:279–283.
198. Salazar SA, Berk SH, Howe D, et al. Ivermectin vs thiabendazole in the treatment of strongyloidiasis. *Infect Med* 1994;11: 50–59.
199. Ashraf M, Gue CL, Baddour LM. Case report: strongyloidiasis refractory to treatment with ivermectin. *Am J Med Sci* 1996; 311:178–179.
200. Daubenton JD, Buys HA, Hartley PS. Disseminated strongyloidiasis in a child with lymphoblastic lymphoma. *J Pediatr Hematol Oncol* 1998;20:260–263.
201. Adenusi AA. Cure by ivermectin of a chronic, persistent, intestinal strongyloidosis. *Acta Trop* 1997;66:163–167.
202. Marti H, Haji HJ, Savioli L, et al. A comparative trial of a single-dose ivermectin versus three days of albendazole for treatment of *Strongyloides stercoralis* and other soil-transmitted helminth infections in children. *Am J Trop Med Hyg* 1996;55:477–481.
203. Albonico M, Crompton DW, Savioli L. Control strategies for human intestinal nematode infections. *Adv Parasitol* 1999;42: 277–341.
204. Menan EI, Nebavi NG, Adjetey TA, et al. Profile of intestinal helminthiases in school-aged children in the city of Abidjan. *Bull Soc Pathol Exot* 1997;90:51–54.
205. Taranto NJ, Bonomi de Filippi H, Orione O. Prevalence of *Strongyloides stercoralis* infection in childhood, Oran, Salta, Argentina. *Bol Chil Parasitol* 1993;48: 49–51.
206. Borda CE, Rea MJ, Rosa JR, et al. Intestinal parasitism in San Cayetano, Corrientes, Argentina. *Bull Pan Am Health Organ* 1996;30:227–233.
207. Cimerman S, Cimerman B, Lewi DS. Prevalence of intestinal parasitic infections in patients with acquired immunodeficiency syndrome in Brazil. *Int J Infect Dis* 1999;3:203–206.
208. Machado ER, Costa-Cruz JM. *Strongyloides stercoralis* and other enteroparasites in children at Uberlandia city, state of Minas Gerais, Brazil. *Mem Inst Oswaldo Cruz* 1998;93:161–164.
209. Fontanet AL, Sahlu T, Rinke de Wit T, et al. Epidemiology of infections with intestinal parasites and human immunodeficiency virus (HIV) among sugar-estate residents in Ethiopia. *Ann Trop Med Parasitol* 2000;94:269–278.
210. Gyorkos TW, Camara B, Kokoskin E, et al. Survey of parasitic prevalence in school-aged children in Guinea (1995). *Sante* 1996;6:377–381.
211. Huminer D, Symon K, Groskopf I, et al. Seroepidemiologic study of toxocariasis and strongyloidiasis in institutionalized mentally retarded adults. *Am J Trop Med Hyg* 1992;46:278–281.
212. Joyce T, McGuigan KG, Elmore-Meegan M, et al. Prevalence of enteropathogens in stools of rural Maasai children under five years of age in the Maasailand region of the Kenyan Rift Valley. *East Afr Med J* 1996;73:59–62.
213. Vannachone B, Kobayashi J, Nambanya S, et al. An epidemiological survey on intestinal parasite infection in Khammouane Province, Lao PDR, with special reference to *Strongyloides* infection. *Southeast Asian J Trop Med Public Health* 1998;29:717–722.
214. Guarner J, Matilde-Nava T, Villasenor-Flores R, et al. Frequency of intestinal parasites in adult cancer patients in Mexico. *Med Res* 1997;28:219–222.
215. Agi PI. Comparative helminth infections of man in two rural communities of the Niger Delta, Nigeria. *West Afr J Med* 1997; 16:232–236.

216. Panaitescu D, Capraru T, Bugarin V. Study of the incidence of intestinal and systemic parasitoses in a group of children with handicaps. *Roum Arch Microbiol Immunol* 1995;54: 65–74.
217. Gbakima AA, Sahr F. Intestinal parasitic infections among rural farming communities in eastern Sierra Leone. *Afr J Med Med Sci* 1995;24:195–200.
218. Magambo JK, Zeyhle E, Wachira TM. Prevalence of intestinal parasites among children in southern Sudan. *East Afr Med J* 1998;75:288–290.
219. Kasuya S, Khamboonruang C, Amano K, et al. Intestinal parasitic infections among schoolchildren in Chiang Mai, northern Thailand: an analysis of the present situation. *J Trop Med* Hyg 1989;92:360–364.

71

SCHISTOSOMIASIS

CHRISTOPHER L. KING
ADEL A. F. MAHMOUD

Human infection with several species of schistosome (1) may result in considerable morbidity in the gastrointestinal tract and liver. In some cases, death may occur because of elevation in portal pressure or liver failure. In many endemic communities, high prevalence of infection results in schistosomiasis being the leading cause of gastrointestinal disease. Between 200 and 300 million people are estimated to be infected throughout tropical and subtropical regions of the world, and death directly attributable to this illness may be in excess of 20,000 to 40,000 annually (2). Its impact on health is more insidious, however, and individuals may suffer chronic sequelae or children may suffer impaired growth and development.

In endemic areas, infection is usually acquired early in life as children experience contact with freshwater bodies that contain the infective cercariae. Peak prevalence and intensity are generally seen in adolescents between 12 and 18 years of age (3). Disease sequelae may occur in association with peak intensity of infection or later in life. Gastrointestinal and liver disease are caused by infection with *Schistosoma mansoni, Schistosoma japonicum, Schistosoma mekongi,* or *Schistosoma. intercalatum*. The other major human *Schistosome* species, *S. haematobium,* involves the bladder and urinary tract; whether it contributes to liver or gastrointestinal disease is controversial.

BIOLOGY

The schistosomes are flat worms (Platyhelminth). They differ from all other flukes that infect humans by differentiating into separate sex adult worms in the definitive host (Fig. 71.1). The complicated life cycle of the schistosomes alternates between parasitic and free-living forms, and between intermediate and definitive hosts (Fig. 71.2). Humans (definitive host) acquire infection while in contact with freshwater-contaminated with cercariae. These free-living forms are capable of penetrating intact human skin and transforming into the first stage of parasitic life in the definitive host. Following skin penetration, cercariae transform into schistosomula, which adapt to the hostile environment of the host through a series of membrane biochemical and antigenic changes (4).

Schistosomula remain in the subcutaneous tissue for 2 to 3 days and then travel to the lungs where they undergo a period of development that lasts several days, adapting them for onward intravascular migration. These changes involve elongation and loss of midbody spines in order to facilitate travel along the lumina of capillaries. The migrating larvae are in a semiquiescent metabolic state (5) with reduced levels of protein synthesis, possibly as an adaptation to prevent premature maturation in the wrong site. Larvae leave the lungs in venous blood and are distributed to all organs via the left side of the heart, in proportion to cardiac output (6). Most larvae eventually reach the liver where they attain sexual maturity in 4 to 6 weeks and descend into the portal venous system. Adult worms mate, remain "in copula" as shown in the Figure 71.1, and the female periodically travels downstream to deposit ova. *Schistosoma mansoni* eggs are usually deposited as single ova, whereas *S. japonicum* eggs are deposited as nests of multiple ova. The schistosome eggs migrate from the small venules, where they were deposited, to the lumen of the gut and ultimately pass to the outside environment with feces. This passage of ova from within venules, through the interstitial space and intestinal mucosa, and into the gut is generally thought to require the host inflammatory response to antigenic molecules secreted by the viable organisms (7). Ova may also release proteases to help disrupt tissue barriers and facilitate their release (8). In the process, not all ova successfully reach the gut lumen. Some are retained in the local tissues and others are carried to the liver in the portal system to become lodged in the hepatic presinusoidal spaces. Due to promiscuous defeca-

C. L. King: Division of Geographic Medicine, Department of Medicine, Case Western Reserve University and University Hospitals, Cleveland, Ohio

A. A. F. Mahmoud: Merck Vaccines, Merck & Co., Inc., Whitehouse Station, New Jersey

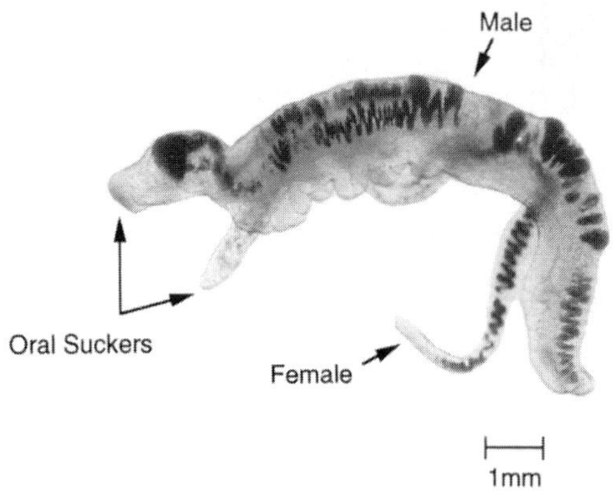

FIGURE 71.1. Male and female schistosomes. Female worm (thinner worm) rests in the gynecophoral canal of the male (×35).

tion in the canals and water bodies of endemic areas, eggs reach freshwater, hatch, and release free-living miracidia. The miracidia search for their specific intermediate host, a snail, in which they penetrate the snail's internal structures and undergo tremendous multiplication, and, finally, transform into cercariae. These forms are shed into fresh water, completing the life cycle of the helminth.

Human infection results in exposure of the host to a multitude of schistosome stages and antigens during the life cycle of the parasite. Disease may occur at each of the major steps of the parasite life cycle: cercarial invasion, schistosomula migration and maturation, and finally egg deposition and retention in tissue (9). Furthermore, the host immunopathologic responses and attempts toward healing result in the major chronic sequelae of infection: granuloma formation and fibrosis.

EPIDEMIOLOGY

The epidemiology of schistosomiasis in nonendemic areas such as North America or Europe differs from its features in endemic communities. Individuals (usually adults) from nonendemic areas are exposed to infection because of a lack of understanding of its mode of transmission. Contact with freshwater bodies in endemic areas, whether stationary, slow, or fast flowing, is the source of infection. This mode of transmission results in infection of individual travelers or,

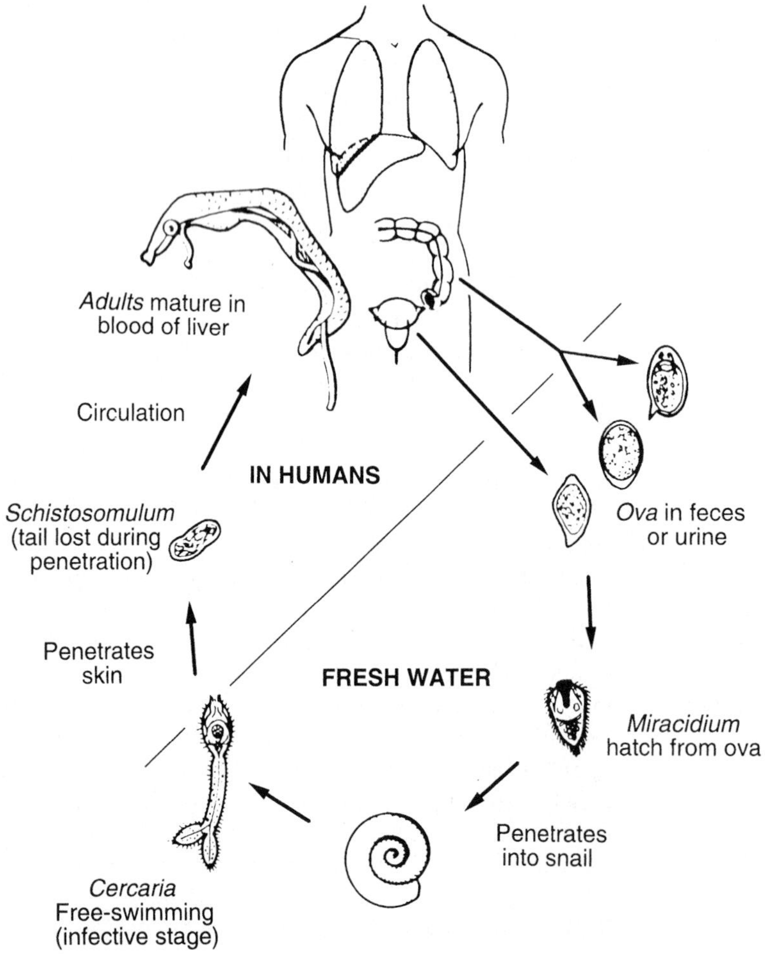

FIGURE 71.2. Life cycle of schistosomiasis.

rarely, a group traveling together, most of them with no previous exposure. Invariably, disease manifestations occur upon return to the nonendemic areas, thus providing a diagnostic and management challenge to an unfamiliar medical profession. Occasionally, several individuals are exposed simultaneously, resulting in a "mini" epidemic, which presents with the acute manifestations of disease.

In endemic areas, exposure to infection usually occurs at a younger age. The prevalence and intensity of infection increase with age up to 15 to 20 years (10). Beyond 30 years of age, prevalence may decline, and intensity of infection decreases significantly. This age-specific pattern of intensity raises important issues related to the ecology of schistosomiasis, patterns of water contact, and the role of acquired immunity in regulating parasite burdens in infected individuals.

Like for other worm infections, the distribution of parasite load in an endemic community does not follow a bell-shaped curve (3,11). Rather, there is an overdispersion of the parasite in the human population with a majority of infected individuals harboring low worm burdens while only a small minority demonstrates high worm and egg counts. This pattern of distribution poses several important clinical, biologic, and epidemiologic issues. Because disease in schistosomiasis is related to the intensity of infection, the group with heavy worm load is at exceptionally high risk for development of disease. Furthermore, this group is responsible for contamination of the environment with parasite eggs and perpetuation of parasite transmission. Finally, the reasons for such an aggregation of infection are unclear; whether it is due to the pattern of exposure, variable host susceptibility to infection and disease, or a combination of factors remains an unanswered question.

PATHOGENESIS

The parasite eggs, produced by adult worms that live in the mesenteric plexus, are the principal cause of chronic pathology in humans. Daily, each female worm deposits hundreds of eggs into the bloodstream. Although the parasite does not self-replicate within the host, it produces eggs continuously throughout the course of its lifespan, which lasts 5 to 10 years. Deposited eggs lodge in the intestinal wall or are carried by venous blood to liver, lungs, and other tissues. The live embryo within each egg secretes antigenic material through ultramicroscopic pores in the shell. These antigens are released for 2 to 4 weeks and induce host sensitization and recruitment of macrophages, lymphocytes, epithelioid and occasional giant cells, fibroblasts, and numerous eosinophils to comprise the host granulomatous response (9). Antigen secretion stops when the embryo within the eggs die; granuloma then undergoes a healing process with deposition of fibrous tissue. Fibrosis of the liver or other tissues can cause portal hypertension, varices, cor pulmonale, and other complications. The mechanisms that initiate, maintain, and immunomodulate the granulomatous response are different from those that regulate the development of fibrosis and are discussed separately.

Granuloma

The function of the granuloma has been postulated to encase the egg and prevent secretion of potentially deleterious antigenic substances by ova (Fig. 71.3). Additionally, the granulomatous response facilitates ova excretion. It also enhances killing of the ova and destruction of its shell. Most of our understanding of how the granuloma is formed and modulated derives from detailed studies of animal models.

Animal Models of Granuloma Formation

Murine experimental models of schistosomiasis have been extensively used to demonstrate the immunologic response to schistosomiasis and mechanisms of granuloma formation and fibrosis (9). Granuloma formation in infected mice occurs after worm maturation and onset of egg deposition at approximately 8 weeks in *S. mansoni* infection. Granulomas reach maximal size and cellularity by 12 weeks and then shrink in size by 20 to 24 weeks (12). A similar pattern of granuloma formation and modulation was observed in murine infection with *S. japonicum*; however, the kinetics are accelerated because of the earlier maturation of these worms. Portal pressure elevates with the increase in granuloma size and diminishes as the granulomas are down-modulated. Initially, studies of the mechanisms of granuloma formation were hindered by the long duration and asynchronous development of granulomas. To avoid these difficulties, viable eggs were isolated from the livers of infected animals and injected intravenously, resulting in well-delineated primary lung granulomas by 16 days. Granuloma formation was found to be T-cell mediated and could be accel-

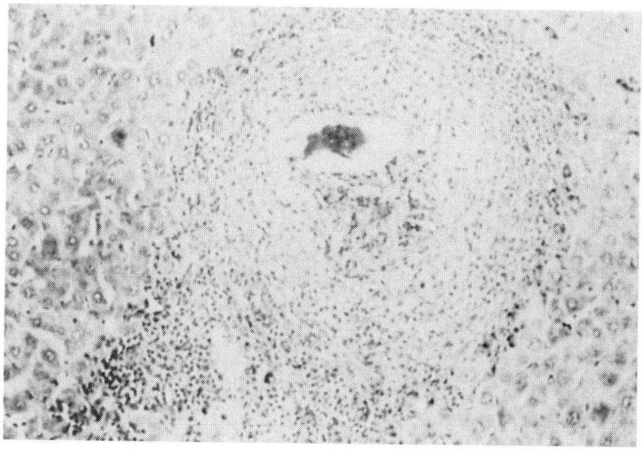

FIGURE 71.3. Schistosome granuloma in liver (*Schistosoma mansoni*). The structureless mass in the center is an ovum.

erated and enhanced by sensitizing mice to egg antigens before intravenous challenge with viable ova. The accelerated granulomatous response could be adoptively transferred by lymphocytes and not serum. This pulmonary model has been widely used to study the immune regulation of schistosome granuloma formation. However, care must be made in extrapolating these finding to granulomas formed in the liver or intestine, because immune cells resident in any particular tissue may have important influences on the mechanisms and dynamics of granuloma formation (14).

The sequence of molecular events involved in the development of schistosome granuloma is shown in Figure 71.4. As the egg becomes trapped in tissues, inflammatory cells are detectable within 48 hours (15). At this point, the granuloma contains multiple populations of rapidly proliferating cells. The initial cell types in the granuloma are phagocytic cells followed by T cells, eosinophils, and finally B cells. The predominant cell type within the maturing granulomas are CD4+ cells, although some CD8+ cells are present. Neutrophils are also observed in the schistosome granuloma, but never exceed 10% of the cellular population. The sequential influx of cells into the granuloma likely reflects both the antigens secreted by the parasite embryo and cytokines and chemokines produced by immune cells in the granuloma.

The initiation, maintenance, and modulation of the granuloma is controlled by series of counterregulating cytokines, chemokines, and cell adhesion molecules, and expression of their associated receptors, which remain to be fully understood. Following egg deposition, T cells initially enter tissues surrounding the eggs, perhaps by adhesion to LFA-1 to ICAM-2, which are constitutively expressed on all endothelial cells (Fig. 71.4). If schistosome Ag-specific T cells recognize egg antigens, they become activated to produce cytokines such as tumor necrosis factor (TNF)-α and interleukin (IL)-4, which activates endothelial cells to express E-selectin, VCAM-1, and ICAM-1 and to produce chemokines such MIP-1α and MIP-1β. These chemokines, in turn, activate T cells to further express adhesion molecules such as VLA-4 and LFA-1, which bind with greater avidity to endothelial cells and in process recruit more activated or effector T cells to antigen secreting ova. At the same time, monocytes are recruited to these sites by adhesion to E-selectin, and they are activated to generate additional chemokines such as eotaxin, MCP-2, and MCP-3 (16). All are ligands for CCR3, a receptor that is strongly expressed on eosinophils (17) and considered important for eosinophil recruitment. Increased production of the chemokine TCA-3 has been observed in schistosome granuloma and is a ligand for CCR8, which also is expressed by Th2 cells and may aid in their recruitment (18). The TNF-α and interferon (IFN)-γ molecules released by activated T cells act synergistically to shape endothelial cells, allowing increased blood flow, greater vascular permeability, and further emigration of leukocytes to form the initial granuloma. Certain neurokines and components of the activated complement cascade may also participate in cell recruitment to the granuloma.

Proposed mechanisms of granuloma modulation are illustrated in Figure 71.5. Cell anergy, death, or emigration reduces cell number in the granuloma. The production of antiinflammatory cytokines such as IL-10 and TGF-β inhibit expression of proinflammatory adhesion molecules, and decreased production of chemokines or their receptors by target cells may prevent cell recruitment and proliferation. Ultimately, ova death produces resolution of the granuloma. Cytotoxic T cells or eosinophils may accelerate ova

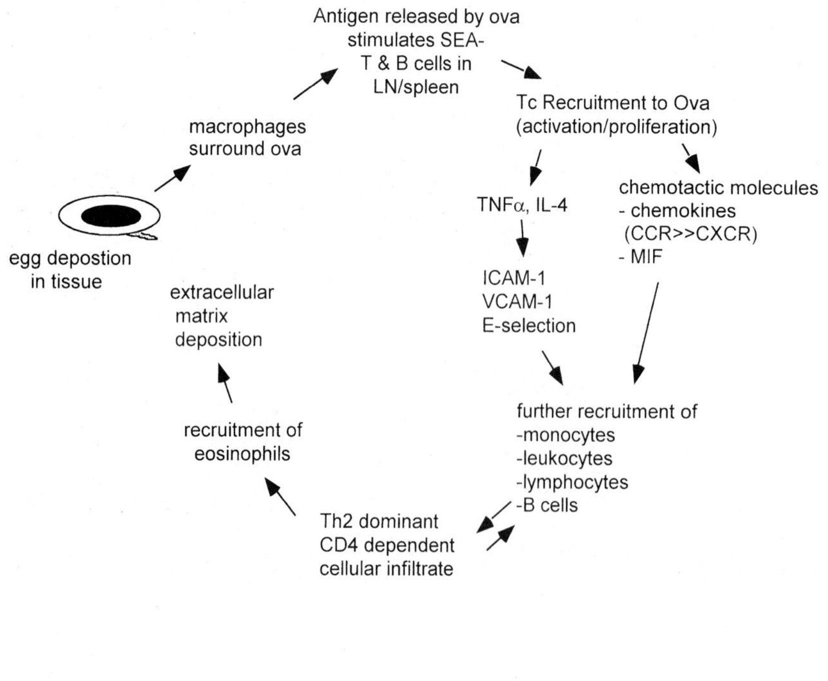

FIGURE 71.4. Molecular events associated with initial granuloma formation.

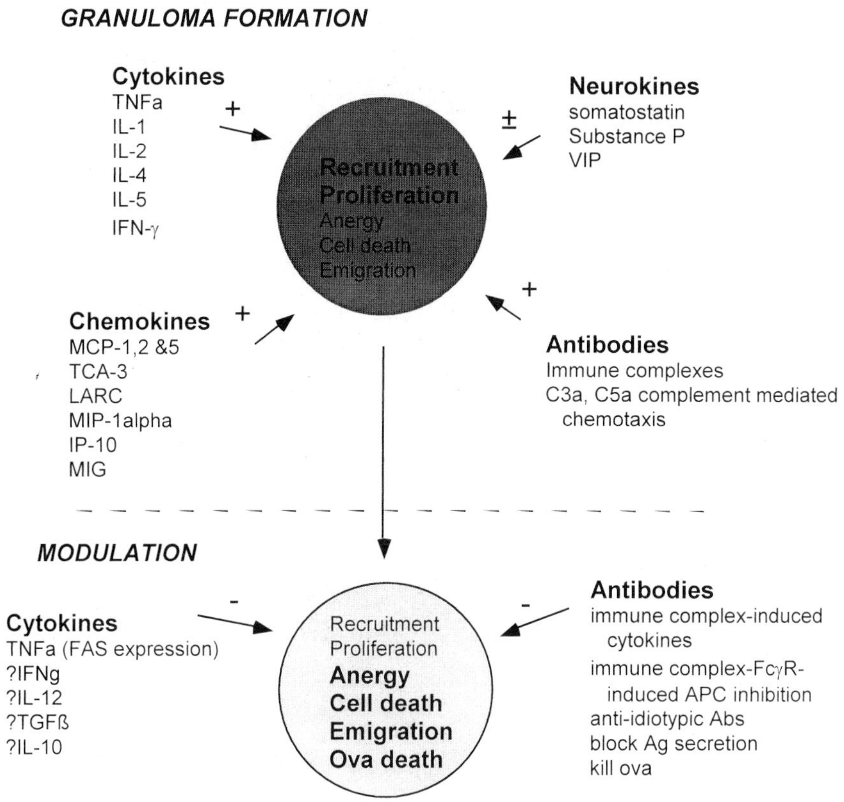

FIGURE 71.5. Molecular signals that control granuloma formation and its subsequent modulation.

death. Antibodies also contribute to granuloma modulation. This may occur by accelerated killing of the ova or by blocking release of their antigens.

DYNAMICS AND REGULATION OF FIBROSIS

Liver and intestinal fibrosis is the major sequelae of granulomatous reactions in schistosomiasis. In addition to the T-cell–mediated inflammatory focus that occurs around schistosome eggs, fibrous healing contributes to the portal and periportal fibrosis (See Color Figure 71.6). Initially, fibrosis was viewed as a static consequence of the dying embryo within the schistosome egg. It is currently recognized that fibrosis is a dynamic process involving mesenchymal cells that respond to a series of molecular signals generated by a variety of cell types (Fig. 71.7). The fundamental process of scar formation that occurs in parallel to that of lymphocyte infiltration into the granuloma includes (a) hyperplasia of the fibroblast population, (b) increased synthesis and deposition of extracellular matrix constituents, particularly collagen, and (c) remodeling of the extracellular matrix by degradative enzymes. Changes in the relative production of collagen isotypes also occur during the course of infection (19,20). As the infection progresses, collagen deposition becomes more pronounced with increased amounts of type I relative to type III, and by 20 weeks, high levels of both types I and III collagen, as well as some type IV collagen, are present. Type I collagen is more heavily cross-linked and degradation resistant and may be correlated with enhanced morbidity. Conversely, in animal models that modulate granuloma formation, a shift from a predominantly type I to type III collagen is observed. These changes in the quantity and makeup of extracellular collagen may ameliorate or exacerbate disease and may enhance or diminish the potential of reversing fibrosis.

T lymphocytes within granuloma that react to egg antigens elaborate cytokines and other molecules such as fibrosin that stimulate fibrosis (Fig. 71.7). IL-13, IL-4, IL-2 and TGF-β are prefibrotic, whereas IFN-γ and IL-12 can inhibit fibrosis (21). Granulomatous inflammation and fibrosis are independently regulated (22). This is highlighted by the lack of spatial relationship of fibrosis to granulomas in humans and nonhuman primates. Periportal fibrosis often develops in the absence of observable granulomas. This implies that soluble factors released from the granulomas can induce fibrosis in locations removed from the granuloma itself.

In most individuals infected with schistosomiasis, clinically significant fibrosis does not develop. The risk factors responsible for development of periportal fibrosis remain poorly understood. Heavy and chronic infection is considered the major risk factors. Other factors may include repeated exposures, duration of infection, age, and the fail-

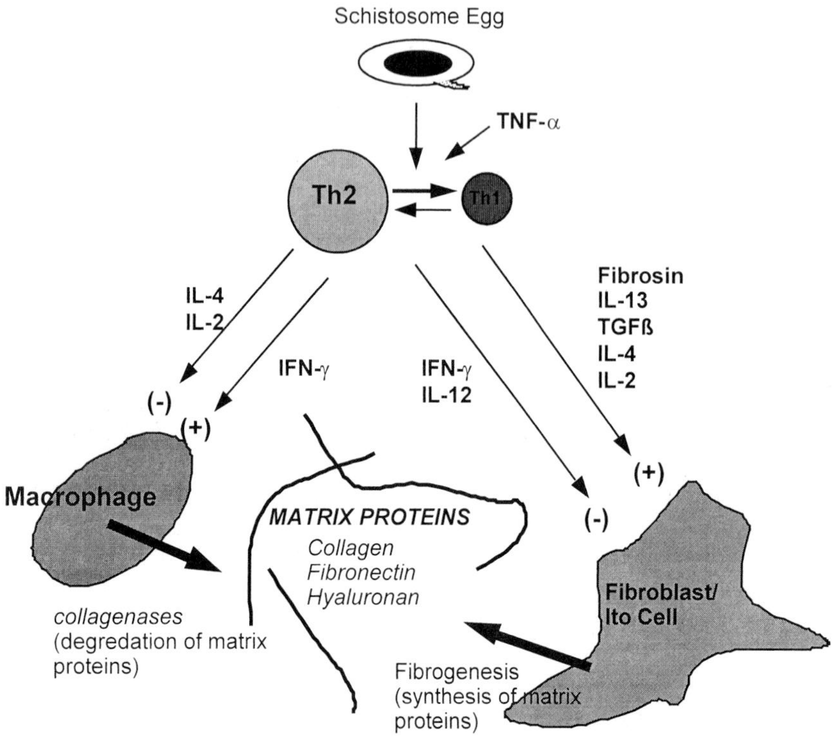

FIGURE 71.7. Cytokine control of hepatic fibrosis.

ure of immunologic modulation. Genetic factors may also contribute as demonstrated by the large variation in the amount of fibrosis observed among different strains of mice. Severe hepatic fibrosis in human *Schistosoma mansoni* infection has been found to be associated with a major locus that is closely linked to the IFN-γ receptor (24). Because IFN-γ can inhibit fibrosis (Fig. 71.7), polymorphisms within the IFN-γ R1 gene could determine severe hepatic disease.

IMMUNITY

During the course of natural infection in fully permissive animal models (mice, baboons) and the semipermissive rat model, acquired immunity develops to reinfection (25). Acquired immunity also develops in chronically infected humans; however, the magnitude and duration of this immunity remain controversial. Although these studies provided an impetus for production of a vaccine, an acceptable candidate vaccine has yet to be developed. This failure in developing a human vaccine results from an inadequate understanding of the mechanisms inducing acquired immunity in humans. Moreover, it has been difficult to extrapolate the multiplicity of immune mechanisms identified in the different animal models to humans.

Immunity to schistosomiasis requires CD4+ lymphocytes and involves both humoral and cell-mediated responses. Because eosinophilia and IgE production are the immunologic hallmarks of schistosome infections in humans and many animal models, it has been postulated that these responses are important effector mechanisms in immunity against parasitic worms. However, other effector cells such as neutrophils, platelets, mast cells, and macrophages may participate in parasite killing.

Acquired immunity has been most completely studied in mice and to lesser extent in nonhuman primates, particularly baboons. In the naturally acquired immunity model, partial resistance to challenge infection after onset of egg deposition develops in chronically infected mice. Egg deposition is necessary for development of this immunity because single-sex infections do not induce immunity in mice. Acquired immunity has also been observed in the rhesus monkey, although the effector mechanisms have not been well defined. In the baboon, which is fully permissive for schistosomiasis, repeated infection and treatment of established infection can enhance immunity to parasite challenge; this protection correlates with elevated levels of parasite-specific IgE (26).

Studies of acquired immunity in humans have been difficult because measurements of exposure and worm burden are imprecise. A striking feature of the epidemiology of schistosomiasis is the linear increase (with increasing age) in both prevalence and intensity of infection, up to the time of early adolescence, after which the average intensity and prevalence of infection declines with age. Although a decline in exposure may partially account for a decline in infection with age (27,28), many epidemiologic studies that have controlled for these confounding variables strongly indicate that part of this decline in prevalence and intensity of infection is a consequence of acquired immunity. Prospective cohort studies in humans based on evaluating rates of reinfection after parasitologic cure provide further evidence that acquired immunity develops in humans. Following treatment, the extent to which reinfection subsequently occurs is strongly age dependent. In areas of continued transmission, young children (12 years or younger) rapidly become heavily reinfected; in some cases, infections develop that reach 50% of pretreatment within 1 year. Moreover, children who are heavily infected before treatment generally reacquire heavy infections and those with light infections become lightly infected again. In contrast, older children and adults become reinfected, if at all, only with low intensity.

The components of the human immune response in host protection remain poorly defined (25). In early studies, passive transfer of serum from presumably immune adults to susceptible children residing in hyperendemic areas failed to show any evidence of protection (27). Many studies suggest a variety of effector mechanisms capable of killing schistosomula *in vitro* primarily by antibody-dependent cell-mediated killing. Macrophages, platelets, neutrophils, and eosinophils all kill schistosomula in the presence of parasite-specific IgG or IgE antibodies. These *in vitro* studies may bear little relationship to human immunity *in vivo*. In children and adults who appear to be partially protected from reinfection, serum levels of parasite-specific IgE correlate with protection (30). Conversely, serum parasite-specific IgG4 levels are higher among susceptible individuals. Because IgG4 recognizes many of the same antigenic epitopes that IgE does, it may act as a blocking antibody to prevent engagement of effector cells coated with IgE. Cellular immunity, such as elevated serum levels of parasite antigen-induced IL-4 and IL-5, has been shown to correlate with protection from reinfection after treatment (31).

Based on the understanding of immune mechanisms in animals and humans, efforts are underway to induce resistance against schistosomiasis using defined antigens. Many recombinant antigens have been cloned and identified particularly for *S. mansoni*. Despite some initially promising results, none of the existing candidate antigens have consistently provided more than the 40% protection necessary in animal models necessary to advance the application to nonhuman primate or human studies.

CLINICAL FEATURES

Infection with any of the intestinal schistosomes may result in gastrointestinal or hepatic disease. These manifestations are seen in association with the established chronic stages of infection. Disease is often appreciated in a small group of infected individuals, usually the young with heavy infection or genetic susceptibility. In contrast, individuals from nonendemic areas often present early with signs and symptoms related to acute schistosomiasis (35). Physicians in North America, Europe, and other nonendemic areas also may encounter disease due to established infection in immigrants.

Pathologic lesions are demonstrated in the gastrointestinal tract and found in most infected individuals. Eggs of *S. mansoni* are mainly deposited in the veins of the inferior mesenteric system, whereas those of *S. japonicum* are usually seen in the distribution of the superior mesenteric vein. Granuloma formation, subsequent scarring, and occasionally colonic polyposis are the main pathologic features. Clinically, infection may be associated with symptoms such as crampy abdominal pain, diarrhea, and passage of blood with stool (32). Colonic polyposis is a specific syndrome described in Egypt (33) but not in other *S. mansoni* endemic areas. Similar lesions have been described in China in association with *S. japonicum* infection. Colonic polyposis may cause bleeding, but the association with colorectal carcinoma is not known. In individuals with chronic infection and portal hypertension due to liver fibrosis, portosystemic varices may develop at the lower end of esophagus and rectum and around the umbilicus (caput medusa). Esophageal varices may result in considerable bleeding, which may be the first serious manifestation of hepatic schistosomiasis and its hemodynamic sequelae. Usually, patients with schistosomal portal hypertension tolerate several bleeding episodes from esophageal varices without going into hepatic encephalopathy. This is because of the retention of a reasonable oxygenation level of hepatocytes due to arterialization of the blood supply of the liver.

In cases of moderate or heavy exposure, an acute febrile reaction can occur approximately 4 to 8 weeks after infection lasting for several days to weeks, which has been referred to as *Katayama fever*. This is seen most often with *S. japonicum* infection and less often with *S. mansoni*. The fever occurs at the time of egg deposition and results from immune complex formation between egg and adult worm antigens that complex with the rapidly increasing antibody levels (36).

Liver disease represents the major morbidity associated with schistosomiasis (see Color Figure 71.6). The first manifestation of liver disease is hepatomegaly, which may be seen in most individuals with heavy infection as well as in others. Hepatomegaly correlates with the intensity of infection in children. With hepatomegaly, there is very little change in liver function tests. As the infection progresses, hepatic fibrosis develops in some individuals, usually 5 to 10 years following the time of peak prevalence of infection. As fibrosis develops, it may take the form of diffuse or clay pipe stem patterns. The nature and dynamics of fibrosis follow a slow course that preserves liver parenchymal architecture and total hepatic blood flow. This occurs because of the shift of total hepatic blood flow from mainly portal to arte-

TABLE 71.1. QUALITATIVE PATTERNS OF HEPATIC FIBROSIS

Pattern	Description
A	Normal
B	Rounded lucencies; increased evidence of walls around portal and subsegmental branches; some lumina occluded
C	Ring echoes around vessels in cross section; pipe stems parallel with portal vessels
D	Echogenic ruff around portal bifurcation and main stem; thickening of walls of main portal branches
E	Hyperechogenic patches expanding into parenchyma
F	Echogenic bands and streaks expanding from main portal vein; bifurcation to liver surface where they retract organ surface
X	Cirrhosis
Y	Fatty liver

From World Health Organization. Ultrasound in schistosomiasis: a practical guide to the standardized use of ultrasonography for assessment of schistosomiasis-related morbidity. Niamey, Niger: World Health Organization, 2000.

rial, thus maintaining hepatocyte oxygenation and function. Decompensation occurs late in course of disease or it may result from additional insults to the liver, such as viral infections or nutritional deficiencies that lead to hepatic encephalopathy. Evaluations of these patients may demonstrate normal hepatic wedge pressure. In the late stages of liver disease, enlargement of the organ may not be detected because of extensive fibrosis. In most of these patients, extensive splenomegaly, esophageal varices, and ascites may be appreciated. At this point in disease, there is little association between intensity of infection and severity of disease, probably because of the delay between infection and the development of disease.

The ability to identify the different stages of liver disease has been greatly enhanced by ultrasonography (38). Recently, a standardized and accepted set of criteria have become available to accurately and specifically determine the extent of disease progression due to schistosomiasis (38). The echoic patterns by ultrasound can usually differentiate liver fibrosis as a consequence of schistosomiasis from that of viral hepatitis or other etiologies (Table 71.1). More advanced disease (e.g., cirrhosis and fatty liver) may not be distinguished for other causes of fibrosis.

DIAGNOSIS AND MANAGEMENT

Individuals who are suspected of having schistosomal gastrointestinal or hepatic disease should be evaluated for geographic history and duration and intensity of infection. Thorough physical examination and laboratory evaluations are mandatory. Definitive diagnosis depends on demonstrating parasite eggs in stool specimens (see Color Figure 71.8). On rare occasions, rectal biopsies may demonstrate the eggs and surrounding granulomatous response. Serologic testing is helpful, especially in individuals living in nonendemic areas who are suspected of having schistosomiasis. Interpretation of serologic testing in endemic areas is difficult because of the frequent exposure to the parasite. Furthermore, once schistosome eggs are demonstrated in feces, quantification of infection and determination of the viability of eggs are recommended.

The drug of choice for all types of human schistosomiasis is praziquantel (39). For *S. mansoni* or *S. haematobium* infection, treatment includes a total oral dose of 40 mg/kg body weight given in divided doses 12 hours apart. For *S. japonicum* or *S. mekongi* infection, the dose is increased to 60 mg/kg body weight, given in divided doses. The drug causes minimal side effects that do not interfere with treatment. Praziquantel administration results in parasitologic cure in approximately 80% to 85% of cases and 95% to 99% reduction in fecal egg counts. Praziquantel may eradicate adult worms, but not developing larvae. Therefore, it is important to confirm cure in several weeks after treatment. When given to adolescents and young adults, praziquantel reverses pathology and diminishes hepatomegaly. In patients with chronic sequelae, specific chemotherapy does not reverse pathologic lesions. Patients with portal hypertension, esophageal varices, or liver failure are treated with the standard surgical and medical regimens. Care should be taken in prescribing immediate surgical intervention for the first bleeding episode from esophageal varices. These patients usually tolerate several bleeding episodes and do not go into hepatic encephalopathy from one or two hematemesis attacks. Because surgery is associated with major complications and does not reverse the pathologic sequences, it should reserved for selected cases of recurrent bleeding.

Drug resistance in schistosomes to praziquantel has been much feared but difficult to document. Several reports have isolated worms from individuals who failed repeated treatment with praziquantel and have demonstrated relative *in vivo* resistance in mice (40), which may presage resistance in the future. Currently, most evidence indicates that praziquantel remains efficacious (41).

Prevention and control of schistosomiasis are complex medical, social, and economic problems (42). For the individual who is traveling to an endemic area, avoidance of contact with freshwater bodies is sufficient. No other practical measure exists as yet. Control programs that have attempted parasite eradication have met with little success. A more realistic goal may be reduction in transmission and morbidity. This may be accomplished by using targeted chemotherapy and focal mollusiciding when appropriate. Such approaches have shown good results that can be maintained. In endemic countries where resources are scarce, studies are currently underway to determine optimal intervals for treatment. Annual treatment may not be necessary in all instances, and treatment of school-aged children at the time of peak intensity of infection indicates long-term benefits of early treatment. The ultimate control strategy should be educational and economic development. An efficacious vaccine would certainly make an impact, but one will not be available soon (44).

REFERENCES

1. Mahmoud AAF. Schistosomiasis and other trematode infections. In: Braunwald E, et al., eds. *Harrison's principles of internal medicine,* fifteenth edition. New York: McGraw-Hill, 2001: 1242–1248.
2. Davis A. The Professor Gerald Webbe Memorial Lecture: global control of schistosomiasis. *Trans R Soc Trop Med Hyg* 2000;94: 609–615.
3. King CH. Epidemiology of schistosomiasis: determinants of transmission of infection. In: Mahmoud A, et al., eds. *Schistosomiasis: tropical medicine science and practice,* vol 3. London: Imperial College Press, 2001:115–132.
4. Hockley DJ, McLaren DJ. Schistosoma mansoni: changes in the outer membrane of the tegument during development from cercaria to adult worm. *Int J Parasitol* 1973;3:13–25.
5. Blanton RE, Licate LS. Developmental regulation of protein synthesis in schistosomes. *Mol Biochem Parasitol* 1992;51:201–208.
6. Sturrock RF. The schistosomes and their intermediate hosts. In: Mahmoud A, et al., eds. *Schistosomiasis: tropical medicine science and practice,* vol 3, London: Imperial College Press, 2001:497–510.
7. Doenhoff M, Musallam R, Bain J, et al. Studies on the host-parasite relationship in *Schistosoma mansoni*-infected mice: the immunological dependence of parasite egg excretion. *Immunology* 1978;35:771–778.
8. Bloch EH, Wahab MF, Warren KS. *In vivo* microscopic observations of the pathogenesis and pathophysiology of hepatosplenic schistosomiasis in the mouse liver. *Am J Trop Med Hyg* 1972;21: 546–557.
9. King CL. Initiation and regulation of disease in schistosomiasis. In: Mahmoud A, et al., eds. *Schistosomiasis: tropical medicine science and practice,* vol 3, London: Imperial College Press, 2001: 213–264.
10. Arap Siongok TK, Mahmoud AA, Ouma JH, et al. Morbidity in schistosomiasis mansoni in relation to intensity of infection: study of a community in Machakos, Kenya. *Am J Trop Med Hyg* 1976;25:273–284.
11. Woolhouse ME, Dye C, Etard JF, et al. Heterogeneities in the transmission of infectious agents: implications for the design of control programs. *Proc Natl Acad Sci U S A* 1997;94:338–342.
12. Boros DL, Pelley RP, Warren KS. Spontaneous modulation of granulomatous hypersensitivity in schistosomiasis mansoni. *J Immunol* 1975;114:1437–1441.
13. Warren KS, Domingo EO, Cohen RBT. Granuloma formation around schistosome eggs as a manifestation of delayed hypersensitivity. *Am J Pathol* 1967;51:735–756.
14. Weinstock JV, Boros DL. Organ-dependent differences in composition and function observed in hepatic and intestinal granulomas isolated from mice with schistosomiasis mansoni. *J Immunol* 1983;130:418–422.
15. Boros DL, Warren KS. Delayed hypersensitivity-type granuloma formation and dermal reaction induced and elicited by a soluble factor isolated from *Schistosoma mansoni* eggs. *J Exp Med* 1970;132:488–507.
16. Qiu B, Frait KA, Reich F, et al. Chemokine expression dynamics in mycobacterial (type-1) and schistosomal (type-2) antigen-elicited pulmonary granuloma formation. *Am J Pathol* 2001;158: 1503–1515.
17. Ponath PD, Qin S, Ringler DJ, et al. Cloning of the human eosinophil chemoattractant, eotaxin. Expression, receptor binding, and functional properties suggest a mechanism for the selective recruitment of eosinophils. *J Clin Invest* 1996;97:604–612.
18. Chensue SW, Lukacs NW, Yang TY, et al. Aberrant *in vivo* T helper type 2 cell response and impaired eosinophil recruitment in CC chemokine receptor 8 knockout mice. *J Exp Med* 2001; 193:573–584.
19. Olds GR, el Meneza S, Mahmound AAF, et al. Differential immunoregulation of granulomatous inflammation, portal hypertension, and hepatic fibrosis in murine schistosomiasis mansoni. *J Immunol* 1989;142:3605–3611.
20. Olds G, Griffith A, Kresina T. Dynamics of collagen accumulation and polymorphism in murine *Schistosoma japonicum. Gastroenterology* 1985;89:617–624.
21. Chiaramonte MG, Donaldson DD, Cheever AW, et al. An IL-13 inhibitor blocks the development of hepatic fibrosis during a T-helper type 2-dominated inflammatory response. *J Clin Invest* 1999;104:777–785.
22. Cheever A, Yap G. Immunologic basis of disease and disease regulation in schistosomiasis. In: Freedman DO, ed. *Immunopathogenetic aspects of disease induced by helminth parasites,* vol 66. Basel: Karger, 1997:159–176.
23. Farah IO, Mola PW, Kariuki TM, et al. Repeated exposure induces periportal fibrosis in *Schistosoma mansoni*-infected baboons: role of TGF-beta and IL-4. *J Immunol* 2000;164: 5337–5343.
24. Dessein AJ, Hillaire D, Elwali NE, et al. Severe hepatic fibrosis in *Schistosoma mansoni* infection is controlled by a major locus that is closely linked to the interferon-gamma receptor gene. *Am J Hum Genet* 1999;65:709–721.
25. Dunne D, Mountford A. Resistance to infection in humans and animal models. In: Mahmoud A, et al., eds. *Schistosomiasis: tropical medicine science and practice,* vol 3. London: Imperial College Press, 2001:133–212.
26. Nyindo M, Kariuki TM, Mola PW, et al. Role of adult worm antigen-specific immunoglobulin E in acquired immunity to *Schistosoma mansoni* infection in baboons. *Infect Immun* 1999; 67:636–642.
27. Ouma JH, Fulford AJ, Kariuki HC, et al. The development of schistosomiasis mansoni in an immunologically naive immigrant population in Masongaleni, Kenya. *Parasitology* 1998;117: 123–132.
28. Butterworth AE, Dunne DW, Fulford AJ, et al. Human immunity to *Schistosoma mansoni*: observations on mechanisms, and implications for control. *Immunol Invest* 1992;21:391–408.
29. Cook JA, Warren KS, Jordan P. Passive transfer of immunity in human schistosomiasis mansoni: attempt to prevent infection by repeated injections of hyperimmune antischistosome gamma globulin. *Trans R Soc Trop Med Hyg* 1972;66:777–780.
30. Hagan P, Blumenthal UJ, Dunn D, et al. Human IgE, IgG4 and resistance to reinfection with *Schistosoma haematobium. Nature* 1991;349:243–245.
31. Roberts M, Butterworth AE, Kimani G, et al. Immunity after treatment of human schistosomiasis: association between cellular responses and resistance to reinfection. *Infect Immun* 1993;61: 4984–4993.
32. Prata A. Disease in schistosomiasis mansoni in Brazil. In: Mahmoud A, et al., eds. *Schistosomiasis: tropical medicine science and practice,* vol 3. London: Imperial College Press, 2001:297–332.
33. Ouma F, El-Khoby T, Fenwick A, et al. Disease in schistosomiasis mansoni in Africa. In: Mahmoud A, et al., eds. *Schistosomiasis: tropical medicine science and practice,* vol 3. London: Imperial College Press, 2001:333–360.

34. Olveda MO. Disease in schistosomiasis japonica. In: Mahmoud A, et al., eds. *Schistosomiasis: tropical medicine science and practice,* vol 3. London: Imperial College Press, 2001:361–389.
35. Lambertucci JR. Acute schistosomiasis: clinical, diagnostic and therapeutic features. *Rev Inst Med Trop Sao Paulo* 1993;35: 399–404.
36. Hiatt RA, Ottesen EA, Sotomayor ZR, et al. Serial observations of circulating immune complexes in patients with acute schistosomiasis. *J Infect Dis* 1980;142:665–670.
37. Kariuki HC, Mbugua G, Magak P, et al. Prevalence and familial aggregation of schistosomal liver morbidity in Kenya: evaluation by new ultrasound criteria. *J Infect Dis* 2001;183:960–966.
38. World Health Organization. Ultrasound in schistosomiasis: a practical guide to the standardized use of ultrasonography for assessment of schistosomiasis-related morbidity. Niamey, Niger: World Health Organization, 2000.
39. King CH, Mahmoud AA. Drugs five years later: praziquantel. *Ann Intern Med* 1989;110:290–296.
40. Ismail M, Botros S, Metwally A, et al. Bennett JL. Resistance to praziquantel: direct evidence from *Schistosoma mansoni* isolated from Egyptian villagers. *Am J Trop Med Hyg* 1999;60: 932–935.
41. King CH, Muchiri EM, Ouma JH. Evidence against rapid emergence of praziquantel resistance in *Schistosoma haematobium,* Kenya. *Emerg Infect Dis* 2000;6:585–594.
42. Bergquist R. Strategies for control of infection and disease: current practice and future potential. In: Mahmoud A, et al., eds. *Schistosomiasis: tropical medicine science and practice,* vol 3. London: Imperial College Press, 2001:413–467.
43. Mahmoud AA, Siongok TA, Ouma J, et al. Effect of targeted mass treatment on intensity of infection and morbidity in schistosomiasis mansoni. 3-Year follow-up of a community in Machakos, Kenya. *Lancet*1983;1:849–851.
44. James SL, Colley DG. Progress in vaccine development. In: Mahmoud A, et al., eds. *Schistosomiasis: tropical medicine science and practice,* vol 3. London: Imperial College Press, 2001:469–495.

72

USE OF THE PARASITOLOGY LABORATORY IN THE DIAGNOSIS OF GASTROINTESTINAL INFECTIONS

RICHARD A. OBERHELMAN

Parasitic infections of the gastrointestinal (GI) tract are a major cause of morbidity in developing countries and are increasingly important in certain populations from developed countries, particularly in patients with AIDS (1). In contrast to bacterial and viral infections, parasitic infections of the GI tract may be diagnosed rapidly by direct microscopic examination of clinical specimens. However, the diagnosis of parasitic infections still presents at least four challenges for the clinician and the laboratory technician. First, excretion of parasitic pathogens in stool may be intermittent, requiring examination of several specimens collected at different times (2). Second, identification of various morphologic stages of parasites and differentiation between potential pathogens and commensal parasites requires expertise, which may be insufficient in laboratories that handle few specimens. Third, the presence of multiple parasites in a single specimen may make it difficult to determine whether disease is caused by one or more than one pathogen. Finally, the correlation between the presence of parasitic pathogens in stool and clinical disease is not always straightforward, particularly in persons from developing countries who may harbor potential pathogens asymptomatically for prolonged periods.

COMMON CLINICAL SYNDROMES CAUSED BY PARASITIC PATHOGENS OF THE GI TRACT

Diarrhea is the most common clinical syndrome associated with parasitic infections of the GI tract. Common parasitic pathogens associated with diarrhea and other GI tract syndromes are shown in Table 72.1. Although the distinction between bloody diarrhea ("dysentery") and watery diarrhea is often useful, because these clinical syndromes are associated with different parasitic pathogens, many parasites that cause dysentery by disruption or invasion of the enteric mucosa may also cause watery diarrhea. Thus, the differen-

TABLE 72.1. COMMON CLINICAL SYNDROMES CAUSED BY PARASITIC INFECTIONS IN THE GI TRACT

A. Diarrhea
   1. Bloody diarrhea ("dysentery")
      Entamoeba histolytica
      Balantidium coli
      Trichuris trichiura
      Schistosoma sp.
      Strongyloides stercoralis
   2. Watery diarrhea
      Giardia lamblia
      Cryptosporidium parvum
      Cyclospora spp. ("Cyanobacterium-like bodies")
      Isospora belli
      Microsporidium sp.
B. Abdominal pain (often not associated with diarrhea)
      Ascaris lumbricoides
      Strongyloides stercoralis
      Hookworm
      Schistosoma sp.
      Taeniasis
C. Failure to thrive (weight-for-height deficit)
   1. Parasitic infections frequently associated with diarrhea
      Giardia lamblia
      Trichuris trichiura
      Entamoeba histolytica
      Cryptosporidium parvum
      Isospora belli
   2. Parasitic infections *in*frequently associated with diarrhea
      Ascaris lumbricoides
      Strongyloides stercoralis
      Hookworm
      Taeniasis
D. GI blood loss/anemia
      Hookworm (*Necator* sp., *Ancylostoma* sp.)

R.A. Oberhelman: Departments of Tropical Medicine and Pediatrics, Tulane School of Public Health and Tropical Medicine, New Orleans, Louisiana tial diagnosis of diarrhea due to parasitic infection of the GI tract also depends on epidemiologic factors such as geographic location, age of the patient, and whether the patient is native to the region, an expatriate resident, or a traveler (3). A thoughtful assessment of the differential diagnosis should be the first step in the laboratory evaluation, because many potential pathogens can be ruled out on clinical and epidemiologic grounds, allowing the laboratory to focus on the techniques most likely to yield positive results.

Other clinical syndromes associated with parasitic infections of the GI tract are abdominal pain, failure to thrive, and GI tract blood loss/anemia. Abdominal pain is a frequent symptom in patients with diarrhea, but it may also be a presenting symptom of parasitic infection of the GI tract in the absence of diarrhea. "Failure to thrive" is the euphemism for malnutrition commonly used in the United States. Malnutrition due to chronic diarrhea, malabsorption, or both may result from parasitic infections of the GI tract, and both wasting (weight-for-height deficit) and stunting (height-for-age deficit) have been associated with parasitic infections (particularly helminthic infections) among children in developing countries (4–6). The relationship between parasitic infections of the GI tract and malnutrition is multifactorial, and parasitic infection of the GI tract in a child with malnutrition does not necessarily indicate a cause-and-effect relationship. Fecal blood loss may produce anemia from chronic dysentery due to parasitic infection, although severe anemia from parasites is usually due to hookworm infection.

DIAGNOSTIC TECHNIQUES FOR PARASITIC INFECTIONS OF THE GI TRACT

The decision to obtain laboratory studies for parasitic pathogens in patients with these syndromes should be based in part on clinical and epidemiologic features. For example, a child from an urban area in the United States with watery diarrhea presenting during the same week as other children with confirmed rotaviral infection should not ordinarily be evaluated for parasitic infection of the GI tract. Factors that would suggest a parasitic etiology of diarrhea include illness lasting more than 10 days, contact with known cases of parasitic infection (such as outbreaks of giardiasis in a day care center), impaired host immunity (particularly patients with HIV or AIDS), and recent travel to developing countries (3). When parasitic infection of the GI tract is a logical consideration, the most reasonable approach is to start with direct microscopy, because of its low cost and potentially high yield. If direct microscopy does not provide a diagnosis, other tests that should be considered based on the clinical history include concentration techniques, special stains, antigen detection tests, and serologic techniques (see the flowchart under "Summary").

Specimen Collection

Stool Specimens

Examination of stool specimens allows for the diagnosis of 35 species of pathogenic parasites (7) and is the initial method of choice for detection of parasites in patients with all of the clinical syndromes listed above. If the initial stool specimen does not reveal a diagnosis, due to intermittent passage of organisms and fluctuating numbers of parasites, it is useful to collect an additional two or three specimens over 7 to 10 days. Although excretion of nematodes is usually continuous, certain protozoans (such as *Giardia* and *Entamoeba histolytica*) and helminths (such as schistosomes) are intermittently excreted and may be missed if a single specimen is examined (8). Stool specimens should be collected in clean, labeled containers free of water and urine that could lyse trophozoite forms of protozoal parasites (7). Specimens collected from toilet bowls or from soil or grass should not be used, because they may contain contaminating parasites. Stools with a mushy, liquid consistency are most likely to contain short-lived trophozoite forms, and these should optimally be examined within 30 minutes of collection. With refrigeration, protozoal cysts remain intact for several days and helminth eggs can be identified for at least a week after specimen collection. However, stool specimens for parasites should never be frozen, because cysts and eggs are often destroyed at temperatures less than 0°C. Although purgatives may increase detection of some parasites, preparations with mineral oil, magnesia, or bismuth should be avoided before stool collection, because they interfere with parasite identification (2). Barium contrast material also interferes with stool examination and should not be administered for 2 weeks before stool collection. Certain antibiotics such as tetracycline may also eliminate or reduce the number of some parasites in the stool for weeks.

Stool preservatives are useful for stool specimens that cannot be examined immediately. The choice of preservative will vary in different clinical settings, because all solutions present certain benefits and limitations. Most stool preservatives are poisonous to humans if ingested and should therefore be stored in places where they are inaccessible to children and animals. Ten percent formalin (4% formaldehyde) in saline is the least expensive preservative available, but it is not suitable for trophozoites (9). Preservation is accomplished by emulsifying 1 to 2 g of stool in 5 mL of 10% formalin. Protozoal cysts are well preserved in 10% formalin for many months. A sodium acetate–acetic acid–formalin fixative offers many of the benefits of 10% formalin while preserving trophozoites, although the quality of the smears can be inconsistent. Merthiolate–iodine–formalin (MIF) fixative is a more complex formalin mixture that preserves trophozoites, cysts, eggs, and larvae for several weeks. MIF fixative is a convenient preservative for processing large numbers of specimens in the field, and the iodine in MIF fixative allows for easy interpretation of temporary smears without further staining. However, the instability of the Lugol iodine solution in MIF results in a short shelf life for this preparation (good for several weeks if stored in a dark, well-stoppered bottle). Concentration of specimens in 10% formalin and MIF can be performed by sedimentation, but not by routine flotation procedures. Polyvinyl alcohol (PVA) fixative is the best preservative for trophozoites and is stable for 6 to 12 months (9). Preservation is accomplished by mixing one part stool with nine parts PVA. The resin in PVA provides additional stability and prevents collapse of fragile protozoal forms. Unlike MIF, PVA-preserved specimens require staining for microscopy and cannot be easily screened in the field. Schaudinn's fixative is also excellent for preservation of all stages of protozoans and helminths, and like PVA, it can be used to prepare permanent smears (9). Unlike PVA, it does not contain resin to promote adhesiveness for mucoid specimens. Both PVA and Schaudinn's fixative contain mercuric chloride, a particularly poisonous and environmentally hazardous solution. Mercuric chloride must be "washed out" of the preserved specimen by immersing fixed slides in 70% ethanol–iodine solution for 3 to 5 minutes to prevent crystalline precipitation; longer washout periods may adversely affect staining of organisms (10). Fixatives and solutions containing mercuric chloride should be handled as hazardous waste and should be disposed of in well-sealed containers according to the Occupational Safety and Health Administration regulations.

Duodenal Contents

Examination of duodenal contents may be useful in some patients with suspected *Giardia* or *Strongyloides* infection when stool specimens are unrevealing. Fresh specimens can be obtained by duodenal intubation with a weighted flexible feeding tube, and parasites may be observed directly by wet mount. An alternative method for obtaining duodenal fluid is with an Entero-Test capsule or a locally constructed string capsule device (Fig. 72.1) (2). The Entero-Test capsule is a gelatin capsule with a weight on one end and nylon thread wrapped inside. The nylon yarn protruding from one end of the string is taped to the patient's cheek, and the capsule is swallowed. After 3 to 4 hours, when the end of the string has reached the duodenum, the string is removed. The presence of green, bile-stained fluid with a pH level higher than 7 by test paper confirms the presence of duodenal fluid, which can then be examined by wet mount. *Duodenal biopsies* may be useful in some patients with chronic diarrhea when extensive evaluations are unrevealing, although this procedure requires more extensive technical expertise and should not be included in an initial evaluation. Biopsy specimens may reveal organisms such as *Isospora belli, Cryptosporidium parvum, Giardia lamblia,* and *Strongyloides stercoralis.*

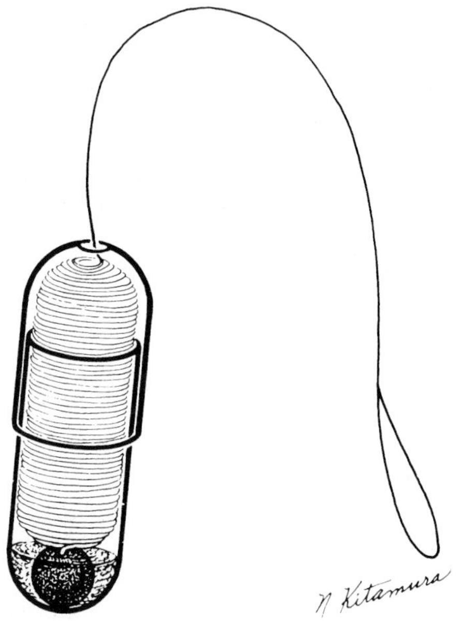

FIGURE 72.1. The Entero-Test capsule, for collection of duodenal secretions. (Illustration by Nobuko Kitamura. Image courtesy of L. Garcia and D. Bruckner.)

Serum Specimens

Serologic evaluation of patients with diarrheal diseases is of limited benefit because antibody tests do not distinguish between recent and old infections. Utility is greatest in nonendemic areas, in which the positive predictive value is greater. Blood for antibody detection should be collected in a sterile container to obtain serum for antibody testing. Serum is usually stored at −20°C or −70°C and may be kept at 4°C for shorter times (days to 1 to 2 weeks). Repeated freezing and thawing should be avoided to prevent degradation of antibodies.

Macroscopic Examination Of Stool And Perianal Secretions

Ascaris lumbricoides can often be observed directly in the stool of infected children, and they are easily identified by size (15 to 40 cm) and shape. *Enterobius vermicularis* eggs (50 to 60 × 20 to 30 μm) and adults (3 to 5 cm) are rarely visualized in the stool but can be detected on the perianal area using the Scotch tape slide test (see Chapter 67).

Biochemical And Microscopic Examination Of Stool And Duodenal Secretions

Cytologic and biochemical analysis of stool specimens may provide additional information to support the diagnosis of particular parasitic infections. The presence of either *gross* or *occult* blood in the stool should be determined in most patients with symptoms that are possibly related to parasitic infection of the GI tract. Blood in the stool may indicate disruption of the mucous membrane or frank dysentery produced by pathogens that either invade or erode the intestinal mucosa. Lower GI tract bleeding may produce gross blood in the stool, although occult GI bleeding is more common and can only be detected biochemically. Parasites associated with bloody diarrhea include *E. histolytica, Trichuris trichiura,* and *Balantidium coli;* less common causes include *S. stercoralis* and *Schistosoma* species (Katayama fever). Other causes of blood in the stool should also be considered, including bacterial causes of dysentery and noninfectious causes of bleeding (e.g., diverticulitis, colonic polyps and cancers, and hemorrhoids). Occult blood can be detected by reaction with guaiac solution, either as liquid suspension or by commercial test kits (e.g., Hemoccult cards). Tests for occult blood are very sensitive, but particularly in the case of liquid guaiac reagent, they lack specificity. Tests for occult blood in stool may produce false-positive results from myoglobin in ingested meats (1).

Detection of microscopic *fecal fat* (steatorrhea) is an indication of fat malabsorption. Parasitic infections that are commonly associated with steatorrhea include giardiasis and strongyloidiasis. Excessive fecal fat produces a frothy appearance on gross examination and clear liquid fat droplets that may be observed on microscopic examination without special stains. Sudan stain may reveal needle-like crystals of fatty acids that are normal or large 10- to 75-µm orange globules suggestive of malabsorption (11). *Fecal leukocytes* indicate an inflammatory process in the GI tract and are commonly observed in bloody stool specimens from patients with dysentery. Although the significance of scant numbers of fecal leukocytes may be questionable, the presence of large numbers (conventionally more than 20 high-power field [HPF]) is suggestive of dysentery produced by parasites such as *E. histolytica, T. trichiura,* or *B. coli* or by bacterial pathogens such as *Shigella* species. One study demonstrated that fecal leukocytes were less numerous in the stools of patients with amebic dysentery (average 39 ± 6 HPF) than in specimens from patients with bacillary dysentery (average 81 ± 6 HPF), reflecting the greater extent of mucosal disease seen histologically in patents with shigellosis (12). In addition, neutrophils are lysed by *E. histolytica* trophozoites (see Chapter 60). *Charcot–Leyden crystals* (see Color Figure 72.2) are breakdown products of eosinophils seen in the stool of patients with amebiasis, *Isospora* infections, and helminthic infections (*Trichuris,* hookworm) (13). These crystals are needle-like and variable in size and appear red-purple with trichrome stain. Charcot–Leyden crystals may be seen in stool specimens of patients with *Trichuris* infection even before worms or eggs appear in the stool (11). In cases of heavy infection with hookworms, these crystals may persist in the stool for several weeks after treatment.

Direct Microscopic Examination Of Stool And Duodenal Secretions

Direct visualization of parasites in stool is the easiest and most definitive way to diagnose parasitic infections of the GI tract. The simplest and most inexpensive technique is a *saline preparation,* which is the method of choice for detection of motile trophozoites and flagellates (9). Helminth eggs may also be seen by this technique in patients with moderate to heavy infections. Saline preparations are performed by mixing a small amount of stool with a drop of physiologic saline, and covering with a coverslip. Lugol solution or D'Antoni iodine may be added to enhance the distinctive morphology of parasites (see Color Figure 72.3). However, iodine kills organisms and eradicates motility, so the slide should first be examined without staining. Proper technique requires an emulsion thin enough to be able to read newsprint through the slide; thicker solutions interfere with the ability to detect organisms. The *thick smear* or *Kato preparation* is particularly useful for detection of small numbers of helminth eggs, especially for patients with suspected schistosomiasis (9). Thick smears do not permit detection of helminth larvae or protozoans. The advantage of this technique is that large amounts of stool (40 to 50 g) can be examined without concentration. Thick smears are performed by covering the fecal mass on a slide with a wettable cellophane strip that has been immersed in aqueous solution of glycerin (50%) with malachite green. After incubation for 1 hour, the glycerin solution clears the fecal material, allowing for easy detection of helminth eggs. The disadvantage of the thick smear is that it requires a fresh specimen or a specimen that has been preserved soon after collection with sodium azide (3 mg/g of stool).

Stains of fecal smears may enhance detection of parasitic pathogens in certain cases. Although many laboratories in developed countries use stains routinely for all specimens, this technique is not cost-effective for developing countries (14). Stains are most useful for detection of fragile trophozoite stages, for examination of specimens from patients with diarrhea, or to clarify parasite morphology when mixed infections are suspected. *Dientamoeba fragilis* is most easily detected in stained smears, because it does not exist in a cyst stage. Trichrome stain (see Color Figure 72.4) is the most widely used technique because it is simple and sensitive. Although traditional methods required prolonged incubation periods for staining, new trichome staining techniques can be completed in 8 to 12 minutes (9). Nuclei of protozoans stain red to pink with trichome stain, with the exception of *Entamoeba coli* (purple staining). The *iron–hematoxylin stain* (Fig. 72.5; see Color Figure 72.6) permits visualization of more detail, but it is also more complex and time consuming than the trichrome stain. Organisms stain darker and with greater contrast than with trichrome, allowing for easy detection of parasites while

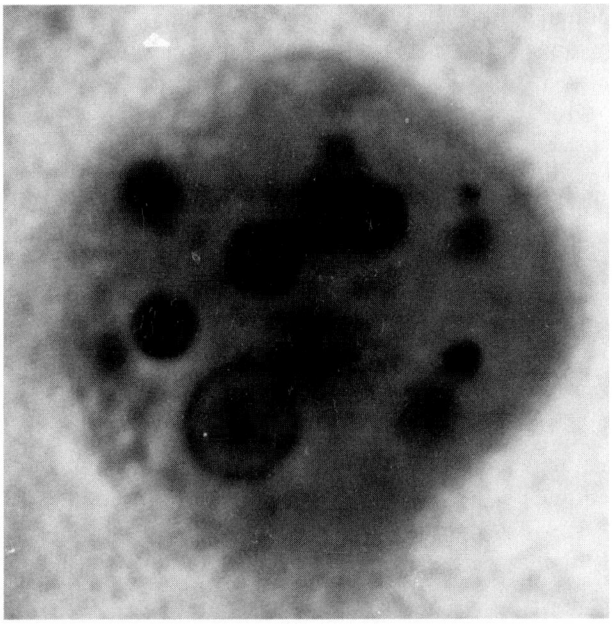

FIGURE 72.5. *Entamoeba histolytica* trophozoite; iron and hematoxylin stain. In contrast to the example shown in Color Figure 72.4, ingested red blood cells stain dark blue or black with iron and hematoxylin stain. (Courtesy of L. Garcia and D. Bruckner.)

scanning at ×40 magnification. The combination of preservation with PVA and iron–hematoxylin staining is probably the best technique for detection of *E. histolytica* trophozoites, as demonstrated in studies comparing this technique with other staining and concentration procedures (14). When looking for trophozoites, one should always evaluate stained unconcentrated specimens, because concentration techniques often destroy these fragile organisms. Proper procedures must be followed to wash out PVA when specimens are stained with iron–hematoxylin, to prevent the dissolution of PVA in aqueous solution, causing the release of the stool specimen from the slide.

Quantitation of Parasitic Infections by Egg Counts

In some cases, quantitation of helminth eggs may provide clinically useful information. These techniques are most applicable for cases of schistosomiasis or infections with soil-transmitted nematodes (e.g., *Ascaris, Trichuris,* hookworm). Egg counts provide a rough estimate of worm burdens in population surveys conducted before and after interventions (such as drug therapy), and they may aid the clinician managing an individual patient. Quantitation techniques have been standardized only for helminth eggs; assessment of parasite burdens for other GI tract organisms is less useful. Egg counts are always suspect due to the nature of the test. Results may be affected by characteristics of the specimen (e.g., consistency), parasite factors (e.g., duration of infection and presence of multiple parasites), and host factors (e.g., intermittent excretion and immunologic responses).

The *Stoll egg count* is the most widely used technique in reference laboratories (9). Although this method is relatively precise, it is of limited use in developing countries because it requires a special apparatus (Stoll flask or another stoppered, calibrated flask). In brief, 4 mL of stool is added to 56 mL of 0.1 normal sodium hydroxide solution in a stoppered flask containing small beads (about 5 mm diameter). After the flask has been allowed to stand 12 to 24 hours with intermittent agitation, a −0.075-mL (75-μL) sample is removed and placed on a microscope slide for examination. Eggs counted on the slide are multiplied by 200 to determine the number of eggs per gram of stool. The *direct smear egg count* is less precise but more adaptable to laboratories with limited resources. This technique is based on the preparation of standardized smears containing 1 or 2 mg of stool and counting all eggs on the smear in a standardized fashion. Because most laboratories are not able to make standard smears, many technicians estimate a 2-mg specimen for quantitation. This technique provides a rough estimate of worm burden when performed by experienced technicians, although practical limitations prevent reading smears made with excessively large amounts of stool (a 3-mg specimen will make the smear too thick to read). Egg counts per gram of stool are estimated by using the appropriate mathematical conversion factor, that is, the number of eggs in direct smear (≈2 mg) × 500 = eggs per gram.

Interpretation of egg counts depends on the infecting organism. An adult female *Ascaris* produces an average of 2,000 eggs per gram of stool, and adult female hookworm and *Trichuris* produce about 50 eggs per gram (9). "Light" infections with *Ascaris* are generally those with egg counts of less than 20,000 per gram, "moderate" infections are those with egg counts between 20,000 and 100,000 per gram, and "heavy" infections are those with more than 100,000 eggs per gram of stool. However, these counts must be interpreted with caution because any *Ascaris* infection can produce serious disease due to the potential effects of adult worms. Light infections with hookworm and *Trichuris* have egg counts of less than 5,000 per gram, "moderate" infections are those between 5,000 and 25,000 per gram, and "heavy" infections are those exceeding 25,000 per gram. Hookworm infections may produce symptoms with relatively low egg counts (above 2,500 per gram), whereas *Trichuris* rarely produces symptoms when egg counts are less than 20,000 per gram.

Concentration Techniques For Diagnosis Of Parasitic Infections

Concentration techniques are useful for detecting small numbers of parasites that may not be seen on direct smears, although trophozoites are destroyed by most concentration procedures (9). Concentration is based on the separation of other elements of stool that differ from parasites by size or density, and it is achieved either by sedimentation (removal of lighter elements in the supernatant) or by flotation (lifting of parasites out of a mass of denser objects). *Formalin ether* and *formalin–ethyl acetate sedimentation* are common techniques performed in very similar ways. Ethyl acetate has been used more frequently than ether in recent years because it is less explosive (9). The ethyl acetate technique is better than ether for visualization of *Giardia* cysts or *Taenia* eggs, although ethyl acetate is less effective than ether for dissolution of fat and mucus in stool specimens. Formalin–ethyl acetate sedimentation is performed by mixing stool with 10% formalin and normal saline and centrifugation, after which this procedure is repeated with addition of ethyl acetate to the formalin solution. Variations of this technique are described for stool specimens preserved in PVA, MIF, and other solutions. *Gravity sedimentation* is the simplest concentration technique, allowing for concentration of eggs, cysts, and larvae without a centrifuge or expensive equipment. The disadvantage of this technique is that parasites may be difficult to visualize because it also concentrates fecal debris. Gravity sedimentation is performed by mixing 10 g of stool in 50 to 100 mL of water, straining through gauze, and decanting the supernatant after allowing fecal material to settle in solution. This procedure is repeated until the supernatant is clear. Sedimentation can be enhanced by adding glycerin to the water (0.5% solution), and a 0.85% saline solution should be used instead of water if *Schistosoma* infection is suspected (schistosome eggs will hatch in water). The *Baermann larval extraction procedure* (Fig. 72.7) is another procedure used for concentration of nematode larvae, particularly *Strongyloides* (15). A wire mesh covered with a piece of gauze is placed over a closed funnel filled with water, and the stool specimen to be tested is placed on a filter paper and inverted specimen side down on the gauze. Larvae migrate from the stool and are concentrated at the bottom of the funnel. This technique can also be used to recover larvae from soil and tissue samples.

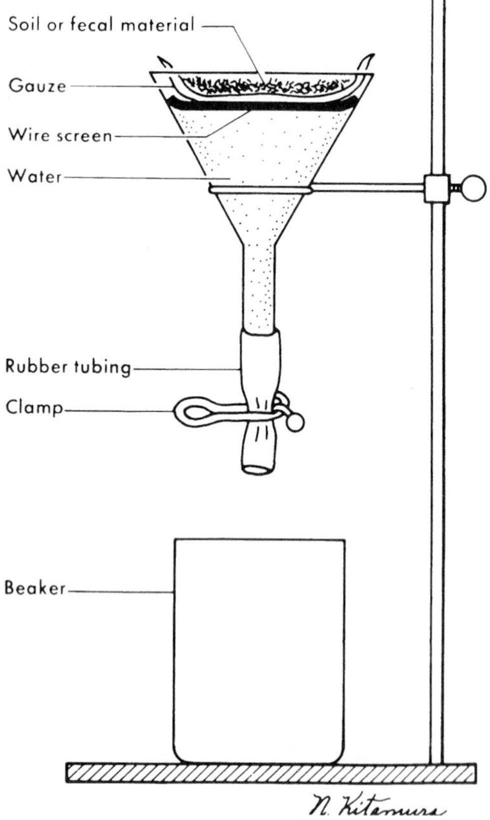

FIGURE 72.7. The Baermann larval extraction apparatus. (Illustration by Nobuko Kitamura. Image courtesy of L. Garcia and D. Bruckner.)

Flotation techniques provide cleaner specimens than sedimentation procedures, although they have the disadvantage of distorting some organisms in dense solutions. The *zinc sulfate flotation technique* is widely used to concentrate protozoal cysts and helminth eggs, but it is not suitable for concentrating fatty stool specimens or for detecting the eggs of trematodes (e.g., schistosomes) or most cestodes (e.g., tapeworms). Stool specimens to be examined are mixed in water and zinc sulfate solution, and after centrifugation, the center of the surface film is stained and examined microscopically. *Sheather sugar flotation technique* is particularly suited for the detection of *Cryptosporidium* species in fresh or formalin-preserved specimens, although these can also be seen in zinc sulfate preparations. Some investigators report that *Cryptosporidium* oocysts are more refractile and easier to visualize by sugar flotation than by zinc sulfate flotation (8).

Special Staining Techniques For Parasite Identification

Certain parasitic infections of the GI tract require special staining procedures for diagnosis. *Cryptosporidium parvum,* unlike other coccidian parasites such as *I. belli,* does not stain by trichrome or iron–hematoxylin techniques. Cryptosporidia are generally diagnosed by a modified *Ziehl–Neelsen acid-fast stain* (see Color Figure 72.8). Several modifications of the Ziehl–Neelsen staining techniques that can be used to stain either fresh specimens or formalin-fixed specimens include the modified acid-fast stain (requires heat) and the Kinyoun carbol fuchsin stain, whereas the dimethyl sulfoxide (DMSO)-modified acid-fast stain can only be performed on fresh specimens (9). *Cryptosporidium* oocysts stain an intense red color with black granules inside, whereas *Isospora* species generally demonstrate a red inner germinal mass (sporoblast) with only an outline of red around the cyst wall. Acid-fast stains have also been used to detect *Cyclospora cayetanensis,* another coccidian parasite resembling *Cryptosporidium* that is associated with diarrheal disease in humans (16). *Cyclospora* species are distinguished from *Cryptosporidium* primarily by their larger size (8 to 10 μm vs. 4 to 5 μm) and the presence of paired sporozoites in two distinct sporocysts, but *Cyclospora* organisms stain variably with Kinyoun acid-fast stain and may be confused with blue-green algae or other similarly sized organisms. Therefore, some laboratories have advocated other methods to confirm the presence of *Cyclospora,* including a modified safranin stain and *in vitro* sporulation assays (17). The latter test requires 5 days to 2 weeks to complete, so it is not practical for diagnostic laboratories.

Auramine–rhodamine fluorescent staining is also useful for detection of acid-fast organisms, but some organisms (notably *Cyclospora*) stain only weakly and the technique is limited by the need for a fluorescence microscope (18). *Cyclospora* and *Isospora* organisms are notable because they autofluoresce, demonstrating a neon-blue glow under ultraviolet light with epifluorescence microscopy, but without the use of specific florescent antibodies or markers (19). This technique provides a quick and easy way to confirm the identity of *Cyclospora* and *Isospora* when florescence microscopy is available.

Microsporidia organisms, in particular *Enterocytozoon bieneusi,* are an increasingly important cause of diarrheal diseases in persons infected with HIV (20). These small organisms are very difficult to visualize in stool specimens, although many laboratories have improved detection of microsporidians by using a modified trichrome stain with a high concentration of chromotrope 2R (21), which stains the microsporidians pink and surrounding bacteria green, or by using fluorescent dyes or optical brightening agents that stain the chitinous layers of the organisms (19). The latter method also stains fungal spores, which must be distinguished from microsporidians by size. Microsporidians are usually seen on small-intestine biopsy specimens using Giemsa stain. Intestinal biopsies stained with Giemsa may also reveal other parasitic pathogens, such as *G. lamblia.*

Antibody Detection (Serologic Techniques)

Serologic tests are available for many enteric parasitic pathogens, although the usefulness of these tests is limited. The major problems of serologic diagnosis are that serum antibodies may not reach high levels when infections are limited to the GI tract, and that it is often difficult to distinguish between recent and past infections. Serum antibody responses are produced in many cases of giardiasis, and *Giardia* immunoglobulin M (IgM) assays available in some research laboratories may be useful to detect recent infection. Commercial kits for detection of *Giardia*-specific antibodies are not available. Serologic tests for amebiasis are most useful for the detection of invasive disease, particularly for cases of liver abscess, for example, indirect hemagglutination (IHA) titers exceed 1 : 128 in 95% of liver abscess cases and 85% of dysentery cases (22). However, serologic responses to *E. histolytica* remain positive for years, and 10% to 35% of persons living in endemic areas are seropositive, so confirmation of amebic disease by serology is more difficult in endemic areas (23). The IHA assay has greater sensitivity and specificity than other assays, such as counterimmunoelectrophoresis (CIE) and enzyme immunoassay (EIA), although titers do not correlate with severity of disease. Antibodies to *Cryptosporidium* may be detected by EIA for parasite-specific immunoglobulin G (IgG) and IgM, and these assays have been used as diagnostic tools for outbreaks (18). However, experience with these assays is limited and they are only available through research laboratories.

Antigen Detection Tests

Antigen detection tests for stool testing are available commercially for *Giardia* and *Cryptosporidium.* Several EIA kits can be used to detect *Giardia* from both fresh and formalin-preserved specimens, with sensitivities ranging from 90% to 98% and specificities from 87% to 100% (24). Some EIAs cannot be performed on specimens in stool preservatives, and several EIA for *C. parvum* cross-react with nonhuman (non-*parvum*) species. This is not a problem for testing human specimens, but it can have an impact on testing of environmental samples (25). Immunofluorescent antibody (IFA) assays have also been used to detect *Giardia* cysts in frozen stool specimens, where cyst integrity may be distorted by freezing and thawing (21). One product is a combined IFA with monoclonal antibodies for *Giardia* cysts and *Cryptosporidium* oocysts for water testing purposes and testing of high-risk populations.

Several EIA antigen detection tests for *E. histolytica* in stool are commercially available, but most of these are limited by their inability to distinguish between *E. histolytica* and *Entamoeba dispar* infections (23). This is problematic because the World Health Organization recommends that intestinal amebiasis be diagnosed with an *E. histolytica*-specific test, and *E. dispar* infection is several-fold more common than *E. histolytica* infection. At least one commercially available EIA (Techlab, Blacksburg, VA) is specific for *E. histolytica* detection (23).

Molecular Biologic Approaches

The use of molecular technology has revolutionized the diagnosis of infectious diseases, and some DNA probes and polymerase chain reaction (PCR) assays have been developed for parasitic pathogens in the GI tract. *C. parvum* has been diagnosed by PCR in fixed paraffin-embedded tissues, but this technique has not been reported for the diagnosis of *Cryptosporidium* in stool (26). The presence of abundant genetic material from the fecal bacterial flora in stool requires the use of highly specific PCR assays, to prevent false-positive reactions. PCR assays for *Cyclospora* in stool have been limited by a relatively low sensitivity, even though their specificity approaches 100% (17). DNA probes have been developed for *E. histolytica*, and some studies have shown close to 100% sensitivity of detection in stool with small numbers of samples (14). DNA probes (with or without PCR) provide the added advantage of specific antigen (gene) detection, a feature that has been applied to the differentiation of pathogenic and nonpathogenic *E. histolytica* at the molecular level (27). The advantages of DNA probes and PCR are that they can be used to process large numbers of specimens rapidly, results can be provided quickly, and with refinement, they may be very cost effective (14). Limitations of a molecular technique include their restricted availability and the lack of sensitivity of some DNA probe tests. Further refinement will be necessary for these tests to become widely available and useful for most clinicians.

Culture Techniques

Culture of parasitic pathogens of the GI tract is labor intensive and rarely, if ever, indicated in medical practice. Culture techniques are best described for *E. histolytica* (28). Because these techniques require a very fresh specimen, they are not useful for processing specimens received in the mail. Several culture media for *E. histolytica* have been developed, such as the Cleveland and Collier's liver extract and the modified Boeck and Drbohlav's Locke-egg-serum medium. Specimens are incubated in culture media at 37°C, and fluid from the bottom of the flask is examined microscopically at 24 to 48 hours. Maintenance of viable cultures requires the inoculation of fresh media every 2 to 3 days, and an aseptic technique is critical because bacterial contamination will kill the parasites. Culture methods have also been used to distinguish between pathogenic and nonpathogenic *E. histolytica* by enzymatic assays. The morphology of *E. histolytica* trophozoites in culture is essentially identical to that seen in stool; cyst forms do not develop in liquid culture. Techniques for axenic cultivation of *Giardia* have also been described, although this procedure is rarely useful for diagnostic purposes.

SUMMARY AND OVERALL APPROACH TO THE PATIENT WHO MAY HAVE A PARASITIC INFECTION OF THE GI TRACT

Although parasites have figured prominently on lists of emerging infectious agents causing GI tract diseases, all patients with diarrhea do not require screening tests for intestinal parasites. Surveys in several U.S. hospitals over the last 10 years showed that less than 1% of stools tested were positive for parasites, and nonpathogenic parasites accounted for about one-half of all organisms detected (8).

TABLE 72.2. APPROACH TO THE DIAGNOSIS OF PARASITIC PATHOGENS IN THE PATIENT WITH ABDOMINAL PAIN OR FAILURE TO THRIVE[a]

Clinical features suggestive of a parasitic etiology:
Altered host immunity (particularly HIV positive)
Recent travel to developing country
Frequent etiologies shown in Table 72.1
Specimen collection:
a. Unpreserved stool—for saline smear, egg counts, Baermann concentration, some antigen detection tests
b. Preserved stool—
For cysts and eggs: 10% formalin
For cysts, eggs, and trophozoites: PVA, MIF Schaudinn's (SAF)[b]
First-order evaluation
Biochemical/cytologic evaluation:
a. Occult blood—Hemetest
b. Fecal leukocytes—methylene blue stain
c. Charcot—Leyden crystals
d. Fecal fat—Sudan's Stain
Direct microscopy
Saline smear for motile trophozoites
Stained smear: trichrome or iron–hematoxylin
Second-order evaluation
Thick smear: if suspect helminth infection (particularly *Schistosoma*)
Concentration techniques
Formalin—ethyl acetate: for most cysts and eggs
Zinc sulfate flotation: for most cysts and eggs (except *Strongyloides* and tapeworms)
Baermann's extraction: if *Strongyloides* is suspected
Sheather's sugar flotation: if suspect *Cryptosporidium*
Autofluorescence assay: for *Cyclospora* and *Isospora*
Special stains
Acid-fast or rhodamine–auramine stain: if suspect Cryptosporidium, *Isospora*, or *Cyclospora*
Antigen detection tests
for *Giardia:* EI, CIE, IFA
for *Cryptosporidium:* IFA
(for *Entamoeba histolytica:* EIA)[b]
Third-order evaluation
Serologic evaluation[b]
Potentially useful serologies:
for *E. histolytica:* IHA, (CIE, EIA)
for *Giardia:* (EIA)
for *Cryptosporidium:* (EIA)
Culture techniques
Molecular techniques

Note: EI, enzyme immunoassay; CIE, counterimmunoelectrophoresis; IFA, immunofluorescence assay.
[a]Flowcharts indicate the usual sequence for obtaining specific tests, based on the progression from the initial first-order evaluation to more sophisticated and directed studies. Differences in common diagnostic techniques for dysentery and watery diarrhea are shown. Most diagnostic evaluations do not require that all tests listed be performed; the extent of the diagnostic workup will depend on the results of preliminary diagnostic tests, the clinical picture, and the need for a definitive diagnosis.
[b]Choices shown in parentheses are generally less optimal than other choices.

TABLE 72.3. APPROACH TO THE DIAGNOSIS OF PARASITIC PATHOGENS IN THE PATIENT WITH DIARRHEA[a]

Clinical features suggestive of a parasitic etiology:
- a. Duration of illness >10 days
- b. Recent travel to developing countries
- c. Consistent epidemiologic pattern (e.g., out-breaks in day care centers)
- d. Altered host immunity (particularly HIV positive)

Specimen collection:
- a. Unpreserved stool—for saline smear, egg counts, Baermann's concentration, some antigen detection tests
- b. Preserved stool—
  for cysts and eggs: 10% formalin
  for cysts, eggs, and trophozoites: PVA, MIF
  Schaudinn's (SAF)[b]

First-order evaluation

Biochemical/cytologic evaluation:
- a. Occult blood—Hemetest
- b. Fecal leukocytes—methylene blue stain
- c. Charcot–Leyden crystals
- d. Fecal fat—Sudan stain

Dysenteric (Bloody)	Nondysenteric (watery)
Small volume, abundant mucus	Large volume scant mucus
Soft consistency	Liquid consistency
+ Fecal leukocytes	– Fecal leukocytes
+ Occult blood	– Occult blood
± Fecal fat	± Fecal fat
± Charcot–Leyden[c]	± Charcot–Leyden[d]
Frequent etiologies shown in Table 72.1	Frequent etiologies shown in Table 72.1

Dysenteric (Bloody):

Direct microscopy
- Saline smear for motile trophozoites
- Stained smear: trichrome or iron–hematoxylin

Nondysenteric (watery):

Direct microscopy
- Saline smear for motile trophozoites
- Stained smear: trichrome or iron–hematoxylin

Second-order evaluation

Thick smear if suspect helminth infection (particularly *Schistosoma*):

Dysenteric (Bloody):

Concentration techniques
- Formalin–ethyl acetate: for most cysts and eggs
- Zinc sulfate flotation: for most cysts and eggs (except *Strongyloides* and tapeworms)
- Baermann's extraction: if *Strongyloides* is suspected

Nondysenteric (watery):

Concentration techniques
- Formalin–ethyl acetate: for most cysts and eggs
- Zinc sulfate flotation: for most cysts and eggs

Sheather's sugar flotation: if suspect *Cryptosporidium*

Special Stains
- Acid-fast or rhodamine–auramine stain: if suspect *Cryptosporidium, Isospora,* or *Cyclospora*
- Giemsa stain: if suspect *Microsporidium*

Antigen detection tests
- for *Giardia:* EIA, CIE, IFA
- for *Cryptosporidium:* IFA
- (for *Entamoeba histolytica:* EIA)[b]

Third-order evaluation

Dysenteric (Bloody):

Serologic evaluation[b]
- Potentially useful serologies: for *E. histolytica:* IHA, (CIE, EIA)

Culture techniques

Molecular techniques

Nondysenteric (watery):

Serologic evaluation[b]
- Potentially useful serologies:
  - for *Giardia:* (EIA)
  - for *Cryptosporidium:* (EIA)

Culture techniques

Molecular techniques

Note: IHA, indirect hemagglutination; CIE, counterimmunoelectrophoresis; EIA, enzyme immunoassay; IFA, immunofluorescent assay.

[a]Flow charts indicate the usual sequence for obtaining specific tests, based on the progression from the initial first-order evaluation to more sophisticated and directed studies. Differences in common diagnostic techniques for dysentery and watery diarrhea are shown. Most diagnostic evaluations do not require that all tests listed be performed; the extent of the diagnostic workup will depend on the results of preliminary diagnostic tests, the clinical picture, and the need for a definitive diagnosis.

[b]Choices shown in parentheses are generally less optimal than other choices.

[c]Charcot–Leyden crystals are characteristically seen in cases of dysentery due to *E. histolytica* and *Trichuris trichiura*

[d]Charcot–Leyden crystals seen in cases of watery diarrhea are often associated with *Isospora belli* infection.

In a hospital-based study in the United States, Sigel et al. (29) found that most stool specimens with intestinal parasites were from outpatients or from patients hospitalized for less than 3 days. As a result of similar findings by other investigators, many U.S. hospitals have instituted policies to reject stools for ova and parasites from patients hospitalized for more than 3 days unless there are other risk factors, resulting in a significant reduction in laboratory time evaluating negative specimens. However, these guidelines do not apply to all U.S. hospital populations, and characteristics of the referral population (including socioeconomic level, proportion of immigrants and refugees from areas with higher rates of parasitic infections, and proportion of persons with predisposing immunodeficiencies) must be considered in designing screening strategies for ova and parasite examinations.

Once a decision is made to evaluate a patient with diarrhea for parasites, the initial diagnostic evaluation must be guided by several factors, including the medical history, severity of disease, extent of medical evaluation for nonparasitic diseases, and cost-effectiveness of the tests. Model algorithms for the evaluation of patients with diarrhea and other GI tract symptoms are shown in Tables 72.2 and 72.3. In general, the evaluation of the patient with diarrhea should follow a directed approach using diagnostic tools that are simple, inexpensive, and potentially useful for diagnosis of various pathogens. These would include the biochemical and cytologic tests described in this chapter and direct microscopic examination for parasites, along with selected tests for bacterial and viral pathogens (e.g., stool culture and rotaviral EIAs). Some "special stains" are often included in the initial battery of tests, such as an acid-fast stain for the detection of *Cryptosporidium.*

For patients with prolonged diarrhea or other risk factors for parasitic infection whose initial evaluation is nonproductive, a second order of diagnostic tests may be useful. These tests should be selected based on the likely presence of particular parasites, because many tests are organism specific or are limited in diagnostic scope. Second-order tests include thick fecal smears, concentration techniques (e.g., sucrose or zinc sulfate flotation for *Cryptosporidium,* and Baermann extraction for *Strongyloides*), special stains (e.g., acid-fast stain for *Cryptosporidium*), and antigen detection tests (e.g., CIE or EIA for *Giardia*). The decision regarding which second-order tests to perform also depends on available laboratory resources, cost, and clinical usefulness of the information (e.g., can the infection that would be diagnosed be treated?). Although thick smears, concentration techniques, and special stains are usually not expensive tests, the limited experience of many diagnostic laboratories with these techniques may reduce the yield. When the receiving laboratory is inexperienced with techniques requested, these assays should be performed in a reference laboratory. Antigen detection tests may be more costly than other second-order tests, and their use should generally be limited to more complicated cases in which the results will affect therapeutic decisions.

A third order of tests may be indicated for a few patients with severe disease or when unusual presentations of parasitic diseases are a diagnostic consideration. These tests would include serology, molecular approaches, and culture techniques. In addition to the considerations mentioned for second-order tests, one must also consider lag time from test submission to results, particularly for tests sent to reference laboratories that may perform such tests infrequently. In addition, in the case of serologic tests, one must consider whether the test result will distinguish between past and recent infection and the degree of test standardization. The cost of most third-order tests is justified only in a limited number of patients.

ACKNOWLEDGMENTS

The author thanks Dr. M. D. Little and Dr. Antonio D'Alessandro for their valuable help in preparing this manuscript.

REFERENCES

1. Guerrant RL, Bobak DA. Bacterial and protozoal gastroenteritis. *N Engl J Med* 1991;325:327–340.
2. Carroll MJ. Routine procedures for examination of stool and blood for parasites. *Pediatr Clin North Am* 1985;32:1041–1046.
3. Guerrant RL, Hughes JM, Lima NL, et al. Diarrhea in developed and developing countries: magnitude, special settings, and etiologies. *Rev Infect Dis* 1990;12[Suppl 1]:S41–S50.
4. Thein-Hliang, Thane-Toe, Than-Saw, et al. A controlled chemotherapeutic intervention trial on the relationship between *Ascaris lumbricoides* infection and malnutrition in children. *Trans Royal Soc Trop Med Hyg* 1991;85:523–528.
5. Stephenson L, Latham MC, Kurz KM, et al. Treatment with a single dose of albendazole improves growth of Kenyan schoolchildren with hookworm, *Trichuris trichiura,* and *Ascaris lumbricoides* infections. *Am J Trop Med Hyg* 1989;41:78–87.
6. Stephenson LS, Crompton DWT, Latham MC, et al. Relationships between *Ascaris* infection and growth of malnourished preschool children in Kenya. *Am J Clin Nutr* 1980;33:1165–1172.
7. Desowitz RS. Fecal, blood, and urine examinations in parasitology. In: Goldsmith R, Heyneman D, eds. *Tropical medicine and parasitology.* Norwalk, CT: Appleton & Lange, 1989:866–875.
8. Koontz F, Weinstock JV. The approach to stool examination for parasites. *Gastroenterol Clin North Am* 1996;25:435–449.
9. Ash LR, Orihel TC. *Parasites: a guide to laboratory procedures and identification.* Chicago: American Society of Clinical Pathologists Press, 1987.
10. Garcia LS, Bruckner DA. Macroscopic and microscopic examination of fecal specimens. In: *Diagnostic medical parasitology,* second edition. Washington, DC: American Society for Microbiology, 1993.
11. Guerrant RL. Principles and syndromes of enteric infection. In: Mandell GL, Douglas RG Jr, Bennett JE, eds. *Principles and practice of infectious diseases.* New York: Churchill Livingstone, 1990.

12. Speelman P, McGaughlin R, Kabir I, et al. Differential clinical features and stool findings in shigellosis and amoebic dysentery. *Trans Royal Soc Trop Med Hyg* 1987;81:549–551.
13. Beaver PC, Jung RC, Cupp EW. Examination of specimens for parasites. In: *Clinical parasitology,* ninth edition. Philadelphia, PA: Lea & Febiger, 1984:733–758.
14. Proctor EM. Laboratory diagnosis of amebiasis. *Clin Lab Med* 1991;11:829–859.
15. Garcia LS. Special laboratory examinations for parasitic infections. *Pediatr Clin North Am* 1985;32:1047–1061.
16. Ortega YR, Sterling CR, Gilman RH, et al. *Cyclospora* species—a new protozoan pathogen of humans. *N Engl J Med* 1993;328:1308–1312.
17. Eberhard ML, Pieniazek NJ, Arrowood MJ. Laboratory diagnosis of *Cyclospora* infections. *Arch Pathol Lab Med* 1997;121:792–797.
18. Current WL, Garcia LS. Cryptosporidiosis. *Clin Microbiol Rev* 1991;4:325–358.
19. Curry A, Smith HV. Emerging pathogens: *Isospora, Cyclospora* and microsporidia. *Parasitology* 1998;117:S143–S159.
20. Schattenkerk J, Van Gool T, Van Ketel R, et al. Clinical significance of small intestinal microsporidiosis in HIV-1 infected individuals. *Lancet* 1991;337:895–898.
21. Weber R, Bryan RT, Owen RL, et al. Improved light-microscopical detection of *Microsporidia* spores in stool and duodenal aspirates. *N Engl J Med* 1992;326:161–166.
22. Botero D. Amebiasis. In: Goldsmith R, Heyneman D, eds. *Tropical medicine and parasitology.* Norwalk, CT: Appleton & Lange, 1989:224–228.
23. Petri WA, Singh U. Diagnosis and management of amebiasis. *Clin Infect Dis* 1999;29:1117–1125.
24. Wolfe MS. Giardiasis. *Clin Microbiol Rev* 1992;5:93–100.
25. Clark DP. New insights into human cryptosporidiosis. *Clin Microbiol Rev* 1999;12:554–563.
26. Laxer MA, D'Nicuola ME, Patel RJ. Detection of *Cryptosporidium parvum* DNA in fixed, paraffin-embedded tissue by the polymerase chain reaction. *Am J Trop Med Hyg* 1992;47:450–455.
27. Ambroise-Thomas P. Les sondes moléculaires dans l'étude et le diagnostique des maladies parasitaires. *Ann Parasitol Hum Comp* 1990;65[Suppl 1]:83–88.
28. Beaver PC, Jung RC, Cupp EW. Culture methods. In: *Clinical parasitology,* ninth edition. Philadelphia, PA: Lea & Febiger, 1984:759–775.
29. Sigel DL, Edelstein PH, Nachamkin I. Inappropriate testing for diarrheal diseases in the hospital. *JAMA* 1990;263:979.

73

ROLE OF ENDOSCOPY IN THE EVALUATION OF GASTROINTESTINAL INFECTIONS

GEORGE TRIADAFILOPOULOS
ROY SOETIKNO
JOHN CELLO
HARVEY S. YOUNG

The widespread use of flexible endoscopies has dramatically changed the way that gastrointestinal (GI) tract infections are evaluated and managed. The plethora of opportunistic GI infections seen in immunosuppressed patients has further expanded the utility of endoscopy. This chapter addresses the impact of endoscopy in the management of infections affecting the GI tract, the pancreas, and the biliary system. The clinical syndromes of these infections are covered in detail elsewhere in this book. This chapter concentrates on the diagnostic and therapeutic potential of endoscopy in these infections. Finally, this chapter discusses nosocomial infections induced by endoscopy and methods for preventing these infections.

ROLE OF ESOPHAGOGASTRODUODENOSCOPY IN INFECTIONS OF THE ESOPHAGUS, STOMACH, AND DUODENUM

Esophagogastroduodenoscopy (EGD) provides a simple, safe, and direct examination of the mucosa from the esophagus to the duodenum. This procedure is a convenient method for gathering tissue, cell, and fluid samples in order to identify the specific pathogen potentially responsible for an upper GI infection.

G. Triadafilopoulos and **R. Soetikno:** Division of Gastroenterology and Hepatology, Stanford University School of Medicine, Stanford, California; Section of Gastroenterology, Palo Alto VA Health Care System, Palo Alto, California

J. Cello: Departments of Medicine and Surgery, University of California, San Francisco School of Medicine, San Francisco, California

H. S. Young: Department of Medicine, Stanford University School of Medicine, Stanford, California

Bacterial Infections

Helicobacter pylori

H. pylori has a well-established role in the pathogenesis of chronic gastritis as well as gastric and duodenal ulceration. *H. pylori* infection can be found in 90% to 100% of duodenal ulcers and in 70% of gastric ulcers (1,2) and gastric cancer. Its association with gastric carcinoma and lymphoma has also been strongly suggested (1,3–5).

The endoscopic appearance of *H. pylori* infection varies. Most commonly, infected patients have chronic gastritis, with mucosal erythema and sometimes gastroduodenal erosions (2,3,6) (see Color Figure 73.1). The mucosal erythema may be diffuse, focal, or in the form of linear streaks. These changes are usually most prominent in the antrum. These endoscopic changes may also be seen in gastritis induced by nonsteroidal antiinflammatory drugs (NSAIDs). Gastric ulcers associated with *H. pylori* infection occur mostly in older people, whereas in the duodenum, single ulcers are associated with *H. pylori* infection and multiple ulcers are more frequent in the non–*H. pylori*, non–NSAID–using patients (7). However, the gastric mucosa may also appear entirely normal and still harbor the bacteria in endoscopic biopsy specimens (2). Therefore, the endoscopic appearance alone cannot predict the presence or absence of *H. pylori*.

Antral nodularity may also be seen in *H. pylori* gastritis, and most of these antral nodules harbor intestinal metaplasia, a premalignant condition to gastric adenocarcinoma (see Color Figure 73.2). Resolution of antral nodularity correlates with *H. pylori* eradication but not necessarily to resolution of intestinal metaplasia (8).

The normal esophagus does not appear to be affected by *H. pylori*. However, *H. pylori* organisms can be found in up to 62% of patients with columnar metaplasia in which a portion of the esophagus is replaced columnar-lined, gastric-type epithelium. The presence of bacteria in these patients is not associated with esophagitis (6). *H. pylori* has also been found in dental plaque (9) and in heterotopic gastric mucosa (10).

During endoscopy, biopsies or rapid urease testing are necessary to confirm the presence of *H. pylori*. Biopsy specimens should be obtained from both the antrum and the fundus. The organism is commonly found at both sites, but can be found in the fundus alone or, more frequently, in the antrum alone (2,3,11). Based on small studies, obtaining biopsy specimens from either the antrum or fundus alone yields positive results in 80% to 90% of cases, but biopsy specimens from both sites increase the yield to nearly 100%. Because the presence of *H. pylori* may be patchy, two biopsy specimens should be taken in each area (12). The rapid urease tests provide immediate information and have a sensitivity of 91% to 98% with a specificity of 100% compared with histology (1,13). Urease tests are also inexpensive. Histology adds the benefit of assessing microscopic evidence of inflammation, intestinal metaplasia, lymphoid aggregation, cancer, or lymphoma. Culture of biopsy specimens is not routinely performed because it is relatively insensitive and difficult to perform (1,2,3,11–13).

At present, endoscopic biopsy with either the rapid urease testing or histologic examination, or both, is the most common method used to establish the diagnosis of active *H. pylori* infection. Newer noninvasive methods such as serology and breath and fecal antigen tests probably will replace endoscopy in this function (see chapter 34). However, endoscopy will remain the method of choice for the diagnosis of *H. pylori*–related conditions, such as gastric adenocarcinoma or mucosa-associated lymphoid tissue lymphoma.

Whipple Disease

Whipple disease is rare and may affect many organ systems. It is caused by a gram-positive bacillus that has been identified using molecular genetic techniques, but has not yet been cultured *in vitro* (15) (see Chapter 51). The symptoms are protean and may include diarrhea, weight loss, fever, migratory arthritis, and central nervous system symptoms.

The small bowel is involved during the course of the illness in most patients, and the diagnosis is most commonly established after examination and biopsy of the postbulbar duodenal mucosa. The characteristic duodenal abnormality is a pale, yellow, shaggy mucosa alternating with erythematous, erosive, or friable mucosa (16,17) (see Color Figure 73.3). Alternatively, only yellow-white plaques or erosions may be seen. However, the affected mucosa may also appear normal. These endoscopic findings cannot be easily distinguished from infection of the small bowel by *Mycobacterium avium* complex (MAC). The endoscopic lesions correspond to the histologic finding of periodic acid-Schiff (PAS)–positive macrophages within the lamina propria of the villi. The stomach may occasionally show endoscopic abnormalities, typically erosive or atrophic gastritis (18).

The diagnosis is suggested when duodenal biopsies show blunted villi packed with PAS-positive macrophages. These histologic findings also occur in patients with MAC infection. Special stains for mycobacteria should therefore be performed. When mucosal abnormalities are noted in the stomach, gastric biopsies may also show PAS-positive macrophages. Granulomas are also seen in histologic specimens in 10% of patients (19). Rarely, the esophagus or the colon may be involved by pale, plaquelike, smooth-surface nodules that correspond histologically to the presence of abundant PAS-positive macrophages.

The mucosal abnormalities regress with treatment, although biopsies may still show the presence of macrophages. With clinical relapse of the disease, the endoscopic lesions usually return.

Whipple disease is often diagnosed late in its course, because it is rare and often produces a confusing clinical picture. When the diagnosis is being considered, early endoscopy with multiple duodenal biopsies should be performed.

Bacterial Esophagitis

Bacterial esophagitis is an unusual cause of infectious esophagitis that occurs almost exclusively in immunocompromised patients (21–23). In the past, it was mistakenly believed that bacteria simply colonize an esophagus already damaged by other factors, but it has become clear that bacterial invasion of the esophagus can occur without underlying esophageal damage. Bacterial esophagitis may be noted in 12% to 16% of immunocompromised patients undergoing endoscopy for dysphagia (21,22). The most common organisms implicated are orally derived gram-positive cocci or gram-positive bacilli (21,22,24,25). Gram-negative bacilli are less commonly seen.

The endoscopic appearance ranges from mucosal erythema to frank circular or linear ulcerations with exudate, to pseudomembrane formation (see Color Figure 73.4). It appears that pseudomembranes, which indicate extensive epithelial destruction, are most commonly seen in severe cases, and these patients have an increased likelihood of associated bacteremia (21). The type of organism involved, however, cannot be predicted by the endoscopic appearance. Indeed, the endoscopic appearance of bacterial esophagitis can easily be mistaken for *Candida* or herpes simplex virus (HSV) esophagitis. However, bacterial colonization of herpetic and candidal ulcers should not be equated with true bacterial esophagitis (26). Bacterial invasion should be seen within the mucosa or deeper layers of the esophageal wall when biopsy specimens are examined, and no concomitant viral or fungal infections of the esophagus should be present (21). Therefore, endoscopy with biopsy and culture is crucial in establishing the diagnosis of bacterial esophagitis.

Phlegmonous Gastritis

Phlegmonous gastritis is a rare bacterial infection of the gastric wall. Gram-positive organisms are most commonly implicated in the disease, with alpha-hemolytic *Streptococcus* found in 70% of cases (27). *Escherichia coli*, *Proteus* species *Enterobacter*, *Staphylococcus* species, and *Clostridium* species are other organisms that have been isolated (27,28). The infection extends from the submucosa to the serosa of the gastric wall, sparing the mucosa (27,29).

Endoscopically, phlegmonous gastritis appears as edematous and reddened gastric mucosa with or without a mass effect, mostly in the gastric antrum. Endoscopic ultrasonography shows thickening of the gastric wall and occasionally hypoechoic masses in the gastric antrum, representing fluid or pus collections (30). These collections may be drained using a transendoscopic fine needle. Most patients present with an acute abdomen and undergo exploratory laparotomy for diagnosis. Surgical findings include edematous gastric mucosa and thickened, rigid gastric folds. The gastric lumen may be narrowed, suggesting the presence of a submucosal mass (31,32). Sometimes pus can be seen. The antrum is most commonly involved, but the whole stomach may be affected. The infection does not usually extend beyond the pylorus or proximal to the esophagogastric junction (27).

The demonstration of air in the gastric wall or edematous gastric folds by plain abdominal films helps in establishing the diagnosis of phlegmonous gastritis preoperatively (32,33). Upper GI barium study or abdominal computed tomography (CT) scan may also show thickened gastric folds (28,32,33).

These surgical and radiologic changes should be evident during an endoscopic examination. However, the role of endoscopy in phlegmonous gastritis has not been defined because the disease is rare and the presentation acute. Because early surgical intervention is indicated for both diagnosis and definitive treatment, endoscopic examination may not be important. However, if the diagnosis is unclear, demonstration of bacteria by endoscopic biopsy should help to confirm the diagnosis (32).

Viral Infections

Herpes Simplex

HSV infection of the GI tract is typically seen in immunocompromised patients, but it has also been described in healthy subjects (22,26,34–37). In the upper GI tract, the esophagus is the most commonly involved site and the stomach is affected infrequently.

The natural evolution of HSV involvement of the esophagus has not been well documented, but it is generally believed that the infection advances through several stages (38). Early in its course, endoscopy reveals discrete vesicular lesions, but these short-lived vesicles are quickly replaced by superficial ulcerations (26,39,40). By the time endoscopy is usually performed, the appearance is that of single or multiple discrete punched-out ulcerations with normal intervening mucosa (26,35,41) (see Color Figure 73.5). The ulcerations are often less than 5 mm in diameter, but they can be up to 1.5 to 2.0 cm in size. In later stages of the illness, they can become confluent. The ulcers may have the characteristic raised yellow rims of exudate, the so-called volcano ulcers (26,42,43). In later stages, HSV esophagitis may be indistinguishable from *Candida* esophagitis with nonspecific diffuse exudative erosions and ulcerations (34,42).

Endoscopy with tissue sampling is the only way to confirm the diagnosis (26). Because HSV infects epithelial cells, biopsy specimens must be taken from the ulcer margins in order to display the typical cell changes under microscopic examination (40). Biopsy specimens taken from the ulcer center usually yield only inflammatory changes. Cultures of specimens should also be sent. The sensitivity of a viral culture alone is approximately 76% to 89%, whereas histology alone is sensitive in 70% to 75% of cases. Frequently, only one of the two techniques may yield a positive result, but performing both tests increases the diagnostic yield substantially (38,39,44). Endoscopic brushing specimens have been shown in one limited retrospective study to be as accurate as biopsies for microscopic examination, but they have a less diagnostic yield than biopsies when the material is used for culture (38).

Other less invasive diagnostic tests for HSV infections are available but they are inferior to endoscopy. Barium studies of the esophagus may show variable mucosal abnormalities but cannot delineate between HSV infection and other mucosal abnormalities (41,42). A positive serologic test for HSV does not imply active infection and is of no diagnostic value (41). The absence of active or past HSV stomatitis does not exclude HSV esophagitis. In fact, up to 80% of patients with well-documented HSV esophagitis do not even give a history of previous HSV stomatitis (38,39). It is logical to presume the diagnosis of HSV esophagitis in a patient with active HSV stomatitis and esophageal symptoms, but data validating this presumption are not available. Endoscopy with tissue sampling is the preferred method of establishing the diagnosis of HSV infection in the upper GI tract.

Cytomegalovirus

GI cytomegalovirus (CMV) disease is another opportunistic infection frequently seen in immunocompromised patients (44). CMV-infected cells, characteristically, are enlarged cells with intranuclear inclusions that can occur anywhere in the GI tract (45,46). The endoscopic appearance is often characterized by ulcerations with sharp borders, which may be very deep and large (47). The ulcerations are rarely heaped up at their borders (48) and, in general, have little or no ulcer membrane or plaque. The intervening mucosa is typically normal (22). However, ulcerations are not a universal finding in GI CMV and the endoscopic appearance can be quite varied. Other endoscopic findings include gastric erythema with erosions, gastric nodules or polyps, and duodenal erythema (45,49,50) (see Color Figure 73.6). In the upper GI tract, the distal esophagus, stomach, and duodenum are often affected. It is important to note that the ulcerations induced by CMV cannot be reliably distinguished from peptic ulcers, nor can they be positively differentiated from other infectious ulcerations based on endoscopic appearance (22).

Endoscopic biopsies early in the course of suspected infection should be performed to confirm the presence of CMV (48). Unlike HSV, CMV infects the stromal cells. CMV inclusion bodies are found in the granulation tissue of the ulcer base rather than in the tissue adjacent to the ulcer (48). Biopsy samples should therefore be taken from the ulcer bed and not near the ulcer borders. Biopsy samples from the edge of the ulceration are likely to show only inflammation (51). Similarly, if nonulcerated tissue is biopsied in the upper GI tract, it is unlikely that superficial biopsy samples will establish a diagnosis. Sampling of deeper lamina propria tissue is necessary (48). However, because ulcers caused by CMV may not be easily distinguishable from those induced by HSV, biopsy specimens should be obtained from both the edge and the center of the ulcer crater. Up to 10 biopsy specimens are needed to diagnose CMV esophagitis. In one study on HIV-infected patients, the sensitivity of three biopsy specimens for the diagnosis of CMV esophagitis was 80%, for six biopsy specimens was 90%, and for 10 biopsy specimens was 99% (52). Some investigators have found that examination of biopsy specimens for inclusion bodies is the most sensitive and specific technique for diagnosing CMV infection (48). Others believe that cultures of brushing or biopsy specimens are more sensitive (44,47), even though cultures often take weeks to become positive. The sensitivities of the two techniques vary widely in different studies. Biopsy specimens for histologic examination and cultures of biopsy specimens should be considered complementary, and both should be sent.

Brushings for cytologic examination have yielded poor results in GI CMV infection (22,44). In one study of AIDS patients with CMV esophagitis, brushings for cytology were positive in only 3% of cases (47). Similarly, serologic tests are unreliable in that they are often positive in the absence of clinical disease.

After a course of ganciclovir or foscarnet treatment for GI CMV, endoscopy with biopsies should be repeated to document the healing of the CMV-associated lesions. If CMV is still present in biopsy specimens, treatment may need to be continued (45).

Other Viral Infections

Varicella zoster can cause infection of the upper GI tract, often in patients with associated cutaneous herpes zoster lesions (53–55). Endoscopic findings are similar to those seen with HSV, with vesicles, erosions, and ulcerations involving the esophagus or stomach. The GI lesions seem to improve with the skin lesions.

Esophageal ulcerations occurring evanescently with HIV seroconversion have been described (56,57). Endoscopy reveals multiple discrete shallow ulcerations that may be distributed over the length of the esophagus. The intervening mucosa is normal. Light microscopy and cultures of biopsy specimens are nonrevealing, but electron microscopy of biopsy specimens shows retrovirus particles.

Epstein-Barr virus has also been reported to be a cause of esophageal ulceration in immunosuppressed patients (58).

Fungal Infections

Candida

Candida esophagitis is one of the most common causes of dysphagia or odynophagia in immunocompromised patients. The infection may also account for cases of acute or subacute dysphagia or odynophagia in patients with underlying motility disorders of the esophagus, notably esophageal achalasia and scleroderma. These conditions significantly impair esophageal clearance, leading to stasis (59). *Candida* esophagitis can also occur in patients without other predisposing illnesses (26,60,61). Although it most commonly affects the esophagus, all regions of the upper GI tract can be involved. Infection of both the stomach and small bowel has been described.

The classic endoscopic appearance of esophageal candidiasis is that of multiple raised white plaques, usually less than 1 cm in diameter (26,61,62). The surrounding mucosa is erythematous and friable (43,60). The plaques can become confluent and nodular, and can be associated with ulcerations (see Color Figure 73.7). Typically, the plaques are adherent to the mucosa and cannot easily be washed off. Although the presence of plaques is strongly suggestive of candidiasis, the endoscopic appearance can be mistaken for other diseases, including reflux esophagitis and other infectious diseases. Therefore, specimens should be obtained to confirm the presence of *Candida* (43). Gastric candidiasis may appear as erythematous mucosa with overlying patchy white exudate. It may also take on a nodular form, with small nodular projections against an inflamed mucosa, or an ulcerative form, with multiple gastric ulcerations (60,63). Similar findings can occur in the duodenum.

Endoscopic brushing smears or biopsies are the preferred method to confirm the diagnosis of *Candida* esophagitis (26,43,64). The cytology brush with its overlying protective sheath is placed through the biopsy channel of the endoscope, and brushing is carried out under endoscopic visualization. The brush is extended from the sheath and the brush is moved back and forth over the mucosa. The brush is then withdrawn into the sheath, and the two are pulled out together through the channel of the endoscope. The specimen should then be immediately smeared onto the slide for fixation. Brushing of the lesions has been shown in a number of studies to be superior to biopsy in the diagnosis of esophageal candidiasis (43,64–66). Brushing allows sampling of a larger surface area than does biopsy alone, and it is thought that the fixation process may destroy or wash away some of the superficial hyphae in biopsy specimens (34). Cytologic examination of esophageal brushing smears has a sensitivity of up to 100%, whereas histologic examination of biopsy specimens is sensitive in only 10% to 75% of cases (61,64,66,67).

Blind brushing of the esophagus to establish the diagnosis of esophageal candidiasis has been studied in AIDS patients (65). Brushing is performed by placement of a sterile brush through an oroesophageal tube. The sensitivity and specificity of blind brushing techniques are 87% to 96% and 87% to 100%, respectively, with false-positive results thought to be due to contamination of the nasogastric tube by oral thrush (65,68,69).

Barium esophagrams may be sensitive in up to 88% of cases, but the specificity is relatively low (70). The radiographs may show a shaggy, irregular mucosa or ulcerations, but the abnormalities do not distinguish between candidiasis and other types of infections (22,41,43,60,62).

Oral thrush is not a reliable predictor of *Candida* esophagitis. Approximately 70% to 80% of patients with symptomatic *Candida* esophagitis also have oral thrush (65). However, 20% of patients with oral thrush do not have *Candida* as a cause of their esophagitis (64,65,68).

Early endoscopy with brushing is currently the preferred method to confirm the diagnosis of *Candida* infection in the upper GI tract. Although the blind brushing technique appears to be an accurate tool for the diagnosis of *Candida* esophagitis in AIDS patients, its ability to exclude other concomitant infection has not been established. In some centers with a large population of AIDS patients, an empirical trial of antifungal therapy using fluconazole is often given to these patients with mild symptoms of dysphagia without performing endoscopy (41,64). If the patient's symptoms do not improve after 7 to 10 days of therapy, endoscopy is performed. This approach is often taken even if oropharyngeal candidiasis is not seen, and its justification is based on the fact that esophageal candidiasis is the most common esophageal disease in these patients (41). In other immunosuppressed patients, such as transplant recipients, or in normal hosts in whom the diagnosis of candidiasis is being entertained, early endoscopy to confirm the *Candida* infection and exclude the presence of other serious infections is still the standard of care.

Other Fungal Infections

Histoplasmosis is a well-recognized infection of the esophagus, stomach, and small bowel, with endoscopic findings ranging from ulcerations to multiple small submucosal nodules to mass lesions (71). *Aspergillus* species can affect the GI tract and can cause ulcerations of variable configurations and mass lesions (72). The lesions may be segmental. Transmural infarction of the small bowel can occur due to vascular occlusion by *Aspergillus* organisms. *Torulopsis glabrata* has been described as causing focal esophageal ulcerations in immunocompromised patients (73).

In these and other fungal infections, it is important to recognize that the endoscopic features are not diagnostic, and biopsies and brushings should be performed.

Parasitic Infections

Anisakiasis

Anisakiasis is caused by the ingestion of *Anisakis* larvae in undercooked contaminated salt water fish. The worm burrows into the gastric or intestinal mucosa causing severe abdominal symptoms. The stomach is affected in 75% of cases and the small or large bowel in 25% (74, 75). A worm penetrating the gastric mucosa may be found by endoscopy (see Color Figure 73.8). The worm is surrounded by mucosal edema in 86% of cases, and a surrounding mass is seen in 43% of cases (74,75). In the stomach, the worm can be found in any area, but is most commonly located in the fundus.

Endoscopy is the main tool used for the diagnosis and treatment of anisakiasis. The disease is confirmed by locating the worm during endoscopy. Immunologic assays for *Anisakis* antigens may be helpful when the worm cannot be recovered easily, but these assays are not currently available in routine clinical laboratories (76,77). Early endoscopic removal of the worm with biopsy forceps abates the symptoms and prevents the characteristic eosinophilic tissue reaction to the degenerating larvae. Therefore, early endoscopy is indicated in patients suspected to have anisakiasis as the definitive treatment for the infection (74–76).

Giardia lamblia

Giardia lamblia is the most common parasite implicated in GI illness in the world (78–80). *Giardia* cysts are ingested and passed into the duodenum where they produce trophozoites, which, in turn, colonize the upper intestine (79). The host may be asymptomatic during the course of the infection, or acute or chronic intestinal symptoms may develop.

Because endoscopic findings are nonspecific, endoscopy is not the first avenue of investigation for the diagnosis of giardiasis. Inflammation, erosion, or nodularity of the duodenal mucosa may be seen (81). However, the mucosa may also appear entirely normal and still harbor the parasite. Cysts have also been found in gastric biopsy specimens, but only in the presence of chronic atrophic gastritis (82). It is thought that decreased gastric acidity may be necessary for colonization of the parasite in the stomach.

There is no gold standard for the diagnosis of *Giardia* infection. The most widely used method of diagnosis is the microscopic detection of cysts or trophozoites in multiple concentrated stool specimens (78). However, the sensitivity of this method is only 50% to 70% (79,83). There are a number of antigen detection assays, such as enzyme-linked immunosorbent assay (ELISA), to detect *Giardia* antigen in fecal material (79,83,84–86). These use sera from animals immunized with *Giardia* trophozoites in order to detect *Giardia* antigen in stool specimens, and appear to be quite accurate (83). The sensitivity and specificity of these systems are each approximately 90% to 99% in cases of giardiasis proven by microscopic examination of stool specimens (84–86).

If stool testing is negative and the clinical suspicion for *Giardia* infection is high, endoscopy with small-bowel biopsy or aspiration of duodenal fluid can be considered (87). Biopsies of the small bowel for microscopic examination yield positive results in 66% of cases (88). Endoscopic biopsy is as effective as the older peroral suction biopsy technique and is better tolerated (89,90). Although animal studies suggest that the midjejunum may be more heavily colonized with the organism than the duodenum (80), duodenal biopsies are adequate (90). Aspiration of duodenal fluid is sensitive in detecting the protozoan in up to 80% of cases. Duodenal aspirates can be obtained by instilling 10 to 20 mL of normal saline into the duodenum through the endoscope, then aspirating into a sterile trap. Normal saline should be used because the trophozoites undergo lysis in tap water (91). Passing a nasogastric tube into the duodenum to obtain an aspirate is often unsuccessful and is uncomfortable. Similarly, the Entero-Test duodenal capsule (string test) is as sensitive as duodenal aspiration (88), but is often unsuccessful in reaching the duodenum (76). Endoscopic brush cytology has also yielded good results in two small studies (89,92). These patients had negative small-bowel biopsies and stool studies for *Giardia*, but brush cytology of the duodenum showed the organism.

There are no studies directly comparing the sensitivities of antigen detection assays on fecal samples and small-bowel biopsy or aspiration in diagnosing *Giardia* infection. It may be true that the detection of *Giardia* antigen in fecal samples may become the new gold standard, because the sensitivity and specificity of this technique appear to be quite high. It is unlikely that endoscopy will reveal many cases of giardiasis missed by antigen studies, and it should be considered a second-line investigative technique in the diagnosis of giardiasis. The major role of endoscopy may be in excluding other diseases that mimic *Giardia* infection.

Cryptosporidium *and* Isospora belli

Coccidian parasites such as *Cryptosporidium parvum* and *Isospora belli* are commonly seen in severely immunocompromised patients with AIDS, usually with CD4 counts less than 100/mm^3 Both can cause a debilitating GI syndrome characterized by diarrhea, abdominal pain, and weight loss. Although the parasites typically affect the small bowel, they can be found anywhere in the GI tract, from the pharynx to the rectum (93).

There are no gross endoscopic features thought to be specific for these protozoa (94). Biopsies of infected tissue may show nonspecific changes, such as atrophic mucosa and shortened villi in the small bowel (93). *Cryptosporidium* parasites may be seen along the intestinal epithelial surface.

Stool analysis is the main avenue of investigation for the diagnosis of *Cryptosporidium* and *Isospora* (96, 97). In one study of 28 patients with *Cryptosporidium* infection, stool studies were positive in 71% of cases, with endoscopic biopsies positive in 29% (94). In another study of nine patients with *Cryptosporidium* detected in stool samples, only three had positive biopsies (97).

The role of endoscopy in the evaluation of these infections is primarily to exclude other possible infections affecting immunosuppressed patients. Endoscopy with biopsy has been shown to be of benefit in detecting CMV, MAC, and other infections in AIDS patients (94,97,98) who may present with similar symptoms of diarrhea, weight loss, and abdominal pain. Furthermore, a pathogen isolated in the stool is not necessarily the principal cause of the patient's illness, and other pathogens may be coexistent (94,98,99).

Other Parasitic Infections

Parasites occasionally discovered by upper endoscopy include hookworms, tapeworms, and ascaris (100–104) (see Color Figure 73.9). Schistosomal infection of the stomach and small bowel can occur, although the colon is more often involved (105,106). With schistosomal infection, endoscopy may show nonspecific inflammation and microulcerations of the mucosa, and biopsies show live or degenerating ova (81,105).

Examination of stool samples is the main diagnostic modality in the evaluation of most parasitic diseases of the GI tract (107). Barium radiographs have also been useful and may reveal filling defects or barium in the worm's alimentary tract, suggesting the diagnosis of parasitic infection (81). Endoscopy is mainly performed to exclude other causes of abdominal symptoms when stool studies for parasites have been unrevealing.

Mycobacterial Infections

Mycobacterium tuberculosis

GI tuberculosis is rare, especially in the absence of pulmonary tuberculosis. Its diagnosis is therefore often delayed. The mycobacteria can affect the entire GI tract, from the esophagus to the anus, but the most common site of involvement is the ileocecal region (108,109). The esophagus, stomach, and proximal small bowel are less commonly involved. The duodenum, for example, is infected 30 times less than the ileocecal region (110,111). Involvement of the stomach occurs in only 0.5% to 3% of tuberculous GI infections (112). However, if preexisting lesions exist in the upper GI tract, such as esophagitis, ulceration, or carcinoma, implantation of acid-fast bacilli in these areas occurs more easily (113,114).

Esophageal tuberculosis is most often a consequence of spread from adjacent lymph nodes (115). The most common site affected is therefore the midesophagus just above the carina, where the mediastinal lymph nodes are located (113,115,117). In the stomach, the pylorus and lesser curvature of the antrum are most commonly involved, often leading to gastric outlet obstruction (118–120). The small bowel is often segmentally involved, which may lead to the mistaken diagnosis of Crohn's disease. Small-bowel involvement commonly manifests as intestinal obstruction secondary to stricture or mass formation (110,111,120–124). In one study, 75% of patients with duodenal tuberculosis presented with gastric outlet or intestinal obstruction (110).

The endoscopic appearance of upper GI tuberculosis is variable, but usually takes one of three forms: ulcerative, hypertrophic, or granular (113,115,117). The ulcerative form is the most common (119). The ulcers may be single or multiple, longitudinal or transverse, and often have irregular ("geographic") borders with a gray shallow base (108, 113,122). The adjacent mucosa may be normal or may be erythematous (117). The hypertrophic form is caused by a fibrotic reaction of the mycobacteria (often called *tuberculoma*) and can mistakenly lead to a diagnosis of carcinoma (115). This form can cause obstruction and narrowing of the lumen. Finally, the least common type is the granular form. These are small, miliary tubercles on the mucosa. Strictures, fistulas, and sinuses may occur, and probing of hypertrophic masses or ulcers may uncover deep tracts to adjacent structures (114,117).

The endoscopic appearance is not diagnostic, and biopsy specimens must be obtained. Because the acid-fast bacilli are mostly submucosal, superficial biopsy samples may only show inflammation (109,111,112,117,119,121). Even with deeper specimens, acid-fast bacilli and granulomas may not be identified on direct smear, but the yield is increased in the deeper specimens (109). At best, acid-fast bacilli can be identified only in approximately 50% of biopsy specimens, which is similar to the yield of gastric aspirates (110,115). Tissue should always be sent for mycobacterial culture.

Radiologic studies are not pathognomonic in diagnosing GI tuberculosis. The findings of ulcers, strictures, pseudotumor masses, or even fistulas are nonspecific and may be confused with Crohn's disease, tumor, or acid peptic disease (5,113,114).

Although endoscopy with biopsy is the procedure of choice (114), the limitations of endoscopy in the diagnosis of GI tuberculosis must be emphasized (121). Entertaining the diagnosis even in the absence of clear exposure to tuberculosis is critical. Biopsy specimens should be sent for histologic study, acid-fast bacilli staining, and culture. Surgical exploration is often performed when the diagnosis of tuberculosis is not made preoperatively (120).

Colonoscopy may be the best endoscopic diagnostic tool. The cecum and the ileocecal valve are often deformed and contracted, 8- to 10-cm segments of nodules and ulcers may be present, and nodular strictures and ulcers with or without pseudopolypoid folds may obstruct the lumen.

Mycobacterium avium *complex*

GI infection with MAC is seen in the context of systemic infection in immunocompromised hosts (126,127). It may affect the entire GI tract but commonly affects the duodenum. Endoscopic findings in the duodenum include the presence of fine white nodules thought to be characteristic of this infection (127) (see Color Figure 73.10). However, the endoscopic appearance can be easily mistaken as Whipple disease. Ulcerations and fistulas have also been described (126,127,129). Even with normal-appearing mucosa, MAC can be found in biopsy specimens.

In one study of 35 AIDS patients, biopsies were positive for acid-fast bacilli smear in up to 65% of patients with GI MAC infection, and cultures of biopsy specimens were positive in up to 85% (127,129). Biopsy specimens for histologic study, acid-fast bacilli smear, and culture should be submitted in patients with suspected MAC infection.

ROLE OF ENTEROSCOPY IN SMALL INTESTINE INFECTIONS

Currently, two types of endoscopes are available for examination of the small intestine. The Sonde-type enteroscopy involves the passage of a thin and long endoscope transnasally into the patient's duodenum. Peristalsis then carries the endoscope to the terminal ileum in approximately 80% of cases (130). This phase of the procedure takes from 6 to 8 hours. The small intestine is then examined upon withdrawal of the endoscope. However, this instrument lacks the ability to obtain tissue specimen or aspirates. The push-type enteroscopy is similar to routine upper endoscopy, but a special 240-cm long endoscope is used (131). This instrument can be advanced to the midjejunum and can be used to obtain tissue samples. The procedure can be performed in 1 to 2 hours.

Although a large number of common bacterial, viral, and parasitic infections affect the small intestine and typically result in diarrhea, enteroscopy is seldom needed to make the diagnosis. Stool studies, clinical characteristics, and epidemiologic considerations are generally more valuable in establishing the diagnosis of these infections. In developing countries, using this technique in patients with obscure GI bleeding, *Ascaris lumbricoides* and ankylostoma duodenale have been found, producing multiple erosions and bleeding points in the jejunum. In patients with chronic diarrhea, push-type enteroscopy may reveal tropical sprue, *Giardia lamblia*, or strongyloidiasis.

Opportunistic infections of the small intestine in immunocompromised patients can often be detected by examination of the duodenum by routine upper endoscopy. The role of enteroscopy in these patients is yet to be defined, but it is likely of minor importance.

ROLE OF FLEXIBLE SIGMOIDOSCOPY AND COLONOSCOPY IN INFECTIONS OF THE COLON AND TERMINAL ILEUM

Endoscopic examinations of the entire colon by colonoscopy, or to a limited extent by flexible sigmoidoscopy, are well tolerated. Intubation of the terminal ileum through the ileocecal valve is a routine maneuver during colonoscopy and has a success rate of more than 80%. Endoscopic tissue sampling again plays an important role in the management of infectious processes affecting these regions. The colon is a frequent site of GI complications in patients with HIV infection, and these colonic disorders increase in frequency as immunodeficiency worsens, usually with CD4 cells less than 100/mm^3. The most common clinical manifestations of colonic disease in AIDS are diarrhea, lower GI bleeding, and abdominal pain. Toxic megacolon, intussusception, typhlitis, idiopathic colonic ulcer, and pneumatosis intestinalis have been diagnosed and treated by colonoscopy. In the HIV-infected patient with preserved immunity, the most common cause of colitis is bacterial, but as the degree of immunodeficiency worsens, opportunistic pathogens (CMV, protozoa, mycobacteria, fungi) and neoplasms become more frequent. The frequent use of antibiotics, chemotherapeutic agents, and frequent hospitalization increase the susceptibility to *Clostridium difficile* colitis. Colonoscopy plays an integral role in the management of many colonic disorders in AIDS.

Bacterial Infections

Acute Bacterial Colitis

Common pathogens isolated from stool cultures in patients with acute bacterial colitis include *Campylobacter, Salmonella, Shigella*, toxigenic *E. coli* O157:H7, and *C. difficile*. These organisms can cause a spectrum of clinical illness, ranging from an asymptomatic carrier state to acute hemorrhagic colitis. *C. difficile* causes pseudomembranous colitis and is discussed separately.

There is a wide range of endoscopic findings in infectious colitis. Findings include edematous mucosa with loss of the normal vascular pattern, erythema, friability, ulcerations, and the presence of luminal exudate (134–136) (see Color Figure 73.11). Ulcerations may be small or several centimeters in size, and are of variable configuration (134, 137). Pseudomembranes may also be found in a minority of cases associated with *E. coli* O157:H7 (138).

The endoscopic findings are variable depending on when endoscopy is performed in the course of the illness. The evolution of endoscopic findings was studied in a group of patients with acute shigellosis (137). During the first week after presentation, edema was the dominant finding on colonoscopy. In the second and third weeks, slightly raised mucosal hemorrhages appearing as punctate spots, ulcerations, and friability were prominent. The punctate spots persisted after the other endoscopic abnormalities and clinical symptoms improved. Erythema was also present through the course of the disease, with diffuse involvement in early weeks and patchy involvement in later weeks. Luminal pus, mucus, and blood were maximal in the first 3 weeks. The endoscopic abnormalities lasted an average of 39 days, whereas the clinical symptoms lasted 23 days. Of importance, normal-appearing mucosa eventually developed in all patients. Although this study was performed in patients with shigellosis, similar endoscopic changes are probably seen in acute colitis caused by other common pathogens (134,137,139). It is not possible to predict the bacterial organism involved on the basis of endoscopic examination.

The mucosal abnormalities may be segmental or continuous (134,139). Normal-appearing rectal mucosa on proctoscopy does not exclude an infectious colitis, and indeed normal proctoscopies were noted in 10 of 19 patients with *Campylobacter* isolated from stool samples in one study (140). The endoscopic findings of *E. coli* O157:H7–associated colitis are especially prominent in the right colon, although the whole large bowel can be involved (138, 141–143). Either the cecum or the ascending colon has endoscopic abnormalities in most cases, whereas the sigmoid colon is abnormal less than one-half of the time and the rectum less than one-third of the time (144). There appears to be a gradation of endoscopic abnormalities from the cecum to the rectum, with the rectosigmoid often being normal or showing only moderate hyperemia (138,144).

One of the major concerns in a patient presenting with bloody diarrhea is differentiating an acute, self-limited, and presumably infectious colitis from idiopathic inflammatory bowel disease. Clinically, the symptoms may be identical. The endoscopic appearance is also generally not helpful (139,140,145). The presence of mucosal granularity has been suggested to be indicative of inflammatory bowel disease (137), but it can be seen in infectious colitis as well (134,135,139,145).

Biopsy specimens for histologic examination may be helpful in differentiating between acute infectious colitis and inflammatory bowel disease. Although many histologic features are seen in both illnesses, some features seem to be more specific for inflammatory bowel disease. One retrospective evaluation of rectal biopsy specimens from patients with either acute self-limited colitis or inflammatory bowel disease revealed that seven features were seen commonly in inflammatory bowel disease but rarely in acute self-limited colitis (146). These features included distorted crypt architecture, increased number of mononuclear cells and neutrophils in the lamina propria, a villous surface, epithelioid granulomas, crypt atrophy, basal lymphoid aggregates, and basally located giant cells. The predictive probability of each of these features in diagnosing inflammatory bowel disease ranges from 79% to 100%.

In another study of colorectal biopsy specimens obtained from patients with bloody diarrhea within 4 days of presentation, the presence of crypt distortion and plasmacytosis in the lamina propria was diagnostic of ulcerative colitis, whereas edema, neutrophilic infiltration in the lamina propria, and crypts were diagnostic of acute self-limited colitis (145). The histologic features in patients with acute self-limited colitis did not differ with the type of bacterial organisms isolated from the stool. However, as the histologic changes in acute self-limited colitis rapidly evolve, biopsy specimens obtained later than 4 days after the onset of bloody diarrhea were not diagnostic.

Stool cultures should be the first tests performed in the evaluation of what is presumed to be an acute infectious diarrhea. In only 42% to 58% of patients with acute self-limited colitis, however, are stool studies positive (145). When patients present with severe symptoms of colitis and rapid institution of treatment is necessary, sigmoidoscopy with biopsy should be performed to help differentiate between idiopathic inflammatory bowel disease and an infectious colitis. If the sigmoidoscopy is nondiagnostic, a colonoscopy should be considered, with concomitant examination of the terminal ileum.

Clostridium difficile–*Associated Colitis*

C. difficile is the most common cause of pseudomembranous colitis. Although the name implies the presence of pseudomembranes, the endoscopic appearance of *C. difficile* colitis takes on many forms, and pseudomembranes may not be seen in mild cases (147–149). The mucosa may appear only mildly granular, friable, or erythematous (148, 149) before the appearance of pseudomembranes. The endoscopic appearance, as well as the pseudomembranes, seem to go through stages as the disease evolves (see Color Figure 73.12). Within the first few days after diarrheal symptoms begin, small 1- to 2-mm round yellowish spots dotting the colonic mucosa have been described (150). They appear as tiny lesions with erythematous bases and central yellow plaques, and may be confused with aphthous ulcerations or even mucus. Biopsies of these lesions confirm the presence of early pseudomembranes. The pseudomembranes later appear as elevated adherent yellow, white, or gray plaques. They are usually 2 to 5 mm in size at this stage, but can become confluent and extend several centimeters (151). The intervening mucosa may be normal, but can also be edematous and hyperemic.

Endoscopy often quickly establishes the diagnosis of *C. difficile* colitis. Proctoscopy alone is insufficient and misses 23% to 70% of cases (152–155), because rectal sparing is common. Although flexible sigmoidoscopy reveals abnormalities in most cases, up to 10% may be missed with sigmoidoscopy alone (153). In a prospective study of 22 patients with pseudomembranous colitis, 91% of cases could be diagnosed with sigmoidoscopy to 60 cm from the anus (153) with the remaining 9% having localized proximal colonic disease. The disease is limited to the colon, and even if there is proximal colonic involvement, there is usually an abrupt termination of the disease at the ileocecal valve (151). Toxic megacolon due to *C. difficile* infection is increasingly recognized (156). In these instances, diagnostic and decompressive colonoscopy with intraluminal administration of vancomycin may be considered (157). It has been suggested that colonic biopsies are not entirely necessary if pseudomembranes are seen, because the diagnosis of pseudomembranous colitis can be established on visual grounds by an experienced observer. However, other endoscopic abnormalities can be mistaken for pseudomembranes, and confirmation of pseudomembranes by histologic examination is useful. In addition, even if pseudomembranes are not seen, biopsies of inflamed or granular mucosa may show the classic pseudomembranes microscopically (volcano or summit lesion) (138,148,149,158). Biopsies should be performed routinely if pseudomembranous colitis is being considered.

The colitis is a result of two potent toxins (enterotoxin A and cytotoxin B) elaborated by the organism (148). These toxins are the basis of diagnostic tests used in the evaluation of pseudomembranous colitis. The toxins are detected in stool samples. Although the tests are specific, the sensitivity of these tests is quite variable (148,149, 159). Rapid ELISAs that detect toxin A appear to have a sensitivity of 80% to 90% (148,160). Recently, the polymerase chain reaction (PCR) technique has been used to identify the toxigenic *C. difficile* in stool specimens (161, 162). This technique appears to be quite sensitive but is not in widespread clinical use.

C. difficile can be cultured from stool specimens in up to 97% of patients who meet clinical criteria for *C. difficile*–associated colitis (159). However, as many as 20% of hospitalized asymptomatic patients harbor *C. difficile* in their stools without having colitis (148, 149,163). In one study, only 11% of hospitalized patients with diarrhea who were culture-positive and cytotoxin-negative had pseudomembranes on sigmoidoscopy (163). Therefore, clinical correlation and possibly endoscopic confirmation is important when a positive culture is obtained in patients with negative *C. difficile* toxins (160). Toxin A-negative, toxin B-positive strains have recently been described and account for some cases of pseudomembranous colitis with negative stool ELISA assays (164).

The approach to a patient with suspected *C. difficile* infection is to first send stool for *C. difficile* toxin examination. Stool for culture may also be sent. If patients are severely ill and require a rapid diagnosis or if clinical suspicion is high when toxin and culture results are negative, endoscopy should be performed. Sigmoidoscopy identifies most cases, but colonoscopy is necessary in the 10% of cases in which the disease is limited to the proximal colon.

Viral Infections

Cytomegalovirus Colitis

There has been a steady increase in the number of cases of CMV colitis with the increased number of transplant patients and patients with the AIDS (165,166). It is estimated that CMV GI disease will develop in approximately 20% of AIDS patients at some time (167).

As with upper GI CMV infection, the endoscopic appearance of CMV colitis is one of mucosal ulcerations (165,168). The ulcers are discrete and can be quite large. Focal ulcerations occur, but in severe cases, ulcers may be found throughout the colon. The surrounding mucosa may be edematous, erythematous, granular, and friable, and the changes may be continuous or discontinuous (168). In early stages, the mucosa may show only punctate submucosal hemorrhages or superficial ulcerations. The colonic mucosa may appear entirely normal and still harbor CMV inclusion bodies in biopsy specimens (166). In one study, 25% of AIDS patients with CMV infection of the colon had normal-appearing colonic mucosa with biopsies showing CMV inclusion bodies (166).

Localized CMV colitis has been described to be more common in the right colon (166,169), with a tendency toward sparing of the transverse and left colon. However, it has been noted that the rectosigmoid region is commonly involved in AIDS patients (166). Distal small-bowel involvement is rare, comprising only 1.4% of all cases of GI CMV infection (169). Even with diffuse colitis, the disease often stops abruptly at the ileocecal valve, although isolated ileal CMV has also been reported (169). If colonoscopy is negative, passage of the colonoscope into the terminal ileum should be attempted.

Because the endoscopic changes are not specific for CMV, biopsy specimens must be obtained to establish the diagnosis. If ulcers are present, specimens should be obtained from the base of the ulcer (48). Even if the mucosa is normal, however, random samples should be obtained if CMV colitis is being considered, such as in AIDS patients with diarrhea. The biopsy specimens are more likely to show inclusion bodies if they are obtained from the right colon rather than the left (46). It also appears that examination of colonic biopsy specimens for inclusion bodies is more likely to yield a positive diagnosis than examination of biopsy specimens of the upper GI tract, because the highest number of inclusion bodies is found in colonic biopsy specimens (46). In a patient suspected of having CMV colitis, three random samples should be obtained from the cecum, transverse colon, and rectosigmoid colon (166).

Viral cultures of biopsy specimens may take weeks to become positive; therefore, histologic examination using routine hematoxylin and eosin stains remains the mainstay of diagnosis. Stool cultures for CMV are unlikely to show CMV and are of no diagnostic value (166).

In patients with suspected CMV colitis, early endoscopic evaluation is warranted. Flexible sigmoidoscopy with biopsies should be performed as the initial study. If the examination is unrevealing, a colonoscopy is indicated because the disease is often localized in the proximal colon. Even with normal-appearing mucosa, random biopsy samples should be obtained to exclude the presence of inclusion bodies.

Herpes Simplex Colitis

Herpes simplex infection of the proximal colon is rare, although it is a common cause of ulcerative proctitis in homosexual men. It is usually seen in immunocompromised patients but can occur in immunocompetent hosts as well (170). Colonoscopic findings include erythematous, friable mucosa, aphthous ulcerations, and multiple necrotic ulcers (170,171) (see Color Figure 73.13). Anorectal ulcers caused by HSV are exquisitely tender; endoscopic examination of the infected anorectal area may require general anesthesia. It is probable that the evolution of mucosal changes is similar to that theorized in upper GI tract infection, with short-lived vesicles quickly evolving to form ulcerations. The entire colon may be involved with HSV colitis. As with HSV infection of the upper GI tract, biopsy specimens should be obtained from the margin of the ulcers and sent for both histologic examination and culture.

Fungal Infections

Candida

GI candidiasis usually affects the upper GI tract, most notably the esophagus and stomach. In an autopsy series of patients with GI *Candida* infection, the colon was involved in less than 4% of cases (172). Even with the prolonged survival of immunosuppressed patients and the high prevalence of *Candida* esophagitis in these patients, there does not seem to be an increase in invasive *Candida* infections of the lower GI tract (98,173). When the lower GI tract is involved, findings include small erosions and ulcerations, sometimes with overlying plaque (173).

Candida has been isolated from the stool in normal hosts and is thought to be nonpathogenic in these individuals. In hospitalized, debilitated patients with diarrhea, GI candidiasis has been implicated as, but not conclusively proven to be, a cause of the symptoms. In one report of 10 ill patients with diarrhea who had positive stool cultures for *Candida* species, there was a response to treatment with oral nystatin (173). Colonoscopies with biopsy in these patients were normal, suggesting a possible noninvasive role of *Candida* in the diarrheal illness. Based on this limited study, colonoscopy does not appear to play a significant role in patients with diarrhea and *Candida* isolated from stool cultures.

Parasitic Infections

Entamoeba histolytica

The clinical symptoms of amebic colitis can mimic other causes of diarrhea. Therefore, amebiasis should be considered in the differential diagnosis of any patient with symptoms suggestive of inflammatory bowel disease or bacterial colitis. Like inflammatory bowel disease, the symptoms may occur intermittently over years (174). It is important to recognize that the disease may be present in people without obvious risk factors, such as recent travel to endemic areas (175,176). Ten percent of the world population (177) and 5% of the U. S. population (176) harbor *E. histolytica*, although up to 90% of these individuals are asymptomatic.

Endoscopic findings are nonspecific, and the colonic abnormalities are easily mistaken for acute idiopathic inflammatory bowel disease (174–176,178). Diffuse inflammatory changes and multiple ulcerations can be seen (176,179). The ulcers are typically shallow, discrete, and round, with surrounding mucosal elevation (174,178). They are of variable size, from a few millimeters to 2 cm and are usually covered by a white or yellow exudate. The intervening mucosa can be normal or inflamed and granular. Aphthous ulcers can also commonly be seen (174). The rectum is involved in most cases, although the entire colon can be involved. The right colon can show isolated abnormalities in approximately 10% of cases (174,180). Endoscopic ulcerations may persist for several weeks to months after clinical symptoms have resolved (175). Amebomas, manifesting as polypoid mass lesions, have also been described (181). These uncommon lesions occur mainly in the cecum and represent areas of the bowel in which the amebae have infiltrated the wall, causing the inflamed mucosa to bulge into the lumen. In asymptomatic carriers of *E. histolytica*, the colonic mucosa appears grossly normal (177).

A definitive diagnosis of amebiasis is made by identifying amebic trophozoites and flask-shaped ulcers in colonic biopsy specimens (178). To increase the yield of finding the ameba, biopsy specimens should be obtained from the ulcer margins at the interface between the normal and ulcerated tissue. Even with adequate biopsy specimens, however, the ameba may easily be missed or may not be present in the specimen because of sampling error (179). One study suggests that as many as two-thirds of biopsy specimens will be nondiagnostic in detecting ameba (178). Even so, histologic examination of biopsy specimens is more sensitive than examination of fecal specimens (174,178). Cathartics and enemas given before endoscopic evaluation may decrease the sensitivity of histologic examination, because they can wash away and lyse the trophozoites (178). For this reason, some clinicians have recommended that no colonic preparation be given before endoscopic examination. Immediate microscopic examination of material aspirated or scraped from rectal lesions seen on proctoscopy has also been used to identify the parasite.

Stool studies for detection of amebic cysts have a high false-negative rate (176,180). The sensitivity of stool studies ranges from 50% to 60% (174,176,180). However, stool studies should be a routine test performed in patients being evaluated for possible infectious diarrhea. A stool ELISA test has been developed to detect *E. histolytica* infection and appears to differentiate between pathogenic and nonpathogenic forms (182). In a small study, the sensitivity and specificity of identifying pathogenic *E. histolytica* were 97% and 100%, respectively (182). This test is not yet available clinically.

Serologic tests are positive in 85% to 95% of patients with invasive amebiasis (178,180), whereas asymptomatic cyst carriers usually have a negative serology (176). However, serologic tests do not differentiate between past and present disease (177,180). The indirect hemagglutination test, for example, may remain elevated for as long as 20 years after the disease is cured (176,178). Serologic testing should be correlated with clinical and endoscopic findings. Acute and convalescent serologic titers should be sent 2 to 4 weeks apart, because false-negative tests can occur as a result of delayed seroconversion (176).

Stool studies and serologic tests should be sent in any patient with new clinical symptoms suggestive of amebic colitis. Given the limitations of these tests, endoscopic examination of the colonic mucosa with biopsy sampling is an important part of the evaluation.

Schistosomiasis

Colonic involvement of schistosomiasis (usually *Schistosoma mansoni* or *Schistosoma mekongi*) often manifests with bleeding and diarrhea, but can also manifest with an abdominal mass (183). Colonoscopic findings include scattered mucosal erosions, edema, and erythema (184,185). Rectal mucosal nodularity and polyps can also occur (183, 185–187). Mucosal vascular alterations thought to be highly suggestive of schistosomiasis include loss of the reticular structure of blood vessels, vessel interruption, corkscrew vessels, and petechiae (185,188). Hypertrophy and fibrosis of the mucosa due to an inflammatory reaction to the submucosal schistosomal ova can cause formation of large masses simulating tumor (183). However, in 35% to 50% of patients, the mucosa appears normal but biopsies demonstrate the presence of *Schistosoma* ova (184,186).

Biopsy specimens show granulomas containing *Schistosoma* ova (183) and are superior to stool examination. Biopsy specimens should be obtained from abnormal mucosal lesions for the best yield, but random specimens may still show the ova.

Stool examinations for ova and parasites were positive in only 11% of cases in which colonoscopic biopsies were positive for *S. mansoni* (184,186). Serologic tests were positive in 53%, but the use of serology is limited because it does not distinguish between active and past infection. Therefore, colonoscopy with biopsy is a superior method for diagnosing intestinal schistosomiasis.

Mycobacterium Infections

Colonic Tuberculosis

Intestinal tuberculosis continues to present a diagnostic challenge, especially in the United States, where it is relatively uncommon. Although endoscopic and radiologic findings have been well described, none are pathognomonic, and the diagnosis is still established by surgical intervention in many cases.

The ileocecal area is the most common site of infection with GI tuberculosis (108,111,189). In patients with colonic tuberculosis, the cecum is involved in up to 90% of cases, with the rectum involved the least often (190). However, segmental involvement of the colon without cecal lesions is being described more frequently (191). Typically, 4- to 8-cm segments of disease are seen with segmental tuberculosis (192,193), and, in approximately 30% of patients, two or more segments of the colon are involved (193).

The colonic abnormalities usually take on an ulcerative form, a nodular hypertrophic form, or both (189–192, 194–195). Ulcers appear as multiple linear or round lesions with granular necrotic bases and edematous, elevated borders (189,194,195). Ulcers may be only a few millimeters deep, but can be several centimeters in dimension (193). Nodules and hypertrophic mucosa are also commonly seen. The nodules are typically 2 to 6 mm in diameter and can be densely packed (193). Ulcers are often interspersed among the nodules. Stricture formation is common. The ileocecal valve is characteristically deformed and edematous, and is associated with nodular mucosa and ulcerations in most cases (189,190). Early colonoscopic abnormalities were described in 11 patients with pulmonary tuberculosis whose barium enema results were normal (190). Findings included small nodules resembling polyps in 70% of patients, and multiple small superficial ulcers in 30%. Biopsies were positive for acid-fast bacilli in all 11 patients. The cecum was also involved without ileal involvement in four cases, suggesting that cecal infection begins first, followed by ileal infection as the disease progresses.

Diagnosis requires histopathologic demonstration of acid-fast bacilli or granulomas, or culture of *Mycobacterium* from tissue specimens. Unfortunately, histologic examination of endoscopic biopsy specimens has a poor diagnostic yield, partly because of the submucosal location of the *Mycobacterium* (189). Even with multiple biopsy specimens obtained from the same site to allow deeper sampling, histology is unrevealing in 20% to 60% of cases (189,191,193,194). Biopsy specimens are more frequently diagnostic if obtained from an ulcerated lesion rather than a nodular lesion (48% versus 25% in one series) (193). Some cases of intestinal tuberculosis have been diagnosed not by histology of biopsy specimens but by obtaining endoscopic fine-needle aspiration cytology samples from ileocecal nodules. The smears showed acid-fast bacilli and may have had an increased yield because submucosal tissue was obtained. In another study of nine consecutive patients suspected of having intestinal tuberculosis, only two of nine biopsy samples showed acid-fast bacilli, whereas eight of nine brushing specimens showed acid-fast bacilli (196). The brushings were taken from a deep well where multiple biopsy samples had been obtained first at the same site.

Culture of biopsy material is helpful, although it may take many weeks to become positive. Culture is positive in only approximately 40% of cases. However, the combination of histologic examination and culture of biopsy specimens yields a positive diagnosis in approximately 60% of cases (193).

Radiologic studies may suggest the diagnosis, but the findings are nonspecific (189,192,193). The role of colonoscopy in the diagnosis of colonic tuberculosis is well established and should be performed in any patient suspected of having the disease. However, emphasis is placed on the difficulty in ascertaining the diagnosis despite extensive biopsy sampling.

ROLE OF ENDOSCOPIC RETROGRADE CHOLANGIOPANCREATOGRAPHY IN INFECTIONS OF THE PANCREATICOBILIARY SYSTEM

Endoscopic retrograde cholangiopancreatography (ERCP) is currently the most definitive imaging technique for examining the biliary and pancreatic ducts. Although technically challenging, in experienced hands, this method of examination of the pancreaticobiliary system is successful in more than 90% of cases. ERCP not only plays a role in obtaining tissue samples, but, when combined with sphincterotomy or stent placement, it also plays an important role in treating infections of the pancreaticobiliary system by providing drainage of obstructed ducts.

Bacterial Infection

Bacterial Cholangitis

The most common cause of acute bacterial cholangitis is bile duct obstruction resulting from choledocholithiasis.

Malignant or benign biliary strictures are important but less frequent causes of cholangitis. The patient's clinical presentation, laboratory data, and abdominal ultrasound or CT scan provide enough information to establish the proper diagnosis in most cases. ERCP is seldom needed for diagnostic purposes in these patients.

However, in approximately 30% of patients with acute cholangitis, treatment with antibiotics alone is not adequate and urgent decompression of pus of the biliary tract is warranted (197) (see Color Figure 73.14). In experienced hands, ERCP can delineate the cause of bile duct obstruction in more than 90% of cases (197,198). In addition, decompression of the bile duct by endoscopic sphincterotomy with stone extraction or by stent placement through a stricture has a success rate of greater than 85%. In a prospective study of patients with severe acute cholangitis due to choledocholithiasis, the mortality rate of patients who underwent emergency endoscopic drainage was 10% (199). This was significantly lower than the 32% rate observed in the group who underwent emergency surgical decompression. Endoscopic biliary drainage is also probably preferable to percutaneous transhepatic biliary drainage. Prospective comparison of these two techniques in relieving malignant biliary obstruction suggested that the transhepatic approach was associated with a higher complication rate resulting from intraperitoneal bile leak and hepatic bleed (200). However, direct comparison of these two drainage techniques in acute cholangitis has not been studied.

Viral Infections

HIV

AIDS cholangiopathy is a well-recognized entity. Endoscopic cholangiogram demonstrates biliary ductal abnormalities, including strictures, dilation, sclerosis, and papillary stenosis. Although opportunistic infections such as CMV, cryptosporidiosis, and microsporidiosis are often implicated as etiologic factors of hepatobiliary pathology in these patients, in 30% to 55% of cases, no pathogen is identified (201,202). This has been called AIDS cholangiopathy and it is considered to be directly related to local HIV infection. Some studies suggest that intrahepatic ductal irregularity is more indicative of concomitant infection with CMV or *Cryptosporidium* (203). Endoscopic sphincterotomy has been reported to provide long-term pain relief in these patients (203–205).

Cytomegalovirus

As much as 28% of AIDS-related cholangitis has been documented to be secondary to CMV infection (206). The predominant clinical complaint at presentation is abdominal pain. Diagnosis of CMV infection is usually made in other regions of the body and is associated with disseminated infection. Endoscopic sphincterotomy relieves pain in more than 85% of these patients (206).

Fungal Infections

Pancreaticobiliary infection caused by fungal organisms has been infrequently reported. *Candida albicans* is the predominant organism noted (207,208). ERCP has been helpful in establishing the diagnosis in some cases by demonstrating ductal filling defects (207–209). Surgery has been the treatment of choice to date (209–211). The role of endoscopic management of these patients has yet to be defined.

Parasitic Infections

Cryptosporidia and Microsporidia

These organisms are the other common pathogens associated with cholangiopathy in AIDS patients (202,212,213). The cholangiographic abnormalities cannot be differentiated from those induced by CMV (203). Endoscopic sphincterotomy also provides pain relief.

Ascaris

Ascaris lumbricoides is a major cause of acute obstructive cholangitis and pancreatitis throughout the world. In one region of India, ascariasis was considered to be an etiologic factor in 23% of patients presenting with acute pancreatitis (214). ERCP is effective in identifying and extracting worms from both the biliary and pancreatic ducts with rapid relief of symptoms (215,216). Concomitant treatment with oral antihelminthic therapy is indicated for successful eradication of the parasite (214).

Echinococcus

Hydatid cysts of the liver are usually diagnosed after obtaining a clinical history, serology, and radiologic examination, including plain film of the abdomen, ultrasound, and CT scan. Surgical resection of the cyst with concomitant antihelminthic therapy with either mebendazole or albendazole has been the standard of treatment. Percutaneous drainage with hypertonic saline lavage of the cavity has also been advocated and offers a promising alternative to surgery (217). Intrabiliary rupture of a hepatic hydatid cyst occurs in 8% to 17% of cases and can lead to bile duct obstruction (218–221). ERCP is an effective diagnostic tool in this situation (222–224). Cholangiogram often demonstrates irregularly shaped mobile filling defects, displacement and distortion of intrahepatic bile ducts by the hepatic cysts, and dilation of the pancreatic duct (225). Treatment options include sphincterotomy to facilitate drainage of cyst material, as well as lavage of the bile ducts and cysts with hypotonic or hypertonic saline via a nasobiliary tube (223,

226). Effective lavage of the cyst cavity requires continued communication with the biliary tree. These techniques have obviated the need for surgery in some cases, and long-term follow-up from 6 months to 1 year has demonstrated excellent results in most of these cases (225,227,228).

Liver Flukes

Clonorchis senensis, Opisthorchis viverrini, and *Fasciola hepatica* follow similar patterns of existence within the bile ducts of a human host. Diagnosis, treatment, and management can be accomplished by examination of the stools without the use of ERCP. The latter modality is employed when such complications as stricture or bacterial superinfection arise. These organisms may remain in the biliary tract decades after immigration outside endemic area.

Mycobacterial Infections

Mycobacterium tuberculosis and MAC infections of the pancreaticobiliary system are rare. In addition to direct bile ductal infection, duct obstruction may occur by porta hepatic node compression. Frequently, tuberculosis of the pancreas is diagnosed postmortem (229). Because symptoms of these infections are predominantly related to other organs or organ systems, ERCP usually does not afford any earlier or greater diagnostic accuracy. Stenosis of the pancreatic duct secondary to tuberculosis diagnosed by ERCP in the setting of generalized *M. tuberculosis* infection has been reported (230).

ROLE OF ENDOSCOPY IN NOSOCOMIAL INFECTIONS

Nosocomial infections associated with endoscopy can be divided into three categories: (a) transmission of exogenous microorganisms to the patient by contaminated equipment, (b) infection caused by the patient's endogenous enteric microorganisms that are introduced during endoscopy, and (c) transmission of infection from an infected patient to endoscopy personnel. The incidences of these events, the sources and types of microorganisms involved, and the methods for preventing these infections are discussed in this section. This topic has been reviewed extensively in several recent reports (231–233).

Transmission of Infection by Contaminated Equipment

Incidence

The true incidence of transmission of pathogens by endoscopy is unknown. The number of reported cases of this event is remarkably small. Earlier reports on the incidence of patient infections due to endoscopy found rates for upper endoscopy, ERCP, colonoscopy, and colonoscopy plus polypectomy to be 0.008%, 0%, 0.01%, and 0.06%, respectively (234). More than 250 cases of infection transmitted by endoscopy have been reported (231,232). Twenty-eight cases were reported between 1988 and 1992. Because approximately 40 million endoscopies were performed in this 4-year period, a crude and likely underestimate of incidence of infection transmitted by any endoscopy is therefore 1:1.8 million, or 0.000055% (231).

Types of Pathogens

Transmission of various species of *Salmonella* by either upper or lower endoscopy has been documented in 84 patients (235–241). Forty-five cases of *Pseudomonas aeruginosa* transmission were reported (242–252). Most of these cases were associated with ERCP. Other bacterial organisms reported include *E. coli, Enterobacter cloacae, Enterobacter aerogenes* (251,253), *Staphylococcus epidermidis, Klebsiella* (254), *Serratia marcescens* (255), and *Helicobacter pylori* (256).

There is only one reported case of endoscopic transmission of hepatitis B (257). Several studies have demonstrated no transmission of hepatitis B in endemic areas where seronegative patients underwent endoscopies with equipment that had been used on hepatitis B surface and e-antigen–positive patients (258–260). There have been at least two likely endoscopic transmissions of hepatitis C. Bronowicki and colleagues (261) reported a probable transmission of hepatitis C infection from a seropositive patient to a husband and wife at the time of colonoscopy. They sequenced the viral isolates recovered from the donor and recipients and found nucleotide homology among the sequenced segment, suggesting that hepatitis C was transmitted during colonoscopy. Other reports of possible transmission of hepatitis C during upper endoscopy, endoscopic retrograde cholangiography, and colonoscopy have included potential chronologic evidence (262). We are not aware of any reported cases of HIV, CMV, or HSV infection related to GI endoscopy.

Two cases of endoscopic transmission of fungus (263,264) and one case of *Strongyloides stercoralis* transmission (265) have also been reported. Transmission of *Mycobacterium* through GI endoscopy has not been documented.

Sources of Pathogens

Transmission of pathogens by endoscopy is invariably due to inadequately decontaminated endoscopic equipment. In a review of 28 cases of endoscopic transmissions with waterborne, enteric, or cutaneous bacteria that had been reported since the introduction of specific guidelines for endoscopic cleaning and disinfection, there was a breach in the recommended cleaning or disinfecting procedures, or there was contamination of an automated endoscope reprocessor or accessories in each of the 28 reported cases (266,267).

Contamination of equipment may be secondary to inadequate removal of debris before disinfection, ineffective cleaning or disinfecting agents (241,242,268,269), incomplete drying of equipment before storage (246), improper use of or poor design of automated cleaning machines (242,270,271), rinsing of equipment with tap water after disinfection (272), or handling of equipment by personnel before use.

Method of Prevention

The critical measure to prevent transmission of pathogens by endoscopy is proper decontamination and cleaning of equipment. High-level disinfection of endoscopes is perhaps most widely practiced. This can be achieved by thorough manual cleaning of the equipment followed by soaking of the equipment in liquid chemical disinfectants. The recommended and most commonly used liquid disinfectant is 2% activated alkaline glutaraldehyde. Immersion of endoscopes in this solution for 5 to 10 minutes eliminates all viral, fungal, and bacterial pathogens such as hepatitis B virus (HBV), HIV, HSV, *Candida*, *Salmonella*, and *Pseudomonas*. Longer immersion time is needed to kill mycobacterial organisms. Bacterial spores are especially resistant to glutaraldehyde, but transmission of these organisms by endoscopy has not been reported. The current standard of care is a 20-minute soak at room temperature using a 2% glutaraldehyde solution that has been properly tested to ensure adequacy of germicidal concentrations and is without surfactant or stabilizing additives. Sterilization using peroxyacetic acid in Steris systems is also used in many endoscopy units in the United States. The Steris system, however, cannot be used for ultrasound endoscopes. Sterilization of all endoscopes and accessories using gas sterilization with ethylene oxide is too time consuming, and autoclaving damages the endoscope.

The first and most important step in the prevention of transmission of pathogens by endoscopy is mechanical cleaning. This step is personnel-dependent and heavily depends on training and quality control. The next step is high-level disinfection, commonly achieved using glutaraldehyde-based formulations utilizing manual or automated processors. The third part involves rinsing and drying of the endoscope and its channels. Rinsing requires flushing large volumes of water in order to completely flush the disinfectants. Drying is important to prevent proliferation of residual bacteria and fungi during storage. Drying is accomplished with forced air and by storing the endoscope in an upright hanging position. Certain endoscopes, such as the endoscopic retrograde cholangiopancreatography endoscopes require a 70% alcohol flushing after the water rinse. Detailed guidelines for proper reprocessing of endoscopes have been published (273).

An alternative approach to minimize transmission of pathogens by endoscopy is to use disposable equipment. Disposable accessories such as biopsy forceps and cannulas have been widely used in recent years. Although disposable endoscopes have been developed, their use has been limited (232). The potential benefit of further reducing the small risk of infection transmission and the elimination of the cost of reprocessing equipment must be balanced against the expenses associated with equipment disposal and environmental impact.

Strict adherence to equipment disinfection protocols is the best safeguard against transmission of infection by endoscopy. Adaptation of these disinfection guidelines may have contributed to the apparent decrease in reported transmission of infection by endoscopy since 1988. However, recent surveys suggested a 30% to 70% rate of noncompliance to recommended cleaning protocols by health care personnel (232). Further improvements in compliance with these guidelines by health care providers are needed.

Infections Caused by Endogenous Gastrointestinal Flora

Transient bacteremia occurs with routine daily activity such as chewing hard candy (17%) and brushing one's teeth (25%), and does not lead to systemic infection (274). It is important to keep this in mind when examining data regarding procedure-induced bacteremia because systemic infection is rare.

A wide range of endoscopy-induced bacteremia rates have been reported. Colonoscopy, sigmoidoscopy, and upper endoscopy are associated with lower rates of bacteremia, ranging from 0% to 19% (275–280). Biopsy during the procedure does not increase the incidence of bacteremia. More invasive procedures such as dilation of esophageal strictures, endoscopic laser therapy, injection sclerotherapy, and therapeutic ERCP may have bacteremia rates as high as 30% to 45% (280–282). However, much lower rates of bacteremia associated with these procedures have also been reported. Oropharyngeal flora such as *Streptococcus* and *Staphylococcus* species are the most common organisms isolated (274,276,277,280).

Despite the apparently high rate of bacteremia induced by various endoscopic procedures, the incidence of clinically significant infections as a result of these procedures is extremely low. Only a few cases of endocarditis and perinephric and brain abscesses have been reported (283,286–288). The risk of infectious complication in immunocompromised patients undergoing endoscopy is also not significantly different from that of patients with normal immune systems (287,288).

Use of prophylactic antibiotics before endoscopic procedures is a logical method to prevent serious infectious complications. However, there are no prospective controlled trials that have shown that antibiotic prophylaxis prevents bacterial endocarditis (273). The low risk of infection from most GI endoscopic procedures makes such a trial difficult to conduct in that only a very large randomized trial could demonstrate the efficacy of prophylactic antibiotics. Because of the serious consequences of endocarditis, prophylactic antibiotics before endoscopy are recommended based on the patient's risk for development of endocarditis and the type of procedure to be performed. Patients with a history of endocarditis, prosthetic cardiac valve placement, systemic-pulmonary surgical shunts, cyanotic congenital heart disease, or synthetic vascular grafts less than 1 year old are considered to have the highest risk for endocarditis. These patients are recommended to have prophylaxis before undergoing procedures considered to have the greatest risk of inducing bacteremia: esophageal stricture dilation, variceal sclerotherapy, and cholangiography with biliary obstruction. The American Society of Gastrointestinal Endoscopy guidelines suggest that prophylaxis be individualized when high-risk patients undergo lower risk procedures. The American Heart Association guidelines suggest prophylaxis also be given to those patients undergoing higher risk procedures who have moderate risk cardiac lesions: rheumatic valvular dysfunction, mitral valve prolapse with insufficiency, hypertrophic cardiomyopathy, and most congenital cardiac lesions (289). Prophylaxis is not recommended for patients with moderate risk cardiac lesions undergoing low risk procedures or for patients with low risk cardiac lesions (history of coronary bypass grafting, pacemakers, implantable defibrillators) or prosthetic joints undergoing any procedure. Prophylaxis against soft-tissue infection is recommended for all patients undergoing percutaneous endoscopic gastrostomy placement. Prophylaxis to reduce the incidence of cholangitis is recommended in patients with biliary obstruction undergoing endoscopic retrograde cholangiography. For other situations, including that of immunocompromised patients, the decision to use prophylactic antibiotics should be individualized.

Transmission of Infections from Infected Patient to Endoscopy Personnel

Endoscopy personnel are at risk of acquiring infections transmitted directly from the patient or from contaminated equipment. The incidence of these events is unknown. The endoscopist may have a small risk of acquiring HBV when performing procedures in infected patients (290). Transmission of *H. pylori* during endoscopy has been implicated by the observation that the incidence of *H. pylori* infection in gastroenterologists (52%) appears to be higher than that in other endoscopy personnel, general practitioners, and age-matched control subjects (21%) (291).

Endoscopy personnel must exercise universal precautions in terms of protecting themselves against infections because the patient's infection status may be unknown at the time of endoscopy. Use of protective measures such as gloves, gowns, masks, and eye coverings are recommended, especially when extensive contact with blood or other body fluid is anticipated. Handwashing must be done after each procedure even when gloves have been worn. Infection prevention guidelines during endoscopic procedures and endoscopy cleaning must be followed to maximize safety (292). In addition, vaccination against HBV in endoscopy personnel is appropriate.

Summary

Nosocomial infections caused by GI endoscopy are exceedingly rare, even allowing for possible underreporting of these events. The majority of the cases of infection transmission by endoscopy can be attributed to either inadequate disinfection protocols or noncompliance to these protocols. When proper adjustments in protocol are made, infection outbreaks are effectively terminated. Current standards of cleaning and disinfection, therefore, make GI endoscopy a safe diagnostic and therapeutic tool in the management of GI disease.

REFERENCES

1. Dooley CP, Cohen J. The clinical significance of *Campylobacter pylori*. *Ann Intern Med* 1988;108:70–79.
2. Strauss RM, Wang TC, Kelsey PB, et al. Association of *Helicobacter pylori* infection with dyspeptic symptoms in patients undergoing gastroduodenoscopy. *Am J Med* 1990;89:464–469.
3. Dooley CP, Cohen H, Fitzgibbons PL, et al. Prevalence of *Helicobacter pylori* infection and histologic gastritis in asymptomatic persons. *N Engl J Med* 1989;321:1562–1566.
4. Parsonnet J. *Helicobacter pylori* and gastric cancer. *Gastroenterol Clin North Am* 1993;22:89–104.
5. Parsonnett J, Hansen S, Rodriquez L, et al. *Helicobacter pylori* infection and gastric lymphoma. *N Engl J Med* 1994;330: 1267–1271.
6. Loffeld RJLF, Ten Tije BJ, Arends JW. Prevalence and significance of *Helicobacter pylori* in patients with Barrett's esophagus. *Am J Gastroenterol* 1992;87:1598–1600.
7. Xia HH, Phung N, Kalantar JS, et al. Demographic and endoscopic characteristics of patients with *Helicobacter pylori* positive and negative peptic ulcer disease. *Med J Aus* 2000;173: 515–519.
8. Bujanover Y, Konikoff F, Baratz M. Nodular gastritis and *Helicobacter pylori*. *J Pediatr Gastroenterol Nutr* 1990;11:41–44.
9. Nguyen AH, Engstrand L, Genta RM, et al. Detection of *Helicobacter pylori* in dental plaque by reverse transcription-polymerase chain reaction. *J Clin Microbiol* 1993;31:783–787.
10. Borhan-Manesh F, Farnum JB. Study of *Helicobacter pylori* colonization of patches of heterotopic gastric mucosa (HGM) at the upper esophagus. *Dig Dis Sci* 1993;38:142–146.
11. Hazell SL, Hennessy WR, Borody TJ, et al. *Campylobacter pyloridis* gastritis II: distribution of bacteria and associated inflammation in the gastroduodenal environment. *Am J Gastroenterol* 1987;82:297–301.
12. Goodwin CS, Worsley BW. Microbiology of *Helicobacter pylori* *Gastroenterol Clin North Am* 1993;22:5–19.
13. Brown KE, Peura DA. Diagnosis of *Helicobacter pylori* infection. *Gastroenterol Clin North Am* 1993;22:105–115.

14. Eck M, Greiner A, Schmausser B, et al. Evaluation of *Helicobacter pylori* in gastric MALT-type lymphoma: differences between histological and serological diagnosis. *Mod. Pathol* 1999;12:1148–1151.
15. Relman DA, Schmidt TM, MacDermott RP, et al. Identification of the uncultured bacillus of Whipple's disease. *N Engl J Med* 1992;327:293–301.
16. Crane S, Schlippert W. Duodenoscopic findings in Whipple's disease. *Gastrointest Endosc* 1978;24:248–249.
17. Geboes K, Ectors N, Heidbuchel H, et al. Whipple's disease: endoscopic aspects before and after therapy. *Gastrointest Endosc* 1990;36:247–252.
18. Silverstein FE, Tytgat GNJ. Atlas of gastrointestinal endoscopy. Philadelphia: WB Saunders, 1987.
19. Ectors N, Geboes K, Wynants P, et al. Granulomatous gastritis and Whipple's disease. *Am J Gastroenterol* 1992;87:509–513.
20. Marcial MA, Villafana M. Whipple's disease with esophageal and colonic involvement: endoscopic and histopathologic findings. *Gastrointest Endosc* 1997;46:263–266.
21. Walsh TJ, Bekutsis NJ, Hamilton SR. Bacterial esophagitis in immunocompromised patients. *Arch Intern Med* 1986;146: 1345–1348.
22. Mcdonald GB, Sharma P, Hackman RC, et al. Esophageal infections in immunosuppressed patients after marrow transplantation. *Gastroenterology* 1985;88:1111–1117.
23. Ezzell JH, Bremer J, Adamec TA. Bacterial esophagitis: an often forgotten cause of odynophagia. *Am J Gastroenterol* 1990;85: 296–298.
24. Mcmanus JPA, Webb JN. A yeast-like infection of the esophagus caused by *Lactobacillus acidophilus. Gastroenterology* 1975; 68:583–586.
25. Howlett SA. Acute streptococcal esophagitis. *Gastrointest Endosc* 1979;25:150–151.
26. Goff JS. Infectious causes of esophagitis. *Annu Rev Med* 1988; 39:163–169.
27. Nicholson BW, Maull KI, Scher LA. Phlegmonous gastritis: clinical presentation and surgical management. *South Med J* 1980;73:875–877.
28. Turner MA, Beachley MC, Stanley D. Phlegmonous gastritis. *AJR Am J Roentgenol* 1979;133:527–528.
29. Lifton LJ, Schlossberg D. Phlegmonous gastritis after endoscopic polypectomy. *Ann Intern Med* 1982;97:373–374.
30. Iwakiri Y, Kabemura T, Yasuda D, et al. A case of acute phlegmonous gastritis successfully treated with antibiotics. *J Clin Gastroenterol* 1999;28:175–177.
31. Stein LB, Greenberg RE, Ilardi CR, et al. Acute necrotizing gastritis in a patient with peptic ulcer disease. *Am J Gastroenterol* 1989;84:1552–1554.
32. Miller AI, Smith B, Rogers AI. Phlegmonous gastritis. *Gastroenterology* 1975;68:231–238.
33. Cruz FO, Soffia PS, Del Rio PM, et al. Acute phlegmonous gastritis with mural abscess: CT diagnosis. *AJR Am J Roentgenol* 1992;159:767–768.
34. Cardillo MR, Forte F. Brush cytology in the diagnosis of herpetic esophagitis. A case report. *Endoscopy*1988;20:156–157.
35. Solammadevi SV, Patwardhan R. Herpes esophagitis. *Am J Gastroenterol* 1982;77:48–50.
36. McDonald GB, Shulman HM, Sullivan KM, et al. Intestinal and hepatic complications of human bone marrow transplantation. Part I. *Gastroenterology* 1986;90:460–477.
37. McDonald GB, Shulman HM, Sullivan KM, et al. Intestinal and hepatic complications of human bone marrow transplantation. Part II. *Gastroenterology* 1986;90:770–784.
38. McBane RD, Gross JB. Herpes esophagitis: clinical syndrome, endoscopic appearance, and diagnosis in 23 patients. *Gastrointest Endosc* 1991;37:600–603.
39. McBane RD, Gross JB. Herpes esophagitis: review of the clinical syndrome, endoscopic appearance, and diagnosis in 21 patients. *Gastrointest Endosc* 1990;36:192–193.
40. Agha FP, Lee HH, Nostrant TT. Herpetic esophagitis: a diagnostic challenge in immunocompromised patients. *Am J Gastroenterol* 1986;81:246–253.
41. Wilcox CM. Esophageal disease in the acquired immunodeficiency syndrome: etiology, diagnosis, and management. *Am J Med* 1992;92:412–421.
42. Brady CE, Hover AR. Esophagitis in immunocompromised patients: a diagnostic challenge. *South Med J* 1983;76:1538–1541.
43. Wheller RR, Peacock JE, Cruz JM, et al. Esophagitis in the immunocompromised host: role of esophagoscopy in diagnosis. *Rev Infect Dis* 1987;9:88–96.
44. Alexander JA, Brouillette DE, Chien M-C, et al. Infectious esophagitis following liver and renal transplantation. *Dig Dis Sci* 1988;33:1121–1126.
45. Kaplan CS, Petersen EA, Icenogle TB, et al. Gastrointestinal cytomegalovirus infection in heart and heart-lung transplant recipients. *Arch Intern Med* 1989;149:2095–2100.
46. Hinnant KL, Rotterdam HZ, Bell ET, et al. Cytomegalovirus infection of the alimentary tract: a clinicopathological correlation. *Am J Gastroenterol* 1986;81:944–950.
47. Bonacini M, Young T, Laine L. The causes of esophageal symptoms in human immunodeficiency virus infection. *Arch Intern Med* 1991;151:1567–1572.
48. Culpepper-Morgan JA, Kotler DP, Scholes JV, et al. Evaluation of diagnostic criteria for mucosal cytomegalic inclusion disease in the acquired immune deficiency syndrome. *Am J Gastroenterol* 1987;82:1264–1270.
49. Jacobson MA, Mills J. Serious cytomegalovirus disease in the acquired immunodeficiency syndrome (AIDS). *Ann Intern Med* 1988;108:585–594.
50. Freedman PG, Weiner BC, Balthazar EJ. Cytomegalovirus esophagogastritis in a patient with acquired immunodeficiency syndrome. *Am J Gastroenterol* 1985;80:434–437.
51. Theise ND, Rotterdam H, Dieterich D. Cytomegalovirus esophagitis in AIDS: diagnosis by endoscopic biopsy. *Am J Gastroenterol* 1991;86:1123–1126.
52. Wilcox CM, Straub RF, Schwartz DA. Prospective evaluation of biopsy number for the diagnosis of viral esophagitis in HIV infection. *Gastrointest Endosc* 1995;41:359(abst).
53. Gill RA, Gebhard RL, Dozeman RL, Sumner HW. Shingles esophagitis: endoscopic diagnosis in two patients. *Gastrointest Endosc* 1984;30:26–27.
54. Wisloff F, Bull-Berg J, Myron J. Herpes zoster of the stomach. *Lancet* 1979;2:953.
55. Artigas JMG, Saumell CB, Faure RA, et al. Herpes zoster of upper gastrointestinal tract. *Lancet* 1980;2:43.
56. Bartelsman JFWM, Lange JMA, Van Leeuwen R, et al. Acute primary HIV-esophagitis. *Endoscopy* 1990;22:184–185.
57. Rabeneck L, Popovic M, Gartner S, et al. Acute HIV infection presenting with painful swallowing and esophageal ulcers. *JAMA* 1990;17:2318–2322.
58. Kitchen VS, Helbert M, Francis ND, et al. Epstein-Barr virus associated oesophageal ulcers in AIDS. *Gut* 1990;31:1223–1225.
59. Das K, Kochlar R, Goenka MK, et al. Obstruction, not cancer is responsible for esophageal candidal overgrowth. *J Clin Gastroenterol* 1995;20:330–331.
60. Trier JS, Bjorkman DJ. Esophageal, gastric and intestinal candidiasis. *Am J Med* 1984;76:39–43.
61. Kodsi BE, Wickremesinghe PC, Kozinn PF, et al. *Candida* esophagitis. A prospective study of 27 cases. *Gastroenterology* 1976;71:715–719.

62. Mathieson R, Dutta SK. *Candida* esophagitis. *Dig Dis Sci* 1983; 28:365–370.
63. Minoli G, Terruzzi V, Butti G, et al. Gastric candidiasis: an endoscopic and histological study in 26 patients. *Gastrointest Endosc* 1982;28:59–61.
64. Porro GB, Parente F, Cernuschi M. The diagnosis of esophageal candidiasis in patients with acquired immune deficiency syndrome: is endoscopy always necessary? *Am J Gastroenterol* 1989; 84:143–146.
65. Bonacini M, Laine L, Gal AA, et al. Prospective evaluation of blind brushing of the esophagus for *Candida* esophagitis in patients with human immunodeficiency virus infection. *Am J Gastroenterol* 1990;85:385–389.
66. Young JA, Elias E. Gastro-oesophageal candidiasis: diagnosis by brush cytology. *J Clin Pathol* 1985;38:293–296.
67. Debongnie JC, Beyaert C, Legros G. Touch cytology, a useful diagnostic method for diagnosis of upper gastrointestinal tract infections. *Dig Dis Sci* 1989;34:1025–1027.
68. Rosario MT, Raso CL, Comer GM, et al. Transnasal brush cytology for the diagnosis of *Candida* esophagitis in the acquired immunodeficiency syndrome. *Gastrointest Endosc* 1989;35:102–103.
69. Korlipara AP, Shrinpreis MN, Luk GD, et al. Blind cytology brushing as a method of diagnosis of esophageal candidiasis. *Gastrointest Endosc* 1988;34:205.
70. Levine MS, Macones AJ Jr, Laufer I. *Candida* esophagitis: accuracy of radiographic diagnosis. *Radiology* 1985;154:581–587.
71. Forsmark CE, Wilcox CM, Darragh TM, et al. Disseminated histoplasmosis in AIDS: an unusual case of esophageal involvement and gastrointestinal bleeding. *Gastrointest Endosc* 1990; 36:604–605.
72. Prescott RJ, Harris M, Banerjee SS. Fungal infections of the small and large intestine. *J Clin Pathol* 1992;45:806–811.
73. Tom W, Aaron JS. Esophageal ulcers caused by *Torulopsis glabrata* in a patient with acquired immune deficiency syndrome. *Am J Gastroenterol* 1987;82:766–768.
74. Ikeda K, Kumashiro R, Kifune T. Nine cases of acute gastric anisakiasis. *Gastrointest Endosc* 1989;35:304–308.
75. Sugimachi K, Inokuchi K, Ooiwa T, et al. Acute gastric anisakiasis. Analysis of 178 cases. *JAMA* 1985;253:1012–1013.
76. Sakanari JA, Loinaz M, Deardorff TL, et al. Intestinal anisakiasis. A case diagnosed by morphologic and immunologic methods. *Am J Clin Pathol* 1988;90:107–113.
77. Sakanari JA, McKerrow JH. Anisakiasis. *Clin Microbiol Rev* 1989;2:278–284.
78. McHenry R, Bartlett MS, Lehman GA, et al. The yield of routine duodenal aspiration for *Giardia lamblia* during esophagogastroduodenoscopy. *Gastrointest Endosc* 1987;33:425–426.
79. Flanagan PA. *Giardia*—diagnosis, clinical course and epidemiology. A review. *Epidemiol Infect* 1992;109:1–22.
80. Oberhuber G, Stolte M. Giardiasis: analysis of histological changes in biopsy specimens of 80 patients. *J Clin Pathol* 1990; 43:641–643.
81. El Sheikh Mohemed AR, Al Karawi MA, Yasawy MI. Modern techniques in the diagnosis and treatment of gastrointestinal and biliary tree parasites. *Hepatogastroenterology* 1991;38: 180–188.
82. Doglioni C, De Boni M, Ciclo R, et al. Gastric giardiasis. *J Clin Pathol* 1992;45:964–967.
83. Knisley CV, Engelkirk PG, Pickering LK, et al. Rapid detection of *Giardia* antigen in stool with the use of enzyme immunoassays. *Am J Clin Pathol* 1989;91:704–708.
84. Green EL, Miles MA, Warhurst DC. Immunodiagnostic detection of *Giardia* antigen in faeces by a rapid visual enzyme-linked immunosorbent assay. *Lancet* 1985;2:691–693.
85. Ungar BLP, Yolken RH, Nash TE, et al. Enzyme-linked immunosorbent assay for the detection of *Giardia lamblia* in fecal specimens. *J Infect Dis* 1984;149:90–97.
86. Janoff EN, Craft JC, Pickering LK, et al. Diagnosis of *Giardia lamblia* infections by detection of parasite-specific antigens. *J Clin Microbiol* 1989;27:431–435.
87. Kamath KR, Murugasu R. A comparative study of four methods for detecting *Giardia lamblia* in children with diarrheal disease and malabsorption. *Gastroenterology*1974;66:16–21.
88. Rosenthal P, Liebman WM. Comparative study of stool examinations, duodenal aspiration, and pediatric Entero-Test for giardiasis in children. *J Pediatr* 1980;96:278–279.
89. Bendig DW. Diagnosis of giardiasis in infants and children by endoscopic brush cytology. *J Pediatr Gastroenterol Nutr* 1989;8: 204–206.
90. Achkar E, Carey WD, Petras R, et al. Comparison of suction capsule and endoscopic biopsy of small bowel mucosa. *Gastrointest Endosc* 1986;32:278–281.
91. Korman SH. Endoscopic duodenal aspiration for diagnosis of giardiasis. *Gastrointest Endosc* 1989;35:354–355.
92. Marshall JB, Kelley DH, Vogele KA. Giardiasis: diagnosis by endoscopic brush cytology of the duodenum. *Am J Gastroenterol* 1984;79:517–519.
93. Gellin BG, Soave R. Coccidian infections in AIDS. Toxoplasmosis, cryptosporidiosis and isosporiasis. *Med Clin North Am* 1992;76:205–234.
94. Rene E, Marche C, Regnier B, et al. Intestinal infections in patients with acquired immunodeficiency syndrome. A pros pective study in 132 patients. *Dig Dis Sci* 1989;34:773–780.
95. Edwards P, Wodak A, Cooper DA, et al. The gastrointestinal manifestations of AIDS. *Aust N Z J Med* 1990;20:141–148.
96. Angus KW. Cryptosporidiosis and AIDS. *Bailliere Clin Gastroenterol* 1990;4:425–441.
97. Connolly GM, Forbes A, Gleeson JA, et al. The value of barium enema and colonoscopy in patients infected with HIV. *AIDS* 1990;4:687–689.
98. Ullrich R, Heise W, Bergs C, et al. Gastrointestinal symptoms in patients infected with human immunodeficiency virus: relevance of infective agents isolated from gastrointestinal tract. *Gut* 1992;33:1080–1084.
99. Cello JP. Evaluation of AIDS-related diarrhea. *Hosp Prac* 1993; 28:95–102.
100. Dumont A, Seferian V, Barbier P. Endoscopic discovery and capture of *Necator americanus* in the stomach. *Endoscopy* 1983; 15:65–66.
101. Genta RM, Woods KL. Endoscopic diagnosis of hookworm infection. *Gastrointest Endosc* 1991;37:476–478.
102. Descombes P, Dupas JL, Capron JP. Endoscopic discovery and capture of *Taenia saginata*. *Endoscopy* 1981;13:44–45.
103. Jacob GS, Nakib A, Ruwaih AA. Ascariasis producing upper gastrointestinal hemorrhage. *Endoscopy* 1983;15:67.
104. Hamed AD, Akinola O. Intestinal ascariasis in the differential diagnosis of peptic ulcer disease. *Trop Geogr Med* 1990;42: 37–40.
105. Contractor QQ, Benson L, Schulz TB, et al. Duodenal involvement in *Schistosoma mansoni* infection. *Gut* 1988;29:1011–1012.
106. Webbe G. Schistosomiasis: some advances. *BMJ* 1981;283: 1104–1106.
107. Salas SD, Heifetz R, Barrett-Connor E. Intestinal parasites in Central American immigrants in the United States. *Arch Intern Med* 1990;150:1514–1516.
108. Weissman D, Gumaste VV, Dave PB, et al. Bleeding from a tuberculous gastric ulcer. *Am J Gastrolenterol* 1990;85:742–744.
109. Abel ME, Chiu YS, Russell TR, et al. Gastrointestinal tuberculosis. Report of four cases. *Dis Colon Rectum* 1990;33: 886–889.

110. Vijayraghavan M, Arunabh, Sarda AK, et al. Duodenal tuberculosis: a review of the clinicopathologic features and management of twelve cases. *Jpn J Surg* 1990;20:526–529.
111. Nair KV, Pai CG, Rajagopal KP, Ghat VN, Thomas M. Unusual presentations of duodenal tuberculosis. *Am J Gastroenterol* 1991;86:756–760.
112. Salpeter SR, Shapiro RM, Gasman JD. Gastric tuberculosis presenting as fever of unknown origin. *West J Med* 1991;155: 412–413.
113. Eng J, Sabanathan S. Tuberculosis of the esophagus. *Dig Dis Sci* 1991;36:536–540.
114. Rosario MT, Raso CL, Comer GM. Esophageal tuberculosis. *Dig Dis Sci* 1989;34:1281–1284.
115. Tornieporth N, Lorenzo R, Gain T, et al. An unusual case of active tuberculosis of the oesophagus in an adult. *Endoscopy* 1991;23:294–296.
116. Tornieporth N, Lorenz R, Gain T, et al. An unusual case of active tuberculosis of the oesophagus in an adult. *Endoscopy* 1991;23:294–296.
117. Gordon AH, Marshal JB. Esophageal tuberculosis: definitive diagnosis by endoscopy. *Am J Gastroenterol* 1990;85:174–177.
118. Gupta B, Mathew S, Bhalla S. Pyloric obstruction due to gastric tuberculosis and endoscopic diagnosis. *Postgrad Med J* 1990; 66:63–65.
119. Tromba JL, Inglese R, Rieders B, et al. Primary gastric tuberculosis presenting as pyloric outlet obstruction. *Am J Gastroenterol* 1991;86:1820–1822.
120. Subei I, Attar B, Schmitt G, et al. Primary gastric tuberculosis: a case report and literature review. *Am J Gastroenterol* 1987; 82:769–772.
121. Regan F, Tran T. Duodenal tuberculosis—a continuing diagnostic challenge. *Postgrad Med J* 1990;66:787–791.
122. Sivasubramanian S, Senapaati MK. Tuberculosis of the stomach. *Trop Doctor* 1992;22:132–133.
123. Fukuya T, Yoshimitsu K, Kitagawa S, et al. Single tuberculous stricture in the jejunum: report of 2 cases. *Gastrointest Radiol* 1989;14:300–304.
124. Rosario Mt, Raso CL, Comer GM. Esophageal tuberculosis. *Dig Dis Sci* 1989;34:1281–1284.
125. Horvath KD, Whelan RL. Intestinal tuberculosis: Return of an old disease. *Am J Gastroenterol* 1998;93:692–696.
126. De Silva R, Stoopack PM, Raufman J-P. Esophageal fistulas associated with mycobacterial infection in patients at risk for AIDS. *Radiology* 1990;175:449–453.
127. Gray JR, Rabeneck L. Atypical mycobacterial infection of the gastrointestinal tract in AIDS patients. *Am J Gastroenterol* 1989; 84:1521–1524.
128. Cappell MS, Philogene C. The endoscopic appearance of severe intestinal *Mycobacterium avium* complex infection as a coarsely granular mucosa due to massive infiltration and expansion of intestinal villi without mucosal exudation. *J Clin Gastroenterol* 1995;21:323–326.
129. Cotton PB, Tytgat GNJ, Williams CB. *Slide atlas of gastrointestinal endoscopy.* London: Current Science, 1992.
130. Lewis BS, Kornbluth A, Waye JD. Small bowel tumours: yield of enteroscopy. *Gut*1991;32:763–765.
131. Barkin JS, Lewis BS, Reiner DK, et al. Diagnostic and therapeutic jejunoscopy with a new, longer enteroscope. *Gastrointest Endosc* 1992;38:55–58.
132. Sharma BC, Bhasin DK, Makharia G, et al. Diagnostic value of push-type enteroscopy: a report from India. *Am J Gastroenterol* 2000;95:137–140.
133. Monkemuller KE, Wilcox CM. Diagnosis and treatment of colonic disease in AIDS. *Gastrointest Endosc Clin North Am* 1998;8:889–911.
134. Loss RW, Mangla JC, Pereira M. *Campylobacter* colitis presenting as inflammatory bowel disease with segmental colonic ulcerations. *Gastroenterology* 1980;79:138–140.
135. Lambert ME, Schofield PF, Ironside AG, et al. *Campylobacter* colitis. *BMJ* 1979;1:857–859.
136. Blaser MJ, Parsons RB, Wang W-LL. Acute colitis caused by *Campylobacter fetus* ss. *jejuni. Gastroenterology* 1980;78:448–453.
137. Khuro MS, Mahajan R, Zargar SA, et al. The colon in shigellosis: serial colonoscopic appearances in *Shigella dysenteriae* I. *Endoscopy* 1990;22:35–38.
138. Kelly J, Oryshak A, Wenetsek M, et al. The colonic pathology of *Escherichia coli* O157:H7 infection. *Am J Surg Pathol* 1990;14:87–92.
139. Fry RD. Infectious enteritis. A collective review. *Dis Colon Rectum* 1990;33:520–527.
140. Drake AA, Gilchrist MJR, Washington JA, et al. Diarrhea due to *Campylobacter fetus* subspecies *jejuni.* A clinical review of 63 cases. *Mayo Clin Proc* 1981;56:414–423.
141. Griffin PM, Ostroff SM, Tauxe RV, et al. Illnesses associated with *Escherichia coli* O157:H7 infections. A broad clinical spectrum. *Ann Intern Med* 1988;109:705–712.
142. Shortsleeve MJ, Wilson ME. Finklestein M, et al. Radiologic findings in hemorrhagic colitis due to *Escherichia coli* O157:H7. *Gastrointest Radiol* 1989;14:341–344.
143. Remis RS, MacDonald KL, Riley LW, et al. Sporadic cases of hemorrhagic colitis associated with *Escherichia coli* O157:H7. *Ann Intern Med* 1984;101:624–626.
144. Griffin PM, Olmsteasd LC, Petras RE. *Escherichia coli* O157:H7-associated colitis. A clinical and histological study of 11 cases. *Gastroenterology* 1990;90:142–149.
145. Nastrant TT, Kumar NB, Appelman HD. Histopathology differentiates acute self-limited colitis from ulcerative colitis. *Gastroenterology* 1987;92:318–328.
146. Surawicz CM, Belic L. Rectal biopsy helps to distinguish acute self-limited colitis from idiopathic inflammatory bowel disease. *Gastroenterology*1984;86:104–113.
147. Gerding DN. Disease associated with *Clostridium difficile* infection. *Ann Intern Med* 1989;110:255–257.
148. Fekety R, Shah AB. Diagnosis and treatment of *Clostridium difficile* colitis. *JAMA* 1993;269:71–75.
149. Pounder RE, Allison MC, Dhillon AP. *Colour atlas of the digestive system.* London: Wolfe Publishing, 1989.
150. Gebhard RL, Gerding DN, Olson MM, et al. Clinical and endoscopic findings in patients early in the course of *Clostridium difficile*-associated pseudomembranous colitis. *Am J Med* 1985;78:45–48.
151. Tedesco FJ. Pseudomembranous colitis: pathogenesis and therapy. *Med Clin North Am* 1982;66:655–663.
152. Talbot RW, Walker RC, Beart RW Jr. Changing epidemiology, diagnosis, and treatment of *Clostridium difficile* toxin-associated colitis. *Br J Surg* 1986;73:457–460.
153. Tedesco FJ, Corless JK, Brownstein RE. Rectal sparing in antibiotic-associated pseudomembranous colitis: a prospective study. *Gastroenterology* 1982;83:1259–1260.
154. Seppala K, Hjelt L, Sipponen P. Colonoscopy in the diagnosis of antibiotic-associated colitis. A prospective study. *Scand J Gastroenterol* 1981;16:465–468.
155. Tedesco FJ. Antibiotic associated pseudomembranous colitis with negative proctosigmoidoscopy examination. *Gastroenterology* 1979;77:295–297.
156. Triadafilopoulos G, Hallstone AE. Acute abdomen as the initial presentation of pseudomembranous colitis. *Gastroenterology* 1991;101:685–691.
157. Shetler K, Nieuwenhuis R, Wren SM, et al. Decompressive colonoscopy with intracolonic vancomycin administration for the treatment of severe pseudomembranous colitis. *Surg Endosc* 2001;15:653–659.

158. Price AB, Davies DR. Pseudomembranous colitis. *J Clin Pathol* 1977;30:1–12.
159. Peterson LR, Olson MM, Shanholtzer CH, et al. Results of a prospective, 18-month clinical evaluation of culture, cytotoxin testing, and Culturette brand (CDT) latex testing in the diagnosis of *Clostridium difficile*-associated diarrhea. *Diagn Microbiol Infect Dis* 1988;10:85–91.
160. Lashner BA, Todorczuk J, Sahm DF, et al. *Clostridium difficile* culture-positive toxin-negative diarrhea. *Am J Gastroenterol* 1986;81:940–943.
161. Gumerlock PH, Tang YJ, Weiss JB, et al. Specific detection of toxigenic strains of *Clostridium difficile* in stool specimens. *J Clin Microbiol* 1993;31:507–511.
162. Kato N, Ou C-Y, Kato H, et al. Detection of toxigenic *Clostridium difficile* in stool specimens by the polymerase chain reaction. *J Infect Dis* 1993;167:455–458.
163. Gerding DN, Olson MM, Peterson LR, et al. *Clostridium difficile*-associated diarrhea and colitis in adults. A prospective case-controlled epidemiologic study. *Arch Intern Med* 1986;146: 95–100.
164. Brazier JS, Stubbs SL, Duerden BI. Prevalence of toxin A-negative/B-positive *Clostridium difficile* strains. *J Hosp Infect* 1999; 42:248–249.
165. Foucar E, Mukai K, Foucar K, et al. Colonic ulceration in lethal cytomegalovirus infection. *Am J Clin Pathol* 1981;76:788–801.
166. Dieterich DT, Rahmin M. Cytomegalovirus colitis in AIDS: presentation of 44 patients and a review of the literature. *J AIDS* 1991;4[Suppl 1]:S29–S35.
167. Dieterich DT, Kotler DP, Busch DF, et al. Gangiclovir treatment of cytomegalovirus colitis in AIDS: a randomized, double-blind, placebo-controlled multicenter study. *J Infect Dis* 1993;167:278–282.
168. Rene E, Marche C, Chevalier T, et al. Cytomegalovirus colitis in patients with acquired immunodeficiency syndrome. *Dig Dis Sci* 1988;33:741–750.
169. Weber FH, Frierson JF, Myers BM. Cytomegalovirus as a cause of isolated severe ileal bleeding. *J Clin Gastroenterol* 1992; 14:52–55.
170. Colemont LJ, Pen JH, Peickmans PA, et al. Herpes simplex virus type 1 colitis: an unusual cause of diarrhea. *Am J Gastroenterol* 1990;85:1182–1185.
171. Kinnaert R, Vereerstraeten P, Toussaint C. Diffuse herpes simplex virus colitis in a kidney transplant recipient successfully treated with acyclovir. *Transplantation* 1987;43:919–921.
172. Eras P, Goldstein MJ, Sherlock P. *Candida* infection of the gastrointestinal tract. *Medicine* 1972;51:367–379.
173. Gupta TP, Ehrinpreis MN. *Candida*-associated diarrhea in hospitalized patients. *Gastroenterology* 1990;98:780–785.
174. Matsui T, Iida M, Tada S, et al. The value of double-contrast barium enema in amebic colitis. *Gastrointest Radiol* 1989;14: 73–78.
175. Sanderson IR, Walker-Smith JA. Indigenous amoebiasis: an important differential diagnosis of chronic inflammatory bowel disease. *BMJ* 1984;289:823.
176. Patel AS, DeRidder PH. Amebic colitis masquerading as acute inflammatory bowel disease: the role of serology in its diagnosis. *J Clin Gastroenterology* 1989;11:407–410.
177. Variyam EP, Gogate P, Hassan M, et al. Nondysenteric intestinal amebiasis. Colonic morphology and search for *Entamoeba histolytica* adherence and invasion. *Dig Dis Sci* 1989;34:732–740.
178. Blumencranz H, Kasen L, Romeu J, et al. The role of endoscopy in suspected amebiasis. *Am J Gastroenterol* 1983;78: 15–18.
179. Rozen P, Baratz M, Rattan J. Rectal bleeding due to amebic colitis diagnosed by multiple endoscopic biopsies: report of two cases. *Dis Colon Rectum* 1981;24:127–129.
180. Patterson M, Healy GR, Shabot JM. Serologic testing for amoebiasis. *Gastroenterology* 1980;78:1236–1241.
181. Luterman L, Alsumait AR, Daly DS, et al. Colonoscopic features of cecal amebomas. *Gastrointest Endosc* 1985;31:204–206.
182. Haque R, Kress K, Wood S, et al. Diagnosis of pathogenic *Entamoeba histolytica* infection using a stool ELISA based on monoclonal antibodies to the galactose-specific adhesin. *J Infect Dis* 1993;167:247–249.
183. Zimbalist E, Gettenberg G, Brejt H. Ileocolonic schistosomiasis presenting as lymphoma. *Am J Gastroenerol* 1987;82: 476–478.
184. Yasawy MI, El Shiekh Mohamed AR, Al Karawi MA. Comparison between stool examination, serology and large bowel biopsy in diagnosing *Schistosoma mansoni*. *Trop Doctor* 1989;19: 132–134.
185. Raddawi JM, Nazer H, Ilahi F. Unusual patterns of schistosomal disease of the colon. *Gastrointest Endosc* 1989;35:256–258.
186. El-Shiek Mohamad AR, Al Karawi MA, Yasawy MI. Schistosomal colonic disease. *Gut* 1990;31:439–442.
187. Radhakrishnan S, Al Nakib B, Shaikh H, et al. The value of colonoscopy in schistosomal, tuberculous and amebic colitis. Two-year experience. *Dis Colon Rectum* 1986;29:891–895.
188. Sanguino J, Peixe R, Guerra J, et al. Schistosomiasis and vascular alterations of the colonic mucosa. *Hepatogastroenterology* 1993; 40:184–187.
189. Kochhar R, Rajwanshi A, Goenka MK, et al. Colonoscopic fine needle aspiration cytology in the diagnosis of ileocecal tuberculosis. *Am J Gastroenterol* 1991;86:102–104.
190. Pettengell KE, Pirie D, Simjee AE. Colonoscopic features of early intestinal tuberculosis. Report of 11 cases. *South Afr Med J* 1990;79:279–280.
191. Shah S, Thomas V, Mathan M, et al. Colonoscopic study of 50 patients with colonic tuberculosis. *Gut* 1992;33:347–351.
192. Medina E, Orti E, Tome A, et al. Segmental tuberculosis of the colon diagnosed by colonoscopy. *Endoscopy* 1990;22:188–190.
193. Bhargava DK, Kushwaha AKS, Dasarathy S, et al. Endoscopic diagnosis of segmental colonic tuberculosis. *Gastrointest Endosc* 1992;38:571–574.
194. Morgante PE, Gandara MA, Sterle E. The endoscopic diagnosis of colonic tuberculosis. *Gastrointest Endosc* 1989;35: 115–118.
195. Breiter JR, Hajjar J-J. Segmental tuberculosis of the colon diagnosed by colonoscopy *Am J Gastroenterol* 1981;76:369–373.
196. Bhasin DK, Roy P, Sharma M, et al. Acid-fast bacilli in colonoscopic brushings. *Lancet* 1991;338:184–185.
197. Leung JWC, Chung SCS, Sung JJY, et al. Urgent endoscopic drainage for acute suppurative cholangitis. *Lancet* 1989;1:1307.
198. Ott DJ, Gilliam JH III, Zagoria RJ, et al. Interventional endoscopy of the biliary and pancreatic ducts: current indications and methods. *AJR Am J Roentgenol* 1992;158:243–250.
199. Lai EC, Mok FP, Tan ES, et al. Endoscopic biliary drainage for severe acute cholangitis. *N Engl J Med* 1992;326:1626–1628.
200. Speer AG, Russell RC, Hatfield ARW, et al. Randomised trial of endoscopic versus percutaneous stent insertion in malignant obstructive jaundice. *Lancet* 1987;2:57.
201. Cello JP. Acquired immunodeficiency syndrome cholangiopathy: spectrum of disease. *Am J Med* 1989;86:539–546.
202. Pol S, Romana CA, Richard S, et al. Microsporidia infection in patients with the human immunodeficiency virus and unexplained cholangitis. *N Engl J Med* 1993;328:95–99.
203. Benhamou Y, Caumes E, et al. AIDS-related cholangiopathy. Critical analysis of a prospective series of 26 patients. *Dig Dis Sci* 1993;38:1113–1118.
204. Dowsett JF, Miller R, et al. Sclerosing cholangitis in acquired immunodeficiency syndrome. Case reports and review of the literature. *Scand J Gastroenterol* 1988;23:1267–1274.

205. Schneiderman DJ, Cello JP, Laing FC. Papillary stenosis and sclerosing cholangitis in the acquired immunodeficiency syndrome. *Ann Intern Med* 1987;106:546–549.
206. Bouche H, Housset C, et al. AIDS-related cholangitis: diagnostic features and course in 15 patients. *J Hepatol* 1993;17:34–39.
207. Chung RT, Schapiro RH, Warshaw AL. Intraluminal pancreatic candidiasis presenting as recurrent pancreatitis. *Gastroenterology* 1993;104:1532–1543.
208. Ryan ME, Kirchner JP, Sell T, et al. Cholangitis due to *Blastomyces dermatitidis*. *Gastroenterology* 1989;96:1346–1349.
209. Ho F, Snape WJ Jr, Venegas R, et al. Choledochal fungal ball. An unusual cause of biliary obstruction. *Dig Dis Sci* 1988;33: 1030–1034.
210. Magnussen CR, Olson JP, Ona FV, et al. *Candida* fungus balls in the common bile duct. Unusual manifestation of disseminated candidiasis. *Arch Intern Med* 1979;139:821–822.
211. Carstensen H, Nilsson KO, Nettelblad SC, et al. Common bile duct obstruction due to an intraluminal mass of candidiasis in a previously healthy child. *Pediatrics* 1986;77:858–861.
212. Pol S, Romana C, Richard S, et al. *Enterocytozoon bieneusi* infection in acquired immunodeficiency syndrome-related sclerosing cholangitis. *Gastroenterology* 1992;102:1778–1781.
213. Girard PM, Rozenbaum W, et al. Cholangiopathy associated with microsporidia infection of the common bile duct mucosa in a patient with HIV infection. *Ann Intern Med* 1992;117: 401–402.
214. Khuroo MS, Zargar SA, et al. Ascaris-induced acute pancreatitis. *Br J Surg* 1992;79:1335–1338.
215. el Sheikh Mohamed AR, al Karawi MA, et al. Modern techniques in the diagnosis and treatment of gastrointestinal and biliary tree parasites. *Hepatogastroenterology* 1991;38:180–188.
216. Krige JE, Lewis G, Bornman PC. Recurrent pancreatitis caused by a calcified ascaris in the duct of Wirsung. *Am J Gastroenterol* 1987;82:256–257.
217. Acunas B, Rozanes I, et al. Purely cystic hydatid disease of the liver: treatment with percutaneous aspiration and injection of hypertonic saline. *Radiology* 1992;182:541–543.
218. Xu MQ. Diagnosis and management of hepatic hydatidosis complicated with biliary fistula. *Chin Med J* 1992;105:69–72.
219. Aktan AO, Yalin R, et al. Surgical treatment of hepatic hydatid cysts. *Acta Chir Belg* 1993;93:151–153.
220. Ozmen V, Igci A, et al. Surgical treatment of hepatic hydatid disease. *Can J Surg* 1992;34:423–427.
221. Bilge A, Sozuer EM. Diagnosis and surgical treatment of hepatic hydatid disease. *HPB Surg* 1992;6:57–64.
222. Radin DR, Johnson MB. *Candida* cholangitis in a diabetic woman. *AJR Am J Roentgenol* 1992;158:1029–1030.
223. al Karawi MA, Yasawy MI, el Shiekh Mohamed AR. Endoscopic management of biliary hydatid disease: report on six cases. *Endoscopy* 1991;23:278–281.
224. al Karawi MA, el Shiekh Mohamed AR, Yasawy MI. Advances in diagnosis and management of hydatid disease. *Hepatogastroenterology* 1990;37:327–331.
225. Van Steenbergen W, Fevery J, et al. Hepatic echinococcosis ruptured into the biliary tract. Clinical, radiological and therapeutic features during five episodes of spontaneous biliary rupture in three patients with hepatic hydatidosis. *J Hepatol* 1987;4: 133–139.
226. al Karawi MA, Mohamed AR, et al. Non-surgical endoscopic trans-papillary treatment of ruptured echinococcus liver cyst obstructing the biliary tree. *Endoscopy* 1987;19:81–83.
227. Magistrelli P, Masetti R, et al. Value of ERCP in the diagnosis and management of pre- and postoperative biliary complications in hydatid disease of the liver. *Gastrointest Radiol* 1989;14: 315–320.
228. Vignote ML, Mino G, et al. Endoscopic sphincterotomy in hepatic hydatid disease open to the biliary tree. *Br J Surg* 1990; 77:30–31.
229. Ezratty A, Gumaste V, et al. Pancreatic tuberculosis: a frequently fatal but potentially curable disease. *J Clin Gastroenterol* 1990;12:74–77.
230. Stock KP, Riemann W, et al. Tuberculosis of the pancreas. *Endoscopy* 1981;13:178–80.
231. Transmission of infection by gastrointestinal endoscopy. ASGE Technology Assessment Position Paper, April 1993.
232. Spach DH, Silverstein FE, Stamm WE. Transmission of infection by gastrointestinal endoscopy and bronchoscopy. *Ann Intern Med* 1993;118:117–128.
233. Standards of Practice Committee of the American Society for Gastrointestinal Endoscopy. Infection control during gastrointestinal endoscopy. *Gastrointest Endosc* 1999;49:836–841.
234. Silvis SE, Nebel O, et al. Endoscopic complications. Results of the 1974 American Society for Gastrointestinal Endoscopy Survey. *JAMA* 1976;235:928–930.
235. Beecham HJ, Cohen ML, Parking WE. *Salmonella typhimurium*: transmission by fiberoptic upper gastrointestinal endoscopy. *JAMA* 1979; 241:1013–1015.
236. Chmel H, Armstron D. *Salmonella oslo*: a focal outbreak in a hospital. *Am J Med* 1976;60:203–208.
237. Dean AG. Transmission of *Salmonella typhi* by fiberoptic endoscopy. *Lancet* 1977;2:134.
238. Dwyer DM, Klein EG, et al. *Salmonella newport* infections transmitted by fiberoptic colonoscopy. *Gastrointest Endosc* 1987;33:84–87.
239. Holmberg SD, Osterholm MT, et al. Drug-resistant *Salmonella* from animals fed antimicrobials. *N Engl J Med* 1984;311: 617–622.
240. Schliessler KH, Rozendaal B, et al. Outbreak of *Salmonella agona* infection after upper intestinal fiberoptic endoscopy. *Lancet* 1980;2:1246.
241. Tuffnell PG. *Salmonella* infections transmitted by a gastroscope. *Can J Public Health* 1976;67:141–142.
242. Struelens MJ, Rost F, et al. *Pseudomonas aeruginosa* and Enterobacteriaceae bacteremia after biliary endoscopy: an outbreak investigation using DNA macrorestriction analysis. *Am J Med* 1993;95:489–498.
243. Deviere J, Motte S, et al. Septicemia after endoscopic retrograde cholangiopancreatography. *Endoscopy* 1990;22:72–75.
244. Siegman-Igra Y, Isakov A, et al. *Pseudomonas aeruginosa* septicemia following endoscopic retrograde cholangiopancreatography, with a contaminated endoscope. *Scan J Infect Dis* 1987; 19:527–530.
245. Davion T, Braillon A, et al. *Pseudomonas aeruginosa* liver abscesses following endoscopic retrograde cholangiopancreatography. Report of a case without biliary tract disease. *Dig Dis Sci* 1987;32:1044–1046.
246. Allen JI, Allen MO, et al. *Pseudomonas* infection of the biliary system resulting from use of a contaminated endoscope. *Gastroenterology* 1987;92:759–763.
247. Cryan EM, Falkiner FR, et al. *Pseudomonas aeruginosa* cross-infection following endoscopic retrograde cholangiopancreatography. *J Hosp Infect* 1984;5:371–376.
248. Schousboe M, Carte A, Sheppard PS. Endoscopic retrograde cholangiopancreatography: related nosocomial infections. *N Z Med J* 1980;92:275–277.
249. Doherty DE, Falko JM, et al. *Pseudomonas aeruginosa* sepsis following retrograde cholangiopancreatography (ERCP). *Dig Dis Sci* 1982;27:169–170.
250. Earnshaw JJ, Clark AW, et al. Outbreak of *Pseudomonas aeruginosa* following endoscopic retrograde cholangiopancreatography. *J Hosp Infect* 1985;6:95–97.
251. Elson CO, Hattori K, Balckstone MO. Polymicrobial sepsis fol-

lowing endoscopic retrograde cholangiopancreatography. *Gastroenterology* 1975;69:507–510.

252. Schoutens-Serruys E, Rost F, et al. The significance of bacterial contamination of fiberoptic endoscopes. *J Hosp Infect* 1981;2: 392–394.
253. Noy MF, Harrison L, et al. The significance of bacterial contamination of fiberoptic endoscopes. *J Hosp Infect* 1980;1:53–61.
254. Parker HW, Geenen JE, et al. A prospective analysis of fever and bacteremia following ERCP. *Gastrointest Endosc* 1979;25: 102–103.
255. Godiwala T, Andry M, et al. Consecutive *Serratia marcescens* infections following endoscopic retrograde cholangiopancreatography. *Gastrointest Endosc* 1988;34:345–347.
256. Langenberg W, Rauws EA, et al. Patient-to-patient transmission of *Campylobacter pylori* infection by fiberoptic gastroduodenoscopy and biopsy. *J Infect Dis* 1990;161:507–511.
257. Birnie GG, Quigley Em, et al. Endoscopic transmission of hepatitis B virus. *Gut* 1983;24:171–174.
258. Chiaramonte M, Farini R, et al. Risk of hepatitis B virus infection following upper gastrointestinal endoscopy: a prospective study in an endemic area. *Hepatogastroenterology* 1983;30:189–191.
259. Hoofnagle JH, Blake J, et al. Lack of transmission of type B hepatitis by fiberoptic upper endoscopy. *J Clin Gastroenterol* 1980;2:65–69.
260. Ayoola EA. The risk of type B hepatitis infection in flexible fiberoptic endoscopy. *Gastrointest Endosc* 1981;27:60–62.
261. Bronowicki J-P, Venard V, Botte C, et al. Patient-to-patient transmission of hepatitis C virus during colonoscopy. *N Engl J Med* 1997;337:237–240.
262. Delwaide J, Gerard C, Vaira D, et al. Hepatitis C virus transmission following invasive medical procedures. *J Intern Med* 1999;245:107–108.
263. Stuart D, Orelowitz J, et al. Fungemia with *Torulopsis glabrata* after endoscopic biliary stent replacement. *Am J Gastroenterol* 1992;87:883–885.
264. Ito M, Kato T, et al. Disseminated *Candida tropicalis* infection following endoscopic retrograde cholangiopancreatography. *J Infect* 1991;23:77–80.
265. Mandelstram P, Sugawa C, et al. Complications associated with esophagogastroduodenoscopy and with esophageal dilation. *Gastrointest Endosc* 1976;23:16–19.
266. American Society for Gastrointestinal Endoscopy Ad Hoc Committee on Disinfection. Reprocessing of flexible gastrointestinal endoscopes. *Gastrointest Endosc* 1996;43:540–546.
267. Kozarek RA. Transmission of hepatitis C virus during colonoscopy. *N Engl J Med* 1997;337:1848–1849.
268. Axon AT, Phillips I, et al. Disinfection of gastrointestinal fiber endoscopes. *Lancet* 1974;1:656–658.
269. Hanson PJV, Gor D, et al. Contamination of endoscopes used in AIDS patients. *Lancet* 1989;2:86–88.
270. Struelens MJ, Rost F, et al. Septicemia after ERCP: outbreak linked to an automatic endoscopic disinfecting machine. 3rd International Conference on Nosocomial Infections, Atlanta, GA, 1990:32.
271. Alvarado CJ, Stoltz SM, Maki DG. Nosocomial infections from contaminated endoscopes: a flawed automatic endoscope washer. An investigation using molecular epidemiology. *Am J Med* 1991;91[Suppl 3B]:272s–280s.
272. Low DE, Micflikier AB, et al. Infectious complications of endoscopic retrograde cholangiopancreatography. *Arch Intern Med* 1980;140:1076–1077.
273. Standards of Practice Committee of the American Society for Gastrointestinal Endoscopy. Infection control during gastrointestinal endoscopy. *Gastrointest Endosc* 1999;49:836–841.
274. Kullman E, Borch K, Lindstrom E, et al. Bacteremia following diagnostic and therapeutic ERCP. *Gastrointest Endosc* 1992;38: 444–449.
275. LeFrock J, Ellis C, Turchik J, et al. Transient bacteremia associated with sigmoidoscopy *N Engl J Med* 1973;289:102–104.
276. Baltch A, Buhac I, Agrawal A, et al. Bacteremia after upper gastrointestinal endoscopy. *Arch Intern Med* 1977;137:594–597.
277. Mellow M, Lewis R. Endoscopy-related bacteremia. *Arch Intern Med* 1976;136:667–669.
278. Norfleet R, Mulholland D, Mitchell P, et al. Does bacteremia follow colonoscopy? *Gastroenterology* 1976;70:20–21.
279. Norfleet R, Mitchell P, Mulholland D, et al. Does bacteremia follow upper gastrointestinal endoscopy? *Am J Gastroenterol* 1981;76:420–422.
280. Schembre D, Bjorkman D. Review article: endoscopy related infections. *Aliment Pharmacol Ther* 1993;7:347–355.
281. Botoman V, Surawics C. Bacteremia with gastrointestinal endoscopic procedures. *Gastrointest Endosc* 1986;32:342–346.
282. Yin T, Ellis R, Dellipiani A. The incidence of bacteremia after outpatient Hurst bougienage in the management of benign esophageal stricture. *Endoscopy* 1983;15:289–290.
283. Infection control during gastrointestinal endoscopy. Guidelines for clinical application, ASGE publication No. 1018. *Gastrointest Endosc* 1988;34[Suppl]:37s–40s.
284. Wang WM, Chen CY, et al. Central nervous system infection after endoscopic injection sclerotherapy. *Am J Gastroenterol* 1990;85:865–867.
285. Tai DI, Lan CK, Hen HJ. Brain abscess following endoscopic injection sclerotherapy: report of a case. *J Formos Med Assoc* 1991;90:857–859.
286. Ritchie MT, Lightdale CJ, Botet JF. Bilateral perinephric abscesses: a complication of endoscopic injection sclerotherapy. *Am J Gastroenterol* 1987;82:670–673.
287. Kaw M, Przepiorka D, Sekas G. Infectious complications of endoscopic procedures in bone marrow transplant recipients. *Dig Dis Sci* 1993;38:71–74.
288. Bianco J, Sullivan P, Higano C, et al. Prevalence of clinically relevant bacteremia after upper gastrointestinal endoscopy in bone marrow transplant recipients. *Am J Med* 1990;89:134–136.
289. Dajani AS, Tabuert KA, Wilson W, et al. Prevention of bacterial endocarditis: recommendations by the American Heart Association. *JAMA* 1997;277:1794–1801.
290. Koretz RL, Chin K, Gitnick G. The endoscopists' risks from endoscopic transmission of hepatitis. *Gastroenterology* 1985;88: 1454.
291. Mitchell H, Lee A, Carrick J. Increased incidence of *Campylobacter pylori* infection in gastroenterologists: further evidence to support person-to-person transmission of *C. pylori*. *Scan J Gastroenterol* 1989;24:396–400.
292. Martin MA, Reichelderfer M. APIC guidelines for infection prevention and control in flexible endoscopy. Association for Professionals in Infection Control and Epidemiology, Inc. 1991, 1992, and 1993 APIC Guidelines Committee. *Am J Infect Cont* 1994;22:19–38.

74

DIAGNOSTIC IMAGING IN THE DIAGNOSIS OF GASTROINTESTINAL INFECTIONS

DESIREE E. MORGAN

Radiology plays an important role in the detection and assessment of many gastrointestinal infections. Barium studies have for years been the most effective primary radiographic method, but computed tomography (CT) and, to a lesser extent, ultrasonography (US) are increasingly useful, particularly in the evaluation of colonic infections and the evaluation of immunocompromised patients.

The double-contrast esophagram is especially helpful in the detection and characterization of infectious esophagitis. The pattern of radiologic abnormalities differs predictably from one infectious agent to another and can often suggest a specific etiology. Even small, superficial erosions can be detected in most patients when good double-contrast technique is employed. In infections of the stomach, duodenum, and small intestine, radiologic assessment plays a less important role than other diagnostic modalities. The gastric infections that cause gross morphologic alterations of the stomach, principally tuberculosis, syphilis, and histoplasmosis, are rare. Most infections of the small intestine are brief and self-limited, leaving little role for radiologic studies. Infections of the small bowel in immunocompromised individuals may have radiologic manifestations, but such findings are usually nonspecific and do not indicate the etiologic agent. Radiologic methods have more to contribute to the evaluation and assessment of colonic infections. Single- and double-contrast barium enema findings are diagnostic in several colonic infections. CT has become the mainstay in the radiologic assessment of suspected appendicitis and colonic diverticulitis. In patients with diverticulitis, CT allows confirmation of the disease and provides information regarding the presence of associated abscess or fistula, which helps guide management.

D. E. Morgan: Department of Diagnostic Radiology, University of Alabama at Birmingham, Birmingham, Alabama

ESOPHAGUS

Infections of the esophagus occur most commonly in immunocompromised patients with hematologic malignancy, AIDS, or pharmacologic immunosuppression to prevent organ transplant rejection. To a lesser extent, esophageal infections also occur in patients with esophageal stasis. Infectious esophagitis is rare in otherwise healthy persons. Compared with the single-contrast barium esophagram, the double-contrast barium esophagram facilitates better radiologic recognition of the superficial mucosal abnormalities that occur in these diseases. In esophagitis due to *Candida albicans*, for example, the sensitivity of the double-contrast esophagram is approximately 90% (1). Typical radiologic features support a decision to treat before or without endoscopic confirmation.

Candida

Candida esophagitis has a spectrum of radiographic findings. Mild disease is associated with widespread discrete, irregular mucosal plaques (2). This particular pattern is seen most often in patients immunocompromised by diseases other than AIDS (3). In patients with moderate disease, the plaques coalesce. Combined with the debris of necrotic epithelium, the plaques develop a more irregular mucosal outline. In its most severe stage, *Candida* esophagitis causes the esophageal mucosa to look shaggy with marked irregularity caused by plaques, ulcers, and pseudomembranes (4) (Fig. 74.1). This fulminant form of *Candida* esophagitis occurs most often in patients with AIDS (3).

Uncommon radiologic presentations of *Candida* esophagitis include focal mucosal changes (5), stricture, complete obstruction with or without fungus ball, and perforation. Dramatic regression of the radiographic features of *Candida* esophagitis often occurs after treatment, but disappearance of the radiographic abnormalities may lag behind the clinical recovery. Because the infection may lead

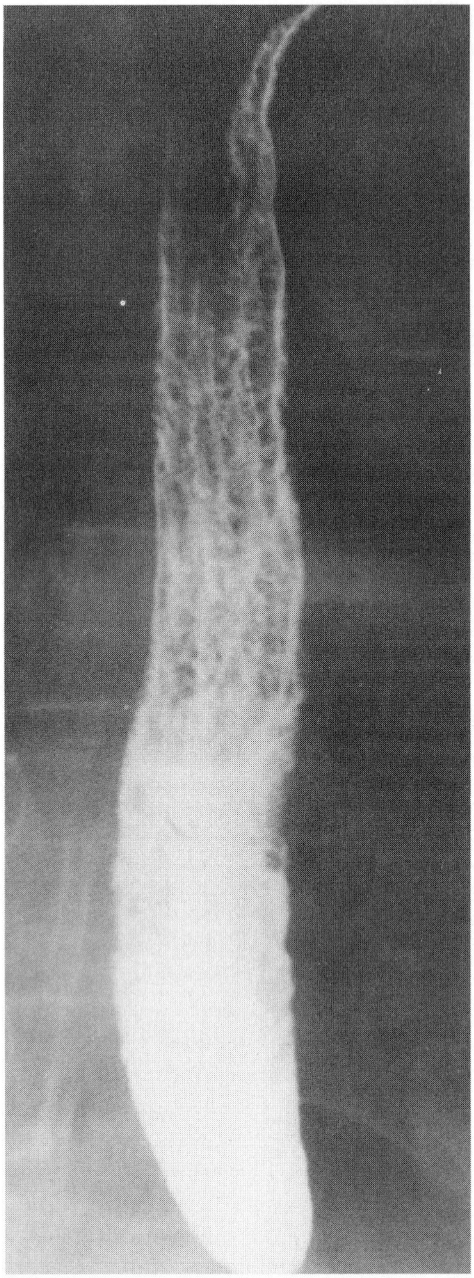

FIGURE 74.1. Severe *Candida* esophagitis in an elderly man receiving steroids for chronic obstructive pulmonary disease. The diffuse shaggy irregularity of the mucosa in this double-contrast esophagram is typical for monilial infection.

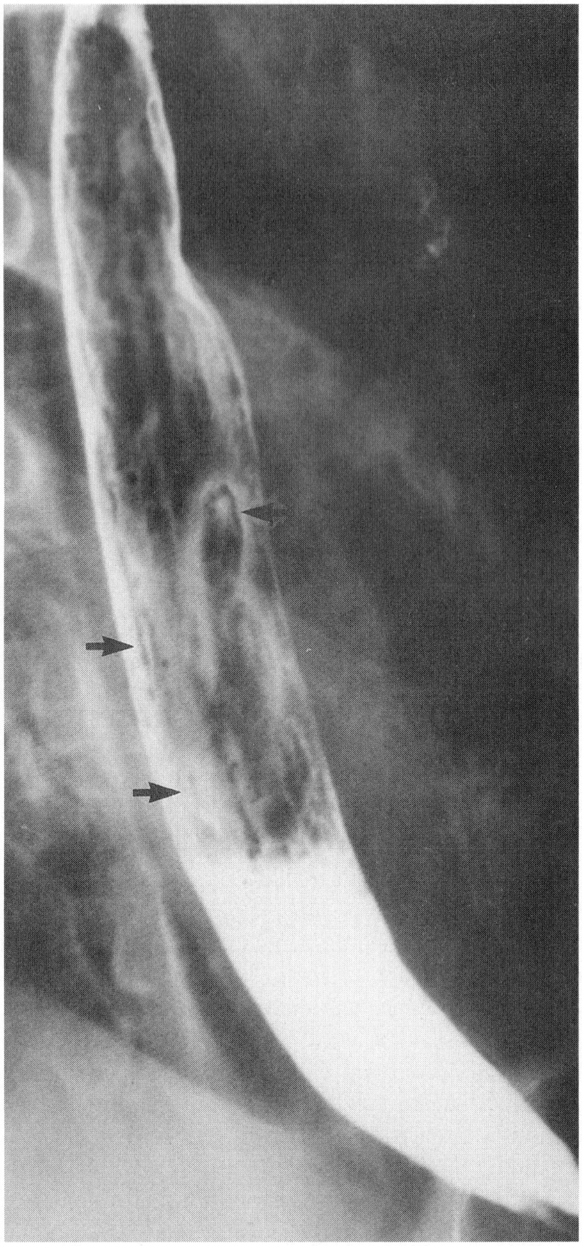

FIGURE 74.2.. Herpes simplex virus infection in an HIV-1–infected man with odynophagia. Numerous linear and punctate ulcers (*arrows*) appear as white barium collections surrounded by a darker halo of edematous tissue.

to permanent stricture or scarring, follow-up double-contrast esophagram has been recommended (6).

Herpes Simplex Virus

Esophagitis caused by herpes simplex virus (HSV) typically presents as small, discrete, punctate ulcers with a linear or stellate shape clustered in the midesophagus (Fig. 74.2) (6) or as multiple small, often diamond-shaped ulcers scattered throughout the esophagus. The ulcers are usually surrounded by normal appearing mucosa (3). Because the radiographic appearance of HSV esophagitis is not as specific as that of *Candida* esophagitis and because treatment carries more risk, biopsy confirmation of the radiologic findings is warranted (4). An acute transient form of HSV esophagitis occurs infrequently in immunocompetent persons, typically localizing in the midesophagus near the level of the left main bronchus (7). Advanced HSV esophagitis may also produce a diffusely shaggy esophagus, but concomitant *Candida* infection is usually present.

Cytomegalovirus

Cytomegalovirus (CMV) esophagitis occurs most often in patients with AIDS. The infection is characterized by one or more large (up to 2 cm), flat ulcers in the distal esophagus (Fig. 74.3). The surrounding mucosa usually appears normal. The radiographic features depend on the severity of the disease. Milder CMV infection presents as segmental areas of granular mucosa with superficial erosions and shallow, poorly defined ulcers (8,9).

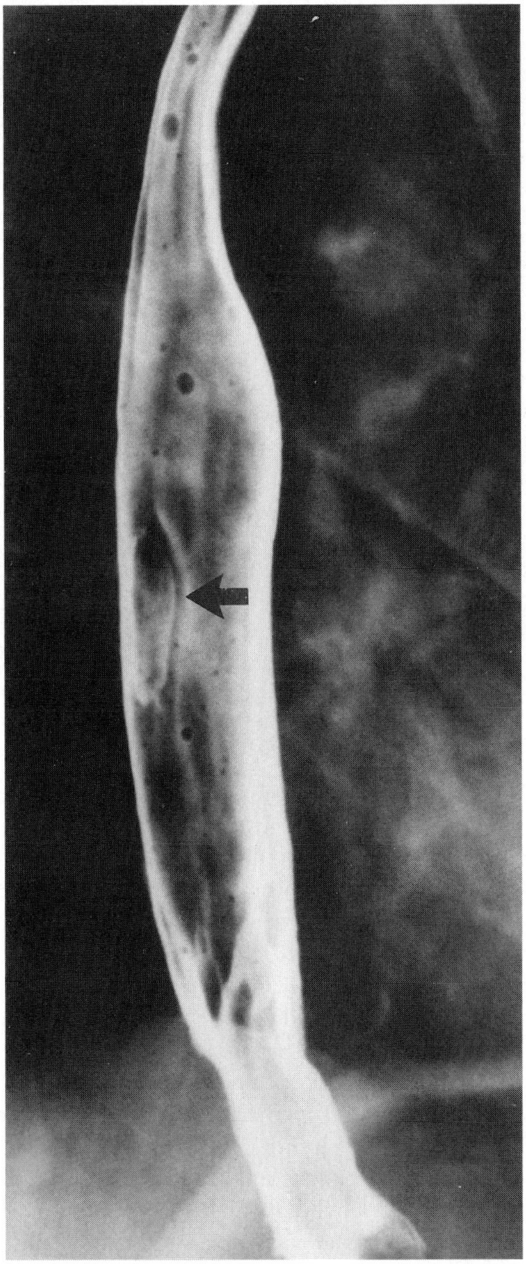

FIGURE 74.3. A large esophageal ulcer due to cytomegalovirus in a young male patient with AIDS. Cytomegalovirus may also cause shallow, longitudinally oriented, ovoid ulcers (*arrow*).

Other Esophageal Infections

Human immunodeficiency virus-1 (HIV-1) itself has also been associated with esophagitis, usually occurring within weeks of seroconversion but also in later stages of the disease. The typical presentation is that of large, shallow, isolated (or less commonly multifocal) ulcers in the mid or dis-

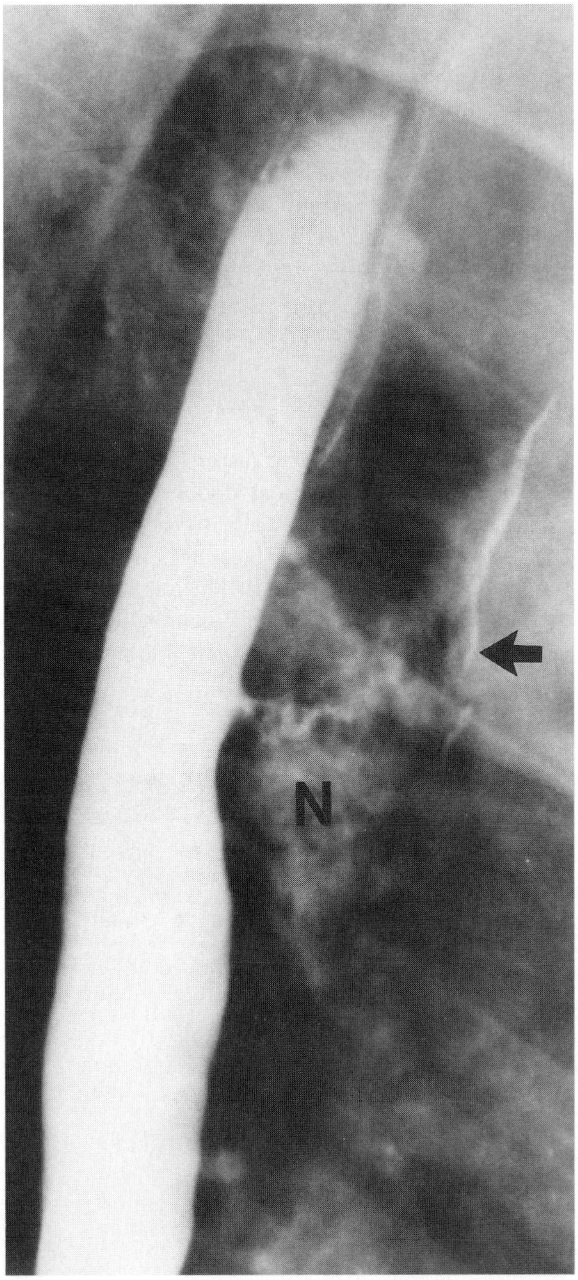

FIGURE 74.4. Tracheoesophageal fistula due to *Histoplasma capsulatum*. This 54-year-old man described a sensation of air passing from one portion of his chest to another when he lay on his left side. A single-contrast esophagram shows a pinpoint fistula filled with barium extending from the esophageal lumen through an enlarged, mediastinal, calcified lymph node (N) into the trachea (*arrow*).

tal esophagus (10). The appearance may be radiographically indistinguishable from that of CMV disease (11). One study of 100 HIV-1–infected patients found that the incidence of HIV-1 and CMV esophageal ulcers was nearly equal. In general, endoscopic evaluation with biopsy is necessary to establish a histologic diagnosis and institute therapy (12).

Uncommon infectious causes of esophagitis include *Mycobacterium avium* complex (MAC), which causes discrete ulceration of the esophagus (13), and *Mycobacterium tuberculosis*. *M. tuberculosis* usually arises from contiguous, infected, mediastinal lymph nodes that have become necrotic, causing transmural inflammation that may lead to deep ulceration, intramural dissection, and bronchial fistula (14). Other granulomatous infections may produce similar findings. A small esophagobronchial fistula that passes through a calcified mediastinal lymph node is typical of infection with *Histoplasma capsulatum* (Fig. 74.4).

STOMACH

Helicobacter pylori

In recent years, the radiographic features of *H. pylori* infection have been described using double-contrast barium studies. Enlargement of the areae gastricae and thickened gastric folds in the antrum or body region are the most common findings (15) (Fig. 74.5). The role of the radiologist in the evaluation of dyspepsia should be to suggest the presence of *H. pylori* when radiographic findings characteristic of *H. pylori* infection are present (16,17). An important complication of chronic *H. pylori* infection is the development of low-grade mucosa-associated lymphoid tumors (MALT lymphomas, or MALTomas). These tumors are identified radiographically by the presence of multiple rounded and often confluent gastric mucosal nodules on barium studies (18,19) or by extensive, nodular wall thickening by CT (Fig. 74.6). Treatment for *H. pylori* infection has been shown to induce dramatic resolution of the lesions.

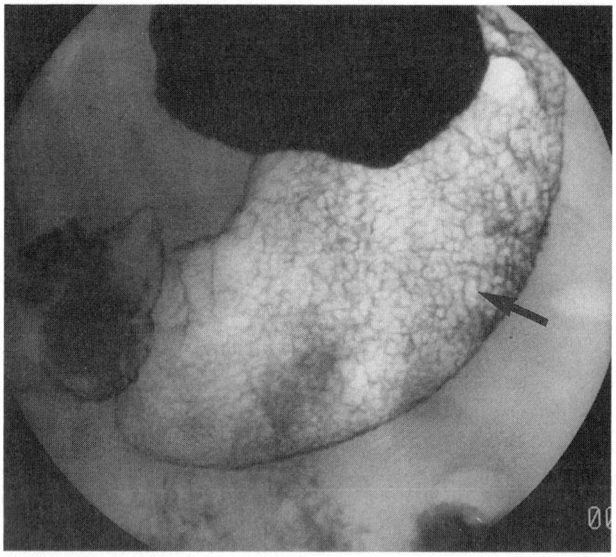

FIGURE 74.5. *Helicobacter pylori* infection. Double-contrast spot radiograph from an upper gastrointestinal series in a 69-year-old man with epigastric pain shows enlargement of the areae gastricae pattern, typical of *H. pylori* infection. No frank ulceration is noted. (Courtesy of Dr. Cheri L Canon.)

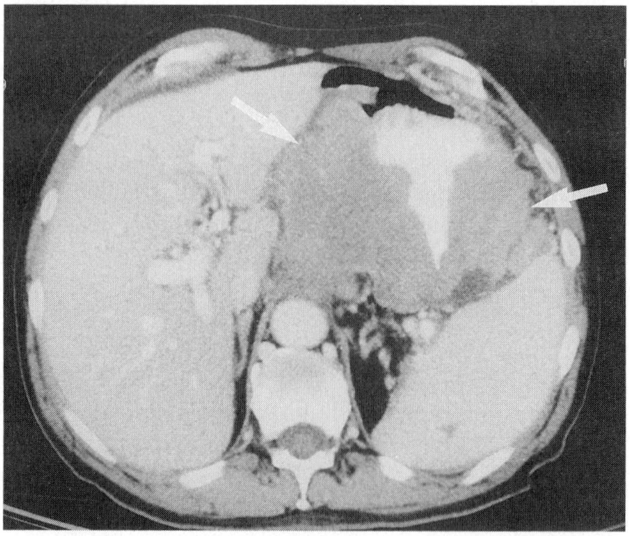

FIGURE 74.6. A 73-year-old man with abdominal pain and mucosa-associated lymphoid tumors (MALT) lymphoma. Oral and intravenous contrast-enhanced abdominal computed tomography scan shows marked, heterogeneous gastric wall thickening; histology showed MALT lymphoma. (Courtesy of Dr. Cheri L. Canon).

Other Gastric Infections

The radiographic differentiation of infectious diseases of the stomach is difficult because of the nonspecificity and variability of findings with double-contrast radiographic examination. Reports in the radiologic literature describe aphthous ulcers or superficial erosions in the stomach resulting from fungal and viral infection (20), antral narrowing resulting from *Toxoplasma gondii* infection (21), and thickened rugal folds caused by CMV infection. The radiologic appearance of *Cryptosporidium* and *T. gondii* infection in AIDS patients has also been described and includes gastric fold thickening, superficial aphthous ulcers, deep ulcers, and fistula formation (22). The varied radiographic features of tuberculous infection of the stomach include an ulcerative form and a hyperplastic form; the latter produces thickening of the antrum and pylorus. Gastric syphilis (Fig. 74.7), most often a manifestation of the tertiary stage of the disease, causes thickening of the gastric wall with an intact mucosa, leading to funnel-shaped narrowing of the antrum,

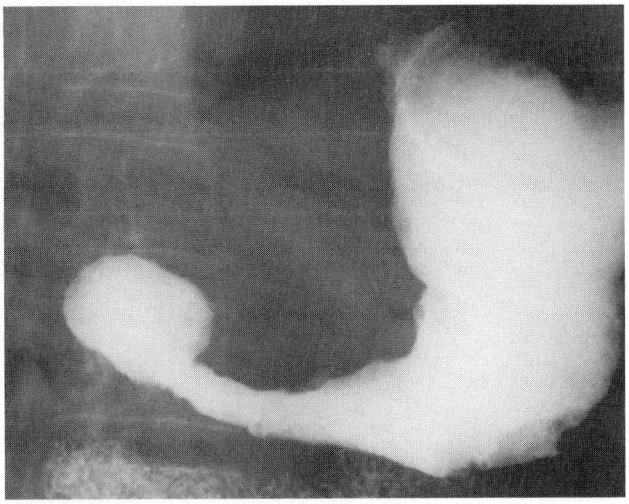

FIGURE 74.7. Linitis plastica due to gastric syphilis in an 82-year-old Haitian male with a positive VDRL (Venereal Disease Research Laboratory) and 15-pound weight loss during the preceding year. (Courtesy of Dr. Jack Farman.)

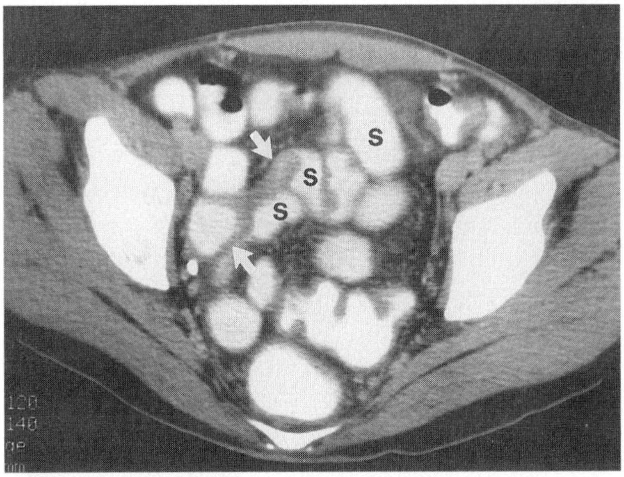

FIGURE 74.8. Cryptosporidiosis in a 28-year-old man with AIDS and diarrhea. Computed tomography (CT) scan at the level of the pelvis shows focal thickening (*arrows*) of the wall of the small intestine (S).

fold effacement, and decreased peristaltic activity (23). Endoscopic biopsy is required to determine the etiology of radiologically detected gastric infections (20).

SMALL INTESTINE

Radiographic studies are used to detect mucosal abnormalities that suggest a specific pathogen and to define the location and extent of disease for biopsy planning. The barium small-bowel follow-through may be used in screening patients at risk for small-bowel infections, with enteroclysis reserved for more difficult cases. However, given the potential for multiorgan system involvement in immunocompromised patients, contrast-enhanced abdominal CT scanning should be considered early in the evaluation (24).

AIDS-Associated Infections

In patients with AIDS or other immunocompromising conditions, one of the most common small-bowel infections is cryptosporidiosis (Fig. 74.8). The radiographic features of this parasitic infection include pronounced fold thickening, predominantly in the duodenum and jejunum, and increased fluid content in the bowel lumen (25,26). In chronic infection, ileal and even colonic involvement occur (27). Infections with *Isospora belli* and microsporidia produce clinical and radiographic findings indistinguishable from cryptosporidiosis (24).

MAC infection causes a variety of findings on barium studies of the small bowel, including irregular fold thickening and mild dilatation of the distal jejunum and ileum in a pattern similar to that of Whipple's disease (28). Enlarged lymph nodes may separate small-bowel segments on barium studies; the enlarged nodes may be readily detected by CT (Fig. 74.9). MAC-induced lymphadenopathy is usually more extensive in the mesentery than in the retroperitoneum (4,29) and is accompanied by hepatosplenomegaly on CT (30). Lymph nodes may vary from small (1.0 to 1.5 cm) to large, bulky masses (27,30). Because granulomas rarely form in MAC disease, most patients show adenopathy with soft tissue attenuation by CT, in contrast to the low attenuation of necrotic adenopathy characteristic of *M. tuberculosis* infection (24,31).

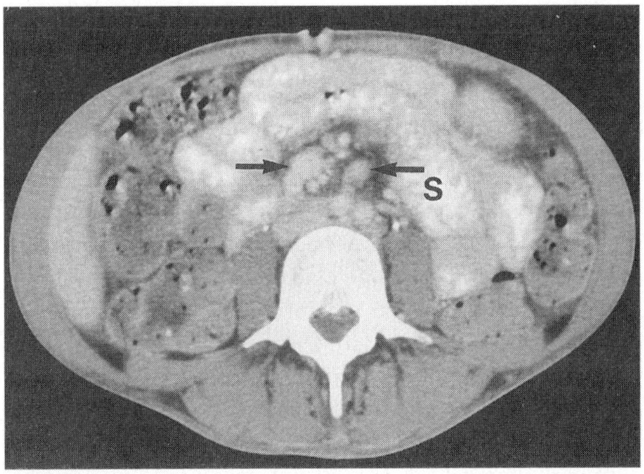

FIGURE 74.9. Infectious enteritis due to cytomegalovirus (CMV), *Mycobacterium avium* complex (MAC), and *Cryptosporidium* in a 37-year-old HIV-1–positive male with abdominal pain. Computed tomography scan through the midabdomen shows enlarged mesenteric lymph nodes (*arrows*) and diffuse thickening of the valvulae conniventes and wall of the small intestine (S). The enlarged mesenteric nodes are consistent with MAC infection, and the small intestinal thickening is likely related to the cryptosporidiosis or CMV infection.

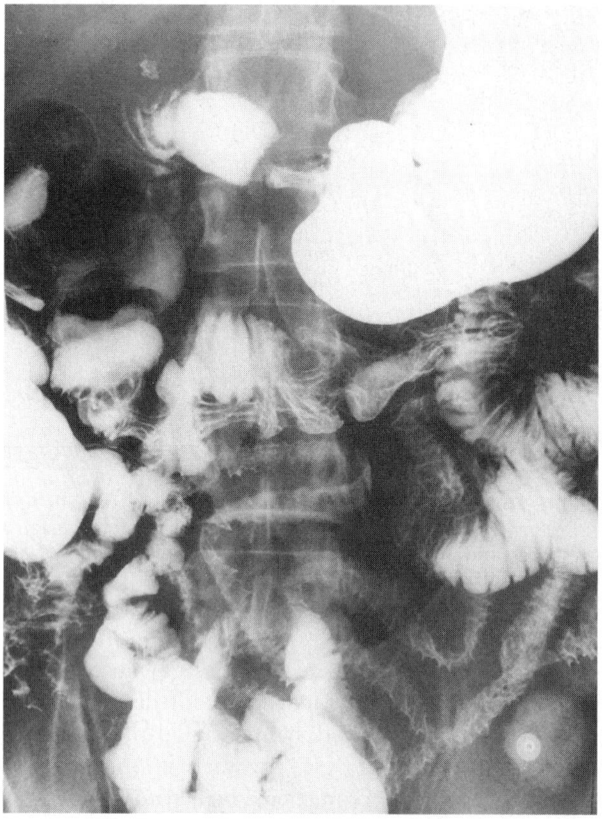

FIGURE 74.10. Cytomegalovirus infection of the jejunum in a 36-year-old HIV-1–infected man. Barium small bowel series demonstrates long segments of jejunum with extensive mucosal and mural thickening.

CMV infection of the small bowel (Fig. 74.10) may cause diffuse ulcers that can perforate or bleed (25). Multifocal disease of the bowel, especially when the duodenum is involved, should suggest underlying AIDS (32).

Bacterial Infections

Bacterial infections of the small intestine are associated with an array of radiologic findings, some of which may suggest a specific pathogen. However, most findings are nonspecific, necessitating microbiologic evaluation.

The radiologic features of ileocecal tuberculosis resemble those of Crohn's disease. However, tuberculosis can be suspected when the cecum is more extensively involved than terminal ileum, the ileocecal junction is straightened (due to retraction of the cecum superiorly), the transition from normal to diseased bowel is abrupt, mesenteric adenopathy is present, and high-density ascites is also present. Tuberculosis should also be in the differential diagnosis when transaxial, oval ulcers are present, rather than the linear, longitudinal ulcers typical of Crohn's disease (25). On contrast-enhanced CT scan, necrotic low attenuation adenopathy is typical (31,33). Tuberculous of the duodenum, which occurs most often in association with gastric tuberculosis, may give rise to nodular mucosal thickening and small-bowel obstruction. The presence of enteroliths should also suggest tuberculosis (23).

Yersinia enterocolitica infection affects the terminal ileum, producing ulcers acutely and bowel wall and nodu-

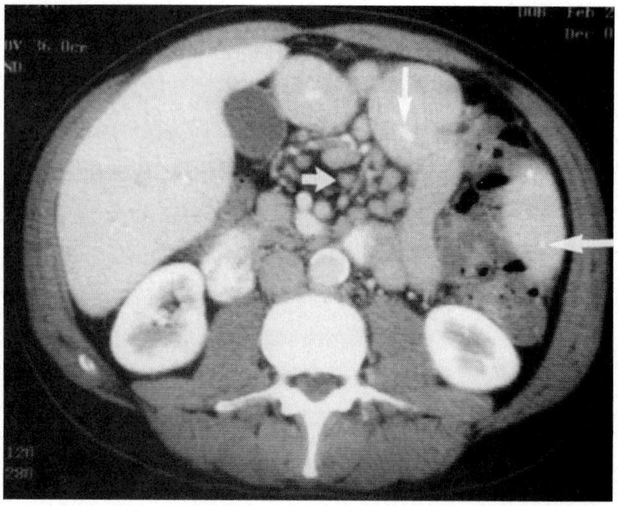

FIGURE 74.11. A 79-year-old male world traveler with acute shigellosis. Oral and intravenous contrasted abdominal computed tomography scan shows marked jejunal mural thickening, producing a pinpoint bowel lumen (*arrows*). Adenopathy (*arrowheads*) is also present.

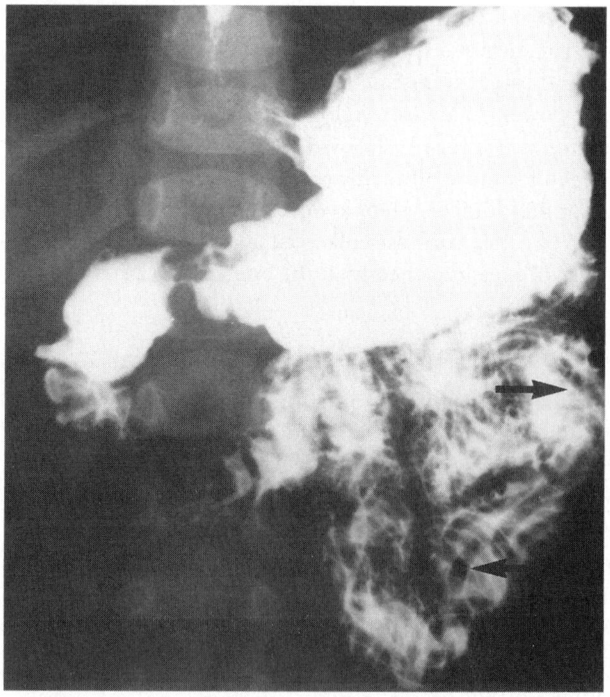

FIGURE 74.12. Ascariasis in a 10-year-old child with recurrent asthmatic attacks. Numerous worms appear as linear filling defects (*arrows*) in the proximal jejunum in this small bowel barium follow-through study. (Courtesy of the Department of Radiology, Children's Hospital of Alabama.)

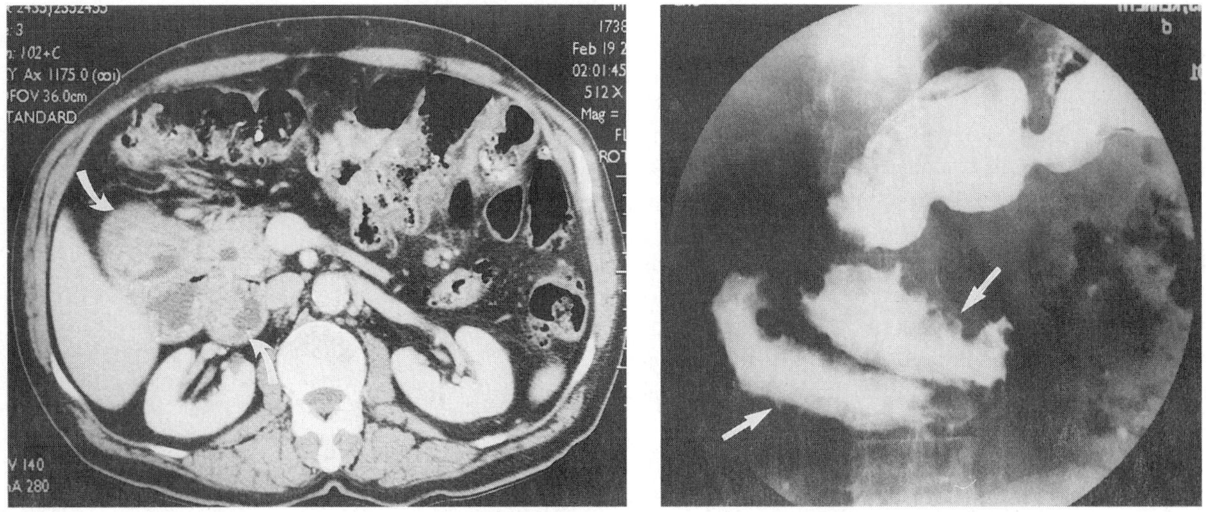

A B

FIGURE 74.13. Strongyloides infection in a 61-year-old immunocompetent man with abdominal pain of 6 months' duration. **A:** Intravenous contrast-enhanced abdominal computed tomography scan with water used as an oral contrast agent shows nonrotation of the bowel and irregular thickening of the duodenum and proximal jejunum around a normal pancreatic head. **B:** Spot radiograph of the duodenum from a barium small bowel series shows irregular mucosal thickening and ulceration of the duodenum and proximal jejunum. Note the absence of normal ligament of Treitz position. (Courtesy of Dr. Sean Fell.)

lar fold thickening later. *Salmonella* infection manifests radiographically as gaseous distention of the small bowel without fluid levels on plain films. Barium studies can show dilatation and fold thickening in the jejunum and fine ulceration of the terminal ileum. Intestinal transit is usually delayed. Infection of the small intestine by *Shigella* species (Fig.74.11) is also characterized by mucosal edema, hypersecretion, and hypermotility with rapid intestinal transit. Radiologic studies are usually not performed during acute enterocolitis, but such studies may demonstrate complications such as perforation of the terminal ileum in typhoid fever, when water-soluble contrast medium should be used.

Parasitic Infections

Parasitic infestations of the small intestine produce interesting and often characteristic radiographic findings. Giardiasis may result in thickening, blunting, and distortion of valvulae conniventes, predominantly in the duodenum and proximal jejunum. Accompanying spasm and irritability, rapid bowel transit, and increased luminal secretions may also be seen (23).

Because of the growing popularity of eating raw fish, the radiologic manifestations of anisakiasis have come to attention. The findings on conventional small-bowel follow-through are similar to those of Crohn's disease. Ultrasonographic features of anisakiasis include marked thickening of bowel loops and mucosal fold edema with decreased peristalsis. Small amounts of ascites adjacent to the affected loops may also be present (34).

During helminthic infections, worms may be identified by barium radiography. In ascariasis, the worms appear as linear filling defects (Fig. 74.12) and may show ingested barium within their own gastrointestinal tracts. The radiologic features of strongyloidiasis are similar to those of giardiasis and include prominent duodenal folds (Fig. 74.13), excess mucous secretion, and such rapid transit time that the proximal small bowel can be difficult to evaluate. More extensive strongyloidiasis affects larger portions of the small intestine with dilatation and slower transit resulting from paralytic ileus (23).

COLON

A wide range of colonic infections have radiologic manifestations. The standard radiographic method for the evaluation of colitis is the double-contrast barium enema. Contraindications to barium enema include suspected perforation, toxic megacolon, and severe or fulminant colitis. In these situations, it is safer to rely on a diagnostic enema performed with water-soluble contrast material (25% solution of sodium diatrizoate) or to treat the patient based on nonradiologic findings and consider barium enema at a later time if still needed. In immunocompromised patients, abdominal CT scan is often the initial radiologic test because of its ability to demonstrate solid visceral disease and adenopathy, as well as bowel abnormalities. Pericolonic inflammatory changes related to diverticulitis and appendicitis are also more effectively evaluated by CT.

Common Protozoal and Bacterial Infections of the Colon

Amebiasis may present as haustral fold thickening due to mucosal edema (Fig. 74.14). In addition, ulcerations in the cecum and ascending colon, along with rigidity and bowel wall thickening, may be present. Disease may progress to the characteristic flask-shaped, undermined ulceration or fulminating colitis (toxic megacolon with deep ulcerations and perforation). Amebomas are readily detected radiographically. These tumor-like lesions occur within or adjacent to the colon wall and are caused by direct transmural extension of amebic infection and accompanying bacterial infection (Fig. 74.15). Amebomas typically produce irregular, long, tapering strictures in the cecum and flexure regions.

Tuberculosis of the colon most commonly involves the ileocecal region, but the infection may also cause multifocal colitis and strictures with partial obstruction (23). A localized tuberculoma can mimic an annular carcinoma of the colon.

Yersinia, Campylobacter, Salmonella, and *Shigella* (Fig. 74.16) cause diffuse colitis in which the mucosa has a granular texture caused by mucosal edema, or the infections can cause fine ulcerations. The same findings may be demonstrated radiographically by enterohemorrhagic *Escherichia coli* infection, although diffuse colonic wall thickening with thumbprinting and spasm have also been noted. On contrast-enhanced abdominal CT, low-density diffuse colon wall thickening produced by marked edema has been reported (35).

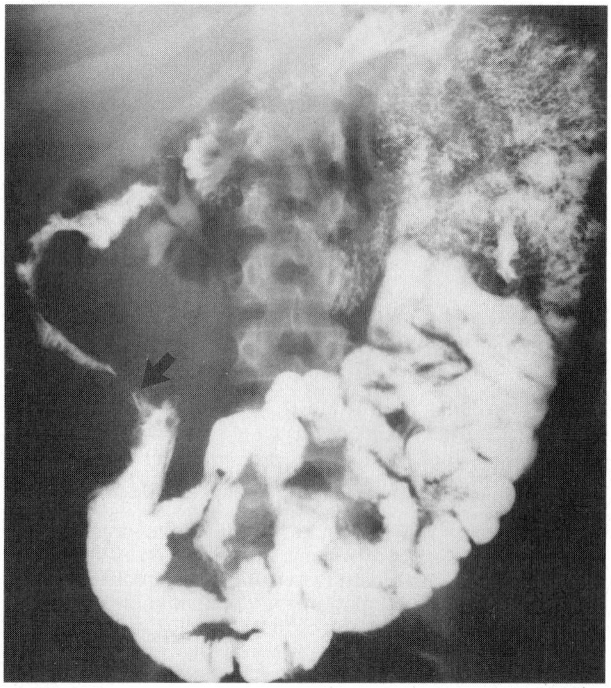

FIGURE 74.15. Marked narrowing of the ascending colon (*arrow*) in a patient with amebic colitis. The displacement of the small intestine from the right midabdomen is due to the large inflammatory mass (ameboma) surrounding the affected right colon.

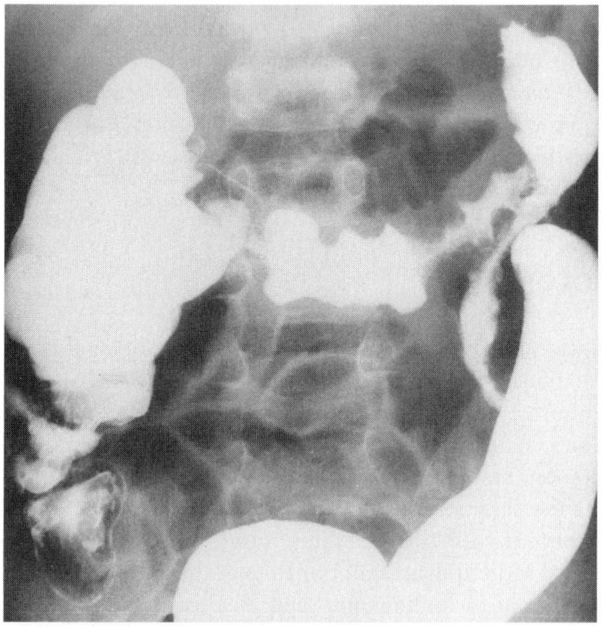

FIGURE 74.14. A 10-year-old boy with crampy abdominal pain and diarrhea of 5 days' duration and stool specimens positive for *Entamoeba histolytica* and *Salmonella* species. Single-column barium enema performed in the acute phase shows marked edema and spasm in the region of the splenic flexure. (Courtesy of the Department of Radiology, The Children's Hospital of Alabama.)

Pseudomembranous Colitis

Therapy with broad-spectrum antibiotics can lead to overgrowth of *Clostridium difficile* and pseudomembranous colitis, manifesting on plain radiographs as diffuse dilation of the small and large intestine with characteristic transverse banding of the colon (Fig. 74.17). The transverse bands represent thickened haustral folds, which appear radiographically as broad bands of soft tissue traversing the air-filled lumen of the colon (36,37). On barium enema, mucosal edema and plaquelike lesions (pseudomembranes) may be seen (4). Occasionally, rectal sparing or focal involvement is noted (38). US can also be used to demonstrate a thickened and echogenic colonic wall with effacement of the lumen (39). CT findings are often the most helpful in identifying this disease (40–42). Characteristic features include circumferential, irregular, diffuse colonic wall thickening with eccentric polypoid folds and the relative absence of pericolonic inflammatory changes (41) (Fig. 74.18). These CT findings are relatively specific, and, in the proper clinical setting, the diagnosis of pseudomembranous colitis can be confidently suggested. The accordion pattern

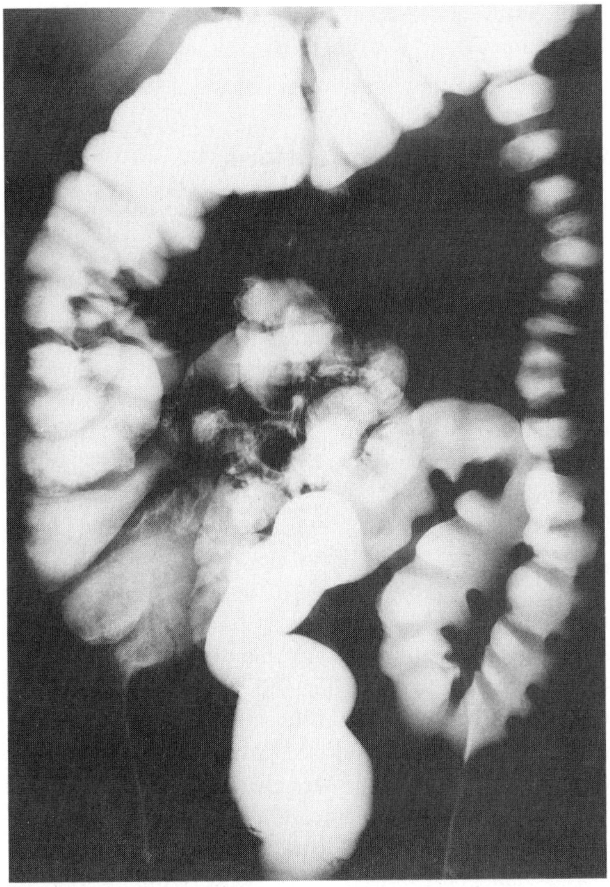

FIGURE 74.16. Acute shigellosis. Barium enema shows the intrahaustral folds in the left colon are diffusely thickened by colonic edema, but no ulceration or other mucosal irregularities are seen.

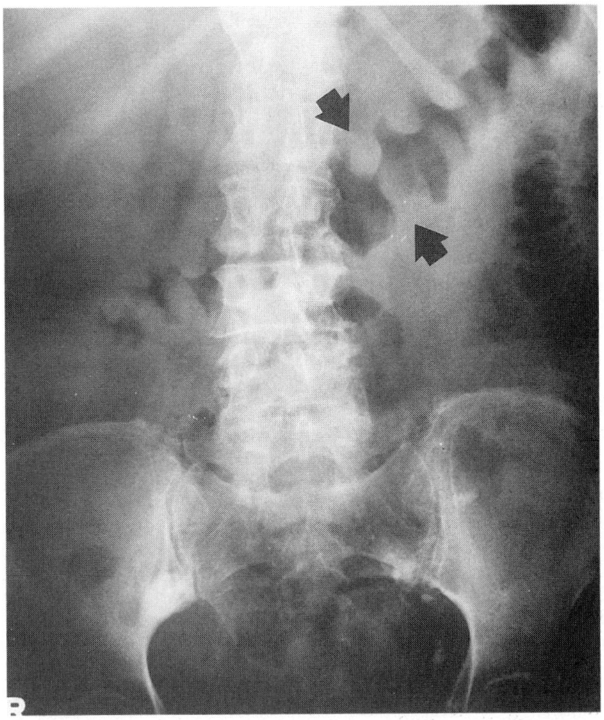

FIGURE 74.17. Abdominal radiograph without contrast in a patient with severe pseudomembranous colitis. Pronounced thickening of the intrahaustral folds (*arrows*) is seen in the transverse colon.

of wall thickening on CT was initially described in patients with pseudomembranous colitis (43), but this pattern has since been shown to be a relatively nonspecific sign of bowel wall edema associated with a variety of colonic diseases, notably ischemia.

Typhlitis

Typhlitis or neutropenic colitis is an inflammatory process affecting the cecum and sometimes the terminal ileum or appendix that was first described in patients with leukopathic conditions (44). The process may be detected on conventional abdominal radiographs as a right lower quadrant soft tissue mass with a dilated, fluid-filled cecum (25). CT may allow differentiation of typhlitis from pseudomembranous colitis. Typhlitis is limited to the cecum and produces mucosal edema and wall thickening in addition to pericolonic inflammatory fluid and thickening of fascial planes (4) (Fig. 74.19). Pneumatosis and subtle perforation may also be readily demonstrated by CT.

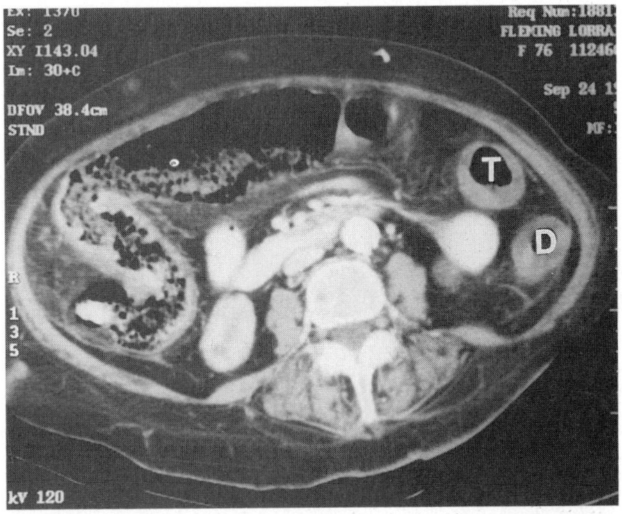

FIGURE 74.18. Pseudomembranous colitis. Oral and intravenous contrast-enhanced abdominal computed tomography scan in a 74-year-old woman recently on antibiotics shows irregular ascending colonic wall thickening (*arrow*), which corresponds with pseudomembranes observed during colonoscopy. Circumferential thickening of the transverse (T) and descending (D) colonic wall is also present in this patient with pancolitis.

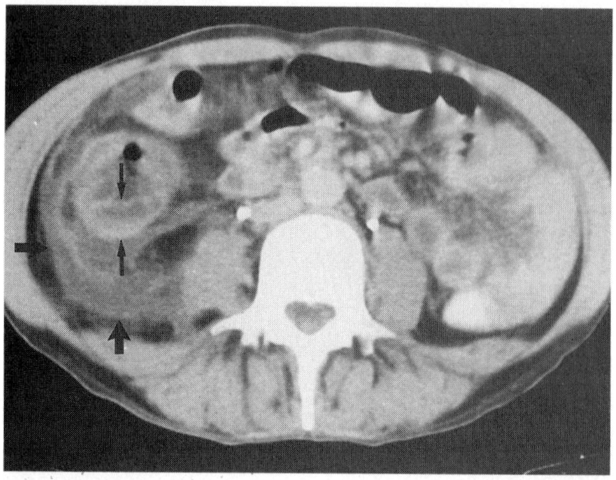

FIGURE 74.19. Typhlitis in a 56-year-old man receiving chemotherapy for acute myelogenous leukemia. The patient presented with right lower quadrant abdominal pain and neutropenia. Computed tomography shows marked thickening of the wall (*small arrows*) of the ascending colon with markedly edematous pericolic fat (*arrows*).

Cytomegalovirus Colitis

CMV colitis occurs most commonly in patients with AIDS and organ transplant recipients. On CT scan, CMV infection is seen as diffuse or, less commonly, segmental thickening of the bowel wall (Fig. 74.20). The colon wall often shows low attenuation due to edema (45). CMV colitis is sometimes difficult to distinguish from pseudomembranous colitis by CT. With barium examination, fine mucosal nodularity in a pattern suggestive of lymphoid nodular hyperplasia may be seen in early CMV infection (4). This may progress to diffuse aphthous ulceration and deep ulcerations in severe disease. When CMV colitis is confined to the cecum (4), it is differentiated from typhlitis by the absence of pericolonic changes.

AIDS-associated Infections

In addition to the previously described colonic infections, *H. capsulatum* and possibly HIV-1 itself can cause radiographic changes in the colon. Colonic histoplasmosis can mimic colon carcinoma, with one or more segmental areas of circumferential wall thickening accompanied by regional adenopathy (46). One report suggests that HIV-1 can cause colitis, resulting in multiple small ulcers acutely and segmental ahaustral narrowing chronically (47). However, the ability of HIV-1 to cause colitis awaits confirmation by other groups.

Proctitis

Infectious proctitis occurs often, but not exclusively, in homosexual men and is usually due to infection with *Neisseria gonococcus* and HSV (Fig. 74.21). In mild gonococcal proctitis, the barium enema is normal. In more severe infection, diffuse ulceration, spasm, loss of distensibility, and widening of the presacral space are seen on barium enema. HSV proctitis, which is uncommon, shows identical features and is limited to the distal 10 cm of the rectum.

The radiographic features of acute lymphogranuloma venereum (LGV) are primarily diffuse ulceration, spasm, and fistula formation; long, featureless, or granular strictures (Fig. 74.22) are noted in severe persistent disease (23,48). LGV, as well as gonococcal and HSV infections, may produce nonspecific CT signs of focal thickening of the rectal wall with abnormal soft tissue infiltration of the perirectal space.

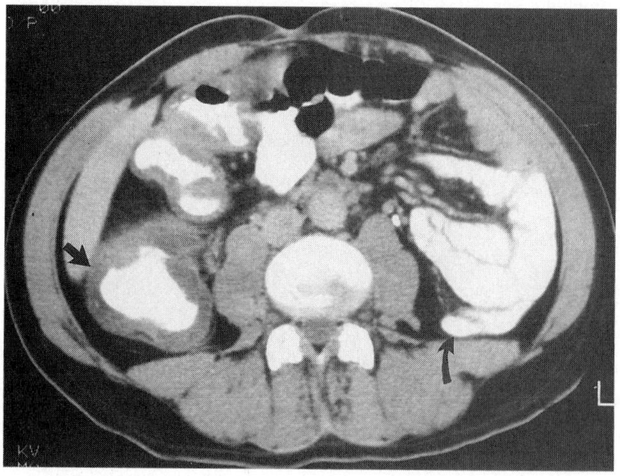

FIGURE 74.20. Severe cytomegalovirus colitis in a 38-year-old man with AIDS and diarrhea. Note thickening of the wall of the ascending colon (*straight arrow*) and a normal descending colon (*curved arrow*) in this computed tomography scan with contrast.

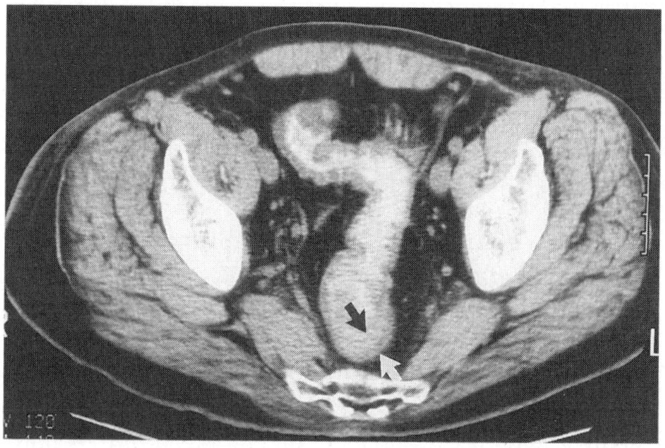

FIGURE 74.21. Proctocolitis due to herpes simplex virus infection in a 40-year-old HIV-1–negative male with diabetic ketoacidosis and candidal sepsis. Computed tomography shows severe thickening (*arrows*) of the rectosigmoid colon where friable mucosa with punctate ulcers and mucosal edema was observed during colonoscopy.

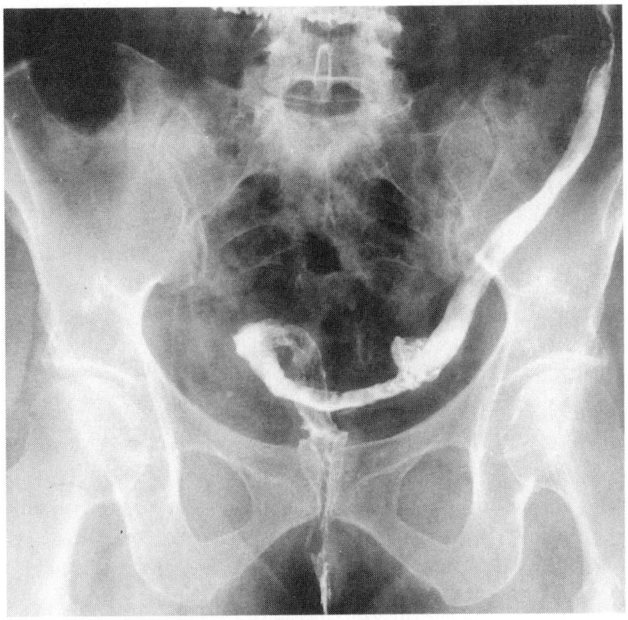

FIGURE 74.22. Lymphogranuloma venereum infection of the rectum and sigmoid colon. The long stricture shown in this barium enema is typical of the late stages of this disease.

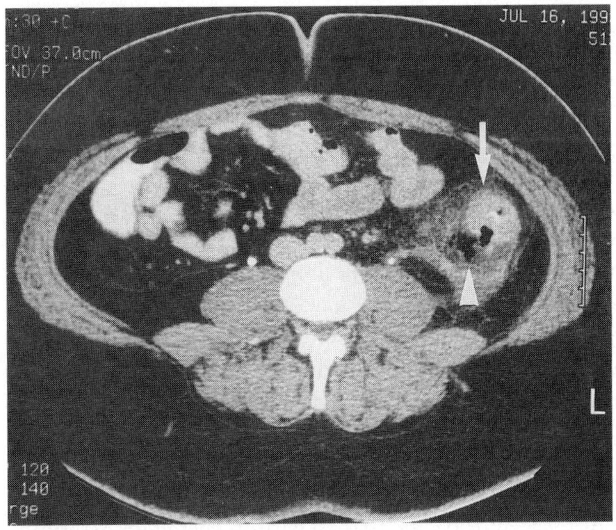

FIGURE 74.23. Diverticulitis of the descending colon in a 37-year-old man who presented with left lower abdominal pain. Computed tomography shows marked thickening of the wall of the descending colon (*arrow*) and extraluminal gas (*arrowhead*) in the inflamed paracolic soft tissues, consistent with a contained perforation.

Rarely, amebic and *Shigella* proctitis occur and may extend to the sigmoid and descending colon, respectively, and show scattered areas of superficial and later deep, collar button ulceration on barium enema examination (23).

Diverticulitis

The radiologic evaluation of suspected diverticulitis should begin with an intravenous contrast-enhanced abdominal CT scan using oral and rectal contrast (3% meglumine diatrizoate solution). Whereas barium enema was the main radiologic test used in the past to document diverticulitis, CT is more effective in demonstrating the extent and complications of diverticular inflammation for both right- and left-sided disease (49–52). When allergy or renal function precludes the use of intravenous contrast material, noncontrast CT is still effective for identifying bowel wall thickening, mesenteric inflammatory change, and extraluminal air in patients with suspected diverticulosis. Sonographic identification of gut wall thickening, diverticula, pericolic and intramural fluid collections, and edema of the pericolic fat have been described (53,54). Although the accuracy of CT and US for diagnosing diverticulitis was recently reported to be equivalent (55), in most centers, CT is the diagnostic test of choice because of its greater sensitivity and specificity. The CT criteria for diverticulitis include the presence of colonic diverticula, localized inflammatory infiltration of the pericolic fat, focal thickening of colon wall, intramural sinus tract, pelvic or abdominal abscess associated with an inflamed segment of colon, and fistula formation (especially sigmoid-vesical fistula) (56).

Radiographic stages of diverticulitis have been established to facilitate optimal treatment planning. Stage 0 is the most common form of diverticulitis, occurring when diverticular inflammation is contained with the serosa. This stage produces only thickening of the colon wall on CT scan and is usually responsive to antibiotic therapy alone. Stage I diverticulitis is defined by the presence of small (up to 3 cm) abscesses or phlegmon confined to the mesentery (Fig. 74.23). This stage is also usually responsive to antibiotic therapy. In stage II diverticulitis, an abscess spreads beyond the mesentery and is frequently walled off by pelvic structures, such as the small intestine or omentum. Such abscesses are often suited for percutaneous CT-guided drainage. Stage III is characterized by the spread of disease to other parts of the peritoneal cavity or retroperitoneum. Percutaneous drainage may allow surgery to be delayed until the patient is able to tolerate an operation (57). Stage IV diverticulitis is indistinguishable on CT from stage III but is accompanied by acute peritonitis and life-threatening sepsis (56).

When the CT findings of diverticulitis are unclear, barium enema examination may be helpful. Patients with perforated colon carcinoma occasionally present with clinical and radiographic findings similar to those of diverticulitis, so it is prudent to perform a follow-up barium examination or colonoscopy 4 to 6 weeks after resolution of symptoms to evaluate the colonic mucosa for tumor.

Appendicitis

In the past, patients with signs and symptoms of acute appendicitis often underwent operation without a preoperative radiologic workup. Presently, patients with typical as well as atypical presentations are commonly evaluated before determination of therapy. CT and, in some patients, US have replaced barium enema as the most useful initial radiologic examination. In children, sonography of the right lower quadrant with graded compression is often the only preoperative imaging study performed (58). Whereas sonography is also useful in thin adults (59–61), operator performance variability and limitations due to body habitus and abdominal guarding have thus far limited the widespread application of this noninvasive method. CT has the added capability of routinely demonstrating the normal appendix and thus excluding the possibility of acute appendicitis; the normal noninflamed appendix cannot be seen by US (62).

Similar to the evaluation of diverticulitis, CT has greater sensitivity and specificity than barium enema for determining the extent and complications of appendicitis. The accuracy of barium enema ranges between 50% and 84% and depends on the demonstration of a nonfilling appendix and an extrinsic mass on the medial cecal wall (63). Previously, the sensitivity and specificity of CT for the diagnosis of appendicitis ranged between 79% and 94% (60,64), but, in recent years, thin-slice (5 mm) helical scanning techniques and aggressive retrograde filling of the colon have increased the sensitivity to 97% to 98% and specificity to 94% to 98% (65,66). Although authors agree on the benefit of thin-slice helical scanning, there is less agreement regarding the use of intravenous-, oral-, or rectal-only contrast.

Uncomplicated appendicitis is characterized on CT by appendiceal wall thickening and periappendiceal edema and inflammation (64,67). The abnormal appendix (Fig. 74.24) is seen in nearly all cases (68). Additional findings on CT include focal indentation or eccentric thickening of the posteromedial cecum; thickening of the distal small bowel, anterior renal fascia, lateroconal fascia, and abdominal wall muscles; and enlargement and blurring of the right psoas muscle. In addition, CT often shows appendicoliths not visible on plain abdominal radiographs (Fig. 74.25). This is an important finding because appendicoliths are present in a higher percentage of patients with complicated rather than uncomplicated appendicitis (69).

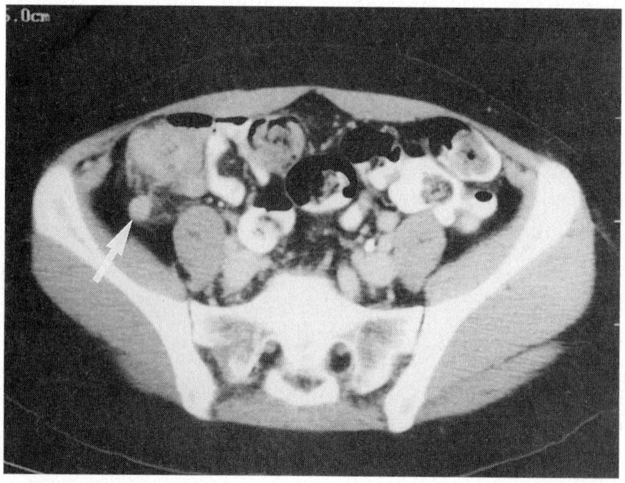

FIGURE 74.24. Acute, early, nonperforated appendicitis. Abdominal computed tomography scan with oral, rectal, and intravenous contrast shows a thickened appendiceal wall (*arrow*) in cross section with mild surrounding mesenteric inflammation.

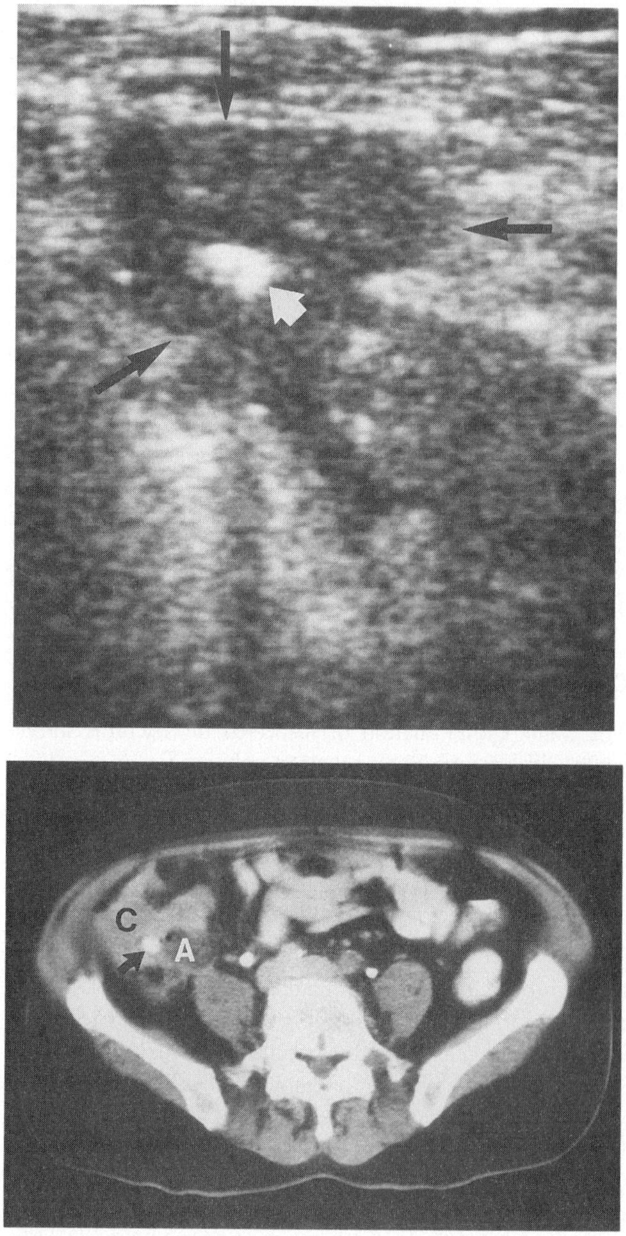

A

B

FIGURE 74.25. A 64-year-old man with acute appendicitis. **A:** Ultrasonogram shows a right lower quadrant fluid collection (*arrows*) containing a calcified appendicolith (*arrowhead*). **B:** Computed tomography scan shows thickened cecal wall (C) and the appendicolith (*arrow*), which was not visible on the barium enema scout radiograph. An adjacent periappendiceal abscess (A) contains fluid and a single bubble of gas.

Periappendiceal phlegmon or abscess can be located in the right lower quadrant, medial to the cecum, in the right anterior pararenal space, posterior to the right colon, or elsewhere in the abdomen, and can be accurately detected by CT. Complications such as hepatic abscess or pylephlebitis are also easily shown (64,70). Although right colonic diverticulitis, perforated right colonic neoplasm, and mucocele of the appendix occasionally mimic appendicitis on CT, it is usually possible to at least identify patients with an inflammatory or neoplastic process severe enough to warrant surgical intervention, even when an accurate preoperative diagnosis is not possible. A potentially important role for CT in patients with atypical appendicitis is the detection of other (nonappendiceal) abdominal pathology giving rise to the patient's symptoms. In recent studies, an alternative diagnosis for abdominal pain was discovered by CT in 54% to 62% of patients with a normal appendix (65,66).

SUMMARY

Contrast-enhanced CT is a key diagnostic imaging test for the evaluation of patients with certain gastrointestinal infections. Excellent delineation of bowel wall thickening, extent and distribution of disease, presence of adenopathy, and the presence of complications, such as abscess and perforation, is possible with this single diagnostic modality. Although some CT findings may be nonspecific, CT findings often guide further workup and diagnostic considerations. For the definition of mucosal detail, carefully performed double-contrast barium techniques provide more specificity. Together with US, these diagnostic imaging tests play important roles in the evaluation of many gastrointestinal tract infections.

REFERENCES

1. Levine MS, Macones AJ, Laufer I. *Candida* esophagitis: accuracy of radiographic diagnosis. *Radiology* 1986;158:597–603.
2. Levine MS. Radiology of esophagitis: a pattern approach. *Radiology*1991;179:1–7.
3. Levine MS, Woldenbrg R, Herlinger H, et al. Opportunistic esophagitis in AIDS: radiographic diagnosis. *Radiology* 1987; 165:815–820.
4. Jones B, Wall SD. Gastrointestinal disease in the immunocompromised host. In: Federle MP, ed. Radiology of the immunocompromised host. *Radiol Clin North Am* 1992;30:555–557.
5. Farman J, Tavitian A, Rosenthan LE, et al. Focal esophageal candidiasis in acquired immunodeficiency syndrome (AIDS). *Gastrointest Radiol* 1986;11:213–217.
6. Levine MS. *Radiology of the esophagus.* Philadelphia: WB Saunders, 1989.
7. Shortsleeve MJ, Levine MS. Herpes esophagitis in otherwise healthy patients: clinical and radiographic findings. *Radiology* 1992;182:859–861.
8. Balthazar EJ, Megibow AJ, Hulnick D, et al. Cytomegalovirus esophagitis in AIDS: radiographic features in 16 patients. *AJR Am J Roentgenol* 1987;149:919–923.
9. Balthazar EJ, Megibow AJ, Hulnick DH. Cytomegalovirus esophagitis and gastritis in AIDS. *AJR Am J Roentgenol* 1985;144: 1201–1204.
10. Levine MS, Loercher G, Katzka DA, et al. Giant, human immunodeficiency virus-related ulcers in the esophagus. *Radiology* 1991;180:323–326.
11. Sor S, Levine MS, Kowalski TE, et al. Giant ulcers of the esophagus in patients with human immunodeficiency virus: clinical, radiographic, and pathologic findings. *Radiology* 1995;194: 447–451.
12. Wilcox CM, Schwartz DA, Clark WS. Esophageal ulceration in human immunodeficiency virus infection. *Ann Intern Med* 1995; 122:143–149.
13. Goodman P, Pinero SS, Rance RM, et al. Mycobacterial esophagitis in AIDS. *Gastrointest Radiol* 1989;14:103–105.
14. De Silva R, Stoopack PM, Raufman J. Esophageal fistulas associated with mycobacterial infection in patients at risk for AIDS. *Radiology* 1990;175:449–453.
15. Sohn J, Levine MS, Furth EE, et al. *Helicobacter pylori* gastritis; radiographic findings. *Radiology* 1995;195:763–767.
16. Pattison CP, Combs MJ, Marshall BJ. *Helicobacter pylori* and peptic ulcer disease: evolution to revolution to resolution. *AJR Am J Roentgenol* 1997;168:1415–1420.
17. NIH Consensus Development Conference. *Helicobacter pylori* in peptic ulcer disease. *JAMA* 1994;272:65–69.
18. Levine MS, Elma N, Furth EE. *Helicobacter pylori* and gastric MALT lymphoma. *AJR Am J Roentgenol* 1996;166:85–86.
19. Yoo CC, Levine MS, Furth EE, et al. Gastric mucosa-associated lymphoid tissue lymphoma: radiographic findings in six patients. *Radiology* 1998;208:239–243.
20. Falcone S, Murphy J, Weinfeld A. Gastric manifestations of AIDS: radiographic findings on upper gastrointestinal examination. *Gastrointest Radiol* 1991;16:95–98.
21. Smart PE, Weinfeld A, Thompson NE, et al. Toxoplasmosis of the stomach: a cause of antral narrowing. *Radiology* 1990;174: 369–370.
22. Farman J, Lerner ME, Ng C, et al. Cytomegalovirus gastritis: protean radiologic features. *Gastrointest Radiol* 1992;17:202–206.
23. Margulis AR, Burhenne HJ, eds. *Alimentary tract radiology,* fourth edition. St. Louis: CV Mosby, 1989.
24. Redvanly RD, Silverstein JE. Intra-abdominal manifestations of AIDS. In: Goodman PC, ed. Imaging of the patient with AIDS. *Radiol Clin North Am* 1997;35:1087–1103.
25. Laufer I, Levine MS. *Double contrast gastrointestinal radiology,* second edition. Philadelphia: WB Saunders, 1992.
26. Goodgame RW. Understanding intestinal spore-forming protozoa: cryptosporidia, microsporidia, isospora and cylcospora. *Ann Intern Med* 1996;124:429–441.
27. Wall SD, Jones B. Gastrointestinal tract in the immunocompromised host: opportunistic infections and other complications. *Radiology* 1992;185:327–335.
28. Vincent ME, Robbins AH. *Mycobacterium avium-intracellulare* complex enteritis: pseudo-Whipple's disease in AIDS. *AJR Am J Roentgenol* 1985;144:921–927.
29. Marshall JB. Tuberculosis of the gastrointestinal tract and peritoneum. *Am J Gastroenterol* 1993;88:989–999.
30. Jeffrey RB Jr, Nyberg DA, Bottles K, et al. Abdominal CT in acquired immunodeficiency syndrome. *AJR Am J Roentgenol* 1986;146:7–13.
31. Radin DR. Intraabdominal *Mycobacterium tuberculosis* vs. *Mycobacterium avium-intracellulare* infections in patients with AIDS: distinction based on CT findings. *AJR Am J Roentgenol* 1991;156:487–491.
32. Wall SD, Ominsky S, Altman DF, et al. Multifocal abnormalities

of the gastrointestinal tract in AIDS. *AJR Am J Roentgenol* 1986; 146:1–5.
33. Hulmick DH, Megibow AJ, Naidich DP, et al. Abdominal tuberculosis: CT evaluation. *Radiology* 1985;157:199–204.
34. Shirahama M, Koga T, Ishibashi H, et al. Intestinal anisakiasis: US in diagnosis. *Radiology* 1992;185:789–793.
35. Fan KT, Whitman GJ, Chew FS. Enterohemorrhagic *Escherichia coli* colitis. *AJR Am J Roentgenol* 1996;166;788.
36. Stanley RJ, Melson GL, Tedesco FJ. The spectrum of radiographic findings in antibiotic-related pseudomembranous colitis. *Radiology* 1974;111:519–524.
37. Stanley RJ, Melson GL, Tedesco FJ. Plain-film findings in severe pseudomembranous colitis. *Radiology* 1976;118:7–11.
38. Rubesin SE, Levine MS, Glick SN. Pseudomembranous colitis with rectosigmoid sparing on barium studies. *Radiology* 1989; 170:811–815.
39. Downey DB, Wilson S. Pseudomembranous colitis: sonographic features. *Radiology* 1991;180:61–64.
40. Fishman EK, Kavuru M, Jones B, et al Pseudomembranous colitis: CT evaluation of 26 cases. *Radiology* 1991;180:57–60.
41. Merine D, Fishman EK, Jones B. Pseudomembranous colitis: CT evaluation. *J Comput Assist Tomogr* 1987;11:1017–1020.
42. Ros PR, Beutow PC, Pantograg-Brown L, et al. Pseudomembranous colitis. *Radiology* 1996;198:1–9.
43. Boland GW, Lee MJ, Cats AM, et al. Antibiotic-induced diarrhea: specificity of abdominal CT for the diagnosis of *Clostridium difficile* disease. *Radiology* 1994;191:103–108.
44. Amronin GD, Solomon RD. Necrotizing enteropathy: complications of treated leukemia or lymphoma patients. *JAMA* 1961; 192:23–27.
45. Balthazar EJ, Megibow AJ, Fazzini E, et al. Cytomegalovirus colitis in AIDS: radiographic findings in 11 patients. *Radiology* 1985;155:585–589.
46. Balthazar EJ, Megibow AJ, Barry M, et al. Histoplasmosis of the colon in patients with AIDS: imaging findings in four cases. *AJR Am J Roentgenol* 1993;161:585–587.
47. Solomon JA, Levine MS, O'Brien CO, et al. HIV colitis: clinical and radiographic findings. *AJR Am J Roentgenol* 1997;168: 681–682.
48. Sider L, Mintzer RA, Mendelson EB, et al. Radiographic findings of infectious proctitis in homosexual men. *AJR Am J Roentgenol* 1982;139:667–671.
49. Cho KC, Morehouse HT, Alterman DD, et al. Sigmoid diverticulitis: diagnostic role of CT-comparison with barium enema studies. *Radiology* 1990;176:111–115.
50. Katx DS, Lane MJ, Ross BA, et al. Diverticulitis of the right colon revisited. *AJR Am J Roentgenol* 1998;171:151–156.
51. Oudenhoven LFIJ, Koumans RK, Puylaert JBCM. Right colonic diverticulitis: US and CT findings-new insights about frequency and natural history. *Radiology* 1998;208:611–618.
52. Molitch HI. Septic thrombophlebitis of the inferior mesenteric vein complicating sigmoid diverticulitis: CT findings. *AJR Am J Roentgenol* 1996;167:1014–1016.
53. Wilson SR, Toi A. The value of sonography in the diagnosis of acute diverticulitis of the colon. *AJR Am J Roentgenol* 1990;154: 1199–1202.
54. Wada M, Kikuchi Y, Doy M. Uncomplicated acute diverticulitis of the cecum and ascending colon: sonographic findings in 18 patients. *AJR Am J Roentgenol* 1990;155:283–287.
55. Pradel JA, Adell JF, Taourel P, et al. Acute colonic diverticulitis: prospective comparative evaluation with US and CT. *Radiology* 1997;205:503–512.
56. Neff CC, van Sonnenberg E. CT of diverticulitis. In: Gore RM, ed. CT of the gastrointestinal tract. *Radiol Clin North Am*. 1989; 27:743–752.
57. Neff CC, van Sonnenberg E, Casola G, et al. Diverticular abscesses: percutaneous drainage. *Radiology* 1987;163:15–18.
58. Patriquin HB, Garcier JM, Lafortune M, et al. Appendicitis in children and young adults: Doppler sonographic-pathologic correlation. *AJR Am J Roentgenol* 1996;166:629–633.
59. Puylaert JBCM. Acute appendicitis: US evaluation using graded compression. *Radiology* 1986;158:355–360.
60. Abu-Yousef MM, Bleicher JJ, Maher JW, et al. High-resolution sonography of acute appendicitis. *AJR Am J Roentgenol* 1987; 149:53–58.
61. Jeffrey RB, Laing FC, Lewis FR. Acute appendicitis: high-resolution real-time US findings. *Radiology* 1987;163:11–14.
62. Balthazar EJ, Birnbaum BA, Yee J, et al. Acute appendicitis: CT and US correlation in 100 patients. *Radiology* 1994;190:31–35.
63. Fedyshin P, Kelvin FM, Rice RP. Nonspecificity of barium enema findings in acute appendicitis. *AJR Am J Roentgenol* 1984;143: 99–102.
64. Balthazar EJ, Megibow AJ, Hulnick D, et al. CT of appendicitis. *AJR Am J Roentgenol* 1986;147:705–710.
65. Rao PM, Rhea JT, Novelline RA, et al. Helical CT combined with contrast material administered only through the colon for imaging of suspected appendicitis. *AJR Am J Roentgenol* 1997; 169:1275–1280.
66. Funaki B, Grosskreutz SR, Funaki CN. Using unenhanced helical CT with enteric contrast material for suspected appendicitis in patients treated at a community hospital. *AJR Am J Roentgenol* 1998;171:997–1001.
67. Fisher JK, Findly T. Diagnosing appendicitis by computed tomography. *Mo Med* 1988;85:15–20.
68. Balthazar EJ, Megibow AJ, Gordon RB, et al. Computed tomography of the abnormal appendix. *J Comput Assist Tomogr* 1988; 12:595–601.
69. Gale ME, Birnbaum S, Gerzof SG. CT of appendicitis and its local complications. *J Comput Assist Tomogr* 1985;9:34–37.
70. Feldberg MAM, Hendriks MJ, van Waes PFGM. Computed tomography in complicated acute appendicitis. *Gastrointest Radiol* 1985;10:289–295.

75

ADVANCES IN THE CLINICAL MICROBIOLOGY OF ENTERIC INFECTIONS

YI-WEI TANG
DAVID H. PERSING

The role of diagnostic microbiology in gastroenterology is to determine whether suspected pathogenic microorganisms are present in test specimens collected from stool, blood, tissue, and other secretions of patients, and, if present, to identify them. The digestive system, in health or disease, is a microbial milieu of unsurpassed variety and complexity. It varies in degree of colonization from the "buggiest" parts of the body, at both ends, to the nearly sterile environment of the small intestine and accessory glands. A community of at least 400 distinct species of bacteria, fungi, and protozoa have been identified in the resident flora of the normal gastrointestinal tract, and many more remain to be discovered by molecular approaches. The detection and differentiation of human pathogens from the large numbers and varieties of environmental flora represents a major challenge to the clinical laboratory.

A microorganism from a test sample collected from the gastrointestinal tract can be detected and identified in any of four possible ways: (a) Cultivation of microorganisms using artificial media or living hosts, (b) direct microscopic examination, (c) measurement of microorganism-specific immune responses, and (d) detection of microorganism-specific macromolecules, especially nucleic acids. The contrast of these techniques is summarized in Table 75.1. Technologic revolutions in microbiology, immunology, and molecular biology have significantly expanded and improved the capabilities of diagnostic microbiology. For example, while cultivation of pathogenic bacteria in stools remains the gold standard for detecting pathogens causing diarrhea, the urea breath test has emerged as a quick and noninvasive test for detecting *Helicobacter pylori* infections and monitoring therapy efficacy (1,2). Polymerase chain reaction (PCR) has dramatically changed the way infectious agents are detected and characterized (3–5).

This chapter emphasizes the advanced techniques developed in the past decade for laboratory diagnosis and monitoring of the gastrointestinal tract infections. The application of these diagnostic techniques are elucidated through citation of specific diseases or syndromes encountered in gastroenterology. For detailed descriptions of diagnostic techniques and procedures, refer to protocols from commercially available systems (6–9).

ADVANCES IN DIAGNOSTIC TOOLS

Until the early 1970s, definitive laboratory diagnoses of infectious diseases were largely accomplished through the use of cumbersome, costly, time-consuming, and often subjective techniques. However, in the 1980s and 1990s, diagnostic technology evolved rapidly. Some of these advanced techniques have been widely used in the diagnosis and monitoring of gastrointestinal tract infections. The physical structure of laboratories, staffing patterns, and workflow have all been influenced profoundly by technical advances (10). These methods have not only decreased the turnaround time for the patient results but have also increased the clinical relevance of the information provided by the laboratory.

Phenotypic Techniques

Detection of Metabolic Products

The causal relationship between *H. pylori* colonization of the gastric mucosa and gastritis has been proven (11). *H. pylori* produces large amounts of extracellular urease, which

Y. W. Tang: Departments of Medicine and Pathology, Vanderbilt University School of Medicine; and Molecular Infectious Disease Laboratory, Vanderbilt University Hospital, Nashville, Tennessee

D. H. Persing: Department of Molecular Biology, Corixa Corporation; and Infectious Disease Research Institute, Seattle, Washington

TABLE 75.1. METHODS USED FOR LABORATORY DIAGNOSIS OF ENTERIC INFECTIONS

Test	Ease of Performance	Turnaround Time	Result Interpretation	Advantages	Disadvantages	Examples (References)
Direct examination	Could be performed in routine clinical lab and in nurse station	1–3 h	Direct if correlated with symptoms	Rapid	Poor sensitivity and specificity; special skills are needed for interpretation	Direct EIA for rotavirus detection (14); urea breath test for *H. pylori* detection and monitoring (1,2)
Culture	Could be performed in sophisticated clinical lab and in research lab	2–14 days	Definite	For phenotypic drug susceptibility testing	Time-consuming; poor sensitivity; limited micro-organisms are culturable	Cultivation and confirmation of diarrhea and food poisoning pathogens (18,20)
Serology	Could be performed in larger and sophisticated clinical lab	4–6 h	Indirect	Automation	Results are generally retrospective; immunosupressed host may be unable to mount a response	Detection and monitoring of hepatitis infections (15,16)
Molecular diagnostics	Could be performed in only a few very sophisticated research and clinical lab	1–2 days	Direct without knowing microbial viability	High sensitivity and specificity	Facility requirement; false-positive results due to carryover contamination and false-negative results due to inhibitors in specimen	VRE typing (88); identification of Whipple disease (65–67); hepatitis virus quantitation (37,49,50)

EIA, enzyme immunoassay; VRE, vancomycin-resistant enterococci.

hydrolyses urea to form ammonia and soluble carbon dioxide. This is detectable within hours in human breath specimens. The noninvasive urea breath test, originally described by Graham and colleagues (1), has enabled the direct detection of *H. pylori* infections without endoscopy. However, the urea breath test was not widely accepted in the routine clinical microbiology laboratory until a commercial, nonradioactive ^{13}C-based kit (Meretek Diagnostics) was approved by the U. S. Food and Drug Administration (FDA) in 1996. The urea breath test has excellent sensitivity and specificity for the initial diagnosis of active infection in untreated patients and for treatment follow-up after therapy. It has been recommended as the method of choice to establish or exclude *H. pylori* infection without endoscopy (2).

Rapid Antigen Detection

Using a specific antibody in an enzyme immunoassay (EIA) format to directly detect microbial antigens is widely used in laboratory identification of diarrhea-causing pathogens in stools, including toxin-producing *Clostridium difficile* (12). EIAs are also available for the detection of *Giardia lamblia* and *Cryptosporidium parvum* in feces (13). The direct detection of rotavirus antigen in stools is critical and practical because this agent yields relatively large numbers in the intestinal tract and is difficult to recover in culture. A solid-phase EIA kit is commercially available from Abbott Laboratories for rotavirus antigen detection (14). Incorporated by highly sensitive and specific monoclonal antibodies, some of these direct pathogen antigen detection kits are quite accurate. The obvious advantages of these antigen tests are ease of use and significantly improved test turnaround time, which is critical in clinical intervention.

Advanced Serologic Techniques

Serologic tests measure the host's humoral immune response to a microorganism infection. Serologic tests are important for diagnosing certain microorganism infections whenever recovery of those organisms in culture is difficult or impossible. The best examples applied in the gastrointestinal tract infections are EIA and recombinant immunoblot assays for diagnosis of hepatitis C virus (HCV), the leading infectious cause of hepatitis in the United States (15,16). The EIA provides a sensitive and quick method for screening all serum specimens collected from patients with suspected hepatitis, and, if positive, the specificity of a serologic test is determined largely by the antigen used to capture the antibody in direct test formats (Western blot). Recently, several rapid tests, such as the strip immunoblot assay for *H. pylori* antibody detection (17), have been developed for the detection of specific antibodies in clinical specimens. Like rapid antigen tests, these assays are simple to perform, require less technologist training, and can provide a result within 30 minutes, allowing on-the-spot treatment of patients.

Enhancement of Pathogen Isolation

Isolation and cultivation of a microbial pathogen is still the predominant technique for laboratory diagnosis of diarrheogenic pathogenic microorganisms in stool specimens. Although selective culture media have been used to maximally inhibit indigenous flora, the isolation procedure is, in general, poorly sensitive and specific. In addition, the number of pathogenic microorganisms present in food or stools may be low. Several processes, such as immunomagnetic separation and immunoaffinity concentration, have been used for the enhancement of microbial pathogen isolation and detection (18,19). Isolation and recovery of verocytotoxin-producing *Escherichia coli* O157 has be significantly enhanced by applying magnetic beads coated with an antibody against *E. coli* O157 to the crude clinical specimen before inoculating it onto a medium plate. The O157-specific beads, available from Dynal, Inc., enhance the detection of *E. coli* O157 from patients with a hemolytic uremic syndrome, patients presenting an extended period of time after the onset of illness, asymptomatic carriers, or specimens that have been stored or transported improperly (18,20).

Automated Instrument-Assisted Blood Culture System

One complication of gastrointestinal infections is sepsis, resulting from microbial pathogens growing in the blood. Currently, the isolation and identification of a bacterial microorganism in blood has been significantly improved by introducing an automated instrument-assisted blood culture system, which has significantly improved the sensitivity and specificity for detecting all pathogens by virtue of automation, eliminating the hands-on time for detection of positive cultures. Automatic blood culture and identification systems, including Bactec 9240 (Becton Dickinson), BacT/Alert (Organon Teknika), Vital (bioMérieux Vitek), and ESP (Difco), have been approved by the FDA (21).

Molecular Diagnosis and Monitoring

Polymerase Chain Reaction

Probably the greatest advance in the field of diagnostic microbiology has been in the area of nucleic acid detection (Table 75.2). As one technologic milestone in biotechnol-

TABLE 75.2. NUCLEIC ACID AMPLIFICATION METHODS

Amplification Method	Amplification Category	Manufacturer/ License	Enzymes Used	Temperature Requirement	Nucleic Acid Target	Main Reference(s)
Polymerase chain reaction (PCR)	Target	Roche Molecular System, Inc., Branchburg, NJ	*Taq* DNA polymerase	Thermal cycler	DNA (RNA)	(22,23)
Transcription mediated amplification (TMA)	Target	Gen-Probe, Inc., San Diego, CA	Reverse transcriptase, (RNase H), RNA polymerase,	Isothermal	RNA or DNA	(30)
Nucleic acid sequence–based amplification (NASBA)	Target	bioMérieux Corp. (Organon-Teknika, Corp.), Durham, NC	Reverse transcriptase, RNA polymerase, RNase H	Isothermal	RNA or DNA	(28,29)
Strand displacement amplification (SDA)	Target	Becton-Dickinson Microbiology Systems, Sparks, MD	Restrictive endonucleonase, DNA polymerase	Isothermal	DNA	(31)
Qβ replicase (QβR)	Probe	Gene-Trak Systems, Framingham, MA	Qβ replicase	Isothermal	DNA or RNA	(108)
Cycling probe technology (CPT)	Probe	ID Biomedical, Vancouver, Canada	RNase H	Isothermal	DNA (RNA)	(33)
Ligase chain reaction (LCR)	Probe	Abbott Laboratories, Abbott Park, IL	DNA ligase	Thermal cycler	DNA	(32)
Hybrid capture system	Signal	DiGene Diagnostics, Inc., Silver Spring, MD	None	Isothermal	DNA	(34)
Branched DNA (bDNA)	Signal	Bayer Corp., Emeryville, CA	None	Isothermal	DNA or RNA	(35,36)

ogy, PCR has simplified and accelerated the *in vitro* process of nucleic acid amplification and significantly broadened the microbiologist's diagnostic arsenal (3,5,22,23). PCR is based on the ability of DNA polymerase to copy a strand of DNA. The enzyme initiates elongation at the 3′ end of a short (primer) sequence bound to a longer (target) strand of DNA. When two primers bind to complementary strands of target DNA, the sequence between the two primer binding sites is amplified exponentially with each cycle of PCR (5,8,10). Each cycle consists of three steps: a DNA denaturation step, a primer annealing step, and an extension step. At the end of each cycle, which consists of the three steps, the PCR products are theoretically doubled. PCR techniques are widely used because of their simplicity and flexibility.

Since Roche Diagnostics Systems, Inc., purchased the patent rights in 1992 to develop PCR-based kits for the diagnosis of genetic and infectious diseases, semiautomated and automated systems for detection and quantitation of several organisms have been manufactured by Roche. These organisms include HCV and hepatitis B virus (HBV) for the diagnosis of viral hepatitis. In addition, numerous user-developed PCR-based DNA amplification techniques have been developed and applied to the detection of microbial pathogens (24), the identification of clinical isolates (25), and strain subtyping (26,27) for gastroenterologists. PCR-derived techniques, such as reverse transcriptase (RT)-PCR, nested PCR, multiplex PCR, arbitrary primed PCR, and broad-range PCR, have collectively expanded the flexibility and power of these methods in laboratories around the world.

Other Nucleic Acid Amplification Techniques

Given the patent restrictions on PCR and the expanding interest in nucleic acid–based diagnosis, alternative amplification methods have been sought. Another target amplification system, transcription-mediated amplification (TMA) or nucleic acid sequence-based amplification (NASBA), begins with the synthesis of a DNA molecule complementary to the target nucleic acid (usually RNA). This technique involves several enzymes and a complex series of reactions that all take place simultaneously at the same temperature and in the same buffer (28–30). The advantages include very rapid kinetics and the lack of requirement for a thermocycler. Isothermal conditions in a single tube with a rapidly degradable product (RNA) help minimize (but may not eliminate) contamination risks. Amplification of RNA not only makes it possible to detect RNA viruses but also increases the sensitivity of detecting bacterial and fungal pathogens by targeting high copy number RNA templates. Other amplification systems included strand displacement amplification (31), ligase chain reaction (32), cycling probe technology (33), hybrid capture system (34), and branched DNA (bDNA) technology (35,36) (Table 75.2). The bDNA technology, increasing the signal generated by a fixed amount of probe hybridized to a fixed amount of specific target, may be extremely useful for histopathology diagnosis. By targeting a certain pathogen in tissues by a bDNA probe, it will not only detect the pathogen but also visualize the location of the pathogen.

Microorganism Quantitation

Recently, there has been a growing demand for the quantitation of nucleic acid targets. Microbial load data are used to monitor therapeutic responses and provide prognostic information for patients infected with HCV (37) and HBV (35) in the field of gastrointestinal infections. Because the amplification technique yields products in an exponential manner until a plateau is reached, any factors interfering with the exponential nature of the amplification process would thereby affect the result of the quantitative assay. To overcome this problem, a competitive RT-PCR has been

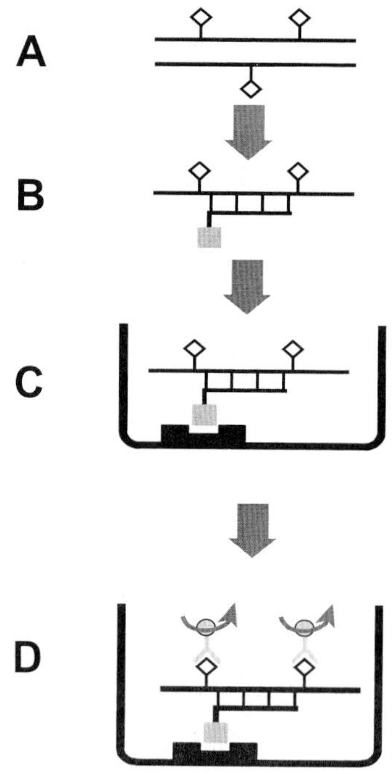

FIGURE 75.1. Detection of digoxigenin-labeled polymerase chain reaction (PCR) product with the Roche PCR ELISA (digoxigenin detection) kit. **A:** During PCR amplification, *Taq* DNA polymerase incorporates digoxigenin-11-dUTP into the target DNA. **B:** A biotin-labeled oligonucleotide probe captures the digoxigenin-labeled PCR product. **C:** The probe-PCR product hybrid is immobilized on a streptavidin-coated microtiter plate. **D:** The immobilized probe-PCR product hybrid is detected with peroxidase-conjugated antidigoxigenin antibody and colorimetric substrate. (Adapted from Tang Y W, Mitchell PS, Espy MJ, et al. Molecular diagnosis of herpes simplex virus infections in the central nervous system. *J Clin Microbiol* 1999;37:2127–2136, with permission.

developed based on coamplification of an internal competitor with the target sequence (38). This approach forms the basis of the Amplicor Monitor kits manufactured by Roche, which are now widely used in HIV-1 and HCV quantitation. Other quantitation techniques are based on either NASBA or bDNA techniques, which have been routinely used for quantitation and therapeutic response monitoring of HCV and HBV.

Amplification Product Identification

There have been significant technique advances in "visualizing" products. The classic means of detection and characterization of the PCR product is agarose gel electrophoresis with or without Southern blotting and DNA probe hybridization. Several user-friendly, rapid techniques have been adopted to enhance the test sensitivity and specificity

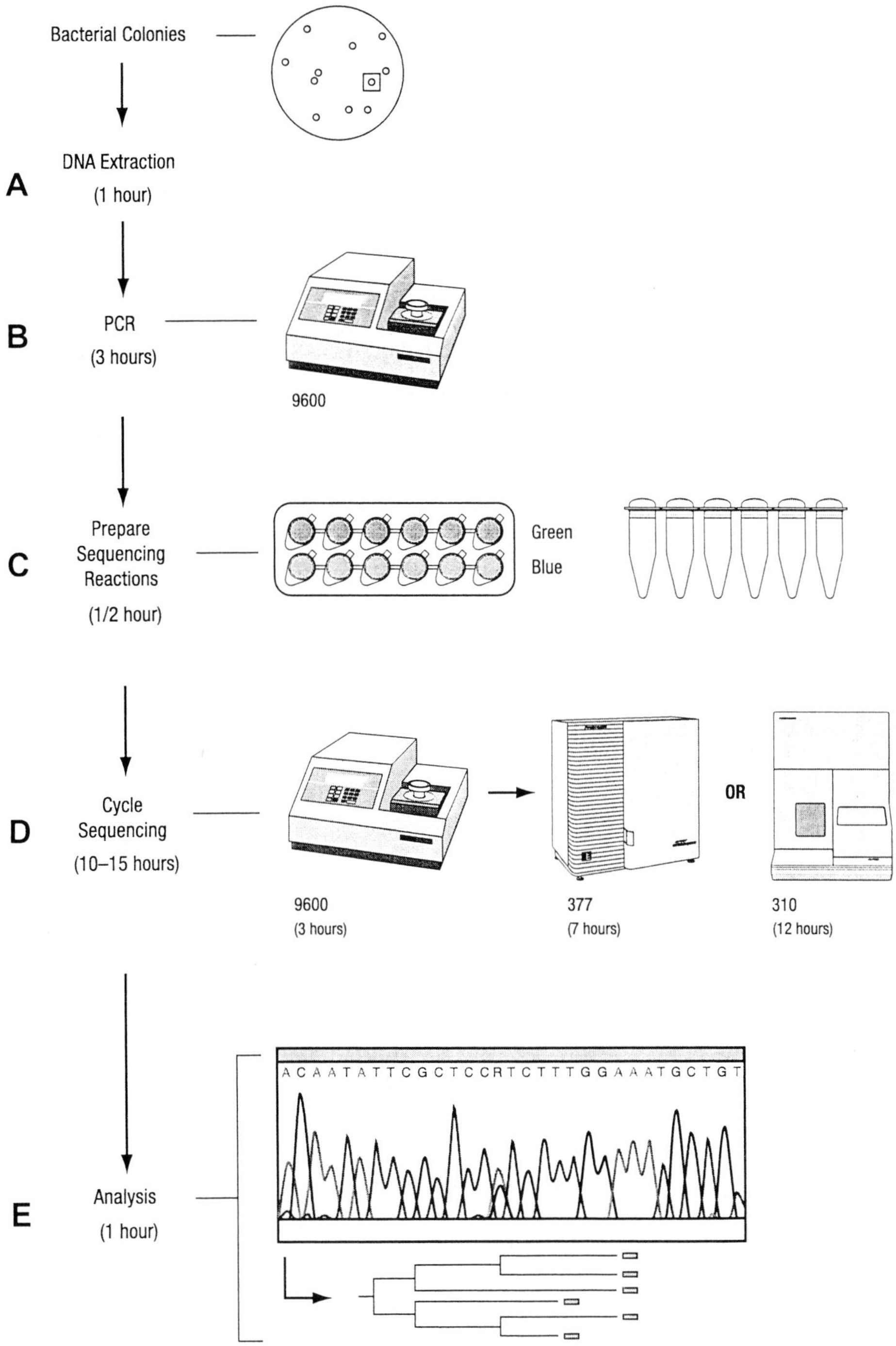

FIGURE 75.2. Flowchart of microorganism identification based on 16S rRNA gene sequence analysis. The total identification time was 15.5 to 18.5 hours, comprising bacterial DNA extraction **(A)**, PCR **(B)**, sequencing reaction preparation **(C)**, cycle sequencing **(D)**, and analysis **(E)**. The time for each step is in parentheses. (Adapted from Tang YW, Ellis NM, Hopkins MK, et al. Comparison of phenotypic and genotypic techniques for identification of unusual pathogenic aerobic gram-negative bacilli. *J Clin Microbiol* 1998;36:3674–3679, with permission.)

as well as test turnaround time. One method gaining popularity is colorimetric microtiter plate detection, which has been used for detecting *H. pylori* DNA in gastric biopsy specimens (24). In a microtiter plate, hybridization and detection of PCR products can be performed using an enzyme-linked immunosorbent assay procedure with color formation read on a spectrophotometer (39,40). One such system, illustrated in Figure 75.1, in combination with rapid extraction and thermal cycling profiles, allows same-day test results and is adapted to automation (41).

Genotypic Identification of Microorganisms

Microbial identification remains a mainstay of diagnostic microbiology, and genotypic identification is emerging as an alternative or a complement to established phenotypic methods. Broad-range PCR primers are designed to recognize conserved sequences in the phylogenetically informative gene of a variety of bacteria, and highly variable regions between the primer binding sites are amplified by PCR. The amplified segment is sequenced and compared with known databases to identify a close relative (42). The most successful example is the small-subunit (16S) rRNA gene sequence-based microbial identification system, which includes the extraction of nucleic acids, PCR-mediated gene amplification, sequence determination, and computer-aided analysis (Fig. 75.2). At present, the time and effort associated with data analysis and its cost are major limitations. The capital investment is high, particularly for automated analysis. With improved automation and decreased cost, as well as the establishment of a complete 16S rRNA gene sequence database, such systems may become established in many diagnostic microbiology laboratories (43).

Simultaneous Amplification and Detection

Another technical advance in molecular diagnosis is the innovation of rapid thermocycling with a real-time detection (real-time PCR) system. The conventional DNA detection system includes a PCR amplification followed by a separate identification of PCR products. With the introduction of a fluorescence resonance energy transfer (44), the thermocycling, detection, and probe confirmation of PCR products can be accomplished simultaneously and rapidly in the real-time PCR system. Such real-time PCR systems are commercially available from Applied Biosystems (TaqMan) and Roche (LightCycler), respectively. The latter, which was originally developed by Idaho Technology, Inc., (Idaho Falls, Idaho), has incorporated air-driven, disposable thin-walled glass capillaries to facilitate heat exchange in the reaction mixture, which makes the rapid thermocycling steps feasible (45). Unlike PCR performed using conventional thermocyclers, the real-time PCR system is "closed" and therefore avoids the important concerns of carryover contamination with the previous product. In addition, the detection of nucleic acid products can be monitored in real time after each cycle of amplification. As a result of shorter thermocycling and simultaneous product detection, the turnaround time for results has been significantly shortened. This technique has been successfully used for identifying new disease targets, detecting single nucleotide polymorphisms, and quantifying gene expression. In the field of gastrointestinal infection diagnosis, it has been described for determining clarithromycin sensitivity in *H. pylori* (46), detecting and following up *Toxoplasma* reactivation (47), and quantifying HCV and HBV viral loads (48–50). It is predicted that the real-time PCR system will maintain test sensitivity and specificity and decrease result turnaround time and cost, which translates into improved patient care.

APPLICATIONS OF CLINICAL MICROBIOLOGY IN DIAGNOSIS AND MONITORING OF ENTERIC INFECTIONS

Detecting Unculturable, Slow-Grown Microorganisms

The rapid, *in vitro* enzymatic amplification characteristic of PCR indicates its primary application in the field of clinical microbiology for detection of unculturable or slow-growing microorganisms. Microbial DNA/RNA extracted from a clinical specimen may be analyzed for the presence of various organism-specific nucleic acid sequences regardless of the physiologic requirements or viability of the organism (51,52). For example, the inability to culture and analyze the principal etiologic agent of non-A, non-B hepatitis limits medical advances in this area. Using various molecular methods, investigators have been able to isolate HCV nucleic acid (53). Analysis and cloning of the HCV genome has provided the viral antigens necessary for the development of specific serologic tests (16,54). Similar molecular techniques have been described for detection of other microbial agents such as hepatitis G virus (55) and TT virus (56).

Another good example is the identification of pathogens causing gastroenteritis. Several microorganisms can cause debilitating gastroenteritis in immunocompromised hosts. Some of these pathogens are either unculturable or slow growing in routine culture systems. Immunomagnetic separation and immunoaffinity concentration have been successfully applied for enhancement of microbial pathogen isolation and detection (18,19). Development of a rapid PCR-based assay for *Yersinia* species detection and differentiation has been important in preventing food-borne transmission of the bacteria (57). Several PCR-based assays have been described for the detection and strain typing of various diarrheogenic pathogens, including *Campylobacter* (25), *Salmonella* (27), *Shigella* (58), *Yersinia*

(59), *E. coli* O157:H7 (60), *Cryptosporidium* (61), *Microsporidium* (62), and *Cyclospora* (63). PCR-based techniques have made clinical diagnosis of these infections possible.

Identifying Etiologic Agents

Nucleotide sequence analysis of the small-subunit (16S) bacterial rRNA gene has greatly expanded our understanding of phylogenetic relationships among members of the bacterial kingdom (52,64). This approach also allows characterization of previously unrecognized species. *Tropheryma whippelii,* the causative agent of Whipple's disease (65–67), is an unculturable microbe that was initially identified by PCR with broad-range primers and sequence analysis of 16S rRNA genes. Because of the inability of this organism to grow on conventional media and the lack of a serologic test, the diagnosis of Whipple's disease is usually based on clinical and biopsy findings in which small-bowel biopsies reveal characteristic foamy histiocytes, which fill the lamina propria. The definitive diagnosis is made with the identification of non–acid-fast, periodic-acid shift–positive, diastase-resistant bacillary forms within the histiocytes. Extraintestinal Whipple's disease, principally arthritis and central nervous system involvement, may be missed entirely unless there is a high index of suspicion. Advances in the molecular detection of *T. whippelii* by amplifying and sequencing the universal bacterial 16S rRNA gene have resolved this dilemma (65–67).

Another intriguing application is the study of the relationship between *Mycobacterium paratuberculosis* infection and chronic idiopathic inflammatory bowel disease (IBD), which encompasses ulcerative colitis and Crohn's disease. An association of IBD with mycobacteria has been postulated since the original description of terminal ileitis. This idea has been resurrected by the recovery of an unclassified acid-fast organism from IBD tissues (68). Detection and isolation of mycobacteria in tissues by immunochemistry and culture have met with limited success and the use of PCR has increased the sensitivity to detect *M. paratuberculosis*-specific DNA sequences in tissues (69). In one study performed by Sanderson and colleagues (70), the *M. paratuberculosis*-specific gene was detected in 65% of involved Crohn's disease tissues compared with 4% in patients with ulcerative colitis and 12% in control subjects. These mycobacterial DNAs can be amplified from granulomatous tissue. Although not yet conclusive, the possible association with *M. paratuberculosis* has led to new ideas in treatment; the experimental use of antileprosy treatment has been reported to yield good results in some patients (71).

Subtyping Microorganisms

Subtyping using amplification-based techniques has important implications for infectious disease prognosis and therapy. It has been described that pathogenic diversity exists between *cagA*-positive and *cagA*-negative *H. pylori.* Infection with a *cagA*-positive strain increases the risk for development of gastric ulcer and gastric cancer (11,72). Two different species of *Entamoeba* have been demonstrated—one pathogenic, *E. histolytica,* and one nonpathogenic, *E. dispar*—and differences in the genomic sequence have been identified between these two species (73). PCR-based assays were subsequently developed that target the small subunit rRNA gene to detect and differentiate between *E. histolytica* and *E. dispar* (74,75). The entire procedure can be performed at room temperature within 24 hours, which is significantly faster than previous methods.

Subtyping of viral infections may also have prognostic value. In the field of gastrointestinal infections, different HCV genotypes have distinct profiles of pathogenicity, infectivity, and response to antiviral therapy (76). Specific primer sets for the detection of the 5′-untranslated or NS5 regions are designed to allow differentiation of genotypes (77). Using PCR followed by automated sequencing, several studies have revealed that the most common genotypes of HCV in the United States and western Europe are 1a and 1b, whereas other genotypes, including 2a, 2b, 3, 4, 5, and 6, have their own distinct global distributions and prognostic significances (78–80). In the United States, infection with type 1b is associated with a longer duration of infection, which perhaps accounts for the finding in some studies of an overrepresentation of this subtype in liver cancer cases (80).

Quantifying Microorganisms

In recent years, there has been growing demand for the quantitation of nucleic acid targets, which has been used to monitor therapeutic response and provide prognostic information for HCV (37,48,50,81) and HBV (35,49) in the field of gastroenterology. The task of quantitative amplification remains problematic (82) because the amplification techniques yield products in an exponential manner until a plateau is reached; any factor interfering with the exponential nature of the amplification process would thereby affect the result of the quantitative assay. To overcome this problem, a competitive RT-PCR has been developed based on coamplification of an internal competitor with the target sequence (38). Quantitation of viral load currently is based primarily on (a) target amplification, which includes both PCR- and NASBA-based techniques and (b) bDNA-based signal amplification. Kit-based technologies make it possible for many laboratories to carry out quantitative analysis.

As discussed earlier, real-time PCR-based systems represent a significant advance and are being adapted to various applications. The unique, characteristic, simultaneous, cycle-by-cycle detection of PCR products has made possible a rapid, high-throughput quantitation of nucleic acid sequences (83,84). The TaqMan system has been successfully applied to HBV DNA quantitation (49). Takeuchi and co-workers (50) have reported using the same system for the quantification of the HCV genome. This real-time PCR system can detect as few as 10 copies of the genome, and the quantitation range is between 10 and 10^8 copies/mL (50). The establishment of a real-time detection system enables a more accurate diagnosis of infection and the monitoring of viral load in interferon-treated HCV patients via quantitation of the viral genome.

Determining Antimicrobial Drug Resistance

Antimicrobial susceptibility testing is one of the most important tasks in the clinical microbiology laboratory, which provides an *in vitro* estimate of the probability that an infection will respond to therapy *in vivo*. Molecular techniques are starting to play a role in the rapid detection of resistance. In some cases, such techniques offer the opportunity to reduce the time required for the institution of definitive therapy, thus reducing the use of inappropriate antibiotics (85). Rapid detection may also allow early recognition of carriers infected by resistant organisms and the appropriate implementation of isolation, epidemiologic investigation, and integrated infection control practices.

Detecting antimicrobial drug resistance by genotypic methods is extremely important in the field of gastroenterology for monitoring therapy. The emergence of clarithromycin-resistant *H. pylori* has been an obstacle to efficiently curing *H. pylori* infections (46). Extended spectrum β-lactamase (ESBL) has emerged in several Enterobacteriaceae, mainly *Klebsiella pneumoniae* and *E. coli* (86). Most recently, different genotypes of HCV infections have been demonstrated to be associated with differing IFN-α therapeutic responses (78,79). The phenotypic techniques for determining these resistances or varied responses are either unavailable or limited to research laboratories. PCR-based genotypic methods for accessing antimicrobial resistance have been developed and are being used in the field of diagnostic microbiology (Table 75.3). Clearly, the advent of these technologies makes it possible to imagine numerous diagnostic applications in the future.

Enhancing Infection Control

The investigation and control of nosocomial infections is complex. The efforts of both the microbiologist and the hospital epidemiologist are facilitated by the availability of new molecular typing techniques. Molecular diagnostic

TABLE 75.3. EXAMPLES OF GENOTYPIC METHODS FOR ASSESSING ANTIMICROBIAL RESISTANCE IN GASTROINTESTINAL TRACT

Resistance	Resistance Basis	Genotypic Methods (Reference)	Clinical Application	Remarks
Vancomycin-resistant enterococci	Novel genes, including *vanA, vanB, vanC,* and *vanD*	PCR-RFLP (88)	Detection and typing	Current phenotypic methods may not identify low-level resistance due to *vanC* genes
Quinolone-resistant Salmonella	Mutations in the gyrase gene (*gyrA*)	PCR-DNA sequencing (109)	Detection and therapy monitoring	This resistance happens to other bacteria as well, such as *Acinetobacter baumannii* and *Escherichia coli*
Clarithromycin-resistant *Helicobacter pylori*	Point mutation in the 23S rRNA gene	PCR-FRET (46)	Detection and therapy monitoring	Current phenotypic methods are not routinely available
Extended spectrum β-lactamase	Mutations in TEM, SHV, and other β-lactamase genes	PCR-RFLP (86)	Detection and therapy monitoring	DNA sequencing is the gold standard for analyzing novel ESBL gene
Macrolides-resistant *Mycobacterium avium* complex	Mutations in the 23S rRNA gene	PCR-NIRCA (110)	Detection and therapy monitoring	Current phenotypic methods may take weeks due to the slow growth of the organism
Ganciclovir-resistant cytomegalovirus	Mutations in the UL97 and UL54 genes	PCR-DNA sequencing (111)	Therapy monitoring	Other mechanisms causing ganciclovir-resistance are also reported
Hepatitis C virus with differing interferon response	Sequence variance in the 5′ non-coding region	RT-PCR-DNA sequencing (78,79)	Genotyping and therapy monitoring	No phenotypic methods are currently available
Antiretroviral drug-resistant HIV-1	Multiple mutations in the protease and RT genes	PCR-DNA sequencing (112)	Detection and therapy monitoring	Time-consuming phenotypic methods are only available in research laboratories

NIRCA, nonisotopic RNase cleavage assay; RFLP, restriction fragment length polymorphism; FRET, fluorescence resonance energy transfer; PCR, polymerase chain reaction; RT, reverse transcriptase.

techniques have been successful in the investigation and control of classic and emerging nosocomial pathogens. These methods combined with clinical epidemiologic analysis were successfully used to investigate an outbreak of *Mycobacterium abscessus* pseudoinfection. Environmental and all 15 case patient isolates had identical genomic DNA patterns assessed by pulsed-field gel electrophoresis (PFGE). An automated endoscope washer was implicated as the source of the pseudoepidemic (87).

Vancomycin-resistant enterococci (VRE) have emerged as important nosocomial pathogens. Consequently, it is important to understand the distribution of VRE within and between hospitals to implement appropriate infection control measures. Bacteremia caused by VRE can be endogenously acquired from the gastrointestinal tract where enterococci are part of the normal flora. Several molecular techniques, including PFGE and PCR *vanA*, *vanB*, and *vanC* genotyping (88), have been used for demonstrating the dissemination of VRE outbreaks within hospital units, between units within hospitals, and between hospitals (89–91). Rapid detection and typing of VRE would permit prevention measures including the isolation of infected patients to reduce the possibility of transmission of VRE to other hospitalized patients.

FUTURE DIRECTIONS

A Gastrointestinal "Chip"

Molecular screening of at-risk populations for a group of possible pathogens is an exciting area of development in molecular microbiology. This idea is very important for quick isolation and identification of various microbial pathogens causing diarrhea. There are numerous etiologic agents that can cause debilitating gastroenteritis in immunosuppressed patient populations, including mycobacteria (e.g., *M. avium* complex and *M. genavense*), parasites (e.g., *Cryptosporidium*, *Microsporidium*), viruses (e.g., rotavirus, Norwalk agent), and typical bacterial pathogens (e.g., *E. coli* variants, *Salmonella*, *Shigella*, *Campylobacter*). Traditionally, different methods of detection are employed for each group of pathogens. This requires special media, equipment, and expensive facilities for the culture of mycobacteria, expertise in the identification of parasites in ova and parasite stool preparations, virology facilities, and the special media for bacterial enteric pathogens.

Molecular techniques can screen a clinical specimen from panels of probable pathogens. One of the PCR "cousins," multiplex PCR, uses numerous primers within a single reaction tube in order to amplify nucleic acid fragments from different targets. Nucleic acids extracted from the stools of patients with gastroenteritis are added into the multiplex PCR reactions. Specific nucleic acid amplification should occur if the appropriate target DNA is present in the sample tested. After PCR amplification, a special gastrointestinal DNA chip, which includes an array of specific oligonucleotide probes, is used to identify the microorganism-specific PCR products (92).

Determine Host Susceptibility to Gastrointestinal Diseases

Enhanced by the human genome programs, clinical microbiology laboratories started to do something beyond microorganisms to help physicians manage infectious diseases. According to human genome sequence information revealed so far, humans appear to be heterogeneous for approximately 1% to 10% of the nucleotides in their DNA. Different forms of a host gene that are sustained in a stable manner at the same chromosomal site within a population are termed *alleles*. Polymorphisms in various alleles in several host immunogenetic factors have been described that influence the host immune response to infectious agents, thereby determining the host susceptibility to certain diseases and pathologic conditions. Mutations in the IFN-γ receptor alleles predispose to severe disseminated mycobacterial infections (93) including fatal infection with Bacille Calmette-Guerin, the tuberculosis vaccine used worldwide (94). Similarly, complete deficiencies or specified polymorphisms in the IL-12 receptor gene have been associated with severe tuberculosis and *Salmonella* infection (95,96). Genetic polymorphisms also affect the entry, multiplication, and survival of *Plasmodium falciparum* and confer resistance to malarial infection (97). Resistance to HIV-1 infection, both *in vitro* and *in vivo* has been associated with an internal 32 base-pair deletion in the human chemokine receptor CCR-5 gene (98,99). The absence of a specific red blood cell antigen among inbred human subpopulations confers absolute resistance to infection by parvovirus B19 (100). Mutations existing in the exon 1 of mannose binding lectin gene is associated with increased susceptibility to Mollaret's meningitis (101).

In the field of gastroenterology, several G to A polymorphisms in the TNF-α promoter region are associated with increased susceptibility to persistent hepatitis B and C infections (102,103). Detection of host polymorphisms in the IL-10 promoter has been used for predicting initial response of chronic hepatitis C to IFN-α (104). Epidemiologic studies have demonstrated that a multistep and multifactorial process is involved in gastric carcinogenesis, and *H. pylori* has been identified as the first bacterial pathogen causing such cancers (11). A recent study reported that IL-1 gene cluster polymorphisms suspected of enhancing the production of IL-1β are associated with an increased risk of both hypochlorhydria induced by *H. pylori* and gastric cancer (105). These data indicated that host genetic factors that affect the level of IL-1β production may determine why gastric cancer develops in some individuals infected with *H. pylori* and not in others. If infections, especially chronic infections, can be viewed as horizontally acquired genetic diseases, it makes sense to view pathogen and host as an integrated system. Enhanced by the ongoing human genome project, the detection of infection-related host gene polymorphism may become an increasingly important role in clinical microbiology laboratories in the future.

Laboratory-Physician Communication

Exchange of relevant information between the clinician and the laboratory is essential to good patient care. During the interval until the identification of a pathogen causing diarrhea, the laboratory would appreciate learning from physicians their clinical "priorities" instead of blindly choosing from an available test menu. By knowing the initial, fragmentary results yielded in the laboratory, physicians would be better able to modify their clinical impression. By enhancing the dialogue between the laboratory and the physician, inappropriate specimens and irrelevant tests can be avoided. Traditional communication formats include structured letters, telephone contact, and face-to-face discussion.

Laboratory-physician communication has been significantly facilitated by the development of the Internet, the immense collection of independent but cooperating computer networks (106). The Internet is rapidly becoming an important source of medical information and many people already have access to the Internet for a variety of purposes. Therefore, laboratory-physician communications are no longer limited to the traditional communication formats. Laboratory-to-physician communications, which used to be limited to the transfer of test results, alert values, and interpretation, have been dramatically expanded. New Internet-related communications include on-line access for physicians to all laboratory test requesting procedures, replacing (or in addition to) the standard booklet usually distributed by the laboratory of test panels, interpretations, and disease trend analysis based on laboratory test results. On the other hand, physician-to-laboratory communication should continue for the transmission of test requests, possible requirements for STAT results, and to indicate patient medication status, which might interfere with laboratory determinations (107). The widespread availability of computer-generated data interpretation of clinical laboratory determinations, new advances in technology, and the measurement of disease markers on a molecular basis have added a new dimension to the field of diagnostic microbiology.

REFERENCES

1. Graham DY, Klein PD, Evans DJ Jr, et al. *Campylobacter pylori* detected noninvasively by the 13C-urea breath test. *Lancet* 1987;1:1174–1177.
2. Slomianski A, Schubert T, Cutler AF. [13C]urea breath test to confirm eradication of *Helicobacter pylori*. *Am J Gastroenterol* 1995;90:224–226.
3. Eisenstein BI. The polymerase chain reaction. A new method of using molecular genetics for medical diagnosis. *N Engl J Med* 1990;322:178–183.
4. Guyer RL, Koshland DE, Jr. The molecule of the year. *Science* 1989;246:1543–1546.
5. Tang YW, Procop GW, Persing DH. Molecular diagnosis of infectious diseases. *Clin Chem* 1997;43:2021–2038.
6. Isenberg HD. *Essential procedures for clinical microbiology.* Washington, DC: American Society for Microbiology, 1998.
7. Murray PR, Baron EJ, Pfaller MA, et al. *Manual of clinical microbiology,* seventh edition. Washington, DC: American Society for Microbiology, 1999.
8. Persing DH, Smith TF, Tenover FC, et al. *Diagnostic molecular microbiology: principles and applications.* Washington, DC: American Society for Microbiology, 1993.
9. Persing DH. *PCR protocols for emerging infectious diseases.* Washington, DC: American Society for Microbiology, 1996.
10. Tang YW, Persing DH. Molecular detection and identification of microorganisms. In: Murray PR, Jo Baron E, Pfaller MA, et al., eds. *Manual of clinical microbiology,* seventh edition. Washington, DC: American Society for Microbiology, 1999: 215–244.
11. Blaser MJ. *Helicobacter pylori* and gastric diseases. *BMJ* 1998; 316:1507–1510.
12. Fekety R, Shah AB. Diagnosis and treatment of *Clostridium difficile* colitis. *JAMA* 1993;269:71–75.
13. Alles AJ, Waldron MA, Sierra LS, et al. Prospective comparison of direct immunofluorescence and conventional staining methods for detection of *Giardia* and *Cryptosporidium* spp. in human fecal specimens. *J Clin Microbiol* 1995;33:1632–1634.
14. Chernesky M, Castriciano S, Mahony J, et al. Ability of TESTPACK ROTAVIRUS enzyme immunoassay to diagnose rotavirus gastroenteritis. *J Clin Microbiol* 1988;26:2459–2461.
15. Ebeling F, Naukkarinen R, Leikola J. Recombinant immunoblot assay for hepatitis C virus antibody as predictor of infectivity. *Lancet* 1990;335:982–983.
16. Kuo G, Choo QL, Alter HJ, et al. An assay for circulating antibodies to a major etiologic virus of human non-A, non-B hepatitis. *Science* 1989;244:362–364.
17. Nilsson I, Lindgren S, Eriksson S, et al. Serum antibodies to *Helicobacter hepaticus* and *Helicobacter pylori* in patients with chronic liver disease. *Gut* 2000;46:410–414.
18. Cubbon MD, Coia JE, Hanson MF, et al. A comparison of immunomagnetic separation, direct culture and polymerase chain reaction for the detection of verocytotoxin-producing *Escherichia coli* O157 in human faeces. *J Clin Microbiol* 1996; 44:219–222.
19. Schwab KJ, De Leon R, Sobsey MD. Immunoaffinity concentration and purification of waterborne enteric viruses for detection by reverse transcriptase PCR. *Appl Environ Microbiol* 1996;62:2086–2094.
20. Karch H, Janetzki-Mittmann C, Aleksic S, et al. Isolation of enterohemorrhagic *Escherichia coli* O157 strains from patients with hemolytic-uremic syndrome by using immunomagnetic separation, DNA-based methods, and direct culture. *J Clin Microbiol* 1996;34:516–519.
21. Reimer LG, Wilson ML, Weinstein MP. Update on detection of bacteremia and fungemia. *Clin Microbiol Rev* 1997;10:444–465.
22. Mullis KB. The unusual origin of the polymerase chain reaction. *Sci Am* 1990;262:56–65.
23. Saiki RK, Gelfand DH, Stoffel S, et al. Primer-directed enzymatic amplification of DNA with a thermostable DNA polymerase. *Science* 1988;239:487–491.

24. Lage AP, Fauconnier A, Burette A, et al. Rapid colorimetric hybridization assay for detecting amplified *Helicobacter pylori* DNA in gastric biopsy specimens. *J Clin Microbiol* 1996;34:530–533.
25. Cardarelli-Leite P, Blom K, Patton CM, et al. Rapid identification of *Campylobacter* species by restriction fragment length polymorphism analysis of a PCR-amplified fragment of the gene coding for 16S rRNA. *J Clin Microbiol* 1996;34:62–67.
26. Arola A, Santti J, Ruuskanen O, et al. Identification of enteroviruses in clinical specimens by competitive PCR followed by genetic typing using sequence analysis. *J Clin Microbiol* 1996;34:313–318.
27. Hermans PW, Saha SK, van Leeuwen WJ, et al. Molecular typing of *Salmonella typhi* strains from Dhaka (Bangladesh) and development of DNA probes identifying plasmid-encoded multidrug-resistant isolates. *J Clin Microbiol* 1996;34:1373–1379.
28. Compton J. Nucleic acid sequence-based amplification. *Nature* 1991;350:91–92.
29. Guatelli JC, Whitfield KM, Kwoh DY, et al. Isothermal, *in vitro* amplification of nucleic acids by a multienzyme reaction modeled after retroviral replication. *Proc Natl Acad Sci U S A* 1990;87:1874–1878.
30. Kwoh DY, Davis GR, Whitfield KM, et al. Transcription-based amplification system and detection of amplified human immunodeficiency virus type 1 with a bead-based sandwich hybridization format. *Proc Natl Acad Sci U S A* 1989;86:1173–1177.
31. Walker GT, Little MC, Nadeau JG, et al. Isothermal *in vitro* amplification of DNA by a restriction enzyme/DNA polymerase system. *Proc Natl Acad Sci U S A* 1992;89:392–396.
32. Wu DY, Wallace RB. The ligation amplification reaction (LAR)—amplification of specific DNA sequences using sequential rounds of template-dependent ligation. *Genomics* 1989;4:560–569.
33. Bekkaoui F, Poisson I, Crosby W, et al. Cycling probe technology with RNase H attached to an oligonucleotide. *Biotechniques* 1996;20:240–248.
34. Morrison EA, Ho GY, Vermund SH, et al. Human papillomavirus infection and other risk factors for cervical neoplasia: a case-control study. *Int J Cancer* 1991;49:6–13.
35. Hendricks DA, Stowe BJ, Hoo BS, et al. Quantitation of HBV DNA in human serum using a branched DNA (bDNA) signal amplification assay. *Am J Clin Pathol* 1995;104:537–546.
36. Urdea MS, Horn T, Fultz TJ, et al. Branched DNA amplification multimers for the sensitive, direct detection of human hepatitis viruses. *Nucleic Acids Symp Series* 1991;24:197–200.
37. Jacob S, Baudy D, Jones E, et al. Comparison of quantitative HCV RNA assays in chronic hepatitis C. *Am J Clin Pathol* 1997;107:362–367.
38. Becker-Andre M, Hahlbrock K. Absolute mRNA quantification using the polymerase chain reaction (PCR). A novel approach by a PCR aided transcript titration assay (PATTY). *Nucleic Acids Res* 1989;17:9437–9446.
39. Mantero G, Zonaro A, Albertini A, et al. DNA enzyme immunoassay: general method for detecting products of polymerase chain reaction. *Clin Chem* 1991;37:422–429.
40. Poljak M, Seme K. Rapid detection and typing of human papillomaviruses by consensus polymerase chain reaction and enzyme-linked immunosorbent assay. *J Virol Methods* 1996;56:231–238.
41. Tang YW, Rys PN, Rutledge BJ, et al. Comparative evaluation of colorimetric microtiter plate systems for detection of herpes simplex virus in cerebrospinal fluid. *J Clin Microbiol* 1998;36:2714–2717.
42. Fredericks DN, Relman DA. Sequence-based identification of microbial pathogens: a reconsideration of Koch's postulates. *Clin Microbiol Rev* 1996;9:18–33.
43. Tang YW, Ellis NM, Hopkins MK, et al. Comparison of phenotypic and genotypic techniques for identification of unusual pathogenic aerobic gram-negative bacilli. *J Clin Microbiol* 1998;36:3674–3679.
44. Cardullo RA, Agrawal S, Flores C, et al. Detection of nucleic acid hybridization by nonradiative fluorescence resonance energy transfer. *Proc Natl Acad Sci U S A* 1988;85:8790–8794.
45. Wittwer CT, Ririe KM, Andrew RV, et al. The LightCycler: a microvolume multisample fluorimeter with rapid temperature control. *Biotechniques* 1997;22:176–181.
46. Gibson JR, Saunders NA, Burke B, et al. Novel method for rapid determination of clarithromycin sensitivity in *Helicobacter pylori*. *J Clin Microbiol.* 1999;37:3746–3748.
47. Costa JM, Pautas C, Ernault P, et al. Real-time PCR for diagnosis and follow-up of *Toxoplasma* reactivation after allogeneic stem cell transplantation using fluorescence resonance energy transfer hybridization probes. *J Clin Microbiol* 2000;38:2929–2932.
48. Morris T, Robertson B, Gallagher M. Rapid reverse transcription-PCR detection of hepatitis C virus RNA in serum by using the TaqMan fluorogenic detection system. *J Clin Microbiol* 1996;34:2933–2936.
49. Pas SD, Fries E, De Man RA, et al. Development of a quantitative real-time detection assay for hepatitis B virus DNA and comparison with two commercial assays. *J Clin Microbiol* 2000;38:2897–2901.
50. Takeuchi T, Katsume A, Tanaka T, et al. Real-time detection system for quantification of hepatitis C virus genome. *Gastroenterology* 1999;116:636–642.
51. Falkow S. Perspectives series: host/pathogen interactions. Invasion and intracellular sorting of bacteria: searching for bacterial genes expressed during host/pathogen interactions. *J Clin Invest* 1997;100:239–243.
52. Monteiro L, Bonnemaison D, Vekris A, et al. Complex polysaccharides as PCR inhibitors in feces: *Helicobacter pylori* model. *J Clin Microbiol* 1997;35:995–998.
53. Choo QL, Kuo G, Weiner AJ, et al. Isolation of a cDNA clone derived from a blood-borne non-A, non-B viral hepatitis genome. *Science* 1989;244:359–362.
54. Aach RD, Stevens CE, Hollinger FB, et al. Hepatitis C virus infection in post-transfusion hepatitis. An analysis with first- and second-generation assays. *N Engl J Med* 1991;325:1325–1329.
55. Schlueter V, Schmolke S, Stark K, et al. Reverse transcription-PCR detection of hepatitis G virus. *J Clin Microbiol* 1996;34:2660–2664.
56. Nishizawa T, Okamoto H, Konishi K, et al. A novel DNA virus (TTV) associated with elevated transaminase levels in post-transfusion hepatitis of unknown etiology. *Biochem Biophys Res Commun* 1997;241:92–97.
57. Kapperud G, Vardund T, Skjerve E, et al. Detection of pathogenic *Yersinia enterocolitica* in foods and water by immunomagnetic separation, nested polymerase chain reactions, and colorimetric detection of amplified DNA. *Appl Environ Microbiol* 1993;59:2938–2944.
58. Frankel G, Riley L, Giron JA, et al. Detection of *Shigella* in feces using DNA amplification. *J Infect Dis* 1990;161:1252–1256.
59. Weynants V, Jadot V, Denoel PA, et al. Detection of *Yersinia enterocolitica* serogroup O:3 by a PCR method. *J Clin Microbiol* 1996;34:1224–1227.
60. Fratamico PM, Sackitey SK, Wiedmann M, et al. Detection of *Escherichia coli* O157:H7 by multiplex PCR. *J Clin Microbiol* 1995;33:2188–2191.
61. Laxer MA, D'Nicuola ME, Patel RJ. Detection of *Cryptosporid-*

ium parvum DNA in fixed, paraffin-embedded tissue by the polymerase chain reaction. *Am J Trop Med Hyg* 1992;47: 450–455.
62. Fedorko DP, Nelson NA, Cartwright CP. Identification of microsporidia in stool specimens by using PCR and restriction endonucleases. *J Clin Microbiol* 1995;33:1739–1741.
63. Relman DA, Schmidt TM, Gajadhar A, et al. Molecular phylogenetic analysis of *Cyclospora*, the human intestinal pathogen, suggests that it is closely related to *Eimeria* species. *J Infect Dis* 1996;173:440–445.
64. Woese CR. Bacterial evolution. *Microbiol Rev* 1987;51: 221–271.
65. Ramzan NN, Loftus E Jr, Burgart LJ, et al. Diagnosis and monitoring of Whipple disease by polymerase chain reaction. *Ann Intern Med* 1997;126:520–527.
66. Relman DA, Schmidt TM, MacDermott RP, et al. Identification of the uncultured bacillus of Whipple's disease. *N Engl J Med* 1992;327:293–301.
67. von Herbay A, Ditton HJ, Maiwald M. Diagnostic application of a polymerase chain reaction assay for the Whipple's disease bacterium to intestinal biopsies. *Gastroenterology* 1996;110: 1735–1743.
68. Chiodini RJ, Van Kruiningen HJ, Thayer WR, et al. Possible role of mycobacteria in inflammatory bowel disease. I. An unclassified *Mycobacterium* species isolated from patients with Crohn's disease. *Dig Dis Sci* 1984;29:1073–1079.
69. Dell'Isola B, Poyart C, Goulet O, et al. Detection of *Mycobacterium paratuberculosis* by polymerase chain reaction in children with Crohn's disease. *J Infect Dis* 1994;169:449–451.
70. Sanderson JD, Moss MT, Tizard ML, et al. *Mycobacterium paratuberculosis* DNA in Crohn's disease tissue. *Gut* 1992;33: 890–896.
71. Bateson MC. Advances in gastroenterology and hepatology. *Postgrad Med J* 2000;76:328–332.
72. Covacci A, Censini S, Bugnoli M, et al. Molecular characterization of the 128-kDa immunodominant antigen of *Helicobacter pylori* associated with cytotoxicity and duodenal ulcer. *Proc Natl Acad Sci U S A* 1993;90:5791–5795.
73. Clark CG, Diamond LS. Ribosomal RNA genes of "pathogenic" and "nonpathogenic" *Entamoeba histolytica* are distinct. *Mol Biochem Parasitol* 1991;49:297–302.
74. Acuna-Soto R, Samuelson J, De Girolami P, et al. Application of the polymerase chain reaction to the epidemiology of pathogenic and nonpathogenic *Entamoeba histolytica*. *Am J Trop Med Hyg* 1993;48:58–70.
75. Katzwinkel-Wladarsch S, Loscher T, Rinder H. Direct amplification and differentiation of pathogenic and nonpathogenic *Entamoeba histolytica* DNA from stool specimens. *Am J Trop Med Hyg* 1994;51:115–118.
76. Choo QL, Richman KH, Han JH, et al. Genetic organization and diversity of the hepatitis C virus. *Proc Natl Acad Sci U S A* 1991;88:2451–2455.
77. McOmish F, Yap PL, Dow BC, et al. Geographical distribution of hepatitis C virus genotypes in blood donors: an international collaborative survey. *J Clin Microbiol* 1994;32:884–892.
78. Germer JJ, Rys PN, Thorvilson JN, et al. Determination of hepatitis C virus genotype by direct sequence analysis of products generated with the Amplicor HCV test. *J Clin Microbiol* 1999;37:2625–2630.
79. Yoshioka K, Kakumu S, Wakita T, et al. Detection of hepatitis C virus by polymerase chain reaction and response to interferon-alpha therapy: relationship to genotypes of hepatitis C virus. *Hepatology* 1992;16:293–299.
80. Zein NN, Rakela J, Krawitt EL, et al. Hepatitis C virus genotypes in the United States: epidemiology, pathogenicity, and response to interferon therapy. *Ann Intern Med* 1996;125:634–639.
81. Detmer J, Lagier R, Flynn J, et al. Accurate quantification of hepatitis C virus (HCV) RNA from all HCV genotypes by using branched-DNA technology. *J Clin Microbiol* 1996;34:901–907.
82. Crotty PL, Staggs RA, Porter PT, et al. Quantitative analysis in molecular diagnostics. *Hum Pathol* 1994;25:572–579.
83. Gibson UE, Heid CA, Williams PM. A novel method for real time quantitative RT-PCR. *Genome Res* 1996;6:995–1001.
84. Heid CA, Stevens J, Livak KJ, et al. Real time quantitative PCR. *Genome Res* 1996;6:986–994.
85. Pfaller MA, Cormican MG. Role of the microbiology laboratory in monitoring and identifying resistance: use of molecular biology. *New Horizons* 1996;4:361–369.
86. Nuesch-Inderbinen MT, Hachler H, Kayser FH. Detection of genes coding for extended-spectrum SHV beta-lactamases in clinical isolates by a molecular genetic method, and comparison with the E test. *Eur J Clin Microbiol Infect Dis* 1996;15:398–402.
87. Maloney S, Welbel S, Daves B, et al. *Mycobacterium abscessus* pseudoinfection traced to an automated endoscope washer: utility of epidemiologic and laboratory investigation. *J Infect Dis* 1994;169:1166–1169.
88. Patel R, Uhl JR, Kohner P, et al. Multiplex PCR detection of vanA, vanB, vanC-1, and vanC-2/3 genes in enterococci. *J Clin Microbiol* 1997;35:703–707.
89. Bopp LH, Schoonmaker DJ, Baltch AL, et al. Molecular epidemiology of vancomycin-resistant enterococci from 6 hospitals in New York State. *Am J Infect Control* 1999;27:411–417.
90. D'Agata EM, Li H, Gouldin C, et al. Characterization of vancomycin-resistant *Enterococcus faecium* strains during endemicity. *Clin Infect Dis* 2001;33:511–516.
91. Kirkpatrick BD, Harrington SM, Smith D, et al. An outbreak of vancomycin-dependent *Enterococcus faecium* in a bone marrow transplant unit. *Clin Infect Dis* 1999;29:1268–1273.
92. Fodor SP, Rava RP, Huang XC, et al. Multiplexed biochemical assays with biological chips. *Nature* 1993;364:555–556.
93. Newport MJ, Huxley CM, Huston S, et al. A mutation in the interferon-gamma-receptor gene and susceptibility to mycobacterial infection. *N Engl J Med* 1996;335:1941–1949.
94. Jouanguy E, Altare F, Lamhamedi S, et al. Interferon-gamma-receptor deficiency in an infant with fatal bacille Calmette-Guerin infection. *N Engl J Med* 1996;335:1956–1961.
95. Altare F, Jurandy A, Lammas D, et al. Impairment of mycobacterial immunity in human interleukin-12 receptor deficiency. *Science* 1998;280:1432–1435.
96. de Jong R, Altare F, Haagen IA, et al. Severe mycobacterial and salmonella infections in interleukin-12 receptor-deficient patients. *Science* 1998;280:1435–1438.
97. Miller LH, Mason SJ, Dvorak JA, et al. Erythrocyte receptors for (*Plasmodium knowlesi*) malaria: Duffy blood group determinants. *Science* 1975;189:561–563.
98. Dean M, Carrington M, Winkler C, et al. Genetic restriction of HIV-1 infection and progression to AIDS by a deletion allele of the CKR5 structural gene. *Science* 1996;273:1856–1862.
99. Samson M, Libert F, Doranz BJ, et al. Resistance to HIV-1 infection in Caucasian individuals bearing mutant alleles of the CCR-5 chemokine receptor gene. *Nature* 1996;382:722–725.
100. Brown KE, Hibbs JR, Gallinella G, et al. Resistance to parvovirus B19 infection due to lack of virus receptor (erythrocyte P antigen). *N Engl J Med* 1994;330:1192–1196.
101. Tang YW, Cleavinger PJ, Li HJ, et al. Analysis of candidate-host immunogenetic determinants in herpes simplex virus-associated Mollaret's meningitis. *Clin Infect Dis* 2000;30:176–178.
102. Hohler T, Kruger A, Gerken G, et al. Tumor necrosis factor alpha promoter polymorphism at position -238 is associated with chronic active hepatitis C infection. *J Med Virol* 1998; 54:173–177.
103. Hohler T, Kruger A, Gerken G, et al. A tumor necrosis factor-

alpha (TNF-alpha) promoter polymorphism is associated with chronic hepatitis B infection. *Clin Exp Immunol* 1998;111:579–582.

104. Edwards-Smith CJ, Jonsson JR, Purdie DM, et al. Interleukin-10 promoter polymorphism predicts initial response of chronic hepatitis C to interferon alpha. *Hepatology* 1999;30:526–530.
105. El-Omar EM, Carrington M, Chow WH, et al. Interleukin-1 polymorphisms associated with increased risk of gastric cancer. *Nature* 2000;404:398–402.
106. Kassirer JP. The next transformation in the delivery of health care. *N Engl J Med* 1995;332:52–54.
107. Zinder O. New directions in laboratory-clinician communications. *Clin Chim Acta* 1998;278:83–94.
108. Kramer FR, Lizardi PM. Replicatable RNA reporters. *Nature* 1989;339:401–402.
109. Griggs DJ, Gensberg K, Piddock LJ. Mutations in gyrA gene of quinolone-resistant *Salmonella* serotypes isolated from humans and animals. *Antimicrob Agents Chemother* 1996;40:1009–1013.
110. Nash KA, Inderlied CB. Rapid detection of mutations associated with macrolide resistance in *Mycobacterium avium* complex. *Antimicrob Agents Chemother* 1996;40:1748–1750.
111. Smith IL, Cherrington JM, Jiles RE, et al. High-level resistance of cytomegalovirus to ganciclovir is associated with alterations in both the UL97 and DNA polymerase genes. *J Infect Dis* 1997;176:69–77.
112. Hirsch MS, Brun-Vezinet F, D'Aquila RT, et al. Antiretroviral drug resistance testing in adult HIV-1 infection: recommendations of an International AIDS Society-USA Panel. *JAMA* 2000;283:2417–2426.

76

PROPHYLAXIS FOR GASTROINTESTINAL SURGERY

DOUGLAS S. KERNODLE
ALLEN B. KAISER

Advances in anesthesia and antisepsis during the late 1800s ushered in the modern era of surgery. Abdominal surgery, in particular, underwent dramatic changes, with the development of procedures to treat common acute and oftentimes fatal illnesses such as appendicitis. Also, surgical procedures became important in the management of chronic illnesses for which medical therapy alone had proved ineffective. So swift were the changes in general surgery that most of today's basic surgical procedures involving the gastrointestinal (GI) tract had been developed by World War I (1), predating the discovery and clinical use of antibiotics.

The surgical advances during that earlier era are even the more remarkable considering that many of these procedures involve portions of the GI tract that are heavily colonized with bacteria. In 1920, Lord Moynihan wrote that "every operation in surgery is an experiment in bacteriology" (2). Nowhere is this statement more relevant than in surgery involving the GI tract. For example, in the descending colon, as many as 10^{12} bacteria are present per gram of stool (3,4). Before antibiotic prophylaxis became an accepted part of surgical management, procedures involving the colon were associated with infection rates of 30% to 60% (5). The infecting bacteria, usually *Escherichia coli* and *Bacteroides* species, generally were derived from the patient's endogenous flora.

The high incidence of wound infections in the preantibiotic era would be considered unacceptable by today's standards. Despite the relatively late acceptance of antibiotic prophylaxis as the standard of care in surgical practice (6), it is difficult to imagine modern GI surgery without it. And in spite of its routine use, postoperative infections are still a major cause of surgical morbidity.

D. S. Kernodle: Department of Medicine, Vanderbilt University School of Medicine; Infectious Diseases Section, Nashville VA Medical Center, Nashville, Tennessee

A. B. Kaiser: Department of Medicine, Vanderbilt University School of Medicine, Nashville, Tennessee

PATHOGENESIS OF SURGICAL WOUND INFECTIONS AND THE RATIONALE FOR ANTIBIOTIC PROPHYLAXIS

General Concepts

Based on the risk of bacterial contamination of the operative site, surgical wounds have been divided into several categories (7,8). Clean wounds are nontraumatic wounds in which no inflammation is encountered, no break in aseptic technique occurs, and the alimentary, respiratory, and urinary tracts are not entered. Clean-contaminated wounds are nontraumatic wounds in which a minor break in technique occurs or in which the GI, respiratory, or urinary tracts are entered into without significant spillage. This category includes cholecystectomy and appendectomy "in passing" in the absence of acute inflammation. Contaminated wounds are associated with procedures in which acute inflammation is encountered or there is visible spillage of material from a hollow viscus. Included in this category are procedures involving the biliary system in the presence of infected bile and surgery involving trauma, fecal contamination, a devitalized viscus, or pus from any source. Dirty wounds refer to surgery performed under conditions in which there is preexisting infection, for example, drainage of an abscess and surgical creation of a diverting colostomy after perforation of the colon. The use of antibiotics in this clinical setting is considered "therapeutic," rather than "prophylactic" (6). Several studies have demonstrated a correlation between the density of bacteria at the operative site and the subsequent risk of infection (9,10).

Although these categories historically have been useful in defining the epidemiology and risk of infectious complications, there is enough variance in the infection rates associated with different procedures within the same category to make procedure-specific infection rates a superior indicator for hospital surveillance. Also, newer algorithms based on both patient and procedure-related risk factors appear to have better predictive value (11,12). Current

TABLE 76.1. INFECTION RATES OF GASTROINTESTINAL SURGICAL PROCEDURES, 1992–1998[a]

<table>
<tr><th></th><th colspan="5">Risk Index Category[b]</th></tr>
<tr><th>Operation</th><th>M/0-Yes</th><th>0/0-No</th><th>1</th><th>2</th><th>3</th></tr>
<tr><td>Cholecystectomy</td><td>0.49[c]</td><td>0.69[c]</td><td>2.0</td><td>3.5</td><td>6.6</td></tr>
<tr><td>Colon Surgery</td><td>0.69[c]</td><td>4.3[c]</td><td>6.2</td><td>9.6</td><td>13.0</td></tr>
<tr><td>Appendectomy</td><td>0.56[d]</td><td>1.4[d]</td><td>3.2</td><td colspan="2">5.8</td></tr>
<tr><td>Gastric Surgery</td><td>0.49[d]</td><td>2.7[d]</td><td>5.1</td><td colspan="2">10.7</td></tr>
<tr><td>Laparotomy</td><td>—</td><td>1.7</td><td>3.2</td><td>5.4</td><td>8.0</td></tr>
<tr><td>Small Bowel</td><td>—</td><td>5.6</td><td>7.5</td><td>9.8</td><td>14.8</td></tr>
<tr><td>Liver/pancreas</td><td>—</td><td>3.2</td><td colspan="3">7.0</td></tr>
<tr><td>Other digestive surgery</td><td>—</td><td colspan="2">3.2</td><td colspan="2">8.1</td></tr>
</table>

[a]Adapted from Centers for Disease Control and Prevention. Semiannual report: aggregated data from the National Nosocomial Infection Surveillance (NNIS) System. December 1999. Available at: www.cdc.gov/ncidod/hip/NNIS/dec99sar.pdf, with permission. Data reported as number of infections per 100 procedures.
[b]Risk index category designates whether 0, 1, 2, or 3 risk factors were present. Risk factors include an American Society of Anesthesiologists score of 3, 4, or 5; duration of surgery >75th percentile for the procedure; or contaminated/dirty wound class (12). The data for cholecystectomy, colon surgery, appendectomy, and gastric surgery use a modified risk index that incorporates the influence of laparoscope or endoscope on wound infection rates. Risk factor groups were merged when the differences between them were not statistically significant.
[c]For cholecystectomy and colon surgery, the number 1 was subtracted from the number of risk factors when the procedure was done laparoscopically. When the number of risk factors was zero, this led to a new category called *minus-1* or *M*.
[d]For appendectomy and gastric surgery, procedures with zero risk factors were grouped as *0-Yes* and *0-No* based on whether or not a laparoscope was used.

infection rates for major GI surgical procedures are shown in Table 76.1 (13).

Risk Factors For Infection

Various host and technique-related variables have been identified as risk factors for the development of a surgical wound infection.

Host Factors

Host risk factors for infection are summarized in Table 76.2 (14–15).

TABLE 76.2. HOST RISK FACTORS FOR WOUND INFECTION AFTER GASTROINTESTINAL SURGERY

Extremes of age (i.e., very old or very young)
Diabetes
Cigarette smoking
Prior irradiation of the operative site
Steroids and other immunosuppressive therapy
Severe obesity
Malnutrition
Cutaneous anergy
Low expression of human leukocyte antigen DR on monocytes
Remote infection at the time of surgery (e.g., urinary tract infection)
Long duration of hospitalization before surgery
Gastric achlorhydria (gastroduodenal surgery)
Obstruction or perforation of viscus
Preoperative assessment score of 3, 4, or 5 (American Society of Anesthesiologists)

Surgical Technique

Operative risk factors for infection are summarized in Table 76.3. The maintenance of adequate tissue perfusion in the postoperative period is of critical importance and in part reflects the care with which the surgeon handles body tissues and achieves hemostasis during the procedure. Tissue devitalization at a gross or microscopic level provides a niche wherein inoculated bacteria may grow in relative isolation from host defense mechanisms. Good surgical technique is one of the most important determinants of whether a wound becomes infected and is reflected in the "traditional surgical view that untidy operative techniques

TABLE 76.3. OPERATIVE RISK FACTORS FOR WOUND INFECTION AFTER GASTROINTESTINAL SURGERY

No preoperative shower or inadequate preparation of skin with antiseptics
Shaving the operative site on the day before surgery
Prolonged length of procedure
Intraoperative contamination
Homologous blood transfusion
Excessive use of an electrosurgical knife
Poor hemostasis
Use of foreign material
Use of prophylactic abdominal drains
Injection of epinephrine into the wound
Appendectomy in passing added to elective cholecystectomy
Inadequate preparation of the colon (colorectal surgery)

predispose to infection" (16). Other technical factors, including the method of preoperative hair removal (i.e., clipping or shaving), topical antisepsis, the choice of suture material, the use of electrocautery, whether or not a drain is placed during surgery, and if so its position (i.e., exiting via the incision vs. a separate site and distance from an intestinal anastomotic site), and the use of intraoperative irrigation, also have been correlated with the risk of wound infection (15,17).

Unique Risk Factors Among Gastrointestinal Procedures

Some GI procedures have unique risks not shared by other surgical procedures. An "appendectomy in passing" added to elective cholecystectomy increases the infection rate from 1.4% to 4.5% (18). Gastric achlorhydria or the use of histamine (H_2) blocking agents has been associated with an increased risk of infection after gastric procedures (19,20). This is believed to be related to an increased number of bacteria in the stomach at the time of surgery stemming from the loss of the normal antibacterial effect of a low gastric pH level. In a canine model, vagotomy is associated with hypochlorhydria and a marked increase in the coliform population of the stomach (21). Obstruction or perforation of a viscus is a strong predictor of subsequent infection. Inadequate preparation of the colon with the retention of intestinal fluid and feces at the time of surgery is a strong risk factor for several types of septic complications, including dehiscence of the anastomotic site (22,23). Abdominoperineal rectal resections have a greater risk of infection than intraperitoneal resections (24,25).

Blood Transfusion

The transfusion of homologous blood is an independent risk factor for infection in patients undergoing elective intraabdominal surgery, with most of the infections occurring at sites other than the surgical wound (26–28). Homologous blood transfusions suppress cellular immunity. In contrast, autologous blood transfusion does not appear to increase the risk of infection after surgery.

Interrelationship Of Risk Factors

Some risk factors for infection are interrelated, with a patient exhibiting one factor also being likely to have others. Haley et al. (11) described an index to ascertain the risk of postoperative infection, which involves combining a traditional assessment of the wound category (i.e., clean, clean contaminated, or contaminated) with three patient- and procedure-related factors. These include an operation involving the abdomen, a procedure lasting longer than 2 hours, and the presence of three or more underlying diagnoses (as a surrogate for identifying the complicated patient). Subsequently, this model for identifying patients at risk for infection has been further simplified: (a) a patient with an American Society of Anesthesiologists preoperative assessment score of 3, 4, or 5; (b) an operation classified as contaminated or dirty infected; and (c) an operation lasting longer than *T* hours, where *T* depends on the procedure (12). In clean surgery, the importance of the duration of the operation appears diminished in studies in which antibiotic prophylaxis is readministered intraoperatively during long procedures (29). These observations suggest that the duration-related risk may be due to the lack of adequate antibiotic concentrations in the blood and tissues with longer surgical procedures, and that the risk of wound infection may be reduced by more aggressive prophylaxis.

The "Decisive Interval"

Whether or not a wound becomes infected is largely determined at the time of surgery. In experimental models, maneuvers initiated several hours after the inoculation of bacteria into the wound do not influence whether or not infection occurs (30,31). The demonstration that the efficacy of antibiotics in preventing wound infection is limited to only a few hours after the moment of bacterial inoculation implies that the wound microenvironment is not static. However, the changes that occur during this "decisive interval" are poorly understood. Elucidation of the pathophysiology of the decisive interval will likely have a profound effect on developing strategies for preventing infection. The clinical relevance of the decisive interval in the prophylaxis of surgery has been established in clinical trials, in which the risk of infection is higher for patients who have prophylaxis initiated in the late intraoperative or postoperative period than in the immediate preoperative period (32,33).

Host Defenses And The Wound Microenvironment

Because of the large serosal surface of the peritoneum and the relative ease with which infection at the incision site of a viscus may track to other parts of the abdomen and pelvis, it is important to consider the peritoneal defense systems in addition to the defenses of the skin and soft tissues through which the surgical incision was made. Three forms of peritoneal responses to bacterial challenge have been described: (a) direct absorption of bacteria into the lymphatic stomas under the diaphragm, (b) the destruction of bacteria by phagocytosis, and (c) the localization of bacteria within an abscess (4,34).

Cellular and humoral factors contribute to the bacterial eradication from the peritoneum and the surgical wound site. In animal models, the initial clearing of a bacterial challenge to the peritoneum is mediated by macrophages, followed by the mobilization of neutrophils (35,36). Failure of peripheral monocytes to express the class II antigen human leukocyte antigen DR, which is critical for the recognition of foreign antigens and the T-lymphocyte proliferative response, has been associated with an increased incidence of infection and death among patients who have undergone surgery and trauma (37,38). Whereas neutrophils can kill *Bacteroides fragilis* in the presence of serum, serum alone is not bactericidal (39). Immunoglobulins and the alternative complement pathways facilitate the opsonophagocytosis of *B. fragilis* (40). An anaerobic environment does not appear to adversely affect the microbicidal activity of neutrophils (41,42).

Microbial attachment to the wound tissues is believed to be important in the pathogenesis of wound infection. Coliforms and *B. fragilis* organisms adhere to the peritoneal serosal mesothelium (43). The use of fibrinolytic agents inhibits abscess formation in investigational models (44), which is consistent with the hypothesis that the adherence of bacteria to fibrinous exudates is an essential step in wound infection pathogenesis.

Surgery and trauma induce systemic and local changes in the immune defense mechanisms of the host. Major surgery causes defects in T-lymphocyte proliferation and cytokine secretion (45). It also impairs neutrophil function and serum opsonizing capacity (46–48). Neutrophils from an unfavorable wound environment can be stimulated to premature activation and degranulation in the absence of a bacterial stimulus more readily than can neutrophils from a well-perfused wound (47). Immunostimulating agents that enhance neutrophil function have shown benefit in clinical trials (49). Furthermore, laparoscopic surgery is less traumatic to host tissues than open procedures and is associated with better preservation of immune function (50).

The formation of an abscess after intraabdominal surgery is a complex process that appears to require lymphocytes. Renal transplant recipients with lymphopenia who undergo appendectomy have a high incidence of bacteremia with *B. fragilis* without abscess formation (51). The capsule of *B. fragilis* promotes abscess formation, even when the bacteria are not viable (52). After experimental inoculation of *B. fragilis,* antibiotics with good activity fail to prevent abscesses from developing, but the combination of antibiotics with cell-free splenic extracts of animals previously challenged with *B. fragilis* prevents abscess formation (53). Furthermore, immunization against capsular polysaccharide protects by a T-cell-dependent mechanism against abscess formation after *B. fragilis* inoculation (54,55). However, this protection can be reduced by the presence of foreign material.

Fecal roughage has a strong adjuvant effect on the ability of intestinal bacteria to induce abscess formation. The mechanism is believed to involve complement activation by the roughage and the depletion of complement-derived opsonins, with reduced opsonization of abscess-inducing bacteria (56). Roughage may also provide a niche wherein bacteria grow in relative isolation from the host defense mechanisms in much the same manner as described earlier for devitalized tissue.

Normal Flora And Wound Pathogens Of The Gastrointestinal Tract

For most GI procedures, the major wound pathogens come from the viscus entered during surgery, and an understanding of the GI flora during health and disease is fundamental to effective surgical prophylaxis. This topic is covered in more detail in Chapter 4.

The flora of the esophagus and stomach reflect what is swallowed from the mouth; however, gastric acid has a potent antibacterial effect and renders the stomach nearly sterile under normal conditions (57). *Helicobacter pylori* and related organisms, the only known bacterial species adapted for living in the human stomach, are discussed elsewhere (Chapters 33 through 35) and these fastidious organisms do not appear to be wound pathogens.

During the postprandial period, persons with a full stomach and relatively high gastric pH levels have oral bacteria counts of up to 10^5 colony-forming units (CFU) per milliliter (58). The quantitative gastric flora also increase under circumstances of hypochlorhydria and obstruction (19). The predominant species include streptococci, staphylococci, and lactobacilli (4); however, *B. fragilis* can be recovered from patients with achlorhydria or gastric carcinoma (4).

The biliary tract is normally sterile, and even in the setting of surgery for cholelithiasis, most patients have sterile bile (59). Infected bile from patients with acute cholecystitis and other biliary tract diseases from different institutions, geographic locations, and comprising different demographic populations shows marked variability in the aerobic and anaerobic organisms isolated (60,61). In general, aerobes are more common than anaerobes. Anaerobic cocci or *Clostridium perfringens* are the most frequently recovered anaerobes. *B. fragilis* usually is not isolated; in one study it was recovered from 29% of elderly patients, however (62). Human bile acids normally inhibit the growth of *B. fragilis,* but among patients with gallstones, the inhibitory properties of bile are diminished (63). In septicemia after cholecystectomy, the most common pathogens include *E. coli, Klebsiella* species, *Proteus* species, streptococci, and enterococci (64).

Although studies based on culturing fluid from the small intestine at autopsy or via peroral tubes suggest a complex microbial flora (4,65), aspirates obtained from living patients at the time of surgery show that the duodenum and jejunum are usually sterile or contain small numbers of ingested bacteria that are passing through (66). Heavier colonization occurs under conditions of gastric hypochlorhydria, intestinal stasis, cholelithiasis, and deficiencies in the secretion of pancreatic enzymes or bile acids (4,67).

The microflora of the colon include hundreds of different bacterial species, but only a few have the propensity to cause infection (3,15). In the descending colon, bacterial counts are as high as 10^{12} CFU/g and bacteria account for

40% of the volume of stool (3,4). In the colon, 99.9% of the flora are anaerobic (3).

The patient's endogenous GI flora are the major reservoir of pathogens causing postoperative infection. Polymicrobial infections are common, particularly among patients undergoing procedures involving the appendix or colon. For example, patients undergoing surgery for perforated or gangrenous appendicitis have an average of 11 bacterial species—3 aerobic and 8 anaerobic—isolated from the operative specimen (68). *E. coli* and *B. fragilis* are the most common aerobic and anaerobic pathogens, respectively. Despite the predominance of the intestinal flora, *Staphylococcus aureus,* the prototypic clean-wound pathogen, is also commonly recovered from wound infections complicating colorectal surgery when the prophylactic regimen does not have activity against gram-positive pathogens (69). Presumably, they are derived either from the patient's endogenous skin or stool flora or exogenously from personnel involved in the procedure (70). Also, *S. aureus* has been recovered from 6% of wound infections and 12% of gastric secretions of patients undergoing gastric operations, demonstrating its pathogenic potential in surgery of the upper GI tract (71). Staphylococci also have been problematic in studies when no prophylaxis was used in low-risk patients undergoing cholecystectomy (72) and are believed to come from the skin, rather than the bile.

Concepts Of Effective Prophylaxis

Spectrum Of Activity

It is a basic tenet of antimicrobial prophylaxis that the regimen should be active against the major pathogens, and it is not necessary to cover those species among the normal flora that have little pathogenic potential. For potentially contaminated procedures involving the appendix, colon, or rectum, prophylaxis should be directed primarily against *B. fragilis* and the organisms belonging to the Enterobacteriaceae family, in particular, *E. coli.* Anaerobic coverage appears to be less important for gastroduodenal and biliary tract procedures. Activity against *S. aureus,* which presumably is inoculated into the wound from the patient's endogenous skin flora or exogenously from operating department personnel, also has been recommended (15,69).

Whether resistant gram-negative pathogens such as *Pseudomonas aeruginosa* should be covered in the prophylactic regimen is controversial (73). Similarly, although enterococcal species including *Enterococcus faecalis* and *Enterococcus faecium* are commonly recovered from abdominal wound infections, the importance of providing coverage in the prophylactic regimen remains controversial. Animal model studies and clinical experience showing that polymicrobial infections, which include enterococci, can be eradicated successfully using antibiotics that have poor activity against enterococci argue against the need for including a specific anti-enterococcal agent in the prophylactic regimen (4,74,75). On the other hand, enterococci increase the size of abscesses caused by other bacteria and can independently establish abscesses in animal models (4,76). In one study, postoperative enterococcal bacteremia was associated with increased patient morbidity (77). Among patients with prosthetic heart valves or with other risk factors for endocarditis, anti-enterococcal coverage with gentamicin plus either ampicillin or vancomycin should be given (78). Routine prophylaxis for preventing wound infection does not protect against endocarditis.

There are several recent changes in the antibiotic susceptibility patterns of wound pathogens that may affect the efficacy of current routine prophylactic regimens. Isolates of *E. coli* and *Klebsiella* species that are resistant to the third-generation cephalosporins, because of the production of extended-spectrum β-lactamases (ESBLs), are becoming more common (79,80). ESBLs generally are susceptible to inhibition by β-lactamase inhibitors including clavulanic acid, sulbactam, and tazobactam (81). Also, ESBLs are less active against the anti-anaerobic second-generation cephalosporins including cefoxitin, cefotetan, and cefmetazole; such agents maintain activity against most ESBL-producing strains. The emergence of vancomycin-resistant isolates of *E. faecium,* as well as the widespread dissemination of methicillin-resistant strains of *S. aureus,* (79) also may have implications for surgical prophylaxis.

Route Of Administration

The principle on which most systemic antibiotic prophylaxis is based is the belief that antibiotics in the host tissues can augment natural immune defense mechanisms and help to kill bacteria that are inoculated into the wound. In some studies, topical and incisional administration of the antibiotic has yielded good results (82,83).

The rationale for the administration of oral antibiotics before colonic surgery differs because although some agents are absorbed systemically (e.g., erythromycin and metronidazole, but not neomycin), the primary goal is to reduce the potential pathogens among the normal gut flora at the time of surgery. Oral sulfanilamide was the first perioperative prophylactic antibiotic, being used for colorectal surgery in 1939 (84) and gastroduodenal surgery in 1941 (85). Oral prophylaxis is generally combined with mechanical preparation of the bowel to reduce colonic flora, including cathartics and isotonic lavage solutions (86,87).

Timing And Duration Of Prophylaxis

For systemic prophylaxis, every effort should be made to ensure that free antibiotic levels are maintained at a level higher than the minimal inhibitory concentration (MIC) of common wound pathogens throughout the duration of the surgical procedure (15,88). Initiation of intravenous antibiotics in the operating room just before the induction of anesthesia provides time for the agent to distribute to body tissues before incision and avoids the premature administration associated with "on-call" dosing. To prevent the serum and tissue concentrations of antibiotic from falling too low during long procedures, agents with a short half-life need to be dosed again intraoperatively. Although a number of studies have indicated that prolonged surgical procedures are associated with a higher infection rate (24,89), it is unclear whether a long procedure is truly a risk factor for infection or whether this association reflects inadequate intraoperative repeated dosing.

For nonemergent colorectal procedures, an oral antibiotic regimen should be started on the afternoon before surgery in conjunction with isotonic lavage. Supplemental prophylaxis with a parenteral agent should be given when the duration of the procedure exceeds 3.5 hours (24,89,90). Also, the timing of the administration of oral regimens is critical, and delays in the start of surgery from the originally scheduled time may diminish the efficacy of the oral regimen; under such circumstances, a systemic agent should be added.

In the setting of emergency surgery after abdominal trauma, parenteral prophylaxis should begin preoperatively and the duration of postsurgical antibiotic therapy should be based on the findings at the time of surgery. Thadepalli and Mandal (4) have recommended discontinuation of antibiotics if there is no hollow viscus injury; 48- to 72-hour coverage if the stomach, duodenum, or jejunum have been injured; and 7 days of therapy for colonic injuries.

Antibiotic Penetration

Under normal circumstances, the biliary concentrations of various antibiotics in the bile are markedly different (91–94). In the presence of cystic or common bile duct obstruction, however, the biliary concentration of most antibiotics falls dramatically (94–97). In general, antibiotic concentration in the bile does not correlate with prophylactic efficacy (98). Gentamicin, for example, is an effective prophylactic agent for biliary surgery even though MICs are rarely achieved in the bile (99,100). Other antibiotics, including erythromycin, chloramphenicol, metronidazole, and clindamycin, are primarily excreted or detoxified in the liver (94,101). Caution should be exercised in the administration of these agents to patients with hepatic dysfunction.

Most antibiotics exhibit poor penetration into pancreatic secretions (94). An exception is chloramphenicol, which exhibits about 50% of its serum concentration in pancreatic juice. The "blood–pancreatic barrier" is reduced for some agents in the setting of acute pancreatitis (4,94,102,103).

Some of the common mistakes associated with antibiotic prophylaxis of GI procedures are summarized in Table 76.4.

TABLE 76.4. COMMON ERRORS IN THE ADMINISTRATION OF SYSTEMIC PERIOPERATIVE PROPHYLAXIS

Selection of an antibiotic that is not active against the important pathogens
Administering the initial dose too early ("on call") or too late
Failure to administer additional intraoperative doses during long operations
Continuing prophylaxis for longer than necessary

Adverse Effects

Complications of perioperative prophylaxis for the patient include pseudomembranous colitis from overgrowth of *Clostridium difficile,* allergic reactions, and bleeding problems induced by the methylthiotetrazole side chain of some of the cephalosporin antibiotics (94,104). The routine use of prophylaxis also has implications for the entire hospital and appears to correlate with the development of increased resistance among common nosocomial pathogens. Not surprisingly, antibiotic prophylaxis increases the prevalence and quantity of antibiotic-resistant bacteria among the patient's skin and GI flora (105–107).

ANIMAL MODEL STUDIES OF PROPHYLAXIS AND EARLY THERAPY

The role of coliforms and anaerobes in abdominal sepsis has been elucidated in a rat model that simulates sepsis after colonic perforation and involves an intraperitoneal challenge with pooled cecal contents in a gelatin capsule placed via a midline abdominal incision (108–110). Without treatment, acute peritonitis and septicemia from coliforms caused rapid death in 35% to 45% of the animals, and all survivors developed abscesses with anaerobes as the predominant organisms. Different antibiotics, started 4 hours after inoculation and continued for 10 days, vary markedly in the ability to prevent early peritonitis or mortality versus abscess formation. In general, agents active against *E. coli* and other coliforms prevent early peritonitis and death, whereas drugs active against *B. fragilis* reduce abscess formation. Optimal results have been observed with regimens active against both coliforms and *B. fragilis.*

SUMMARY OF CLINICAL TRIALS AND RECOMMENDATIONS

Gastroduodenal Surgery

Pathogens including *E. coli, Klebsiella* species, enterococci, *S. aureus,* and anaerobes frequently can be isolated from the gastric lumen of patients at the time of gastric surgery. In one study, 90% of patients with gastric carcinoma or gastric ulcers were colonized, compared with only 17% of patients

TABLE 76.5. RECOMMENDATIONS FOR PROPHYLACTIC ANTIBIOTICS IN GASTROINTESTINAL SURGERY

Operative Site	Indication	Antibiotic	Dose, Route, and Duration[a]
Gastroduodenal	All patients[b]	Cefazolin	1–2 g; preinduction of anesthesia
Biliary	High-risk patient[c]	Cefazolin	1–2 g; preinduction of anesthesia
Appendectomy	All patients	Cefoxitin, cefotetan, or cefmetazole	1–2 g; preinduction of anesthesia
Colorectal	Elective[d]	Neomycin and erythromycin base	1 g of each at 1, 2, and 11 p.m. on the day before surgery
	Emergency, trauma, or for patients unable to take by mouth, Cefoxitin, cefotetan, or cefmetazole		1–2 g initially; postoperative doses may be given if surgical findings suggest infection

[a]Intraoperative doses of parenteral agents should be administered during long procedures.
[b]Efficacy established only for "high-risk" patients with abnormalities in gastrointestinal motility or gastric acidity, including gastric carcinoma or ulcer, obstruction, bleeding, achlorhydria, or hypochlorhydria.
[c]Includes patients older than 60 years or with acute cholecystitis, obstructive jaundice, or common duct stones.
[d]See Table 76.6 for conditions for which systemic antibiotics should be added to oral prophylaxis.

undergoing surgery for duodenal ulcers (71). In general, the greatest risk factor for wound infection after gastroduodenal surgery is a breakdown in normal gastric acid secretion, and prophylaxis is clearly indicated for patients with clinical conditions associated with decreased gastric acidity or abnormal motility (111). Patients undergoing gastric bypass surgery for morbid obesity also have high wound infection rates, which can be reduced with cefazolin prophylaxis (112). Although the benefit of giving prophylaxis to patients outside of these risk groups is unproven, it is commonly done. The prophylactic regimen should be directed primarily against coliforms; however, activity against gram-positive anaerobes and aerobes, including *S. aureus,* has been emphasized (24,111,113). Cefazolin, cefamandole, and cefuroxime appear to be as effective as antibiotics with activity against *B. fragilis* (114,115) (Table 76.5).

Biliary Tract Surgery

Although bile usually is sterile, 17% to 48% of patients undergoing biliary tract surgery have bacteria isolated from intraoperative cultures (64,98,116,117), and 90% of all wound infections occur in patients with infected bile (118). The major pathogens are aerobic, including *E. coli, Klebsiella* species, *Proteus* species, streptococci, and enterococci. Anaerobes are isolated infrequently, although *C. perfringens* is occasionally found. There is a strong correlation between the bacterial species isolated from preoperative bile cultures and blood cultures among patients with postcholecystectomy septicemia (98).

Historically, the decision to administer prophylactic antibiotics in biliary surgery has been based on risk stratification for the likelihood of positive bile cultures (15). Patients are at higher risk of infection at ages older than 60 years or with previous biliary tract surgery, common duct stones, and acute symptoms or laboratory abnormalities (e.g., elevated serum bilirubin level or white blood cell count) (119,120). In this setting, the preoperative administration of an antibiotic with activity against aerobic flora, such as cefazolin, reduces the risk of infection (98,119, 121). The risk of infection without antibiotic prophylaxis among uncomplicated patients undergoing elective cholecystectomy is small and routine prophylaxis has not been shown to be beneficial (60,119,122); however, many surgeons now routinely administer antibiotics to all patients undergoing biliary tract surgery regardless of risk (15).

Although the studies are not completely consistent, expanding the spectrum of coverage to include anaerobic bacteria or enterococci does not appear to reduce the risk of infection further. Most studies comparing cefazolin, cephalothin, or cefamandole with cefoxitin, cefotetan, or newer agents with broad antibacterial activity have demonstrated equivalent efficacy (114,121). The efficacy of single-dose regimens and that of multiple-dose regimens are equivalent in most studies (121). Gentamicin is also effective and may be administered to patients who are allergic to β-lactams (99).

Whether antibiotic prophylaxis is needed during the postoperative manipulation of T tubes remaining in the biliary tract has not been evaluated prospectively. The bile is usually colonized with *E. coli, Klebsiella pneumoniae,* or enterococci in this clinical setting, however, and septicemia with the same species occurs in up to 9% of patients undergoing postoperative T-tube cholangiography (123,124). Culturing the bile before performing cholangiography and tailoring the prophylaxis to cover the bacterial strains that are isolated appear to be prudent precautions in this setting.

Laparoscopic cholecystectomy has been increasingly performed. A retrospective analysis of 77,604 procedures identified damage to the bile ducts as the major complication, and infection appears to be uncommon (125). The role of antibiotic prophylaxis has not been established (50). Furthermore, the clinical consequences of trocar wound infection are less than those of infection of a large laparotomy incision, providing a strong rationale for giving prophylaxis only to high-risk patients.

Appendectomy

Antibiotics are clearly efficacious in patients undergoing surgery for appendicitis with perforation; in this setting, the patient already has established infection and the antibiotic course should be regarded as therapeutic, rather than prophylactic (126,127). Although the benefits to the patient of perioperative antibiotics for appendicitis without perforation are less clear (128–130), such controversy is rendered academic by the imprecision of clinical discrimination before surgery between disease with perforation and that without perforation (126,131). The current standard of care is to provide prophylaxis to all patients undergoing surgery for possible appendicitis. Because such surgery usually is performed under emergent conditions, peroral prophylaxis is not feasible and parenteral agents should be used. The antibiotic regimen should have activity against both aerobic and anaerobic bacteria, and various regimens have been shown to be efficacious (126,132,133). A regimen of one to three doses is appropriate, unless there is evidence of gangrenous appendicitis or abscess formation at surgery; in which case, a therapeutic course of antibiotics to treat active infection should be continued for at least 3 to 5 days.

Colorectal Surgery

Although colorectal surgery without antibiotic prophylaxis or with inappropriate agents is associated with infection rates up to 30% to 60%, fewer than 10% of patients receiving appropriate prophylaxis develop infection (5,126). Three basic approaches to prophylaxis are accepted for routine use: oral agents in combination with mechanical cleansing, parenteral prophylaxis, or a combination of both. The regimen should have activity against both aerobic and anaerobic bacteria (126,134).

Mechanical preparation of the colon and the use of oral antibiotics, together with mechanical cleansing, have been in practice longer than the routine use of systemic perioperative prophylaxis. Sulfanilamide was employed in colonic surgery by the late 1930s (84), at least 20 years before the pioneering work of Miles et al. (30) and Burke (31) that led to the widespread acceptance of systemic antibiotic prophylaxis in surgery. Effective preparation of the colon is essential to the success of the oral prophylactic regimens; however, mechanical preparation without antibiotics reduces fecal bulk without altering the concentration of bacteria in the colon (135). Older procedures included the use of liquid diets, cathartics, and enemas for up to 3 days; however, the more recent use of isotonic lavage appears comparable in its ability to remove feces and fluid (86,87).

A recent evaluation of the studies that employed a randomized, prospective design and that included a sufficient number of patients to achieve statistical validity concluded that the lowest infection rates, from 3% to 9%, were observed among the trials that included an oral regimen, with or without systemic prophylaxis (126). The oral regimens are appropriate only for nonemergent procedures in which antibiotics can be administered on the afternoon and evening before the surgery and for which sufficient time is available for mechanical cleansing of the colon by cathartics, enemas, or isotonic lavage. Although the combination of erythromycin and neomycin (1 g of each component at 1 p.m., 2 p.m., and 11 p.m. the day before surgery) is the most carefully evaluated regimen in the United States (136–138), kanamycin has been substituted for neomycin, and metronidazole for erythromycin, with apparently similar efficacy (139–141). The addition of a systemic cephalosporin to oral erythromycin–neomycin is particularly indicated in certain clinical settings (Table 76.6) (126). Several parenteral regimens have been shown to be efficacious, including cefoxitin, cefotetan, and cefmetazole (89,142–146). Single-dose systemic prophylaxis appears to be just as efficacious as multiple-dose regimens, except among patients with inflammatory bowel disease (144,145,147).

TABLE 76.6. CONDITIONS FOR WHICH SYSTEMIC ANTIBIOTICS SHOULD BE ADDED TO ORAL PROPHYLAXIS IN COLORECTAL SURGERY

The mechanical preparation is incomplete
Surgery lasting longer than 3.5 h
Surgery has been delayed substantially
Procedures involving rectal resection
Intestinal contents spill during the procedure
Surgery involving a site distal to an established colostomy[a]

[a]Oral antibiotics do not reach high intraluminal concentrations at sites distal to the colostomy.

Prophylaxis For Other Gastrointestinal Surgery And Procedures

Laparotomy

Data are not available to recommend prophylaxis for laparotomy, the division of adhesions, and other abdominal surgery in which a hollow viscus is not opened.

Small-bowel Surgery

Although the duodenum, jejunum, and upper ileum are normally sterile, fecal organisms can be found in large numbers in the setting of obstruction. Although randomized prospective studies to establish the efficacy of prophylaxis in this clinical setting have not been performed, it appears prudent to administer systemic antibiotics that cover both aerobic and anaerobic bacteria (148).

Percutaneous Endoscopic Gastrostomy

Cefazolin appears to be superior to placebo in preventing peristomal wound infections after percutaneous endoscopic gastrostomy (149). Single-dose prophylaxis is sufficient (150).

Liver Transplantation

During the first few weeks after liver transplantation, patients are at high risk for the development of infections caused by aerobic gram-negative bacilli and *Candida* species (151,152). In an effort to reduce the incidence of infection below that achieved with perioperative systemic prophylaxis alone, selective decontamination of the GI flora with nonabsorbable oral antibiotics such as gentamicin, polymyxin, and nystatin has been advocated (153–155). However, no controlled trials have been done to study the efficacy of such regimens in preventing infection in patients undergoing liver transplantation. Because it may take days to weeks to achieve selective bowel decontamination and because of the impairment of gut peristalsis by surgery, it appears prudent to begin administering the oral regimen several days before the transplant liver is obtained (153). Perioperative systemic prophylaxis should have broad activity against coliforms. Cefotaxime (2 g intravenously starting immediately before surgery and repeated every 6 hours during and every 8 hours after surgery for 48 hours) is an acceptable regimen (153).

Cost Considerations

The primary reason for administering prophylactic antibiotics in surgery is to prevent wound infection. Aside from this obvious benefit to the patient, however, the routine employment of prophylaxis has important cost implications for the institution.

Any assessment of the economic impact of surgical prophylaxis must balance the costs involved in purchasing and administering antibiotics with the costs of managing the infections that would have occurred if prophylaxis had not been given (156). The cost of antibiotic prophylaxis is considerable: It is estimated that one-third of all inpatient antibiotic use is for surgical prophylaxis (157,158).

In addition, surgical infections are costly. Surgical wound infections account for about 25% of all nosocomial infections yet are responsible for 50% of infection-related costs (156). As many as 71% of all nosocomial infections occur in patients who have undergone surgery (159). For patients undergoing uncomplicated GI surgery, the extra expenses attributable to the management of nosocomial infection represent 6.8% of all patient-related costs (160).

There is a general consensus that the benefits of perioperative prophylaxis in the selected operations in which it is efficacious far outweigh the costs and consequences of this practice (156,171).

REFERENCES

1. Lyons AS, Petrucelli RJ II. *Medicine: an illustrated history.* New York: Abradale Press, Harry N. Abrams Inc, Publishers, 1987.
2. Bucknall TE. Factors affecting the development of surgical wound infections: a surgeon's view. *J Hosp Infect* 1985;6:1–8.
3. Bartlett JG. Anaerobic bacteria: general concepts. In: Mandell GL, Douglas RG, Bennett JE, eds. *Principles and practice of infectious diseases,* third edition. New York: Churchill Livingstone, 1990;1828–1842.
4. Thadepalli H, Mandal AK. *Antimicrobial therapy in abdominal surgery: precepts and practices.* Boca Raton, FL: CRC Press, 1991.
5. Baum ML, Anish DS, Chalmers TC, et al. A survey of clinical trials of antibiotic prophylaxis in colon surgery: evidence against further use of no-treatment controls. *N Engl J Med* 1981;305: 795–799.
6. Kaiser AB. Antimicrobial prophylaxis in surgery. *N Engl J Med* 1986;315:1129–1138.
7. Altemeier WA, Burke JF, Pluitt BA Jr, et al. *Manual on control of infection in surgical patients.* Philadelphia: JB Lippincott Co, 1976.
8. Simmons BP. CDC guidelines on infection control. *Infect Control* 1982;3:187–196.
9. Raahave D, Friis-Moller A, Bjerre-Jepsen K, et al. The infective dose of aerobic and anaerobic bacteria in postoperative wound sepsis. *Arch Surg* 1986;121:924–929.
10. Houang ET, Ahmet Z. Intraoperative wound contamination during abdominal hysterectomy. *J Hosp Infect* 1991;19:181–189.
11. Haley RW, Culver DH, Morgan WM, et al. Identifying patients at high risk of surgical wound infection: a simple multivariate index of patient susceptibility and wound contamination. *Am J Epidemiol* 1985;121:206–215.
12. Culver DH, Horan TC, Gaynes RP, et al. Surgical wound infection rates by wound class, operative procedure, and patient risk index. *Am J Med* 1991;91[Suppl 3B]:152S–157S.
13. Centers for Disease Control and Prevention. Semiannual report: aggregated data from the National Nosocomial Infection Surveillance (NNIS) System. December 1999. Available at: www.cdc.gov/ncidod/hip/NNIS/dec99sar.pdf.
14. Siegman-Igra Y, Rozin R, Simchen E. Determinants of wound infections in gastrointestinal operations: the Israeli study of surgical infections. *J Clin Epidemiol* 1993;46:133–140.
15. Page CP, Bohnen JMA, Fletcher JR, et al. Antimicrobial prophylaxis for surgical wounds: guidelines for clinical care. *Arch Surg* 1993;128:79–88.
16. Elek SD, Conen PE. The virulence of *Staphylococcus pyogenes* for man. A study of the problems of wound infection. *Br J Exp Pathol* 1958;38:573–586.
17. Kernodle DS, Kaiser AB. Postoperative infections and antimicrobial prophylaxis. In: Mandell GL, Bennett JE, Dolin R, eds. *Mandell, Douglas, and Bennett's principles and practice of infectious diseases,* fifth edition. New York: Churchill Livingstone, 2000:3177–3191.
18. Cruse PJE, Foord R. The epidemiology of wound infection: a ten-year prospective study of 63,939 wounds. *Surg Clin North Am* 1980;60:187–196.
19. Nichols RL, Smith JW. Intragastric microbial colonization in common disease states of the stomach and duodenum. *Ann Surg* 1975;182:557–561.
20. Gatehouse D, Dimock F, Burdon DW, et al. Prediction of wound sepsis following gastric operations. *Br J Surg* 1978;65:551–554.
21. Broido PW, Gorbach SL, Condon RE, et al. Upper intestinal microflora control, effects of gastric acid and vagal denervation on bacterial concentrations. *Arch Surg* 1973;106:90–93.

22. Irvin TT, Goligher JC. Aetiology of disruption of intestinal anastomosis. *Br J Surg* 1973;60:461–464.
23. Cohen SR, Cornell CN, Collins MH, et al. Healing of ischemic colonic anastomoses in the rat: role of antibiotic preparation. *Surgery* 1985;4:443–447.
24. Coppa GF, Eng K, Gough TH, et al. Parenteral and oral antibiotics in elective and rectal surgery. A prospective, randomized trial. *Am J Surg* 1983;145:62–65.
25. Tartter PI. Determinants of postoperative stay in patients with colorectal cancer. Implications for diagnostic-related groups. *Dis Colon Rectum* 1988;31:694–698.
26. Pinto V, Baldonedo R, Nicolas C, et al. Relationship of transfusion and infectious complications after gastric carcinoma operations. *Transfusion* 1991;31:114–118.
27. Mezrow CK, Bergstein I, Tartter PI. Postoperative infection following autologous and homologous blood transfusions. *Transfusion* 1992;32:27–30.
28. Blumberg N, Heal JM. The transfusion immunomodulation theory: the Th1/Th2 paradigm and an analogy with pregnancy as a unifying mechanism. *Semin Hematol* 1996;33:329–340.
29. Nagachinta T, Stephens M, Reitz B. Risk factors for surgical-wound infection following cardiac surgery. *J Infect Dis* 1987; 156:967–973.
30. Miles AA, Miles EM, Burke J. The value and duration of defense mechanisms to the primary lodgement of bacteria. *Br J Exp Pathol* 1957;38:79–86.
31. Burke JF. The effective period of preventive antibiotic action in experimental incisions and dermal lesions. *Surgery* 1961;50: 161–168.
32. Stone HH, Hooper CA, Kolb LD, et al. Antibiotic prophylaxis in gastric, biliary and colonic surgery. *Ann Surg* 1976;184: 443–452.
33. Classen DCM, Evans RS, Pestotnik SL, et al. The timing of prophylactic administration of antibiotics and the risk of surgical-wound infection. *N Engl J Med* 1992;326:281–286.
34. Hau T. Bacteria, toxins and the peritoneum. *World J Surg* 1990; 14:167–175.
35. Skau T, Nystrom PO, Ohman L, et al. The kinetics of peritoneal clearance of *Escherichia coli* and *Bacteroides fragilis* and participating defense mechanisms. *Arch Surg* 1986;121: 1033–1039.
36. Dunn DL, Berke RA, Ewald DC, et al. Macrophages and translymphatic absorption represent the first line of host defense of the peritoneal cavity. *Arch Surg* 1987;122:105–110.
37. Hershman MJ, Cheadle WG, Kuftinec D, et al. An outcome predictive score for sepsis and death following trauma. *Injury* 1988;19:263–266.
38. Cheadle WG, Hershman MJ, Wellhausen SR, et al. HLA-DR antigen expression on peripheral blood monocytes correlates with surgical infection. *Am J Surg* 1991;161:639–645.
39. Bjornson AB, Altemeier WA, Bjornson SH. Comparison of the in vitro bactericidal activity of human serum and leukocytes against *Bacteroides fragilis* and *Fusobacterium mortiferum* in aerobic and anaerobic environments. *Infect Immun* 1976;14: 843–847.
40. Bjornson AB, Bjornson HS. Participation of immunoglobulin and the alternative complement pathway in opsonization of *Bacteroides fragilis* and *Bacteroides thetaiotaomicron. J Infect Dis* 1978;138:351–358.
41. Mandell GL. Bactericidal activity of aerobic and anaerobic polymorphonuclear neutrophils. *Infect Immun* 1974;9:337–341.
42. Wetherall BL, Pruull H, McDonald PJ. Oxygen-independent killing of *Bacteroides fragilis* by granule extracts from human polymorphonuclear leukocytes. *Infect Immun* 1984;43: 1080–1084.
43. Edmiston CE, Gohen MP, Kornhall S, et al. Fecal peritonitis: microbial adherence to serosal mesothelium and resistance to peritoneal lavage. *World J Surg* 1990;14:176–183.
44. Rotstein OD, Kao J. Prevention of intra-abdominal abscesses by fibrinolysis using recombinant tissue plasminogen activator. *J Infect Dis* 1988;158:766–772.
45. Hensler T, Heckler H, Heeg K, et al. Distinct mechanisms of immunosuppression as a consequence of major surgery. *Infect Immun* 1997;65:2283–2291.
46. El-Maallem H, Fletcher J. Effects of surgery on neutrophil granulocyte function. *Infect Immun* 1981;32:38–41.
47. Moelleken BRW, Mathes SJ, Amerhauser A, et al. An adverse wound environment activates leukocytes prematurely. *Arch Surg* 1991;126:225–230.
48. Galandiuk S, Appel SH, Polk HC Jr. A biologic basis for altered host defenses in surgically infected abscesses. *Ann Surg* 1993; 217:624–633.
49. Dellinger EP, Babineau TJ, Bleicher P, et al. Effect of PGG-glucan on the rate of serious postoperative infection or death observed after high-risk gastrointestinal operations. *Arch Surg* 1999;134:977–983.
50. Targarona EM, Balagué C, Knook MM, et al. Laparoscopic surgery and surgical infection. *Br J Surg* 2000;87:536–544.
51. Fisher MC, Balurate HJ, Long SS. Bacteremia due to *Bacteroides fragilis* after elective appendectomy in renal transplant recipients. *J Infect Dis* 1981;143:635–638.
52. McConville JH, Snyder MJ, Calia FM, et al. Model of intraabdominal abscess in mice. *Infect Immun* 1981;31:507–509.
53. Gollapudi SV, Gupta A, Thadepalli H, et al. Use of lymphokines in treatment of experimental intra-abdominal abscess caused by *Bacteroides fragilis. Infect Immun* 1988;56: 2369–2372.
54. Onderdonk AB, Markham RB, Zaleznik DF, et al. Evidence of T cell-dependent immunity to *Bacteroides fragilis* in an intraabdominal abscess model. *J Clin Invest* 1982;69:9–16.
55. Zaleznik DF, Finberg RW, Shapiro ME, et al. A soluble suppressor T cell factor protects against experimental intraabdominal abscesses. *J Clin Invest* 1985;75:1023–1027.
56. Finlay-Jones JJ, Kenney PA, Nulsen MF, et al. Pathogenesis of intraabdominal abscess formation: abscess-potentiating agents and inhibition of complement-dependent opsonization of abscess-inducing bacteria. *J Infect Dis* 1991;164:1173–1179.
57. Giannella RP, Broitman SA, Zamcheck N. Gastric acid barrier to ingested microorganisms in man: studies *in vivo* and *in vitro. Gut* 1972;13:251–256.
58. Drasar BS, Hill MJ. *Human intestinal flora.* London: Academic Press, 1974.
59. Lou MA, Mandal AK, Alexander JL, et al. Bacteriology of the human biliary tract and the duodenum. *Arch Surg* 1977;112: 965–967.
60. Farnell MB, van Heerden JA, Beart RW Jr. Elective cholecystectomy. The role of biliary bacteriology and administration of antibiotics. *Arch Surg* 1981;116:537–540.
61. Claesson BE, Holmlund DEW, Matzsch TW. Microflora of the gallbladder related to duration of acute cholecystitis. *Surg Gynecol Obstet* 1986;162:531–535.
62. Shimada K, Inamatsu T, Yamashiro M. Anaerobic bacteria in biliary disease in elderly patients. *J Infect Dis* 1977;135:850–854.
63. Thadepalli H, Chuah SK, Bansal MB, et al. The effect of human bile on *Bacteroides fragilis* in health and disease. *Microbios* 1988;55:17–24.
64. Willis RG, Lawson WC, Hoare EM, et al. Are bile bacteria relevant to septic complications following biliary surgery? *Br J Surg* 1984;71:845–849.
65. Gorbach SL, Plaut AG, Nahas L, et al. Studies of intestinal microflora, II. Microorganisms of the small intestine and their relations to oral and fecal flora. *Gastroenterology* 1967;53:856–867.

66. Thadepalli H, Lou MA, Bach VT, et al. Microflora of the human small intestine. *Am J Surg* 1979;138:845–850.
67. Sykes PA, Boulter KH, Schofield PF. Alterations in small-bowel microflora in acute intestinal obstruction. *J Med Microbiol* 1976;9:13–22.
68. Bennion RS, Thompson JE, Baron EJ, et al. Gangrenous and perforated appendicitis with peritonitis: treatment and bacteriology. *Clin Ther* 1990;12[Suppl C]:31–44.
69. Morris DL, Rodgers Wilson S, Pain J, et al. A comparison of aztreonam/metronidazole and cefotaxime/metronidazole in elective colorectal surgery: antimicrobial prophylaxis must include gram-positive cover. *J Antimicrob Chemother* 1990;25:673–678.
70. Calia FM, Wolinsky E, Mortimer EA Jr, et al. Importance of the carrier state as a source of *Staphylococcus aureus* in wound sepsis. *J Hyg (London)* 1969;67:49–57.
71. Stone HH. Gastric surgery. *South Med J* 1977;70:35–37.
72. Morran C, McNaught W, McArdle CS. Prophylactic cotrimoxazole in biliary surgery. *Br Med J* 1978;2:462–464.
73. Yellin AE, Heseltine PN, Berne TV, et al. The role of *Pseudomonas* species in patients treated with ampicillin and sulbactam for gangrenous and perforated appendicitis. *Surg Gynecol Obstet* 1985;161:303–307.
74. Willey SH, Hindes RG, Eliopoulos GM, et al. Effects of clindamycin and gentamicin and other antimicrobial combinations against enterococci in an experimental model of intra-abdominal abscess. *Surg Gynecol Obstet* 1989;169:199–202.
75. Gorbach SL, Thadepalli H. Clindamycin in pure and mixed anaerobic infections. *Arch Intern Med* 1974;134:87–92.
76. Matlow AG, Bohnen JMA, Nohr C, et al. Pathogenicity of enterococci in a rat model of fecal peritonitis. *J Infect Dis* 1989; 160:142–145.
77. Garrison RN, Fry DE, Berberich S, et al. Enterococcal bacteremia: clinical implications and determinants of death. *Ann Surg* 1983;196:43–47.
78. Dajani AS, Bisno AL, Chung KJ, et al. Prevention of bacterial endocarditis. Recommendations by the American Heart Association. *JAMA* 1990;264:2919–2922.
79. Sahm DF, Tenover FC. Surveillance for the emergence and dissemination of antimicrobial resistance in bacteria. *Infect Dis Clin North Am* December 1997;11(4):767–783.
80. Coudron PE, Moland ES, Sanders CC. Occurrence and detection of extended-spectrum β-lactamases in members of the family Enterobacteriaceae at a veterans medical center: seek and you may find. *J Clin Microbiol* 1997;35:2593–2597.
81. Rice LB, Yao JDC, Klimm K, et al. Efficacy of different β-lactams against an extended-spectrum β-lactamase-producing *Klebsiella pneumoniae* strain in the rat intra-abdominal abscess model. *Antimicrob Agents Chemother* 1991;35:1243–1244.
82. Pitt HA, Postier RG, Gadacz TR, et al. The role of topical antibiotics in "high-risk" biliary surgery. *Surgery* 1982;91:518–524.
83. Freischlag J, McGrattan M, Busuttil RW. Topical versus systemic cephalosporin administration in elective biliary operations. *Surgery* 1984;96:686–693.
84. Garlock JH, Seley GP. The use of sulfanilamide in surgery of the colon and rectum. Preliminary report. *Surgery* 1939;5:787–790.
85. Seley GP, Colp R. The bacteriology of peptic ulcers and gastric malignancies: possible bearing on complications following gastric surgery. *Surgery* 1941;10:369–380.
86. Soballe PW, Greif JM. Preoperative whole-gut lavage vs. traditional three-day bowel preparation in left colon surgery. *Mil Med* 1989;154:198–201.
87. Fleites RA, Marshall JB, Eckhauser ML, et al. The efficacy of polyethylene glycol-electrolyte lavage solution versus traditional mechanical bowel preparation for elective colonic surgery: a randomized, prospective, blinded clinical trial. *Surgery* 1985;98: 708–717.
88. Redington J, Ebert SC, Craig WA. Role of antimicrobial pharmacokinetics and pharmacodynamics in surgical prophylaxis. *Rev Infect Dis* 1991;13[Suppl 10]:S790–S799.
89. Kaiser AB, Herrington JL Jr, Jacobs JK, et al. Cefoxitin versus erythromycin, neomycin, and cefazolin in colorectal operations: importance of the duration of the surgical procedure. *Ann Surg* 1983;198:525–530.
90. Ehrenkranz NJ. Antimicrobial prophylaxis in surgery: mechanisms, misconceptions, and mischief. *Infect Control Hosp Epidemiol* 1993;14:99–106.
91. Brogard JM, Dorner M, Pinget M, et al. The biliary excretion of cefazolin. *J Infect Dis* 1975;131:625–633.
92. Pitt HA, Roberts RB, Johnson WD Jr. Gentamicin levels in the human biliary tract. *J Infect Dis* 1979;127:299–302.
93. Hansbrough JF, Clark JE. Concentrations of cefoxitin in gallbladder bile of cholecystectomy patients. *Antimicrob Agents Chemother* 1982;22:709–710.
94. Kucers A, Bennett NMcK. *The use of antibiotics: a comprehensive review with clinical emphasis,* fourth edition. Philadelphia: JB Lippincott Co, 1987.
95. McLeish AR, Strachan CJL, Powis SJA, et al. The influence of biliary disease on the excretion of cefazolin in human bile. *Surgery* 1977;81:426–430.
96. Brown RB, Martyak SN, Barza M, et al. Penetration of clindamycin phosphate into the abnormal human biliary tract. *Ann Intern Med* 1976;84:168–170.
97. Mortimer PR, Mackie DB, Haynes S. Ampicillin levels in human bile in the presence of biliary tract disease. *Br Med J* 1969;3:88–89.
98. Kanter MA, Geelhoed GW. Biliary antibiotics; clinical utility in biliary surgery. *South Med J* 1987;80:1007–1015.
99. Keighley MRB, Baddeley RM, Burden DW, et al. A controlled trial of parenteral prophylactic gentamicin therapy in biliary surgery. *Br J Surg* 1975;62:275–279.
100. Kaufman Z, Engelberg M, Eliashiv A, et al. Systemic prophylactic antibiotics in elective biliary surgery. *Arch Surg* 1984;119: 1002–1004.
101. Davey PG. Pharmacokinetics in liver disease. *J Antimicrob Chemother* 1988;21:1–5.
102. Burns GP, Stein TA, Kabnick LS. Blood–pancreatic juice barrier to antibiotic excretion. *Am J Surg* 1986;151:205–208.
103. Trudel JL, Mutch DO, Brown PR, et al. Antibiotic therapy for pancreatic sepsis: differences in bioactive blood and tissue levels. *Surg Forum* 1982;33:26.
104. Block BS, Mercer LJ, Ismail MA, et al. *Clostridium difficile*-associated diarrhea follows perioperative prophylaxis with cefoxitin. *Am J Obstet Gynecol* 1986;153:835–838.
105. Roberts NJ Jr, Douglas RG Jr. Gentamicin use and *Pseudomonas* and *Serratia* resistance: effect of a surgical prophylaxis regimen. *Antimicrob Agents Chemother* 1978;13:214–220.
106. Archer GL, Armstrong BC. Alteration of staphylococcal flora in cardiac surgery patients receiving antibiotic prophylaxis. *J Infect Dis* 1983;147:642–649.
107. Kernodle DS, Barg NL, Kaiser AB. Low-level colonization of hospitalized patients with methicillin-resistant coagulase-negative staphylococci and emergence of the organisms during surgical antimicrobial prophylaxis. *Antimicrob Agents Chemother* 1988;32:202–208.
108. Weinstein WM, Onderdonk AB, Bartlett JG, et al. Experimental intra-abdominal abscesses in rats: development of an experimental model. *Infect Immun* 1974;10:1250–1255.
109. Onderdonk AB, Bartlett JG, Louie T, et al. Microbial synergy in experimental abscess. *Infect Immun* 1976;13:22–26.
110. Bartlett JG, Louie TJ, Gorbach SL, et al. Therapeutic efficacy of 29 antimicrobial regimens in experimental intraabdominal sepsis. *Rev Infect Dis* 1981;3:535–542.

111. Nichols RL, Webb WR, Jones JW, et al. Efficacy of antibiotic prophylaxis in high risk gastroduodenal operations. *Am J Surg* 1982;143:94–98.
112. Pories WL, van Rij AM, Burlingham BT, et al. Prophylactic cefazolin in gastric bypass surgery. *Surgery* 1981;90:426–432.
113. Lewis RT, Allan CM, Goodall RG, et al. Discriminate use of antibiotic prophylaxis in gastroduodenal surgery. *Am J Surg* 1979;138:640–643.
114. Leaper DJ, Cooper MJ, Turner A. A comparative trial between cefotetan and cephazolin for wound sepsis prophylaxis during penetration into the obstructed biliary tree. *J Hosp Infect* 1986; 7:269–276.
115. Morris DL, Young D, Burdon DW, et al. Prospective randomized trial of single dose cefuroxime against mezlocillin in elective gastric surgery. *J Hosp Infect* 1984;5:200–204.
116. Mason GR. Bacteriology and antibiotic selection in biliary tract surgery. *Arch Surg* 1968;97:533–537.
117. Pyrtek LJ, Bartus SA. An evaluation of antibiotics in biliary tract surgery. *Surg Gynecol Obstet* 1967;125:101–105.
118. Nielsen ML, Moesgaard F, Justesen T, et al. Wound sepsis after elective cholecystectomy: restriction of prophylactic antibiotics to risk groups. *Scand J Gastroenterol* 1981;16:937–940.
119. Elliott DW. Biliary tract surgery. *South Med J* 1977;70:31–35.
120. Thompson JE Jr, Bennion RS, Doty JE, et al. Predictive factors for bactibilia in acute cholecystitis. *Arch Surg* 1990;125: 261–264.
121. Meijer WS, Schmitz PIM, Jeekel J. Meta-analysis of randomized, controlled clinical trials of antibiotic prophylaxis in biliary tract surgery. *Br J Surg* 1990;77:283–290.
122. Chetlin SH, Elliot DW. Preoperative antibiotics in biliary surgery. *Arch Surg* 1973;107:319–323.
123. Keighley MRB, Lister DM, Jacobs SI, et al. Hazards of surgical treatment due to microorganisms in the bile. *Surgery* 1974; 75:578–583.
124. Pitt HA, Postier RG, Cameron JL. Postoperative T-tube cholangiography: is antibiotic coverage necessary? *Ann Surg* 1980; 191:30–34.
125. Deziel DJ, Millikan KW, Economou SG, et al. Complications of laparoscopic cholecystectomy: a national survey of 4,292 hospitals and an analysis of 77, 604 cases. *Am J Surg* 1993;165: 9–14.
126. Gorbach SL. Antimicrobial prophylaxis for appendectomy and colorectal surgery. *Rev Infect Dis* 1991;13[Suppl 10]: S815–S820.
127. Krukowski ZH. Preventing wound infection after appendicectomy: a review. *Br J Surg* 1988;75:1023–1033.
128. Lewis FR, Holcroft JW, Boey J, et al. Appendicitis—a critical review of diagnosis and treatment in 1000 cases. *Arch Surg* 1975;110:677.
129. Fine M, Busuttil RW. Acute appendicitis: efficacy of prophylactic pre-operative antibiotics in the reduction of septic morbidity. *Am J Surg* 1978;135:210–212.
130. Coleman RJ, Blackwood JM, Swan KG. Role of antibiotic prophylaxis in surgery for nonperforated appendicitis. *Am Surg* 1987;53:584–586.
131. Browder W, Smith JW, Vivoda LM, et al. Nonperforative appendicitis: a continuing surgical dilemma. *J Infect Dis* 1989; 159:1088–1094.
132. Flannigan GM, Clifford RP, Carver RA, et al. Antibiotic prophylaxis in acute appendicitis. *Surg Gynecol Obstet* 1983;156: 209–211.
133. Foster MC, Kapila L, Morris DL, et al. A randomized comparative study of sulbactam plus ampicillin vs. metronidazole plus cefotaxime in the management of acute appendicitis in children. *Rev Infect Dis* 1986;8[Suppl 5]:S634–S638.
134. The Norwegian Study Group for Colorectal Surgery. Should antimicrobial prophylaxis in colorectal surgery include agents effective against both anaerobic and aerobic microorganisms? A double-blind, multi-center study. *Surgery* 1985;97:402–407.
135. Nichols RL, Broido P, Condon RE, et al. Effect of preoperative neomycin-erythromycin intestinal preparation on the incidence of infection complications following colon surgery. *Ann Surg* 1973;178:453–462.
136. Clarke JS, Condon RE, Bartlett JG, et al. Preoperative oral antibiotics reduce septic complications of colon operations: results of a prospective randomized, double-blind clinical study. *Ann Surg* 1977;186:251–259.
137. Bartlett JG, Condon RE, Gorbach SL, et al. Veterans Administration Cooperative Study on bowel preparation for elective colorectal operations: impact of oral antibiotic regimen on colonic flora, wound irrigation cultures and bacteriology of septic complications. *Ann Surg* 1978;188:249–254.
138. Condon RE, Bartlett JG, Greenlee H, et al. Efficacy of oral and systemic antibiotic prophylaxis in colorectal operations. *Arch Surg* 1983;118:496–502.
139. Wapnick S, Guinto R, Reizis I, et al. Reduction of postoperative infection in elective colon surgery with preoperative administration of kanamycin and erythromycin. *Surgery* 1979;85: 317–321.
140. Vergnes D, Moatti N. Pre-operative colonic preparation using kanamycin and metronidazole: qualitative and quantitative effects on the bacterial flora of the intestine. *J Antimicrob Chemother* 1980;6:709–716.
141. Washington JA II, Dearing WH, Jedd ES, et al. Effect of preoperative antibiotic regimen on development of infection after intestinal surgery. Prospective, randomized, double-blind study. *Ann Surg* 1974;4:567–572.
142. McDonald PJ, Karran SJ. A comparison of intravenous cefoxitin and a combination of gentamicin and metronidazole as prophylaxis in colorectal surgery. *Dis Colon Rectum* 1983;26: 661–664.
143. Hoffman CEJ, McDonald PJ, Watts JM. Use of preoperative cefoxitin to prevent infection after colonic and rectal surgery. *Ann Surg* 1981;193:353–356.
144. Periti P, Mazzei T, Tonelli F. Single-dose cefotetan vs. multiple-dose cefoxitin—antimicrobial prophylaxis in colorectal surgery. Results of a prospective, multicenter, randomized study. *Dis Colon Rectum* 1989;32:121–127.
145. Jagelman DG, Fabian TC, Nichols RL, et al. Single dose cefotetan versus multiple-dose cefoxitin as prophylaxis in colorectal surgery. *Am J Surg* 1988;155:71–76.
146. Griffith DL, Novak E, Greenwald CA, et al. Clinical experience with cefmetazole sodium in the United States: an overview. *J Antimicrob Chemother* 1989;23[Suppl D]:21–33.
147. Juul P, Klaaborg KE, Kronberg O. Single or multiple doses of metronidazole and ampicillin in elective colorectal surgery. A randomized trial. *Dis Colon Rectum* 1987;30:526–528.
148. Condon RE. Rational use of prophylactic antibiotics in gastrointestinal surgery. *Surg Clin North Am* 1975;55:1309–1318.
149. Jain NK, Larson DE, Schroeder KW, et al. Antibiotic prophylaxis for percutaneous endoscopic gastrostomy: a prospective, randomized, double-blind clinical study. *Ann Intern Med* 1987; 107:824–828.
150. Hollands MJ, Fletcher JP, Young J. Percutaneous feeding gastrostomy. *Med J Aust* 1989;151:328–331.
151. Colonna JO II, Winston DH, Brill JE, et al. Infectious complications in liver transplantation. *Arch Surg* 1988;123:360–364.
152. Kusne SJ, Dummer JS, Singh N, et al. Infections after liver transplantation: an analysis of 101 consecutive cases. *Medicine (Baltimore)* 1988;67:132–143.

153. Arnow PM, Furmaga K, Flaherty JP, et al. Microbiological efficacy and pharmacokinetics of prophylactic antibiotics in liver transplant patients. *Antimicrob Agents Chemother* 1992;36:2125–2130.
154. van Zeijl JH, Kroes ACM, Metselaar HJ, et al. Infections after auxiliary partial liver transplantation. Experiences in the first ten patients. *Infection* 1990;18:146–151.
155. Wiesner RH, Hermans PE, Rakela J, et al. Selective bowel decontamination to decrease gram-negative aerobic bacterial and *Candida* colonization and prevent infection after orthotopic liver transplantation. *Transplantation* 1988;45:570–574.
156. McGowan JE Jr. Cost and benefit of perioperative antimicrobial prophylaxis: methods for economic analysis. *Rev Infect Dis* 1991;13[Suppl 10]:S879–S889.
157. Shapiro M, Townsend TR, Rosner B, et al. Use of antimicrobial drugs in general hospitals: patterns of prophylaxis. *N Engl J Med* 1979;301:351–355.
158. Kaiser AB. Overview of cephalosporin prophylaxis. *Am J Surg* 1988;155[Suppl 5A]:52–55.
159. Tetteroo GWM, Wagenvoort JHT, Bruining HA. Role of selective decontamination in surgery. *Br J Surg* 1992;79:300–304.
160. Fabry J, Meynet R, Joron MT, et al. Cost of nosocomial infections: analysis of 512 digestive surgery patients. *World J Surg* 1982;6:362–365.
161. Liss RH, Batchelor FR. Economic evaluations of antibiotic use and resistance—a perspective: report of Task Force 6. *Rev Infect Dis* 1987;9[Suppl 3]:S297–S312.

77

PHARMACOLOGY OF AGENTS OTHER THAN ANTIMICROBIALS USED IN GASTROINTESTINAL INFECTIONS

RONALD D. SOLTIS

Infections of the hollow gastrointestinal (GI) tract—the esophagus, stomach, small intestine, and colon—may cause various symptoms. Infections of the esophagus may cause painful swallowing (odynophagia) and difficulty swallowing (dysphagia), along with pyrosis (heartburn) and regurgitation. Gastric infections may be associated with nausea and vomiting, epigastric pain, and early satiety due to gastric retention. Infections of the small intestine usually produce diarrhea and abdominal cramping and may result in weight loss due to malabsorption. Colonic infections usually result in diarrhea and lower abdominal cramping and may be associated with hematochezia and tenesmus. Anorectal pain may also be associated with various infections either due to the primary infection or secondary to diarrhea.

Specific therapy of the causative infection is obviously the primary goal in treating these conditions. When this is not possible or when symptomatic response is expected to be delayed, a number of pharmacologic agents are available to treat these symptoms. An understanding of the pathophysiology of these symptoms is important when choosing the appropriate pharmacotherapy.

PATHOPHYSIOLOGY OF GASTROINTESTINAL SYMPTOMS

Systemic Symptoms

The primary role of the GI tract is as a portal of entry for fluids and nutrients and the efficient recovery of these nutrients and the 6 to 10 L of ingested fluids and GI secretions that pass through each day. Diminished fluid intake due to anorexia or nausea or increased fluid loss due to vomiting, diarrhea, or fever may result in dehydration (1). Symptoms and signs of dehydration are classified as mild, moderate, or severe. In mild dehydration, symptoms include thirst and restlessness, with normal physical findings such as pulse and skin turgor. The mucous membranes remain moist. The fluid deficit is less than 50 mL/kg of body weight. Moderate dehydration produces thirst and lethargy. The pulse is weak and rapid, skin turgor is decreased, the urine is dark, respirations are rapid, and mucous membranes are dry. The fluid deficit is between 50 and 80 mL/kg of body weight. Severe dehydration is characterized by lethargy, cyanosis of the extremities, dry mucous membranes, poor skin turgor, and deep rapid respirations. Urine output is nonexistent. Fluid deficit in severe dehydration is often more than 80 mL/kg of body weight (2).

The most important goal in treating dehydration is restoration of fluid and electrolyte balance. The preferable route is oral, using various rehydration solutions that have been developed for this purpose. When this is not feasible or the patient is in shock, intravenous rehydration is mandatory.

Nausea And Vomiting

Nausea and vomiting occur in a variety of GI tract infections. In addition to being unpleasant symptoms, they may lead to complications such as aspiration pneumonia, Mallory–Weiss tears, esophageal rupture, fluid and electrolyte depletion, and malnutrition. GI tract infections may lead to nausea and vomiting through two mechanisms: (a) gastric mucosal irritation due to ingested toxins and inflammatory products and (b) functional or mechanical obstruction of the gastroduodenal outlet.

Three components are recognized: nausea, retching, and vomiting, each associated with changes in GI tract motility. Nausea often precedes vomiting (3). The neural pathways that mediate nausea are not known, but evidence suggests that they are the same pathways that mediate vomiting. Gastric tone is diminished during nausea and gastric peristalsis is diminished or absent, whereas duodenal and prox-

R. D. Soltis: Department of Medicine, University of Minnesota Medical School, Minneapolis, Minnesota imal jejunal tone are increased, resulting in reflux of duodenal contents into the stomach. Retching consists of coordinated contractions of the abdominal wall muscles and opposing spasmodic respiratory movements of the chest wall and diaphragm with the glottis closed. The antrum of the stomach contracts while the fundus and cardia relax. Gastroduodenal contents move retrograde into the esophagus, but the closed glottis prevents vomiting. Vomiting occurs as gastroduodenal contents are ejected through the mouth due to forceful contractions of the abdominal muscles and diaphragm when the cardia of the stomach is raised and the pylorus is contracted (4).

Vomiting involves a complex group of activities controlled by a central neurologic "vomiting center," located in the lateral reticular formation of the medulla. This is most likely a pharmacologic, rather than an anatomic, entity. Afferent impulses to this center are transmitted via the vagus and sympathetic nerves (5,6). A second center in the brainstem, the chemoreceptor trigger zone (CTZ), is located in the area postrema of the medulla in the floor of the fourth ventricle (5–9). Various stimuli induce vomiting by stimulating the CTZ, which activates the vomiting center. The vomiting center, but not the CTZ, is responsive to electrical stimuli. The CTZ responds to a variety of emetic stimuli in the circulation, including enterotoxin derived from gram-positive bacteria, because the blood–brain barrier is virtually nonexistent in the region of the CTZ.

Dopamine, acting through dopamine D_2 receptors in the CTZ or vomiting center, plays a role in mediating vomiting. Thus dopamine receptor antagonists, such as metoclopramide, domperidone, and haloperidol, are effective antiemetics. In addition to dopamine, many other ligands such as neurotransmitters and neuropeptides stimulate the CTZ by binding to specific receptors. One of these ligands, serotonin (5-hydroxytryptamine [5-HT]), binds to 5-HT_3 receptors in the area postrema and the CTZ, inducing vomiting. Orally administered 5-HT_3-receptor antagonists, such as ondansetron and granisetron, are very effective at controlling nausea and vomiting induced by chemotherapy.

The act of vomiting is initiated in the vomiting center, regardless of the stimulus, and efferent pathways include the vagus, phrenic nerves, and the spinal nerves that supply the abdominal muscles.

Dysphagia, Odynophagia, Pyrosis, and Dyspepsia

Infection of the esophagus may result in dysphagia, the sensation of food sticking in the esophagus. This may be mechanical, either from luminal narrowing due to edema or from an esophageal smooth muscle spasm due to inflammation. Severe inflammation of the esophagus, from infections with cytomegalovirus (CMV), herpesvirus, candida, or deep esophageal ulcers associated with AIDS, may produce odynophagia, pain with swallowing.

Helicobacter pylori is the most common gastric infection. In the absence of associated gastric or duodenal ulcers or gastric lymphoma, the chronic infection is asymptomatic. The acute infection may be associated with nausea, vomiting, epigastric pain, and transient achlorhydria, an entity described by Sir William Osler as "acute epidemic achlorhydria." Other bacterial infections of the stomach (phlegmonous gastritis), fungal infections, and mycobacterial infections are rare. In the immunocompromised host, gastric and duodenal infection with CMV may be associated with nausea, vomiting, epigastric pain, or dyspepsia (indigestion) and pyrosis (heartburn) due to gastroesophageal reflux.

Pill-induced esophagitis may cause dysphagia and odynophagia. Medications such as tetracycline, doxycycline, azidothymidine, potassium supplements, nonsteroidal antiinflammatory drugs (NSAIDs), and bisphosphonates are all capable of causing esophageal inflammation, particularly when ingested in the supine position or without adequate fluid intake.

Symptomatic treatment of odynophagia includes the frequent use of liquid antacids and lidocaine (viscous Xylocaine). Secondary acid-peptic injury can be minimized by the use of antacids and gastric antisecretory drugs, along with measures designed to minimize gastroesophageal reflux, such as elevating the head of the bed and avoiding late and large meals. Deep esophageal ulcers associated with AIDS have been responsive to frequent sucralfate slurries (10).

Diarrhea

To the patient, diarrhea is the passage of loose or frequent stools. Pathophysiologically, diarrhea has traditionally been defined as passage of more than 150 to 200 g of stool per day, depending on dietary fiber intake. This definition has been challenged on the grounds that stool consistency best relates to the water-holding capacity of insoluble solids compared with total water content (11). From the practical standpoint, clinically significant loss of water from the intestine is usually readily apparent. Diarrhea results from either increased intestinal water secretion or decreased intestinal water absorption. On average, 9 L of fluid enters the GI tract each day: 2 L from oral intake and 7 L from GI tract secretions. The small intestine absorbs all but about 1,800 to 2,000 mL per day, and the colon absorbs all but about 150 to 200 mL per day. Excess water entering the colon from the small bowel or colonic secretion and/or not absorbed by the colon results in diarrhea.

GI tract infections cause diarrhea by several mechanisms. Acute bacterial diarrhea may be toxigenic, where enterotoxin is the major pathogenic agent, or invasive, where the organism penetrates the mucosal cell surface, but enterotoxins may be produced as well. Diarrheal toxins can be classified as cytotonic, leading to cellular fluid secretion by activation of intracellular enzymes such as adenylate cyclase without damaging the cell surface, or cytotoxic, inducing cell injury and fluid secretion, but not primarily by activating cyclic nucleotides (12). The prototype of toxigenic diarrhea is infection due to *Vibrio cholerae* and enterotoxigenic *Escherichia coli.* (ETEC). These organisms do not invade the mucosa but stick to the cell surface, elaborating an enterotoxin that induces secretion of water, particularly from the duodenum and proximal jejunum where the enterotoxin is most active. Colonic mucosa is unaffected, and colonic water absorption continues but is overwhelmed by the volume of fluid entering it. By contrast, the enterotoxins produced by *Clostridium perfringens,* a common cause of bacterial food poisoning, exerts its maximal effect in the ileum, inhibits glucose transport, damages the intestinal epithelium, and induces protein loss into the lumen, features not seen with *V. cholerae* enterotoxin.

In contrast to toxigenic pathogens, invasive pathogens cause mucosal ulceration with an acute inflammatory infiltrate in the lamina propria. Whereas toxigenic organisms typically exert their effect in the upper small intestine, invasive organisms typically target the distal ileum and colon. *Salmonella, Shigella,* invasive *E. coli, Campylobacter,* and *Yersinia* are the most common pathogens in this class. Three theories have been proposed to explain the mechanism of fluid production in these infections (13):

1. An enterotoxin may be involved, at least in the early phase of the illness.
2. Invasive organisms increase local synthesis of prostaglandins at the sites of intense inflammation, which may induce fluid secretion.
3. Epithelial cell surface damage may prevent reabsorption of fluid from the gut lumen.

Gastroenteritis viruses cause diarrhea not only by inhibiting intestinal epithelial cell fluid absorption due to cell damage, but also in severe forms of infection such as with rotavirus by producing denuded villi and flattening of the mucosa in the upper intestine (14). These changes are accompanied by diminished D-xylose absorption and decreased levels of disaccharidases such as lactase. Transient lactase deficiency is common in viral gastroenteritis and ingestion of lactose during the illness may worsen and prolong the diarrhea due to the osmotic effect of malabsorbed lactose in the colon.

Malabsorption of fatty acids occurs in some GI tract infections with pathogens such as Norwalk virus and *Giardia duodenalis.* In these infections, ingested triglyceride is digested to fatty acids by pancreatic lipase but is not absorbed. In the colon, malabsorbed fatty acids are hydroxylated by colonic bacteria forming hydroxyfatty acids such as ricinoleic acid, potent cathartics that inhibit colonic water absorption and stimulate water secretion. Restriction of dietary fat ingestion often diminishes the diarrhea in these conditions.

Anorectal Disorders

Diarrhea due to GI tract infections may be associated with tenesmus, rectal pain, perianal excoriation, and discomfort. Sexually transmitted diseases of the intestine are associated with anal pain, tenesmus, and rectal bleeding. Perianal condylomata are often painful with minor trauma. Herpetic lesions of the sacral dermatomes may be associated with vesicles and pain in the perianal area.

PHARMACOLOGY AND USE OF SPECIFIC THERAPIES

Antiemetic Drugs

Ideally, treatment of nausea and vomiting should target the cause. When this is not possible or when results of specific therapy are delayed, antiemetic drugs are employed (Table 77.1).

5-HT$_3$-receptor Antagonists

Ondansetron and granisetron exert their effect by blocking 5-HT, both peripherally and on vagal nerve terminals and centrally in the CTZ. Ondansetron can be administered both orally and by intravenous infusion. Effective blood levels appear within 60 minutes after administration. Granisetron is easier to administer. Its onset of action is within 3 minutes

TABLE 77.1. ANTIEMETIC DRUGS

Drug	Adult Dose
Serotonin antagonists	
Ondansetron (Zofran)	32 mg IV in divided dose or 4–8 mg tid PO
Granisetron (Kytril)	10 μg/kg IV or 1 mg bid PO
Phenothiazines	
Prochlorperazine (Compazine)	2.5–10 mg tid or qid PO, IM, or IV
Promethazine (Phenergan)	25 mg bid rectally 12.5–25 mg q4h PO, IM, or IV
Chlorpromazine (Thorazine)	10–25 mg q4-6h PO
Thiethylperazine (Torecan, Norzine)	10 mg 1–3 times daily PO, IM, or rectally
Substituted benzamides	
Trimethobenzamide (Tigan)	250 mg tid or qid PO 200 mg tid or qid IM or rectally
Metoclopramide (Reglan)	5–10 mg qid PO
Cannabinoids	
Dronabinol (Marinol)	5–7.5 mg/m^2 q2-4h PO
Nabilone (Cesamet)	1–2 mg bid or tid PO
Butyrophenones	
Haloperidol (Haldol)	1–5 mg q12h PO, IM, or IV
Droperidol (Inapsine)	2.5–5.0 mg q4-6h IM or IV
Other antiemetics	
Diphenidol (Vontrol)	25–50 mg q4h PO

IV, intravenously; tid, three times a day; PO, orally; bid, twice a day; qid, four times a day; IM, intramuscularly.

of administration. Side effects are minimal, consisting of headache, constipation, diarrhea, and transient elevation in liver enzymes. Although primarily used to treat chemotherapy-induced nausea and vomiting, often in combination with corticosteroids, they have found increasing use in the treatment of nausea and vomiting due to various causes.

Phenothiazines

Prochlorperazine, chlorpromazine, promethazine, and thiethylperazine are effective in treating nausea and vomiting induced by drugs, radiation, and gastroenteritis. They have both anticholinergic and antihistaminic effects, and they block dopamine D_3 receptors in the CTZ and reduce afferent signals to the vomiting center. Sedation is the most common side effect. Extrapyramidal effects (dystonia, torticollis, oculogyric crises, akathisia, and gait disturbances) have been reported with all the phenothiazines.

Substituted Benzamines

Trimethobenzamide is structurally related to the antihistamines but exhibits only weak antihistaminic activity. It appears to directly inhibit stimuli at the CTZ without inhibiting impulses to the vomiting center. Side effects are infrequent. Metoclopramide, a substituted benzamine dopamine D_2 receptor antagonist, is discussed below.

Diphenidol

Diphenidol is an antiemetic agent that is structurally unrelated to the antihistamines and phenothiazines. It is believed to inhibit the CTZ. Because it may cause hallucinations, disorientation, and confusion, its use should be restricted to hospitalized patients or others under close medical supervision.

Cannabinoids

Most often self-prescribed in the form of marijuana, derivatives of tetrahydrocannabinol (dronabinol and nabilone) are moderately effective antiemetics. Hallucinations, mood changes, and disorientation limit their effectiveness. They are rarely indicated in the treatment of acute self-limited nausea and vomiting.

Antacids And Antisecretory Drugs

Gastric parietal cells secrete acid both in the basal state and secondary to a number of stimuli, the most common being food. The basolateral membrane of the parietal cell contains at least four receptors: one each for histamine, gastrin, acetylcholine, and prostaglandin. Binding of these agents to their receptor stimulates acid secretion. At the luminal surface of the parietal cell are proton pumps (H^+, K^+-ATPase), which exchange potassium ions for hydrogen ions, which are then secreted into the gastric lumen. Reduction in gastric acidity can be accomplished by neutralizing secreted acid, by blocking receptors on the parietal cells, or by blocking the H^+, K^+-ATPase pumps.

Antacids

Antacids are classified as either absorbable (calcium carbonate) or nonabsorbable (magnesium hydroxide, aluminum hydroxide, and aluminum phosphate). Calcium-containing antacids, taken in doses sufficient to raise gastric pH levels, may cause hypercalcuria and acid rebound due to stimulation of gastrin release and are rarely prescribed as antacids. Magnesium-containing antacids tend to cause diarrhea, whereas aluminum-containing antacids are constipating. For this reason, most liquid antacids contain a combination of the two. Although classified as nonabsorbable, small amounts of magnesium and aluminum are absorbed, creating potential problems in patients with renal insufficiency.

Although antacids are widely available and inexpensive, the need for frequent dosing and potential side effects have limited their use. They are infrequently used as primary therapy for upper GI tract symptoms.

H_2-receptor Antagonists

Of the four receptors on the parietal cell, only the histamine receptor can be effectively blocked. Histamine binds to the H_2 receptor, stimulating acid secretion. H_2-receptor antagonists block these receptors, resulting in diminished acid secretion. For many years the mainstay of acid antisecretory therapy, three of these four oral agents are now available as over-the-counter medications. The available agents are shown in Table 77.2. Three of these (cimetidine, ranitidine, and famotidine) are available as intravenous formulations, used primarily in the critically ill patient to prevent stress-related mucosal damage.

Still widely used to treat acid-related disorders, these drugs are indicated for patients who do not require the

TABLE 77.2. GASTRIC ANTISECRETORY DRUGS

Drug	Adult Dose
H_2 receptor antagonists	
Cimetidine (Tagamet)	400 mg bid or 800 mg hs
Ranitidine (Zantac)	150 mg bid or 300 mg hs
Famotidine (Pepcid)	20 mg bid or 40 mg hs
Nizatidine (Axid)	150 mg bid or 300 mg hs
Proton pump inhibitors	
Omeprazole (Prilosec)	20 mg qd
Lansoprazole (Prevacid)	30 mg qd
Rabeprazole (Aciphex)	20 mg qd
Pantoprazole (Protonix)	40 mg qd
Esomeprazole (Nexium)	40 mg qd

bid, twice daily; hs, at bedtime; qd, every day.

higher degree of acid suppression afforded by proton pump inhibitors (PPIs) and are considerably less expensive.

Cimetidine binds to hepatic cytochrome P-450 enzymes (mainly CYP 1A2) and may inhibit the metabolism of several drugs. The most important of these are phenytoin, theophylline, and warfarin. Ranitidine causes fewer drug interactions and these are of little clinical significance. Drug interactions with famotidine and nizatidine are rare.

Proton Pump Inhibitors

PPIs are weak bases that permeate the parietal cell and accumulate in the strongly acidic environment of the secretory canaliculus. After acid-induced activation, PPIs bind to the sulfhydryl groups of the proton pump and inhibit the final step of acid secretion. These drugs are the most potent inhibitors of both basal and meal-stimulated acid secretion. Five (Table 77.2) oral preparations are available. They differ slightly in onset of action and duration of acid suppression. Pantoprazole is available in an intravenous formulation, indicated for the short-term treatment of patients with gastroesophageal reflux disease who are unable to take oral medications.

Side effects are rare (headaches, abdominal pain, and diarrhea in some). Although PPIs are safe and highly effective, a few concerns have been raised concerning long-term use. These relate to the fact that gastric acid, long considered the demon of the GI tract, may in fact play some beneficial roles. Some drugs (e.g., ketoconazole and iron salts) are best absorbed in an acidic environment. Dietary vitamin B_{12}, bound to protein, must be cleaved by acid to be absorbed. Whether long-term use of PPIs, particularly in the elderly with diminished hydrochloride secretion, will eventually result in vitamin B_{12} deficiency remains to be seen. Gastric acid appears to be the most important mechanism to maintain upper GI tract sterility. Bacterial colonization of the stomach in patients in the intensive care unit on H_2-receptor antagonists, potentially leading to nosocomial aspiration pneumonia, has been well documented (15). Bacterial overgrowth of the small bowel, with resultant malabsorption, is an increasingly recognized complication of long-term PPI therapy.

Clinically significant drug interactions with PPIs are uncommon. Omeprazole has more interactions with the cytochrome P-450 system than the other PPIs. These interactions may include decreased clearance of carbamazepine, diazepam, and phenytoin and inhibition of metabolism of warfarin. Lansoprazole may modestly increase theophylline levels.

Cytoprotective Drugs

Sucralfate

Sucralfate is an aluminum salt of octasulfated sucrose that is insoluble in water. Approximately 5% is absorbed as the aluminum base and sucrose octasulfate, which is excreted unchanged in the urine. The remaining 95% is excreted in the stool unchanged. In the stomach, sucralfate forms a polymerized gel that binds to damaged mucosa for several hours and binds pepsin and bile salts, reducing their deleterious effects. As a cytoprotective agent, sucralfate concentrates growth factors at ulcer sites, stimulates mucosal release of prostaglandins, and stimulates bicarbonate and mucus release.

For treating gastric and duodenal ulcers, sucralfate is as effective as the H_2-receptor antagonists. Used as a suspension, it has been useful in treating esophageal ulcers, including giant HIV-associated ulcers (10). It is well tolerated with minimal side effects. Clinically significant drug interactions are uncommon. It may bind to quinidine, quinolones, and tetracycline, diminishing their absorption. This can be avoided by administering the drugs at different times.

Misoprostol

Misoprostol is a synthetic prostaglandin E_1 analogue, a 20-carbon oxygenated fatty acid. At low doses, it acts as a cytoprotective agent, stimulating cell proliferation and mucus and bicarbonate secretion, as well as increasing mucosal blood flow. At higher doses, misoprostol inhibits acid secretion. It is primarily used to prevent ulcers due to NSAID use. The major side effect is diarrhea, which is dose dependent. No significant drug interactions have been reported.

Prokinetic Agents

Prokinetic agents are drugs that stimulate GI tract motility and accelerate gut transit. These drugs may be useful in patients with GI tract infections accompanied by esophageal, gastric, and intestinal dysmotility symptoms. Those with central antidopaminergic action often have antiemetic effects as well. The recent withdrawal of cisapride from the market and the failure of domperidone to gain Food and Drug Administration approval before the patent expired have left few effective drugs in this class.

Bethanecol

Bethanecol is a cholinergic agent that acts on muscarinic receptors. It increases esophageal emptying and lower esophageal sphincter pressure but does not increase gastric emptying. Common side effects including abdominal pain, sweating, and flushing of the skin, along with its lack of central antiemetic effects, have limited its usefulness.

Erythromycin

The antibiotic erythromycin has long been known to cause upper abdominal pain, presumably by causing forceful antral contractions. This explains its ability to enhance gastric emptying, by stimulating motilin receptors. It is used primarily in the short-term treatment of gastroparesis. Intravenous erythromycin (16) is usually more effective than the oral form. Prolonged use often leads to tachyphylaxis.

Metoclopramide

Metoclopramide exerts a cholinomimetic effect on the upper GI tract, increasing lower esophageal sphincter pressure and antral peristaltic activity. Because of its central antidopaminergic effect, metoclopramide also acts as an antiemetic. Side effects, due to its crossing the blood–brain barrier, are common and limit its use. These include drowsiness, confusion, dystonic reactions, tardive dyskinesia, and other parkinsonian symptoms. Hyperprolactinemia may also occur. The usual adult dose is 5 to 10 mg four times a day.

Domperidone, a similar antidopaminergic agent, is a more potent prokinetic agent. Because it does not cross the blood–brain barrier, it has none of the central nervous system (CNS) side effects of metoclopramide. Because of its action on the CTZ, it is equally effective as an antiemetic. The only significant side effect is occasional hyperprolactinemia. The usual dose is 20 mg four times a day. Domperidone is available throughout the world except in the United States, although many U.S. patients have been able to obtain it from Canada.

Tegaserod

Tegaserod is a newly released 5-HT receptor partial agonist, which binds to 5-HT_4 receptors, stimulating GI tract peristalsis (17). Approved for the treatment of constipation-predominant irritable bowel syndrome, it stimulates motility in the esophagus, stomach, and small intestine, as well as in the colon. It may become an important agent for diffuse GI tract hypomotility disorders.

Antidiarrheal Agents

Antidiarrheal agents and their doses are given in Table 77.3.

Opiates And Their Synthetic Analogues

Opium has been used for 2,500 years to control diarrhea, and natural and synthetic opiates remain the most effective antidiarrheals. Tinctures of opium and paregoric, the camphorated opium preparation, have been available since the fifteenth century. Morphine is the most active component of these preparations and can control most cases of diarrhea except high-volume secretory states. Because of the potential for abuse, these drugs are controlled substances. In reality, patients rarely abuse these drugs and their short-term use in controlling infectious diarrhea rarely leads to dependence. Diphenoxylate, a synthetic opiate, is combined with atropine to discourage abuse. It has minimal central effects.

TABLE 77.3. ANTIDIARRHEAL AGENTS

Drug	Adult Dose
Opiates	
Tincture of opium	0.3–1.0 mL qid PO
Codeine sulfate	30 mg qid PO
Diphenoxylate with Atropine (Lomotil)	5 mg (two tablets) qid PO
Loperamide (Imodium)	4 mg initially, 2 mg PO after each loose stool up to 16 mg/d
Octreotide (Sandostatin)	0.1–1.8 mg/d in two to four divided doses SC
Racecadotril	1.5 mg/kg tid PO
Cholestyramine (Questran)	4 g (one packet) one to two times/d PO
Bismuth subsalicylate (Pepto-Bismol)	524 mg (15 mL or one caplet) q30–60 min up to eight times/d

qid, four times a day; PO, orally; SC, subcutaneously; tid, three times a day.

Loperamide, another synthetic opiate, is two to three times as potent as diphenoxylate. It has even less ability to cross the blood–brain barrier and has no abuse potential. For this reason, it is not a controlled substance and is available without prescription.

These drugs decrease diarrhea primarily by slowing intestinal transit (18), thereby increasing contact time between luminal contents and the mucosa, facilitating water absorption. Tincture of opium and paregoric are the most effective, codeine is somewhat less effective, and diphenoxylate and loperamide are clearly less potent but are generally used first before resorting to more potent drugs.

No significant drug interactions have been reported with loperamide. The other opioid preparations have the potential for CNS depression and should be used with caution in patients taking other CNS depressants such as barbiturates, benzodiazepines, phenothiazines, and tricyclic antidepressants. Because of the risk of toxic megacolon, these antimotility agents should generally not be used in patients with invasive GI tract infections.

Octreotide

Octreotide, a synthetic cyclic octapeptide analogue of somatostatin, has numerous effects on the GI tract. It inhibits gastric, pancreatic, and intestinal secretion and diminishes motility in the stomach and gallbladder. It diminishes local and circulating concentrations of a number of gut peptides including gastrin, secretin, cholecystokinin, vasoactive intestinal peptide, glucagon, and motilin. It has been successful in controlling secretory diarrhea associated with pancreatic tumors, such as VIPoma, and the carcinoid syndrome. It has had more limited success in patients with pathogen-negative AIDS-associated diarrhea (19) and some patients with microsporidiosis (20). Side effects include local irritation at injection sites, nausea, abdominal cramping, and bloating.

Long-term use may be associated with an increased risk of gallstones, due to hypomotility of the gallbladder, and suppression of pituitary and thyroid function. Because of its cost and the need for injection, its use is usually reserved for those not responding to opiate antidiarrheals.

Racecadotril

Racecadotril (Acetorphan) is a specific inhibitor of enkephalinase, a cell membrane peptidase located in the epithelium of the small intestine (21). This enzyme serves to digest both exogenous peptides from dietary sources and endogenous peptides such as enkephalins, neurokinin, and substance P (22). Racecadotril, given orally, is effective against the secretory diarrhea caused by cholera toxin and castor oil (23–25). It does not increase intestinal transit (26) but instead acts by a selective antisecretory action (27–28). Studies both in adults and children with acute diarrhea have shown a reduction in stool volume up to 50% with no significant side effects (24,26,29). It is likely to play a role as an effective and safe adjunct to oral rehydration therapy in adults and children with acute infectious diarrhea.

Bismuth Compounds

Bismuth compounds have been used since the eighteenth century to treat GI symptoms. Modern-day medical interest in these compounds increased during the 1980s when they were recognized to play an important role in regimens to treat *H. pylori* infection. Their efficacy in treating nausea, vomiting, abdominal cramping, and diarrhea has been well documented (30,31). The only bismuth compound available in the United States is bismuth subsalicylate (BSS) (Pepto-Bismol). In the stomach, it dissociates, allowing for approximately 95% absorption of the salicylate moiety from the proximal small bowel. Salicylate toxicity is possible, particularly in patients ingesting other salicylate compounds such as aspirin. Although poorly absorbed, the bismuth moiety may lead to bismuth encephalopathy (32) when these compounds are taken in high doses.

BSS is effective in treating acute infectious diarrhea, reducing the number of stools by about 50% compared with placebo (33). It is the salicylate moiety, through its antisecretory action, that results in diminished diarrhea (34,35). The drug also has antimicrobial properties, which may explain its efficacy in preventing traveler's diarrhea (36,37). *In vitro,* it exhibits bactericidal activity against ETEC and binds to cholera toxin. BSS appears to be the most effective agent in treating vomiting associated with viral gastroenteritis, such as with the Norwalk agent (38).

Cholestyramine And Colestipol

These drugs are high-molecular-weight anion exchange resins that bind bile salts in the lumen, prevent their absorption in the terminal ileum, and when bile salts are present in the colon, prevent their stimulation of water secretion. They are used primarily to treat bile salt-induced diarrhea and cholestatic liver diseases, as well as to lower serum cholesterol levels. *In vitro,* they bind *Clostridium difficile* toxin and decrease diarrhea associated with pseudomembranous colitis. These agents bind to a number of drugs, thereby decreasing their absorption. They should be given 4 hours before or 1 hour after other drugs.

Anticholinergic Agents

Atropine, hyoscyamine, scopolamine, and the synthetic agents dicyclomine and propantheline are antimuscarinic agents that slow intestinal motility and in theory should facilitate intestinal water absorption, thereby improving diarrhea. In clinical practice, the side effects (gastric retention and ileus) usually preclude their use in treating acute infectious diarrhea.

Intraluminal Agents

Dietary fiber, which represents the noncellulose polysaccharides comprising the indigestible portion of the plant cell wall, and fiber supplements, such as psyllium, absorb excess water in the colon, thus symptomatically improving diarrhea by increasing stool consistency. Because they do not decrease loss of water in the stool, their role in treating infectious diarrhea is mainly cosmetic.

Combinations of kaolin (hydrated aluminum silicate) and pectin (a polymer of polygalacturonic acid) act as an absorbent of water, a variety of drugs, bacteria, and toxins. Like fiber, they may increase stool consistency but do not decrease fecal water excretion. Widely used and available without prescription (such as Kaopectate), there are only limited equivocal data to support their efficacy in diarrhea due to GI tract infections.

Dietary Therapy And Dietary Supplements

Transient lactase deficiency is common in infections of the small intestine, especially with reovirus and parvovirus infections. Avoiding lactose during the infection and for a week after, when lactase activity usually returns, will help minimize the diarrhea. Other osmotically active carbohydrates such as sorbitol and fructose, found in many fruits, soft drinks, and reduced-calorie foods and sweets, should also be restricted. Transient malabsorption of fatty acids may occur in some viral and protozoal infections of the small intestine. Restriction of dietary fat may lessen the diarrhea in these cases.

The use of "probiotics" in the treatment of GI tract infections remains controversial (39). *Lactobacillus acidophilus* and *Lactobacillus bulgaricus* ferment carbohydrate to lactic acid, thereby creating an environment unfavorable to the overgrowth of potentially pathogenic bacteria and favorable to the growth of beneficial flora in the colon. Although used for many years to treat antibiotic-associated diarrhea due to alterations in colonic bacterial flora, well-designed controlled trials to support their efficacy are lacking. Commonly used preparations include Lactinex granules and tablets, acidophilus milk, and active culture yogurt. Ingestion of the nonpathogenic yeast *Saccharomyces boulardii,* by inhibiting the growth of various pathogenic bacteria, has been suggested to have the ability to prevent relapse of *C. difficile* colitis (40).

Care Of Anorectal Disorders

Perineal Care

Diarrhea and attempts to clean the perineum with frequent wiping often result in local tissue irritation and abrasion. Control of diarrhea, either through specific antimicrobial therapy or through the use of antidiarrheals, will usually resolve these problems. Sitz baths, immersing the buttocks in warm water for 10 minutes two or three times a day, followed by gentle drying with absorbent cotton, will help maintain perineal hygiene. Soaps should be avoided because they cause further irritation. A similar protocol should be followed after bowel movements. Toilet paper and paper towels should be avoided, because they tend to be abrasive.

Short-term use of topical agents applied to the perineum may afford relief in more severe cases. Hydrocortisone cream, witch hazel, and Desitin ointment (40% zinc oxide in a petroleum jelly base, used to treat diaper rash) may be useful. Topical anesthetics are not recommended and may lead to sensitization.

Rectal Suppositories

In cases of chronic proctitis due to infections such as herpes simplex, CMV, and chlamydia, rectal suppositories, foams, or enemas containing hydrocortisone or mesalamine (5-aminosalicylic acid) may exert an antiinflammatory effect and relieve symptoms such as tenesmus and hematochezia.

REFERENCES

1. Sartor R. Cytokines in intestinal inflammation: pathophysiological and clinical considerations. *Gastroenterology* 1994;106: 533–539.
2. Banwell J. Treatment of traveler's diarrhea: fluid and dietary management. *Infect Dis* 1986;8[Suppl 2]:S182–S187.
3. Melzack R, Rosberger Z, Hollingsworth ML, et al. New approaches to measuring nausea. *Can Med Assoc J* 1985;133: 755–758.
4. Lee M, Feldman M. Nausea and vomiting. In: Feldman M, Scharschmidt BF, Sleisenger MH, eds. *Sleisenger and Fordtran's gastrointestinal and liver disease,* sixth edition. Philadelphia: WB Saunders, 1998:117–127.
5. Miller AD. Neuroanatomy and physiology. In: Sleisenger MH, ed. *The handbook of nausea and vomiting.* New York: Parthenon, 1993:1–9.
6. Carpenter DO. Neural mechanisms of emesis. *Can J Physiol Pharmacol* 1990;68:230–236.
7. Borison HL, Borison R, McCarthy LE. Role of the area postrema in vomiting and related functions. *Fed Proc* 1984;43:2955–2958.
8. Borison HL, Wang SC. Physiology and pharmacology of vomiting. *Pharmacol Rev* 1953;5:193–230.
9. Baker PCH, Bernat JL. The neuroanatomy of vomiting in man: association of projectile vomiting with a solitary metastasis in the lateral tegmentum of the pons and the middle cerebellar peduncle. *J Neurol Neurosurg Psychiatry* 1985;48:1165–1168.
10. Baehr P, McDonald G. Esophageal infections: risk factors, presentation, diagnosis, and treatment. *Gastroenterology* 1994;106: 509–532.
11. Wenzl HH, Fine KD, Schiller LR, et al. Determinants of decreased fecal consistency in patients with diarrhea. *Gastroenterology* 1995;108:1729–1738.
12. Keusch GT, Donta ST. Classification of enterotoxins on the basis of activity in cell culture. *J Infect Dis* 1975;131:58–63.
13. Hamer DH, Gorbach SL. Infectious diarrhea and bacterial food poisoning. In: Feldman M, Scharschmidt BF, Sleisenger MH, eds. *Sleisenger and Fordtran's gastrointestinal and liver disease,* sixth edition. Philadelphia: WB Saunders, 1998:1594–1632.
14. Schreiber DS, Blacklow NR, Trier JS. The mucosal lesion of the proximal small intestine in acute infectious nonbacterial gastroenteritis. *N Engl J Med* 1973;288:1318–1323.
15. Driks MR, Craven DE, Celli BR, et al. Nosocomial pneumonia in intubated patients given sucralfate as compared with antacids or histamine type 2 blockers. The role of gastric colonization. *N Engl J Med* 1987;317:1376–1382.
16. Reynolds J, Putnam P. Prokinetic agents. *Gastroenterol Clin North Am* 1992;21(3):567–596.
17. Scott LJ, Perry CM. Tegaserod. *Drugs* 1999;58(3):491–496.
18. Awouters F, Niemegeers C, Janssen P. Pharmacology of antidiarrheal drugs. *Annu Rev Pharmacol Toxicol* 1983;23:279–301.
19. Schiller LR. Review article: anti-diarrhoeal pharmacology and therapeutics. *Aliment Pharmacol Ther* 1995;9:87–106.
20. Simon D, Weiss L, Tanowitz H, et al. Light microscopic diagnosis of human microsporidiosis and variable response to octreotide. *Gastroenterology* 1991;100:271–273.
21. Kenny J. Twin brush border metalloendopeptidases. In: Lentze MJ, Sterat EE, eds. *Mammalian brush border membrane proteins.* Stuttgart, Germany: Thieme-Verlag, 1990:75–88.
22. Primi MP, Bueno L, Baumer P, et al. Racecadotril demonstrates intestinal antisecretory activity *in vivo. Aliment Pharmacol Ther* 1999;13[Suppl 6]:3–7.
23. Hinterleitner TA, Petritsch W, Dimsity G, et al. Acetorphan prevents cholera toxin-induced water and electrolyte secretion in the human jejunum. *Gastroenterology* 1997;9:887–891.
24. Baumer P, Danquechin-Dorval E, Bertrand J, et al. Effects of Acetorphan, an enkephalinase inhibitor, on experimental and acute diarrhoea. *Gut* 1992;33:753–758.
25. Marcais-Collado H, Uchida G, Costentin J, et al. Naloxone reversible antidiarrheal effect of enkephalinase inhibitors. *Eur J Pharmacol* 1987;144:125–132.
26. Hamza H, Ben Khalifa H, Baumer P, et al. Racecadotril versus placebo in the treatment of acute diarrhea in adults. *Aliment Pharmacol Ther* 1999;13[Suppl 6]:15–19.
27. Shook JE, Lemcke PK, Gehrig CA, et al. Antidiarrheal properties of supraspinal mu and delta and peripheral mu, delta and kappa opioid receptors: inhibition of diarrhea without constipation. *J Pharmacol Exp Ther* 1989;249:83–90.
28. Salazar-Lindo E, Santisteban-Ponce J, Chea-Woo E, et al. Racecadotril in the treatment of acute watery diarrhea in young boys. *N Engl J Med* 2000;343:463–467.

29. Cezard JP, Duhamel JF, Meyer M, et al. Efficacy and tolerability of racecadotril in acute diarrhea in children. *Gastroenterology* 2001;120:799–805.
30. Hailey F, Newsom J. Evaluation of bismuth subsalicylate in relieving symptoms of indigestion. *Arch Intern Med* 1984;144:269–272.
31. Marshall B. The use of bismuth in gastroenterology. *Am J Gastroenterol* 1991;86(1):16–25.
32. Mendelowitz P, Hoffman R, Weber S. Bismuth absorption and myoclonic encephalopathy during bismuth subsalicylate therapy. *Ann Intern Med* 1990;112:140–141.
33. DuPont H, Sullivan P, Pickering L, et al. Symptomatic treatment of diarrhea with bismuth subsalicylate among students attending a Mexican university. *Gastroenterology* 1977;73:715–718.
34. Ericsson C, Evans D, DuPont H, et al. Bismuth subsalicylate inhibits activity of crude toxins of *Escherichia coli* and *Vibrio cholerae. J Infect Dis* 1977;136:693–696.
35. Powell D, Tapper E, Morris S. Aspirin-stimulated intestinal electrolyte transport in rabbit ileum *in vitro. Gastroenterology* 1979; 76:1429–1437.
36. DuPont H, Ericsson C, Johnson P, et al. Prevention of travelers' diarrhea by the tablet formulation of bismuth subsalicylate. *JAMA* 1987;257:1347–1350.
37. Graham D, Esres, M, Gentry L. Double-blind comparison of bismuth subsalicylate and placebo in the prevention and treatment of enterotoxigenic *Escherichia coli. Gastroenterology* 1983; 85:1017–1022.
38. Steinhoff M, Douglass RJ, Greenberg H, et al. Bismuth subsalicylate therapy of viral gastroenteritis. *Gastroenterology* 1980;78: 1495–1499.
39. Shanahan F. Probiotics: science or snake oil? *Clin Perspect Gastroenterol* 2001;4:47–50.
40. Pothoulakis C, Kelly C, Joshi M, et al. *Saccharomyces boulardii* inhibits *Clostridium difficile* toxin A binding and enterotoxicity in rat ileum. *Gastroenterology* 1993;104:1108–1115.

78

THERAPY FOR DIARRHEAL ILLNESS IN CHILDREN

LARRY K. PICKERING
THOMAS G. CLEARY

Enteric infections generally are self-limited conditions that require fluid and electrolyte therapy (1,2). In some instances, specific antimicrobial therapy may eradicate fecal shedding of the causative organism, prevent transmission of the enteropathogen, abbreviate clinical symptoms, or prevent future complications. The number of enteropathogens capable of producing gastroenteritis is large, and the response of each to therapy varies. Organisms that commonly cause dehydration are the enteric viruses, *Vibrio cholerae,* and enterotoxigenic *Escherichia coli.* Invasive bacterial enteropathogens, including *Campylobacter jejuni coli, Shigella* species, *Salmonella* species, shigatoxin producing *E. coli, Yersinia enterocolitica,* and *Clostridium difficile,* may produce complications other than dehydration. Guidelines and primers have been published to assist in managing patients with infectious diarrhea (1–5).

Major considerations for children with gastroenteritis include (a) fluid and electrolyte replacement, (b) dietary intake, (c) nonspecific therapy with antidiarrheal compounds, (d) specific therapy with antimicrobial agents, and (e) prevention of disease.

PRINCIPLES OF TREATING CHILDREN

Several basic principles underlie treatment of children with acute infectious gastroenteritis.

1. Fluid and electrolyte therapy is the most important therapeutic consideration.
2. Many bacterial, viral, and parasitic enteropathogens are capable of causing gastroenteritis. These organisms have varying degrees of response to antimicrobial agents (Table 78.1).
3. Enteropathogens are acquired through the fecal-oral route by contaminated food or water or are spread from person to person. In certain instances, antimicrobial therapy will reduce the potential of person-to-person transmission.
4. Infections in children with primary or secondary immune deficiencies, including HIV, are often severe, commonly disseminate, require prolonged therapy, and frequently relapse when therapy is stopped.
5. Diagnostic assays for several enteropathogens are cumbersome, costly, and available only in research or reference laboratories.
6. Development of resistance to antimicrobial agents by bacterial enteropathogens is an increasing problem.
7. *In vitro* drug susceptibility results do not always predict *in vivo* clinical response.
8. Safety factors and side effects generally preclude the use in children of certain antimicrobial agents (e.g., the fluoroquinolones and tetracyclines) that are approved for administration to adults. There is a need for systematic assessment of drugs in children, rather than extrapolation of findings of studies in adults.
9. There are public health consequences of infection with several enteropathogens.

The increased number of persons who are immunodeficient has led to recognition of uncommonly encountered organisms, such as *Isospora, Enterocytozoon bieneusi, Encephalitozoon intestinalis* (formerly *Septata intestinale*), and several enteric viruses, as causes of diarrhea (6–8). These agents have expanded the list of potential causes of diarrhea in immunodeficient patients and treatment of these patients may be difficult because their course of illness often is severe, prolonged, or recurrent.

L. K. Pickering: National Immunization Program, Centers for Disease Control and Prevention.

T. G. Cleary: Division of Infectious Diseases, Department of Pediatrics, University of Texas Medical School, Houston, Texas.

TABLE 78.1. POTENTIAL BENEFITS OF ANTIMICROBIAL THERAPY FOR ENTEROPATHOGENS OR DISEASES PRODUCED BY ENTEROPATHOGENS

Potential Benefit	Enteropathogen or Disease
Established benefit	Amebiasis
	Antimicrobial associated colitis (*Clostridium difficile*)
	Cholera
	Cyclosporiasis
	Enteroinvasive *Escherichia coli*
	Enterotoxigenic *Escherichia coli*
	Giardiasis
	Isosporiasis
	Shigella species
	Strongyloidiasis
	Any bacterium that produces bacteremia (e.g., *Salmonella typhi*)
Limited or unknown	*Aeromonas* species
	Blastocystis hominis
	Campylobacter jejuni coli
	Cryptosporidiosis
	Encephalitozoon intestinalis
	Intestinal salmonellosis
	Yersinia enterocolitica
Therapy not available	Enteric viruses
	Enterocytozoon bieneusi
Therapy may be harmful	Shigatoxin producing *Escherichia coli*

ANTIDIARRHEAL COMPOUNDS

Most available antidiarrheal compounds are not approved for children younger than 2 or 3 years (2). These compounds may be classified by their mechanisms of action, which include alteration of intestinal motility, adsorption of fluid or toxins, alteration of intestinal microflora, and alteration of fluid and electrolyte secretion (Table 78.2) (9–34).

Many persons with diarrhea medicate themselves or their children before they seek medical care. Although self-medication usually results in no harm, several problems may occur if antidiarrheal compounds are used. First, adverse effects may develop, including worsening of diarrhea because of slowing of intestinal motility by agents that alter intestinal function (9–11), salicylate or bismuth absorption from bismuth subsalicylate (BSS) preparations (18–20), or prevention of absorption of medicines or nutrients in the gastrointestinal (GI) tract when they come in contact with adsorbents. Second, these compounds may interfere with identification of enteropathogens by microscopy, enzyme immunoassay (EIA), culture, or other diagnostic assays. Third, patients may have a false sense of security after using a compound with no therapeutic benefit.

TABLE 78.2. MEDICATIONS USED TO RELIEVE SYMPTOMS IN PATIENTS WITH ACUTE DIARRHEA

Category	Generic Names
Alteration of intestinal motility	Loperamide
	Difenoxin HCl and atropine sulfate
	Diphenoxylate and atropine
	Tincture of opium
Adsorption of toxins and water	Attapulgite
	Calcium polycarbophil
Alteration of intestinal microflora	Prebiotics (fructooligosaccharides)
	Probiotics (*Lactobacillus*, *Bifidobacterium*)
Alteration of secretion	Bismuth subsalicylate
	Octreotide
	Racecadotril

Drugs that alter intestinal motility usually have a rapid onset of action by producing segmental contractions of the intestine (30–32,34), which serve to retard movement of intestinal contents responsible for diarrhea and to restrict the intestinal distention responsible for pain. These agents also may inhibit intestinal secretion. Side effects include dizziness, dry mouth, drowsiness, tachycardia, constipation, and vomiting. These drugs should be avoided in patients with fever, toxemia, or bloody stools. They can worsen the clinical course of shigellosis (9), *C. difficile* (26), and *E. coli* O157:H7 (35,36). Because of concern about safety in children, including the potential for overdose, use of these compounds is not recommended in children (2,10,11).

Several antidiarrheal compounds are used as adsorbents (12,13) and are reported to work by adsorbing bacterial toxins and water to improve symptoms of diarrhea. Most currently available compounds in this category contain activated attapulgite, which is a clay that acts as an adsorbent. These compounds relieve diarrhea by reducing the number of bowel movements and improving stool consistency. Although attapulgite has been shown to be effective in animals (27), controlled studies showing the effectiveness of adsorbents in reducing the duration of diarrhea or the loss of fluid and electrolytes in humans need to be conducted. Potential disadvantages include adsorption of nutrients, enzymes, and antibiotics in the intestine, particularly with prolonged use.

Addition of biotherapeutic agents, which include probiotics (lactic acid-producing bacteria such as lactobacilli) and prebiotics (nondigestible food ingredients that promote growth and/or metabolic activity of certain bacteria in the colon) to the diet of an infant or child has been shown to reduce or prevent diarrhea of unknown etiology or diarrhea due to specific organisms (23–25). These preparations are administered to re-colonize the intestine with saccharolytic flora and to lower the intestinal pH level to deter potential pathogens. Lactobacillus preparations available as antidiarrheal compounds have not been shown to be effective in the symptomatic treatment of diarrhea (14–16,37). Studies are needed to better define and standardize the optimal probiotic and prebiotic agents needed for prevention and treatment of various diseases and conditions, as well as the optimal combination of organisms or agents in the probiotic and prebiotic preparations. Information on the properties of microorganisms that enables them to interfere with pathogenic species is needed (23).

BSS, bismuth subnitrate, and bismuth subgallate are used as adjunctive therapy for acute diarrhea. The mechanism of action of these compounds is uncertain, although laboratory studies have shown that BSS inhibits intestinal secretion caused by *E. coli* and cholera toxins (17). BSS in both liquid and tablet forms has been shown to be effective in the prevention and treatment of acute diarrhea among adult students in Mexico (38,39). Controlled trials of BSS demonstrate reduced frequency of unformed stools and increased stool consistency among adult volunteers receiving the Norwalk virus, as well as a decreased duration of naturally occurring diarrhea among children (23,40). Salicylate absorption has been reported after ingestion of BSS (18,19). Bismuth-associated encephalopathy and other toxicities have been reported from chronic administration of high doses of bismuth-containing compounds (20). Racecadotril (acetorphan) is an enkephalinase inhibitor that decreases intestinal hypersecretion but not motility in animals and humans by preventing breakdown of endogenous enkephalins in the GI tract. Racecadotril has been shown in children with watery diarrhea to decrease 48-hour stool output, median duration of diarrhea, and intake of oral rehydration solution (21).

Octreotide acetate (Sandostatin) is a long-acting octapeptide that mimics the natural hormone somatostatin by inhibiting secretion of various endocrine and exocrine hormones, including growth hormone, thyroid-stimulating hormone, adrenocorticotropic hormone, insulin, glucagon, gastrin, secretin, pancreozymin, and pepsin (21). Octreotide is approved by the Food and Drug Administration (FDA) for symptomatic treatment of patients with metastatic carcinoid tumors because it suppresses or inhibits the severe diarrhea and flushing episodes associated with this disease. Octreotide also reduces the profuse, watery diarrhea associated with vasoactive intestinal peptide-secreting tumors. Octreotide has been used in patients with cryptosporidial infection (28), but it has not been approved by the FDA for this purpose.

The addition of other nonspecific compounds to the diet of children with acute infectious diarrhea, including zinc, vitamin A, and amino acids, has been shown to produce reductions in the duration and severity of diarrhea (29).

ANTIMICROBIAL THERAPY

Antimicrobial therapy will not benefit most children with acute infectious diarrhea. Antimicrobial agents are not effective for the treatment of gastroenteritis caused by viral enteropathogens that include rotavirus, enteric adenovirus, calicivirus, including the Norwalk virus, astrovirus, and unclassified viruses or by *E. bieneusi.* Patients with diarrhea associated with certain bacterial and protozoal agents may benefit from therapy (Table 78.1). Because resistance among enteric bacteria follows widespread use of antimicrobial agents in humans and animals, and because resistant organisms can spread rapidly due to mobility of the world population, constant monitoring of susceptibility of bacterial isolates is critical for selection of appropriate antimicrobial agents for therapy (41).

Bacteria

Antimicrobial-associated Colitis

One aspect of *C. difficile* infection in infants and children is that this group is more likely to carry *C. difficile* asymptomatically in the GI tract than adults (42). Approximately 15% to 63% of neonates, 3% to 33% of infants and toddlers younger than 2 years, and up to 8% of children older than 2 years are asymptomatic carriers (43). Because the rates of symptomatic carriage (coexisting diarrhea) are not dissimilar to those for asymptomatic carriage (43), establishment of a clear role for *C. difficile* as a cause of mild GI tract disease in children is difficult. In addition, *C. difficile* may be found in stools of children in association with other enteric pathogens, such as *Salmonella* species, *Campylobacter* species, *Giardia lamblia,* or rotavirus, regardless of whether antibiotics have been administered recently (43). Most episodes of antimicrobial agent-associated diarrhea in children and adults are not due to *C. difficile* (42,44).

In patients with antimicrobial-associated colitis (AAC), the most important aspects of therapy are discontinuation of the antimicrobial or antineoplastic agent and replacement of fluid and electrolytes (42). Approximately 25% of patients with mild disease may respond to these measures (45). If symptoms persist or worsen, or if the disease is severe, patients will require specific therapy. Metronidazole, vancomycin, teicoplanin, and fusidic acid are all effective therapeutic agents (46), but most experience has been with metronidazole and vancomycin (45,47). Metronidazole is considered the initial drug of choice because of clinical efficacy similar to vancomycin, lower cost, bitter taste of vancomycin, and concern of vancomycin resistance to other pathogens such as enterococci (Table 78.3). Oral vancomycin is used only for seriously ill patients or those who do not respond to metronidazole (45,48,49). All strains of *C. difficile* are susceptible to vancomycin, whereas resistance to metronidazole has been reported (50). Bacitracin has been used to treat patients with *C. difficile* disease, but this compound has a slower and less certain response rate than vancomycin (51–53) and is not approved by the FDA for this condition. Bacitracin can be toxic if absorbed from an inflamed intestine.

Relapses occur in 10% to 20% of patients treated with vancomycin, metronidazole, or bacitracin (45,49,53), gen-

TABLE 78.3. ANTIMICROBIAL THERAPY FOR GASTROENTERITIS CAUSED BY BACTERIAL PATHOGENS

Organism	Antimicrobial Agent	Days of Therapy
Clostridium difficile	Metronidazole or vancomycin	7
Campylobacter jejuni	Erythromycin or	5–7
	azithromycin or	5–7
	ciprofloxacin[a]	5
Vibrio cholerae O1	Tetracycline or	3
	doxycycline or	1
	TMP-SMX	3
V. cholerae O139[b]	Tetracycline	3
	Doxycycline	1
Yersinia enterocolitica	None	
Vibrio parahaemolyticus	None	
Enterotoxigenic *Escherichia coli*	TMP-SMX or ciprofloxacin[a]	3–5
Enteroinvasive *Escherichia coli*	See Table 78.5	Same as for shigellosis
Plesiomonas shigelloides	TMP-SMX or ciprofloxacin[a]	3–5

[a]Not approved by the Food and Drug Administration for individuals younger than 18 years.
[b]See text for alternatives.
TMP-SMX, trimethoprim-sulfamethoxazole.

erally 1 to 4 weeks after treatment has been discontinued. Recurrences are due to either germination of *C. difficile* spores that persist despite treatment or reinfection with *C. difficile* acquired from human or environmental exposure. Stool should be tested to document a reinfection or relapse, both of which generally respond to a second course of metronidazole or vancomycin.

Teicoplanin, a glycopeptide antibiotic, has been used successfully to treat patients with AAC (46). Cholestyramine and other anion exchange resins were used in the past for treatment of patients with AAC when the cause was less clear and when bile acids were considered to be causative (54). Other modes of therapy include dietary carbohydrate reduction and administration of prebiotics to allow normal flora to reestablish (55,56). Both the American College of Gastroenterology and the Society of Healthcare Epidemiology have published practice guidelines for prevention and control of *C. difficile* infection in adults (42). Similar guidelines have not been published for children.

Salmonella

The type of syndrome produced by *Salmonella* dictates the selection and duration of antimicrobial therapy (Table 78.4). Antibiotics have been shown to prolong symptoms and increase the risk of complications among persons who are nontyphoidal *Salmonella* carriers or in patients who have mild gastroenteritis. Several randomized studies have demonstrated no difference between treated and untreated patients (57). Antimicrobial therapy may convert intestinal carriage to systemic disease with bacteremia (58), produce a bacteriologic and symptomatic relapse (59–61), encourage

TABLE 78.4. ANTIMICROBIAL THERAPY FOR *SALMONELLA* INFECTIONS IN CHILDREN

Clinical Manifestation	Antimicrobial Agent	Days of Therapy
Carrier state with *Salmonella typhi*	Amoxicillin with probenecid	42
Acute gastroenteritis	Generally none	
Bacteremia or enteric fever or both[a,b]	Ceftriaxone or cefotaxime or ampicillin[c] or chloramphenicol[c] or TMP-SMX[c]	14
Dissemination with localized suppuration (e.g., osteomyelitis)	Same as above for bacteremia	4–6 wk

[a]Fluoroquinolones are effective but not approved for people younger than 18 years.
[b]Azithromycin and cefixime have been used with success in developing countries.
[c]Can be used if organism is susceptible.
TMP-SMX, trimethoprim-sulfamethoxazole.

development or selection of resistant strains, or prolong fecal excretion (59,61,62).

Antibiotic treatment of patients with *Salmonella* infection generally is restricted to those with (a) typhoid fever, including patients with clinical illness and carriers; (b) bacteremia from nontyphoidal strains; and (c) dissemination with localized suppuration. Antimicrobial therapy also should be considered in infants younger than 3 to 6 months and in patients with enterocolitis who have an underlying condition or disease that impairs host resistance, such as AIDS, hemoglobinopathy including sickle cell anemia, lymphoma, leukemia, immunosuppression, congenital heart disease, valvular heart disease, prostheses, or uremia (3). Recommended antimicrobial agents include ampicillin, chloramphenicol, trimethoprim-sulfamethoxazole (TMP-SMX), ceftriaxone, cefotaxime, or a fluoroquinolone, which is only approved for people older than 17 years (63,64). Ciprofloxacin, azithromycin, and cefixime are active *in vitro* against *Salmonella,* including *Salmonella* serotype Typhi, and have been used clinically with success (65–71). Many other antibiotics are active *in vitro* against *Salmonella* strains, including *Salmonella* serotype Typhi, but susceptibility correlates poorly with *in vivo* response (72). Corticosteroids can be beneficial in patients with typhoid fever in whom prompt relief of manifestations of toxemia might be lifesaving (73), but they may increase the relapse rate (74). In the United States, attention has focused on resistance of nontyphoidal *Salmonella* strains, which have their major reservoir in animals (75–81). Several outbreaks of multidrug-resistant *Salmonella* infection have been traced to animal sources in the United States and are a major problem in other parts of the world (77–79,81–83). Human isolates of *Salmonella* should have susceptibility testing performed to guide therapy.

Since the mid 1960s, the incidence of infections due to *Salmonella* serotype Typhi in the United States has been stable, at approximately 400 cases per year, but the percentage of cases diagnosed in the United States that were acquired abroad has increased from 33% from 1967 through 1972 to 72% from 1985 through 1994 to 81% from 1996 through 1997 (84). Because of the high rate of *Salmonella* serotype Typhi transmission, together with widespread indiscriminate use of antimicrobial agents in some areas of the world, an increase in resistance patterns to ampicillin, chloramphenicol, and TMP-SMX has occurred (85). The proportion of typhoid cases attributed to exposure in Mexico decreased from 46% in 1985 to 6% in 1996 and 1997, whereas the number due to exposure in the Indian subcontinent increased from 25% in 1985 to 57% in 1996 and 1997 (84). Overall in 1996 and 1997, 17% of *Salmonella* serotype Typhi isolates in the United States had multiple resistance patterns to ampicillin, chloramphenicol, and TMP-SMX with the highest rates occurring in isolates from the Indian subcontinent, Vietnam, and Tajikistan. Because of this high rate of resistance in *Salmonella* serotype Typhi strains imported by travelers (62), empiric treatment of *Salmonella* serotype Typhi should be provided with ceftriaxone, cefotaxime, or fluoroquinolones if the patient is older than 17 years. Ampicillin, chloramphenicol, and TMP-SMX should be reserved for domestically acquired cases or persons from whom susceptibility testing of the causative organism has shown susceptibility. Resistance of *Salmonella* serotype Typhi to ceftriaxone and fluoroquinolones has been reported and is uncommon but needs to be monitored (65,79,85,86). In areas of the world where *Salmonella* serotype Typhi strains with reduced susceptibility to fluoroquinolones have been reported, azithromycin was effective for the treatment of people with enteric fever (65,66,69), as was cefixime (67,68). In a prospective randomized study of children and adults with confirmed typhoid fever, ceftriaxone administered for 5 days was as effective and safe as a 2- to 3- week course of chloramphenicol (87), but in another study, short-course therapy failed (88). First- and second-generation cephalosporin antibiotics have been less effective than expanded-spectrum cephalosporin antibiotics and should not be used.

Antibiotics listed in Table 78.4 can be used for treatment of *Salmonella.* Patients with defective host defense mechanisms, such as individuals with AIDS, should be treated with ampicillin or an expanded-spectrum cephalosporin (89–91). Ciprofloxacin has been reported to be effective in the treatment of acute diarrhea due to *Salmonella* (92–94), recurrent *Salmonella* sepsis (95), and brain abscesses in a neonate (96). Duration of therapy is influenced by the site of infection and by the host. Patients with bacteremia without a localized infection should be treated for 14 days, whereas those with localized infection, such as osteomyelitis or endocarditis, or patients with AIDS and bacteremia should receive at least 4 to 6 weeks of therapy (88). In most cases, chronic carriage of *Salmonella* serotype Typhi is associated with gallbladder disease. The presence of cholelithiasis may have a significant impact on the efficacy of therapy. When gallbladder disease is present, the failure rate of ampicillin is about 75% (97). In patients without gallbladder disease, ampicillin with probenecid or amoxicillin administered for 6 weeks is the treatment of choice for chronic enteric carriers (98,99). Norfloxacin (100) and ciprofloxacin (101) also have been reported to be successful in eradicating *Salmonella* serotype Typhi in adult chronic carriers. Resistance of clinical isolates and failure of treatment with ciprofloxacin have been noted in patients infected with *Salmonella* serotype Typhi (102). Ceftriaxone resistance of nontyphoidal strains of *Salmonella* have been reported in the United States at a rate of 0.5% in 1998 (86).

Shigella

In the United States, 60% of reported cases of diarrhea associated with *Shigella* are due to *Shigella sonnei; Shigella flexneri* serotypes account for most of the remaining cases. *Shigella dysenteriae* and *Shigella boydii* are uncommon causes of diarrhea in the United States. Table 78.5 outlines suggested antimicrobial therapy for children who have presumed shigellosis or in whom *Shigella* has been isolated from stool. *Shigella* strains have become progressively resistant to multiple antimicrobial agents, initially to sulfonamides, shortly after they became commercially available, then to tetracycline, chloramphenicol, and streptomycin less than 10 years after each was introduced, and subsequently to ampicillin, kanamycin, and TMP-SMX (103, 104). In certain Native American populations and in a study from Oregon, TMP-SMX resistance to *Shigella* is common (104,105). In Oregon, 59% of *Shigella* isolates were resistant to TMP-SMX and 63% were resistant to ampicillin (104). In children with TMP-SMX-susceptible or ampicillin-susceptible strains, either of these antibiotics is an accepted treatment (106–110), but neither should be used as empiric therapy due to increasing resistance. Amoxicillin is not as effective as ampicillin and should not be used (111). Furazolidone has been shown to be effective in children infected with susceptible strains (112,113). Patients who are transient symptom-free carriers may be managed without antimicrobial therapy if they employ excellent standards of personal and public hygiene. Treatment of these patients, however, will reduce fecal shedding of the organism and may prevent spread of infection.

Parenterally and orally administered extended-spectrum cephalosporins have been used successfully in the treatment of children with shigellosis (114–116). Two-day (115) and 5-day (116) courses of ceftriaxone were effective in eradication of *Shigella* from stool and reduction of duration of diarrhea. In one study, a single parenteral dose of ceftriaxone produced a moderate reduction in diarrhea but failed to eradicate *Shigella* strains from stools (117). Previous studies of first- and second-generation cephalosporins for treatment of shigellosis have demonstrated them to be ineffective (118–120). Cefixime administered orally has been shown to be therapeutic for children and adolescents whose isolates were resistant to TMP-SMX (114), although it is not approved by the FDA for this condition. Ceftibuten, an orally administered third-generation cephalosporin, has shown good *in vitro* activity against various enteric pathogens and promising clinical efficacy in patients with shigellosis (121).

Ciprofloxacin, norfloxacin, and enoxacin have been used successfully to treat adults with shigellosis, even those infected with resistant strains (94,122–125). In a study evaluating dosing of ciprofloxacin in adults, ten 1-g doses (5 days) were an effective therapy for patients infected with *S. dysenteriae* type 1. For other *Shigella* species, a single 1-g dose was sufficient (124). Ciprofloxacin is FDA approved for treatment of GI tract infections caused by *S. sonnei* and *S. flexneri.* In a randomized double-blinded study of 120 children age 2 to 15 years with shigellosis, ciprofloxacin and pivmecillinam given for 5 days were successful in providing a clinical cure and eradicating the organism from stool (123). Ciprofloxacin was not associated with the development of arthropathy in children in this study. The fluoroquinolones, such as ofloxacin and ciprofloxacin, have greater activity against gram-negative bacteria than do the older DNA gyrase inhibitors such as nalidixic acid. However, reduced susceptibility to ciprofloxacin and ofloxacin, probably due to mutation in the DNA gyrase subunit A gene, has been noted in *S. sonnei* strains isolated from patients with dysentery (126). Nalidixic acid can be used as an alternative drug (127), although resistance has been described (103,128,129). A comparative study of a 5-day course of either azithromycin or ciprofloxacin in adults with shigellosis showed comparable clinical and bacteriologic results (122).

Campylobacter

C. jejuni strains generally are susceptible to a wide variety of antimicrobial agents, including erythromycin, furazolidone, quinolones, aminoglycosides, tetracycline, chloramphenicol, imipenem, and clindamycin; by contrast, penicillin, ampicillin, and the cephalosporins are relatively inactive (130–133). Isolation of *Campylobacter* from stool does not mandate antibiotic therapy; the decision to institute therapy should be made on clinical grounds. In patients with *Campylobacter* enteritis, erythromycin or azithromycin represent the agents of choice (134,135). Ciprofloxacin has been approved by the FDA as treatment of *C. jejuni* enteritis in persons older than 17 years, as detailed below, but resistance is increasing. In double-blinded, placebo-controlled trials of the treatment of patients with *Campylobacter* enteritis, erythromycin promptly eradicated *Campylobacter* from feces but did not

TABLE 78.5. ANTIMICROBIAL THERAPY FOR SHIGELLOSIS

Antimicrobial Agent[a]	Days of Therapy	Comment
Azithromycin	5	Evaluated in adults
Ciprofloxacin or ofloxacin	3–5	Drugs of choice for adults; not approved for persons under 18 yrs of age
Ceftriaxone	3	Resistant strains; not FDA approved for this purpose
Cefixime	5	Resistant strains; not FDA approved for this purpose

[a]Ampicillin and trimethoprim-sulfamethoxazole are effective if strain is susceptible.

alter the natural course of enteritis when administered 4 days or longer after the onset of symptoms. Studies in which therapy was initiated early in the course of illness gave conflicting results with regard to clinical resolution, although *C. jejuni* was eliminated from stools significantly faster in the treatment groups of both studies (136,137). Clindamycin or amoxicillin plus clavulanate is an alternative choice in children, but studies supporting the effectiveness of these drugs are limited. The treatment of choice for patients with septicemia due to *C. jejuni* appears to be parenterally administered gentamicin or ciprofloxacin in adults, although chloramphenicol, tetracycline, and erythromycin are alternative choices (134). Therapy of septicemia due to *C. fetus* is either imipenem, meropenem, or gentamicin (134,138).

The frequency of isolation of erythromycin-resistant *Campylobacter* strains ranges from less than 1% in Canada and the United Kingdom (132,139–142) to 8% in Belgium, and 10% in Sweden (143,144). In one study from the United States, 3% of *Campylobacter* strains from human sources were resistant to erythromycin (145). In this and other studies, a higher frequency of erythromycin resistance was noted in hog isolates, most of which were *C. coli* (145–147). In Spain, resistance of *C. coli* to erythromycin was 81% in hog isolates, 35% in human isolates, and less than 1% in broiler isolates (146). Other studies have reported that the frequency of resistance in *C. coli* is much higher than in *C. jejuni* (130,145,146,148,149). This resistance may be due to production of RNA methylase or a mutational change of a ribosomal protein gene (139). Strains of *C. jejuni* and *C. coli* that show high-level resistance to erythromycin also appear to be resistant to clarithromycin and azithromycin (150). Development of resistance to ciprofloxacin in *Campylobacter* species has been reported in several studies (146,151–158,160,161). These high rates have been related to the introduction of fluoroquinolones in animal feed (158,159). Resistance by *C. jejuni* (162) and *C. fetus* (155) to ciprofloxacin has developed in people during therapy with ciprofloxacin.

Shiga Toxin-producing Escherichia coli

The role of antimicrobial therapy in patients with hemorrhagic colitis caused by Shiga toxin-producing *E. coli* (STEC), including *E. coli* O157:H7 or other STEC, has undergone a transition. Initially, the fact that treatment of patients infected with *E. coli* O157:H7 may be harmful was raised by several observations. When *E. coli* O157:H7 was cultured with subinhibitory concentrations of certain antibiotics, including TMP-SMX, the intracellular and extracellular concentrations of Shiga toxin increased (163,164). Because hemolytic–uremic syndrome (HUS) and thrombotic thrombocytopenic purpura are thought to be mediated by Shiga toxin, certain antibiotics may increase the amount of toxin released in the intestine, resulting in an increased risk of systemic sequelae. In nonrandomized studies of residents in an institution for the mentally retarded, five of eight individuals with HUS had received TMP-SMX, compared with none of seven who had no subsequent complications (165). In another study, nursing home patients with *E. coli* O157:H7 infections who were treated with antimicrobial agents had an increased risk of death (166). An issue with these two clinical reports of antimicrobial use in patients with diarrhea due to *E. coli* O157:H7 is that antimicrobial agents were not administered in a randomized fashion and patients who had more severe illness were likely to have received medication (35,167). Therefore, the outcome of treatment was more likely to be associated with poor outcome because the prognosis was worse at the onset of therapy (165). In contrast to these observations, in one prospective controlled trial, which evaluated the effect of TMP-SMX in children with proven *E. coli* O157:H7 enteritis, treatment had no effect on the progression of symptoms, fecal pathogen excretion, or incidence of HUS (168), indicating that antibiotics were neither helpful nor harmful to children with infection due to STEC, but the sample size in this study was small.

In 2000, a cohort study of 71 children younger than 10 years who had diarrhea caused by *E. coli* O157:H7 was published. This study showed an increase in the risk of HUS in the 9 children treated with antimicrobial agents, compared with the 62 children who did not receive antibiotic therapy (56% vs. 8%; $p < .002$, respectively (169). Therefore, antimicrobial therapy is not recommended for children with STEC infection.

This occurrence of HUS after antimicrobial therapy of patients with STEC infection may depend on the number of organisms present, the environmental conditions of those organisms, their bactericidal activity or ability to induce toxin gene expression. Toxin synthesis by STEC appears to be co-regulated through induction of the integrated bacteriophage that encodes the toxin gene. Phage production is linked to induction of bacterial distress response, which is a ubiquitous response to DNA damage. Induction of toxin gene expression occurs upon exposure to distress-inducing antimicrobial agents, particularly the fluoroquinolones, TMP, and furazolidone (170). The fluoroquinolones and TMP are the most potent distress inducers. Mitomycin C, another potent distress inducer, is known to increase Shiga toxin levels *in vitro* (171) and has been associated with HUS in humans with cancer (172). Distress induction occurs with several β-lactams but appears to be inhibited by imipenem (170). A distress-inducing effect was not detected with fosfomycin, gentamicin, chloramphenicol, doxycycline, and erythromycin under various incubation conditions (170). A study in mice showed that animals treated with fosfomycin did not have an increase in free fecal Shiga toxin and death, compared with animals treated with ciprofloxacin (173). In addition, ciprofloxacin, but not fosfomycin, caused Shiga toxin-encoding bacteriophage induction and enhanced Shiga toxin production from *E. coli* O157:H7 *in vitro.* Interestingly, in 1996 in an outbreak of STEC infection in Japan associated with white radish sprouts, fosfomycin was associated with prevention of HUS (174). These data indicate that agents with distress-inducing activity including fluoroquinolones, TMP, furazolidone, and most β-lactams should not be used in patients with STEC. The potential benefit and safety of non-distress inducers, such as macrolides, in infection due to STEC is not known. Additional studies are needed to determine whether non-distress-inducing antibiotics are safe and effective therapy for patients with STEC.

Vibrio cholerae

Diarrhea caused by infection with *V. cholerae* O1 is uncommon in the United States, although the organism is endemic along the Gulf Coast (175). In addition, since appearing in Peru in 1991, *V. cholerae* has spread to most countries in South and North America. Oral fluid and electrolyte therapy is essential for patients with cholera. Antimicrobial therapy for gastroenteritis from cholera will shorten the duration of diarrhea and reduce fluid losses but is not a substitute for prompt fluid and electrolyte replacement. For most patients, either tetracycline or single-dose doxycycline is the drug of choice (Table 78.3) (176–179). Other effective antimicrobial agents are TMP-SMX, ciprofloxacin, and ofloxacin, but the fluoroquinolones are not approved for use in individuals younger than 18 years (177,180,181). The use of tetracycline or doxycycline is not recommended for children younger than 9 years; however, in severe cholera infections, one of these agents is the drug of choice. *V. cholerae* has remained relatively susceptible to antibiotics, most likely because only a few plasmid types are stable in these organisms. Nevertheless, resistance to tetracycline, streptomycin, chloramphenicol, sulfonamides, ampicillin, kanamycin, TMP-SMX, and the fluoroquinolones has been reported (103,182).

V. cholerae O139 was first identified during a large outbreak of cholera-like disease in 1992 in southern India (183) and rapidly spread to all cholera endemic areas in India and neighboring countries (184). This organism has been shown to be susceptible to tetracycline, ampicillin, chloramphenicol, erythromycin, and ciprofloxacin, but not to TMP-SMX and furazolidone, two agents used to treat cholera in children (183). The drugs of choice for the treatment of this organism in children and adults are doxycycline or tetracycline.

Other Bacteria

Other bacteria that infrequently produce diarrhea in children in the United States are *E. coli* other than *E. coli* O157:H7, *Y. enterocolitica,* and *Vibrio parahaemolyticus. Y. enterocolitica* appears to be a common cause of diarrhea among children in Europe and Canada (185). Infection occurs infrequently in the United States but has been reported in young children during the winter holidays after ingestion of chitterlings (186). This organism usually is susceptible *in vitro* to aminoglycosides, chloramphenicol, tetracycline, TMP-SMX, extended-spectrum cephalosporins, quinolones, imipenem, and aztreonam (185,187). Strains are often resistant to penicillin, ampicillin, and first-generation cephalosporins. There are no data to support the use of antimicrobial agents in diarrhea caused by this organism (188). Patients with *Y. enterocolitica*-induced septicemia should be treated with TMP-SMX, gentamicin, tobramycin, ceftriaxone, or cefotaxime. In adults, doxycycline or a fluoroquinolone has been shown to be effective (185,189). Despite treatment, the mortality rate for this condition approaches 50%. *V. parahaemolyticus* GI tract infection is self-limited and can be effectively treated with oral rehydration alone. Antimicrobial therapy shortens neither the clinical course nor the duration of fecal excretion of the organism (190).

Diarrhea caused by enterotoxigenic *E. coli* (ETEC) usually is self-limited, but studies have shown that antimicrobial agents such as TMP-SMX or ciprofloxacin are effective (94,109,110), depending on susceptibility patterns. Ciprofloxacin is FDA approved for treatment of persons with diarrhea due to ETEC and has been shown to be effective in adult travelers with diarrhea due to enteroaggregative *E. coli* (191). Little is known about the treatment of enteroinvasive *E. coli* infection because the diagnosis usually is not established. Antimicrobial therapy should be similar to that administered to patients with shigellosis. Susceptibility studies should be performed if an organism is isolated.

Evidence suggests that some aeromonads cause gastroenteritis, but it is uncertain whether many of the strains isolated from stool cause diarrheal disease (192). *In vitro* studies have shown that more than 90% of 131 strains of *Aeromonas* species were susceptible to aminoglycosides, ureidopenicillins, extended-spectrum cephalosporin antibiotics, aztreonam, quinolones, tetracycline, and chloramphenicol; more than 75% were susceptible to TMP-SMX; and all strains were resistant to ampicillin (193). Differences in susceptibility patterns may exist among geographic areas and within species of *Aeromonas* (192). Invasive strains generally are treated with gentamicin, tobramycin, imipenem, or a fluoroquinolone if the patient is older than 17 years (194). Infections of the GI tract may respond to TMP-SMX or ciprofloxacin, which is approved only for patients older than 17 years.

Plesiomonas shigelloides has been identified as a cause of endemic and traveler's diarrhea. These organisms are susceptible to TMP-SMX, ciprofloxacin, extended-spectrum cephalosporins, and imipenem (195). Many strains are resistant to aminoglycosides.

Protozoal Agents

Because patients with AIDS frequently develop persistent diarrhea, there has been a renewed interest in parasitic

TABLE 78.6. ANTIMICROBIAL THERAPY FOR GIARDIASIS

Antimicrobial Agent	Days of Therapy	Common Side Effects	Comment
Furazolidone (Furoxone)	7–10	Nausea, vomiting, diarrhea, brown urine, disulfiram reaction with alcohol	Available in liquid form
Metronidazole[a] (Flagyl)	5	Nausea, headache, dry mouth, metallic taste, disulfiram-like reaction with alcohol	Mutagenic in bacteria carcinogenic in mice and rats at high doses over prolonged time
Quinacrine HCl (Atabrine)	5	Dizziness, headache, vomiting, diarrhea, yellow-orange skin color	Not available commercially but can be obtained[b]
Paromomycin[a] (Humatin)	7	Gastrointestinal tract disturbance	Not absorbed and not very effective; may be useful for treatment of giardiasis in pregnancy
Albendazole[a]	5	Anorexia, constipation	Clinical trials have shown mixed results

[a]Not a U.S. Food and Drug Administration approved indication.
[b]Medical Center Pharmacy, New Haven, CT, 203-785-6818 or Panorama Compounding Pharmacy, 800-247-9767.

infections involving the GI tract. In immunocompetent patients, infections with these organisms are generally of short duration and respond to therapy when available; however, the clinical course may be protracted in children with AIDS (7). Parasitic diseases of the GI tract that fulfill the Centers for Disease Control and Prevention surveillance definition for AIDS are those caused by *Cryptosporidium* and *Isospora* (196). Tables 78.6 through 78.8 show the recommended therapy for infection with enteric parasitic organisms (197). Several of these compounds have severe adverse effects that should be considered against the potential benefit of therapy.

Giardia lamblia

Differences in studies make comparison of the clinical efficacy of drugs used to treat giardiasis difficult. Metronidazole, furazolidone, quinacrine hydrochloride, and albendazole are effective in treating patients with infection caused by *G. lamblia* (198). Metronidazole may be better tolerated than quinacrine, but it is more expensive and may be slightly less effective. In addition, metronidazole is carcinogenic in rodents and mutagenic in bacteria and is considered an investigational drug for this condition by the FDA. Quinacrine hydrochloride may produce a yellow discoloration of the skin, which disappears after the drug is stopped (199). Quinacrine is not available commercially but as a service can be compounded (Table 78.6). Furazolidone is the only one of these three compounds available in liquid form; like quinacrine, it is less expensive than metronidazole. Furazolidone can be used in children (200) if compliance is a problem with quinacrine and metronidazole, both of which have an objectionable taste. Clinical trials using albendazole to treat people with giardiasis have produced mixed results (198). Treatment of children with albendazole for 5 days (201) but not 3 days (201–203) has been effective. Toxicity of albendazole is low and this compound is effective against many helminths, making it useful for treatment when multiple intestinal parasites are identified or suspected. Paromomycin is a nonabsorbable aminoglycoside that may be useful for the treatment of giardiasis in pregnancy. The dosage schedule for children and adults is given in Table 78.6. Outside the United States, tinidazole and ornidazole also are used to treat giardiasis. Tinidazole

TABLE 78.7. ANTIMICROBIAL THERAPY FOR AMEBIASIS

Clinical Manifestations	Antimicrobial Agent	Days of Therapy	Comment
Asymptomatic cyst excretor	Iodoquinol (Yodoxin)	20	Do not exceed maximum dose, because of possibility of optic neuritis
	or		
	Paromomycin (Humatin) or	7	Non-absorable aminoglycoside
	Diloxanide furoate (Furamide)[a]	10	Available from the Centers for Disease Control and Prevention Drug Service
Mild-to-moderate intestinal disease	Metronidazole (Flagyl) first	10	Not recommended for pregnant women, especially in first trimester
	followed by iodoquinol	20	
	or paromomycin	7	
Severe intestinal disease and extra-intestinal disease	Metronidazole first,	7	
	followed by iodoquinol	20	
	or paromomycin	7	

[a]Telephone number 404-639-3670 or 639-2888.

TABLE 78.8. ANTIMICROBIAL THERAPY FOR ENTERIC PARASITES IN CHILDREN

Organism	Antimicrobial Agent	Days of Therapy	Comments
Cryptosporidium	Paromomycin	Two to four doses	Disease is self-limited in immunocompetent persons; not curative in immunocompromised persons; combination with azithromycin has been effective
Isospora belli	TMP/SMX	10 then every 12 h/3 wk	Considered an investigational drug for this condition by the Food and Drug Administration; studies lacking in children
Encephalitozoon intestinalis	Albendazole		Octreotide (Sandostatin) has provided symptomatic relief
or *Enterocytozoon bieneusi*	Albendazole		No effect or minimal effect
Strongyloides	Ivermectin or thiabendazole	1–2 2	In immunocompromised persons or disseminated disease, repeated or prolonged therapy may be necessary
Blastocystis hominis	Metronidazole or iodoquiniol	10 20	Controlled studies not available; clinical significance of this organism is unknown
Cyclospora	TMP/SMX	7	HIV-infected persons may need higher doses and long-term maintenance; no studies in children

For *Giardia lamblia* see Table 78.6; for *Entamoeba histolytica* see Table 78.7.

and ornidazole are nitroimidazoles similar to metronidazole and appear to be as effective as metronidazole and better tolerated (198).

Entamoeba histolytica

Entamoeba histolytica, a protozoal parasite, can invade the intestinal mucosa and spread to other organs, particularly the liver (204). Iodoquinol is the recommended drug to eradicate both cysts and trophozoites of *E. histolytica* in the lumen of the GI tract (Table 78.7). Invasive amebiasis of the intestine, liver, or other organs necessitates additional use of tissue amebicides such as metronidazole. Table 78.7 shows the recommended drugs for the treatment of children with various forms of amebiasis (197).

Cryptosporidium

Infection with *Cryptosporidium* is self-limited in immunocompetent individuals; however, patients with AIDS may have large volume, intractable diarrhea (205). There is no curative therapy for cryptosporidiosis, despite *in vitro* and *in vivo* testing of hundreds of compounds. In immunocompetent children and adults, no specific therapy is indicated due to the self-limited nature of the disease. In persons with persistent disease, an underlying immunodeficiency should be considered. Recommended antimicrobial therapy for *Cryptosporidium* infection is paromomycin, which may be effective in rapid resolution of chronic diarrhea (206–208). Spiramycin has been used but is ineffective (209). Paromomycin also has been shown to inhibit *Cryptosporidium* infection of a human enterocyte cell line (210). In a prospective, randomized, double-blinded, placebo-controlled trial in the treatment of adults with AIDS and symptomatic cryptosporidiosis (211), paromomycin was not effective, although inadequate statistical power prevented definitive rejection of the usefulness of paromomycin as therapy for this infection. In dexamethasone-immunosuppressed rats, azithromycin consistently prevented ileal infection with *Cryptosporidium parvum* in a dose-related manner (212). Azithromycin has been shown to be effective in the treatment of two children with cancer who had severe diarrhea due to *Cryptosporidium* (213). Combination therapy with paromomycin and azithromycin has been effective in some patients with AIDS and chronic cryptosporidiosis (214). Nitazoxanide (an investigational drug in the United States) may be used as an alternative (*www.romarklaboratories.com*) (197). Orally administered bovine transfer factor, hyperimmune colostrum, monoclonal antibody, cow milk immunoglobulin, and human serum immunoglobulin have all been evaluated with varying success (215–220). Octreotide (Sandostatin) may control the severe diarrhea that occurs in patients with AIDS, as it has in patients with scleroderma (221), although it has no effect on the infection (28,221, 222). The combination of clarithromycin and rifabutin, but not azithromycin alone, was highly protective against the development of cryptosporidiosis in immunosuppressed HIV-infected adults (223). The best approach to prevention of cryptosporidiosis in HIV-infected people is maintenance of immune system function by using highly active antiretroviral therapy, because chronic cryptosporidiosis occurs only in severely immunocompromised people.

Isospora

Isospora species can cause serious disease in humans and nursing pigs, and rarely in primates, dogs, and cats (224). Unlike *Cryptosporidium, Isospora* organisms respond to treatment with TMP-SMX (Table 78.8) (225). However, symptomatic disease recurs in 50% of patients (226). Pyrimethamine-sulfadoxine has been used less frequently than TMP-SMX but also gives clinical response and eliminates the parasite (224). Recurrent disease may be prevented by prophylaxis with TMP-SMX or weekly doses of pyrimethamine-sulfadoxine (Fansidar). Both of these compounds are considered investigational by the FDA for isosporiasis. In sulfonamide-sensitive patients, including people with AIDS, pyrimethamine has been effective in adults (227). In immunocompromised patients, therapy may need to be continued indefinitely. Patients who receive TMP-SMX or pyrimethamine-sulfadoxine should be monitored carefully for bone marrow suppression, skin reactions, and allergic manifestations.

Strongyloides stercoralis

Persons infected with *Strongyloides stercoralis* should be treated with ivermectin or alternatively thiabendazole (228,229). In disseminated strongyloidiasis, ivermectin or thiabendazole therapy should be continued for at least 5 days. In immunocompromised patients or persons with *Strongyloides* hyperinfection, longer therapy may be necessary (230); however, the mortality rate is high despite therapy. A thorough examination should be performed before immunosuppressive therapy is given to a patient with a history of infection with *S. stercoralis.*

Microsporidia

Based on *in vitro* studies, several drugs have been used to treat microsporidial infections in humans, but successful treatment with any of them in humans is limited (231). Microsporidians that infect the GI tract include *E. bieneusi* and *E. intestinalis* (231–236). Therapy with anti-parasitic drugs, diet alteration, and antidiarrheal medications often fails to relieve diarrhea and malabsorption associated with microsporidiosis, although octreotide may provide symptomatic relief (222) and diet modification to include medium-chain triglyceride-based diets has produced clinical improvement (237). *In vitro* studies have shown that *E. intestinalis* is susceptible to albendazole (238,239). Albendazole has been reported to stop diarrhea and weight loss, as well as promote weight gain, in persons infected with *E. intestinalis* (233,235,236,240), although improvement has not been uniform. Infections due to *E. bieneusi* are much more difficult to treat and there is no acceptable treatment. Albendazole treatment of patients infected with *E. bieneusi* has shown improvement in 50% of patients in some studies, lower response rates in other studies, and persistence of the organism in most (231).

Blastocystis hominis

The clinical significance of *Blastocystis hominis* remains unclear. Few studies have considered the treatment of large numbers of patients, and case–control studies are lacking (241). Use of metronidazole or iodoquinol in the same dose used for mild to moderate intestinal disease from *E. histolytica* (Table 78.7) has been reported to be effective in uncontrolled studies (241,242), and these drugs are the recommended drugs of choice. TMP-SMX or paromomycin may be the most appropriate second choice drugs (241). Treatment should be provided with caution, only after a thorough clinical review of other possible causes of symptoms has been performed.

Cyclospora

Cyclospora cayetanensis is a coccidian parasite that causes moderate to severe self-limited diarrhea by injuring the small bowel (243). Illness in immunocompetent people is often prolonged but ultimately self-limited. Infection in HIV-infected people has been reported and can range from asymptomatic to a severe illness and can include ascending infection of the biliary tract (244). A 7-day course of TMP-SMX is the recommended therapy (245,246); although ciprofloxacin is not as effective as TMP-SMX, it is acceptable for patients who cannot tolerate TMP-SMX (245).

PROTRACTED VIRAL INFECTIONS IN THE IMMUNOCOMPROMISED CHILD

Occasionally, a clinician will face the challenge of treating an immunocompromised child with protracted diarrhea associated with continual excretion of rotavirus, calicivirus, astrovirus, or other enteric viruses. The diarrhea in these children may be unremitting and fatal. Factors important for clearing viral infection in these individuals include an intact cellular immune system and the presence of specific neutralizing antibody. In these special situations, the administration of immunoglobulins enterically, as milk, colostrum, or specific immunoglobulin preparations, may reduce the burden of illness (247,248). These preparations usually are not standardized for level of antibody to any enteric virus and multiple agents frequently infect the child simultaneously. Therefore, choice and dose of therapy frequently are empiric. However, in a tertiary care facility, immune electron microscopy, EIAs, or neutralization tests may be available to evaluate the potency of antibody preparations and the virologic response to therapy.

PREVENTION OF ACUTE INFECTIOUS GASTROENTERITIS IN CHILDREN

Issues relating to prevention of GI tract illness in children can be considered in several major categories, which include child health issues, interrupting transmission, epidemic control, and immunization. Child health issues encompass the promotion and implementation of exclusive breastfeeding for approximately the first 6 months of life to continue to 1 year of age and beyond with the addition of supplemental foods as recommended by the American Academy of Pediatrics (249). Other preventive health issues relating to children need to be implemented, including adhering to the recommended childhood immunization schedule.

Interrupting the transmission of enteropathogens involves availability of a clean water supply and sanitation facilities, as well as promotion of personal and domestic hygiene. Many GI tract illnesses can be prevented by following personal hygiene practices including hand washing and safe food preparation. Select populations with immunodeficient conditions may require additional education about food safety and animal exposure (250,251). Individuals who are immunodeficient are more susceptible to infection with a variety of enteric pathogens and may be more likely to develop severe illness and complications once infected. Immunodeficient persons can reduce their risk by being educated about and following safe food handling and preparation practices and adhering to appropriate animal exposure practices (4,5,250). In addition, instructions about safe travel habits should be provided (252).

Epidemic control includes surveillance, investigation, reporting, and control. Children in child care centers, hospitals, and extended-care facilities are at an increased risk for enteric infection because of close contact, need for hands-on contact, immature immune systems, and lack of appropriate hygiene practices. Reporting of outbreaks to public health officials may be critical to interrupting transmission and preventing disease.

The only vaccine against diarrheal diseases that is available in the United States includes a vaccine against typhoid fever, which is an uncommon cause of disease in the United States (84). The vaccine available in the United States against cholera has been removed from the market, as has the typhoid vaccine for children younger than 2 years. The rotavirus vaccine, which made a brief appearance in the United States, has been withdrawn because of the association with intussusception (253). Vaccines against several enteric pathogens are in various phases of testing. Currently, oral rehydration, breast-feeding, adherence to appropriate sanitation practices, adequate surveillance systems for disease, and availability of clean water supplies and sanitation facilities are paramount for disease prevention.

SUMMARY

Many organisms in multiple microbiologic classes cause acute infectious gastroenteritis among children. The diversity of etiologic agents is associated with differences in response to therapy, complexity in the diagnosis of specific causes of infection, and complexity of treatment options, particularly because of the increasing prevalence of strains resistant to antimicrobial agents. With a few exceptions, the constellation of symptoms associated with diarrhea is remarkably uniform. Because these agents usually are spread by the fecal-oral route, the potential for polymicrobial infection is real. Multiple agents should be suspected, particularly in the immunocompromised host and when the response to specific therapy for a detected pathogen is delayed. The discovery of a large number of emerging enteric pathogens will provide opportunities for fruitful and careful investigations of treatment and prevention over the next several years.

REFERENCES

1. Duggan C, Santosham M, Glass RI. The management of acute diarrhea in children: oral rehydration, maintenance, and nutritional therapy. *MMWR Morb Mortal Wkly Rep* 1992;41(RR-16):1–19.
2. American Academy of Pediatrics, Provisional Committee on Quality Improvement, Subcommittee on Acute Gastroenteritis. Practice parameter: the management of acute gastroenteritis in young children. *Pediatrics* 1996;97:424–435.
3. Guerrant RL, VanGilder T, Steiner TS, et al. Practice guidelines for the management of infectious diarrhea. *Clin Infect Dis* 2001; 32:331–350.
4. Centers for Disease Control and Prevention. Diagnosis and management of foodborne illnesses. A primer for physicians. *MMWR Morb Mortal Wkly Rep* 2001;50(RR-2):1–54.
5. Centers for Disease Control and Prevention. Surveillance for waterborne disease outbreaks—United States, 1997–1998. *MMWR Morb Mortal Wkly Rep* 2000;49(SS-4):1–32.
6. Grohmann GS, Glass RI, Pereira HG, et al. Enteric viruses and diarrhea in HIV-infected patients. *N Engl J Med* 1993;329: 14–20.
7. Mitchell DK, Snyder J, Pickering LK. Gastrointestinal infections. In: Pizzo PA, Wilfert CM, eds. *Pediatric AIDS: the challenge of HIV infection in infants, children and adolescents,* third edition. Baltimore, MD: Williams & Wilkins, 1999:267–291.
8. Arbo A, Santos JI. Diarrheal disease in the immunocompromised host. *Pediatr Infect Dis J* 1987;6:894–906.
9. DuPont HL, Hornick RB. Adverse effect on Lomotil therapy in shigellosis. *JAMA* 1973;226:1525–1528.
10. Ginsburg CM. Lomotil (diphenoxylate and atropine) intoxication. *Am J Dis Child* 1973;125:241–242.
11. Rumack BH, Temple AR. Lomotil poisoning. *Pediatrics* 1974; 53:495–500.
12. McClung HJ, Beck RD, Powers P. The effect of kaolin-pectin adsorbent on stool losses of sodium, potassium, and fat during a lactose-intolerance diarrhea in rats. *J Pediatr* 1980;96: 769–771.
13. Portnoy BL, DuPont HL, Pruitt D, et al. Antidiarrheal agents in the treatment of acute diarrhea in children. *JAMA* 1976; 236:844–846.
14. Clements ML, Levine MM, Black RE, et al. Lactobacillus prophylaxis for diarrhea due to enterotoxigenic *Escherichia coli. Antimicrob Agents Chemother* 1981;20:104–108.
15. Levine MM, Hornick RB. Lactulose therapy in *Shigella* carrier state and dysentery. *Antimicrob Agents Chemother* 1975;8: 581–584.
16. Pearce JL, Hamilton JR. Controlled trial of orally administered lactobacilli in acute infantile diarrhea. *J Pediatr* 1974;84: 261–262.
17. Ericsson CD, DuPont HL, Evans DG, et al. Bismuth subsalicy-

late inhibits activity of crude toxins of *Escherichia coli* and *Vibrio cholerae. J Infect Dis* 1977;136:693–696.
18. Feldman S, Chen SL, Pickering LK, et al. Salicylate absorption from a bismuth subsalicylate anti-diarrheal preparation (Pepto-Bismol). *Clin Pharmacol Ther* 1981;29:788–792.
19. Pickering LK, Feldman S, Ericsson CD, et al. Absorption of salicylate and bismuth from a bismuth subsalicylate containing compound (Pepto-Bismol). *J Pediatr* 1981;99:654–656.
20. Mendelowitz PC, Hoffman RS, Weber S. Bismuth absorption and myoclonic encephalopathy during bismuth subsalicylate therapy. *Ann Intern Med* 1990;112:140–141.
21. Salazar-Lindo E, Santisteban-Ponce J, Chea-Woo E, et al. Racecadotril in the treatment of acute watery diarrhea in children. *N Engl J Med* 2000;343:463–467.
22. Lamberts SWJ, van der Lely A-J, de Herder WW, et al. Drug therapy. Octreotide. *N Engl J Med* 1996;334:246–254.
23. Pickering LK. Biotherapeutic agents and disease in infants. In: Newburg DS, ed. *Bioactive substances in human milk.* Plenum Publishing 2001;365–373.
24. Vanderhoff JA, Whitney DB, Antonson DL, et al. Lactobacillus GG in the prevention of antibiotic-associated diarrhea in children. *J Pediatr* 1999;135:564–568.
25. Oberhelman RA, Gilman RH, Sheen P, et al. A placebo-controlled trial of *Lactobacillus* GG to prevent diarrhea in undernourished Peruvian children. *J Pediatr* 1999;134:15–20.
26. Novak E, Lee JG, Seckman CE, et al. Unfavorable effect of atropine-diphenoxylate (Lomotil) therapy in lincomycin-caused diarrhea. *JAMA* 1976;235:1451–1454.
27. Rateau JG, Morgant G, Droy-Priot MT, et al. A histological, enzymatic and water-electrolyte study of the action of smectite, a mucoprotective clay, on experimental infectious diarrhoea in the rabbit. *Curr Med Res Opin* 1982;8:233–241.
28. Cook DJ, Kelton JG, Stanisz AM, et al. Somatostatin treatment for cryptosporidial diarrhea in a patient with the acquired immunodeficiency syndrome (AIDS). *Ann Intern Med* 1988;108:708–709.
29. Zinc Investigators' Collaborative Group. Prevention of diarrhea and pneumonia by zinc supplementation in children in developing countries: pooled analysis of randomized controlled trials. *J Pediatr* 1999;135:689–697.
30. Diarrhoeal Diseases Study Group (UK). Loperamide in acute diarrhoea in childhood: results of a double-blind, placebo-controlled multicentre clinical trial. *Br Med J* 1984;289:1263–1267.
31. Vesikari T, Isolauri E. A comparative trial of cholestyramine and loperamide for acute diarrhoea in infants treated as outpatients. *Acta Paediatr Scand* 1985;74:650–654.
32. Bergstrom T, Alestig K, Thoron K, et al. Symptomatic treatment of acute infectious diarrhoea: loperamide versus placebo in a double-blind trial. *J Infect Dis* 1986;12:35–38.
33. Soriano-Brucher HE, Avendano P, O'Ryan M, et al. Use of bismuth subsalicylate in acute diarrhea in children. *Rev Infect Dis* 1990;12:S51–S56.
34. Ericsson CD, DuPont HL, Mathewson JJ, et al. Treatment of travelers' diarrhea with sulfamethoxazole and trimethoprim and loperamide. *JAMA* 1990;263:257–261.
35. Cimolai N, Carter JE, Morrison BJ, et al. Risk factors for the progression of *Escherichia coli* O157:H7 enteritis to hemolytic–uremic syndrome. *J Pediatr* 1990;116:589–592.
36. Cimolai N, Carter JE, Morrison BJ, et al. The progression of *Escherichia coli* O157:H7 enteritis to hemolytic uremic syndrome: anti-diarrheal agent use and age as risk factors? *Clin Invest Med* 1988;11[Suppl]:C71.
37. Reuman PD, Duckworth DH, Smith KL, et al. Lack of effect of *Lactobacillus* on gastrointestinal bacterial colonization in premature infants. *Pediatr Infect Dis* 1986;5:663–668.
38. DuPont HL, Ericsson CD, Johnson PC, et al. Prevention of travelers' diarrhea by the table formulation of bismuth subsalicylate. *JAMA* 1987;257:1347–1350.
39. DuPont HL, Sullivan P, Pickering LK, et al. Symptomatic treatment of diarrhea with bismuth subsalicylate among students attending a Mexican university. *Gastroenterology* 1977;73:715–718.
40. Figueroa-Quintanilla D, Salazar-Lindo E, Sack RB, et al. A controlled trial of bismuth subsalicylate in infants with acute watery diarrheal disease. *N Engl J Med* 1993;328:1653–1658.
41. Kunin CM. Resistance to antimicrobial drugs-a worldwide calamity. *Ann Intern Med* 1993;118:557–561.
42. Johnson S, Gerding DN. *Clostridium difficile*-associated diarrhea. *Clin Infect Dis* 1998;26:1027–1036.
43. Cerquetti M, Luzzi I, Caprioli A, et al. Role of *Clostridium difficile* in childhood diarrhea. *Pediatr Infect Dis J* 1995;14:598–603.
44. Mitchell DK, Van R, Mason EH, et al. Prospective study of toxigenic *Clostridium difficile* in children given amoxicillin/clavulanate for otitis media. *Pediatr Infect Dis J* 15:514–519, 1996.
45. Teasley PG, Gerding DN, Olson MM, et al. Prospective randomized trial of metronidazole versus vancomycin for *Clostridium difficile*-associated diarrhea and colitis. *Lancet* 1983;2:1043–1046.
46. Wenisch C, Parschalk B, Hasenhundl M, et al. Comparison of vancomycin, teicoplanin, metronidazole, and fusidic acid for the treatment of *Clostridium difficile*-associated diarrhea. *Clin Infect Dis* 1996;22:813–818.
47. Cherry RD, Portnoy D, Jabbari M, et al. Metronidazole: an alternate therapy for antibiotic associated colitis. *Gastroenterology* 1982;82:849–851.
48. Batts DH, Martin D, Holmes R, et al. Treatment of antibiotic-associated *Clostridium difficile* diarrhea with oral vancomycin. *J Pediatr* 1980;97:151–153.
49. Fekety R, Silva J, Kauffman C, et al. Treatment of *Clostridium difficile* antibiotic-associated colitis with oral vancomycin. Comparison of two dosage regimens. *Am J Med* 1989;86:15–19.
50. Fekety R, Silva J, Toshniwal R, et al. Antibiotic-associated colitis: effects of antibiotics on the disease in hamsters. *Rev Infect Dis* 1979;1:386–396.
51. Tedesco FJ. Bacitracin therapy in antibiotic associated pseudomembranous colitis. *Dig Dis Sci* 1980;25:783.
52. Young GP, Ward PB, Bayley N, et al. Antibiotic associated colitis due to *Clostridium difficile:* double-blind comparison of vancomycin with bacitracin. *Gastroenterology* 1985;89:1038–1045.
53. Dudley MN, McLaughlin JC, Carrington G, et al. Oral bacitracin vs. vancomycin therapy for *Clostridium difficile*-induced diarrhea. A randomized double-blind trial. *Arch Intern Med* 1986;146:1101–1104.
54. Burbige BJ, Milligan FD. Pseudomembranous colitis: association with antibiotics and therapy with cholestyramine. *JAMA* 1975;231:1157–1158.
55. Högenauer C, Hammer HF, Krejs GJ, et al. Mechanisms and management of antibiotic-associated diarrhea. *Clin Infect Dis* 1998;27:702–710.
56. Surawizc CM, McFarland LV, Greenberg RN, et al. The search for a better treatment for recurrent *Clostridium difficile* disease: use of high-dose vancomycin combined with *Saccharomyces boulardii. Clin Infect Dis* 2000;31:1012–1017.
57. Sanchez C, Garcia-Restoy E, Garau J, et al. Ciprofloxacin and trimethoprim/sulfamethoxazole versus placebo in acute uncomplicated *Salmonella* enteritis: a double-blind trial. *J Infect Dis* 1993;168:1304–1307.
58. Rosenthal SL. Exacerbation of *Salmonella* enteritis due to ampicillin. *N Engl J Med* 1969;280:147–148.

59. Aserkoff B, Bennett JV. Effect of antibiotic therapy in acute salmonellosis on the fecal excretion of salmonellae. *N Engl J Med* 1969;281:636–640.
60. Nelson JD, Kusmiesz H, Jackson LH, et al. Treatment of *Salmonella* gastroenteritis with ampicillin, amoxicillin, or placebo. *Pediatrics* 1980;65:1125–1130.
61. Neill MA, Opal SM, Heelan J, et al. Failure of ciprofloxacin to eradicate convalescent fecal excretion after acute salmonellosis: experience during an outbreak in health care workers. *Ann Intern Med* 1991;114:195–199.
62. Mourad AS, Metwally M, El Deen A, et al. Multiple-drug-resistant *Salmonella typhi. Clin Infect Dis* 1993;17:135–136.
63. Pillay N, Adams EB, Coombes DN. Comparative trial of amoxicillin and chloramphenicol in treatment of typhoid fever in adults. *Lancet* 1975;2:333–334.
64. Robertson RP, Wahab MFA, Raasch FO. Evaluation of chloramphenicol and ampicillin in *Salmonella* enteric fever. *N Engl J Med* 1968;278:171–176.
65. Chinh NT, Parry CM, Ly NT, et al. A randomized controlled comparison of azithromycin and ofloxacin for treatment of multidrug-resistant or nalidixic acid-resistant enteric fever. *Antimicrob Agents Chemother* 2000;44:1855–1859.
66. Girgis NI, Butler T, Frenck RW, et al. Azithromycin versus ciprofloxacin for treatment of uncomplicated typhoid fever in a randomized trial in Egypt that included patients with multidrug resistance. *Antimicrob Agents Chemother* 1999;43:1441–1444.
67. Memon IA, Billoo AG, Memon HI. Cefixime: an oral option for the treatment of multi-drug-resistant enteric fever in children. *South Med J* 1997;90:1204–1207.
68. Phuong CXT, Kneen R, Anh NT, et al. A comparative study of ofloxacin and cefixime for treatment of typhoid fever in children. *Pediatr Infect Dis J* 1999;18:245–248.
69. Frenck RW Jr, Nakhla I, Sultan Y, et al. Azithromycin versus ceftriaxone for the treatment of uncomplicated typhoid fever in children. *Clin Infect Dis* 2000;31:1134–1138.
70. Dutta P, Rasaily R, Saha MR, et al. Ciprofloxacin for treatment of severe typhoid fever in children. *Antimicrob Agents Chemother* 1993;37:1197–1199.
71. Limson BM, Littana RT. Ciprofloxacin vs. co-trimoxazole in *Salmonella* enteric fever. *Infection* 1989;17:105–106.
72. Kaye D, Marselis JG, Hook EW. Susceptibility of *Salmonella* species to four antibiotics. *N Engl J Med* 1963;269:1084–1086.
73. Cooles P. Adjuvant steroids and relapse of typhoid fever. *J Trop Med Hyg* 1986;89:229–231.
74. Hoffman SL, Punjabi NH, Kumala S, et al. Reduction of mortality in chloramphenicol-treated severe typhoid fever by high dose dexamethasone. *N Engl J Med* 1984;310:82–88.
75. Hakaken A, Kotilainen P, Jalava J, et al. Detection of decreased fluoroquinolone susceptibility in salmonellas and validation of nalidixic acid screening test. *J Clin Microbiol* 1999;37:3572–3577.
76. Herikstad H, Hayes P, Mokhtar M, et al. Emerging quinolone-resistant *Salmonella* in the United States. *Emerging Infect Dis* 1997;3:371–372.
77. Glynn MK, Bopp C, Dewitt W, et al. Emergence of multidrug-resistant *Salmonella enterica* serotype Typhimurium DT104 infections in the United States. *N Engl J Med* 1998;338: 1333–1338.
78. Molbak K, Baggesen DL, Aarestrup FM, et al. An outbreak of multidrug resistant *Salmonella enterica* serotype Typhimurium DT104. *N Engl J Med* 1999;341:1420–1425.
79. Murdoch DA, Banatvala NA, Bone A, et al. Epidemic ciprofloxacin-resistant *Salmonella typhi* in Tajikistan. *Lancet* 1998;351:339.
80. Gebreyes WA, Davies PR, Morrow WEM, et al. Antimicrobial resistance of *Salmonella* isolates from swine. *J Clin Microbiol* 2000;38:4633–4636.
81. Davis MA, Hancock DD, Besser TE, et al. Changes in antimicrobial resistance among *Salmonella enterica* serovar Typhimurium isolates from humans and cattle in the northwestern United States, 1982–1997. *Emerging Infect Dis* 1999;5: 802–806.
82. Munoz P, Diaz MD, Rodriguez-Creixems M, et al. Antimicrobial resistance of *Salmonella* isolates in a Spanish hospital. *Antimicrob Agents Chemother* 1993;37:1200–1202.
83. Maiorioni E, Lopez EL, Morrow AL, et al. Multiply resistant non-typhoidal *Salmonella* gastroenteritis in children. *Pediatr Infect Dis J* 1993;12:139–144.
84. Ackers M-L, Puhr ND, Tauxe RV. Laboratory-based surveillance of *Salmonella* serotype Typhi infections in the United States. Antimicrobial resistance on the rise. *JAMA* 2000;283: 2668–2673.
85. Rowe B, Ward LR, Threlfall EJ. Multidrug-resistant *Salmonella typhi:* a worldwide epidemic. *Clin Infect Dis* 1997;24[Suppl 1]:S106–S109.
86. Dunne EF, Fey PD, Kludt P, et al. Emergence of domestically acquired ceftriaxone-resistant salmonella infections associated with AmpC β-lactamase. *JAMA* 2000;284:3151–3156.
87. Islam A, Butler T, Kabir I, et al. Treatment of typhoid fever with ceftriaxone for 5 days or chloramphenicol for 14 days: a randomized clinical trial. *Antimicrob Agents Chemother* 1993;37: 1572–1575.
88. Bhutta ZA, Khan IA, Shadmani M. Failure of short-course ceftriaxone chemotherapy for multidrug-resistant typhoid fever in children: a randomized controlled trial in Pakistan. *Antimicrob Agents Chemother* 2000;44:450–452.
89. Jacobs JL, Gold JWM, Murray HW, et al. *Salmonella* infections in patients with the acquired immunodeficiency syndrome. *Ann Intern Med* 1985;102:186–188.
90. Galser JB, Morton-Kute L, Berger SR, et al. Recurrent *Salmonella typhimurium* bacteremia associated with the acquired immunodeficiency syndrome. *Ann Intern Med* 1985;102: 189–193.
91. Smith PD, Macher AM, Bookman AM, et al. *Salmonella typhimurium* enteritis and bacteremia in the acquired immunodeficiency syndrome. *Ann Intern Med* 1985;102:207–209.
92. Pichler H, Divide G, Wolf D. Ciprofloxacin in the treatment of acute bacterial diarrhea: a double-blind study. *Eur J Clin Microbiol* 1986;5:241–243.
93. Pichler HET, Divide G, Stickler K, et al. Clinical efficacy of ciprofloxacin compared with placebo in bacterial diarrhea. *Am J Med* 1987;82[Suppl 4a]:329–332.
94. Ericsson CD, Johnson PC, DuPont HL, et al. Ciprofloxacin or trimethoprim/sulfamethoxazole as initial therapy for travelers' diarrhea. *Ann Intern Med* 1987;106:216–220.
95. Connolly MJ, Snow MH, Ingham HR. Ciprofloxacin treatment of recurrent *Salmonella* septicaemia in a patient with acquired immune deficiency syndrome. *J Antimicrob Chemother* 1986;18:647–648.
96. Wessalowski R, Thomas L, Kivit J, et al. Multiple brain abscesses caused by *Salmonella* enteritis in a neonate: successful treatment with ciprofloxacin. *Pediatr Infect Dis J* 1993;12: 683–688.
97. Johnson WD Jr, Hook EW, Lindsey E, et al. Treatment of chronic typhoid carriers with ampicillin. *Antimicrob Agents Chemother* 1973;3:439–440.
98. Phillips WE. Treatment of chronic typhoid carriers with ampicillin. *JAMA* 1971;217:913.
99. Nolan CM, White PC Jr. Treatment of typhoid carriers with amoxicillin. *JAMA* 1978;239:2352–2354.
100. Gotuzzo E, Guerra JG, Benavente L, et al. Use of norfloxacin to treat chronic typhoid carriers. *J Infect Dis* 1988;157:1221–1225.

101. Ferreccio C, Morriss G, Valdivieso C, et al. Efficacy of ciprofloxacin in the treatment of chronic typhoid carriers. *J Infect Dis* 1988;157:1235–1239.
102. Piddock LJV, Griggs DJ, Hall MC, et al. Ciprofloxacin resistance in clinical isolates of *Salmonella typhimurium* obtained from two patients. *Antimicrob Agents Chemother* 1993;37:662–666.
103. Murray BE. Problems and mechanisms of antimicrobial resistance. *Infect Dis Clin North Am* 1990;3:423–439.
104. Replogle ML, Fleming DW, Cieslak PR. Emergence of antimicrobial-resistant shigellosis in Oregon. *Clin Infect Dis J* 2000;30:515–519.
105. Griffin PM, Tauxe R, Redd SC, et al. Emergence of highly trimethoprim/sulfamethoxazole-resistant *Shigella* in a Native American population: an epidemiologic study. *Am J Epidemiol* 1989;129:1042–1051.
106. Nelson JD, Kusmiesz H, Jackson LH. Comparison of trimethoprim/sulfamethoxazole and ampicillin therapy for shigellosis in ambulatory patients. *J Pediatr* 1976;89:491–493.
107. Nelson JD, Kusmiesz H, Jackson LH, et al. Trimethoprim/sulfamethoxazole therapy for shigellosis. *JAMA* 1976;235:1239–1244.
108. Barada FA Jr, Guerrant RL. Sulfamethoxazole/trimethoprim versus ampicillin in treatment of acute invasive diarrhea in adults. *Antimicrob Agents Chemother* 1980;17:961–964.
109. DuPont HL, Reves RR, Galindo E, et al. Treatment of travelers' diarrhea with trimethoprim/sulfamethoxazole and with trimethoprim alone. *N Engl J Med* 1982;307:841–844.
110. Oberhelman RA, de la Cabada FJ, Garibay EV, et al. Efficacy of trimethoprim/sulfamethoxazole in treatment of acute diarrhea in a Mexican pediatric population. *J Pediatr* 1987;110:960–965.
111. Nelson JD, Haltalin KC. Amoxicillin less effective than ampicillin against *Shigella in vitro* and *in vivo:* relationship of efficacy to activity in serum. *J Infect Dis* 1974;129:S222–S227.
112. Lexomboon U, Mansuwan P, Duangmani C, et al. Clinical evaluation of co-trimoxazole and furazolidone in treatment of shigellosis in children. *Br Med J* 1972;3:23–26.
113. DuPont HL, Ericsson CD, Galindo E, et al. Furazolidone versus ampicillin in the treatment of travelers' diarrhea. *Antimicrob Agents Chemother* 1984;26:160–163.
114. Ashkenazi S, Amir J, Waisman Y, et al. A randomized, double-blind study comparing cefixime and trimethoprim/sulfamethoxazole in the treatment of childhood shigellosis. *J Pediatr* 1993;123:817–821.
115. Eidlitz-Marcus T, Cohen YH, Nussinovitch M, et al. Comparative efficacy of two-and five-day courses of ceftriaxone for treatment of severe shigellosis in children. *J Pediatr* 1993;123:822–824.
116. Varsano I, Eidlitz-Marcus T, Nussinovitch M, et al. Comparative efficacy of ceftriaxone and ampicillin for treatment of severe shigellosis in children. *J Pediatr* 1991;118:627–632.
117. Kabir I, Butler T, Khanam A. Comparative efficacies of single intravenous doses of ceftriaxone and ampicillin for shigellosis in a placebo-controlled trial. *Antimicrob Agents Chemother* 1986;29:645–648.
118. Ostrower VG. Comparison of cefaclor and ampicillin in the treatment of shigellosis. *Postgrad Med J* 1979;55:82–84.
119. Orenstein WA, Ross L, Overturf GD, et al. Antibiotic treatment of acute shigellosis: failure of cefamandole compared to trimethoprim/sulfamethoxazole and ampicillin. *Am J Med Sci* 1981;282:27–33.
120. Nelson JD, Haltalin KC. Comparative efficacy of cephalexin and ampicillin for shigellosis and other types of acute diarrhea in infants and children. *Antimicrob Agents Chemother* 1975;7:415–420.
121. Prado D, Lopez E, Liu H, et al. Ceftibuten and trimethoprim/sulfamethoxazole for treatment of *Shigella* and enteroinvasive *Escherichia coli* disease. *Pediatr Infect Dis J* 1992;11:644–647.
122. Khan WA, Seas C, Dhar U, et al. Treatment of shigellosis, V: comparison of azithromycin and ciprofloxacin. *Ann Intern Med* 1997;126:697–703.
123. Salam MA, Dhar U, Khan WA, et al. Randomised comparison of ciprofloxacin suspension and pivmecillinam for childhood shigellosis. *Lancet* 1998;352:522–527.
124. Bennish ML, Salam MA, Khan WA, et al. Treatment of shigellosis, III: comparison of one-or two-dose ciprofloxacin with standard 5-day therapy. *Ann Intern Med* 1992;117:727–734.
125. Gotuzzo E, Oberhelman RA, Maguila C, et al. Comparison of single-dose treatment with norfloxacin with standard 5 day treatment with trimethoprim/sulfamethoxazole for acute shigellosis in adults. *Antimicrob Agents Chemother* 1989;33:1101–1104.
126. Horiuchi S, Inagaki Y, Yamamoto N, et al. Reduced susceptibilities of *Shigella sonnei* strains isolated from patients with dysentery to fluoroquinolones. *Antimicrob Agents Chemother* 1993;37:2486–2489.
127. Salam MA, Bennish ML. Therapy for shigellosis, I: Randomized, double-blind trial of nalidixic acid in childhood shigellosis. *J Pediatr* 1988;113:901–907.
128. Bennish ML, Salam MA, Hossain MA, et al. Antimicrobial resistance of *Shigella* isolates in Bangladesh, 1983–1990: increasing frequency of strains multiply resistant to ampicillin, trimethoprim/sulfamethoxazole, and nalidixic acid. *Clin Infect Dis* 1992;14:1055–1060.
129. Burstein S, Regalli G. *In vitro* susceptibility of *Shigella* strains isolated from stool cultures of dysenteric patients. *Scand J Gastroenterol* 1989;24[Suppl]:34–38.
130. LaChance N, Gaudreau C, Lamothe F, et al. Susceptibilities of beta-lactamase-positive and -negative strains of *Campylobacter coli* to beta-lactam agents. *Antimicrob Agents Chemother* 1993;37:1174–1176.
131. Chow AW, Pattern V, Bednorz D. Susceptibility of *Campylobacter fetus* to twenty-two antimicrobial agents. *Antimicrob Agents Chemother* 1978;13:416–418.
132. Karmali MA, DeGrandis S, Fleming PC. Antimicrobial susceptibility of *Campylobacter jejuni* with special reference to resistance patterns of Canadian isolates. *Antimicrob Agents Chemother* 1981;19:593–597.
133. Taylor DE, Courvalin P. Mechanisms of antibiotic resistance in *Campylobacter* species. *Antimicrob Agents Chemother* 1988;32:1107–1112.
134. The choice of anti-bacterial drugs. *Med Lett* 2001;43:69–78.
135. Kuschner RA, Trofa AF, Thomas RJ, et al. Use of azithromycin for the treatment of *Campylobacter* enteritis in travelers to Thailand, an area where ciprofloxacin resistance is prevalent. *Clin Infect Dis J* 1995;21:536–541.
136. Salazar-Lindo E, Sack B, Chea-Woo E, et al. Early treatment with erythromycin of *Campylobacter jejuni*-associated dysentery in children. *J Pediatr* 1986;109:355–360.
137. Williams D, Schorling J, Barrett LJ, et al. Early treatment of *Campylobacter jejuni* enteritis. *Antimicrob Agents Chemother* 1989;33:248–250.
138. Tremblay C, Gaudreau C. Antimicrobial susceptible testing of 59 strains of *Campylobacter fetus* subsp. *fetus. Antimicrob Agents Chemother* 1998;42:1847–1849.
139. Yan W, Taylor DE. Characterization of erythromycin resistance in *Campylobacter jejuni* and *Campylobacter coli. Antimicrob Agents Chemother* 1991;35:1989–1996.
140. Brunton WAT, Wilson AAM, Macrae RM. Erythromycin-resistant campylobacters. *Lancet* 1978;2:1385.

141. Taylor DE, Chang N, Garner RS, et al. Incidence of antibiotic resistance and characterization of plasmids in *Campylobacter jejuni* strains isolated from clinical sources in Alberta, Canada. *Can J Microbiol* 1986;32:28–32.
142. Gaudreau C, Gilbert H. Antimicrobial resistance of clinical strains of *Campylobacter jejuni* isolated from 1985 to 1997 in Quebec, Canada. *Antimicrob Agents Chemother* 1998;42:2106–2108.
143. Vanhoof R, Vanderlinden MP, Dierickx R, et al. Susceptibility of *Campylobacter fetus* subsp. *jejuni* to twenty-nine antimicrobial agents. *Antimicrob Agents Chemother* 1978;14:553–556.
144. Walder M, Forgren A. Erythromycin-resistant campylobacters. *Lancet* 1978;2:1201.
145. Wang WLL, Reller LB, Blaser MJ. Comparison of antimicrobial susceptibility patterns of *Campylobacter jejuni* and *Campylobacter coli. Antimicrob Agents Chemother* 1984;26:351–353.
146. Saenz Y, Zarazaga M, Lantero M, et al. Antibiotic resistance in *Campylobacter* strains isolated from animals, foods, and humans in Spain in 1997–1998. *Antimicrob Agents Chemother* 2000;44:267–271.
147. Jensen LB, Aarestrup FM. Macrolide resistance in *Campylobacter coli* of animal origin in Denmark. *Antimicrob Agents Chemother* 2001;45:371–372.
148. Taylor DN, Blaser MJ, Echeverria PE, et al. Erythromycin-resistant *Campylobacter* infections in Thailand. *Antimicrob Agents Chemother* 1987;31:438–442.
149. Sagara H, Mochizuki A, Okamura N, et al. Antimicrobial resistance of *Campylobacter jejuni* and *Campylobacter coli* with special reference to plasmid profiles of Japanese clinical isolates. *Antimicrob Agents Chemother* 1987;31:713–719.
150. Taylor DE, Chang N. *In vitro* susceptibilities of *Campylobacter jejuni* and *Campylobacter coli* to azithromycin and erythromycin. *Antimicrob Agents Chemother* 1991;35:1917–1918.
151. Reina J, Alomar P. Fluoroquinolone-resistance in thermophilic *Campylobacter* spp. isolated from stools of Spanish patients. *Lancet* 1990;336:186.
152. Rautelin H, Renkonen O-V, Kosunen TU. Emergence of fluoroquinolone resistance in *Campylobacter jejuni* and *Campylobacter coli* in subjects from Finland. *Antimicrob Agents Chemother* 1991;35:2065–2069.
153. Endtz HP, Mouton RP, van der Reyden T, et al. Fluoroquinolone resistance in *Campylobacter* spp isolated from human stools and poultry products. *Lancet* 1990;335:787.
154. Navarro F, Miro E, Fuentes I, et al. *Campylobacter* species: identification and resistance to quinolones. *Clin Infect Dis J* 1993;17:815–816.
155. Meier PA, Dooley DP, Jorgensen JH, et al. Development of quinolone-resistant *Campylobacter fetus* bacteremia in human immunodeficiency virus-infected patients. *J Infect Dis* 1998;177:951–954.
156. Zirnstein G, Li Y, Swaminathan B, et al. Ciprofloxacin resistance in *Campylobacter jejuni* isolates: detection of *gyrA* resistance mutations by mismatch amplification mutation assay PCR and DNA sequence analysis. *J Clin Microbiol* 1999;37:3276–3280.
157. Wilson DL, Abner SR, Newman TC, et al. Identification of ciprofloxacin-resistant *Campylobacter jejuni* by use of a fluorogenic PCR assay. *J Clin Microbiol* 2000;38:3971–3978.
158. Talsma E, Goettsch WG, Nieste HLJ, et al. Resistance of *Campylobacter* species: increased resistance to fluoroquinolones and seasonal variation. *Clin Infect Dis J* 1999;29:845–848.
159. Smith, KE, Besser JM, Hedberg CW. Quinolone-resistant *Campylobacter jejuni* infections in Minnesota, 1992–1998. *N Engl J Med* 1999;340:1525–1532.
160. Gibreel Am, Sjogren E, Kaijser B, et al. Rapid emergency of high-level resistance to quinolones in *Campylobacter jejuni* associated with mutational changes in *gyrA* and *parC. Antimicrob Agents Chemother* 1998;42:3276–3278.
161. Sanchez R, Fernandez-Baca V, Diaz MD, et al. Evolution of susceptibilities of *Campylobacter* spp. to quinolones and macrolides. *Antimicrob Agents Chemother* 1994;38:1879–1882.
162. Segreti J, Gootz TD, Goodman LJ, et al. High-level quinolone resistance in clinical isolates of *Campylobacter jejuni. J Infect Dis* 1992;165:667–670.
163. Karch H. Growth of *Escherichia coli* in the presence of trimethoprim/sulfamethoxazole facilitates detection of Shiga-like toxin producing strains by colony blot assay. *FEMS Microbiol Lett* 1986;35:141–145.
164. Walterspiel JN, Ashkenazi S, Morrow AL, et al. Effect of subinhibitory concentrations of antibiotics on the release of Shiga-like toxin I. *Infection* 1992;20:25–29.
165. Pavia AT, Nichols CR, Green DP, et al. Hemolytic–uremic syndrome during an outbreak of *Escherichia coli* O157:H7 infections in institutions for mentally retarded persons: clinical and epidemiologic observations. *J Pediatr* 1990;116:544–551.
166. Carter AO, Borczyk AA, Carlson JAK, et al. A severe outbreak of *Escherichia coli* O157:H7-associated hemorrhagic colitis in a nursing home. *N Engl J Med* 1987;317:1496–1500.
167. Butler T, Islam MR, Azad MAK, et al. Risk factors for development of hemolytic uremic syndrome during shigellosis. *J Pediatr* 1987;110:894–897.
168. Prouix F, Turgeon JP, Delage G, et al. Randomized, controlled trial of antibiotic therapy for *Escherichia coli* O157:H7 enteritis. *J Pediatr* 1992;121:299–303.
169. Wong CS, Jelacic S, Habeeb RL, et al. The risk of the hemolytic–uremic syndrome after antibiotic treatment of *Escherichia coli* O157:H7 infections. *N Engl J Med* 2000;342:1930–1936.
170. Kimmitt PT, Harwood CR, Barer MR. Toxin gene expression by Shiga toxin-producing *Escherichia coli:* the role of antibiotics and the bacterial SOS response. *Emerging Infect Dis* 2000;6:458–465.
171. Yee AJ, DeGrandis S, Gyles CL. Mitomycin-induced synthesis of a Shiga-like toxin from enteropathogenic *Escherichia coli* H.I.8. *Infect Immun* 1993;61:4510–4513.
172. Lesesne JB, Rothschild N, Erickson B, et al. Cancer-associated hemolytic-uremic syndrome: analysis of 85 cases from a national registry. *J Clin Oncol* 1989;115:781–789.
173. Zhang X, McDaniel AD, Wolf LE, et al. Quinolone antibiotics induce Shiga toxin-encoding bacteriophages, toxin production and death in mice. *J Infect Dis* 2000;181:664–670.
174. Ikeda K, Ida O, Kimoto K, et al. Effect of early fosfomycin treatment on prevention of hemolytic uremic syndrome accompanying *Escherichia coli* O157:H7 infection. *Clin Nephrol* 1999;52:357–362.
175. Blake PA, Allegra DT, Snyder JD, et al. Cholera—a possible endemic focus in the United States. *N Engl J Med* 1980;302:305–309.
176. Kobari K, Uylangco C, Vasco J, et al. Observations on cholera treated orally and intravenously with antibiotics: with particular reference to the number of vibrios excreted in the stool. *Bull World Health Organ* 1967;37:751–772.
177. Khan WA, Bennish ML, Seas C, et al. Randomised controlled comparison of single-dose ciprofloxacin and doxycycline for cholera caused by *Vibrio cholerae* O1 and O139. *Lancet* 1996;348:296–300.
178. Rahaman MM, Majid MA, Alam AKM, et al. Effects of doxycycline in actively purging cholera patients. A double-blind clinical trial. *Antimicrob Agents Chemother* 1976;10:610–612.
179. Sack DA, Islam S, Rabbani H, et al. Single-dose doxycycline for cholera. *Antimicrob Agents Chemother* 1978;14:462–464.
180. Gotuzzo E, Seas C, Echevarria J, et al. Ciprofloxacin for the

treatment of cholera: a randomized, double-blind, controlled clinical trial of a single dose in Peruvian adults. *Clin Infect Dis* 1995;20:1485–1490.
181. Swerdlow DL, Ries AA. Cholera in the Americas: guidelines for the clinician. *JAMA* 1992;267:1495–1499.
182. Mukhopadhyay AK, Basu I, Bhattacharya SK, et al. Emergence of fluoroquinolone resistance in strains of *Vibrio cholerae* isolated from hospitalized patients with acute diarrhea in Calcutta, India. *Antimicrob Agents Chemother* 1998;42:206–207.
183. Cholera Working Group. Large epidemic of cholera-like disease in Bangladesh caused by *Vibrio cholerae* O139 synonym Bengal. *Lancet* 1993;342:387–390.
184. Basu A, Garg P, Datta S, et al. *Vibrio cholerae* O139 in Calcutta, 1992–1998: incidence, antibiograms, and genotypes. *Emerging Infect Dis* 2000;6:139–147.
185. Bottone EJ. *Yersinia enterocolitica:* the charisma continues. *Clin Microbiol Rev* 1997;10:257–276.
186. Abdel-Haq NM, Asmar BI, Abuhammour WM, et al. *Yersinia enterocolitica* infection in children. *Pediatr Infect Dis J* 2000; 19:954–948.
187. Hoogkamp-Korstanje JAA. Antibiotics in *Yersinia enterocolitica* infections. *J Antimicrob Chemother* 1987;20:123–131.
188. Pai CH, Gillis F, Tuomanen E, et al. Placebo-controlled double-blind evaluation of trimethoprim-sulfamethoxazole treatment of *Yersinia enterocolitica* gastroenteritis. *J Pediatr* 1994;104:308–311.
189. Gayraud M, Scavizzi MR, Mollaret HH, et al. Antibiotic treatment of *Yersinia enterocolitica* septicemia: a retrospective review of 43 cases. *Clin Infect Dis* 1993;17:405–410.
190. Daniels NA, Ray B, Easton A, et al. Emergence of a new *Vibrio parahaemolyticus* serotype in raw oysters. *JAMA* 2000;284: 1541–1545.
191. Glandt M, Adachi JA, Mathewson JJ, et al. Enteroaggregative *E. coli* as a cause of travelers' diarrhea: clinical response to ciprofloxacin. *Clin Infect Dis* 1999;29:335–338.
192. Janda JM, Abbott SL. Evolving concepts regarding the genus *Aeromonas:* an expanding panorama of species, disease presentations, and unanswered questions. *Clin Infect Dis* 1998;27: 332–344.
193. Koehler JM, Ashdown LR. *In vitro* susceptibilities of tropical strains of *Aeromonas* species from Queensland, Australia, to 22 antimicrobial agents. *Antimicrob Agents Chemother* 1993;37: 905–907.
194. Parras F, Diaz MD, Reina J, et al. Meningitis due to *Aeromonas* species: case report and review. *Clin Infect Dis* 1993;17: 1058–1060.
195. Kain KC, Kelly MT. Clinical features, epidemiology, and treatment of *Plesiomonas shigelloides* diarrhea. *J Clin Microbiol* 1989; 27:998–1001.
196. Castro KG, Ward JW, Slutsker L, et al. 1993 revised classification system for HIV infection and expanded surveillance case definition for AIDS among adolescents and adults. *Clin Infect Dis* 1993;17:802–810.
197. Drugs for parasitic infections. [duplicate publication of American Academy of Pediatrics. Drugs for parasitic infections. In: Pickering LK, ed. 2000 Red Book: report of the committee on infectious diseases, 25th edition. Elk Grove Village, IL: American Academy of Pediatrics, 2000:683–725.]. *Med Lett* [Serial Online]. 2000. Available at: *www.medicalletter.org.*
198. Gardner TB, Hill DR. Treatment of giardiasis. *Clin Microbiol Rev* 2001;14:114–128.
199. Sokol RJ, Lichtenstein PK, Farrell MK. Quinacrine hydrochloride-induced yellow discoloration of the skin in children. *Pediatrics* 1982;69:232–233.
200. Craft JC, Murphy T, Nelson JD. Furazolidone and quinacrine: comparative study of therapy for giardiasis in children. *Am J Dis Child* 1981;135:164–166.
201. Hall A, Nahar Q. Albendazole as a treatment for infections with *Giardia duodenalis* in children in Bangladesh. *Trans Royal Soc Trop Med Hyg* 1993;87:84–86.
202. Pungpak S, Singhasivanon V, Bunnag D, et al. Albendazole as a treatment for *Giardia* infection. *Ann Trop Med Parasitol* 1996; 90:563–565.
203. Pengsaa K, Sirivichayakul C, Pojjaroen-anant C, et al. Albendazole treatment of *Giardia intestinalis* infections in school children. *S Asian J Trop Med Public Health* 1999;30:78–83.
204. Petri WA Jr, Singh U. Diagnosis and management of amebiasis. *Clin Infect Dis* 1999;29:117–125.
205. Clark DP. New insights into human cryptosporidiosis. *Clin Microbiol Rev* 1999;12:554–563.
206. Armitage K, Flanigan T, Carey J, et al. Treatment of cryptosporidiosis with paromomycin. *Arch Intern Med* 1992;152: 2497–2499.
207. Fichtenbaum CJ, Ritchie DJ, Powderly WG. Use of paromomycin for treatment of cryptosporidiosis in patients with AIDS. *Clin Infect Dis* 1993;16:298–300.
208. Wallace MR, Nguyen M-T, Newton JA Jr. Use of paromomycin for the treatment of cryptosporidiosis in patients with AIDS. *Clin Infect Dis* 1993;17:1070–1071.
209. Pilla AM, Rybak MJ, Chandrasekar PH. Spiramycin in the treatment of cryptosporidiosis. *Pharmacotherapy* 1987;7: 188–190.
210. Marshall RJ, Flanigan TP. Paromomycin inhibits *Cryptosporidium* infection of a human enterocyte cell line. *J Infect Dis* 1992; 165:772–774.
211. Hewitt RG, Yiannoutsos CT, Higgs ES, et al. Paromomycin: no more effective than placebo for treatment of cryptosporidiosis in patients with advanced human immunodeficiency virus infection. *Clin Infect Dis* 2000;31:1084–1092.
212. Rehg JE. Activity of azithromycin against cryptosporidia in immunosuppressed rats. *J Infect Dis* 1991;163:1293–1296.
213. Vargas SL, Shenep JL, Flynn PM, et al. Azithromycin for treatment of severe *Cryptosporidium* diarrhea in two children with cancer. *J Pediatr* 1993;123:154–156.
214. Smith NH, Cron S, Valdez LM, et al. Combination drug therapy for cryptosporidiosis in AIDS. *J Infect Dis* 1998;178: 900–903.
215. Perryman LE, Riggs MW, Mason PH, et al. Kinetics of *Cryptosporidium parvum* sporozoite neutralization by monoclonal antibodies, immune bovine serum, and immune bovine colostrum. *Infect Immun* 1990;58:257–259.
216. Borowitz SM, Saulsbury FT. Treatment of chronic cryptosporidial infection with orally administered human serum immune globulin. *J Pediatr* 1991;119:593–595.
217. Bjorneby JM, Hunsaker BD, Riggs MW, et al. Monoclonal antibody immunotherapy in nude mice persistently infected with *Cryptosporidium parvum. Infect Immun* 1991;59:1172–1176.
218. Louie E, Borkowsky W, Klesius PH, et al. Treatment of cryptosporidiosis with oral bovine transfer factor. *J Clin Immunol Pathol* 1987;44:329–334.
219. Tzipori S, Robertson D, Chapman C. Remission of diarrhea due to cryptosporidiosis in an immunodeficient child treated with hyperimmune bovine colostrum. *Br Med J* 1986;293: 1276.
220. Perryman LE, Kegerreis KA, Mason PH. Effect of orally administered monoclonal antibody on persistent *Cryptosporidium parvum* infection in SCID mice. *Infect Immun* 1993;61: 4906–4908.
221. Soudah HC, Hasler WL, Owyang C. Effect of octreotide on intestinal motility and bacterial overgrowth in scleroderma. *N Engl J Med* 1991;325:1461–1467.
222. Cello JP, Grendell JH, Basuk P, et al. Effect of octreotide on

refractory AIDS-associated diarrhea: a prospective multicenter clinical trial. *Ann Intern Med* 1991;115:705–710.

223. Holmberg SD, Moorman AC, VonBargen JC, et al. Possible effectiveness of clarithromycin and rifabutin for cryptosporidiosis chemoprophylaxis in HIV disease. *JAMA* 1998;279: 384–386.
224. Lindsay DS, Dubey JP, Blagburn BL. Biology of *Isospora* spp. From humans, non-human primates, and domestic animals. *Clin Microbiol Rev* 1997;10:19–34.
225. Pape JW, Verdier R-I, Johnson WD Jr. Treatment and prophylaxis of *Isospora belli* infection in patients with the acquired immunodeficiency syndrome. *N Engl J Med* 1989;320: 1044–1047.
226. DeHovitz JA, Page JW, Boney M, et al. Clinical manifestations and therapy of *Isospora belli* infection in patients with the acquired immunodeficiency syndrome. *N Engl J Med* 1986; 315:87–90.
227. Weiss LM, Perlman DC, Sherman J, et al. *Isospora belli* infection: treatment with pyrimethamine. *Ann Intern Med* 1988; 109:474–475.
228. Lyagoubi M, Datry A, Mayorga R, et al. Chronic persistent strongyloidiasis cured by ivermectin. *Trans Royal Soc Trop Med Hyg* 1992;86:541.
229. Naguira C, Jiminez G, Guerra JG, et al. Ivermectin for human strongyloidiasis and other intestinal helminths. *Am J Trop Med Hyg* 1989;40:304–309.
230. Lessnau KD, Can S, Talavera W. Disseminated *Strongyloides stercoralis* in human immunodeficiency virus-infected patients: treatment failure and a review of the literature. *Chest* 1993;104: 119–122.
231. Franzen C, Muller A. Molecular techniques for detection, species differentiation, and phylogenetic analysis of microsporidia. *Clin Microbiol Rev* 1999;12:243–285.
232. Rijpstra AC, Canning EU, Van-Ketel RJ, et al. Use of light microscopy to diagnose small intestinal microsporidiosis in patients with AIDS. *J Infect Dis* 1988;157:827–831.
233. Dieterich DT, Lew EA, Kotler DP, et al. Treatment with albendazole for intestinal disease due to *Enterocytozoon bieneusi* in patients with AIDS. *J Infect Dis* 1994;169:178–183.
234. Molina JM, Sarfati C, Beauvais B, et al. Intestinal microsporidiosis in human immunodeficiency virus-infected patients with chronic unexplained diarrhea: prevalence and clinical biologic features. *J Infect Dis* 1993;167:217–221.
235. Cali A, Kotler DP, Orenstein JM. *Septata intestinalis* n.g., n.sp., an intestinal microsporidian associated with chronic diarrhea and dissemination in AIDS patients. *J Eukaryot Microbiol* 1993; 40:101–112.
236. Blanshard C, Ellis DS, Tovey DG, et al. Treatment of intestinal microsporidiosis with albendazole in patients with AIDS. *AIDS* 1992;6:311–313.
237. Wanke CA, Plesko D, DeGirolami PC, et al. A medium chain triglyceride-based diet in patients with HIV and chronic diarrhea reduces diarrhea and malabsorption: a prospective, controlled trial. *Nutrition* 1996;12:766–771.
238. Ridoux O, Drancourt M. *In vitro* susceptibilities of the microsporidia *Encephalitozoon cuniculi, Encephalitozoon hellem,* and *E. intestinalis* to albendazole and its sulfoxide and sulfone metabolites. *Antimicrob Agents Chemother* 1998;42:3301–3303.
239. Katiyar SK, Edlind TD. *In vitro* susceptibilities of the AIDS-associated microsporidian *Encephalitozoon intestinalis* to albendazole, its sulfoxide metabolite, 12 additional benzimidazole derivatives. *Antimicrob Agents Chemother* 1997;41:2729–2732.
240. Molina J-M, Chastang C, Goguel J, et al. Albendazole for treatment and prophylaxis of microsporidiosis due to *Encephalitozoon intestinalis* in patients with AIDS: a randomized double-blind controlled trial. *J Infect Dis* 1998;177:1373–1377.
241. Stenzel DJ, Boreham PFL. *Blastomycosis hominis* revisited. *Clin Microbiol Rev*1996;9:563–584.
242. Boreham PF, Stenzel D. *Blastocystis* in humans and animals: morphology, biology, and epizootiology. *Adv Parasitol* 1993; 32:1–70.
243. Connor BA, Shlim DR, Scholes JV, et al. Pathologic changes in the small bowel in nine patients with diarrhea associated with a coccidia-like body. *Ann Intern Med* 1993;119:377–382.
244. Herwaldt BL. *Cyclospora cayetanensis:* a review, focusing on the outbreaks of cyclosporiasis in the 1990s. *Clin Infect Dis* 2000;31:1040–1057.
245. Verdier R-I, Fitzgerald DW, Johnson WD, et al. Trimethoprim/sulfamethoxazole compared with ciprofloxacin for treatment and prophylaxis of *Isospora belli* and *Cyclospora cayetanensis* infection in HIV-infected patients. A randomized controlled trial. *Ann Intern Med* 2000;132:885–888.
246. Madico G, Gilman RH, Miranda E, et al. Treatment of *Cyclospora* infections with co-trimoxazole. *Lancet* 1993;342: 122–123.
247. Yolken R, Kinney J, Wilde J, et al. Immunoglobulins and other modalities for the prevention and treatment of enteric viral infections. *J Clin Immunol* 1990;10:80S–87S.
248. Losonsky GA, Johnson JP, Winkelstein JA, et al. Oral administration of human serum immunoglobulin in immunodeficient patients with viral gastroenteritis. *J Clin Invest* 1985;76: 2362–2367.
249. American Academy of Pediatrics, Work Group on Breastfeeding. Breastfeeding and the use of human milk.*Pediatrics* 1997; 100:1035–1039.
250. Centers for Disease Control and Prevention. 1999 USPHS/IDSA guidelines for the prevention of opportunistic infections in persons infected with human immunodeficiency virus. *MMWR Morb Mortal Wkly Rep* 1999;48(RR-19):1–59.
251. Centers for Disease Control and Prevention. Guidelines for preventing opportunistic infections among hematopoietic stem cell transplant recipients. Recommendations of CDC, the Infectious Disease Society of America, and the American Society of Blood and Marrow Transplantation. *MMWR Morb Mortal Wkly Rep* 2000;49(RR-10):1–94.
252. Ryan ET, Kain KC. Health advice and immunization for travelers. *N Engl J Med* 2000;342:1716–1725.
253. Murphy TV, Gargiullo PM, Mehan MS, et al. Intussusception among infants given an oral rotavirus vaccine. *N Engl J Med* 2001;344:564–572.

79

ORAL THERAPY FOR DIARRHEA

JOHN D. SNYDER

Diarrhea continues to be a major problem in developing and developed countries. The greatest impact from diarrhea is in developing countries, where approximately 1.5 billion diarrheal episodes and 4 million deaths occur each year in children younger than 5 years (1). The impact of diarrheal illness is not so overwhelming in the United States but is still a major problem. Outpatient visits for diarrhea account for as many a 20% of acute care visits by young children at large urban hospitals (2), and approximately 9% of hospital admissions for children younger than 5 years are due to diarrhea (3). Diarrhea accounts for approximately 300 deaths in children younger than 5 years in the United States each year, which is about 10% of the potentially preventable deaths in this age-group (4). Hospitalization and outpatient care for diarrhea in children in the United States is estimated to result in direct costs of more than $2 billion per year (5,6).

The critical element of effective therapy for acute diarrhea is the replacement of fluid and electrolyte losses. For more than 50 years, intravenous (IV) therapy has been a successful method of administration of the fluid and electrolytes lost during diarrhea. Efforts to find a less expensive and more easily administered therapy have led to the development of effective oral therapy for acute diarrhea (7). This therapy is a rare but important example of the reverse transfer of technology from developing to developed countries. The initial clinical trials of oral therapy were performed primarily in less-developed countries where its effectiveness was established in children and adults with acute diarrhea from many etiologies (8–10). Although industrialized countries have been slow to adopt the use of oral therapy (11,12), its use is now endorsed by organizations such as the American Academy of Pediatrics (AAP), the U.S. Centers for Disease Control and Prevention (CDC), and the European Society for Pediatric Gastroenterology and Nutrition (13–15).

Oral therapy has evolved over the past 25 years to include oral rehydration solutions (ORSs) of fluid and electrolytes and appropriate early feeding and is the major focus of this chapter. This chapter also briefly discusses the use of antimicrobial therapy and antidiarrheal agents.

J. D. Snyder: Department of Pediatrics, GI/Nutrition Division, University of California Medical Center, San Francisco, California

HISTORY OF ORAL THERAPY

Oral Rehydration Solution

The first studies of the optimal method to replace fluid and electrolyte losses from diarrhea began about 175 years ago (16). These initial efforts during cholera epidemics were associated with high mortality rates until investigators eventually documented that stool losses of water, sodium, potassium, chloride, and base must be restored to ensure the most effective rehydration (17). Early attempts at parenteral administration of therapy were largely failures because of inadequate aseptic technique, primitive equipment, and limited understanding of mechanisms of maintaining intravascular volume (18). Approximately 50 years ago, IV therapy became the first successful method of administration of fluid and electrolytes and was widely accepted as the standard for rehydration therapy (19). The success of IV therapy increased with the realization of the importance of correcting acidosis with administration of base and subsequently with the appreciation of the importance of replacing potassium (19).

However, several important limitations of IV therapy stimulated the search for simpler, less-expensive methods to rehydrate patients with diarrhea and dehydration. These limitations, which are particularly important in developing countries where the burden of diarrhea is greatest, include the expense for large amounts of sterile solutions, needles, and tubing; the need for administration by skilled health workers; and the requirement for specialized facilities (7).

The initial efforts to develop effective orally administered fluid and electrolyte solutions were begun by Harrison at Johns Hopkins and Darrow at Yale in the early 1950s (11). Harrison et al. (20) included sodium (60 mmol/L), potassium (20 mmol/L), chloride (54 mmol/L), and lactate (33 mmol/L) and added 3.3 g/L of glucose for protein-sparing purposes. The first commercial oral glucose-electrolyte solution was introduced shortly thereafter, but this solution had a much higher carbohydrate content and osmolality than the solution used by Harrison and colleagues. An important setback to the development of oral therapy for diarrhea then occurred when an outbreak of hypernatremic dehydration coincided with the introduction of the hyperosmolar commercial solution (21). Several other factors contributed in large part to this epidemic, including the incorrect mixing of home-prepared sugar and salt preparations, inappropriate administration of the early forms of IV solutions, and the recommended use of boiled skim milk, a very hypertonic solution (21). At the time, the epidemic was incorrectly attributed to the sodium content of the solutions, rather than to their excessive carbohydrate concentrations and osmolality (21). These misconceptions influenced a generation of pediatricians and slowed the acceptance of the physiologically based ORSs that followed.

Physiologic Principles

The discovery of the coupled transport of sodium with glucose, amino acids, or short-chain polypeptides in the early 1960s is the foundation on which effective oral rehydration therapy (ORT) was developed (22). Coupled transport causes enhanced absorption of salt and water from the intestinal lumen across the epithelium and is effective even during intestinal inflammation caused by enteritis (7).

A large number of controlled clinical trials in adults and children began just after the discovery of coupled transport and have demonstrated the safety and efficacy of ORSs for all types of diarrhea (1,7,9,10,23,24). Several formulations have been studied and used, but by far the most widely and successfully used of these ORS solutions has been the World Health Organization (WHO)–United Nations Children's Fund (UNICEF) formulation (1,7). This solution contains glucose (20 g/L) and three salts: sodium chloride (3.5 g/L), potassium chloride (1.5 g/L), and either trisodium citrate (2.9 g/L) or sodium bicarbonate (2.5 g/L) (Table 79.1). For maximum co-transport of electrolytes, sugar, and water, the ratio of carbohydrate to sodium should approach 1 : 1 (7).

Clinical trials of ORS in health facilities and communities have consistently demonstrated its ability to successfully rehydrate 90% or more of patients with dehydration from all causes of acute diarrhea (1,7), to reduce significant case-fatality ratios (1,25), to be substantially less expensive than IV therapy (26), and to be administered safely and effectively by family members, even with little or no formal education (25). ORSs are usually packaged in aluminum foil packets, which give them a long shelf-life even in hot and humid conditions.

Feeding

Interest in the role of feeding during diarrhea has been present for many years. Some of the earliest studies of feeding during diarrhea were carried out by Chung and Viscerova (27,28) in the late 1940s. They demonstrated in careful nutrient balance experiments that effective intestinal absorption occurs during diarrhea and that absorption is roughly proportional to intake (27,28). However, these observations had little effect on the common practice in this and many countries and cultures of withholding feedings until the diarrhea stopped (29). The rationale for withholding food during diarrhea was based primarily on the concern for malabsorption, which can occur because of an altered intestinal mucosa, decreased brush border enzymes, and more rapid intestinal transit time (29).

More recently, the several important potential benefits of early feeding became a strong stimulus for studies of safety and efficacy (29). These benefits include the chance to provide nutritional therapy to malnourished patients with diarrhea, particularly in developing countries. In addition, nutrient uptake plays an important role in intestinal repair (30).

TABLE 79.1. COMPOSITION OF REPRESENTATIVE GLUCOSE ELECTROLYTE SOLUTION

	Concentration (mmol/L)				
	CHO	Na	K	Base	Osmolality
Naturalyte (Unlimited Beverages)	140	45	20	48	265
Pediatric Electrolyte (NutraMax)	140	45	20	30	250
Pedialyte (Ross)	140	45	20	30	250
KaoLectrolyte (Pharmacia & Upjohn)	140	48	20	28	240
Infalyte (Mead Johnson)	70	50	25	30	200
Rehydralyte (Ross)	140	75	20	30	301
Cera-lyte	80	70	20	30	235
Reduced osmolar ORS (WHO/UNICEF)	75	75	20	30	245
WHO/UNICEF ORS	111	90	20	30	310

CHO, carbohydrate; ORS, oral rehydration solution; WHO, World Health Organization; UNICEF, United Nation's Children's Fund.

Physiologic Principles

Although some element of malabsorption is often associated with diarrhea, it is rarely complete and substantial amounts of nutrients can be absorbed (27,29,31,32). In considering the impact of diarrhea on digestion and absorption, these processes can be divided into luminal and mucosal components. The luminal component is usually less affected because the concentrations of amylases and pancreatic enzymes are largely unaffected during diarrhea (31). These conditions are particularly favorable for the digestion and absorption of complex carbohydrates and simple proteins in staple foods. As much as 90% of complex carbohydrates and 70% of protein is digested during diarrhea (27,32). Fat digestion, which is a complex process involving multiple factors including bile salts, fatty acid-binding protein, and apolipoprotein, as well as pancreatic lipase, is the most affected of the macronutrients in the luminal phase. The coefficient of absorption of fat is about 50% to 60% in most studies (31–34).

The negative effect of diarrhea is greater on the mucosal phase of digestion and absorption (31,33). This is particularly true when diarrhea is associated with an altered absorptive surface due to damaged enterocytes.

Carbohydrate digestion can be affected because of the decreased levels of brush border disaccharidases. Lactase levels are decreased most during diarrhea, followed by sucrase, and the effect is least on glucoamylase (35). The relative preservation of glucoamylase levels provides an important reason why starches have proven to be so successful in ORS and appropriate early feeding (36).

Although lactase enzyme levels are often decreased in diarrhea, clinically important lactose intolerance is uncommon, indicating that substantial quantities of lactose can be digested (37). The effect of diarrhea on monosaccharide absorption depends on the extent of injury, but even in severe cases, this mechanism is often very effective (38).

The brush border peptidase enzymes are also decreased during diarrhea, particularly when invasive mucosal lesions are present (31). The combined effect of diarrhea on luminal and mucosal digestion results in a coefficient of absorption of protein at a level intermediate between carbohydrate and fat (27,32).

The impact of diarrhea on the mucosal phase of fat digestion also depends on the amount of mucosal damage (31). When severe injury has occurred, fewer enterocytes are available for triglyceride resynthesis and chylomicron formation.

Concern has also been raised that feeding during diarrhea could result in increased macromolecular uptake across the damaged mucosa, leading to intestinal allergy (39). A review of many clinical studies demonstrates that this theoretic risk has never been shown to be of practical importance in diarrhea (39).

Other factors that influence the success of feeding include the age of the child, the etiology of the diarrhea, the severity of the stooling, and the composition of the diet (29).

CURRENT PRACTICES OF OPTIMAL ORAL THERAPY

Oral Rehydration Therapy And Appropriate Early Feeding

Oral Rehydration Solution

Based on the data from the many controlled clinical trials conducted in the first decade after the introduction of glucose-electrolyte solutions, the WHO/UNICEF incorporated ORS as the cornerstone of their child survival efforts beginning in 1978 (1,7). Further trials confirming the safety and efficacy of ORS, most often using the WHO/UNICEF formulation, have now been carried out in nearly every country in the world (1,7). In the United States, several commercial solutions similar to the WHO/UNICEF solution are widely available (Table 79.1). In controlled trials in this country, solutions with sodium concentrations of 45 to 90 mmol/L and glucose concentrations of up to 140 mmol/L have proven effective in the treatment of well-nourished children with mild to severe dehydration (26,40–42).

Glucose-electrolyte solutions formulated on physiologic principles must be distinguished from other popular liquids that have been used inappropriately to treat diarrhea (Table 79.2). Unfortunately, the use of these nonphysiologic solutions is still widespread (43).

Enhanced Oral Rehydration Solution

Although ORS has been hailed as "potentially the most important medical advance this century" (44) and has been credited with saving an estimated one million lives each year (1), it has limitations. Perhaps the most important is that although it is extremely effective at replacing fluid and electrolyte losses, glucose-electrolyte ORS has no beneficial effect on the volume or duration of diarrhea.

Several methods have been used to improve the absorptive capabilities of ORS and to decrease stool output. The evolution of these attempts has included the use of addi-

TABLE 79.2. COMPOSITION OF REPRESENTATIVE CLEAR LIQUIDS

	(Concentrations in mmol/L)				
Liquid	CHO	Na	K	Base	Osmolality
Cola	700 (F,G)	2	0	13	750
Apple juice	690 (F,G,S)	3	32	0	730
Chicken broth	0	250	8	0	500
Sports beverage	255 (S,G)	20	3	3	330

CHO, carbohydrate; F, fructose; G, glucose; K, potassium; Na, sodium; S, sucrose.
From Editorial, Oral glucose/electrolyte therapy for acute diarrhea. *Lancet* 1975;1:79–80, with permission.

tional co-transport molecules such as amino acids, polymers of glucose and short-chain polypeptides, and cereal-based solutions; the incorporation of early, effective feeding; and the use of hypoosmolar solutions.

Additional Co-transport Molecules

The first attempt at incorporating additional co-transport molecules was the use of amino acids. However, clinical trials in children showed that these solutions offered little or no benefit over standard ORS and had important limitations such as increased urine output, the development of metabolic abnormalities, and instability during storage (45,46).

Polymers of glucose and amino acids were promising because of their effective co-transport properties and lower osmolality (36) but in their purified form are very expensive. However, naturally occurring foods, particularly grains, are inexpensive and contain polymers of starch and simple proteins, which can also provide more co-transport molecules without exacting an osmotic penalty (36). The greatest success with enhanced ORT formulations has been with cereal-based solutions in less-developed countries (7). By far the most experience has been with rice-based solutions (36,47), but successful use of maize, wheat, and sorghum has also been reported (36). Cereal-based solutions can reduce stool volume by more than 30% in children with toxigenic diarrhea and by close to 20% in those with nontoxigenic diarrhea when compared with standard WHO ORSs (47). However, further development of cereal-based ORS has been limited because of the success of early, aggressive nutritional therapy (48). Clinical trials have demonstrated that glucose-electrolyte ORS, plus early appropriate feeding, is as effective as the use of cereal-based ORS and provides obvious nutritional advantages (48,49).

Incorporation Of Early Effective Feeding

The recommendation to include feeding along with ORS as an important component of oral therapy for diarrhea is a more recent development in the evolution of optimal therapy. In the mid 1980s, the validity of withholding feedings during diarrhea began to be rigorously questioned (29). An increasing volume of literature indicates that feeding can have a direct beneficial effect on the outcome of acute diarrhea (29,46). The most important benefit of feeding is to offer nutritional rehabilitation to the patient with diarrhea, particularly in developing countries. In addition, intestinal nutrient uptake has long been known to be an important factor involved in repair after injury (30,50).

As discussed earlier, some element of malabsorption is often associated with diarrhea, but it is rarely complete, and substantial percentages of dietary carbohydrate, fats, and protein are absorbed (31,32). Various early feeding regimens have been studied including breast milk (51,52), dilute or full-strength animal milk or animal milk formulas (52,53), dilute and full-strength lactose-free formulas (52,54,55), and staple food diets with milk (53,56–58). These studies have demonstrated that an unrestricted diet does not affect the course or symptoms in children with mild diarrhea (52,56). In fact, appropriate early feeding can help reduce stool output (32,51,54,57,58) and duration of diarrhea (52,54,56), compared with the use of ORS or IV therapy alone. Perhaps most importantly, early feeding can also result in improved initial nutritional outcome (54,55).

Cereal-based diets appear to be particularly effective during diarrhea (57,58), but if cereals or legumes are the sole source of protein, an incomplete amino acid profile, deficient in essential amino acids, is likely to result (59). Also, a greater proportion of protein may be required in cereal or legume-based diets because of their digestibility (59). A potential solution to this problem is to include milk, a more complete protein source, with cereals to improve the amino acid profile and digestibility.

The amount of lactose that can be tolerated by children with diarrhea is still subject to controversy, but several principles have become clear (37). Breast-fed infants who receive a higher concentration of lactose than children receiving cow's milk or cow's milk formula can be fed safely through diarrhea (29). Full-strength animal milk or animal milk formula is usually well tolerated by children who have mild self-limited diarrhea, which is very common in the United States (52). A recent metaanalysis on the use of lactose in children with acute diarrhea found that most can safely tolerate full-strength animal milk (37). As long as children are carefully monitored to identify the few who will develop signs of intolerance, full-strength milk should be used as part of appropriate early feeding (37).

Combining milk with staple foods such as cereals is well tolerated by children who normally take solid foods (56–58). These mixed diets are better tolerated than milk alone (58) and are thought to be successful in part because of the smaller total lactose load and because solid foods help delay gastric emptying and thus slow transit time (60).

Recent studies of diets such as chicken and cereal (34,61), cereal and milk (57,61) and, cereal and legumes (58,61) have confirmed that a substantial proportion of nutrients can be absorbed from mixed diets by young children and infants with acute diarrhea. These studies indicate that diets of naturally occurring, culturally acceptable inexpensive foods can be effective in diarrhea. The implications of these findings are enormous from a health policy standpoint because they provide hope that the important ingredients of successful feeding therapy are already present, even in developing countries.

Hypoosmolar Solutions

Another area of active research in ORT has been the study of hypoosmolar solutions. Renewed interest in oral hypoosmolar solutions for treatment of diarrhea stems from perfusion studies in animals and humans, which show a significant inverse correlation between ORS osmolality and water absorption (62). Clinical trials have demonstrated that hypoosmolar ORT formulations can result in lower stool output and less need for IV therapy for failures of ORS in children with noncholera diarrhea compared with standard ORS (63–65). The most widely studied of these formulations have an osmolality range of 224 to 250 and glucose and sodium concentrations of 75 to 90 mmol/L and 60 to 75 mmol/L, respectively (Table 79.1). These formulations may be particularly beneficial in developed countries where ORS solutions with sodium concentrations lower than that of the standard WHO/UNICEF ORS have been advocated because low rates of breast-feeding and low frequency of malnutrition increase the risk of hypernatremia during diarrhea (15).

Indications For Use

The WHO and AAP recommend the use of ORS to treat all degrees of dehydration and provide maintenance fluid and electrolytes for all cases of diarrhea and dehydration (1,13). In cases of severe dehydration (≥10% fluid deficit, shock, or near shock) IV (or intraosseous) rehydration should be started immediately if available. In patients who can tolerate enteral solutions, ORS can be used to treat severe dehydration if parenteral therapy is not available (1,13). ORS is effective in treating all types of diarrhea including those caused by invasive, adherent, or toxin-producing organisms (7,13).

Contraindications To Use

ORS can be used for almost all cases of diarrhea, but several important limitations to its use must be remembered. ORS should not be used in unconscious persons or those with ileus (13). Monosaccharide malabsorption occurs in only about 1% of acute diarrhea cases but would obviate the use of ORS (13). Patients suspected of glucose malabsorption should be treated with IV therapy.

ORS can be used effectively in cases of dysentery to replace fluid and electrolyte losses, but antimicrobial therapy should also be used for shigellosis and *Clostridium difficile* and *Entomoeba histolytica* colitis (13).

Vomiting commonly accompanies diarrhea, and more than 90% of patients with diarrhea and vomiting can be treated with ORS if it is given frequently in small volumes (7,13). However, severe intractable vomiting occurs rarely but may require parenteral therapy.

Efforts To Increase Use

ORS is estimated to be used in about 25% to 30% of the cases who could benefit from its use in the United States and in developing countries (1,11). The reasons for this relative underuse include the logistic and economic difficulties in producing and supplying prepackaged ORS to families in the developing world, the need for labor-intensive administration, and the difficulty in overcoming the reliance on the longtime successful practice of IV therapy (11).

The substantial impact of ORS on the morbidity and mortality of diarrhea may increase with the growing awareness of the effectiveness of ORS and continued success of the promotional activities of organizations such as the WHO and UNICEF (1,7). The further evolution of oral therapy to include treatment that can reduce stool volume and diarrhea duration will also likely have a major impact of its use. The appreciation that locally available, culturally acceptable ingredients can be used to make oral therapy effective may also increase its use.

Applications Beyond Diarrhea

In addition to diarrhea, ORT can be used in other conditions associated with fluid and electrolyte losses, such as burns (11). Because the gastrointestinal tract is usually intact in burn patients, ORS can have an important role, particularly in patients in whom IV access is difficult. The use of the oral rather than the IV route helps to reduce the risk of infection in these patients who have an altered skin barrier.

The efforts to improve oral therapy to include effective feeding regimens may be very beneficial in diseases with an important component of malnutrition. For example, these regimens may prove helpful in patients with AIDS who often have some element of altered intestinal function and malnutrition (66).

THERAPEUTIC GUIDELINES

The specific guidelines for oral therapy of children with diarrhea are related to the degree of dehydration. The clinical assessment of dehydration is critical to effective oral therapy.

Evaluation

A careful history is essential to guiding and focusing the evaluation process. The history should seek information of an associated illness including meningitis, sepsis, pneumonia, otitis media, or urinary tract infection, which can cause similar symptoms. The history should also evaluate possible risk factors for a causative agent such as travel to lesser developed countries, use of untreated water, exposure to animals, involvement in a day care setting, or recent use of antibiotics. The dietary history is also important, because food allergies and excessive intake of juice can cause diarrhea in infants and young children (67).

The physical examination must include an accurate body weight measurement as part of the assessment of

TABLE 79.3. ASSESSMENT OF DEHYDRATION

	Mild (<5%)	Moderate (5–9%)	Severe (>10%)
Blood pressure	Normal	Decreased	Moderately to severely decreased
Heart rate	Normal	Normal to increased	Tachycardia
Skin turgor	Normal	Decreased	Decreased
Fontanelle	Normal	Sunken	Sunken
Mucous membranes	Slightly dry	Dry	Dry
Eyes	Normal	Sunken orbits	Sunken orbits
Extremities	Perfused	Delayed capillary refill	Cool, mottled
Mental status	Normal	Lethargy	Lethargy, coma
Urine output	Slightly decreased	Decreased	Absent
Thirst	Increased	Moderately increased	Greatly increased

From Duggan C, Santosham M, Glass R. The management of acute diarrhea in children: oral rehydration, maintenance and nutritional therapy. *MMWR Morb Mortal Wkly Rep* 1992;41:1–20, with permission.

hydration. The assessment of hydration also includes evaluation of the skin turgor, moisture of the mucous membranes, firmness of the orbits, mental status, and presence or absence of postural changes in the heart rate or blood pressure (Table 79.3). The fullness of the anterior fontanelle should also be assessed in young infants. In addition, tenting of the skin, rapid deep breathing (evidence of acidosis), and delayed capillary refill time can be particularly helpful in determining the severity of dehydration (68,69). The physical examination can also be helpful in detecting electrolyte abnormalities. Altered sensorium should raise the possibility of hypernatremia, and abnormal neuromuscular states can be seen with hypokalemia. Hyperkalemia can cause cardiac arrhythmias. In general, the other portions of the physical examination are not helpful in evaluating the severity or etiology of the diarrhea.

The laboratory evaluation is only rarely required in the immunocompetent child with acute diarrhea. Serum chemistries are usually not helpful, although electrolytes should be obtained when clinical signs and symptoms of sodium or potassium abnormalities are present (14). A microscopic stool evaluation using either a Wright or a Gram stain identifies the presence of red or white blood cells in the stool. Stool cultures have a very low yield of enteric pathogens when red and white cells are not present (70).

Therapeutic Recommendations

No Dehydration

ORS is recommended to replace the ongoing stool and emesis losses (13,14). Stool losses are replaced with 10 mL/kg for each stool and emesis losses are replaced using one-half cup increments (14). However, children with no dehydration are the least likely to take ORS, in part because of the slightly salty taste of the solutions. Fortunately, if the stool output remains modest, ORS may not be required. If no dehydration develops, which is the case in most diarrhea cases in the United States, continued age-appropriate feeding is the only therapy required. Nonweaned infants should receive breast milk or continued use of the regular formula. The formula does not require dilution if the diarrhea remains mild. If a diluted formula is used, the concentration should be increased rapidly if the diarrhea does not worsen. Weaned infants and children should have their regular diet continued, emphasizing complex carbohydrates (such as rice, wheat, and potatoes), meats (particularly chicken), and the child's regular milk of formula. Foods high in simple sugars and fats should be avoided (13,14).

Mild Dehydration (<5%)

Dehydration should be corrected by giving 50 ml/kg of ORS over four to six hours (13,14). Rapid restoration of the circulating blood volume helps to correct acidosis and improves tissue perfusion, which aids the early refeeding process. Replacement of continuing stool and emesis losses is accomplished as outlined above. As soon as the dehydration is corrected, feeding should begin following the guidelines given above.

Moderate Dehydration (5–9%)

Dehydration is corrected by giving 100 mL of ORS per kilogram of body weight over 4 to 6 hours. At the end of each hour of rehydration, continuing stool losses and emesis volume should be calculated and the total added to the amount remaining to be given.

When rehydration is complete, feeding is continued after the guidelines above.

Severe Dehydration (>10%)

By definition, severe dehydration designates shock or a near-shocklike condition (13,14) and should be treated as a true medical emergency. A large-bore catheter should be used for the infusion of Ringer lactate, normal saline, or similar solution and boluses of 20 to 40 mL/kg should be administered until signs of shock resolve. Fluid and electrolyte resuscitation may require more than one IV site and the use of alternative access sites including venous cutdown, femoral vein, or interosseous locations may be needed (13,14). As the level of consciousness improves, ORS can be instituted. The hydration status must be frequently reassessed to monitor the effectiveness of the therapy.

When rehydration is complete, feeding is continued as above.

ANTIMICROBIAL THERAPY

Because most episodes of diarrhea are self-limited, antimicrobial agents are not generally recommended (14,71). In fact, the use of antibiotics in infections such as salmonella may actually lead to a prolonged carrier state and an increased risk of bacteriologic and symptomatic relapse (72). However, antibiotics do have a role in cholera, *Shigella* dysentery, and *C. difficile*-induced disease (71). Other causes of dysentery such as *Campylobacter* are usually self-limited and do not benefit from therapy. Anti-parasitic agents have long been recommended for treatment of *Giardia* and are critically important in the treatment of amebiasis (71).

ANTIDIARRHEAL AGENTS

The three major categories of antidiarrheal drugs are antimotility, antisecretory, and adsorbent agents. They are intended to decrease the frequency and volume of diarrheal stools. In general, these agents have been shown to have little impact on episodes of acute diarrhea, although consumers continue to pay hundreds of millions of dollars for them each year (71).

Antimotility agents are primarily opioids that work by inhibiting smooth muscle contractions (13,73). In controlled trials, these agents have been shown to slow transit time and to shorten the duration of diarrhea (13). However, they have little or no effect on total stool volume and can have important side effects including nausea, vomiting, drowsiness, and ileus. Antisecretory agents attempt to decrease intestinal secretion, which is a major cause of watery stool. The two agents most completely studied and available, aspirin and bismuth subsalicylate, have been shown to have a modest clinical impact (13,74). Often, however, such large volumes of drugs and frequent administration are required that they are of little practical use (71). In children, concern for salicylate toxicity and for the statistic association of salicylate use and Reye syndrome have limited the use of these agents (74).

Commonly used adsorbent agents such as kaolin, pectin, and charcoal act by binding to bacterial toxins. They usually have little effect on stool weight and water content, although they may improve stool form (13). Cholestyramine, an exchange resin that can bind bacterial toxins and bile acids, has been shown to reduce the duration of diarrhea but can cause acidosis, hyperchloremia, and intestinal obstruction in patients not properly rehydrated (13). Young children are probably the least responsive patients.

These adjunctive therapies have little evidence to support their effectiveness, can have important side effects, and are costly. Because their use is unlikely to be of benefit and may divert attention and resources away from optimal oral therapy, the use of antidiarrheal drugs is not recommended by the AAP, the CDC, or the WHO for the treatment of acute diarrhea (13,14,71).

REFERENCES

1. Cleason M, Merson MH. Global progress in the control of diarrheal diseases. *Pediatr Infect Dis J* 1990;9:345–355.
2. Koloff KL, Wasserman SS, Steciak JY, et al. Acute diarrhea in Baltimore children attending an outpatient clinic. *Pediatr Infect Dis J* 1988;7:753–759.
3. Cicirello, Glass RI. Current concepts of the epidemiology of diarrheal diseases. *Semin Pediatr Infect Dis* 1994;5:163–167.
4. Ho MS, Glass RI, Pinsky PF. Diarrheal deaths in American children: are they preventable? *JAMA* 1988;260:3281.
5. Avendano P, Matson DO, Long J, et al. Costs associated with office visits for diarrhea in infants and toddlers. *Pediatr Infect Dis J* 1993;12:897–902.
6. Matson DO, Estes MK. Impact of rotavirus infection at a large pediatric hospital. *J Infect Dis* 1990;162:598–604.
7. Hirschhorn N, Greenough WB III. Progress in oral rehydration therapy. *Sci Am* 1991;264:50–56.
8. Phillips RA. Water and electrolyte losses in cholera. *Fed Proc* 1964;23:705–712.
9. Hirschhorn NB, Kinzie JL, Sachar DB, et al. Decrease in net stool output in cholera during intestinal perfusion with glucose-containing solutions. *N Engl J Med* 1968;279:174–181.
10. Pierce NF, Sack RB, Mitra RC, et al. Replacement of water and electrolyte losses in cholera by an oral glucose-electrolyte solution. *Ann Intern Med* 1969;70:1173.
11. Avery ME, Snyder JD. Oral therapy for acute diarrhea: the underused simple solution. *N Engl J Med* 1990;323:891–894.
12. Hirschhorn N. The treatment of acute diarrhea in children: an historical and physiological perspective. *Am J Clin Nutr* 1980;33:637–663.
13. Subcommittee on Acute Gastroenteritis. Practice parameter: the management of acute gastroenteritis in young children. *Pediatrics* 1996;97:424–435.
14. Duggan C, Santosham M, Glass R. The management of acute diarrhea in children: oral rehydration, maintenance and nutritional therapy. *MMWR Morb Mortal Wkly Rep* 1992;41:1–20.
15. ESPGAN Working Group. Recommendations for composition of oral rehydration solutions for the children of Europe. *J Pediatr Gastroenterol Nutr* 1992;14:113.
16. O'Shaughnessy WB. Proposal for a new method of treating the blue epidemic cholera. *Lancet* 1830;1:366.
17. Phillip RA. Water and electrolyte losses in cholera. *Fed Proc* 1964;23:705–712.
18. Cosnett JE. The origins of intravenous fluid therapy. *Lancet* 1989;1:768–771.

19. Finberg L. The role of oral electrolyte-glucose solutions in hydration for children: international and domestic aspects. *J Pediatr* 1980;96:51–54.
20. Harrison HE. The treatment of diarrhea in infancy. *Pediatr Clin North Am* 1954;1:335–348.
21. Paneth N. Hypernatremic dehydration in infancy: an epidemiologic review. *Am J Dis Child* 1980;134:785–791.
22. Curran PF. NaCl and water transport by rat ileum in vitro. *J Gen Physiol* 1960;43:1137–1148.
23. Nalin DR, Cash RA. Oral or nasogastric maintenance therapy in pediatric cholera patients. *J Pediatr* 1971;78:355–358.
24. Hirschhorn NB, et al. Oral fluid therapy of Apache children with infectious diarrhea. *Lancet* 1971;2:15.
25. Mahalanalis D, Choudri AB, Bagchi NG, et al. Oral fluid therapy of cholera among Bangladesh refugees. *Johns Hopkins Med J* 1973;132:197–205.
26. Listernik R, Zieseri E, Davis AT. Outpatient oral rehydration in the United States. *Am J Dis Child* 1986;140:211–215.
27. Chung AW. The effect of oral feeding at different levels on the absorption of foodstuffs in infantile diarrhea. *J Pediatr* 1948;33:14–22.
28. Chung AW, Viscerova B. The effect of early oral feeding versus early oral starvation on the course of infantile diarrhea. *J Pediatr* 1948;33:14–22.
29. Brown KH, MacLean WL Jr. Nutritional management of acute diarrhea; an appraisal of the alternatives. *Pediatrics* 1984;73:119–128.
30. Vanderhoof JA, Langnas AN. Short-bowel syndrome in children and adults. *Gastroenterology* 1997;113:1767–1778.
31. Thobani S, Molla AM, Snyder JD. Nutritional therapy for persistent diarrhea. In: Baker S, Baker R, Davis A, eds. *Pediatric enteral nutrition.* New York: Rhineholt Publishers, 1994.
32. Molla A, Molla AM, Sarker S, et al. Absorption of nutrients during diarrhea due to *V. cholerae, E. coli*, rotavirus and shigella. In: Chen LC, Scrimshaw HA, eds. *Diarrhea and malnutrition: interactions, mechanisms and interventions.* New York: Plenum Publishing, 1981:114–123.
33. Fine KD, Kreijs GJ, Fordtran JS. Diarrhea. In: Sleisenger MH, Fordtran JS, eds. *Gastrointestinal disease: pathophysiology, diagnosis and management.* Philadelphia: WB Saunders, 1989.
34. Molla A, Molla AM, Sarker S, et al. Effects of acute diarrhea on absorption of macronutrients during disease and after recovery. *Scand J Gastro* 1983;18:537–543.
35. Barnes Gl, Townley RW. Duodenal mucosal damage in 31 infants with gastroenteritis. *Arch Dis Child* 1973;48:343–349.
36. Carpenter CCJ, Greenough WB, Pierce NF. Oral rehydration therapy—the role of polymeric substrates. *N Engl J Med* 1988;319:1346–1348.
37. Brown KH, Peerson JM, Fontaine O. Use of non-human milks in the dietary management of young children with acute diarrhea: a meta-analysis of clinical trials. *Pediatrics* 1994;93:17–27.
38. Hirschhorn N. The treatment of acute diarrhea in children: an historical and physiological perspective. *Am J Clin Nutr* 1980;33:637–663.
39. Snyder JD. Dietary protein sensitivity: Is it an important risk factor for persistent diarrhea? *Acta Paediatr* 1992;81[S381]:78–81.
40. Santosham M, Daum RS, Dillman L, et al. Oral rehydration therapy of infantile diarrhea: a controlled study of well-nourished children hospitalized in the United States and Panama. *N Engl J Med* 1982;306:1070–1076.
41. Tamer AM, Friedman LB, Maxwell SRW, et al. Oral rehydration of infants in a large urban U.S. Medical center. *J Pediatr* 1986;107:14–19.
42. Santosham M, Burns B, Nadkarni V, et al. Oral rehydration therapy for acute diarrhea in ambulatory children in the United States: a double-blind comparison of four different solutions. *Pediatrics* 1985;76:159–166.
43. Snyder JD. Use and misuse of oral therapy for diarrhea: comparison of U.S. practices with American Academy of Pediatrics recommendations. *Pediatrics* 1991;87:28–33.
44. Editorial. Oral glucose/electrolyte therapy for acute diarrhea. *Lancet* 1975;1:79–80.
45. Santosham M, Burns BA, Reid R, et al. Glycine-based oral rehydration solution: reassessment of safety and efficacy. *J Pediatr* 1986;109:795–801.
46. Ribeiro HD Jr, Lifshitz F. Alanine-based oral rehydration therapy for infants with acute diarrhea. *J Pediatr* 1991;118:S86–S90.
47. Gore SM, Fontaine O, Pierce NF. Impact of rice based oral rehydration solution on stool output and duration of diarrhoea: meta-analysis of 13 clinical trials. *Br Med J* 1992;304:287–291.
48. Santosham M, Fayad I, Hashem M, et al. A comparison of rice-based oral rehydration solution and "early feeding" for the treatment of acute diarrhea in infants. *J Pediatr* 1990;116:868–875.
49. Snyder JD. The continuing evolution of oral therapy for diarrhea. *Semin Pediatr Infect Dis* 1994;5:231–235.
50. Isolauri E, Juntunen M, Wiren S, et al. Intestinal permeability changes in acute gastroenteritis: effects of clinical factors and nutritional management. *J Pediatr Gastroenterol Nutr* 1989;8:466–473.
51. Khin Maung U, Nyunt-Nyunt W, Myo Khon, et al. Effect of clinical outcome of breast feeding during acute diarrhoea. *Br Med J* 1985;290:587–589.
52. Margolis PA, Litteer T. Effects of unrestricted diet on mild infantile diarrhea. *Am J Dis Child* 1990;144:162–164.
53. Placzek M, Walker-Smith JA. Comparison of two feeding regimens following acute gastroenteritis in infancy. *J Pediatr Gastroenterol Nutr* 1984;3:245–248.
54. Santosham M, Foster S, Reid R, et al. Role of soy-based, lactose-free formula during treatment of acute diarrhea. *Pediatrics* 1985;76:292–298.
55. Brown KH, Gastanaduy AS, Saaverdra JM, et al. Effect of continued oral feeding on clinical and nutritional outcomes of acute diarrhea in children. *J Pediatr* 1988;112:191–200.
56. Hjelt K, Paerregard A, Petersen W, et al. Rapid versus gradual refeeding in acute gastroenteritis in childhood: energy intake and weight gain. *J Pediatr Gastroenterol Nutr* 1989;8:75–80.
57. Brown KH, Perez F, Gastanaduy AS. Clinical trial of modified whole milk, lactose-hydrolyzed whole milk, or cereal-milk mixtures for the dietary management of acute childhood diarrhea. *J Pediatr Gastroenterol Nutr* 1991;12:340–350.
58. Alarcon P, Montoya R, Perez F, et al. Clinical trial of home available, mixed diets versus a lactose-free, soy-protein formula for the dietary management of acute childhood diarrhea. *J Pediatr Gastroenterol Nutr* 1991;12:224–232.
59. Brown KH. Appropriate diets for the rehabilitation of malnourished children in the community setting. *Acta Paediatr Scand* 1991;374S:151–159.
60. Martini MC, Savaiano DA. Reduced intolerance symptoms from lactose consumed during a meal. *Am J Clin Nutr* 1988;47:57–60.
61. International Working Group on Persistent Diarrhoea. Evaluation of an algorithm for the treatment of persistent diarrhoea: a multicentre study. *Bull World Health Organ* 1996;74:479–489.
62. Thillainayagam AV, Hunt JB, Farthing MJG. Enhancing clinical efficacy of oral rehydration therapy: Is low osmolality the key? *Gastroenterology* 1998;114:197–210.
63. El-Mougi M, El-Akkad N, Hendawi A, et al. Is a low-osmolarity ORS solution more efficacious than standard WHO ORS solution? *J Paediatr Gastroenterol Nutr* 1994;19:83–86.
64. International Study Group on Reduced Osmolarity ORS Solution. Multicentre evaluation of reduced-osmolarity oral rehydration salts solution. *Lancet* 1995;345:282–285.

65. Faruque ASG, Mahalanabis D. Reduced osmolarity oral rehydration salt in cholera. *Scand J Infect Dis* 1996;28:87–90.
66. Greenson JK, Belitsos PC, Yardly JH, et al. AIDS enteropathy: occult enteric infections and duodenal mucosal alterations in chronic diarrhea. *Ann Intern Med* 1991;114:366–372.
67. Hyams JS, Leichner AM. Apple juice: an unappreciated cause of chronic diarrhea. *Am J Dis Child* 1985;139:503–505.
68. Saavedra JM, Harris GD, Li S, et al. Capillary refilling (skin turgor) in the assessment of dehydration. *Am J Dis Child* 1991;145: 296–298.
69. Schriger DL, Baraff L. Defining normal capillary refill: variation with age, sex and temperature. *Ann Emerg Med* 1988;17: 932–935.
70. Guerrant RL, Bobak DA. Bacterial and protozoal gastroenteritis. *N Engl J Med* 1991;325:327–340.
71. World Health Organization. *The rational use of drugs in the management of acute diarrhoea in children.* Geneva: World Health Organization, 1990.
72. Nelson JD, Kusmiesz H, Jackson LH, et al. Treatment of *Salmonella* gastroenteritis with ampicillin, amoxicillin, or placebo. *Pediatrics* 1980;65:1125–1130.
73. Kassen AS, Madkour AA, Massoud BZ, et al. Loperamide in acute childhood diarrhea: a double blind controlled trial. *J Diarrhoeal Dis Res* 1983;1:10–16.
74. Snyder JD. Can bismuth improve the simple solution for diarrhea? *N Engl J Med* 1993;383:1705–1706.

80

BACTERIAL ENTERIC VACCINES

MYRON M. LEVINE

GLOBAL DISEASE BURDEN, THE ROLE OF BACTERIAL PATHOGENS, AND VACCINE PRIORITIES

Infections of the gastrointestinal (GI) tract, including diarrheal diseases, dysenteries, and enteric fevers, constitute an important public health problem worldwide. The populations at greatest risk include infants and young children in less-developed countries and travelers from industrialized countries who visit less-developed areas of the world. Within industrialized countries, infants and the elderly suffer much higher incidence rates of diarrheal disease than other segments of the population. In North America, diarrheal illness is also a recognized problem among children attending day care centers, patients in custodial institutions for the mentally retarded and psychotic, and native Americans on some tribal reservations.

Before the mid 1970s, a specific etiologic agent could not be ascribed to most cases of infectious diarrhea. Without knowledge of the infectious agents responsible for GI infections in high-risk populations, it was neither possible to undertake the development of vaccines nor in that era was there reason to predict that immunoprophylaxis might one day represent a feasible and rational approach to the control of diarrheal disease. However, since the early 1970s, a plethora of viral, bacterial, and protozoal agents have been identified as causes of diarrhea. Indeed, the list of diarrheal pathogens has lengthened so markedly in the past 20 years that, at first glance, one might wonder whether a score of distinct vaccines might be necessary to prevent and control GI tract infections. Fortunately, this is not the case because only a relative handful of etiologic agents account for the vast majority of infections of clinical and epidemiologic importance.

The relative importance of the various diarrheal agents can be assessed from several different perspectives, including (a) association with severe or complicated disease (including dehydration) that requires treatment at health centers or hospitals; (b) association with a high incidence mild diarrhea; (c) propensity to cause explosive epidemics and pandemics of severe disease; (d) association with adverse nutritional consequences; and (e) frequency as agents of traveler's diarrhea. By this analysis, a small number of bacterial agents, including enterotoxigenic *Escherichia coli* (ETEC), enteropathogenic *E. coli* (EPEC), *Shigella,* and *Vibrio cholerae* (O1 and O139), as well as a single virus, rotavirus, combine to cause a major proportion of the diarrheal illness of public health importance (1). Similarly, *Salmonella enterica* serovar Typhi is by far the leading cause of enteric fever. Several of these pathogens have been targeted by the World Health Organization (WHO) as priorities for the development of new or improved vaccines, including *V. cholerae* O1 and O139 (causes of epidemic and pandemic dehydrating diarrhea), *Shigella* (the most common etiologic agent of dysentery), ETEC (the second most common cause of dehydrating infant diarrhea, after rotavirus), and *S. enterica* serovar Typhi (*Salmonella typhi,* the etiologic agent of typhoid fever) (1). If such new and improved vaccines could be developed and delivered to the population at risk in developing countries, the global burden of enteric infections could be greatly diminished.

Other than *Shigella,* the above-mentioned bacterial enteric infections rarely pose a problem for children or adults in industrialized countries, unless they travel to developing areas of the world. On the other hand, as a consequence of animal husbandry, mass food processing and fast-food practices in industrialized countries, three other bacterial pathogens have emerged as enteric disease agents of public health importance, including enterohemorrhagic *E. coli* (EHEC) (also called Shiga toxin [Stx]-producing *E. coli* [STEC]), *Campylobacter jejuni,* and nontyphoidal *Salmonella* (in particular *S. enterica* serovar Enteritidis). Although the targets for use of an EHEC vaccine remain controversial, a few EHEC vaccines are in early development (2–4). Efforts to develop a *C. jejuni* vaccine have been driven by the high rate of traveler's diarrhea among U.S. military personnel deployed to certain areas of the world, particularly Southeast Asia.

M. M. Levine: Divisions of Geographic Medicine and Infectious Diseases and Tropical Pediatrics, and Center for Vaccine Development, University of Maryland School of Medicine, Baltimore, Maryland

THE VACCINE DEVELOPMENT PARADIGM

Candidate vaccines are evaluated in a stepwise fashion, with success in the previous step serving as a prerequisite for entering the next phase. Phase 1 studies preliminarily test the safety and immunogenicity of a candidate vaccine. Even if the ultimate target for immunization is children or infants, phase 1 studies typically begin in older subjects before moving to young children. Phase 2 studies, which involve larger numbers of subjects, yield more substantial data on safety and immune response and identify the likely dose and immunization schedule. Issues such as shedding (excretion) and potential transmissibility of live vaccines are usually addressed in phase 2 trials. Phase 3 trials that assess the efficacy of a vaccine use a refined formulation of the vaccine that can be scaled up for large-scale manufacture and typically involve large numbers of subjects (often thousands or tens of thousands). Modern clinical trials are conducted according to the tenets of good clinical practice and are quite expensive. The vaccine development paradigm is characterized by considerable attrition among candidates in the pipeline. Most vaccine candidates do not even progress beyond phase 1, only a small proportion reach the point of phase 3 efficacy trials, and only a fraction of those become licensed vaccines. This attrition must be borne in mind. One must also appreciate the influence of antigenic complexity. Pathogens for which only one or a few antigenic types need be targeted (e.g., typhoid and cholera vaccines) are easier problems to tackle. In contrast, vaccines that must incorporate a strategy to cope with a diverse array of relevant serotypes or antigenic types, such as vaccines to prevent shigellosis and ETEC diarrhea, generally progress more slowly.

VACCINES AGAINST TYPHOID FEVER

Target Populations

Target populations for the use of typhoid vaccines include preschool-aged and school-aged children in developing countries where typhoid fever is endemic or epidemic, travelers from industrialized countries who visit such areas, and clinical microbiology technicians (5,6). In most endemic areas, the peak incidence of typhoid fever occurs in school-aged children. However, in a few instances in which systematic blood culture surveys of febrile toddlers and preschool-aged children have been undertaken, a high incidence of bacteremic *S. typhi* disease has been observed (7,8). The clinical disease is often milder in these young children (7,9). Since 1990, strains of *S. typhi* that carry a plasmid encoding resistance to most of the clinically important antibiotics have emerged and disseminated throughout Asia and Northeast Africa (10,11). Consequences of this in affected areas include increased case-fatality rates, more costly treatment, and a rekindling of interest in typhoid vaccines.

Currently Available Typhoid Vaccines

The parenteral heat-inactivated phenol-preserved whole-cell typhoid vaccine that was developed at the end of the nineteenth century was shown in the 1960s in randomized placebo-controlled field trials sponsored by the WHO to confer a moderate level of protection (60% to 67% vaccine efficacy) that endures for at least 7 years (6,12) (Table 80.1). However, this vaccine was never an acceptable public health tool because it so frequently elicits severe adverse reactions. Approximately 25% of recipients of inactivated whole-cell vaccine develop high fever and malaise, leading to absenteeism from school or work in approximately 15% of vaccinees. In the 1980s, two new well-tolerated licensed typhoid vaccines, attenuated *S. typhi* strain Ty21a live oral vaccine and purified Vi capsular polysaccharide parenteral vaccine, came to replace the highly reactogenic heat-inactivated phenol-preserved whole-cell vaccine (5,13) (Table 80.1). In randomized controlled field trials of efficacy that mainly involved school-aged children, both vaccines were shown to confer a moderate level of protection (14–19). In field tri-

TABLE 80.1. TYPHOID VACCINES THAT ARE LICENSED AND CANDIDATE VACCINES THAT ARE IN CLINICAL TRIALS

Vaccine	Type	Route	Doses	Status	Reference No.
Heat-inactivated, phenol-preserved	Killed whole cell	IM	2	Licensed	6,12
Vi polysaccharide	Subunit	IM	1	Licensed	5,13
Vi conjugated to exotoxin A	Conjugate	IM	2, 21 days apart	Phase 3 completed	31
Ty21a, enteric coated capsules	Mutagenized live strain	PO	3–4	Licensed	5,13
Ty21a, liquid formulation	Mutagenized live strain	PO	3	Licensed*	5,13
CVD 908-*htrA*	Engineered live strain	PO	1	Phase 2	41,42
CVD 909	Engineered live strain	PO	1	Phase 1	59
Ty800	Engineered live strain	PO	1	Phase 1	45
X4073	Engineered live strain	PO	1	Phase 1	47
MicroTyZH9	Engineered live strain	PO	1	Phase 1	S. Chatfield (personal communication)

*In multiple countries, including Canada, but not in the United States.
IM, intramuscularly; PO, orally.

als in Santiago, Chile, three doses of an enteric-coated capsule formulation of Ty21a conferred 62% protection through 7 years of follow-up and a liquid formulation provided 78% protection for 5 years of surveillance (20). In a field trial in South Africa, a single dose of Vi conferred 55% protection for 3 years of follow-up (21).

Although the Ty21a and Vi vaccines both represent improvements over the old killed whole-cell parenteral vaccine, neither of these vaccines is ideal. Moreover, although they are amenable to school-based immunization (5,16,22), neither is adapted for immunization of infants. Consequently, in developing countries, it has not been possible to administer them through the routine immunization services along with other infant vaccines.

The Vi polysaccharide and the Ty21a vaccine each confers significant protection by eliciting quite distinct immune mechanisms. Vi stimulates serum immunoglobulin G (IgG) Vi antibody (17,18,21), whereas Ty21a, a mutant strain that does not express Vi, induces a panoply of humoral and cell-mediated immune responses, but not Vi antibody (13,23–26). Improved typhoid vaccines aim to enhance these immune responses, particularly for infants and toddlers.

Parenteral Vi Conjugate Vaccine

Vi polysaccharide is markedly less immunogenic in young infants in whom it functions as a T-cell–independent antigen giving rise to weak, short-lived serologic responses (13). In contrast, when conjugated to a carrier protein, Vi behaves as a T-cell–dependent antigen, stimulating higher antibody levels and boostable immunologic memory (27–30).

A vaccine consisting of Vi conjugated to recombinant *Pseudomonas aeruginosa* exotoxin A was well tolerated and highly immunogenic in 2- to 4-year-olds (30), as well as in adults and school-aged children. At least two spaced parenteral immunizations must be administered to glean the enhanced immunogenicity of the Vi conjugate (Table 80.1). The efficacy conferred by a two-dose (6 weeks apart) immunization schedule of this Vi conjugate was evaluated in a large-scale, randomized, controlled field trial in Vietnam in children age 2 to 5 years (31). In total, 5,525 children received two doses of Vi conjugate and 5,566 received placebo. During 27 months of follow-up, active surveillance was carried out to detect cases of typhoid fever by visiting children weekly, eliciting a symptom history, and recording their axillary temperature. Subjects who had a temperature of 37.5°C or higher for at least 3 days were referred to a health center where 5 mL of blood was drawn for bacteriologic culture. Typhoid fever was diagnosed in 4 of 5,525 vaccinees and 47 of 5,566 controls, demonstrating an efficacy of 91.5% (95% confidence interval, 77.1–96.6%) (31). The level of efficacy did not vary by year of age among these 2- to 5-year-olds, and it did not appear to wane during the second year of surveillance.

A nested immunogenicity study documented the serologic response to the Vi conjugate. Before the first injection, the geometric mean IgG Vi antibody level (enzyme-linked immunosorbent assay units) was 0.11 in vaccinees and 0.15 in controls (31). Four weeks after the second injection, the geometric mean titer (GMT) in vaccinees was 72.9 and in controls was 0.27. Every vaccinee increased their Vi antibody level by at least a factor of 10.

New-generation Live Oral Vaccines

Five attenuated strains of *S. typhi,* all derived from wild-type strain Ty2 (the parent of Ty21a), have shown promising results in clinical trials. By extrapolation from clinical trials with Ty21a, clinical trials of the new live oral typhoid vaccines include measurements of immunoglobulin A (IgA) O antibody-secreting cells (ASCs) and serum IgG O antibody as part of the assessment of immunogenicity. The reason is that in trials with Ty21a, the magnitude of the gut-derived IgA O-antigen ASC response (detected among peripheral blood mononuclear cells) and the serum IgG O antibody response were stronger in those formulations and immunization schedules that exhibited higher levels of protective efficacy in field trials (13,24,32).

CVD 908

This strain harbors precise deletion mutations in *aroC* and *aroD* that encode enzymes in the aromatic amino acid biosynthesis pathway, rendering the strain nutritionally dependent on substrates (*p*-aminobenzoic acid and 2,3-dihydroxybenzoate) that are not available in sufficient quantity in human tissues (33). When administered to young adults in phase 1 dose–response safety–immunogenicity trials, a single oral dose of CVD 908 was well tolerated in doses as high as 5×10^8 colony forming units (CFU) and excretion was short-lived (≤3 days) (34,35). The vaccine elicited strong serum IgG and gut-derived IgA ASC responses against *S. typhi* O (lipopolysaccharide [LPS]) and H (flagellar) antigens (35), lymphoproliferation and interferon-γ secretion in the presence of *S. typhi* antigens (25), and cytotoxic lymphocytes that recognized targets bearing *S. typhi* antigen (26). Although this vaccine was clinically well tolerated, blood cultures on days 4 to 8 after vaccination detected silent self-limited vaccinemias in 50% of subjects who ingested the highest doses ($5 \times 10^{7-8}$ CFU) (35). The blood cultures were collected systematically from all subjects within a few hours after ingesting CVD 908 and then on days 2, 4, 5, 7, 8, 10, 14, 27, and 60. No culture was positive before day 4 or after day 8, and the clinically silent vaccinemias disappeared spontaneously without antibiotics (35). It is believed that these blood cultures were detecting vaccine organisms en route to the reticuloendothelial system (36,37), analogous to the silent primary bacteremia of typhoid fever (as opposed to the symptomatic secondary bacteremia that occurs later). These silent vaccinemias were considered an impediment for continued evaluation of CVD 908, even though several useful vaccines such as type 2 Sabin attenuated poliovirus and RA27/3 attenuated rubella virus routinely cause silent vaccinemia.

CVD 908-htrA

Chatfield et al. (38) found that mutations in *htrA* (encoding a stress protein that functions as a serine protease) attenuated *S. typhimurium* for mice and such mutants served well as live oral vaccines. A precise *htrA* deletion mutation was introduced into CVD 908, resulting in strain CVD 908-*htrA* (39–41). CVD 908-*htrA* was administered to more than 120 young adult subjects in phase 1 and 2 clinical trials (41,42) (Table 80.1). In single-dose levels up to 10^9 CFU, CVD 908-*htrA* proved to be as well tolerated as CVD 908, was likewise excreted for only 3 days, and was similarly immunogenic (41,42). However, in contrast with CVD 908, CVD 908-*htrA* did not cause silent vaccinemia in any subject.

Ty800

The two-component regulatory system *phoP-phoQ* is essential for *Salmonella* to survive within phagosomes of macrophages and *phoP-phoQ* mutants of *S. typhimurium* are attenuated in mice (43,44). *S. typhi* strain Ty800, harboring a deletion mutation in *phoP-phoQ*, was evaluated in a dose–response phase 1 clinical trial in young adults in which it proved to be generally well tolerated and quite immunogenic in eliciting serum IgG O and H antibody and IgA O ASCs (45) (Table 80.1).

X4073

This construct harbors mutations in the *cya,crp* global regulatory system and in *cdt* that is involved with dissemination of *Salmonella* from gut-associated lymphoid tissue to deep organs (46). X4073 was well tolerated in a phase 1 clinical trial but was less immunogenic than CVD 908-*htrA* and Ty800 (47) (Table 80.1).

CVD 909

Parenteral Vi, polysaccharide vaccine and live oral Ty21a each protect by distinct immune mechanisms, the former by means of serum Vi antibody and the latter by humoral and cellular immune mechanisms other than Vi antibodies (Ty21a does not express Vi). Consequently, it is reasonable to expect that a higher level of protection may be achieved if both serum Vi antibody and the other humoral and cellular responses can be concomitantly elicited (32). Disappointingly, although they can express Vi *in vitro,* the CVD 908, CVD 908-*htrA,* Ty800, and X4073 live oral vaccine strains (described above) have failed to consistently stimulate serum Vi antibodies or IgA Vi ASCs when administered as oral vaccines (34,35,41,42,45,47). This is not entirely surprising because only 20% of patients with acute typhoid fever develop serum Vi antibodies (48,49). On the other hand, infection with *S. typhi* can stimulate serum Vi antibodies, because chronic gallbladder carriers of *S. typhi* typically manifest high titers of serum Vi antibody (49,50). An explanation for these somewhat contradictory observations may stem from the fact that the expression of Vi is highly regulated in relation to certain environmental signals such as osmolarity, and at least two separate two-component systems are involved in this regulation (51,52). It is presumed that Vi expression ensues when typhoid bacilli reside in certain extracellular environments such as blood and bile to protect them from complement-mediated O antibody-dependent bacterial killing (53,54–56) but is turned off when the bacteria gain their intracellular niche within macrophages. If Vi expression by a live oral vaccine strain can be rendered constitutive so that it is expressed continuously, this may allow the stimulation of serum IgG Vi antibodies in orally vaccinated subjects, thereby enhancing the protection against typhoid fever. The *viaB* locus of *S. typhi* contains the genes required for synthesis, surface transport, and anchoring of Vi (57,58). Replacement of the promoter of *tviA,* the most upstream gene in the *viaB* locus of CVD 908-*htrA,* with a strong constitutive promoter resulted in strain CVD 909, which expresses Vi constitutively (59). To test the hypothesis, a single dose of CVD 909 was fed to small groups of healthy adult North Americans in increasing dose levels from 10^5 to 10^9 CFU in a phase 1 clinical trial. The vaccine was well tolerated, elicited IgA Vi ASC responses in the vast majority of subjects and serum IgG Vi antibody in a proportion of recipients of the higher dose levels.

NEW VACCINES AGAINST CHOLERA

Target Populations

Of the more than 100 O serogroups of *V. cholerae,* until the early 1990s, only serogroup O1 was recognized as the cause of explosive epidemics and pandemics of severe dehydrating diarrhea (60). Cholera gravis, the clinically severe form of cholera, can rapidly and fatally dehydrate adults and children. Besides its clinical severity in the individual patient, cholera is one of the few bacterial diseases that is capable of true pandemic spread. Since the seventh pandemic caused by *V. cholerae* O1 biotype El Tor began on the island of Sulawesi in 1961, El Tor cholera has progressively extended to all the inhabited continents.

Several epidemiologic events in the last decade of the twentieth century illustrate why cholera commands special attention among public health authorities. These include (a) the return of cholera to Latin America in 1991, after a century of absence, and its rapid dissemination, leading to more than one million cases by 1994 (61); (b) the explosive outbreak of El Tor cholera among Rwandan refugees in Goma, Zaire, in 1994, resulting in circa 70,000 cases and 12,000 deaths (62); (c) the appearance in 1992 to 1993 of epidemic cholera in the Indian subcontinent caused for the first time by a *V. cholerae* serogroup other than O1, so-called O139 Bengal (63,64).

Potential target populations for the use of the cholera vaccines include individuals of all ages who reside in high-risk areas during cholera epidemics (e.g., refugees), children (and perhaps adults) living in areas of very high endemicity, and travelers from industrialized countries who visit areas of the developing world where cholera is endemic or epidemic.

Oral Cholera Vaccines

Two modern oral cholera vaccines have been licensed by regulatory authorities in a number of countries (Table 80.2). One is a nonliving vaccine consisting of inactivated *V. cholerae* O1 administered in combination with B subunit (BS) of cholera toxin (CT), so-called BS-WCV (65). The other vaccine is a genetically engineered attenuated strain of *V. cholerae* O1, CVD 103-HgR, which is used as a single-dose live oral vaccine (66).

BS-WCV

This nonliving oral vaccine contains 10^{11} heat-inactivated and formalin-inactivated *V. cholerae* O1, consisting of a mixture of classic Inaba, classic Ogawa, El Tor Inaba, and El Tor Ogawa organisms, coadministered with 1.0 mg of BS, along with buffer. Three spaced doses of an early formulation of the vaccine (distinct from the current commercial formulation) conferred 85% protection during the initial 6 months of surveillance, and 50% protection over 3 years of follow-up in a large-scale randomized field trial in Bangladesh in the mid 1980s (67). One of the largest seasonal cholera epidemics ever recorded in the Matlab Bazar field area occurred shortly after completion of the vaccination, thereby allowing a definitive assessment of the efficacy of that early formulation of the BS-WCV. The positive results gave support to the concept of mucosal immunization.

The current commercial formulation, rBS-WCV, which uses a recombinant BS (to help diminish production costs), is well tolerated by adults and children when administered as a two-dose immunization regimen, 10 to 14 days apart (68). There have been three randomized, double-blinded, controlled trials undertaken to assess the efficacy of the two-dose regimen of the commercial formulation and one trial that provides data on the protective efficacy of an unusual three-dose regimen (with booster doses given at 2 weeks and 12 months after the initial dose) of the commercial formulation. Two doses of the rBS-WC vaccine given 2 weeks apart conferred on a small group of Peruvian soldiers (710 vaccinees, 714 placebo controls) a high degree of short-term protection (86% protective efficacy) against epidemic cholera in the face of exposure to a common source vehicle of transmission (encountered shortly after vaccination) that resulted in a high rate of cholera among placebo recipients (69). In contrast, in a large placebo-controlled field trial of efficacy in Lima, Peru, that included children and adults,

TABLE 80.2. LICENSED CHOLERA VACCINES AND CANDIDATE VACCINES THAT ARE IN CLINICAL TRIALS

Vaccine	Type	Antigens	Route	Doses	Status	Reference No.
Whole-cell vaccine	Killed O1 vibrios	Mixture of O1 classical Inaba and Ogawa	Intramuscularly	2	Licensed	
B subunit/WCV	Killed whole-cell plus B subunit combination	Mixture of O1 classical and El Tor biotypes and Inaba and Ogawa serotypes	Oral	2	Licensed[a]	69,183
B subunit/O1 and O139 WCV	Killed whole-cell plus B subunit combination	Above O1 strains + O139 strain	Oral	2	Phase 1	72
CVD 103-HgR	Engineered live strain	O1 classical Inaba	Oral	1	Licensed[b]	66,88
CVD 111/CVD 103-HgR	Engineered live strain	O1 El Tor Ogawa + classical Inaba	Oral	1	Phase 2	105,106
Peru-15	Engineered live strain	O1 El Tor Inaba	Oral	1	Phase 2	110,112
638	Engineered live strain	O1 El Tor Ogawa	Oral	1	Phase 1	114
CVD 112	Engineered live strain	O139	Oral	1	Phase 1	115
Bengal-15	Engineered live strain	O139	Oral	1	Phase 1	117
Lipopolysaccharide conjugate	Conjugate	Inaba lipopolysaccharide conjugated to hydrazine-treated cholera toxin	Parenteral	2	Phase 1	120

[a]Manufactured by SBL Vaccin AB, Sweden, and marketed in Latin America, Sweden, and Norway under the trade names Dukoral or Colorvac.
[b]Manufactured by Berna Biotech, Switzerland, and marketed in Switzerland, Canada, Philippines, Australia and several other countries under the trade names Mutacol or Orochol.

two doses of the rBS-WC vaccine given 2 weeks apart did not provide significant protection (0% efficacy) against either hospitalized cases (detected by passive surveillance) or field cases (detected by active surveillance) during a 12-month follow-up (70). However, after the administration of a third dose of vaccine 1 year later, significant (61%) protection was observed over the next year of observation, including against both hospitalized cases (82% efficacy) and field cases (49% efficacy) (70).

Another large-scale field trial of the two-dose regimen of the commercial formulation of rBS-WCV was carried out in Arequipa, Peru, a city that had experienced high rates of cholera in the previous three years prior to the initiation of the field trial. During the first two years of follow-up after vaccination, almost no cases of cholera were observed, precluding any assessment of vaccine efficacy. Cholera then returned to Arequipa with several dozen cases of cholera occurring in the field trial participants in the third year after vaccination. Analysis of the cases showed no evidence of vaccine efficacy in this situation (71) (C. Lanata, personal communication).

The rBS-WC vaccine, which is manufactured by SBL Vaccin AB, Stockholm, Sweden, and marketed under the names Dukoral or Colorvac, is licensed in six Latin American countries and in Sweden and Norway. The vaccine, which is administered in a glass of water with an alkaline buffer, is given in two doses 2 weeks apart; a booster dose is recommended after 1 or 2 years.

Bivalent O1-O139 rBS-WCV

An oral bivalent BS O1/O139 whole-cell cholera vaccine has been prepared by adding formalin-inactivated *V. cholerae* O139 to the oral recombinant O1 rBS-WCV (72). When tested in a phase 1 trial in Swedish adults, a two-dose regimen of the bivalent vaccine was well tolerated and elicited intestinal secretory IgA (sIgA) antibody responses to CT in all nine subjects and to both O1 and O139 antigen in seven of nine (Table 80.2). All subjects mounted serum antibody responses to both O1 and O139.

CVD 103-HgR

Single-dose recombinant live oral cholera vaccine CVD 103-HgR was engineered by deleting from wild-type *V. cholerae* O1 classic Inaba strain 569B 94% of the gene encoding the alpha subunit of CT and by inserting into the hemolysin A locus a gene encoding resistance to mercury ions (73,74). CVD 103-HgR is a licensed vaccine available in Canada under the name Mutacol and in a number of European and Asian countries under the trade name Orochol.

The safety and immunogenicity of a single oral dose of this vaccine in subjects as young as 3 months and as old as 65 years, including HIV-positive subjects, has been established in a large number of randomized, placebo-controlled, double-blinded clinical trials with active surveillance (involving more than 7,000 subjects). These clinical trials were carried out in Asia, Latin America, Africa, Europe, and North America (75–85). CVD 103-HgR was licensed based on evidence of efficacy from experimental cholera challenge studies in adult volunteers in North America. A single dose of CVD 103-HgR conferred on adult volunteers significant protection against experimental challenge with pathogenic *V. cholerae* O1 of either biotype or serotype (74,86–88). Notably, almost complete protection (>95%) was conferred against moderate and severe diarrhea caused by either El Tor or classical biotype. In these experimental challenge studies, protection (against wild-type *V. cholerae* O1 of either El Tor or classical biotype) was evident as early as 8 days after vaccination and lasted for at least 6 months (the shortest and longest intervals tested) (86,87). The single-dose efficacy and rapid onset of protection are attractive characteristics of CVD 103-HgR.

Heretofore, only one large-scale, randomized, placebo-controlled, double-blinded field trial has been carried out in a developing country to assess the efficacy of a single dose of CVD 103-HgR in preventing cholera under natural challenge conditions in an endemic area. In that trial in North Jakarta, Indonesia, 67,508 pediatric and adult subjects received a single dose of vaccine or identically appearing placebo (89). Overall, during 4 years of follow-up, the vaccine did not confer significant long-term protection in this venue (13.5% vaccine efficacy overall). Unfortunately, too few cases occurred during the first 4 months of follow-up after vaccination to allow a valid comparison with the experimental challenge studies (seven total: five in controls and two in vaccinees; vaccine efficacy, 60%). The disparity is that all but one of the experimental challenge studies had been carried out less than 4 months after vaccination. Some evidence of long-term efficacy in the Jakarta trial was seen in an analysis in relation to blood group. In an "intent to vaccinate" analysis assessing vaccine efficacy in relation to blood group, persons of blood group O were modestly protected by vaccine ($p = .06$; vaccine efficacy = 45%) (89).

It is unclear why a single dose of CVD 103-HgR did not confer long-term protection in the Jakarta trial when a high level of short-term protection was observed in North American volunteers participating in experimental challenge studies. An important clue may reside in the fact that much lower vibriocidal antibody responses have been observed in subjects vaccinated with CVD 103-HgR in developing countries versus subjects vaccinated in industrialized countries; this has been a remarkably consistent observation (77,78,84). Factors that have been shown to modulate the vibriocidal antibody response include (Table 80.3): (a) blood group O; persons of blood group O (an important host risk factor for the development of cholera gravis) (90,91) mount a stronger response, particularly among immunologically naive persons lacking prior contact with

TABLE 80.3. SOME PARAMETERS THAT AFFECT THE SERUM VIBRIOCIDAL RESPONSE AFTER IMMUNIZATION WITH A SINGLE DOSE OF LIVE ORAL CHOLERA VACCINE

Parameter	Effect	Reference No.
Dose of viable vaccine organisms	Seroconversion rate increases as dosage (CFU) increases	77,84,92
Type of buffer	Better buffering increases serologic response	111
Baseline vibriocidal titer	High baseline titer mutes seroconversion	77,84,92
Blood group	Increased geometric mean titer in persons of blood group O	81
Small-bowel bacterial overgrowth (SBBO)	SBBO diminishes vibriocidal response	98
Age	Lower peak titers in infants and young children	77,78,82,83
Impoverished, unsanitary living conditions	Lower responses in persons living in underprivileged conditions	84,92

V. cholerae O1 (81); (b) prior exposure to *V. cholerae* O1; subjects with high baseline titers usually do not undergo boosts in titer (77,78,80,84,92); (c) socioeconomic level; populations living in underprivileged conditions manifest lower GMTs, independent of blood group or prior contact with *V. cholerae* O1 (84,92). Several live oral viral vaccines, including Sabin polio and RIT bovine rotavirus vaccines, are less immunogenic when given to young children living in low socioeconomic conditions in less-developed countries than children in industrialized countries (93,94). Possible explanations for this diminished immunogenicity include interference from enteroviruses, sIgA antibodies in breast milk, and an unreliable cold chain, resulting in loss of vaccine potency. This phenomenon was also observed in phase 2 studies of live oral cholera vaccine CVD 103-HgR in adults and children living in underprivileged conditions in Asia and Latin America (77,84,92). To achieve high seroconversion rates of vibriocidal antibody in Indonesian children and Peruvian adults living in underprivileged conditions, it was necessary to give a 10-fold higher dose (5×10^9 CFU) of CVD 103-HgR (77,84) than the dose (5×10^8 CFU) that is consistently immunogenic in North Americans and Europeans (75,76). Thus, there exists a poorly understood "barrier" to successful intestinal immunization of children in less-developed countries by live oral vaccines.

Two factors that can contribute to this barrier include small-bowel bacterial overgrowth (SBBO) and heavy intestinal helminth infection (Table 80.3). Persons living in poverty in developing countries endure fecally contaminated environments. Young children often develop SBBO and "environmental enteropathy" (95–97). The relationship between SBBO and vibriocidal response to CVD 103-HgR was investigated in Chilean school children age 5 to 9 years who had lactulose breath H_2 tests to detect proximal small-bowel bacteria, one day before ingesting CVD 103-HgR (98). Logistic regression analysis revealed a clear inverse relationship between H_2 production in the small bowel and the propensity for vibriocidal antibody seroconversion (98).

Short-chain fatty acids elaborated by SBBO flora may inhibit *V. cholerae* O1 (99), thereby blunting the vibriocidal response to CVD 103-HgR. Alternatively, the abnormal intestinal architecture (95,96) and increased lymphocytes in the mucosa (95,96) of children with SBBO, indicating an immunologically "tolerant" gut, may indirectly mute immune responses.

Cooper et al. (100) investigated the hypothesis that heavy infestation with intestinal helminths may contribute to the diminished vibriocidal antibody response observed in persons living in underprivileged conditions in less-developed countries. Ecuadorian school children with documented heavy *Ascaris lumbricoides* infection were randomly allocated two courses of albendazole antihelminthic or placebo before receiving a single 5×10^8 CFU dose CVD 103-HgR. In subjects of blood group O, there was no difference in the vibriocidal responses observed in the albendazole versus the placebo groups. However, for subjects of non-O blood groups, those treated with albendazole had a significantly higher vibriocidal antibody response than those given placebo.

Live oral vaccines that have been licensed in various countries include Sabin trivalent poliovirus (101), Ty21a live oral typhoid (15), quadrivalent rhesus reassortant rotavirus (102), and CVD 103-HgR live oral cholera vaccines (66). CVD 103-HgR is unique among these in having a single-dose immunization schedule. Therefore, CVD 103-HgR was used to explore immunization of Chilean infants and toddlers with a single-dose oral vaccine in a safety–immunogenicity study undertaken successively in 12- to 17-month-olds (N = 104), 7-to 11-month-olds (N = 106), and 3- to 5-month-olds (N = 102) (83). One-half of the subjects were randomly allocated to receive vaccine and the other one-half placebo, in double-blinded fashion. After 2 weeks of double-blinded follow-up, all subjects received a dose of vaccine. Vibriocidal antibody titers were measured at baseline and 2 weeks after each dose. The formulation of CVD 103-HgR, which consists of two sachets, one containing lyophilized vaccine and the other buffer powder, was modeled after the "liquid" formulation of Ty21a live oral typhoid vaccine, which demonstrated clear advantages over the enteric-coated capsule formulation in its practicality for immunizing preschool-aged children and its greater efficacy in the field (16,19,103). This formulation of CVD 103-HgR was practical for immunizing preschool-aged children in Chile, Indonesia, and Peru (78,82). However, in the toddler and infant age-groups, palatability was clearly an issue (83). One-fourth of the toddlers and older infants (age 7 to 11 months) and fully 71% of the young infants (age 3 to 5 months) failed to imbibe at least 70 mL of the 100-mL vaccine cocktail (the criterion defining "fully vaccinated"). This was a function of individual infant preference because a strong predictor of whether an infant or toddler would ingest at least 70 mL of the second dose was whether that subject had imbibed at least 70 mL of the first dose.

CVD 103-HgR was well tolerated in Chilean infants and toddlers; adverse reactions did not occur more frequently in vaccine versus placebo recipients. Because the seroconversion of vibriocidal antibody after ingestion of a single dose of CVD 103-HgR was similar in fully vaccinated infants and toddlers (66%) versus those who ingested a smaller fraction of the vaccine "cocktail" (63%), there was apparently no practical consequence to the poor palatability. Thus, in infants the ingestion of a partial dose of CVD 103-HgR is as likely to result in seroconversion as if 70% or more of the dose is consumed. It appears that in infants and toddlers the dose of vaccine organisms necessary to immunize is likely far less than the 5×10^9 CFU present in the full vaccine cocktail (83).

A salient feature of vaccination with CVD 103-HgR is that moderate or high rates of vibriocidal seroconversion are observed in vaccinees who show low rates of excretion of the vaccine strain (75,77,78,82,84). In the clinical trial in infants in Chile, a second dose of vaccine was given to one-half of the subjects 2 weeks later. Whereas 5 of 118 vaccinated infants and toddlers had positive stool cultures on day 7 after the first dose, 0 of these 118 had positive stool cultures after the second dose of vaccine ($p < .025$)(83). This suggests that the first dose stimulated local intestinal immune mechanisms that reduced colonization of the intestine upon reexposure to the vaccine strain.

CVD 111/CVD 103-HgR Bivalent Vaccine

Attenuated *V. cholerae* O1 vaccine strain CVD 111, derived from an El Tor Ogawa wild-type parent, was shown to be well tolerated, immunogenic, and protective against experimental challenge in small clinical trials in volunteers CVD 111 (104). A combined CVD 111/CVD 103-HgR bivalent vaccine was evaluated in a phase 2 trial in several hundred U.S. military personnel in Panama (105) and Peruvian adults (106), in whom it was shown to be well tolerated and to elicit both anti-Inaba and anti-Ogawa antibodies.

Coadministration Of Ty21a And CVD 103-HgR

Sachets containing lyophilized CVD 103-HgR and Ty21a can be mixed in the same cup containing 100 mL of water to prepare a combined cholera–typhoid vaccine cocktail (107,108). Thereafter, the remaining two doses of the three-dose immunization regimen of liquid Ty21a are administered alone. The vibriocidal antibody response and the serum IgG anti-*S. typhi* O antibody responses are as good as those when these vaccines are administered separately.

Peru-15

V. cholerae O1 Inaba vaccine strain Peru-15 (109) has a deletion of the CT virulence cassette, along with the attRS1 insertion-like sequences. The gene encoding the CT BS under control of a heat shock promoter is inserted into *recA* in Peru-15. Peru-15 also has an undefined mutation, resulting in diminished motility compared with its parent, Peru-5. In randomized, double-blinded, controlled phase 2 vaccine trials, single doses of Peru-15 have been well tolerated, have elicited strong vibriocidal antibody responses, and have conferred 100% protection against moderate and severe cholera in challenge studies (110–112) (Table 80.2).

El Tor Ogawa 638

A nontoxigenic hemagglutinin/protease-deficient mutant, strain 638, was derived by Cuban investigators from a wild-type *V. cholerae* O1 El Tor Ogawa strain isolated in Peru (113,114). In small phase 1 clinical trials, 638 gave promising preliminary results (Table 80.2). The vaccine was generally well tolerated (4 of 42 subjects developed mild diarrhea) and elicited moderate serum vibriocidal antibody responses in more than 80% of vaccinees (114).

Vaccines To Prevent Cholera Caused By *V. cholerae* O139

Beginning in late 1992 and in early 1993 in India and Bangladesh, there appeared epidemic cholera caused by a *V. cholerae* strain of a serogroup other than O1. This new epidemic strain, *V. cholerae* O139 Bengal (63,64), initially appeared to have pandemic potential, as cases of O139 cholera were documented in Thailand, China, Malaysia, Pakistan, and Kazakhstan and travel-associated cases were reported in the United States and the United Kingdom. In cholera-endemic areas of Bangladesh, attack rates for O1 cholera are highest in young children and decrease in older age groups, indicative of acquisition of immunity from repeated antigenic contact. Attack rates for O139 cholera were initially high in adults compared with children, suggesting that antibacterial and antitoxic immunity elicited by *V. cholerae* O1 does not provide cross-protection against *V. cholerae* O139. Fearing that the early epidemiologic behavior of *V. cholerae* O139 might constitute the harbinger of an eighth pandemic of cholera, the WHO encouraged the accelerated development of vaccines against O139 cholera.

In the course of establishing an O139 experimental challenge model in volunteers, investigators at the University of Maryland documented the virulence of wild-type O139 strain AI1837 and demonstrated that an initial clinical diarrheal infection conferred significant protection against subsequent challenge with O139 (115). This observation provided a rationale for hypothesizing that moderate levels of protective immunity may also be achieved by means of O139 live oral vaccine candidates.

The scientific approaches to develop O139 vaccines follow the same strategies for developing vaccines against O1 cholera. Investigators at the University of Goteborg prepared an oral nonliving antigen vaccine consisting of inactivated *V. cholerae* O139 in combination with the BS of CT (72) (Table 80.2). In contrast, investigators at the Center for Vaccine Development of the University of Maryland and at Harvard University constructed live oral vaccine candidates (Table 80.2), as described in more detail below.

Live Oral Vaccines Against O139 Cholera

Investigators at the Center for Vaccine Development (115) engineered an attenuated *V. cholerae* O139 vaccine candidate by deleting from volunteer-tested wild-type strain AI1837 the entire "virulence cassette" region of the chromosome that includes the genes encoding CT, zonula occludens toxin (Zot), accessory cholera toxin (Ace), and the core encoded pili. A gene encoding resistance to Hg^{2+} and the gene encoding the BS under control of its native promoter was introduced into the chromosome in the *hlyA* locus, thereby inactivating the hemolysin cytotoxin enterotoxin as well. The resultant vaccine candidate is designated CVD 112. A further derivative, CVD 112RM, harbors a deletion mutation in *recA,* thereby diminishing the ability of the vibrio to recombine foreign DNA into its chromosome. The *recA* mutation serves to diminish even further the already unlikely possibility of reacquisition of the virulence cassette by a recombinational event with wild-type *V. cholerae* O1 or O139 (115). In phase 1 clinical trials, these O139 vaccine candidates, CVD 112 and CVD 112RM, were fairly well tolerated and immunogenic and provided vaccinated subjects with 84% protection against experimental challenge with virulent *V. cholerae* O139 (115).

Waldor and Mekalanos (116) constructed attenuated O139 vaccine candidates, starting from wild-type strain MO10 (117). Their attenuated strains have deletions of the virulence cassette that contains *ctxAB, zot, ace,* and *cep,* as well as RS1 and *attRS1* (factors that are involved in virulence cassette site specific and homologous recombination). A recombinant gene encoding the BS under control of the promoter from heat shock gene *htpG* is inserted into *recA,* resulting in inactivation of that gene. Prototype vaccine strain Bengal-3 expresses 25-fold more BS than its wild-type parent, MO10 (116). Bengal-15 is a stable spontaneous nonmotile mutant of Bengal-3 (117). In phase 1 clinical trials with Bengal-3 and Bengal-15, Bengal-15 was generally well tolerated, immunogenic, and conferred 83% protective efficacy against experimental challenge with wild-type *V. cholerae* O139 (117) (Table 80.2).

Parenteral Conjugate Vaccines

Recognizing that serum vibriocidal antibodies constitute a correlate of protection against O1 cholera, some investigators have prepared candidate conjugate vaccines consisting of different forms of O1 or O139 O polysaccharide covalently linked to carrier proteins (118,119). Two of these conjugates, consisting of hydrazine-treated O1 Inaba LPS conjugated to CT variants CT-1 and CT-2, were tested in a phase 1 trial in U.S. adults (120) (Table 80.2). These conjugates were well tolerated and elicited strong vibriocidal responses that endured longer than vibriocidal antibody stimulated by killed whole-cell vaccine (120).

NEW VACCINES AGAINST SHIGELLA

Target Populations

There is increasing awareness of *Shigella* as an important public health problem (121). In part this is due to the success of oral rehydration therapy, which has diminished pediatric mortality from dehydrating diarrhea. As a consequence, *Shigella,* which causes bacillary dysentery, a clinical syndrome that is little affected by oral rehydration, has increased in relative importance. The annual number of *Shigella* episodes that occur throughout the world is estimated to be about 165 million, including 163 million cases in developing countries (1.3 million of which result in death) and 1.5 million cases in industrialized countries (121). Children younger than 5 years account for 69% of all episodes and 61% of all deaths attributable to shigellosis; the peak incidence is seen in children age 1 to 4 years. Of the four species or groups of *Shigella,* including *Shigella dysenteriae* (group A), *Shigella flexneri* (group B), *Shigella boydii* (group C), and *Shigella sonnei* (group D), all except *S. sonnei* contain multiple serotypes and subtypes. This antigenic diversity complicates vaccine development efforts. *Shigella* is spread by person-to-person fecal-oral contact involving a minute inoculum (122). Thus, shigellosis (almost entirely caused by *S. sonnei*) remains a problem in certain subpopulations in industrialized countries that manifest primitive hygienic practices, such as preschool-aged children in day care centers and mentally retarded or psychotic persons in custodial institutions. In many studies of traveler's diarrhea, *Shigella* is the second most common pathogen, following ETEC, and typically causes a more severe clinical disease (123,124).

S. dysenteriae type 1, the Shiga bacillus, is unique among the serotypes in that it causes particularly severe clinical disease accompanied by grave complications such as hemolytic–uremic syndrome (HUS), elaborates Stx (a potent cytotoxin), and has the propensity to cause extended pandemics that spread through many countries over several years. Recent epidemics of Shiga dysentery in Africa and Asia have been caused by strains that carry resistance to most clinically useful antibiotics (125).

Target populations for *Shigella* vaccines include toddlers and preschool-aged children in developing countries, travelers, and certain high-risk groups in industrialized countries such as children in day care centers where shigellosis has been endemic (121). A practical and effective vaccine is also needed to control epidemic Shiga dysentery.

Achieving Broad-spectrum Protection Against *Shigella*

A globally useful *Shigella* vaccine will have to protect against *S. dysenteriae* type 1 (cause of severe epidemic disease in the least developed countries), all 15 serotypes of *S. flexneri* (the main serotypes responsible for endemic disease in developing countries), and *S. sonnei* (the most frequent serotype associated with traveler's shigellosis and the most common serotype causing disease in industrialized countries). Infection-derived immunity against *Shigella* appears to be directed toward O antigens. Based on the distribution of shared O antigens among the 15 *S. flexneri* serotypes, Noriega et al. (126) hypothesized that a vaccine containing *S. flexneri* types 2a, 3a, and 6 O antigens could provide broad protection against all 15 *S. flexneri* serotypes. By means of challenge studies in guinea pigs, Noriega et al. (126) generated preclinical evidence supporting this hypothesis. Pursuing this strategy, investigators at the Center for Vaccine Development have designed a multivalent *Shigella* vaccine that includes O antigens of five carefully selected serotypes: *S. dysenteriae* type 1, *S. flexneri* type 2a, *S. flexneri* type 3a, *S. flexneri* type 6, and *S. sonnei.* This pentavalent vaccine should provide broad coverage against the most important *Shigella* serotypes that cause disease worldwide (126,127).

Strains with Mutations in *iuc* and *icsA* (*virG*)

The xylose rhamnose region of the *Shigella* chromosome contains the *iucABCD* operon responsible for production of the hydroxamate siderophore aerobactin and *iutA*, which encodes the 76-kd receptor protein located on the bacterial outer membrane. Nassif et al. (128) reported that although *iuc* mutants of *S. flexneri* remain invasive for epithelial cells and their growth within such cells resembles wild-type *Shigella,* such mutants are attenuated in their capacity to cause keratoconjunctivitis in guinea pigs and to cause fluid accumulation after inoculation into the lumen of rabbit ileal loops. It appears that *iuc* mutants are limited in their capacity to grow in extracellular environments, but once they attain an intracellular niche, they are able to scavenge sufficient iron to maintain normal bacterial growth.

Located on the large invasiveness plasmid of *Shigella, virG* (also known as *icsA*) encodes a 120-kd protein (so-called VirG or IcsA) that is involved in intracellular spread of the bacteria, as well as cell-to-cell spread. This protein is secreted as a 95-kd protein in the outer membrane, following a carboxyl terminus cleavage of the 120-kd moiety.

Investigators at the Pasteur Institute, Paris engineered candidate *S. flexneri* type 2a vaccine strain SC602 by introducing mutations in *iuc, iut,* and *icsA* (129). In phase 1 clinical trials of SC602 performed in U.S. adults (130),

TABLE 80.4. STATUS OF CANDIDATE *SHIGELLA* AND ENTEROTOXIGENIC *ESCHERICHIA COLI* VACCINES

Vaccine	Type	Route	Doses	Status	Reference No.
Shigella O polysaccharide conjugated to carrier protein	*Shigella sonnei* and *Shigella flexneri* conjugates	IM	2	Phase 2 and 3	143–145
SC602 and related *iuc, iut, icsA* mutants	Engineered *S. flexneri* 2a strain	PO	2–3	Phase 2	130
WRSS1 *virG* mutant	Engineered *S. sonnei* strain	PO	1–2	Phase 1	131
CVD 1207 (deletions in *virG, guaBA, set & sen*)	Engineered *S. flexneri* 2a strain	PO	2	Phase 2	136
CVD 1208 (deletions in *guaBA, set* and *sen*)	Engineered *S. flexneri* 2a strain	PO	2	Phase 1	71
Shigella proteosomes	*S. sonnei* or *S. flexneri* 2a LPS noncovalently linked to group B *Neisseria meningitidis* outer membrane protein	PO or intranasal		Phase 2	139
ETEC BS-WCV	Five inactivated ETEC strains cumulatively expressing CFA/I and CS1–CS6 in combination with cholera toxin B subunit	PO	2	Phase 3	159–161
Multivalent *Shigella*/ETEC hybrid vaccine	Five attenuated *Shigella* strains (*Shigella dysenteriae* 1, *S. flexneri* 2a, 3a, and 6, and *S. sonnei*), each carrying a stable plasmid encoding two ETEC fimbrial antigens (cumulatively expressing CFA/I, CS1–CS6) and an LTh antigen	PO	2	Phase 1	71,126,169, 170

ETEC, enterotoxigenic *Escherichia coli;* LPS, lipopolysaccharide; CFA, colonization factor antigens; CS, colony surface factor; IM, intramuscularly; PO, orally.

some subjects developed shigellosis-like adverse reactions at higher dose levels. Lower doses were less reactogenic and protective against severe dysentery after experimental challenge. Phase 2 trials with SC602 are underway in pediatric subjects in Bangladesh (Table 80.4).

WRSS1 is a derivative of *S. sonnei* strain Mosley that harbors a 212-bp deletion in *virG*. WRSS1 is invasive for epithelial cells (a function of invasion plasmid antigens) but does not form plaques (i.e., deficient in VirG) (131). In a phase 1 clinical trial, WRSS1 was mildly reactogenic in doses ranging from 10^3 to 10^6 CFU but was highly immunogenic, eliciting strong IgA anti-LPS ASCs and moderate serum IgG anti-LPS responses. Based on these encouraging preliminary data, further clinical trials with WRSS1 are planned.

Strains With *virG* And *aro* Or *guaBA* Mutations

Swedish investigators showed that deletion of a gene encoding a critical enzyme in the aromatic amino acid biosynthesis pathway partially attenuated *S. flexneri* type 2a (132). Further attenuation of *S. flexneri* type 2a was achieved by introducing a mutation in *virG* to limit intracellular and intercellular spread, in addition to an aromatic pathway mutation, resulting in strain CVD 1203 (133). In phase 1 studies, CVD 1203 was well tolerated and immunogenic (134) at low and mid dose levels but induced self-limited reactogenicity at high dose levels.

Introducing mutations in *guaBA* (which impairs guanine nucleotide synthesis) was found to be highly attenuating for *Shigella* (135). Building on *guaBA* as a basic attenuating mutation, a series of additional attenuating mutations were introduced in stepwise fashion, resulting in a bevy of isogenic vaccine candidates of increasing complexity. A strain bearing the full gamut of attenuating mutations, CVD 1207, which harbors deletion mutations in *guaBA* (impairing nucleotide synthesis), *virG* (thereby limiting intracellular spread), and *set* and *sen* (encoding enterotoxins), was well tolerated in phase 1 trials even at high dose levels (136). Phase 1 clinical trials are also beginning with strain CVD 1208, which has mutations in *guaBA, set,* and *sen.*

A multivalent *Shigella* vaccine that includes attenuated *S. dysenteriae* type 1, *S. flexneri* types 2a, 3a, and 6, and *S. sonnei* strains is being prepared (71,126). By means of cross-protection, this multivalent vaccine, containing five carefully selected *Shigella* serotypes, may be able to provide broad coverage against the most important serotypes that cause shigellosis worldwide (121).

Mucosal Proteosome Vaccines

Complexes of the LPSs of *S. sonnei* and *S. flexneri* type 2a noncovalently bound to proteosomes (vesicles composed of the outer membrane protein of group B *Neisseria meningitidis* [137–139]). Results of clinical trials with intranasal vaccine are particularly interesting. Two intranasal spray doses were administered 14 days apart with 0.1, 0.4, 1.0, or 1.5-mg doses of the *Shigella* proteosomes. The vaccine was generally well tolerated, except for some rhinorrhea or nasal stuffiness. Notably, the intranasal vaccine elicited strong anti-LPS IgA ASC responses and rises in fecal and urinary IgA anti-LPS antibodies (139).

O Polysaccharide Carrier Protein Conjugate Parenteral Vaccines

One *Shigella* vaccine approach that is being followed is to prepare conjugate vaccines for parenteral administration by covalently linking O polysaccharides of the most prevalent *Shigella* serotypes to carrier proteins (140,141). The assumption is that the transudation of vaccine-induced serum IgG antibodies onto the mucosal surface mediates protection by eliminating the ingested bacterial inoculum, nipping infection in the bud (142). A parenteral vaccine consisting of *S. sonnei* O polysaccharide conjugated to *P. aeruginosa* exotoxin A was well tolerated and highly immunogenic in eliciting serum IgG anti-O antibodies in young Israeli soldiers (143,144). In a small randomized, controlled, double-blinded phase 3 efficacy trial involving several hundred soldiers, a single dose of the conjugate vaccine conferred 74% protection against *S. sonnei* disease in the course of an outbreak (143).

Phase 2 trials to assess the safety and immunogenicity of *S. sonnei* and *S. flexneri* type 2a conjugate vaccines have been carried out in children age 4 to 7 years in Israel (145). A two-dose immunization schedule was used in these pediatric studies, with doses spaced 6 weeks apart. The first injection of each vaccine stimulated a significant rise in homologous serum IgG antibodies. The second injection stimulated a booster response in the *S. flexneri* type 2a vaccine recipients but not in those who received the *S. sonnei* vaccine. A phase 3 trial of these vaccines is underway in pediatric subjects in Israel. Two important issues that this trial will address include whether parenteral conjugate *Shigella* vaccines can elicit protection in immunologically naive children and what duration of efficacy will be conferred.

VACCINES AGAINST ENTEROTOXIGENIC *E. COLI*

Target Populations

ETEC is a major cause of dehydrating infant diarrhea in the developing world and is the most common cause of traveler's diarrhea. In endemic areas, infants and toddlers typically suffer three to five episodes of ETEC diarrhea over the first 2 to 3 years of life (146). Target populations for ETEC vaccines include young infants in endemic areas and travelers who visit less-developed countries.

Antigenic Diversity Among Human Enterotoxigenic *E. coli* Pathogens

Analysis of the antigenic structure of ETEC strains from endemic areas shows many different O:H serotypes, at least 10 distinct antigenic types of fimbrial colonization factor antigens (CFAs) (of which the most common are CFA/I and colony surface factors 1 through 6 [CS1 through CS6]) and three different toxin phenotypes (heat-labile toxin [LT], heat-stable toxin [ST], and a combination [LT/ST]) (147,148). Most authorities agree that to provide broad-spectrum protection against human ETEC infections, a vaccine will have to contain fimbrial antigens representative of the most prevalent ETEC pathogens. The most common fimbrial CFAs of human ETEC are CFA/I, the CFA/II family, and the CFA/IV family of antigens. CFA/I is a single antigenic moiety. *E. coli* CS1, CS2, and CS3 antigens constitute the CFA/II family of antigens. All CFA/II strains express CS3, either alone or in conjunction with CS1 or CS2. CS4, CS5, and CS6 comprise the CFA/IV family of antigens. All CFA/IV strains express CS6, either alone or in conjunction with CS4 or CS5. Other fimbrial colonization factors are much less frequent. Carriage of the genes that encode expression of a particular fimbrial colonization factor is closely correlated with O:H serotype and with toxin phenotype.

Analysis of ETEC isolates from diverse geographic areas shows that CFA/I and CS1 through CS6 are found on most isolates. Approximately 80% to 90% of isolates that elaborate both LT and ST enterotoxins express these CFAs, whereas they are found on 60% of ST-only strains. Generally, less than 10% of LT-only strains bear these CFAs. Thus, if a multivalent ETEC vaccine contained just CFA/I and CS1 through CS6, it could theoretically provide protection against approximately 50% to 80% of ETEC strains in most geographic areas. If an LT toxoid (such as the BS of LT) were included, and if such a vaccine were well tolerated and efficacious, the multivalent vaccine might provide relatively broad protection against 80% to 90% of ETEC strains worldwide. Inclusion of the less frequent fimbrial antigens in a multivalent vaccine (that would also include LTB) could potentially expand the spectrum of coverage to more than 90% of ETEC strains.

Infection-derived Immunity

Despite the antigenic heterogeneity of ETEC, evidence from both volunteer studies and epidemiologic surveys shows that prior infection with ETEC confers immunity (149–151). In endemic areas, multiple infections with distinct strains bearing different fimbrial CFAs and of different toxin phenotypes must occur in order for broad-spectrum immunity to be elicited. In less-developed countries, infants and young children experience up to three separate clinical ETEC infections per year during the first 3 years of life, after which the incidence of ETEC diarrhea drastically falls (150). It is obvious that this lower incidence in older individuals is due to acquired immunity, rather than to other age-related host factors, because adult travelers from industrialized countries who visit less-developed countries where ETEC pediatric diarrhea is endemic suffer high attack rates of ETEC traveler's diarrhea. Fortunately, from the perspective of vaccine development, the antigenic makeup of strains that cause endemic pediatric diarrhea and those that cause traveler's diarrhea, including O:H serotypes and fimbrial antigenic types, is the same.

Travelers from industrialized countries who remain in less-developed countries for at least a year and travelers who arrive from other less-developed countries suffer significantly lower incidence rates of ETEC diarrhea than newly arrived travelers from industrialized countries (151). These data support the concept of acquired immunity. A few prospective epidemiologic field studies provide direct evidence that acquired immunity is largely directed at fimbrial colonization factors of ETEC (152).

Passive Protection With Oral Immunoglobulin

Tacket et al. (153) immunized cows with ETEC strains expressing different fimbrial antigens including CFA/I. A bovine immunoglobulin concentrate was prepared from the milk of cows. In a randomized, placebo-controlled, double-blinded clinical trial in volunteers, all 10 subjects who received the ETEC milk immunoglobulin concentrate were completely protected against challenge with a wild-type ETEC strain that expresses CFA/I, LT, and ST and that caused diarrhea in 90% of the 10 volunteers who received the control preparation. Although passive protection is neither practical nor economical for long-term immunoprophylaxis, the results generate optimism for the concept of prevention of ETEC diarrhea. If active immunization with oral vaccines can succeed in eliciting high titers of intestinal antibody, it may be possible to confer protection that will be more enduring.

Killed Enterotoxigenic *E. coli* Whole-Cell/Cholera BS Combination Vaccine

By far the vaccine furthest along is one that consists of inactivated ETEC administered in combination with the BS of CT. The prototype inactivated whole-cell ETEC vaccine was developed by Evans et al. (154) who used ETEC inactivated with colicin E1, which did not damage the fimbrial protein antigens. Oral immunization with such colicin E1-inactivated ETEC induced intestinal IgA antibody response against the homologous CFA (and against LT) and protected volunteers against experimental challenge with wild-type ETEC. However, further development of the colicin-inactivated vaccine was not pursued. In the late 1980s, a prototype oral ETEC vaccine was developed, consisting of CT BS in combination with formalin-killed ETEC strains expressing the most important CFAs. Cholera BS was included because this antigen (as an oral killed whole-cell/BS combination vaccine) had conferred significant protection for several months against LT-producing ETEC, both among subjects in an endemic area and among vaccinated travelers (155,156).

The initial prototype vaccine was subsequently replaced by an oral ETEC vaccine containing recombinant cholera BS (rBS) in combination with five different formalin-inactivated *E. coli* strains expressing CFA/I and CS1 through CS6. Inactivation by formalin-treatment killed the ETEC without major loss in antigenicity of the different CFAs. Phase 1 and 2 trials of this ETEC-rBS vaccine in Swedish, Bangladeshi, American, and Egyptian volunteers showed that the vaccine is well tolerated and stimulates intestinal immune responses against the different vaccine CFAs in most subjects (157–160). Clinical trials for safety and immunogenicity were carried out with this inactivated-ETEC vaccine in Egyptian preschool-aged children; the vaccine was well tolerated and immunogenic (161). Two doses of vaccine or placebo (inactivated *E. coli* K12) were administered given 2 weeks apart to 97 children age 2 to 5 years. Serum IgA and IgG antitoxin and antifimbrial responses were also measured in the adult, school-aged, and preschool-aged subjects in the phase 2 trials of this vaccine in Egypt. Significant rises in antibody (defined as more than or equal to twofold by the investigators) to CT BS were found in about 95% of subjects; 44% to 75% of children and 25% to 81% of adults exhibited significant rises in IgG antibody to the fimbrial antigens (160).

Studies on the protective efficacy of the ETEC-rBS vaccine are underway in European and American travelers and a field trial of the efficacy of this vaccine is underway in Egypt in children age 6 to 18 months.

Polylactide-polyglycolide Microspheres

Edelman et al. (162) incorporated purified CFA/I fimbriae into biodegradable polymer microspheres composed of poly(D,L-lactide-co-glycolide). Rabbits were immunized orally with these microspheres or with native purified CFA/I. Only rabbits immunized with the CFA/I delivered in microspheres exhibited high titers of serum CFA/I antibody, suggesting that the microspheres protected the fimbriae from the deleterious effects of gastric juice.

Reid et al. (163) incorporated a CFA/II (CS1/CS3) fimbrial vaccine into poly(D,L-lactide-co-glycolide) microspheres. Preliminary clinical trials investigated the utility of this antigen delivery system in humans. A feasibility clinical trial was carried out in volunteers by Tacket et al. (164), who administered CS1/CS3 purified fimbriae vaccine in microspheres directly via intestinal tube. The vaccine was well tolerated by 10 subjects. Gut-derived IgA ASCs that make specific antibody when stimulated by CS1/CS3 antigen were detected in peripheral blood in five volunteers and five developed significant levels of jejunal fluid sIgA antibody to CS1/CS3 fimbrial antigen.

Attenuated *E. coli* As Live Oral Vaccines Against Enterotoxigenic *E. coli*

E. coli E1392-75-2A is a CFA/II-positive mutant that was derived in the Central Public Health Laboratory, Colindale, wherein the genes encoding LT and ST spontaneously deleted from the CFA/II plasmid. Consequently, E1392-75-2A, which expresses CS1 and CS3 fimbrial antigens, is negative when tested with toxin assays and gene probes for LT and ST. Levine et al. (165–167) used strain E1392-75-2A to explore fundamental questions of anti-colonization immunity in the absence of antitoxic immunity. All volunteers who were fed 10^{10}-CFU doses of strain E1392-75-2A developed significant rises in intestinal fluid sIgA antibody to CS1 and CS3 fimbriae. The GMT of antifimbrial CS1 and CS3 sIgA antibody in these volunteers was 10-fold higher than the peak postvaccination GMT of volunteers who received enteral immunization with multiple doses of purified CS1 and CS3 fimbriae.

A group of vaccinees, who were immunized with a single 5- $\times 10^{10}$-CFU dose of E1392-75-2A with buffer, were challenged 1 month later, along with un-immunized control volunteers. The pathogenic ETEC challenge strain used, E24377A, was of a heterologous serotype O139:H28 but expressed CS1 and CS3 and elaborated LT and ST. The vaccinees were significantly protected ($p < .005$; 75% vaccine efficacy) against ETEC diarrhea (165). By means of bacteriologic studies, it was shown that anti-colonization immunity was responsible for the protection. In the challenge study, all participants, both vaccinees and un-immunized controls, excreted the ETEC challenge strain and there was no difference between the groups in the mean number of ETEC per gram of stool. In contrast, a striking difference was found in duodenal cultures that monitored colonization of the proximal small intestine, the critical site of ETEC–host interaction. The challenge strain was recovered from duodenal cultures of 5 of 6 controls (mean 7×10^3 CFU/mL) versus only 1 of 12 vaccinees (10^1 CFU/mL) ($p < .004$). The interpretation by Levine et al. (165) states that anti-CS1 and anti-CS3 fimbrial sIgA antibody in the proximal intestine prevented the challenge of ETEC from colonizing the proximal small intestine. Because the immune response was not bactericidal, the ETEC organisms were carried by peristalsis to the large intestine, where they could colonize without causing diarrheal illness.

Although the E1392-75-2A strain provided invaluable information when used as a prototype live oral vaccine, it caused mild diarrhea in approximately 15% of the recipients who ingested it, an unacceptable rate of adverse reactions. Therefore, research is ongoing to prepare a live oral ETEC vaccine that will be acceptably immunogenic and efficacious without causing mild diarrhea or other adverse reactions. One approach being taken by British investigators is to introduce specific attenuating mutations into E1392-75-2A in an attempt to make it less reactogenic while retaining its immunogenicity. Once an acceptable set of attenuating mutations is identified for E1392-75-2A, these mutations would then be introduced into strains expressing other CFAs.

Attenuated *Shigella* Strains Expressing Enterotoxigenic *E. coli* Antigens

Investigators at the Center for Vaccine Development have shown that attenuated *Shigella* can be used as live vector vaccines to express ETEC fimbrial antigens and LT toxoids and deliver them to the immune system, resulting in antifimbrial and anti-LT sIgA responses (168–170). The utility of attenuated *Shigella* as live vectors to coexpress CFA/I and CS3 fimbriae of ETEC (a combination never found in nature), and to elicit mucosal sIgA antibody responses to those antigens has been clearly demonstrated in a guinea pig model. Similarly, in this model a bivalent *Shigella* live vector CS2 and CS3 vaccine elicited strong anti-CS2 and anti-CS3 mucosal sIgA responses (170). Plasmids have been constructed that carry operons both for fimbrial biogenesis and for either mutant LTh or LT BS expression (169) so that both antifimbrial and antitoxin antibodies can be stimulated. Preclinical studies with these constructs are paving the way for proof-of-principle clinical trials. Pursuing this strategy, a multivalent live oral vaccine against both *Shigella* and ETEC is being developed based on the hypothesis that protection can be achieved if attenuated *Shigella* express ETEC fimbrial colonization factors and an appropriate LTh antigen. In its final form, the multivalent *Shigella*/ETEC vaccine will contain five attenuated *Shigella* serotype strains (*S. dysenteriae* type 1, *S. flexneri* types 2a and 3a, and *S. sonnei*), each expressing two different ETEC CFAs and either mutant LTh or LTB subunit (50,167,194). Notably, expression of the ETEC fimbriae and mutant LT does not diminish the capacity of the vector strain to protect against challenge with *Shigella* in a guinea pig model (169).

VACCINES AGAINST ENTEROPATHOGENIC *E. COLI*

Target Populations

It is during the first 12 months of life, and in the first 6 months, in particular, that EPEC poses a notable disease risk. Although EPEC vaccines are technologically achievable, the epidemiologic need to immunize neonates or very young infants to protect during the period of high risk has generally discouraged vaccine development efforts.

Vaccine Development Strategies

EPEC was the first category of *E. coli* to be incriminated as a cause of diarrhea, beginning in the 1940s (171). Originally, they were defined only by their O:H serotypes, and somewhat later by serotype and lack of LT and ST production and absence of *Shigella*-like invasiveness properties (171).

Studies of molecular pathogenesis have identified several antigens that constitute potential immunogens. It is hypothesized that the stimulation of intestinal immune responses against these antigens could elicit protective immunity against EPEC disease. The antigens of interest include (a) the bundle-forming pili (BFP) encoded by the EPEC adherence factor plasmid (172); (b) intimin, the 94-kd protein encoded by *eaeA,* a chromosomal gene (173); and (c) the product of *espB* (previously referred to as *eaeB*) (174). sIgA intestinal antibody to BFP may interfere with bacterial binding or initial attachment of EPEC, whereas anti-intimin should prevent intimate attachment. sIgA antibodies against the gene product of *espB* may prevent signal transduction that ultimately culminates in secretion. Moreover, these immune responses could work synergistically to enhance the protection that would be achieved by immunity to any single one of the antigens.

VACCINES AGAINST ENTEROHEMORRHAGIC *E. COLI*

Target Populations

The epidemiologic importance in some human populations of HUS, hemorrhagic colitis, and milder forms of diarrheal illness caused by EHEC (defined as a subset of STEC) that carry a specific circa 65-Md virulence plasmid, in addition to harboring *stx* phages that encode Stxs, and that often also have the *LEE* chromosomal locus encoding enterocyte effacement), has led some authorities to propose immunologic means to prevent infection, disease, or complications of disease.

Possible high-risk groups that might serve as targets for EHEC vaccines might include abattoir workers, veterinarians, farm workers, and forest rangers in endemic areas. However, identifying other target populations for the possible broader use of EHEC vaccines is a subject of considerable controversy. Even if one or more EHEC vaccines proved safe and efficacious, there would be important hurdles to their licensure and more importantly, for their recommendations for implementation. For example, in the parts of North America where the incidence of HUS is relatively high (e.g., the Pacific Northwest), the disease burden is distributed throughout childhood and adult ages, even though the highest incidence is in young children. This implies that immunization would have to be universal, to have a strong impact. If the U.S. population were to be immunized against EHEC because of the "danger" posed by consumption of U.S. meat products and other foods, would it then not be necessary and appropriate to recommend that visitors to the United States be immunized? Could the United States continue to export beef to other countries if it deemed it necessary to protect its own population by immunization? What effect would this have on world trade and the U.S. agricultural economy? Clearly, there is enormous complexity to the public health, economic, and public policy issues that would ensue from any attempt to implement widely an anti-EHEC vaccine in human populations.

Vaccine Development Strategies

One point of intervention in the immunoprophylaxis of EHEC disease could be the active immunization of at-risk humans to prevent infection and disease. Immunization with antigens such as intimin (or its carboxyl terminus) that promote colonization would aim at preventing infection, whereas immunization with Stx BS, Stx toxoids, or peptides representing toxin-neutralizing epitopes would prevent the pathologic effects of toxin-mediated, clinically severe forms of disease.

Conjugate Vaccines

Although a precedent has been established to show that parenteral conjugate vaccines consisting of a capsular polysaccharide or O polysaccharide of LPS covalently linked to a carrier protein can successfully prevent other bacterial enteric infections, including typhoid fever and *S. sonnei* shigellosis (31,143), there is not a strong pathogenetic rationale for expecting anti-O antibodies to be protective against O157:H7.

Early O157 conjugates prepared by Konadu et al. (2) used recombinant exotoxin of *P. aeruginosa*. However, a subsequent decision to link the O157 polysaccharide to the BS of Stx-1 and Stx-2 appears wise, because such conjugates can induce neutralizing antitoxin, which by itself may prove protective against complications and severe forms of disease; moreover, antitoxin may be synergistic with any protective effect of O antibody.

Live Vector Vaccines

One of the most popular approaches in modern vaccine development is the use of attenuated strains of bacteria or viruses as carriers or live vectors in which to express foreign protective antigens and deliver them to the immune system. Attenuated *V. cholerae* live vectors have been used with success to express the BS of Stx-1 and have elicited neutralizing antitoxin in rabbits after oral immunization. Butterton et al. (4) have also expressed the *eaeA* gene product in *V. cholerae* from *eaeA* carried on a plasmid or integrated into the *V. cholerae* chromosome. This group has successfully used the hemolysin A export system to achieve extracellular secretion of foreign antigens in *V. cholerae*. Other live vector systems such as attenuated *Salmonella* have been employed by various other investigators to express STEC antigens.

Toxoid Vaccine

A bivalent toxoid vaccine containing Stx-1 and Stx-2 antigens that could stimulate neutralizing antitoxin presumably would not prevent infection with EHEC but would prevent the severe consequences of infection such as HUS and hemorrhagic colitis.

VACCINES AGAINST *CAMPYLOBACTER JEJUNI*

Target Population

Although *C. jejuni* is incriminated as a cause of diarrheal disease in young infants, the disease burden and severity are not considered to be sufficiently compelling to warrant specific control by vaccines. However, among some travelers (e.g., U.S. military troops deployed in some tropical areas such as southeast Asia), *C. jejuni* is deemed to be an important cause of traveler's diarrhea. The impetus behind current *C. jejuni* vaccine development efforts is being driven by the perceived need to prevent disease in such travelers.

Vaccine Development Strategies

In an experimental infection model in adult volunteers, an initial clinical diarrheal infection caused by *C. jejuni* strain 81-176 stimulated significant protection against diarrhea upon homologous rechallenge (175), thereby providing a rationale for vaccine development. Investigators in the U.S. Department of Defense have since developed and tested in phase 1 clinical trials an inactivated whole-cell *C. jejuni* strain 81-176 oral vaccine administered with mutant LT R192G as a mucosal adjuvant (176,177). Subjects ingested two doses of inactivated vaccine containing 10^5, 10^7, 10^9, or 10^{11} killed bacteria alone or coadministered with 25 μg of mutant LT. Anti-*Campylobacter* immune responses were increased in groups that received vaccine with the mucosal adjuvant (178). The two-dose regimen was unable to protect volunteers from a stringent experimental challenge with wild-type *C. jejuni* strain 81-176 (178). The protective capacity of a four-dose immunization schedule is currently under investigation.

The development of some types of *C. jejuni* vaccines is impeded by a fundamental safety question related to a rare neurologic complication of *C. jejuni* infection. *C. jejuni* infection has been associated with the Guillain–Barré syndrome of ascending paralysis, including the Miller Fisher clinical variant characterized by ataxia, areflexia, and ophthalmoplegia. IgG antibodies to GQ_{1b} and GT_{1a} gangliosides are found in more than 90% of patients suffering from this acute demyelinating disease. Certain strains of *C. jejuni* isolated from infected patients with this acute neurologic syndrome exhibit ganglioside-like epitopes in their LPS, which elicit immunopathologic responses based on molecular mimicry with GQ_{1b}/GT_{1a} gangliosides. Considerable evidence implicates these antibodies as being responsible for damage to motor-nerve terminals in susceptible hosts. Because of this association, serious regulatory concerns have been raised over certain *C. jejuni* vaccine candidates (179). If precise putatively protective antigens that do not cross-react with gangliosides could be identified for use as vaccine antigens, this could provide a safer alternative to the whole-cell vaccine approach.

VACCINES AGAINST *HELICOBACTER PYLORI*

Target Populations

In some individuals, infection with *H. pylori* is associated with the development, decades later, of duodenal ulcers and gastric carcinoma. Two broad approaches to the use of *H. pylori* vaccines are being proposed. One is to use vaccines in persons with established *H. pylori* infection to help eradicate chronic infection and thereby preclude the progression to severe consequences such as gastritis, duodenal ulcer, and gastric carcinoma. For this approach, individuals (mainly adults) with established infection detected by some form of screening would be the target.

The second approach is to use the vaccine as a primary prevention of infection for individuals at relatively high risk. In the least developed countries, *H. pylori* infection is virtually universal by age 6 years. In contrast, in industrialized countries, most of the population remains seronegative and infection, when it occurs, tends to transpire later in childhood. The prophylactic use of *H. pylori* vaccines would likely be targeted mainly at young children in newly industrializing or transitional developing countries.

Vaccine Strategies

Multiple *H. pylori* vaccine development efforts are underway with candidate vaccines that include purified antigens (e.g., urease) (180), live vectors expressing *H. pylori* antigens (181), and inactivated whole bacteria or sonicates (182), typically administered with a powerful adjuvant such as LT or mutant LT. Despite the extensive body of preclinical data demonstrating the efficacy of both therapeutic and prophylactic vaccines in animal models, there have been only a few clinical trials with *H. pylori* vaccine candidates. Marchetti et al. (180) administered recombinant urease plus wild-type LT to *H. pylori*-infected adults. Although infection was not cleared, the density of *H. pylori* in gastric biopsies decreased significantly. Kotloff et al. (182) gave multiple oral doses of formalin-inactivated *H. pylori* whole-cell vaccine plus R192G mutant LT to *H. pylori*-infected adults. Although immune responses were observed, their *H. pylori* carriage was not eradicated.

NONTYPHOIDAL *SALMONELLA*

Although nontyphoidal *Salmonella* such as *S. enterica* serovar Enteritidis and Typhimurium are common causes of food-borne gastroenteritis in humans, control of human infections through immunoprophylaxis is not generally considered to be a rational cost-effective strategy. Rather, because these infections derive from infection of food animals and their contaminated products, the primary strategies for control of these infections is through animal husbandry, food hygiene, and health education practices. Where immunoprophylaxis may play an increasingly important role in the future is in the vaccination of animals.

REFERENCES

1. Levine MM. Modern vaccines. Enteric infections. Lancet 1990;335:958–961.
2. Konadu EY, Parke JCJ, Tran HT, et al. Investigational vaccine for *Escherichia coli* O157: phase 1 study of O157 O-specific polysaccharide-*Pseudomonas aeruginosa* recombinant exoprotein A conjugates in adults. *J Infect Dis* 1998;177:383–387.
3. Acheson DWK, Levine MM, Kaper JB, et al. Protective immunity to Shiga-like toxin I following oral immunization with Shiga-like toxin I B-subunit-producing *Vibrio cholerae* CVD 103-HgR. *Infect Immun* 1996;64:355–357.
4. Butterton JR, Ryan ET, Acheson DW, et al. Coexpression of the β subunit of Shiga toxin 1 and EaeA from enterohemorrhagic *Escherichia coli* in *Vibrio cholerae* vaccine strains. *Infect Immun* 1997;65:2127–2135.
5. Levine MM, Taylor DN, Ferreccio C. Typhoid vaccines come of age. Pediatr Infect Dis J 1989;8:374–381.
6. Ivanoff B, Levine MM, Lambert PH. Vaccination against typhoid fever: present status. Bull World Health Organ 1994; 72:957–971.
7. Ferreccio C, Levine MM, Manterola A et al. Benign bacteremia caused by *Salmonella typhi* and paratyphi in children younger than 2 years. J Pediatr 1984;104:899–901.
8. Sinha A, Sazawal S, Kumar R, et al. Typhoid fever in children aged less than 5 years. *Lancet* 1999;354:734–737.
9. Mahle WT, Levine MM. *Salmonella typhi* infection in children younger than five years of age. *Pediatr Infect Dis J* 1993;12: 627–631.
10. Bhutta ZA, Naqvi SH, Razzaq RA, et al. Multidrug-resistant typhoid in children: presentation and clinical features. Rev Infect Dis 1991;13:832–836.
11. Rowe B, Ward LR, Threlfall EJ. Multidrug-resistant *Salmonella typhi*: a worldwide epidemic. Clin Infect Dis 1997;24[Suppl 1]: S106–S109.
12. Levine MM. Typhoid fever vaccines. In: Plotkin SA, Mortimer E Jr, eds. *Vaccines,* second edition. Philadelphia: WB Saunders, 1994:597–633.
13. Levine MM. Typhoid fever vaccines. In: Plotkin SA, Orenstein WA, eds. *Vaccines,* third edition. Philadelphia: WB Saunders, 1999:781–814.
14. Wahdan MH, Serie C, Cerisier Y, et al. A controlled field trial of live *Salmonella typhi* strain Ty21a oral vaccine against typhoid: three year results. *J Infect Dis* 1982;145:292–296.
15. Levine MM, Ferreccio C, Black RE, et al, and the Chilean Typhoid Committee. Large-scale field trial of Ty21a live oral typhoid vaccine in enteric-coated capsule formulation. *Lancet* 1987;1:1049–1052.
16. Levine MM, Ferreccio C, Cryz S, et al. Comparison of enteric-coated capsules and liquid formulation of Ty21a typhoid vaccine in randomised controlled field trial. *Lancet* 1990;336:891–894.
17. Acharya VI, Lowe CU, Thapa R, et al. Prevention of typhoid fever in Nepal with the Vi capsular polysaccharide of *Salmonella*

typhi. A preliminary report. *N Engl J Med* 1987;317:1101–1104.
18. Klugman K, Gilbertson IT, Kornhoff HJ, et al. Protective activity of Vi polysaccharide vaccine against typhoid fever. *Lancet* 1987;2:1165–1169.
19. Simanjuntak C, Paleologo F, Punjabi N, et al. Oral immunisation against typhoid fever in Indonesia with Ty21a vaccine. *Lancet* 1991;338:1055–1059.
20. Levine MM, Ferreccio C, Abrego P, et al. Duration of efficacy of Ty21a, attenuated salmonella typhi live oral vaccine. *Vaccine* 1999;17[Suppl 2]:S22–S27.
21. Klugman KP, Koornhof HJ, Robbins JB, et al. Immunogenicity, efficacy and serological correlate of protection of *Salmonella typhi* Vi capsular polysaccharide vaccine three years after immunization. *Vaccine* 1996;14:435–438.
22. Ferreccio C, Levine MM, Rodriguez H, et al. Comparative efficacy of two, three, or four doses of Ty21a live oral typhoid vaccine in enteric-coated capsules: a field trial in an endemic area. *J Infect Dis* 1989;159:766–769.
23. Forrest BD, LaBrooy JT, Dearlove CE, et al. The human humoral immune response to *Salmonella typhi* Ty21a. *J Infect Dis* 1991;163:336–345.
24. Kantele A. Antibody-secreting cells in the evaluation of the immunogenicity of an oral vaccine. *Vaccine* 1990;8:321–326.
25. Sztein MB, Wasserman SS, Tacket CO, et al. Cytokine production patterns and lymphoproliferative responses in volunteers orally immunized with attenuated vaccine strains of *Salmonella typhi. J Infect Dis* 1994;170:1508–1517.
26. Sztein MB, Tanner MK, Polotsky Y, et al. Cytotoxic T lymphocytes after oral immunization with attenuated vaccine strains of *Salmonella typhi* in humans. *J Immunol* 1995;155:3987–3993.
27. Szu SC, Stone AL, Robbins JD, et al. Vi capsular polysaccharide-protein conjugates for prevention of typhoid fever. Preparation, characterization, and immunogenicity in laboratory animals. *J Exp Med* 1987;166:1510–1524.
28. Szu SC, Li XR, Stone AL, et al. Relation between structure and immunologic properties of the Vi capsular polysaccharide. *Infect Immun* 1991;59:4555–4561.
29. Szu SC, Taylor DN, Trofa AC, et al. Laboratory and preliminary clinical characterization of Vi capsular polysaccharide-protein conjugate vaccines. *Infect Immun* 1994;62:4440–4444.
30. Kossaczka Z, Lin FY, Ho VA, et al. Safety and immunogenicity of Vi conjugate vaccines for typhoid fever in adults, teenagers, and 2- to 4-year-old children in Vietnam. *Infect Immun* 1999;67:5806–5810.
31. Lin FYC, Ho VA, Khiem HB, et al. The efficacy of a *Salmonella typhi* Vi conjugate vaccine in two-to-five-year-old children. *N Engl J Med* 2001;344:1263–1268.
32. Levine MM, Ferreccio C, Black RE, et al. Progress in vaccines against typhoid fever. *Rev Infect Dis* 1989;2[Suppl 3]:S552–S567.
33. Hone DM, Harris AM, Chatfield S, et al. Construction of genetically-defined double *aro* mutants of *Salmonella typhi. Vaccine* 1991;9:810–816.
34. Tacket CO, Hone DM, Curtiss RI, et al. Comparison of the safety and immunogenicity of *aroC, aroD* and *cya,crp Salmonella typhi* strains in adult volunteers. *Infect Immun* 1992;60:536–541.
35. Tacket CO, Hone DM, Losonsky GA, et al. Clinical acceptability and immunogenicity of CVD 908 *Salmonella typhi* vaccine strain. *Vaccine* 1992;10:443–446.
36. Balfour HH, Groth KE, Edelman CK, et al. Rubella viremia and antibody responses after rubella vaccination and reimmunization. *Lancet* 1981;1:1078–1080.
37. Horstmann DM, Opton EM, Klemperer R, et al. Viremia in infants vaccinated with oral poliovirus vaccine (Sabin). *Am J Hyg* 1964;79:47–63.
38. Chatfield SN, Strahan K, Pickard D, et al. Evaluation of *Salmonella typhimurium* strains harbouring defined mutations in *htrA* and *aroA* in the murine salmonellosis model. *Microb Pathog* 1992;12:145–151.
39. Levine MM, Galen J, Barry E, et al. Attenuated *Salmonella* as live oral vaccines against typhoid fever and as live vectors. *J Biotechnol* 1995;44:193–196.
40. Levine MM, Galen J, Barry E, et al. Attenuated *Salmonella typhi* and *Shigella* as live oral vaccines and as live vectors. *Behring Inst Mitt* 1997;120–123.
41. Tacket CO, Sztein MB, Losonsky GA, et al. Safety of live oral *Salmonella typhi* vaccine strains with deletions in *htrA* and *aroC aroD* and immune response in humans. *Infect Immun* 1997;65:452–456.
42. Tacket CO, Sztein MB, Wasserman SS, et al. Phase 2 clinical trial of attenuated *Salmonella enterica* serovar Typhi oral live vector vaccine CVD 908-*htrA* in U.S. volunteers. *Infect Immun* 2000;68:1196–1201.
43. Miller SI, Pulkkinen WS, Selsted ME, et al. Characterization of defensin resistance phenotypes associated with mutations in the phoP-virulence regulon of *Salmonella typhimurium. Infect Immun* 1990;58:3706–3710.
44. Miller SI, Kukral AM, Mekalanos JJ. A two-component regulatory system (phoP phoQ) controls *Salmonella typhimurium* virulence. *Proc Natl Acad Sci U S A* 1989;86:5054–5058.
45. Hohmann EL, Oletta CA, Killeen KP, et al. *phoP/phoQ*-deleted *Salmonella typhi* (Ty800) is a safe and immunogenic single-dose typhoid fever vaccine in volunteers. *J Infect Dis* 1996;173:1408–1414.
46. Curtiss R III, Kelly SM, Tinge SA, et al. Recombinant *Salmonella* vectors in vaccine development. *Develop Biol Standard* 1994;82:23–33.
47. Tacket CO, Kelly SM, Schodel F, et al. Safety and immunogenicity in humans of an attenuated *Salmonella typhi* vaccine vector strain expressing plasmid-encoded hepatitis B antigens stabilized by the ASD balanced lethal system. *Infect Immun* 1997;65:3381–3385.
48. Lanata CF, Levine MM, Ristori C, et al. Vi serology in detection of chronic *Salmonella typhi* carriers in an endemic area. *Lancet* 1983;2:441–443.
49. Losonsky GA, Ferreccio C, Kotloff KL, et al. Development and evaluation of an enzyme-linked immunosorbent assay for serum Vi antibodies for detection of chronic *Salmonella typhi* carriers. *J Clin Microbiol* 1987;25:2266–2269.
50. Levine MM, Black RE, Lanata C, and the Chilean Typhoid Committee. Precise estimation of the numbers of chronic carriers of *Salmonella typhi* in Santiago, Chile, an endemic area. *J Infect Dis* 1982;146:724–726.
51. Pickard D, Li J, Roberts M, et al. Characterization of defined *ompR* mutants of *Salmonella typhi: ompR* is involved in the regulation of Vi polysaccharide expression. *Infect Immun* 1994;62:3984–3993.
52. Arricau N, Hermant D, Waxin H, et al. The RcsB-RcsC regulatory system of *Salmonella typhi* differentially modulates the expression of invasion proteins, flagellin and Vi antigen in response to osmolarity. *Mol Microbiol* 1998;29:835–850.
53. Felix A, Pitt R. Virulence of *B. typhosus* and resistance to O antibody. *J Pathol Bacteriol* 1934;38:409–420.
54. Felix A, Pitt R. The pathogenic and immunogenic activities of *Salmonella typhi* in relation to its antigenic constituents. *J Hyg (Cambridge)* 1951;49:92–109.
55. Felix A, Bhatnagar SS. Further observations on the properties of the Vi antigen of *B. typhosus* and its corresponding antibody. *Br J Exp Pathol* 1935;16:422–434.
56. Robbins J, Robbins J. Reexamination of the protective role of the capsular polysaccharide Vi antigen of *Salmonella typhi. J Infect Dis* 1984;150:436–449.

57. Virlogeux I, Waxin H, Ecobichon C, et al. Role of the *viaB* locus in synthesis, transport and expression of *Salmonella typhi* Vi antigen. *Microbiology* 1995;141:3039–3047.
58. Virlogeux I, Waxin H, Ecobichon C, et al. Characterization of the *rcsA* and *rcsB* genes from *Salmonella typhi: rcsB* through *tviA* is involved in regulation of Vi antigen synthesis. *J Bacteriol* 1996;178:1691–1698.
59. Wang JY, Noriega FR, Galen JE, et al. Constitutive expression of the Vi polysaccharide capsular antigen in attenuated *Salmonella enterica* serovar Typhi oral vaccine strain CVD 909. *Infect Immun* 2000.
60. Kaper JB, Morris JG Jr, Levine MM. Cholera. *Clin Microbiol Rev* 1995;8:48–86.
61. Mintz ED, Tauxe RV, Levine MM. The global resurgence of cholera. In: Noah N, Mahoney M, eds. *Communicable disease: epidemiology and control.* Chichester: John Wiley and Sons, 1998;63–104.
62. Goma Epidemiology Group. Public health impact of Rwandan refugee crisis: what happened in Goma, Zaire, in July, 1994? *Lancet* 1995;345:339–344.
63. Nair GB, Shimada T, Kurazono H, et al. Characterization of phenotypic, serological, and toxigenic traits of *Vibrio cholerae* O139 Bengal. *J Clin Microbiol* 1994;32:2775–2779.
64. Cholera Working Group IcfDDRB. Large epidemic of cholera-like disease in Bangladesh caused by *Vibrio cholerae* O139 synonym Bengal. *Lancet* 1993;342:387–390.
65. Holmgren J, Svennerholm A-M, Jertborn M, et al. An oral β subunit: whole cell vaccine against cholera. *Vaccine* 1992;10: 911–914.
66. Levine MM, Kaper JB. Live oral cholera vaccine: from principle to product. *Bull Inst Pasteur* 1995;93:243–253.
67. Clemens JD, Sack DA, Harris JR, et al. Field trial of cholera vaccines in Bangladesh: results from three year follow-up. *Lancet* 1990;335:270–273.
68. Sanchez J, Holmgren J. Recombinant system for overexpression of cholera toxin β subunit in *Vibrio cholerae* as a basis for vaccine development. *Proc Natl Acad Sci U S A* 1989;86:481–485.
69. Sanchez JL, Vasquez B, Begue RE, et al. Protective efficacy of oral whole-cell/recombinant-β-subunit cholera vaccine in Peruvian military recruits. *Lancet* 1994;344:1273–1276.
70. Taylor DN, Cardenas V, Sanchez JL, et al. Two year study of the protective efficacy of the oral whole cell plus recombinant β subunit (WC/rBS) cholera vaccine in Peru. *J Infect Dis* 2000; 181:1667–1673.
71. Levine MM. Immunization against bacterial diseases of the intestine. *J Pediatr Gastroenterol Nutr* 2000;31:336–355.
72. Jertborn M, Svennerholm AM, Holmgren J. Intestinal and systemic immune responses in humans after oral immunization with a bivalent β subunit-O1/O139 whole cell cholera vaccine. *Vaccine* 1996;14:1459–1465.
73. Ketley JM, Michalski J, Galen J, et al. Construction of genetically marked *Vibrio cholerae* O1 vaccine strains. *FEMS Microbiol Lett* 1993;111:15–21.
74. Levine MM, Kaper JB, Herrington D, et al. Safety, immunogenicity, and efficacy of recombinant live oral cholera vaccines, CVD 103 and CVD 103-HgR. *Lancet* 1988;2:467–470.
75. Kotloff KL, Wasserman SS, O'Donnell S, et al. Safety and immunogenicity in North Americans of a single dose of live oral cholera vaccine CVD 103-HgR: results of a randomized, placebo-controlled, double-blind crossover trial. *Infect Immun* 1992;60:4430–4432.
76. Cryz SJ, Levine MM, Kaper JB, et al. Randomized double-blind placebo controlled trial to evaluate the safety and immunogenicity of the live oral cholera vaccine strain CVD 103-HgR in Swiss adults. *Vaccine* 1990;8:577–580.
77. Suharyono, Simanjuntak C, Witham N, et al. Safety and immunogenicity of single-dose live oral cholera vaccine CVD 103-HgR in 5-9-year-old Indonesian children. *Lancet* 1992; 340:689–694.
78. Simanjuntak CH, O'Hanley P, Punjabi NH, et al. The safety, immunogenicity, and transmissibility of single-dose live oral cholera vaccine CVD 103-HgR in 24 to 59 month old Indonesian children. *J Infect Dis* 1993;168:1169–1176.
79. Migasena S, Pitisuttitham P, Prayurahong P, et al. Preliminary assessment of the safety and immunogenicity of live oral cholera vaccine strain CVD 103-HgR in healthy Thai adults. *Infect Immun* 1989;57:3261–3264.
80. Lagos R, Avendano A, Horwitz I, et al. Tolerancia e inmunogenicidad de una dosis oral de la cepa de *Vibrio cholerae* O1, viva-atenuada, CVD 103-HgR: estudio de doble ciego en adultos Chilenos. *Rev Med Chile* 1993;121:857–863.
81. Lagos R, Avendano A, Prado V, et al. Attenuated live oral cholera vaccine strain CVD 103-HgR elicits significantly higher serum vibriocidal antibody titers in persons of blood group O. *Infect Immun* 1995;63:707–709.
82. Lagos R, Losonsky G, Abrego P, et al. Tolerancia, immunogenicidad, excresión y transmisión de la vacuna anti-colera oral viva-atenuada, CVD 103-HgR, estudio pareado de doble ciego en niños Chilenos de 24 a 59 meses. *Bol Hosp Infant Mex* 1996; 53:214–220.
83. Lagos R, San Martin O, Wasserman SS, et al. Palatability, reactogenicity and immunogenicity of engineered live oral cholera vaccine CVD 103-HgR in Chilean infants and toddlers. *Pediatr Infect Dis J* 1999;18:624–630.
84. Gotuzzo E, Butron B, Seas C, et al. Safety, immunogenicity, and excretion pattern of single-dose live oral cholera vaccine CVD 103-HgR in Peruvian adults of high and low socioeconomic levels. *Infect Immun* 1993;61:3994–3997.
85. Perry RT, Plowe CV, Koumaré B, et al. A single dose of live oral cholera vaccine CVD 103-HgR is safe and immunogenic in HIV-infected and non-infected adults in Mali. *Bull World Health Organ* 1998;76:63–71.
86. Tacket CO, Losonsky G, Nataro JP, et al. Onset and duration of protective immunity in challenged volunteers after vaccination with live oral cholera vaccine CVD 103-HgR. *J Infect Dis* 1992;166:837–841.
87. Levine MM, Tacket CO. Live oral vaccines against cholera. In: Ala'Aldeen DAA, Hormaeche CE, eds. *Molecular and clinical aspects of bacterial vaccine development.* Chichester: John Wiley and Sons, 1995;233–258.
88. Tacket CO, Cohen MB, Wasserman SS, et al. Randomized, double-blind, placebo-controlled, multicentered trial of the efficacy of a single dose of live oral cholera vaccine CVD 103-HgR in preventing cholera following challenge with vibrio cholerae O1 El Tor Inaba three months after vaccination. *Infect Immun* 1999;67:6341–6345.
89. Richie E, Punjabi NH, Sidharta Y, et al. Efficacy trial of single-dose live oral cholera vaccine CVD 103-HgR in North Jakarta, Indonesia, a cholera-endemic area. *Vaccine* 2000;18: 2399–2410.
90. Glass RI, Holmgren J, Haley CE, et al. Predisposition for cholera of individuals with O blood group. Possible evolutionary significance. *Am J Epidemiol* 1985;121:791–796.
91. Tacket CO, Losonsky G, Nataro JP, et al. Extension of the volunteer challenge model to study South American cholera in a population of volunteers predominantly with blood group antigen O. *Trans Royal Soc Trop Med Hyg* 1995;89:75–77.
92. Su-Arehawaratana P, Singharaj P, Taylor DN, et al. Safety and immunogenicity of different immunization regimens of CVD 103-HgR live oral cholera vaccine in soldiers and civilians in Thailand. *J Infect Dis* 1992;165:1042–1048.
93. Patriarca PA, Wright PF, John TJ. Factors affecting the

immunogenicity of oral poliovirus vaccine in developing countries: review. *Rev Infect Dis* 1991;13:926–929.
94. Hanlon P, Hanlon L, Marsh V, et al. Trial of an attenuated bovine rotavirus vaccine (RIT 4237) in Gambian infants. *Lancet* 1987;1:1342–1345.
95. Fagundes-Neto U, Viaro T, Wehba J, et al. Tropical enteropathy (environmental enteropathy) in early childhood: a syndrome caused by contaminated environment. *J Trop Pediatr* 1984;30: 204–209.
96. Fagundes Neto U, Martins MC, Lima FL, et al. Asymptomatic environmental enteropathy among slum-dwelling infants. *J Am Coll Nutr* 1994;13:51–56.
97. Khin-Maung-U, Bolin TD, Duncombe VM, et al. Epidemiology of small bowel bacterial overgrowth and rice carbohydrate malabsorption in Burmese (Myanmar) village children. *Am J Trop Med Hyg* 1992;47:298–304.
98. Lagos R, Fasano A, Wasserman SS, et al. Effect of small bowel bacterial overgrowth on the immunogenicity of single-dose live oral cholera vaccine CVD 103-HgR. *J Infect Dis* 1999;180: 1709–1712.
99. Shedlofsky S, Freter R. Synergism between ecologic and immunologic control mechanisms of intestinal flora. *J Infect Dis* 1974;129:296–303.
100. Cooper PJ, Chico ME, Losonsky G, et al. Albendazole treatment of children with ascariasis enhances the vibriocidal antibody response to the live attenuated oral cholera vaccine CVD 103-HgR. *J Infect Dis* 2000;182:1199–1206.
101. Sabin AB. Oral poliovirus vaccine. History of its development and prospects for eradication of poliomyelitis. *JAMA* 1965;194: 130–134.
102. Kapikian AZ, Hoshino Y, Chanock RM, et al. Efficacy of a quadrivalent rhesus rotavirus-based human rotavirus vaccine aimed at preventing severe rotavirus diarrhea in infants and young children. *J Infect Dis* 1996;174[Suppl 1]:S65–S72.
103. Olanratmanee T, Levine MM, Losonsky G, et al. Safety and immunogenicity of *Salmonella typhi* Ty21a liquid formulation vaccine in 4- to 6-year old Thai children. *J Infect Dis* 1992; 166:451–452.
104. Tacket CO, Kotloff KL, Losonsky G, et al. Volunteer studies investigating the safety and efficacy of live oral El Tor *Vibrio cholerae* O1 vaccine strain CVD 111. *Am J Trop Med Hyg* 1997; 56:533–537.
105. Taylor DN, Sanchez JL, Castro JM, et al. Expanded safety and immunogenicity of a bivalent, oral, attenuated cholera vaccine, CVD 103-HgR plus CVD 111, in United States military personnel stationed in Panama. *Infect Immun* 1999;67:2030–2034.
106. Taylor DN, Tacket CO, Losonsky G, et al. Evaluation of a bivalent (CVD 103-HgR/CVD 111) live oral cholera vaccine in adult volunteers from the United States and Peru. *Infect Immun* 1997;65:3852–3856.
107. Cryz SJ Jr, Que JU, Levine MM, et al. Safety and immunogenicity of a live oral bivalent typhoid fever (*Salmonella typhi* Ty21a)-cholera (*Vibrio cholerae* CVD 103-HgR) vaccine in healthy adults. *Infect Immun* 1995;63:1336–1339.
108. Kollaritsch H, Furer E, Herzog C, et al. Randomized, double-blind placebo-controlled trial to evaluate the safety and immunogenicity of combined *Salmonella typhi* Ty21a and *Vibrio cholerae* CVD 103-HgR live oral vaccines. *Infect Immun* 1996;64:1454–1457.
109. Kenner JR, Coster TS, Taylor DN, et al. Peru-15, an improved live attenuated oral vaccine candidate for *Vibrio cholerae* O1. *J Infect Dis* 1995;172:1126–1129.
110. Sack DA, Sack RB, Shimko J, et al. Evaluation of Peru-15, a new live oral vaccine for cholera, in volunteers. *J Infect Dis* 1997;176:201–205.
111. Sack DA, Shimko J, Sack RB et al. Comparison of alternative buffers for use with a new live oral cholera vaccine, Peru-15, in outpatient volunteers. Infect Immun 1997;65:2107–2111.
112. Cohen MB, Bean J, Gianella RA, et al. Randomized, double-blind, placebo-controlled trial of a single-dose of live oral cholera vaccine Peru-15 in preventing cholera following challenge with *Vibrio cholerae* O1 El Tor Inaba approximately three months after vaccination. 2002 *J Infect Dis* (in press).
113. Valle E, Ledon T, Cedre B, et al. Construction and characterization of a nonproliferative El Tor cholera vaccine candidate derived from strain 638. *Infect Immun* 2000;68:6411–6418.
114. Benitez JA, Garcia L, Silva A, et al. Preliminary assessment of the safety and immunogenicity of a new CTXPhi-negative, hemagglutinin/protease-defective El Tor strain as a cholera vaccine candidate. *Infect Immun* 1999;67:539–545.
115. Tacket CO, Losonsky G, Nataro JP, et al. Initial clinical studies of CVD 112 *Vibrio cholerae* O139 live oral vaccine: safety and efficacy against experimental challenge. *J Infect Dis* 1995;172: 883–886.
116. Waldor MK, Mekalanos JJ. Emergence of a new cholera pandemic: molecular analysis of virulence determinants in *Vibrio cholerae* O139 and development of a live vaccine prototype. *J Infect Dis* 1994;170:278–283.
117. Coster TS, Killeen KP, Waldor MK, et al. Safety, immunogenicity, and efficacy of live attenuated *Vibrio cholerae* O139 vaccine prototype. *Lancet* 1995;345:949–952.
118. Kossaczka Z, Shiloach J, Johnson V, et al. *Vibrio cholerae* O139 conjugate vaccines: synthesis and immunogenicity of *V. cholerae* O139 capsular polysaccharide conjugates with recombinant diphtheria toxin mutant in mice. *Infect Immun* 2000;68: 5037–5043.
119. Boutonnier A, Villeneuve S, Nato F, et al. Preparation, immunogenicity, and protective efficacy, in a murine model, of a conjugate vaccine composed of the polysaccharide moiety of the lipopolysaccharide of *Vibrio cholerae* O139 bound to tetanus toxoid. *Infect Immun* 2001;69:3488–3493.
120. Gupta RK, Taylor DN, Bryla DA, et al. Phase 1 evaluation of *Vibrio cholerae* O1, serotype Inaba, polysaccharide-cholera toxin conjugates in adult volunteers. *Infect Immun* 1998;66: 3095–3099.
121. Kotloff KL, Winickoff JP, Ivanoff B, et al. Global burden of *Shigella* infections: implications for vaccine development and implementation of control strategies. *Bull World Health Organ* 1999;77:651–666.
122. DuPont HL, Levine MM, Hornick RB, et al. Inoculum size in shigellosis and implications for expected mode of transmission. *J Infect Dis* 1989;159:1126–1128.
123. Hyams KC, Bourgeois AL, Merrell BR, et al. Diarrheal disease during Operation Desert Shield. *N Engl J Med* 1991;325: 1423–1428.
124. Sharp TW, Thornton SA, Wallace MR, et al. Diarrheal disease among military personnel during Operation Restore Hope, Somalia, 1992–1993. *Am J Trop Med Hyg* 1995;52:188–193.
125. Ries AA, Wells JG, Olivola D, et al. Epidemic *Shigella dysenteriae* type 1 in Burundi: panresistance and implications for prevention. *J Infect Dis* 1994;169:1035–1041.
126. Noriega FR, Liao FM, Maneval DR, et al. Strategy for cross-protection among *Shigella flexneri* serotypes. *Infect Immun* 1999;67:782–788.
127. Kotloff KL, Winickoff JP, Ivanoff B, et al. Global burden of *Shigella* infections: implications for vaccine development and implementation of control strategies. *Bull World Health Organ* 1999;77:651–666.
128. Nassif X, Mazert MC, Mounier J, et al. Evaluation with an iuc::Tn10 mutant of the role of aerobactin production in the virulence of *Shigella flexneri*. *Infect Immun* 1987;55:1963–1969.
129. Barzu S, Arondel J, Guillot S, et al. Immunogenicity of IpaC-

hybrid proteins expressed in the *Shigella flexneri* 2a vaccine candidate SC602. *Infect Immun* 1998;66:77–82.
130. Coster TS, Hoge CW, VanDeVerg LL, et al. Vaccination against shigellosis with attenuated *Shigella flexneri* 2a strain SC602. *Infect Immun* 1999;67:3437–3443.
131. Kotloff K, Taylor D, Losonsky G, et al. Phase 1 evaluation of a *vriG* deleted *Shigella sonnei* live, attenuated vaccine (strain WRSS1) in healthy adult volunteers. 2002 *Infect Immun* (in press).
132. Karnell A, Li A, Zhao CR, et al. Safety and immunogenicity study of the auxotrophic *Shigella flexneri* 2a vaccine SFL1070 with a deleted *aroD* gene in adult Swedish volunteers. *Vaccine* 1995;13:88–89.
133. Noriega FR, Wang JY, Losonsky G, et al. Construction and characterization of attenuated Δ*aroA* Δ*virG Shigella flexneri* 2a strain CVD 1203, a prototype live oral vaccine. *Infect Immun* 1995;65:5168–5172.
134. Kotloff KL, Noriega F, Losonsky GA, et al. Safety, immunogenicity, and transmissibility in humans of CVD 1203, a live oral *Shigella flexneri* 2a vaccine candidate attenuated by deletions in *aroA* and *virG. Infect Immun* 1996;64:4542–4548.
135. Noriega FR, Losonsky G, Lauderbaugh C, et al. Engineered Δ*guaB-A,* Δ*virG Shigella flexneri* 2a strain CVD 1205: construction, safety, immunogenicity and potential efficacy as a mucosal vaccine. *Infect Immun* 1996;64:3055–3061.
136. Kotloff KL, Noriega FR, Samandari T, et al. *Shigella flexneri* 2a strain CVD 1207, with specific deletions in *virG, sen, set,* and *guaBA,* is highly attenuated in humans. *Infect Immun* 2000; 68:1034–1039.
137. Orr N, Arnon R, Rubin G, et al. Enhancement of anti-*Shigella* lipopolysaccharide (LPS) response by addition of the cholera toxin β subunit to oral and intranasal proteosome-*Shigella flexneri* 2a LPS vaccines. *Infect Immun* 1994;62:5198–5200.
138. Mallett CP, Hale TL, Kaminski RW, et al. Intranasal or intragastric immunization with proteosome-*Shigella* lipopolysaccharide vaccines protects against lethal pneumonia in a murine model of *Shigella* infection. *Infect Immun* 1995;63:2382–2386.
139. Fries LF, Montemarano AD, Mallett CP, et al. Safety and Immunogenicity of a proteosome-*Shigella flexneri* 2a lipopolysaccharide vaccine administered intranasally to healthy adults. *Infect Immun* 2001;69:4545–4553.
140. Polotsky YE, Robbins JB, Bryla D, et al. Comparison of conjugates composed of lipopolysaccharide from *Shigella flexneri* type 2a detoxified by two methods and bound to tetanus toxoid. *Infect Immun* 1994;62:210–214.
141. Robbins JB, Schneerson R. Polysaccharide-protein conjugates: a new generation of vaccines. *J Infect Dis* 1990;161:821–832.
142. Robbins JB, Chu C, Schneerson R. Hypothesis for the vaccine development: protective immunity to enteric diseases caused by non-typhoidal salmonellae and shigellae may be conferred by serum IgG antibodies to the O-specific polysaccharides of their lipopolysaccharides. *Clin Infect Dis* 1992;15:346–351.
143. Cohen D, Ashkenazi S, Green MS, et al. Double-blind vaccine-controlled randomised efficacy trial of an investigational *Shigella sonnei* conjugate vaccine in young adults. *Lancet* 1997; 349:155–159.
144. Cohen D, Ashkenazi S, Green M, et al. Safety and immunogenicity of investigational Shigella conjugate vaccines in Israeli volunteers. *Infect Immun* 1996;64:4074–4077.
145. Ashkenazi S, Passwell JH, Harlev E, et al. Safety and immunogenicity of *Shigella sonnei* and *Shigella flexneri* 2a O-specific polysaccharide conjugates in children. *J Infect Dis* 1999;179: 1565–1568.
146. Black RE, Brown KH, Becker S, et al. Longitudinal studies of infectious diseases and physical growth in rural Bangladesh, II: incidence of diarrhea and association with known pathogens. *Am J Epidemiol* 1982;115:315–324.
147. Levine MM, Ferreccio C, Prado V, et al. Epidemiologic studies of *Escherichia coli* infections in a low socioeconomic level periurban community in Santiago, Chile. *Am J Epidemiol* 1993; 138:849–869.
148. Levine MM, Giron JA, Noriega F. Fimbrial vaccines. In: Klemm P, ed. *Fimbriae: adhesion, biogenics, genetics and vaccines.* Boca Raton: CRC Press, 1994.
149. Levine MM, Nalin DR, Hoover DL, et al. Immunity to enterotoxigenic *Escherichia coli. Infect Immun* 1979;23:729–736.
150. Black RE, Merson MH, Rowe B, et al. Enterotoxigenic *Escherichia coli* diarrhoea: acquired immunity and transmission in an endemic area. *Bull World Health Organ* 1981;59:263–268.
151. DuPont HL, Olarte J, Evans DG, et al. Comparative susceptibility of Latin American and United States students to enteric pathogens. *N Engl J Med* 1976;285:1520–1521.
152. Cravioto A, Reyes RE, Ortega R, et al. Prospective study of diarrhoeal disease in a cohort of rural Mexican children: incidence and isolated pathogens during the first two years of life. *Epidemiol Infect* 1988;101:123–134.
153. Tacket CO, Losonsky G, Link H, et al. Protection by milk immunoglobulin concentrate against oral challenge with enterotoxigenic *Escherichia coli. N Engl J Med* 1988;318: 1240–1243.
154. Evans DG, Evans DJ Jr, Opekun A, et al. Non-replicating whole cell vaccine protective against enterotoxigenic *Escherichia coli* (ETEC) diarrhea: stimulation of anti-CFA (CFA/I) and anti-enterotoxin (anti-LT) intestinal IgA and protection against challenge with ETEC belonging to heterologous serotypes. *FEMS Microbiol Lett* 1988;47:117–125.
155. Clemens JD, Sack DA, Harris JR, et al. Cross-protection by β subunit-whole cell cholera vaccine against diarrhea associated with heat-labile toxin-producing enterotoxigenic *Escherichia coli:* results of a large-scale field trial. *J Infect Dis* 1988;158: 372–377.
156. Peltola H, Siitonen A, Kyrönseppä H, et al. Prevention of travellers' diarrhoea by oral β-subunit/whole-cell cholera vaccine. *Lancet* 1991;338:1285–1289.
157. Svennerholm A-M, Ahren C, Jertborn M. Oral inactivated vaccine against enterotoxigenic *Escherichia coli.* In: Levine MM, Woodrow GC, Kaper JB, et al, eds. *New generation vaccines,* second edition. New York: Marcel Dekker Inc, 1997:865–874.
158. Ahren C, Jertborn M, Svennerholm AM. Intestinal immune responses to an inactivated oral enterotoxigenic *Escherichia coli* vaccine and associated immunoglobulin A responses in blood. *Infect Immun* 1998;66:3311–3316.
159. Savarino SJ, Brown FM, Hall E, et al. Safety and immunogenicity of an oral, killed enterotoxigenic *Escherichia coli*-cholera toxin β subunit vaccine in Egyptian adults. *J Infect Dis* 1998;177:796–799.
160. Hall ER, Wierzba TF, Ahren C, et al. Induction of systemic antifimbria and antitoxin antibody responses in Egyptian children and adults by an oral, killed enterotoxigenic *Escherichia coli* plus cholera toxin B subunit vaccine. *Infect Immun* 2001; 69:2853–2857.
161. Savarino SJ, Hall ER, Bassily S, et al. Oral, inactivated, whole cell enterotoxigenic *Escherichia coli* plus cholera toxin β subunit vaccine: results of the initial evaluation in children. PRIDE Study Group. *J Infect Dis* 1999;179:107–114.
162. Edelman R, Russel RG, Losonsky GA, et al. Immunization of rabbits with enterotoxigenic *E. coli* colonization factor antigen (CFA/I) encapsulated in biodegradable microspheres of poly (lactide-co-glycolide). *Vaccine* 1993;11:155–158.
163. Reid RH, Boedeker EC, McQueen CE, et al. Preclinical evalu-

ation of microencapsulated CFA/II oral vaccine against enterotoxigenic *E. coli. Vaccine* 1993;11:159–167.

164. Tacket CO, Reid RH, Boedeker EC, et al. Enteral immunization and challenge of volunteers given enterotoxigenic *E. coli* CFA/II encapsulated in biodegradable microspheres. *Vaccine* 1994;12:1270–1274.
165. Levine MM. *Escherichia coli* that cause diarrhea: enterotoxigenic, enteropathogenic, enteroinvasive, enterohemorrhagic, and enteroadherent. *J Infect Dis* 1987;155:377–389.
166. Levine MM, Black RE, Clements ML, et al. Prevention of enterotoxigenic *Escherichia coli* diarrheal infection by vaccines that stimulate antiadhesion (antipili) immunity. In: Boedeker EC, ed. *Attachment of organisms to the gut mucosa.* Boca Raton: CRC Press, 1984:223–244.
167. Levine MM. Travellers' diarrhoea: prospects for successful immunoprophylaxis. *Scand J Gastroenterol* 1983;84[Suppl]: 121–134.
168. Noriega FR, Losonsky G, Wang JY, et al. Further characterization of Δ*aroA,* ΔvirG Shigella flexneri 2a strain CVD 1203 as a mucosal *Shigella* vaccine and as a live vector vaccine for delivering antigens of enterotoxigenic *Escherichia coli. Infect Immun* 1996;64:23–27.
169. Koprowski H, Levine MM, Anderson RJ, Losonsky G, Pizza M, Barry EM. Attenuated *Shigella flexneri* 2a vaccine strain CVD 1204 expressing colonization factor antigen I and mutant heat-labile enterotoxin of enterotoxigenic *Escherichia coli. Infect Immun* 2000;68:4884–4892.
170. Altboum Z, Barry EM, Losonsky G, et al. Attenuated *Shigella flexneri* 2a delta *guaBA* strain CVD 1204 expressing enterotoxigenic *Escherichia coli* (ETEC) CS2 and CS3 fimbriae as a live mucosal vaccine against *Shigella* and ETEC infection. *Infect Immun* 2001;69:3150–3158.
171. Levine MM, Edelman R. Enteropathogenic *Escherichia coli* of classic serotypes associated with infant diarrhea: epidemiology and pathogenesis. *Epidemiol Rev* 1984;6:31–51.
172. Giron JA, Ho ASY, Schoolnik GK. An inducible bundle-forming pilus of enteropathogenic *Escherichia coli. Science* 1991; 254:710–713.
173. Jerse AE, Yu J, Tall BD, et al. A genetic locus of enteropathogenic *Escherichia coli* necessary for the production of attaching and effacing lesions on tissue culture cells. *Proc Natl Acad Sci U S A* 1990;87:7839–7843.
174. Rabinowitz RP, Lai LC, Jarvis K, et al. Attaching and effacing of host cells by enteropathogenic *Escherichia coli* in the absence of detectable tyrosine kinase mediated signal transduction. *Microb Pathog* 1996;21:157–171.
175. Black RE, Levine MM, Clements ML, et al. Experimental *Campylobacter jejuni* infection in humans. *J Infect Dis* 1988; 157:472–479.
176. Baqar S, Bourgeois AL, Schultheiss PJ, et al. Safety and immunogenicity of a prototype oral whole-cell killed *Campylobacter* vaccine administered with a mucosal adjuvant in non-human primates. *Vaccine* 1995;13:22–28.
177. Scott DA. Vaccines against *Campylobacter jejuni. J Infect Dis* 1997;176[Suppl 2]:S183–S188.
178. Tribble DR, Baqar S, Scott DA, et al. Clinical development of an inactivated whole cell *Campylobacter* vaccine candidate. 2001 *(unpublished work).*
179. Kopecko DJ. Regulatory considerations for *Campylobacter* vaccine development. *J Infect Dis* 1997;176[Suppl 2]:S189–S191.
180. Marchetti M, Rossi M, Giannelli V, et al. Protection against *Helicobacter pylori* infection in mice by intragastric vaccination with *H. pylori* antigens is achieved using a non-toxic mutant of *E. coli* heat-labile enterotoxin (LT) as adjuvant. *Vaccine* 1998;16:33–37.
181. Angelakopoulos H, Hohmann EL. Pilot study of *phoP/phoQ*-deleted *Salmonella enterica* serovar Typhimurium expressing *Helicobacter pylori* urease in adult volunteers. *Infect Immun* 2000;68:2135–2141.
182. Kotloff KL, Sztein MB, Wasserman SS, et al. Safety and immunogenicity of oral inactivated whole-cell *Helicobacter pylori* vaccine with adjuvant among volunteers with or without subclinical infection. *Infect Immun* 2001;69:3581–3590.
183. Holmgren J, Jertborn M, Svennerholm A-M. Oral β subunit killed whole-cell cholera vaccine. In: Levine MM, Woodrow GC, Kaper JB, et al, eds. *New generation vaccines,* second edition. New York: Marcel Dekker Inc, 1997:459–468.

81

PREVENTION AND CONTROL OF NOSOCOMIAL ENTERIC INFECTIONS

WILLIAM SCHAFFNER
ANNE M. ANGLIM
BARRY M. FARR

Nosocomial gastrointestinal tract infections cause substantial additional morbidity, mortality, and hospital costs (1). A case definition has been formulated by the Centers for Disease Control and Prevention (CDC), enabling standardized surveillance and reporting of nosocomial infections (2). Use of this definition should allow comparison among studies and analysis of secular trends. The CDC definition of nosocomial gastroenteritis requires either of the following:

1. The acute onset of diarrhea in a hospitalized patient, characterized by liquid stool for more than 12 hours, with or without vomiting and/or fever (higher than 38°C).

or

2. Two of the following symptoms with no other recognized cause: nausea, vomiting, abdominal pain, or headache. These symptoms must occur in conjunction with objective evidence of enteric infection, obtained by either stool culture, antigen or antibody assay of feces or blood, routine or electron microscopic examination of stool, or toxin assay.

The amount of time the patient has been hospitalized before the onset of symptoms and the incubation period of the particular etiology of gastroenteritis are used to differentiate community-acquired from nosocomial illness (Table 81.1). Three days after admission is a frequently used cut point for distinguishing nosocomial from community-acquired infections. It may, however, be deceptive for pathogens with longer or shorter average incubation periods. Moreover, the incubation period of a particular infection can be longer than expected; altered immunologic function may also result in development of symptoms from a previously inactive infection. Hospital spread of pathogens from the community can result from hospital employees working while ill. Visitors can also bring in pathogens from the community. Finally, the workup of nosocomial diarrhea in patients with AIDS or those in developing countries is particularly difficult because of the high endemic rate of enteric disease in these populations and the wide variety of pathogens known to infect these patients.

The hospitalized patient who develops diarrhea should be evaluated for non-infectious conditions. Inflammatory bowel disease, endocrine disturbances, exocrine deficiencies, or mechanical processes such as fecal impaction can be detected by history, physical examination, and supplemental laboratory tests. Medications are another potential cause of diarrhea in the hospitalized patient, with laxatives, cathartics, antacids, quinidine, and digoxin being frequently implicated. Cytotoxic chemotherapeutic drugs, antibiotics, and enteral nutritional formulas not only cause non-infectious diarrhea but also increase the risk for infectious gastroenteritis.

IMPORTANCE OF NOSOCOMIAL GASTROENTERITIS

The CDC's National Nosocomial Infections Surveillance (NNIS) program (3), a voluntary network of participating hospitals that report data on nosocomial infections, has provided much of the data regarding nosocomial gastroenteritis. The most current available surveillance data are from 1985 to 1994. During those years, the crude rate of gastroenteritis was 10.5 per 10,000 discharges, an apparent eightfold increase over rates from 1980 to 1984 (4). This increase could be due to a combination of improved surveillance and reporting techniques, advances in diagnostic technology, or a true increase in infection.

A. M. Anglim and **B. M. Farr:** University of Virginia Health Sciences Center, Charlottesville, Virginia.

W. Schaffner: Vanderbilt University School of Medicine, Nashville, Tennessee.

TABLE 81.1. PATHOGENS IN NOSOCOMIAL GASTROENTERITIS

Agent	Incubation Period	Modes of Transmission	Duration of Illness[a]
Adenovirus	8–10 d	Unknown	8 d
Aeromonas species	Unknown	Food ingestion	1–7 d
Bascillus cereus	1–6 hr (short) 8–16 hr (long)	Food ingestion	<24 hr
Campylobacter jejuni	3–5 d	Food ingestion, direct contact	2–10 d
Clostridium botulinum	18–36 hr	Food ingestion	Weeks to months
Clostridium difficile	Unknown	Direct/indirect contact	5 d to 10 wk[b]
Clostridium perfringens	8–16 hr	Food ingestion	24–72 hr
Cryptosporidium	2–14 d	Food/water ingestion, direct and indirect contact	Weeks to months
Entamoeba histolytica	7–14 d	Food/water ingestion, direct and indirect contact	Variable
Escherichia coli			
ETEC	16–72 hr	Food/water ingestion	3–5 d
EPEC	16–48 hr	Food/water ingestion, direct and indirect contact	5–15 d
EIEC	16–48 hr	?Food/water ingestion	2–7 d
EHEC	72–120 hr	Food ingestion, direct and indirect contact	2–12 d
Giardia lamblia	7–14 d	Food/water ingestion, direct and indirect contact	Weeks to months
Listeria monocytogenes	3–70 d	Food ingestion, ?direct or indirect contact	Variable
Norwalk agent(s)	24–48 hr	Food/water ingestion, direct and indirect contact, ?aerosol	24–48 hr
Rotavirus	24–72 hr	Direct and indirect contact, ?aerosol	4–6 d
Salmonellae	16–72 hr	Food ingestion, direct and indirect contact	2–7 d
Shigellae	16–72 hr	Food/water ingestion, direct and indirect contact	2–7 d
Staphylococcus aureus	1–6 hr	Food ingestion	<24 hr
Yersinia enterocolitica	3–7 d	Food ingestion, direct contact	1–3 wk

[a]Course of illness without antimicrobial therapy.
[b]After stopping antibiotics.

Modifications in case finding can substantially alter rates of nosocomial gastroenteritis. This is exemplified by cases of nosocomial infectious diarrhea increasing 150- to 200-fold at the University of Virginia Hospital after the Clinical Microbiology Laboratory was requested to notify infection control personnel of all positive *Clostridium difficile* results (1). Stool ova and parasite examinations and bacterial cultures for *Salmonella, Shigella,* and *Campylobacter* species yield so few diagnoses in the evaluation of sporadic nosocomial diarrhea that they are not recommended for routine use (5,6). *C. difficile* and rotavirus have been the most frequent causes of nosocomial diarrhea (Table 81.2).

A study from a children's hospital found that infections of the gastrointestinal (GI) tract were exceeded only by those of the respiratory tract as causes of nosocomial infection (9); these infections were confirmed to be viral by stool electron microscopy. The study suggested that the availability and use of testing capabilities for viral pathogens may explain some of the increase in rates of nosocomial GI tract infections that has been evident in the past decade.

Rates of nosocomial gastroenteritis several hundred times higher than the NNIS data have been found in surveillance studies conducted in several hospitals. A study observing an adult medical intensive care unit and two pediatric wards found a rate of nosocomial diarrhea of 2.6 per 100 admissions, with a pathogen identified in about 40% of cases (11). In these particular wards, nosocomial diarrhea was the most frequently identified nosocomial infection, occurring in 7.7 and 2.3 per 100 admissions in adults and children, respectively.

NNIS data suggest that most infections occur in the elderly, with 64% involving patients 60 years or older (4). Such a finding may reflect a relative lack of viral diagnostic capabilities or infrequent testing for viral pathogens in sporadic diarrhea in hospitals that have facilities. Viral nosocomial diarrhea has been most frequently documented in children (6–8).

Although accounting for less than 1% of nosocomial infections reported from NNIS hospitals during the 1970s (17), gastroenteritis, primarily due to *Salmonella* species and enteropathogenic *Escherichia coli* (EPEC) made up 21% of nosocomial epidemics investigated by the CDC from 1956 to 1979 (18). In contrast, GI tract disease made up only 7.4% of nosocomial epidemics investigated by the CDC between 1980 and 1991 (4), perhaps because there are fewer hospital epidemics due to gastroenteritis. Just as plausibly, hospitals and local health departments may be managing more outbreaks without requesting CDC assistance.

Recent studies have examined the mortality attributable to nosocomial gastroenteritis. Zaidi et al. (19) prospectively evaluated adult patients in a Mexico City referral hospital, finding an 18% mortality rate in patients with nosocomial diarrhea compared with 5% in matched controls. Also evident was a 7% complication rate from diarrhea, such as volume depletion, GI bleeding, and candidemia. A study of bone marrow transplant recipients also found a significantly

TABLE 81.2. PATHOGENS ISOLATED IN ENDEMIC NOSOCOMIAL GASTROENTERITIS

Etiologic Agent	Study (References)	Number of Positive Cultures	Total Number Tested	Relative Frequency
Viral				
Rotavirus	6–14	343	919	0.37
Adenovirus	6,8,9,15	31	413	0.08
Calicivirus	8	13	80	0.16
Astrovirus	8	11	80	0.14
Minireovirus	8	10	80	0.13
Coxsackievirus	12	4	78	0.05
Coronavirus	9	2	65	0.03
Norwalk agent	8	2	80	0.03
Other viruses	9	11	65	0.17
Bacterial				
Clostridium difficile	6,10–12,15	94	324	0.29
Salmonellae	10,11,16	13	435	0.03
Shigellae	10,16	15	405	0.04
Fungal				
Candida species	10	19	45	0.42[a]

[a]Yeast was identified in the stool cultures of 55% of control patients.

increased mortality rate in patients with nosocomial gastroenteritis (12). Those infected with viral pathogens or *C. difficile* had a 55% case-fatality rate over the 9-month study period, versus 13% in matched controls. Patients with GI infections also had an average duration of hospitalization of 66 days, compared with 46 days for the controls.

Some have proposed that an increased risk for other nosocomial infections after nosocomial gastroenteritis may contribute to increased mortality. Lima et al. (20) found that nosocomial diarrhea was a significant risk factor for nosocomial urinary tract infections (UTIs), which were 10 times more common in patients with preceding diarrhea than in those without diarrhea. This may occur as a result of colonization of the urethral meatus with enteric flora during the diarrhea (21–24).

MECHANISMS OF SPREAD

The transmission of hospital-acquired GI tract infections has been clarified by newly developed techniques in molecular epidemiology (25). Transmission can occur by any of the following:

1. Spread among patients by contaminated hands of hospital workers
2. Direct patient-to-patient contact
3. Dissemination by a vehicle such as contaminated medical equipment, food, or water
4. Environmental contamination and subsequent direct or indirect spread

Nosocomial gastroenteritis is usually spread by the hands of hospital personnel. Contamination of hands has been documented in 59% of health care workers after routine contact with patients colonized with *C. difficile;* contamination was also demonstrable after handling patient charts (26). Another study showed a significant reduction of nosocomial transmission of *C. difficile* by the routine use of gloves (27). Accentuating the need for consistent use of barrier precautions is the finding that 21% of asymptomatic patients in one Veterans Administration Hospital study were colonized with *C. difficile* (28).

The use of molecular markers has proved useful in defining transmission patterns of *C. difficile.* Serogroup analysis of one outbreak found clusters of infection on hospital wards and provided a gauge of efficacy of infection control measures (29). The technique allowed discrimination of serotypes with tendencies for epidemic spread. Hospital-wide transmission has been documented with such procedures as restriction endonuclease analysis of chromosomal DNA, which in one instance was able to identify one clone as the cause of nosocomial diarrhea on several wards of a hospital (29).

Acquisition and transmission of sporadic *C. difficile* cases have been studied using immunoblot typing (26). On one ward, 22.7% of patients acquired *C. difficile,* with 37% of these developing diarrhea. Thus, it was suggested that most hospitalized patients who develop *C. difficile* disease become infected with the organism in the hospital. This method also showed person-to-person spread, with spatial clustering of affected patients and caregivers. Positive cultures were still evident in 82% of infected patients at the time of discharge.

McFarland et al. (26) have suggested that asymptomatic carriers are an important mechanism for the spread of *C. difficile*-associated diarrhea (CDAD) (26). Of 92 initially culture-negative patients, 23 (25%) acquired *C. difficile* from exposure to a roommate with a positive culture. Asymptomatic roommates were the source of *C. difficile* colonization in 14 (61%) of these 23 patients. Symptomatic patients were more likely to harbor toxigenic strains and excrete greater organism loads, theoretically increasing the possibility of transmission (29).

Contamination of the hospital environment has a potential role in the spread of nosocomial enteric disease (30,31). *C. difficile* spores can remain viable for 5 months on inanimate surfaces (31). One study showed that 8% of cultures of surfaces such as bed rails, commodes, floors, call buttons, bedpans, and windowsills were positive in the rooms of uninfected patients; 29% were positive in the rooms of patients with asymptomatic carriage. Of those cultures taken from rooms of patients with CDAD, 49% were positive (26). The occurrence of *C. difficile* on the hands of health care providers increases with the level of environmental contamination with the organism (32).

Nosocomial *Salmonella* gastroenteritis is characteristically associated with food-borne epidemics (33). In the developed world, point-source outbreaks due to contaminated food comprise most hospital-acquired *Salmonella* disease. After entry into the hospital, a sustained period of secondary person-to-person spread of *Salmonella* may result (34), aided by employees who transmit organisms on their hands (35). Asymptomatic carriers may also be vectors of spread (36). Susceptibility to infection can be increased by achlorhydria, malignancy, HIV infection, hemoglobinopathies, or prior antibiotic treatment. As a result of these multiple routes of spread, an originally food-borne epidemic continued for 5 years (36), maintained by food handlers, medical personnel, or patients who were colonized and/or infected with the organism.

Foods most often associated with nosocomial salmonellosis have included eggs, poultry, meat, and protein supplements. Pharmacologic agents and blood products have also been found to cause outbreaks (37). Contaminated animal extracts of pancreas, thyroid, pituitary, or liver were documented to occur in the years before the breakthrough of recombinant technology (33). The contamination of such objects as a delivery room suction apparatus (33) and endoscopy equipment (38) has also been responsible for outbreaks. A *Salmonella hadar* outbreak in a nursing home demonstrated spread from patients to laundry workers handling linens soiled by incontinent infected patients (39).

In the developing world, nosocomial salmonellosis has illustrated the consequences of liberal antibiotic utilization. In many regions, hospitals have become abundant sources of multiply resistant organisms (40). Multiply resistant *Salmonella* species have been linked to several hospital outbreaks that have had considerable mortality rates (35). In a Tunisian special care nursery, an outbreak of *Salmonella wien* that was marked by significant secondary spread had a 33% case-fatality rate (35). The development of a *Salmonella* species with plasmids carrying the extended-spectrum β-lactamase SHV-2 was likely fostered by extensive use of cefotaxime. Its subsequent spread was accelerated by casual adherence to the hospital's infection control policies.

Gastroenteritis of viral etiology frequently spreads within hospitals by contact with contaminated hands. There are anecdotal reports suggesting an additional route of spread by aerosol, possibly by movement of contaminated laundry (41,42) or by vomiting (43). Assessment of the importance of both the aerosol route and the health care worker in transmission of viral gastroenteritis warrants further study.

Of epidemics investigated by the CDC from 1956 to 1975, 11% were false outbreaks. The GI tract was involved in 20% of these pseudoepidemics, the second most common site involved (44). Specimen processing mistakes, misdiagnosis, and misinterpretation of surveillance findings produced false spatial and temporal relationships of alleged infections. A group of "infections" were due to *Salmonella saint-paul* contamination of a saline solution used for specimen processing in a hospital laboratory. Two other outbreaks were reported because of improper discrimination between community-acquired and nosocomial infection. A nursery outbreak, thought to be due to *Staphylococcus aureus,* resulted from dependence on positive stool cultures in the absence of clinical evaluation. Judicious analysis of epidemiologic findings can prevent wasting resources on investigation of pseudoepidemics.

The indigenous flora of the intestinal tract may provide a source for the development and spread of bacteria resistant to antimicrobial agents. Studies have demonstrated increased fecal colonization in both hospitalized patients and those in community surveys, irrespective of whether antimicrobials were administered (45–47). Similarly, diapered children in day care centers have been shown to harbor trimethoprim-resistant and multiresistant *E. coli* in their stools. Carriage in that setting was not correlated with recent antibiotic use (48). Extended courses of ampicillin for UTI have, however, been associated with the development of resistant *E. coli* (49). Studies in volunteers have shown an association between the administration of oral glycopeptides and the development of glycopeptide-resistant enterococci in fecal flora (50). The spread of vancomycin-resistant enterococci has produced the suggestion that the equally effective and considerably less expensive oral metronidazole should replace vancomycin as the treatment of choice for *C. difficile* colitis (51). The relationship between antimicrobials, indigenous gut flora, and the emergence of antimicrobial resistance merits further study.

ENVIRONMENTAL DETERMINANTS OF INFECTION

Risk for nosocomial GI tract infection is the aggregate of an intricate relationship between host defenses and exposure to pathogens in the hospital environment. An understanding of the environmental factors that influence the development of nosocomial diarrhea provides the basis for measures that prevent acquisition of infection. Extrinsic factors predisposing to nosocomial GI tract infections include nasogastric intubation, which allows introduction of bacteria into the GI tract (52), and enteral feeding (19). Although bacterial contamination of nutritional formulas has occasionally been reported to produce a nosocomial GI illness (53), diarrhea from enteral supplements is usually an osmotic process. Zaidi et al. (19), however, found that patients with nosocomial diarrhea were 67 times more likely to have received enteral feeding supplementation and identified pathogenic organisms in 59% of cases.

Transmission of nosocomial gastroenteritis can occur by cross-infection in crowded hospital environments. Ford-Jones et al. (8) found an association between nosocomial gastroenteritis and the number of patients in a room. Infection rates of 15.7 cases per 1,000 patient-days were found for rooms with one patient, 27.7 cases per 1,000 for rooms with two to three patients, and 45.2 cases per 1,000 for rooms with four or more patients. Diaper use was associated with a fivefold increased risk of nosocomial gastroenteritis.

Several studies of nosocomial gastroenteritis have linked prior antimicrobial use to an increased incidence of infection presumably by effects on the resident intestinal microflora (54). Thibault et al. (55) found that the risk of CDAD increased with the number of antibiotics administered to a patient. Risk was further magnified depending on the type of antibiotic used, with the highest odds ratio found with clindamycin usage.

INSTITUTIONAL FOOD-BORNE DISEASES

Patients in hospitals, nursing homes, and custodial facilities are predisposed to acquire and suffer serious effects of food-borne GI tract disease. Thus, institutional food services are challenged with procuring quality food at a low cost, appropriately storing food items before consumption, adequately preparing and cooking for large numbers of patients, and serving it before spoilage occurs.

Of food-borne outbreaks documented by the CDC during a 12-year period, hospitals and nursing homes were the settings for 3% of the outbreaks and 5% of total cases. These locations contributed 24% of deaths due to epidemic food-borne disease (56). The grave consequences of these outbreaks are illustrated by a 35% mortality rate in one nursing home outbreak of *E. coli* O157:H7, linked to sandwiches (57). Most institutional epidemics, however, have less serious outcomes. Salmonellosis in nursing homes has historically been a major determinant of food-borne morbidity and mortality. *Salmonella* accounted for 52% of outbreaks and 81% of deaths in outbreaks of confirmed etiology in 1975 to 1987, resulting in a case-fatality rate of 3.8% (58).

In institutions, food-borne GI illness typically follows a biphasic epidemic pattern, with a primary source—contaminated food—that infects many patients rapidly. Subsequent transmission generally follows (59), with a characteristically more sluggish course, consequent to cross-infection among patients and health care workers.

Nosocomial food-borne epidemics most often are caused by *Salmonella* species, *S. aureus,* and *Clostridium perfringens* (56). Because clinical laboratories commonly lack the diagnostic testing abilities for such entities as Norwalk and related agents and many *E. coli,* their relative importance in institutional food-borne illness is not well defined.

Epidemics may be caused by many different food vehicles. *Salmonella* species are associated with poultry, meat loaf, and egg-based foods, such as eggnog and scrambled eggs. Recipes made with meat are frequent vehicles of *C. perfringens* gastroenteritis. Although bacterial contamination of feeding formulas appears to be a relatively rare phenomenon, enteral feeding supplements have occasionally been found to be responsible for disease due to agents such as *Enterobacter sakazakii* (53) and other *Enterobacter* species.

Numerous food preparation errors have produced outbreaks of gastroenteritis. Most often cited have been food storage problems, such as inadequate refrigeration. Other frequently reported difficulties have included substandard hygienic practices by food workers, equipment contamination, incomplete cooking, and use of food that was contaminated during the initial processing (56). The prevention of food-borne nosocomial infection must concentrate on proper food preparation, storage, and distribution, as well as the health and hygiene of food service personnel. Regulations in these areas are provided by the Joint Commission on Accreditation of Healthcare Organizations (JCAHO).

COMMON PATHOGENS THAT CAUSE NOSOCOMIAL GASTROENTERITIS

Aerobic Gram-negative Organisms

Escherichia coli

E. coli is an important etiology of noninflammatory diarrhea in developing countries and the leading cause of traveler's diarrhea. In contrast, the incidence of nosocomial diarrhea due to the pathogenic *E. coli* is perceived to be low, although routine testing for such organisms is not possible in many clinical laboratories. Several noteworthy institutional epidemics nonetheless reveal this organism's relevance as a nosocomial pathogen.

Enterohemorrhagic *E. coli* (EHEC) serotype O157:H7 is now recognized as the causative pathogen in a four-state outbreak that affected more than 500 people. Linked to undercooked hamburger meat from a national chain of fast-food restaurants, infection was often marked by hemorrhagic colitis. Forty cases were complicated by hemolytic–uremic syndrome (HUS), resulting in four deaths (60). Both citizens and public officials were explicitly shown the necessity for strict food hygiene standards to protect the nation's food supply (61).

Hospital epidemics due to EHEC have not been reported, although nursing home outbreaks have been noted (57,62). One reported an attack rate of 32.5% among patients (57). Twelve residents developed HUS, with 11 resultant deaths. Nineteen residents died, resulting in a case-fatality rate of 35%. The epidemic showed a biphasic pattern, with secondary person-to-person spread including the nursing home staff. It is possible that indolent outbreaks, as well as sporadic cases of EHEC gastroenteritis, may be detected by the submission of stool cultures for patients with thrombotic thrombocytopenic purpura or HUS (63).

Decades ago, EPEC was associated with epidemic infantile diarrhea. Numerous outbreaks, both in the hospital and in the community, were ascribed to EPEC between 1940 and 1970 (64). Nosocomial infantile diarrhea was a frequent occurrence in nurseries, with outbreaks marked by high attack rates and case-fatality rates of 50%, usually from sepsis, shock, and acidosis (65). Children were usually afebrile, with poor feeding and watery diarrhea ensuing for more than 3 to 6 days (66). For reasons that have been ascribed to altered virulence of the organism, improved rehydration techniques, and antibiotic therapy, cases in recent years have been substantially milder (67).

Despite its departure from the United States and western Europe (68,69), institutional diarrhea caused by EPEC is an ongoing challenge in the developing nations of Africa, Asia, and South America (70).

Enterotoxigenic *E. coli* (ETEC) has been the cause of two documented nosocomial outbreaks (71,72). One 9-month-long outbreak, spread by contaminated enteral feedings, was linked to a strain elaborating a heat-stable enterotoxin. This serotype was seemingly unable to colonize adults despite its prevalence in the special care nursery (71). In addition, the responsible strain was unique because a common plasmid carried resistance genes for multiple antibiotics as well as the enterotoxin gene (73).

Salmonella

Salmonella species remain prominent causes of nosocomial disease. *Salmonella* accounts for 81% of deaths from food-borne disease in nursing homes (58). About 50% of nosocomial salmonellosis occurs in neonatal and pediatric wards (74). Unlike infections in adults, which often stem from consumption of a food vehicle, cross-infection is the primary mode of spread of pediatric infection. Nursery outbreaks have followed admission of a parturient patient with diarrhea due to *Salmonella* (75).

Most nosocomial outbreaks due to *Salmonella* have been due to a common source (18). Vehicles that have been linked to these epidemics include diagnostic agents, blood products, medications, banked human milk, and enteral feeding supplements containing yeast or raw egg. Contaminated equipment such as endoscopes (76) and suction apparatuses have also been implicated (34). The food sources most often cited are dairy products, poultry, and eggs.

Those who asymptomatically excrete the organism are not thought to be important sources of nosocomial transmission. Convalescent shedding of *Salmonella* is evident for a median of 5 weeks after overt disease (77,78). The use of enteric precautions with rigorous hand washing (79) is indicated.

Hospital employees recuperating from salmonellosis must nonetheless be considered a potential risk for nosocomial transmission and those with contact with patients or food should be confirmed to be culture-negative on two consecutive cultures before returning to such duties. *Salmonella* excretion can be intermittent, however, and positive stool cultures have been found after four to nine consecutive negative cultures in 17% of patients (77). Rectal swabs, which are unable to reliably detect fewer than 10^3 organisms per gram of feces, are not recommended because of poor sensitivity (80).

Because of the problems in demonstrating clearance of *Salmonella* and the erratic ability of antibiotics to eliminate carriage, a reasonable and cost-effective strategy is advocating uniform hand washing by all employees in patient care and food service positions. Those who show evidence of ongoing *Salmonella* carriage must not have direct patient or food contact. A trial of ampicillin therapy can be considered in some employees. The administration of 4 to 5 g of ampicillin daily for 4 to 6 weeks has been able to eradicate *Salmonella* from chronic excreters of ampicillin-susceptible organisms. Another study demonstrated success in 70% of 17 carriers without cholelithiasis. Negative cultures were obtained in only 23% of patients with biliary stones, however (81). The use of ampicillin eliminated *Salmonella* in 13 (87%) of the long-term excreters who were observed for 7 to 54 months (82). The frequency of adverse drug effects in the study sample was remarkable: 53% of patients reported loose stools, 40% rash, and 20% eosinophilia. Fluoroquinolones also have been evaluated. One study documented that 10 (83%) of 12 patients who finished 4 weeks of ciprofloxacin had negative cultures after 1 year (83). Reinforcing the low risk of transmission, a food-borne outbreak of salmonellosis affecting 203 nurses showed no evidence of spread to patients in spite of 77 nurses working 120 shifts while symptomatic (84).

The use of antibiotics can prolong bacterial shedding (85) and foster the development of resistance to antimicrobial agents. Moreover, antibiotic therapy has also been shown to increase the risk of infection (86).

Nosocomial salmonellosis is more frequently seen in the developing world. In Africa, South America, and Asia, hospitals have been identified as wellsprings for evolution and spread of multiply resistant *Salmonella* (40,87).

Shigella

Shigella species are an exceedingly uncommon cause of hospital-acquired diarrhea. Shigellosis was reported in only 1 of 3,363 patients with nosocomial gastroenteritis recorded by the NNIS program between 1986 and 1989, although *Shigella* has been regarded as one of the most infectious of bacterial agents, with a dose of 100 organisms sufficient to produce disease (88).

Scattered outbreaks have been reported in custodial care facilities (89) and nurseries (90). The likely mode of spread has been postulated to be the hands of employees with caregiving duties (91). The low incidence of hospital spread of *Shigella* was shown in a Kenyan study, where the organism is endemic and frequently present in newly admitted patients (16).

Yersinia enterocolitica

Yersinia enterocolitica as a nosocomial pathogen has become more apparent in the last 10 years. Although less common than *Campylobacter jejuni, Y. enterocolitica* is a common cause of community-acquired gastroenteritis in industrialized nations, particularly in the countries of northern Europe. Of the 50 known serotypes, most illness in humans results from infection with O8, O9, O27, and particularly O3 (92). Because of the prevalence of nonpathogenic serotypes, any *Y. enterocolitica* strain isolated from a clinical specimen should undergo serotyping. This will help to associate pathogen with illness and to establish any epidemiologic link between cases (93). Community outbreaks have been traced to milk (94), chitterlings (95), tofu packed in spring water (96), and bean sprouts packed in well water (97), with foods produced from pigs most often incriminated (97,98).

Instances of nosocomial bloodstream infection, caused by transfusion of contaminated packed red blood cells producing a sepsis syndrome due to *Y. enterocolitica,* have received significant publicity. Ten reported cases in nine states had a case-fatality rate of 70%. Almost half of the donors of the implicated blood had GI symptoms within 3 weeks before donation but were asymptomatic at the time of donation. All donors demonstrated evidence of recent *Yersinia* infection by serologic testing (99,100).

A few clusters of nosocomial gastroenteritis due to *Yersinia* have been documented (101,102). A study by Cannon and Linnemann (103) analyzed 4 years of surveillance. They determined that five patients had hospital-acquired *Yersinia* infection. They concluded that the infections usually originated from a patient with community-acquired yersiniosis and that nosocomial spread only would occur to one subsequent patient, suggesting that direct transmission of *Y. enterocolitica* seems to occur rarely.

Campylobacter jejuni

C. jejuni is increasingly recognized as an important cause of invasive gastroenteritis. More frequent than *Salmonella* or *Shigella,* it is perhaps the most common cause of bacterial diarrhea in the developed world (104). Population studies have shown a bimodal distribution of age-specific incidence, with the first peak in children younger than 1 year and the second occurring in patients 15 to 29 years (105,106).

Nosocomial transmission of *C. jejuni* has been documented only rarely. Food-borne illness has been confirmed in nursing homes, with milk the reported vehicle (58). Reports of a case of bacteremia from a contaminated blood transfusion (107) and vertically transmitted cases of enteritis in neonates have been published (108). Asymptomatic excreters of *Campylobacter* do not seem to disseminate the disease (104).

Aeromonas *Species and Other Gram-negative Bacteria*

In addition to EPEC, other Enterobacteriaceae are known to cause epidemic infantile diarrhea, particularly *Klebsiella* and *Citrobacter* species (109). One diarrheal outbreak was caused by multiple species using a common enterotoxin, likely disseminated by a plasmid or bacteriophage (110). Such noteworthy events are seldom detected using the facilities in most hospital laboratories.

Aeromonas species are controversial pathogens, which only recently have been found to cause GI tract illness. They appear, however, unable to produce disease in healthy adults (111); in volunteer studies, even large bacterial challenges did not cause symptoms (112). The mechanisms by which *Aeromonas* causes disease are not yet well defined but include a heat-labile cytotonic enterotoxin (113) and another enterotoxin that cross-reacts with cholera toxin (114) and has enteroinvasive traits (115).

Both seasonal and geographic associations have been reported with *Aeromonas* infections (116). *Aeromonas* species have been recovered from 52.8% of Peruvian infants hospitalized with diarrhea, versus 8.7% of controls (117). In Australia, only rotavirus is a more common cause of endemic diarrhea in pediatric populations (118). In contrast, a study evaluating diarrhea in Brazilian children did not isolate *Aeromonas* in a single culture (119).

Isolation of *Aeromonas* species from hospital water sources (120) implies a possibility for nosocomial epidemics. Actual reports, however, have been rare. One described respiratory colonization with resultant pneumonia or extrapulmonary infections (but not diarrhea) in 19 patients (121). Another apparent outbreak of *Aeromonas* occurred in a nursing home where 17 patients developed a brief illness of nonbloody diarrhea over a 3-day period (122). Of 11 cultures submitted, four grew *Aeromonas hydrophila.* In neither outbreak was a common source found, nor were cultures tested for the presence of a toxin.

Gram-positive Aerobic Bacteria

Listeria monocytogenes

Listeria monocytogenes is a motile, nonspore-forming gram-positive rod that is ubiquitous in the environment and among animals (123). Approximately 20% of sporadic cases (124) and many large outbreaks have been traced to contaminated food. Common sources of major outbreaks have been pasteurized milk (125), cheese (126), coleslaw (127), and undercooked meats (124). It also has frequently been isolated from commercially prepared foods intended for instant use, with a number of products recalled or not released as a result (128).

The spectrum of clinical manifestations caused by *Listeria* ranges from transient, asymptomatic carriage (123) to sepsis and meningoencephalitis (129). One-third of patients with listeriosis in a large British survey were infected during pregnancy (130), most often as a nonspecific febrile illness. Transplacental transmission can be inconsequential (131) or catastrophic, with stillbirth, prematurity, and neonatal sepsis/meningitis resulting (130). The reporting of GI symptoms before the development of invasive listeriosis has roused speculation that the organism may be damaging the intestinal mucosa and allowing the invasion of *Listeria* (132).

Only 10% to 30% of patients have no identifiable predisposition for infection (129). Invasive disease in the general population is rare, with a risk for adults of 0.5 per 100,000 population (128), despite point prevalence gut colonization rates of 0.6% to 16% in the general population and longitudinal studies showing transient carriage occurring in 70% of people (133).

Hospital-associated outbreaks of listeriosis are rare. One outbreak in 1979, traced to raw vegetables, affected 20 patients in eight Boston-area hospitals. Ten of these patients were immunosuppressed (134). An unusual epidemic in a Costa Rican nursery documented cross-infection from an infant with neonatal listeriosis, via a contaminated bottle of mineral oil that was used on other infants (135). Although not associated with gastroenteritis, it should be emphasized that no other food-borne illness has a higher case-fatality rate; non-perinatal cases of listeriosis reported in a nationwide survey in 1986 had a case-fatality rate of 35% (128).

L. monocytogenes requires temperatures of at least 70°C to kill the organism (123). The agent can also grow at temperatures near the freezing point, which allows for "cold enrichment" techniques and facilitates its isolation in the microbiology laboratory (123). Person-to-person transmission of infection has not yet been firmly described, with a few reports of small outbreaks suggesting spread by fomites or hospital workers (136,137).

Staphylococci

Staphylococcal food-borne disease is a common institutional occurrence. Food-borne *S. aureus* outbreaks made up 8% of hospital and 23% of nursing home outbreaks reported to the CDC from 1975 to 1987 (56). Although mortality is rare, with a 0.4% case-fatality rate in the CDC nursing home survey (58), morbidity can be considerable.

The source of epidemic staphylococcal food poisoning is often a food handler colonized with *S. aureus*. Disease can ensue if food prepared by the carrier is stored at an improper temperature or not served promptly. Interruption of this chain of events can be accomplished by (a) conscientious employee hygiene with hand washing, the use of gloves, or the exclusion of food handlers with skin infections; (b) proper refrigeration of foods at temperatures below 4°C, especially after partial cooking (138); and (c) rapid serving of food kept at room temperature.

In the last decade methicillin-resistant *S. aureus* (MRSA) have received widespread attention as increasingly important nosocomial pathogens. Despite a reputation as primarily a bloodstream and wound pathogen, a single report has implicated MRSA as a cause of food-borne disease (139).

Anaerobic Organisms

Clostridium difficile

A gram-positive, spore-forming, obligate anaerobe, *C. difficile* has been shown to be the predominant microbial etiology of nosocomial diarrhea. In early experiments, hamsters given antibiotics were noted to develop severe colitis (140), providing insight into the pathogenesis of antibiotic-associated pseudomembranous colitis. A cytotoxin neutralized by *Clostridium sordelli* antitoxin was identified in the hamster feces (141). It was subsequently associated with *C. difficile* and is now known as toxin B (142). An enterotoxin (toxin A) is also elaborated by *C. difficile,* producing intestinal fluid secretion and hemorrhage in an animal model (143). Although toxin A is thought to express the clinical symptoms, most strains of *C. difficile* produce both toxins (144).

Until recently, tissue culture assay to detect cytopathic effects of toxin B had been considered the gold standard for diagnosis of antibiotic-associated colitis. Used independently, it was reported to have a sensitivity between 67% (145) and 100% (146) and a specificity of 99% (145,147, 148). However, this test is technically difficult to perform. Several commercial enzyme immunoassay (EIA) tests are available that can detect toxin A, B, or both. Latex agglutination tests have also been developed. They are rapid and simple, but sensitivities have ranged from 71% to 92% when compared with a cytotoxin assay (148). Many of these kits have either insufficient sensitivity or an excessive number of indeterminate results to allow use as a definitive test (10,146,149). Other diagnostic tests such as a polymerase chain reaction (PCR) that uses primers from both toxins A and B have shown promise (150,151).

Techniques for culturing *C. difficile* commonly use a selective egg-yolk agar base medium with cycloserine, cefoxitin, and fructose (CCFA) (152). Because the rate of asymptomatic *C. difficile* carriage in hospitalized patients is about 16% (26), culture alone should not be used for the diagnosis of CDAD. To facilitate epidemiologic studies, 0.1% sodium taurocholate can be added to CCFA to increase recovery of *C. difficile* from environmental sources by increasing spore germination (153). Likewise, alcohol shock enrichment also seems to increase yield from cultures of suspected *C. difficile* carriers (154,155). Because of the high rate of asymptomatic carriage of *C. difficile* in hospitalized patients, the evaluation of antibiotic-associated colitis must use both clinical and laboratory criteria (28,145).

Follow-up cultures to document cure do not seem to be helpful in patients with CDAD. After treatment, high rates of asymptomatic colonization persist (156). Although transmission may occur from an asymptomatic excreter, eradication of *C. difficile* carriage usually has not been successful and is not advised. One recent study found that the use of metronidazole had no effect on excretion and vancomycin had only a temporary influence on excretion rates (157). Therefore, the recommended measures to interrupt nosocomial outbreaks of CDAD are use of enteric precautions, glove and gown use, hand washing, and use of private rooms and cohorting if patient hygiene is poor. Contaminated electronic thermometers have been linked to an outbreak of CDAD. Discontinuation of their use was temporally associated with cessation of the outbreak (158).

Clostridium perfringens

Nosocomial gastroenteritis due to *C. perfringens* is the third most common food-borne illness in hospitals and nursing homes (56). After an incubation period of 6 to 24 hours, diarrhea and abdominal cramps develop, usually in the absence of systemic toxicity. The illness lasts up to 24 hours and resolves without therapy (159). Although typically benign, deaths due to *C. perfringens* food poisoning have been reported (58).

Toxigenic strains of *C. perfringens* are usually found in meats, stews, poultry, gravies, and meat pies (160) that become contaminated during prolonged cooling and storage at room temperature (161). Heat-stable spores are able to survive cooking and germinate with cooling. Optimal growth in meat occurs at a temperature of 43°C to 47°C (160). Thus, it is the storage of food at inappropriate temperatures that will most likely favor the growth of *C. perfringens.* Cooked foods must therefore be promptly refrigerated at a temperature of no greater than 4°C and, if reheated, cooked to a temperature of at least 100°C, which will inactivate both the toxin and *C. perfringens* spores that might have germinated due to insufficient refrigeration (162).

Syndromes other than food-borne gastroenteritis have been associated with *C. perfringens.* Sporadic diarrhea has been reported and shown to be independent of contaminated food ingestion. This illness follows a protracted clinical course, akin to that of *Salmonella* or *Campylobacter* species (163). Cases of antibiotic-associated diarrhea have also been reported (164). *C. perfringens* (165) and *Clostridium butyricum* (166) have both been implicated in the pathogenesis of infant necrotizing enterocolitis (NEC). The discovery that *C. perfringens* type C was the etiologic agent in pigbel (167) (a syndrome of necrotizing enteritis described in highland natives of New Guinea, which classically occurs after ritual consumption of a large pork meal), suggested that NEC may be caused by a bacterial toxin.

Viral Pathogens

Rotavirus

Rotavirus is the major worldwide cause of childhood diarrhea, producing substantial mortality in the children of developing nations (168). In the United States and western Europe, diarrheal mortality is rare, but 35% of wintertime pediatric hospital admissions for gastroenteritis are due to rotavirus (169). Children between age 6 months and 2 years experience the majority of disease, with 62% of children having had at least one infection by age 2 years (170). Hospitalization rates for children have been reported to be as high as 8.5 admissions per 1,000 children (171).

After an incubation period of 48 to 72 hours, there is the onset of fever and vomiting that generally lasts about 2 days. A watery diarrhea that is devoid of blood and leukocytes follows, subsiding within 8 days (4). Viral shedding in the feces is usual from the third to the eighth day of illness. Although clinically inapparent infection can occur in any age-group, it is most common in adults. In contrast, children age 6 to 24 months often have pronounced symptoms (172). Infected patients may excrete 10^{12} organisms per gram of feces (173).

Rotavirus has been found to exist on environmental surfaces for up to 10 days (174). A simian rotavirus can survive acid and alkaline exposures, freeze thawing, ether, and chloroform (175), as well as chlorhexidine (176). The most effective disinfectant has been found to be 95% ethanol (177), with glutaraldehyde and povidone iodine also useful (176).

The infectious nature of rotavirus has been shown in household studies that describe a 40% seroconversion rate in parents of children with rotavirus gastroenteritis (178). The development of electron microscopy in the 1970s allowed diarrheal illness to be correlated with demonstration of the virus in stool specimens. The first outbreaks were reported from nurseries in England (179), Australia (180), and the United States (181). These accounts described high attack rates, but with only a fraction of infected infants having detectable symptoms.

Transmission is thought to be horizontal, supported by the detection of rotavirus in the hand washings of asymptomatic caregivers of patients with diarrhea (182). Emphasizing the practical importance of person-to-person spread, several institutions have ended outbreaks by cohorting infected patients and caregivers (181,183). In contrast, one study was unable to find efficacy by using early screening of symptomatic patients with enzyme-linked immunoassay (ELISA) testing and isolation. This very small study found no difference in transmission rates from cases identified during two separate 5-week surveillance periods, occurring before and after the introduction of rapid testing for rotavirus (13).

Although solid data are lacking, conjecture has been raised about the potential for aerosol spread (184,185). The frequent occurrence of simultaneous respiratory symptoms with rotavirus gastroenteritis implies a need for further investigation of this possible mode of transmission.

Nosocomial rotavirus gastroenteritis has been documented in adults, with multiple outbreaks reported among elderly patients (183,186). One outbreak affected 19 out of 34 patients, with six severe cases of gastroenteritis and two deaths (187). Yolken et al. (12) studied adult bone marrow transplant recipients and found that 9 of 31 patients with infectious diarrhea had disease due to rotavirus. Other studies have found this entity to be the etiologic agent in 1% to 4% of nosocomial gastroenteritis in adults (68).

In some populations, rotavirus infection may be more severe. Immunodeficient patients may experience chronic diarrhea and prolonged viral shedding (188). Potential for more serious illness with protracted infectivity likewise exists for elderly patients (187) and transplant recipients (12,189).

The epidemiologic study of rotavirus has greatly been facilitated by improved diagnostic technologies. The use of ELISA testing has made case-finding rapid, inexpensive, and simple. These commercially available kits can detect rotavirus inner capsid antigen in stools with a sensitivity early in the illness equivalent to that of virus isolation and visualization by electron microscopy (190). Latex agglutination tests, although less sensitive than ELISA (191), are also rapid and readily available. The use of PCR can detect rotavirus antigen at concentrations 1,000 times lower than electron microscopy or immunoassay methods (192).

Polyacrylamide gel electrophoresis (PAGE) has been used to differentiate rotavirus strains. Using variations in migration patterns of the RNA segments in the virus genome to define strains, PAGE (or "electropherotyping") is a powerful technique for epidemiologic analysis (193, 194). Its ability to classify rotaviruses or analyze organisms over time or in widely separated outbreaks is limited by the fact that a given electropherotype does not always correlate with DNA hybridization patterns or serotype (195,196). Despite these shortcomings, electropherotyping is useful in the study of individual outbreaks. It has shown infant-to-infant transmission, with involvement of multiple strains in an outbreak (197). One outbreak with an initial predominance of one electropherotype had subsequent appearance of highly variable RNA segments by PAGE (198), suggesting that a rotavirus strain may evolve during an epidemic, either by genetic reassortment ("antigenic drift") or by introduction of other strains with multiple infections.

Efforts to prevent nosocomial rotavirus infection should concentrate on diagnosing patients newly admitted with diarrhea and early isolation using enteric precautions, those shown to be the most important sources of nosocomial rotavirus outbreaks (199). Other efforts should include strengthening of hygienic practices, particularly hand washing, among hospital staff, who have also been implicated in nosocomial spread of rotavirus (181). Regular disinfection of communal play toys also is important (200).

Adenovirus

The role of adenoviruses in childhood enteric disease is now firmly established after their first identification by electron microscopy in the stools of infants with diarrhea in 1975 (201,202). Strains linked to gastroenteritis are called enteric adenoviruses and belong to serogroups 40 and 41 (203). These strains are often referred to as uncultivable adenoviruses because of fastidious growth requirements in cell culture.

For children younger than 2 years, only rotavirus is a more common cause of community-acquired gastroenteritis (204,205). Serologic evidence of prior infection is present in 50% of children by age 4 years (206). Unlike rotavirus, there is no seasonal variability in infection rates (205,207). Person-to-person transmission is the probable route of spread (208), although spread to adults is uncommon (205,207). The prevalence of latent infection is illustrated by a prospective study that found that 46% of infected children were asymptomatic (204). Infection appears to confer long-term immunity.

Nosocomial acquisition of adenovirus was first reported by Flewett et al. (201). They described a diarrheal illness of 24- to 48-hours' duration affecting 6 of 19 children and one nurse in a pediatric ward. Adenovirus-like particles were found on stool electron microscopy in four of six ill children and the nurse, but none of the well children (201). In another study, Yolken et al. (209) described adenovirus in the stools of 14 (52%) of 27 hospitalized infants with gastroenteritis, with 13 (93%) of the 14 affected patients having concurrent respiratory symptoms. Nosocomial acquisition was suggested by the fact that 5 of the 14 children with gastroenteritis were not excreting adenovirus at the time of admission (209). Only one of 72 asymptomatic children had adenovirus detectable on stool examination. Another prospective study of hospitalized children younger than 2 years determined that adenovirus was the third most common cause of nosocomial diarrhea in this age-group, causing 6.2% of cases (210). A study of bone marrow transplant recipients with a mean age of 21 years discovered that the incidence of gastroenteritis due to adenovirus was equal to that of *C. difficile* and was associated with a 45% mortality rate (12).

Small, Round Structured Viruses (Norwalk and Other Agents)

A syndrome of acute nausea and vomiting commonly occurs during the winters in temperate climates. This illness aggregates in families, usually affecting children 1 to 10 years of age, but not sparing adults. Until recently, this illness was identified as "winter vomiting disease" (211), reflecting the lack of a known etiology.

Investigation of a large outbreak of winter vomiting disease in Norwalk, Ohio (212), revealed the first of a collection of small (20 to 35 nm), round structured viral agents that were subsequently linked to gastroenteritis (213). Of the outbreaks of acute nonbacterial gastroenteritis investigated by the CDC from 1976 to 1981, 42% were caused by the Norwalk and related entities (214).

These viruses are generally identified either by immune electron microscopy or by paired serology. Other methods have been developed, such as an ELISA (215) and PCR (216) for the Norwalk agent, and ELISA for both the calicivirus (217) and astrovirus (218), but routine use is limited by availability of reagents.

Most Norwalk-related outbreaks result from such contaminated vehicles as water (219), salad (220), or shellfish (214). Nursing homes have been the most common sites for institutional epidemics. In fact, it was the study of an outbreak in a California nursing home that initially recognized the Marin County agent (221). High attack rates have been reported; another nursing home epidemic affected 64% of its 120 residents and 29% of the staff (222). Nine (12%) of the residents required hospitalization, and two deaths occurred. Documentation of this outbreak was incomplete; stool electron microscopy was not performed and a vehicle for the outbreak was not found.

Person-to-person spread seems to perpetuate some outbreaks (223). Investigators in an emergency department found some ill patients and staff without any history of direct contact with other ill patients. It was theorized that movement of infectious laundry extended the area where virus could be spread (42). Despite conjecture regarding an aerosol route in this instance, as well as another nursing home outbreak (41), confirmation of this route for the spread of GI illness remains forthcoming.

Testing for this class of viruses is not commonly done in clinical laboratories. Therefore, without prospective surveillance, recognition of early outbreaks and sporadic cases is unlikely. Also complicating investigations is the short duration of the illness. Stool and blood must be obtained in the presence of symptoms. Specimens must then be evaluated quickly for best results using immune electron microscopy, serology, or PCR (208).

Other viruses have been associated with nosocomial gastroenteritis. They include coronaviruses, echoviruses, and coxsackieviruses. These agents have primarily been linked to outbreaks in infants.

Protozoans

Cryptosporidium

The correlation of infection with *Cryptosporidium* and human disease was first reported in 1976 by two investigators (224,225). This organism produces an illness in which both the severity and the duration of illness are modified by the competence of the patient's immune system (226). An intractable, frequently fatal, diarrhea occurs in AIDS patients, with less severe disease in healthy hosts (227). The illness can result from exposure to infected animals and humans, in addition to consumption of water (228). Nosocomial transmission between patients and from infected patients to hospital personnel has been reported (229–232). One outbreak affected all six patients in a bone marrow transplantation unit after a recently admitted patient shared a room with a patient with cryptosporidiosis on another unit (230). Convalescent shedding of organisms can persist after cessation of symptoms but will generally subside within 2 weeks (233).

Cryptosporidium oocysts are extremely difficult to inactivate. They survive the chlorination in public water supplies, as well as such common disinfectants as iodophors, hypochlorite, and 5% formaldehyde. Heat (≥60°C), formalin (≥10%), and ammonia (≥50%) appear to be effective in killing the organism (228,234–237). Even concentrated to 100%, hypochlorite alone appears to be only partially effective in eradicating oocysts.

Laboratory diagnosis is most often made by microscopic examination of stool using a Kinyoun acid-fast stain looking for oocysts (238,239). Because oocyst shedding is not always continuous, evaluation of multiple specimens may increase yield (233). Recently available is an EIA kit, shown in one study to have a sensitivity and a specificity of 100% compared with a standard of immunofluorescence (240). Concentration methods (241) may assist in epidemic investigation by evaluating suspected nosocomial cases and detecting oocysts in water and other environmental samples. Serologic methods, such as ELISA, have a 95% sensitivity when both immunoglobulin M and immunoglobulin G antibodies are used (242). As in other pathogens, efforts to control institutional spread must rely on aggressive identification of infected patients and strict enteric precautions.

Entamoeba histolytica

Although it is a known cause of diarrhea in custodial institutions (243) and in AIDS patients (244), *Entamoeba histolytica* is a rare nosocomial pathogen. One noteworthy outbreak of amebiasis, however, was connected to an improperly maintained colonic irrigation machine in a chiropractor's office. Over 2½ years, 36 cases of the illness, including 6 deaths, were reported (245).

Although hospital-acquired amebiasis occurs in developing countries (19), it is generally thought to be a reactivation illness. Not only do affected patients appear to lack identifiable risk factors for recent acquisition of infection, but no geographic or spatial clustering of cases is evident. Most patients had received prior corticosteroids or chemotherapy, with resultant suppression of cell-mediated immunity permitting recrudescence of dormant infection. If there is ever a concern regarding possible nosocomial transmission of *E. histolytica,* methods such as DNA hybridization (246) and PCR (247) may be useful in elucidating modes of transmission.

Giardia lamblia *(Giardia duodenalis)*

Currently the most frequently identified intestinal parasite in the United States, *Giardia lamblia* has caused numerous large waterborne community outbreaks (248,249). *G. lamblia* also is a well-known cause of diarrhea in both day care centers (250) and custodial institutions (251). One outbreak in a nursing home has also been documented (252). The ingestion of water contaminated by cysts is a characteristic route of acquisition, with person-to-person spread next in frequency. Indirect transmission of *Giardia* cysts can occur, resulting from their survival on environmental surfaces (253) and resistance to many disinfectants (254).

Children in day care centers may excrete cysts for as long as 6 months in the absence of overt symptoms (250). Up to 50% of children younger than 3 years demonstrate silent fecal shedding of cysts. Other studies have found that 25% of family members of children in day care have evidence of *Giardia* infection (255). Hand washing is nonetheless effective in curtailing spread of this agent in the day care center (256).

The organism is visible on either a saline wet-mount examination of a fresh stool specimen or a preserved sample that is stained with trichrome or hematoxylin. Some recommend use of a concentration method (257), sampling of duodenal contents by a string test (258), or endoscopy with brushings/biopsy (259) if initial stool microscopy is unproductive. The use of an ELISA that can detect *Giardia* in stool with a sensitivity and specificity of more than 90% may assist epidemiologic study (260). The PCR could add power to such investigation by virtue of its ability to distinguish subgroups of *G. lamblia* (261).

Fungal Pathogens

Candida *species*

The isolation of *Candida* from 65% of stool specimens from healthy persons (262) has confounded efforts to understand the potential of *Candida* to cause serious enteric nosocomial disease. The organism's role beyond that of a saprophyte has nonetheless grown, largely as a result of the increasing use of immunosuppressive and cytotoxic agents as well as the expansion of the AIDS epidemic. GI candidiasis may manifest as invasive enteritis in immunocompromised hosts or a non-invasive overgrowth syndrome (263).

Case–control studies show that colonization with *Candida* is a risk factor for the development of candidemia (264,265), which carries a mortality rate as high as 38% (266). It has been demonstrated by restriction endonuclease digestion with fungal DNA that colonizing strains are identical to those that appear in the blood (267). It is postulated that fungal invasion of the GI tract mucosa leads to the organism's subsequent hematogenous spread (268). A healthy human volunteer developed fever and rigors hours after swallowing a saline suspension containing 10^{12} *Candida albicans* cells and was documented to have candidemia and candiduria (269).

Although its pathogenesis is unclear, an illness of watery diarrhea, with *Candida* overgrowth in the absence of mucosal invasion, has been documented (270). Some suggest a toxin-mediated process produces the disease (271). In contrast, deranged small intestinal brush border enzyme activity is felt by others to be the primary lesion (272). This syndrome has been described most commonly in neonates (273) and debilitated patients (270), with a uniformly positive response to oral nystatin (270,274).

Despite their use being almost exclusively in research centers, serotyping techniques have contributed to an understanding of the acquisition and transmission of *Candida* (275). Doebbling et al. (276) have used contour-clamped homogeneous electric-field electrophoresis to demonstrate hand carriage of *Candida* in health care personnel, thus implying a potential for direct spread. DNA fingerprinting and biotyping have been used together, producing precise discrimination among clinical specimens (277). Unfortunately, early and reliable diagnosis of invasive candidiasis in the clinical setting is still difficult, generally necessitating blood culture and biopsy of appropriate anatomic sites. New rapid tests for *Candida* species, applying EIA to detect either cell wall (278) or cytoplasmic (279) antigens, have shown potential in selected samples but seem to be limited by poor specificity in patient groups at a lesser risk for candidiasis (280).

OUTBREAK DETECTION AND MANAGEMENT

Institutions can effectively perform surveillance for nosocomial gastroenteritis by routine review of positive stool results, coupled with periodic observation of high-risk wards, such as the newborn and special care nurseries, intensive care units, and oncology wards. This method incorporates aspects of laboratory surveillance and selective chart review (281,283). Such use of surveillance to detect sporadic cases of CDAD has been demonstrated to be useful in decreasing spread of that organism within the hospital (29). Rapid interpretation of positive stool assays for *C. difficile* can permit early institution of procedures to limit nosocomial spread, including glove use with patient contact, gowns if soiling is likely, and a private room if the patient's hygiene is poor.

After confirmation of a nosocomial outbreak of gastroenteritis, epidemiologic investigation should begin, with initial isolation measures being undertaken concurrent with the gathering of preliminary data. If a large number of persons appear to be affected, cohorting of patients and caregivers should be considered. Prompt notification of the local or state health department is required. The health department can perform serotyping or test for such organisms as pathogenic *E. coli* or Norwalk and related agents, as well as provide epidemiologic support.

PREVENTION OF NOSOCOMIAL GASTROENTERITIS

Prevention of GI tract infections in hospitalized patients lies with the awareness that these diseases are fundamentally spread by the fecal-oral route. Subsequently, transmission to others may occur by direct physical contact or indirectly by the hands of caregivers or contact with inanimate surfaces. GI pathogens may also be acquired by a contaminated common vehicle such as food, water, medication, or equipment. Thus, approaches to control these infections require incorporation of these concepts.

Of paramount importance is hand washing between patient and food contact, as well as the use of enteric precautions. The use of universal precautions (284) reduces nosocomial transmission of agents such as *C. difficile.* In one medical center, the institution of an employee educational program that urged glove use for contact with any moist body substance resulted in an 80% decrease in the incidence of CDAD (27). Hand washing after all patient contact (285) and changing gloves between patients should be urged (286). Strategies must improve hand-washing compliance rates estimated to be 40% in one intensive care unit survey (287,288).

Contamination of such equipment as endoscopy and respiratory therapy devices has been found to be associated with institutional spread of enteric diseases, notably *C. difficile, Salmonella* species, and *Helicobacter pylori* (31,32,38, 76,289,290). Most implicated equipment is classified as "semicritical" (291), needing a minimum of high-level disinfection due their close proximity to non-intact skin or mucous membranes. One nationwide sample found a significant heterogeneity in protocols used for disinfection of endoscopic devices (292). In addition, manual cleaning, the first and essential step in proper disinfection, is complicated by the intricate design and fragility of endoscopes (293). An inadequate performance of this step makes prolonged chemical disinfection with high-potency germicides necessary. Such an alternative can include either a 20-minute treatment in 2% glutaraldehyde or ethylene oxide sterilization as another option (294). Incomplete rinsing of devices after exposure to such agents has been documented to cause a dermatitis in employees and, in patients, a chemical colitis with an endoscopic appearance similar to pseudomembranous colitis (295). Automated washers do not totally eliminate potential for contamination of devices. Alvarado et al. (296) reported nosocomial *Pseudomonas aeruginosa* infections originating from an endoscope washer that was contaminated with the same strain. The internal components were noted to be colonized with *Pseudomonas,* with positive cultures of rinse-cycle water seen over a 1-year period. The washer's self-operating decontamination procedure had failed to eliminate the organism. Colonization was successfully eradicated by the addition of a step after machine cleansing and disinfection: rinsing external surfaces and endoscope channels using 70% alcohol and subsequent drying with forced air. In situations in which the source of contamination is unknown, sterilization with ethylene oxide can be used if infections seem to be occurring due to problems with high-level disinfection.

Clinical thermometers are also a semicritical item and should undergo high-level disinfection, most easily done with 70% to 90% isopropyl alcohol (294). Outbreaks of *C. difficile* have been associated with electronic rectal thermometers, with their successful cessation by substituting disposable thermometers (158). A crossover study comparing disposable thermometers with electronic thermometers demonstrated a 64% reduction in rates of *C. difficile* infection with the use of the disposable device (297).

Disinfection of environmental surfaces is a relatively uncomplicated procedure. Any of a number of agents, such as 70% to 90% isopropyl alcohol, sodium hypochlorite, or detergents with phenol, iodophor, or ammonia (294), can be used for low-level disinfection of noncritical items (those coming in contact with intact skin) and surfaces.

Prevention should also center on patients. Established risk factors for nosocomial diarrhea should be minimized to lessen the chance of its development. These strategies can include reducing antimicrobial utilization, using sucralfate instead of antacids or H_2 blockers if ulcer prophylaxis is needed, limiting enema use, and reducing duration of nasogastric tube use. Some innovative approaches have been tried, with uneven results. The administration of nonpathogenic bacteria and yeasts has been attempted in an effort to prevent antibiotic-associated diarrhea. One study demonstrated a significant decrease in the incidence of antibiotic-associated diarrhea by using a saprophytic yeast *Saccharomyces boulardii.* The yeast, however, had no impact on the colonization of *C. difficile* as well as the toxin (298).

Hospital and food service employee education should emphasize relevant aspects of personal health. The Study on the Efficacy of Nosocomial Infection Control project addressed the attitudes of hospital employees toward their own illnesses (299). It was discovered that infection control nurses often had negligible authority to mandate suspension from patient contact for employees with communicable diseases. The study also reported that 68% of nurses believed that working with diarrheal symptoms was acceptable, in comparison to 4% in the presence of fever and sore throat. Outbreaks of gastroenteritis due to Norwalk and related agents have been traced to health care providers working in the presence of GI symptoms (43). The customarily brief course of gastroenteritis can permit an ill employee to spread the infection at work and experience subsequent cessation of symptoms, evading the notice of supervisors, employee health, or infection control personnel. To avert this type of scenario, the institution's employee health service, perhaps with infection control, must take on a more proactive approach. Illness should promptly be identified. Educational interventions must stress that patient contact must be avoided in the presence of illness, in spite of notions that a condition is minor. Finally, the success of such interventions rests on the certainty that employees will not receive financial penalty for time lost from duty due to illness (300).

Employees with gastroenteritis should be evaluated and released from direct patient or food contact until symptoms subside. Most of these illnesses will only require supportive treatment. If there is concern over an invasive illness or a possible institutional outbreak, more thorough evaluation is indicated, with stool samples submitted for bacterial culture and perhaps ova and parasite examination. In this way, a specific diagnosis can be made to not only guide treatment but also estimate the risk for further dissemination (301). A significant concern is to consider those entities that are likely to be excreted for a prolonged interval after recovery from acute illness. For nontyphoidal *Salmonella* or *Shigella* infections, an asymptomatic employee should have at least two negative stool cultures before resuming duties (302). For the most valid results, stool specimens should be collected at least 24 hours apart and at least 48 hours after discontinuation of antibiotics. More than 50% of those having salmonellosis will have negative cultures within 5 weeks after the illness, with 90% by 9 weeks (77). A health care worker with disease due to most agents may resume work after cessation of symptoms, with explicit advice to use universal precautions and hand washing.

Prevention of institutional food-borne disease must focus on maintaining hygienic food storage and preparation procedures. Kitchen surfaces and equipment should be kept fastidiously clean. Food should be sought from reliable sources, avoiding unpasteurized products. Appropriate temperatures, either above 60°C or below 7°C, must be used for storage of food. Thawing must be complete before cooking, optimally done while the food is refrigerated. Although modified ultraviolet lamps have been used to eradicate *Salmonella* species on culture plates (303), the technique is not currently applicable to food disinfection. Proper training of food service personnel cannot be overemphasized, because they are most able to prevent food-borne disease spread.

REFERENCES

1. Farr BM. Diarrhea: a neglected nosocomial hazard [Editorial]? *Infect Control Hosp Epidemiol* 1991;12:343–344.
2. Garner JS, Jarvis WR, Emori TG, et al. CDC definitions for nosocomial infections. *Am J Infect Control* 1988;16:128–140.
3. Emori TG, Culver DH, Horan TC, et al. National nosocomial infections surveillance system (NNIS): description of surveillance methods. *Am J Infect Control* 1991;19:19–35.
4. Cookson ST, Hughes JM, Jarvis WR. Nosocomial gastrointestinal infections. In: Wenzel R, ed. *Prevention and control of nosocomial infections.* Baltimore: Williams & Wilkins, 1997:925–975.
5. Zaidi AKM, Macone A, Goldmann D. Impact of simple screening criteria on utilization of low-yield bacterial stool cultures in a children's hospital. *Pediatr* 1999;103:1189–1192.
6. Ozerek AE, Rao GG. Is routine screening for conventional enteric pathogens necessary in sporadic hospital acquired diarrhoea? *J Hosp Infect* 1999;41:159–163.
7. Lam BCC, Tam J, Ng MH, et al. Nosocomial gastroenteritis in pediatric patients. *J Hosp Infect* 1989;14:351–355.
8. Ford-Jones EL, Mindorff CM, Gold R, et al. The incidence of viral-associated diarrhea after admission to a pediatric hospital. *Am J Epidemiol* 1990;131:711–718.
9. Welliver RC, McLaughlin S. Unique epidemiology of nosocomial infection in a children's hospital. *Am J Dis Child* 1984;138:131–135.
10. Lima NL, Farr BM, Lima MEF, et al. Etiologies of nosocomial diarrhea at a university hospital in northeastern Brazil. In: Programs and abstracts of the 33rd Interscience Conference on Antimicrobial Agents and Chemotherapy; October 17–20, 1993; New Orleans, Louisiana. Abstract 1297.
11. Guerrant RL, Hughes JM, Lima NL, et al. Diarrhea in developed and developing countries: magnitude, special settings, and etiologies. *Rev Infect Dis* 1990;12[Suppl]:S41–S50.
12. Yolken RH, Bishop CA, Townsend TR, et al. Infectious gastroenteritis in bone marrow transplant recipients. *N Engl J Med* 1982;306:1009–1012.
13. Dennehy PH, Tenle WE, Fisher DJ, et al. Lack of impact of rapid identification of rotavirus-infected patients on nosocomial rotavirus infections. *Pediatr Infect Dis J* 1989;8:290–296.
14. Cone R, Mohan K, Thouless M, et al. Nosocomial transmission of rotavirus infection. *Pediatr Infect Dis J* 1988;7(2):103–109.
15. Yannelli B, Qurevich I, Schoch PE, et al. Yield of stool cultures, ova and parasite tests, and *Clostridium difficile* determinations in nosocomial diarrheas. *Am J Infect Control* 1988;16:246–249.
16. Paton S, Nicolle L, Mwongera M, et al. *Salmonella* and *Shigella* gastroenteritis at a public teaching hospital in Nairobi, Kenya. *Infect Control Hosp Epidemiol* 1991;12:710–717.
17. Hughes JM, Jarvis WR. Nosocomial gastrointestinal infections. In: Wenzel R, ed. *Prevention and control of nosocomial infections.* Baltimore: Williams & Wilkins, 1987:405–439.
18. Stamm WE, Weinstein RA, Dixon RE. Comparison of endemic and epidemic nosocomial infections. *Am J Med* 1981;70:393–397.
19. Zaidi M, Ponce de Leon S, Ortiz RM, et al. Hospital-acquired diarrhea in adults: a prospective case–controlled study in Mexico. *Infect Control Hosp Epidemiol* 1991;12:349–355.
20. Lima NL, Guerrant RL, Kaiser DL, et al. A retrospective cohort study of nosocomial diarrhea as a risk factor for nosocomial infection. *J Infect Dis* 1990;161:948–952.
21. Garibaldi RA, Burke J, Britt MR, et al. Meatal colonization and catheter-associated bacteriuria. *N Engl J Med* 1980;303:316–318.
22. Schaeffer AJ, Chmiel J. Urethral meatal colonization in the pathogenesis of catheter-associated bacteriuria. *J Urol* 1983;130:1096–1099.
23. Daifuku R, Stamm WE. Association of rectal and urethral colonization with urinary tract infection in patients with indwelling catheters. *JAMA* 1984;252:2028–2030.
24. Monti S, Opal SM, Palardy JE, et al. Nosocomial *C. difficile* diarrhea: risk factors, complications, and cost [Abstract]. In: Programs in abstracts of the second annual SHEA Meeting; April 12–14, 1992; Baltimore, Maryland.

25. Eisenstein BI. New molecular techniques for microbial epidemiology and the diagnosis of infectious diseases. *J Infect Dis* 1990;161:595–602.
26. McFarland LV, Mulligan ME, Kwok RYY, et al. Nosocomial acquisition of *Clostridium difficile* infection. *N Engl J Med* 1989;320:204–210.
27. Johnson S, Gerding DN, Olson MM, et al. Prospective controlled study of vinyl glove use to interrupt *Clostridium difficile* nosocomial transmission. *Am J Med* 1990;88:137–140.
28. Gerding DN, Olson MM, Peterson LR, et al. *Clostridium difficile* associated diarrhea and colitis in adults. A prospective case–controlled epidemiologic study. *Arch Intern Med* 1986;146:95–100.
29. Struelens MJ, Maas A, Nonhoff C, et al. Control of nosocomial transmission of *Clostridium difficile* based on sporadic case surveillance. *Am J Med* 1991;91[Suppl 3B]:138S–144S.
30. Kaatz GW, Gitlin SD, Schaberg DR, et al. Acquisition of *Clostridium difficile* from the hospital environment. *Am J Epidemiol* 1988;127:1289–1294.
31. Fekety R, Kim KH, Brown D, et al. Epidemiology of antibiotic-associated colitis. Isolation of *Clostridium difficile* from the hospital environment. *Am J Med* 1981;70:906–908.
32. Samore MH, Venkataraman L, De Girolami PC, et al. Clinical and molecular epidemiology of sporadic and clustered cases of nosocomial *Clostridium difficile* diarrhea. *Am J Med* 1996;100:32–40.
33. Baine WB, Gangarosa EJ, Bennett JV, et al. Institutional salmonellosis. *J Infect Dis* 1973;128:357–360.
34. Rice PA, Craven PC, Wells JG. *Salmonella heidelberg* enteritis and bacteria: an epidemic on two pediatric wards. *Am J Med* 1976;60:509–516.
35. Hammami A, Arlet G, Ben Redjeb S, et al. Nosocomial outbreak of acute gastroenteritis in a neonatal intensive care unit in Tunisia caused by multiply drug resistant *Salmonella wien* producing SHV-2 beta-lactamase. *Eur J Clin Microbiol Infect Dis* 1991;10:641–646.
36. Linnemann CC Jr, Cannon CG, Staneck JL, et al. Prolonged epidemic of salmonellosis: use of trimethoprim-sulfamethoxazole for control. *Infect Control* 1985;6:221–225.
37. Haley CE, Guerrant RL. Institutional salmonellosis. *Asepsis* 1982;4:7–12.
38. Dwyer DW, Klein EG, Istre GR, et al. *Salmonella newport* infections transmitted by fiberoptic colonoscopy. *Gastrointest Endosc* 1987;33:84–87.
39. Standaert SM, Hutcheson RH, Schaffner W. Nosocomial transmission of salmonella gastroenteritis to laundry workers in a nursing home. *Infect Control Hosp Epidemiol* 1994;15:22–26.
40. Riley LW, Ceballos O, Tabuls LR, et al. The significance of hospitals as reservoirs for epidemic multiresistant *Salmonella typhimurium* causing infection in urban Brazilian children. *J Infect Dis* 1984;150:236–241.
41. Gellert GA, Waterman SH, Ewert D, et al. An outbreak of acute gastroenteritis caused by a small round structured virus in a geriatric convalescent facility. *Infect Control Hosp Epidemiol* 1990;11:459–464.
42. Sawyer LA, Murphy JJ, Kaplan JE, et al. 25- to 30-nm particle associated with a hospital outbreak of acute gastroenteritis with evidence for airborne transmission. *Am J Epidemiol* 1988;127:1261–1271.
43. Aitken C, Jeffries DJ. Nosocomial spread of viral disease. *Clin Microb Rev* 2001;14:528–546.
44. Weinstein RA, Stamm WE. Pseudoepidemics in hospital. *Lancet* 1977;2:862–864.
45. Datta N. Drug resistance and R factor in the bowel bacteria of London patients before and after admission to hospital. *Br Med J* 1969;2:407–411.
46. McGowan JE. Antimicrobial resistance in hospital organisms and its relation to antibiotic use. *Rev Infect Dis* 1983;5:1033–1048.
47. Isameel NA. Resistance of bacteria from human faecal flora to antimicrobial agents. *J Trop Med Hyg* 1993;96:51–55.
48. Reves RR, Fong M, Pickering LK, et al. Risk factors for fecal colonization with trimethoprim-resistant and multiresistant *E coli* among children in day-care centers in Houston, Texas. *Antimicrob Agent Chemother* 1990;34:1429–1434.
49. Datta N, Faiers MC, Reeves WS, et al. R-factors in *Escherichia coli* in faeces after oral chemotherapy in general practice. *Lancet* 1971;1:312–315.
50. Van der Auwesa P, Defresne N, Grenier P, et al. Emergence of resistant (R) *Enterococcus faecium* and coagulase negative staphylococci (CNS) in fecal flora of volunteers receiving teicoplanin. In: Programs and abstracts of the 30th Interscience Conference of Antimicrobial Agents and Chemotherapy; 1990; Atlanta, Georgia. Abstract 258.
51. Spera RV Jr, Farber BF. Multiply-resistant *Enterococcus faecium*. The nosocomial pathogen of the 1990s. *JAMA* 1992;268(18):2563–2564.
52. Brown E, Talbot GH, Axelrod P, et al. Risk factors for *Clostridium difficile* toxin-associated diarrhea. *Infect Control Hosp Epidemiol* 1990;11:283–290.
53. Simmons BP, Gelfand MS, Haas M, et al. *Enterobacter sakazakii* infections in neonates associated with intrinsic contamination of a powdered infant formula. *Infect Control Hosp Epidemiol* 1989;10:398–401.
54. Mentzing LO, Ringertz O. *Salmonella* infection in tourists, II: prophylaxis against salmonellosis. *Acta Pathol Microbiol Scand* 1968;74:405–413.
55. Thibault A, Miller MA, Gaese C. Risk factors for the development of *Clostridium difficile*-associated diarrhea during a hospital outbreak. *Infect Control Hosp Epidemiol* 1991;12:345–348.
56. Slutsker L, Villarino ME, Jarvis WR, et al. Foodborne disease prevention in healthcare facilities. In: Bennett JV, Brachman PS, eds. *Hospital infections.* Philadelphia: Lippincott–Raven Publishers, 1998:333–341.
57. Carter AO, Borezyk AA, Carlson JAK, et al. A severe outbreak of *Escherichia coli* O157:H7-associated hemorrhagic colitis in a nursing home. *N Engl J Med* 1987;327:1496–1500.
58. Levine WC, Smart JF, Archer DL, et al. Foodborne disease outbreaks in nursing homes, 1975 through 1987. *JAMA* 1991;266:2105–2109.
59. Steere AC, Craven PJ, Hall WJ III, et al. Person-to-person spread of *Salmonella typhimurium* after a hospital common-source outbreak. *Lancet* 1975;1:319–321.
60. Centers for Disease Control and Prevention. Update: multistate outbreak of *Escherichia coli* O157:H7 infections from hamburgers—western United States, 1992–1993. *MMWR Morb Mortal Wkly Rep* 1993;42:258–263.
61. MacDonald KL, Osterholm MT. The emergence of *Escherichia coli* O157:H7 infection in the United States. The changing epidemiology of foodborne disease. *JAMA* 1993;269:2264–2266.
62. Ryan CA, Tauxe RV, Hosek GW, et al. *Escherichia coli* O157:H7 diarrhea in a nursing home: clinical, epidemiological, and pathological findings. *J Infect Dis* 1986;154:631–638.
63. Ostroff SM, Griffin PM, Tauxe RV, et al. A statewide outbreak of *Escherichia coli* O157:H7 infections in Washington State. *Am J Epidemiol* 1990;132:239–247.
64. Levine MM, Edelman R. Enteropathogenic *Escherichia coli* of classic subtypes associated with infant diarrhea: epidemiology and pathogenesis. *Epidemiol Rev* 1984;6:31–51.
65. Giles C, Sangster G, Smith J. Epidemic gastroenteritis of infants in Aberdeen during 1947. *Arch Dis Child* 1949;24:45–53.
66. Levine MM, Bergquist EJ, Nalin DR, et al. *Escherichia coli* strains that cause diarrhea but do not produce heat-labile or

heat-stable enterotoxins and are non-invasive. *Lancet* 1978;1: 1119–1122.

67. Bower JR, Congeni BL, Cleary TG, et al. *Escherichia coli* O114: nonmotile as a pathogen in an outbreak of severe diarrhea associated with a day care center. *J Infect Dis* 1989;160:243–247.
68. DuPont HL, Ribner BS. Infectious gastroenteritis. In: Bennett J, Brachman PS, eds. *Hospital infections.* Philadelphia: Lippincott–Raven Publishers, 1998:537–550.
69. Morris KJ, Rao GG. Conventional screening for enteropathogenic *Escherichia coli* in the U.K. Is it appropriate or necessary? *J Hosp Infect* 1992;21:163–167.
70. Western KA, St. John RK, Shearer LA. Hospital infection control—an international perspective [Editorial]. *Infect Control* 1982;3:453–455.
71. Ryder RW, Wachsmuth IK, Buxton AE, et al. Infantile diarrhea produced by heat-stable enterotoxigenic *E. coli. N Engl J Med* 1976;295:849–853.
72. Gross RJ, Rowe B, Henderson A, et al. A new *Escherichia coli* O-group, O159, associated with outbreaks of enteritis in infants. *Scand J Infect Dis* 1976;8:195–198.
73. Wachsmuth IK, Falkow S, Ryder RW. Plasmid-mediated properties of a heat-stable enterotoxin-producing *Escherichia coli* associated with infantile diarrhea. *Infect Immun* 1976;14:403–407.
74. DuPont HL. Nosocomial salmonellosis and shigellosis. *Infect Control Hosp Epidemiol* 1991;12:707–709.
75. Lyons RW, Samples CL, DeSilva HN, et al. An epidemic of resistant *Salmonella* in a nursery. *JAMA* 1980;243:346–347.
76. Chmel H, Armstrong D. *Salmonella oslo:* a focal outbreak in a hospital. *Am J Med* 1976;60:203–208.
77. Buchwald DS, Blaser MJ. A review of human salmonellosis, II: duration of excretion following infection with nontyphi *Salmonella. Rev Infect Dis* 1984;6:345–356.
78. Musher DM, Rubenstein AD. Permanent carriers of nontyphoidal salmonellae. *Arch Intern Med* 1973;132:869–872.
79. Pether JVS, Scott RHD. *Salmonella* carriers: are they dangerous? A study to identify finger contamination with salmonellae by convalescent carriers. *J Infect* 1982;5:81–88.
80. McCall CE, Martin WT, Boring JR. Efficiency of cultures of rectal swabs and fecal specimens in detecting *Salmonella* carriers: correlation with numbers of salmonellae excreted. *J Hyg (London)* 1966;64:261–269.
81. Perkins JC, Devetski RL, Dowling HF. Ampicillin in the treatment of *Salmonella* carriers. Report of six cases and summary of the literature. *Arch Intern Med* 1966;118:528–533.
82. Simon HJ, Miller RC. Ampicillin in the treatment of chronic typhoid carriers. Report of fifteen treated cases and a review of the literature. *N Engl J Med* 1966;274:807–815.
83. Ferreccio C, Morris JG Jr, Valdivieso C, et al. Efficacy of ciprofloxacin in the treatment of chronic typhoid carriers. *J Infect Dis* 1988;157:1235–1239.
84. Tauxe RV, Hassan FL, Findeisen KO, et al. Salmonellosis in nurses: lack of transmission to patients. *J Infect Dis* 1988;157: 370–373.
85. Askerkoff B, Bennett JV. Effect of antibiotic therapy in acute salmonellosis in the fecal excretion of salmonellae. *N Engl J Med* 1969;281:636–640.
86. Pavia AT, Shipman LD, Wells JG, et al. Epidemiologic evidence that prior antimicrobial exposure decreases resistance to infection by antimicrobial-sensitive *Salmonella. J Infect Dis* 1990; 161:255–260.
87. Maiorini E, Lopez EL, Morrow AL, et al. Multiply resistant nontyphoidal *Salmonella* gastroenteritis in children. *Pediatr Infect Dis* 1993;12:139–143.
88. DuPont HL, Levine MM, Hornick RB, et al. Inoculum size in shigellosis and implications for expected mode of transmission. *J Infect Dis* 1989;159:1126–1128.
89. DuPont HL, Gangarosa EJ, Reller LB, et al. Shigellosis in custodial institutions. *Am J Epidemiol* 1970;92:172–179.
90. Salzman TC, Scher CD, Moss R. Shigellae with transferable drug resistance: outbreak in a nursery for premature infants. *Pediatr Res* 1967;71:21–26.
91. Weissman JB, Hutcheson RH. Shigellosis transmitted by nurses. *South Med J* 1976;69:1341–1346.
92. Lee LA, Taylor J, Carter GP, et al. *Yersinia enterocolitica* O:3: an emerging cause of pediatric gastroenteritis in the United States. *J Infect Dis* 1991;163:660–663.
93. Jarvis WR. *Yersinia enterocolitica:* a new or unrecognized nosocomial pathogen [Editorial]? *Infect Control Hosp Epidemiol* 1992;13:137–138.
94. Shayegani M, Morse D, DeForge I, et al. Microbiology of a major foodborne outbreak of gastroenteritis caused by *Yersinia enterocolitica* serogroup O:8. *J Clin Microbiol* 1983;17:35–40.
95. Lee LA, Gerber AR, Lonsway DR, et al. *Yersinia enterocolitica* O:3 infections in infants and children associated with household preparation of chitterlings. *N Engl J Med* 1990;322: 984–987.
96. Tacket CO, Ballard J, Harris N, et al. An outbreak of *Yersinia enterocolitica* infections caused by contaminated tofu (soybean curd). *Am J Epidemiol* 1985;121:705–711.
97. Aber RC, McCarthy MA, Berman R, et al. An outbreak of *Yersinia enterocolitica* gastrointestinal illness among members of a Brownie troop in Centre County, Pennsylvania. In: Programs and abstracts of the 22nd Interscience Conference on Antimicrobial Agents and Chemotherapy; October 4–6, 1982; Miami Beach, Florida. Abstract 860.
98. Tauxe RV, Vandepitte J, Wauters G, et al. *Yersinia enterocolitica* infections and pork: the missing link. *Lancet* 1987;1:1129–1132.
99. Tipple MA, Bland LA, Murphy JJ, et al. Sepsis associated with transfusion of red cells contaminated with *Yersinia enterocolitica. Transfusion* 1990;30:207–213.
100. Centers for Disease Control and Prevention. *Yersinia enterocolitica* bacteremia and endotoxin shock associated with red blood cell transfusions—United States, 1991. *MMWR Morb Mortal Wkly Rep* 1991;40:176–178.
101. Rutnam S, Mercer E, Picco B, et al. A nosocomial outbreak of diarrheal disease due to *Yersinia enterocolitica* serotype O:5; biotype 1. *J Infect Dis* 1982;145:242–247.
102. Toivanen P, Toivanen A, Olkkonen L, et al. Hospital outbreak of *Yersinia enterocolitica* infections. *Lancet* 1973;1:801–803.
103. Cannon CG, Linnemann CC Jr. *Yersinia enterocolitica* infections in hospitalized patients: the problem of hospital-acquired infections. *Infect Control Hosp Epidemiol* 1992;13:139–143.
104. Blaser MJ, Wells JG, Feldman RA, et al., Group CDDS. *Campylobacter enteritis* in the United States: a multicenter study. *Ann Intern Med* 1983;98:360–365.
105. Riley LW, Finch MJ. Results of a first year of surveillance of *Campylobacter* infections in the United States. *J Infect Dis* 1985;151:956–959.
106. Tauxe RV, Deming MS, Blake PA. *Campylobacter jejuni* infections on college campuses: a national survey. *Am J Public Health* 1985;75:659–660.
107. Pepersack F, Prigogyne T, Butzler JP, et al. *Campylobacter jejuni* post-transfusional septicaemia [Letter]. *Lancet* 1979;2:911.
108. Karmali MA, Norrish B, Lior H, et al. *Campylobacter* enteritis in a neonatal nursery. *J Infect Dis* 1984;149:847–877.
109. Guarino A, Capano G, Malamisura B, et al. Production of *Escherichia coli* STa-like heat-stable enterotoxin by *Citrobacter freundii* isolated from humans. *J Med Microbiol* 1987;25: 110–114.
110. Guerrant RL, Dickens MD, Wenzel RP, et al. Toxigenic bacterial diarrhea: nursery outbreak involving multiple bacterial strains. *J Pediatr* 1976;89:885–891.

111. Moyer NP. Clinical significance of *Aeromonas* species isolated from patients with diarrhea. *J Clin Microbiol* 1987;25: 2044–2048.
112. Morgan DR, Johnson PC, DuPont HL, et al. Lack of correlation between known virulence properties of *Aeromonas hydrophila* and enteropathogenicity for humans. *Infect Immun* 1985;50:62–65.
113. Chakraborty T, Montenegro MA, Sanyal SC, et al. Cloning of the enterotoxin gene from *Aeromonas hydrophila* provides conclusive evidence of production of a cytotonic cytotoxin. *Infect Immun* 1984;46:435–441.
114. Shimada T, Sakazaki R, Horigome K, et al. Production of cholera-like enterotoxin by *Aeromonas hydrophila. Jpn J Med Sci Biol* 1984;37:141–144.
115. Pazzaglia G, Sack RB, Bourgeois AL, et al. Diarrhea and intestinal invasiveness of *Aeromonas* strains in the removable intestinal tie rabbit model. *Infect Immun* 1990;58:1924–1931.
116. Altwegg M, Geiss HK. *Aeromonas* as a human pathogen. *Crit Rev Microbiol* 1989;16:253–286.
117. Pazzaglia G, Sack RB, Salazar E, et al. High frequency of coinfecting enteropathogens in *Aeromonas*-associated diarrhea of hospitalized Peruvian infants. *J Clin Microbiol* 1991;29:1151–1156.
118. Hazen TC, Fliermans CB, Hirsch RP, et al. Prevalence and distribution of *Aeromonas hydrophila* in the United States. *Appl Environ Microbiol* 1978;36:731–738.
119. Schorling JB, Wanke CA, Schorling SK, et al. A prospective study of persistent diarrhea among children in an urban Brazilian slum. *Am J Epidemiol* 1990;132:144–156.
120. Millership SE, Stephenson JR, Tabaqchalis S. Epidemiology of *Aeromonas* species in a hospital. *J Hosp Infect* 1988;11:169–175.
121. Mellersh AR, Norman P, Smith GH. *Aeromonas hydrophila:* an outbreak of hospital infection. *J Hosp Infect* 1984;5:425–430.
122. Bloom HG, Bottone EJ. *Aeromonas hydrophila* diarrhea in a long-term care setting. *J Am Geriatr Soc* 1990;38:804–806.
123. Farber JM, Peterkin PI. *Listeria monocytogenes:* a foodborne pathogen. *Microbiol Rev* 1991;55:476–511.
124. Schwartz B, Ciesielski CA, Broome CV, et al. Association of sporadic listeriosis with consumption of uncooked hot dogs and undercooked chicken. *Lancet* 1988;2:779–782.
125. Fleming DW, Cochi SL, MacDonald KL, et al. Pasteurized milk as a vehicle of infection in an outbreak of listeriosis. *N Engl J Med* 1985;312:404–407.
126. Linnan MJ, Mascola L, Lou XD, et al. Epidemic listeriosis associated with Mexican-style cheese. *N Engl J Med* 1988;319: 823–829.
127. Schlech WF III, Lavigne PM, Bortolussi RA, et al. Epidemic listeriosis—evidence for transmission by food. *N Engl J Med* 1983;308:203–206.
128. Gellin BG, Broome CV, Bibb WF, et al. The epidemiology of listeriosis in the United States—1986. *Am J Epidemiol* 1991; 133:392–401.
129. Nieman RE, Lorber B. Listeriosis in adults: a changing pattern. Report of eight cases and review of the literature, 1968–1978. *Rev Infect Dis* 1980;2:207–227.
130. McLauchlin J. Human listeriosis in Britain 1967–1985: a summary of 772 cases, 1: listeriosis during pregnancy and in the newborn. *Epidemiol Infect* 1990;104:181–189.
131. MacGowan AP, Cartlidge PH, MacLeod F, et al. Maternal listeriosis in pregnancy without fetal or neonatal infection. *J Infect* 1991;22:55–57.
132. Schwartz B, Hexter D, Broome DV, et al. Investigation of an outbreak of listeriosis: a new hypothesis for the etiology of epidemic *Listeria monocytogenes* infections. *J Infect Dis* 1989;159: 680–685.
133. Lamont RJ, Postlethwaite R, MacGowan AP. *Listeria monocytogenes* and its role in human infection. *J Infect* 1988;17:7–28.
134. Ho JL, Shands KN, Friedland G, et al. An outbreak of type 4b *Listeria monocytogenes* infection involving patients from eight Boston hospitals. *Arch Intern Med* 1986;146:520–524.
135. Schuchat A, Lizano C, Broome CV, et al. Outbreak of neonatal listeriosis associated with mineral oil. *Pediatr Infect Dis J* 1991;10:183–189.
136. Nelson KE, Warren D, Tomasi AM, et al. Transmission of neonatal listeriosis in a delivery room. *Am J Dis Child* 1985; 139:903–905.
137. Bibb WF, Schwartz B, Gellin BG, et al. Analysis of *Listeria monocytogenes* by multilocus enzyme electrophoresis and application of the method to epidemiologic investigations. *Int J Food Microbiol* 1989;8:233–239.
138. Bryan FL. What the sanitarian should know about staphylococci and salmonellae in non-dairy products, 1: staphylococci. *J Milk Food Technol* 1968;31:110–116.
139. Jones TF, Kellum ME, Porter SS, et al. An outbreak of community-acquired foodborne illness caused by methicillin-resistant *Staphylococcus aureus. Emerging Infect Dis* 2002;8:82–84.
140. Lusk RH, Fekety R, Silva J, et al. Clindamycin-induced enterocolitis in hamsters. *J Infect Dis* 1978;137:464–475.
141. Rifkin GD, Fekety FR, Silva J, et al. Antibiotic-associated colitis: implication of a toxin neutralized by *Clostridium sordelli* antitoxin. *Lancet* 1977;2:1103–1106.
142. Bartlett JG. Antibiotic-associated pseudomembranous colitis. *Rev Infect Dis* 1979;1:530–539.
143. Lima AAM, Lyerly DM, Wilkins TD, et al. Effects of *Clostridium difficile* toxins A and B in rabbit small and large intestine in vivo and on cultured cells in vitro. *Infect Immun* 1988;56: 582–588.
144. Bartlett JG. Antibiotic-associated diarrhea. *Clin Infect Dis* 1992;15:573–581.
145. Peterson LR, Olson MM, Shanholtzer CJ, et al. Results of a prospective, 18-month clinical evaluation of culture, cytotoxin testing, and Culturette brand (CDT) latex testing in the diagnosis of *Clostridium difficile*-associated diarrhea. *Diagn Microbiol Infect Dis* 1988;10:85–91.
146. Shanholtzer CJ, Willard KE, Holter JJ, et al. Comparison of VIDAS *C. difficile* toxin A immunoassay (CDA) with *C. difficile* culture, cytotoxin, and latex test. *J Clin Microbiol* 1992;30: 1837–1840.
147. Barbut F, Kajzer C, Planas N, et al. Comparison of three enzyme immunoassays, a cytotoxicity assay and toxigenic culture for the diagnosis of *Clostridium difficile*-associated diarrhea. *J Clin Microbiol* 1993;31:963–967.
148. Peterson LR, Kelly PJ. Role of the clinical microbiology laboratory in the management of *Clostridium difficile*-associated diarrhea. *Infect Dis Clin North Am* 1993;7:277–293.
149. Doern GV, Coughlin RT, Wu L. Laboratory diagnosis of *Clostridium difficile*-associated gastrointestinal disease: comparison of monoclonal antibody enzyme immunoassay for toxins A and B with a monoclonal antibody enzyme immunoassay for toxin A only and two cytotoxicity assays. *J Clin Microbiol* 1992;30:2042–2046.
150. Kato N, Ou C-Y, Kato H, et al. Identification of toxigenic *Clostridium difficile* in stool specimens by the polymerase chain reaction. *J Infect Dis* 1993;162:455–458.
151. Gumerlock PH, Tary YJ, Weiss JB, et al. Specific detection of toxigenic strains of *Clostridium difficile* in stool specimens. *J Clin Microbiol* 1993;31:507–511.
152. George WL, Sutter VL, Citron D, et al. Selective and differential medium for isolation of *Clostridium difficile. J Clin Microbiol* 1979;9:214–219.
153. Wilson KH, Kennedy MJ, Fekety R. Use of sodium taurocholate to enhance spore recovery on a medium selective for *Clostridium difficile. J Clin Microbiol* 1982;15:443–446.

154. Clabots CR, Gerding SJ, Olson MM, et al. Detection of asymptomatic *Clostridium difficile* carriage by an alcohol shock procedure. *J Clin Microbiol* 1989;27:2386–2387.
155. Riley TV, Brazier JS, Hassan H, et al. Comparison of alcohol shock enrichment and selective enrichment for the isolation of *Clostridium difficile. Epidemiol Infect* 1987;99:355–359.
156. Teasley DG, Gerding DN, Olson MM, et al. Prospective randomized trial of metronidazole versus vancomycin for *Clostridium difficile*-associated diarrhoea and colitis. *Lancet* 1983;2: 1043–1046.
157. Johnson S, Homann SR, Bettin KM, et al. Treatment of asymptomatic *Clostridium difficile* carriers (fecal excreters) with vancomycin or metronidazole. A randomized, placebo controlled trial. *Ann Intern Med* 1992;117:297–302.
158. Brooks SE, Veal RO, Kramer M, et al. Reduction in the incidence of *Clostridium difficile*-associated diarrhea in an acute care hospital and a skilled nursing facility following replacement of electronic thermometers with single-use disposables. *Infect Control Hosp Epidemiol* 1992;13:98–103.
159. Shandera WX, Tacket CO, Blake PA. Food poisoning due to *Clostridium perfringens* in the United States. *J Infect Dis* 1983; 147:167–170.
160. Hall HE, Angelotti R. *Clostridium perfringens* in meat and meat products. *Appl Microbiol* 1965;13:352–357.
161. Peterson LR, Musher R, Cooper GH, et al. A large *Clostridium perfringens* foodborne outbreak with an unusual attack rate pattern. *Am J Epidemiol* 1988;127:605–611.
162. Hobbs BC. *Clostridium perfringens* and *Bacillus cereus* infections. In: Riemann H, ed. *Foodborne infections and intoxications.* New York: Academic Press, 1969;131–173.
163. Larson HE, Borriello SP. Infectious diarrhea due to *Clostridium perfringens. J Infect Dis* 1988;157:390–391.
164. Schwartz JN, Hamilton JP, Fekety R, et al. Ampicillin-induced enterocolitis: implication of toxigenic *Clostridium perfringens* type C. *J Pediatr* 1980;97:661–663.
165. Kosloske AM, Ball WS Jr, Umland E, et al. Clostridial necrotizing enterocolitis. *J Pediatr Surg* 1985;20:155–159.
166. Sturm R, Staneck JL, Stauffer LR, et al. Neonatal necrotizing enterocolitis associated with penicillin-resistant, toxigenic *Clostridium butyricum. Pediatrics* 1980;66:928–931.
167. Murrell TGC, Egerton JR, Rampling A, et al. The ecology and epidemiology of the pig-bel syndrome in man in New Guinea. *J Hyg (London)* 1966;64:375–396.
168. Guerrant RL, Kirchoff LV, Shields DS, et al. Prospective study of diarrheal diseases in northeastern Brazil: patterns of disease, nutritional impact, and risk factors. *J Infect Dis* 1983;148: 986–997.
169. Ho MS, Glass RI, Pinsky PF, et al. Rotavirus as a cause of diarrheal morbidity and mortality in the United States. *J Infect Dis* 1988;158:1112–1116.
170. Gurwith M, Wenman W, Hinde D, et al. A prospective study of rotavirus infection in infants and young children. *J Infect Dis* 1981;144:218–224.
171. Matson DO, Estes MK. Impact of rotavirus at a large pediatric hospital. *J Infect Dis* 1990;162:598–604.
172. Wenman WM, Hinde D, Feltham S. Rotavirus in adults: results of a prospective family study. *N Engl J Med* 1979;301:303–306.
173. Flewett TH. Rotavirus in the home and hospital nursery. *Br Med J* 1983;287:568–569.
174. Sattar SA, Lloyd-Evans N, Springthorpe VA. Institutional outbreaks of rotavirus diarrhoea: potential role of fomites and environmental surfaces as vehicles for virus transmission. *J Hyg (London)* 1986;96:277–289.
175. Estes MK, Palmer EL, Obijeski JF. Rotaviruses: a review. *Curr Top Microbiol Immunol* 1983;105:123–184.
176. Sattar SA, Raphael RA, Lochnan H, et al. Rotavirus inactivation by chemical disinfectants and antiseptics used in hospitals. *Can J Microbiol* 1983;29:1464–1469.
177. Tan JA, Schnagel RD. Inactivation of a rotavirus by disinfectants. *Med J Aust* 1981;1:19–23.
178. Haug KW, Orstavik I, Kuelstad G. Rotavirus infections in families. *Scand J Infect Dis* 1978;10:265–269.
179. Chrystie IL, Totterdell BM, Banatvala JE. Asymptomatic endemic rotavirus infection in the newborn. *Lancet* 1978;1: 1176–1178.
180. Bishop RI, Hewstone AS, Davidson GP, et al. An epidemic of diarrhoea in human neonates involving a reovirus-like agent and "enteropathogenic" serotypes of *E. coli. J Clin Pathol* 1976; 29:46–49.
181. Rodriguez WJ, Kim HW, Brandt CD, et al. Rotavirus: a cause of nosocomial infection in the nursery. *J Pediatr* 1982;101: 274–277.
182. Samadi AR, Huq MI, Ahmed OS. Detection of rotavirus in handwashings of attendants of children with diarrhoea. *Br Med J* 1983;286:188.
183. Cubitt WD, Holzel H. Outbreak of rotavirus infection in a long-stay ward of a geriatric hospital. *J Clin Pathol* 1980;33: 306–308.
184. Stals F, Walther FJ, Bruggeman CA. Faecal and pharyngeal shedding of rotavirus and rotavirus IgA in children with diarrhea. *J Med Virol* 1984;14:333–339.
185. Santosham M, Yolken RN, Quiroz E, et al. Detection of rotavirus in respiratory secretions of children with pneumonia. *J Pediatr* 1983;103:583–585.
186. Holzel H, Cubitt DW, McSwiggen DA, et al. An outbreak of rotavirus infection among adults in a cardiology ward. *J Infect* 1980;2:33–37.
187. Marrie TJ, Lee SHS, Faulkner RS, et al. Rotavirus infection in a geriatric population. *Arch Intern Med* 1982;142:313–316.
188. Saulsbury FT, Winkelstein JA, Yolken RH. Chronic rotavirus infection in immunodeficiency. *J Pediatr* 1980;97:61–65.
189. Peigue-Lafeuille H, Henquell C, Chambon M, et al. Nosocomial rotavirus infections in adult renal transplant recipients. *J Hosp Infect* 1991;18:67–70.
190. Miotti PG, Eiden J, Yolken RH. Comparative efficacy of commercial immunoassays for the diagnosis of rotavirus gastroenteritis during the course of infection. *J Clin Microbiol* 1985;22:693–698.
191. Doern GV, Herrmann JE, Henderson P. Detection of rotavirus with a new polyclonal antibody enzyme immunoassay (Rotazyme II) and a commercial latex agglutination test (Rotalex): comparison with a monoclonal antibody enzyme immunoassay. *J Clin Microbiol* 1986;23:226–229.
192. Wilde J, Yolken RH, Willoughby R, et al. Improved detection of rotavirus shedding by polymerase chain reaction. *Lancet* 1991;337:323–326.
193. Spencer E, Avendano LF, Araya M. Characteristics and analysis of electropherotypes of human rotavirus isolated in Chile. *J Infect Dis* 1983;148:41–48.
194. Steele HM, Garnham S, Beards GM, et al. Investigation of an outbreak of rotavirus infection in geriatric patients by serotyping and polyacrylamide gel electrophoresis (PAGE). *J Med Virol* 1992;37:132–136.
195. Chanock SJ, Wenske EA, Fields BN. Human rotaviruses and genomic RNA [Editorial]. *J Infect Dis* 1983;48:49–50.
196. Clark IN, McCrae MA. Structural analysis of electrophoretic variation in the genomic profiles of rotavirus field isolates. *Infect Immun* 1982;36:492–497.
197. Rodriguez WJ, Kim HW, Brandt CD, et al. The use of electrophoresis of RNA from human rotavirus to establish identity of strains involved in outbreaks in a tertiary care nursery. *J Infect Dis* 1983;148:34–40.

198. Konno T, Sato T, Suzuki H, et al. Changing RNA patterns in rotavirus of human origin: demonstration of a single dominant pattern at the start of an epidemic and various patterns thereafter. *J Infect Dis* 1984;149:683–687.
199. Gaggero A, Avendano LF, Fernandex J, et al. Nosocomial transmission of rotavirus from patients admitted with diarrhea. *J Clin Microbiol* 1992;30:3294–3297.
200. Rogers M, Weinstock DM, Eagan J, et al. Rotavirus outbreak on a pediatric oncology floor: possible association with toys. *Am J Infect Cont* 2000;28:378–380.
201. Flewett TH, Bryden AS, Davies H, et al. Epidemic viral enteritis in a long-stay children's ward. *Lancet* 1975;1:4–5.
202. Uhnoo I, Wadell G, Svensson L, et al. Importance of enteric adenoviruses 40 and 41 in acute gastroenteritis in infants and young children. *J Clin Microbiol* 1984;20:365–372.
203. Horwitz MS. Adenoviruses. In: Fields B, Knipe D, eds. *Virology.* New York: Raven Press, 1990:1723–1740.
204. Van R, Wun C-C, O'Ryan ML, et al. Outbreaks of human enteric adenovirus types 40 and 41 in Houston day care centers. *J Pediatr* 1992;120:516–521.
205. Brandt CD, Kim HW, Rodriguez WJ, et al. Adenovirus and pediatric gastroenteritis. *J Infect Dis* 1983;151:437–443.
206. Shinozak T, Araki K, Ushijima H, et al. Antibody response to enteric adenovirus types 40 and 41 in sera of various age groups. *J Clin Microbiol* 1987;25:1679–1682.
207. Rodriguez WJ, Kim HW, Brandt CD, et al. Fecal adenoviruses from a longitudinal study of families in metropolitan Washington, DC: laboratory, clinical and epidemiologic observations. *J Pediatr* 1985;107:514–520.
208. Centers for Disease Control and Prevention. Viral agents of gastroenteritis: public health importance and outbreak management. *MMWR Morb Mortal Wkly Rep* 1990;39(RR-5):1–24.
209. Yolken RH, Lawrence F, Leister F, et al. Gastroenteritis with enteric type adenovirus in hospitalized infants. *J Pediatr* 1982; 101:21–26.
210. Kotloff KL, Losonsky GA, Morris JG Jr, et al. Enteric adenovirus infection and childhood diarrhea: an epidemiologic study in three clinical settings. *Pediatrics* 1989;84:219–225.
211. Zahorsky J. Hyperemesis hiemis or the winter vomiting disease. *Arch Pediatr* 1929;46:391–395.
212. Adler JL, Zickl R. Winter vomiting disease. *J Infect Dis* 1969;119:668–673.
213. Kapikian AZ, Wyatt RG, Dolin R, et al. Visualization by immune electron microscopy of a 27nm particle associated with acute infectious nonbacterial gastroenteritis. *J Virol* 1972;10: 1075–1081.
214. Kaplan JE, Gary GW, Baron RC, et al. Epidemiology of Norwalk gastroenteritis and the role of Norwalk virus in outbreaks of acute nonbacterial gastroenteritis. *Ann Intern Med* 1982; 96:756–761.
215. Herrmann JE, Nowak NA, Blacklow NR. Detection of Norwalk virus in stools by enzyme immunoassay. *J Med Virol* 1985; 17:127–133.
216. DeLeon R, Matsui SM, Barrie RS, et al. Detection of Norwalk virus in stool specimens by reverse transcriptase polymerase chain reaction and nonradioactive oligoprobes. *J Clin Microbiol* 1992;30:3151–3157.
217. Nakata S, Estes MK, Chiba S. Detection of human calicivirus antigen and antibody by enzyme-linked immunosorbent assays. *J Clin Microbiol* 1988;26:2001–2005.
218. Herrmann JE, Nowak NA, Perron-Henry DM, et al. Diagnosis of astrovirus gastroenteritis by antigen detection with monoclonal antibodies. *J Infect Dis* 1990;161:226–229.
219. Taylor JW, Gary GW Jr, Greenberg HB. Norwalk-related viral gastroenteritis due to contaminated drinking water. *Am J Epidemiol* 1981;114:584–592.
220. Griffin MR, Surowiec JJ, McCloskey DI, et al. Foodborne Norwalk virus. *Am J Epidemiol* 1982;115:178–184.
221. Oshiro LS, Haley CE, Roberto RR, et al. A 27nm virus isolated during an outbreak of acute infectious nonbacterial gastroenteritis in a convalescent hospital: a possible new serotype. *J Infect Dis* 1981;143:791–795.
222. Pegues DA, Woernle CH. An outbreak of acute nonbacterial gastroenteritis in a nursing home. *Infect Control Hosp Epidemiol* 1993;14:87–94.
223. Kaplan J, Schonberger L, Varano G, et al. An outbreak of acute nonbacterial gastroenteritis in a nursing home. Demonstration of person-to-person transmission by temporal clustering of cases. *Am J Epidemiol* 1982;116:940–948.
224. Nime FA, Burek JD, Page DL, et al. Acute enterocolitis in a human being infected with the protozoan *Cryptosporidium. Gastroenterology* 1976;70:592–598.
225. Meisel JL, Perea DR, Meligro C, et al. Overwhelming watery diarrhea associated with a *Cryptosporidium* in an immunosuppressed patient. *Gastroenterology* 1976;70:1156–1160.
226. Soave R, Armstrong D. *Cryptosporidium* and cryptosporidiosis. *Rev Infect Dis* 1986;8:1012–1023.
227. Current WL, Reese NC, Ernst JV, et al. Human cryptosporidiosis in immunocompetent and immunodeficient persons: studies of an outbreak and experimental transmission. *N Engl J Med* 1983;308:1252–1257.
228. Fayer R, Ungar BLP. *Cryptosporidium* spp. and cryptosporidiosis. *Microbiol Rev* 1986;50:458–483.
229. Baxby D, Hart CA, Taylor C. Human cryptosporidiosis: a possible cause of hospital infection. *Br Med J* 1983;287:1760–1761.
230. Martino P, Gentile G, Caprioli A, et al. Hospital-acquired cryptosporidiosis in a bone marrow transplantation unit. *J Infect Dis* 1988;158:647–649.
231. Koch KL, Phillips DJ, Aber R, et al. Cryptosporidiosis in hospital personnel: evidence for person-to-person transmission. *Ann Intern Med* 1985;102:593–596.
232. Dryjanski J, Gold JW, Ritchie MT, et al. Cryptosporidiosis: case report in health team worker. *Am J Med* 1986;1986:751–752.
233. Jokipii L, Jokipii AMM. Timing of symptoms and oocyst excretion in human cryptosporidiosis. *N Engl J Med* 1986;315: 1643–1647.
234. Tzipori S. *Cryptosporidium* in animals and humans. *Microbiol Rev* 1983;47:84–96.
235. Tzipori S. Cryptosporidiosis in humans and animals. *Microbiol Rev* 1983;47:84–86.
236. Sundermann CA, Lindsay DS, Blagburn BL. Evaluation of disinfectants for ability to kill avian *Cryptospordium* oocysts. *Companion Anim Pract* 1987;2:36–39.
237. Campbell I, Tzipori S, Hutchinson G, et al. Effect of disinfectants on survival of cryptosporidial oocysts. *Vet Rec* 1982; 111:414–415.
238. Henricksen SA, Pohlenz JFL. Staining of cryptosporidia by a modified Ziehl-Neelson technique. *Acta Vet Scand* 1981;22: 594–596.
239. Ma P, Soave R. Three-step stool examination for cryptosporidiosis in 10 homosexual men with protracted watery diarrhea. *J Infect Dis* 1983;147:824–828.
240. Siddons CA, Chapman PS, Rush BA. Evaluation of an enzyme immunoassay kit for detecting *Cryptosporidium* in faeces and environmental samples. *J Clin Pathol* 1992;45:479–482.
241. Weber R, Bryan RT, Juranek DD. Improved stool concentration procedure for detection of cryptosporidium oocysts in fecal specimens. *J Clin Microbiol* 1992;30:2869–2873.
242. Ungar BL, Soave R, Fayer R, et al. Enzyme immunoassay detection of immunoglobulin M and G antibodies to *Cryptosporidium* in immunocompetent and immunocompromised patients. *J Infect Dis* 1986;153:570–578.

243. Petri WA Jr, Ravdin JI. Amebiasis in institutionalized populations. In: Ravdin JI, ed. *Amebiasis.* New York: Wiley, 1988: 576–581.
244. Smith PD, Lane HC, Gill VJ, et al. Intestinal infections in patients with the acquired immunodeficiency syndrome (AIDS). *Ann Intern Med* 1988;108:328–333.
245. Istre GR, Kreiss K, Hopkins RS, et al. An outbreak of amebiasis spread by colonic irrigation at a chiropractic clinic. *N Engl J Med* 1982;307:339–341.
246. Samuelson J, Acuna-Soto R, Reed S, et al. DNA hybridization probe for clinical diagnosis of *Entamoeba histolytica. J Clin Microbiol* 1989;27:671–676.
247. Acuna-Soto R, Samuelson J, De Giralami P, et al. Application of polymerase chain reaction to the epidemiology of pathogenic and nonpathogenic *Entamoeba histolytica. Am J Trop Med Hyg* 1993;48:58–70.
248. Craun GF. Waterborne giardiasis in the United States 1965–1984. *Lancet* 1986;2:513–514.
249. Kent GP, Greenspan JR, Herndon JL, et al. Epidemic giardiasis caused by a contaminated public water supply. *Am J Public Health* 1988;78:139–143.
250. Pickering LK, Woodward WE, DuPont HL, et al. Occurrence of *Giardia lamblia* in children in day care centers. *J Pediatr* 1984;104:522–526.
251. Yoeli M, Most H, Hammond J, et al. Parasitic infection in a closed community: results of a 10 year survey in Willowbrook State Hospital. *Trans R Soc Trop Med Hyg* 1972;66:764–776.
252. White KE, Hedber CW, Edmonson LM, et al. An outbreak of giardiasis in a nursing home with evidence for multiple modes of transmission. *J Infect Dis* 1989;160:298–304.
253. Flanagan PA. Giardiasis—diagnosis, clinical course and epidemiology. A review. *Epidemiol Infect* 1992;109:1–22.
254. Hoff JC. *Inactivation of microbial agents by chemical disinfectants.* Cincinnati, OH: Water Engineering Research Laboratory, US Environmental Protection Agency; 1986. EPA-600/2-86-067.
255. Black RE, Dykes AC, Sinclair SP, et al. Giardiasis in day-care centers: evidence of person-to-person transmission. *Pediatrics* 1977;60:486–491.
256. Black RE, Dykes AC, Anderson KE, et al. Handwashing to prevent diarrhea in day care centers. *Am J Epidemiol* 1982;113: 445–451.
257. Paerregaard A, Kjelt K, Krasilnikoff PA. The diagnosis of childhood giardiasis. *J Pediatr Gastroenterol Nutr* 1990;10:275.
258. Bezjak B. Evaluation of a new technic for sampling duodenal contents in parasitologic diagnosis. *Am J Dig Dis* 1972;17: 848–850.
259. Bendig DW. Diagnosis of giardiasis in infants and children by endoscopic brush cytology. *J Pediatr Gastroenterol Nutr* 1989;8: 204–206.
260. Knisley CV, Engelkirk PG, Pickering LK, et al. Rapid detection of *Giardia* antigen in stool with the use of enzyme immunoassays. *Am J Clin Pathol* 1989;91:704–708.
261. Weiss JB, van Keulen H, Nash TE. Classification of subgroups of *Giardia lamblia* based on ribosomal DNA gene sequence using polymerase chain reaction. *Mol Biochem Parasitol* 1992;54:73–86.
262. Cohen R, Roth FJ, Delgado E, et al. Fungal flora of the normal human small and large intestine. *N Engl J Med* 1969;208: 638–641.
263. Chretien JH, Garagusi VF. Current management of fungal enteritis. *Med Clin North Am* 1982;66:675–687.
264. Karabinis A, Hill C, Leclercq B, et al. Risk factors for candidemia in cancer patients: a case–control study. *J Clin Microbiol* 1988;126:429–432.
265. Wey SB, Mori M, Pfaller MA, et al. Risk factors for hospital-acquired candidemia. A matched case–control study. *Arch Intern Med* 1989;149:2349–2353.
266. Wey SB, Mori M, Pfaller MA, et al. Hospital-acquired candidemia: the attributable mortality and excess length of stay. *Arch Intern Med* 1988;148:2642–2645.
267. Regan DR, Pfaller MA, Hollis RJ, et al. Characterization of the sequence of colonization and nosocomial candidemia using DNA fingerprinting and a DNA probe. *J Clin Microbiol* 1990; 28:2733–2738.
268. Stone HH, Kolb LD, Currie CA, et al. *Candida* sepsis: pathogenesis and principles of treatment. *Ann Surg* 1974;179:697–711.
269. Krause W, Matheis H, Wulf K. Fungaemia and funguria after oral administration of *Candida albicans. Lancet* 1969;1:598–599.
270. Gupta T, Ehrinpreis MN. *Candida*-associated diarrhea in hospitalized patients. *Gastroenterology* 1990;98:780–785.
271. Cutler JE, Friedman L, Milner KC. Biological and chemical characterization of toxic substances from *Candida albicans. Infect Immun* 1972;6:616–627.
272. Barnes GL, Bishop RF, Townley RRW. Microbial flora and disaccharidase depression in infantile gastroenteritis. *Acta Pediatr Scand* 1974;63:423–426.
273. Kozinn PJ, Taschdjian CL. Enteric candidiasis. *Pediatrics* 1962;30:71–85.
274. Margolis BD, Tsang T-K, Kuo D. Persistent diarrhea secondary to *Candida* overgrowth [Letter]. *Am J Gastroenterol* 1990;85: 329–330.
275. Pfaller MA. Epidemiological typing methods for mycoses. *Clin Infect Dis* 1992;14[Suppl]S4–S10.
276. Doebbling BN, Hollis RJ, Wenzel RP, et al. Method of *Candida* typing by contour-clamped homogeneous electric fields electrophoresis (CHEF) [Abstract]. In: Programs and abstracts of the Interscience Conference on Antimicrobial Agents and Chemotherapy; October 11–14, 1992; Anaheim, California.
277. Pfaller MA, Cabezudo I, Hollis RJ, et al. The use of biotyping and DNA fingerprinting in typing *Candida albicans* from hospitalized patients. *Diagn Microbiol Infect Dis* 1990;13:481–489.
278. Pfaller MA, Cabezudo I, Buschelman B, et al. Value of the Hybritech ICON *Candida* assay in the diagnosis of invasive candidiasis in high-risk patients. *Diagn Microbiol Infect Dis* 1993;16:53–60.
279. Walsh TJ, Hathorn JW, Sobel JD, et al. Detection of circulating *Candida* enolase by immunoassay in patients with cancer and invasive candidiasis. *N Engl J Med* 1991;324:1026–1031.
280. Kealey GD, Heinle JA, Lewis RW II, et al. Value of *Candida* antigen assay in the diagnosis of systemic candidiasis in burn patients. *J Trauma* 1992;32:285–288.
281. Centers for Disease Control and Prevention. Outline for surveillance and control of nosocomial infections. February 1981.
282. Wenzel RP, Osterman CA, Hunting KJ, et al. Hospital-acquired infections, I: surveillance in a university hospital. *Am J Epidemiol* 1976;103:251–259.
283. Lima NL, Periera CRB, Souza IC, et al. Selective surveillance for nosocomial infections in a Brazilian hospital. *Infect Control Hosp Epidemiol* 1993;14:197–202.
284. Centers for Disease Control and Prevention. Recommendations for precautions of HIV transmission in health care settings. *MMWR Morb Mortal Wkly Rep* 1987;36:S3–S18.
285. Conley JM, Hill S, Ross J, et al. Handwashing practices in an intensive care unit: the effects of an educational program and its relationship to infection rates. *Am J Infect Control* 1989;17: 303–339.
286. Doebbling BN, Pfaller MA, Houston AK, et al. Removal of nosocomial pathogens from the contaminated glove: implications for glove reuse and handwashing. *Ann Intern Med* 1988; 109:394–398.
287. Doebbling BN, Stanley GL, Sheetz CT, et al. Comparative efficacy of alternative hand-washing agents in reducing nosocomial infections in intensive care units. *N Engl J Med* 1992;327:88–93.

288. Simmons B, Bryant J, Neiman K, et al. The role of handwashing in prevention of endemic intensive care unit infections. *Infect Control Hosp Epidemiol* 1990;11:589–594.
289. Katoh M, Saito D, Noda T, et al. *Helicobacter pylori* may be transmitted through gastrofiberscope even after manual Hyamine washing. *Jpn J Cancer Res* 1993;84:117–119.
290. Langenberg W, Rauws EAJ, Oudbier JH, et al. Patient-to-patient transmission of *Campylobacter pylori* infection by fiberscopic gastroduodenoscopy and biopsy. *J Infect Dis* 1990;161:507–511.
291. Spaulding EH. Chemical disinfection of medical and surgical materials. In: Lawrence C, Block S, eds. *Disinfection, sterilization and preservation.* Philadelphia: Lea & Febiger, 1968:517–531.
292. Gorse GJ, Messner RL. Infection control practices in gastrointestinal endoscopy in the United States. *Infect Control Hosp Epidemiol* 1991;12:289–296.
293. Favero MS. Strategies for disinfection and sterilization of endoscopes: the gap between basic principles and actual practice. *Infect Control Hosp Epidemiol* 1991;12:279–281.
294. Rutala WA. APIC guideline for selection and use of disinfectant. *Am J Infect Control* 1990;18:99–117.
295. Jonas G, Mahoney A, Murray J, et al. Chemical colitis due to endoscope cleaning solutions: a mimic of pseudomembranous colitis. *Gastroenterology* 1988;95:1403–1408.
296. Alvarado CJ, Stolz SM, Maki DG. Nosocomial infections from contaminated endoscopes: a flawed automated endoscope washer: an investigation using molecular epidemiology. *Am J Med* 1991;91[Suppl 3B]:272S–280S.
297. Jernigan JA, Giuliano K, Guerrant RL, et al. Effect of disposable thermometer use on rates of nosocomial *Clostridium difficile* diarrhea and total nosocomial infections: a randomized controlled study. In: Programs and abstracts of the 33rd Interscience Conference on Antimicrobial Agents and Chemotherapy; October 17–20, 1993; New Orleans, Louisiana. Abstract 62.
298. Surawicz CM, Elmer GW, Speelman P, et al. Prevention of antibiotic associated diarrhea by *Saccharomyces boulardii:* a prospective study. *Gastroenterology* 1989;96:981–988.
299. Haley R, Emori T. The employee health service and infection control in U.S. hospitals, 1976–1977 II. *JAMA* 1981;246: 962–966.
300. Valenti WM. Employee work restrictions for infection control. *Infect Control* 1984;5:583–584.
301. Williams WW. Guideline for infection control in hospital personnel. *Infect Control* 1983;4:326–349.
302. Benenson AS. *Control of communicable diseases in man,* 15th ed. Washington, DC: American Public Health Association, 1990.
303. Bank HL, John JF, Atkins LM, et al. Bactericidal action of modulated ultraviolet light on six groups of *Salmonella. Infect Control Hosp Epidemiol* 1991;12:486–489.

SUBJECT INDEX

Note: Page numbers followed by f refer to figures; page numbers followed by t refer to tables.

D

E

F

I

K

N

O

P

W

X

Y